Medicine
q BP 8
2015-R

Rubin's Pathology

CLINICOPATHOLOGIC FOUNDATIONS OF MEDICINE

SEVENTH EDITION

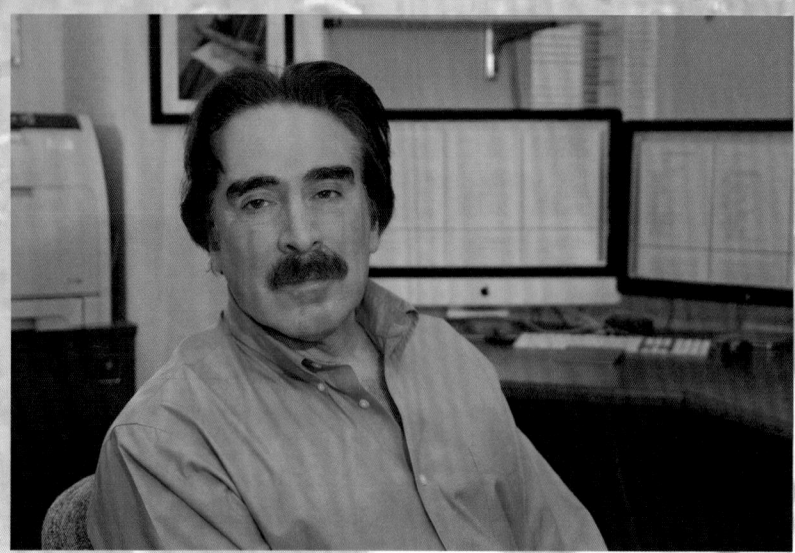

Editor David S. Strayer, MD, PhD

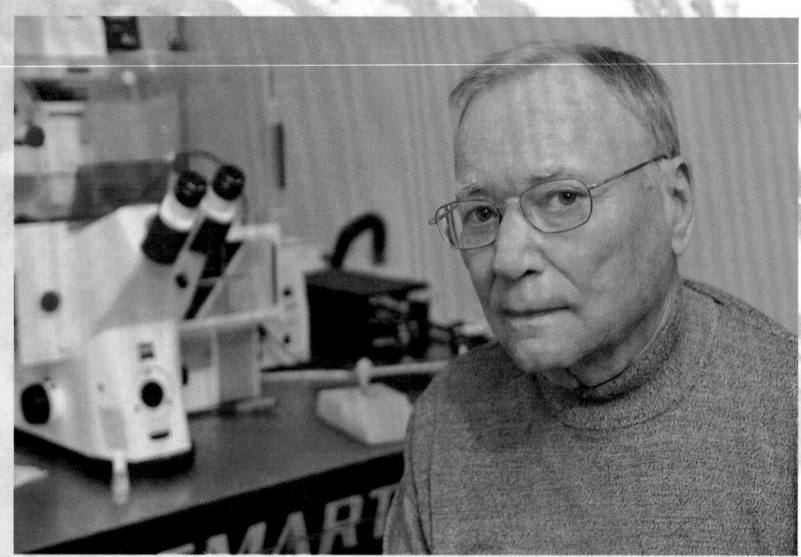

Founder and Contributing Editor Emanuel Rubin, MD

Rubin's Pathology

CLINICOPATHOLOGIC FOUNDATIONS OF MEDICINE

SEVENTH EDITION

EDITOR

David S. Strayer, MD, PhD

Professor of Pathology
Department of Pathology and Cell Biology
Jefferson Medical College of Thomas Jefferson University
Philadelphia, Pennsylvania

FOUNDER AND CONTRIBUTING EDITOR

Emanuel Rubin, MD

Gonzalo Aponte Distinguished Professor of Pathology
Chairman Emeritus of the Department of Pathology and Cell Biology
Jefferson Medical College of Thomas Jefferson University
Philadelphia, Pennsylvania

ASSOCIATE EDITORS

Jeffrey E. Saffitz, MD, PhD

Mallinckrodt Professor of Medicine
Harvard Medical School
Chairman, Department of Pathology
Beth Israel Deaconess Medical Center
Boston, Massachusetts

Alan L. Schiller, MD

Professor and Chairman
Department of Pathology
John A. Burns School of Medicine
University of Hawaii
Honolulu, Hawaii

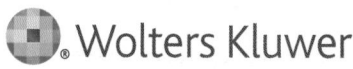

Wolters Kluwer

Philadelphia • Baltimore • New York • London
Buenos Aires • Hong Kong • Sydney • Tokyo

Publisher: Michael Tully
Acquisitions Editor: Sirkka Howes
Product Development Editor: Stacey Sebring
Marketing Manager: Joy Fisher-Williams
Production Project Manager: Alicia Jackson
Manufacturing Manager: Margie Orzech
Designer: Steve Druding
Medical Illustrator: Holly R. Fischer, MFA
Compositor: Aptara, Inc.

Seventh Edition
Copyright © 2015 Wolters Kluwer Health

2012, 2008, 2005, 2001, 1995, 1989 Lippincott Williams & Wilkins, a Wolters Kluwer business.

351 West Camden Street   Two Commerce Square
Baltimore, MD 21201   2001 Market Street
                             Philadelphia, PA 19103

Printed in China

9 8 7 6 5 4 3 2 1

Library of Congress Cataloging-in-Publication Data
Rubin's pathology : clinicopathologic foundations of medicine / editor, David S. Strayer; founder and contributing editor, Emanuel Rubin; associate editors, Jeffrey E. Saffitz, Alan L. Schiller.—Seventh edition.
    p. ; cm.
  Pathology : clinicopathologic foundations of medicine
  Includes bibliographical references and index.
  ISBN 978-1-4511-8390-0 (alk. paper)
  I. Strayer, David S. (David Sheldon), 1949- editor. II. Rubin, Emanuel, 1928- editor.
III. Saffitz, Jeffrey E., editor. IV. Schiller, Alan L., editor. V. Title: Pathology : clinicopathologic foundations of medicine.
  [DNLM: 1. Pathologic Processes. QZ 4]
  RB111
  616.07—dc23   2014016625

We dedicate this book to our wives and families, whose tolerance, love and support sustained us throughout this endeavor; to our colleagues, from whom we have learned so much; to our chapter authors, who have given so much of themselves to produce this new edition; and to students everywhere, upon whose curiosity and energy the future of medical science depends.

This 7th edition is also specially dedicated to the memory of Raphael Rubin, MD, who was associate editor of the 4th edition and who co-edited the 5th and 6th editions. There are no words to express either our happiness that he was part of our lives, or our feelings of loss at his untimely death. We are grateful to him for his courage and grace in the face of terrible disease and for his essential goodness, which permeated everything he did.

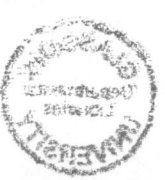

CONTRIBUTORS

Ronnie Abraham, MD
Department of Pathology
Hospital of the University of Pennsylvania
Philadelphia, Pennsylvania

Michael F. Allard, MD
Professor of Pathology and Laboratory Medicine
University of British Columbia
Cardiovascular Pathologist
Department of Pathology and Laboratory Medicine
The iCAPTURE Centre
St. Paul's Hospital
Vancouver, British Columbia, Canada

Mary Beth Beasley, MD
Associate Professor of Pathology
Mount Sinai Medical Center
New York, New York

Thomas W. Bouldin, MD
Professor of Pathology and Laboratory Medicine
Chair for Faculty and Trainee Development
University of North Carolina at Chapel Hill
Director of Neuropathology
McLendon Clinical Laboratories
University of North Carolina Hospitals
Chapel Hill, North Carolina

Linda A. Cannizzaro, PhD
Professor of Pathology
Albert Einstein College of Medicine
Director of Cytogenetics
Montefiore Medical Center
Bronx, New York

Diane L. Carlson, MD
Assistant Attending
Department of Pathology
Memorial Sloan-Kettering Cancer Center
New York, New York

Emily Y. Chu, MD, PhD
Department of Dermatology
Hospital of the University of Pennsylvania
Perelman Center for Advanced Medicine
Philadelphia, Pennsylvania

Philip L. Cohen, MD
Professor of Medicine
Temple University School of Medicine
Chief, Section of Rheumatology
Temple University Hospital
Philadelphia, Pennsylvania

Ivan Damjanov, MD, PhD
Professor of Pathology
The University of Kansas School of Medicine
Pathologist
Department of Pathology
University of Kansas Medical Center
Kansas City, Kansas

Jeffrey M. Davidson, PhD
Professor of Pathology
Vanderbilt University School of Medicine
Senior Research Career Scientist
Medical Research Service
Veterans Affairs Tennessee Valley Healthcare
    System
Nashville, Tennessee

Elizabeth G. Demicco, MD, PhD
Assistant Professor of Pathology
Icahn School of Medicine at Mount Sinai
Pathologist
Mount Sinai Hospital
New York, New York

Alina Dulau Florea, MD
Assistant Professor of Pathology
Thomas Jefferson University
Philadelphia, Pennsylvania

David E. Elder, MD, ChB, FRCPA
Professor of Pathology and Laboratory Medicine
University of Pennsylvania School of Medicine
Director of Anatomic Pathology
Hospital of the University of Pennsylvania
Philadelphia, Pennsylvania

Gregory N. Fuller, MD, PhD
Professor of Pathology
Chief of Neuropathology
The University of Texas M.D. Anderson
    Cancer Center
Houston, Texas

Roberto A. Garcia, MD
Assistant Professor of Pathology
Mount Sinai School of Medicine
Chief of Orthopaedic and Soft Tissue Pathology
Mount Sinai Hospital
New York, New York

J. Clay Goodman, MD
Professor of Pathology and Neurology
Walter Henrick Moursund Chair in Neuropathology
Associate Dean of Undergraduate Medical Education
Baylor College of Medicine
Houston, Texas

Avrum I. Gotlieb, MD, CM, FRCP
Professor of Laboratory Medicine and Pathology
University of Toronto
Staff Pathologist
Laboratory Medicine Program
University Health Network
Toronto, Ontario, Canada

Leana A. Guerin, MD
Assistant Professor of Pathology
University of Iowa Hospitals and Clinics
Iowa City, Iowa

Philip N. Hawkins, PhD, FRCP, FRCPath, FMedSci
Professor of Medicine
Centre for Amyloidosis and Acute Phase Proteins
University College London Medical School
Head, National Amyloidosis Centre
Royal Free Hospital
London, England, United Kingdom

Kendra Iskander, MD
Department of Surgery
Boston Medical Center
Boston, Massachusetts

J. Charles Jennette, MD
Brinkhous Distinguished Professor and Chair of Pathology
    and Laboratory Medicine
University of North Carolina, School of Medicine
Chief of Service
Department of Pathology and Laboratory Medicine
University of North Carolina Hospitals
Chapel Hill, North Carolina

Sergio A. Jimenez, MD
Professor and Co-Director
Jefferson Institute of Molecular Medicine
Director of Connective Tissue Diseases
Director of Scleroderma Center
Department of Dermatology and Cutaneous Biology
Thomas Jefferson University
Philadelphia, Pennsylvania

Lawrence C. Kenyon, MD, PhD
Associate Professor of Pathology, Anatomy and Cell
    Biology
Thomas Jefferson University
Pathologist and Neuropathologist
Department of Pathology, Anatomy and Cell Biology
Thomas Jefferson University Hospital
Philadelphia, Pennsylvania

Michael J. Klein, MD
Professor of Pathology and Laboratory Medicine
Weill Medical College of Cornell University
Pathologist-in-Chief and Director of Pathology and
    Laboratory Medicine
Hospital for Special Surgery
New York, New York

David S. Klimstra, MD
Chief of Surgical Pathology
Department of Pathology
Memorial Sloan-Kettering Cancer Center
New York, New York

Gordon K. Klintworth, MD, PhD
Professor of Pathology
Joseph A.C. Wadsworth Research Professor
    of Ophthalmology
Duke University
Durham, North Carolina

Shauying Li, MD
Assistant Professor
Department of Pathology, Microbiology and Immunology
Vanderbilt University Medical Center
Nashville, Tennessee

Amber Chang Liu, MSc
Harvard Medical School
Resident Physician
Department of Anesthesiology, Critical Care and
    Pain Medicine
Massachusetts General Hospital
Boston, Massachusetts

David Benner Lombard, MD, PhD
Assistant Professor of Pathology
Department of Pathology and Institute of Gerontology
Staff Pathologist
Department of Pathology
University of Michigan
Ann Arbor, Michigan

Peter A. McCue, MD
Professor of Pathology
Thomas Jefferson University
Director of Anatomic Pathology
Thomas Jefferson University Hospital
Philadelphia, Pennsylvania

Bruce McManus, MD, PhD, FRSC
Professor of Pathology and Laboratory Medicine
University of British Columbia
Director, Providence Heart and Lung Institute
St. Paul's Hospital
Vancouver, British Columbia, Canada

Maria J. Merino, MD
Chief of Translational Pathology
Department of Pathology
National Cancer Institute
Bethesda, Maryland

Marc S. Micozzi, MD, PhD
Private Practice, Forensic Medicine
Policy Institute for Integrative Medicine
Bethesda, Maryland

Frank Mitros, MD
Frederic W. Stamler Professor
Department of Pathology
University of Iowa
Iowa City, Iowa

Anna Marie Mulligan, MB, MSc, FRCPath
Assistant Professor of Laboratory Medicine and Pathobiology
University of Toronto
Anatomic Pathologist
Department of Laboratory Medicine
St. Michael's Hospital
Toronto, Ontario, Canada

Hedwig S. Murphy, MD, PhD
Associate Professor of Pathology
University of Michigan
Staff Pathologist
Department of Pathology and Laboratory Medicine
Veterans Affairs Ann Arbor Health System
Ann Arbor, Michigan

George L. Mutter, MD
Associate Professor of Pathology
Harvard Medical School
Pathologist
Department of Pathology
Brigham and Women's Hospital
Boston, Massachusetts

Frances P. O'Malley, MB, FRCPC
Professor of Laboratory Medicine and Pathobiology
University of Toronto
Staff Pathologist
Department of Pathology and Laboratory Medicine
Mount Sinai Hospital
Toronto, Ontario, Canada

Jaime Prat, MD, PhD, FRCPath
Professor of Pathology
Director of Pathology
Autonomous University of Barcelona
Director of Pathology
Hospital de la Santa Creu i Sant Pau
Barcelona, Spain

Daniel G. Remick, MD
Chair and Professor, Department of Pathology and
    Laboratory Medicine
Boston University School of Medicine
Chief of Pathology, Department of Pathology and
    Laboratory Medicine
Boston Medical Center
Boston, Massachusetts

Emanuel Rubin, MD
Gonzalo Aponte Distinguished Professor of Pathology
Chairman Emeritus of the Department of Pathology and
    Cell Biology
Jefferson Medical College of Thomas Jefferson University
Philadelphia, Pennsylvania

Jeffrey E. Saffitz, MD, PhD
Mallinckrodt Professor of Medicine
Harvard Medical School
Chairman, Department of Pathology
Beth Israel Deaconess Medical Center
Boston, Massachusetts

Alan L. Schiller, MD
Professor and Chairman
Department of Pathology
John A. Burns School of Medicine
University of Hawaii
Honolulu, Hawaii

David A. Schwartz, MD, MSHyg, FCAP
Pathologist
Atlanta, Georgia

Gregory C. Sephel, PhD
Associate Professor of Pathology
Vanderbilt University School of Medicine
Nashville, Tennessee

Elias S. Siraj, MD
Associate Professor of Medicine
Section of Endocrinology
Temple University School of Medicine
Program Director, Endocrinology Fellowship
Temple University Hospital
Philadelphia, Pennsylvania

Edward B. Stelow, MD
Associate Professor of Pathology
University of Virginia
Charlottesville, Virginia

Arief A. Suriawinata, MD
Associate Professor of Pathology
Geisel School of Medicine at Dartmouth
Hanover, New Hampshire
Section Chief of Anatomic Pathology
Dartmouth-Hitchcock Medical Center
Lebanon, New Hampshire

Swan N. Thung, MD
Professor of Pathology
Mount Sinai School of Medicine
Director, Division of Liver Pathology
Mount Sinai Medical Center
New York, New York

William D. Travis, MD
Professor of Pathology
Weill Medical College of Cornell University
Attending Thoracic Pathologist
Memorial Sloan Kettering Cancer Center
New York, New York

Riccardo Valdez, MD
Assistant Professor of Pathology
Section Head, Hematopathology
Department of Laboratory Medicine and
    Pathology
Mayo Clinic
Scottsdale, Arizona

Jeffrey S. Warren, MD
Aldred S. Warthin Endowed Professor of
    Pathology
Director, Division of Clinical Pathology
University of Michigan Medical School
University of Michigan Hospitals
Ann Arbor, Michigan

Kevin Jon Williams, MD
Professor of Medicine
Chief, Section of Endocrinology, Diabetes and
    Metabolism
Temple University School of Medicine
Philadelphia, Pennsylvania

Robert Yanagawa, MD, PhD
Division of Cardiac Surgery
University of Toronto, Faculty of Medicine
Toronto, Ontario, Canada

Mary M. Zutter, MD
Professor of Pathology and Cancer Biology
Vanderbilt University
Director of Hematopathology
Vanderbilt University Medical Center
Nashville, Tennessee

Students and instructors have complementary roles and needs as participants in the educational process. This book is intended to help modern medical students learn—and to help instructors teach—pathology as a foundation of clinical medicine.

So much has happened to change what and how medical students are taught. Medicine is rapidly being transformed, in part by the pace of scientific advance, and in part by the world around us. These forces reshape the subject matter and how it is presented. They also require that we consider carefully what we expect students of medicine to master.

Thus, this book's purpose is to teach pathology and disease pathogenesis to medical students. It is not geared to residents or fellows in pathology, nor to bench scientists. *Our goal is to prepare future medical practitioners—cardiologists, pediatricians, gerontologists and so forth—for their specialties, not for ours.* We do this by helping them to understand how diseases happen and how they appear. We provide a foundation on which future clinicians of all specialties can build and, we hope, a sense of excitement for medical advances yet to come.

Perhaps the hardest—and at the same time the most important—challenge facing us in preparing this textbook is determining what should not be stressed, that is, what is better left for more specialized texts in biochemistry, molecular biology, pathology subspecialities and so on. Even as we try to avoid such superfluities as unproven hypotheses, abstruse discussions, medical minutiae and details of scientific experiments that fill some other textbooks, the amount of information remains overwhelming. We therefore applied a filter throughout this book, a question we asked both in writing our own chapters (Chapters 1, 5 and 8) and in editing the work of our superb contributors: what do students of medicine *need* to know in order to be good doctors, to prepare them for a lifetime of professional learning and to understand how advances in the medical sciences will affect their patients?

We stress the interrelatedness of the many medical disciplines. Traditional pathology texts have a section of basic principles, followed by a section covering each of the several organs in turn. This is no longer enough. Many processes and diseases affect multiple organ systems and are best understood and taught as such. It does not suffice, for example, only to describe aging as a series of separate effects on cells in culture or on the brain or on the cardiovascular system. As we can attest from personal experience, aging—apart from the very dubious wisdom that some people believe accompanies it—affects almost everything an individual does and can do. Its impact on one organ system is inextricably linked to its effects on others. It, and similar processes that affect multiple organ systems, is thus best approached against the background of the whole person, not just individual organs.

Accordingly, we have added a new section on systemic conditions: processes that affect whole human beings, not just their kidneys, lungs or joints. These include new chapters on aging (Chapter 10), autoimmune diseases (Chapter 11),

sepsis (Chapter 12) and pregnancy (Chapter 14), plus amyloidosis (Chapter 15) and obesity, diabetes and metabolic syndrome (Chapter 13), which appeared in past editions. These are among the most important processes that doctors will have to understand in approaching patients. These integrated presentations should greatly facilitate how these topics are taught and, hopefully, understood. Organ-specific chapters still cover respective manifestations of these processes.

Understanding systemic processes is thus fundamental to this book and our approach to presenting pathology. Pathology is not just a compilation of burdensome, isolated facts or abstruse and arcane pathways to be memorized and promptly forgotten. It is the drama of human frailty and mortality, which we present as concepts to understand and principles to apply.

We also include a new chapter, which we feel adds excitement to the study of pathology: pathology in forensic investigation. This addition illustrates the relevance and sophistication of pathology as it interfaces with patient care and relates to the world outside of medicine.

Education in general is changing. Traditional, printed textbooks are being replaced by texts viewed on portable devices such as tablet computers. These versatile devices offer many more opportunities for interactive learning, including self-quizzing, animated illustrations, virtual microscopy, networking and many more. Many such ancillaries are part of the instructional package that begins with this textbook. Because students have become increasingly sophisticated and exacting, our presentations encompass the full range of instructional aids and are based on the principle that pathology and pathogenesis are inseparable and are fundamental to all clinical medicine.

These teaching adjuncts underscore the fact that *the real challenge is to identify what students should understand, and then decide how best to aid that understanding*—not to apply the maximum number of electronic (or other) embellishments, or to use these tools to add yet more facts to the mountains of information that already burden students. Appreciating what a good doctor must understand, and the limits of students' time and energy, we have not tried to be comprehensive, preferring instead to be useful.

Consequently, this new edition is much different from its predecessors. The reorganization of this textbook, described above, is an attempt to help students learn about complex issues in modern medicine in a more unified way. Many chapters are rewritten or extensively revised. New authors in Chapters 6, 10, 11, 12, 14, 19, 20, 26, 28 and 34 join the outstanding authors whose continuing contributions are so valuable, and exemplify this goal. The diligent and selfless work of all these authors is the backbone of this textbook.

We emphasize what is understood but also describe the limits of our current knowledge. Hopefully, inquisitive minds will find in this textbook a springboard to further exploration, and students and colleagues will share the excitement of discovery that we have been privileged to experience in our education and careers.

What is the role of a textbook in an era when most medical school courses prepare their own syllabi, when online information and other resources are abundantly available to students and when many faculty may feel their time and energy are more profitably invested in other pursuits? This volume was designed to gather experts from around the world, to have them present to students a thorough but digestible understanding of how diseases occur and to provide for faculty an educational program that facilitates instruction. *Rubin's Pathology* is characterized by its stylistic uniformity and readability, its strikingly visual presentation, its focus on clinical relevance in all material presented, the dedication of its authors to maintaining the currency of the material and the desire of the entire production team to providing textual material and instructional ancillaries that help students to learn and that help teachers to teach. The determination to achieve these goals is, we believe, an important contribution to medical education that can only be provided in this format.

This is the 25th anniversary of the first edition of this textbook, and the occasion lends itself to recounting one of the most amusing anecdotes from editions past. Thus, we recall that one chapter author for the first edition had prepared elaborate hand-drawn figures ready to be sent for rendering by the illustrator. One night, he fell asleep on the couch, with his precious illustrations scattered on the surrounding floor. It just so happened that he was paper-training a new puppy at the time. Unaware of the significance of the papers, and not appreciating their contents, the puppy dutifully used the papers as it had been trained. The author, when he awoke, wiped the results of the dog's training from the sheets of paper and sent them to us. Picture our perplexity when we received a sheath of papers decorated with brown smears of some unknown type!! We only found out the reason later.

Finally, we remember with humility and deep enduring affection Raphael Rubin, a previous coeditor of *Rubin's Pathology*. His death in September 2011, at age 55, was an incalculable professional and personal loss for us both. We have tried to memorialize Raph in our dedication of this 7th edition. He is with us in our hearts, and we trust that this new edition would have made him proud.

David S. Strayer, MD, PhD
Emanuel Rubin, MD
Philadelphia, 2014

Many dedicated people, too numerous to list, provided insight that made this 7th edition of *Rubin's Pathology* possible. The editors would like especially to thank the managing and editorial staff at Lippincott Williams & Wilkins and in particular Sirkka Howes and Stacey Sebring whose encouragement and support throughout all phases of this endeavor have not only touched us greatly personally but also been a key to the successful publication of this text and its ancillaries.

The editors also acknowledge contributions made by our colleagues who participated in writing previous editions and those who offered suggestions and ideas for the current edition.

Stuart A. Aaronson
Mohammad Alomari
Adam Bagg
Karoly Balogh
Sue Bartow
Douglas P. Bennett
Marluce Bibbo
Hugh Bonner
Patrick J. Buckley
Stephen W. Chensue
Daniel H. Connor
Jeffrey Cossman
John E. Craighead
Mary Cunnane
Giulia DeFalco
Hormuz Ehya
Joseph C. Fantone
John L. Farber
Kevin Furlong
Antonio Giordano

Barry J. Goldstein
Stanley R. Hamiliton
Terrence J. Harrist
Arthur P. Hays
Steven K. Herrine
Serge Jabbour
Robert B. Jennings
Kent J. Johnson
Anthony A. Killeen
Robert Kisilevsky
William D. Kocher
Robert J. Kurman
Ernest A. Lack
Antonio Martinez-Hernandez
Steven McKenzie
Wolfgang J. Mergner
Victor J. Navarro
Adebeye O. Osunkoya
Juan Palazzo
Stephen Peiper

Robert O. Peterson
Roger J. Pomerantz
Martha Quezado
Timothy R. Quinn
Stanley J. Robboy
Brian Schapiro
Roland Schwarting
Stephen M. Schwartz
Benjamin H. Spargo
Charles Steenbergen, Jr.
Craig A. Storm
Steven L. Teitelbaum
Ann D. Thor
John Q. Trojanowski
Benjamin F. Trump
Beverly Y. Wang
Jianzhou Wang
Bruce M. Wenig

CONTENTS

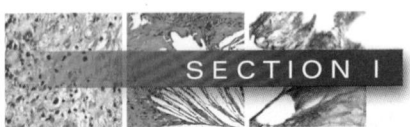
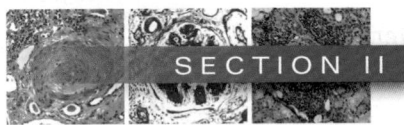

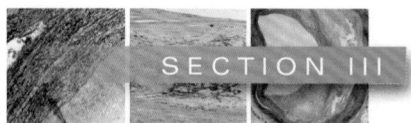

DISEASES OF INDIVIDUAL ORGAN SYSTEMS

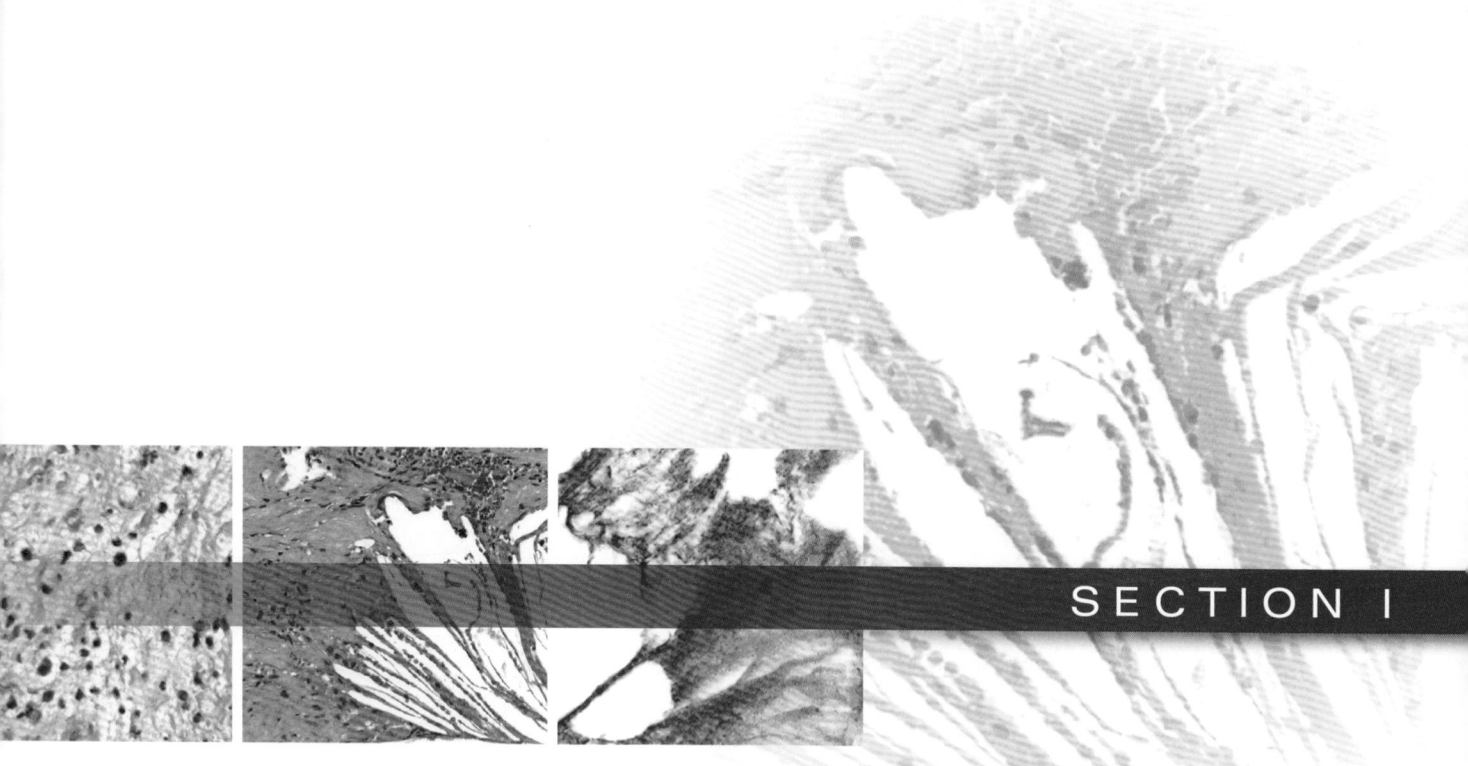

Mechanisms of Disease

SECTION II

Mechanisms of Disease

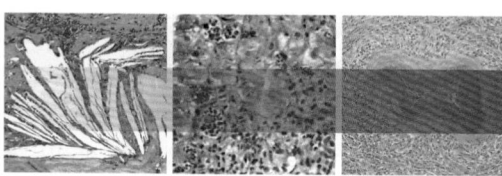

Cell Adaptation, Injury and Death

David S. Strayer ▪ Emanuel Rubin

MECHANISMS AND MORPHOLOGY OF CELL INJURY
Hydropic Swelling
Ischemic Cell Injury
Oxidative Stress
Antioxidant Defenses
Role of p53 in Oxidative Injury
Intracellular Storage
Calcification
Hyaline
Hyperplasia
Metaplasia
Dysplasia

Reactions to Persistent Stress and Cell Injury
Atrophy and Hypertrophy
Normal Homeostasis
Atrophy and Hypertrophy as Inverses
Signaling in Atrophy and Hypertrophy

Loss of Muscle Mass
Turnover of Postmitotic Cells

Ubiquitin and Ubiquitin–Proteasome System
Ubiquitin and Ubiquitination
Proteasomes and Cell Homeostasis
UPS and Pathogens
UPS and Disease
Autophagy
Molecular Chaperones and Chaperonopathies
Nonlethal Mutations That Impair Cell Function

CELL DEATH

Morphology of Cell Death
Pathology of Necrotic Cell Death
Pathology of Apoptotic Cell Death
Active Cell Death

Necrosis
Ischemic Injury and Reperfusion

Programmed Cell Death
Apoptosis

Mechanisms of Apoptosis
Apoptosis Signaling Pathways
Extrinsic Pathway of Apoptosis
Intrinsic Pathway of Apoptosis
Endoplasmic Reticulum Ca^{2+} Release and Apoptosis
Role of Mitochondrial Proteins in Apoptosis
Apoptosis in Disease

Other Forms of Programmed Cell Death
Autophagy and Cell Death
Necroptosis
Anoikis
Granzymes and Apoptosis
Pyroptosis
NETosis
Entosis

Pathology *is the study of structural and functional abnormalities that manifest as diseases of organs and systems.* Classic theories attributed disease to imbalances or noxious effects of "humors." In the 19th century, Rudolf Virchow, often called the father of modern pathology, proposed that injury to cells, the smallest living units in the body, is the basis of all disease. To this day, this concept underlies all of pathology.

To understand cell injury, it is useful to consider how cells sustain themselves in a hostile environment.[1] To remain viable, the cell must generate energy. This process requires it to establish a structural and functional barrier between its internal milieu and the outside. The **plasma membrane** does this in several ways:

- It maintains a constant internal ionic composition against very large chemical gradients between interior and exterior compartments.
- It selectively admits some molecules while excluding or extruding others.
- It provides a structural envelope to contain the cell's informational, synthetic and catabolic constituents. Thus, it creates an environment to house signal transduction molecules that communicate between each other and between the external and internal milieus.

Cells must also be able to adapt to fluctuating environmental conditions, such as changes in temperature, solute concentrations, oxygen supply, noxious agents and so on. The evolution of multicellular organisms eased the precarious lot of individual cells by establishing a controlled extracellular environment, in which temperature, oxygen availability, ionic content and nutrient supply remain

---

[1]Facts can only be established by observation (i.e., without imposing an external logical framework suggesting that certain functions or abilities evolved in order to achieve a particular goal). However, teleology—the study of design or purpose in nature—can be a useful tool to help in framing questions, even though it is not accepted as a legitimate part of scientific investigation.

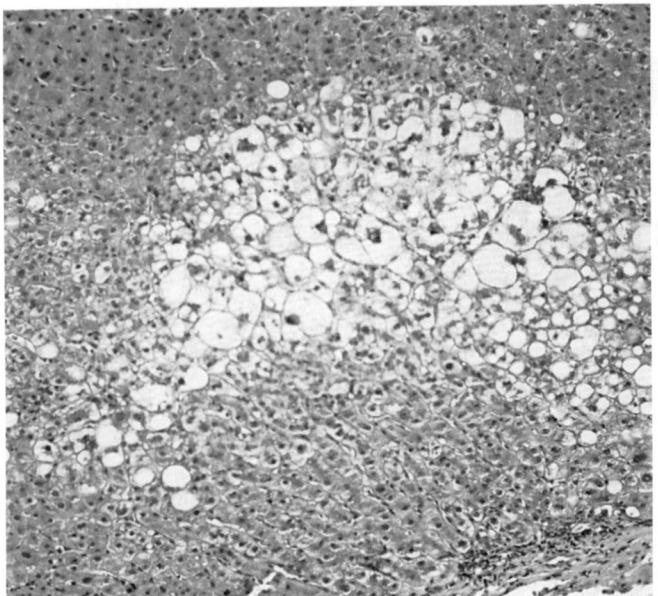

FIGURE 1-1. Hydropic swelling. The liver of a patient with toxic hepatic injury shows severe hydropic swelling in the centrilobular zone. Affected hepatocytes exhibit central nuclei and cytoplasm distended by excess fluid.

Mechanisms and Morphology of Cell Injury

All cells have efficient mechanisms to deal with shifts in environmental conditions. Thus, ion channels open or close, harmful chemicals are detoxified, metabolic stores such as fat or glycogen may be mobilized and catabolic processes lead to the segregation of internal particulate materials. When environmental changes exceed the cell's capacity to maintain normal homeostasis, we recognize acute cell injury. If the stress is removed in time or if the cell can withstand the assault, the damage is reversible, and complete structural and functional integrity is restored. For example, when circulation to the heart is interrupted for less than 30 minutes, all structural and functional alterations prove to be reversible. The cell can also be exposed to persistent sublethal stress, as in mechanical irritation of the skin or exposure of the bronchial mucosa to tobacco smoke. Cells have time to adapt to reversible injury in a number of ways, each of which has a morphologic counterpart. On the other hand, if the stress is sufficiently severe, irreversible injury leads to cell death. The moment when reversible injury becomes irreversible injury, the "point of no return," is not known at present.

Hydropic Swelling Is a Reversible Increase in Cell Volume

Hydropic swelling is characterized by a large, pale cytoplasm and a normally located nucleus (Fig. 1-1). The greater volume is caused by increased water content and reflects acute, reversible cell injury. It may result from such varied causes as chemical and biological toxins, viral or bacterial infections, ischemia, excessive heat or cold and so on.

By electron microscopy, the number of organelles is unchanged, although they appear dispersed in a larger volume. The excess fluid accumulates preferentially in cisternae of the endoplasmic reticulum, which are conspicuously dilated, presumably because of ionic shifts into this compartment (Fig. 1-2).

Hydropic swelling results from impairment of cellular volume regulation, a process that controls ionic concentrations in the cytoplasm. This regulation, particularly for sodium, involves three components: (1) the plasma

relatively constant. It also permitted the luxury of cell differentiation for such diverse functions as energy storage (glycogen in hepatocytes, lipids in adipocytes), communication (neurons), contractile activity (heart muscle), protein synthesis for export (pancreas, endocrine cells), absorption (intestine) and defenses from foreign invaders (immune system).

These adaptations notwithstanding, changes in an organism's internal and external environments strain the tranquility of its constituent cells. *Patterns of response to such stresses make up the cellular basis of disease.* If an injury exceeds a cell's adaptive capacity, that cell dies. A cell exposed to persistent sublethal injury has limited available responses, expression of which we interpret as cell injury. *Thus, pathology is the study of injury to cells and organs and of their capacity to adapt to such injury.* The science of disease (pathology) is thus an application of normal biological principles.

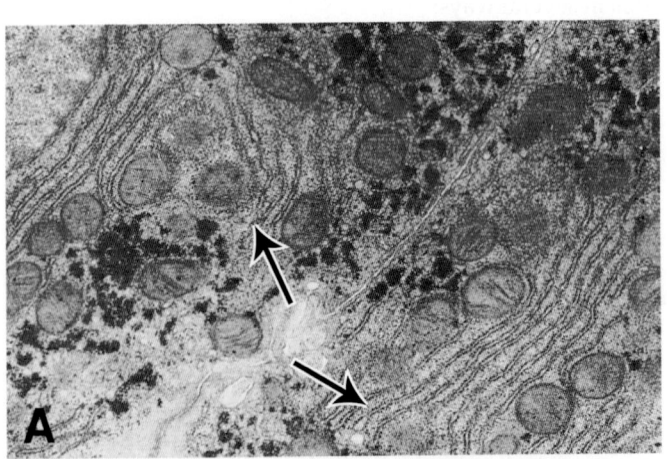

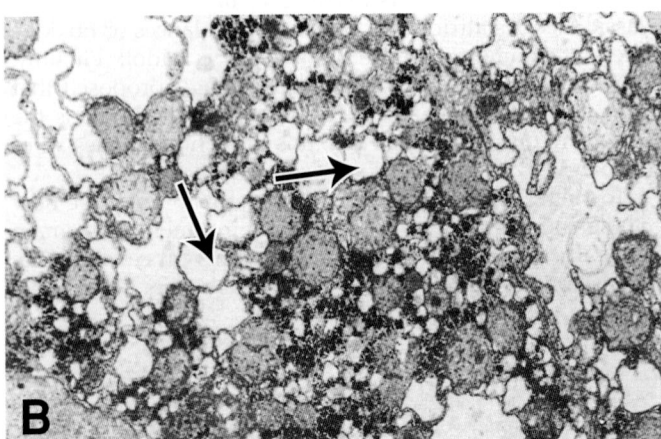

FIGURE 1-2. Ultrastructure of hydropic swelling. A. Two apposed normal hepatocytes contain tightly organized, parallel arrays of rough endoplasmic reticulum (*arrows*). **B.** Swollen hepatocytes show dilations of the cisternae of the endoplasmic reticulum by excess fluid (*arrows*).

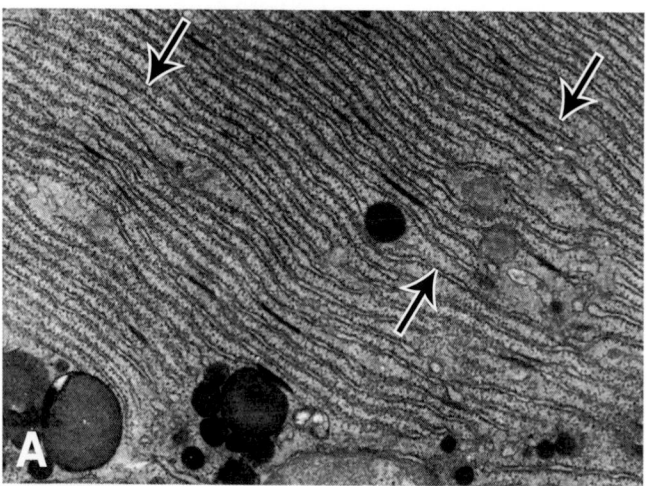 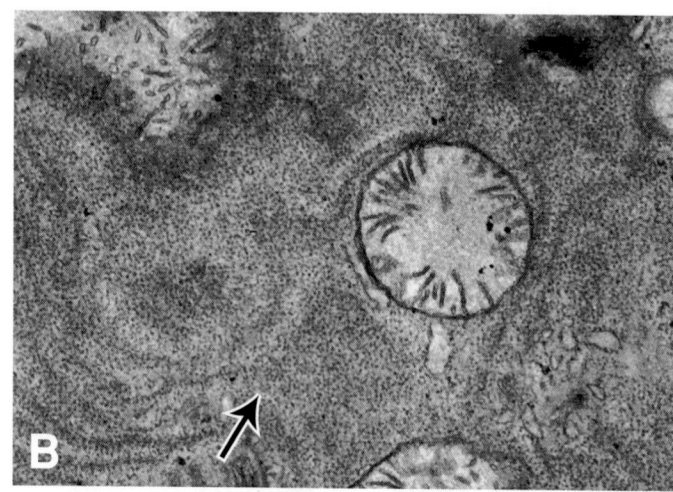

FIGURE 1-3. Disaggregation of membrane-bound ribosomes in acute, reversible liver injury. A. The profiles of endoplasmic reticulum (*arrows*) in a normal hepatocyte are studded with ribosomes. **B.** An injured hepatocyte shows detachment of ribosomes from the membranes of the endoplasmic reticulum and accumulation of free ribosomes in the cytoplasm (*arrow*).

membrane, (2) the plasma membrane sodium (Na$^+$) pump and (3) adenosine triphosphate (ATP). The plasma membrane prevents two gradient-driven ion flows: the flow of Na$^+$ from the extracellular fluid into the cell, and the flow of potassium (K$^+$) out of the cell. The barrier to sodium is imperfect and its relative leakiness permits some passive entry of sodium into the cell. To compensate for this intrusion, the energy-dependent, plasma membrane sodium pump (Na$^+$/K$^+$-ATPase), which is fueled by ATP, extrudes sodium from the cell. Noxious agents may interfere with this membrane-regulated process by (1) increasing plasma membrane permeability to Na$^+$, thereby exceeding the capacity of the pump to extrude the ion; (2) damaging the pump directly; or (3) interfering with ATP synthesis, and so depriving the pump of its fuel. In any event, accumulation of sodium in the cell leads to increased intracellular water to maintain isosmotic conditions. The cell then swells.

Subcellular Changes in Reversibly Injured Cells

- **Endoplasmic reticulum (ER):** The cisternae of the ER are distended by fluid in hydropic swelling (Fig. 1-2). Membrane-bound polysomes may disaggregate and detach from the surface of the rough endoplasmic reticulum (Fig. 1-3).
- **Mitochondria:** In some forms of acute injury, particularly ischemia (lack of adequate blood flow; see below), mitochondria swell (Fig. 1-4). This enlargement is due to dissipation of the mitochondrial energy gradient (membrane potential), impairing volume control.

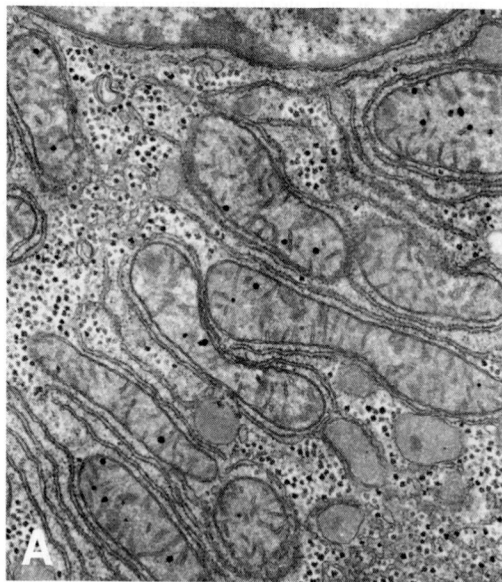 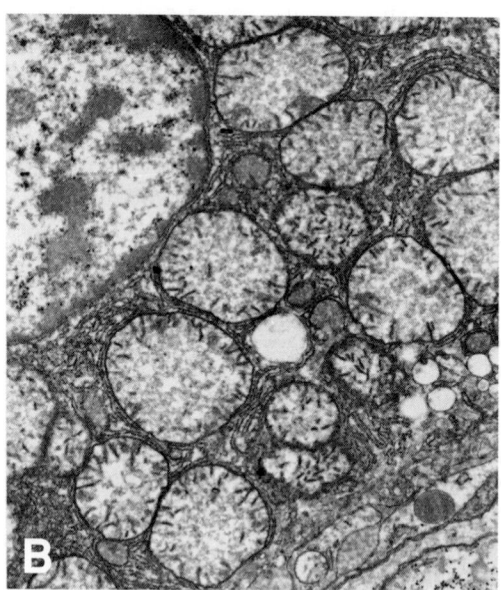

FIGURE 1-4. Mitochondrial swelling in acute ischemic cell injury. A. Normal hepatocyte mitochondria are elongated and display prominent cristae, which traverse the mitochondrial matrix. **B.** Mitochondria from an ischemic cell are swollen and round and exhibit a decreased matrix density. The cristae are less prominent than in the normal organelle.

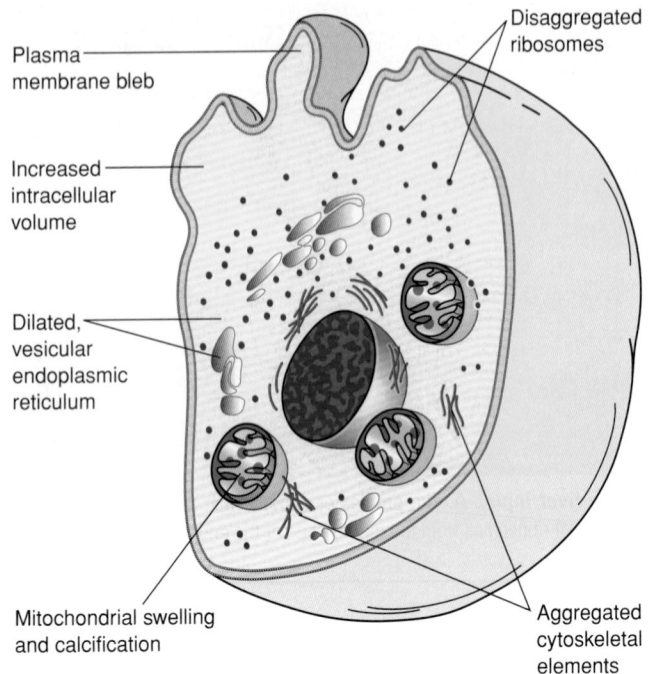

FIGURE 1-5. Ultrastructural features of reversible cell injury.

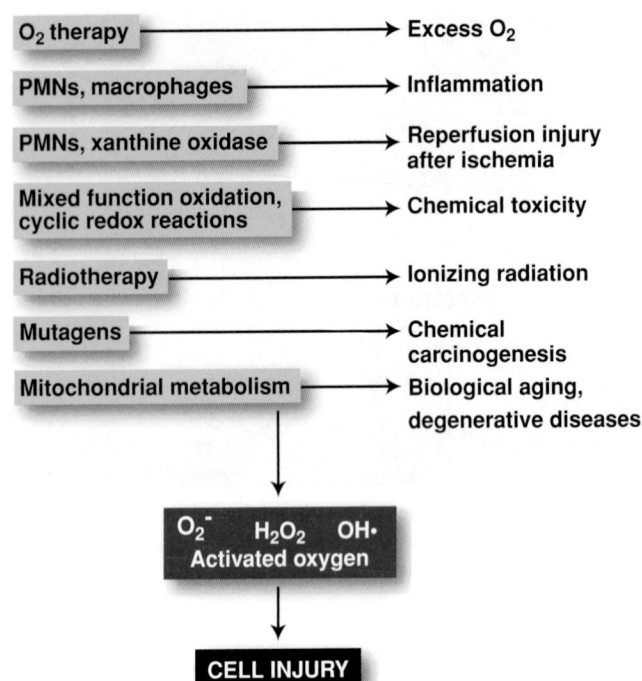

FIGURE 1-6. The role of activated oxygen species in cell injury. H_2O_2 = hydrogen peroxide; O_2 = oxygen; O_2^- = superoxide; $OH\bullet$ = hydroxyl radical; *PMNs* = polymorphonuclear neutrophils.

Amorphous densities rich in phospholipid may appear in the mitochondria, but these effects are fully reversible on recovery.

- **Plasma membrane:** Blebs of plasma membrane—that is, focal extrusions of the cytoplasm—are occasionally noted. These can detach from the membrane into the external environment without loss of cell viability.
- **Nucleus:** Reversible injury of the nucleus is reflected mainly by segregation of the fibrillar and granular components of the nucleolus. Alternatively, the granular component may be diminished, leaving only a fibrillar core.

These changes in cell organelles (Fig. 1-5) are reflected in functional derangements (e.g., reduced protein synthesis, impaired energy production). *After withdrawal of the stress that caused the reversible cell injury, by definition, the cell returns to its normal state.*

Ischemic Cell Injury Results from Obstruction to the Flow of Blood

When tissues are deprived of oxygen, ATP cannot be produced by aerobic metabolism and is instead made inefficiently by anaerobic metabolism. Ischemia initiates a series of chemical and pH imbalances, which are accompanied by increased generation of injurious free radical species. The damage produced by short periods of ischemia tends to be reversible if circulation is restored. However, long periods of ischemia lead to irreversible cell injury and death. The mechanisms of cell damage are discussed below.

Oxidative Stress Is a Key Trigger for Cell and Tissue Injury and Adaptive Responses

For human life, oxygen is both a blessing and a curse. Without it, life is impossible, but some of its derivatives are partially reduced oxygen species that can react with, and damage, virtually any molecule they reach.

Reactive Oxygen Species

Reactive oxygen species (ROS) are the likely causes of cell and tissue injury in many settings (Fig. 1-6). Oxygen (O_2) has a major role as the terminal electron acceptor in mitochondria. It is reduced from O_2 to H_2O, and resultant energy is harnessed as an electrochemical potential across the mitochondrial inner membrane.

Conversion of O_2 to H_2O entails transfer of four electrons. Three partially reduced species, representing transfers of varying numbers of electrons, are intermediate between O_2 and H_2O (Fig. 1-7). These are O_2^-, superoxide (one electron); H_2O_2, hydrogen peroxide (two electrons); and $OH\bullet$, the hydroxyl radical (three electrons). Under physiologic conditions these ROS come from several sources, including leaks in mitochondrial electron transport and mixed-function oxygenases (P450). In addition, ROS are important cellular signaling intermediates. The major forms of ROS are listed in Table 1-1. Importantly, excessive ROS levels both cause and aggravate many disorders (Fig. 1-6).

Superoxide

The superoxide anion (O_2^-) is produced mainly by leaks in mitochondrial electron transport or as part of inflammatory responses. In the first case, the promiscuity of coenzyme Q (CoQ) and other imperfections in the electron transport chain allow transfer of electrons to O_2 to yield O_2^-. In phagocytic inflammatory cells, activation of a plasma membrane oxidase produces O_2^-, which is then converted to H_2O_2 and eventually to other ROS (Fig. 1-8). These ROS

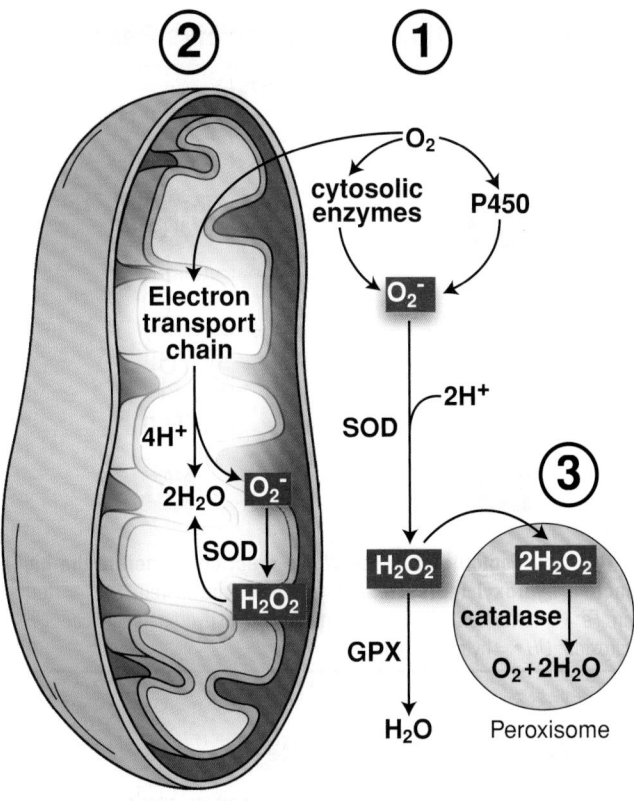

FIGURE 1-7. Mechanisms by which reactive oxygen radicals are generated from molecular oxygen and then detoxified by cellular enzymes. Circulating oxygen delivered to the cell may follow one of three paths: **1.** Molecular O_2 is converted to O_2^- in the cytosol. O_2^- is reduced to H_2O_2 by cytosolic superoxide dismutase (Cu/Zn SOD), and finally to water. **2.** O_2 enters the mitochondria, where inefficiencies in electron transport result in conversion of O_2 to O_2^-. This superoxide is rendered less reactive by further reduction to H_2O_2, via mitochondrial SOD (MnSOD). This H_2O_2 is then converted to H_2O by GPX. **3.** Cytosolic H_2O_2 enters peroxisomes where it is detoxified to H_2O by catalase. *CoQ* = coenzyme Q; *GPX* = glutathione peroxidase; *H^+* = hydrogen ion; *H_2O* = water; *H_2O_2* = hydrogen peroxide; *O_2* = oxygen; *O_2^-* = superoxide; *SOD* = superoxide dismutase.

TABLE 1-1
REACTIVE OXYGEN SPECIES (ROS)

Molecule	Attributes
Hydrogen peroxide (H_2O_2)	Forms free radicals via Fe^{2+}-catalyzed Fenton reaction Diffuses widely within the cell
Superoxide anion (O_2^-)	Generated by leaks in the electron transport chain and some cytosolic reactions Produces other ROS Does not readily diffuse far from its origin
Hydroxyl radical (OH•)	Generated from H_2O_2 by Fe^{2+}-catalyzed Fenton reaction The intracellular radical most responsible for attack on macromolecules
Peroxynitrite (ONOO•)	Formed from the reaction of nitric oxide (NO) with O_2^- Damages macromolecules
Lipid peroxide radicals (RCOO•)	Organic radicals produced during lipid peroxidation
Hypochlorous acid (HOCl)	Produced by macrophages and neutrophils during respiratory burst that accompanies phagocytosis Dissociates to yield hypochlorite radical (OCl⁻)

Fe^{2+} = ferrous iron.

within peroxisomes and (2) glutathione peroxidase (GPX) in both the cytosol and mitochondria (Fig. 1-7). GPX uses reduced glutathione (GSH) as a cofactor in a reaction yielding oxidized glutathione (GSSG). Because it is membrane permeable, H_2O_2 generated in mitochondria affects the oxidant balance, not only in mitochondria but also in other cellular compartments.

Hydroxyl Radical

Hydroxyl radicals (OH•) are formed by (1) radiolysis of water, (2) reaction of H_2O_2 with ferrous iron (Fe^{2+}) or cuprous copper (Cu^{1+}) (Fenton reaction) and (3) conversion of O_2^- with H_2O_2 (Haber-Weiss reaction) (Fig. 1-9). *The hydroxyl radical is the most reactive ROS*, and there are several mechanisms by which it can damage macromolecules.

Iron is often an active participant in oxidative damage to cells (see below) by virtue of the Fenton reaction. In a number of different cell types, H_2O_2 stimulates iron uptake and so increases production of hydroxyl radicals.

■ **Lipid peroxidation:** The hydroxyl radical removes a hydrogen atom from unsaturated fatty acids in membrane phospholipids, a process that forms a free lipid radical (Fig. 1-10). The lipid radical then reacts with molecular oxygen to generate a lipid peroxide radical. Subsequently, lipid peroxides act as initiators, removing a hydrogen atom from a second unsaturated fatty acid, to yield a lipid peroxide and a new lipid radical, initiating

have generally been viewed as key effectors of cellular defenses that destroy pathogens, fragments of necrotic cells or other phagocytosed material (see Chapter 2). ROS acting as signaling intermediates elicit the release of proteolytic and other degradative enzymes, which are critical effectors of neutrophil-mediated destruction of bacteria and other foreign materials.

Hydrogen Peroxide

O_2^- anions are converted by superoxide dismutase (SOD) to H_2O_2. Hydrogen peroxide is also produced directly by a number of oxidases in cytoplasmic peroxisomes (Fig. 1-7). By itself, H_2O_2 is not particularly injurious, and it is largely metabolized to H_2O by catalase. However, when produced in excess, it is converted to highly reactive OH•. In neutrophils, myeloperoxidase transforms H_2O_2 to a potent radical, hypochlorite (OCl⁻), which is lethal for microorganisms and, if released extracellularly, can kill cells.

Most cells have efficient mechanisms for removing H_2O_2. Two different enzymes reduce H_2O_2 to water: (1) catalase

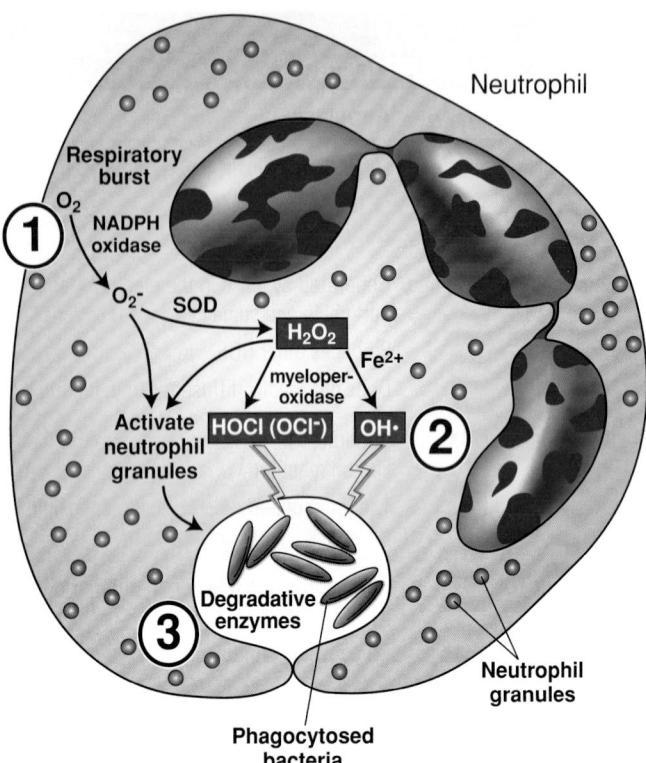

FIGURE 1-8. Generation of reactive oxygen species in neutrophils as a result of phagocytosis of bacteria. 1. The respiratory burst in neutrophils begins with reduction of O_2 to O_2^- by NADPH oxidase. In turn, O_2^- is converted to H_2O_2 by SOD. **2.** Reactive oxygen species (ROS) (HOCl, OH●) are produced from H_2O_2 by myeloperoxidase. Concurrently, O_2^- and H_2O_2 activate neutrophil granules to release degradative enzymes. **3.** Bacteria are engulfed by neutrophils, where they are destroyed by ROS and degradative enzymes. Fe^{2+} = ferrous iron; H_2O_2 = hydrogen peroxide; $HOCl$ = hypochlorous acid; $NADPH$ = reduced nicotinamide adenine dinucleotide phosphate; OCl^- = hypochlorite radical; $OH●$ = hydroxyl radical; SOD = superoxide dismutase.

a chain reaction. Lipid peroxides are unstable and break down into smaller molecules. Destruction of unsaturated fatty acids of phospholipids results in a loss of membrane integrity.

- **Protein interactions:** Hydroxyl radicals may also attack proteins. The sulfur-containing amino acids cysteine and methionine, as well as the nitrogen-containing moieties arginine, histidine and proline, are especially vulnerable to attack by OH●. As a result of oxidative damage, proteins undergo fragmentation, cross-linking, aggregation and eventually degradation (see below).
- **Sugars:** OH● can attack a variety of sugars and other carbohydrates to generate reactive intermediates that modify proteins to form injurious compounds, called advanced glycation end-products (AGEs).
- **DNA damage:** The hydroxyl radical causes diverse structural alterations in DNA, including strand breaks, modified bases and cross-links between strands. The integrity of the genome can usually be reconstituted by the various DNA repair pathways. However, if oxidative damage to DNA is sufficiently extensive, permanent DNA mutations or cell death may result.

Fig. 1-11 summarizes the mechanisms of cell injury by ROS.

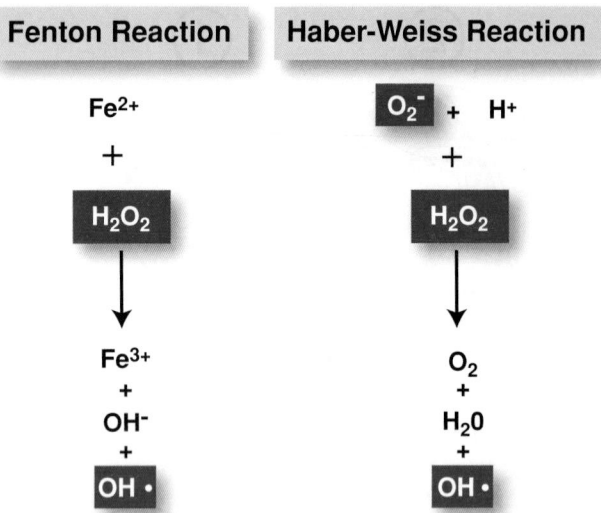

FIGURE 1-9. Fenton and Haber-Weiss reactions generate the highly reactive hydroxyl radical. Reactive species are in red. Fe^{2+} = ferrous iron; Fe^{3+} = ferric iron; H^+ = hydrogen ion; H_2O_2 = hydrogen peroxide; OH^- = hydroxide; $OH●$ = hydroxyl radical.

Nitric Oxide and Peroxynitrite

Nitric oxide (NO) is a reactive nitrogen molecule that is found in many cells and has a half-life measured in seconds. It is the product of nitric oxide synthase (NOS), a ubiquitous enzyme that comes in two flavors: inducible NOS (iNOS) and constitutive NOSs that are found in several tissues. NO has diverse signaling properties and may be harmful or protective to cells, depending on the circumstances. As a free radical, NO reacts with many molecular targets and activates or inhibits numerous cell functions.

When NO and oxygen interact, production of other free radicals results. These secondary radicals may nitrosate amines or modify other available groups, such as sulfurs on some amino acids. In addition, NO can react with

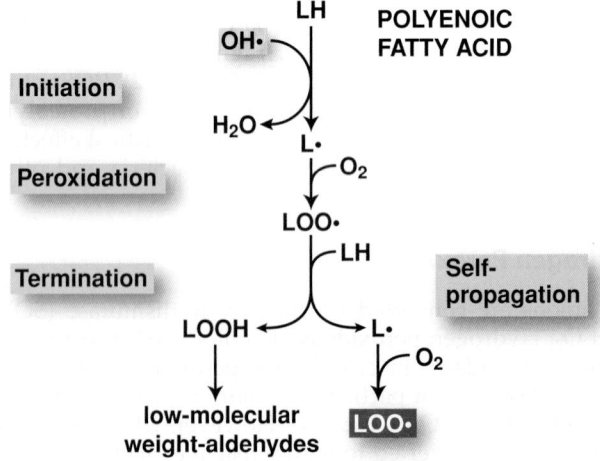

FIGURE 1-10. Lipid peroxidation initiated by the hydroxyl radical (OH●). Unsaturated fatty acids are converted to lipid radicals by OH●, which in turn reacts with molecular oxygen to form lipid peroxides. H_2O = water; O_2 = oxygen; $L●$ = lipid radical; $LOO●$ = lipid peroxy radical; $LOOH$ = lipid peroxide.

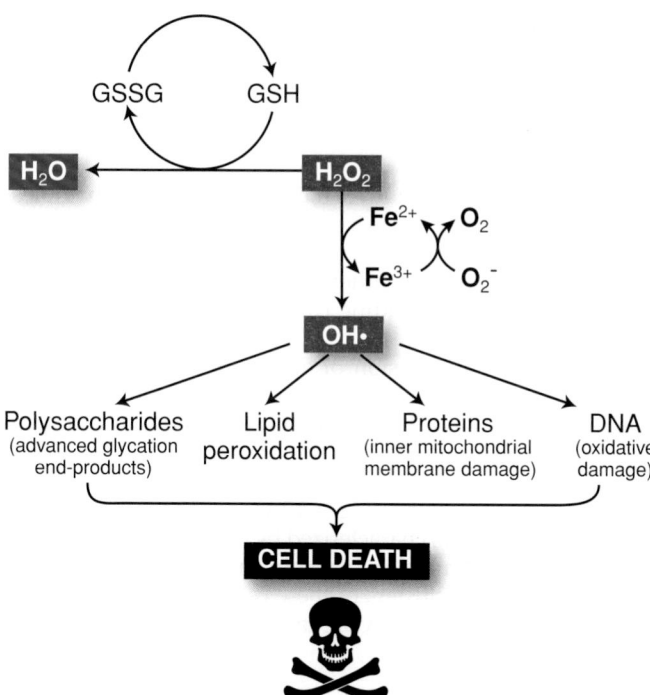

FIGURE 1-11. Mechanisms of cell injury by activated oxygen species. Fe^{2+} = ferrous iron; Fe^{3+} = ferric iron; GSH = glutathione; $GSSG$ = oxidized glutathione; H_2O_2 = hydrogen peroxide; O_2 = oxygen; O_2^- = superoxide anion; $OH\bullet$ = hydroxyl radical.

superoxide to form another free radical, namely, peroxynitrite ($ONOO^-$):

$$NO\bullet + O_2^- \rightarrow ONOO^-.$$

Peroxynitrite attacks many important cellular molecules, including lipids, proteins and DNA. Its actions may be beneficial or harmful, depending on the context.

Miscellaneous ROS

Recent data suggest that other ROS, particularly singlet oxygen ($O\bullet$) and carbonyl radical ($CO_3^-\bullet$), may play important roles in oxidative stress.

The Effectiveness of Cellular Defenses May Determine the Outcome of ROS-Mediated Injury

Cells possess potent antioxidant defenses, including detoxifying enzymes and exogenous free radical scavengers (e.g., vitamins). The major enzymes that convert ROS to less reactive molecules are SOD, catalase and GPX.

Detoxifying Enzymes

- **SOD** is the first line of defense against O_2^-, converting it to H_2O_2 and O_2 ($2O_2^- + 2H^+O_2 + H_2O_2$).
- **Catalase,** mainly located in peroxisomes, is one of two enzymes that complete the detoxification of O_2^- by converting H_2O_2 to water, thereby, preventing its conversion to $OH\bullet$ ($2H_2O_2 \rightarrow 2H_2O + O_2$).
- **GPX** catalyzes the reduction of H_2O_2 and lipid peroxides in mitochondria and the cytosol ($H_2O_2 + 2GSH \rightarrow 2H_2O + GSSG$).

Scavengers of ROS

- **Vitamin E (α-tocopherol)** is a terminal electron acceptor that aborts free radical chain reactions. As it is fat soluble, α-tocopherol protects membranes from lipid peroxidation.
- **Vitamin C (ascorbate)** is water soluble and reacts directly with O_2, $OH\bullet$ and some products of lipid peroxidation. It also serves to regenerate the reduced form of vitamin E.
- **Retinoids,** the precursors of vitamin A, are lipid soluble and act as chain-breaking antioxidants.
- **NO•** may scavenge ROS, principally by chelation of iron and combination with other free radicals.

Extracellular Oxidants and Antioxidants

Many intracellular processes generate ROS that diffuse or are transported outside cells, where they then may act as precursors of further oxidants. Such molecules include H_2O_2, lipid hydroperoxides, halogenated species such as hypochlorous acid (HOCl) derived from myeloperoxidase and related enzymes, as well as other compounds. Extracellular molecules that act as antioxidants include albumin, glutathione, ascorbate (vitamin C), α-tocopherol (vitamin E) and an extracellular form of SOD.

Although the consequences of oxidative stress in the extracellular matrix (ECM) are not well understood, matrix proteins such as collagen, elastin, fibronectin and laminin are damaged. Nonprotein ECM constituents (glycosaminoglycans, chondroitin sulfate, hyaluronan, etc.) may also be altered. Damage to these ECM molecules may lead to functional impairments in skin, bone and cartilage. Basement membranes throughout the body are also affected, particularly in the kidney and lungs.

p53 May Enhance or Inhibit Oxidative Damage

p53 is a versatile actor that plays diverse roles in the drama of cell survival and death (see later and Chapter 5). On the one hand, p53 helps to prevent and repair DNA damage, thereby rescuing cells from injury due to many endogenous and exogenous sources. On the other hand, if DNA damage is irreparable, p53 activates cell death programs (see below). In addition to these activities, p53 orchestrates cellular metabolic activity in response to levels of oxidative stress.

Under normal conditions with low oxidant stress and normal levels of metabolic activity, this protein maintains expression of many antioxidant genes, thus promoting cell survival. In the face of severe oxidant stress, p53 performs an about-face and activates a different suite of target genes that impair oxidant defenses, allow cellular damage to accumulate and eventuate in cell death. In addition to these effects on gene transcription, p53 directs metabolic pathways that reinforce its transcriptional activity.

Intracellular Storage Is Retention of Materials within the Cell

Substances that accumulate within cells may be normal or abnormal, endogenous or exogenous, harmful or innocuous.

- **Nutrients,** such as fat, glycogen, vitamins and minerals, are stored for later use.
- **Degraded phospholipids,** from the turnover of endogenous membranes, are engulfed in lysosomes and may be recycled.

- **Substances that are not metabolized** accumulate in cells. These include (1) endogenous substrates that are not further processed because a key enzyme is missing (hereditary storage diseases), (2) insoluble endogenous pigments (e.g., lipofuscin, melanin), (3) aggregates of normal or abnormal proteins and (4) foreign particulates, such as inhaled silica or carbon or injected tattoo pigments.
- **Overload of normal body constituents,** including iron, copper and cholesterol, injures a variety of cells.
- **Abnormal forms of proteins** may be toxic if they are retained within cells (e.g., Lewy bodies in Parkinson disease and mutant α_1-antitrypsin; see below).

Fat

Bacteria and other unicellular organisms continuously ingest nutrients. By contrast, mammals do not need to eat continuously. They eat periodically and can survive a prolonged fast because they store nutrients in specialized cells for later use—fat in adipocytes and glycogen in the liver, heart and muscle.

Abnormal accumulation of fat is most conspicuous in the liver (see Chapter 20). Briefly, hepatocytes always contain some fat, because they take up free fatty acids released from adipose tissue and convert them to triglycerides. Most such newly synthesized triglycerides are secreted by the liver as lipoproteins. If delivery of free fatty acids to the liver increases, as in diabetes, or intrahepatic lipid metabolism is disturbed, as in alcoholism, triglycerides accumulate in liver cells. Fatty liver is visualized as lipid globules in the cytoplasm. Other organs, including the heart, kidney and skeletal muscle, also store fat. *Fat storage is always reversible and there is no evidence that excess fat in the cytoplasm per se interferes with cell function.*

Glycogen

Glycogen is a long-chain polymer of glucose, formed and largely stored in the liver and to a lesser extent in muscles. It is depolymerized to glucose and liberated as needed. Glycogen is degraded in steps by a series of enzymes, each of which may be deficient because of an inborn error of metabolism. Regardless of the specific enzyme deficiency, the result is a glycogen storage disease (see Chapter 6). These inherited disorders affect the liver, heart and skeletal muscle and range from mild and asymptomatic conditions to inexorably progressive and fatal diseases (see Chapters 11, 20 and 31).

Glycogen storage in cells is normally regulated by blood glucose concentration, and hyperglycemic states are associated with increased glycogen stores. Thus, in uncontrolled diabetes, hepatocytes and epithelial cells of the renal proximal tubules are enlarged by excess glycogen.

Inherited Lysosomal Storage Diseases

As with glycogen, catabolism of certain complex lipids and mucopolysaccharides (glycosaminoglycans) takes place by a sequence of enzymatic steps. Since these enzymes are located in the lysosomes, their absence results in lysosomal storage of incompletely degraded lipids, such as cerebrosides (Gaucher disease) and gangliosides (Tay-Sachs disease) or products of mucopolysaccharide catabolism (Hurler and Hunter syndromes). Although these disorders are all progressive, their manifestations vary from asymptomatic organomegaly to rapidly fatal brain disease (see Chapter 6 for the metabolic bases of these disorders and Chapters 30 and 32 for specific organ pathology).

Cholesterol

The human body has a love–hate relationship with cholesterol. On the one hand, it is a critical component of all plasma membranes. On the other hand, when stored in excess, it is closely associated with atherosclerosis and cardiovascular disease, which is the leading cause of death in the Western world (see Chapter 16).

Briefly, the initial lesion of atherosclerosis (fatty streak) reflects accumulation of cholesterol and cholesterol esters in macrophages within the arterial intima. As the disease progresses, smooth muscle cells also store cholesterol. Advanced lesions of atherosclerosis are characterized by extracellular deposition of cholesterol (Fig. 1-12A).

In some disorders characterized by elevated blood levels of cholesterol (e.g., familial hypercholesterolemia), macrophages store cholesterol. If clusters of these cells in subcutaneous tissues are grossly visible, they are called **xanthomas** (Fig. 1-12B).

Lipofuscin

Lipofuscin is a mixture of lipids and proteins that appears as a golden-brown pigment and has been termed "wear and tear" pigment. **It tends to accumulate by accretion of peroxidized unsaturated lipids and oxidized, cross-linked proteins. It is indigestible** and has been compared to production of linoleum by oxidation of linseed oil. This process causes the unsaturated lipids in the oil progressively to solidify, turn brown and become less soluble. Lipofuscin accumulates mainly in postmitotic cells (e.g., neurons, cardiac myocytes) or in cells that cycle infrequently (e.g., hepatocytes) (Fig. 1-12C) and increases with age. In fact, measurement of lipofuscin in optic neurons has been used by fisheries to estimate age in lobsters and other crustaceans. It is often more conspicuous in conditions associated with atrophy of an organ.

Although it was previously thought to be benign, there is increasing evidence that lipofuscin may be both a result and a cause of increasing oxidant stress in cells. It may impair both proteasomal function and lysosomal degradation of senescent or poorly functioning organelles, and so promote cellular oxidant injury. Inefficient or misfunctioning mitochondria may accumulate, make more ROS and continue the cycle.

Melanin

Melanin is an insoluble, brown-black pigment found principally in epidermal cells of the skin, but also in the eye and other organs (Fig. 1-12D). It is located in intracellular organelles known as melanosomes and results from polymerization of certain oxidation products of tyrosine. The amount of melanin is responsible for the differences in skin color among the various races, as well as the color of the eyes. It serves a protective function owing to its ability to absorb ultraviolet light. In white persons, exposure to sunlight increases melanin formation (tanning). The hereditary inability to produce melanin is known as **albinism**. The presence of melanin is also a marker of cancers that arise from melanocytes (melanoma). Melanin is discussed in detail in Chapter 28.

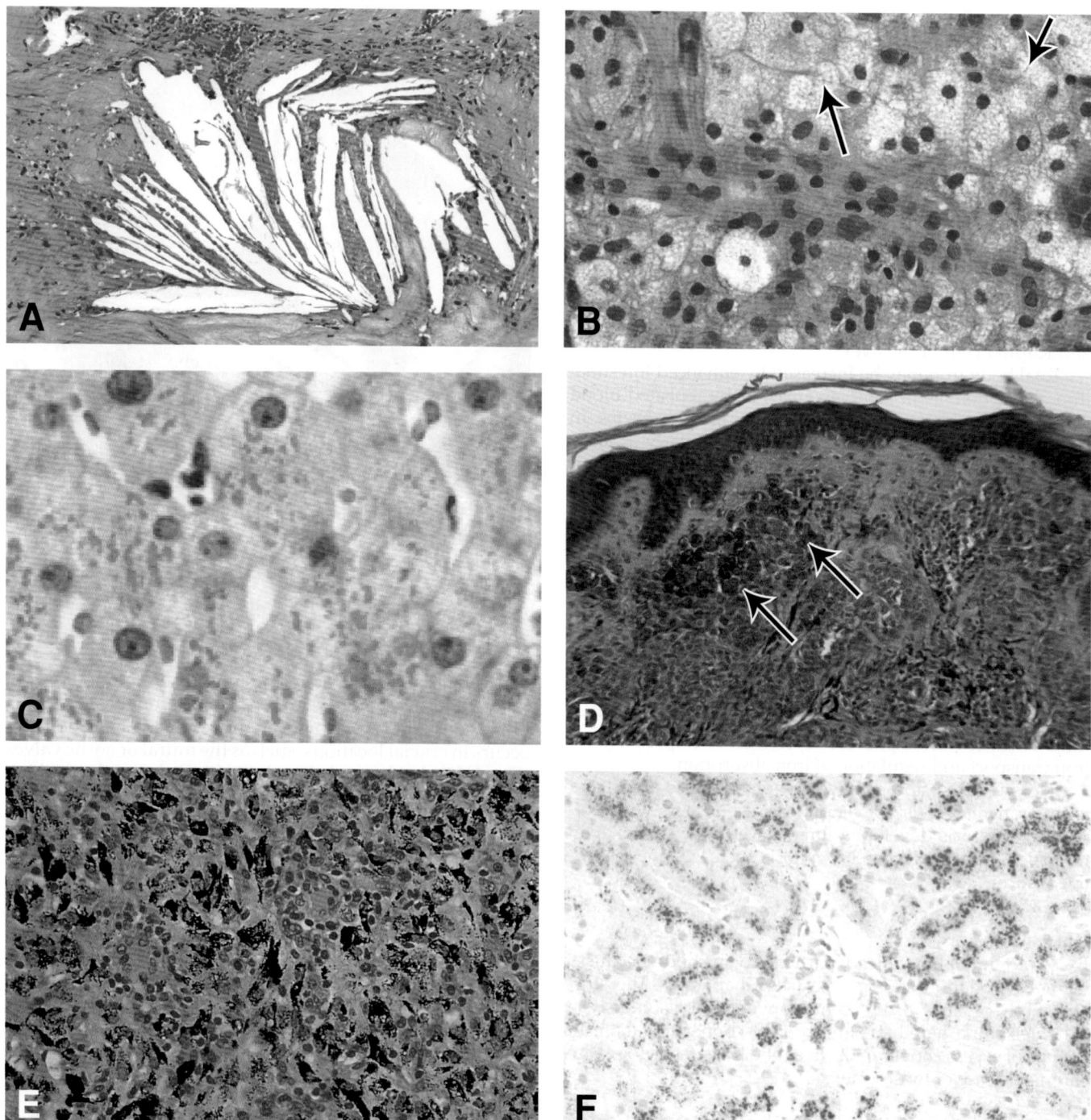

FIGURE 1-12. Abnormal intracellular storage. A. Abnormal cholesterol accumulation is characterized by transparent clefts, shown here in an atherosclerotic plaque. **B.** Lipid is stored in macrophages (*arrows*) in a cutaneous xanthoma. **C.** Lipofuscin in the liver from an 80-year-old man appears as golden cytoplasmic granules in lysosomes. **D.** Melanin (*arrows*) is stored in the cells of an intradermal nevus. **E.** Carbon pigment storage. A mediastinal lymph node, which drains the lungs, exhibits numerous macrophages that contain black anthracotic (carbon) pigment. This material was inhaled and originally deposited in the lungs. **F.** Iron storage in hereditary hemochromatosis. Prussian blue stain of the liver reveals large deposits of iron within hepatocellular lysosomes.

Exogenous Pigments

Anthracosis refers to storage of carbon particles in the lung and regional lymph nodes (Fig. 1-12E). Virtually all urban dwellers inhale particulates of organic carbon generated by the burning of fossil fuels. These particles accumulate in alveolar macrophages and are also transported to hilar and mediastinal lymph nodes, where the indigestible material is stored indefinitely within macrophages. Although the gross appearance of the lungs of persons with anthracosis may be alarming, the condition is innocuous.

Tattoos (from the Samoan, "tatou") reflect the introduction of insoluble metallic and vegetable pigments into the skin, where they are principally engulfed by dermal macrophages and persist for a lifetime.

Iron and Other Metals

Iron

About 25% of the body's total iron content is in an intracellular storage pool composed of the iron-storage proteins **ferritin** and **hemosiderin**. The liver and bone marrow are particularly rich in ferritin, although it is present in virtually all cells. Hemosiderin is a partially denatured form of ferritin that aggregates easily and is recognized microscopically as yellow-brown granules in the cytoplasm. Normally, hemosiderin is found mainly in the spleen, bone marrow and Kupffer cells of the liver.

Total body iron may be increased by enhanced intestinal iron absorption, as in some anemias, or by repeated blood transfusions, which include iron-containing erythrocytes. In either case, the excess iron is stored intracellularly as ferritin and hemosiderin. Increasing the body's total iron content leads to progressive accumulation of hemosiderin, which is called **hemosiderosis**. In this case, iron is present throughout the body, including the skin, pancreas, heart, kidneys and endocrine organs. However, by definition, intracellular accumulation of iron in hemosiderosis does not injure cells.

If, contrariwise, the increase in total body iron is extreme, it damages vital organs—the heart, liver, testes and pancreas. Iron overload can result from a genetic abnormality in iron absorption, namely, **hereditary hemochromatosis (HH)** (Fig. 1-12F). Tissue injury in HH most likely reflects iron-generated oxidative stress, as described above. In HH, mutations occur in one of the several genes responsible for iron transport and regulation of iron absorption.

Excessive iron storage in some organs is also associated with an increased risk of cancer. Metal polishers with pulmonary siderosis developed lung cancer with greater than normal frequency. Hemochromatosis increases the risk of liver cancer.

Other Metals

Excess accumulation of lead, particularly in children, causes mental retardation and anemia (see Chapter 8). The storage of other metals also presents dangers. In Wilson disease (Chapter 20), a hereditary disorder of copper metabolism, storage of excess copper in the liver and brain leads to severe chronic disease of those organs.

Calcification May Reflect Normal Development or an Abnormal Process

The deposition of mineral salts of calcium is, of course, a normal part of the formation of bone from cartilage. Calcium enters dead or dying cells because such cells cannot maintain a steep calcium gradient (see below). This cellular calcification is not ordinarily visible except as inclusions within mitochondria.

In "dystrophic" calcification macroscopic calcium salt deposits occur in injured tissues. This process does not simply represent accumulation of calcium derived from the bodies of dead cells but rather is caused by extracellular deposition of calcium from the circulation or interstitial fluid. Dystrophic calcification apparently requires the

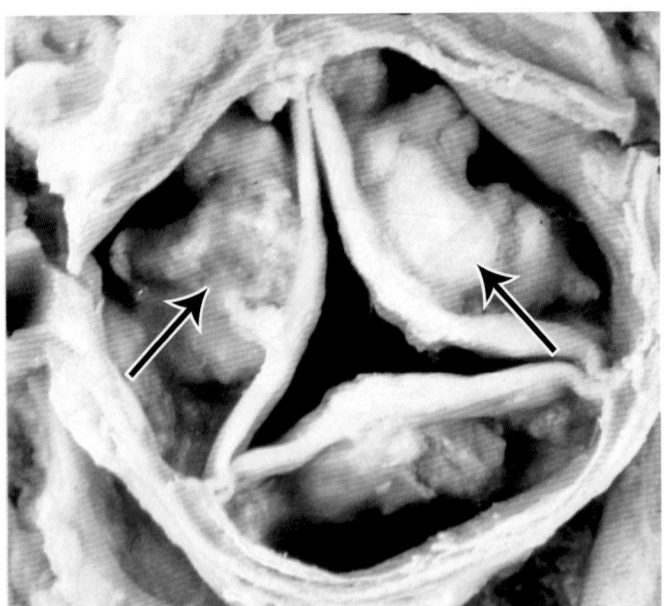

FIGURE 1-13. Calcific aortic stenosis. Deposits of solid calcium salts (*arrows*) are seen in the cusps and the free margins of the thickened aortic valve, viewed from above.

persistence of necrotic tissue; it is often visible to the naked eye and ranges from gritty, sand-like grains to firm, rock-hard material. Often, as in the lung or lymph nodes with tuberculous caseous necrosis, calcification has no functional consequences. However, dystrophic calcification that occurs in crucial locations, such as the mitral or aortic valves (Fig. 1-13), leads to obstruction of blood flow by making valve leaflets rigid and narrowing valve orifices (mitral and aortic stenosis). Dystrophic calcification in atherosclerotic coronary arteries contributes to narrowing of those vessels. Although molecules that participate in physiologic calcium deposition in bone (e.g., osteopontin, osteonectin and osteocalcin) are reported in association with dystrophic calcification, the mechanisms underlying this process remain obscure.

Dystrophic calcification also plays a role in diagnostic radiography. For example, mammography is based largely on the detection of small calcifications in breast cancers; congenital toxoplasmosis, an infection involving the central nervous system, is suggested when calcification is visualized in an infant's brain.

Unlike dystrophic calcification, which has its origin in cell injury, "metastatic" calcification reflects deranged calcium metabolism and is associated with increased serum calcium concentrations (**hypercalcemia**). In general, almost any disorder that increases blood calcium levels can lead to calcification in such inappropriate locations as pulmonary alveolar septa, renal tubules and blood vessels. Metastatic calcification is seen in various disorders, including chronic renal failure, vitamin D intoxication and hyperparathyroidism.

The formation of calcium-containing stones in sites such as the gallbladder, renal pelvis, bladder and pancreatic duct is another form of pathologic calcification. Under certain circumstances, the mineral salts precipitate from solution and crystallize about foci of organic material. Those who have suffered the agony of gallbladder or renal colic will attest to the unpleasant consequences of this type of calcification.

Hyaline Refers to Any Reddish, Homogeneous Material That Stains with Eosin

The term **hyaline** was used in classic descriptions of diverse and unrelated lesions, such as hyaline arteriolosclerosis, alcoholic hyaline in the liver, hyaline membranes in the lung and hyaline droplets in various cells. The various lesions called hyaline have nothing in common. Alcoholic hyaline is composed of cytoskeletal filaments; the hyaline found in arterioles of the kidney is derived from basement membranes; and hyaline membranes in the lung consist of plasma proteins deposited in alveoli. The term is anachronistic but is still used as a morphologic descriptor.

Hyperplasia Is an Increase in Cell Numbers in an Organ or Tissue

Stimuli that induce hyperplasia and the mechanisms by which they act vary greatly from one tissue and cell type to the next. An agent that elicits hyperplastic responses in one tissue either may not do so in another or may do so via mechanisms that are totally distinct. In response to such stimuli, cells divide to generate an organ or tissue that contains more than its usual complement of those cells (hypercellular). The dividing cells may derive from cells that are already cycling or from resting progenitors. This process may occur as a response to an altered endocrine milieu, increased functional demand or chronic injury. Hypertrophy (an increase in organ and/or cell size; see below) may occur simultaneously with hyperplasia.

Hormonal Stimulation

Changes in hormone concentrations can elicit proliferation of responsive cells. These changes may reflect developmental, pharmacologic or pathologic influences. For example, the normal increase in estrogens at puberty or early in the menstrual cycle leads to increased numbers of endometrial and uterine stromal cells. Estrogen administration to postmenopausal women has the same effect. Enlargement of the male breast, called gynecomastia, may occur in men with excess estrogens (e.g., following estrogen therapy for prostate cancer or when the liver's inability to metabolize endogenous estrogens leads to their accumulation, as in liver failure). Ectopic hormone production may be a tumor's first presenting symptom (e.g., erythropoietin secretion by renal tumors leads to hyperplasia of erythrocytes in the bone marrow).

Increased Functional Demand

Increased physiologic requirements may result in hyperplasia. For example, at high altitudes, low atmospheric oxygen tension causes compensatory hyperplasia of erythroid precursors in the bone marrow and increased blood erythrocytes (secondary polycythemia) (Fig. 1-14). In this fashion, increased numbers of cells compensate for the decreased oxygen carried by each erythrocyte. The number of red blood cells promptly falls to normal on return to sea level. Similarly, chronic blood loss, as in excessive menstrual bleeding, also causes hyperplasia of erythrocytic elements.

Immune responsiveness to many antigens may lead to lymphoid hyperplasia (e.g., the enlarged tonsils and swollen lymph nodes that occur with streptococcal pharyngitis). The hypocalcemia that occurs in chronic renal failure produces increased demand for parathyroid hormone in order to augment blood calcium. The result is hyperplasia of the parathyroid glands.

Chronic Injury

Persistent injury may result in hyperplasia. Long-standing inflammation or chronic physical or chemical injury is often accompanied by a hyperplastic response. For instance, pressure from ill-fitting shoes causes hyperplasia of the skin of the foot, so-called corns or calluses. Resultant thickening of the skin protects it from the continued pressure. Chronic inflammation of the bladder (chronic cystitis) often causes hyperplasia of the bladder epithelium, visible as white plaques on the bladder lining.

Inappropriate hyperplasia can itself be harmful—witness the unpleasant consequences of psoriasis, which is characterized by conspicuous hyperplasia of the skin (Fig. 1-14D). Excessive estrogen stimulation, whether from endogenous sources or from medication, may eventuate in endometrial hyperplasia.

The variety of cellular and molecular mechanisms responsible for the increased mitotic activity that characterizes hyperplastic responses clearly relates to altered control of cell proliferation. These topics are discussed in Chapters 3 and 5.

Metaplasia Is Conversion of One Differentiated Cell Type to Another

Metaplasia is usually an adaptive response to persistent injury. That is, a tissue will assume a phenotype that protects it best from the insult. Most often, glandular epithelium is replaced by squamous epithelium. Columnar or cuboidal lining cells that are committed to mucus production may not be adequately resistant to the effects of chronic irritation or a pernicious chemical. For example, prolonged exposure of bronchial epithelium to tobacco smoke leads to squamous metaplasia. A similar response is associated with chronic infection in the endocervix (Fig. 1-15). Whether metaplasia results from altered differentiation of maturing cells or a change in the commitment of tissue stem cells to one lineage rather than another remains unknown.

The process is not restricted to squamous differentiation. When highly acidic gastric contents reflux chronically into the lower esophagus, the squamous epithelium of the esophagus may be replaced by glandular mucosa (**Barrett esophagus**). This effect can be thought of as an adaptation to protect the esophagus from injury by gastric acid and pepsin, to which the glandular mucosa is more resistant.

Metaplasia may also consist of replacement of one glandular epithelium by another. In chronic gastritis, chronic inflammation causes atrophic stomach glands to be replaced by cells resembling those of the small intestine. The adaptive value of such intestinal metaplasia is not clear. Metaplasia of transitional epithelium to glandular epithelium occurs when the bladder is chronically inflamed (cystitis glandularis).

Although metaplasia may be thought of as adaptive, it is not necessarily innocuous. For example, squamous metaplasia may protect a bronchus from tobacco smoke, but it also impairs mucus production and ciliary clearance. Cancers

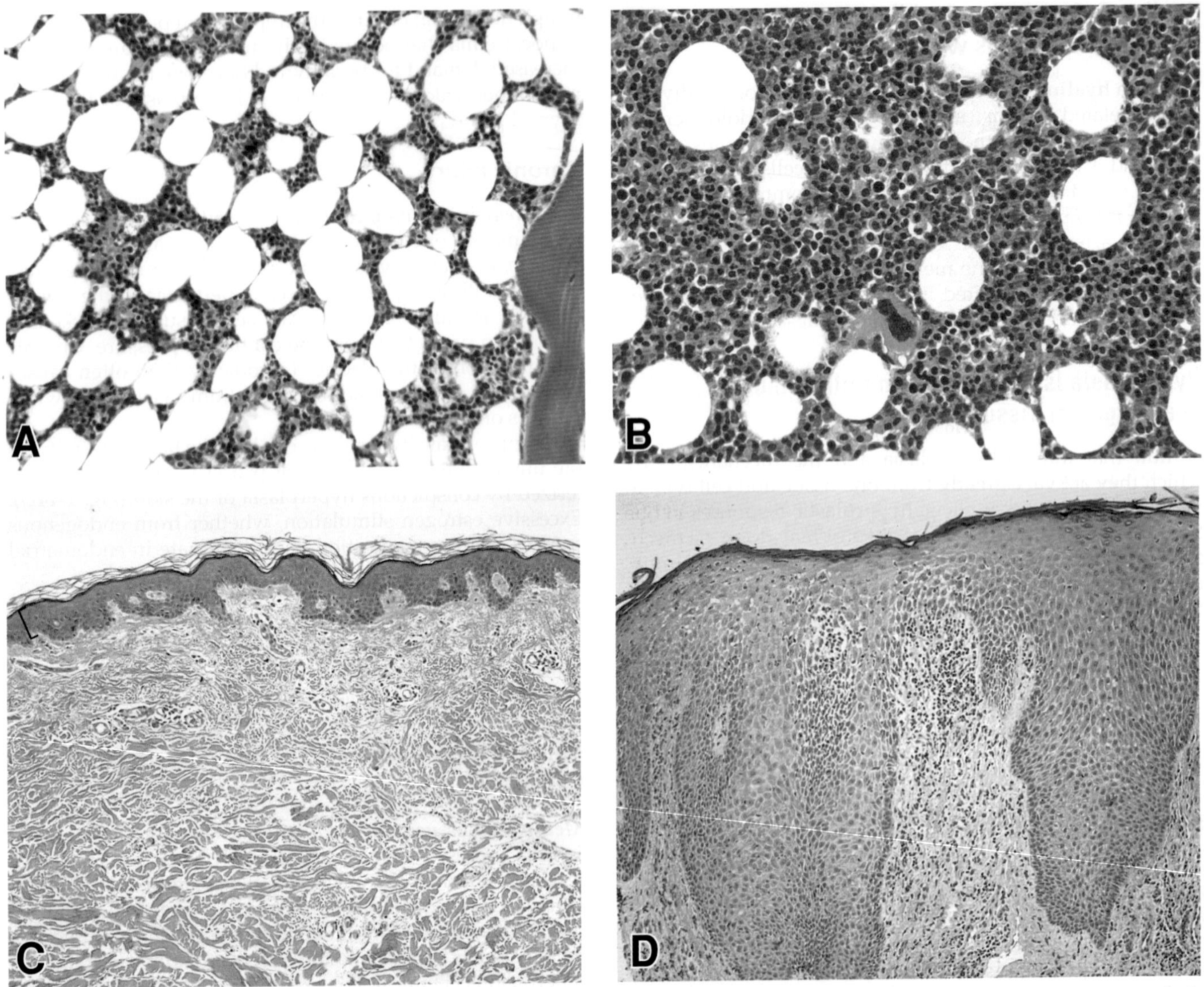

FIGURE 1-14. Hyperplasia. A. Normal adult bone marrow. Normocellular bone marrow shows the usual ratio of fat to hematopoietic cells. **B. Hyperplasia** of the bone marrow. Cellularity is increased; fat is relatively decreased. **C. Normal epidermis.** Epidermal thickness is modest (*bracket*) compared to the dermis (below). **D. Epidermal hyperplasia** in psoriasis is shown at the same magnification as in C. The epidermis is thickened owing to an increase in the number of squamous cells.

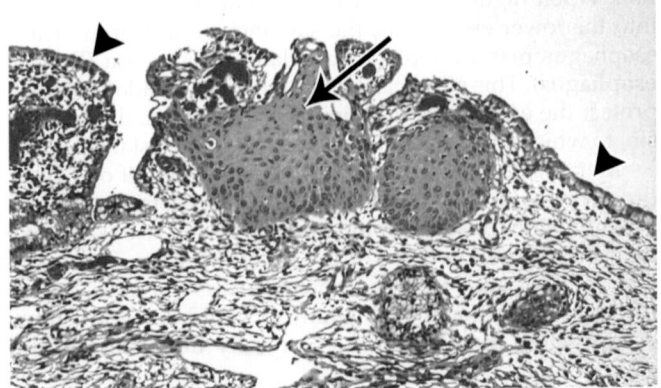

FIGURE 1-15. Squamous metaplasia. A section of endocervix shows the normal columnar epithelium at both margins (*arrowheads*) and a focus of squamous metaplasia in the center (*arrow*).

may develop in metaplastic epithelium; malignancies of the lung, cervix, stomach and bladder often arise in such areas. However, if the chronic injury ceases, there is little stimulus for cells to proliferate, and the epithelium does not become cancerous.

Metaplasia is usually fully reversible. If the noxious stimulus is removed (e.g., when one stops smoking), the metaplastic epithelium eventually returns to normal.

Dysplasia Is Disordered Cellular Growth and Maturation

The cells that compose an epithelium normally exhibit uniformity of size, shape and nuclei. Moreover, they are arranged in a regular fashion; for example, a squamous epithelium progresses from plump basal cells to flat superficial cells. In dysplasia, this pattern is disturbed by (1) variation

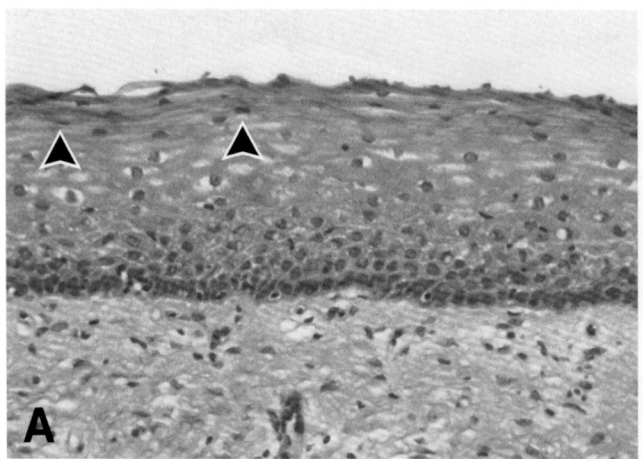
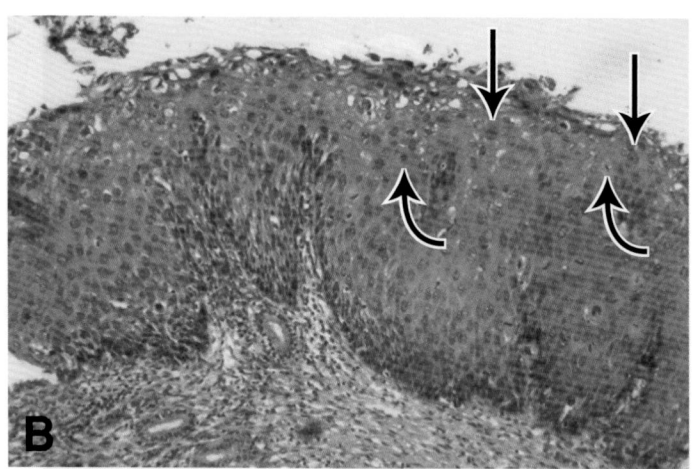

FIGURE 1-16. Dysplasia. A. Nondysplastic cervical epithelium. Normal cervix shows no mitotic activity above the most basal layers, but rather shows epithelial maturation, with flattening of the cells and progressive diminution of nuclei (*arrowheads*). **B.** At the same magnification, dysplastic epithelium of the uterine cervix lacks normal polarity, and individual cells show hyperchromatic nuclei and a greater than normal nucleus-to-cytoplasm ratio. Compare, for example, the size and hyperchromaticity of nuclei in the dysplastic cells (*straight arrows*) with the characteristics of normal counterparts at comparable height in the normal cervix. In contrast to normal cervix, cellular arrangement in dysplastic epithelium is disorderly, largely lacking appropriate histologic maturation, from the basal layers to the surface. Mitotic figures far above the basal layers (*curved arrows*) are common.

in cell size and shape; (2) nuclear enlargement, irregularity and hyperchromatism; and (3) disorderly arrangement of cells in the epithelium (Fig. 1-16). Dysplasia occurs most often in hyperplastic squamous epithelium, as in epidermal actinic keratosis (caused by sunlight), and in areas of squamous metaplasia, such as in the bronchus or the cervix. It is not, however, exclusive to squamous epithelium. For example, dysplastic changes occur in the columnar mucosal cells of the colon in ulcerative colitis, in metaplastic epithelium of Barrett esophagus (see Chapter 19), in prostate glands of prostatic intraepithelial neoplasia and in the urothelium of the bladder (see Chapter 23).

Like metaplasia, dysplasia is a response to persistent injury and will usually regress, for example, if smoking ceases or if human papilloma virus disappears from the cervix. However, dysplasia shares many cytologic features with cancer, and the line between the two may be very fine indeed. It may be difficult to distinguish severe dysplasia from early cancer of the cervix by appearance. ***Dysplasia is a preneoplastic lesion, in that it is a necessary stage in the multistep cellular evolution to cancer.*** In fact, dysplasia is included in morphologic classifications of the stages of intraepithelial neoplasia in several organs (e.g., cervix, prostate, bladder). Severe dysplasia is considered an indication for aggressive preventive therapy to (1) cure the underlying cause, (2) eliminate a noxious agent or (3) surgically remove the offending tissue.

As in the development of cancer (see Chapter 5), dysplasia results from sequential mutations in a proliferating cell population. The fidelity of DNA replication is imperfect, and occasional mutations are inevitable. When a particular mutation confers a growth or survival advantage, the progeny of the mutant cell will tend to predominate. In turn, their continued proliferation provides a greater opportunity for additional mutations. Accumulation of such mutations progressively distances the cell from normal regulatory constraints. ***Dysplasia is the morphologic expression of a disturbance in growth regulation.*** However, unlike cancer cells, dysplastic cells are not entirely autonomous, and with intervention, the tissue may still revert to normal.

REACTIONS TO PERSISTENT STRESS AND CELL INJURY

Persistent stress often requires that a cell either die or adapt. At the *cellular level,* then, it is more appropriate to speak of chronic adaptation than of chronic injury. The major adaptive responses are atrophy, hypertrophy, hyperplasia, metaplasia, dysplasia and intracellular storage. In some settings, as noted, neoplasia may follow adaptive responses.

Atrophy and Hypertrophy Are Two Sides of the Same Coin

Atrophy

Atrophy is the decreased size or function of cells or organs and occurs in both pathologic and physiologic settings. Thus, for example, atrophy may result from disuse of skeletal muscle or from loss of hormonal signals following menopause. It may also be an adaptive response whereby a cell accommodates changes in its environment, all the while remaining viable. However, most commonly atrophy reflects harmful processes, like those involved in some chronic diseases and biological aging (see below).

Atrophy of an organ differs from cellular atrophy. Reduction in an organ's size may be caused either by reversible cell shrinkage or by irreversible loss of cells. For example, renewing physical activity of a disused limb may cause atrophic muscle cells to resume their usual size and function. By contrast, atrophy of the brain in Alzheimer disease[2] is due to

---

[2]A note about eponymous diseases (i.e., diseases named after a person). In common usage, diseases bearing the names of Alzheimer, Parkinson, Cushing and so forth are cited as possessives (e.g., Alzheimer's disease, Parkinson's disease), but medical convention requires these diseases to be identified *without the possessive proper noun* ("Classification and nomenclature of morphological defects", *Lancet* 1975;1:513). Like many other journals and texts, we honor this convention.

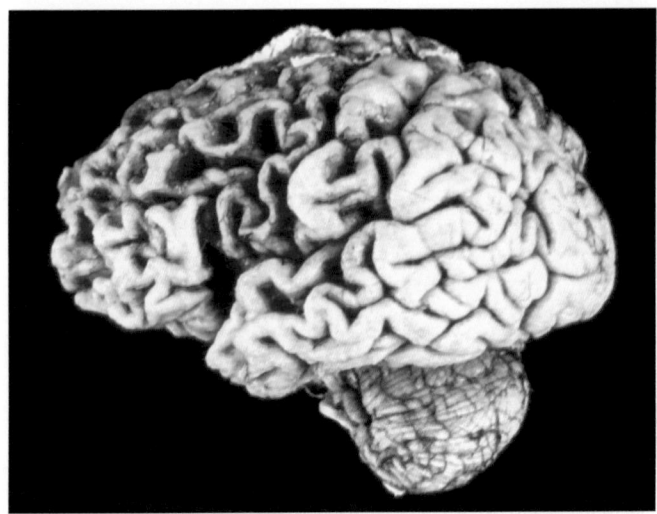

FIGURE 1-17. Atrophy of the brain. Marked atrophy of the frontal lobe is characterized by thinned gyri and widened sulci.

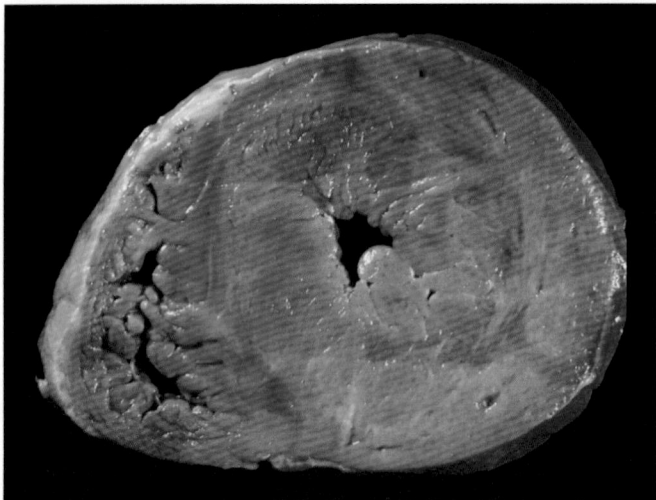

FIGURE 1-18. Myocardial hypertrophy. Cross-section of the heart of a patient with long-standing hypertension shows pronounced, concentric left ventricular hypertrophy.

extensive cell death; the size of the organ cannot be restored (Fig. 1-17). Atrophy occurs under a variety of conditions as outlined in Table 1-2.

Hypertrophy

Hypertrophy is an increase in cell or organ size and functional capacity. When trophic signals or functional demands increase, adaptive changes to satisfy these needs lead to larger cells (hypertrophy) and, in some cases, increased cell number (hyperplasia; see above). In several organs (e.g., heart, skeletal muscle), such adaptive responses are achieved mainly by increased cell size, which leads to increased organ

TABLE 1-2

CONDITIONS ASSOCIATED WITH ATROPHY

Disease or Condition	Examples of Conditions in Which Atrophy Occurs
Aging	Most organs that do not continuously turn over; most common setting for atrophy to occur
Chronic disease	Prototype for atrophy occurring in chronic disease is cancer; also seen in congestive heart failure, chronic obstructive pulmonary disease, cirrhosis of the liver and AIDS
Ischemia	Hypoxia, decreased nutrient availability, renal artery stenosis
Malnutrition	Generalized atrophy
Decreased functional demand	Limb immobilization, as in a fracture
Interruption of trophic signals	Denervation atrophy following nerve injury; menopause effect on the endometrium and other organs
Increased pressure	Decubitus ulcers, passive congestion of the liver

mass (Fig. 1-18). In other organs (e.g., kidney), cell numbers and cell size may both increase.

Normal Homeostasis Determines Individual Cell Mass

Cell size reflects an equilibrium between anabolic and catabolic forces. Although many different cell types are capable of atrophy and hypertrophy, skeletal muscle is the tissue most extensively studied, and it will be used as the paradigm of these mechanisms. In this organ, myocytes can adapt to increased functional demand by increasing synthesis of muscle proteins and downregulating their degradation. Conversely, muscle atrophy (wasting) may have many causes and leads to reduced synthesis and increased degradation of contractile proteins. Within a cell, the signaling pathways that control hypertrophy and atrophy are closely interconnected.

Conditions That Cause Atrophy Are Often the Inverse of Those That Stimulate Hypertrophy

Conditions Leading to Atrophy

Reduced Functional Demand
A common form of atrophy follows reduced functional demand. For example, after immobilization of a limb in a cast as treatment for a bone fracture, the limb's muscle cells lose mass, and strength is correspondingly reduced.

Inadequate Supply of Oxygen
Interference with blood supply to tissues, called ischemia, causes oxygen deprivation. If the ischemia is not sufficient to kill cells, affected cells may be viable but functionally impaired. In such settings, cell atrophy is common. It is frequently seen around the inadequately perfused margins of areas of ischemic necrosis (infarcts) in the heart, brain and kidneys after a vascular occlusion affecting these organs.

Insufficient Nutrients
Starvation or malnutrition leads to wasting (decreased mass) of skeletal muscle and adipose tissue. Microscopically this

appears as cell atrophy. Decreased size is prominent in cells (e.g., myocytes and adipocytes) that are not vital to the survival of the organism.

Interruption of Trophic Signals

The activities of many cells depend on signals triggered by chemical mediators (e.g., hormonal or neuromuscular transmission), which place functional demands on them. If the source of the signal is removed (e.g., via ablation of an endocrine gland or denervation), cells dependent on that stimulus will atrophy. If the anterior pituitary is surgically resected or lost to ischemia (e.g., Sheehan syndrome; see Chapter 14), deficiency of thyroid-stimulating hormone (TSH), adrenocorticotropic hormone (ACTH, also called corticotropin) and follicle-stimulating hormone (FSH) results in atrophy of the thyroid, adrenal cortex and ovaries, respectively.

Atrophy due to changes in hormone levels is not restricted to pathologic conditions; the endometrium atrophies when estrogen levels decrease after menopause (Fig. 1-19). Even certain cancer cells may undergo atrophy, at least to some extent, following hormonal deprivation. Androgen-dependent prostatic cancers and estrogen receptor–expressing breast cancers regress partially after administration of hormone antagonists. If neurologic damage (e.g., from traumatic spinal cord injury) leads to denervation of muscle, the affected muscles atrophy.

Persistent Cell Injury

Persistent cell injury may occur in prolonged viral or bacterial infections or via inflammation in immunologic and granulomatous disorders. Thus, atrophy of the gastric mucosa occurs during chronic gastritis, and small intestinal villous atrophy accompanies the chronic inflammation of celiac disease (see Chapter 19).

Increased Pressure

Even physical injury, such as prolonged pressure in inappropriate locations, produces atrophy. Prolonged bed rest may create sustained pressure on the skin, causing atrophy of the skin and consequent decubitus ulcers (bed sores).

Also, the cells in the center of the liver lobule atrophy when poor venous return from the liver in congestive heart failure increases the pressure within hepatic sinusoids.

Aging

In addition to conspicuous loss of skeletal muscle and adipose tissue, one of the hallmarks of aging (see Chapter 10) is decreased size and/or number of nonreplicating cells, such as those of the brain and heart. The mass of all parenchymal organs decreases with age. Brain size is invariably diminished, and in the very aged the heart may be so small that the term **senile atrophy** has been used.

Chronic Disease

People afflicted with wasting chronic diseases (see below), such as cancer, congestive heart failure or AIDS, often show generalized atrophy of many tissues. Tissue loss exceeds what can be attributed to decreased caloric intake and reflects alterations in cytokines and other mediators.

Conditions Leading to Hypertrophy

The situations that are associated with increased cell and organ mass are in many, but not all, cases the converse of those that lead to atrophy. Thus, increased functional demand or increased trophic signaling (see below) results in adaptive increases in cell or organ size. Unfortunately for many of us, even though nutrient deprivation may lead to atrophy of both muscle and fat, excess nutrient intake only causes increased fat.

Increased Functional Demand

Human skeletal muscle is composed of a mixture of slow-twitch (type I) and fast-twitch (type II) fibers. Each responds to different types of increased functional demand. A marathon runner undergoing endurance training with light loads will increase the strength of type I fibers. This is not usually associated with increased muscle mass (see below). For proper function, type I fibers depend principally on aerobic metabolism, mediated by mitochondria.

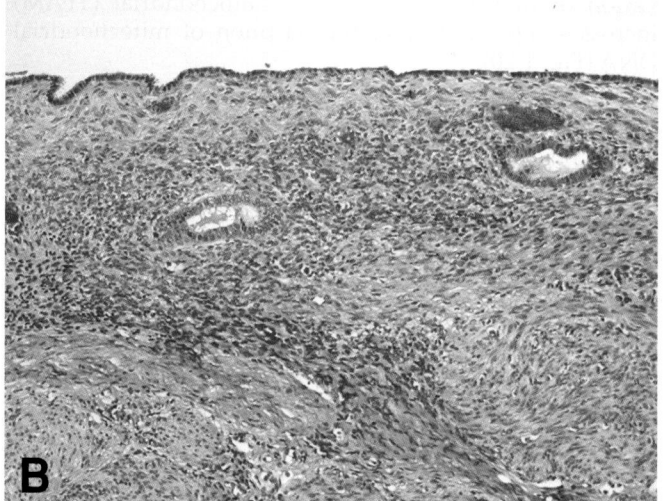

FIGURE 1-19. Atrophy of the endometrium. A. A section of the normal uterus from a woman of reproductive age reveals a thick endometrium composed of proliferative glands in an abundant stroma. **B.** The endometrium of a 75-year-old woman (shown at the same magnification) is thin and contains only a few atrophic and cystic glands.

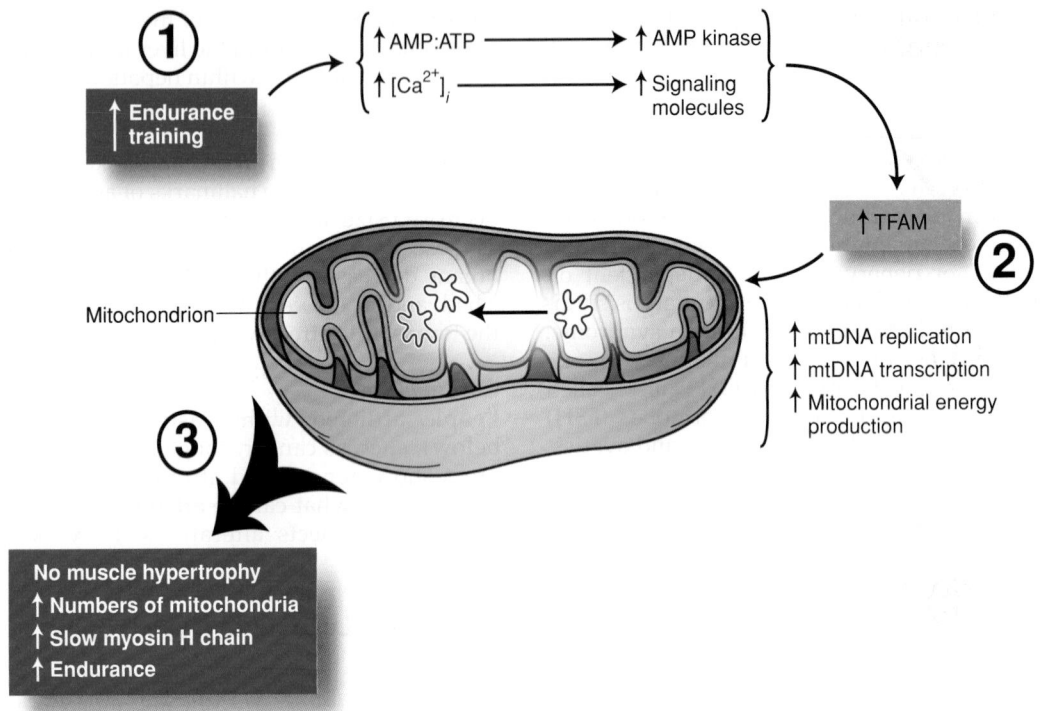

FIGURE 1-20. **Mechanisms involved in muscle hypertrophy: Endurance training. 1.** Muscle strengthening for endurance entails repeated or prolonged exercise with small loads and raises the adenosine monophosphate–to–adenosine triphosphate (AMP:ATP) ratio, stimulating AMP kinase activity. Such training also increases cytosolic calcium concentration ($[Ca^{2+}]_i$), which triggers a number of cellular signaling intermediates. **2.** Consequent peroxisome activation triggers TFAM (transcription factor–activating mitochondrial transcription), which in turn leads to both replication and transcription of mitochondrial DNA. **3.** The consequence is augmentation of muscle content of slow myosin H chains, increased numbers of mitochondria and improved endurance without muscle cell hypertrophy.

Thus, endurance training increases aerobic activity of type I fibers and, therefore, oxygen consumption (Fig. 1-20). Endurance training augments ATP consumption and Ca^{2+} release from the sarcoplasmic reticulum, both leading to activation of adenosine monophosphate (AMP) kinase and resulting phosphorylation of AMP. Consequent activation of transcription factor-A, mitochondrial (TFAM) increases replication and transcription of mitochondrial DNA (Fig. 1-20).

By contrast, weightlifting with large weight loads leads to hypertrophy of type II fibers and increases muscle mass. These fibers favor anaerobic glycolysis. Mechanisms that mediate type II fiber hypertrophy are more complex than for type I fibers and bear directly on the equilibrium between hypertrophy and atrophy (see Fig. 1-21, below).

Increased Trophic Signals
Cells and organs that respond to soluble mediators, such as the thyroid (TSH) or the breast (estrogens and progestins), undergo hypertrophy when levels of trophic hormones increase.

Puberty
Just as aging is associated with muscle atrophy, the onset of puberty, especially in boys, leads to greater muscle mass. The surge in androgens and growth hormone (GH) raises levels of downstream mediators (see below) and consequently increases the mass of muscle and other tissues.

Mechanisms of Cellular Hypertrophy

Whether the stimulus to enlarge is increased workload or response to endocrine or neuroendocrine mediators, there are certain processes that usually contribute to generating cellular hypertrophy.

When cells are stimulated to enlarge, one of the first responses is accelerated degradation of selected cellular proteins (see proteasomes, below). Specifically, proteins that do not contribute to the need for hypertrophy are removed, even as production of proteins that promote hypertrophy tends to increase.

Signaling Mechanisms in Hypertrophy
Although signals that elicit hypertrophic responses vary depending on cell type and circumstances, the example of skeletal muscle hypertrophy illustrates some critical general principles that apply to many cell types:

- **Growth factor stimulation:** Each tissue responds to different signals. As previously noted, certain growth factors are key initiators of hypertrophy (e.g., insulin-like growth factor-I [IGF-I] in muscle; see below).
- **Neuroendocrine stimulation:** In some tissues, especially the heart, adrenergic signaling may be important in initiating or facilitating hypertrophy.
- **Ion channels:** Ion fluxes may activate adaptation to increased demand. Calcium channel activity, in particular, may stimulate a host of downstream enzymes

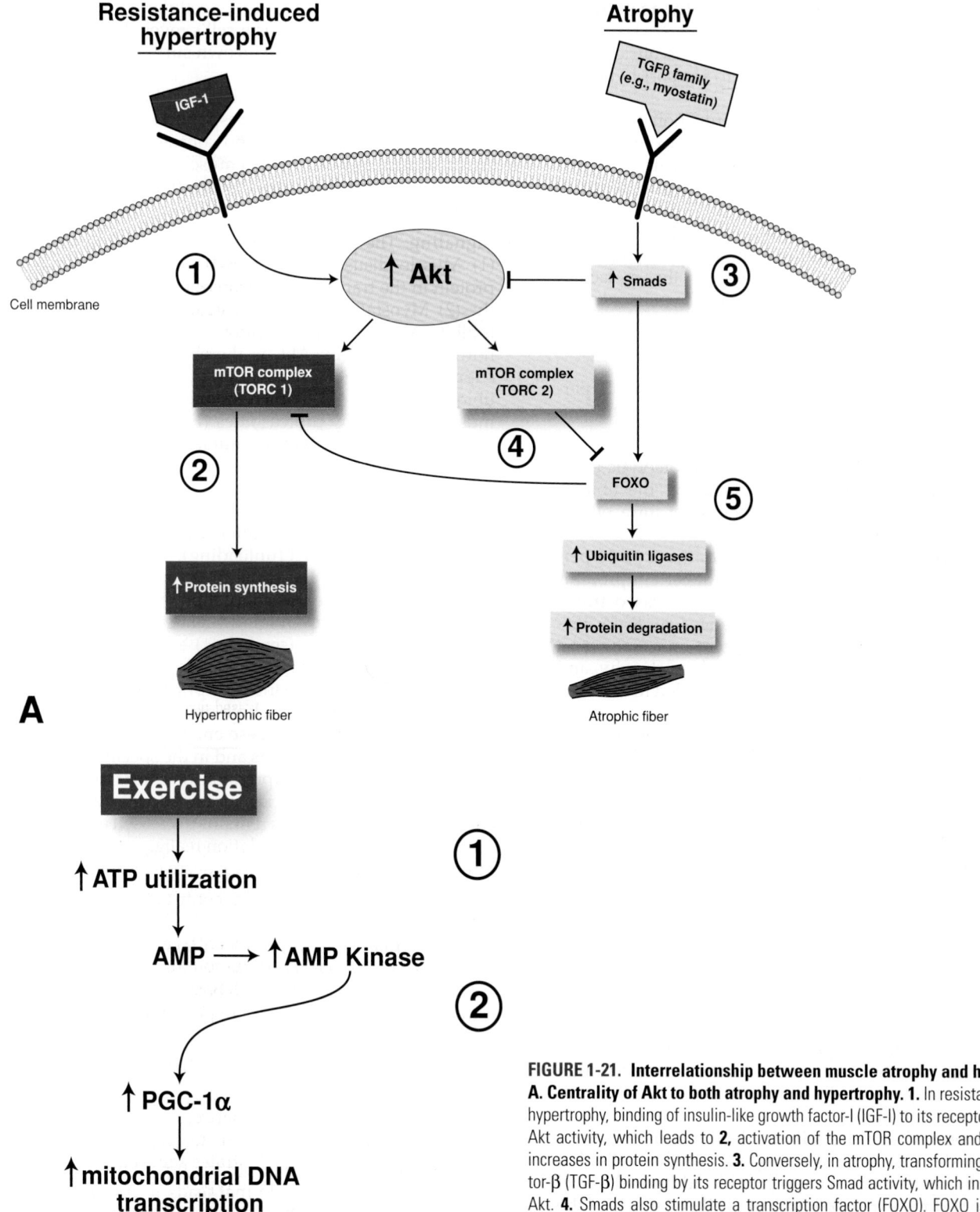

FIGURE 1-21. Interrelationship between muscle atrophy and hypertrophy.
A. Centrality of Akt to both atrophy and hypertrophy. 1. In resistance-induced
hypertrophy, binding of insulin-like growth factor-I (IGF-I) to its receptor stimulates
Akt activity, which leads to **2,** activation of the mTOR complex and consequent
increases in protein synthesis. **3.** Conversely, in atrophy, transforming growth factor-β (TGF-β) binding by its receptor triggers Smad activity, which in turn inhibits
Akt. **4.** Smads also stimulate a transcription factor (FOXO). FOXO is also inhibited by the Akt-activated mTOR complex, TORC2. Blocking of FOXO relieves its
inhibition of the mTORC complex, TORC1, thereby leading to greater protein production during hypertrophy. **5.** Concurrently, FOXO increases protein degradation,
which is characteristic of atrophy. **B. Akt-independent mechanism of muscle
hypertrophy and prevention of atrophy. 1.** Exercise requires adenosine triphosphate (ATP), which is then converted to adenosine monophosphate (AMP), in turn
stimulating AMP kinase. **2.** AMP kinase activates PGC-1α (a transcription factor
coactivator that upregulates energy production), leading to increased transcription
of mitochondrial DNA. **3.** The final result is an increased number of mitochondria.

(e.g., calcineurin) to produce hypertrophy, again in the heart.

- **Other chemical mediators:** Such factors as nitric oxide, angiotensin II and bradykinin tend to support hypertrophic responses in some tissues.
- **Oxygen supply:** Clearly increased functional demand requires increased energy supply. If a tissue oxygen deficit is sensed, angiogenesis is stimulated, and with it oxygen delivery. Angiogenesis is a key component in adaptive hypertrophy.
- **Hypertrophy antagonists:** Just as some mechanisms foster cellular hypertrophy, others inhibit it. Atrial natriuretic factors and high concentrations of NO• and other molecules either brake or prevent cell adaptation by hypertrophy.

Effector Pathways in Hypertrophy

Whatever mechanisms initiate signaling to stimulate hypertrophy, there are a limited number of downstream pathways that mediate the effects of such signaling:

- **Increased protein degradation:** Several proteolytic pathways contribute to hypertrophy, including the ubiquitin–proteasome system (UPS), activation of intracellular proteases and autophagy (see below).
- **Increased protein translation:** Shortly after a prohypertrophic signal is received, production of certain proteins increases. This occurs very quickly via increased translational efficiency, and without changes in RNA levels. Activities of translational initiators and elongation factors are often stimulated early in hypertrophy and quickly raise levels of specific proteins needed to meet the increased functional demand.
- **Increased gene expression:** Concentrations of key proteins are also elevated by transcriptional upregulation of their genes. Many signaling pathways activated by cytokines, neurotransmitters and so forth in turn activate an array of transcription factors. Thus, for example, the phosphatase calcineurin dephosphorylates transcription factor NFAT (*nuclear factor of activated T cells*), thereby facilitating its movement to the nucleus to stimulate transcription of target genes. Hypertrophy may also involve increased transcription of genes encoding growth-promoting transcription factors, such as Fos and Myc.
- **Survival:** During hypertrophy, cell death is inhibited. Stimulation of specific receptors activates several enzymes (e.g., Akt, PI3K; see below) that promote cell survival, largely by inhibiting programmed cell death (see below).
- **Extracellular matrix:** In some situations hypertrophy involves changes in a cell's environment, such as remodeling extracellular matrix.
- **Recruitment of satellite cells:** Skeletal muscle hypertrophy includes recruiting perimuscular satellite cells that fuse with myocyte syncytia to provide additional nuclei that support the expanded protein synthetic needs of the enlarging muscle.

Atrophy and Hypertrophy Impact on Similar Signaling Pathways

Molecular Mechanisms in Atrophy

The size of cells and organs reflects an equilibrium between anabolic and catabolic processes and involves changes in both production and destruction of cellular constituents. In its most basic sense, atrophy is a cell's reversible restructuring of its activities to facilitate its own survival and adapt to conditions of diminished use.

Atrophy has been most extensively studied in adipose tissue and skeletal muscle, which respond rapidly to changes in demand for energy storage and contractile force, respectively. In skeletal muscle, when a muscle is immobilized, the need for contraction decreases ("unloading") and myocytes activate adaptive mechanisms:

- **Signaling:** The protein kinase Akt is central to atrophy. (1) Muscle disuse increases extracellular myostatin, a protein in the transforming growth factor-β (TGF-β) family. (2) Myostatin binding activates its receptor, which inhibits Akt. (3) A transcription factor, FOXO, which is normally curbed by Akt, is thereby released from that suppression. (4) FOXO activation increases production of ubiquitin ligases (E3), which mediate the degradation of muscle proteins by proteasomes (Fig. 1-21A, right side). In this context, inactivating mutations of the myostatin gene in cattle are characterized by massively increased muscle mass (double muscling), underscoring the interplay of atrophy and hypertrophy.
- **Protein synthesis:** Shortly after a muscle is relieved of its obligation to contract (unloading), synthesis of certain proteins declines; at the same time, production of other proteins that mediate this adaptation may increase.
- **Protein degradation:** Ubiquitin-related specific protein degradation pathways (see below) are activated as part of atrophic responses. Proteasomal degradation of muscle actomyosin is greatly enhanced by prior actomyosin cleavage by caspase-3 or calpain, both of which also participate in apoptosis (see below). These enzymes cause decreases in certain contractile proteins and in the specific transcription factors that drive expression of contractile protein genes. If the atrophic state is maintained, cells reach a new equilibrium in which mass remains decreased and rates of protein synthesis and degradation realign.
- **Energy utilization:** A selective decrease in use of free fatty acids (as opposed to glucose) as an energy source for muscle occurs during response to unloading.

Atrophy is thus an active, specific adaptive response rather than a passive shutdown of cellular processes. It is also reversible; if the environment that existed before atrophy developed is restored, myocytes reassume their prior size and function.

Molecular Mechanisms in Hypertrophy

At the fulcrum of the balance between atrophy and hypertrophy sits the protein kinase Akt. With resistance training, synthesis of extracellular IGF-I is increased. When IGF-I binds to its cell membrane receptor on type II muscle fibers, it initiates a signaling cascade that leads to Akt activation. This event stimulates mTOR (mammalian target of rapamycin), which upregulates protein synthesis (Fig. 1-21, left side; also see below).

In addition to Akt-related hypertrophy/atrophy mechanisms, an Akt-independent system involves PGC-1α. This molecule is a regulator of transcription factors and a master integrator of exogenous signals that elicit mitochondrial biogenesis. Exercise upregulates PGC-1α, which then induces factors that stimulate production of mitochondrial DNA, thereby increasing mitochondrial biogenesis (Fig. 1-21B). In the delicate equilibrium between atrophy and hypertrophy, this anabolic response also serves as a countermeasure to prevent development of atrophy.

In this way, atrophy and hypertrophy, although phenotypically presenting as polar opposites, affect the same molecular intermediates.

Loss of Muscle Mass Commonly Results from Disease

Loss of 40% of body mass is usually fatal, but even a decrease of 5% in lean body mass can impair function. A number of conditions are characterized by such loss, and the pathways that are implicated in that result differ among various settings.

Cancer-Related Weight Loss and Cross-Talk between Adipose Tissue and Muscle

Over 80% of patients with gastric and pancreatic cancers lose weight, as do half of those with lung and colorectal cancers. Loss of adipose tissue and muscle is seen in cachexia (wasting), such as occurs in patients with advanced cancers. Tumor-induced lipolysis and energy utilization from adipose tissue release cytokines that initiate muscle atrophy. If such lipolysis is prevented experimentally, muscle mass is preserved.

Other Diseases Characterized by Weight Loss

Other chronic conditions in which weight loss occurs include:

- **Congestive heart failure (CHF):** In cardiac cachexia, type I (mitochondria-rich) muscle fibers are most affected. This unique susceptibility of type I fibers in CHF occurs because impaired oxygen delivery results in the sacrifice of those muscle fibers that use the most oxygen.
- **Chronic obstructive pulmonary disease (COPD).**
- **AIDS:** Before the introduction of effective antiretroviral therapy, wasting was the initial defining presentation in AIDS in 1/3 of patients. This association may reflect the energy expenditure needed to mount continuous acute phase inflammatory responses (see Chapter 2), including ongoing production of inflammatory mediators and decreased hepatic IGF-I production.
- **Rheumatoid arthritis (RA):** RA, the most common adult autoimmune disease (see Chapter 11), is associated with increased production of many catabolic cytokines (e.g., tumor necrosis factor-α [TNF-α], interleukin-1β [IL-1β], IL-6; see Chapters 2 and 4).
- **Aging:** Loss of muscle mass in aging, or **sarcopenia,** is universal and distinct from disease-related cachexia. Unlike the predominant loss of type I fibers in CHF, aging-related sarcopenia affects type II (fast-twitch) muscle fibers. The pathogenesis of sarcopenia is poorly understood, but includes (1) reduced protein synthesis, (2) loss of spinal cord motor units and (3) altered production of and response to anabolic hormones and cytokines. Interestingly, treating elderly patients with inhibitors of angiotensin-converting enzyme (see Chapters 2 and 8)—but not other types of antihypertensive agents—tends to preserve muscle strength, suggesting that the angiotensin system may play a role in sarcopenia.

Postmitotic Cells May Turn Over

Historically, neurons, cardiac myocytes and skeletal muscle cells were considered to be incapable of mitosis and essentially static throughout their life span. This view was generally interpreted to imply that such cells cannot be replaced, and therefore that their respective tissues cannot respond to cell loss or increased demand by adding cells. This conclusion is now considered only partially correct.

The Concept of Postmitotic Cells and Terminal Differentiation

Neurons and cardiac myocytes may not undergo mitosis, but committed progenitor cells in the brain and heart can proliferate and differentiate in response to cell loss and injury or, in the case of striated muscle, increased functional demand. Thus, there is a natural, albeit low, rate of cell loss and replacement among cells that were once considered irreplaceable. If the kinetics of such replacement favor cell loss, organ atrophy results, as in the heart, muscle and brain of the very aged. If progenitor cell activity predominates (e.g., in the skeletal muscle), hypertrophy may result.

UBIQUITIN AND THE UBIQUITIN–PROTEASOME SYSTEM

Ubiquitin and Ubiquitination Initiate Protein Degradation

Ubiquitin (Ub) is an evolutionarily conserved 76-amino-acid protein that is central to multiple cellular functions. These activities are accomplished via reversible Ub conjugation with target proteins and can be divided into proteolytic and nonproteolytic (trafficking) pathways. The Ub molecule contains seven lysine residues, and functional selectivity is provided by diverse patterns of protein linkage to these amino acids. Linkage to some lysines leads to passage of the tagged protein to the proteasome for degradation. However, other patterns of Ub linkage direct proteins to numerous other functions (Fig. 1-22). The fate of Ub-conjugated proteins among the several pathways is determined by the number of Ub moieties conjugated and the site of the conjugation linkages on the Ub molecule. Among the diverse functions of Ub-directed protein sorting are the following:

- Endocytosis
- Intracellular trafficking
- Regulation of histones and transcription
- Cell cycle control
- Autophagy (see below)
- Repair of DNA damage
- Cellular signaling

Further elucidation of these Ub-related mechanisms is beyond the scope of this discussion. We focus here on the proteolysis-related Ub pathway, which involves targeting proteins to degradative proteasomes (Fig. 1-23).

Mechanisms of Ub Conjugation to Proteins

Ub attachment to proteins occurs via a sequence of enzymatic reactions. A Ub-activating enzyme, E1, binds to Ub and then transfers it to one of dozens of Ub-conjugating enzymes (E2). These act together with one of about 800 different Ub-ligating enzymes (E3) to add Ub to a lysine on

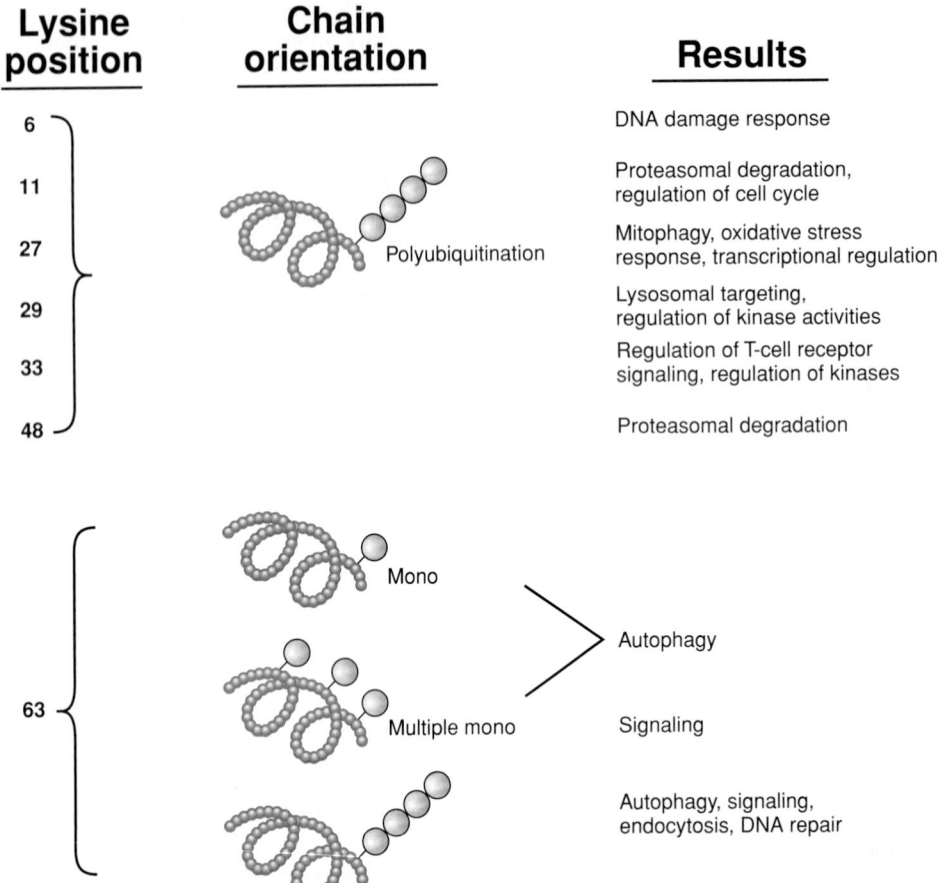

FIGURE 1-22. The diversity of ubiquitination and its consequences. The several lysines of the Ub (ubiquitin) molecule can be used either to form poly-Ub chains or for mono- or oligoubiquitination. Ubiquitination of different lysine residues (represented here by *K*) imparts different functions to the target protein.

the doomed protein (Fig. 1-23). Additional Ub moieties are added to the original Ub, forming a polyubiquitin chain (at least four Ubs). The specificity of the process for the targeted protein resides in the combinations of E2 and E3 enzymes. E3 Ub ligases control many cellular processes, including cell cycle, transcription, life and death, as well as normal cellular homeostasis (see below and Chapter 5).

Proteasomes Are Key Participants in Cell Homeostasis

Cellular responses to altered environments were once studied exclusively by analyzing changes in gene expression and protein production. Protein degradation was either ignored or relegated to the nonspecific proteolytic activities of lysosomes. However, it is now clear that cellular homeostasis requires mechanisms that allow the cell to destroy proteins selectively. Although more than one such pathway exists, the best-understood setting in which specific proteins are eliminated is the proteasomal apparatus.

Proteasomes

Proteasomes are highly conserved organelles in the cytoplasm and possibly the nucleus. They are barrel-shaped complexes whose main (but not only) function is to digest polyubiquitinated proteins. There are two types of

proteasomes: 20S and 26S. The degradative unit of both is a 20S destruction chamber, to which, in the 26S proteasome, two 19S "caps" are attached, as shown in Fig. 1-23. The caps at the entrance to the proteolytic core regulate entry. The 20S proteasomes lack these caps.

Proteins targeted for destruction are modified as described below and recognized by one 19S cap. They are then degraded in the proteolytic core. This process produces peptides of 3 to 25 amino acids, which are released through the lower 19S subunit. These peptides may then be further degraded by cytosolic proteases.

The importance of proteasomes is underscored by the fact that they make up 1–2% of the total mass of the cell. *Mutations that interfere with normal proteasomal function are lethal.* The 20S proteasomes are important in degradation of **oxidized proteins** (see below). In 26S proteasomes, **polyubiquitinated proteins** are degraded. A type of proteasome, the immunoproteasome, is formed when cells produce interferon-γ (IFN-γ) and is important in processing protein antigens into peptides that attach to major histocompatibility complex (MHC) type I for presentation to the immune system (see Chapter 4).

Proteasomes are charged with eliminating proteins that have been incorrectly folded, damaged, reached the end of their usefulness or need to be destroyed for some other reason. They are, then, key to regulating cell cycle transit, in that they degrade progrowth proteins after they accomplish

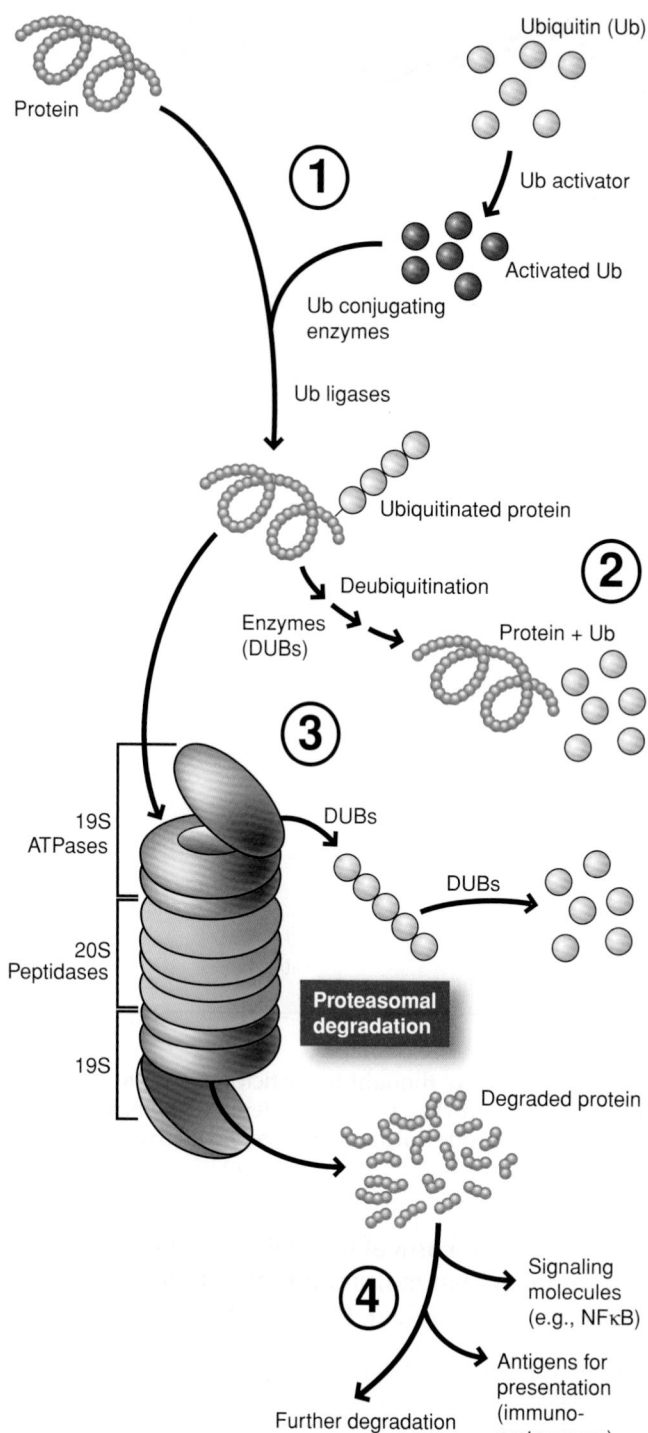

their objectives. Proteasomes also maintain the balance of life and death in favor of cell survival by specifically eliminating proapoptotic molecules (such as p53; see below). On balance, these structures maintain and protect cellular viability. Thus, a proteasome inhibitor (bortezomib) is now used in routine clinical practice to treat patients with certain malignancies.

Deubiquitinating Enzymes

Deubiquitinating enzymes (DUBs) are proteases that remove Ubs from poly-Ub chains and their partner proteins. Once a protein's doom is sealed for degradation in a proteasome or lysosome (see below), recycling of the Ub that determines this fate is economically advantageous. However, deubiquitination can also commute a protein's death sentence and enhance its stability. DUBs are critical to the function of Ub-regulated cellular switches in that they counteract the ubiquitination of specific protein targets. As many as 100 DUBs are known that reverse the effects of ubiquitination on many cellular processes, including (1) protein degradation, (2) cell cycle regulation, (3) gene expression, (4) signaling pathways and (5) DNA repair.

Some Pathogens Can Manipulate the Ubiquitin System

Some pathogens can control Ub/DUB pathways at multiple points. Certain bacterial proteins, called effectors, resemble E3 Ub ligases and activate ubiquitination, allowing exquisite exploitation of host cells to facilitate invasion and pathogenicity. Other bacteria (e.g., *Salmonella typhimurium*, *Chlamydia trachomatis*) and viruses (e.g., herpes simplex virus) encode proteins that act as DUBs, suggesting that interference with cellular ubiquitination may confer a selective advantage to these pathogens.

Some modifications of proteins may protect them from ubiquitination. For example, when the tumor suppressor protein p53 is phosphorylated in response to DNA damage, it is protected from Ub-mediated degradation.

There are a number of proteins that resemble Ub but are structurally and functionally distinct from it, and that subserve somewhat different functions. Such proteins (e.g., SUMO and NEDD8) may participate in forming some E3 complexes. Their polymeric chains may direct protein localization and diverse protein activities.

Ubiquitination and Deubiquitination Are Key to Many Diseases

Ubiquitination and specific protein elimination not only are important for normal cellular homeostasis but also are critical to cellular adaptation to stress and injury. Mutations in Ub pathway constituents can cause specific diseases, and in many cases altered UPS activity is important in disease pathogenesis (Table 1-3). For example, defective ubiquitination is involved in several important neurodegenerative diseases. Mutation in parkin, a ubiquitin ligase, is implicated in the pathogenesis of some hereditary forms of Parkinson disease, in which undegraded parkin accumulates as Lewy bodies (see Chapter 32).

Regulation of ubiquitination may be important in tumor development. Thus, human papillomavirus strains that are associated with human cervical cancer (see Chapters 5 and 24)

FIGURE 1-23. Ubiquitin–proteasome pathways. Ub (ubiquitin) targets proteins for specific elimination in proteasomes. **1.** Ub is activated by E1 ubiquitin-activating enzyme, after which it is transferred to an E2 ubiquitin-conjugating enzyme. The E2–Ub complex interacts with an E3 ubiquitin ligase to bind a particular protein. The process may be repeated multiple times to append a chain of Ub moieties. There follows a choice: **2.** These complexes may be deubiquitinated by deubiquitinating enzymes (DUBs). **3.** If degradation is to proceed, 26S proteasomes recognize the poly-Ub-conjugated protein via their 19S subunit and degrade it into oligopeptides. In the process, Ub moieties are returned to the cell pool of Ub monomers by DUBs. **4.** After release from the proteasome, partially degraded proteins may follow alternative fates.

TABLE 1-3

INVOLVEMENT OF THE UBIQUITIN–PROTEASOME SYSTEM IN DISEASE

Disease	Ubiquitin–Proteasome System Activity	Anatomic Effect
Neurologic Diseases (Diseases Associated with Neuron Loss)		
Parkinson disease	Decreased	Lewy bodies
Alzheimer disease	Decreased	Amyloid plaques, neurofibrillary tangles
Amyotrophic lateral sclerosis	Decreased	Superoxide dismutase aggregates in motor neurons
Huntington disease	Decreased	Polyglutamine inclusions
Autoimmune Diseases		
Sjögren syndrome	Decreased	Chronic inflammation
Metabolic Diseases		
Type 2 diabetes mellitus	Increased	Insulin insensitivity
Cataract formation	Decreased	Aggregated oxidized proteins
Muscle Wasting		
Aging	Increased	Atrophy
Cancer and other chronic disease	Increased	Atrophy
Cardiovascular		
Ischemia/reperfusion	Decreased	Myocyte apoptosis
Pressure overload	Decreased	Myocyte apoptosis

produce E6 protein, which inactivates the p53 tumor suppressor. E6 accomplishes this by binding an E3 (ubiquitin ligase) and facilitating its association with p53. Such increased ubiquitination of p53 accelerates its degradation, and the loss of its activity is implicated in the genesis of cervical cancer. Impaired ubiquitination may also contribute to cellular degenerative changes in aging and to a variety of storage diseases.

Ubiquitination also plays a role in gene expression. Nuclear factor-κB (NFκB) is an important transcriptional activator that is activated in two different ways by the UPS. The active form of NFκB is a heterodimer (i.e., it is composed of two different protein subunits). Inactive precursor forms of the two NFκB subunits are ubiquitinated and cleaved to their active forms in proteasomes. *This is an example of incomplete protein degradation by the UPS.* Also, the inhibitor of NFκB, called IκB, is degraded by ubiquitination. This step releases active NFκB, which mediates expression of genes that promote cell survival. Proteasome inhibition permits persistence of the IκB–NFκB complex and so decreases NFκB-induced transcriptional activation. In the case of cancer cells, inhibiting proteasome function would impair tumor cell survival and is consequently a target for pharmaceutical manipulation.

Virtually anything that ubiquitination can do, deubiquitination can undo or prevent. DUBs are critical to gene expression and influence a wide variety of distinct mechanisms. They have been shown to activate tumor suppressor proteins and are likely to be important in tumorigenesis. In this way, DUBs are thought to participate in diverse protein interaction networks. Their involvement in major disease pathways may offer attractive targets for pharmacological intervention.

Autophagy Is a Form of Controlled Cellular Cannibalism That Is Crucial to the Balance Between Cell Survival, Death and Adaptation

Autophagy (Greek: "auto," *self;* "phagy," *eating*) is a highly conserved catabolic process by which cytoplasmic targets are recognized and delivered to lysosomes for digestion. Autophagic degradation is generally divided into three categories, based on both the cargoes involved and how they arrive at lysosomes. **Macroautophagy** is responsible for handling bulk portions of cytoplasm, and both macroautophagy and **microautophagy** target damaged cellular organelles, aggregated proteins and other potentially injurious materials. In addition, some defective proteins require interaction with molecular chaperones (see below) and enter the autophagic system via **chaperone-mediated autophagy** (CMA) (Fig. 1-24).

It is important to appreciate that autophagy systems operate continuously and are obligatory for cell homeostasis and survival. Bulk autophagy, the most primitive form of the process, protects cells when nutrients are lacking, as in starvation or compromised blood supply. Other forms of autophagy maintain functional homeostasis among cellular

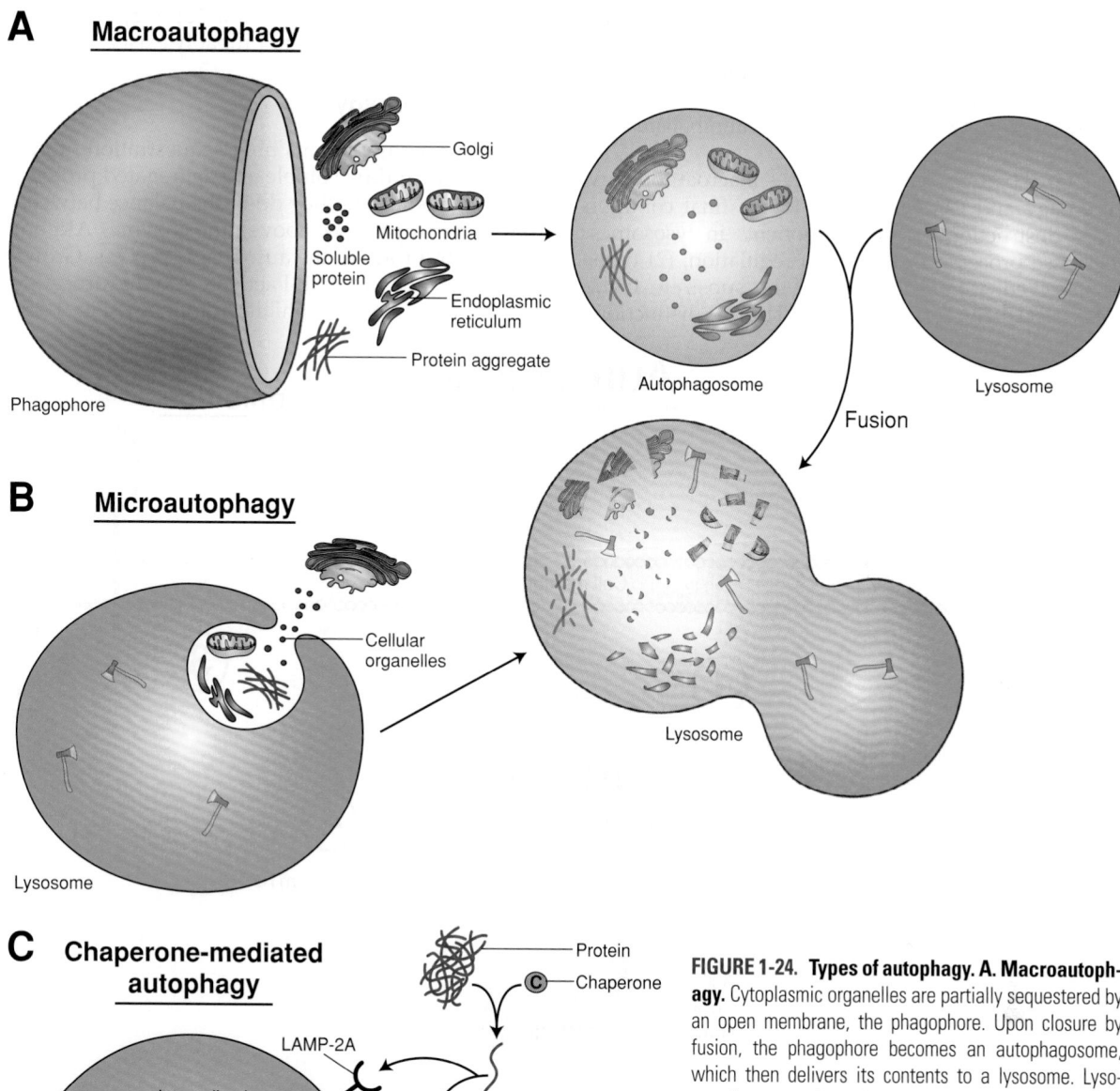

FIGURE 1-24. Types of autophagy. A. Macroautophagy. Cytoplasmic organelles are partially sequestered by an open membrane, the phagophore. Upon closure by fusion, the phagophore becomes an autophagosome, which then delivers its contents to a lysosome. Lysosomal enzymes degrade the contents to small molecules for reutilization. **B. Microautophagy.** Cytosolic cargoes are engulfed by invagination of the lysosomal membrane. The contents are then degraded by lysosomal enzymes. **C. Chaperone-mediated autophagy.** Proteins conjugated to chaperones (e.g., Hsc70) are recognized by lysosomal receptor proteins (LAMP-2A) and translocated to the lysosomal interior, where they are received by a second chaperone and then degraded. The original, extralysosomal chaperone survives to work further.

proteins and organelles in normal settings and in times of stress. Autophagic pathways act as ongoing physiologic quality control mechanisms protecting from, for example, excess production of ROS by inefficient or damaged mitochondria. Autophagy in its various forms is thus essential both for basal cellular physiology and for adaptation to adversity, as illustrated by this abbreviated list of its functions and of circumstances in which it protects the cell:

- Starvation
- Ischemia
- Recycling nutrients from cellular organelles and macromolecules

- Clearance of misfolded or damaged proteins and organelles
- Antigen presentation
- Protection from tumorigenesis
- Protection from neurodegeneration

The following sections illustrate the mechanisms of autophagy, their interrelationships with other systems, their role in maintaining health and their involvement in disease. Since continuous maintenance of intracellular components is necessary for cell survival, impairment of any form of autophagy may lead to accumulation of abnormal proteins and defective organelles. The result may be cell death or disease.

Autophagy is basically a series of processes that are obligatory for normal cell function and that make it possible for a cell to remain viable in hostile environments. It is thus a form of "programmed cell survival." Under some circumstances, however, it may give rise to self-cannibalism as a form of cell death (see below).

The principal pathways of autophagy—macroautophagy, microautophagy and CMA—all lead to the final common pathway of destruction of cell components in lysosomes. However, these processes differ in (1) regulation, (2) types of cargo involved, (3) recognition of the substrate to be degraded and (4) delivery to lysosomes. The fine distinctions

between the various forms of autophagy remain somewhat blurred, and some overlap probably exists.

Macroautophagy

Macroautophagy entails bulk sequestration of cytoplasmic contents, including soluble and aggregated proteins and cellular organelles. As they do in the balance between atrophy and hypertrophy (see above), the enzymes **Akt** and **mTOR** play central roles in the autophagic process. Growth factors such as insulin and IGF-I activate Akt. In turn, Akt activates mTOR, which in turn inhibits autophagy (Fig. 1-25).

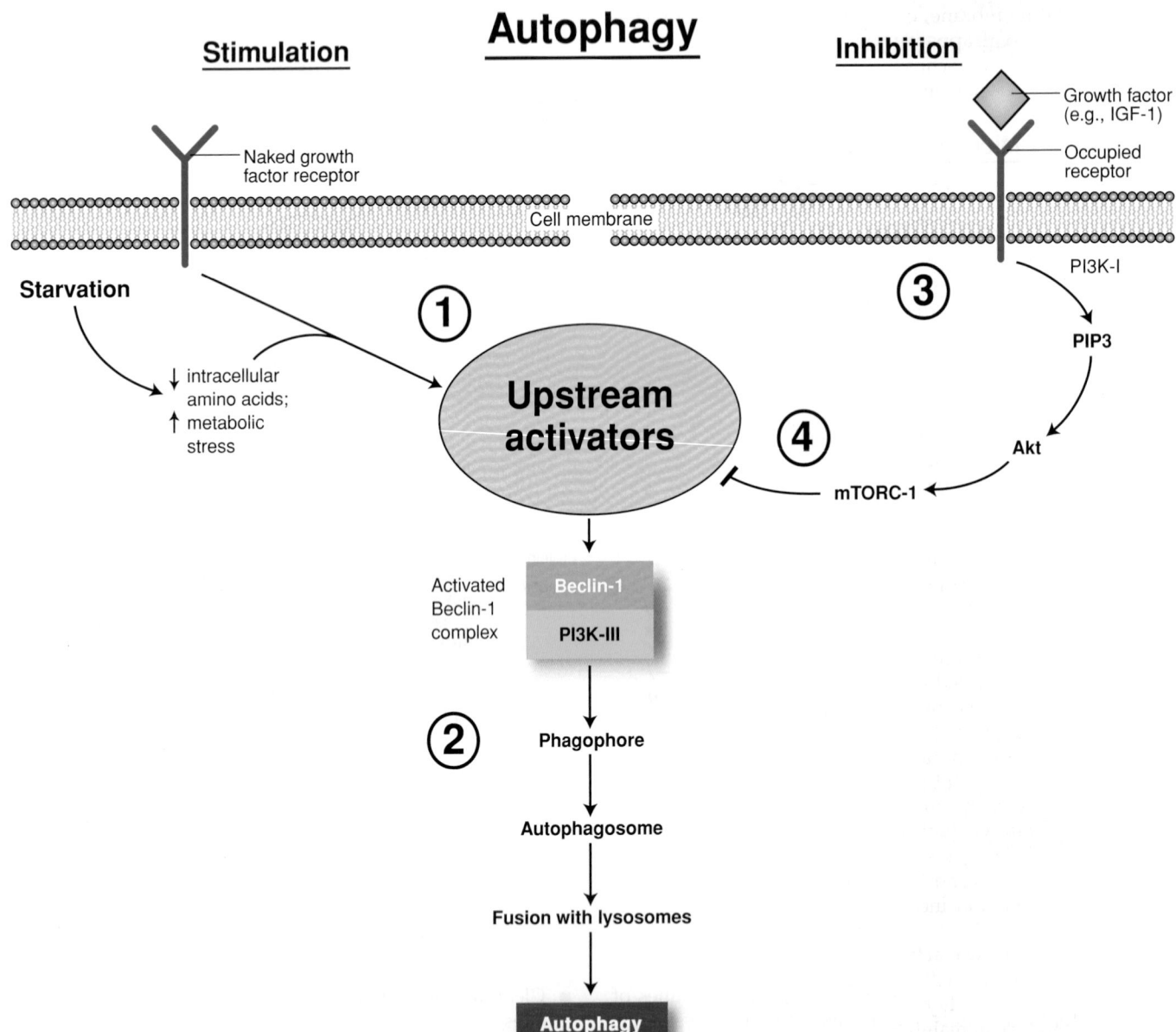

FIGURE 1-25. Triggering and inhibiting autophagy. Stimulation (left). 1. In the setting of starvation or other initiators of autophagy, lack of growth factors leads to depletion of nutrients and hence metabolic stress. A consortium of upstream molecules is triggered. **2.** As a result, an autophagy-activating complex containing Beclin-1 and class III phosphatidylinositol-3-kinase (PI3K-III) is formed. This complex triggers autophagy, from the phagophore to the fusion of the phagosome with the lysosome. **Inhibition (right). 3.** Autophagy is inhibited when nutrients or other stimuli elicit growth factors (e.g., insulin-like growth factor-I [IGF-I], insulin), which bind to their cell membrane receptors. This process activates class I PI3K (PI3K-I), which produces phosphatidylinositol-tris-phosphate (PIP3). **4.** PIP3 then recruits Akt to the cell membrane, where it is activated and in turn stimulates the mTOR-related complex, mTORC1. The latter directly blocks the autophagy cascade, including Beclin-1, to prevent autophagy.

However, in a situation such as starvation, cellular sensors detect a scarcity of amino acid reserves, and production of endocrine and paracrine growth factors declines. This removes mTOR-mediated inhibition and stimulates autophagy. In the process, Beclin-1 and PI3K (phosphatidylinositol-3-kinase) form a complex, which is then activated and sets the autophagic pathway in motion (Fig. 1-25). Thereafter, bulk cytoplasm, containing cytoplasmic organelles and including proteins, lipids and other constituents, is partially sequestered by a membrane (the **phagophore**). The latter fuses at its ends to enclose a structure, the **autophagosome**. Autophagosome membranes may derive from several cytoplasmic sources, including the outer mitochondrial membrane, endoplasmic reticulum, plasma membrane or Golgi apparatus. The autophagosome then fuses with lysosomes, whose enzymes reduce autophagosome contents to small molecules for reutilization by the cell (Fig. 1-25).

Identifying Targets in Macroautophagy

Starvation-related autophagy is mostly nonselective for soluble cytoplasmic constituents and organelles, although even in this setting, recycling of cell contents is not totally random. Macroautophagy also handles damaged cytoplasmic organelles and aggregated proteins, for both of which specific recognition is needed.

In such circumstances, target identification depends on the nature of the dysfunction. For example, a damaged mitochondrion that produces excess reactive oxygen species from dysfunctional electron transport suffers altered membrane potential, thereby causing a cytosolic protein, Nix, to bind to the outer mitochondrial membrane. This complex recruits a protein called **parkin** (for its likely involvement in Parkinson disease). In turn, parkin binds to several members of a series of Ub-like (**UBL**; see below) recognition proteins, which are termed autophagy-related proteins, or **Atgs**. A bridge protein, **p62**, recognizes these UBLs and attaches the damaged mitochondrion to the interior of the developing phagophore (Fig. 1-26).

Protein aggregates are usually concretions of misfolded proteins and are handled by a parallel, but different, pathway. Misfolding may occur at the time of translation or from acquired (e.g., oxidative) damage. Resultant exposure of hydrophobic residues that are normally hidden in the interior of proteins leads to both their recognition by the Ub system and attachment of poly-Ub chains by E3 Ub ligases. In some cases Atgs are also conjugated to these masses of proteins. However, these aggregates are too large to pass through proteasomes, and so Ubs and UBLs are recognized by the same p62 bridge protein and incorporated into autophagosomes (Fig. 1-26).

Macroautophagy was at first considered to be a nonspecific response to stress, especially starvation. It is now recognized that the continuous quality control exerted by this process is of great importance in maintaining cellular integrity.

Microautophagy

Microautophagy (Fig. 1-24) is a process by which cytosolic cargoes are directly engulfed by invagination of lysosomal membranes, then transferred into the interior of lysosomes for degradation. This process is largely constitutive and is important for continuous turnover of membranes and organelles and for maintaining organelle size and composition.

Chaperone-Mediated Autophagy

CMA (Fig. 1-24) is characterized by the fact that all of its targets are recognized selectively by chaperone proteins. Targets are translocated via receptor recognition across lysosomal membranes, without phagosome intermediates. Like an adult chaperone at a teenage dance, who is responsible for maintaining decorum in conduct and for removing incorrigible violators, cytosolic molecular chaperones preside over correct folding of nascent proteins and destruction of misfolded or damaged proteins via CMA. There is a modest level of constitutive CMA, but this pathway can be further activated when the cell is stressed (e.g., starvation, oxidant stress, toxic exposures, etc.).

Crosstalk Among Degradative Pathways

Some branches of the autophagic pathway are regulated by sequential enzymatic activation of Ub and UBLs, the latter resembling the activation cascade of the UPS (see above). Short-lived proteins are generally specifically digested by the UPS, whereas autophagy tends to remove longer-lived proteins selectively. This division of labor is not rigid: if one system is compromised, the other may compensate, at least in part. The UPS cannot handle protein aggregates or large cytoplasmic structures, like organelles or endocytosed foreign matter (e.g., bacteria). These systems thus complement each other. In addition, there are molecular interactions among the different types of autophagy, and impairment of one such pathway may lead to compensatory activation of another.

Both the autophagic pathway and the UPS operate continuously, and inhibition of either often has harmful consequences. Although autophagy can act as a bulk recycling mechanism for nutrients in times of starvation, both systems can be remarkably selective. This specificity reflects the participation of many molecules in the process of selective identification of materials for degradation. This ability to accommodate diverse targets is reminiscent of the body's antigen recognition and drug-metabolizing (P450) systems. The Ub pathway contains over 1000 proteins that confer comparable precision in target selection. Autophagy relies on the diversity of the Ub system and the parallel Atg proteins to maintain a similarly broad scope and accuracy. As mentioned above, conjugation of either Ub or Atg proteins to aggregated proteins or organelles can lead to recognition of the doomed structure by the p62 linker protein, followed by transport to phagophores to complete autophagic and degradative processes.

Why is selectivity important? A significant proportion of newly synthesized proteins are translated or folded incorrectly. Oxidative damage further increases the cell's load of defective proteins. Such molecules must be removed, lest the cell risk continuing to accumulate proteins that can form large, insoluble aggregates that lead to abnormal protein–protein interactions or exhibit other poisonous properties.

Autophagy and Disease

Autophagy maintains cellular homeostasis during starvation and removes obsolete or damaged cell constituents, whose retention could lead to diverse harmful consequences (cancer, infection, etc.). It may be for this reason that periodic fasting, which activates autophagy, has been practiced by many cultures.

The links between autophagy and many diseases are such that considerable energy is now being invested to develop

Damaged mitochondria

Damaged proteins

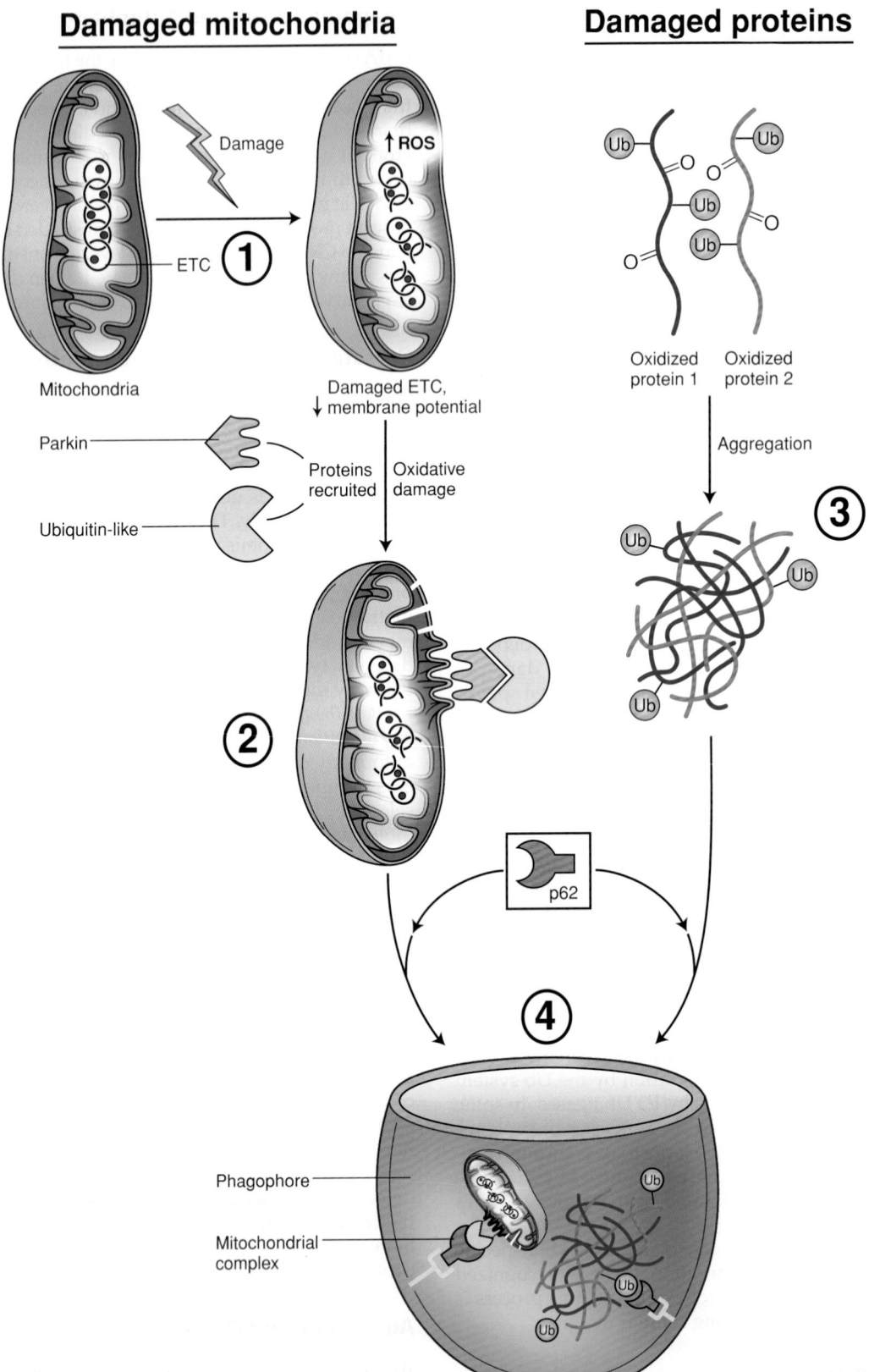

FIGURE 1-26. Role of autophagy in handling damaged cellular organelles and protein aggregates. Damaged cellular organelles (left). 1. Damage (here) to mitochondria disrupts electron transport and dissipates the electrochemical gradient across the mitochondrial membrane. Increased ROS result and produce oxidative damage. This leads to recruitment of cytosolic proteins, parkin and a UBL. **2.** The complex of fragmented mitochondria–parkin–UBL binds to p62. **3.** Proteins that have sustained oxidative damage are conjugated to Ub or a UBL and form aggregates, which are then bound by p62. **4.** The p62-bound complexes with damaged mitochondria or aggregated proteins are recognized by a specific receptor in the phagophore, thereby leading to autophagy. *ETC* = electron transport chain; *ROS* = reactive oxygen species; *Ub* = ubiquitin; *UBL* = Ub-like protein.

ways to manipulate the process pharmacologically. Autophagy and defective autophagy contribute to:

- **Neurodegenerative diseases:** Many inherited neurodegenerative diseases involve mutations in proteins of the autophagic pathways, as do many lysosomal storage diseases. In some cases, like Alzheimer and Parkinson diseases, autophagy may fail to keep pace with the pace at which protein aggregates accrue. This may be due in part to age-related decreases in Beclin-1 synthesis.
- **Aging:** Macroautophagy and CMA decline with age, in parallel with Beclin-1 and certain lysosomal membrane proteins. This type of dysfunction in autophagy may account for age-related changes in organ systems such as the central nervous system (CNS), heart and so forth.
- **Pancreatitis:** There is evidence that impaired autophagy in this necroinflammatory disease may be responsible for inappropriate conversion of trypsinogen to trypsin, thereby creating autodigestion of the pancreas.
- **Infectious diseases:** Autophagy generally represents an important host defense mechanism against pathogens. Not surprisingly, many invasive organisms have developed ways to evade or subvert this process. A microorganism may inhibit the autophagic pathway, thereby avoiding a gruesome death. Other bacteria may interfere with phagosome–lysosome fusion, a strategy exploited by, for example, *Mycobacterium tuberculosis* and *Shigella flexneri*, to survive and replicate unmolested. Herpes simplex virus type 1 (HSV-1) encodes a protein that inactivates Beclin-1, thereby protecting the virus from autophagic degradation. Conversely, some viruses, particularly RNA viruses such as poliovirus and hepatitis C virus, benefit from increased autophagy; autophagic vesicles serve as membrane scaffolds for their replication.
- **Crohn disease:** There is a robust association between the occurrence of mutations in two genes and the risk of Crohn disease. Mutations in both genes, which normally facilitate autophagic clearance of invasive bacteria, impair bacterial clearance and promote increased production of molecules that stimulate inflammation.
- **Cancer:** The involvement of autophagy in the development and progression of cancer is complex and represents a double-edged sword. Several autophagy genes (e.g., Beclin-1 and some Atg genes) act as tumor suppressors (see Chapter 5) and are deleted or mutated in many human tumors. Autophagy can also protect cancer cells if they are deprived of nutrients or oxygen because of therapy or insufficient blood supply.
- **Miscellaneous:** Mutations in genes that encode proteins involved in autophagosome–lysosome fusion are linked to a disease of skeletal muscle (inclusion body myopathy), Paget disease of bone and frontotemporal dementia. Autophagy has been implicated in other diseases (cardiac ischemia and ischemia/reperfusion injury [see later], type II diabetes [see Chapter 13], stroke, etc.), but its role is not well defined.

Molecular Chaperones Establish and Maintain Functional Protein Conformations

Nascent proteins must assume particular three-dimensional configurations by folding appropriately as they exit ribosomes. Left to their own devices, newly produced proteins are in great danger of folding abnormally and then aggregating, thereby potentially overwhelming the cell with harmful species. To prevent such a disaster, cells have evolved a network of supervisory molecules that use ingenious approaches to ensure and maintain appropriate folding. Molecular chaperones are proteins that associate with client proteins and help them assume their final, functional, three-dimensional configurations. Some chaperones also help to sustain that conformation over time, thereby preventing accumulation of abnormal proteins.

The ongoing process of quality control by chaperones is called **proteostasis**. The folding-energy landscape of cells is complex, and ATP-dependent chaperones are needed to help other proteins navigate it successfully in a crowded intracellular environment. There are several hundred chaperone proteins, which are organized into distinct families based on structural homologies. Many of these molecules are induced by stress and are called heat shock proteins (Hsp). These are now grouped into clans based on prototypical members. They were originally designated by molecular weight (e.g., Hsp70, Hsp90), although terminologies are in transition and each subserves different functions, including acting as cofactors for other heat shock proteins.

As they exit ribosomes, nascent proteins are met by one or more chaperones, which direct their folding. If the resulting conformation is sufficient for functionality, the chaperone and the new protein dissociate, and the latter proceeds to its appropriate location (Fig. 1-27). However, some proteins behave like unruly children and require additional education. In that case, they are encapsulated by cylindrical channels called chaperonins, which provide an environment that fosters their final tertiary structures.

The chaperone system consists of a proteostasis hub that influences many cellular functions, including cell cycle progression, apoptosis (see below), telomere maintenance (see Chapter 5), intracellular transport, innate immunity and specific degradation of proteins. This mechanism collaborates closely with the UPS and with autophagy machinery to establish an integrated proteostasis network (Fig. 1-28). The circuitry of this network provides cradle-to-grave care for proteins. It (1) guides conversion of single polypeptide chains into proteins, (2) maintains active three-dimensional structures and (3) at the appropriate juncture, presides over their destruction.

Chaperonopathies

Defects in molecular chaperones are implicated in several disorders, called "chaperonopathies." These diseases are characterized by defects, excesses or mistakes in chaperone proteins.

Genetic chaperonopathies, which mainly reflect inherited germline mutations in one or another of the molecular chaperones, have been implicated in developmental disorders, neuropathies, dilated cardiomyopathy and polycystic liver and kidney diseases. A mutation in a chaperone cofactor causes a form of X-linked retinitis pigmentosa. Hereditary spastic paraplegia is related to a mutation in Hsp60, a mitochondrial chaperone. If von Hippel-Lindau protein (VHL) is mutated, it may bind its chaperone poorly, leading to its being misfolded and inactive as a tumor suppressor. Affected people develop tumors of the adrenal, kidney and brain. Moreover, mutant chaperone genes are responsible for certain types of cancer.

Acquired chaperonopathies arise for several reasons. Impairment of stress responses may result in inadequate amounts of chaperone proteins. By contrast, high levels of substrate (misfolded or degraded) proteins may exceed the capacity of the chaperone system. Chaperone molecules

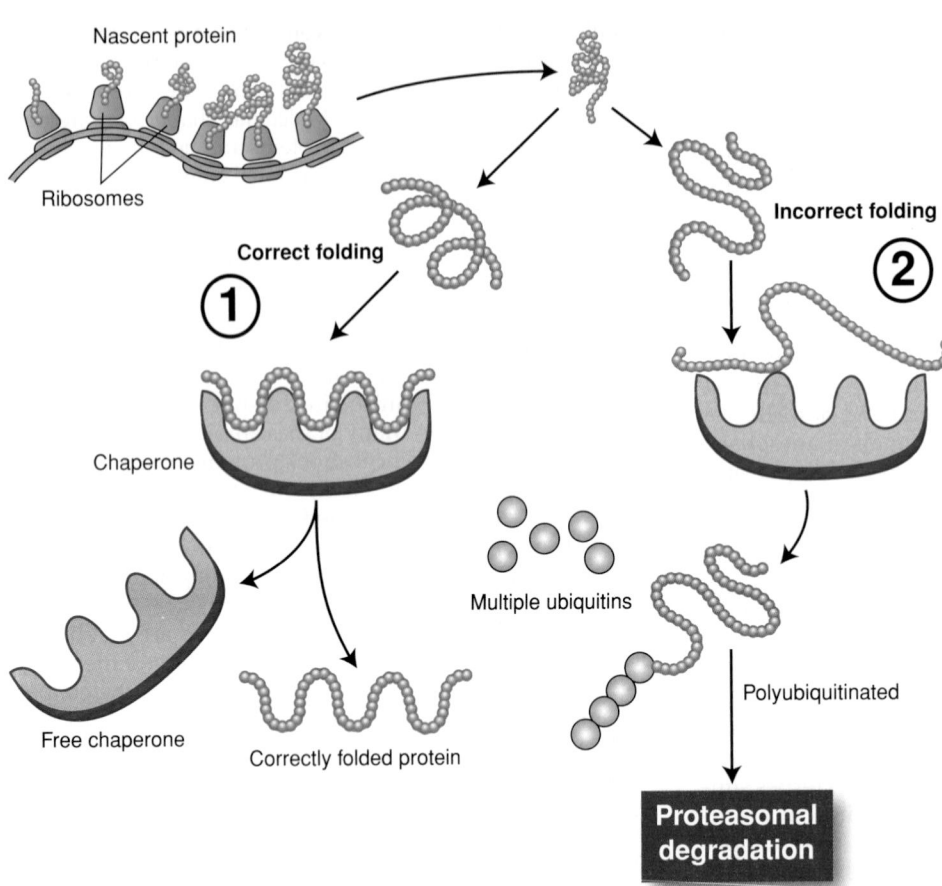

FIGURE 1-27. Differential handling of protein that is (1) correctly folded and protein that is (2) incorrectly folded. Correctly folded proteins are chaperoned from the ribosomes that produce them to their ultimate cellular destination. Incorrectly folded proteins are polyubiquitinated, which directs them to proteasomes, where they are degraded.

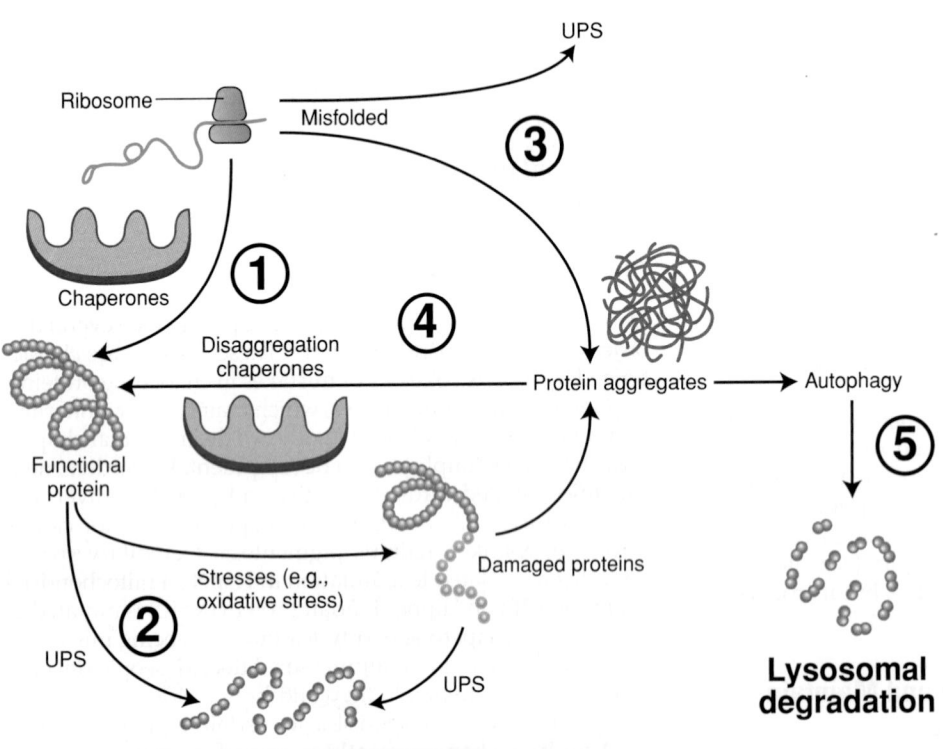

FIGURE 1-28. The fate of proteins: the roles of chaperones, stress-related modifications and autophagy. 1. Nascent polypeptides are folded into functional proteins with the assistance of chaperones. **2.** A small proportion of proteins originate in a misfolded state and may be degraded by the ubiquitin–proteasome system (UPS) directly, or they may form aggregates. **3.** The correctly folded protein may experience one of three fates. It may (a) continue as a functional protein, (b) reach the end of the cell's need for it and then be degraded by the UPS or (c) be damaged by a variety of stresses. In the last event, if protein conformations are distorted because of oxidative or other stresses, the tertiary structures of these proteins can be deformed. They may then be degraded by the UPS or aggregate in the cytosol. **4.** Chaperones may also mediate disaggregation of agglutinated proteins, thereby preventing accumulation of toxic particulates and so allowing proteins to resume productive functionality. **5.** Protein aggregates may also undergo autophagy, with consequent degradation in lysosomes.

may also be sequestered in protein deposits or inactivated by exogenous toxins (e.g., an enzyme from a virulent strain of *E. coli* cleaves Hsp70). Chaperones may also contribute to tumorigenesis through effects on proteins that regulate the cell cycle and cell death (see below). Acquired chaperonopathies are also implicated in biological aging and in cardiovascular and neurodegenerative diseases.

Mutations May Impair Cell Function without Causing Cell Death

Although mutations in genes that encode a variety of proteins may be responsible for a wide array of clinical syndromes, they do not necessarily involve the death of affected cells. Increasingly, such mutations provide pathogenetic links among seemingly unrelated diseases.

Channelopathies

Channelopathies are inherited or acquired disorders of ion channels. Ion channels are transmembrane pore-forming proteins that allow ions, such as Na^+, K^+, Ca^{2+} and Cl^-, to enter or exit cells. Such ion traffic is critical for control of heartbeat, muscle contraction and relaxation, regulation of insulin secretion in pancreatic β cells and many other functions. For example, activation and inactivation of Na^+ and K^+ channels determine the action potential in neurons, and Ca^{2+} channels are important in contraction and relaxation of cardiac and skeletal muscle. Mutations in many ion channel genes cause a variety of diseases, including cardiac arrhythmias (e.g., short and long QT syndromes) and neuromuscular syndromes (e.g., myotonias, familial periodic paralysis). Several inherited human disorders affecting skeletal muscle contraction, heart rhythm and nervous system function are due to mutations in genes that encode voltage-gated Na^+ channels. Channelopathies are also implicated in certain pediatric epilepsy syndromes.

In addition, nonexcitable tissues may also be affected. Cystic fibrosis, which is caused by a mutation in a chloride channel, is a channelopathy affecting mucus- and sweat-secreting cells of various organs. In pancreatic β cells, ATP-sensitive K^+ channels regulate insulin secretion, and mutations in these channel genes lead to certain forms of diabetes. Some types of retinitis pigmentosa are attributed to mutations in ion channels. It deserves mention that mutations in gap junctions, channels that provide direct communication between cells, are also associated with a variety of inherited diseases.

Channelopathies may reflect gains (epilepsy, myotonia) or losses (weakness) of ion channel function. Different mutations that affect the same ion channel may result in different disorders. For instance, inherited mutations in a single Na^+ channel in skeletal muscle can lead to either hyperkalemic or hypokalemic periodic paralysis. By contrast, sometimes mutations in different genes may give rise to the same phenotype; mutations in different skeletal muscle Na^+ channels all cause hyperkalemic periodic paralysis.

Acquired channelopathies have also been identified in various other disorders, including the evolution of some cancers (see Chapter 5) and autoimmune neurologic conditions. Autoantibodies (see Chapter 4) may cause disorders of both ligand-gated ion channels (receptors) and voltage-gated ones. In this context, myasthenia gravis and autoimmune neuropathy have been related to autoantibodies versus nicotinic acetylcholine receptors, which control ion channels. Autoantibodies against voltage-gated Ca^{2+} and K^+ channels are also responsible for diverse neuromuscular disorders. Ion channels are involved in cell cycle progression and may play a role in tumor development.

Channelopathies are not merely esoteric diseases, but often are matters of life and death. Up to 20% of sudden unexplained deaths and 10% of sudden infant death syndrome (SIDS; see Chapter 6) are attributable to cardiac arrhythmias associated with mutations in the Na^+ channel responsible for long-QT syndrome. Remarkably, a large majority of patients with mucolipidosis type IV, as well as those with autosomal dominant polycystic kidney disease, have mutations in cell membrane Ca^{2+} channels.

Abnormal Proteins

Many acquired and inherited diseases are characterized by intracellular accumulation of abnormal proteins. A protein's deviant tertiary structure may result from a mutation that alters the amino acid sequence or may reflect an acquired defect in protein folding. The following are a few examples:

- **α₁-Antitrypsin deficiency** is a heritable disorder in which mutations in the gene coding for α₁-antitrypsin yield an insoluble protein that is not easily exported. It accumulates in liver cells (Fig. 1-29), thereby causing cell injury and eventually cirrhosis (see Chapter 19).
- **Prion diseases** are neurodegenerative disorders (spongiform encephalopathies) caused by accumulation of abnormally folded prion proteins. The normal α-helical structure is changed to a β-pleated sheet. Abnormal prion proteins may result from inherited mutations or from exposure to the aberrant form of the protein (see Chapter 32). The function of the normal prion protein is unclear, but data suggest several activities, including a role in myelination, antioxidant (SOD-like) activity, a role in T-lymphocyte–dendritic cell interactions, enhancing neural progenitor proliferation and a key role in development of long-term memory.
- **Lewy bodies** (α-synuclein) are seen in neurons of the substantia nigra in Parkinson disease (see Chapter 32).
- **Neurofibrillary tangles** (tau protein) characterize cortical neurons in Alzheimer disease (see Chapter 32).
- **Mallory bodies** (intermediate filaments) are hepatocellular inclusions in alcoholic liver injury (see Chapter 20).

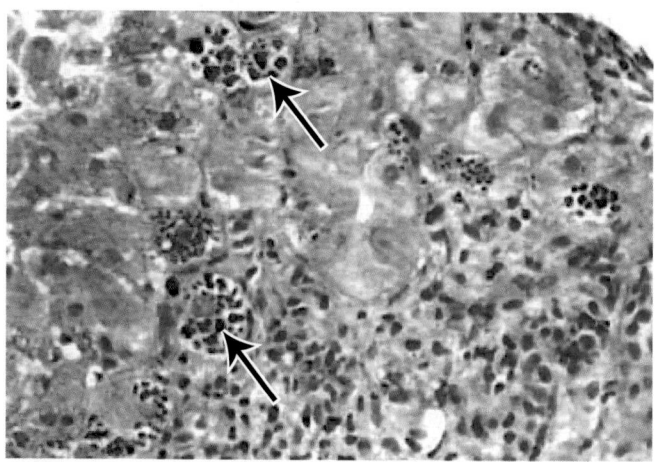

FIGURE 1-29. Storage of abnormal, mutant α₁-antitrypsin in the liver. Periodic acid–Schiff stain after diastase treatment to remove glycogen highlights the aggregates of α₁-antitrypsin protein (*arrows*).

MOLECULAR PATHOGENESIS: As discussed above, when ribosomes translate messenger RNA (mRNA), they make a linear chain of amino acids without a defined three-dimensional structure. Curiously, it is energetically more favorable for cells to produce many foldings, even abnormal ones, and then edit the protein repertoire than to construct only a single correct conformation. Thus, protein misfolding is an intrinsic tendency of proteins and occurs continuously. However, there is an escape valve, because evolutionary preference for energy conservation has dictated that a substantial proportion of newly formed proteins are rogues unsuitable for the society of civilized cells. Protein synthesis presents a number of possible outcomes:

- The primary sequence is correct and proper folding into the appropriate functional conformation occurs.
- The primary sequence may be correct but the protein does not fold correctly, owing to random energetic fluctuations.
- A mutant protein (with an incorrect amino acid sequence) folds incorrectly.
- A conformationally correct protein may become unfolded or misfolded due to an unfavorable environment (e.g., altered pH, high ionic strength, oxidation, etc.). The protein quality control system may fail because of a malfunction of protein quality control or overload of this mechanism. In either case, misfolded proteins accumulate as amorphous aggregates or fibrils and may cause cell injury by (1) decreasing a necessary activity **(loss of function)** or (2) a harmful increase in a cellular enterprise that alters a delicate balance of forces within the cell **(gain of function)**.
- **Loss of function:** Some mutations prevent correct folding of crucial proteins, which then do not function properly or cannot be incorporated into the correct site. For example, abnormal cystic fibrosis proteins are misfolded chloride ion channels, which are then degraded. The protein does not reach its intended destination at the cell membrane, creating a defect in Cl⁻ transport that produces the disease. Other examples of loss of function include mutations of the low-density lipoprotein (LDL) receptor in certain types of hypercholesterolemia and mutations of a copper-transporting ATPase in Wilson disease.
- **Formation of toxic protein aggregates:** Defects in protein structure may be acquired as well as genetic. Thus, particularly in nondividing cells, impairment of cellular antioxidant defenses is accompanied by protein oxidation, which alters protein tertiary structure and exposes interior hydrophobic amino acids that are normally hidden. In situations of mild to moderate oxidative stress, 20S proteasomes recognize the exposed hydrophobic moieties and degrade these proteins. However, if oxidative stress is severe, these proteins aggregate by virtue of a combination of hydrophobic and ionic bonds (Fig. 1-30). Such proteins may form disordered aggregates, which are insoluble and tend to sequester Fe^{2+} ions. In turn, Fe^{2+} helps to produce additional ROS (see above), further increasing aggregate size. Disordered aggregates may be degraded (e.g., by autophagy; see above) or may become partially ordered into denser structures in which the normal α-helical protein conformation is transformed

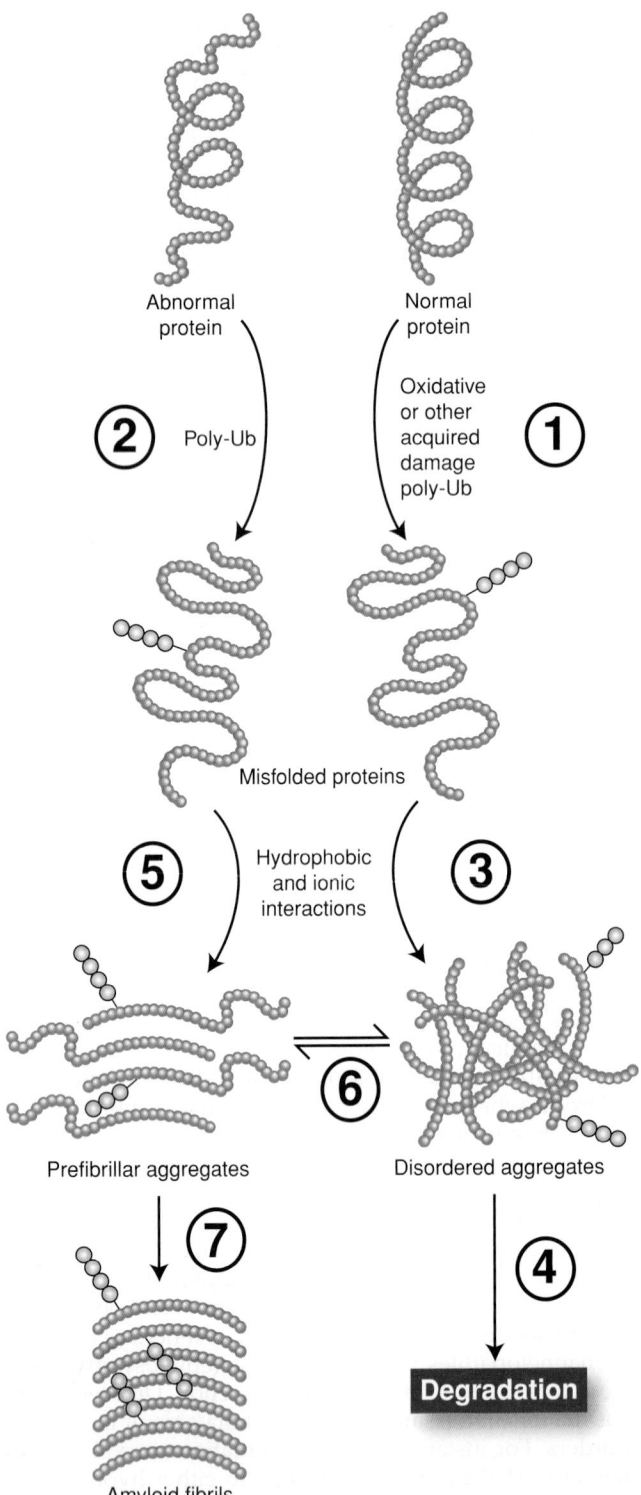

FIGURE 1-30. Formation of toxic protein aggregates. 1. Normal proteins can become damaged by exposure to reactive oxygen species and other stresses. **2.** Nonnative proteins may result from genetic mutations or translational errors. In any event, the resulting abnormal proteins may become misfolded and polyubiquitinated, after which two paths are open. **3.** Some of the misfolded proteins may become disordered aggregates, which can be degraded **(4)**. Alternatively **(5)**, the normal α-helical structure may be transformed into less soluble forms, consisting, to a variable extent, of β-pleated sheets (prefibrillar aggregates). The latter may exist to some extent **(6)** in equilibrium with disordered aggregates or they may evolve irreversibly into insoluble amyloid fibrils **(7)**. *Ub* = ubiquitin.

to a variable degree into insoluble fibrillar β-pleated sheet structures. These latter tend to accumulate as indigestible agglomerations, which may resemble amyloid (see **Chapter 21**). Any Ub bound to them is lost, which may cause a cellular deficit in Ub and impair protein degradation in general. By virtue of both their generation of toxic ROS and their inhibition of proteasomal degradation, these aggregates may lead to cell death. Accumulation of β-amyloid protein in Alzheimer disease and α-synuclein in Parkinson disease may occur by this type of mechanism.

- **Retention of secretory proteins:** Many proteins that are destined to be secreted by the cell must be correctly folded to be transported through cellular compartments and released at the cell membrane. Mutations in genes that encode such proteins (e.g., α_1-antitrypsin) lead to cell injury because of massive accumulation of misfolded proteins within the cell. Failure to secrete this antiprotease into the circulation also leads to unregulated proteolysis of connective tissue in the lung and loss of pulmonary parenchyma (emphysema).

- **Extracellular deposition of aggregated proteins:** Misfolded proteins tend to assume β-pleated conformations in place of random coils or α-helices. These abnormal proteins often form insoluble aggregates, which may be deposited extracellularly, the appearance depending on the specific disease. These accumulations often assume the forms of various types of amyloid and produce cell injury in systemic amyloidoses (see **Chapter 15**) and a variety of neurodegenerative diseases (see **Chapter 32**).

Cell Death

"To be or not to be–that is the question
Whether 'tis nobler in the mind to suffer
The slings and arrows of outrageous fortune
Or to take arms against a sea of troubles
And by opposing end them. To die . . ." (*Hamlet, III:i*)

Throughout recorded history, death has been considered as tragic, especially when youth has been cut short. Similarly, traditional concepts viewed cell death simply as the endpoint of disease processes. However, it is now clear that a cell's death is often needed for an organism to live; it is crucial for both development and survival of multicellular organisms. Just as the grim reaper himself assumes many guises, so cell death takes diverse forms. In some cases it represents the consequences of nonphysiologic and unregulated injury, but in others, complex intracellular molecular pathways respond to external and internal triggers to cause the cell's demise. Such programmed cell death oversees the size and diversity of many tissue compartments by eliminating obsolescent cells, as in the gastrointestinal tract, skin and hematopoietic system. Not all such mechanisms eliminate only older, senescent cells; in some cases younger upstarts, like autoreactive lymphocyte clones, may be targeted for destruction.

In addition to the unplanned murder of a cell by external violence, which is called necrosis, diverse suicide programs have been identified: apoptosis, autophagic cell death, necroptosis, NETosis and so forth. To further complicate

matters, many of these programmed pathways interrelate extensively, so that clear-cut distinctions are not always possible. The outcomes of such overlapping mechanisms are parallel, but on occasion they are opposite. For example, while autophagy may impede malignant transformation, it also protects malignant cells from the effects of chemotherapy. In its many forms, programmed cell death is integral to many disease processes.

The multiplicity and connectivity of the various networks are confusing and challenge the student to understand how processes whose consequences seem so different can be tightly linked. The field of cell death is evolving rapidly, and the following discussion is necessarily limited to those issues about which there is a consensus and that are important for an appreciation of disease development.

Understanding cell death is not simply an academic exercise; manipulation of cell viability is currently a major area of research. For example, if we understand the biochemistry of ischemic death of cardiac myocytes, which is responsible for the leading cause of death in the Western world, we may be able to prolong myocyte survival after a coronary occlusion until circulation is restored.

Once upon a time, all cell death was referred to as necrosis. Now, we know better. Three main avenues leading to cell death have been delineated: necrosis, apoptosis and autophagy. Other, more specialized forms of cell death are also described (see below). These processes had formerly been viewed as separate, nonintersecting roads. Necrosis was defined as an accidental form of cell death caused by a hostile environment to which a cell could not adapt effectively. It was thus seen as a passive process in which the cell was more sinned against than sinning itself. By contrast, apoptosis is a form of cellular suicide in which the cell participates actively in its own demise. It is a mechanism by which individual cells activate their own signaling systems to sacrifice themselves for the preservation of the organism. Autophagy (see above) is also an active signaling process that is elicited when a stressful environment requires autodigestion of a portion of the cell's macromolecular constituents. Since the principal pathways of cell death may overlap, it is important to understand how the processes manifest morphologically.

MORPHOLOGY OF CELL DEATH

Necrosis Is Reflected in Geographic Areas of Cell Death

Necrosis occurs when hostile external forces overwhelm cells' adaptive abilities. Diverse insults can cause necrotic cell death, which typically affects geographically localized groups of cells. The response to this process is usually acute inflammation, which itself may generate further cell injury (see Chapter 2). The stimuli that initiate pathways leading to necrosis are highly variable and produce diverse and recognizable histologic and cytologic patterns.

Coagulative Necrosis

Coagulative necrosis refers to specific light microscopic appearances of dead or dying cells (Fig. 1-31). Shortly after a cell's death, its outline is maintained. When stained with

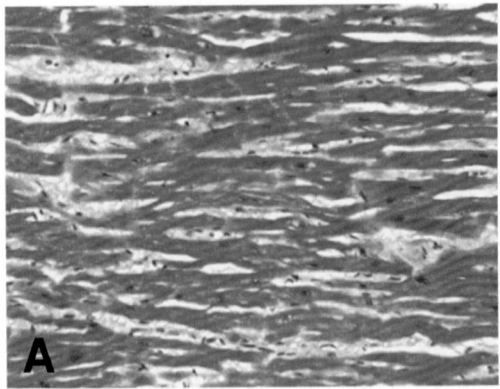
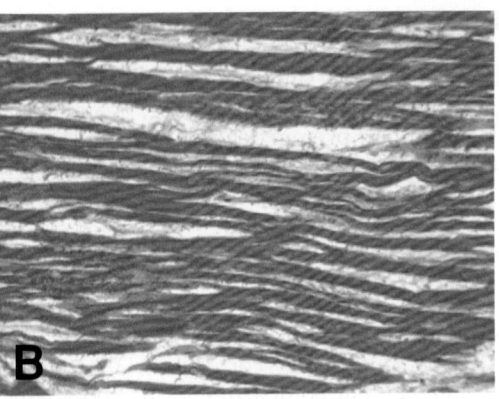

FIGURE 1-31. Coagulative necrosis. A. Normal heart. All myocytes are nucleated, and striations are clear. **B. Myocardial infarction.** The heart from a patient following acute myocardial infarction. The necrotic cells are deeply eosinophilic and most have lost their nuclei.

the usual combination of hematoxylin and eosin, the cytoplasm of a necrotic cell is more deeply eosinophilic than usual. Nuclear chromatin is initially clumped and then redistributes along the nuclear membrane. Three morphologic changes follow:

- **Pyknosis:** The nucleus becomes smaller and stains deeply basophilic as chromatin clumping continues.
- **Karyorrhexis:** The pyknotic nucleus breaks up into many smaller fragments scattered about the cytoplasm.
- **Karyolysis:** The pyknotic nucleus may be extruded from the cell or it may progressively lose chromatin staining.

Early ultrastructural changes in a dying or dead cell reflect an extension of alterations associated with reversible cell injury (Figs. 1-3 and 1-4). In addition to the nuclear changes described above, the dead cell features dilated endoplasmic reticulum, disaggregated ribosomes, swollen and calcified mitochondria, aggregated cytoskeletal elements and plasma membrane blebs.

After a variable time, depending on the tissue and circumstances, the lytic activity of intracellular and extracellular enzymes causes the cell to disintegrate. This is particularly the case when necrotic cells have elicited an acute inflammatory response.

The appearance of necrotic tissue has traditionally been described as **coagulative necrosis** because it resembles the coagulation of proteins that occurs upon heating. This term, while based on obsolete concepts, remains useful as a morphologic descriptor.

Liquefactive Necrosis

When the rate at which necrotic cells dissolve greatly exceeds the rate of repair, the resulting appearance is termed **liquefactive necrosis**. Polymorphonuclear leukocytes of the acute inflammatory reaction contain potent hydrolases capable of digesting dead cells. A sharply localized collection of these acute inflammatory cells, generally in response to bacterial infection, produces rapid cell death and tissue dissolution. The result is often an **abscess** (Fig. 1-32), a cavity formed by liquefactive necrosis in a solid tissue. In time, the abscess is walled off by a fibrous capsule that contains its contents.

Coagulative necrosis of the brain may occur after cerebral artery occlusion and is often followed by rapid dissolution—liquefactive necrosis—of the dead tissue by a mechanism that cannot be attributed to the action of an

acute inflammatory response. It is not clear why coagulative necrosis in the brain and not elsewhere is followed by the disappearance of necrotic cells, but the abundant lysosomal enzymes, or different hydrolases specific to cells of the CNS, may be responsible. Liquefactive necrosis of large areas of the CNS can lead to an actual cavity or cyst that persists for the life of the person.

Fat Necrosis

Fat necrosis specifically affects adipose tissue and most commonly results from pancreatitis or trauma (Fig. 1-33). The unique feature determining this type of necrosis is the presence of triglycerides in adipose tissue. In the peripancreatic fat, for example, the process begins when digestive enzymes that are normally found only in the pancreatic duct and small intestine lumen are released from injured pancreatic acinar cells and ducts into extracellular spaces. Upon extracellular activation, these enzymes digest both the pancreas itself and surrounding tissues, including adipocytes.

1. Phospholipases and proteases attack plasma membranes of adipocytes, releasing their stored triglycerides.

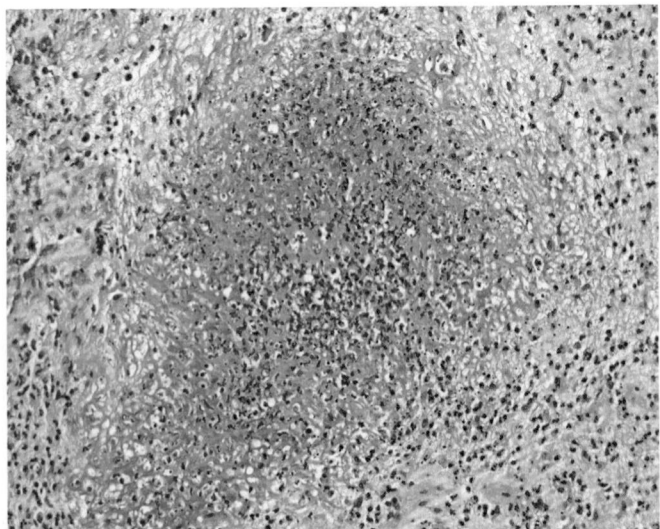

FIGURE 1-32. Liquefactive necrosis in an abscess of the skin. The abscess cavity is filled with polymorphonuclear leukocytes.

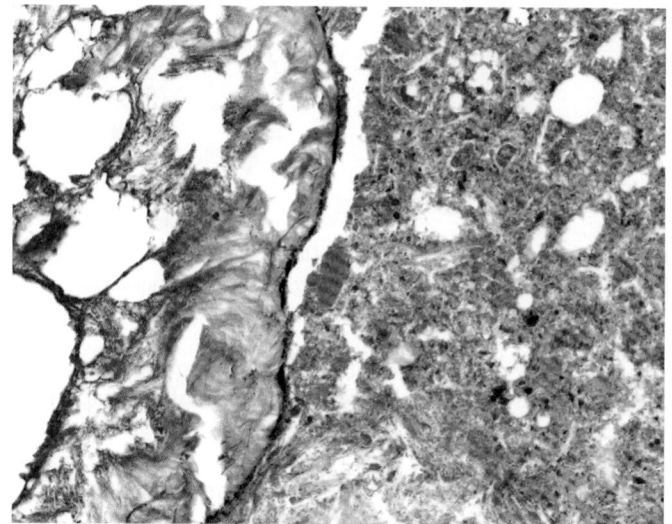

FIGURE 1-33. Fat necrosis. Peripancreatic adipose tissue from a patient with acute pancreatitis shows fatty acids precipitated as calcium soaps, which appear as amorphous, basophilic deposits **(left)**. These appear at the periphery of the irregular island of necrotic adipocytes **(right)**.

2. Pancreatic lipase hydrolyzes the triglycerides, which produces free fatty acids.
3. Free fatty acids bind Ca^{2+} and precipitate as soaps. These appear as amorphous, basophilic deposits at the edges of irregular islands of necrotic adipocytes.

Grossly, fat necrosis appears as an irregular, chalky white area embedded in otherwise normal adipose tissue. In the case of traumatic fat necrosis, triglycerides and lipases are released from the injured adipocytes. In the breast, fat necrosis due to trauma is common and may mimic a tumor, particularly if calcification has occurred.

Caseous Necrosis

Caseous necrosis is characteristic of tuberculosis and is seen, less often, in other settings as well. The lesions of tuberculosis are granulomas, or tubercles (Fig. 1-34). In the center of such granulomas, the accumulated mononuclear cells that mediate a chronic inflammatory reaction to the offending mycobacteria are killed. Unlike coagulative necrosis, the necrotic cells in granulomas lose their cellular outlines. They do not disappear by lysis, however, as in liquefactive necrosis. Rather, the dead cells persist indefinitely as amorphous, coarsely granular, eosinophilic debris. Grossly, this material is grayish white, soft and friable. It resembles clumpy cheese, hence the name **caseous necrosis**. This distinctive type of necrosis is generally attributed to the toxic effects of mycobacterial cell walls, which contain complex waxes (peptidoglycolipids) that exert potent biological effects. Recent work suggests that granuloma formation may actually be orchestrated by mycobacteria and may in fact facilitate the organism's survival in the face of host immune responsiveness.

Fibrinoid Necrosis

Fibrinoid necrosis is an alteration of injured blood vessels, in which insudation and accumulation of plasma proteins cause the wall to stain intensely with eosin (Fig. 1-35). The term is a misnomer, however, as the eosinophilia of the accumulated plasma proteins obscures the underlying alterations in the blood vessel, making it difficult, if not impossible, to determine whether there truly is necrosis in the vascular wall.

Apoptosis Produces Individual Cell Death Amidst Viable Cells

Morphology of Apoptosis

Apoptosis is a pattern of cell death that is triggered by a variety of extracellular and intracellular stimuli and is carried to its conclusion by organized cellular signaling cascades. Apoptotic cells are recognized by nuclear fragmentation and pyknosis, generally against a background of viable cells. Importantly, apoptosis occurs in single cells or small groups of cells, whereas necrosis characteristically involves larger geographic areas of cell death. Ultrastructural features of apoptotic cells include (1) nuclear

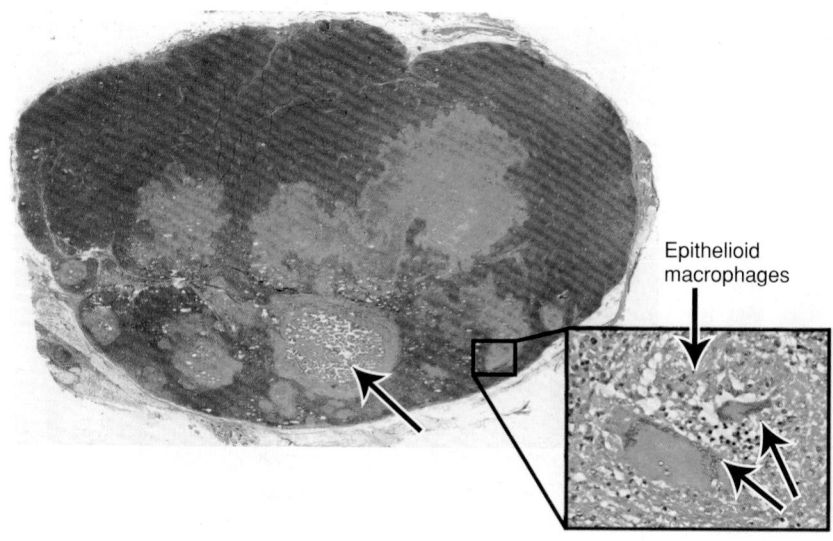

Epithelioid macrophages

FIGURE 1-34. Caseous necrosis in a tuberculous lymph node. Hilar lymph node from a patient with active tuberculosis. Irregular pink areas of caseous necrosis (*arrow*) are evident against a background of lymphocytes. **Inset:** Granulomas on the periphery of necrotic areas show epithelioid macrophages and multinucleated giant (Langhans) cells (*arrows*).

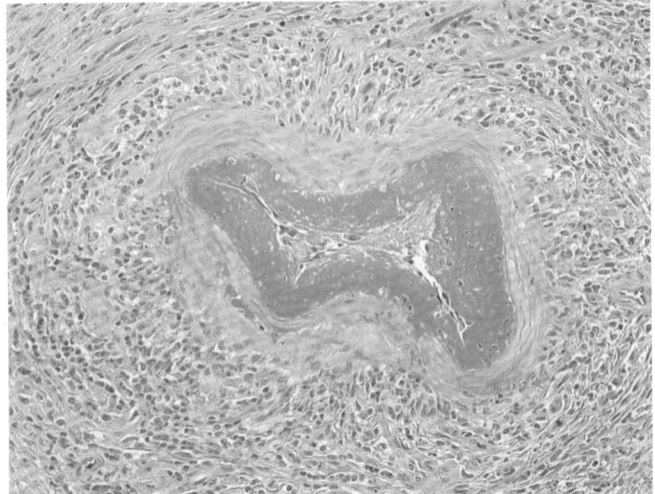

FIGURE 1-35. Fibrinoid necrosis. An inflamed muscular artery in a patient with systemic arteritis shows a sharply demarcated, homogeneous, deeply eosinophilic zone of necrosis.

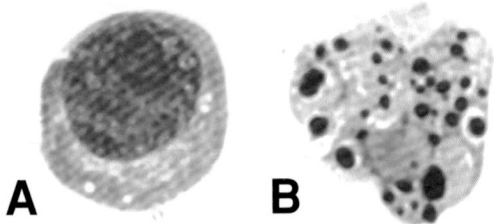

FIGURE 1-36. Apoptosis. A viable cell **(A)** contrasts with an apoptotic cell **(B)** in which the nucleus has undergone condensation and fragmentation.

condensation and fragmentation, (2) segregation of cytoplasmic organelles into distinct regions, (3) blebs of the plasma membrane and (4) membrane-bound cellular fragments, which often lack nuclei (Fig. 1-36).

Removal of Apoptotic Cells

Once the self-destructive process of apoptosis has propelled a cell to DNA fragmentation and cytoskeletal dissolution, the final phase, the *apoptotic body*, remains. Apoptotic bodies are phagocytosed by tissue macrophages.

Phosphatidylserine (PS), a phospholipid that is normally on the interior aspect of the cell membrane, is externalized in cells undergoing apoptosis. PS is recognized by macrophages and activates ingestion of an apoptotic cell's mortal remains without release of intracellular constituents, thus avoiding an inflammatory reaction (Fig. 1-37). Mononuclear phagocytes ingest the debris from apoptotic cells, but recruitment of neutrophils or lymphocytes is rare. This situation is unlike that of cells that undergo necrotic cell death, which tends to elicit acute inflammatory responses (see Chapter 2).

Cells May Participate Actively in Their Own Death

There is increasing agreement that the various forms of cell death are not strictly separate, but rather share molecular effectors and signaling pathways. Cell processes incriminated in one may be co-conspirators with the others, and a particular cell's death may involve combinations of two, or all, of these mechanisms. For the sake of clarity, mechanisms of cell death by necrosis, apoptosis and autophagy are presented separately, but it is important to understand that all of these processes involve signaling, borrow from one another and collaborate with each other.

NECROSIS

Ischemia Injures Cells during Both Deprivation and Restoration of Oxygen Supply

Ischemic Injury

As noted above, ischemia is the interruption of blood flow (e.g., myocardial infarction, stroke). Loss of blood flow leads to decreased O_2 and key nutrients, such as glucose, and increased CO_2 in cells. A number of deleterious events

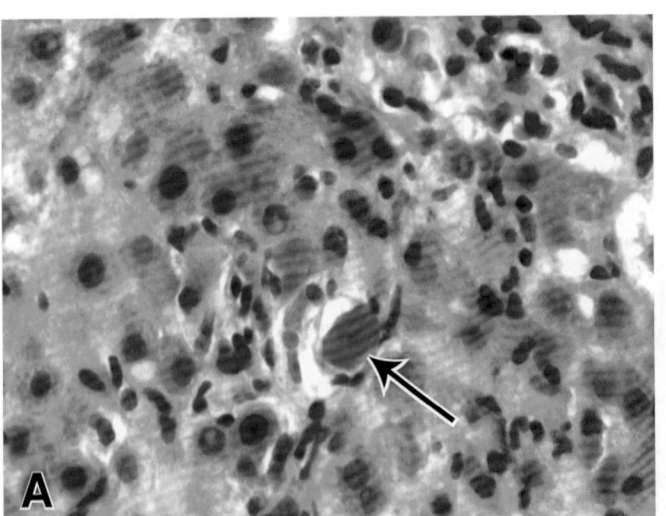

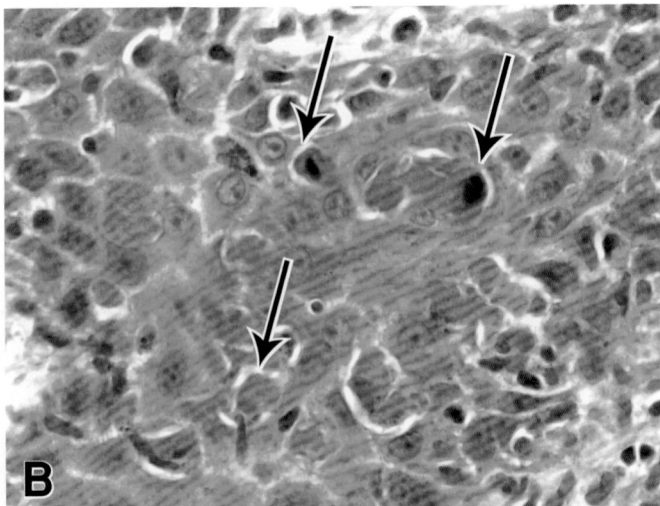

FIGURE 1-37. Apoptosis in the liver in viral hepatitis (A) and in the skin in erythema multiforme (B). Apoptotic cells are indicated by *arrows.*

occur, including acidosis, generation of ROS, loss of glycogen stores, disruption of intracellular Ca^{2+} homeostasis, increased intracellular Ca^{2+}, mitochondrial injury and DNA damage.

Ischemic Cell Death

Myocardial infarction and stroke together represent the most common cause of mortality in the Western world and are both due to ischemic cell death. Thus, mechanisms of cellular injury and death due to ischemia represent the most important example of necrosis.

Cells exist in a skewed equilibrium with their external environment. The extracellular fluid is separated from the internal cellular milieu by the plasma membrane. Extracellular levels of Na^+ and Ca^{2+} are normally orders of magnitude more than intracellular concentrations. The opposite holds for K^+. This selective ion permeability requires (1) considerable energy (ATP), (2) structural integrity of the lipid bilayer, (3) intact ion channel proteins and (4) normal association of the membrane with cytoskeleton. Whatever the lethal insult, cell necrosis is heralded by loss of the plasma membrane's permeability barrier function. If ischemia is incomplete or if the episode of ischemia is brief, normal ionic equilibrium can be re-established without tissue damage. However, if one or more of the elements mentioned above is severely damaged, the resulting disturbance of ionic balance is thought to represent the "point of no return" for the injured cell. Thus, ischemic cell injury and death share the same pathophysiologic spectrum.

The role of calcium in the pathogenesis of cell death deserves special mention. Ca^{2+} concentration in extracellular fluids is in the millimolar range (10^{-3} M). By contrast, cytosolic Ca^{2+} concentration is 1/10,000 of that outside the cell (i.e., about 10^{-7} M). Many crucial cell functions are exquisitely regulated by minute fluctuations in cytosolic free calcium concentration ($[Ca^{2+}]_i$). Thus, **massive influx of Ca^{2+} through a damaged plasma membrane is key to ischemic cell damage** and may ensure loss of viability.

The processes of cell death by necrosis vary according to the cause, organ and cell type. The best-studied and most clinically important example is ischemic necrosis of cardiac myocytes. The mechanisms underlying the death of these cells are in part unique, but the basic processes involved are comparable to those in other organs. Some of these events may occur simultaneously; others may be sequential (Fig. 1-38).

1. **Interruption of blood supply decreases delivery of O_2 and glucose.** For most cells, but especially for cardiac myocytes and neurons, which do not store much energy, this combined insult is formidable.
2. **Anaerobic glycolysis leads to overproduction of lactate and decreased intracellular pH.** The lack of O_2 during myocardial ischemia both blocks ATP production and inhibits mitochondrial oxidation of pyruvate. Instead of entering the citric acid cycle, pyruvate is reduced to lactate in the cytosol, a process called anaerobic glycolysis. Lactate accumulation lowers cytosol pH (acidification), thus initiating a spiral of events that propels the cell downward toward disaster.
3. **Distortion of the activities of pumps in the plasma membrane skews the ionic balance of the cell.** Na^+ accumulates because lack of ATP impairs the Na^+/K^+ ion exchanger. This effect leads to activation of the Na^+/H^+ ion exchanger. This pump is normally quiescent, but when intracellular

acidosis threatens, it pumps H^+ out of the cell in exchange for Na^+ to maintain proper intracellular pH. The resulting increase in intracellular sodium activates the Na^+/Ca^{2+} ion exchanger, which increases calcium entry. Ordinarily, excess intracellular Ca^{2+} is extruded by an ATP-dependent calcium pump. However, with ATP in very short supply, Ca^{2+} accumulates in the cell.

4. **Activation of phospholipase A_2 (PLA_2) and proteases disrupts the plasma membrane and cytoskeleton.** Elevated $[Ca^{2+}]_i$ in an ischemic cell activates PLA_2, leading to degradation of membrane phospholipids and consequent release of free fatty acids and lysophospholipids. The latter act as detergents that solubilize cell membranes. Both fatty acids and lysophospholipids are also potent mediators of inflammation (see Chapter 2), an effect that may further disrupt the integrity of the already compromised cell.

   Calcium also activates a series of proteases that attack the cytoskeleton and its attachments to the cell membrane. As cohesion between cytoskeletal proteins and the plasma membrane is disrupted, membrane blebs form, causing the cell's shape to change. The combination of electrolyte imbalance and increased cell membrane permeability makes the cell swell, often a morphologic prelude to its dissolution.
5. **Lack of O_2 impairs mitochondrial electron transport, thereby decreasing ATP synthesis and facilitating production of ROS.** Normally, 1–3% of oxygen entering mitochondria is converted to ROS, because of inefficiencies in the electron transport chain. During ischemia, generation of ROS increases because of damage to ROS detoxification mechanisms and impaired processing of reactive oxygen intermediates. ROS cause peroxidation of cardiolipin, a membrane phospholipid that is unique to mitochondria and is sensitive to oxidative damage by virtue of its high content of unsaturated fatty acids. This attack inhibits the function of the electron transport chain and decreases its ability to produce ATP.
6. **Mitochondrial damage promotes release of cytochrome c (Cyt c) to the cytosol.** In normal cells the mitochondrial permeability transition pore (MPTP) opens and closes sporadically. Ischemic injury to mitochondria causes sustained opening of the MPTP. Resulting loss of Cyt c from the electron transport chain further diminishes ATP synthesis and may also trigger apoptotic cell death (see below).
7. **The cell dies.** When a cell can no longer maintain itself as a metabolic unit, it dies. The line between reversible and irreversible cell injury (i.e., the "point of no return") is not precisely defined.

Reperfusion Injury

Reperfusion is the restoration of blood flow after a period of ischemia. Although reperfusion is beneficial in salvaging cells that have remained viable, the process itself can cause damage, to which the term "reperfusion injury" is applied. Such injury occurs most often in settings of organ ischemia, such as myocardial infarction, but also in other situations (e.g., organ transplantation).

Reperfusion injury reflects the interplay of transient ischemia, consequent tissue damage and exposure of damaged tissue to the oxygen that arrives when blood flow is re-established (reperfusion). Lethal reperfusion injury is significant. In the heart, it may account for up to half of the final size of myocardial infarcts. Initially, ischemic cellular damage

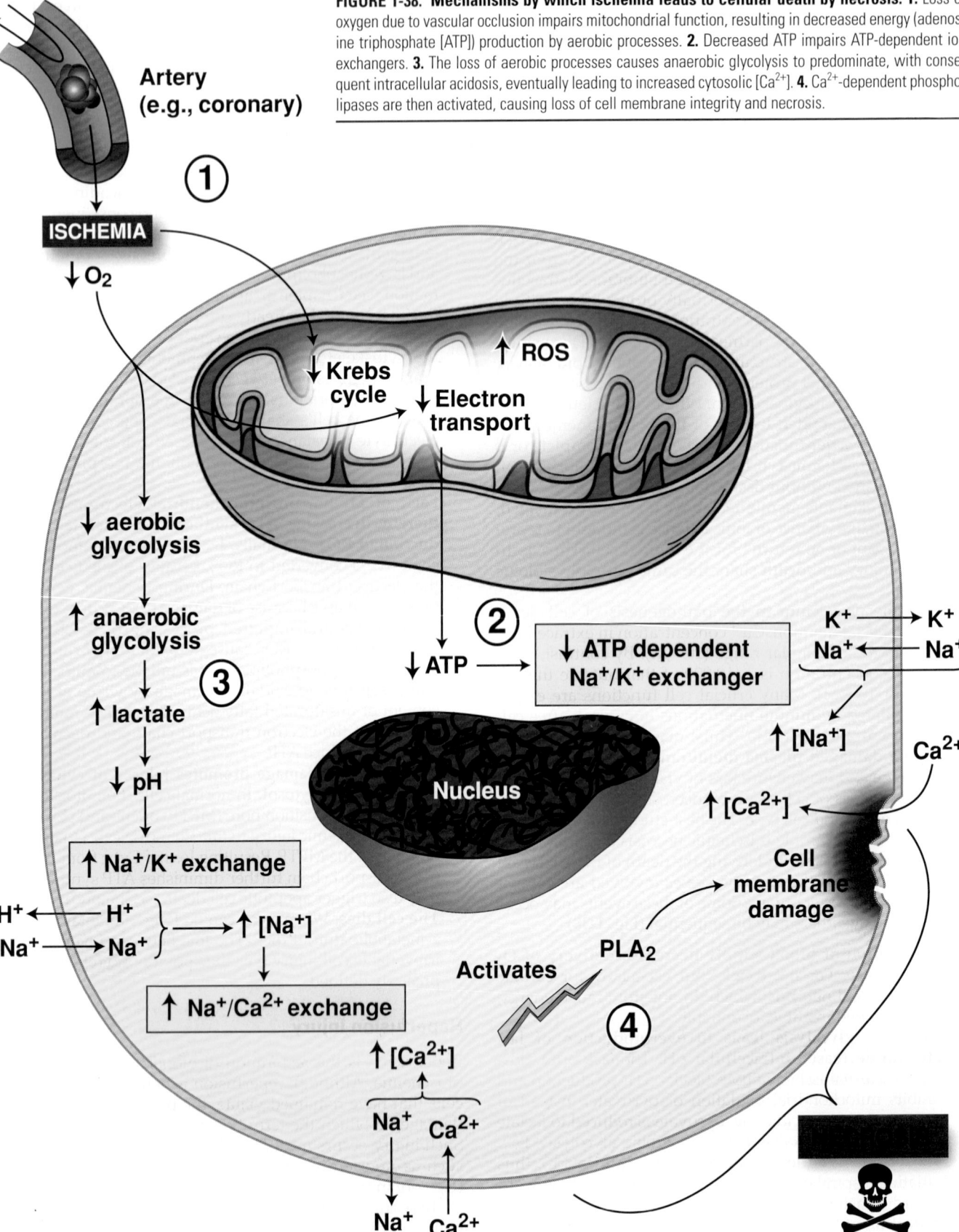

FIGURE 1-38. Mechanisms by which ischemia leads to cellular death by necrosis. 1. Loss of oxygen due to vascular occlusion impairs mitochondrial function, resulting in decreased energy (adenosine triphosphate [ATP]) production by aerobic processes. **2.** Decreased ATP impairs ATP-dependent ion exchangers. **3.** The loss of aerobic processes causes anaerobic glycolysis to predominate, with consequent intracellular acidosis, eventually leading to increased cytosolic [Ca^{2+}]. **4.** Ca^{2+}-dependent phospholipases are then activated, causing loss of cell membrane integrity and necrosis.

leads to generation of free radical species (see above). Reperfusion then provides abundant molecular O_2 to combine with free radicals to form additional ROS. The evolution of reperfusion injury also involves many other factors, including inflammatory mediators, platelet-activating factor (PAF), NOS and NO•, intercellular adhesion molecules, dysregulation of Ca^{2+} homeostasis and many more.

Xanthine Oxidase
Xanthine oxidase activity, particularly in vascular endothelium, increases during ischemia. The enzyme converts ATP-derived xanthine into uric acid in an oxygen-requiring reaction, producing superoxide in the process. On reperfusion, oxygen returns and the abundant purines derived from ATP catabolism during ischemia become substrates for xanthine oxidase. Since this enzyme requires oxygen, restoration of oxygen supply during reperfusion leads to a sudden increase in ROS. This occurs after ischemia-related impairment leaves mitochondrial antioxidant systems ill-prepared for the sudden increase in ROS. Mitochondrial oxidant stress is further magnified by two events. One is the sudden increase in electron transport, which is driven by the renewed availability of oxygen. The other is changes in pH and calcium concentrations (see below).

The Role of Neutrophils
An additional source of ROS during reperfusion is the neutrophil. Reperfusion prompts endothelial cells to move preformed P-selectin to the cell surface, increasing neutrophil binding to intercellular adhesion molecule-1 (ICAM-1) at the endothelial cell membrane (see Chapter 2). Neutrophils release large quantities of ROS and hydrolytic enzymes, both of which further injure the previously ischemic cells.

Ion Fluxes During Reperfusion
Ischemia changes cellular ion transporter activities, which become even more problematic with reperfusion. When blood flow is re-established, cellular pH is suddenly rectified. The Ca^{2+} overload that began during ischemia is then exacerbated by reversal of the Na^+/Ca^{2+} exchanger. Increased $[Ca^{2+}]_i$ activates Ca^{2+}-dependent proteases and increases ROS generation. It also acts in concert with increased mitochondrial ROS to open the MPTP and triggers mitochondria-related cell death programs (see below).

The Role of Nitric Oxide and Nitric Oxide Synthase
NO is generated from arginine by both constitutive and inducible NOSs. NO exerts a protective effect, dilating microvasculature by relaxing smooth muscle, inhibiting platelet aggregation and decreasing leukocyte adhesion to endothelial cells. NO also decreases transferrin-mediated iron uptake, limiting the amount of iron available to generate OH• from other ROS. These activities largely reflect the ability of NO to decrease cytosolic Ca^{2+} by extruding it from the cell and by sequestering it within intracellular stores.

NO and NOS are double-edged swords, however. In the setting of ischemia-triggered ATP depletion, Ca^{2+} overload and nutrient deprivation, mitochondrial NOS tends to produce NO. NO• also reacts with O_2^- to form $ONOO^-$, a highly reactive species. Normally, O_2^- is detoxified by SOD and little $ONOO^-$ is produced. However, reperfusion both inactivates SOD and provides abundant O_2^-, which together favor production of $ONOO^-$. This free radical gives rise to DNA strand breaks and lipid peroxidation in cell membranes.

Inflammatory Cytokines
Reperfusion injury is complicated by the release of cytokines, which both promote inflammation and modulate its severity. Proinflammatory cytokines such as TNF-α, IL-1 and IL-6 are key. These (1) promote vasoconstriction, (2) stimulate adherence of neutrophils and platelets to endothelium and (3) have effects at sites distant from the ischemic insult itself.

Platelets
Platelets adhere to the microvasculature of injured tissue and release a number of factors that play a role in both tissue damage and cytoprotection. These include cytokines, TGF-β, serotonin and NO•.

Complement
Activation of the complement system (see Chapter 2) during reperfusion leads to deposition of membrane attack complexes and elaboration of chemotactic agents and proinflammatory cytokines. The net result is recruitment and adhesion of neutrophils.

Summary of Ischemia and Reperfusion Injury
We can put reperfusion injury in perspective by emphasizing that there are three different degrees of cell injury, depending on the duration of the ischemia:

- With short periods of ischemia, reperfusion (and, thus, the resupply of oxygen) completely restores the cell's structural and functional integrity. Cell injury in this case is completely reversible.
- With longer periods of ischemia, reperfusion is associated with cell deterioration and death. In this case, lethal cell injury occurs during the period of reperfusion.
- Lethal cell injury may develop during the period of ischemia itself, in which case reperfusion need not be a factor. A longer period of ischemia is required to produce this third type of cell injury.

Processes involved in reperfusion injury are summarized in Table 1-4.

Ischemic Preconditioning
Sudden and complete ischemia may cause cell death before adaptive mechanisms can come into play, but repeated episodes of ischemia, as in recurrent angina due to coronary artery disease, stimulate adaptive responses. In the heart, these are collectively called **ischemic preconditioning**. The transcription factor hypoxia-inducible factor-1α (HIF-1α) is the master regulator of transcriptional responses to low O_2 tension. HIF-1α activates genes whose protein products limit production of ROS, Ca^{2+} accumulation and ATP depletion. As a result, HIF-1α tends to protect against mitochondrial injury, DNA damage and oxidative stress, and so facilitates survival of the ischemic cell.

PROGRAMMED CELL DEATH

Programmed cell death (PCD) refers to processes that are lethal to individual cells and are regulated by pre-existing signaling pathways. It was first observed 170 years ago and was thought to represent a passive form of cell death. However, we now recognize various forms of PCD that entail activation of cellular signaling cascades.

PCD is part of the balance between the life and death of cells and determines that a cell dies when it is no longer useful or when its survival may be harmful to the larger

TABLE 1-4

CELL INJURY MECHANISMS ACTIVE IN REPERFUSION INJURY

Formation of reactive oxygen species

Generated by xanthine oxidase

Produced by neutrophils

Made by mitochondria

Altered ionic composition

Rapid pH normalization following period at acidic pH

Increased [Na^+]

Increased [Ca^{2+}]

Abnormalities of nitric oxide metabolism

Decreased endothelial cell NOS with subsequent vasoconstriction, increased **platelet aggregation and neutrophil recruitment**

ONOO generation

Altered vascular function and inflammation

Vasoconstriction and inhibition of vasodilatation

Increase in proinflammatory cytokines

High cell membrane levels of adhesion molecules

Clumping of platelets

Migration of neutrophils

Complement

Cell death

Opening of MPTP

Activation of apoptosis

Activation of autophagy

MPTP = mitochondrial permeability transition pore; NOS = nitric oxide synthase; ONOO = peroxynitrite.

organism. Without programmed cell death to limit the size of bodily compartments, it is estimated that two tons of bone marrow and lymph nodes and 16 km (10 miles) of intestines would have accumulated by age 80. PCD is also a self-defense mechanism: cells that are infected with pathogens or that sustain genomic alterations are destroyed.

Classification of PCD

Recent work in this field has uncovered a bewildering variety of mechanisms that eventuate in PCD. Originally, this term was synonymous with apoptosis. However, mutant mice lacking the key elements of the apoptotic machinery develop almost normally. This observation indicated that alternatives to apoptosis exist. Thus, a number of mechanisms of PCD have been identified:

- Apoptosis
- Autophagy-associated cell death
- Necroptosis
- Pyroptosis
- Anoikis
- NETosis
- Pyrosis
- Entosis

The fact that nonapoptotic PCD pathways are best studied when apoptosis is inhibited does not mean that other mechanisms are subordinate to apoptosis. Rather, each seems to predominate in specific circumstances. The various cell death networks do not function in isolation from each other, and there are interconnections between them. As a result, multiple PCD mechanisms may contribute to cell death in any given situation. Detailed discussion of all these processes is beyond the scope of this chapter, and we focus here on the highlights of the major pathways: apoptosis, autophagy and necroptosis. The other more restricted forms of PCD are mentioned briefly.

There is ambiguity in the nomenclature of PCD, so that the same or similar phenomena may be labeled differently by different authors. Intersecting signaling among cell death pathways is a further source of confusion. For the sake of clarity, we use the term "apoptosis" for PCD involving caspase signaling (see below). "Necroptosis" refers to a cell death resembling necrosis that entails programmed signaling pathways.

APOPTOSIS IS A FORM OF PCD THAT RELIES EXCLUSIVELY ON THE CASPASE CASCADE

Apoptosis is a highly conserved cell death process that depends on a family of cysteine proteases (caspases) as crucial signaling intermediates and as executioners.

Apoptosis in Development and Physiology

Fetal development involves the sequential appearance and regression of many evolutionary relics. Some aortic arches do not persist. The pronephros and mesonephros regress in favor of the metanephros. Structures required by only one sex disappear in embryos of the other sex. Thus, the müllerian duct, the progenitor of the uterus, is deleted in males, and the wolffian duct, which forms part of the male genital tract, disappears in females. In some organs, such as the brain and ovaries, cells are overproduced, then culled by apoptosis. Apoptosis also mediates the disappearance of interdigital tissues to yield discrete fingers and toes, converts solid primordia to hollow tubes (e.g., gastrointestinal tract), produces the four-chamber heart and mediates other body-sculpting activities. Lymphocyte clones that recognize self-antigens are deleted by apoptosis, thereby avoiding potentially dangerous autoimmune disease.

Physiologic apoptosis principally affects progeny of stem cells that are constantly dividing (e.g., stem cells of the hematopoietic system, gastrointestinal mucosa and epidermis). Apoptosis of mature cells in these organs prevents overpopulation of the respective cell compartments by removing excess cells. Thus, normal organ size and architecture are maintained (Fig. 1-39).

Apoptosis Eliminates Obsolescent Cells

Cell turnover is essential to maintaining the size and function of many organs. For example, as cells are continuously supplied to the circulating blood, older and less functional white blood cells must be eliminated to maintain the normal complement of the cells. Indeed, pathologic accumulation of polymorphonuclear leukocytes in chronic myeloid leukemia results from a mutation that inhibits apoptosis and so

Sculpting

Deletion of structures

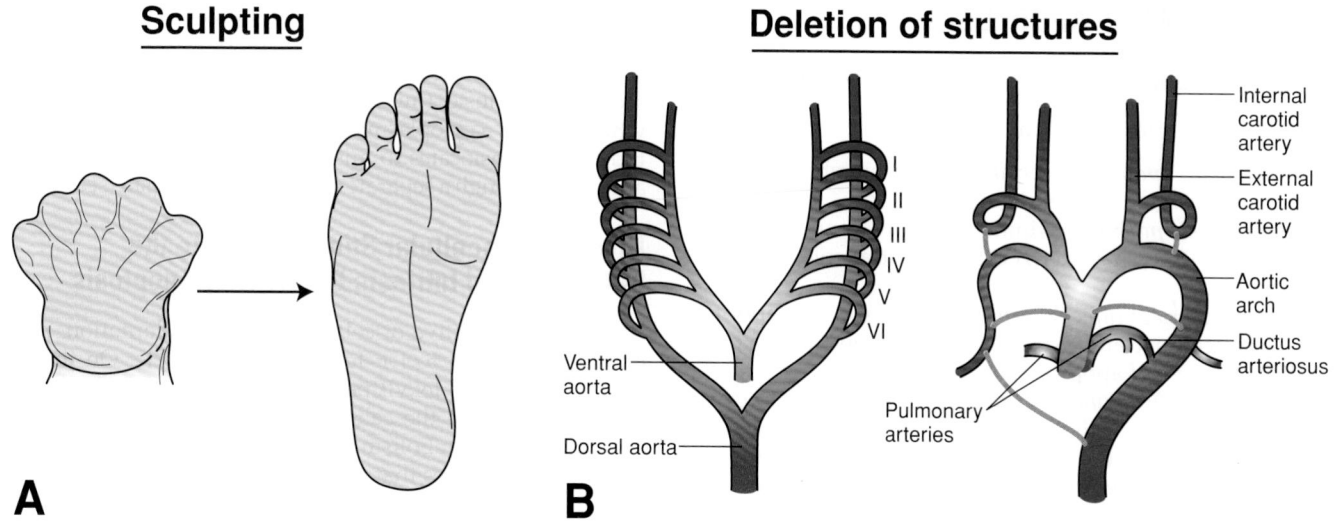

Removing dangerous cells

Regulating cell number

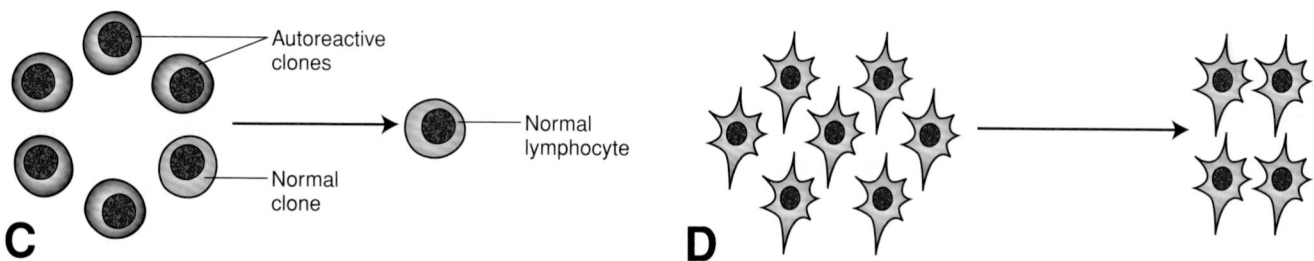

FIGURE 1-39. Activities of apoptosis during embryonic development. A. Sculpting. Apoptosis eliminates interdigital tissue. **B. Aortic arches.** Multiple embryonic aortic arches **(left)**, which are evolutionary relics, are eliminated and transformed by apoptosis into the eventual adult circulatory system **(right). C. Dangerous cells.** Autoreactive lymphocytes and other errant cells are eliminated by apoptosis. **D. Population control.** Excessive numbers of diverse cell types, such as central nervous system neurons, are pruned by apoptosis.

allows these cells to persist. In the small intestine mucosa, cells migrate from the depths of the crypts to the tips of the villi, where they undergo apoptosis and are sloughed into the lumen.

Apoptosis also maintains the balance of cellularity in organs that respond to trophic stimuli, such as hormones, as in the regression of lactational hyperplasia of the breast in women who have stopped nursing their infants. Later in life, postmenopausal atrophy of the endometrium follows loss of hormonal support.

An interesting facet of apoptosis is its impact on gametogenesis. Adult men produce about 1000 new spermatozoa per second, of which most undergo apoptosis because of intrinsic defects or external damage. Excessive apoptosis among spermatozoa has been implicated in some forms of male infertility. An analogous effect occurs in females, in whom 99% of neonatal ovarian oocytes are eventually deleted by apoptosis.

Apoptosis Deletes Mutant Cells

The integrity of an organism requires that damaged cells be eliminated. There is a finite, albeit low, error rate in DNA replication, owing to the imperfect fidelity of DNA polymerases. Environmental stresses such as ultraviolet (UV) light, ionizing radiation and DNA-binding chemicals may also alter DNA structure. There are several means, the most important of which probably involve p53, by which cells recognize genomic abnormalities and "assess" whether or not they can be repaired. If the DNA damage is too severe to be repaired, a cascade of events leads to apoptosis. This process protects an organism from the consequences of a nonfunctional cell or one that cannot control its own proliferation (e.g., a cancer cell). Perversely, cancer cells often evolve mechanisms to circumvent apoptosis that might otherwise eliminate them (see Chapter 5).

Apoptosis as a Defense Against Dissemination of Infection

When a cell "detects" nonchromosomal DNA replication, as in a viral infection, it tends to initiate apoptosis. In destroying infected cells, the body limits the spread of the virus. Many viruses have evolved mechanisms that manipulate cellular apoptosis. Many viruses are known to carry genes whose products inhibit apoptosis. Some of these viral proteins bind and inactivate cellular proteins (e.g., p53) that are important in triggering apoptosis. Others may interfere with the signaling pathways that activate apoptosis.

MECHANISMS OF APOPTOSIS

Apoptosis Comprises Several Signaling Pathways

The several apoptosis pathways include:

- In *extrinsic apoptosis*, certain plasma membrane receptors are activated by their ligands.
- The *intrinsic pathway* is initiated by diverse intracellular stresses and is characterized by a central role for mitochondria.
- *Inflammatory or infectious processes* may lead to apoptosis. Intracellular and extracellular infectious agents both elicit this type of apoptosis, by diverse routes.
- The *perforin/granzyme pathway* is triggered when cytotoxic T cells attack their cellular targets, with transfer of granzyme B from the killer cell to its intended victim.
- *p53-activated apoptosis* occurs in response to cellular stress or DNA damage.
- The *endoplasmic reticulum* may elicit apoptosis in which calcium signaling plays a central role.

These pathways are not rigid categories, but rather are paradigms of varied signaling mechanisms that lead to apoptosis. In fact, the different routes to apoptosis intersect and overlap.

A family of cysteine proteases, called caspases, is central to apoptosis. Sequential activation of these enzymes, which entails conversion from proenzyme forms to catalytically effective enzymes, is central to apoptotic pathways. Some 14 caspases are now known, of which about half are important participants in apoptotic signaling (other functions, unrelated to apoptosis, are also known; see below).

Although the various pathways to apoptosis may start differently and signal via different members of this enzyme family, these diverse roads all generally lead to the killer enzymes: caspases-3, -6 and -7.

Extrinsic Apoptosis Is Triggered by Receptor–Ligand Interactions at the Cell Membrane

Prominent examples of initiation of apoptosis at the cell membrane are the binding of TNF-α to its receptor (TNFR) and the recognition of FasL (Fas ligand) by its receptor, Fas. TNF-α is a soluble cytokine, whereas FasL is found at the plasma membrane of certain cells, such as cytotoxic effector lymphocytes.

At the cell surface, TNFR and Fas become activated upon binding their ligands. Specific amino acid sequences in the cytoplasmic tails of these transmembrane receptors, called death domains, act as docking sites for the corresponding death domains of other proteins (Fig. 1-40). After binding to the ligand-activated receptors, the docking proteins stimulate downstream signaling molecules, especially procaspases-8 and -10, which are converted to their operational forms, caspases-8 and -10. In turn, these caspases activate downstream caspases in the apoptosis pathway.

The ultimate caspases in this process are "effector," or "executioner," caspases-3, -6 and -7. Caspase-3 is the most commonly activated effector caspase. It stimulates enzymes that cause nuclear fragmentation (e.g., caspase-activated DNase [CAD], which degrades chromosomal DNA). Caspase-3 also destabilizes the cytoskeleton as the cell begins to fragment into apoptotic bodies.

Notably, TNFR activation by TNF-α may also stimulate the antiapoptotic protein NFκB, a transcription factor that directs production of proteins that inhibit apoptosis. This is described in more detail below, in the discussion of necroptosis.

The extrinsic (death receptor) pathway of apoptosis intersects the intrinsic (mitochondrial) pathway via caspase-8, which cleaves a cytoplasmic protein, Bid (Fig. 1-41). Truncated Bid (tBid) translocates to mitochondria, where it can activate apoptosis through a separate signaling mechanism (see below).

Diverse Intracellular Stimuli Activate the Mitochondrial Intrinsic Pathway of Apoptosis

From the perspective of cell survival and adaptation, mitochondria are akin to Dr. Jekyll and Mr. Hyde. On the one hand, in their Dr. Jekyll persona, they generate the energy needed to sustain the cell and participate in carbohydrate and fatty acid metabolism. On the other hand, as Mr. Hyde, they store molecules that can lead to cell death.

Current understanding of this route of apoptosis can be viewed as involving two sequential series of events. The specific order of events is not completely understood, and some steps presented below may occur simultaneously or in a different sequence.

Mitochondrial Matrix and Inner Membrane Pathways

The components of the mitochondrial matrix, which is the interior of these organelles, are constrained by the impermeability of the inner mitochondrial membrane. This barrier is traversed by the MPTP, which is closed under normal circumstances. Attached to the inner membrane are several molecules that play key roles as the apoptotic drama unfolds. These molecules include Cyt c (a member of the electron transport chain), Smac/diablo (second mitochondria-derived activator of caspases, which promotes caspase activation; see below), apoptosis-inducing factor (AIF) and others. There is an electrochemical potential ($\Delta\Psi_m$) across the inner membrane, with the interior of the mitochondrion charged negatively and the exterior positively. Thus:

1. If mitochondria accumulate Ca^{2+} or generate excessive ROS or if $\Delta\Psi_m$ or mitochondrial pH decrease, the MPTP opens (Fig. 1-42).
2. MPTP opening lets water, protons (H^+) and salts into the mitochondrial matrix.
3. The influx of H^+, water and solutes collapses $\Delta\Psi_m$, and the loss of membrane potential impairs mitochondrial ATP production.
4. In parallel, the entry of large amounts of water causes mitochondria to swell.
5. The outer mitochondrial membrane then becomes more permeable, either due to its rupture or to the opening of outer membrane pores.
6. Consequent release of inner membrane constituents (AIF, Smac/diablo, Cyt c, etc.) into the cytosol has two important effects. First, there are metabolic consequences relating to these proteins exiting the mitochondria. Second, released mitochondrial constituents activate the next phase of apoptotic signaling.

The Outer Membrane Components

The normal constituents of the outer mitochondrial membrane include both proapoptotic and antiapoptotic proteins of the Bcl-2 family.

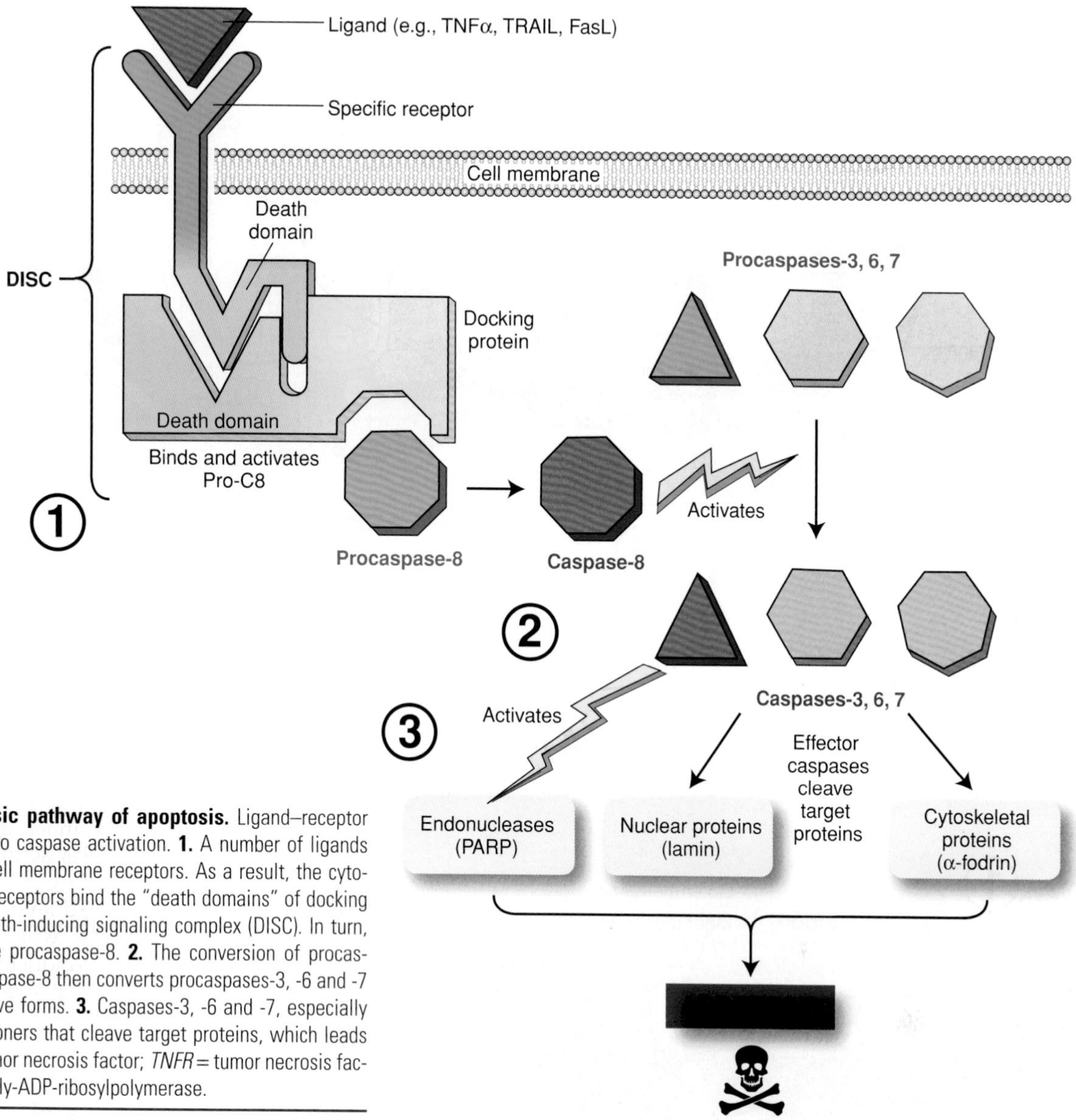

FIGURE 1-40. Extrinsic pathway of apoptosis. Ligand–receptor interactions that lead to caspase activation. **1.** A number of ligands bind their respective cell membrane receptors. As a result, the cytoplasmic tails of these receptors bind the "death domains" of docking proteins, to form a death-inducing signaling complex (DISC). In turn, these proteins activate procaspase-8. **2.** The conversion of procaspase-8 to activated caspase-8 then converts procaspases-3, -6 and -7 to their respective active forms. **3.** Caspases-3, -6 and -7, especially caspase-3, are executioners that cleave target proteins, which leads to apoptosis. *TNF* = tumor necrosis factor; *TNFR* = tumor necrosis factor receptor; *PARP* = poly-ADP-ribosylpolymerase.

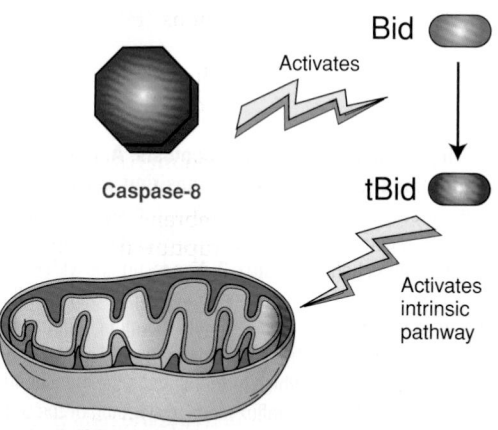

FIGURE 1-41. Intersection of the extrinsic and intrinsic pathways of apoptosis. Caspase-8, activated by, for example, a receptor–ligand interaction such as in Fig. 1-40, may in turn cleave cytosolic Bid to yield a truncated derivative, tBid. In turn, tBid translocates to mitochondria, thereby activating the intrinsic (mitochondrial) pathway of apoptosis.

The Bcl-2 Family as the Life/Death Switch of the Cell

The members of the Bcl-2 family can be viewed as belonging to one of three subfamilies, depending on the number of Bcl-2 homology (BH) domains (Fig. 1-43).

1. The antiapoptotic (i.e., prosurvival) members have four BH domains (labeled BH1, BH2, etc.) and are often referred to as multi-BH domain proteins. These include Bcl-2, Bcl-xL, Mcl-1 and others.
2. Proapoptotic (antisurvival) members are divided into two groups:
   a. One group contains three BH domains (Fig. 1-43). The key members of this group are Bak and Bax. A third member, Bok, is less well understood. Bak is mainly a mitochondrial protein, while Bax is largely cytoplasmic.
   b. A larger group of proapoptotic proteins, BH3-only proteins, carry a single BH3 domain. These include Bim, Bid, Bik, Bad and others. Different BH3-only proteins can elicit apoptosis by inactivating prosurvival functions of Bcl-2 family members or by directly stimulating death-inducing properties of Bax and Bak.

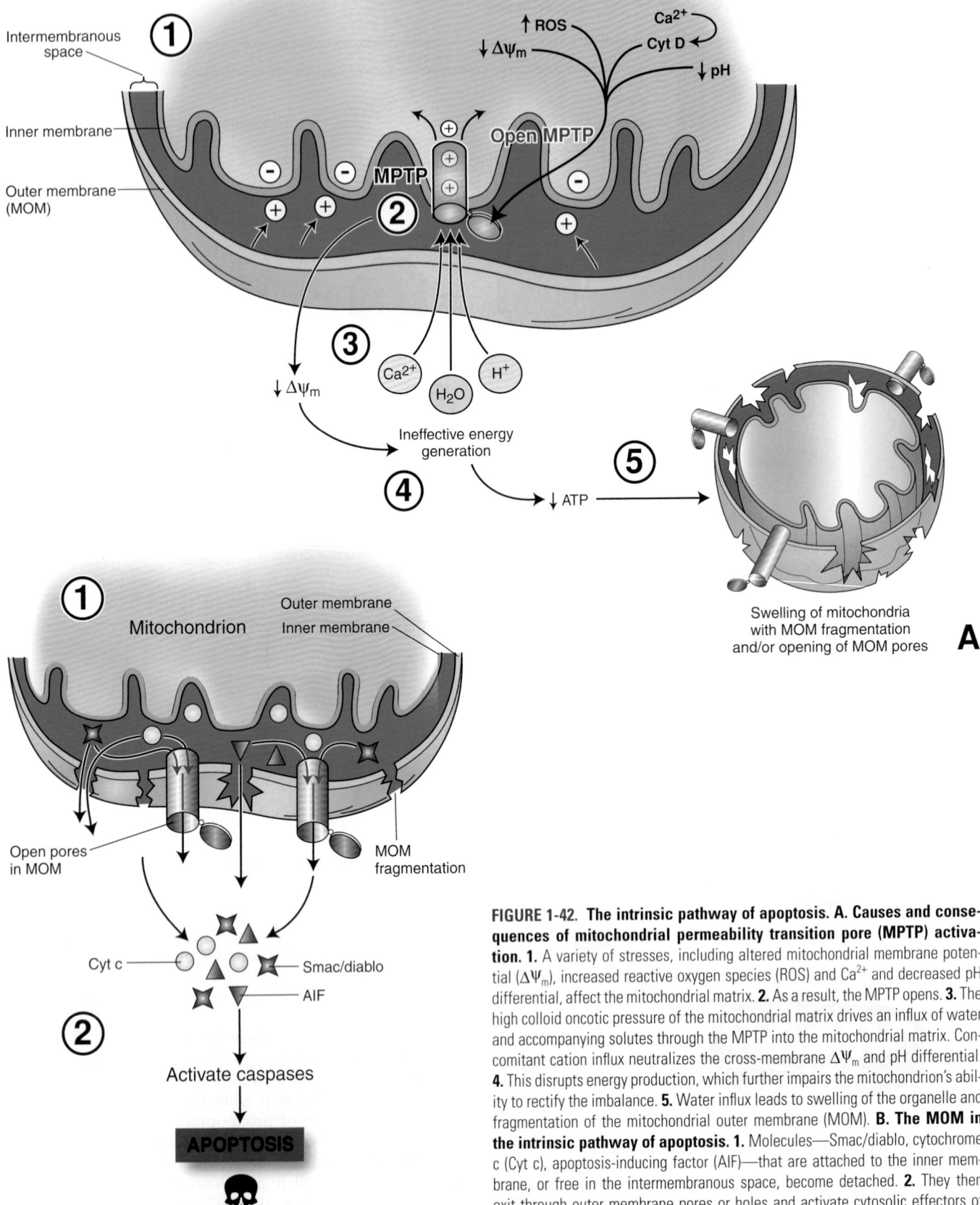

FIGURE 1-42. The intrinsic pathway of apoptosis. A. Causes and consequences of mitochondrial permeability transition pore (MPTP) activation. 1. A variety of stresses, including altered mitochondrial membrane potential ($\Delta\Psi_m$), increased reactive oxygen species (ROS) and Ca^{2+} and decreased pH differential, affect the mitochondrial matrix. **2.** As a result, the MPTP opens. **3.** The high colloid oncotic pressure of the mitochondrial matrix drives an influx of water and accompanying solutes through the MPTP into the mitochondrial matrix. Concomitant cation influx neutralizes the cross-membrane $\Delta\Psi_m$ and pH differential. **4.** This disrupts energy production, which further impairs the mitochondrion's ability to rectify the imbalance. **5.** Water influx leads to swelling of the organelle and fragmentation of the mitochondrial outer membrane (MOM). **B. The MOM in the intrinsic pathway of apoptosis. 1.** Molecules—Smac/diablo, cytochrome c (Cyt c), apoptosis-inducing factor (AIF)—that are attached to the inner membrane, or free in the intermembranous space, become detached. **2.** They then exit through outer membrane pores or holes and activate cytosolic effectors of apoptosis.

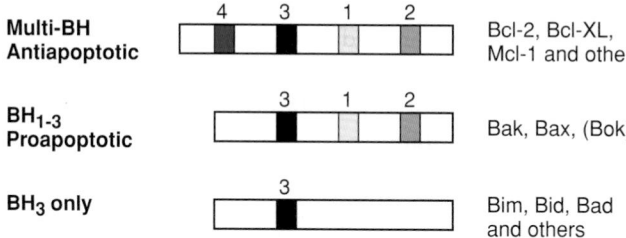

FIGURE 1-43. Bcl-2 family of apoptosis-related proteins. These proteins are divided into three groups, differentiated by structure and function. This division reflects the numbers of Bcl-2 homology (BH) domains in the protein. The presence of the BH4 domain characterizes the antiapoptotic family members. By contrast, proapoptotic Bcl-2 family members lack the BH4 domain and may have BH1-3 or only BH3. The latter are referred to as BH3-only proteins.

Mechanisms That Control the Intrinsic Pathway

The Normal Mitochondrion
Among other proteins, Cyt c and Smac/diablo are attached to the inner mitochondrial membrane, facing the intermembranous space. Opposite these, and attached to the outer membrane, are complexes of Bax and/or Bak bound to antiapoptotic Bcl-2 family members. In this peaceful equilibrium, Bcl-2 (Bcl-xL, Mcl-1, etc.) inhibits proapoptotic functions of Bax/Bak, and the mitochondrial default setting is prosurvival.

Triggering the Intrinsic Pathway of Apoptosis via the Bcl-2 Family of Proteins
Many intracellular agent provocateurs, often involving stress or injury, act via BH3-only family members. Such actions may include increasing concentrations of some BH3-only proteins (e.g., by activating transcription), altering their conformations from quiescent to active, modifying enzymes and so forth. The now-active BH3-only molecules may interpose themselves into Bcl-2 (Bcl-xL, etc.) complexes with Bak and Bax, causing these complexes to dissociate, and thus liberate Bax and Bak to form channels in the outer mitochondrial membrane. These channels, called mitochondrial apoptosis-induced channels (MACs), allow release of toxic mitochondrial proteins (Cyt c, Smac/diablo, etc.) into the cytosol (Fig. 1-44). Free Bax can also be directly activated by BH3-only proteins to form MACs.

Apoptosis Activated by p53

Cells are continually perched on a precipice between life and death. p53 is pivotal to the outcome of that balancing act. It may maintain vital functions and repair injury, thereby sustaining life. Alternatively, it may push the cell toward death. This discussion focuses on the role of p53 in cell death. (p53 is discussed in greater detail in Chapter 5.)

Homeostasis of p53
Normally, p53 is present in very small amounts, mostly in the cytosol, where it is bound mainly to Mdm2, an E3 Ub ligase. Mdm2 promotes p53 degradation via polyubiquitination. Even so constrained, p53 can foster cell health and effective responses to stress.

When a cell is injured or its equilibrium is disturbed, p53 undergoes diverse molecular modifications. These include phosphorylation, monoubiquitination at multiple sites (i.e., adding single Ub moieties at several points on p53 protein, rather than polymeric Ub chains at a single site) and others.

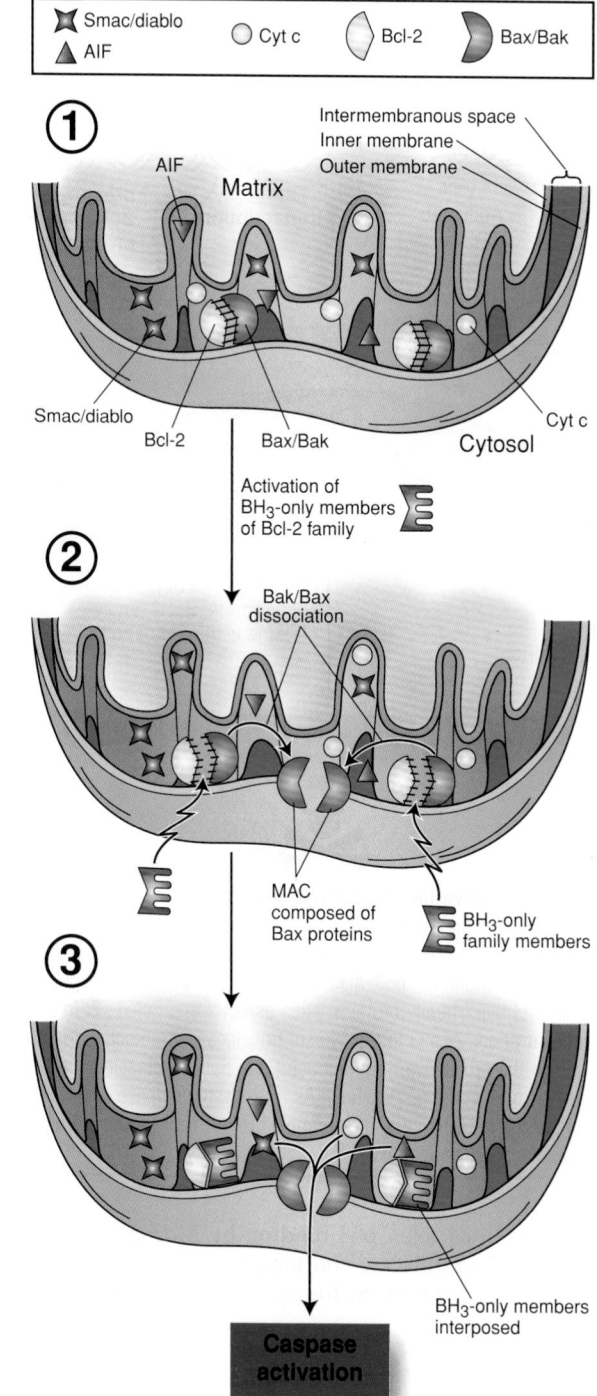

FIGURE 1-44. Formation of pores in the outer mitochondrial membrane during activation of the intrinsic pathway of apoptosis. 1. At equilibrium, Cyt c, Smac/diablo and apoptosis-inducing factor (AIF) either are attached to the mitochondrial inner membrane or float in the intermembranous space. The complex of oligomeric Bak/Bax with antiapoptotic Bcl-2 family cousins resides at the outer membrane. **2.** When BH3-only members of the Bcl-2 clan are activated, they interpose themselves between their prosurvival relatives and Bak/Bax, thereby freeing Bak/Bax proteins. The latter then form a pore (MAC) in the outer mitochondrial membrane. **3.** Proapoptotic proteins Cyt c, Smac/diablo, AIF and others exit from the mitochondrion via the MAC pore. Once in the cytosol, these proteins facilitate activation of the caspase cascade and so cause apoptosis. *Cyt c* = cytochrome C; *MAC* = mitochondrial apoptosis-induced channel.

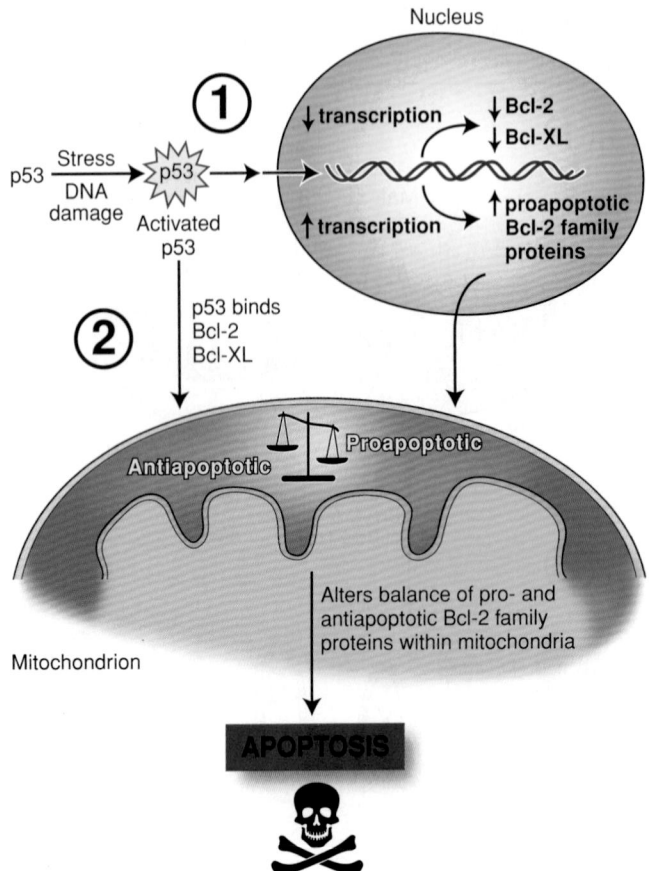

FIGURE 1-45. Activation of p53 and apoptosis. When p53 is activated (e.g., by DNA damage), it translocates to the nucleus. **1.** If DNA damage is irreparable, p53 promotes transcription of proapoptotic proteins, which then migrate to mitochondria. p53 also decreases transcription of prosurvival (antiapoptotic) Bcl-2 family proteins, such as Bcl-2 and Bcl-xL. **2.** In parallel, high concentrations of p53 in the cytosol translocate to mitochondria, where they bind to the prosurvival proteins Bcl-2 and Bcl-xL, releasing their bound proapoptotic partners (e.g., Bax/Bak). As a result, the balance of Bcl-2 family members at the mitochondrial membrane shifts to favor proapoptotic forces, and the cell undergoes apoptosis.

These alterations relax p53 binding by Mdm2, which both allows p53 to accumulate and targets it to the mitochondria or nucleus, depending on the specific molecular modification (Fig. 1-45).

Apoptosis-Related Activities of p53

Within the nucleus, p53 is both a transcriptional activator and a repressor, depending on the target gene. It activates transcription of many proapoptotic proteins, such as Bad, Bax, NOXA, PUMA and others, while simultaneously repressing transcription of prosurvival proteins, including Bcl-2, Bcl-xL and Mcl-1.

Protein–protein interactions between p53 and Bcl-2 family members also enhance induction of apoptosis. Cytosolic p53 may directly activate Bax, whereupon Bax relocates to mitochondria to cause apoptosis via release of mitochondrial proteins (see above). Mitochondria-targeted (i.e., [poly]-monoubiquitinated) p53 acts as a functional BH3-only protein. In this mode, it disrupts complexes between Bak and its inhibitor, Mcl-1, and tips the mitochondrial Bcl-2 family equilibrium to favor apoptosis.

p53 also regulates cell cycle, metabolism and many other cell functions. These are addressed more fully in Chapter 5.

Ca^{2+} Release by the Endoplasmic Reticulum May Elicit Apoptosis

Cells maintain a large calcium concentration ([Ca^{2+}]) gradient relative to the extracellular space, which has about four orders of magnitude higher [Ca^{2+}] than does the cytosol. Ligand-induced and other changes in cytosolic Ca^{2+} concentration ([Ca^{2+}]$_i$) are often secondary signals in many cellular processes. However, excessive changes in [Ca^{2+}]$_i$ may also induce apoptosis. The ER stores considerable calcium, which may be released in response to various stimuli (stress response). When ER Ca^{2+} is released, and particularly if Ca^{2+} release is prolonged, apoptosis ensues.

The proximity of the ER to mitochondria is key to this process. Ca^{2+} released by the ER may be taken up by mitochondria, especially where the two organelles meet. Resulting increases in mitochondrial [Ca^{2+}] cause the MPTP to open, releasing Cyt c and activating downstream apoptosis pathways.

Sustained release of Ca^{2+} from ER stores also promotes release of caspase-12. This protein, which is normally bound to the ER membrane, becomes activated upon its release. Activated caspase-12 then activates caspase-9 in the apoptosome (see below), in turn triggering the executioner caspases (mainly caspase-3).

Metabolic Factors in the Mitochondrial Apoptosis Pathway

Just as effective mitochondrial functioning is fundamental to cell survival, its loss can contribute to the mitochondrial mechanism of apoptosis. Thus:

- Because Cyt c, AIF and other mitochondrial proteins released into the cytosol are also integral to the electron transport chain, their loss impairs mitochondrial ATP generation. The cell's ability to repair injury is consequently suboptimal. If the causative insult is limited or transient, remaining functional mitochondria may compensate for the temporary loss of energy generation and sustain repair.
- Bax alters mitochondrial metabolism, directly and indirectly, to both increase generation and decrease detoxification of ROS, which in turn magnify mitochondrial injury. ROS increase the release of Cyt c and other proteins.
- Caspase-3 directly impairs parts of the electron transport complex.
- Antioxidant defenses are weakened, both because of decreased production of antioxidant enzymes (related to p53) and because the defects in electron transport allow increased ROS generation.
- Imbalances in Ca^{2+} metabolism affect mitochondria. Increases in [Ca^{2+}] (e.g., in excitable cells like neurons and myocytes) may be transient, coinciding with stimulated release from the ER and leading to brief MPTP opening, which does not impair cell viability. However, if Ca^{2+} influx into mitochondria is prolonged, increases in mitochondrial ROS and other factors can lead to sustained, fatal MPTP opening.
- p53 may promote mitochondrial respiration, which, when electron transport is impaired (see above), generates more ROS. The harmful consequences of this phenomenon

may be further exacerbated by p53-related transcriptional repression of SOD, which decreases antioxidant protection.

It should be noted that ATP, even depleted by the events mentioned above, is required for apoptosome activity (see below). Thus, if MPTP opening is prolonged and ATP supply is exhausted, a cell may undergo necrotic, rather than apoptotic, death.

Proteins Released from Mitochondria Lead to Apoptosis via Several Pathways

As noted above, permeabilization of the outer mitochondrial membrane causes several mitochondrial molecules—Cyt c,

Smac/diablo, AIF and others—to exit into the cytosol. Once in the cytosol, Cyt c binds cytosolic Apaf-1 (apoptotic protease-activating factor) and procaspase-9 to form the **apoptosome**. This structure releases activated caspase-9, which then cleaves procaspases-3, -6 and -7, resulting in cell death (Fig. 1-46, left side).

The enzymes, caspases-3, -7 and -9, may be inactivated by a family of E3 ubiquitin ligases, called inhibitors of apoptosis (IAPs). Smac/diablo, and other similar proteins, bind IAPs and free caspases from IAP-mediated inhibition, thereby allowing them to execute the cell (Fig. 1-46, right side).

In addition, AIF and other proteins that are released from mitochondria through MACs can initiate apoptosis directly. They do so by activating the destructive enzymes (including

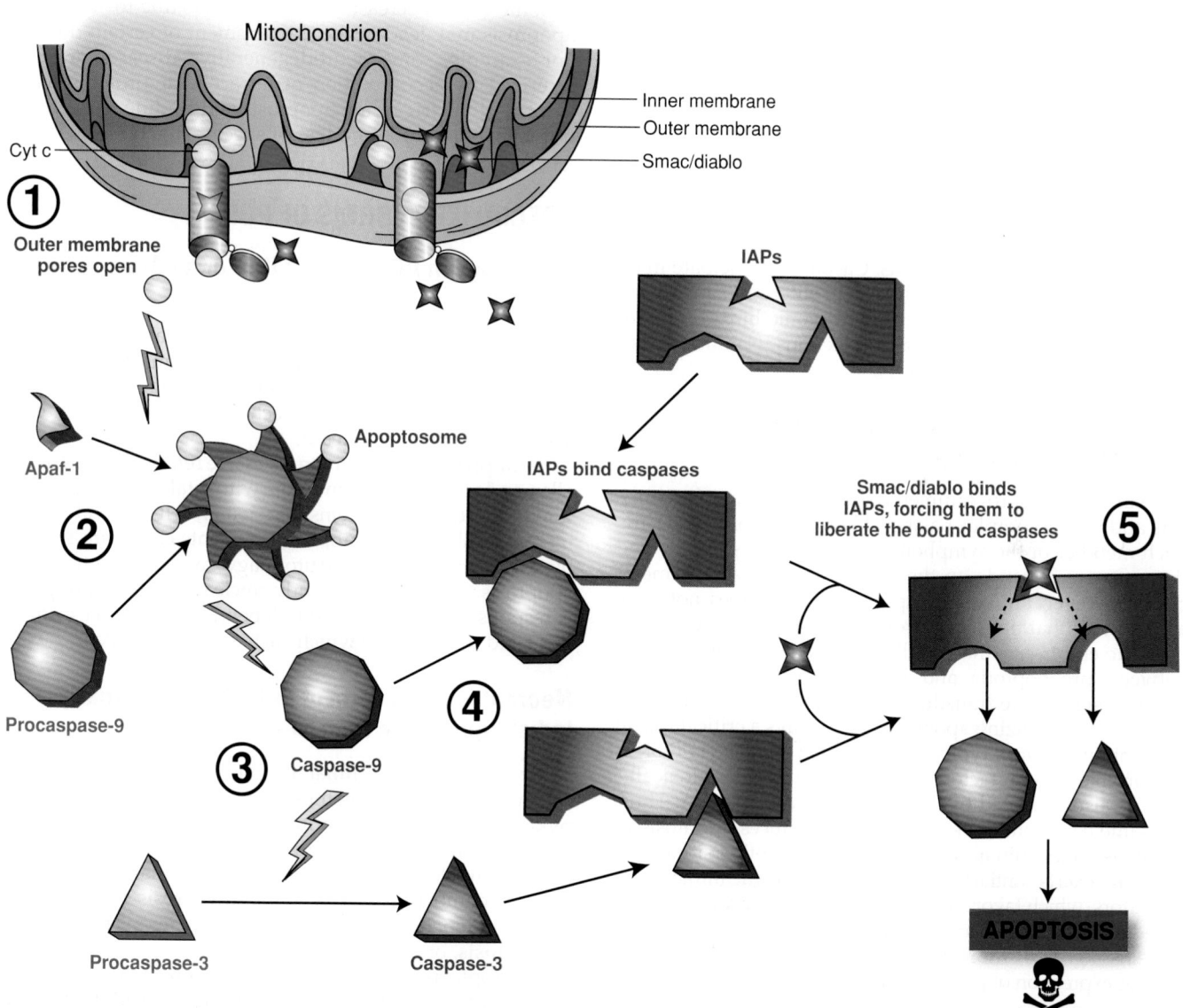

FIGURE 1-46. Opening of the mitochondrial outer membrane, leading to Apaf-1 activation, thereby triggering the apoptotic cascade. 1. Upon triggering by proapoptotic stimuli, pores in the outer membrane open and release proapoptotic proteins. **2.** Cyt c activates multiple molecules of Apaf-1 and both together recruit procaspase-9 to form a structure called the apoptosome, in which the procaspase is activated to caspase-9. Two sets of events may then occur to caspase-9. **3.** It may activate the effector caspases, particularly caspase-3. **4.** As well, IAPs may bind and sequester active forms of several caspases, including caspase-3 and -9. In so doing, IAPs impede apoptosis. **5.** However, Smac/diablo and other mitochondrial proteins that are released when apoptosis is triggered may bind IAPs, causing them to release their bound caspases. The latter then cause the cell to undergo apoptosis. *Apaf-1* = apoptosis-activating factor; *Cyt c* = cytochrome c; *IAP* = inhibitor of apoptosis.

CAD; see above) that cause nuclear condensation and DNA fragmentation, thus generating a *caspase-independent form of programmed cell death.*

Pathways That Regulate Apoptosis

As discussed above, multiple specific mechanisms give rise to and prevent apoptosis. These are, in turn, regulated by many other cellular pathways. For example, the ubiquitin–proteasome system can target proapoptotic proteins, such as caspases, for degradation. This may occur via the IAP family of proteins or by other means. Ubiquitination in turn is controlled by deubiquitinating enzymes and other modulators. The balance between apoptosis and cell survival is influenced by the interplay between inducers and inhibitors of apoptosis, heat shock proteins, protein kinases that may alter caspases or other enzymatic activities and a host of other factors. Recent studies have also implicated microRNAs in regulating intracellular levels of many of these proteins and, consequently, the cell's survival. *Whether or not a cell lives is therefore not determined solely by unique apoptosis-related mechanisms, but rather by a complex array of pathways whose functions converge on that single point.*

Other Functions of Caspases

It is important to recognize that the caspase family has many functions unrelated to apoptosis. Caspases participate in (1) inflammation and immunity, (2) cell proliferation and differentiation in embryonic and extraembryonic life, (3) remodeling of cellular structures and projections, (4) mitogenesis and (5) many other processes.

The Equilibrium between Proapoptotic and Antiapoptotic Signals

Cell survival and programmed cell death are part of an intricate and highly complex balance, like a symphony orchestra. Each member of the symphony has many parts to play and the outcome depends on the coordination of all the members. However, unlike a symphony, the cell does not have a conductor that tightly controls its music. In this vein, it is useful to emphasize that a cell's fate is driven by the balance between proapoptotic and prosurvival influences. Some survival signals are transduced through receptors linked to PI3K. By antagonizing apoptosis, PI3K plays a critical role in cell viability. A prototypical receptor that signals via PI3K is insulin-like growth factor-I receptor (IGF-IR). Paradoxically, PI3K is also activated by TNFR after binding TNF-α. Thus, the same cell membrane receptor that induces apoptosis in some cases may initiate survival signaling in other situations.

PI3K exerts antiapoptotic effects through intracellular mediators, which favor survival by activating a protein kinase, called Akt. The latter inactivates several important proapoptotic proteins (e.g., Bad). More importantly, Akt activates NFκB, thus driving expression of prosurvival proteins (Bcl-xL and A1).

Apoptosis Is Central to Many Disease Processes

When regulation of apoptosis goes awry, there is the devil to pay. Apoptosis is vital for correct progression of embryologic development, elimination of self-reactive B- and T-lymphocyte clones and many other normal functions. Apoptosis guards against uncontrolled cell proliferation (e.g., cancer) due to mutations in DNA (see Chapter 5).

Insufficient Apoptosis

If a major protein that mediates the defense of the organism, such as p53, is mutated, the protection afforded by apoptosis is compromised. Further mutations may then accumulate unhindered. Such pathways are commonly considered to be important in tumor development and progression (see Chapter 5). As another example, the ability of some viruses to block apoptosis allows those pathogens to replicate with less interference, and so to disseminate more widely than would otherwise be possible. Oncogenic viruses often inhibit apoptosis (e.g., human papillomavirus inactivates p53), increasing susceptibility of infected cells to progress to cancer.

Excessive Apoptosis

In some cases, decreases in cell numbers due to "excessive" apoptosis may lead to the development of certain diseases. For example, some neurodegenerative diseases are characterized by accumulation of intracellular proteins within neurons, thus triggering apoptosis and leading to decreased numbers of neurons and loss of specific functions.

SPECIALIZED FORMS OF PCD

Autophagy in PCD: Is It a Killer or an Accomplice?

Autophagy plays an important prosurvival role in cell adaptation to stress and injury, as described above. The function of autophagy as an independent form of cell death is unclear. There is a body of evidence that suggests—but does not prove—that autophagic mechanisms may also represent a separate form of cell death.

Autophagy may promote excessive removal of cell organelles, and so irrevocably interfere with vital cellular functions. It may also destroy proteins that sustain cell survival. Experimental inhibition of autophagy prevents cell death induced by a variety of agents. Autophagy can also contribute to apoptosis. Thus, it is currently unclear whether autophagy is responsible for cell death independently of other forms of PCD and the extent to which such events may occur.

Necroptosis Is a Form of PCD Morphologically Indistinguishable from Necrosis

As discussed above, cellular morphology in necrosis involves cell swelling, plasma membrane fragmentation and nuclear pyknosis, followed by an inflammatory response. Apoptosis, by contrast, is characterized by plasma membrane blebbing and nuclear fragmentation without inflammation. Cells may succumb to a fate resembling necrosis (see above) if a PCD independent of caspases is activated. This is called **necroptosis,** or signaled necrosis.

Necroptosis can be initiated in several ways, but commonly begins when Fas ligand (FasL) or TNF-α binds to its respective receptors. This leads to receptor-bound complexes that incorporate caspase-8; two IAP proteins (E3 Ub ligases), along with several other proteins; and the receptor-interacting proteins (RIP1, RIP3). This complex sits on the knife edge of several alternative fates, but activation of RIP1 and RIP3 leads to cell death by necroptosis.

RIP3 is the epicenter of this process (Fig. 1-47). It leads to increased cytosolic Ca^{2+}, which activates calpain and other

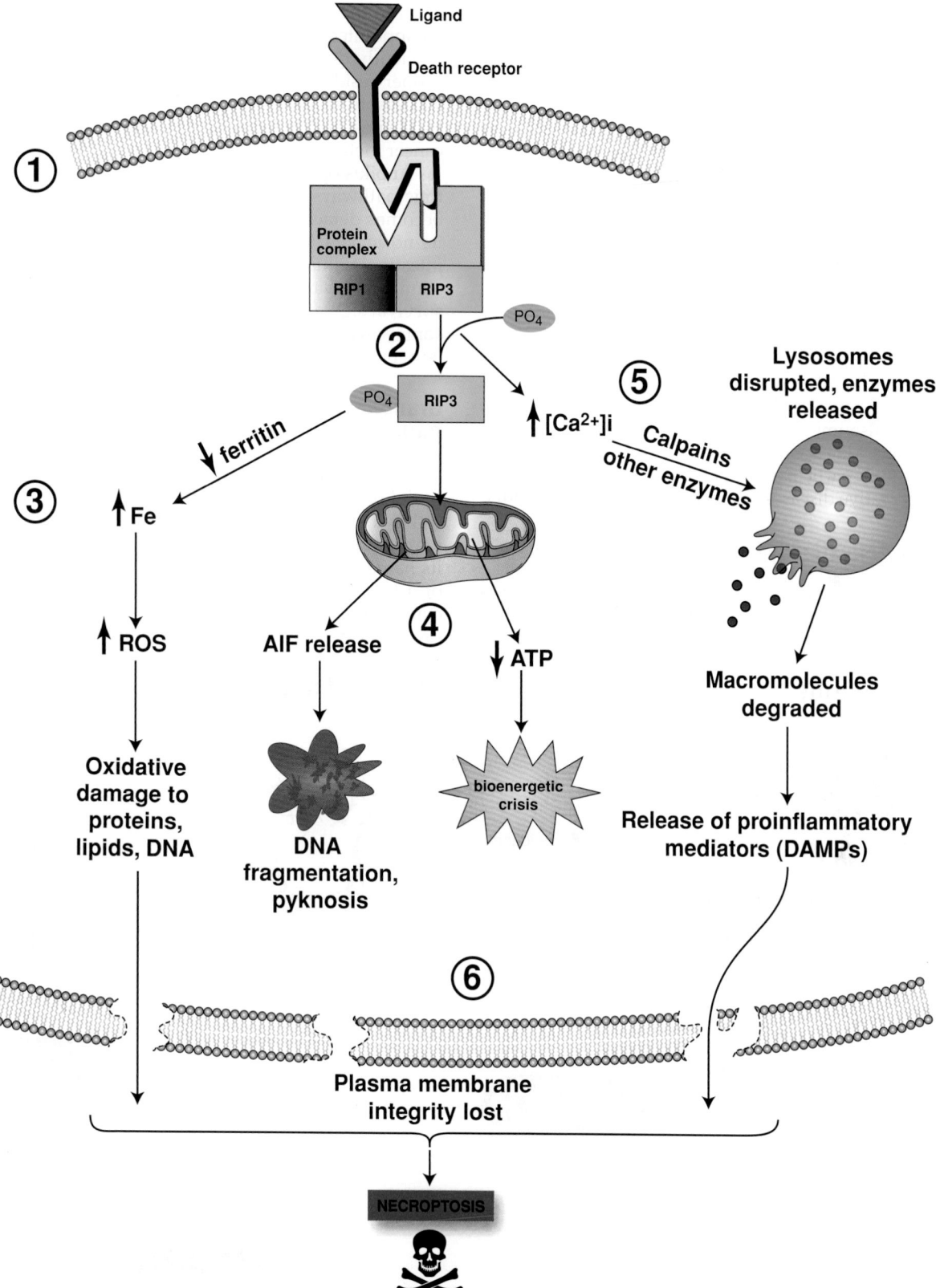

FIGURE 1-47. Pathways leading to necroptosis. 1. Binding of a ligand to a death receptor results in formation of a protein complex that binds RIPs. **2.** As a result, RIP3 is phosphorylated, which leads to necroptosis by several paths. **3.** Phosphorylated RIP3 increases free iron and so increases reactive oxygen species (ROS). **4.** Damage to mitochondria leads to apoptosis-inducing factor (AIF) release and also impairs adenosine triphosphate (ATP) production. **5.** Also, increased [Ca^{2+}] leads to activation of Ca^{2+}-dependent degradative enzymes, which disrupt lysosomes and release lysosomal enzymes that degrade cellular macromolecules. **6.** The final steps in each of these pathways consist of necroptosis: AIF triggers DNase activity and leads to nuclear pyknosis; loss of ATP precipitates a bioenergetic crisis; and plasma membrane damage due to oxidative disruption of membrane lipids produces holes in the cell membrane and leads to release of macromolecular breakdown products that stimulate inflammation (DAMPS). *DAMPs* = damage-associated molecular products; *RIP* = receptor-interacting protein.

degradative enzymes, which attack lysosome membranes and cause release of lysosomal hydrolases into the cytosol. Calpain also damages mitochondria, precipitating metabolic dysfunction with impaired ATP generation and iron release, with consequent increases in ROS (see Fenton and Haber-Weiss reactions above) and damage to proteins, lipids and DNA. At the same time, mitochondria release AIF (see above), which enters the nucleus and activates DNA degradation. A bioenergetic crisis with the morphologic features of necrosis ensues. Cells then release molecules (called damage-associated molecular patterns; see Chapter 2) that provoke inflammation.

Under physiologic circumstances, necroptosis participates in development, particularly at the bone growth plate. It is also active normally in some adult tissues such as the lower portion of the intestinal crypts. If physiologic apoptosis is unavailable to cells, necroptosis may become the default cell death pathway. In this mode, it may be an important mechanism of PCD in cancer cells in which apoptotic pathways are blocked. It is also important in limiting the spread of certain viral infections. Like apoptosis, necroptosis is a double-edged sword and may participate in pathologic processes such as neurodegenerative diseases and ischemia/reperfusion injury.

Anoikis Is Activated by Loss of Cell Attachments

Anoikis (Greek: "homelessness") is a variety of apoptosis that occurs in epithelial cells and is caused by loss of cell adhesion or inappropriate cell adhesion. Correct binding of a cell to the ECM helps to determine whether that cell is in its appointed location. The significance of anoikis is that it efficiently deletes cells that have been displaced from their proper residence. Thus, it prevents wandering cells or cell clusters from developing colonies at distant or improper ECM sites, and so helps protect against the development of cancer metastases.

Anoikis operates via intrinsic or extrinsic classical apoptotic pathways, both of which are upregulated when a cell becomes detached (Fig. 1-48). A cell that loses contact with its normal ECM, like one that is pushed off the tip of an intestinal villus by proliferating cells deeper in the crypts, is stimulated to undergo anoikis by loss of integrin-mediated survival signaling. Similarly, if a detached cancer cell makes contact with inappropriate ECM components, anoikis may be activated (see Chapter 5).

Granzymes Released by Lymphocytes Kill Cells via Apoptosis

Activation of caspase signaling also occurs when cytotoxic T lymphocytes (CTLs) and natural killer (NK) cells recognize a cell as foreign. These lymphocytes release two major molecular species, namely, perforin and granzymes. Perforin, as its name suggests, punches a hole in the plasma membrane of a target cell, through which proteins from the lymphocyte enter. Granzymes are a family of multifunctional serine proteases, among which the best understood is granzyme B.

Bound integrins

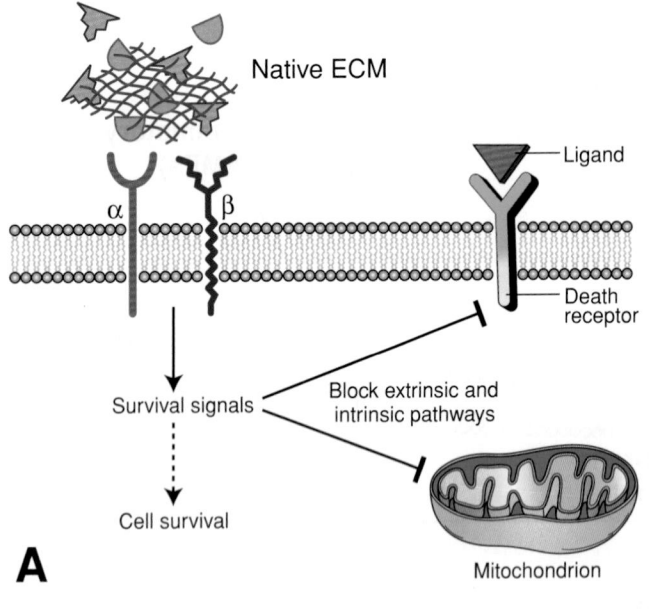

Unbound integrins

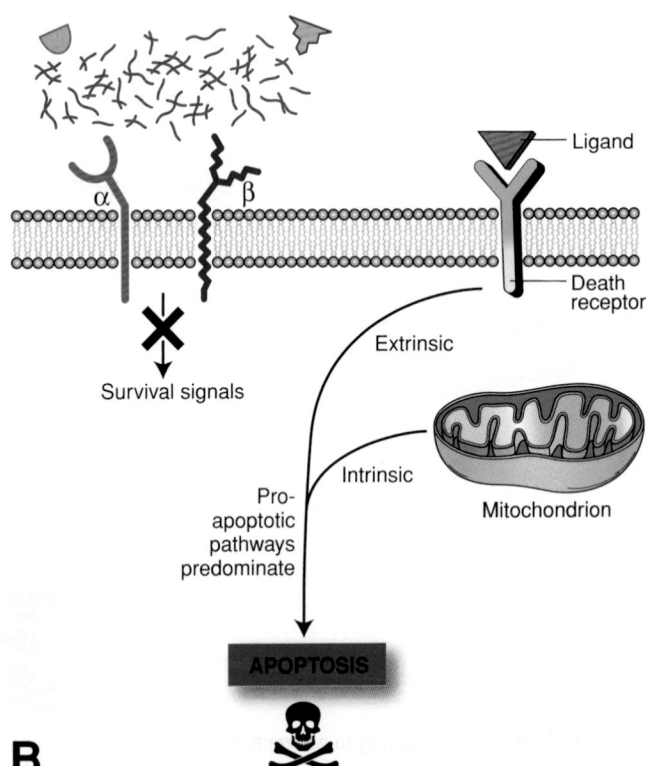

FIGURE 1-48. Mechanisms of anoikis. A. Normal. Under normal circumstances, epithelial cells are bound to their native ECM by transmembrane molecules, including α- and β-integrins. These molecules activate survival signals and block both intrinsic and extrinsic apoptotic signaling pathways. **B. Loss of attachment.** When the cell's integrins are not bound, or not bound by the appropriate ECM moieties, their survival signals are eliminated. Then, activation of apoptosis by death receptor signaling is no longer blocked, and apoptosis may proceed. *ECM* = extracellular matrix.

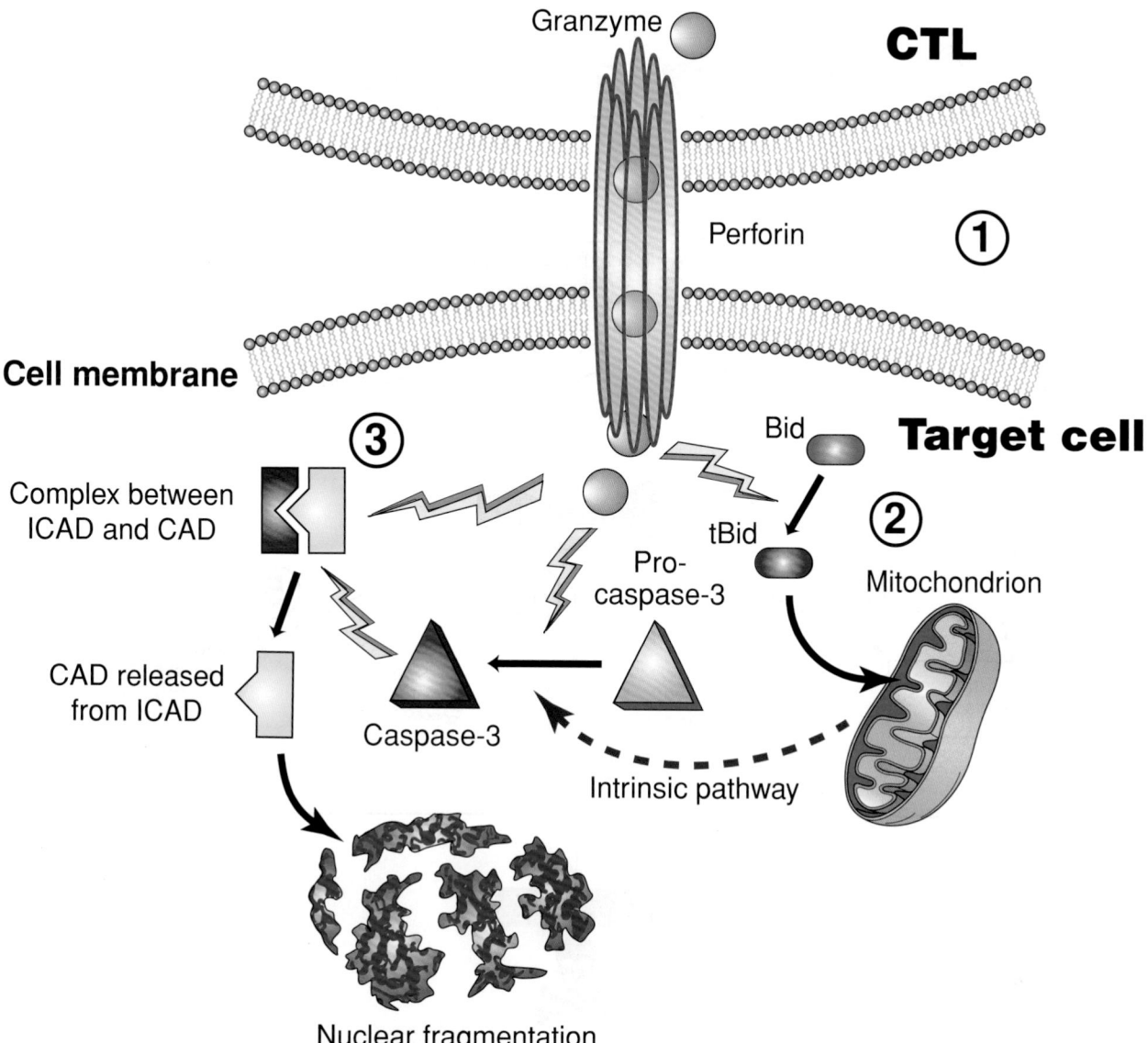

FIGURE 1-49. Cell death caused by CTLs. 1. Granzyme and perforin are two molecules made, mainly, by CTLs and natural killer (NK) cells. After a CTL binds its cellular victim, perforin molecules combine to create an intercellular channel through which granzyme enters the target cell. **2.** Granzyme cleaves cytoplasmic Bid to its active form, tBid, which translocates into mitochondria and triggers the intrinsic pathway of apoptosis. It also activates procaspase-3 to caspase-3, via which apoptosis may proceed. **3.** Granzyme may also disrupt the complex between CAD and its inhibitor, ICAD. This effect releases the DNase (CAD) to elicit a caspase-independent form of apoptosis. The CAD–ICAD complex may also be cleaved by caspase-3. *CAD* = caspase-activated DNase; *CTL* = cytotoxic T lymphocyte; *ICAD* = inhibitor of CAD.

This protease activates cytosolic Bid, a BH3-only protein, by cleaving it to tBid (Fig. 1-49). In turn, tBid increases mitochondrial release of Cyt c and other cell death effector proteins. It also converts several procaspases (notably pro-caspase-3) to active caspases.

Granzyme A is also released by NK cells and CTLs into target cells. Granzymes A and B together induce cell death by caspase-independent mechanisms. They activate the DNA nicking enzyme, CAD (see above), which degrades genomic DNA (Fig. 1-49).

Pyroptosis Contributes to Innate Immune Defenses

Pyroptosis is a cell death program that relies on caspase-1 (previously called IL-1β–converting enzyme). Many infectious agents, particularly viruses, but also bacteria and others, stimulate inflammatory reactions by interacting with members of a group of cell membrane receptors called **pattern recognition receptors** (see Chapters 2 and 4).

Although caspase-1 is a cysteine protease involved in PCD, it is independent of apoptotic signaling, and its activation does not bring about apoptosis (Fig. 1-50). Instead, caspase-1 is a proinflammatory protease that is produced by a structure called an inflammasome (Fig. 1-50). Once activated, caspase-1 cleaves select cellular molecules, including enzymes that are important for glycolysis, thereby depleting cellular energy. It also produces ion-permeable plasma pores, allowing influx of water and solutes to provoke cell swelling and then death. Furthermore, by activating a number of proinflammatory cytokines, the dead cell elicits inflammation.

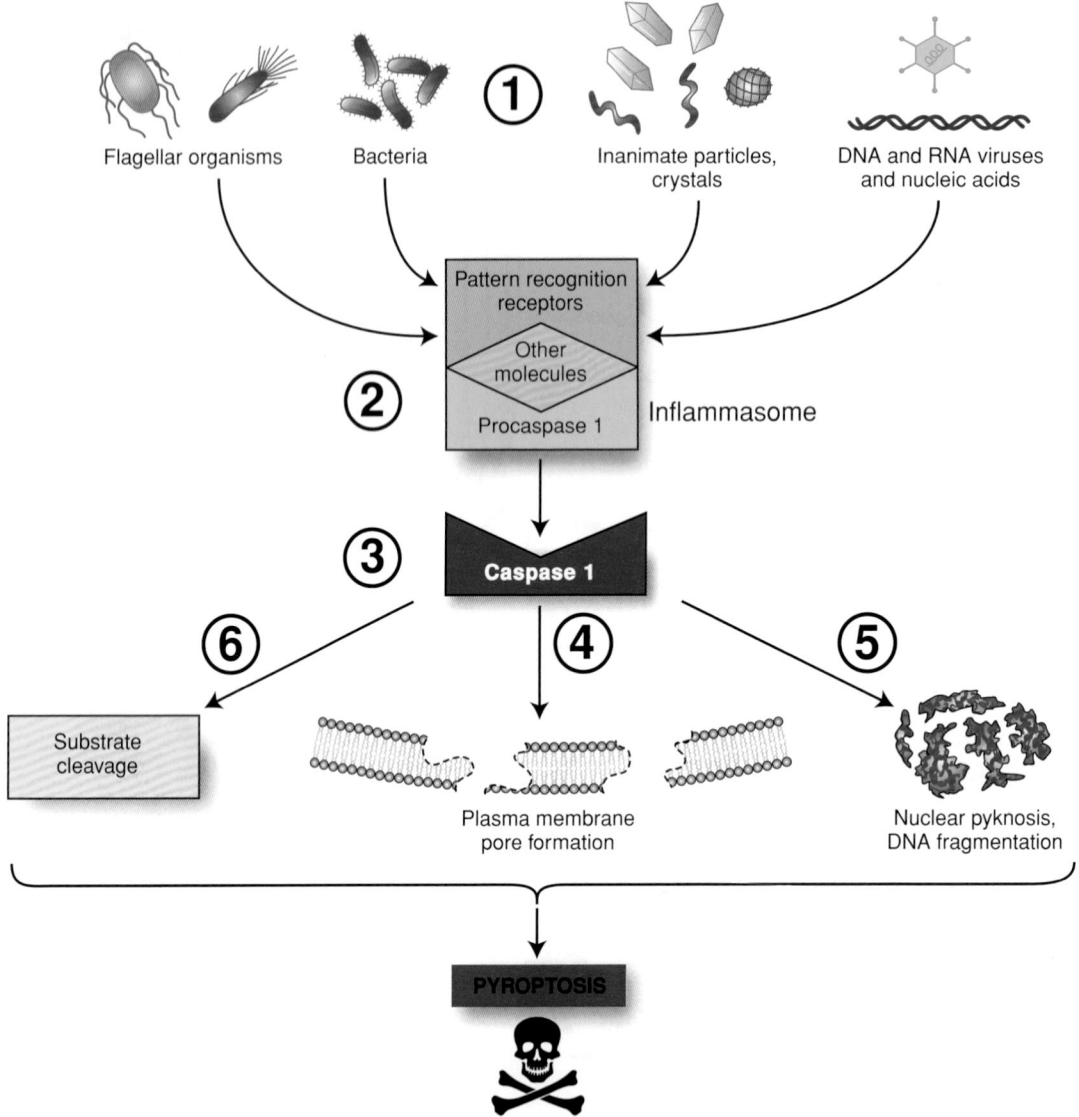

FIGURE 1-50. Pyroptosis. 1. The cell is exposed to injurious agents, both infectious and irritative (e.g., mineral crystals). **2.** Complexes called inflammasomes recognize these exogenous agents via diverse pattern recognition receptors. Inflammasomes contain procaspase-1. **3.** When inflammasome-linked receptors are activated, procaspase-1 is converted to its active form, caspase-1, which has several consequences. **4.** Caspase-1 forms pores in the plasma membrane, allowing intracellular components to leak out of the dying cell. **5.** At the same time, the nucleus is damaged, and **(6)** important intracellular substrates, including cytoskeleton, chaperones, glycolytic proteins and caspase-7, are cleaved. **7.** All these effects contribute to pyroptotic cell death.

In addition to its host-protective role in encounters with nefarious pathogens, pyroptosis has been implicated in the pathogenesis of metabolic syndrome and the etiology of type 2 diabetes mellitus (see Chapter 13).

NETosis Reflects the Action of a Potent Antimicrobial Defense Mechanism

Neutrophil extracellular traps (NETs) are structures produced by polymorphonuclear granulocytes. NETs function as chromatin traps for bacteria and other pathogens and contain antimicrobial cell products. These formations can kill bacterial, fungal and protozoal pathogens, and so constitute an important host defense from infection.

NETs result from activation of a cell death program, mainly in neutrophils, but also including eosinophils and mast cells. This program is called NETosis. Interestingly, NETs may be composed of either nuclear or mitochondrial chromatin and do not necessarily need self-sacrifice of the neutrophil that contributes the chromatin.

NETosis requires both autophagy and nicotinamide adenine dinucleotide phosphate (NADPH) oxidase activity and is characterized by destruction of the cell's nuclear envelope and the membranes of most cytoplasmic granules (Fig. 1-51). Chromatin disaggregation results, and the cell extrudes a NET containing both chromatin and strongly microbicidal histones and histone cleavage products.

Unlike apoptotic cells, neutrophils and other NETosis-susceptible cells do not present the "eat me" signals (cell membrane phosphatidyl serine; see above) that are characteristic of apoptosis. Lacking such signals, NETotic cells are not preemptively removed by macrophages and are able to stimulate inflammatory responses.

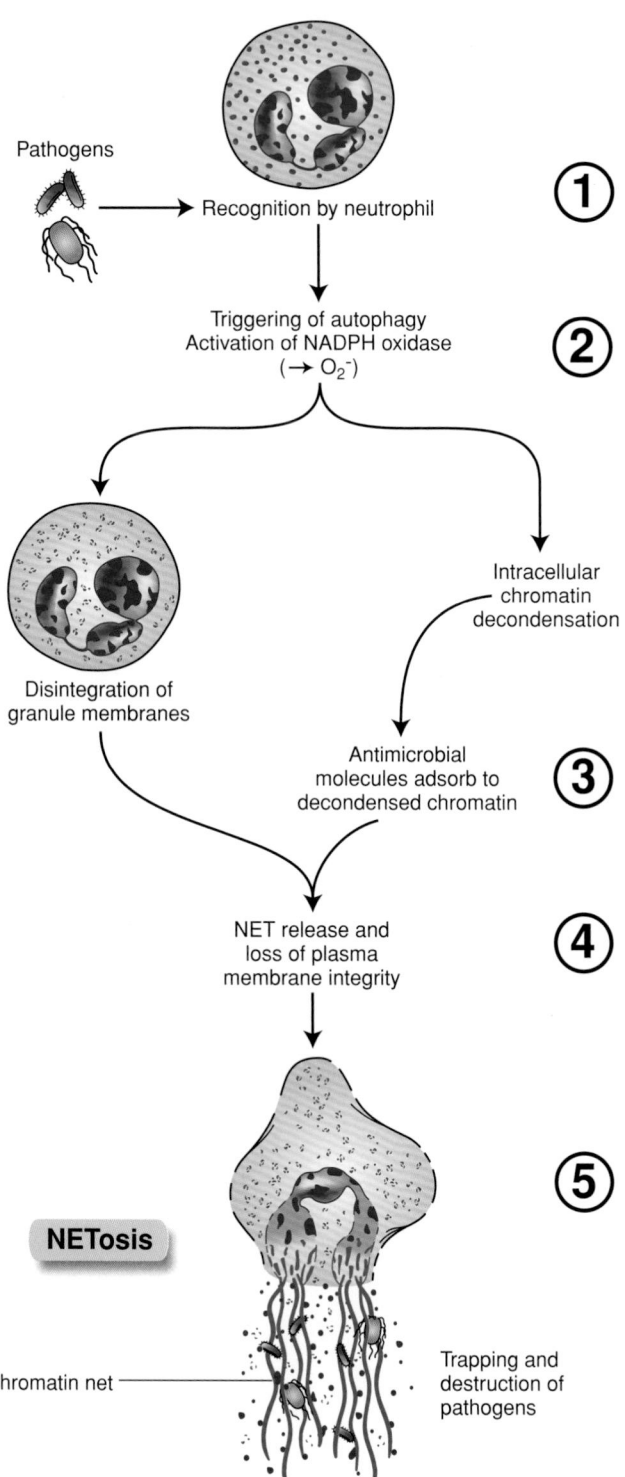

Entosis Is a Cell-Eat-Cell Form of Cell Death

Entosis is a type of cellular cannibalism in which cells that are not professional phagocytes engulf nearby living cells. Aggressor cells may engulf cells of either the same or other lineages. For example, hepatocytes may ingest and destroy autoreactive T lymphocytes, thus inhibiting experimental autoimmune liver disease. More often, entosis is seen in tumors.

Vacuoles containing cells undergoing entosis may fuse with lysosomes, in which case target cells usually die, although death is not an inevitable outcome. The cannibalized cell, or parts thereof, may survive the process. Its nuclear material may become part of the aggressor cell, leading to multinucleate cells, polyploidy or aneuploidy. Some engulfed cells actually escape their captors and re-emerge unscathed. Mechanisms governing entosis are largely obscure.

FIGURE 1-51. NETosis. 1. Neutrophils recognize pathogens, after which **(2)** autophagy and NADPH oxidase are activated, the latter yielding reactive oxygen species (ROS). **3.** As a result, intracellular chromatin becomes dispersed and membranes of cytoplasmic granules disintegrate. **4.** NETotic activity leads to release of neutrophil chromatin traps containing antimicrobial cellular products. **5.** These traps then catch and destroy pathogens.

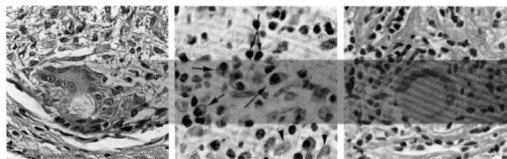

Inflammation

Hedwig S. Murphy

DEVELOPMENT OF THE CONCEPT OF INFLAMMATION

Inflammation is a systemic and local reaction of tissues and microcirculation to a pathogenic insult. It is characterized by elaboration of inflammatory mediators and movement of fluid and leukocytes from the blood into extravascular tissues. This response localizes and eliminates altered cells, foreign particles, microorganisms and antigens and paves the way for a return to normal structure and function.

The clinical signs of inflammation, called *phlogosis* by the Greek physician Galen, and *inflammation* in Latin, were described in classical times. In the first century AD, the Roman encyclopedist Aulus Celsus described the four cardinal signs of inflammation: **rubor** (redness), **calor** (heat), **tumor** (swelling) and **dolor** (pain). These features correspond to inflammatory events of vasodilation, edema and tissue damage. According to medieval concepts, inflammation was an imbalance of various "humors," including blood, mucus and bile. Modern understanding that inflammation had a vascular basis began in the 18th century with John Hunter, who noted blood vessel dilation and appreciated that pus was accumulated material derived from the blood. Rudolf Virchow first described inflammation as a reaction to prior tissue injury. To Celsus' four cardinal signs Virchow added a fifth: **functio laesa** (loss of function). His pupil Julius Cohnheim first associated inflammation with emigration of leukocytes through microvasculature walls. At the end of the 19th century, the role of phagocytosis in inflammation was emphasized by the eminent Russian zoologist Eli Metchnikoff. Finally, Thomas Lewis described the importance of chemical mediators in 1927, showing that histamine and other substances increased vascular permeability and caused leukocytes to migrate into extravascular spaces. More recent studies have elucidated the molecular and genetic bases of acute and chronic inflammation.

OVERVIEW OF INFLAMMATION

The primary function of the inflammatory response is to eliminate a pathogenic insult and remove injured tissue components, thus allowing tissue repair to take place. In teleologic terms, the body attempts to contain or eliminate offending agents to protect tissues, organs and, ultimately,

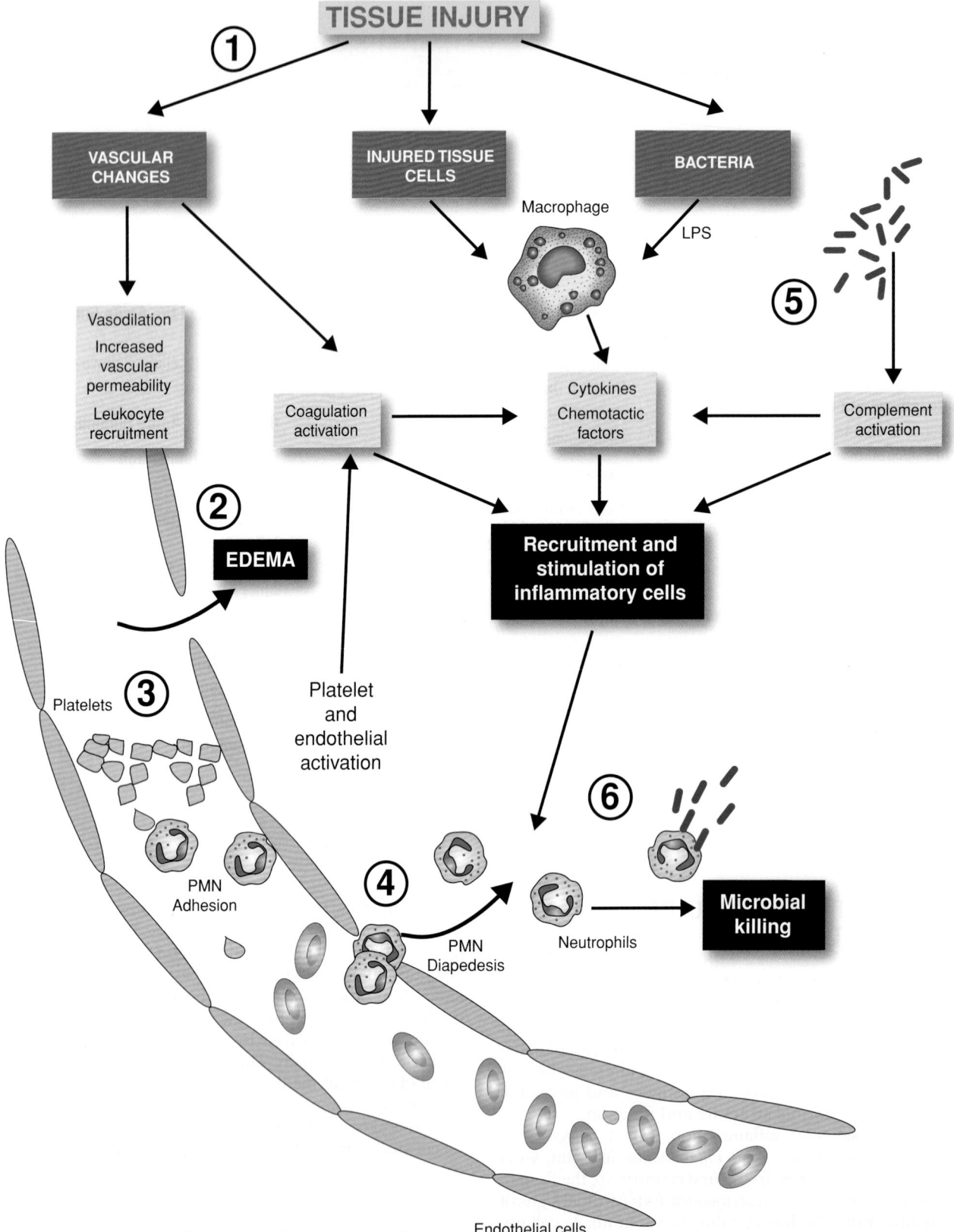

FIGURE 2-1. The inflammatory response to injury. 1. Tissue injury results in immediate and prolonged vascular changes. Chemical mediators and damaged tissue cells stimulate vasodilation and vascular injury, leading to **(2)** leakage of fluid into tissues (edema). **3.** Platelets are activated to initiate clot formation and hemostasis and to increase vascular permeability via histamine release. **4.** Vascular endothelial cells contribute to clot formation, anchor circulating neutrophils via their upregulated adhesion molecules and retract to allow increased vascular permeability to plasma and to inflammatory cells. At the same time, microbes (*red rods*) **(5)** initiate activation of the complement cascade, which, along with soluble mediators from macrophages, **(6)** recruits neutrophils to the site of tissue injury. Neutrophils and macrophages eliminate microbes and remove damaged tissue so that repair can begin. *PMN* = polymorphonuclear leukocyte.

the whole body from damage. Specific cells are imported to attack and destroy injurious agents (e.g., infectious organisms, toxins or foreign material), enzymatically digest and remove them, or wall them off. In the process, damaged cells and tissues are digested and removed to allow repair to occur. Responses to many damaging agents are immediate and stereotypic. The character of the inflammatory response is "modulated," depending on several factors, including the nature of the offending agent, duration of the insult, extent of tissue damage and microenvironment.

- **Initiation** of an inflammatory response results in activation of soluble mediators and recruitment of inflammatory cells to the area. Molecules released from the offending agent, damaged cells and extracellular matrix alter the permeability of nearby blood vessels to plasma, soluble molecules and circulating inflammatory cells. This stereotypic immediate response leads to rapid flooding of injured tissues with fluid, coagulation factors, cytokines, chemokines, platelets and inflammatory cells, neutrophils in particular (Figs. 2-1 and 2-2). This overall process is **acute inflammation**.
- **Amplification** depends on the extent of injury and activation of mediators such as kinins and complement components. Additional leukocytes and macrophages are recruited to the area.
- **Destruction** of the damaging agent brings the process under control. Enzymatic digestion and phagocytosis reduce or eliminate foreign material or infectious organisms. At the same time, damaged tissue components are also removed and debris is cleared, paving the way for repair to begin (see Chapter 3).
- **Termination** of the inflammatory response is mediated by intrinsic anti-inflammatory mechanisms that limit tissue damage and allow repair and a return to normal physiologic function. Alternatively, depending on the nature of

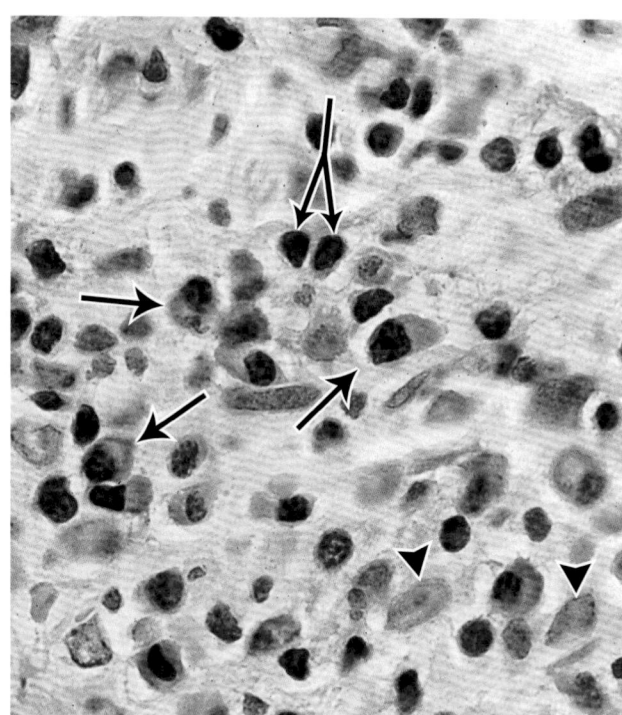

FIGURE 2-3. Chronic inflammation. Lymphocytes (*double-headed arrow*), plasma cells (*arrows*) and a few macrophages (*arrowheads*) are present.

the injury and specific inflammatory and repair responses, a scar may develop in place of normal tissue. Importantly, intrinsic mechanisms terminate the inflammatory process; prevent further influx of fluid, mediators and inflammatory cells; and prevent damage to normal cells and tissue.

Some types of injury trigger sustained immune and inflammatory responses if injured tissue and foreign agents are not cleared. Such persistent responses are called **chronic inflammation**. Chronic inflammatory infiltrates are largely lymphocytes, plasma cells and macrophages (Fig. 2-3). Acute and chronic inflammatory infiltrates often coexist.

Inflammation usually works to defend the body but may also be harmful. Acute inflammatory responses may be exaggerated or sustained, with or without clearance of the offending agent. Tissue damage may result; witness the ravages of bacterial pneumonia due to acute inflammation or joint destruction in septic arthritis. Chronic inflammation may also damage tissue and cause scarring and loss of function. Indeed, chronic inflammation is the basis for many degenerative diseases.

Weak inflammatory responses may lead to uncontrolled infection, as in immunocompromised hosts. In several congenital diseases, deficient inflammation is due to defects in inflammatory cell function or immunity.

ACUTE INFLAMMATION OFTEN BEGINS WITH TISSUE INJURY

Direct injury or stimulation of cellular or structural components of a tissue includes:

- Parenchymal cells
- Microvasculature

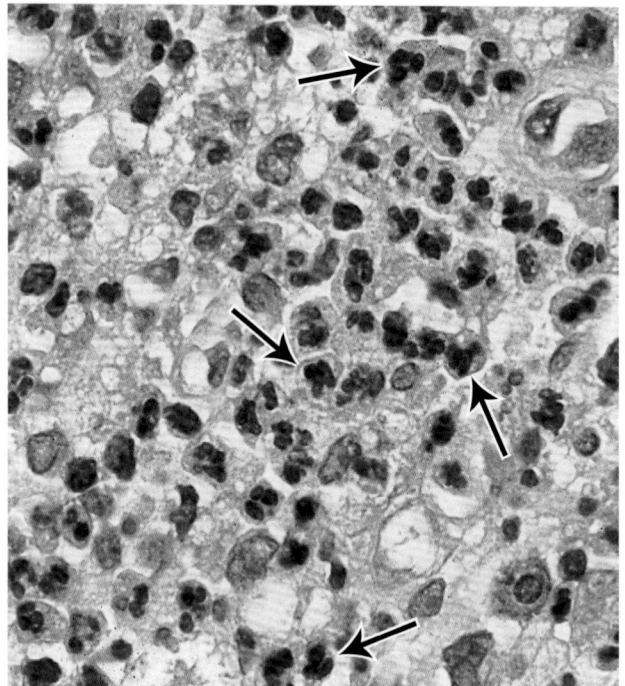

FIGURE 2-2. Acute inflammation. Densely packed polymorphonuclear leukocytes (PMNs) with multilobed nuclei (*arrows*).

- Tissue macrophages and mast cells
- Mesenchymal cells (e.g., fibroblasts)
- Extracellular matrix (ECM)

A Sequence of Events Follows Initiation of Acute Inflammation

- *As the immediate response to injury or insult, blood vessels rapidly and transiently constrict and then dilate.* Under the influence of nitric oxide (NO), histamine and other soluble agents, vasodilation allows increased blood flow and expansion of the capillary bed.
- *Increased vascular permeability allows fluid and plasma components to accumulate in affected tissues.* Normally, the endothelium is a permeability barrier as fluid moves between intravascular and extravascular spaces. Endothelial cells are connected to each other by tight junctions and separated from the tissue by a limiting basement membrane (Fig. 2-4A). *Disruption of this barrier function is a hallmark of acute inflammation.* Shortly after

tissue injury, specific inflammatory mediators are produced at the site of injury that directly increase permeability of capillaries and postcapillary venules. Vascular leakage reflects endothelial cell contraction, endothelial cell retraction and alterations in transcytosis. Endothelial cells are also damaged, either by direct injury to the cells or indirectly by leukocytes. Thus, there may be extensive loss of the permeability barrier, so that fluid and cells leak into the extravascular space, which is called **edema** (Fig. 2-4B, C).

- *Soluble mediators stimulate intravascular platelets and inflammatory cells.* These include kinins and complement. Components of the coagulation cascade are activated (Figs. 2-1 and 2-5), causing more vascular permeability and edema.
- *Neutrophils are recruited to the injured site.* All these vascular changes, vasodilation and edema increase the concentration of red blood cells and leukocytes within the capillary network. Chemotactic factors then recruit leukocytes, especially neutrophils, from the vascular

A NORMAL VENULE

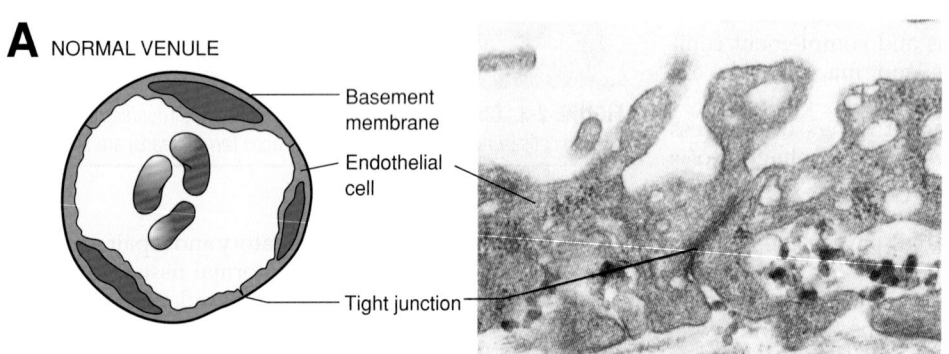

B VASOACTIVE MEDIATOR-INDUCED INJURY

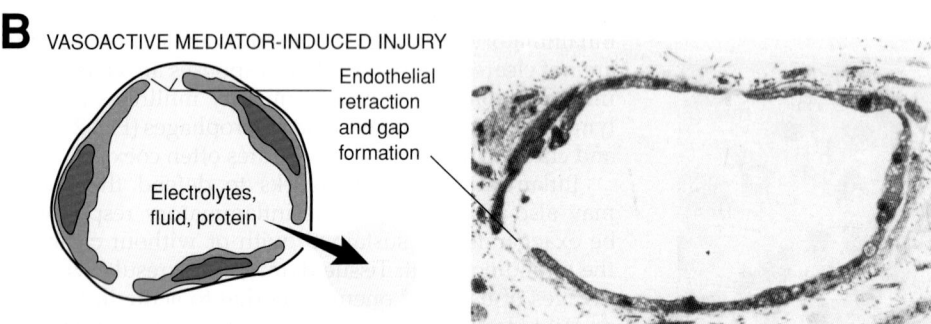
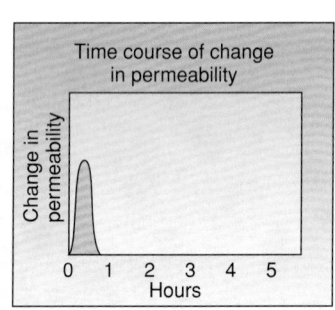

C DIRECT INJURY TO ENDOTHELIUM

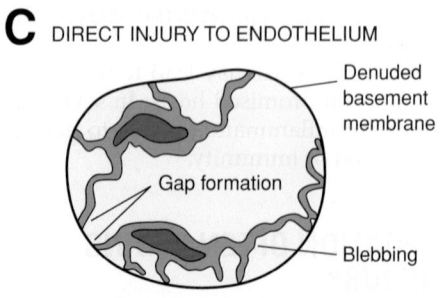
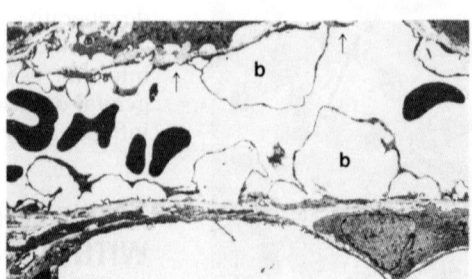
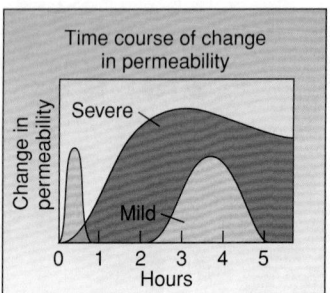

FIGURE 2-4. Responses of the microvasculature to injury. A. The wall of the normal venule is sealed by tight junctions between adjacent endothelial cells. **B.** During mild vasoactive mediator-induced injury, the endothelial cells separate and permit the passage of the fluid constituents of the blood. **C.** With severe direct injury, the endothelial cells form blebs (*b*) and separate from the underlying basement membrane. Areas of denuded basement membrane (*arrows*) allow a prolonged escape of fluid elements from the microvasculature.

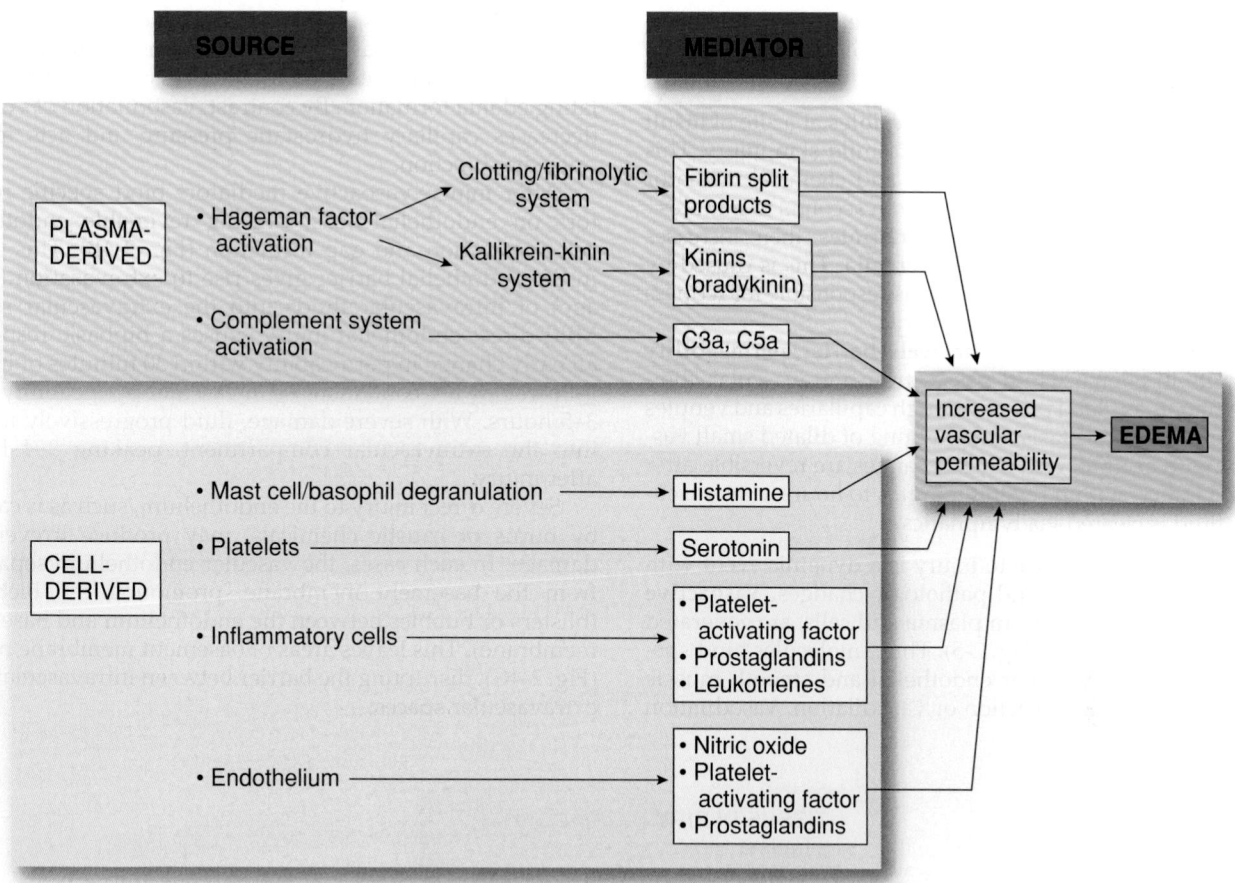

FIGURE 2-5. Inflammatory mediators of increased vascular permeability. Plasma and cell-derived products generate potent vasoactive mediators.

compartment into the injured tissue (Figs. 2-1 and 2-2). Once in tissues, these leukocytes start attacking offending agents so damaged components can be removed and tissue repair can commence. These cells secrete additional mediators, which either enhance or inhibit the inflammatory response.

Intravascular and Tissue Fluid Levels Are Regulated by a Balance of Forces

Normally, there is continual movement of fluid from the intravascular compartment to the extravascular space. Fluid in the extravascular space is cleared via lymphatics and returned to the circulation. Regulation of fluid transport across vascular walls is described in part by the **Starling principle**. According to this law, fluid interchange between vascular and extravascular compartments reflects a balance of forces that draw fluid into vascular spaces or out into tissues (see Chapter 7). These forces include:

- **Hydrostatic pressure** from blood flow and plasma volume. Increased hydrostatic pressure forces fluid out of the vasculature.
- **Oncotic pressure,** due to plasma proteins, draws fluid into vessels.
- **Osmotic pressure** reflects relative amounts of sodium and water in vascular and tissue spaces.
- **Lymph flow,** the passage of fluid through lymphatics, continuously drains fluid out of tissues and into lymphatic spaces.

Noninflammatory Edema

If the balance of forces controlling fluid transport is altered, flow into the extravascular compartment or clearance through lymphatics is disrupted. The net result is fluid accumulation in interstitial spaces **(edema)**. This excess fluid expands spaces between cells and the extracellular matrix and causes tissue swelling. Many clinical conditions, whether systemic or organ specific, lead to edema. For example, obstruction of venous outflow **(thrombosis)** or decreased right ventricular function (congestive heart failure) causes back-pressure in the vasculature, thus increasing hydrostatic pressure (see Chapter 7). Loss of albumin (kidney disorders) or decreased synthesis of plasma proteins (liver disease, malnutrition) reduces plasma oncotic pressure. Any abnormality of sodium or water retention alters osmotic pressure and the balance of fluid forces. Finally, **lymphedema** may result from obstruction to lymphatic flow, most often due to surgical removal of lymph nodes, radiation or obstruction by tumor.

Inflammatory Edema

Among the earliest responses to tissue injury are changes in microvasculature anatomy and function, which may allow fluid to accumulate in tissues (Figs. 2-4 and 2-5). These changes are characteristic of the classic "triple response" first described by Sir Thomas Lewis in 1924. In the original experiments, a dull red line developed at the site of mild trauma to skin, followed by a **flare** (red halo) and then a **wheal** (swelling). Lewis postulated that a vasoactive mediator caused vasodilation and increased vascular permeability at the site of injury. The triple response can be explained as follows:

1. **Transient vasoconstriction of arterioles** at a site of insult is the earliest vascular response to mild skin injury. This process is caused by neurogenic and chemical mediator systems and usually resolves within seconds to minutes.
2. **Vasodilation of precapillary arterioles** then increases blood flow to the tissue, or **hyperemia**. This is caused by release of specific mediators and is responsible for redness and warmth at sites of tissue injury.
3. **An increase in endothelial cell barrier permeability** results in edema. Fluid passes from intravascular compartments as blood passes through capillaries and venules to produce local stasis and plugging of dilated small vessels with erythrocytes. These changes are reversible after mild injury; within several minutes to hours, extravascular fluid is cleared via lymphatics.

The vascular response to injury is a dynamic event with sequential physiologic and pathologic changes. **Vasoactive mediators,** originating from plasma and cells, are generated at sites of tissue injury (Fig. 2-5). These molecules bind specific receptors on vascular endothelial and smooth muscle cells, causing vasoconstriction or vasodilation. Vasodilation of arterioles increases blood flow and exacerbates fluid leakage into the tissue. Vasoconstriction of postcapillary venules increases capillary bed hydrostatic pressure, further stimulating edema formation. By contrast, vasodilation of venules decreases capillary hydrostatic pressure and acts in the opposite direction.

After injury, vasoactive mediators bind specific receptors on endothelial cells, causing reversible endothelial cell contraction and gap formation (Fig. 2-4B). This break in the endothelial barrier gives rise to extravasation (leakage) of intravascular fluids into the extravascular space. Mild direct endothelial injury causes a biphasic response: an early change in permeability within 30 minutes of injury, followed by a second increase in vascular permeability after 3–5 hours. With severe damage, fluid progressively moves into the extravascular compartment, peaking 3–4 hours after injury.

Severe direct injury to the endothelium, such as is caused by burns or caustic chemicals, may produce irreversible damage. In such cases, the vascular endothelium separates from the basement membrane, promoting cell blebbing (blisters or bubbles between the endothelium and basement membrane). This leaves areas of basement membrane naked (Fig. 2-4C), disrupting the barrier between intravascular and extravascular spaces.

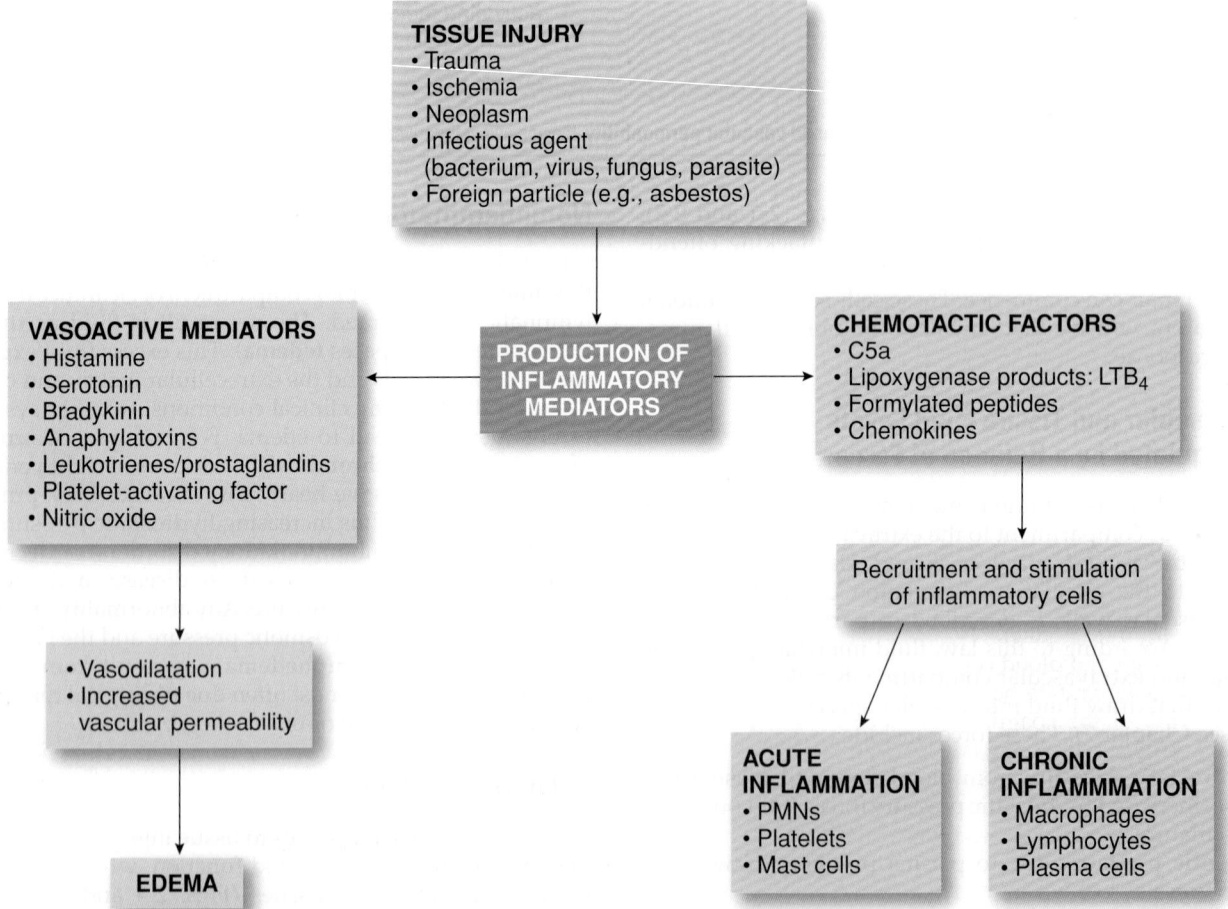

FIGURE 2-6. Mediators of the inflammatory response. Tissue injury stimulates the production of inflammatory mediators in plasma and released into the circulation. Additional factors are generated by tissue cells and inflammatory cells. These vasoactive and chemotactic mediators promote edema and recruit inflammatory cells to the site of injury. *PMNs* = polymorphonuclear leukocytes.

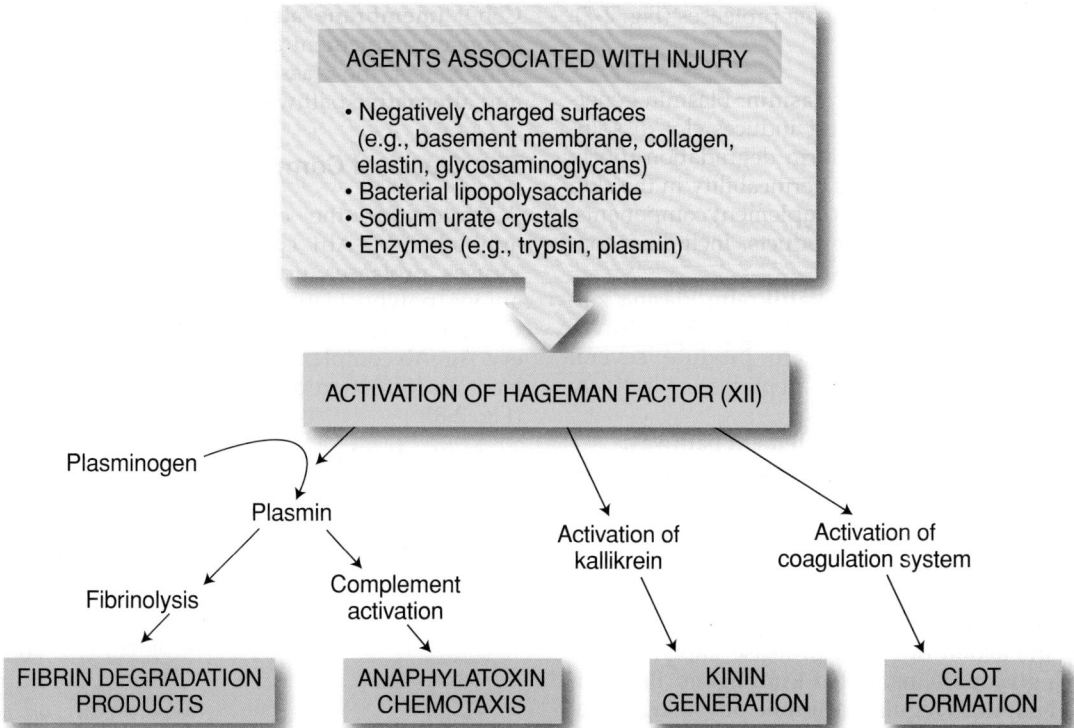

FIGURE 2-7. Hageman factor activation and inflammatory mediator production. Hageman factor activation is a key event leading to conversion of plasminogen to plasmin, resulting in generation of fibrin split products and active complement products. Activation of kallikrein produces kinins and activation of the coagulation system results in clot formation.

Several definitions help in the understanding of the consequences of inflammation:

- **Edema** is accumulation of fluid in the extravascular space and interstitial tissues.
- An **effusion** is excess fluid in body cavities (e.g., peritoneum or pleura).
- A **transudate** is edema fluid with a low protein content (specific gravity <1.015).
- An **exudate** is edema fluid with a high protein concentration (specific gravity >1.015), which frequently contains inflammatory cells. Exudates are seen early in acute inflammation and are produced by mild injuries, such as sunburn or traumatic blisters.
- A **serous exudate,** or **effusion,** is characterized by the absence of a prominent cellular response and has a yellow, straw-like color.
- **Serosanguineous** refers to a serous exudate, or effusion, that contains red blood cells and has a reddish tinge.
- A **fibrinous exudate** has large amounts of fibrin, due to activation of the coagulation system. When a fibrinous exudate occurs on a serosal surface, such as the pleura or pericardium, it is termed "fibrinous pleuritis" or "fibrinous pericarditis."
- **A purulent exudate or effusion** contains prominent cellular components. Purulent exudates and effusions are often associated with pathologic conditions, such as pyogenic bacterial infections, in which polymorphonuclear neutrophils (PMNs) predominate.
- In **suppurative inflammation,** a purulent exudate is accompanied by significant liquefactive necrosis; **it is the equivalent of pus.**

PLASMA-DERIVED MEDIATORS OF INFLAMMATION

Many chemical mediators help to trigger, amplify and terminate inflammatory processes (Fig. 2-6). Cell- and plasma-derived mediators work in concert to activate cells by binding specific receptors, activating cells, recruiting cells to sites of injury and stimulating release of additional soluble mediators. These mediators themselves are short-lived or are inhibited by intrinsic mechanisms, effectively turning off the response and allowing the process to resolve. Thus, these are important "on" and "off" control mechanisms of inflammation. Cell-derived mediators are considered below.

Plasma contains the elements of three major enzyme cascades, each composed of a series of proteases. Sequential activation of proteases results in release of important chemical mediators. These interrelated systems include (1) the **coagulation cascade,** (2) **kinins** and (3) the **complement system** (Fig. 2-7). The coagulation cascade is discussed in Chapters 16 and 26; the kinin and complement systems are presented here.

Hageman Factor Is a Key Initiator of Vasoactive Responses

Hageman factor (clotting factor XII), generated within the plasma, is activated by exposure to negatively charged surfaces, such as basement membranes, proteolytic enzymes, bacterial lipopolysaccharides and foreign materials. It triggers activation of additional plasma proteases (Fig. 2-7), leading to:

- **Conversion of plasminogen to plasmin:** Plasmin generated by activated Hageman factor induces clot dissolution (fibrinolysis). Products of fibrin degradation (fibrin split products) increase vascular permeability in the skin and lung. Plasmin also cleaves complement components, generating biologically active products, including anaphylatoxins, C3a and C5a.
- **Conversion of prekallikrein to kallikrein:** Plasma kallikrein, also generated by activated factor XII, cleaves high–molecular-weight kininogen to produce several vasoactive low–molecular-weight peptides, collectively called **kinins.**
- **Activation of the alternative complement pathway.**
- **Activation of the coagulation system** (see Chapters 16 and 26).

Kinins Amplify the Inflammatory Response

Kinins are potent inflammatory agents formed in plasma and tissue by the action of serine protease kallikreins on specific plasma glycoproteins, called **kininogens.** Bradykinin and related peptides regulate multiple physiologic processes, including blood pressure, contraction and relaxation of smooth muscle, plasma extravasation, cell migration, inflammatory cell activation and inflammatory-mediated pain responses. The immediate effects of kinins are mediated by B_1 and B_2 receptors. The former are induced by inflammatory mediators and selectively activated by bradykinin metabolites. B_2 receptors are expressed constitutively and widely.

Kinins act quickly and then are rapidly inactivated by kininases. Perhaps the most significant function of kinins is their ability to amplify inflammatory responses by stimulating local tissue cells and inflammatory cells to generate additional mediators, such as prostanoids, cytokines (e.g., tumor necrosis factor-α [TNF-α] and interleukins), NO and tachykinins.

Complement Is Activated through Three Pathways to Form the Membrane Attack Complex

The complement system is a group of proteins found in plasma and on cell surfaces. Its main function is defense against microbes. First identified as a heat-labile serum factor that kills bacteria and "complements" antibodies, the complement system has over 30 proteins, including plasma enzymes, regulatory proteins and cell lysis proteins. They are mainly made in the liver and are activated in sequence.

Physiologic activities of the complement system include (1) defense against pyogenic bacterial infection by opsonization, chemotaxis, activation of leukocytes and lysis of bacteria and cells; (2) bridging innate and adaptive immunity to defend against microbial agents by augmenting antibody responses and enhancing immune memory; and (3) disposal of immune products and products of inflammatory injury by clearing immune complexes from tissues and removing apoptotic cells. Certain complement components, **anaphylatoxins,** are vasoactive mediators. Others fix opsonins to cell surfaces. Still others lyse cells by generating a lytic complex,

C5b-9 (**membrane attack complex [MAC]**). Proteins that activate complement are themselves activated by 3 convergent routes: the **classical, mannose-binding lectin (MBL)** and **alternative** pathways.

The Classical Complement Pathway

Activators of the classical pathway include antigen–antibody (Ag–Ab) complexes, products of bacteria and viruses, proteases, urate crystals, apoptotic cells and polyanions (polynucleotides). This pathway includes C1 through C9, the nomenclature following historical order of discovery. Ag–Ab complexes activate C1, triggering a cascade that leads to formation of the MAC and proceeding as follows (Fig. 2-8):

1. **Antibodies bound to antigens on bacterial cell surfaces bind the C1 complex.** The C1 complex consists of C1q, 2 molecules of C1r and 2 molecules of C1s. Antibodies in immune complexes bind C1q, eliciting activation of C1r and C1s.

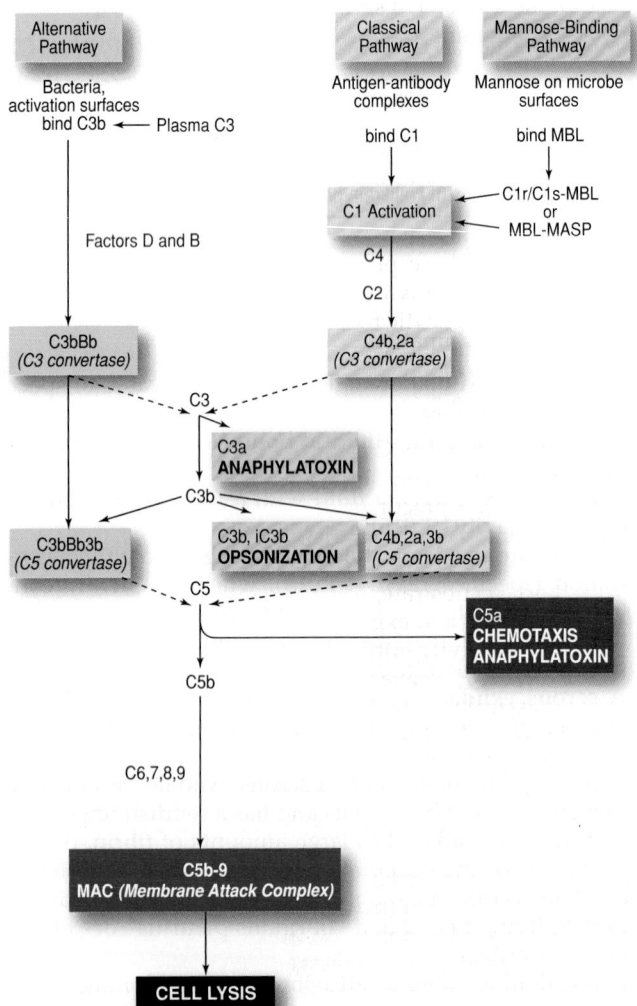

FIGURE 2-8. Complement activation. The alternative, classical and mannose-binding pathways lead to generation of the complement cascade of inflammatory mediators and to cell lysis by the membrane attack complex (MAC). *MBL* = mannose-binding lectin; *MBL-MASP* = MBL-associated serine protease.

2. **C1s cleaves C4, which binds the bacterial surface, then cleaves C2.** Resulting split molecules form the C4b2a enzyme complex, also called **C3 convertase,** which remains covalently bound to the bacterial surface. This effect anchors the complement system at specific tissue sites. If a covalent bond is not formed, the complex is inactivated, thus aborting the cascade in normal host cells or tissues.

3. **C3 convertase cleaves C3 into C3a and C3b.** This is a critical step. C3a is released as an **anaphylatoxin.** C3b reacts with cell proteins to localize, or "fix," on the cell surface. C3b and its degradation products, especially iC3b, on the surface of pathogens, enhance phagocytosis. This process of coating a pathogen with a molecule that enhances phagocytosis is called **opsonization,** and the molecule that does this is an **opsonin.**

4. **The complex of C4b, C2a and C3b (termed C5 convertase) cleaves C5 into C5a and C5b.** C5a also is an anaphylatoxin, and C5b acts as the nidus for subsequent sequential binding of C6, C7 and C8 to form the MAC.

5. **The MAC assembles on target cells.** The MAC directly inserts into the plasma membrane by hydrophobic binding of C7 to the lipid bilayer. The resulting cylindrical transmembrane channel disrupts the barrier function of the plasma membrane and leads to cell lysis.

The Mannose-Binding Pathway

The mannose- or lectin-binding pathway shares some elements with the classical pathway. It begins when microbes with terminal mannose groups bind MBL, one of the family of calcium-dependent lectins, or **collectins.** This multifunctional acute phase protein resembles immunoglobulin M (IgM) (it binds many oligosaccharide structures), IgG (it interacts with phagocytic receptors) and C1q. This last property enables it to interact with C1r-C1s or with a serine protease called MASP (*MBL-a*ssociated *s*erine *p*rotease) to activate complement (Fig. 2-8):

1. **MBL interacts with C1r and C1s to elicit C1 esterase activity.** Alternatively and preferentially, MBL forms a complex with a precursor of the serine protease, MASP. MBL and MASP bind to mannose groups on glycoproteins or carbohydrates on bacterial cell surfaces. After MBL binds a substrate, the MASP proenzyme is cleaved into two chains and expresses a C1-esterase activity.

2. **C1-esterase activity, either from C1r/C1s–MBL interaction or MBL–MASP, cleaves C4 and C2, leading to assembly of the classical pathway C3 convertase.** The complement cascade then continues as described for the classical pathway.

The Alternative Pathway

This pathway is initiated by derivative products of microorganisms, like endotoxin (from bacterial cell surfaces), zymosan (yeast cell walls), polysaccharides, cobra venom factor, viruses, tumor cells and foreign materials. Alternative pathway members are "factors," followed by a letter. Activation of this pathway proceeds as follows (Fig. 2-8):

1. **A small amount of C3 in plasma cleaves to C3a and C3b.** This C3b is covalently bound to carbohydrates and proteins on microbial cell surfaces. It binds factor B and factor D to form the alternative pathway C3 convertase, C3bBb. This C3 convertase is stabilized by **properdin.**

2. **C3 convertase generates additional C3b and C3a.** Binding of a second C3b molecule to C3 convertase converts it to a C5 convertase, C3bBb3b.

3. **As in the classical pathway, cleavage of C5 by C5 convertase generates C5b and C5a and leads to assembly of the MAC.**

The Complement System Is Tightly Regulated to Generate Proinflammatory Molecules

Biological Activities of Complement Components

The endpoint of complement activation is MAC formation and cell lysis. Cleavage products generated at each step both catalyze the next step in the cascade and have supporting roles as important inflammatory molecules (Fig. 2-9):

- **Anaphylatoxins** (C3a, C4a, C5a): These proinflammatory molecules mediate smooth muscle contraction and increase vascular permeability.
- **Opsonins** (C3b, iC3b): In bacterial opsonization, a specific molecule (e.g., IgG or C3b) binds the surface of a bacterium. The process enhances phagocytosis by allowing receptors on phagocytic cell membranes (e.g., Fc receptor or C3b receptor) to recognize and bind the opsonized bacterium. Viruses, parasites and transformed cells also activate complement similarly, which leads to their inactivation or death.
- **Proinflammatory molecules** (MAC, C5a): These chemotactic factors also activate leukocytes and tissue cells to generate oxidants and cytokines and induce mast cell and basophil degranulation.
- **Lysis** (MAC): C5b binds C6 and C7, and subsequently C8 to the target cell; C9 polymerization is catalyzed to lyse the cell membrane.

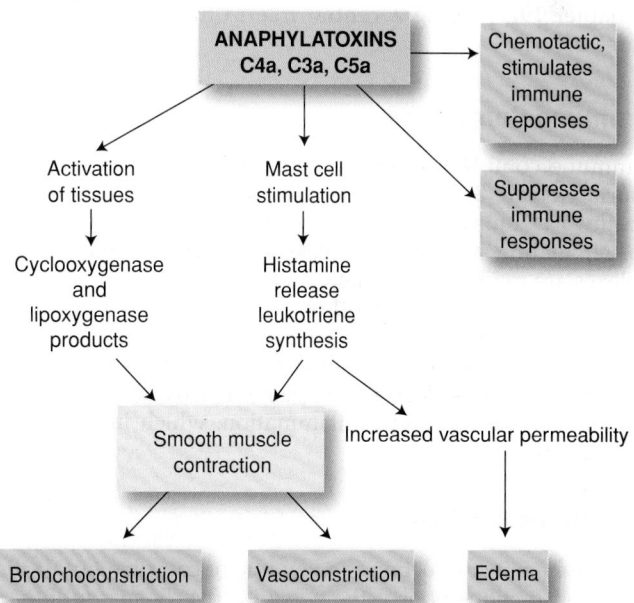

FIGURE 2-9. Biological activity of the anaphylatoxins. Complement activation products, generated during activation of the complement cascade, regulate vascular permeability, cell recruitment and smooth muscle contraction.

Regulation of the Complement System

Proteins in serum and on cell surfaces protect the host from indiscriminate injury by regulating complement activation. Four major mechanisms mediate this effect:

- **Spontaneous decay:** C4b2a and C3bBb and their cleavage products, C3b and C4b, decrease by decay.
- **Proteolytic inactivation:** Plasma inhibitors include factor I (an inhibitor of C3b and C4b) and serum carboxypeptidase N (SCPN). SCPN removes a carboxy-terminal arginine from anaphylatoxins C4a, C3a and C5a. Deleting this single amino acid markedly decreases their biological activities.
- **Binding active components:** C1 esterase inhibitor (C1 INA) binds C1r and C1s to form an irreversibly inactive complex. Other binding proteins in the plasma include factor H– and C4b-binding protein. These complex with C3b and C4b, respectively, increasing their susceptibility to proteolytic cleavage by factor I.
- **Cell membrane–associated molecules:** Two proteins linked to the cell membrane by glycophosphoinositol (GPI) anchors are decay-accelerating factor (DAF) and protectin (CD59). DAF breaks down the alternative pathway C3 convertase; CD59 (membrane cofactor protein, protectin) binds membrane-associated C4b and C3b, promotes its inactivation by factor I and prevents formation of the MAC.

The Complement System Is Finely Focused to Target Microorganisms and Avoid Normal Cells and Tissues

When the mechanisms regulating this balance malfunction or are deficient because of mutation, resulting imbalances in complement activity can cause tissue injury. Uncontrolled systemic activation of complement may occur in sepsis (see Chapter 19), playing a central role in the development of septic shock.

Immune Complexes

Immune complexes (Ag–Ab complexes) form on bacterial surfaces and associate with C1q, activating the classical pathway. Complement then promotes physiologic clearance of circulating immune complexes. However, if these complexes are made continuously and in excess (e.g., in chronic immune responses), relentless activation consumes, and therefore depletes, complement. Complement inefficiency, whether due to complement depletion, deficient complement binding or defects in complement activation, results in immune deposition and inflammation, which in turn may trigger autoimmunity.

Infectious Disease

Defense against infection is a key role of complement. If the system functions poorly, the person is overly susceptible to infection.

- Defects in antibody production, complement proteins or phagocyte function increase susceptibility to pyogenic infections with organisms such as *Haemophilus influenzae* and *Streptococcus pneumoniae*.

- Deficiencies in MAC formation lead to increased infections, particularly with meningococci.
- Deficiency of complement MBL results in recurrent infections in young children.

Thick capsules may protect some bacteria from lysis by complement. Some bacterial enzymes can also inhibit the effects of complement components, especially C5a. Or, they can also increase catabolism of components, such as C3b, thus reducing formation of C3 convertase. Viruses, on the other hand, may use cell-bound components and receptors to facilitate cell entry. *Mycobacterium tuberculosis*, Epstein-Barr virus, measles virus, picornaviruses, HIV and flaviviruses use complement components to target inflammatory or epithelial cells.

Inflammation and Necrosis

The complement system amplifies the inflammatory response. Anaphylatoxins C5a and C3a activate leukocytes, and C5a and MAC stimulate endothelial cells, thus inducing excess generation of oxidants and cytokines that injure tissues (see Chapter 1). Nonviable or damaged tissues cannot regulate complement normally.

Complement Deficiencies

The importance of an intact and appropriately regulated complement system is exemplified in people with acquired or congenital deficiencies of specific complement components or regulatory proteins (Table 2-1). The most common congenital defect is a C2 deficiency, inherited as an autosomal codominant trait.

Acquired deficiencies of early complement components occur in patients with some autoimmune diseases, especially those associated with circulating immune complexes. These include certain forms of membranous glomerulonephritis and systemic lupus erythematosus (SLE). Deficiencies in early components of complement (e.g., C1q, C1r, C1s, C4) are strongly associated with susceptibility to SLE.

Patients lacking the middle (C3, C5) components are prone to recurrent pyogenic infections, membranoproliferative

TABLE 2-1	
HEREDITARY COMPLEMENT DEFICIENCIES	
Complement Deficiency	**Clinical Association**
C3b, iC3b, C5, MBL	Pyogenic bacterial infections
	Membranoproliferative glomerulonephritis
C3, properdin, MAC proteins	Neisserial infection
C1 inhibitor	Hereditary angioedema
CD59	Hemolysis, thrombosis
C1q, C1r and C1s, C4, C2	Systemic lupus erythematosus
Factor H and factor I	Hemolytic–uremic syndrome
	Membranoproliferative glomerulonephritis

MAC = membrane attack complex; MBL = mannose-binding lectin.

glomerulonephritis and rashes. Those who lack terminal complement components (C6, C7 or C8) are vulnerable to infections with *Neisseria* species. Such differences in susceptibility underscore the roles of individual complement components in protecting from specific bacteria. Congenital defects in proteins that regulate the complement system (e.g., C1 inhibitor, SCPN) lead to chronic complement activation. Lack of C1 inhibitor is associated with hereditary angioedema.

CELL-DERIVED INFLAMMATORY MEDIATORS

Platelets, basophils, PMNs, endothelial cells, monocyte/macrophages, tissue mast cells and the injured tissue itself may all potentially generate vasoactive and inflammatory mediators. These molecules are (1) derived from metabolism of phospholipids and arachidonic acid (e.g., prostaglandins, thromboxanes, leukotrienes, lipoxins, platelet-activating factor [PAF]), (2) preformed and stored in cytoplasmic granules (e.g., histamine, serotonin, lysosomal hydrolases) or (3) derived from altered production of normal regulators of vascular function (e.g., nitric oxide and neurokinins).

Arachidonic Acid and Platelet-Activating Factor Are Derived from Membrane Phospholipids

Phospholipids and fatty acid derivatives released from plasma membranes are metabolized into mediators and homeostatic regulators by inflammatory cells and injured tissues (Fig. 2-10). As part of a complex regulatory network, prostanoids, leukotrienes and lipoxins, which are derivatives of arachidonic acid, both promote and inhibit inflammation (Table 2-2). The net impact depends on several factors, including levels and profiles of prostanoid production, both of which change during an inflammatory response.

Arachidonic Acid

Depending on the specific inflammatory cell and nature of the stimulus, activated cells generate arachidonic acid by one of two routes (Fig. 2-10). In one pathway, arachidonic acid is liberated from the glycerol of cell membrane phospholipids

TABLE 2-2
BIOLOGICAL ACTIVITIES OF ARACHIDONIC ACID METABOLITES

Metabolite	Biological Activity
PGE_2, PDG_2	Induce vasodilation, bronchodilation; inhibit inflammatory cell function
PGI_2	Induces vasodilation, bronchodilation; inhibits inflammatory cell function
$PGF_{2\alpha}$	Induces vasodilation, bronchoconstriction
TXA_2	Induces vasoconstriction, bronchoconstriction; enhances inflammatory cell functions (esp. platelets)
LTB_4	Chemotactic for phagocytic cells; stimulates phagocytic cell adherence; enhances microvascular permeability
LTC_4, LTD_4, LTE_4	Induce smooth muscle contraction; constrict pulmonary airways; increase microvascular permeability

PG . . . = prostaglandin; LT . . . = leukotriene; TXA_2 = thromboxane A_2.

(in particular, phosphatidylcholine) by stimulus-induced activation of phospholipase A_2 (PLA_2). The pathway is phospholipase C cleavage of phosphatidylinositol phosphates to diacylglycerol and inositol phosphates. Diacylglycerol lipase then cleaves arachidonic acid from diacylglycerol. This arachidonic acid is further metabolized by either (1) **cyclooxygenation,** to produce prostaglandins and thromboxanes, or (2) **lipoxygenation,** to leukotrienes and lipoxins (Fig. 2-11).

Corticosteroids are widely used to suppress tissue destruction associated with many inflammatory diseases, including allergic responses, rheumatoid arthritis and SLE. They induce synthesis of an inhibitor of PLA_2 and block arachidonic acid release by inflammatory cells. However, prolonged corticosteroid use can be quite harmful and lead to increased risk of infection and damage to connective tissue.

Platelet-Activating Factor

PAF is another potent inflammatory mediator derived from membrane phospholipids. It is synthesized by virtually all activated inflammatory cells, endothelial cells and injured tissue cells. During inflammatory and allergic responses, PAF is derived from choline-containing glycerophospholipids in the cell membrane, initially by the catalytic action of PLA_2, followed by acetylation by an acetyltransferase (Fig. 2-10). In plasma, PAF-acetylhydrolase regulates PAF activity.

PAF has many functions. It stimulates platelets, monocyte/macrophages, neutrophils, endothelial cells and vascular smooth muscle cells. It also induces platelet aggregation and degranulation at sites of tissue injury and enhances release of serotonin, thereby altering vascular permeability. Since PAF primes leukocytes, it promotes functional responses (e.g., O_2 production, degranulation) to a second stimulus and induces adhesion molecule expression, specifically of integrins. It is also a very potent vasodilator, augmenting permeability of microvasculature at sites of tissue

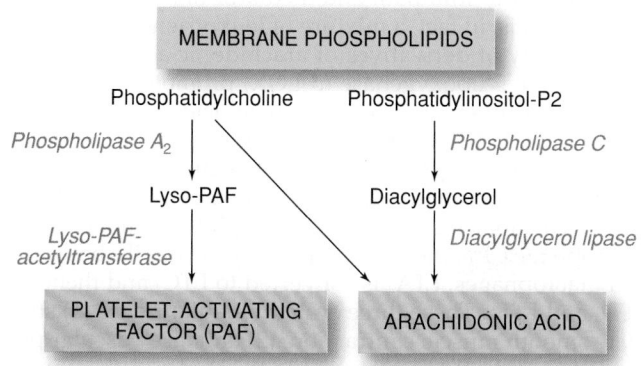

FIGURE 2-10. Cell membrane–derived mediators. Platelet-activating factor (PAF) is derived from choline-containing glycerophospholipids in the membrane. Arachidonic acid derives from phosphatidylinositol phosphates and from phosphatidyl choline.

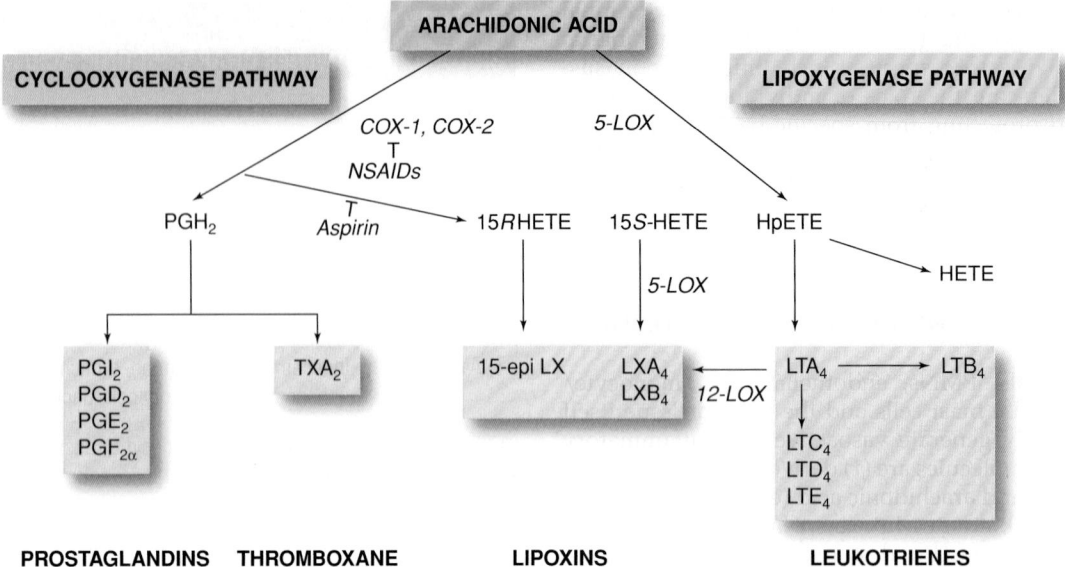

FIGURE 2-11. Biologically active arachidonic acid metabolites. The cyclooxygenase (COX) pathway of arachidonic acid metabolism generates prostaglandins (PG…) and thromboxane (TXA_2). The lipoxygenase (LOX) pathway forms lipoxins (LX…) and leukotrienes (LT…). Aspirin (acetylsalicylic acid) blocks the formation of 5-HETE (*HETE* = hydroxyicosatetraenoic acid). NSAIDs (non-steroidal anti-inflammatory drugs) block COX-1 and COX-2. *HpETE* = 5-hydroperoxyeicosatetraenoic acid.

injury. PAF generated by endothelial cells cooperates with P-selectin. When P-selectin lightly tethers a leukocyte to an endothelial cell, PAF from the endothelial cell binds its receptor on the leukocyte and induces intracellular signaling.

Prostanoids, Leukotrienes and Lipoxins Are Biologically Active Metabolites of Arachidonic Acid

Prostanoids

Arachidonic acid is further metabolized by cyclooxygenases 1 and 2 (COX-1, COX-2) to generate prostanoids (Fig. 2-11). **COX-1** is constitutively expressed by most cells and increases upon cell activation. It is a key enzyme in the synthesis of prostaglandins, which in turn (1) protect the gut mucosa, (2) regulate water/electrolyte balance, (3) stimulate platelet aggregation to maintain normal hemostasis and (4) maintain resistance to thrombosis on vascular endothelial cell surfaces. **COX-2** expression is generally low or undetectable but increases substantially upon stimulation to yield metabolites that are important in inducing pain and inflammation.

The early inflammatory prostanoid response is COX-1 dependent. As inflammation proceeds, COX-2 takes over as the major source of prostanoids. Both COX isoforms generate prostaglandin H_2 (PGH_2), which is the substrate for production of prostacyclin (PGI_2), PGD_2, PGE_2, $PGF_{2\alpha}$ and TXA_2 (thromboxane). The quantity and variety of prostaglandins produced during inflammation depends in part on the cells present and their state of activation. Thus, mast cells make mostly PGD_2; macrophages generate PGE_2 and TXA_2; platelets are the major source of TXA_2; and endothelial cells secrete PGI_2. Prostanoids affect immune cell function by binding G-protein–coupled cell surface receptors, triggering many intracellular signaling pathways in immune cells and

resident tissue cells. The repertoire of prostanoid receptors on various immune cells differs, so the functional responses of these cells may be different, according to the prostanoids present.

Inhibition of COX is one mechanism by which nonsteroidal anti-inflammatory drugs (NSAIDs), including aspirin, indomethacin and ibuprofen, exert potent analgesic and anti-inflammatory effects. NSAIDs block COX-2–induced formation of prostaglandins, and so mitigate pain and inflammation. However, they also affect COX-1, decreasing homeostatic functions and affecting the stomach and kidneys adversely. This complication has led to the development of COX-2–specific inhibitors.

Leukotrienes

Slow-reacting substance of anaphylaxis (SRS-A) is a smooth muscle stimulant and mediator of hypersensitivity reactions. It is, in fact, a mixture of leukotrienes, the second major family of derivatives of arachidonic acid (Fig. 2-11). The enzyme 5-lipoxygenase (5-LOX) promotes the synthesis of 5-hydroperoxyeicosatetraenoic acid (5-HpETE) and leukotriene A_4 (LTA_4) from arachidonic acid; the latter is a precursor for other leukotrienes. In neutrophils and some macrophage populations, LTA_4 is metabolized to LTB_4, a potent chemotactic agent for neutrophils, monocytes and macrophages. In other cells, especially mast cells, basophils and macrophages, LTA_4 is converted to LTC_4 and thence to LTD_4 and LTE_4. These three cysteinyl-leukotrienes (1) stimulate smooth muscle contraction, (2) enhance vascular permeability and (3) are responsible for many of the clinical symptoms associated with allergic-type reactions. Thus, they play a pivotal role in the development of asthma. Leukotrienes exert their action through high-affinity specific receptors that may prove to be important targets of drug therapy.

Interleukins	Growth Factors	Chemokines	Interferons	Pro-Inflammatory Cytokines
IL-1 IL-6 IL-8 IL-13 IL-10	GM-CSF M-CSF	CC CXC XC CX3C	IFNα IFNβ IFNγ	TNFα
• Inflammatory cell activation	• Macrophage • Bactericidal activity • NK and dendritic cell function	• Leukocyte chemotaxis • Leukocyte activation	• Antiviral • Leukocyte activation	• Fever • Anorexia • Shock • Cytotoxicity • Cytokine induction • Activation of endothelial cells and tissue cells

FIGURE 2-12. Cytokines important in inflammation. *GM-CSF* = granulocyte–macrophage colony-stimulating factor; *IL* = interleukin; *NK* = natural killer; *IFN* = interferon; *TNF* = tumor necrosis factor.

INFLAMMATION

Lipoxins

Lipoxins, the third class of arachidonic acid products, are made in the vascular lumen by cell–cell interactions (Fig. 2-11). They are proinflammatory, trihydroxytetraene-containing eicosanoids, generated during inflammation, atherosclerosis and thrombosis. Several cell types synthesize lipoxins from leukotrienes. LTA_4, released by activated leukocytes, is available for transcellular enzymatic conversion by nearby cells. When platelets adhere to neutrophils, LTA_4 from neutrophils is converted by platelet 12-lipoxygenase to lipoxin A_4 and B_4 (LXA_4 and LXB_4). Monocytes, eosinophils and airway epithelial cells generate 15S-hydroxyeicosatetraenoic acid (15S-HETE), which is taken up by neutrophils and converted to lipoxins via 5-LOX. Activation of this pathway can also inhibit leukotriene biosynthesis, thus regulating the whole process.

Aspirin initiates transcellular biosynthesis of a group of lipoxins termed "aspirin-triggered lipoxins," or 15-epimeric-lipoxins (15-epi-LXs). When aspirin is given in the presence of inflammatory mediators, 15R-HETE is generated by COX-2. Activated neutrophils convert 15R-HETE to 15-epi-LXs, which are anti-inflammatory lipid mediators. Thus, this is another pathway in which aspirin exerts a beneficial effect.

Cytokines Are Low–Molecular-Weight Proteins Secreted by Cells

Many different cytokines, including interleukins, growth factors, colony-stimulating factors, interferons and chemokines, are produced at sites of inflammation (Fig. 2-12).

Cytokines

Cytokines are low–molecular-weight proteins secreted by activated cells. They are produced at sites of tissue injury and regulate inflammatory responses from initial changes in vascular permeability to resolution and restoration of tissue integrity. Cytokines are inflammatory hormones that act in several modes (Fig. 2-13): **autocrine,** affecting cells that make them; **paracrine,** affecting neighboring cells; and **endocrine,**

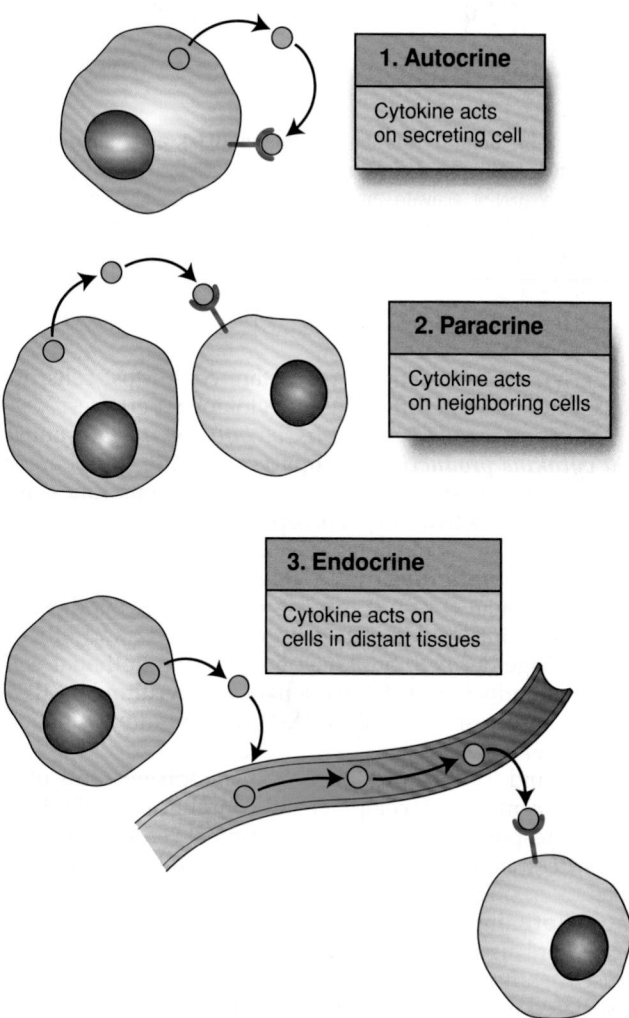

1. Autocrine
Cytokine acts on secreting cell

2. Paracrine
Cytokine acts on neighboring cells

3. Endocrine
Cytokine acts on cells in distant tissues

FIGURE 2-13. Types of cytokine signaling. 1. Autocrine signaling occurs when secreted products act through receptors on the secreting cell. **2.** Paracrine signaling occurs when secreted products act on nearby cells. **3.** In endocrine signaling, products are carried in the vascular system to act on distant cells.

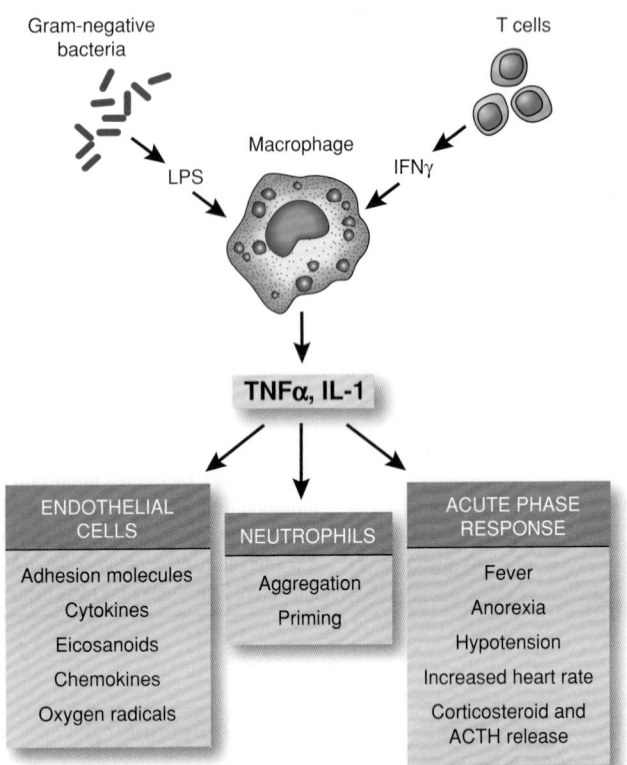

FIGURE 2-14. Central role of interleukin (IL)-1 and tumor necrosis factor (TNF)-α in inflammation. Lipopolysaccharide (LPS) and interferon-γ (IFN-γ) activate macrophages to release inflammatory cytokines, principally IL-1 and TNF-α, responsible for directing local and systemic inflammatory responses. *ACTH* = adrenocorticotrophic hormone.

acting via the bloodstream on distant cells. Most cells produce cytokines but differ in their cytokine repertoires.

Macrophages orchestrate tissue inflammatory responses via cytokine production. **Lipopolysaccharide** (LPS), a constituent of gram-negative bacterial outer membranes, is a highly potent activator of macrophages, as well as of endothelial cells and leukocytes (Fig. 2-14). LPS binds specific cellular receptors directly, or after binding a serum LPS-binding protein (LBP). It triggers macrophage synthesis of TNF-α and interleukins (IL-1, IL-6, IL-8, IL-12 and others). Macrophage-derived cytokines modulate endothelial cell–leukocyte adhesion (TNF-α), leukocyte recruitment (IL-8), acute phase responses (IL-6, IL-1) and immune functions (IL-1, IL-6, IL-12).

IL-1 and TNF-α, produced by macrophages and other cells, are central to development and amplification of inflammatory responses. These cytokines activate endothelial cells to express adhesion molecules and then release cytokines, chemokines and reactive oxygen species (ROS). TNF-α causes priming and aggregation of neutrophils. IL-1 and TNF-α are also among the mediators of fever, catabolism of muscle, shifts in protein synthesis and hemodynamic effects associated with inflammatory states (Fig. 2-14).

Interferon-γ (IFN-γ), another potent stimulus for macrophage activation and cytokine production, is produced by a subset of T lymphocytes as part of the immune response (see Chapter 4). It is also synthesized by natural killer (NK) cells in the primary host response to intracellular

pathogens (e.g., *Listeria monocytogenes*) and certain viruses. NK cells migrate to tissues at sites of injury where, when exposed to IL-12 and TNF-α, they produce IFN-γ. Thus, there is an amplification pathway by which activated tissue macrophages produce TNF-α and IL-12, stimulating IFN-γ production by NK cells, with subsequent activation of additional macrophages.

Chemokines Regulate Cell Trafficking and Activation

There are more than 50 known cytokines that participate in inflammation and immunity. Chemotactic cytokines, or chemokines, stimulate cell activation, hematopoiesis and angiogenesis. Accumulation of inflammatory cells at sites of tissue injury requires their migration from vascular spaces into extravascular tissue. The most important chemotactic factors for PMNs are:

- C5a, derived from complement
- Bacterial and mitochondrial products, particularly low–molecular-weight N-formylated peptides (e.g., *N*-formyl-methionyl-leucyl-phenylalanine [FMLP])
- Products of arachidonic acid metabolism, especially LTB$_4$
- Chemokines

Chemokines are small secreted molecules that bind G-protein–coupled receptors on target cells. They are produced by a variety of cell types, either constitutively or after induction, and differ widely in biological action. This diversity is based on specific cell types targeted, specific receptor activation and differences in intracellular signaling.

There are two functional classes of chemokines: **inflammatory chemokines** and **homing chemokines**. Inflammatory chemokines are elicited by bacterial toxins and inflammatory cytokines (especially IL-1, TNF-α and IFN-γ) by a variety of tissue cells and by leukocytes themselves. They recruit leukocytes during host inflammatory responses. Homing chemokines are constitutively expressed and upregulated in disease. They direct trafficking and homing of lymphocytes and dendritic cells to lymphoid tissues during an immune response (see Chapter 4).

Structure and Nomenclature of Chemokines

Chemokines are synthesized as secretory proteins, consisting of 70–130 amino acids, with four conserved cysteines linked by disulfide bonds. The two major subpopulations, termed CXC or CC chemokines (formerly called α and β chemokines), are distinguished by the position of the first two cysteines, which are either separated by one amino acid (CXC) or are adjacent (CC). Two additional classes of chemokines, each with a single member, have been identified. Lymphotactin has two, instead of four, conserved cysteines (XC), and fractaline (or neurotactin) has three amino acids between the first two cysteines (CX$_3$C). Chemokines are named according to their structure, followed by "L" and the number of their gene (CCL1, CXCL1, etc.). However, many of the traditional names for chemokines persist in current usage. Chemokine receptors are named according to their structure, "R," and a number (CCR1, CXCR1, etc.); most receptors recognize more than one chemokine and most chemokines bind more than one receptor. Receptor binding by chemokines may lead to agonistic or antagonistic activity. In fact, the same chemokine may act as an agonist at one receptor and an antagonist at another. Combinations of these agonistic and antagonistic activities and the profile of chemokines at a site dictate the attraction and activation of specific resident and inflammatory cell types.

Anchoring and Activity of Chemokines

Chemokines may be either immobilized or soluble molecules, controlling leukocyte motility and localization within extravascular tissues by establishing a chemotactic gradient. They generate this gradient by binding ECM proteoglycans or cell surfaces. As a result, high concentrations of chemokines persist at sites of tissue injury. Specific receptors on the surface of migrating leukocytes recognize matrix-bound chemokines and associated adhesion molecules, causing cells to move along the chemotactic gradient to a site of injury. The process of responding to matrix-bound chemoattractants is **haptotaxis**. During this migration, the cell extends a pseudopod toward increasing chemokine concentrations. At the leading front of the pseudopod, marked changes in levels of intracellular calcium are associated with assembly and contraction of cytoskeleton proteins. This pulls the rest of the cell along the chemical gradient. Chemokines are also displayed on cytokine-activated vascular endothelial cells. This process can augment very late antigen-4 (VLA-4) integrin-dependent adhesion of leukocytes, resulting in their firm arrest. The variety and combinations of chemokine receptors on cells allow for diverse biological functions. Neutrophils, monocytes, eosinophils and basophils share some receptors but express other receptors exclusively. Thus, specific chemokine combinations can recruit selective cell populations.

Chemokines in Disease

Chemokines are implicated in many acute and chronic diseases. In disorders with a pronounced inflammatory component, multiple chemokines are expressed in inflamed tissues. Examples are rheumatoid arthritis, ulcerative colitis, Crohn disease, pulmonary inflammation (chronic bronchitis, asthma), autoimmune diseases (multiple sclerosis, rheumatoid arthritis, SLE) and vascular diseases, including atherosclerosis.

Reactive Oxygen Species Are Signal-Transducing, Bactericidal and Cytotoxic Molecules

ROS are chemically reactive molecules derived from oxygen. Normally, they are rapidly inactivated, but they can be toxic to cells if generated inappropriately (see Chapters 1 and 5). ROS activate signal transduction pathways and combine with proteins, lipids and DNA, which can impair cell function and kill cells. Leukocyte-derived ROS, released within phagosomes, are bactericidal. Key ROS in inflammation include superoxide (O_2^-), nitric oxide (NO, or NO•), hydrogen peroxide (H_2O_2) and hydroxyl radical (OH•) (Fig. 2-15).

Superoxide

Molecular oxygen is converted to superoxide anion (O_2^-) (1) within cells, where O_2^- is generated spontaneously by the inner mitochondrial membrane; (2) in vascular endothelium, when it is produced by flavoenzymes, such as xanthine oxidase, lipoxygenase and cyclooxygenase; and (3) during inflammation, by leukocytes as well as endothelial cells using a nicotinamide adenine dinucleotide phosphate (NADPH) oxidase to produce O_2^-.

In endothelial cells, xanthine oxidase, a purine-metabolizing enzyme, converts xanthine and hypoxanthine to uric acid, thus generating O_2^-. This pathway is a major intracellular source of O_2^- in neutrophil-mediated cell injury. Proinflammatory mediators, including leukocyte elastase and several cytokines, convert xanthine dehydrogenase to the active xanthine oxidase. Intracellular O_2^- interacts with nuclear factor-κB (NFκB), activating protein-1 (AP-1) and other molecules during signal transduction. It is converted to other free radicals, particularly OH•, which contribute to inflammation-related cell injury.

NADPH oxidase in phagocytic cells, neutrophils and macrophages is a multicomponent enzyme complex that generates high concentrations of extracellular and intracellular O_2^-, mainly for bactericidal and cytotoxic functions. This oxidase uses nicotinamide adenine dinucleotide (NADH) and NADPH to transfer electrons to molecular oxygen. A similar enzyme complex in endothelial cells generates significant, albeit lower, concentrations of O_2^-.

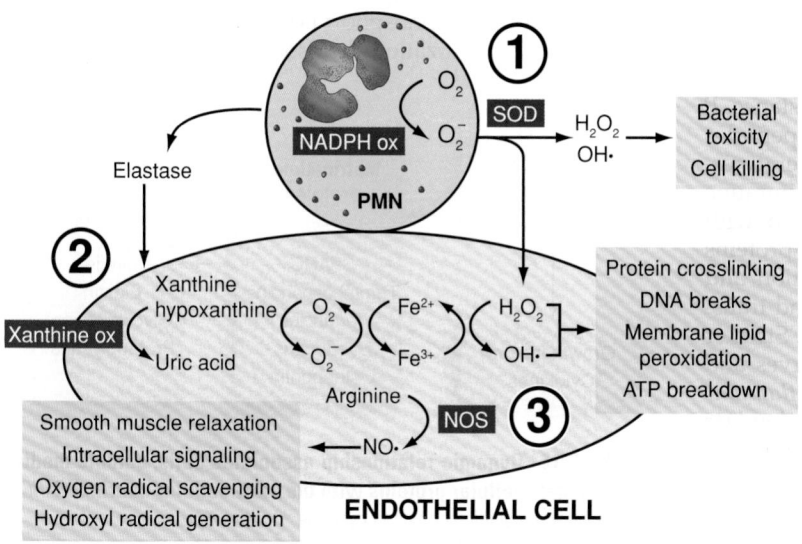

FIGURE 2-15. Biochemical events in neutrophil–endothelial cell interactions. When neutrophils are in firm contact with endothelial cells, oxygen radicals and other active molecules generated by both cells interact. **1.** Superoxide (O_2^-) generated by the neutrophil nicotinamide adenine dinucleotide phosphate oxidase (NADPHox) is converted to toxic hydrogen peroxide (H_2O_2) and hydroxyl radical (OH•). **2.** Within the endothelial cell xanthine oxidase (xanthine ox) converts xanthine to uric acid, ultimately generating O_2^- from molecular oxygen. **3.** Nitric oxide synthase (NOS) generates nitric oxide (NO•) from arginine. Reactive oxygen species contribute to numerous cellular events. *ATP* = adenosine triphosphate; *Fe²⁺* = ferrous iron; *Fe³⁺* = ferric iron; *PMN* = polymorphonuclear neutrophil.

Nitric Oxide

NO is produced by nitric oxide synthase (NOS), which oxides the guanidino nitrogen of L-arginine in the presence of O_2. There are three main NOS isoforms: constitutively expressed **neuronal** (nNOS) and **endothelial** (eNOS) forms and **inducible NOS** (iNOS). Inflammatory cytokines increase expression of iNOS, generating intracellular and extracellular NO, which has many roles in vascular physiology and pathophysiology:

- NO generated by eNOS is **endothelium-derived relaxing factor** (EDRF), mediating vascular smooth muscle relaxation.
- In physiologic concentrations, it—alone and in balance with O_2^-—is an intracellular messenger.
- NO prevents platelet adherence and aggregation at sites of vascular injury, reduces leukocyte recruitment and scavenges oxygen radicals.
- Excessive NO production, especially in parallel with O_2^-, generates the highly reactive and cytotoxic species, peroxynitrite ($ONOO^-$).

Stress Proteins Protect from Inflammatory Injury

When cells are stressed, many suffer irreversible injury and die. Others may be severely damaged. However, mild heat treatment prior to potentially lethal injury provides tolerance to subsequent injury (see Chapter 1). This phenomenon reflects increased expression of the heat shock family of stress proteins (HSPs). Stress proteins belong to multigene families and are named according to molecular size (e.g., Hsp27, Hsp70, Hsp90). They are upregulated by diverse threats, such as oxidative/ischemic stress and inflammation, and are associated with protection during sepsis and metabolic stress. Protein damage and misfolded proteins are common denominators in injury and disease (see Chapter 1). Protection from many kinds of nonlethal stresses is mediated by HSPs, which are molecular chaperones, increasing protein expression by guiding folding of nascent proteins and preventing misfolding. Potential functions of stress proteins include suppression of proinflammatory cytokines and NADPH oxidase, increased nitric oxide–mediated cytoprotection and enhanced collagen synthesis.

Neurokinins Link the Endocrine, Nervous and Immune Systems

The neurokinin family of peptides includes substance P (SP) and neurokinins A (NKA) and B (NKB). These peptides are distributed throughout the central and peripheral nervous systems and link the endocrine, nervous and immune systems. Diverse biological processes are associated with these peptides, including extravasation of plasma proteins and edema, vasodilation, smooth muscle contraction and relaxation, salivary secretion, airway contraction and transmission of nociceptive responses. As early as 1876, Stricker noted an association between sensory afferent nerves and inflammation. *Injury to nerve terminals during inflammation evokes an increase in neurokinins that in turn stimulate production of inflammatory mediators, such as histamine, NO and kinins.* The actions of neurokinins are mediated by activation of at least three classes of receptors—NK1, NK2 and NK3—which are widely distributed in the body. The neurokinin system is linked to inflammation in the following settings:

- **Edema formation:** SP, NKA and NKB induce edema by promoting release of histamine and serotonin from mast cells.
- **Thermal injury:** SP and NKA cause edema right after thermal injury.
- **Arthritis:** SP is widespread in nerves in joints and increases vascular permeability. SP and NKA modulate tasks of inflammatory and immune cells.
- **Airway inflammation:** SP and NKA mediate bronchoconstriction, mucosal edema, leukocyte adhesion and activation and vascular permeability.

EXTRACELLULAR MATRIX MEDIATORS

Interactions of cells and ECM regulate tissue responses to inflammation. The extracellular environment consists of macromolecular matrices specific for each tissue. During injury, resident inflammatory cells interact with the ECM, using this scaffolding for migration along a chemokine gradient. Collagen, elastic fibers, basement membrane proteins, glycoproteins and proteoglycans are among the ECM components (see Chapter 3). Matricellular proteins are secreted macromolecules that link cells to the ECM or that disrupt cell–ECM interactions. Cytokines and growth factors influence associations among cells, the ECM and matricellular proteins (Fig. 2-16). Matricellular proteins include:

- **SPARC (secreted protein acidic and rich in cysteine)** is a multifunctional glycoprotein that organizes ECM components and modulates growth factor activity. It affects cell proliferation, migration and differentiation and is counteradhesive, especially for endothelial cells.
- **Thrombospondins** are secreted glycoproteins that affect cell–matrix interactions, influence platelet aggregation and support neutrophil chemotaxis and adhesion.
- **Tenascins C, X and R** are counteradhesive proteins expressed during development, tissue injury and wound healing.
- **Syndecans** are heparan sulfate proteoglycans implicated in coagulation, growth factor signaling, cell adhesion to the ECM and tumorigenesis.
- **Osteopontin** is a phosphorylated glycoprotein important in bone mineralization. It also (1) mediates cell–matrix

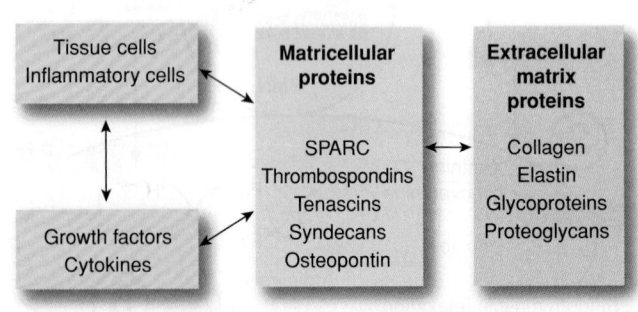

FIGURE 2-16. Dynamic relationship associates cells, soluble mediators and matricellular proteins with the extracellular matrix. *SPARC* = secreted protein acidic and rich in cysteine.

interactions, (2) activates cell signaling (mainly in T cells), (3) is chemotactic for and supports adhesion of leukocytes and (4) has anti-inflammatory effects via regulation of macrophage function.

CELLS OF INFLAMMATION

Leukocytes are the major cellular participants in inflammation and include neutrophils, T and B lymphocytes, monocytes, macrophages, eosinophils, mast cells and basophils. Each cell type has specific functions, but they overlap and change as inflammation progresses. *Inflammatory cells and*

resident tissue cells interact with each other in a continuous response during inflammation.

Neutrophils

PMNs predominate in acute inflammation. They are stored in bone marrow, circulate in the blood and rapidly accumulate at sites of injury or infection (Figs. 2-17A and 2-18). PMNs have granulated cytoplasm and a 2- to 4-lobed nucleus. Neutrophil receptors recognize the Fc portion of IgG and IgM; complement components C5a, C3b and iC3b; arachidonic acid metabolites; chemotactic factors; and cytokines. In tissues, PMNs phagocytose, invading microbes and

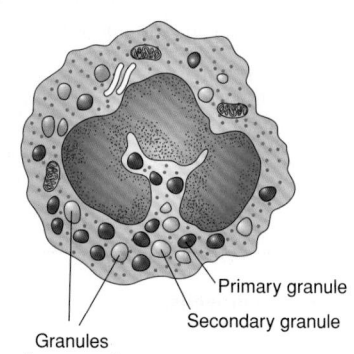

POLYMORPHONUCLEAR LEUKOCYTE

CHARACTERISTICS AND FUNCTIONS
• Central to acute inflammation
• Phagocytosis of microorganisms and tissue debris
• Mediates tissue injury

PRIMARY INFLAMMATORY MEDIATORS
• Reactive oxygen metabolites
• Lysosomal granule contents

Primary granules	Secondary granules
Myeloperoxidase	Lysozyme
Lysozyme	Lactoferrin
Defensins	Collagenase
Bactericidal/permeability increasing protein	Complement activator Phospholipase A$_2$
Elastase	CD11b/CD18
Cathepsins protease 3	CD11c/CD18
Glucuronidase	Laminin
Mannosidase	
Phospholipase A2	**Tertiary granules**
	Gelatinase
	Plasminogen activator
	Cathepsins
	Glucuronidase
	Mannosidase

Primary granule
Secondary granule
Granules (lysosomes)
A

ENDOTHELIAL CELL

CHARACTERISTICS AND FUNCTIONS
• Maintains vascular integrity
• Regulates platelet aggregation
• Regulates vascular contraction and relaxation
• Mediates leukocyte recruitment in inflammation

PRIMARY INFLAMMATORY MEDIATORS
• von Willebrand factor
• Nitric oxide
• Endothelins
• Prostanoids

B
Capillary lumen

MONOCYTE/MACROPHAGE

CHARACTERISTICS AND FUNCTIONS
• Regulates acute and chronic inflammatory response
• Regulates coagulation/fibrinolytic pathway
• Regulates immune response (see Chapter 4)

PRIMARY INFLAMMATORY MEDIATORS
• Enzymes
• Proteins
• Complement proteins
• Chemokines
• Cytokines
• Reactive oxygen species
• Antioxidants
• Coagulation factors
• Bioactive lipids

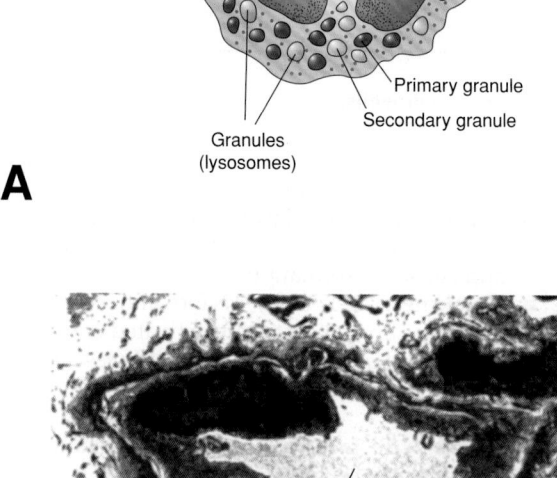

Lysosome
Phagocytic vacuole
C

FIGURE 2-17. Cells of inflammation: morphology and function. A. Neutrophil. **B.** Endothelial cell. **C.** Monocyte/macrophage.

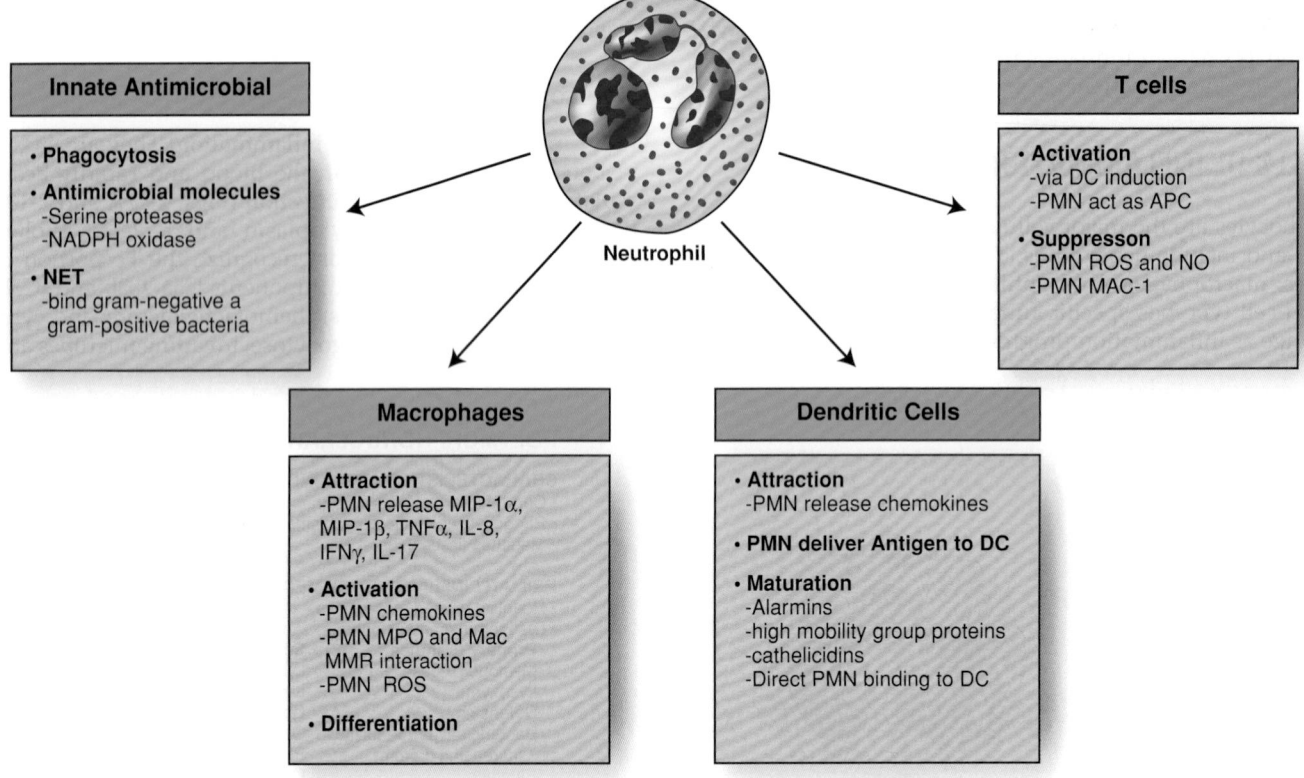

FIGURE 2-18. Effector functions of neutrophils.

dead tissue, then undergo apoptosis, largely during the resolution phase of acute inflammation. They exhibit NETosis (see Chapter 1), a unique mechanism of trapping and killing microbial invaders, while at the same time dying themselves. In addition to microbicidal and proinflammatory properties, PMNs affect dendritic cells, T cells and macrophages.

Endothelial Cells

Endothelial cells line blood vessels as a monolayer and help separate intravascular and extravascular spaces. They produce antiplatelet and antithrombotic agents that maintain blood vessel patency and secrete vasodilators and vasoconstrictors that regulate vascular tone. Injury to a vessel wall interrupts the endothelial barrier and exposes local procoagulant signals (Fig. 2-17B).

Endothelial cells are gatekeepers in inflammatory cell recruitment; they may promote or inhibit tissue perfusion and inflammatory cell influx. Inflammatory agents such as bradykinin and histamine, endotoxins and cytokines induce endothelial cells to show adhesion molecules that anchor and activate leukocytes, causing them to present major histocompatibility complex (MHC) class I and II molecules, and generate key vasoactive and inflammatory mediators. These mediators include:

- **NO:** Nitric oxide is a low–molecular-weight vasodilator that inhibits platelet aggregation, regulates vascular tone by stimulating smooth muscle relaxation and reacts with ROS to create highly reactive radical species (see above).
- **Endothelins:** Endothelins-1, -2 and -3 are low–molecular-weight peptides made by endothelial cells. They are potent vasoconstrictor and pressor agents, which induce prolonged vasoconstriction of vascular smooth muscle.
- **Arachidonic acid–derived contraction factors:** Oxygen radicals generated by the hydroperoxidase activity

of cyclooxygenase and prostanoids, such as TXA_2 and PGH_2, induce smooth muscle contraction.
- **Arachidonic acid–derived relaxing factors:** The biological opponent of TXA_2, PGI_2 inhibits platelet aggregation and causes vasodilation.
- **Cytokines:** IL-1, IL-6, TNF-α and other inflammatory cytokines are generated by activated endothelial cells.
- **Anticoagulants:** Heparin-like molecules and thrombomodulin inactivate the coagulation cascade (see Chapters 16 and 26).
- **Fibrinolytic factors:** Tissue-type plasminogen activator (t-PA) promotes fibrinolytic activity.
- **Prothrombotic agents:** von Willebrand factor facilitates adhesion of platelets, and tissue factor activates the extrinsic clotting cascade.

Monocyte/Macrophages

Circulating monocytes (Fig. 2-17C) are bone marrow–derived cells that have a single lobed or kidney-shaped nucleus. They may exit the circulation to migrate into tissue and become resident macrophages that accumulate at sites of acute inflammation and clear pathogens, cell debris and apoptotic cells. Monocytes/macrophages produce potent phlogistic mediators, influencing initiation, progression and resolution of acute inflammatory responses. They also have a central role in regulating progression to, and maintenance of, chronic inflammation. Macrophages respond to inflammatory stimuli by phagocytosis of cell debris and microorganisms, chemotaxis, antigen processing and presentation, and secretion immunomodulatory factors. A large repertoire of surface receptors mediate these various macrophage functions; some immune receptors are macrophage specific, but others are shared with PMNs and lymphocytes.

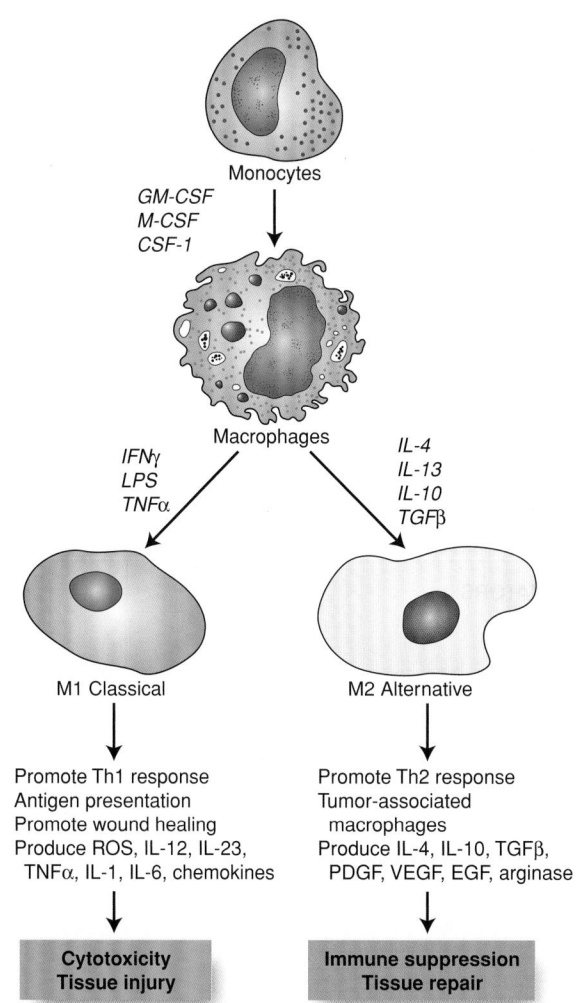

Classically activated macrophages (Figs. 2-19 and 2-20) are driven by IFN-γ, TNF-α and LPS to promote proinflammatory responses and release ROS and immune defense cytokines. Alternatively, activated macrophages respond to IL-4 and IL-13 to help clear parasitic infections. Macrophages also respond to cytokines such as IL-10 and transforming growth factor-β (TGF-β) to promote resolution of inflammation or switch acute to chronic inflammatory responses.

Like PMNs, macrophages are phagocytes and, like dendritic cells, are crucial in antigen processing and presentation. Members of this mononuclear phagocyte system are functionally diverse and include bone marrow macrophages, alveolar macrophages (lung), Kupffer cells (liver), microglial cells (CNS), Langerhans cells (skin), mesangial cells (kidney) and tissue macrophages throughout the body. Tumor-associated macrophages (TAMs) can recognize and lyse tumor cells.

Dendritic Cells

Dendritic cells are derived from bone marrow progenitors, circulate in the blood as immature precursors, then settle widely in tissues, where they differentiate. They are highly efficient, antigen-presenting cells and stimulate naive T cells. Antigens bind to MHC class II on dendritic cells and are presented to lymphocytes, which are subsequently activated (see Chapter 4).

Mast Cells and Basophils

Basophils (Fig. 2-21A) are the least common leukocyte in the blood and can migrate into tissue to participate in immunologic responses. Functionally similar mast cells are long-lived and reside in all supporting tissues. They are important in regulating vascular permeability and bronchial smooth muscle tone, especially in hypersensitivity reactions (see Chapter 4). Mast cells are seen in connective tissues and

FIGURE 2-19. Macrophage activation states.

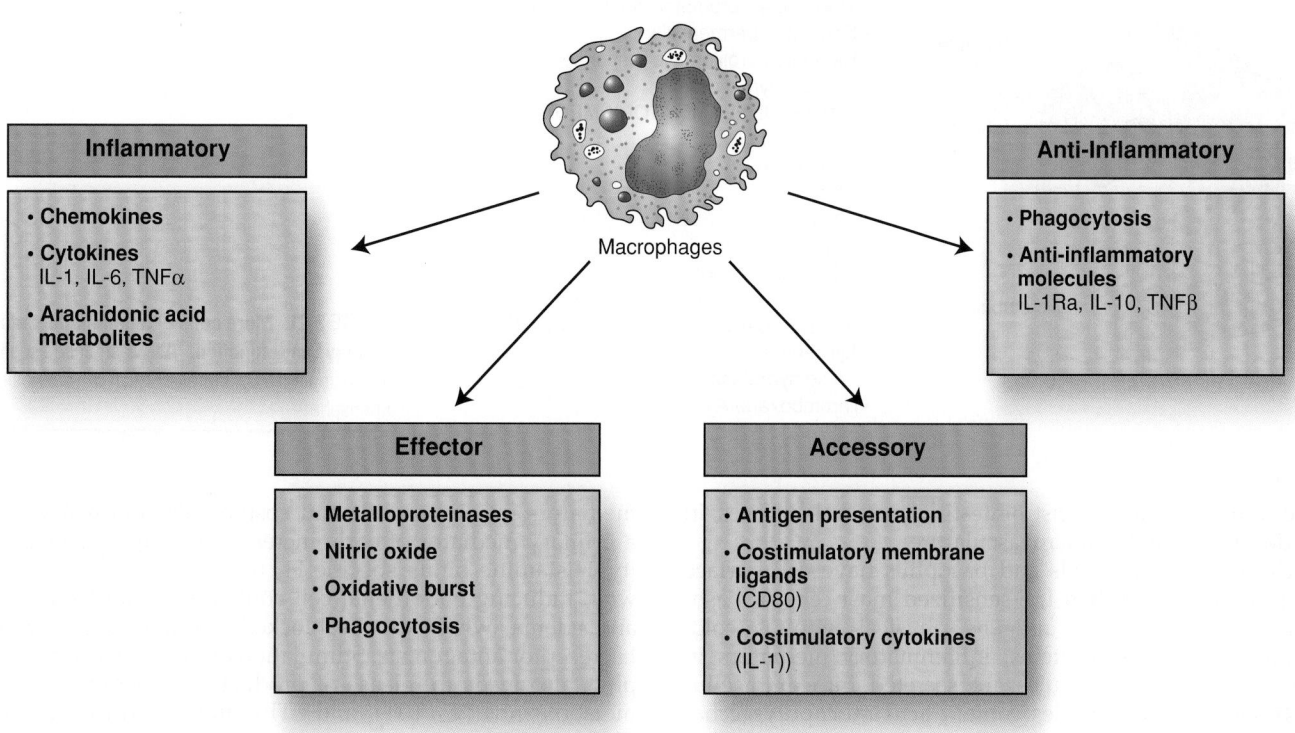

FIGURE 2-20. Effector functions of macrophages.

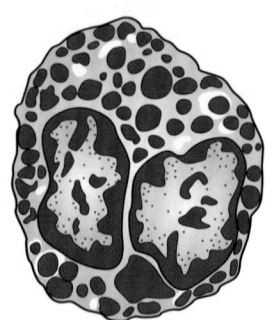

A

MAST CELL (BASOPHIL)

CHARACTERISTICS AND FUNCTIONS
• Binds IgE molecules
• Contains electron-dense granules

PRIMARY INFLAMMATORY MEDIATORS
• Histamine
• Leukotrienes (LTC, LTD, LTE)
• Platelet-activating factor
• Eosinophil chemotactic factors
• Cytokines (e.g., TNF-α IL-4)

EOSINOPHIL
CHARACTERISTICS AND FUNCTIONS
• Associated with:
  -Allergic reactions
  -Parasite-associated inflammatory reactions
  -Chronic inflammation
• Modulates mast cell-mediated reactions

PRIMARY INFLAMMATORY MEDIATORS
• Reactive oxygen metabolites
• Lysosomal granule enzymes
  (primary crystalloid granules)
  -Major basic protein
  -Eosinophil cationic protein
  -Eosinophil peroxidase
  -Acid phosphatase
  -β-glucuronidase
  -Arylsulfatase B
  -Histaminase
• Phospholipase D
• Prostaglandins of E series
• Cytokines

Granules

B

PLATELET
CHARACTERISTICS AND FUNCTIONS
• Thrombosis; promotes clot formation
• Regulates permeability
• Regulates proliferative response of
  mesenchymal cells
PRIMARY INFLAMMATORY MEDIATORS
• Dense granules
  -Serotonin
  -Ca^{2+}
  -ADP
• α-granules
  -Cationic proteins
  -Fibrinogen and coagulation proteins
  -Platelet-derived growth factor (PDGF)
• Lysosomes
  -Acid hydrolases
•Thromboxane A_2

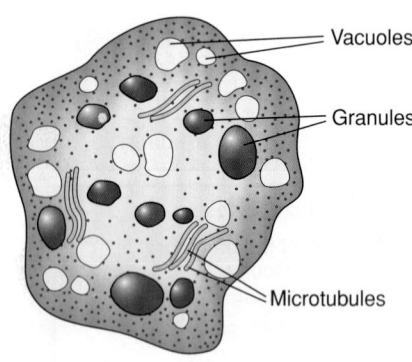

Vacuoles

Granules

Microtubules

C

FIGURE 2-21. More cells of inflammation: morphology and function. A. Mast cell/basophil. **B.** Eosinophil. **C.** Platelet. *ADP* = adenosine diphosphate.

especially on lung and gastrointestinal mucosal surfaces, in the dermis and in the microvasculature.

Granulated mast cells and basophils have cell surface receptors for IgE. When IgE-sensitized mast cells or basophils are stimulated by antigens, physical agonists (cold, trauma) or cationic proteins, inflammatory mediators in dense cytoplasmic granules are secreted into extracellular tissues. These granules contain acid mucopolysaccharides (including heparin), serine proteases, chemotactic mediators for neutrophils and eosinophils, and histamine, a primary mediator of early increased vascular permeability. Histamine binds specific H_1 receptors in the vascular wall, inducing endothelial cell contraction, gap formation and edema, which can be blocked pharmacologically by H_1-receptor antagonists. Stimulation of mast cells and basophils also leads to release of products of arachidonic acid metabolism (LTC_4, LTD_4 and LTE_4) and cytokines, such as TNF-α and IL-4.

Eosinophils

Eosinophils (Fig. 2-21B) circulate in blood and are recruited to tissue similarly to PMNs. They are often seen in settings of IgE-mediated reactions, such as allergy and asthma. Eosinophils contain leukotrienes and PAF, acid phosphatase and peroxidase. They express IgA receptors and exhibit large granules that contain eosinophil major basic protein, both of which are involved in defense against parasites (see Chapter 4).

Platelets

Platelets (Fig. 2-21C) play a primary role in normal homeostasis and in initiating and regulating clotting (see Chapter 26). They produce inflammatory mediators, such as potent vasoactive substances and growth factors that modulate mesenchymal cell proliferation. Platelets are small (about 2 mm), lack nuclei and have three types of inclusions: (1) **dense granules,** rich in serotonin, histamine, calcium and adenosine diphosphate (ADP); (2) **α-granules,** containing fibrinogen, coagulation proteins, platelet-derived growth factor (PDGF) and other peptides and proteins; and (3) **lysosomes,** which sequester acid hydrolases.

Platelets adhere, aggregate and degranulate when they contact fibrillar collagen (e.g., after vascular injury that exposes interstitial matrix proteins) or thrombin (after activation of the coagulation system) (Fig. 2-22). Degranulation releases serotonin (5-hydroxytryptamine), which, like histamine, directly increases vascular permeability. In addition, the platelet arachidonic acid metabolite TXA$_2$ plays a key

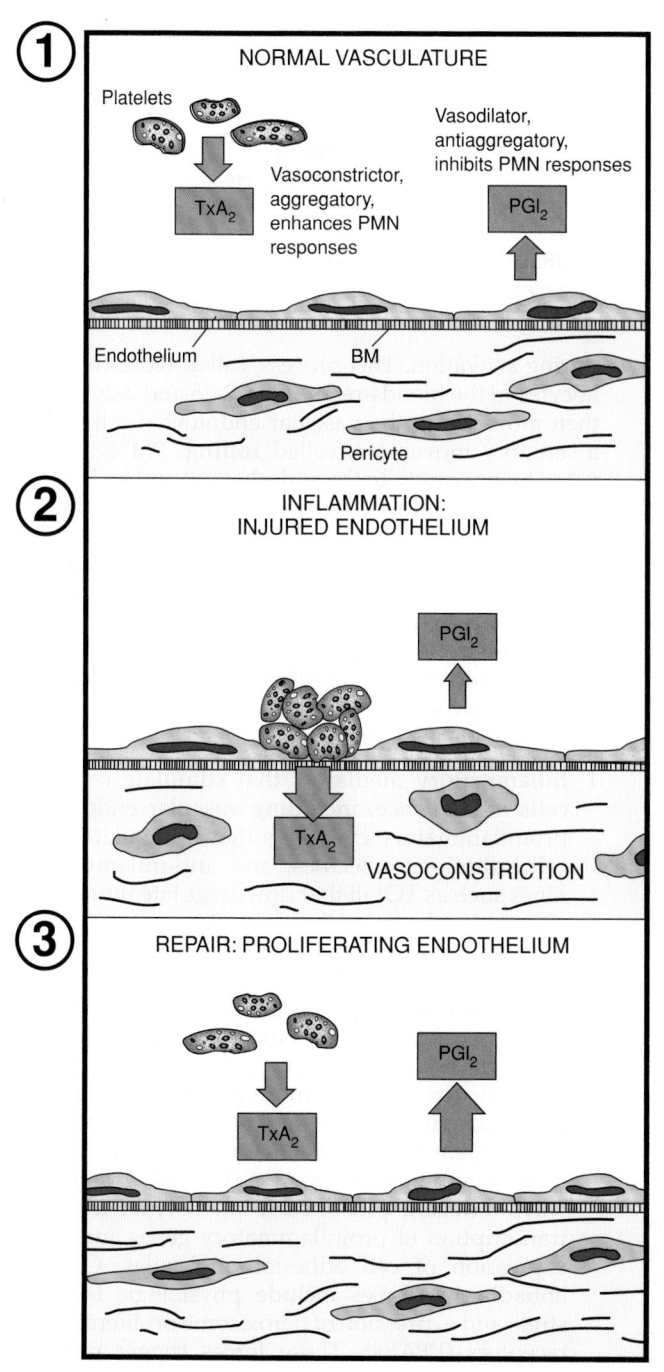

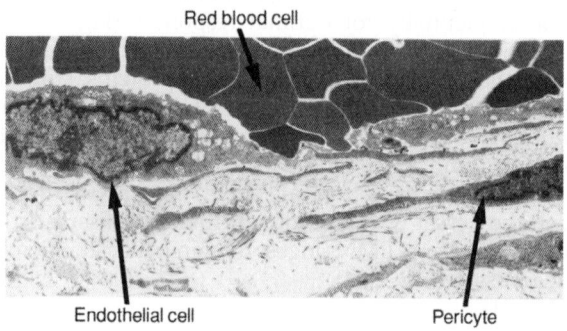

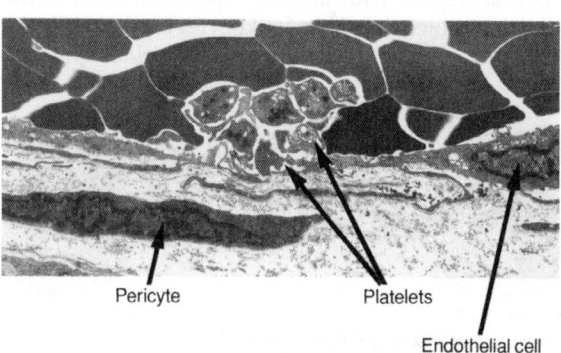

FIGURE 2-22. Regulation of platelet and endothelial cell interactions by thromboxane A$_2$ (TXA$_2$) and prostaglandin I$_2$ (PGI$_2$). 1. Platelet-derived TXA$_2$ and endothelial-derived PGI$_2$ maintain vasodilation and vasoconstriction in balance. **2.** During inflammation, the normal balance is shifted to vasoconstriction, increased vascular permeability, platelet aggregation and polymorphonuclear neutrophil (PMN) responses. **3.** During repair, the prostaglandin effects predominate, inhibiting PMN responses and promoting normal blood flow. *BM* = basement membrane.

role in the second wave of platelet aggregation and mediates smooth muscle constriction. On activation, platelets, as well as phagocytic cells, secrete cationic proteins that neutralize the negative charges on endothelium and promote increased permeability.

LEUKOCYTE RECRUITMENT IN ACUTE INFLAMMATION

An essential feature of inflammation is leukocyte accumulation, especially PMNs, in affected tissues. Swift recruitment requires a response orchestrated by chemoattractants that induce directed cell migration. In several models of neutrophil recruitment, lipid mediators, eicosanoids (such as LTB_4 interacting with neutrophil receptor BLT1), serum proteins (complement products C3a, C5a, cytokines) and chemokines function sequentially for optimal responses (Fig. 2-23). A variety of inflammatory stimuli, including proinflammatory cytokines, bacterial endotoxins and viral proteins, stimulate endothelial cells, resulting in loss of barrier function and recruitment of leukocytes. Leukocytes adhere to activated endothelium and are themselves activated in the process. They then flatten and migrate from the vascular space, through the vessel wall and into surrounding tissue. In the extravascular tissue, PMNs ingest foreign material, microbes and dead tissue (Fig. 2-24).

Leukocyte Adhesion to Endothelium Reflects Interaction of Complementary Adhesion Molecules

Leukocyte recruitment in postcapillary venules is a multistep process that begins with altered expression of endothelial cell adhesion molecules. Then leukocytes bind to endothelial cell selectins, which redistribute to endothelial cell surfaces

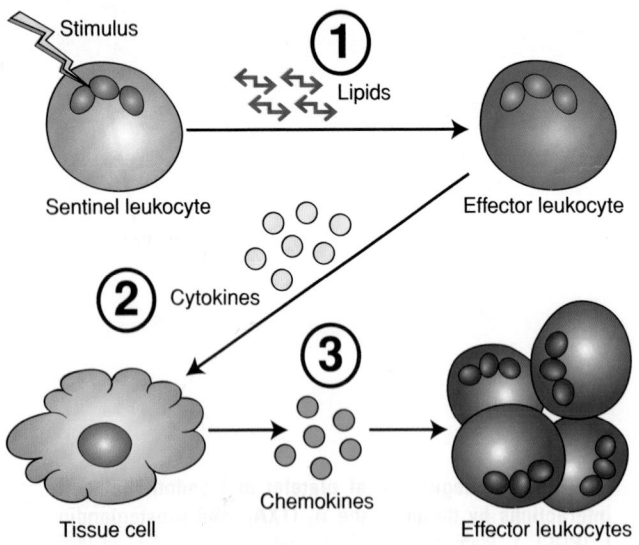

FIGURE 2-23. A schema of orchestrated initiation of inflammatory responses. 1. Lipid mediators (eicosanoids) are released from activated cells, resulting in early recruitment of inflammatory cells from bone marrow into the vascular system. **2.** Proinflammatory cytokines activate resident tissue cells, which in turn **(3)** release chemokines to amplify inflammatory cell recruitment.

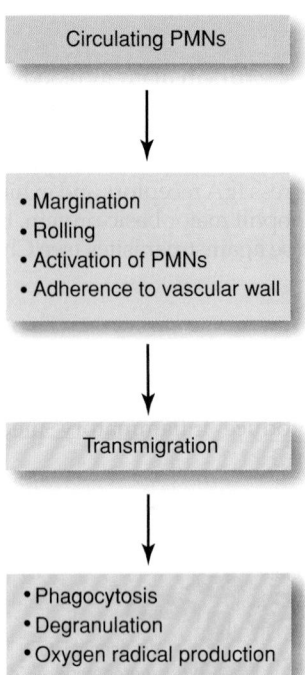

FIGURE 2-24. Leukocyte recruitment and activation. *PMNs* = polymorphonuclear neutrophils.

during activation. This process, called **tethering,** slows leukocytes in the bloodstream (Figs. 2-25 and 2-26). Leukocytes then move along the vascular endothelial cell surface with a saltatory movement, called **rolling.** PMNs become activated by proximity to the endothelium and by inflammatory mediators and adhere strongly to intercellular adhesion molecules (ICAMs) on the endothelium **(leukocyte arrest).** As endothelial cells separate, leukocytes **transmigrate** through the vessel wall and, under the influence of chemotactic factors, migrate to the site of injury.

Events in leukocyte recruitment are regulated by a temporal and spatial distribution of forces. Pro- and anti-inflammatory effects of healthy and diseased tissue microenvironments include:

1. Inflammatory mediators that stimulate resident tissue cells in sequence, including vascular endothelial cells; proinflammatory cytokines that upregulate endothelial cell adhesion molecules; and anti-inflammatory cytokines such as TGF-β that downregulate these same adhesion molecules as well as proinflammatory cytokines.
2. Chemotactic factors, which attract leukocytes along a chemical gradient to the site of injury (Fig. 2-25).
3. Expression of adhesion molecules on vascular endothelial cell surfaces, which bind to reciprocal molecules on the surfaces of circulating leukocytes. Endothelial cells are activated by exposure to proinflammatory cytokines and vasoactive peptides and by blood flow patterns, such as turbulent flow or oscillatory shear stress. NFκB and c-Jun N-terminal kinase-AP-1 (JNK-AP-1) signaling pathways induce a proadhesive phenotype, with increased transcription of proinflammatory genes and augmented expression of cell adhesion molecules. Counteracting antiadhesive forces include physiologic laminar shear stress and expression of peroxisome proliferator-activated receptors (PPARs). These forces trigger production of

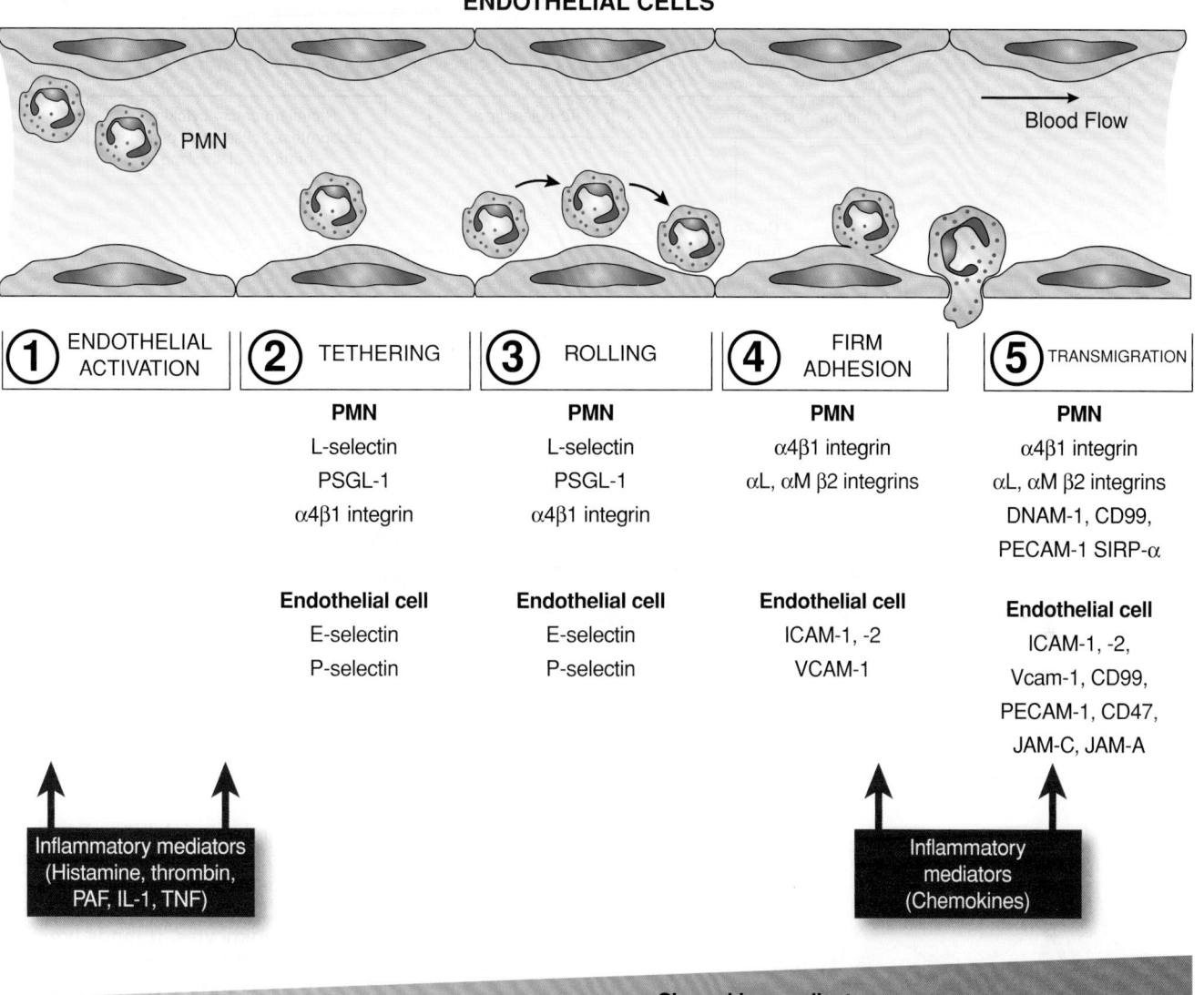

ENDOTHELIAL CELLS

FIGURE 2-25. Neutrophil adhesion and extravasation. 1. Inflammatory mediators activate endothelial cells to increase expression of adhesion molecules. Sialyl-Lewis X on neutrophil P-selectin glycoprotein-1 (PSGL-1) and E-selectin ligand (ESL-1) binds to P- and E-selectins to facilitate **(2)** tethering and **(3)** rolling of neutrophils. Increased integrins on activated neutrophils bind to intercellular adhesion molecule-1 (ICAM-1) on endothelial cells to form **(4)** a firm attachment. **5.** Endothelial cell attachments to one another are released and neutrophils then pass between separated cells to enter the tissue. *EC* = endothelial cell; *IL* = interleukin; *PAF* = platelet-activating factor; *PMN* = polymorphonuclear neutrophil; *TNF* = tumor necrosis factor.

superoxide dismutase (SOD) and NO, thus reducing O_2^- and oxidative stress, inhibiting proinflammatory cytokine expression and suppressing formation of specific adhesion molecules (Fig. 2-26).

Adhesion Molecules

Four molecular families of adhesion molecules are involved in leukocyte recruitment: selectins, addressins, integrins and immunoglobulins (Fig. 2-27).

Selectins

The selectin family includes P-selectin, E-selectin and L-selectin. They are expressed respectively on platelets and endothelial and leukocyte surfaces. Selectins share a

similar molecular structure: a chain of transmembrane glycoproteins with an extracellular lectin-binding domain. This calcium-dependent, or C-type, lectin binds sialylated oligosaccharides, specifically the sialyl-Lewis X moiety, on addressins, which allows rapid cell attachment and rolling.

P-selectin (CD62P, GMP-140, PADGEM) is preformed and stored in Weibel-Palade bodies of endothelial cells and α-granules of platelets. On stimulation with histamine, thrombin or specific inflammatory cytokines, P-selectin moves rapidly to the cell surface, where it binds sialyl-Lewis X on leukocyte surfaces. Preformed P-selectin can be delivered quickly to the cell surface, allowing rapid adhesive interaction between endothelial cells and leukocytes.

E-selectin (CD62E, ELAM-1) is not normally expressed on endothelial cell surfaces but is induced by inflammatory

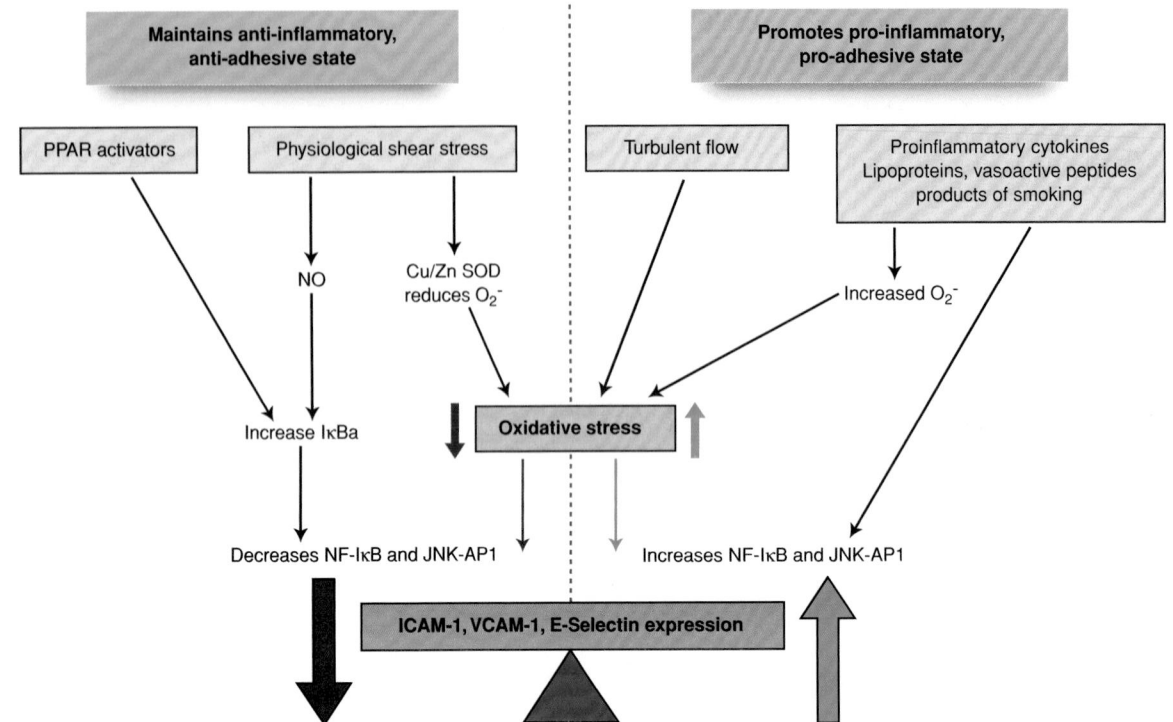

FIGURE 2-26. Balance of pro- and antiadhesive forces in vascular endothelial cells. Under physiologic conditions of vascular flow and expression of peroxisome proliferator-activated receptors (PPARs), oxidative stress and adhesion molecule expression are held in check. In the presence of proinflammatory mediators and turbulent flow or oscillatory shear stress, oxidative stress increases, followed by increased transcription of proinflammatory genes and enhanced expression of adhesion molecules.

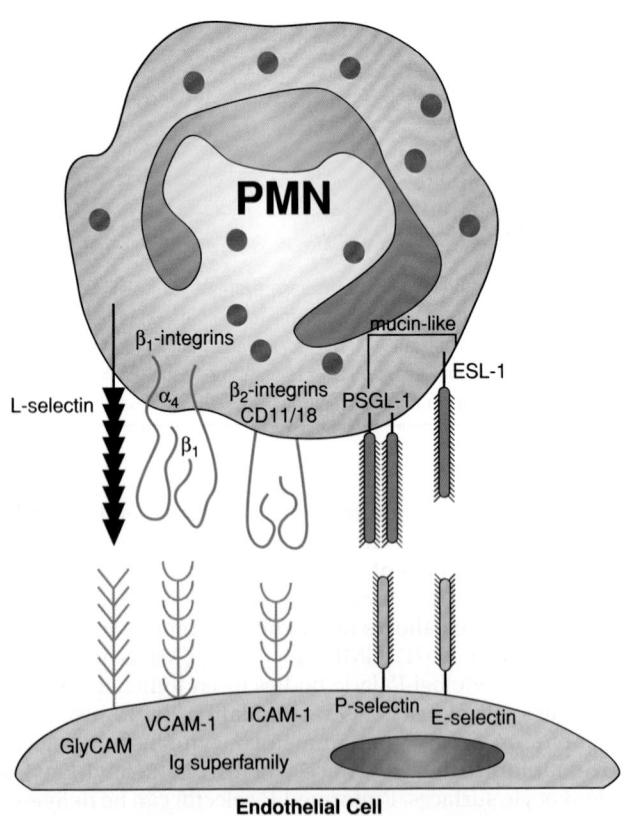

FIGURE 2-27. Leukocyte and endothelial cell adhesion molecules. *GlyCAM* = glycan-bearing cell adhesion molecule; *ICAM-1* = intercellular adhesion molecule-1; *VCAM* = vascular cell adhesion molecule.

mediators, such as cytokines or bacterial LPSs. E-selectin mediates adhesion of neutrophils, monocytes and certain lymphocytes by binding to Lewis X or Lewis A.

L-selectin (CD62L, LAM-1, Leu-8) is a "homing" molecule found on many types of leukocytes. It binds lymphocytes to high endothelial venules (HEVs) in lymphoid tissues, thus regulating trafficking. It also binds glycan-bearing cell adhesion molecule-1 (GlyCAM-1), mucosal addressin cell adhesion molecule-1 (MadCAM-1) and CD34.

This selectin-mediated interaction of PMNs and endothelial cells in turn enhances G-protein–mediated activation by endothelial chemokines. The chemokine-induced adhesion involves actin reorganization and α-integrins on neutrophil surfaces.

Addressins

Vascular addressins are mucin-like glycoproteins including GlyCAM-1, P-selectin glycoprotein-1 (PSGL-1), E-selectin ligand (ESL-1) and CD34. They possess sialyl-Lewis X, which binds the lectin domain of selectins. Addressins are expressed at leukocyte and endothelium surfaces. They regulate localization of leukocyte subpopulations and are involved in lymphocyte activation.

Integrins

Chemokines, lipid mediators and proinflammatory molecules activate cells to express integrin adhesion molecules (see Chapter 3). Integrins have transmembrane α- and β-chains arranged as heterodimers. They participate in cell–cell interactions, cell–ECM binding and leukocyte recruitment. *Very late activation* (VLA) molecules include VLA-4 ($\alpha_4\beta_1$) on leukocytes and lymphocytes, which bind vascular cell adhesion molecule-1 (VCAM-1) on endothelial cells. The β2 (CD18) integrins form molecules by association with α-integrin chains: $\alpha_l\beta_2$ and $\alpha_m\beta_2$ (CD11b/CD18 or Mac-1) bind ICAM-1 and ICAM-2, respectively. Leukocyte integrins exist in a low-affinity state but are converted to a high-affinity state via a G-protein–mediated conformational change when these cells are activated. This results in a transition from leukocyte rolling to firm adhesion.

Immunoglobulins

Adhesion molecules of the Ig superfamily include ICAM-1, ICAM-2 and VCAM-1, all of which interact with integrins on leukocytes to mediate recruitment. They are expressed at the surfaces of cytokine-stimulated endothelial cells and some leukocytes, as well as certain epithelial cells, such as pulmonary alveolar cells.

Junctional adhesion molecules (JAMs) are also proteins of the Ig superfamily. JAM-A, JAM-B and JAM-C are found on endothelial cells, leukocytes and platelets. JAM-A binds the integrin LFA-1; VLA-4 binds to JAM-B; MAC1 connects with JAM-C.

Adhesion Molecules Mediating Endothelial Barrier Function and Leukocyte Recruitment

Endothelial cells adhere to one another to seal off the vascular space from adjacent tissue. The vascular endothelial–cadherin complex forms adherens junctions, and occludin, claudins and JAMs, PECAM-1 (platelet endothelial cell adhesion molecule) and CD99, each adherent to homologous molecules on adjacent endothelial cells, form tight junctions. Together, these molecules create a barrier to transmigration of cells from the vascular space (Fig. 2-28A).

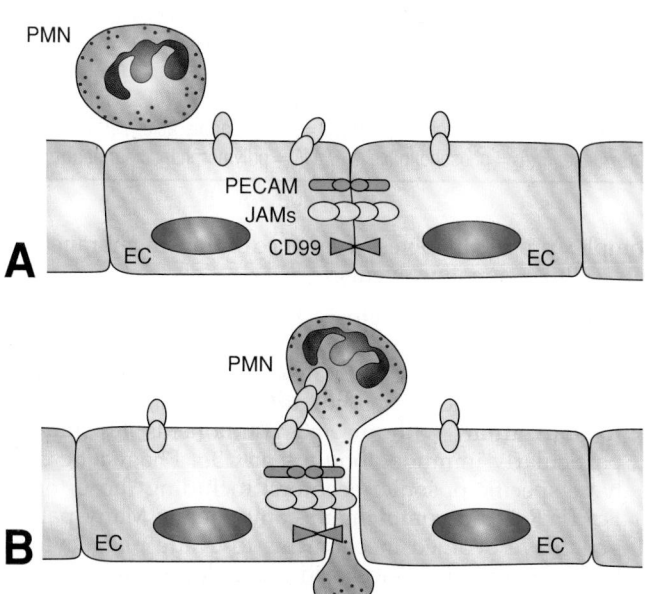

FIGURE 2-28. Endothelial cell junctional molecules participate in leukocyte recruitment. A. Junctional molecules contribute to cell–cell adhesion and maintenance of endothelial barrier function. **B.** These same molecules regulate paracellular transmigration of leukocytes. *PMN* = polymorphonuclear neutrophil; *EC* = endothelial cell; *PECAM* = platelet endothelial cell adhesion molecule, CD31; *JAMs* = junctional adhesion molecules.

Tethering, Rolling and Firm Adhesion Are Prerequisites for Leukocyte Recruitment into Tissues

Endothelial cells are activated by blood flow patterns and exposure to proinflammatory cytokines and vasoactive peptides. These trigger NFκB and JNK-AP-1 signaling to elicit a proadhesive phenotype, with increased surface cell adhesion molecules (Fig. 2-26). Cytokines or chemokines specific to the inflammatory process induce adhesion molecules on endothelium and leukocytes and change their affinity for their ligands.

For a rolling cell to adhere, there is a selectin-dependent reduction in rolling velocity. Early increases in rolling depend on P-selectin, whereas cytokine-induced E-selectin initiates early adhesion. Integrin family members function cooperatively with selectins to facilitate rolling and subsequent firm adhesion of leukocytes. Leukocyte β_1 and β_2 integrins bind their counterreceptors, the Ig superfamily of ligands (VCAM-1, ICAM-1, ICAM-2, JAMs), on endothelium. This process further slows leukocytes and increases the exposure time for each leukocyte to endothelium. Simultaneously, engagement of adhesion molecules activates intracellular signal transduction. As a result, leukocytes and endothelial cells are further activated, with subsequent upregulation of L-selectin and integrin binding. The net result is firm adhesion.

Recruitment of specific subsets of leukocytes to areas of inflammation results from unique patterns or relative densities of adhesion molecules on cell surfaces. For subsets of leukocytes, each cell type can express specific adhesion molecules. Leukocyte adherence to arterioles and capillaries also has different requirements, as hydrodynamic forces in these vessels differ. Regional recruitment is also influenced by vascular flow conditions, which alter expression of adhesion molecules and leukocyte transmigration.

Chemotactic Molecules Direct Neutrophils to Sites of Injury

Leukocytes must be accurately positioned at sites of inflammatory injury to function correctly. For the right subsets of leukocytes to arrive in a timely fashion, they must get very specific directions. *Leukocytes are guided through vascular and extravascular spaces by a complex interaction of attractants, repellants and adhesion molecules.* **Chemotaxis** is a dynamic and energy-dependent process of directed cell migration. Blood leukocytes are recruited by chemoattractants released by endothelial cells. They migrate from the endothelium toward the target tissue, down a gradient of one chemoattractant in response to a second, more distal chemoattractant gradient.

PMNs must integrate the various signals to arrive at the correct site at the correct time for their assigned tasks. Their most important chemotactic factors are C5a, bacterial and mitochondrial products (particularly low–molecular-weight N-formylated peptides such as FMLP), products of arachidonic acid metabolism (especially LTB$_4$), products of ECM degradation and chemokines. The latter represent a key mechanism of leukocyte recruitment because they generate a chemotactic gradient by binding to ECM proteoglycans. As a result, high concentrations of chemokines persist at sites of tissue injury. In turn, specific receptors on migrating leukocytes bind matrix-bound chemokines, moving cells along the chemotactic gradient to the site of injury.

Chemotactic factors for other cell types, including lymphocytes, basophils and eosinophils, are also produced at sites of tissue injury and may be secreted by activated endothelial cells, tissue parenchymal cells or other inflammatory cells. They include PAF, TGF-β, neutrophilic cationic proteins and lymphokines. *The cocktail of chemokines within a tissue largely determines the types of leukocytes that come to the site.* When cells arrive at their destination, they must then be able to stop there. Contact guidance, regulated adhesion molecules or inhibitory signals determine the final arrest of specific cells in specific tissue locations.

Leukocytes Traverse the Endothelium to Gain Access to Tissues

Leukocytes adherent to the endothelium emigrate by **paracellular diapedesis** (i.e., passing between adjacent endothelial cells). Responding to chemokine gradients, neutrophils extend pseudopods and insinuate themselves between the endothelial cells, then out of the intravascular space.

Several adhesion molecules, expressed intercellularly, contribute to tight adhesion between endothelial cells. However, they may also release during leukocyte transmigration or redistribute to cell surfaces to facilitate leukocyte recruitment (Fig. 2-28). JAMs are proteins of the immunoglobulin superfamily. JAM-A, JAM-B and JAM-C are expressed on endothelial cells, leukocytes and platelets. JAMs, CD99 and PECAM-1 (CD31, platelet endothelial cell adhesion molecule) on endothelial cell surfaces bind to each other to keep cells together. These junctions separate under the influence of inflammatory mediators, intracellular signals generated by adhesion molecule engagement and signals from the adherent neutrophils. Neutrophils mobilize elastase to their pseudopod membranes, inducing endothelial cells to retract and separate at the advancing edge of the neutrophil, a process facilitated by PMN-elicited increases in endothelial cell intracellular calcium. At the same time, JAMs and particularly CD99 and PECAM are integral to neutrophil adhesion to endothelial cells during this process of transmigration.

A little-understood method of migration of neutrophils through endothelial cells is **transcellular diapedesis**. In tissues with fenestrated microvessels, such as gut mucosa and secretory glands, PMNs may traverse thin regions of endothelium, called **fenestrae**, without damaging endothelial cells. In nonfenestrated microvessels, PMNs may cross the endothelium using endothelial cell caveolae or pinocytotic vesicles, which form small, membrane-bound passageways across the cell.

INFLAMMATORY CELL FUNCTIONS IN ACUTE INFLAMMATION

Phagocytosis of Microorganisms and Tissue Debris

Many inflammatory cells—including monocytes, tissue macrophages, dendritic cells and neutrophils—recognize, internalize and digest foreign material, microorganisms or cellular debris by **phagocytosis**. This term, first used over a century ago by Elie Metchnikoff, is now defined as ingestion by eukaryotic cells of large (usually >0.5 μm) insoluble particles and microorganisms. **Phagocytes** are effector cells. The

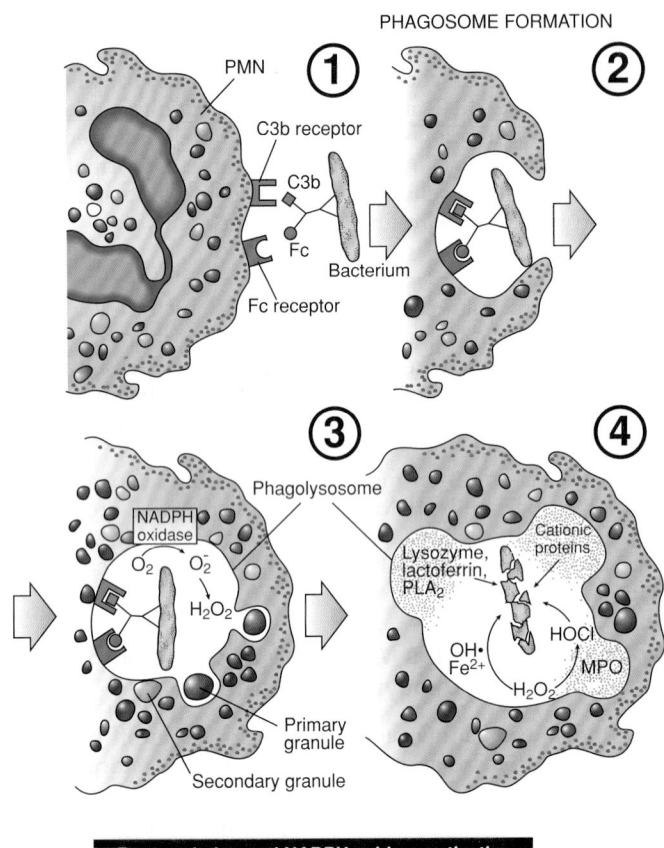

PHAGOSOME FORMATION

- Degranulation and NADPH oxidase activation
- Bacterial killing and digestion

FIGURE 2-29. Mechanisms of neutrophil bacterial phagocytosis and cell killing. 1. Opsonins such as C3b coat the surface of microbes, allowing recognition by the neutrophil C3b receptor. **2.** Receptor clustering triggers intracellular signaling and actin assembly within the neutrophil. Pseudopods form around the microbe to enclose it within a phagosome. **3.** Lysosomal granules fuse with the phagosome to form a phagolysosome, into which the lysosomal enzymes and oxygen radicals are released to **(4)** kill and degrade the microbe. Fe^{2+} = ferrous iron; HOCl = hypochlorous acid; MPO = myeloperoxidase; PLA_2 = phospholipase A_2; PMN = polymorphonuclear neutrophil.

complex process involves a sequence of transmembrane and intracellular signaling events:

1. **Recognition:** Phagocytosis is initiated when specific receptors on the surface of phagocytic cells recognize their targets (Fig. 2-29). Phagocytosis of most biological agents is enhanced by, if not dependent on, their coating (**opsonization**) with plasma components (**opsonins**), particularly immunoglobulins or C3b. Phagocytic cells have specific opsonic receptors, including those for Ig Fcγ (FcRs) and complement components. Many pathogens have evolved mechanisms to evade phagocytosis by leukocytes. Polysaccharide capsules, protein A, protein M or peptidoglycans around bacteria can prevent complement deposition or antigen recognition and receptor binding.

2. **Signaling:** Clumping of opsonins at bacterial surfaces causes phagocyte plasma membrane Fcγ receptors to cluster. Subsequent phosphorylation of immunoreceptor, tyrosine-based, activation motifs (ITAMs), in the cytosolic domain or γ subunit of the receptor, triggers intracellular

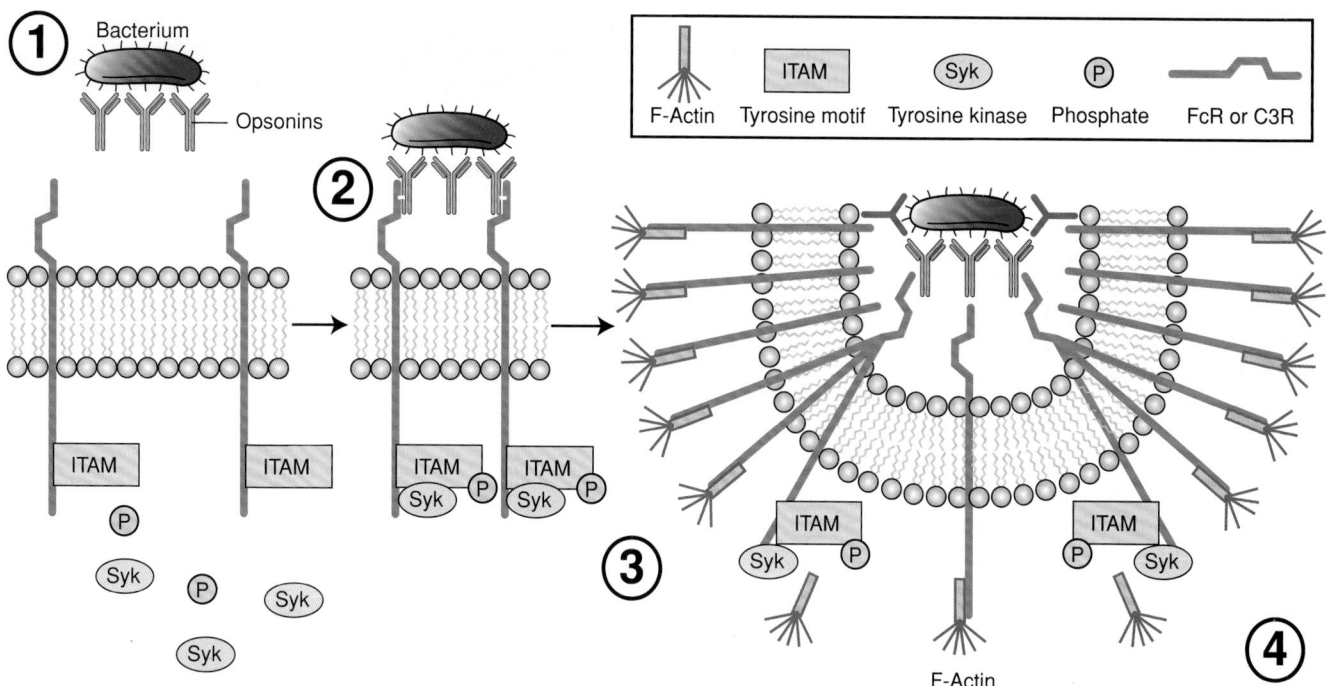

FIGURE 2-30. Intracellular signaling during leukocyte phagocytosis. 1. Opsonins coating the surface of microbes or foreign material are recognized by the neutrophil C3b receptor. **2.** Receptor clustering triggers **(3)** phosphorylation of immunoreceptor tyrosine-based activation motifs (ITAMs) on the receptor, and tyrosine kinases initiate intracellular signaling. **4.** Polymerized actin filament aggregates beneath the plasma membrane to form a pseudopod to enclose the foreign agent.

signaling via tyrosine kinases that associate with the Fcγ receptor (Fig. 2-30).

3. **Internalization:** For Fcγ receptor or CR3, actin assembly occurs directly under the phagocytosed target. Polymerized actin filaments push the plasma membrane forward. The plasma membrane remodels to increase surface area and to form pseudopods surrounding the foreign material. The resulting phagocytic cup engulfs the foreign agent. The membrane then "zippers" around the opsonized particle to enclose it in a vacuole called a **phagosome** (Fig. 2-29).

4. **Digestion:** The phagosome with the foreign material fuses to cytoplasmic lysosomes to form a **phagolysosome,** into which lysosomal enzymes are released. The acid pH in the phagolysosome activates these hydrolytic enzymes, which then degrade the phagocytosed material. Some microorganisms have evolved mechanisms for evading killing by neutrophils by preventing lysosomal degranulation or inhibiting neutrophil enzymes.

Inflammatory Cell Enzymes Provide Antimicrobial Defense and Debridement

PMNs and macrophages are critical for degrading microbes and cell debris but may also cause tissue injury (Fig. 2-31): release of PMN granule contents at sites of injury is a double-edged sword. On the one hand, debridement of damaged tissue by proteolytic breakdown facilitates tissue repair. On the other hand, degradative enzymes can damage endothelial and epithelial cells and degrade connective tissue.

Inflammatory cells possess the armamentarium of enzymes used to degrade microbes and tissue. Neutrophil primary, secondary and tertiary granules are morphologically

and biochemically distinct; each has unique activities (Fig. 2-17).

■ **Primary granules (azurophilic granules):** Antimicrobial and proteinase activity of these granules can directly activate other inflammatory cells. Potent acid hydrolases and

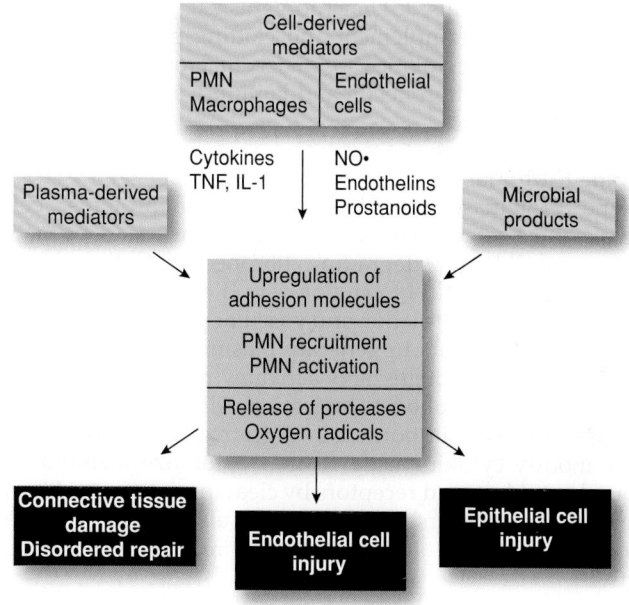

FIGURE 2-31. Mechanisms of cell and tissue damage. *IL* = interleukin; *LPS* = lipopolysaccharide; *NO•* = nitric oxide; *PMN* = polymorphonuclear neutrophil; *TNF* = tumor necrosis factor.

neutral serine proteases digest diverse macromolecules. Lysozyme and PLA_2 degrade bacterial cell walls and biological membranes and are important in killing bacteria. Myeloperoxidase, a key enzyme in the metabolism of hydrogen peroxide, generates toxic ROS.

- **Secondary granules (specific granules):** These contain PLA_2, lysozyme and proteins that initiate killing of specific cells. In addition, their contents include the cationic lactoferrin, a vitamin B_{12}–binding protein and matrix metalloproteinase (collagenase) specific for type IV collagen.
- **Tertiary granules (small storage granules, C granules):** These granules are released at the leading front of neutrophils during chemotaxis. They are the source of enzymes that promote migration of cells through basement membranes and tissues, including proteinases, cathepsin, gelatinase and urokinase-type plasminogen activator (u-PA).

In the macrophage, the specific array of agents released varies, depending on the role of the macrophage as pro- or anti-inflammatory (Figs. 2-17C and 2-20).

Proteinases

Proteolytic enzymes (proteinases) are stored in cytoplasmic granules and secretory vesicles of neutrophils. They cleave peptide bonds in polypeptides. As PMNs leave the circulation, they release proteinases that enable them to penetrate the ECM and migrate to sites of injury, there to degrade matrix, cell debris and pathogens. Neutrophils are not the only source of proteinases, however. Monocytes, eosinophils, basophils, mast cells, lymphocytes and tissue cells, including endothelium, also produce proteinases.

Proteinases are grouped by their catalytic activity: serine proteinases and metalloproteinases are neutral enzymes that work in extracellular spaces; cysteine proteinases and aspartic proteinases are acidic and act in the acidic milieu of lysosomes (Table 2-3). These enzymes target many intracellular and extracellular proteins, such as (1) inflammatory products; (2) debris from damaged cells, microbial proteins and matrix proteins; (3) microorganisms; (4) plasma proteins, including complement and clotting proteins, immunoglobulins and cytokines; (5) matrix macromolecules (e.g., collagen, elastin, fibronectin and laminin); and (6) lymphocytes and platelets.

Serine Proteinases
Serine proteinases degrade extracellular proteins, cell debris and bacteria. Human leukocyte elastase is primarily responsible for degrading fibronectin. Cathepsin G converts angiotensin I to angiotensin II, thereby mediating smooth muscle contraction and vascular permeability. u-PA dissolves fibrin clots to generate plasmin at wound sites, degrades ECM proteins and activates procollagenases to create a path for leukocyte migration. Although serine proteinases are most important in digesting ECM molecules, they modify cytokine activity; they solubilize membrane-bound cytokines and receptors by cleaving active cytokines from inactive precursors as well. They also detach cytokine receptors from cell surfaces, thereby regulating cytokine activity.

Metalloproteinases
At least 25 metalloproteinases are known (see Chapter 3). Matrix metalloproteinases (**MMPs**, matrixins) degrade all ECM components, including basement membranes. They

TABLE 2-3
PROTEINASES IN INFLAMMATION

Enzyme Class	Examples
Neutral Proteinases	
Serine proteinases	Human leukocyte elastase
	Cathepsin G
	Proteinase 3
	Urokinase-type plasminogen
	Activator
Metalloproteinase	Collagenases (MMP-1, MMP-8, MMP-13)
	Gelatinases (MMP-7, MMP-9)
	Stromelysins (MMP-3, MMP-10, MMP-11)
	Matrilysin (MMP-7)
	Metalloelastase (MMP-12)
	ADAMs-7, -9, -15, -17
Acidic Proteinases	
Cysteine proteinases	Cathepsins, S, L, B, H
Aspartic proteinases	Cathepsin D

MMP = matrix metalloproteinase; ADAM = *A* protein with *d*isintegrin and *m*etalloproteinase domains.

are subgrouped by substrate specificity into interstitial collagenases, gelatinases, stromelysins, metalloelastases and matrilysin. Proteins with metalloproteinase and disintegrin domains (ADAMs) regulate neutrophil infiltration by targeting disintegrins, polypeptides that disrupt integrin-mediated binding of cells to each other and to the ECM.

Cysteine Proteinases and Aspartic Proteinases
These acid proteinases function primarily within lysosomes of leukocytes to degrade intracellular proteins.

Proteinase Inhibitors

The proteolytic environment is regulated by a battery of inhibitors. During wound healing, these antiproteases protect from tissue damage by limiting protease activity. ECM remodeling entails a balance between enzymes and their inhibitors. In chronic wounds, ongoing influx of neutrophils, with their proteases and ROS, may overwhelm and inactivate these inhibitors, allowing continuation of proteolysis (see Chapter 3). Known proteinase inhibitors include:

- α_2-**Macroglobulin:** Nonspecific inhibitor of all classes of proteinases, primarily found in plasma
- **Serpins:** The major inhibitors of serine proteinases
- α_1-**Antiproteases (α_1-antitrypsin, α_1-antichymotrypsin):** Inhibit human leukocyte elastase and cathepsin G
- **Secretory leukocyte proteinase inhibitor (SLPI), Elafin:** Inhibit proteinase 3
- **Plasminogen activator inhibitors (PAIs):** Inhibit u-PA
- **Tissue inhibitors of metalloproteinases (TIMP-1s):** Specific for tissue matrix metalloproteinases

Inflammatory Cells Kill Bacteria by ROS- and Non-ROS-Mediated Mechanisms

Bacterial Killing by Oxygen Species

Phagocytosis is accompanied by metabolic reactions in inflammatory cells that lead to production of oxygen metabolites (see Chapter 1). These ROS are more reactive than oxygen itself and contribute to the killing of ingested bacteria (Fig. 2-29).

- **Superoxide anion** (O_2^-): Phagocytosis activates an NADPH oxidase in PMN cell membranes. NADPH oxidase is a multicomponent electron transport complex that reduces molecular oxygen to O_2^-. Activation of this enzyme is enhanced by prior exposure of cells to a chemotactic stimulus or LPS. NADPH oxidase increases oxygen consumption and stimulates the hexose monophosphate shunt. Together, these cell responses are the **respiratory burst**.
- **Hydrogen peroxide** (H_2O_2): O_2^- is rapidly converted to H_2O_2 at the cell surface and in phagolysosomes by SOD. H_2O_2 is stable and is a source for generating additional reactive oxidants.
- **Hypochlorous acid** (HOCl): Myeloperoxidase (MPO), a neutrophil product with a very strong cationic charge, is secreted from granules during exocytosis. In the presence of a halide, usually chlorine, MPO catalyzes conversion of H_2O_2 to HOCl. This powerful oxidant is a major bactericidal agent made by phagocytic cells. It also helps activate neutrophil-derived collagenase and gelatinase, both of which are secreted as latent enzymes. HOCl also inactivates α_1-antitrypsin.
- **Hydroxyl radical** (OH•): Reduction of H_2O_2 via the Haber-Weiss reaction, forms the highly reactive OH•. This occurs slowly at physiologic pH, but if ferrous iron (Fe^{2+}) is present, the Fenton reaction rapidly converts H_2O_2 to OH•, which is a potent bactericidal agent. Further reduction of OH• yields H_2O (see Chapter 1).
- **Nitric oxide** (NO•): Phagocytes and endothelial cells produce NO• and its derivatives, which have many physiologic and nonphysiologic effects. NO• and other free radicals interact with one another to balance their cytotoxic and cytoprotective effects. NO• can react with oxygen radicals to form toxic molecules such as peroxynitrite and *S*-nitrosothiols, or it can scavenge O_2^-, thus reducing the amount of toxic radicals.

Monocytes, macrophages and eosinophils also make oxygen radicals, depending on their state of activation and the stimulus to which they are exposed. Production of ROS by these cells contributes to their bactericidal and fungicidal activity and to their ability to kill certain parasites. The importance of oxygen-dependent bacterial killing is exemplified in **chronic granulomatous disease** of childhood, a hereditary deficiency of NADPH oxidase. Affected patients fail to produce O_2^- and H_2O_2 during phagocytosis and so are prone to recurrent infections, especially with gram-positive cocci. Patients with a related genetic deficiency in MPO cannot produce HOCl and are excessively susceptible to fungal infections with *Candida* (Table 2-4).

Nonoxidative Bacterial Killing

Phagocytes, particularly PMNs and monocytes/macrophages, have substantial oxygen-independent antimicrobial

TABLE 2-4

CONGENITAL DISEASES OF DEFECTIVE PHAGOCYTIC CELL FUNCTION CHARACTERIZED BY RECURRENT BACTERIAL INFECTIONS

Disease	Defect
Leukocyte adhesion deficiency (LAD)	LAD-1 (defective β_2-integrin expression or function [CD11/CD18]) LAD-2 (defective fucosylation, selectin binding)
Hyper-IgE-recurrent infection, (Job) syndrome	Poor chemotaxis
Chediak-Higashi syndrome	Defective lysosomal granules, poor chemotaxis
Neutrophil-specific granule deficiency	Absent neutrophil granules
Chronic granulomatous disease	Deficient NADPH oxidase, with absent H_2O_2 production
Myeloperoxidase deficiency	Deficient HOCl production

H_2O_2 = hydrogen peroxide; HOCl = hypochlorous acid; Ig = immunoglobulin; NADPH = nicotinamide adenine dinucleotide phosphate.

activity. This activity mainly involves bactericidal proteins in cytoplasmic granules, such as lysosomal acid hydrolases and specialized noncatalytic proteins unique to inflammatory cells.

- **Lysosomal hydrolases:** Primary and secondary granules in PMNs and lysosomes of mononuclear phagocytes contain hydrolases, such as sulfatases, phosphatases and other enzymes that can digest polysaccharides and DNA.
- **Bactericidal/permeability-increasing protein (BPI):** This cationic protein in PMN primary granules can kill many gram-negative bacteria but is not toxic to gram-positive bacteria or eukaryotic cells. BPI inserts into bacterial envelope outer membranes and increases their permeability. Activation of certain phospholipases and enzymes then degrades bacterial peptidylglycans.
- **Defensins:** Primary granules of PMNs and lysosomes of some mononuclear phagocytes contain these cationic proteins, which kill many gram-positive and gram-negative bacteria, fungi and some enveloped viruses. Some also kill host cells. Defensins are chemotactic for phagocytes, immature dendritic cells and lymphocytes and so help mobilize and amplify antimicrobial immunity.
- **Lactoferrin:** Lactoferrin is an iron-binding glycoprotein in neutrophil secondary granules and in most body secretory fluids. It chelates iron and so competes with bacteria for iron. It may help generate OH• for oxidative killing of bacteria.
- **Lysozyme:** This bactericidal enzyme is found in many tissues and body fluids, in primary and secondary granules of PMNs and in lysosomes of mononuclear phagocytes. Peptidoglycans of gram-positive bacterial cell walls are sensitive to degradation by lysozyme; gram-negative bacteria are usually resistant to it.
- **Eosinophils' bactericidal proteins:** Eosinophils have several granule-bound cationic proteins, the most important

of which are major basic protein (MBP) and eosinophilic cationic protein. Both are potent killers of many parasites, though not bacteria. MBP accounts for half of the total protein of eosinophil granules.

Defects in Leukocyte Function

The importance of acute inflammatory cells in protection from infection is underscored by the frequency and severity of infections when PMNs are depleted or defective. *The most common such deficit is iatrogenic neutropenia due to cancer chemotherapy.* Functional impairment of phagocytes may occur at any step in the sequence: adherence, emigration, chemotaxis, phagocytosis or killing. These disorders may be acquired or congenital. Acquired diseases, such as leukemia, diabetes, malnutrition, viral infections and sepsis, often entail defects in inflammatory cell function. Table 2-4 shows representative examples of congenital diseases linked to defective phagocytic function.

REGULATION OF THE ACUTE INFLAMMATORY RESPONSE

Infection, foreign agents and injured tissue are triggers for acute inflammation. The specificity and intensity of inflammatory mediators, both humoral and cellular, affect tissue responses to the offending agents. Left unchecked, acute inflammation can cause serious tissue injury and death. However, genetic and biochemical regulation mitigates "bystander" effects of acute inflammation, thus allowing resolution and repair. Positive and negative regulation and modulation of these responses occurs at several levels, including (1) release of pro- or anti-inflammatory mediators, (2) expression of surface molecules, (3) intracellular signaling pathways with positive and negative feedback loops and (4) gene expression of molecules involved in the inflammatory process.

Soluble Mediators Activate Common Intracellular Pathways

Plasma- and cell-derived proinflammatory mediators amplify tissue responses in a positive feedback loop, with progressive amplification and resultant tissue injury. Complement, proinflammatory cytokines and, in some cases, immune complexes activate signal transduction pathways that control expression of proinflammatory mediators, including TNF-α, IL-1, chemokines and adhesion molecules. Secreted cytokines then propagate responses by activating other cell types via these and similar pathways. The process by which diverse stimuli lead to functional inflammatory responses is **stimulus–response coupling**. Stimuli include microbial products and the many plasma- or cell-derived inflammatory mediators described in this chapter. Although intracellular signaling pathways are complex and vary with cell type and stimulus, some common intracellular pathways are associated with inflammatory cell activation by soluble mediators, including G-protein, TNF receptor (TNFR) and JAK-STAT pathways (Janus kinase–signal transducer and activator of transcription) (Figs. 2-32, 2-33, and 2-34, respectively).

The inflammatory response is also regulated so as to contain the cascade described above and to limit tissue damage.

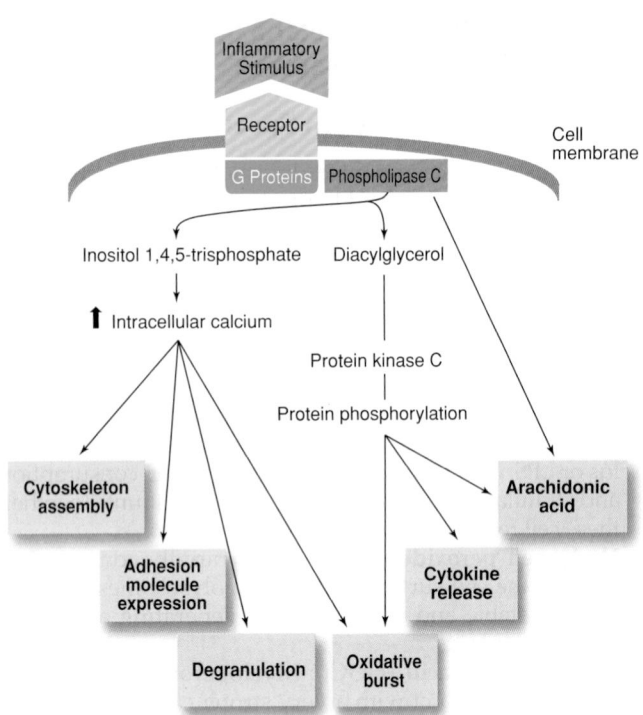

FIGURE 2-32. G-protein–mediated intracellular signal transduction pathway common to many inflammatory stimuli.

Inducible cytokines, like IL-4, IL-10 and IL-12, block NFκB activation by stabilizing its inhibitor, Iκb, thus reducing the response. Protease inhibitors, such as secreted leukocyte protease inhibitor (SLPI); inhibitors of metalloproteases (e.g., tissue inhibitor of MMPs [TIMPs]); antioxidant enzymes (e.g., peroxide dismutase); lipoxins; glucocorticoids and phosphatases; and transcriptional regulatory factors, including suppressor of cytokine signaling (SOC), inhibit the activation of proinflammatory factors, oxidants and signaling pathways.

G-Protein Pathways

Many chemokines, hormones, neurotransmitters and other mediators signal via G-binding proteins (Fig. 2-32). G proteins

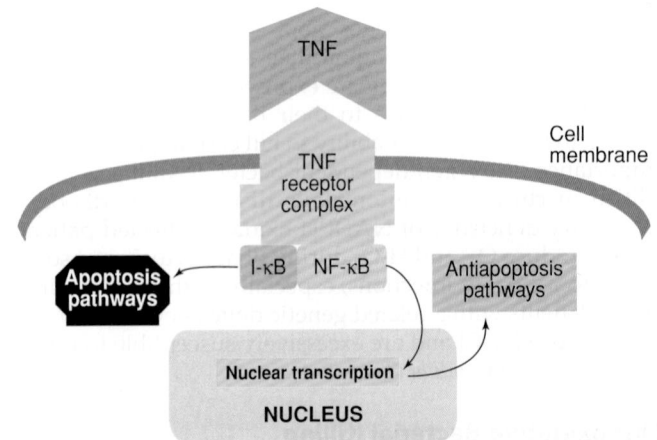

FIGURE 2-33. Tumor necrosis factor (TNF) receptor–mediated intracellular signal transduction pathway.

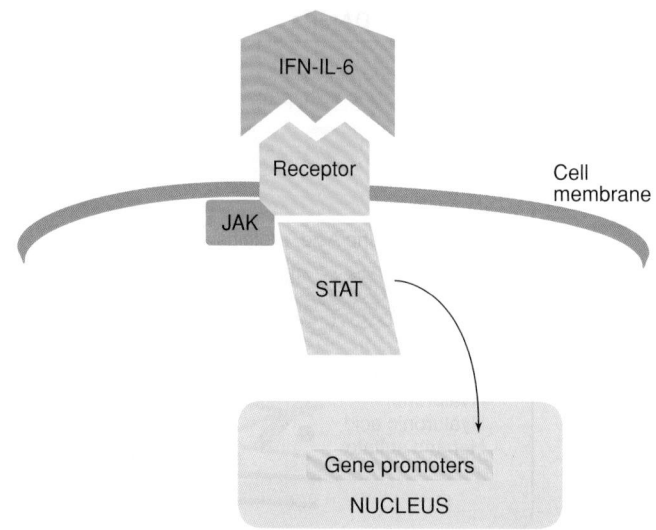

FIGURE 2-34. JAK-STAT–mediated intracellular transduction pathway. *IFN* = interferon; *IL* = interleukin.

vary in downstream intracellular signaling pathways, but common activities include:

- **Ligand–receptor binding:** Binding of a stimulatory factor to a specific cell membrane receptor creates a ligand–receptor complex. Exchange of guanosine diphosphate (GDP) for guanosine triphosphate (GTP) activates the G protein, which dissociates into subunits that, in turn, activate phospholipase C (PLC) and phosphatidylinositol-3-kinase (PI3K).
- **Phospholipid metabolism of cell membranes:** PLC hydrolyzes a plasma membrane phosphoinositide (phosphatidylinositol bisphosphate [PIP$_2$]) to generate diacylglycerol and inositol trisphosphate (IP$_3$).
- **Elevated cytosolic free calcium:** IP$_3$ induces release of stored intracellular Ca^{2+}. Together with influx of Ca^{2+} from the extracellular fluid, IP$_3$ increases cytosolic free calcium, a key event in inflammatory cell activation.
- **Protein phosphorylation and dephosphorylation:** Specific tyrosine kinases bind the ligand–receptor complex and initiate a series of protein phosphorylations.
- **Protein kinase C activation:** Protein kinase C (PKC) and other protein kinases activate intracellular signaling pathways, often activating gene transcription.

Tumor Necrosis Factor Receptor Pathways

TNF-α is central to the development of inflammation and its symptoms. It induces tumor cell apoptosis and regulates immune functions (Fig. 2-33). TNF-α and related proteins bind two cell surface receptors to form a multiprotein-signaling complex at the cell membrane. This complex can trigger (1) apoptosis-related enzymes (i.e., **caspases**) (see Chapter 1), (2) inhibitors of apoptosis or (3) the transcription factor **NFκB**. NFκB activity is regulated by association with, and disassociation from, the NFκB inhibitor, IκB. If IκB is bound to NFκB, the latter cannot translocate to the nucleus, where it can act as a transcriptional activator. This latter pathway is critical to regulation of TNF-mediated events during inflammation.

JAK-STAT Pathway

This pathway provides a direct route from extracellular polypeptides (e.g., growth factors) or cytokines (e.g., interferons or interleukins) through cell receptors to gene promoters in the nucleus. Ligand–receptor interactions elicit transcription complexes of JAK-STAT. STAT proteins translocate to the nucleus, where they regulate gene promoters (Fig. 2-34).

Pathogens and Damaged Cells Regulate Gene Expression

Four phases of gene expression in inflammation are shown in Fig. 2-35.

1. **Initiation** of an inflammatory response, often by microbial products
2. **Gene activation** to induce proinflammatory mediators
3. **Reprogramming** to silence acute proinflammatory genes and activate anti-inflammatory mediators
4. **Gene silencing** to promote resolution of inflammatory responses and allow tissue to recover its integrity

Initiation of Inflammation

Infectious agents or damaged cells trigger signaling pathways, leading to an innate or adaptive immune response. In the setting of infection, **pathogen-associated microbial patterns** (PAMPs) of microorganisms are recognized by membrane-bound or endosomal families of **pattern-recognition receptors** (PRRs). **Danger (damage)-associated molecular patterns** (DAMPs) derived from damaged cells are released extracellularly after tissue injury and are also recognized by PRRs located on cell surfaces and intracellularly. Together, they activate intracellular cascades to drive a coordinated immune response (Figs. 2-36 and 2-37).

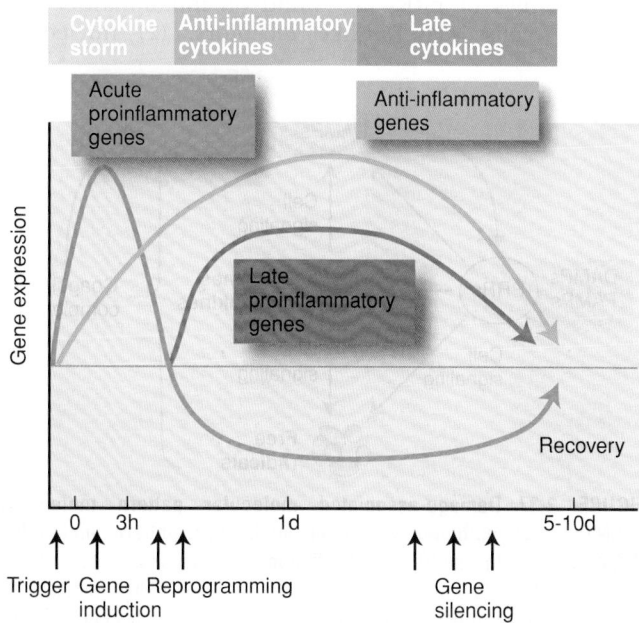

FIGURE 2-35. Time course of gene expression in the activation and regulation phases of the acute inflammatory response.

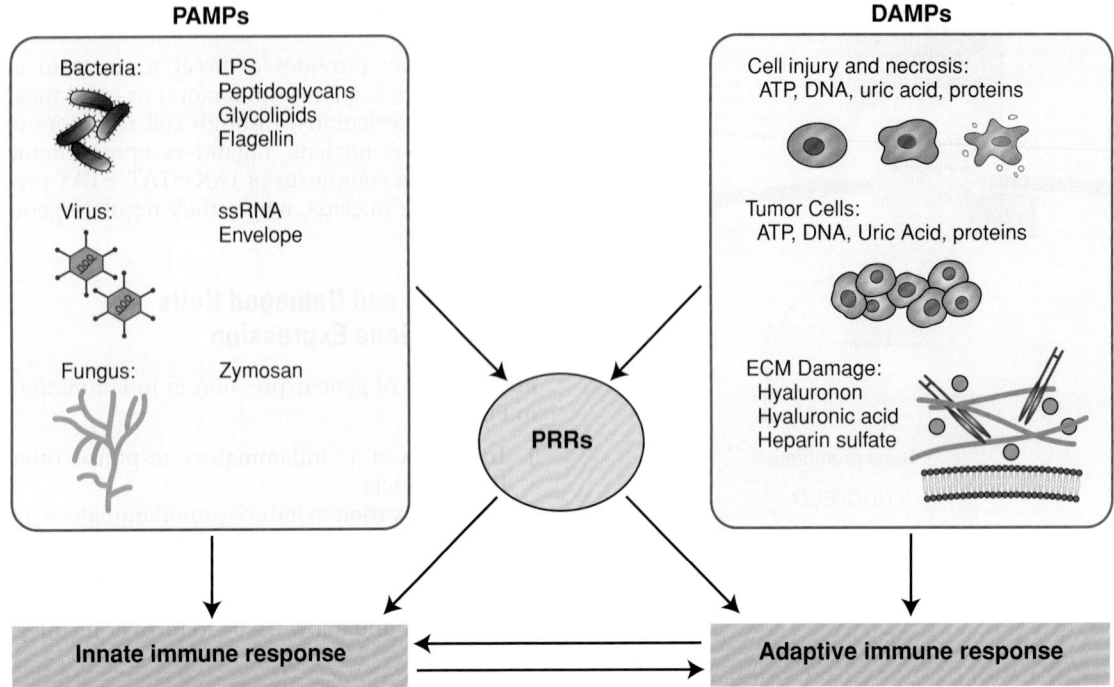

FIGURE 2-36. Pathogen-associated molecular pattern molecules (PAMPS) and damage-associated molecular pattern molecules (DAMPS) initiate adaptive and innate immune responses. Microbes release PAMPs. Damaged cells and tissue release DAMPS. Binding to receptors belonging to the family of pattern recognition receptors (PRRs) mediates innate and adaptive immune responses.

With activation, the multifaceted inflammatory response commences and is amplified by (1) release of cytokines and chemokines, (2) activation of coagulation and complement cascades and (3) release of free radical products (Fig. 2-37).

Pattern-Recognition Receptors

Four families of PRRs are found on inflammatory and immune cells: (1) Toll-like receptors, (2) nucleotide

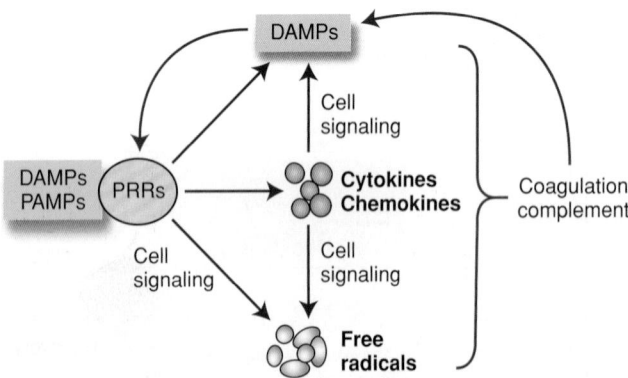

FIGURE 2-37. Damage-associated molecular pattern molecules (DAMPs) and pathogen-associated molecular pattern molecules (PAMPs) drive the multifaceted inflammatory response. Interaction of PAMPs and DAMPS with pattern recognition receptors (PRRs) initiates cell signaling, leading to enhanced activation of inflammatory mediators. These inflammatory signals can lead to further release of DAMPs and maintenance of the inflammatory response.

oligomerization domain leucine-rich repeat proteins (NOD-like receptors), (3) cytoplasmic caspase activation and recruitment domain helicases and (4) C-type lectin receptors.

Toll-like Receptors

Toll-like receptors (TLRs) are a major class of PRRs found on immune, inflammatory and tissue cells, including macrophages, endothelial cells and epithelial cells (Table 2-5). TLRs on the cell surface recognize bacterial cell wall components and viruses. Genetic polymorphisms of TLRs are related to specific cellular responses. Thus, specific TLRs recognize lipid and carbohydrates on gram-positive bacteria, fungi, LPS of gram-negative bacteria and viral RNA. Although TLR engagement activates intracellular pathways to defend against microbial organisms, it may lead to excessive activation of cytokine cascades, notably contributing to septic shock (see Chapter 20). Thus, IL-1 and TLR signaling participate in many inflammatory and infectious diseases, which has prompted development of TLR antagonists.

NOD-like Receptors

These intracellular soluble proteins are sensors for microbes (PAMPs) and cell injury (DAMPs). They form large molecular complexes, **inflammasomes,** that are linked to the proteolytic activation of proinflammatory cytokines.

Cytoplasmic Caspase Activation and Recruitment Domain Helicases

This large family includes receptors such as retinoic acid inducible gene-1–like receptors (RIG-1-like receptors) expressed by macrophages, dendritic cells and fibroblasts.

TABLE 2-5
PATHOGEN RECOGNITION RECEPTORS

Toll-like Receptor	Cell Expression	Pathogen Recognized
TLR1	Macrophages Neutrophils	Lipid and carbohydrates from gram-positive bacteria
TLR2	Macrophages Basophils Neutrophils	Lipid and carbohydrates from gram-positive bacteria Fungal organisms
TLR3	Macrophages	Nucleic acid and derivatives Double-stranded RNA (viral DNA)
TLR4	Macrophages Basophils Neutrophils	LPS from gram-negative bacteria
TLR5	Macrophages Neutrophils	Bacterial flagellin
TLR6	Macrophages Neutrophils	Lipid and carbohydrates from gram-positive bacteria
TLR7	Macrophages Neutrophils	Nucleic acid and derivatives (viral DNA)
TLR8	Macrophages Neutrophils	Nucleic acid and derivatives (viral DNA)
TLR9	Macrophages Neutrophils	Nucleic acid and derivatives Bacterial DNA containing unmethylated CpG motifs
TLR10	Macrophages Neutrophils	Ligand unknown
TLR11 (pseudogene)	Macrophages Neutrophils	Bacterial profilin

LPS = lipopolysaccharide.

They are cytoplasmic RNA helicases that survey for microbes and recognize viral RNA in the cytoplasm.

C-Type Lectin Receptors

Glycosylated proteins have pathogen recognition functions in addition to their role in cell adhesion. Mainly expressed on macrophages and dendritic cells, these receptors participate in fungal recognition and modulation of innate immunity. Members include the mannose receptor, dendritic cell–specific ICAM-3–grabbing nonintegrin (DC-SIGN), dectin-1, dectin-2 and the collectins. When pathogens bind these receptors on epithelial and endothelial cells, additional DAMPS are released. This stimulates inflammatory cells and amplifies activation of coagulation and complement cascades. These, in turn, positively feed back to drive production of inflammatory mediators (i.e., cytokine, chemokines and DAMPS) (Fig. 2-37).

Gene Activation

The primary function of PRRs is to activate three major signaling pathways:

1. NFκB pathway
2. Mitogen-activated protein kinase/activator protein-1 (MAPK/AP-1) pathway
3. Interferon regulatory factor (IRF) pathway

Activation of NFκB promotes induction of proinflammatory cytokines. MAPK activates AP-1, which induces proinflammatory cytokines. IRFs activate type 1 IFNs and proinflammatory mediators. Via these signal transduction pathways, microbial recognition activates transcription factors, which in turn bind specific sequences in gene promoters. TLRs engage microbes and activate immune cells by signaling from the plasma membrane via NFκB and AP-1. TLRs also signal from endosomes via activation of IRFs to induce type 1 interferons. Activation of RIG-1 by binding to cytoplasmic viral RNA activates NFκB and IRF3 to increase interferon transcription. The soluble cytoplasmic retinoic acid inducible gene-1–like receptors (RLRs) activate NFκB, thus increasing IFN and inflammatory cytokine production.

Negative Regulators of Acute Inflammation

The natural resolution of acute inflammation involves removal of the initial stimulus and subsequent apoptosis of inflammatory cells. Decreased proinflammatory mediators and increased anti-inflammatory mediators brake the process. Removal of damaged tissue and cell debris allows proper healing to take place.

The response to injury is, however, variable. Genetics and the sex and age of a patient determine the response to injury, extent of healing and, especially, progression to chronic inflammatory disease. Negative regulators of inflammation include:

- **Gene silencing and reprogramming:** Inflammation is associated with gene reprogramming, which (1) silences acute proinflammatory gene expression, (2) increases anti-inflammatory gene expression and (3) allows the inflammatory process to start to resolve. Notably, TNF-α, IL-1β and other proinflammatory genes are repressed. At the same time, expression of anti-inflammatory factors, like IL-1 receptor antagonist (IL-1RA), TNF-α receptors, IL-6 and IL-10, increases.
- **Cytokines:** Several interleukins (IL-6, IL-10, IL-11, IL-12, IL-13) limit inflammation by reducing production of TNF-α. This may occur by preserving IκB, thus blocking cell activation and release of inflammatory mediators.
- **Protease inhibitors:** Secretory leukocyte proteinase inhibitor (SLPI) and TIMP-2 are important in reducing the responses of a variety of cell types, including macrophages and endothelial cells, and in decreasing connective tissue damage.
- **Lipoxins:** Lipoxins and aspirin-triggered lipoxins are anti-inflammatory lipid mediators that inhibit leukotriene biosynthesis.
- **Glucocorticoids:** Stimulating the hypothalamic–pituitary–adrenal axis increases release of immunosuppressive glucocorticoids. These have transcriptional and posttranscriptional suppressive effects on inflammatory response genes.
- **Kininases:** Kininases in plasma and blood degrade the potent proinflammatory mediator bradykinin.

■ **Phosphatases:** A signal transduction mechanism that commonly regulates inflammatory cell signaling is rapid and reversible protein phosphorylation. Phosphatases and associated proteins balance the effect via dephosphorylation.

■ **Transforming growth factor-β (TGF-β).** Apoptotic cells, particularly PMNs, induce TGF-β expression. TGF-β suppresses proinflammatory cytokines and chemokines, switches arachidonic acid–derived mediators to favor production of lipoxin and resolvin (resolution phase interaction products; omega-3 unsaturated fatty acid), causes recognition and clearance of apoptotic cells and debris by macrophages and stimulates anti-inflammatory cytokines and fibrosis.

OUTCOMES OF ACUTE INFLAMMATION

A combination of regulatory activities and the short life span of neutrophils limit the duration of acute inflammatory reactions. As the source of tissue injury is eliminated, inflammation recedes and normal tissue architecture and physiologic function are restored. How the inflammation ends depends on the balance between cell recruitment, cell division, cell emigration and cell death. If a tissue is to return to normal, the inflammatory process must be reversed: the stimulus to injury must be removed, proinflammatory signals turned off, acute inflammatory cell influx ended, tissue fluid balance restored, cell and tissue debris removed, normal vascular function restored, epithelial barriers repaired and the ECM regenerated. As signals for acute inflammation wane, apoptosis of PMNs limits the immune response and resolution begins.

However, inflammatory responses can lead to other outcomes (Fig. 2-38):

■ **Scar:** Although the body may eliminate the offending agent, if a tissue is irreversibly injured, normal architecture is often replaced by a scar (see Chapter 3).

■ **Abscess:** If the area of acute inflammation is walled off by inflammatory cells and fibrosis, PMN products destroy the tissue, leaving an abscess (see Chapter 1).

■ **Lymphadenitis:** Localized acute and chronic inflammation may cause secondary inflammation of lymphatic channels **(lymphangitis)** and lymph nodes **(lymphadenitis)**. These inflamed lymphatic channels appear as red streaks, and lymph nodes are enlarged and painful. Affected lymph nodes show lymphoid follicle hyperplasia and proliferation of mononuclear phagocytes in the sinuses **(sinus histiocytosis)**.

■ **Persistent inflammation:** If an insulting agent persists or resolution is incomplete, inflammation may persist. This may be a prolonged acute response, with continued influx of neutrophils and tissue destruction, or, more commonly, chronic inflammation.

CHRONIC INFLAMMATION

In chronic inflammation, inflammatory cells persist, the stroma becomes hyperplastic and tissue destruction and scarring may lead to organ dysfunction. The process may be localized, but it often progresses to disabling diseases, such as chronic lung disease, rheumatoid arthritis, ulcerative colitis, granulomatous diseases, autoimmune diseases and chronic dermatitis. Acute and chronic inflammation are ends of a dynamic continuum with overlapping morphologies: (1) inflammation that features continued recruitment of chronic inflammatory cells is followed by (2) tissue injury due to a prolonged inflammatory response and (3) an often

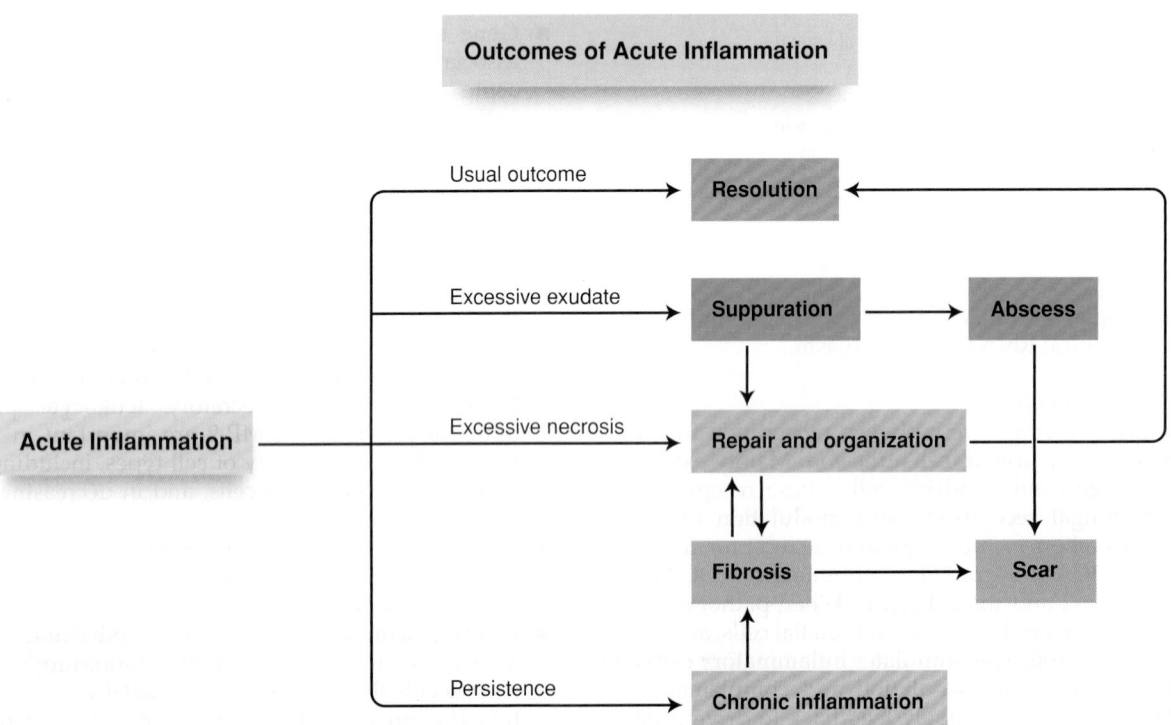

FIGURE 2-38. Outcomes of acute inflammation.

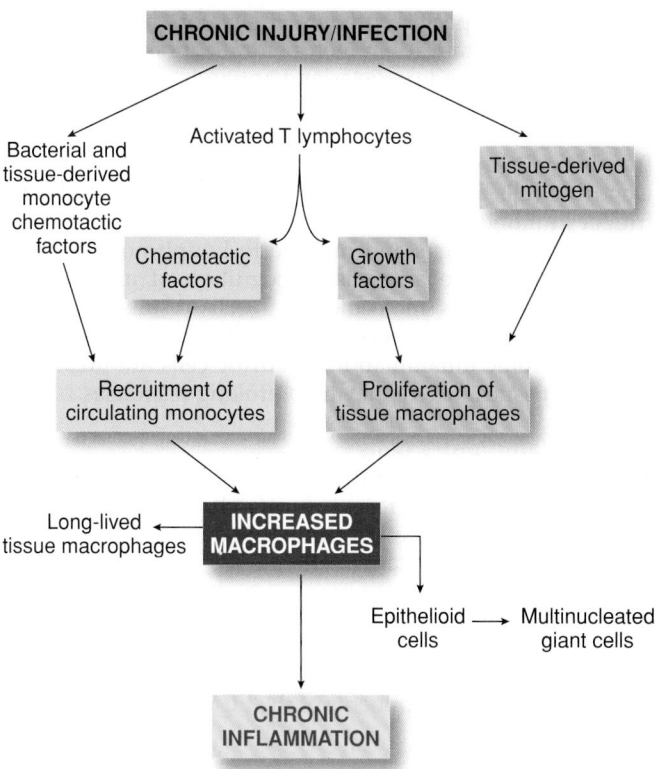

FIGURE 2-39. Accumulation of macrophages is central to development of chronic inflammation.

disordered attempt to restore tissue integrity. Macrophages are key determinants of the outcome (Fig. 2-39).

The events leading to amplified inflammatory responses resemble those of acute inflammation in several ways:

- **Specific triggers,** microbial products or injury, initiate the response.
- **Chemical mediators** direct recruitment, activation and interaction of inflammatory cells. Activation of coagulation and complement generates small peptides that act to prolong the inflammatory response. Cytokines, specifically IL-6 and RANTES, regulate a switch in chemokines, so that mononuclear cells are directed to the site. Other cytokines (e.g., IFN-γ) then promote macrophage proliferation and activation.
- **Inflammatory cells** come in from the blood. Interactions between lymphocytes, macrophages, dendritic cells and fibroblasts generate antigen-specific responses. Macrophages have a central, controlling role, producing inflammatory mediators that activate other macrophages, lymphocytes and tissue fibroblasts (Fig. 2-39) either to promote resolution or to perpetuate injury.
- **DAMPs and PAMPs drive multifaceted inflammatory responses.** Interaction of PAMPs, DAMPS and PRRs increases activation of inflammatory mediators. This can cause more release of DAMPs and subsequent maintenance of the inflammatory response, even after the initial inciting event has passed (Fig. 2-37).
- **Stromal cell activation and extracellular matrix** remodeling occur, both of which affect cellular immune responses. Variable fibrosis may result, depending on the extent of tissue injury and the persistence of injury and inflammation.

Chronic inflammation is not synonymous with chronic infection, but if an inflammatory response does not eliminate an injurious agent, infection may persist. Chronic inflammation does not necessarily require infection: it may follow an acute inflammatory or immune response to a foreign antigen. Signals that lead to an extended response include:

- **Bacteria, viruses and parasites:** These agents can provide signals to support persistent inflammatory responses, which may be directed toward isolating the invader from the host.
- **Apoptosis:** As apoptotic PMNs induce an anti-inflammatory reaction, defects in recognizing or responding to PMN remnants may lead to chronic inflammation.
- **Defective gene silencing:** Delayed or persistent expression of late proinflammatory genes helps to perpetuate the inflammatory environment. In this case, a gene silencing phase does not occur, cytokine onslaught persists and pathologic inflammation develops.
- **Trauma:** Extensive tissue damage releases mediators that prolong the inflammatory environment.
- **Cancer:** Chronic inflammatory cells, especially macrophages and T lymphocytes, may be recruited by tumors to feed and stimulate tumor cell growth (see Chapter 5). Chemotherapy may limit inflammation and increase susceptibility to infection.
- **Immune factors:** In many autoimmune diseases, including rheumatoid arthritis, chronic thyroiditis and primary biliary cirrhosis, chronic inflammatory responses occur in affected tissues. There may be associated activation of antibody-dependent and cell-mediated immunity (see Chapter 4). Such autoimmune abnormalities may lead to persistent injury in affected organs.

Mononuclear Cells Are Mainly Those Involved in Chronic Inflammation

The cellular participants in chronic inflammatory responses are recruited from the circulation (macrophages, lymphocytes, plasma cells, dendritic cells and eosinophils) and affected tissues (fibroblasts, endothelial cells).

Monocytes/Macrophages

Activated macrophages and their cytokines are central to inflammation and prolonging responses that lead to chronic inflammation. Tissue macrophages are stimulated and proliferate as circulating monocytes are recruited and differentiate into tissue macrophages (Fig. 2-39). Under the influence of the microenvironment, resident tissue macrophages become phenotypically polarized into classically activated M1 macrophages and alternatively activated M2 macrophages (Figs. 2-19 and 2-20). Macrophages produce inflammatory and immunologic mediators and regulate reactions leading to chronic inflammation. They also regulate lymphocyte responses to antigens and secrete other mediators that modulate proliferation of fibroblasts and endothelial cell proliferation and their activities.

Within different tissues, resident macrophages differ in their armamentarium of enzymes and responses to local inflammatory signals. Granules of circulating monocytes contain serine proteinases, like those in PMNs. Blood monocytes synthesize additional enzymes, particularly MMPs. When monocytes enter tissue and differentiate into macrophages, they acquire the ability to make additional MMPs and cysteine proteinases but lose the capacity to produce serine proteinases. The activities of these enzymes are central to the tissue destruction that may occur in chronic inflammation. For example, in the case of emphysema, resident macrophages generate proteinases, particularly MMPs with elastolytic activity, which destroy alveolar walls and recruit blood monocytes into the lung. *Other macrophage products include oxygen metabolites, chemotactic factors, cytokines and growth factors* (Fig. 2-17C).

Lymphocytes

Naive lymphocytes home to secondary lymphoid organs, where they encounter antigen-presenting cells and become antigen-specific lymphocytes. Plasma cells and T cells leave secondary lymphoid organs and circulate in the vascular system, from which they are recruited to peripheral tissues.

T cells regulate macrophage activation and recruitment by secreting specific mediators (lymphokines), modulate antibody production and cell-mediated cytotoxicity and maintain immunologic memory (Fig. 2-40A). NK cells, as well as other lymphocyte subtypes, help defend against viral and bacterial infections.

Plasma Cells

Plasma cells are rich in rough endoplasmic reticulum and are the primary source of antibodies (Fig. 2-40B). Production of antibody to specific antigens at sites of chronic inflammation is important in antigen neutralization, clearance of foreign antigens and particles and antibody-dependent cell-mediated cytotoxicity (see Chapter 4).

Dendritic Cells

Dendritic cells are professional antigen-presenting cells that trigger immune responses to antigens (see Chapter 4). They phagocytose antigens and migrate to lymph nodes, where they present those antigens. Recognition of antigen and other costimulatory molecules by T cells results in recruitment of specific cell subsets to the inflammatory process. During chronic inflammation, dendritic cells are present in inflamed tissues, where they help prolong responses.

Acute Inflammatory Cells

Neutrophils characteristically participate in acute inflammation but may also be present during chronic inflammation if there is ongoing infection and tissue damage. Eosinophils are particularly prominent in allergic reactions and parasitic infestations.

Fibroblasts

Fibroblasts are long-lived, ubiquitous cells, whose chief function is to produce components of the ECM (Fig. 2-40C). They

A

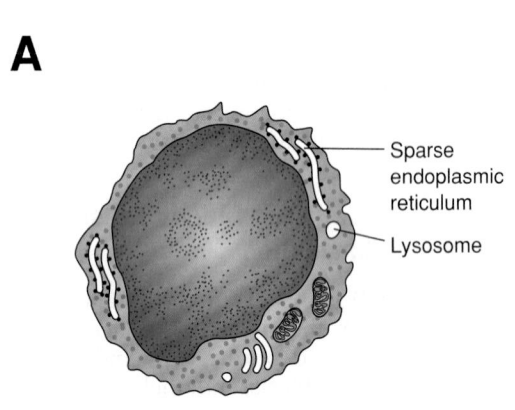

Sparse endoplasmic reticulum

Lysosome

LYMPHOCYTE

CHARACTERISTICS AND FUNCTIONS

- Associated with chronic inflammation
- Key cells in humoral and cell-mediated immune responses
- Cytokine production
- Multiple subtypes:

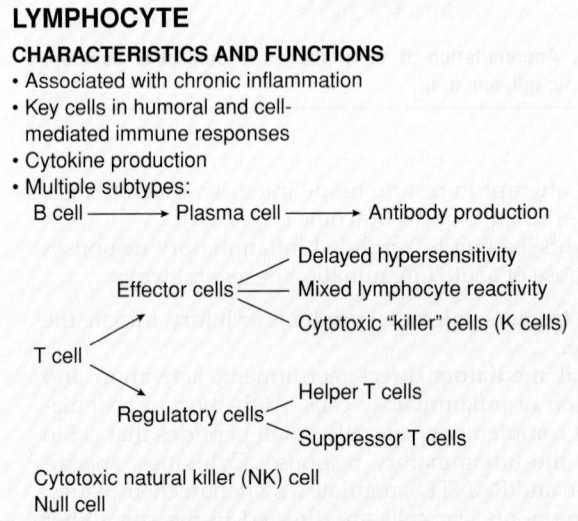

B cell ⟶ Plasma cell ⟶ Antibody production

Effector cells — Delayed hypersensitivity
— Mixed lymphocyte reactivity
— Cytotoxic "killer" cells (K cells)

T cell

Regulatory cells — Helper T cells
— Suppressor T cells

Cytotoxic natural killer (NK) cell
Null cell

B

Endoplasmic reticulum

Golgi apparatus

Peripheral chromatin

PLASMA CELL

CHARACTERISTICS AND FUNCTIONS

- Associated with:
  - Antibody synthesis and secretion
  - Chronic inflammation
- Derived from B lymphocytes

C

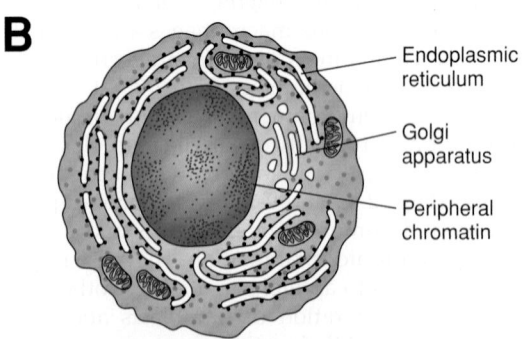

FIBROBLAST

CHARACTERISTICS AND FUNCTIONS

- Produces extracellular matrix proteins
- Mediates chronic inflammation and wound healing

PRIMARY INFLAMMATORY MEDIATORS

- IL-6
- IL-8
- Cyclooxygenase-2
- Hyaluronan
- PGE$_2$
- CD40 expression
- Matricellular proteins
- Extracellular proteins

FIGURE 2-40. More cells of inflammation: morphology and function. A. Lymphocyte. **B.** Plasma cell. **C.** Fibroblast.

are derived from mesoderm or neural crest and can differentiate into other connective tissue cells (e.g., chondrocytes, adipocytes, osteocytes and smooth muscle cells). Fibroblasts are the construction workers of tissue, rebuilding the scaffolding of the ECM upon which tissue is re-established.

Fibroblasts not only respond to immune signals that induce their proliferation and activation but also actively function in immune responses. They interact with inflammatory cells, particularly lymphocytes, via surface molecules and receptors on both cells. For example, when CD40 on fibroblasts binds its ligand on lymphocytes, both cells are activated. Activated fibroblasts produce cytokines, chemokines and prostanoids, creating a tissue microenvironment that further regulates the behavior of inflammatory cells in the damaged tissue. This process results in resolution and subsequent wound healing or chronic persistent inflammation (see Chapter 3).

INJURY AND REPAIR IN CHRONIC INFLAMMATION

Chronic inflammation is mediated by immunologic and nonimmunologic mechanisms and often occurs with reparative responses, namely, granulation tissue and fibrosis.

Extended Inflammatory Responses May Lead to Persistent Injury

The primary role of PMNs in inflammation is host defense and debridement of damaged tissue. The neutrophil response, however, is both yin and yang. PMN products protect the host from foreign invaders and help debride damaged tissues, but if they are not well regulated, these same products may prolong tissue damage and promote chronic inflammation. PMN enzymes are beneficial when they digest phagocytosed organisms intracellularly, but these same enzymes can be destructive if they are released extracellularly. Thus, when PMNs accumulate, connective tissue may be digested by their enzymes.

Persistent tissue injury due to inflammatory cells is important in the pathogenesis of several diseases (e.g., emphysema, rheumatoid arthritis, some immune complex diseases, gout and acute respiratory distress syndrome). Phagocytic cell adherence, escape of ROS and release of lysosomal enzymes together enhance cytotoxicity and tissue degradation. Proteinase activity is significantly elevated in chronic wounds, creating a proteolytic environment that prevents healing.

Altered Repair Mechanisms Prevent Resolution

Repair processes initiated as part of inflammation can restore normal architecture and function. However, if inflammation is prolonged or exaggerated, repair may be ineffective, alter tissue architecture and cause tissue dysfunction (Fig. 2-38). Thus:

- Ongoing proliferation of epithelial cells can cause metaplasia (see Chapter 1). Goblet cell metaplasia, for example, is seen in the airways of smokers.
- Fibroblast proliferation and activation lead to increased ECM. Because ECM components such as collagen now occupy space normally devoted to tissue cells, organ function is altered (see Chapter 3).

- The ECM may be altered. Matrix degradation and production change the normal mix of extracellular proteins. Thus, elastin degradation is important in the development of emphysema.
- Altered ECM (e.g., fibronectin) can be a chemoattractant for inflammatory cells and present an altered scaffolding to cells.

GRANULOMATOUS INFLAMMATION

PMNs ordinarily remove agents that incite acute inflammatory responses. However, sometimes these cells cannot digest those substances. Such a situation is potentially dangerous, because it can lead to a vicious circle of (1) phagocytosis, (2) failure of digestion, (3) death of the PMN, (4) release of undigested provoking agents and (5) rephagocytosis by a newly recruited PMN (Fig. 2-41). *Granuloma formation is a protective response to chronic infection (e.g., some fungi, tuberculosis) or the presence of foreign material (e.g., suture or talc). It isolates a persistent offending agent, preventing it from disseminating and restricting inflammation, thus protecting the host.* Some autoimmune diseases are also associated with granulomas (e.g., Crohn disease). In some granulomatous disorders such as sarcoidosis, no inciting agent has yet been identified.

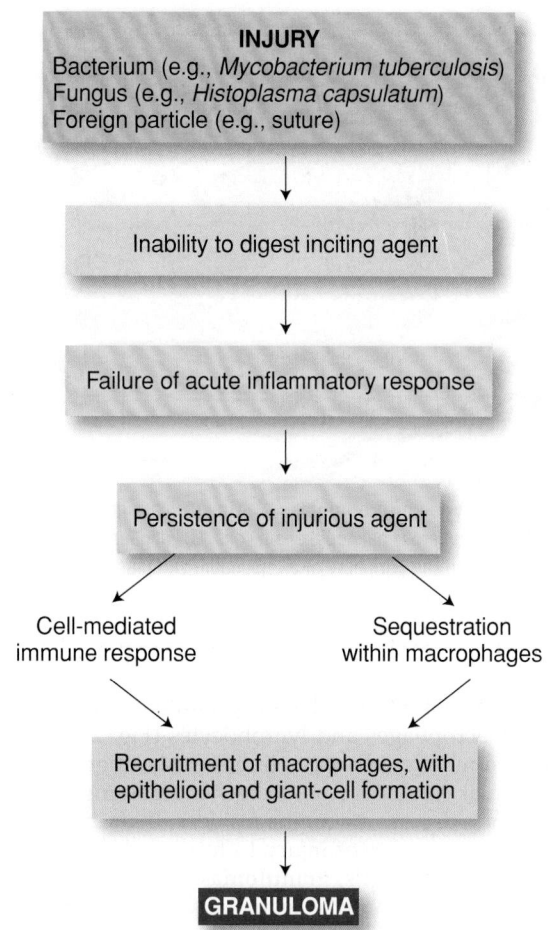

FIGURE 2-41. Mechanism of granuloma formation.

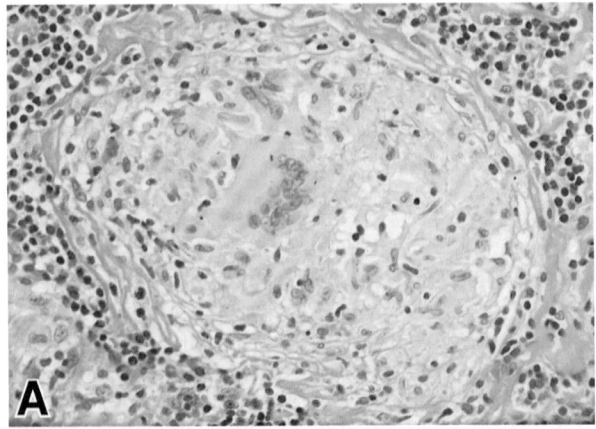

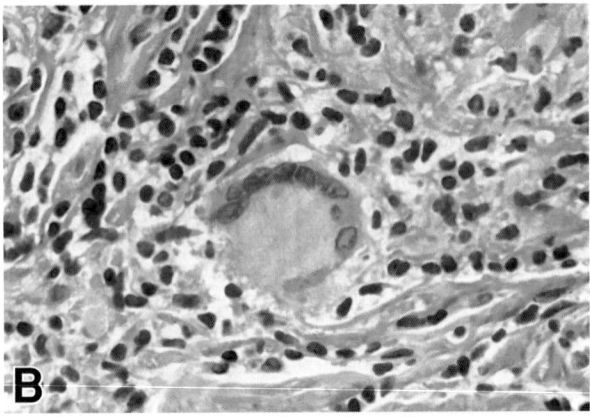

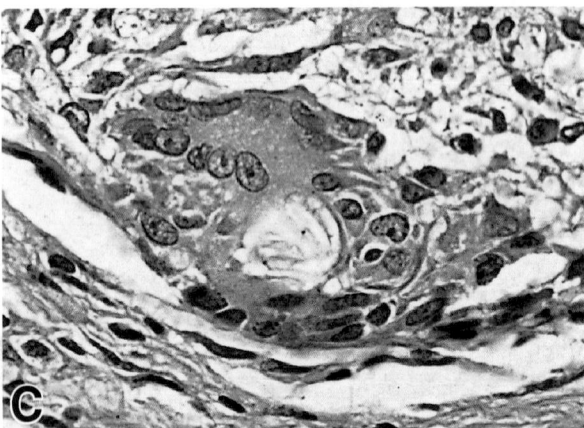

FIGURE 2-42. Types of granulomas. A. Granuloma with a multinucleated giant cell amid numerous pale epithelioid cells. **B.** Langhans giant cell shows nuclei arranged on the periphery of an abundant cytoplasm. **C.** Foreign body giant cell with numerous nuclei randomly arranged in the cytoplasm and foreign material in the center.

The principal cells involved in granulomatous inflammation are macrophages and lymphocytes (Fig. 2-42). Macrophages are mobile cells that continuously migrate through extravascular connective tissues. After amassing substances they cannot digest, macrophages lose their motility and accumulate at the site of injury to form nodular collections of pale, epithelioid cells, **granulomas**. Multinucleated giant cells are formed by cytoplasmic fusion of macrophages. When the nuclei of such giant cells are arranged around the periphery of the cytoplasm in a horseshoe pattern, the cell is called a **Langhans giant cell** (Fig. 2-42B). A foreign agent (e.g., silica or a *Histoplasma* spore) or other indigestible

material persists in the cytoplasm of a multinucleated giant cell, in which case the term **foreign body giant cell** is used (Fig. 2-42C). Foreign body giant cells tend to have more central nuclei. Granulomas are further classified by the presence or absence of necrosis. Certain infectious agents, such as *Mycobacterium tuberculosis*, characteristically produce necrotizing granulomas, the centers of which are filled with an amorphous mixture of debris and dead microorganisms and cells. In other diseases, such as sarcoidosis, granulomas characteristically lack necrosis.

Immune granulomas, formed during delayed-type hypersensitivity responses, contain activated T cells and macrophages, which initiate granuloma formation. CD4+ T cells then recruit and organize cells at the site. They use CXCL chemokines to develop Th1-type granulomas and CCL chemokines to develop Th2-type granulomas. Several T-cell cytokines stimulate macrophage function (e.g., IFN-γ), whereas others inhibit macrophage activation (e.g., IL-4, IL-10). Thus, lymphocytes are vital for regulating development and resolution of inflammatory responses.

The outcome of granulomatous reactions depends on the immunogenicity and toxicity of the inciting agent. Cell-mediated immune responses may modify granulomatous reactions by recruiting and activating more macrophages and lymphocytes. Under the influence of T-cell cytokines, such as IL-13 and TGF-β, a granuloma may burn out and become a fibrotic nodule.

CHRONIC INFLAMMATION AND TUMORIGENESIS

Several chronic infectious diseases are associated with development of malignancies such that chronic inflammation may enable tumorigenesis. For example, schistosomiasis in the urinary bladder leads to squamous cell carcinoma of that organ. Inflammation that is not specifically linked to infection may also be a risk factor for cancer. Patients with reflux esophagitis or ulcerative colitis are at higher risk for adenocarcinoma in those organs. An environment created by chronic inflammation promotes malignant transformation by several mechanisms (see Chapter 5):

- **Increased cell proliferation:** Chronically stimulated cell division increases the likelihood of transforming mutations in proliferating cells.
- **Oxygen and NO• metabolites:** Inflammatory metabolites, such as nitrosamines, may cause genomic damage (see Chapter 5).
- **Chronic immune activation:** Chronic antigen exposure alters the cytokine milieu by suppressing cell-mediated immune responses. This creates a more permissive environment for malignant growth.
- **Angiogenesis:** Growth of new vessels is associated with inflammation and wound healing and is important in sustaining cancers.
- **Inhibition of apoptosis:** Chronic inflammation suppresses apoptosis. Increased cell division and decreased apoptosis favor survival and expansion of mutated cell populations.

SYSTEMIC MANIFESTATIONS OF INFLAMMATION

An effective inflammatory response will (1) limit the area of injury, (2) clear the inciting pathologic agent and damaged tissue and (3) restore tissue function. However, local injury may cause prominent systemic consequences that may themselves be debilitating. These effects may result when a pathogen enters the bloodstream, a separate condition acts synergistically and the combination of a local and a systemic insult directly or indirectly causes both local and systemic effects of inflammation. The symptoms associated with inflammation, including fever, myalgia, arthralgia, anorexia and somnolence, are attributable to these cytokines. The most prominent systemic manifestations of inflammation, termed the **systemic inflammatory response syndrome (SIRS),** are activation of the hypothalamic–pituitary–adrenal axis, leukocytosis and the acute phase response, fever and shock.

Hypothalamic–Pituitary–Adrenal Axis

Many of the systemic effects of inflammation are mediated via the hypothalamic–pituitary–adrenal axis, a key component in the response to chronic inflammation and chronic immune disease. Inflammation results in release of anti-inflammatory glucocorticoids from the adrenal cortex. Thus, loss of adrenal function can increase the severity of inflammation.

Leukocytosis

Leukocytosis is an increase in circulating leukocytes. It commonly accompanies acute inflammation. Immature PMNs ("band" forms) may also be seen in the peripheral blood (see Chapter 26). Leukocytosis is most commonly associated with bacterial infections and tissue injury and is caused by release of specific mediators from macrophages and perhaps other cells. These mediators accelerate release of PMNs, even immature ones, from the bone marrow. Subsequently, macrophages and T lymphocytes are stimulated to produce a group of proteins (colony-stimulating factors) that induce proliferation of bone marrow hematopoietic precursor cells. Occasionally, circulating levels of PMNs and their precursors may be very high, a condition known as a **leukemoid (i.e., leukemia-like) reaction,** which may be confused with leukemia (see Chapter 26).

In contrast to bacterial infections, viral infections (including infectious mononucleosis) are characterized by **lymphocytosis,** an increase in the number of circulating lymphocytes. Parasitic infestations and certain allergic reactions cause eosinophilia (i.e., increased blood eosinophils).

Leukopenia

Leukopenia is an absolute decrease in circulating white cells. It happens occasionally during chronic inflammation, especially in patients who are malnourished or who suffer from a chronic debilitating disease such as disseminated cancer. Leukopenia may also be caused by typhoid fever and certain viral and rickettsial infections.

Acute Phase Response

The acute phase response is a regulated physiologic reaction that occurs in inflammatory conditions. It is characterized clinically by fever, leukocytosis, decreased appetite and altered sleep patterns, and chemically by changes in plasma levels of acute phase proteins. These molecules (Table 2-6) are synthesized primarily by the liver and released in large quantities into the circulation in response to an acute inflammatory challenge. Changes in plasma levels of acute phase proteins are mediated primarily by IL-1, IL-6 and TNF-α. Increased plasma levels of some acute phase proteins

TABLE 2-6 ACUTE PHASE PROTEINS	
Protein	**Function**
Mannose-binding protein	Opsonization/complement activation
C-reactive protein	Opsonization
α_1-Antitrypsin	Serine protease inhibitor
Haptoglobin	Binds hemoglobin
Ceruloplasmin	Antioxidant, binds copper
Fibrinogen	Coagulation
Serum amyloid A protein	Apolipoprotein
α_2-Macroglobulin	Antiprotease
Cysteine protease inhibitor	Antiprotease

increase the **erythrocyte sedimentation rate** (ESR), which is a qualitative index used clinically to monitor the activity of many inflammatory diseases.

Fever

Fever is a clinical hallmark of inflammation. Release of **pyrogens** (molecules that cause fever) by bacteria, viruses or injured cells may directly affect hypothalamic thermoregulation. More importantly, they stimulate production of endogenous pyrogens, namely, cytokines (IL-1α, -1β and -6 and TNF-α) and interferons. IL-1 stimulates prostaglandin synthesis in hypothalamic thermoregulatory centers, thus altering the "thermostat" that controls body temperature. Inhibitors of cyclooxygenase (e.g., aspirin) block the fever response by inhibiting IL-1–stimulated PGE_2 synthesis in the hypothalamus. TNF-α and IL-6 also increase body temperature by a direct action on the hypothalamus. Chills (the sensation of cold), rigor (profound chills with shivering and piloerection) and sweats (to allow heat dissipation) are symptoms associated with fever.

Pain

Pain in acute phase reactions is associated with (1) **nociception** (i.e., detection of noxious stimuli and transmission of this information to the brain), (2) pain perception and (3) suffering and pain behavior. Nociception is mainly a neural response initiated in injured tissues by specific nociceptors, which are high-threshold receptors for thermal, chemical and mechanical stimuli. Most chemical mediators of inflammation described in this chapter—including ions, kinins, histamine, NO, prostanoids, cytokines and growth factors—activate peripheral nociceptors directly or indirectly. Kinins, especially bradykinin, are formed after tissue trauma and during inflammation; they activate primary sensory neurons via B_2 receptors to mediate pain transmission. Another kinin, des-arg bradykinin, activates B_1 receptors to produce pain only during inflammation. Cytokines, particularly TNF-α and IL-1, -6 and -8, produce pain hypersensitivity to mechanical and thermal stimuli. Prostaglandins and growth factors may directly activate nociceptors but appear to act mostly by enhancing nociceptor sensitivity. Pain perception and subsequent behavior arise in response to this enhanced sensitivity to both noxious and normally innocuous stimuli.

Shock

If tissue injury is massive or infection spreads to the blood (sepsis), huge quantities of cytokines, especially TNF-α, and other chemical mediators of inflammation are poured into the circulation. Their persistence affects the heart and peripheral vascular system by causing generalized vasodilation; increasing vascular permeability, intravascular volume loss and myocardial depression; and decreasing cardiac output (SIRS) (see Chapter 7). Cardiac output may then not satisfy the body's need for oxygen and nutrients **(cardiac decompensation)**. In severe cases, activation of coagulation pathways causes microthrombi throughout the body, consuming clotting components and predisposing to bleeding. This condition is **disseminated intravascular coagulation**. The net result is multisystem organ dysfunction syndrome (MODS) and death (see Chapter 20).

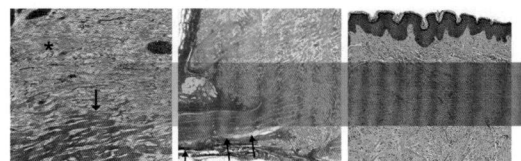

Repair, Regeneration and Fibrosis

Gregory C. Sephel ▪ Jeffrey M. Davidson

From scarring to regeneration, damaged tissue heals in ways that ensure the immediate survival of the organism. Observations regarding the repair of wounds (i.e., wound healing) date to physicians in ancient Egypt and battle surgeons in classic Greece. The clotting of blood to prevent exsanguination was recognized as the first necessary event in wound healing. With the advent of the microscope, studies of wound infection led to the discovery that inflammatory cells are primary actors in the repair process. The importance of antisepsis to wound healing is now taken for granted. From the 2nd-century Greco-Roman physician Galen to the works of Pasteur and Lister at the end of the 19th century, the presence of pus at a wound site was praised and even referred to as "laudable pus." In 1876, British physician Joseph Lister was invited to serve as president of the Surgical Section of the International Medical Congress in Philadelphia. Five years later, President Garfield died after being shot by an assassin, succumbing not to damage from the bullet but several months later to pus and sepsis, the result of tissue probing by physicians leery of the germ theory and antiseptic methods. The importance of extracellular matrix, specifically collagen, in tissue integrity and wound healing was first recognized through study of scurvy, a disease that claimed the lives of millions (see Chapter 8). In 1747, Dr. James Lind, a surgeon in England's Royal Navy, conducted what is thought to be the first controlled clinical trial. Aboard the HMS Salisbury, he separated scurvy-ridden sailors into six treatment groups and observed that sailors given oranges and lemons derived the greatest benefit by preventing the reopening of wounds and loss of teeth. In 1907, the role of vitamin C began to be clarified when Norwegians Axel Holst and Theodor Frolich discovered that guinea pigs, like humans, were unable to synthesize vitamin C (ascorbic acid). Ascorbate was eventually found necessary for the action of prolyl hydroxylase, an enzyme required for proper folding and stabilization of the collagen triple helix, an important step in establishing tissue integrity and building a strong scar.

The topic of regeneration elicits thoughts of flatworms, starfish and amphibians. However, the regeneration of the human liver was the basis of the Greek myth of Prometheus, whose liver regenerated daily. Modern concepts of regeneration and cell differentiation progressed in the latter half of the 20th century. In the 1950s, Sir John Gurdon determined that even somatic cell nuclei transplanted into a Xenopus egg could form a normal adult organism, and his work was a progenitor of current technologies that yield inducible pluripotent stem cells from many tissues. Current studies on epigenetic control of gene expression, stem and progenitor cell biology and directed control of differentiation patterns in cells are rapidly advancing the fields of regenerative healing and tissue engineering.

The study of wound healing now encompasses a variety of cells, matrix proteins, growth factors and cytokines, which regulate and modulate the repair process. Nearly every stage in the repair process is redundantly controlled, and there is no one rate-limiting factor, except uncontrolled infection. Extracellular matrix will be presented here in some detail as it occupies a central role in both repair and regeneration. Matrix deposition is a key process in tissue repair and fibrosis, and matrix composition is an important functional factor in both the niche environment that maintains stem and progenitor cells in an undifferentiated state during regeneration and in the tissue microenvironments in which these cells differentiate. In the adult, *successful healing maintains tissue function and repairs tissue barriers, preventing blood loss and infection, but it is usually accomplished through collagen deposition or scarring (fibrosis).* Advances in our understanding of critical factors—growth factors, extracellular matrix and stem cell biology—are improving healing, and they offer the possibility of restoring injured tissues to their normal architecture and of engineering replacement tissues.

Successful repair relies on a crucial balance between the *yin* of tissue formation and the *yang* of tissue remodeling. *Regeneration is favored when matrix composition and architecture are preserved.* Thus, wounds that do not heal may reflect excess proteinase activity, reduced signaling, decreased matrix accumulation or altered matrix assembly. Conversely, fibrosis and scarring may result from inadequate proteinase activity or increased matrix production. Although formation of new collagen during repair is essential for increased strength of the healing site, fibrosis is a major complication of diseases that involve chronic injury.

THE BASIC PROCESSES OF HEALING

Many of the basic cellular and molecular mechanisms required for wound healing participate in other processes that involve dynamic tissue changes, such as development and tumor growth. Three key cellular mechanisms are necessary for wound healing once hemostasis is achieved:

- Cellular migration
- Extracellular matrix organization and remodeling
- Cell proliferation

Migration of Cells Initiates Repair

Cells That Migrate to the Wound

Migration of cells into a wound and activation of local cells are initiated by changes in the mechanical environment and mediators that are either expressed de novo by resident cells or released from preformed reserves stored in granules of **platelets** and **basophils**. These granules contain cytokines, chemoattractants, proteases and mediators of inflammation, which together control vascular supply, degrade damaged tissue and initiate the repair cascade. Platelets are activated when bound to collagen exposed at sites of endothelial damage. Their ensuing aggregation, in combination with fibrin cross-linking, limits blood loss. Activated platelets release platelet-derived growth factor (PDGF) and many other molecules that facilitate adhesion, coagulation, vasoconstriction, cell proliferation and clot resorption. **Mast cells** are bone marrow–derived cells whose granules contain high concentrations of heparin, histamine and proteinases. They reside in connective tissue near small blood vessels and respond to foreign antigens by releasing the contents of their granules, many of which are angiogenic. **Resident macrophages,** tissue-fixed mesenchymal cells and epithelial cells also release mediators that contribute to and perpetuate the early response. The cellularity of wound sites increases through proliferation and recruitment to sites of injury (Fig. 3-1). *Cell types characteristic of skin wounds are:*

- **Leukocytes** arrive at the wound site early by adherence to activated endothelium, exit from the circulation and rapidly migrate into tissue by forming small focal adhesions with matrix molecules such as fibrin, fibronectin and collagen. A family of small peptide chemoattractants **(chemokines)** mediates both restricted and broad recruitment of particular leukocyte subtypes (see Chapter 2).
- **Polymorphonuclear leukocytes** from the bone marrow invade the wound site within hours. They degrade and destroy nonviable tissue and infectious organisms by releasing their granular contents and generating reactive oxygen species, before undergoing apoptosis and digestion by macrophages.

- **Monocytes/macrophages** maintain a basal resident population in tissues; they are recruited transiently in larger numbers from bone marrow and spleen shortly after neutrophil entry. During their more extended residence time in wounds, macrophages phagocytose debris and orchestrate the developing granulation tissue and healing by releasing cytokines and chemoattractants.
- **Dendritic cells** are resident antigen-presenting cells that regulate innate and adaptive immunity. They can proliferate in some tissues, such as skin, and they are also recruited from bone marrow or differentiated from closely related macrophages.
- **Fibroblasts, myofibroblasts, pericytes and smooth muscle cells** represent a spectrum of mesenchymal cells that are recruited locally and are also populated from mesenchymal progenitors in bone marrow. They migrate and propagate via signals from growth factors and matrix degradation products, populating a skin wound by day 3 or 4. These cells mediate synthesis of connective tissue (fibroplasia), tissue remodeling, vascular integrity, wound contraction and wound strength.
- **Endothelial cells** sprout from existing postcapillary venules and are also seeded by circulating bone marrow progenitors. Nascent capillaries form in response to growth factors and are visible in wound granulation tissue, together with fibroblasts, beyond day 3. Development of capillaries is critical for gas exchange, delivery of nutrients and influx of inflammatory cells.
- **Epidermal cells** move across the surface of a skin wound (Fig. 3-1.5). Reepithelialization is delayed if the migrating epithelial cells must reconstitute a damaged basement membrane. In open wounds, keratinocytes migrate between provisional matrix (see below) and preexisting or newly formed stromal collagen, which is coated with plasma glycoproteins, fibrinogen and fibronectin. The phenotype of the epithelial layer is altered if basement membrane is lacking.
- **Stem cells** from bone marrow, or in the skin, stem cells or **progenitor cells** in the hair follicle and within the basal epidermal layer, provide renewable sources of epidermal and dermal cells capable of differentiation, proliferation and migration. Stem cells for epidermal regeneration reside in the bulge region of the hair follicle and the interfollicular epidermis (Fig. 3-1.4). Dermal progenitors are also associated with the lower hair shaft and the follicular bulb. Marrow-derived, multipotential progenitors of fibroblasts and endothelium are recruited to sites of injury (Fig. 3-1.1) as well, although they appear to play a temporary role in repair. These cells aid in forming new blood vessels and new epithelium and regenerate skin structures, such as hair follicles and sebaceous glands.

Mechanisms of Cell Migration

Cell migration uses the most important mechanisms of wound healing, receptor-mediated responses to chemical signals **(cytokines)** and insoluble substrates of the extracellular matrix. Ameboid locomotion powers the rapidly migrating leukocytes via wave-like membrane extensions called **lamellipodia.** Slower-moving cells, such as fibroblasts, extend narrower, finger-like membrane protrusions called **filopodia.** Growth factors or chemokines bind to specific receptors on cell surfaces to trigger cell polarization and

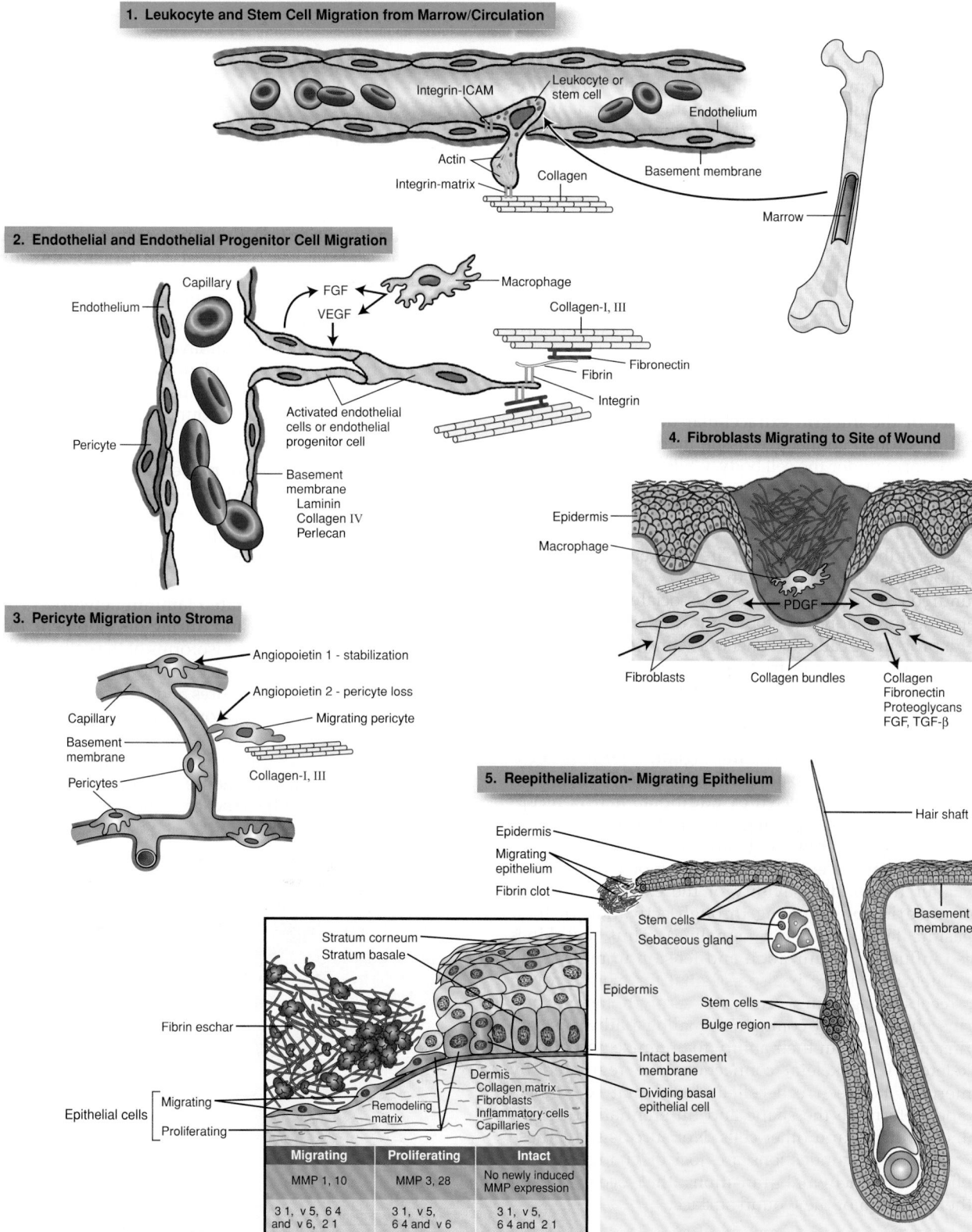

1. Leukocyte and Stem Cell Migration from Marrow/Circulation

Integrin-ICAM
Leukocyte or stem cell
Endothelium
Actin
Integrin-matrix
Collagen
Basement membrane
Marrow

2. Endothelial and Endothelial Progenitor Cell Migration

Capillary
Endothelium
FGF
VEGF
Macrophage
Collagen-I, III
Fibronectin
Fibrin
Integrin
Pericyte
Activated endothelial cells or endothelial progenitor cell
Basement membrane
Laminin
Collagen IV
Perlecan

3. Pericyte Migration into Stroma

Angiopoietin 1 - stabilization
Angiopoietin 2 - pericyte loss
Capillary
Migrating pericyte
Basement membrane
Pericytes
Collagen-I, III

4. Fibroblasts Migrating to Site of Wound

Epidermis
Macrophage
PDGF
Fibroblasts
Collagen bundles
Collagen
Fibronectin
Proteoglycans
FGF, TGF-β

5. Reepithelialization- Migrating Epithelium

Hair shaft
Epidermis
Migrating epithelium
Fibrin clot
Stem cells
Sebaceous gland
Basement membrane
Epidermis
Stem cells
Bulge region
Intact basement membrane
Dividing basal epithelial cell

Stratum corneum
Stratum basale
Fibrin eschar
Epithelial cells
Migrating
Proliferating
Remodeling matrix
Dermis
Collagen matrix
Fibroblasts
Inflammatory cells
Capillaries

Migrating	Proliferating	Intact
MMP 1, 10	MMP 3, 28	No newly induced MMP expression
3 1, v 5, 6 4 and v 6, 2 1	3 1, v 5, 6 4 and v 6	3 1, v 5, 6 4 and 2 1

FIGURE 3-1. Resident and migrating cells initiate repair and regeneration. 1. After cytokine activation of capillary endothelium, leukocytes and bone marrow–derived circulating stem cells attach to, and migrate between, capillary endothelial cells; penetrate the basement membrane; and enter the interstitial matrix in response to chemotactic signals. **2.** Under the influence of locally released angiogenic factors, capillary endothelial cells lose their connection with the basement membrane and extend through the provisional matrix to form new capillaries. Pericytes and basement membranes are required to stabilize new and existing capillary structures. **3.** Pericytes detach from capillary endothelial cells and their basement membranes to migrate into the matrix. **4.** Under the influence of growth factors such as platelet-derived growth factor (PDGF), fibroblasts become bipolar and migrate through the matrix to the site of injury where transforming growth factor-β (TGF-β) can cause differentiation into smooth muscle actin-containing myofibroblasts. These then become bipolar and migrate through the matrix to the site of injury. **5.** During reepithelialization, groups of basal keratinocytes at the wound edge release from underlying basement membrane, take on a migratory behavior and penetrate between the fibrin eschar (if present) and the granulation tissue that generates wound dermis. Migrating cells switch to a different display of integrin matrix receptors that recognize provisional matrix and stromal collagen (type I) and to different metalloproteinases that favor migration and matrix remodeling. *FGF* = fibroblast growth factor; *VEGF* = vascular endothelial growth factor.

membrane extensions. **Actin fibrils** polymerize and form a network at the membrane's leading edge, thereby propelling lamellipodia and filopodia forward, with traction achieved by engaging extracellular matrix substrate. Actin-related proteins modulate actin assembly, and numerous actin-binding proteins act like molecular tinkertoys, rapidly constructing, stabilizing and destabilizing actin networks.

The leading edge of the cell membrane impinges upon adjacent extracellular matrix and adheres to it through allosterically activated, transmembrane adhesion receptors called **integrins** (see Chapter 2). These molecules show significant redundancy; many of the 24 known vertebrate integrin heterodimer combinations recognize the same matrix components (e.g., collagen, laminin, fibronectin), yet they show specificity in distinguishing basement membrane, provisional and stromal matrices. Focal contacts develop via adherence of the integrin extracellular domain to the provisional or stromal connective tissue matrix. In vitro, focal adhesions form under the cell body, while smaller focal contacts form at the leading edges of migrating cells. The focal contact anchors actin stress fibers, against which myosins pull to extend or contract the cell body. As cells move forward, older adhesions at the rear are weakened or destabilized, allowing the trailing edge to retract.

Hundreds of proteins have been associated with formation of adhesion plaques. Cytoplasmic domains of integrins trigger a protein cascade that anchors actin stress fibers. The Rho family of guanosine triphosphatases (GTPases; Rho, Rac, Cdc42) are molecular switches that interact with surface receptors to regulate matrix assembly, generate focal adhesions and organize the actin cytoskeleton.

Integrins transmit intracellular signals that also regulate cellular survival, proliferation and differentiation. Integrin functions are affected by additional matrix receptors, such as collagen-binding discoidin domain receptors (DDRs), tetraspanins and other cell activators (e.g., growth factors and chemokines). These molecules allosterically alter the binding avidity of the extracellular portion of integrins by signaling through activation of their cytoplasmic tails (inside-out signaling). Thus, cytokines can also influence organization and tension in matrix and tissue. Integrin binding is also essential for many growth factor receptor signaling processes. Growth factors and integrins share several common signaling pathways, but integrins are unique in their ability to organize and anchor cytoskeleton. Cytoskeletal connections are regulated by the interplay between cell–cell and cell–matrix connections and determine the shape and differentiation of epithelial, endothelial and other cells. Not surprisingly, these same cytoskeletal connections are foci of change during epithelial-to-mesenchymal transitions that occur during reepithelialization of the wound surface.

Extracellular Matrix Sustains the Repair Process

Extracellular matrix is presented in some depth since it is critical for repair and regeneration by providing the key components of scar tissue and the stem cell niche. Three types of extracellular matrix contribute to the organization, physical properties and function of tissue:

- **Basement membrane**
- **Provisional matrix**
- **Connective tissue (interstitial matrix or stroma)**

Basement Membrane

Basement membrane, also called **basal lamina,** is a thin, well-defined layer of specialized extracellular matrix that separates cells that synthesize it from adjacent interstitial connective tissue (Fig. 3-2). It is a supportive and biological boundary important in development, healing and regeneration, providing key signals for cell differentiation and polarity and contributing to tissue organization. Basement membrane is also a key structural and functional feature of the neuromuscular synapse. It appears as a thin lamina that stains by the periodic acid–Schiff (PAS) stain, owing to its high glycoprotein content. Unique basement membranes form under different epithelial layers and around epithelial ducts and tubules of skin and organs and around adipocytes, cover smooth and skeletal muscle cells and peripheral nerve Schwann cells and surround capillary endothelium and associated pericytes.

- Basement membranes are made from special extracellular matrix molecules, including isoforms of collagen IV, isoforms of the glycoprotein laminin, entactin/nidogen and perlecan, a heparan sulfate proteoglycan (Table 3-1). They self-assemble into a sandwich-like structure with a covalently associated type IV collagen lattice built upon the noncovalently associated laminin network.
- Within different tissues and during development, expression of unique members or isoforms of the collagen IV and laminin families imparts diversity to the basement membrane and the many structures and _functions it supports.
- Basement membranes support cellular differentiation and act as filters, cellular anchors and a surface for migrating epidermal cells after injury. They also help re-form neuromuscular junctions after nerve damage. Basement membranes determine cell shape, contribute to developmental

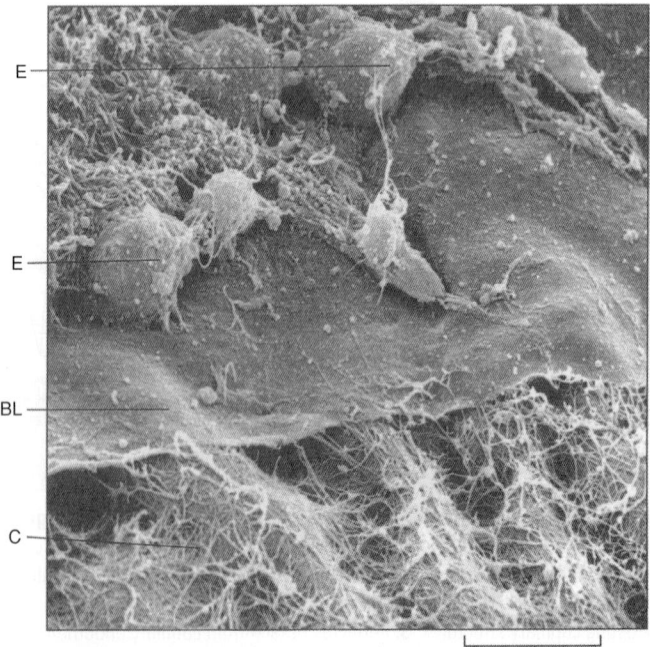

10 μm

FIGURE 3-2. Scanning electron micrographs of basement membrane. The basement membrane (BL, basal lamina) separates chick embryo corneal epithelial cells (E) from underlying stromal connective tissue with collagen fibrils.

TABLE 3-1
BASEMENT MEMBRANE CONSTITUENTS AND ORGANIZATION

Basement Membrane Components	Chains	Molecular Structure	Molecular Associations	Basement Membrane Aggregate Form
Perlecan (heparan sulfate proteoglycan)	1 protein core 3 heparan sulfate GAG chains	GAG chains	Laminin, collagen IV, fibronectin, growth factors (VEGF, FGF), chemokines	
Laminin	16 isoforms Heterotrimers with α-, β-, γ-chains 5 α-chains, 3 β-chains, 3 γ-chains	α β γ	Integrin, dystroglycan and other receptors on a variety of cells (epithelium, endothelium, muscle, Schwann cells, adipocytes) Forms self-associated noncovalent network that organizes basement membranes Laminin, nidogen/entactin, perlecan, agrin, fibulin	
Nidogen/ entactin	2-member family monomeric		Collagen IV, laminin, perlecan, fibulin Stabilizes basement membrane through association of laminin and collagen IV networks	
Collagen IV	≥3-member family Heterotrimers Chains selected from 2 or 3 of 6 unique α-chains	3 single chains form α-helical tail of collagenous regions and association of the 3 globular regions	Integrin receptors on many cells Forms covalent self-associated network Collagen IV, perlecan nidogen/entactin, SPARC	

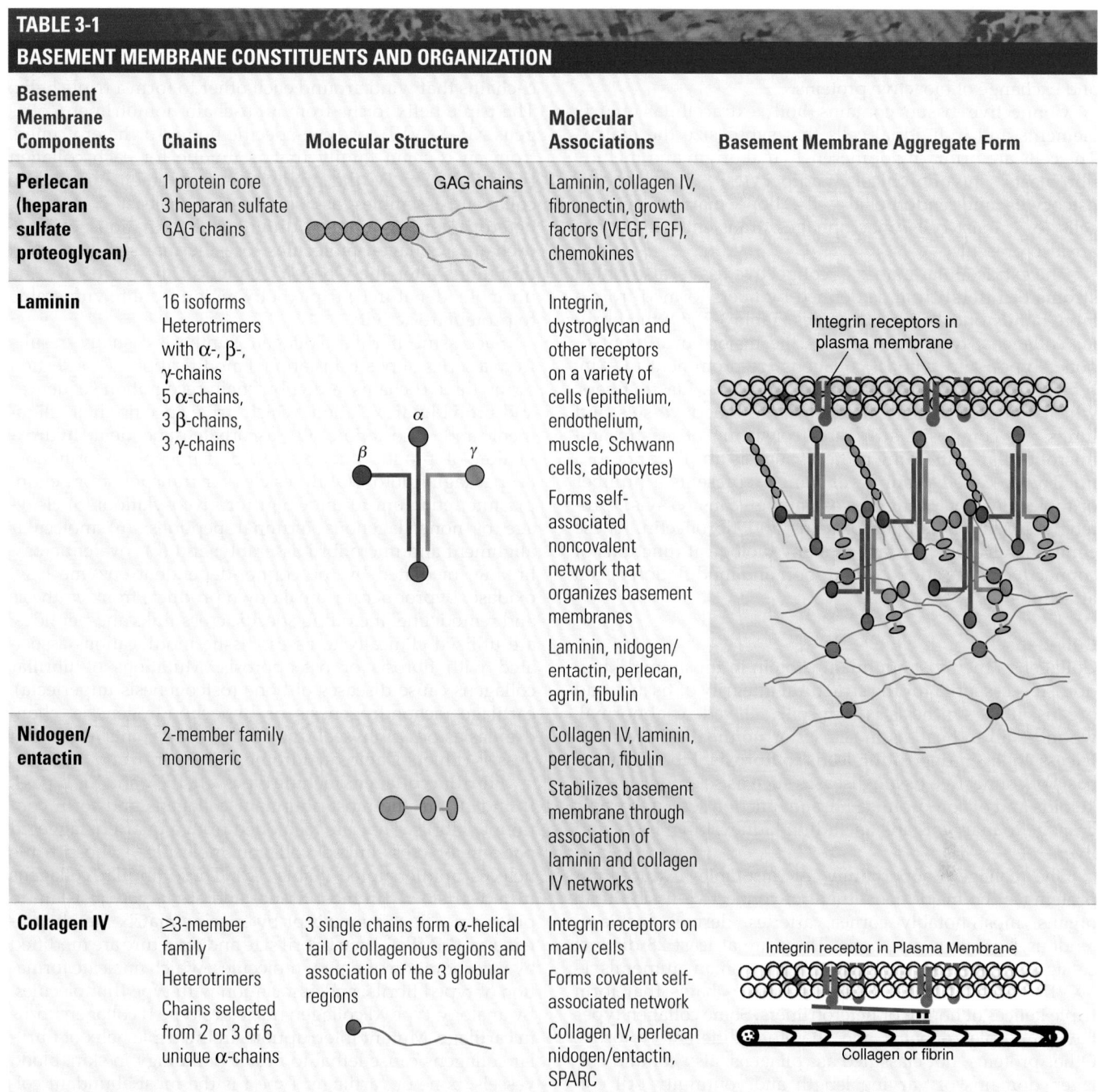

FGF = fibroblast growth factor; GAG = glycosaminoglycan; SPARC = secreted protein acidic and rich and cysteine; VEGF = vascular endothelial growth factor.

morphogenesis and, notably, provide a repository for growth factors and chemotactic peptides.

Provisional Matrix

Provisional matrix is the temporary extracellular organization of plasma-derived matrix proteins and tissue-derived components that accumulate at sites of injury (e.g., hyaluronan, tenascin and fibronectin). These molecules associate with pre-existing stromal matrix and serve to stop blood or fluid loss. Provisional matrix supports migration of leukocytes, endothelial cells and fibroblasts to the wound site. *Plasma-derived provisional matrix proteins include fibrinogen, fibronectin,* *thrombospondin and vitronectin.* The platelet thrombus also contains several growth factors, most prominently PDGF. Insoluble fibrin is generated through the clotting cascade, and the provisional matrix is internally stabilized and bound to the adjacent stromal matrix by transglutaminase (factor XIII)-generated cross-links. In addition to factor XIII stabilization of the fibrin clot, tissue transglutaminases 1 and 2 are also active in wound remodeling and cutaneous regeneration.

Stromal (Interstitial Connective Tissue) Matrix

Connective tissue forms a continuum between tissue elements such as epithelia, nerves and blood vessels and provides physical protection by conferring resistance to compression or tension. Connective tissue stroma is also important for cell migration and as a medium for storage and exchange of bioactive proteins.

Connective tissue contains both extracellular matrix elements and individual cells that synthesize the matrix. The cells are primarily of mesenchymal origin and include fibroblasts, myofibroblasts, adipocytes, chondrocytes, osteocytes and endothelial cells. Bone marrow–derived cells (e.g., mast cells, macrophages, transient leukocytes) are also present.

The extracellular matrix of connective tissue, also called **stroma** or **interstitium,** is defined by fibers formed from a large family of collagen molecules (Table 3-2). Of the fibrillar collagens, type I collagen is the major constituent of bone. Type I and type III collagens are prominent in skin; type II collagen is predominant in cartilage. Elastic fibers, which impart elasticity to skin, large blood vessels and lungs, are composite structures consisting of elastin and microfibrillar scaffolding proteins such as fibrillin and fibulin. The so-called **ground substance** represents a number of molecules, including glycosaminoglycans (GAGs), proteoglycans, matricellular proteins and fibronectin. These components are important in many biological functions of connective tissue and in the support and modulation of cell attachment.

Collagens

Collagen is the most abundant protein in the animal kingdom; it is essential for the structural integrity of tissues and organs. If its synthesis is reduced, delayed or abnormal, wounds fail to heal, as in scurvy or **nonhealing wounds**. Excess collagen deposition leads to **fibrosis**. Fibrosis is the basis of connective tissue diseases such as scleroderma and keloids and of compromised tissue function seen in chronic damage to many organs, including kidney, lung, heart and liver.

The collagen superfamily of insoluble extracellular proteins is the major constituent of connective tissue in all organs, most notably cornea, arteries, dermis, cartilage, tendons, ligaments and bone. There are at least 28 distinct collagen molecules (designated with Roman numerals I–XXVIII), each formed by type-specific α-chains that form triple helices of homo- or heterotrimers. Some collagen types have multiple α-chains and therefore different isoforms. Other proteins, not classified as collagens, also contain collagen domains of varying length and continuity. All collagen α-chains have at least one domain with a repeating α-helical segment, largely composed of glycine, proline and hydroxyproline, in which every third amino acid is glycine (Gly-X-Y). Formation of the triple helical structure depends on this primordial collagen domain with its glycine repeat and on ascorbate-dependent posttranslational formation of hydroxyproline. Residues of lysine, hydroxylysine and histidine form tissue-specific intramolecular and intermolecular, covalent cross-links. A continuous, uninterrupted, triple helical organization of α-chains is the predominant structure of the rigid, stiff, fibrillar collagens. Nonfibrillar collagens contain interrupting, flexible, noncollagenous domains that may even be the major portion of the protein. Collagen family members have important structural functions, but they also affect cell differentiation, growth, migration and matrix morphogenesis through interaction with integrin and discoidin domain transmembrane receptors.

Collagen synthesis exemplifies the complexity of posttranslational protein modification. Each molecule is made by self-association of three homotypic or heterotypic α-chains that wind around each other to form a triple helix. The triple helix forms from an α-chain homotrimer (collagens XII–XXVIII), or type-specific homo- or heterotrimers from an α-chain family that is unique for each collagen type. Collagen IV, the predominant basement membrane collagen, assembles as isoforms of at least 3 different heterotrimers containing different combinations of its 6 α-chains. Collagen molecules lose thermal stability when mutations alter the Gly-X-Y sequence, in which case the unstable (denatured) triple helix region is more vulnerable to proteinase activity.

Successful fibrillar collagen synthesis usually results from a series of posttranslational modifications: (1) selection of the three α-chains, aided by chain recognition sequences and prolyl hydroxylation, which drive specific chain alignment and association; (2) ascorbate-dependent hydroxylation of proline and lysine; (3) triple helix formation; (4) packaging into COPII vesicles for transport from endoplasmic reticulum to the Golgi for glycosylation; (5) cleavage of noncollagenous terminal peptides; (6) molecular alignment and microfibril assembly; and (7) covalent cross-linking, mediated by the copper-dependent enzyme lysyl oxidase. Byproducts or breakdown products from synthesis and remodeling, including specific cross-links and peptides, are utilized clinically to assess tissue modifications associated with fibrosis or osteoporosis. Mutations of fibrillar collagens cause diseases of bone (osteogenesis imperfecta), cartilage (achondrogenesis or hypochondrogenesis, chondroplasias or epiphyseal dysplasias), skin, joints and blood vessels (Ehlers-Danlos syndrome) (Chapters 6 and 30).

Fibrillar collagens include types I, II, III, V and XI. Types I, II and III are the most abundant collagens and form continuous fibrils. They are fashioned from a quarter-staggered packing of cross-linked collagen molecules, whose triple helix is uninterrupted (Table 3-2). These fibrillar collagens turn over slowly in most tissues and are largely resistant to proteinase digestion, except by specific matrix metalloproteinases (MMPs). Type I fibril size and structure are modified by incorporation of type V molecules, which nucleate formation of type I fibrils, and association with type III molecules. By analogy, type XI collagen nucleates type II collagen fibrils in cartilage. Mutant interruptions in the triple helix of fibrillar collagens cause lethal to minor pathology in skin, blood vessels, bone or cartilage. Type I is the most abundant collagen, and mutations in the genes for this molecule cause assembly defects in the triple helix that can lead to increased bone fractures, hyperextensible ligaments and dermis or easy bruising (Chapter 6).

Nonfibrillar collagens (Table 3-2) contain a mixture of globular and triple helical domains. The interruption of the triple helical domains confers structural diversity and molecular flexibility not possessed by fibrillar collagens. Nonhelical domains enable small collagens (IX, XII) to associate with fibrillar collagens, thereby modulating fiber packing of a linear collagen. Collagen VI, which forms beaded filament structures (VI) that encircle fibrillar collagens I and II, is found close to cells and associates with elastin in elastic fibers; mutations are associated with certain myopathies and muscular dystrophy, as collagen VI helps connect muscle cells to basement membrane. Other nonfibrillar collagens act as **transmembrane** proteins (XVII) in hemidesmosomes

TABLE 3-2
COLLAGEN MOLECULAR COMPOSITION AND STRUCTURE

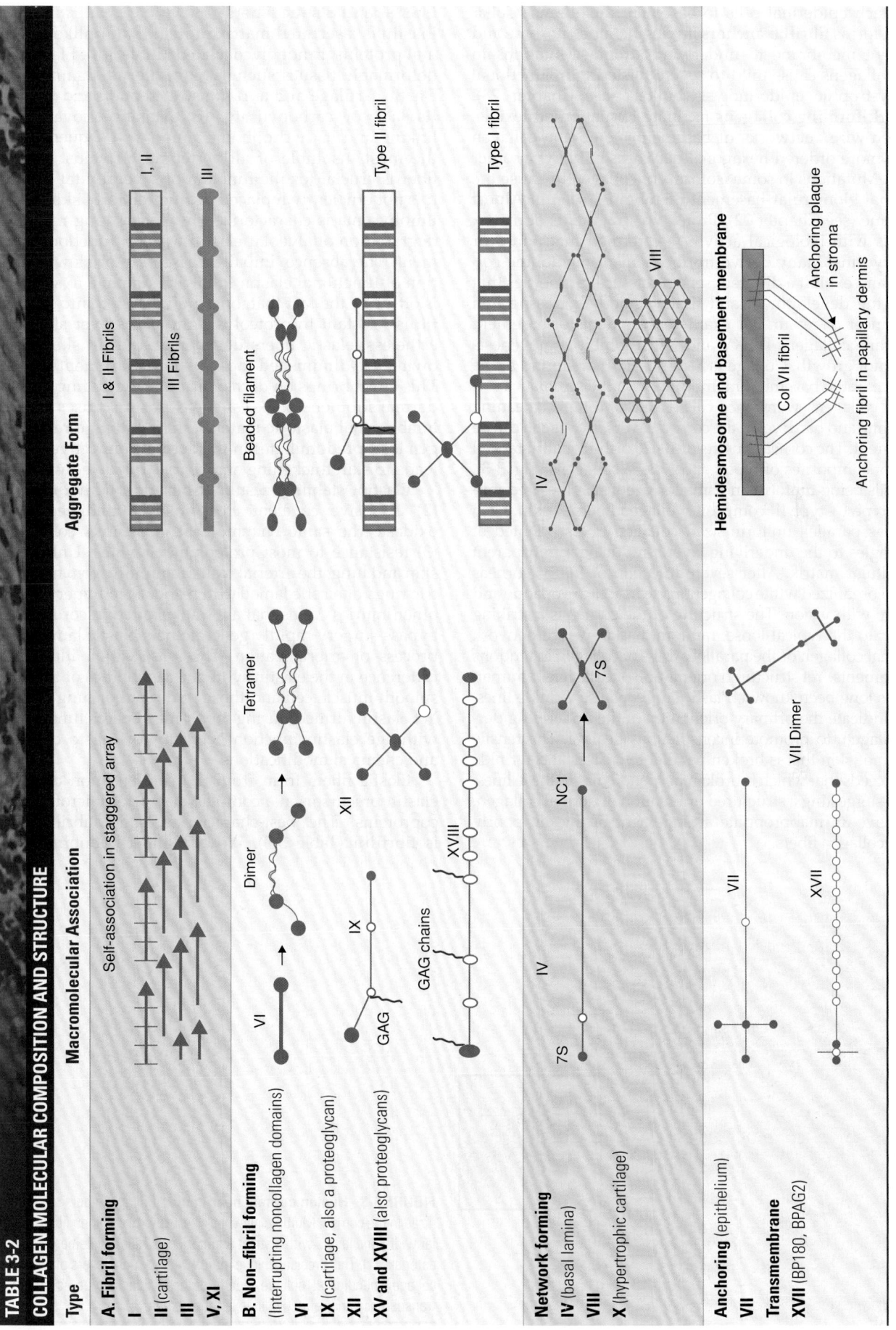

Type	Macromolecular Association	Aggregate Form
A. Fibril forming	Self-association in staggered array	I & II Fibrils III Fibrils I, II III
I		
II (cartilage)		
III		
V, XI		
B. Non–fibril forming (Interrupting noncollagen domains)	Dimer Tetramer	Beaded filament
VI		
IX (cartilage, also a proteoglycan)	GAG XII	Type II fibril
XII		
XV and XVIII (also proteoglycans)	GAG chains XVIII	Type I fibril
Network forming	7S NC1 7S IV	IV VIII
IV (basal lamina)		
VIII		
X (hypertrophic cartilage)		
Anchoring (epithelium)	VII VII Dimer	Hemidesmosome and basement membrane
VII		Col VII fibril Anchoring plaque in stroma Anchoring fibril in papillary dermis
Transmembrane	XVII	
XVII (BP180, BPAG2)		

that attach epidermal cells to basement membrane. Collagen VII forms **fibrillar anchors** linking hemidesmosome and basement membrane to underlying stroma. Mutations in these collagens cause mild to severe blistering in junctional and dystrophic epidermolysis bullosa (see Chapter 28). **Network-forming collagens** facilitate formation of flexible, "chicken-wire" networks of basement membrane collagen (IV) or more ordered hexagonal networks (VIII, X) in other tissues. Mutations in some isoforms of collagen IV cause the abnormal glomerular basement membranes seen in Alport syndrome (see Chapter 22). Proteolytic fragments of matrix proteins with biological activity are termed matrikines or matricryptins. Many derive from basement membrane collagens and exhibit a different set of biological properties that act during development and tissue remodeling associated with cancer or repair. For example, fragments of basement membrane collagens IV, XV and XVIII inhibit angiogenesis and tumor growth. Collagens XV and XVIII are found at the interface of the basement membrane with the stroma.

The collagens were once called **scleroproteins,** meaning both white and hard; yet in the cornea, layers of collagen can be transparent. The cornea consists of 10–20 orthogonally stacked layers of composites of type I and type V collagens (Fig. 3-3), the fibrils being uniform and smaller sized than the predominantly type I + type III composite collagen fibers in skin. Each layer has parallel, uniform-sized collagen fibers oriented at right angles to the underlying layer, producing a transparent extracellular matrix. After severe infection or injury, corneas form disorganized white collagenous scars that are opaque and interfere with vision. The structure of the cornea is a striking contrast to the typical loose, random, basket-weave network of dermal collagen or the parallel arrays of collagen in tendons and ligaments. Yet structured orientation of collagen in human skin has long been known. Plastic surgeons use wrinkle lines, which indicate the primary orientation of the underlying dermal collagen, to promote inconspicuous healing. The tensile strength of skin that is broken parallel to creases and wrinkle lines exceeds that which is broken perpendicular to these lines, further suggesting a structured orientation of dermal collagen. Scars have an inappropriate arrangement of thicker, poorly woven collagen fibers.

Elastin and Elastic Fibers

Elastin is a secreted matrix protein that, unlike other stromal proteins, is not glycosylated (Table 3-3). Elastin allows deformable tissues such as skin, uterus, ligaments, lung, elastic cartilage and aorta to stretch and bend with recoil. Its lack of carbohydrate, its extensive covalent cross-linking and its hydrophobic amino acid sequence make it the most insoluble of all vertebrate proteins. The elastic fiber is crucial for the function of several vital tissues, yet it is not efficiently replaced during repair of skin and lung. Emphysema is characterized by loss of lung recoil due to degradation of alveolar elastin without functional replacement. The absence, impaired assembly or slow accumulation of functional elastin following damage to skin or lung is offset by the fact that, once polymerized into fibers, elastin is resistant to proteolysis and turns over slowly. Nevertheless, elastic fibers degenerate and, in skin, decrease owing to a diminished capacity for replacement with aging. This effect brings on dermal atrophy, wrinkling and loss of dermal suppleness. Excess sun exposure causes an increase in abnormal elastotic material that, with age-related collagen loss, predominates in the dermal connective tissue and leads to skin thickening and coarse, furrowed wrinkles.

Elastin stability results from its (1) hydrophobicity, (2) extensive covalent cross-linking (mediated by lysyl oxidase, the same enzyme that cross-links collagen) and (3) resistance to most proteolytic enzymes. Unlike injured skin and lung, the arterial wall can rapidly form new concentric rings of elastic lamellae in response to hypertension and other injuries. Veins that are transplanted in coronary artery bypass surgery rapidly generate new elastic lamellae in the process of arterialization. This observation illustrates the difference in the elastin synthetic capabilities of the vascular smooth muscle cell and those of dermal or lung fibroblasts. Yet elastin formed during repair may be less functional, and with age elastin function decreases owing to degradation and chemical modifications.

Elastic fibers form from the condensation of a soluble elastin precursor on a complex of several microfibrillar glycoproteins. The best-characterized microfibrillar protein is **fibrillin** (Table 3-3). When mutated, abnormal fibrillin

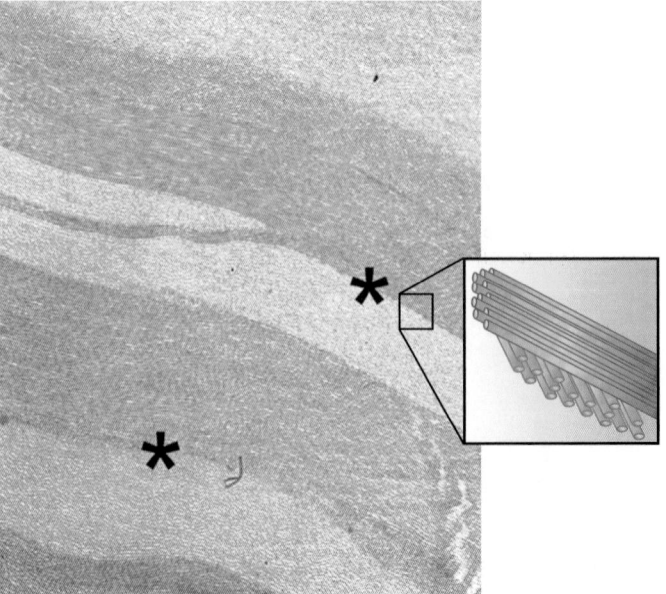

FIGURE 3-3. Human cornea, near center. Collagen fibers are highly organized in the cornea. Multiple plywood-like arrays of collagen fibers are of similar width and layers with distinct orientation are sharply demarcated between asterisks (*). This precise, unique matrix organization, layers of highly ordered collagen bundles at oblique, nearly perpendicular angles, is critical to the transparency and refractive index of the cornea.

TABLE 3-3
NONCOLLAGENOUS MATRIX CONSTITUENTS OF STROMA

Stromal Connective Tissue Components	Chains	Molecular Structure	Molecular Associations	Tissue Structures
Fibronectin	Dimeric protein Chains chosen from ~20 splice variants of one gene	 fibrin collagen heparin fibrin heparin cells RGD N C	Integrin receptors of many cells (RGD-binding site) Plasma fibronectin is soluble Cellular fibronectin can self-associate into fibrils at cell surface and also binds collagen, heparin, decorin, fibrin, certain bacteria (opsonin), LTBPs	 Cell cytoplasm Integrin receptor in plasma membrane Collagen or fibrin
Elastin	Monomer with several splice variants, 1 gene	 Elastin cross-links to form fiber	Self-association to form cross-linked amorphous fibers Formed on scaffold of microfibrillar polymers	 Elastin fiber with microfibril polymers
Fibrillins	Large glycoproteins—most common microfibrils needed for elastin fiber assembly		Forms beaded polymer Other microfibrillar proteins: LTBPs, fibulins, emilins, MAGP 1 and 2, lysyl oxidase	
Versican (hyaluronan-binding proteoglycans)	Family of 4 related genes Aggrecan found in cartilage Protein core decorated with 10–30 chondroitin sulfate and dermatan sulfate GAG chains	 CS	Proteoglycans linked to hyaluronan via link protein to form very large composite structure	 Hyaluronan
Decorin (small leucine-rich proteoglycans)	1 protein core, 1 gene 1 chondroitin sulfate or dermatan sulfate GAG chain Biglycan and fibromodulin structurally related, genetically distinct		Collagen I and II, fibronectin, TGF-β, thrombospondin	 Collagen I or II

GAG = glycosaminoglycan; LTBPs = latent transforming growth factor-β–binding proteins; MAGP = microfibril-associated growth protein; RGD = Arg-Gly-Asp; TGF-β = transforming growth factor-β.

demonstrates decreased binding and reduced activation of transforming growth factor-β (TGF-β). The result is Marfan syndrome, with pleomorphic manifestations that include dissecting aortic aneurysm (Chapter 6). Mutations in **fibulin** can result in the generalized elastin defect, cutis laxa.

Matrix Glycoproteins

Matrix glycoproteins, sometimes referred to as matricellular proteins, contribute essential biological functions to basement membrane and stromal connective tissue. In general, these are large (150,000–1,000,000 kd) multimeric and multidomain macromolecules, with long arms that bind other matrix molecules and support or modulate cell attachment. Matrix glycoproteins help to (1) organize tissue topography, (2) support cell migration, (3) orient cells and (4) induce cell behavior. The principal matrix glycoprotein of basement membrane is **laminin,** and that of stromal connective tissue is **fibronectin**.

LAMININS: The laminins are a versatile family of basement membrane glycoproteins whose cross-like structure is formed by products of three related gene subfamilies to form α, β and γ heterotrimers (Table 3-1). There are 18 known laminin isoforms, which assemble intracellularly from varying combinations of the five α-, three β- and three γ-chains. Once secreted, some laminin trimers are further processed by proteinases. Laminin molecules self-polymerize into sheets that initiate basement membrane formation by association with type IV collagen sheets and other basement membrane molecules. Expression of laminin isoforms in specific tissues contributes to the heterogeneity of tissue morphology and functions, in part, by supporting cell attachment via binding to membrane sulfated glycolipids and transmembrane receptors. The cell attachments concentrate laminin and construct the lattice on which other basement membrane molecules accumulate. Laminin binds to both heparan sulfate proteoglycans in basement membranes and to heparan sulfate chains on syndecan receptors. Cells also bind to laminin via several integrins, as well as muscle dystroglycan and Lutheran blood grouping receptors, which on red cells may be involved in the release from bone marrow during hematopoiesis. The muscle cell dystroglycan receptor complex binds basement membrane laminin, and mutations in either the receptor or laminin account for different forms of muscular dystrophy (see Chapter 31). The appropriate proteolytic processing of the epidermal laminin isoform is critical for normal epidermal function and reepithelialization of wounds. Epidermal integrity is stabilized at the basal surface by hemidesmosomes, which develop from the binding of basement membrane laminin to epithelial integrin (integrin $\alpha_6\beta_4$) and involve collagen XVII and collagen VII. The latter forms the anchoring fibril that connects the epidermal cell and basement membrane to the dermal connective tissue. Mutations in epidermal laminin or the appropriate integrin, or the previously mentioned collagen VII or collagen XVII, produce different forms of a potentially fatal skin blistering disease, termed **epidermolysis bullosa**.

FIBRONECTINS: Fibronectins are versatile, adhesive glycoproteins that are widely distributed in stromal connective tissue and deposited in wound provisional matrix (Table 3-3). Fibronectin chains form a V-shaped homo- or heterodimer linked at the C terminus by two disulfide bonds. Specific fibronectin domains bind bacteria, collagen, heparin, fibrin, fibrinogen and the cell matrix receptor integrin.

Indeed, the integrin receptor family has been partly defined by studies showing its specific binding to fibronectin. The multifunctional dimer links matrix molecules to one another or to cells. Thrombi support cell migration owing to the high concentration of plasma-derived fibronectin that connects fibrin strands. The complex is further stabilized by cross-linking of factor XIII (transglutaminase) to other provisional and dermal matrix components.

Two classes of fibronectin are encoded by a single gene but from different sources: (1) the insoluble, cellular form; and (2) a hepatocyte-derived, soluble form in plasma. As many as 24 fibronectin variants may be formed by alternative splicing. Clot-bound fibronectin supports platelet adhesion. It can also interact with collagen to promote keratinocyte attachment and migration during reepithelialization of corneal and cutaneous wounds by aiding collagen. Fibronectin synthesized by mesenchymal cells such as fibroblasts is assembled into insoluble fibrils with the aid of integrin receptors and collagen fibrils. Polymerized cellular fibronectin is found in granulation tissue and loose connective tissue. Excisional wound clotting and reepithelialization are unaffected by experimentally knocking out plasma fibronectin, suggesting that cellular fibronectin and other factors can compensate for its absence.

Glycosaminoglycans

Glycosaminoglycans (historically known as mucopolysaccharides) are long, linear polymers of specific repeating disaccharides, each containing a uronic acid. GAG chains are distinguished by the disaccharide subunits in the polymer. The chains are negatively charged, owing to the presence of carboxylate groups and, save for hyaluronan, by modification with N- or O-linked sulfate groups. GAGs have the potential for exceptional diversity and biological specificity because of epimerization and variability in modifications (e.g., acetylation and sulfation). When sulfated GAG chains are O-linked to serine residues of protein cores, the structures are called **proteoglycans** (see below). GAG storage disorders result from autosomal recessive (or X-linked) deficiency of one of several lysosomal hydrolases that degrade GAGs, causing intracellular accumulation within lysosomes. The 12 known mucopolysaccharidoses are slowly evolving disorders of connective tissue that significantly decrease life expectancy; affect ossification of cartilage, skeletal structure, stature and facies; and may cause psychomotor problems or even mild retardation.

Hyaluronan

Hyaluronan, the only GAG not covalently linked to a protein, is a linear polymer of 2000–25,000 disaccharides of glucosamine and glucuronic acid. Its charge content makes hyaluronan very hydrophilic. Hyaluronan can associate with protein cores of proteoglycans (defined below) that contain hyaluronan-binding regions and with hyaluronan-binding proteins at the cell surface. Certain proteoglycans bind noncovalently along the hyaluronan backbone via a link protein to form large, space-filling, hydrophilic hyaluronan/proteoglycan composites. These are **aggrecan** and **versican** (Table 3-3), molecules found in cartilage and stromal tissues, respectively. The viscosity of free hyaluronan in solution imparts resilience and lubrication to joints and connective tissue, and pericellular accumulation of these molecules as part of the glycocalyx facilitates cell migration through the extracellular matrix. Hyaluronan is highly prevalent in the stroma during embryonic development, and it is an early addition to the provisional matrix. The negatively charged carboxylate backbone of hyaluronan binds large amounts of water, creating a viscous gel that produces turgor in the matrix. As a biomaterial, hyaluronan can be chemically modified to act as a temporary dermal filler, joint lubricant or replacement for vitreous humor. Unlike other secreted macromolecules, hyaluronan synthesis occurs at the cell surface, and cells also express several types of hyaluronan receptors. Concentrations of pericellular hyaluronan are higher during dynamic tissue remodeling associated with inflammation, wound repair, morphogenesis or cancer. Resolution of the wound healing process relies on inflammatory monocytes with CD44 receptors to bind to and remove the pericellular hyaluronan matrix and excess hyaluronan in matrix, in concert with the action of hyaluronidases. Reduced hyaluronidase activity in fetal wounds may reduce inflammation and favor less scar formation.

Proteoglycans

Proteoglycans are a diverse family of proteins with varying numbers, types and sizes of attached glycosaminoglycan chains linked by O-glycosidic bonds to serines or threonines. They have a higher carbohydrate content than matrix glycoproteins and, though not branched, show substantial diversity through numerous carbohydrate modifications, such as sulfation, unique linkages and varying sequences. Individual proteoglycans whose names are designated by the core protein can differ widely in number and choice of GAG chains, as well as tissue distribution.

Proteoglycans participate in matrix organization, structural integrity and cell attachment. Though their protein core often has biological activity, the properties of several proteoglycans are largely mediated by the GAG chains themselves. The strongly charged heparan sulfate GAG chains of basement membrane (perlecan, collagen XVIII) and cell receptor proteoglycans (syndecan, glypican) modulate the availability and actions of heparin-binding growth factors, such as vascular endothelial growth factor (VEGF), fibroblast growth factor (FGF) and heparin-binding epidermal growth factor (HB-EGF). PDGF is also more weakly bound to these highly charged molecules. A group of small proteoglycans, which share a core protein domain of leucine-rich repeats, regulates TGF-β activity and fibril formation in collagens I and II (Table 3-3). Sequestered growth factors are released when proteoglycans are degraded by heparanase and other hydrolases.

Tissue expression of extracellular matrix proteins and proteoglycans is shown in Table 3-4.

Remodeling Is the Long-Lasting Phase of Repair

As repair proceeds, inflammatory cells become fewer in number and capillary formation is completed. In remodeling, fibroblast numbers rapidly rise and then fall as an equilibrium between collagen deposition and degradation is restored. MMPs are the main remodeling enzymes, but neutrophil cathepsins and serine proteases are also present at the early phase of wound debridement. Unlike the inflammatory cell proteinases, MMP and ADAM protease activity is highly localized. The superfamily of proteinases with the presence of zinc at the catalytic site (metzincins) includes the MMPs and other subfamilies including ADAM (a disintegrin and metalloproteinase) and ADAM

with thrombospondin motifs (ADAMTS). Members of the metzincin superfamily are key regulators in tissue during times of change such as development or remodeling. The activity of these proteases is controlled, in part, by a family of tissue-based molecules known as tissue inhibitors of metalloproteinases (TIMPs).

MMPs are a large family of 25 proteinases with overlapping specificities. They enable cells to migrate through stroma by degrading matrix proteins and so are central to wound healing (Table 3-3). They participate in cell–cell communication and activation or inactivation of bioactive molecules (e.g., immune system components, matrix fragments, growth factors) and influence cell growth and apoptosis. MMPs are synthesized as inactive proenzymes (zymogens), and many secreted MMPs require extracellular activation by already activated MMPs, such as MMP-3, MMP-14 or serine proteinases. The six membrane-anchored MMPs are activated prior to locating at the cell surface. They are attached via a small cytoplasmic tail or, for two of them, via a glycosylphosphatidylinositol (GPI) anchor. Secreted MMPs are named sequentially (e.g., MMP-1, MMP-2), and membrane-type MMPs also have a secondary designation (e.g., MT1-MMP, MT2-MMP). The cell surface activities of MT1- and MT2-MMPs are important for cell migration and invasion. Originally, MMPs were named by their matrix substrates (e.g., collagenase, stromelysin and gelatinase). However, MMPs cleave diverse extracellular substrates, many of which are degraded by more than one MMP. As with integrins, such redundancy emphasizes the importance of these molecules in regulatory control through activating, deactivating and shedding of substrates. *The list of molecules needed for wound healing is indistinguishable from the list of MMP substrates.* These include:

- Clotting factors
- Extracellular matrix proteins
- Latent growth factors and growth factor–binding proteins
- Receptors for matrix molecules and cell–cell adhesion molecules
- Immune system components
- Other MMPs, other proteinases and proteinase inhibitors
- Chemotactic molecules

Most MMPs are closely regulated at the transcriptional level, except for MMP-2 (gelatinase A), which is often constitutively expressed and activated at the cell surface by MT1-MMP (MMP-14). Transcription is regulated by (1) integrin signaling, (2) cytokine and growth factor signaling, (3) binding to certain matrix proteins or (4) tensional force on a cell. MMPs have a number of activities that support the remodeling and resolution phases of wound healing. MT1-MMP and MT2-MMP may associate with integrins to aid cell migration and invasion or activate TGF-β. MMP-1 associates with $\alpha_2\beta_1$ integrin, facilitating cell migration of dermal keratinocytes on collagen during the reepithelialization of the wound surface. The integrin binds the cell to the collagen substrate and the MMP-1 cleaves collagen to enable cell release and migration. Membrane-associated proteoglycans (syndecans, CD44) also store and regulate the availability and activity of MMPs. In addition to affecting cell–cell adhesion and release, MMPs activate or inactivate bioactive molecules stored in the matrix. These include growth factors, chemokines, growth factor–binding proteins, angiogenic/antiangiogenic factors and bioactive

TABLE 3-4

TISSUE EXPRESSION OF EXTRACELLULAR MATRIX MOLECULES

Tissue or Body Fluid	Primary Mesodermal Cell	Prominent Collagen Types	Noncollagenous Matrix Proteins	Glycosaminoglycans Proteoglycans (PGs)
Plasma			Fibronectin, fibrinogen, vitronectin	Hyaluronan
Dermis Reticular/papillary Epidermal junction	Fibroblast	I, III, V, VI, XII, XXIV, XXIX, VII, XVII (BP 180), anchoring fibrils, hemidesmosome	Fibronectin, elastin, fibrillin	Hyaluronan, decorin, biglycan, versican
Muscle	Muscle cell	I, III, V, VI, VIII, XII, XV, XXII	Fibronectin, elastin, fibrillin	Aggrecan, biglycan, decorin, fibromodulin
Peri-, epimysium Aortic media/ adventitia	Fibroblast			
Tendon	Fibroblast	I, III, V, VI, XII, XXII	Fibronectin, tenascin (myotendon junction), elastin, fibrillin	Decorin, biglycan, fibromodulin, lumican, versican
Ligament	Fibroblast	I, III, V, VI	Fibronectin, elastin, fibrillin	Decorin, biglycan, versican
Cornea	Fibroblast	I, II, III, V, VI, XII, XXIV		Lumican, keratocan, mimecan, biglycan, decorin
Cartilage	Chondrocyte hypertrophic cartilage	II, IX, VI, VIII, X, XI, XXVII	Anchorin CII, fibronectin, tenascin	Hyaluronan, aggrecan, biglycan, decorin, fibromodulin, lumican, perlecan (minor)
Bone	Osteocyte	I, V, XXIV, XIII	Osteocalcin, osteopontin, bone sialoprotein, SPARC (osteonectin)	Decorin, fibromodulin, biglycan
Nervous system: CNS, PNS (including Schwann cell basement membrane)	Neurons, neurologic cells	I–IX; XI–XIX; XXI–XXIII; XXV, XXVII, XXVIII, XXIX	Laminins, nidogen/entactin, tenascin, thrombospondin	Chondroitin sulfate containing proteoglycans, heparan sulfate containing proteoglycans (agrin, perlecan)
Basement membrane zones	Epithelial (most organs, e.g., kidney), endothelial (capillaries) adipocytes, Schwann cell, muscle cells (endomysium), pericytes, neuromuscular junction	IV, XV, XVIII	Laminins, nidogen/entactin	Heparan sulfate proteoglycans, perlecan Collagen XVIII (vascular), agrin (neuromuscular junctions)

CNS = central nervous system; PNS = peripheral nervous system; SPARC = secreted protein acidic and rich in cysteine.

cryptic fragments of collagens and proteoglycans. The fragments are released when their parent matrix molecules are degraded **(matrikines).**

Once secreted, MMPs act largely near the cell surface, its activity confined by diffusion/sequestration, reduced activation, substrate specificity and peptide inhibitors. The last group includes the family of TIMPs and the general, plasma-derived proteinase inhibitor, α_2-macroglobulin. The ADAMs function to shed ectodomains of growth factors, chemokines and receptors on cell or neighboring cell surfaces. The ADAMTS family members are released and activated through cleavage of the thrombospondin (TS) domain, thereby generating the cleavage of substrates such as aggrecan, a large proteoglycan of cartilage, and von Willebrand factor.

Cell Proliferation Is Evoked by Cytokines and Matrix

Early in tissue injury, there is a dramatic, transient increase in cellularity that elevates immune surveillance and replaces (some) damaged cells. Cell proliferation and migration initiate and perpetuate **granulation tissue,** a specialized, highly vascularized tissue that forms transiently during repair (see below). Cells of granulation tissue derive from ephemeral cell populations, including circulating leukocytes, and from adjacent, resident capillary endothelial and mesenchymal cells (fibroblasts, myofibroblasts, pericytes and smooth muscle cells). Local and marrow-derived progenitor cells, which share some properties of leukocytes, can also populate wounds, potentially differentiating into (transient) endothelial and fibroblast populations. Terminally differentiated cells (e.g., cardiac myocytes, neurons) do not for the most part contribute to repair or regeneration (discussed below).

Growth factors and small chemotactic peptides (chemokines) provide soluble autocrine and paracrine signals for cell proliferation, differentiation and migration. Signals from soluble factors and extracellular matrix also work collectively to influence cell behavior.

Behaviors of cells in healing wounds—proliferation, migration and altered gene expression—are largely initiated by three receptor systems that share integrated signaling pathways:

- **Protein tyrosine kinase receptors** for peptide growth factors
- **G-protein–coupled receptors** for chemokines and other factors
- **Integrin receptors** for extracellular matrix

Tyrosine kinase receptors, growth factor matrix integrin receptors and G-protein–coupled receptors act in concert to direct cell behavior. Primarily through integrin-mediated binding to the extracellular matrix, these distinct receptor families are influenced by the mechanical environment. Although they bind distinct ligands, they transmit signals within a network of cascading and intersecting intracellular signaling pathways. These routes amplify the messages, often activating similar processes that affect cytoskeletal organization and gene expression. Even different processes, such as proliferation, differentiation and migration, may share signals, such as those that initiate cytoskeletal changes. The myriad intracellular signaling mechanisms that regulate cell growth, survival and proliferation are beyond the scope of the current discussion. It is important to recognize that tissue responses are governed by integration of signals from all these systems.

REPAIR

Outcomes of Injury Include Repair with Restoration or Regeneration

Repair and restoration follow inflammatory responses, inflammation itself being the primary response to tissue injury (see Chapter 2). To understand how inflammation influences repair, it is useful to review the various possible outcomes of acute inflammation. *Transient* acute inflammation may resolve completely, with locally injured parenchymal elements regenerating without significant scarring. Thus, after a moderate sunburn, occasional acute inflammatory cells accompany transient vasodilation under solar-injured epidermis. By contrast, *progressive* acute inflammation, with eventual macrophage-predominant infiltrates, is central to the sequence of collagen elaboration and repair. Complete regeneration—as opposed to the more usual restoration

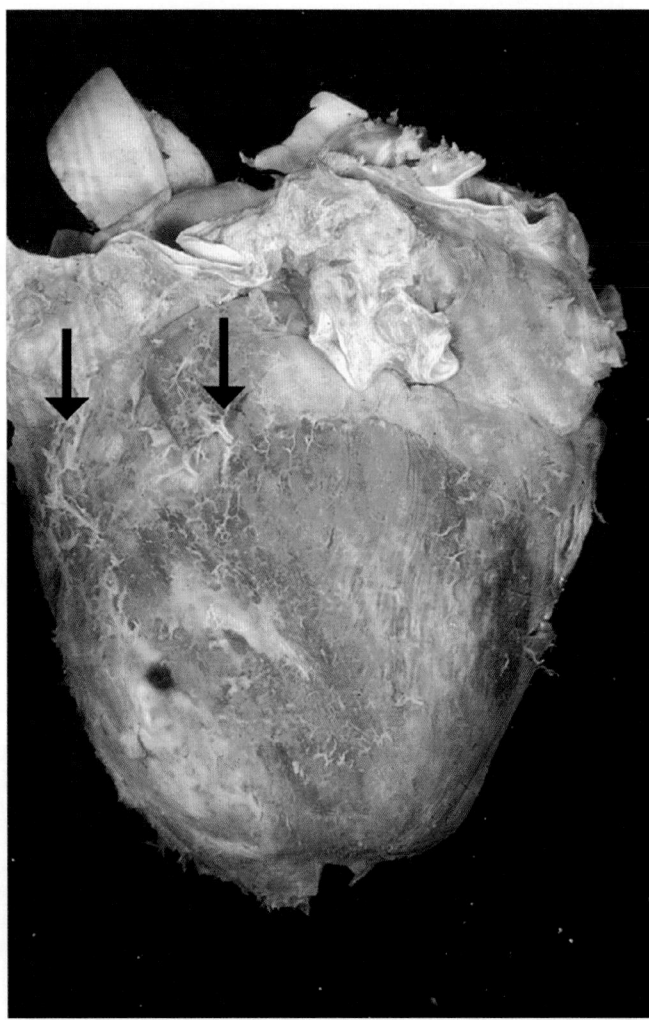

FIGURE 3-4. Organized strands of collagen in constrictive pericarditis (*arrows*). Excess collagen distorts the biomechanical properties of the heart.

during adult repair—may occur with injury to liver or bone: that is, normal hepatic structure is replaced after many self-limited hepatic insults.

Organization is a pathologic outcome of fibrinogen leakage from blood vessels during an inflammatory response. It occurs in serous cavities, like the peritoneum, when fibrin strands are not degraded and form a provisional matrix. Conversion of the provisional matrix to fibrous (granulation) tissue occurs following invasion of connective tissue cells, inflammatory cells and capillaries. In pericarditis, fibroblasts invade the provisional fibrin matrix and secrete and organize a collagenous extracellular matrix among fibrin strands, thus binding visceral and parietal pericardium together (Fig. 3-4). This constricts ventricular filling of the heart and may require surgical intervention. Fibrin strands may become organized in the peritoneal cavity after intra-abdominal surgery. Such adhesions (threads of collagen) can trap loops of bowel and cause intestinal obstruction.

Wound Healing Exhibits a Defined Sequence

Wound healing that results in scar formation remains the predominant mode of adult repair. Given that wounds in the skin and extremities are easily accessible, they have been extensively

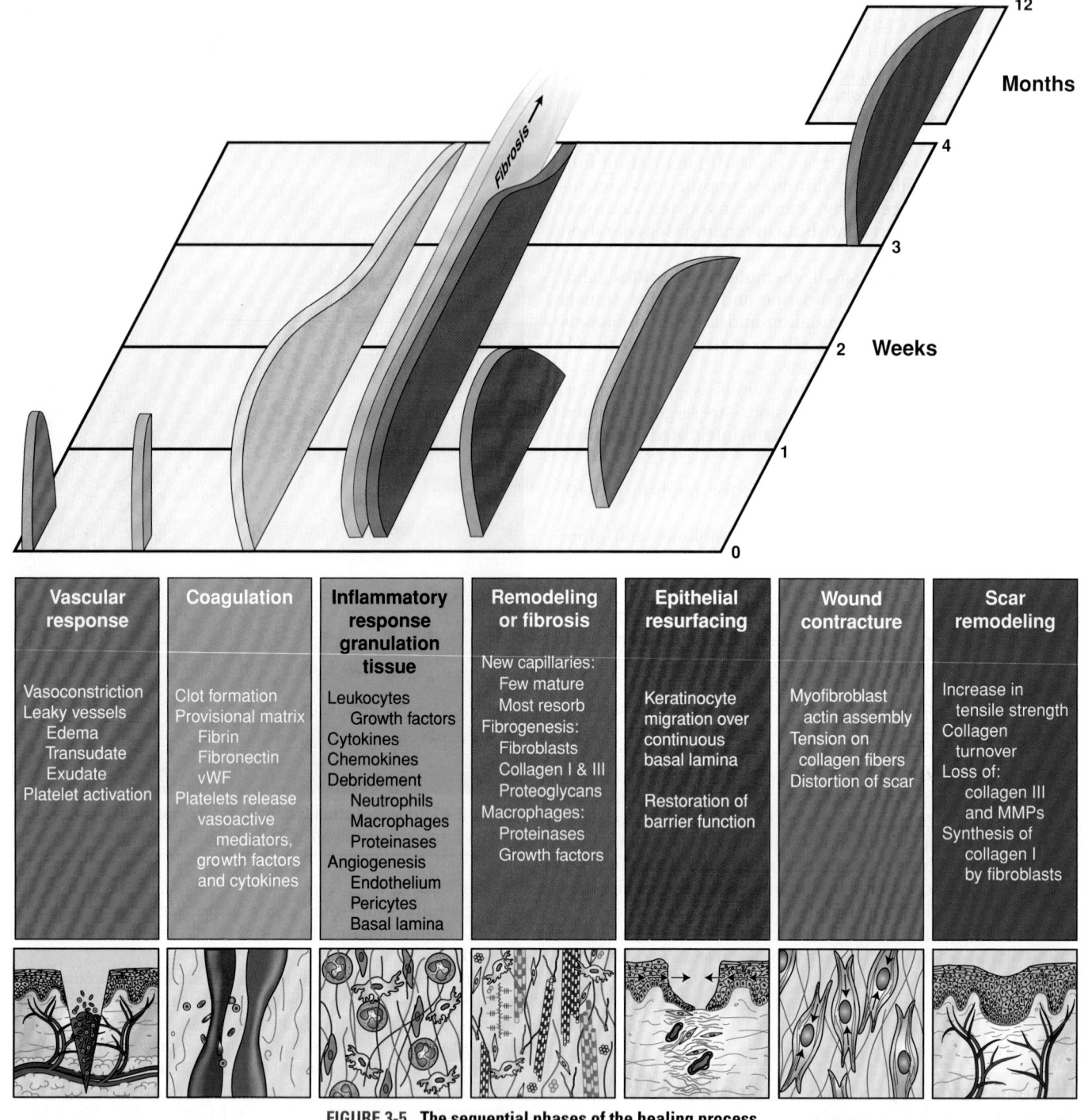

FIGURE 3-5. The sequential phases of the healing process.

studied as models. Healing within hollow viscera and body cavities, though less accessible for study, generally parallels the repair sequence in skin, as illustrated in Figs. 3-5 and 3-6.

Thrombosis

A thrombus (clot)—a **scab** or **eschar** after it dries atop a surface wound—forms a barrier on wounded skin to invading microorganisms. The formation of the fibrin clot is essential to prevent loss of plasma and tissue fluid. Although the clot/thrombus is predominantly plasma fibrin, the thrombus is also rich in the adhesive protein fibronectin. The thrombus

also contains contracting platelets, whose aggregation produces an initial burst of stored growth factors. At the site of injury, fibrin is bound to fibronectin and is progressively cross-linked by factor XIII (FXIII), a transglutaminase that forms glutamyl-lysine cross-links between proteins that form the clot and extracellular matrix proteins. Cross-linking aids clot retraction. Transglutaminase 2 (tissue transglutaminase) fosters cell adhesion, cell migration and organization of wound extracellular matrix by (1) interlinking matrix proteins such as fibrinogen, fibronectin, collagen and vitronectin; (2) providing local tensile strength; and (3) maintaining closure during the evolution of new extracellular

2–4 Days

Thrombus

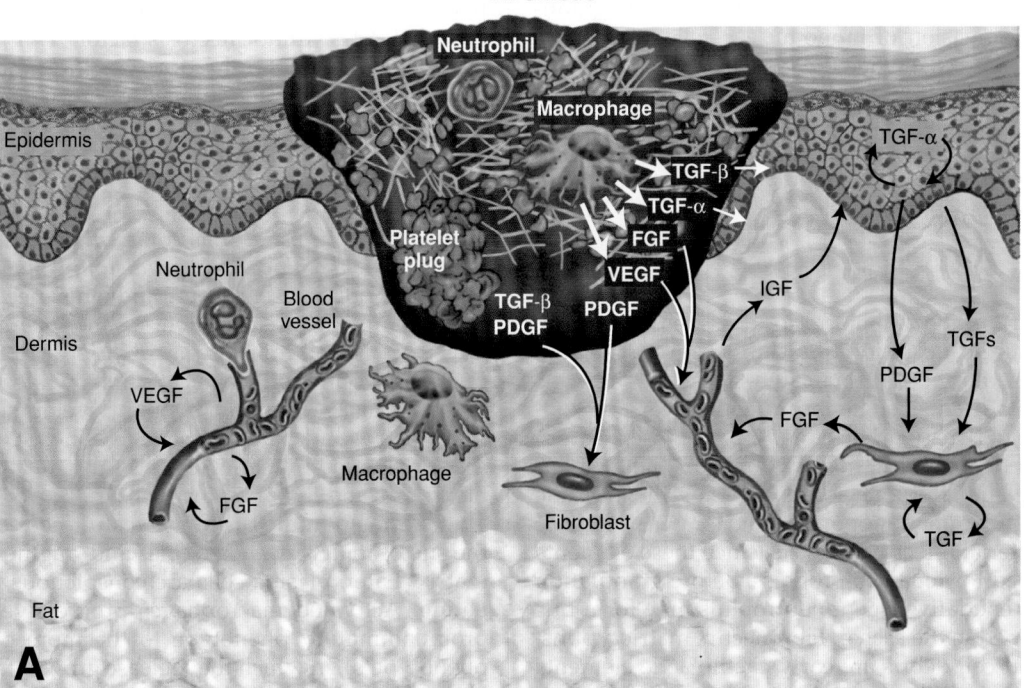

4–8 Days

Thrombus

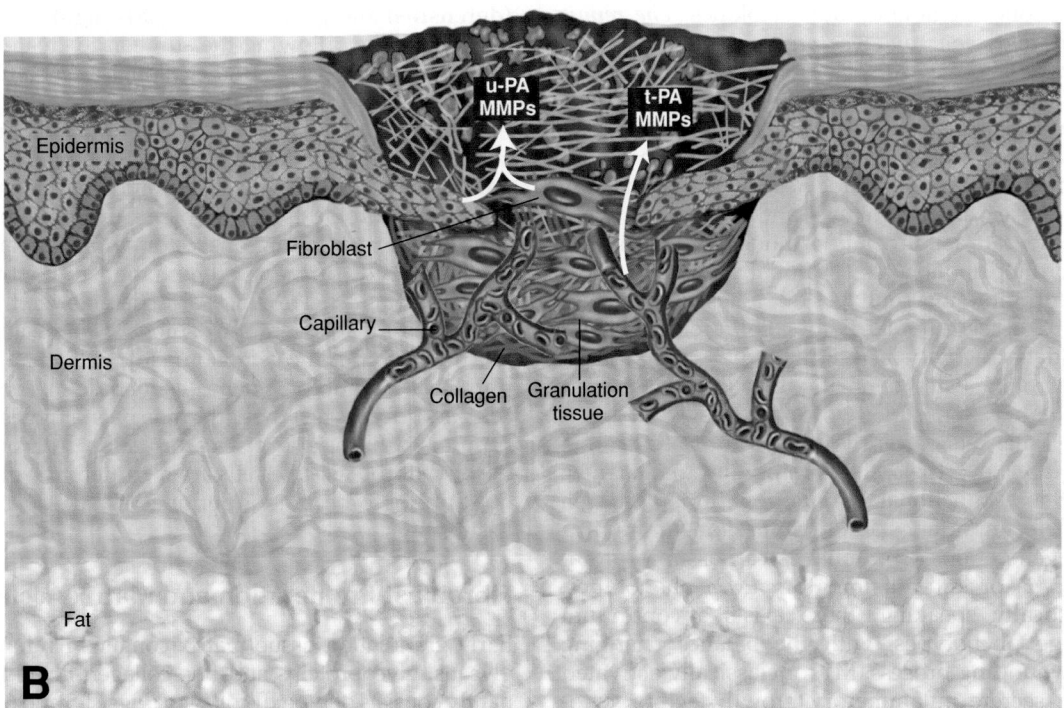

FIGURE 3-6. Cutaneous wound healing. A. 2–4 days. Growth factors controlling migration of cells are illustrated. Extensive redundancy is present, and no single growth factor is rate limiting. Most factors have multiple effects, as listed in Table 3-6. Growth factor signals first arise from degranulating platelets, but activated macrophages, resident tissue cells, injured epidermis and the matrix itself release a complex interplay of interacting signals. **B. 4–8 days.** Capillary blood vessels invade and proliferate within the provisional matrix, and the epidermal keratinocytes advance along the granulation tissue below the thrombus. The upper, acellular portion of the wound site will become an eschar or scab. Fibroblasts deposit a collagen-rich matrix. *FGF* = fibroblast growth factor; *IGF* = insulin-like growth factor; *MMPs* = matrix metalloproteinases; *PDGF* = platelet-derived growth factor; *TGF-β* = transforming growth factor-β; *t-PA* = tissue plasminogen activator; *u-PA* = urokinase-type plasminogen activator; *VEGF* = vascular endothelial growth factor.

matrix. Excess transglutaminase may cause undue scarring. By contrast, factor XIII deficiencies are associated with poor wound healing and bleeding. The internal (nondesiccated) portion of the provisional matrix is transformed into granulation tissue by invasion of mononuclear cells, connective tissue and vascular cells, while the outer portion (eschar) is a temporary repository for spent neutrophils and killed bacteria. As the granulation tissue is partitioned from the eschar by migrating epidermis during normal healing, the portion of the thrombus that is not repopulated by new tissue is digested. The scab then detaches.

Inflammation

Repair sites vary in the amount of local tissue destruction. For example, surgical excision of a skin lesion leaves little or no devitalized tissue. Demarcated, localized necrosis accompanies medium-sized myocardial infarcts. By contrast, widespread, irregularly defined necrosis is a feature of a large third-degree burn. Initially, an acute, neutrophil-dominated, inflammatory response liquefies the necrotic tissue. Acute inflammation persists as long as necrotic material or bacterial infection persists, since these elements must be removed for repair to progress. Before granulation tissue appears, exudative, spent neutrophils may form pus or become trapped in the eschar. Fibronectin, matricryptins, chemokines and cell debris are early chemotactic elements for macrophages and fibroblasts (Figs. 3-5 and 3-7). In epithelial tissues such as skin, a resident population of γδT cells, called dendritic epidermal T cells (DETCs), recognizes adjacent injury and helps initiate the cellular response. It also supports keratinocyte proliferation and survival by secreting growth factors, chemokines and cytokines. *The repair process begins when macrophages predominate at the site of injury (Fig. 3-8).* Local tissue macrophages are reported to be capable of proliferation in some tissue settings. However, inflammation triggers significant recruitment of inflammatory cells, including monocyte macrophages. Chemokines facilitate the mobilization of monocytes from bone marrow and a splenic reserve. Chemokines and neutrophil granule contents then attract circulating monocytes to the site of injury. Recruited monocytes (1) initially move into tissue, (2) transform into macrophages, (3) ingest remnants of neutrophils and (4) secrete matrix metalloproteinases, with further degradative activity facilitating liquefaction. Classification of macrophage and dendritic cell subtypes, or even the distribution between these two cells types, is problematic, as the cell markers currently utilized for classification schemes overlap. Nevertheless, it is important to recognize the plasticity and functional variation within these cell types and their importance in inflammation, immunity, repair and regeneration. Macrophages can assume proinflammatory (M1) or anti-inflammatory (M2) phenotypes, though, practically speaking, there exists a continuum of macrophage phenotypes, with the balance changing through the wounding process. M1, or classically activated macrophages, secrete inflammatory growth factors, cytokines, chemokines and MMPs. M2, or alternatively activated anti-inflammatory macrophages, secrete factors that stimulate fibroblast proliferation, collagen secretion, neovascularization and wound resolution. Macrophage phagocytosis of apoptotic neutrophils favors their inflammatory to anti-inflammatory transition. Regulatory dendritic cells or regulatory macrophages, which may derive from M2

macrophages, suppress the inflammatory response further, supporting wound resolution. Classic dendritic cells are also recruited from bone marrow and migrate to lymph nodes, where they present antigen and activate T helper cells. TIP-DCs (tumor necrosis factor [TNF]- and inducible nitric oxide [NO] synthase–producing inflammatory dendritic cells [DCs]) differentiate from recruited inflammatory macrophages.

Granulation Tissue

Granulation tissue is the transient, specialized organ of repair, which replaces the provisional matrix. Like a placenta, it is only present where and when needed. It is deceptively simple, with a glistening and pebbled appearance (Fig. 3-9). Microscopically, a mixture of fibroblasts, mononuclear cells and red blood cells first invades the provisional matrix. This is followed by the development of extracellular matrix and patent, single cell-lined capillaries, which are surrounded by pericytes and provide a blood supply to fibroblasts and inflammatory cells.

A key step in the process is recruitment of monocytes to the site of injury by chemokines and fragments of damaged matrix. Later, plasma cells are conspicuous, even predominating. Activated macrophages progressively shift from a proinflammatory phenotype to the more constructive M2 phenotype(s), in which they release growth factors and cytokines (Table 3-5, and see below) that direct angiogenesis, activate fibroblasts to form new stroma and continue the degradation and removal of the provisional matrix.

Granulation tissue is fluid-rich, and its cellular constituents supply immunoglobulins, antibacterial peptides **(defensins)** and growth factors. It is highly resistant to bacterial infection, allowing the surgeon to create anastomoses at such nonsterile sites as the colon, in which fully one third of the fecal contents consist of bacteria.

Fibroblasts are also early responders to injury. These collagen-secreting cells (Fig. 3-10) are activated by cytokines, particularly PDGF, FGF, TGF-β and the biochemical environment. Fibroblasts are involved in inflammatory, proliferative and remodeling phases of wound repair. These cells are capable of further differentiation to contractile myofibroblasts (Fig. 3-11), which are characterized by abundant actin stress fibers containing smooth muscle actin. The bone marrow also produces mononuclear cells that can take on a fibroblast phenotype. Such cells include mesenchymal stem cells and fibrocytes; the latter has been suggested as a contributor to fibrosis and scar formation. Although marrow-derived fibroblast-like cells are recruited to wounds, they do not appear to become a permanent part of the connective tissue.

Fibroblast Proliferation and Matrix Accumulation

Early granulation tissue matrix contains hyaluronan, proteoglycans, glycoproteins and fine collagen fibers that predominantly consists of type III collagen (Figs. 3-5 and 3-6). Cytokines released by cells in the damaged area cause vascular leakage and attract both inflammatory cells and vascular endothelial cells. About 2–3 days after injury, activated fibroblasts and capillary sprouts are seen. Fibroblasts in the wound change from oval to bipolar, as they begin to produce collagen (Figs. 3-7 and 3-10) and other matrix proteins, such as fibronectin, and develop contractile properties. Secretion of type III collagen is

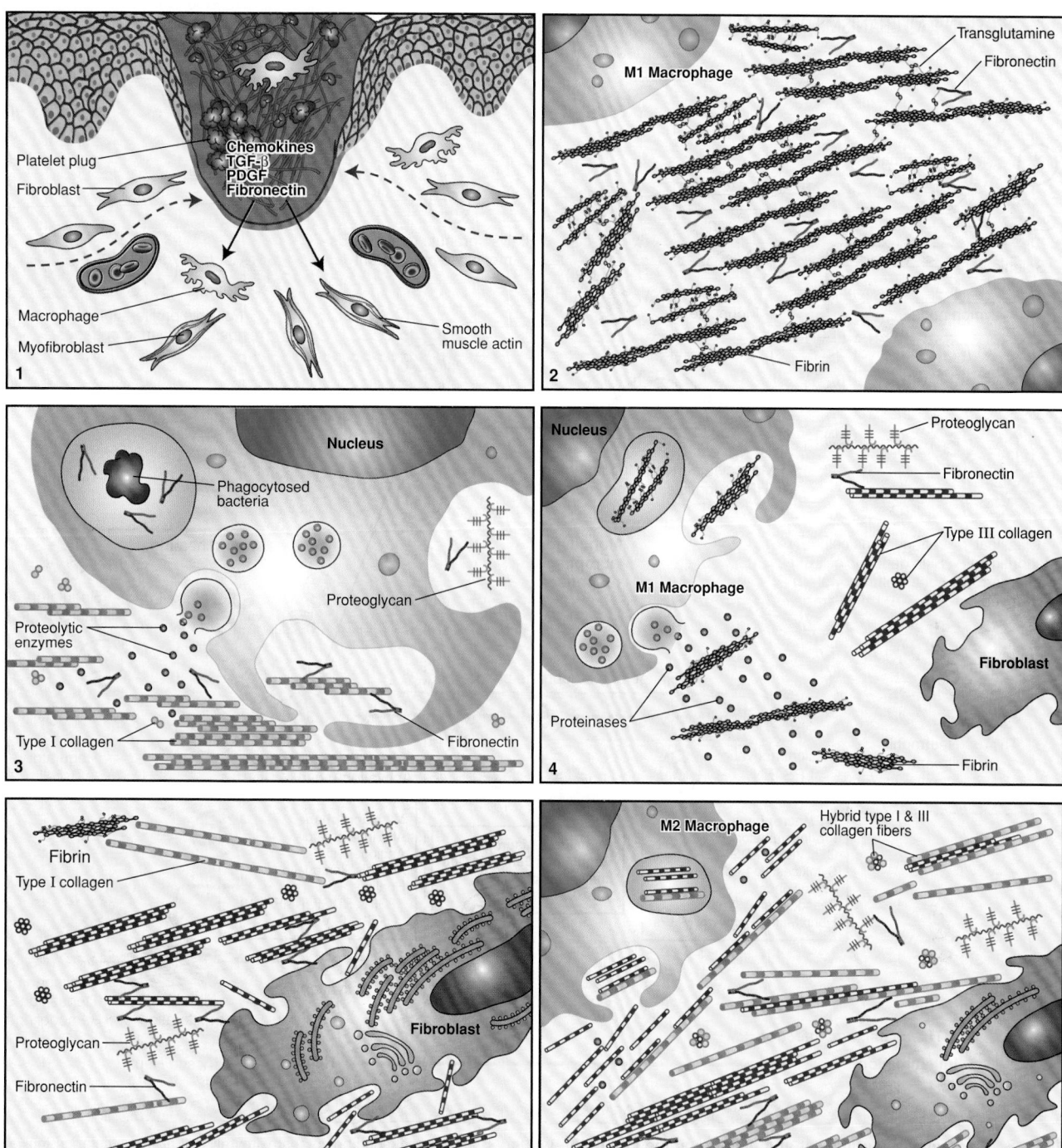

FIGURE 3-7. Summary of the healing process. 1. Inflammatory cell migration. A low-power view of the wound site depicts the mobilization of macrophages, fibroblasts and smooth muscle actin-containing myofibroblasts as they migrate to the wound from the surrounding tissue into the provisional matrix. Fibronectin, growth factors, chemokines, cell debris and bacterial products are chemoattractants for a variety of cells that are recruited to the wound site (2–4 days). The initial phase of the repair reaction typically begins with hemorrhage into the tissues. **2.** A **fibrin clot** forms from plasma and platelets, and it fills the gap created by the wound. Fibronectin from the extravasated plasma binds fibrin, collagen and other extracellular matrix components within fibrin strands that are cross-linked by the action of transglutaminase (factor XIII). This cross-linking provides a provisional mechanical stabilization of the wound (0–4 hours) and a substrate for integrin-dependent cell migration. Neutrophils rapidly infiltrate in the presence of chemotactic signals from bacteria or damaged tissue. **3. Macrophages** recruited to the wound area further process cell remnants and damaged extracellular matrix. The binding of fibronectin to cell membranes, collagens, proteoglycans, DNA and bacteria (opsonization) facilitates phagocytosis by these macrophages and contributes to the removal of debris (1–3 days). **4.** During the intermediate phase of the repair reaction, recruited **fibroblasts** deposit a new extracellular matrix at the wound site that is initially enriched in type III collagen and hence finer collagen fibers. Concurrently, the fibrin clot is cleared by a combination of extracellular proteolysis and phagocytosis (2–4 days). **5.** Together with fibrin removal by macrophages, there is continued fibroblast production of a **temporary matrix** including proteoglycans, glycoproteins such as polymerized cellular fibronectin and fibers enriched in type III collagen (2–5 days). Integrin receptors aid in the assembly of fibronectin complexes, and both integrins and fibronectin help assemble collagen fibrils. **6. Final phase of the repair reaction.** Fibroblasts progressively convert to production of thicker, stiffer collagen fibers that are enriched in type I collagen and the temporary, thinner collagen III–enriched fibers are turned over, leading to the stronger definitive matrix (5 days to weeks). Many other matrix molecules are involved in the assembly of the collagen network.

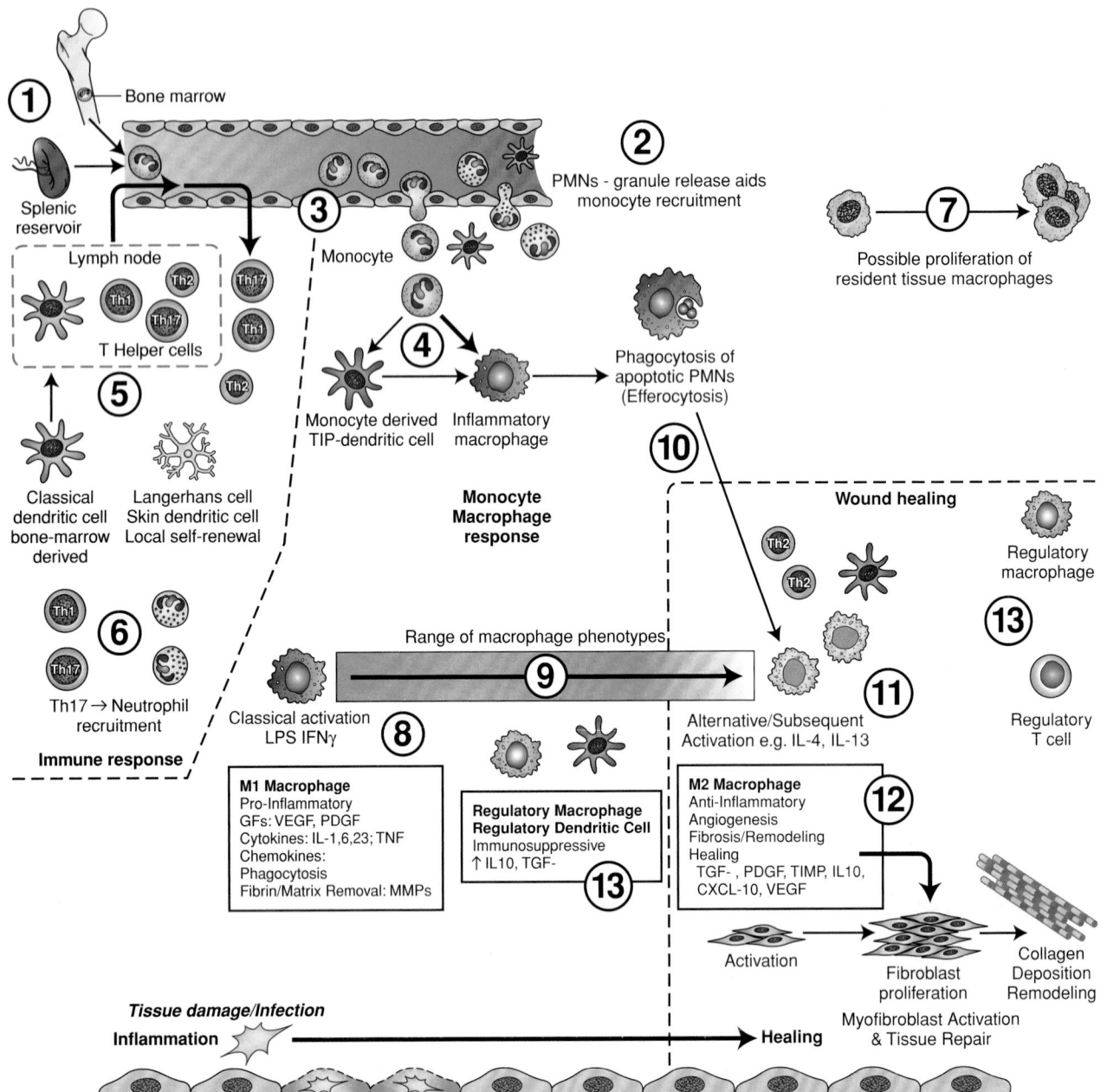

FIGURE 3-8. Macrophage recruitment and function at the site of the wound. Under normal conditions, approximately 5% of the circulating leukocytes are monocytic, some of which crawl along vascular endothelium, apparently patrolling tissue vasculature for injury. Chemokine release, caused by inflammation, stimulates release of neutrophils and monocytes from bone marrow (1). Monocytes may also be recruited from a reservoir in the subcapsular red pulp of the spleen (1). Neutrophil granule release aids in attracting monocytes to the site of injury (2). Monocytes and dendritic cells (DCs) have separate and shared paths of differentiation and often have shared markers but different functions; plasticity is a feature of both cell types. Classic dendritic cells populate tissue from bone marrow. In skin resides a resident population of dendritic cells called Langerhans cells, which resemble resident tissue macrophages and arise prenatally from a macrophage population. Dendritic cells renew locally and are not as likely to migrate to lymph nodes as classic DCs unless activated by antigen. Monocytes entering tissue (3) develop the phenotype of an inflammatory/M1 macrophage or TIP-DCs (tumor necrosis factor– and inducible nitric oxide synthase–producing inflammatory DCs) (4). As part of the innate immune response, dendritic cells phagocytose antigen and migrate (5) to a local lymph node where they encounter hundreds of T lymphocytes, activating those able to recognize the antigen. The T helper/effector cells (Th1 or Th17) then return to the tissue to aid in the immune response. During the early response, Th17 cells secrete interleukin-17, attracting more neutrophils (6). Resident tissue macrophages have been shown to proliferate in some tissues (7); however, the bulk of macrophages migrate from the circulation to the site of injury. Recruited macrophages are M1 macrophages, activated by interferon and infectious particles. They are proinflammatory and secrete cytokines, growth factors, chemokines and matrix metalloproteinases (8) to attract more inflammatory cells and stimulate breakdown and removal of infectious agents and debris. The macrophages at the wound site are a mixture of transitional (9) phenotypes, with M1 cells predominating during early phases (8). As macrophages phagocytose apoptotic neutrophils (10) and the cytokine environment transitions from inflammatory cytokines to immunosuppressive cytokines while growth factors increase, an anti-inflammatory, M2, macrophage (11) begins to predominate. Under this influence, angiogenesis and fibrogenesis prevail as the restorative process initiates. Fibroblasts accumulate, and under the influence of macrophage-derived transforming growth factor-β (TGF-β), a portion of these cells transform into myofibroblasts, leading to increased collagen and matrix synthesis, mechanical tension and contraction of the wound (12). Regulatory T cells and macrophages (13) aid in development and maintenance of an immunosuppressive phenotype in the presence of interleukin-10 (IL-10) and TGF-β, and the wound transitions to remodeling of the early matrix.

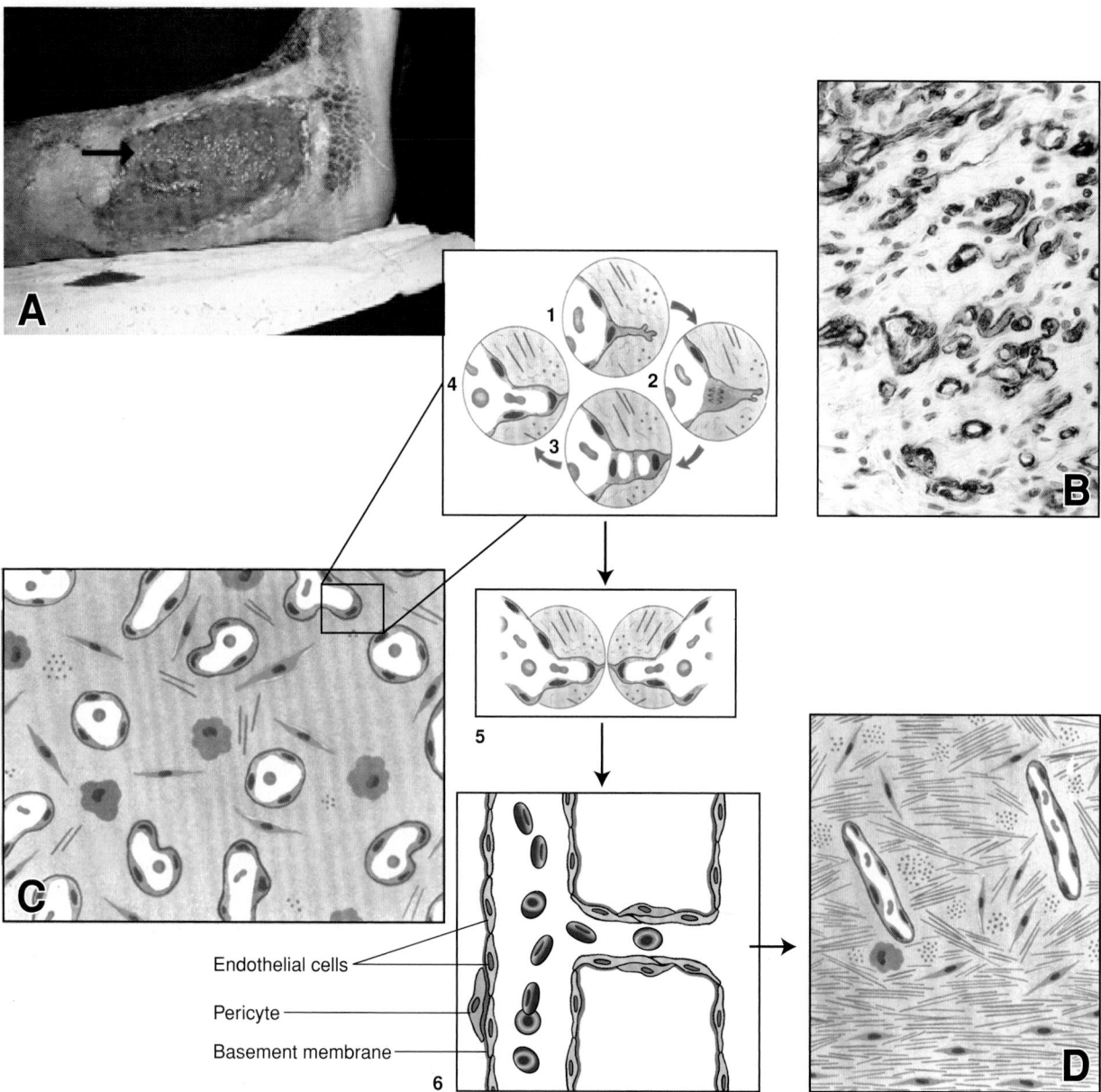

FIGURE 3-9. Granulation tissue. A. A venous stasis leg ulcer illustrates the cobbled appearance of exposed granulation tissue. **B.** A photomicrograph of granulation tissue shows thin-walled capillary sprouts immunostained to highlight the basement membrane collagens. The infiltrating capillaries penetrate a loose connective tissue matrix containing mesenchymal cells and occasional inflammatory cells. **C.** Granulation tissue has two major components: stromal cells and proliferating capillaries. Initially, capillary sprouts of granulation tissue are a key feature, growing in a loose matrix in the presence of fibroblasts, myofibroblasts and macrophages. The macrophages are derived from monocyte migration to the wound site. The fibroblasts derive from adjacent connective tissue or possibly from circulating fibrocytes and mesenchymal stem cells; myofibroblasts derive from fibroblasts, fibrocytes or pericytes; and the capillaries arise primarily from adjacent vessels by division of the lining endothelial cells (steps 1–6), in a process termed **_angiogenesis_**. Endothelial cells put out cell extensions, called **_pseudopodia_**, that grow toward the wound site. Cytoplasmic flow enlarges the pseudopodia, and eventually the cells divide. Vacuoles formed in the daughter cells eventually fuse to create a new lumen. The entire process continues until the sprout encounters another capillary sprout, with which it will connect. At its peak, granulation tissue is the most richly vascularized tissue in the body. **D.** Once repair has been achieved, most of the newly formed capillaries undergo apoptosis, leaving a pale, avascular scar rich in collagen.

rapidly overwhelmed by type I collagen, which promotes the assembly of larger-diameter fibrils with greater tensile strength. Eventually, the matrix resumes its original composition of predominantly type I collagen and 15%–20% type III collagen.

The rate of matrix accumulation peaks at 5–7 days, depending on the tissue. This process is strongly influenced by the production of TGF-β, which increases synthesis of collagen, fibronectin, TIMPs and other matrix proteins, while

decreasing MMP transcription and matrix degradation. Extracellular cross-linking of newly synthesized collagen progressively increases wound strength.

Growth Factors and Fibroplasia

The discovery of epidermal growth factor (EGF) and later identification of at least 20 other growth factors have helped

TABLE 3-5

EXTRACELLULAR SIGNALS IN WOUND REPAIR

Phase	Factor(s)	Source	Effects
Coagulation	XIIIa	Plasma	Cross-linking of fibrin thrombus
	TGF-α, TGF-β, PDGF, ECGF, FGF	Platelets	Chemoattraction and activation of subsequent cells
Inflammation	TGF-β, chemokines	Neutrophil, M1 macrophages, endothelial cells	Attract monocytes and fibroblasts; differentiate fibroblasts and stem cells
	TNF-α, IL-1, IL-6, CXCL12, CX3CL1, PDGF		
Granulation tissue formation	FGF-2, TGF-β, HGF	Keratinocytes, monocytes then fibroblasts	Various factors are bound to proteoglycan matrix
Angiogenesis	VEGFs, FGFs, HGF, angioprotein-1/-2	Monocytes, macrophages, fibroblasts, endothelial cells	Development of blood vessels
	PDGF		Pericyte growth
Contraction	TGF-β1, β2	Macrophages, fibroblasts, keratinocytes	Myofibroblasts differentiate, bind to each other and to collagen and contract
Reepithelialization	KGF (FGF-7), HGF, EGF, HB-EGF, TGF-α, activin, TGF-β3, CXCL10, CXCL11	Macrophages, platelets, fibroblasts, keratinocytes, endothelial cells	Epithelial proliferation, migration and differentiation
Maturation, fibroplasia, arrest of proliferation	TGF-β1, PDGF, CTGF, IL-27, IL-4, CX3CL1, thrombospondin	M2 macrophages, fibroblasts, keratinocytes	Accumulation of extracellular matrix, fibrosis, tensile strength
	Heparan sulfate proteoglycan (HSPG)	Endothelium	HSPG: Capture of TGF-β, VEGF and basic FGF in basement membrane
		Secretory fibroblasts	
	Decorin proteoglycan		Decorin: Capture of TGF-β, stabilization of collagen structure, downregulation of migration, proliferation
	Interferon, CXCL10, CXCL11	Plasma monocytes	Suppresses proliferation of fibroblasts and endothelial cells and accumulation of collagen
	Increased local oxygen, decreased mechanotransduction	Repair process	Suppression of release of cytokines
Resolution and remodeling	PDGF-FGF, TGF-β, interleukins	Platelets, fibroblasts, keratinocytes, macrophages	Regulation of MMPs and TIMPs
			Remodeling by restructuring of ECM (e.g., collagen III replaced by collagen I)
	MMPs, t-PAs, u-PAs	Sprouted capillaries, epithelial cells, fibroblasts	
	Tissue inhibitors of MMPs	Local, not further defined	Balance the effects of MMPs in the evolving repair site
	Signals for arrest:	Basal keratinocytes	
	CXCL11 or IP-9,	Neovascular endothelium	Reduce cellularity CXCR3 signals
	CXCL10 or IP-10		Reduced migration and proliferation of fibroblasts, endothelial cells, increased migration of keratinocytes

CTGF = connective tissue growth factor; CXCL10 and 11 = chemokine CXC-type ligand 10 and 11; IP = interferon-γ–induced protein; ECGF = endothelial cell growth factor; ECM = extracellular matrix; EGF = epidermal growth factor; FGF = fibroblast growth factor; HB-EGF = heparin-binding EGF; HGF = hepatocyte growth factor; IL = interleukin; KGF = keratinocyte growth factor (FGF-7); MMPs = matrix metalloproteinases; PDGF = platelet-derived growth factor; SDF-1 = stromal cell–derived factor-1; TIMP = tissue inhibitor of metalloproteinase; TGF = transforming growth factor; TNF = tumor necrosis factor; t-PA = tissue plasminogen activator; u-PA = urokinase-type plasminogen activator; VEGF = vascular endothelial growth factor.

define the signaling mechanisms that rapidly change the course of repair and restoration. The interactions among growth factors, other cytokines and MMPs are illustrated in Tables 3-6 and 3-7. Each signal has a predominant function in repair, but gene deletion studies in mice have revealed the redundancy of many pathways. Frequently, conditional gene deletion is needed because of the essential role of a factor during fetal development. Specificity derives from (1) selective expression from members of large families (e.g., FGF and TGF-β), (2) temporal expression of different

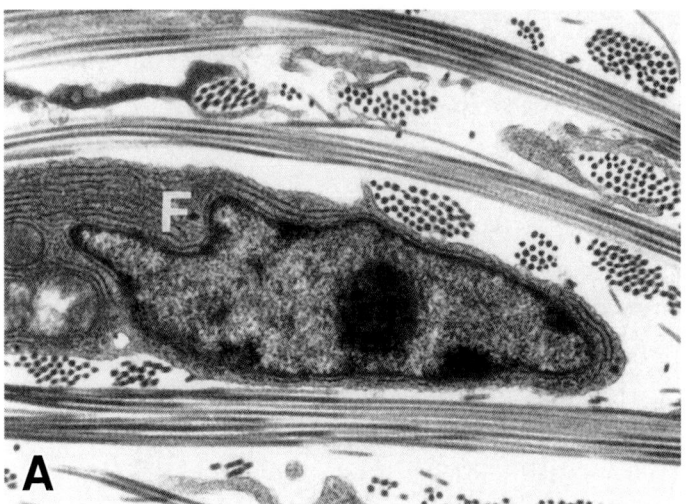
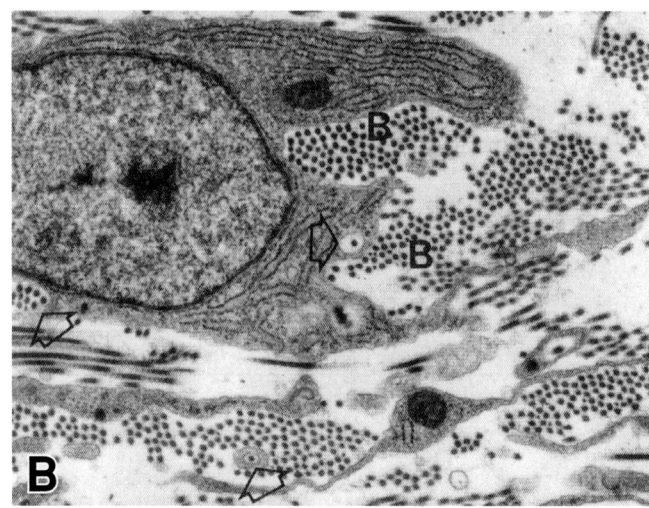

FIGURE 3-10. Fibroblasts and collagen fibers. Electron micrographs. A. Chick embryo fibroblast (F) lying between collagen fibers. The collagen fibers are seen as crosswise strands traversing the field and along the long axis, at a right angle, as dots. **B.** A chick embryo dermal fibroblast with abundant endoplasmic reticulum consistent with secretory activity and cell surface–associated collagen fibril bundles (B); some bundles are enveloped by fibroblast membrane and cytoplasm, indicating that collagen fibers can be assembled and extruded from long cellular processes (fibropositors; *arrows*). The fibrils are visualized in cross-section as dots.

tyrosine kinase receptors and isotypes in unrelated cell populations, (3) variation in response pathways or intensity by distinct receptors and (4) latency or activation of growth factors (Table 3-5). Tables 3-6 and 3-7 show how growth factors control specific events in repair.

Several growth factor ligands are presented to their (tyrosine kinase) receptors by local release from extracellular matrix components, such as heparan sulfate proteoglycan and matricellular and microfibrillar proteins. There are some domains in matrix molecules in the laminin, collagen, tenascin and decorin families that bind weakly to growth factor

TABLE 3-6
GROWTH FACTORS CONTROL VARIOUS STAGES IN REPAIR

Attraction of Monocytes/Macrophages	PDGFs, FGFs, TGF-β, MCP-1 (CCL2)
Attraction of fibroblasts	PDGFs, FGFs, TGF-β, CTGF, EGFs, SDF-1
Proliferation of fibroblasts	PDGFs, FGFs, EGFs, IGF, CTGF
Angiogenesis	VEGFs, FGFs, HGF
Collagen synthesis	TGF-β, PDGFs, IGF, CTGF
Collagen secretion	PDGFs, FGFs, CTGF
Epithelial migration and proliferation	KGF, TGF-α, HGF, IGF of epithelium–epidermis
Resolution of repair	IP-9 (CXCL11), IP-10 (CXCL10)

CCL2 = C-type chemokine ligand 2; CXCL 10 and 11 = CXC-type chemokine ligand 10 and 11; CTGF = connective tissue growth factor; EGF = epidermal growth factor; FGF = fibroblast growth factor; HGF = hepatocyte growth factor; IGF = insulin-like growth factor; IP-9/10 = interferon-γ–inducible protein 9/10; KGF = keratinocyte growth factor; MCP-1 = macrophage chemotactic protein-1; PDGF = platelet-derived growth factor; SDF-1 = stromal cell–derived factor-1; TGF = transforming growth factor; VEGF = vascular endothelial growth factor.

TABLE 3-7
GROWTH FACTORS, ENZYMES AND OTHER FACTORS REGULATE PROGRESSION OF REPAIR AND FIBROSIS

Secretion of Collagenase	PDGF, EGF, IL-1, TNF, Proteases
Movement of surface and stromal cells	t-PA (tissue plasminogen activator)
	u-PA (urokinase-type plasminogen activator)
	Elastase
	MMPs (matrix metalloproteinases)
	MMP-1 (collagenase 1)
	MMP-2 (gelatinase A)
	MMP-3 (stromelysin 1)
	MMP-8 (collagenase 2)
	MMP-9 (gelatinase B)
	MMP-13 (collagenase 3)
	MT1-MMP (MMP-14; membrane bound)
	MMP-19
Maturation or stabilization of blood vessels	Angiopoietins (Ang1, Ang2); PDGF; HIF-1
Inhibition of collagenase production	TGF-β
Increase of TIMP production	
Reduction in collagen production and turnover	Reduction in mechanotransduction feedback and release/activation of latent TGF-β
Collagen cross-linking and maturation	Lysyl oxidase, integrin receptors, fibronectin polymers, small proteoglycans

EGF = epidermal growth factor; HIF-1 = hypoxia-inducible factor 1; IL = interleukin; PDGF = platelet-derived growth factor; TGF = transforming growth factor; TIMP = tissue inhibitor of metalloproteinases; TNF = tumor necrosis factor.

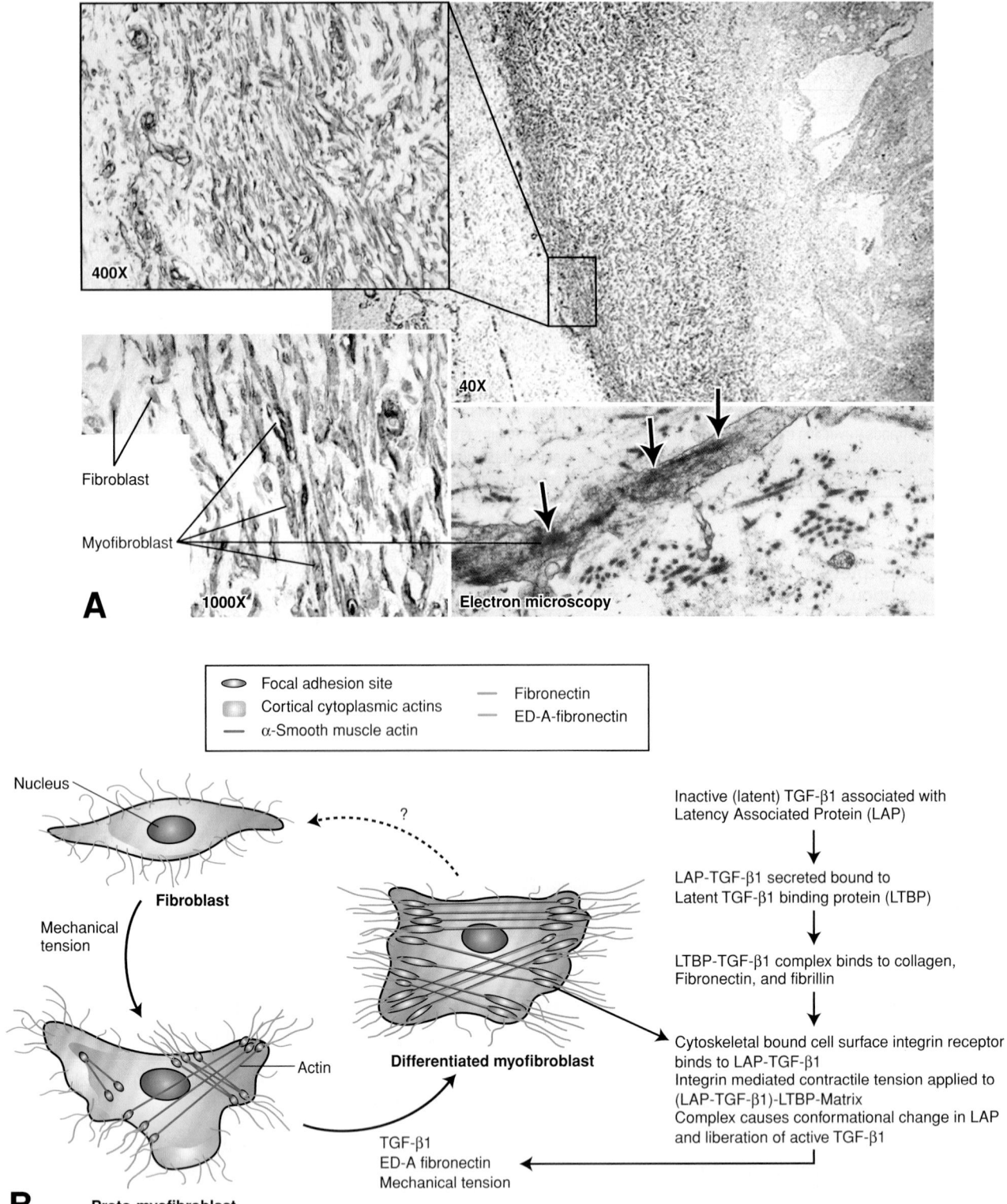

FIGURE 3-11. Myofibroblasts. Myofibroblasts have an important role in the repair reaction. These cells derive from pericytes or fibroblasts, with features intermediate between those of smooth muscle cells and fibroblasts, and they are characterized by the presence of discrete bundles of α-smooth muscle actin in the cytoplasm (*arrows*). Their clustered integrin receptors adhere tightly to and aid in formation of insoluble fibrils of cellular fibronectin, which align the cytoskeleton and bind collagen fibers, generating contractile forces important in wound contraction. **A. Myofibroblasts stained with anti–smooth muscle actin** can be viewed by light microscope at different magnifications. A band of cells (nuclei stain blue, α-smooth muscle actin stains brown) are stained in the papillary dermis of an ulcerated skin wound. Pericytes that surround capillaries also contain α-smooth muscle actin. α-Smooth muscle actin is seen in dense bundles by electron microscopy (*arrows*). **B. Development of myofibroblasts** from fibroblast and a model involving increased matrix production and matrix stiffness, leading to increased cytoskeletal contractility that activates matrix-bound latent transforming growth factor-β (TGF-β), hence creating a positive feedback system that magnifies matrix deposition and contractility. It is thought that this loop is normally interrupted by the phenomenon of tensional homeostasis, a biochemical set point.

receptors. Equally important in growth factor signaling is the presence of cell surface proteoglycans, which weakly tether the signal molecule, and integrins that place receptor binding into a biochemical context by linking the extracellular matrix (ECM) with the cell interior. Unlike hormones, the signals generated by these interactions are confined, persistent and concentrated.

Growth factors expressed or mobilized early in wound responses (VEGF, FGF, PDGF, EGF, keratinocyte growth factor [KGF, FGF7] and others) support migration, recruitment and proliferation of cells involved in fibroplasia, reepithelialization and angiogenesis. Growth factors that peak later (TGF-β, insulin-like growth factor-I [IGF-I]) sustain the maturation phase, growth and remodeling of granulation tissue. Tissue restoration is driven by complex, interactive signaling networks, which, in cooperation with matrix, support self-renewal, maintenance and differentiation of progenitor cells.

Wound outcomes can be improved after various exogenous growth factors are added to experimental wounds. PDGF is clinically effective in accelerating healing in neuropathic diabetic foot ulcers. However, topical application of a single growth factor in a bolus form generally does not prevent scars and does not consistently speed up or improve healing in all problem wounds when compared to accepted methods of chronic wound management. Limited success results, in part, from the lack of responsiveness of the target tissue and wound diagnosis. Progress in cell culture, matrix and growth factor biology has sped the engineering of cultured skin substitutes that express or can be genetically engineered to express many growth factors, which—in combination—can improve clinical outcomes in chronic wounds.

Growth factor participation in the early phases of repair is reasonably well understood, but the mechanisms for limiting and terminating repair are not well defined. Diminishing anoxia as repair progresses and reduced matrix turnover may trigger the denouement of the repair process. Recent evidence suggests that cytokines that bind to the CXCR3 receptor may be important for regression of granulation tissue and limiting scarring. Finally, increased storage and decreased release of growth factors may stabilize the matrix, which may then transmit mechanical signals that reduce the effects of growth factors. Granulation tissue eventually becomes scar tissue, as the equilibrium between collagen synthesis and breakdown comes into balance within weeks of injury. Fibroblasts continue to alter scar appearance for several years.

Angiogenesis

The Growth of Capillaries
At its peak, granulation tissue has more capillaries per unit volume than any other tissue. New capillary growth is essential for delivery of oxygen and nutrients. New capillaries form by angiogenesis (i.e., sprouting of endothelial cells from preexisting capillary venules) (Fig. 3-9) and create the granular appearance for which the tissue is named. Less often, new blood vessels form de novo from angioblasts (endothelial progenitor cells [EPCs]). The latter process, known as **vasculogenesis,** is primarily associated with ontogeny.

Angiogenesis in wound repair is tightly regulated. Quiescent capillary endothelial cells are activated by loss of basement membrane and local release of cytokines and growth factors. Disruption or paucity of basement membranes surrounding endothelial cells and surrounding pericytes precedes or predicts sites of endothelial cells sprouting into the provisional matrix. Endothelial passage through the matrix is an invasive process that requires the cooperation of plasminogen activators, matrix MMPs and integrin receptors. The growth of new capillaries is supported by proliferation and assembly of endothelial cells (Fig. 3-9). There is also a possible contribution of limited numbers of mononuclear, bone marrow–derived endothelial progenitor cells, recruited, at least transiently, to support growing vessels.

Migration of cells into a wound site is directed by soluble ligands. It proceeds as cells follow cytokine signals (by **chemotaxis**) on and inherent signals from matrix substrates (by **haptotaxis**), together with adhesive and mechanical signals from matrix (**durotaxis** or **mechanotaxis**). Once capillary endothelial cells are immobilized, cell–cell contacts form, and an organized basement membrane develops on the exterior of the nascent capillary. Interplay between endothelial cells and pericytes occurs during angiogenesis. Endothelial association with pericytes and signals from angiopoietin I, TGF-β and PDGF are essential to establish a mature vessel phenotype of nonleaky capillaries. New capillaries that have not matured are leaky, create hemorrhage or edema and may undergo apoptosis.

Experimentally, stimulation of angiogenesis in cell culture requires extracellular matrix and growth factors, mainly VEGF. Loss of even one VEGF allele causes lethal defects in embryonic vasculature. In vivo, angiogenesis is initiated by hypoxia and a redundancy of cytokines, growth factors and various lipids, which stimulate or regulate VEGF. The transcription factor HIF-1α (see Chapter 1), whose stability is exquisitely regulated by tissue oxygen tension, is the main trigger for VEGF expression. MicroRNA (miRNA) expression is directly and indirectly influenced by wounding and levels of tissue oxygenation, varying with healing phases in ways that may be specific to cell and tissue. Activated granulation tissue macrophages and endothelial cells produce basic FGF (FGF-2) and VEGF, and wound epidermal cells release VEGF in response to KGF (FGF-7) that is expressed by dermal cells. Because the chief target of VEGF is endothelial cells, this molecule is critical for embryonic vascular development and angiogenesis, endothelial survival, differentiation and migration. Splice variants of VEGF concentrate along soluble and matrix-bound gradients to ensure appropriate vessel branching.

The binding of angiogenic growth factors to heparan sulfate containing GAG chains on proteoglycans of basement membrane and syndecan receptors is crucial to angiogenesis. Association with heparan sulfate chains affects the availability and action of growth factors and vessel pattern formation by (1) creating a storage reservoir of VEGF and basic FGF in capillary basement membranes and (2) using cell surface proteoglycan receptors to regulate VEGF and FGF receptor congregation, as well as signal delivery and intensity.

Angiogenesis and Receptor Crosstalk
Surface integrin receptors sense changes in extracellular matrix and can react by modulating cellular responses to growth factors. This crosstalk is possible because integrin and growth factor signal cascades converge to trigger many of the processes that support cell survival, proliferation, differentiation and migration. Unlike growth factors, integrin receptors drive cell locomotion by organizing

cytoskeletal changes at the membrane. When exposed to growth factors or the loss of an organized basement membrane, quiescent endothelial cells express new integrins that modulate their migration on provisional matrix proteins. Capillary sprouting relies principally on β_1-type integrins. Survival and spatial organization of the capillary network are regulated by other integrins, such as $\alpha_v\beta_3$, which respond to the composition and structure of their extracellular matrix ligands. Without appropriate matrix or sufficient growth factor signaling, endothelial cells are vulnerable to apoptotic cues.

Reepithelialization

The epidermis constantly renews itself by the mitosis of keratinocyte stem cells in the basal layer. The squamous cells then cornify or keratinize as they mature, move toward the surface and are shed a few days later. Maturation requires an intact layer of basal cells that are in direct contact with one another and the basement membrane (Fig. 3-1.5). If cell–cell contact is disrupted, basal epidermal cells migrate laterally and divide to reestablish contact with other basal cells. In partial-thickness skin wounds where the epidermis is destroyed, specialized progenitor cells in the hair follicle become a primary source of regenerating epithelium (Fig. 3-1.5). Once reestablished, the epidermal barrier demarcates the scab from the newly formed granulation tissue. When epithelial continuity is reestablished, the epidermis resumes its normal cycle of maturation and shedding.

Epidermal integrity protects against infection and fluid loss. Epithelial cells in the skin and many hollow organs cover or close wounds either by migrating to cover the damaged surface or, less often in minor abrasions, by a cinching process called **purse-string closure,** augmenting fibroblast/myofibroblast-mediated wound contraction. Skin provides an intensively studied example of epithelial repair, since there are complex differentiation patterns in the epidermal surface itself, the hair follicle and the sweat glands. The basal layer **epidermal keratinocytes** contribute important cytokines (interleukin-1 [IL-1], VEGF, TGF-α, PDGF, TGF-β) that initiate healing and local immune responses as part of the innate immune system. To begin migration, keratinocytes, like capillary endothelium, must transiently differentiate into a migratory cell phenotype before forming a new covering over the wound. These cells normally bind laminin in the underlying basement membrane by hemidesmosome protein complexes containing $\alpha_6\beta_4$ integrin. Several members of the collagen family, namely, type XVII collagen (BP-180) and collagen type VII, also termed **anchoring fibril** (Table 3-2), are associated with the hemidesmosome complex. The anchoring fibril connects the hemidesmosome–basement membrane complex to the dermal connective tissue collagen fibers. Mutations in collagen XVII, epidermal basement membrane laminin, integrin $\alpha_6\beta_4$ or collagen VII produce a potentially fatal skin blistering disease, termed **epidermolysis bullosa.** Autoantibodies against the transmembrane collagen XVII (BP180, BPAG2) cause acquired blistering disorders like **bullous pemphigoid** (see Chapter 28).

Epithelial cells are connected at their lateral edges by **tight junctions** and **adherens junctions** composed of cadherin receptors. Cadherins are calcium-dependent, integral membrane proteins that form extracellular cell–cell connections and anchor intracellular cytoskeletal connections. In adherens junctions, they bind stable actin bundles to a cytoplasmic complex of α-, β- and γ-catenins. The layer of actin that encircles the epithelial cytoplasm creates lateral tension and strength and is called the **adhesion belt.** *The shape and strength of epithelial sheets result from the tension of cytoskeletal connections to basement membrane and cell-to-cell connections.*

Cellular migration is the predominant means by which wound surfaces are reepithelialized. Groups of basal and suprabasal keratinocytes originate at the margin of a wound and migrate along the provisional matrix. At the same time, adjacent progenitor cells in the basal layer, hair follicles or sweat glands undergo mitosis, resulting in a thickened (hypertrophic) and less differentiated epidermis. If the basement membrane is lost, cells come in contact with unfamiliar stromal or provisional matrix components, which stimulates cell locomotion and proteinase expression. As a result, β_1 integrins that recognize stromal collagens shift from the lateral to the basal epithelial surface. Keratinocytes at the leading edge of the wound margin become migratory and secrete MMPs. These enzymes facilitate their detachment from the basement membrane and remodeling of the granulation tissue surface. Cells migrate along a soluble chemical gradient **(chemotaxis),** owing to matrix concentration or adhesion **(haptotaxis)** and matrix pliability or stiffness **(durotaxis).**

Epithelial motility is activated by assembly of actin fibers at focal adhesions organized by integrin receptors. Distinct sets of integrins bind to components of the wound, namely, stromal or basement membrane matrices, and direct the migrating cells along the margin of viable dermis. Movement through cross-linked fibrin apposed to the granulation tissue also requires activation of plasmin from plasminogen to degrade fibrin. In addition to degrading fibrinogen and fibrin, plasmin activates specific MMPs. Proteolytic cleavage of stromal collagens I and III and laminin at focal adhesion contacts can release cell adhesion or enable keratinocyte migration. Migrating keratinocytes that have undergone this **epithelial-mesenchymal transition** (EMT) (see Chapter 5) eventually resume their normal phenotype. They become less hypertrophic after re-forming a confluent layer and attaching to their newly formed basement membrane.

Wound Contraction

Open wounds contract and deform as they heal, depending on the degree of attachment to underlying connective tissue structures. A central role in wound contraction and fibrosis in particular is played by a specialized cell of granulation tissue, the **myofibroblast** (Fig. 3-11). Without special immunostaining, this modified fibroblast-like cell is indistinguishable from collagen-secreting fibroblasts. Myofibroblasts contain abundant actin stress fibers (often α-smooth muscle actin), desmin, vimentin and a particular fibronectin splice variant (ED-A) that forms polymerized cellular fibronectin. Myofibroblasts respond to physical or mechanical forces and agents that cause smooth muscle cells to contract or relax. In short, they look like fibroblasts but behave like smooth muscle cells. In addition to differentiating from fibroblasts, the wound myofibroblast has been postulated to derive from circulating, marrow-derived fibrocytes and by EMT in the lung and kidney. Myofibroblasts may also arise from closely related cells in the wound environment, such as perivascular- or perisinusoidal-like pericytes, mesangial cells in the glomerulus and stellate cells in the liver. *Together with fibroblasts, myofibroblasts contribute to normal wound contraction and become more prevalent in deforming, pathologic wound contracture.* Myofibroblasts usually appear about the third day of wound healing, in parallel with the sudden appearance of contractile forces, which then gradually diminish over the next several weeks. These cells are associated with an increase in type I collagen and are prevalent in fibrosis and hypertrophic scars, particularly burn scars. Myofibroblasts and fibroblasts (and other mesenchymal cells) sense the stress exerted by the stiffness of the extracellular matrix on the integrin receptors. This effect triggers contraction in myofibroblasts via intracellular actin stress fibers. The action of cell contraction on the ECM through integrins facilitates the activation of TGF-β, which then reinforces the fibrotic response. Myofibroblasts extend their contractile effects through specific cell–cell interconnections, while fibroblasts are widely distributed in the extracellular matrix. The latter cells lack α-smooth muscle actin and are surrounded by collagen fibers, but with less of the ED-A fibronectin variant.

Wound Strength

Skin incisions and surgical anastomoses in hollow viscera ultimately develop 75% of the strength of the unwounded site. Despite a rapid increase in tensile strength at 7–14 days, by the end of 2 weeks the wound still has a high proportion of type III collagen and has only about 20% of its ultimate strength. Most of the strength of the healed wound results from synthesis and intermolecular cross-linking of type I collagen during the remodeling phase. A 2-month-old incision, although healed, is still obvious. Incision lines and suture marks are distinct, vascular and red. By 1 year, the incision is white and avascular, but usually still identifiable. As the scar fades further, it is often slowly deformed into an irregular line by stresses in the skin.

REGENERATION

Regeneration returns an injured tissue or lost appendage to its original state. Both regeneration and tissue maintenance require a population of stem or progenitor cells that can replicate and differentiate.

The adult human body is composed of several hundred types of well-differentiated cells, yet it maintains the remarkable potential to sustain its form and function by replenishing dying cells. It also heals itself by recruiting or activating cells that repair or regenerate injured tissue. Epithelial cells in the skin and gastrointestinal tract turn over rapidly, but for the most part tissue remodeling is much slower in other adult tissues. Some forms of regeneration may be viewed as partially recapitulating embryonic morphogenesis from pluripotent stem cells. In most cases, regeneration appears to be overwhelmed in the adult by inflammation and fibrosis. The power to replenish or regenerate tissue is derived from a small number of long-lived, unspecialized **stem cells,** unique in their slow replication rate, capacity for self-renewal and production of clonal progeny that rapidly divide and differentiate into more specialized cell types. Stem cells in most tissues, including bone marrow, epidermis, intestine and liver, maintain sufficient developmental plasticity to orchestrate tissue-specific regeneration.

Embryonic and Adult Stem Cells Are Key to Regeneration

Embryonic stem (ES) cells, up to the stage of the preimplantation blastocyst, can differentiate into all cells of the adult organism *and* preserve small populations of more restricted stem cells. Hence, these cells are pluripotent. Postnatal progenitor/stem cells, which are able to divide indefinitely without terminally differentiating, inhabit many adult tissues, and they have been identified even in tissues not known to regenerate. These **adult stem cells** may inhabit a specific tissue or be recruited to sites of injury from circulating cells of bone marrow origin. Either way, the recently appreciated presence of stem cells in many tissues underscores the importance of a permissive and supportive environment for stem cell–driven regeneration (Table 3-8). Multipotential stem cells of adult tissues have a more restricted range of cell differentiation than ES cells and can be isolated from autologous tissue, reducing concerns of immunologic rejection after implantation. More recently, regulators of transcription patterns active in embryonic stem cells have been used to restore pluripotency in differentiated cells of adult tissues (induced pluripotential stem [iPS] cell).

Adult stems cells are challenging to identify and categorize because (1) any organ or tissue may contain more than one type of stem cell, (2) similar stem cells may be found in different organs and (3) a stem cell found in tissue may have originated in the bone marrow. Stem cells may be generally defined by common properties that reflect their exquisite regulation, including:

- Ability to divide without limit, avoid senescence and maintain genomic integrity
- Capacity to intermittently undergo division or to remain quiescent
- Ability to propagate by self-renewal and differentiation of daughter cells
- Absence of lineage markers
- In some cases, specific anatomic localization
- Shared presence of growth and transcription markers common to uncommitted cells

Self-Renewal

Self-renewal is the defining property of adult stem cells and of early ES cells in vivo. The definition of a stem cell depends on the ability of the cell to differentiate into multiple cell types, in vitro or in vivo. Stem cells achieve self-renewal by asymmetric cell division, which produces a new stem cell and a daughter cell that is able to proliferate transiently and to differentiate. In contrast to stem cells, these **progenitor** cells (transit amplifying cells) have little or no capability for self-renewal.

Stem Cell Differentiation Potential

The ability of ES cells to differentiate into all lineages diminishes as the embryo develops. Cells from the zygote and the first few divisions of the fertilized egg are **totipotent;** they can form any of approximately 200 different cell types in the adult body and the cells of the placenta. Nuclei of adult somatic cells can be totipotent, as dramatically proven by nuclear transplantation cloning experiments in amphibians and now several species of domesticated mammals.

TABLE 3-8

ADULT STEM CELLS DESCRIBED IN MAMMALS

Cell Type	Cell Source and Stability	Tissue Stem Cell and Role
Bone marrow–derived stem cells	Hematopoietic stem cells (HSCs) Mesenchymal stem cells (MSCs)	HSC—Hematopoiesis, formation of all blood system cells MSC—Replenish non-blood cells of bone and bone marrow, provide HSC niche and potential source of progenitor cells for certain other tissues
Adult tissue stem cells except connective tissue (some may be bone marrow derived)	*Constantly renewing (labile) cells* –Epithelial and epithelial-like cells of epidermis and gut (ectoderm or endoderm derived) *Persistent (stable) cells in tissues with less turnover* –Epithelial, parenchyma, neural (endoderm or ectoderm derived)	*Epidermis:* unipotent basal keratinocyte basal stem cell and multipotent stem cells of hair follicle bulge and sebaceous gland *Gut:* multipotent columnar cells of small and large intestine crypt base *Cornea:* corneal epithelial stem cells are located in the basal layer of the limbus between the cornea and the conjunctiva (corneal stromal stem cells are similarly located but beneath the epithelial basement membrane) *Liver:* compensatory hepatocyte hyperplasia for maintenance, for regeneration and in response to surgical resection (other liver cells also divide); hepatic stem cells, DNA markers in label retention studies are seen in cells in the canals of Hering, intralobular bile duct cells, peribiliary null cells and peribiliary hepatocytes *Lung:* putative lung bronchioalveolar progenitor or stem cells that form bronchiolar Clara cells and possibly alveolar cells. Some evidence for alveolar epithelial type II progenitor cells *Ear:* mammalian cochlea are not known to regenerate sensory hair cells, though some nonmammalian vertebrates do. Human mesenchymal stem cells have been differentiated to hair cells and auditory neurons in vitro *Neural stem cells:* multipotent, thought to be ependymal cells or astrocytes; subventricular zone of the lateral ventricle (possibly inactive in adult humans); subgranular zone of dentate gyrus of the hippocampus. Other potential sites are the olfactory bulb and subcallosal zone under the corpus callosum.
Connective tissue or mesenchymal stem cells outside bone marrow	*Mesoderm derived* Progenitors of connective tissue cells; isolated from several tissues, although bone marrow origin cannot be excluded *Muscle cells*	*Skeletal:* satellite cells—between sarcolemma and overlying basement membrane of myofiber—also derived from pericytes or bone marrow mesenchymal stem cells *Adipose:* fat is a rich source of multipotential mesenchymal cells *Kidney:* there are findings supportive of kidney renal tubular and parietal epithelial podocyte (Bowman capsule) stem/progenitor cells. Cells of the kidney are of mesodermal origin, with the possible exception of the endothelial cell *Cardiac:* cardiac progenitor or stem cells—multipotent cardiomyocytes capable of maintaining homeostasis, limited differentiation and proliferation after ischemic injury; bone marrow mesenchymal stem cells

[a]These may be the same as multipotent adult progenitor cells (MAPCs), which represent bone marrow stromal cells whose differentiation is influenced by in vitro growth conditions. These cells are capable of seeding tissues outside the bone marrow by one or more several possible processes: (1) specific progenitors or multipotent progenitors, (b) transdifferentiation, (c) cell fusion and (d) dedifferentiation.

However, this should not be confused with stem cell potency. Somatic cells can now be converted into the totipotent iPS cell with the potential to supply new tissues from the same individual. Postembryonically, implanted ES cells can also form teratomas owing to unregulated differentiation. ES cells that are derived from the inner cell mass of the blastocyst are **pluripotent,** meaning they may differentiate into nearly all cell lineages within any of the three germ layers. Pluripotent stem cells of the postfertilization zygote, such as neural crest cells, may differentiate into many cell types,

but they are not totipotent. Those adult cells that must self-renew throughout the lifetime of the organism are generally **multipotent,** or able to differentiate into several cell types within one lineage or one of the germ layers. Hematopoietic stem cells, for example, are lineage restricted; they can form all the cells found in blood (Table 3-8). Marrow stromal cells (also known as mesenchymal stem cells [MSCs]) are multipotent stem cells within bone marrow that can mobilize into the bloodstream and be recruited to (injured) organs. MSCs can be induced to differentiate into multiple cell types in vitro (adipocytes, chondrocytes, osteoblasts, myoblasts, fibroblasts) derived from a single cell lineage, the mesoderm germ layer. Mesenchymal stem cells have also been isolated from cord blood and many other connective tissues.

Tissue-specific cells support renewal as multipotent stem cells or as progenitor cells. Progenitor cells are **stable cells** that are distinguished from stem cells by their incapacity for self-renewal; however, they maintain the potential for differentiation and rapid proliferation. They are sometimes referred to as **unipotent** stem cells, as exemplified by the interfollicular basal keratinocyte of skin, although other skin cells may be multipotent or oligopotent. An example is the more versatile bulge stem cells of the hair follicle, which are able to reconstitute the hair follicle and sebaceous gland and contribute to repair of epidermis.

In addition to normal differentiation pathways within a single tissue, cells of one tissue can **transdifferentiate** into cells of another tissue. In the adult, injured epithelium (renal tubules, pulmonary) may have the ability to transform into fibroblasts under the influence of cytokines such as TGF-β, adding to scarring and fibrosis; cardiac endothelial cells may have the same capacity.

Bone marrow contains hematopoietic, mesenchymal and endothelial stem cells, providing a multifaceted regenerative capacity. Bone marrow stem cells, which are set aside during embryonic development, replenish the bone marrow mesenchyme and hematopoietic population. Endothelial progenitor cells from bone marrow have been implicated in tissue angiogenesis and may supplement endothelial hyperplasia during regeneration of blood vessels. Likewise, bone marrow–derived mesenchymal stem cells can populate repairing tissues in many distant sites (Table 3-8).

Cornified skin epithelium and hair follicles regenerate from stem cells in basal epidermis and the bulge region of the hair follicle. Intestinal epithelium turns over rapidly and is replenished by intestinal stem cells that reside in the crypts of Lieberkühn. Liver reconstitution after partial hepatectomy is a hyperplastic response by mature differentiated hepatocytes of the remaining lobes and is not thought to involve stem cells. However, there is evidence for stem, or progenitor, cell–driven liver regeneration when hepatocytes are damaged by viral hepatitis or toxins. This regeneration is thought to arise from "oval cells" in the small bile ducts. These putative stem cells have characteristics of both hepatocytes (α-fetoprotein and albumin) and bile duct cells (γ-glutamyl transferase and duct cytokeratins) and may reside in terminal ductal cells in the canal of Hering.

Influence of Environment on Stem Cells

Stem cells exist in **microenvironments** or **niches** that provide sustaining signals from extracellular matrix and neighboring cells to limit their differentiation and to ensure their perpetuation, while providing feedback mechanisms that control cell number, fate and motility. Important features of several stem cell niches are basement membrane matrix molecules and proximity of mesenchymal cells, chemokines and specific growth and differentiation factors. The mere presence of adult stem cells or progenitor cells is not sufficient for tissue regeneration when tissue is damaged. Many tissues contain resident progenitor cells, yet do not heal by regeneration. The method of repair is also influenced by the environment of the injury, that is, the growth factors,

cytokines, proteinases and composition of the extracellular matrix. Whether a wound is repaired by regeneration or scarring and fibrosis is at least partly determined by the concentration, duration and composition of environmental signals present during inflammation. Maintenance regeneration of adult epidermis or intestinal epithelium generally occurs without inflammation and within an innate extracellular matrix. In such instances, normal structures and architecture are assembled in the absence of fibrosis or scarring. Wounds eventually shift to an inflammatory response and a matrix expression profile that places emphasis on protection (scarring) rather than perfection (regeneration). Spinal cord injury, as an example, provides a particularly difficult challenge. Injury-induced cellular reactions lead to death of neurons, glial cells and oligodendrocytes. Further inflammatory damage results in glial scar development by astrocytes, which release chondroitin sulfate proteoglycans and proteins that block axonal growth. The current strategies for regeneration rest upon the possibility that transplantation of an appropriate stem cell population might reestablish normal tissue function and prevent scarring. Fibrosis, an urgent response to preserve mechanical integrity after tissue damage, is a key impediment to regeneration.

Differentiated Cells Can Revert to Pluripotency

Cell differentiation involves controlled regulation of gene expression within an existing DNA sequence. This occurs via (1) **epigenetic modification** to DNA without changing or rearranging the sequence; (2) reduced expression of pluripotency-limiting genes, including the Polycomb group proteins; and (3) increased expression of lineage development genes. Epigenetic modifications include nucleic acid modifications within the DNA sequence, such as methylation, expression of microRNAs and remodeling of chromatin organization by chromatin-associated proteins and modification of histone proteins (see Chapter 5).

Epigenetic modifiers stabilize and restrict transcriptional states as necessary for cell differentiation and are heritable by progeny (monoallelic alteration inherited from egg or sperm is called **imprinting**). Interplay between epigenetic modifiers and lineage-determining transcription factors is necessary for the progressive differentiation states in a cell lineage. Differentiation is controlled at many levels. It may involve cell–cell contact and extracellular signals, but coactivation and coregulation of transcription factors associated with potency or lineage and epigenetic modifications are also key to the final state of a cell.

Cells Can Be Classified by Their Proliferative Potential

Cell populations divide at different rates. Some mature cells do not divide at all, while others cycle repeatedly.

LABILE CELLS: Labile cells are found in tissues that are in a constant state of renewal. Tissues in which more than 1.5% of the cells are in mitosis at any one time are composed of labile cells. However, stable cells are also constituents of labile tissues with high rates of cell turnover. Labile epithelial tissues that typically form physical barriers between the body and the external environment self-renew constantly. Examples include epithelia of the gut, skin, cornea, respiratory tract, reproductive tract and urinary tract. Hematopoietic cells of the bone marrow and lymphoid organs involved in immune defense are also labile. Polymorphonuclear nucleocytes and reticulocytes are terminally differentiated cells that are rapidly renewed. *Under appropriate conditions, tissues composed of labile cells regenerate after injury, provided enough stem cells remain.*

STABLE CELLS: Stable cells populate tissues that normally are renewed very slowly but are populated with progenitor cells capable of more rapid renewal after tissue loss. Liver, bone and proximal renal tubules are examples of stable cell populations. Stable cells populate tissues in which less than 1.5% of cells are in mitosis. Stable tissues (e.g., endocrine glands, endothelium and liver) do not have conspicuous stem cells. Rather, their cells require an appropriate stimulus to divide. *The potential to replicate, not the actual number of steady state mitoses, determines the ability of an organ to regenerate.* For example, the liver, a stable tissue with less than one mitosis for every 15,000 cells, rapidly recovers through hepatocyte hyperplasia after loss of up to 75% of its mass.

PERMANENT CELLS: Permanent cells are terminally differentiated, have lost all capacity for regeneration and do not enter the cell cycle. Traditionally, neurons, chondrocytes, cardiac myocytes and cells of the lens were considered permanent cells. If lost, cardiac myocytes and neurons may be replaced from progenitors, but not from division of existing cardiac myocytes or mature neurons. Permanent cells do not divide, but do renew their organelles. The extreme example of permanent cells is the lens of the eye. Every lens cell generated during embryonic development and postnatal life is preserved in the adult without turnover of its constituents.

CONDITIONS THAT MODIFY REPAIR

Local Factors May Influence Healing

Location of the Wound

In addition to its size and shape, the location of a wound also affects healing. In sites where scant tissue separates skin and bone (e.g., over the anterior tibia), a wound in the skin cannot contract. Skin lesions in such areas, particularly burns, often require skin grafts because their edges cannot be apposed. Complications or other treatments, like infection, obesity, diabetes, chemotherapy, glucocorticoids or ionizing radiation, also slow repair processes.

Blood Supply

Lower extremity wounds of diabetics often heal poorly or may even require amputation because advanced atherosclerosis in the legs (peripheral vascular disease) and defective angiogenesis compromise blood supply and impede repair. Varicose veins of the legs, due to failure of the venous valves to ensure venous return, can cause edema, formation of thick (fibrin) cuffs around microvessels, ulceration and nonhealing (venous stasis ulcers). Bed/pressure sores (decubitus ulcers) result from prolonged, localized, dependent pressure, which diminishes both arterial and venous blood flow and results in intermittent ischemia. Joint (articular) cartilage is largely avascular and has limited diffusion capacity. Often it cannot mount a vigorous inflammatory response, so that articular cartilage repairs poorly in the face of progressive, age-related wear and tear.

Systemic Factors

No specific effect of age alone on repair has been found, although there is evidence that stem cell reserves are reduced with aging (see Chapter 10). Scarring peaks during adolescence and diminishes with age. Healing also declines in postmenopausal women. Although reduced collagen and elastin may make the skin of a 90-year-old person fragile and thus heal slowly, that person's colon resection or cataract extraction heals normally because the bowel and eye are practically unaffected by age.

Coagulation defects, thrombocytopenia and anemia impede repair. Local thrombosis decreases platelet activation, reducing the supply of growth factors and limiting the healing cascade. The decrease in tissue oxygen that accompanies severe anemia also interferes with repair. Exogenous corticosteroids retard wound repair by inhibiting collagen and protein synthesis and by suppressing both destructive and constructive aspects of inflammation.

Fibrosis and Scarring Contrasted

Successful wound repair that leads to localized, transient scarring promotes rapid resolution of local injury. Scars reflect altered deposition of matrix compared to normal, surrounding tissue. Scars may vary in size and may be larger than the wound site, depending on the nature of the wound or its treatment. This occurs particularly where there exists greater mechanical movement and tension, such as over limb joints. Scarring is a typical response to tissue ischemia or infarction, where resident cells cannot be replaced. By contrast, in many chronic diseases of skin and parenchymal organs, including many autoimmune diseases (e.g., scleroderma), inflammation persists. It then progresses to diffuse and progressive **fibrosis**, or **continued and excessive deposition of matrix** proteins, particularly collagen. Inhaled smoke or inhaled silica particles induce chronic inflammation in the lung, while other disturbances of alveolar epithelial type II cell homeostasis foreshadow development of life-threatening idiopathic pulmonary fibrosis. Innate and adaptive immune-mediated inflammation, such as that of joints in rheumatoid arthritis, leads to differentiation and activation of fibroblasts. Both inflammatory and noninflammatory factors cause cardiac, hepatic, lung and kidney fibrosis. By example, glomerulosclerosis in the kidney results from infection, hypertension or diabetes.

Ongoing insult or inflammation, mediated via the interplay of M1 macrophages and T helper (Th2, Th17) lymphocytes, results in persistently high levels of cytokines (IL-1β, IL-6, TNF-α), fibrogenic growth factors (TGF-β) and locally destructive enzymes, such as matrix metalloproteinases. Resolution of a fibrogenic response is associated with M2 macrophages and, in some studies, Th1 and T regulatory cells. The fibrotic reaction, once initiated, may resolve with early removal of the inflammatory or noninflammatory triggers. Fibrosis itself further alters matrix composition, stiffness and mechanical stress, propagating fibroblast conversion to myofibroblasts and further matrix production. The composition of matrix changes from provisional matrix during fibrogenesis and remodeling, providing opportunities for a matrix that supports continued fibrosis. Uncontrolled fibrosis self-perpetuates, despite absence of continued inflammation; it features myofibroblast production of extracellular matrix.

The protein osteonectin/BM-40/SPARC (secreted protein acidic and rich in cysteine) is a nonstructural extracellular matrix protein secreted into the extracellular space (matricellular protein) during development and during fibrosis. SPARC dissociates collagen from the cell surface by competing with binding of fibrillar collagens to the cellular discoidin domain receptor, and it may encourage further collagen secretion and deposition. Similarly, osteopontin is associated with persistent fibrosis in several organs. Regardless of the underlying mechanism, fibrosis of parenchymal organs such as the heart, lungs, kidney or liver disrupts normal architecture and impedes function. The functional unit (smooth muscle, alveolus, hepatic lobule or renal glomerulus or tubule) is replaced by disordered collagen. Such fibrosis and resulting dysfunction are largely irreversible. Correction requires removing the inciting stimulus by treatment, as in rheumatoid arthritis, to suppress inflammation and so minimize tissue damage. Otherwise, tissue architecture and mechanics are so impaired that regenerative processes cannot reverse the injury.

Fibrosis is the pathologic consequence of persistent injury and causes loss of function. Fibrosis is an abnormal process that develops from persistent or impaired normal processes. Often it is the final common result of diverse diseases or injuries, the causes of which cannot be ascertained from the end result. As an example, in scars of former glomeruli damaged following bacterial or immunologic injury to the kidney, the specific cause is no longer identifiable. Scarring, however, is often beneficial; it restores structural (if not necessarily functional) integrity to the injured area.

Prevention of fibrosis requires either blocking the stimulus of matrix production or increasing the level of matrix degradation. TGF-β and connective tissue growth factor (CTGF, CCN-2) are regulators of matrix production and have been associated with fibrotic connective tissue diseases. The process is also regulated by cytokines, growth factors, Wnt/β-catenin signaling and microRNAs. Approaches to controlling fibrotic progression to end-stage kidney disease have targeted profibrotic factors such as TGF-β and plasminogen activator inhibitor-1 (PAI-1). Inhibition of PAI-1 elicits activation of plasminogen. As a result, plasmin degradation of extracellular matrix is increased, directly or through activating MMPs. Matrix deposition in the glomerulus is reduced, protecting the glomerulus from scarring and obliteration. Interestingly, inhibition of PAI could also reduce the incidence of **intra-abdominal adhesions,** a persistent problem of abdominal surgery and an important cause of intestinal obstruction. These adhesions are initiated by fibrin deposition when mesothelial lining is disrupted or heals ineffectively. If the fibrin matrix is not dissolved by plasmin within a few days, the provisional matrix is invaded by fibroblasts and eventually transformed into a permanent fibrotic adhesion, with collagen, capillaries and nerves.

There is accumulating evidence that resolution of the fibrotic process may not derive merely from reducing activating signals or developing an appropriate level of tensile strength and elasticity. Members of the CXCL3 family of cytokines, which includes interferon-γ–inducible protein 9 (IP-9 or CXCL11) and IP-10 (or CXCL10), are produced by fibroblasts and epithelial cells, among other cell types. Increases in these proteins are associated with reduced fibrosis, while their absence can lead to exaggerated scarring.

Specific Sites Exhibit Different Repair Patterns

Skin

Healing in the skin involves repair, primarily dermal scarring, and regeneration, principally of the epidermis and its appendages, innervation and vasculature. The salient features of primary and secondary healing are provided in Fig. 3-12.

Primary healing occurs when the surgeon closely approximates the edges of a wound. The actions of myofibroblasts are minimized owing to the lack of mechanical strain, and regeneration of the epidermis is optimal, since epidermal cells need migrate only a minimal distance.

Secondary healing proceeds when a large area of hemorrhage and necrosis cannot be totally corrected surgically. In this situation, myofibroblasts contract the wound and reinforce healing with extensive ECM. Resultant scarring repairs the defect.

The success and method of healing following a burn wound depends on the depth of the injury. If it is superficial or does not extend beyond the upper dermis, stem cells from sweat glands and hair follicles regenerate the epidermis. If deep dermis is involved, the regenerative elements are destroyed and surgery with epidermal or keratinocyte grafts is necessary to cover or heal the wound site and reduce scarring and severe contractures. In this case, epidermal appendages (follicles, sweat glands) are not regenerated, but cytokines produced by the grafted epidermis may contribute to the improved outcome.

Cornea

The cornea differs from skin in its stromal organization, vascularity and cellularity. Like skin, corneal stratified squamous epithelium is continually renewed by a stem cell population, at the periphery of the corneal limbus. Epithelial damage that does not involve stroma heals by keratinocyte migration and replication without scarring. Chemical, infectious, surgical or traumatic injury to the cornea results in scarring, owing to the distortion of the precisely arranged collagen fibers, effectively blinding the eye. Parenthetically, the cornea, because of its relative avascularity, was the first organ or anatomic structure to be successfully transplanted. Trachoma, an infectious human disease caused by an inflammatory response to *Chlamydia trachomatis*, is the world's most common cause of blindness, resulting from scarring and opacity of the cornea (see Fig. 33-1).

Liver

The liver has tremendous regenerative capacity, even though the normal liver almost totally lacks mitoses and virtually all hepatocytes are in cell cycle phase G_0. After resection, liver regenerates by compensatory hyperplasia of hepatocytes. The necessary conditions for hepatic regeneration are complex (see Chapter 20). Suffice it to say here that regeneration ceases when the normal ratio of liver to total body weight is reestablished; the molecular switch that regulates this ratio is unknown but may involve the *Hippo* pathway, a kinase cascade that controls organ size.

Acute chemical injury or fulminant viral hepatitis causes widespread necrosis of hepatocytes. However, if the connective tissue stroma, vasculature and bile ducts survive, liver parenchyma regenerates, and normal form and function

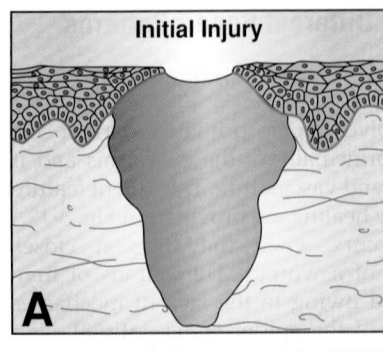
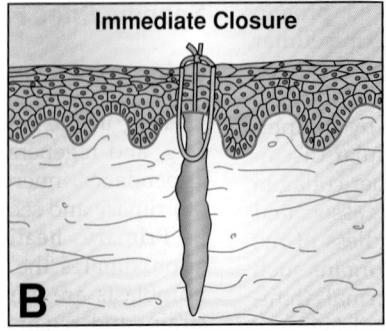
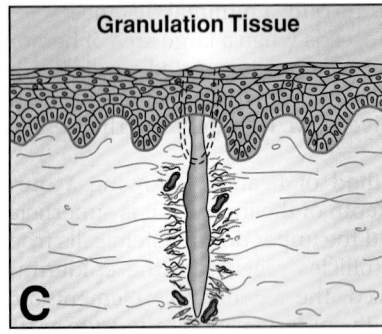
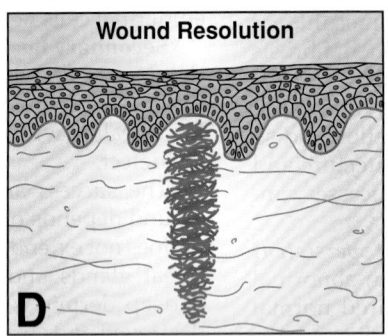

HEALING BY PRIMARY INTENTION (WOUNDS WITH APPOSED EDGES)

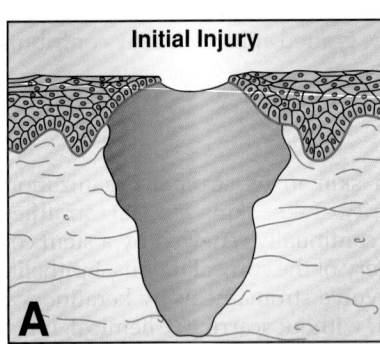
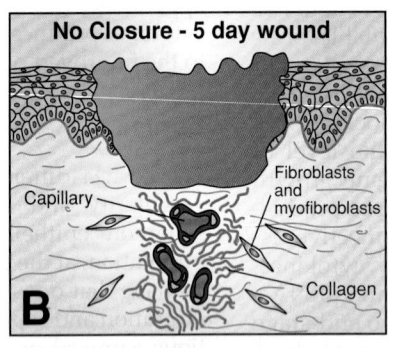
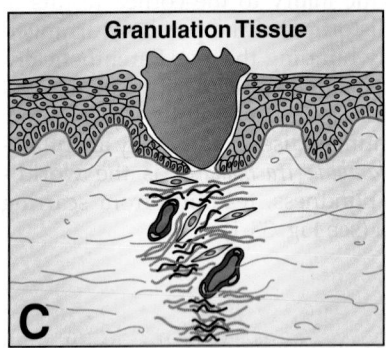
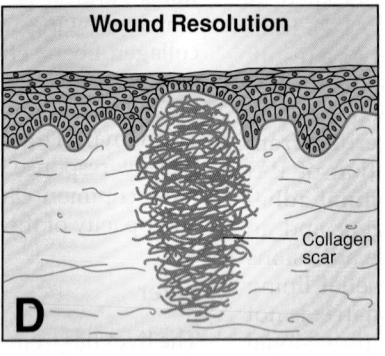

HEALING BY SECONDARY INTENTION (WOUNDS WITH SEPARATED EDGES)

FIGURE 3-12. Top. Healing by primary intention. **A.** An initial open, incised wound **(B)** with closely apposed wound edges is held together with a suture, leading to minimal tissue gaping or loss. **C.** There is decreased granulation tissue. Such a wound requires only minimal cell proliferation and neovascularization to heal. **D.** The result is a narrow, linear scar. **Bottom. Healing by secondary intention. A.** A gouged wound that remains or is left to remain open. The edges remain far apart and there is substantial tissue loss. **B.** The healing process requires wound contraction (mechanical strain), extensive cell proliferation, matrix accumulation and neovascularization (granulation tissue) to heal. **C.** The wound is reepithelialized from the margins, and collagen fibers are deposited throughout the granulation tissue. **D.** Granulation tissue is eventually resorbed, leaving a large collagenous scar that is functionally and esthetically imperfect.

are restored. There is evidence for liver stem cells capable of supporting regeneration at the canal of Hering, within or peripheral to intralobular bile ducts, and among peribiliary hepatocytes (Table 3-8). By contrast, in chronic injury, viral hepatitis or alcoholism, broad collagenous scars develop within the hepatic parenchyma, termed **cirrhosis** of the liver (Fig. 3-13). Hepatocytes form regenerative nodules that lack central veins and expand to obstruct blood vessels and bile flow. Despite adequate numbers of regenerated hepatocytes, architectural disarray impairs liver function and patients eventually suffer hepatic insufficiency.

Kidney

Although the kidney has limited regenerative capacity, removal of one kidney (nephrectomy) is followed by compensatory hypertrophy of the remaining kidney. If renal injury, such as acute kidney injury due to nephrotoxins or ischemia, is not extensive and the extracellular matrix framework, in particular the basement membrane, is not destroyed, tubular epithelium will regenerate. In most renal diseases, however, the matrix is disrupted, leading to incomplete regeneration with scar formation. The regenerative capacity of renal tissue

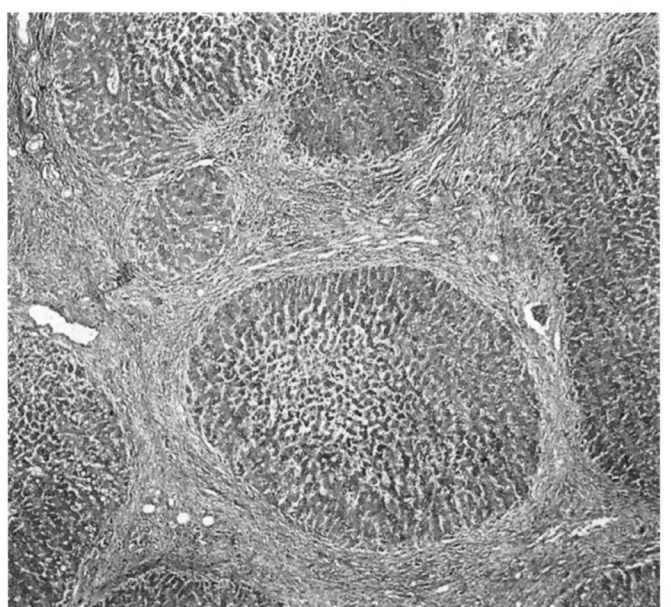

FIGURE 3-13. Cirrhosis of the liver. The consequence of chronic hepatic injury is the formation of regenerating nodules separated by fibrous bands. A microscopic section shows regenerating nodules (*red*) surrounded by bands of connective tissue (*blue*).

is maximal in cortical tubules and less in medullary tubules. Podocyte hypertrophy or regeneration appears to be a possibility in some diseases like diabetes or chronic nephropathy, in which scarring and disease are reversed with pancreatic transplants or inhibition of angiotensin-converting enzyme. Recent data suggest that tubule repair occurs not from bone marrow–derived cells but as a result of proliferation of endogenous, multipotent tubular stem cells.

Cortical Renal Tubules

Tubular epithelium normally turns over and cells are shed into the urine. No reserve cell has been identified, and simple division accomplishes replacement. The outcome of injury hinges on the integrity of the tubular basement membrane. As long as the basement membrane is continuous, surviving tubular cells in the vicinity of a wound flatten, acquire a squamous-like appearance and migrate into the injured area

along the basement membrane. Mitoses are frequent, and occasional clusters of epithelial cells project into the lumen. The flattened cells soon become more cuboidal, and differentiated cytoplasmic elements appear. Tubular morphology and function return to normal in 3–4 weeks.

Tubulorrhexis

Following tubulorrhexis, or rupture of the tubular basement membrane, events resemble those in tubular damage with an intact basement membrane, except that interstitial changes are more prominent. Fibroblasts proliferate, increased extracellular matrix is deposited and tubular lumina collapse. Some tubules will regenerate and others will become fibrotic, with consequent focal losses of functional nephrons.

Medullary Renal Tubules

Medullary diseases of the kidney are often associated with extensive necrosis, which involves tubules, interstitium and blood vessels. The necrotic tissue sloughs into the urine. Healing by fibrosis produces urinary obstruction within the kidney. Although there is some epithelial proliferation, there is no significant regeneration.

Glomeruli

Unlike tubules, glomeruli do not regenerate. Necrosis of glomerular endothelial or epithelial cells, whether focal, segmental or diffuse, heals by scarring (Fig. 3-14). Mesangial cells are related to smooth muscle cells and seem to have some capacity for regeneration. Following unilateral nephrectomy, glomeruli in the remaining kidney enlarge by both hypertrophy and hyperplasia. Podocyte progenitor cells in the Bowman capsule may replace lost podocytes.

Lung

The epithelium lining the respiratory tract can regenerate to some degree, if the underlying extracellular matrix framework is not destroyed. Superficial injuries to tracheal and bronchial epithelia heal by regeneration from adjacent epithelium. The progenitor cell has not been clearly identified, although bronchioalveolar stem cells have been proposed, and there is evidence for an alveolar epithelial type II progenitor. Bone marrow–derived stem cells may

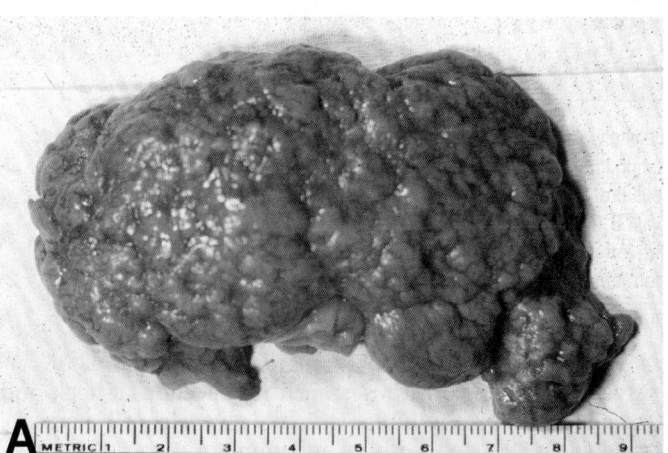

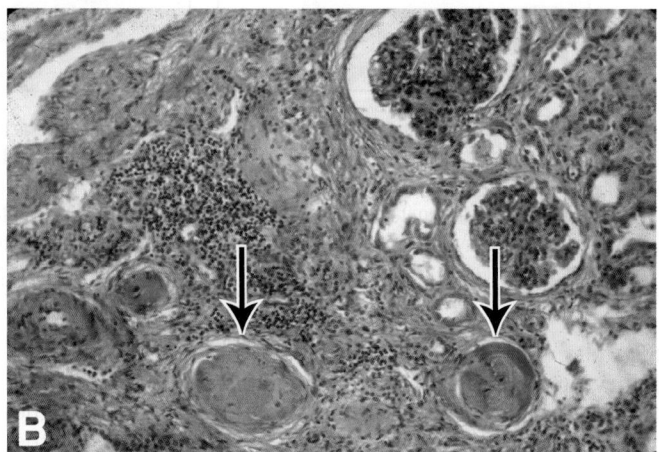

FIGURE 3-14. Scarred kidney. A. Repeated bacterial urinary tract infections have scarred the kidney. **B.** Many glomeruli have been destroyed and appear as circular scars (*arrows*).

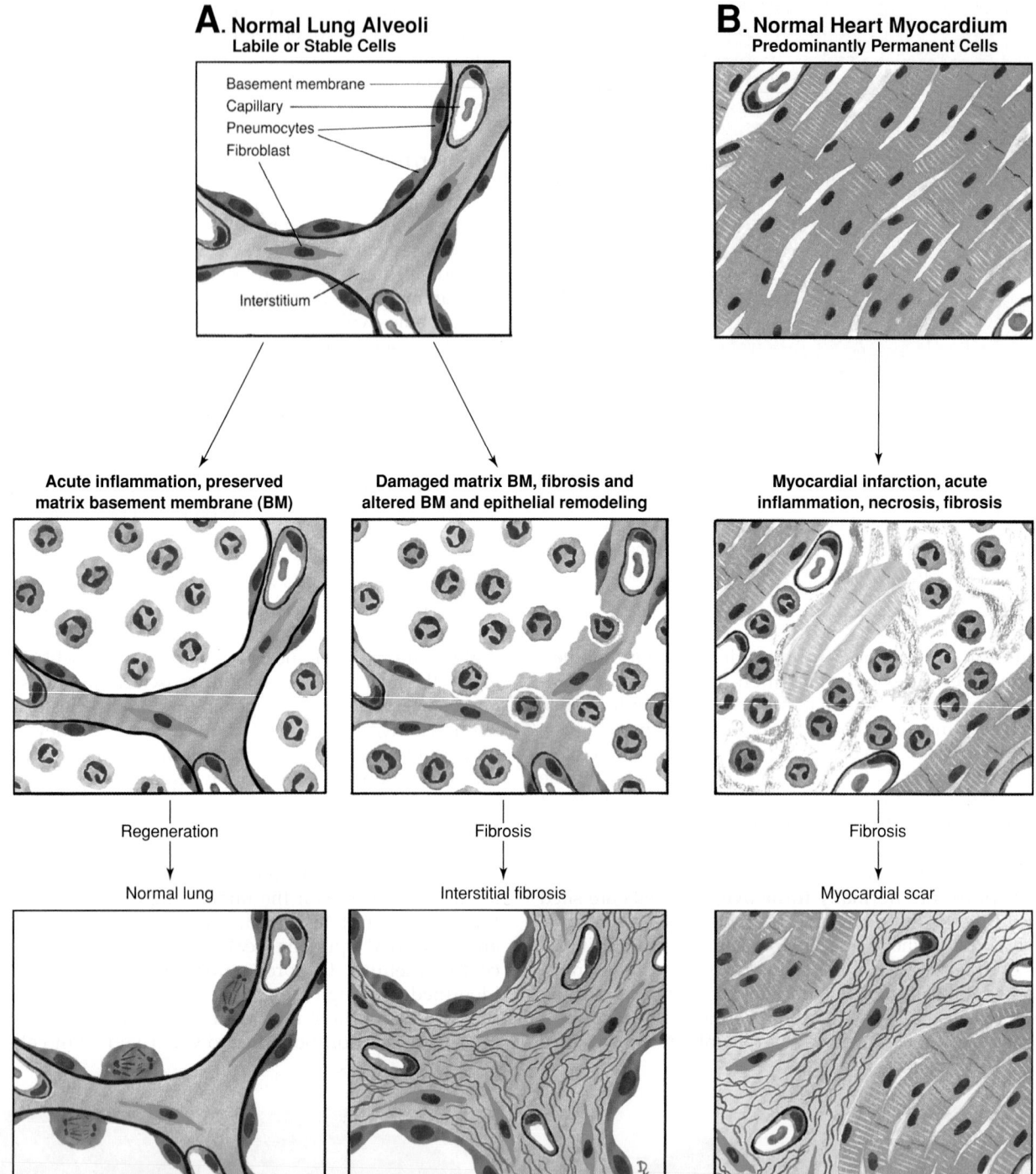

FIGURE 3-15. Examples of fibrotic and regenerative repair. A. The lung alveoli are lined with type I and type II epithelial cells (pneumocytes) that lie on a basement membrane. If the basement membrane remains intact following lung damage, there is rapid reepithelialization and return to normal lung architecture. If the basement membrane is damaged, type II epithelial cells proliferate on the underlying extracellular matrix, and fibroblasts and myofibroblasts are recruited to deposit a collagen-rich matrix, leading to fibrosis. **B.** Though small numbers of cardiac stem cells have been described, regeneration of myocardium is rarely observed. By and large cardiomyocytes are terminally differentiated and not capable of renewal. Myocardial damage due to infarction and acute inflammation is repaired by fibrosis and scar formation, increasing chances of arrhythmia or heart failure.

also take residence in the lung. The outcome of alveolar injury ranges from complete regeneration of structure and function to incapacitating fibrosis. As with the liver, the degree of cell necrosis and the extent of the damage to the extracellular matrix framework determine the outcome (Fig. 3-15).

Alveolar Injury with Intact Basement Membranes
Alveolar injury from causes such as infections, shock and oxygen toxicity produces variable alveolar cell necrosis. Alveoli are flooded with an inflammatory exudate rich in plasma proteins. As long as the alveolar basement membrane is intact, healing can occur by regeneration. Neutrophils and

macrophages clear the alveolar exudate, but if they fail to do so, it is organized by granulation tissue, and intra-alveolar fibrosis results. Alveolar type II epithelial cells or pneumocytes (the alveolar reserve cells) migrate to denuded areas and divide to form cells with features intermediate between type I and type II pneumocytes. These cells cover the alveolar surface and establish contact with other epithelial cells. Mitosis then stops and the cells differentiate into type I pneumocytes. Bone marrow–derived cells or putative lung bronchioalveolar progenitor or stem cells may participate by differentiating into bronchiolar Clara cells and alveolar cells (Table 3-8).

Alveolar Injury with Disrupted Basement Membranes
Extensive damage to alveolar basement membranes evokes scarring and fibrosis. Mesenchymal cells from alveolar septa proliferate and differentiate into fibroblasts and myofibroblasts. The role of macrophage products in inducing fibroblast proliferation in the lung is well documented. The myofibroblasts and fibroblasts migrate into the alveolar spaces, where they secrete extracellular matrix components, mainly type I collagen and proteoglycans, to produce pulmonary fibrosis. The most common chronic pulmonary disease is emphysema, which involves airspace enlargement and the destruction of alveolar walls. Ineffective replacement of elastin in this condition is associated with irreversible loss of tissue resiliency and function.

Heart

Cardiac myocytes had long been considered permanent, nondividing, terminally differentiated cells. There is recent evidence that cardiomyocytes, while not able to sufficiently repair damaged myocardium, are able to regenerate at a very low rate and maintain myocyte homeostasis during the low rates of myocyte turnover. The origin of these cells, whether they reside in the myocardium as cardiomyocyte progenitors or migrate there from bone marrow or sites unknown, is not resolved. For practical purposes, myocardial necrosis, from whatever cause, heals by the formation of granulation tissue and eventual scarring (Figs. 3-15 and 3-16). Not only does myocardial scarring result in the loss of contractile elements, but also the fibrotic tissue decreases the effectiveness of contraction in the surviving myocardium. With ischemia or infarction in the heart, as is often the case in other organs,

healing results in scarring despite the presence in the tissue of stem or progenitor cells.

Nervous System

Mature neurons have been historically considered as permanent and postmitotic cells. There is limited regenerative capacity in the brain from stem cells, derived from bone marrow and perhaps other sources. Nonetheless, the poor reparative capabilities of the nervous system are well documented. Following trauma, only regrowth and reorganization of the surviving neuronal cell processes can reestablish neural connections. Although the peripheral nervous system can regenerate axonals, the central nervous system cannot. The olfactory bulb and hippocampal dentate gyrus regions of adult mammalian brain are now known to regenerate via neural precursor or stem cells. Multipotent precursor cells have also been seen elsewhere in the brain, raising hope that repair of neural circuitry may eventually be possible (Table 3-8).

Central Nervous System
Damage to the brain or spinal cord is followed by growth of capillaries and gliosis (i.e., inflammatory immune cell response, proliferation of astrocytes and microglia). Gliosis in the central nervous system is the equivalent of scar formation elsewhere; once established, it is permanent. In spinal cord injuries, axonal outgrowth can be seen up to 2 weeks after injury. After 2 weeks, gliosis has taken place and attempts at axonal regeneration end, having been inhibited by release of molecules such as myelin-associated glycoprotein and chondroitin sulfate proteoglycans. In the central nervous system, axonal regeneration occurs only in the hypothalamo-hypophysial region, where glial and capillary barriers do not interfere.

Peripheral Nervous System
Neurons in the peripheral nervous system can regenerate axons, and under ideal circumstances, interruption in the continuity of a peripheral nerve may result in complete functional recovery. However, if cut ends are not in perfect alignment or are prevented from establishing continuity by inflammation or a scar, a traumatic neuroma results (Fig. 3-17). This bulbous lesion consists of disorganized

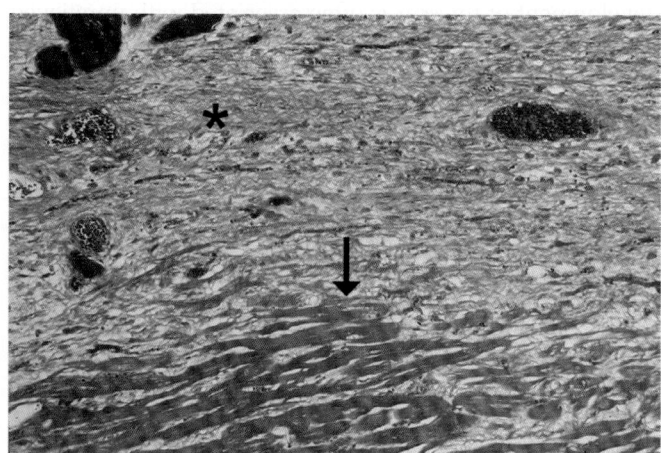

FIGURE 3-16. Myocardial infarction. A section through a healed myocardial infarct shows mature fibrosis (*) and disrupted myocardial fibers (*arrow*).

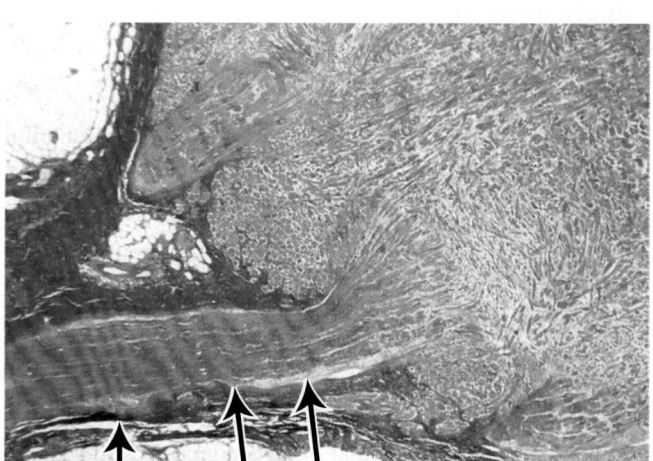

FIGURE 3-17. Traumatic neuroma. In this photomicrograph, the original nerve (*arrows*) enters the neuroma. The nerve is surrounded by dense collagenous tissue, which appears dark blue with this trichrome stain. Excessive repair obstructs axonal reconnection.

axons and proliferating Schwann cells and fibroblasts. The regenerative capacity of the peripheral nervous system can be ascribed to (1) the fact that the blood-nerve barrier, which insulates peripheral axons from extracellular fluids, is not restored for 2–3 months, and (2) the presence of Schwann cells with basement membranes. Laminin, a basement membrane component, and nerve growth factor (NGF) guide and stimulate neurite growth.

Effects of Scarring

In the absence of the ability to form scars, mammalian survival would hardly be possible. Yet scarring in parenchymal organs modifies their complex structure and never improves their function. For example, in the heart, the scar of a myocardial infarction serves to prevent rupture of the heart, but it reduces the amount of contractile tissue. If extensive enough, it may cause congestive heart failure or lead to a ventricular aneurysm (see Chapter 17). Similarly, an aorta that is weakened and scarred by atherosclerosis is prone to dilate as an aneurysm (see Chapter 16). Scarred mitral and aortic valves injured by rheumatic fever are often stenotic, regurgitant or both, leading to congestive heart failure. Persistent inflammation within the pericardium produces fibrous adhesions, which result in constrictive pericarditis and heart failure.

Pulmonary alveolar fibrosis causes respiratory failure. Infection in the peritoneum or even surgical exploration may create adhesions and intestinal obstruction. Immunologic injury generates replacement of renal glomeruli by collagenous scars and, if it is extensive, renal failure. Scarring in the skin after burns or surgery produces unsatisfactory cosmetic results and may severely limit mobility. An important goal of therapeutic intervention is to create optimum conditions for "constructive" scarring and prevent pathologic "overshoot" of this process.

Wound Repair Is Often Suboptimal

Abnormalities in any of the three healing processes—repair, contraction and regeneration—result in unsuccessful or prolonged wound healing. The skill of the surgeon is often of critical importance.

Deficient Scar Formation

Inadequate formation of granulation tissue or an inability to form a suitable extracellular matrix gives rise to deficient scar formation and its complications.

Wound Dehiscence and Incisional Hernias

Dehiscence (a wound splitting open) is most frequent after abdominal surgery and can be life-threatening. Increased mechanical stress on an abdominal wound from vomiting, coughing, pathologic obesity or bowel obstruction may cause dehiscence of that wound. Systemic factors predisposing to dehiscence include metabolic deficiency, hypoproteinemia and the general inanition that often accompanies metastatic cancer. **Incisional hernias** of the abdominal wall are defects caused by weak surgical scars owing to insufficient deposition of extracellular matrix or inadequate cross-linking in the collagen matrix. Loops of intestine may be trapped within incisional hernias.

Ulceration

Wounds can ulcerate if an intrinsic blood supply is inadequate or if vascularization is insufficient during healing. Failure of the venous valves in the lower leg leads to tissue edema, the formation of pericapillary fibrin cuffs and the generation of venous stasis ulcers, often on the inner aspect of the lower leg. This is the most prevalent chronic wound in Western society. Severe atherosclerosis or peripheral arterial disease can evoke the formation of arterial ulcers on the outer part of the lower leg or the foot. Diabetic foot ulcers are brought about by a combination of poor arterial and capillary blood supply that may be accompanied by a **diabetic peripheral neuropathy** that renders the patient insensitive to the progressing ulcer. Diabetes also reduces expression of and cellular responsiveness to growth factors, making it difficult to stimulate the healing process. This form of ulceration, if left unchecked, proceeds to infection of the underlying bone **(osteomyelitis)** and progressive loss of the extremity. Nonhealing wounds also develop in areas devoid of sensation because of trauma or pressure. Such **decubitus ulcers** are commonly seen in patients who are immobilized in either beds or wheelchairs. Constant pressure on the skin over a bony process can produce a local infarct in as little as 2–3 hours. These ulcers can be both broad and deep, with infection penetrating deep into connective tissue.

Excessive Scar Formation in the Skin

Excessive deposition of extracellular matrix, mostly excessive collagen, at the wound site results in hypertrophic scars and keloids. **Keloids** are exuberant scars that tend to progress beyond the site of initial injury and recur after excision (Fig. 3-18), thus having properties akin to a benign tumor. Keloids are unsightly, and attempts at surgical repair are always problematic, the outcome likely being a still larger keloid. Keloids are generally restricted to adolescence and early adulthood and to the upper trunk, neck and head, with the exception of the scalp. This aspect reflects the (epigenetic) heterogeneity of fibroblast populations in different locations. Dark-skinned persons are more frequently affected, suggesting a genetic basis for this condition. Unlike normal scars, these keloids do not reduce collagen synthesis if glucocorticoids are administered.

By contrast, **hypertrophic scars** are not associated with race or heredity, but the severity of scarring can decline with age. The scar is confined within the wound margins, and the development of the scar is often associated with unrelieved mechanical stress. Hypertrophic scars often have a reddened appearance indicative of hypervascularity, and they are pruritic, which suggests activation of mast cells producing histamine. Histologically, both types of scars exhibit broad and irregular collagen bundles, with more capillaries and fibroblasts than is normal for a scar of the same age. The rate of collagen synthesis and number of reducible cross-links remain high. This situation suggests a "maturation arrest," or block, in the healing process, a hypothesis that is supported by the overexpression of fibronectin.

Excessive Contraction

A decrease in the size of a wound depends on the presence of fibroblasts and myofibroblasts, development of cell–cell contacts and sustained cell contraction. An exaggeration of these processes is termed **contracture** and results in severe deformity of a wound and surrounding tissues. Interestingly,

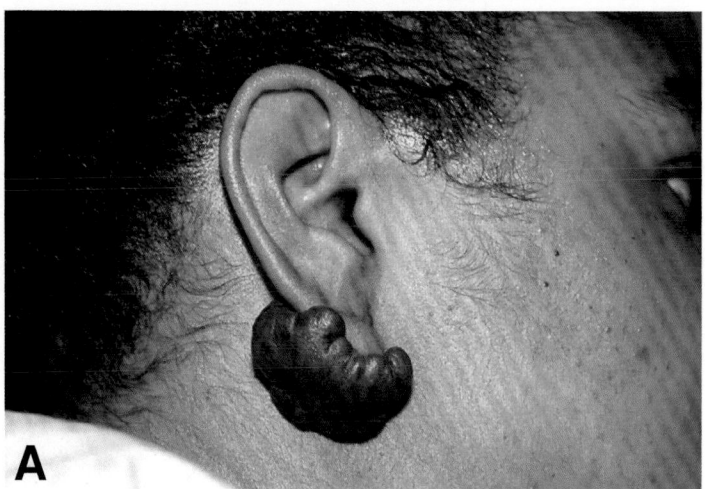 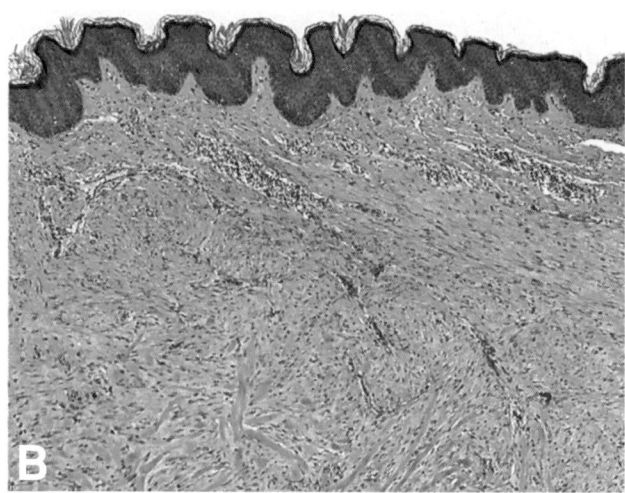

FIGURE 3-18. Keloid. A. A light-skinned black woman developed a keloid as a reaction to having her earlobe pierced. **B.** Microscopically, the dermis is markedly thickened by the presence of collagen bundles with random orientation and abundant cells.

regions that normally show minimal wound contraction (e.g., the palms, soles and anterior aspect of the thorax) are often prone to contractures. Contractures are particularly conspicuous when serious burns heal, and they can be severe enough to compromise the movement of joints. In the alimentary tract, a contracture (stricture) can obstruct the passage of food in the esophagus or block the flow of intestinal contents.

Several diseases are characterized by contracture and irreversible fibrosis of the superficial fascia, including Dupuytren contracture (palmar contracture), Lederhosen disease (plantar contracture) and Peyronie disease (contracture of the cavernous tissues of the penis). In these diseases, there is no known precipitating injury, even though the basic process is similar to contracture in wound healing.

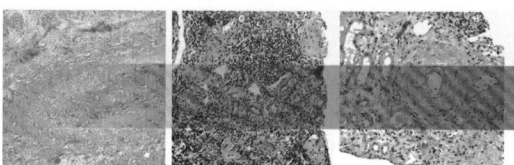

Immunopathology

Jeffrey S. Warren ▪ David S. Strayer

The Biology of the Immune System

The multifaceted, integrated immune system of higher vertebrates has evolved to protect the host from invasion by foreign agents. Toxins, chemicals, drugs, viruses, microorganisms, multicellular parasites and transplanted foreign tissues can all elicit immunity. Responses are characterized by their capacity to distinguish self from nonself, discriminate among invaders (specificity) and generate immune memory and amplification loops (i.e., to recall previous exposures and mount an intensified—**anamnestic**—response on subsequent exposures).

INNATE AND ADAPTIVE IMMUNITY

Humans possess barriers such as regionally adapted epithelia (e.g., thick keratinized skin, ciliated respiratory epithelium), chemical-mechanical surface coatings (e.g., antibacterial peptides, mucus) and indigenous microbial flora that compete with potential pathogens. Patterned responses, cell surface and soluble mediator systems (e.g., complement) and phagocytes (e.g., neutrophils) that bind targets through mechanisms not dependent on specific antigen recognition are integral to **host defense** (see Chapter 2). Host defenses that are not antigen specific constitute the **innate immune system**.

Antigen-specific or **adaptive** immunity encompasses specialized antigen-presenting cells (APCs) (e.g., dendritic cells), clonal lymphocytes (B and T cells) that express and/or secrete molecules (T-cell receptor [TCR]), antibodies that specifically bind foreign structures, and many cell surface and soluble regulatory mediators. The adaptive system also encompasses generative lymphoid organs (bone marrow, thymus) that produce immune cells, secondary lymphoid structures (lymph nodes, spleen, regionally adapted lymphoid tissues) that facilitate the colocalization and concentrated exposure of foreign antigens to immune cells via a system of cell trafficking and recirculation (via the lymphatics and vascular system) orchestrated by soluble chemotactic factors, and location-specific intercellular adhesion molecules. These integrated systems enable the relatively few lymphocytes that express a particular antigen receptor to efficiently interact with individual specific target molecules among the wide variety of incoming antigens. The abilities of APCs to interact with T cells to stimulate immune responses and of antigen-specific cytotoxic T effector cells to kill (e.g., virus-infected) host cells are mediated by cell surface **histocompatibility molecules** (human leukocyte antigens) encoded by genes of the **major histocompatibility complex (MHC)**.

It is important to consider components of the immune system under the general rubrics of acute and chronic inflammation, cell injury and cell death (see Chapter 2). Immune responses are involved in tissue- and organ-specific pathology whether in the context of infections, hypersensitivity reactions, autoimmune diseases or transplantation.

Innate Immunity Entails Pattern Recognition Responses

The innate immune system is the "first line" defense against foreign agents. Unlike adaptive responses, which develop over a period of several days, cells and soluble mediators of the innate system are either already completely functional or rapidly activated (minutes to hours) upon exposure to invaders. The innate system appeared early in evolution and evolved in concert with microorganisms as the latter developed novel mechanisms to circumvent host defenses. Innate immunity is multilayered. Epithelial barriers and surface defense molecules retard microbial entry into the host. Both resident and recruited phagocytes respond quickly to agents that have penetrated the outer defense, and a redundant set of soluble mediators and circulating phagocytes attack agents that have entered. The innate system distinguishes self from nonself in a manner that is far less fine-tuned than occurs in adaptive immunity. Germline-encoded receptors recognize and bind to categories of structures (**pathogen-associated molecular patterns [PAMPs]**) present on the surfaces of microbes but not on host cells. **Pattern recognition receptors (PRRs)** exhibit far less diversity (hundreds of patterns) than antibodies and TCRs (many thousands of specificities) and are not clonal (i.e., each is identical on all cell types). PRRs of the innate system are diverse, are redundant, and have evolved to counter both extracellular and intracellular invaders. Finally, the innate system is functionally linked to many levels of the adaptive system.

As noted, the first levels of innate immunity encompass mechanical epithelial barriers, chemical defenses and resident host defense cells. Whether cutaneous, respiratory, gastrointestinal or urothelial, barrier epithelial cells are held together by tight junctions and exhibit region-specific adaptations (e.g., keratin layers, cilia and mucus production) that enhance their defense functions. Chemical defenses include low pH (e.g., skin and gastric juice) as well as secreted **defensins** and **cathelicidins**. Defensins are 18- to 45-amino-acid cationic peptides, classified into α, β and θ families based on the locations of six conserved cysteine residues that form internal disulfide bonds. They are produced by a variety of leukocytes and epithelial cells (skin, respiratory, gastrointestinal) and bind microbes in which they form pore-like surface defects. Cathelicidins are 12- to 80-amino-acid peptides made by neutrophils and activated macrophages and barrier cells. The physical and chemical barriers of innate immunity are backed by phagocytes (neutrophils, monocytes, macrophages and antigen-presenting cells [e.g., dendritic cells]) as well as nonphagocytic natural killer (NK) cells, mast cells and specialized lymphocytes with limited antigen receptor diversity. Lymphocytes that exhibit less antigen receptor diversity than do the B and T lymphocytes include γδ T cells, intraepithelial T cells with α/β TCRs, NK T cells, B1 B cells and marginal zone B cells.

PRRs recognize PAMPs. These are biochemical moieties expressed by microbes but not by mammalian cells and thus "seen" as nonself (Table 4-1). A separate set of endogenous moieties, produced by injured or dying host cells, are the **damage-associated molecular patterns (DAMPs)** (Table 4-1). Receptors among the heterogeneous group of PRRs recognize

TABLE 4-1		
PATHOGEN-ASSOCIATED (PAMPs) AND DAMAGE-ASSOCIATED MOLECULAR PATTERNS (DAMPs)		
	Molecular Moiety (Examples)	**Microbe Type**
PAMPs		
Cell wall lipids	Lipopolysaccharide (LPS)	Gram-negative bacteria
	Teichoic acid	Gram-positive bacteria
Cell wall carbohydrates	Mannans	Fungi
	Glucans	
Cell surface proteins	Flagellin	Bacteria
	Pilin	
Microbial nucleic acids	ssRNA	Viruses
	dsRNA	Microorganisms
	CpG sequences	
DAMPs		
Stress-induced proteins	Heat-shock proteins (HSPs)	N/A
Nuclear proteins	High-mobility group box 1	N/A
Crystals (foreign)	Monosodium urate	N/A

CpG = cytidine-guanidine dinucleotide; dsRNA = double-stranded RNA; N/A = not applicable; ssRNA = single-stranded RNA.

PAMPs and/or DAMPs. PRRs are encoded by nonrecombinatory germline genes that, in contrast to immunoglobulins and TCRs, exhibit limited structural variability and thus exhibit a more limited repertoire of specificities. For example, a particular PRR might recognize most or all lipopolysaccharides. Various lipopolysaccharides exhibit chemical differences, but all have a similar categorical structure and are found on the surfaces of essentially all gram-negative bacteria. DAMPs are revealed by injured or dying cells whether the result of infection, trauma or other injury. In addition to their varied structures, PRRs may be soluble, external cell membrane associated, endosomal membrane associated or cytosolic (Table 4-2). This anatomic distribution of PRRs reflects their varied roles in innate host defense. Soluble and extracellular PRRs provide defense against extracellular microorganisms (e.g., pyogenic bacteria), while endosomal or cytosolic PRRs play important roles in defense against viruses and intracellular bacteria. The relationships between cellular locations of PRRs and various types of infections (e.g., pyogenic bacterial vs. viral) are reflected by the types of infections observed among patients with various immunodeficiency disorders.

Toll-like Receptors

Toll-like receptors (TLRs) are leucine-rich transmembrane receptors found throughout the animal kingdom (Fig. 4-1). There are nine human TLRs. Toll-like receptors form

TABLE 4-2
PATTERN RECOGNITION MOLECULES

	Cellular/Anatomic Location	Examples
Membrane Associated		
Toll-like receptors (TLRs)	Plasma membranes	TLR1, -2, -4, -5, -6
	Endosomal membranes	TLR3, -7, -8, -9
C-type lectin-like receptors	Plasma membrane	Mannose receptor
Scavenger receptors	Plasma membrane	CD36 (Platelet gpIIIb)
N-formyl peptide receptors	Plasma membrane	N-formyl peptide receptor
Cytosolic		
NOD-like receptors (NLRs)	Cytosol	NOD1/2
RIG-like receptors (RLRs)	Cytosol	RIG-1
Soluble		
Natural antibodies (IgM)	Plasma	IgM antiphosphorylcholine
Complement	Plasma	C3, C1qrs[a]
Pentraxins	Plasma	C-reactive protein
Collectins	Plasma/alveoli	Mannose-binding lectin
		Surfactant protein, SP-A
Ficolins	Plasma	Ficolin

[a]C1qrs binds to span two Fc domains of fixed immunoglobulin molecules and directly to some pattern-associated molecular patterns.

IgM = immunoglobulin M; NOD = nucleotide oligomerization domain–containing protein; RIG = retinoic acid–inducible gene.

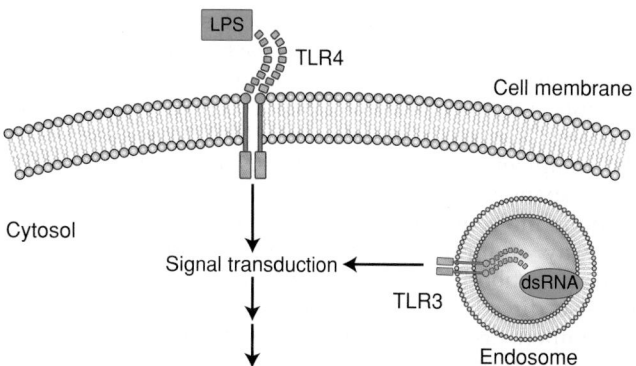

FIGURE 4-1. Toll-like receptors (TLRs) form transmembrane dimers that bind pathogen-associated molecular patterns (PAMPs) on the outer surfaces of cells and on the inner surfaces of phagocyte endosomes. Plasma membrane TLRs (e.g., TLR4) mediate defense against extracellular pathogens (e.g., pyogenic bacteria) and endosomal TLRs (e.g., TLR3) mediate defense against intracellular pathogens (e.g., viruses). In both cases, signal transduction leads to a variety of proinflammatory and/or antiviral cellular responses. The extracellular and intraendosomal TLR domains that recognize and bind PAMPs contain leucine-rich repeat sequences.

dimers that recognize PAMPs and, as noted in Table 4-2, are expressed specifically on either plasma or endosomal membranes. Plasma membrane TLRs (TLR1, -2, -4, -5, -6) recognize surface moieties of extracellular microbes (e.g., bacterial lipopeptides, lipopolysaccharides, flagellin, bacterial peptidoglycan), while endosomal TLRs (TLR3, -7, -8, -9) recognize microbial nucleic acid moieties (e.g., double-stranded RNA [dsRNA], single-stranded RNA [ssRNA], CpG DNA). In turn, engagement of TLRs by foreign invaders, whether extracellular or intracellular, leads to signal transduction events that culminate in the expression of proinflammatory genes (e.g., cytokines, chemokines, endothelial adhesion molecules, costimulatory molecules) and/or antiviral genes (e.g., type I interferons). In some cases, TLR-mediated cell activation by a PAMP is enhanced by accessory molecules (e.g., lipopolysaccharide-binding protein, CD14 and MD2).

Several additional categories of cell surface PRRs participate in innate host defense. C-type lectin receptors, through a calcium-dependent mechanism, bind to carbohydrate moieties (e.g., β-glucans, mannose, glucose, N-acetylglucosamine) characteristic of microorganisms but not mammals, thus conferring distinction of nonself from self. The best-studied C-type lectin receptors are dectin-1, dectin-2 and the mannose receptor (CD206). Dectin-1 and dectin-2 bind β-glucan and mannose-rich oligosaccharides, which are expressed by the yeast and hyphal forms, respectively, of *Candida albicans*. Diverse scavenger receptors bind a range of cell surface moieties, mediate uptake of oxidized lipoproteins and carry out microbe phagocytosis. Finally, N-formyl peptide receptors are guanosine triphosphate (GTP)-binding proteins expressed by phagocytes. N-formyl peptides are produced only by bacteria (and within mitochondria). Engagement of these receptors induces cell activation and chemotaxis.

NOD-like and RIG-like Receptors

NOD-like (nucleotide oligomerization domain–containing protein) and RIG-like (retinoic acid–inducible gene I) receptors for PAMPs and DAMPs are cytosolic receptors that are distinct from cell surface and endosomal receptors. They monitor the cytosolic compartment (Table 4-2) and are linked to activation pathways for inflammation and/or type I interferon generation. Nearly two dozen NOD-like receptors (NLRs), grouped into three subfamilies, have been identified. Most NLR proteins have a leucine-rich microbial recognition domain like TLRs. Other functional domains allow formation of oligomers and the formation of multiunit signaling complexes. NOD1 and NOD2 (expressed in gastrointestinal epithelial cells and phagocytes) play important roles in innate responses to the gastrointestinal pathogens *Helicobacter pylori* and *Listeria monocytogenes*. Mutations that affect the pyrin effector domain of NOD-like receptor P3 (NLRP3) are associated with hereditary periodic fever syndromes. Finally, some crystalline substances like monosodium urate also act via NLRs to trigger an inflammatory response and assembly and activation of the "inflammosome" (see Chapter 1). RIG-like receptors (RLRs) sense cytosolic viral RNA and mediate generation of antiviral type I interferons.

Table 4-2 also lists five groups of soluble pattern recognition molecules. Members of each group are active in plasma and extracellular tissue fluid, possess high molecular weights and contain several extended PAMP ligand-binding domains. **Natural immunoglobulin M (IgM) antibodies** and the complement protein complex C1qrs are most familiar. C1qrs spans adjacent Fc domains of surface-bound immunoglobulin molecules, thus initiating the classical complement pathway and functionally linking the adaptive immune system (antibodies) to the complement system. **C1qrs and C3** also directly bind microbial structures and thus serve as components of innate immunity. **Pentraxins,** including C-reactive protein, contain five extended binding domains. **Collectins** include mannose-binding lectin, a key mediator of the third complement pathway (nonclassical, nonalternative) and the pulmonary alveolar surfactant proteins, SP-A and SP-D. **Ficolins** possess structural homology to both C1qrs and collectins and bind to a variety of PAMPs found on the surfaces of gram-positive bacteria.

Activated innate system pathways facilitate the acute inflammatory response, which plays an important role in host defense. Acute inflammation is characterized by a stereotyped set of vascular changes including vasodilatation, slowing of blood flow, leakage of fluid into the extravascular space, concentration of leukocytes and an ordered set of leukocyte-endothelial activation, binding and recruitment/extravasation events (see Chapter 2). The innate immune system also participates in host defense via the antiviral response. A variety of PRRs, including several TLRs, NLRs and RLRs, mediate the production of type I interferons. Interferons-α and -β are classified as type I interferons. Type I interferons upregulate class I MHC molecules on potential target cells for cytotoxic T lymphocytes, increase the cytotoxic activities of NK cells and cytotoxic T lymphocytes, facilitate the conversion of naive T cells to Th1 helper cells, increase intranodal lymphocyte sequestration and, via the type I interferon receptor, induce host cell resistance to viral infection. Finally, the activated innate immune system also facilitates the adaptive immune response through induction of the "second signal" (e.g., CD80 [B7-1], CD86 [B7-2]) needed in antigen-induced responses, through the conversion of naive T helper cells into Th1 and Th17 effector cells and through the stimulation of proliferation and differentiation of lymphocytes via the induction of various cytokines.

CELLS AND TISSUES OF THE IMMUNE SYSTEM

The cells of the immune and hematopoietic systems are derived from multipotent **hematopoietic stem cells** (HSCs). Near the end of the first month of embryogenesis, HSCs appear in the extraembryonic erythropoietic islands adjacent to the yolk sac. At 6 weeks, the primary site of hematopoiesis shifts to fetal liver and then to bone marrow. The latter process begins at 2 months and by 6 months has completely shifted to bone marrow. While sequential changes in the primary site of hematopoiesis are well defined, there are periods of overlap. By 8 weeks' gestation, **lymphoid progenitors** derived from HSCs circulate to the thymus where they differentiate into mature but naive T lymphocytes. ("Naive" indicates that the lymphocytes have not been exposed to foreign antigens.) Lymphoid progenitors destined to become B cells differentiate first within fetal liver (8 weeks) and later within bone marrow (12 weeks). In both

thymus-derived T-lymphocyte and bone marrow–derived B-lymphocyte development, microenvironment (e.g., thymic epithelium, bone marrow stromal cells and growth factors) is critical. Thymus and bone marrow are "generative" lymphoid organs, while peripheral lymphoid tissues (lymph nodes, spleen and regionally adapted areas) are "secondary." Mature lymphocytes exit the thymus and bone marrow and "home" to peripheral lymphoid tissues (e.g., lymph nodes, spleen, skin and mucosa). The colonization of peripheral lymphoid tissues by mature B and T lymphocytes and the rapid deployment and recirculation of mature lymphocytes to different, often remote, parts of the immune system is anatomically specific. **Lymphocyte homing and recirculation** are orchestrated by a series of complementary leukocyte and endothelial surface molecules that include site-specific **selectins** and **addressins** (see below). The processes of lymphocyte development and homing/recirculation are important in understanding immune responses, immunodeficiency states, regional host defense and the underpinnings of modern therapeutics (e.g., HSC transplantation).

Cells of the immune system express a vast array of surface molecules important in differentiation and cell-to-cell communication. These surface molecules also serve as markers of cell identity. The International Workshop on Human Leukocyte Differentiation Antigens is responsible for nomenclature and assigns so-called **cluster of differentiation** or **cluster designation (CD)** numbers. Currently, 300 different molecules have been assigned CD numbers.

HSCs Are the Progenitors for the Cells of the Immune System

Multipotent HSCs account for 0.01%–0.1% of nucleated bone marrow cells, exhibit characteristic light-scattering properties as assessed by flow cytometry, can self-renew, usually express CD34 and c-KIT cell surface proteins and lack cell surface molecules that characterize more mature lymphocyte subpopulations (e.g., CD2, CD3 and others). The absence of lineage-specific molecules is referred to as "LIN–." HSCs differentially express more than 2000 genes involved in a variety of cellular functions. It is clear that stem cells cycle, replicate and give rise to progenitor cells. As progenitor cells differentiate into lymphocytes, red blood cells, neutrophils and so forth, they lose proliferative capacity (Fig. 4-2). Prevailing models of hematopoiesis/lymphopoiesis suggest that primitive stem cells give rise to committed progenitors (the **hierarchical model**) or that stem cells can develop either into progenitor cells or back to stem cells (the **cell cycle or continuum model**).

Circulating CD34$^+$ HSCs account for 0.01%–0.1% of peripheral blood mononuclear cells. Bone marrow and blood HSCs are heterogeneous in terms of lymphocyte marker expression, myeloid markers, activation antigens and capacity to engraft bone marrow. Infusion of sufficient numbers of peripheral blood HSCs into transplant recipients leads to faster marrow recovery than occurs in recipients of marrow-derived HSCs. In clinical HSC transplantation, it is current practice for donors to receive recombinant growth factors prior to HSC harvest. This practice leads to higher yields of harvested HSCs, decreased time to engraftment and improved engraftment rates. The overall efficacy of peripheral blood HSCs versus marrow preparations in patients with leukemia is still being debated.

Mature hematopoietic and lymphoid cells are derived from a common population of multipotential HSCs (Fig. 4-2).

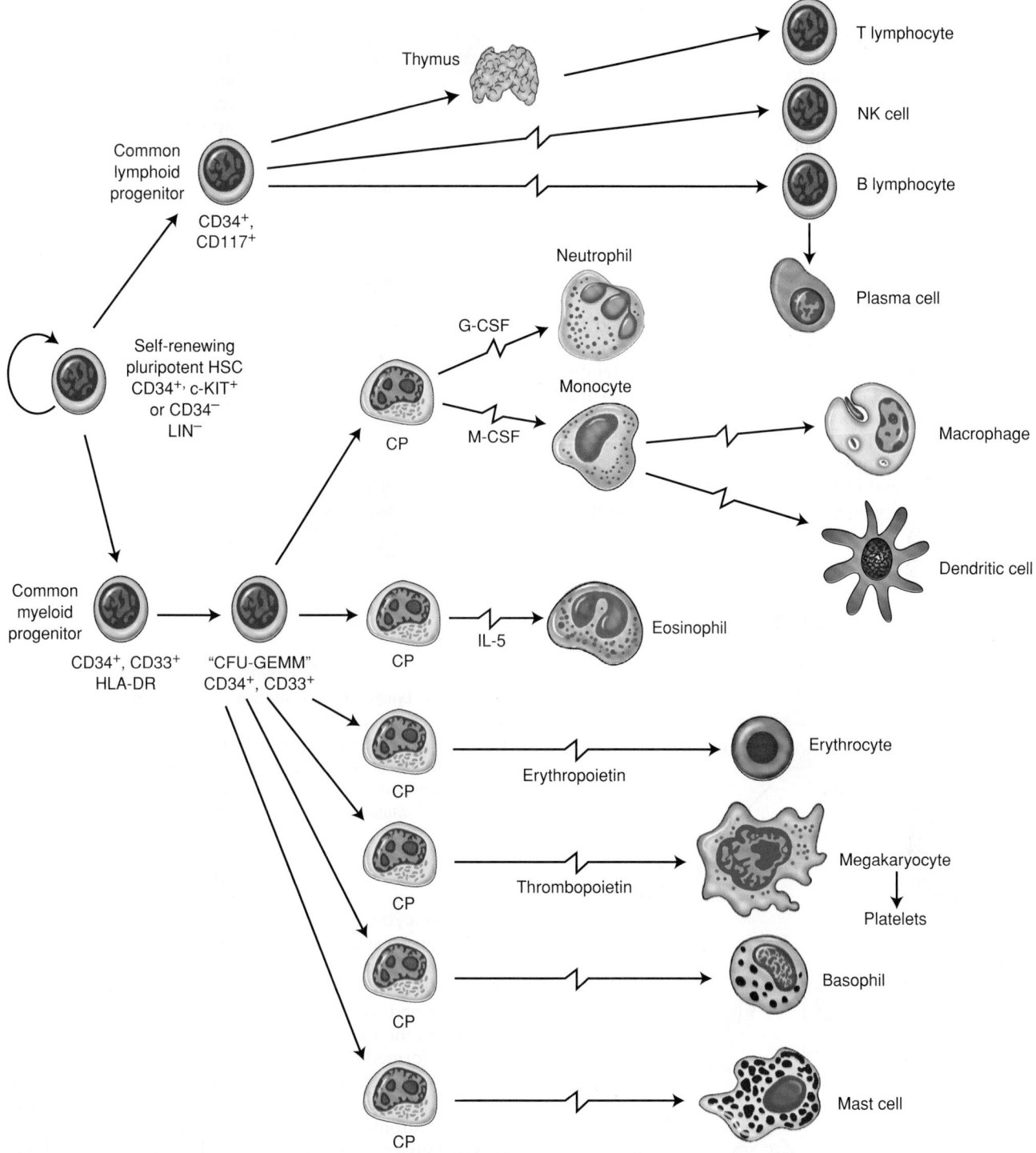

FIGURE 4-2. Pluripotent hematopoietic stem cells (HSCs) differentiate into either common lymphoid or myeloid progenitors and, in the case of myeloid cells, into lineage-specific colony-forming units (CFUs). Under the influence of an appropriate microenvironment and growth factors, committed precursors (CPs) give rise to definitive cell types. Lymphoid progenitors are precursors of natural killer (NK) cells, T lymphocytes and B lymphocytes. B lymphocytes give rise to plasma cells. *Lin–* = lineage-negative; *CD* = cluster designation; *CFU-GEMM* = granulocytic, erythroid, monocytic-dendritic and megakaryocytic colony-forming units; *HLA* = human leukocyte antigen. "Colony-forming unit" refers to an in vitro bioassay.

The primary branch point in differentiation is between lymphoid and myeloid progenitors. The former ultimately give rise to T lymphocytes, B lymphocytes and NK cells, while the latter develop into granulocytic, erythroid, monocytic-dendritic and megakaryocytic colony-forming units (GEMM-CFUs). Colony-forming units (CFUs) are the cells that give rise to specified populations of derivative cells, such as granulocytes, monocytes and so forth. Downstream CFUs become increasingly lineage specific: for example, CFU-GM (granulocyte-monocyte), CFU-Eo (eosinophil) and CFU-E (erythrocyte).

Lymphocytes

Committed lymphoid progenitor (CLP) cells, derived from HSCs, in turn give rise to B lymphocytes, T lymphocytes and NK cells (Fig. 4-3). There are three major types of lymphocytes—T cells, B cells and NK cells—which together make up 25% of peripheral blood leukocytes. Blood lymphocytes are about 80% T cells, 10% B cells and 10% NK cells. The relative proportions of lymphocytes in the peripheral blood and central and peripheral lymphoid tissues vary. In contrast to blood, only 30%–40% of splenic and bone marrow lymphocytes are T cells.

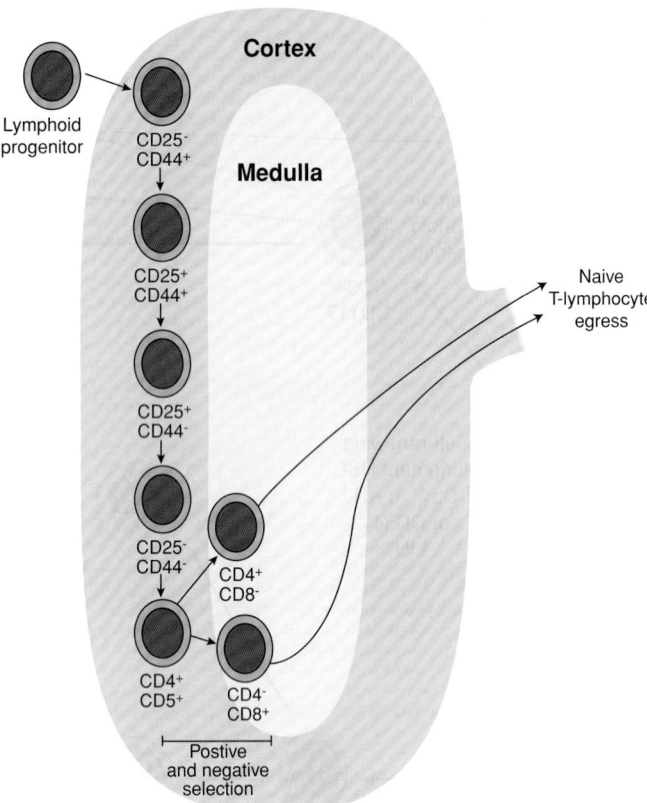

Thymus

FIGURE 4-4. Lymphoid progenitors give rise to mature but naive T lymphocytes. Lymphocytes destined to become T lymphocytes migrate to the thymus where they become either α/β or γ/δ T cells. As thymocytes percolate through the cortex and then medulla, they are positively and negatively selected. Most α/β T lymphocytes emerge as either CD4⁺/CD8⁻ helper cells or CD4⁻/CD8⁺ cytotoxic cells.

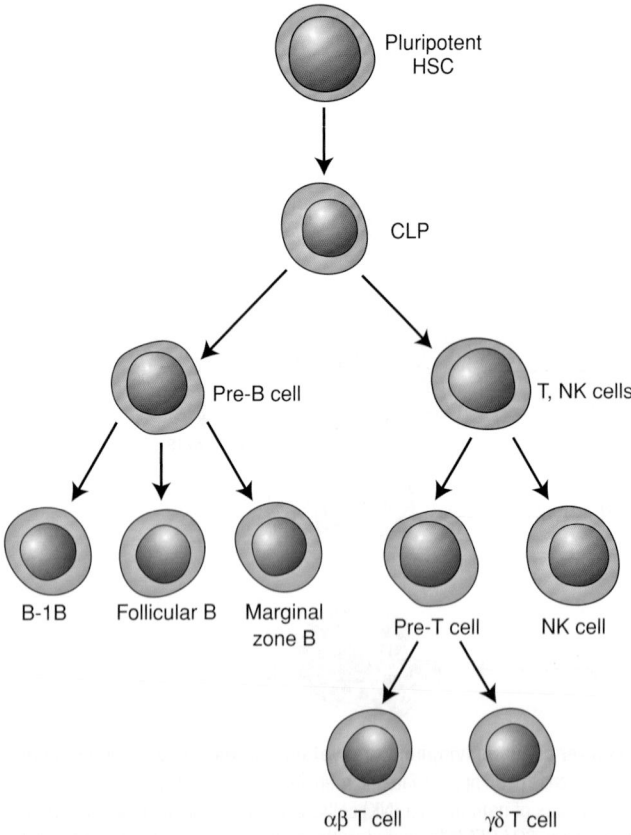

FIGURE 4-3. Pluripotent hematopoietic stem cells (HSCs) give rise to B and T lymphocytes—including their subsets. The common lymphoid progenitor (CLP) gives rise to B lymphocytes, T lymphocytes and NK cells. (See Fig. 4-2 to see how HSCs and CLPs fit into the larger hematopoietic and lymphopoietic development schemes.) Key transcription factors are listed within dashed-line circles. Commitment of CLPs to the B-lymphocyte lineage is triggered by *E2A* and *EBF* transcription factors followed by *Pax5*. In turn, commitment of T and NK progenitor cells to T lymphocytes is triggered by *Notch 1, GATA3* and other (not shown) transcription factors.

T Lymphocytes

T cells can be subdivided into subpopulations by virtue of their specialized functions, surface CD molecules and, in some cases, morphologic features. Lymphoid progenitor cells destined to become T cells exit the bone marrow and migrate to the thymus. There, both α/β and γ/δ T lymphocytes are formed (Fig. 4-4), referring to the two major classes of heterodimeric TCRs that specifically recognize and bind antigens. The thymic microenvironment is determined by its epithelial stroma. The early thymus is colonized by progenitors that give rise to T cells, macrophages and dendritic cells. The thymic cortex is composed of a meshwork of epithelial cell processes that surround groups of immature thymocytes that bear *both* CD4⁺ and CD8⁺ surface molecules. As T lymphocytes mature, they percolate into thymic medulla where, in close proximity to nested groups of epithelial cells, they form more mature cells that are *either* CD4⁺ or CD8⁺ (Fig. 4-4).

The thymic corticomedullary junction contains marrow HSC-derived macrophages and dendritic cells. Much of the **positive selection** of thymocytes occurs in the cortex; **negative selection** tends to occur through exposure of developing thymocytes to corticomedullary dendritic cells. In positive thymic selection, transient, low-affinity binding of cell surface TCRs to a person's own MHC class I or II molecules *prevents* cell death. Negative thymic selection is the converse process in which high-affinity TCR-mediated binding to one's own MHC class I or II molecules results in cell death by apoptosis. These complementary processes are pivotal to T lymphocyte development, so that T cells can interact with the host's own cells but not in a manner that results in excessive self-reactivity (see below).

Lineage-specific differentiation and thymic selection of T lymphocytes are fundamental to understanding the immune response and autoimmunity, respectively. Thymic T-lymphocyte maturation includes several processes. Developing T cells recombine dispersed gene segments that encode the heterodimeric α/β or γ/δ TCRs. α/β T lymphocytes progress through stages of development that are characterized as $CD4^-/CD8^-$, then $CD4^+/CD8^+$ and then *either* $CD4^+/CD8^-$ *or* $CD4^-/CD8^+$ (Fig. 4-4). Most $CD4^+/CD8^-$ T cells act as **helper cells**, while most $CD4^-/CD8^+$ T cells are **cytotoxic**.

Naive T lymphocytes exit the thymus and populate secondary lymphoid tissues. In the thymus, antigen-specific TCRs are formed and expressed in conjunction with CD3, an essential accessory molecule. Nearly 95% of circulating T lymphocytes express α/β TCRs plus either CD4 or CD8. A smaller population (5%) of T cells express γ/δ TCRs and CD3 but neither CD4 nor CD8.

B Lymphocytes

The maturation of B cells from CLP cells occurs in the bone marrow where several maturation stages can be identified. These include, in sequence, pro-B lymphocytes, which exhibit unrecombined (germline) DNA and no surface immunoglobulin; pre-B lymphocytes, which express an "early" antigen receptor (μ heavy chain plus an invariant surrogate light chain); immature B cells, which express a recombined H chain gene plus κ or λ messenger RNA (mRNA) and membrane IgM κ or λ; and finally, mature but naive B lymphocytes, which coexpress surface IgM **and** IgD. B-1 and marginal zone B cells develop from immature B lymphocytes via a different program than do B cells that coexpress IgM and IgD. B cells differentiate in the bone marrow into mature B cells and in some cases further into antibody-secreting plasma cells. Similar to T-lymphocyte development, the microenvironments of fetal liver and bone marrow are critical to B-cell development. In both sites, only B lymphocytes that survive pass through the multiple steps necessary to produce surface immunoglobulin. Conversely, when surface immunoglobulin binds too avidly to self-antigens, developing B cells are negatively selected and eliminated.

Analogous to T cells, B lymphocytes express a surface antigen-binding receptor, **membrane immunoglobulin (mIg)**, with the same antigen-binding specificity as the soluble immunoglobulin that will ultimately be secreted by the corresponding terminally differentiated plasma cells. Like T cells, B lymphocytes are also heterogeneous (e.g., $CD5^+$ [B1] and $CD5^-$ [B2]). TCRs, along with immunoglobulins and MHC class I and class II molecules (see below), confer specificity to the immune system by virtue of their capacity to bind specifically to foreign antigens and interact with histocompatible self-cells. TCRs, Ig and a portion of the MHC class I molecule are encoded by members of the immunoglobulin supergene family (Fig. 4-5). The structural variability and, in turn, great specificity of TCRs and Igs are achieved by recombination of TCR and Ig genes. An individual TCR is a heterodimer that forms an antigen-binding

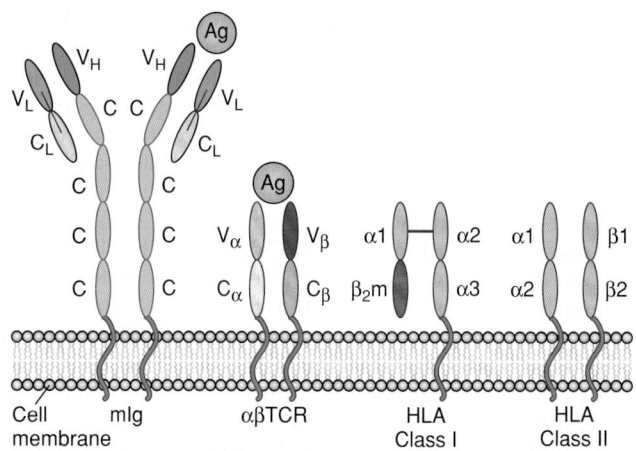

FIGURE 4-5. Alignment of two N-terminal variable domains of membrane immunoglobulin and two N-terminal variable domains of T-cell receptors (TCRs) forms the respective antigen-binding sites of B lymphocytes and T lymphocytes, respectively. Each variable (V) domain is derived from disparate recombined gene segments. The antigen-binding grooves of human leukocyte antigen (HLA) molecules are formed by the alignments of α_1 and α_2 domains in class I and α_1 and β_1 domains in class II. β_2m is β_2–microglobulin, which is encoded outside of the major histocompatibility complex (MHC).

site (Fig. 4-5). TCRs and Igs each possess an amino-terminal antigen-binding variable (V) domain and a carboxy-terminal constant (C) domain (Fig. 4-5). TCRs anchor antigen to the cell surface, while Igs either anchor the receptor to the B-cell surface as mIg or, in the case of soluble Ig, mediate its biological function.

NK Cells

NK cells recognize target cells mainly via antigen-independent mechanisms. They form in both thymus and bone marrow and bear several types of receptors that bind class I MHC molecules. NK receptors *inhibit* the cell's capacity to secrete cytolytic products. Certain tumor cells and virus-infected cells express reduced numbers of MHC class I molecules and thus fail to inhibit NK cells. Such NK cells engage virus-infected or tumor cells and secrete a complex of complement-like pore-forming cytolytic proteins (perforin), as well as granzymes A and B and other lytic molecules. NK cells also secrete granulysin, a cationic protein that induces target cell apoptosis.

In another example of linkage between different facets of the immune system, NK cells can also lyse target cells via antibody-dependent cellular cytotoxicity (ADCC). In ADCC, NK-cell Fc receptors engage the Fc domain of IgG that has specifically bound to antigen on surfaces of target cells. As with T and B cells, NK cells exhibit a degree of heterogeneity (e.g., $CD16^+$, $CD16^-$).

Mononuclear Phagocytes, Antigen-Presenting Cells and Dendritic Cells

Mononuclear phagocytes, chiefly **monocytes,** make up 10% of white blood cells. Circulating monocytes give rise to resident tissue macrophages including, among others, Kupffer cells (liver), alveolar macrophages (lung) and microglial cells (brain). Monocytes and macrophages express specific cell surface host defense molecules. These include MHC class II molecules, CD14 (which binds bacterial lipopolysaccharide and can trigger cell activation), several types of Fc Ig receptors, TLRs and other PRRs, adhesion molecules and a variety of cytokine receptors that participate in regulating monocyte/macrophage function. Activated macrophages produce a variety of cytokines and soluble mediators of host defense (e.g., interferon [IFN-γ], interleukin-1β [IL-1β], tumor necrosis factor-α [TNF-α] and complement components).

Antigen-presenting cells (APCs), defined by their function and derived from HSCs, acquire the capacity to present antigen to T lymphocytes in the context of histocompatibility, after cytokine-driven upregulation of MHC class II molecules. Monocytes, macrophages, dendritic cells and, under certain conditions, B lymphocytes, endothelial cells and epithelial cells can function as APCs. In some locations, APCs are highly specialized for this function. For instance, in B-cell–rich follicles of lymph nodes and spleen, specialized APCs are termed follicular dendritic cells. In these sites, through engagement of antibody and complement via Fc and C3b receptors, APCs trap antigen–antibody complexes. In the case of lymph nodes, immune complexes arrive via afferent lymphatics, and in spleen, via blood. Antigen presentation by follicular dendritic cells leads to generation of memory B lymphocytes.

Dendritic cells are specialized APCs whose name, "dendritic," reflects their spider-like appearance. They are present in B-lymphocyte–rich lymphoid follicles, thymic medulla and many peripheral sites, including intestinal lamina propria, lung, genitourinary tract and skin. Peripherally located dendritic cells are less mature than APCs found in lymphoid follicles and express lower levels of accessory cell activation molecules (CD80 [B7-1], CD86 [B7-2]) than do mature dendritic cells. An example of a peripheral APC is the epidermal Langerhans cell. Upon exposure, Langerhans cells engulf antigen, migrate to regional lymph nodes through afferent lymphatics and differentiate into more mature dendritic cells. Langerhans cell–derived dendritic cells express high densities of MHC class I and II molecules and costimulatory molecules (CD80, CD86) and present antigens efficiently to T cells. This latter act occurs through TCRs in the context of histocompatibility determined by MHC class II molecules.

The Structure of the Tissues of the Immune System Plays a Key Role in the Biology of the Adaptive Immune System

Lymph Nodes

Lymph nodes are distributed throughout the body along thin-walled lymphatic vessels that ultimately drain into the vascular system via the superior vena cava. Individual nodes are encapsulated, vascularized and internally structured in a manner that facilitates antigen processing and presentation by follicular dendritic cells to B cells in the B-lymphocyte–rich cortical follicles and by dendritic cells to T cells in the T-lymphocyte–rich parafollicular cortex. The anatomic organization of the B-cell–rich and T-cell–rich areas of a lymph node is dictated by the region-specific structure of reticular fibers, the composition of stromal cells and complementary sets of locally produced chemokines and lymphocyte-specific chemokine receptors. Naive B and T cells circulate to a lymph node, exit the vascular space through high endothelial venules (HEVs) and then migrate to their designated

areas. Lymphocytes home to HEVs where they engage in specific receptor–ligand binding interactions (see below). Naive B cells express a chemokine receptor, CXCR5 ("R" denotes receptor), which binds specifically to chemokine CXCL13 ("L" denotes ligand) that is produced by follicular dendritic cells. B lymphocytes follow the follicle-centric CXCL13 gradient and are thus concentrated in this region. In an analogous process, naive T cells express CCR7, which binds CCL19 and CCL21 produced by stromal and dendritic cells in the paracortical T region.

Antigen processing in lymph nodes is initiated by an ingenious size-dependent sorting process that is dependent on microanatomic features depicted in Fig. 4-6. First, dendritic cells that have phagocytized proteins, microbes and so forth elsewhere (e.g., skin) migrate via afferent lymphatics into regional lymph nodes and then to the T-cell zone of the node where antigens are processed and presented. Soluble lymph-borne substances such as intact viruses or high–molecular-weight particles/molecules also enter lymph nodes via afferent lymphatics. Within the subcapsular sinus, viruses, particles and high–molecular-weight molecules are engulfed by macrophages/dendritic cells that process and present antigen to cortical B cells that make antibody. Finally, lower–molecular-weight molecules (which cannot penetrate the impermeable lymph node sinus floor) flow down tubular

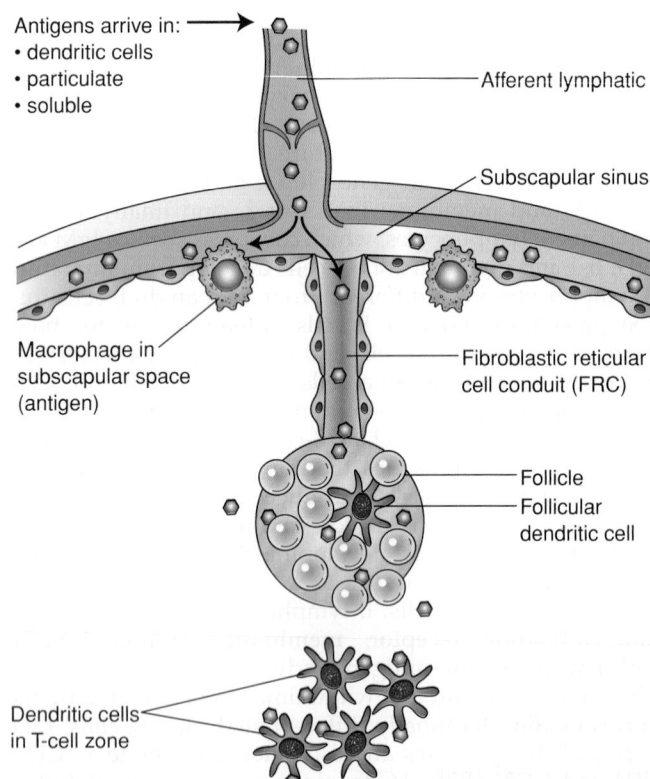

FIGURE 4-6. Potential antigens (viruses, higher–molecular-weight particles/molecules and lower–molecular-weight molecules) enter lymph nodes via afferent lymphatic vessels. Entry may occur via migratory dendritic cells or as free soluble structures. Within the subcapsular sinus, higher–molecular-weight particles/molecules are engulfed by subcapsular macrophage/dendritic cells, while lower–molecular-weight molecules flow down fibroblastic reticular cell conduits (FRCs) where they are pinocytosed dendritic cell processes.

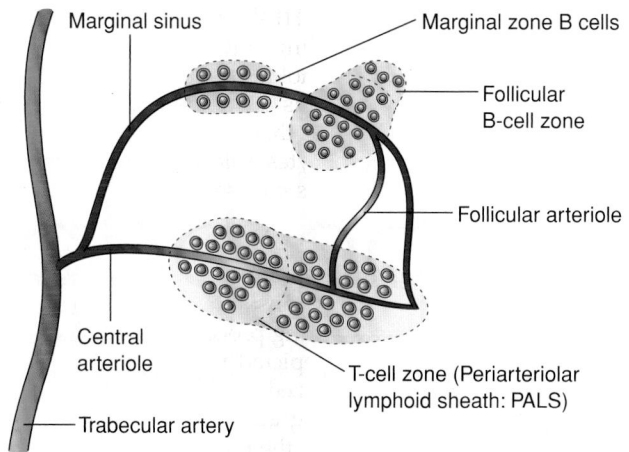

Marginal sinus

Marginal zone B cells

Follicular B-cell zone

Follicular arteriole

Central arteriole

T-cell zone (Periarteriolar lymphoid sheath: PALS)

Trabecular artery

FIGURE 4-7. Splenic white pulp includes a sheath of T lymphocytes wrapped around and along the central arteriole, collections of B lymphocytes around and along the marginal sinuses (marginal zone B cells) and follicular B-cell aggregates.

structures called fibroblastic reticular cell (FRC) conduits where they encounter dendritic cell processes intercalated between FRC cells along the conduits. Here, molecules are taken up, processed by the dendritic cells and presented to T lymphocytes (Fig. 4-6). The structure and function of lymph nodes allows the "sorting" of incoming agents/molecules in a manner that optimizes antigen presentation to either B or T cells, which, in turn, constitute key pivot points to the development of adaptive immune responses.

Spleen

The spleen initiates adaptive immune responses to blood-borne antigens and removes aged and damaged red blood cells, circulating immune complexes and opsonized microbes. As evidenced by the increased susceptibility of asplenic patients to infection by encapsulated bacteria, the spleen is particularly important to the development of antibody-mediated immunity. Induction of adaptive immunity in the spleen occurs in the lymphocyte-rich white pulp, while particle clearance occurs within the red pulp (Fig. 4-7). White pulp lymphocyte aggregates are organized into T-cell– and B-cell–rich zones based on the local stromal cell and APC elaboration of the same chemokines (CXCL13 for B cells, CCL19 and CCL21 for T cells) that direct analogous lymph node structure. Periarteriolar T-cell zones of the splenic white pulp contain filtration conduits lined by FRC-like cells. Marginal zone B cells have a limited antigen receptor repertoire, while follicular B cells possess the whole range of receptor antibody diversity. Blood-borne particles (including microbes) may be delivered to marginal zone B cells via circulating plasmacytoid dendritic cells, and soluble antigens (particularly polysaccharides) may bind marginal zone macrophages directly and then are engaged by nearby B cells.

Thymus

The bilobed thymus is located in the anterior mediastinum before it undergoes involution during puberty. As noted above, the thymus is the site of T-lymphocyte maturation.

Individual thymic lobules are organized into highly cellular cortical areas and less cellular medullary areas. Thymic lymphocytes (thymocytes) originate from the bone marrow as progenitors committed to T-lymphocyte development. Maturation occurs as the cells percolate first through the cortex and then the medulla before egress.

Antibodies and T-Cell Receptors Mediate Adaptive Immunity

Antibodies

Antibody function was recognized over a century ago when serum from animals previously exposed to attenuated diphtheria toxin specifically protected naive animals from diphtheroid bacteria. Secreted by plasma cells and B lymphocytes, soluble Ig molecules bind a wide variety of complementary antigens with high degrees of specificity and affinity. They recognize a variety of biological (and nonbiological) molecules including proteins, carbohydrates, lipids, nucleic acids and others. The portion of an antigen that is bound by an Ig molecule is called an "epitope." Antibody–antigen interactions differ from TCR–antigen interactions in that the latter, with few exceptions, involve only protein antigens and occur in the context of MHC molecule compatibility. The various Ig isotypes exhibit different effector functions. Membrane-bound Igs serve as receptors that can mediate B-lymphocyte activation upon antigen binding. Both secreted and membrane Igs consist of paired light chains and heavy chains that together form antigen-binding sites (Fig. 4-8). An individual's repertoire of Ig molecules entails tremendous ranges of antigen-binding specificity (10^7–10^9) and binding affinity ($K_d = 10^{-7}$–10^{-11} M). The broad range of specificities is determined by hypervariablity of amino acid sequence

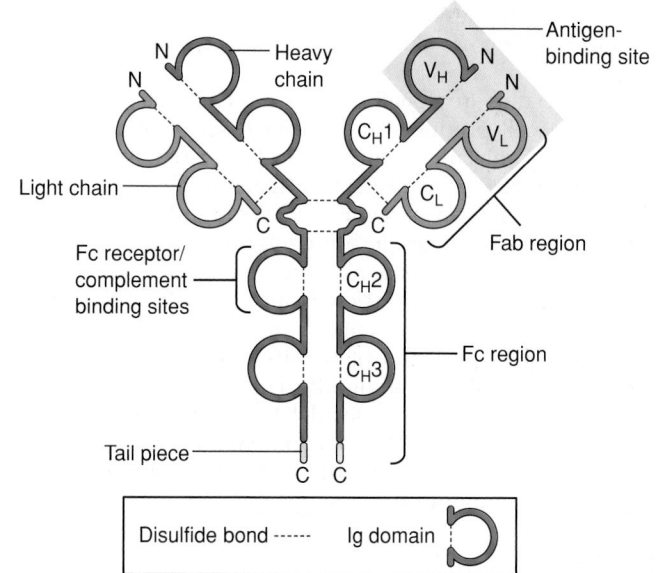

N — Heavy chain

N — Antigen-binding site

V_H

C_H1 V_L

Light chain

C_L

C   C — Fab region

Fc receptor/ complement binding sites

C_H2

C_H3 — Fc region

Tail piece

C   C

Disulfide bond ------   Ig domain

FIGURE 4-8. Schematic structure of immunoglobulin molecule (IgG). Immunoglobulin molecules consist of disulfide-linked pairs of heavy chains and light chains. Antigen-binding sites (2 for IgG) are determined by the highly variable VH and CH Ig domains located at the N-terminal portions of the structure. "Fab" refers to antigen-binding fragment and "Fc" refers to crystallizable fragment.

IMMUNOPATHOLOGY

TABLE 4-3
IMMUNOGLOBULIN ISOTYPES AND FUNCTIONS

Isotype	Subtypes	Secreted Form	Functions
IgG	IgG 1, 2, 3, 4	Monomer	Complement fixation Opsonization ADCC Neutralization
IgA	IgA 1, 2	Dimer, monomer	Mucosal immunity
IgM	None	Pentamer	Naive B cell Complement fixation
IgE	None	Monomer	Immediate hypersensitivity
IgD	None	Not secreted	Naive BCR

ADCC = antibody-dependent cellular cytotoxicity; BCR = B-cell receptor;
Ig = immunoglobulin.

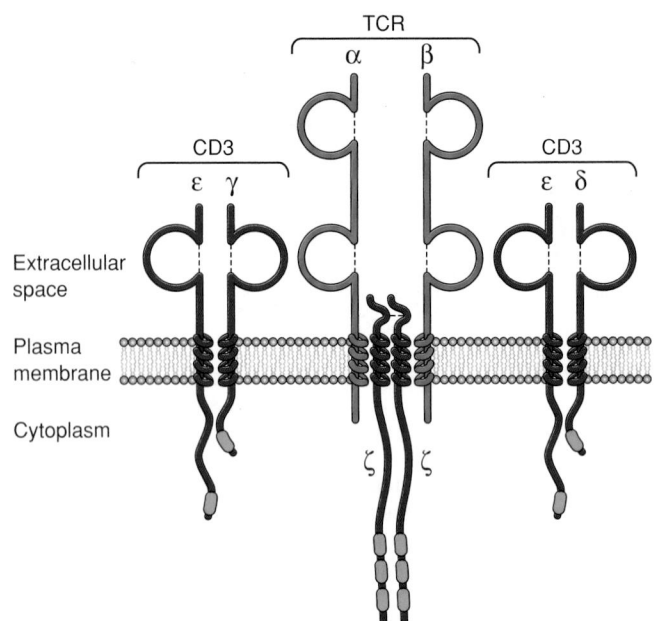

FIGURE 4-9. The T-cell receptor (TCR) consists of noncovalently linked α- and β-chains that each contain a transmembrane domain. The TCR complex includes two ζ-chains and two CD3 subunits ε/γ and ε/δ. TCRs recognize antigen presented in the context of class I human leukocyte antigen (HLA) or class II HLA.

within the so-called complementarity-determining regions (CDRs) of the antigen-binding V_L and V_H domains (Fig. 4-8). The high degree of variability is made possible through the highly regulated and stereotyped somatic recombination of physically separated germline segments of DNA that encode different portions of the variable domains. Additional variability is generated by addition and/or deletion of nucleotides at sites where the above-mentioned gene segments are joined together.

Ig isotypes include IgG, IgA, IgM, IgE and IgD, which are each determined by their heavy-chain gene segments. Antibodies also include light chains, either κ or λ, which are determined by light-chain gene segments (Table 4-3). Heavy chains guide function (and isotype) (Table 4-3). The role of secreted antibodies (e.g., complement fixation, Fc receptor binding, etc.) is determined by Fc region interactions (Fig. 4-8).

Ig molecules are clonally expressed. That is, a given B cell or plasma cell produces one identical set of intact immunoglobulin molecules. During T-cell–dependent humoral immune responses to protein antigens, high-affinity antibody molecules can be generated through somatic mutation of V-region genes in antigen-stimulated B cells. As a humoral immune response evolves, subsets of B lymphocytes that bind a particular antigen with high affinity proliferate and differentiate into plasma cells. Thus, the subsequent selection of B cells (via antigen binding) produces high-affinity antibody. This process results in a population of antibody molecules that exhibit higher average affinity over time. This phenomenon is called "affinity maturation" and is important in the development of an effective humoral immune response.

T Cells

Most TCRs consist of paired α- and β-chains that each have an N-terminal variable (V) domain, a constant (C) region, a transmembrane region and a cytosolic C-terminus (Fig. 4-9). TCRs bind peptide–MHC complexes where the Vα and Vβ domains of the TCR recognize and bind peptide (antigen), which fits into the $α_1/α_2$ peptide–binding cleft of MHC class I molecules or the $α_1/β_1$ peptide-binding cleft of MHC class II molecules. (As noted above, CD4+ T cells bind processed peptide presented by an APC in the context of MHC class II and CD8+ T cells bind surface peptide presented by a target cell in the context of MHC class I.) In turn, the **TCR complex** is composed of the TCR α- and β-chains, which contribute to antigen recognition and the CD3 γ, δ and ε signaling chains as well as the ζ homodimer. Engagement of the TCR complex leads to signal transduction and cell activation.

Lymphocyte Trafficking and Recirculation

The segments of DNA that encode antigen-binding domains of TCRs and Ig are rearranged in developing T cells and B cells, respectively, to form "new" genes. Through this combinatorial process and several other diversity-generating mechanisms, a large number of different antigen receptors is generated. Adults possess about 10^{12} lymphocytes, of which only 10% are in circulation at a given time. Despite the large aggregate number of lymphocytes, the subset with any specific antigen receptor is relatively small. Body surfaces that serve as portals of entry for foreign invaders are very large (e.g., skin, 2 m²; respiratory tract, 100 m²; gastrointestinal tract, 400 m²). Lymphocyte trafficking is a necessary aspect of host defense because it allows relatively small numbers of any subset of antigen-specific lymphocytes to move to sites of "need." Lymphocyte trafficking, which entails homing and recirculation, has evolved to provide rapid, flexible and widespread distribution of lymphocytes and a means of focusing specific immunologic processes in anatomically discrete sites (e.g., lymph node cortex). Lymphocyte trafficking is a high-flux process whereby individual lymphocytes pass through each lymph node, on average, one time per day!

Following completion of early development, naive B and T lymphocytes circulate via the vascular system to secondary lymphoid tissues (e.g., spleen, lymph nodes and mucosa-associated lymphoid tissues [e.g., Peyer patches]). Lymphocyte trafficking through lymph nodes occurs through specialized postcapillary **high endothelial venules** so-named because of the high cuboidal shape of the endothelial cells (Fig. 4-6). HEVs express cellular adhesion molecules that mediate lymphocyte binding. The cuboidal shape of HEV cells reduces flow-mediated shear forces, and specialized intercellular connections facilitate egress of lymphocytes from the vascular space. Lymphocytes that do not find their cognate antigen as they percolate through secondary lymphoid tissues reenter the circulation through efferent lymphatics and the thoracic duct. Naive lymphocytes have a finite life span maintained by receptor-mediated signals. For example, B cells are engaged via B-cell receptors (surface Ig) and BAFF receptors. (BAFF is B-cell activity factor, a member of the TNF family.)

In contrast, lymphocytes that have engaged an antigen leave the secondary lymphoid tissue, enter the circulation via lymphatics and thoracic duct and then preferentially bind and migrate into peripheral tissues (e.g., lymph nodes or mucosa-associated lymphoid tissue) from which the activating antigen was introduced. Hence, there are at least two major circuits, namely, lymph node and mucosa associated. Within the mucosa-associated system, nonnaive lymphocytes can distinguish among the gastrointestinal, respiratory and genitourinary tracts. Lymphocyte (and neutrophil) homing into sites of inflammation is mediated by different sets of leukocyte and endothelial cell adhesion molecules (see Chapter 2). The best-understood adhesion molecules involved in lymphocyte-lymphoid tissue trafficking include L-selectins (on lymphocytes) and peripheral lymph node addressin (PNAds) that serve as attachment sites for lymphocytes. Among others, the addressins include mucosal addressin cell adhesion molecule-1 (MadCAM-1), glycosylation-dependent cell adhesion molecule-1 (GlyCAM-1) and CD34.

MAJOR HISTOCOMPATIBILITY COMPLEX

The discovery that sera of multiparous women and multiply transfused patients contain antibodies against foreign blood leukocytes led to identification of a system of cell surface proteins known as **human leukocyte antigens (HLAs)** because they were first identified on leukocytes and are expressed in high concentrations on lymphocytes.

HLAs (also known as **histocompatibility** antigens) orchestrate many cell–cell interactions fundamental to immune responses. Conversely, these antigens are major immunogens and thus targets in transplant rejection. The MHC encodes these cell surface proteins, which include class I, II and III antigens. (Class III antigens represent certain complement components and are not histocompatibility antigens per se.)

Molecules structurally like "traditional" MHC class I and II molecules are encoded beyond the specific MHC region on the short arm of chromosome 6. Among these, MHC-1b and CD1d can activate so-called NK T cells. The latter resemble both NK cells and T lymphocytes. Other nontraditional MHC class I molecules (e.g., HLA-E, -F and -G) are not well understood. They may regulate NK-cell activity.

Class I MHC Molecules Are Encoded by A, B and C MHC Regions

Class I MHC loci (Fig. 4-10) encode similarly structured molecules that are expressed in virtually all tissues. Class I molecules are heterodimers consisting of a 44-kd polymorphic transmembrane glycoprotein and a 12-kd nonpolymorphic molecule, β_2-microglobulin. The latter lacks a membrane component and is noncovalently associated with the larger heavy chain. Structural polymorphism occurs primarily in the extracellular domains of the α-chain. *MHC class I alleles are codominantly expressed,* so tissues bear class I molecules inherited from each parent. Antigens are recognized by cytotoxic T cells during graft rejection and T-lymphocyte–mediated killing of virus-infected host cells in the context of histocompatibility.

Class II MHC Molecules Are Encoded in MHC D

Multiple MHC D region loci encode class II MHC: DP, DN, DM, DO, DQ and DR. These are structurally similar molecules expressed primarily on cells involved in antigen presentation. Noted above, APCs include monocytes, macrophages, dendritic cells and B lymphocytes. Class II molecules, also called "Ia" (immunity-associated) antigens, are heterodimers of two noncovalently linked transmembrane glycoproteins. A 29-kd α-chain has two disulfide bonds. The 34-kd β-chain has a single disulfide bond; its extracellular domain is the major site of class II variability. Like class I antigens, D alleles are codominantly expressed.

Nomenclature for MHC genes and antigens was revised by the World Health Organization (WHO) in 2010, to allow high-resolution designations. For example, the old HLA-B27 became B*2701-2725, where B*2701, B*2702, B*2703, . . . encompass 25 different B27 molecules.

IMMUNE CELL EFFECTOR MECHANISMS

Cell-Mediated Immunity

Cellular immunity encompasses adaptive responses triggered by microorganisms within host cells. These responses are mediated by CD4$^+$ and CD8$^+$ T cells. CD4$^+$ Th17 cells recognize microbial antigens and in turn secrete cytokines (interferon-γ) that activate macrophages. Activated macrophages ingest microorganisms and kill through a series of chemical reactions that involve enzymes and both reactive oxygen and nitrogen intermediates. CD4$^+$ T$_H$2 cells recognize microbial (and other) antigens and promote B-cell differentiation and immunoglobulin production, immunoglobulin isotype switching and the production of IgE. Finally, CD4$^+$ Th17 cells induce a neutrophilic response whereby the neutrophils kill microorganisms by phagocytosis, enzymatic digestion and reactive oxygen species. CD8$^+$ cytotoxic T cells (CTLs) kill host target cells that express surface foreign antigen (in MHC I context). CTL-mediated killing occurs via the perforin/granzyme pathway and/or via IFN-γ production and subsequent macrophage activation (see above).

Humoral Immunity

Antibodies produced by B lymphocytes and plasma cells are integral to the effector branch of humoral immunity. Antibodies exhibit very high degrees of antigen specificity and

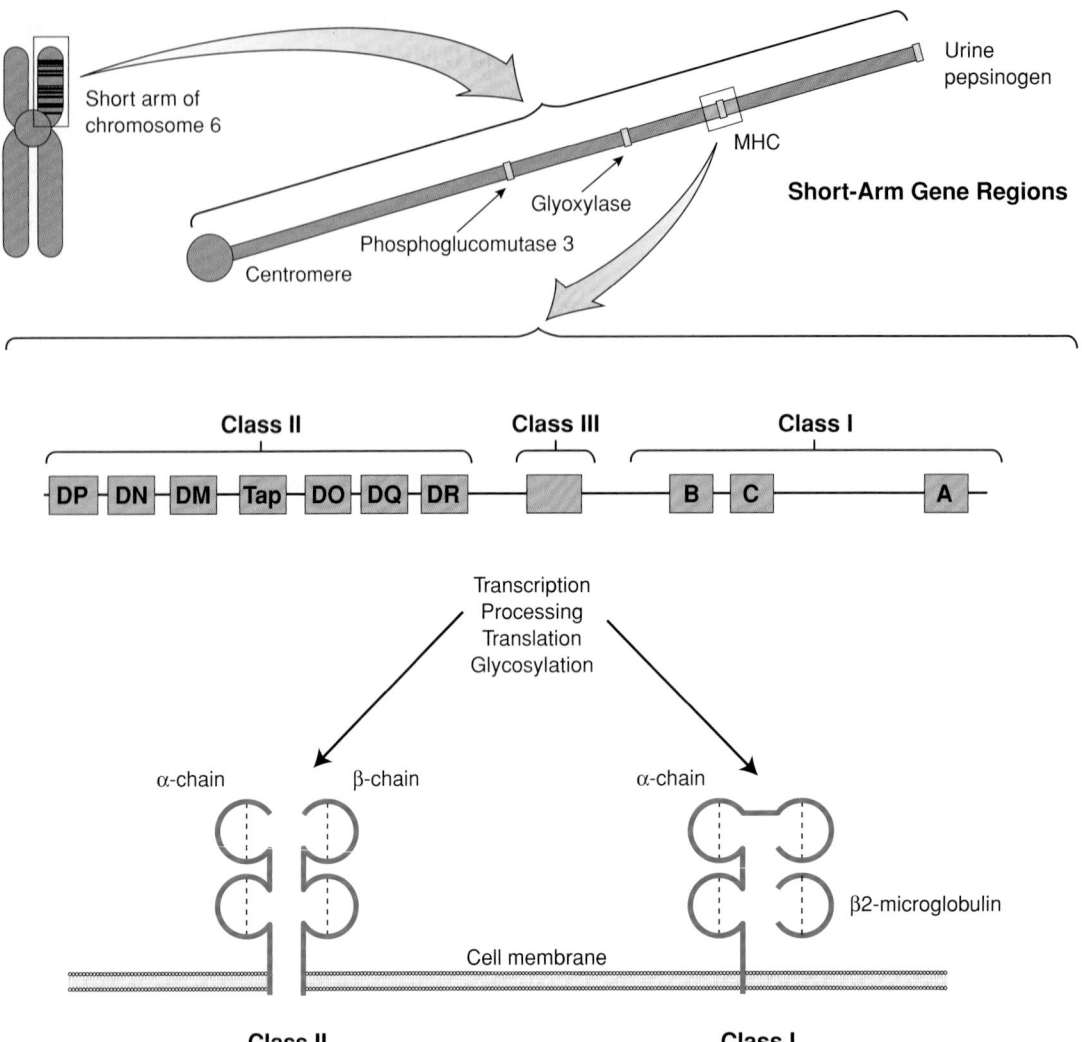

Short-Arm Gene Regions

FIGURE 4-10. The highly polymorphic loci that encode major histocompatibility antigens are located on the short arm of chromosome 6. Class I and class II molecules exhibit different structures, but each participates in fundamentally important cell–cell interactions. Class III genes encode some complement components that are not formally histocompatibility antigens.

binding affinity. As noted, the various immunoglobulin isotypes determine effector function (Table 4-3). Immunoglobulin effector functions include steric blockade (e.g., antibody to human immunodeficiency virus type 1 prevents binding to CD4 molecules on T cells), binding and Fc-mediated clearance by the mononuclear phagocyte system, binding and Fc-mediated ADCC, Fc binding and cell activation (e.g., IgE antibody tightly bound to most cells via Fcε receptor) and mast cell activation triggered by allergen binding to cytophilic IgE and immunoglobulin/antibody-mediated complement fixation. Pentavalent IgM and properly spaced IgG molecules (IgG subclasses 1, 2 and 3) effectively bind (fix) C1qrs, leading to activation of the classical complement cascade and generation of its attendant proinflammatory mediators (e.g., C3a, C3b, C5a, membrane attack complex).

INTEGRATED IMMUNE RESPONSES

T-Lymphocyte Interactions

T lymphocytes recognize specific antigens, usually proteins or haptens bound to proteins. T cells undergo activation when engaged via the TCR in the context of antigen presentation by a histocompatible (i.e., MHC-matched) APC. Exogenous signals are delivered by cytokines. CD4+ and CD8+ T-cell subsets exhibit a variety of regulatory and effector functions. Regulatory functions include augmentation or suppression of immune responses, usually via secretion of specific helper or suppressor cytokines. Effector functions include secretion of proinflammatory cytokines and killing of cells that express foreign or altered membrane antigens.

CD4+ T cells, and possibly CD8+ T cells, can be further distinguished by the types of cytokines they produce. Helper type 1, or "Th1," cells produce IFN-γ and IL-2, while helper type 2, or "Th2," cells secrete IL-4, IL-5 and IL-10. Th1 lymphocytes have been associated with cell-mediated phenomena and Th2 cells with allergic responses. In general, CD4+ T cells promote antibody and inflammatory responses. CD8+ T cells largely exert suppressor and/or cytotoxic functions. Suppressor cells inhibit the activation phase of immune responses; cytotoxic cells kill target cells that express foreign antigens. However, there is some overlap, as some CD8+ T cells secrete helper cytokines and CD4+ Th1 and Th2 cells can exhibit cross-regulatory suppression.

A key aspect of T-cell antigen recognition is the requirement for antigen to be presented on the surfaces of other cells in association with a histocompatible membrane protein (Figs. 4-5, 4-9 and 4-10). As noted, T cells bear membrane receptor complexes (α/β TCRs plus CD3 accessory molecules) on their surfaces (Figs. 4-5 and 4-9). For maximal immune response, the TCR–CD3 complex must interact with a foreign antigen in the context of cell-to-cell histocompatibility. Antigens may also be presented to T cells by cells that do not "present" antigens but rather express on their surface a foreign or altered self-protein in association with an appropriate histocompatibility molecule.

CD8$^+$ cells (cytotoxic T cells) recognize antigens in conjunction with HLA class I molecules, while CD4$^+$ cells (T helper cells) recognize antigens together with class II molecules. The membrane CD4 and CD8 molecules of α/β T cells help stabilize binding interactions. γ/δ T cells may also acquire CD8 outside the thymus and then use class I antigens for binding target cells. Foreign class I and class II molecules, which are histoincompatible with the host (e.g., histocompatibility molecules in transplanted tissues), are themselves potent immunogens and can be recognized by host T cells. *This is why optimal tissue transplantation requires that donor and recipient be HLA matched.* In addition to binding foreign peptides presented by MHC molecules to the TCR complex, several other receptor–ligand interactions must occur for maximal lymphocyte activation. A CD4$^+$ T cell becomes an activated effector cell when stimulated via the TCR complex and "accessory" receptors (CD28 and cytotoxic lymphoid line [CTLL]-4), which engage costimulatory molecules (e.g., CD80 [B-7.1] and CD86 [B-7.2]). In turn, an activated T helper cell recognizes an antigen-specific B cell via its receptor. The T helper cell then provides costimulatory and regulatory signals, such as CD40 ligand and "helper" cytokines (e.g., IL-4, IL-5).

B-Lymphocyte Interactions

Mature B cells exist primarily in a resting state, awaiting activation by foreign antigens. Activation requires cross-linking of mIg receptors via antigens presented by accessory cells and/or interactions with membrane molecules of helper T cells via a mechanism called cognate T-cell–B-cell help. The initial stimulus leads to B-cell proliferation and clonal expansion, a process amplified by cytokines from both accessory cells and T cells. If an insufficient additional signal is provided, proliferating B cells return to a resting state and enter the memory cell pool. These events take place largely in lymphoid tissues. B-lymphocyte proliferation can be seen as germinal centers, within which B cells undergo further somatic gene rearrangements to generate cells that produce the various immunoglobulin isotypes and subclasses (Table 4-3). T cells also influence B-cell differentiation. In the presence of antigen, T cells produce helper cytokines that stimulate isotype switching or induce proliferation of previously committed isotype populations. For example, IL-4 induces switching to the IgE isotype.

The final stage of B-cell differentiation into antibody-synthesizing plasma cells requires exposure to additional products of T lymphocytes (e.g., IL-5, IL-6), especially in the case of protein antigens. However, some polyvalent agents directly induce B-cell proliferation and differentiation into plasma cells, bypassing the requirements for B cell growth and differentiation factors. Such agents are called "polyclonal B-cell activators" because they do not interact with antigen-binding sites; they are not specific antigens. Such polyclonal B-cell activators include bacterial products (lipopolysaccharide, *Staphylococcus* protein A) and certain viruses (Epstein-Barr virus [EBV], cytomegalovirus [CMV]).

The predominant type of Ig produced during an immune response changes with age. Newborns produce mainly IgM. Older children and adults initially produce IgM following antigenic challenge but rapidly shift toward IgG synthesis.

IMMUNOLOGICALLY MEDIATED TISSUE INJURY

There are many diseases in which an immunologically triggered inflammatory response attacks the body's own tissues. A variety of foreign substances (e.g., dust, pollen, viruses, bacteria) provoke protective responses. In certain situations, the protective effects of an immune response lead to harmful consequences, which can range from temporary discomfort to substantial injury. For example, in the process of ingesting and destroying bacteria, phagocytic cells (neutrophils and macrophages) often cause injury to surrounding tissue. An immune response that leads to tissue injury is broadly called a **hypersensitivity** reaction. Many diseases are categorized as immune disorders or immunologically mediated conditions, in which an immune response to a foreign or self-antigen causes injury. Immune- or hypersensitivity-mediated diseases are common and include hives (urticaria), asthma, hay fever, hepatitis, glomerulonephritis and arthritis.

Hypersensitivity reactions are classified according to immune mechanism (Table 4-4). Type I, II and III hypersensitivity reactions all involve antibodies specific for exogenous (foreign) or endogenous (self) antigens. (An exception includes a subset of type I reactions.) Antibody isotype influences the mechanism of tissue injury.

- **Type I, or immediate-type hypersensitivity, reactions:** IgE antibody is formed and binds high-affinity receptors on mast cells and/or basophils via its Fc domain. Subsequent antigen binding and cross-linking of IgE trigger rapid (immediate) release of products from these cells, leading to the characteristic manifestations of urticaria, asthma and anaphylaxis.
- **Type II hypersensitivity reactions:** IgM or IgG antibody is formed against an antigen, usually a cell surface protein. Less commonly, the antigen is an intrinsic structural component of the extracellular matrix (e.g., basement membrane). Such antigen–antibody coupling activates complement, which in turn lyses the cell (cytotoxicity) or damages the extracellular matrix. In some type II reactions, other antibody-mediated effects are operative.
- **Type III hypersensitivity reactions:** The antibody responsible for tissue injury is also usually IgM or IgG, but the mechanism of tissue injury differs. Antigen circulates in the vascular compartment until it is bound by antibody. Resulting immune complexes deposit in tissue where complement activation leads to recruitment of leukocytes, which mediate tissue injury. In some type III reactions, antigen is bound by antibody in situ.
- **Type IV, cell-mediated** or **delayed-type, hypersensitivity reactions:** Antigen activation of T lymphocytes, usually with the help of macrophages, causes release of products by these cells, leading to tissue injury.

TABLE 4-4

MODIFIED CELL AND COOMBS CLASSIFICATION OF HYPERSENSITIVITY REACTIONS

Type	Mechanism	Examples
Type 1 (anaphylactic type): immediate hypersensitivity	IgE antibody–mediated mast cell activation and degranulation Non–Ig mediated	Hay fever, asthma, hives, anaphylaxis Physical urticarias
Type II (cytotoxic type): cytotoxic antibodies	Cytotoxic (IgG, IgM) antibodies formed against cell surface antigens; complement usually involved Noncytotoxic antibodies against cell surface receptors	Autoimmune hemolytic anemias, Goodpasture disease Graves disease
Type III (immune complex type): immune complex disease	Antibodies (IgG, IgM, IgA) formed against exogenous or endogenous antigens; complement and leukocytes (neutrophils, macrophages) often involved	Autoimmune diseases (SLE, rheumatoid arthritis), many types of glomerulonephritis
Type IV (cell-mediated type): delayed-type hypersensitivity	Mononuclear cells (T lymphocytes, macrophages) with interleukin and lymphokine production	Granulomatous disease (tuberculosis), delayed skin reactions (poison ivy)

Ig = immunoglobulin; SLE = systemic lupus erythematosus.

Many immunologic diseases are mediated by more than one type of hypersensitivity reaction. For example, in hypersensitivity pneumonitis, lung injury from inhaled fungal antigens involves types I, III and IV reactions.

IgE-Mediated Hypersensitivity Reactions (Type I)

Immediate-type hypersensitivity entails localized or generalized reactions that occur immediately (within minutes) after exposure to an antigen or "allergen" to which the person has been previously sensitized. Clinical manifestations depend on the site of antigen exposure and extent of sensitization. For example, when a reaction involves the skin, the characteristic local reaction is a "wheal and flare," or urticaria. When the conjunctiva and upper respiratory tract are involved, sneezing and conjunctivitis result and we speak of hay fever (allergic rhinitis). In its generalized and most severe form, immediate hypersensitivity reactions are associated with bronchoconstriction, airway obstruction and circulatory collapse, as seen in anaphylactic shock. There is a high degree of genetically determined variability in susceptibility to type I hypersensitivity reactions, and susceptible individuals are said to be "atopic."

Type I reactions usually feature IgE antibodies formed by a CD4+, Th2 T-cell–dependent mechanism that bind avidly to Fcε receptors on mast cells and basophils. High avidity ($K_d = 10^{-15}$ M) of IgE binding accounts for the term **cytophilic** antibody. Once exposed to a specific allergen that elicits IgE, a person is sensitized; subsequent exposures to that allergen or a cross-reacting epitope induce immediate hypersensitivity reactions. Once IgE is elicited, repeat exposure to antigen typically induces additional IgE antibody, rather than antibodies of other classes.

Bound to Fcε receptors on mast cells and basophils, IgE can persist for years. Upon reexposure, recognition of the soluble antigen or allergen by IgE coupled to its surface Fcε receptor activates the mast cell or basophil. Released inflammatory mediators cause type I hypersensitivity reactions. As shown in Fig. 4-11, the antigen (allergen) binds the Fab region of the IgE antibody. To activate the cell, antigen must cross-link at least two adjacent IgE antibody molecules.

Mast cells and basophils can also be activated by agents other than antibodies. For example, some individuals develop urticaria after exposure to an ice cube (physical urticaria) or pressure (dermographism). The complement-derived anaphylatoxic peptides, C3a and C5a, can directly stimulate mast cells by a different receptor-mediated process (Fig. 4-11). These cell-activating events trigger release of stored granule constituents and rapid synthesis and release of other mediators. Some compounds, such as melittin (from bee venom), and some drugs (e.g., morphine) activate mast cells directly.

Regardless of how mast cell activation is initiated, a rise in cytosolic free calcium triggers an increase in cyclic adenosine monophosphate (cAMP), activation of several metabolic pathways within the mast cell and subsequent secretion of both preformed and newly synthesized products. Stored in granules, mediators are released within minutes and act rapidly. Of the granule constituents listed in Fig. 4-11, histamine is particularly important. It induces constriction of vascular and nonvascular smooth muscle, causes microvascular dilation and increases venule permeability. These effects are largely mediated through H_1 histamine receptors. Histamine also increases gastric acid secretion through H_2 histamine receptors and provokes the cutaneous wheal-and-flare reaction. In the lungs, it causes the early manifestations of immediate hypersensitivity, including bronchospasm, vascular congestion and edema. Other preformed products released from mast cell granules include heparin, a series of neutral proteases (trypsin, chymotrypsin carboxypeptidase and acid hydrolases) and both neutrophil and eosinophil chemotactic factors. The latter is responsible for the accumulation of eosinophils, a characteristic finding in immediate hypersensitivity. The synthesis and secretion of cytokines by mast cells, by other recruited inflammatory cells and even by indigenous cells (e.g., epithelium) are important in the so-called "late-phase" reaction of immediate hypersensitivity. Late-phase responses typically last 2–24 hours, are marked by a mixed inflammatory infiltrate and are mediated by many cytokines including IL-1, IL-3, IL-4, IL-5, IL-6, TNF, granulocyte-macrophage colony-stimulating factor (GM-CSF) and macrophage inflammatory protein (MIP)-1α and MIP-1β.

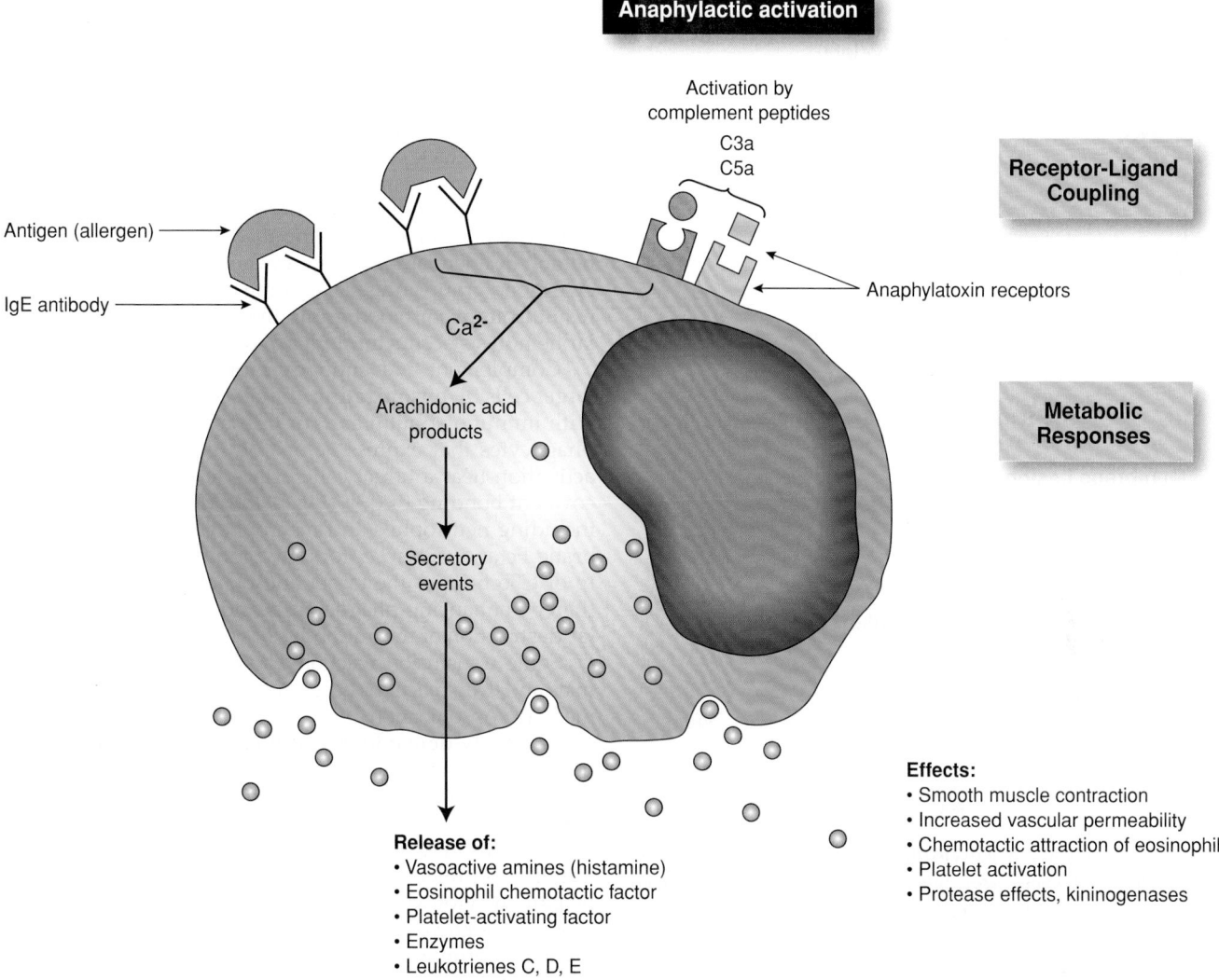

Anaphylactic activation

Activation by
complement peptides
C3a
C5a

**Receptor-Ligand
Coupling**

Antigen (allergen)

IgE antibody

Anaphylatoxin receptors

Ca^{2-}

Arachidonic acid
products

**Metabolic
Responses**

Secretory
events

Release of:
- Vasoactive amines (histamine)
- Eosinophil chemotactic factor
- Platelet-activating factor
- Enzymes
- Leukotrienes C, D, E
- Prostaglandin PGD_2, thromboxane

Effects:
- Smooth muscle contraction
- Increased vascular permeability
- Chemotactic attraction of eosinophils
- Platelet activation
- Protease effects, kininogenases

FIGURE 4-11. In a type I hypersensitivity reaction, antigen (allergen) binds to cytophilic surface IgE antibody on a mast cell or basophil and triggers cell activation and the release of a cascade of proinflammatory mediators. Mast cells and basophils can also be activated by anaphylatoxins like C3a and C5a, as well as some physical stimuli (e.g., cold). These mediators are responsible for smooth muscle contraction, edema formation and the recruitment of eosinophils. Ca^{2+} = calcium ion; Ig = immunoglobulin; PGD_2 = prostaglandin D_2.

Mast cell activation also increases synthesis of arachidonic acid pathway products formed after activation of phospholipase A_2. Products of cyclooxygenase (prostaglandins D_2, E_2 and F_2 and thromboxane) and lipoxygenase (leukotrienes B_4, C_4, D_4, E_4) are also produced. Arachidonic acid derivatives, generated by a variety of cell types, induce smooth muscle contraction, vasodilation and edema. Leukotrienes C_4, D_4 and E_4, previously known as "slow-reacting substances of anaphylaxis" (SRS-As), are important in the delayed bronchoconstriction phase of anaphylaxis. Leukotriene B_4 is a potent chemotactic factor for neutrophils, macrophages and eosinophils.

Another inflammatory mediator synthesized by mast cells is **platelet-activating factor** (PAF), a lipid derived from membrane phospholipids. PAF is a potent inducer of platelet aggregation and release of vasoactive amines as well as a potent neutrophil chemotaxin. PAF can activate all types of phagocytic cells.

Activated T cells, specifically Th2 cells, produce cytokines that have important roles in allergic responses. This subset releases IL-4, IL-5 and IL-13, leading to IgE production and increased numbers of mast cells and eosinophils. In allergy-prone people, a similar response occurs via T cells that produce IL-4, IL-6 and IL-2, concentrations of which are also increased in allergic individuals. These individuals also have reduced levels of IFN-γ, which suppresses development of Th2 cells and subsequent production of IgE.

In summary, type I (immediate) hypersensitivity reactions are characterized by specific cytophilic antibody (IgE) that binds to high-affinity Fcε receptors on basophils and mast cells and reacts with a specific antigen (allergen). Activated mast cells and basophils release preformed (granule) products and synthesize mediators that cause the classic manifestations of immediate hypersensitivity and the late-phase reaction.

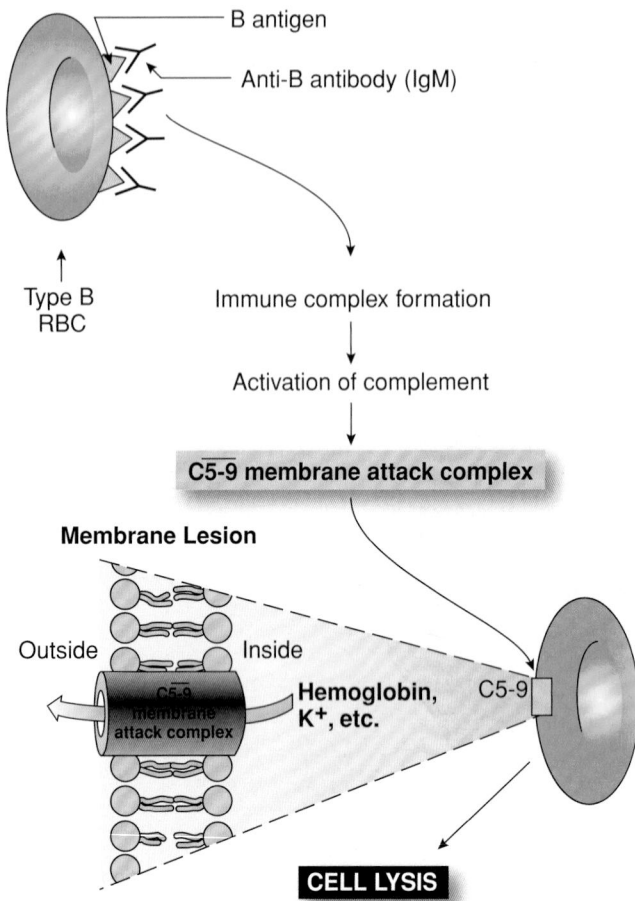

FIGURE 4-12. In a type II hypersensitivity reaction, binding of IgG or IgM antibody to an immobilized antigen promotes complement fixation. Activation of complement leads to amplification of the inflammatory response and membrane attack complex (MAC)-mediated cell lysis. *Ig* = immunoglobulin; K^+ = potassium ion; *RBC* = red blood cell.

Non-IgE Antibody-Mediated Hypersensitivity Reactions (Type II)

IgM and IgG mediate most type II reactions. These Ig isotypes activate complement via their Fc domains. There are several antibody-dependent mechanisms of tissue injury.

Prototypic antibody-mediated erythrocyte cytotoxicity is illustrated in Fig. 4-12. IgM or IgG antibody binds an antigen on the erythrocyte membrane. At sufficient density, bound Ig fixes complement via C1q and the classical pathway (see Chapter 2). Activated complement can destroy target cells directly, via C5b-9 complexes (Fig. 4-12). The C5b-9 **membrane attack complex** inserts like the staves of a barrel into the plasma membrane and forms holes or ion channels, destroying the permeability barrier and inducing cell lysis. This type of cell lysis is exemplified by certain autoimmune hemolytic anemias resulting from antibodies against erythrocyte blood group antigens. In some transfusion reactions that result from major blood group incompatibilities, intravascular hemolysis occurs through activation of complement.

Complement and antibody molecules can also destroy target cells by **opsonization**. Target cells coated (opsonized) with immunoglobulin and/or C3b molecules are bound by phagocytes that express Fc or C3b receptors. Complement activation near a target cell surface leads to formation and covalent bonding of C3b (Fig. 4-13). Many phagocytic cells, including neutrophils and macrophages, express cell membrane Fc and C3b receptors. By binding to these receptors, Ig or C3b bridges the target and effector (phagocytic) cells, thereby enhancing phagocytosis and subsequent intracellular destruction of the antibody- or complement-coated cell.

Some transfusion reactions, autoimmune hemolytic anemias and drug reactions occur via antibody- and complement-mediated opsonization.

Antibody-dependent cell-mediated cytotoxicity does not require complement, but rather involves cytolytic leukocytes that attack antibody-coated target cells after binding via Fc receptors. Phagocytic cells and NK cells can act as effector cells in ADCC. Effector cells synthesize homologs of terminal complement proteins (e.g., perforins), which participate in cytotoxic events (see preceding discussion of NK cells). *Only rarely is antibody alone directly cytotoxic.* In cases involving primarily lymphoid cells, apoptosis is activated. ADCC is implicated in the pathogenesis of some autoimmune diseases (e.g., autoimmune thyroiditis).

In some type II reactions, antibody binding to a specific target cell receptor does not lead to cell death but rather to change in function. For example, in Graves disease and myasthenia gravis, autoantibodies against cell surface hormone receptors and postsynaptic neurotransmitter receptors, respectively (Fig. 4-14), may activate or inhibit cell activation

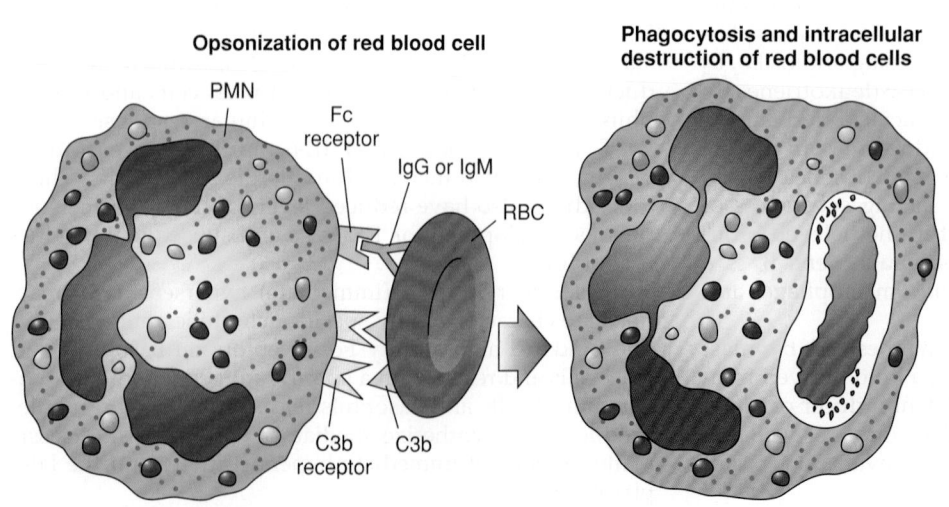

FIGURE 4-13. In a type II hypersensitivity reaction, opsonization by antibody or complement leads to phagocytosis via either Fc or C3b receptors, respectively. *Ig* = immunoglobulin; *PMN* = polymorphonuclear leukocyte; *RBC* = red blood cell.

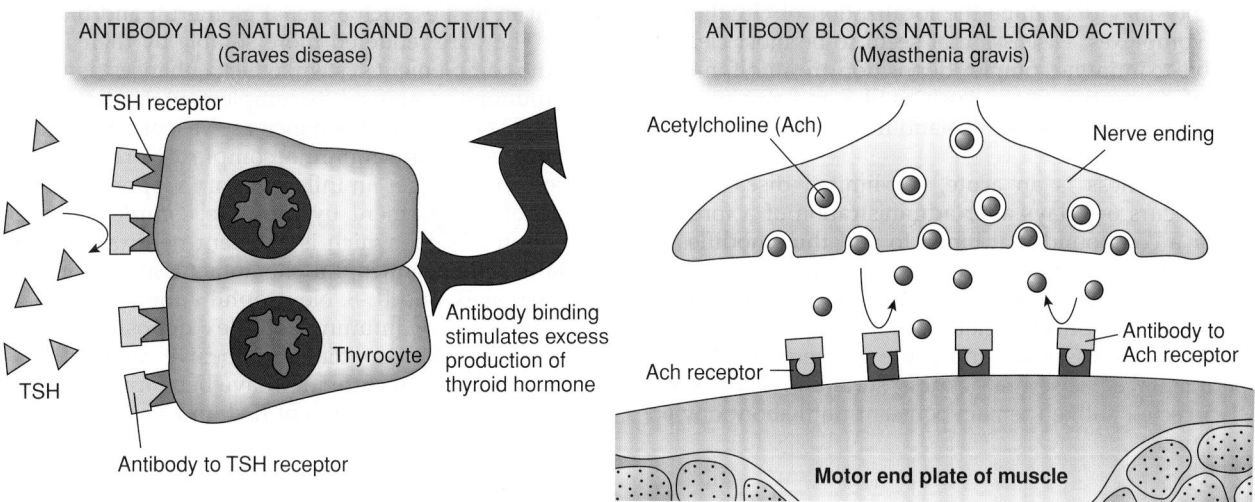

ANTIRECEPTOR ANTIBODY

FIGURE 4-14. In a type II hypersensitivity reaction, antibodies bind to a cell surface receptor and induce activation (e.g., thyroid-stimulating hormone [TSH] receptors in Graves disease) or inhibition/destruction (e.g., acetylcholine receptors in myasthenia gravis).

(see below). In Graves disease, autoantibody against thyroid-stimulating hormone (TSH) receptors elicits thyroxin production, leading to thyrotoxicosis. In myasthenia gravis, autoantibodies to acetylcholine receptors on postsynaptic membranes block acetylcholine binding and/or mediate internalization or destruction of receptors, thereby preventing effective synaptic transmission. Patients with myasthenia gravis suffer from muscle fatigue.

Some type II reactions result from antibody against a structural connective tissue component. Classic examples are Goodpasture syndrome and the bullous skin diseases, pemphigus and pemphigoid. In these disorders, circulating antibodies bind intrinsic connective tissue antigens and evoke destructive local inflammatory responses. In Goodpasture syndrome, antibody binds the noncollagenous domain of type IV collagen, which is a major structural component of pulmonary and glomerular basement membranes (Fig. 4-15). Local complement activation results in neutrophil chemotaxis and activation, tissue injury and pulmonary hemorrhage and glomerulonephritis. Direct complement-mediated damage to glomerular and alveolar basement membranes via membrane attack complexes may also be involved.

In summary, type II hypersensitivity reactions are directly or indirectly cytotoxic through action of antibodies against antigens on cell surfaces or in connective tissues. Complement participates in many of these events. It may directly mediate lysis, or it may act indirectly by opsonization and phagocytosis or chemotactic attraction of phagocytic cells, which produce a variety of tissue-damaging products. Complement-independent reactions, such as ADCC, also play a role in type II hypersensitivity.

Immune Complex Reactions (Type III)

IgM, IgG and occasionally IgA against a circulating antigen that deposits or is planted in a tissue can cause a type III response. Physicochemical characteristics of the immune complexes, such as size, charge and solubility, in addition to Ig isotype, determine whether an immune complex deposits in tissue and fixes complement. "Phlogistic" (inflammatory) immune complexes elicit inflammatory responses by activating complement, thus recruiting neutrophils and monocytes. These activated phagocytes release tissue damage mediators, such as proteases and reactive oxygen species.

Immune complexes have been implicated in many human diseases. The most compelling cases are those in which demonstration of immune complexes in injured tissue correlates with development of injury. Examples include cryoglobulinemic vasculitis associated with hepatitis C infection, Henoch-Schönlein purpura (in which IgA deposits are found at sites of vasculitis) and systemic lupus erythematous (SLE) (anti–double-stranded DNA in vasculitic lesions). In many diseases, immune complexes can be detected in plasma but

FIGURE 4-15. Goodpasture syndrome involves a type II hypersensitivity reaction in which antibody binds to a structural antigen, activates the complement system and leads to the recruitment of tissue-damaging inflammatory cells. Several complement-derived peptides (e.g., C5a) are potent chemotactic factors. *GBM* = glomerular basement membrane; *PMN* = polymorphonuclear leukocyte.

are not associated with tissue injury. The physicochemical properties of circulating immune complexes frequently differ from those deposited in tissues. In some cases, vascular permeability may determine the localization of circulating immune complexes. Diseases that seem to be most clearly attributable to immune complex deposition are autoimmune diseases of connective tissue, such as SLE and rheumatoid arthritis, some types of vasculitis and many varieties of glomerulonephritis.

Serum sickness is an acute, self-limited disease that typically occurs 6–8 days after administration of a foreign protein or a compound that binds to and thus modifies a native protein. Human serum sickness is uncommon but can occur in patients given foreign proteins as a therapeutic agent (e.g., antilymphocyte globulin). It is characterized by fever, arthralgias, vasculitis and acute glomerulonephritis. In experimental acute serum sickness, serum levels of exogenously injected antigen remain constant until about day 6,

after which they fall rapidly (Fig. 4-16). At the same time, immune complexes (containing IgM or IgG bound to antigen) appear in the circulation. Some circulating complexes deposit in tissues such as renal glomeruli and blood vessel walls. They are rendered more soluble by their interaction with the complement system, which enhances tissue deposition. Immune complexes fix complement, leading to generation of C3a and C5a, which increase vascular permeability.

Once phlogistic immune complexes are deposited in tissues, they trigger an inflammatory response. Local activation of complement by immune complexes results in formation of C5a, which is a potent neutrophil chemoattractant. Other neutrophil chemotactic mediators include leukotriene B_4 and IL-8. Neutrophil adherence and migration into sites of immune complex deposition involve a series of cytokine-mediated adhesive interactions (see Chapter 2). Several cytokines have been implicated in this response. Early production of IL-1 and TNF-α upregulates

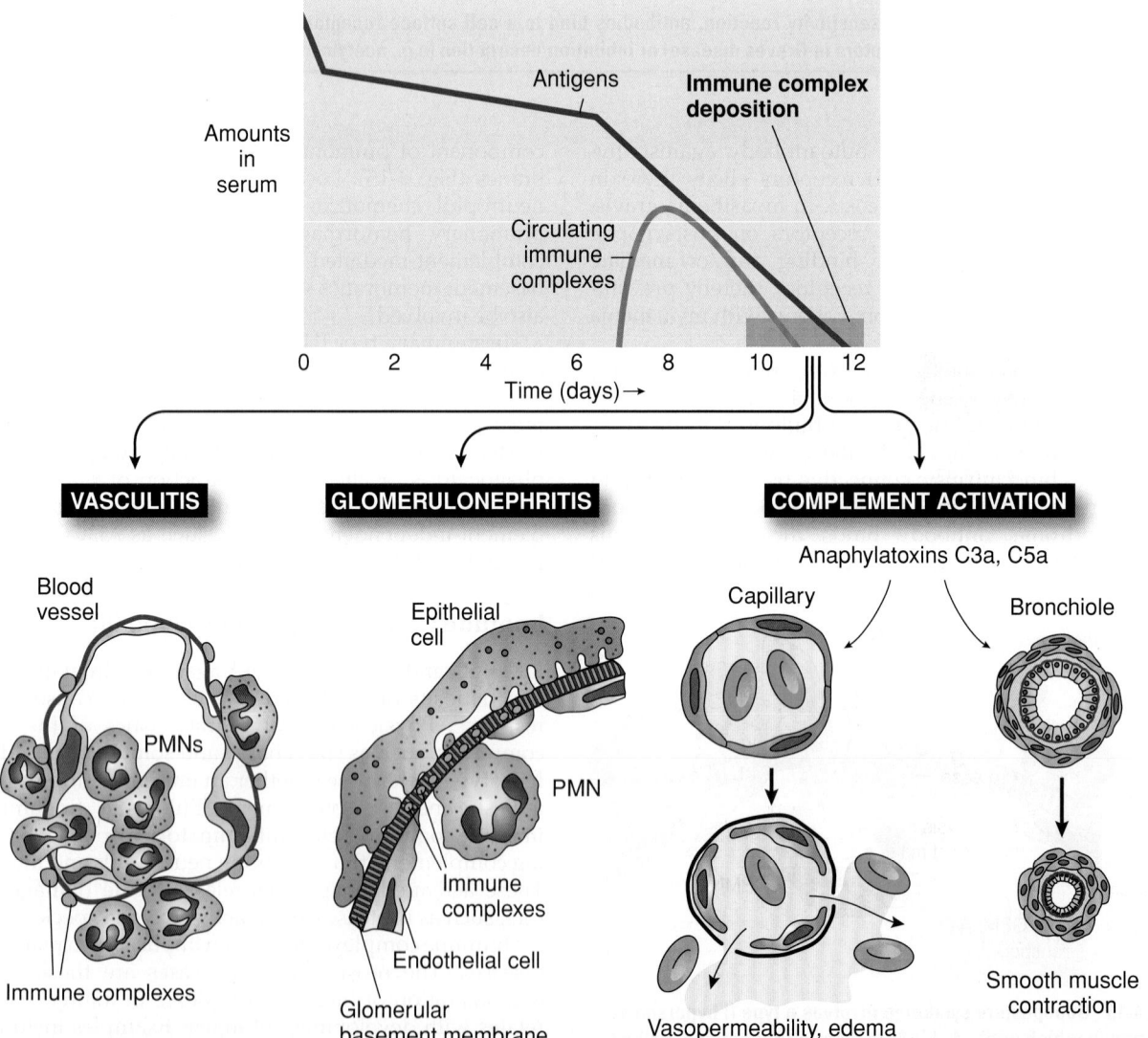

FIGURE 4-16. In type III hypersensitivity, immune complexes are deposited and can lead to complement activation and the recruitment of tissue-damaging inflammatory cells. This schematic illustrates the series of events that occur in acute serum sickness. The ability of immune complexes to mediate tissue injury depends on size, solubility, net charge and ability to fix complement. *PMN* = polymorphonuclear leukocyte.

adhesion molecules on endothelial cells and production of other proinflammatory cytokines that include platelet-derived growth factor (PDGF); transforming growth factor-β (TGF-β); and IL-4, IL-6 and IL-10, which modulate activation of leukocytes and fibroblasts. Not all cytokines are proinflammatory; IL-10, in particular, downregulates inflammatory responses.

Recruited neutrophils are activated through contact with, and ingestion of, immune complexes. Activated cells release inflammatory mediators, including proteases, reactive oxygen intermediates and arachidonic acid products, which collectively produce tissue injury. Tissue injury associated with experimental serum sickness mimics that seen in human vasculitis and glomerulonephritis.

The **Arthus reaction** has been studied using an experimental model of vasculitis in which localized injury is induced by immune complexes (Fig. 4-17). This reaction is classically seen in dermal blood vessels after local injection

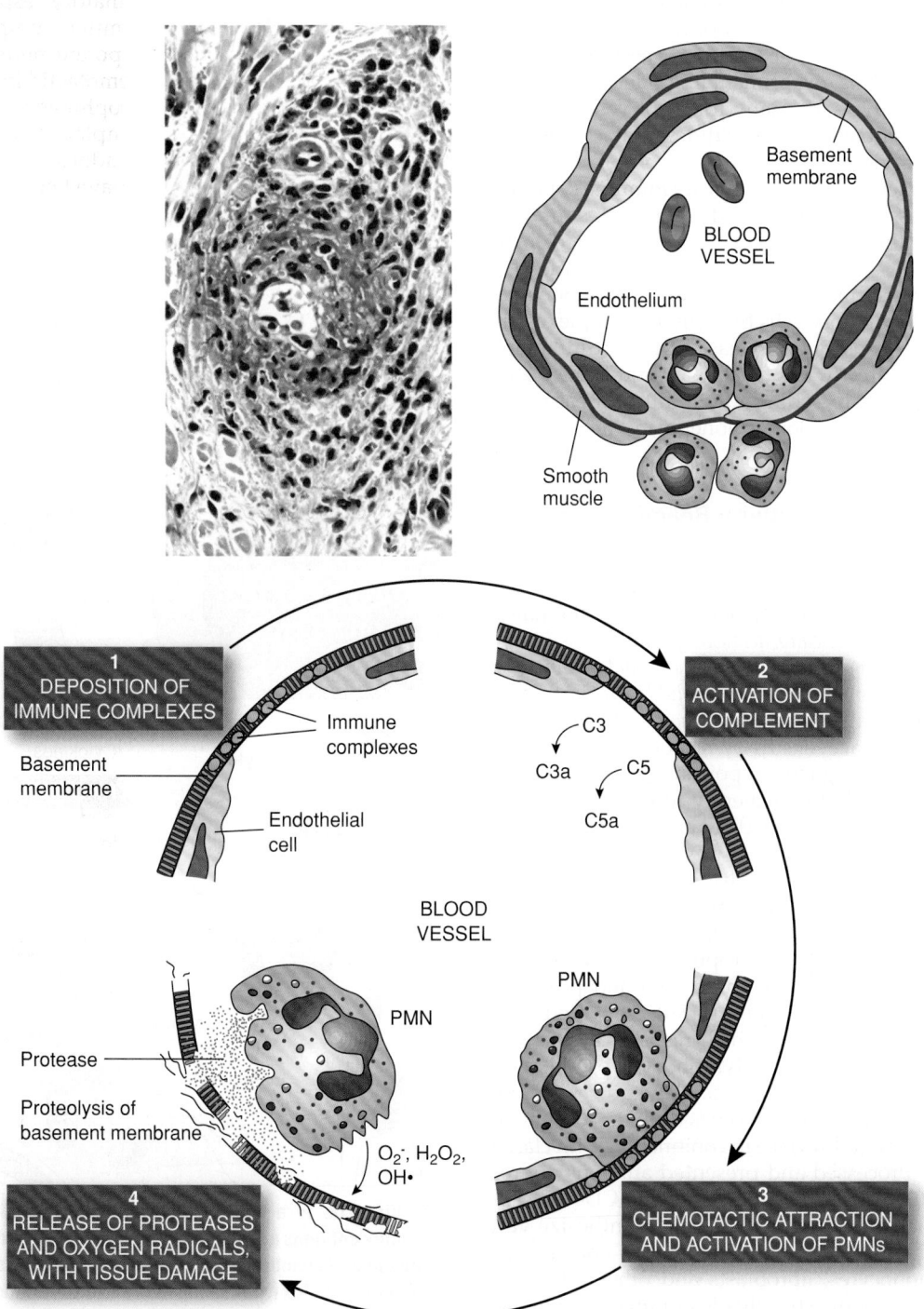

FIGURE 4-17. The Arthus reaction is a type III hypersensitivity reaction characterized by the deposition of immune complexes and the induction of an acute inflammatory response within blood vessel walls. Some vasculitic lesions exhibit fibrinoid necrosis. H_2O_2 = hydrogen peroxide; O_2^- = superoxide anion; $OH\bullet$ = hydroxyl radical; *PMN* = polymorphonuclear leukocyte.

of an antigen to which an individual was previously sensitized. The circulating antibody and locally injected antigen diffuse down concentration gradients toward each other to form complex deposits in walls of small blood vessels. Resulting vascular injury is mediated by complement activation, recruited neutrophils and their proinflammatory mediators. In contrast to type I (immediate) hypersensitivity, these lesions develop over a period of 2–10 hours. Walls of affected vessels contain numerous neutrophils and show evidence of damage, with edema and hemorrhage into surrounding tissue. The presence of fibrin creates the classic appearance of immune complex–induced vasculitis, namely, fibrinoid necrosis. This experimental model of localized vasculitis is a prototype for many forms of vasculitis seen in humans (e.g., cutaneous vasculitides that characterize certain drug reactions).

Type III hypersensitivity reactions are immune complex–mediated injuries. Antigen–antibody complexes may be formed either in the circulation and then deposited in the tissues, or in situ. Immune complexes fix complement, which leads to recruitment of neutrophils and monocytes. Activation of inflammatory cells by immune complexes and complement, with consequent release of potent inflammatory mediators, is directly responsible for injury (Fig. 4-17). Many human diseases, including autoimmune diseases such as SLE and many types of glomerulonephritis, are mediated by this mechanism.

Cell-Mediated Hypersensitivity Reactions (Type IV)

Type IV reactions often occur together with antibody reactions, which can make it difficult to distinguish them. The type of tissue response is largely determined by the nature of the inciting agent. *Classically, delayed-type hypersensitivity is a tissue reaction, mainly involving lymphocytes and mononuclear phagocytes, occurring in response to a soluble protein antigen and reaching peak intensity after 24–48 hours.* A classic type IV reaction is the contact sensitivity response to poison ivy. Although the chemical ligands in poison ivy (e.g., urushiol) are not proteins, they bind covalently to cell proteins, the products of which are recognized by antigen-specific lymphocytes.

In delayed-type hypersensitivity reactions (Fig. 4-18), foreign protein antigens or chemical ligands first interact with accessory cells that express class II HLA molecules (Fig. 4-18A). Accessory cells (macrophages, dendritic cells) secrete IL-12, which, along with processed and presented antigen, activate CD4$^+$ T cells (Fig. 4-18B). Activated CD4$^+$ T cells secrete IFN-γ and IL-2, which respectively activate more macrophages and elicit T-lymphocyte proliferation (Fig. 4-18C). Protein antigens are actively processed into short peptides within phagolysosomes of the macrophages and presented on the cell surface in conjunction with class II HLA molecules. Processed and presented antigens are recognized by MHC-restricted, antigen-specific CD4$^+$ T cells, which become activated and, as Th1 cells, synthesize various cytokines. In turn, the cytokines recruit and activate lymphocytes, monocytes, fibroblasts and other inflammatory cells. If the antigenic stimulus is eliminated, the reaction spontaneously resolves after about 48 hours. If the stimulus persists (e.g., poorly biodegradable mycobacterial cell wall components), an attempt to sequester the inciting agent may result in a granulomatous reaction.

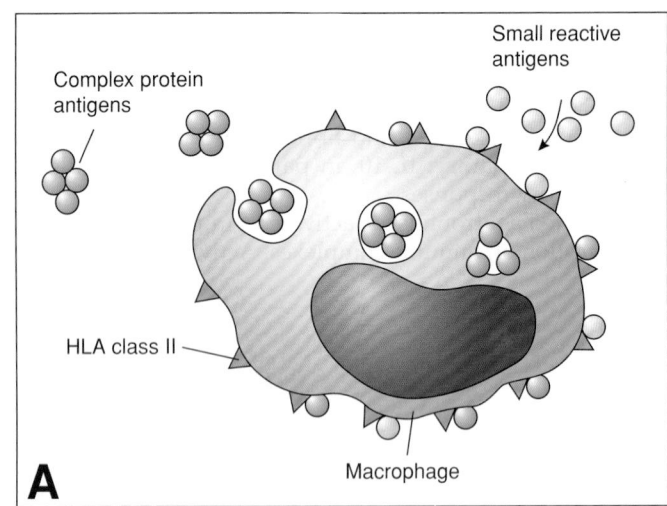

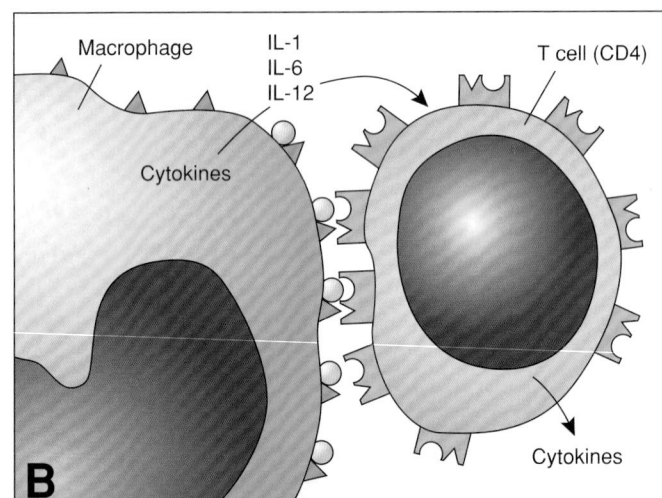

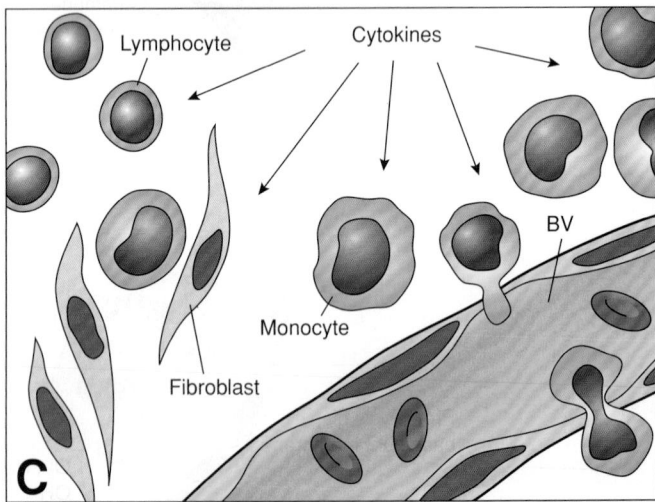

FIGURE 4-18. In a type IV (delayed-type) hypersensitivity reaction, complex antigens are phagocytized, processed and presented on macrophage cell membranes in conjunction with class II major histocompatibility complex (MHC) antigens. Antigens are in turn recognized via T-cell receptors (TCRs) expressed on histocompatible T lymphocytes. **A.** Antigen-specific, histocompatible, cytotoxic T lymphocytes bind presented antigens and are activated. **B, C.** Activated cytotoxic T cells secrete cytokines that amplify the response. *BV* = blood vessel.

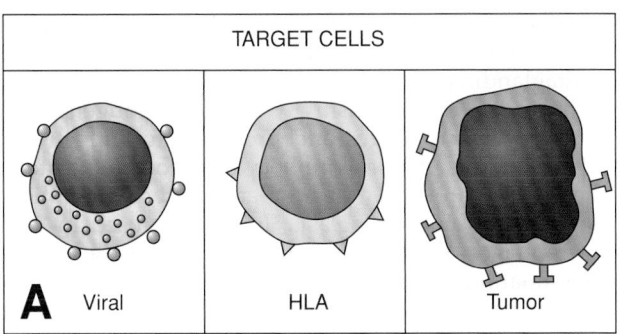

TARGET CELLS

A — Viral — HLA — Tumor

TARGET ANTIGENS
• Virally coded membrane antigen
• Foreign or modified histocompatibility antigen
• Tumor-specific membrane antigens

B — T-helper (CD4) — T-Cytotoxic (CD8)

RECOGNITION OF ANTIGEN BY T CELLS
• T-helper cells recognize antigen plus class II molecules
• T-cytotoxic/killer cells recognize antigen plus class I molecules

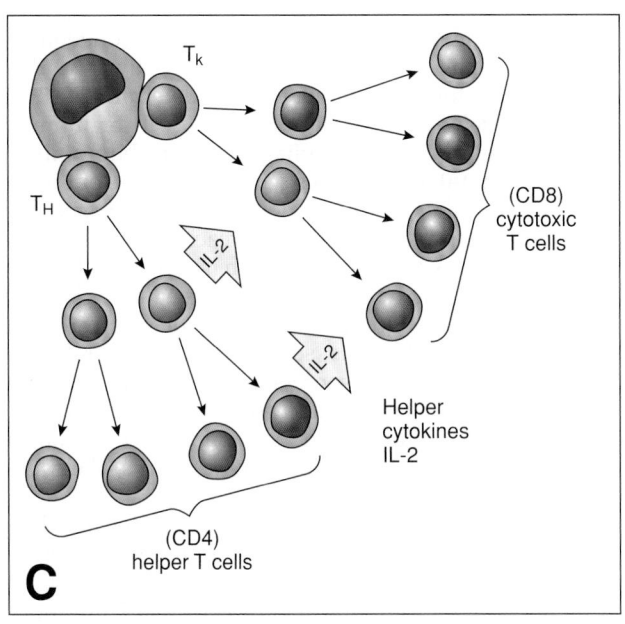

T_k
T_H
IL-2
(CD8) cytotoxic T cells
Helper cytokines IL-2
IL-2
(CD4) helper T cells
C

ACTIVATION AND AMPLIFICATION
• T-helper cells activate and proliferate, releasing helper molecules (e.g., IL-2)
• T-cytotoxic/killer cells proliferate in response to helper molecules

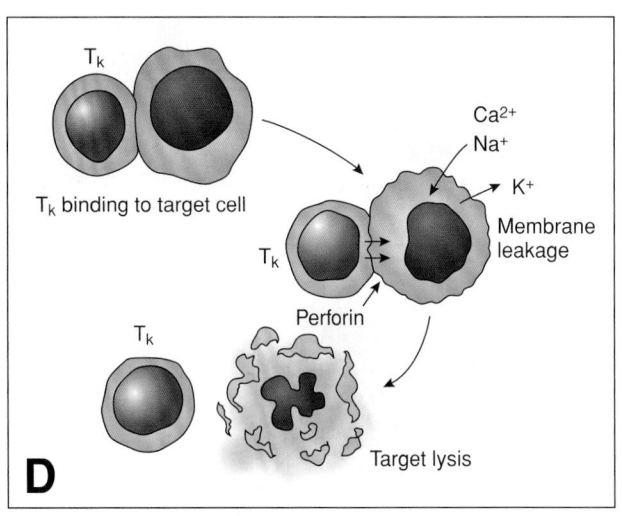

T_k
T_k binding to target cell
Ca^{2+}
Na^+
K^+
Membrane leakage
T_k
Perforin
T_k
Target lysis
D

TARGET CELL KILLING
• T-cytotoxic/killer cells bind to target cell
• Killing signals perforin release and target cell loses membrane integrity
• Target cell undergoes lysis

FIGURE 4-19. In T-cell–mediated cytotoxicity, potential target cells include (A) virus-infected host cells, malignant host cells and foreign **(histoincompatible transplanted) cells. B.** Cytotoxic T lymphocytes recognize foreign antigens in the context of human leukocyte antigen (HLA) class I molecules. **C.** Activated T cells secrete lytic compounds (e.g., perforin and other mediators) and cytokines that amplify the response. **D.** Apoptosis (target cell killing) is mediated by perforin and involves influx of Ca^{2+} (calcium ion) and Na^+ (sodium ion) and efflux of K^+ (potassium ion). *IL* = interleukin.

Another mechanism by which T cells (especially CD8$^+$) mediate tissue damage is direct lysis of target cells (Fig. 4-19). This mechanism is important in destroying and eliminating cells infected by viruses, transplanted tissues and, possibly, tumor cells.

In contrast to delayed-type hypersensitivity reactions, cytotoxic CD8$^+$ T cells specifically recognize target antigens in the context of class I MHC molecules. Foreign antigens are actively presented together with self-MHC antigens. In graft rejection, foreign MHC antigens are themselves potent activators of CD8$^+$ T cells. Once activated by antigen, cytotoxic cell proliferation is aided by helper cells and mediated by soluble growth factors such as IL-2 (Fig. 4-19C), and the

population of antigen-specific cytotoxic cells thus expands. Cell killing occurs via several mechanisms (Fig. 4-19D; see also Chapter 1). Cytolytic T cells (CTLs) secrete perforins that form pores in target cell membranes and introduce granzymes that activate intracellular caspases, leading to apoptosis. CTLs can also kill targets by engaging Fas ligand (FasL, on the CTL) and Fas (on the target). FasL–Fas interaction triggers apoptosis of the Fas-bearing cell.

The defining characteristics of NK cells have been described, but the extent to which they participate in tissue-damaging reactions is unclear. Some evidence indicates that NK cells exert both effector and immunoregulatory functions. Fig. 4-20 illustrates target cell killing by an NK cell. NK

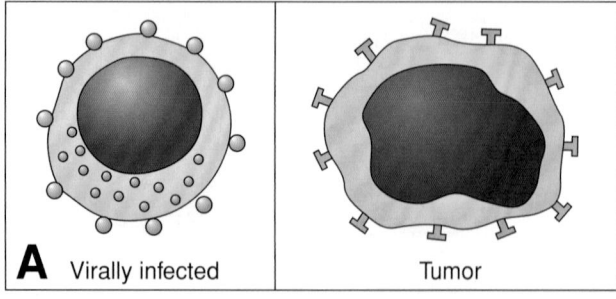

A Virally infected — Tumor

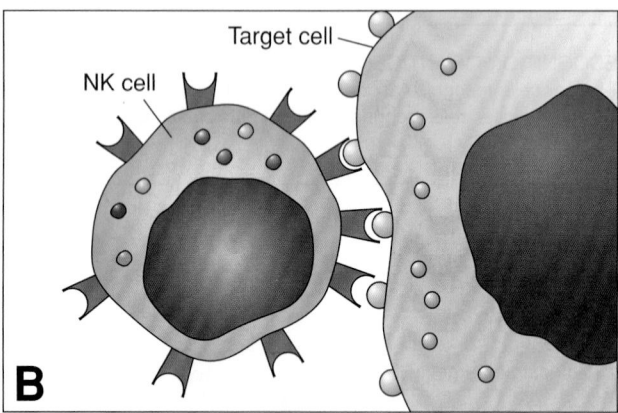

B

Target cell

NK cell

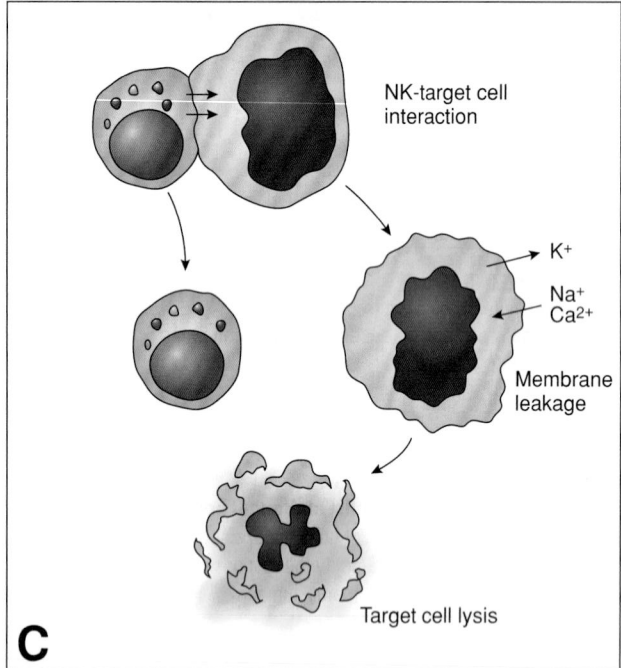

C

NK-target cell
interaction

K⁺

Na⁺
Ca²⁺

Membrane
leakage

Target cell lysis

FIGURE 4-20. In natural killer (NK)-cell–mediated cytotoxicity, potential target cells include virus-infected and neoplastic cells. NK cells bind target cells **(A)**, are activated **(B)**, and secrete lytic compounds **(C)**. NK cells bind to target cells that express decreased numbers of surface human leukocyte antigen (HLA) class I molecules. Ca^{2+} = calcium ion; K^+ = potassium ion; Na^+ = sodium ion.

cells can recognize a variety of targets including membrane glycoproteins expressed by some virus-infected cells and tumor cells. Similar to events described for cytotoxic T cells, NK cells bind to target cells through membrane receptors and deliver molecular signals that result in lysis. NK cells also express membrane Fc receptors, which can bind antibodies that mediate cell killing by ADCC. NK cell activity

is influenced by a variety of mediators. For example, it is increased by IL-2, IL-12 and IFN-γ and decreased by several prostaglandins.

In type IV hypersensitivity reactions, antigens are processed by macrophages and presented to antigen-specific T lymphocytes. These lymphocytes become activated and release mediators that recruit and activate lymphocytes, macrophages and fibroblasts. Injury is caused by T cells, macrophages or both. No antibodies are involved. Chronic inflammation associated with autoimmune diseases—including type 1 diabetes, chronic thyroiditis, Sjögren syndrome and primary biliary cirrhosis—is largely the result of type IV hypersensitivity.

IMMUNODEFICIENCY DISEASES

Immunodeficiency diseases are classified as congenital (primary) or acquired (secondary), and by defective host defense system. The former are genetically determined. **Primary immunodeficiencies are classified as B cell or humoral, T cell or cellular, defects of phagocytes or abnormalities of the complement system.** This scheme is useful, but it should be recognized that a primary defect within one aspect of the immune system may have farther-reaching effects. Complement deficiencies are associated with recurrent and/or severe bacterial infections (encapsulated pyogens and *Neisseria*) as well as lupus-like disorders. Phagocyte defects are generally associated with cutaneous, soft tissue and visceral bacterial and fungal infections. Disorders of complement and primary defects of phagocytes are discussed in detail elsewhere (see Chapter 2). In contrast to the low prevalence of congenital immunodeficiencies, acquired immune deficits, like AIDS, are common.

Functional defects in lymphocytes can be localized to particular stages in the ontogeny of the immune system, or the interruption of discrete immune activation events (Fig. 4-21). A detailed classification scheme for primary immunodeficiency disorders is available via the WHO.

People with Antibody Deficiency Diseases Are Inordinately Susceptible to Recurrent Bacterial Infections

Several specific types of viral infections may also occur (e.g., central nervous system [CNS] echovirus infections in patients with Bruton agammaglobulinemia) and subnormal serum concentrations of either all or specific isotypes of Igs. There are a variety of immunoglobulin isotype and subclass deficiencies including selective deletions of immunoglobulin heavy chains and selective loss of light-chain expression (Table 4-5). Some patients have normal immunoglobulin levels but fail to make antibodies against specific antigens, usually polysaccharides. The clinical manifestations of these entities are highly variable; some patients suffer from life-threatening bacterial infections, varying from meningitis to mucosal infections, while other patients are asymptomatic.

Bruton X-Linked Agammaglobulinemia

Bruton X-linked agammaglobulinemia (XLA) often presents in boys younger than 1 year old, when protective maternal antibody levels have declined. Up to 10% of XLA patients do

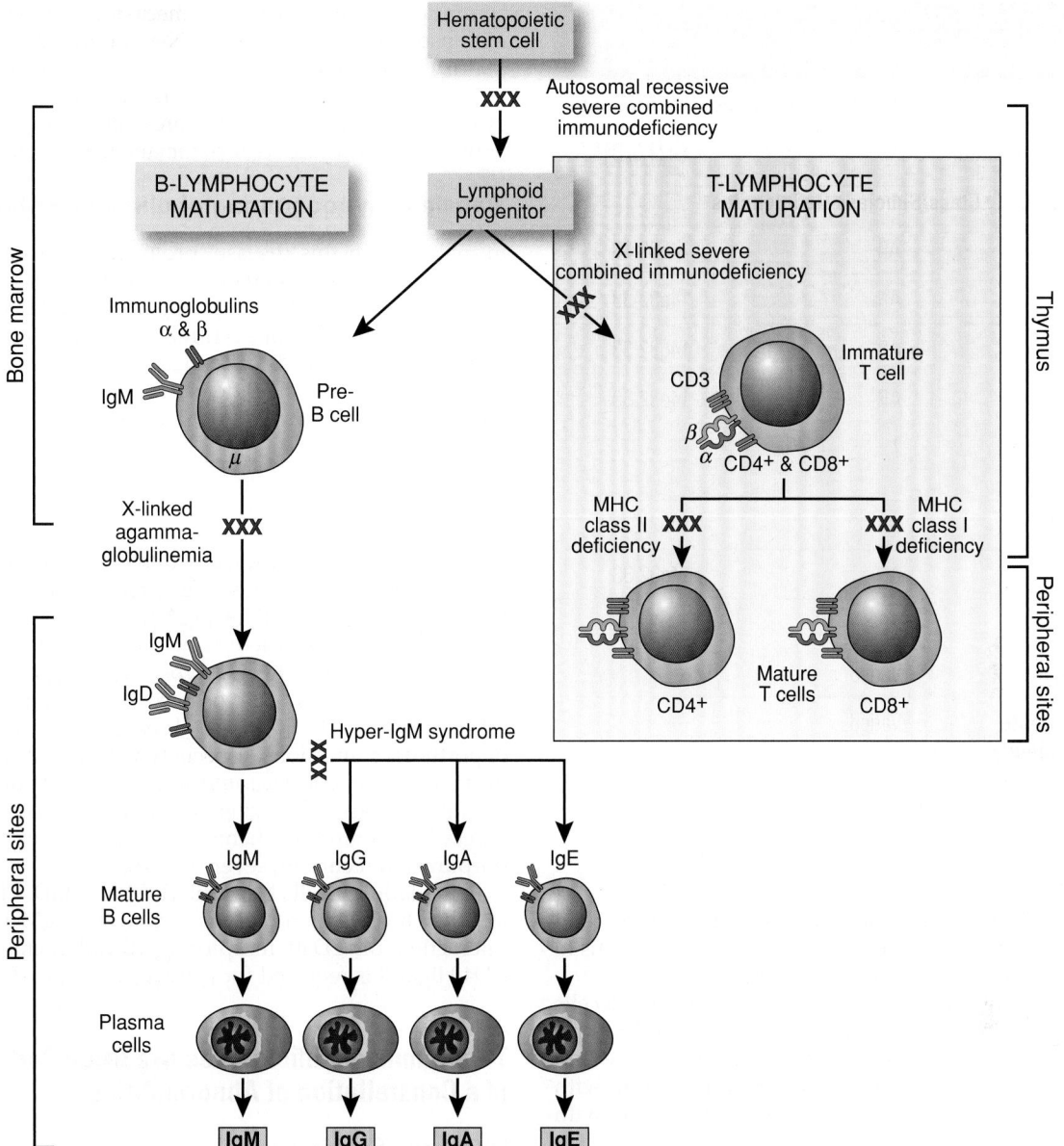

FIGURE 4-21. Hematopoietic stem cells give rise to lymphoid progenitor cells that, in a predetermined manner, populate either the bone marrow or thymus. More than 100 primary immunodeficiency disorders have been characterized at the genetic and/or molecular levels. In a number of immunodeficiency disorders, a discrete molecular defect results in a form of "maturational arrest" in the development of fully differentiated and functional lymphocytes. The identification of specific molecular lesions has hastened diagnostic evaluation and mechanistic understanding.

not present until they are teenagers, and recent studies suggest that perhaps 10% of adults diagnosed with "common variable immunodeficiency (CVID)" (see below) actually have XLA. Patients develop recurrent infections of mucosal surfaces (e.g., sinusitis, bronchitis), pyoderma, meningitis and septicemia. Severe hypogammaglobulinemia involves all Ig isotypes. Some patients develop viral hepatitis or chronic enterovirus infections of the CNS or large joints. Immunization with live attenuated poliovirus can lead to paralytic poliomyelitis. About 1/3 of XLA patients suffer from a poorly understood form of arthritis, possibly caused by enteroviruses or *Ureaplasma.*

There are no mature B cells in peripheral blood or plasma cells in lymphoid tissues. Pre-B cells, however, can be

detected. The genetic defect, on the long arm of the X chromosomes (Xq21.22), inactivates the gene for B-cell tyrosine kinase (Bruton tyrosine kinase), an enzyme critical to B-lymphocyte maturation (Table 4-5).

Selective IgA Deficiency

This is the most common primary immunodeficiency syndrome. It is characterized by normal serum levels of IgM and IgG and low serum (<7 mg/dL) and secretory concentrations of IgA. Incidence ranges from 1:18,000 in Japan to 1:400 among northern Europeans. Patients are often asymptomatic but may present with chronic or recurrent respiratory or gastrointestinal infections. They often develop allergies,

TABLE 4-5

PRIMARY HUMORAL IMMUNODEFICIENCY DISORDERS

Disease	Mode of Inheritance	Locus/Gene
Agammaglobulinemia	XL	Xq21.3/BTK
Selective Antibody Class/Subclass Deficiencies		
γ1 isotype	AR	14q32.33
γ2 isotype	AR	14q32.33
Partial γ3 isotype	AR	14q32.33
γ4 isotype	AR	14q32.33
IgG subclass ± IgA deficiency	?	
α1 isotype	AR	14q32.33
α2 isotype	AR	14q32.33
ε isotype	AR	14q32.33
IgA Deficiency	Varied	—
Common Variable Immunodeficiency	Varied	—

AR = autosomal recessive; *BTK* = Bruton tyrosine kinase; Ig = immunoglobulin; XL = X-linked.

autoimmune diseases and collagen vascular disorders and are at risk for allergic, occasionally anaphylactic, reactions to IgA-containing transfused blood products.

Patients with IgA deficiency have peripheral blood B cells that coexpress IgA, IgM and IgD; their varied and poorly understood defects result in an inability to synthesize and secrete IgA (Table 4-5). There may be a common origin with CVID (see below). Some cases have been associated with drug exposures (e.g., phenytoin, D-penicillamine) and some with deletions or defects in chromosome 18. Patients with concomitant IgG subclass deficiencies are more likely to be clinically affected.

Common Variable Immunodeficiency

CVID is a heterogenous group of disorders with severe hypogammaglobulinemia and attendant infections (Table 4-5), apparently due to a variety of defects in B-lymphocyte maturation or T cells that regulate B-lymphocyte maturation. Some relatives of patients with CVID have selective IgA deficiency. Affected patients present with recurrent severe pyogenic infections, especially pneumonia and diarrhea, the latter often due to infection with *Giardia lamblia*. Recurrent attacks of herpes simplex virus are common; herpes zoster develops in 1/5 of patients. CVID appears years to decades after birth, with a mean age at onset of 25 years. It occurs in between 1:50,000 and 1:200,000 people. Inheritance patterns vary. CVID features several maturational and regulatory defects of the immune system. Cancers are increased in CVID, including a 50-fold greater incidence of gastric cancer. Interestingly, lymphoma is 300 times more

common in women with this disease than in affected men. Malabsorption due to lymphoid hyperplasia and inflammatory bowel diseases occurs more frequently than in the general population. Patients are also more susceptible to other autoimmune disorders, including hemolytic anemia, neutropenia, thrombocytopenia and pernicious anemia.

Transient Hypogammaglobulinemia of Infancy

In infants with this disease, prolonged hypogammaglobulinemia occurs once maternal antibodies reach their nadir. Some affected children develop recurrent infections and require therapy, but all eventually produce antibodies. The infants have mature B cells that are temporarily unable to produce antibodies. The defect is not well understood but may represent delayed helper T-cell signal-generating capacity.

Hyper-IgM Syndrome

Hyper-IgM (HIM) syndrome is often classified as a humoral immunodeficiency because Ig production is disordered. Patients have subnormal IgG, IgA and IgE levels and elevated IgM concentrations. There is an X-linked form that results from defects in CD40 ligand (type 1 hyper-IgM) and an autosomal recessive form due to defects in CD40 (type 3 hyper-IgM). Infants with X-linked disease suffer pyogenic and opportunistic infections, especially with *Pneumocystis jiroveci* (formerly *Pneumocystis carinii*), and also tend to develop autoimmune diseases involving the formed elements of blood, especially autoimmune hemolytic anemia, thrombocytopenic purpura and recurrent, severe neutropenia.

Circulating B cells bear only IgM and IgD. The "switch" to other heavy-chain isotypes from IgD/IgM is defective. Interaction of CD40 receptor on B-cell membranes with CD40 ligand is required for isotype switching (Fig. 4-21).

T-Cell Immunodeficiencies Are Often Part of a Constellation of Abnormalities

DiGeorge Syndrome

In its complete form, DiGeorge syndrome is a severe T-cell immunodeficiency disorder in which serum Igs are reduced due to lack of T-helper activity. Although variable, some infants present with conotruncal great vessel and cardiac defects and severe hypocalcemia (due to hypoparathyroidism). Others show characteristically abnormal facial features. Infants who survive the neonatal period are subject to recurrent and/or chronic viral, bacterial, fungal and protozoal infections.

DiGeorge syndrome is caused by defective development of the third and fourth pharyngeal pouches, which give rise to thymic epithelium and parathyroid glands and influence conotruncal cardiac development. Most patients have a deletion in the long arm of chromosome 22; thus, DiGeorge syndrome is considered to be a form of the "22q11 deletion syndrome." In the absence of functional thymus, T-cell maturation is interrupted at the pre–T-cell stage. The immunologic defect has been corrected by transplanting thymic tissue. Most affected patients have "partial" DiGeorge syndrome, in which a small remnant of thymus is present. With time, many individuals recover T-cell function without treatment. Some individuals with 22q11 mutations suffer only from conotruncal cardiac defects.

Chronic Mucocutaneous Candidiasis

This disease results from impaired T-cell function and is characterized by susceptibility to candidal infections and endocrinopathy (hypoparathyroidism, Addison disease, diabetes mellitus). Most T-cell functions are intact, but the response to *Candida* antigens is deficient.

A series of defects in T-cell development underlie this syndrome. Patients with this disorder react to *Candida* antigens differently from normal individuals. Unlike normal responses in which Th1 (IL-2/IFN-γ) cells predominate and effectively control candidal infections, affected patients mount a Th2 (IL-4/IL-6) helper cell response, which is ineffective in resisting the organism.

Combined Immunodeficiency Diseases Vary in Severity

Severe combined immunodeficiencies are conspicuously heterogenous and are often life-threatening (Table 4-6).

Severe Combined Immunodeficiency

Severe combined immunodeficiency (SCID) encompasses over 20 disorders associated by deficiencies in T-cell and B-cell development and function. Affected patients present in the first few months of life with recurrent, often severe infections, diarrhea and failure to thrive. Some forms of SCID have nonimmunologic developmental defects. SCID is usually fatal within the first year of life unless an immune system can be provided by HSC transplantation.

SCID is consistently marked by defective T-cell development and/or function. In some types, B-cell development is also affected. Since B cells require T-cell–derived signals for optimal antibody production, most patients have defective cellular and humoral immunity. NK-cell development and function are variably affected. Current classifications of SCID include several categories (Table 4-6).

The most common form of SCID in the United States (50% of cases) is due to mutations within *IL2RG*; *IL2RG* encodes the cytokine receptor common γ-chain, which is shared by receptors for IL-2, IL-4, IL-7, IL-9, IL-15 and IL-21. Defects result in complete absence of T cells and NK cells (90% of cases) but normal numbers of B cells. Immunoglobulin production is severely impaired because of the T-cell defect. Signaling downstream of the IL receptors with the common γ-chain requires activation of JAK3 tyrosine kinase (Janus kinase 3). Not surprisingly, T−/−B+/−NK− SCID patients with mutations in *JAK3* have been identified.

MOLECULAR PATHOGENESIS: More than a dozen molecular lesions have been described in T−/−B+/−NK+ SCID patients. For instance, mutations in genes (*CD3D, CD3E, CD3G*) that encode each subunit (δ, ε, γ) of the TCR-associated CD3 complex have been described. These patients all show defects in T-lymphocyte function, but clinical features have varied. Another group of

TABLE 4-6	
SEVERE COMBINED IMMUNODEFICIENCY (SCID): MOLECULAR LESIONS[a]	
Disease	**Locus/Gene**
T−/−B+/−NK−/−	
IL2RG	Cytokine receptor common γ-chain
JAK3	Tyrosine kinase JAK3
T−/−B+/−NK+/−	
CD3D	CD3 complex, δ subunit
CD3E	CD3 complex, ε subunit
CD3G	CD3 complex, γ subunit
CIITA	MHC class II transactivator
RFXANK	MHC class II transactivator
FRX5	MHC class II transactivator
RXAP	MHC class II transactivator
ZAP70	TCR-associated protein of 70 kd
TAP1	Transporter-associated antigen processing 1
TAP2	Transporter-associated antigen processing 2
T−/−B−/−NK−/−	
ADA	Adenosine deaminase
PNP	Purine nucleoside phosphoacylase
T−/−B−/−NK+/−	
RAG1	Recombinase-activating gene 1
RAG2	Recombinase-activating gene 2

[a]This is a partial list of SCID disorders.
MHC = major histocompatibility complex; TCR = T-cell receptor.

T−/−B+/−NK+ SCID patients lack CD4+ T cells in association with various defects in expression of MHC class II molecules. Yet another group of T−/−B+/−NK+ SCID patients are deficient in CD8+ T cells. Among this group of patients, mutations in *ZAP70, TAP1* and *TAP2* have been described. *ZAP70* (TCR-associated protein of 70 kd) is a tyrosine kinase involved in TCR signaling; *TAP1* and *TAP2* are required for shuttling of cytosolic peptide onto naive HLA class I molecules for subsequent presentation to TCRs.

Mutations in the genes for enzymes in the purine nucleotide salvage pathway, adenosine deaminase (*ADA*) and purine nucleoside phosphorylase (*PNP*), result in T−/−B−/−NK− SCID. Accumulation of toxic purine metabolites leads to death of immature, proliferating lymphocytes (and other cell types). ADA deficiency accounts for 15% of all SCID patients in the United States. PNP deficiency is very rare.

Rare patients with T−/−B−/−NK+ SCID possess mutations within genes for DNA-binding proteins involved in

Ig and TCR gene rearrangement. Some patients suffer from radiation sensitivity in addition to immunodeficiency.

Molecular lesions are identified in approximately 95% of patients with SCID, suggesting that additional molecular lesions account for the remaining 5%.

AUTOIMMUNITY

The Occurrence of Autoimmune Disease Implies That the Immune System Fails to Discriminate Adequately between Self and Nonself

Once considered an abnormal response that invariably caused disease, autoimmunity is in fact a physiologic process that helps regulate the immune system. When "normal" regulatory mechanisms are in some way disrupted, uncontrolled autoantibody production or abnormal cell–cell recognition leads to tissue injury and autoimmune disease. Specific autoantibodies may be present and useful in diagnosing autoimmune diseases, but in order to conclude causality, an autoimmune reaction (humoral or cellular) must be integral to the disease process. Autoimmune diseases may be organ specific or generalized. Relatively few diseases (e.g., Hashimoto thyroiditis, type 1 diabetes, SLE) clearly fit this rigorous criterion.

Immune tolerance occurs when there is no measurable (or clinically deleterious) immune response to specific (usually self) antigen. An abnormal or injurious autoimmune response to self-antigens implies loss of immune tolerance. Tolerance to self-antigens appears to be an active process and requires contact between self-antigens and immune cells. In fetal life, tolerance is readily established to antigens that trigger vigorous immune responses in adults. Several mechanisms induce and maintain tolerance, actively and continuously. Thus, in tolerance, potentially harmful immune responses are constantly blocked or aborted. Induction of tolerance to an antigen is partly related to the dose of antigen to which cells are exposed.

Central and peripheral mechanisms both participate. In **central tolerance,** self-reactive immature T and B lymphocytes are "deleted" or changed during their maturation in the "central" thymus and bone marrow, respectively. Developing T cells that recognize self-peptides in the context of compatible MHC molecules with high binding affinity undergo apoptosis. These T cells are said to have been "negatively selected." The AIRE protein (autoimmune regulator) is involved in expression of peripheral tissue-restricted self-antigens within the thymus, and so is important in central expression of peripheral self-antigens to which the individual becomes tolerant. Mutations in *AIRE* cause an autoimmune polyendocrinopathy.

In the bone marrow, a similar negative selection process involves B cells. In addition, engagement of self-antigens by developing marrow B cells can reset antigen receptor gene rearrangement through a process called "receptor editing." These reprogrammed B cells thus do not recognize self. CD4+ regulatory T cells also develop. **Peripheral tolerance** is important in regulating T cells that escape intrathymic negative selection. Mature T lymphocytes are held in check in the periphery via **anergy,** suppression and/or activation-induced cell death. Anergy occurs when T lymphocytes bind antigen presented by APCs in the absence of the "second

signal," which is normally provided by CD80/B7-1 and CD86/B7-2 on the APC and CD28 on the T cell. Downstream T-cell inactivation/unresponsiveness (anergy) is mediated by at least two mechanisms. Immune responses are suppressed by the population of regulatory T cells (T_{reg}, noted above) generated in response to exposure to self-antigens. These T_{reg}s are CD4+, constitutively express CD25 (β-chain of high-affinity IL-2 receptor) and express FOXp3 transcription factor. Mutations and polymorphisms affecting *CD25*, IL-2 or FOXp3 result in autoimmune disorders. Finally, CD4+ T cells and self-reactive B cells can be deleted by several activation-initiated mechanisms.

Theories of Autoimmunity

There are multiple explanations for the development of autoimmune disease, which are not mutually exclusive.

Inaccessible Self-Antigens
An immune reaction may develop against self-antigens not normally "accessible" to the immune system. Intracellular antigens are generally not exposed or released until infection and/or tissue injury "releases" or "exposes" them. At that time, an immune response develops (e.g., antibodies against spermatozoa, lens tissue and myelin). Whether such autoantibodies directly induce injury is another matter. For example, there is no evidence that antisperm antibodies induce generalized injury, aside from a localized orchitis. Thus, autoantibodies may form against normally "sequestered" antigens but appear to be pathogenic infrequently.

Abnormal T-Cell Function
Autoimmune reactions may develop due to T-cell abnormalities. As noted above, several mutations and/or polymorphisms are linked to autoimmune disease. Altered numbers or functional activities of helper or suppressor T cells could thus influence one's ability to mount an immune response. Defects, particularly in suppressor T cells, occur in many autoimmune diseases (see above). Lymphocytotropic antibodies also occur in patients with SLE. Abnormal suppressor T-cell function characterizes other autoimmune diseases, including primary biliary cirrhosis, thyroiditis, multiple sclerosis, myasthenia gravis, rheumatoid arthritis and scleroderma. The key question is whether these alterations in suppressor T-cell function cause these diseases or are epiphenomena. Defects in suppressor T-cell activity also occur in people who do not have any evidence of autoimmune disease.

Helper T cells are defined by their role in antigen-specific B-cell activation, and their function may also be abnormal in autoimmune disease. Helper T-cell tolerance is most likely induced by low doses of antigen. These cells become autoreactive in autoimmune diseases.

Epigenetic modulation, as in DNA hypomethylation caused by drugs and other agents, is a type of environmentally influenced upregulation of leukocyte function antigen-1 (LFA-1) and B-cell activation and is independent of antigen. An example of T-cell autoreactivity and loss of antigen specificity is drug-induced lupus. It is also possible to "break" tolerance by altering an antigen, so that helper cells are activated and trigger B cells. This occurs when an antigen is modified by partial degradation or by complexing with a carrier protein. In some rheumatic diseases, antibodies recognize partially degraded connective tissue proteins such as collagen or elastin. In some drug-induced hemolytic anemias, antibody against the drug causes hemolysis when the drug binds to erythrocyte membranes.

Molecular Mimicry

Helper T-cell tolerance may also be overcome if foreign antigens elicit antibodies that cross-react with self-antigens. In this case, helper T cells act "correctly": they do not induce autoantibodies. Rather, the efferent limb of the immune response is abnormal. Thus, in rheumatic heart disease, antibodies against streptococcal bacterial antigens cross-react with antigens from cardiac muscle, which is called **molecular mimicry**.

Polyclonal B-Cell Activation

In polyclonal B-cell activation, B lymphocytes are directly activated by complex substances that contain many antigenic sites (e.g., bacterial cell walls and viruses). Bacterial, viral and parasitic infections may thus stimulate development of rheumatoid factor in rheumatoid arthritis, anti-DNA antibodies in SLE and other autoantibodies. Such scattergun stimulation of antibody responses may also lead to autoantibodies.

Tissue Injury in Autoimmune Diseases

Autoimmune diseases have traditionally been considered to be prototypical immune complex diseases, with immune complexes forming in the circulation or in tissues. Thus, type II (cytotoxic) and type III (immune complex) hypersensitivity reactions are implicated in tissue injury in many. These hypersensitivity reactions explain most autoimmune tissue injury, but of course the story is more complicated. In some autoimmune diseases, T cells sensitized to self-antigens (such as thyroglobulin) cause tissue injury directly (type IV reaction), but the extent is not clear.

In addition, in ADCC, antibodies against an antigen expressed at the cell membrane lead to destruction of that cell. Thus, antibodies against parietal cell H^+/K^+-ATPase contribute to the pathogenesis of atrophic gastritis. However, many people have antiparietal cell antibodies but not gastritis.

Not all autoantibodies cause disease via cytotoxicity. In **antireceptor antibody diseases,** such as Graves disease and myasthenia gravis, antibody binds a receptor but the disease process reflects either activation or inactivation of the receptor, rather than cell loss. In Graves disease, autoantibody against the TSH receptor acts as an agonist to simulate thyroid hormone production, while in myasthenia gravis the autoantibody either prevents acetylcholine binding to its receptor or leads to damage of the receptor, thereby impairing neuromuscular synaptic transmission. Anti-insulin receptor antibodies in acanthosis nigricans and ataxia telangiectasia cause some patients to develop diabetes that entails extreme insulin resistance.

Type III hypersensitivity reactions (immune complex disease) explain tissue injury in some autoimmune diseases (e.g., SLE). DNA–anti-DNA complexes formed in the circulation (or at local sites) deposit in tissues, where they induce inflammation and injury (e.g., vasculitis, glomerulonephritis). Similarly, rheumatoid arthritis, scleroderma, polymyositis/dermatomyositis and Sjögren syndrome are all characterized by immune phenomena and classified as "collagen vascular diseases" (see Chapter 11). Their clinical manifestations are systemic, and many organs and tissues are typically involved. By contrast, cytotoxic (type II–mediated) autoimmune reactions are, for the most part, organ specific.

TRANSPLANTATION IMMUNOLOGY

Donor MHC-encoded antigens are immunogenic molecules that can stimulate rejection of transplanted tissues. Optimal graft survival occurs when recipient and donor are closely matched for histocompatibility antigens. In practice, an exact HLA match is uncommon, except between monozygotic twins. Thus, immunosuppressive therapy and vigilant monitoring of graft function are required after organ transplantation. Therapeutic advances have greatly improved transplant success rates, even when there is a degree of histoincompatibility. When host-versus-graft immune reactions (rejection) occur, a combination of immune mechanisms may injure the graft.

Both T-cell–mediated and antibody-mediated reactions participate in transplant rejection. Within the graft, antigen-presenting cells, specifically those bearing foreign MHC molecules, are recognized by host CD8+ cytotoxic T lymphocytes, which mediate tissue injury, and host CD4+ T helper cells, which augment antibody production, induce IFN-γ production and activate macrophages. In turn, IFN-γ enhances MHC expression, amplifying the immune response and resulting tissue injury. Host APCs also process foreign donor antigens, leading to CD4+-mediated delayed-type hypersensitivity and CD4+-mediated antibody production.

Solid organ transplant rejection reactions are usually categorized as "hyperacute," "acute" and "chronic" based on the clinical tempo of the response and pathophysiologic mechanism involved. However, in practice, features often overlap, creating diagnostic ambiguity. Categorization of transplant rejection is further complicated by the toxicity of immunosuppressive drugs, the potential for mechanical problems (e.g., vascular thrombosis) and recurrence of original disease (e.g., some types of glomerulonephritis). The next sections illustrate rejection in the context of renal transplantation. Similar responses occur in other transplanted tissues, although rejection as applied to each tissue type has its own unique features.

Hyperacute Rejection Is a Sudden Reaction That Occurs within Minutes of Transplantation

Hyperacute rejection of a kidney may be so rapid as to occur intraoperatively and manifests as a sudden cessation of urine output, darkening of the graft and rapid development of fever and pain at the graft site. This form of rejection is mediated by preformed anti-HLA antibodies and complement activation products, including chemotactic and other inflammatory mediators. Hyperacute rejection is catastrophic, necessitating prompt surgical removal of the grafted kidney. Histologic features include vascular congestion, fibrin–platelet thrombi within capillaries, neutrophilic vasculitis with fibrinoid necrosis, prominent interstitial edema and neutrophil infiltrates (Fig. 4-22A). Fortunately, hyperacute rejection is distinctly uncommon when appropriate pretransplantation antibody screening has been performed.

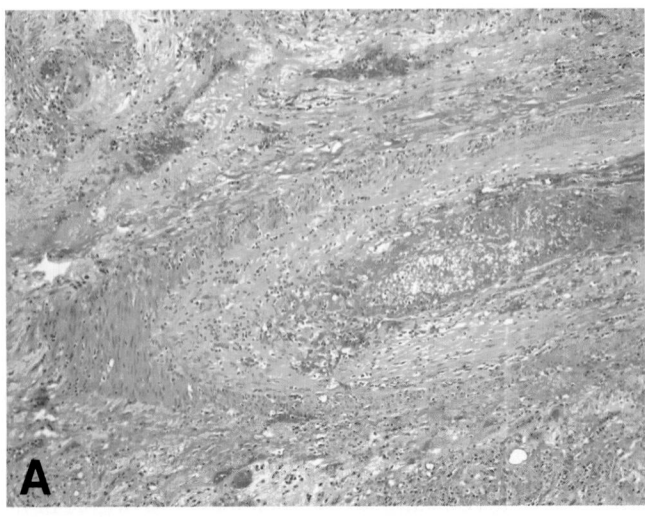

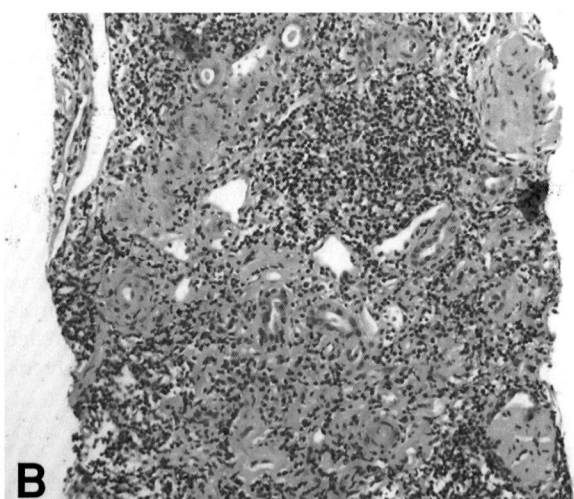

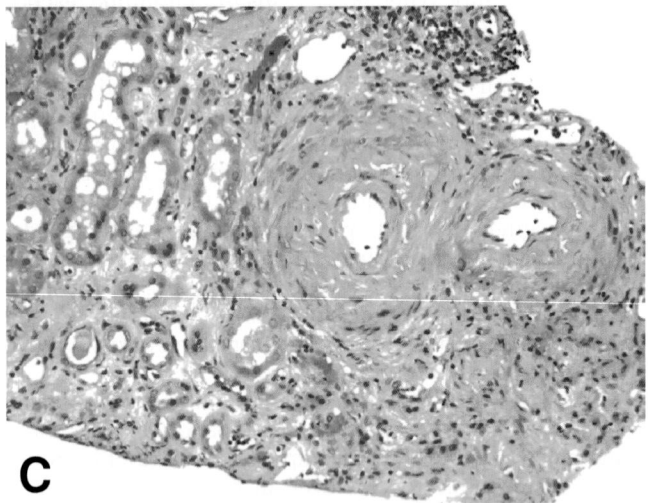

FIGURE 4-22. There are three major forms of renal transplant rejection. A. Hyperacute rejection occurs within minutes to hours after transplantation and is characterized, in part, by neutrophilic vasculitis, intravascular fibrin thrombi and neutrophilic infiltrates. **B.** Acute cellular rejection occurs within weeks to months after transplantation and is characterized by tubular damage and mononuclear leukocyte infiltration. **C.** Chronic rejection is observed months to years after transplantation and is characterized by tubular atrophy, patchy interstitial mononuclear cell infiltrates and fibrosis. In this example, arteries show fibrointimal thickening.

Acute Rejection Usually Occurs Weeks to Months after Organ Transplantation

It is characterized by the abrupt onset of azotemia and oliguria, which may be associated with fever and graft tenderness. Acute rejection typically involves both cell-mediated and humoral mechanisms of tissue damage. If detected early, acute rejection can be reversed with immunosuppressive therapy. Needle biopsy is often needed to differentiate acute rejection from acute tubular necrosis or toxicity associated with immunosuppressive drugs. Findings vary depending on whether the process is mainly cellular or humoral. In acute cellular rejection, interstitial lymphocyte and macrophage infiltration, edema, lymphocytic tubulitis and tubular necrosis occur (Fig. 4-22B). In the acute humoral form, which is sometimes called "rejection vasculitis," vascular damage predominates, with arteritis, fibrinoid necrosis and thrombosis. Blood vessel involvement is an ominous sign since it usually signifies resistance to therapy.

Chronic Rejection Follows Transplantation by Months to Years

Affected patients typically develop progressive azotemia, oliguria, hypertension and weight gain over a period of

months. Chronic rejection may be due to repeated episodes of cellular rejection, either asymptomatic or clinically apparent. Arterial and arteriolar intimal thickening cause vascular stenosis or obstruction, thickened glomerular capillary walls, tubular atrophy and interstitial fibrosis (Fig. 4-22C). There are scattered interstitial mononuclear infiltrates. Tubules contain proteinaceous casts. Chronic rejection represents an advanced state of organ injury and does not respond to therapy. Acute and chronic rejection may overlap histologically and they may vary in degree, so that unambiguous pathologic distinction may not be possible.

In Graft-Versus-Host Disease, Donor Lymphocytes React against the Graft Recipient

The advent of transplantation of allogeneic (donor) bone marrow or HSCs harvested from peripheral blood makes possible treatment of diseases that had previously been considered terminal or untreatable. In order for the transplanted marrow/HSCs to engraft in the new host, the recipient's bone marrow and immune system must be "conditioned" (usually ablated) by cytotoxic drugs, sometimes plus radiation. If the graft includes immunocompetent lymphocytes, these donor cells may react to—"reject"—host tissues, causing graft-versus-host disease (GVHD). GVHD can also occur if a severely immunodeficient patient receives a solid organ containing many "passenger" lymphocytes or is transfused with blood products containing viable HLA-incompatible lymphocytes.

The major organs affected in GVHD are skin, gastrointestinal tract and liver. The skin and intestine show mononuclear cell infiltrates and epithelial cell necrosis. The liver displays periportal inflammation, damaged bile ducts and liver cell injury. Clinically, acute GVHD manifests as rash, diarrhea, abdominal cramps, anemia and liver dysfunction. Chronic GVHD is characterized by dermal sclerosis, sicca syndrome (see above: dry eyes and mouth due to chronic inflammation of lacrimal and salivary glands) and immunodeficiency. Treatment of GVHD requires immunosuppression. Patients, especially those with chronic GVHD, may be at a higher risk for potentially life-threatening opportunistic infections (e.g., invasive aspergillosis).

Human Immunodeficiency Virus and Acquired Immunodeficiency Syndrome

THE APPEARANCE OF AIDS

AIDS is the most common immunodeficiency state worldwide. It is mainly caused by human immunodeficiency virus type 1 (HIV-1), although a small minority of patients, primarily in western Africa, are infected with HIV-2. People infected with HIV-1, if untreated, develop many immunologic defects, the most devastating of which is severely impaired cellular immunity, leading to catastrophic opportunistic infections. HIV-1 infection progresses from an initial asymptomatic state to severe immune depletion in overt AIDS. This continuum is called HIV/AIDS. Infection of CD4$^+$ (helper) T lymphocytes by HIV-1 causes depletion of this cell population, leading to impaired immune function and dysregulation. Because they cannot mount new immune responses, especially cell-mediated immune responses, patients with AIDS usually die of opportunistic infections, principally with mycobacteria, viruses or fungi. There is also a high incidence of malignant tumors, mainly B-cell lymphomas and Kaposi sarcoma. Finally, HIV-1 infection in the CNS causes HIV-associated neurologic disease (HAND), which ranges from minor cognitive or motor disorders to frank dementia.

Early Human HIV Infections Were Unreported

The onset of this human epidemic is uncertain, but unreported human HIV infections almost certainly occurred at least as early as 1902. The North American epidemic probably began in Haiti in 1966 and a single transmission event led to its spread to the United States about 5 years later. By the late 1970s, clusters of strange infectious diseases in New York and Miami among men who have sex with men (MSM), intravenous drug users and Haitians are now recognized as having been caused by HIV. AIDS was first reported in the United States in 1981, as *P. carinii* (now called *P. jiroveci*) pneumonia in MSM. By 1982, these unusual infections were linked to Kaposi sarcoma (KS) and understood to reflect an acquired immune defect. Thus, "AIDS" was coined.

It became clear that AIDS was spread by contact with blood or body fluids from infected people: largely MSM and intravenous drug users who shared needles, but also recipients of blood and blood products, especially hemophiliacs, and heterosexual contacts and infants born to female drug users. Once the responsible virus, now called HIV-1, was identified (1983), it became possible to develop a serologic test to detect antibodies to HIV-1 (1985), which in turn allowed accurate diagnosis and screening of donated blood to prevent transmission by blood and its derivatives.

 **EPIDEMIOLOGY:** AIDS originated in sub-Saharan Africa, and at least 3 different viral strains were transmitted from chimpanzees to humans. It is now a worldwide pandemic due to the ease of international travel and enhanced population mobility, which in many societies coincided with a rapid increase in sexual activity and sexually transmitted diseases. Presently, the WHO estimates that 34 million people carry HIV worldwide, with 2.7 million new infections and 1.8 million deaths yearly. The death rate peaked in 2005 and has declined since then. Annual new infections peaked in 1997, at 3.3 million, and have dropped subsequently. As antiretroviral therapy (ART) reaches more people, the total number of people living with HIV infection continues to increase.

The highest prevalence is in sub-Saharan Africa, but no country is free of HIV-1. MSM once were by far the largest group of HIV-positive people in the United States and still account for most newly infected cases. In some other parts of the world, transmission may be largely by heterosexual contact or via intravenous drug users. Most AIDS patients in the United States are men, although the prevalence of HIV-1 infection in women continues to increase.

Sub-Saharan Africa, which has suffered more from the ravages of AIDS than other regions, has made progress in lowering the rate of new infections and AIDS-related deaths. However, in some parts of sub-Saharan Africa, 20% of the population is HIV positive. African patients largely acquire HIV infection by heterosexual intercourse or via maternal–child transmission.

Further, although new HIV infections and HIV-related deaths have declined in the Western world and sub-Saharan Africa, the AIDS epidemic continues to grow in the Middle East, Eastern Europe and parts of central and eastern Asia. Multiple factors contribute to the sustained increases in HIV/AIDS in these areas.

As the epidemic matures and stabilizes in many parts of the world, new issues arise. Thus, the affected (i.e., infected) populations are aging. Already, 15% of new infections occur in people over 50, and by 2015, it is estimated that half of HIV-positive patients will be 50 years old or older. These changing demographics, which reflect both lifestyles and improvements in therapies, present their own challenges as CNS infections and therapy-related complications become increasingly important.

HIV Is Transmitted by Contact with Blood and Certain Body Fluids, and through Sexual Activity

HIV is present in blood, semen, vaginal secretions, breast milk and cerebrospinal fluid of infected patients. HIV is present in most of these fluids in lymphocytes and as free virus. It is transmitted via these fluids to sexual partners, drug users who share needles and recipients of blood products and via breast milk to nursing infants.

Infection is transmitted by a single virus or virus-infected cell in about 80% of cases, the remainder of new infections reflecting multiple viruses or infected cells. Virus in semen enters through tears in the rectal mucosa, particularly in anal-receptive MSM partners. It can also infect rectal epithelial cells directly. In heterosexual contact, male-to-female transmission is more likely than the reverse, perhaps because there is more HIV in semen than in vaginal fluid. Additionally, genital lesions facilitate virus entry. HIV infections are lower in circumcised men, perhaps because the foreskin is less well keratinized than other parts of the penis and has a higher concentration of cutaneous dendritic cells (Langerhans cells).

HIV-1 is not transmitted by nonsexual, casual exposure to infected people. Further, fewer than 1% of health care workers who sustained "needle sticks" or other accidental exposures to blood from HIV-positive patients became infected with HIV-1. Immediate postexposure antiretroviral prophylaxis is available (see http://www.cdc.gov/hiv/resources/guidelines for details).

HIV-1 BIOLOGY AND BEHAVIOR

The Biology of HIV-1 Determines Its Success as a Pathogen

 **MOLECULAR PATHOGENESIS:** HIV-1 is a member of the lentivirus family of retroviruses. Animal lentiviruses have been recognized for a century, but human lentiviruses have been known for less than three decades.

HIV-1 virions carry two identical 9.7-kb copies of the virus single-stranded RNA genome plus some key enzymes, such as reverse transcriptase (RNA-dependent DNA polymerase, RT) and integrase (IN), that are needed early in the infectious cycle (see below). These are packaged in a core of viral proteins. The outermost layer, the envelope, is derived from the host cell membrane, in which are found virally encoded Env glycoproteins (gp120 and gp41). In addition to the *gag*, *pol* and *env* genes present in all replication-competent RNA viruses, HIV-1 has six other genes that code for proteins that control viral replication and certain host cell functions. Mononuclear phagocytes and CD4+ helper T lymphocytes are the virus's main targets, although B lymphocytes, astrocytes, endothelial cells and intestinal epithelium can also be infected.

The replicative cycle of HIV-1 is depicted in Fig. 4-23.

1. **Binding:** Free HIV or an infected lymphocyte can transmit the virus to an uninfected cell. HIV gp120, either on a free virus or on the surface of an infected cell, binds the CD4 molecule on the surface of helper T lymphocytes and other cells, plus specific β-chemokine receptors. The most important of these chemokine receptors are CCR5 (on many phagocytic cells) and CXCR4 (on T lymphocytes). Virus binding to both CD4 and a chemokine receptor mediates HIV entry. However, HIV-1 can enter dendritic cells (DCs) via C-type lectin receptors (e.g., DC-SIGN). There is also evidence that CCR3 may be important in HIV-1 infection in the CNS (see below) and elsewhere.

2. **Internalization:** Upon binding to CD4, gp120 undergoes a conformational change, to uncover its CCR5 (or CXCR4) binding domain. Thereupon, viral gp41 forms a loop, fusing virus and cell membranes. The virus capsid, genome and those enzymes needed for the early phase of the infectious cycle enter the cell.

3. **DNA synthesis:** The virus genome and viral RT and IN enter the cytosol and reverse transcription occurs. HIV-1 RT has several functions and is a key target for ART. It reverse-transcribes HIV-1 RNA into a complementary DNA (cDNA) copy. As it does this, it digests the RNA it has just reverse-transcribed. RT then acts as a DNA-dependent DNA polymerase and synthesizes a second DNA strand complementary to the first. The resulting double-stranded DNA version of the HIV-1 genome is called the provirus. *One critical function that this versatile RT lacks is an editing capacity. There is, consequently, a very high error rate in this whole process.* Consequently, viral replication entails an extremely high mutation rate. While this results in a high percentage of defective or noninfectious virus particles, it also results in rapid viral adaptation—and so resistance—to therapies. This characteristic of HIV also leads to rapid evolution of the virus after it enters the host. Thus, coreceptor usage, envelope antigenicity and other features of the virus may change substantially, allowing adaptation to a changing host environment.

4. **Integration:** Once proviral DNA has entered the nucleus, HIV-1 IN catalyzes provirus cDNA integration into the host genome. HIV-1 genomes therefore remain in the cell as long as the cell survives and are replicated along with host chromosomes. As tissue phagocytes and memory T cells are very long-lived, some experts estimate that even if total suppression of HIV-1 replication were achieved, over 60 years would be needed for infected cells to die off. Also, some replication occurs even with the most effective ART regiments.

5. **Replication:** Viral RNA is reproduced by transcriptional activation of the integrated HIV provirus, a process that, for example, for T cells, requires "activation" of the infected cell plus certain inducible host transcription factors, especially nuclear factor-κB (NFκB).

6. **Dissemination:** To complete its cycle, nascent virus is assembled in the cytoplasm just beneath the cell membrane and disseminated to other target cells. This is accomplished either by fusion of an infected cell with an uninfected one or by budding of virions from the plasma membrane of infected cells (Fig. 4-24).

The mechanism by which HIV kills infected T lymphocytes is incompletely understood. Virus-induced apoptosis and autophagy may be involved. Other possibilities include immune clearance of infected cells and the actions of secondary mediators such as cytokines. Whatever the mechanism(s), there is a clear association between increasing viral burden and declining CD4+ lymphocyte counts.

HIV-1 persists, effectively, for the lifetime of the host. Even in the face of low or undetectable plasma virus levels (see below), a latent or quiescent form of the virus remains

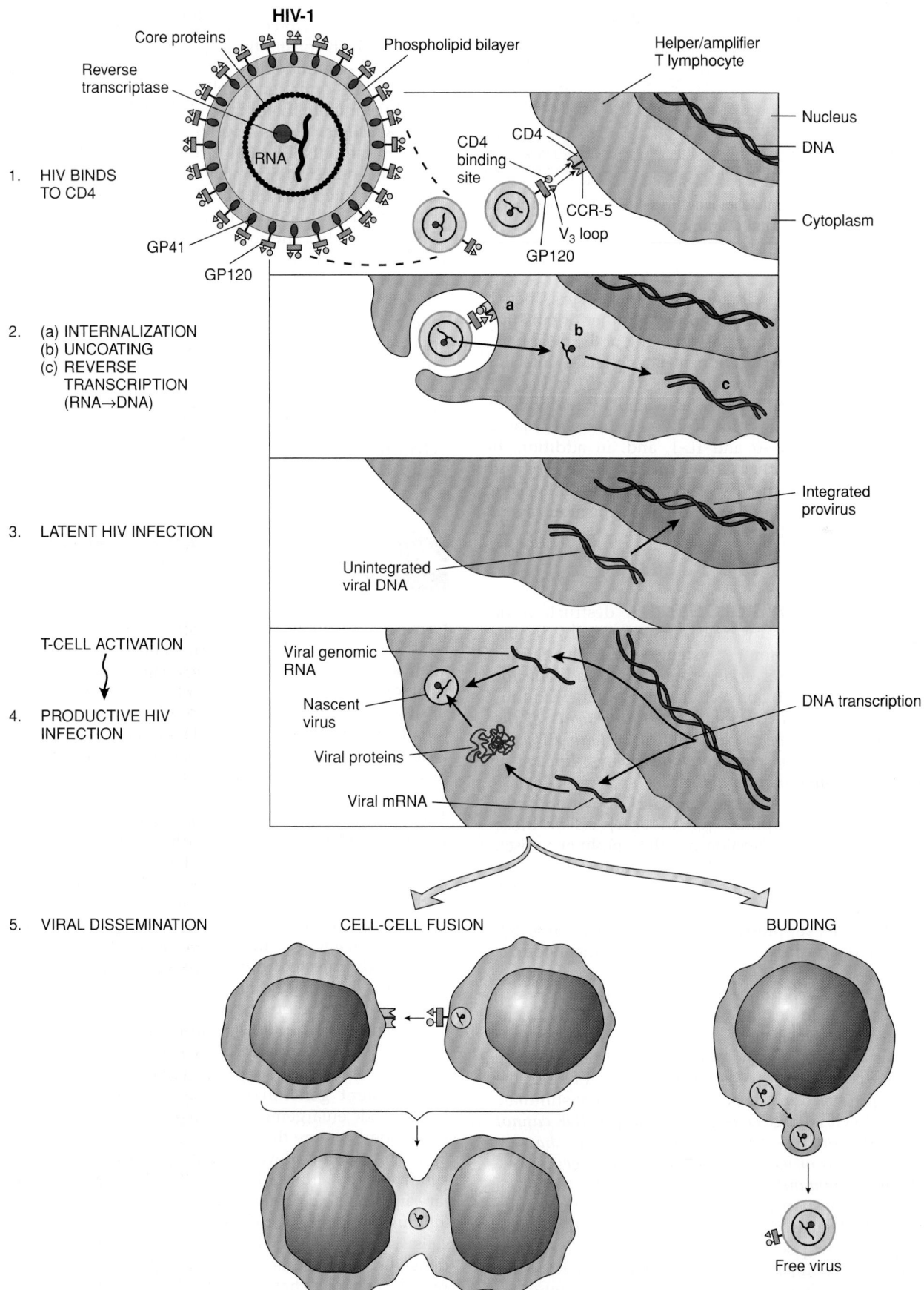

FIGURE 4-23. **The life cycle of human immunodeficiency virus-1 (HIV-1) is a multistep process that includes (1) binding CD4 receptor in conjunction with chemokine receptor (e.g., CCR5); (2) internalization, uncoating and reverse transcription; (3) integration into host DNA as a provirus where it persists in a state of latency; (4) replication in concert with host T-cell activation; and (5) dissemination.**

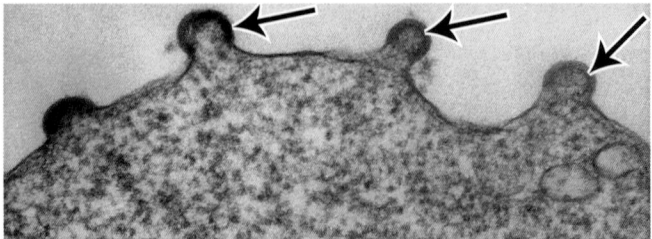

FIGURE 4-24. Human immunodeficiency virus-1 (HIV-1) virions can be seen budding from infected cells (*arrows*).

in long-lived memory T cells and tissue phagocytes. There is also evidence that the CNS and possibly other organs may serve as a reservoir for potential reseeding of the periphery.

Initiation of viral replication in latent HIV-1 infection depends on induction of host proteins during T-cell activation. Viral transcription may be activated by many T-cell mitogens and cytokines produced by monocyte/macrophages, including TNF-α and IL-1, and, in addition, by proteins produced by other viruses that infect patients with AIDS, such as herpesvirus, EBV, adenovirus and CMV. Thus, immune system activation by a variety of infectious agents may promote HIV replication.

PATHOPHYSIOLOGY: The destruction of CD4+ T cells by HIV-1 can essentially disable the entire immune system because this subset of lymphocytes exerts critical regulatory and effector functions that involve both cellular and humoral immunity. *Thus, in typical AIDS patients, all elements of the immune system are eventually crippled, including T cells, B cells, NK cells, the monocyte/macrophage lineage of cells and immunoglobulin production.*

Of the two functional types of CD4+ T lymphocytes (i.e., helper and amplifier [or inducer] cells), those affected first in HIV infection are the amplifier subset. Eventually, total CD4+ lymphocyte counts fall to less than 500 cells/μL, and helper-to-suppressor T-cell ratios decline from a normal of 2.0 to as little as 0.5. Numbers of CD8+ (cytotoxic/suppressor) cells are variable, although in AIDS, most of these cells seem to be of the cytotoxic variety.

Defects in T-cell function are manifested by weak responses in skin testing with a variety of antigens (delayed hypersensitivity) and impaired proliferative responses to mitogens and antigens in vitro. Moreover, the deficiency of CD4+ cells reduces levels of IL-2, the cytokine produced in response to antigens that stimulate cytotoxic T-cell killing. *Thus, patients with AIDS cannot generate the antigen-specific cytotoxic T cells that are required to clear viruses and other infectious agents.*

Humoral immunity is also abnormal. Production of antibodies in response to specific antigenic stimulation is markedly decreased, often to less than 10% of normal. B cells also show poor proliferative responses in vitro to mitogens and antigens. Yet, sera of patients with AIDS usually show high levels of polyclonal immunoglobulins, autoantibodies and immune complexes. This apparent paradox is probably explained by the concurrent infection

with polyclonal B-cell–activating viruses (e.g., EBV or CMV), which constantly stimulate B cells nonspecifically to produce immunoglobulins. Lack of CD4+ lymphocytes impairs the cytotoxic T-cell proliferation that normally would eliminate B cells infected with EBV.

NK-cell activity is severely decreased in AIDS as well. Since these cells kill both virus-infected cells and tumor cells, this defect may contribute to the malignant tumors and viral infections that plague these patients. Suppression of NK-cell activity is related both to a decrease in NK-cell number and to reduction in IL-2 levels, owing to a loss of CD4+ cells.

Lentiviruses tend to target macrophages, and infected macrophages may serve as reservoirs for dissemination of the virus. Interestingly, some macrophages express CD4 on their surfaces. Unlike T lymphocytes, which are killed by HIV, infected macrophages generally survive. Macrophages from patients with AIDS phagocytose immune complexes and opsonized particles poorly and show impaired chemotaxis and responsiveness to antigenic challenges.

  PATHOLOGY; CLINICAL FEATURES: Patients recently infected with HIV-1 may have an acute, usually self-limited flu-like illness termed the **acute retroviral syndrome**. It clinically resembles infectious mononucleosis. This occurs 2–3 weeks after exposure to HIV, before appearance of antibodies against the virus. Less commonly, patients present with neurologic symptoms that suggest encephalitis, aseptic meningitis or a neuropathy. Fever, myalgia, lymphadenopathy, sore throat and a macular rash are common. Most of these symptoms resolve within 2–3 weeks, although lymphadenopathy, fever and myalgia may persist for a few months. Seroconversion occurs 1–10 weeks after the onset of this acute illness. Thus, the standard HIV-1 enzyme immunoassay (EIA) and Western blot testing, which depends on the presence of anti–HIV-1 *gag* antibodies, is negative during the initial stage of the infection. Most patients recover from this initial illness as their immune system mounts a cytotoxic T-cell counterattack, although a small percentage progress rapidly to frank AIDS within a few months. After the initial acute syndrome, most newly infected individuals enter a period of latency and slow immune system decline that averages approximately 10 years before they reach a state of serious immune compromise. If symptoms go unrecognized or untreated, the outcome will eventually be fulminant immunodeficiency and its fatal complications (Fig. 4-25).

Persistent generalized lymphadenopathy is palpable lymph node enlargement at two or more extrainguinal sites, persisting for more than 3 months in a person infected with HIV. The disorder develops either as part of the acute HIV syndrome or within a few months of seroconversion. Axillary, inguinal and posterior cervical nodes are most affected, although any group of lymph nodes can be involved. Many cells within the affected lymph nodes, especially follicular dendritic cells, harbor actively replicating virus. Biopsy reveals reactive changes with follicular hyperplasia, but these are not diagnostic. Persistent generalized lymphadenopathy does not have any prognostic significance with respect to progression of HIV infection to AIDS. The ability

IMMUNOPATHOLOGY

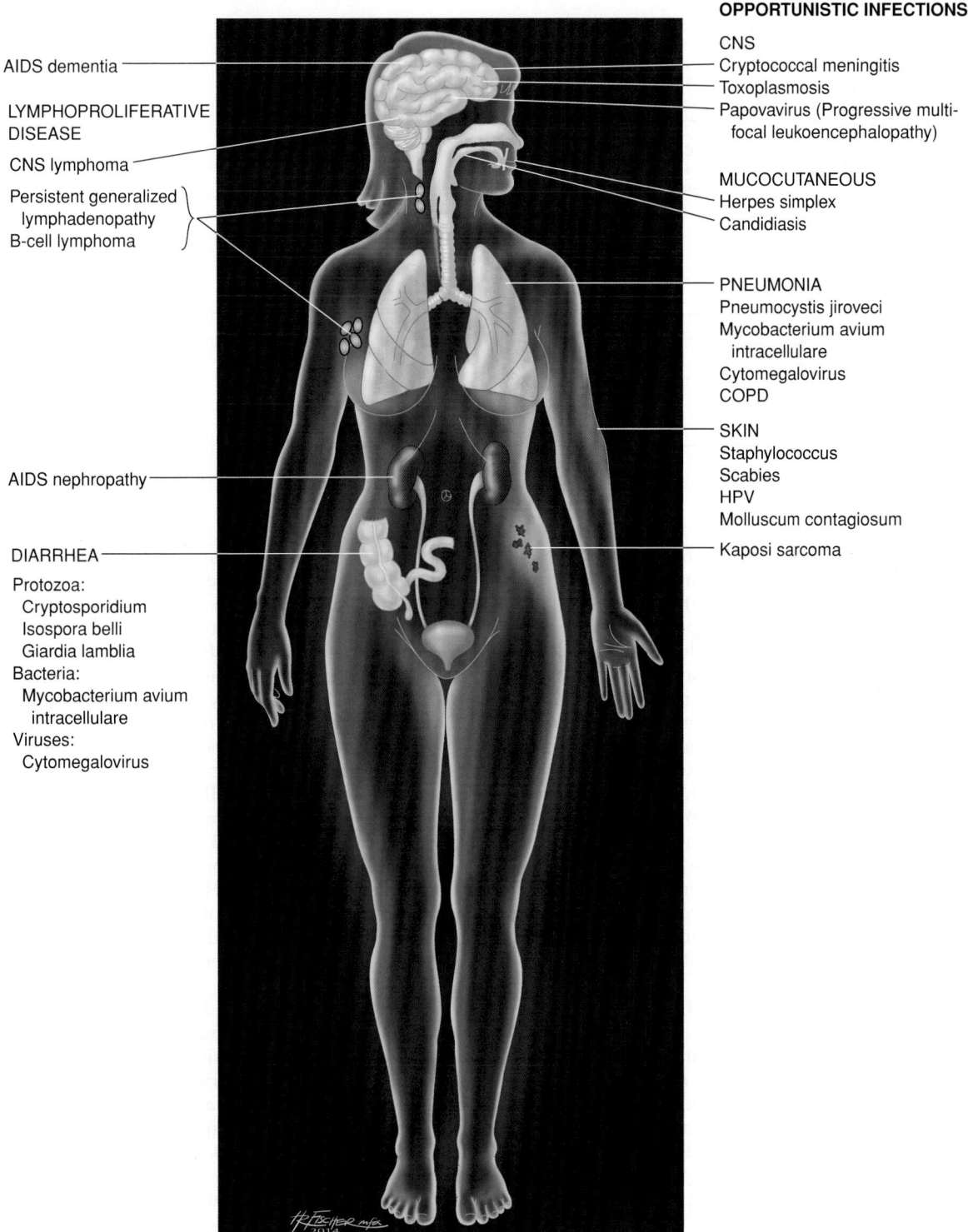

OPPORTUNISTIC INFECTIONS

AIDS dementia

LYMPHOPROLIFERATIVE
DISEASE

CNS lymphoma

Persistent generalized
lymphadenopathy
B-cell lymphoma

AIDS nephropathy

DIARRHEA

Protozoa:
  Cryptosporidium
  Isospora belli
  Giardia lamblia
Bacteria:
  Mycobacterium avium
   intracellulare
Viruses:
  Cytomegalovirus

CNS
Cryptococcal meningitis
Toxoplasmosis
Papovavirus (Progressive multi-
  focal leukoencephalopathy)

MUCOCUTANEOUS
Herpes simplex
Candidiasis

PNEUMONIA
Pneumocystis jiroveci
Mycobacterium avium
  intracellulare
Cytomegalovirus
COPD

SKIN
Staphylococcus
Scabies
HPV
Molluscum contagiosum

Kaposi sarcoma

FIGURE 4-25. Human immunodeficiency virus-1 (HIV-1)-mediated destruction of the cellular immune system results in AIDS.
The infectious and neoplastic complications of AIDS can affect practically every organ system. *CNS* = central nervous system; *HPV* = human papilloma virus.

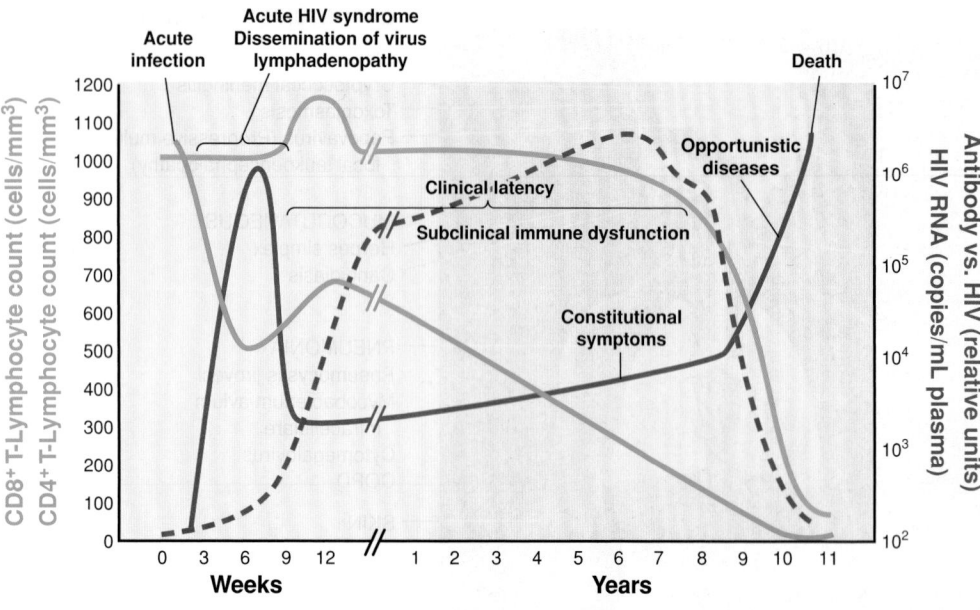

FIGURE 4-26. **Generalized time course of human immunodeficiency virus-1 (HIV-1) infection.** Important events in the development of HIV-1 infection are shown, including the clinical syndrome, virus loads and CD4+ and CD8+ lymphocyte population dynamics over time.

to persist and elicit ongoing lymphoproliferative responses is responsible for much of the long-term effects of HIV, even in patients treated with ART (see below).

Most patients infected with HIV express detectable viral antigens and antibodies within 6 months. Patients will generally experience an initial period of intense viremia with very high viral loads during the acute retroviral syndrome and a corresponding sharp drop in their absolute number of CD4+ T cells (Fig. 4-26). As a patient's immune system begins to recognize the new infection, viral load drops and CD4+ T-cell count begins to climb. This control of HIV-1 infection occurs via a vigorous cytotoxic T-cell response. Viral replication continues but is constrained by the immune response. The immune system and the HIV-1 load eventually enter into a sort of uneasy equilibrium, during which the HIV-1 viral RNA load stays fairly constant at the "viral set point." During this time infected individuals are generally asymptomatic. However, the rapidity with which HIV-1 evolves within each host ensures that it represents a continually moving antigenic target for the body's immune system.

The long interval between HIV-1 entry and the appearance of clinical symptoms of AIDS is related to the small number of infected T lymphocytes and viral latency and, it is now becoming clear, extensive virus replication away from the circulation in the gut-associated lymphoid tissue (GALT), and perhaps elsewhere. During this asymptomatic period, only 0.01%–0.001% of circulating T cells actively transcribe the HIV-1 genome, even though 1% contain integrated proviral DNA. Moreover, virus replication continues apace in the GALT, consuming certain CD4+ T-cell populations, particularly memory T cells. When this depletion eventually exceeds the body's ability to replenish these cells, systemic HIV-1 replication supervenes.

At some time CD4+ T cell counts start to decrease. Patients generally remain asymptomatic until their CD4+ counts fall below 500/μL. Nonspecific constitutional symptoms may appear, along with opportunistic infections. Once CD4+ levels are under 150/μL and CD4:CD8 ratios less than 0.8, the disease progresses rapidly. A variety of bacteria, viruses and

fungi attack immunocompromised patients. KS and lymphoproliferative disorders, especially virus-related lymphoproliferative disorders (see Chapter 26), may appear, and neurologic disease is common.

Symptoms of CNS dysfunction occur in 1/3 of AIDS patients. Postmortem studies of patients who have died of AIDS reveal CNS pathology in more than 3/4 of cases. HIV is thought to enter the brain via infected blood monocytes shortly after it enters the body. It resides there in microglial cells and perivascular macrophages. HIV infection of neurons is not common, but HIV gene products produced by infected brain phagocytes are very toxic for neurons and cause apoptosis via several mechanisms. ART drugs cross the blood-brain barrier poorly, so CNS HIV-1 infection can progress independently of HIV-1 infection outside the CNS, and despite good control of HIV-1 in the periphery. Longer survival among the HIV-positive population has led to greater numbers of patients with discernible neurologic deficits.

About 1% of whites are homozygous for asymptomatic major deletions in the CCR5 gene (the major mutation being a 32-base-pair deletion, causing a frameshift leading to a premature stop codon and a truncated, inactive protein product). *These people may remain uninfected despite extensive exposure to the virus.* Heterozygosity for the mutant CCR5 allele provides partial protection against HIV infection, and if infections do occur, they usually progress more slowly. Carriage of the mutant allele is found in up to 20% of whites but is largely absent in blacks and Asians.

Opportunistic Infections, Particularly Polymicrobial Infections, Are Common in Patients with AIDS

Discussion of the diversity of infectious agents that ravage patients with AIDS is beyond the scope of this chapter, and only a few representative examples are mentioned. It is important to recognize that while most immunocompetent patients will have only one infection at a time, HIV-1–infected patients can develop multiple severe infections simultaneously.

The majority of patients with HIV-1/AIDS suffer from opportunistic pulmonary infections, although this has been greatly reduced through the use of prophylactic antibiotics. *P. jiroveci* (formerly *P. carinii*) pneumonia may occur in patients with advanced HIV-1 disease. Lung infections with CMV and *M. avium-intracellulare* are less common. Patients with AIDS are also susceptible to *Legionella* infections.

Diarrhea occurs in over 75% of patients, often representing simultaneous infections with more than one organism. The most frequent pathogens are protozoans, including *Cryptosporidium, Isospora belli* and *Giardia lamblia. M. avium-intracellulare* and *Salmonella* species are the most common bacterial causes of diarrhea in AIDS patients. CMV infection of the gastrointestinal tract can manifest as a colitis associated with watery diarrhea in patients whose CD4 counts are under 50 cells/mm^3.

Cryptococcal meningitis is a devastating complication and represents 5%–8% of all opportunistic infections in patients with AIDS. Other CNS infectious complications include cerebral toxoplasmosis; primary CNS lymphoma; encephalitis caused by herpes simplex, varicella or CMV; and progressive multifocal leukoencephalopathy, which is due to JC virus (see Chapter 32).

Virtually all patients with AIDS develop some form of skin disease, infections being the most prominent. *Staphylococcus aureus* is the most common, causing bullous impetigo, deeper purulent lesions (ecthyma) and folliculitis. Chronic mucocutaneous herpes simplex infection is so characteristic of AIDS that it is considered an index infection in establishing the diagnosis. Skin lesions produced by *Molluscum contagiosum* and human papilloma virus (HPV) are also common, as are scabies and infections with *Candida* species. A varicella zoster eruption in someone under the age of 50 should raise the question of a possible occult HIV-1 infection.

Among the most common causes of death in patients with HIV/AIDS is hepatitis C virus (HCV) infection (see Chapter 20). In some studies, over 1/4 of deaths among HIV-positive individuals are from hepatitis C. A very high percentage of HIV-positive intravenous drug abusers are also infected with HCV. There is evidence that coinfection with HIV and HCV accelerates the course of disease with both viruses.

Kaposi sarcoma is an otherwise rare, multicentric, malignant neoplasm (see Chapters 5 and 28). It is characterized by cutaneous and (less commonly) visceral nodules, in which endothelium-lined channels and vascular spaces are admixed with spindle-shaped cells (see Chapter 24). Patients with AIDS, especially MSM rather than intravenous drug users, are at very high risk for KS. In fact, KS in an otherwise healthy person under age 60 is strong evidence of AIDS. Unlike the classic indolent variety of KS, the tumor in AIDS is usually aggressive, often involving viscera such as the gastrointestinal tract or lungs. Lung involvement frequently leads to death.

A strain of herpesvirus—human herpes virus 8 (HHV8)—is implicated in all forms of KS, including that associated with AIDS. HHV8 is also thought to be the cause of a peculiar lymphoma associated with AIDS (**primary effusion lymphoma**) and of **AIDS-associated Castleman disease** (see Chapter 26). The virus has been detected in both KS spindle cells and endothelial cells. The finding of HHV8 in the blood strongly predicts later development of KS. In fact, 75% of HIV-infected people with HHV8 in the blood developed KS within 5 years. It is thought that HHV8 is sexually transmitted, as almost all MSM HIV carriers are infected, but only 1/4 of heterosexual drug users with HIV infection harbor HHV8.

B-cell lymphoproliferative diseases are common in AIDS patients. Congenital and acquired immunodeficiency states are associated with B-cell hyperplasia, usually manifested as generalized lymphadenopathy. This lymphoproliferative syndrome may be followed by the appearance of high-grade B-cell lymphomas. In fact, patients who have been subjected to immunosuppressive therapy for renal transplants are at a 35-times-greater risk of developing lymphoma, and in 1/3 of these cases the tumor is confined to the CNS. Lymphomas in chronically immunodeficient patients may manifest as invasive polyclonal B-cell proliferations or monoclonal B-cell lymphomas. EBV infection has been closely associated with these lesions.

B-cell hyperplasia and generalized lymphadenopathy precede malignant lymphoproliferative disease. HIV-associated lymphomas are usually the large cell variety, as in other immunodeficiency conditions, although small cell lymphomas are sometimes seen. A conspicuous feature of AIDS-associated lymphomas is their preference for extranodal primary sites, particularly the brain, gastrointestinal tract, liver and bone marrow. The EBV genome has also been demonstrated in many AIDS-related lymphomas, especially in the CNS.

Efforts at Immunization to Prevent HIV-1 Infection Have to Date Been Unsuccessful

Enormous energy and resources have been applied to developing a vaccine to protect from HIV-1 infection. To date, no approach to vaccination has provided more than a glimmer of hope. Many approaches have been tried, from killed whole virus, to isolated viral proteins, to gene delivery of viral proteins using various vectors. None has yet been successful. This failure reflects many factors, including the antigenic diversity of HIV-1 strains (Fig. 4-27). To further complicate the task, since spontaneous recovery from HIV-1 infection has not been documented, it is unclear what effective immunity to HIV-1 would look like—what part(s) of the immune system would mediate resistance and what their immunologic target(s) would be. More mundane measures, such as careful screening of transfused blood products, condoms, male circumcision (see above) and prophylactic ART treatment of babies born to HIV-positive mothers, have helped to slow the spread of the virus.

HIV-2 Causes a Clinical Syndrome Like That Caused by HIV-1

In 1985, otherwise healthy prostitutes in Senegal were discovered to harbor antibodies that cross-reacted with a monkey retrovirus, now termed **simian immunodeficiency virus** (SIV). A year later, a retrovirus similar to HIV-1 was isolated from West African patients with AIDS who were negative for antibodies against HIV-1. Antibodies to this new retrovirus, now termed HIV-2, also cross-reacted with SIV antigens. Frozen sera from West Africa dating to the 1960s have been shown to contain antibodies to HIV-2. In Guinea-Bissau, infection with HIV-2 has been shown in 8% of pregnant women, 10% of male blood donors and more than 1/3 of prostitutes. The infection has

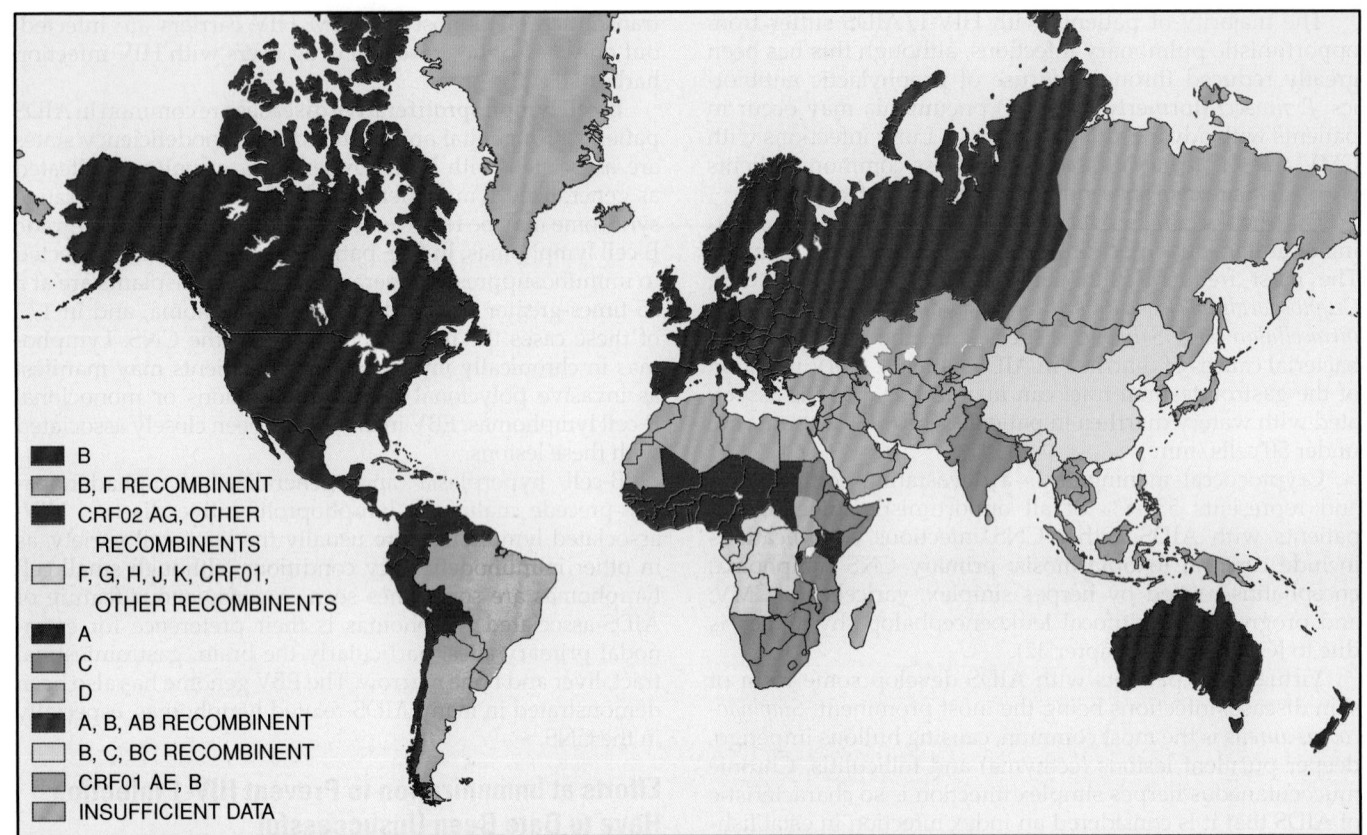

FIGURE 4-27. Diversity of human immunodeficiency virus-1 (HIV-1) antigens worldwide. The dominant HIV-1 serotypes (clades), by country; 2005 figures from the World Health Organization (WHO).

Legend:
- B
- B, F RECOMBINENT
- CRF02 AG, OTHER RECOMBINENTS
- F, G, H, J, K, CRF01, OTHER RECOMBINENTS
- A
- C
- D
- A, B, AB RECOMBINENT
- B, C, BC RECOMBINENT
- CRF01 AE, B
- INSUFFICIENT DATA

now also been reported from other parts of Africa, Europe and the United States.

HIV-2 is morphologically similar to HIV-1, and the immunodeficiency state associated with HIV-2 infection is indistinguishable from AIDS caused by HIV-1. The risk factors for infection in both diseases seem to be similar. However, HIV-2 is felt to be derived from a different nonhuman primate virus from HIV-1 and is more difficult to transmit than HIV-1. People infected with HIV-2 tend to progress to AIDS more slowly than those infected with HIV-1.

ANTIRETROVIRAL THERAPY AND ITS CONSEQUENCES

The Introduction of Combination Antiretroviral Therapy Has Helped Many HIV-Positive People Live Longer and Healthier Lives

HIV infection represents a novel challenge in treatment. Human lentivirus infections have not been therapeutic targets in the past. Thus, new strategies have had to be developed to treat patients with HIV/AIDS. Therapy focuses on HIV proteins that are obligatory for HIV replication and sufficiently different from normal cellular proteins to offer clear targets for pharmacotherapy. Initial agents were designed to inhibit the function of HIV RT and protease (PR). Combining compounds that inhibit RT with drugs that inhibit PR has been the mainstay of ART. Use of ART revolutionized AIDS

treatment, reducing AIDS-related mortality and increasing all indices of health in HIV-1–infected patients. Newer medications that target CCR5 and HIV-1 IN and other HIV-1–related functions have been added to the antiretroviral therapeutic armamentarium.

As mentioned above, HIV-1 RT lacks an editing function, so that HIV mutates much more often than most other viruses. This high mutation rate facilitates avoidance of immune attack and enhances its ability to generate functional mutations that are resistant to ART. Although combining three or more drugs in most ART regimens depresses viral replication, HIV mutants resistant to multiple chemotherapeutic agents contribute now a high percentage of primary HIV isolates in the United States. Further, ART drugs do not cross the blood-brain barrier well and are less effective in inhibiting HIV-1 persistence in macrophages. Thus, the CNS and other organs—especially mononuclear phagocytes in other organs like the gut and lung—may be sanctuaries for the virus (see above). Thus, continuing development of antiretrovirals is needed to stay ahead of the virus's adaptability to the evolving therapeutic environment.

Immune Reconstitution Inflammatory Syndrome

The introduction of effective antiretroviral therapy has led to an unanticipated consequence: the complications of sudden widespread suppression of HIV-1 replication, reconstitution of immune function. This syndrome affects about 1/6 of patients, usually shortly after ART begins.

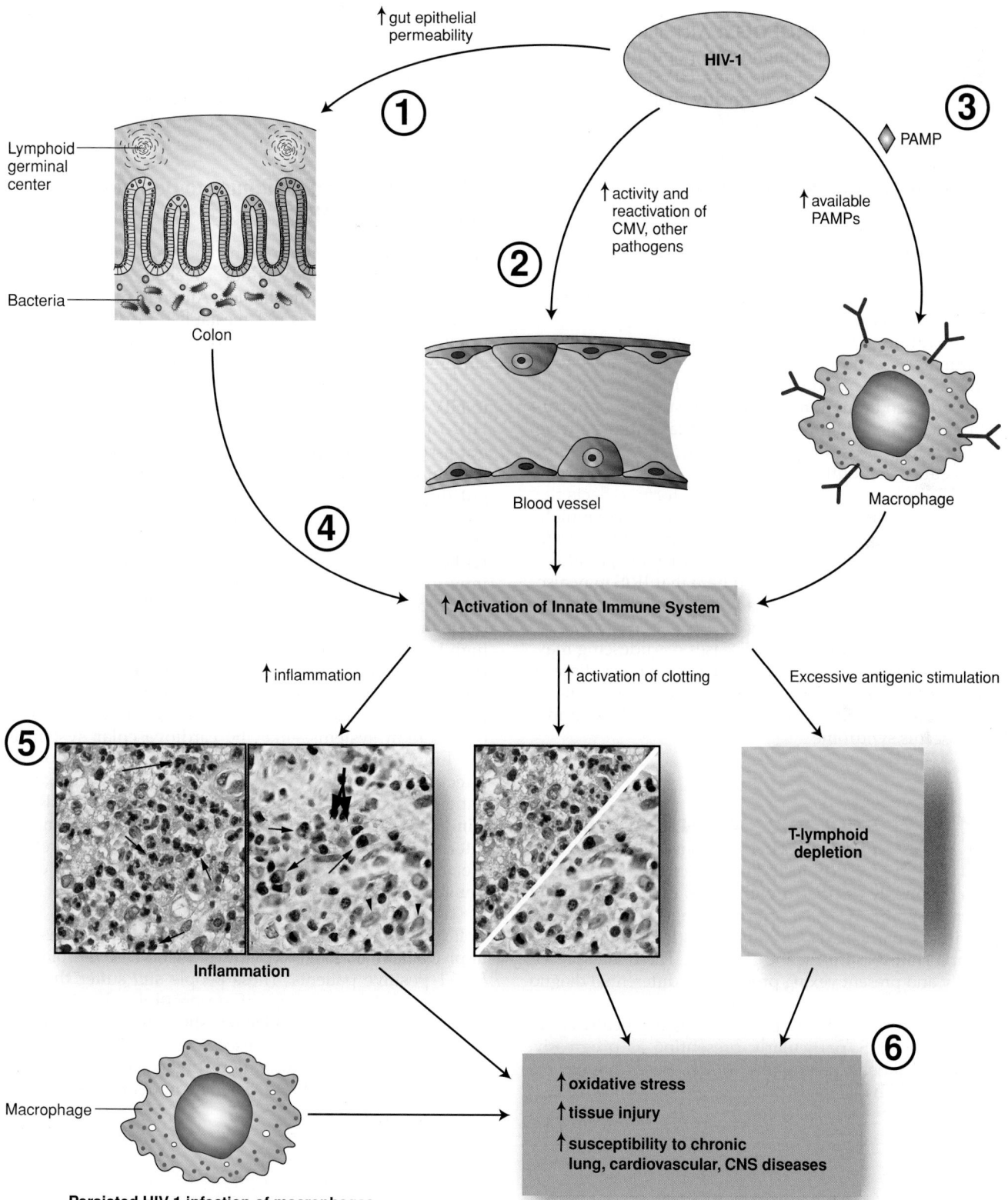

FIGURE 4-28. Probable pathogenesis of long-term complications of human immunodeficiency virus-1 (HIV-1) infection in the antiretroviral therapy (ART) era. 1. HIV-1 infection impairs the barrier function of the gut epithelium, leading to chronic antigenic stimulation by bacteria and other microbes in the gastrointestinal lumen. **2.** Impairment of ongoing surveillance immunity against resident pathogens, such as cytomegalovirus (CMV), leads to reactivation, in this case, within vasculature. **3.** Increased circulating microbial antigens present macrophages and other cells of the innate immune system with excessive levels of pathogen-associated molecular patterns (PAMPs) that stimulate their receptors (PRRs) on these cells. **4.** These factors all combine to activate the innate immune system excessively. **5.** As a consequence, systemic levels of inflammatory responses, tissue factor triggering of clotting and T-cell compartment exhaustion all contribute to tissue injury. **6.** A combination of these factors (5) with persistent macrophage infection by HIV-1, with continuing production of HIV-1 antigens and virus particles, leads to increased oxidative stress, depleting antioxidant reserves and accelerating the types of tissue injury (e.g., cardiovascular, pulmonary, etc.) most often associated with degenerative diseases of the elderly.

 **PATHOPHYSIOLOGY:** ART allows recovery of peripheral lymphocyte populations, especially memory T cells, from HIV-1–caused suppression. These cells increase greatly in the circulation between 3 and 6 months after ART starts. This sudden increase in both CD4 and CD8 memory cells can be dangerous, as, being memory cells, their repertoire reflects previous contact with foreign antigens. The presence of unresolved infections (see below) then magnifies these populations, leading to exaggerated immune responses. A defect in immunoregulatory T_{reg} cells has been postulated, as the ensuing clinical course reflects exaggerated activation of preexisting memory cells and their conversion into effector cells.

The lurking triggers for immune reconstitution inflammatory syndrome (IRIS) are largely infectious agents. So-called paradoxical IRIS occurs in the face of what had been thought to be effectively treated opportunistic infections, when residual microbial antigens drive the T-cell responses noted above. Typically, this type of IRIS occurs 3–6 months after ART begins. A second type of IRIS, which is called the unmasking form, reflects the ability of a previously unsuspected infection to stimulate the unrestrained inflammation. In general, IRIS due to undiagnosed pathogens occurs sooner than the paradoxical form. (It should be mentioned here that IRIS may also complicate recovery of patients with hematologic malignancies, without HIV-1 infection.)

Additionally, autoimmune diseases recrudescing may trigger IRIS. The most common of these is Graves disease (see Chapter 27), but other autoimmune diseases have also been implicated. Sarcoidosis may also act as an initiator for this syndrome.

 **ETIOLOGIC AGENTS, CLINICAL FEATURES:** Pathogens often responsible for IRIS include many of the opportunistic villains commonly associated with AIDS: mycobacteria, both *M. tuberculosis* and *M. avium* complex; fungi such as *C. neoformans*; viruses, particularly CMV, hepatitis B virus and herpes zoster and simplex viruses; and *P. jiroveci*. These may present atypically and present vexing problems in differential diagnosis.

Among the most difficult problems diagnostically is IRIS involving the CNS, particularly presenting as progressive multifocal leukoencephalopathy (PML, see Chapter 32), which is caused by JC virus.

As mentioned above, IRIS often presents atypically and may not be suspected. It tends to affect more severely those whose circulating CD4+ T-cell counts were lowest and whose peripheral viral loads were highest. Although IRIS, properly handled, is rarely fatal, a high index of suspicion should be exercised in patients who present with deteriorating clinical pictures within 6 months after ART is initiated.

HIV-1 Persists and Continues to Deplete T Cells Despite ART

HIV-positive cells remain in the body, so that eradication of the virus from the body is not a realistic expectation with therapies currently available. Among therapy-adherent patients, about 1/3 do not reestablish normal CD4+ T-cell numbers in the blood, despite complete or almost complete suppression of virus in the circulation.

Further, even if CD4+ T-cell levels reach normal and even if HIV-1 replication is not detectable in circulating cells, HIV-1 persists and replicates. Viral replication continues in gut-associated lymphoid tissue and elsewhere. Gastrointestinal epithelial dysfunction leads to ongoing leakage of gut microbes and their antigens into the lymphoid tissues and beyond. This generates a state of continued antigenic stimulation, adding to that caused by persistent HIV-1 replication and release of antigens. High-level, persistent immune responses so generated have several important consequences: (1) exhaustion of CD4+ T-cell reserves, whether by telomere depletion or other mechanisms; (2) ongoing high levels of oxidative stress with depletion of antioxidant reserves; (3) increased susceptibility to infections, such as CMV and EBV, that occur and tend to recur in settings of poor defenses; and (4) accelerated degenerative changes in other organ systems—like the cardiovascular system and the lung—that may not be directly attributable to HIV-1 infection but that may reflect the state of chronic excessive antigenic stimulation (Fig. 4-28). Finally, although ART may eliminate HIV-positive cells from the blood, even temporary interruption of therapy invariably leads to viral rebound (i.e., reactivation of HIV from reservoirs outside the circulation to produce a high circulating viral load).

Therefore, we have achieved tremendous success in controlling blood HIV-1 levels in most patients and consequent improvement in longevity and reduction in morbidity for HIV-1–positive patients. These people still suffer the consequences of their ongoing—if suppressed—HIV-1 infection, continued long-term antigenic stimulation and immune depletion that result, chronic excessive oxidative stress with its harmful consequences for various organs and the still intractable problem of HIV-1–associated neurodegenerative disease.

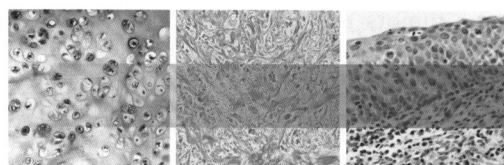

Neoplasia

David S. Strayer ▪ Emanuel Rubin

The Pathology of Neoplasia

A **neoplasm** (Greek, *neo,* "new," + *plasma,* "thing formed") is the autonomous growth of tissues that have escaped normal restraints on cell proliferation and accumulation and exhibit varying degrees of fidelity to their precursors. As well, some tumors (e.g., promyelocytic leukemia) involve impaired maturation, even if the tumor cells are committed to a specific line of differentiation. Neoplastic cells' resemblance to their cells of origin usually enables conclusions about tumors' sources and potential behavior. As most neoplasms occupy space, they are often called **tumors** (Gr., *swelling*). Tumors that remain localized are considered **benign,** while those that spread to distant sites are called **malignant,** or **cancer**. The neoplastic process entails not only cell proliferation but also variable modification of the differentiation of the involved cell types. Thus, in a sense, cancer may be viewed as a burlesque of normal development.

Cancer is an ancient disease. Evidence of bone tumors has been found in prehistoric remains, and the disease is mentioned in early writings from India, Egypt, Babylonia and Greece. Hippocrates is reported to have distinguished benign from malignant growths. He also introduced the term *karkinos*, from which our term **carcinoma** is derived. In particular, Hippocrates described cancer of the breast, and in the 2nd century AD, Paul of Aegina commented on its frequency.

The incidence of neoplastic disease increases with age, and longer life spans in modern times enlarge the population at risk. In previous centuries, humans did not live long enough to develop many cancers that are particularly common in middle and old age, such as those of the prostate, colon, pancreas and kidney. If all cancer deaths caused by tobacco smoke are removed from the statistics, the overall age-adjusted cancer death rate has been decreasing. In part, this stability and decline in cancer death rates reflects improved early detection techniques (e.g., Pap smears, colonoscopy).

Neoplasms are derived from cells that normally can multiply. Thus, mature neurons and cardiac myocytes do not give rise to tumors. A tumor may mimic its tissue of origin to a variable degree. Some closely resemble their parent structures (e.g., hepatic adenomas), while others seem to be collections of cells that are so primitive that the tumor's origin cannot be identified.

BENIGN VERSUS MALIGNANT TUMORS

Although exceptions are known, benign tumors basically do not penetrate (invade) adjacent tissue borders, nor do they spread (metastasize) to distant sites. They remain as localized overgrowths in the area in which they arise. Benign tumors tend to be more differentiated than malignant ones—that is, they more closely resemble their tissue of origin. *By contrast, malignant tumors or cancers, invade contiguous tissues and metastasize to distant sites, where subpopulations of malignant cells take up residence, grow a new and again grow into surrounding areas.*

In common usage, **the terms "benign" and "malignant" refer to a tumor's overall biological behavior rather than its morphologic characteristics**. In most circumstances, malignant tumors have the capacity to kill, while benign ones spare the host. However, so-called benign tumors in critical locations can be deadly. For example, a benign intracranial tumor of the meninges (meningioma) can kill by exerting pressure on the brain. A minute benign tumor of the ependymal cells of the third ventricle (ependymoma) can block the circulation of cerebrospinal fluid, resulting in lethal hydrocephalus. A benign mesenchymal tumor of the left atrium (myxoma) may cause sudden death by blocking the mitral valve orifice. In certain locations, erosion of a benign tumor of smooth muscle can lead to serious hemorrhage—witness the peptic ulceration of a stromal tumor in the gastric wall. On rare occasions, a functioning, benign endocrine adenoma can be life-threatening, as in the case of the sudden hypoglycemia associated with an insulinoma of the pancreas or the hypertensive crisis produced by a pheochromocytoma of the adrenal medulla. Conversely, certain types of malignant tumors are so indolent that they pose no threat to life. In this category there are many cancers of the breast and prostate.

Tumors can usually be identified as benign or malignant by virtue of their microscopic morphologic characteristics. However, the biological behavior of some types of tumors may not necessarily reflect, or correlate with, pathologic appearance. Some tumors that look histologically malignant may not metastasize or be able to kill a patient. Thus, basal cell carcinomas of the skin may invade subjacent structures locally but rarely metastasize and are not life-threatening. On the other hand, some tumors showing benign histologic characteristics may be lethal. Aggressive meningiomas do not metastasize, but their local invasiveness may cause death by compromising vital structures. For many endocrine tumors (e.g., islet cell tumors of the pancreas) metastatic potential is not predictable from histology, and a tumor's benign or malignant nature can only be determined retrospectively, based on the presence or absence of metastases.

CLASSIFICATION OF NEOPLASMS

In any language, the classification of objects and concepts is pragmatic and useful only insofar as its general acceptance permits effective prognostication. Similarly, the nosology of tumors reflects historical concepts, technical jargon, location, origin, descriptive modifiers and predictors of biological behavior. Although the language of tumor classification is neither rigidly logical nor consistent, it still serves as a reasonable mode of communication.

HISTOLOGIC DIAGNOSIS OF MALIGNANCY

Essentially, labeling a tumor as benign or malignant is a prediction of its eventual biological behavior and clinical outcome. In effect, the criteria used to assess the true biological nature of any tumor are based not on scientific principles but rather on accumulated experience and historical correlations between histologic and cytologic patterns and clinical courses. In most cases, the differentiation between benign and malignant tumors poses few problems; in a few, additional study is required before an accurate diagnosis is secure. However, there will always be tumors that defy the diagnostic skills and experience of any pathologist; in these cases, the correct diagnosis must await the clinical outcome. *Remember that the definition of a benign tumor resides above all in its inability to invade adjacent tissue and to metastasize.*

The Primary Descriptors of All Tumors Are Their Cells of Origin

Although historically the suffix "oma" referred to benign tumors, current terminology is so varied that tumor names do not specify biological behavior with any precision. For example, tumors called melanomas, mesotheliomas and seminomas are all highly malignant even though they carry the suffix "oma." Growths called hamartomas are not even true neoplasms but disorganized developmental medleys of multiple structures. Nevertheless, by definition, the term "carcinoma" describes a malignant proliferation of epithelial cells and "sarcoma" refers to malignancies of mesenchymal origin. These terms are not necessarily all-inclusive, as most malignant proliferations of the blood-forming organs are called leukemias and those of the lymphoid system are lymphomas. Finally, tumors in which historically the histogenesis was poorly understood are often given an eponym—for example, Hodgkin disease or Ewing sarcoma.

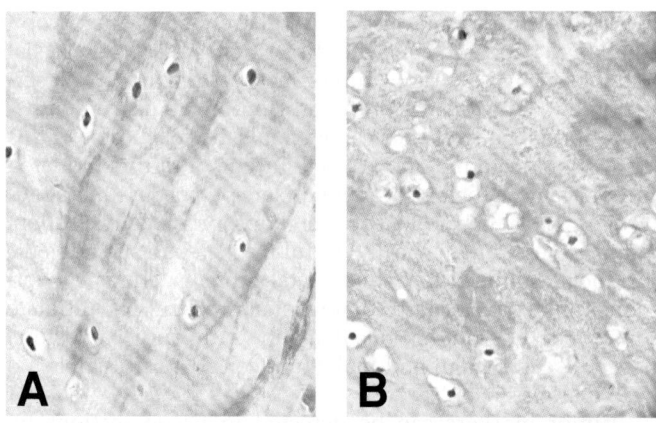

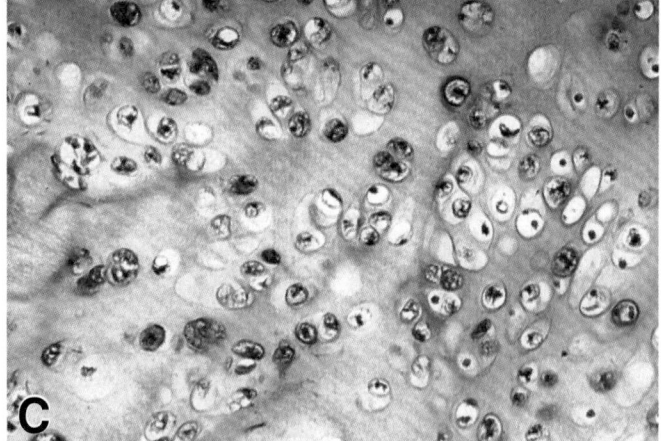

FIGURE 5-1. Cartilaginous lesions. A. Normal cartilage. **B.** A benign chondroma closely resembles normal cartilage. **C.** Chondrosarcoma of bone. The tumor is composed of malignant chondrocytes, which have bizarre shapes and irregular hyperchromatic nuclei, embedded in a cartilaginous matrix. Compare with **A** and **B**.

Some of the histologic features that are considered in distinguishing benign from malignant tumors include the following:

- **Degree of cellular atypia:** This term refers to the extent to which the tumor departs from the appearance of its normal tissue or cellular counterparts (Fig. 5-1). An example is the difference between normal cartilage, a benign chondroma and a malignant chondrosarcoma. In general, the magnitude of cellular atypia (also called **anaplasia**) correlates with the aggressiveness of the tumor. Cytologic evidence of anaplasia includes (1) variation in size and shape of cells and cell nuclei **(pleomorphism)**, (2) enlarged and hyperchromatic nuclei with coarsely clumped chromatin and prominent nucleoli, (3) atypical mitoses and (4) bizarre cells, including tumor giant cells (Fig. 5-2).

- **Mitotic activity:** Many malignant tumors show high mitotic rates. For some tumors (e.g., leiomyosarcomas), a diagnosis of malignancy is based on finding even a few mitoses. Nonetheless, such obvious proliferative activity is not obligatory to consider a tumor malignant in all situations.

- **Growth pattern:** In common with many benign tumors, malignant neoplasms often exhibit disorganized growth, which may be expressed as sheets of cells, arrangements around blood vessels, papillary structures, whorls, rosettes and so forth. Malignant tumors often suffer from compromised blood supply and show ischemic necrosis.

- **Invasion:** Malignancy is proved by the demonstration of invasion, particularly of blood vessels and lymphatics. In some circumstances (e.g., squamous carcinoma of the cervix or carcinoma arising in an adenomatous polyp), the diagnosis of malignant transformation is made mainly on the basis of local invasion.

- **Metastases:** The presence of metastases identifies a tumor as malignant. If a metastatic tumor was not preceded by a diagnosed primary cancer, the site of origin may not be readily apparent from histologic characteristics alone. In such cases, electron microscopy and demonstration of specific tumor markers may establish the correct origin.

General criteria for malignancy are recognized but must be used cautiously in specific cases. For example, **nodular fasciitis,** a reactive proliferation of connective tissue cells (Fig. 5-3), appears more alarming histologically than many fibrosarcomas, and misdiagnosis can lead to unnecessary surgery. Conversely, well-differentiated endocrine adenocarcinomas may be pathologically identical to benign adenomas.

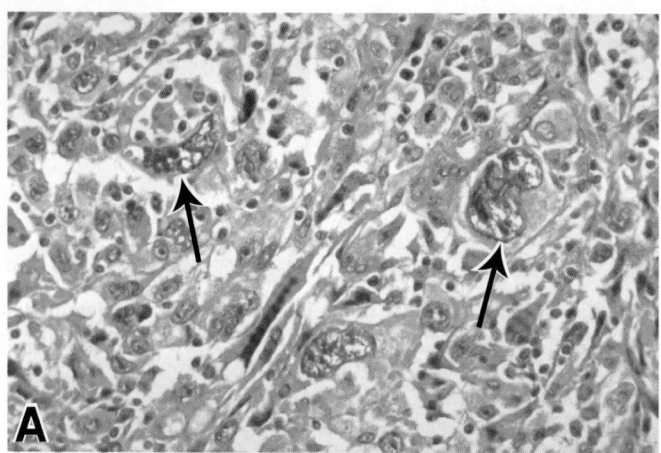

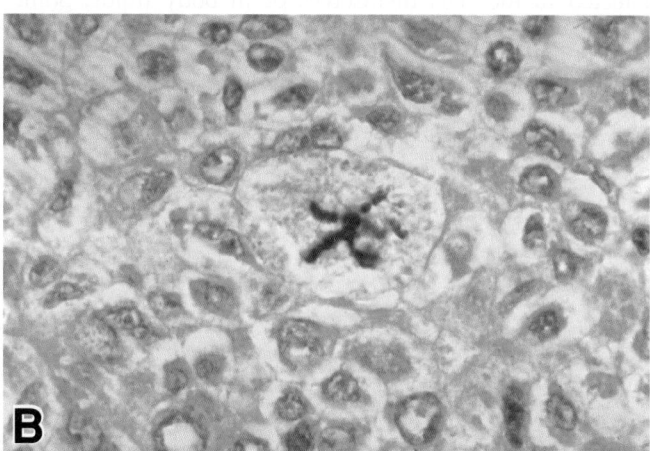

FIGURE 5-2. Anaplastic features of malignant tumors. A. The cells of this anaplastic carcinoma are highly pleomorphic (i.e., they vary in size and shape). The nuclei are hyperchromatic and are large relative to the cytoplasm. Multinucleated tumor giant cells are present (*arrows*). **B.** A malignant cell in metaphase exhibits an abnormal mitotic figure.

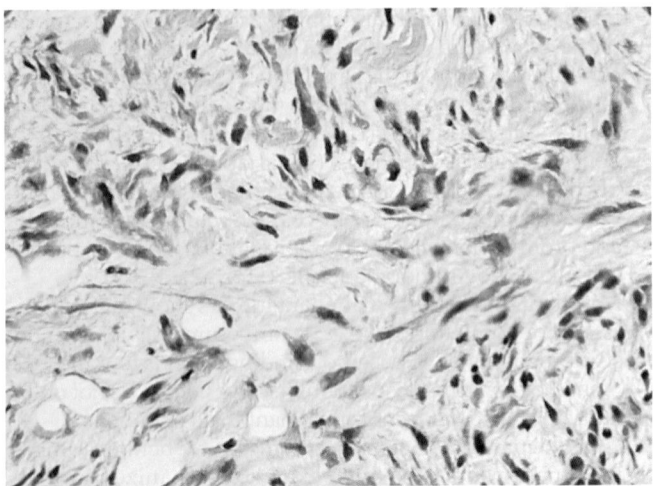

FIGURE 5-3. Nodular fasciitis. This cellular reactive lesion contains a typical and bizarre fibroblasts, which may be mistaken for a fibrosarcoma.

Marker Studies Are Used to Identify Tumor Origin

Electron Microscopy

There are no specific determinants of malignancy or even of neoplasia itself that can be detected by electron microscopy. Although this technique may aid in identifying poorly differentiated cancers whose classification is problematic by routine light microscopy, electron microscopy has largely been supplanted in tumor diagnosis by immunohistochemical staining. Nonetheless, carcinomas often contain desmosomes and specialized junctional complexes, structures that are not typical of sarcomas or lymphomas. The presence of melanosomes or premelanosomes signifies a melanoma, and small, membrane-bound granules with dense cores are features of endocrine neoplasms (Fig. 5-4). Another diagnostically useful granule is the characteristic crystal-containing granule of an insulinoma derived from the pancreatic islets.

Tumor Markers

Tumor markers are products of neoplasms that can be detected in the cells themselves or in body fluids. Some

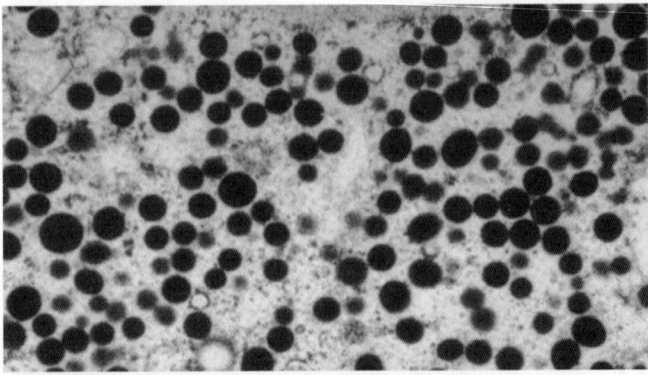

FIGURE 5-4. Electron micrograph of a metastatic cancer of the adrenal medulla (pheochromocytoma). The neuroendocrine origin of this poorly differentiated tumor was identified by the presence of characteristic cytoplasmic secretory granules.

metastatic tumors may be so undifferentiated microscopically as to preclude even the distinction between epithelial and mesenchymal origin. Tumor markers rely on the preservation of characteristics of the progenitor cell or the synthesis of specialized substances by neoplastic cells to make this distinction. Determination of cell lineage of undifferentiated tumors is more than an academic exercise, because therapeutic decisions may be based on their appropriate identification. Among these diagnostically useful markers are such diverse products as immunoglobulins, fetal proteins, enzymes, hormones and cytoskeletal and junctional proteins. The ultimate tumor marker would be one that allows unequivocal distinction between benign and malignant cells. Unfortunately, no such marker exists.

Tumor markers can be detected in tissue sections by immunologic (immunohistochemistry, immunofluorescence) techniques (Fig. 5-5) and by molecular studies (in situ hybridization). Table 5-1 contains examples of marker studies that are used to identify the tissue of origin of tumors.

In addition to their use in identifying the lineages of malignancies, tumor-associated antigens are also used in

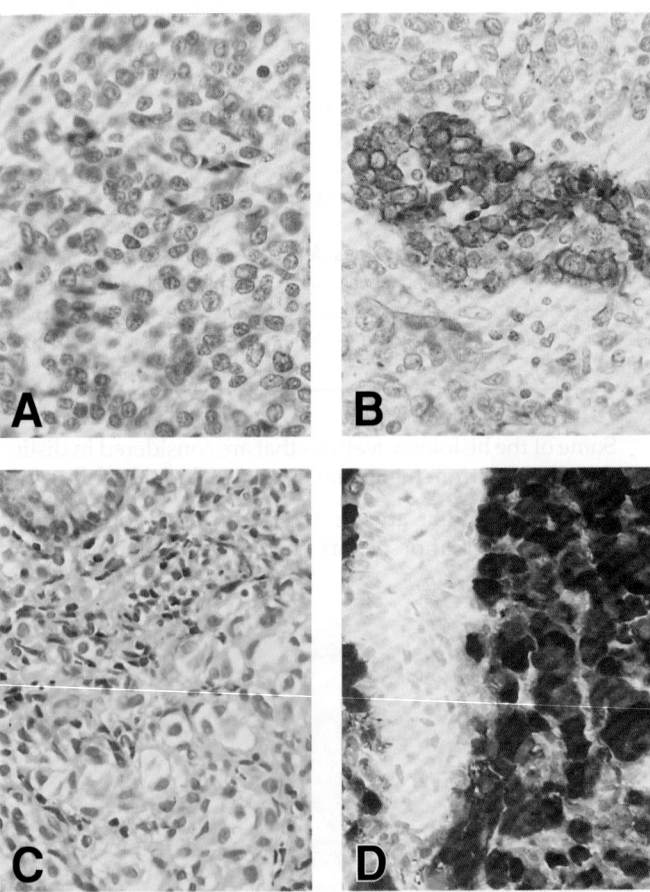

FIGURE 5-5. Tumor markers in the identification of undifferentiated neoplasms. A. A poorly differentiated metastatic bladder cancer is difficult to identify as a carcinoma with the hematoxylin and eosin stain. **B.** A section of the tumor depicted in **A** is positive for cytokeratin with an immunoperoxidase stain and is identified as carcinoma. **C.** A metastasis to the colon of an undifferentiated malignant melanoma is not pigmented, and its origin is unclear. **D.** An immunoperoxidase stain of the tumor shown in **C** reveals numerous cells positive for S-100 protein, a commonly used marker for cells of melanocytic origin.

TABLE 5-1

FREQUENTLY USED MARKERS TO IDENTIFY TUMORS

Marker	Target Cells
Epithelial Cells	
Cytokeratins (CKs)	Carcinomas, mesothelioma
CK7	Many nongastrointestinal adenocarcinomas
CK20	Gastrointestinal and ovarian carcinomas, urothelial carcinomas, Merkel cell tumor
Epithelial membrane antigen (EMA)	Carcinomas, mesothelioma, some large cell lymphomas
Ber-Ep4	Most carcinomas, but not in mesothelioma
B72.3 (tumor associated)	Many adenocarcinomas, but not in mesothelioma
Carcinoembryonic antigen (CEA)	Many adenocarcinomas of endodermal origin but not in others (e.g., renal, mesothelioma)
Mesothelial Cells	
Cytokeratins CK5/6	Mesothelioma
Vimentin	Mesothelioma
HBME	Mesothelioma, thyroid tumors
Calretinin	Mesothelioma
Melanocytes	
HMB-45	Malignant melanoma
S-100 protein	Malignant melanoma, glial cells
Mel A	Malignant melanoma
Neuroendocrine and Neural Cells	
Chromogranins, particularly chromogranin A	Neuroendocrine tumors
Synaptophysin	Neuroendocrine tumors
CD57	Neuroendocrine tumors, T and NK cells, Schwann cells
Glial Cells	
Glial fibrillary acidic protein (GFAP)	Astrocytoma and other glial tumors
Mesenchymal Cells	
Vimentin	Most sarcomas
Desmin	All types of muscle tumors
Muscle-specific actin	Muscle tumors, myofibroblast tumors
CD99	Ewing sarcoma, peripheral neuroectodermal tumors (PNETs), acute lymphoid and myeloid leukemias

Marker	Target Cells
Specific Organs	
Prostate-specific antigen (PSA)	Prostatic cancer
Prostate-specific alkaline phosphatase (PSAP)	Prostate cancer
Thyroglobulin	Thyroid cancer
α-Fetoprotein (AFP)	Hepatocellular carcinoma, yolk sac tumor
HepPar1	Hepatocellular carcinoma
WT1	Wilms tumor, some mesotheliomas
Placental alkaline phosphatase (PLAP)	Seminoma, embryonal carcinoma
Human chorionic gonadotropin (hCG)	Trophoblastic tumors
CA19-9	Pancreatic and gastrointestinal carcinomas
CA125	Ovarian carcinoma, endometrial carcinoma, some other nongynecologic tumors (pancreas, mesothelioma)
Calcitonin	Medullary carcinoma of the thyroid
CD Markers	
CD1	Some T-cell leukemias, Langerhans cell proliferations
CD2	T cells, T-cell malignancies
CD3	T cells, T-cell malignancies
CD4	T cells, T-cell malignancies, monocytes, monocytic malignancies
CD5	T cells, some B-cell malignancies
CD8	Suppressor T cells, some T-cell malignancies
CD10 (common ALL antigen, CALLA)	Acute lymphoblastic leukemia, some B-cell lymphomas, renal cell carcinomas
CD15	Reed-Sternberg cells, some T cells, some myeloid leukemias, many adenocarcinomas, but not in mesothelioma
CD19	B cells, B-cell malignancies
CD20	B cells, B-cell malignancies
CD30	Hodgkin disease, anaplastic large cell lymphoma
CD33	Myeloid leukemias

(continued)

TABLE 5-1	
FREQUENTLY USED MARKERS TO IDENTIFY TUMORS (*Continued*)	

Marker	Target Cells	Marker	Target Cells
CD34	Acute myeloid or lymphoblastic leukemias, some spindle cell tumors	von Willebrand factor (vWF)	Vascular neoplasms
CD117 (c-Kit)	Chronic myeloid leukemia, gastrointestinal stromal tumors, seminomas, also tumors of lung, breast, endometrium, urinary bladder	CD31	Vascular neoplasms, endothelial cells
Non-CD Leukemia/Lymphoma Markers		CD34	Bone marrow stem cells, vascular neoplasms (endothelial cells)
κ Light chain	B-cell malignancies	Lectins	Vascular neoplasms
λ Light chain	B-cell malignancies	CD43	Almost all leukocytes
TdT	Acute lymphoblastic leukemia	CD56	NK cells
Bcl-1 and cyclin D1	Mantle cell lymphoma		

CA = cancer antigen; CD = cluster designation; NK = natural killer; TdT = terminal deoxynucleotidyl transferase.

other ways. Blood levels of tumor antigens are helpful in following the development of metastases and progression of the tumor after the primary neoplasm has been treated. Representative examples include carcinoembryonic antigen (CEA) for gastrointestinal tumors, cancer antigen (CA) 125 for ovarian carcinoma and prostate-specific antigen (PSA) for prostate cancer. Tumor markers can be detected in blood using immunoassays (e.g., enzyme-linked immunosorbent assay [ELISA]) on serum, immunologic analyses of circulating blood cells (flow cytometry), electrophoretic separation of blood proteins and other methodologies. As effective as analysis of blood levels for tumor-produced substances may be in following a tumor's course, application of such analyses to screening for tumors has generally met with little success.

Some tumor antigens may also be used to make important therapeutic decisions (e.g., estrogen/progesterone receptors and HER2/neu in breast cancer, epidermal growth factor receptor [EGFR] for lung cancer and c-kit for gastrointestinal stromal tumors). Tumor antigens may also be useful therapeutic targets, as illustrated by HER2/neu for breast cancer and CD20 for B-cell lymphoma.

INVASION AND METASTASIS

Two properties that are unique to cancer cells are the ability to invade locally and the capacity to metastasize to distant sites. These characteristics are responsible for the vast majority of deaths from cancer; the primary tumor itself (e.g., breast or colon cancer) is generally amenable to surgical resection.

Direct Extension Damages Involved Organs and Adjacent Tissues

Most carcinomas begin as localized growths confined to the epithelium where they arise. As long as these early cancers do not penetrate the basement membrane on which the epithelium rests, such tumors are called **carcinoma in situ** (Fig. 5-6). In this stage, it

is unfortunate that in situ tumors are asymptomatic, because they are invariably curable. When in situ tumors acquire invasive potential and extend through the underlying basement membrane, they can compromise neighboring tissues and metastasize. In situations in which cancer arises from cells that are not confined by a basement membrane—such as connective tissue cells, lymphoid elements and hepatocytes—an in situ stage is not defined.

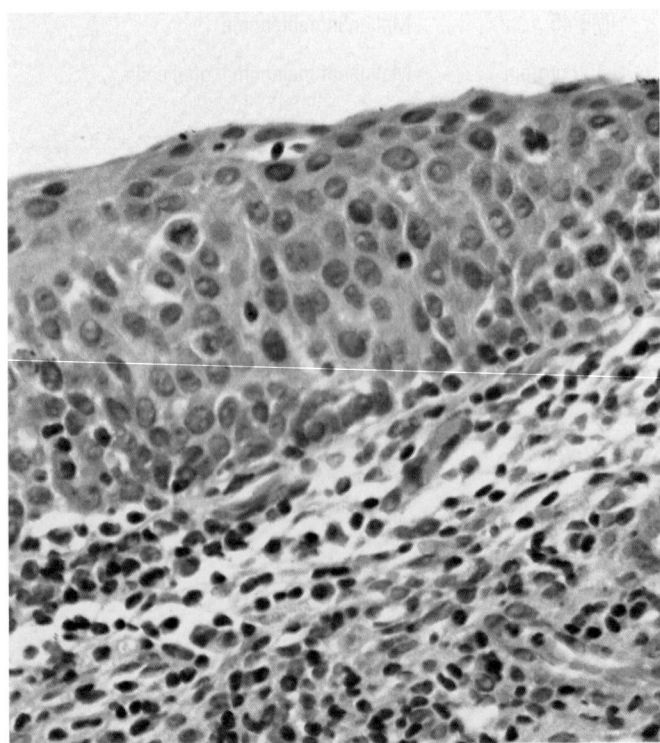

FIGURE 5-6. Carcinoma in situ. A section of the uterine cervix shows neoplastic squamous cells occupying the full thickness of the epithelium and confined to the mucosa by the underlying basement membrane.

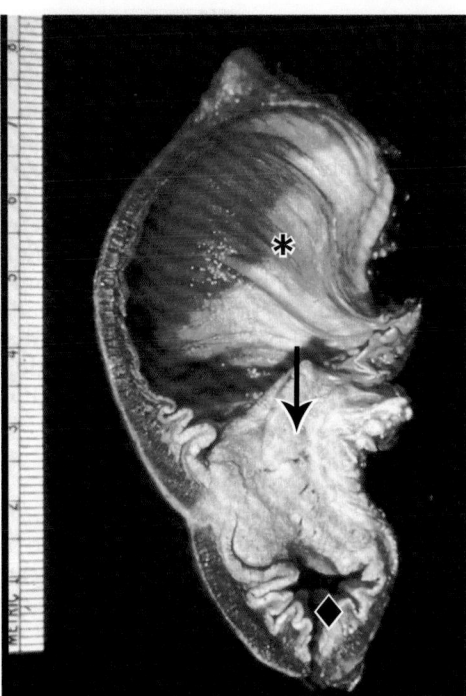

FIGURE 5-7. Adenocarcinoma of the colon with intestinal obstruction. The lumen of the colon at the site of the cancer is narrow (*arrow*). The colon above the obstruction is dilated (*). The colon distal to the stricture is normal caliber (♦).

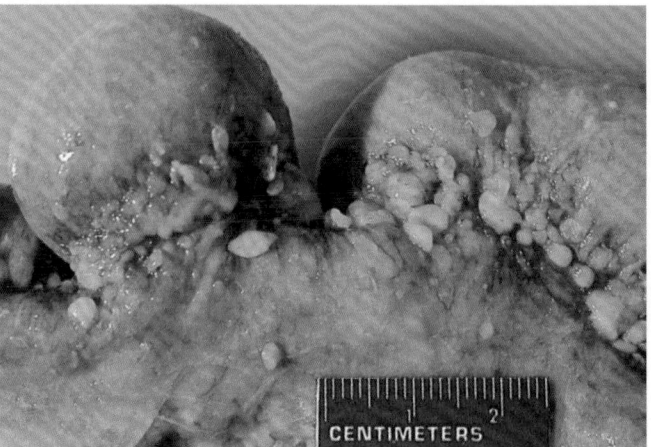

FIGURE 5-8. Peritoneal carcinomatosis. The mesentery attached to a loop of small bowel is studded with small nodules of metastatic ovarian carcinoma.

Malignant tumors growing within the tissue of origin may also extend beyond the confines of that organ to involve adjacent tissues. The growth of the cancer is occasionally so extensive that replacement of the normal tissue results in functional insufficiency of the organ. Such a situation is not uncommon in primary liver cancer. Brain tumors, such as astrocytomas, infiltrate the brain until they compromise vital regions. The direct extension of malignant tumors within an organ may also be life-threatening because of their location. A common example is intestinal obstruction produced by colon cancer (Fig. 5-7).

The invasive growth pattern of cancers may secondarily impair the function of an adjacent organ. Squamous carcinoma of the cervix frequently grows beyond the genital tract to obstruct the ureters or produce vesicovaginal fistulas. Neglected cases of breast cancer are often complicated by extensive skin ulceration. Even small tumors can produce severe consequences when they invade vital structures. A small lung cancer can cause a bronchopleural fistula when it penetrates the bronchus or exsanguinating hemorrhage when it erodes a blood vessel. The agonizing pain of pancreatic carcinoma results from direct extension of the tumor to the celiac nerve plexus. Tumor cells that reach serous cavities (e.g., those of the peritoneum or pleura) spread easily by direct extension or can be carried by the fluid to new locations on the serous membranes. The most common example is the seeding of the peritoneal cavity by certain types of ovarian cancer (Fig. 5-8).

Metastatic Spread Is the Most Common Cause of Cancer Deaths

Metastasis (Greek, "displacement") is the migration of malignant cells from one site to another noncontiguous site. The invasive

properties of malignant tumors bring them into contact with blood and lymphatic vessels, which they can also penetrate, and through which they disseminate to distant sites. They may also reach body cavities (e.g., pleural space), and so spread via those routes as well.

Hematogenous Metastases

Cancer cells often invade capillaries and venules, but thicker-walled arterioles and arteries are relatively resistant to their attack. Before they can form viable metastases, circulating tumor cells must lodge in the vascular bed of the metastatic site (Fig. 5-9). Here they attach to, and then traverse, blood vessel and lymphatic walls. Often, the location of a primary tumor with regard to blood or lymph flow determines the distribution of the initial metastases from that tumor. Thus, abdominal tumors that seed the hepatic portal system may cause liver metastases; other tumors penetrate systemic veins that eventually drain into the vena cava and hence to the lungs. Breast cancers first metastasize to regional lymph

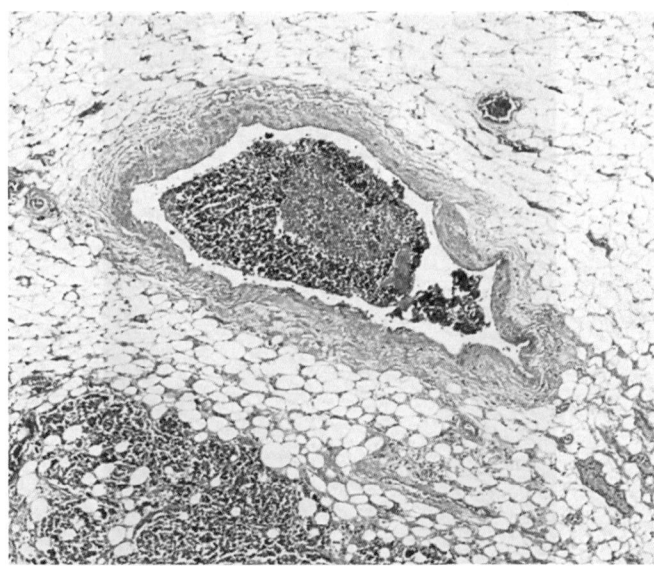

FIGURE 5-9. Hematogenous spread of cancer. A malignant tumor (*bottom*) has invaded adipose tissue and penetrated into a small vein.

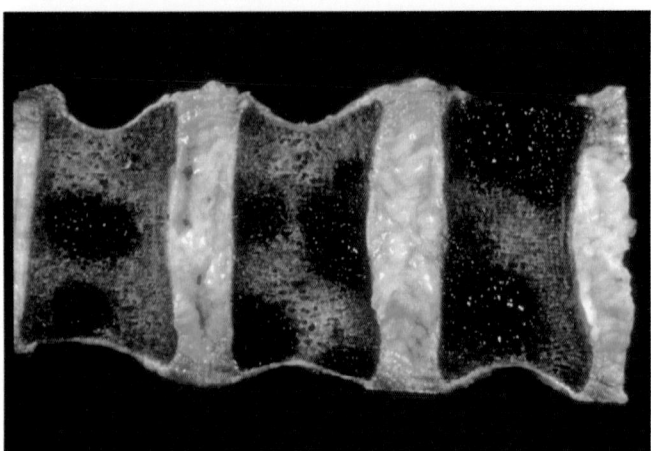

FIGURE 5-10. Multiple pigmented metastases in the vertebral bodies in a patient who died of malignant melanoma.

nodes because of the direction of lymphatic flow. More widespread metastatic disease may result from extensive early dissemination of tumor cells or from secondary spread from early metastatic foci (Fig. 5-10).

Lymphatic Metastases

Basement membranes envelop only large lymphatic channels; lymphatic capillaries lack them. Once in lymphatic vessels, itinerant tumor cells are carried to regional draining lymph nodes. There, they first lodge in the marginal sinus and then extend throughout the node. Lymph nodes bearing metastatic deposits may be enlarged to many times their normal size, often exceeding the diameter of the primary lesion (Fig. 5-11).

The regional lymphatic pattern of metastasis is most prominently exemplified by breast cancer. The initial metastases are almost always lymphatic, and these regional lymphatic metastases have considerable prognostic significance. Cancers that arise in the lateral aspect of the breast

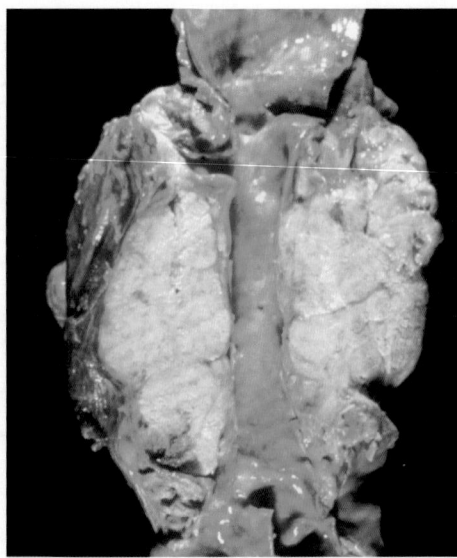

FIGURE 5-11. Metastatic carcinoma in periaortic lymph nodes. The aorta has been opened and the nodes bisected.

characteristically spread to axillary lymph nodes; those arising in the medial portion drain to the internal mammary thoracic lymph nodes.

Lymphatic metastases are occasionally found in lymph nodes far from the primary tumor site. For example, the first sign of some abdominal cancers may be an enlarged supraclavicular node. A graphic example of the relationship of lymphatic anatomy to the spread of malignant tumors is afforded by cancers of the testis. Rather than metastasizing to inguinal nodes, as do other tumors of the male external genitalia, testicular cancers typically involve the draining abdominal periaortic nodes. The explanation lies in the descent of the testis from an intra-abdominal site to the scrotum, during which it is accompanied by its own lymphatic supply.

Seeding of Body Cavities

Malignant tumors that arise in organs adjacent to body cavities (e.g., ovaries, gastrointestinal tract and lung) may shed malignant cells into these spaces. Such body cavities principally include the peritoneal and pleural cavities, although occasional seeding of the pericardial cavity, joint space and subarachnoid space is observed. Similar to tissue culture, tumors in these sites grow in masses and often produce fluid (e.g., ascites, pleural fluid), sometimes in very large quantities. Mucinous adenocarcinoma may also secrete copious amounts of mucin in these locations.

Organ Tropisms of Metastases

It was recognized more than a century ago that the distribution of metastases in breast cancer is not random. In 1889, Paget proposed that the spread of tumor cells to specific secondary sites depends on compatibility between the tumor cells (the seed) and favorable microenvironmental factors in the secondary site (the soil). For example, cancers of the breast, prostate and thyroid metastasize to bone, a tropism that suggests a favored "soil." Conversely, despite their size and abundant blood flow, neither the spleen nor skeletal muscle is a common site of metastases. There is evidence that tumor-associated stromal cells in fact "plow the road" for tumor spread to particular sites that are suitable to the metastatic survival of implants from that tumor (see below).

STAGING AND GRADING OF CANCERS

Cancer Staging Describes the Extent of Spread

In an attempt to predict the clinical behavior of a malignant tumor and to establish criteria for therapy, many cancers are staged: they are assessed using specific protocols that help determine the detectable extent of their spread.

The choice of surgical approach, or the selection of treatment modalities, is influenced by the stage of a cancer. Moreover, most statistical data related to cancer survival are also based on this criterion. The significant criteria used for staging vary with different organs. Commonly used criteria include:

- Tumor size
- Extent of local growth, whether within or out of the organ
- Presence of lymph node metastases
- Presence of distant metastases

These patterns have been codified in the international **TNM cancer staging system,** in which "T" refers to the size and local extent of the primary tumor, "N" to the level of regional node metastases and "M" to the presence of distant metastases. Thus, for example, a breast cancer that is staged at T3N2M0 is a large primary tumor (T3) that has involved axillary lymph nodes moderately (N2) but has not detectably spread to distant sites (M0). The specific definitions of each T, N or M number vary among different tumors. As well, some tumor types, like central nervous system (CNS) tumors and hematologic malignancies, are staged according to different systems.

Cancer Grading Reflects the Architecture and Cytology of Tumors

Well-differentiated tumors are referred to as low grade, and poorly differentiated neoplasms are regarded as high grade. Cytologic and histologic grading, which are necessarily subjective and at best semiquantitative, are based on the degree of anaplasia and on the number of proliferating cells. The degree of anaplasia is determined from the shape and regularity of the cells and from the presence of distinct differentiated features, such as functioning gland-like structures in adenocarcinomas or epithelial pearls in squamous carcinomas. The presence of such characteristics identifies a tumor as well differentiated. By contrast, the cells of poorly differentiated malignancies bear little resemblance to their normal counterparts. Evidence of rapid growth is provided by (1) large numbers of mitoses, (2) atypical mitoses, (3) nuclear pleomorphism and (4) tumor giant cells. Most grading schemes classify tumors into three or four grades of increasing malignancy (Fig. 5-12). The general correlation between the cytologic grade and the biological behavior of a neoplasm is not invariable: there are many examples of tumors of low cytologic grades that exhibit substantial malignant properties. Thus, in most cases, staging is a more important criterion in predicting a tumor's course and influencing therapeutic decisions than is grading.

The Biology and Molecular Pathogenesis of Cancer

Normal cells, even those that divide the most rapidly (e.g., myelocytes, intestinal mucosal cells), are exquisitely controlled in the rate and location of their proliferation and accumulation. Cancer arises with accumulated DNA mutations within a single cell. When enough mutations have occurred, the cell escapes growth control and eventually acquires additional mutations that permit local invasion and subsequent spread through vascular and lymphatic channels.

For most of recorded history, cancer was considered to be simply due to a mysterious act of God. That is, the causation of cancer was not inherently comprehensible. However, in the late 18th century, specific causes of cancer were first identified. At that time, John Hill of London proposed that exposure to tobacco caused cancer. Shortly thereafter, in 1775, Sir Percival Pott described scrotal cancer caused by soot among chimney sweeps in London. More than a century later, bladder cancer was reported in aniline dye workers in Germany.

In modern times, major events in our understanding of oncogenesis include:

- 1911: F. Peyton Rous first described an avian cancer as being caused by a filterable agent (virus).
- 1920s: Human exposure to x-rays via fluoroscopy led to cancer.
- 1941: Berenblum first proposed the two-step (initiation/promotion) theory of chemical carcinogenesis.
- 1953: Watson and Crick identified DNA as the genetic material of cells and elucidated the structure of DNA.
- 1971: A. G. Knudson reported the involvement of two mutated alleles of the retinoblastoma (Rb) gene in the development of retinoblastomas and named these genes tumor suppressors.
- 1974: The gene responsible for defective DNA repair in the skin disease xeroderma pigmentosum was linked to visceral cancers.

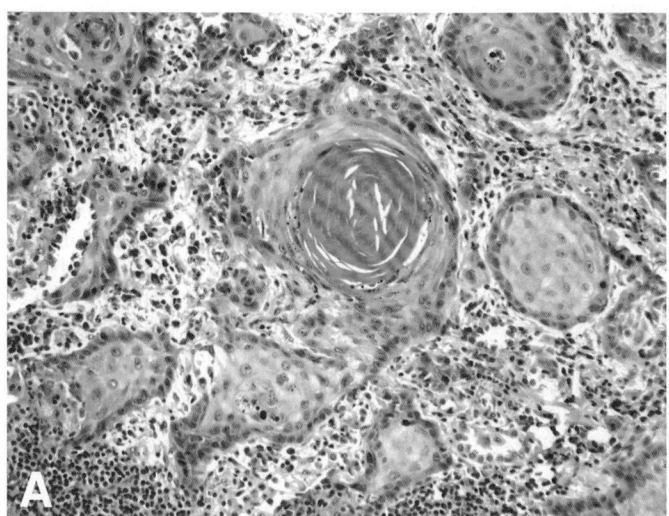
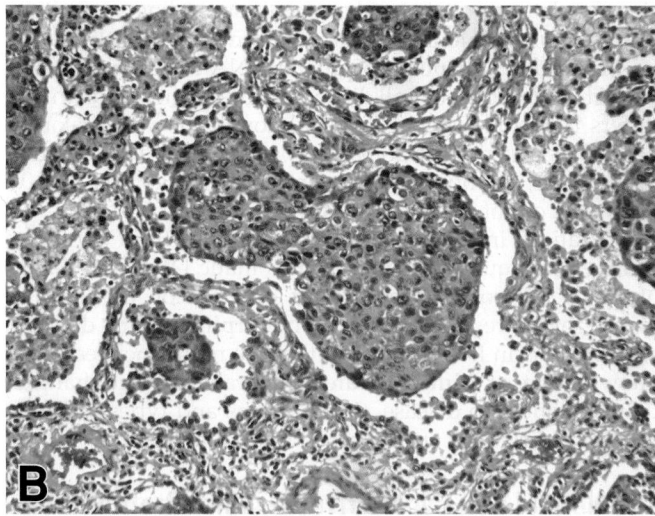

FIGURE 5-12. Cytologic grading of squamous cell carcinoma of the lung. A. Well-differentiated (grade 1) squamous cell carcinoma. The tumor cells bear a strong resemblance to normal squamous cells and synthesize keratin, as evidenced by epithelial pearls. **B.** Poorly differentiated (grade 3) squamous cell carcinoma. The malignant cells are difficult to identify as being of squamous origin.

- 1976: Bishop and Varmus demonstrated mammalian genetic homologs, called **proto-oncogenes,** of viral transforming genes **(oncogenes)**. When mutated, these cellular genes may become growth-promoting genes that can lead to cancer.

Substantial progress has been made in understanding neoplasia by the study of human tumors. Nonetheless, much of our appreciation of the processes involved in cancer development and spread has been derived from experiments in cells in culture, laboratory animals and genetically modified species. The applicability of those studies to oncogenesis in people should not always be assumed.

NORMAL PROCESSES THAT REGULATE CELLS AND INHIBIT ONCOGENESIS

As we will see shortly, cancer develops as a consequence of genetic changes in cells, leading to development, and often spread, of a tumor that is potentially fatal. Several critical cellular processes protect the organism and prevent tumor development. These processes are closely related, and intertwined: cell cycle regulation, DNA repair and telomerase activity. The next several pages describe how these cellular defenses operate and open the door to an understanding as to how they can be, and are, subverted during oncogenesis. As we will see, these defense mechanisms offer clues as to approaches to attacking tumors.

What is a gene? A century before the discovery of the structure of DNA, Gregor Mendel described discrete units of heredity that were later called genes. With the elucidation of the genetic code, the term "gene" came to signify a DNA string that defined the amino acid sequence of a protein. However, the idea of a gene is now being reexamined because regions of the genome previously thought to be "noncoding" are now known to produce new classes of RNAs that influence gene expression. Moreover, regulatory DNA sequences may be located adjacent to, at a large distance from and even within the protein-coding sequences. The contemporary notion of a gene entails interdependent structures and layers and webs of control involving DNA sequences, RNA species, regulatory proteins and a complex signaling apparatus. Thus, the precise definition of a gene remains unsettled.

Mutations and polymorphism: DNA replication is not perfect, and with each cell division about 1 nucleotide in 10^9 differs from the original. Thus, although the vast majority (99.6%) of base pairs in somatic cells are identical within the human race, two humans differ on average by about 2.4×10^7 base pairs out of 6×10^9 base pairs.

Variations in DNA sequences may result from germline changes or acquired alterations in somatic DNA as a result of single nucleotide substitutions or insertion or deletion of one or more nucleotides. **Polymorphisms** are defined as variations in DNA sequence that are not associated with known diseases. **Mutations** are comparable genetic changes that contribute to disease. (Mechanisms and types of DNA sequence variations are described in Chapter 6.)

The Normal Cell Cycle Drives Cellular Proliferation

Since most cancers are characterized by uncontrolled cellular proliferation, an understanding of the normal cell cycle is important. We focus here only on those aspects of the

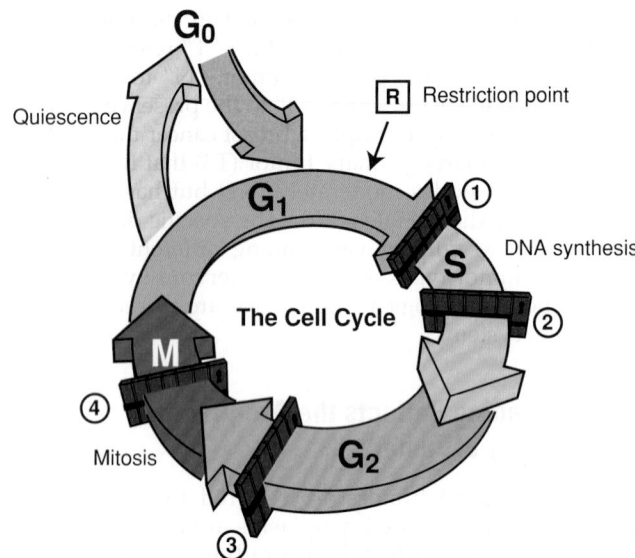

FIGURE 5-13. Normal cell cycle. The phases of the cell cycle, with key checkpoints indicated. R = restriction point.

cell cycle that are commonly aberrant in the pathogenesis of cancers.

Phases of the Cell Cycle

Cells may be cycling or quiescent. Those that replicate continuously (e.g., intestinal mucosa, hematopoietic progenitor cells) always transition from mitosis (M phase) to G_1, which is the antechamber to further cell division. By contrast, cells that replicate infrequently (e.g., hepatocytes) are in a quiescent phase, G_0. Cells in G_0 may be propelled to enter G_1 by various stimuli. They then replicate their DNA in S phase and proceed to G_2 and ultimately M (Fig. 5-13). When they are in an actively dividing mode, cells progress directly from M phase into G_1 by diverse stimuli. Thereafter, they initiate DNA replication, which occurs in S phase. G_2 follows S, and ultimately cells undergo mitosis (M phase). Following mitosis, cells again enter G_1 if they are in an actively dividing mode.

Cyclins and Cyclin-Dependent Kinases Driving Cell Cycle Progression

A cell's progress through the proliferative cycle is dependent on two important classes of regulatory molecules, **cyclins** and **cyclin-dependent kinases (CDKs)** (Fig. 5-14). These form a series of dimeric complexes that propel cell proliferation. Once a cell is stimulated to divide (e.g., by growth factors), D-type cyclins are activated first and form complexes of two CDKs (4 and 6). These cyclin D–CDK complexes play key roles in inactivating the retinoblastoma protein (pRb; see below). Together with cyclin E–CDK2 complexes they drive the cell into S phase. Other cyclins, A and then B, bind to CDKs (1 and 2), then push the cycle to completion.

Regulation of Cyclins and CDKs Provides Critical Protection against Tumor Development

Considering their importance in driving cell proliferation, it is not surprising that the activities of cyclins and CDKs

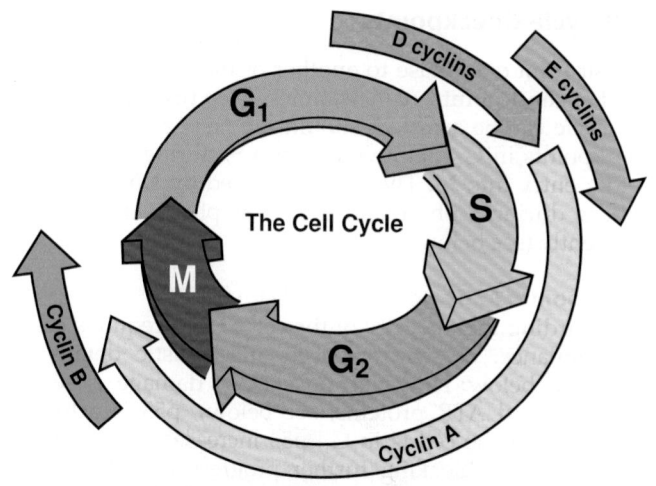

FIGURE 5-14. Activities of the cyclins and cyclin-dependent kinases (CDKs) in the cell cycle. The D cyclins mediate passage through G_1 and into early S phase. The E cyclins overlap D cyclins early in S phase. Cyclin A shepherds the cell through S and G_2 phases, into M phase. Finally, cyclin B overlaps cyclin A in late G_2 phase and directs the cell through mitosis (M phase).

are carefully controlled. Restraint of the cyclin–CDK system occurs in several ways (Fig. 5-15).

Decreasing Cyclin Availability

CDKs require activation by cyclins. Thus, the availability of cyclins limits the activity of CDKs. Levels of most cyclins fluctuate with the cell cycle: most are synthesized only when needed, and then, when the cell has traversed that part of the cycle for which a particular cyclin is required, that cyclin is ubiquitinated and degraded by the ubiquitin–proteasome system (UPS; see Chapter 1).

CDK Inhibitors

Several families of CDK inhibitors (CKIs) strongly inhibit cell proliferation and so collectively represent an important protective mechanism against oncogenesis. Not surprisingly, then, CKIs are commonly mutated in human cancers. CKIs mostly act by either binding the binary cyclin–CDK complexes or themselves binding with CDKs and preventing CDK activation by cyclins. The three major families of CKIs are:

- **INK4** proteins bind and inhibit CDKs 4 and 6 (*in*hibit cd*k4*), and prevent them from forming complexes with cyclin D. INK4 CKIs thus block cell cycle progression in G_1. There are several INK4 proteins: p15, p16, p18 and p19. As well, p14^{ARF} is encoded by the same gene as p16^{INK4a} but is an alternate reading frame (i.e., ARF). These proteins play important roles in regulating both CDKs and MDM2 (see Chapter 1 and below).
- **Cip/Kip** proteins bind and strongly block CDK2 and, to a lesser extent, CDK1. Thus, they take up where the INK4 family leaves off and inhibit the rest of the cell cycle. The best understood of the Cip/Kip proteins is p21^{CIP} (also called p21^{WAF1}).
- **Rb** family members (see below) also target CDK2.

Expression of CKIs can be induced by senescence, contact inhibition, extracellular antimitogenic factors (e.g.,

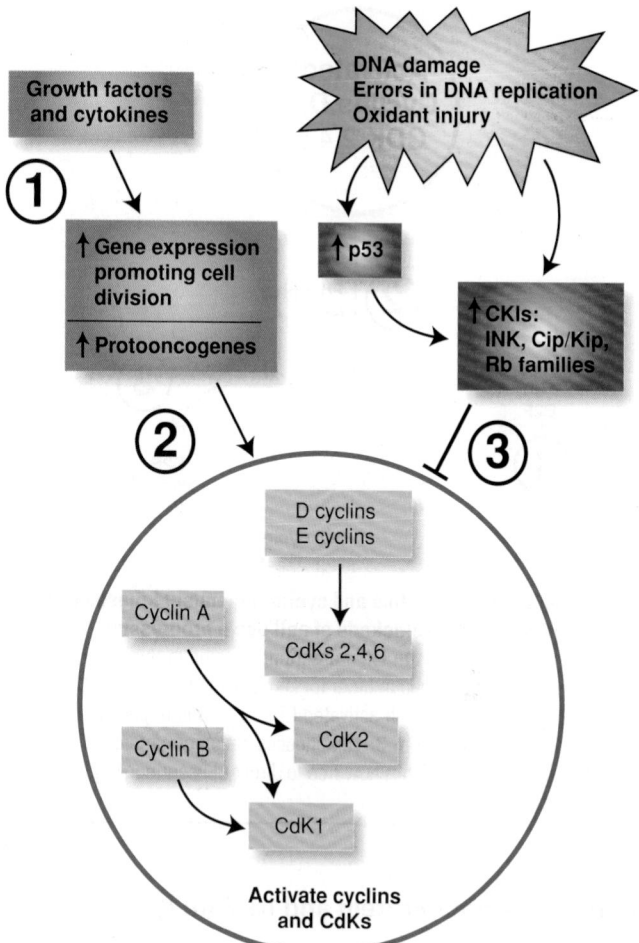

FIGURE 5-15. Activation and inhibition of the cyclins. 1. Activation. Cells receive signals via growth factors, cytokines and so forth that trigger the process of cell division. This leads to increased expression of genes that promote cell cycle progression, including a number of proto-oncogenes. **2. Actions of the early-phase cyclins.** D and E cyclins increase activity of cyclin-dependent kinases (CDKs) 2, 4 and 6. In addition, cyclin A activates CDKs 2 and 1, while cyclin B activates the latter. These CDKs drive cell cycle progression. **3. Inhibition.** Diverse stimuli, including errors in DNA replication, DNA damage and inhibitory signals of many kinds, may counteract the activating signals in **1.** These may do so by activating p53. Whether via p53 action or directly, these inhibitor stimuli increase production and activity of cyclin kinase inhibitors (CKIs), such as the INK family of proteins, CIP and KIP, as well as Rb. These families of CKIs block all the steps listed in **2.**

transforming growth factor-β [TGF-β]) and the tumor suppressor protein p53 (see below).

Other Forms of Inhibition of Cyclin–CDK Activities

In addition to mechanisms mentioned above, cells limit the ability of cyclin–CDK complexes to drive proliferation by selective posttranslational modification, largely phosphorylation, to inactivate some CDKs. Specific nuclear export systems also prevent cyclin–CDK dimers from accumulating in the nucleus, which is their site of activity. Both of these mechanisms support regulation supplied by other modalities mentioned above.

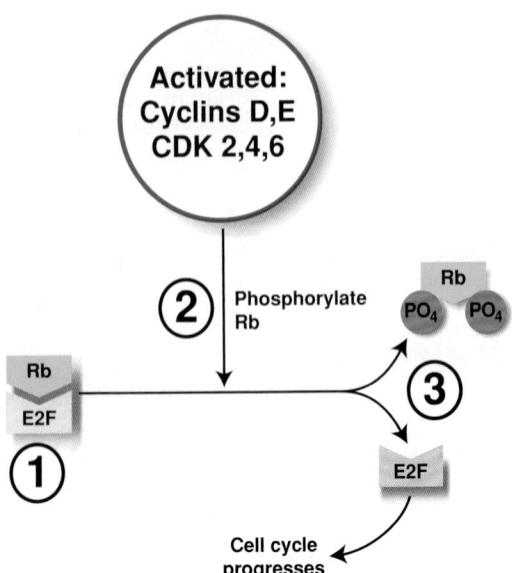

FIGURE 5-16. Role of cyclins and cyclin-dependent kinases (CDKs) in removing Rb-mediated blockade of cell cycle progression. 1. Normally Rb protein is complexed with E2F transcription factor. In this complex, E2F is inactive, yet it must be freed in order for cell division to proceed. **2.** Activated cyclins D and E, together with activated CDKs 2, 4 and 6, phosphorylate and then hyperphosphorylate Rb. **3.** This induces a conformational change that makes Rb release E2F, which is now free to direct transcription of proteins that help cell division to proceed.

Retinoblastoma Protein and Its Family

One of the most important mechanisms regulating the cell's commitment to division involves the family of retinoblastoma proteins, which principally act near the $G_1 \rightarrow S$ boundary. The prototype of these related proteins is p105^{Rb} (pRb). Other members are related structurally and functionally, and for simplicity, we refer here only to pRb. pRb inhibits progression of the cell cycle by binding members of the **E2F** family of transcription factors. These E2F factors mediate cell entry into, and transit through, S phase by increasing transcription of downstream cyclins (A and E), as well as other proteins that promote DNA replication.

Binding of E2F by pRb blocks E2F activity. Phosphorylation of pRb by the complex of cyclin D–CDK4/6 (see above) alters pRb conformation, releasing E2F. E2F-mediated upregulation of other cyclins (A and E; see above), which, complexed to CDK2, again phosphorylate pRb, allows the cell cycle to progress (Fig. 5-16). The Rb system thus integrates many signals that control cell cycle progression.

Interestingly, Rb resumes its cell cycle inhibitory activity as cell division culminates. In anaphase, a protein phosphatase (PP1) dephosphorylates pRb, allowing it to bind E2F again, thus preventing further division.

Landmark Transitions in the Cell Cycle

The major cell cycle transitions are $G_1 \rightarrow S$ and $G_2 \rightarrow M$. Passage from $G_1 \rightarrow S$ occurs when the activity of complexes involving cyclins A and E overwhelm inhibition by the Cip/Kip family of inhibitors. Cells progress from $G_2 \rightarrow M$ when cyclin B–CDK1 complexes are activated by removing inhibitory phosphorylation of CDK1.

Cell Cycle Checkpoints

Transit from one phase to another of the cell cycle is regulated at **checkpoints,** namely, times when progression in the cell cycle can be arrested, should the need arise. There are checkpoints in G_1, before entry into S, during S and in G_2 before entry into M. These are activated by DNA damage. Others, during S phase and during M phase, are activated differently (see below).

Checkpoints Activated by DNA Damage
Safeguarding the integrity of the cell's DNA requires ceaseless vigilance, of which specific mechanistic details are discussed below. However, once DNA damage is sensed (by ATM and ATR proteins; see below), p53 is activated (Fig. 5-17). If the cell is in G_1, p53 increases production of Cip/Kip CKIs, blocking further progress in cell division. If the cell is in G_2, there are two means by which cycling is stopped. One involves p53-mediated downregulation of cyclin B and CDK1. The other involves two related enzymes called checkpoint kinases (**chk1, chk2;** see below), which block cell cycle progression immediately. These kinases are also responsible for blocking the cycle at the S phase DNA damage checkpoint as well.

Restriction Point
During G_1, the cell commits itself to enter S phase at the **restriction point (R)**. Here, the cell crosses the Rubicon and decides whether to proceed with mitosis or not. Past the R point, external forces driving or inhibiting mitosis no longer come into play (i.e., cell proliferation is determined only by intracellular mechanisms). The R point is activated by cyclin D–CDK4/6 phosphorylation of pRb, with consequent release of E2F (see above) to facilitate mitosis. *Loss of R-point control occurs in many cancers and deregulates progression through the cell cycle.*

Other Checkpoints
The duration of the proliferative cycle is finite. On occasion, the cell dawdles (usually because of exposure to a

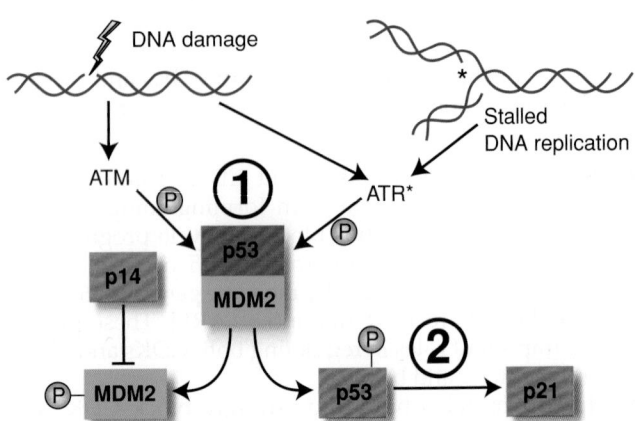

FIGURE 5-17. Linkage of DNA damage and replication stress to cell cycle arrest, via p53. 1. Both DNA damage and other interference with DNA replication activate the kinases ATM (ataxia telangiectasia mutated) and ATR (ATM and Rad3 related). These kinases phosphorylate p53, releasing it from binding to its inhibitor, MDM2. **2.** Activated p53 stimulates p21 (also called p21$^{CIP1/WAF1}$).

toxic agent) in S phase. Should that happen, nature loses its patience and activates chk1 to block mitotic separation of incompletely duplicated chromosomes. This is called the **replication checkpoint**.

During M phase, there are elaborate controls to ensure that daughter cells each receive the correct complement of chromosomes. Thus, sensors at the points (kinetochores) where chromosomes attach to the mitotic spindle may activate a **spindle integrity checkpoint** if they sense that the segregation process is unbalanced or inaccurate. An additional mechanism involves an important enzyme, **Aurora B kinase,** which ensures that the kinetochore binds effectively and the mitotic spindle is effective, and so prevents improper segregation of chromosomes.

p53 in the Cell Cycle

As mentioned in Chapter 1, p53 has been called "the guardian of the genome." It coordinates cellular responses to DNA damage, mediates activation of G_1/S and G_2/M checkpoints and initiates apoptosis. Mechanisms underlying p53 activities include:

1. Normally, p53 is maintained at low levels by MDM2 (murine double minute), an E3 ubiquitin (Ub) ligase that conjugates p53 to Ub and triggers its proteasomal degradation (Fig. 5-18A; see Chapter 1).

2. The protein kinases **ATM** (ataxia telangiectasia mutated) and **ATR** (ATM and Rad3 related) recognize DNA damage and, in combination with chk1 and chk2 kinases, phosphorylate, and therefore activate, p53. Activation of p53 through these kinases or via telomere dysfunction (see Chapter 1 and below) contributes to cell cycle arrest (Fig. 5-17).

3. Activation of a cell cycle checkpoint requires a period of arrest to permit DNA repair. When p53 is phosphorylated, it dissociates from MDM2 and translocates to the nucleus.

4. In this location, p53 further promotes cell cycle arrest by stimulating production of p21^{Cip1}, one of the Cip/Kip family of CKIs (Fig. 5-18B).

5. If DNA is repaired, the block is removed and the cell cycle proceeds (Fig. 5-18B).

6. If DNA cannot be repaired, p53 triggers apoptosis (Fig. 5-18C).

It is important to appreciate that tumor cells often have mutations in genes that control cell cycle transit and that, whether these genes are mutated or not, many antineoplastic agents target cell cycle–related genes to try to limit the ability of cancer cells to divide. Mutations in cyclins or CDKs, for example, may render them impervious to the regulatory activities described above. Other alterations, in regulatory proteins like Cip/Kip CKIs or pRb, may eliminate one or another aspect of their ability to limit cell cycle progression.

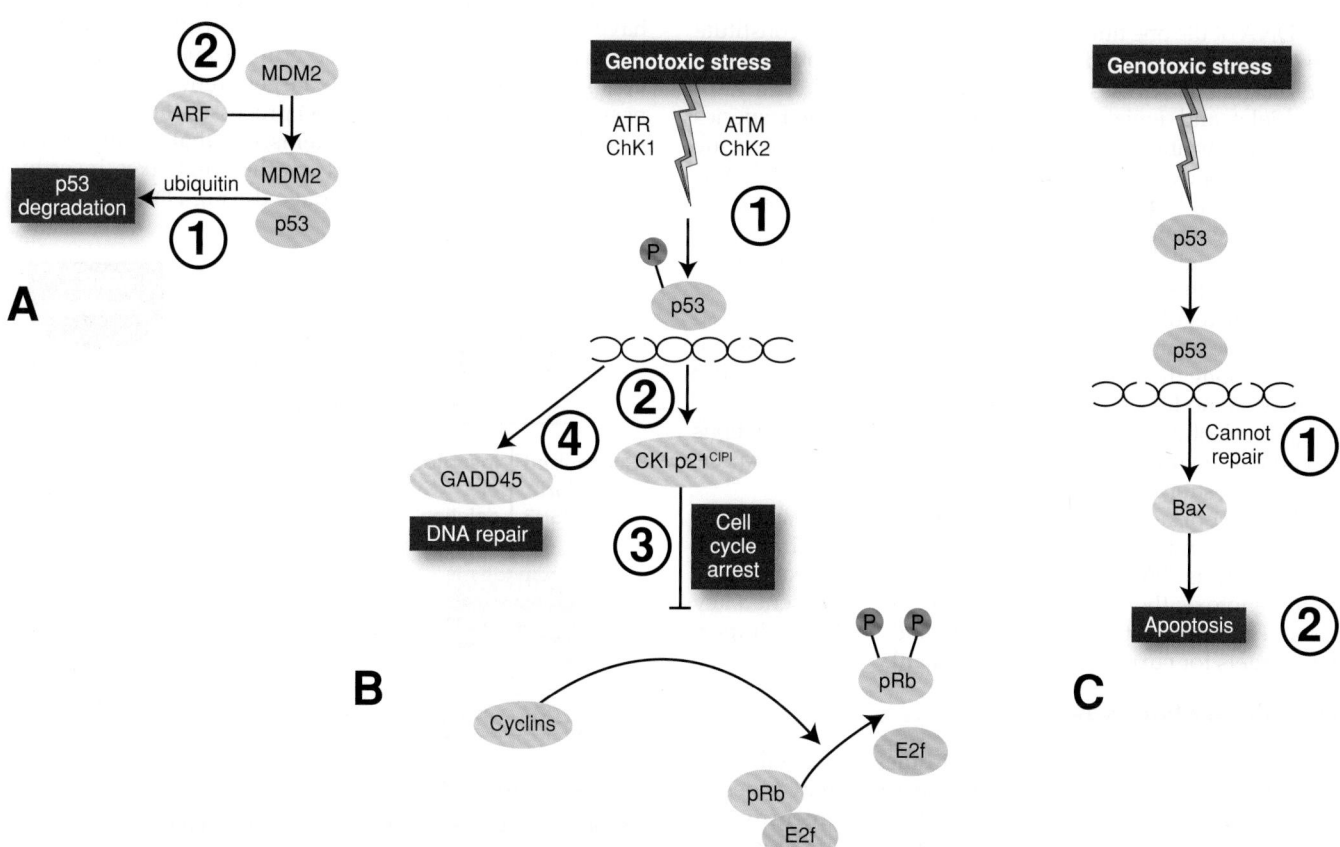

FIGURE 5-18.   A. Regulation of p53 and MDM2 (murine double minute). 1. MDM2 is an E3 ubiquitin ligase that binds to and directs the inactivation of p53. **2.** MDM2 activity is inhibited by the tumor suppress p14^{ARF}. **B. 1.** In response to genotoxic stress (e.g., ionizing radiation, carcinogens, mutagens), ATR (ATM and Rad3 related) and ATM (ataxia telangiectasia mutated) increase p53, which does two things. **2.** It binds to DNA and upregulates transcription of several genes, including cyclin kinase inhibitor (CKI) p21$^{CIP1/WAF1}$. **3.** It also induces cell cycle arrest by preventing release of E2F from retinoblastoma protein (pRB). **4.** GADD45 promotes DNA repair. **C. 1.** Should DNA repair not be possible, p53 directs increased transcription of the proapoptotic protein Bax. **2.** Increased Bax triggers apoptosis.

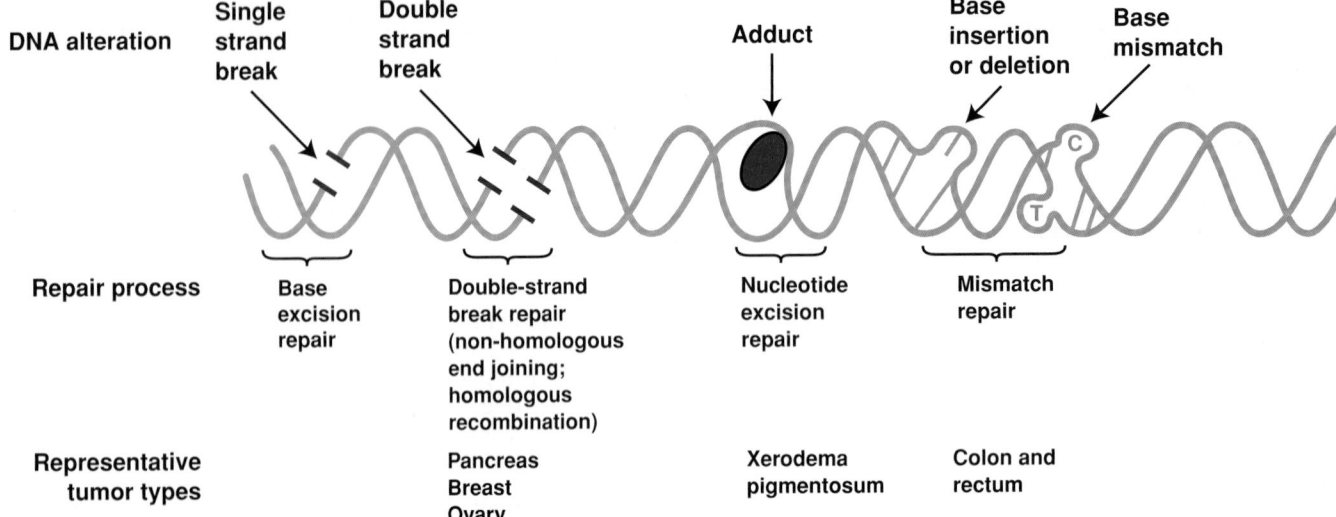

FIGURE 5-19. DNA damage and the mechanisms that repair DNA damage. Most forms of localized DNA damage are either (1) single-strand breaks, (2) double-strand breaks, (3) DNA adducts, (4) base insertions or deletions or (5) base mismatches. The mechanisms that repair these insults are, respectively, (1) base excision repair, (2) double-strand break repair, (3) nucleotide excision repair, and (4) and (5) mismatch repair. Some tumor types that arise from dysfunctional DNA repair mechanisms are indicated in conjunction with the mechanisms that tend to malfunction in those tumors.

DNA Repair Protects Cellular Genomes from Genotoxic Stresses

The DNA of the one hundred trillion (10^{14}) cells that constitute the human body is under relentless assault by both internal and exogenous stresses, including environmental chemicals, ultraviolet and ionizing radiation, reactive oxygen species (ROS) and an intracellular milieu that may break down the chemical bonds that hold DNA together. Cellular DNA is further at risk from the infidelity of DNA polymerases. Cells maintain genomic stability via diverse mechanisms that are ceaselessly vigilant in detecting and repairing such damage. In addition, these systems also communicate with cell cycle checkpoint regulators (see above) and apoptosis triggers, so that mutations are not transmitted to daughter cells. Collaborations among diverse proteins restore genomic integrity after such DNA modifications as single- and double-strand breaks, single nucleotide substitutions, base insertions and deletions of variable lengths and other perturbations of orderly and correct double-stranded DNA structure.

The importance of understanding these mechanisms extends beyond their roles in homeostasis and, if impaired, tumorigenesis. DNA repair systems may also protect tumors from genotoxic therapies. In this sense, they represent a key facet of tumor resistance to treatment and, therefore, important targets for current drug development.

DNA Repair Pathways

DNA damage may occur at different times in the cell cycle, be caused by diverse insults and reflect different types of alterations in DNA structure. Maintaining the integrity of a cell's genome thus requires multiple DNA repair processes, illustrated in Fig. 5-19.

Mismatch Repair
This pathway is mainly involved in repairing errors in DNA replication. From one somatic cell division to the next, the error rate in duplicating the genome is 1 miscopied base

per 10^9 bases. In germ cells, it is even lower, 1 miscopied base in 10^{11}. The two polymerases that replicate human DNA (called Pol δ and ε) possess editing functions that have error rates of 1 base/10^{4-5}. The difference between the error rates of polymerase editing and the final product, 4–5 orders of magnitude, largely reflects the effectiveness of mismatch repair (MMR) processes (Fig. 5-20). MMR includes two overlapping systems, one that mainly corrects single base mismatches and another that fixes insertions and deletions caused by slippage during DNA replication.

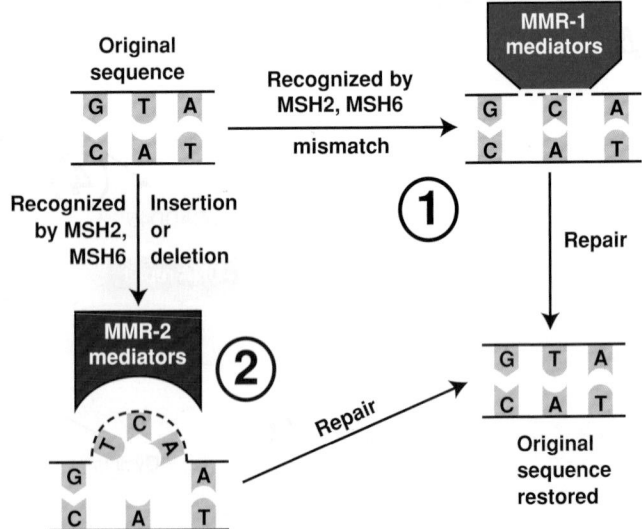

FIGURE 5-20. Mediators of mismatch repair (MMR). 1. A DNA single base mismatch (here, a C is present where a T should be) is recognized by two proteins, MSH2 and MSH6. These recruit a group of MMR repair enzymes, which correct the defect. **2.** If the mispairing is the result of a small insertion or deletion, a second group of MMR enzymes, MSH2 and MSH3, recognize the mistake and recruit another group of MMR mediators to correct the defect and restore the correct sequence.

Errors are recognized and repaired by a family of enzymes (e.g., MSH6, MSH2, MLH1; Fig. 5-20) that stop DNA replication at the G_2/M checkpoint, correct the mistake and then allow replication to continue. If the damage is irreparable, MMR enzymes activate apoptosis.

Defective MMR may be inherited or acquired. Acquired defects in MMR may reflect either mutations that develop over time in somatic cells or epigenetic silencing (see below) of a component of the MMR system. An important indicator of defective MMR is **microsatellite instability**. Microsatellites are short sequences of up to 6 base pairs that may be repeated as many as 100 times. They are common in the human genome and are inordinately prone to mutation, including changes in numbers of repeats. Microsatellite mutations are usually detected and repaired by MMR enzymes. If, however, they escape repair in germline or somatic cells, microsatellite mutations may indicate the likelihood of cancer developing (see below).

Nucleotide Excision and Repair

This process corrects distortions of DNA helical structure, such as are caused by bulky DNA adducts, by base oxidation by ROS derived from mitochondria or other sources or by ultraviolet (UV) and ionizing radiation (Table 5-2). Nucleotide excision and repair (NER) searches for DNA damage in two ways. One constantly scans the genome and the other identifies alterations that interfere with RNA transcription. Inherited defects in these NER detection systems are associated with human cancer syndromes. The first (scanning) pathway is deficient in **xeroderma pigmentosum,** and the second (transcription coupled) in **Cockayne syndrome**.

Once either NER system recognizes a defect, both pathways repair it similarly, via an enzyme called ERCC1. This enzyme is of considerable practical therapeutic importance. As mentioned above, effective DNA repair by tumor cells helps to protect them from chemotherapies that target DNA. For certain types of tumor, the activity (or lack thereof) of ERCC1 helps to predict the sensitivity of cancer cells to chemotherapy with such DNA-damaging agents as *cis*-platinum.

Base Excision Repair

Base excision repair (BER) is related to NER, and the two overlap somewhat in the types of DNA damage for which they are responsible (Table 5-2). BER mostly repairs chemical injury to DNA bases, such as hydrolysis of base–sugar bonds, single-strand breaks and small chemical changes in base structure. Such alterations occur 10^4 times/cell/day. Insults leading to BER are mostly caused by environmental and other chemicals, ROS and UV and ionizing radiation. Inherited defects in BER have not been described.

Double-Strand Break Repair

Double-strand breaks (DSBs) may be caused by ROS or ionizing radiation, or during DNA replication if replication is stalled at a single-strand break (Table 5-2). Such DNA lesions commonly lead to chromosome rearrangements, particularly when they occur, as they often do, in clusters.

Two related enzymes, ATM and ATR (see above, Fig. 5-17), are the sensors for DSBs, and each recognizes different types of DSBs. ATM identifies those that result from DNA damage (e.g., ionizing radiation). Once activated, ATM recruits chk2. ATR detects single-stranded DNA at stalled replication forks, whereupon it in turn activates chk1 (see above).

TABLE 5-2

TYPES OF DNA DAMAGE, THEIR COMMON CAUSES AND THE RESPECTIVE REPAIR PATHWAYS

Type of Damage	Causes	Repair Pathway
Base oxidation	Mitochondrial ROS	NER, BER
	Phagocyte-generated oxidants	
	UV and ionizing radiation	
	Smoking	
Other base modifications	Chemotherapeutic drugs	BER
	Neutrophil bactericidal enzymes	
	Cigarette smoke	
	Other environmental chemicals	
Alterations Perturbing DNA Architecture		
Additions	Errors in transcription, ROS	NER
	UV light	
Interstrand DNA cross-links	Ionizing radiation	Other[a]
	Arrested DNA replication	
	Environmental chemicals	
Single-strand nicks	ROS	BER, NER
	Ionizing radiation	
	Spontaneous loss of sugar–phosphate bonding	
Double-strand breaks	Arrested DNA replication	HR, NHEJ
	Ionizing radiation	
	Chemical damage	

[a]Other mechanisms include Fanconi-related repair pathways.
BER = base excision repair; HR = homologous recombination; NER = nucleotide excision repair; NHEJ = nonhomologous end-joining; ROS = reactive oxygen species; UV = ultraviolet.

Both resulting complexes, ATM/chk2 and ATR/chk1, phosphorylate p53 and so activate cell cycle checkpoints, halting cell division until the break is fixed. DSBs are repaired either by **nonhomologous end-joining (NHEJ)** or by **homologous recombination (HR)**.

In HR, which is mostly active in S and G_2, the sister chromatid or the homologous chromosome is used as a template, to reproduce the original sequence. However, in so doing, two major types of genome alterations may result. If HR uses the homologous chromosome as a template for DNA repair, allelic differences between the two chromosomes may be lost (**loss of heterozygosity [LOH];** see below). As well, because repetitive sequences are abundant throughout the human genome, HR repair of a break that happens to occur in repetitive sequences in one chromosome may lead to use of an identical repetitive sequence on a nonhomologous chromosome as a template for recombination, thus generating a translocation. Several genes (e.g., BRCA1, BRCA2, PALB2) whose protein products are important for HR are often mutated or inactivated in many human tumors. This may occur (see below) either as part of inherited cancer susceptibility syndromes or epigenetically during oncogenesis.

By contrast, NHEJ repairs DSBs by rejoining the broken ends. NHEJ thus restores DNA integrity but may not reproduce the original sequence (depending on the nature of the break). Furthermore, there is no guarantee that the ends that are so joined are in fact the broken ends of the same chromatid, in which case, translocations may result.

Unlike HR, NHEJ operates throughout the cell cycle. It is more efficient than HR and uses the Ku proteins (Ku70, Ku80), which are among the most abundant protein species within cells. NHEJ is the mechanism behind V(D)J recombination to generate diversity in B lymphocytes.

NHEJ generally functions well, and without many errors. However, it does not easily account for the original base order of the DNA sequences it joins. In settings in which there are multiple, clustered DSBs, NHEJ may link non-contiguous DNAs. It should be noted that defective NHEJ is not associated with any known inherited predispositions to developing cancer, nor is it commonly associated with oncogenesis.

HALLMARKS OF CANCER

Tumor development generally requires accumulation of changes in cellular behavior, many of which occur via mutation. Extensive and ongoing analyses of human tumors have uncovered a great many mutations. Not all changes so identified are equally important for tumor development and spread: some are more equal than others.

A relatively small number of genetic changes are fundamental to oncogenesis. These are called **"drivers."** It should be stressed that **driver mutations** may affect both DNA sequences that encode proteins and so-called noncoding sequences, since altered sequences and levels of untranslated RNAs (see below) and of regulatory regions may drive oncogenesis. Thus, the idea of driver mutations should be inclusive and should accommodate the complexities of regulation of gene expression and action.

Other mutations—"passengers" or "hitchhikers"—seem to be along for the ride. How they affect tumor development and progression, if at all, is unknown.

What is clear is that there are several basic activities that distinguish cells of solid malignancies from their normal counterparts. (Hematologic cancers develop and spread differently, and so share some, though not all, of these characteristics.) To understand oncogenesis and how cancer-related processes are being targeted therapeutically, the following hallmarks or attributes of malignant tumors should be appreciated:

- **Unregulated cellular proliferation:** In normal tissues, progression through the cell cycle (see above) is carefully regulated. However, cancer cells have acquired the ability to determine their own destinies, independently of normal restraints to multiplication.
- **Cellular immortalization:** While normal cells in culture have a limited potential for replication, cancer cells can multiply indefinitely. Thus, malignant cells circumvent the process of senescence and retain youthful vigor and ability to reproduce.
- **Evasion of programmed cell death (PCD):** Programmed cell death (see Chapter 1) can be activated by such factors

as genomic instability and inhospitable cellular microenvironments. Cancer cells often develop strategies that circumvent destruction via such suicide programs.
- **Stimulation of vascular proliferation:** Expansion of solid tumors requires increased supplies of nutrients and oxygen. This, in turn, necessitates proliferation of blood vessels. Thus, tumor cells secrete signaling molecules that stimulate **angiogenesis** (i.e., formation of new blood vessels).
- **Invasion and metastasis:** Death from cancers is usually caused by tumor dissemination (metastasis). To accomplish such spread, tumor cells must be able to surmount anatomic barriers such as basement membrane, traverse intervening connective tissues, enter blood vessels and lymphatics, identify fertile sites for implantation, exit the vasculature and then establish colonies far from their origin.
- **Inactivation of tumor suppressors:** Many strong influences normally limit cell cycle transit, maintain genomic stability and regulate other key functions. These restraints affect most of the key attributes mentioned above, as well as associated facilitating processes described below. If a tumor is to be successful, these endogenous tumor suppressors must be evaded or inactivated.

Additional Processes Facilitate Tumor Cell Growth and Spread

Some mechanisms play supporting roles in developing and maintaining many cancers but are not yet generally accepted as being obligatory to tumor development.

- **Genomic instability:** Most human cancer cells show increased susceptibility to random mutation. This allows tumor cells to evolve quickly and to achieve genotypes that favor cancer maintenance and progression.
- **Altered epigenetic regulation:** Epigenetics refers to management of gene function by mechanisms independent of the DNA base sequences whose activities are being controlled. Among the modalities involved are covalent modifications of DNA and DNA-associated proteins (such as histones), noncoding RNAs, altered messenger RNA (mRNA) translation and posttranslational modifications of gene products.
- **Altered bioenergenetics:** Generally, cancer cells favor glycolysis over oxidative phosphorylation for adenosine triphosphate (ATP) generation. This metabolic change requires increased glucose utilization, which has many consequences for the cell's metabolic needs and products.
- **Immune avoidance:** A body of clinical and experimental evidence suggests that the immune system may protect from tumor production and progression. However, the nature of the interactions between tumors and host immunity remains uncertain.
- **Inflammation:** Inflammatory cells infiltrate most developing solid tumors and secrete diverse factors that facilitate tumor development and progression.

Most cancers develop because multiple mutations accumulate in dividing cells. Incipient tumors become malignant by undergoing serial genetic changes that lead to their acquiring hallmarks of cancers, as listed above. The order in which these changes arise may vary from tumor to tumor, but eventually a tumor amasses all of them.

These basic tumor attributes and contributing factors are interdependent mechanistically, and a single altered protein or gene may contribute to more than one characteristic, and no one trait operates in isolation. Interrelated though they are, cancer hallmarks are conceptually distinct. Further, every tumor evolves differently. Thus, certain attributes and genes may contribute to one tumor but not to others, or may suppress oncogenesis in one context but encourage it in another. The discussion of neoplasia that ensues follows the sequence of essential tumor characteristics and contributing factors listed above.

Tumor Cells Elude Processes That Normally Regulate Proliferation

Tumor cell escape from controlled proliferation occurs as a result of mutations that have the effects of both activating and inactivating certain genes. Generally, activating mutations stimulate passage through the cell cycle. The genes affected by such mutations have traditionally been called oncogenes. Inactivating mutations, by contrast, usually prevent the inhibitory influences of tumor suppressor genes (see below).

The Concept of Oncogenes

Early research on transforming retroviruses showed that some viral genes could impart a neoplastic phenotype to

normal cells. It was later found that transfer of specific genes from human cancer cells (oncogenes) in vitro could also impart a transformed phenotype to normal recipient cells. Some such transforming human tumor genes were found to be mutant versions of normal genes (proto-oncogenes) that stimulated cellular proliferation. Transforming retroviral genes were designated with a *v*- (e.g., *v-myb*), and their cellular counterparts with a *c*- (e.g., *c-myb*).

Mechanisms by Which Cell Proliferation Is Driven

Among the key genes often altered during oncogenesis are those that stimulate cell multiplication. They are in the biochemical pathways that guide entry into the cell cycle. These include the following (Fig. 5-21):

- Growth factors
- Cell surface receptors
- Intracellular signal transduction pathways
- DNA-binding nuclear proteins (transcription factors)

Growth Factor–Related Signaling and Oncogenesis

Cell proliferation normally reflects a balance between forces driving cells to divide and, on the other hand, the cell cycle regulators discussed above. In acquiring the

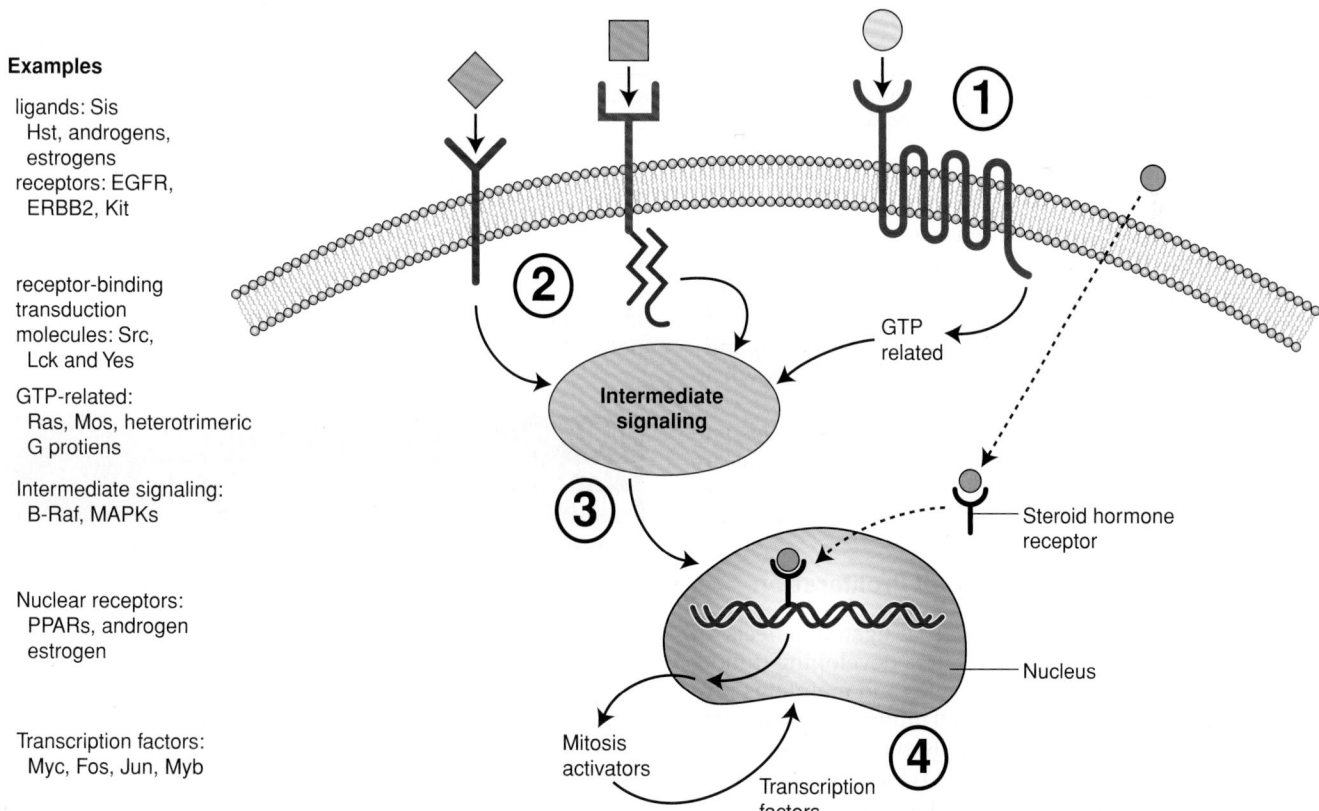

FIGURE 5-21. Signaling paradigms in cellular transformation. 1. Extracellular ligands bind to cell membrane receptors. **2.** One of several pathways of signaling is then activated. The receptor itself can activate intracellular signaling (*left*). A protein that binds to the activated receptor may trigger intracellular signaling (*center*). The receptor may be a G-protein–coupled receptor, which stimulates guanine nucleotide–related signaling. Or, the ligand may traverse the cell membrane to activate receptors within the cytosol directly, without a cell membrane intermediate (*far right*). **3.** In the first three cases, cellular intermediates of many types are activated. **4.** The end result for all pathways is activation of transcription, particularly of proteins that help take the cell through the cell cycle. Shown at the *left* are examples of proto-oncogenes and other cellular products that act in each capacity.

TABLE 5-3
COMMON PROTEINS THAT DRIVE CELL PROLIFERATION, THEIR ACTIVITIES AND ACTIVATION

Activity	Name of Protein	Nature of Mutation	Explanation
Ligand	Hst	Amplification	Growth factor in FGF family
	Sis	Derepression (autocrine stimulation)	PDGF, β subunit
	FGF3	Amplification	
RTK	Kit	Activating point mutation	Receptor for stem cell factor
	Her2/neu (ErbB2)	Amplification	Constitutively activated
	EGFR	Mutations, amplification	Constitutively activated
	Met	Translocation	HGF receptor
	Ret	Point mutation, translocation	Constitutively activated
Intracellular signaling intermediate	Ras (K-Ras, N-Ras, H-Ras)	Point mutation	GTP binding protein, three different *RAS* genes, activated in different settings
	B-Raf	Point mutation	Tyrosine kinase
	Src	Point mutation	Tyrosine kinase
	Abl	Translocation	Mutant protein, Bcr-Abl
Transcription factor	Myc (c-Myc, N-Myc, L-Myc)	Amplification, translocation	Directs transcription of up to 15% of human genes
	Fos	Amplification	Part of AP-1, with Jun
	Myb	Point mutations	Promotes hematopoietic stem cell proliferation
	Rel	Amplification, point mutations	Member of NFκB family, expressed mainly in lymphocytes
	Ets	Translocation	Large family; fusion products may drive tumorigenesis

AP-1 = activation protein-1; EGFR = epidermal growth factor receptor; FGF = fibroblast growth factor; GTP = guanosine triphosphate; HGF = human growth factor; NF = nuclear factor; PDGF = platelet-derived growth factor; RTK = receptor tyrosine kinase.

ability to multiply without restraint, cancer cells must be able to circumvent dependence on outside stimulatory influences. They usually do this by mimicking those influences. To understand how this occurs, one must first review how receptor–ligand interactions drive cells into mitosis. A general schematic relating the roles of ligand–receptor interactions in tumor development is shown in Fig. 5-21.

Tumor-driving mutations may occur at any step of this process. The consequence of such mutations is that proteins are produced that drive cellular proliferation without the normal restraints that match cell numbers to the body's needs.

Ligands, Their Receptors and Cell Proliferation

Ligands. In general, the role of external ligands reflects an ongoing need of normal cells and, often, developing tumors for exogenous stimulation that activates and maintains proliferation. Some ligands may drive cell multiplication in early stages of oncogenesis, with tumor cells eventually becoming independent of those ligands, owing to changes in, for example, receptors or other molecules. Sometimes, the developing (or developed) tumor cell itself undertakes production of these ligands, which amounts to an autocrine trigger to cell division. Some such stimulatory molecules occasionally act as oncoproteins being overexpressed, mostly by virtue of gene amplification (Table 5-3).

Receptors. There are several basic classes of receptors that may stimulate or inhibit cell proliferation. These are listed in Table 5-4. Except for the steroid hormone receptors, these are cell membrane molecules that respond to ligands produced by other cells. Usually, receptor–ligand interactions cause changes in the receptors, leading to their serving as docking sites for one or more intracellular signaling networks.

TABLE 5-4
TYPES OF SIGNAL-TRANSDUCING RECEPTORS IMPORTANT IN TUMORIGENESIS

Receptor Category	Prototypical Ligands
Tyrosine kinase (RTK)	EGF, IGF-I, insulin
G-protein–coupled receptor (GPCR)	Prostaglandins, RANTES, SDF-1
Nuclear receptors	Androgens, estrogens, other steroid hormones
Serine/threonine kinases	TGF-β
Kinase-associated receptors	GH, TCR, IL-2
Extracellular matrix receptors	Fibronectin, collagen, laminin

EGF = epidermal growth factor; GH = growth hormone; IGF-I = insulin-like growth factor-1; IL-2 = interleukin-2; RANTES = CCL5, a ligand for CCR5; SDF-1 = CXCL12, stromal-derived factor-1 (CXCR4 ligand); TCR = T-cell receptor; TGF-β = transforming growth factor-β.

The changes that ligands elicit in receptors reflect the specifics of the receptor:

- **Receptor tyrosine kinases (RTKs)** possess intrinsic tyrosine kinase activity that causes the receptor to phosphorylate itself, and perhaps other molecules as well, after recognizing its ligand.
- **Nonkinase receptors** include many that undergo structural rearrangements, making them receptive to initiating downstream signaling (see below). These types of receptors often associate with nonreceptor tyrosine kinases (**NRTKs;** see below), which mediate further signaling.
- **G-protein–coupled receptors (GPCRs)** are the most common type of membrane receptors. Upon binding their ligands—which include very diverse types of molecules—GPCRs change conformation. In so doing, they activate guanosine triphosphate (GTP)-related nucleotide exchange factors (GEFs; see below). Some GPCRs transduce mitogenic signals triggered by such ligands as prostaglandins, endothelin and thrombin. GPCRs may be amplified in cancers or they may mediate stimulatory autocrine or paracrine signals.

The nature of signaling elicited by receptor–ligand interaction varies. Many activated RTKs and nonkinase receptors serve as platforms for other proteins, including NRTKs. The latter often phosphorylate the nonkinase receptor, as well as the NRTKs themselves. In these settings, a cell membrane complex is formed, which recruits signaling intermediates and activates diverse downstream signaling pathways.

Receptor proteins are among the most important transforming proteins. They are widely implicated in oncogenesis (Table 5-3), *often driving tumor formation via mutations that render them constitutively active, independently of their ligands.*

Signaling after Receptor Activation

Once a receptor binds to its ligand, downstream signaling pathways are stimulated. If an RTK or NRTK is involved, the phosphorylated tyrosine is recognized by the next cadre of signaling intermediates via specialized structures, called SH2 (for Src-homology-2) domains, on these intermediates. These domains bind phosphotyrosines. They also are specific for individual proteins bearing the phosphotyrosines.

What follows depends on many factors, including the type of receptor activated, if its activation entails tyrosine kinase activity and the molecular species that immediately follow. Pathways that may be set in motion include:

- **Ras:** The three members of the Ras family (K-Ras, N-Ras, H-Ras) are small guanine nucleotide-binding proteins that may be activated by tyrosine kinases via a linker protein, usually Grb2. To understand activated Ras and Ras-related oncogenesis, the Ras cycle should be appreciated (Fig. 5-22). Ras binds guanosine diphosphate (GDP) and GTP. In the GTP-bound state, Ras is active. GTP binding is catalyzed by a GEF (see above), which is in turn activated when Grb2 recognizes phosphorylated tyrosines (see above). A GTPase activating protein (GAP) directs the GTPase activity of Ras, thus activating downstream signaling, converting Ras–GTP to Ras–GDP and returning Ras to its quiescent resting state.

  Many malignant tumors possess a mutated form of Ras. Such mutated Ras does not undergo the deactivation step and is constitutively turned on.

  Activation of many GPCRs stimulates a similar type of response, but by a different group of proteins, called heterotrimeric G proteins. Unlike Ras, these G proteins tend not to be mutated in cancers. Rather, they may be overexpressed, achieving a comparable effect (i.e., constitutive activation of downstream signaling).
- **Phosphatidylinositol-3 (PI3) kinase:** This family of enzymes is generally activated by RTKs and GPCRs. Family members add a phosphate group to a phosphatidylinositol lipid to create the small molecule phosphatidylinositol-3-phosphate [PI(3)P], as well as more heavily phosphorylated derivatives such as PI(3,4,5)P₃. These

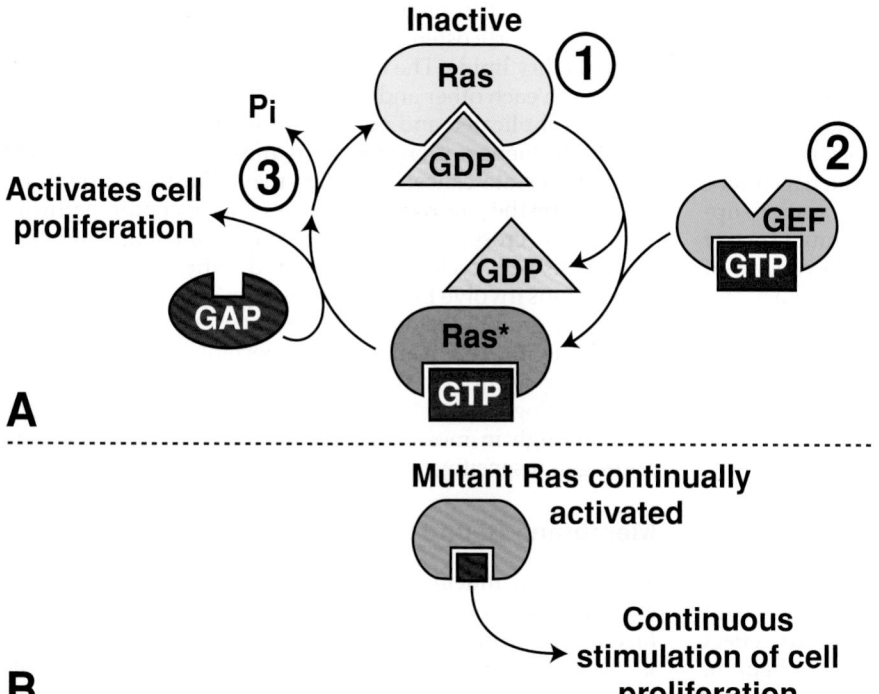

A

B

FIGURE 5-22. Mechanism of action of Ras. A (upper). Normal. The Ras protein, p21^{Ras}, exists in two conformational states, determined by the binding of either guanosine diphosphate (GDP) or guanosine triphosphate (GTP). **1.** Normally, most of the p21^{Ras} is in the inactive GDP-bound state. **2.** An external stimulus, or signal, triggers the exchange of GTP for GDP, an event that converts Ras to the active state. **3.** Activated p21^{Ras}, which is associated with the plasma membrane, binds GTPase-activating protein (GAP) from the cytosol. The binding of GAP has two consequences. In association with other plasma membrane constituents, it initiates the effector response. At the same time, the binding of GAP to Ras GTP stimulates by about 100-fold the intrinsic GTPase activity of Ras, promoting hydrolysis of GTP to GDP and the return of Ras to its inactive state. **B (lower).** Mutated Ras protein is locked into the active GTP-bound state because of an insensitivity of its intrinsic GTPase to GAP or because of a lack of the GTPase activity itself. As a result, the effector response is exaggerated, and the cell is transformed.

mediate many proliferation-related (see below) and cell survival reactions.

- **Phospholipase C:** This family of enzymes is commonly activated by diverse types of receptors, especially GPCRs, but also others. They cleave certain phospholipids and so participate in generation of inositol phosphate signaling intermediates and diacylglycerol. These both may drive cellular multiplication via (respectively) calcium signaling pathways and protein kinase C.
- **Mitogen-activated protein kinases (MAPKs):** These enzymes mediate many different types of signaling reactions, leading to cell proliferation. MAPKs may be triggered by upstream proteins such as Ras (after RTK activation), GPCRs or other mechanisms. Some very important driver mutations for malignancy (e.g., b-Raf) occur among these proteins, frequently leading to constitutive activation. Typically, MAPK cascades involve three sequential species, one activating the next. The consequences of MAPK stimulation are diverse, and there is extensive cross-talk between these and other signaling intermediates.

Transforming Growth Factor-β and Other Cytokines

TGF-β, an extracellular cytokine in the microenvironment of cancer cells that triggers important regulatory pathways, is an example of a cell communication mediator that strongly influences the pathogenesis of tumors. Its role in the genesis of cancer appears to be important, although cell and tissue responses to this cytokine are highly contextual. Normally, TGF-β tends mainly to suppress tumor development by modulating cell proliferation, survival, adhesion and differentiation. It also inhibits mitogenesis induced by constituents of the extracellular matrix (see above).

However, frankly malignant cells often acquire the capacity to evade or even to manipulate TGF-β pathways for their own wicked ends. Abnormal signaling in the TGF-β pathway can actually stimulate proliferation of tumor cells, facilitate their evasion of host defense mechanisms (see below) and foster invasion and metastasis.

Cancer cells may develop the ability to circumvent TGF-β–related suppressive activity via mutations in genes for TGF-β receptors or by interfering with downstream signaling by mutation or by promoter methylation of key proteins. Under these circumstances, cancer cells can hijack the regulatory activities of TGF-β to further their needs, such as tumor growth, invasion and metastasis. The loss of the tumor suppressor function of TGF-β through inactivating mutations of genes in its core pathway has been described in cancers of the colon, prostate, stomach, breast, pancreas and ovary and many others. A summary of the effects of TGF-β in cancer is presented in Table 5-5.

Other cytokines (e.g., granulocyte/monocyte colony-stimulating factor [GM-CSF] and interleukin-3 [IL-3]) may contribute to tumor development simply by overexpression, especially for hematopoietic malignancies.

Steroid Hormones

Some three centuries ago, the Italian physician Ramazzini observed that nuns had a particularly high incidence of breast cancer. This curiosity is now recognized to reflect the unopposed estrogen stimulation of breast epithelium, uninterrupted by pregnancy and lactation. Both estrogens

---

TABLE 5-5

TRANSFORMING GROWTH FACTOR-β (TGF-β) AND CANCER

Promotes	Inhibits
Normal Tumor-Suppressive Effects	
Apoptosis	Inflammation
Differentiation	Mitogenesis induced by extracellular matrix
Maintenance of cell number	
Failure of Tumor Suppression	
Autocrine mitogens	Immune surveillance
Motility	
Invasion and Metastasis	
Recruitment of myofibroblasts	
Malignant cell extravasation	
Modification of microenvironment	
Mobilization of osteoclasts	

Normally, TGF-β compels homeostasis and exerts tumor-suppressive activity through effects on the target cells themselves or the extracellular matrix.

Failure of this activity by TGF-β permits production of growth factors, evasion of immune surveillance and establishment of factors that facilitate tumor cell invasion and metastasis.

---

and progesterone bind to specific cytoplasmic receptors. The resulting hormone–receptor complexes are then translocated to the nucleus, where they act as transcription factors that foster proliferation of responsive cells. Antiestrogen therapy for hormone receptor–positive tumors reduces the risk of recurrence after surgery. Other nuclear receptors have been identified in breast cancer, including those that bind androgens, corticosteroids, vitamins A and D, fatty acids and some dietary lipids. The interactions of these signaling pathways with each other and with other signaling pathways are highly complicated and not well understood.

The influence of androgens is most conspicuous in the case of prostate cancer, in which they stimulate growth by binding to the androgen receptor. This receptor pathway engages in cross-talk with other important pathways that affect the cell cycle, apoptosis and differentiation. Such interactions involve EGF, insulin-like growth factor-I (IGF-I), fibroblast growth factor (FGF), vascular endothelial growth factor (VEGF), TGF-β and other important signaling species. Removing androgen stimulation, whether by surgical or pharmacologic means, inhibits the growth of prostate cancer, although in most cases the tumors eventually become androgen insensitive.

Membrane-Bound Mucins

Traditionally, mucins have been thought to be exclusively extracellular molecules charged with establishing an interface between many epithelial surfaces and the exterior. It is now recognized that membrane-bound mucins comprise a large family of glycoproteins that are frequently

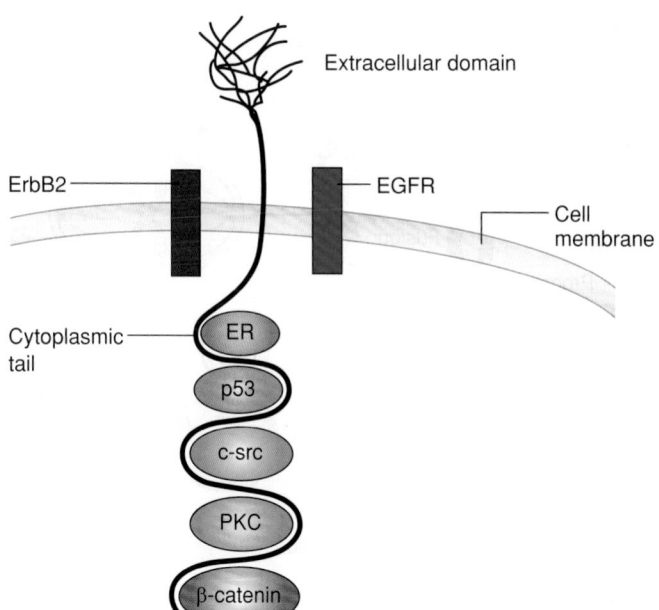

FIGURE 5-23. Membrane-bound mucins with important signaling molecules. *ER* = estrogen receptor; *PKC* = protein kinase C.

overproduced in a variety of cancers. Extracellular domains of these membrane-bound mucins (MUCs) lubricate and protect the cell surface. The cytoplasmic domains of these transmembrane glycoproteins function as scaffolds for interaction with signaling molecules that influence cell proliferation and survival (Fig. 5-23). In this context, MUC1 is overexpressed in the large majority of breast cancers, and often in malignancies of the colon, ovary, pancreas and lungs.

Interaction among Intermediate Signaling Pathways

Whether elicited by receptor–ligand interactions or by constitutively activating driver mutation, the signaling avenues discussed above, and many others, interconnect extensively. This fact endows them with baffling complexity and challenges both those seeking to understand how cells sustain proliferation and those seeking specific targets for therapy. In this context, it should be emphasized that the results of unrestrained activation of a given gene are not always predictable. A mutant protein may drive proliferation in one cell type, apoptosis in another and differentiation in a third.

Transcriptional Activation

In the end, a key element of the ability of cancer cells to proliferate without restraint is the array of genes whose transcriptional activities are turned on or off. Thus, whatever upstream driver mutations there are, transcription factors sit at the end of the afferent limb of the processes that push cancer cells to undergo uncontrolled mitosis. When transcription factors drive oncogenesis, the genetic changes responsible usually entail increased production of wild-type proteins. Thus, driver mutations of transcription factors generally entail, for example, translocations that place them under the control of more vigorous promoters. Many transcription factors are

implicated in oncogenesis. Among the best known and most often inculpated are:

- **Myc:** A ubiquitous transcription factor that may control transcription of as many as 10%–15% of all human genes, c-Myc and its cousins, N-Myc and L-Myc, are key to development of many tumors. Among its functions, Myc pushes cellular proliferation, favors stemness (see Cancer Stem Cells, below), increases energy production and facilitates tumor cell invasiveness. It is of interest that Myc may also activate cell death programs in cells with intact p53 and other cell death effectors.

- **Fos and Jun:** Together, these proteins form the **AP-1** (activation protein-1) transcription factor. Increased AP-1 activity promotes cellular proliferation and survival (Fig. 5-24) and is generally a result of increased signaling via several pathways, including MAPK and the protein kinase C family (PKC; see above). AP-1 also represses expression of such tumor proteins as p53 (see below).

- **Androgen and estrogen receptors:** These cytoplasmic receptor proteins act both as receptors and as transcription factors. They translocate to the nucleus upon binding their cognate ligands. Once in the nucleus, they act as transcription factors. Depending on the cell type, these steroid sex hormone receptors may stimulate cell proliferation. Thus, estrogen receptors stimulate mammary epithelial cell proliferation and are important in the progression of many breast cancers. In many prostate cancers, similarly, androgens cause prostatic tumor cells to proliferate.

As noted above, however, cell proliferation mediated by these and similar receptors need not necessarily require exogenous hormones. Autocrine stimulation may occur when the tumor cells themselves produce the requisite androgen or estrogen. The ability of the tumor to progress thus becomes independent of exogenous sources of the stimulatory hormone and the tumor is resistant to hormone antagonist therapies.

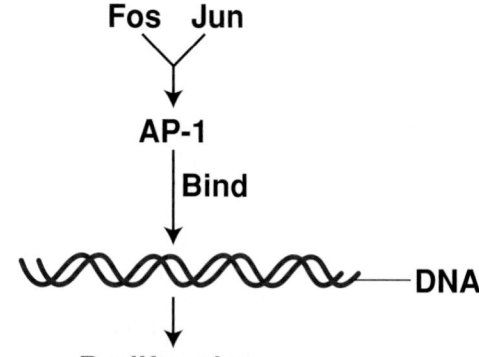

FIGURE 5-24. Activating protein-1 (AP-1) complex. The AP-1 transcription factor complex is formed by the protein products of two proto-oncogenes, Fos and Jun. When these factors form a heterodimer, they bind DNA and direct transcription of genes whose products are involved in cell proliferation, tumor cell invasion and metastasis, angiogenesis and inhibiting apoptosis.

Thus, whether by gene amplification, point mutation, translocation or other mechanisms (see genomic instability, below), tumors are characterized by cellular proliferation that is unshackled by the regulatory chains that limit normal cells. They must still, however, escape other restraints.

Cellular Senescence Helps Prevent Cancer

Senescence is a process that maintains cell viability when a cell can no longer contribute by cell division to continued homeostasis. Senescent cells are growth arrested and viable but remain unable to proliferate.

This state was reported initially in cultured normal human fibroblasts. After a certain number of mitoses (usually 40–45), they stopped dividing but remained alive. The upper limit of the number of mitoses is called the Hayflick limit, after its original discoverer. It largely reflects the effects of telomere depletion in preventing cell cycling when a cell's telomeres become very short (see below).

Mediators of Cellular Senescence

Clearly, a mechanism that limits the number of mitoses a cell may undergo must be neutralized for malignant cells to indulge in endless proliferation. The senescent phenotype entails increased formation of heterochromatin (senescence-associated heterochromatin formation [SAHF]), in which certain proteins are modified, leading them to bind chromosomal DNA and impede transcription of E2F-activated genes such as mediate cell multiplication (see above). Several effectors of senescence are involved:

- **The DNA damage response (DDR):** As noted above, once telomeres have shortened to a certain point, they elicit DDR. DNA damage-sensing proteins activate p53 and cdc25, and the cell stops dividing until either the offending DNA damage is fixed or the cell is directed into senescence or apoptosis pathways. This mechanism is critical to oncogene-induced senescence (OIS; see below).
- **Tumor suppressors:** The intimacy between several critical proteins and cell cycle blockage is important in forcing cells into a senescent phenotype. Key among these proteins are p16^{INK4a} and Rb, which induce certain proteins to associate with the cell's DNA. This results in SAHF and gene silencing.
- **Oxidative stress:** In cultured cells, senescence can be delayed by decreasing ambient oxygen. Conversely, it can be hastened by adding oxidants like H_2O_2 to the culture. Activation of some oncogenes, like RAS, increases oxidative stress. Resulting increases in ROS may trigger p38 MAPK signaling and activate ATM.
- **Cytokines:** Cells secrete factors, including IL-6 and IL-8, that help trigger the senescent phenotype. Together with their receptors, they help to establish and maintain the senescence. Their participation led to the descriptive designation, secretion-associated senescent phenotype (SASP). Transcriptional regulation that these cytokines elicit inhibits cellular proliferation and promotes senescence.

Telomere Stability and Tumorigenesis

Telomeres are tandem repeats of the sequence TTAGGG, at the 3' ends of each DNA strand. They serve as docks for protein caps that bind the ends of DNA sequences and

Breakage-Fusion-Bridge Cycle

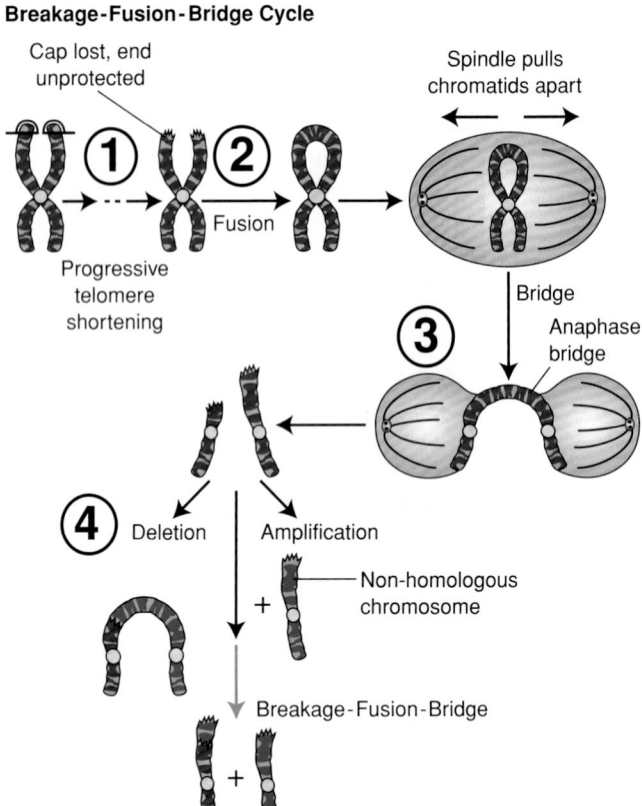

FIGURE 5-25. The genesis of telomere-related chromosome breakage. 1. In the absence of telomerase, extensive cell proliferation leads to unprotected telomere ends. **2.** These are "repaired" by fusion of telomeres between sister chromatids, creating a bridged structure like a tongs. **3.** During anaphase, the spindles attached to the two centromeres pull the now-attached chromatids apart, resulting in abnormal chromosomes. **4.** Further production of chromosome ends without telomeres may cause the cycle to repeat itself.

prevent them from being used in NHEJ (see above) reactions. Because DNA polymerases "fall off" as they approach the ends of chromosomes, telomere lengths decrease with each cell division. When telomeres are reduced beyond a critical size, they become uncapped and are subject to NHEJ. Resulting NHEJ may fuse the ends of either two sister chromatids or nonhomologous chromosomes. As the cell cycle progresses, this fusion generates a chromosome "bridge" as the fused DNA strands are pulled apart during anaphase. The force of chromosome separation may then lead to chromosomal breakage, which can lead to further recombination (Fig. 5-25).

This process can be prevented in several ways. In normal cells, where p53 and pRb pathways are intact, shortened telomeres activate cell cycle checkpoints and cell division ceases. This is called replicative senescence (Fig. 5-26). The cell then remains in G_0 or dies. Alternatively, many cells that replicate frequently (e.g., colon crypt epithelium) express **telomerase,** a ribonucleoprotein enzyme that lengthens telomeres and so maintains genomic stability in the face of continuing cell proliferation.

Oncogene-Induced Cellular Senescence

The vast majority of cells sustaining oncogenic mutations never become cancers. In the human body, such mutations occur several times per minute, which contrasts with

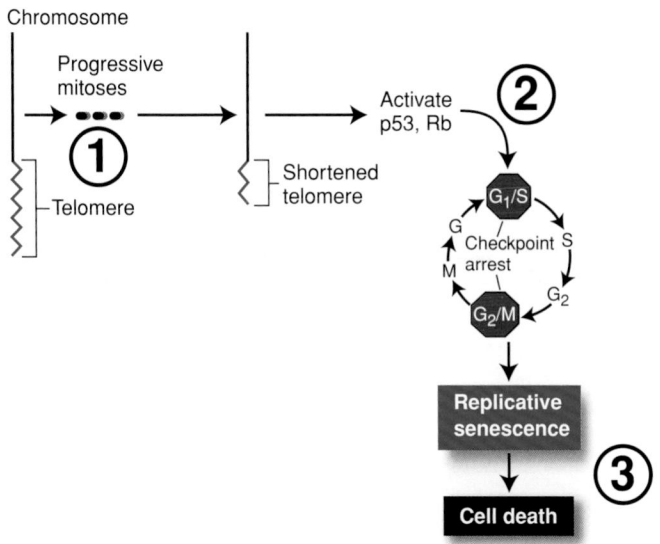

FIGURE 5-26. The sequence of events resulting from DNA instability as a result of telomere shortening and leading to cell death. This sequence occurs when the tumor suppressors p53 and Rb are intact. **1.** Progressive telomere shortening activates p53 and Rb. **2.** This leads to cell cycle arrest at the G_1/S and G_2/M checkpoints. **3.** Consequent replicative senescence triggers cell death programs.

the relative infrequency of cancer in a human life span. A major barrier to the development of cancer appears to be OIS (Fig. 5-27). OIS has been shown to constrain tumor development for many types of cancer. Consistent with this role for OIS, oncogene activation stimulates tumor suppressors such as p53 and Rb.

Earlier studies showed that after activated Ras enhanced proliferation of affected cells, an irreversible

growth arrest (i.e., senescence) occurred. This senescence could be avoided by crippling p53 and Rb pathways, suggesting that such OIS actually evolved as a means to prevent tumors (Fig. 5-27). Activating alterations in other oncogenes also induce OIS in vivo. The ability to undergo OIS is a major distinction between many benign and malignant tumors, as well as between "premalignant" cell proliferations and frankly malignant ones. That is, benign tumors can senesce, but advanced malignant tumors do not. For example, benign tumors may show heightened responsiveness to IL-8 (see above), which is lost in malignancy. Thus, OIS prevents benign cell proliferations from progressing to cancers.

Evading Senescence

If critical shortening and uncapping of telomeres occur in the context of acquired loss of cell cycle checkpoint regulation (e.g., mutations in $p16^{INK4a}$ or p53), chromosomes become susceptible to instability resulting from the types of rearrangements mentioned above (breakpoint–fusion–bridge cycles). Such instability promotes carcinogenesis by facilitating chromosomal rearrangements, which in turn can lead to aneuploidy, translocations, amplifications and deletions. Thus, telomere attrition leads to sufficient genomic instability to set the stage for the development of mutations in sufficient numbers for cells to cross the borderline from benign to malignant.

Cancer cells may solve this problem, as indicated above, via telomerase. In normal human cells, levels of this enzyme are insufficient to maintain telomere length, and each cell division therefore leads to progressive telomere attrition. However, in normal cells that divide frequently, telomerase makes a DNA copy of an RNA telomere template and affixes it to the 3' end of the replicating DNA strand. In this way, the

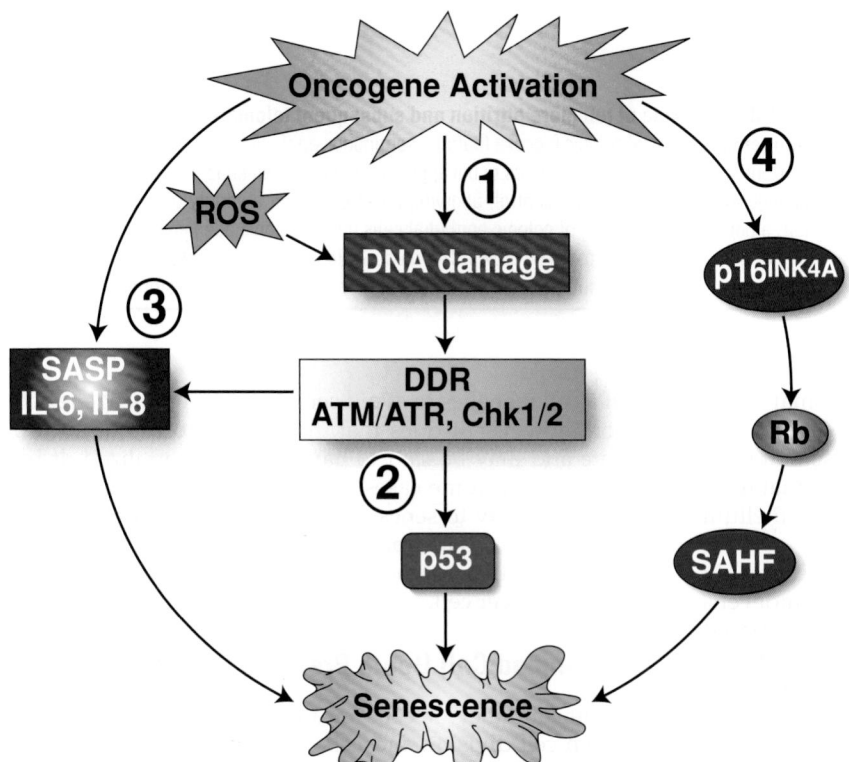

FIGURE 5-27. Oncogene-induced senescence (OIS). Oncogenic stress can elicit cellular responses that eventuate in cellular senescence. **1.** Excessive cell division, a result of oncogene activation, for example, causes oxidative stress and DNA damage to accumulate. **2.** As a consequence, the DNA damage response (DDR) is activated, with p53 expression blocking cell cycle progression. **3.** The same DDR may also activate the senescence-associated secretory phenotype (SASP), which leads affected cells to secrete cytokines that maintain the senescent state (interleukin-6 [IL-6], IL-8). SASP can also be activated directly by the excessive oncogene activity. **4.** Oncogene activation may directly activate the tumor suppressor $p16^{INK4A}$, which in turn activates Rb. This leads to the formation of senescence-associated heterochromatin (SAHF), which restricts expression of cell cycle drivers.

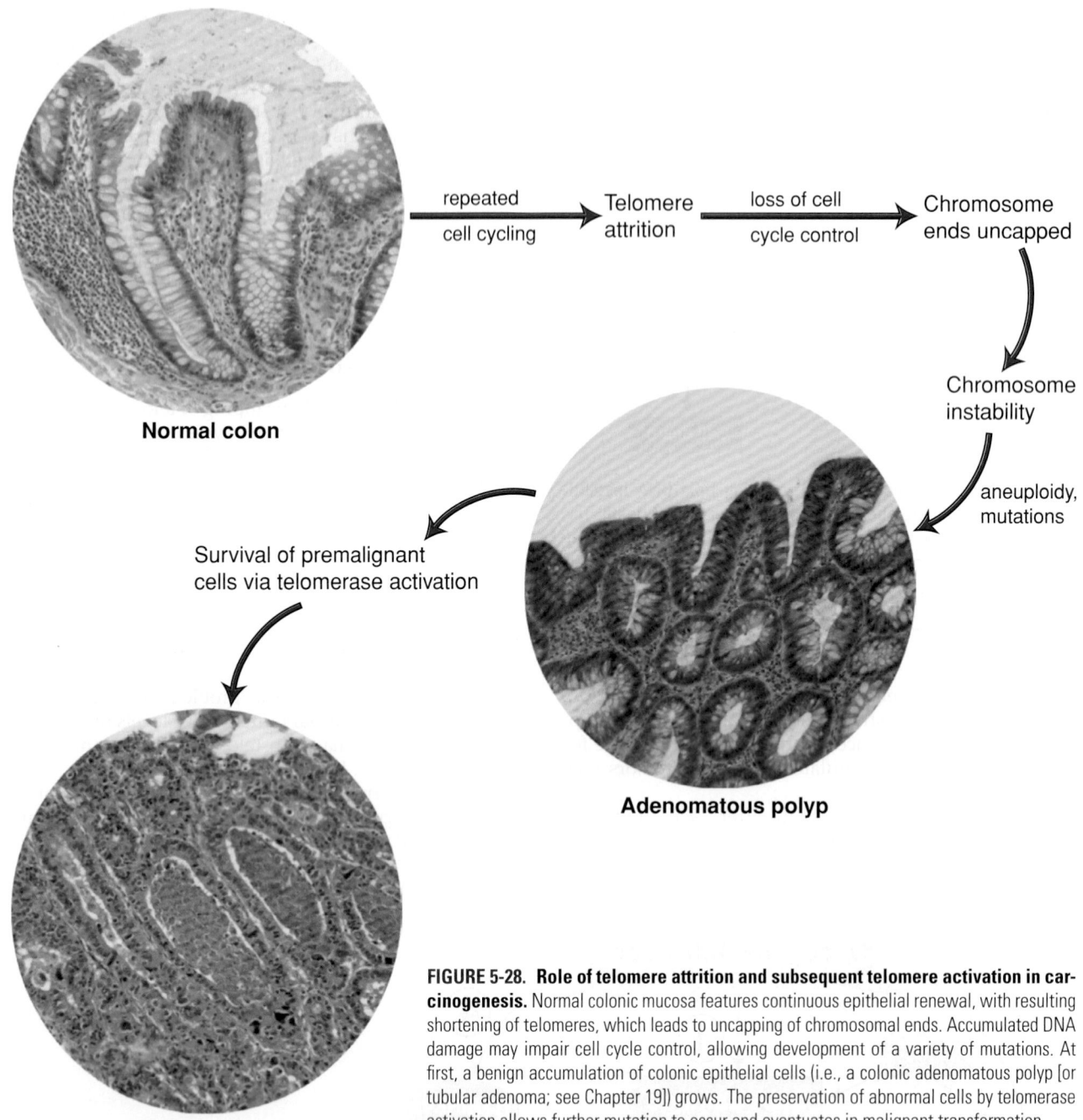

Normal colon

repeated cell cycling → Telomere attrition

loss of cell cycle control → Chromosome ends uncapped

Chromosome instability

aneuploidy, mutations

Survival of premalignant cells via telomerase activation

Adenomatous polyp

Invasive colon carcinoma

FIGURE 5-28. Role of telomere attrition and subsequent telomere activation in carcinogenesis. Normal colonic mucosa features continuous epithelial renewal, with resulting shortening of telomeres, which leads to uncapping of chromosomal ends. Accumulated DNA damage may impair cell cycle control, allowing development of a variety of mutations. At first, a benign accumulation of colonic epithelial cells (i.e., a colonic adenomatous polyp [or tubular adenoma; see Chapter 19]) grows. The preservation of abnormal cells by telomerase activation allows further mutation to occur and eventuates in malignant transformation.

enzyme preserves telomere length and chromosomal integrity despite continuing cell division. Not surprisingly, then, normal cells that express telomerase include those that need to continue to divide for the lifetime of the individual (e.g., hematopoietic progenitor cells, gastrointestinal epithelium and germ cells).

The cancer cell takes a page from that book. Presumably as a protective adaptation to genomic instability, tumor cells reactivate telomerase: 80% of human tumors show increased telomerase activity. A high level of this activity actually protects the cancer cell by suppressing the development of further, potentially lethal, chromosomal instability. *Thus, telomerase activation permits—but does not directly cause—the emergence of cancer* (Fig. 5-28).

If a cell manages to avoid senescence after oncogene activation, however it does that, the cell can continue to proliferate and may be said to have been immortalized. It has been shown in some cases that benign human tumors may retain the ability to senesce, while their malignant counterparts have lost that capacity. Thus, loss of tumor suppressor activities that promote senescence is important for the emerging cancer cell.

Programmed Cell Death Prevents Oncogenesis

The total number of cells in any organ reflects a balance between cell division and cell death. Interference with this intricate equilibrium can lead to tumor development. Cell death programs encompass several different pathways (see Chapter 1), dysfunction of which is often a fundamental requirement for tumor development. The best understood of these is apoptosis and its cousin, anoikis.

Apoptosis as an Inhibitor of Cancer

As mentioned above and in Chapter 1, apoptosis eliminates damaged or abnormal cells. Apoptotic pathways are activated by errors in DNA replication or repair, detected genetic or metabolic instability, loss of anchoring connections to the extracellular matrix (ECM) **(anoikis)** and other stimuli. Since many triggers for apoptosis are among the attributes of tumor cells, it is not surprising that those cells often evolve mechanisms to disable it. There are many known pro- and antiapoptotic proteins that interact in a head-spinning number of ways. To make this topic understandable, we present illustrative examples. Thus, cancers may avoid PCD by impairing proapoptotic activities and/or by augmenting prosurvival functions.

Fighting for Survival Against the Forces of Death

There are many participants in the programs of cell death. The best known is p53, and it is no surprise that the gene for this protein, *TP53*, is mutated in over half of human cancers (see below). As the key angel of cell death, p53 is activated when oncogenic danger is sensed, for example, if damage to cellular DNA cannot be repaired (see Chapter 1). Wearing several of its many hats, activated p53 upregulates transcription of proapoptotic Bcl-2–like proteins and downregulates their prosurvival cousins. In addition, it is a BH3-only protein (see Chapter 1) and so may meddle directly in Bcl-2 family affairs by binding, for example, prosurvival Bcl-2 or Bcl-X_L to force them to release proapoptotic Bad and Bax. The latter activate effector caspases and cause the cell to die. It is worth recalling that apoptosis does not elicit florid, cytokine-rich inflammatory responses, but rather that apoptotic cells pass from the world not with a bang but with a whimper—they are quietly removed by macrophages.

Along similar lines, anoikis is form of apoptosis that is activated with epithelial cell membrane integrins that no longer bind their appropriate ECM partners. Integrins mediate prosurvival signals. Their detachment from their extracellular ligands leaves cells excessively susceptible to all manners of proapoptotic stimuli. Also, unligated integrins may activate caspase-8 directly. However, in some cancer cells, unbound integrins can maintain survival signaling and so protect from PCD.

The prototypical example of the effectiveness of inhibiting apoptosis in human cancer is follicular lymphoma (see Chapter 26). There, the prosurvival protein, Bcl-2, is constitutively activated by a translocation [t(14:8)] that places its expression under the control of the immunoglobulin heavy-chain promoter. As a result, the normal equilibrium between the life and death of B lymphocytes is altered in favor of the former, thus allowing accumulation—or, perhaps, more to the point, insufficient elimination—of excess neoplastic B cells.

Some other tumor types, including lung cancer and non-Hodgkin lymphoma, also express excess Bcl-2. Chromosomal translocation is not the only mechanism by which tumor cells increase Bcl-2 expression. They may show methylation and suppression of microRNAs (miRNAs) that repress Bcl-2 expression. Similarly, any impairment of p53

function can increase Bcl-2 production and decrease expression of proapoptotic Bcl-2 binding partners (see Chapter 1) and, in so doing, promote tumor formation.

The issue of PCD and cancer is further complicated by **oncogene-mediated apoptosis**. For example, although the transcription factor Myc is generally considered to be oncogenic, if PCD pathways are intact, Myc overproduction induces a default apoptosis pathway. Thus, promotion of cell proliferation by deregulated production of Myc is usually balanced by increased apoptosis. Induction of apoptosis by Myc acts as a molecular safety valve to block cancer development. If Myc-stimulated tumors are to develop, some cells overproducing Myc must also inactivate PCD, whether by overexpressing antiapoptotic proteins or by inactivating apoptosis mediators like p53.

This example illustrates the complexity inherent in the control of the on/off switch of apoptosis in cancer development.

Tumors Stimulate New Blood Vessel Formation (Angiogenesis)

Angiogenesis is the formation of new blood vessels from preexisting small blood vessels. In order to grow beyond about 2 mm in diameter, tumors need more nutrient and oxygen supply than preexisting blood vessels can provide. Most tumors experience hypoxia, which induces expression of **hypoxia-induced factors (HIFs),** especially **HIF-1α.** In turn, HIF-1α elicits production of angiogenic growth factors, which stimulate formation of new tumor-associated blood vessels. This process is obligatory for a primary tumor to grow and metastasize.

Under homeostatic conditions, there is a fine equilibrium between factors favoring new blood vessel formation and those impeding it. Consequently, endothelial cells turn over slowly, renewing themselves over the course of months or years. Solid tumors often disrupt this equilibrium in favor of new blood vessel formation.

Steps in the Formation of New Blood Vessels

Tumor angiogenesis begins when existing cells (e.g., tumor cells or attendant stromal cells) secrete substances (see below) that stimulate new blood vessel formation. The process triggered by these chemicals resembles vasculogenesis in embryonic development and follows several steps:

1. Proteolytic enzymes perforate postcapillary venule basement membranes.
2. Endothelial cells in the area of the interrupted basement membrane proliferate and migrate toward the source of the angiogenic cytokines.
3. A lumen develops in the advancing cell mass.
4. These immature capillaries are invested with a basement membrane.
5. The cells in the vanguard of the developing structure ("tip cells") join to other similar tip cells to produce a capillary network.

Under some circumstances, and for some tumor types, tumor vessels may form differently—directly from the tumor cells themselves. The end result, however the blood vessels are generated, is not always well-formed vasculature. Tumor-associated vessels may differ from their non-tumor-associated counterparts in several ways.

Tumor-associated capillaries may be variably invested by pericytes and basement membranes. They may vary in size and shape, leak blood components excessively, display excessive tortuosity and be distributed inhomogeneously. Excessive leakiness of tumor blood vessels may increase tissue hydrostatic pressure and so retard diffusion of soluble materials into tissues. Consequently, some areas of tumors may be richly supplied with oxygen and nutrients while other areas may go begging.

Mediators of Tumor Angiogenesis

Three main groups of factors may mediate tumor angiogenesis: (1) the family of VEGFs, (2) angiopoietins and (3) other agents that stimulate tumor-associated blood vessels to proliferate. These are assisted by a bevy of associated helpers including TGF-β (see below), several interleukins (IL-6, IL-8) and steroid sex hormones. The multiplicity—some might suggest redundancy—of stimulating and interacting factors has important implications for the efficacy of tumor therapies that preferentially target one or another.

VEGF

This term actually represents a family of related proteins, the best understood of which is VEGF-A, which has several isoforms. The family will be referred to collectively as VEGF, but the multiplicity of VEGFs should be borne in mind. VEGF is a major mediator of tumor angiogenesis and is made by the cells of most tumors. However, quantities of VEGF capable of stimulating tumor angiogenesis may also be produced by other cells, chiefly platelets and connective tissue cells. A related family of mediators, platelet-derived growth factors (PDGFs), has a similar spectrum of activities. In addition to stimulating new blood vessel formation, VEGF also enhances capillary permeability, promotes endothelial cell survival and mobilizes progenitor cells (e.g., from the bone marrow) to participate in angiogenesis.

VEGF Mechanisms of Action

As noted above, tumor cells produce HIF-1α when they sense insufficient oxygen. HIF-1α is a transcription factor that upregulates diverse genes, including the VEGFs. The family of VEGFs bind a family of receptors on endothelial cells, the most important of which is VEGFR2. VEGF–VEGFR2 interaction activates several signaling pathways (Fig. 5-29). Consequences of VEGFR2 activation include endothelial cell proliferation, protection from PCD, enhanced cell migration and increased vascular permeability. The latter function leads to leakage of such blood components as fibrinogen into the area. Once outside blood vessels, fibrinogen generates a fibrin matrix that facilitates endothelial cell migration and angiogenesis. VEGFR2-positive progenitors from the blood are also recruited to the site. Several members of the VEGF family also mediate proliferation of lymphatic vessels.

Angiopoietins

Of the several known angiopoietins, angiopoietin-2 contributes the most to tumor blood vessel formation. It acts principally to stabilize growing blood vessels and stimulate pericytes to surround the developing structures.

Other Angiogenic Factors

Other important stimuli include cytokines (e.g., IL-6), androgens and estrogens, as well as diverse growth factors. These

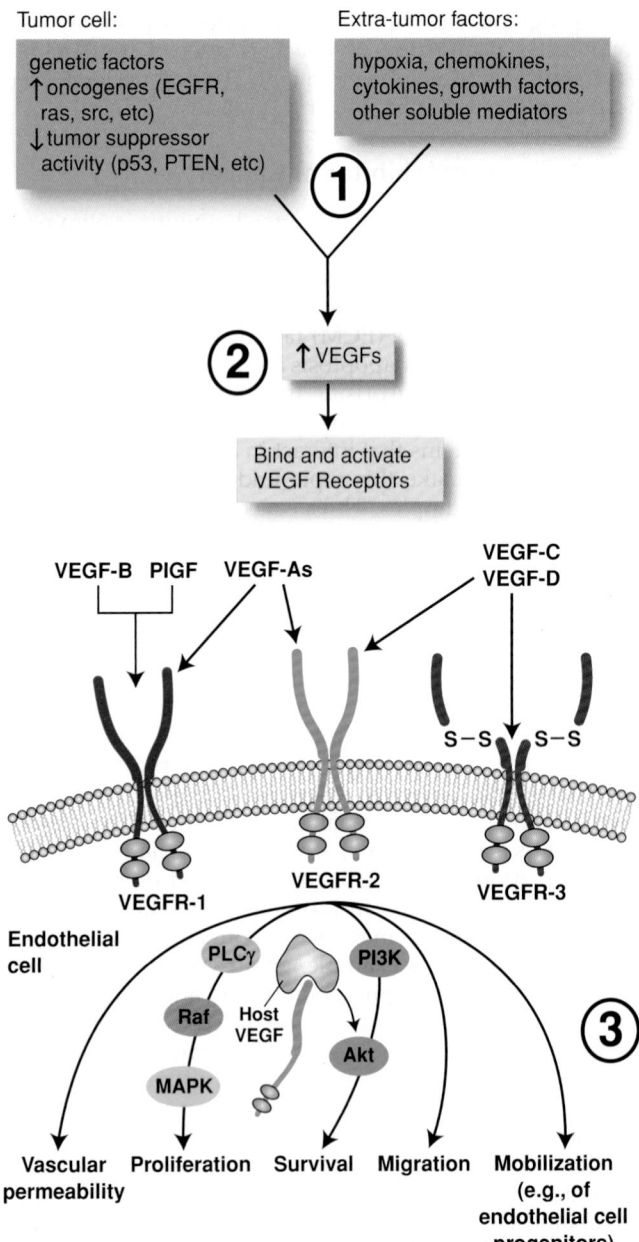

FIGURE 5-29. The vascular endothelial growth factor (VEGF) system and its effects. 1. Under the influence of factors generated by tumor cells (*left;* increased expression of certain oncogenes or decreased activity or tumor suppressors) or coming from other sources (tumor-related stroma, external environment, etc.), several VEGFs are produced. **2.** These bind the several VEGF receptors (VEGFRs), the principal of which is VEGFR-2. **3.** Downstream signaling from these receptors has diverse effects on vascular endothelium, including increasing vascular permeability, activating cell proliferation and survival mechanisms, inducing in-migration of endothelial cells and mobilizing progenitor cells to the area, to help form new blood vessels. PIGF = placental growth factor.

serve diverse functions, including eliciting VEGF production. Mutations in several important oncogenes, including *src, EGFR* and *ras,* may increase VEGF secretion by tumor cells, as may impairment of activities of certain tumor suppressor genes (see below).

The multiplicity of proangiogenic activities includes such factors as basic FGF (bFGF), PDGF, VEGF homologs and isoforms and others. These may augment blood vessel growth

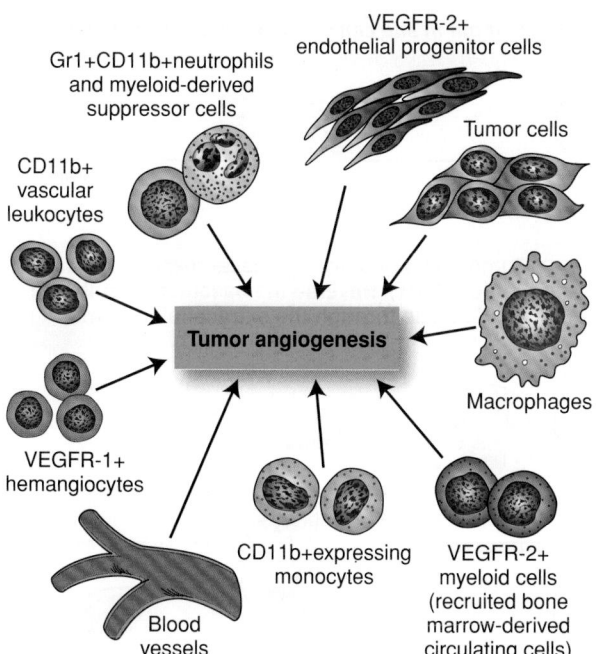

FIGURE 5-30. Diverse populations of bone marrow–derived cells that participate in angiogenesis. Circulating cells derived from bone marrow progenitors contribute to the development of tumor-related blood vessels. These include macrophages, early cells in the myeloid (neutrophil) series, neutrophils and myeloid-derived suppressor cells, endothelial progenitor cells and tumor cells themselves.

that is triggered by primary factors such as FGF2 or angiopoietin. This breadth of tumor angiogenic factors, combined with the likelihood that at least some tumor cells may differentiate into tumor blood vessels, frustrates attempts at effective tumor treatment by targeting individual VEGFs or VEGFRs.

Inflammatory Cytokines and Chemokines

Bone marrow–derived immune and inflammatory cells, including macrophages, neutrophils, natural killer cells, dendritic cells and myeloid precursor cells, all produce numerous soluble angiogenic factors and stimulators, and some may even differentiate into endothelial cells (Fig. 5-30). Equally important are tumor-associated stromal fibroblasts. The contributions of these cells to tumor blood vessel growth reflects the context of the tumor. In some settings, these cells assume a Dr. Jekyll–like antineoplastic phenotype and produce antitumor and antiangiogenic activities. In other settings, they become Mr. Hyde and generate proangiogenic and protumor microenvironments. As if this were not sufficiently complex, cells such as dendritic cells and myeloid-derived suppressor cells are capable of trans-differentiating into endothelial cells.

Invasion and Metastasis Are Multistep Events

The lethality of cancer resides in its ability to spread. Over 90% of patients who die of cancer succumb to metastatic disease. While we have accumulated considerable understanding of tumorigenesis, our appreciation of the basic principles of metastasis remains rudimentary. What is clear is that tumor spread is a multistep process, with each step

potentially representing major genetic and epigenetic modifications in tumor cells and their behavior.

Malignant cells go through several steps to establish a metastasis (Fig. 5-31):

1. Invasion of the basement membrane underlying the tumor
2. Movement through extracellular matrix
3. Penetration of vascular or lymphatic channels
4. Survival within circulating blood or lymph
5. Homing to a new site and exiting from the circulation there
6. Establishment of a micrometastasis

A final step, growth of micrometastatic foci into sizeable tumor masses, culminates this progression and represents the ultimate lethality of almost all malignancies.

Cancer cells develop at a given location, comfortable in their native environments, owing in part to their interactions with tumor-associated matrix constituents and stromal and inflammatory cells (see below). The latter may either be present in the extracellular matrix or be recruited from the bone marrow. In order to metastasize, cancer cells must also establish a comparably commodious ecosystem at a distant site. This is no small undertaking.

As the discussion below will demonstrate, some—perhaps most—of the traits necessary for tumors to metastasize are quite distinct from those needed for tumors to establish themselves at their sites of origin. It bears mention that it is not clear how the traits required for metastatic behavior are selected in primary tumors. While some traits needed for tumorigenesis may overlap the needs of metastases, other do not. Further, as one climbs the ladder of steps needed for metastasis, it is not known how cells that carry a phenotype that allows them to succeed at one rung are in a position to select for characteristics that facilitate success at the next rung.

The practical upshot of these philosophical ruminations is that *once a primary tumor has been removed, metastatic deposits are already in place.* The goal of subsequent therapy is to limit the growth of metastases that already exist.

Tumor cells start to disseminate early in oncogenesis. Many tumor cells enter the circulation daily (it is estimated to be 10^6 cells per gram of tumor per day). Taking out a gross primary tumor does not, therefore, "get it all out": micrometastases already exist.

Invasion and Tumor Cell Motility

For solid tumors, invasion requires that the previously stationary cell become motile. It must also become capable of disrupting and penetrating the underlying basement membrane, and then passing through the ECM. Orchestrating movement through the ECM requires proteases secreted by cancer cells and nonmalignant tumor-associated cells (see below). Cancer cells develop protrusions that contain an actin core and integrins. These projections, called **invadopodia,** express **matrix metalloproteinases (MMPs;** see below) and other proteases. Integrins in the ECM may not only act as mechanical anchors but also promote development of invadopodia. The invadopodia help to degrade the ECM and offer a guide to the perplexed cell in navigating its microenvironment via exploration of cell–cell and cell–matrix adhesions and by sensing chemoattractive molecules.

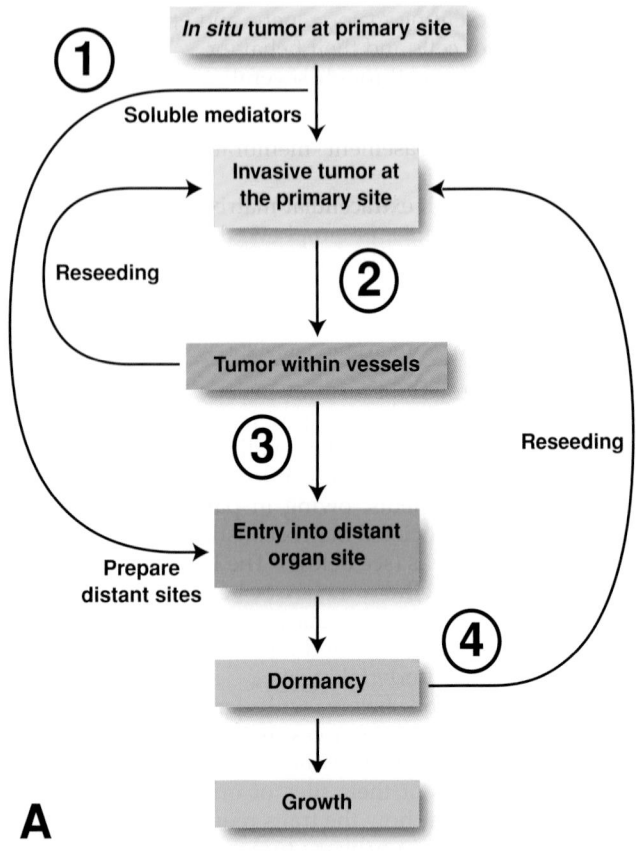

A

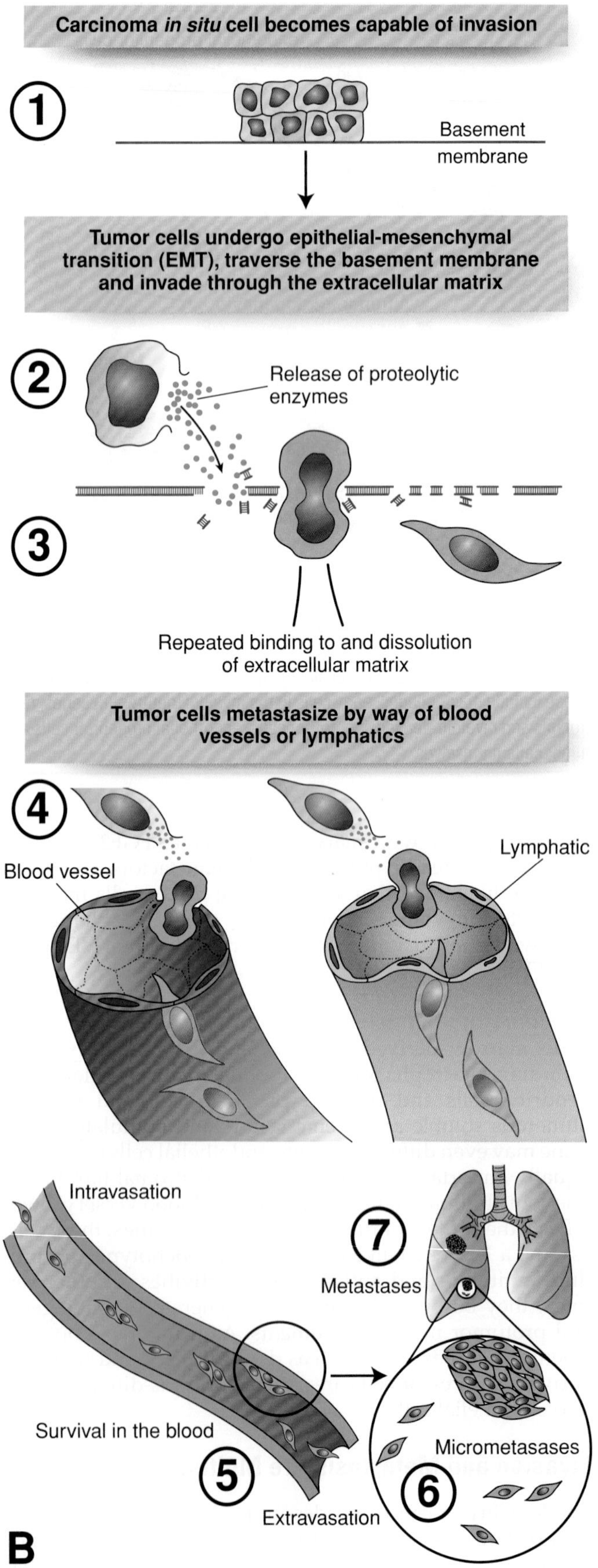

B

FIGURE 5-31. Mechanisms of tumor invasion and metastasis. The mechanism by which a malignant tumor initially penetrates a confining basement membrane and then invades the surrounding extracellular environment involves several steps. **1.** The tumor first acquires the ability to bind components of the extracellular matrix. These interactions are mediated by the expression of a number of adhesion molecules. **2.** The tumor undergoes epithelial–mesenchymal transition (EMT) and traverses the basement membrane. **3.** Proteolytic enzymes are then released from the tumor cells, and the extracellular matrix is degraded. **4.** After moving through the extracellular environment, the invading cancer penetrates blood vessels and lymphatics by the same mechanisms. **5.** After survival in blood vessels or lymphatics, the tumor exits the vascular system. **6.** It establishes micrometastases at the site where it leaves the vasculature. **7.** These micrometastases grow into gross masses of metastatic tumor.

Epithelial–Mesenchymal Transition

To escape the confines of the mucosa in which they originate, the epithelial cancer cells assume a phenotype that permits enhanced motility. The tumor cells, which are nonmotile and are encased in cell collectives via cell–cell tight junctions, disrupt these bonds and assume a new guise as single, nonpolarized mobile mesenchymal cells. This chameleon-like **epithelial–mesenchymal transition (EMT)** is reversible and temporary.

What Elicits EMT?

Many factors contribute to EMT (see below), but diverse stimuli probably can trigger this function. Among these, hypoxia is felt to be critical. Since the diffusion radii of glucose and oxygen are limited to 100–150 μ, tumors growing in situ (e.g., comedo-type breast intraductal carcinomas; see Chapter 25) may show central necrosis. Hypoxia induces HIF-1α (see above), which itself regulates many genes. Among these are the proteases, MMP1 and MMP2, and lysyl oxidase (LOX). (Other HIF-1α functions are discussed below.) MMP2 degrades basement membrane, and MMP1 and LOX help to digest ECM to clear a path for the tumor cell.

EMT also entails the activation of a series of transcription factors that promote a mesenchymal phenotype. These factors—colorfully named Slug, Snail, Twist and ZEB1—were once active in mediating cell mobility during embryogenesis. They are reactivated to make adult epithelial cells act like their mesenchymal embryonic forbearers. Snail and Twist downregulate expression of E-cadherin (see below), a glycoprotein that anchors epithelial cells to each other and suppresses motility. In addition, Twist and ZEB1 downregulate the antiproliferative proteins p16^{INK4a} and p21^{CIP1}. Freed of their E-cadherin shackle, epithelial cells can then invade. Proteases clear the way.

Tumor-Associated Cells

Nonneoplastic cells associated with tumors constitute about half of all cells within tumor masses. They include macrophages, leukocytes, fibroblasts, vascular endothelial cells, neuronal cells and fat cells (Fig. 5-32). Many of these resided originally in the ECM, but others are of bone marrow origin and are recruited to the site of the expanding tumor. All of these nontumor cells can influence the behavior of the cancer, both at its site of origin and at locations of metastases.

The Contributions of Tumor Stroma

Stimulation of tumor cell invasiveness by nearby stromal elements plays an important role in the ability of cancer cells to breach the basement membrane and traverse underlying connective tissues. Tumors co-opt normal stromal cell functions, trigger inflammatory reactions and recruit additional cells to the area of the developing malignancy to further subvert anatomic and other barriers to invasion. Perversely, components of inflammatory and wound repair processes (see Chapters 2, 3 and 4) that protect against, for example, pathogens are then brought to bear to render the individual susceptible to cancer cell invasiveness. It is important to appreciate that *the players in inflammatory and wound healing that are observed in nearby tumors are orchestrated by the developing cancers themselves* (Fig. 5-33) *and should not be misconstrued as protecting the host:*

- **MMPs:** The MMPs are a family of endopeptidases that are normally regulated by tissue inhibitors of MMPs (TIMPs). MMPs are synthesized and secreted by normal cells during physiologic tissue remodeling, at which times the balance between MMPs and TIMPs is strictly regulated. By contrast, invasive and metastatic phenotypes of cancer cells are characterized by dysregulation of the MMP–TIMP balance.

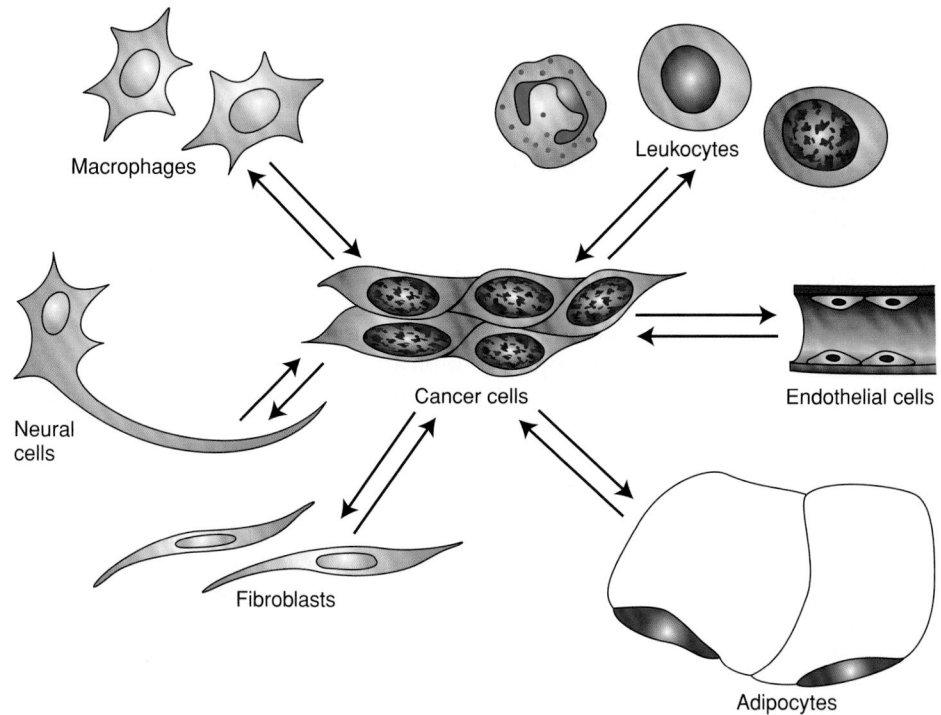

FIGURE 5-32. The cancer cell ecosystem. The developing tumor cells interact with the nonmalignant cells in their environment, via production of soluble and other mediators.

Macrophages

Leukocytes

Neural cells

Cancer cells

Endothelial cells

Fibroblasts

Adipocytes

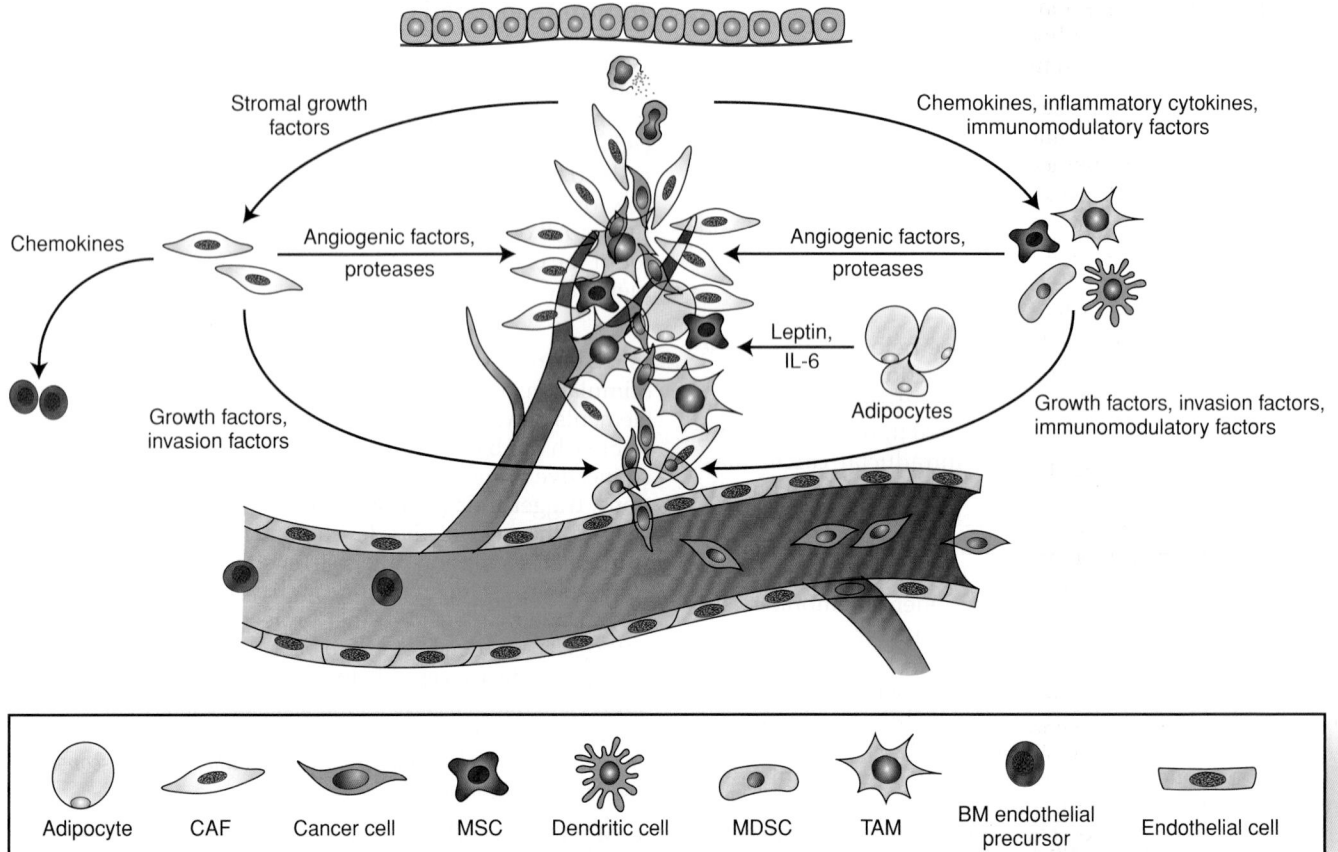

FIGURE 5-33. Tumor cell–stromal interactions involved in invasion and metastasis. Stroma adjacent to tumor is critical to the survival of tumor cells in place and to their dissemination. Such "cancerized stroma" contains bone marrow–derived elements (Fig. 5-30), including myeloid-derived suppressor cells (MDSCs), dendritic cells, tumor-associated macrophages (TAMs), fibroblasts, adipocytes and endothelial cells. Cytokines, chemokines and other mediators produced by tumor cells, as well as influences of tissue destruction and hypoxia, recruit TAMs, MDSCs, cancer-associated fibroblasts (CAFs) and mesenchymal stem cells (MSCs). MDSCs and TAMs are present at the invading tumor front—points where the basement membrane is being broken down and the tumor cells are infiltrating the stroma. These cells produce angiogenic factors, proteases and other factors that promote tumor invasion. CAFs produce similar facilitators and bring marrow–derived blood vessel precursor cells to generate new blood vessels.

In many tumors, invasiveness correlates directly with increased MMP expression. In many of these same tumors, TIMPs are decreased. MMPs in invading cancers may be produced by the tumor cells themselves, by surrounding stromal cells or both, depending on the particular neoplasm. MMPs secreted by stromal cells may be bound to integrins on the surface of the tumor cells, thus providing particularly high local concentrations of protease activity precisely where the tumor needs it in order to invade. Deregulated MMP activity permits cancer cells to enter and traverse the ECM.

Tumor cell motility is enhanced by upregulation of CXCR4 chemokine receptors in cancer cells at the invasion front. Interestingly, the invading cells induce nearby stromal cells to secrete SDF-1 (also called CXCL12), the ligand for this receptor.

- **Marrow-derived suppressor cells (MDSCs):** Tumors recruit these cells from the blood and bone marrow. They are at the edges of developing tumors and affect host responses to tumors (see below). MDSCs also secrete MMPs, which help to degrade basement membrane and ECM. They stimulate angiogenesis by secreting VEGF and PDGF.

- **Tumor-associated macrophages (TAMs):** These cells congregate at areas in which the basement membrane is breaking down. Like MDSCs, they secrete proteases, particularly urokinase plasminogen activator (uPA), which converts plasminogen to plasmin. The latter, in turn, helps digest type IV collagen in basement membranes. TAMs also produce cathepsin proteases in response to IL-4 made by tumor cells, further augmenting tumor invasiveness.

- **Carcinoma-associated fibroblasts (CAFs):** Like TAMs, CAFs produce proteases that facilitate tumor cell invasion. They also synthesize growth factors and angiogenic factors, and recruit precursor cells from the marrow, to become vascular endothelium.

- **Adipocytes:** The stroma in which many tumors arise contains adipocytes. Cross-talk between these cells and tumor cells facilitates early stromal invasion by the malignant cells. Fat cells near tumors often express a particular MMP that assists cancer cells in traversing surrounding connective tissues. Adipocyte-derived IL-6 stimulates tumor cell invasiveness. Leptin produced by adipocytes (see Chapter 13) induces macrophages to secrete proinflammatory cytokines, which, in turn, promote invasion and metastasis.

- **Lymphocytes:** T cells may facilitate tumor invasiveness via TAMs. CD4$^+$ lymphocyte-activated TAMs can elicit EGFR-related activation in some types of cancers.

The combination of these and other elements by developing tumors is sometimes called cancerized stroma. It should be noted that many interactions between invading cancer cells and their stromal accessories in crime constitute a positive feedback loop: tumors recruit and activate stromal cells, which repay the favor by magnifying the tumor's invasive tendencies.

Following their invasion of surrounding tissue, malignant cells may spread to distant sites by a process that includes a number of steps.

Invasion of the Circulation

Malignant cells penetrate lymphatic or vascular channels. Solitary cells that have already undergone EMT represent only a small component of the entire primary tumor. As lone travelers, however, these cells move more rapidly than do cell clusters and **intravasate** (penetrate) into blood vessels, which provide a route for migration to far-away body sites. Tumor-associated capillaries stimulated by tumor-produced VEGF and related angiogenic factors (see above) are not completely invested by pericytes. Tumor blood vessels are constantly being remodeled, and so are less well formed than their physiologic cousins. The angiogenesis initiator, VEGF, increases vascular permeability. In addition, TAMs produce EGF and tumor cells secrete colony stimulating factor-1 (CSF-1), both enhancing intravasation. MMP1 and MMP2, as well as other tumor and stromal cell products, increase the leakiness of tumor-induced blood vessels and facilitate their invasion by cancer cells.

By contrast, compact cell collections preferentially transfer to the lymph nodes, where they generally remain in place. Collective cell migration to lymph nodes appears to be independent of spread through blood vessels, and each may be the preferred mode of dissemination for specific tumors. However, metastases may in turn metastasize and single cells may exfiltrate and disseminate widely via the bloodstream. This phenomenon is the basis of currently used assays to quantitate single tumor cells in the peripheral blood, the results of which are used both as prognostic indicators and to guide choice of chemotherapy.

In lymph nodes, communications between lymphatics and venous tributaries allow the cells access to the systemic circulation. Most tumor cells do not survive their journey in the bloodstream, and a tiny percentage remain to establish a new colony.

Survival in the Vascular System

Once in the circulation, tumor cells have two main tasks: to survive and to find a new home. **Circulating tumor cells (CTCs)** are unlikely to spend long in the vascular system. Their size (20–30 μ on average) far exceeds the diameter of pulmonary capillaries (about 8 μ). A single passage through the pulmonary circulation should filter the vast majority from the blood.

To remain viable when detached from their native ECM, CTCs must be able to avoid anoikis (see Chapter 1), a form of apoptosis that is triggered by loss of the ECM anchors that constitute a cell's native environment. In some cases, this is achieved by activating TrkB, a suppressor of anoikis.

Preparing the Soil

It has been known for many years that metastasis is not random, that is, that certain types of tumors specifically tend to colonize particular organs. The molecular basis for some of these patterns of cancer spread is beginning to be understood.

There are certain general mechanisms that, even before a tumor begins to disseminate, help to prepare distant sites in ways that make the wandering tumor comfortable. Secretion of angiogenesis factors, VEGF and its cousin, placental growth factor (PlGF), with variable cocktails of other growth factors generated by tumor cells and their stroma causes hematopoietic progenitor myeloid cells (HPCs) to leave the bone marrow. These cells home to specific organs and set up a microenvironment there that accommodates the needs of the soon-to-arrive metastatic tumor cells. These so-called premetastatic niches undergo repeated remodeling by cytokines and enzymes produced by the marrow-derived cells. Inflammatory cells recruited from organ stroma and from the blood produce cytokines and enzymes (such as MMPs and LOX) that make the distant environment even more homey for metastatic colonization. The result is like a prefabricated house, just waiting for its future occupants.

Tumor Cell Arrest in the Circulation

While circulating, tumor cells associate with diverse formed constituents in the blood, including neutrophils, immune cells and platelets. These blood cells protect tumor cells from shear, immune and other stresses in the circulation. Such associations are mediated by adhesion molecules such as integrins, selectins (see Chapter 2) and a glycoprotein (CD44) at the surface of tumor cells. Tumor cells produce a factor that activates platelets via production of thrombin, and including fibrin and von Willebrand factor as bridging proteins. The binding of tumor cells to platelets requires P-selectin and platelet integrins, which recognize tumor cell CD44 via von Willebrand factor and fibrin. Similar interactions mediate tumor cell recognition and tethering to endothelial cells and to endothelial-bound leukocytes (Figs. 5-34A,B).

Leaving the Circulation

After arrest in the bloodstream, tumor cells and their fellow travelers mediate the process of extravasation. This is a bit more complex than its obverse—intravasation—earlier in the cancer cells' odyssey, because blood vessels at the tumor cells' destination are well constructed and anatomically complete, rather than new, poorly formed tumor-induced blood vessels. Extravasation appears to be relatively organ specific, so that the factors that are involved in extravasation of one tumor type into the lung, for example, differ from those that help the same or other tumor types exit the circulation elsewhere.

With that caveat in mind, the ability of tumor cells to enter the lung has been ascribed to a small number of proteins that increase vascular permeability, degrade tight junctions between endothelial cells and promote tumor cell escape from the circulation. These include several MMPs and VEGFs, cyclooxygenase-2 (COX-2), the EGFR ligand epiregulin and a protein called **angiopoietin-like 4 (Angptl4)**. This latter cytokine is particularly important for dissolving tight junctions between endothelial cells, thus facilitating tumor cell migration through vascular walls.

A. Tumor cell adhesion to surface - anchored platelets

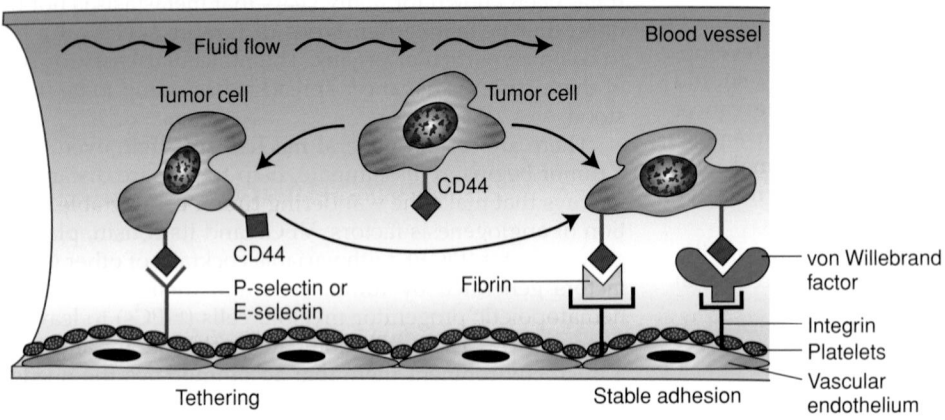

B. Adhesion of tumor cells to activated endothelial cells and endothelium-adherent leukocytes

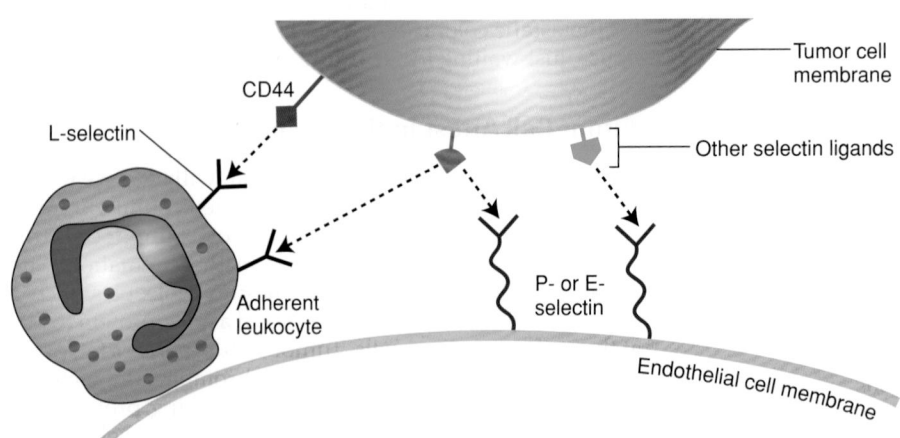

Figure 5-34. Mechanisms of tumor cell arrest in the circulation. A. Tumor cell adhesion to surface-anchored platelets. B. Adhesion of tumor cells to activated endothelial cells and endothelium-adherent leukocytes.

Establishing Micrometastases

The process of establishing colonies distant from primary tumors requires complex synchronization of the biochemistry, matrix and cellular composition of the soon-to-be metastatic site with the circulating tumor cells. Micrometastases may survive but never grow. Or they may not survive. Prospective micrometastatic foci must cope with issues relating to the suitability of the ECM, blood supply and stromal cells for tumor growth. More often than not, individual tumor cells or small clusters of tumor cells either become dormant in distant sites (see below) or die. For example, extravasated carcinoma cells may be unable to connect adequately with adhesion processes at foreign locations. Among the factors that enable micrometastatic foci to persist is the recruitment of bone marrow–derived HPCs to help guide tumor cells and stimulate their growth. SDF-1, derived from such cells, binds its receptor, CXCR4, on the tumor cells and stimulates proliferation. Active signaling through Src (see above) is important in ensuring continued survival of nascent micrometastases.

The Inefficiency of Metastasis

Tumor cells circulate in large numbers in cancer patients. It has been estimated that for every gram of tumor mass, 10^6 tumor cells are released into the circulation daily. CTCs can be detected even before the primary tumor becomes pathologically invasive. Furthermore, patients who inadvertently developed very high CTC levels because of a peritoneal-vascular shunt developed metastatic disease only infrequently.

What accounts for the inefficiency of metastasis is not clear. Mechanisms that suppress it (see below), both inherent to and outside tumor cells, undoubtedly contribute. Until we better understand these mechanisms and how tumors evade them, our effectiveness in treating metastatic solid tumors is likely to be limited.

Tumor Dormancy and Evolution of Micrometastases

What happens to all those CTCs that never become gross metastatic deposits? Some surely die, whether by apoptosis, anoikis, immune elimination or some other mechanism. Many, though, establish a dormant state. It is well known that metastases may become clinically apparent many years, even decades, after a primary tumor mass is removed. This is particularly the case in breast cancers and malignant melanomas. Such deposits were clearly derived from the original tumor yet remained below the clinical radar for long periods of time.

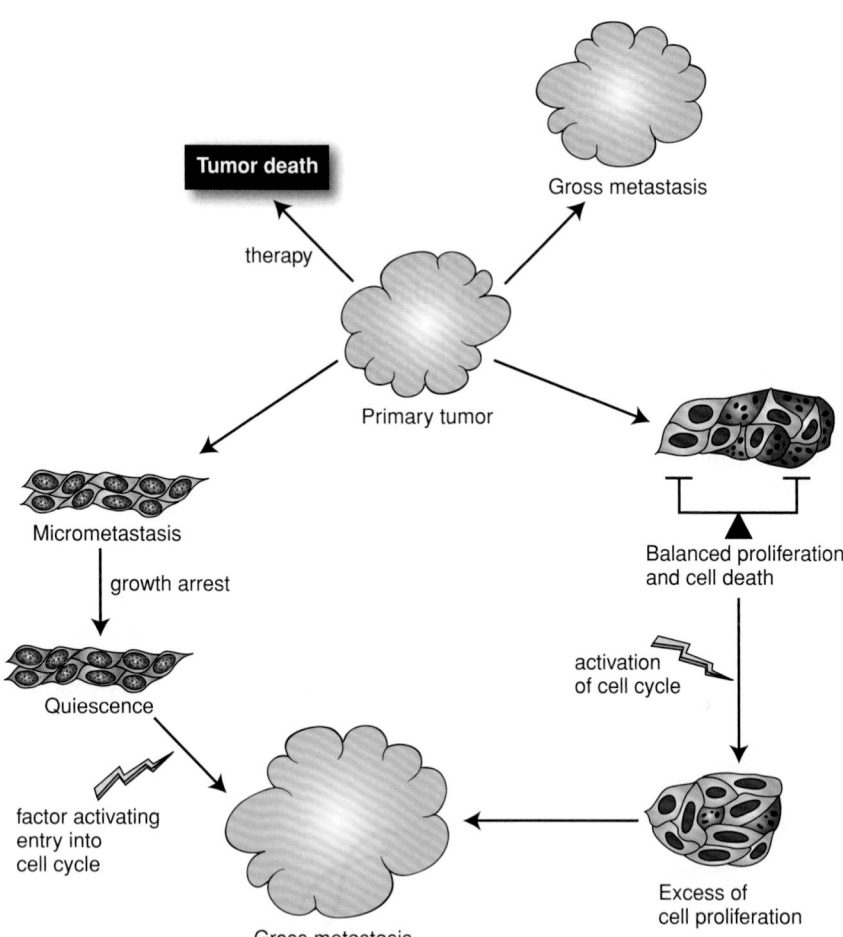

FIGURE 5-35. The fate of foci of cancer micrometastases. A primary cancer may be killed by therapies, such as radiation or chemotherapy, or it may be surgically removed. The tumor may produce a grossly evident metastasis. A number of factors may cause minute, clinically inapparent, metastatic foci of tumor cells to enter G_0 (*green*), but may be reactivated to enter the cell cycle (*blue*) and form a clinically detectable metastasis. Micrometastasis may also entail a balance between cell proliferation (*blue*) and cell death (*red*). If this equilibrium is disturbed in favor of tumor cell proliferation, the result may be a grossly evident mass of metastatic tumor.

It is also clear that some primary tumors may exist for many years before they are detected clinically. The presence of cancers, whether primary or metastatic, that do not enlarge to the point of being clinically detectable is **tumor dormancy**.

Growth of both the primary tumor and metastases is not necessarily exponential. Rather, it is often interrupted by quiescent intervals. As a result, the time needed for a tumor to grow into a clinically detectable mass is highly variable, likely reflecting fluctuations in stimulating or permissive signals on the one hand, the actions of inhibitory factors on the other or both.

Although tumor dormancy is a well-established observation, the mechanisms underlying this phenomenon are poorly understood. Factors that have been implicated in tumor dormancy and in escape from somnolence include angiogenesis, immune surveillance, apoptosis after oncogene inactivation (in cells that are oncogene addicted; see above), local processes such as inflammation, activation of cancer stem cells and adhesion molecules such as integrins. Sometimes, dormant tumor foci may represent a highly dynamic state—an equilibrium between cell proliferation and cell loss. At other times, the tumor cells are hypnotized into a somnolent state, in which they remain in the G_0 phase of the cell cycle (Fig. 5-35).

There are many **metastasis suppressor genes** that prevent various segments of the metastatic pathway. Thus, tumor dormancy has many faces, as reflected by the panoply of pathways by which tumor cells may be blocked from

propagating and may be subsequently awakened by a still unrecognized Prince Charming (Fig. 5-35).

Currently, resection of many tumors in patients without evidence of distant metastases is often followed by adjuvant therapies that are directed against undetected micrometastases. Such treatments are usually of short duration and are often aimed at rapidly proliferating tumor cells. If metastases are dormant, these types of therapies may not affect somnolent tumor foci. Future cancer therapies may need to be able to exploit the characteristics of tumor dormancy (e.g., by altering the equilibrium that sustains dormancy in favor of cell death or by forcing dormant foci into more active cycling to facilitate their targeting by more conventional chemotherapy).

TUMOR SUPPRESSORS

Tumor suppressors are a very large and diverse group of cellular functions, carried out via many different pathways and mediators. Suppressors exist for all the cancer attributes mentioned above (immortalization, evading PCD, etc.) and those companion tumor characteristics (genomic instability, altered metabolism, etc.) described below. This section highlights how tumor suppression works and the nature of many different molecules, and the diverse types of molecules, that carry the burden of these functions. It is organized according to the tumor attributes listed above and illustrates how some processes counteract those attributes.

Tumor suppression is an amalgam of processes. Some of these processes are inherent in particular cellular molecules (e.g., cell cycle regulation and Rb, or the intrinsic pathway of apoptosis and Bax). It is tempting to confuse the function with the mediators of that function, a logical jump that is made all the time. But, just like that extra scoop of ice cream, this temptation should be resisted, and the student would do well to remember that tumor suppression is defined by function, not by structure. One tumor suppressor function may be executed by several different molecules, and any one molecule may have multiple functions.

There are almost infinite variations on the themes of tumor suppression. Many tumor suppressors only inhibit development and spread of some types of tumors. Still others (e.g., WT1) are tumor suppressors in some circumstances but act as oncogenes in others. Some molecules may execute their duties in some settings, but not always. Further, some mutated tumor suppressors (like p53) not only fail to inhibit tumor development but also may actively facilitate it and inactivate other tumor suppressors. This fluidity should be kept in mind. We present tumor suppressors as static structures (e.g., PTEN, VHL, etc.) as a means to aid in understanding how they work, the processes they antagonize and what goes awry when they are mutated or inactivated.

The student should be mindful of this complexity, as it may come in handy when dealing with one of nature's most vexing principles, the law of unintended consequences. That is, it may help in appreciating that, for example, therapeutic manipulations conceived with ironclad theoretical logic so as to produce a particular result may yield consequences quite different from expectations.

Tumor Suppressor Mechanisms Protect from Oncogenesis by Inhibiting Every Tumor Attribute

Cells possess complex mechanisms that guard against tumor development. The molecular guardians responsible for this protection are called tumor suppressors, and the genes that encode them, tumor suppressor genes (TSGs). Major activities of tumor suppressors are illustrated in Fig. 5-36. If an incipient tumor is to develop successfully, it must generally inactivate one or more TSGs or their products.

There are many TSGs, with diverse targets, functions and mechanisms of action. Some tumor suppressors have multiple functions and targets. Some are not proteins, but may be untranslated RNA species (see below). And some are part-time tumor suppressors and part-time oncogenes. In light of this considerable complexity, we focus here on key concepts

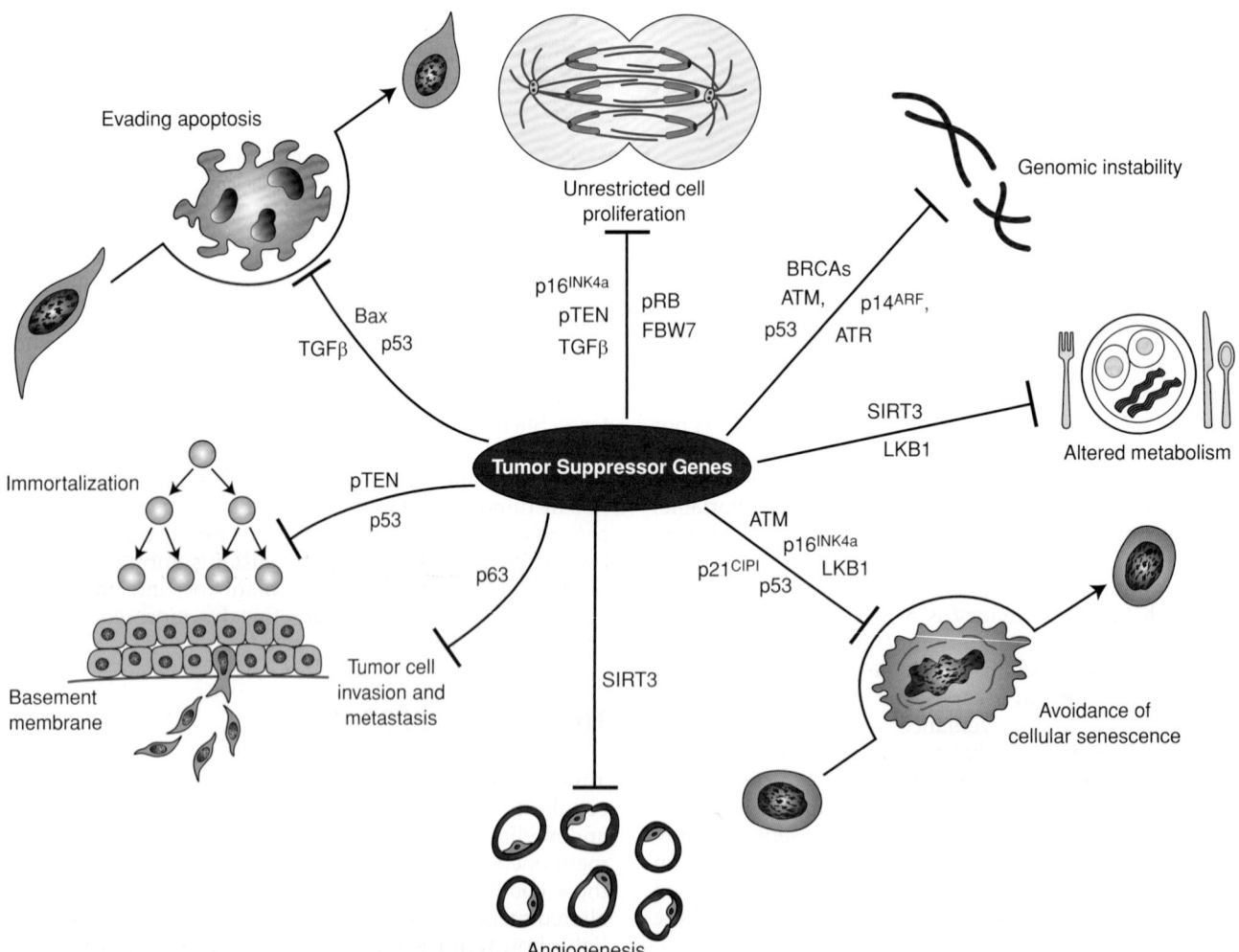

FIGURE 5-36. Tumor-related activities that are targeted by important tumor suppressor genes and representative tumor suppressors involved. The major hallmarks of malignant tumors each is antagonized by multiple tumor suppressor gene products. Those hallmarks, and the tumor suppressor activities that work against them, are illustrated here.

in understanding how important aspects of tumor suppression work, the ways in which tumor suppressors are circumvented and how tumors arise once TSG activities go awry. The protective activities of tumor suppressors are illustrated below for each of the major cancer attributes (see above).

Tumor Suppressors Regulate Cellular Proliferation

In normal settings, there are several important mechanisms that limit cell division. As noted previously, interactions between extracellular molecules and their cell membrane receptors trigger intracellular signaling via multiple pathways (Fig. 5-37). These include activation of PI-3 kinase (PI-3K; see above), which phosphorylates phosphatidylinositol-4,5-bisphosphate (PIP2) to produce phosphatidylinositol-3,4,5-trisphosphate (PIP3). PIP3 then activates downstream signaling via Akt and mTOR to drive cell division. A key tumor suppressor protein, PTEN, dephosphorylates PIP3, and so impedes cell activation initiated by mitogenic extracellular signaling (Fig. 5-38). PTEN is a major tumor suppressor, second only to p53 in the frequency with which loss of a tumor suppressor function is observed in human cancers.

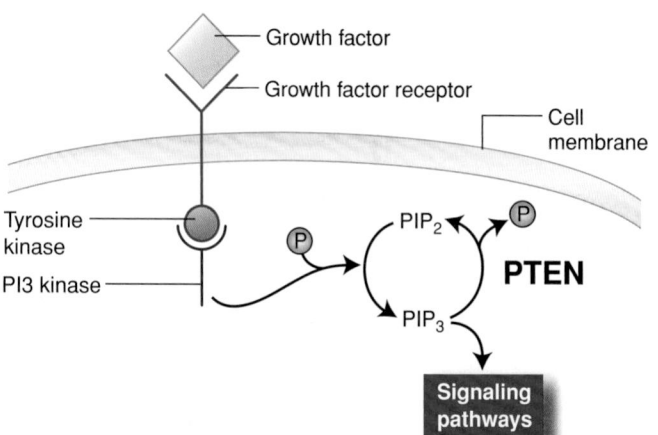

FIGURE 5-38. Signaling function of PTEN. Normal binding of a growth factor to its receptor leads to phosphorylation of phosphatidylinositol-4,5-bisphosphate (PIP2) to produce the important signaling molecule phosphatidylinositol-3,4,5-trisphosphate (PIP3). The level of PIP3 is regulated by its dephosphorylation by PTEN.

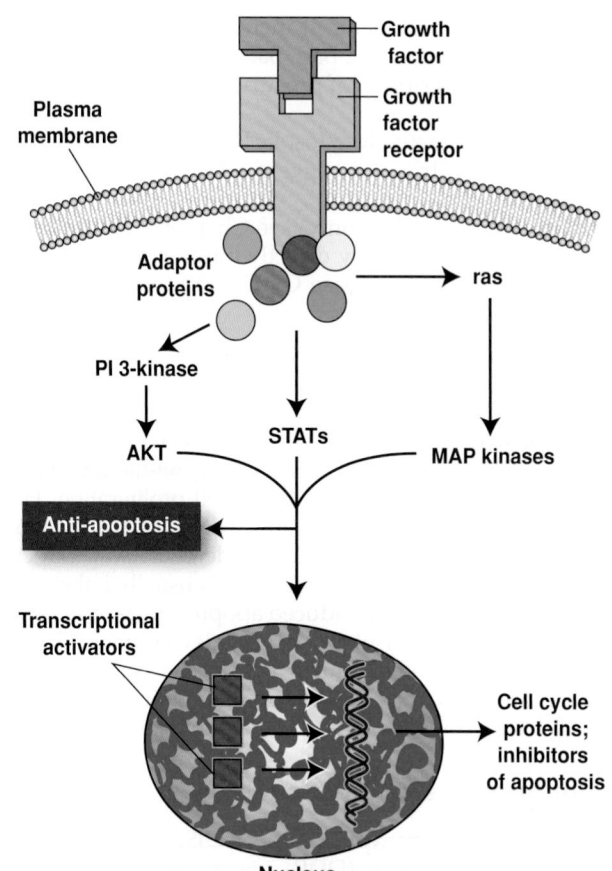

FIGURE 5-37. Signaling pathways controlling proliferation and apoptosis. The activation of growth factor receptors by their ligands causes the binding of adaptor proteins and the activation of a series of intracellular signaling molecules, leading to transcriptional activation, the induction of cell cycle proteins and inhibition of apoptosis. Key targets include *ras*, mitogen-activated protein (MAP) kinases, signal transducer and activator transcription factors (STATs), phosphatidylinositol-3-kinase (PI3-kinase) and the serine/threonine kinase Akt.

Many tumor suppressors act downstream from receptor–ligand interactions. Key tumor suppressor targets include the various transitions in the cell cycle (see above) and activation/inactivation of gene transcription. Thus, pRb blocks cell cycle transit, unless it is hyperphosphorylated, to release the E2F transcription factor that drives cell division. The enzymes that phosphorylate pRb (CDKs 2, 4 and 6, complexed with various cyclins; see above) are inhibited by the tumor suppressors p16INK4a and p21WAF1. Once pRb is phosphorylated, however, it may be dephosphorylated. Thus (see above), pRb can be dephosphorylated to restore its ability to inhibit E2F.

E2F-mediated transcription of many genes that drive cell division (e.g., c-myc) is powerfully inhibited by TGF-β. TGF-β binds its receptor to activate a series of intermediary signaling molecules called Smads (Fig. 5-39A). Smad4 is a key effector of TGF-β–induced transcriptional activity. It first blocks transcription of the c-myc proto-oncogene, thus inhibiting cell cycle transit and allowing Smad4 to upregulate expression of genes that block cell division, p16INK4a and p21WAF1 (Fig. 5-39B). TGF-β signaling is among the most potent endogenous mechanisms that inhibit cell division and is commonly mutated in human cancers.

Tumor suppressors also inhibit cell division at stages that follow transcriptional activation or repression. Thus, TGF-β signaling activates molecules that impede translation of mRNAs for proteins that drive cell cycle progression. Another tumor suppressor, FBW7, is part of a ubiquitin ligase complex that eliminates many proteins that drive cell division, such as Myc, cyclin E and Jun.

Many other tumor suppressors, far too numerous to mention, also regulate cell division. The above descriptions illustrate the diversity of mechanisms that protect the organism from runaway cell proliferation.

Programmed Cell Death Destroys Cells at the Cusp of Becoming Dangerous

The several signaling networks that culminate in cell death have been described in Chapter 1. They are all relevant to

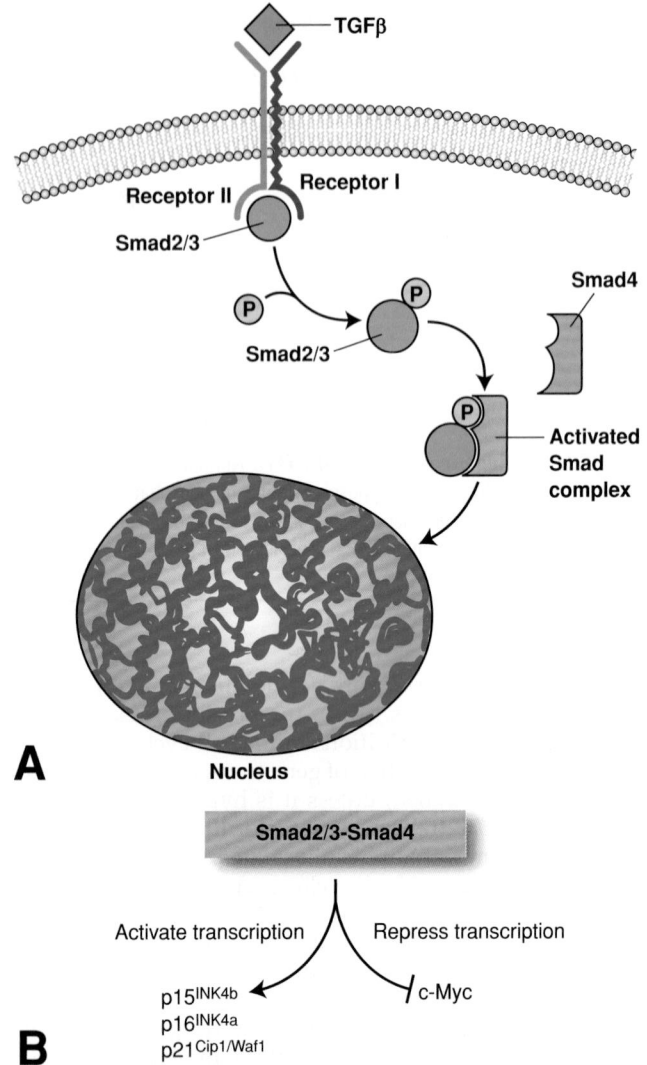

A

B

FIGURE 5-39. Transforming growth factor-β (TGF-β) as a tumor suppressor. A. Signaling. TGF-β binds its heteromeric receptor to phosphorylate and so activates Smads 2 and 3. These bind Smad4, to form an activated Smad complex that translocates to the nucleus to mediate transcriptional activation and repression. **B. Consequences.** The Smad2/3–Smad4 complex activates transcription of cell cycle suppressors, as shown, and represses transcription of the proliferation activator *c-Myc*.

protecting from tumor development, but the most critical of these is the PCD pathway that is activated by altered DNA structure. This pathway, in which there are several key participants—including ATM and ATR (see above) and, most critically, p53—is illustrated in Figs. 5-17 and 5-18.

The p53 tumor suppressor is a principal mediator of growth arrest, senescence and apoptosis (Figs. 5-17 and 5-18). In response to DNA damage, oncogenic activation of other proteins and other stresses (e.g., hypoxia), p53 levels rise and prevent cells from entering the S phase of the cell cycle, thus allowing time for DNA repair to take place. p53 thus acts as a "guardian of the genome" by restricting uncontrolled cellular proliferation under circumstances in which cells with abnormal DNA might propagate.

Acquired mismatches in DNA bases are detected by ATM if they occur in resting cells damaged by, for example, radiation or by ATR if they occur during DNA replication

(see above). These proteins then activate one of two kinases, Chk2 or Chk1, respectively. The latter phosphorylates p53 (see above and Fig. 5-17), causing it to dissociate from its inhibitor, MDM2, and activating the p53 damage response.

p53 protein is a transcription factor that promotes expression of other genes involved in controlling cell cycle progression and apoptosis. DNA damage and other stresses (e.g., hypoxia) upregulate the expression of *p53*, which in turn enhances the synthesis of CKIs. The latter inactivates cyclin/CDK complexes, thus leading to cell arrest at the G_1/S checkpoint. Cells arrested at this checkpoint may either repair the DNA damage and then reenter the cycle, or undergo apoptosis. The stimulation of gene transcription by p53 results in the synthesis of proteins (CIP1, GADD45) (Fig. 5-18B) that enhance DNA repair by binding to proliferating cell nuclear antigen (PCNA; see above). Thus, *upregulation of p53 as a tumor suppressor has two important and related consequences: arrest of cell cycle progression and promotion of DNA repair.*

If it is not possible to return the cell's DNA to its correct sequence, p53 may then trigger cell death. It may do this in several ways (see Chapter 1). Largely, p53 induces apoptosis by activating the intrinsic apoptosis pathway. It does this in the following ways:

- As a transcription factor, it increases production of proapoptotic proteins (e.g., Bad, Bax, PUMA and others) and represses transcription of prosurvival proteins (e.g., Bcl-2, Bcl-xL, Mcl-1).
- It may directly activate cytosolic Bax, which in turn moves into mitochondria and triggers release of cytochrome C (CytC).
- p53 may act as a BH3-only (see Chapter 1), proapoptotic Bcl-2 family member by directly binding to Mcl-1, therefore freeing Bak to release CytC and other proapoptotic mitochondrial proteins.

By whatever means p53 activates apoptosis, the cell death program is executed by caspases, especially caspases-3, -6 and -7 (see Chapter 1).

The issue of apoptosis and protection from cancer is further complicated by the phenomenon of **oncogene-mediated apoptosis.** Myc transcription factor drives cell proliferation. However, activated Myc can be a blessing in disguise. It also induces a default apoptosis pathway. That is, deregulated production of Myc promotes cell proliferation but is usually balanced by increased apoptosis. Myc-induced apoptosis acts as a "molecular safety valve" that blocks cancer development. If Myc-stimulated tumor development is to occur, cells producing Myc at high levels must also overcome PCD-inducing mechanisms by overexpressing Bcl-2 or other antiapoptotic proteins.

Tumor Suppressors and Senescence

No single paradigm explains all of OIS. The centrality of DNA damage response (DDR) via Rb and p53 is generally accepted, but senescence entails complex signaling (Fig. 5-27), and perturbation of any member of this could facilitate development of malignancy.

As described above, ongoing telomere shortening in normal cells eventually leads to senescence. Tumor suppressor activities that elicit senescence are critical defenses against oncogenesis. They include components of the DDR system, such as ATM, ATR, Chk 1 and 2, the cell cycle regulators p53 and Rb and many others.

Inhibitors of Tumor Angiogenesis Limit Tumor Growth

There are many potent endogenous suppressors of tumor-related blood vessel growth:

- **VHL:** This protein is part of a ubiquitin ligase that targets transcription factors, called HIFs (see Chapter 1), for degradation. Inactivation of the *VHL* gene leads to a defect in Ub conjugation, which leads to increased HIF-1α (see above), an angiogenic factor that activates transcription of genes important in cellular responses to low oxygen environments. These include those that (1) increase cellular intake of glucose for anaerobic glycolysis, (2) stimulate angiogenesis (VEGF; see Chapter 16) and (3) activate several critical growth factors.

    The carcinogenicity associated with the inactivation of VHL is caused in large part by the action of HIF-1α in promoting tumor growth. Interestingly, similar activation of HIF-1α occurs in the often oxygen-starved cores of many tumors, even in the absence of *VHL* mutation. In those settings, HIF-1α degradation is impaired by decreased activity of a cofactor for the ubiquitination reaction.

    The normal VHL protein has additional tumor suppressor activities independent of HIF-1α. These include (1) promoting apoptosis, (2) increasing cellular immobilization by adherence to matrix proteins and (3) repressing certain cell activation responses.

- **NOTCH:** Although it is an important stimulator of embryonic blood vessel development, the NOTCH family of endothelial cell receptors, together with their cognate cell surface–bound ligands (especially DLL4), inhibits tumor angiogenesis. In fact, VEGF stimulation elicits DLL4 production as a negative feedback mechanism. Its conversion to angiogenesis inhibitor in postembryonic life notwithstanding, the NOTCH/DLL4 system is thought to represent a mechanism by which tumors outwit VEGF-targeted antiangiogenic therapies.

- **ECM and other angiogenesis inhibitors:** ECM constituents and clotting factors, and their breakdown products, all suppress tumor angiogenesis. **Thrombospondin** (TSP-1), derived from a large ECM glycoprotein, is a powerful inhibitor of blood vessel formation. **Angiostatin,** a breakdown product of plasminogen, and numerous fragments of ECM constituents (endostatin, inhibin and many others) restrain tumor-related blood vessel growth as well.

- **p53:** While p53 is not known to interfere with tumor angiogenesis itself, it upregulates TSP-1 expression, as noted above, and so has a strong antitumor angiogenic function. TSP-1 inhibition of tumor angiogenesis is a casualty of loss of p53.

- **SIRT:** Sirtuin deacetylases are important in stress responses and longevity. One of the sirtuins, SIRT3, increases the mitochondrial antioxidant, manganese superoxide dismutase (MnSOD; see Chapter 1). As a result, mitochondria produce less reactive oxygen species (ROS), causing decreased HIF-1 activity and thus less angiogenesis.

For Each Step of Invasion and Metastasis, There Are Antagonists That Hinder the Ability of Tumors to Spread

Just as the body arrays its defenses to prevent cancers from arising, it has developed mechanisms to impede every step of the process of invasion and metastasis. Metastasis inhibitors are conceptually distinct from tumor suppressors. To qualify as a metastasis suppressor, a molecule must impede one of the invasion- or metastasis-related processes without necessarily affecting growth and survival of the primary lesion. To date, about 30 metastasis suppressor proteins are known, plus an increasing family of miRNAs that show metastasis suppressor activity. Some suppressors act at multiple steps, while others are known to act at only one. Also, some molecules may inhibit certain processes in some tumors or tumor types but have the opposite effects in others. Finally, there are some metastasis suppressors that have additional, separate activities directed against the primary tumor (e.g., pro-apoptotic, antiproliferative).

Impairing EMT

Cadherins are a family of cell–cell adhesion molecules, the best characterized of which is E-cadherin. It is expressed on the surface of all epithelia and mediates cell–cell adhesion by mutual **zipper** interactions. Catenins (α, β and γ) are proteins that interact with the intracellular domain of E-cadherin and create a mechanical linkage between that molecule and the cytoskeleton, which is essential for effective epithelial cell interactions. Overall, cadherins and catenins are paramount in the suppression of invasion and metastasis. Expression of both E-cadherin and catenins is reduced or lost in most carcinomas, owing in large part to downregulation by the transcription factors mentioned above, Snail, ZEB1 and so forth. The miRNAs, miR-101 and the miR-200 family, help maintain the epithelial phenotype. The latter does so by repressing ZEB1 and ZEB2 levels, thus relieving their repression of E-cadherin levels (see above). (Nothing, of course, is so simple: the ZEBs also downregulate miR-200.)

Not to be outdone, TGF-β, which is an inhibitor of tumorigenesis, is also a promoter of metastasis. It acts in part by downregulating miR-200s. As a result, in most carcinomas, loss of E-cadherin is associated with the development of an invasive and aggressive phenotype. Clinically, there is an inverse correlation of levels of E-cadherin with tumor grade and patient mortality. Interestingly, β-catenin also binds to the APC gene product, an effect that is independent of its interaction with E-cadherin and α-catenin. Mutations in either the APC or β-catenin gene are implicated in the development of colon cancer (see later and Chapter 19).

Inhibitors of Tumor Cell Invasiveness

Nm23-H1. This was the first metastasis suppressor discovered. Its mechanism of action is still not fully understood, but it is known to inhibit tumor cell motility. Nm23-H1 achieves this by blocking cellular mobility signaled by Ras-related cell activation pathways.

p63. This member of the p53 family of tumor suppressors (see below) helps to restrain cellular invasiveness. p63 is often expressed in some in situ carcinomas, such as those of the prostate and breast. It is often repressed or lost in aggressive, metastatic carcinomas. Furthermore, mutants of p53 (see below) may bind and inactivate p63 by forming heterotetramer aggregates. Acting as a transcriptional regulator, p63 also upregulates expression of certain genes that inhibit metastasis (e.g., miR-130B).

Movement through connective tissue is a key function of tumor cells after EMT. This passage depends on the ability of cells to wiggle through the ECM, which in turn depends on integrin-α5 as a mediator of EMT and RhoA, which helps to direct ameboid movement. These invasive characteristics are inhibited by miR-31 (see below).

Suppressors of Intravasation

Notch is a key inhibitor of tumor angiogenesis (see above). Mechanisms that impede intravasation also involve Notch. Thus, a protein called Aes (for amino-terminal enhancer of split) helps to inhibit migration of tumor cells through vascular walls via signaling networks that include Notch activation.

Limiting Tumor Cell Survival in the Circulation

Life for a tumor cell as a vagabond is no simple matter. Anoikis (see Chapter 1) is a form of apoptotic cell death triggered by loss of cells' usual liaisons with familiar ECM constituents. To add to the dangers of a cell's metastatic pilgrimage, many endothelial cells express the Duffy blood group glycoprotein, **DARC**. Upon recognizing KAI1 on tumor cell membranes, DARC triggers senescence programs, thus condemning the wandering tumor cell to a short, sterile existence. In addition, cells of the innate immune system can trigger cell death programs via TRAIL and CD95 (see Chapter 1).

As mentioned above, tumor cells tend to be significantly larger than the caliber of many vascular spaces they encounter. This disparity can stimulate the cells lining liver sinusoids to secrete nitric oxide (NO). NO triggers apoptosis in the overly large tumor cells trying to slog their way through channels that are too small for them.

Impeding Extravasation

The versatile miR-31 (see above), which inhibits tumor cell invasiveness, also blocks extravasation. This miRNA targets both integrin-5α and RhoA in the process.

Metastatic Colonization

Colonization and subsequent growth may be the major rate-limiting process in tumor metastasis. Several documented and likely metastasis suppressors act at this point, including KISS1 and its receptor, KISS1R. This pair derives their names from their discovery in Hershey, PA, home of chocolate kisses. KISS1, made by tumor cells, binds its cell membrane receptor, KISS1R. The result of this interaction is tumor cell apoptosis.

Other suppressors of metastatic colonization include GATA3 in breast cancers, which promotes cellular differentiation and impedes multiplication, and Psap in prostate cancers, which induces stromal cell production of the antiangiogenic substance thrombospondin-1 (see above). MiR-31, which has multiple antimetastatic activities, also inhibits the ability of cancer cells to colonize distant sites effectively.

Many metastasis suppressors have documented antimetastatic function, but the mechanisms by which these properties are exerted are uncertain. Once a primary tumor is removed, almost all therapy is aimed at suppressing metastases. Thus, it is not surprising that activating endogenous metastasis suppressive functions and trying to mimic them pharmacologically represent key targets of pharmaceutical investigation.

Diverse Mechanisms Participate in Compromising the Effectiveness of Tumor Suppressors

Of course, despite the body's best efforts, tumors still develop. In order to do so, they must either inactivate or circumvent the formidable defenses described above. There are a number of mechanisms by which this treachery occurs:

- **Loss of heterozygosity**
- **Spontaneous mutation**
- **Dominant negative mutations**
- **Fragile site translocations**
- **Altered levels or activities of tumor suppressor proteins**
- **Functional blockade by other related proteins**
- **Epigenetic changes that alter tumor suppressor expression or function**

These mechanisms are described and illustrated below. Epigenetic changes in cancer are discussed in a subsequent section.

Retinoblastoma Gene and Loss of Heterozygosity

Inactivation of tumor suppression may occur in many ways and is incriminated in the pathogenesis of both hereditary and spontaneous cancers in humans. It should be kept in mind that inherited defects in tumor suppression are fortunately rare. However, they help to identify tumor suppressors, to delineate how the affected tumor suppressor gene (TSG) products act and to identify mechanisms of tumor suppressor inactivation. Acquired impairments in tumor suppression are common.

Many more TSGs are known than can be described here, and their numbers are increasing. In addition, inherited mutations in TSGs are responsible for many named tumor susceptibility syndromes, some of which are listed in Table 5-6 (see below).

Retinoblastoma Gene

Retinoblastoma is a rare childhood cancer, about 40% of which reflect a germline mutation; the remainder are not hereditary. In patients with the hereditary form, all somatic cells carry a single missing or mutated allele of a gene (the *Rb* gene) on the long arm of chromosome 13. In the retinoblastoma tumors they develop, however, both alleles of the *Rb* gene are inactive. As mentioned above, the protein product of this *Rb* gene, p105^{Rb}, *is a critical checkpoint in the cell cycle, and inactive* Rb *proteins permit unregulated cell proliferation.*

Knudson's Two-Hit Hypothesis

A child with hereditary retinoblastoma is heterozygous at the *Rb* locus. The child inherits one defective *Rb* allele, plus one normal allele (Fig. 5-40). This heterozygous state is not associated with any observable changes in the retina, because 50% of the *Rb* gene product in the heterozygous child is sufficient to prevent a retinoblastoma. However, heterozygosity in some TSGs is unstable, because a subsequent, randomly acquired deletion or mutation may inactivate the remaining normal *Rb* allele. If that occurs, there is no residual Rb tumor suppressor function remaining to protect from unregulated cell proliferation. The child then develops a retinoblastoma. Thus, even though the child inherits a heterozygous Rb genotype, susceptibility to retinoblastoma is inherited in a dominant fashion: it is the heterozygote who develops the tumor.

Precisely the same susceptibility to LOH occurs when there is an acquired mutation in *Rb*. Cells carrying the newly

NEOPLASIA

TABLE 5-6

SELECTED HEREDITARY CONDITIONS ASSOCIATED WITH AN INCREASED RISK OF CANCER

Syndrome	Gene	Predominant Malignancies	Gene Function	Inheritance[a]
Chromosomal Instability Syndromes				
Bloom syndrome	*BLM*	Many sites	DNA repair	R
Fanconi anemia	?	Acute myelogenous leukemia	DNA repair	R
Hereditary Skin Cancer				
Familial melanoma	*CDKN2 (p16)*	Malignant melanoma	Cell cycle regulation	D
Xeroderma pigmentosum	*XP group*	Squamous cell carcinoma of skin; malignant melanoma	DNA repair	R
Endocrine System				
Hereditary paraganglioma and pheochromocytoma	*SDHD*	Paraganglioma; pheochromocytoma	Oxygen sensing and signaling	D
Multiple endocrine neoplasia (MEN) type 1	*MEN1*	Pancreatic islet cell tumors	Transcriptional regulation	D
MEN type 2	*RET*	Thyroid medullary carcinoma; pheochromocytoma (MEN type 2A)	Receptor tyrosine kinase; cell cycle regulation	D
Breast Cancer				
Breast/ovary cancer syndrome	*BRCA1*	Carcinomas of ovary, breast, fallopian tube and prostate	DNA repair	D
Site-specific breast cancer	*BRCA2*	Female and male breast carcinoma; carcinomas of prostate, pancreas and ovary	DNA repair (Fanconi pathway)	D/R
Breast cancer	*PALB2*	Breast, pancreas	DNA repair (Fanconi pathway)	D/R
Nervous System				
Retinoblastoma	*RB*	Retinoblastoma	Cell cycle regulation	D
Phacomatoses				
Neurofibromatosis type 1	*NF1*	Neurofibrosarcomas; astrocytomas; malignant melanomas	Regulator of ras-mediated signaling	D
Neurofibromatosis type 2	*NF2*	Meningiomas; schwannomas	Regulator of cytoskeleton	D
Tuberous sclerosis	*TSC1*	Renal cell carcinoma; astrocytoma	Regulator of cytoskeleton	D
Gastrointestinal System				
Familial adenomatous polyposis	*APC*	Colorectal carcinoma	Cell cycle regulation; migration and adhesion	D
Hereditary nonpolyposis colorectal carcinoma (HNPCC; Lynch syndrome)	*hMSH2, hMSH6, MLH1, hPMS1, hPMS2*	Carcinomas of colon, endometrium, ovary and bladder; malignant melanoma	DNA repair	D
Juvenile polyposis coli	*DPC4/Smad4*	Colorectal carcinoma; endometrial carcinoma	TGF-β signaling	D
Peutz-Jeghers syndrome	*LKB1/STK11*	Stomach, small bowel and colon carcinomas	Serine threonine kinase	D
Kidney				
Hereditary papillary renal cell carcinoma	*MET*	Papillary renal cell carcinoma	Receptor tyrosine kinase; cell cycle regulation	D
Wilms tumor	*WT*	Wilms tumor	Transcriptional regulation	D
Von Hippel-Lindau	*VHL*	Renal cell carcinoma	Regulator of adhesion	D
Multiple Sites				
Carney complex	*PRKARIA*	Testicular neoplasms; thyroid carcinoma	cAMP signaling	D
Cowden syndrome	*PTEN*	Colorectal, breast and thyroid carcinomas	Protein tyrosine phosphatase	D
Li-Fraumeni syndrome	*TP53*	Breast carcinoma; soft tissue sarcomas; brain tumors; leukemia	Transcriptional regulation	D
Werner syndrome	*WRN*	Soft tissue sarcomas	DNA repair	R
Ataxia-telangiectasia	*ATM*	Lymphoma; leukemia	Cell signaling and DNA repair	R

[a]D = autosomal dominant; R = autosomal recessive.

ATM = mutated AT (gene); cAMP = cyclic adenosine 3′,5′-monophosphate; PTEN = phosphatase and tensin homolog; TGF-β = transforming growth factor-β.

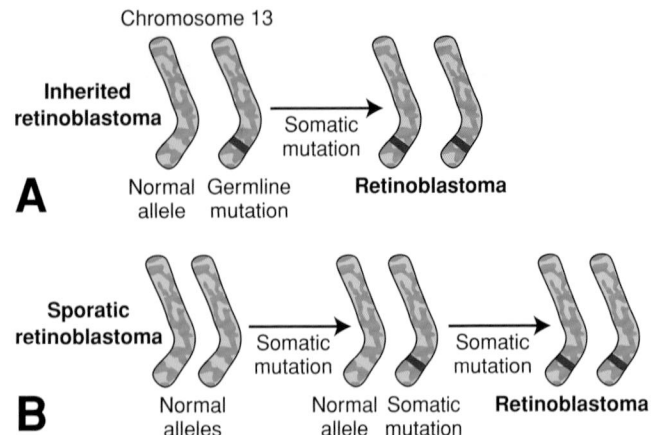

FIGURE 5-40. The "two-hit" origin of retinoblastoma. A. A child with the inherited form of retinoblastoma is born with a germline mutation in one allele of the retinoblastoma gene located on the long arm of chromosome 13. This mutation is not sufficient for tumorigenesis, but the absence of two wild-type alleles weakens protection from tumor development in the event that the remaining allele becomes altered. Then, a second somatic mutation in the retina leads to the inactivation of the functioning *RB* allele and the subsequent development of a retinoblastoma. **B.** In sporadic cases of retinoblastoma, the child is born with two normal *RB* alleles. It requires two independent somatic mutations to inactivate *RB* gene function and allow the appearance of a neoplastic clone.

acquired mutation become similarly susceptible to inactivation of the remaining *Rb* allele.

The principle, then, is that the presence of one mutant *Rb* TSG predisposes to eventual LOH and consequent development of malignancy. A mutation in one allele (whether inherited or acquired) facilitates clonal expansion of cells bearing a mutation in the other allele. This fact underscores an essential paradox of tumor suppressor genes: even if a wild-type phenotype is dominant, heterozygous cells are at high risk for LOH and becoming homozygous mutant cells, with tumor development likely to ensue.

While Rb is named for its signature tumor, an inherited *Rb* mutation affects every cell in the body and confers a more general increase in malignancies. Such patients have a 200-fold increased risk of developing mesenchymal tumors in early adult life. As well, *Rb* is not infrequently mutated in sporadic tumors, including 70% of cases of osteosarcoma and in many instances of small cell lung cancer; carcinomas of the breast, bladder and pancreas; and other organs.

Many types of *Rb* mutations have been described, including point mutations, insertions, deletions and translocations. Epigenetic events, such as promoter hypermethylation (see below), may also decrease *Rb* expression and contribute to a tumorigenic phenotype.

p53, Acquired Point Mutations and Dominant Negative Mutants

The *TP53* gene is located on the short arm of chromosome 17, and its protein product, p53, is present in virtually all normal tissues. *TP53* is deleted or mutated in 75% of human colorectal cancers and frequently in carcinomas of the breast, lung (small cell), liver, brain (astrocytomas) and many others. *In fact, mutations of* TP53 *are the most common genetic change in human cancer.* Inactivating mutations found in human cancers are largely missense mutations that impair the ability

of p53 to bind to DNA (Fig. 5-41A). Affected cells may then progress through the cell cycle despite having damaged DNA. While in some cancers both *TP53* alleles are inactivated by the mechanism described above, this is not always the case. Often, one mutant *TP53* gene is sufficient.

The active form of p53 protein is a homotetramer (i.e., a composite of four individual p53 proteins) (Fig. 5-41B). For the complex to be functional, all four p53 monomers must be functional. Mutant p53 subunits therefore can inactivate the whole tetramer (Fig. 5-41C). When the protein product of a mutant allele inactivates that of the wild-type allele, the mutant is said be a **dominant negative**. A cell carrying one mutant *TP53* allele (i.e., a heterozygote) should have a growth advantage over normal cells, and so predominate in vivo with a high risk of then becoming cancerous.

Additional Mechanisms of Inactivating p53

Because p53 is so intensively studied, much of the diversity of mechanisms by which tumor suppression can be inactivated has been uncovered for this protein. Normally, p53 activity is regulated by its binding to the E3 ubiquitin ligase, MDM2. The MDM2–p53 complex prevents p53 from functioning and targets it for degradation via the ubiquitin–proteasome pathway. In turn, MDM2 is inhibited (see above) by binding p14^ARF. Any oncogenic stimulus (e.g., *myc*, *ras*) upregulates the p14^ARF tumor suppressor protein, which in turn induces Rb phosphorylation.

Some cancers in which both *p53* alleles are structurally normal may overexpress MDM2, consequently increasing p53 degradation. Other tumors in which p53 is intact do not express functional p14^ARF, and so allow unopposed MDM2-mediated proteolysis of p53. As in the case of *Rb*, certain DNA viral products in tumors (e.g., human papillomavirus [HPV] E6, see below) bind to p53 and promote its degradation. In addition to numerous feedback loops, there are posttranslational modifications (phosphorylation, acetylation, etc.), natural antisense transcripts, binding proteins and small regulatory RNAs. It is no surprise, then, that *most human cancers display either inactivating mutations of p53 or abnormalities in the proteins that regulate p53 activity.*

p53 directs cell cycle arrest, apoptosis and cellular senescence, but these activities are only a part of a more complex tapestry of p53 functions. p53 also regulates responses to metabolic stress; regulation of autophagy and the redox state; production of ROS; and both promotion and limitation of longevity.

The p53 Family

Like a gathering of relations among whom one is the most boisterous, the family of p53-like proteins has largely been dominated by its most conspicuous member—that is, p53. However, there are several important cousins, p63 and p73, as well as some derivative proteins that deserve mention. Just as the region on chromosome 17 that encodes p53 is often mutated or deleted in human cancers, so are the regions on chromosomes 1 and 3 where p73 and p63 reside, respectively. If p63 and p73 are intact, they may partly compensate for loss of p53. Both are now considered to be a tumor suppressor in their own rights, with functions that partly overlap, and that are partly distinct from, those of p53. p63 is a transcriptional regulator, directly increasing levels of the proapoptotic proteins, CD95 (FasR; see Chapter 1) and Bax. It is also important for effective chemotherapy using agents like *cis*-platinum.

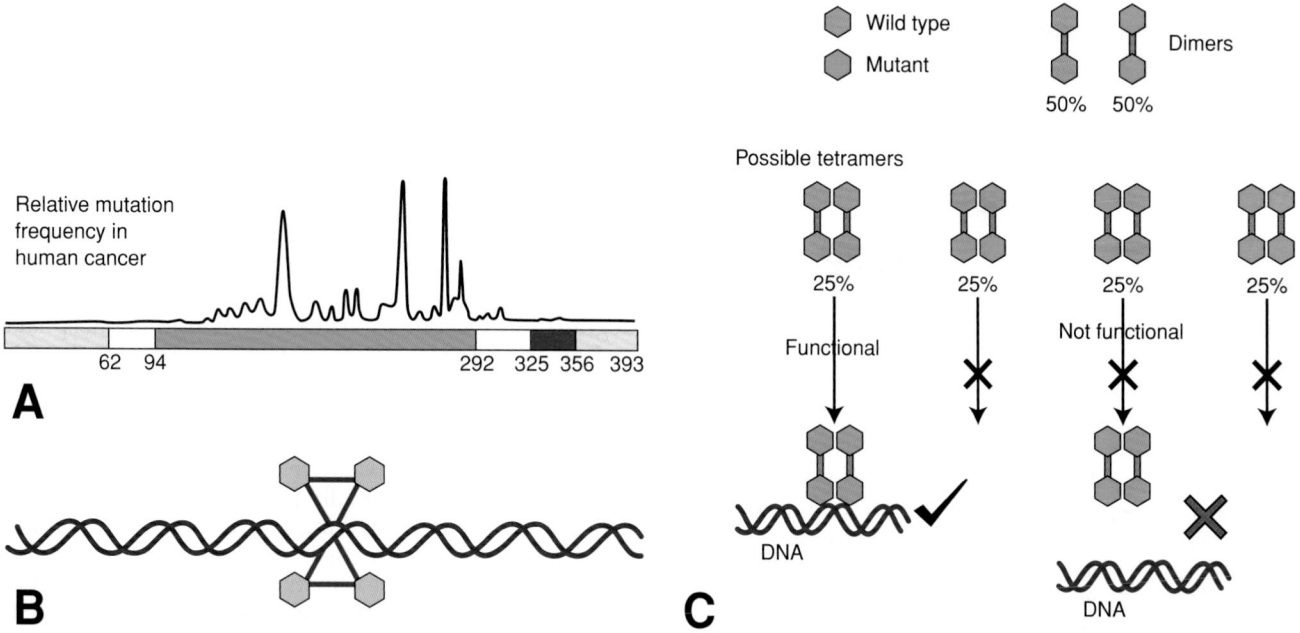

FIGURE 5-41. Mutations in TP53 and stoichiometry of impaired function of p53 tumor suppressor. A. Locations and frequency of mutations in different p53 protein regions. There are multiple domains of the p53 protein. The largest domain is the DNA-binding domain, which is where the vast majority of known mutations in p53 are located. **B. p53 binding to DNA.** To regulate transcription, p53 binds DNA as a tetramer. The tetramer is composed of two dimers. Each dimer is the product of one of the two alleles of the *TP53* gene. **C. Consequences of heterozygous mutation in *TP53* gene.** If one of the two alleles of the p53 gene is mutant, the result is that one dimer is completely mutant (and hence inactive) and the other is wild type (and hence active). However, as p53 transcriptional activity requires a fully functional tetramer, and as the sorting of the dimers into a tetramer is random, 3/4 of the resulting tetramers will be inactive, as shown. Thus, one mutant allele of p53 inactivates 3/4 of p53 activity.

There are many variants of each of these proteins. These may affect the protection afforded by these three proteins in diverse ways (see below).

Treacherous Mutant p53

Interestingly, the mischief of mutant p53 molecules extends far beyond simple inactivation of tumor suppressor function. The aberrant protein also functions as an oncogene, modulating gene transcription. In addition, it protects cells from apoptosis. Mutant p53 also activates proinflammatory cytokines and extracellular matrix modulators. It blocks ATM-mediated (see above) protection against double-stranded DNA breaks. A common denominator underlying the effects of mutant p53 is its widespread stimulation of genes involved with cell proliferation. Moreover, mutant p53 activates cellular mechanisms that are responsible for resistance to chemotherapeutic drugs. In many cases, including tumors of the hematopoietic system, breast, urinary bladder and head and neck, mutant p53 is associated with a poorer prognosis. Along these lines, it should be noted that some splice variants of p53 and p73, particularly those lacking the N-terminal domains, appear to inhibit aspects of their tumor suppressor activities and to act in part as oncogenes.

Fragile Site Translocation

The human genome contains a number of more or less universally shared **common fragile sites** (CFSs) that are inordinately structurally unstable. (Small percentages, 5% or less, of the population also possess rare fragile sites that are prone to the same fragility.) Gene amplification, chromosomal translocations, sister chromatid exchanges, deletions and other kinds of chromosomal malfunctions occur inordinately often at these sites. This instability may be implicated in tumor development, via resultant loss of TSG integrity.

The most active CFS is called FRA3B, and deletions or translocations there are associated with many human malignancies, including solid tumors and leukemias. A gene that is often inactivated or deleted in that setting is the **fragile histidine triad (FHIT)** tumor suppressor. It encodes a protein that cleaves certain nucleotides into adenosine monophosphate (AMP) and adenosine diphosphate (ADP), but it is not clear how much its tumor suppressor activity relates to this enzymatic function. Unlike most tumor suppressors except for APC, the FHIT protein does not bind DNA. Rather, it (like APC) enhances microtubule assembly. It is also felt to promote apoptosis via caspase-8 activation (see Chapter 1). Lack of *FHIT* expression is associated with enhanced resistance to apoptosis. FRA3B alterations are particularly common in human cancers associated with environmental carcinogens.

Other important tumor suppressors that are commonly inactivated during genomic alterations involving CFSs include Wwox, Parkin and caveolin-1. The gene encoding Wwox spans the FRA16D common fragile site. Wwox is important in growth regulation and some forms of apoptosis. Levels of this protein are decreased in most human malignancies. Parkin, an E3 ubiquitin ligase, plays an important role in autophagy (see later and Chapter 1) and is often lost in certain solid tumors. **Caveolin-1** is one of two tumor suppressors (the other being testin) located at FRA7G. Caveolins regulate several cellular functions, including signal transduction. This site is often lost in diverse human cancers, both solid and hematopoietic tumors.

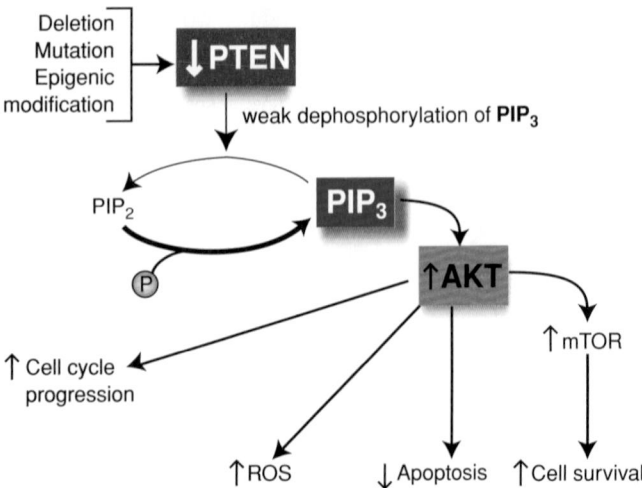

FIGURE 5-42. The consequences of decreased PTEN activity. If activity of PTEN is decreased by mutation or by epigenetic means, phosphatidylinositol-3,4,5-trisphosphate (PIP3) accumulates, activating Akt, a central signaling intermediate. As a result, certain regulators—p27, Bad and FOXO—are not activated, thus promoting cell cycle progression and decreasing apoptosis. At the same time, activation of mTOR (mammalian target of rapamycin) stimulates cell survival. Loss of PTEN activity therefore facilitates the development of uncontrolled cell proliferation and cancer.

Altered Levels of Tumor Suppressor Proteins and/or Activity

It would be tempting to understand loss of effective tumor suppression as basically a matter of altered TSG structure, or LOH, as above. It would also be wrong. For some important tumor suppressors, the critical parameter is the level of tumor suppressor activity, the presence or absence of mutations being important mainly insofar as it determines protein level. Such a tumor suppressor is PTEN (phosphatase and tensin homolog detected on chromosome 10).

PTEN Function

PTEN is a phosphatase that dephosphorylates both proteins and lipids. It regulates the many signals that connect growth factor–triggered signals from receptors at the cell surface to nuclear transcription factors that mediate many cellular functions. PTEN dephosphorylates the highly active signaling intermediate, PIP3, to its inactive 3,4-bisphosphate (PIP2) form. In so doing, PTEN inhibits the AKT-mTOR pathway (Figs. 5-38 and 5-42). As well, PTEN and p53 physically interact and regulate each other. PTEN may be necessary for p53 to be functional and protects p53 from MDM2-mediated degradation. Overall, by virtue of both its lipid phosphatase and other activities, PTEN protein is critical for the DNA damage repair response, apoptosis, regulation of cell cycle progression, maintenance of epithelial polarity and inhibition of EMT. It also regulates cell metabolism to limit glycolysis, as opposed to oxidative phosphorylation (see later).

PTEN protein is normally maintained at a steady, high concentration. Thus, anything that changes PTEN protein levels even slightly, whether inactivation of one or both alleles, altered promoter activity or other epigenetic or posttranslational change, may lower the concentration of the protein to a point where it is unable to modulate levels of PIP3 effectively. Decreased PTEN activity permits PIP3 to accumulate and constitutively activate a variety of signaling pathways involved in cell proliferation and survival, which are key in cancer development.

Alterations in PTEN Levels and Function

PTEN is the second most frequently mutated gene in human cancers, after p53. However, it is the level of PTEN activity that is the key to its tumor suppressor activity, and even small decreases in PTEN activity may allow some tumors to develop.

There are many mechanisms, and many points in the pathway from gene to functional PTEN activity, at which the levels of that activity are subject to upregulation or, mostly, downregulation (Fig. 5-43):

■ **Regulation of transcription:** Several epigenetic mechanisms (see below) are known to decrease levels of

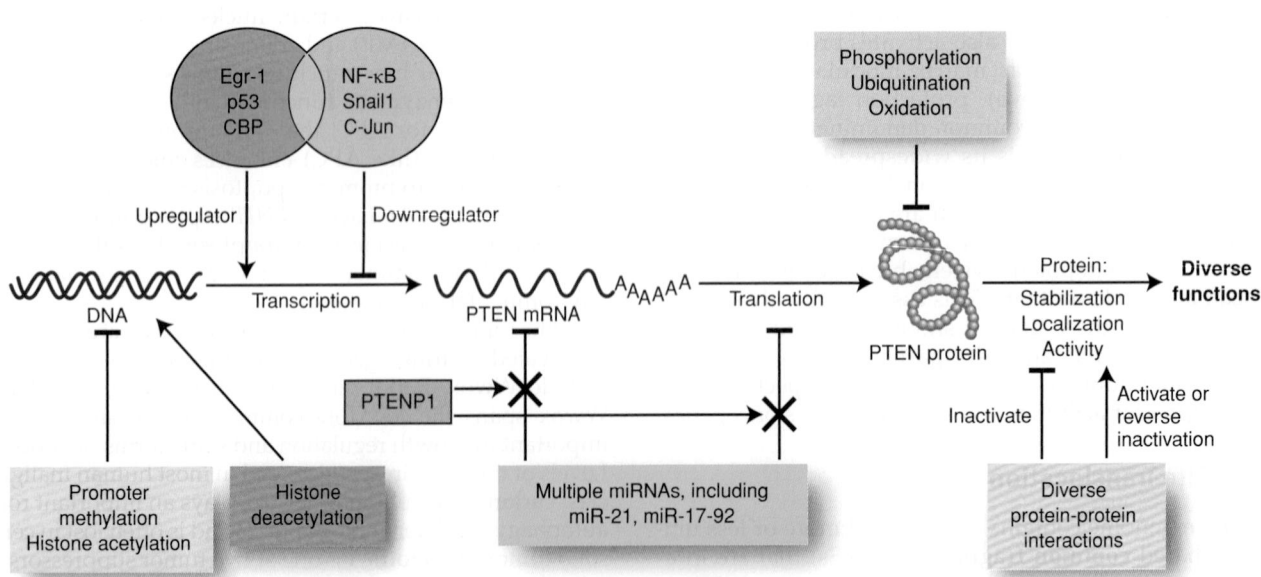

FIGURE 5-43. Regulation of levels of PTEN expression and activity. PTEN is a fundamental regulator of many cellular activities involved in oncogenesis (Fig. 5-42). The levels of PTEN expression and activity are crucial to cellular homeostasis. PTEN can be regulated by multiple mechanisms, as illustrated here, from altered transcription to messenger RNA (mRNA) stability to protein modifications.

transcription of the *PTEN* gene. These include altered histone structure and promoter DNA methylation. Concentrations of proteins that increase or decrease promoter activity are also important.

- **miRNAs:** MicroRNAs (see below) bind mainly the 3' untranslated region of the PTEN transcript and may cause that mRNA to be degraded, or may prevent its translation.

- **Pseudogene transcripts as decoys:** A gene, called *PTENP1*, which does not code for a protein, produces an untranslated RNA that closely resembles PTEN mRNA. This transcript is representative of a class of transcripts called **competing endogenous RNAs (ceRNAs)**. Sequence homology between the PTENP1 ceRNA and the PTEN mRNA allows the former to bind to miRNAs that would otherwise target and inhibit PTEN transcripts. The likely significance of this decoy to tumor suppression is illustrated by the fact that the *PTENP1* gene is commonly lost in some human cancers, leading to lower PTEN protein levels in such tumors.

- **Protein modifications:** Known posttranslational modifications of PTEN protein can inactivate it (acetylation, oxidation), target it for degradation (polyubiquitination), direct it to subcellular sites where its activity is particularly needed (monoubiquitination) or reverse inactivating modifications (e.g., SIRT1 deacetylates PTEN).

This intricacy and diversity of systems that control amounts of active PTEN protein maintain its functionality in normal tissues within very narrow tolerances. Data suggest that a decrease of only 20% in PTEN levels contributes to oncogenesis. In this context, some tissues (e.g., endometrium, hematopoietic) are more susceptible than others (e.g., prostate) to tumorigenesis when PTEN activity is slightly reduced. These observations underscore two important facts: (1) loss of protective tumor suppressor function may occur when levels of a tumor suppressor protein are reduced by as little as 20%, in the absence of an inactivating mutation in the TSG itself; and (2) different tissues vary greatly in their susceptibility (see below) to oncogenic stimuli—be they decreased tumor suppression or increased tumor promotion.

PTEN is not the only such protein to which these conclusions apply. Protection afforded by several tumor suppressors, like the breast cancer susceptibility proteins BRCA1 and BRCA2, is impaired when one allele is mutant while the other is still active, and so does not necessarily require LOH.

Effects of Alternate or Aberrant Forms of Tumor Suppressors

Mechanisms

A single gene may encode multiple proteins, independent of alterations in DNA structure. Among the most important of these are alternate splicing and the activities of multiple promoters (Fig. 5-44 frames 1,2). About 95% of human genes with multiple exons are known to be spliced in multiple ways, generating proteins of different sizes, often containing different amino acid sequences and having diverse functions.

Two characteristically important aspects of alternative splicing are shown in Fig. 5-44 frames 3,4. What is important here is that the same genomic DNA sequence is responsible for generating multiple variants of an individual protein. Alternative splice donor and acceptor sites may cause an entirely, or partially, different protein to be

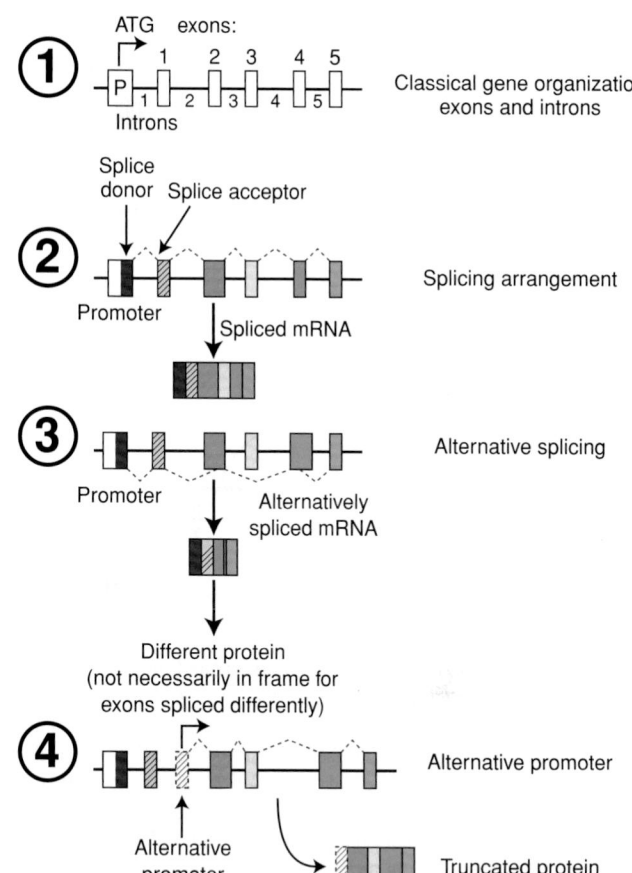

FIGURE 5-44. How alternate splicing affects a gene's products and their activities. RNA splicing is an important mechanism by which gene activity is controlled. It is illustrated here. **1.** The organization of exons and introns in a hypothetical gene is shown. **2.** Transcribed RNAs are spliced; that is, a splice "donor" site at the 3' end of one exon is linked to a splice "acceptor" site at the 5' end of the following exon, with the RNA corresponding to the intervening intron removed. The result is a messenger RNA (mRNA) that is exported from the nucleus for translation by ribosomes. **3.** However, there may be alternative splice donor and acceptor sites at different points within the several exons, so that an entirely different mRNA may be generated. The resulting protein may have variable sequence homology to the protein produced in **2**, depending on whether the alternate splice sites result in an mRNA that is in frame with the original or not. **4.** Another strategy for generating a different protein from the same gene is alternate promoters. In this situation, a promoter different from the promoter in **2** mediates transcriptional activation, and transcription begins from a completely different site in the DNA sequence. The result may be a partial protein, a protein that is spliced differently from the original (in **2**) and thus potentially completely different or some variation thereof.

produced, depending on whether the resulting splicing is in frame or not, compared to the original, "classical," transcript and its derivative protein.

Alternatively, transcription may be initiated from a second promoter (often designated P2). This may yield a protein homologous to the "classical protein," yet truncated at its amino terminus. Such amino terminal variants are often designated ΔN. Of course, these two mechanisms may operate in tandem to produce an array of variant proteins of different sizes, compositions and degrees of homology.

The factors that determine how splicing occurs, what sites are suitable donors and acceptors and so forth are quite complex. They involve many participant molecules. Some of

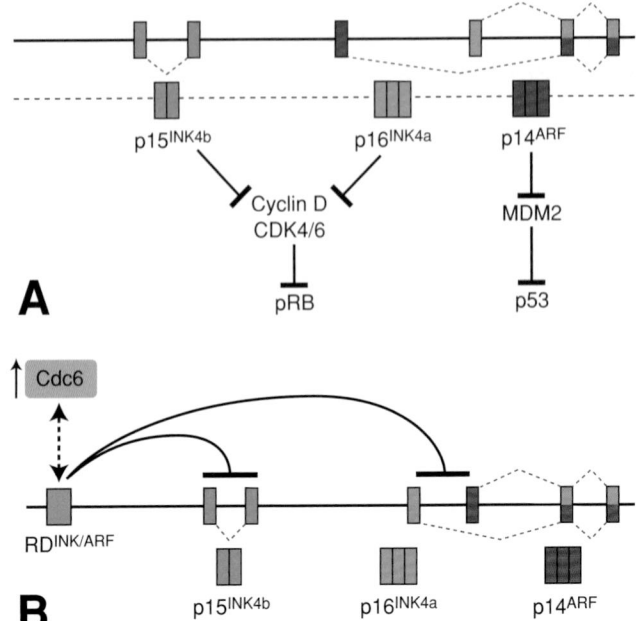

A

B

**FIGURE 5-45. Multiple tumor suppressors from one locus. A. The orga-
nization of the INK/ARF locus.** This gene encodes three major and different
tumor suppressors, as shown. p15^{INK4b} and p16^{INK4a} are both critical regulators
of cyclin D and cyclin-dependent kinases (CDKs) 4 and 6. p15 is transcribed
separately from p16. However, p16 and p14^{ARF} (ARF stands for alternate reading frame) coding sequences overlap. Owing to alternate splicing (Fig. 5-44),
their coding sequences are totally different. The functions of p16 and p14 are
also distinct, as shown. **B.** The area RD$^{INK/ARF}$ represents a region 5' to the
transcriptional start sites that is the target for Cdc6-mediated transcriptional
silencing of all of these proteins. All three tumor suppressors are silenced
by Cdc6, however, as Cdc6 binds the promoter for p15 and recruits histone
deacetylases to the entire gene complex, inhibiting transcription of all three
tumor suppressors.

these are tissue specific, so that different mRNA alternatives
and resulting variant proteins may be dissimilar in different
cell or tissue types.

Alternative Splicing, Tumor Suppression and Interference with Tumor Suppression

Alternative splicing, etc., is important in generating specific tumor suppressor proteins, in determining their ability to protect from cancer and the spread of cancer, in
regulating tumor suppression and in escape from tumor
suppression.

The ARF-INK4 Locus. One of nature's more impres-
sive mistakes was to have concentrated three major
(and several minor) tumor suppressors at the same locus
(Fig. 5-45A). This renders them all simultaneously susceptible to elimination with a single deletion event. Even
worse, these tumor suppressors can all be turned off by a
single interaction between a repressor protein and one specific area in the gene complex. Thus, p14^{ARF}, p15^{INK4b} and
p16^{INK4a} (see above) are all encoded on chromosome 9p21.
Loss of this locus is very common in human cancers and
leads to deregulation of Rb-related cell cycle control and
excessive inhibition of p53 (Fig. 5-45A).

The tumor suppressor transcripts are all driven by different promoters, p15^{INK4b} being upstream of the others. However, some of the exons for p14^{ARF} and p16^{INK4a} are shared

(Fig. 5-45A). The shared coding sequences are in different
reading frames, though, so that the two proteins have no
sequence homology.

Despite having different promoters, these three open
reading frames all share a common repressor site (Fig.
5-45B). The protein, Cdc6, binds a common site prepressor
and can simultaneously extinguish expression of the three
critical tumor suppressors.

An additional mechanism of tumor suppression is
exemplified at this locus, that is, **long, noncoding RNAs**
(**lncRNAs**; see below). An important lncRNA, called *ANRIL,*
suppresses expression of p15^{INK4b} and is particularly important in some leukemias and prostate cancers.

p53 and Its Cousins. As mentioned above, p53 is the most
prominent member of a family of tumor suppressors with
diverse functions. All of them are transcriptional activators
and repressors, and all inhibit one or more cancer attributes
(see above). Like p53, p63 and p73 are active in this mode
as homotetramers. The p53/p63/p73 story is more complex
than that, however. Each of these genes gives rise to multiple
transcripts, for which diverse, sometimes antagonistic, functions have been identified.

The best understood of these variants are shortened
transcripts, generated by alternative splicing and/or different internal promoters. These variant mRNAs encode proteins lacking variable amounts of the full-length proteins.
Transcriptionally deficient forms of each family are known:
ΔNp53, ΔNp63, ΔNp73. Many splice variants, designated
with α, β and so forth, are also known. These ΔN and splice
variants may oligomerize with the full-length proteins to
form transcriptionally inactive tetramers. Furthermore,
these variants, especially the ΔN variants, can bind to promoters normally activated by the full-length proteins (e.g.,
proapoptotic proteins such as Bax, Puma) and block access
to these promoters (Fig. 5-46). The presence of multiple additional promoters and many splice variants for each protein
further complicates matters.

Nonetheless, ratios of full-length:ΔN variants are tightly
regulated in normal tissues. Although the genes for p63

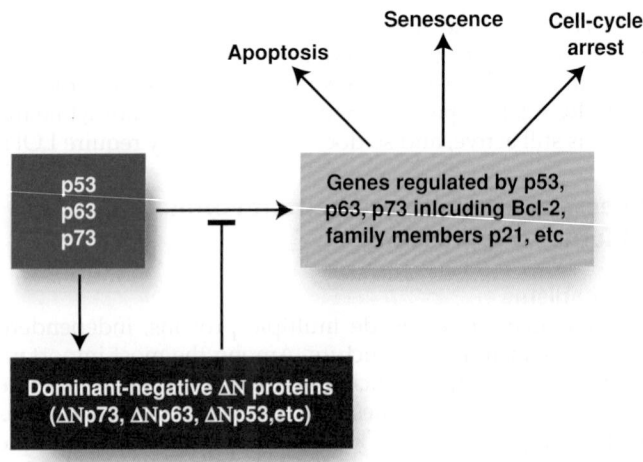

**FIGURE 5-46. The isoforms of the members of the p53 family and their
interactions.** All members of the p53 tumor suppressor protein family have
alternate isoforms deleted at their amino termini (ΔN), which act as dominant
negative proteins, and impede the transcriptional and other activities of the
full-length p53, p63 and p73.

and p73 are not often mutated in cancers, the ΔN forms of p53 family member proteins are upregulated—or ΔN:full-length ratios altered—in many tumors. For example, ΔNp63 predominance is associated with poor response to certain chemotherapies that target DNA and may portend poor prognosis.

Thus, complex as it is, the availability of alternate transcripts, and resulting variants or different proteins, encoded by the same locus represents an important means by which cancers can evade tumor suppression mechanisms.

INHERITED CANCER SYNDROMES

Cancer syndromes attributed to inherited mutations make up only 1% of cancers. These mutations principally involve tumor suppressor and DNA repair genes. As previously discussed for *Rb*, inheritance of a single mutated allele of a tumor suppressor gene results in a heterozygous state and high risk for LOH (i.e., inactivation of the normal allele). What is inherited in this setting is a high degree of susceptibility to developing cancer. Although the germline genotype of such people is heterozygous, both tumor suppressor alleles are inactivated in the tumors that develop in these individuals.

Hereditary tumor syndromes can be arbitrarily divided into three categories:

1. Inherited malignant tumors (e.g., Rb, WT, many endocrine tumors)
2. Inherited tumors that remain benign or have a malignant potential (e.g., APC)
3. Inherited syndromes associated with a high risk of malignant tumors (e.g., Bloom syndrome, ataxia telangiectasia)

These syndromes highlight tumor suppressor activities and the genes that cause them. However, many inherited syndromes entail a different spectrum of tumors than the significance of the mutated gene(s) would suggest. For example, decreased PTEN is very common in many malignancies (see above), but germline loss of PTEN (Cowden syndrome) is mainly associated with benign hamartomas.

Most of these are discussed in chapters dealing with specific organs, and selected examples are given in Table 5-6.

Some disorders, called **phacomatoses** (e.g., tuberous sclerosis, neurofibromatosis), are difficult to classify. These have both developmental and neoplastic features. Tumors associated with these syndromes mostly involve the nervous system.

Only a small proportion of all cancers show Mendelian inheritance, but certain malignancies undeniably tend to run in families. For many tumors, other family members of an affected person have a twofold to threefold increased risk of developing that type of cancer. This predisposition is particularly marked for cancers of the breast and colon, but is also exemplified in the interplay of heredity and environment. Thus, smokers who are closely related to someone with lung cancer have a higher risk of developing lung cancer than do smokers without this familial background.

Organ Specificity in Inherited Cancer Syndromes

Many of the inherited germline mutations cited above (e.g., *BRCA1* or *VHL* genes) lead to specific tumor syndromes. However, it remains unclear why alterations in certain genes tend to affect some organs but not others. Thus, the importance of BRCA1 in repair of DNA double-strand breaks is well established, but it is obscure why germline *BRCA1* mutations lead mainly to breast and ovarian cancers and not other types of cancer, and why women are so profoundly affected, as compared to men.

EPIGENETIC MECHANISMS AND CANCER

Structural changes in the coding sequences of genes, the study of which is called **genomics,** are important determinants of cancer development. It has, however, become clear that tumorigenesis and tumor suppression cannot be understood solely in terms of changes in DNA sequence leading either to dysfunctional proteins or loss of proteins entirely. Rather, regulation of the amounts of proteins in cells influences cell behavior at least as profoundly as the DNA sequences that encode those proteins. **Epigenetics** is the umbrella term for the mechanisms that control gene expression, independently of DNA base sequences.

The most important epigenetic mechanisms that are involved in neoplasia, to suppress tumor development, to facilitate it or both, are listed in Table 5-7. Some were mentioned above. These are physiologic processes that are obligatory parts of normal cellular equilibrium. *It is when these processes go awry that problems, including cancer, develop. Thus, no individual modality is necessarily cancer promoting or cancer suppressing, but may act both to inhibit tumor development and to promote it, the net result depending on the specific genes involved and how they are affected.* These mechanisms interact with each other, so that effects of one may require others to participate.

DNA Methylation at CpGs Regulates Promoter Activity

The amounts of a protein in a cell can be at least as important as the structure of that protein in determining how effectively it, for example, repairs DNA or restrains cell proliferation. The level of transcription of a gene is among the most basic determinants of how much protein is made. Transcription, in turn, depends on promoter activity. The promoters of many genes contain disproportionate concentrations of CpG dinucleotides, called "**CpG islands.**" (The *p* represents the interbase phosphodiester bond.) These islands are inhomogeneously distributed in the genome. They predominate in

TABLE 5-7

MAJOR MECHANISMS OF EPIGENETIC REGULATION THAT AFFECT ONCOGENESIS

Mechanism	Example
Covalent modifications of DNA	CpG methylation
Covalent modifications of histones	Acetylation
Remodeling/repositioning of nucleosomes	Incorporation of histone variants
Small noncoding RNAs	MicroRNAs
Long noncoding RNAs	Pseudogene transcripts

the promoter regions of many genes and in repetitive DNA sequences, particularly transposable elements (see below).

DNA Hypermethylation. DNA methylation is the work of a family of enzymes called DNA methyl transferases (DNMTs). DNMTs, especially DNMT3A, are recruited in part by modified histones (see below) to the specific CpG islands to be methylated. Methylation of cytosines at promoter CpGs generally silences the gene immediately downstream. This occurs both because CpG methylation prevents transcription factors from binding the promoter and because methylation may recruit transcriptional suppressors to the site. In many cancers, methylation inactivates TSG activity and is generally more common as a means by which tumors evade suppression than TSG mutations. Some genes, especially p15^{INK4b}, FHIT and BRCA1 (see above), are highly susceptible to downregulation by promoter methylation. CpG methylation may also complement mutation, to complete the inactivation of both of a pair of TSG alleles. Thus, if one allele of the DNA mismatch-repair gene *MLH1* is mutated in a colon cancer, the other is likely to be inactivated by promoter methylation.

It should be noted that DNA methylation patterns are not automatically transmitted to both daughter cells after mitosis. A special enzyme, DNMT1, is responsible for perpetuating parental cellular DNA methylation patterns to mitotic progeny. This enzyme is lost or impaired in some tumors.

Hypomethylation: On average, the DNA of most cancer cells is hypomethylated, compared to their normal tissue counterparts. This occurs in repetitive DNA sequences, as well as in exons and introns of protein-encoding genes. The extent of DNA hypomethylation may increase as oncogenesis advances from a benign proliferation to a malignant tumor. Undermethylation destabilizes DNA structure and favors recombination during mitosis, leading to increased deletions, translocations, chromosomal rearrangements and aneuploidy, all of which contribute to malignant progression. Transposable DNA sequences are particularly prone to undergo translocation when hypomethylated. Decreased methylation of genes associated with cell proliferation may increase transcription of such genes. The same principle applies to latent human tumor viruses (e.g., HPV, Epstein-Barr virus), hypomethylation of which may lead to tumor development.

Mechanisms of Methylation and Demethylation

Lest the above appear too straightforward, reality is always more complex. In fact, even though tumors may benefit from overall hypomethylation, in fact, levels of CpG methylation vary considerably, from one gene to the next. Some genes' promoters are hypermethylated (often TSGs), while others, such as oncogenes, transposable sequences and other repetitive DNA stretches, are likely to be hypomethylated.

Demethylation may also occur, although it tends to be more complex and may involve nonenzymatic reactions (see below), increased oxidation and removal of affected cytosines by DNA damage repair pathways.

DNMTs are also not immune to tumor-related genomic instability. Mutations in DNMT3A are important in allowing leukemic hematopoietic stem cells to proliferate, and so are also associated with poor prognosis. Thus, *the basic alteration is **aberrant methylation** and is site specific. CpG methylation patterns in every tumor and every gene are different.*

MicroRNAs May Act as Oncogenes and as Tumor Suppressors

Not too long ago, researchers noticed that a specific area in a B-lymphocytic leukemia (see Chapter 26) tended to be disrupted, but the affected region did not code for any known protein. On further analysis, they determined that the disrupted gene encoded not a protein, but a tiny RNA species that acted as a tumor suppressor. Loss of that miRNA tumor suppressor was linked to development of that type of leukemia. Since then, over 1000 miRNAs have been discovered. Functions relating to neoplasia have been ascribed to many of these (Table 5-8).

TABLE 5-8

EXAMPLES OF MICRORNAS (miRNAs) THAT ACT AS ONCOGENES, TUMOR SUPPRESSORS OR BOTH, AND THE TUMOR TYPES FOR WHICH THEY DISPLAY THOSE ACTIVITIES

Oncogenic miRNAs		Tumor Suppressor miRNAs		miRNAs That Act as Both Suppressors and Oncogenes	
miRNA	Organ	miRNA	Organ	miRNA	Organ
miR-21	Breast, CLL, colorectal, esophagus, glioblastoma, liver, lung, pancreas, prostate	miR-143	Breast, CLL, colorectal, lung, prostate	miR-23 group	Bladder (o), breast (o), CLL (o), prostate (s)
miR-23	Bladder, breast, CLL	let-7group[a]	ALL, breast, CLL colorectal, lung, pancreas	miR-23 group	Bladder (o), breast (o), CLL (o), prostate (s)
miR-221	AML, bladder, CLL, glioblastoma, liver, pancreas, prostate, thyroid	miR-145	Bladder, breast, colorectal, lung, ovary, prostate	miR-181 group	ALL (o), AML (s), breast (o), CLL (s), glioblastoma (s), pancreas (o), prostate (o), thyroid (o)
miR-17–92 cluster[b]	ALL, CML, colorectal, lung, ovary			miR-125 group	ALL (o, s), AML (o), breast (s), glioblastoma (s), liver (s), ovary (s), pancreas (o), prostate (s), thyroid (s)

[a]The let-7 group includes let-7-a-a1 through -a3, -b through -g, -i and miR-98.
[b]The miR17-92 cluster includes structurally homologous miRs 17-3p, 17-5p, 18a, 19a, 19b-1, 20a and 92a-1.
ALL = acute lymphoblastic leukemia; AML = acute myeloblastic leukemia; CLL = chronic lymphocytic leukemia; CML = chronic myeloid leukemia.

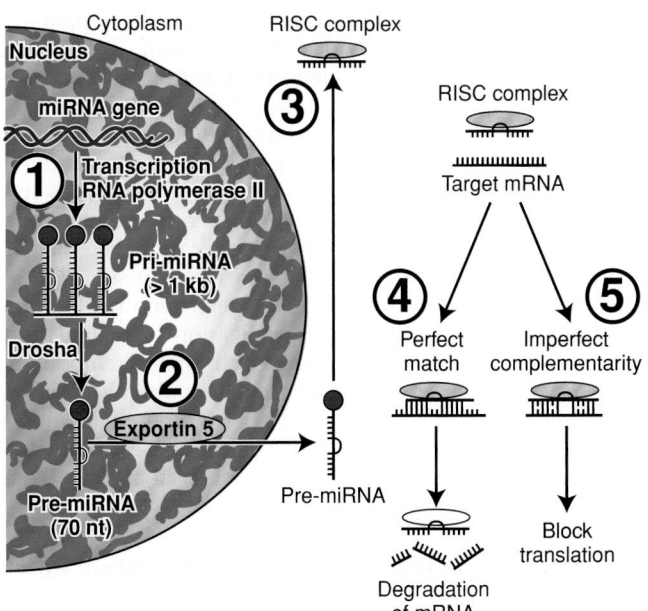

FIGURE 5-47. Production, modification and activities of microRNAs (miRNAs). 1. Most miRNAs are transcribed by RNA polymerase II, the same enzyme that transcribes messenger RNAs (mRNAs) for protein production. **2.** However, the original transcript, which is often more than 1 kb in length, is processed by an enzyme, Drosha, to a shorter form, which is called a pre-miRNA. **3.** This form is exported from the nucleus. In the cytosol, it joins an RNA-induced silencing complex (RISC), where the pre-miRNA is tailored further to the final miRNA by an enzyme called Dicer. A member of this complex, a protein called Argonaute, or Ago, can cleave targeted mRNAs. The nature of the effect of miRNAs depends on the extent of complementarity with a particular mRNA. **4.** If the nucleotides 2–8 of the miRNA align with the 3′-untranslated region of a target perfectly, the target is digested and degraded. **5.** If, on the other hand, the complementarity is imperfect, the miRNA inhibits translation of the target mRNA.

Generation and Actions of miRNAs

MicroRNAs may be encoded anywhere in the genome: intergenic DNA, introns, exons, 3′ untranslated regions (UTRs) and so forth. They are usually transcribed by RNA polymerase II (pol II), the same enzyme that transcribes protein-encoding genes. The initial transcripts that will eventually become miRNAs are often long (>1 kb). These are processed to precursor miRNAs about 70 bases long, which are exported (Fig. 5-47) to the cytosol. There, they are processed further and incorporated as single strands about 22 bases long into an RNA-induced silencing complex **(RISC)**. RISC includes an enzyme (Argonaute, or Ago) that can cleave target mRNAs.

If the recognition sequence (bases 2–8) of an miRNA matches an mRNA—usually the 3′ UTR—perfectly or nearly perfectly, Ago may degrade the targeted transcript. If miRNA complementarity for an mRNA is imperfect, translation of the latter is blocked without degrading the target. miRNAs are thus promiscuous, and any individual miRNA may regulate many different transcripts.

miRNAs and Cancer

miRNAs are critical controllers of many activities, such as embryogenesis and development, cell cycling, differentiation,

apoptosis and maintaining stem cell pluripotency ("stemness"). They also regulate many steps in oncogenesis.

miRNAs may inhibit tumor suppressor proteins or may themselves act as tumor suppressors. In the latter case, they may perform several functions, including directly targeting oncogene transcripts. They may also upregulate cell proliferation, and so act as oncogenes. In some cases, one miRNA species, or clusters of related species, may promote tumor development in some tissues but suppress it in others. This context dependence recalls the ambidexterity of some proteins that may be tumor suppressors sometimes and tumor activators at other times (see above). Examples of cancer-related activities for a small number of the more than 1000 known miRNAs are shown in Table 5-8.

miRNAs That Promote Oncogenesis

The cluster of homologous miRNAs designated miR-17–92 is commonly increased in certain hematologic cancers. Expression of these miRNAs is induced by c-Myc. The miR-17–92 cluster protects cells from oncogene-induced apoptosis (see above) in several ways, including by tightly regulating Myc-induced proliferation and downregulating the proapoptotic protein Bim (see Chapter 1). These miRNAs also inhibit the tumor suppressor PTEN and the cell cycle regulator p21$^{WAF1/CIF1}$ (see above).

MiR-21 also restricts apoptosis and other tumor suppressor functions. It downregulates p53 and proteins important in mitochondrial apoptosis. MiR-21 also targets key regulators of cell proliferation, such as TGF-β signaling and PTEN pathways (see above). In various tumor types, miR-21 reduces other tumor suppressor and proapoptotic activities, underscoring both the context dependence and promiscuity of miRNA actions. This miRNA is overexpressed in many human tumors, including those in lung, pancreas and colon cancers.

Tumor Suppression by miRNAs

The let-7 family of miRNAs contains 12 highly conserved members. They have overlapping specificities and target ranges, especially downregulating proteins that activate cell proliferation, such as K-Ras, N-Ras and Myc. miRNAs of this group also target CDK6 and CDC25A, thus blocking cell cycle transit through $G_1 \to S$ transition. Levels of let-7 members are reduced in many human tumors, especially lung cancers.

Important miRNAs that target the prosurvival (antiapoptotic) branch of the Bcl-2 family include the cluster of miR-15/16 species. These directly inhibit Bcl-2, the main mitochondrial antiapoptotic protein (see above, Chapter 1). They also block production of important cell cycle drivers, including cyclins D and E. MiR-15/16 are often decreased or absent in solid tumors and certain lymphomas.

Histone Modifications Alter the Ability of Nonhistone Regulators to Reach the DNA

Chromatin is a complex of DNA and proteins that promotes DNA stability and allows it to fit in a small space (the nucleus). It contains repeating units, **nucleosomes,** periodically spaced structures that consist of a combination of 4 histone proteins (H2A, H2B, H3, H4), wrapped in DNA. Covalent alterations to histones include methylation, acetylation, ubiquitination, phosphorylation and others. These occur via specific histone-modifying enzymes, and are reversible. The operation of histone methylases can be undone by histone demethylases. The work of histone acetylases (HACs) can be reversed by histone deacetylases (HDACs). Covalent changes to histone structure control such gene activities as transcription, DNA repair and DNA replication. Not surprisingly, then, the enzymes that acetylate or deacetylate and methylate or demethylate histones are key regulators of many activities, including oncogenesis.

Histone methylation. Lysines are the principal targets of histone modifications, including acetylation and methylation. However, there are many lysines on several histone species, so the consequences of histone methylation (etc.) depend on where (on which histone, on what amino acids and near what gene) and how much the histone is methylated. In some cases, a specific transcriptional repressor complex, the **polycomb repressor complex-2** (PRC2), is recruited to promoters that are to be inactivated. This complex methylates a specific residue on H3 and silences transcription. If, by different means, a different H3 lysine is methylated, the opposite effect (transcriptional activation) occurs. The histone methylating enzyme, EZH2, is part of PRC2. Altered expression of EZH2 occurs in many cancers and has been associated with a poor prognosis. Cells may gain or lose EZH2 function by mutation or by altered levels of a miRNA that inhibits it (miR-101).

Histone acetylation. Histone acetylation tends to open chromatin and is generally associated with increased transcriptional activity. Histone deacetylation causes chromatin condensation, making it inaccessible for transcription, and so is associated with transcriptional silencing. HDACs are often dysregulated in cancers, causing both silencing of tumor suppressor genes and derepression of oncogenes. The combination of histone modifications and DNA methylation constitutes an intricate regulatory network whose disruption plays an important role in oncogenesis.

The role of histone acetylation status in regulation cannot, apparently, be overestimated. A recent report indicates that histone acetylation is a key determinant of monogamous mating behaviors in prairie voles. Apparently, monogamy in these animals occurs (at least in part) because of histone acetylation near oxytocin and vasopressin receptor genes in the nucleus accumbens in their brains.

Modified Histones and DNA Methylation

As indicated above, the acetylation state of histones affects the transcriptional activity of the gene in question. Histone methylation and DNA methylation also regulate transcription. Histone methylases may directly recruit DNMTs to a gene to be silenced. DNMTs, in turn, can bring HDACs to these sites to deacetylate histones and silence expression. These relationships are complex, however. In some cases, DNA methylation appears to precede histone methylation and deacetylation, and vice versa. Thus, the three processes are linked, but the sequence of events and the final status of the DNA and histones at a site are probably all specific for individual genes.

Nucleosome Positioning and Histone Composition Influence Gene Activity

Chromatin structure is dynamic and varies with a cell's needs at the moment. Nucleosomes tend to leave open those parts of genes where the transcriptional apparatus binds

to start gene expression, and again where that apparatus releases the DNA at the end of transcription. Remodeling complexes busily modify nucleosome position and composition, causing nucleosomes to slide or be removed as needed to tailor gene expression to changing cellular circumstances.

The process of synchronizing nucleosome positioning entails incorporation of modified or variant histones into chromatin. These also substitute for their more conventional cousins on an ongoing basis and strongly influence the susceptibility or resistance of associated DNA to silencing by methylation. Such histones help to determine nucleosome positioning itself. Continued modification of histone proteins, as well, is part of the dynamic of chromatin remodeling. For every histone acetylating, methylating, ubiquitinating or phosphorylating an enzyme, there is another that undoes these modifications. As we will see below, these modifiers of histone structure, as well as the mechanisms that sense them, are often central to tumor development.

Long Noncoding RNAs Play Major Regulatory Roles

About 3% of the human genome encodes proteins. Not long ago, it was thought that most of the rest was inactive, or "junk" DNA. Nothing could be further from the truth. It is now clear that over 90% of the human genome is actively transcribed, almost all of it as transcripts that do not make proteins. Furthermore, many DNA sequence changes associated with cancer and other diseases occur within the regions that encode these untranslated RNAs.

These RNAs are called **long noncoding RNAs,** *which are defined as RNAs, either primary or spliced transcripts, that do not fit into recognized classes such as structural, protein-coding or small RNAs.* DNA sequences almost anywhere can encode lncRNAs, including intergenic regions, introns, exons and even antisense to coding regions. LncRNAs may be quite large, often 1000s or 10,000s of bases. About 5000 are currently cataloged, and over 20,000 different species may exist. However many there are, they are very low in abundance, poorly understood and almost completely uncharacterized. They do, though, play many important regulatory epigenetic roles, including processing of small RNAs, controlling transcription and acting as organizers, decoys, signal transducers and scaffolds that bind to proteins, DNA or other RNAs. For example, inactivation of one of the pair of X chromosomes in females is the work of an lncRNA called Xist. LncRNAs also help direct chromatin remodeling and DNA methylation and determine the stability and fate of protein-coding RNAs.

We have mentioned lncRNAs in several contexts (above), including as the products of pseudogenes (e.g., PTENP1). These pseudogene lncRNAs may act as decoys for regulatory miRNAs (i.e., as alternative targets for degradative miRNAs), allowing their protein-coding tumor suppressor cousin (here, PTEN mRNA) to survive unmolested. Examples of lncRNAs involved in cancer are shown in Table 5-9.

Epigenetic Regulators Are Distorted in Cancers

The intricacy of epigenetic control over normal cellular processes should be abundantly evident, as should the limitations of our understanding of it. Tumor development, progression and dissemination all entail extensive disequilibrium at every level of epigenetic activity. The explanations above touch on many of these, both in principle and specifically. *It should be emphasized, in summarizing this topic,*

TABLE 5-9

REPRESENTATIVE LONG NONCODING RNAs (lncRNAs) THAT ARE ALTERED IN CANCERS

lncRNA	Tumor Type	Alteration	Function/Consequence
MALAT1	NSCLC, colorectal	↑	Tumor progression and dissemination
ANRIL	Prostate, leukemias	↑	Silences TSG p15^{INK5b} by recruiting PRC2 to methylate promoter
PTENP1	Lung, prostate, endometrium	↓	Pseudogene decoy protecting PTEN mRNA from miRNA-mediated destruction
HOTAIR	Pancreas, colorectal, breast, liver	↑	Recurrence; metastasis; recruits PRC2 to silence tumor suppressors
HULUC	Liver	↑	Represses expression of tumor suppressor miR-372

miRNA = microRNA; mRNA = messenger RNA' NSCLC = non–small cell lung cancer; PRC2 = Polycomb repressor complex-2; TSG = tumor suppressor gene.

that the devil is always in the details, and that overarching generalizations about how tumors develop may be conceptually useful but often break down when one attempts to apply them to specific situations. Thus, a transcriptional activating function may be overactive in a tumor and so upregulate an oncogene, but the same function may be blocked with respect to a tumor suppressor in the same cancer. With that caveat, it is reasonable to summarize the impact of epigenetics on cancer as follows:

- **DNA methylation:** Generally, cancer cell genomes are hypomethylated. This causes general genomic instability and extensive derepression of transcription affecting many genes, especially oncogenes. At the same time, site-specific hypermethylation (e.g., of tumor suppressor genes) also characterizes cancers. The role of PRC2 (see above) is emerging as fundamental to these changes.
- **Histone modifications:** Many tumors show general loss of histone acetylation, especially associated with silencing of TSGs. HDAC overexpression is common in cancers. This has stimulated development of therapeutic HDAC inhibitors. However, HACs are also often abnormal in cancers, and it is the specific interplay of both HACs and HDACs relative to tumor suppressor genes and oncogenes that determines the end result: which genes are activated and which repressed. Other types of histone-modifying enzymes, such as the methylating enzyme EZH2, are also often involved in silencing tumor suppressor genes.
- **Nucleosome positioning:** Altered chromatin structure in cancer accompanies changes in DNA methylation and histone derivatives. Thus, nucleosome localization in tumor cells differs from that in their nonmalignant cellular counterparts.
- **Noncoding RNAs:** Levels of specific noncoding RNAs, both short and long noncoding RNA species, in cancer differ greatly from those in normal cells. These disturbances of normal equilibrium play central roles in regulating almost all facets of cancer cell behavior.

Environmental Stimuli Shape Epigenetic Regulators

The epigenome is highly dynamic and responds to modulation by nutrition, stress, pharmacologic and toxic agents and other influences. For example, identical twins diverge increasingly over time in patterns of DNA methylation. In fact, patterns of CpG methylation of specific genes change over the course of years in any given individual. The ways in which the cellular milieu influences epigenetic regulation are largely obscure. But what is known suggests that this impact may be fundamental to the processes by which tumors originate and spread.

Epigenetic Remodeling as a Function of Metabolism

Tumor cell metabolism is fundamentally different from that of normal cells (see below). The key differences known to affect epigenetic regulation are (1) reliance on glycolysis for energy (as opposed to oxidative phosphorylation), (2) increased levels of HIF-1α, (3) a highly oxidant-rich environment, (4) mutations in key enzymes in the Krebs cycle and (5) abnormally high levels of fatty acid biosynthesis. These factors influence epigenetic regulators as follows:

- **Histone acetylation:** The net result of HACs' and HDACs' actions on histones largely determines gene expression (see above). The acetyl donor for acetylation is acetyl-coenzyme A (CoA). A combination of decreased Krebs cycle effectiveness, via mutations and other means, and high need for acetyl-CoA for fatty acid synthesis reduces the pool of acetyl-CoA available for histone acetylation. This may increase transcriptional repression, especially of TSGs.
- **Histone deacetylation:** A key class of HDACs (class III) are sirtuins, which use NAD^+ to deacetylate histones. Cancer cells' excessive reliance on glycolysis decreases the pool of available NAD^+, restraining this group of HDACs and causing further disequilibrium in histone acetylation. This situation is exacerbated further by metabolic consequences of HIF-1α upregulation, which occurs often in tumors and further limits NAD^+ availability.
- **Methylation:** DNMTs and histone methyl transferases (HMTs) require S-adenosylmetionine (SAM) as a methyl group donor. High levels of oxidative stress in transformed cells lower SAM levels in several ways and accelerate its conversion to other species (especially the antioxidant glutathione). Reduced SAM availability unbalances both histone and DNA methylation.
- **Base changes and oxidation:** Several changes associated with DNA oxidation and modification may result in base changes, particularly affecting CpGs. Thus, methylated cytosine (5-methylcytosine) can undergo two changes that alter DNA structure. It may be spontaneously deaminated to thymine, thus creating a C→T base change transition. In an oxidant-rich environment, it may also be oxidized to 5-(hydroxymethyl) cytosine. This reaction, catalyzed by an enzyme called **Tet methylcytosine dioxygenase (TET2)**, is of note because the *TET2* gene is specifically mutated in certain hematologic malignancies and premalignant conditions. TET2 activity is also affected by certain metabolic aberrations (see below). The added hydroxyl group may then be further oxidized to a carboxyl group, which is enzymatically removed to regenerate the original, unmethylated, cytosine.

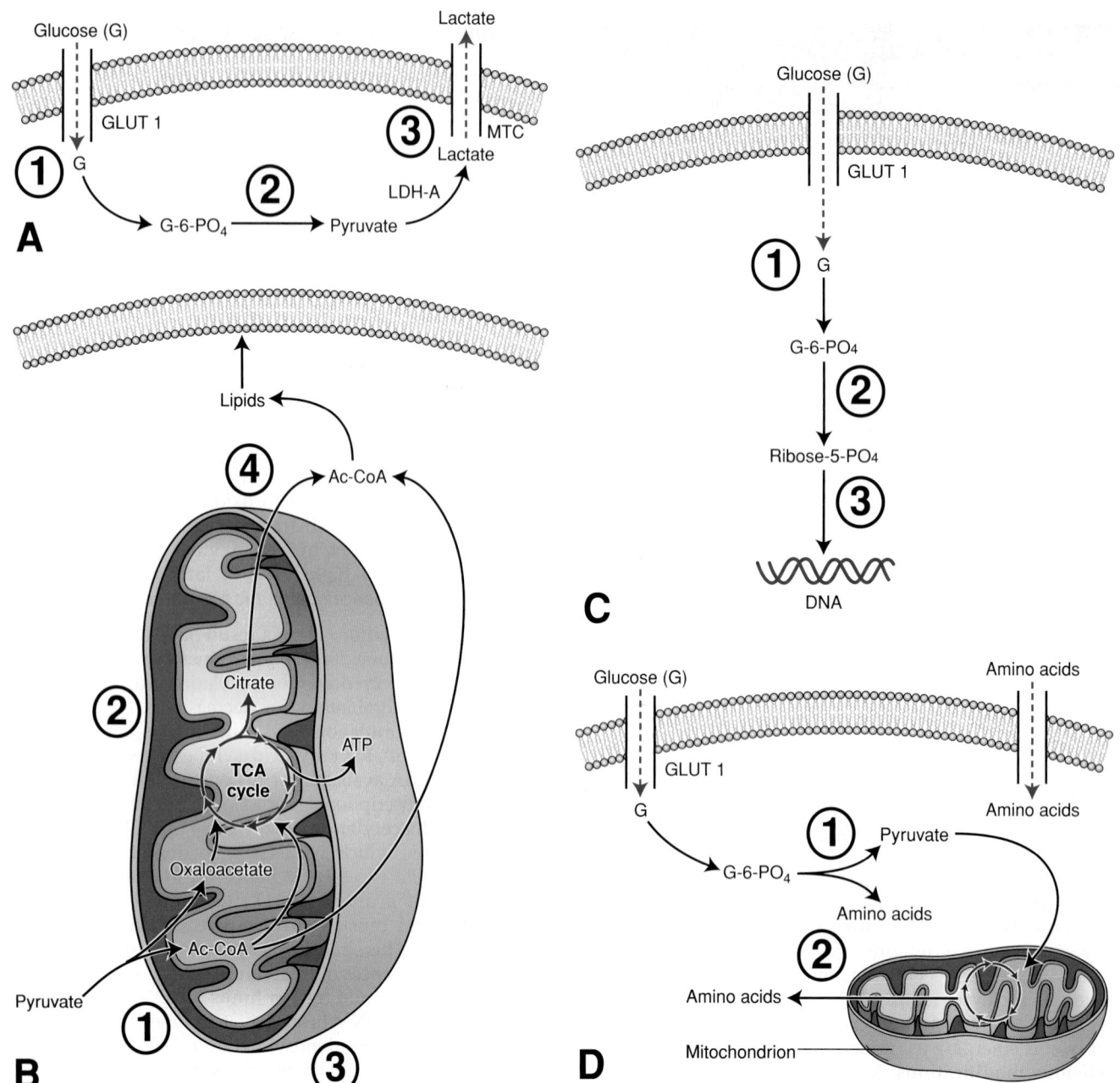

FIGURE 5-48. Cell metabolism. A. Glucose entry. 1. Entry of glucose (G) into the cell is mediated by the glucose transporter, GLUT1. Upon entry, it is converted to glucose-6-phosphate. **2.** Most of the glucose-6-phosphate is metabolized by glycolysis, which leads to production of pyruvate. Pyruvate, in turn, is converted by lactic dehydrogenase-A (LDH-A) to lactate. **3.** Lactate is exported from the cell by a transporter called MTC. **B. Pyruvate utilization in mitochondria. 1.** Some of the pyruvate generated from glucose metabolism enters mitochondria, to become oxaloacetate and to join the tricarboxylic acid (TCA) cycle, which drives oxidative phosphorylation to produce adenosine triphosphate (ATP). **3.** Pyruvate may be converted as well to acetyl-coenzyme A (acetyl-CoA). **4.** Either this acetyl-CoA or citrate from the TCA cycle is exported to the cytosol, where it is incorporated into lipids. **C. Incorporation into DNA. 1.** Glucose-6-phosphate undergoes a number of enzymatic alterations. **2.** It is a precursor for ribose-5-phosphate (ribose-5-PO_4). **3.** Ribose-5-PO_4 enters the nucleus and is an important building block in nucleic acid synthesis. **D. Incorporation into amino acids. 1.** Glucose-6-phosphate metabolism products may be directly converted into certain amino acids. **2.** Alternatively, after pyruvate enters mitochondria, products of the TCA cycle may be converted into amino acids.

As well, oxidation of the G in CpGs may produce 8-oxoguanine. Not only does this disrupt CpG methylation, but also it is highly mutagenic, because 8-oxo-G may be read by polymerases as either G or A.

Therefore, epigenetic regulators are central to normal cellular equilibrium. They become unbalanced during carcinogenesis, but unevenly so: opposite changes in these regulators affect tumor suppressors as compared to oncogenes. Thus, epigenetics is both important and complex: as central as it is to tumor development and spread, there is as yet no single general principle that applies to all aspects of epigenetic regulation.

CANCER CELL METABOLISM

All cells must engage in several critical activities, including to generate energy; produce and repair DNA, RNA, membrane and other lipids; make proteins; and so forth. The proportions of the substrates that cells import or synthesize and that the cell devotes to these different pursuits depends on what the cell does. Most of these functions begin with a source of carbon, which is used to generate energy and build cellular constituents.

Normal Cell Metabolism Favors ATP Generation

Normal cells utilize glucose as their main (but not only; see below) carbon source, both to produce ATP and to synthesize macromolecules. Energy production from glucose includes the following (Fig. 5-48):

- **Glucose entry:** Glucose enters cells via transporters, the best understood being GLUT1 (Fig. 5-48A), although GLUT2, GLUT3 and GLUT4 may also participate.
- **Aerobic glycolysis:** These enzymatic reactions transform glucose to pyruvate and generate 2 net ATPs.
- **Pyruvate:** This product of aerobic glycolysis is the lynchpin of metabolism in normal and malignant cells. Pyruvate enters mitochondria, where it may become acetyl-CoA, in a reaction catalyzed by pyruvate dehydrogenase (PDH; see below). Pyruvate may enter the tricarboxylic acid (TCA) cycle in two ways—after conversion to oxaloacetate or after conversion to acetyl-CoA (Fig. 5-48B).
- **Ribose-5-phosphate:** This sugar is produced from a product of the first reaction that is performed upon glucose after it enters the cell (i.e., its conversion to glucose-6-phosphate). Ribose-5-phosphate is then incorporated into nucleic acids (Fig. 5-48C).
- **Acetyl-CoA:** Pyruvate enters mitochondria and is converted to acetyl-CoA by PDH. This step allows entry into the TCA cycle, which eventually produces 36 ATPs (Fig. 5-48D). Acetyl-CoA can also exit mitochondria to participate in lipid biosynthesis.
- **Amino acid synthesis:** Many amino acids enter the cell via cell membrane transporters. Some are so-called essential amino acids, which humans cannot synthesize and need to derive from foodstuffs. Other amino acids, however, can be synthesized by cells from pyruvate or its metabolites that are part of, for example, the TCA cycle.

Therefore, glucose metabolism provides the cell with much more than just energy. It furnishes key building blocks required for virtually all types of cellular structural and functional constituents.

Glucose Uptake Helps Determine Cellular Metabolism

Cells import glucose (and other carbon sources; see below) in response to both intracellular and extracellular signals. Many of these signals are significantly altered in cancers, contributing to tumor cells' deviant metabolism.

Exogenous signals. The key outside regulators of cellular metabolism are insulin and IGF-I. Upon binding their receptors, these hormones activate intracellular signals that drive many of the processes and mediators that participate in oncogenesis.

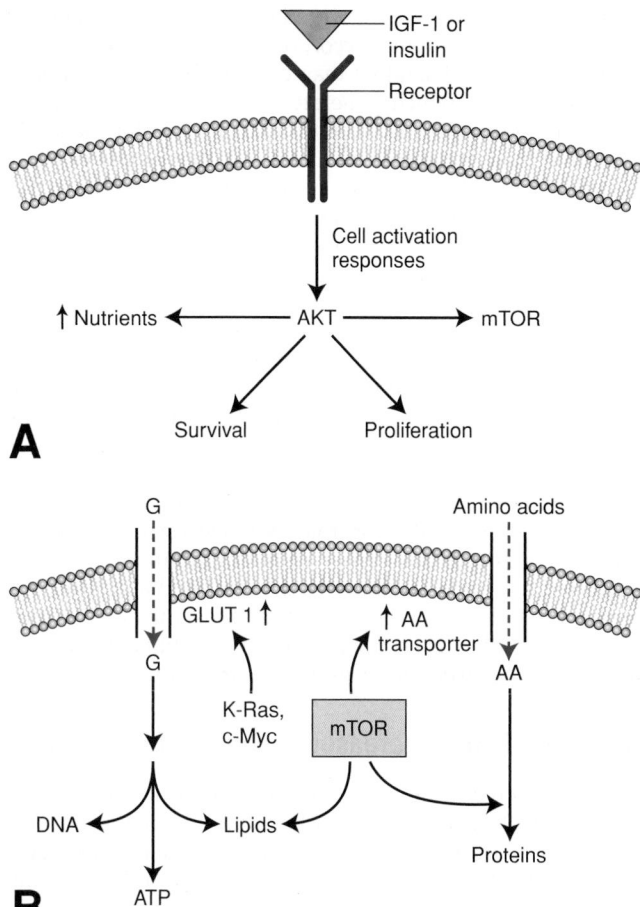

FIGURE 5-49. Effects of metabolic activation on cancer cell metabolism. A. Insulin-like growth factor-I (IGF-I) activation. When IGF-I or insulin binds its receptor, it activates Akt, which in turn elicits many downstream responses. Among the key mediators of Akt effects on cancer cell metabolism is mTOR. **B. Consequences of mTOR activation for cancer cell metabolism.** Operating in tandem with K-Ras– and c-Myc– activated increases in the GLUT1 glucose transporter, mTOR increases synthesis of lipids. It also increases the activity of cell membrane transporters so that increased amino acids are available to support the increased proteosynthetic needs of cancer cells.

Endogenous mediators. At the center of the intracellular response is Akt (Fig. 5-49A). By virtue of the many pathways downstream from Akt (see above and Chapter 1), the cell is protected from apoptosis, stimulated to proliferate and so forth. Akt function is antagonized by the PTEN tumor suppressor. In terms of metabolism, the key downstream effector of Akt is mTOR. This protein stimulates production of amino acid transporters and uptake of amino acids (Fig. 5-49B). It also causes increased lipid and protein synthesis. C-Myc, also upregulated by IGF-I, increases production of GLUT1 and importation of glucose.

Metabolism in Cancer Cells

Cancer cells have different needs from normal cells. As their proliferative rate generally far exceeds that of their normal cousins, they must produce the structural components of their soon-to-be daughter cells at a rate that sustains their mitotic activity. Thus, synthesis of protein, lipid and so forth must march to a much faster drummer than normal.

In 1930, Otto Warburg observed that tumor cells generated energy mainly by aerobic glycolysis in the cytosol, producing pyruvate and 2 ATPs, rather than by mitochondrial oxidative phosphorylation, which generates 36 ATPs, CO_2 and H_2O. The seeming paradox between tumor cells' greater metabolic needs and their preference for a pathway that produces much less energy may be resolved, at least in part, by noting that pyruvate contributes to protein, lipid and other macromolecular synthesis. Furthermore, lactate generated by LDH from pyruvate (Fig. 5-48) may be exported via a special cell membrane channel (monocarbohydrate transporter [MCT]).

Like an athlete who uses an array of different power bars, tumor cells can also generate energy from multiple carbon sources. Lactate, excreted via the MCT by some tumor cells after aerobic glycolysis, may be imported via the same channel. LDH converts this lactate back into pyruvate, for use in any of the several ways described above. Acetate may also be taken up by tumor cells, where it can be made into acetyl-CoA, to be used mostly for lipid synthesis. Another important energy source for cancer cells is glutamine, which is converted to α-ketoglutarate, a TCA intermediate. Although normal cells, depending on their functions, may also exploit these other molecules similarly, cancer cells have turned this multiplicity of carbon sources into an art form.

Cancer Cells Use Increased Amounts of Glucose

As noted above, cells import more glucose in response to stimulation by exogenous insulin. This phenomenon may explain in part the increased cancer incidence in obese patients with high levels of circulating insulin. Many studies relate both the hyperglycemia and the hyperinsulinemia of type 2 diabetes mellitus (Chapter 13) to worse prognosis for diverse tumors. However, GLUT1, the main glucose importer, is upregulated by several oncoproteins, especially c-Myc, B-Raf and K-Ras. Interestingly, c-Myc also increases glutamine transport into cancer cells and upregulates LDH, which catalyzes the (bidirectional) interconversion of lactate and pyruvate. Myc-dependent tumors are often inhibited if LDH or glutamine is decreased.

HIF-1α helps mediate increased metabolism in cancer cells. It upregulates GLUT1, increases cellular importation of glutamine and stimulates glycolysis. It also inhibits movement of pyruvate into mitochondria by blocking PDH, thus favoring glycolysis over the TCA cycle in energy production. HIF-1α is increased when oxygen tension is low or when its inhibitor, the tumor suppressor VHL, is lost. Activation of mTOR, even in the absence of hypoxia, also augments HIF-1α levels.

Tumor Suppressors Regulate Metabolism

The ability of oncoproteins to accelerate anabolism is normally balanced by the effectiveness of tumor suppressors in preventing runaway metabolism:

- **VHL:** This E3 ubiquitin ligase component is responsible for directing polyubiquitination—and thence degradation—of HIF-1α. VHL thus prevents HIF-1α from redirecting the cell's energy production toward glycolysis.
- **PTEN:** Activation of mTOR, leading to enhanced glycolysis, among other things, is a direct consequence of increased Akt triggering of PI3K (see above). PTEN strongly inhibits PI3K. It decreases mTOR activity, reduces HIF-1α and limits GLUT1 production (Fig. 5-50).

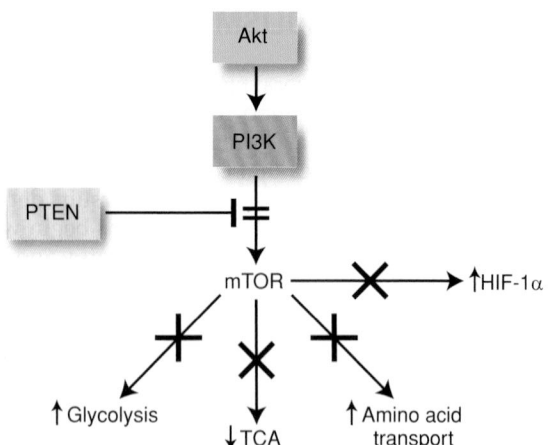

FIGURE 5-50. PTEN controls cellular metabolism and is a suppressor of the metabolic changes that power cancer cell activity. PTEN downregulates mTOR by dephosphorylating phosphatidylinositol-3,4,5-trisphosphate (PIP3) (Fig. 5-38). All downstream effects of mTOR are thus restricted: upregulation of hypoxia-induced factor-1α (HIF-1α), increased glycolysis, increased amino acid transport and decreased tricarboxylic acid (TCA) activity. Thus, PTEN's regulation of mTOR makes it impossible for cancer cells to generate the biosynthetic building blocks they need to sustain proliferation.

Because it inhibits HIF-1α, PTEN also prevents HIF-1α–induced blockage of mitochondrial use of pyruvate to drive the TCA cycle forward.

- **p53:** In addition to its many other regulatory functions, p53 controls and directs cellular metabolism. It has been suggested, in fact, that the main reason for the Warburg phenomenon is that many tumors inactivate p53. The actions of p53 in orchestrating cellular metabolism are summarized in Fig. 5-51 and described below. *It is instructive not only to view p53 activities as directing certain energy-producing functions but also to appreciate how loss of p53 activity (e.g., by mutation) affects all of these activities.* p53 is activated by AMPK in response to metabolic stress. As a result, p53:
  - upregulates a glycolysis regulator, **TIGAR** (TP53-induced glycolysis regulator) that blocks aerobic glycolysis and shunts its intermediates to other pathways;
  - decreases glucose transporter (mainly GLUT1) synthesis and so impedes glucose entry into cells;
  - blocks nuclear factor-κB (NFκB), thus hindering its direct and indirect activation of glycolysis (NFκB upregulates HIF-1α);
  - increases the synthesis of a stimulator of cytochrome oxidase, **SCO_2,** which then increases mitochondrial electron transport and thus
  - increases pyruvate and glutamine importation into mitochondria and incorporation into the TCA cycle by upregulating PDH;
  - lowers c-Myc levels by activating miR-145, a direct inhibitor of c-Myc; this, in turn, decreases c-Myc-stimulated HIF-1α production and increases oxidative phosphorylation;
  - indirectly impedes fatty acid biosynthesis; and
  - upregulates intermediate molecules that can trigger autophagy (see below).

The net metabolic effect of p53, acting in all of these ways, is to shunt energy production away from glycolysis and toward oxidative phosphorylation. Thus, loss of p53 leads directly to the Warburg phenomenon.

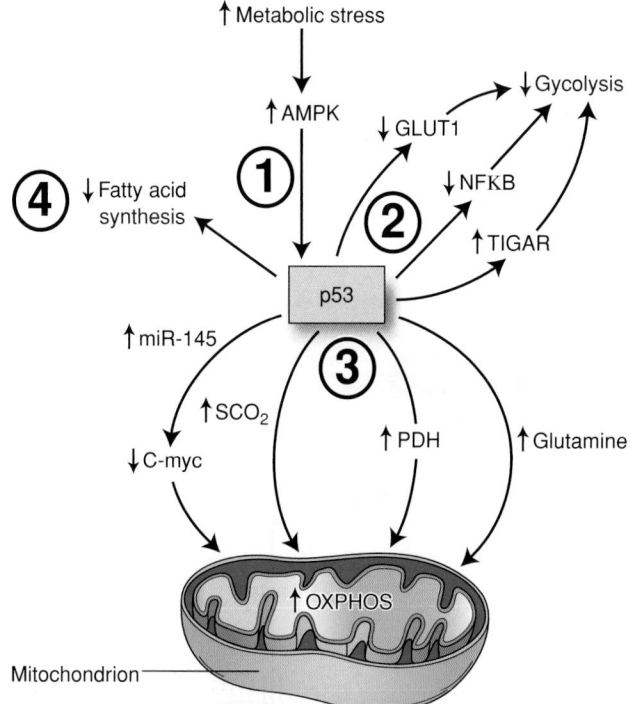

FIGURE 5-51. p53 regulation of cellular metabolism. In addition to its other functions, p53 is a critical metabolic regulator. It prevents cancer cells from achieving their malignant potential by multiple pathways. **1.** p53 is activated by the increased metabolic stress attendant to increased cellular proliferation. This activates adenosine monophosphate (AMP)-protein kinase (AMPK), which in turn activates p53. **2.** p53 directly downregulates transcription of GLUT1 and nuclear factor-κB (NFκB). It also upregulates TIGAR (TP53-induced glycolysis regulator), which impedes glycolysis and directs glycolytic intermediates into other pathways. **3.** It increases TCA cycle activity in several ways. p53 upregulates SCO$_2$, a stimulator of cytochrome oxidase that directly increases mitochondrial electron transport. It also increases pyruvate and glutamine incorporation into the tricarboxylic acid (TCA) by upregulating pyruvate dehydrogenase (PDH). As well, it upregulates miR-145, which directly downregulates c-Myc and so prevents Myc-mediated metabolic effects (Fig. 5-49). **4.** As well, p53 downregulates a key enzyme that mediates fatty acid synthesis.

It is worth noting in this context that p53-related metabolic protection is triggered by a sequence of events in which AMPK is activated. AMPK directly inhibits mTOR (see above), and pharmacologic stimulation of AMPK (e.g., with metformin) has been used in tumor therapy.

- **Isocitrate dehydrogenase (IDH):** This TCA enzyme has turned out to be a potent tumor suppressor. One allele of IDH is mutated in a high percentage of malignant gliomas (see Chapter 32) and in myelodysplastic syndromes (MDSs; see Chapter 26). The oncogenic mutation results in a gain-of-function alteration, which leads to generation of large amounts of a new product (called **R-2-hydroxyglutarate, or R2HG**). R2HG directly inhibits the TET family of DNA hydroxylases and also a family of histone demethylases (see above). The result is that TET2-related histone demethylation and 5-methylcytosine hydroxylation (see above) are not available to undo the downregulation of tumor suppressor gene promoters by CpG and histone methylation, such as occurs during oncogenesis. This inactivation of TET tumor suppressors facilitates tumor development.

Tumor-Associated Stroma Supports Cancer Cell Metabolism

The Warburg effect, which is based on observations of cultured cancer cells, is generally accepted as reflecting cancer cell metabolism. It may not, however, be the whole story. In vivo, cancers contain tumor cells and stromal cells. These latter both strongly influence, and are strongly influenced by, the metabolism of their malignant neighbors.

Stromal Cell Responses to Tumor Cell–Derived Triggers

Tumor cells create a milieu of oxidative stress. Stromal fibroblasts respond to this in a sequence of events that involves impaired mitochondrial function. This, in turn, increases their ROS levels. Increased ROS further damages stromal cells' mitochondria, which leads to increased ROS and even greater impairment of mitochondrial function, in a vicious cycle (Fig. 5-52A). Resulting ROS generated by the stromal cells affect adjacent tumor cells by promoting even greater destabilizing changes in their already destabilized cancer cell DNA.

The mitochondrial injury that stromal cells sustain in this process eventually leads to autophagic destruction of the damaged organelles (mitophagy; see Chapter 1). Deprived of much of the machinery of oxidative phosphorylation, stromal cells engage in more aerobic glycolysis. They therefore produce and export more lactate (see above), which is used as a source of energy and a biosynthetic substrate by nearby cancer cells, as detailed above (Fig. 5-52B). Therefore, tumor cells induce metabolic alterations in their nonmalignant stromal neighbors that cause them to undergo oxidant injury and autophagy, and to supply tumor cells with abundant lactate for use in sustaining multiple nefarious cancer cell activities.

Autophagy Is Closely Regulated in Cancer Cells

Autophagy (see Chapter 1) is a process of recycling and removing, mostly of cellular constituents. It was first noted to be a cellular response to supplying metabolic needs in times of stress (e.g., starvation). As such, it might be of considerable utility to tumors that experience episodic depletion of energy and metabolic substrates. However, perhaps counterintuitively, the key activator of autophagy, Beclin-1, is among the genes most commonly mutated in human cancers. Mice with one or both Beclin-1 genes deleted develop far more cancers than do animals with both genes intact.

Why? To date, the best understanding of the explanation focuses on functions of autophagy not directly related to cellular nutrition. Autophagy is a key means by which oxidant-damaged cell proteins and organelles are recognized and removed. If autophagy is impaired, oxidant injury accumulates, with two important consequences. First, oxidatively damaged cellular molecules can accumulate, aggregate and mediate further oxidant injury (see Chapter 1), eventually increasing the DNA mutation rate and leading to genomic instability (see below). Accumulation of damaged cell constituents relies on the autophagy-related protein, p62 (see Chapter 1). p62 is in fact central to tumorigenesis and is overexpressed in many human tumors. Without it, the oxidized aggregates do not form and resultant oxidant genetic damage does not occur.

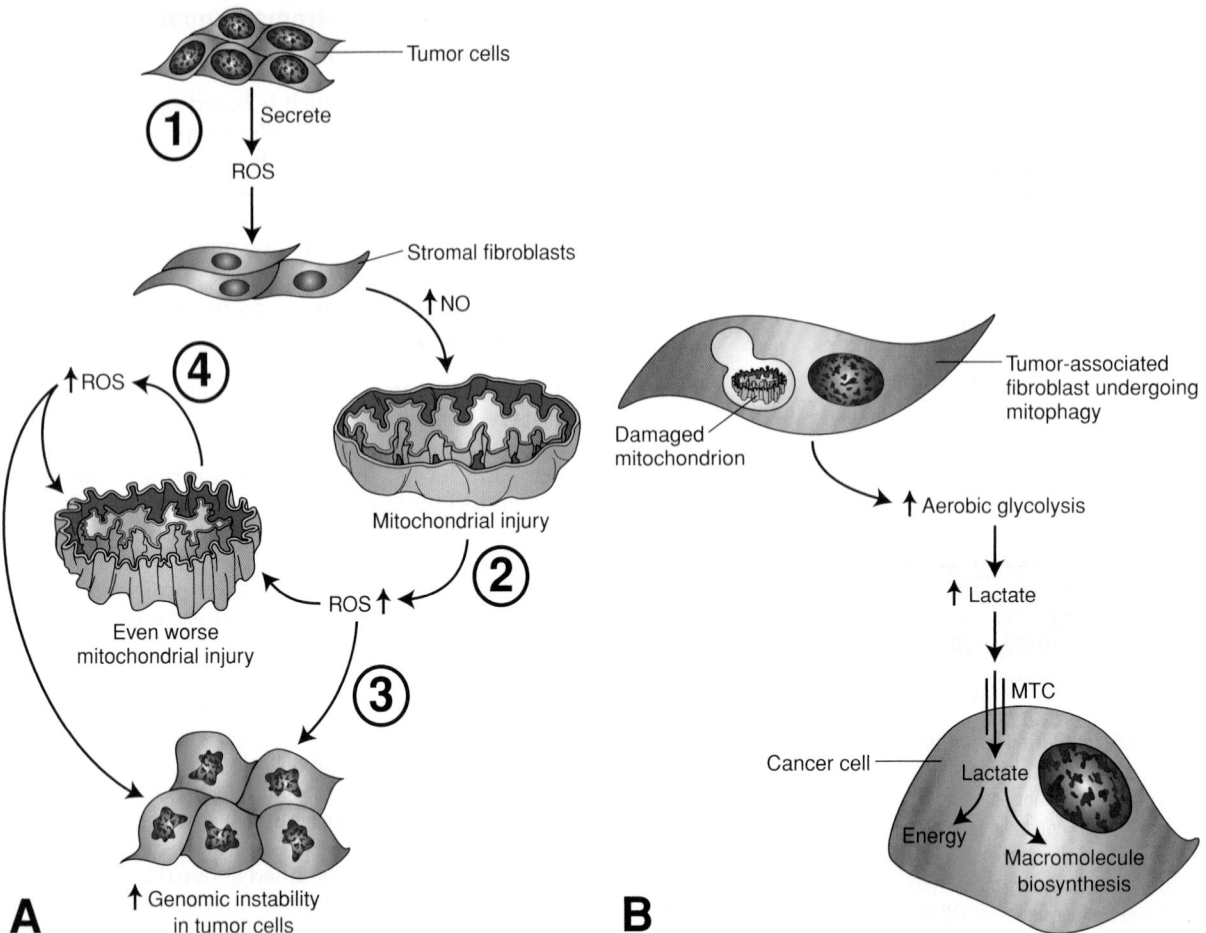

FIGURE 5-52. Stromal cell responses to tumor cell–derived signals. A. Role of reactive oxygen species (ROS). Tumor cells manipulate stromal cells so as to augment tumor cell metabolic activity. **1.** ROS elaborated by tumor cells stimulate stromal cells to increase their production of nitric oxide (NO). This NO causes mitochondrial injury in the stromal cells. **2.** As a result, stromal cells generate excessive ROS. **3.** Increased stromal cell ROS generates more oxidative injury in neighboring cancer cells, leading to increased genomic instability in the tumor. **4.** Increased stromal cell ROS also increases stromal cell mitochondrial injury, creating a vicious circle and magnifying tumor cell genomic instability. **B. Altered metabolism in tumor-associated fibroblasts.** Mitochondrial damage in tumor-associated fibroblasts leads to autophagy of damaged mitochondria (mitophagy). Resulting loss of mitochondria directs more fibroblast metabolism toward glycolysis, producing lactate, which is secreted by the stromal cells. Lactate is taken up by tumor cells, via MTC, and used for macromolecule biosynthesis and other tumor cell metabolic activities.

Second, if autophagy is impaired, accumulation of damaged and damaging cell components will lead to cell death. But p53-dependent apoptosis in such settings requires that the process of autophagy is intact. As a consequence, the cell dies, not by apoptosis, but by necrosis. Unlike apoptosis, necrotic cell death elicits inflammatory responses, including such shady characters as tumor-associated macrophages that facilitate and further tumorigenesis (see above).

Many tumor suppressors, such as PTEN and the tuberous sclerosis proteins (TSC1, TSC2), constitutively facilitate autophagy. The supreme tumor suppressor, p53, has an ambiguous relationship with autophagy, stimulating it in some ways and inhibiting it in others. Several oncogenic proteins (Akt, Bcl-2, mTOR) impair autophagy, underscoring its importance as an antioncogenic process. Important genes involved in autophagy, such as Beclin-1, are commonly mutated in many human cancers. Interestingly, several antineoplastic medications strongly promote autophagy. Although the connection between autophagy and cancer is not fully understood, impairment of the tumor suppressor function of autophagy may result in accumulation of

materials within the cell that cause chromosomal instability, which ultimately may lead to cancer development.

GENETIC INSTABILITY IN CANCER

The pathogenesis of cancer involves multiple genetic—and, undoubtedly, epigenetic—changes, and genomic instability is a key contributor to these processes. Although not universal in tumors, **chromosomal instability (CI)** entails additions or deletions of entire chromosomes, or portions thereof, to yield variable cellular karyotypes. CI may result in **aneuploidy** (abnormal chromosome number), **gene amplification** (increased copy number of a gene) and **loss of heterozygosity** (loss of one allele out of a pair). LOH may reflect loss of a whole chromosome, deletion of a bit of DNA bearing the gene in question or inactivation of that gene. As a result, the remaining allele is the only one for that locus and controls the phenotype. If that remaining allele is rendered abnormal, the lack of a second allele to counterbalance it means that its abnormal phenotype is unopposed. Moreover, the phenotype of the remaining allele may promote the development of cancer. Typically, about one fourth of alleles are lost in malignancies.

Mechanisms of Altered Activation of Cellular Genes

There are three general mechanisms by which proto-oncogenes become activated:

- A mutation in a proto-oncogene leads to **constitutive production of an abnormal protein.**
- Increased expression of a proto-oncogene causes **overproduction of a normal gene product**.
- Activation or expression of proto-oncogenes is regulated by numerous auto-inhibitory mechanisms that safeguard against inappropriate activity. Many mutations in proto-oncogenes render them **insensitive to normal auto-inhibitory and regulatory constraints** and lead to constitutive activation.

The converse processes apply to inactivation of tumor suppressors (see above). That is, (1) they may suffer mutations that increase production of an abnormal protein that either lacks or interferes with tumor suppression; (2) their effectiveness is rendered useless when a regulatory target is overexpressed, overwhelming a normally expressed suppressor; or (3) their expression is impaired, whether by an inactivating mutation or epigenetic inactivation.

Multiple Mechanisms Generate Genetic Instability

Several mechanisms of genetic instability contribute to tumorigenesis. These include (1) point mutations, (2) translocations, (3) amplifications and deletions, (4) loss or gain of whole chromosomes and (5) epigenetic changes. These types of instability occur in many ways. Among the most important is the loss—whether by inheritance, mutation or epigenetic inactivation—of proteins that protect the cell from mutations. These include cell cycle regulatory proteins (checkpoints, proofreaders, mitosis-related chromosomal sorting proteins, etc.) and proteins that mediate DNA repair functions.

Role of Defects in DNA Repair Systems

An understanding of how defects in DNA repair contribute to oncogenesis was derived in part from observations made in familial cancer syndromes. For example, a type of colon cancer syndrome, hereditary nonpolyposis colon cancer (HNPCC, Lynch syndrome), entails a 75% lifetime risk for colon cancer. The large majority of HNPCC patients have mutations in MLH1 or MSH2 DNA mismatch repair enzymes (see above).

Xeroderma pigmentosum (XP), a hereditary syndrome characterized by enhanced sensitivity to UV light and development of skin cancer, reflects defects in nucleotide excision repair (NER) enzymes. In some common types of spontaneous lung cancer, a majority of cases exhibit mutant proteins involved in NER.

Double-Strand Break Repair and Cancer

As mentioned above, detection of DSBs and initiation of repair processes involve the ATM protein. Mutations in ATM and other enzymes involved in DSB repair are associated with a high frequency of malignant tumors.

Point Mutations

Although humans have evolved highly efficient mechanisms to recognize and repair DNA base changes, single base changes do occur normally, at the rate of 10^{-9}/base/cell division in somatic cells and 10^{-11} in germ cells. Application of advanced DNA sequencing techniques has allowed detection of many of these single base changes—called single nucleotide polymorphisms, or SNPs—in tumors.

Activation by Point Mutation

Conversion of proto-oncogenes into oncogenes may involve (1) point mutations, (2) deletions or (3) chromosomal translocations. The first oncogene identified in a human tumor was activated *HRAS* in a bladder cancer. This gene had a remarkably subtle alteration—a point mutation in codon 12. This change led to the substitution of valine for glycine in the H-ras protein. Subsequent studies of other cancers have revealed point mutations involving other codons of the *ras* gene, suggesting that these positions are critical for the normal function of the ras protein. Since the discovery of mutations in *HRAS*, alterations in other growth-regulatory genes have been described.

Activating, or gain-of-function, mutations in proto-oncogenes are usually somatic rather than germline alterations. Germline mutations in proto-oncogenes, which are known to be important regulators of growth during development, are ordinarily lethal in utero. There are several exceptions to this rule. For example, c-*ret* is incriminated in the pathogenesis of certain heritable endocrine cancers, and c-*met*, which encodes the receptor for hepatocyte growth factor, is associated with a hereditary form of renal cancer.

Chromosomal Translocation

Chromosomal translocations involve joining of a piece of one chromosome with a part of another. These rearrangements generally contribute to tumorigenesis in one of two ways. Sometimes they place a normal gene, like a proto-oncogene, under the control of a promoter that is regulated less effectively than the native proto-oncogene promoter.

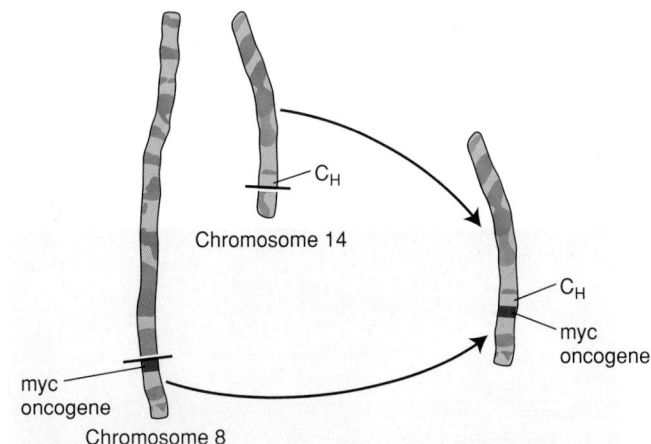

FIGURE 5-53. Schematic representation of the t(8;14) translocation in Burkitt lymphoma. In this disorder, chromosomal breaks involve the long arms of chromosomes 8 and 14. The c-*myc* gene on chromosome 8 is translocated to a region on chromosome 14 adjacent to the gene coding for the constant region of an immunoglobulin heavy chain (C$_H$). The expression of c-*myc* is enhanced by its association with the promoter/enhancer regions of the actively transcribed immunoglobulin genes.

In 75% of patients with Burkitt lymphoma (see below and Chapter 26), there is a translocation of c-*myc*, a proto-oncogene involved in cell cycle progression, from its site on chromosome 8 to a position on chromosome 14 (Fig. 5-53). This translocation places c-*myc* adjacent to genes that control transcription of the immunoglobulin heavy chains. As a result, the c-*myc* proto-oncogene is activated by the promoter/enhancer sequences of these immunoglobulin genes and is consequently expressed constitutively rather than in a regulated manner. In 25% of patients with Burkitt lymphoma, the c-*myc* proto-oncogene remains on chromosome 8 but is activated by translocation of immunoglobulin light-chain genes from chromosome 2 or 22 to the 3′ end of the c-*myc* gene. In either case, a chromosomal translocation does not create a novel chimeric protein but stimulates the overproduction of a normal gene product. In Burkitt lymphoma, the excessive amount of the normal c-*myc* product, probably in association with other genetic alterations, leads to the emergence of a dominant clone of B cells, driven relentlessly to proliferate as a monoclonal neoplasm. Many other hematopoietic malignancies, lymphomas and solid tumors reflect activation of oncogenes by chromosomal translocation. Although some malignant conditions are **initiated** by chromosomal translocations, during the **progression** of many cancers, myriad chromosomal abnormalities take place (translocations, breaks, aneuploidy, etc.).

Activation by Chromosomal Translocation

In addition, chromosomal translocation may lead to production of a new, abnormal, protein. Thus, a part of one chromosome including part or all of the coding region from a protein (e.g., a proto-oncogene) moves to another chromosome, into the coding region of another gene. The result is a new protein, sharing sequence homology with the original ones, but active in driving oncogenesis in a way that the originals are not.

This process has been implicated in the pathogenesis of several human leukemias and lymphomas. The first and still the best-known example of an acquired chromosomal translocation in a human cancer is the **Philadelphia chromosome**, which is found in 95% of patients with chronic myelogenous leukemia (CML; Fig. 5-54). The c-*abl* proto-oncogene

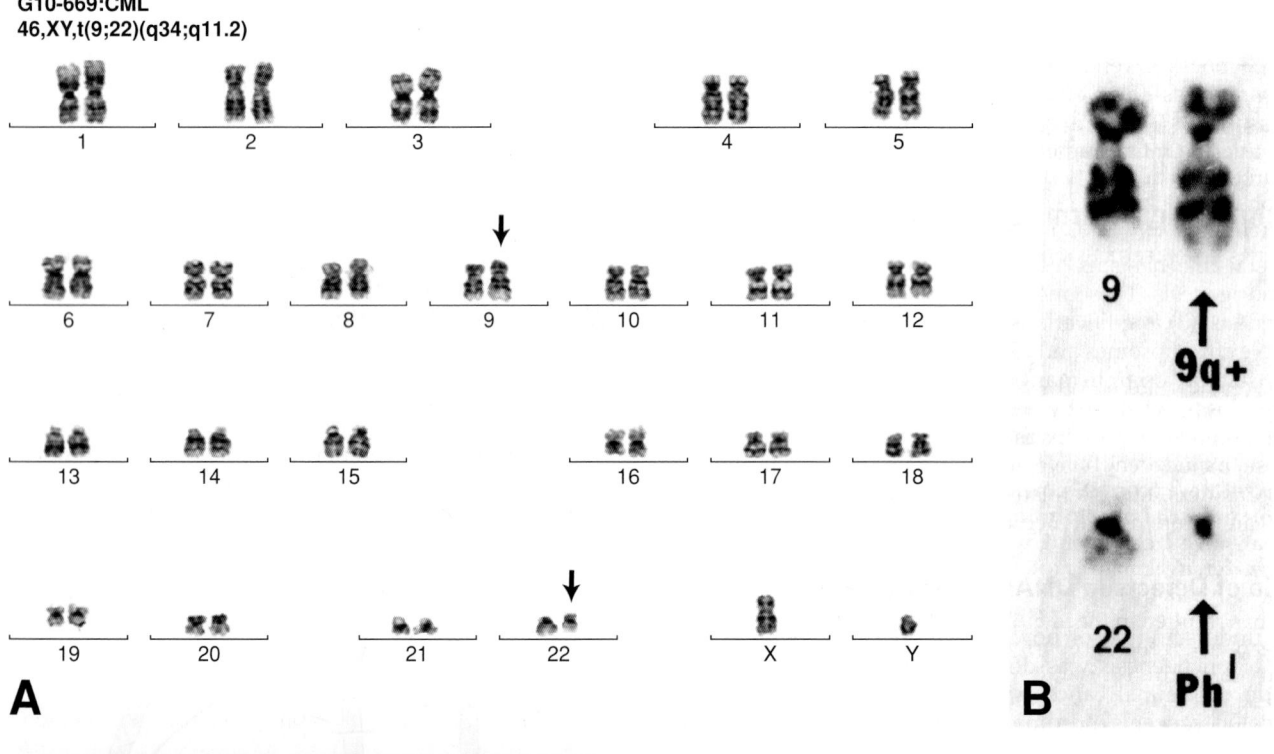

G10-669:CML
46,XY,t(9;22)(q34;q11.2)

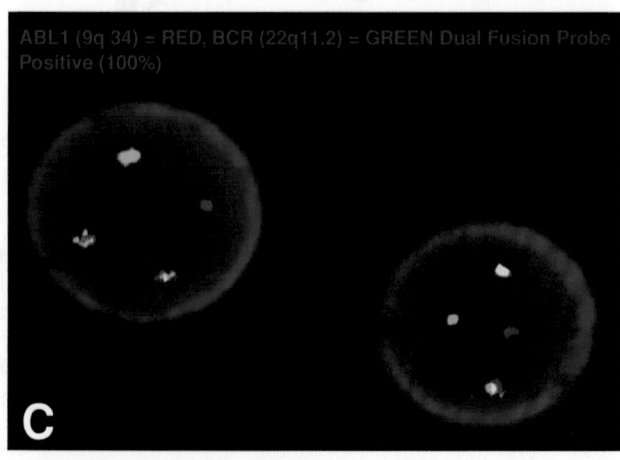

FIGURE 5-54. The t(9;22) translocation in chronic myelogenous leukemia. A. Abnormal karyotype with the shortened chromosome 22 and the longer chromosome 9 highlighted. B. Higher magnification of the translocated chromosomes. C. Fluorescence in situ hybridization (FISH). This assay demonstrates the fusion chromosome using a red ABL chromosome 9 probe and a green BCR chromosome 22 probe, the joining of which yields a yellow signal. Two tumor cells are shown. Each has one normal chromosome 9 and one normal chromosome 22.

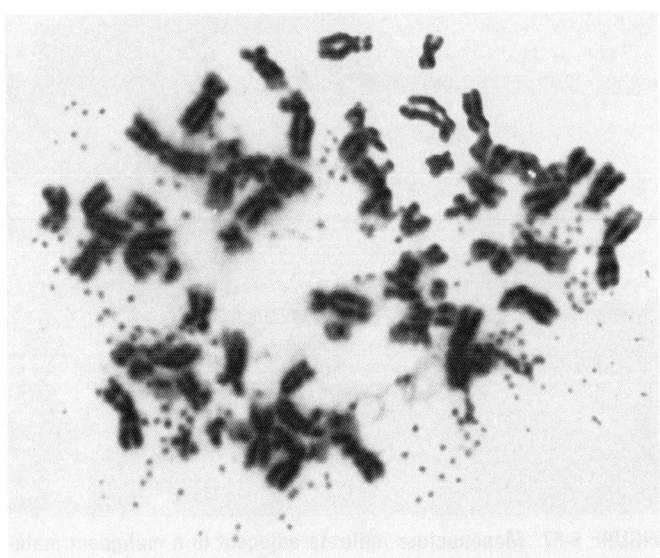

FIGURE 5-55. Double minutes in human cancers. Double minutes in a karyotype of a soft tissue sarcoma appear as multiple small bodies.

on chromosome 9 is translocated to chromosome 22, where it is placed in juxtaposition to a site known as the breakpoint cluster region (*bcr*). The c-*abl* gene and *bcr* region unite to produce a hybrid oncogene that codes for an aberrant protein with very high tyrosine kinase activity, which generates mitogenic and antiapoptotic signals. The chromosomal translocation that produces the Philadelphia chromosome is an example of oncogene activation by formation of a chimeric (fusion) protein. Inhibition of the resulting abnormal kinase by imatinib causes long-term remissions in CML.

Amplifications and Deletions

Genetic amplifications are duplications of variable-sized regions of chromosomes. Cytogenetically, such modifications appear as small DNA fragments that are not part of any chromosome, called "double minutes" (Fig. 5-55), or as increased signal intensity when fluorescent probes for specific regions hybridize with chromosomes. These changes not infrequently affect oncogenes, drug resistance genes or related nefarious characters along with adjacent genomic fragments.

Activation by Gene Amplification
The *ERBB2* proto-oncogene is amplified in up to a third of breast and ovarian cancers. The *ERBB2* gene (also called *HER2/neu*) encodes a receptor-type tyrosine kinase that structurally resembles the EGF receptor. Amplification of *ERBB2* in breast and ovarian cancer (Fig. 5-56) may be associated with poor overall survival and decreased time to relapse. In this context, an antibody targeted against *HER2/neu* (trastuzumab) is now used as adjunctive therapy for breast cancers that overexpress this protein.

Inactivation by Deletion
Deletions, naturally, are lost chromatin. These can vary from tiny pieces to whole arms of chromosomes. Just as amplifications tend to occur at sites of oncogenes, deletions that come to our attention in cancer cells tend to affect tumor suppressor genes.

Alterations in Chromosome Number

Addition or loss of whole chromosomes generally occurs during mitosis and is thought to reflect defects in binding of the mitotic spindle to chromosomal kinetochores (see above), possibly due to malfunctioning of the Aurora B kinase apparatus (see above). As a consequence, chromosomes attach too avidly to mitotic spindles and fail to separate and segregate appropriately.

Almost all solid tumors have abnormal karyotypes. Commonly, tumors lose one copy of a chromosome 10, where the gene for PTEN (see above) resides, or possess extra copies of chromosomes that carry particular oncogenes.

A tumor with a normal karyotype may still have experienced chromosomal loss, however. One parental chromosome of any particular pair may be lost, only to be replaced by a reduplicated copy of the copy of that chromosome derived from the other parent. That is, one parent's copy of a chromosome may be replaced by a duplicated copy of the other parent's chromosome of the same number. The resulting so-called copy-neutral loss of heterozygosity (CN-LOH) is called **uniparental disomy**, and is common in many malignancies. CN-LOH has prognostic significance in several cancer types, such as acute myeloid leukemias.

Epigenetic Modifiers in Cancer Genomic Instability

There are, as discussed above, many heritable factors that can affect gene expression without necessarily changing DNA base sequence. The scope of epigenetic alterations in human cancers is barely understood, but all evidence to date indicates that such modifications impact cancer development and progression profoundly.

A mutation in a gene that participates in chromatin remodeling is seen in most malignant rhabdoid tumors. This mutation occurs in diploid cells without obvious genomic

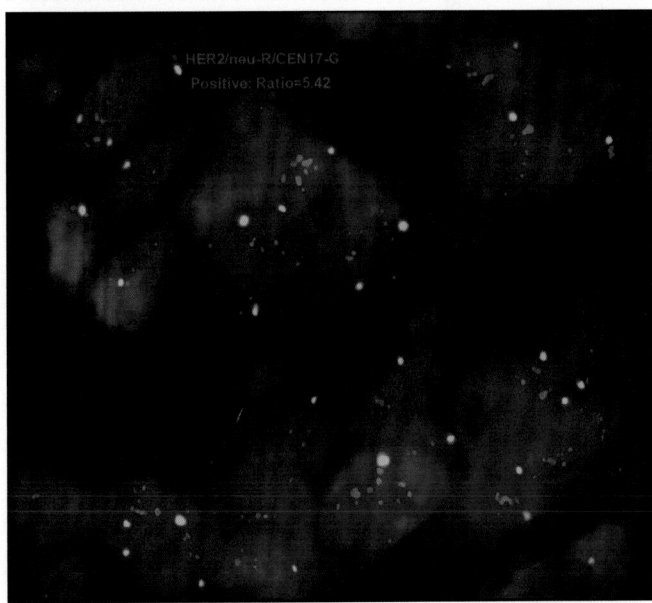

FIGURE 5-56. *ERBB2* amplification in human cancers. ERBB2 also called HER2/neu amplification in a human breast cancer (fluorescence in situ hybridization [FISH]), showing the multiple copies (red fluorescence) as minute bodies. As a chromosome control, a green probe for chromosome 17 is shown.

alterations or gene amplifications/deletions. It is, however, associated with profound changes in gene expression.

Epigenetic modifiers need not only involve direct mechanisms of cell proliferation. They may, for example, affect cellular sensitivity to chemotherapeutic agents or provide escape routes if an enabling mutation is targeted by a particular drug.

The Role of the Immune System in Carcinogenesis Is Unclear

The immune system distinguishes self from nonself molecules and is very effective in combating infectious agents. The notion that it plays a role in suppressing tumor development is rooted in the concept of tumors as nonself entities, with unique "tumor-specific antigens" that can elicit protective immunologic responses. This principle has been extensively demonstrated in experimental animals.

Experimental systems in which tumors are induced by powerful chemical carcinogens have shown that such tumors may be highly immunogenic, particularly when transplanted into immunocompetent recipients. Mice with defects, whether in innate or adaptive immunity (see Chapter 4), develop tumors more often than immunocompetent animals. Similarly, people with immune deficiencies, such as patients with AIDS, are also more prone to cancers than are immunocompetent individuals.

The tumors that develop in these settings, however, bear little resemblance to most human cancers. Potent carcinogens are powerful mutagens and can cause new tumor antigens to arise because of substantial genetic alterations. There is little evidence that spontaneous human tumors bear such antigens. As well, the tumors that occur in immunocompromised humans and animals are almost always virus induced and, again, dissimilar to the tumors that normally afflict people (lung, colon, etc.) that are not connected to infectious agents. The immune deficits thus can be seen as defects in virus clearance (or removal of virus-infected cells), rather than as antitumor surveillance or defense mechanisms.

Inflammatory Cells Nearby Tumors: Friends or Foes?

Pathologists have observed for many years that mononuclear inflammatory cells often accompany cancers (Fig. 5-57). Once an understanding of the role of lymphocytes in immune function had developed, it was a short step to conclude that these lymphocytes (and other cells) were part of a host response to the presence of tumor. The conclusion that tumors produced antigens that elicited such a response was seemingly inescapable.

There are reports that, for certain kinds of tumors, abundant mononuclear infiltration near the tumor may correlate with a good prognosis. Such observations led to many attempts at "immunotherapy," either to elicit or to magnify immune responses against tumors. Immunotherapy was particularly attempted for tumors for which such infiltrates were common, if not invariable, concomitants. Melanomas are an example. To date, immunotherapy of any type of tumor remains experimental, with effectiveness as a treatment modality still unproven.

Even the presence of mononuclear infiltrates near tumors does not necessarily mean that those mononuclear

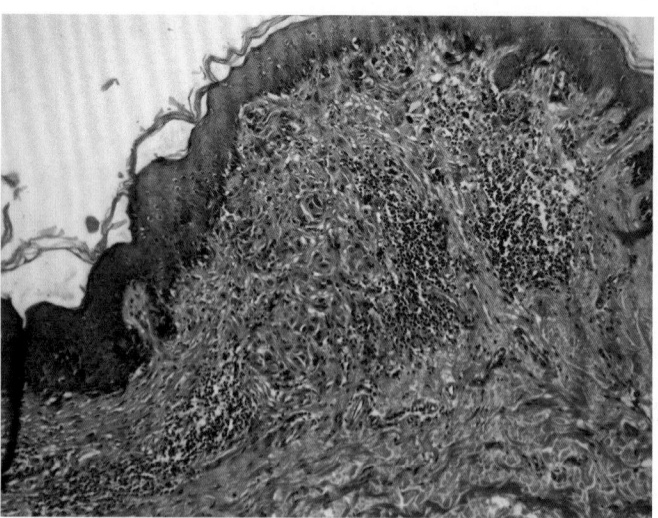

FIGURE 5-57. Mononuclear infiltrate adjacent to a malignant melanoma. Extensive mononuclear cell (mostly lymphocytes) near a primary malignant melanoma in the skin. The significance of the mononuclear cells, traditionally considered to represent host immune responses to the presence of a "foreign tumor antigen", is unclear.

cells signify host immunity against the tumor. Tumor-associated mononuclear infiltrates may not, in fact, be inflammatory. Rather, as indicated above, such cells—far from representing host defenses against a foreign invader—often actually serve the purposes of developing tumors. In short, the function of tumor-associated mononuclear infiltrates is not settled.

Tumor Antigens

Most human cancers reflect somatic mutations that may theoretically produce mutant proteins, which in turn serve as targets of the immune system. In addition, normal proteins may be overexpressed, and posttranslational modifications of normal proteins may produce altered antigens. Tumor antigens not associated with oncogenic viruses may be categorized as follows:

- **Tumor-specific antigens (TSAs):** These represent somatic mutations or alterations in protein (and other) processing, unique to tumors.
- **Tumor-associated antigens (TAAs):** These reflect the production of normal proteins, either in excess or in a setting different from their normal expression.

Tumor-Specific Antigens

Most tumor-related mutations occur in intracellular proteins, which could theoretically offer immunologic targets. However, most TSAs tend to be specific for individual patients' tumors, and not for tumor types, making immunologic targeting for therapy complicated and highly personalized. Nevertheless, since TSAs are expressed only by the cancer cells and not in normal tissues, there should be no preexisting immune tolerance to them and they are theoretically excellent candidates for tumor immunotherapy. These conclusions hold true for normal proteins that undergo aberrant posttranslational modifications, such as altered glycosylation, lipid association and so forth.

Tumor-Associated Antigens

TAAs are molecules that are shared between cancer cells and normal cells and include:

- **Oncospermatogonial antigens:** These molecules are normally only seen in testicular germ cells but may be produced by malignant cells. Since the testis is an immunologically privileged site, such molecules are not normally exposed to the immune system. However, immune reactivity of both cell- and antibody-mediated limbs to these antigens tends to be weak.
- **Differentiation antigens:** These molecules are seen on normal cells of the same derivation as the cancer cells. As an example, CD20, which is a normal B-cell differentiation antigen, is expressed by some lymphomas, and anti-CD20 antibody (rituximab) is effective treatment for such tumors.
- **Oncofetal antigens:** These antigens are made by normal embryonic and fetal structures and by several cancers (e.g., carcinoembryonic antigen, α-fetoprotein).
- **Overexpressed antigens:** These are normal proteins that are overproduced in certain malignant cells (e.g., prostate-specific antigen, HER2/neu).

Since TAAs represent a class of antigens that is principally recognized as "self" by the immune system, and so have elicited tolerance, they do not lead to effective immunologic responses.

To date, the evidence for natural control of neoplasia by immunologically mediated mechanisms (immune surveillance) in humans is scanty. Most interest in this area is directed toward possible therapeutic applications.

The potential development of effective cancer immunotherapy is complicated by tumor mechanisms to evade immunologically mediated destruction (Table 5-10). Among tumors' escape routes from immune attack are production of immunosuppressive cytokines, resistance to lysis by cytotoxic lymphocytes, inhibition of apoptotic signaling and changes in antigenic profiles. Interestingly, there is substantial evidence implicating mutant p53 as protecting cancer cells from granzyme-mediated apoptosis (see Chapter 1) caused by cytotoxic T lymphocytes (CTLs).

Another effect of cancer immunotherapy that must be overcome is related to tumor heterogeneity. Antibodies or CTLs directed against tumor antigens may lead to selective emergence of malignant clones that have lost these antigens. Nevertheless, major efforts to develop new immune therapies for cancer continue.

CANCER STEM CELLS AND TUMOR HETEROGENEITY

Most Cancers Are of Monoclonal Origin

Studies of human and experimental tumors indicate that most cancers arise from single transformed cells. This conclusion is best established for proliferative disorders of the lymphoid system, in which clonality is easiest to assess. Neoplastic plasma cells in multiple myeloma produce a single immunoglobulin species, unique to each individual patient and consistent in that patient over time. Monoclonal T-cell receptor and immunoglobulin gene rearrangement, as well as monoclonal cell surface markers, establish a monoclonal origin for many lymphoid malignancies. The cells of B-cell lymphomas

TABLE 5-10

POTENTIAL PATHWAYS FOR TUMOR CELL AVOIDANCE OF IMMUNOLOGICALLY MEDIATED DESTRUCTION

Related to CTLs

Development of immune tolerance

Failure of helper T cells

Low numbers of sensitized CTLs

Lack of specificity for malignant cells

Barriers to entry of CTLs into tumor environment

Impairment of signal transduction in T cells

Deficiencies in CTL cytolytic activity

Regulatory T cells block antitumor activity

Related to Tumor Cells

Failure of tumor cells to stimulate latent lymphocyte reactivity

Low levels of tumor antigen production

Weak immunogenicity of tumor antigens

Decreased MHC antigens on tumor cell membranes

Elaboration of immunosuppressive molecules by tumors

Resistance of cancer cells to apoptosis and other cell death mechanisms

Tumor cells cause CTLs to undergo apoptosis

CTL = cytotoxic T lymphocyte; MHC = major histocompatibility complex.

exclusively display either κ or λ light chains on their surfaces, while polyclonal lymphoid proliferations—which are almost always benign—contain a mixture of cells, some with κ, and some with λ, light chains.

Monoclonality has also been demonstrated for many solid tumors. One of the best examples of this principle utilized glucose-6-phosphate dehydrogenase in women who were heterozygous for its two isozymes, A and B (Fig. 5-58). These isozymes are encoded by genes located on the X chromosome. Since one X chromosome is randomly inactivated, only one of the two alleles is expressed in any given cell. Thus, although the genotypes of all cells are the same, half of cells express only A; the rest express only B. Examination of benign uterine smooth muscle tumors (leiomyomas, or "fibroids") revealed that in any individual tumor all cells expressed either A or B. No tumor included a mixture of A-expressing cells and B-expressing cells. Thus, each tumor was derived from a single progenitor cell. Oligoclonal tumors have been described, but they are rare and are usually caused by infection with oncogenic viruses (see below).

Cancer Stem Cells Are Primordial Malignant Cells from Which Tumors Arose and Which Can Generate, and Regenerate, the Tumors

Only a minute proportion of the cells in a malignant tumor can produce a new tumor when they are transplanted

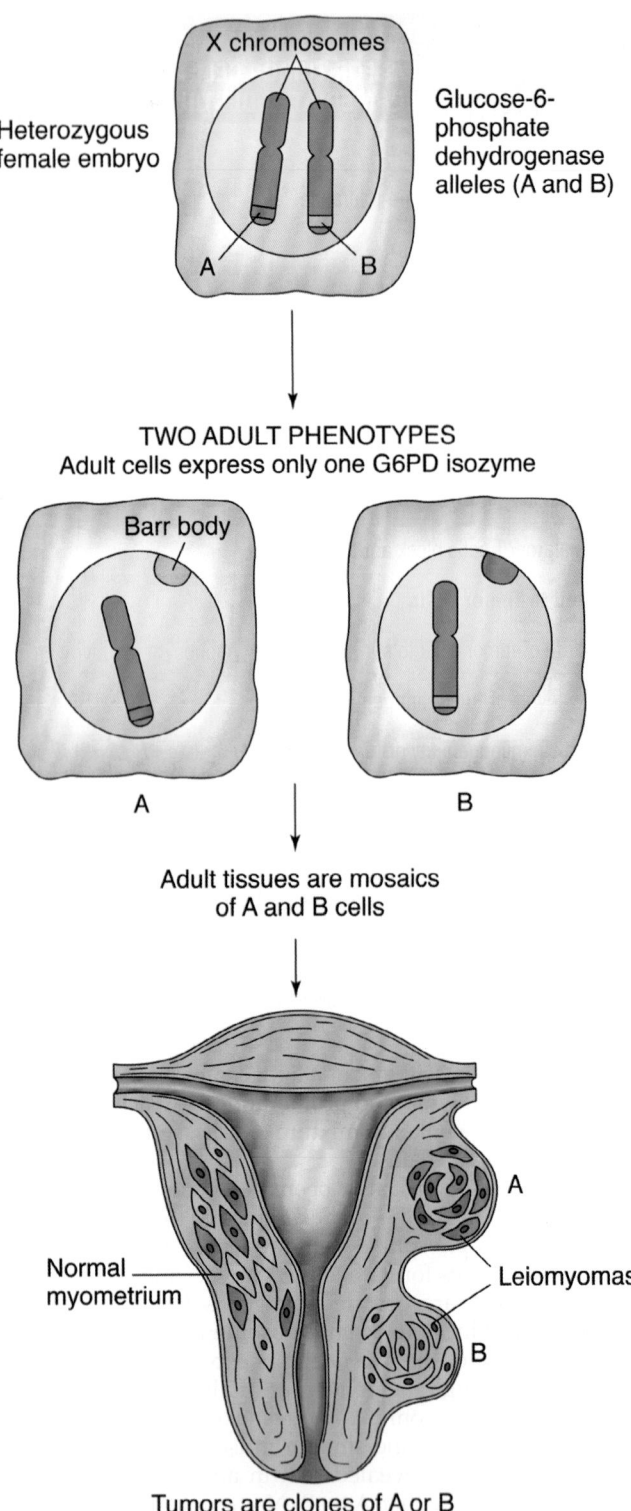

FIGURE 5-58. Monoclonal origin of human tumors. Some females are heterozygous for the two alleles of glucose-6-phosphate dehydrogenase (G6PD) on the long arm of the X chromosome. Early in embryogenesis, one of the X chromosomes is randomly inactivated in every somatic cell and appears cytologically as a Barr body attached to the nuclear membrane. As a result, the tissues are a mosaic of cells that express either the A or the B isozyme of G6PD. Leiomyomas of the uterus have been shown to contain one or the other isozyme (A or B) but not both, a finding that demonstrates the monoclonal origin of the tumors.

into immunologically deficient animals. Normal tissues contain pluripotent somatic stem cells, which can both replenish their own numbers (self-renewal) and differentiate into more mature derivative cells. Cancers also have a small population of malignant cells with such capabilities. These are called **cancer stem cells (CSCs)**. Their existence has been most convincingly demonstrated in hematologic malignancies like acute myeloblastic leukemia (AML), but there is also strong evidence for their existence in an increasing number of solid tumors.

In AML, far less than 1% of leukemic cells express hematopoietic stem cell membrane markers (CD34+, CD38−). Only these cells among the entire leukemic population can reestablish leukemia in an appropriate transplant recipient host. Comparable, but not identical, data have been obtained from studies of cancers of the breast, colon and brain, in which different markers identify CSC-rich cell populations and exclude the vast majority of tumor cells, which cannot recapitulate tumorigenesis. CSCs are defined functionally. The respective markers allow us to identify populations that are enriched for stem cells, but not pure CSCs. Only some of the cells in those populations function as cancer stem cells.

Derivation of CSCs

The origins of CSCs are murky. In some cases, they may derive from the pluripotent somatic stem cells of the affected organ, for example, hematopoietic stem cells in the case of AML (Fig. 5-59A). In other cases, lineage-committed progenitor cells may be the culprits. Such cells are multipotent, but not pluripotent, at the time of transformation. They may reacquire a degree of "stemness," allowing them both to repopulate their own numbers and to differentiate into more committed cells (Fig. 5-59B). Therefore, it is most likely that CSCs can arise both from tissue stem cells and from slightly differentiated immediate progeny of these tissue stem cells. Lurking within the tumor, they function as a reservoir of cells that continue to provide more differentiated tumor cells and that can regenerate the entire tumor, should that become necessary.

Tumor Cells Derived from CSCs

Although almost all tumors begin as single clones of neoplastic cells, as they grow, their cells show considerable variation in appearance (Fig. 5-60) and behavior. Diversity of cells among a tumor population has broad implications for tumor progression and dissemination, as well as for responses to chemotherapy and the development of resistance to these agents. Several theories, which are not necessarily mutually exclusive, and which all may be correct in some cases, have been proposed to account for the development of phenotypic diversity of cells in tumors.

It is critical to understand that the overwhelming majority of tumor bulk is composed of these derivative cells. Treatments that reduce tumor volume mostly target these cells, and consequent reduced tumor volume reflects the susceptibility of these cells—not CSCs—to the therapies employed. However, as will become clear (see below), reduced tumor volume does not equate with elimination of CSCs, nor does it necessarily affect the ability of CSCs to regenerate the tumor after treatment.

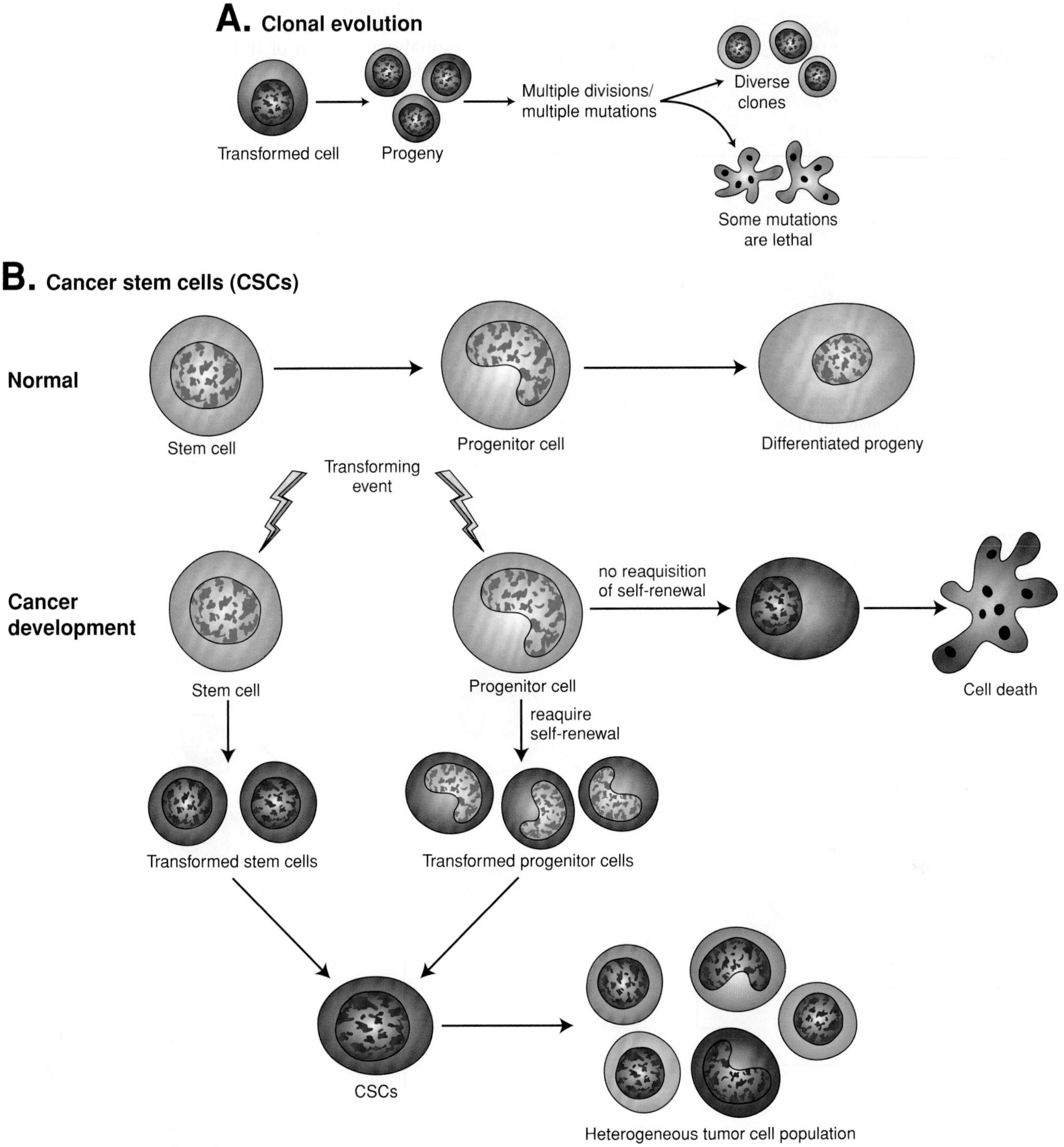

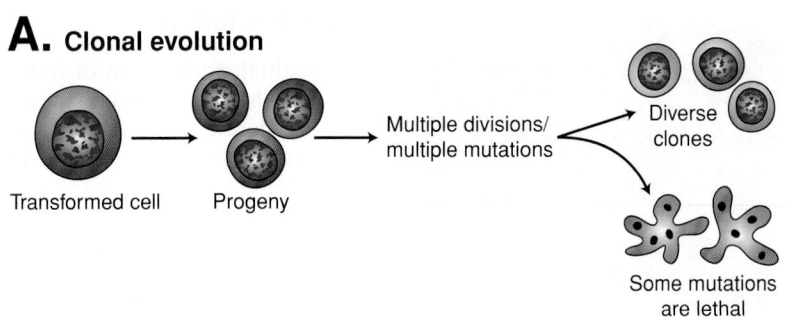

A. Clonal evolution

Transformed cell   Progeny   Multiple divisions/ multiple mutations   Diverse clones

Some mutations are lethal

B. Cancer stem cells (CSCs)

Normal

Stem cell   Progenitor cell   Differentiated progeny

Transforming event

Cancer development

Stem cell   Progenitor cell   no reaquisition of self-renewal   Cell death

reaquire self-renewal

Transformed stem cells   Transformed progenitor cells

CSCs

Heterogeneous tumor cell population

FIGURE 5-59. Tumor stem cells and tumor heterogeneity. A. Linear progression of tumor clonal evolution. Proliferating cancer progenitor cells eventually develop a variety of mutations, with different individual cells acquiring different mutations, leading to heterogeneity in the tumor cell population. Some such mutations are inconsistent with cell survival, while others facilitate cancer progression. This model is most consistent with critical enabling primordial mutations in a stem cell that must be retained throughout subsequent tumor evolution. **B. Cancer stem cells and progenitor cells.** Normally (*above*) stem cells give rise to committed progenitor cells. These then produce terminally differentiated cells. An oncogenic stimulus (*below*) to a stem cell may lead to an expanded pool of transformed stem cells. These become cancer stem cells (CSCs). Alternatively, the oncogenic stimulus may affect a committed progenitor cell. If the latter recapitulates a program of self-renewal, the resulting transformed progenitor may become a CSC. If it does not activate the self-renewal program, resulting differentiated progeny will be produced and eventually die. CSCs generated either via transformation of stem cells or transformation of committed progenitors may then be the antecedents of a heterogeneous malignant cell population.

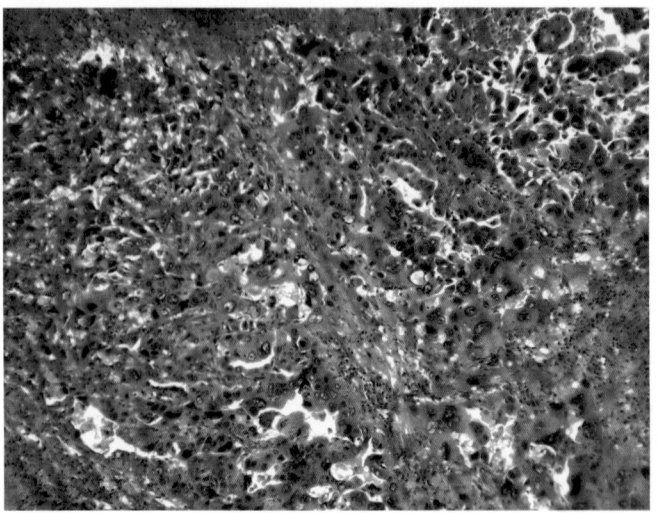

FIGURE 5-60. Phenotypic diversity in human tumors. Human tumor cells show great heterogeneity in their appearance, proliferative activity and so forth. Thus, most human tumors are mixtures of small and large cells, often with diverse shapes, varying nuclear appearances and differences in mitotic activity.

Clonal Evolution

The original explanation of tumor heterogeneity holds that tumor cells progressively accumulate new mutations as they proliferate. A tumor in which many cells are dividing can thus, over time, generate a diverse population of genetically different cells. Some of these cells may be destined for ignominious death, while others may flourish as genetically distinct subclones of the original malignant cells (Fig. 5-59A). Darwinian-style selection—whether due to localized hypoxia, differences in proliferation rates, potential for invasion and metastasis, therapy and so forth—governs which subclones will succeed and which will perish, which will metastasize and which will remain localized.

Epigenetic Cancer Cell Plasticity

Cancer's evil machinations have led to even more devious ways for tumors to maintain themselves and to grow and spread. Thus, for some tumors (e.g., malignant melanomas), tumors adapt to the progressive challenges to survival and dissemination via epigenetic changes (e.g., noncoding RNAs, or expression of proteins that modify histones) (Fig. 5-61). A mass of slowly proliferating tumor cells may alternate among

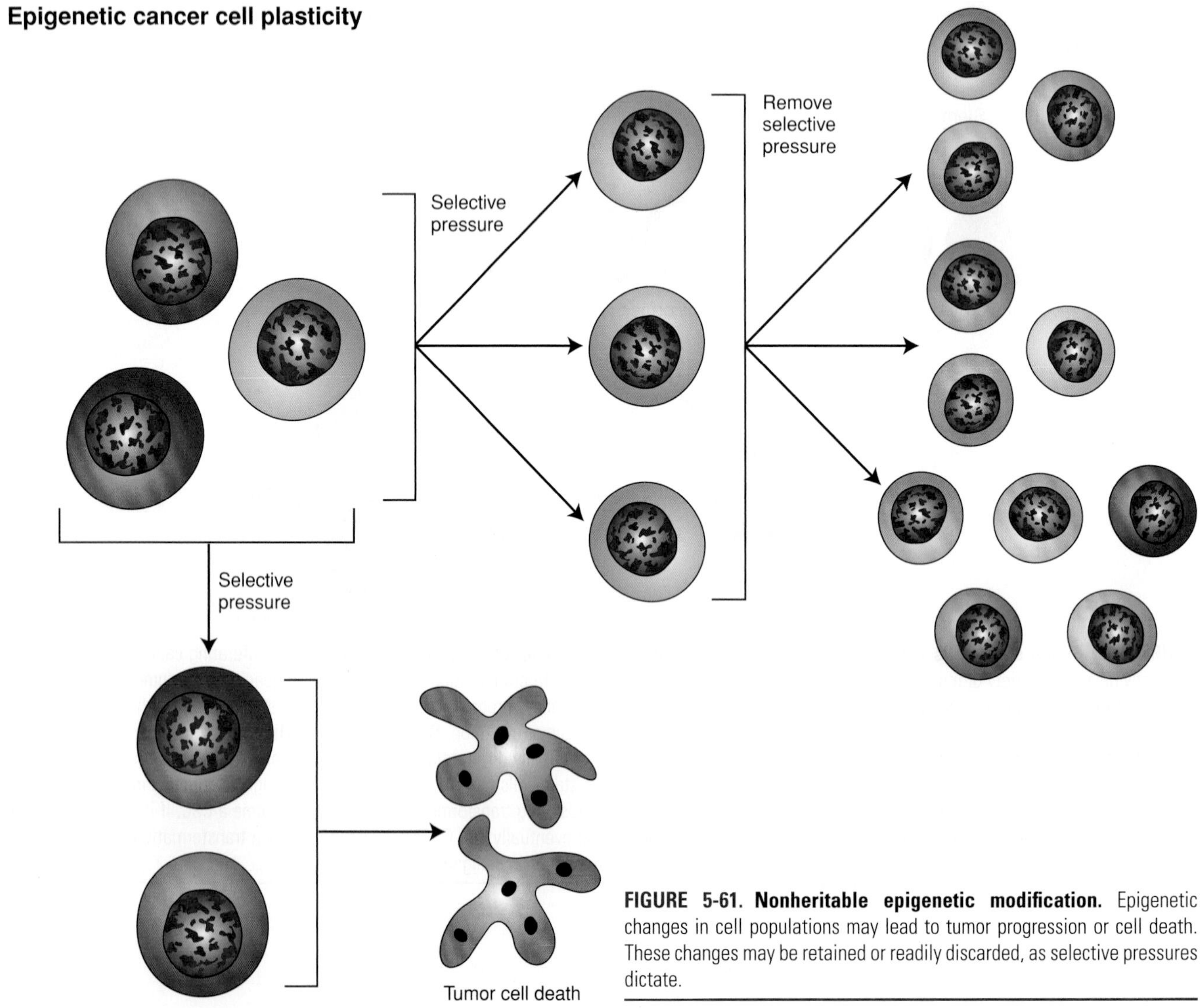

Epigenetic cancer cell plasticity

Selective pressure

Remove selective pressure

Selective pressure

Tumor cell death

FIGURE 5-61. Nonheritable epigenetic modification. Epigenetic changes in cell populations may lead to tumor progression or cell death. These changes may be retained or readily discarded, as selective pressures dictate.

different epigenetic states, and so fluctuate between the ability to reconstitute a tumor (stem cell–like) and the lack of such ability. This type of deviousness allows for diverse populations of tumor cells to alternate between stemness—slowly dividing, tumor-reconstituting cells—and rapidly dividing, nonreconstituting cells. Furthermore, tumor cells may achieve such metamorphoses without incurring further mutations.

The implications of this phenomenon are substantial. Some malignant tumors may represent constantly shifting therapeutic targets, with incredible plasticity in adapting to a changing chemotherapeutic milieu via the ability to shift phenotypes rapidly to evade antineoplastic drugs, and then to shift back to reemerge from a defensive posture and reassert an aggressive nature.

The Significance of CSCs

CSCs are not merely an experimental curiosity. They are the cells from which many human tumors arise. They divide infrequently, which allows them to evade destruction by cytotoxic chemotherapeutic agents that preferentially kill rapidly dividing cells. Thus, while chemotherapy may destroy the bulk of the rapidly dividing cells in a malignant tumor mass, residual CSCs may survive to regenerate the cancer.

Even more significantly, CSCs in many ways are closer to their normal tissue counterparts than to the cells that make up the bulk of the tumor. They may be far more capable of, for example, repairing DNA damage than their more differentiated malignant derivative cells. Also, because they proliferate less, they rely less on mutant cell activation signaling pathways and resemble normal cells more than do their highly mitotically active progeny. Thus, the main determinants of their survival make them more likely to persevere through treatments, even kinase inhibitors, that kill the rapidly dividing cells that make up the vast majority of the tumor. Radiation of glioblastomas may kill the great majority of the tumor cells, but CSCs are radioresistant. Their numbers, as a percentage of remaining viable tumor cells, increase after radiation. They survive and repopulate the tumor. In this sense, therapy may destroy 99.9%, or 99.99%, of a tumor, shrinking its mass correspondingly, but may do little more than buy the patient a few months more of life.

CSCs have evolved to evade apoptosis and senescence and therefore are likely to be less sensitive to cancer therapies than their normal tissue counterparts. Thus, tumor stem cells are better suited to survive cytotoxic therapy that is likely to kill the normal tissue stem cells from which the CSCs probably derived.

It is therefore critical to bear in mind that the goal of tumor therapy is not to eliminate the bulk of the tumor, but to save the patient's life. This requires approaches that are effective against CSCs because it is these cells, and not the aggregate of their highly proliferating progeny, that will regenerate the tumor after cytoreductive or other therapy. The CSCs, then, are the true enemies; it is they that will kill the patient.

Tumors Are Heterogeneous

We have alluded above to phenotypic heterogeneity in tumor cell morphology and to divergent evolution after tumor cells arise from CSCs (Fig. 5-62). In fact, however, the term "tumor heterogeneity" has two basic and different meanings. **Intertumor heterogeneity** describes the variation (genetic, epigenetic, phenotypic) between tumors that

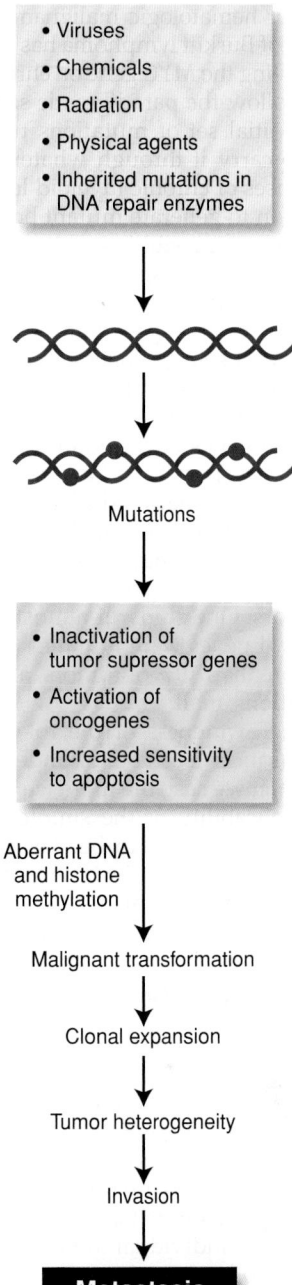

FIGURE 5-62. Summary of the general mechanisms of cancer.

develop in one patient and those that arise in others. **Intratumor heterogeneity** refers to variation in the same parameters among different tumor cells and areas, and between a primary tumor and its metastases, within one patient.

Intertumor Heterogeneity

Walter Donovan: "…We're on the verge of completing a quest that began [many] years ago. We're just one step away."
Indiana Jones: "That's usually when the ground falls out from underneath your feet."
Indiana Jones and the Last Crusade

There are distinct patterns of alterations that are both characteristic of certain tumor types and that offer useful therapeutic targets, at least for hematologic malignancies. For example, almost every case of Burkitt lymphoma has chromosome rearrangements involving the *MYC* gene on chromosome 8. These tumors seem to follow the paradigmatic sequence shown in Fig. 5-59A: one initial set of mutations triggers the tumor and is needed to carry it through whatever follows. Similarly, almost all cases of chronic myeloid leukemia show the t(9;22) translocation to generate mutant bcr-abl protein. The successful targeting of bcr-abl is emblematic of the goal of developing agents that are specific for mutations that are necessary for tumor survival.

As comforting as this paradigm is for hematologic malignancies (at least selected ones), the situation for characteristic mutations in solid tumors has been more problematic. Even though some studies that have focused on selected individual genes have found mutational patterns, these studies in retrospect may have exercised such high levels of selectivity that many other, perhaps more important, mutations were not detected. More extensive genetic analysis of the protein-coding parts of the genome (whole exome sequencing) have shown wide diversity among individual solid tumors. One study of almost 200 lung cancers showed that only 4 genes were mutated (all SNPs or point mutations) in more than 10% of tumors, and 15% of tumors showed no mutations at all.

Our increasing awareness of the roles of untranslated RNAs in human cancer (see above) underscores this problem. The wider a net we cast, the more we find and the more restricted the applicability of the simple step-wise model shown in Fig. 5-59A appears to be. The extensive tumor-to-tumor diversity (e.g., Fig. 5-61) in patterns of genetic changes in solid tumors underscores the potential complexity of developing effective targeted therapies.

Intratumor Heterogeneity

In addition to variability of one tumor type from one person's tumor to someone else's tumor, all models predict that there will be variability within the tumor of a single individual. If a stochastic (i.e., random) mutation model (e.g., Fig. 5-61) applies to solid tumor evolution, rather than a linear step-wise model in which all cells are progressively derived from identically altered progenitors (as in Fig. 5-59A), one would expect the cells of any individual tumor to be highly heterogeneous, one to the other.

Although only a few such studies have been reported, they generally confirm our worst fears along these lines. It is clear that, at least for some solid tumors, variability is enormous. In one study of renal cell carcinomas, multiple biopsies of a single tumor mass showed that only 34% of protein-coding genetic alterations were concordant *between different pieces of that one tumor mass*. When analyses also included metastases, or comparison of pre- and posttreatment tumor samples, concordance was even lower.

Therefore, sophisticated tools to analyze tumors have not exactly allowed us to impose a man-made paradigm—either analytical or therapeutic—on the field of cancer biology. Rather, these technologies have illuminated the fact that cancers, especially solid ones, are highly diverse genetically and that each patient's individual tumor presents a vast, nonuniform array of mutations. When patient-to-patient variations in tumor genotypes are considered, it is clear that tumors are incredibly more complicated than we had imagined. We are only beginning to lift the veil on that heterogeneity.

Agents Implicated in Causing Cancer

VIRUSES AND HUMAN CANCER

Despite the existence of viral oncogenes and many viruses that are known to cause cancers in mice and other animals, only a few viruses demonstrably cause human cancers. Thus, viral infections are responsible for an estimated 15% of human cancers. The strongest associations between specific viruses and tumors in humans involve:

- Human T-cell leukemia virus type I (HTLV-I) **(RNA retrovirus)** and T-cell leukemia/lymphoma
- Hepatitis B virus (HBV, **DNA**) and hepatitis C virus (HCV, **RNA**) and primary hepatocellular carcinoma
- HPV **(DNA)** and carcinomas of the cervix, anus and vulva, and some oropharyngeal cancers
- Epstein-Barr virus (EBV, DNA) and certain forms of lymphoma and nasopharyngeal carcinoma
- Human herpes virus 8 (HHV8, **DNA**) and Kaposi sarcoma

Worldwide, infections with hepatitis B and C viruses and HPVs alone account for 80% of all virus-associated human cancers.

Human T-Cell Leukemia Virus Type I Is Lymphotropic

The one human cancer that has been firmly linked to infection with an RNA retrovirus is the rare adult T-cell leukemia, which is endemic in southern Japan and the Caribbean basin and occurs sporadically elsewhere. The etiologic agent, HTLV-I, is tropic for CD4$^+$ T lymphocytes and has also been incriminated in the pathogenesis of a number of neurologic disorders. It is estimated that leukemia develops in 3%–5% of people infected with HTLV-I and then only after a latency period of 30–50 years. A closely related virus, HTLV-II, has been associated with only a few cases of lymphoproliferative disorders.

The HTLV-I genome contains no known oncogene and does not integrate at specific sites in the host DNA. Viral oncogenicity appears to be mediated mainly by the viral transcriptional activator Tax. This protein not only drives transcription of the viral genome but also promotes the activity of other genes involved in cell proliferation, such as NFκB and IL-2 receptor. Tax also downregulates the cell cycle control protein, p16^{INK4a} and p53. Lymphocyte transformation in vitro by HTLV-I is initially polyclonal and only later monoclonal. Tax therefore probably initiates transformation, but additional genetic events are required for the complete malignant phenotype.

Hepatitis B and C Viruses Are Responsible for Liver Carcinomas

Epidemiologic studies have established a strong link between primary hepatocellular carcinoma and chronic infection with HBV, a DNA virus, and HCV, an RNA virus (see Chapter 20). Two mechanisms have been invoked to explain the mechanism of carcinogenesis in virus-related liver cancer. One theory holds that the inability of some people to clear these infections leads to continued hepatocyte proliferation owing to ongoing liver injury, and eventually causes malignant transformation. However, a small subset of patients with HBV infection develop hepatocellular carcinomas in noncirrhotic livers. A second theory implicates a virally encoded protein in the pathogenesis of HBV-induced liver cancer. Transgenic mice expressing HBx, a small viral regulatory protein, also develop liver cancer, but without evident preexisting liver cell injury and inflammation. The *HBx* gene product upregulates a number of cellular genes. It also binds to and inactivates p53. The underlying mechanisms in HBV-induced carcinogenesis are still controversial and require further investigation.

It has not been shown that HCV is directly oncogenic. Tumors, when they develop in HCV-infected patients, tend to do so 20 or more years after primary infection, and then usually in the context of cirrhosis and chronic liver injury. However, some data suggest that expression of HCV core protein may contribute to the pathogenesis of hepatocellular carcinoma, and one of the HCV nonstructural proteins activates NFκB.

DNA Viruses Encode Proteins That Bind Regulatory Proteins

Four DNA viruses (HPV, EBV, HBV, HHV8) are incriminated in human cancers. The transforming genes of oncogenic DNA viruses exhibit virtually no homology with cellular genes, but those of animal RNA retroviruses (oncogenes) are derived from, and are homologous with, their cellular counterparts (proto-oncogenes). As discussed above, oncogenic DNA viruses have genes that encode protein products that bind to, and inactivate, the products of tumor suppressor genes (e.g., *Rb, p53*).

Human Papilloma Virus

HPVs induce lesions in humans that progress to squamous cell carcinoma. They manifest a pronounced tropism for epithelial tissues, and their full productive life cycle occurs only in squamous cells. More than 140 distinct HPVs have been identified, and most are associated with benign lesions of squamous epithelium, including warts, laryngeal papillomas and condylomata acuminata (genital warts) of the vulva, penis and perianal region. Occasionally, condylomata acuminata and laryngeal papillomas undergo malignant transformation to squamous cell carcinoma. Although warts of the skin invariably remain benign, in a rare hereditary disease called **epidermodysplasia verruciformis,** HPV produces benign flat warts that commonly progress to squamous carcinoma. At least 20 HPV types are associated with cancer of the uterine cervix, especially HPV types 16 and 18 (see Chapter 18). This association holds for both ectocervical squamous carcinoma and endocervical adenocarcinoma. A newly available vaccine protects against infection with most oncogenic HPV types and is expected to reduce the incidence of cervical cancer.

In recent years, HPV, especially HPV-16, has been identified in many head and neck squamous cell carcinomas, especially those of the tonsils and oropharynx (see Chapter 29). Similar colocalization has been reported for non–small cell lung carcinomas. Some of these tumor types are also associated with cigarette smoking, and tumors that are HPV positive may also occur in smokers. In addition, high-risk strains of HPV are involved in about 6% of lung cancers that arise in smokers.

The major oncoproteins encoded by HPV are E5, E6 and E7. E6 binds to p53 and targets it for degradation. It also activates telomerase expression and promotes tumor development via other mechanisms that are independent of p53. E7 binds to Rb, thus releasing its inhibitory effect on E2F transcriptional activity and allowing cell cycle progression. E6 and E7 of non-cancer-causing strains of HPV do not have these activities. E5 has been shown to activate the epidermal growth factor receptor. During the last half century, a cell line derived from cervical cancer, *HeLa cells,* has maintained worldwide popularity in the study of cancer. Interestingly, these cells have been found to express HPV-18 E6 and E7, and inactivation of these oncoproteins results in growth arrest. Thus, after many years growing in vitro in innumerable laboratories, these cancer cells remain dependent on the expression of HPV proteins.

Epstein-Barr Virus

EBV is a human herpesvirus that is so widely disseminated that 95% of adults in the world have antibodies to it. EBV infects B lymphocytes, transforming them into lymphoblasts. In a small proportion of primary infections with EBV, this lymphoblastoid transformation is manifested as infectious mononucleosis (see Chapter 9), a short-lived benign lymphoproliferative disease. However, EBV is also intimately associated with the development of certain human cancers. A number of EBV genes are implicated in lymphocyte immortalization, including Epstein-Barr nuclear antigens (EBNAs); certain untranslated nuclear EBV RNAs, called EBER1 and EBER2; and latency-associated membrane proteins (LMPs). As well, about 40 miRNAs are encoded by EBV, some of which activate or repress specific cellular genes. LMP1 interacts with cellular proteins that normally transduce signals from the tumor necrosis factor (TNF) receptor, but it does not trigger apoptosis. Rather, it activates NFκB and other cell division–associated signaling molecules. Generally, EBV-related tumors are ascribed to the activities of the virus's latency-associated genes.

EBV-induced tumors tend to reflect the establishment of patterns of gene expression associated with viral latency. This may happen even in acute infection. EBV, in fact, is unusual in that virus-related lymphomas (see below) can occur during primary exposure. The known three different patterns of EBV latency (called latency I, II and III) have different associations with human malignancies. However, the human tumors that develop as a result all appear to entail viral orchestration of the same types of cancer hallmark traits (see above) that characterize sporadic cancers that occur independently of such infections.

BURKITT LYMPHOMA: EBV was the first virus to be unequivocally linked to the development of a human tumor. In 1958, Denis Burkitt described a form of childhood lymphoma in a geographical belt across equatorial Africa, which he suggested might have a viral etiology. A few years later, Epstein and Barr discovered viral particles in cell lines cultured from patients with Burkitt lymphoma (BL).

African BL is a B-cell tumor, in which the neoplastic lymphocytes invariably contain EBV and manifest EBV-related antigens (see Chapter 26). The tumor has also been recognized in non-African populations, but in those cases only about 20% carry EBV genomes. The localization of BL to equatorial Africa is not understood, but prolonged stimulation of the immune system by endemic malaria may be important. Normally, EBV-stimulated B-cell proliferation is controlled by suppressor T cells. The lack of an adequate T-cell response often reported in chronic malarial infections might result in uncontrolled B-cell proliferation, thus providing a context for further genetic changes that may lead to the development of lymphoma. One of these is a translocation in which c-myc is being brought into proximity to an immunoglobulin promoter. In addition, EBV proteins inhibit apoptosis and activate signaling pathways involved in cell proliferation. Therefore, the multistep pathogenesis of African BL may be viewed as follows:

1. Infection and polyclonal lymphoblastoid transformation of B cells by EBV
2. Proliferation of B cells and inhibition of suppressor T cells induced by malaria
3. Deregulation of c-myc by translocation in a single transformed B cell, with effects on other signaling pathways
4. Uncontrolled proliferation of a malignant clone of B lymphocytes

NASOPHARYNGEAL CARCINOMA: Nasopharyngeal carcinoma is a variant of squamous cell carcinoma that is particularly common in certain parts of Asia. EBV DNA and EBNA are present in virtually all of these cancers. Epithelial cells may be exposed to EBV via infected lymphocytes traveling through lymphoid-rich epithelium. One of the EBV proteins in this tumor has been shown to activate the EGFR signaling. Fortunately, 70% of patients with this disease are cured by radiation therapy alone.

OTHER EBV-ASSOCIATED TUMORS: EBV markers have been identified in about half of cases of classical Hodgkin lymphoma, in which the virus infects Reed-Sternberg cells. A number of T-cell and NK lymphomas have also been found to harbor EBV, as well as 5% of gastric carcinomas.

POLYCLONAL LYMPHOPROLIFERATION IN IMMUNODEFICIENT STATES: Congenital or acquired immunodeficiency states can be complicated by the development of EBV-induced B-cell proliferative disorders. These lesions are clinically and pathologically indistinguishable from true malignant lymphomas, but most of them are polyclonal. Lymphoid neoplasia occurs in immunosuppressed renal transplant recipients 30–50 times more often than in the general population. Almost all congenital or acquired immunodeficiencies (especially AIDS) and lymphoproliferative diseases associated with organ transplantation involve EBV. Occasionally, a true monoclonal lymphoma may develop in the background of an EBV-induced lymphoproliferative disorder.

Human Herpesvirus 8

Kaposi sarcoma (KS) is a vascular tumor that was originally described in elderly eastern European men and later observed in sub-Saharan Africa (see Chapter 16). Kaposi sarcoma is today the most common neoplasm associated with AIDS. The neoplastic cells contain sequences of a novel herpesvirus, HHV8, also known as KS-associated herpesvirus (KSHV). HHV8 is present in virtually all specimens of Kaposi sarcoma, whether from HIV-positive or HIV-negative patients, and appears to be necessary—but not sufficient—for development of KS.

Other, unidentified, factors contribute. Many more people are HHV8 positive than ever develop KS. In the United States, about 6% of the population carries HHV8, and 60%–80% of the black population in sub-Saharan Africa is seropositive for HHV 8, but the risk of developing KS is miniscule compared to these percentages. Furthermore, among HIV-1–positive people, the risk of KS is greatest when HIV-1 infection was acquired via sexual transmission, rather than by transfusion or by a baby from an infected mother.

In addition to infecting the spindle cells of Kaposi sarcoma, HHV8 is lymphotropic and has been implicated in two uncommon B-cell lymphoid malignancies, namely, **primary effusion lymphoma** and **multicentric Castleman disease** (see Chapter 26).

Like other DNA viruses, the HHV8 viral genome encodes proteins that interfere with the p53 and Rb tumor suppressor pathways. Some viral proteins also inhibit apoptosis and act in multiple ways to accelerate cell cycle transit. HHV8 encodes an inhibitor of the normal regulator of NFκB (i.e., IκB). As a result, HHV8 infection is associated with unrestrained activation of NFκB. Development and progression of KS seems to entail interdependence between lytic HHV8 infection and latently infected cells. Thus, antiviral drugs that inhibit HHV8 lytic infection provide strong protection from the development of KS.

Other DNA Viruses

There have been intriguing claims that a recently discovered virus, **Merkel cell polyoma virus** (MCV), causes a very uncommon skin tumor, Merkel cell carcinoma. MCV genomes integrated into cellular DNA have been identified in 70% of these tumors. However, serologic evidence indicates that MCV infection is widespread in the general population, so the nature of the association of the virus with the rare tumor that gives MCV its name remains uncertain.

Other viruses have been claimed to be associated with human cancers over the years, but with little or no verifiable data to substantiate those assertions. SV40, which does cause tumors in some rodents, is a case in point. However, after extensive study, there are no reproducible experimental or epidemiologic data to support the contention that SV40 is oncogenic for humans.

Enormous interspecies differences in susceptibility to oncogenicity, and past experience, reinforce concern as to the dangers of falling prey to excessive gullibility and accepting seeming reasonableness as a substitute for hard data. One should be skeptical about such contentions and demand careful studies and independent verification before inculpating any agent as a cause of human cancer.

CHEMICAL CARCINOGENESIS

The field of chemical carcinogenesis originated some two centuries ago in descriptions of an occupational disease (this was not the first recognition of an occupation-related cancer, since a specific predisposition of nuns to breast cancer was appreciated even earlier). The English physician Sir Percival Pott gets credit for relating cancer of the scrotum in chimney sweeps to a specific chemical exposure, namely, soot. Today we realize that other products of the combustion of organic materials are responsible for a man-made epidemic of cancer, namely, lung cancer in cigarette smokers.

The experimental production of cancer by chemicals dates to 1915, when Japanese investigators produced skin cancers in rabbits with coal tar. Since that time, the list of organic and inorganic carcinogens has grown exponentially. Yet a curious paradox existed for many years. Many compounds known to be potent carcinogens are relatively inert in terms of chemical reactivity. *The solution to this riddle became apparent in the early 1960s, when it was shown that most, although not all, chemical carcinogens require metabolic activation before they can react with cell constituents.* On the basis of those observations and the close correlation between mutagenicity and carcinogenicity, an in vitro assay using *Salmonella* organisms for screening potential chemical carcinogens— the Ames test—was developed a decade later. Subsequently, a variety of genotoxicity assays have been developed and are still used to screen chemicals and new drugs for potential carcinogenicity.

Chemical Carcinogens Are Mostly Mutagens

Associations between exposure to a specific chemical and human cancers have historically been established on the basis of epidemiologic investigations. These studies have numerous inherent disadvantages, including uncertainties in estimated doses, variability of the population, long and variable latency and dependence on clinical and public health records of questionable accuracy. As an alternative to epidemiologic studies, investigators turned to the use of studies involving animals. Indeed, such studies are legally required before the introduction of a new drug. Yet the logarithmic increase in the number of chemicals synthesized every year makes even this method prohibitively cumbersome and expensive. The search for rapid, reproducible and reliable screening assays for potential carcinogenic activity has centered on the relationship between carcinogenicity and mutagenicity.

A **mutagen** *is an agent that can permanently alter the genetic constitution of a cell.* The Ames test uses the appearance of frameshift mutations and base-pair substitutions in a culture of bacteria of a *Salmonella* sp. Mutations, unscheduled DNA synthesis and DNA strand breaks are also detected in rat hepatocytes, mouse lymphoma cells and Chinese hamster ovary cells. Cultured human cells are now used increasingly for assays of mutagenicity. About 90% of known carcinogens are mutagenic in these systems. Moreover, most, but not all, mutagens are carcinogenic. This close correlation between carcinogenicity and mutagenicity presumably occurs because both reflect damage to DNA. Although not infallible, in vitro mutagenicity assays have proved to be valuable tools in screening for the carcinogenic potential of chemicals.

Chemical Carcinogenesis Is a Multistep Process

Studies of chemical carcinogenesis in experimental animals have shed light on the distinct stages in the progression of normal cells to cancer. Long before the genetic basis of cancer was appreciated, it was demonstrated that a single application of a carcinogen to the skin of a mouse was not, by itself, sufficient to produce cancer. However, when a proliferative stimulus was then applied locally, in the form of a second, noncarcinogenic, irritating chemical (e.g., a phorbol ester), tumors appeared. The first effect was called **initiation**. The action of the second, noncarcinogenic chemical was called **promotion**. Subsequently, further experiments in rodent models of a variety of organ-specific cancers (liver, skin, lung, pancreas, colon, etc.) expanded the concept of a two-stage mechanism to our present understanding of *carcinogenesis as a multistep process that involves numerous mutations.*

From these studies, one can abstract four stages of chemical carcinogenesis:

1. **Initiation** likely represents a mutation in a single cell.
2. **Promotion** reflects the clonal expansion of the initiated cell, in which the mutation has conferred a growth advantage. During promotion, the altered cells remain dependent on the continued presence of the promoting stimulus. This stimulus may be an exogenous chemical or physical agent or may reflect an endogenous mechanism (e.g., hormonal stimulation [breast, prostate] or the effect of bile salts [colon]).
3. **Progression** is the stage in which growth becomes autonomous (i.e., independent of the carcinogen or the promoter). By this time, sufficient mutations have accumulated to immortalize cells.
4. **Cancer,** the end result of the entire sequence, is established when the cells acquire the capacity to invade and metastasize.

The morphologic changes that reflect multistep carcinogenesis in humans are best exemplified in epithelia, such as those of the skin, cervix and colon. Although initiation has no morphologic counterpart, *promotion and progression are represented by the sequence of hyperplasia, dysplasia and carcinoma in situ.*

Chemical Carcinogens Usually Undergo Metabolic Activation

The International Agency for Research in Cancer (IARC) has listed about 75 chemicals as human carcinogens. Chemicals cause cancer either directly or, more often, after metabolic activation. The direct-acting carcinogens are inherently reactive enough to bind covalently to cellular macromolecules. A number of organic compounds, such as nitrogen mustard, *bis*(chloromethyl)ether and benzyl chloride, as well as certain metals are included in this category. Most organic carcinogens, however, require conversion to an ultimate, more reactive compound. This conversion is enzymatic and, for the most part, is effected by the cellular systems involved in drug metabolism and detoxification. Many cells in the body, particularly liver cells, possess enzyme systems that can convert procarcinogens to their active forms. Yet each carcinogen has its own spectrum of target tissues, often limited to a single organ. The basis for organ specificity in chemical carcinogenesis is not well understood.

POLYCYCLIC AROMATIC HYDROCARBONS: The polycyclic aromatic hydrocarbons, originally derived from coal tar, are among the most extensively studied carcinogens. In this class are such model compounds as benzo(a)pyrene, 3-methylcholanthrene and dibenzanthracene. These compounds have a broad range of target organs and generally produce cancers at the site of application. The specific type of cancer produced varies with the route of administration and includes tumors of the skin, soft tissues and breast. Polycyclic hydrocarbons have been identified in cigarette smoke, and so it has been suggested, but not proved, that they are involved in the production of lung cancer.

Polycyclic hydrocarbons are metabolized by cytochrome P450–dependent mixed function oxidases to electrophilic epoxides, which in turn react with proteins and nucleic acids. The formation of the epoxide depends on the presence of an unsaturated carbon–carbon bond. For example, vinyl chloride, the simple two-carbon molecule from which the widely used plastic polyvinyl chloride is synthesized, is metabolized to an epoxide, which is responsible for its carcinogenic properties. Workers exposed to the vinyl chloride monomer in the ambient atmosphere later developed hepatic angiosarcomas.

ALKYLATING AGENTS: Many chemotherapeutic drugs (e.g., cyclophosphamide, cisplatin, busulfan) are alkylating agents that transfer alkyl groups (methyl, ethyl, etc.) to macromolecules, including guanines within DNA. Although such drugs destroy cancer cells by damaging DNA, they also injure normal cells. Thus, alkylating chemotherapy carries a significant risk of solid and hematologic malignancies at a later time.

AFLATOXIN: Aflatoxin B_1 is a natural product of the fungus *Aspergillus flavus.* Like the polycyclic aromatic hydrocarbons, aflatoxin B_1 is metabolized to an epoxide, which can bind covalently to DNA. Aflatoxin B_1 is among the most potent liver carcinogens recognized, producing tumors in fish, birds, rodents and primates. Since *Aspergillus* sp. are ubiquitous, contamination of vegetable foods exposed to the warm moist conditions, particularly peanuts and grains, may result in the formation of significant amounts of aflatoxin B_1. It has been suggested that in addition to hepatitis B and C, aflatoxin-rich foods may contribute to the high incidence of cancer of the liver in parts of Africa and Asia. In rodents exposed to aflatoxin B_1, the resulting liver tumors exhibit a specific inactivating mutation in the *p53* gene (G:C→T:A transversion at codon 249). Interestingly, human liver cancers in areas of high dietary concentrations of aflatoxin carry the same *p53* mutation.

AROMATIC AMINES AND AZO DYES: Aromatic amines and azo dyes, in contrast to the polycyclic aromatic hydrocarbons, are not ordinarily carcinogenic at the point of application. However, they commonly produce bladder and liver tumors, respectively, when fed to experimental animals. Both aromatic amines and azo dyes are primarily metabolized in the liver. The activation reaction undergone by aromatic amines is N-hydroxylation to form the hydroxylamino derivatives, which are then detoxified by conjugation with glucuronic acid. In the bladder, hydrolysis of the glucuronide releases the reactive hydroxylamine. Occupational exposure to aromatic amines in the form of aniline dyes has resulted in bladder cancer.

NITROSAMINES: Carcinogenic nitrosamines are a subject of considerable study because it is suspected that they may play a role in human gastrointestinal neoplasms and possibly other cancers. The simplest nitrosamine, dimethylnitrosamine, produces kidney and liver tumors in rodents. Nitrosamines are also potent carcinogens in primates, although unambiguous evidence of cancer induction in humans is lacking. However, the extremely high incidence of esophageal carcinoma in the Hunan province of China (100 times higher than in other areas) has been correlated with the high nitrosamine content of the diet. There is concern that nitrosamines may also be implicated in other gastrointestinal cancers because nitrites, commonly added to preserve processed meats and other foods, may react with other dietary components to form nitrosamines. In addition, tobacco-specific nitrosamines have been identified, although a contribution to carcinogenesis has not been proved. Nitrosamines are activated by hydroxylation, followed by formation of a reactive alkyl carbonium ion.

METALS: A number of metals or metal compounds can induce cancer, but the carcinogenic mechanisms are unknown. Divalent metal cations, such as nickel (Ni^{2+}), lead (Pb^{2+}), cadmium (Cd^{2+}), cobalt (Co^{2+}) and beryllium (Be^{2+}), are electrophilic and can, therefore, react with macromolecules. In addition, metal ions react with guanine and phosphate groups of DNA. A metal ion such as Ni^{2+} can depolymerize polynucleotides. Some metals can bind to purine and pyrimidine bases through covalent bonds or pi electrons of the bases. These reactions all occur in vitro, and the extent to which they occur in vivo is not known. Most metal-induced cancers occur in an occupational setting (see Chapter 8).

Endogenous and Environmental Factors Influence Chemical Carcinogenesis

Chemical carcinogenesis in experimental animals involves consideration of genetic aspects (species and strain, age and sex of the animal), hormonal status, diet and the presence or absence of inducers of drug-metabolizing systems and tumor promoters. A similar role for such factors in humans has been postulated on the basis of epidemiologic studies.

METABOLISM OF CARCINOGENS: Mixed-function oxidases are enzymes whose activities are genetically determined, and a correlation has been observed between the levels of these enzymes in various strains of mice and their sensitivity to chemical carcinogens. Since most chemical carcinogens require metabolic activation, agents that enhance the activation of procarcinogens to ultimate carcinogens should lead to greater carcinogenicity, while those that augment the detoxification pathways should reduce the incidence of cancer. In general, this is the case experimentally. Since humans are exposed to many chemicals in the diet and environment, such interactions are potentially significant.

SEX AND HORMONAL STATUS: These factors are important determinants of susceptibility to chemical carcinogens but are highly variable and in many instances not readily predictable. In experimental animals, there is sex-linked susceptibility to the carcinogenicity of certain chemicals. However, the effects of sex and hormonal status on chemical carcinogenesis in humans are not clear.

DIET: The composition of the diet can affect the level of drug-metabolizing enzymes. Experimentally, a low-protein diet, which reduces the hepatic activity of mixed-function oxidases, is associated with decreased sensitivity to hepatocarcinogens. In the case of dimethylnitrosamine, the decreased incidence of liver tumors is accompanied by an increased incidence of kidney tumors, an observation that emphasizes the fact that the metabolism of carcinogens may be regulated differently in different tissues.

PHYSICAL CARCINOGENESIS

The physical agents of carcinogenesis discussed here are UV light, asbestos and foreign bodies. Radiation carcinogenesis is discussed in Chapter 8.

Ultraviolet Radiation Causes Skin Cancers

Among fair-skinned people, a glowing tan is commonly considered the mark of a successful holiday. However, this overt manifestation of the alleged healthful effects of the sun conceals underlying tissue damage. The harmful effects of solar radiation were recognized by ladies of a bygone era, who shielded themselves from the sun with parasols to maintain a "roses-and-milk" complexion and to prevent wrinkles. The more recent fad for a tanned complexion has been accompanied not only by cosmetic deterioration of facial skin but also by an increased incidence of the major skin cancers.

Cancers attributed to sun exposure, namely, basal cell carcinoma, squamous carcinoma and melanoma, occur predominantly in people of the white race. The skin of people of the darker races is protected by the increased concentration of melanin pigment, which absorbs UV radiation. In fair-skinned people, the areas exposed to the sun are most prone to develop skin cancer. Moreover, there is a direct correlation between total exposure to sunlight and the incidence of skin cancer.

UV radiation is the short-wavelength portion of the electromagnetic spectrum adjacent to the violet region of visible light. It appears that only certain portions of the UV spectrum are associated with tissue damage, and a carcinogenic effect occurs at wavelengths between 290 and 320 nm. *The effects of UV radiation on cells include enzyme inactivation, inhibition of cell division, mutagenesis, cell death and cancer.*

The most important biochemical effect of UV radiation is the formation of **pyrimidine dimers** in DNA, a type of DNA damage that is not seen with any other carcinogen. Pyrimidine dimers may form between thymine and thymine, between thymine and cytosine or between cytosine pairs alone. Dimer formation leads to a cyclobutane ring, which distorts the phosphodiester backbone of the double helix in the region of each dimer. Unless efficiently eliminated by the nucleotide excision repair pathway, genomic injury produced by UV radiation is mutagenic and carcinogenic.

Xeroderma pigmentosum, an autosomal recessive disease, exemplifies the importance of DNA repair in protecting against the harmful effects of UV radiation. In this rare disorder, sensitivity to sunlight is accompanied by a high incidence of skin cancers, including basal cell carcinoma, squamous cell carcinoma and melanoma. Both the neoplastic and nonneoplastic disorders of the skin in xeroderma pigmentosum are attributed to an impairment in the excision of UV-damaged DNA.

Asbestos Causes Mesothelioma

Pulmonary asbestosis and asbestosis-associated neoplasms are discussed in Chapter 12. Here we review possible mechanisms of carcinogenesis attributed to asbestos. In this context, it is not conclusively established whether the cancers related to asbestos exposure should be considered examples of chemical carcinogenesis or of physically induced tumors, or both.

Asbestos, a material widely used in construction, insulation and manufacturing, is a family of related fibrous silicates, which are classed as "serpentines" or "amphiboles." Serpentines, of which chrysotile is the only example of commercial importance, occur as flexible fibers; the amphiboles, represented principally by crocidolite and amosite, are firm narrow rods.

*The characteristic tumor associated with asbestos exposure is **malignant mesothelioma** of the pleural and peritoneal cavities.* This cancer, which is exceedingly rare in the general population, has been reported to occur in 2%–3% (in some studies even more) of heavily exposed workers. The latent period (i.e., the interval between exposure and the appearance of a tumor) is usually about 20 years but may be twice that figure. It is reasonable to surmise that mesotheliomas of both pleura and peritoneum reflect the close contact of these membranes with asbestos fibers transported to them by lymphatic channels.

The pathogenesis of asbestos-associated mesotheliomas is obscure. Thin crocidolite fibers are associated with a considerably greater risk of mesothelioma than shorter and thicker chrysotile fibers. There is increasing evidence that the surface properties of asbestos fibers are important in their carcinogenic properties.

An association between cancer of the lung and asbestos exposure is clearly established in smokers. A slight increase in the prevalence of lung cancer has been reported in nonsmokers exposed to asbestos, but the small number of cases renders an association questionable. Claims that exposure to asbestos increases the risk of gastrointestinal cancer have not withstood statistical analysis of the collected data. In any case, the widespread adoption of strict safety standards will undoubtedly relegate the hazards of asbestos to historical interest.

Foreign Bodies Produce Experimental Cancer

The implantation of inert materials induces sarcomas in certain experimental animals. However, *humans are resistant to foreign body carcinogenesis, as evidenced by the lack of cancers following the implantation of prostheses constructed of plastics and metals.* A few reports of cancer developing in the vicinity of foreign bodies in humans probably reflect scar formation, which in some organs seems to be associated with an increased incidence of cancers. Despite numerous contrary claims in lawsuits, there is no evidence that a single traumatic injury can lead to any form of cancer.

The general mechanisms underlying the development of neoplasia are summarized in Fig. 5-62.

Dietary Influences on Cancer Development Are Highly Controversial

About a quarter of a century ago, respected epidemiologists suggested that approximately one third of cancers in the United States could be prevented by changes in diet. Numerous epidemiologic studies have attempted to identify possible relationships between dietary factors and the occurrence of a variety of cancers. Such investigations have particularly emphasized the roles of dietary fats, red meat and fiber. The results of studies comparing different ethnic groups or societies across international borders have often not been accepted as accurate and in fact have sometimes yielded misleading conclusions. Prospective, cohort studies comparing like populations are usually more reliable.

Some such cohort studies have indicated correlations between consumption of animal (but not vegetable) fat and increased risk of breast cancer. This relationship was limited to premenopausal women, and there is a suggestion that nonlipid components of food containing animal fats may be involved.

In the case of colon cancer, consumption of red meat has been associated with increased risk; total fat and animal fat intake are not correlated independently of red meat intake. At one time, it was thought that intake of dietary fiber protected from colorectal cancer and other malignancies, but these conclusions have not withstood the test of time.

An association between the risk of aggressive (but not indolent) prostate cancer and the consumption of red meat has been claimed. However, further studies of this matter are needed.

Despite claims that eating fruits and vegetables helps to prevent cancer, there is little evidence that these dietary constituents protect from tumor development. Although there is a popular notion that high intake and blood concentrations of vitamin D may be associated with a lower incidence of some cancers, a recent review indicates that this is not the case. Several epidemiologic studies have provided preliminary data suggesting that a folate-rich diet decreases the risk of colorectal cancer.

In conclusion, the beneficial effects of dietary constituents on cancer risk are at best limited and are often controversial. The consequences of a specific type of diet on longevity are largely limited to reduced cardiovascular disease.

Physical activity and obesity are closely correlated with diet, and the dissection of independent effects of these influences by epidemiologic techniques has proven to be exceedingly difficult. The best evidence that physical activity decreases the risk of developing cancer exists for breast and colon malignancies. The same is true for obesity, which adds risk for endometrial, esophageal and kidney cancer. However, it is generally agreed that the evidence for these associations is not sufficient to allow for specific recommendations for changes in lifestyle in order to decrease cancer risk.

SYSTEMIC EFFECTS OF CANCER ON THE HOST

The symptoms of cancer are, for the most part, referable to local effects of the primary tumor or its metastases. However, in a minority of patients, cancer produces remote effects that are not attributable to tumor invasion or to metastasis, and are collectively called **paraneoplastic syndromes**. Such effects are rarely lethal, but in some cases they dominate the clinical course. It is important to recognize these syndromes for several reasons. First, signs and symptoms of the paraneoplastic syndrome may be the first clinical manifestation of a malignant tumor. Second, the syndromes may be mistaken for those produced by advanced metastatic disease and may, therefore, lead to inappropriate therapy. Third, the paraneoplastic syndrome itself may be disabling, and treatment that alleviates those symptoms may have important palliative effects. Finally, certain tumor products that result in paraneoplastic syndromes provide a means of monitoring recurrence of the cancer in patients who have had surgical resections or are undergoing chemotherapy or radiation therapy.

We discuss here systemic paraneoplastic manifestations. Those mainly manifesting as involvement of one or another organ are addressed in the chapters specific for individual organs.

Fever

It is not uncommon for cancer patients to present initially with fever of unknown origin that cannot be explained by an infectious disease. Fever attributed to cancer correlates with tumor growth, disappears after treatment and reappears on recurrence. The cancers in which this most commonly occurs are Hodgkin disease, renal cell carcinoma and osteogenic sarcoma, although many other tumors are occasionally complicated by fever. Tumor cells may themselves release pyrogens or the inflammatory cells in the tumor stroma can produce IL-1.

Anorexia and Weight Loss

A paraneoplastic syndrome of anorexia, weight loss and cachexia is very common in patients with cancer, often appearing before its malignant cause becomes apparent. For example, a small asymptomatic pancreatic cancer may be suspected only on the basis of progressive and unexplained weight loss. Although cancer patients often decrease their caloric intake because of anorexia and abnormalities of taste, restricted food intake does not explain the profound wasting so common among them. The mechanisms responsible for this phenomenon are poorly understood. It is known, however, that unlike starvation, which is associated with a lowered metabolic rate, cancer is often accompanied by an elevated metabolic rate. It has been demonstrated that TNF-α and other cytokines (interferons, IL-6) can produce a wasting syndrome in experimental animals.

EPIDEMIOLOGY OF CANCER

The mere compilation of raw epidemiologic data is of little use unless they are subjected to careful analysis. In evaluating the relevance of epidemiologic observations to cancer causation, the Hill criteria are germane:

- Strength of the association
- Consistency under different circumstances
- Specificity
- Temporality (i.e., the cause must precede the effect)
- Biological gradient (i.e., there is a dose-response relationship)
- Plausibility
- Coherence (i.e., a cause-and-effect relationship does not violate basic biological principles)
- Analogy to other known associations

It is not mandatory that a valid epidemiologic study satisfy all these criteria, nor does adherence to them guarantee that the hypothesis derived from the data is necessarily true. However, as a guideline they remain useful.

Cancer accounts for one fifth of the total mortality in the United States and is the second-leading cause of death after ischemic cardiovascular diseases. For most cancers, death rates in the United States have largely remained flat for more than half a century, with some notable exceptions (Fig. 5-63). The death rate from cancer of the lung among men has risen dramatically from 1930, when it was an uncommon tumor, to the present, when it is by far the most common cause of death from cancer in men. As discussed in Chapter 8, the entire epidemic of lung cancer deaths is attributable to smoking. Among women, smoking did not become fashionable until World War II. Considering the time lag needed between starting to smoke and the development of cancer of the lung, it is not surprising that the increased death rate from lung cancer in women did not become significant until after 1965. In the United States, the death rate from lung cancer in women now exceeds that for breast cancer, and it is now, as in men, the most common fatal cancer. By contrast, for reasons difficult to fathom, cancer of the stomach, which in 1930 was by far the most common cancer in men and was more

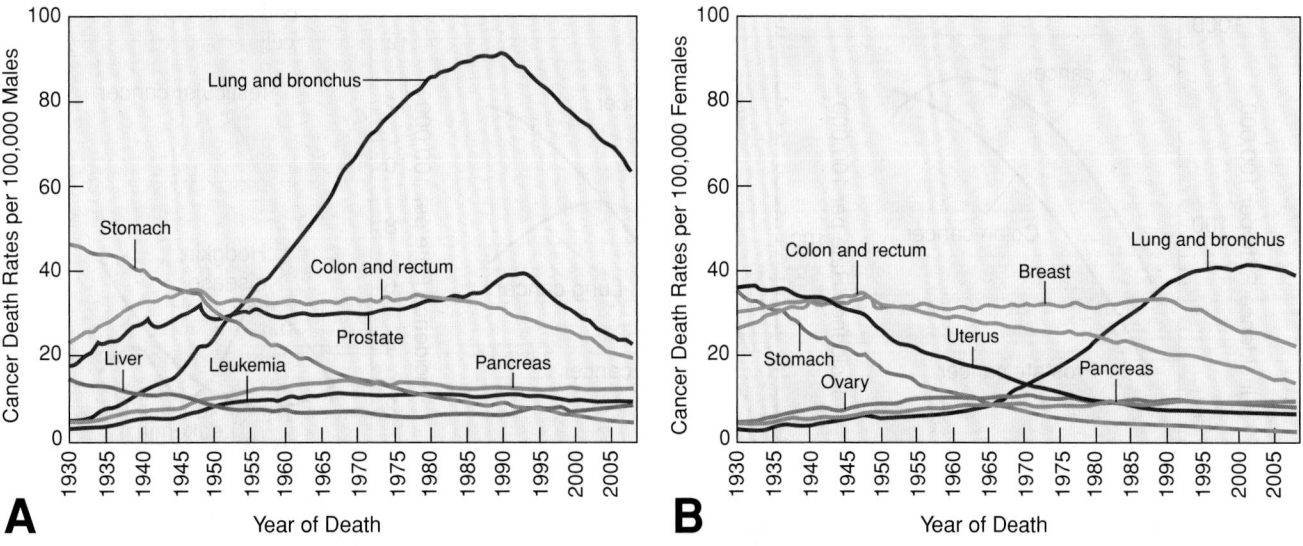

FIGURE 5-63. Cancer death rates in the United States, 1930–2009, among men (**A**) and women (**B**).

common than breast cancer in women, has shown a remarkable and sustained decline in frequency. Similarly, there has been a conspicuous decline in the death rate from cancer of the uterine corpus and cervix, possibly explained by better screening, diagnostic techniques and therapeutic methods. Overall, after decades of steady increases, the age-adjusted mortality as a result of all cancers has now reached a plateau. The ranking of the incidence of tumors in men and women in the United States is shown in Table 5-11.

Individual cancers have their own age-related profiles, but for most, increased age is associated with an increased incidence. The most striking example of the dependency on age is carcinoma of the prostate, in which the incidence increases 30-fold between men ages 50 and 85 years. Certain neoplastic diseases, such as acute lymphoblastic leukemia in children and testicular cancer in young adults, show different age-related peaks of incidence (Fig. 5-64).

Geographic and Ethnic Differences Influence Cancer Incidence

NASOPHARYNGEAL CANCER: Nasopharyngeal cancer is rare in most of the world except for certain regions of China, Hong Kong and Singapore.

ESOPHAGEAL CARCINOMA: The range in incidence of esophageal carcinoma varies from extremely low in Mormon women in Utah to a value some 300 times higher in the female population of northern Iran. Particularly high rates of esophageal cancer are noted in a so-called Asian esophageal cancer belt, which includes the great land mass stretching from Turkey to eastern China. Interestingly, throughout this region, as the incidence rises, the proportional excess in males decreases; in some of the areas of highest incidence there is even a female excess. The disease is also more common in certain regions of sub-Saharan Africa and among blacks in the United States. The causes of esophageal cancer are obscure, but it is known that it disproportionately affects the poor in many areas of the world, and the combination of alcohol abuse and smoking is associated with a particularly high risk.

STOMACH CANCER: The highest incidence of stomach cancer occurs in Japan, where the disease is almost 10 times as frequent as it is among American whites. A high incidence has also been observed in Latin American countries, particularly Chile. Stomach cancer is also common in Iceland and eastern Europe.

COLORECTAL CANCER: The highest incidence of colorectal cancer is found in the United States, where it is three or four times more common than in Japan, India, Africa and Latin America. It had been theorized that the high fiber content of the diet in low-risk areas and the high fat content in the United States are related to this difference, but this concept has been seriously questioned.

TABLE 5-11			
MOST COMMON TUMOR TYPES IN MEN AND WOMEN			
Tumor Type	**% of Cases**	**Tumor Type**	**% of Cases**
Men		**Women**	
Prostate	29	Breast	29
Lung and bronchus	14	Lung and bronchus	14
Colon and rectum	9	Colon and rectum	9
Urinary bladder	7	Uterine corpus	6
Melanoma (cutaneous)	5	Thyroid	5
Kidney and renal pelvis	5	Melanoma (cutaneous)	4
Non-Hodgkin lymphoma	4	Non-Hodgkin lymphoma	4
Oral cavity	3	Kidney and renal pelvis	3
Leukemia	3	Ovary	3
Pancreas	3	Pancreas	3
All other sites	18	All other sites	20

Source: American Cancer Society, estimates for 2012.

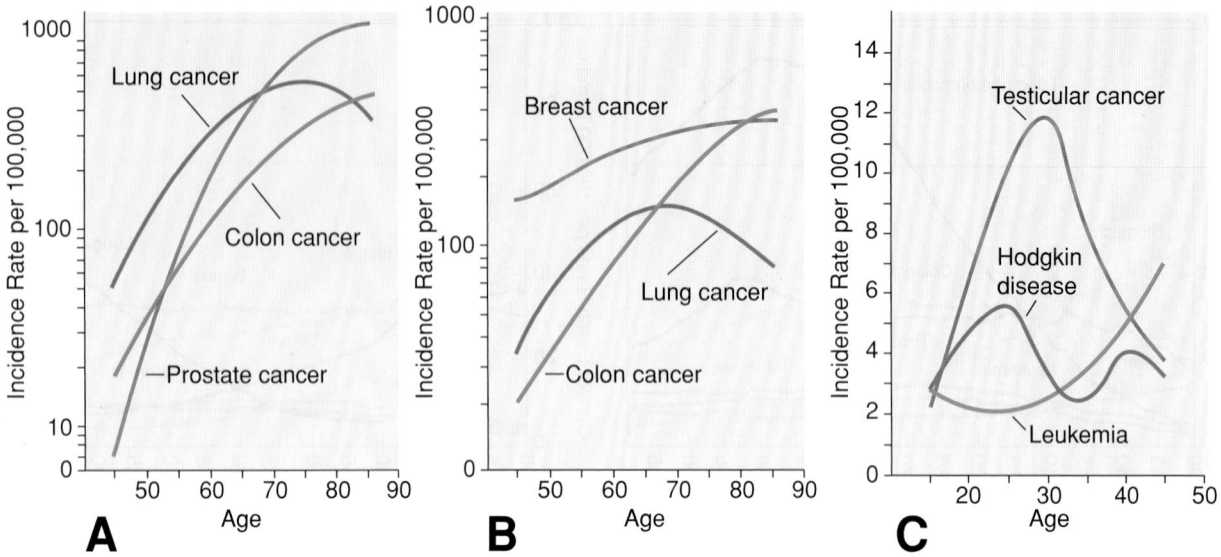

FIGURE 5-64. Incidence of specific cancers as a function of age. A. Men. **B.** Women. **C.** Testicular cancer in men and Hodgkin disease and leukemia in both sexes. The incidence of these cancers in **C** peaks at younger ages than do those in **A** and **B**.

LIVER CANCER: There is a strong correlation between the incidence of primary hepatocellular carcinoma and the prevalence of hepatitis B and C. Endemic regions for both diseases include large parts of sub-Saharan Africa and most of Asia, Indonesia and the Philippines. It must be remembered that levels of aflatoxin B_1 are high in the staple diets of many of the high-risk areas.

SKIN CANCER: As noted above, the rates for skin cancers vary with skin color and exposure to the sun. Thus, particularly high rates have been reported in northern Australia, where the population is principally of English origin and sun exposure is intense. Increased rates of skin cancer have also been noted among the white population of the American Southwest. The lowest rates are found among people with pigmented skin (e.g., Japanese, Chinese and Indians). The rates for African blacks, despite their heavily pigmented skin, are occasionally higher than those for Asians because of the higher incidence of melanomas of the soles and palms in the former population.

BREAST CANCER: Adenocarcinoma of the breast, the most common female cancer in many parts of Europe and North America, shows considerable geographic variation. The rates in African and Asian populations are only one fifth to one sixth of those prevailing in Europe and the United States. Epidemiologic studies have contributed little to our understanding of the etiology of breast cancer.

CERVICAL CARCINOMA: Striking differences in the incidence of squamous carcinoma of the cervix exist between ethnic groups and different socioeconomic levels. For instance, the very low rate in Ashkenazi Jews of Israel contrasts with a 25 times greater rate in the Hispanic population of Texas. In general, groups of low socioeconomic status have a higher incidence of cervical cancer than the more prosperous and better educated. This cancer is also directly correlated with early sexual activity and multiparity, and is rare among women who are not sexually active, such as nuns. It is also uncommon among women whose husbands are circumcised. A strong association with infection by HPVs has been demonstrated, and cervical cancer should be classed as a venereal disease.

CHORIOCARCINOMA: Choriocarcinoma, an uncommon cancer of trophoblastic differentiation, is found principally in women, following a pregnancy, although it can occur in men as a testicular tumor. The rates of this disease are particularly high in the Pacific rim of Asia (Singapore, Hong Kong, Japan and the Philippines).

PROSTATIC CANCER: Very low incidences of prostatic cancer are reported for Asian populations, particularly Japanese, while the highest rates described are in American blacks, in whom the disease occurs some 25 times more often. The incidence in American and European whites is intermediate.

TESTICULAR CANCER: An unusual aspect of testicular cancer is its universal rarity among black populations. Interestingly, although the rate in American blacks is only about one-fourth that in whites, it is still considerably higher than the rate among African blacks.

CANCER OF THE PENIS: This squamous carcinoma is virtually nonexistent among circumcised men of any race but is common in many parts of Africa and Asia. It is usually associated with HPV infection.

CANCER OF THE URINARY BLADDER: The rates for transitional cell carcinoma of the bladder are fairly uniform. Squamous carcinoma of the bladder, however, is a special case. Ordinarily far less common than transitional cell carcinoma, it has a high incidence in areas where schistosomal infestation of the bladder (bilharziasis) is endemic.

BURKITT LYMPHOMA: Burkitt lymphoma, a disease of children, was first described in Uganda, where it accounts for half of all childhood tumors. Since then, a high frequency has been observed in other African countries, particularly in hot, humid lowlands. It has been noted that these are areas where malaria is also endemic. High rates have been recorded in other tropical areas, such as Malaysia and New Guinea, but European and American cases are encountered only sporadically.

MULTIPLE MYELOMA: This malignant tumor of plasma cells is uncommon among American whites but displays a three to four times higher incidence in American and South African blacks.

CHRONIC LYMPHOCYTIC LEUKEMIA: Chronic lymphocytic leukemia is common among elderly people in Europe and North America but is considerably less common in Japan.

Studies of Migrant Populations Give Clues to Cancer Development

Although planned experiments on the etiology of human cancer are hardly feasible, certain populations have unwittingly performed such experiments by migrating from one environment to another. Initially at least, the genetic characteristics of such people remained the same, but the new environment differed in climate, diet, infectious agents, occupations and so on. *Consequently, epidemiologic studies of migrant populations have provided many intriguing clues to the factors that may influence the pathogenesis of cancer.* The United States, which has been the destination of one of the greatest population movements of all time, is the source of most of the important data in this field.

COLORECTAL, BREAST, ENDOMETRIAL, OVARIAN AND PROSTATIC CANCERS: Emigrants from low-risk areas in Europe and Japan to the United States exhibit an increased risk of colorectal cancer in the United States. Moreover, their offspring continue at higher risk and reach the incidence levels of the general American population. This rule for colorectal cancer also prevails for cancers of the breast, endometrium, ovary and prostate.

CANCER OF THE LIVER: As noted above, primary hepatocellular carcinoma is common in Asia and Africa, where it has been associated with hepatitis B and C. In American blacks and Asians, however, the neoplasm is no more common than in American whites, a situation that presumably reflects the relatively low prevalence of chronic viral hepatitis in the United States.

HODGKIN DISEASE: In general, in poorly developed countries the childhood form of Hodgkin disease is the one reported most often. In developed Western countries, by contrast, the disease is most common among young adults, except in Japan. Such a pattern is characteristic of certain viral infections. Further evidence for an environmental influence is the higher incidence of Hodgkin disease in Americans of Japanese descent than that in Japan.

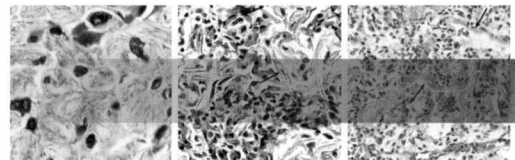

6

Developmental and Genetic Diseases

Linda A. Cannizzaro

GLOSSARY

The following terms are used in the text or figures of this chapter:

Allele—One of multiple forms of a physical genetic locus on a specific chromosome.

Alternative splicing—A mechanism by which variations in the assembly of a gene's exons, or coding regions, create different forms of mature messenger RNAs (mRNAs) from the same gene, leading to production of more than one related protein, or isoform.

Autosomes—Any chromosome other than a sex chromosome; autosomes normally occur in pairs in somatic cells and singly in gametes.

Base pair (bp)—The association of nucleotide bases of opposite strands of DNA within a chromosome. Adenine (A) pairs with thymine (T); cytosine (C) pairs with guanine (G) in a DNA double helix. An attached number (e.g., 12 bp) denotes the size of a sequence of DNA.

Centromere—The nonstaining primary constricted region of a chromosome, which is the point of attachment to the spindle fiber.

Codon—Three consecutive nucleotides of DNA or RNA that specify a single amino acid to be incorporated into a protein or serve as a termination signal.

Epigenetic—Regulation of the expression of gene activity without alteration of the DNA nucleotide sequence, such as methylation of regulatory sequences and histone modification.

Exon—A region of a gene that codes for mature messenger RNA, which is then translated into a protein.

Frame-shift mutation—Addition or deletion of a number of DNA bases not a multiple of 3 that disrupts boundaries of nucleotides in codons, thus shifting the reading frame of the gene. Codons downstream from the mutation are changed. The resulting protein is abnormal. Introduction of a premature stop codon or removal of a normal translational termination may alter protein size.

Gain-of-function mutation—A mutation that produces a protein that takes on a new or enhanced function.

Gene—A functional unit of heredity that occupies a specific place (locus) on a chromosome.

Genomics—The study of the functions and interactions of all the genes in the genome, including their interactions with environmental factors.

Genotype—An individual's complete genetic constitution at one or more gene loci.

Haplotype—A group of physically linked genes on one chromosome that are inherited together.

Hemizygous—Having a gene on one chromosome for which there is no counterpart on the opposite chromosome.

Heterochromatin—Chromatin that remains densely packed throughout the cell cycle. It includes satellite DNA in centromeres; acrocentric short arms; 1qh, 9qh, 16qh, and Yqh (all constitutive heterochromatin); and the inactive X chromosome (facultative heterochromatin).

Heterozygous—Having two different alleles at a specified locus.

Homozygous—Having two identical alleles at a specified locus.

Intron—A region of a gene in the intervening sequences between exons. Introns are transcribed into RNA but are spliced out of the mature mRNA that is translated into protein. Thus, introns do not contribute to the open reading frame that encodes a protein.

Linkage disequilibrium—The nonrandom occurrence of alleles at two or more loci (i.e., when two loci are not independent of each other). It implies a group of markers that are inherited coordinately.

Loss-of-function mutation—A mutation that decreases/inactivates a protein's production and/or function.

Missense mutation—A change in one DNA base that alters the amino acid encoded by a codon.

Monogenic—A trait or disease governed by the action of a single gene.

Multifactorial disease—Caused by the interaction of several genes and the environment.

Nonsense mutation—A 1-bp change resulting in the introduction of a stop codon, which causes premature truncation of a protein.

Penetrance—The likelihood of an altered phenotype in a person with a certain mutant gene.

Phenotype—The appearance or other characteristics of an individual resulting from a specific gene(s) or interactions of their genetic constitution with the environment.

Point mutation—The substitution of a single DNA base in the normal DNA sequence.

Regulatory gene—A gene that codes for an RNA or protein molecule that regulates expression of other genes.

Repeat sequence—DNA sequences present in multiple identical copies in the genome.

Silent mutation—Substitution of a single DNA base, typically in the third position of a codon, that produces no change in the amino acid sequence of the encoded protein.

Single-nucleotide polymorphism (SNP/"Snip")—A variation (substitution, deletion or insertion) in DNA sequence in which a single nucleotide alteration occurs at a site in the genome that is different among members of a species. The majority of SNPs have only two alleles.

Termination (stop) codon—One of three codons (UAG, UAA, UGA) that terminate synthesis of a polypeptide.

INTRODUCTION

Our understanding of developmental, genetic and neoplastic disorders has increased dramatically since 2003 when the Human Genome Project provided the first draft of the roughly 3 billion nucleotides in a human genome. The human genome contains about 23,000 protein-coding genes, but these constitute only less than 2% of the whole genome. Furthermore, most of the protein-coding genes in the human genome are found in genomes of other organisms including lower life forms such as yeast. It is the remaining 98% of the human genome that adds the remarkable complexity that ultimately determines the human species. This remaining 98% includes many non-protein-coding genes that are transcribed into RNA molecules such as microRNAs and long noncoding RNAs, which are increasingly being recognized to fulfill important regulatory functions.

Advances in molecular genetics and cytogenetics technologies have greatly improved clinical characterization of the genetic basis of human disease. It is also now possible to target drugs to specific genetic loci responsible for disease susceptibility and prevention. The modern field of pharmacogenomics seeks to create new classes of medicines targeting specific variants in gene and protein structure, to provide highly specific therapies with fewer side effects than occur in many of today's medicines. Gene therapies also hold great potential for treating genetic and acquired diseases.

Diseases that manifest during the perinatal period may be caused solely by factors in the fetal environment, solely by genomic abnormalities or by interactions between genetic defects and environmental influences. For example, in phenylketonuria (PKU), a genetic deficiency of phenylalanine hydroxylase causes mental retardation only if an affected infant is exposed to dietary phenylalanine.

Each year, about one quarter of a million babies in the United States are born with a birth defect. Worldwide, at least 1 in 50 newborns has a major congenital anomaly, 1 in 100 has a defect that can be attributed to a single-gene abnormality and 1 in 200 has a major chromosomal abnormality. At the same time, it has been estimated that the genomes of *healthy* individuals contain at least 400 protein-damaging sequence variants and at least 2 bona fide disease mutations. Thus, simply having a potential disease-causing mutation does not inevitably produce disease. As we will see in this chapter, disease expression ultimately depends on complex interactions among genetic, epigenetic and environmental factors.

A specific cause is not apparent in more than 2/3 of all birth defects (Fig. 6-1). No more than 6% can be attributed to uterine factors; maternal disorders such as metabolic imbalances or infections during pregnancy; or environmental exposures (drugs, chemicals, radiation). Others are caused by genomic defects (inherited traits or spontaneous mutations) and only a small number by chromosomal abnormalities. Currently about 70% have no known genetic or other cause.

Up to 50% of fetuses spontaneously aborted early in pregnancy have chromosomal abnormalities. *The incidence of specific numerical chromosomal abnormalities in abortuses is several times higher than in term infants, indicating that most such chromosomal defects are lethal.* Thus, only a small number of children with cytogenetic abnormalities are born alive.

In Western countries, developmental and genetic birth defects account for half of deaths in infancy and childhood. By contrast, 95% of infant mortality in less developed countries is due to environmental causes such as infectious diseases and malnutrition. Ongoing reductions in the incidence of birth anomalies will require genetic counseling, early prenatal diagnosis, identification of high-risk pregnancies, avoidance of potential teratogens and implementation of preventive measures. For example, introduction of prenatal dietary folic acid supplements has significantly reduced the incidence of congenital neural tube defects.

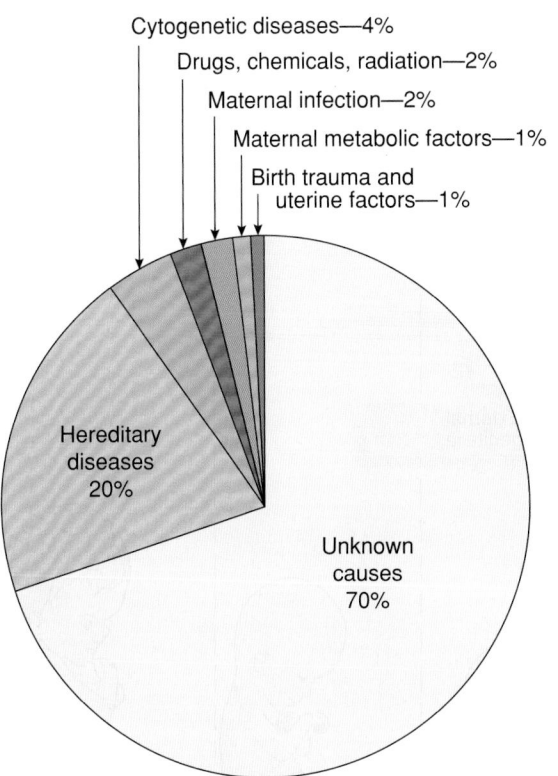

FIGURE 6-1. Causes of birth defects in humans. Most birth defects have unknown causes.

PRINCIPLES OF TERATOLOGY

Teratology is the study of developmental anomalies (Greek *teraton*, "monster"). **Teratogens** are chemical, physical and biological agents that cause developmental anomalies. Although only a relatively few teratogens have been *proven* in humans, many drugs and chemicals are teratogenic in animals and should thus be considered potentially dangerous for humans.

Malformations are morphologic defects or abnormalities of an organ, part of an organ or anatomic region due to perturbed morphogenesis. Exposure to a teratogen may result in a malformation, but not invariably. Such observations have led to the formulation of general principles of teratology:

- **Susceptibility to teratogens is variable.** Key determinants are the genotypes of the fetus and mother, but other factors play a role. For example, the fetal alcohol syndrome (FAS) affects some children of alcoholic mothers but not others. An infant of an alcoholic mother born with characteristic facial features, small size and central nervous system (CNS) damage may be diagnosed with FAS, but alcoholic mothers often abuse other substances and self-reporting of alcohol intake may be inaccurate. Thus, conclusions as to the teratogenic effects of prenatal alcohol exposure may be confounded by many variables.
- **Susceptibility to teratogens is specific for each embryologic stage.** Most agents are teratogenic only at particular times in development (Fig. 6-2). Thus, maternal rubella infection can cause congenital rubella syndrome (CRS) but only if the mother is infected within the first 20 weeks of pregnancy.

- **Mechanisms of teratogenesis are specific for each agent.** Teratogenic drugs may inhibit crucial enzymes or receptors, interfere with formation of mitotic spindles or impair energy production, thus inhibiting metabolic steps critical for normal morphogenesis. Many drugs and viruses affect specific tissues and damage some developing organs more than others.
- **Teratogenesis is dose dependent and may be idiosyncratic.** Thus, an absolutely safe dose cannot be predicted for every woman.
- **Teratogens produce death, growth retardation, malformation or functional impairment.** The outcome depends on complex interactions between a teratogen, the maternal organism and the fetal–placental unit.

Human teratogens can be identified by (1) population surveys, (2) prospective and/or retrospective studies of single malformations and (3) investigation of adverse effects of drugs or other chemicals. Proven teratogens include most cytotoxic drugs, alcohol, some antiepileptic drugs, heavy metals and thalidomide. Many drugs and chemicals have been declared safe for use during pregnancy because they were not teratogenic in laboratory animals, but the fact that a drug is not teratogenic for mice or rabbits does not necessarily mean that it is innocuous for humans. For example, thalidomide is not teratogenic in mice and rats, but it caused complex malformations when many pregnant women used it as an antiemetic during the first trimester of pregnancy. Antiviral medications to treat herpes simplex and zoster, proton pump inhibitors to treat gastroesophageal reflux and antiepileptic medications have been studied in large numbers of pregnant women with relatively reassuring results, but whether they are always safe in pregnancy is unknown. Some vaccines recommended during pregnancy to prevent infections in mothers and infants have been tested in clinical trials that specifically excluded pregnant women; thus, evaluation of their safety depends entirely on observational studies. Without adequate, well-controlled data, it is necessary to weigh the benefits of medications or vaccines with potential risks to the embryo or fetus.

Developmental and genetic disorders are classified as follows:

- **Errors of morphogenesis**
- **Chromosomal abnormalities**
- **Single-gene defects**
- **Polygenic inherited diseases**

A fetus may also be injured by **adverse transplacental influences** or deformities and injuries caused by intrauterine trauma or during parturition. After birth, acquired diseases of infancy and childhood are also important causes of morbidity and mortality.

ERRORS OF MORPHOGENESIS

Normal intrauterine and postnatal development depends on sequential activation and repression of genes. A fertilized ovum (zygote) has all the genes of an adult, but most of them are inactive. As zygotes enter cleavage stages of development, individual genes or sets of genes are specifically activated at different stages of embryogenesis. Thus, *abnormal gene activation in early embryonic cells can cause death.*

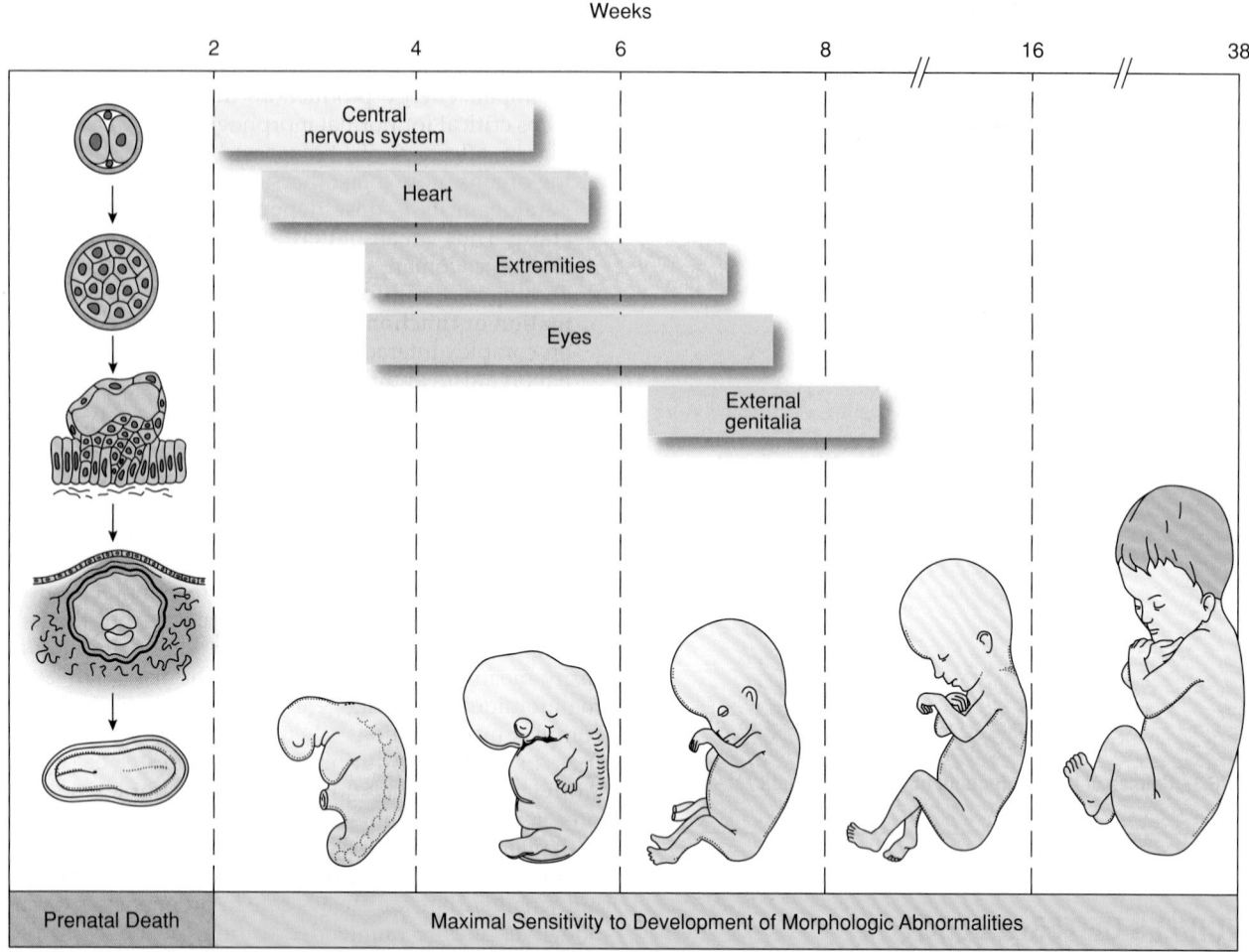

FIGURE 6-2. Sensitivity of specific organs to teratogenic agents at critical stages of human embryogenesis. Exposure to adverse influences in preimplantation and early postimplantation stages of development (*far left*) leads to prenatal death. Periods of maximal sensitivity to teratogens (*horizontal bars*) vary for different organ systems but overall are limited to the first 8 weeks of pregnancy.

Cells that form two- and four-cell embryos (blastomeres) are equipotent: each can give rise to an adult organism. If such cells separate at this stage, identical twins or quadruplets can result. Since blastomeres are equipotent and interchangeable, loss of a single blastomere at this stage does not have serious consequences. But, if one blastomere carries lethal genes, the others probably do as well. Activation of such genes is invariably fatal. Similarly, noxious exogenous agents typically affect all blastomeres and cause death. *As a rule, exogenous toxins acting on preimplantation embryos do not produce errors of morphogenesis or malformations* (Fig. 6-2). *The most common consequence is death of the embryo, which often goes unnoticed or is perceived as heavy, delayed, menstrual bleeding.*

Injury during the first 8–10 days after fertilization may cause incomplete separation of blastomeres, to yield conjoined twins ("Siamese twins") linked at the head (craniopagus), thorax (thoracopagus) or rump (ischiopagus). Conjoined twins may be asymmetric; one is well developed and the other rudimentary or hypoplastic. The latter is always abnormal and may reside within the body of the better-developed sibling (fetus in fetu). Some congenital teratomas, especially in the sacrococcygeal area, are actually asymmetric monsters.

Complex developmental abnormalities affecting multiple organ systems are usually due to injuries during early organogenesis. This period is characterized by formation of so-called **developmental fields,** in which rapidly dividing cells interact to determine their developmental fate through irreversible differentiation of groups of cells. Complex morphologic movements form organ primordia (anlage), and organs are then interconnected in functionally active systems. *The developmental stage of primordial organ system formation is most susceptible to teratogenesis owing to faulty gene activity or effects of exogenous toxins* (Fig. 6-2). Impaired morphogenesis may affect (1) cells and tissues, (2) organs or organ systems and (3) anatomic regions.

■ **Agenesis** is complete absence of an organ primordium. It may manifest as (1) total lack of an organ (e.g., unilateral or bilateral renal agenesis); (2) absence of part of an organ, such as agenesis of the corpus callosum of the brain; or (3) lack of specific cell types in an organ, such as absence of testicular germ cells in congenital Sertoli cell–only syndrome. This unusual syndrome is characterized by severely reduced or absent spermatogenesis despite the presence of both Sertoli and Leydig cells. Microdeletions in the Yq11 region of the Y chromosome, known as the AZF (azoospermia factor) region, have been implicated.

- **Aplasia** is persistence of an organ anlage or rudiment, without the mature organ. In pulmonary aplasia, for example, the main bronchus ends blindly in a nondescript mass of rudimentary ducts and connective tissue.
- **Hypoplasia** is reduced size due to incomplete development of all or part of an organ, as in micrognathia (small jaw) and microcephaly (small brain and head).
- **Dysraphic anomalies** are defects caused by failure of apposed structures to fuse. In spina bifida, the spinal canal does not close completely, and overlying bone and skin do not fuse, leaving a midline defect.
- **Involution failures** denote persistence of embryonic or fetal structures that normally involute during development. Thus, a persistent thyroglossal duct results from incomplete involution of the tract that connects the base of the tongue with the developing thyroid.
- **Division failures** are caused by incomplete programmed cell death in embryonic tissues (see Chapter 1). Fingers and toes are formed at the distal ends of limb buds by loss of cells between cartilage-containing primordia. If these cells do not undergo apoptosis, fingers are conjoined or incompletely separated (syndactyly).
- **Atresia** reflects incomplete formation of a normal body orifice or tubular passage. Many hollow organs originate as cell strands and cords whose centers undergo programmed cell death to yield a central cavity or lumen. Esophageal atresia is characterized by localized absence of the lumen, which was not fully established in embryogenesis.
- **Dysplasia** is caused by abnormal histogenesis. (This context is different from "dysplasia" in precancerous epithelial lesions [see Chapters 1 and 5]). In tuberous sclerosis, for example, aggregates of normally developed cells are arranged into grossly visible "tubers."
- **Ectopia, or heterotopia,** denotes a normally formed organ outside of its normal anatomic location. Thus, heterotopic parathyroid glands may arise within the thymus in the anterior mediastinum.
- **Dystopia** is inadequate migration of an organ from its site of development to its normal location. Thus, kidneys originate in the pelvis and then move in a cephalad direction. Dystopic kidneys remain in the pelvis. Dystopic testes remain in the inguinal canal and do not enter the scrotum (cryptorchidism).

Developmental anomalies due to interference with morphogenesis are often multiple:

- A **polytopic effect** occurs when an injurious agent affects several organs at once during a critical stage of development.
- A **monotopic effect** is a single localized anomaly that results in a cascade of pathogenetic events.
- A **developmental sequence anomaly** (anomalad or complex anomaly) is a pattern of defects arising from a single anomaly or pathogenetic mechanism. In the Potter complex (Fig. 6-3), pulmonary hypoplasia, external signs of intrauterine fetal compression and morphologic changes of the amnion are all related to oligohydramnios (severely reduced amount of amniotic fluid). The features of Potter complex occur regardless of the cause of oligohydramnios.

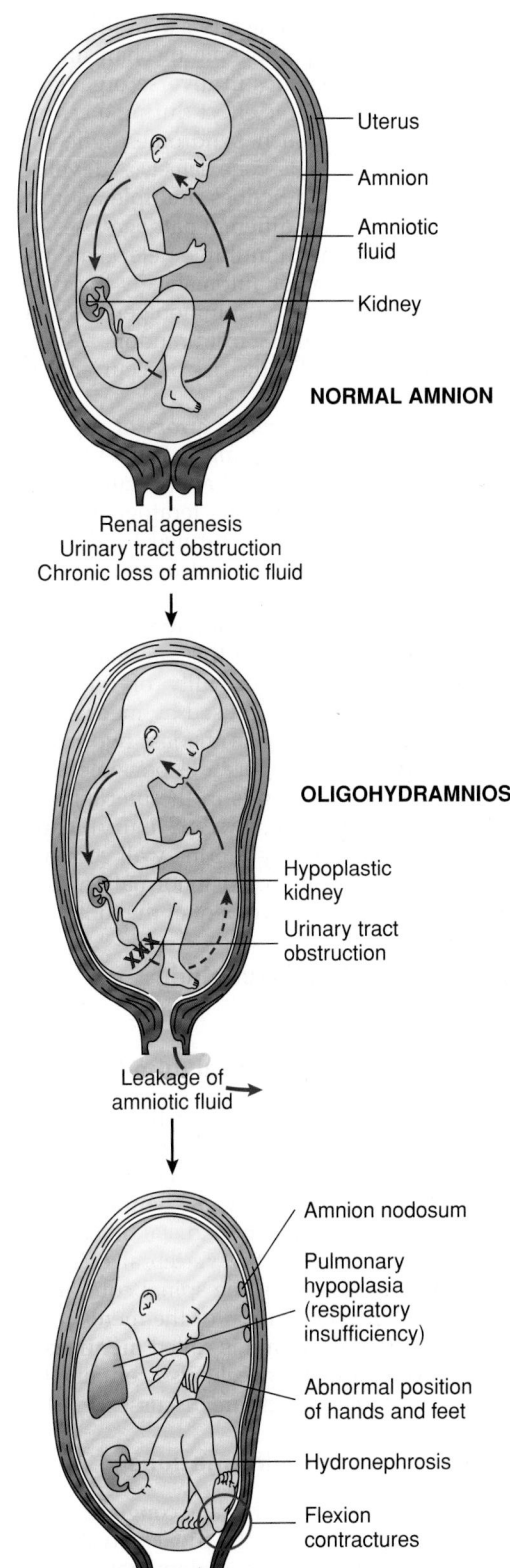

FIGURE 6-3. Potter complex. The fetus normally swallows amniotic fluid and, in turn, excretes urine, thus maintaining a normal volume of amniotic fluid. In the face of urinary tract disease (e.g., renal agenesis or urinary tract obstruction) or leakage of amniotic fluid, the volume of amniotic fluid becomes reduced, a situation called **oligohydramnios**. Oligohydramnios results in a spectrum of congenital abnormalities called **Potter sequence,** which includes pulmonary hypoplasia and contractures of the limbs. The amnion has a nodular appearance.

A **developmental syndrome** refers to multiple anomalies arising from a common pathogenic mechanism. The term **syndrome** indicates anomalies in diverse organs that have been damaged by a polytopic effect during a critical developmental period. Many such syndromes reflect chromosomal abnormalities or single-gene defects. A **developmental association,** or **syntropy,** describes multiple anomalies that arise concurrently but have different pathogeneses. Congenital anomalies in a child with multiple defects are not necessarily interrelated and do not automatically imply exposure to an exogenous teratogen or a common genetic defect. Distinguishing specific syndromes from random associations is required to accurately predict the risk of recurrence in subsequent offspring.

Teratogens rarely cause major errors of morphogenesis after the third month of pregnancy. However, functional and, to a lesser degree, structural abnormalities may occur in children exposed to exogenous teratogens during later trimesters. Although organs are formed by the end of the first trimester, most continue to restructure and mature at prescribed rates. For example, the CNS attains functional maturity several years after birth and remains susceptible to adverse exogenous influences for this interval.

A **deformation** is an abnormality of form, shape or position of a part of the body caused by mechanical forces. Most anatomic defects arising in the last two trimesters of pregnancy fall into this category. Responsible forces may be external (e.g., amniotic bands in the uterus) or intrinsic (e.g., fetal hypomobility caused by CNS injury). Thus, equinovarus foot may be caused by uterine wall compression in oligohydramnios or by spinal cord abnormalities that lead to defective innervation and movement of the foot.

All Organ Systems Are Susceptible to Malformations

Anencephaly and Other Neural Tube Defects

Anencephaly is congenital absence of the cranial vault. In this dysraphic defect of neural tube closure, cerebral hemispheres are completely missing or reduced to small masses at the base of the skull. Normally, the neural tube closes in a craniocaudad direction, so a more distal defect in this process causes abnormalities of the vertebral column. **Spina bifida** is incomplete closure of the spinal cord and/or vertebral column or both. Protrusion of the meninges through a defect in the vertebral column is called **meningocele.** In a **myelomeningocele,** a meningocele also contains herniated spinal cord. Neural tube defects are discussed in Chapter 32.

Thalidomide-Induced Malformations

Limb reduction deformities are rare congenital defects of mostly obscure origin that affect 1 in 5000 liveborn infants. They have been known for ages. A depiction of an affected infant by the 18th-century Spanish painter Goya was used in medical texts to illustrate this condition. In the 1960s, a dramatic increase in the incidence of limb reduction deformities in Germany and England was linked to maternal ingestion of a sedative, thalidomide, early in pregnancy. This derivative of glutamic acid is teratogenic between the 28th and 50th days of pregnancy. Many children born to mothers exposed to thalidomide had skeletal deformities and pleomorphic defects in other organs, mostly the ears

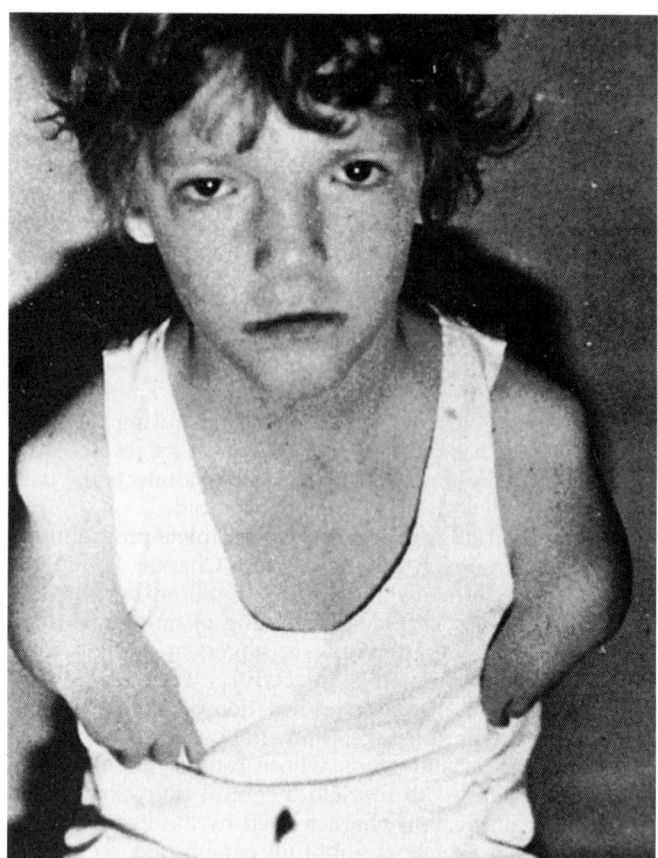

FIGURE 6-4. Thalidomide-induced deformity of the arms.

(**microtia** and **anotia**) and heart. Typically, their arms were short and malformed (Fig. 6-4), resembling the flippers of a seal **(phocomelia),** or sometimes even completely missing **(amelia).** The CNS was unaffected, and these children had normal intelligence. Once the link between phocomelia and thalidomide was established, the drug was banned (1962), but not before an estimated 3000 such children had been born. Thalidomide impairs limb growth by blocking angiogenesis and, perhaps, by inducing caspase-8–dependent apoptosis. The same properties make it useful in treating certain malignancies.

Fetal Hydantoin Syndrome

Ten percent of children born to mothers taking antiepileptic drugs, such as hydantoin, during pregnancy show characteristic facial features, hypoplasia of nails and digits and various congenital heart defects. This syndrome also occurs in children born to untreated epileptic mothers, raising a question about the adverse effects of the drug. Nevertheless, susceptibility to this disorder appears to correlate with fetal levels of the microsomal detoxifying enzyme epoxide hydrolase, suggesting that accumulation of reactive intermediates of hydantoin metabolism may be teratogenic.

Fetal Alcohol Syndrome

Fetal alcohol syndrome is a complex of abnormalities caused by maternal consumption of alcoholic beverages during pregnancy. It includes (1) growth retardation, (2) CNS abnormalities and (3) characteristic facial dysmorphology. Not all children harmed by maternal alcohol abuse show the full spectrum of abnormalities. In such cases, the term **fetal alcohol effect** is used.

  **EPIDEMIOLOGY AND ETIOLOGIC FACTORS:** Harm caused by intrauterine exposure to alcohol was noted in biblical times and was reported during the historic London gin epidemic (1720–1750). However, a specific syndrome was not defined until 1968. The incidence of fetal alcohol syndrome ranges from 0.2 to 2.0 cases per 1000 live births in the United States, but may be as high as 20–150 cases per 1000 in populations with high rates of alcoholism, such as some tribes of Native Americans. *Mild mental deficiency and emotional disorders related to fetal alcohol effect are far more common than full-blown fetal alcohol syndrome.* The minimum amount of alcohol that causes fetal injury is not well established. Children with the full syndrome are usually born to mothers who are chronic alcoholics. Heavy alcohol consumption during the first trimester of pregnancy is particularly dangerous. The mechanism by which alcohol damages the developing fetus is poorly understood.

  PATHOLOGY AND CLINICAL FEATURES: Infants born to alcoholic mothers often show prenatal growth retardation, which continues after birth. They may also have microcephaly, epicanthal folds, short palpebral fissures, maxillary hypoplasia, thin upper lip, micrognathia and a poorly developed philtrum. One third may have cardiac septal defects, which often close spontaneously. Minor abnormalities of joints and limbs may occur.

Fetal alcohol syndrome is the most common cause of acquired but preventable mental retardation. One fifth of children with fetal alcohol syndrome have intelligence quotients (IQs) below 70, and 40% are between 70 and 85. Even with normal IQ, these children tend to have short memory spans and exhibit impulsive behavior and emotional instability (see Chapter 8).

TORCH Complex

TORCH refers to a complex of signs and symptoms produced by fetal or neonatal infection with *Toxoplasma* (T), rubella (R), cytomegalovirus (C) or herpes simplex virus (H). The "O" in TORCH represents "others" including syphilis, varicella-zoster virus (chicken pox), fifth disease (parvovirus B19) and HIV. The term reminds pediatricians that these fetal and newborn infections may be indistinguishable from one another and testing for all TORCH agents should be done in suspected cases (Fig. 6-5).

Infections with TORCH agents affect 1%–5% of all live-born infants in the United States. They are major causes of neonatal morbidity and mortality. Suspicion of congenital infection and awareness of its prominent features help facilitate early diagnosis. Severe damage due to these organisms is largely irreparable, and prevention is the best approach. The specific organisms of the TORCH complex are discussed in detail in Chapter 9.

 PATHOLOGY: Clinical and pathologic findings in symptomatic newborns vary. Only a minority show the entire spectrum of abnormalities (Table 6-1).

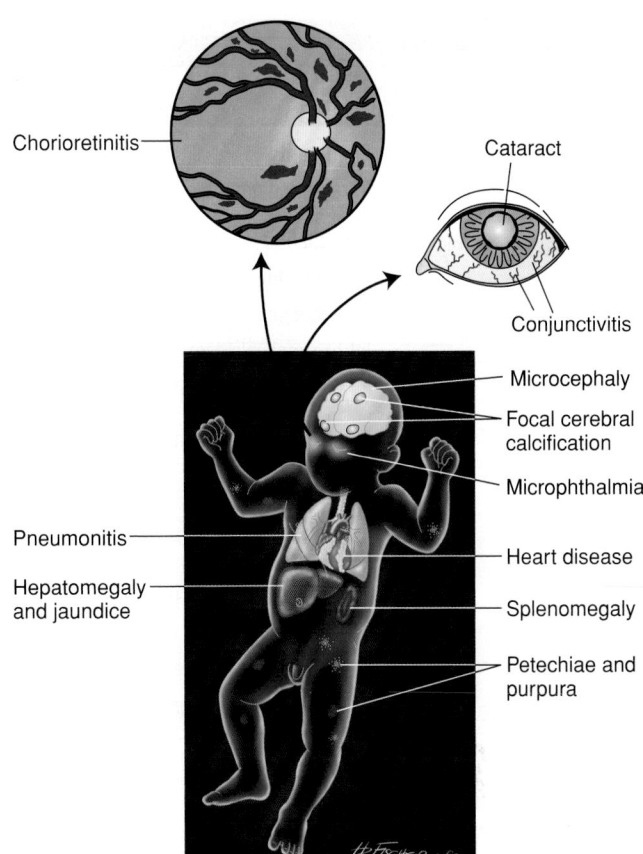

FIGURE 6-5. TORCH complex. Children infected in utero with *Toxoplasma*, rubella virus, cytomegalovirus or herpes simplex virus show remarkably similar effects.

Growth retardation and abnormalities of the brain, eyes, liver, hematopoietic system and heart are common.

CNS lesions are the most serious changes in TORCH-infected children. In acute encephalitis, foci of necrosis are initially surrounded by inflammatory cells. Later these lesions calcify, most prominently in congenital toxoplasmosis. Microcephaly, hydrocephalus and abnormally shaped gyri and sulci (microgyria) are common. Radiologically, abnormal cerebral cavities (porencephaly), missing olfactory bulbs and other major brain defects may occur. Severe CNS injury may entail psychomotor retardation, neurologic defects and seizures.

Ocular defects may also be prominent, particularly with rubella, in which over 2/3 of patients have cataracts and microphthalmia. Glaucoma and retinal malformations (coloboma) may occur. Choroidoretinitis, usually bilateral, is common with rubella, *Toxoplasma* and CMV. Keratoconjunctivitis is the most common eye lesion in neonatal herpes infection.

Cardiac anomalies occur in many children with the TORCH complex, mostly in congenital rubella, patent ductus arteriosus and septal defects. Pulmonary artery stenosis and complex cardiac anomalies are occasionally seen.

Congenital Syphilis

The organism that causes syphilis, *Treponema pallidum,* is transmitted to the fetus by a mother who had been infected

TABLE 6-1

PATHOLOGIC FINDINGS IN THE FETUS AND NEWBORN INFECTED WITH TORCH AGENTS

General	Prematurity
	Intrauterine growth retardation
Central nervous system	Encephalitis
	Microcephaly
	Hydrocephaly
	Intracranial calcifications
	Psychomotor retardation
Ear	Inner ear damage with hearing loss
Eye	Microphthalmia (R)
	Chorioretinitis (TCH)
	Pigmented retina (R)
	Keratoconjunctivitis (H)
	Cataracts (RH)
	Glaucoma (R)
	Visual impairment (TRCH)
Liver	Hepatomegaly
	Liver calcifications (R)
	Jaundice
Hematopoietic system	Hemolytic and other anemias
	Thrombocytopenia
	Splenomegaly
Skin and mucosae	Vesicular or ulcerative lesions (H)
	Petechiae and ecchymoses
Cardiopulmonary system	Pneumonitis
	Myocarditis
	Congenital heart disease
Skeleton	Various bone lesions

R = rubella virus; C = cytomegalovirus; H = herpesvirus; T = *Toxoplasma.*

during pregnancy or, potentially, within 2 years before the pregnancy. About 1 in 2000 liveborn infants in the United States have congenital syphilis. One third of pregnancies in syphilitic women end in stillbirth, and the remainder in term infants with congenital syphilis. *T. pallidum* may invade a fetus any time in pregnancy. Early infections mostly cause abortion, but 50%–80% of neonates surviving early vertical transmission show congenital infection. Grossly visible signs of congenital syphilis appear only in fetuses infected after the 16th week of pregnancy. As spirochetes grow in all fetal tissues, clinical presentations vary.

Children with congenital syphilis may appear normal at first or show changes of the TORCH complex. Early lesions teem with spirochetes. They show perivascular infiltrates of lymphocytes and plasma cells, and granuloma-like lesions, called **gummas.** Many infants are asymptomatic and only develop stigmata of congenital syphilis in the first few years of life. Late symptoms of congenital syphilis appear many

years later and reflect slowly evolving tissue destruction and repair:

- **Rhinitis:** A conspicuous mucopurulent nasal discharge, "snuffles," is almost always present as an early sign of congenital syphilis. The nasal mucosa is edematous and tends to ulcerate, leading to nosebleeds. Destruction of the nasal bridge eventually results in flattening of the nose, so-called **saddle nose.**
- **Skin:** A maculopapular rash is common early in congenital syphilis. It usually affects palms and soles (as in secondary syphilis of adults), although it may cover the entire body or any part of it. Cracks and fissures **(rhagades)** occur around the mouth, anus and vulva. Flat raised plaques **(condylomata lata)** around the anus and female genitalia may develop early or after a few years.
- **Visceral organs:** A distinctive pneumonitis, with pale hypocrepitant lungs **(pneumonia alba),** may develop in the neonatal period. Hepatosplenomegaly, anemia and lymphadenopathy may also occur in early congenital syphilis.
- **Teeth:** Buds of incisors and sixth-year molars develop early in postnatal life, at a time when congenital syphilis is particularly aggressive. Thus, permanent incisors may be notched **(Hutchinson teeth)** and molars malformed **(mulberry molars).**
- **Bones:** Periosteal inflammation with new bone formation **(periostitis)** is common, especially in the anterior tibia. This causes a distinctive outward curving **(saber shins).**
- **Eye:** Progressive corneal vascularization **(interstitial keratitis)** is an especially vexing complication of congenital syphilis, occurring as early as 4 years and as late as 20 years of age. The cornea eventually scars and becomes opaque.
- **Nervous system:** The nervous system is commonly involved, with symptoms starting in infancy or after 1 year. **Meningitis** predominates in early congenital syphilis, causing convulsions, mild hydrocephalus and mental retardation. **Meningovascular syphilis** is common later and may lead to deafness, mental retardation, paresis and other complications. **Hutchinson triad** is a combination of deafness, interstitial keratitis and notched incisor teeth.

Appropriate clinical findings, plus a history of maternal infection, suggest the diagnosis, but serologic testing to confirm active infection may not be definitive since newborns, in addition to receiving the treponeme, carry transplacentally transferred maternal immunoglobulin G (IgG). Penicillin is the drug of choice for intrauterine and postnatal syphilis. If given during intrauterine life or the first 2 years of postnatal life, prognosis can be excellent, and most symptoms of congenital syphilis are prevented.

CYTOGENETICS AND CHROMOSOMES

Cytogenetics is the study of chromosomes and their abnormalities. The current classification is the International System for Human Cytogenetic Nomenclature (ISCN, 2013). A normal human has 46 chromosomes: 2 sex chromosomes (XX or XY) plus 44 nonsex chromosomes, or autosomes.

Cytogenetic studies can be done on any cell type undergoing mitotic division. Lymphocytes are most often used as they are easily stimulated to divide. Proliferating cells are arrested in metaphase, then spread onto glass slides to

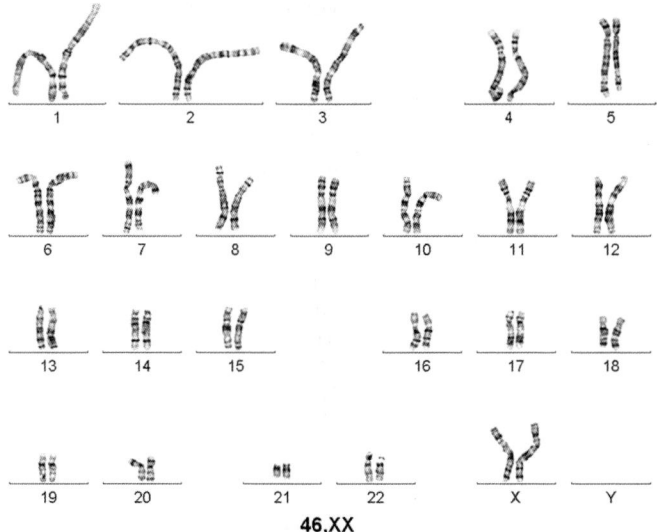

FIGURE 6-6. G-banded normal female karyotype. Chromosomes are grouped as shown: #1-3 are group A; #4, 5, group B; #6-12, group C; #13-15, group D; #16-18, group E; #19, 20, group F; #21, 22, group G.

disperse the chromosomes. Staining, usually with Giemsa trypsin, facilitates identification of chromosomes by generating distinctive band patterns (Fig. 6-6).

Chromosome Structure

Accurate detection of specific chromosome abnormalities depends on defined methods to identify normal chromosomes. Chromosomes are classified by length and centromere position—the point at which two identical strands of chromosomal DNA, the sister chromatids, attach to each other during mitosis. Centromere location identifies them as metacentric, submetacentric or acrocentric. Metacentric chromosomes (1, 3, 19, 20) have centromeres in their middle. Although these chromosomes are divided into two equal parts, the top part is defined as the p (from French, *petit*) short arm and the bottom is called q, the long arm. In submetacentric chromosomes (2, 4 through 12, 16, 17,18, X), centromeres produce two arms of unequal length, of which the q arm is longer than the upper p arm. Acrocentric chromosomes (13, 14, 15, 21, 22, Y) have very short p arms containing stalks and satellites attached to eccentrically located centromeres. In a **karyotype,** chromosomes are lined up according to their size

and centromere position and classified into several groups (A to G from largest to smallest) (Fig. 6-6).

Chromosomal Banding

Special stains delineate specific bands unique to each chromosome. *This makes it possible to recognize each chromosome, pair homologous chromosomes and identify defects on each segment of a chromosome.* Chromosome bands are labeled as follows:

- **G bands** are highlighted using Giemsa stain (hence "G").
- **Q bands** stain with Giemsa and fluoresce when treated with quinacrine (thus, "Q").
- **R bands** are reverse (hence "R") images of G and Q bands such that dark G bands are light R bands and vice versa.
- **C banding** stains centromeres (hence "C") and other portions of chromosomes containing **constitutive heterochromatin,** highly condensed, repetitive DNA sequences that are transcriptionally silent. By contrast, **facultative heterochromatin,** which forms the inactive X chromosome (Barr body), is not repetitive but it shares the condensed structure of constitutive heterochromatin.
- **Nucleolar organizing region (NOR) staining** demonstrates secondary constrictions (stalks) of chromosomes with satellites.
- **T banding** stains chromosome termini/telomeric (hence "T") ends.

Clinical cytogenetics laboratories mostly use G banding to distinguish normal and abnormal chromosome patterns. However, each of these stains identifies DNA sequences with different structure and function along each chromosome. In centromeric DNA, most sequences are long repeats, while very short repeating units of DNA make up each chromosome's telomere region.

Fluorescence in Situ Hybridization Uses DNA Probes to Identify Specific Chromosome Regions

Fluorophore-labeled DNA probes vary in size from individual genes to small chromosome regions. They are used in fluorescence in situ hybridization (FISH) to determine if genetic material is lost, gained or rearranged. Probes with different fluorophores can identify chromosomal translocations. In multicolor FISH, or spectral karyotyping, such probes hybridize to whole chromosomes, to facilitate detection of gross abnormalities (Fig. 6-7).

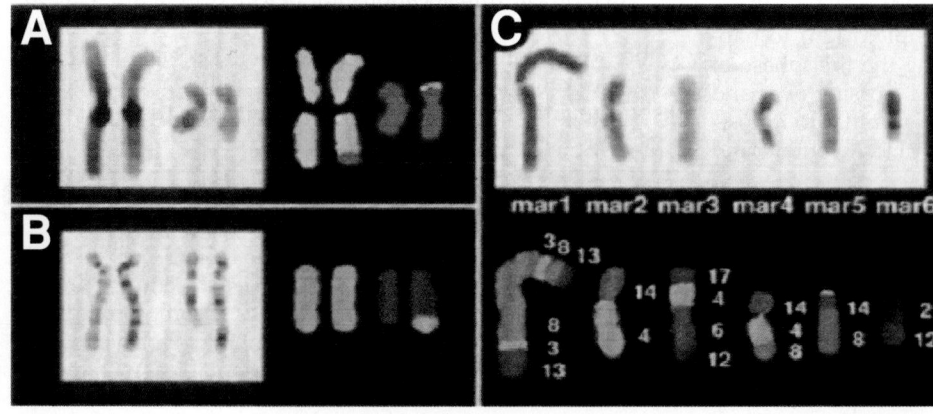

FIGURE 6-7. Translocations in human chromosomes demonstrated by spectral karyotyping. A. Balanced translocation: t(1;11). **B.** Unbalanced karyotype: derivative chromosome 12 with chromosome 4 material attached (partial trisomy for 4p and partial monosomy for 12q). **C.** Characterization of marker chromosomes from an aneuploid breast cancer showing multiple translocations.

Structural Chromosomal Abnormalities May Arise During Somatic Cell Division (Mitosis) or Gametogenesis (Meiosis)

The frequency of structural abnormalities varies considerably in different situations. Spontaneous abortions show the highest frequency, and newborns, the lowest. In part, this reflects early fetal loss, particularly in cases with significant unbalanced rearrangements. To understand how structural chromosome abnormalities arise, it is important to understand how cells undergo division. Somatic cells undergo mitosis, while gametes undergo meiosis.

Cell Division

Mitotic cell division in somatic cells results in two daughter cells identical to the original parent cell in chromosome number and genetic content. Mitosis results in a diploid (2n) number of chromosomes in the daughter cells.

Meiosis only occurs in male and female germline cells, resulting in gametes with half the diploid chromosome content (23 chromosomes, plus either an X or a Y sex chromosome). This is the haploid number (n) of chromosomes.

Mitosis

Mitosis is divided into five stages: prophase, prometaphase, metaphase, anaphase and telophase. In the resting stage, interphase, the chromosomes are in their most decondensed state and exist as long, thread-like structures in the nucleus. As mitosis approaches, chromosomes thicken and condense, allowing them to be visualized by light microscopy at prometaphase and metaphase stages. Centromeres of each chromosome attach to the spindle and are pulled to opposite poles of the dividing cell during anaphase. Chromosomes congregate at opposite ends at telophase, while the cell constricts into two daughter cells, each with the same amount of DNA as the parent cell. Colcemid, a colchicine derivative, added to a culture of dividing cells depolymerizes microtubules that form the spindle and arrests mitosis in prometaphase/metaphase.

Meiosis

Structural chromosomal abnormalities arising during gametogenesis are transmitted to all somatic cells of an individual's offspring and may cause heritable diseases. During normal meiosis, homologous chromosomes (i.e., the copies of each chromosome inherited from both parents) form pairs, called **bivalents**. Meiosis has two stages. Meiosis I results in the halving of the DNA content from diploid (2n) to haploid (n) number of chromosomes. During the first phase of meiosis, sister chromatids may engage in crossing over and so exchange genetic material. Meiosis II is similar to mitosis and gives rise to gametes haploid (n) in DNA content and with 23 chromosomes.

Structural Chromosome Alterations Occur Once in 375 Live Births

These alterations result from breakage and reunion of homologous and nonhomologous autosomal and sex chromosome segments. Chromosome breakage can occur spontaneously or result from exposure to clastogenic agents, such as viruses, radiation or various chemicals.

Chromosome Translocations

A **chromosome translocation** is an abnormal process in which *nonhomologous* chromosomes (e.g., chromosomes 11 and 22) cross over and exchange genetic material. This exchange of chromosome material can be balanced or unbalanced.

Chromosomal translocations are classified according to the International System for Human Cytogenetic Nomenclature. For example, translocation between chromosomes "11" and "22" is written as t(11;22). Sites of the translocation are further defined by Giemsa bands. Thus, t(11;22)(q23;q11) means that the region of the chromosome 11 long arm broken at band q23 translocated to the long arm of chromosome 22 at band q11, and the region from 22q11 is now part of the long arm at 11q23.

The two major types of translocations are reciprocal and robertsonian.

Reciprocal Translocations

A reciprocal translocation is exchange of chromosomal segments between different (nonhomologous) chromosomes (Fig. 6-8). Reciprocal translocations are **balanced** if there is no net loss of genetic material; each chromosomal segment is translocated in its entirety. If this occurs in gametes (sperm or ova), all somatic cells in the progeny inherit the abnormal chromosomal structure. Balanced translocations identified by cytogenetics testing are not usually associated with loss of genes or disruption of vital gene loci, so most carriers of balanced translocations are phenotypically normal. Balanced reciprocal translocations can be inherited for many generations.

Nevertheless, offspring of carriers of balanced translocations can have unbalanced karyotypes and may show severe phenotypic abnormalities (Fig. 6-9). The abnormal positions of exchanged chromosome segments may disturb meiosis and lead to abnormal segregation of chromosomes. Formation of bivalents may also be disturbed. Complete pairing of translocated segments can result in formation of a cross-like structure (quadriradial) between the two chromosomes containing the translocations and their two normal homologs. Unlike a normal bivalent, which typically resolves as each chromosome migrates to opposite poles, a quadriradial can divide along several different planes potentially yielding gametes with unbalanced chromosomes. On fertilization, the resulting zygotes may exhibit partial trisomy and monosomy for segments of the translocated chromosomes (Fig. 6-9).

Reciprocal translocations are detected in about 1 in 965 liveborn infants. Most patients with balanced translocations are asymptomatic, but 6% have an associated disorder, such as autism, decreased intellectual ability and congenital abnormalities, which are likely to result from disruption of a gene at the translocation breakpoint.

Robertsonian Translocations

Robertsonian translocations (centric fusion) result from fusion of centromere regions of two acrocentric chromosomes (Fig. 6-8). When nonhomologous chromosomes break near the centromere, the two arms combine to form one large chromosome. A small acentric chromosomal fragment is also formed and because it lacks a centromere, it is usually lost in

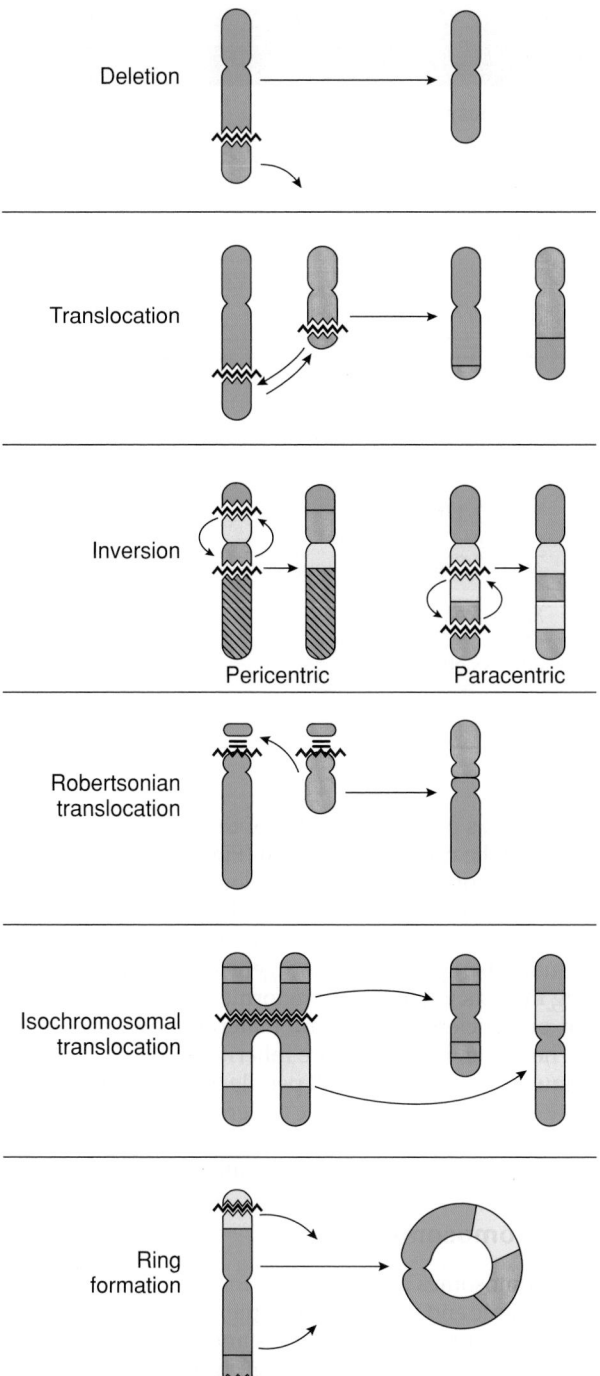

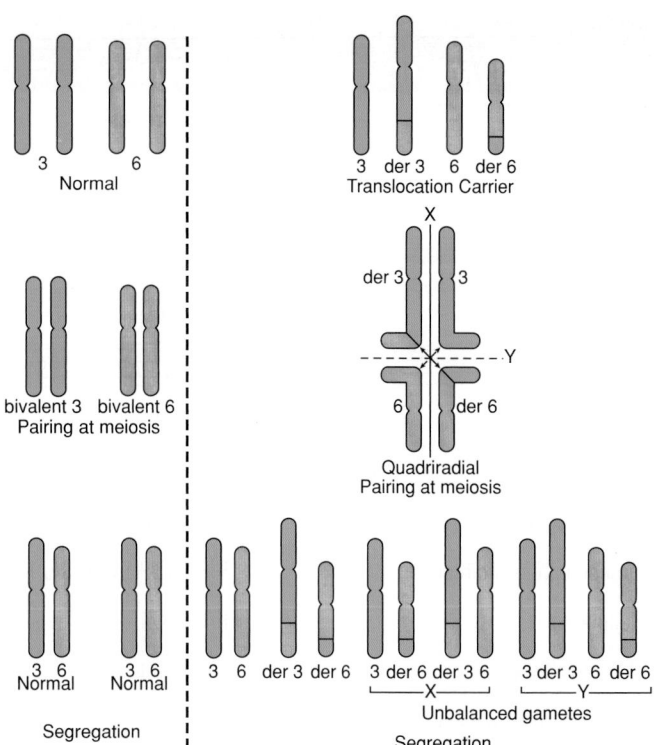

FIGURE 6-9. Meiotic segregation in a reciprocal balanced translocation involving chromosomes 3 and 6. The pairing of homologous chromosomes 3 and 6 in normal meiosis forms bivalents, which then segregate uniformly to create two gametes, each of which carries a single chromosome 3 and chromosome 6. Here the translocation carrier bears a balanced exchange of portions of the long arms of chromosomes 3 and 6. The chromosomes that carry the translocated genetic material are called **derivative chromosomes** (der3 and der6). Diploid germ cells contain pairs of homologous chromosomes 3 and 6, each of which consists of one normal chromosome and one that carries a translocation. During meiosis, instead of the normal pairing into two bivalents, a quadriradial structure, containing all four chromosomes, is formed. In this circumstance, the chromosomes can segregate along several different planes of cleavage, shown as *X* and *Y*. In addition, the chromosomes can segregate diagonally (*arrows*). As a result, six different gametes can be produced, four of which are unbalanced and can result in congenital abnormalities.

FIGURE 6-8. Structural abnormalities of human chromosomes. The **deletion** of a portion of a chromosome leads to the loss of genetic material and a shortened chromosome. A **reciprocal translocation** involves breaks on two nonhomologous chromosomes, with exchange of the acentric segments. An **inversion** requires two breaks in a single chromosome. If the breaks are on opposite sides of the centromere, the inversion is **pericentric;** it is **paracentric** if the breaks are on the same arm. A **robertsonian translocation** occurs when two nonhomologous acrocentric chromosomes break near their centromeres, after which the long arms fuse to form one large metacentric chromosome. **Isochromosomes** arise from faulty centromere division, which leads to duplication of the long arm (iso q) and deletion of the short arm, or the reverse (iso p). **Ring chromosomes** involve breaks of both telomeric portions of a chromosome, deletion of the acentric fragments and fusion of the remaining centric portion.

subsequent divisions. As in reciprocal translocations, a robertsonian translocation is balanced if there is no loss of genetic material. The carrier is also usually phenotypically normal but may be infertile because a robertsonian translocation can reduce the number of chromosomes, which are then asymmetrically segregated during meiosis. If a carrier is fertile, however, his or her gametes may produce unbalanced translocations, in which case offspring may have congenital malformations.

Robertsonian translocations of chromosomes 13 and 14 are most common and are seen in about 1 in 1000 newborns. A robertsonian translocation of chromosome 21 imparts a significantly greater risk of having a child with Down/trisomy 21 syndrome. In this case, maternal transmission is more common than paternal.

Chromosomal Deletions

A deletion is loss of any portion of a chromosome. By definition, such chromosome alterations are unbalanced with the loss of one or multiple genes from within the deleted chromosome segment.

TABLE 6-2

FISH ANALYSIS FOR MICRODELETION SYNDROMES

Syndrome	DNA Probes	Chromosome Location	Abnormality Detected
1p36 microdeletion	p58/LSI 1q25	1p36/1q25	1p36 deletion
Wolf Hirschhorn	WHS/CEP4	4p16.3/cen 4	4p16.3 deletion
Cri du chat	D5S23/D5S721	5p15.2	5p15.2 deletion
Williams	ELN/D7S486	7q11.23/7q31	7q11.23 deletion
Prader-Willi	SNRPN/GARB3/D15S10	15q11–13	15q11.2 deletion
Angelman	SNRPN/GARB3/D15S10	15q11–13	15q11.2 deletion
Miller Dieker	LIS1/RARA	17p13.3/17q21.1	17p13.3 deletion
Smith Magenis	SMS/RARA	17p11.2/17p21.1	17p11.2 deletion
DiGeorge/velocardiofacial	HIRA/TUPLE1/ARSA/ N25	22q11.2/22q13	22q11.2 deletion
Kallmann	KAL/DXZ1	Xp22.3/cen X	Xp22.3 deletion
X-linked ichthyosis	STS/DXZ1	Xp22.3/cen X	Xp22.3 deletion
Sex reversal/ambiguous genitalia	SRY	Yp11.3	Yp11.3 deletion

FISH = fluorescence in situ hybridization.

Chromatid breaks during mitosis in somatic cells may generate chromosomal fragments that do not recombine with any other chromosome and are lost in subsequent cell divisions. Deletions may also result from unequal crossover during meiosis. Deletions of specific genes or chromosomal regions can be detected by FISH and such higher-resolution techniques as array comparative genomic hybridization (aCGH), which detects gene copy number variations related to ploidy. aCGH can help to profile whole genomes to detect very small or cryptic deletions in unidentified regions. These minute cryptic deletions, or microdeletions, involve definitive genes in specific chromosomes (Table 6-2). Several microdeletion syndromes have been characterized using unique sequence DNA probes for the specific gene involved, such as the ELN gene (elastin). Deletion of this gene in chromosome region 7q11.2, which leads to Williams syndrome, is too small to be detected by routine chromosome analysis. It is readily detected by FISH and aCGH (Table 6-2). Prader-Willi and Angelman syndromes entail microdeletions of the long arm of chromosome 15 (see below).

Chromosome deletions play a role in the pathogenesis of cancer, including several hereditary forms. Familial **retinoblastomas** are associated with deletions in the long arm of chromosome 13 containing the RB1 gene locus at 13q14.1-q14.2.

People with chromosome 11 deletions may have **Wilms tumor aniridia syndrome** (WAGR), which includes Wilms tumor, aniridia, genitourinary malformations and mental retardation. The gene specific for WAGR syndrome, WT1, is a tumor suppressor gene in region 11p13.

Chromosomal Inversions

In chromosomal inversions, a chromosome breaks at two points and a segment inverts and then reattaches. **Pericentric inversions** result from breaks on opposite sides of the centromere and include the centromere; **paracentric inversions** involve breaks on the same arm of the chromosome and do not involve the centromere region (Fig. 6-8). During meiosis, crossing over of segments in homologous chromosomes that carry inversions does not occur as readily as in normal chromosomes, owing to formation of inversion loops. Inversions are usually benign because no genetic material is lost, but during meiosis when loops are formed, gametes with duplication or deficiency of genetic material may arise. In most cases, however, inversions are inherited with no phenotypic consequences. Up to 1% of all people have the most common inversion, a small pericentric inversion of chromosome 9 [inv(9)(p11q12)]. This classic benign inversion is considered a normal polymorphism in most families.

Ring Chromosomes

Ring chromosomes are rare. They form by breaks involving both telomeric ends of a chromosome, deletion of the acentric (without a centromere) fragments and end-to-end fusion of the remaining centric portion of the chromosome (Fig. 6-8). If the ring contains a centromere, it is usually somewhat stable. However, because of its abnormal shape, it may be lost during meiotic cell division. Any phenotype depends primarily on the amount of genetic material lost because of the break. The chromosome abnormality is often of no consequence. However, ring chromosomes have been reported in patients with epilepsy (chromosome 20); mental retardation and dysmorphic facies (chromosomes 13 and 14); mental retardation, dwarfism and microcephaly (chromosome 15); and Turner syndrome (chromosome X).

Isochromosomes

Isochromosomes are formed by faulty centromere division. Normally, centromeres divide in a plane parallel to a chromosome's long axis, to give two identical hemichromosomes.

If, instead, a centromere divides in a plane transverse to the long axis, pairs of isochromosomes result (Fig. 6-8). One pair contains the short arms bound to the upper part of the centromere and the other has the long arms with the lower part of the centromere.

The most important clinical condition involving isochromosomes is **Turner syndrome:** 15% of those affected have an isochromosome of chromosome X. Thus, a woman with a normal X chromosome and an isochromosome made of long arms of the X chromosome is monosomic for all genes on the missing short arm because the other isochromosome was lost during meiotic division. She also has 3 copies of the genes on the long arm. The absence of the genes from the short arm leads to abnormal development and Turner syndrome.

The Causes of Numerical Chromosome Abnormalities Are Obscure

Several terms help in understanding developmental defects with abnormal chromosome numbers:

- **Haploid:** A single set of each chromosome (23 in humans). Normally, only germ cells have a haploid number (n) of chromosomes.
- **Diploid:** A double set of each of the chromosomes (46 in humans). Somatic cells have a diploid number (2n) of chromosomes.
- **Euploid:** Any multiple (from n to 8n) of the haploid number of chromosomes. For example, many normal liver cells have 2 times (4n) the diploid DNA content of somatic cells and so are euploid or, more specifically, tetraploid. If the multiple is greater than 2n (i.e., greater than diploid), the karyotype is **polyploid**.
- **Aneuploid:** Karyotypes that are not exact multiples of the haploid number. Many cancer cells are aneuploid, which often corresponds to aggressive cell division (see Chapter 5).
- **Monosomy:** Absence in a somatic cell of one chromosome of a homologous pair. Thus, in Turner syndrome, there is a single X chromosome (45,X).
- **Trisomy:** Presence of an extra copy of a normally paired chromosome. For example, in Down syndrome, there are three chromosomes 21 (47,XX,+21).

Genesis of Numerical Aberrations

The causes of chromosomal aberrations are obscure. Exogenous factors, such as radiation, viruses and chemicals, can affect mitotic spindles or DNA synthesis, disturb mitosis and meiosis and cause breakage in human chromosomes, all of which increase risk of chromosome alteration. Changes in chromosome numbers arise primarily from nondisjunction, which occurs more commonly in maternal and paternal gametes of older people.

Nondisjunction

Nondisjunction is failure of paired chromosomes or chromatids to separate and move to opposite poles of the spindle at anaphase, during mitosis or meiosis. This leads to aneuploidy if only one pair of chromosomes fails to separate. It results in polyploidy if the entire set does not divide and all the chromosomes are segregated into a single daughter cell. Aneuploidy due to nondisjunction in somatic cells leads to one daughter cell with trisomy (2n + 1) and the other with monosomy (2n − 1) for the affected chromosome pair. Aneuploid germ cells have two copies of the same chromosome (n + 1) or lack the affected chromosome entirely (n − 1).

Chromosomal Aberrations at Various Stages of Pregnancy

Chromosomal abnormalities identified in liveborn infants at birth differ from those in early spontaneous abortions. At birth, the common chromosomal abnormalities are trisomies 21 (most frequent), 18, 13 and X or Y (47,XXX; 47,XXY; and 47,XYY). About 0.3% of all infants have a chromosomal abnormality. The most common chromosomal abnormalities in spontaneous abortions are, in descending order of frequency, 45,X, then trisomies 16, 21 and 22. However, trisomy of almost any chromosome occurs in spontaneous abortions. *Up to 35% of spontaneous abortions have a chromosomal abnormality.* The reason for these differences is presumably related to survival in utero. Very few fetuses with 45,X survive to term, and trisomy 16 is nearly always lethal in utero. A fetus with trisomy 21 has a better chance of surviving to birth.

Effects of Chromosomal Aberrations

Most major chromosomal abnormalities are incompatible with life. They are usually lethal to a developing conceptus and cause early death and spontaneous abortion. Embryos with significant loss of genetic material (e.g., autosomal monosomies) rarely survive pregnancy. Even though X chromosome monosomy (45,X) may be compatible with life, more than 95% of such embryos are lost during pregnancy. Absence of an X chromosome in male fetuses (45,Y) invariably leads to early abortion.

Autosomal trisomies lead to developmental abnormalities. Affected fetuses usually die during pregnancy or shortly after birth. Trisomy 21, which causes Down syndrome, is an exception, and people with Down syndrome survive for years. X chromosome trisomy may result in abnormal development but is not lethal.

Mitotic nondisjunction in embryonic cells early in development results in **mosaicism,** in which chromosomal aberrations are transmitted in some cell lineages but not others. *The body thus has two or more karyotypically different cell lines.* Mosaicism may involve autosomes or sex chromosomes, and the phenotype depends on the chromosome involved and the extent of mosaicism. Autosomal mosaicism was once thought to be rare but probably occurs fairly frequently, and mosaicism involving sex chromosomes is common. Aneuploidy and mosaicism of sex chromosomes are the most important causes of infertility and/or abnormal development. Phenotypes in patients with mosaicism depend on the ratio of abnormal to normal cells and are more severe when the proportion of abnormal cells is higher.

Nomenclature of Chromosomal Aberrations

According to the International System for Human Cytogenetic Nomenclature (Table 6-3), structural and numerical chromosomal abnormalities are classified by:

1. Total number of chromosomes
2. Designation (number) of affected chromosomes
3. Nature and location of the defect on the chromosome

TABLE 6-3
CHROMOSOMAL NOMENCLATURE

Numerical designation of autosomes	1–22
Sex chromosomes	X, Y
Addition of a whole or part of a chromosome	+
Loss of a whole or part of a chromosome	−
Numerical mosaicism (e.g., 46/47)	/
Short arm of chromosome (petite)	p
Long arm of chromosome	q
Isochromosome	i
Ring chromosome	r
Deletion	del
Insertion	ins
Translocation	t
Derivative chromosome (carrying translocation)	der
Terminal	ter

Representative Karyotypes

Male with trisomy 21 (Down syndrome)	47,XY, +21
Female with robertsonian translocation between chromosomes 14 and 21	45,XX,t(14;21) (q10;q10)
Cri du chat syndrome (male) with deletion of a portion of the short arm of chromosome 5	46,XY, del(5p)
Male with ring chromosome 19	46,XY, r(19)
Turner syndrome with monosomy X	45,X
Mosaic Klinefelter syndrome	47,XXY/46,XY

TABLE 6-4
CLINICAL FEATURES OF THE AUTOSOMAL CHROMOSOMAL SYNDROMES[a]

Syndromes	Features
Trisomic Syndromes	
Chromosome 21 (Down syndrome 47,XX or XY, +21)	Epicanthic folds, speckled irides, flat nasal bridge, congenital heart disease, simian crease of palms, Hirschsprung disease, increased risk of leukemia
Chromosome 18 (47,XX or XY, +18)	Female preponderance, micrognathia, congenital heart disease, horseshoe kidney, deformed fingers
Chromosome 13 (47,XX or XY, +13)	Persistent fetal hemoglobin, microcephaly, congenital heart disease, polycystic kidneys, polydactyly, simian crease
Deletion Syndromes	
5p– syndrome (cri du chat 46,XX or XY, 5p–)	Cat-like cry, low birth weight, microcephaly, epicanthic folds, congenital heart disease, short hands and feet, simian crease
11p– syndrome (46,XX or XY, 11p–)	Aniridia, Wilms tumor, gonadoblastoma, male genital ambiguity
13q– syndrome (46,XX or XY, 13q–)	Low birth weight, microcephaly, retinoblastoma, congenital heart disease

[a]All of these syndromes are associated with mental retardation.

CHROMOSOMAL SYNDROMES

Structural alterations that may result in clinical disorders include trisomies, translocations, deletions and chromosomal breakage (Tables 6-3 and 6-4).

Trisomy 21: Down Syndrome

Trisomy 21 is the most common cause of mental retardation. Liveborn infants represent only a fraction of all conceptuses with this defect, as 2/3 abort spontaneously or die in utero. Advances in treating infections, congenital heart defects and leukemia—the leading causes of death in Down syndrome—have increased life expectancy of patients with trisomy 21.

 **EPIDEMIOLOGY:** *The incidence of trisomy 21 rises dramatically with increasing maternal age: older mothers are at increased risk to have children with Down syndrome* (Fig. 6-10). Up to the mid-30s, a woman's risk of giving birth to a trisomic child is about 1 in 300–900 liveborn infants. By age 45, the incidence is 1 in 25. Nevertheless, 80% of children with Down syndrome are born to mothers under 35, perhaps because women in this age group conceive more often and are not usually screened. The risk of a second child with Down syndrome is comparable to the normal population's risk, regardless of maternal age, unless the syndrome is associated with translocation of chromosome 21.

Karyotypes are described sequentially by:

1. Total number of chromosomes
2. Sex chromosome complement
3. Any abnormality

Addition of chromosomal material, either an entire chromosome or a portion, is indicated by a plus sign (+) before the number of the affected chromosome. A minus sign (−) denotes loss of part or all of a chromosome. Deletion of part of a chromosome is designated by **del,** followed by the location of the deleted material on the affected chromosome. Translocations, deletions and duplications may all cause clinical disorders (Table 6-3).

Defining chromosome alterations in patients can be a complicated process. For example, multiple cell lines with different chromosome abnormalities may arise in patients with aggressive cancers. It is important to distinguish primary from secondary alterations to determine which genes are driving the disease and should be targeted for therapy.

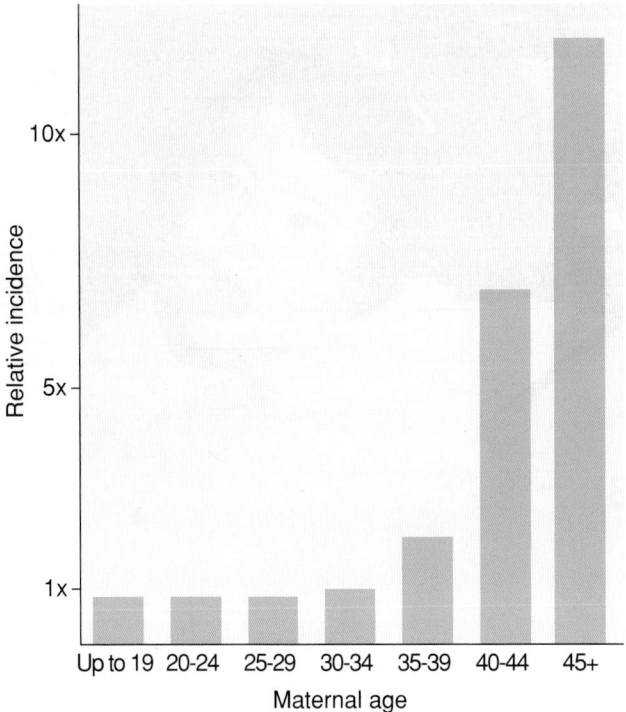

FIGURE 6-10. Incidence of Down syndrome in relation to maternal age. A conspicuous increase in the frequency of this disorder is seen beyond the age of 35 years.

MOLECULAR PATHOGENESIS: Chromosome 21 is the smallest human autosome, containing less than 2% of all human DNA. It is an acrocentric chromosome, and all known functional genes (except ribosomal RNA genes) are on the long arm (21q). It is estimated that chromosome 21 contains 200–250 genes. Studies of inherited translocations, in which only part of chromosome 21 is duplicated, suggest that the region responsible for the full Down syndrome phenotype is in band 21q22.2, a 4-Mb region of DNA, called the **Down syndrome critical region** (DSCR). Genes in DSCR implicated in Down syndrome are designated as DSCR1, DSCR2 and so forth.

Mechanisms explain how 3 copies of DSCR genes occur in somatic cells:

- **Nondisjunction** in the first meiotic division of gametogenesis (meiosis I) accounts for the majority (92%–95%) of patients with trisomy 21. The extra chromosome 21 is maternal in about 95% of such cases. Virtually all maternal nondisjunction seems to occur in meiosis I.
- **Translocation** of an extra long arm of chromosome 21 to another acrocentric chromosome accounts for 5% of cases.
- **Mosaicism** for trisomy 21 is caused by nondisjunction during mitosis of a somatic cell early in embryogenesis (2%).

How maternal age increases the risk of bearing a child with trisomy 21 is poorly understood. The maternal age effect is related to maternal nondisjunction events, usually during maternal meiosis I. Down syndrome due to translocation or mosaicism is not related to maternal age.

Down syndrome caused by translocation of an extra portion of chromosome 21 occurs in two situations. Either parent may be a phenotypically normal carrier of a balanced translocation, or a translocation may arise de novo during gametogenesis. These translocations are typically robertsonian,

tending to involve only acrocentric chromosomes, with short arms consisting of a satellite and stalk (chromosomes 13, 14, 15, 21 and 22). Translocations between these chromosomes are particularly common because they cluster during meiosis and are liable to break and recombine more than other chromosomes. The most common translocation in Down syndrome (50%) is fusion of the long arms of chromosomes 21 and 14, designated rob(14;21)(q10;q10), followed in frequency (40%) by similar fusion involving two chromosomes 21, rob(21;21)(q10;q10).

If the translocation is inherited from a parent, a balanced translocation has been converted to an unbalanced one (Fig. 6-7B shows an example of this involving chromosomes 4 and 12). Then, one would expect a 1 in 3 chance of Down syndrome among offspring of a carrier of a balanced robertsonian translocation. However, early loss of most embryos with trisomy 21 means that the actual incidence is only 10%–15% with a maternal translocation and less than 5% if the father is the carrier.

  PATHOLOGY AND CLINICAL FEATURES: Down syndrome is ordinarily diagnosed at birth based on the infant's flaccid state and characteristic appearance. Diagnoses are confirmed by cytogenetics or FISH analyses. Over time, a typical constellation of abnormalities appears (Fig. 6-11).

- **Mental status:** Children with Down syndrome are invariably mentally retarded; their average IQ is usually 30–60. With stimulation programs, such children can graduate high school and work at paid jobs. Some attend postsecondary school. Still, many Down syndrome children have severe mental disability. Their cognitive skills decrease as they grow older and they are at higher risk for Alzheimer disease.
- **Craniofacial features:** Face and occiput tend to be flat, with a low-bridged nose, reduced interpupillary distance and oblique palpebral fissures. Epicanthal folds of the eyes impart an Asian appearance, which accounts for the obsolete term **mongolism**. Irides are speckled with **Brushfield spots**. Ears are enlarged, low set and malformed. A prominent tongue, typically lacking a central fissure, protrudes through an open mouth.
- **Heart:** One third of children with Down syndrome have cardiac malformations. The incidence is even higher in aborted fetuses. Anomalies include atrioventricular canal, ventricular and atrial septal defects; tetralogy of Fallot; and patent ductus arteriosus (see Chapter 17).
- **Skeleton:** These children tend to be small, owing to shorter than normal bones of the ribs, pelvis and extremities. Their hands are broad and short with a "simian crease," a single transverse crease across the palm. The middle phalanx of the fifth finger is hypoplastic and curves inward.
- **Gastrointestinal (GI) tract:** Duodenal stenosis or atresia, imperforate anus and Hirschsprung disease (megacolon) occur in 2%–3% of these children (see Chapter 19).
- **Reproductive system:** Men are invariably sterile, owing to arrested spermatogenesis. A few women with Down syndrome have given birth to children, 40% of which had trisomy 21.
- **Immune system:** Affected children are unusually susceptible to respiratory and other infections, although there is no clear pattern of immune defects.

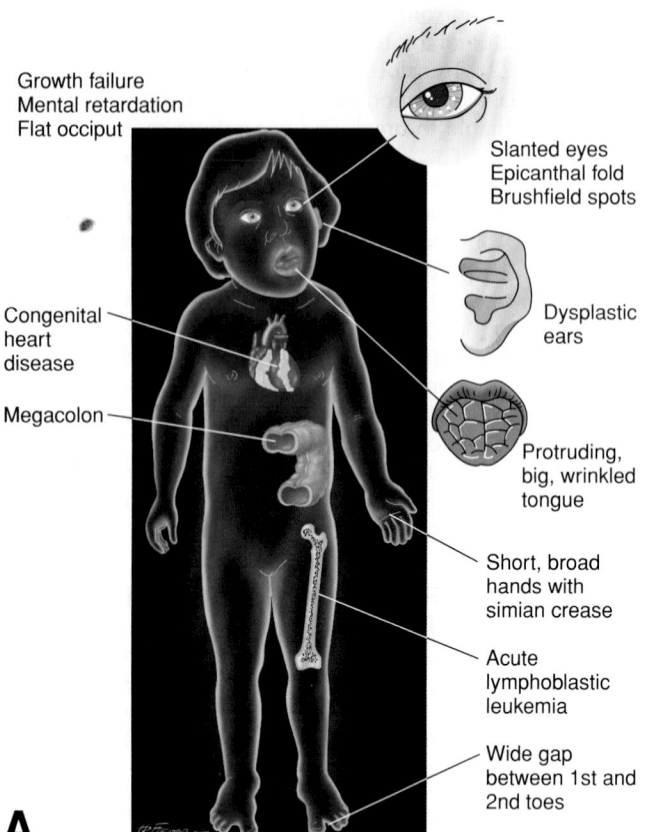

A

Growth failure
Mental retardation
Flat occiput

Slanted eyes
Epicanthal fold
Brushfield spots

Dysplastic
ears

Congenital
heart
disease

Megacolon

Protruding,
big, wrinkled
tongue

Short, broad
hands with
simian crease

Acute
lymphoblastic
leukemia

Wide gap
between 1st and
2nd toes

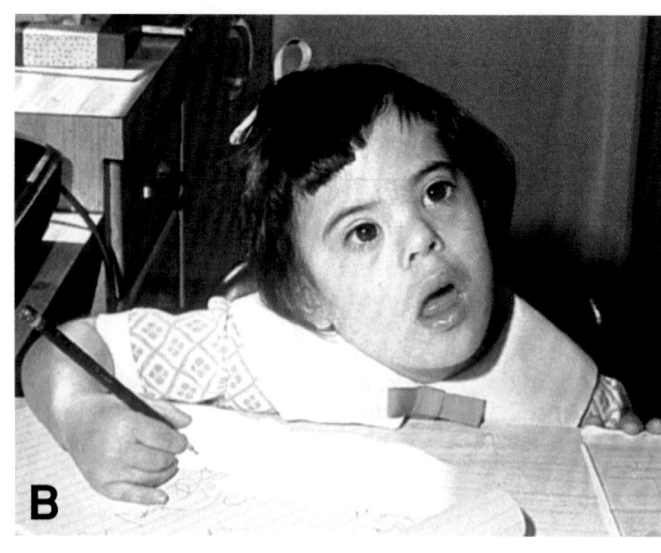

B

FIGURE 6-11. A. Clinical features of Down syndrome. **B.** A young girl with the facial features of Down syndrome.

■ **Hematologic disorders:** Patients with Down syndrome have a particularly high risk of developing leukemia at all ages. *The risk of leukemia in Down syndrome children under 15 years is 10–20-fold higher than normal.* In children under 4 years of age, acute myeloid leukemia (AML) predominates. Therapy for these children is less intensive than standard AML therapy, and outcomes are generally good. Down syndrome children over 4 years of age with AML have a significantly worse prognosis and usually receive standard AML regimens. In older individuals, leukemias are usually acute lymphoblastic leukemias. The basis for the high incidence of leukemia is unknown, but leukemoid reactions (transient pronounced neutrophilia) are common in newborns with Down syndrome.

■ **Neurologic disorders:** There is no clear pattern of neuropathology in Down syndrome, nor are there characteristic changes on the electroencephalogram. Nevertheless, electrophysiologic properties and other parameters are altered in cultured neurons from infants with Down syndrome. *The association of Down syndrome with Alzheimer disease* has been known for more than half a century. By age 35, characteristic Alzheimer lesions are universal in these patients, including granulovacuolar degeneration, neurofibrillary tangles, senile plaques and loss of neurons (see Chapter 32). Senile plaques and cerebral blood vessels in both Alzheimer disease and Down syndrome always contain β-amyloid protein. These similarities are mirrored in the appearance of dementia in 1/4 to 1/2 of older patients with Down syndrome and progressive loss of intellectual functions beyond that attributable to mental retardation alone. Alzheimer disease causes the sharp decline in survival in Down syndrome subjects over 45 years of age.

Only about 25% live to be more than 60 years old, and most have Alzheimer disease.

■ **Life expectancy:** In the first decade of life, the presence or absence of congenital heart disease largely determines survival in Down syndrome. Only 5% of those with normal hearts die before age 10, but 1/4 of those with heart disease die by then. Life expectancy in patients who reach age 10 is about 55 years, which is 20 years or more lower than that of the general population. Only 10% reach age 70.

Trisomy of Chromosomes 18 and 13

Trisomy 18, or Edwards syndrome, occurs in 1 of 3000–8000 live births and is the second most common autosomal trisomy syndrome. It causes mental retardation and affects females 3 times more often than males. Virtually all infants with trisomy 18 have severe cardiac malformations and survival of a few months is rare. Other anomalies include clenched hands with overlap of fingers, intrauterine growth retardation (IUGR), rocker bottom feet, micrognathia, prominent occiput, micro-ophthalmia, low-set ears and renal anomalies. Given the severe anomalies, about 95% abort spontaneously. About 50% of trisomy 18 patients die within 1 week, and 90% die within a year. Risk of bearing a fetus with trisomy 18 is higher in women older than 35 years. This trisomy may occur as a mosaic with more moderate phenotypic expression.

Trisomy 13, or Patau syndrome, is rare. It occurs in 1 in 20,000–25,000 births and is associated with severe mental and growth retardation. Significant malformations include cleft lip and cleft palate, plus severe nervous system and cardiac malformations. This syndrome is also associated with increased maternal age. Trisomy 21, trisomy 18 and trisomy 13 are the only known trisomies in liveborn infants.

Chromosomal Deletion Syndromes Almost Always Involve Deletion of Parts of One or More Chromosomes

Deletion of an entire autosomal chromosome (i.e., monosomy) is usually not compatible with life. However, several syndromes arise from deletions of parts of several chromosomes (Tables 6-2 and 6-4). Most of these congenital syndromes are sporadic, but in a few instances, reciprocal translocations occur in the parents. Virtually all of these deletion syndromes have phenotypes including low birth weight, mental retardation, microcephaly and craniofacial and skeletal abnormalities. Cardiac and urogenital malformations are also common.

- **5p– syndrome (cri du chat):** This is the best-known deletion syndrome, because the high-pitched cry of the infant is like that of a kitten and calls attention to the disorder. It features intellectual disability and delayed development, microcephaly, low birth weight and hypotonia in infancy. These patients also have distinctive facial features, with widely set eyes (hypertelorism), low-set ears, a small jaw and a rounded face. Some are born with heart defects. Most cases are sporadic; reciprocal translocations occur in 10%–15% of the parents. The size of the 5p deletions varies among affected individuals; larger deletions tend to cause more severe intellectual disability and developmental delay. Loss of a specific gene, *CTNND2*, on the short arm of chromosome 5 is associated with severe intellectual disability in some people with this condition.
- **Microdeletion syndromes:** These syndromes are characterized by small deletions (<5 Mb) of a chromosomal segment spanning contiguous multiple disease genes that contribute independently to the phenotype. High-resolution karyotyping (2–5 Mb) rarely detects such microdeletions, but FISH using probes for the critical deleted interval can make the diagnosis. Selected microdeletion syndromes and their respective chromosome deletions are listed in Tables 6-2 and 6-4.
- **Deletions and rearrangements of telomeric/subtelomeric sequences:** Telomeres are specialized protein–DNA complexes at the ends of chromosomes (see Chapter 5) that prevent chromosomal degradation and end-to-end fusion. Telomeric DNA has 3–20 kb of TTAGGG repeats. *Subtelomeres,* segments of DNA adjacent to telomeric caps, are rich in genes. Deletions and rearrangements of these regions, demonstrated by FISH, are major causes of mild to severe mental retardation and dysmorphic features.

Translocation Syndromes May Cause Partial Trisomies

The prototypical translocation that causes partial trisomy is Down syndrome, but many other partial trisomies are known. The best documented is 9p trisomy, in which the short arm of chromosome 9 may be translocated to one of several autosomes. Many kindreds with this syndrome have been described. Carriers of a balanced chromosome 9 translocation are asymptomatic but may pass an unbalanced

translocation to their offspring. The disorder is characterized by mental retardation, microcephaly and other craniofacial abnormalities.

A reciprocal translocation between the long arms of chromosomes 11 and 22 is the most common translocation in the general population. Offspring of carriers may have an extra chromosome with parts of both 11 and 22, and so may have partial trisomy of both chromosomes, leading to microcephaly and other anomalies.

Chromosomal Breakage Syndromes Typically Show Autosomal Recessive Inheritance

These include xeroderma pigmentosum, Bloom syndrome, ataxia telangiectasia and Fanconi anemia (constitutional aplastic pancytopenia). These disorders are characterized by defects in DNA repair or genomic instability. Affected patients show increased predisposition to cancer (see Chapters 5 and 26), and their cells exhibit elevated chromosomal breakage or instability, leading to chromosomal rearrangements. Fortunately, these breakage syndromes are relatively rare, but they occur in high rates in specific ethnic groups.

Numerical Aberrations of Sex Chromosomes Usually Cause Less Severe Clinical Syndromes Than Aberrations in Autosomes

The reasons are not entirely clear, but additional sex chromosomes (Fig. 6-12) cause less severe clinical manifestations than do extra autosomes and are less likely to disturb critical stages of development. Additional X chromosomes probably cause less severe phenotypes because of **lyonization,** a normal process in which each cell only has one active X chromosome.

The contrast between the X and Y chromosomes is striking: the X chromosome is one of the larger chromosomes, containing about 2000 genes, but the much smaller Y chromosome has only 78 genes, one of which is the testis-determining gene (*SRY*). About 95% of the human Y chromosome is unable to recombine; only the tip of the Y chromosome, called the **pseudoautosomal region,** recombines with the X chromosome. The rest of the Y chromosome is passed on to the next generation relatively intact. For this reason, the Y chromosome is used for investigating male human evolution.

The Y Chromosome

In humans, genes on the Y chromosome are key determinants of gender phenotype. Thus, people who are XXY (Klinefelter syndrome; see below) have a male phenotype, and those who are XO (Turner syndrome) are female. The intronless SRY gene near the end of the short arm of the Y chromosome at Yp11.3 encodes a transcription factor that belongs to the SOX (SRY-like box) gene family of DNA-binding proteins. It is the therian testis determining factor (TDF), also called the **sex-determining region Y protein** or **SRY protein,** that initiates male sex determination. Mutations in *SRY* lead to XY females, while translocations that add *SRY* to an X chromosome produce XX males.

A small proportion of infertile men with azoospermia or severe oligospermia have small deletions in parts of the Y chromosome. The sizes and locations of these deletions vary and do not correlate with the severity of spermatogenic failure.

Gametes Sperm / Ovum	X	Y	XY	O
X	46,XX Normal ♀ 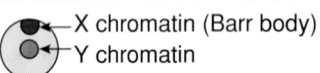	46,XY Normal ♂	47,XXY Klinefelter ♂	45,X Turner ♀
XX	47,XXX ♀	47,XXY Klinefelter ♂	48,XXXY Klinefelter ♂	46,XX Normal ♀
XXX	48,XXXX ♀	48,XXXY Klinefelter ♂	49,XXXXY Klinefelter ♂	47,XXX Triple X ♀
O	45,X Turner ♀	45,Y LETHAL	46,XY LETHAL	44 LETHAL

● ←X chromatin (Barr body)
◉ ←Y chromatin

FIGURE 6-12. Numerical aberrations of sex chromosomes. Nondisjunction in either the male or female gamete is the principal cause of these abnormalities.

The X Chromosome

Males carry only one X chromosome but have the same amount of X chromosome gene products as do females. This seeming discrepancy is explained by the **Lyon effect:**

- In females, one X chromosome is irreversibly inactivated early in embryogenesis and is detectable in interphase nuclei as a clump of heterochromatin attached to the inner nuclear membrane, the **Barr body**. The inactive X chromosome is extensively methylated at gene control regions and transcriptionally repressed. Nevertheless, a significant minority of X-linked genes escape inactivation and continue to be expressed by both X chromosomes. The probability that an X chromosome is inactive seems to correlate with levels of *XIST*, an X-linked non-protein-coding RNA gene expressed only by the inactive partner.
- Either the paternal or maternal X chromosome is inactivated randomly.
- Inactivation of the X chromosome is virtually complete.
- X chromosome inactivation is permanent and transmitted to progeny cells, so paternally or maternally derived X chromosomes are propagated clonally. *All females are thus mosaic for paternal and maternal X chromosomes.* Mosaicism in females for glucose-6-phosphate dehydrogenase was key in demonstrating the monoclonal origin of neoplasms (see Chapter 5).

The issue is not quite so simple, however. If one X chromosome is entirely nonfunctional, individuals with XXY (Klinefelter) or XO (Turner) karyotypes should be phenotypically normal. They are not, which indicates that inactivated X chromosomes still function, at least in part. Indeed, a part of the X chromosome short arm is known to escape inactivation. This pseudoautosomal region can pair with a homologous region on the short arm of the Y chromosome and undergo meiotic recombination. Genes in this location are present in two functional copies in both males and females. Thus, patients with Turner syndrome (45,X) are haploinsufficient for these genes, and those with more than two X chromosomes (e.g., Klinefelter patients) have more than two functional copies. A gene in this region, *SHOX*, is associated

with height, and its haploinsufficiency in Turner syndrome may explain the short stature of Turner patients. Extra copies of *SHOX* may explain the increased stature in other sex chromosome aneuploidy conditions such as 47,XXX; 47,XYY; 47,XXY; 48,XXYY; and so forth. Several other genes outside the pseudoautosomal region also escape X inactivation. *Mental retardation in phenotypic boys and girls with extra X chromosomes correlates roughly with the number of X chromosomes.*

Klinefelter Syndrome (47,XXY)

In Klinefelter syndrome, males have a Y chromosome plus 2 more X chromosomes. This is the most important clinical condition involving trisomy of sex chromosomes (Fig. 6-13). It is a prominent cause of male hypogonadism and infertility.

MOLECULAR PATHOGENESIS: Most men with Klinefelter syndrome (80%) have one extra X chromosome (47,XXY). A minority are mosaics (46,XY/47,XXY) or have more than two X chromosomes (48,XXXY). *Regardless of the number of supernumerary X chromosomes (even up to 4), the Y chromosome ensures a male phenotype.* Additional X chromosomes correlate with more abnormal phenotypes, despite inactivation of the extra X chromosomes. Presumably, the same genes that escape inactivation in normal females are functional in Klinefelter syndrome.

Klinefelter syndrome occurs in 1 per 1000 male newborns, about the incidence of Down syndrome. Interestingly, half of all 47,XXY conceptuses are miscarried. The additional X chromosome(s) results from meiotic nondisjunction during gametogenesis. In half of cases, nondisjunction in paternal meiosis I leads to sperm with both X and Y chromosomes. Fertilization of a normal egg by such a sperm yields a 47,XXY karyotype.

PATHOLOGY: After puberty, the intrinsically abnormal testes do not respond to gonadotropin stimulation and show later regressive changes.

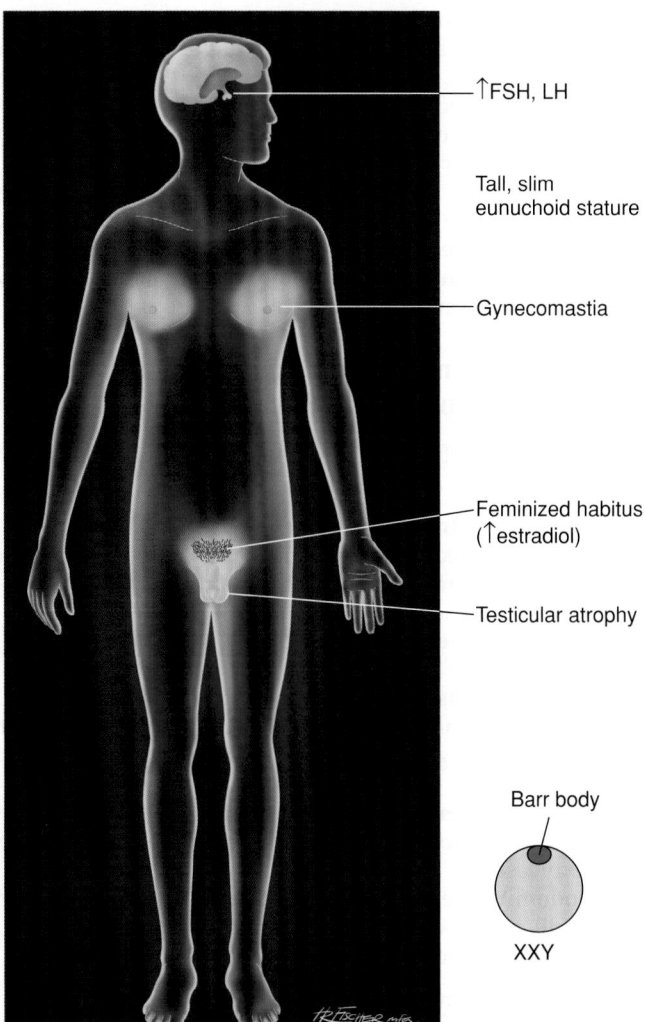

↑FSH, LH

Tall, slim eunuchoid stature

Gynecomastia

Feminized habitus (↑estradiol)

Testicular atrophy

Barr body

XXY

FIGURE 6-13. Clinical features of Klinefelter syndrome. *FSH* = follicle-stimulating hormone; *LH* = leuteinizing hormone.

Seminiferous tubules display atrophy, hyalinization and peritubular fibrosis. Germ cells and Sertoli cells are usually absent and the tubules become dense cords of collagen. Leydig cells are usually increased in number and are functionally impaired, as evidenced by low testosterone levels in the face of elevated luteinizing hormone (LH) levels.

 CLINICAL FEATURES: The diagnosis of Klinefelter syndrome is usually made after puberty, since the main manifestations of the disorder during childhood are behavioral and psychiatric. Gross mental retardation is uncommon, but average IQ is probably somewhat reduced. As the syndrome is so common, it should be suspected in all boys with some mental deficiency and/or severe behavioral problems.

Children with Klinefelter syndrome tend to be tall and thin, with relatively long legs (eunuchoid body habitus). Normal testicular growth and masculinization do not occur at puberty, and testes and penis remain small. Feminine characteristics include a high-pitched voice, gynecomastia and a female pattern of pubic hair (female escutcheon). Azoospermia results in infertility. These changes reflect hypogonadism and a resulting lack of androgens. Serum testosterone

is low to normal, but LH and FSH are quite high, indicating normal pituitary function. High circulating estradiol levels increase the estradiol-to-testosterone ratio, which determines the degree of feminization. Treatment with testosterone will virilize these patients but does not restore fertility.

The XYY Male

Interest in the XYY phenotype (1 in 1000 male newborns) comes from studies suggesting that this karyotype is significantly more prevalent in male prisoners than in the general population. However, the idea that XYY "supermales" show antisocial behavior because of an extra Y chromosome has not been substantiated and the topic remains controversial. Acknowledged features of the XYY phenotype are tall stature, a tendency toward cystic acne and some problems in motor and language development. Y chromosome aneuploidy results from meiotic nondisjunction in the father.

Turner Syndrome

Turner syndrome is the spectrum of abnormalities that derives from **complete or partial X chromosome monosomy in a phenotypic female**. It occurs in 1 in 5000 females. In 3/4 of cases, the single X chromosome is of maternal origin, suggesting that the meiotic error tends to be paternal. The incidence of Turner syndrome does not correlate with maternal age, and the risk of producing a second affected female infant is not increased.

The 45,X karyotype is one of the most common aneuploids in human conceptuses, but almost all are aborted spontaneously. As Turner patients survive normally after birth, it is unclear why the missing X chromosome is lethal during fetal development. It is believed that homologs of Y genes in the pseudoautosomal region of the X chromosome escape inactivation and are critical for survival of female embryos.

About half of Turner patients lack an entire X chromosome (monosomy X). The remainder are mosaics or have structural X chromosome aberrations, such as isochromosome of the long arm, translocations and deletions. Mosaics with a 45,X/46,XX karyotype tend to have a milder phenotype and may even be fertile. In about 5% of patients, the mosaic karyotype is 45,X/46,XY, in which case an original male zygote was subsequently modified by a mitotic nondisjunction. Such individuals have a 20% risk of developing a germ cell cancer and should have prophylactic removal of the abnormal gonads.

  PATHOLOGY AND CLINICAL FEATURES: The clinical hallmarks of Turner syndrome are sexual infantilism with primary amenorrhea and sterility (Fig. 6-14). The disorder is usually discovered when absence of menarche brings the child to medical attention. Virtually all of these women are under 5 ft (152 cm) tall. Other clinical features include a short, webbed neck (pterygium coli); low posterior hairline; wide carrying angle of the arms (cubitus valgus); broad chest with widely spaced nipples; and hyperconvex fingernails. Half of patients have renal anomalies, the most common being horseshoe kidney and malrotation. Many have facial abnormalities, including a small mandible, prominent ears and epicanthal folds. Defective hearing and vision are common, and up to 20% may be mentally retarded. Pigmented nevi

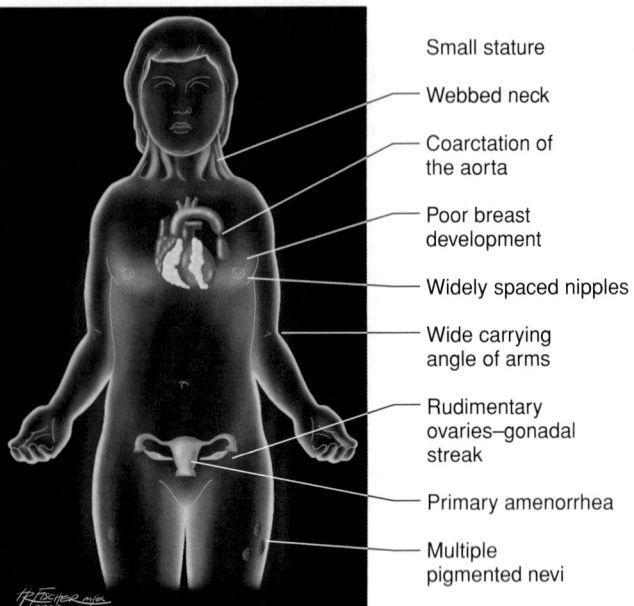

FIGURE 6-14. Clinical features of Turner syndrome.

become prominent with age. For unknown reasons, women with Turner syndrome are at a greater risk for chronic autoimmune thyroiditis and goiter.

Cardiovascular anomalies occur in almost half of Turner patients: coarctation of the aorta in 15% and a bicuspid aortic valve in up to 1/3. Essential hypertension occurs in some patients, and dissecting aneurysm of the aorta may occasionally cause death.

Ovaries of women with Turner syndrome show a curious acceleration of normal aging. Normal female fetal ovaries initially contain 7 million oocytes each, less than half of which survive until birth. Relentless loss of oocytes continues, so that by menarche only about 5% (400,000) remain. At menopause 0.1% survive. Ovaries of fetuses with Turner syndrome contain oocytes at first but lose them rapidly. None remain by 2 years of age. The ovaries become fibrous streaks, but the uterus, fallopian tubes and vagina develop normally. Thus, menopause in children with Turner syndrome may be considered to occur long before menarche.

Interestingly, there are families in which several women develop menopause prematurely and show deletions of portions of the long arm of one X chromosome. These data, with observations of Turner syndrome, further support the idea that genes controlling ovarian development and function in the inactivated X chromosome continue to be expressed in normal females.

Children with Turner syndrome are treated with growth hormone and estrogens and enjoy an excellent prognosis for a normal, albeit infertile, life.

Syndromes in Females with Multiple X Chromosomes

One extra X chromosome in a phenotypic female (i.e., a 47,XXX karyotype) is the most frequent abnormality of sex chromosomes in women. It occurs at about the same rate as Klinefelter syndrome. Most of these women are of normal intelligence but may have some difficulty in speech, learning and emotional responses. Minor physical

anomalies are seen, such as epicanthal folds and clinodactyly (inward curvature of the fifth finger). These women are usually fertile, but their children are more susceptible to congenital defects.

Women with four and five X chromosomes have also been reported. Virtually all have been mentally retarded. They superficially resemble women with Down syndrome and do not mature sexually. Women with supernumerary X chromosomes have additional Barr bodies, indicating inactivation of all but one X chromosome. Clearly, some genes on inactivated X chromosomes are still expressed.

Single-Gene Abnormalities Confer Traits That Segregate Sharply within Families

The classic laws of mendelian inheritance, named in honor of Gregor Mendel, are:

- **A mendelian trait** is determined by two copies of the same gene, called alleles, situated at the same locus on two homologous chromosomes. In the case of the X and Y chromosomes in males, a trait is determined by just one allele.
- **Autosomal genes** are those located on one of the 22 autosomes.
- **Sex-linked traits** are encoded by loci on the X chromosome.
- **A dominant phenotypic trait** requires only one allele of a homologous gene pair and is expressed whether the allelic genes are homozygous or heterozygous.
- **A recessive phenotypic trait** demands that both alleles be identical (i.e., homozygous) in order for the phenotype to be expressed.
- In **codominance,** both alleles in a heterozygous gene pair are fully expressed and contribute to the phenotype (e.g., the AB blood group genes).

Mendelian traits are classified as:

1. **Autosomal dominant**
2. **Autosomal recessive**
3. **Sex-linked dominant**
4. **Sex-linked recessive**

Diseases due to sex-linked dominant genes are rare and of little practical significance.

Mutations

To make proteins, DNA is transcribed into RNA, which is processed into mRNA. This, in turn, is translated into protein by ribosomes. Changes in DNA can lead to corresponding changes in the amino acid sequence of its encoded protein or to interference with its synthesis.

A mutation is a stable heritable change in DNA. The consequences of mutations are highly variable. Some have no functional consequences, but others are lethal and so are not transmitted to the next generation. Between these extremes is a broad range of DNA changes that account for the genetic diversity of any species. *About 1 in 1000 base pairs is polymorphic in the human genome,* and evolution is based on the accumulation over time of such nonlethal mutations that alter the ability of a species to adapt to its environment. The genetics of human disease focuses on mutations that impair protein function detectably. The major types of mutations (Fig. 6-15) are:

- **Point mutations** occur when one base replaces another. If it is in the coding region (the part of the gene that is

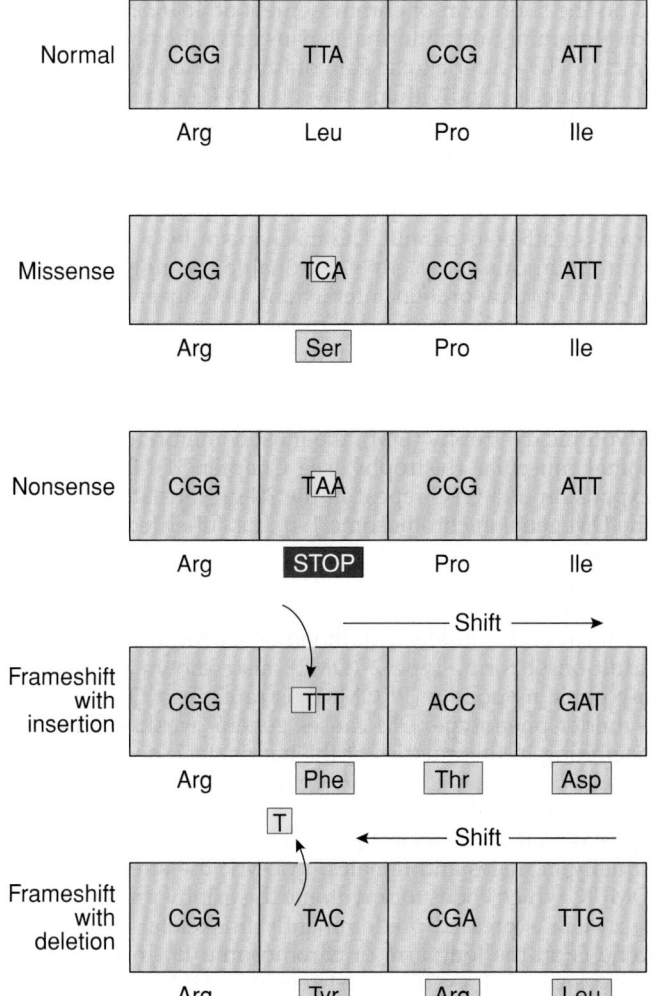

FIGURE 6-15. Point mutations that alter the reading frame of DNA. A variety of mutations in the second codon of a normal sequence of four amino acids is depicted. With a missense mutation, a change from T to C substitutes serine (Ser) for leucine (Leu). With a nonsense mutation, a change from T to A converts the leucine codon to a stop codon. A shift in the reading frame to the right results from insertion of a T, thus changing the sequence of all subsequent amino acids. Conversely, deletion of a T shifts the reading frame one base to the left and also changes the sequence of subsequent amino acids. *Arg* = arginine; *Asp* = aspartate; *Ile* = isoleucine; *Phe* = phenylalanine; *Pro* = proline; *Thr* = threonine; *Tyr* = tyrosine.

translated into a protein), a point mutation has three possible consequences:

1. A **synonymous mutation** occurs when the altered codon still encodes the same amino acid. For example, CGA and CGC both code for arginine.
2. A **missense mutation** (three fourths of base changes in the coding region) occurs when the new codon codes for a different amino acid. In sickle cell anemia, an adenine-to-thymine change in the β-globin gene replaces glutamic acid (GAG) with valine (GUG).
3. A **nonsense mutation** (4%) stops translation; that is, a codon for an amino acid is changed to a termination codon, yielding a truncated protein. For example, TAT codes for tyrosine, but TAA is a stop codon.

- **Frameshift mutations:** Amino acids are encoded by trinucleotide sequences. If the number of bases in a gene is changed by insertion or deletion, and if the number of bases added or lost is not a multiple of 3, *the reading frame of the message is changed.* Then, although the downstream sequence is the same, it will encode a different amino acid sequence and an unscheduled termination signal. Frameshift mutations can also alter transcription, splicing or mRNA processing.
- **Large deletions:** When a large segment of DNA is deleted, the coding region of a gene may be entirely removed, in which case the protein product is absent. A large deletion may also appose coding regions of nearby genes, giving rise to a fused gene that yields a hybrid protein in which part or all of one protein is followed by part or all of another.
- **Expansion of unstable trinucleotide repeat sequences:** The human genome contains many tandem trinucleotide repeats, some of which are associated with disease. The number of copies of some such repeats varies among individuals, representing allelic polymorphism of the genes in which they are found. As a rule, the number of repeats below a particular threshold does not change during mitosis or meiosis; but above this threshold, the number of repeats can contract or, more commonly, expand. A number of distinct trinucleotide expansions have been identified in human disease (Table 6-5).

Identification of a family of genetic diseases resulting from expansion of trinucleotide repeats has generated a new molecular category of disease. The number of these

TABLE 6-5					
REPRESENTATIVE DISEASES ASSOCIATED WITH TRINUCLEOTIDE REPEATS					
Disease	**Location**	**Sequence**	**Normal Length**	**Premutation**	**Full Mutation**
Huntington disease	4p16.3	CAG	10–30	—	40–100
Kennedy disease	Xq21	CAG	15–25	—	40–55
Spinocerebellar ataxia	6p23	CAG	20–35	—	45–80
Fragile X syndrome	Xq27.3	CGG	5–44	50–200	200–1000
Myotonic dystrophy	19q13	CTG	5–35	37–50	50–2000
Friedreich ataxia	9q13	GAA	7–30	—	120–1700

repeats increases with each successive generation, as does the severity of the disease and a younger age at onset. This mechanism is known as **genetic anticipation**. Most trinucleotide repeat diseases result from expansions of a CAG codon, which encodes glutamine, in the open reading frame of the gene, resulting in polyglutamine tracts in the protein product. All of these disorders are associated with neuronal degeneration.

Fragile X Syndrome: Loss of Protein Function

The prototypic trinucleotide repeat disease is fragile X syndrome (FXS), in which the number of trinucleotide CGG repeats is increased. It is transmitted as an X-linked dominant trait with variable penetrance and is *the most common cause of inherited mental retardation*. Expansion of the CGG trinucleotide repeat affects the fragile X mental retardation 1 (FMR1) gene on the X chromosome, causing failure to express the fragile X mental retardation protein (FMRP) that is required for normal neural development. Depending on the length of the CGG repeat, an allele may be classified as normal (unaffected by the syndrome; 5–44 CGG repeats), a premutation (considered to be 50–200 repeats) or full mutation (affected by the syndrome, with >200 CGG repeats). A definitive diagnosis of fragile X syndrome is made through genetic testing to determine the number of CGG repeats. Testing for premutation carriers can also be performed for genetic counseling purposes.

The abnormal repeat is also associated with an inducible "fragile site" on the X chromosome, which appears as a nonstaining gap or an apparent chromosomal break at region Xq23.1 (Fig. 6-16). The phenotype includes slow intellectual development and physical abnormalities, such as an elongated face and prominent ears.

FXS occurs in about 1 in 3600 males and 1 in 4000–6000 females. Although CGG repeat expansion accounts for over 98% of cases, FXS can also occur as a result of point mutations affecting the FMR1 gene.

Huntington Disease

Huntington disease (HD) is the most common genetic cause of chorea. It is also associated with abnormalities of muscle coordination and psychomotor and cognitive functions. The disease, transmitted as an autosomal dominant trait, is caused by expansion of a CAG repeat within the HTT/IT15 gene, which encodes the protein **huntingtin**. The HTT gene

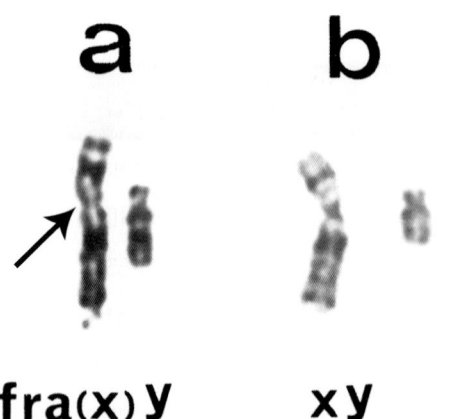

FIGURE 6-16. Fragile X chromosome. The arrow shows the nonstaining gap at Xq23.1.

is on the short arm of chromosome 4 at 4p16.3. CAG codes for glutamine and abnormal expansion of the polyglutamine tract in HD confer a toxic gain of function to huntingtin.

Unaffected individuals have 10–26 CAG repeats, while those affected by the disease have 36 or more. In 3% of cases, a new HD mutation can occur by further expansion of CAG in offspring of individuals with a premutation between 27 and 35 repeats. In 97% of these, the HD mutation is inherited from an affected parent. The mechanism by which mutant huntingtin causes selective neuronal loss is not known, but altered protein–protein interactions have been implicated. Expanded CAG repeats determine several other neurodegenerative disorders in addition to HD (Table 6-5).

Myotonic Dystrophy

Myotonic dystrophy (DM), the most common form of autosomal muscular dystrophy (see Chapter 31), is caused by expansion of a CTG repeat in the 3′-untranslated region of the DM gene on chromosome 19q. It is inherited as an autosomal dominant trait.

Two types of myotonic dystrophy exist. Type 1 (DM1), also known as Steinert disease, has a severe congenital form and a milder childhood-onset form as well as an adult-onset form. Type 2 (DM2), also known as proximal myotonic myopathy (PROMM), is rarer than DM1 and has a milder phenotype. DM causes general weakness, usually beginning in the muscles of the hands, feet, neck or face. It slowly progresses to involve other muscle groups, including the heart. DM affects a wide variety of other organ systems as well. It occurs in 1 per 7000–8000 people worldwide, equally in males and females. In DM1, the affected gene is DMPK, which codes for myotonic dystrophy protein kinase, a protein expressed predominantly in skeletal muscle. The gene is on the long arm of chromosome 19. In DM1, there is expansion of a CTG triplet repeat in *DMPK*. Individuals with 5–37 repeats are considered normal, while those with 38–49 repeats are considered to have a premutation and are at risk of having children with further expanded repeats and thus symptomatic disease. People with more than 50 repeats are usually symptomatic. Longer repeats are associated with earlier onset and more severe disease.

DM2 is caused by a defect of the *ZNF9* gene on chromosome 3 between 3q13.3-q24. ZNF9 protein is believed to be an RNA-binding protein. The specific defect is a repeat of the CCTG tetranucleotide in the *ZNF9* gene. Thus, DM2 is not a trinucleotide repeat disorder, but rather a tetranucleotide repeat disorder. The repeat expansion for DM2 is much larger than for DM1, ranging from 75 to over 11,000 repeats. Unlike DM1, the size of the repeated DNA expansion in DM2 does not appear to make a difference in the age of onset or disease severity. In both cases, prenatal diagnosis is now available with molecular testing for the tri- and tetranucleotide repeats.

Friedreich Ataxia

Friedrich ataxia (FA) is an autosomal recessive degenerative disease associated with expansion of a GAA repeat. It affects the CNS and is also characterized by cardiomyopathy and type 2 diabetes. FA is the most common inherited ataxia, affecting 1 in 50,000 people in the United States, with males and females affected equally. The estimated carrier prevalence is 1 in 110. Because the defect is in an intron (which is removed from the mRNA transcript between transcription and translation), abnormal frataxin (FXN) protein is not produced. Instead, it causes gene silencing and loss of function of the frataxin gene protein product (see Chapter 32). Affected individuals have 200–1700 repeats in the first intron of the FXN gene.

Functional Consequences of Mutations

A biochemical pathway represents the sequential actions of a series of enzymes, which are encoded by specific genes. A typical pathway can be represented by the conversion of a substrate (A) through intermediate metabolites (B and C) to a final product (D).

$$A \rightarrow B \rightarrow C \rightarrow D$$
initial　　intermediary　end-products
substrate　　metabolites

A single gene defect can have several consequences:

- **Failure to complete a metabolic pathway:** The end-product (D) is not formed since an enzyme needed to complete a metabolic sequence is missing:

$$A \rightarrow B \rightarrow C - // \rightarrow (D) (\downarrow)$$

An example of failure to complete a metabolic pathway is **albinism,** a pigment disorder caused by a deficiency of tyrosinase. Tyrosinase converts tyrosine to melanin (via intermediate formation of dihydroxyphenylalanine [DOPA]). Without tyrosinase, the melanin end-product is not formed, and an affected person (an "albino") has no pigment in all organs that normally contain it, primarily the eyes and skin.

- **Accumulation of unmetabolized substrate:** The enzyme that converts the initial substrate to the first intermediary metabolite may be missing, so the initial substrate accumulates in excess.

$$A (\rightarrow)^- // \rightarrow (B) (\downarrow) (C) (\downarrow) (D) (\downarrow)$$

Thus, in **phenylketonuria,** an inborn deficiency of phenylalanine hydroxylase causes dietary phenylalanine to accumulate and reach toxic concentrations that interfere with postnatal brain development and cause severe mental retardation.

- **Storage of an intermediary metabolite:** An intermediary metabolite, which is normally quickly processed into the final product and so is usually present only in minute amounts, accumulates in large quantities if the enzyme for its metabolism is lacking.

$$A \rightarrow B(\rightarrow)^- \rightarrow // \rightarrow C (\downarrow) D (\downarrow)$$

This type of genetic disorder is exemplified by glycogen storage disease type I (GSD I), a glycogen storage disease due to a deficiency of glucose-6-phosphatase. The inability to convert glucose-6-phosphate into glucose leads to its alternative conversion to glycogen.

- **Formation of an abnormal end-product:** A mutant gene encodes an abnormal protein. In sickle cell anemia, valine replaces glutamate in β-globin.

Mutation Hotspots

Certain regions of the genome mutate at a much higher rate than average. These hotspots are usually DNA sequences with inherent instability. They have an increased tendency toward unequal crossing over, or may be predisposed to

FIGURE 6-17. **5-Methylcytosine is formed from cytosine.** Spontaneous deamination of 5-methylcytosine produces thymine.

single nucleotide substitutions. The best-characterized hotspot is the dinucleotide CG or CpG sites. These sites are regions of DNA where a cytosine nucleotide occurs next to a guanine in the linear sequence of bases along its length. "CpG" is shorthand for "—C—PO_4—G—" (i.e., C and G separated by a PO_4); phosphate links any two nucleosides together in DNA.

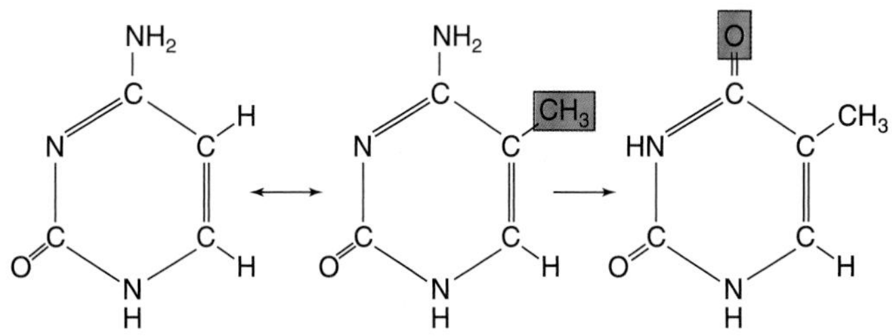

The Cs in CpG dinucleotides can be methylated to 5-methylcytosine. In mammals, CpG methylation may alter the gene's transcription. Such *epigenetic* changes affect gene expression by mechanisms other than changes in DNA base sequence (see Chapter 5). CpG methylation commonly represses gene expression. Such 5-methylcytosines can undergo spontaneous deamination to thymine (Fig. 6-17). If this occurs in a gamete, it can become a fixed, heritable trait in the offspring.

Regions of the genome that have higher concentrations of CpGs are known as **CpG islands**. Many mammalian genes have CpG islands in their promoter regions. CpG methylation within promoters regions may, for example, silence tumor suppressor genes in malignancies (see Chapter 5). By contrast, hypomethylation of CpG sites is associated with overexpression of oncogenes in cancer cells.

Copy Number Variation

The term "copy number variation" (CNV) is a genetic change that results in an abnormal number of copies of one or more regions of DNA. It involves sequences over 1000 base pairs in length but less than 5 megabases. CNVs can arise from duplications, deletions, translocations and inversions. Roughly 12% of human genomic DNA shows CNVs.

CNVs can affect a single gene or a contiguous set of genes. They can lead to too many or too few copies of dosage-sensitive genes, which may account for significant phenotypic variability, complex behavioral traits and disease susceptibility.

There are two types of CNVs. The first category, called copy number polymorphisms (CNPs), is relatively common in the general population, with an overall frequency of greater than 1%. CNPs are typically small (most are less than 10 kilobases in length). The second class of CNVs consist of relatively rare variants that are much longer than CNPs, ranging from hundreds of thousands of base pairs to over 1 million base pairs in length. They are also called microdeletions and microduplications, and are believed to arise during gametogenesis. They have been observed disproportionately in patients with mental retardation, developmental delay, schizophrenia and autism, leading to speculation that large, rare CNVs may be more important in neurocognitive diseases than other forms of inherited mutations.

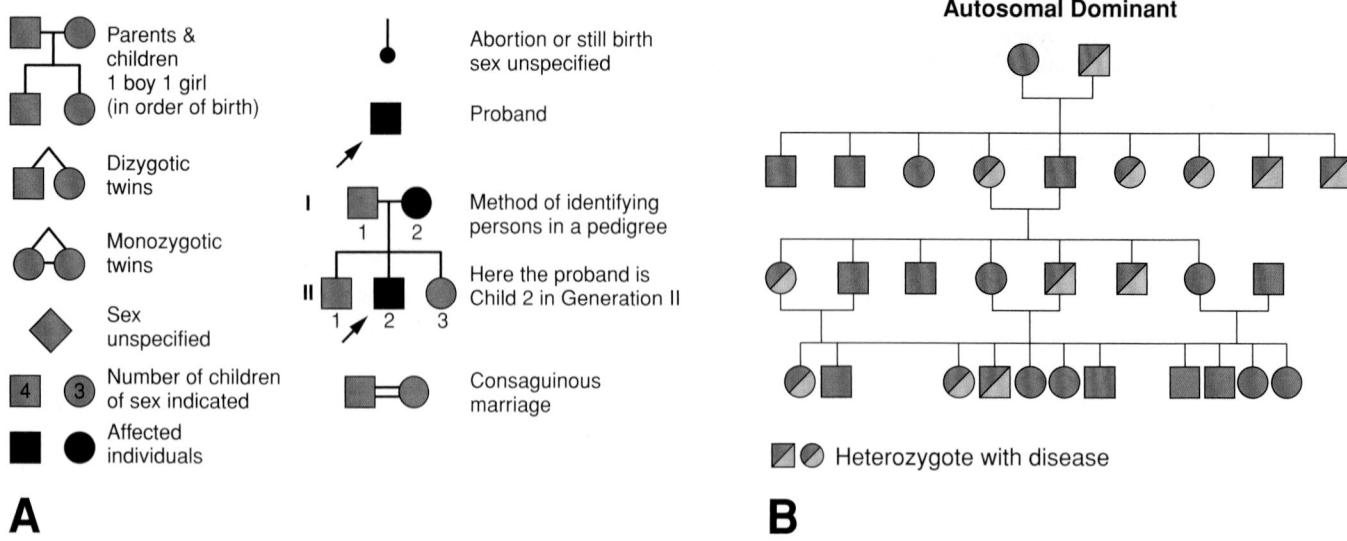

FIGURE 6-18. A. Definition of symbols in a pedigree. Males = squares; females = circles. A line drawn between a square and a circle represents a mating of that male and female. Two lines drawn between a square and a circle indicate a consanguineous mating in which the two individuals are related, usually as second cousins. Children of a mating are connected to a horizontal line, called the sibship line, by short vertical lines. The children of a sibship are always listed in order of birth, the oldest being on the left. Other conventions concerning twins and identification of probands and affected individuals are shown in the figure. **B. Autosomal dominant inheritance.** Only symptomatic individuals transmit the trait to the next generation, and heterozygotes are symptomatic. Both males and females are affected.

AUTOSOMAL DOMINANT DISORDERS ARE EXPRESSED IN HETEROZYGOTES

If only one mutated allele is sufficient to cause disease when its paired allele on the homologous autosome is normal, the mutant trait is considered to be dominant. The features of autosomal dominant traits are (Fig. 6-18):

- Males and females are affected equally, as the mutant gene is on an autosome. Thus, father-to-son transmission (which is absent in X-linked disorders) may occur.
- The trait encoded by the mutant gene can be transmitted to successive generations (unless reproductive capacity is compromised).
- Unaffected members of a family do not transmit the trait to their offspring. Unless the disease represents a new mutation, everyone with the disease has an affected parent.
- Proportions of normal and diseased offspring of patients with the disorder are about equal, since most affected people are heterozygous, and their normal mates do not carry the defective gene.

New Mutations versus Inherited Mutations

As noted above, autosomal dominant diseases may result from a new mutation rather than transmission from an affected parent. Nevertheless, offspring of patients with a new dominant mutation have a 50% risk for the disease. *With autosomal dominant disorders, the ratio of new mutations to transmitted ones varies with the effect of the disease on fertility.* The more a disease impairs reproduction, the greater the proportion of affected people who represent new mutations. A dominant mutation causing 100% infertility would have to be a new mutation. If reproductive capacity is only partly impaired, the proportion of new mutations is lower. Thus, in **tuberous sclerosis,** an autosomal dominant condition in which mental retardation limits reproductive potential, new

mutations account for 80% of cases. If a dominant disease has little effect on fertility (e.g., familial hypercholesterolemia), virtually all affected people will have pedigrees showing classic vertical transmission of the disorder.

Biochemical Basis of Autosomal Dominant Disorders

There are several major mechanisms by which a single mutant allele may cause disease even when the other allele is normal.

- If the gene product is rate limiting in a complex metabolic network (e.g., a receptor or an enzyme), having half of the normal amount of gene product may be insufficient for a normal phenotype. This is known as **haploinsufficiency.** For example, familial hypercholesterolemia is caused by inadequate low-density lipoprotein (LDL) uptake receptors on hepatocytes.
- In some diseases, the presence of an extra copy of an allele gives rise to a phenotype. An example of this is Charcot-Marie-Tooth disease type IA, which is caused by duplication of the peripheral myelin protein-22 gene.
- A mutant protein may be insensitive to normal regulation. For example, mutations in the *RET* proto-oncogene in families with multiple endocrine neoplasia type 2 increase activity of a tyrosine kinase that stimulates cell proliferation.
- Mutations in genes for structural proteins (e.g., collagens, cytoskeletal constituents) cause abnormal molecular interactions and disrupt normal morphologic patterns. Such a situation is exemplified by osteogenesis imperfecta and hereditary spherocytosis.

More than 1000 human diseases are inherited as autosomal dominant traits, although most are rare. Examples of human autosomal dominant diseases are shown in Table 6-6.

TABLE 6-6
REPRESENTATIVE AUTOSOMAL DOMINANT DISORDERS

Disease	Frequency	Chromosome
Familial hypercholesterolemia	1/500	19p
von Willebrand disease	1/8000	12p
Hereditary spherocytosis (major forms)	1/5000	14, 8
Hereditary elliptocytosis (all forms)	1/2500	1, 1p, 2q, 14
Osteogenesis imperfecta (types I–IV)	1/10,000	17q, 7q
Ehlers-Danlos syndrome (all types)	1/5000	2q
Marfan syndrome	1/5000	15q
Neurofibromatosis type 1	1/3500	17q
Huntington chorea	1/15,000	4p
Retinoblastoma	1/14,000	13q
Wilms tumor	1/10,000	11p
Familial adenomatous polyposis	1/10,000	5q
Acute intermittent porphyria	1/15,000	11q
Hereditary amyloidosis	1/100,000	18q
Adult polycystic kidney disease	1/1000	16p

Inherited Connective Tissue Diseases Are Often Autosomal Dominant Traits

This discussion is limited to three of the most common and best-studied diseases of connective tissue: Marfan syndrome, Ehlers-Danlos syndrome and osteogenesis imperfecta. Even in these well-delineated disorders, clinical phenotypes often overlap. Thus, some patients in a family may develop the joint dislocations typical of Ehlers-Danlos syndrome, while others suffer from multiple fractures characteristic of osteogenesis imperfecta, and still others, with the same genetic defect, may have no symptoms. Thus, current classifications based on clinical criteria will eventually be replaced by references to specific gene defects, as with the hemoglobinopathies.

Marfan Syndrome

Marfan syndrome is an autosomal dominant disorder of connective tissue affecting many organs, including the heart, aorta, skeleton, eyes and skin. Fifteen to 30% are de novo mutations occurring once in 20,000 live births. Marfan syndrome affects males and females equally and shows no ethnic or geographical bias. About 1 in 3000–5000 individuals have Marfan syndrome.

 MOLECULAR PATHOGENESIS: The cause of Marfan syndrome is a missense mutation in the gene for *fibrillin-1 (FBN1)*, on the long arm of chromosome 15 (15q21.1). **Fibrillins** are a family of collagen-like connective tissue proteins. There are now about a dozen genetically

distinct fibrillins, and over 100 mutations are known. They are present in many tissues, in the form of **microfibrils,** thread-like filaments that form larger fibers and are organized into rods, sheets and interlaced networks. These fibers are scaffolds for elastin deposition during embryonic development, after which they remain as a component of elastic tissues (e.g., elastin is deposited on lamellae of microfibrillar fibers in the concentric rings of elastin in the aortic wall). Abnormal microfibrillar fibers can be visualized by immunofluorescent microscopy in all tissues affected in Marfan syndrome.

Fibrillin-1 is a large, cysteine-rich glycoprotein that forms 10-nm microfibrils in the extracellular matrix of many tissues. Interestingly, the ciliary zonules that suspend the lens of the eye are devoid of elastin but consist almost exclusively of fibrillin. Dislocation of the lens is characteristic of Marfan syndrome.

Deficiencies in the amount and distribution of microfibrillar fibers occur in skin, which renders the elastic fibers incompetent to resist normal stress. Fibrillin also binds to transforming growth factor-β (TGF-β), a multifunctional protein that regulates cell proliferation and is upregulated in a variety of inflammatory diseases (see Chapters 2, 4 and 5). Patients with Marfan syndrome have increased TGF-β in their aortas, cardiac valves and lungs, possibly because of decreased fibrillin-1, which normally sequesters this cytokine. Treating fibrillin-1–deficient mice with a TGF-β antagonist decreases the severity of their "Marfan phenotype," suggesting a potential therapeutic approach in this disease that does not directly target the genetic mutation.

 PATHOLOGY AND CLINICAL FEATURES: People with Marfan syndrome are usually (but not always) tall, with greater lower body length (pubis to sole) than upper body length. They are slender in habitus reflecting a paucity of subcutaneous fat and have long, thin extremities and fingers (arachnodactyly/spider fingers) (Fig. 6-19).

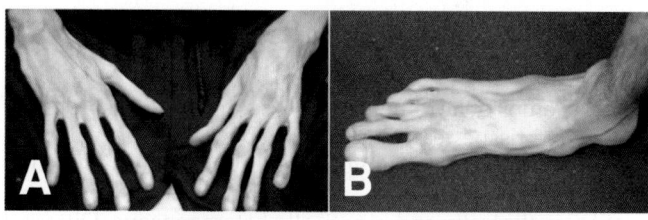

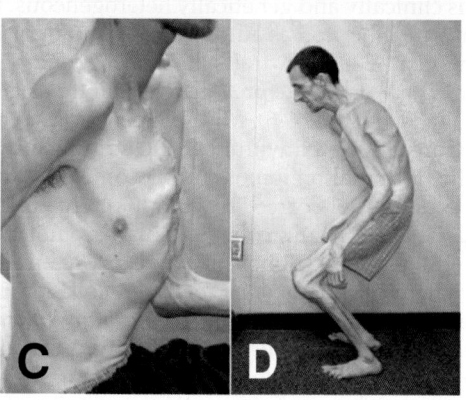

FIGURE 6-19. Features of Marfan syndrome. A, B. Long, slender digits (arachnodactyly). **C, D.** Tall slender build with disproportionately long arms, legs, fingers and toes and a breastbone that protrudes outward or dips inward.

- **Skeletal system:** The skull in Marfan syndrome is usually long (dolichocephalic), with prominent frontal eminences. Disorders of the ribs causing pectus excavatum (concave sternum) and pectus carinatum (pigeon breast) are conspicuous. Tendons, ligaments and joint capsules are weak, leading to hyperextensibility of the joints (double-jointedness), dislocations, hernias and often severe kyphoscoliosis.
- **Cardiovascular system:** *The most important defect is in the aorta, where the tunica media is weak.* This leads to variable dilation of the ascending aorta and a high incidence of dissecting aneurysms, usually of the ascending aorta. These may rupture into the pericardial cavity or extend down the aorta and rupture into the retroperitoneal space. Dilation of the aortic ring results in aortic regurgitation, which may be severe enough to produce angina pectoris and congestive heart failure. The mitral valve typically has redundant leaflets and chordae tendineae—leading to mitral valve prolapse syndrome (see Chapter 16). Patients most often die of cardiovascular disorders.

  The aorta shows marked fragmentation and loss of elastic fibers, with increased metachromatic mucopolysaccharide, which may accumulate in discrete pools. These features are sometimes called cystic medial necrosis of the aorta. Smooth muscle cells are enlarged and lose their orderly circumferential arrangement.
- **Eyes:** Ocular changes are common in Marfan syndrome. These include dislocation of the lens (ectopia lentis), severe myopia due to elongation of the eye and retinal detachment.

Untreated men with Marfan syndrome usually die in their 30s, and untreated women often die in their 40s. There is no cure, but life expectancy has increased significantly over the past few decades and now approaches that of the average person. Antihypertensive therapy and replacement of the ascending aorta and aortic valve with prosthetic grafts have significantly improved longevity.

Ehlers-Danlos Syndromes

Ehlers-Danlos syndromes (EDSs) are inherited disorders of connective tissue featuring remarkable hyperelasticity and fragility of the skin, joint hypermobility and often a bleeding diathesis.

EDS is clinically and genetically heterogeneous. Different forms may be inherited as autosomal dominant or recessive (autosomal or X-linked) traits depending on the specific mutation. The worldwide prevalence of all types is approximately 1 in 5000 (Table 6-6). Multiple genes on several chromosomes are associated with EDS, including the *ADAMTS2* gene at the terminal region of chromosome 5q. Procollagen cannot be processed correctly without an enzyme encoded by this gene. As a result, collagen fibrils are not assembled properly; they appear ribbon-like and disorganized. Cross-links, or chemical interactions, between collagen fibrils are also affected. *Whatever the underlying biochemical defect, the result is deficient or defective collagen.* Depending on the type of EDS, these molecular lesions are associated with conspicuous weakness of supporting structures of the skin, joints, arteries and viscera.

Classical EDS types 1 and 2 occur in 1 in 20,000–50,000 people. Both are autosomal dominant and affect types I and

V collagen. Type 1 EDS typically presents with severe skin involvement, but in type 2 disease, the skin is only mildly to moderately affected. More than 50% of classical EDS is caused by mutations in the *COL5A1* gene at 9q34.2-q34.3 and some by mutations in *COL5A2* at 2q14-q32. Mutations in *COL1A1* on chromosome 17q21.33 are also responsible for the classic types of EDS. These gene mutations cause significant changes in the structure of connective tissue, which elicits the characteristic features of the classic types of EDS.

Hypermobility EDS type 3 affects 1 in 10,000–15,000 and can be either autosomal dominant or autosomal recessive. Joint hypermobility and chronic musculoskeletal pain are the most prominent features of EDS type 3; skin manifestations are less severe. Mutations of *TNXB* located at 6p21.3 prevent production of tenascin-X protein, which disrupts the normal organization of collagen fibrils and elastic fibers and leads to hypermobility.

Vascular EDS type 4 affects 1 in 100,000–250,000 individuals. Vascular EDS patients exhibit characteristic facial features (small chin, thin nose and lips, sunken cheeks), slight body habitus and translucent skin, through which veins appear prominently. This form of EDS is more serious than other types because autosomal dominant mutations in *COL3A1* at 2q31 produce a defect in type III collagen, resulting in fragile blood vessels that are liable to rupture. About 25% of patients with EDS type 4 experience significant complications by age 20, and more than 75% have life-threatening problems before age 40.

EDS type 6 is rare and causes severe kyphoscoliosis, blindness from retinal hemorrhage or rupture of the globe, and death from aortic rupture. Mutations in the *PLOD1* gene at 1p36.22 cause type 6 EDS. Other very rare types include EDS type 8 characterized by severe periodontal disease and loss of teeth by the third decade, and EDS type 9 with skeletal deformities and bladder diverticula during childhood, with a danger of bladder rupture.

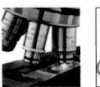 **PATHOLOGY AND CLINICAL FEATURES:** All types of EDS show soft, fragile, hyperextensible skin. Patients typically can stretch their skin many centimeters and trivial injuries can lead to serious wounds. Sutures do not hold well, so surgical incisions often dehisce (burst open). Joint hypermobility allows unusual extension and flexion (e.g., as in the "human pretzel" and other contortionists), which may lead to subluxation or dislocation of joints. EDS type 4 is the most dangerous variety, owing to a tendency of the large arteries, bowel and gravid uterus to spontaneously rupture. Death from such complications is common in the third and fourth decades of life.

Many people with clinical abnormalities suggesting EDS do not match any of the documented types of this disorder. Further characterization of such cases is likely to expand the classification of EDS.

Osteogenesis Imperfecta

Osteogenesis imperfecta (OI), or brittle bone disease, is a group of inherited disorders in which a generalized abnormality of connective tissue is expressed principally as fragility of bone. OI is inherited as an autosomal dominant trait, although rare cases are transmitted as autosomal recessives.

MOLECULAR PATHOGENESIS: *Genetic defects in the 8 types of OI are heterogeneous, but all affect type I collagen synthesis, helical structure or, rarely, other structural proteins in bone.* The genes most commonly involved are *COL1A1* and *COL1A2,* which are required to form mature type I collagen. Point mutations may disrupt the α-helical structure of type I collagen by converting glycines that occur at every third amino acid position into bulkier amino acids. Or, alterations in the C-terminus and certain deletions can disrupt formation of mature type I collagen fibrils. Some patients have no family history and represent founders resulting from a sporadic mutation. The combined incidence of all forms is 1 in 20,000 live births in the United States.

PATHOLOGY AND CLINICAL FEATURES:

- **Type I** OI is characterized by a normal appearance at birth, but fractures of many bones occur during infancy and at the time the child learns to walk. Such patients have been described as being as "fragile as a china doll." Children with type I OI typically have blue sclerae as the deficiency in collagen fibers makes sclerae translucent so that choroidal veins are visible. Fractures and fusion of the bones of the middle ear restrict their mobility and often cause hearing loss. Type I collagen is normal, but the quantity is reduced by half (haploinsufficiency).
- **Type II** OI is usually fatal in utero or shortly after birth. Affected infants have a characteristic facies and skeletal abnormalities. Those who are born alive usually die of respiratory failure within their first month. Abnormal forms of collagen are the result of glycine substitution.
- **Type III** OI causes progressive deformities. It is ordinarily detected at birth by the baby's short stature and misshapenness caused by fractures in utero. Dental defects and hearing loss are common. Unlike other OI types, type III is often inherited as an autosomal recessive trait.
- **Type IV** OI resembles type I, but sclerae are normal and the phenotype is more variable.

Neurofibromatosis

The neurofibromatoses include two distinct autosomal dominant disorders characterized by development of multiple neurofibromas, which are benign Schwann cell tumors of peripheral nerves. These disorders involve all cells derived from the neural crest, including melanocytes in addition to Schwann cells and endoneurial fibroblasts. Thus, type 1 includes disorders of pigmentation as well as neural tumors.

Neurofibromatosis Type I (von Recklinghausen Disease)

Neurofibromatosis type I (NF1) is characterized by (1) disfiguring neurofibromas, (2) areas of dark pigmentation of the skin (café au lait spots), (3) pigmented lesions of the iris (Lisch nodules), (4) freckles in the groin or axilla, (5) optic nerve gliomas and (6) skeletal abnormalities, including thinning of the cortices of long bones (Fig. 6-20). It is one of the more common autosomal dominant disorders, occurring once in 4000 people of all races. The *NF1* gene has a very high rate of mutation, and over 500 mutations are known. Half of cases are sporadic rather than familial. NF1 was first described in 1882 by von Recklinghausen, but references to it can be found as early as the 13th century.

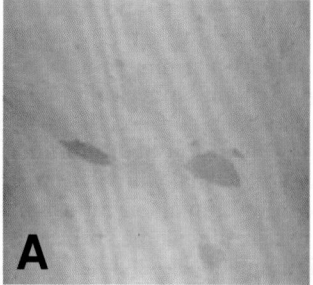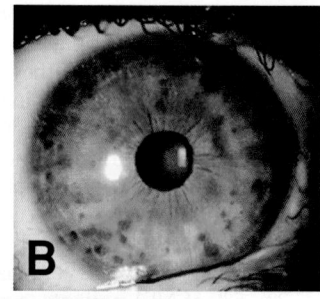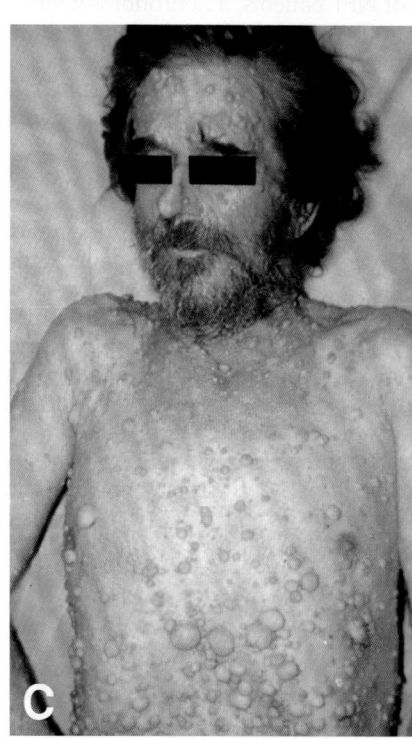

FIGURE 6-20. Features of neurofibromatosis type 1. A. Café au lait spots. **B.** Lisch nodules. **C.** Multiple cutaneous neurofibromas on the face and trunk.

MOLECULAR PATHOGENESIS: Germline mutations in the *NF1* gene, on the long arm of chromosome 17 (17q11.2), include deletions, missense mutations and nonsense mutations. The gene product, *neurofibromin,* belongs to a family of guanosine triphosphatase (GTPase)-activating proteins (GAPs), which inactivate the ras protein (see Chapter 5). In this sense, NF1 is a classic tumor suppressor. The loss of GAP activity permits uncontrolled ras activation, which greatly increases the risk of developing neoplasia in the form of neurofibromas. The high mutation rate for the *NF1* gene may reflect its large size (estimated to be 286 Kb). More than 250 mutations leading to protein truncation have been identified. The spontaneous mutation rate is 100 times greater than for many genes, and such mutations contribute to 30%–50% of neurofibromatosis cases. A more severe phenotype occurs in patients with complete gene deletion.

PATHOLOGY AND CLINICAL FEATURES: Clinical manifestations of NF1 are highly variable and include:

- **Neurofibromas:** Over 90% of patients with NF1 have cutaneous and subcutaneous neurofibromas by late childhood or adolescence. These tumors may exceed 500 and appear as soft, pedunculated masses, usually about 1 cm (Fig. 6-20). On occasion, however, they may reach alarming proportions (up to 25 cm) and dominate a patient's physical appearance. Subcutaneous neurofibromas are soft nodules along the course of peripheral nerves. **Plexiform neurofibromas** only occur in the context of NF1 and usually involve larger peripheral nerves or occasionally cranial or intraspinal nerves. Plexiform neurofibromas are often large, infiltrative tumors that cause severe disfigurement (see Chapter 32). In 3%–5% of NF1 patients, a neurofibrosarcoma will develop in a neurofibroma, usually a larger plexiform one. Other neurogenic tumors, such as meningiomas, optic gliomas and pheochromocytomas, occur more often in NF1.

- **Café au lait spots:** Although normal people may have occasional light brown patches on the skin, greater than 95% of people with NF1 have 6 or more such lesions. These are over 5 mm before puberty and exceed 1.5 cm thereafter (Fig. 6-20). Café au lait spots tend to be ovoid, with the longer axis parallel to a cutaneous nerve. Numerous freckles, particularly in the axilla, are also common.
- **Lisch nodules:** Over 90% of patients with NF1 have pigmented nodules of the iris. These are masses of melanocytes (Fig. 6-20) and are felt to be hamartomas.
- **Skeletal lesions:** Bone lesions occur frequently in NF1. These include malformations of the sphenoid bone and thinning of the cortices of the long bones, with bowing and pseudarthrosis of the tibia, bone cysts and scoliosis.
- **Mental status:** Mild, but not severe, intellectual impairment is common in NF1.
- **Leukemia:** The risk of myeloid leukemias in children with NF1 is 200–500 times normal. In some patients, both alleles of the NF1 gene are inactivated in leukemic cells.

Neurofibromatosis Type II (Central Neurofibromatosis)

NF2 is a syndrome defined by bilateral tumors of the eighth cranial nerve (acoustic neuromas) and, commonly, by meningiomas and gliomas. NF2 is much less common than NF1, occurring in 1 in 40,000–45,000 people. Most patients have bilateral acoustic neuromas, but the condition can be diagnosed if a unilateral eighth nerve tumor occurs with two or more of the following: neurofibroma, meningioma, glioma, schwannoma or juvenile posterior lenticular opacity.

 **MOLECULAR PATHOGENESIS:** Despite their superficial similarities, NF1 and NF2 are not variants of the same disease and have separate genetic origins. The *NF2* gene is on the long arm of chromosome 22 (22q,11.1-13.1). Unlike NF1, tumors in NF2 often show deletions or loss of heterozygous DNA markers in the affected chromosome. *NF2* encodes a tumor suppressor, **merlin** or **schwannomin,** a member of a superfamily of proteins that link the cytoskeleton to the cell membrane. This family also includes ezrin, moesin, radixin, talin and protein 4.1. Merlin is detectable in most differentiated tissues, including Schwann cells.

Achondroplastic Dwarfism

This is an autosomal dominant, hereditary disease of epiphyseal chondroblastic development that leads to inadequate enchondral bone formation (see Chapter 30). This distinctive form of dwarfism is characterized by short limbs with a normal head and trunk. Affected individuals have abnormal growth of the facial bones, which results in a small face, a bulging forehead and a deeply indented bridge of the nose. Achondroplastic dwarfism occurs once in 25,000 live births in all ethnic groups and is the most common type of short-limbed dwarfism.

 **MOLECULAR PATHOGENESIS:** Achondroplasia reflects mutations in the basic fibroblast growth factor receptor 3 gene (*FGFR3*) with 75% arising de novo owing to advanced paternal age. This inactivating mutation removes the negative regulatory activity of this receptor on bone growth, resulting in abnormal cartilage formation and increased osteogenesis. Achondroplasia is discussed in Chapter 30.

Familial Hypercholesterolemia

Familial hypercholesterolemia is an autosomal dominant disorder characterized by high levels of LDLs in the blood and cholesterol deposition in arteries, tendons and skin. It is one of the most common autosomal dominant disorders, affecting 1 in 500 adults in the United States in its heterozygous form. Only 1 person in 1 million is homozygous for the disease. In this disease, there is a striking acceleration of atherosclerosis and its complications.

 **MOLECULAR PATHOGENESIS:** The gene on the short arm of chromosome 19 that encodes the cell surface receptor for low-density lipoprotein (LDLR) is mutated in familial hypercholesterolemia. The LDL receptor removes LDL from the blood, a process that occurs mainly in the liver. Over 150 different mutations are known. The LDL receptor is made in the endoplasmic reticulum (ER), transferred to the Golgi and transported to the cell surface, where it resides in clathrin-coated pits. Once it binds LDL, the receptor and its ligand are internalized by receptor-mediated endocytosis and processed in lysosomes. Genetic defects in each step are known:

- **Class 1:** This, the most common defect, leads to failure to synthesize nascent LDLR protein in the ER, mostly owing to large deletions in the gene (null alleles).
- **Class 2:** These mutations impede transfer of nascent receptors from the ER to the Golgi (transport-defective alleles), preventing it from reaching the cell surface.
- **Class 3:** LDL receptors of class 3 mutations are expressed on the cell surface but are defective in the ligand-binding domain (binding-defective alleles).
- **Class 4:** These are rare mutations. LDL binds normally to its receptor, but the receptor does not cluster in coated pits. Thus, receptor internalization by endocytosis is blocked (internalization-defective alleles).
- **Class 5:** Internalized LDL–receptor complexes remain in endosomes, and receptors do not recycle to the plasma membrane (recycling-defective alleles).

Hepatocytes are the main cells that express LDLR, and roughly 70% of LDL is removed from the blood by the liver. After LDLs bind the receptor, they are internalized and processed in lysosomes, freeing cholesterol for further metabolism. If LDL receptor function is impaired, high levels of LDLs circulate and are taken up by tissue macrophages, which accumulate to form occlusive arterial plaques (atheromas), papules or nodules of lipid-laden macrophages (xanthomas; see Chapter 16).

CLINICAL FEATURES: Heterozygous and homozygous familial hypercholesterolemia are distinct clinical syndromes, reflecting a clear gene–dosage effect. In heterozygotes, total blood cholesterol (mean, 350 mg/dL; normal, <200 mg/dL in adults) is elevated at birth. Tendon xanthomas develop in half of the patients before age 30, and symptoms of coronary heart disease often occur before age 40. In homozygotes, blood cholesterol content is extremely high (600–1200 mg/dL), and virtually all patients have tendon xanthomas and generalized atherosclerosis in childhood. Untreated homozygotes typically die of myocardial infarction before age 30. Treatment of heterozygotes with statins has significantly reduced mortality and morbidity due to coronary heart disease to a level equivalent to that seen in the general population.

AUTOSOMAL RECESSIVE DISORDERS

Most genetic metabolic diseases show autosomal recessive inheritance (Fig. 6-21; Table 6-7). The fact that recessive genes are uncommon and the need for two mutant alleles to cause clinical disease determine the key characteristics of autosomal recessive inheritance. Some of the salient features of these disorders are:

■ The more infrequent the mutant gene in the general population, the lower the chance that unrelated parents carry the trait. *Rare autosomal recessive disorders often occur in offspring of consanguineous parents.*
■ Both parents are usually heterozygous for the trait and are clinically normal.
■ Symptoms appear in about 25% of their children. Half of all offspring are heterozygous for the trait and are asymptomatic. Thus, 2/3 of unaffected offspring are heterozygous carriers.
■ Autosomal recessive traits are transmitted equally to males and females.
■ Symptoms of autosomal recessive disorders tend to be more consistent than in autosomal dominant diseases. Recessive traits therefore present more commonly in childhood, while dominant disorders may initially appear in adults.

TABLE 6-7
REPRESENTATIVE AUTOSOMAL RECESSIVE DISORDERS

Disease	Frequency	Chromosome
Cystic fibrosis	1/2500	7q
α-Thalassemia	High	16p
β-Thalassemia	High	11p
Sickle cell anemia	High	11p
Myeloperoxidase deficiency	1/2000	17q
Phenylketonuria	1/10,000	12q
Gaucher disease	1/50,000	1q
Tay-Sachs disease	1/300,000	15q
Hurler syndrome	1/100,000	22p
Glycogen storage disease Ia (von Gierke disease)	1/100,000	17
Wilson disease	1/50,000	13q
Hereditary hemochromatosis	1/1000	6p
α1-Antitrypsin deficiency	1/7000	14q
Oculocutaneous albinism	1/20,000	11q
Alkaptonuria	<1/100,000	3q
Metachromatic leukodystrophy	1/100,000	22q

■ Variability in clinical expression of some autosomal recessive diseases may reflect residual functionality of the affected protein. Such variability manifests in (1) different degrees of clinical severity, (2) age at onset or (3) the existence of acute and chronic forms of the specific disease.

Most mutant genes responsible for autosomal recessive disorders are rare in the general population, since those homozygous for the trait often die before reproductive age. However, a few autosomal recessive diseases, such as sickle cell anemia and cystic fibrosis (CF), are common. New mutations for recessive diseases are difficult to identify clinically because heterozygotes are asymptomatic. Nonconsanguineous mating of two such heterozygotes would occur by chance, and many generations later, if at all.

Biochemical Basis of Autosomal Recessive Disorders

Autosomal recessive diseases are usually due to deficiencies in enzymes rather than structural proteins. A mutation that inactivates an enzyme rarely causes an abnormal phenotype in heterozygotes: most cellular enzymes operate at substrate concentrations well below saturation, so an enzyme deficiency is easily corrected simply by increasing the amount of substrate. In autosomal recessive diseases caused by impaired catabolism of dietary substances (e.g., phenylketonuria, galactosemia) or cellular constituents (e.g., Tay-Sachs, Hurler),

Autosomal Recessive

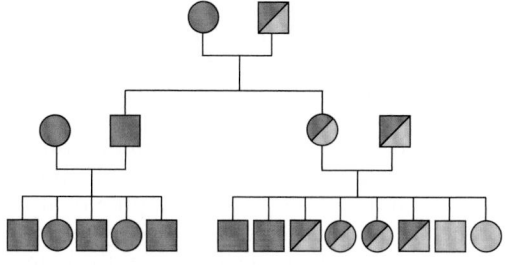

☐○ Homozygote with disease

◪◨ Heterozygote without disease (silent carrier)

FIGURE 6-21. Autosomal recessive inheritance. Symptoms of the disease appear only in homozygotes, male or female. Heterozygotes are asymptomatic carriers. Symptomatic homozygotes result from the mating of asymptomatic heterozygotes.

increased substrate concentrations in heterozygotes overcome partial lack of the enzyme. By contrast, loss of both alleles in a homozygote results in complete loss of enzyme activity, which cannot be corrected by such mechanisms.

Cystic Fibrosis is the Most Common Lethal Autosomal Recessive Disorder in the Caucasian Population

CF is characterized by (1) chronic pulmonary disease; (2) deficient exocrine pancreatic function; and (3) other complications of inspissated/thickened mucus in several organs, including the small intestine, liver and reproductive tract. A defective chloride channel, the cystic fibrosis transmembrane conductance regulator (CFTR), is responsible.

 **EPIDEMIOLOGY:** Cystic fibrosis is most common among whites. Among white Americans, about 1 in 29 people carry a mutation of the CF gene. One in 46 Hispanic Americans, 1 in 65 black Americans and 1 in 90 Asian Americans carry a CF gene mutation.

 MOLECULAR PATHOGENESIS: The *CFTR* gene is on the long arm of chromosome 7 (7q31.2) (Table 6-7). It encodes a protein of 1480 amino acids that functions as a halide ion transporter in most epithelial cells. Its two adenosine triphosphate (ATP)-hydrolyzing domains drive transporter function. It also has two domains that anchor the transporter as a transmembrane spanning protein. Two R domains with phosphorylation sites for cyclic adenosine 3',5'-monophosphate (cAMP)-dependent protein kinase A (PKA) regulate chloride channel activity.

CFTR activity is regulated by the balance between kinase and phosphatase activities (i.e., phosphorylation and dephosphorylation). Phosphorylation of the R domains, mostly by PKA, stimulates chloride channel activity. Secretion of chloride anions by mucus-secreting epithelial cells controls the parallel secretion of fluid and, thus, the viscosity of the mucus. In normal mucus-secreting epithelia, cAMP activates PKA, which phosphorylates the regulatory domains of CFTR and permits channel opening. Mutations in CFTR perturb this process. The most common mutation in the white population is loss of 3 base pairs, which deletes a phenylalanine (F) residue (ΔF_{508}), producing an abnormally folded protein that is degraded. ΔF_{508} accounts for 70% of CFTR mutations among whites. Mutations in the *CFTR* gene that disturb chloride channel function fall into several functional groupings (Fig. 6-22):

- **Failure of CFTR synthesis:** Mutations that result in premature termination signals interfere with synthesis of the full-length CFTR protein. As a result, no CFTR-mediated chloride secretion occurs in involved epithelia.
- **Failure of CFTR transport to the plasma membrane:** Some mutations prevent proper folding of the nascent protein, so it is then targeted for proteasomal degradation rather than for transport to the plasma membrane. The ΔF_{508} mutation is of this class.
- **Defective ATP binding to CFTR:** Certain mutations allow CFTR proteins to reach the plasma membrane but affect ATP-binding domains, thus interfering with channel regulation and limiting, but not abolishing, chloride secretion.
- **Defective chloride secretion by mutant CFTR:** Mutations in the channel pore inhibit chloride secretion.

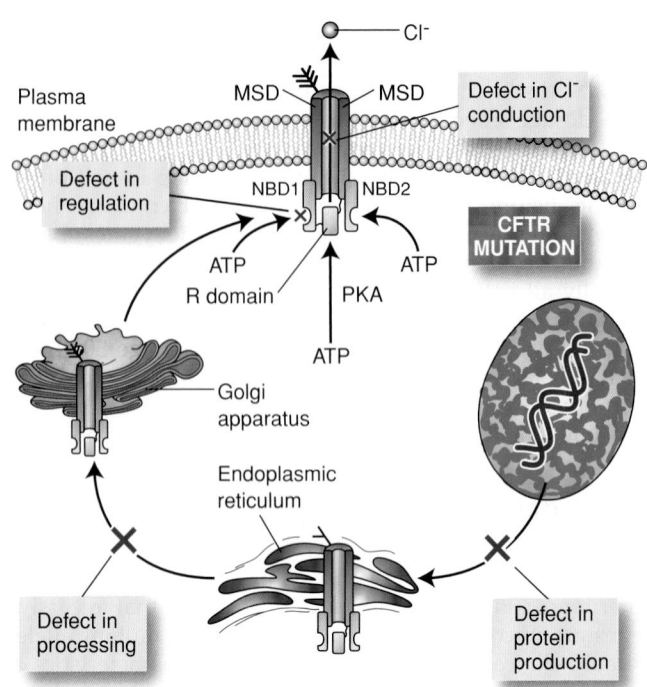

FIGURE 6-22. Cellular sites of disruption in the synthesis and function of the cystic fibrosis transmembrane conductance regulator (CFTR) in cystic fibrosis. *ATP* = adenosine triphosphate; *Cl–* = chloride ion; *MSD* = membrane-spanning domain; *NBD* = nucleotide-binding domain; *PKA* = protein kinase A.

The relationship between these genotypes (more than 1500 mutations are known) and the clinical severity of CF is complicated and not always consistent. The best correlation relates to pancreatic insufficiency. Severe symptoms are generally found in those with pancreatic insufficiency (85% of cases), while in milder cases pancreatic function is preserved. Class I and class II mutations are generally found among severely affected patients. By contrast, milder forms of CF have class III and class IV mutations.

Pathologic consequences of CF arise from abnormally thick mucus, which obstructs airway lumina, pancreatic and biliary ducts and the fetal intestine. CF was once called mucoviscidosis. Normal CFTR corrects the defect in chloride secretion in cultured cells from CF patients.

 PATHOLOGY: CF affects many organs that produce exocrine secretions (Fig. 6-23).

RESPIRATORY TRACT: Lung disease causes most morbidity and mortality in CF. The earliest lesion is obstruction of bronchioles by mucus, with secondary infection and inflammation of bronchiolar walls. Recurrent cycles of obstruction and infection result in **chronic bronchiolitis** and **bronchitis,** which increase in severity as the disease progresses, and may lead to secondary pulmonary hypertension. Bronchial mucous glands undergo hypertrophy and hyperplasia, and airways are distended by thick, tenacious secretions. Widespread **bronchiectasis** is apparent by age 10 and often earlier. Late in the disease, large bronchiectatic cysts and lung abscesses are common.

PANCREAS: Most patients (85%) with CF have a form of **chronic pancreatitis,** and in long-standing cases, little or no functional exocrine pancreas remains. Inspissated secretions in central pancreatic ducts produce secondary dilation and cystic change of the distal ducts (Fig. 6-24). Recurrent pancreatitis leads to loss of acinar cells and extensive fibrosis so

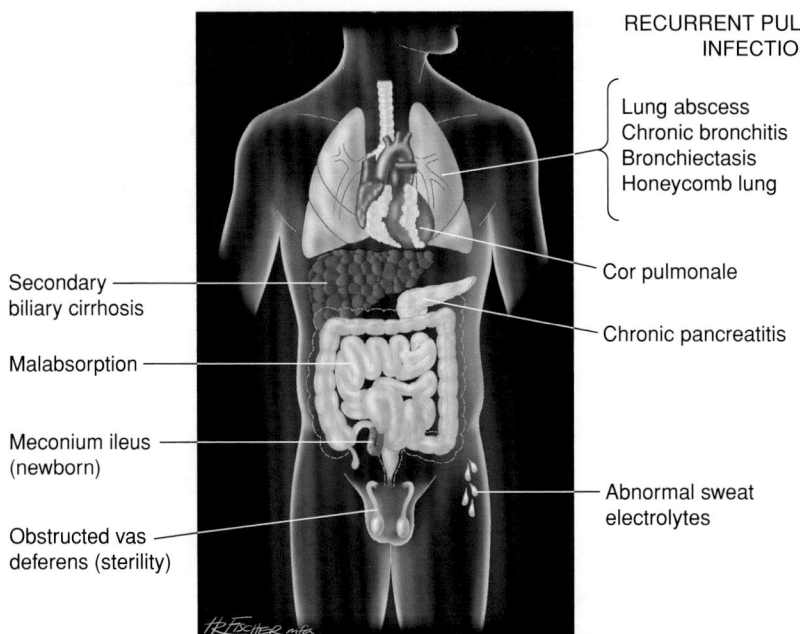

RECURRENT PULMONARY INFECTION

Lung abscess
Chronic bronchitis
Bronchiectasis
Honeycomb lung

Cor pulmonale

Chronic pancreatitis

Secondary biliary cirrhosis

Malabsorption

Meconium ileus (newborn)

Obstructed vas deferens (sterility)

Abnormal sweat electrolytes

FIGURE 6-23. Clinical features of cystic fibrosis.

that the pancreas may become simply cystic fibroadipose tissue containing islets of Langerhans. The finding of pancreatic cysts and fibrosis led to the original name of cystic fibrosis.

LIVER: Inspissated mucous secretions in the intrahepatic biliary system obstruct bile flow in draining areas of the affected ducts and lead to focal **secondary biliary cirrhosis**. This is seen in 1/4 of patients at autopsy. Inspissated concretions clog bile ducts and ductules. Sometimes (<5%), hepatic lesions, which include chronic portal inflammation and septal fibrosis, are sufficiently widespread to lead to the clinical manifestations of biliary cirrhosis.

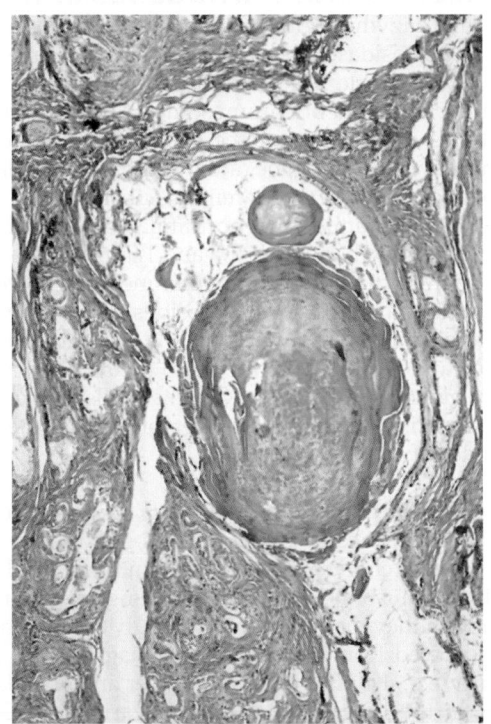

FIGURE 6-24. Intraductal concretion and acinar atrophy in the pancreas of a patient with cystic fibrosis.

GASTROINTESTINAL TRACT: Shortly after birth, a normal newborn passes the intestinal contents that have accumulated in utero (meconium). The most important lesion of the gut in CF is small bowel obstruction in newborns, **meconium ileus,** which is due to failure to pass meconium in the immediate postpartum period. This occurs in 5%–10% of newborns with CF and reflects the failure of pancreatic secretions to digest meconium, possibly augmented by the greater viscosity of small bowel secretions.

REPRODUCTIVE TRACT: Almost all boys with CF have atrophy or fibrosis of the reproductive duct system, including the vas deferens, epididymis and seminal vesicles. These lesions are due to luminal obstruction by inspissated secretions early in life and even in utero. Thus, only 2%–3% of males are fertile, with spermatozoa absent from the semen in the rest.

A minority of women with CF are fertile. Many suffer from anovulatory cycles as a result of poor nutrition and chronic infections. Moreover, the cervical mucous plug is abnormally thick and tenacious.

 CLINICAL FEATURES: *The diagnosis of CF is most reliably made by detecting increased electrolyte concentrations in the sweat and by genetic studies that show disease-causing mutations.* Decreased chloride conductance in CF results in failure of chloride reabsorption by cells of sweat gland ducts and thus to accumulation of sodium chloride in the sweat. The skin in children with CF is salty and may even display salt crystals after vigorous sweating.

Pulmonary symptoms of CF begin with cough, which becomes productive of large amounts of tenacious and purulent sputum. Repeated bouts of infectious bronchitis and bronchopneumonia become progressively more frequent, and eventually dyspnea develops. Respiratory failure and cardiac complications of pulmonary hypertension (cor pulmonale) occur late.

The most common organisms that infect the respiratory tract in CF are *Staphylococcus* and *Pseudomonas* spp. As the disease advances, *Pseudomonas* may be the only organism cultured from the lung. *In fact, recovery of* Pseudomonas *sp., particularly the mucoid variety, from the lungs of a child with chronic pulmonary disease is virtually diagnostic of CF.* Infection with *Burkholderia cepacia* is associated with **cepacia syndrome,** a very severe pulmonary infection that is highly resistant to antibiotics and is commonly fatal.

Failure of pancreatic exocrine secretion leads to fat and protein malabsorption, causing bulky, foul-smelling stools (steatorrhea), nutritional deficiencies and growth retardation. Postural drainage of airways, antibiotic therapy and pancreatic enzyme supplementation are mainstays of treatment. Molecular prenatal diagnosis of CF is now accurate in 95% of cases.

In 1959, children with CF in the United States rarely survived for 1 year. With improved therapies, life expectancy has increased to 40 years.

Lysosomal Storage Diseases Are Enzyme Deficiencies That Cause Abnormal Accumulation of Substances within Lysosomes

Lysosomes are membrane-bound collections of hydrolytic enzymes that digest macromolecules (see Chapter 1). Lysosomal digestive enzymes are called "acid hydrolases" since their optimal activities occur at acidic pHs (pH 3.5–5.5). This environment is maintained by an ATP-dependent proton pump in the lysosomal membrane. These enzymes degrade virtually all types of biological macromolecules including lipids, glycoproteins and mucopolysaccharides. Extracellular macromolecules that are internalized by endocytosis or phagocytosis and intracellular constituents that are subjected to autophagy are digested in lysosomes to their basic components. End-products may be transported across lysosomal membranes into the cytosol, where they are reused in the synthesis of new macromolecules.

Virtually all lysosomal storage diseases result from mutations in genes for lysosomal hydrolases. Acid hydrolases may be nucleases, proteases, glycosidases, lipases, phosphatases, sulfatases and phospholipases; they make up lysosomes' 50 or so degradative enzymes. Deficiency in one of these acid hydrolases can prevent catabolism the normal macromolecular substrate of that enzyme. As a result, undigested substrates accumulate in, and engorge, lysosomes, expanding the lysosomal compartment of the cell. Resulting lysosomal distention impairs other critical cellular activities, particularly in the brain and heart, and can lead to poor cellular function or cell death.

Lysosomal storage diseases are classified by the material retained in the lysosomes. Thus, when accumulated substrates are sphingolipids, they are **sphingolipidoses.** Storage of mucopolysaccharides (glycosaminoglycans) leads to the **mucopolysaccharidoses.** Over 50 lysosomal storage diseases are known, but we limit our discussion to the more important ones.

Sphingolipidoses are lysosomal storage diseases characterized by accumulation of lipids derived from the turnover of obsolete cell membranes. Cerebrosides, gangliosides, sphingomyelin and sulfatides are all sphingolipid components of membranes of a variety of cells. These substances are degraded within lysosomes by complex pathways producing sphingosine and fatty acids (Fig. 6-25). Deficiencies of acid hydrolases that mediate specific steps in these pathways lead to accumulation of undigested intermediate substrates in lysosomes and hence a metabolic disorder.

Gaucher Disease

Gaucher disease is characterized by accumulation of glucosylceramide, mainly in macrophage lysosomes.

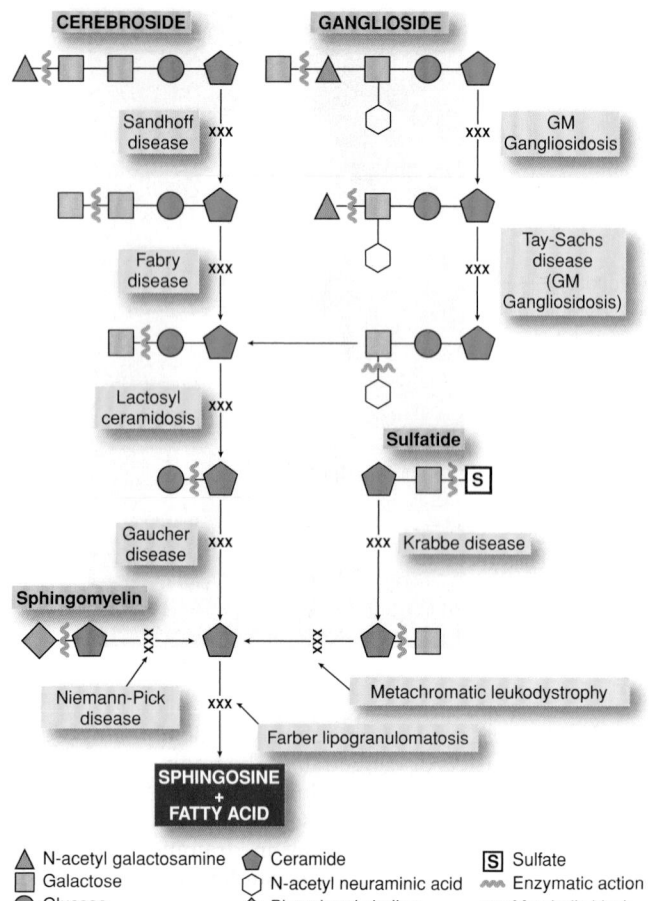

FIGURE 6-25. Disturbances of lipid metabolism in various sphingolipidoses.

 MOLECULAR PATHOGENESIS: The abnormal enzyme is glucocerebrosidase, a lysosomal acid β-glucosidase. The enzyme deficiency can be traced to a variety of single base mutations in the β-glucosidase gene, on the long arm of chromosome 1 (1q21). Each of the clinical types of the disease (see below) exhibits heterogeneous mutations in this gene, although the molecular basis for the phenotypic differences remains unclear.

The glucosylceramide that accumulates in Gaucher cells of the spleen, liver, bone marrow and lymph nodes derives principally from catabolism of membranes of senescent leukocytes, which are rich in cerebrosides. When membrane degradation is blocked by a lack of glucocerebrosidase, glucosylceramide, the intermediate metabolite, accumulates. The glucosylceramide of Gaucher cells in the brain is believed to originate from turnover of plasma membrane gangliosides of cells in the CNS.

PATHOLOGY: The hallmark of this disorder is the presence of **Gaucher cells,** lipid-laden macrophages characteristically seen in the red pulp of the spleen, liver sinusoids, lymph nodes, lungs and bone marrow, although they may appear in virtually any organ. These cells are derived from resident macrophages in the respective organs (e.g., Kupffer cells in the liver and alveolar macrophages in the lung). In uncommon variants of Gaucher disease with CNS involvement, Gaucher cells originate from periadventitial cells in Virchow-Robin spaces.

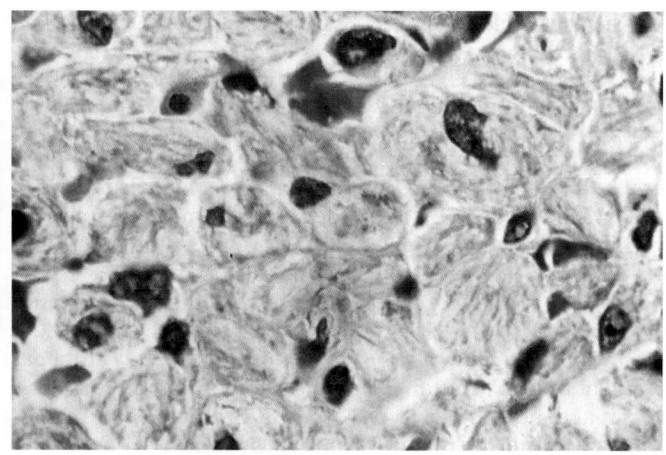

FIGURE 6-26. The spleen in Gaucher disease. Typical Gaucher cells have foamy cytoplasm and eccentrically located nuclei.

Gaucher cells are large (20–100 μm), with eccentric nuclei and clear cytoplasm (Fig. 6-26) that has a characteristic fibrillar appearance, which has been likened to "wrinkled tissue paper" and is intensely positive with periodic acid–Schiff (PAS) stain. The material is stored in enlarged lysosomes and appears as parallel layers of tubular structures.

Splenomegaly is virtually universal in Gaucher disease. In the adult form of the disorder, spleens may weigh up to 10 kg. The cut surface of the enlarged spleen is firm and pale and often contains sharply demarcated infarcts. The red pulp shows nodular and diffuse infiltrates of Gaucher cells and moderate fibrosis.

The liver is usually enlarged by Gaucher cells within sinusoids, but hepatocytes are not affected. In severe cases, hepatic fibrosis and even cirrhosis may ensue. Bone marrow involvement varies but leads to radiologic abnormalities in 50%–75% of cases.

Gaucher cells may also be found in many other organs, including lymph nodes, lungs, endocrine glands, skin, GI tract and kidneys, but symptoms referable to involvement of these organs are uncommon.

In the infantile (neuronopathic) form of the disease, Gaucher cells are also seen in the brain parenchyma, where they may stimulate gliosis and microglial nodules.

 CLINICAL FEATURES: Gaucher disease is classified into three distinct forms, based on the age at onset and degree of neurologic involvement:

- **Type 1 (chronic nonneuronopathic):** This variant is the most common of the lysosomal storage diseases. It occurs in 1 in 40,000–60,000 in the general population and in 1 in 500–800 of those with Ashkenazi Jewish ancestry. Thus, the carrier rate is 1 in 12 Ashkenazi Jews. Age at onset is variable; some cases are diagnosed in infants and others at age 70. The severity of clinical manifestations also varies widely. Most cases are diagnosed as adults and present initially as painless splenomegaly and complications of hypersplenism including anemia, leukopenia and thrombocytopenia. Hepatomegaly is common, but clinical liver disease is infrequent. Bone involvement, manifesting as pain and pathologic fractures, can cause disability severe enough to confine a patient to a wheelchair.

  The life expectancy of most patients with type 1 Gaucher disease is normal. The disease is now treated by administering modified acid glucose cerebrosidase, although its high cost limits its use. Marrow transplantation is also effective but is little used because of the attendant risks. Prenatal diagnosis is based on β-glucosidase activity in amniotic fluid or chorionic villi. Prenatal DNA testing is now routinely available. As there are numerous mutations, sequencing of the affected gene is sometimes necessary to confirm the diagnosis.

- **Type 2 (acute neuronopathic):** Type 2 Gaucher disease is rare and quite different from type 1 in age at onset and clinical presentation. It usually presents by age 3 months with hepatosplenomegaly and has no ethnic predilection. Within a few months, infants show neurologic signs, with a classic triad of trismus, strabismus and backward flexion of the neck. Further neurologic deterioration rapidly ensues. Most patients die by age 3 years.

- **Type 3 (subacute neuronopathic):** This form is also rare and combines features of types 1 and 2. Neurologic deterioration starts later than in type 2 and progresses more slowly, with most living until about age 30.

Tay-Sachs Disease (GM₂ Gangliosidosis Type 1)

Tay-Sachs disease is a catastrophic infantile form of a class of lysosomal storage diseases known as the GM₂ gangliosidoses, in which this ganglioside is deposited in CNS neurons, owing to a failure of lysosomal degradation. The association of a "cherry-red spot" in the retina and profound mental and physical retardation was first pointed out in 1881 by Warren Tay, a British ophthalmologist. Fifteen years later, Bernard Sachs, an American neurologist, described the pathology of the disorder and coined the term "amaurotic (blind) family idiocy." Tay-Sachs disease is inherited as an autosomal recessive trait and is mainly seen in Ashkenazi Jews, among whom the carrier rate is about 1 in 30, with homozygotes seen in 1 in 4000 live newborns. By contrast, incidence in non–Jewish American populations is less than 1 in 100,000. Tay-Sachs disease is caused by a genetic mutation in the hexosaminidase A (HEXA) gene on (human) chromosome 15. Numerous HEXA mutations have been reported with significant frequencies in specific populations. The carrier frequency in French Canadians is similar to that in Ashkenazi Jews, but with different mutations. Interestingly, Cajuns of southern Louisiana carry the mutation seen most commonly in Ashkenazi Jews, which has been traced back to a founder couple in 18th-century France. Screening programs for heterozygous Ashkenazi Jews have reduced disease incidence by 90%. The other GM₂ gangliosidoses are very rare.

MOLECULAR PATHOGENESIS: Gangliosides are glycosphingolipids with a ceramide and an oligosaccharide chain that contains N-acetyl-neuraminic acid (Fig. 6-25). They are located in the outer leaflet of the plasma membrane of animal cells, particularly in brain neurons.

Lysosomal catabolism of ganglioside GM₂, 1 of the 12 known gangliosides in the brain, requires β-hexosaminidases (A and B), which have α- and β-subunits and need GM₂-activator protein. Deficiency in any of these components results in clinical disease.

Tay-Sachs disease (also known as hexosaminidase α-subunit deficiency) results from about 50 different mutations in the gene on chromosome 15q23–24 that codes for the α-subunit of hexosaminidase A (HEXA), with a resulting defect in the synthesis of this enzyme. An insertion of four

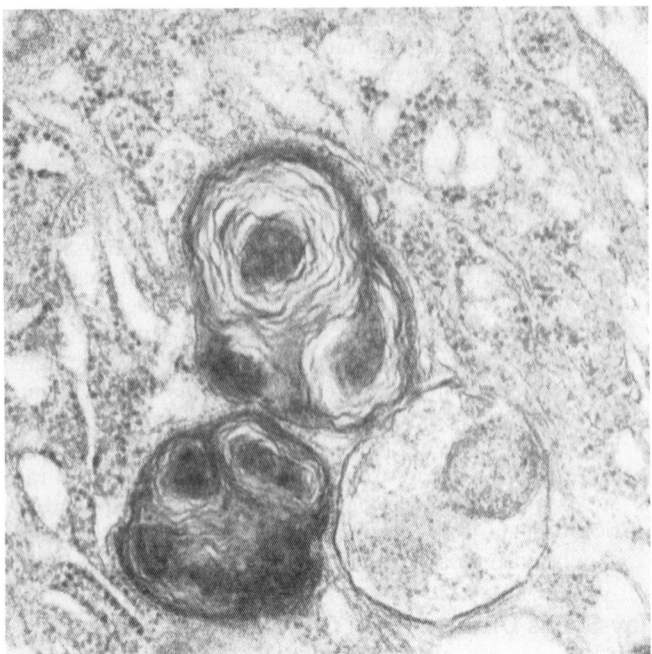

FIGURE 6-27. Tay-Sachs disease. A neuron contains lysosomes filled with whorled membranes.

nucleotides in exon 11 accounts for over 2/3 of the carriers among Ashkenazi Jews (i.e., about 2% of that population). The β-subunits are synthesized normally and associate to form hexosaminidase B dimers, levels of which are normal or even increased in Tay-Sachs disease.

Sandhoff disease is caused by a mutation in the gene for the β-subunit on chromosome 5 and leads to deficiencies of both hexosaminidases A and B.

A third, rare variant is the result of a defect in the synthesis of the GM$_2$-activator protein (chromosome 5) in the face of normal activities of the hexosaminidases.

 PATHOLOGY: GM$_2$ ganglioside accumulates in lysosomes of all organs in Tay-Sachs disease, but it is most prominent in brain neurons and cells of the retina. The size of the brain varies with the length of survival of affected infants. Early cases are marked by brain atrophy, but the organ weight may be as much as doubled in those who survive beyond a year. Neurons are markedly distended with stored lipids. By electron microscopy, neurons are stuffed with "membranous cytoplasmic bodies," composed of concentric whorls of lamellar structures (Fig. 6-27). As disease progresses, neurons are lost and many lipid-laden macrophages are conspicuous in the cortical gray matter. Eventually, gliosis becomes prominent and myelin and axons in the white matter die. The pathologies of the other forms of GM$_2$ gangliosidosis are similar to those of Tay-Sachs disease, but usually less severe.

 CLINICAL FEATURES: Tay-Sachs disease presents between 6 and 10 months of age with progressive weakness, hypotonia and decreased attentiveness. Motor and mental deterioration, often with generalized seizures, follow rapidly. Vision is seriously impaired. Retinal ganglion cell involvement is detected by ophthalmoscopy as a **cherry-red spot** in the macula. This feature reflects the pallor of the affected cells, which enhances the prominence of blood vessels underlying the central fovea. Most children with Tay-Sachs disease die before 4 years of age.

Niemann-Pick Disease

Niemann-Pick disease (NPD) is a form of sphingolipidosis involving dysfunctional catabolism of cell membrane sphingolipids. Macrophage lysosomes in many cells, especially in the liver and the brain, store **sphingomyelin**. There are several NPD variants; types A and B are caused by mutations in the *SMPD1* gene, which encodes the enzyme acid sphingomyelinase; type C is caused by mutations in the *NPC1* and *NPC2* genes, which encode lipid transport proteins.

Type A NPD appears in infancy, with hepatosplenomegaly and progressive neurodegeneration. Death occurs by 3 years of age. Type B NPD is more variable, with hepatosplenomegaly, minimal neurologic symptomatology and survival to adulthood. Type C NPD is biochemically, genetically and clinically distinct from types A and B NPD.

 **EPIDEMIOLOGY:** The incidence of type A NPD is 1 in 40,000 among Ashkenazi Jews. In all other populations, both types A and B NPD occur in 1 in 250,000. For type C, incidence is 1 in 100,000. Total incidence for all types in the general population is thus 1 in 100,000.

 **MOLECULAR PATHOGENESIS:** Sphingomyelin is a membrane phospholipid composed of phosphorylcholine, sphingosine (a long-chain amino alcohol) and a fatty acid (Fig. 6-25). It is especially abundant in myelin sheaths of nerve axons. It accounts for up to 14% of phospholipids of the liver, spleen and brain. The metabolic defect in NPD reflects 12 different mutations in the gene (11p15.1–15.4) for **sphingomyelinase,** the lysosomal enzyme that hydrolyzes sphingomyelin to ceramide and phosphorylcholine. In types A and B, this enzyme is completely or partially lacking. In type C, the protein product of the major mutated gene *NPC1* is not an enzyme but appears to function as a transporter in the endosomal-lysosomal system, which moves large water-insoluble molecules through the cell. The protein encoded by the *NPC2* gene more closely resembles an enzyme structurally but seems to cooperate with the NPC1 protein in transporting molecules in the cell. Disruption of this transport system causes cholesterol and glycolipids to accumulate in lysosomes.

 PATHOLOGY: The characteristic storage cell in NPD is a foam cell, that is, an enlarged (20–90 μm) macrophage whose cytoplasm is distended by uniform vacuoles containing sphingomyelin and cholesterol. By electron microscopy, whorls of concentrically arranged lamellar structures distend lysosomes.

Foam cells are particularly abundant in the spleen, lymph nodes and bone marrow but also occur in the liver, lungs and GI tract. The spleen is enlarged, often massively, with foam cells distributed diffusely throughout the red pulp. Lymph nodes enlarged by foam cells are seen in many locations. Hematopoietic tissues in bone marrow may be displaced by aggregates of foam cells. The liver is enlarged by stored sphingomyelin and cholesterol in lysosomes of both Kupffer cells and hepatocytes.

The brain is the most important organ involved in type A NPD, and neurologic damage is the usual cause of death. Such brains are atrophied and in severe cases may be 1/2 of normal weight. Neurons are distended by vacuoles containing the same stored lipids found elsewhere in the body. In advanced cases, neuron loss is severe and may be accompanied by demyelination. Half of children with type A disease have cherry-red retinal spots, as in Tay-Sachs disease.

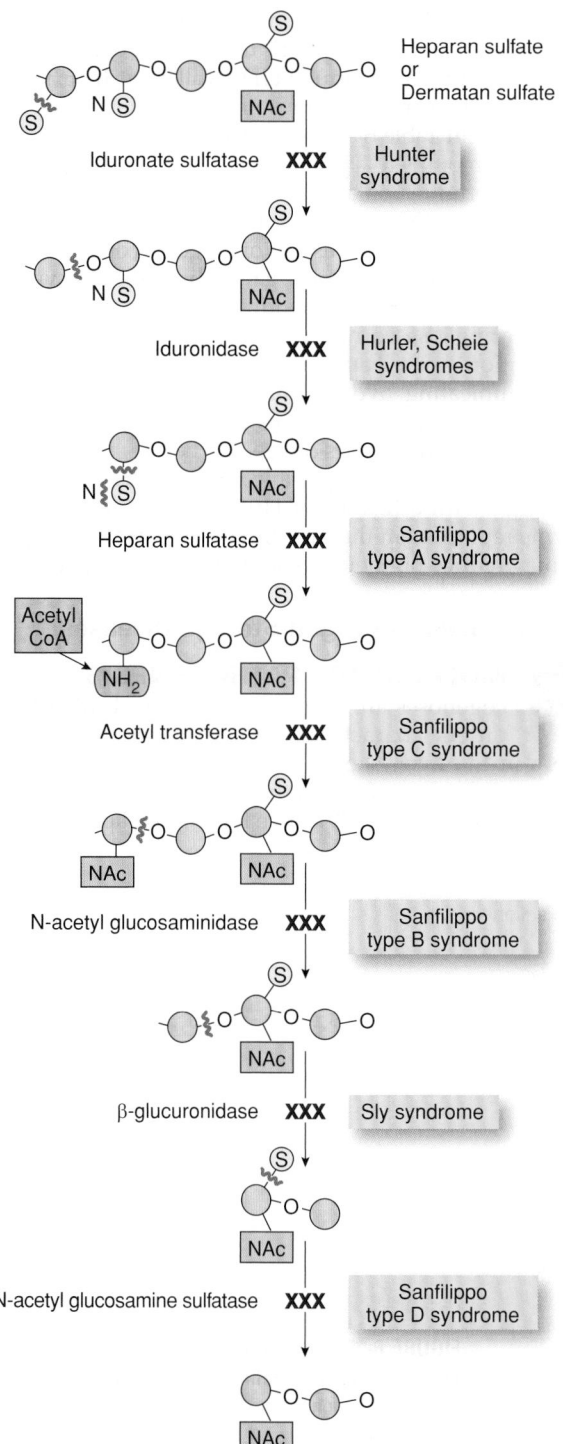

§ -Site of enzymatic action   **XXX** Metabolic block

FIGURE 6-28. Metabolic blocks in various mucopolysaccharidoses that affect the degradation of heparan sulfate and dermatan sulfate with resulting syndromes. *Acetyl CoA* = acetyl coenzyme A; *Nac* = N-acetyl moiety.

TABLE 6-8
MUCOPOLYSACCHARIDOSES

Type	Eponym	Location of Gene	Clinical Features
I H	Hurler	4p16.3	Organomegaly, cardiac lesions, dysostosis multiplex, corneal clouding, death in childhood
I S	Scheie	4p16.3	Stiff joints, corneal clouding, normal intelligence, longevity
II	Hunter	X	Organomegaly, dysostosis multiplex, mental retardation, death earlier than 15 years of age
III	Sanfilippo	12q14	Mental retardation
IV	Morquio	16q24	Skeletal deformities, corneal clouding
V	Obsolete	—	—
VI	Maroteaux Lamy	5q13–14	Dysostosis multiplex, corneal clouding, death in second decade
VII	Sly	7q21.1–22	Hepatosplenomegaly, dysostosis multiplex

eventually impairs respiratory function. However, these patients have few neurologic symptoms and may survive for years. Progressive neurologic disease is the hallmark of Niemann–Pick type C disease and causes disability and early death in all cases beyond early childhood.

Mucopolysaccharidoses

Mucopolysaccharidoses (MPSs) are lysosomal diseases in which **glycosaminoglycans (mucopolysaccharides)** accumulate in many organs. All are inherited as autosomal recessive traits, except for Hunter syndrome, which is X-linked recessive. These rare diseases are caused by deficiencies in any of the 12 lysosomal enzymes that catabolize glycosaminoglycans (Fig. 6-28). Six abnormal phenotypes are described, each varying with the specific enzyme deficiency (Table 6-8).

 **MOLECULAR PATHOGENESIS:** Glycosaminoglycans (GAGs) are large polymers of repeating disaccharide units containing *N*-acetylhexosamine and a hexose or hexuronic acid. Either disaccharide may be sulfated. The accumulated GAGs (dermatan sulfate, heparan sulfate, keratan sulfate and chondroitin sulfate) in MPSs all derive from cleavage of proteoglycans, which are important extracellular matrix constituents. GAGs are degraded stepwise by removing sulfates or sugar residues. Thus, a deficiency in any one of the glycosidases or sulfatases causes undegraded GAGs to accumulate. A special case is deficiency of an *N*-acetyltransferase, which leads to deposition of heparan sulfate in Sanfilippo C disease.

 PATHOLOGY: Although the severity and location of lesions in MPSs vary with the specific enzyme deficiency, most of these syndromes share common features. Undegraded GAGs tend to accumulate in

CLINICAL FEATURES: Type A NPD manifests in early infancy with conspicuous spleen and liver enlargement and psychomotor retardation. Motor and intellectual function are lost over time. Children usually die before 3 years of age. Most type B patients present in childhood with marked hepatosplenomegaly. Pulmonary infiltration with sphingomyelin-laden macrophages

connective tissue cells, mononuclear phagocytes (including Kupffer cells), endothelial cells, neurons and hepatocytes. Affected cells are swollen with clear cytoplasm. Stains for metachromasia confirm the presence of GAGs. Electron microscopy shows enlarged lysosomes containing granular or striped material. The most critical lesions involve the CNS, skeleton and heart, although hepatosplenomegaly and corneal clouding are common.

■ Initially, the **CNS** only accumulates GAGs, but as the disease advances, extensive neurons die and gliosis occurs, leading to cortical atrophy. Communicating hydrocephalus, due to meningeal involvement, is common.
■ **Skeletal deformities** result from CAG accumulation in chondrocytes, a process that eventually interferes with normal endochondral ossification. Abnormal foci of osteoid and woven bone are common in the deformed skeleton.
■ **Cardiac** involvement is often severe, with thickening and distortion of valve leaflets, chordae tendineae and endocardium. Coronary arteries are frequently narrowed owing to proliferation of intimal smooth muscle cells containing GAG deposits.
■ **Hepatosplenomegaly** is secondary to distention of Kupffer cells and hepatocytes and accumulation of GAG-filled macrophages in the spleen.

 CLINICAL FEATURES: Hurler syndrome (MPS I) is the most severe clinical form of MPS and is the prototype for these syndromes. Deficiency of α-L

iduronidase (IDUA) results in buildup of heparin sulfate and dermatan sulfate in various tissues (Fig. 6-28). Parents of affected children carry a mutant IDUA allele, at 4p16.3 on chromosome 4. The clinical features of other varieties of MPS are summarized in Table 6-8. The symptoms of Hurler syndrome appear at 6 months to 2 years of age. Children typically show skeletal deformities, enlarged livers and spleens, characteristic facies and joint stiffness. The combination of coarse facial features and dwarfism reminiscent of gargoyles on Gothic cathedrals accounts for the old term, **gargoylism,** for this syndrome.

Children with Hurler syndrome suffer developmental delay, hearing loss, corneal clouding and progressive mental deterioration, as well as increased intracranial pressure, due to communicating hydrocephalus. Most patients die from recurrent pulmonary infections and cardiac complications before they reach 10 years of age.

Prenatal diagnosis is possible for the MPSs and is routine in families with a history of Hurler or Hunter syndromes. Enzyme replacement therapy and bone marrow transplantation may reduce nonneurologic symptoms and pain.

Glycogenoses (Glycogen Storage Diseases)

 **MOLECULAR PATHOGENESIS:** The glycogenoses are a group of at least 14 inherited disorders characterized by glycogen accumulation, mainly in the liver, skeletal muscle and heart. Each entity reflects a deficiency of one of the enzymes involved in glycogen metabolism (Fig. 6-29). Save for X-linked phosphorylase

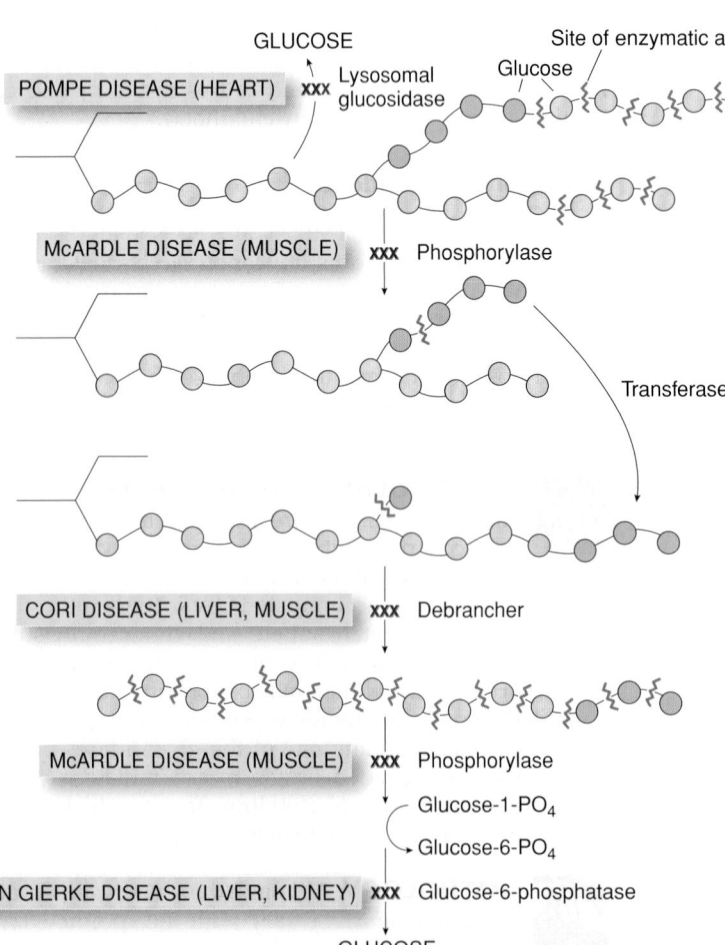

FIGURE 6-29. Sequential catabolism of glycogen and enzymes that are deficient in various glycogenoses. Glycogen is a long-chain branched polymer of glucose residues connected by α-1,4 linkages, except at branch points, where an α-1,6 linkage is present. Phosphorylase hydrolyzes α-1,4 linkages to a point three glucose residues distal to an α-1,6–linked sugar. These three glucose residues are transferred to the chain linked by α-1,4 bonds, by the bifunctional debrancher enzyme amylo-1,6-glucosidase. Subsequently, the same enzyme removes the α-1,6–linked sugar at the original branch point. This creates a linear α-1,4 chain, which is degraded by phosphorylase to glucose-1-phosphate. Following the conversion to glucose-6-phosphate, glucose is released by the action of glucose-6-phosphatase. A small proportion of glycogen is totally degraded within lysosomes by acid α-glucosidase. Red x's indicate a metabolic block and its associated glycogen storage disease.

kinase deficiency, all glycogen storage diseases are autosomal recessive traits. In the United States, they occur once in 20,000–25,000 births.

Glycogen is a large glucose polymer (20,000–30,000 glucose units per molecule) that is stored in most cells as a ready source of energy during fasting, although its function is different in each organ. Liver and muscle are particularly rich in glycogen. The liver stores glycogen not for its own use but rather to supply glucose to the blood quickly, particularly to benefit the brain. By contrast, glycogen in skeletal muscle is used as a local fuel when oxygen or glucose supplies fall. Glycogen is made and degraded by several enzymes, deficiency in any of which leads to accumulation of glycogen. Significant organ involvement varies with the specific enzyme defect. Some mainly affect the liver, while others principally cause cardiac or skeletal muscle dysfunction. Symptoms of glycogenosis may reflect accumulation of glycogen itself (Pompe disease, Andersen disease) or lack of the glucose normally derived from glycogen degradation (von Gierke disease, McArdle disease). We discuss only several representative examples of the known glycogenoses.

VON GIERKE DISEASE (TYPE IA GLYCOGENOSIS): In von Gierke disease, glucose-6-phosphatase is lacking. Glycogen accumulates in the liver, and symptoms reflect the inability of the liver to convert glycogen to glucose, leading to hepatomegaly and hypoglycemia. The disorder usually presents in infancy or early childhood. Growth is commonly stunted, but with treatment, the prognosis for normal mental development and longevity are generally good.

POMPE DISEASE (TYPE II GLYCOGENOSIS): Pompe disease is a lysosomal storage disease that involves virtually all organs and results in death from heart failure before the age of 2. Juvenile and adult variants are less common and have a better prognosis. The incidence of the disease is 1 in 140,000 for infantile GSD II and 1 in 60,000 for adult GSD II. Normally, a small proportion of cytoplasmic glycogen is degraded within lysosomes after an autophagic sequence. Type II glycogenosis is caused by a mutation in the gene for the lysosomal enzyme acid maltase/acid α-glucosidase (GAA) located on the long arm of chromosome 17 at 17q25.2-q25.3. It leads to inexorable accumulation of undegraded glycogen in lysosomes of many different cells. Patients do not develop hypoglycemia, because cytoplasmic metabolic pathways of glycogen synthesis and degradation are intact.

Without enzyme replacement therapy, the hearts of babies with infantile-onset Pompe disease progressively thicken and enlarge. These babies die before 1 year of age from cardiorespiratory failure or respiratory infection. For individuals with late-onset Pompe disease, prognosis depends on the age of onset. In general, the later the age of onset, the slower the disease progresses. Ultimately, prognosis depends on the extent of respiratory muscle involvement.

ANDERSEN DISEASE (TYPE IV GLYCOGENOSIS): Andersen disease is a very rare condition in which the branching enzyme (amyloglucantransferase; at 3p12) that creates the branch points in normal glycogen molecules is lacking. The absence of the branching enzyme leads to formation and accumulation of an abnormal, toxic form of glycogen, **amylopectin**. This starch-like material is deposited, mostly in the liver but also in the heart, skeletal muscles and nervous system. Children with this disease typically die between 2 and 4 years of age from **cirrhosis of the liver**. Liver transplantation is curative. After a liver transplant, cardiac and other extrahepatic deposits of amylopectin are greatly reduced by an unknown mechanism.

McARDLE DISEASE (TYPE V GLYCOGENOSIS): In McArdle disease, glycogen accumulates in skeletal muscles, owing to a lack of muscle phosphorylase, the enzyme that releases glucose-1-phosphate from glycogen. There are two autosomal recessive forms of this disease, childhood onset and adult onset. The gene for myophosphorylase, *PYGM* (the muscle type of the glycogen phosphorylase gene), is on chromosome 11q13. Nearly 100 different mutations, which vary among ethnic groups, have been implicated. Symptoms usually appear in adolescence or early adulthood and consist of muscle cramps and spasms during exercise, which may lead to myocytolysis and myoglobinuria. Aerobic exercise and high-protein diets have been effective therapies in some patients.

Cystinosis

Cystinosis is a lysosomal storage disease that occurs in 1 per 100,000–200,000 live births, in which crystalline cystine accumulates in lysosomes. **Cystinosin,** a transmembrane cystine transporter, is lacking. The affected gene is at chromosome 17p13. It is characterized by renal Fanconi syndrome (polydipsia, excretion of large amounts of dilute urine, dehydration, electrolyte imbalances, growth retardation and rickets) starting at 6–12 months of age. Untreated, cystinosis progresses to renal failure, often in childhood. Lung and brain function are often impaired in older patients. Cystine crystals are seen in almost all cells and organs. Renal transplantation can be used to treat the kidney disease. The use of cysteamine to decrease lysosomal cystine greatly slows disease progression and improves survival.

Inborn Errors of Amino Acid Metabolism Vary Greatly in Severity

Heritable disorders of the metabolism of many amino acids have been described (Table 6-9). Some are lethal in early childhood; others are clinically insignificant. Some of these are addressed in chapters on specific organs. This discussion

TABLE 6-9

REPRESENTATIVE INHERITED DISORDERS OF AMINO ACID METABOLISM

Phenylketonuria (hyperphenylalaninemia)
Tyrosinemia
Histidinemia
Ornithine transcarbamylase deficiency (ammonia intoxication)
Carbamyl phosphate synthetase deficiency (ammonia intoxication)
Maple syrup urine disease (branched-chain ketoacidemia)
Arginase deficiency
Arginosuccinic acid synthetase deficiency (citrulline accumulation)

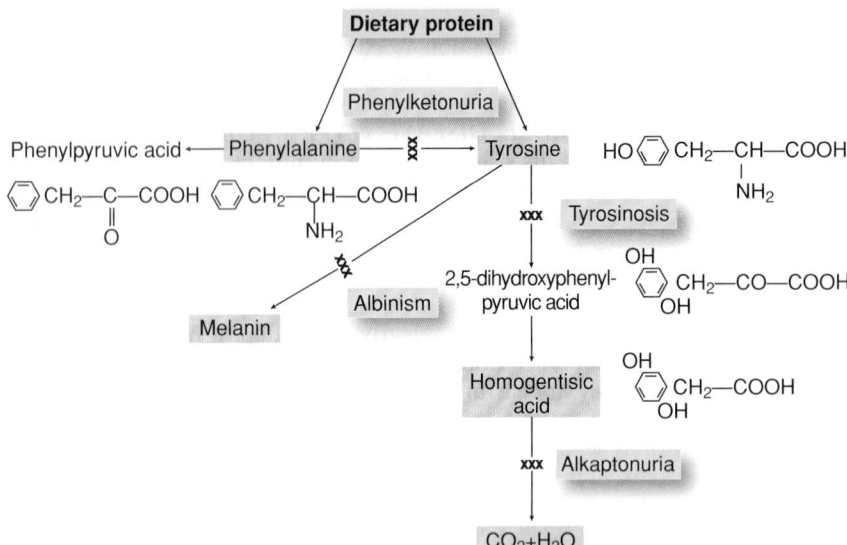

FIGURE 6-30. Diseases caused by disturbances of phenylalanine and tyrosine metabolism.

focuses on examples provided by defects in the metabolism of phenylalanine and tyrosine (Fig. 6-30).

Phenylketonuria

PKU **(hyperphenylalaninemia)** is an autosomal recessive deficiency of the hepatic enzyme phenylalanine hydroxylase. There are high circulating levels of phenylalanine, which leads to progressive mental deterioration in the first few years of life. The incidence of PKU is 1 per 10,000 in white and Asian populations, but it varies widely across different geographic areas. It is most frequent (1 in 5000) in Ireland and western Scotland and among Yemenite Jews.

MOLECULAR PATHOGENESIS: Phenylalanine is an essential amino acid derived exclusively from the diet. It is oxidized in the liver to tyrosine by phenylalanine hydroxylase (PAH). Deficiency in PAH causes hyperphenylalaninemia and formation of phenylketones by the transamination of phenylalanine. Phenylpyruvic acid and its derivatives are excreted in the urine, but phenylalanine itself, rather than its metabolites, causes the neurologic damage central to this disease. Thus, hyperphenylalaninemia is actually a more appropriate name than PKU.

Classic PKU is caused by mutations in the *PAH* gene on the long arm of chromosome 12 (12q22–24.1). Up to 400 mutations are known, most causing deficiency in PAH.

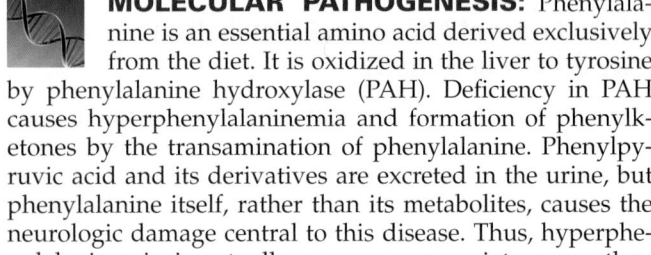

PATHOPHYSIOLOGY: The mechanism of neurotoxicity in hyperphenylalaninemia in infancy is not clear. Several processes have been implicated: competitive interference with amino acid transport systems in the brain, inhibition of neurotransmitter synthesis and disturbance of other metabolic processes. These effects presumably impair neuronal development and myelin synthesis.

PAH activity is not always totally lacking, and forms milder than classic PKU are known. In such cases, phenylpyruvic acid is not excreted in the urine. Patients with less than 1% of the normal PAH activity generally have a PKU phenotype, but those with more than 5% exhibit non-PKU hyperphenylalaninemia, do not suffer neurologic damage and develop normally. Non-PKU hyperphenylalaninemia is probably caused by mutations different from those in classic PKU.

Malignant hyperphenylalaninemia occurs in fewer than 5% of infants with the disease. In this case, dietary restriction of phenylalanine does not arrest neurologic deterioration. These patients have a deficiency in tetrahydrobiopterin (BH$_4$), a cofactor required for hydroxylation of phenylalanine by PAH. Sometimes this defect results from failure to regenerate BH$_4$, due to a lack of dihydropteridine reductase (DHPR), the enzyme that reduces dihydrobiopterin (BH$_2$) to the tetrahydro form (BH$_4$). The mutant *DHPR* gene is on the short arm of chromosome 4, and so is distinct from the *PAH* gene. Alternatively, in some cases synthesis of BH$_4$ is impaired. Infants with malignant hyperphenylalaninemia are phenotypically indistinguishable from those with classic PKU at first, but BH$_4$ deficiency also interferes with synthesis of the neurotransmitters dopamine (tyrosine hydroxylase dependent) and serotonin (tryptophan hydroxylase dependent). Thus, brain damage in malignant hyperphenylalaninemia most likely involves more than a simple elevation in phenylalanine levels.

CLINICAL FEATURES: Phenylketonuria illustrates the interaction between genetic and environmental factors in the pathogenesis of disease. It is caused by a genetic defect, but its expression requires a dietary constituent. Affected infants appear normal at birth, but mental retardation is evident within a few months. By 12 months, untreated infants have lost about 50 IQ points, which means that a child who would otherwise have normal intelligence has become severely retarded. Infants with PKU tend to have fair skin, blond hair and blue eyes, because the inability to convert phenylalanine to tyrosine leads to reduced melanin synthesis. They exude a "mousy" or "musty" odor, owing to the phenylacetic acid they make.

The main treatment for classic PKU patients is a strict phenylalanine-restricted diet supplemented by a medical formula containing amino acids and other nutrients. In the United States, the current recommendation is that the PKU diet should be maintained for life. Patients who are diagnosed early and maintain a strict diet can have a normal life span with normal mental development. However, recent studies suggest that neurocognitive and psychosocial development and growth are slightly suboptimal if the diet is not supplemented with amino acids.

In developed countries, the clinical phenotype of classical PKU is now more of historical interest than a significant concern. About 10 million newborns worldwide are screened annually for hyperphenylalaninemia by a simple blood test (Guthrie test), and new cases are promptly treated. The success of newborn PKU screening and the prompt use of a low-phenylalanine diet allow many PKU homozygotes to live normal lives and to reproduce. Expectant mothers homozygous for PKU (maternal PKU) must restrict phenylalanine intake while pregnant for the fetus to avoid complications of maternal hyperphenylalaninemia. Infants exposed to high levels of phenylalanine in utero show microcephaly, mental and growth retardation and cardiac anomalies. In other words, high levels of phenylalanine are teratogenic.

Tyrosinemia

There are three types of tyrosinemia. The most severe is type I, a rare (1 in 100,000) autosomal recessive inborn error of tyrosine catabolism caused by a shortage of the enzyme fumarylacetoacetate hydrolase (FAH). It manifests as acute liver disease in early infancy or as a more chronic disease of the liver, kidneys and brain in children.

 MOLECULAR PATHOGENESIS: Blood levels of tyrosine and its metabolites are elevated. Fumarylacetoacetate hydrolase (15q23–25), the last enzyme in the catabolic pathway that converts tyrosine to fumarate and acetoacetate, is deficient in both acute and chronic forms of type I tyrosinemia. In the acute form, there is no enzyme activity, while children with chronic disease have variable residual activity. Cell injury in hereditary tyrosinemia is attributed to abnormal toxic metabolites, succinylacetone and succinylacetoacetate.

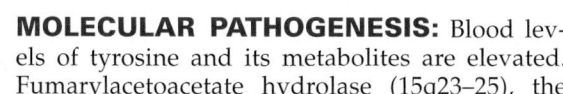 **CLINICAL FEATURES:** Acute tyrosinemia manifests in the first few months of life as hepatomegaly, edema, failure to thrive and a cabbage-like odor. Within a few months, infants die of hepatic failure.

Chronic tyrosinemia is characterized by cirrhosis of the liver, renal tubular dysfunction (Fanconi syndrome) and neurologic abnormalities. Hepatocellular carcinoma occurs in more than a third of these patients. Most children die before the age of 10. Liver transplantation corrects hepatic metabolic abnormalities and prevents the neurologic crises. Combined liver–kidney transplants have also been performed. Analysis of amniotic fluid for succinylacetone or of fetal cells for FAH establishes the diagnosis prenatally.

Alkaptonuria (Ochronosis)

This is a rare autosomal recessive disease affecting 1 in 250,000–1,000,000 people worldwide. It is more frequent in Slovakia and the Dominican Republic. Alkaptonuria

has greater historical significance than clinical importance: reports of Garrod and others 100 years ago of the inheritance of alkaptonuria helped define the idea of hereditary inborn errors of metabolism.

 PATHOPHYSIOLOGY: Alkaptonuria is due to a defect in the enzyme homogentisate 1,2-dioxygenase (HGD), which participates in tyrosine degradation. This deficiency prevents catabolism of homogentisic acid, an intermediate gene product in phenylalanine and tyrosine metabolism. As a result, homogentisic acid and its oxide, alkapton, accumulate in the blood and are excreted in urine in large amounts. Excessive homogentisic acid causes damage to cartilage (ochronosis, leading to osteoarthritis) and heart valves as well as precipitating as kidney stones.

  PATHOLOGY AND CLINICAL FEATURES: Patients with alkaptonuria excrete urine that darkens rapidly on standing, owing to formation of a pigment on the nonenzymatic oxidation of homogentisic acid (Fig. 6-31). In longstanding alkaptonuria, a similar pigment is deposited in numerous tissues, particularly the sclerae, cartilage in many areas (ribs, larynx, trachea), tendons and synovial membranes. Although the pigment is bluish black on gross examination, it is brown under the microscope, hence the term **ochronosis** (color of ocher) coined by Virchow. A degenerative and frequently disabling **arthropathy** ("ochronotic arthritis") often develops after years of alkaptonuria. It is tempting to ascribe the joint disease to the pigment deposition, but this is not proven. Despite affecting many organs, alkaptonuria does not reduce longevity.

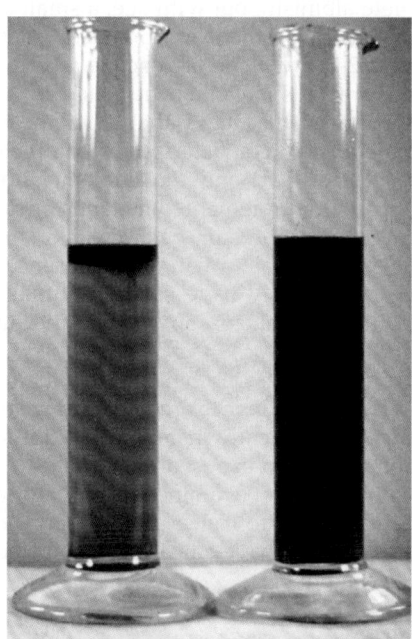

FIGURE 6-31. Urine from a patient with alkaptonuria. The specimen on the left, which has been standing for 15 minutes, shows some darkening at the surface, owing to the oxidation of homogentisic acid. After 2 hours (*right*), the urine is entirely black.

Albinism

Albinism is a heterogeneous group of at least 10 inherited disorders in which absent or reduced biosynthesis of melanin causes hypopigmentation. It is found throughout the animal kingdom (from insects to humans). Type 1 albinism is caused by defects in production of melanin pigment. Type 2 albinism is due to a defect in the "P" gene, which interferes with metabolism of tyrosine, a precursor of melanin. People with this type have slight coloring at birth.

Hermansky-Pudlak syndrome (HPS) is a form of oculocutaneous albinism caused by recessive mutations in various genes. Depending on the affected gene, it can occur with a bleeding disorder, immunodeficiency and/or lung and bowel diseases. Other complex diseases may lead to loss of coloring in only a certain area (localized albinism). These conditions include Chediak-Higashi syndrome (lack of coloring all over the skin, but not complete; see Chapter 2); tuberous sclerosis (small areas without skin coloring; see Chapter 5); Waardenburg syndrome (often a lock of hair that grows on the forehead, or no coloring in one or both irises).

The most common type is oculocutaneous albinism (OCA), a family of closely related diseases that (with one rare exception) are autosomal recessive traits. In OCA, melanin pigment is absent or reduced in the skin, hair follicles and eyes. The frequency of OCA in whites is 1 per 18,000 in the United States and 1 in 10,000 in Ireland. Blacks have the same high frequency of OCA as the Irish.

PATHOPHYSIOLOGY: Two major forms of OCA are distinguished by the presence or absence of tyrosinase, the first enzyme in the biosynthetic pathway that converts tyrosine to melanin (Fig. 6-30).

Tyrosinase-positive OCA is the most common type of albinism in whites and blacks. Patients typically begin life with complete albinism, but with age, a small amount of clinically detectable pigment accumulates. A defect in the *P* gene (15q11.2-13), which may encode a tyrosine transport protein, prevents melanin synthesis.

Tyrosinase-negative OCA is the second most common type of albinism and is characterized by complete absence of tyrosinase (11q14-21) and melanin: melanocytes are present but contain unpigmented melanosomes. Affected people have snow-white hair, pale pink skin, blue irides and prominent red pupils, owing to an absence of retinal pigment. They typically have severe ophthalmic problems, including photophobia, strabismus, nystagmus and poor visual acuity.

The skin of all types of albinos is strikingly sensitive to sunlight. Exposed skin areas require strong sunscreens. These patients have greatly increased risk for squamous cell carcinomas of sun-exposed skin. In fact, among a group of more than 500 albinos in equatorial Africa, nearly all succumbed to cancer before age 40. Interestingly, albinos seem to have a below-normal frequency of malignant melanoma.

X-LINKED DISORDERS

Expression of X-linked disorders (Fig. 6-32) is different in males and females. Females, with two X chromosomes, may be

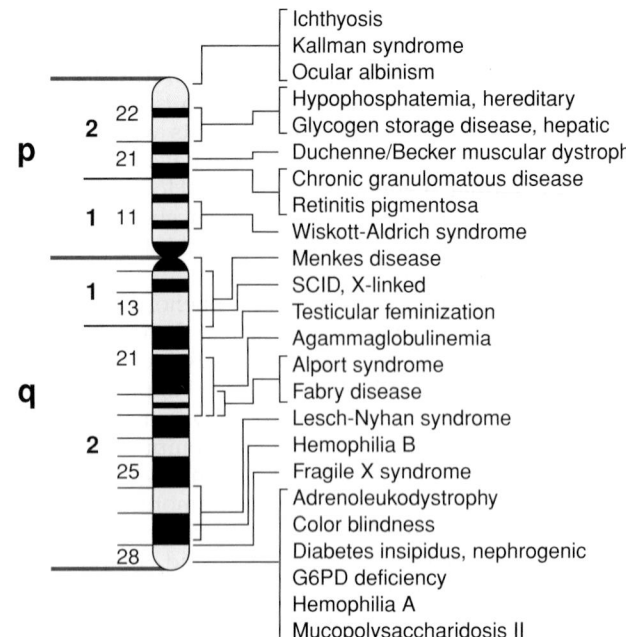

FIGURE 6-32. Localization of representative inherited diseases on the X chromosome. *G6PD* = glucose-6-phosphate dehydrogenase; *SCID* = severe combined immunodeficiency (syndrome).

homozygous or heterozygous for a given trait. It follows that clinical expression of the trait in a female is variable, depending on whether it is dominant or recessive. Males, having one X chromosome, are hemizygous for that trait and express it regardless of whether the trait is dominant or recessive.

X-linked traits are not transmitted from father to son: a symptomatic father donates only a normal Y chromosome to his male offspring. By contrast, he always donates his abnormal X chromosome to his daughters, who are thus obligate carriers of the trait. The disease thus skips a generation in males, as female carriers transmit it to grandsons of a symptomatic male.

X-Linked Dominant Traits

MOLECULAR PATHOGENESIS: X-linked dominance refers to expression of a trait only in females, since the hemizygous state in males precludes distinction between dominant and recessive inheritance (Fig. 6-33). The distinctive features of X-linked dominant disorders are:

- Females are affected twice as often as males.
- Heterozygous women transmit disease to half their children, both male and female.
- A man with a dominant X-linked disorder transmits it only to his daughters.
- Clinical expression of disease tends to be less severe and more variable in heterozygous females than in hemizygous males.

Only a few X-linked dominant disorders are known, including familial hypophosphatemic rickets and ornithine transcarbamylase deficiency. Phenotypic variation in these traits in females may reflect, at least in part, the Lyon effect (i.e., inactivation of one X chromosome), which produces mosaicism for the mutant allele, and inconstant expression of the trait.

X-LINKED DOMINANT

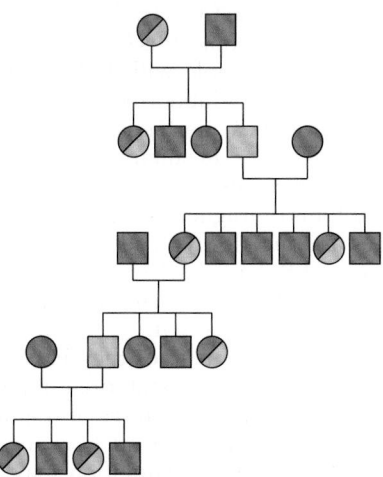

- 🔵 🟥 Unaffected female and male
- ◐ Affected heterozygous female
- ◻ Affected hemizygous male

FIGURE 6-33. X-linked dominant inheritance. A heterozygous woman transmits the trait equally to males and females; men transmit the trait only to their daughters. Asymptomatic males and females do not carry the trait.

TABLE 6-10	
REPRESENTATIVE X-LINKED RECESSIVE DISEASES	
Disease	**Frequency in Males**
Fragile X syndrome	1/4000
Hemophilia A (factor VIII deficiency)	1/10,000
Hemophilia B (factor IX deficiency)	1/70,000
Duchenne-Becker muscular dystrophy	1/3500
Glucose-6-phosphate dehydrogenase deficiency	Up to 30%
Lesch-Nyhan syndrome (HPRT deficiency)	1/10,000
Chronic granulomatous disease	Not rare
X-linked agammaglobulinemia	Not rare
X-linked severe combined immunodeficiency	Rare
Fabry disease	1/40,000
Hunter syndrome	1/70,000
Adrenoleukodystrophy	1/100,000
Menkes disease	1/100,000

HPRT = hypoxanthine-guanine phosphoribosyltransferase.

Table 6-10 lists representative X-linked recessive disorders.

X-Linked Recessive Traits

Most X-linked traits are recessive; that is, heterozygous females do not manifest clinical disease (Fig. 6-34). The characteristics of this mode of inheritance are:

- Sons of women who are carriers have a 50% chance of inheriting the disease. Daughters are not symptomatic, but 50% of daughters will also be carriers.
- All daughters of affected men are asymptomatic carriers, but the sons of these men do not have the trait and cannot transmit it to their children.
- Symptomatic homozygous females can result from a rare mating of an affected man with an asymptomatic, heterozygous woman. Or, lyonization may preferentially inactivate the normal X chromosome, which, in extreme cases, may lead to an affected heterozygous female.
- The trait tends to occur in maternal uncles and in male cousins descended from the mother's sisters.

X-Linked (Duchenne and Becker) Muscular Dystrophies

The muscular dystrophies are devastating muscle diseases. Most are X-linked, although a few are autosomal recessive. The X-linked muscular dystrophies are among the most common human genetic diseases, occurring in 1 per 3500 boys, an incidence approaching that of CF. The most common X-linked recessive disorders include *Duchenne muscular dystrophy (DMD)* and *Becker muscular dystrophy (BMD)*. DMD, the most common variant, is a fatal progressive degeneration of muscle that appears before the age of 4 years. It is associated with mutations in the dystrophin gene, the largest gene on the X chromosome, and characterized by rapid progression

X-LINKED RECESSIVE

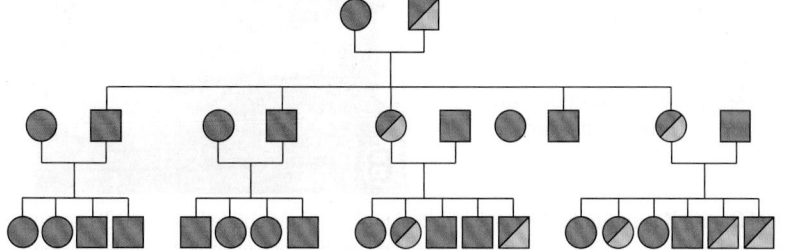

- ▨ Affected male
- ◐ Heterozygous female without disease (silent carrier)

FIGURE 6-34. X-linked recessive inheritance. Only males are affected; daughters of affected men are all asymptomatic carriers. Asymptomatic men do not transmit the trait. Clinical expression of the disease skips a generation.

of muscle degeneration, with eventual loss of skeletal muscle control, respiratory failure and death. BMD is allelic with DMD but is milder and causes slowly progressive muscle weakness of the legs and pelvis (see Chapter 31).

Hemophilia A (Factor VIII Deficiency)

Hemophilia A (see Chapter 26) is an X-linked recessive disorder of blood clotting that results in spontaneous bleeding, mainly into joints, muscles and internal organs. It is caused by deficiency of factor VIII due to a mutation in the factor VIII gene.

Red-Green Color Blindness

Red-green color blindness is a very common trait in humans. Between 7% and 10% of men and 0.49% and 1% of women are affected. It is most commonly inherited as an X-linked recessive condition, but mutations involving as many as 19 chromosomes and 56 genes have been implicated in rare forms of this disorder.

Fragile X Syndrome

Fully 20% of heritable mental retardation is due to X-linked disorders, and 1/5 of these reflect an inducible fragile site on the X chromosome. A **fragile site** represents a specific locus, or band, on a chromosome that breaks easily under certain conditions. Fragile X syndrome (FXS) is second only to Down syndrome as a genetic cause of mental retardation. The prevalence of FXS in males is 1 in 3600–4000 and in females is 1 in 4000–6000.

MOLECULAR PATHOGENESIS: Mutations in the *FMR1* gene (Xq27.2) cause fragile X syndrome. This gene encodes a protein called fragile X mental retardation 1 protein, or FMRP, which helps regulate production of other proteins and plays a role in synapse development. Nearly all cases of fragile X syndrome are caused by a mutation in which DNA in the 5' untranslated region, known as the CGG triplet repeat, is expanded within *FMR1*. In normal people, this DNA segment is repeated from 5 to 45 times. In people with FXS, however, it is repeated over 200 times. The abnormally expanded CGG silences the gene through a mechanism involving methylation of selected nucleotides. Resultant loss or deficiency of the protein disrupts nervous system functions, leading to the signs and symptoms of fragile X syndrome.

Males and females with 50–200 repeats of the CGG segment are said to have *FMR1* gene **premutation**. About 1 in 260 females and 1 in 800 males are carriers of fragile X premutation. Most people with premutation are intellectually normal, although sometimes they have lower than normal amounts of FMRP. As a result, premutation may cause mild versions of the physical features of fragile X syndrome and lead to emotional problems such as anxiety or depression. Some children with a premutation may have learning disabilities or autistic-like behavior.

Fragile sites are detected in cytogenetic preparations as a nonstaining gap or constriction (Fig. 6-16). When the cells in culture are treated to impair DNA synthesis (e.g., with methotrexate, floxuridine), fragile sites are revealed. Most people have at least 11, and possibly up to 50, fragile sites, on autosomes and on the X chromosome. However, the locus at Xq27.2 is associated with mental retardation and other clinical findings that characterize fragile X syndrome. As discussed, the fragile site at Xq27 is a distinct kind of mutation characterized by amplification of a CGG repeat.

Within fragile X families, the probability of being affected is related to position in the pedigree: later generations are more likely than earlier ones to be affected **(Sherman paradox** or **genetic anticipation).** This is due to progressive triplet repeat expansion (Fig. 6-35). Chromosomes with more than about 52 repeats can increase the number of repeats—so-called expansion. Small expansions tend to be asymptomatic but can

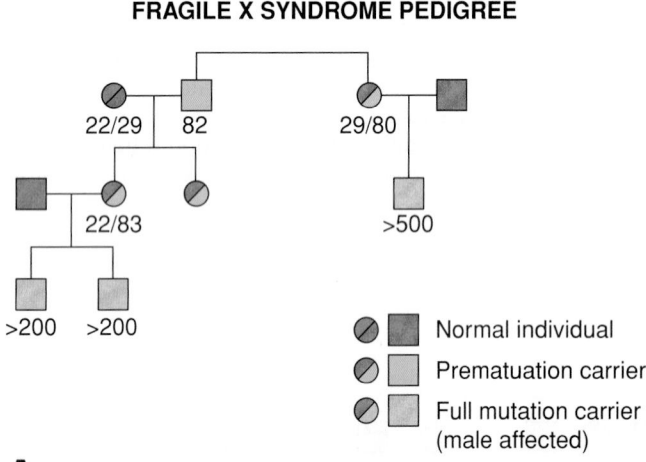

FRAGILE X SYNDROME PEDIGREE

22/29   82   29/80

22/83

>500

>200   >200

Normal individual

Prematuation carrier

Full mutation carrier
(male affected)

A

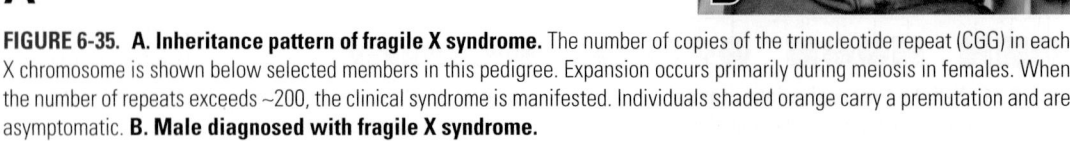

B

FIGURE 6-35. A. Inheritance pattern of fragile X syndrome. The number of copies of the trinucleotide repeat (CGG) in each X chromosome is shown below selected members in this pedigree. Expansion occurs primarily during meiosis in females. When the number of repeats exceeds ~200, the clinical syndrome is manifested. Individuals shaded orange carry a premutation and are asymptomatic. **B. Male diagnosed with fragile X syndrome.**

enlarge, particularly during meiosis in females, leading to larger expansions in successive generations. Expansions with over 200 repeats are associated with mental retardation and are considered full mutations of the FMR1 gene locus. Expansion of a premutation to a full mutation during gametogenesis occurs only in females (Fig. 6-35). Thus, daughters of men with premutations (carriers) are never clinically symptomatic but always harbor the premutation. However, sisters of transmitting males occasionally produce affected daughters. *The frequency of conversion of a premutation to a full mutation in such women (i.e., the probability that their sons will have fragile X syndrome) varies with the length of the expanded tract.* Premutations with more than 90 repeats are almost always converted to full mutations. Hence, the risk of the disorder increases in succeeding generations of fragile X families. As the syndrome is recessive, most daughters of carrier males transmit mental retardation to 50% of their sons.

 CLINICAL FEATURES: A male newborn with FXS appears normal, but during childhood, typical features appear, including increased head circumference and elongated face, large protruding ears (Fig. 6-35B), joint hyperextensibility, enlarged testes and hypotonia. Mental retardation is profound: IQ scores vary from 20 to 60. Interestingly, a significant proportion of autistic boys have a fragile X chromosome. Among mentally handicapped female carriers, the severity of the impairment varies from a learning disability with normal IQ to serious retardation. About 80% of males with the Xq27.2 fragile site are mentally retarded; the others have expansions of less than 200 copies and are clinically normal but can transmit the trait.

A syndrome characterized by tremors, ataxia and declining cognitive abilities has been described in elderly men with fragile X premutations. This disorder has some clinical similarities to Parkinson disease and Alzheimer disease and has been called fragile X tremor ataxia syndrome (FTAXS).

Two thirds of females who carry a fragile X chromosome (obligate carriers) are intellectually normal, and the fragile site on the X chromosome cannot be demonstrated. By contrast, virtually all the 1/3 of female carriers who are mentally retarded display a fragile Xq27.2 locus. This phenotypic variability in females may relate to the pattern of X chromosome inactivation.

Molecular DNA diagnostic testing is now available to identify fragile X premutation carriers and those with the full fragile X syndrome mutation.

Fabry Disease

Fabry disease is an X-linked lysosomal storage disease. The X-linked recessive mutations cause deficiency of α-galactosidase A, which leads to accumulation of globotriaosylceramide and other glycosphingolipids in endothelial and smooth muscle cells throughout the vasculature, especially in coronary arteries, renal glomeruli, cardiac myocytes and components of the cardiac conduction system. A particular type of tumor, angiokeratoma, is a characteristic cutaneous manifestation of Fabry disease. Functionally affected microvasculature becomes increasingly compromised, causing progressive vascular insufficiency with cerebral, renal and cardiac infarcts. Patients die in early adulthood from complications of their vascular disease. Therapy with recombinant α-D-galactosidase A shows promise in arresting the disease.

MITOCHONDRIAL DISEASES

 **MOLECULAR PATHOGENESIS:** Proteins in mitochondria are encoded by both nuclear and mitochondrial genes. Most mitochondrial respiratory chain proteins are encoded by nuclear genes, but 13 such proteins are products of the mitochondrial genome. The remaining 1500 or so proteins in mitochondria are nuclear encoded. A few rare, autosomal recessive (mendelian) disorders are caused by defects in nuclear-encoded mitochondrial proteins. Defects in nuclear-encoded mitochondrial proteins have also been associated with complex (i.e., polygenic rather than mendelian) disorders such as anemia, hypertension, dementia and neurodevelopmental disorder. However, most inherited defects in mitochondrial function result from mutations in the mitochondrial genome itself.

To understand these conditions, an explanation of the unique genetics of the mitochondria is needed. These features include:

- **Maternal inheritance:** All vertebrate mitochondria are inherited from the mother via the ovum, which has up to 300,000 copies of mitochondrial DNA (mtDNA).
- **Variability of mtDNA copies:** The number of mitochondria and the number of copies of mtDNA per mitochondrion vary in different tissues. Each mitochondrion has 2–10 mtDNA copies, and varying tissue needs for ATP correlate with the DNA content per mitochondrion.
- **Threshold effect:** Since any given cell has many mitochondria and thus hundreds or thousands of mtDNA copies, mutations in mtDNA lead to mixed populations of mutant and normal mitochondrial genomes, a situation called **heteroplasmy**. The phenotype of mtDNA mutations reflects the severity of the mutation, the proportion of mutant genomes and the tissue's demand for ATP. Different tissues need different amounts of ATP to sustain their metabolism; the brain, heart and skeletal muscle have particularly high energy demands.
- **High mutation rate:** The rate of mtDNA mutation is much higher than that of nuclear DNA, owing (at least in part) to less DNA repair capacity.

Diseases caused by mutations in the mitochondrial genome mainly affect the nervous system, heart and skeletal muscle. Functional deficits in all of these disorders are traced to impaired oxidative phosphorylation (OXPHOS). **OXPHOS diseases** are divided into several classes: I, nuclear mutations; II, mtDNA point mutations; III, mtDNA deletions; and IV, undefined defects.

All inherited mitochondrial diseases are rare and have variable clinical presentations for the reasons discussed above. Many diseases of aging are caused by defects in mitochondrial function. Since mitochondria process oxygen and convert constituents of foods into energy for essential cellular functions, mitochondrial dysfunction can contribute to complex diseases in adults including type 2 diabetes, Parkinson disease, atherosclerotic heart disease, stroke, Alzheimer disease and cancer. The first human mtDNA disease described was **Leber hereditary optic neuropathy,** which is characterized by progressive loss of vision. Various mitochondrial myopathies (skeletal and cardiac) and encephalomyopathies are known (see Chapter 31).

GENETIC IMPRINTING

MOLECULAR PATHOGENESIS: Phenotypes associated with some genes differ, depending on whether the allele is inherited from the mother or father. This phenomenon is called **genetic imprinting**. For imprinted genes, either the maternal or paternal allele is maintained in an inactive state. This normal physiologic process results from CpG methylation (see above) in regulatory regions of imprinted allele, such that the nonimprinted allele provides the sole biological function for that locus. If the nonimprinted allele is disrupted via mutation, the imprinted allele remains inactive and cannot compensate for the missing function. *Imprinting occurs in meiosis during gametogenesis, and the pattern of imprinting is maintained to variable degrees in different tissues. It is reset during meiosis in the next generation, so the selection of a given allele for imprinting can vary from one generation to the next.*

In extreme cases, experimental (nonhuman) embryos that obtain both sets of chromosomes exclusively from either the mother or the father never survive to term. A less severe manifestation of genetic imprinting is seen in **uniparental disomy,** in which both members of a single chromosome pair are inherited from the same parent. The pair of chromosomes may be copies of one parental chromosome (uniparental isodisomy) or may be the same pair found in one parent (uniparental heterodisomy). Uniparental disomy is rare but is implicated in unexpected inheritance patterns of genetic traits. Thus, a child with uniparental isodisomy may show a recessive disease when only one parent carries the trait, which has been observed in a few cases of cystic fibrosis and hemophilia A. Loss of a chromosome from a trisomy or duplication of a chromosome in the case of a monosomy can lead to uniparental disomy. Up to 1% of viable pregnancies carry uniparental disomy for at least one chromosome.

Genetic imprinting is illustrated by certain hereditary diseases whose phenotype is determined by the parental source of the mutant allele. Prader-Willi syndrome (PWS) and Angelman syndrome (AS) provide excellent examples of the effect of imprinting on genetic diseases. Both disorders are associated with (heterozygous) deletion in the region of 15(q11-13). In PWS, the deletion is in the paternal chromosome and critical genes in this region of the maternal chromosome are expressed but epigenetically silenced. By contrast, in AS, the same region of the maternal chromosome 15 is affected; critical genes in the paternal chromosome are expressed and epigenetically silenced.

The phenotypes of these disorders are remarkably different. PWS features hypotonia, hyperphagia with obesity, hypogonadism, mental retardation and characteristic facies. By contrast, AS patients are hyperactive, display inappropriate laughter, have different facies from that in PWS and suffer from seizures.

Prader-Willi syndrome develops because critical genes in the maternal locus are normally silenced by imprinting and the same region on the paternal chromosome is deleted, resulting in lack of expression. The converse applies in Angelman syndrome: the paternal gene is normally imprinted and silenced, and the maternal locus is inactivated by mutation or deletion. Critical genes silenced by methylation in the maternal 15q11-13 include *SNRPN* (encoding small nuclear ribonucleoprotein polypeptide), *NDN* (encoding necdin) and a cluster of small nucleolar RNAs (snoRNAs). In AS, *UBE3A*, which encodes a ubiquitin ligase, is mutated or deleted in the maternal chromosome and epigenetically silenced (in the paternal chromosome).

Each of these disorders is now routinely diagnosed by FISH or array CGH to detect the microdeletion of genes in 15q11-13 and by DNA methylation studies to detect uniparental disomy of maternal/paternal genes. This pattern is similar to loss of heterozygosity in tumor suppressor genes by aberrant methylation in some cases of cancer (see Chapter 5).

Genetic imprinting is implicated in a number of other situations relevant to human disease. In some childhood cancers, such as Wilms tumor, osteosarcoma, bilateral retinoblastoma and embryonal rhabdomyosarcoma, the maternal allele of a putative tumor suppressor gene is lost and the remaining allele is on a chromosome of paternal origin. In the case of familial glomus tumor, an adult neoplasm, both males and females may carry the trait, but it is transmitted only through the male. Thus, the responsible gene is active only when it is located on the paternal autosome. Finally, as noted above, premutation in fragile X syndrome expands to full mutation only during female gametogenesis, indicating that the trinucleotide repeat is treated differently on passage through the female than in the male.

MULTIFACTORIAL INHERITANCE

Most normal human traits reflect such complexities and are not inherited as simple dominant or recessive mendelian attributes. Many result from interplay between multiple genes and environmental, epigenetic and other factors. These reflect multifactorial inheritance. Thus, such inheritance determines height, skin color and body habitus. Similarly, most chronic disorders of adults—diabetes, atherosclerosis, many forms of cancer, arthritis and hypertension—are diseases that are understood to "run in families" but in which inheritance does not follow simple patterns. Many birth defects (e.g., cleft lip and palate, pyloric stenosis and congenital heart disease) are also transmitted via such complex mechanisms (Table 6-11).

TABLE 6-11

REPRESENTATIVE DISEASES ASSOCIATED WITH MULTIFACTORIAL INHERITANCE

Adults	Children
Hypertension	Pyloric stenosis
Atherosclerosis	Cleft lip and palate
Diabetes, type 2	Congenital heart disease
Allergic diathesis	Meningomyelocele
Psoriasis	Anencephaly
Schizophrenia	Hypospadias
Ankylosing spondylitis	Congenital hip dislocation
Gout	Hirschsprung disease

Multifactorial inheritance entails multiple genes interacting with each other and with environmental factors to produce disease in an individual. Such inheritance leads to familial aggregation that does not obey simple mendelian rules. Thus, inheritance of polygenic diseases is studied by population genetics, rather than by analysis of individual families.

The number of involved genes for any such disease is not known. Thus, in an individual case, the risk of a particular disorder cannot be quantified. The probability of disease can only be suggested from the numbers of relatives affected, the severity of their disease and statistical projections based on population analyses. While monogenic inheritance implies a specific risk of disease (e.g., 25%, 50%), the probability of symptoms in first-degree relatives of someone with a polygenic disease is usually only about 5%–10%.

The basis of polygenic inheritance is that over 1/4 of all genes in normal humans have polymorphic alleles. Such heterogeneity leads to wide variability in susceptibility to many diseases, made yet more complex by interactions with the environment.

- **Expression of symptoms is proportional to the number of mutant genes.** Close relatives of an affected person have more mutant genes than the population at large and more chance of expressing the disease. The probability of disease is highest in identical twins.
- **Environmental factors influence expression of the trait.** Thus, concordance for the disease may occur in only 1/3 of monozygotic twins.
- **Risk in first-degree relatives (parents, siblings, children) is the same (5%–10%).** The probability of disease is much lower in second-degree relatives.
- **The likelihood of a trait's expression in later offspring is influenced by its expression in earlier siblings.** If one or more children are born with a multifactorial defect, the chance it will recur in later offspring is doubled. For simple mendelian traits, by contrast, the probability is independent of the number of affected siblings.
- **The more severe the defect, the greater the risk of transmitting it to offspring.** Patients with more severe polygenic defects probably have more mutant genes. Their children thus will more likely inherit more abnormal genes than offspring of less severely affected parents.
- **Some diseases with multifactorial inheritance also show gender predilection.** Thus, pyloric stenosis is more common in males, while congenital hip dislocation is more common in females. Such differential susceptibility is thought to reflect different thresholds for expression of mutant genes in the two sexes, so that if the number of mutant genes required for pyloric stenosis in males is A, it may require 4A in the female. If so, a woman who had pyloric stenosis as an infant has more mutant genes to transmit to her children than does a similarly afflicted man. Indeed, sons of such women have a 25% chance of having pyloric stenosis, compared to a 4% risk for the son of an affected man. *As a rule, if there is an altered sex ratio in the incidence of a polygenic defect, a member of the less commonly affected sex has a much greater probability of transmitting the defect.*

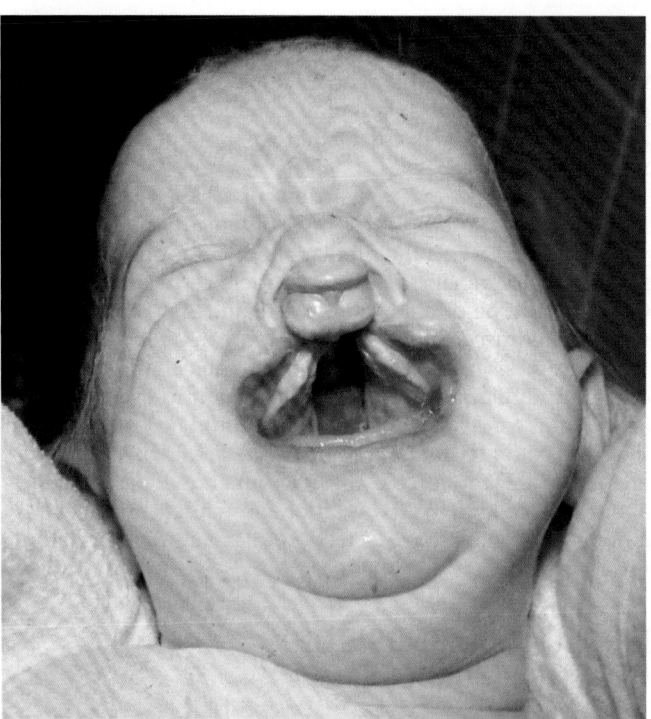

FIGURE 6-36. Cleft lip and palate in an infant.

Cleft Lip and Cleft Palate Exemplify Multifactorial Inheritance

At the 35th day of gestation, the frontal prominence fuses with the maxillary process to form the upper lip. This process is under the control of many genes, and disturbances in gene expression (hereditary or environmental) at this time interfere with proper fusion, resulting in cleft lip, with or without cleft palate (Fig. 6-36). This anomaly may also be part of a systemic malformation syndrome caused by teratogens (e.g., rubella, anticonvulsants) and often occurs in children with chromosomal abnormalities.

Incidence of cleft lip, with or without cleft palate, is 10 per 10,000 live births. The incidence of cleft palate alone is 6 per 10,000 live births. If one child is born with a cleft lip, the chances are 4% that a second child will have the same defect. If the first two children are affected, the risk of cleft lip in the third child increases to 9%. The more severe the defect, the greater the probability of transmitting cleft lip will be. While 75% of cases of cleft lip occur in boys, the sons of women with cleft lip have a 4-fold higher risk for the defect than do sons of affected fathers.

SCREENING FOR CARRIERS OF GENETIC DISORDERS

Until recently, screening for carriers of genetic diseases was not common. Among Ashkenazi Jews, screening to identify carriers of Tay-Sachs disease, an autosomal recessive disease, was done because of the relatively high frequency of the disease in that group. A number of other inherited conditions are also included in a so-called Ashkenazi screen. The goal is to identify couples in which both members are heterozygous carriers and who thus have a 25% risk of being affected. These couples can be offered prenatal diagnosis to determine the genetic status of their fetus. In vitro fertilization combined with preimplantation genetic diagnosis is available in some centers to ensure that an implanted embryo will not have this disease.

Prenatal screening for carriers of CF has been recommended by national professional organizations for several years and represents the first large-scale adoption of testing for carriers of genetic diseases. Guidelines recommend that CF screening be offered to all white and Ashkenazi Jewish women because of the relatively high frequency of CF in these groups. The CF screening test detects 23 relatively common mutations, plus 9 other less common mutations. If a woman is a CF carrier, her partner should be tested to see if the couple is at risk of having an affected child. Because there are many CF mutations, the recommended panel detects about 88% of known CF mutations in whites, but over 94% among Ashkenazi Jews. Detection rates among other ethnic groups are lower.

PRENATAL DIAGNOSIS OF GENETIC DISORDERS

Amniocentesis and chorionic villus biopsy are the most important diagnostic tools for genetic or developmental disorders. Both procedures are safe, reliable and easily done. Indications for performing them are:

- **Age 35 years old and over:** The likelihood of having a child with Down syndrome is about 1 in 1250 for a mother age 25, compared with 1 in 100 for a 40-year-old. Risk increases even more with advanced maternal age.
- **Previous chromosomal abnormality:** The risk of Down syndrome recurring in a later child of a woman who has already had an infant with trisomy 21 is 1%.
- **Translocation carrier:** Estimates of risks to the offspring of translocation carriers are from 3% to 15%. *Carriers of balanced translocations are more likely to produce children with unbalanced karyotypes and resulting phenotypic abnormalities.*
- **History of familial inborn error of metabolism:** Recessive inborn errors of metabolism have a 25% risk for each child if both parents are heterozygous for the trait. Newborn screening can identify disorders for which a biochemical diagnosis can be made.
- **Identified heterozygotes:** Carrier detection projects (e.g., Tay-Sachs Disease Prevention Program) identify couples in which both spouses are carriers of the same recessive gene. Each of their pregnancies has a 25% risk of an affected child and diagnosis can be made prenatally.
- **Family history of X-linked disorders:** Fetal sex determination, using amniotic cells, can be offered to women known to be carriers of X-linked disorders. Diagnosis of some of these conditions can be established biochemically by amniotic fluid analysis.

Gene-specific DNA probes have been developed for many genetic diseases, including hemophilia A and B, the hemoglobinopathies, phenylketonuria and α_1-antitrypsin deficiency. Most heterozygous carriers for Duchenne and Becker muscular dystrophies, Huntington chorea and cystic fibrosis can be identified by such techniques.

DISEASES OF INFANCY AND CHILDHOOD

The period from birth to puberty has been traditionally subdivided into several stages.

- Neonatal age (the first 4 weeks)
- Infancy (the first year)
- Early childhood (1–4 years)
- Late childhood (5–14 years)

Each of these periods has its own anatomic, physiologic and immunologic characteristics, which determine which diseases occur and how they manifest. Causes and mechanisms of morbidity and mortality in the neonatal period differ greatly from those in infancy and childhood. Infants and children are not simply "small adults," and they may be afflicted by diseases unique to their particular age group.

PREMATURITY AND INTRAUTERINE GROWTH RETARDATION

Human pregnancy normally lasts 40 ± 2 weeks, and most newborns weigh 3300 ± 600 g. The World Health Organization defines prematurity as a gestational age under 37 weeks (timed from the first day of the last menstrual period). Traditionally, prematurity signified a birth weight below 2500 g, regardless of gestational age. However, since full-term infants may weigh under 2500 g because of intrauterine growth retardation rather than prematurity, **low–birth-weight infants** (<2500 g) are either appropriate for gestational age (AGA) or small for gestational age (SGA).

The frequency of low birth weight in the United States has recently risen to 8.3% owing to increased numbers of multiple births. Two thirds of such infants are premature (AGA). By contrast, when the frequency of low–birth-weight infants exceeds 10%, as it does for blacks (>13%), most newborns suffer from IUGR and are considered SGA.

About 1% of infants born in the United States weigh under 1500 g and are classified as **very-low-birth-weight infants**. These represent half of neonatal deaths, and their survival is related to birth weight. If they are cared for in neonatal intensive care units, 90% of infants over 750 g survive. From 500 g to 750 g, 45% survive. Of these, over half develop normally.

 **ETIOLOGIC FACTORS:** Factors that predispose to premature birth of an infant (AGA) include (1) maternal illness, (2) uterine incompetence, (3) fetal disorders and (4) placental abnormalities (see Chapter 14). If the life of a fetus is threatened by such conditions, it may be necessary to induce premature delivery to save the infant. In many AGA infants, the cause of premature birth is unknown. Intrauterine growth retardation and the resulting birth of SGA infants are associated with disorders that impair maternal health and nutrition, interfere with placental circulation or function or disturb fetal growth or development (see Chapter 14).

 CLINICAL FEATURES: Complications of prematurity itself (AGA) and of IUGR (SGA) overlap. However, certain general principles apply. Prematurity is often associated with severe respiratory distress, metabolic disturbances (e.g., hypoglycemia, hypocalcemia, hyperbilirubinemia), circulatory problems (anemia, hypothermia, hypotension) and bacterial sepsis. By contrast, SGA infants are a much more heterogeneous group, including many with congenital anomalies and infections acquired in utero. Even when these causes of intrauterine growth retardation are excluded, neonatal complications in SGA infants reflect gestational age more than birth weight. In addition to problems related to prematurity, SGA infants often suffer from perinatal asphyxia, meconium aspiration, necrotizing enterocolitis, pulmonary hemorrhage and sequelae of birth defects or inherited diseases.

Organ Immaturity Is a Cause of Neonatal Problems

The maturity of the newborn can be defined in both anatomic and physiologic terms. Organ maturation in infants born prematurely differs from that in term infants, even as total maturation of many organs may require days (lungs) to years (brain) after birth.

LUNGS: Pulmonary immaturity is a common and immediate threat to the viability of low–birth-weight infants. Fetal alveolar lining cels do not differentiate into type I and type II pneumocytes until late in pregnancy. Amniotic fluid fills fetal alveoli and drains from the lungs at birth. Sometimes respiratory movements of immature infants are sluggish and do not fully expel amniotic fluid from their lungs. Respiratory embarrassment may ensue, a syndrome called **amniotic fluid aspiration,** but that actually represents retained amniotic fluid. Air passages contain desquamated squamous cells **(squames)** and lanugo hair from the fetal skin and protein-rich amniotic fluid (Fig. 6-37; see Chapter 18).

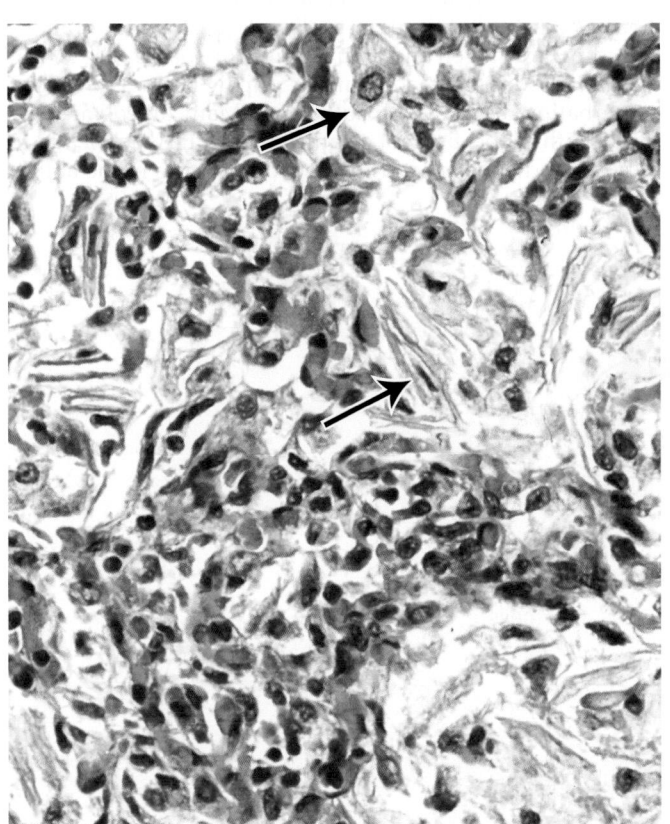

FIGURE 6-37. Retention of amniotic fluid in the lung of a premature newborn. The incompletely expanded lung contains squames (*arrows*) consisting of squamous epithelial cells shed into the amniotic fluid from the fetal skin.

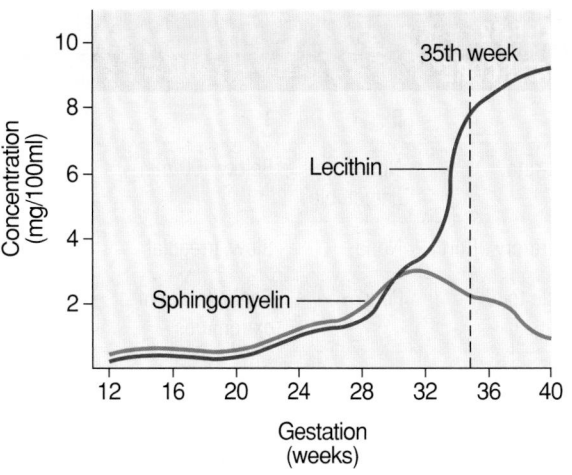

FIGURE 6-38. Changes in amniotic fluid composition during pregnancy.

The ability of alveoli to remain expanded during the respiratory cycle (i.e., not to collapse during expiration) is due largely to **pulmonary surfactant,** which reduces intra-alveolar surface tension. Surfactant, produced by type II pneumocytes, is a complex mixture of 10% proteins and 90% mixed phospholipids, the latter including 75% phosphatidylcholine (lecithin) and 10% phosphatidylglycerol. Surfactant composition changes as a fetus matures: (1) lecithin increases at the start of the third trimester and then rises rapidly to peak near term (Fig. 6-38); (2) most lecithin in the mature lung is dipalmitoyl phosphatidylcholine, but in the immature lung it is a less-surface-active α-palmitoyl, α-myristoyl species; (3) phosphatidylglycerol is not present in the lungs before the 36th week of pregnancy; and (4) before the 35th week, immature surfactant contains a higher proportion of sphingomyelin than adult surfactant.

The protein constituents of surfactant, though they make up a small proportion of its total weight, are important in facilitating the surface activity of the mixture and serve other functions as well. Two highly hydrophobic surfactant-associated proteins (SPs), SP-B and SP-C, are critical for surface activity. Two more hydrophilic proteins, SP-A and SP-D, fulfill additional functions, thought to include regulating surfactant secretion, antimicrobial protection and others.

Pulmonary surfactant is released into the amniotic fluid, which can be sampled by amniocentesis to assess fetal lung maturity. A lecithin-to-sphingomyelin ratio above 2:1 predicts extrauterine survival without respiratory distress syndrome (see below). After the 35th week, the appearance of phosphatidylglycerol in the amniotic fluid is the best proof of fetal lung maturity.

LIVER: The liver of premature infants is morphologically similar to that of adults, except for conspicuous extramedullary hematopoiesis. However, the hepatocytes tend to be functionally immature. Fetal liver is deficient in glucuronyl transferase. The liver's resulting inability to conjugate bilirubin often leads to **neonatal jaundice** (see Chapter 20). This enzyme deficiency is aggravated by the rapid destruction of fetal erythrocytes, a process that increases supply of bilirubin.

BRAIN: The brain of immature newborns differs from that of the adult, morphologically and functionally, but this difference is rarely fatal. Still, incomplete CNS development

TABLE 6-12
APGAR SCORE[a]

Sign	0	1	2
Heart rate	Not detectable	Below 100/min	Over 100/min
Respiratory effort	None	Slow, irregular	Good, crying
Muscle tone	Poor	Some flexion of extremities	Active motion
Response to catheter in nostril	No response	Grimace	Cough or sneeze
Color	Blue, pale	Body pink, extremities blue	Completely pink

[a]Sixty seconds after the completion of birth, these five objective signs are evaluated, and each is given a score of 0, 1, or 2. A maximum score of 10 is assigned to infants in the best possible condition.

often contributes to poor vasomotor control, hypothermia, feeding difficulties and recurrent apnea.

The Apgar Score

Clinical assessments of neonatal maturity in general are usually performed 1 minute and 5 minutes after delivery, and certain parameters are scored according to the criteria recommended by Virginia Apgar (Table 6-12). In general, the higher the **Apgar score,** the better the clinical condition of the infant. The score taken at 1 minute is an index of asphyxia and the need for assisted ventilation. The 5-minute score is a more accurate indication of impending death or likelihood of persistent neurologic damage. For example, newborns under 2000 g whose 5-minute Apgar scores are 9 or 10 have

a 95% chance of surviving their first month. This declines to 20% if the 5-minute Apgar score is 3 or less.

Neonatal Respiratory Distress Syndrome Is Due to Deficiency of Surfactant

Neonatal respiratory distress syndrome (RDS) is the leading cause of morbidity and mortality among premature infants, accounting for half of neonatal deaths in the United States. Its incidence varies inversely with gestational age and birth weight. Over half of infants born younger than 28 weeks' gestational age develop RDS, compared with 1/5 of infants born between 32 and 36 weeks. Additional risk factors for RDS include (1) neonatal asphyxia, (2) maternal diabetes, (3) delivery by cesarean section, (4) precipitous delivery and (5) twin pregnancy.

 ETIOLOGIC FACTORS: *The pathogenesis of RDS of the newborn is intimately linked to surfactant deficiency* (Fig. 6-39). When a newborn starts breathing, type II cells release their surfactant stores. Surfactant reduces surface tension by decreasing the affinity of alveolar surfaces for each other. This allows alveoli to remain open when the baby exhales and reduces resistance to reinflating the lungs. If surfactant function is inadequate, as it is in many premature infants with immature lungs, alveoli collapse when the baby exhales and resist expansion with the next breath. The energy required for the second breath must then overcome the stickiness within alveoli. Inspiration therefore requires considerable effort, and the alveolar lining becomes damaged when adherent alveolar walls pull apart. As a result, injured alveoli leak plasma constituents, including fibrinogen and albumin, into airspaces. These proteins bind surfactant and further impair its function, thus exacerbating respiratory insufficiency. Many alveoli are perfused with blood but not ventilated by air, which leads to hypoxia and acidosis and further compromise in the ability

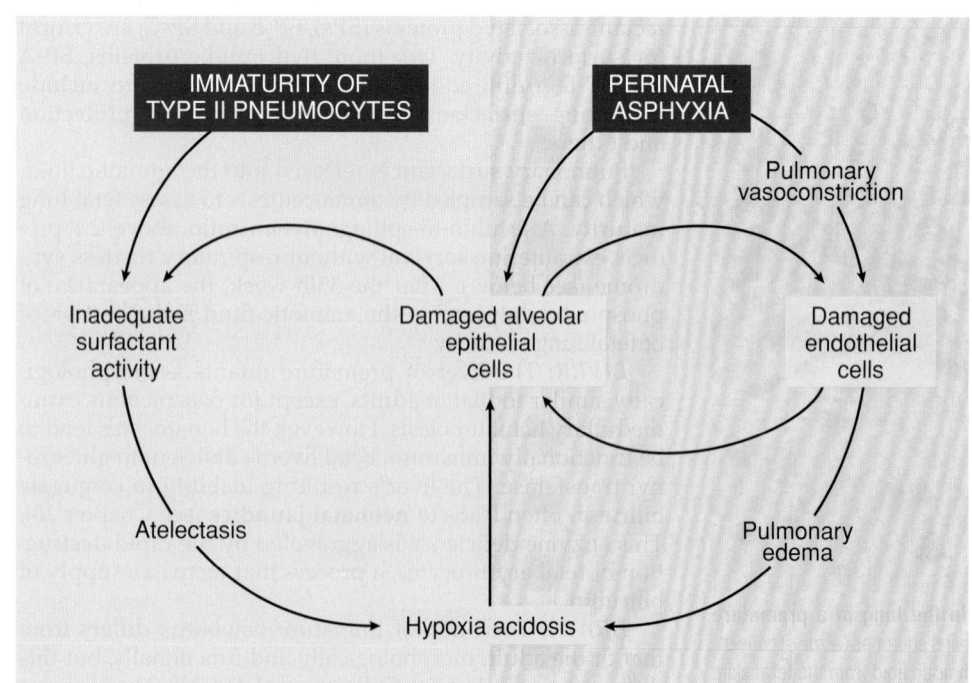

FIGURE 6-39. Pathogenesis of respiratory distress syndrome in the neonate. Immaturity of the lungs and perinatal asphyxia are the major pathogenetic factors.

of type II pneumocytes to produce surfactant. Intra-alveolar hypoxia induces pulmonary arterial vasoconstriction, thus increasing right-to-left shunting through the ductus arteriosus, through the foramen ovale and within the lung itself. Resulting pulmonary ischemia further aggravates alveolar epithelial damage and injures alveolar capillary endothelium. Leak of protein-rich fluid into alveolar spaces from the injured vascular bed contributes to the typical clinical and pathologic features of RDS.

The course of RDS is further complicated by the need to expose the infant to high concentrations of inspired oxygen (FiO_2) to maintain adequate arterial oxygen levels. Although respiratory support has improved greatly, the damage caused by high FiO_2 levels (see ROS-mediated damage, Chapter 1) adds to the already ongoing lung injury.

 PATHOLOGY: The lungs in neonatal RDS are dark red, solid in consistency and airless. Alveoli are collapsed. Alveolar ducts and respiratory bronchioles are dilated and contain cellular debris, proteinaceous edema fluid and erythrocytes. Alveolar ducts are lined by conspicuous, eosinophilic, fibrin-rich, amorphous structures, called **hyaline membranes,** hence the original term **hyaline membrane disease** (Fig. 6-40). Collapsed alveoli have thick walls, capillaries are congested and lymphatics are filled with proteinaceous material.

 CLINICAL FEATURES: Most newborns destined to develop RDS appear normal at birth and have high Apgar scores. The first symptom, appearing usually within an hour of birth, is increased respiratory effort, with forceful intercostal retraction and the use of accessory neck muscles. Respiratory rate increases to more than 100 breaths per minute, and the baby becomes cyanotic. Chest radiographs show a characteristic "ground-glass" granularity, and in terminal stages the fluid-filled alveoli appear as complete "white-out" of the lungs. In severe cases, infants become progressively obtunded and flaccid. Long periods of apnea ensue; infants eventually die of asphyxia.

Therapeutic advances in recent decades have improved survival in infants with RDS, allowed survival of very young premature babies who previously would have had almost no chance of living and decreased the incidence of many complications of RDS (see below). It is generally accepted that if labor threatens a preterm pregnancy, administration of corticosteroids to mothers hastens fetal lung maturation and decreases the incidence of RDS in preterm babies. Use of animal-derived surfactants (porcine or bovine), combined with improved ventilatory therapy, has dramatically improved the survival of infants with RDS. Currently, even very small premature infants have an 85%–90% chance of survival.

The major complications of RDS relate to anoxia and acidosis and include:

- **Intraventricular cerebral hemorrhage:** The periventricular germinal matrix in the newborn brain is particularly vulnerable to hemorrhage because the dilated, thin-walled veins in this area rupture easily (Fig. 6-41). The pathogenesis of this complication is not fully understood but is believed to reflect anoxic injury to the periventricular capillaries, venous sludging and thrombosis and impaired vascular autoregulation.
- **Persistent patent ductus arteriosus:** The ductus arteriosus remains patent in almost 1/3 of newborns who survive RDS. With recovery from the pulmonary disease, pulmonary arterial pressure declines, and the higher pressure in the aorta reverses the direction of blood flow in the ductus, thus creating a persistent left-to-right

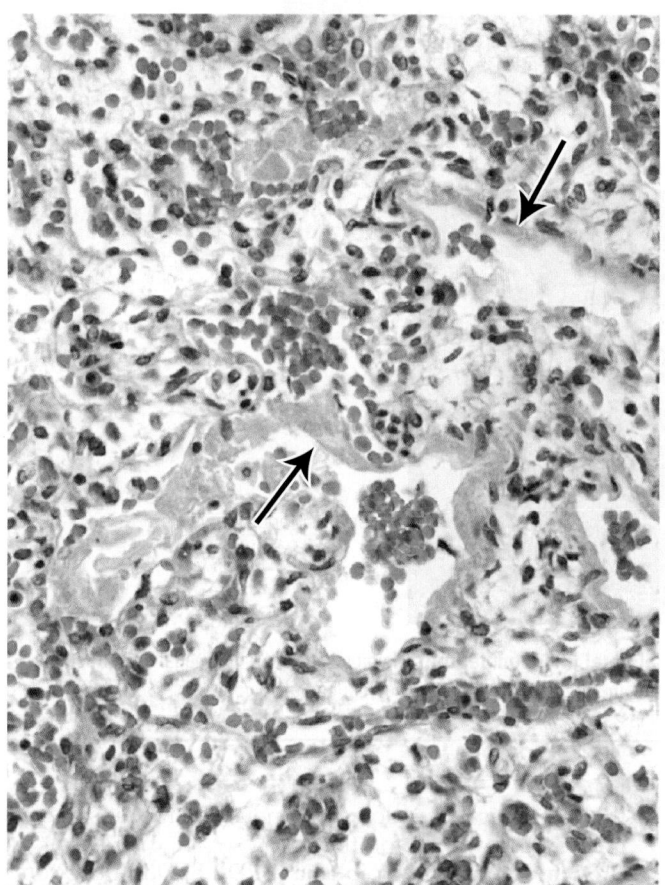

FIGURE 6-40. The lung in respiratory distress syndrome of the neonate. Alveoli are atelectatic, and dilated alveolar ducts are lined by fibrin-rich hyaline membranes (*arrows*).

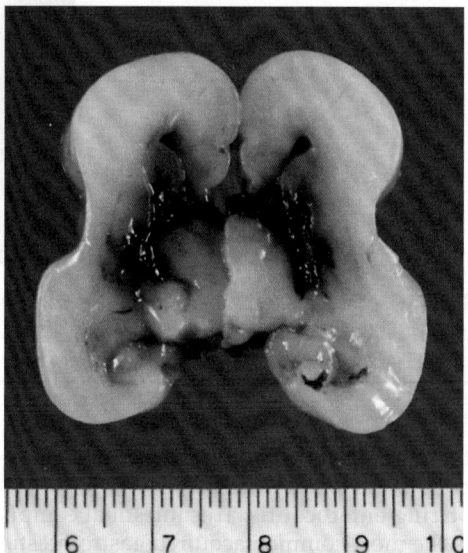

FIGURE 6-41. Intraventricular hemorrhage in a premature infant suffering from respiratory distress syndrome of the neonate.

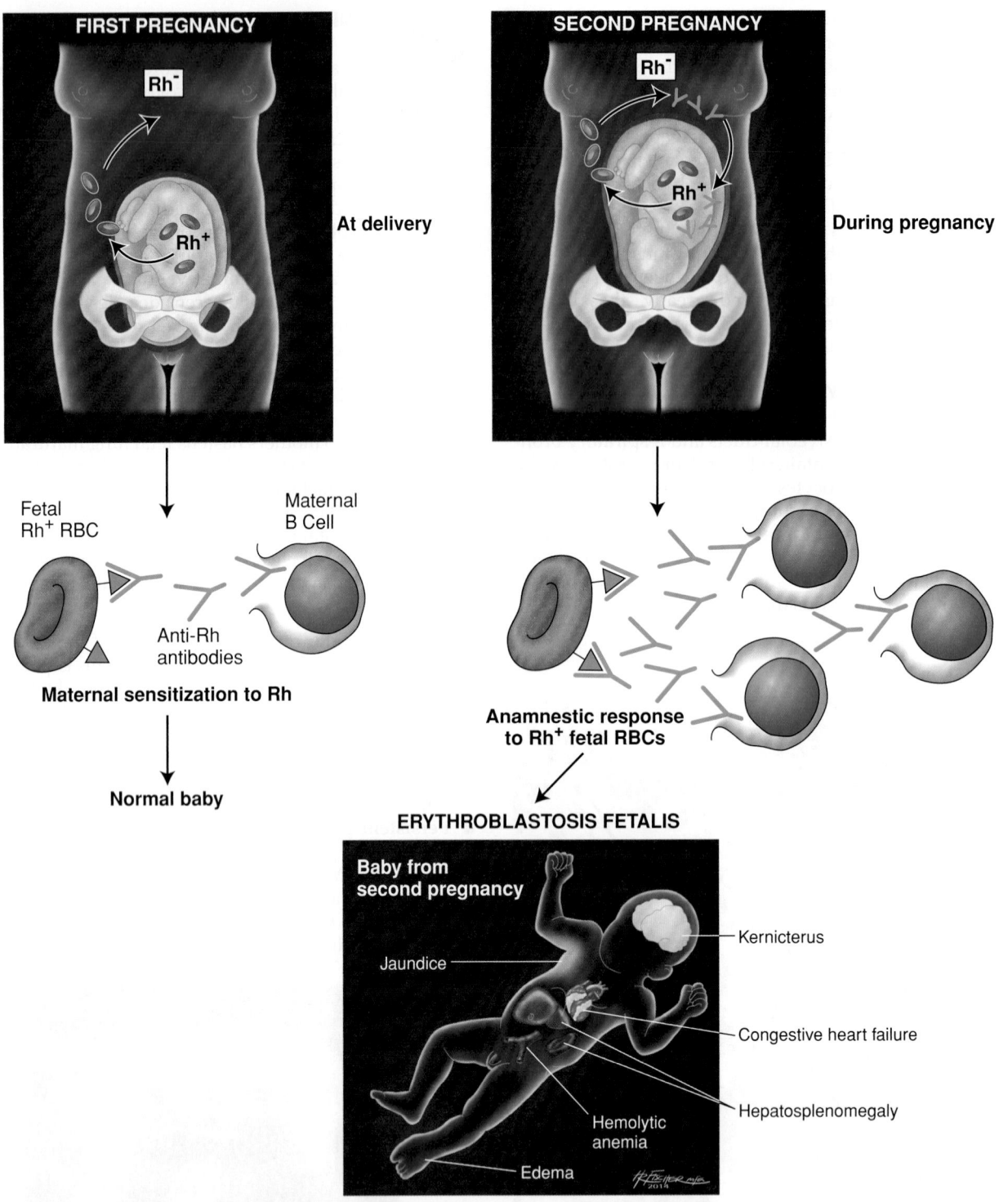

FIGURE 6-42. Pathogenesis of erythroblastosis fetalis due to maternal–fetal Rh incompatibility. Immunization of an Rh-negative mother with Rh-positive erythrocytes in the first pregnancy leads to formation of anti-Rh antibodies of the immunoglobulin (Ig) G type. These antibodies cross the placenta and damage the Rh-positive fetus in subsequent pregnancies.

shunt. Congestive heart failure may ensue and necessitate correction of the patent ductus.

■ **Necrotizing enterocolitis:** This intestinal complication of RDS is the most common acquired gastrointestinal emergency in newborns. It is thought to be related to ischemia of the intestinal mucosa, which leads to bacterial colonization, usually with *Clostridium difficile*. Lesions vary from

those of typical pseudomembranous enterocolitis to gangrene and bowel perforation.

■ **Bronchopulmonary dysplasia (BPD):** BPD is a late complication of RDS usually in infants who weigh less than 1500 g and were maintained on positive-pressure respirators with high FiO_2. BPD affects about 1/3 of RDS survivors and is manifest by continuing need for increased

FiO$_2$ beyond 1 month postnatal age. In older infants, it probably results from oxygen toxicity superimposed on RDS. However, the BPD that occurs in very young premature infants (25–28 weeks' gestation) may differ in pathogenesis and be related, at least in part, to inadequate maturation of lung architecture. In such patients, respiratory distress persists after the third or fourth day and is reflected in hypoxia, acidosis, oxygen dependency and onset of right-sided heart failure. Radiographs of the lungs show a change from almost complete opacification to a sponge-like appearance, with small lucent areas alternating with denser foci. The bronchiolar epithelium is hyperplastic, with squamous metaplasia in the bronchi and bronchioles. Atelectasis, interstitial edema and thickening of alveolar basement membranes are also seen. BPD is a chronic disease; affected infants may continue to require oxygen supplementation into their second or third years of life, and some degree of respiratory impairment may persist, even into adolescence and beyond.

It should be noted that RDS may occur in term or near-term infants. Clinically, this syndrome mimics that seen in premature infants who lack adequate surfactant. A high proportion of term infants with RDS suffer from genetic deficiencies of one of the hydrophobic surfactant proteins (SP-B or SP-C) or have mutations in the ATP-binding cassette transporter (ABCA3) responsible for transporting surfactant phospholipids and proteins to the alveolar space.

Erythroblastosis Fetalis Is a Hemolytic Disease Caused by Maternal Antibodies against Fetal Erythrocytes

The disorder was first recognized by Hippocrates but was not explained until 1940, when Rh (Rhesus) antigen on erythrocytes was identified. More than 60 antigens on red blood cell membranes can elicit antibody responses, but only antibodies to Rh D and ABO antigens cause substantial hemolytic disease.

Rh Incompatibility

The distribution of Rh antigens among ethnic groups varies. In American whites, 15% are Rh negative (Rh D–); only 8% of blacks are Rh D–. Japanese, Chinese and Native Americans are essentially all Rh D+. By contrast, 35% of Basque people, among whom the Rh D– phenotype may have arisen, are Rh D–.

 PATHOPHYSIOLOGY: The Rh blood group system consists of some 25 components, of which only the alleles cde/CDE need be considered here. Antibodies against D cause 90% of erythroblastosis fetalis related to Rh incompatibility; the remaining cases involve C or E. Rh-positive fetal erythrocytes (in >1 mL fetal blood) enter the circulation of an Rh-negative mother at the time of delivery and elicit maternal antibodies to the fetus's D antigen (Fig. 6-42). As the fetal blood required to sensitize a mother is introduced into her circulation only at the time of delivery, the disease does not ordinarily affect her first fetus. However, at subsequent pregnancies, when a now sensitized mother again carries an Rh-positive fetus, much smaller quantities of fetal

D antigen boost antibody titer. Resulting IgG antibodies cross the placenta and thus cause hemolysis in the fetus. This cycle is magnified in multiparous women, the severity of erythroblastosis increasing progressively with each subsequent pregnancy.

About 15% of white women are Rh D–. Since they have an 85% chance of marrying an Rh D+ man, 13% of marriages are theoretically at risk for maternal–fetal Rh incompatibility. The actual incidence of erythroblastosis fetalis is much lower because (1) more than half of Rh-positive men are heterozygous (D/d), and thus only half of their offspring express Rh D antigen; (2) only half of all pregnancies have large enough fetal-to-maternal transfusions to sensitize the mother; and (3) even in those Rh-negative women who are exposed to significant amounts of fetal Rh-positive blood, many do not mount a substantial immune response. Even after multiple pregnancies, only 5% of Rh-negative women ever deliver infants with erythroblastosis fetalis.

 PATHOLOGY AND CLINICAL FEATURES: The severity of hemolysis in erythroblastosis fetalis varies from mild to fatal anemia, the pathology being determined by disease severity.

■ **Death in utero** occurs in the most extreme form of the disease, and severe maceration is evident on delivery. Many erythroblasts are seen in organs that are not extensively autolyzed.

■ **Hydrops fetalis** is the most serious form of erythroblastosis fetalis (Fig. 6-43) in liveborn infants. *It is characterized by severe edema due to congestive heart failure caused by*

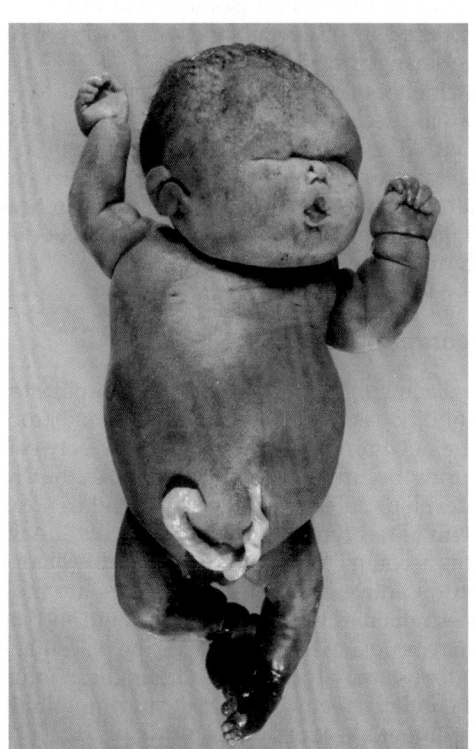

FIGURE 6-43. Hydrops fetalis. The infant shows severe anasarca.

severe anemia. Affected infants generally die unless adequate exchange transfusions with Rh-negative cells correct the anemia and treat the hemolysis. Infants are not jaundiced at birth but rapidly develop progressive hyperbilirubinemia. Those who die have hepatosplenomegaly and bile-stained organs, erythroblastic hyperplasia in the bone marrow and extramedullary hematopoiesis in the liver, spleen, lymph nodes and other sites.

- **Kernicterus,** or **bilirubin encephalopathy,** is a neurologic condition associated with severe jaundice and characterized by bile staining of the brain, particularly the basal ganglia, pontine nuclei and cerebellar dentate nuclei. Although brain damage in jaundiced newborns was first noted in the 15th century, its association with elevated unconjugated bilirubin levels was first appreciated in 1952. Kernicterus (from the German *kern,* "nucleus") is largely limited to infants with severe unconjugated hyperbilirubinemia, as in erythroblastosis. Bilirubin from destruction of erythrocytes and catabolism of the released heme is poorly conjugated by the immature liver, which is deficient in glucuronyl transferase.

Kernicterus directly reflects levels of unconjugated bilirubin. It is rare in term infants if serum bilirubin levels are below 20 mg/dL. Premature infants are more vulnerable to hyperbilirubinemia and may develop kernicterus at levels as low as 12 mg/dL. Bilirubin is thought to injure the cells of the brain by interfering with mitochondrial function. Severe kernicterus leads initially to loss of the startle reflex and athetoid movements and progresses to lethargy and death in 75%. Most surviving infants have severe choreoathetosis and mental retardation; a minority have varying degrees of intellectual and motor retardation.

PREVENTION AND TREATMENT: Exchange transfusions may keep the maximum serum bilirubin at an acceptable level. However, phototherapy converts toxic unconjugated bilirubin into isomers that are nontoxic and can be excreted in the urine, and has greatly reduced the need for exchange transfusions.

The incidence of erythroblastosis fetalis due to Rh incompatibility has declined (to <1% of women at risk) when human anti-D globulin (RhoGAM) is given to mothers within 72 hours of delivery. RhoGAM neutralizes antigenicity of fetal cells that may have entered the maternal circulation during delivery and prevents development of maternal anti-Rh D antibodies.

ABO Incompatibility

With the decline in Rh-incompatible erythroblastosis, ABO incompatibility has become the main cause of hemolytic disease of the newborn. ABO incompatibility between mother and offspring occurs in 1/4 of pregnancies, but hemolytic disease develops in only 10% of such children, usually in infants with blood type A. Low antigenicity of ABO factors in the fetus accounts for the mildness of ABO hemolytic disease. Natural anti-A and anti-B antibodies are mostly IgM, which does not cross the placenta, but some antibodies to A antigen may be IgG, which does cross the placenta. ABO isoimmune disease may thus be seen in firstborn infants. Most cases of hemolytic anemia from ABO incompatibility follow a prior incompatible pregnancy.

Most infants with ABO incompatibility have mild jaundice as the only clinical feature. The extreme complications of erythroblastosis in cases of Rh incompatibility are unusual with ABO disease. Kernicterus occurs, but rarely.

Injury at Birth Ranges from Mechanical Trauma to Anoxic Damage

Some birth injuries relate to obstetric manipulation, but many are due to unavoidable events in routine delivery. Birth injuries occur in 5 per 1000 live births. Predisposing factors include cephalopelvic disproportion, dystocia (difficult labor), prematurity and breech presentation.

Cranial Injury

- **Caput succedaneum** is scalp edema caused by trauma to the head during passage through the birth canal. Swelling disappears rapidly and is of little clinical concern.
- **Cephalohematoma** is subperiosteal hemorrhage of a single cranial bone. It becomes apparent within a few hours after birth and may be associated with a linear fracture of the underlying bone. Most cephalohematomas resolve without complication and require no treatment.
- **Skull fractures** during birth result from the impact of the head on the pelvic bones or pressure from obstetric forceps. Linear fractures, the most common variety, are asymptomatic and do not require treatment. Depressed fractures are usually caused by trauma from forceps. Although many depressed fractures do not initially produce symptoms, they may require mechanical elevation to avoid underlying cranial trauma from persistent pressure. Unlike most cranial fractures, those of the occipital bone often extend through the underlying venous sinuses and may produce fatal hemorrhage.
- **Intracranial hemorrhage** is one of the most dangerous birth injuries and may be traumatic, secondary to asphyxia or a result of an underlying bleeding diathesis. Traumatic intracranial hemorrhage occurs in settings of (1) significant cephalopelvic disproportion, (2) precipitous delivery, (3) breech presentation, (4) prolonged labor or (5) inappropriate use of forceps. These traumas can result in **subdural or subarachnoid hemorrhage,** often due to lacerations of the falx cerebri or tentorium cerebelli that involve the vein of Galen or the venous sinuses. As noted above, anoxic injury from asphyxia, particularly in premature infants, is often associated with intraventricular hemorrhage.

The prognosis for newborns with intracranial hemorrhage depends on its extent. Massive hemorrhage is often rapidly fatal. Surviving infants may recover completely or have long-term impairment, usually in the form of cerebral palsy or hydrocephalus. However, many cases of cerebral palsy have been shown by ultrasound studies to be related to brain damage 2 weeks or more prior to birth rather than from birth trauma.

Peripheral Nerve Injury

- **Brachial palsy,** with varying degrees of paralysis of the arm, is caused by excessive traction on the head and neck or shoulders during delivery. If the nerves are severed, impairment may be permanent. Function may return within a few months if the palsy results from edema and hemorrhage.

- **Phrenic nerve paralysis** and associated paralysis of a hemidiaphragm may be associated with brachial palsy and lead to breathing difficulties. It generally resolves spontaneously within a few months.
- **Facial nerve palsy** usually presents as unilateral flaccid paralysis of the face caused by injury to the seventh cranial nerve during labor or delivery, especially with forceps. If severe, the entire affected side of the face is paralyzed and even the eyelid cannot be closed. Prognosis depends on the extent of nerve injury.

Fractures

The **clavicle** is most vulnerable to fracture during delivery, and there may be associated fracture of the **humerus**. Immobilization of the arm and shoulder usually allows for complete healing. Fractures of other long bones and the nose occasionally occur during birth but heal easily.

Rupture of the Liver

The liver is the only internal organ other than the brain that is injured with any frequency during labor and delivery. Mechanical pressure during difficult or premature births is responsible. Hepatic rupture may cause a hematoma large enough to be palpable and to cause anemia; surgical repair of the laceration may be required.

Sudden Infant Death Syndrome Is an Important Cause of Postperinatal Death

Sudden infant death syndrome (SIDS), also known as "crib death" or "cot death," is defined as "sudden death of an infant or young child which is unexpected by history and in which a thorough postmortem examination fails to demonstrate an adequate cause of death."[1] A diagnosis of SIDS is made only after excluding other specific causes of sudden death, such as infection, hemorrhage, aspiration and so forth. Homicide must be eliminated as a potential cause of SIDS, especially in settings in which more than one sibling has died of apparent SIDS. Descriptions of apparent SIDS date to the Bible, and the syndrome was noted in the American colonies in 1686. However, modern attention to the disorder dates to the late 1960s.

Typically, victims of SIDS are apparently healthy young infants who went to sleep without any hint of the impending calamity but did not wake up. As more predisposing factors and environmental, biochemical, structural and genetic contributors are identified, the number of deaths that truly have no identifiable pathogenesis has diminished. Nevertheless, many authorities still embrace a more inclusive definition of this syndrome.

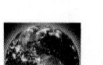 **EPIDEMIOLOGY:** After the neonatal period, SIDS is the leading cause of death in the first year of life, accounting for more than 1/3 of deaths in this period. Its incidence in the United States has decreased from 1.2 in 1000 live births in 1992 to 0.5 in 1000 live births in 2006 but has not changed much since then. SIDS is still responsible for over 2000 infant deaths annually in the United States.

Most (90%) cases occur before 6 months of age, although infants up to 1 year are included in currently accepted criteria. Reducing the risk of SIDS remains an important public health priority.

The majority of deaths from SIDS occur during the winter months, and a significantly higher percentage of infants dying of SIDS are reported to have experienced upper respiratory infections within the previous 4 weeks. However, deaths involving active infections are by definition excluded. Most deaths occur at night or during periods associated with sleep. Once it was determined that infants who slept prone or on their sides had much a higher incidence of SIDS than those who slept supine, a worldwide "Back to Sleep" campaign that encouraged parents to place infants on their backs for sleeping reduced the incidence of SIDS by about half.

Risk factors for SIDS are difficult to ascertain, and much of what is known is based on retrospective studies. There are both maternal and infant risk factors. The strongest **maternal risk factors** are:

- Low socioeconomic status (poor education, unmarried mother, poor prenatal care)
- Black or Native American parentage (in the United States, and independent of economic status; in other countries indigenous populations, like Maoris in New Zealand and Aborigines in Australia, are also at higher risk)
- Age younger than 20 years at first pregnancy
- Maternal cigarette smoking and/or alcohol consumption during and after pregnancy
- Use of illicit drugs during pregnancy
- Increased parity

Risk factors for the infant are more controversial. The consensus includes:

- Low birth weight.
- Prematurity.
- An illness, often respiratory, within the last 4 weeks before death.
- Subsequent siblings of SIDS victims.
- Survivors of an apparent life-threatening event (i.e., an episode of some combination of apnea, color change, marked alteration in muscle tone and choking or gagging). A definite cause, such as seizures or aspiration after vomiting, is known in only half the cases of an apparent life-threatening event.

 **PATHOPHYSIOLOGY AND ETIOLOGIC FACTORS:** Studies of the etiology and pathogenesis of SIDS have provided important insight into the factors that contribute to this syndrome and, in some instances, the molecular bases for sudden infant death. While the original definition of SIDS excludes from the diagnosis known causes, we use a more expansive definition here because of our improved understanding of both molecular and environmental factors involved.

Channelopathies, inherited abnormalities in cell membrane ion channels (see Chapters 1 and 16), are felt to be responsible for 10%–12% of cases of SIDS, although this percentage may be higher (up to about 30%) in SIDS deaths between 6 and 12 months. Various inherited arrhythmia syndromes have been implicated in sudden infant death.

[1]Willinger M, James LS, Catz C. Defining the sudden infant death syndrome (SIDS): deliberations of an expert panel convened by the National Institute of Child Health and Human Development. Pediatr Pathol 1991;11:677–684.

All involve more than one different mutation, producing clustered phenotypes.

The most common of these is long QT syndrome, which is mostly due to loss-of-function mutations in cardiac potassium channels (*KCNQ1, KCNH2*), but mutations in other ion channel proteins have also been identified in some cases, including sodium channel (*SCN5A*) and L-type calcium channel (*CACNA1C*). Long QT syndrome is characterized by prolonged QT intervals on the surface electrocardiogram and is seen in about 10% of SIDS deaths.

Other channelopathies associated with SIDS include catecholaminergic polymorphic ventricular tachycardia (CPVT, mostly due to mutations in ryanodine receptor 2), Brugada syndrome (involving different mutations in the *SCN5A* sodium channel, and also mutations in calcium channels) and short QT syndrome (gain-of-function mutations in cardiac potassium channels, causing accelerated repolarization of cardiac muscle). While these mutations are seen disproportionately in SIDS deaths, the great majority of individuals with ion channelopathies survive infancy. Some experience sudden death in adolescence or later. Others may never be symptomatic.

Now that SIDS relating to prone sleeping position has diminished greatly, **maternal smoking during pregnancy is the most important single etiologic factor in SIDS,** accounting for 80% or more of SIDS deaths. The key factor appears to be exposure to nicotine in utero. There is a dose-response effect: the likelihood of an infant developing SIDS is a direct function of the number of cigarettes smoked by the mother during pregnancy. Babies born to women who smoked 20+ cigarettes daily while pregnant have a greater than 5-fold increased risk of SIDS, compared to children of nonsmokers.

Significant abnormalities have been detected in the brains of infants dying of SIDS. These include hypoplasia of the arcuate nucleus, decreased serotonin receptors and decreased muscarinic cholinergic activity in favor of increased, abnormal nicotinic activity. Comparable abnormalities are seen in experimental animals exposed to nicotine in utero and are associated with depressed ventilatory responses to hypercarbia and hypoxia. Low levels of serotonin, a brain chemical involved in regulating breathing and other vital functions, have been found in the brain stems of SIDS victims. Further, prospective studies of babies who later died of SIDS demonstrated abnormal autonomic nervous system physiology, including depressed gasping reflexes and abnormal regulation of heart rhythm.

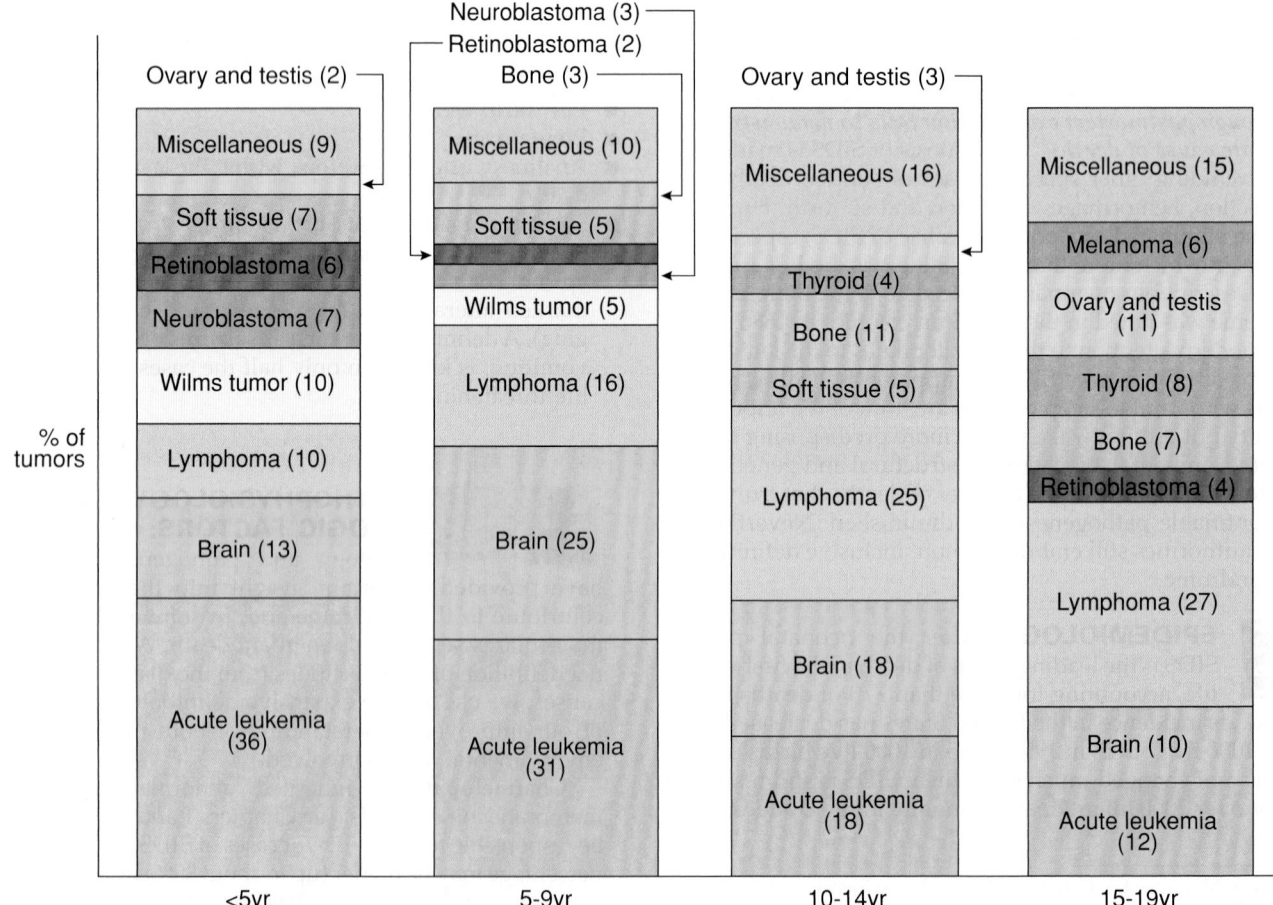

FIGURE 6-44. Distribution of childhood tumors according to age and primary site.

PATHOLOGY: At autopsy, several morphologic alterations have been noted in victims of SIDS, some of which may bear on SIDS pathogenesis, while the significance of others remains unclear. These include arcuate nucleus hypoplasia and brainstem gliosis. Medial hypertrophy of small pulmonary arteries, persistence of extramedullary hematopoiesis in the liver, right ventricular hypertrophy and increased periadrenal brown fat have also been seen and suggest a degree of chronic hypoxia. However, except for brainstem pathologies, none of these changes occurs with any regularity. Petechiae on the surfaces of the lungs, heart, pleura and thymus are reported in most infants dying of SIDS but probably reflect terminal events attributed to negative intrathoracic pressure produced by respiratory efforts.

NEOPLASMS OF INFANCY AND CHILDHOOD

Malignancies in children 1–15 years old are uncommon, but cancer remains the leading cause of death from disease in this age group. Ten percent of deaths in children are due to cancer, exceeded only by accidental trauma. Unlike adults, in whom most cancers are of epithelial origin (e.g., carcinomas of the lung, breast and GI tract), most malignant tumors in children arise from hematopoietic, nervous and soft tissues (Fig. 6-44). Many childhood cancers are part of developmental complexes (Table 6-4). Examples include short arm deletions of chromosome 11, especially 11p13, causing Wilms tumor associated with aniridia, genitourinary malformations and mental retardation (WAGR complex); hemihypertrophy of the body with Wilms tumor, hepatoblastoma and adrenal carcinoma; and tuberous sclerosis with renal tumors and cardiac rhabdomyomas. Loss of the long arm of chromosome 13 is associated with retinoblastoma due to the loss of the *Rb* tumor suppressor gene. Some tumors are evident at birth and so obviously develop in utero. In addition, abnormally developed organs, persistent organ primordia and displaced organ rests are all liable to neoplastic transformation.

Individual cancers of childhood are discussed in detail in chapters on the respective organs, and the principles of neoplasia and carcinogenesis are discussed in Chapter 5. FISH is used to identify specific genetic abnormalities in both childhood and adult cancers including amplifications, deletions and rearrangements involving specific oncogenes and/or tumor suppressors. Examples are listed in Table 6-13.

Tumor-Like Conditions Involve Displaced Tissues and Cells

HAMARTOMAS: These lesions are focal, benign overgrowths of one or more mature cellular elements of a normal tissue, often arranged irregularly. Many hamartomas are clonal and have defined DNA rearrangements, and so may be classified as true neoplasms.

CHORISTOMAS: Also called **heterotopias,** choristomas are tiny aggregates of normal tissue components in aberrant locations. They are not true tumors. Examples include pancreatic rests in the walls of gastrointestinal organs, and adrenal tissue in the renal cortex.

TABLE 6-13
FISH ANALYSIS OF TUMORS IN CHILDREN AND ADULTS

Tumor Type	DNA Probes	Chromosome Location	Abnormality Detected
Breast cancer (FDA approved)	D17Z1/HER-2/neu	Centromere 17 and 17q11.2-12	HER-2/neu amplification
Bladder cancer and cholangiocarcinoma (FDA approved)	D3Z1/D7Z1/D17Z1/p16	Centromere 3, 7, 17 and 9p21	Loss of centromere 3, 7, 17 and p16 loci
Lung cancer	D5S23/D5S721/D6Z1/EGFR/C-MYC	5p15.2/centromere 6/7p12/8q24	Loss or gain of 5p15.2/centromere 6/7p12/8q24
Retinoblastoma	RB1	13q14	Deletion of 13q14
Neuroblastoma	NMYC	2p24.1	NMYC amplification
Burkitt lymphoma	C-MYC	8q24	8q24 rearrangement
Ewing sarcoma	EWSR1	22q12	22q12/ t(11;22)(q24;q12) rearrangement
Oligodendroglioma	LSI 1p36 (TP73)/1p25(ABL2) LSI 19q13(ZNF)/19p13(CRX)	1p36/1p25/19q13/19p13	1p36 and 19q13 deletions
Gliomas	PTEN	10q23	10q23 deletion
Synovial sarcoma	SYT	18q11.2	18q11.2 rearrangement
Myxoid/round cell liposarcoma	CHOP	12q13	12q13 rearrangement
Alveolar rhabdomyosarcoma	FKHR	13q14	13q14 rearrangement

FDA = Food and Drug Administration; FISH = fluorescence in situ hybridization.

Benign Childhood Tumors of Vascular Origin Are Common

HEMANGIOMAS: These lesions, of varying size and in diverse locations, are the most common tumors in childhood. Whether they are true neoplasms is unclear, but half are present at birth and most regress with age. Large, rapidly growing hemangiomas, especially on the head or neck, may occasionally cause serious problems. **Port wine stains** are congenital capillary hemangiomas of the skin of the face and scalp. They are often disfiguring, giving the affected area a dark purple color. Unlike many small hemangiomas, they persist for life.

LYMPHANGIOMAS: Also called **cystic hygromas,** these are poorly circumscribed swellings that are usually present at birth and thereafter rapidly increase in size. Most occur on the head and neck, but the floor of the mouth, mediastinum and buttocks are not uncommon sites. Some authorities consider lymphangiomas to be developmental malformations; others call them neoplasms. They may be unilocular or multilocular and have thin, transparent walls and contain straw-colored fluid. Myriad dilated lymphatic channels are separated by fibrous septa. Unlike hemangiomas, these lesions do not regress spontaneously and should be resected.

SACROCOCCYGEAL TERATOMAS: These rare germ cell tumors, which occur in 1 in 40,000 live births, are the most common solid neoplasms in the newborn. Over 75% of sacrococcygeal teratomas occur in girls, and a substantial number are seen in twins. They are usually noticed at birth as masses near the sacrum and buttocks. They may be large, lobulated tumors, sometimes as large as the infant's head. One half grow externally and may be connected to the body by a stalk. Some have both external and intrapelvic components, and a few grow entirely in the pelvis. Sacrococcygeal teratomas contain multiple tissues, particularly of neural origin. Most (90%) detected before the age of 2 months are benign, but up to half of those found later in life are malignant. Associated congenital anomalies of vertebrae, the genitourinary system and the anorectum are common. These lesions should be resected promptly.

Pediatric Malignancies Are Mostly of Mesodermal Origin

The incidence of childhood cancer is 1.3 per 10,000 per year in children younger than 15. Mortality is determined by the intrinsic behavior of the tumor and its response to therapy, but overall, the death rate for childhood cancer is 1/3 of the incidence. Almost half of all such malignancies are acute leukemias and lymphomas. The former, particularly acute lymphoblastic leukemia, make up 1/3 of childhood cancers. Most of the rest are neuroblastomas, brain tumors, Wilms tumors, retinoblastomas, bone cancers and soft tissue sarcomas.

Genetic influences in the development of childhood tumors are well studied in the case of retinoblastoma, Wilms tumor and osteosarcoma. Interactions of heritable factors and environmental influences in the pathogenesis of malignant tumors in both children and adults are discussed in Chapter 5.

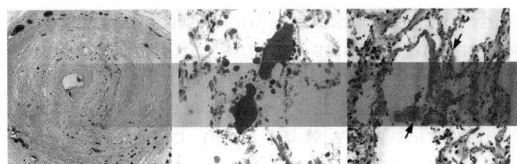

Hemodynamic Disorders

Bruce M. McManus ▪ Michael F. Allard ▪ Robert Yanagawa

NORMAL CIRCULATION

Normal function and metabolism of organs and cells depend on an intact circulatory system for continuous delivery of oxygen, nutrients, hormones, electrolytes and water, as well as for removal of metabolic waste and carbon dioxide. The circulatory system is a vascular conduit made of a muscular pump connected to tubes (or blood vessels) that deliver blood to organs and tissues and return it to the heart to complete the circuit. Delivery and elimination at the cellular level are controlled by exchanges between the intravascular space, interstitial space, cellular space and lymphatic space, which occur via the smallest-diameter blood vessels in the body (the microcirculation).

The Heart Is a Two-Sided Pump with Vascular Circuits in Series

In this series circuit, the amount of blood handled by the right ventricle, which pumps blood to the lungs (pulmonary circulation), must, over time, exactly equal the amount of blood going through the left ventricle, which distributes blood to the body (systemic circulation). The hemodynamically important parameters are cardiac output, perfusion pressure and peripheral vascular resistance.

- **Cardiac output** is the volume of blood pumped by each ventricle per minute and represents the total blood flow in pulmonary and systemic circuits. Cardiac output is the product of heart rate and stroke volume and, as the **cardiac index,** is often adjusted for body surface area (in square meters) as an indicator of ventricular function.

- **Perfusion pressure** (also called **driving pressure**) is the difference in dynamic pressure between two points along a blood vessel. Blood flow to any segment of the circulation ultimately depends on arterial driving pressure. However, each organ can autoregulate flow and so determine the amount of blood it receives from the circulation. Such local control of perfusion depends on continuous modulation of microvascular beds by hormonal, neural, metabolic and hemodynamic factors.

- **Peripheral vascular resistance** is the sum of the factors that determine regional blood flow in each organ. Two thirds of the resistance in the systemic vasculature is determined by the arterioles.

The sum of all regional flows equals the **venous return,** which in turn determines the cardiac output. Assessment of the heart's response to inflow (preload) and outflow (afterload) relies on cardiac reflexes as well as cardiac muscle integrity and neurohormonal regulation.

The Aorta and Arteries Are Conducting Vessels

The major functions of the aorta and arteries are to transport blood to the organs and convert pulsatile flow into sustained regular flow. The latter function derives from the elastic properties of the aorta and the resistance produced by the arteriolar sphincters.

The Microcirculation Includes Arterioles, Capillaries and Venules

The blood vessels of the microcirculation are less than 100 μM in diameter. Blood from an arteriole enters capillaries, which

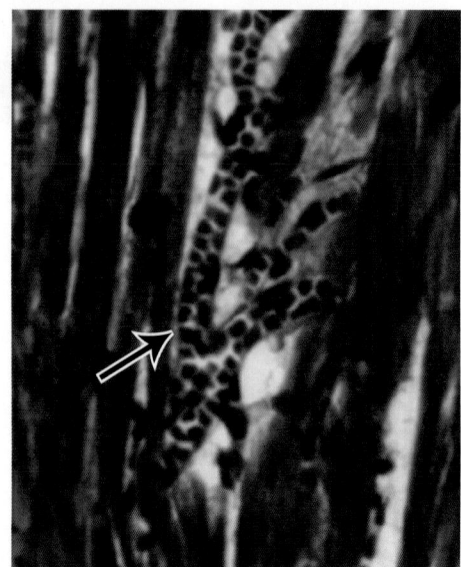

FIGURE 7-1. Microcirculation. Photomicrograph of myocardium showing capillaries and venules (*arrow*).

freely anastomose with each other (Fig. 7-1), either directly or through metarterioles. Capillary length, measured from terminal arteriole to collecting venule, ranges from 0.1 to 3 mm, averaging 1 mm. However, the path length by which blood cells traverse capillaries may actually be longer because of their extensive anastomoses. This fact is likely an important factor with respect to microvascular exchange of substances such as oxygen because it increases the time available for such exchange to take place. The large aggregate surface area of capillaries determines that velocity is low, which further enhances microvascular exchange (Fig. 7-2). The density of capillaries in a tissue also influences microvascular exchange by affecting the diffusion distance. For example, in

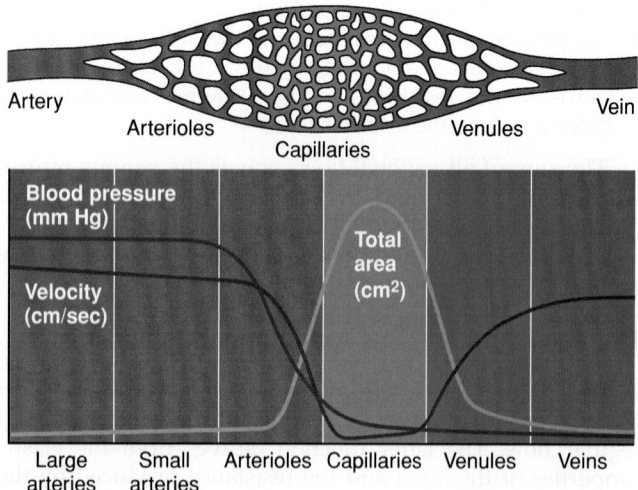

FIGURE 7-2. Blood pressure, velocity and total area within the circulatory system. Note that the higher resistance due to diameter reduction in the arterioles results in a drop in perfusion pressure, the capillary network constitutes the vast majority of vascular surface area and the venous system is a low-pressure, high-capacitance structure with a series of valves to prevent retrograde flow.

tissues with high oxygen demands, such as the heart, capillary density is very high. Entry into the capillary system is guarded by precapillary sphincters, except for **thoroughfare channels,** which bypass capillaries and are always open. Since not all capillaries are always open, blood flow to a structure can be increased by recruiting additional capillaries. The sum of blood flow through the capillary bed, the thoroughfare channels and the arteriovenous anastomoses determines the regional blood flow.

The exact means by which an organ regulates blood flow according to its metabolic needs are still debated, but there is a link between oxygen demand and blood flow. In the heart, blood flow is adjusted on a second-to-second basis. Factors that mediate and link metabolic vasodilation to cellular metabolism include adenosine, other nucleotides, nitric oxide, certain prostaglandins, carbon dioxide and pH. The microcirculation is an important contributor to all forms of hyperemia and edema, and is a target in septic shock (see below). Vasoregulation in conducting arteries, resistance arteries and veins relies on delicate interactions between blood, endothelium, smooth muscle cells and surrounding stroma.

The Endothelium Provides a Continuous Partition between Blood and Tissues

Endothelial cells play important roles in anticoagulation, facilitation of migration of substances from blood to tissue and back, regulation of vessel tone (particularly that of resistance arteries) and regulation of vasopermeability (see Chapters 2 and 16).

Veins and Venules Return Blood to the Heart

Blood from the capillaries enters venules and eventually veins on its route back to the heart. Veins not only serve as a conduit for blood but also act as a blood reservoir; 64% of the total blood volume resides in the venous system.

The Interstitium Represents 15% of Total Body Volume

The interstitial fluid between cells provides a means for the delivery of nutrients and the elimination of waste. Most interstitial water is bound to a dense network of glycosaminoglycans.

Lymphatics Reabsorb Interstitial Fluid

Interstitial fluid is reabsorbed into the circulation at the venous end of the capillary, and a small portion is drained through lymphatics. Lymphatic capillaries conduct lymph from the periphery to the central venous system via the thoracic duct. Normal oscillatory constrictions and relaxations of lymphatic vessels contribute to the steady return of lymph fluid to the central circulation. Lymph is a solvent for large molecules that cannot return to the circulation through blood capillaries.

DISORDERS OF PERFUSION

Hemodynamic disorders are characterized by disturbed perfusion that results in organ and cellular injury.

Hyperemia Is an Excess of Blood in an Organ

Hyperemia may be caused either by an increased supply of blood from the arterial system **(active hyperemia)** or by impaired exit of blood through venous pathways **(passive hyperemia or congestion)**.

Active Hyperemia

Active hyperemia is augmented supply of blood to an organ. It is usually a physiologic response to increased functional demand, as in the heart and skeletal muscle during exercise. Neurogenic and hormonal influences play a role in active hyperemia (e.g., the blushing bride and the menopausal flush). Although the utility of vasodilation in these examples is not clear, cutaneous hyperemia in febrile states serves to dissipate heat. In addition, skeletal muscle may increase its blood flow (and thus oxygen delivery) 20-fold during exercise. The increased blood supply occurs by arteriolar dilation and recruitment of unperfused capillaries.

The most striking active hyperemia occurs in association with inflammation. Vasoactive materials released by inflammatory cells (see Chapter 2) cause dilation of blood vessels; in the skin this contributes to classic "tumor, rubor and calor" of inflammation. In pneumonia, for example, alveolar capillaries are engorged with erythrocytes as a hyperemic response to inflammation. Because inflammation can also damage endothelial cells and increase capillary permeability, inflammatory hyperemia is often accompanied by edema and local extravasation of erythrocytes.

Reactive hyperemia occurs after temporary interruption of blood supply (ischemia). The release of the obstruction is followed by active hyperemia, probably due to ischemic tissue injury and release of inflammatory agents such as histamine. The degree and duration of hyperemia is proportional to the period of occlusion until a plateau of hyperemic response is reached.

Passive Hyperemia (Congestion)

Passive hyperemia, or congestion, is engorgement of an organ with venous blood. Acute passive congestion is clinically a consequence of acute left or right ventricular failure. Regarding the former, resultant venous engorgement of the lungs leads to accumulation of a transudate in the alveoli, which is called **pulmonary edema**. With acute failure of the right ventricle, the liver can become severely congested.

Generalized increases in venous pressure, typically from chronic heart failure, lead to slower blood flow and a consequent increase in blood volume in many organs, including liver, spleen and kidneys. In the past, heart failure from rheumatic mitral stenosis was a common cause of generalized venous congestion, but with the decline in the prevalence of rheumatic fever and the advent of surgical valve replacement, such cases are unusual. Congestive heart failure secondary to coronary artery disease and hypertension and right-sided failure due to pulmonary disease are now more common.

Passive congestion may also be confined to a limb or an organ as a result of more-localized obstruction to venous drainage. Examples include deep venous thrombosis of the leg veins, with resulting edema of the lower extremity, and thrombosis of hepatic veins (Budd-Chiari syndrome), with secondary chronic passive congestion of the liver.

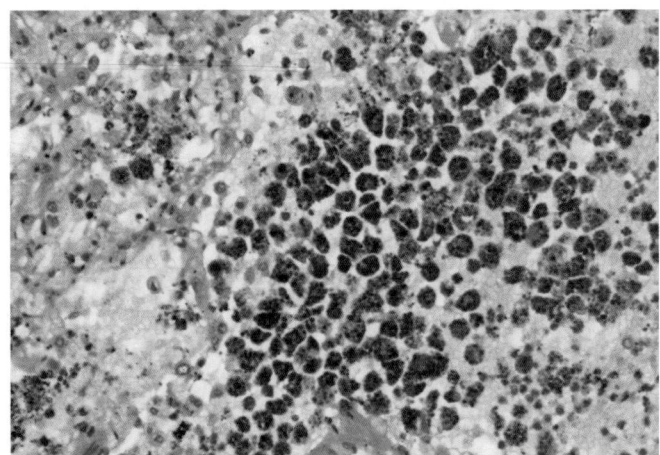

FIGURE 7-3. Passive congestion of lung. Hemosiderin-laden macrophages in the lung of a patient with congestive heart failure.

LUNGS: Chronic left ventricular failure impedes blood flow out of the lungs and gives rise to chronic passive pulmonary congestion. As a result, pressure in alveolar capillaries increases, and these vessels become engorged with blood. Increased pressure in the alveolar capillaries has four major consequences:

- Microhemorrhages release erythrocytes into alveolar spaces, where they are phagocytosed and degraded by alveolar macrophages. The released iron, in the form of hemosiderin, remains in these macrophages, which are then called "heart failure cells" (Fig. 7-3).
- Fluid is forced from the blood into the alveolar airspaces, resulting in pulmonary edema (Fig. 7-4), which interferes with gas exchange in the lung.
- Fibrosis increases in the interstitium of the lung. The presence of fibrosis and iron is viewed grossly as a firm, brown lung **(brown induration)**.
- **Pulmonary hypertension** occurs when the pressure is transmitted to the pulmonary arterial system. This may lead to right-sided heart failure and consequent generalized systemic venous congestion.

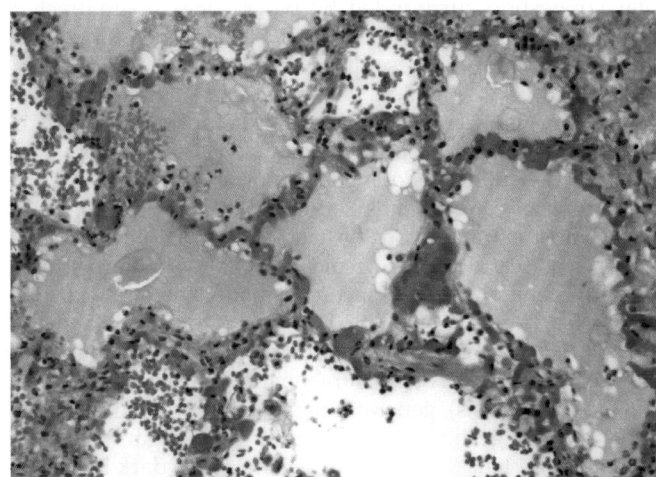

FIGURE 7-4. Pulmonary edema. A patient with congestive heart failure shows pink-staining fluid in the alveoli.

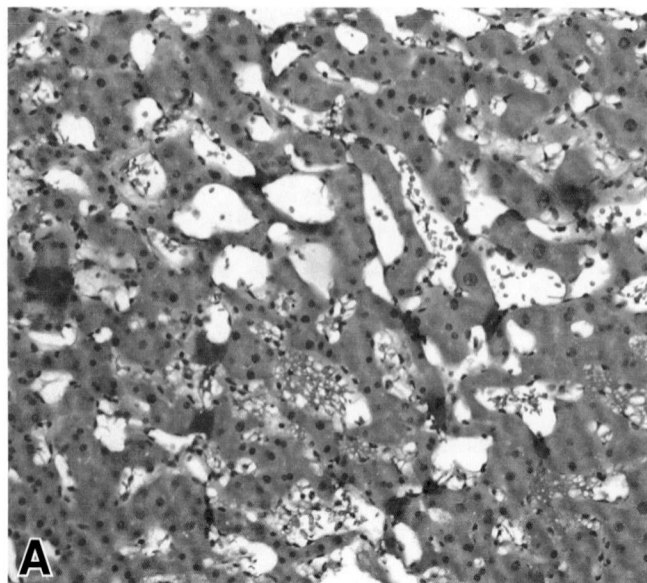

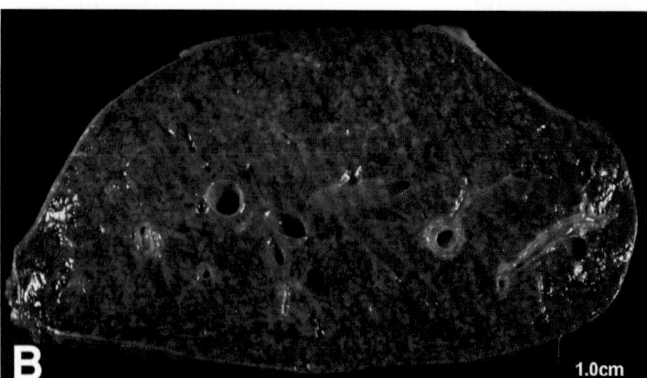

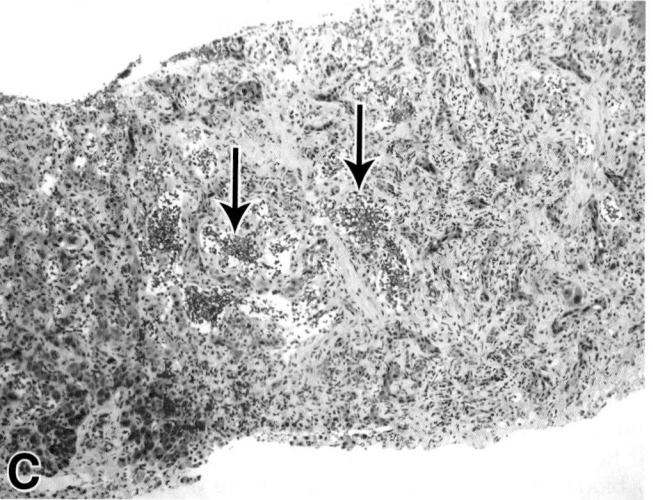

FIGURE 7-5. **Passive congestion of liver. A.** A photomicrograph of liver shows dilated centrilobular sinusoids. The intervening plates of hepatocytes exhibit pressure atrophy. **B.** A gross photograph of liver shows nutmeg appearance, reflecting congestive failure of the right ventricle. **C.** Late changes in chronic passive congestion characterized by dilated sinusoids (*arrows*) and fibrosis (note the blue staining of collagen in this trichrome stain). Proliferated bile ducts are on the right.

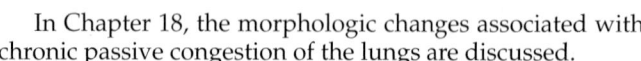

In Chapter 18, the morphologic changes associated with chronic passive congestion of the lungs are discussed.

LIVER: The hepatic veins empty into the vena cava just inferior to the heart, so the liver is particularly vulnerable to acute or chronic passive congestion (see Chapter 20). The central veins of hepatic lobules become dilated. The increased venous pressure is transmitted to the sinusoids, which dilate, and centrilobular hepatocytes undergo pressure atrophy (Fig. 7-5A). Grossly, the cut surface of a chronically congested liver exhibits dark foci of centrilobular congestion surrounded by paler zones of unaffected peripheral portions of the lobules. The result is a reticulated appearance that resembles a cross-section of a nutmeg ("nutmeg liver") (Fig. 7-5). In extreme cases associated with acute right ventricular failure, frank hemorrhagic necrosis of hepatocytes in the centrilobular zones is conspicuous. Prolonged hepatic venous congestion eventually leads to thickening of central veins and centrilobular fibrosis. Only in the most extreme cases of venous congestion (e.g., constrictive pericarditis or tricuspid stenosis) is the fibrosis sufficiently generalized and severe to justify the label **cardiac cirrhosis**.

SPLEEN: Increased intravascular pressure in the liver, from cardiac failure or an intrahepatic obstruction to blood flow (e.g., cirrhosis), generates higher pressure in the splenic vein and congestion of the spleen. The organ becomes enlarged and tense, and the cut section oozes dark blood. In long-standing congestion, diffuse splenic fibrosis develops, as do iron-containing, fibrotic and calcified foci of old hemorrhage (Gamna-Gandy bodies). Such a spleen may weigh 250–750 g, compared with a normal weight of 150 g. The enlarged spleen sometimes displays excessive functional activity—**hypersplenism**—which causes hematologic abnormalities (e.g., thrombocytopenia).

EDEMA AND ASCITES: Venous congestion impedes blood flow through the capillaries, thus increasing hydrostatic pressure and promoting edema formation (see below for a discussion of mechanisms of edema formation). Accumulation of edema fluid in heart failure is particularly noticeable in dependent tissues—legs and feet in ambulatory patients and the back in bedridden patients. **Ascites** is accumulation of fluid in the peritoneal space and reflects (among other factors) lack of tissue rigor, a condition in which there is no countervailing external pressure to oppose hydrostatic pressure within the blood vessels.

Hemorrhage Is a Discharge of Blood out of the Vascular Compartment

Blood can be released from the circulation to the exterior of the body or into nonvascular body spaces. The most common and obvious cause is trauma. Severe atherosclerosis may so weaken the wall of the abdominal aorta that it balloons to form an aneurysm, which then may rupture and bleed into the retroperitoneal space (see Chapter 16). In the same way, an aneurysm may complicate a congenitally weak cerebral artery (berry aneurysm) and cause subarachnoid hemorrhage (see Chapter 32). Certain infections (e.g., pulmonary tuberculosis) and invasive neoplasms may erode blood vessels and result in hemorrhage.

Hemorrhage also results from damage to capillaries. For instance, rupture of capillaries by blunt trauma creates a bruise. Increased venous pressure also causes extravasation of blood from pulmonary capillaries. Scurvy is associated with capillary fragility and bleeding, owing to defective supporting connective tissue structures. The capillary barrier by itself does not suffice to contain blood within the intravascular space. The minor trauma imposed on small vessels and capillaries by normal movement requires an intact coagulation system to prevent hemorrhage. Thus, a severe decrease in the number of platelets **(thrombocytopenia)** or deficiency of a coagulation factor (e.g., factor VIII in hemophilia A or von Willebrand factor in von Willebrand disease) is associated with spontaneous hemorrhage without apparent trauma (see Chapters 16).

Someone may exsanguinate into an internal cavity, as in gastrointestinal hemorrhage from a peptic ulcer (arterial hemorrhage) or esophageal varices (venous hemorrhage). In such cases, large amounts of fresh blood fill the entire gastrointestinal tract. Bleeding into a serous cavity can result in accumulation of a large amount of blood, even to the point of exsanguination.

A few definitions are in order:

- **Hematoma:** Hemorrhage into soft tissue. Such collections of blood can be merely painful, as in a muscle bruise, or fatal, if located in the brain.
- **Hemothorax:** Hemorrhage into the pleural cavity.
- **Hemopericardium:** Hemorrhage into the pericardial space.
- **Hemoperitoneum:** Bleeding into the peritoneal cavity.
- **Hemarthrosis:** Bleeding into a joint space.
- **Purpura:** Diffuse superficial hemorrhages in the skin, up to 1 cm in diameter.
- **Ecchymosis:** A large superficial hemorrhage in the skin (Fig. 7-6). It is purple at first, then turns green, then yellow before resolving. This sequence of events reflects progressive oxidation of bilirubin released from the hemoglobin of degraded erythrocytes. A good example of an ecchymosis is a "black eye."
- **Petechiae:** Pinpoint hemorrhages, usually in the skin or conjunctiva (Fig. 7-7). This lesion represents the rupture of a capillary or arteriole and occurs in conjunction with

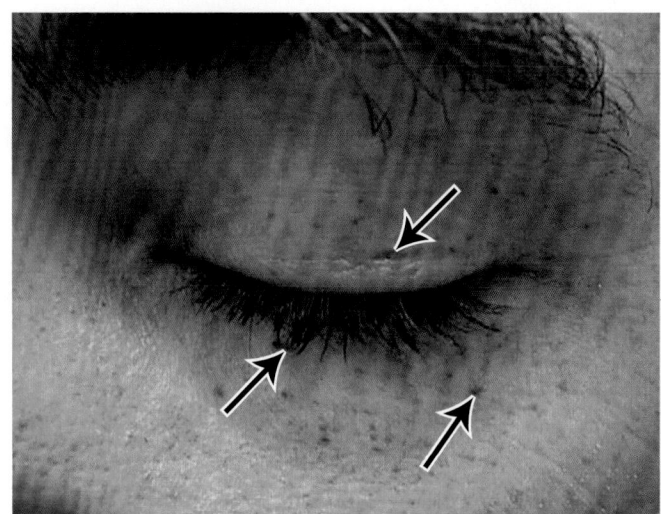

FIGURE 7-7 Petechiae. Periorbital microhemorrhages (*arrows*) appear as punctate red foci.

coagulopathies or vasculitis. Petechiae may also be produced by microemboli from infected heart valves (bacterial endocarditis).

MOLECULAR PATHOGENESIS:

Coagulation

Coagulation has a significant genetic component. Rare, well-characterized, highly penetrant, monogenic causes of coagulopathies include von Willebrand disease and hemophilias. Hereditary factors control the circulating levels of several coagulation cascade proteins, including plasminogen activator inhibitor-1, factor XIII, factor VII, fibrinogen and tissue plasminogen activator.

Pharmacogenetics is the study of individual genetic variations on the action of drugs. Warfarin is an anticoagulant with a narrow therapeutic index and greater than 10-fold variability in dose requirements. Clinically, this necessitates regular measurements of the international normalized ratio (INR). This appears to be dependent on genetic variants of the metabolic enzyme cytochrome P450 2C9 (CYP2C9) and vitamin K epoxide reductase complex 1 (VKORC1). Allelic variants CYP2C9*2 or CYP2C9*3 result in increased metabolic clearance of warfarin. Among several VKORC1 mutations, the -1639G>A is the strongest predictor of warfarin dose requirements. The thienopyridine antiplatelet agent, clopidogrel, is a prodrug requiring hepatic activation by cytochrome P450 (CYP) enzymes. Clopidogrel is susceptible to genetic polymorphisms in CYP2C19, which can result in clopidogrel resistance. On the other hand, newer-generation thienopyridines, such as Ticagrelor, are not CYP dependent and thus have a more rapid and consistent level of activity.

THROMBOSIS

Thrombosis refers to the formation of a thrombus, defined as an aggregate of coagulated blood containing platelets, fibrin and entrapped cellular elements, within a vascular lumen.

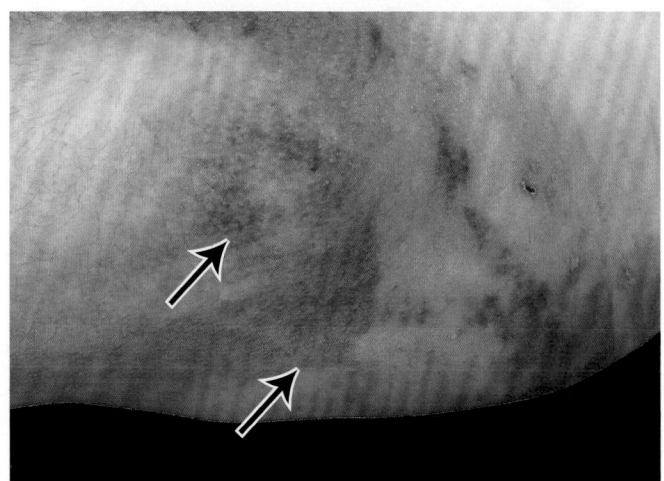

FIGURE 7-6. Ecchymosis. Superficial diffuse hemorrhage (*arrows*) on the thigh caused by blunt force trauma.

A **thrombus** by definition adheres to vascular endothelium and should be distinguished from a simple blood clot, which reflects only activation of the coagulation cascade and can form in vitro or even postmortem. Similarly, a thrombus differs from a hematoma, which results from hemorrhage and subsequent clotting outside the vascular system. Thrombus formation and the coagulation cascade are discussed in more detail in Chapters 16 and 26. Although pathogenesis of venous and arterial thrombosis has been considered distinct, recent epidemiologic evidence has demonstrated commonalities in risk factors and association between these entities, suggesting mechanistic overlap. Here we present the causes and consequences of thrombosis in these different vascular sites.

Thrombosis in the Arterial System Is Usually Due to Atherosclerosis

 **MOLECULAR PATHOGENESIS AND ETIOLOGIC FACTORS:** The vessels most commonly involved in arterial thrombosis are coronary, cerebral, mesenteric and renal arteries and arteries of the lower extremities. Less commonly, arterial thrombosis occurs in other disorders, including inflammation of arteries (arteritis), trauma and blood diseases. Thrombi are common in aneurysms (localized dilations of the lumen) of the aorta and its major branches, in which the distortion of blood flow, combined with intrinsic vascular disease, promotes thrombosis. A major risk factor for thrombosis is immobilization after surgery or after leg casting. Other risk factors include metabolic syndrome, which typically includes obesity, hyperglycemia, insulin resistance, dyslipidemia and hypertension; advanced age; tobacco use; previous thrombosis; and cancer. The pathogenesis of arterial thrombosis involves principally three factors:

- **Damage to endothelium,** usually by atherosclerosis, disturbs the anticoagulant properties of the vessel wall and serves as a nidus for platelet aggregation and fibrin formation.
- **Alterations in blood flow,** whether from turbulence in an aneurysm or at sites of arterial bifurcation, is conducive to thrombosis. Slowing of blood flow in narrowed arteries favors thrombosis.
- **Increased coagulability of the blood,** as seen in polycythemia vera or in association with some cancers, entails an increased risk of thrombosis.

 **MOLECULAR PATHOGENESIS**

Arterial Thromboembolism

Compared with the study of venous thrombosis, for which several mutations in key genes have been identified, genetic studies of arterial thrombosis have not yielded a mutation with a large population-attributable risk. This is likely due to the complex polygenetic and multifactorial nature of an atherosclerotic plaque rupture or erosion. Weak associations have been shown between certain coagulation factors, fibrinolytic factors, inflammatory mediators and others. The most consistent genetic associations with arterial thrombosis are with factor VII and fibrinogen. Hyperhomocysteinemia is also associated with coronary artery disease and cardiac ischemia events.

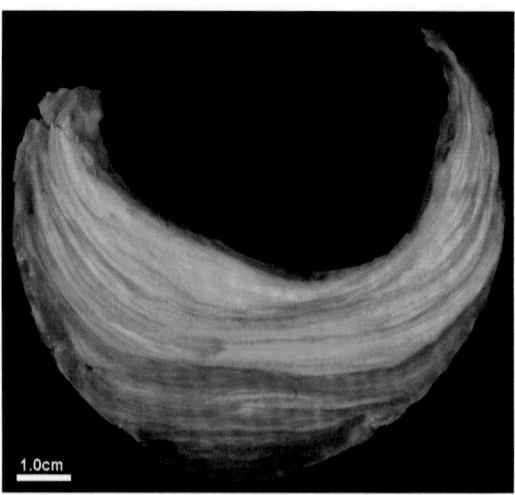

FIGURE 7-8. Arterial thrombus. Gross photograph of a thrombus from an aortic aneurysm shows the laminations of fibrin and platelets known as the lines of Zahn.

 PATHOLOGY: Arterial thrombi attached to vessel walls are soft, friable, and dark red at first, with fine alternating bands of yellowish platelets and fibrin, the lines of Zahn (Fig. 7-8). Then, arterial thrombi have several possible fates.

- **Lysis,** owing to the potent thrombolytic activity of the blood.
- **Propagation** (i.e., increase in size), as the thrombus acts as a focus for further thrombosis.
- **Organization,** the eventual invasion of connective tissue elements, which causes a thrombus to become firm and grayish white.
- **Canalization,** by which new lumina lined by endothelial cells form in an organized thrombus (Fig. 7-9). Its functional significance is often uncertain.
- **Embolization,** when part or all of the thrombus becomes dislodged, travels through the circulation and lodges in a blood vessel some distance from the site of thrombus formation (see below for further discussion).

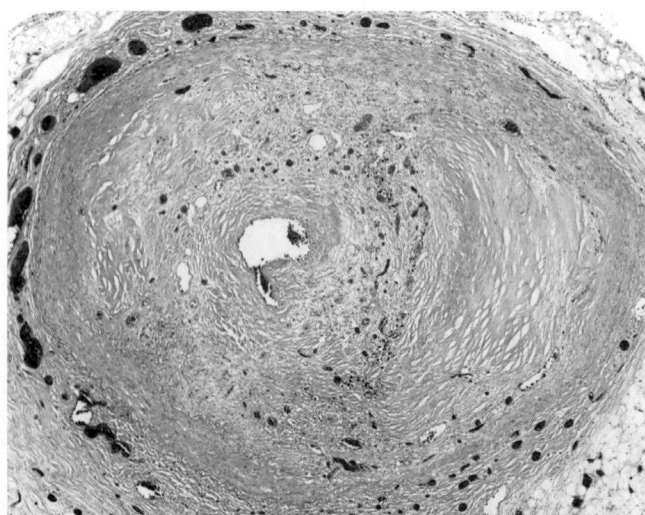

FIGURE 7-9. Canalization of thrombus. Photomicrograph of the left anterior descending coronary artery shows severe atherosclerosis and canalization.

The organized structure of a thrombus reflects a tight interaction between platelets and fibrin and differs in appearance from a postmortem clot or one formed in a test tube. Determination of whether a clot formed during life (antemortem clot) or after death (postmortem clot) is often important in a medical autopsy and in forensic pathology. Lines of Zahn stabilize a thrombus formed during life, while a postmortem clot has a more gelatinous structure. Postmortem clots occur in stagnant blood in which gravity fractionates the blood. The part of the clot containing many red blood cells has a reddish, gelatinous appearance and is referred to as "currant jelly." The overlying clot is firmer and yellow-white, representing coagulated plasma without red blood cells. It is called "chicken fat" because of its color and consistency.

CLINICAL FEATURES: *Arterial thrombosis due to atherosclerosis is the most common cause of death in industrialized countries.* Since most arterial thrombi occlude the vessel, they often lead to ischemic necrosis of tissue supplied by that artery (i.e., an **infarct**). Thus, thrombosis of a coronary or cerebral atherosclerotic plaque (Fig. 7-10) results in **myocardial infarct** (heart attack) or **cerebral infarct** (stroke), respectively. Other end-arteries that are affected often by atherosclerosis and often suffer thrombosis include mesenteric arteries (intestinal infarction), renal arteries (kidney infarcts) and arteries of the leg (ischemic leg and gangrene).

Thrombosis in the Heart Develops on the Endocardium

As in the arterial system, endocardial injury and changes in blood flow in the heart may lead to mural thrombosis (i.e., a thrombus adhering to the underlying wall of the heart). The disorders in which mural thrombosis occurs include:

- **Myocardial infarction:** Mural thrombi adhere to the left ventricular wall, over areas of myocardial infarction, owing to damaged endocardium and alterations in blood flow associated with an akinetic or dyskinetic segment of the myocardium.
- **Atrial fibrillation:** Disordered atrial activity (atrial fibrillation) leads to slower blood flow and impairs left atrial contractility, a situation that predisposes to formation of mural thrombi, most often in the left atrial appendage.
- **Cardiomyopathy:** Primary myocardial diseases are associated with mural thrombi in the left ventricle, presumably because of endocardial injury and altered hemodynamics associated with poor myocardial contractility.
- **Endocarditis:** Small thrombi, **vegetations,** may also develop on cardiac valves, usually mitral or aortic, that are damaged by a bacterial infection (bacterial endocarditis) (Fig. 7-11). Occasionally, vegetations form in the absence of valve infection, on a mitral or tricuspid valve injured by systemic lupus erythematosus (Libman-Sacks endocarditis). In chronic wasting states, as in terminal cancer, large, friable vegetations may appear on cardiac valves (marantic endocarditis), possibly reflecting a hypercoagulable state.

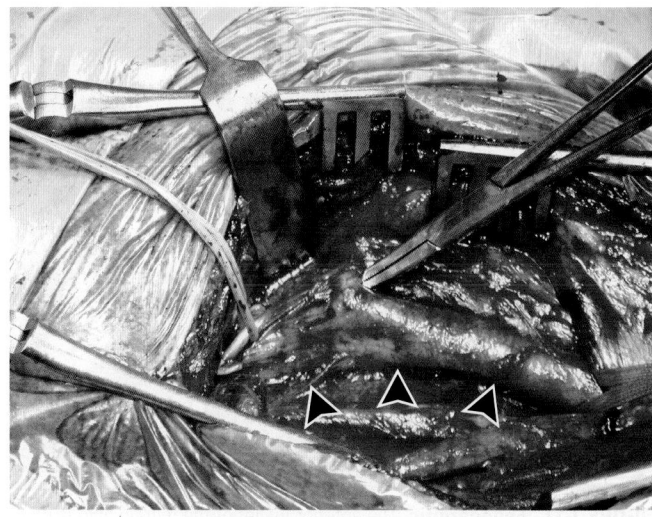

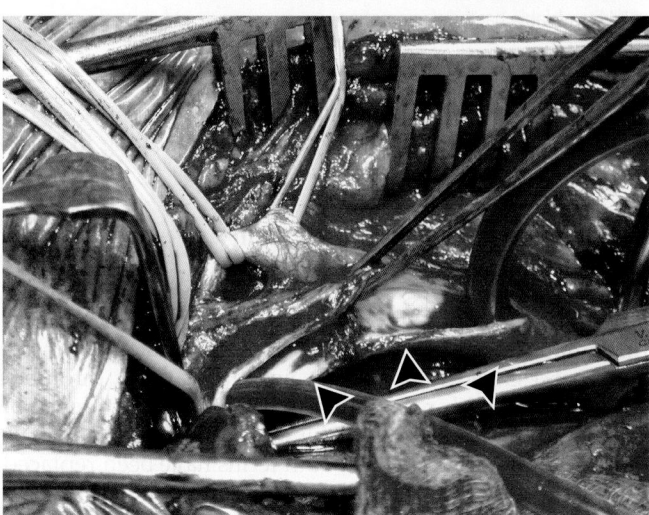

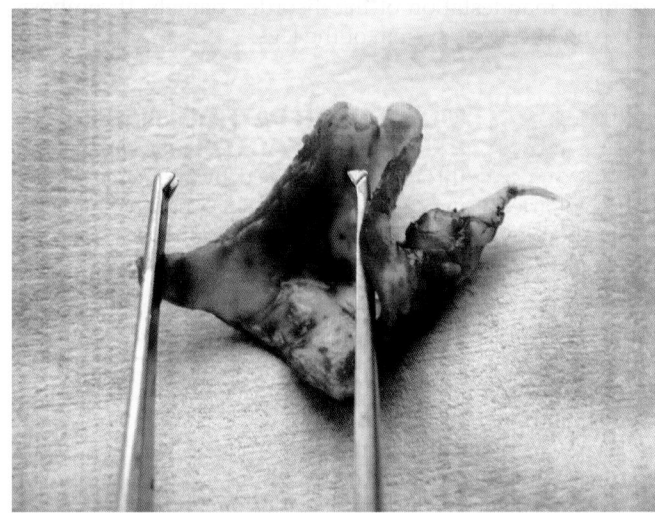

FIGURE 7-10. Endarterectomy. Intraoperative image of a carotid artery (*above, arrowheads*) postarteriotomy displaying a near-occlusive atherosclerotic plaque in situ (*middle, arrowheads*) and the atherosclerotic plaque itself after carotid endarterectomy (*below*).

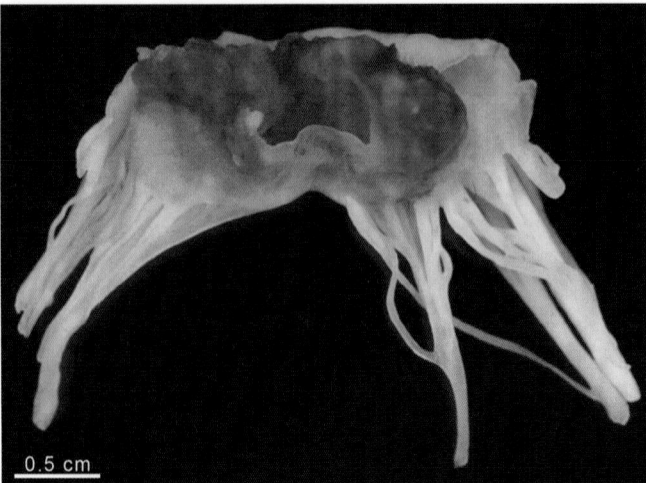

0.5 cm

FIGURE 7-11. Endocarditis. The anterior leaflet of the mitral valve is damaged by a friable bacterial vegetation.

The major complication of thrombi in any location in the heart is detachment of fragments and their lodging in blood vessels at distant sites **(embolization)**.

Thrombosis in the Venous System Is Multifactorial

At one time, venous thrombosis was widely referred to as **thrombophlebitis,** implying that an inflammatory or infectious process had injured the vein, thus causing thrombosis. However, with recognition that there is no evidence of inflammation in most cases, the term **phlebothrombosis** is more accurate. Nevertheless, both terms have been replaced for the most part by the expression **deep venous thrombosis.** This last term is particularly appropriate for the most common manifestation of the disorder, namely, thrombosis of the deep venous system of the legs.

 **MOLECULAR PATHOGENESIS AND ETIOLOGIC FACTORS:** Deep venous thrombosis is caused by the same factors that favor arterial and cardiac thrombosis—endothelial injury, stasis and a hypercoagulable state. Conditions that favor the development of deep venous thrombosis include:

- **Stasis** (heart failure, chronic venous insufficiency, postoperative immobilization, prolonged bed rest, hospitalization and travel)
- **Injury and inflammation** (trauma, surgery, childbirth, infection)
- **Hypercoagulability** (oral contraceptives, late pregnancy, cancer, inherited thrombophilic disorders [see Chapter 26])
- **Advanced age** (venous varicosities, phlebosclerosis)
- **Sickle cell disease** (see Chapter 26)

 **MOLECULAR PATHOGENESIS:**

Venous Thromboembolism

Genetic factors account for 60% of the risk for deep venous thrombosis (DVT) according to twin and family studies.

However, few genetic associations have been consistently identified. Epidemiologic data from the United States demonstrated that blacks are more susceptible to the development of DVT as compared to whites, but Asians and Hispanics are less so. Single nucleotide polymorphisms (SNPs) represent 90% of the common variation in the human genome and are the main focus of disease-related genetic studies. The most common gene variant associated with venous thrombosis is factor V Leiden, which results in a poor inactivation and anticoagulant response to activated protein C. Another common but mild risk factor is the prothrombin G20210A mutation. Deficiencies in proteins C and S and antithrombin are rare but strong risk factors for DVT. Any single SNP or combination of such SNPs can carry an increased risk of venous thromboembolic episodes in childhood and adolescence.

 PATHOLOGY: Most (>90%) venous thromboses occur in deep veins of the legs; the rest usually involve pelvic veins. Most begin in the calf veins, often in the sinuses above venous valves. There, venous thrombi have several potential fates:

- **Lysis:** They may stay small, eventually be lysed and pose no further danger.
- **Organization:** Many undergo organization similar to those of arterial origin. Small, organized venous thrombi may be incorporated into the vessel wall; larger ones may undergo canalization, with partial restoration of venous drainage.
- **Propagation:** Venous thrombi often serve to elicit further thrombosis and so propagate proximally to involve the larger iliofemoral veins (Fig. 7-12).

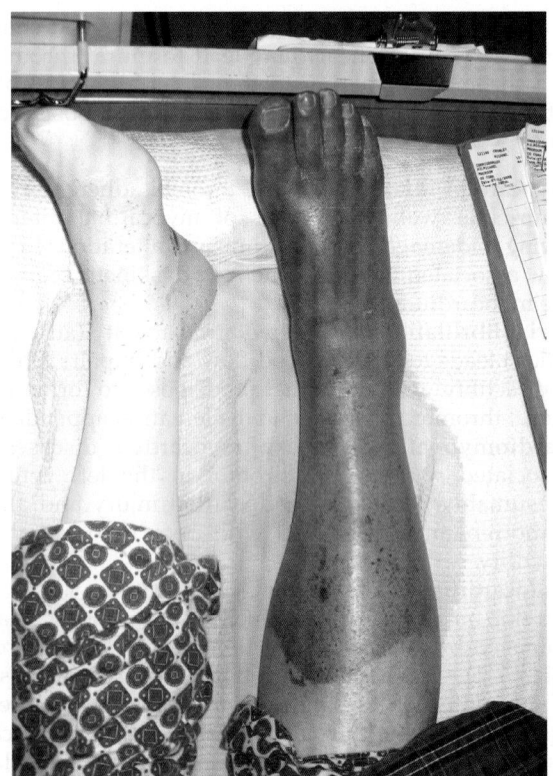

FIGURE 7-12. Phlegmasia cerulea dolens in the right foot. The cause is venous obstruction due to deep vein thrombosis and is associated with cyanosis, edema, swelling and pain.

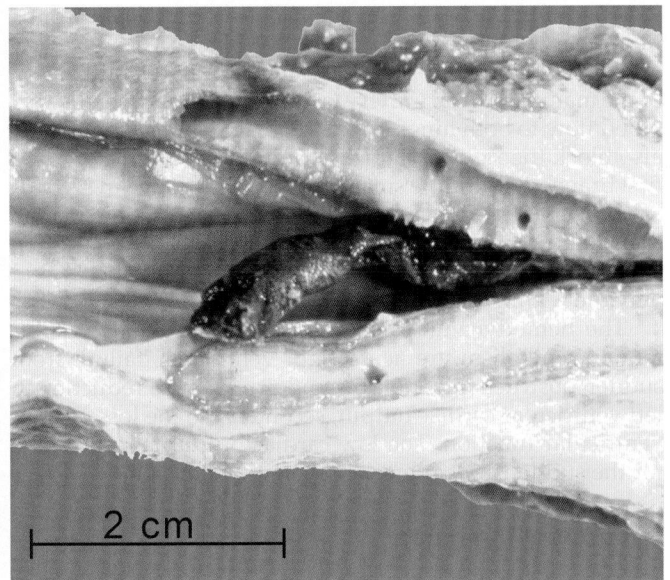

FIGURE 7-13. Venous thrombus. The femoral vein has been opened to reveal a large thrombus within the lumen.

- **Embolization:** Large venous thrombi or those that have propagated proximally represent a significant hazard to life: they may dislodge and be carried to the lungs as pulmonary emboli. In severe cases, complete or near-complete venous obstruction in a limb may result in phlegmasia cerulea dolens, characterized by pain, swelling, edema and cyanosis (Fig. 7-13).

 CLINICAL FEATURES: Small thrombi in the calf veins are ordinarily asymptomatic, and even larger thrombi in the iliofemoral system may cause no symptoms. Some patients have calf tenderness, often associated with forced dorsiflexion of the foot **(Homan sign)**. Occlusive thrombosis of femoral or iliac veins leads to severe congestion, edema and cyanosis of the lower extremity. Symptomatic deep venous thrombosis is treated with systemic anticoagulants, and thrombolytic therapy may be useful in selected cases. In some cases, a filter is inserted into the vena cava to prevent pulmonary embolization.

The function of venous valves is always impaired in a vein subjected to thrombosis and organization. As a result, chronic deep venous insufficiency (i.e., impaired venous drainage) is virtually inevitable. If a lesion is restricted to a small segment of the deep venous system, the condition may remain asymptomatic. However, more extensive involvement leads to pigmentation, edema and induration of leg skin. Ulceration above the medial malleolus can occur and is often difficult to treat.

Venous thrombi elsewhere may also be dangerous. Thrombosis of mesenteric veins can cause hemorrhagic small bowel infarction; thrombosis of cerebral veins may be fatal; hepatic vein thrombosis (Budd-Chiari syndrome) tends to destroy the liver.

Inherited disorders of blood clotting increase susceptibility to these types of events. These diseases are covered in detail in Chapter 26.

EMBOLISM

Embolism is passage through venous or arterial circulations of any material that can lodge in a blood vessel and obstruct its lumen. The most common embolus is a thromboembolus—that is, a thrombus formed in one location that detaches from a vessel wall at its point of origin and travels to a distant site.

Pulmonary Arterial Embolism Is Potentially Fatal

Pulmonary thromboemboli occur in over half of autopsies. As well, this complication occurs in 1%–2% of postoperative patients over the age of 40. The risk of pulmonary embolism after surgery increases with advancing age, obesity, length and type of operative procedure, postoperative infection, cancer and preexisting venous disease.

Most pulmonary emboli (90%) arise from deep veins of the lower extremities; most fatal ones form in iliofemoral veins (Fig. 7-14). Only half of patients with such emboli have signs of deep vein thrombosis. Some thromboemboli arise from the pelvic venous plexus and others from the right side of the heart. Emboli are also derived from thrombi around indwelling lines in the systemic venous system or pulmonary artery. The upper extremities are rarely sources of thromboemboli.

The clinical features of pulmonary embolism are determined by the size of the embolus, the health of the patient

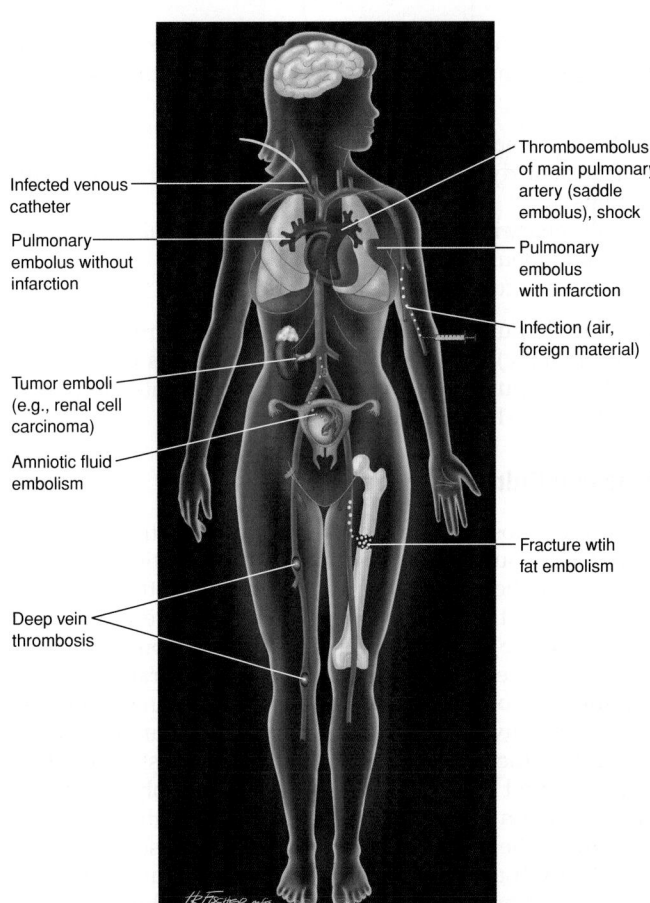

FIGURE 7-14. Sources and effects of venous emboli.

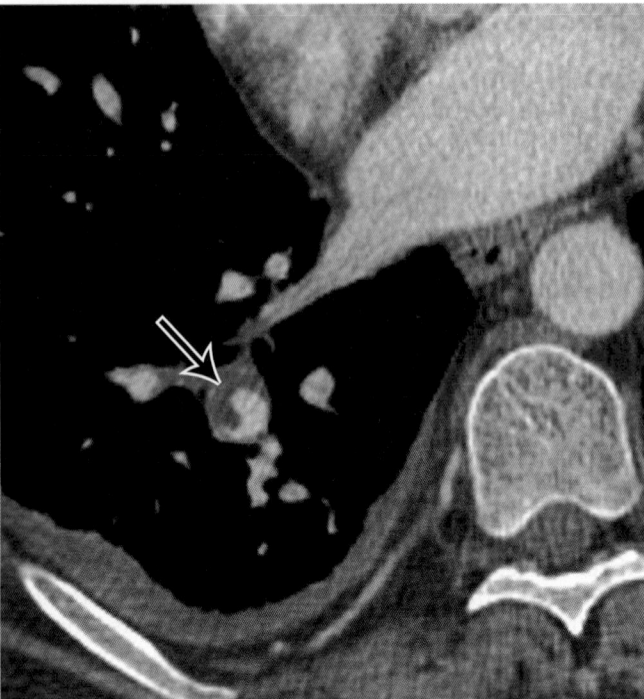

FIGURE 7-15. Contrast-enhanced computed tomographic image of chronic pulmonary embolism. A low attenuation (dark) nonocclusive thrombus is seen in a right segmental pulmonary artery (*arrow*).

and whether embolization occurs acutely or chronically. Acute pulmonary embolism is divided into the following syndromes:

- Asymptomatic small pulmonary emboli
- Transient dyspnea and tachypnea without other symptoms
- Pulmonary infarction, with pleuritic chest pain, hemoptysis and pleural effusion
- Cardiovascular collapse with sudden death

Chronic pulmonary embolism, with numerous (usually asymptomatic) emboli lodged in small arteries of the lung, can lead to pulmonary hypertension and right-sided heart failure (Fig. 7-15; see below).

Massive Pulmonary Embolism

One of the most dramatic calamities complicating hospitalization is the sudden collapse and death of a patient who had appeared to be well on the way to an uneventful recovery. The cause of this catastrophe is often massive pulmonary embolism due to release of a large deep venous thrombus from a lower extremity. Classically, a postoperative patient succumbs upon getting out of bed for the first time. The muscular activity dislodges a thrombus that formed as a result of the stasis from prolonged bed rest. Excluding deaths related to surgery itself, pulmonary embolism is the most common cause of death after major orthopedic surgery and is the most frequent nonobstetric cause of postpartum death. It also is an especially common cause of death in patients who suffer from chronic heart and lung diseases and in those subjected to prolonged immobilization for any reason. Inactivity associated with air travel can also lead to

venous thrombosis and, occasionally, sudden death from a pulmonary embolus.

A large pulmonary embolus may lodge at the bifurcation of the main pulmonary artery **(saddle embolus)** and obstruct blood flow to both lungs (Fig. 7-16). Large lethal emboli may also block the right or left main pulmonary arteries or their first branches. Multiple smaller emboli may lodge in secondary branches and prove fatal. With acute obstruction of more than half of the pulmonary arterial tree, the patient often experiences immediate severe hypotension (or shock) and may die within minutes.

The hemodynamic consequences of such massive pulmonary embolism are acute right ventricular failure from sudden obstruction of outflow and pronounced reduction in left ventricular cardiac output, secondary to the loss of right ventricular function. The low cardiac output is responsible for the sudden appearance of severe hypotension.

Pulmonary Infarction

Small pulmonary emboli are not ordinarily lethal. They tend to lodge in peripheral pulmonary arteries and sometimes (15%–20% of all pulmonary emboli) they produce lung infarcts. Clinically, pulmonary infarction is usually seen in the context of congestive heart failure or chronic lung disease, because the normal dual circulation of the lung ordinarily protects against ischemic necrosis; since the bronchial artery supplies blood to the necrotic area, pulmonary infarcts are typically hemorrhagic. They tend to be pyramidal, with the base of the pyramid on the pleural surface. Patients experience cough, stabbing pleuritic pain, shortness of breath and occasional hemoptysis. Pleural effusion is common and

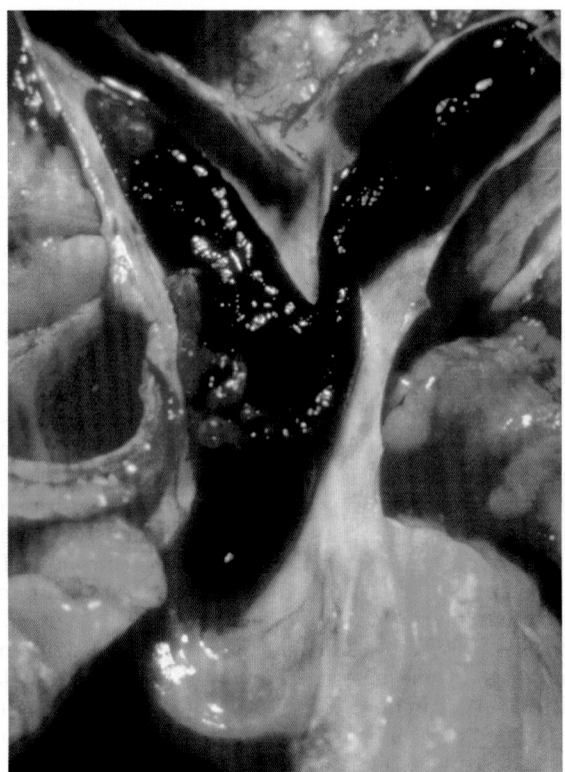

FIGURE 7-16. Pulmonary embolism. The main pulmonary artery and its bifurcation have been opened to reveal a large saddle embolus.

often bloody. With time, the blood in the infarct is resorbed, and the center of the infarct becomes pale. Granulation tissue forms on the edge of the infarct, after which it is organized to form a fibrous scar.

Pulmonary Embolism without Infarction

Since the lung is supplied by both the bronchial arteries and the pulmonary artery, most (75%) small pulmonary emboli do not produce infarcts. Although such emboli usually do not attract clinical attention, a few give rise to a syndrome characterized by dyspnea, cough, chest pain and hypotension. Rarely (3%), recurrent pulmonary emboli cause pulmonary hypertension by mechanical blockage of the arterial bed. In this circumstance, reflex vasoconstriction and bronchial constriction, due to release of vasoactive substances, may contribute to shrinkage of the functional pulmonary vascular bed.

In the clinical syndrome of "partial infarction," patients have the clinical and radiologic findings of pulmonary infarction due to thromboembolism. However, the lesion resolves instead of contracting to leave a scar. In such cases, hemorrhage and necrosis of the lung tissue in the affected area occur, but the tissue framework remains. Collateral circulation maintains tissue viability and enables its regeneration.

Fate of Pulmonary Thromboemboli

Small pulmonary emboli may completely resolve, depending on (1) the embolic load, (2) the adequacy of the pulmonary vascular reserve, (3) the state of the bronchial collateral circulation and (4) the thrombolytic process. Alternatively, thromboemboli may become organized and leave strings of fibrous tissue attached to a vessel wall in the lumen of pulmonary arteries. Radiologic studies have indicated that half of all pulmonary thromboemboli are resorbed and organized within 8 weeks, with little narrowing of the vessels.

Paradoxical Embolism

Paradoxical embolism refers to emboli that arise in the venous circulation and bypass the lungs by traveling through an incompletely closed foramen ovale, subsequently entering the left side of the heart and blocking flow to the systemic arteries. Since left atrial pressure usually exceeds that in the right, most of these cases occur in the context of a right-to-left shunt (see Chapter 17).

Systemic Arterial Embolism Often Causes Infarcts

Thromboembolism

The heart is the most common source of arterial thromboemboli (Fig. 7-17), which usually arise from mural thrombi (Fig. 7-18) or diseased valves. These emboli tend to lodge at points where vessel lumens narrow abruptly (e.g., at bifurcations or near atherosclerotic plaques). The viability of tissue supplied by the vessel depends on the available collateral circulation and the fate of the embolus itself. The thromboembolus may propagate locally and lead to a more severe obstruction, or it may fragment and lyse. Organs that suffer the most from arterial thromboembolism include:

- **Brain:** Arterial emboli to the brain cause ischemic necrosis (strokes).

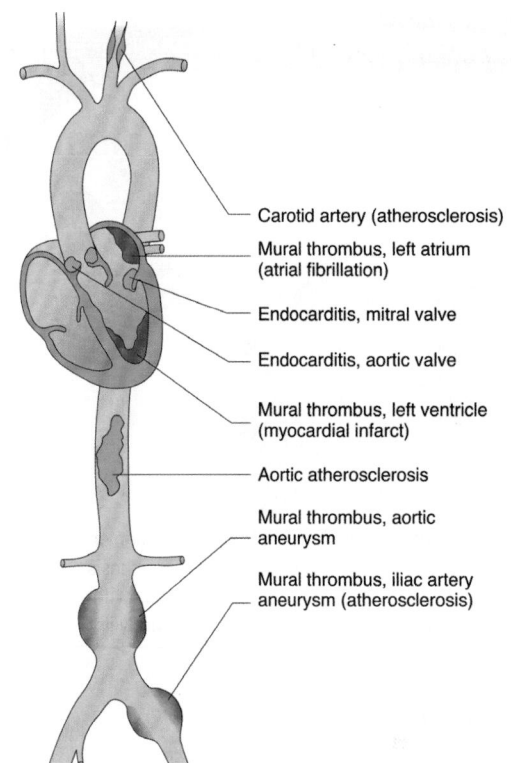

FIGURE 7-17. Sources of arterial emboli.

- Carotid artery (atherosclerosis)
- Mural thrombus, left atrium (atrial fibrillation)
- Endocarditis, mitral valve
- Endocarditis, aortic valve
- Mural thrombus, left ventricle (myocardial infarct)
- Aortic atherosclerosis
- Mural thrombus, aortic aneurysm
- Mural thrombus, iliac artery aneurysm (atherosclerosis)

- **Intestine:** In the mesenteric circulation, emboli cause bowel infarction, which manifests as an acute abdomen and requires immediate surgery.
- **Legs:** Embolism to an artery of the leg leads to sudden pain, absence of pulses and a cold limb (Fig. 7-19). In some cases, the limb may require amputation.
- **Kidney:** Renal artery embolism may infarct an entire kidney but more commonly causes small peripheral infarcts.
- **Heart:** Coronary artery embolism and resulting infarction occur but are rare.

The more common sites of infarction from arterial emboli are shown in Fig. 7-20.

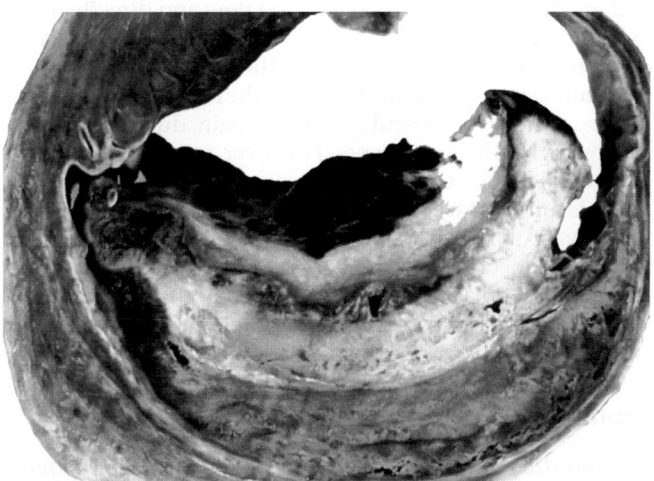

FIGURE 7-18. Mural thrombus of the left ventricle. A laminated thrombus adheres to the endocardium overlying a healed aneurysmal myocardial infarct.

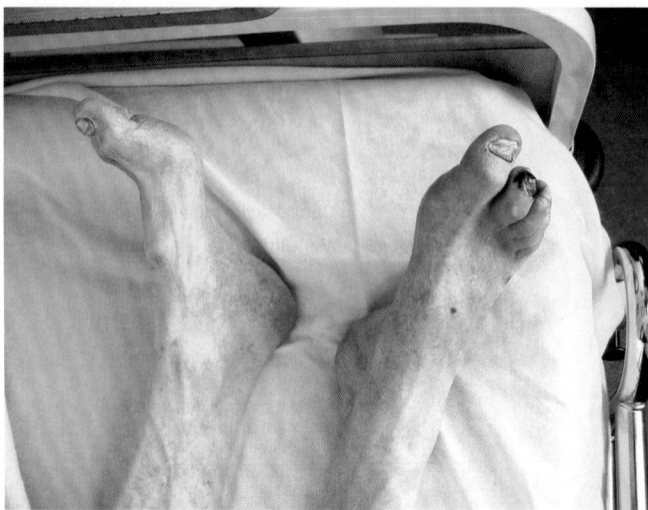

FIGURE 7-19. Acute ischemic right foot. A condition of sudden poor arterial perfusion, usually the consequence of acute thrombosis of an atherosclerotic plaque or embolism. This foot has a red dusky hue with second-toe necrosis. Symptoms may include pain, paresthesia and paralysis.

Air Embolism

Air may enter the venous circulation through neck wounds, thoracentesis or punctures of the great veins during invasive procedures or intraoperatively during cardiac surgery. Small amounts of circulating air in the form of bubbles are of little consequence, but quantities of 100 mL or more can result in sudden death. Air bubbles tend to coalesce and physically obstruct blood flow in the right side of the heart, the pulmonary circulation, and the brain. Histologically, air bubbles appear as empty spaces in capillaries and small vessels of the lung.

People exposed to increased atmospheric pressure, such as scuba divers and workers in underwater occupations (e.g., tunnels, drilling platform construction), are subject to **decompression sickness,** a unique form of gas embolism. During descent, large amounts of inert gas (nitrogen or helium) are dissolved in bodily fluids. When the diver ascends, this gas is released from solution and exhaled. However, if ascent is too rapid, gas bubbles form in the circulation and within tissues, obstructing blood flow and directly injuring cells. Air embolism is the second most common cause of death in sport diving (drowning is first).

Acute decompression sickness, "the bends," is characterized by temporary muscular and joint pain, due to small vessel obstruction in these tissues. However, severe involvement of cerebral blood vessels may cause coma or even death.

Caisson disease refers to decompression sickness in which vascular obstruction causes multiple foci of ischemic (avascular) necrosis of bone, particularly affecting the head of the femur, tibia and humerus. This complication was originally described in construction workers in diving bells (or caissons).

Amniotic Fluid Embolism

In amniotic fluid embolism, amniotic fluid containing fetal cells and debris enters the maternal circulation through open uterine and cervical veins. It is a rare maternal complication of childbirth, but can be catastrophic when it occurs. This

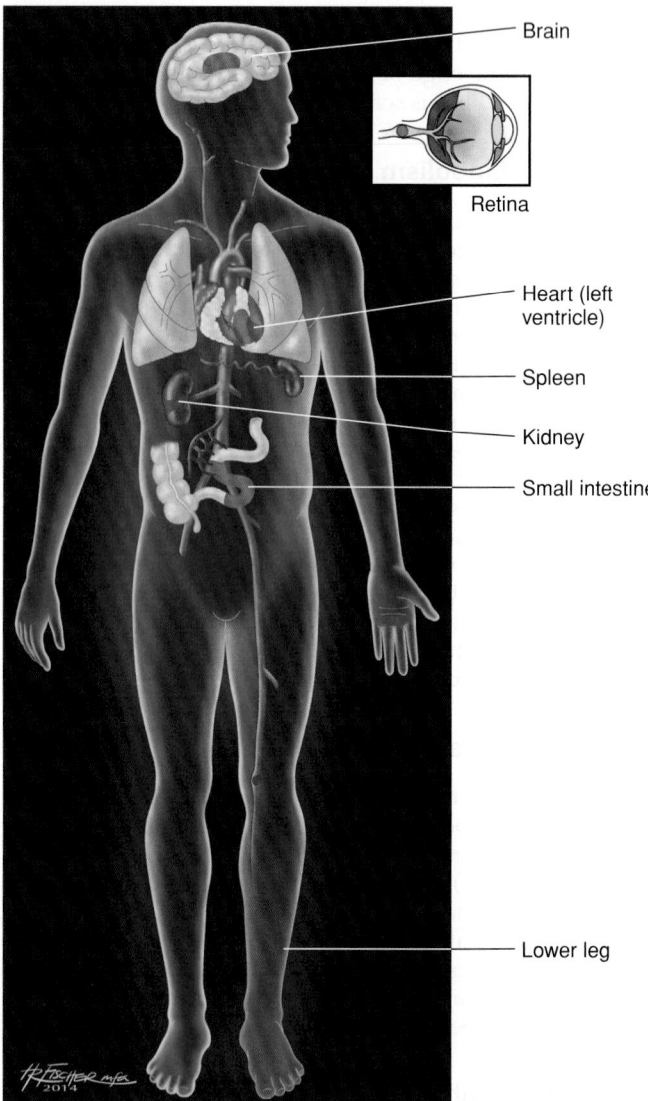

FIGURE 7-20. Common sites of infarction from arterial emboli.

disorder usually occurs at the end of labor when the pulmonary emboli are composed of the solid epithelial constituents (squames) contained in the amniotic fluid (Fig. 7-21). Of greater importance is the initiation of a potentially fatal consumptive coagulopathy caused by the high thromboplastin activity of the amniotic fluid.

The clinical presentation of amniotic fluid embolism can be dramatic, with sudden onset of cyanosis and shock, followed by coma and death. If the mother survives this acute episode, she may die of disseminated intravascular coagulation. Should she overcome this complication, she is at substantial risk of developing **acute respiratory distress syndrome** (see Chapter 18). Minor amniotic fluid embolism is probably common and asymptomatic, since autopsies of mothers who have died of other causes in the perinatal period frequently show evidence of this event.

Fat Embolism

Fat embolism is release of emboli of fatty marrow (Fig. 7-22) into damaged blood vessels following severe trauma to

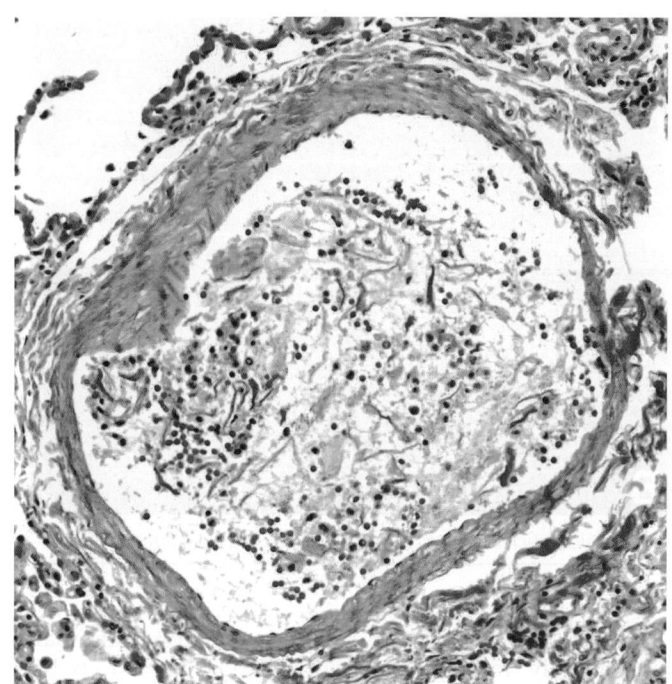

FIGURE 7-21. Amniotic fluid embolism. A section of lung shows a pulmonary artery filled with epithelial squames.

fat-containing tissue, particularly accompanying bone fractures. In most instances, fat embolism is clinically inapparent. However, severe fat embolism induces **fat embolism syndrome** 1–3 days after the injury. In its most severe form, which may be fatal, this syndrome is characterized by respiratory failure, mental changes, thrombocytopenia and widespread petechiae. Chest radiography reveals diffuse opacity of the lungs, which may progress to a "whiteout" typical of acute respiratory distress syndrome. At autopsy,

innumerable fat globules are seen in the microvasculature of the lungs (Fig. 7-22B) and brain and sometimes other organs. Morphologically, the lungs typically exhibit the changes of acute respiratory distress syndrome (see Chapter 18). The lesions in the brain include cerebral edema, small hemorrhages and occasionally microinfarcts.

Fat embolism is usually considered a direct consequence of trauma, with fat entering ruptured capillaries at the site of the fracture. However, this explanation may be too simplistic. It has been suggested that hemorrhage into the marrow and perhaps also into the subcutaneous fat increases interstitial pressure above capillary pressure, so fat is forced into the circulation. Moreover, there is more fat in the pulmonary vascular system than can be accounted for by simple transfer of fat from peripheral depots, and the chemical composition of the fat in the lung differs from that in tissue. Finally, there is a discrepancy between the frequency of fat embolism and bone marrow embolism.

Bone Marrow Embolism

Bone marrow emboli to the lungs, complete with hematopoietic cells and fat, are often encountered at autopsy after cardiac resuscitation, a procedure in which fractures of the sternum and ribs commonly occur. They also occasionally occur after fractures of long bones. In most cases no symptoms are attributed to bone marrow embolism.

Miscellaneous Pulmonary Emboli

Intravenous drug abusers who use talc as a carrier for illicit drugs may introduce it into the lung via the bloodstream. **Talc emboli** produce a granulomatous response in the lungs (Fig. 7-23). **Cotton emboli** are surprisingly common and are due to cleansing of the skin prior to venipuncture. **Schistosomiasis** may be associated with the embolization of ova to the lungs from bladder or gut, in which case they incite

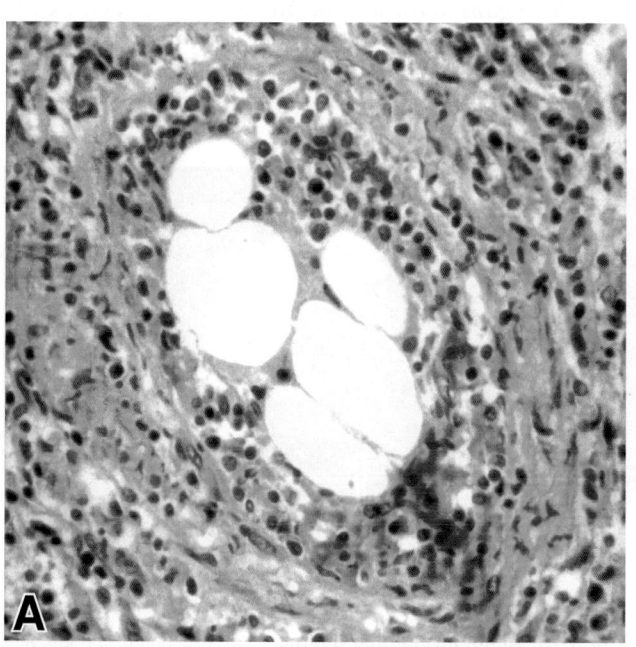

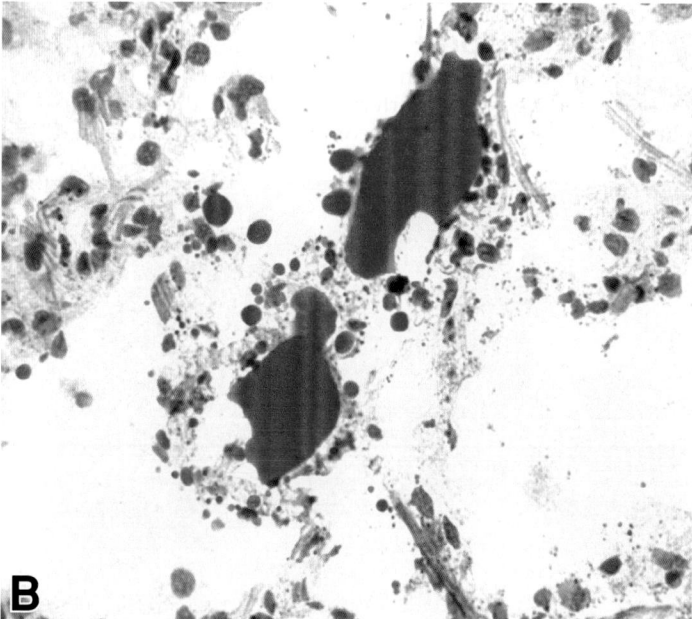

FIGURE 7-22. Fat embolism. A. The lumen of a small pulmonary artery is occluded by a fragment of bone marrow consisting of fat cells and hematopoietic elements. **B.** A frozen section of lung stained with Sudan red shows capillaries occluded by red-staining fat emboli.

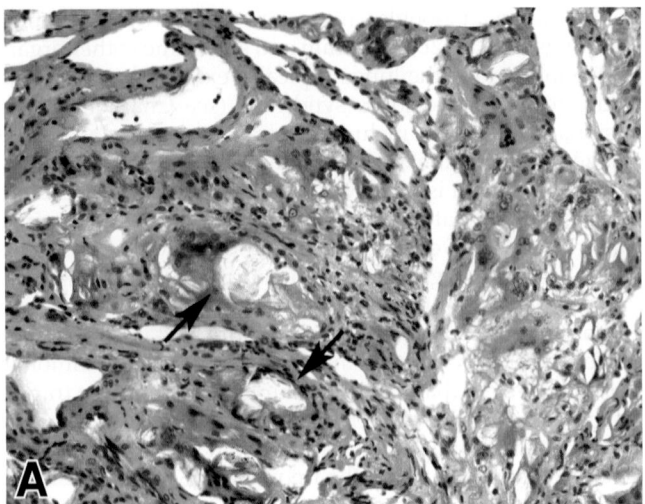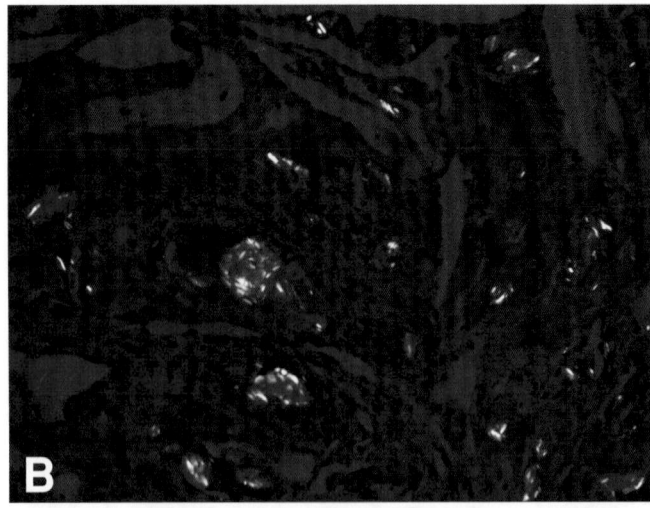

FIGURE 7-23. Talc emboli. A section of lung from an intravenous drug abuser shows talc particles (*arrows*) before **(A)** and after **(B)** polarization of light.

a foreign body granulomatous reaction. **Tumor emboli** are occasionally seen in the lung during hematogenous dissemination of cancer.

INFARCTION

Infarction is the process by which coagulative necrosis develops in an area distal to occlusion of an end-artery. The necrotic zone is an **infarct**. Infarcts of vital organs such as heart, brain and intestine are serious medical conditions and are major causes of morbidity and mortality. If the victim survives, the infarct heals with a scar. Partial arterial occlusion (i.e., stenosis) occasionally causes necrosis, but it more commonly leads to atrophic changes associated with chronic ischemia. For example, in the heart, these changes include vacuolization of cardiac myocytes, atrophy, loss of muscle cell myofibrils and interstitial fibrosis.

PATHOLOGY: The gross and microscopic appearance of an infarct depends on its location and age. Upon arterial occlusion, the area supplied by the vessel rapidly becomes swollen and deep red.

Microscopically, vascular dilation and congestion and occasionally interstitial hemorrhage are noted. Subsequently, several types of infarcts are distinguishable by gross examination.

Pale infarcts are typical in the heart, kidneys and spleen (Fig. 7-24), although certain renal infarcts may be cystic. **Dry gangrene** of the leg due to arterial occlusion (often noted in diabetes) is actually a large pale infarct. Within 1 or 2 days after the initial hyperemia, an infarct becomes soft, sharply delineated and light yellow (Fig. 7-25). The border tends to be dark red, reflecting hemorrhage into surrounding viable tissue. Microscopically, a pale infarct exhibits uniform coagulative necrosis.

Red infarcts may result from either arterial or venous occlusion and are also characterized by coagulative necrosis. However, they are distinguished by bleeding into the affected area from adjacent vessels. *Red infarcts occur mainly in organs with a dual blood supply,* such as the lung, or those with extensive collateral circulation (e.g., the small intestine and brain). In the heart, a red infarct occurs when the infarcted area is reperfused, as may occur after

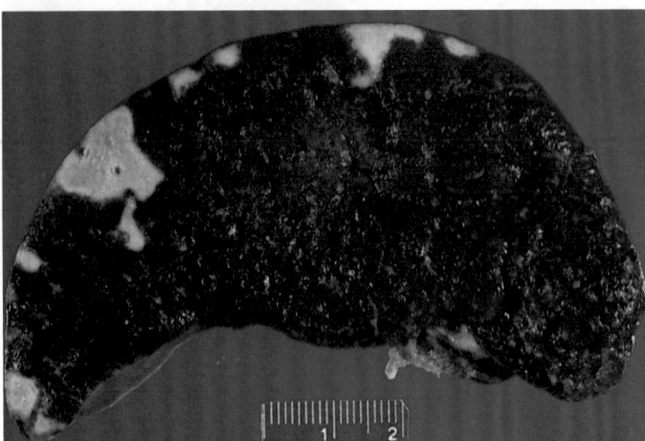

FIGURE 7-24. Spleen infarcts. A cut section of spleen displays multiple pale, wedge-shaped infarcts beneath the capsule.

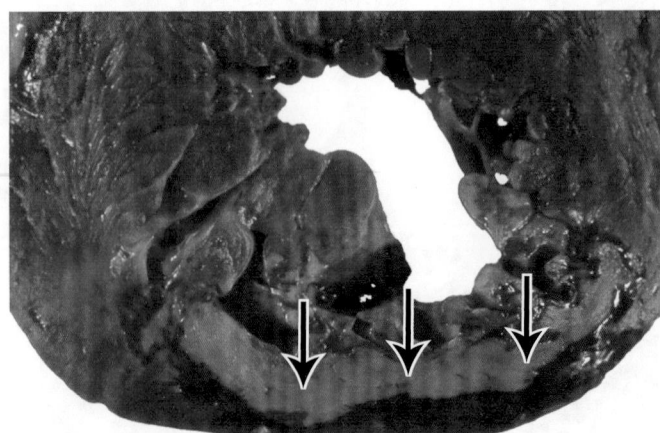

FIGURE 7-25. Acute myocardial infarct. A cross-section of the left ventricle reveals a sharply circumscribed, soft, yellow area of necrosis in the posterior free wall (*arrows*).

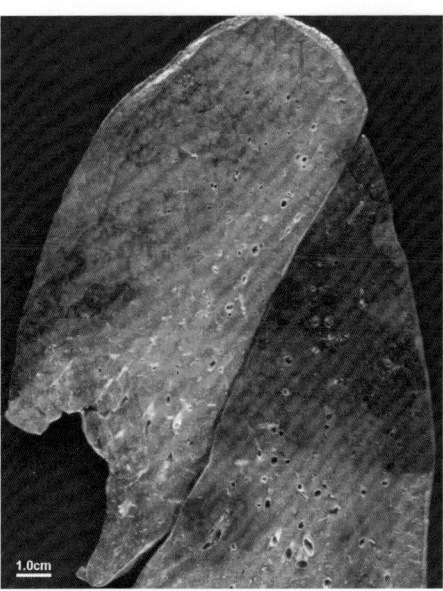

FIGURE 7-26. Red infarct. A sagittal slice of lung shows a hemorrhagic infarct in upper segments of the lower lobe.

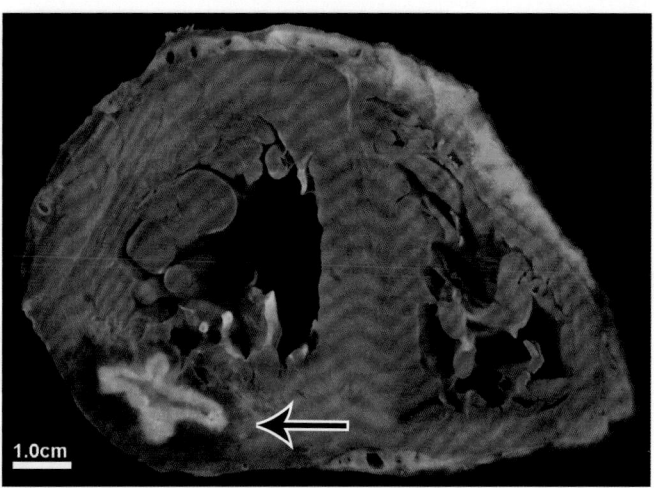

FIGURE 7-28. Septic infarct. A myocardial abscess (*arrow*) within the left ventricular free wall was due to infection with *Staphylococcus aureus.*

spontaneous or therapeutically induced lysis of an occluding thrombus. Red infarcts are sharply circumscribed, firm and dark red to purple (Fig. 7-26). For several days, acute inflammatory cells infiltrate the necrotic area from the viable border. Cellular debris is phagocytosed and digested by neutrophils and later by macrophages. Granulation tissue eventually forms, to be replaced ultimately by a scar. In a large infarct of an organ such as the heart or kidney, the necrotic center may remain inaccessible to the inflammatory exudate and may persist for months. In the brain, an infarct typically undergoes liquefactive necrosis and may become a fluid-filled cyst, which is referred to as a **cystic infarct** (Fig. 7-27).

Septic infarction results when the necrotic tissue of an infarct is seeded by pyogenic bacteria and becomes infected. Pulmonary infarcts are not uncommonly infected, presumably because necrotic tissue offers little resistance to inhaled bacteria. In the case of bacterial endocarditis, the emboli themselves are infected and resulting infarcts are often septic. A septic infarct may become a frank abscess (Fig. 7-28).

Infarction in Specific Locations Is Often Fatal

Myocardial Infarcts

Myocardial infarcts are transmural (through the entire wall) or subendocardial. A transmural infarct results from complete occlusion of a major extramural coronary artery. Subendocardial infarction reflects prolonged ischemia caused by partially occluding, atherosclerotic, stenotic coronary artery lesions when the requirement for oxygen exceeds the supply. This happens in, for example, shock, anoxia or severe tachycardia (rapid pulse). A myocardial infarct may be pale or red, depending on the extent of reflow of blood into the infarcted area (Fig. 7-29).

Pulmonary Infarcts

Only about 10% of pulmonary emboli elicit clinical symptoms referable to pulmonary infarction, usually after occlusion of a middle-sized pulmonary artery. Infarction occurs only if circulation from bronchial arteries is inadequate to compensate for supply lost from the pulmonary arteries. This circumstance is often found in congestive heart failure, although stasis in the pulmonary circulation may contribute. Hemorrhage into the alveolar spaces of the necrotic lining tissue occurs within 48 hours.

Cerebral Infarcts

Infarction of the brain may result from local ischemia or a generalized reduction in blood flow. The latter often results from systemic hypotension, as in shock, and produces infarction in the border zones between the distributions of the major cerebral arteries **(watershed infarct)**. If prolonged, severe hypotension can cause widespread brain necrosis. The occlusion of a single vessel in the brain (e.g., after an embolus has lodged) causes ischemia and necrosis in a well-defined area. This type of cerebral infarct may be pale or red, the latter being common with embolic occlusions. The occlusion of a large artery produces a wide area of necrosis, which may ultimately resolve as a large fluid-filled cavity in the brain (cystic infarct).

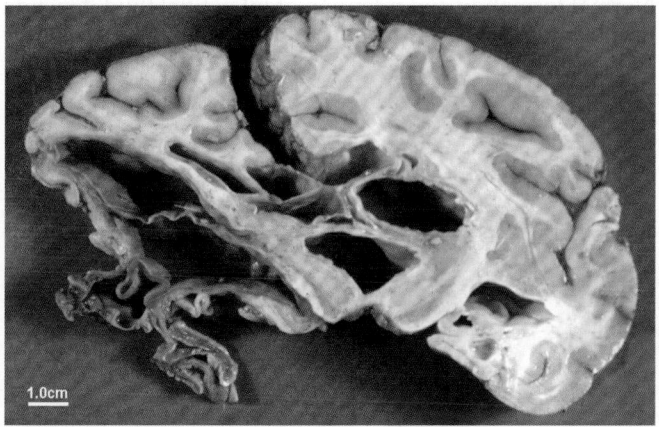

FIGURE 7-27. Cystic infarct. A cross-section of brain in the frontal plane shows a healed cystic infarct.

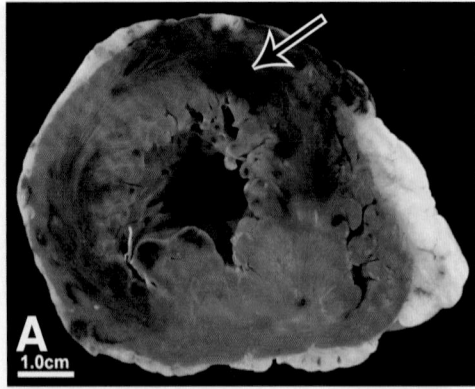

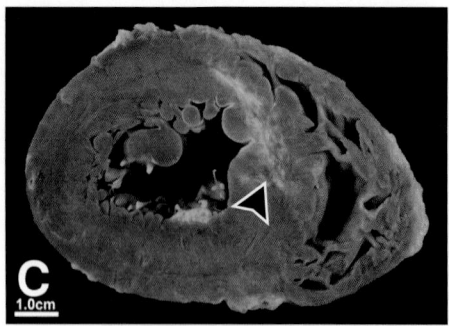

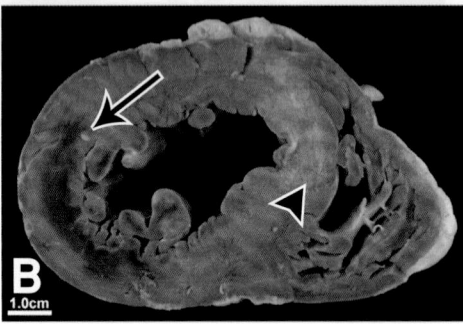

FIGURE 7-29. **Myocardial infarct.** Transverse sections of ventricular myocardium show **(A)** reperfused, **(B)** acute (*arrow*) and healed (*arrowhead*) together and **(C)** healed infarct. Reperfusion is typically associated with hemorrhage as in **A** (*arrow*) and **B** (*arrow*). In **C,** a white scar (*arrowhead*) is evident in the anterior ventricular septum.

Intestinal Infarcts

The earliest tissue changes in intestinal ischemia are necrosis of the tips of the villi in the small intestine and necrosis of the superficial mucosa in the large intestine. In either case, more severe ischemia causes hemorrhagic necrosis of the submucosa and muscularis but not the serosa. Small mucosal infarcts heal within a few days, but more severe injury leads to ulceration. These ulcers can eventually reepithelialize. However, if ulcers are large, they are repaired by scarring, a process that may give rise to strictures. Severe transmural necrosis is associated with massive bleeding or bowel perforation, complications that often result in irreversible shock, sepsis and death.

EDEMA

Edema is excess fluid in interstitial tissue spaces, which may be local or generalized. **Local edema** in most instances occurs with inflammation, the "tumor" of "tumor, rubor and calor." Local edema of a limb, usually the leg, results from

venous or lymphatic obstruction. Burns cause prominent local edema by altering the permeability of local vasculature. Local edema may be a prominent component of an immune reaction, for example, urticaria (hives) or edema of the epiglottis or larynx (angioneurotic edema).

Generalized edema, affecting visceral organs and the skin of the trunk and lower extremities (Fig. 7-30), reflects a global disorder of fluid and electrolyte metabolism, most often due to heart failure. Generalized edema is also seen in certain renal diseases associated with loss of serum proteins into the urine (nephrotic syndrome) and in cirrhosis of the liver. **Anasarca** is extreme generalized edema, a condition evidenced by conspicuous fluid accumulation in subcutaneous tissues, visceral organs and body cavities. Edema fluid may accumulate in body spaces, such as the pleural cavity **(hydrothorax),** peritoneal cavity **(ascites)** or pericardial space **(hydropericardium).**

Normal Capillary Filtration

Normal formation and retention of interstitial fluid depends on filtration and reabsorption at the level of the capillaries

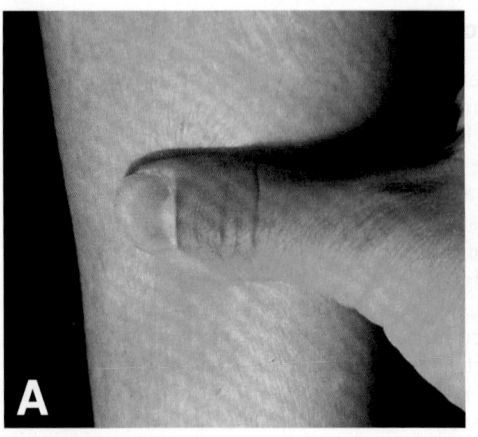

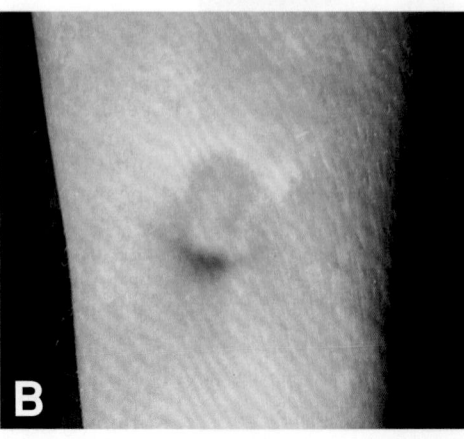

FIGURE 7-30. **Pitting edema of the leg. A.** In a patient with congestive heart failure, severe edema of the leg is demonstrated by applying pressure with a finger. **B.** The resulting "pitting" reflects the inelasticity of the fluid-filled tissue.

(Starling forces). The internal or hydrostatic pressure in the arteriolar segment of the capillary is 32 mm Hg. At the middle of the capillary, it is 20 mm Hg. Since interstitial hydrostatic pressure is only 3 mm Hg, there is an outward fluid filtration of 14 mL/min. Hydrostatic pressure is opposed by plasma oncotic pressure (26 mm Hg), which results in osmotic reabsorption at 12 mL/min at the venous end of the capillary. Thus, interstitial fluid is formed at the rate of 2 mL/min and is reabsorbed by the lymphatics. As a result, in equilibrium there is no net fluid gain or loss in the interstitium.

Sodium and Water Metabolism

Water represents 50%–70% of body weight and is divided between the extracellular and intracellular fluid spaces. Extracellular fluid is further divided into interstitial and vascular compartments. Interstitial fluid constitutes about 75% of the latter.

Total body sodium is the principal determinant of extracellular fluid volume because it is the major cation in the extracellular fluid. In other words, increased total body sodium must be balanced by more extracellular water to maintain constant osmolality. Control of extracellular fluid volume depends to a large extent on regulation of renal sodium excretion, which is influenced by (1) atrial natriuretic factor, (2) the renin–angiotensin system of the juxtaglomerular apparatus and (3) sympathetic nervous system activity (see Chapter 22).

Edema Caused by Increased Hydrostatic Pressure

Unopposed increases in hydrostatic pressure result in greater filtration of fluid into the interstitial space and its retention as edema. Such a situation is particularly prominent in decompensated heart disease, in which back-pressure in the lungs secondary to left ventricular failure causes acute pulmonary edema and right-sided heart failure, and contributes to systemic edema. Similarly, back-pressure caused by venous obstruction in the lower extremity causes edema of the leg. Obstruction to portal blood flow in cirrhosis of the liver contributes to formation of abdominal fluid (ascites).

Edema Caused by Decreased Oncotic Pressure

The difference in pressure between intravascular and interstitial compartments is largely determined by the concentration of plasma proteins, especially albumin. Any condition that lowers plasma albumin levels, whether it is albuminuria in the nephrotic syndrome, reduced albumin synthesis in chronic liver disease or severe malnutrition, tends to promote generalized edema.

Edema Caused by Lymphatic Obstruction

Under normal circumstances, more fluid is filtered into the interstitial spaces than is reabsorbed into the vascular bed. This excess interstitial fluid is removed by lymphatics. Thus, obstruction to lymphatic flow leads to localized edema. Lymphatic channels can be obstructed by (1) malignant neoplasms, (2) fibrosis resulting from inflammation or irradiation and (3) surgical ablation. For instance, the inflammatory response to filarial worms (Bancroftian and Malayan filariasis; see Chapter 9) can result in lymphatic obstruction that produces massive lymphedema of the scrotum and lower

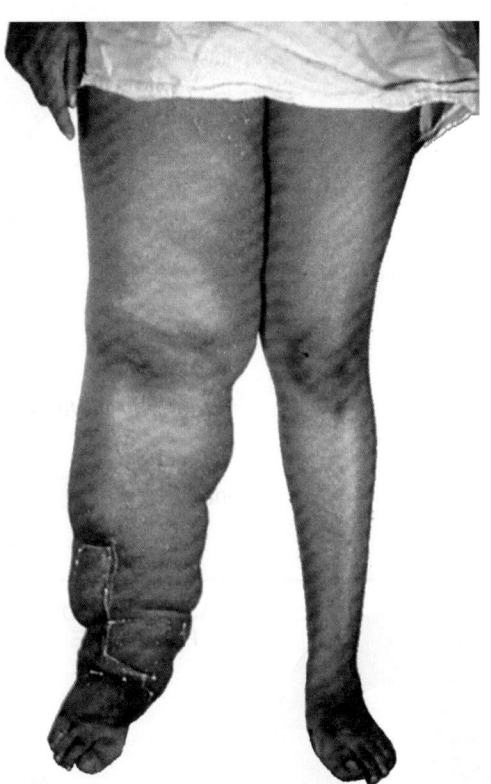

FIGURE 7-31. Edema secondary to lymphatic obstruction. Massive edema of the right lower extremity (elephantiasis) in a patient with obstruction of lymphatic drainage.

extremities **(elephantiasis)** (Fig. 7-31). Lymphedema of the arm often complicates radical mastectomies for breast cancer, owing to removal of axillary lymph nodes and lymphatics.

Lymphatic edema differs from other forms of edema in its high protein content, since lymph is the vehicle by which proteins and interstitial cells are returned to the circulation. The increased protein concentration may be a fibrogenic stimulus in the formation of dermal fibrosis in chronic edema (indurated edema).

The Role of Sodium Retention in Edema

Generalized edema and ascites invariably reflect increased total body sodium, as a consequence of renal sodium retention. When peripheral edema is first detectable clinically, extracellular fluid volume has already expanded by at least 5 L. The most common conditions in which generalized edema is found include congestive heart failure, cirrhosis of the liver, nephrotic syndrome and some cases of chronic renal insufficiency. The mechanisms of edema formation and representative disorders associated with them are summarized in Fig. 7-32 and Table 7-1.

Congestive Heart Failure Is the Consequence of Inadequate Cardiac Output

It is estimated that 5 to 6 million people in the United States suffer congestive heart failure, of whom 15% die annually. Half of all patients with congestive heart failure who require admission to the hospital will die within 1 year. In the United States, this disorder is most commonly associated

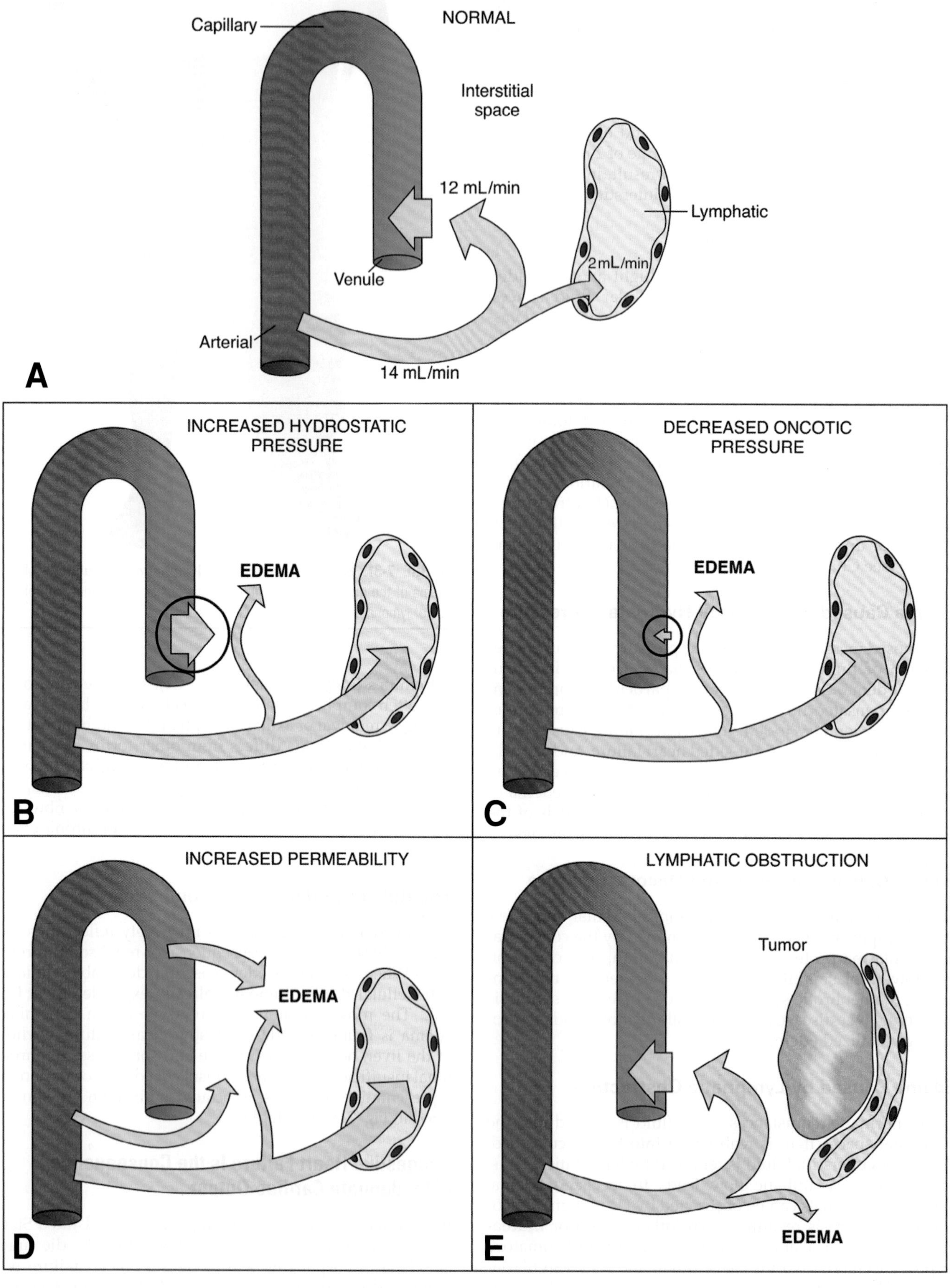

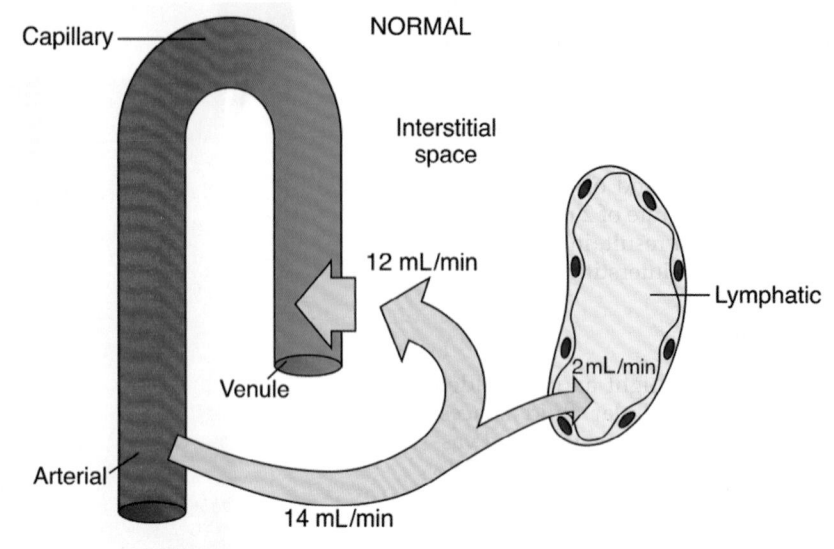

NORMAL

Capillary

Interstitial space

12 mL/min

Lymphatic

Venule

2 mL/min

Arterial

A

14 mL/min

INCREASED HYDROSTATIC PRESSURE

EDEMA

B

DECREASED ONCOTIC PRESSURE

EDEMA

C

INCREASED PERMEABILITY

EDEMA

D

LYMPHATIC OBSTRUCTION

Tumor

EDEMA

E

TABLE 7-1
DISORDERS ASSOCIATED WITH EDEMA

Increased Hydrostatic Pressure

Arteriolar dilation	Inflammation
	Heat
Increased venous pressure	Venous thrombosis
	Congestive heart failure
	Cirrhosis (ascites)
	Postural inactivity (e.g., prolonged standing)
Hypervolemia	Sodium retention (e.g., decreased renal function)

Decreased Oncotic Pressure

Hypoproteinemia	Nephrotic syndrome
	Cirrhosis
	Protein-losing gastroenteropathy
	Malnutrition
Increased Capillary Permeability	Inflammation
	Burns
	Adult respiratory distress syndrome
Lymphatic Obstruction	Cancer
	Postsurgical lymphedema
	Inflammation

with ischemic heart disease, although virtually any chronic cardiac disorder may eventuate in congestive heart failure (see Chapter 17).

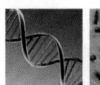 **MOLECULAR PATHOGENESIS AND ETIOLOGIC FACTORS:** The argument regarding the relative contributions of "forward failure" (low cardiac output) versus "backward failure" (venous congestion) in the pathogenesis of edema in congestive heart failure is no longer a burning issue. Both systolic and diastolic dysfunction contribute to the low cardiac output and high ventricular filling pressure characteristic of congestive heart failure. However, systolic dysfunction is more important in most patients.

Inadequate cardiac output in congestive heart failure gives rise to decreased glomerular filtration and increased renin secretion. The latter activates angiotensin, inducing the release of aldosterone, subsequent sodium reabsorption and fluid retention. Furthermore, reduced hepatic blood flow impairs catabolism of aldosterone, thus further raising its concentration in the blood. As a compensatory mechanism, increased fluid volume preserves an adequate intracardiac pressure. In addition, increased sympathetic discharge leads to augmented levels of catecholamines, which stimulate cardiac contractility and further counteract the impairment in cardiac performance. At the same time, distention of the atria by the increased blood volume promotes release of atrial natriuretic peptide, which stimulates renal sodium excretion.

After long-standing heart failure, these compensatory mechanisms fail, in which case renal sodium retention again becomes important. Further expansion of plasma volume increases pulmonary and systemic venous pressure, thus increasing hydrostatic pressure in the respective capillary beds. The increased capillary pressure, together with decreased plasma oncotic pressure, results in the edema of congestive heart failure.

 PATHOLOGY: Failure of the left ventricle is associated principally with passive congestion of the lungs and pulmonary edema (Fig. 7-33). When chronic, these conditions result in pulmonary hypertension and eventual failure of the right ventricle. Right ventricular failure is characterized by generalized subcutaneous edema (most prominent in the dependent portions of the body), ascites and pleural effusions. The liver, spleen and other splanchnic organs are typically congested. At autopsy, the heart is enlarged and its chambers dilated.

 CLINICAL FEATURES: The effects of heart failure depend on which ventricle is failing, recognizing that both may be failing simultaneously. Patients in left-sided heart failure complain of shortness of breath **(dyspnea)** on exertion and when recumbent **(orthopnea)**. They may be awakened from sleep by sudden episodes of shortness of breath **(paroxysmal nocturnal dyspnea)**. Physical examination usually reveals distended jugular veins. People with right-sided failure have pitting edema of the legs and an enlarged and tender liver. When ascites is present, the abdomen is distended. Patients in congestive heart failure with pulmonary edema have crackling breath sounds **(rales)** caused by expansion of fluid-filled alveoli.

In Pulmonary Edema Fluid Fills the Air Spaces and Interstitium of the Lung

Pulmonary edema leads to decreased gas exchange in the lung, causing hypoxia and retention of carbon dioxide **(hypercapnia)**.

FIGURE 7-32. The capillary system and mechanisms of edema formation. A. Normal. The differential between the hydrostatic and oncotic pressures at the arterial end of the capillary system is responsible for the filtration into the interstitial space of approximately 14 mL of fluid per minute. This fluid is reabsorbed at the venous end at the rate of 12 mL/min. It is also drained through the lymphatic capillaries at a rate of 2 mL/min. Proteins are removed by the lymphatics from the interstitial space. **B. Hydrostatic edema.** If the hydrostatic pressure at the venous end of the capillary system is elevated, reabsorption decreases. As long as the lymphatics can drain the surplus fluid, no edema results. If their capacity is exceeded, however, edema fluid accumulates. **C. Oncotic edema.** Edema fluid also accumulates if reabsorption is diminished by decreased oncotic pressure of the vascular bed, owing to a loss of albumin. **D. Inflammatory and traumatic edema.** Edema, either local or systemic, results if the vascular bed becomes leaky following injury to the endothelium. **E. Lymphedema.** Lymphatic obstruction causes the accumulation of interstitial fluid because of insufficient reabsorption and deficient removal of proteins, the latter increasing the oncotic pressure of the fluid in the interstitial space.

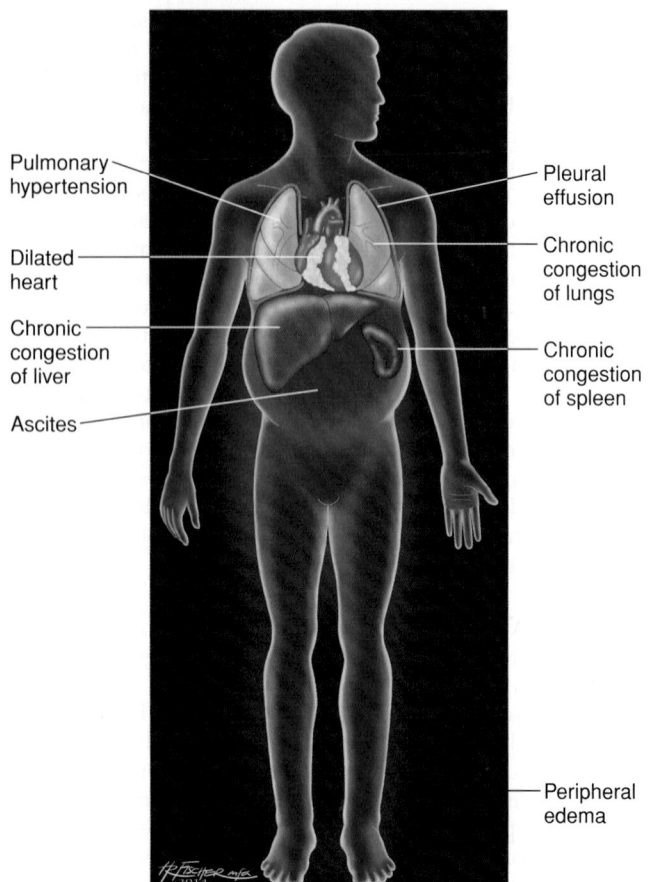

Pulmonary hypertension

Dilated heart

Chronic congestion of liver

Ascites

Pleural effusion

Chronic congestion of lungs

Chronic congestion of spleen

Peripheral edema

FIGURE 7-33. Pathologic consequences of chronic congestive heart failure.

Pulmonary edema may be interstitial or alveolar. Interstitial edema is the earliest phase and is an exaggeration of normal fluid filtration. Lymphatics become distended and fluid accumulates in the interstitium of lobular septa and around veins and bronchovascular bundles. Radiologic examination reveals a reticulonodular pattern, more marked at lung bases. Lobular septa become edematous and produce linear shadows ("Kerley B lines") on chest radiographs. Edema results in shunting of blood flow from the lung bases to the upper lobes, and increased airflow resistance occurs because of edema of the bronchovascular tree. Patients are often asymptomatic in this early stage.

When the fluid can no longer be accommodated in the interstitial space, it spills into the alveoli, which is called **alveolar edema**. At this stage, a radiologic alveolar pattern is seen, usually worse in central portions of the lung and in lower zones. The patient becomes acutely short of breath and bubbly rales are heard. In extreme cases, frothy fluid is coughed up or wells up out of the trachea.

Microscopically, the edematous lung shows severely congested alveolar capillaries and alveoli filled with a homogeneous, pink-staining fluid permeated by air bubbles (Fig. 7-3). If pulmonary edema is caused by alveolar damage, cell debris, fibrin and proteins form films of proteinaceous material in the alveoli, called **hyaline membranes** (Fig. 7-34).

 CLINICAL FEATURES: Fluid accumulation may go unnoticed initially, but eventually dyspnea and coughing become prominent. If edema is severe, large amounts of frothy pink sputum are expectorated. Hypoxemia is manifested as cyanosis.

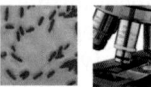 **ETIOLOGIC FACTORS AND PATHOLOGY:** The lung is a loose tissue with little connective tissue support and so requires certain conditions to prevent the development of edema. Among these protective devices are:

- Low perfusion pressure in lung capillaries, due to low right ventricular pressure
- Effective drainage of the interstitial space of the lung by lymphatics, which are under a slightly negative pressure and can accommodate up to 10 times the regular lymph flow
- Tight cellular junctions between endothelial cells, which control capillary permeability

Pulmonary edema results when these protective mechanisms are disturbed. The most common causes of pulmonary edema relate to hemodynamic alterations in the heart that increase perfusion pressure in pulmonary capillaries and block effective lymphatic drainage. These conditions include left ventricular failure (the most common cause), mitral stenosis and mitral insufficiency. Disruption of capillary permeability is the cause of pulmonary edema in acute lung injury associated with adult respiratory distress syndrome, inhalation of toxic gases, aspiration of gastric contents, viral infections and uremia. Acute lung injury is reflected in destruction of endothelial cells or disruption of their tight junctions (see Chapter 18).

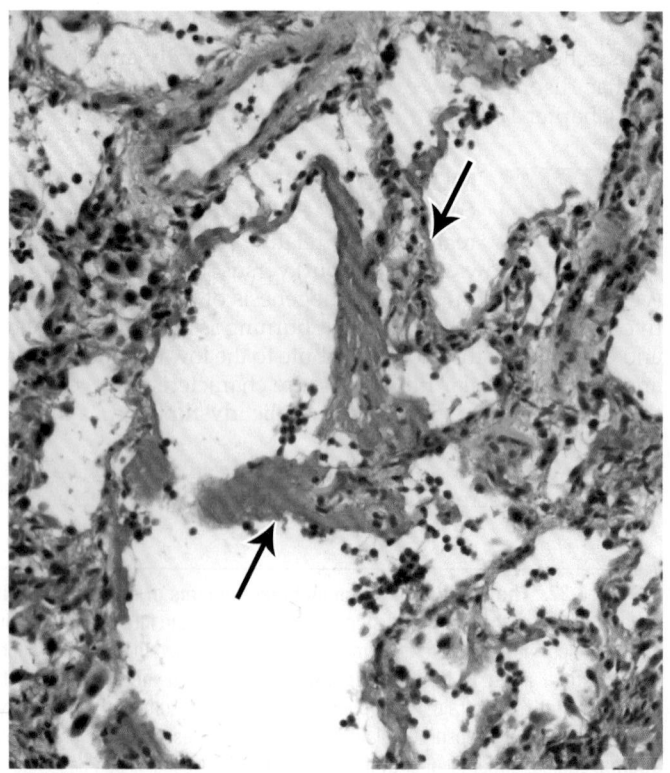

FIGURE 7-34. Pulmonary edema due to diffuse alveolar damage. A section of lung shows hyaline membranes (*arrows*) in alveoli.

Pulmonary function is restricted in severe congestion and in interstitial pulmonary edema because fluid accumulation in the interstitial space causes reduced pulmonary compliance (i.e., stiffening of the lung tissue). Thus, increased respiratory work is required to maintain ventilation. Since alveolar walls are thickened, there is a greater barrier to exchange of oxygen and carbon dioxide. The latter is less affected than the former, resulting in hypoxia with near-normal carbon dioxide levels. Mismatch between ventilation (which is reduced) and perfusion (which persists) contributes to development of hypoxemia in patients with pulmonary edema.

Edema in Cirrhosis of the Liver Is Commonly an End-Stage Condition

Cirrhosis of the liver is often accompanied by ascites and peripheral edema (see Chapter 20). Liver scarring obstructs portal blood flow and leads to portal hypertension and increased hydrostatic pressure in the splanchnic circulation. This situation is compounded by decreased hepatic synthesis of albumin as a result of liver dysfunction. Consequent accumulation of peritoneal fluid causes a lower effective blood volume, which results in renal retention of sodium by mechanisms similar to those operative in congestive heart failure. Alternatively, chronic liver disease itself causes renal retention of sodium. Subsequent expansion of extracellular fluid volume further promotes ascites and edema, thus establishing a vicious circle. In addition, increased transudation of lymph from the liver capsule adds to accumulation of fluid in the abdomen.

The Nephrotic Syndrome Reflects Massive Proteinuria

In the nephrotic syndrome, the magnitude of protein loss in the urine exceeds the rate at which it is replaced by the liver (see Chapter 22). The resulting decline in the concentration of plasma proteins, particularly albumin, reduces plasma oncotic pressure and promotes edema. The ensuing decrease in blood volume stimulates the renin–angiotensin–aldosterone mechanism and causes sodium retention. The edema is generalized but appears preferentially in soft connective tissues, the eyes, the eyelids and subcutaneous tissues. Ascites and pleural effusions also occur.

Cerebral Edema Often Causes a Fatal Increase in Intracranial Pressure

Edema of the brain is dangerous because the rigidity of the cranium allows little room for expansion. Increased intracranial pressure from edema compromises cerebral blood supply, distorts the gross structure of the brain and interferes with central nervous system function (see Chapter 32). Cerebral edema is divided into vasogenic, cytotoxic and interstitial forms.

■ **Vasogenic edema,** the most common variety of edema, is excess fluid in the extracellular space of the brain. It results from increased vascular permeability, mainly in white matter. The tight endothelial junctions of the blood-brain barrier are disrupted and fluid filters into the interstitial space. Disorders causing cerebral vasogenic edema include trauma, neoplasms, encephalitis, abscesses, infarcts, hemorrhage and toxic brain injury (e.g., lead poisoning).

■ **Cytotoxic edema** is equivalent to hydropic cell swelling (i.e., accumulation of intracellular water). It is usually a response to cell injury, such as that produced by ischemia. Cytotoxic cerebral edema preferentially affects the gray matter.

■ **Interstitial edema** is a consequence of hydrocephalus, in which fluid accumulates in the cerebral ventricles and periventricular white matter.

At autopsy, an edematous brain is soft and heavy. Gyri are flattened and sulci narrowed. Because of alterations in brain function, patients with cerebral edema suffer vomiting, disorientation and convulsions. Severe cerebral edema results in herniation of the cerebellar tonsils, ordinarily a lethal event.

Fluid Accumulates in Body Cavities as Extensions of the Interstitial Space

The Pleural Space

Pleural effusion (fluid in the pleural space) is a straw-colored transudate of low specific gravity that contains few cells (mainly exfoliated mesothelial cells). Fluid commonly accumulates as an expression of a generalized tendency to form edema in diseases such as the nephrotic syndrome, cirrhosis of the liver and congestive heart failure. Pleural effusion is also a frequent response to an inflammatory process or tumor in the lung or on the pleural surface.

The Pericardium

Fluid in the pericardial sac may result from either hemorrhage **(hemopericardium)** or injury to the pericardium **(pericardial effusion)**. Pericardial effusions occur with pericardial infections, metastatic neoplasms to the pericardium, uremia and systemic lupus erythematosus. They are also occasionally encountered after cardiac operations **(postpericardiotomy syndrome)** or radiation therapy for cancer.

Pericardial fluid may accumulate rapidly (e.g., with hemorrhage from a ruptured myocardial infarct, dissecting aortic aneurysm or trauma). In these cases, pericardial cavity pressure rises to exceed the filling pressure of the heart, which is called **cardiac tamponade** (Fig. 7-35). The resulting

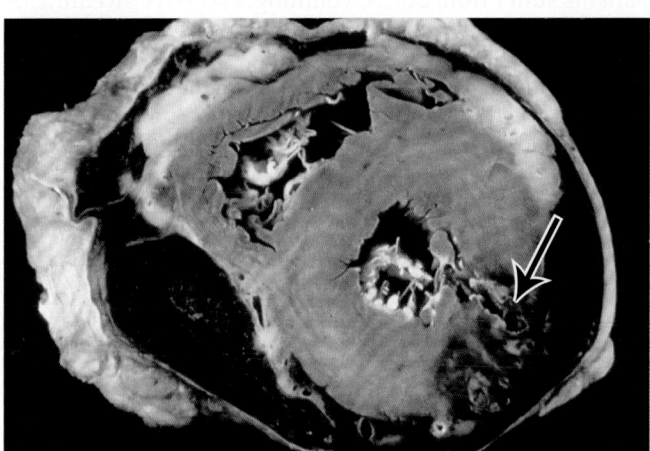

FIGURE 7-35. Cardiac tamponade. A cross-section of the heart shows rupture of a myocardial infarct (*arrow*) with the accumulation of a large quantity of blood in the pericardial cavity.

precipitous decline in cardiac output is often fatal. If pericardial fluid accumulates rapidly, the tolerable limit may be only 90–120 mL, but a liter or more of fluid can be accommodated if the process is gradual.

Peritoneum

Peritoneal effusion, also called **ascites,** is caused mainly by cirrhosis of the liver, abdominal neoplasms, pancreatitis, cardiac failure, the nephrotic syndrome and hepatic venous obstruction (Budd-Chiari syndrome). Obstruction of the thoracic duct by cancer may lead to **chylous ascites,** in which the fluid has a milky appearance and a high fat content. The pathogenesis of ascites in cirrhosis of the liver is discussed above.

Patients with severe ascites accumulate many liters of fluid and have hugely distended abdomens. The complications of ascites derive from increased abdominal pressure and include anorexia and vomiting, reflux esophagitis, dyspnea, ventral hernia and leakage of fluid into the pleural space.

FLUID LOSS AND OVERLOAD

Excessive fluid loss (dehydration) and fluid overload are clinical situations that have potentially grave consequences. Fluid imbalance causes hemodynamic disorders; alterations in osmolality and the quantity of fluid in intravascular, interstitial and cellular spaces may affect perfusion or delivery of substrates, electrolytes or fluids.

Dehydration Features Inadequate Fluid to Fill the Fluid Compartments

Dehydration results from insufficient fluid intake, excessive fluid loss or both. Water loss may exceed intake in cases of vomiting, diarrhea, burns, excessive sweating and diabetes insipidus. When excessive fluid loss occurs, fluid recruited from the interstitial space enters the plasma. Fluids in the cells and within the interstitial and vascular compartments become more concentrated, particularly if there is a preferential loss of water, such as during inappropriate secretion of antidiuretic hormone in diabetes insipidus. When patients suffer from burns, vomiting, excessive sweating or diarrhea, they not only lose fluid but also suffer electrolyte disturbances.

Clinically, only dryness of the skin and mucous membranes is noted initially, but as dehydration progresses, skin turgor is lost. If dehydration persists, **oliguria** (reduced urine output) occurs as a compensation for the fluid loss. More severe fluid loss is accompanied by a shift of water from the intracellular space to the extracellular space, causing severe cell dysfunction, particularly in the brain. Shrinkage of brain tissue may result in the rupture of small vessels and subsequent bleeding. Systemic blood pressure falls with continuous dehydration, and declining perfusion eventually leads to death.

In Overhydration, Fluid Intake Exceeds Renal Excretory Capacity

Overhydration is rare, unless renal injury limits fluid excretion or kidneys cannot properly counterregulate

(e.g., via excessive secretion of antidiuretic hormone). Fluid overload today is mostly caused by administration of excessive amounts of intravenous fluids. The most serious effect of such fluid overload is induction of cerebral edema or congestive heart failure in patients with cardiac dysfunction.

PATHOPHYSIOLOGY:
Blood Pressure Control

Data from twin and family studies indicate that genetics accounts for some 30% of blood pressure (BP) regulation. This finding may also account for the tremendous variation in patient response to BP-lowering medication. Human genetic linkage and whole genome association studies have identified a host of mutations in key blood pressure regulatory processes. Prominent are genes of the renin–angiotensin system, which regulates vasoconstriction and sodium and water balance. SNPs in genes encoding angiotensin, angiotensin-converting enzyme, angiotensin II receptor, renin and renin-binding protein are associated with altered blood pressure control. Hypertension has been associated with SNPs in the vasoconstrictor endothelin and its receptor, the vasodilator nitric oxide synthase and endothelial sodium channel subunits. Polymorphisms of β-adrenergic receptors 1 and 2 have been associated with hypertension and altered response to β-agonists.

SHOCK

Shock is a condition of profound hemodynamic and metabolic disturbance characterized by failure of the circulatory system to maintain an appropriate blood supply to the microcirculation, with consequent inadequate perfusion of vital organs. In this often catastrophic circumstance, tissue perfusion and oxygen delivery fall below levels required to meet normal demands, including failure to remove metabolites adequately. The term **shock** encompasses all the reactions that occur in response to such disturbances. In the course of uncompensated shock, a rapid circulatory collapse leads to impaired cellular metabolism and death. However, in many cases, compensatory mechanisms sustain the patient, at least for a while. When these adaptations fail, shock becomes irreversible. Shock has been a major cause of morbidity and mortality in intensive care units, and despite endeavors to suppress portions of the immune response, the outcome of shock has been unchanged in the past 50 years.

Shock is not synonymous with low blood pressure, although hypotension is often part of shock syndrome. Hypotension is actually a late sign in shock and indicates failure of compensation. At the same time that peripheral blood flow falls below critical levels, extreme vasoconstriction can maintain arterial blood pressure. The distinction between shock and hypotension is important clinically because rapid restoration of systemic blood flow is the primary goal in treating shock. When blood pressure alone is raised with vasopressive drugs, systemic blood flow may actually be diminished.

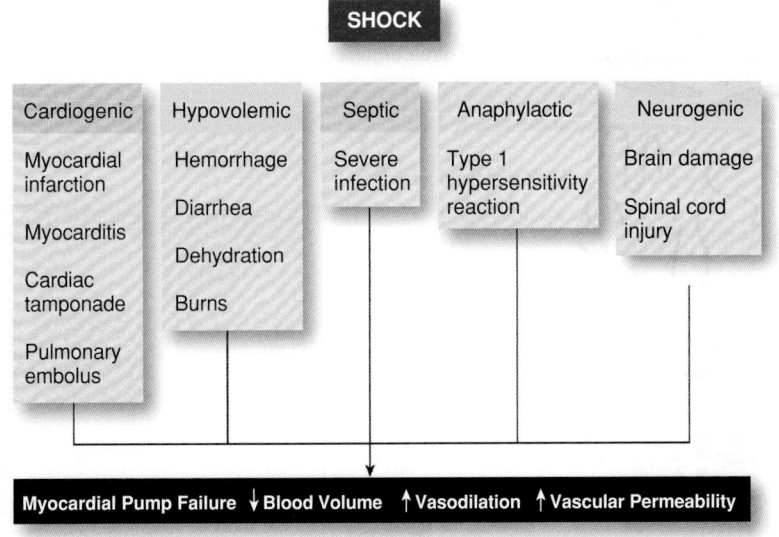

FIGURE 7-36. Classification of shock. Shock results from (1) an inability of the heart to pump adequately (cardiogenic shock), (2) decreased effective blood volume as a consequence of severely reduced blood or plasma volume (hypovolemic shock) or (3) widespread vasodilation (septic, anaphylactic or neurogenic shock). Increased vascular permeability may complicate vasodilation by contributing to reduced effective blood volume.

  **MOLECULAR PATHOGENESIS AND ETIOLOGIC FACTORS:** Decreased perfusion in shock most commonly results from decreased cardiac output, due either to the inability of the heart to pump normal venous return or to decreased effective blood volume that results in decreased venous return. These two mechanisms underlie two of the major types of shock: **cardiogenic** and **hypovolemic** shock. Systemic vasodilation, with or without increased vascular permeability, is responsible for the other broad category of shock, referred to as a **distributive** shock. This condition has several key subcategories: septic, anaphylactic and neurogenic shock (Fig. 7-36).

- **Cardiogenic shock** is caused by myocardial pump failure. It usually arises after massive myocardial infarction, but myocarditis may also be responsible. Disorders that prevent left or right heart filling reduce cardiac output, resulting in "obstructive" shock. Such conditions include pulmonary embolism, cardiac tamponade (Fig. 7-35) and (rarely) atrial myxoma.
- **Hypovolemic shock** occurs owing to pronounced decreases in blood or plasma volume, caused by loss of fluid from the vascular compartment. Hemorrhage, fluid loss from severe burns, diarrhea, excessive urine formation, perspiration and trauma all lead to fluid loss that can trigger hypovolemic shock. Burns or trauma directly damages the microcirculation, increasing vascular permeability.
- **Septic shock** is caused by severe systemic microbial infections. The pathogenesis of septic shock is complex and is discussed in detail below.
- **Anaphylactic shock** is a consequence of a systemic type I hypersensitivity reaction, which generates widespread vasodilation and increased vascular permeability.
- **Neurogenic shock** can follow acute injury to the brain or spinal cord, which impairs neural control of vasomotor tone and causes generalized vasodilation. In the case of both anaphylactic and neurogenic shock, the subsequent redistribution of blood to the periphery, with or without increased vascular permeability, reduces the effective circulating blood and plasma volume. This ultimately leads to the same consequences as in hypovolemic shock.

In hypovolemic and cardiogenic shock, lower cardiac output and resultant decreased tissue perfusion are the key steps in the progression from reversible to irreversible shock. Cellular hypoxia is the common consequence of the initial decrease in tissue perfusion. Although such changes do not initially result in irreversible injury, a vicious circle of decreasing tissue perfusion and further cell injury is perpetuated by several mechanisms:

- Injury to endothelial cells, secondary to hypoxia caused by decreased tissue perfusion and increased vascular permeability, provokes escape of fluid from the vascular compartment.
- Increased exudation of fluid from the circulation reduces (1) blood volume, (2) venous return and (3) cardiac output, thus aggravating hypoxic cell injury.
- Decreased perfusion of kidneys and skeletal muscles results in metabolic acidosis, which in turn further decreases cardiac output and tissue perfusion.
- Decreased perfusion of the heart injures myocardial cells and decreases their ability to pump blood, further reducing cardiac output and tissue perfusion.

Systemic Inflammatory Response Syndrome Characterizes Septic Shock

Systemic inflammatory response syndrome (SIRS) is an exaggerated and generalized manifestation of a local immune or inflammatory reaction, and is often fatal. SIRS is a hypermetabolic state characterized by two or more signs of systemic inflammation. These include fever, tachycardia, tachypnea, leukocytosis or leukopenia, in the setting of a known cause of inflammation. **Septic shock** is defined as clinical SIRS so severe that it causes organ dysfunction and hypotension. Mechanisms leading to septic shock are illustrated in Fig. 7-37. These processes often progress to **multiple organ dysfunction syndrome** (MODS; see Chapter 12), a term used to describe otherwise unexplained abnormalities of organ function in critically ill patients (see below).

The massive inflammatory reaction defined by SIRS results from systemic release of cytokines, the most important being tumor necrosis factor-α (TNF-α), interleukin-1 (IL-1), IL-6 and platelet-activating factor (PAF). Over 30

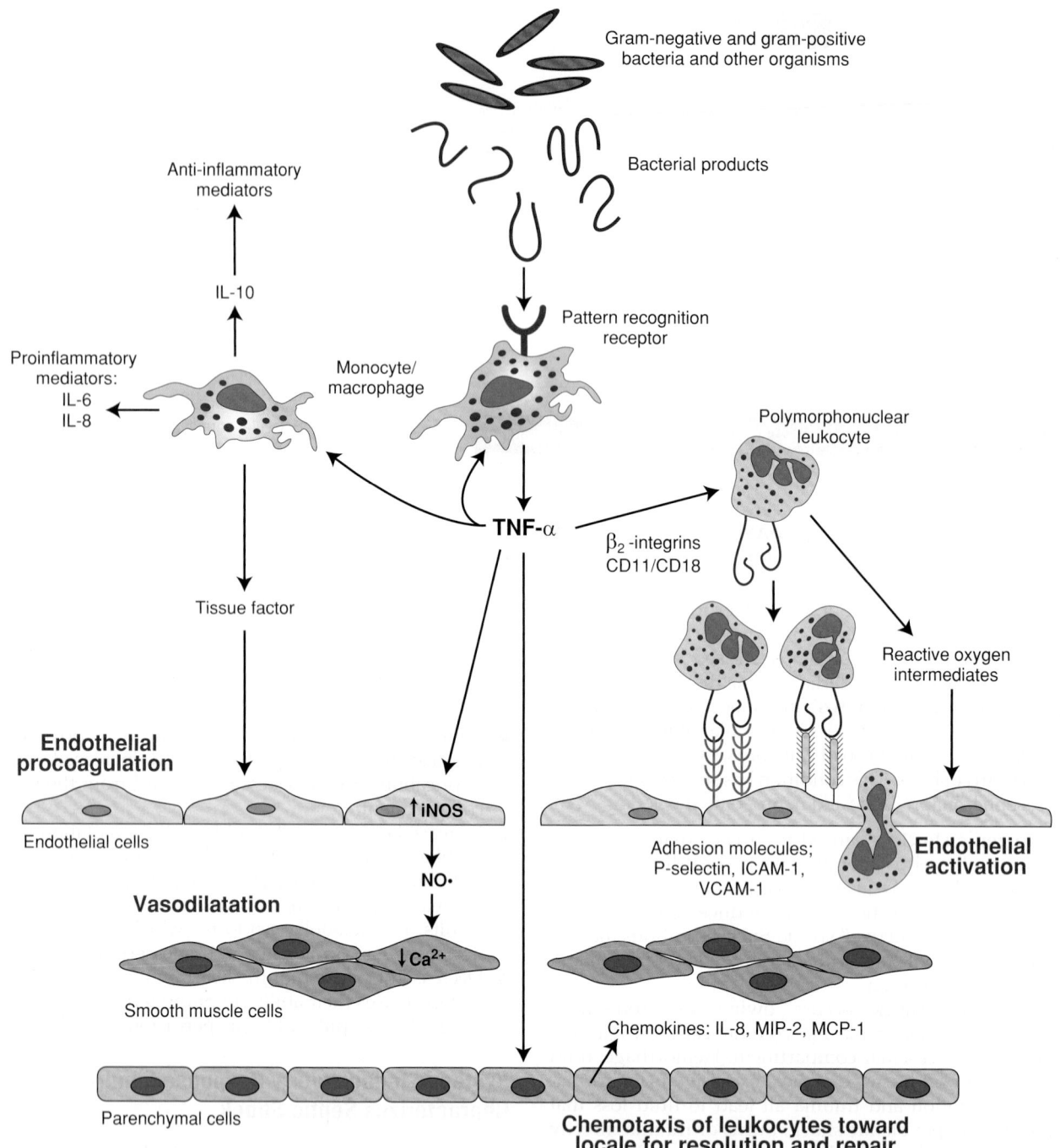

FIGURE 7-37. Pathogenesis of endotoxic shock. Sepsis is caused primarily by gram-negative bacteria and bacterial products such as endotoxin (lipopolysaccharide [LPS]), which is released into the circulation, where it binds to a pattern recognition receptor on the surface of monocyte/macrophages. Such binding stimulates the secretion of substantial quantities of tumor necrosis factor-α (TNF-α). TNF-α mediates septic shock by a number of mechanisms: (1) stimulation of the release of various pro- and anti-inflammatory mediators; (2) induction of endothelial procoagulation by tissue factor, thus leading to thrombosis and local ischemia; (3) direct cytotoxic damage to endothelial cells; (4) endothelial activation, which enhances the adherence of polymorphonuclear leukocytes; (5) stimulation of endothelial cell nitric oxide production and vasodilation; and (6) release of chemokines to attract leukocytes for resolution and repair of tissue injury. Ca^{2+} = calcium ion; *ICAM* = intercellular adhesion molecule; *IL* = interleukin; *iNOS* = inducible nitric oxide synthase; *MCP-1* = monocyte chemotactic protein-1; *MIP-2* = macrophage-inflammatory protein-2; *NO•* = nitric oxide; *VCAM-1* = vascular cell adhesion molecule-1.

endogenous mediators of SIRS have been identified. Their interactions may be important in the pathogenesis of SIRS.

Septicemia with gram-negative organisms is the most common cause of septic shock, followed by gram-positive and fungal infections. The most common primary sources of infection are pulmonary, abdominal and urinary. The invading bacteria release **endotoxin,** a lipopolysaccharide (LPS) whose toxic activity resides in the lipid A component. On entry into the circulation, LPS, via lipid A, binds to LPS-binding protein, after which the complex binds to the CD14 receptor on the surface of monocyte/macrophages. Toll-like receptors (TLRs) are transmembrane pattern recognition receptors (PRRs), which also collectively recognize bacteria, fungi and protozoa on antigen-presenting cells. TLRs trigger (1) downstream myeloid differentiation protein 88 (MyD88), (2) toll-interleukin-1 (TIR) domain-containing adaptor protein, (3) TIR receptor domain-containing adaptor protein-inducing interferon-β (TRIF) and (4) TRIF-related adaptor molecule. They mediate signaling through activation of the transcription factor, nuclear factor-κB (NF-κB), and upregulate TNF expression. LPS binding to TLR-4 causes mononuclear phagocytes to secrete large quantities of cytokines, such as TNF, IL-1, IL-6, IL-8, IL-12, macrophage inhibitory factor and others, all of which mediate a variety of responses. Cytosolic PRRs include the Nod-like receptors, the most extensively studied of which is the NLRP3 inflammasome complex. This structure is a multiprotein caspase-activating complex that triggers downstream IL-1β and IL-19 activation. Importantly, antigen-presenting cells expose CD4 T lymphocytes to microbial antigens to stimulate the adaptive arm of the immune response.

Cytokine activation and subsequent production of nitric oxide (NO) and procoagulant proteins ultimately cause the overwhelming cardiovascular collapse characteristic of septic shock. In this context, activation of inducible NO synthase (iNOS) by TNF upregulates NO synthesis from L-arginine, an effect that is primarily responsible for the drop in blood pressure during sepsis. TNF is also involved in the pathogenesis of shock unassociated with endotoxemia (e.g., cardiogenic shock). LPS is the most potent stimulus for TNF release, but other antigens also promote its secretion. These include toxin-1 of the toxic shock syndrome; enterotoxin; antigens of mycobacteria, fungi, parasites and viruses; and products of complement activation.

Although TNF exerts beneficial effects by enhancing tissue remodeling, wound healing and defense against local infections, when macrophages are exposed to LPS in septic shock, TNF is suddenly released in great excess, often with lethal consequences. Administering anti-TNF antibody before exposing an animal to endotoxin or to gram-negative bacteria completely protects from septic shock. Unfortunately, comparable studies in humans have not been successful.

TNF released by monocyte/macrophages exerts a direct toxic effect on endothelial cells by compromising membrane permeability and inducing endothelial cell apoptosis. It also acts indirectly by (1) initiating a cascade of other mediators that amplify its deleterious effects, (2) promoting the adhesion of polymorphonuclear leukocytes to endothelial surfaces and (3) activating the extrinsic coagulation pathway. The presence of TNF stimulates the release of IL-1 and IL-6, PAF and other eicosanoids that mediate tissue injury. Interestingly, nonlethal doses of TNF become fatal when administered together with IL-1. TNF also increases expression of adhesion molecules, such as intercellular adhesion molecules (ICAMs), vascular cell adhesion molecules (VCAMs), P-selectin and endothelial–leukocyte adhesion molecules (ELAMs) on endothelial surfaces, thus promoting leukocyte adhesion and leukostasis. This mechanism presumably plays a role in the respiratory distress syndrome, in which activated neutrophils are sequestered in the pulmonary circulation and damage the alveoli. Other vasoactive peptides include the vasodilatory prostacyclins and endothelin (ET)-1, a potent vasoconstrictor (Fig. 7-37). Note that the term "septic syndrome" refers to the physiologic and metabolic response characteristic of sepsis in the absence of an infection.

Multiple Organ Dysfunction Syndrome Is the End-Result of Shock

Improvements in the early treatment of shock and sepsis have allowed patients to survive long enough to manifest a new problem, progressive deterioration of organ function. Almost all septic shock patients suffer from dysfunction of at least one organ. However, multiple organ dysfunction occurs in one third of patients with septic shock, trauma or burns, and a quarter of those with acute pancreatitis. Whatever the cause, the clinical deterioration of MODS is held to result from common mechanisms of tissue injury subsumed under the rubric of SIRS. Mortality of SIRS/MODS exceeds 50%, making it responsible for most deaths in noncoronary intensive care units in the United States. In most circumstances, the inflammatory reaction and the progression from sepsis to organ dysfunction reflects a balance between proinflammatory and anti-inflammatory factors. As mentioned above, TNF-α, IL-1 and NO have systemic effects.

Also, reactive oxygen species (ROS) are important triggers of end-organ dysfunction. The acute response to sepsis is characterized by release of adrenocorticotropic hormone (ACTH), cortisol, adrenaline and noradrenaline, vasopressin, glucagon and growth hormone. The net result is shutdown of noncritical systems and an overall catabolic state. Although proinflammatory mediators predominate in SIRS, counterinflammatory factors play an important role in some patients. It is now thought that following bacterial infection, there is an initial response of excessive inflammation and septic shock characteristic of SIRS. Such uncontrolled cytokine induction is preceded by a stage of anergy and immune repression.

Vascular Compensatory Mechanisms

Changes in the macrovascular and microvascular circulation are at least partly responsible for variable organ injury in SIRS. Compensatory mechanisms in shock shift blood flow away from the periphery, so as to maintain flow to the heart and the brain. These responses involve the sympathetic nervous system, release of endogenous vasoconstrictors and hormonal substances, and local vasoregulation. The result is increased cardiac output achieved by increasing heart rate and myocardial contractility while constricting arteries and arterioles.

- **Increased sympathetic discharge** augments catecholamine release by the adrenal medulla. Skeletal muscle, splanchnic bed and skin arterioles respond to increased sympathetic discharge; cardiac and cerebral arterioles are less reactive. Thus, increased sympathetic tone works to shift blood flow from the periphery to the heart and brain. The marked arteriolar vasoconstriction reduces capillary hydrostatic pressure and decreases fluid shifted into the interstitium. This facilitates an osmotic fluid shift from the interstitium to the vascular system. This sympathetic–adrenal response can completely compensate for blood loss of 10% of intravascular volume. With a greater volume deficit, cardiac output and blood pressure are affected and blood flow to tissues is reduced.

- **The renin–angiotensin–aldosterone system** also helps compensate by stimulating sodium and water reabsorption, thus helping to maintain intravascular volume. A similar water-preserving action is provided by pituitary antidiuretic hormone.

■ **Vascular autoregulation** preserves regional blood flow to vital organs, particularly the heart and brain, by vasodilation in the coronary and cerebral circulations in response to hypoxia and acidosis. Vasoconstriction mediated largely by α-adrenergic receptors in mesenteric venules and veins helps maintain cardiac filling and arterial pressure. Circulation to organs such as skin and skeletal muscles, which are less sensitive to hypoxia, does not display such tightly controlled autoregulation.

MOLECULAR PATHOGENESIS:
Genetic Polymorphisms in Toll-Like Receptors and Tumor Necrosis Factor Participate in the Pathogenesis of Sepsis

Epidemiologic studies have shown that death from infection has a higher genetic background than that of cardiovascular disease or cancer. Gene mutations in several cytokines, cell surface receptors and other circulating markers have been associated with susceptibility to sepsis. TLR pattern recognition receptors recognize pathogen-associated microbial patterns and thus are critical in triggering innate immune responses. Toll-like receptor-4 (TLR4) is critical in recognizing LPS of gram-negative bacteria. A mutation of TRL4 (aspartic acid to glycine at amino acid 299) has been associated with patients with septic shock in a number of studies. As mentioned earlier, TLR4 is important in the exacerbation of the endotoxin response, and in sepsis, polymorphisms in TLRs and other PRRs may help explain why patients respond so differently to a given infective agent.

Similarly, recently discovered mutations in the TNF-α gene have improved our understanding of the role of TNF-α in sepsis. A mutation in the TNF-α promoter, TNF2, has been associated with increased susceptibility to sepsis and shock.

Other gene mutations associated with worse prognosis in sepsis are found in IL-1 receptor agonist, CD14 and plasminogen activator inhibitor-1 (PAI-1). Finally, gene profiling studies have found unique molecular signatures in circulating neutrophils and mononuclear cells from patients with sepsis.

PATHOLOGY: Shock is associated with specific changes in a number of organs (Fig. 7-38), including acute renal tubular necrosis, acute respiratory distress syndrome, liver failure, depression of host defense mechanisms and heart failure. Interestingly, paracrine cross-talk from molecules in one injured organ, such as proinflammatory mediators from the lung, can effect distant organ injury.

Heart

Systolic and diastolic dysfunction occurs during sepsis, likely secondary to paracrine injury and possibly hypoperfusion. In sepsis, the heart shows petechial hemorrhages of the epicardium and endocardium. Microscopically, necrotic foci in the myocardium range from loss of single fibers to large areas of necrosis. Prominent contraction bands are visible by light microscopy but are better seen by electron microscopy. Ultrastructurally, flattened areas of the intercalated disk are a sign of cell swelling, and invagination of adjacent cells is considered to be a catecholamine-induced lesion.

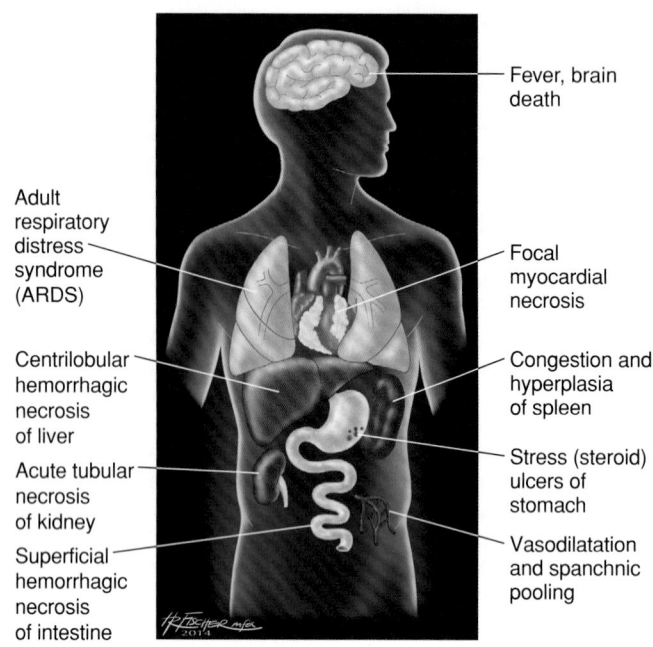

FIGURE 7-38. Complications of shock.

Kidney

Acute tubular necrosis (ATN, acute renal failure), a major complication of shock, has been divided into three phases: (1) **initiation,** from the onset of injury to the beginning of renal failure; (2) **maintenance,** from the onset of renal failure to a stable, reduced renal function; and (3) **recovery**. In those who survive an episode of shock, the recovery phase begins about 10 days after its onset and may last up to 8 weeks.

Renal blood flow is restricted to 1/3 of normal after the acute ischemic phase. This effect is even more severe in the outer cortex. Constriction of arterioles reduces the filtration pressure, thus reducing the amount of filtrate and contributing to oliguria. Interstitial edema occurs, possibly through a process called **backflow**. Excessive vasoconstriction is also related to stimulation of the renin–angiotensin system.

During acute renal failure, the kidney is large, swollen and congested, although the cortex may be pale. A cross-section reveals blood pooling in the outer stripe of the medulla. Microscopically, fully developed acute tubular necrosis is evidenced by dilation of the proximal tubules and focal necrosis of cells (Fig. 7-39). Often, pigmented casts in tubular lumina indicate leakage of hemoglobin or myoglobin. Coarse "ropy" casts are seen in the distal nephron and distal convoluted tubules. Interstitial edema is prominent in the cortex, and mononuclear cells accumulate within tubules and surrounding interstitium. ATN is discussed in more detail in Chapter 22.

Lung

After the onset of severe and prolonged shock, injury to alveolar walls can lead to **shock lung,** which is a cause of **acute respiratory distress syndrome** (ARDS) (see Chapter 18). The sequence of changes is mediated by polymorphonuclear leukocytes and includes interstitial edema, necrosis of endothelial and alveolar epithelial cells and formation of

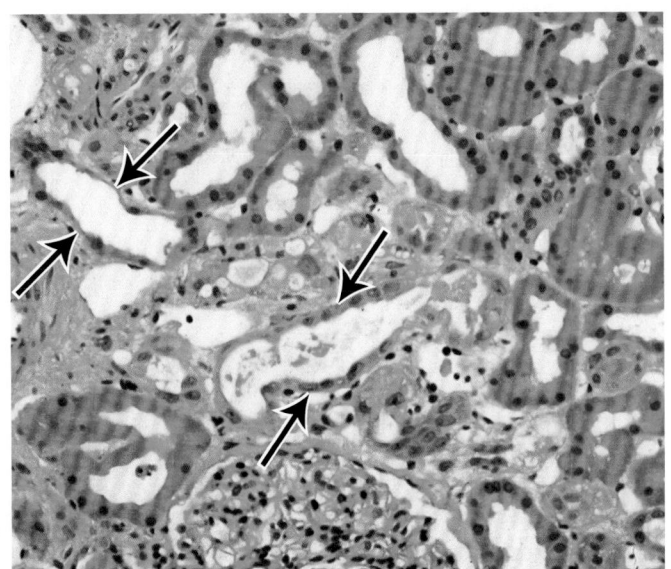

FIGURE 7-39. Acute tubular necrosis. A section of kidney shows swelling and degeneration of tubular epithelium. *Arrows* indicate the thinned and damaged epithelium.

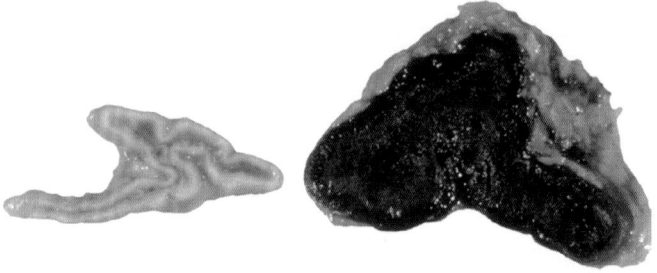

FIGURE 7-40. Waterhouse-Friderichsen syndrome. A normal adrenal gland (*left*) in contrast to an adrenal gland enlarged by extensive hemorrhage (*right*), obtained from a patient who died of meningococcemic shock.

intravascular microthrombi and hyaline membranes lining the alveolar surface.

Macroscopically, the lung is firm and congested and a frothy fluid often exudes from the cut surface. Interstitial edema is first seen around peribronchial connective tissue and lymphatics, subsequently filling the interstitial connective tissue. In this initial period, a large fluid volume drains into the pulmonary lymphatics. If removal of this fluid becomes inadequate, or if the balance of forces that keep the fluid in the interstitial space is disturbed, alveolar edema develops.

Shock-induced lung injury leads to alveolar hyaline membranes (Fig. 7-34), which also frequently line alveolar ducts and terminal bronchioles. These changes may heal entirely, but in half of patients, repair processes cause thickening of the alveolar wall. Type II pneumocytes proliferate to replace damaged type I pneumocytes and line the alveoli. Fibrous tissue proliferation gives rise to organization of the alveolar exudate. These chronic changes may result in persistent respiratory distress and even death. Shock lung and ARDS are more fully discussed in Chapter 18.

Gastrointestinal Tract

Shock often results in diffuse gastrointestinal hemorrhage. Erosions of the gastric mucosa and superficial ischemic necrosis in the intestines are the usual sources of this bleeding. Interruption of the barrier function of the intestine may result in septicemia. More-severe necrotizing lesions contribute to deterioration in the final phase of shock.

Liver

In patients who die in shock, the liver is enlarged and has a mottled cut surface that reflects marked centrilobular pooling of blood. The most prominent histologic lesion is centrilobular congestion and necrosis. The basis for the apparent increased sensitivity of centrilobular hepatocytes to shock may not simply represent their greater distance from the source of blood via the portal tracts, a matter that is not settled (see Chapter 20).

Pancreas

The splanchnic vascular bed, which supplies the pancreas, is particularly affected by impaired circulation during shock. Resulting ischemic damage to the exocrine pancreas unleashes activated catalytic enzymes and causes acute pancreatitis, a complication that further promotes shock.

Brain

Although septic patients often develop clinical encephalopathy, brain lesions are rare in SIRS and shock. Microscopic hemorrhages may be seen, but patients who recover do not ordinarily have neurologic deficits. In severe cases, particularly in people with cerebral atherosclerosis, hemorrhage and necrosis may appear in the overlapping region between the terminal distributions of major arteries, so-called **watershed infarcts** (see Chapter 32).

Adrenals

In severe shock, adrenal glands exhibit conspicuous hemorrhage in the inner cortex. Although the hemorrhage is often focal, it can be massive and accompanied by hemorrhagic necrosis of the entire gland, as seen in the **Waterhouse-Friderichsen syndrome** (Fig. 7-40), typically associated with overwhelming meningococcal septicemia.

Host Defenses

The changes in immune function and host defenses in shock are not well understood, although it is common for patients who survive the acute phase of shock to succumb to subsequent overwhelming infection. It may well be that several factors interact, namely, ischemic colitis, tissue trauma and immune and metabolic suppression of host defenses. Humoral immunity and phagocytic activity by leukocytes and macrophages are both depressed, but the mechanisms underlying these effects are not clear.

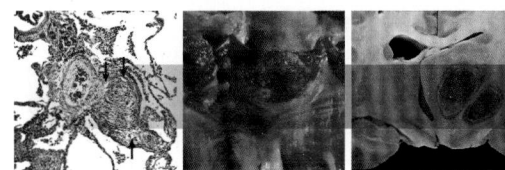

8

Environmental and Nutritional Pathology

David S. Strayer ■ Emanuel Rubin

Smoking
Cardiovascular Disease
Cancer
Nonneoplastic Diseases
Female Reproductive Function
Fetal Tobacco Syndrome
Environmental Tobacco Smoke

Alcoholism
Effects of Alcohol on Organs and Tissues
Fetal Alcohol Syndrome
Alcohol and Cancer
Mechanisms of Alcohol-Related Injury

Drug Abuse
Illicit Drugs
Intravenous Drug Abuse
Drug Addiction during Pregnancy

Iatrogenic Drug Injury

Sex Hormones
Oral Contraceptives
Postmenopausal Hormone Replacement
   Therapy

Environmental Chemicals
Toxicity versus Hypersensitivity
Occupational Exposure
Air Pollution
Biological Toxins

Thermal Regulatory Dysfunction
Hypothermia
Hyperthermia

Altitude-Related Illnesses

Physical Injuries
Contusions
Abrasions
Lacerations
Wounds

Ultraviolet Light

Radiation
Whole-Body Irradiation
Localized Radiation
Radiation and Cancer
Microwave Radiation, Electromagnetic
   Fields and Ultrasound

Nutritional Disorders
Protein-Calorie Malnutrition
Vitamin Deficiencies
Deficiencies of Essential Trace Minerals

Environmental pathology is the study of diseases caused by exposure to harmful external agents and deficiencies of vital substances. With heightened awareness of the fact that chemical agents may mediate tissue changes and recognition that many of these are environmental contaminants, "occupational pathology" has developed. In this chapter we concentrate on diseases caused by (1) exposure to toxic agents, (2) physical damage and (3) nutritional deficiencies.

SMOKING

Smoking tobacco is the single largest preventable cause of death in the United States. *About 480,000 deaths per year—or 1/5 of the total deaths in the United States—occur prematurely because of smoking.* The Surgeon General in 2014[1] incriminates tobacco in 48% of deaths from cancer, 19% of deaths from cardiovascular and metabolic diseases, 61% of deaths from nonmalignant lung diseases and 8% of perinatal deaths. Life expectancy is shortened and overall mortality is proportional to the amount and duration of cigarette smoking, commonly quantitated as "pack-years" (Fig. 8-1).

[1]The Health Consequences of Smoking—50 Years of Progress: A Report of the Surgeon General. 2014. U.S. Department of Health and Human Services, Rockville, MD.

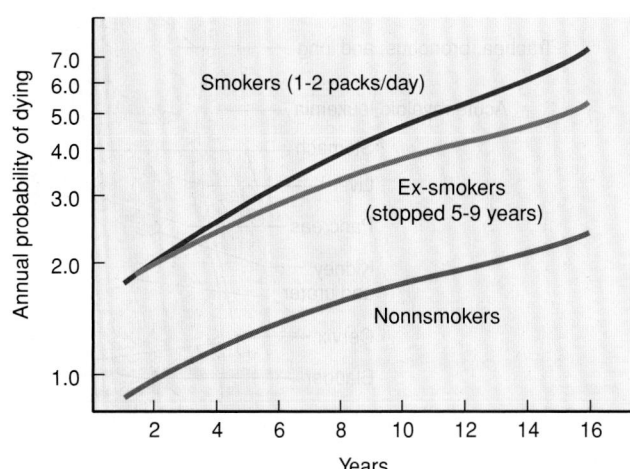

FIGURE 8-1. The risk of dying in smokers and nonsmokers. Note that the annual probability of an individual dying, indicated on the ordinate, is a logarithmic scale. Individuals who have smoked for 1 year have a twofold greater probability of dying than a nonsmoker, while those who have smoked for more than 15 years have more than a threefold greater probability of dying.

For example, a person who smokes two packs of cigarettes a day at the age of 30 years will live an average of 8 years less than a nonsmoker.

As women have taken to smoking as much as men, the previous male preponderance of smoking-related illness has equalized between the sexes. Thus, the development of smoking-related illnesses reflects the amount smoked, not the gender of the smoker. In fact, mortality from lung cancer, almost all of which is related to cigarette smoking, exceeds that from cancers of the breast and prostate, which are the most common cancers of women and men, respectively, in the United States. The excess mortality associated with cigarette smoking declines after one quits smoking: by 15 years of abstinence from cigarettes, mortality in ex-smokers from all causes approaches that of people who have never smoked. Cancer mortality among those who smoke only cigars or pipes is somewhat greater than that of the nonsmoking population. Use of smokeless tobacco (snuff, chewing tobacco) entails little, if any, increased risk of malignancy.

The major diseases responsible for excess mortality reported in cigarette smokers are, in order of frequency, many types of cancers, cardiovascular and metabolic diseases and chronic pulmonary diseases. Cancers of the oral cavity, larynx, esophagus, pancreas, bladder, kidney, colon, liver and cervix are all more common in smokers than in nonsmokers. Also, smokers show excess mortality from tuberculosis, atherosclerotic aortic aneurysms and peptic ulcers. The effects of cigarette smoking on the various organs of smokers are illustrated in Fig. 8-2.

Cardiovascular Disease Is a Major Complication of Smoking

Cigarette smoking is a major independent risk factor for myocardial infarction. It acts synergistically with other risk factors, such as elevated blood pressure and blood cholesterol levels (Fig. 8-3). Smoking precipitates initial myocardial infarction, increases the risk for second heart attacks and diminishes survival after a heart attack among those who continue to smoke. Smoking also increases the incidence of sudden cardiac death: it contributes to development of atherosclerotic plaques and may lead to ischemia and arrhythmias.

Cigarette smoking is an independent risk factor for **ischemic stroke**. The risk correlates with the number of cigarettes smoked and is reduced after cessation of smoking. Tobacco use also increases risk of certain forms of **intracranial hemorrhage**. The combination of smoking and oral contraceptive use in women older than 35 years of age increases the likelihood of **myocardial infarction**. Similarly, use of cigarettes by women who are using oral contraceptives significantly increases their risk of stroke.

Atherosclerosis of the coronary arteries and aorta is more severe and extensive among cigarette smokers than among nonsmokers, and the effect is dose related. As a consequence, cigarette smoking is a strong risk factor for **atherosclerotic aortic aneurysms**. The incidence and severity of **atherosclerotic peripheral vascular disease** are also remarkably increased by smoking. Smoking is also a major risk factor

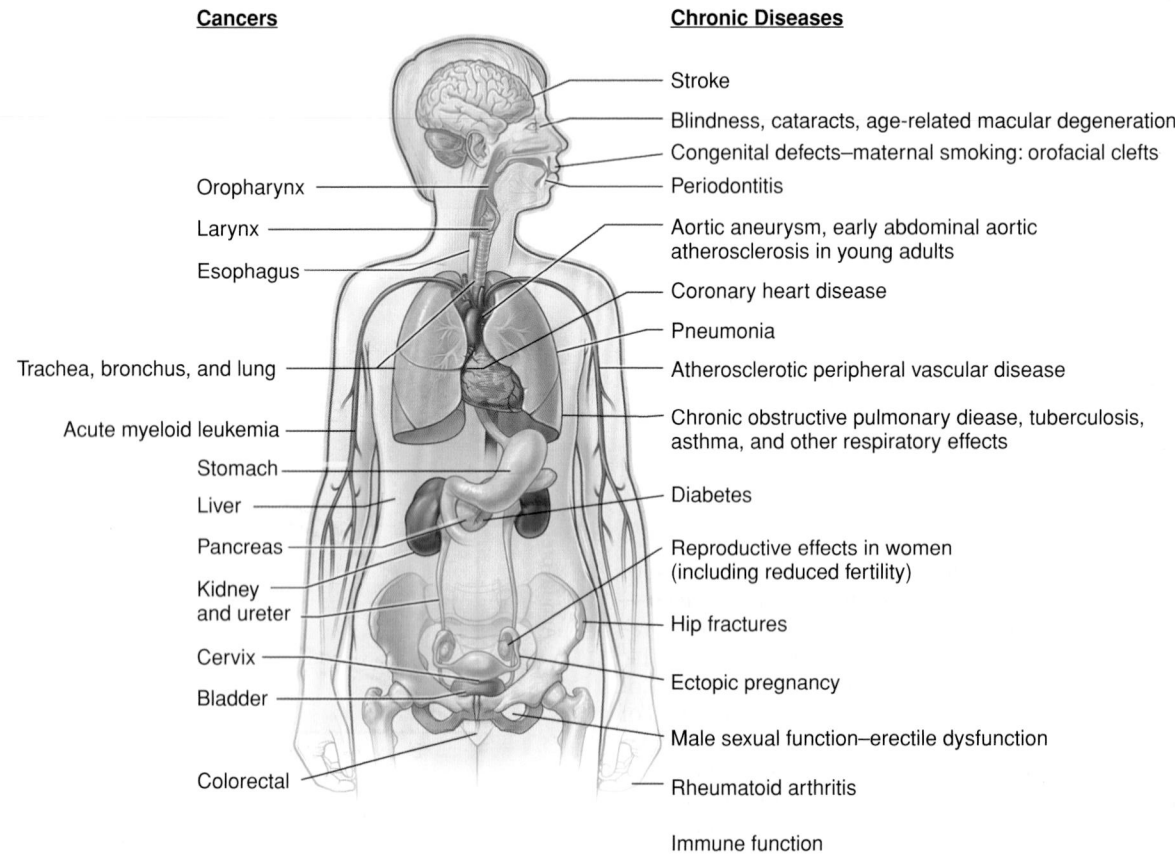

Cancers

- Oropharynx
- Larynx
- Esophagus
- Trachea, bronchus, and lung
- Acute myeloid leukemia
- Stomach
- Liver
- Pancreas
- Kidney and ureter
- Cervix
- Bladder
- Colorectal

Chronic Diseases

- Stroke
- Blindness, cataracts, age-related macular degeneration
- Congenital defects–maternal smoking: orofacial clefts
- Periodontitis
- Aortic aneurysm, early abdominal aortic atherosclerosis in young adults
- Coronary heart disease
- Pneumonia
- Atherosclerotic peripheral vascular disease
- Chronic obstructive pulmonary diease, tuberculosis, asthma, and other respiratory effects
- Diabetes
- Reproductive effects in women (including reduced fertility)
- Hip fractures
- Ectopic pregnancy
- Male sexual function–erectile dysfunction
- Rheumatoid arthritis

Immune function

Overall diminished health

FIGURE 8-2. Organs affected by active cigarette smoking.

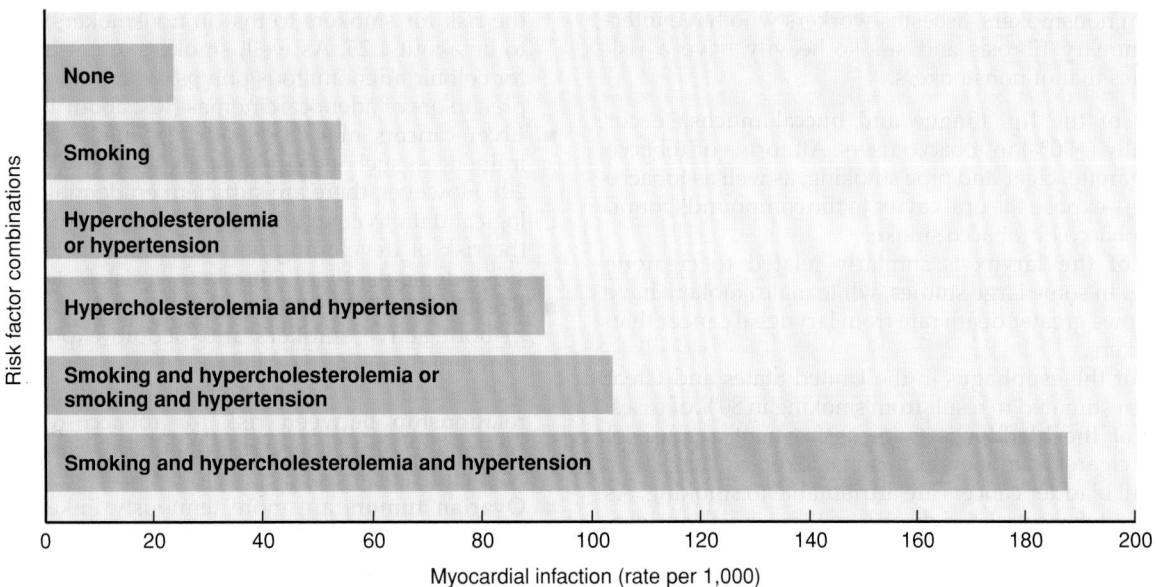

FIGURE 8-3. The risk of myocardial infarction in cigarette smokers. Smoking is an independent risk factor and increases the risk of a myocardial infarction to about the same extent as does hypertension or hypercholesterolemia alone. The effects of smoking are additive to those of these other two risk factors.

for **coronary vasospasm**. It disturbs regional coronary blood flow in patients with coronary artery disease and lowers the threshold for ventricular fibrillation and cardiac arrest in patients with established ischemic heart disease. The pharmacologic actions of nicotine itself, carbon monoxide (CO) inhalation, reduced plasma high-density lipoprotein levels, increased plasma fibrinogen levels and higher leukocyte counts are all consequences of smoking that may predispose to myocardial infarction.

Buerger disease, a peculiar inflammatory and occlusive disease of the lower leg vasculature, occurs almost only in heavy smokers (see Chapter 16).

Lung Cancer Is Largely a Disease of Cigarette Smokers

More than 85% of deaths from lung cancer, the single most common cancer death in both men and women in the United States today, are DUE to cigarette smoking (Fig. 8-4). Although the precise offenders in cigarette smoke have not been identified, clearly cigarette smoke is toxic and carcinogenic to the bronchial mucosa. Passing cigarette smoke through a filter separates it into gas and particulate phases. Cigarette tar, the material deposited on the filter, contains over 3000 compounds, many of which have been identified as carcinogens, mucosal toxins and ciliotoxic agents. Compounds with similar harmful properties are found in the gas phase, but they are fewer. Among smokers, the risk of lung cancer is directly related to the number of cigarettes smoked.

The pathology of lung cancers has changed over the years. Previously, squamous carcinoma was the predominant lung cancer in smokers. This has declined as smoking has become less prevalent. In recent years, adenocarcinoma has become more common. The Surgeon General's report on smoking (2014, see above) links this to changes in the composition and configuration of cigarettes.

Cigarette smoking is also an important factor in the induction of **lung cancer** that is associated with certain occupational exposures. For instance, uranium miners have an increased rate of lung cancer, presumably because of inhalation of radon daughters. The rate of lung cancer among miners who smoke is considerably higher than for nonminers with similar smoking habits. Another example is the case of asbestos workers. While heavy smokers in the general population have a risk of lung cancer some 20 times

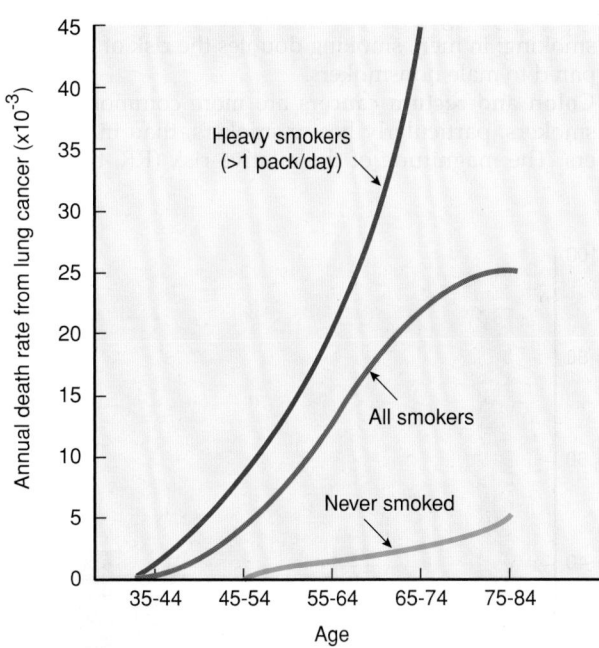

FIGURE 8-4. Death rate from lung cancer among smokers and nonsmokers. Nonsmokers exhibit a small, linear rise in the death rate from lung cancer from the age of 50 onward. By contrast, those who smoke more than one pack per day show an exponential rise in the annual death rate from lung cancer starting at about age 35. By age 70, heavy smokers have about a 20-fold greater death rate from lung cancer than nonsmokers.

greater than nonsmokers, asbestos workers who have interstitial pulmonary fibrosis and smoke heavily have a risk over 60 times that of nonsmokers.

- **Cancers of the lip, tongue and buccal mucosa** occur principally (>90%) in tobacco users. All forms of tobacco use—cigarette, cigar and pipe smoking, as well as tobacco chewing—expose the oral cavity to the compounds found in raw tobacco or tobacco smoke.
- **Cancer of the larynx** is similarly related to cigarette smoking. In some large studies, white male smokers have a 6–13 times greater death rate from laryngeal cancer than nonsmokers.
- **Cancer of the esophagus** in the United States and Great Britain is estimated to result from smoking in 80% of cases.
- **Cancer of the bladder** is twice as frequent a cause of death in cigarette smokers as in nonsmokers. In fact, 30%–40% of all bladder cancers are attributable to smoking. As with most tobacco-related disorders, there is a clear dose-response relationship between incidence of bladder cancer, numbers of cigarettes smoked per day and duration of cigarette smoking.
- **Carcinoma of the kidney** is increased 50%–100% among smokers. A modest increase in cancer of the renal pelvis has also been documented.
- **Cancer of the pancreas** has shown a steady increase in incidence, which is, at least in part, related to cigarette smoking. The risk ratio in male smokers for adenocarcinoma of the pancreas is 2–3, and a dose-response relationship exists. Men who smoke over two packs a day have a five times greater risk of developing pancreatic cancer than nonsmokers.
- **Cancer of the uterine cervix** is significantly increased in women smokers. It has been estimated that about 30% of cervical cancer mortality is associated with this habit.
- **Acute myelogenous leukemia (AML)** is associated with smoking: in men, smoking doubles the risk of AML compared to male nonsmokers.
- **Colon and rectum cancers** are more common in active smokers, particularly heavy smokers, than in nonsmokers. The magnitude of the relative risk (RR, the ratio of

the risk for smokers to that in nonsmokers) is estimated to be about 1.25. As well, smokers are at increased risk for colonic adenomatous polyps, which are premalignant precursors of adenocarcinomas (RR, about 1.5).

- **Liver cancers** may be caused by many environmental influences, such as hepatitis viruses (see Chapters 9 and 20). However, there are sufficient epidemiologic and biological data to conclude that cigarette smoking increases the risk of developing hepatic malignancies (RR, about 1.6) independently of other known risk factors.
- **Breast cancer** has been linked to cigarette smoking in both active smokers and people exposed to environmental smoke (see below). This association is best documented for premenopausal women. There is a relationship between risk for tobacco-related breast cancer and rapid acetylator phenotypes for the enzyme N-acetyltransferase-2.
- **Ovarian tumors** are more tenuously linked to tobacco smoking. A slightly increased incidence of borderline mucinous tumors of the ovary with cigarette smoking is reported. No such relationship is reported for other types of ovarian tumors.

Smokers Are at Higher Risk for Certain Nonneoplastic Diseases

- **Chronic bronchitis and emphysema** occur primarily in cigarette smokers. The incidence of these diseases is a function of the number of cigarettes smoked (Fig. 8-5; see Chapter 18).
- **Peptic ulcers** are 70% more common in male cigarette smokers than in nonsmokers.
- **Diabetes mellitus,** type II, occurs 30%–40% more often in smokers. Several different mechanisms may contribute to this effect, including nicotine-related insulin resistance and beta cell apoptosis, increased central adiposity and altered metabolism of estrogens and androgens in smokers.
- **The course of tuberculosis** is more severe in smokers, who are at increased risk for its recrudescence and for tuberculosis-related death.

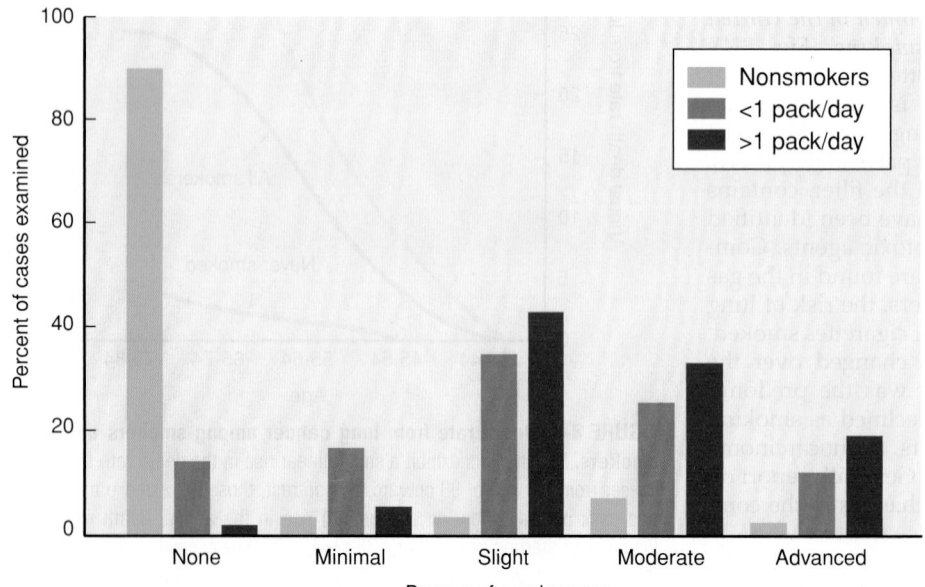

FIGURE 8-5. The association between cigarette smoking and pulmonary emphysema. Some 90% of nonsmokers have no detectable emphysema at autopsy. In contrast, virtually all those who smoke more than one pack per day have morphologic evidence of emphysema at autopsy. Emphysema shows a slight dose dependence on the number of cigarettes smoked. Those who smoke less than one pack per day tend to have less severe emphysema, but 85%–90% of such smokers have some emphysema at autopsy.

- **Asthma** incidence and exacerbations are increased in smokers, compared to nonsmokers.
- **Impaired immune function,** affecting both innate and adaptive arms of the immune system, characterizes smokers. These effects are complex and difficult to summarize briefly. They are mediated via cigarette smoke's pro-oxidant effects, as well as by specific responses induced by individual smoke components. However, although it acts as an irritant, smoke also impairs innate immune system recognition and other responses to pathogens, such that smokers have increased risk of respiratory infections. Cigarette smoke also alters T- and B-cell–mediated immune functions.
- **Seropositive rheumatoid arthritis** can result from cigarette smoking. People who smoke more develop rheumatoid arthritis more often.
- **Osteoporosis** in women is exacerbated by tobacco use. Women who smoke one pack of cigarettes daily during their reproductive period will have a 5%–10% deficit in bone density at menopause. This deficit is enough to increase the risk of bone fractures.
- **Thyroid diseases** are linked to cigarette smoking, especially Graves disease, and particularly when hyperthyroidism is complicated by exophthalmos.
- **Ocular diseases,** particularly macular degeneration and cataracts, are reportedly more frequent in smokers.
- **Brain development** may be impaired by nicotine in adolescent smokers.

Smoking Impairs Reproductive Function

Men who smoke are more susceptible to erectile dysfunction. Smoking women experience an **earlier menopause** than do nonsmokers, possibly because of the effects of tobacco on estrogen metabolism.

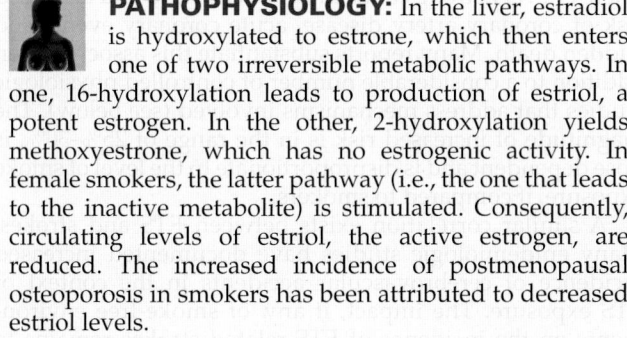

PATHOPHYSIOLOGY: In the liver, estradiol is hydroxylated to estrone, which then enters one of two irreversible metabolic pathways. In one, 16-hydroxylation leads to production of estriol, a potent estrogen. In the other, 2-hydroxylation yields methoxyestrone, which has no estrogenic activity. In female smokers, the latter pathway (i.e., the one that leads to the inactive metabolite) is stimulated. Consequently, circulating levels of estriol, the active estrogen, are reduced. The increased incidence of postmenopausal osteoporosis in smokers has been attributed to decreased estriol levels.

Fetal Tobacco Syndrome Produces Smaller Infants

Maternal cigarette smoking impairs the development of the fetus. Infants born to women who smoke during pregnancy are, on average, 200 g lighter than infants born to comparable women who do not smoke. *These infants are not born preterm but rather are small for gestational age at every stage of pregnancy.* In fact, 20%–40% of the incidence of low birth weight can be attributed to maternal cigarette smoking (Fig. 8-6). Thus, this effect of smoking is not idiosyncratic but reflects a direct retardation of fetal growth.

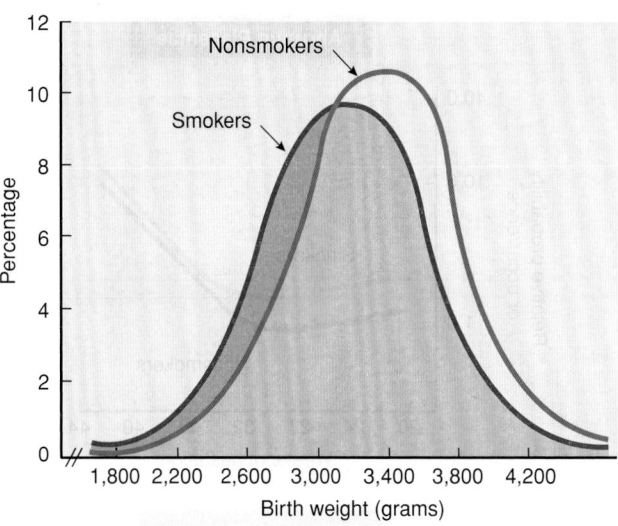

FIGURE 8-6. Effect of smoking on birth weight. Mothers who smoke give birth to smaller infants. In particular, the incidence of babies weighing less than 3000 g is increased significantly by smoking.

The harmful consequences of maternal cigarette smoking on the fetus are illustrated by its effect on the uteroplacental unit. Perinatal mortality is higher among offspring of smokers, the increases ranging from 20% among progeny of women who smoke less than a pack per day to almost 40% among offspring of those who smoke over one pack per day, with the excess mortality reflecting problems related to the uteroplacental system. Incidences of abruptio placentae, placenta previa, uterine bleeding and premature rupture of membranes are all increased (Fig. 8-7; see Chapter 12). These complications of smoking tend to occur at times when the fetus is not viable or is at great risk (i.e., 20–32 weeks of gestation).

Children born of cigarette-smoking mothers have been reported to be more susceptible to several respiratory diseases, including respiratory infections and otitis media.

Substantial evidence indicates that maternal cigarette smoking inflicts lasting harm on children and impairs physical, cognitive and emotional development. Thus, these children showed measurable deficits in physical growth, intellectual maturation and emotional development. In utero exposure to maternal cigarette smoking has been shown to increase severalfold the risk of certain types of attention deficit hyperactivity disorder (ADHD) in children. Deficits in cognitive and auditory function related to smoking during pregnancy may persist for years and are detectable well into adolescence. Boys appear to be generally more vulnerable than girls to many of the psychosocial problems resulting from perinatal exposure to maternal cigarette smoking.

Further, maternal smoking during pregnancy greatly increases (approximately fourfold in a recent study) the risk of sudden infant death syndrome (SIDS; see Chapter 6). This is thought to represent mainly the consequences of prenatal exposure to maternal smoking, since the increase in risk for SIDS if the father smokes, but not the mother, is much less (about 1.5-fold).

In the most comprehensive study to date, 17,000 children born during 1 week in Great Britain were studied at ages 7 and 11 years. Children of mothers who smoked 10 or more cigarettes a day during pregnancy were, on average, 1.0 cm shorter than children of nonsmoking mothers and 3–5 months

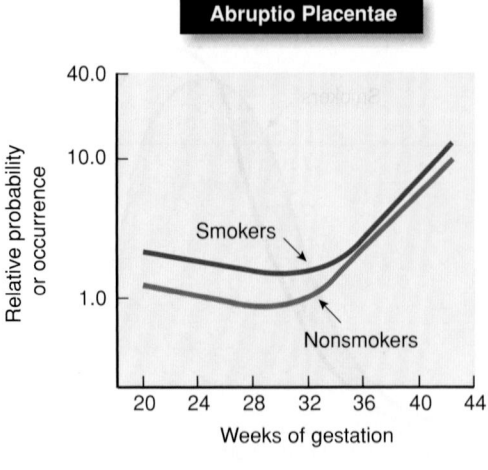

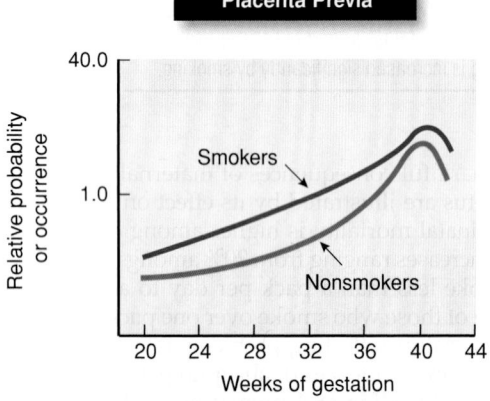

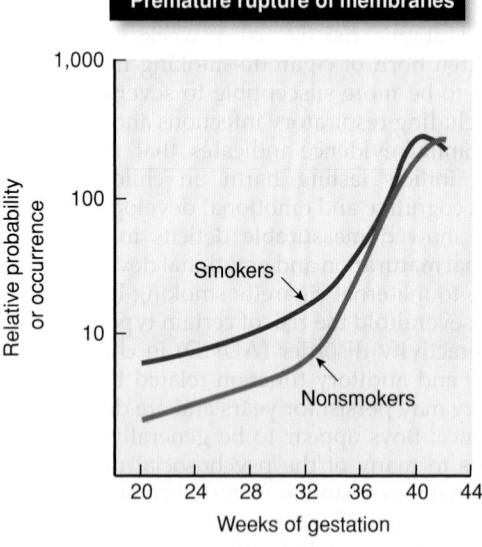

FIGURE 8-7. **Effect of smoking on the incidence of abruptio placentae (*top*), placenta previa (*middle*) and the premature rupture of amniotic membranes (*bottom*).** In each, the ordinate shows the probability of one of three complications of the third trimester of pregnancy. Note that it is a logarithmic scale. Smoking increases the probability of abruptio placentae and premature rupture of the amniotic membranes prior to 34 weeks of gestation, at which time the fetus is still premature. Smoking increases the risk of placenta previa up to 40 weeks of gestation.

behind in reading, mathematics and general intellectual ability. Moreover, the extent of the deficits was proportional to the number of cigarettes smoked during pregnancy.

Environmental Tobacco Smoke Is Harmful to Nonsmokers

Involuntary exposure to tobacco smoke in the environment—which is variably called second-hand smoke, passive smoking or environmental tobacco smoke (ETS)—is a risk factor for some diseases in nonsmokers (Table 8-1). *Nonsmoking spouses of smokers have approximately a 20%–30% increased risk of lung cancer.* The World Health Organization (WHO) and the U.S. Environmental Protection Agency classify ETS as a carcinogen and recognize that it is responsible for some lung cancers occurring in nonsmokers. Data also suggest that ETS is associated with an increased risk of breast cancer in premenopausal women who do not smoke. Data suggest other associations between ETS and human tumors—of the upper respiratory tract and elsewhere—but these connections are more tentative.

An increased incidence of respiratory illnesses and hospitalizations has been reported among infants whose parents smoke, and several studies have reported mild impairment of pulmonary function among children of smokers and exacerbation of preexisting asthma. Reduced indices of pulmonary function are also seen in children of smokers. ETS is associated with an increased risk for SIDS as well (see above).

The range of diseases significantly associated with ETS has been studied in many prospective and retrospective reports, and underlying pathophysiology has been investigated, and continues to be examined. These are illustrated in Fig. 8-8.

ETS, Cardiovascular Disease and Cerebrovascular Disease

There is a very strong connection between ETS and increased risk of coronary artery disease, acute coronary events and sudden death. Many reports substantiate this association, in addition to a considerable number of controlled physiologic studies that address mechanisms involved (see below). The magnitude of increased risk is in the range of 25%–30%, is dose dependent and is disproportionate to the level of smoke exposure, if compared to smokers.

A similar correlation exists between ETS and strokes. Many epidemiologic studies have documented increased incidence of cerebrovascular accidents in the context of ETS exposure. The impact, if any, of smoke-free environments on the incidence of ETS-related strokes remains to be established.

  **ETIOLOGIC FACTORS AND EPIDEMIOLOGY:** The products of cigarette combustion to which active smokers expose passive smokers are not the same as those that active smokers breathe in. Some of the same toxins and carcinogens in mainstream smoke are the same as in ETS. However, unlike mainstream smoke, environmental smoke also includes products of combustion at the ends of lit cigarettes, where hotter temperatures generate higher levels of toxic and carcinogenic combustion products. These include nitrosated and nitrated hydrocarbons and aromatic and polycyclic

TABLE 8-1

HEALTH CONSEQUENCES OF ENVIRONMENTAL TOBACCO SMOKE

Cancer	During Childhood	Cardiac and Vascular	Respiratory and Other	During Pregnancy
Lung	New cases of asthma	Acute myocardial infarction	New cases of asthma	Stillbirth
Breast	Acute otitis media	Ischemic stroke	Pulmonary infections	IUGR
	Pulmonary infections	Sudden cardiac death	COPD	SIDS
		Angina	Stroke	Neurologic and behavioral disorders
				Preterm delivery

COPD = chronic obstructive pulmonary disease; IUGR = intrauterine growth retardation; SIDS = sudden infant death syndrome.

compounds that do not characterize mainstream smoke. There is a documented exposure/risk relationship in ETS-related disease, the magnitude of which differs for men and women. In some studies, women exposed to second-hand smoke for extended periods (e.g., at home) suffer more from acute cardiac events (ACEs) due to ETS. Furthermore, ETS-related ACEs are significantly more likely to predispose to subsequent coronary events; again, the probabilities reflect levels of exposure to ETS.

PATHOPHYSIOLOGY: Although some observers have persisted in arguing otherwise, there is overwhelming pathophysiological mechanistic substantiation that ETS poses considerable danger to the heart and circulation (Table 8-2). The ability of the heart rate to adjust to changes in demand is compromised by short-term (5–60 minutes) exposure to ETS, as is the functionality of the microvasculature and the left ventricle. As a result, exercise tolerance is greatly diminished. Short exposures to sidestream smoke substantially impair antioxidant defenses and similarly hinder parasympathetic adaptive responses to fluctuating demand for cardiac output. Many of these observations have been made in healthy young adults and so point to ETS pathogenicity even in the absence of predisposing conditions.

Platelet and fibrin thrombi are stimulated. ETS also adds to atherogenic mechanisms involving vascular smooth muscle proliferation and oxidant and inflammatory injury to vascular endothelium. At the same time, reparative responses are undermined.

ETS is associated with increased body burden of oxidant stress and with systemic activation of inflammatory responses. Proinflammatory cytokines, circulating

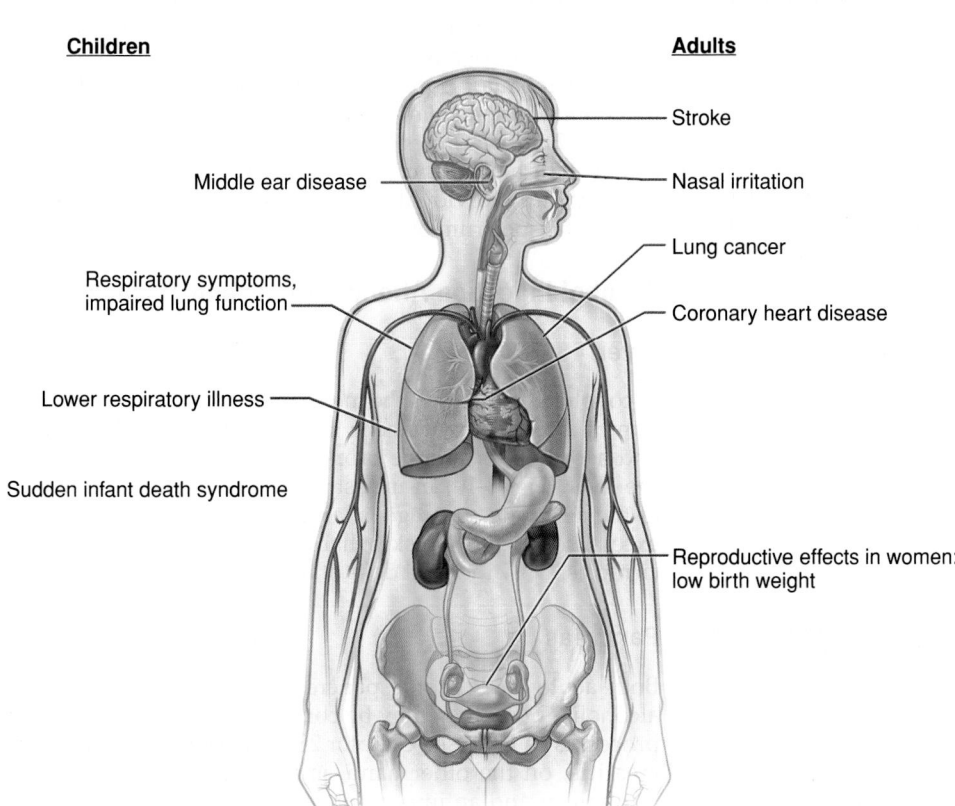

Children

- Middle ear disease
- Respiratory symptoms, impaired lung function
- Lower respiratory illness
- Sudden infant death syndrome

Adults

- Stroke
- Nasal irritation
- Lung cancer
- Coronary heart disease
- Reproductive effects in women: low birth weight

FIGURE 8-8. Complications of environmental tobacco smoke.

TABLE 8-2

EFFECTS OF ENVIRONMENTAL TOBACCO SMOKE ON THE HEART AND BLOOD

Magnification of atherogenesis
    Higher levels of oxidant stress
    Enhanced proliferation of arterial smooth muscle
    Amplification of oxidation of LDL
    Increased WBC adhesion to blood vessel walls

Higher levels of platelet aggregation

Impaired ability to adapt heart rate to fluctuations in demand

Depressed left ventricle function

Heightened inflammatory responses

Intensified platelet activation

Increased thrombogenesis

Poorer exercise tolerance

Reduced ability of arteries to dilate

LDL = low-density lipoprotein; WBC = white blood cell.

white blood cell count, biomarkers of inflammatory activation and indicators of activation of the adaptive immune system are all increased. At the same time, antioxidant defenses and other protective mechanisms are often impaired.

Studies of the consequences of outlawing smoking in public places illustrate the strongest links between ETS and acute coronary morbidity and mortality. In one report, the city of Helena, Montana, banned cigarette smoking in workplaces and public places. This ban was overturned by court order 6 months later. During the interval when the ban was in effect, the number of acute cardiac events leading to hospital admission decreased by 40%. When the ban on smoking was removed, hospital admissions for acute cardiac events rebounded almost to levels seen before the ban was instituted. Many subsequent studies corroborated these basic findings, although the magnitude of the decrease in acute coronary events differs from one study to the next. Both prospective and retrospective analyses have documented that lowering public exposure to ETS reduces acute coronary events by an average of about 15%.

ALCOHOLISM

Chronic alcoholism has been defined as regular intake of sufficient alcohol to injure a person socially, psychologically or physically. It is addiction to ethanol that features dependence and withdrawal symptoms and results in acute and chronic toxic effects of alcohol on the body. There are about 15–18 million alcoholics in the United States, about 1/10 of the population at risk. The proportion is even higher in some other countries. Certain ethnic groups, such as Native Americans and Eskimos, have high rates of alcoholism, while others,

such as Chinese and Jews, are less afflicted. Alcoholism is more common in men, but the number of female alcoholics has been increasing.

Although there are no firm rules, for most people, daily consumption of more than 45 g alcohol should probably be discouraged and 100 g or more a day may be dangerous (10 g alcohol = 1 oz, or 30 mL, of 86 proof [43%] spirits).

The short-term effects of alcohol on the brain are familiar to most people, but the mechanism of inebriation is not understood. Like other anesthetic agents, alcohol is a central nervous system (CNS) depressant. However, it is such a weak anesthetic that it must be drunk by the glassful to exert any significant effect. In a normal person, characteristic behavioral changes can be detected at low alcohol concentrations (below 50 mg/dL). Levels above 80 mg/dL are usually associated with slower reaction times and gross incoordination and in American jurisdictions are considered legal evidence of intoxication while driving a motor vehicle. At levels above 300 mg/dL, most people become comatose, and at concentrations above 400 mg/dL, death from respiratory failure is common. In humans, the LD_{50} (median lethal dose) is about 5 g of alcohol per kilogram of body weight.

The situation is somewhat different in chronic alcoholics, who develop CNS tolerance to alcohol. Such individuals may easily tolerate blood alcohol levels of 100–200 mg/dL; and in fatal automobile accidents, blood levels of 500–600 mg/dL or more have been found by medical examiners. The mechanism underlying tolerance has not been established.

Acute alcohol intoxication is hardly a benign condition. Some 40% of all fatalities from motor vehicle accidents involve alcohol—currently about 14,000 deaths annually in the United States. Alcoholism is also a major contributor to fatal home accidents, death in fires and suicide.

Many chronic diseases associated with alcoholism were once attributed to malnutrition, and some alcoholics do suffer from nutritional deficiencies, such as thiamine deficiency (Wernicke encephalopathy) or folic acid deficiency (megaloblastic anemia). *However, most alcoholics have adequate diets and most alcohol-related disorders should be attributed to the toxic effects of alcohol alone.* The diseases associated with alcoholism are discussed in detail in chapters dealing with individual organs, and we restrict this discussion to the spectrum of disease (Fig. 8-9).

Alcohol Ingestion Affects Organs and Tissues

Liver

Alcoholic liver disease, the most common medical complication of alcoholism, has been known for thousands of years and accounts for a large proportion of cases of cirrhosis of the liver (Fig. 8-10) in industrialized countries. The nature of the alcoholic beverage is largely irrelevant; consumed in excess, beer, wine, whiskey, hard cider and so on all produce cirrhosis. Only the total dose of alcohol itself is relevant.

Pancreas

Both acute and chronic pancreatitis are complications of alcoholism, but they may be consequences of other disease processes as well (see Chapter 23). **Chronic calcifying pancreatitis,** on the other hand, is an unquestioned result of alcoholism and an important cause of incapacitating pain, pancreatic insufficiency and pancreatic stones.

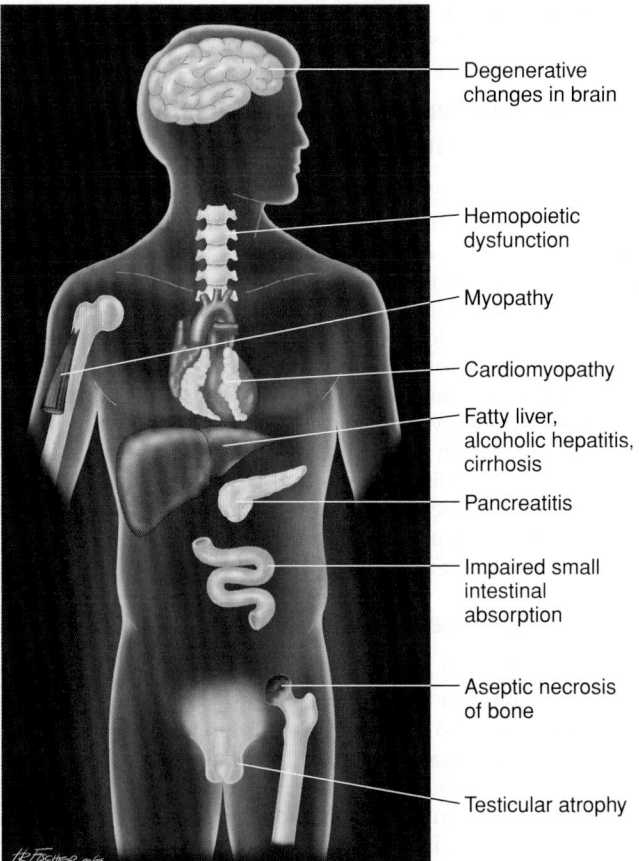

- Degenerative changes in brain
- Hemopoietic dysfunction
- Myopathy
- Cardiomyopathy
- Fatty liver, alcoholic hepatitis, cirrhosis
- Pancreatitis
- Impaired small intestinal absorption
- Aseptic necrosis of bone
- Testicular atrophy

FIGURE 8-9. Complications of chronic alcohol abuse.

Heart

Alcohol-related heart disease was recognized over a century ago in Germany, where it was referred to as "beer-drinker's heart." This degenerative disease of the myocardium is a form of dilated cardiomyopathy, called **alcoholic cardiomyopathy,**

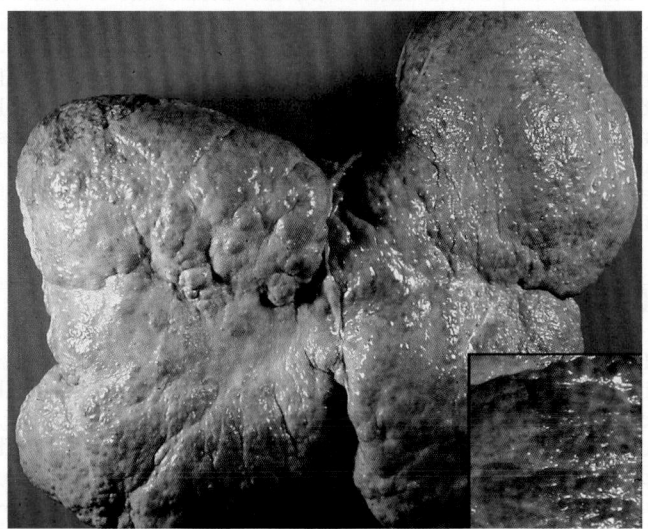

FIGURE 8-10. Cirrhosis of the liver in a chronic alcoholic. The surface displays innumerable small nodules of hepatocytes separated by interconnecting bands of fibrous tissue. These are highlighted in the higher magnification in the inset (lower right).

and leads to low-output congestive heart failure (see Chapter 17). This cardiomyopathy clearly differs from the heart disease associated with thiamine deficiency (beriberi), a disorder characterized by high-output failure. Alcoholics' hearts seem also to be more susceptible to arrhythmias. Many cases of sudden death in alcoholics are probably caused by sudden, fatal arrhythmias.

In this context, moderate alcohol consumption, or "social drinking" (one to two drinks a day), provides significant protection against coronary artery disease (atherosclerosis) and its consequence, myocardial infarction. Similarly, compared with abstainers, social drinkers have a lower incidence of ischemic stroke.

Skeletal Muscle

Muscle weakness, particularly of the proximal muscles, is common in alcoholics (see Chapter 31). A wide range of changes in skeletal muscle occurs in chronic alcoholics, varying from mild alterations in muscle fibers evident only by electron microscopy to severe, debilitating chronic myopathy, with degeneration of muscle fibers and diffuse fibrosis. Rarely, **acute alcoholic rhabdomyolysis**—necrosis of muscle fibers and release of myoglobin into the circulation—occurs. This sudden event can be fatal because of renal failure secondary to myoglobinuria.

Endocrine System

In male alcoholics, feminization and loss of libido and potency are common. Breasts become enlarged (gynecomastia), body hair is lost and a female distribution of pubic hair (female escutcheon) develops. Some of these changes can be attributed to impaired estrogen metabolism due to chronic liver disease, but many of the changes—particularly atrophy of the testes—occur even if there is no liver disease. Chronic alcoholism leads to lower levels of circulating testosterone because of a complex interference with the pituitary–gonadal axis, possibly complicated by accelerated hepatic metabolism of testosterone. Alcohol has a direct toxic effect on the testes; thus, male sexual impairment is one of the prices exacted by alcoholism.

Gastrointestinal Tract

Since the esophagus and stomach may be exposed to 10 M ethanol, it is not surprising that a direct toxic effect on the mucosa of these organs is common. Injury to the mucosa of both organs is potentiated by hypersecretion of gastric hydrochloric acid stimulated by ethanol. **Reflux esophagitis** may be particularly painful and peptic ulcers are also more common in alcoholics. Violent retching may lead to tears at the esophageal–gastric junction **(Mallory-Weiss syndrome),** sometimes severe enough to cause exsanguinating hemorrhage (see Chapter 19). Small intestine mucosal cells are also exposed to circulating alcohol, and a variety of absorptive abnormalities and ultrastructural changes have been demonstrated. Alcohol inhibits active transport of amino acids, thiamine and vitamin B_{12}.

Blood

Megaloblastic anemia is not uncommon in alcoholics and reflects a combination of dietary deficiency of folic acid and the fact that alcohol is a weak folic acid antagonist in humans. Moreover, folate absorption by the small intestine may be decreased in alcoholics. In addition, chronic ethanol intoxication leads directly to an **increase in mean corpuscular volume of erythrocytes**. In the presence of alcoholic cirrhosis, the spleen is often enlarged by portal hypertension; in such cases, **hypersplenism** often causes **hemolytic anemia**. Transient **thrombocytopenia** is common after acute alcohol intoxication and may result in bleeding. Alcohol also interferes with platelet aggregation, thus contributing to bleeding.

Bone

Chronic alcoholics, particularly postmenopausal women, are at increased risk for **osteoporosis**. Although it is well established that alcohol, at least in vitro, inhibits osteoblast function, the precise mechanism responsible for accelerated bone loss is not understood. Interestingly, moderate alcohol intake seems to exert a protective effect against osteoporosis. Male alcoholics exhibit an unusually high incidence of **aseptic necrosis of the head of the femur**. The mechanism for this complication is also obscure.

Immune System

Alcoholics seem to be prone to many infections (particularly pneumonias) with organisms that are unusual in the general population, such as *Haemophilus influenzae*. Experimentally, a number of alcohol-induced effects on immune function have been reported.

Nervous System

General cortical atrophy of the brain is common in alcoholics and may reflect a toxic effect of alcohol (see Chapter 32). By contrast, most of the characteristic brain diseases in alcoholics are probably a result of nutritional deficiency.

- **Wernicke encephalopathy** is caused by thiamine deficiency and is characterized by mental confusion, ataxia, abnormal ocular motility and polyneuropathy, reflecting pathologic changes in the diencephalon and brainstem.
- **Korsakoff psychosis** is characterized by retrograde amnesia and confabulatory symptoms. It was once believed to be pathognomonic of chronic alcoholism but has also been seen in several organic mental syndromes and is considered nonspecific.
- **Alcoholic cerebellar degeneration** differs from other acquired or familial cerebellar degeneration by the uniformity of its manifestations. Progressive unsteadiness of gait, ataxia, incoordination and reduced deep tendon reflex activity are present.
- **Central pontine myelinolysis** is another characteristic change in the brain of alcoholics, apparently caused by electrolyte imbalance—usually after electrolyte therapy, after an alcoholic binge or during withdrawal. In this complication, a progressive weakness of bulbar muscles terminates in respiratory paralysis.
- **Amblyopia** (impaired vision) occurs occasionally in alcoholics. It may reflect alcohol-related decreases in tissue vitamin A, although other vitamin deficiencies may also be involved.
- **Polyneuropathy** is common in chronic alcoholics. It is usually associated with deficiencies of thiamine and other B vitamins, but a direct neurotoxic effect of ethanol

may play a role. The most common complaints include numbness, paresthesias, pain, weakness and ataxia.

Fetal Alcohol Syndrome Results from Alcohol Abuse in Pregnancy

Infants born to mothers who consume excess alcohol during pregnancy may show a cluster of abnormalities that together constitute the fetal alcohol syndrome. These include growth retardation, microcephaly, facial dysmorphology, neurologic dysfunction and other congenital anomalies. About 6% of the offspring of alcoholic mothers are afflicted by the full syndrome. More often, exposure of the fetus to high concentrations of ethanol leads to less severe abnormalities, prominent among which are mental retardation, intrauterine growth retardation and minor dysmorphic features. Alcohol acts as an antagonist of *N*-methyl-D-aspartic acid (NMDA) and γ-aminobutyric acid (GABA)-mimetic neurotransmitters and can trigger neuron apoptosis. Fetal alcohol syndrome is discussed in greater detail in Chapter 6.

Alcohol Increases the Risk of Some Cancers

Cancers of the oral cavity, larynx and esophagus occur more often in alcoholics than in the general population. As most alcoholics are also smokers, the differential contributions of ethanol and cigarette smoke to these observed increases are not well defined. The risk of hepatocellular carcinoma is increased in patients with alcoholic cirrhosis. A number of reports have described increased incidence of breast cancer in alcoholic women, a subject that requires further study.

The Mechanisms by Which Alcohol Injures Tissues Are Not Understood

The pathogenesis of ethanol-induced organ damage remains obscure. In a number of experimental settings, ethanol and its metabolites have been shown to have harmful effects on cells. Among these are changes in redox potential (NAD/NADH ratio). In addition, ethanol may lead to formation of unusual compounds such as the first metabolite of ethanol oxidation, acetaldehyde, protein adducts, fatty acid ethyl esters and phosphatidyl ethanol. It also increases production of reactive oxygen species (ROS; see Chapter 1) and tends to intercalate between phospholipids within biological membranes and so disorders them. Moreover, ethanol has pleiotropic effects on cellular signaling and may promote apoptosis under some circumstances. The relationship of this effect to cell injury requires further study.

DRUG ABUSE

Drug abuse has been defined as "the use of any substance in a manner that deviates from the accepted medical, social or legal patterns within a given society." For the most part, drug abuse involves agents that are used to alter mood and perception. These include (1) derivatives of opium (heroin, morphine); (2) depressants (barbiturates, tranquilizers, alcohol); (3) stimulants (cocaine, amphetamines), marijuana and psychedelic drugs (PCP, lysergic acid diethylamide [LSD]); and (4) inhalants (amyl nitrite, organic solvents such as those in glue). Use of illicit drugs is estimated to cause about 17,000 deaths a year in the United States.

Illicit Drugs Are Responsible for Many Pathologic Syndromes

Heroin

Heroin is a common illicit opiate used to induce euphoria. It is often taken intravenously and in the usual dosage is effective for about 5 hours. Overdoses are characterized by hypothermia, bradycardia and respiratory depression. Other opiates that are subject to abuse include morphine and Dilaudid, but these have been largely replaced by oxycodone and fentanyl. Oxycodone, usually combined with acetaminophen, is an opiate alkaloid with both stimulant and analgesic properties. The strongest effect is achieved by intravenous administration. Fentanyl is an opiate similar to morphine but is up to 100 times more potent. Its illicit use involves injection or oral intake, and it is associated with a high risk of addiction.

Cocaine

Cocaine is an alkaloid derived from South American coca leaves. The freebase form of cocaine is hard and is far more potent than coca leaves. It may be taken by sniffing, smoking, intravenous injection or orally. An even more potent form of cocaine ("crack") is generally smoked. It is hard and is then "cracked" into smaller pieces that are smoked. The half-life of cocaine in the blood is about 1 hour.

Cocaine users report extreme euphoria and heightened sensitivity to a variety of stimuli. However, with addiction, paranoid states and conspicuous emotional lability occur. The mechanism of action of cocaine is related to its interference with the reuptake of the neurotransmitter dopamine.

Cocaine overdose leads to anxiety and delirium and occasionally to seizures. Cardiac arrhythmias and other effects on the heart may cause sudden death in otherwise apparently healthy people. Chronic abuse of cocaine is associated with the occasional development of a characteristic dilated cardiomyopathy, which may be fatal.

Amphetamines

Amphetamines, mainly methamphetamine, are sympathomimetic and resemble cocaine in their effects, although they have a longer duration of action. Methamphetamines are most commonly used as "crystal meth," which is easily produced by hydrogenation of ephedrine or pseudoephedrine. Methamphetamine is often made in home laboratories and is a major public health problem in the United States. The most serious complications of the abuse of amphetamines are seizures, cardiac arrhythmias and hyperthermia. Amphetamine use has been reported to lead to vasculitis of the CNS, and both subarachnoid and intracerebral hemorrhages have been described.

Hallucinogens

Hallucinogens are a group of chemically unrelated drugs that alter perception and sensory experience.

Phencyclidine (PCP) is an anesthetic agent that has psychedelic or hallucinogenic effects. As a recreational drug, it is known as "angel dust" and is taken orally, intranasally or by smoking. The anesthetic properties of phencyclidine effect diminished capacity to perceive pain and, therefore, may lead to self-injury and trauma. Other than the behavioral effects, PCP commonly produces tachycardia and hypertension. High doses result in deep coma, seizures and even decerebrate posturing.

LSD is a hallucinogenic drug whose popularity peaked in the late 1960s and is little used today. It causes perceptual distortion of the senses, interference with logical thought, alteration of time perception and a sense of depersonalization. "Bad trips" are characterized by anxiety and panic and objectively by sympathomimetic effects that include tachycardia, hypertension and hyperthermia. Large overdoses cause coma, convulsions and respiratory arrest.

Organic Solvents

The recreational inhalation of organic solvents is widespread, particularly among adolescents. Various commercial preparations such as fingernail polish, glues, plastic cements and lighter fluid are all sniffed. Among the active ingredients are benzene, carbon tetrachloride, acetone, xylene and toluene. However, many of these compounds are also industrial solvents and reagents and so chronic low-level occupational exposure occurs. These compounds are all CNS depressants, although early effects (e.g., with xylene) may be excitatory. Acute intoxication with organic solvents resembles inebriation with alcohol. Large doses produce nausea and vomiting, hallucinations and eventually coma. Respiratory depression and death may follow. Chronic exposure to, or abuse of, organic solvents may result in damage to the brain, kidneys, liver, lungs and hematopoietic system. Benzene, for example, is a bone marrow toxin and has been associated with the development of acute myelogenous leukemia.

Intravenous Drug Abuse Has Many Medical Complications

Apart from reactions related to pharmacologic or physiologic effects of substance abuse, the most common complications (15% of directly drug-related deaths) are caused by introducing infectious organisms by a parenteral route. Most occur at the site of injection: cutaneous abscesses, cellulitis and ulcers (Fig. 8-11). When these heal, "track marks" persist and these areas may be hypopigmented or hyperpigmented.

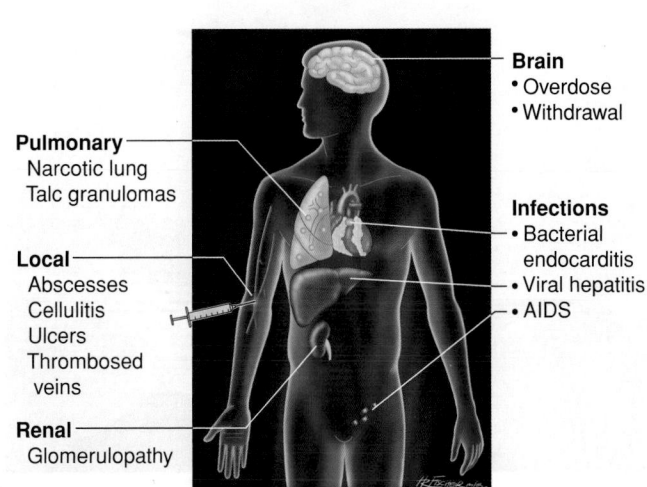

Pulmonary
Narcotic lung
Talc granulomas

Local
Abscesses
Cellulitis
Ulcers
Thrombosed
  veins

Renal
Glomerulopathy

Brain
• Overdose
• Withdrawal

Infections
• Bacterial
  endocarditis
• Viral hepatitis
• AIDS

FIGURE 8-11. Complications of intravenous drug abuse.

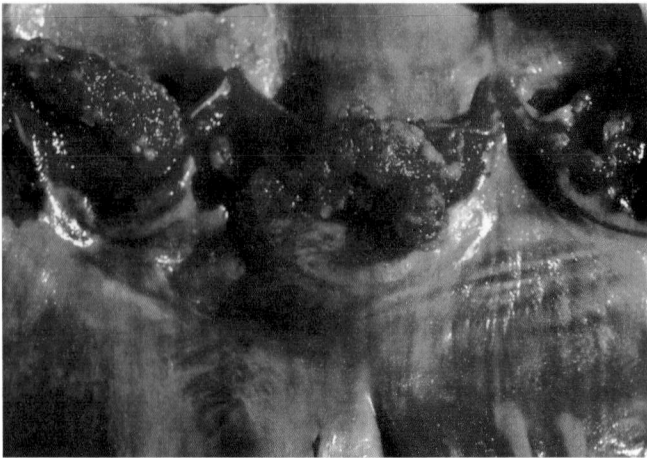

FIGURE 8-12. Bacterial endocarditis. The aortic valve of an intravenous drug abuser displays adherent vegetations.

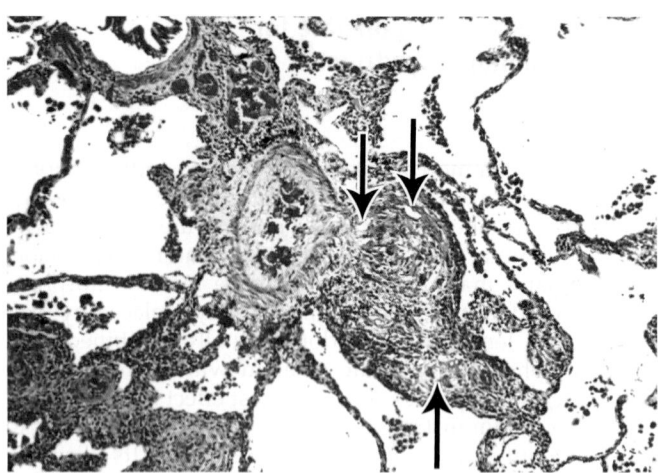

FIGURE 8-14. Talc granulomas in the lung. A section of lung from an intravenous drug abuser viewed under polarized light reveals a granuloma adjacent to a pulmonary artery. The refractile material (*arrows*) is talc that was used to dilute the drug prior to its intravenous injection.

Thrombophlebitis of the veins draining sites of injection is common. Intravenous introduction of bacteria may lead to septic complications in internal organs. Bacterial endocarditis, often involving *Staphylococcus aureus,* occurs on both sides of the heart (Fig. 8-12) and may cause pulmonary, renal and intracranial abscesses; meningitis; osteomyelitis; and mycotic aneurysms (Fig. 8-13).

Intravenous drug abusers are at very high risk for AIDS, as well as hepatitis B and C. These people may also suffer from the complications of viral hepatitis, such as chronic active hepatitis, necrotizing angiitis and glomerulonephritis. A focal glomerulosclerosis ("heroin nephropathy") is characterized by immune complexes and has been ascribed to an immune reaction to impurities that contaminate illicit drugs.

Intravenous injection of talc, which is used to dilute pure drug, is associated with the appearance of foreign body granulomas in the lung (Fig. 8-14). These may be severe enough to lead to interstitial pulmonary fibrosis.

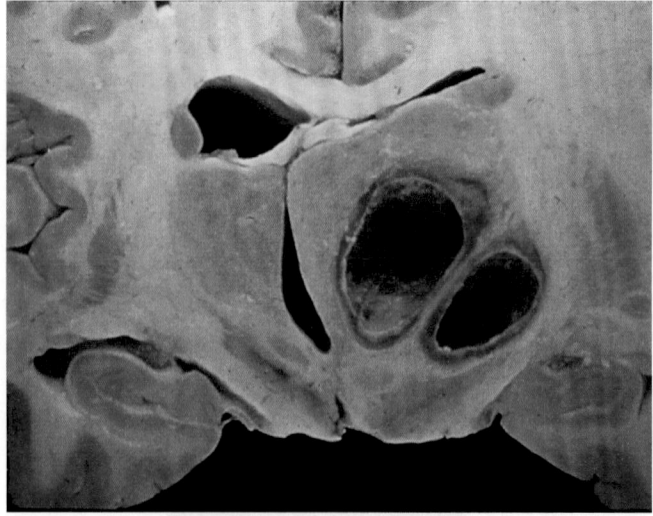

FIGURE 8-13. Brain abscess. Cross-section of the brain from an intravenous drug abuser shows two encapsulated cavities.

Drug Addiction in Pregnant Women Poses Risks for the Fetus

Maternal drug use may cause addiction of newborn infants, who often exhibit a full-blown withdrawal syndrome. Moreover, the appearance of the drug withdrawal syndrome in the fetus during labor may result in excessive fetal movements and increased oxygen demand, a situation that increases the risk of intrapartum hypoxia and meconium aspiration. If labor occurs when maternal drug levels are high, the infant is often born with respiratory depression. Mothers who are addicted to drugs experience higher rates of toxemia of pregnancy and premature labor.

Maternal use of illicit drugs during pregnancy may injure the developing fetus in other ways. Thus, pregnant women who use cocaine more commonly experience placental abruption and premature labor. Infants born to such mothers are prone to be low birth weight, to have one of an array of CNS and other anomalies and to show impaired brain function after birth. Maternal addiction to heroin carries a number of risks of abnormalities of pregnancy and premature birth. It is also associated with a large number of postnatal problems (in addition to heroin withdrawal), including SIDS, neonatal respiratory distress syndrome and developmental retardation. Maternal abuse of other substances (e.g., amphetamines and hallucinogens) also leads to variably severe fetal and postnatal disorders.

IATROGENIC DRUG INJURY

Iatrogenic drug injury refers to the unintended side effects of therapeutic or diagnostic drugs prescribed by physicians. Adverse reactions to pharmaceuticals are surprisingly common. They are seen in 2%–5% of patients hospitalized on medical services; of these reactions, 2%–12% are fatal. The typical hospitalized patient is given about 10 different medications and some receive five times as many. The risk of an adverse reaction increases proportionally with the number of different drugs; for example, the risk of injury is at least 40% when more than 15 drugs are administered.

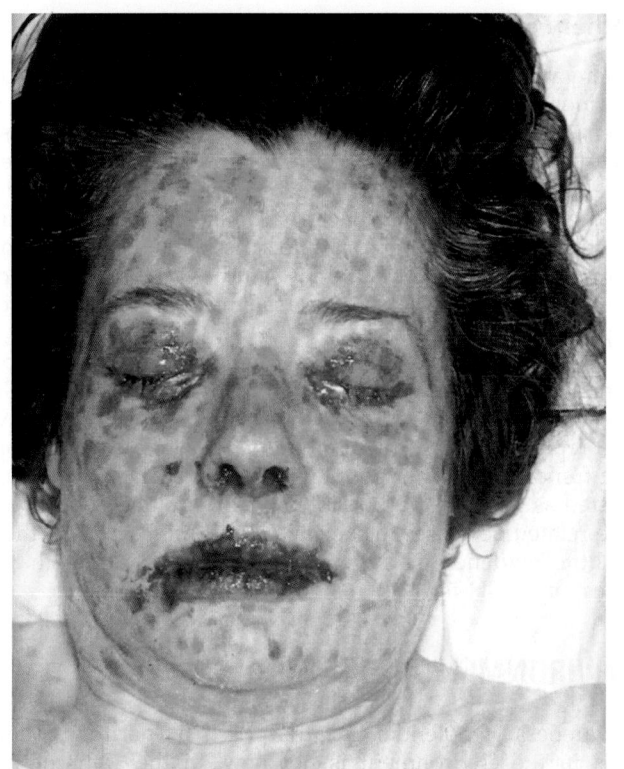

FIGURE 8-15. Erythema multiforme secondary to sulfonamide therapy.

Because they are so ubiquitously prescribed, drugs represent a significant environmental hazard. Untoward effects of drugs result from (1) overdose, (2) exaggerated physiologic responses, (3) a genetic predisposition, (4) hypersensitivity, (5) interactions with other drugs and (6) other unknown factors. The characteristic pathologic changes associated with drug reactions are treated in chapters dealing with specific organs. An example of a drug reaction is illustrated in Fig. 8-15.

SEX HORMONES

Oral Contraceptives Carry a Small Risk of Complications

Orally administered hormonal contraceptives (OCs) are now the most commonly used method of birth control in industrialized countries. Current formulations are combinations of synthetic estrogens and steroids with progesterone-like activity. They act either by inhibiting the gonadotropin surge at midcycle, thus preventing ovulation, or by preventing implantation by altering the phase of the endometrium. Most complications of oral contraceptives involve either the vasculature or reproductive organs (Fig. 8-16).

Vascular Complications

Deep vein thrombosis is a recognized complication of oral contraceptive use, the risk being increased two to three times. As a consequence, the risk of thromboembolism is correspondingly increased. Obesity and smoking magnify the

risk of venous thrombosis attendant to OCs, as do coexisting disorders that increase clotting (thrombophilia).

The risk of arterial thrombotic events in women taking oral contraceptives is also increased. Thus, both myocardial infarction and thrombotic stroke are reported to be increased in some studies.

Neoplastic Complications

Tumors of several of the female reproductive organs, especially ovary, endometrium and breast, are strongly influenced by female hormones. Repeated epidemiologic studies indicate that OC use decreases risk of ovarian and endometrial cancers by about half, presumably because of suppression of the production of pituitary gonadotropins.

There is a small increase in the frequency of breast cancers in OC users. This applies mainly to nonfamilial breast cancers and to women currently taking OCs. The increased risk appears to endure for about 10 years following cessation of OC administration.

Squamous carcinoma of the cervix in women positive for human papilloma virus (HPV) may be somewhat increased in association with long-term (>5 years) OC use.

Benign liver adenomas are rare hepatic neoplasms that are significantly increased in incidence among women who use OCs. The risk of these tumors increases conspicuously with the duration of use, particularly after 5 years.

Several small studies have suggested a small increased risk of **hepatocellular carcinoma** among women using OCs. Fortunately, this cancer is rare in young women without chronic viral hepatitis.

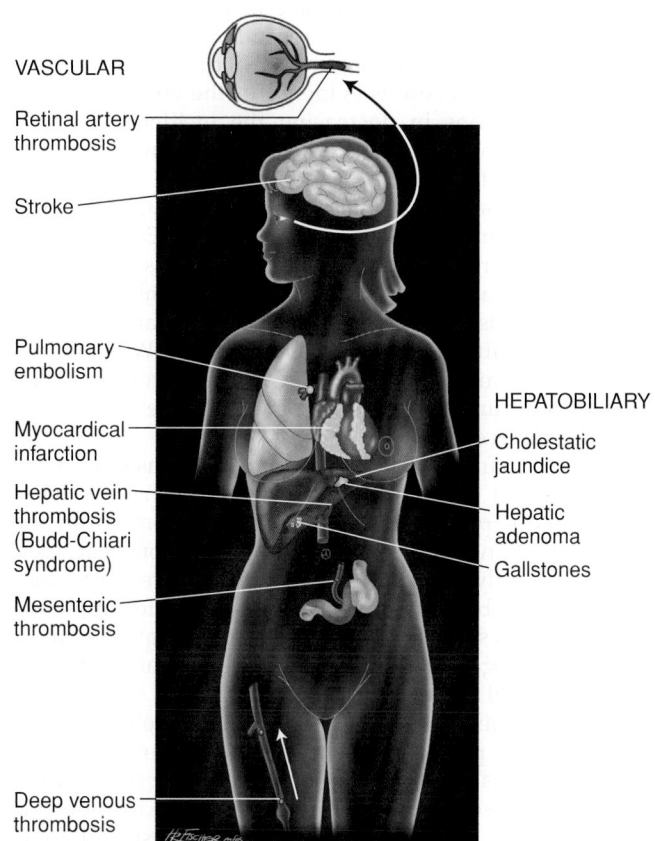

FIGURE 8-16. Complications of oral contraceptives.

Other Complications

For reasons unknown, oral contraceptives may induce an increased pigmentation of the malar eminences, called **chloasma,** which is accentuated by sunlight and persists for a long time after the contraceptives are discontinued.

Cholelithiasis is more frequent (twofold increase) in women who have used OCs for 4 years or less, but its incidence becomes lower than normal after that period of time. Thus, OCs accelerate gallstone formation but do not increase its overall incidence.

Benefits of Oral Contraceptives

In considering the potential side effects of the use of oral contraceptive agents, it is important to recognize that certain benefits accrue. In addition to a significant reduction in the risk of ovarian and endometrial cancers, the use of these agents decreases the risk of pelvic inflammatory disease, uterine leiomyomas, endometriosis and fibrocystic disease of the breast.

The Risks of Postmenopausal Hormone Replacement Therapy Depend on the Formulation, Age at Which Treatment Begins and Duration of Treatment

Hormone replacement (HR) preparations come in many varieties, the most common being oral estrogen only and oral combined estrogen plus progestogen combinations. These are given to women for diverse reasons, including to alleviate distressing symptoms of menopause, protect from osteoporosis and, more recently, protect from cardiovascular, cerebrovascular and CNS diseases that occur in older women. There is evidence of the effectiveness of these preparations in decreasing the incidence of bone fractures and mitigating many of the problems relating to hormone deficits.

However, there are significant risks associated with hormonal replacement following menopause. Estrogen-only and estrogen–progestogen combinations are associated with a slightly increased risk of venous thromboembolism. This increased risk is most common in the first year of HR and declines thereafter, even with continued HR. With the cessation of treatment, the risk of deep vein thrombosis and embolism declines to that in women who never received hormone replacement.

Because many tumors are hormonally sensitive, it has seemed logical that HR would increase the risk of developing tumors, particularly of the breast, endometrium and ovaries. Current data support the conclusion that there is a significantly increased risk of breast cancer in women receiving combined estrogen–progestogen formulations, while there is a slightly increased risk, or none at all, in those receiving estrogens alone. The converse appears to be true for endometrial and ovarian cancers.

There appears to be little overall benefit of either type of preparation in protecting from cardiovascular or cerebrovascular deaths. Women who begin HR more than 6 years after menopause have been reported to have a somewhat higher risk of developing Alzheimer disease, although those who initiate HR during that period appear not to be at risk.

Other Forms of Hormone Replacement

There are scant data regarding the risks of other forms of hormone replacement therapy. Androgen production in men declines with age, resulting in loss of muscle mass, increased adiposity and other problems. However, testosterone replacement therapy for age-related decline in muscular strength, sexual performance and other parameters remains controversial. Although prostate cancer in men is often hormonally sensitive, there are few studies reporting the incidence of prostate or other cancers in men receiving androgen replacement treatments.

Growth hormone (GH) replacement is used in people who lack adequate GH. Although many tumors require GH for their growth, there is no evidence that people who receive GH replacement treatment are more susceptible to developing tumors than other people of their age. GH is being suggested as providing a possible benefit in older people with age-related decreases in skeletal muscle mass. To date, there is little evidence of adverse consequences, although the question of GH-induced insulin resistance remains.

ENVIRONMENTAL CHEMICALS

Awareness of potential hazards posed by harmful chemicals in the environment is not new. In the 12th century Maimonides wrote:

> Comparing the air of cities to the air of deserts is like comparing waters that are befouled and turbid to waters that are fine and pure. In the city, because of the height of its buildings, the narrowness of its streets and all that pours forth from its inhabitants, the air becomes stagnant, turbid, thick, misty and foggy....Wherever the air is altered...men develop dullness of understanding, failure of intelligence and defects of memory.

Humans are surrounded by, breathe in and consume many chemicals that are added to, or appear as contaminants in, foods, water and air. Several important mechanisms govern the effect of toxic agents, including the toxin's absorption, distribution, metabolism and excretion. Absorption (whether via pulmonary, gastrointestinal or cutaneous routes) depends largely on the chemical in question. Thus, the insecticides chlordane and heptachlor are lipid soluble and so rapidly absorbed and stored in body fat. In contrast, the water-soluble herbicide paraquat is readily eliminated.

The storage, distribution and excretion of chemicals control their concentrations in the organism at any given time. Agents stored in adipose tissue may exert prolonged low-level effects, while more water-soluble materials that are easily excreted by the kidney usually have a shorter duration of action.

Among the most important chemical hazards to which humans are exposed are environmental dusts and carcinogens. Inhalation of mineral and organic dusts occurs primarily in occupational settings (e.g., mining, industrial manufacturing, farming) and occasionally as a result of unusual situations (e.g., bird fanciers, pituitary snuff inhalation). Inhaling mineral dusts leads to pulmonary diseases known as **pneumoconioses,** while organic dusts may produce **hypersensitivity pneumonitis.** Pneumoconioses were formerly common, but control of dust exposure

TABLE 8-3

INCREASED MORBIDITY AND MORTALITY AS A FUNCTION OF PARTICULATE AIR POLLUTION (RESULTS OF REPRESENTATIVE STUDIES)

Type of Exposure	Health Consequence	Relative Increase in Incidence of Death and Disease (%)
Acute	Cardiovascular death	0.68[a]
	Ischemic cardiac disease	0.7[a]
	Heart failure	0.8[a]
	Acute attacks of asthma (children)	1.2[a]
	Acute attacks of asthma (adults)	1.1[a]
	Total lung (including asthma and COPD)	0.9[a]
	Acute myocardial infarction	4.5[b]
	Acute myocardial infarction	48[c]
Chronic	Cardiovascular death	12–76[d]
	Atherosclerosis	4[d]
	Venous thromboembolism	70[e]

[a]Per every 10 $\mu g/m^3$ increase in PM_{10}, 1 day before the event.
[b]Per every 10 $\mu g/m^3$ increase in $PM_{2.5}$ acutely.
[c]Per every 25 $\mu g/m^3$ increase in $PM_{2.5}$ acutely.
[d]Per every 10 $\mu g/m^3$ increase in $PM_{2.5}$.
[e]Per every 10 $\mu g/m^3$ increase in PM_{10}.

in the workplace through modifications of manufacturing techniques, improvements in air handling and use of masks has substantially reduced the incidence of these diseases. Because of their importance, pneumoconioses and hypersensitivity pneumonitis are discussed in detail in Chapter 18.

Chemical carcinogens are ubiquitous in the environment. Their potential for causing disease has elicited widespread concern. In particular, exposure to carcinogens in the workplace has been associated epidemiologically with a number of cancers (Table 8-3), which are reviewed in Chapter 5.

Toxic Effects Differ from Hypersensitivity Responses

Many substances predictably elicit disease in a variety of animal species in a dose-dependent manner, with a regular time delay and a reproducible pattern of target organ responses. Furthermore, the morphologic changes in injured tissues are constant and reproducible. By contrast, the actions of other agents are unpredictable, showing (1) great variability in their ability to produce disease, (2) irregular lag times before injury is apparent, (3) no dose dependency and (4) lack of reproducibility. Generally, **predictable dose-response reactions** reflect direct actions of a compound or its metabolite on a tissue—a "toxic" effect. The second, **unpredictable type of reaction** is believed to reflect "hypersensitivity," whether

involving an immunologic response or other type of idiosyncratic side effect.

Chemical Toxicity May Follow Occupational Exposure

Beginning with the industrial revolution, there has been an exponential rise in the number of chemicals manufactured and a corresponding increase in the risk of human exposure. In any consideration of this topic, one must differentiate between acute poisoning and chronic toxicity. One must also distinguish industrial and accidental exposure from that which is likely to occur in the general environment. The lack of adequate quantitative exposure data in humans and the difficulties involved in assessing long-term risks of low-level exposures have led to use of data derived from animal studies to assess toxicities and risks in humans. Such projections can be hazardous because of (1) species differences in sensitivity, (2) differing routes of administration, (3) species-to-species variations in metabolic pathways by which some compounds are modified and (4) extrapolation from very high levels needed to show an effect in a short experimental time frame in animals to low-level exposures over years in humans. These considerations necessarily complicate the need to understand and quantify the potential for human toxicity of a plethora of chemicals.

Except for certain hypersensitivity reactions in susceptible people, acute poisoning by environmental chemicals does not pose a significant threat to the general population. Concentrations necessary to cause acute functional disorders or structural damage occur mainly in the workplace or because of uncommon accidents.

Accidental mass poisonings with the pesticides endrin and parathion have led to as many as 100 deaths in a single event, but long-term sequelae among the survivors have been difficult to document. The experimental literature dealing with the short- and long-term toxicity of industrial chemicals is voluminous and complicated and often contradictory. For this reason we largely restrict the following discussion to documented effects in humans.

Volatile Organic Solvents and Vapors

Volatile organic solvents and vapors are widely used in industry in many capacities. With few exceptions, exposures to these compounds are industrial or accidental and represent short-term dangers rather than long-term toxicity. For the most part, exposure to solvents is by inhalation rather than by ingestion.

- **Chloroform ($CHCl_3$) and carbon tetrachloride (CCl_4):** These solvents are CNS depressants (anesthetics) and impair the heart and blood vessels, but are better known as hepatotoxins. With both, but classically with carbon tetrachloride, large doses lead to acute hepatic necrosis, fatty liver and liver failure. Long-term exposure to carbon tetrachloride does not pertain to humans, as each exposure to it causes recognizable clinical liver injury, so that continued exposure would not be permitted.
- **Trichloroethylene (C_2HCl_3):** A ubiquitous industrial solvent, trichloroethylene in high concentrations depresses the CNS, but hepatotoxicity is minimal. There is no evidence for disease in humans, even after ordinary long-term industrial exposure.

- **Methanol (CH$_3$OH):** Because methanol, unlike ethanol, is not taxed, it is used by some impoverished alcoholics as a substitute for ethanol or by unscrupulous merchants as an adulterant of alcoholic beverages, especially in impoverished areas. In methanol poisoning, inebriation similar to that produced by ethanol is succeeded by gastrointestinal symptoms, visual dysfunction, seizures, coma and death. The major toxicity of methanol is believed to arise from its metabolism, first to formaldehyde and then to formic acid. Metabolic acidosis is common after methanol ingestion. The most characteristic lesion of methanol toxicity is necrosis of retinal ganglion cells and subsequent degeneration of the optic nerve, leading to blindness. Severe poisoning may lead to lesions in the putamen and globus pallidus.
- **Ethylene glycol (HOCH$_2$CH$_2$OH):** Because of its low vapor pressure, toxicity of ethylene glycol chiefly results from ingestion. It is commonly used in antifreeze and has been drunk by chronic alcoholics as a substitute for ethanol for many years. Poisoning with this compound came into prominence when it was used to adulterate wines, owing to its sweet taste and solubility. The toxicity of ethylene glycol is chiefly due to its metabolites, particularly oxalic acid, and occurs within minutes of ingestion. Metabolic acidosis, CNS depression, nausea and vomiting and hypocalcemia-related cardiotoxicity are seen. Oxalate crystals in renal tubules and oxaluria are often noted and may cause renal failure.
- **Gasoline and kerosene:** These fuels are mixtures of aliphatic hydrocarbons and branched, unsaturated and aromatic hydrocarbons. Chronic exposure is by inhalation. Despite prolonged exposure to gasoline by gas station attendants, auto mechanics and so forth, there is no evidence that inhalation of gasoline over the long term is particularly injurious. Acutely, gasoline is an irritant, but really only causes systemic problems if inhaled in very high concentrations. Increased use of kerosene for home heating has led to accidental poisoning of children.
- **Benzene (C$_6$H$_6$):** The prototypic aromatic hydrocarbon is benzene, which must be distinguished from benzine, a mixture of aliphatic hydrocarbons. Benzene is one of the most widely used chemicals in industrial processes, being a starting point for innumerable syntheses and a solvent. It is also a constituent of fuels, accounting for as much as 3% of gasoline. Virtually all cases of acute and chronic benzene toxicity have occurred as industrial exposures (e.g., in shoemakers and workers in shoe manufacturing, occupations that at one time were associated with heavy exposure to benzene-based glues).

  Acute benzene poisoning primarily affects the CNS and death results from respiratory failure. However, it is the long-term effects of benzene exposure that have attracted the most attention. In these cases, the bone marrow is the principal target. Patients who develop hematologic abnormalities characteristically exhibit **hypoplasia** or **aplasia of the bone marrow** and **pancytopenia. Aplastic anemia** usually is seen while the workers are still exposed to high concentrations of benzene. In a substantial proportion of cases of benzene-induced anemias, **myelodysplastic syndromes, acute myeloblastic leukemia, erythroleukemia** or **multiple myeloma** develops during continuing exposure to benzene or after a variable latent period following removal of the worker from the hazardous environment. Some cases of acute leukemia have occurred without a prior history of aplastic anemia. Although instances of chronic myeloid and chronic lymphocytic leukemia have been reported, a cause-and-effect relationship with benzene exposure is less convincing than that with cases of acute leukemia. Overall, the risk of leukemia is increased 60-fold in workers exposed to the highest atmospheric concentrations of benzene. It deserves mention that both gasoline and tobacco smoke contain benzene, and both contribute to increased benzene levels in the urban atmosphere. The consequent contribution of such benzene concentrations to hematologic diseases is speculative.

  The toxic effects of benzene are related to its metabolites, which are the consequence of cytochrome P450 degradation of the parent compound. The closely related compounds toluene and xylenes, also widely used as solvents, have not been incriminated as a cause of hematologic abnormalities, possibly because they are metabolized via different pathways.

Agricultural Chemicals

Pesticides, fungicides, herbicides, fumigants and organic fertilizers are crucial to the productivity of modern agriculture. However, many of these chemicals persist in soil and water and may pose a potential long-term hazard. Acute poisoning with very large concentrations of any of these chemicals has already been mentioned above. It is clear that exposure to industrial concentrations or inadvertently contaminated food can cause severe acute illness. Children are particularly susceptible and may ingest home gardening preparations.

Organochlorine pesticides, such as DDT (dichlorodiphenyltrichloroethane), chlordane and others, have caused concern because they accumulate in soils and in human tissues and break down very slowly. High levels of any such pesticide can be harmful to humans in acute exposures, but the side effects of chronic contact with the materials and their buildup are of greatest interest. Many of these compounds function as weak estrogens, but no harmful effects related to this activity have been documented. Some of these compounds, such as aldrin and dieldrin, have been associated with tumor development, but the acute toxicity of most organochlorine insecticides relates to inhibition of CNS GABA responses.

Symptoms of acute toxicity are often related to the mode of action of the toxin. For example, organophosphate insecticides, which have largely replaced organochlorine compounds, are acetylcholinesterase inhibitors that are readily absorbed through the skin. Thus, acute toxicity in humans mainly involves neuromuscular disorders such as visual disturbances, dyspnea, mucous hypersecretion and bronchoconstriction. Death may come from respiratory failure. In the United States, 30–40 people die annually of acute pesticide poisoning. Long-term exposure to substantial concentrations produces symptoms similar to those of acute exposure.

Human exposure to herbicides is not infrequent. Among the best known of these is paraquat. Occupational paraquat exposure is usually via the skin, although toxicity from ingestion and inhalation are documented. The compound is very corrosive and causes burns or ulcers of whatever it contacts. It is transported actively to the lung, where it can damage the pulmonary epithelium, causing edema and even respiratory failure. High-level exposures may lead to death from cardiovascular collapse, while when lower doses are involved, pulmonary fibrosis may ultimately lead to death.

Aromatic Halogenated Hydrocarbons

The halogenated aromatic hydrocarbons that have received considerable attention include (1) the polychlorinated biphenyls (PCBs); (2) chlorophenols (pentachlorophenol, used as a wood preservative); (3) hexachlorophene, previously used as an antibacterial agent in soaps; and (4) the dioxin TCDD (2,3,7,8-tetrachlorodibenzo-p-dioxin), a byproduct of the synthesis of herbicides and hexachlorophene and, therefore, a contaminant of these preparations that has not been produced intentionally. In 1976, an industrial accident in Seveso, Italy, exposed many people to extremely high concentrations of TCDD. As of 2009, small increases in incidences of breast and lymphoid/hematologic cancers are reported, but these results remain inconclusive. Chronic exposure to PCBs and TCDD does not appear to produce demonstrable toxicity. Serious questions have been raised regarding the danger of long-term exposure to dioxin, and there is now a consensus that at the very least this compound is far more carcinogenic in rodents than in humans. The problem of the presence of PCBs in the environment resembles that of agricultural chemicals: long-term animal toxicity is well documented, but there are no significant increases in the incidence of cancer or other diseases in workers exposed to PCBs. The same situation pertains to hexachlorophene and pentachlorophenol.

Cyanide

Prussic acid (HCN) is the classic murderer's tool in detective fiction, where the smell of bitter almonds (*Prunus amygdalus*) betrays the crime. Cyanide blocks cellular respiration by reversibly binding to mitochondrial cytochrome oxidase, the terminal acceptor in the electron transport chain, which is responsible for reducing molecular oxygen to water. The pathologic consequences are similar to those produced by any acute global anoxia.

Air Pollution Is a Major Cause of Death

The WHO has determined that air pollution is responsible for 8 million lives lost worldwide annually.[2] The most important air pollutants are those generated by combustion of fossil fuels, industrial and agricultural processes and so forth. The principal contributors to human disease among these are particulates, especially carbon particles. In addition, noxious and irritant gasses **sulfur dioxide** (SO_2), **oxides of nitrogen,** CO and **ozone** are important constituents of polluted air.

Carbon Particulates

Considerable evidence implicates carbon **particulates** in urban air and certain industrial settings as responsible for substantial human morbidity and mortality. Although the composition and sources of particulate matter vary widely, exhaust from diesel fuel combustion is the single largest source of carbon particles in urban air.

Particulates vary in size, composition and origin. They generally fall into three categories, according to their aerodynamic diameter (AD): those between 2.5 μm and 10 μm (PM_{10}) are considered coarse particulates; those under 2.5 μm in AD are fine, designated $PM_{2.5}$; and the smallest are $PM_{0.1}$, which are less than 0.1 μm (or 100 nm), ultrafine particles.

The ability of PM to cause disease (see below) is a function of the toxic and carcinogenic combustion products they carry. While polycyclic aromatics (PAHs) were once thought to be the most potent of these, it is now clear that nitrated compounds (nitroarenes) are even more pathogenic. When these chemicals, bound to carbon particles, are breathed in, their disposition is a function of where the particles localize. Carbon particles have different abilities to deliver these toxic chemicals and have different pathogenetic properties based on their size (Fig. 8-17). PM_{10}s mostly settle in the conducting airways of the tracheobronchial tree. Fine particles ($PM_{2.5}$) penetrate more deeply into the lungs because of their smaller size. These find their way to small terminal airways and alveoli. Ultrafine particles ($PM_{0.1}$, <100 nm) penetrate very deeply. They have a high surface area–to–mass ratio (which allows for greater potential delivery of noxious components). These can traverse alveolar walls, pass through alveolar capillaries, enter the bloodstream and disseminate throughout the body (Fig. 8-17).

Many epidemiologic studies establish that both short-term and extended exposures to particulate air pollutants are associated with morbidity and increased mortality. The latter is evident as both

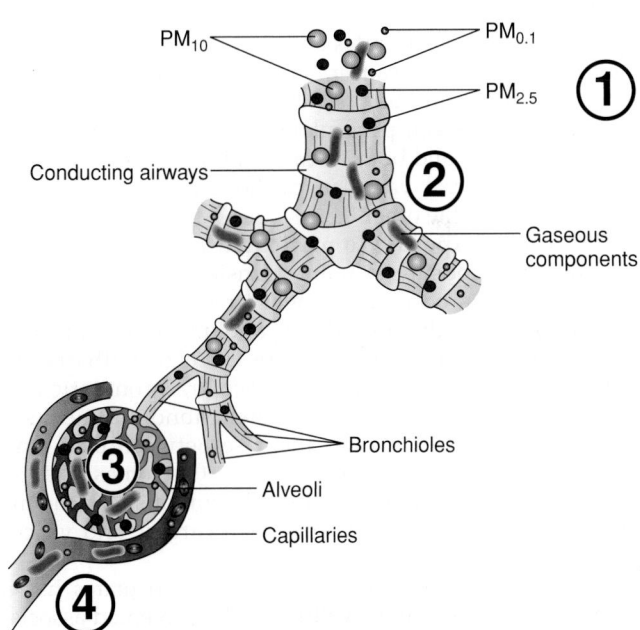

FIGURE 8-17. Fate of inspired pollutant particles. 1. Urban and industrial atmospheric pollution includes gasses and particulate carbon (PM) of various sizes. PM_{10} species (coarse particles) have aerodynamic diameter (AD) between 2.5 μm and 10 μm. $PM_{2.5}$ (fine particles) have AD less than 2.5 μm; and ultrafine particles ($PM_{0.1}$) have AD less than 0.1 μm. **2.** PM_{10} are largely trapped by mucus and cilia in conducting airways. Smaller particles and gasses pass through these airways. **3.** $PM_{2.5}$ deposit in terminal conducting airways and alveoli, where they are commonly engulfed by macrophages and elicit inflammatory responses. **4.** Ultrafine particles ($PM_{0.1}$) and gasses may pass through alveolar walls to enter the capillary circulation and then disseminate throughout the body. $PM_{0.1}$ particles may also deposit in alveolar walls.

---

[2]Estimated 4.3 million deaths from household air pollution and 3.7 million deaths from ambient air pollution for 2012. These deaths include acute lower respiratory disease, chronic obstructive lung disease, ischemic heart disease, stroke and lung cancer, according to WHO, March 24, 2014.

TABLE 8-4

CANCERS ASSOCIATED WITH EXPOSURE TO OCCUPATIONAL CARCINOGENS

Agent or Occupation	Site of Cancer
Arsenic	Lung cancer
Asbestos	Mesothelioma (pleura and peritoneum) Lung cancer (in smokers)
Aromatic amines	Bladder cancer
Benzene	Leukemia, multiple myeloma
bis-(Chloromethyl)ether	Lung cancer
Chromium	Lung cancer
Furniture and shoe manufacturing	Nasal carcinoma
Hematite mining	Lung cancer
Nickel	Lung cancer, paranasal sinus cancer
Tars and oils	Cancers of lung, gastrointestinal tract, bladder and skin
Vinyl chloride	Angiosarcoma of liver

increased overall death rates and more deaths from cardiovascular diseases and cancer. Short- and long-term studies document excess mortality (Table 8-4) and dose-response relationships between particulate concentrations and sizes on the one hand, and both disease and death from cerebrovascular, peripheral vascular, cardiopulmonary and neoplastic causes on the other.

Short-term exposure to particulates. Studies of short-term human exposure examine transient spikes in ambient air pollution occur and, together with particle sizes, are correlated with morbidities and mortality. In such analyses, particulate concentrations correlate with disease and death that involve cardiac, vascular, thrombotic and short-term autonomic nervous system abnormalities (see Fig. 8-18). Daily death rates increase between 0.2% and 0.6% per 10 $\mu g/m^3$ elevation in PM_{10}. Outcomes include acute myocardial infarction, thromboembolism, ischemic stroke, arrhythmias and other related cardiac and vascular diseases.

In addition, short-term exposure to particulates has a strong impact on respiratory illnesses. Documented associations include acute exacerbations of preexisting asthma in children and adults, as well as increased hospital admissions for people who have chronic obstructive pulmonary disease (COPD; see Chapter 18). Particulates measured in these studies were principally PM_{10} and $PM_{2.5}$.

Extended exposure to particulates. Longer-term studies document associations between PM_{10} and $PM_{2.5}$ levels and, for example, lung cancer and more protracted indices of cardiovascular disease. For example, a large study conducted under the auspices of the American Cancer Society showed an average 13% increased risk of lung cancer for each 10-$\mu g/m^3$ increase in $PM_{2.5}$. Increased levels of larger

particulates also correlated with higher rates of lung cancer. Other cancers have been linked as well to occupational exposure to diesel fumes, including bladder tumors and lymphomas.

In addition to neoplastic diseases, long-term studies of the toxicity of particulate pollution have shown increases in, or acceleration of, atherosclerosis and atherogenesis. These nonrespiratory consequences of particulates tend to reflect the ability of ultrafine particles to enter the systemic blood circulation (see below).

PATHOPHYSIOLOGY: The principal mechanisms by which carbon particle pollution exerts these effects appear to relate to inflammation and oxidative stress (Fig. 8-18). Carbon particles are phagocytosed by alveolar macrophages and endothelial cells, thus delivering their toxic and irritative cargoes into cells where they can alter intracellular oxidant concentrations and modify DNA structure. Generalized inflammatory activity is elevated due to delivery of oxidant chemicals, particularly by $PM_{0.1}$ particles.

Lung-related oxidant stress is a product of chemicals bound to larger particles ($PM_{2.5}$, PM_{10}). Postulated mechanisms mediating these pathologies triggered by both short- and longer-term exposures to high levels of particulates are illustrated in Fig. 8-18. Inflammation-mediated activation of clotting, which in this setting often accompanies inhibition of fibrinolysis, plays a large role in these phenomena. For example, ROS facilitate platelet aggregation and fibrin formation at nearby atherosclerotic plaques. Resultant inflammatory cell infiltration can destabilize such plaques and lead to acute cardiac events.

In utero exposure affects developing infants. Intrauterine growth retardation (IUGR) is more common if mothers are exposed to high levels of particulates (PM_{10}, $PM_{2.5}$). Also, increased formation of PAH–DNA adducts occurs in babies born following this kind of exposure. Such adducts are more abundant in newborns who were exposed in utero than in their mothers. This finding suggests that gestating human embryos are more susceptible to chemical DNA alterations than are adults.

MOLECULAR PATHOGENESIS: Genetic polymorphisms—particularly relating to genes encoding antioxidant enzymes—are likely to affect susceptibility to, and development of, diseases related to air pollution. A cohort of asthmatic children in Mexico City, whose disease exacerbations correlated with levels of fine particulates, was found to have mutations in glutathione S-transferase, an enzyme that metabolizes a variety of toxins and that can detoxify reactive oxygen species. Treating these children with antioxidant vitamins C and E led to clinical improvement. Patients with mutations in *GSTP1* and *GSTM1* genes have much higher levels of immunoglobulin E (IgE) and release more histamine in response to allergen challenge during exposure to diesel exhaust.

Mutant forms of other antioxidant enzymes render people increasingly susceptible to airway disease caused by airborne particulates. Among these enzymes is heme oxygenase-1 (*HMOX1*) and NAD(P)H:quinone

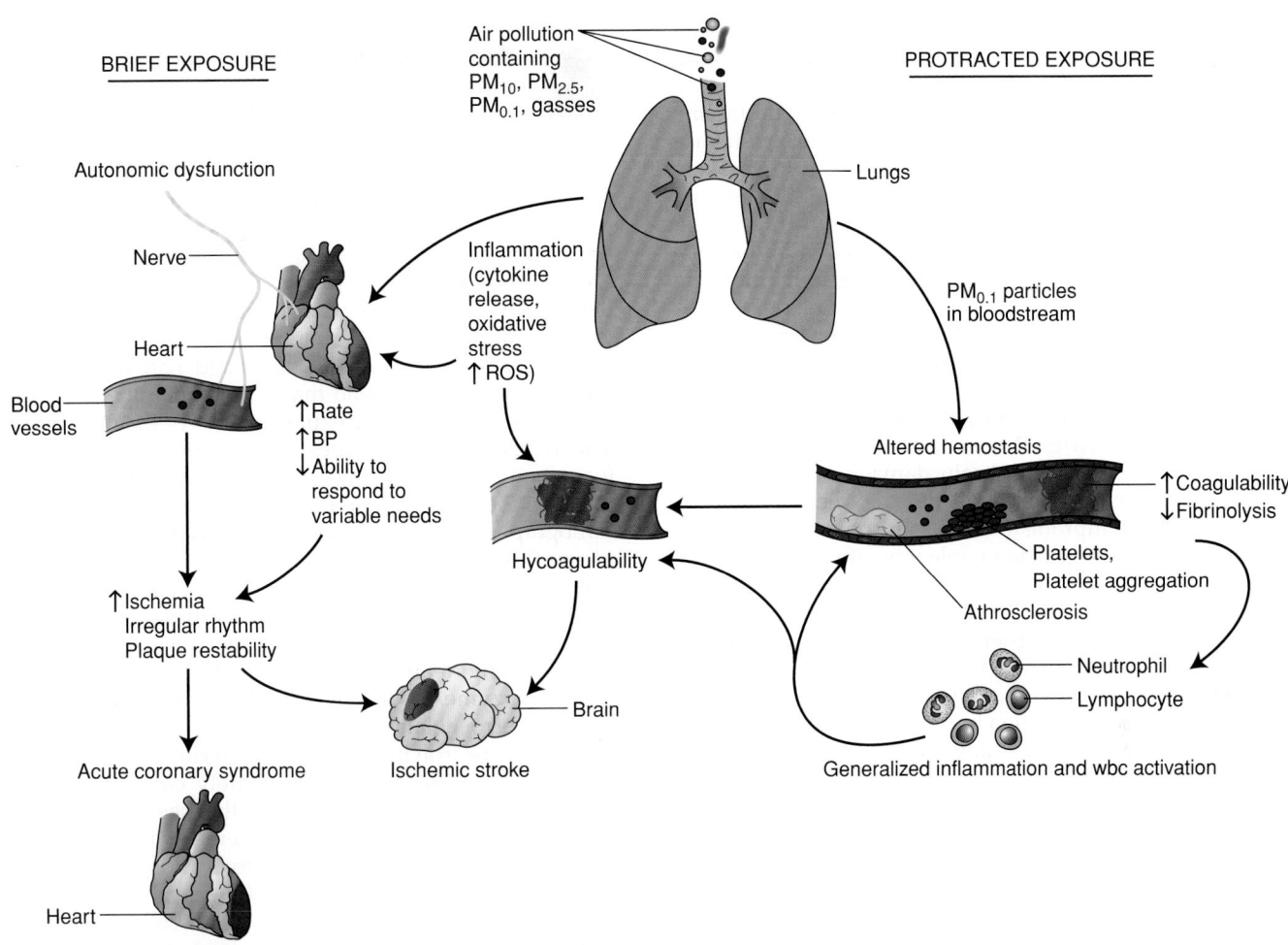

FIGURE 8-18. Pathophysiology relating to cardiovascular and thrombotic consequences of particulate air pollution. These are divided into the consequences of short-term exposure and more extended exposure to particulate air pollution. Carbon particles, especially fine and ultrafine particles, carry toxic and oxidant chemical products of combustion to the distal lungs and the circulation (hence, to blood vessels and the entire body). These affect autonomic responses, elicit inflammation and alter the balance of thrombotic and thrombolytic activities and thus impair hemostasis. The likely pathophysiologic mechanisms mediating the consequences of these derangements after both immediate exposure and protracted exposure are indicated.

oxidoreductase (*NQO1*). Polymorphisms in inflammation-related genes *TLR2* and *TLR4*, encoding toll-like receptors (see Chapters 2 and 4), may also affect the pathogenicity of carbon particulates.

Gasses Associated with Air Pollution

Sulfur Dioxide
Sulfur dioxide (**SO_2**) is highly irritative and may be oxidized to sulfuric acid. SO_2 mainly derives from burning fossil fuels. Acute exposure leads to bronchoconstriction and respiratory tract inflammation. Chronic experimental exposure to high levels of SO_2 may lead to a chronic bronchitis-like syndrome, but it is not clear that there are significant sequelae of human exposure to the concentrations of SO_2 normally found in smog.

Oxides of Nitrogen
Nitrogen oxides are generally written NOx, because they are a mixture of several compounds. They, as well, are derived from burning fossil fuels, especially in generating electricity.

These gases are oxidants and respiratory irritants that induce airway hyperreactivity in acute exposure settings. Adverse effects attributable to chronic atmospheric levels of NOx have not been demonstrated. Tropospheric **ozone** (i.e., ozone near the ground as opposed to in the upper atmosphere) is largely produced by the action of sunlight on NO_2, especially on warm, sunny days. It is a strong oxidant that causes both respiratory (cough, dyspnea) and nonrespiratory (nausea, headache) symptoms on acute exposure. Chronic exposure to ozone in smog is reported to lead to deterioration in pulmonary function and is associated with a slight but significant increase in mortality.

Carbon Monoxide
Carbon monoxide (**CO**) is an odorless and nonirritating gas that results from incomplete combustion of organic substances. Its affinity for hemoglobin is 240 times more than that of oxygen. CO binding to hemoglobin forms carboxyhemoglobin and also increases the affinity of remaining heme moieties for oxygen. Thus, oxygen does not dissociate from such hemoglobin in the tissues as readily

as it should. As a result, hypoxia in CO poisoning is even greater than can be attributed to loss of oxygen-carrying capacity alone.

Atmospheric CO is derived principally from automobile exhaust and does not pose a health problem. Carboxyhemoglobin concentrations under 10% are common in smokers and ordinarily do not produce symptoms. Indoor combustion, however, particularly from space heaters, can generate much higher concentrations of CO, which can be hazardous. Concentrations up to 30% usually cause only headache and mild exertional dyspnea. Higher levels of carboxyhemoglobin lead to confusion and lethargy. Above 50%, coma and convulsions ensue. Levels greater than 60% are usually fatal. In fatal CO poisoning, a characteristic cherry-red color is imparted to the skin by the carboxyhemoglobin in the superficial capillaries. Recovery from severe CO poisoning may be associated with brain damage, which may be manifested as subtle intellectual deficits, memory loss or extrapyramidal symptoms (e.g., parkinsonism). Treatment of acute CO poisoning, as in people who attempt suicide or are trapped in fires, consists principally of the administration of 100% oxygen.

Harmful effects of long-term exposure to low levels of CO have been difficult to substantiate. However, in patients with ischemic heart disease, concentrations of carboxyhemoglobin below 5%–8% (often found in smokers) may accelerate the onset of exertional angina and cause changes in electrocardiograms.

Metals

Metals are an important group of environmental chemicals that have caused disease in humans from ancient times to the present.

Lead

Lead is a ubiquitous heavy metal that is common in the environment of industrialized countries. Before widespread awareness of chronic exposure to lead in the 1950s and 1960s, the classic symptoms of lead poisoning were commonly encountered in children and adults. In the United States, lead poisoning was primarily a pediatric problem related to pica—the habit of chewing on cribs, toys, furniture and woodwork—and eating painted plaster and fallen paint flakes. Most dwellings built before 1940 had lead-containing paint (up to 40% of dry weight) on interior and exterior walls. Children living in dilapidated older homes heavily coated with flaking paint were at significant risk for chronic lead poisoning. To these sources of lead was added a heavy burden of atmospheric lead in the form of dust derived from the combustion of lead-containing gasoline. Children and adults living near point sources of environmental lead contamination, such as smelters, were exposed to even higher levels of lead.

In adults, occupational exposure to lead occurred primarily among those engaged in lead smelting, which releases metal fumes and deposits lead oxide dust in the area. Lead oxide is a constituent of battery grids and an occupational exposure to lead is a hazard in the manufacture and recycling of automobile batteries. Accidental poisonings occasionally occurred from pottery that had been improperly fired with a lead glaze, renovation of old residences heavily coated with lead paint, "moonshine" whiskey made in lead stills or "sniffing" lead-containing gasoline.

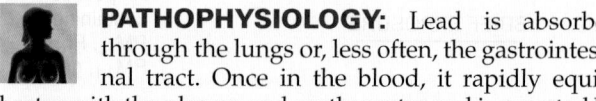

PATHOPHYSIOLOGY: Lead is absorbed through the lungs or, less often, the gastrointestinal tract. Once in the blood, it rapidly equilibrates with the plasma and erythrocytes and is excreted by the kidneys. A portion of blood lead remains freely diffusible. Lead crosses the blood-brain barrier readily, and concentrations in the brain, liver, kidneys and bone marrow are directly related to its toxic effects. It binds sulfhydryl groups and interferes with the activities of zinc (Zn)-dependent enzymes. As well, it interferes with enzymes involved in the synthesis of steroids and cell membranes.

By contrast, bones, teeth, nails and hair represent a tightly bound pool of lead that is not generally regarded as harmful. With chronic exposure, 90% of the total body lead burden is in the bones. During metaphyseal bone formation in children, lead and calcium are deposited to produce the increased bone densities ("lead lines") seen radiographically at the metaphysis, thus providing a simple method of detecting increased body stores of lead in children.

Anemia is a cardinal sign of lead intoxication. Lead disrupts heme synthesis in bone marrow erythroblasts by inhibiting δ-aminolevulinic acid dehydratase, the second enzyme in de novo synthesis of heme. It also inhibits ferrochelatase, which catalyzes the incorporation of ferrous iron into the porphyrin ring. The resulting inability to produce heme adequately causes a microcytic and hypochromic anemia like that seen in iron deficiency (see Chapter 26), in which heme synthesis is also impaired. The anemia of lead intoxication also entails prominent basophilic stippling of erythrocytes, reflecting clustering of ribosomes. Red blood cell life span is decreased; thus, lead intoxication leads to anemia due to ineffective hematopoiesis and accelerated erythrocyte turnover.

PATHOLOGY: Classic lead overexposure, which is rarely seen in the United States today, affects many organs, but its major toxicity involves dysfunction in (1) the nervous system, (2) the kidneys and (3) hematopoiesis (Fig. 8-19).

The brain is the target of lead toxicity in children; adults usually present with manifestation of peripheral neuropathy. Children with lead encephalopathy are typically irritable and ataxic. They may convulse or display altered states of consciousness, from drowsiness to frank coma. Children with blood lead levels above 80 μg/dL, but with concentrations lower than those in children with frank encephalopathy (120 μg/dL), exhibit mild CNS symptoms such as clumsiness, irritability and hyperactivity.

Lead encephalopathy is a condition in which the brain is edematous and displays flattened gyri and compressed ventricles. There may be herniation of the uncus and cerebellar tonsils. Microscopically, congestion, petechial hemorrhages and foci of neuronal necrosis are seen. A diffuse astrocytic proliferation in both the gray and white matter may accompany these changes. Vascular lesions in the brain are particularly prominent, with capillary dilation and proliferation.

Peripheral motor neuropathy is the most common manifestation of lead neurotoxicity in the adult, typically affecting

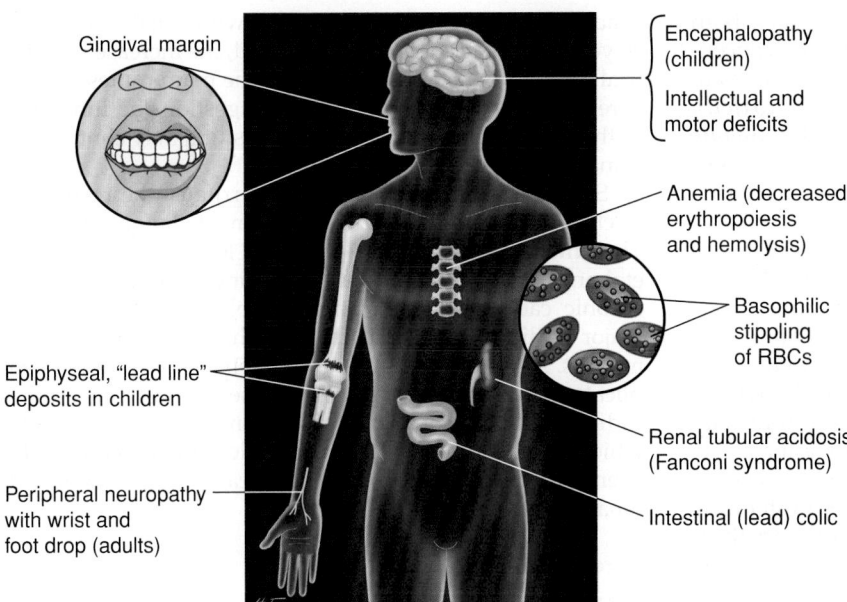

Gingival margin

Encephalopathy (children)

Intellectual and motor deficits

Anemia (decreased erythropoiesis and hemolysis)

Basophilic stippling of RBCs

Epiphyseal, "lead line" deposits in children

Renal tubular acidosis (Fanconi syndrome)

Intestinal (lead) colic

Peripheral neuropathy with wrist and foot drop (adults)

FIGURE 8-19. Complications of lead intoxication.

the radial and peroneal nerves and resulting in **wristdrop** and **footdrop**, respectively. Lead-induced neuropathy is probably also the basis of the paroxysms of gastrointestinal pain known as **lead colic**.

Lead nephropathy reflects the toxic effect of the metal on the proximal tubular cells of the kidney. The resulting dysfunction is characterized by aminoaciduria, glycosuria and hyperphosphaturia (Fanconi syndrome). Such functional alterations are accompanied by the formation of inclusion bodies in the nuclei of the proximal tubular cells. These inclusions are characteristic of lead nephropathy and are composed of a lead–protein complex containing more than 100 times the concentration of lead in the whole kidney.

Lead poisoning is treated with chelating agents such as ethylene diamine tetra-acetic acid (EDTA), either alone or in combination with dimercaprol (BAL). Both the hematologic and renal manifestations of lead intoxication are usually reversible; alterations in the CNS are generally irreversible.

Laboratory diagnosis is made by demonstrating high blood levels of lead and increased free erythrocyte protoporphyrin. Elevated urinary excretion of δ-aminolevulinic acid and decreased levels of aminolevulinic acid dehydratase in erythrocytes are confirmatory.

EFFECTS OF CHRONIC EXPOSURE TO LOW LEAD LEVELS: Owing to the removal of lead from gasoline, improvements in housing, substitution of titanium for lead in paints and control of industrial point sources, ambient levels of lead have fallen significantly: blood levels in the general population of the United States decreased from an average of 16 µg/dL in 1976 to 1.0 µg/dL in 2000. It has been established that cumulative exposure to lead is best measured in bone, rather than blood. The latter lead levels reflect more ongoing exposure. Thus, elevated bone levels of lead have been correlated with adult hypertension, while no relationship has been established with blood levels. The dramatic fall in mean blood lead levels has been accompanied by the near elimination of lead-related childhood fatalities and encephalopathy. However, low lead exposure in children, while not producing recognizable symptoms, may permanently decrease cognitive performance. The regulatory

safe threshold for blood levels of lead in children has been progressively reduced and is now thought to be below 10 µg/dL.

Efforts to reduce environmental lead have led to decreases in the percentage of children in the United States with blood levels of 10 µg/dL of lead or more from 88% in the 1970s to 4.4% in the 1990s. However, high blood lead concentrations remain a problem among poor, mainly urban, children, and vigorous campaigns to address this situation are justified.

Mercury

Inorganic mercury has been used since prehistoric times and has been known to be an occupation-related hazard at least since the Middle Ages, but in recent years it has become recognized that organic mercury represents a greater risk to human health. Although mercury poisoning still occurs in some occupations, there has been increasing concern over the potential health hazards brought about by the contamination of many ecosystems following several well-known outbreaks of methylmercury poisoning. The most widely publicized episodes occurred in Japan, first in Minamata Bay in the 1950s and then in Niigata. In both cases, local inhabitants developed severe, chronic organic mercury intoxication. This poisoning was traced to the consumption of fish contaminated with mercury that had been discharged into the environment in the effluents from a fertilizer and a plastics factory. Children exposed in utero showed delayed developmental milestones and abnormal reflexes, despite the fact that fetal exposure was estimated to be 1/5 to 1/10 that in adults.

Mercury released into the environment may be bioconcentrated and enter the food chain. Bacteria in bays and oceans can convert inorganic mercury compounds from industrial wastes into highly neurotoxic organomercurials. These compounds are then transferred up the food chain and are eventually concentrated in the large predatory fish (e.g., tuna, pike) that make up a substantial part of the diet in many countries.

Although inorganic mercury is not efficiently absorbed in the gastrointestinal tract, organic mercurial compounds are readily taken up because of their lipid solubility. Both inorganic and organic mercury are preferentially concentrated in the kidney and methylmercury also distributes to the brain. *The kidney is the principal target of the toxicity of inorganic mercury, but the brain is damaged by organic mercurials.* Claims that mercuric preservatives in vaccines cause autism or other neurologic complications have been proven false.

NEPHROTOXICITY: At one time, mercuric chloride was widely used as an antiseptic and acute mercuric chloride poisoning was much more common; the compound was ingested by accident or for suicidal purposes. Under such circumstances, **proximal tubular necrosis** was accompanied by oliguric renal failure. Mercurial diuretics were also widely prescribed in the past and chronic mercury nephrotoxicity was a not uncommon complication of their long-term use. Today, chronic mercurial nephrotoxicity is almost always a consequence of long-term industrial exposure. Proteinuria is common in chronic mercurial nephrotoxicity and there may be a nephrotic syndrome with more severe intoxication. Pathologically, there is a membranous glomerulonephritis with subepithelial electron-dense deposits, suggesting immune complex deposition.

NEUROTOXICITY: The neurologic effects of mercury are manifested as a constriction of visual fields, paresthesias, ataxia, dysarthria and hearing loss. Pathologically, there is cerebral and cerebellar atrophy. Microscopically, the cerebellum exhibits atrophy of the granular layer, without loss of Purkinje cells and spongy softenings in the visual cortex and other cortical regions.

Arsenic

The toxic properties of arsenic have been known for centuries. Arsenic-containing compounds have been widely used as insecticides, weed killers and wood preservatives. Arsenicals may also contaminate soil and leach into ground water as a result of naturally occurring arsenic-rich rock formations, from coal burning or from use of arsenical pesticides. As with mercury, there is evidence for the bioaccumulation of arsenic along the food chain.

Acute arsenic poisoning is almost always the result of accidental or homicidal ingestion. Death is due to **CNS toxicity**. Chronic arsenic intoxication affects many organ systems. It is characterized initially by such nonspecific symptoms as malaise and fatigue. Eventually, gastrointestinal, cardiovascular and hematologic dysfunction become evident. Both encephalopathy and peripheral neuropathy develop. The latter is characterized by paresthesias, motor palsies and painful neuritis. On epidemiologic grounds, **cancers of the skin, respiratory tract** and **gastrointestinal tract** have been attributed to industrial and agricultural exposure to arsenic. In some parts of the world, exposure of workers in rice paddies to arsenic in the ground water has been associated with skin cancers. Rare cases of hepatic angiosarcomas have been related to chronic arsenic exposure.

Cadmium

Cadmium is used in ever-increasing quantities in manufacturing alloys, producing rechargeable batteries and electroplating other metals (e.g., automobile parts and musical instruments). It is a plasticizer and a pigment. Cadmium oxide fumes are released in the course of welding steel parts previously plated with a cadmium anticorrosive.

It accumulates in the human body, with a half-life of over 20 years, and since it is rarely recycled, the increase in industrial use of the metal is of concern. The main routes of exposure for the general population are ingestion and inhalation. Both plant- and animal-derived foodstuffs may contain substantial levels of cadmium.

Short-term cadmium inhalation irritates the respiratory tract, with pulmonary edema the most dangerous result. The lungs and the kidneys and, to a lesser extent, the skeletal and vascular systems are the principal target organs of chronic cadmium intoxication. Emphysema has been the major finding in the fatal cases of chronic cadmium pneumonitis. Although the confounding effects of smoking complicate interpretation of some of these studies, inhalation of cadmium does appear to lead to lung cancer. Proteinuria, which reflects tubular rather than glomerular damage, has been the most consistent finding in cadmium workers with renal damage.

Chromium

Chromium (Cr) is used extensively in several industries, including metal plating and some types of manufacturing. Although it occurs in any number of oxidation states, only Cr(III) and Cr(VI) are commonly used industrially. Its toxicity is usually a result of inhalation and the consequences of exposure depend on the solubility of the specific salt. Although acute intoxication is known, it is chronic exposure that is most problematic.

Cr(VI) is highly genotoxic. People who chronically inhale salts of hexavalent chromium have an increased risk of lung cancer and possibly other tumors as well. The less soluble chromate salts are generally more potent pulmonary carcinogens, particularly zinc chromate.

Nickel

Nickel is a widely used metal in electronics, coins, steel alloys, batteries and food processing. Dermatitis ("nickel itch"), the most frequent effect of exposure to nickel, may occur from direct contact with metals containing nickel, such as coins and costume jewelry. The dermatitis is a sensitization reaction; the body reacts to nickel-conjugated proteins formed following the penetration of the epidermis by nickel ions. Exposure to nickel, as to arsenic, increases the risk of development of specific types of cancer. Epidemiologic studies have demonstrated that workers who were occupationally exposed to nickel compounds have an increased incidence of lung cancer and cancer of the nasal cavities.

Iron

Iron-deficiency anemia is a common disease, particularly in premenopausal women. Oral iron preparations contain largely ferrous sulfate, the form absorbed by the gastrointestinal mucosa and then converted to the trivalent form. Acute ferrous sulfate poisoning from accidental ingestion occurs, mainly in children between the ages of 1 and 2 years. As little as 1–2 g of ferrous sulfate may be lethal, but most fatal cases follow ingestion of 3–10 g. Hemorrhagic gastritis and acute liver necrosis have been the most prominent findings at autopsy.

Long-term, excessive dietary intake of iron does not ordinarily lead to abnormal iron accumulation. South African Bantus have a significant incidence of iron overload, which has been attributed to a diet very high in iron, largely derived from iron drums used to prepare home-made beer. The acidic pH of these brews readily solubilizes the iron and their low alcohol content allows large volumes to be consumed. A large proportion of the excess iron is in the liver, and there is a correlation between the degree of siderosis and the presence of cirrhosis. There is also a high incidence of diabetes and heart disease in this "Bantu siderosis."

However, some blacks have shown a similar syndrome, which now is attributed to a mutation in the gene for ferroportin (SLC4A1) that may predispose some people of African descent to iron overload (see Chapter 20).

Cobalt

Acute occupational inhalation of cobalt has led to acute respiratory distress syndrome (see Chapter 18). In addition, excessive intake of cobalt in beer that contained it to enhance foaming qualities was implicated in a degenerative disease of heart muscle (cardiomyopathy; see Chapter 17). When the cobalt was removed from the beer, no further cases of heart disease were reported.

Radioactive Elements

Elements whose radioactive isotopes are potentially hazardous include radium, strontium, uranium, plutonium, thorium and iodine. Chronic toxicities relate principally to radiation-induced carcinogenesis. The individual tumors reflect the organ localization of the elements and are discussed in the chapters that address specific organ pathology.

Biological Toxins Are Organisms and Their Nonviable Components

These toxins are mostly of microbial, algal, plant, protozoan, arthropod or mammalian origin. They include whole organisms, intact particulate or soluble products of those organisms (e.g., exotoxins) and fragments of organisms. Adverse reactions may result from inhalation, ingestion or other contact, and they may reflect infectious, hypersensitivity and toxic effects of those materials. This discussion addresses the latter. Infectious and hypersensitivity reactions to foreign matter are considered in Chapters 9 and 4, respectively, as well as individual organ-specific discussions (e.g., hypersensitivity pneumonitis in Chapter 18).

The toxic effects of microbial products are the best characterized of biological toxicities. **Organic dust toxic syndrome** (ODTS) is a systemic reaction to the direct toxicities of many, mainly fungal, toxins. It consists of flu-like symptoms (fever, malaise, etc.), often with a respiratory component (dyspnea, cough). Unlike hypersensitivity pneumonitis, ODTS appears to reflect cell death and the consequent acute inflammatory reaction. It is usually associated with toxins produced by many common fungi.

Aspergillus, Stachybotrys, Penicillium and *Fusarium* spp. are the most common culprits. These fungi are particularly abundant in water-damaged buildings and moist warm environments. Their mycotoxins include trichothecenes and β-1,3-glucans, which may elicit disease by ingestion and inhalational routes.

One particular toxin produced by *Aspergillus flavus* and *Aspergillus parasiticus,* called **aflatoxin,** is highly hepatotoxic and is recognized as a potent hepatocarcinogen. There are several known varieties of aflatoxin.

Bacterial endotoxins are lipopolysaccharides derived from Gram-negative bacterial cell walls. They are often complexed with proteins and phospholipids. Injected endotoxins are used experimentally to elicit inflammatory and febrile responses characterized by local or systemic macrophage activation. Inhaled, these compounds elicit profuse pulmonary inflammatory responses, involving release of inflammatory mediators (tumor necrosis factor-α [TNF-α], interleukin-1 [IL-1], etc.), causing fever, pneumonitis and pulmonary edema.

The subject of biological toxins is of considerable concern because of possible weaponization for use in biological warfare (see Chapter 9).

THERMAL REGULATORY DYSFUNCTION

Hypothermia Is a Decrease in Body Temperature below 35°C (95°F)

Hypothermia can result in systemic or focal injury, the latter exemplified by **trench foot** or **immersion foot.** In localized hypothermia of these types, actual tissue freezing does not occur. **Frostbite,** by contrast, involves the crystallization of tissue water.

Generalized Hypothermia

Hypothermia may occur in a number of settings, including immersion in cold water and exposure to extremely cold air temperatures, especially after taking agents that impair thermoregulation, such as alcohol and some drugs and pharmacologic agents. Perhaps the best-studied cause of hypothermia is cold water immersion. Acute immersion in water at 4°C–10°C (39.2°F–50°F) reduces central blood flow. Coupled with decreased core body temperature and cooling of the blood perfusing the brain, this results in mental confusion. Tetany makes swimming impossible. Furthermore, increased vagal discharge leads to premature ventricular contractions, ventricular arrhythmias and even fibrillation.

Attempting to increase heat production, the immersed body immediately responds by increasing muscle activity and oxygen consumption. However, there are limits to the sources of energy available for sustained warming. Within 30 minutes, heat loss exceeds heat production because of the combination of high direct conduction of heat from the whole skin surface and altered muscle tone caused by decreased arterial carbon dioxide and exhaustion. Core temperature then begins to fall. Peripheral vasoconstriction is another response to conserve heat. In addition, there is an increased sympathetic neural discharge, resulting in increased heart and basal metabolic rates and shivering. When the core temperature approaches 35°C, this activity may be three to six times above normal. Below 35°C, respiratory rate, heart rate and blood pressure decline because the functional reserve is reduced.

With prolonged cooling, a "cold-induced" diuresis results in increased blood viscosity. As a result, blood flow decreases and oxygen–hemoglobin association is less effective. Cardiac stroke volume decreases and peripheral vascular resistance increases as a direct result of both blood "sludging" and loss of plasma. The most important factor in causing death is cardiac arrhythmia or sudden cardiac arrest. These observations have been confirmed and extended, largely because of the need to induce hypothermia in some patients undergoing open-heart surgery. In fact, with careful pharmacologic control, prolonged periods of lower body temperature can be achieved with no residual harm.

If hypothermia is prolonged, decreased body temperature alters cerebrovascular function. When body core temperature reaches 32°C (89.6°F), the person becomes lethargic, apathetic and withdrawn. A characteristic response is inappropriate behavior, including disrobing, even when cold. If temperature falls further, intermittent "stupor" and eventually coma supervene. If core temperature goes below 28°C (82.4°F), pulse and breathing weaken.

Although there are no specific morphologic changes in those who die from hypothermia, the skin shows red and purple discolorations, ears and hands swell and there is irregular vasoconstriction and vasodilation. Areas of cardiac myocytolysis are seen. Lungs may display pulmonary edema and intra-alveolar, intrabronchial and interstitial hemorrhage.

Focal Thermal Alterations

As discussed above, local reduction in tissue temperature, particularly in the skin, is associated with local vasoconstriction. Tissue water crystallizes if blood circulation is insufficient to counter persistent thermal loss. When freezing occurs slowly, ice crystals form within tissue cells and in the interstitial space. Concomitantly, electrolyte-rich gels are excluded. Injury to cellular organelles reflects the drastic changes in ion concentrations in the excluded volume. Denaturation of macromolecules and physical disruption of cellular membranes by the ice ensue. When freezing is rapid, a gel-like structure forms within the cell that lacks water crystalloids. This water-solid reduces the extent of mechanical and chemical injury. The most significant cellular damage apparently occurs on thawing, when mechanical disruption of membrane structures occurs, perhaps the result of transformation from a gel to a crystal.

The most biologically significant cell injury appears in the endothelial lining of the capillaries and venules, which alters small vessel permeability. This injury initiates extravasation of plasma, formation of localized edema and blisters and an inflammatory reaction. While frostbite results from the actual freezing of water, immersion foot (trench foot) is caused by a prolonged reduction in tissue temperature to a point not low enough to freeze tissue. This cooling causes cellular disruption. Endothelial cell damage leads to local thrombosis and changes caused by altered permeability are prominent. Vascular occlusion often leads to gangrene.

Hyperthermia Means an Increase in Body Temperature

Tissue responses to hyperthermia are similar in some respects to those caused by freezing injuries. In both instances, injury to the vascular endothelium results in altered vascular permeability, edema and blisters. The degree of injury depends on the extent of temperature elevation and how quickly it is reached. Small increases in body temperature increase the metabolic rate. However, above a certain limit, enzymes denature and other proteins precipitate and "melting" of lipid bilayers of cell membranes takes place.

Systemic Hyperthermia

Systemic hyperthermia, or **fever,** is an elevation of body core temperature. It occurs because of (1) increased heat production, (2) decreased elimination of heat from the body (reflecting an aberrant response of the thermal regulatory center) or (3) a disturbance of the thermal regulatory center itself. Hyperthermia can also occur because heat is conducted into the body faster than the system can clear it.

A body temperature above 42.5°C (108.5°F) leads to profound functional disturbances, including general vasodilation, inefficient cardiac function and altered respiration. Isolated heart–lung preparations fail at about the same temperature, suggesting an inherent limitation in the cardiovascular system and perhaps in the myocardial cells themselves. *In general, systemic temperature elevations above 42°C (107.6°F) are not compatible with life.*

During infectious and inflammatory responses, several cytokines, including IL-1, IL-6 and TNF-α, interact with a portion of the hypothalamus at the roof of the third ventricle and apparently reset the body's "thermostat" to permit a higher body core temperature. There is also evidence that for mild pyrogens, parasympathetic activation may be involved.

Few, if any, defined pathologic changes are associated with fever alone. Physical findings include increased heart and respiratory rates, peripheral vasodilation and diaphoresis, all recognized mechanisms for thermal regulation. The CNS may respond with irritability, restlessness and (particularly in children) convulsions. Nocturnal temperature elevations with "night sweats" are a feature of pulmonary granulomatous infection (especially tuberculosis) and are also observed in lymphoproliferative diseases. Prolonged temperature elevation can produce wasting, principally because of an increased metabolic rate.

Malignant hyperthermia is a thermal alteration, accompanied by a hypermetabolic state and often by rhabdomyolysis (muscle necrosis), which occurs after anesthesia in susceptible people. This autosomal dominant disorder is associated with at least 70 different mutations in the gene for the sarcoplasmic reticulum ryanodine receptor (RYR1). A less common mutation causing malignant hyperthermia occurs in the gene for the α-subunit of the L-type voltage-gated calcium channel (CACNA1S). Muscle damage is caused by an abnormally high calcium concentration produced by accelerated release of Ca^{2+} through the mutant calcium release channel. After the introduction of treatment with dantrolene, which binds to the ryanodine receptor, mortality from malignant hyperthermia fell from 80% to less than 10%.

Heat stroke is a form of hyperthermia that occurs under conditions of very high ambient temperatures and is not mediated by endogenous pyrogens. It reflects impaired thermal regulatory cooling responses and characteristically occurs in infants, young children and the very aged. Often the disorder is associated with an underlying chronic illness and use of diuretics, tranquilizers that may affect the hypothalamic thermal regulatory center or drugs that inhibit perspiration. Another form of heat stroke is seen in healthy men during unusually vigorous exercise. Lactic acidosis, hypocalcemia and rhabdomyolysis may be severe problems, and almost 1/3 of patients with exertional heat stroke develop myoglobinuric acute renal failure. Heat stroke is not amenable to treatment with standard antipyretics, and only external cooling and fluid and electrolyte replacement are effective therapy.

Cutaneous Burns

Cutaneous burns are the most common form of localized hyperthermia. Both the elevated temperature and rate of temperature change are important in determining the tissue response. A temperature of 50°C (120°F) may be sustained for 10 minutes or more without cell death, while a temperature of 70°C (158°F) or higher for even several seconds causes necrosis of the entire epidermis.

Cutaneous burns have been separated into full-thickness (previously, third-degree) and partial thickness (previously, first- and second-degree) burns (Fig. 8-20).

■ **Full-thickness burns** char both epidermis and dermis. Histologically, they are carbonized and cellular structure is lost.

FIRST DEGREE

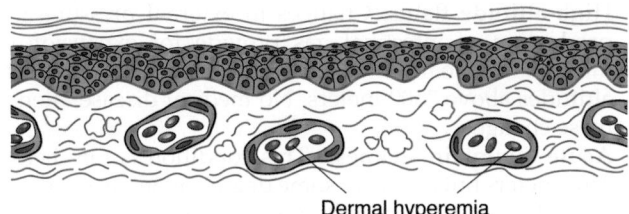

Dermal hyperemia

SECOND DEGREE

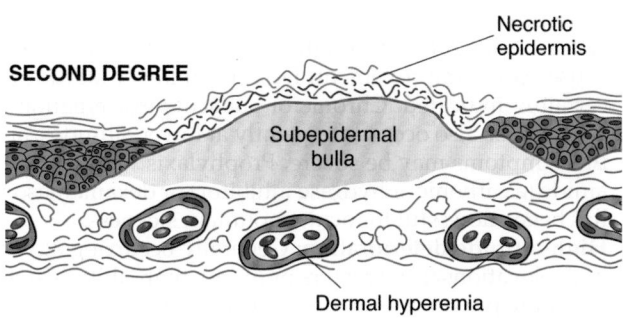

Necrotic epidermis

Subepidermal bulla

Dermal hyperemia

THIRD DEGREE

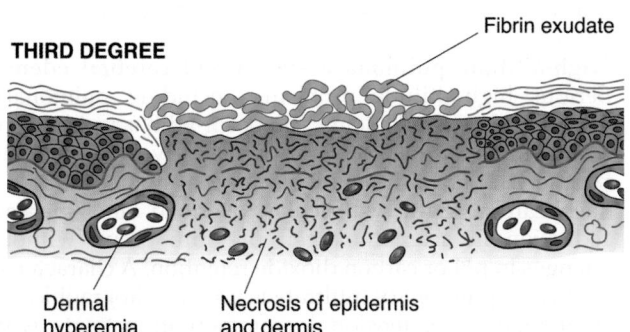

Fibrin exudate

Dermal hyperemia

Necrosis of epidermis and dermis

FIGURE 8-20. The pathology of cutaneous burns. A first-degree skin burn exhibits only dilation of the dermal blood vessels. In a second-degree burn, there is necrosis of the epidermis and subepidermal edema collects under the necrotic epidermis to form a bulla. In a third-degree burn, both the epidermis and dermis are necrotic.

Among the most important functions of the skin are fluid retention and protection from infectious agents. Not surprisingly, then, when skin is severely damaged, its ability to subserve these functions is compromised. One of the most serious systemic disturbances caused by extensive cutaneous burns is fluid loss. Patients with full-thickness burns can lose about 0.3 mL of body water/cm^2 of burned area per day. Resulting hemoconcentration and poor vascular perfusion of the skin and other viscera complicate the recovery of these patients. Many severely burned people, particularly those with more than 70% of their body surface involved with full-thickness burns, develop shock and acute tubular necrosis of the kidneys and mortality is very high. Severely burned patients who survive longer are at great risk of lethal surface infections and sepsis. Even normal skin saprophytes may cause infection of charred tissue and pose another difficulty for healing.

Healing of cutaneous burns is related to the extent of tissue destruction. Mild partial thickness burns, by definition, have little if any cell loss and healing requires only repair or replacement of injured endothelial cells. More severe partial thickness burns also heal without a scar because epidermal basal cells remain and are a source of regenerating cells for the epithelium. Full-thickness burns, in which the entire thickness of the epidermis is destroyed, pose a separate set of problems. If the skin appendages are spared, re-epithelialization can arise from them. Initially, islands of proliferation at the orifices of these glands grow and coalesce to cover the surface. Deeper burns that destroy the skin appendages require new epidermis to be grafted to the débrided area to establish a functional covering. Burned skin that is not replaced by a graft heals with dense scarring. Since this scar tissue lacks the elasticity of normal skin, contractures that limit motion may eventually result.

Inhalation Burns

People trapped in burning buildings and vehicles are exposed to air and aerosolized flammable materials heated to very high temperatures. Inhalation of these noxious fumes injures or destroys respiratory tract epithelium from the oral cavity to the alveoli. If a patient survives the acute episode, acute respiratory distress syndrome (ARDS), which itself may be fatal (see Chapter 18), may develop.

Electrical Burns

Electrical injury produces damage through (1) electrical dysfunction of cardiovascular conduction and the nervous system and (2) conversion of electrical energy to heat energy when the current encounters the resistance of the tissues. *Because electrical energy can potentially disrupt the electrical system within the heart, it frequently causes death through ventricular fibrillation.* The amount of current necessary for such a disruption depends in part on its pathway through the body and its ease in penetrating the skin. Someone who inadvertently touches a 120-V line in a living room may suffer burns on the hand because the skin that contacts the wire has substantial resistance to the flow of electrical current. If that resistance is decreased, as when a person inadvertently touches the same line in a bathtub, the lower resistance increases transmitted current, leading to disordered cardiac electrical activity.

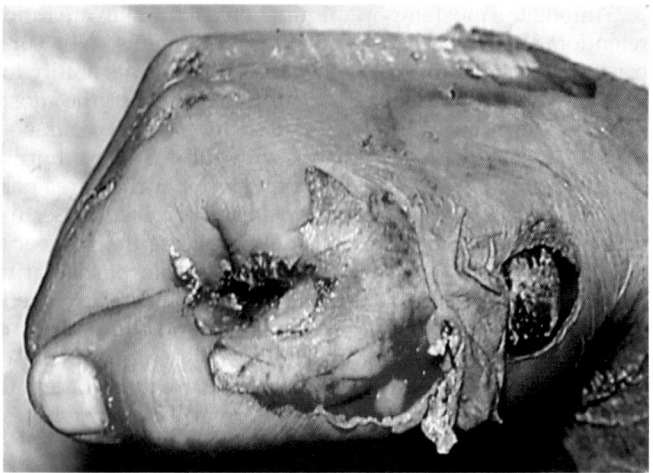

FIGURE 8-21. Electrical burn of the skin. The victim was electrocuted after attempting to stop a fall from a ladder by grasping a high-voltage electrical line.

Electrical burns of the skin reflect the voltage, the area of electrical conductance and the duration of current flow (Fig. 8-21). Very–high-voltage current chars tissue and produces a third-degree burn. On the other hand, broad, moist surfaces exposed to the same flow exhibit less-severe change. With exposure to very–high-voltage currents, the force may be almost "explosive," in which case vaporization of tissue water produces extensive damage.

ALTITUDE-RELATED ILLNESSES

High-altitude illness is rare, in large part because mountain climbers tend to acclimate before extreme altitudes are achieved. However, there is an altitude limit beyond which human life cannot be sustained for prolonged periods. Communities in the Andes succeed at 4000 to 4300 meters (13,124 to 14,108 ft). Inhabitants adapt to the decreased pressure and availability of oxygen by developing elevated hematocrits and large "barrel" chests with increased lung volume. Even those who live in this zone do not survive at elevations above 5500 to 6000 meters (18,045 to 19,686 ft). Prolonged stays at this altitude result in weight loss, difficulty in sleeping and lethargy, perhaps because of the redirection of cellular energy simply for survival. For example, 75%–90% of the oxygen available at 6000 meters is used simply for the effort of inspiration.

The modifications induced by high altitude are related to decreased atmospheric pressure and consequent decreased oxygen availability. Unlike sea level, where activity does not change oxygen saturation, physical activity at these elevations leads to decreased partial pressure of arterial oxygen. At sea level, cardiac output limits exercise; at high altitudes, the diffusing capacity of the lung for oxygen seems to be the determinant.

Acclimation to chronic hypoxia at high altitudes results in a reduced ventilatory drive. Acclimated people exhibit increases in (1) capillaries per unit volume of brain, muscle and myocardium; (2) myoglobin within tissues; (3) mitochondria per cell; and (4) hematocrit. An increase in erythrocyte levels of 2'3'-diphosphoglycerate, which enhances oxygen delivery to tissues, occurs within hours, but

polycythemia takes months. Some of the minor effects of high altitude are systemic edema, retinal hemorrhages and flatulence. The more serious nonfatal diseases are acute and chronic mountain sickness and high-altitude deterioration. Fatal **high-altitude pulmonary edema** and **high-altitude encephalopathy** may ensue.

- **High-altitude systemic edema:** This condition results from asymptomatic increases in vascular permeability, particularly in hands, face and feet and most often at elevations over 3000 meters. It is reflected only in weight gain; on return to lower altitude, diuresis causes the edema to disappear. This disorder may in part reflect endothelial cell responses to hypoxia and is twice as common in women as in men. A calcium channel blocker has been used as treatment.

- **High-altitude retinal hemorrhage:** A critical analysis by funduscopic examination revealed that 30%–60% of those sleeping above 5000 meters had retinal hemorrhages. The initial effect includes retinal vascular engorgement and tortuousness. Optic disc hyperemia is also noted and multiple flame-shaped hemorrhages subsequently occur. These changes are reversible.

- **High-altitude flatus:** Changes in external pressure and production of intestinal gas provide for expansion of intestinal luminal contents and lead to increased flatus at altitudes above 3500 meters. No medical disease attends these changes.

- **Acute mountain sickness:** This condition is rare below 2500 meters but occurs to some degree in nearly everyone at 3000 to 3600 meters. Initial presentation includes headache, lassitude, anorexia, weakness and difficulty sleeping. The underlying pathophysiology is in part related to hypoxia and shifts in plasma fluid to the interstitial space. Adaptation through increased respiratory rate causes some improvement. Descent to lower altitudes is certainly indicated. Chronic or subacute exacerbation of this disease also occurs, frequently at lower altitudes, and the symptoms may be severe. Prophylaxis with acetazolamide (a carbonic anhydrase inhibitor) or dexamethasone has been successful for acute mountain sickness.

- **High-altitude deterioration:** Generally occurring at very high elevations (5500 meters or more), high-altitude deterioration presents as a decrease in physical and mental performance. The combination of chronic hypoxia, inadequate fluid intake, inadequate nutrition, decreased plasma volume and hemoconcentration are aggravating factors.

- **High-altitude pulmonary edema and cerebral edema:** Serious high-altitude problems, including pulmonary edema and cerebral edema, can occur with a rapid ascent to heights over 2500 meters, particularly in susceptible people who have difficulty sleeping at higher altitudes. Tachycardia, right ventricular overload and marked reduction in arterial oxygen pressure occur, without changes in pH or carbon dioxide retention. A characteristic patchy pulmonary infiltrate is noted radiographically. Pulmonary hypertension is common in patients with high-altitude pulmonary edema. Hypoxic vasoconstriction and intravascular thrombosis have been proposed as causes of pulmonary hypertension. Eventually, cardiac output is decreased and systemic blood pressure falls. The precapillary arterioles become dilated, increasing capillary bed pressure and inducing interstitial and alveolar edema. Autopsy findings include severe confluent pulmonary edema, proteinaceous alveolar exudates and hyaline membrane formation. Capillary obstruction by thrombi has been noted. A dilated heart and enlarged pulmonary arteries are commonly found.

- **High-altitude encephalopathy** is characterized by confusion, stupor and coma. Autopsies reveal cerebral edema and vascular congestion. A proposed mechanism is severe cerebral hypoxia, with inhibition of the sodium pump and resultant intracellular edema.

PHYSICAL INJURIES

The effect of mechanical trauma is related to (1) the force transmitted to the tissue, (2) the rate at which the transfer occurs, (3) the surface area to which the force is transferred and (4) the area of the body involved. The compressibility of the tissue adjacent to the transmitted force in part determines its effect. However, transmission of absorbed energy can produce alterations elsewhere in the body. Blows over a hollow viscus can rupture the organ because of compression of the fluid or gas it contains; organs nestled beneath the skin, such as the liver, can be easily ruptured. An impact directly over the heart can even disturb its electrical systems. However, a blow over a large muscle mass, such as the thigh or upper arm, is often less injurious than a direct blow to a poorly shielded bone, such as the anterior tibia. Furthermore, the distribution of the force is important.

A Contusion Is a Localized Mechanical Injury with Focal Hemorrhage

A force with sufficient energy may disrupt capillaries and venules within an organ by physical means alone. The result may be so limited that the only histologic change is hemorrhage in tissue spaces outside the vascular compartment. A discrete extravascular blood pool within the tissue is called a **hematoma**. Initially, the deoxygenated blood renders the area blue to blue-black, as in the classic "black eye." Macrophages ingest the erythrocytes, convert their hemoglobin to bilirubin and so change the color from blue to yellow. Both

mobilization of the pigment by macrophages and further metabolism of bilirubin cause the yellow to fade to yellowish green and then to disappear.

An Abrasion Is a Skin Defect Caused by Crushes or Scrapes

The disruptive force may provide a portal of entry for microorganisms. The impact of the agent and its configuration are frequently seen in these wounds and are of special interest to the forensic pathologist.

A Laceration Is a Split or Tear of the Skin

Lacerations result from an impact stronger than that causing an abrasion and are usually the result of unidirectional displacement. When they have crushed margins, they are called **abraded lacerations**.

Wounds Are Mechanical Disruptions of Tissue Integrity

An incision is a deliberate opening in the skin by a cutting instrument (e.g., a surgeon's scalpel). Incisions have sharp edges and, importantly, spare no tissue to the depth of the wound. **Deep penetrating wounds** made by high-velocity projectiles, such as bullets, are often deceptive, because the energy of the missile as it passes through the body may be released at sites distant from the entrance itself. Bullets, because they rotate, produce a well-defined and usually round entrance wound (Fig. 8-22). Once the projectile enters the flesh, however, it may fragment, tumble, or actually explode, resulting in considerable tissue damage and a large, ragged exit wound.

ULTRAVIOLET LIGHT

Within the large spectrum of electromagnetic radiation emitted by the sun, exposure to ultraviolet (UV) light (100–400 nm) has a number of different effects on the human body. It can damage DNA and is a leading cause of cancer of the skin (see Chapter 5).

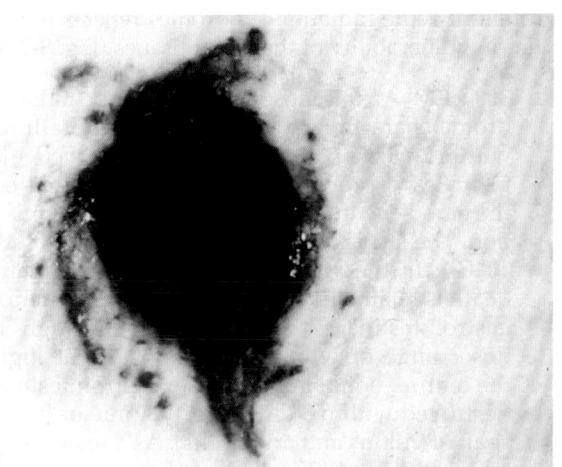
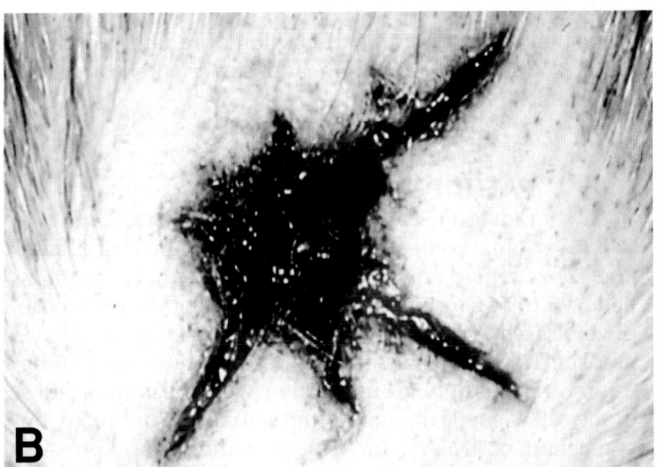

FIGURE 8-22. Bullet wounds. A. The entrance wound is sharply punched out. **B.** The exit wound is irregular with characteristic stellate lacerations.

UV radiation is also absorbed by photoreceptors in the skin, after which substances that suppress cell-mediated immunity may be released. As a consequence, both local and systemic immune functions may be modulated. Recent evidence suggests a beneficial effect of UV light on the severity of some autoimmune diseases, such as multiple sclerosis. Exposure to UV radiation also stimulates endogenous production of vitamin D in the skin (see below). UV wavelengths between 270 nm and 300 nm, called UVB, result in production of a precursor for vitamin D from a cholesterol derivative.

RADIATION

We can define radiation simply as emission of energy by one body, its transmission through an intervening medium and its absorption by another body. By this definition, radiation encompasses the entire electromagnetic spectrum and certain charged particles emitted by radioactive elements. Alpha particles and the beta particles of elements such as tritium (^{3}H) and carbon 14 (^{14}C) are of immense use scientifically and pose few hazards for humans. High-energy radiation, in the form of gamma or x-rays, mediates most of the biological effects discussed here. We do not consider the effects of ultraviolet radiation here; they are discussed in Chapters 5 and 28.

Radiation is quantitated in a number of ways:

- **A roentgen** is a measure of the emission of radiant energy from a source. This unit refers to the amount of ionization produced in air.
- **A rad** measures absorption of radiant energy, which is biologically the more important parameter. A rad defines the energy, expressed as ergs, absorbed by a tissue. One rad equals 100 ergs per gram of tissue.
- **A gray** (Gy) corresponds to 100 rads (1 joule/kg of tissue) and a centigray (cGy) is equivalent to 1 rad.
- **The rem** was introduced to describe the biological effect caused by a rad of high-energy radiation, since low-energy particles produce more biological damage than gamma or x-rays.
- **A sievert** (Sv) is the dose in gray multiplied by an appropriate quality factor Q, so that 1 Sv of radiation is roughly equivalent in biological effectiveness to 1 Gy of gamma rays.

For the purposes of this discussion of radiation-induced pathology, the rad, gray, rem and sievert are considered comparable.

 **PATHOPHYSIOLOGY:** At the cellular level, radiation essentially has two effects: (1) a somatic effect, associated with acute cell killing; and (2) genetic damage. Radiation-induced cell death is believed to be caused by the acute effects of the radiolysis of water (see Chapter 1). The production of activated oxygen species may result in lipid peroxidation, membrane injury and possibly an interaction with macromolecules of the cell. Genetic damage to the cell caused indirectly by a reaction of DNA with oxygen radicals is expressed either as mutation or as reproductive failure. Both mutation and reproductive failure may lead to delayed cell

death, and mutation is involved in development of radiation-induced neoplasia.

Different tissues are differently sensitive to radiation. The vulnerability of a tissue to radiation-induced damage depends on its proliferative rate, which in turn correlates with the natural life span of the constituent cells. For example, the intestine and the hematopoietic bone marrow are far more vulnerable than tissues such as bone and brain. Damage to the DNA of a long-lived, nonproliferating cell does not necessarily impair its function or viability because its reproductive and metabolic functions are separate properties. By contrast, short-lived, proliferating cells, such as intestinal crypt cells or hematopoietic precursors, must be rapidly replaced by division of precursor cells. If radiation-induced DNA damage precludes mitosis of these cells, the mature elements are not replaced and the tissue can no longer function.

It is important to distinguish between whole-body irradiation and localized irradiation. Except for unusual circumstances, as in the high-dose irradiation that precedes bone marrow transplantation, significant levels of whole-body irradiation result only from industrial accidents or from nuclear weapons explosions. By contrast, localized irradiation is an inevitable byproduct of any diagnostic radiologic procedure and it is the intended result of radiation therapy. Rapid somatic cell death occurs only with extremely high doses of radiation, well in excess of 10 Gy. It is morphologically indistinguishable from coagulative necrosis produced by other causes (see Chapter 1). By contrast, irreversible damage to the replicative capacity of cells requires far lower doses, possibly as few as 50 cGy.

Whole-Body Irradiation Injures Many Organs

Fortunately, there have been few instances of human disease caused by whole-body irradiation, and most of our information has been derived from studies of Japanese atom bomb survivors. Further information is now available from the study of the survivors of the much smaller sample of people exposed in the accident at the Chernobyl nuclear power plant in Ukraine in 1986.

Since comparable doses of radiant energy are transmitted to all organs in whole-body irradiation, development of the different acute radiation syndromes reflects the dissimilarities in vulnerability of the target tissues (Fig. 8-23).

- **300 cGy:** At this dose of whole-body radiation, a syndrome characterized by **hematopoietic failure** develops within 2 weeks. After initial depletion of circulating lymphocytes, a progressive decrease in formed elements of the blood eventually leads to bleeding, anemia and infection. The last is often the cause of death.
- **10 Gy:** In the vicinity of this dose, the main cause of death is related to the **gastrointestinal system**. Although gastrointestinal symptoms occur through the entire dose range of whole-body exposure, at higher levels, the entire epithelium of the gastrointestinal tract is destroyed within 3 days (i.e., the time of the normal life span of villous and crypt cells). As a result, fluid homeostasis of the bowel is disrupted and severe diarrhea and dehydration ensue. Moreover, the epithelial barrier to intestinal bacteria is breached; gut organisms invade

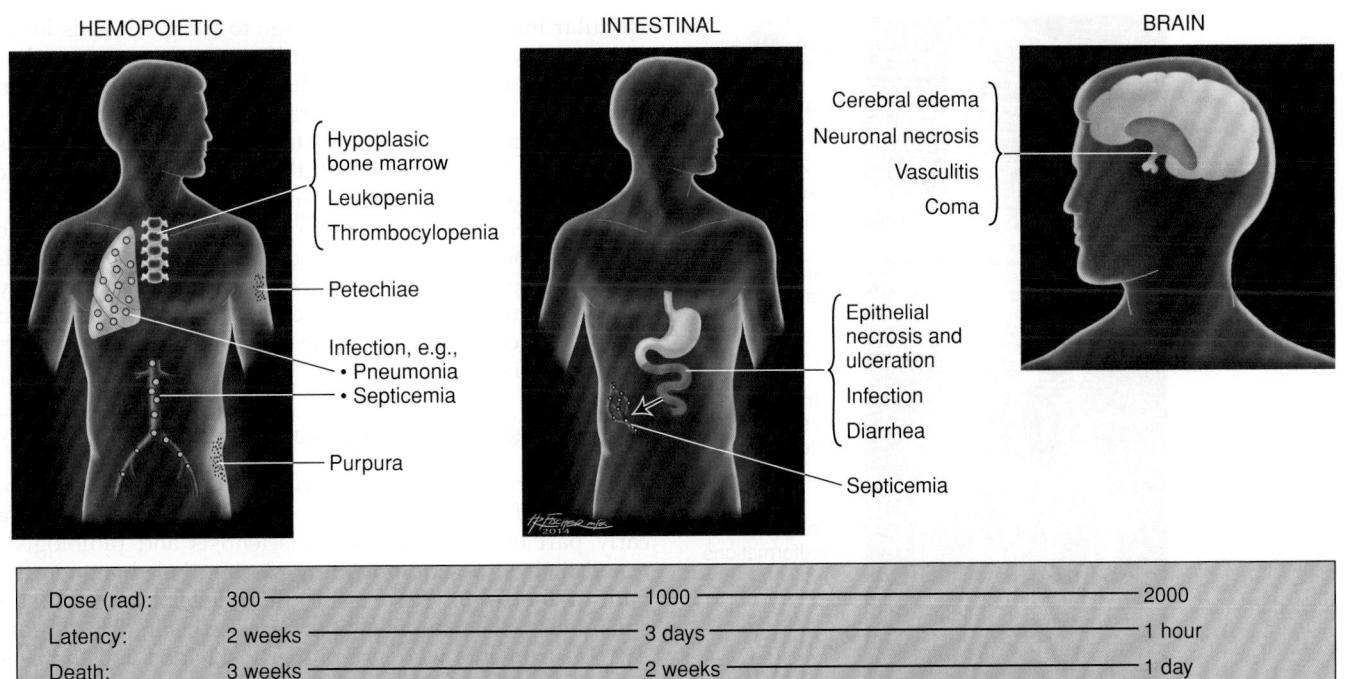

HEMOPOIETIC

Hypoplasic bone marrow
Leukopenia
Thrombocytopenia

Petechiae

Infection, e.g.,
• Pneumonia
• Septicemia

Purpura

INTESTINAL

Epithelial necrosis and ulceration
Infection
Diarrhea

Septicemia

BRAIN

Cerebral edema
Neuronal necrosis
Vasculitis
Coma

Dose (rad):	300	1000	2000
Latency:	2 weeks	3 days	1 hour
Death:	3 weeks	2 weeks	1 day

FIGURE 8-23. Acute radiation syndromes. At a dose of approximately 300 rads of whole-body radiation, a syndrome characterized by hematopoietic failure develops within 2 weeks. In the vicinity of 1000 rads, a gastrointestinal syndrome with a latency of only 3 days is seen. With doses of 2000 rads or more, disease of the central nervous system appears within 1 hour and death ensues rapidly.

and disseminate throughout the body. Septicemia and shock kill the victim.

■ **20 Gy:** With whole-body doses of 20 Gy and above, CNS damage causes death within hours. In most cases, cerebral edema and loss of the integrity of the blood-brain barrier, owing to endothelial injury, predominate. With extreme doses, radiation necrosis of neurons can be expected. Convulsions, coma and death follow.

FETAL EFFECTS: The effects of whole-body irradiation on the human fetus have been documented in studies of Hiroshima nuclear bomb survivors. Pregnant women exposed to 25 cGy or more gave birth to infants with reduced head size, diminished overall growth and mental retardation.

In studies of the clinical status of children exposed to therapeutic doses of radiation between the 3rd and 20th weeks of gestation, growth retardation and microcephaly were observed. Other effects of irradiation in utero include hydrocephaly, microphthalmia, chorioretinitis, blindness, spina bifida, cleft palate, clubfeet and genital abnormalities. Data from experimental and human studies strongly suggest that major congenital malformations are highly unlikely at doses below 20 cGy after day 14 of pregnancy. However, lower doses may produce more-subtle effects, such as a decrease in mental capacity. *To protect against such a possibility, the established maximum permissible dose of radiation to the fetus from exposure of the expectant mother is far below the known teratogenic dose.*

GENETIC EFFECTS: Most data on which predictions of human genetic effects are based are derived from experimental data and analysis of nuclear bomb survivors. *After long-term follow-up, survivors of the nuclear detonations at Hiroshima and Nagasaki have shown no evidence of genetic damage in the form of either congenital abnormalities or heritable diseases in subsequent offspring or their descendants.* In experimental animals, the risk of induced mutation per cGy is at most 0.5%–5% of the risk of spontaneous mutation (the spontaneous risk of mutation in humans is estimated to be 10% of live births). By extension, 20–200 cGy of radiation is necessary to double the spontaneous mutation rate. Consequently, the risk of genetic damage to future generations from radiation appears to be small.

AGING: There is to date no evidence that radiation exposure leads to premature aging. A mortality study of survivors of the nuclear bomb explosions in Japan did not show excess mortality beyond that attributable to neoplasia. Nor is there any evidence of acceleration in disease among the survivors in any part of the age range.

Localized Radiation Injury Complicates Radiation Therapy for Tumors

In the course of radiation therapy for malignant neoplasms, some normal tissue is inevitably irradiated. Although almost any organ can be damaged by radiation, the skin, lungs, heart, kidney, bladder and intestine are susceptible and difficult to shield (Fig. 8-24). Localized damage to the bone marrow is clearly of little functional consequence because of the immense reserve capacity of the hematopoietic system.

 PATHOLOGY: Persistent damage to radiation-exposed tissue can be attributed to (1) compromise of the vascular supply and (2) a fibrotic repair reaction to acute necrosis and chronic ischemia. Radiation-induced tissue injury predominantly affects small arteries and arterioles. The endothelial cells are the most sensitive elements in the blood vessels and in the short term exhibit

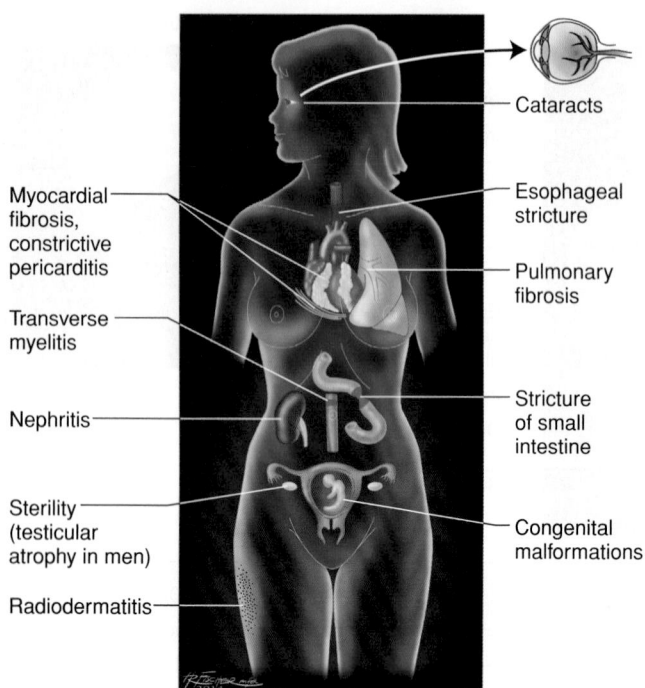

FIGURE 8-24. The nonneoplastic complications of radiation.

swelling and necrosis. With time, vascular walls become thickened by endothelial cell proliferation and subintimal deposition of collagen and other connective tissue elements. Striking vacuolization of intimal cells, so-called foam cells, is typical. Fragmentation of the internal elastic lamina, loss of smooth muscle cells, scarring in the media and fibrosis of the adventitia are seen in the small arteries. Bizarre fibroblasts with large hyperchromatic nuclei are common and probably reflect radiation-induced DNA damage.

CLINICAL FEATURES: Acute necrosis from radiation is represented by such disorders as **radiation pneumonitis, cystitis, dermatitis** and **diarrhea from enteritis**. Chronic disease is characterized by **interstitial fibrosis** in the heart and lungs, **strictures** in the esophagus and small intestine and **constrictive pericarditis**. Chronic **radiation nephritis,** which simulates malignant nephrosclerosis, is primarily a vascular disease that leads to severe hypertension and progressive renal insufficiency.

As radiation therapy inevitably traverses the skin, it often causes **radiation dermatitis**. The initial damage is evidenced by blood vessel dilation, recognized as **erythema**. Necrosis of the skin may follow and linger as **indolent ulcers** that do not heal because the epithelium is unable to regenerate. Impaired wound healing in irradiated tissues may pose serious problems for surgeons operating in those areas. **Poorly healed** or **dehisced wounds** or **persistent ulcers** often require full-thickness skin grafts. **Chronic radiation dermatitis** results from repair and revascularization of the skin and is characterized by atrophy, hyperkeratosis, telangiectasia and hyperpigmentation (Fig. 8-25).

The **gonads,** both testes and ovaries, are similar to other tissues in their dependence on continuous cell cycling and are exquisitely radiosensitive. Acute inhibition of mitosis in the testis results in necrosis of the germinal stem cells, the spermatogonia. The combination of radiation-induced

vascular injury and direct damage to the germ cells leads to progressive atrophy of seminiferous tubules, peritubular fibrosis and loss of reproductive function. Interstitial and Sertoli cells do not cycle rapidly and so persist, thus preserving normal hormonal status. Comparable injury is seen in the irradiated ovary; the follicles become atretic and the organ eventually becomes fibrous and atrophic.

Cataracts (lenticular opacities) may be produced if the eye lies in the path of the radiation beam. **Transverse myelitis** and paraplegia occur when the spinal cord is unavoidably irradiated during treatment of certain thoracic or abdominal tumors. **Vascular damage in the cord** may bring about localized ischemia.

High Doses of Radiation Cause Cancer

The evidence that radiation can lead to cancer is incontrovertible and comes from many sources (Fig. 8-26). In the early part of the 20th century, scientists and radiologists tested their x-ray equipment by placing their hands in the path of the beam. As a result, they developed basal and squamous cell carcinomas of the exposed skin. In addition, early instruments were not properly shielded and the hazards associated with fluoroscopy were not appreciated. The radiologists of that era suffered an unusually high incidence of leukemia. This situation has been rectified with the use of modern shielding and protective equipment.

An unusual occupational exposure to radiation occurred among workers who painted radium-containing material onto watches to create luminous dials. These workers were in the habit of licking their paint brushes to produce a point, which led to their ingesting the radium. Since the

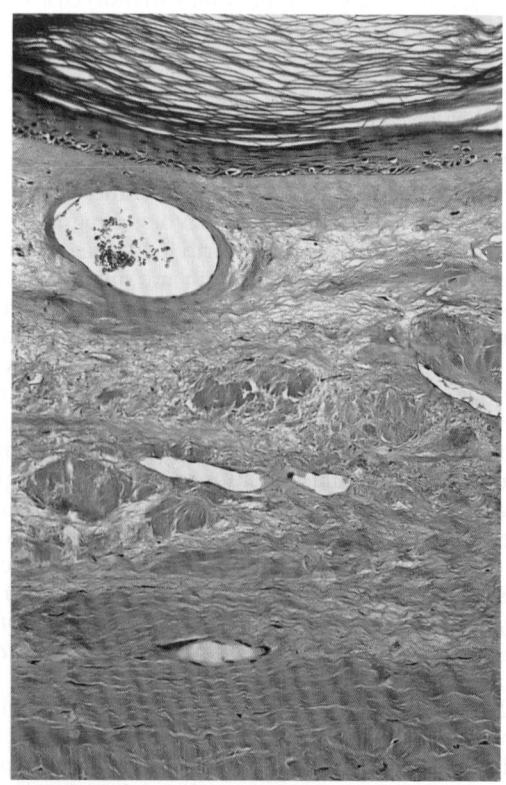

FIGURE 8-25. Chronic radiation dermatitis. The epidermis is atrophic. The dermis is densely fibrotic and contains dilated superficial blood vessels.

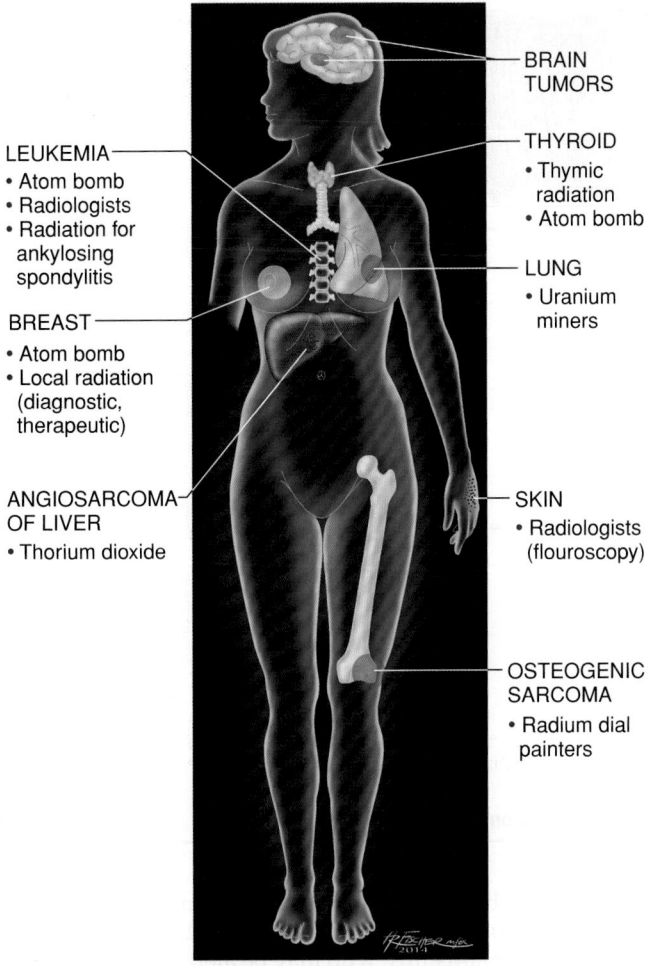

FIGURE 8-26. Radiation-induced cancers.

LEUKEMIA
• Atom bomb
• Radiologists
• Radiation for
  ankylosing
  spondylitis

BREAST
• Atom bomb
• Local radiation
  (diagnostic,
  therapeutic)

ANGIOSARCOMA
OF LIVER
• Thorium dioxide

BRAIN
TUMORS

THYROID
• Thymic
  radiation
• Atom bomb

LUNG
• Uranium
  miners

SKIN
• Radiologists
  (flouroscopy)

OSTEOGENIC
SARCOMA
• Radium dial
  painters

body handles radium as it does calcium, it subsequently localized in their bones, so they were exposed to a long-lived isotope that persisted in their bones indefinitely. These people experienced a high incidence of cancer of the bone and of the paranasal sinuses. Another example of occupational exposure to a radioactive element is the high rate of lung cancer in uranium miners who inhaled radioactive dust and radon gas. Most of these workers also smoked and evidence strongly favors a synergistic effect in lung carcinogenesis.

Iodine is concentrated by the thyroid. If radioactive iodine isotopes are inhaled or ingested, that gland will experience highly concentrated exposure to radioactivity. An explosive increase in the incidence of thyroid cancer among children in geographical areas contaminated by the nuclear catastrophe at Chernobyl in Ukraine in 1986 has been linked to release of radioactive iodine isotopes in that incident.

The risk of **solid tumors**, especially breast cancer, is particularly high among adult women who were treated with thoracic radiation for Hodgkin disease as children. Long-term survivors of childhood Hodgkin disease, who were treated with radiation therapy, have almost a 20-fold increased risk of developing a second neoplasm owing to the radiation. Another example of iatrogenic cancer resulted in Great Britain from widespread use of low-dose spinal irradiation to treat ankylosing spondylitis. These patients later developed aplastic anemia, acute myelogenous leukemia

and other tumors with high frequency. An increase in brain tumors was found in people who had received cranial irradiation for tinea capitis infection of the scalp in childhood. Thorium dioxide (Thorotrast), a material avidly ingested by phagocytic cells, was used a few decades ago for radionuclide imaging. The persistence in the liver of a long-lived radioisotope resulted in development of hepatic angiosarcomas.

The survivors of the nuclear bomb explosions in Japan suffered from a number of cancers. They exhibited a more than 10-fold increase in the incidence of leukemia, which peaked 5–10 years after exposure, then declined to background rates. Two thirds were cases of acute leukemia; the remainder were of chronic myelogenous leukemia. Chronic lymphocytic leukemia, an uncommon disease in Japan, showed no increase in incidence. The risk of multiple myeloma increased fivefold and there was a small increment in the incidence of lymphoma. The frequency of solid tumors, although not as great as that for leukemia, was clearly increased for the breast, lung, thyroid, gastrointestinal tract and urinary tract. The development of malignant tumors, including leukemia, showed a dose-response relationship.

LOW-LEVEL RADIATION AND CANCER: Data from studies of cancer induction in animals, chromosomal damage in human cell cultures, malignant transformation of mammalian cells in vitro and populations exposed to radiation show that the estimates of risk at low radiation doses are very low. The data do not show that the risk of cancer from low-level radiation is zero. There is a general concern that gamma radiation is associated with increased risk of cancer at doses of 5–10 cGy. Although DNA damage appears to occur proportionately to the dose of gamma radiation, there is considerable uncertainty as to the extent to which DNA repair mechanisms may be protective at low radiation doses or dose rates.

RADON: The finding that some homes in the United States are contaminated with radon has elicited considerable public concern. Radon is a radioactive noble gas formed from the decay of uranium 238 (^{238}U), which is found in soil and rock formations. Radon is itself inert. Concern about the environmental hazards of radon focus on its radioactive decay products, which are called radon daughters. These include radioactive isotopes of bismuth, lead and polonium, which are chemically active and which bind to particulates and lung tissues. The half-life of the α-emitting isotope, ^{218}Po, is 103 years.

Previously, studies of the risk of radon gas were done in uranium miners and were not well controlled for smoking as an independent risk factor. More recent large-scale studies indicate that people who dwell in homes containing high concentrations of radon gas have an increased risk of developing lung cancer. The relative risk is by far the greatest for smokers and ex-smokers. However, recent studies also indicate that people who never smoked also have increased risk of lung cancer.

Microwave Radiation, Electromagnetic Fields and Ultrasound Are Not Ionizing

Microwaves, produced by ovens, radar and diathermy, are electromagnetic waves that penetrate tissue but do not produce ionization. Unlike x- and gamma radiation, absorption of microwave energy produces only heat. The activation energy of radiofrequency and microwave radiation is too low to modify chemical bonds or alter DNA. Thus, exposure to microwave radiation under ordinary circumstances is highly unlikely to produce any injury. Moreover, a study of 20,000 radar technicians in the navy who were chronically exposed to high levels of microwave radiation failed to detect any increased incidence of cancer.

Controversy also surrounds possible carcinogenic—especially leukemogenic—effects of exposure to nonionizing electromagnetic fields, such as those encountered in the vicinity of high-voltage electric lines. Recent epidemiologic evidence has led to a consensus that exposure to electromagnetic fields does not raise the incidence of leukemia or other cancers.

Ultrasound, the vibrational waves in air above the audible range, produces mechanical compression but, again, no ionization. Highly focused and energetic ultrasound devices are used to disrupt tissue in vitro for chemical analysis and to clean various surfaces, including teeth. However, there is no reason to believe that diagnostic ultrasound or accidental exposure to any industrial device results in any measurable damage.

NUTRITIONAL DISORDERS

Protein-Calorie Malnutrition Reflects Starvation or Specific Deficiencies

Marasmus is the term used to denote a deficiency of calories from all sources. **Kwashiorkor** is a form of malnutrition in children caused by a diet deficient in protein alone.

Marasmus

Global starvation—that is, a deficiency of all elements of the diet—leads to marasmus. The condition is common throughout the nonindustrialized world, particularly when breast feeding is stopped and a child must subsist on a calorically inadequate diet. Pathologic changes are similar to those in starving adults and include decreased body weight, diminished subcutaneous fat, a protuberant abdomen, muscle wasting and a wrinkled face. In general, the child is a "shrunken old person." Wasting and increased lipofuscin pigment are seen in most visceral organs, especially the heart and the liver. No edema is present. Pulse, blood pressure and temperature are low; diarrhea is common. Since immune responses are impaired, the child suffers from numerous infections. An important consequence of marasmus is **growth failure**. If these children are not provided with adequate food in childhood, they will not reach their full potential stature as adults. Severe marasmus accompanied by iron-deficiency anemia in early childhood, when brain development is under way, may result in permanent intellectual deficits.

Kwashiorkor

Kwashiorkor (Fig. 8-27) results from a **deficiency of protein** in diets relatively high in carbohydrates. It is one of the most common diseases of infancy and childhood in the nonindustrialized world. Like marasmus, it usually occurs after an infant is weaned, when a protein-poor diet, consisting principally of staple carbohydrates, replaces mother's milk. There is generalized growth failure and muscle wasting, as

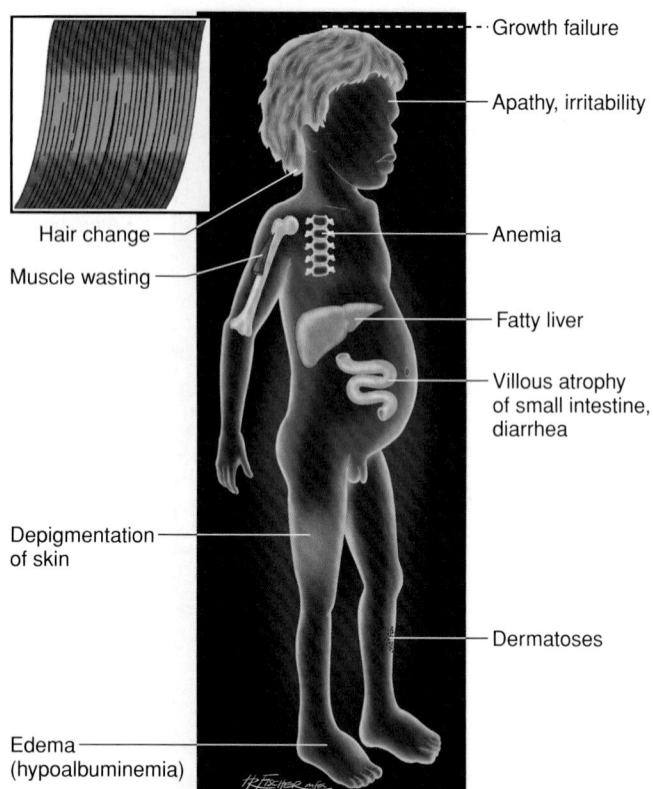

FIGURE 8-27. **Complications of kwashiorkor.**

in marasmus, but subcutaneous fat is normal, since caloric intake is adequate. Extreme apathy is notable, in contrast to children with marasmus, who may be alert. Also in contrast to marasmus, severe edema, hepatomegaly, depigmentation of the skin and dermatoses are usual. "Flaky paint" lesions of the skin on the face, extremities and perineum are dry and hyperkeratotic. Hair becomes a sandy or reddish color; a characteristic linear depigmentation of the hair ("flag sign") provides evidence of particularly severe periods of protein deficiency. The abdomen is distended because of flaccid abdominal muscles, hepatomegaly and ascites due to hypoalbuminemia. Along with general atrophy of the viscera, villous atrophy of the intestine may interfere with nutrient absorption. Diarrhea is common. Anemia is the rule, but it is not generally life-threatening. The nonspecific effects on growth, pulse, temperature and the immune system are similar to those in marasmus. It has been claimed in some studies that kwashiorkor not only impairs physical development but also stunts later intellectual growth.

 PATHOLOGY: Microscopically, the liver in kwashiorkor is conspicuously fatty. Accumulation of lipid within the cytoplasm of the hepatocyte displaces the nucleus to the periphery of the cell. The adequacy of dietary carbohydrate provides lipid for the hepatocyte, but the inadequate protein stores do not permit synthesis of enough apoprotein carrier to transport the lipid from the liver cell. The changes, with the possible exception of mental retardation, are fully reversible when sufficient protein is made available. In fact, the fatty liver reverts to normal after early childhood, even if the diet remains deficient in protein. In any event, hepatic changes are not progressive and do not lead to chronic liver disease.

Vitamins Are Organic Catalysts That Are Both Required for Normal Metabolism and Available Only from Dietary Sources

Thus, vitamins in one species are not necessarily vitamins in another. For example, humans cannot synthesize ascorbic acid (vitamin C) and so require dietary ascorbate to prevent scurvy, but most lower animals can produce their own vitamin C and do not require it as a vitamin.

Vitamin A

Vitamin A is a fat-soluble substance that is important for skeletal maturation and maintenance of specialized epithelial linings and cell membrane structure. In addition, it is an important constituent of the photosensitive pigments in the retina. Vitamin A occurs naturally as **retinoids** or as a precursor, **β-carotene**. The source of the precursor—carotene—is in plants, principally leafy, green vegetables. Fish livers are a particularly rich source of vitamin A itself (retinoids).

Vitamin A appears to be important in immune function and nonimmune defense mechanisms. It has long been known that vitamin A deficiency is associated with poor resistance to infection. Administration of vitamin A to deficient people reduces all overall mortality. In addition, in underdeveloped countries, vitamin A supplementation to pregnant women and their children has reduced infant mortality.

Metabolism

β-Carotene is modified in the intestinal mucosa to retinoids, which are absorbed with chylomicrons. It is stored in the liver, where 90% of the body's vitamin A is located. At times when fat absorption is impaired (e.g., diarrhea), vitamin A absorption decreases.

Vitamin A Deficiency

Although vitamin A deficiency is uncommon in developed countries, it is a significant health problem in poorer regions of the world, including much of Africa, China and Southeast Asia.

 PATHOLOGY: *Deficiency of vitamin A results principally in squamous metaplasia, especially in glandular epithelium* (Fig. 8-28). Thus, keratin debris blocks sweat and tear glands. Squamous metaplasia is common in the trachea and bronchi and bronchopneumonia is a frequent cause of death. The epithelia lining the renal pelvis, pancreatic ducts, uterus and salivary glands are also commonly affected. Epithelial changes in the renal pelvis may be associated with kidney stones. With further diminution of vitamin A stores, squamous metaplasia of conjunctival and tear duct epithelial cells occurs, which leads to **xerophthalmia,** dryness of the cornea and conjunctiva. The cornea becomes softened (**keratomalacia,** Fig. 8-29) and vulnerable to ulceration and bacterial infection, which may lead to blindness. **Follicular hyperkeratosis,** a skin disorder caused by occluded sebaceous glands, is also a feature of this disease.

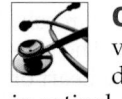 **CLINICAL FEATURES:** The earliest sign of vitamin A deficiency often is diminished vision in dim light. Vitamin A is a necessary component in retinal rod pigment and is active in light transduction.

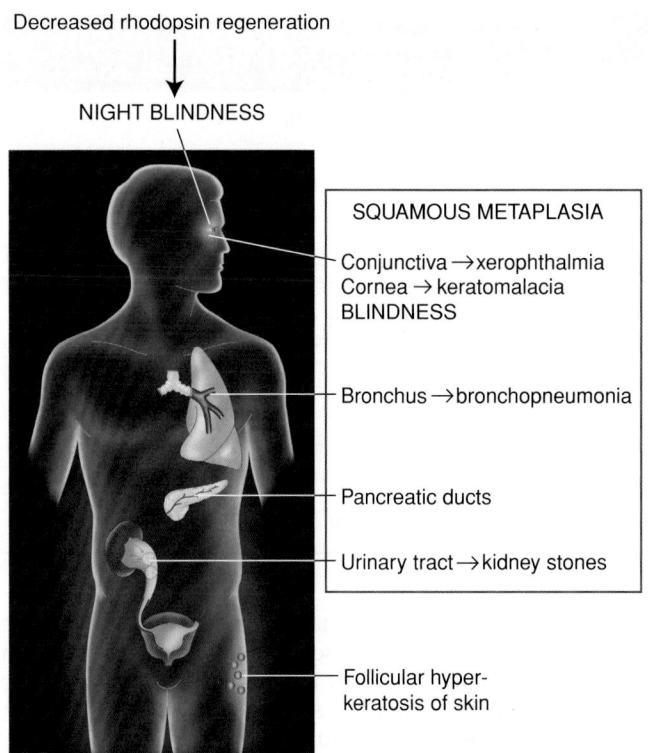

FIGURE 8-28. Complications of vitamin A deficiency.

Because vitamin A aldehyde, retinal, is constantly degraded in generating the light signal, a continuous supply of vitamin A is necessary for night vision.

Vitamin A Toxicity

Vitamin A poisoning is usually caused by overenthusiastic administration of vitamin supplements to children. Early Arctic explorers were said to have experienced vitamin A toxicity because they ate polar bear liver, which is particularly rich in the vitamin. Enlargement of the liver and spleen are common; microscopically, these organs show lipid-laden macrophages. In the liver, vitamin A is also present in hepatocytes, and prolonged hypervitaminosis A has been incriminated in rare cases of cirrhosis. Bone pain and neurologic

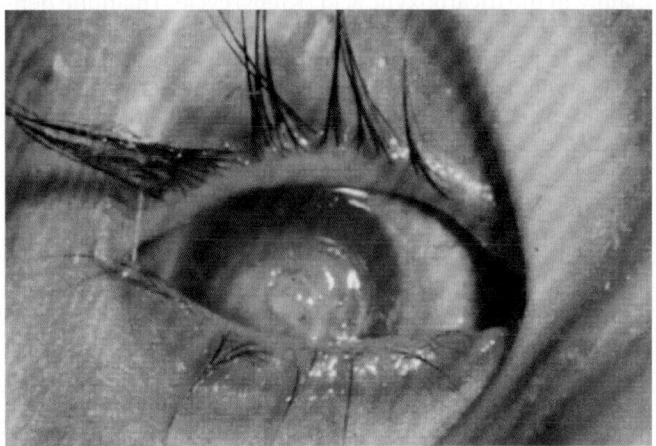

FIGURE 8-29. Keratomalacia in vitamin A deficiency.

TABLE 8-5

B VITAMINS

Vitamin	Biochemical Name
B_1	Thiamine
B_2	Riboflavin
B_3	Niacin
B_5	Pantothenic acid
B_6	Pyridoxine
B_7	Biotin
B_9	Folic acid
B_{12}	Cyanocobalamin

symptoms, such as hyperexcitability and headache, may be the presenting symptoms. Discontinuing the excess vitamin A consumption reverses all or most of the lesions. Excessive carotene intake is benign and simply stains the skin yellow, which may be mistaken for jaundice.

Synthetic derivatives of retinoic acid are now used pharmacologically to alleviate severe acne. Both retinoic acid and a high dietary intake of preformed vitamin A are particularly dangerous in pregnancy because they are potent teratogens. A number of clinical studies have reported that excess intake of vitamin A leads to reduced bone mineral density and consequently increases the incidence of bone fractures.

Vitamin B Complex

Vitamins in the B group of water-soluble vitamins are numbered 1 through 12, but only eight are distinct vitamins (Table 8-5).

Thiamine (B_1)

Thiamine was the active ingredient in the original description of vitamin B, which was defined as a water-soluble extract in rice polishings that cured beriberi (clinical thiamine deficiency). The vitamin is an essential cofactor in the activity of several enzymes crucial to energy metabolism, mainly in the tricarboxylic acid (Krebs) cycle. Thiamine deficiency was classically seen in the Orient, where the staple food was polished rice that had been deprived of its thiamine content by processing. With increased awareness of the disease and improved nutrition in some areas of Asia, the disorder is less common now than in previous generations. In Western countries, the disease occurs in alcoholics, neglected people with poor overall nutrition and food faddists. *The cardinal symptoms of thiamine deficiency are polyneuropathy, edema and cardiac failure* (Fig. 8-30). The deficiency syndrome is classically divided into **dry beriberi,** with symptoms referable to the neuromuscular system, and **wet beriberi,** in which manifestations of cardiac failure predominate.

Thiamine deficiency in chronic alcoholics may be manifested by CNS involvement, in the form of Wernicke syndrome, in which progressive **dementia, ataxia and oph-thalmoplegia** (paralysis of the extraocular muscles) are

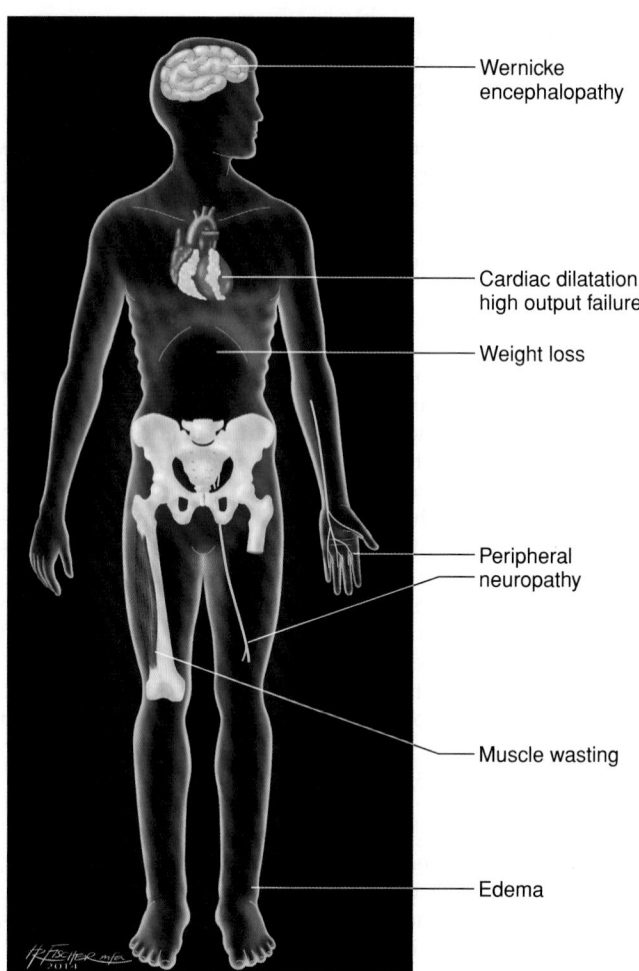

Wernicke encephalopathy

Cardiac dilatation, high output failure

Weight loss

Peripheral neuropathy

Muscle wasting

Edema

FIGURE 8-30. Complications of thiamine deficiency (beriberi).

prominent. Korsakoff syndrome, in which a thought disorder is conspicuous, at one time was attributed solely to thiamine deficiency but is now understood to be seen both in chronic alcoholics and in patients with other organic mental syndromes.

 PATHOLOGY: Pathologic examination of the nervous system in thiamine deficiency has not defined a pathognomonic change in the peripheral nerves, given that similar or identical changes can be seen with other peripheral neuropathies. A characteristic alteration is myelin sheath degeneration, which often begins in the sciatic nerve, then involves other peripheral nerves and sometimes the spinal cord itself. In advanced cases, axon fragmentation may be seen.

The most striking lesions in Wernicke encephalopathy are found in the mamillary bodies and surrounding areas that abut on the third ventricle (see Chapter 32). Indeed, atrophy of the mamillary bodies can be visualized in alcoholics by computed tomography and magnetic resonance imaging. Microscopically, degeneration and loss of ganglion cells, rupture of small blood vessels and ring hemorrhages are seen in the brain.

The changes in the heart are also nonspecific. Grossly, the heart is flabby, dilated and increased in weight. The process may affect either the right or the left side of the heart or both. The microscopic changes are nondescript and include edema, inconsistent fiber hypertrophy and occasional foci of fiber degeneration.

 CLINICAL FEATURES: Patients with dry beriberi present with paresthesias, depressed reflexes and weakness and muscle atrophy in the extremities. Wet beriberi is characterized by generalized edema, a reflection of severe congestive failure. The basic lesion is uncontrolled, generalized vasodilation and significant peripheral arteriovenous shunting. This combination leads to a compensatory increase in cardiac output and eventually to a large dilated heart and congestive heart failure. In a patient without documented metabolic disease (e.g., hyperthyroidism), high output failure and generalized edema strongly suggest thiamine deficiency.

The most reliable diagnostic test for thiamine deficiency is an immediate and dramatic response to parenteral administration of thiamine. Measurements of thiamine in the blood and erythrocyte transketolase activity are also useful.

Riboflavin (B₂)

Riboflavin, a vitamin derived from many plant and animal sources, is important for synthesis of flavin nucleotides, which are important in electron transport and other reactions in which energy transfer is crucial. Riboflavin is converted within the body to flavin mononucleotides and dinucleotides. Clinical symptoms of riboflavin deficiency are uncommon; they are usually seen only in debilitated patients with a variety of diseases and in poorly nourished alcoholics.

Deficiencies of thiamine, riboflavin and niacin are unusual in industrialized countries because bread and cereals are fortified with these vitamins. Occasionally, a mild riboflavin deficiency is seen during pregnancy and lactation, or during a phase of rapid growth in childhood and adolescence, when increased demands are combined with moderate nutritional deprivation.

  PATHOLOGY AND CLINICAL FEATURES: Riboflavin deficiency, when it occurs, is almost always seen in conjunction with deficiencies of other water-soluble vitamins. It is manifested principally by lesions of the facial skin and corneal epithelium. **Cheilosis,** a term used for fissures in the skin at the angles of the mouth, is a characteristic feature (Fig. 8-31). These cracks in the skin may be painful and often become infected.

Hyperkeratosis and a mild mononuclear infiltrate of the skin are noted. **Seborrheic dermatitis,** an inflammation of the skin that exhibits a greasy, scaling appearance, typically involves the cheeks and the areas behind the ears. The tongue is smooth and purplish (magenta), owing to mucosal atrophy. The most troubling lesion may be **corneal interstitial keratitis,** which is followed by opacification of the cornea and eventual ulceration. The localization of the lesions in riboflavin deficiency is not explained biochemically. There is no known toxicity from ingesting large amounts of riboflavin.

Niacin (B₃)

Niacin refers to nicotinic acid. Nicotinic acid is derived from dietary sources or biosynthesized from tryptophan. In the body, nicotinic acid is converted to nicotinamide, which plays a major role in formation of NAD. This compound and its phosphorylated derivative, NADP, are

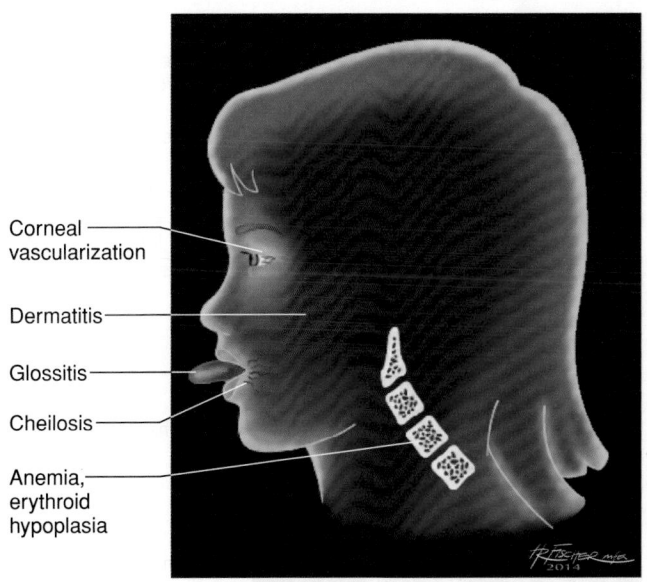

Corneal vascularization

Dermatitis

Glossitis

Cheilosis

Anemia, erythroid hypoplasia

FIGURE 8-31. Complications of riboflavin deficiency.

important in intermediary metabolism and an extensive variety of oxidation–reduction reactions. Animal protein, as found in meat, eggs and milk, is high in tryptophan and is therefore a good source of endogenously synthesized niacin. Niacin itself is available in many types of grain. **Pellagra** is the term for clinical niacin deficiency. It is uncommon today.

 **ETIOLOGIC FACTORS:** Pellagra is seen principally in patients who have been weakened by other diseases and in malnourished alcoholics. Food faddists who do not eat sufficient protein may suffer a deficiency of tryptophan, which in combination with a lack of exogenous niacin may result in mild pellagra. Malabsorption of tryptophan, as in Hartnup disease, or excessive use of tryptophan for serotonin synthesis in the carcinoid syndrome may also lead to mild symptoms of pellagra. Deficiencies of pyridoxine and riboflavin increase the requirement for dietary niacin because both of these cofactors are required for biosynthesis of niacin from tryptophan. Pellagra is particularly prevalent in areas where corn (maize) is the staple food, because the niacin in corn is chemically bound and thus poorly available. Corn is also a poor source of tryptophan.

 PATHOLOGY: Pellagra (Ital., "rough skin") is characterized by the three "Ds" of niacin deficiency: **dermatitis, diarrhea** and **dementia** (Fig. 8-32). Areas exposed to light, such as the face and the hands, and those subjected to pressure, such as the knees and the elbows, exhibit a rough, scaly dermatitis (Fig. 8-33). The involvement of the hands leads to so-called glove dermatitis. The lesions are discrete and show areas of pigmentation and of depigmentation. Microscopically, hyperkeratosis, vascularization and chronic inflammation of the skin are characteristic. Subcutaneous fibrosis and scarring may be seen in late stages. Similar lesions are found in the mucous membranes of the mouth and vagina. In the mouth, inflammation and edema lead to a large, red tongue, which in the chronic stage is fissured and is likened to raw meat. Chronic, watery diarrhea is

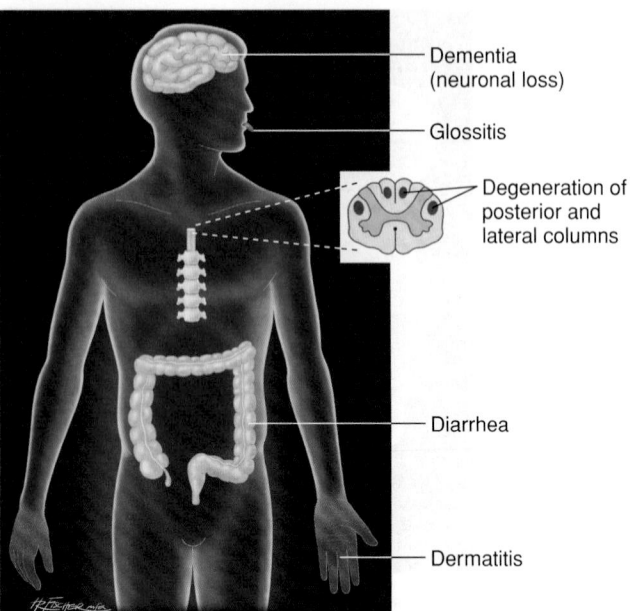

FIGURE 8-32. Complications of niacin deficiency (pellagra).

typical for the disease, presumably due to mucosal atrophy and ulceration in the entire gastrointestinal tract, particularly in the colon. The dementia, characterized by aberrant ideation bordering on psychosis, is represented in the brain by degeneration of ganglion cells in the cortex. Myelin degeneration of tracts in the spinal cord resembles the subacute combined degeneration of vitamin B_{12} deficiency. Severe longstanding pellagra adds another **"D,"** namely, death.

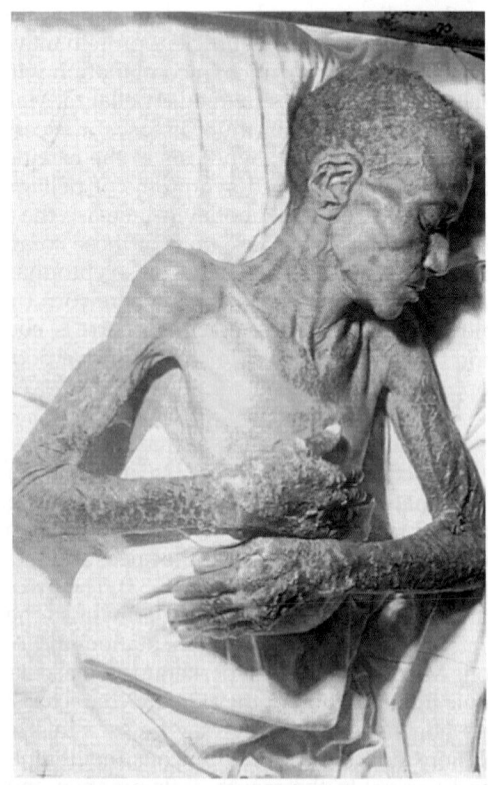

FIGURE 8-33. Pellagra. Dermatitis in sun-exposed areas of the arms and around the neck in this elderly woman is shown.

In pharmacologic doses, niacin supplements decrease levels of low-density lipoprotein (LDL) cholesterol and increase levels of high-density lipoprotein (HDL) cholesterol, thus providing a useful adjunct in preventing atherosclerosis.

Pantothenic Acid (B_5)

Pantothenic acid serves as a component of coenzyme A (CoA) and is an essential cofactor in the biosynthesis of fatty acids and certain peptides. Major sources of pantothenic acid include beef, chicken, liver, eggs, grains and a number of vegetables.

Deficiency of pantothenic acid is distinctly uncommon, except in severe malnutrition. The syndrome is characterized by behavioral, neurologic and gastrointestinal disturbances.

There are no known adverse effects of overconsumption of pantothenic acid.

Pyridoxine (B_6)

Vitamin B_6 activity is found in three related, naturally occurring compounds: pyridoxine, pyridoxal and pyridoxamine. For convenience, they are grouped under the heading pyridoxine. These compounds are widely distributed in vegetable and animal foods. Vitamin B_6 functions as a coenzyme in numerous metabolic pathways, including those related to amino acids, lipids, methylation and decarboxylation, gluconeogenesis, heme and neurotransmitters. Some studies also suggest a role for vitamin B_6 in maintaining normal B- and T-cell immune function.

 EPIDEMIOLOGY: Population studies have incriminated low levels of pyridoxine in increasing risk of atherosclerosis, but the mechanisms for this effect remain obscure. Low blood levels of vitamin B_6 have also been correlated with a number of conditions such as aging, impaired renal function and inflammatory conditions. The relevance of these correlations merits further study.

A recent analysis of prospective studies suggests a 20% lower risk of colorectal cancer when comparing people with high versus low intake of vitamin B_6. The report found that low blood levels of the active form of vitamin B_6, namely, pyridoxal 5-phosphate, correlated with increased risk of developing colorectal cancer.

In the United States, it is estimated that vitamin B_6 intake is inadequate for about 20% of men over age 50 years and for 40% of women in the same age group.

 ETIOLOGIC FACTORS: Pyridoxine is converted to pyridoxal phosphate, a coenzyme for many enzymes, including transaminases and carboxylases. Pyridoxine deficiency is rarely caused by an inadequate diet, although infants who have been fed poorly prepared powdered formula in which pyridoxine was destroyed during preparation have suffered convulsions. A higher demand for the vitamin, as may occur in pregnancy, may lead to a secondary deficiency state. Of particular concern is the deficiency of pyridoxine that follows prolonged medication with a number of drugs, particularly isoniazid, cycloserine and penicillamine. A deficiency state is also occasionally reported in alcoholics.

 CLINICAL FEATURES: There are no clinical manifestations of pyridoxine deficiency that can be considered characteristic or pathognomonic. The usual dermatologic complications of other B vitamin deficiencies occur with pyridoxine deficiency. *The primary expression of the disease is in the CNS, a feature consistent with the role of this vitamin in the formation of pyridoxal-dependent decarboxylase of the neurotransmitter GABA.* In infants and children, diarrhea, anemia and seizures have occurred.

Conditions are encountered in which there is no clinical or biochemical evidence of pyridoxine deficiency, yet large (pharmacologic) doses of the vitamin are useful in treating the disorder. Such diseases are called pyridoxine-dependency syndromes and include anemia, convulsions and homocystinuria caused by cystathionine synthetase deficiency.

Pyridoxine-responsive anemia is hypochromic and microcytic and therefore can be confused with iron-deficiency anemia. Unlike iron-deficiency anemia, however, pyridoxine-responsive anemia is characterized by saturation of iron stores and increased saturation of transferrin. Thus, administration of iron may simply make pyridoxine-responsive anemia worse. By definition, the anemia responds well to massive doses of pyridoxine.

Biotin (B₇)

Most biotin is found in meats and cereals, where it is largely bound to protein. Biotin is an obligatory cofactor for five carboxylases that participate in intermediary metabolism, including the Krebs cycle.

 **ETIOLOGIC FACTORS: Biotin deficiency** is reported in people who consume large amounts of raw eggs, in those with prolonged malabsorption syndrome and in children with severe protein-calorie malnutrition. Chronic administration of anticonvulsant drugs can also lead to biotin depletion.

 CLINICAL FEATURES: Symptoms of biotin deficiency include seborrheic and eczematous skin rash. In adults, neurologic symptoms include lethargy, hallucinations and paresthesias. In infants, hypotonia and developmental delay have been reported.

There are no known adverse consequences of high-dose biotin administration.

Folic Acid (B₉)

Folic acid is a heterocyclic derivative of glutamic acid and serves as a methyl group donor, especially in nucleotide synthesis. Folate, together with vitamin B₁₂ (see below), is a key cofactor in methylation reactions. One of the key reactions in question is the conversion of homocysteine to methionine, which is needed to generate S-adenosylmethionine (SAM). SAM is a key methyl donor in the synthesis of neurotransmitters (norepinephrine to epinephrine), phospholipids (phosphatidylethanolamine to phosphatidylcholine), methylated nucleotides and histones. Folate also is critical in the generation of purine nucleotides and the conversion of uracil to thymidine. The latter reaction is important for understanding the consequences of folate deficiency in causing megaloblastic anemia.

FOLATE DEFICIENCY: Folic acid and vitamin B₁₂ (see below) both participate in the pathway to produce methionine (see above), and the extent of the role of SAM in diverse biochemical reactions explains the extent of the overlap between the manifestations of deficiencies of these two vitamins (e.g., megaloblastic anemia; see Chapter 26). The distinction between deficiencies of these two B vitamins was elucidated by Herbert, who, in 1962, developed megaloblastic anemia following a self-imposed experimental diet lacking only folate.

Folate is present in almost all foods, including meat, dairy products, seafood, cereals and vegetables. Deficiency is thus usually a consequence of a generally poor diet, as is seen in some alcoholics, rather than a diet deficient in any single constituent. Malabsorption syndromes may also result in folate deficiency. Because the settings in which folate deficiency occurs affect many nutrients, isolated folate deficiency is rare.

Folate supplements given during early pregnancy have been shown to decrease the incidence of fetal neural tube defects. This effect is not clearly related to a folate deficiency and may be a pharmacologic benefit. Because neural tube formation occurs before many women know they are pregnant, fortification of cereal and grain products with folic acid has been mandated in the United States since 1998.

Cyanocobalamin (B₁₂)

Deficiency of vitamin B₁₂ is almost always seen in cases of pernicious anemia and results from the lack of secretion of intrinsic factor in the stomach (see Chapter 19), which prevents absorption of the vitamin in the ileum.

 **ETIOLOGIC FACTORS:** Since vitamin B₁₂ is found in almost all animal protein, including meat, milk and eggs, dietary deficiency is seen only in rare cases of extreme vegetarianism and then only after many years of a restricted diet. Parasitization of the small intestine by the fish tapeworm *Diphyllobothrium latum* (from undercooked fish) may lead to vitamin B₁₂ deficiency because the parasite absorbs the vitamin in the gut lumen.

 CLINICAL FEATURES: Deficiency of vitamin B₁₂ is associated with megaloblastic anemia. In addition, pernicious anemia is complicated by a neurologic condition called subacute combined degeneration of the spinal cord. Comprehensive discussions of vitamin B₁₂ deficiency are found in Chapters 26 and 32.

Choline

Choline is an amine that is found in many foods, especially wheat products, peanuts, soybeans, fish and meat. It is incorporated principally into membrane phospholipids and is the major dietary source of methyl groups. Choline is necessary for lipid signaling, transport and metabolism, and for cholinergic neurotransmission. It is also important in reactions involving transfer of methyl groups. Because there is an endogenous pathway for choline biosynthesis, it was not considered to be an essential human nutrient. Recently, however, choline deficiency syndromes have been identified and adequate dietary levels are now established.

Experimentally, a choline-deficient diet led to evidence of liver and muscle damage. Patients maintained on total parenteral nutrition due to short bowel syndrome often develop liver disease, some of which can be prevented by choline supplementation.

Vitamin C (Ascorbic Acid)

The effects of vitamin C deficiency, namely, **scurvy,** were described 5000 years ago in Egyptian hieroglyphs and were mentioned by Hippocrates in 500 BC.

PATHOPHYSIOLOGY: Ascorbic acid is a water-soluble vitamin that is a powerful biological reducing agent involved in many oxidation/reduction reactions and in proton transfer. It is important for chondroitin sulfate synthesis and for proline hydroxylation to form the hydroxyproline of collagen. Ascorbic acid serves many other important functions: it prevents oxidation of tetrahydrofolate and augments absorption of iron from the gut. Without vitamin C, biosynthesis of certain neurotransmitters is impaired, leading to, for example, a reduction in dopamine β-hydroxylase activity. Wound healing and immune functions also involve ascorbic acid. The best dietary sources of vitamin C are citrus fruits, green vegetables and tomatoes.

Scurvy is the clinical vitamin C deficiency state. The first demonstration of the need for this vitamin was the remarkable effect of lime in preventing scurvy among 18th-century British sailors. The distribution of limes in the British navy led to the name "limey" for the seamen. Scurvy is uncommon in the Western world, but is often noted in nonindustrialized countries in which other forms of malnutrition are prevalent. In industrialized countries, scurvy is now a disease of people afflicted with chronic diseases who do not eat well, the neglected aged and malnourished alcoholics. The stress of cold, heat, fever or trauma (accidental or surgical) leads to an increased requirement for vitamin C. Children who are fed only milk for the first year of life develop scurvy, as do alcoholics. Mild depression of ascorbic acid levels also occurs in other conditions, including cigarette smoking, tuberculosis, rheumatic fever and many debilitating disorders. About 3% of the body's ascorbic acid is catabolized per day.

PATHOLOGY: *Most of the events associated with vitamin C deficiency are caused by formation of abnormal collagen that lacks tensile strength* (Fig. 8-34). Within 1–3 months, subperiosteal hemorrhages lead to pain in bones and joints. Petechial hemorrhages, ecchymoses and purpura are common, particularly after mild trauma or at pressure points. Perifollicular hemorrhages in the skin are particularly typical of

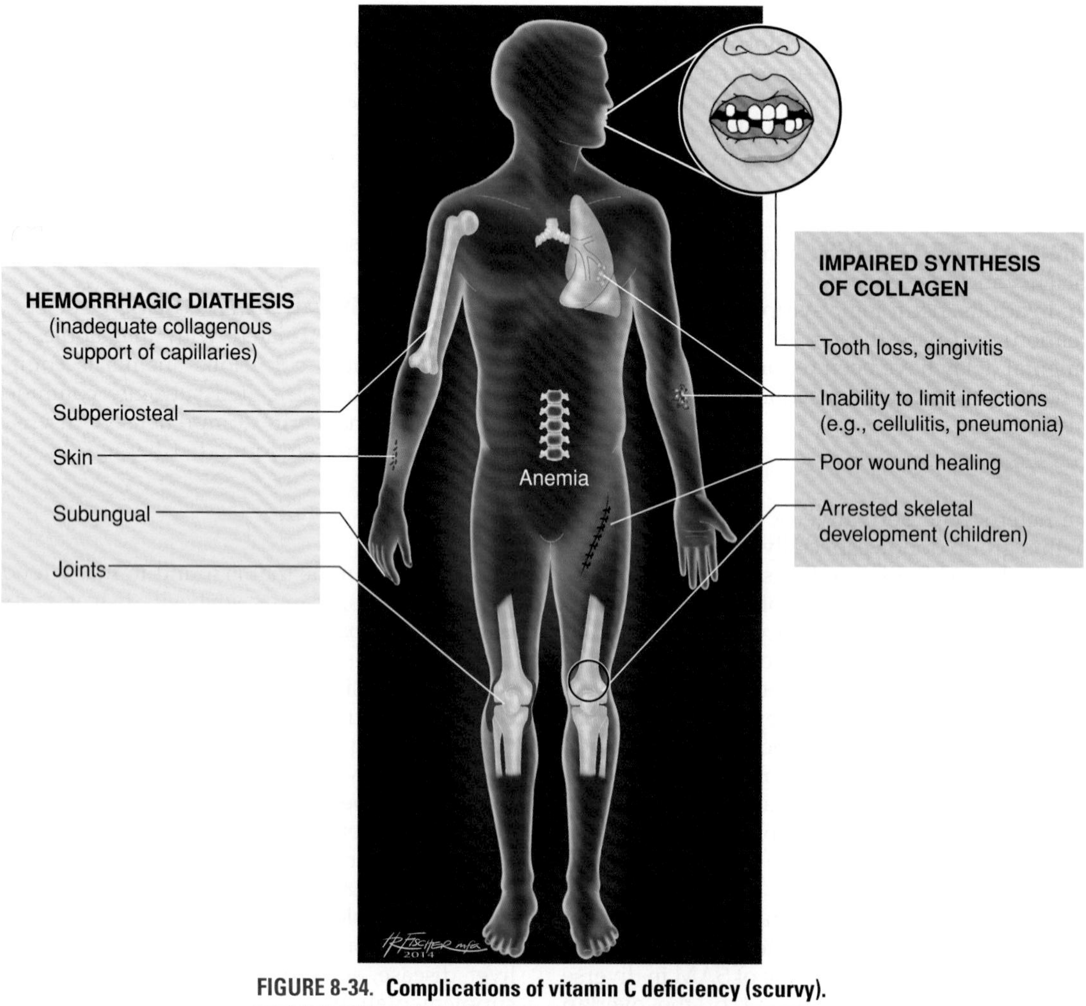

HEMORRHAGIC DIATHESIS
(inadequate collagenous support of capillaries)

Subperiosteal
Skin
Subungual
Joints

Anemia

IMPAIRED SYNTHESIS OF COLLAGEN

Tooth loss, gingivitis
Inability to limit infections (e.g., cellulitis, pneumonia)
Poor wound healing
Arrested skeletal development (children)

FIGURE 8-34. Complications of vitamin C deficiency (scurvy).

scurvy. In advanced cases, swollen, bleeding gums are a classic finding. Alveolar bone resorption results in loss of teeth. Wound healing is poor and dehiscence of previously healed wounds occurs. Anemia may result from prolonged bleeding, impaired iron absorption or associated folic acid deficiency.

In children, vitamin C deficiency leads to growth failure and collagen-rich structures such as teeth, bones and blood vessels develop abnormally. Effects on developing bone are conspicuous and relate principally to impaired function of osteoblasts (see Chapter 30). In addition to poor wound healing, scorbutic patients have difficulty walling off infections to form abscesses, so that infections spread more easily. The diagnosis of scurvy is confirmed by finding low levels of ascorbic acid in the serum.

While the claims that ascorbic acid may help to prevent upper respiratory infections lack substantiation, ingestion of large amounts of vitamin C is not known to be harmful.

Vitamin D

Some 500,000,000 years ago, vitamin D first appeared on Earth in ocean-dwelling phytoplankton, in which it may have functioned to absorb ultraviolet irradiation or act as a photochemical signal. During evolution, terrestrial vertebrates became dependent on vitamin D for the sustenance of their bony skeletons.

Vitamin D is a fat-soluble steroid hormone found in two forms: vitamin D_3 (cholecalciferol) and vitamin D_2 (ergocalciferol), both of which have equal biological potency in humans. Vitamin D_3 is produced in the skin and vitamin D_2 is derived from plant ergosterol. The vitamin is absorbed in the jejunum along with fats and is transported in the blood bound to an α-globulin (vitamin D–binding protein). *To achieve biological potency, vitamin D must be hydroxylated to active metabolites in the liver and kidney. The active form of the vitamin promotes calcium and phosphate absorption from the small intestine and may directly influence mineralization of bone.*

The discovery of nuclear receptors for 1,25(OH)2-vitamin D in various tissues not related to calcium metabolism has led to a search for pharmacologic applications of this vitamin. It may have uses in the treatment of psoriasis, hypertension, possibly certain cancers and multiple sclerosis.

Vitamin D Deficiency

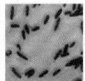 **ETIOLOGIC FACTORS:** *In children, vitamin D deficiency causes rickets; in adults, osteomalacia occurs.* Vitamin D deficiency results from (1) insufficient dietary vitamin D, (2) insufficient production of vitamin D in the skin because of limited sunlight exposure, (3) inadequate absorption of vitamin D from the diet (as in the fat malabsorption syndromes) or (4) abnormal conversion of vitamin D to its bioactive metabolites. The last occurs in liver disease and chronic renal failure.

 CLINICAL FEATURES: The bone lesions of vitamin D deficiency in children (rickets) have been recognized for centuries and were common in the Western industrialized world until recently. It was a disease that affected the urban poor to a much greater extent than their rural counterparts. A partial explanation for this difference lies in the greater exposure of rural residents to

sunlight. Addition of vitamin D to milk and many processed foods, administration of vitamin preparations to young children and generally improved levels of nutrition have made rickets a curiosity in industrialized countries. See Chapter 26 for more details.

Hypervitaminosis D

The most common cause of excess vitamin D is the inordinate consumption of vitamin preparations. Abnormal conversion of vitamin D to biologically active metabolites is occasionally seen in granulomatous diseases such as sarcoidosis. In cases of calcium malabsorption, when the underlying disease is corrected, the sensitivity of target tissues to vitamin D may be increased.

 PATHOLOGY: The initial response to excess vitamin D is **hypercalcemia,** which leads to nonspecific symptoms such as weakness and headaches. Increased renal calcium excretion results in **nephrolithiasis** or **nephrocalcinosis. Ectopic calcification** in other organs, such as blood vessels, heart and lungs, may be seen. Infants are particularly susceptible to excess vitamin D, and if the condition is not corrected, they may develop premature arteriosclerosis, supravalvular aortic stenosis and renal acidosis.

Vitamin E

Vitamin E is an antioxidant that (experimentally at least) protects membrane phospholipids against lipid peroxidation by free radicals formed by cellular metabolism. The activity of this fat-soluble vitamin is found in a number of dietary constituents, principally in α-tocopherol. Corn and soy beans are particularly rich in vitamin E.

Dietary deficiency of vitamin E can occur in children as a result of mutations in the α-tocopherol transfer protein and in adults with various malabsorption syndromes. The deficiency may present clinically as spinocerebellar ataxia, skeletal myopathy and pigmented retinopathy.

In premature infants, hemolytic anemia, thrombocytosis and edema have been associated with vitamin E deficiency. Vitamin E therapy has been reported to improve hemolytic anemia in premature newborns and may reduce the severity but not the incidence of retrolental fibroplasia. Vitamin E is reported to retard development of cirrhosis in infants with congenital biliary atresia. A number of interesting experimental effects are produced by vitamin E, such as inhibition of (1) platelet aggregation, (2) conversion of dietary nitrites to carcinogenic nitrosamines and (3) prostaglandin synthesis. Protection against toxins that exert their activity through production of free radical oxygen species has also been shown. The applicability of these results to humans requires further study.

Attempts to use vitamin E as a pharmacologic agent to prevent cancer and coronary artery disease have been unsuccessful.

Vitamin K

Vitamin K, a fat-soluble material, occurs in two forms: vitamin K_1, from plants, and vitamin K_2, which is principally synthesized by the normal intestinal bacteria. Green leafy vegetables are rich in vitamin K and liver and dairy products contain smaller amounts.

PATHOPHYSIOLOGY: Dietary deficiency is very uncommon in the United States; most cases are associated with other disorders. However, inadequate dietary intake of vitamin K does occasionally occur in conjunction with chronic illness associated with anorexia.

Vitamin K deficiency is common in severe fat malabsorption, as seen in sprue and biliary tract obstruction. Destruction of intestinal flora by antibiotics may also result in vitamin K deficiency. Newborn infants frequently exhibit vitamin K deficiency because the vitamin is not transported well across the placenta and the sterile gut of the newborn does not have bacteria to produce it. Vitamin K confers **calcium-binding properties to certain proteins and is important for the activity of four clotting factors: prothrombin, factor VII, factor IX and factor X. Deficiency of vitamin K can be serious, because it can lead to catastrophic bleeding. Parenteral vitamin K therapy is rapidly effective.**

Amino Acids

Of the 20 amino acids in human proteins, no pathways exist for the synthesis of eight, and possibly nine (the additional amino acid being histidine). These amino acids are required in the diet and are considered to be **essential amino acids**. Another nine amino acids can be synthesized in the human body from simple precursors or from other amino acids. These are called **nonessential amino acids**. Finally, two amino acids (cysteine, tyrosine) are conditionally dispensable because their synthesis is limited under certain conditions or when adequate quantities of precursors are not available. Table 8-6 lists the 20 amino acids and the extent to which they must be acquired in the diet.

Deficiency of essential amino acids is manifest as protein deficiency (kwashiorkor; see above).

Increasing Use of Vitamins

Recent years have witnessed an explosion of interest in potential pharmacologic uses of vitamins, unrelated to treating dietary or other deficiencies. Consequently, many people are consuming certain vitamins in doses that far exceed what is needed to prevent deficiency diseases. It is likely that studies of such people will provide information regarding both the potential beneficial and toxic effects of large doses of vitamins.

Essential Trace Minerals Are Mostly Components of Enzymes and Cofactors

Essential trace minerals include iron, copper, iodine, zinc, cobalt, selenium, manganese, nickel, chromium, tin, molybdenum, vanadium, silicon and fluorine. Dietary deficiencies of these minerals are clinically important in the case of iron and iodine. These are discussed in Chapters 26 and 27, which deal with blood and endocrine diseases, respectively.

Chronic zinc deficiency has been reported in Iran and Egypt to result in hypogonadal dwarfism in boys. The

TABLE 8-6 AMINO ACIDS	
Amino Acid	**Nature of Requirement**
Alanine (A)	Nonessential
Arginine (R)	Nonessential
Asparagine (N)	Nonessential
Aspartic acid (D)	Nonessential
Cysteine (C)	Conditionally essential
Glutamic acid (E)	Nonessential
Glutamine (Q)	Nonessential
Glycine (G)	Nonessential
Histidine (H)	Conditionally essential
Isoleucine (I)	Essential
Leucine (L)	Essential
Lysine (K)	Essential
Methionine (M)	Essential
Phenylalanine (F)	Essential
Proline (P)	Nonessential
Serine (S)	Nonessential
Threonine (T)	Essential
Tryptophan (W)	Essential
Tyrosine (Y)	Conditionally essential
Valine (V)	Essential

children usually are those who eat clay, a substance that may bind zinc, but a deficiency in dietary protein is usually also present. An inherited disorder of zinc metabolism, acrodermatitis enteropathica, which is a chronic form of zinc deficiency, is characterized by diarrhea, rash, hair loss, muscle wasting and mental irritability. Similar symptoms are seen in acute zinc deficiency associated with total parenteral nutrition. Zinc deficiency is also seen in diseases that cause malabsorption, such as Crohn disease, celiac disease, cirrhosis and alcoholism.

Dietary copper deficiency is rare but may occur in certain inherited disorders, in malabsorption syndromes and during total parenteral nutrition. The most common result is microcytic anemia, although megaloblastic changes have also been described.

Manganese deficiency has been described and causes poor growth, skeletal abnormalities, reproductive impairment, ataxia and convulsions. **Industrial exposure to manganese** causes symptoms closely related to those of parkinsonism.

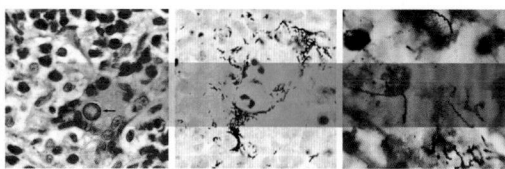

Infectious and Parasitic Diseases

David A. Schwartz

Psittacosis (Ornithosis)

Chlamydia pneumoniae

RICKETTSIAL INFECTIONS

Rocky Mountain Spotted Fever

Epidemic (Louse-Borne) Typhus

Endemic (Murine) Typhus

Scrub Typhus

Q Fever

MYCOPLASMAL INFECTIONS

MYCOBACTERIAL INFECTIONS

Tuberculosis
Primary Tuberculosis
Secondary (Cavitary) Tuberculosis

Leprosy

***Mycobacterium avium-intracellulare* Complex**
Granulomatous Pulmonary Disease
Disseminated Infection in AIDS

Atypical Mycobacteria

FUNGAL INFECTIONS

***Pneumocystis jiroveci* Pneumonia**

Candida

Aspergillosis
Allergic Bronchopulmonary Aspergillosis
Aspergilloma
Invasive Aspergillosis

Mucormycosis (Zygomycosis)

Cryptococcosis

Histoplasmosis

Coccidioidomycosis

Blastomycosis

Paracoccidioidomycosis (South American Blastomycosis)

Sporotrichosis

Chromomycosis

Dermatophyte Infections

Mycetoma

PROTOZOAL INFECTIONS

Malaria

Babesiosis

Toxoplasmosis
Toxoplasma Lymphadenopathy Syndrome
Congenital *Toxoplasma* Infections
Toxoplasmosis in Immunocompromised
    Hosts

Amebiasis
Intestinal Amebiasis
Amebic Liver Abscess

Cryptosporidiosis

Giardiasis

Leishmaniasis
Localized Cutaneous Leishmaniasis
Mucocutaneous Leishmaniasis
Visceral Leishmaniasis (Kala Azar)

Chagas Disease (American Trypanosomiasis)
Acute Chagas Disease
Chronic Chagas Disease

African Trypanosomiasis

Primary Amebic Meningoencephalitis

HELMINTHIC INFECTION

Filarial Nematodes
Lymphatic Filariasis
Onchocerciasis
Loiasis

Intestinal Nematodes
Ascariasis
Trichuriasis
Hookworms
Strongyloidiasis
Pinworm Infection (Enterobiasis)

Tissue Nematodes
Trichinosis
Visceral Larva Migrans (Toxocariasis)
Cutaneous Larva Migrans
Dracunculiasis

Trematodes (Flukes)
Schistosomiasis
Clonorchiasis
Paragonimiasis
Fascioliasis
Fasciolopsiasis

Cestodes: Intestinal Tapeworms
Cysticercosis
Echinococcosis

EMERGING AND REEMERGING INFECTIONS

Agents of Biowarfare

The Toll of Infectious Diseases

Perhaps the greatest scourge to mankind is the diverse group of disorders collectively known as infectious diseases. They have caused more pain, suffering, disability and premature death than any other category of diseases in history. Bacterial and viral diarrheas, bacterial pneumonias, tuberculosis, measles, malaria, hepatitis B, pertussis and tetanus kill more people each year than all cancers and cardiovascular diseases (Table 9-1). The impact of infectious diseases is greatest in less developed countries, where millions of people, mostly children younger than 5 years of age, die of treatable or preventable infectious diseases. Even in the developed countries of Europe and North America,

the mortality, morbidity and loss of economic productivity from infectious diseases is enormous. It is estimated that smallpox alone claimed between 300 million and 500 million human lives during the 20th century alone. Although smallpox has been eradicated from the natural environment, a multitude of other infectious agents continue to claim millions of lives each year. Infectious diseases such as tuberculosis, malaria, childhood diarrhea and acquired immunodeficiency syndrome (AIDS) continue to ravage the developing world, taking millions of lives each year. Even in industrialized nations, the morbidity and mortality from infectious disease is still substantial. In the United States, sepsis alone is responsible for an estimated 200,000 deaths per year (see Chapter 12).

Past accomplishments of individuals illustrate the contributions that can be made in this area to the alleviation of

TABLE 9-1
SOURCES OF GLOBAL DEATHS

Illness	Annual Deaths
Cardiovascular disease	12×10^6
Diarrheal diseases (rotavirus, Norwalk-like viruses, *Salmonella, Shigella,* diarrheagenic *Escherichia coli*)	5×10^6
Cancer	4.8×10^6
Pneumonia	4.8×10^6
Tuberculosis	3×10^6
Chronic obstructive lung disease	2.7×10^6
Measles	1.5×10^6
Malaria	$1-2 \times 10^6$
Hepatitis B	$1-2 \times 10^6$
Tetanus (neonatal)	775×10^3
Pertussis (whooping cough)	500×10^3
Maternal mortality	500×10^3
AIDS (all)	200×10^3
AIDS (children)	28×10^3
Schistosomiasis	200×10^3
Amebiasis	$40-110 \times 10^3$
Hookworm	$50-60 \times 10^3$
Rabies	35×10^3
Typhoid	25×10^3
Yellow fever	25×10^3
African trypanosomiasis (sleeping sickness)	20×10^3
Ascariasis	20×10^3

human suffering: Edward Jenner's use of cowpox (vaccinia) virus in 1798 to immunize against smallpox; John Snow's removal of the Broad Street pump handle, which ended the 1854 cholera outbreak in London; and the discovery in 1843 by Oliver Wendell Holmes, Sr., that simply washing hands between patients could dramatically reduce the incidence of puerperal postpartum fever.

All these discoveries were made before an intelligible theory of causation of these illnesses existed. That theory arrived with the work of Koch, Pasteur, Lister and Ehrlich, who established the field of microbiology. This feat led directly to identification of agents responsible for many infectious diseases, establishment of effective standards of antisepsis and, eventually, the discovery and development of antibiotics to treat common bacterial, fungal, helminthic and protozoal diseases.

By the 1970s, it seemed that infectious diseases would become medical curiosities owing to the development of antibiotics, improved sanitation and immunization. It is instructive that in 1970, the Surgeon General of the United States declared, "The time has come for us to close the book on infectious disease." The fact that we had not conquered infectious diseases and that, in fact, tremendous problems were lurking was illustrated by the discovery of Legionnaires disease in 1976. The end of our naive expectations that infectious diseases were conquered came in 1981, with the first reports of human immunodeficiency virus-1 (HIV-1)/AIDS. Since then, many other infections have emerged (see below), for which we currently have little treatment and no cures: Ebola virus, severe acute respiratory syndrome (SARS), drug-resistant tuberculosis, pandemic strains of influenza virus, carbapenem-resistant Enterobacteriaceae (CRE) and others. The recent concern over these and other infectious diseases underscores the facts that the potential for future infectious threats to human existence is real, animal reservoirs of microbes that can be transmitted to humans are bottomless and vigilance can never be relaxed. Finally, the possibility that people may seek to use infectious agents as weapons of warfare should dispel any complacency that we are safe from these pathogens.

Infectious Diseases Feature Tissue Damage from an Invading Transmissible Agent

Infectious diseases represent many of the familiar taxa: bacteria, fungi, protozoa and various parasitic worms. Yet some infectious agents do not qualify as completely independent organisms. Viruses cannot replicate by themselves and are obligate intracellular parasites that hijack the replicative machinery of susceptible cells. Likewise, prions, the class of proteinaceous infectious agents, lack nucleic acids and clearly represent a different infectious disease paradigm.

There is great diversity in how various infectious diseases are acquired. Many of these maladies, such as influenza, syphilis and tuberculosis, are contagious (i.e., transmissible from person to person). Yet many infectious diseases, such as legionellosis, histoplasmosis and toxoplasmosis, are not contagious but are rather acquired from the environment. *Legionella* bacteria normally replicate in aquatic amebas but can infect humans via aerosolized water or through microaspiration of contaminated water. Other infectious agents come from many diverse sources: animals, insects, soil, air, inanimate objects and the endogenous microbial flora of the human body.

Perhaps the greatest paradox is that certain retroviruses have actually been incorporated into the human genome and are passed from generation to generation. Their function is unclear but their possible activation during placentation has led to speculation that such endogenous retroviruses may have allowed placental mammals to evolve.

INFECTIVITY AND VIRULENCE

Virulence is the complex of properties that allows an organism to establish infection and to cause disease or death. The organism must (1) gain access to the body, (2) avoid multiple host defenses, (3) accommodate to growth in the human milieu and (4) parasitize human resources.

Virulence reflects both the structures inherent to the offending microbe and the interplay of those factors with host defense mechanisms.

HOST DEFENSE MECHANISMS

The means by which the body prevents or contains infections are known as defense mechanisms (Table 9-2). There are major anatomic barriers to infection—the skin and the aerodynamic filtration system of the upper airway—that prevent most organisms from ever penetrating the body. The mucociliary blanket of the airways is also an essential defense, expelling organisms that gain access to the respiratory system. Microbial flora normally resident in the gastrointestinal tract and in various body orifices compete with outside organisms, preventing them from gaining sufficient nutrients or binding sites in the host. The body's orifices are also protected by secretions that possess antimicrobial properties, both nonspecific (e.g., lysozyme and interferon) and specific (secretory immunoglobulin A [IgA]). In addition, gastric acid and bile chemically destroy many ingested organisms.

Heritable Differences in Host Membrane Receptors May Determine Whether an Infection Occurs

The first step in infection is often a highly specific interaction of a binding molecule on an infecting organism with a receptor molecule on the host. If the host lacks a suitable receptor, the organism cannot attach to the target. Thus, *Plasmodium vivax,* one of the organisms that cause human malaria, infects human erythrocytes by using Duffy blood group determinants on the cell surface as receptors. Many people, particularly blacks, lack these determinants and are not susceptible to infection with *P. vivax.* As a result, *P. vivax* malaria is absent from much of Africa. Similar racial or geographic differences in susceptibility are apparent for many infectious agents, including *Coccidioides immitis* and *Coccidioides posadasii,* which are 14 times more common in blacks and 175 times more frequent in Filipinos than in whites.

Age Is Important in Predicting Susceptibility to Many Infections

The effect of age on the outcome of exposure to many infectious agents is well illustrated by infections of the fetus. Some organisms produce more severe disease in utero than in children or adults. Infections of the fetus with cytomegalovirus (CMV), rubella virus, parvovirus B19 and *Toxoplasma gondii* interfere with fetal development. Normally, the fetus is protected by maternal IgG (generated by a specific previous infection) that passively crosses the placenta. In acute infection of a pregnant woman who lacks neutralizing antibody, certain pathogens may cross the placenta. These infections are usually subclinical or produce minimal disease in the mother. Depending on the organism and timing of exposure, fetal infection can produce minimal damage, major congenital abnormalities or death.

Age also affects the course of common illnesses, such as the diverse viral and bacterial diarrheas. In older children and adults, these infections cause discomfort and inconvenience, but rarely severe disease. The outcome can be different in children under 3 years of age, who cannot compensate for rapid volume loss resulting from profuse diarrhea. The World Health Organization (WHO) estimates that acute diarrheal diseases remain the second leading cause of death in children under 5 years of age and kill 1.5 million children yearly.

Other examples include infection with *Mycobacterium tuberculosis,* which produces severe, disseminated tuberculosis in children under the age of 3 years. By contrast, older people tend to fare much better.

Maturity, however, is not always an advantage in infections. Epstein-Barr virus (EBV) is more likely to cause symptomatic infections in adolescents and adults than in younger children. Varicella-zoster virus causes chickenpox in children but produces more severe disease in adults, who are more likely to develop viral pneumonia.

The elderly fare more poorly with almost all infections than younger persons. Common respiratory illnesses such as influenza and pneumococcal pneumonia are more often fatal in those older than 65. An example of the susceptibility of the aged to infectious disease occurred during the 2002–2003 outbreak of the newly emergent SARS coronavirus. The case fatality rate was less than 1% for people younger than 24 years, but was greater than 50% for those over 65 years.

Human Behavior Often Controls Exposure to Infectious Agents

The link between behavior and infection is probably most obvious for sexually transmitted diseases. Syphilis, gonorrhea, urogenital chlamydial infections, AIDS and a number of other infectious diseases are transmitted primarily by sexual contact.

TABLE 9-2
HOST DEFENSES AGAINST INFECTION

Skin
Tears
Normal bacterial flora
Gastric acid
Bile
Salivary and pancreatic secretions
Filtration system of nasopharynx
Mucociliary blanket
Bronchial, cervical, urethral and prostatic secretions
Neutrophils
Monocytes
Complement
Stationary mononuclear phagocyte system
Immunoglobulins
Cell-mediated immunity

Other aspects of behavior also influence the risk of acquiring infections. Humans contract brucellosis and Q fever, which are primarily bacterial diseases of domesticated farm animals, by close contact with infected animals or their secretions. These infections occur in farmers, herders, meat processors and, in the case of brucellosis, people who drink unpasteurized milk. Transmission of a number of parasitic diseases is strongly affected by behavior. Schistosomiasis is acquired when water-borne parasite larvae penetrate the skin of a susceptible host. It is primarily a disease of farmers who work in fields irrigated by infected water. The larvae of hookworm and *Strongyloides stercoralis* live in humid soil and penetrate the skin of the feet in people who walk barefoot. Shoes are probably the single most important factor in limiting infection with soil-transmitted nematodes. Anisakiasis and diphyllobothriasis are helminthic diseases acquired by eating incompletely cooked fish. Toxoplasmosis is a protozoan infection transmitted from animals to humans by ingestion of incompletely cooked, infected meat or by exposure to infected cat feces. Botulism, a food poisoning caused by a bacterial toxin, is contracted by ingestion of improperly canned food that contains the toxin.

As humans change their behavior, they open up new possibilities for infectious diseases. Although the agent of Legionnaires disease is common in the environment, aerosols generated by cooling plants, faucets and humidifiers provide the means for causing human infections. Traditional behaviors are not necessarily health promoting.

People with Compromised Defenses Are More Likely to Contract Infections and to Have More Severe Infections

Disruption or absence of any of the complex host defenses results in increased numbers and severity of infections. Damage to epithelial surfaces by trauma or burns can lead to invasive bacterial or fungal infections. Injury to the airway mucociliary apparatus, as in smoking or influenza, impairs clearance of inhaled microorganisms and gives rise to an increased incidence of bacterial pneumonia. Congenital absence of certain complement components prevents formation of a fully functional membrane attack complex and permits disseminated, and often recurrent, *Neisseria* infections (see Chapter 2). Diseases such as diabetes mellitus and the use of chemotherapeutic drugs and corticosteroids may interfere with neutrophil production or function and increase the likelihood and severity of infections with bacteria or fungi.

Compromised hosts are often attacked by organisms that are innocuous to normal people. For example, patients deficient in neutrophils frequently develop life-threatening bloodstream infections with commensal microorganisms that normally populate the skin and gastrointestinal tract. Such organisms that mainly cause disease in hosts with impaired defenses are **opportunistic pathogens**.

Viral Infections: Introduction

Viruses range from 20 to 300 nm and consist of RNA or DNA surrounded by a protein shell. Some are also enveloped in lipid membranes. *Viruses do not metabolize or reproduce independently. They are obligate intracellular parasites and require living cells in order to replicate.* After invading cells, they divert intracellular biosynthetic and metabolic pathways to synthesizing virus-encoded nucleic acids and proteins.

Viruses often cause disease by killing infected cells, but many do not. For example, rotavirus, a common cause of diarrhea, interferes with the function of infected enterocytes without immediately killing them. It prevents enterocytes from synthesizing proteins that transport molecules from the intestinal lumen, thus causing diarrhea.

Viruses may also promote release of chemical mediators that elicit inflammatory or immunologic responses. The symptoms of the common cold are due to release of bradykinin from infected cells. Other viruses cause cells to proliferate and form tumors. Human papillomaviruses (HPVs), for instance, cause squamous cell proliferative lesions, which include common warts (see Chapter 5).

Some viruses infect and persist in cells without interfering with cellular functions, a process known as **latency**. Latent viruses may emerge to produce disease years after a primary infection. Opportunistic infections may reflect reactivation of latent virus infections. CMV and herpes simplex viruses are commonly present as latent agents and emerge in people with impaired cell-mediated immunity.

Finally, some viruses may reside within cells, either by integrating into their genomes or by remaining episomal. Such viruses can cause those cells to generate tumors. EBV causes endemic Burkitt lymphoma in Africa and other tumors in different settings. Human T-cell leukemia virus-1 (HTLV-1; see Chapter 5) causes a form of T-cell leukemia/lymphoma.

This section is divided into diseases caused by RNA viruses and those caused by DNA viruses. This division reflects fundamental differences in the biology of these agents. Some viruses with highly organ-specific tropisms are not described in detail, but rather are addressed in those chapters that deal with the organs that are principally affected.

Viral Infections: RNA Viruses

RNA viruses generally follow different paths to causing disease than do most DNA viruses. They need different enzymes for their infectious cycles, and many aspects of their biology do not have correlates among DNA viruses. One of the key differences between some RNA viruses and many DNA viruses is that the polymerases of some important pathogenic RNA viruses (e.g., HIV-1, hepatitis C virus [HCV]) do not proofread the strand being synthesized. This has two important consequences. First, the mutation rate—and thus the plasticity of these viruses in circumventing therapies—is very high. Second, a greater proportion of daughter virions is inactive.

RESPIRATORY VIRUSES

The Common Cold Is the Most Common Viral Disease

The common cold (coryza) is an acute, self-limited upper respiratory tract disorder caused by infection with a variety of RNA viruses, including over 110 distinct rhinoviruses and several coronaviruses. Colds are frequent and worldwide in distribution. They spread from person to person via infected secretions. Infection is more likely during winter months in temperate areas and during the rainy seasons in the tropics, when spread is facilitated by indoor crowding. In the United States, children usually suffer six to eight colds per year and adults two to three. Overall, rhinoviruses cause up to 40% of all colds, coronaviruses 20%, and respiratory syncytial virus (RSV) 10%.

Rhinoviruses and coronaviruses have a tropism for respiratory epithelium and optimally reproduce at temperatures well below 37°C (98.6°F). Thus, infection remains confined to the cooler passages of the upper airway. The viruses infect the nasal respiratory epithelial cells, causing increased mucus production and edema. Infected cells release chemical mediators, such as bradykinin, which produce most of the symptoms associated with colds, namely, increased mucus production, nasal congestion and eustachian tube obstruction. Resulting stasis may predispose to secondary bacterial infection and lead to bacterial sinusitis and otitis media. Rhinoviruses and coronaviruses do not destroy respiratory epithelium and produce no visible alterations. Clinically, the common cold is characterized by rhinorrhea, pharyngitis, cough and low-grade fever. Symptoms last about a week.

Influenza May Predispose to Bacterial Pneumonia

Influenza is an acute, usually self-limited, infection of upper and lower airways, caused by influenza virus. These viruses are enveloped and contain single-stranded RNA.

 **EPIDEMIOLOGY:** There are three distinct types of influenza virus—A, B and C—that cause human disease. Influenza A is by far the most common and causes the most severe disease. Ten million to 40 million cases of influenza occur annually in the United States, often accounting for over 40,000 deaths. Influenza is highly contagious, and epidemics frequently spread around the world. New strains emerge regularly, often from animal hosts in parts of the world, largely the far east, where humans and animals, especially fowl, live in close contact. Influenza strains are identified by their type (A, B, C), serotype of their hemagglutinin (H) and neuraminidase (virus subtype), geographic site of origin, strain number and year of isolation (Fig. 9-1). Thus, the avian influenza virus ("bird flu") strain that emerged in 2003 and still continues to spread around the globe is designated A(H5N1). In 2009, a novel influenza A virus, designated H1N1 ("swine flu"), emerged in Veracruz, Mexico, and swiftly spread globally as a pandemic infection. The virulence of the H1N1 strain was underscored by the 10,000 deaths it caused in the United States alone within 7 months of its initial identification and 300,000 identified deaths worldwide by the end of the pandemic in 2009. This strain of influenza A virus has produced significant mortality in infected children and pregnant women. In 2013, a newly emergent and virulent strain of avian flu virus, H7N9, was identified in China. Because epidemic influenza virus antigens change so often, herd immunity that develops during one epidemic rarely protects against the next one.

 **MOLECULAR PATHOGENESIS:** Influenza spreads from person to person by virus-containing respiratory droplets and secretions. When it reaches

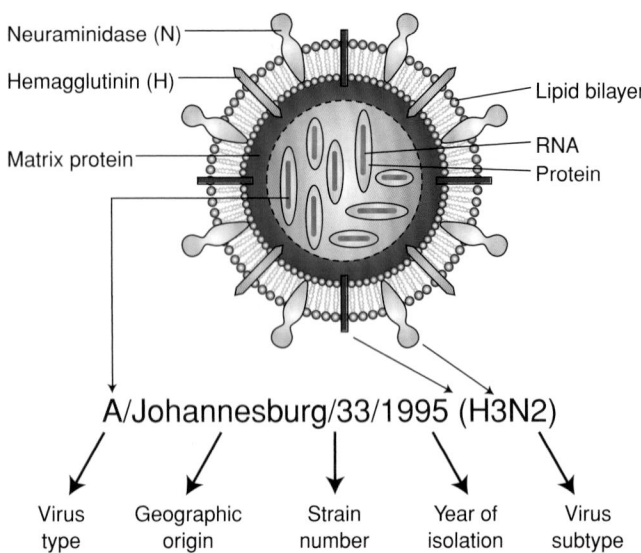

FIGURE 9-1. Nomenclature of influenza virus strains. The virus type (A, B or C) is based on nucleoprotein characteristics encoded by the NP gene of the virus. The H classification is based on the hemagglutinin (most commonly H1, H2 or H3, also H5) encoded by the HA gene. The N classification is based on the type of neuraminidase (N1 or N2) encoded by the NA gene.

the respiratory epithelial cell surface, a viral glycoprotein (hemagglutinin) that binds to sialic acid residues on human respiratory epithelium and the virus binds and enters the cell. Once inside, the virus directs the cell to produce progeny viruses and causes cell death. Infection usually involves both the upper and lower airways. Destruction of ciliated epithelium cripples mucociliary clearance, predisposing to bacterial pneumonia, especially with *Staphylococcus aureus* and *Streptococcus pneumoniae*.

 PATHOLOGY: Influenza virus causes necrosis and desquamation of ciliated respiratory tract epithelium and a predominantly lymphocytic inflammatory infiltrate. Extension of infection to the lungs leads to necrosis, sloughing of alveolar lining cells and the histologic appearance of viral pneumonitis.

 CLINICAL FEATURES: Rapid onset of fever, chills, myalgia, headaches, weakness and nonproductive cough are characteristic. Symptoms may be primarily those of an upper respiratory infection or those of tracheitis, bronchitis and pneumonia. Epidemics are accompanied by deaths from both influenza and its complications, particularly in the elderly and people with underlying cardiopulmonary disease. Prevention by killed viral vaccines specific to epidemic strains is 75% effective.

Parainfluenza Virus Is Associated with Croup

The parainfluenza viruses cause acute upper and lower respiratory tract infections, particularly in young children. The four serotypes of these enveloped, single-stranded RNA viruses belong to the paramyxovirus family. They are the most common cause of croup (laryngotracheobronchitis), which is characterized by stridor on inspiration and a "barking" cough.

 **EPIDEMIOLOGY:** Croup is common in children under the age of 3 years and is characterized by subglottic swelling, airway compression and respiratory distress. The virus spreads from person to person via infectious respiratory aerosols and secretions. Infection is highly contagious; disease is present worldwide. The parainfluenza viruses are isolated from 10% of young children with acute respiratory tract illnesses. While not as well known as influenza virus among the general population, parainfluenza virus infection is the second leading cause of hospitalization of children under 5 years of age for respiratory illness.

 PATHOLOGY: Parainfluenza viruses infect and kill ciliated respiratory epithelial cells and elicit an inflammatory response. In very young children, this process frequently extends into the lower respiratory tract, causing bronchiolitis and pneumonitis. In young children, where the trachea is narrow and the larynx is small, the local edema of laryngotracheitis compresses the upper airway enough to obstruct breathing and cause croup. Parainfluenza infection is associated with fever, hoarseness and cough. A barking cough is characteristic, as is inspiratory stridor. In older children and adults, symptoms are usually mild.

Respiratory Syncytial Virus Causes Bronchiolitis in Infants

 **EPIDEMIOLOGY:** RSV belongs to the same family, Paramyxoviridae, as parainfluenza virus. It spreads rapidly from child to child in respiratory aerosols and secretions, particularly in daycare centers, hospitals and other settings where small children are confined. The virus, which is present worldwide, is highly contagious. In the United States, 60% of infants are infected during their first RSV season, and nearly all will be infected by 2–3 years of age. RSV is the most common cause of bronchiolitis and pneumonia in children younger than 1 year old.

 PATHOLOGY: RSV produces necrosis and sloughing of bronchial, bronchiolar and alveolar epithelium, associated with a predominantly lymphocytic inflammatory infiltrate. Multinucleated syncytial cells are sometimes seen in infected tissues.

 CLINICAL FEATURES: Infants and young children with RSV bronchiolitis or pneumonitis present with wheezing, cough and respiratory distress, sometimes accompanied by fever. The illness is usually self-limited, resolving in 1–2 weeks. In older children and adults, RSV produces much milder disease. Among otherwise healthy young children, mortality from RSV infection is very low, but it rises dramatically, 20%–40%, among hospitalized children with congenital heart disease, chronic lung disease, prematurity or immunosuppression.

Severe Acute Respiratory Syndrome Is an Emergent Viral Disease Causing Outbreaks of Pneumonia

In early 2002, an epidemic of severe pneumonia was traced to Guangdong Province of China. As outbreaks occurred in Hong Kong, Vietnam and Singapore, the disease swept around the globe via international air travel. This emerging clinical disease, SARS, eventually spread to the United States, Canada and Europe. The causative agent is a novel coronavirus, termed the SARS-associated coronavirus (SARS-CoV). This agent is derived from a nonhuman host, now felt most likely to be bats, with civets and other animals as likely intermediate hosts. SARS is a potentially fatal viral respiratory illness, with an incubation period of 2–7 days and symptoms lasting up to 10 days. While this initial pandemic was spreading globally in 2003, there were over 8000 known cases and 775 deaths, a case fatality rate of 9.6%. Although the last infected human case occurred in mid-2003, SARS-CoV has not been eradicated and has the potential to reemerge.

 PATHOLOGY: Lungs of patients who died from SARS show diffuse alveolar damage (see Chapter 18). Multinucleated syncytial cells without viral inclusions have also been observed.

 CLINICAL FEATURES: Clinically, SARS begins with fever and headache, followed shortly by cough and dyspnea. Coryza is often absent and diarrhea is quite common. Some patients develop adult respiratory distress syndrome (ARDS; see Chapter 18) and are at high risk of complications and death. Most patients recover, but mortality may reach 15% in the elderly and in patients with other respiratory disorders. No specific treatment is available, although corticosteroids may offer some benefit.

VIRAL EXANTHEMS

Measles (Rubeola) Is a Highly Contagious Virus That May Cause Fatal Infection

Measles virus is an enveloped, single-stranded RNA paramyxovirus that causes an acute illness, characterized by upper respiratory tract symptoms, fever and rash.

 **EPIDEMIOLOGY:** Measles virus is transmitted to humans by respiratory aerosols and secretions. Among nonimmunized populations, it is primarily a disease of children. Currently available live, attenuated vaccines are highly effective in preventing measles and in eliminating virus spread. Nationwide immunization has made measles uncommon in the United States.

Measles is a particularly severe disease in the very young, the sick or the malnourished. In impoverished countries, it has a high mortality rate (10%–25%). In immunocompromised patients, the fatality rate is approximately 30%. WHO estimates that there were 160,000 deaths worldwide in 2011 due to measles. When measles was first introduced to previously unexposed populations (e.g., Native Americans, Pacific Islanders), resulting widespread infections had devastatingly high mortality rates.

 **PATHOPHYSIOLOGY:** The initial site of infection is the mucous membranes of the nasopharynx and bronchi. Two surface glycoproteins, "H" and "F," mediate viral attachment and fusion with

respiratory epithelium. The virus then spreads to regional lymph nodes and the bloodstream, leading to widespread dissemination and prominent involvement of the skin and lymphoid tissues. The rash results from the action of T lymphocytes on virally infected vascular endothelium.

 PATHOLOGY: Measles virus produces necrosis of infected respiratory epithelium, with a predominantly lymphocytic inflammatory infiltrate, and a vasculitis of small blood vessels in the skin. Lymphoid hyperplasia is often prominent in cervical and mesenteric lymph nodes, spleen and appendix. In lymphoid tissues, the virus sometimes causes fusion of infected cells, producing multinucleated giant cells containing up to 100 nuclei, with both intracytoplasmic and intranuclear inclusions. These cells, **Warthin-Finkeldey giant cells** (Fig. 9-2), are pathognomonic for measles.

CLINICAL FEATURES: Measles first manifests with fever, rhinorrhea, cough and conjunctivitis and progresses to the characteristic mucosal and skin lesions. The mucosal lesions, or "Koplik spots," are minute gray-white dots on a red base that appear on the posterior buccal mucosa. Skin lesions begin on the face as an erythematous maculopapular rash, which usually spreads to involve the trunk and extremities. The rash fades in 3–5 days, and symptoms gradually resolve. The clinical course of measles may be much more severe in those who are very young, malnourished or immunocompromised. The disease often leads to secondary bacterial infections, especially otitis media and pneumonia. Central nervous system invasion is probably a common event, as suggested by changes in electroencephalographic (EEG) readings. Acute encephalitis is rare but does occur. Uncommonly, years after a measles infection, patients can develop subacute sclerosing panencephalitis (SSPE), a slow, chronic neurodegenerative disorder (see Chapter 32). The exact pathophysiology of SSPE is unclear, but prophylactic vaccination against measles has greatly reduced its incidence.

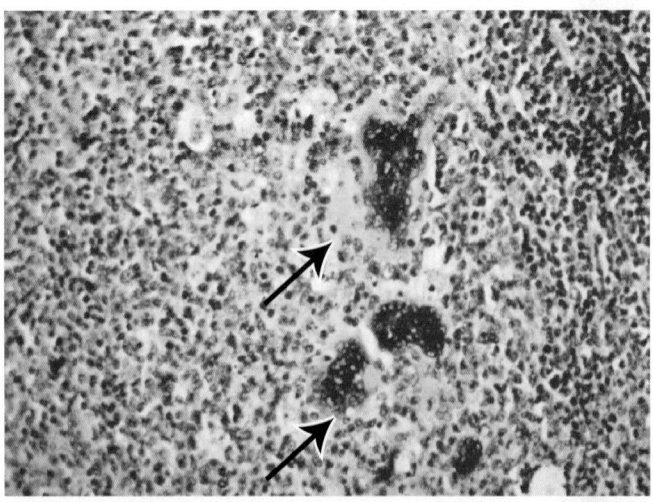

FIGURE 9-2. Warthin-Finkeldey giant cells in measles. A hyperplastic lymph node from a patient with measles shows several multinucleated giant cells (*arrows*).

Rubella Infection in Utero Causes Congenital Anomalies

Rubella virus is an enveloped, single-stranded RNA virus that causes a mild, self-limited systemic disease, usually associated with a rash (also known as "German measles"). Rubella virus is the only member of the genus *Rubivirus* in the family Togaviridae. Many infections are so mild that they go unnoticed. However, in pregnant women, rubella is a destructive fetal pathogen.

 **EPIDEMIOLOGY:** Rubella virus spreads from person to person, primarily by the respiratory route. Infection occurs worldwide. The virus is not highly contagious, and in unvaccinated populations, 10%–15% of young women remain susceptible to infection into their reproductive years. The currently available live attenuated viral vaccine prevents rubella and has largely eliminated the disease from developed countries. Thus, in the Americas, no endemic case has been observed since February 2009.

 **PATHOPHYSIOLOGY:** Rubella infects respiratory epithelium and then disseminates through the bloodstream and lymphatics. The rubella rash is believed to result from an immune response to the disseminated virus. Fetal infection occurs through the placenta during the viremic phase of maternal illness. A congenitally infected fetus remains persistently infected and sheds large amounts of virus in body fluids, even after birth. Maternal infection after 20 weeks' gestation usually does not cause fetal disease.

 PATHOLOGY: In most patients, rubella is a mild, acute febrile illness, with rhinorrhea, conjunctivitis, postauricular lymphadenopathy and a rash that spreads from face to trunk and extremities. The rash resolves within 3 days; complications are rare. As many as 30% of infections are completely asymptomatic.

In the fetus, the heart, eye and brain are the organs most often affected. Cardiac lesions include pulmonary valvular stenosis, pulmonary artery hypoplasia, ventricular septal defects and patent ductus arteriosus (50%). Cataracts, glaucoma, microphthalmia and retinal defects may occur in half of patients. Sensorineural deafness is a common (60%) complication of fetal rubella. Severe brain involvement can produce microcephaly and mental retardation.

MUMPS

Mumps virus is a paramyxovirus, an enveloped, single-stranded RNA virus. It causes an acute, self-limited systemic illness, characterized by parotid gland swelling and meningoencephalitis.

 EPIDEMIOLOGY: Mumps is a worldwide disease, primarily of children. It spreads from person to person via the respiratory route. The virus is highly contagious, and 90% of exposed, susceptible persons become infected, although only 65% develop symptoms. A live attenuated mumps vaccine prevents mumps, and the disease has been largely eliminated from most developed countries.

 PATHOPHYSIOLOGY: Mumps begins as viral infection of respiratory tract epithelium. The virus then disseminates through the blood and lymphatic systems to other sites, most commonly the salivary glands (especially parotids), central nervous system (CNS), pancreas and testes. Over half of infections involve the CNS, with symptomatic disease in 10%. Epididymoorchitis occurs in 20% of males infected after puberty.

 PATHOLOGY: Mumps virus causes necrosis of infected cells, eliciting a predominantly lymphocytic inflammatory infiltrate. Affected salivary glands are swollen, their ducts lined by necrotic epithelium and their interstitium infiltrated with lymphocytes. In mumps epididymoorchitis, the testes swell to three times normal size. The swelling of testicular parenchyma, confined within the tunica albuginea, produces focal infarcts. Mumps orchitis is usually unilateral and, thus, rarely causes sterility.

 CLINICAL FEATURES: Mumps begins with fever and malaise, followed by painful swelling of the salivary glands, usually one or both parotids. Symptomatic meningeal involvement most often manifests as headache, stiff neck and vomiting. Prior to widespread vaccination, mumps was a leading cause of viral meningitis and encephalitis in the United States. Although severe disease of the pancreas is rare in mumps, most patients have elevated serum amylase. Pancreatic infection has been implicated in some cases of type 1 diabetes.

INTESTINAL VIRUS INFECTIONS

Rotavirus Infection Is the Most Common Cause of Severe Diarrhea Worldwide

Rotavirus produces profuse watery diarrhea that can lead to dehydration and death if untreated. There are 5 species (A–E) of this double-stranded RNA member of the family Reoviridae. Type A, the most common, usually infects young children.

 **EPIDEMIOLOGY:** Rotavirus infection spreads from person to person by the oral–fecal route. Infection is most common among children, who shed huge amounts of virus in the stool. Siblings, playmates and parents, as well as food, water and environmental surfaces, readily become contaminated. The peak age of infection is 6 months to 2 years, and virtually all children have been infected by the age of 4 years. In the United States, each year rotavirus causes about 100 deaths in young children, and throughout the world, 500,000 deaths in children under 5 years of age.

 PATHOPHYSIOLOGY: Rotavirus infects enterocytes of the upper small intestine, disrupting absorption of sugars, fats and various ions.

The resulting osmotic load causes a net loss of fluid into the bowel lumen, producing diarrhea and dehydration. Infected cells are shed from intestinal villi, and the regenerating epithelium initially lacks full absorptive capabilities.

 PATHOLOGY: Pathologic changes in rotavirus infection are largely confined to the duodenum and jejunum. The intestinal villi are shortened and there is a mild infiltrate of neutrophils and lymphocytes.

 CLINICAL FEATURES: Rotavirus infection manifests as vomiting, fever, abdominal pain and profuse, watery diarrhea. Vomiting usually lasts for 2–3 days, but diarrhea continues for 5–8 days. Without adequate fluid replacement, diarrhea can produce fatal dehydration in young children.

Norwalk Virus and Other Gastrointestinal Viruses Often Cause Outbreaks of Diarrhea

In addition to rotavirus, many other viruses cause diarrhea. The best understood is the Norwalk family of nonenveloped RNA viruses, a group of caliciviruses whose names derive from the locations of particular outbreaks (e.g., Norwalk virus, Snow Mountain virus, Sapporo virus). Norwalk viruses are responsible for one third of all outbreaks of diarrheal disease. They produce gastroenteritis in children and adults, with self-limited vomiting and diarrhea, similar to that caused by rotavirus. Norwalk viruses infect cells of the upper small bowel and produce changes similar to those that occur with rotavirus.

VIRAL HEMORRHAGIC FEVERS

Viral hemorrhagic fevers are a group of at least 20 distinct viral infections that cause varying degrees of hemorrhage, shock and sometimes death. There are many similar viral hemorrhagic fevers in different parts of the world, usually named for the area where they were first described. Four virus families are involved—the Bunyaviridae, Flaviviridae, Arenaviridae and Filoviridae. On the basis of differences in routes of transmission, vectors and other epidemiologic characteristics, viral hemorrhagic fevers have been divided into four epidemiologic groups (Table 9-3): mosquito-borne; tick-borne; zoonotic; and the filoviruses, Marburg and Ebola virus, in which the route of transmission is unknown.

Yellow Fever May Lead to Fulminant Hepatic Failure

Yellow fever is an acute hemorrhagic fever, sometimes associated with extensive hepatic necrosis and jaundice. It is caused by an insect-borne flavivirus, an enveloped, single-stranded RNA virus. Other pathogenic flaviviruses cause Omsk hemorrhagic fever and Kyasanur Forest disease.

 **EPIDEMIOLOGY:** Yellow fever was first recognized in the New World in the 17th century, but its origins probably were in Africa. Today, the virus is restricted to parts of Africa and South America, including

TABLE 9-3
VIRAL HEMORRHAGIC FEVERS

Vector	Viral Fever
Mosquitoes	Yellow fever
	Rift valley fever
	Dengue hemorrhagic fever
	Chikungunya hemorrhagic fever
Ticks	Omsk hemorrhagic fever
	Crimean hemorrhagic fever
	Kyasanur forest disease
Rodents	Lassa fever
	Bolivian hemorrhagic fever
	Argentine hemorrhagic fever
	Korean hemorrhagic fever
Fruit bats	Ebola virus disease

both jungle and urban settings. Its usual reservoir is tree-dwelling monkeys, which are unaffected by the virus. The agent is passed among them in the forest canopy by mosquitoes. Humans acquire jungle yellow fever by being bitten by infected *Aedes mosquitoes*. Felling trees increases the risk of infection, because mosquitoes are brought down with the tree. On returning to the village or city, the human victim becomes a reservoir for epidemic yellow fever in the urban setting, where *Aedes aegypti* is the vector.

 PATHOPHYSIOLOGY: On inoculation by the mosquito, the virus multiplies within tissue and vascular endothelium, then disseminates through the bloodstream. It has a tropism for liver cells, where it sometimes produces extensive acute hepatocellular destruction. Extensive damage to the endothelium of small blood vessels may lead to the loss of vascular integrity, hemorrhages and shock.

 PATHOLOGY: Yellow fever virus causes coagulative necrosis of hepatocytes, beginning in the middle of hepatic lobules and spreading toward the central veins and portal tracts. The infection sometimes produces confluent necrosis in the middle of the hepatic lobules (i.e., midzonal necrosis). In the most severe cases, entire lobules may be necrotic. Some necrotic hepatocytes lose their nuclei and become intensely eosinophilic. They often dislodge from adjacent hepatocytes and are known as Councilman bodies (recognized today as apoptotic bodies).

 CLINICAL FEATURES: Yellow fever is characterized by abrupt onset of fever, chills, headache, myalgias, nausea and vomiting. After 3–5 days, some patients develop signs of hepatic failure, with jaundice (hence the term "yellow" fever), deficiencies of clotting factors and diffuse hemorrhages. Vomiting of clotted blood ("black vomit") is a classic feature of severe disease.

Patients with massive hepatic failure lapse into a coma and die, usually within 10 days of onset of illness. Overall mortality of yellow fever is 5%, but among those with jaundice, it rises to 30%.

Ebola Hemorrhagic Fever Is a Fatal African Disease

Ebola virus is an RNA virus belonging to the Filoviridae family. It causes a hemorrhagic disease with a **high mortality rate** in humans in several regions of Africa. The only other filovirus pathogenic to humans is Marburg virus, which produces Marburg hemorrhagic fever.

 **EPIDEMIOLOGY:** Ebola virus first emerged in Africa with two major disease outbreaks that occurred almost simultaneously in Zaire and Sudan in 1976. Outbreaks have occurred in Africa up to the present time.

In the wild, the virus infects humans, gorillas, chimpanzees and monkeys. Recent field evidence from Gabon and the Congo area of western Africa has implicated several species of fruit bats as the natural reservoir of Ebola virus. Health care workers and family members have become infected as a result of viral exposure while treating patients with Ebola hemorrhagic fever or during funerary preparation of the bodies of deceased victims. The virus can be transmitted via bodily secretions, blood and used needles.

 **ETIOLOGIC FACTORS AND PATHOLOGY:** *Ebola virus results in the most widespread destructive tissue lesions of all viral hemorrhagic fever agents.* The virus replicates massively in endothelial cells, mononuclear phagocytes and hepatocytes. Necrosis is most severe in the liver, kidneys, gonads, spleen and lymph nodes. The liver characteristically shows hepatocellular necrosis, Kupffer cell hyperplasia, Councilman bodies and microsteatosis. The lungs are usually hemorrhagic. Petechial hemorrhages are seen in the skin, mucous membranes and internal organs. Injury to the microvasculature and increased endothelial permeability are important causes of shock.

 CLINICAL FEATURES: Ebola fever incubates 2–21 days, after which initial symptoms include headache, weakness and fever, followed by diarrhea, nausea and vomiting. Some patients develop overt hemorrhage, including bleeding from injection sites, petechiae, gastrointestinal bleeding and gingival hemorrhage.

West Nile Virus Is Spread by Mosquito Vectors and Birds

 **EPIDEMIOLOGY:** The virus, a member of the family Flaviviridae, is increasing its geographic distribution as a result of spread by infected migratory birds and arthropods transported between continents in pooled water in cargo ships. West Nile virus (WNV) was isolated in 1937 from the blood of a febrile woman in Uganda. It spread rapidly through the Mediterranean and temperate parts of Europe. In 1999, WNV was first identified in the Western Hemisphere when it caused an outbreak of meningoencephalitis (West Nile fever) in New York City and the surrounding metropolitan area. In 2009, 660 cases of WNV infection and 30 fatalities in 34 states in the United

States occurred. By December 2012, WNV had been reported in people, birds or mosquitos from 48 states, with over 5000 human infections, of which half were neuroinvasive and 240 were fatal. WNV has also emerged as a potential threat to the safety of blood products (over 110 positive blood donors in 2009).

 PATHOLOGY: WNV can be recovered from blood for up to 10 days in immunocompetent febrile patients, and as late as 22–28 days after infection in immunocompromised people. Laboratory findings include moderate pleocytosis and elevated protein of the cerebrospinal fluid. Brains show mononuclear meningoencephalitis or encephalitis. The brainstem, particularly the medulla, can be extensively involved, and in some cases the cranial nerve roots show endoneural mononuclear inflammation. There are varying degrees of neuronal necrosis in gray matter, neuronal degeneration and neuronophagia.

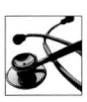 **CLINICAL FEATURES:** Most human WNV infections are subclinical and overt disease occurs in only 1 of 100 cases. The incubation period ranges from 3 to 15 days. Symptoms, if they occur, usually consist of fever, often with rash, lymphadenopathy and polyarthropathy. Patients with severe illness can develop acute aseptic meningitis or encephalitis, convulsions and coma. Anterior myelitis, hepatosplenomegaly, hepatitis, pancreatitis and myocarditis may occur. The probability of severe illness increases with increasing age. CNS infection is associated with 4%–13% mortality and is highest among the elderly.

Viral Infections: DNA Viruses

ADENOVIRUS

Adenoviruses are nonenveloped DNA viruses that are isolated from the respiratory and intestinal tracts of humans and animals. Certain serotypes are common causes of acute respiratory disease and adenovirus pneumonia in military recruits. Some adenoviruses are important causes of chronic pulmonary disease in infants and young children. Adenoviruses spread via direct contact, fecal–oral transmission and occasionally water-borne transmission.

 PATHOLOGY: Pathologic changes include necrotizing bronchitis and bronchiolitis, in which sloughed epithelial cells and inflammatory infiltrate fill damaged bronchioles. Interstitial pneumonitis is characterized by areas of consolidation, with extensive necrosis, hemorrhage and a mononuclear inflammatory infiltrate. Two distinct types of intranuclear inclusions— Cowdry type A inclusions and smudge cells (Fig. 9-3)— involve bronchiolar epithelial cells and alveolar lining cells. Infected cells with intranuclear inclusion bodies may be found. In the early stages of adenovirus infection, cytopathic effects appear as granular, slightly enlarged nuclei containing eosinophilic bodies intermixed with clumped basophilic chromatin. The eosinophilic bodies coalesce, forming larges

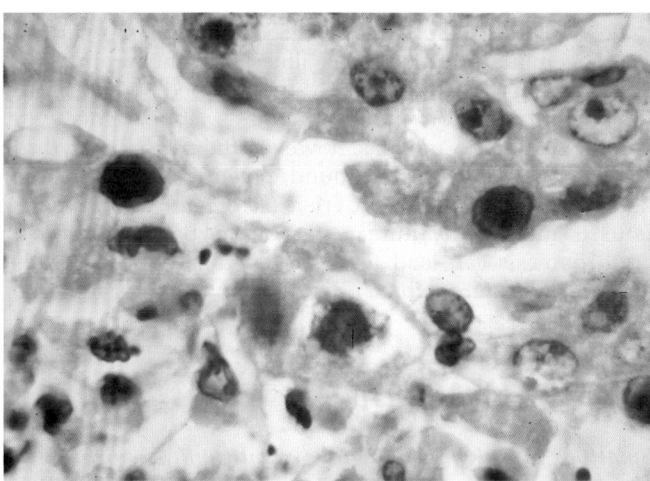

FIGURE 9-3. Adenovirus infection of the liver from a child. The two forms of viral inclusions are present: smudge cells and Cowdry A inclusions.

masses that end as a central, granular, ill-defined mass surrounded by a halo—the so-called Cowdry A inclusions. The second type of inclusion, which is more common and probably corresponds to a late-stage infected cell, is the "smudge cell." The nucleus is rounded or ovoid, large and completely occupied by a granular amphophilic to deeply basophilic mass. There is no halo, and the nuclear membrane and nucleus are indistinct.

Adenoviruses types 40 and 41 infect colonic and small intestinal epithelial cells and may cause diarrhea. People with AIDS are particularly susceptible to urinary tract infections caused by adenovirus type 35. In immunocompromised patients and transplant recipients, adenovirus can cause fulminant or disseminated disease, such as colitis, pneumonitis, pancreatitis, nephritis, meningoencephalitis and hepatitis.

HUMAN PARVOVIRUS (ERYTHROVIRUS) B19

Human parvovirus B19, now called erythrovirus, is a single-stranded DNA virus that causes **erythema infectiosum**, a benign self-limited febrile illness in children. It also produces systemic infections, characterized by rash, arthralgias and transient interruption in erythrocyte production in nonimmune adults.

 ETIOLOGIC FACTORS: The virus spreads from person to person by the respiratory route. Infection is common and occurs in outbreaks, mostly among children. It is not known which cells, other than erythroid precursors, support virus replication, but the agent probably replicates in the respiratory tract before it spreads to erythropoietic cells.

 PATHOLOGY: Human parvovirus B19 gains entry to erythroid precursor cells via the P-erythrocyte antigen and produces characteristic cytopathic effects in those cells. Nuclei of affected cells are enlarged, and chromatin is displaced peripherally by central, glassy, eosinophilic inclusion bodies (giant pronormoblasts).

CLINICAL FEATURES: Most people suffer a mild exanthematous illness, **erythema infectiosum ("fifth disease")**, accompanied by an asymptomatic interruption in erythropoiesis. In patients with chronic hemolytic anemias, however, the pause in erythrocyte production causes profound, potentially fatal anemia, known as **transient aplastic crisis** (see Chapter 26). When a fetus is infected by human parvovirus B19, cessation of erythropoiesis can lead to severe anemia, hydrops fetalis and death in utero, which occurs in about 10% of maternal infections.

SMALLPOX (VARIOLA)

Smallpox is a highly contagious exanthematous viral infection produced by variola virus, a member of the family Poxviridae.

 **EPIDEMIOLOGY:** Smallpox is an ancient disease; a rash resembling smallpox was found in the mummified remains of Egyptian pharaoh Ramses V. In the 6th century, a Swiss bishop named the etiologic agent of smallpox "variola" from the Latin *varius,* meaning "pimple" or "spot." The infection was common in Europe and arrived in the New World with Spanish colonists, where it often decimated native populations. In 1796, Edward Jenner performed the first successful vaccination when he inoculated a child with exudate from the hand of a milkmaid infected with cowpox. Once the cowpox pustule had regressed, Jenner challenged that child with smallpox and demonstrated that he was protected from the disease. In 1967, the WHO began its uniquely successful campaign to eradicate smallpox. The last occurrence of endemic smallpox was in Somalia in 1977, and the last reported human cases were laboratory-acquired infections in 1978. On May 8, 1980, the WHO declared that smallpox had been eradicated. Two known repositories of variola virus remain: one at the Centers for Disease Control and Prevention (CDC) in the United States and one at the Institute for Virus Preparation in Russia. There has been considerable vigilance to its reemergence, either naturally or as a bioweapon.

 **ETIOLOGIC FACTORS:** Smallpox was transmitted between victims and susceptible people via droplets or aerosol of infected saliva. Viral titers in the saliva were highest in the first week of infection. The virus is highly stable and remains infective for long periods outside its human host. Two types of smallpox have been recognized. *Variola major* was prevalent in Asia and parts of Africa and represented the prototypical form of the infection. *Variola minor* was found in Africa, South America and Europe and was distinguished by its milder systemic toxicity and smaller pox lesions.

 PATHOLOGY: Skin vesicles of variola show cellular necrosis and scarce areas of ballooning degeneration. Eosinophilic, intracytoplasmic inclusion bodies (Guarnieri bodies) are seen but are not specific for smallpox since they occur in most poxviral infections. Vesicles also occur in the palate, pharynx, trachea and esophagus. In severe cases of smallpox, there is gastric and intestinal involvement, hepatitis and interstitial nephritis.

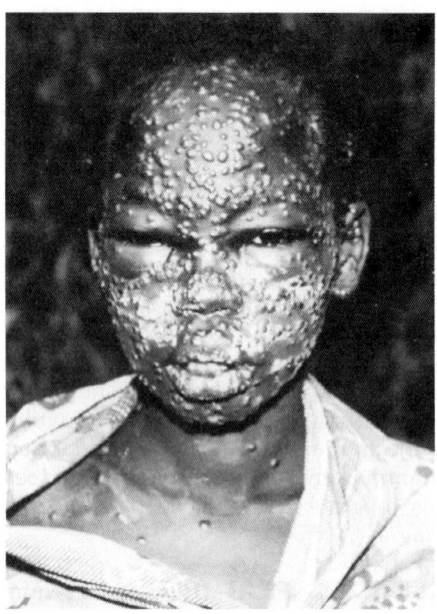

FIGURE 9-4. Child with smallpox, Bangladesh, 1973.

 **CLINICAL FEATURES:** The incubation period of smallpox is 12 days (range, 7–17 days) after exposure. After entering the respiratory tract, variola travels to regional lymph nodes, where it replicates. Viremia follows. Clinical manifestations begin abruptly, with malaise, fever, vomiting and headache. The characteristic rash, most prominent on the face but also involving the hands and forearms, follows in 2–3 days. After subsequent eruptions on the lower extremities, the rash spreads centrally during the next week to the trunk. Lesions progress quickly from macules to papules, then to pustular vesicles (Fig. 9-4), and generally remain synchronous in their stage of development. By 8–14 days after onset, the pustules form scabs, which leave depressed scars on healing after 3–4 weeks. The case fatality rate is 30% in unvaccinated individuals.

MONKEYPOX

Monkeypox, a rare viral disease occurring mostly in Central and Western Africa, and more recently in Sudan, is the only remaining potentially fatal infection of humans to be caused by a member of the Poxviridae.

EPIDEMIOLOGY: The virus was first isolated from monkeys, giving it its name, but it is actually more prevalent in rodents in endemic areas. It is mainly a zoonotic disease in parts of Central and Western Africa. Recent data suggest that since the eradication of smallpox in Africa, residents of the Democratic Republic of the Congo are now 20 times more likely to acquire monkeypox infection than they were in 1986. An outbreak of monkeypox occurred in seven states in the United States in 2003 among 93 people who either owned or had exposure to pet prairie dogs. Infected animals had been exposed to an infected Gambian pouched rat in an exotic pet store. Dormice and squirrels have also been implicated as natural reservoirs of the virus. Human infection can follow a bite from an infected host or contact with its body fluids. Human-to-human transmission is uncommon.

CLINICAL FEATURES: The incubation period in humans is approximately 12 days. Its clinical presentation is similar to that of smallpox, but milder. Illness begins with fever, headache, lymphadenopathy, malaise, muscle ache and backache. Within 1–3 days after onset of fever, a papular rash occurs in the face or other body parts, which ultimately crusts and fall off. Illness typically lasts for 2 weeks. In Africa, the case fatality is as high as 10%.

HERPESVIRUSES

The virus family Herpesviridae includes a large number of enveloped DNA viruses, many of which infect humans. Almost all herpesviruses express some common antigenic determinants, and many produce type A nuclear inclusions (acidophilic bodies surrounded by a halo). The most important pathogenic herpesviruses (HHVs) are varicella-zoster virus (VZV, or HHV-3); herpes simplex virus 1 and 2 (HSV-1 and -2); EBV (HHV-4); HHV6, the cause of roseola; CMV (HHV-5); HHV-7, a cause of exanthema subitum; and Kaposi sarcoma–associated herpesvirus (HHV-8), a human oncovirus causing Kaposi sarcoma, primary effusion lymphoma and some types of Castleman disease. *These viruses are distinguished by their capacity to remain latent for long periods of time.*

Varicella-Zoster Infection Causes Chickenpox and Herpes Zoster

First exposure to VZV produces chickenpox, an acute systemic illness characterized by a generalized vesicular skin eruption (Fig. 9-5). The virus then becomes latent, and its reactivation many years later causes herpes zoster ("shingles"), a localized vesicular skin eruption.

 **ETIOLOGIC FACTORS AND EPIDEMIOLOGY:** VZV is restricted to human hosts and spreads from person to person primarily by the respiratory route. It can also be spread by contact with secretions from skin lesions. The virus is present worldwide and is highly contagious. Most children in the United States were formerly infected by early school age, but an effective vaccine has reduced this incidence.

VZV initially infects the respiratory tract or conjunctival epithelium. There it reproduces and spreads through the blood and lymphatic systems. Many organs are infected during this viremic stage, but skin involvement usually dominates the clinical picture. The virus spreads from the capillary endothelium to the epidermis, where its replication destroys the basal cells. As a result, the upper layers of the epidermis separate from the basal layer to form vesicles.

During primary infection, VZV establishes latent infection in perineuronal satellite cells of the dorsal nerve root ganglia. Transcription of viral genes continues during latency, and viral DNA can be demonstrated years after the initial infection.

Shingles occurs when virus replication occurs in ganglion cells and the agent travels down the sensory nerve from a single dermatome. It then infects the corresponding epidermis, producing a localized, painful vesicular eruption. The risk of shingles in an infected person increases with age, and most cases occur among the elderly. Impaired cell-mediated immunity also increases the risk of VZV reactivation.

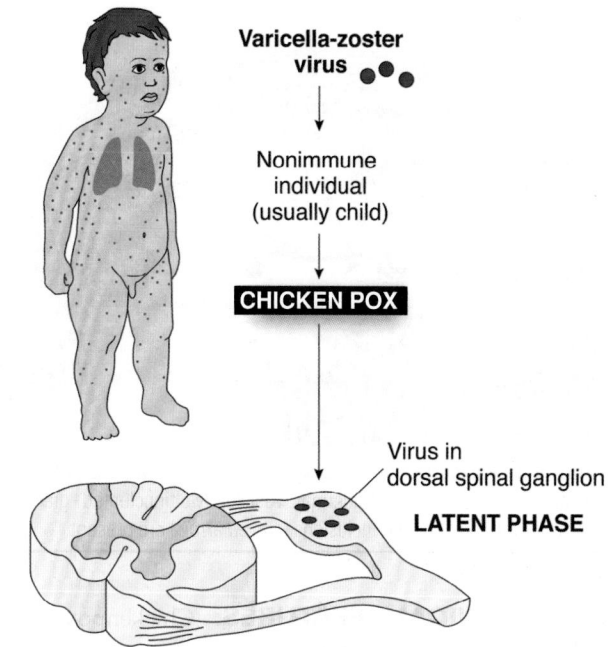

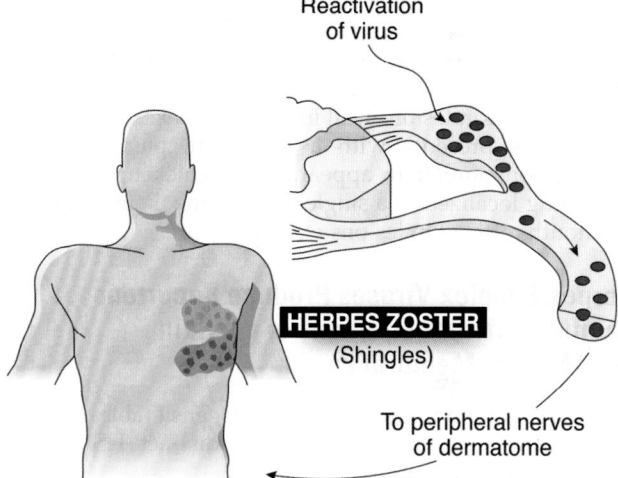

FIGURE 9-5. Varicella (chickenpox) and herpes zoster (shingles). Varicella-zoster virus (VZV) in droplets is inhaled by a nonimmune person (usually a child) and initially causes a "silent" infection of the nasopharynx. This progresses to viremia, seeding of fixed macrophages and dissemination of VZV to skin (chickenpox) and viscera. VZV resides in a dorsal spinal ganglion, where it remains dormant for many years. Latent VZV is reactivated and spreads from ganglia along the sensory nerves to the peripheral nerves of sensory dermatomes, causing shingles.

 PATHOLOGY: The skin lesions of chickenpox and shingles are identical to each other and also to lesions caused by HSV. Vesicles fill with neutrophils, soon erode and become shallow ulcers. In infected cells, VZV produces a characteristic cytopathic effect, with nuclear homogenization and intranuclear inclusions (Cowdry type A). Inclusions are large and eosinophilic and are separated from the nuclear membrane by a clear zone (halo). Multinucleated cells are common (Fig. 9-6). Over several days, vesicles become pustules, which then rupture and heal.

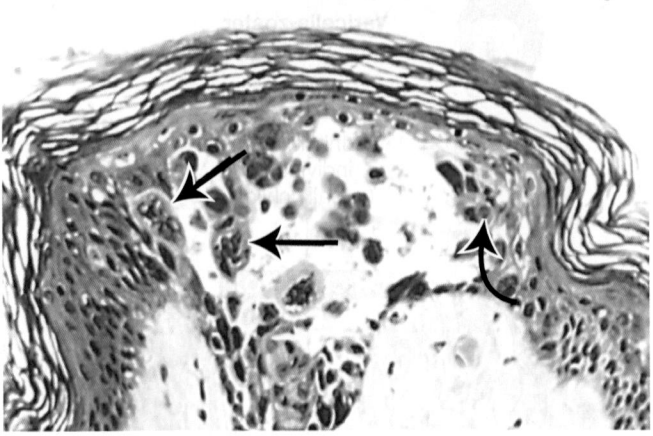

FIGURE 9-6. Varicella. Photomicrograph of the skin from a patient with chickenpox shows an intraepidermal vesicle. Multinucleated giant cells (*straight arrows*) and nuclear inclusions (*curved arrow*) are present.

 **CLINICAL FEATURES:** Chickenpox causes fever, malaise and a distinctive pruritic rash that starts on the head and spreads to the trunk and extremities. Skin lesions begin as maculopapules that rapidly evolve into vesicles, then pustules that soon ulcerate and crust. Vesicles may also appear on mucous membranes, especially the mouth. Fever and systemic symptoms resolve in 3–5 days; skin lesions heal in several weeks.

Shingles presents with a unilateral, painful, vesicular eruption, similar in appearance to chickenpox, usually remaining localized to a single dermatome. Pain can persist for months after skin lesions resolve.

Herpes Simplex Viruses Produce Recurrent Painful Vesicular Eruptions of the Skin and Mucous Membranes

HSVs are common human viral pathogens (Table 9-4). Two antigenically and epidemiologically distinct HSVs cause human disease (Fig. 9-7):

- **HSV-1** is transmitted in oral secretions and typically causes disease "above the waist," including oral, facial and ocular lesions.

TABLE 9-4

HERPES SIMPLEX VIRUS (HSV) DISEASES

Viral Type	Common Presentations	Infrequent Presentations
HSV-1	Oral–labial herpes	Conjunctivitis, keratitis
		Encephalitis
		Herpetic whitlow
		Esophagitis[a]
		Pneumonia[a]
		Disseminated infection[a]
HSV-2	Genital herpes	Perinatal infection
		Disseminated infection[a]

[a]These conditions usually occur in immunocompromised hosts.

- **HSV-2** is transmitted in genital secretions and typically produces genital ulcers and neonatal herpes infection.

 EPIDEMIOLOGY: HSV spreads from person to person, mainly via direct contact with infected secretions or open lesions. HSV-1 spreads in oral secretions, and infection frequently occurs in childhood, most people (50%–90%) being infected by adulthood. HSV-2 spreads by contact with genital lesions and is primarily a venereally transmitted pathogen. Neonatal herpes is acquired when a baby passes through an infected birth canal.

PATHOPHYSIOLOGY: Primary HSV disease occurs at a site of initial viral inoculation, such as the oropharynx, genital mucosa or skin. The virus infects epithelial cells, producing progeny viruses and destroying basal cells in the squamous epithelium, with resulting formation of vesicles. Cell necrosis also elicits an inflammatory response, initially dominated by neutrophils and then followed by lymphocytes. Primary infection resolves when humoral and cell-mediated immunity to the virus develop.

Latent infection is established in a manner analogous to that of VZV. The virus invades sensory nerve endings in the oral or genital mucosa, ascends within axons and establishes a latent infection in sensory neurons within corresponding ganglia. From time to time, the virus awakens from latency and travels back down the nerve to the epithelial site served by the ganglion, where it again infects epithelial cells. Sometimes this secondary infection produces ulcerating vesicular lesions. At other times, the secondary infection does not cause visible tissue destruction, but contagious progeny viruses are shed from the site of infection. Various factors, usually typical for a given person, can induce reactivation of latent HSV infection. These include intense sunlight, emotional stress, febrile illness and, in women, menstruation. Both HSV-1 and HSV-2 can cause severe protracted and disseminated disease in immunocompromised persons.

Herpes encephalitis is a rare (1 in 100,000 HSV infections), but devastating, manifestation of HSV-1 infection. In some instances, it occurs when virus that is latent in the trigeminal ganglion is reactivated and travels retrograde to the brain. However, herpes encephalitis also occurs in people who have no history of "cold sores," and the pathogenesis of the encephalitis in these cases is poorly understood (see Chapter 28). Equally rare is **herpes hepatitis,** which may occur in immunocompromised patients but is also seen in previously healthy pregnant women.

Neonatal herpes is a serious complication of maternal genital herpes. The virus is transmitted to the fetus from the infected birth canal, often the uterine cervix, and readily disseminates in the unprotected newborn child.

Aseptic meningitis without genital involvement may be a manifestation of HSV-2 infection.

 PATHOLOGY: The skin and mucous membranes are the usual sites of HSV infection, but the disease sometimes involves the brain, eye, liver, lungs and other organs. In any location, both HSV-1 and HSV-2 cause

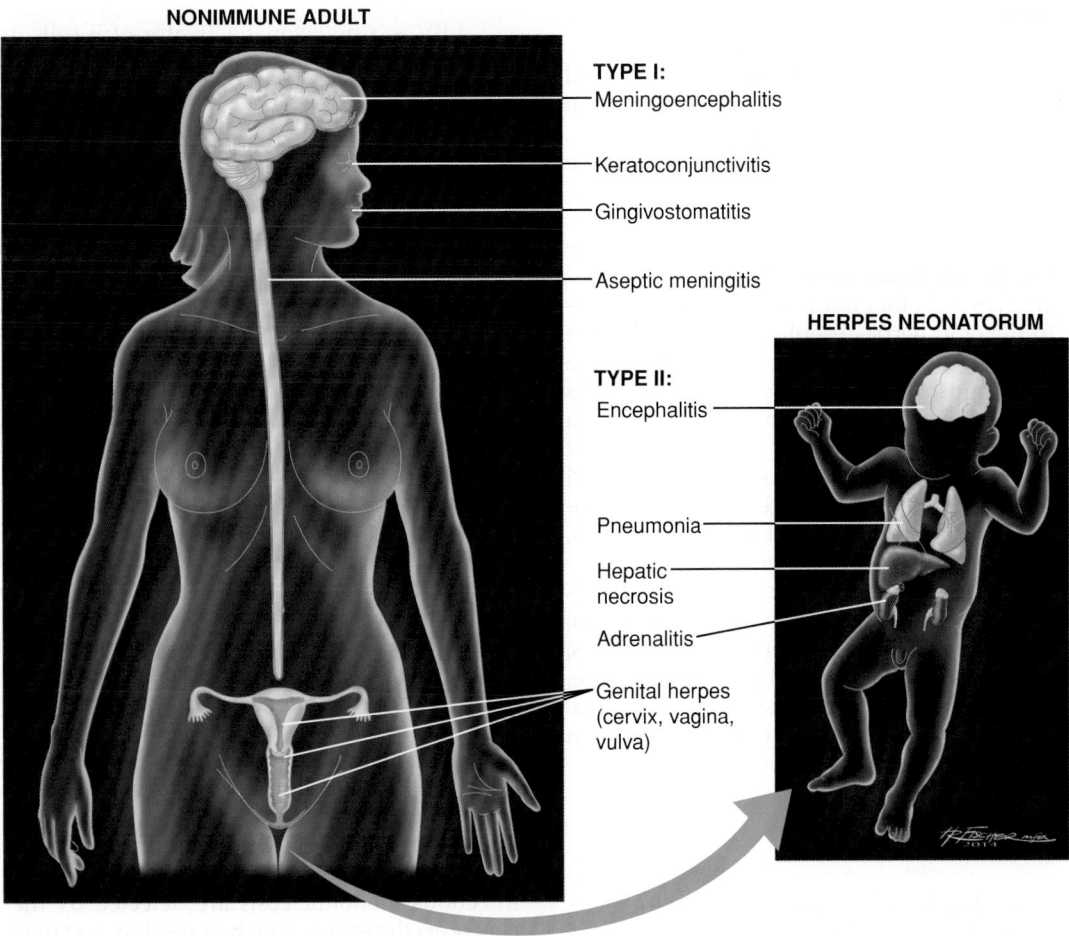

NONIMMUNE ADULT

TYPE I:
— Meningoencephalitis

— Keratoconjunctivitis

— Gingivostomatitis

— Aseptic meningitis

HERPES NEONATORUM

TYPE II:
Encephalitis

Pneumonia

Hepatic
necrosis

Adrenalitis

Genital herpes
(cervix, vagina,
vulva)

FIGURE 9-7. Herpesvirus infections. Herpes simplex virus type 1 (HSV-1) infects a nonimmune adult, causing gingivostomatitis ("fever blister" or "cold sore"), keratoconjunctivitis, meningoencephalitis and aseptic spinal meningitis. HSV-2 infects the genitalia of a nonimmune adult, involving the cervix, vagina and vulva. HSV-2 infects the fetus as it passes through the birth canal of an infected mother. The infant's lack of a mature immune system results in disseminated infection with HSV-1. The infection is often fatal, involving lung, liver, adrenal glands and central nervous system.

necrosis of infected cells, accompanied by a vigorous inflammatory response. Clusters of painful ulcerating vesicular lesions on the skin or mucous membranes are the most frequent manifestation of HSV infection (Fig. 9-8A). These lesions persist for 1–2 weeks and then resolve. The cellular alterations include (1) nuclear homogenization, (2) Cowdry type A intranuclear inclusions and (3) multinucleated giant cells (Fig. 9-8B).

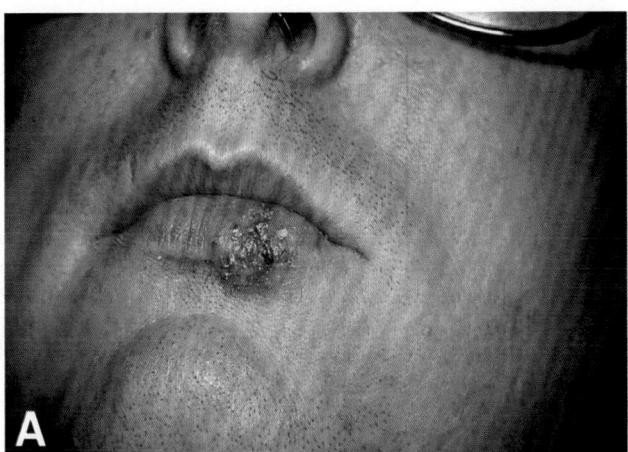

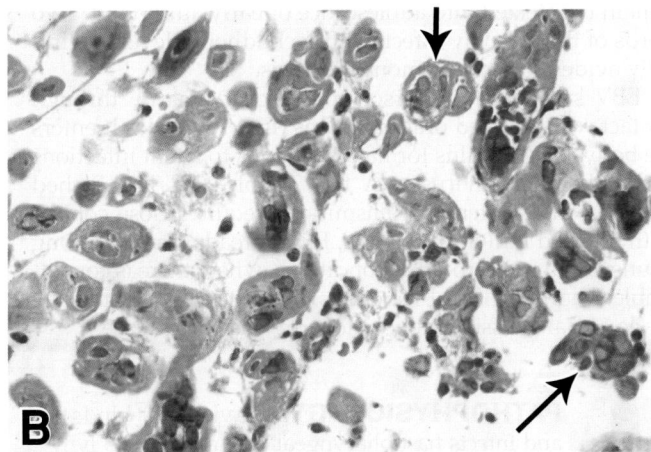

FIGURE 9-8. Herpes simplex virus type 1 (HSV-1). A. Herpetic vesicles are seen on the surface of the lower lip. **B.** Epithelial cells infected with HSV-1 demonstrate Cowdry type A intranuclear inclusions and multinucleated giant cells.

CLINICAL FEATURES: Clinical features of HSV infections vary according to host susceptibility (e.g., neonate, normal host, compromised host), viral type and site of infection. A prodromal "tingling" sensation at the site often precedes the appearance of skin lesions. Recurrent lesions appear weeks, months or years later, at the initial site or at a location subserved by the same nerve ganglion. Recurrent herpetic lesions in the mouth or on the lip, commonly called "cold sores" or "fever blisters," frequently appear after sun exposure, trauma or a febrile illness.

Patients with AIDS and other immunocompromised people are prone to develop herpes esophagitis. Early lesions consist of rounded 1–3-mm vesicles predominantly in the mid- to distal esophagus. As HSV-infected squamous cells slough from these lesions, sharply demarcated ulcers with elevated margins form and coalesce. This process may result in denudation of the esophageal mucosa. Superimposed *Candida* infection is common at this stage. In immunocompromised patients, HSV may also infect the anal mucosa, where it causes painful blisters and ulcers.

Neonatal herpes begins 5–7 days after delivery, with irritability, lethargy and a mucocutaneous vesicular eruption. The infection rapidly spreads to involve multiple organs, including the brain. The infected newborn develops jaundice, bleeding problems, respiratory distress, seizures and coma. Treatment of severe HSV infections with acyclovir is often effective, but neonatal herpes still carries a high mortality.

EPSTEIN-BARR VIRUS

Infectious mononucleosis is a viral disease with fever, pharyngitis, lymphadenopathy and increased circulating lymphocytes. By adulthood, most people have been infected with EBV. Most EBV infections are asymptomatic, but EBV may cause infectious mononucleosis. It is also associated with several cancers, including **African Burkitt lymphoma**, **B-cell lymphoma** in immunosuppressed patients and **nasopharyngeal carcinoma**. These neoplastic complications are discussed in Chapters 5, 26 and 29.

EPIDEMIOLOGY: In areas of the world where children live in crowded conditions, EBV infection usually occurs before 3 years of age, and infectious mononucleosis is rare. In developed countries, many people remain uninfected into adolescence or early adulthood. Two thirds of those newly infected after childhood develop clinically evident infectious mononucleosis.

EBV spreads from person to person primarily through contact with infected oral secretions (Fig. 9-9). Once it enters the body, EBV remains for life, analogous to latent infections with other herpesviruses. A few people (10%–20%) shed the virus intermittently. Transmission requires close contact with infected individuals. Thus, EBV spreads readily among young children in crowded conditions, where there is considerable "sharing" of oral secretions. Kissing is also an effective mode of transmission, hence the term "kissing disease."

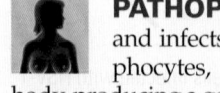

PATHOPHYSIOLOGY: The virus first binds to and infects nasopharyngeal cells and then B lymphocytes, which carry the virus throughout the body, producing a generalized infection of lymphoid tissues.

EBV is a polyclonal activator of B cells. In turn, activated B cells stimulate proliferation of specific killer T lymphocytes and suppressor T cells. The former destroy virally infected B cells, whereas suppressor cells inhibit production of immunoglobulins by B cells.

PATHOLOGY: The pathology of infectious mononucleosis mainly involves the lymph nodes and spleen. In most patients, lymphadenopathy is symmetric and most striking in the neck. The nodes are movable, discrete and tender. General nodal architecture is preserved. Germinal centers are enlarged with indistinct margins, because of proliferation of immunoblasts. Nodes contain occasional large hyperchromatic cells with polylobular nuclei that resemble Reed-Sternberg cells of Hodgkin disease. In fact, lymph node histology may be difficult to distinguish from Hodgkin disease or other lymphomas (see Chapter 26).

The spleen is large and soft owing to hyperplasia of the red pulp, and is susceptible to rupture. Immunoblasts are abundant and infiltrate vessel walls, the trabeculae and the capsule. The liver is almost always involved, with sinusoids and portal tracts containing atypical lymphocytes.

Infectious mononucleosis is characterized by lymphocytosis with **atypical lymphocytes**. These are activated T cells with lobulated, eccentric nuclei and vacuolated cytoplasm that kill EBV-infected B lymphocytes. Patients with infectious mononucleosis develop a specific **heterophile antibody**—an immunoglobulin produced in one species that reacts with antigens of another species. These antibodies in infectious mononucleosis are detected by their affinity for sheep erythrocytes, which is used as a standard diagnostic test for infectious mononucleosis. Specific serologic tests for antibodies against EBV are also available.

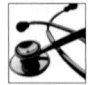

CLINICAL FEATURES: Infectious mononucleosis manifests as fever, malaise, lymphadenopathy, pharyngitis and splenomegaly. Patients usually have elevated leukocyte counts, with a predominance of lymphocytes and monocytes. Treatment is supportive; symptoms usually resolve in 3–4 weeks.

CYTOMEGALOVIRUS

CMV is a congenital and opportunistic pathogen that usually produces asymptomatic infection. However, the fetus and immunocompromised patients are particularly vulnerable to its destructive effects. CMV infects 0.5%–2.0% of all fetuses and injures 10%–20% of those infected, making it the most common congenital pathogen.

EPIDEMIOLOGY: CMV spreads from person to person by contact with infected secretions and bodily fluids and is transmitted to the fetus across the placenta. Children spread it in saliva or urine, while transmission among adolescents and adults is primarily through sexual contact.

ETIOLOGIC FACTORS: CMV infects various human cells, including epithelial cells, lymphocytes and monocytes, and establishes latency in white blood cells. Normal immune responses rapidly control

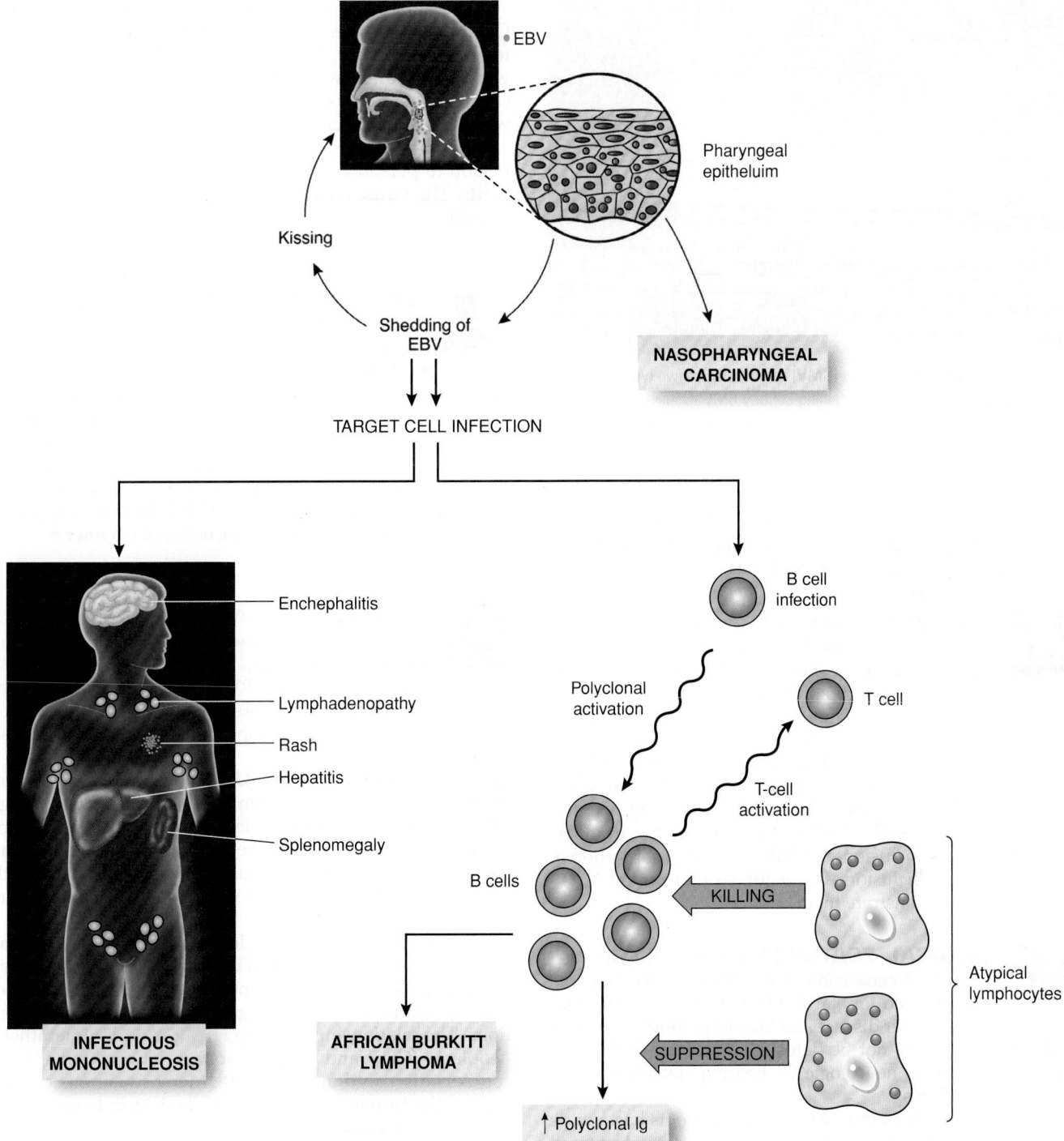

FIGURE 9-9. Role of Epstein-Barr virus (EBV) in infectious mononucleosis, nasopharyngeal carcinoma and Burkitt lymphoma. EBV invades and replicates within the salivary glands or pharyngeal epithelium and is shed into the saliva and respiratory secretions. In some people, the virus transforms pharyngeal epithelial cells, leading to nasopharyngeal carcinoma. In persons who are not immune from childhood exposure, EBV causes infectious mononucleosis. EBV infects B lymphocytes, which undergo polyclonal activation. These B cells stimulate the production of atypical lymphocytes, which kill virally infected B cells and suppress the production of immunoglobulins. Some infected B cells are transformed into immature malignant lymphocytes of Burkitt lymphoma.

infection, and ill effects are rare. However, virus is shed periodically in body secretions. Like other herpesviruses, CMV may remain latent for life.

When an infected pregnant woman passes CMV to her fetus, the fetus is not protected by maternally derived antibodies. As a result, the virus invades fetal cells with little initial immunologic response, causing widespread necrosis and inflammation. CMV produces similar lesions in patients with suppressed cell-mediated immunity.

CMV infection is often symptomatic in immunosuppressed individuals, such as organ transplant recipients. In that setting, the CMV infection usually represents

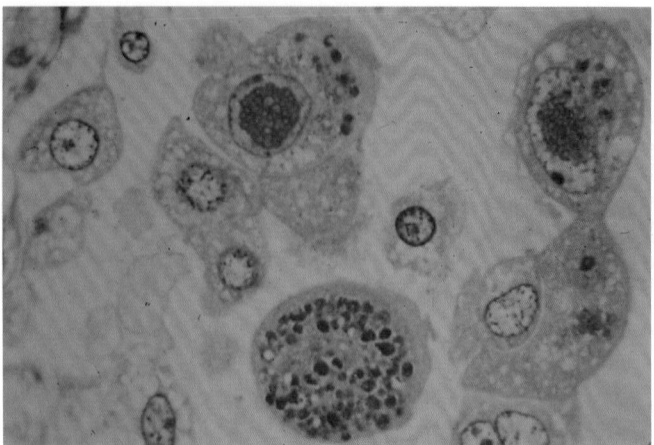

FIGURE 9-10. Cytomegalovirus (CMV) pneumonitis. Two type II pneumocytes display enlarged nuclei containing solitary CMV inclusions surrounded by a clear zone. The cell at the bottom shows numerous intracytoplasmic CMV inclusions.

reactivation of endogenous latent infection, whether the source is the graft or the recipient. Subsequent dissemination may lead to severe systemic disease.

 PATHOLOGY: Fetal CMV disease most commonly involves the brain, inner ears, eyes, liver and bone marrow. Severely affected fetuses may have microcephaly, hydrocephalus, cerebral calcifications, hepatosplenomegaly and jaundice. Lesions of fetal CMV disease show cellular necrosis and a characteristic cytopathic effect, consisting of marked cellular and nuclear enlargement, with nuclear and cytoplasmic inclusions. The giant nucleus, which is usually solitary, contains a large central inclusion surrounded by a clear zone. The smaller, granular intracytoplasmic inclusions of CMV occur after formation of the intranuclear inclusion (Fig. 9-10), so that not all CMV-infected cells demonstrate them.

 CLINICAL FEATURES: Congenital CMV disease has diverse clinical presentations. At its worst, it many lead to fetal death in utero with conspicuous CNS lesions, liver disease and bleeding. Most congenital CMV infection may not be detected until later in life and manifest as subtle neurologic or hearing defects without gross abnormalities.

CMV disease in immunosuppressed patients has a wide range of clinical manifestations. It can lead to decreased visual acuity (chorioretinitis), diarrhea or gastrointestinal hemorrhage (colonic ulcerations), change in mental status (encephalitis), shortness of breath (pneumonitis) or any number of other symptoms.

HUMAN PAPILLOMAVIRUS

HPVs cause proliferative lesions of squamous epithelium, including common warts, flat warts, plantar warts, anogenital warts (condyloma acuminatum) and laryngeal papillomatosis. Some HPV serotypes cause squamous cell dysplasias and squamous cell carcinomas of the genital tract (see Chapters 5 and 24).

HPVs are nonenveloped, double-stranded DNA viruses. Over 100 HPV types are known, different ones causing different lesions. Thus, HPV types 1, 2 and 4 produce common warts and plantar warts. Types 6, 10, 11 and 40 through 45 cause anogenital warts. Types 16, 18 and 31 are associated with squamous carcinomas of the female genital tract.

HPV infection is widespread. It is transmitted by direct person-to-person contact. Most children develop common warts. The viruses that cause genital lesions are transmitted sexually.

 PATHOPHYSIOLOGY: HPV infection begins with viral inoculation into a stratified squamous epithelium, where the virus enters the nuclei of basal cells. Infection stimulates proliferation of the squamous epithelium, producing the various HPV-associated lesions. The rapidly growing squamous epithelium replicates innumerable progeny viruses, which are shed in the degenerating superficial cells. Many HPV lesions resolve spontaneously. Depressed cell-mediated immunity may lead to persistence and spread of HPV lesions. Malignant change in HPV infections is discussed in Chapter 5.

 PATHOLOGY: HPV infections produce squamous proliferations, which vary in appearance and biological behavior. Most show thickening of affected epithelium. Some HPV-infected cells show characteristic **koilocytosis,** with large squamous cells with shrunken nuclei enveloped in large cytoplasmic vacuoles (koilocytes).

CLINICAL FEATURES: Common warts (verruca vulgaris) are firm, circumscribed, raised, rough-surfaced lesions, which usually appear on surfaces subject to trauma, especially the hands (see Chapter 28). **Plantar warts** are similar squamous proliferative lesions on the soles of the feet but are compressed inward by standing and walking.

Anogenital warts (condyloma acuminatum) are soft, raised, fleshy lesions found on the penis, vulva, vaginal wall, cervix or perianal region. When caused by certain HPV types, flat warts can evolve into malignant squamous cell proliferations. The relationship between HPV, cervical intraepithelial neoplasia (CIN) and invasive squamous carcinoma of the cervix is discussed in Chapter 18. Many squamous carcinomas of the upper respiratory tract and lung have recently been shown to harbor HPV.

Prions: A New Disease Paradigm

In the last several decades, it has become clear that infection can be transmitted and propagated solely by proteins, without the participation of nucleic acids. To date, these particles, prions, are only known to cause CNS disease. Prions are essentially misfolded proteins that aggregate in the CNS and cause progressive neurodegeneration. The prion protein (PrP) exists in a normal isoform and in a pathogenic form. The latter is transmissible. Of particular importance is the uncommon persistence of these infectious agents. Normal methods of sterilization do not inactivate them, so they may be transmitted via surgical instruments or electrodes. All prion diseases feature spongiform encephalopathy. The mechanisms of prion-associated diseases are discussed more fully in Chapter 32.

- **Kuru:** Kuru is a progressive neurodegenerative disease only found in the South Fore tribe in the remote highlands of Papua New Guinea. Kuru, the Fore word for "trembling," was transmitted via cannibalism. Once funerary cannibalism among the Fore was eliminated, kuru disappeared within a generation.
- **Sporadic, familial and iatrogenic Creutzfeldt-Jakob disease** (sCJD, fCJD and iCJD): CJD is a rapidly progressive neurodegenerative disorder characterized by myoclonus, behavior changes and dementia (see Chapter 32). With a frequency of 1 in 1,000,000, sCJD is probably the most common human prion disease. Rarely, CJD has resulted from transmission through transplanting such tissues as cornea and dural matter. Before the advent of recombinant protein therapeutics, CJD was also transmitted from human growth hormone isolated by cadaver pituitaries.
- **New variant Creutzfeldt-Jakob disease** (vCJD): One of the more infamous emerging infectious diseases of the last few decades, both vCJD and bovine spongiform encephalopathy (BSE), also known as "mad cow "disease, underscore the interrelatedness of animal and human infectious agents. The use of certain animal products in feeds for domestic ungulates led to a prion disease epidemic in cattle herds of the United Kingdom. Nearly 150 people are known to have been infected with this relentless terminal disease. All patients to date have had an uncommon genetic homozygosity: methionine–methionine at codon 129 of the gene (PRNP) for the prion protein. Presentations have differed from previously recognized forms of CJD in a number of important ways, with age of onset being most notable. Whereas the mean onset of CJD has been 65 years, vCJD has mainly occurred in young adults, with a mean age of 26. Psychiatric signs and symptoms have also been predominant in vCJD. Pathologic changes in vCJD are strikingly similar to those seen in BSE and differ somewhat from changes seen in the sporadic form.
- **Fatal familial insomnia:** This is a rare inherited prion disorder that has as its hallmark a progressive course of insomnia that worsens over time until the patient sleeps barely or not at all. There is also autonomic instability, which usually manifests as increased sympathetic tone. Altered sensorium may also be present, and signs of motor system degeneration follow. Spongiform changes like those seen in other transmissible spongiform encephalopathies are also seen later in the disease.
- **Gerstmann-Sträussler-Scheinker syndrome:** This rare transmissible spongiform encephalopathy is usually familial, although rare sporadic cases have been described. Patients may present with a variety of symptoms, but signs and symptoms of cerebellar degeneration usually predominate. Later, dementia becomes common.

Bacterial Infections

Bacteria, at 0.1–10 μm, are the smallest living cells. They have three basic structural components: nuclear body, cytosol and envelope. The **nuclear body** consists of a single, coiled, circular molecule of double-stranded DNA with associated RNA and proteins. It is not separated from the cytoplasm by a special membrane, a feature that distinguishes bacteria, as prokaryotes, from eukaryotes. The **cytosol** is densely packed with ribosomes, proteins and carbohydrates and lacks the structured organelles, such as mitochondria and Golgi apparatus, of eukaryotic cells. The **bacterial envelope** is a permeability barrier and is also actively involved in transport, protein synthesis, energy generation, DNA synthesis and cell division.

Bacteria are classified by the structural features of their envelope. The simplest envelope is only a phospholipid–protein bilayer membrane. Mycoplasmas have such an envelope. Most bacteria, however, have a rigid cell wall that surrounds the cell membrane. Two types of bacterial cell walls are identified by their Gram stain properties:

- **Gram-positive bacteria** retain iodine–crystal violet complexes when decolorized and appear dark blue. Their cell walls contain teichoic acids and a thick peptidoglycan layer.
- **Gram-negative bacteria** lose the iodine–crystal violet stain when decolorized and appear red with a counterstain. Outer membranes of gram-negative bacteria contain a lipopolysaccharide component, known as endotoxin, which is a potent mediator of the shock that complicates infections with these organisms.

Both gram-positive and gram-negative cell walls may be surrounded by an additional layer of polysaccharide or protein gel, a **capsule**. Capsules aid bacterial attachment and colonization and may protect bacteria from phagocytosis. Because capsules are important in many infections, bacteria may be classified as **encapsulated** or **unencapsulated**.

The cell wall confers rigidity to bacteria and allows them to be distinguished on the basis of shape and pattern of growth in cultures. Round or oval bacteria are **cocci** .Those that grow in clusters are called **staphylococci,** while those that grow in chains are **streptococci**. Elongate bacteria are **rods,** or **bacilli,** and curved ones are **vibrios.** Some spiral-shaped bacteria are named **spirochetes**.

Most bacteria can be cultured on chemical media, and so may be described according to their growth requirements on these media. Bacteria that need high levels of oxygen are called **aerobic,** those that grow best without oxygen are **anaerobic** and those that thrive with limited oxygen are **microaerophilic**. Bacteria that grow well with or without oxygen are **facultative anaerobes**.

BACTERIAL EXOTOXINS: Many bacteria secrete toxins (exotoxins) that damage human cells, either at the site of bacterial growth or at distant sites. These toxins are often named for the site or mechanism of their activity. Thus, those that act on the nervous system are **neurotoxins;** those that affect intestinal cells are **enterotoxins**. Some toxins that kill target cells, such as diphtheria toxin or some of the *Clostridium perfringens* toxins, are known as **cytotoxins.** Others may disturb normal functions of their target cells and damage or kill them, like the diarrheagenic toxin of *Vibrio cholerae* or the neurotoxin of *Clostridium botulinum. C. perfringens* produces over 20 highly diverse toxins.

BACTERIAL ENDOTOXINS: As mentioned above, gram-negative bacteria contain a structural element called **lipopolysaccharide,** or **endotoxin,** in their outer membranes. Lipopolysaccharide activates complement, coagulation, fibrinolysis and bradykinin systems (see Chapter 2). It also causes release of primary inflammatory mediators, including tumor necrosis factor (TNF) and interleukin-1 (IL-1), and various colony-stimulating factors. Endotoxin may cause shock, complement depletion and disseminated intravascular coagulation.

Many bacteria damage tissues by eliciting inflammatory or immune responses. The capsule of *Streptococcus pneumoniae* protects it from phagocytosis while activating a host's inflammatory response. Within the lung, the encapsulated organism causes exudation of fluid and cells that fill alveoli. This inflammation impairs breathing but does not, at least initially, limit the organism's proliferation. *Treponema pallidum,* the spirochete that causes syphilis, persists in the body for years and elicits inflammatory and immune responses that continuously damage host tissues.

Many common bacterial infections (e.g., *Staphylococcus aureus* skin infections) are characterized by purulent exudates, but tissue responses to bacteria are highly variable. In some cases, such as cholera, botulism and tetanus, there is no inflammatory response at critical sites of cellular injury. Other bacterial infections, including syphilis and Lyme disease, lead to a predominantly lymphocytic and plasma cellular response. Still others (e.g., brucellosis) are characterized by granuloma formation.

Many bacterial diseases are caused by organisms that normally inhabit the human body. The gastrointestinal tract, upper respiratory tract, skin and vagina are all home to diverse bacteria. These microorganisms are normally commensal and cause no harm. However, if they gain access to usually sterile sites, or if host defenses are impaired, they can produce extensive destruction. *S. aureus, S. pneumoniae* and *Escherichia coli* are normal flora that are also major human pathogens.

PYOGENIC GRAM-POSITIVE COCCI

Staphylococcus aureus Produces Suppurative Infections

S. aureus is a gram-positive coccus that typically grows in clusters and is among the most common bacterial pathogens. It normally resides on the skin and is readily inoculated into deeper tissues, where it causes suppurative infections. *It is the most common cause of suppurative infections of the skin, joints and bones and is a leading cause of infective endocarditis. S. aureus* is commonly distinguished from other, less virulent staphylococci by the coagulase test. *S. aureus* is coagulase positive; the other staphylococci are coagulase negative.

S. aureus spreads by direct contact with colonized surfaces or persons. Most people are intermittently colonized with *S. aureus* and carry it on the skin, nares or clothing. The organism also survives on inanimate surfaces for long periods.

 PATHOPHYSIOLOGY: Many *S. aureus* infections begin as localized infections of skin and skin appendages, producing cellulitis and abscesses. The organism, equipped with destructive enzymes and toxins, sometimes invades beyond the initial site, spreading by blood or lymphatics to almost any location in the body. Bones, joints and heart valves are the most common sites of metastatic *S. aureus* infections. *S. aureus* also causes several distinct diseases by elaborating toxins that are carried to distant sites.

 PATHOLOGY: When *S. aureus* is introduced into a previously sterile site, infection usually produces suppuration and abscesses. These range from microscopic foci to lesions several centimeters in diameter, which are filled with pus and bacteria.

CLINICAL FEATURES: The clinical manifestations of *S. aureus* disease vary according to the sites and types of infection.

- **Furuncles (boils) and styes:** Deep-seated *S. aureus* infections occur in and around hair follicles, often in a nasal carrier. They localize on hairy surfaces, such as the neck, thighs and buttocks of men and the axillae, pubic area and eyelids of both sexes. Boils begin as nodules at the bases of hair follicles, becoming pimples that remain painful and red for a few days. Yellow apices form and central cores become necrotic and fluctuant. Rupture or incision relieves the pain. **Styes** are boils that involve the sebaceous glands around the eyelid. **Paronychia** are staphylococcal infections of nail beds, and **felons** are the same infections on the palmar side of the fingertips.
- **Carbuncles:** These lesions, mostly on the neck, result from coalescing infections with *S. aureus* around hair follicles and produce draining sinuses (Fig. 9-11).
- **Scalded skin syndrome:** This disease affects infants and children under 3 years, who present with a sunburn-like rash that begins on the face and spreads over the body. Bullae begin to form and even gentle rubbing causes skin to desquamate. The disease begins to resolve in 1–2 weeks, as the skin regenerates. Desquamation is due to systemic effects of a specific exotoxin, and the site of *S. aureus* proliferation is often occult.

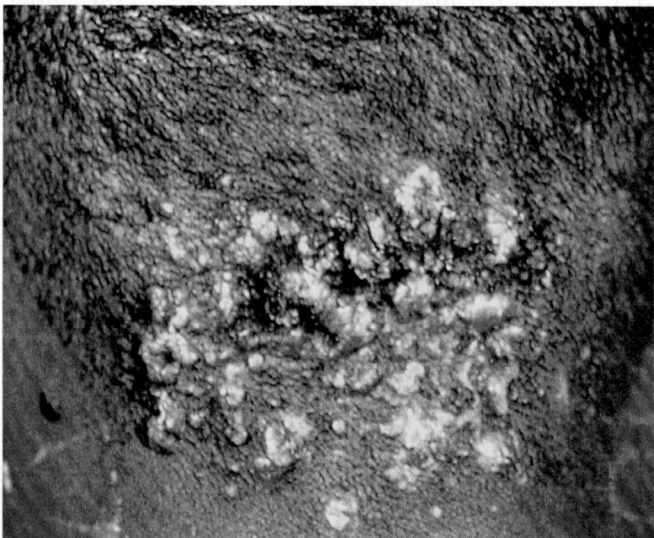

FIGURE 9-11. Staphylococcal carbuncle. The posterior neck is indurated and shows multiple follicular abscesses discharging purulent material.

- **Osteomyelitis:** Acute staphylococcal osteomyelitis, usually in the leg bones, most commonly afflicts boys between 3 and 10 years old. There is usually a history of infection or trauma. If not properly treated, osteomyelitis may become chronic. Adults older than 50 years are more frequently afflicted with vertebral osteomyelitis, which may follow staphylococcal infections of the skin or urinary tract, prostatic surgery or pinning of a fracture.
- **Infections of burns or surgical wounds:** These sites often become infected with *S. aureus* from the patient's own nasal carriage or from medical personnel. Newborns and elderly, malnourished, diabetic and obese persons all have increased susceptibility.
- **Respiratory tract infections:** Staphylococcal respiratory tract infections occur mostly in infants under 2 years, and especially under 2 months. The infection is characterized by ulcers of the upper airway, scattered foci of pneumonia, pleural effusion, empyema and pneumothorax. In adults, staphylococcal pneumonia may follow viral influenza, which destroys the ciliated surface epithelium and leaves the bronchial surface vulnerable to secondary infection.
- **Bacterial arthritis:** *S. aureus* is responsible for half of all septic arthritis, mostly in patients 50–70 years old. Rheumatoid arthritis and corticosteroid therapy are common predisposing conditions.
- **Septicemia:** Septicemia with *S. aureus* afflicts patients with lowered resistance who are in the hospital for other diseases. Some have underlying staphylococcal infections (e.g., septic arthritis, osteomyelitis), some have had surgery (e.g., transurethral prostate resection) and some have infections from an indwelling intravenous catheter. Miliary abscesses and endocarditis are serious complications.
- **Bacterial endocarditis:** This common complication of *S. aureus* septicemia may develop spontaneously on normal valves, on valves damaged by rheumatic fever or on prosthetic valves. Intravenous drug abuse predisposes to staphylococcal endocarditis.
- **Toxic shock syndrome:** This potentially fatal disorder most commonly afflicts menstruating women, who present with high fever, nausea, vomiting, diarrhea and myalgias. Subsequently, they develop shock and within several days a sunburn-like rash. Toxic shock syndrome is associated with use of tampons, particularly hyperabsorbent ones, which provide a site for *S. aureus* replication and toxin elaboration. Toxic shock syndrome occurs rarely in children and men, and is then usually associated with an occult *S. aureus* infection.
- **Staphylococcal food poisoning:** Staphylococcal food poisoning typically begins less than 6 hours after a meal. Nausea and vomiting begin abruptly and usually resolve within 12 hours. This disease is caused by preformed toxin present in the food at the time it is eaten.
- **Antibiotic-resistant *S. aureus:*** One of the most important clinical issues concerning *S. aureus* is the relentless increase in its antibiotic resistance since penicillin was introduced in the early 1940s. *S. aureus* was one of the first important pathogens to become completely resistant to penicillin and, with time, to each subsequent generation of penicillin derivatives. Today, methicillin-resistant *S. aureus* (MRSA) infections are usually acquired in the hospital, in an environment that selects for antibiotic-resistant bacteria. MRSA represents one of the most dreaded of nosocomial infections. Between 1995 and 2004, the percentage of

S. aureus infections due to MRSA in patients in intensive care units doubled to almost two thirds. As of 2007, 0.8% of the U.S. population were colonized with MRSA. MRSA infections in the United States are responsible for 19,000 deaths annually. Community-acquired MRSA appears to be a different strain from hospital-acquired MRSA infections with enhanced virulence and different susceptibility to antibiotics.

Coagulase-Negative Staphylococci Infect Prosthetic Devices

Coagulase-negative staphylococci are the major cause of infections involving medical devices, including intravenous catheters, prosthetic heart valves, heart pacemakers, orthopedic prostheses, cerebrospinal fluid shunts and peritoneal catheters.

Disease caused by coagulase-negative staphylococci usually derives from the normal bacterial flora. Of the more than 20 known species of coagulase-negative staphylococci, 10 are normal residents of human skin and mucosal surfaces. Staphylococcus epidermidis *is the most frequent cause of infections associated with medical devices.* Another species, *Staphylococcus saprophyticus*, causes 10%–20% of acute urinary tract infections in young women.

 PATHOPHYSIOLOGY: Coagulase-negative staphylococci readily contaminate foreign bodies, on which they proliferate slowly, inducing inflammatory responses that damage adjacent tissue. Bacteria present on an intravascular surface, such as the tip of an intravascular catheter, can spread through the bloodstream to cause metastatic infections. Coagulase-negative staphylococci lack the enzymes and toxins that permit *S. aureus* to cause extensive local tissue destruction. Some strains of coagulase-negative staphylococci produce a polysaccharide gel biofilm, which enhances their adherence to foreign objects and protects them from host antimicrobial defenses and from many antibiotics.

 PATHOLOGY: Medical devices infected with coagulase-negative staphylococci are usually thinly coated with tan, fibrinous material. Coagulase-negative staphylococcal infections usually do not produce extensive local tissue necrosis or large quantities of pus. Microscopic examination of infected devices shows clusters of gram-positive bacteria embedded in fibrin and cellular debris, with an associated acute inflammatory infiltrate.

 CLINICAL FEATURES: Coagulase-negative staphylococcal infections usually have subtle clinical presentations, and the only symptom of infection may be persistent low-grade fever. Infection of orthopedic prostheses frequently causes progressive loosening and dysfunction of the devices. These infections are usually indolent, but in compromised hosts, they may be fatal. Treatment usually requires replacement of any infected foreign object and appropriate antibiotic therapy. Nosocomial strains of coagulase-negative *Staphylococcus* are often multidrug resistant. Some 80% of such hospital-acquired isolates have

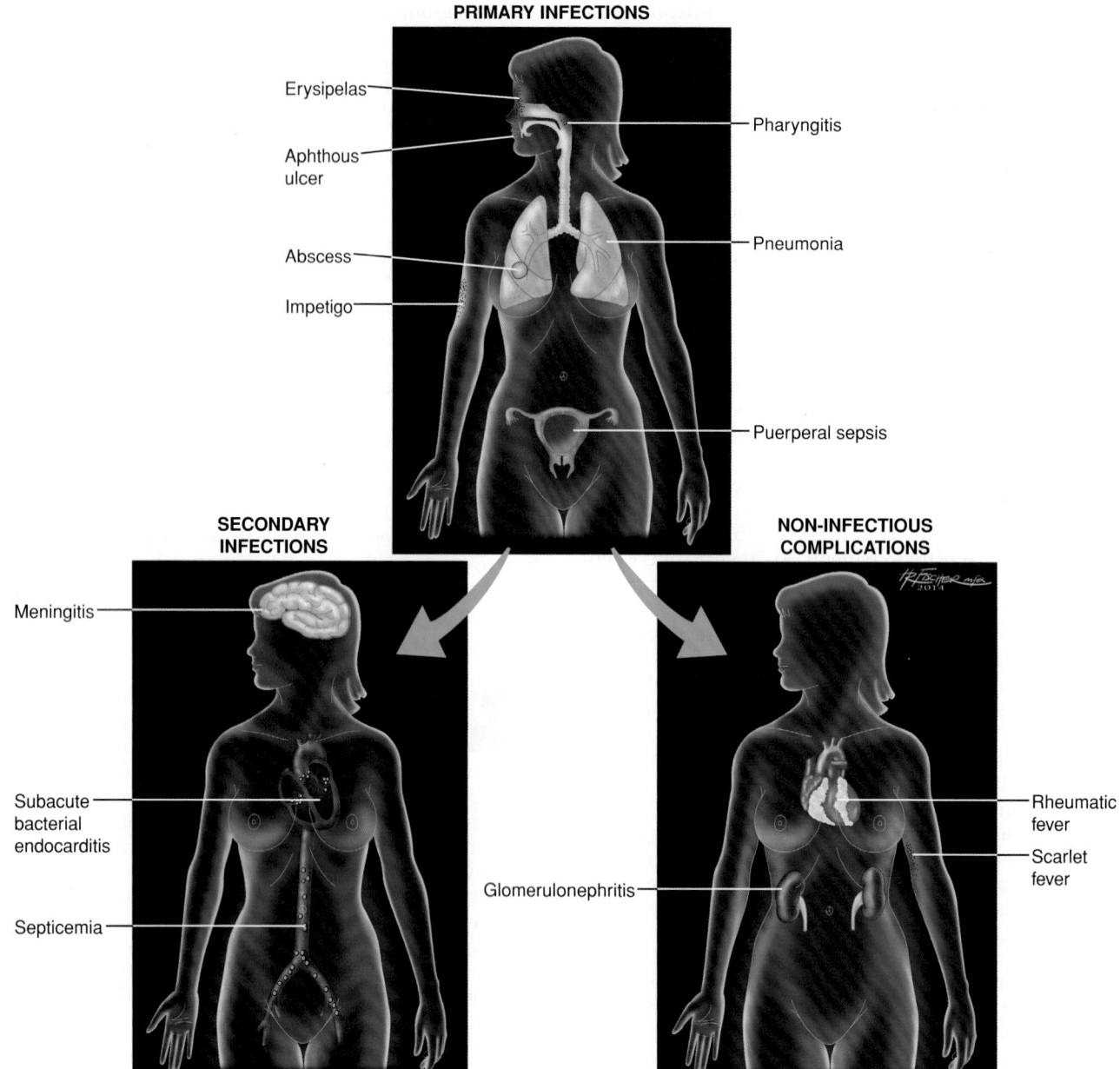

PRIMARY INFECTIONS

Erysipelas

Aphthous ulcer

Abscess

Impetigo

Pharyngitis

Pneumonia

Puerperal sepsis

SECONDARY INFECTIONS

Meningitis

Subacute bacterial endocarditis

Septicemia

NON-INFECTIOUS COMPLICATIONS

Rheumatic fever

Scarlet fever

Glomerulonephritis

FIGURE 9-12. Streptococcal diseases.

the *mecA* gene, which encodes resistance to all classes of β-lactam antibiotics.

Streptococcus pyogenes Causes Suppurative, Toxin-Related and Immunologic Reactions

Streptococcus pyogenes, *also known as group A streptococcus, is one of the most common human pathogens, causing diseases of diverse organ systems, from acute self-limited pharyngitis to major illnesses such as rheumatic fever* (Fig. 9-12). This gram-positive coccus is frequently part of the endogenous flora of the skin and oropharynx.

Diseases caused by *S. pyogenes* may be suppurative or nonsuppurative. The former occur at sites of bacterial invasion and consequent tissue necrosis and usually involve acute inflammatory responses. Suppurative *S. pyogenes* infections include pharyngitis, impetigo, cellulitis, myositis,

pneumonia and puerperal sepsis. By contrast, the locations of nonsuppurative diseases caused by *S. pyogenes* are remote from the site of bacterial invasion. The two major nonsuppurative complications of *S. pyogenes* are rheumatic fever and acute poststreptococcal glomerulonephritis. These involve (1) organs far from the sites of streptococcal invasion, (2) a time delay after the acute infection and (3) immune reactions. Rheumatic fever is discussed in Chapter 17 and poststreptococcal glomerulonephritis in Chapter 22.

S. pyogenes elaborates several exotoxins, including erythrogenic toxins and cytolytic toxins **(streptolysins S and O).** Erythrogenic toxins cause the rash of scarlet fever. Streptolysin S lyses bacterial protoplasts (L forms) and probably destroys neutrophils after they ingest *S. pyogenes*. Streptolysin O induces a persistently high antibody titer, an effect that provides a useful marker for the diagnosis of *S. pyogenes* infections and their nonsuppurative complications.

Streptococcal Pharyngitis ("Strep Throat")

S. pyogenes, the common bacterial cause of pharyngitis, spreads from person to person by direct contact with oral or respiratory secretions. "Strep throat" occurs worldwide, predominantly affecting children and adolescents.

 MOLECULAR PATHOGENESIS: *S. pyogenes* attaches to epithelial cells by binding to fibronectin on their surface. The bacterium produces hemolysins, DNAase, hyaluronidase and streptokinase, which allow it to damage and invade human tissues. *S. pyogenes* also has cell wall components that protect it from the inflammatory response. One of these, **M protein,** protrudes from cell walls of virulent strains and prevents complement deposition, thereby protecting bacteria from phagocytosis. Another surface protein destroys C5a, blocking its opsonizing effect and inhibiting phagocytosis. The invading organism elicits acute inflammation, often producing an exudate of neutrophils in the tonsillar fossae.

CLINICAL FEATURES: "Strep throat" is a sore throat with fever, malaise, headache and elevated leukocyte count. It usually lasts 3–5 days. *In a few cases, streptococcal pharyngitis leads to rheumatic fever or acute poststreptococcal glomerulonephritis.* Penicillin treatment shortens the course of strep throat and, more importantly, prevents nonsuppurative sequelae.

Scarlet Fever

Scarlet fever **(scarlatina)** describes a punctate red rash on the skin and mucous membranes in some suppurative *S. pyogenes* infections, most commonly pharyngitis. It usually begins on the chest and spreads to the extremities. The tongue may develop a yellow-white coating, which sheds to reveal a "beefy-red" surface. Scarlet fever is caused by an erythrogenic toxin.

Erysipelas

Erysipelas is an erythematous swelling of the skin caused chiefly by *S. pyogenes* (Fig. 9-13). This disorder is common in warm climates but is not often seen before the age of 20 years. It usually begins on the face and spreads rapidly. A

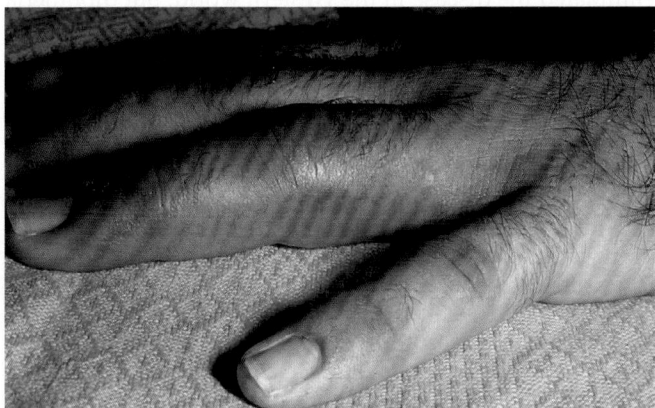
FIGURE 9-13. Erysipelas. Streptoccocal infection of the skin has resulted in an erythematous and swollen finger.

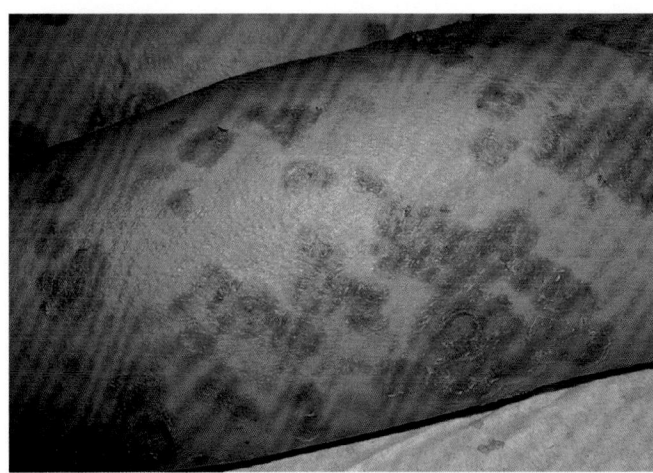
FIGURE 9-14. Streptococcal impetigo. The lower extremities exhibit numerous erythematous papules, with central ulceration and the formation of crusts.

diffuse, edematous, acute inflammatory reaction in the epidermis and dermis extends into subcutaneous tissues. The inflammatory infiltrate is principally composed of neutrophils and is most intense around vessels and adnexa of the skin. Cutaneous microabscesses and small foci of necrosis are common.

Impetigo

Impetigo **(pyoderma)** is a localized, intraepidermal infection caused by *S. pyogenes* or *S. aureus.* Strains of *S. pyogenes* that cause impetigo are antigenically and epidemiologically distinct from those that cause pharyngitis.

Impetigo spreads from person to person by direct contact and most commonly affects children aged 2–5 years. Infection begins with skin colonization with the causative organism. Minor trauma or an insect bite then inoculates the bacteria into the skin, where they form an intraepidermal pustule, which ruptures and leaks a purulent exudate.

Lesions begin on exposed body surfaces as localized erythematous papules (Fig. 9-14). These become pustules, which erode within a few days to form a thick honey-colored crust. Impetigo sometimes leads to poststreptococcal glomerulonephritis, but it does not give rise to rheumatic fever.

Streptococcal Cellulitis

S. pyogenes causes an acute spreading infection of the loose connective tissue of the deeper layers of the dermis. This suppurative process results from traumatic inoculation of microorganisms into the skin and frequently occurs on the extremities in the context of impaired lymphatic drainage. Cellulitis usually begins at sites of unnoticed injury and appears as spreading areas of redness, warmth and swelling.

Puerperal Sepsis

Puerperal sepsis is postpartum infection of the uterine cavity by *S. pyogenes.* The disease was once common but is now rare in developed countries. It is spread by the contaminated hands of attendants at delivery.

Streptococcus pneumoniae Infection Is a Major Cause of Lobar Pneumonia

S. pneumoniae, often called **pneumococcus,** causes pyogenic infections, primarily of the lungs **(pneumonia)**, middle ear **(otitis media)**, sinuses **(sinusitis)** and meninges **(meningitis)**. *It is one of the most common human bacterial pathogens. Most children in the world have had at least one episode of pneumococcal disease (usually otitis media) by the age of 5 years.*

S. pneumoniae is an aerobic, gram-positive diplococcus. Most strains that cause clinical disease have a capsule, although nonserotypeable isolates are a known cause of epidemic conjunctivitis. There are over 80 antigenically distinct serotypes of pneumococcus; antibody to one does not protect from infection with another. These are commensal organisms in the oropharynx, and virtually everyone has been colonized at some time.

PATHOPHYSIOLOGY: Pneumococcal disease begins when the organism gains access to sterile sites, usually those in proximity to its normal residence in the oropharynx. Pneumococcal sinusitis and otitis media are usually preceded by a viral illness, such as the common cold, which injures the protective ciliated epithelium and fills affected air spaces with fluid. Pneumococci then thrive in the nutrient-rich tissue fluid. Infection of the sinuses or middle ear can spread to the adjacent meninges.

Pneumococcal pneumonia arises in a similar fashion. The lower respiratory tract is protected by the mucociliary blanket and cough response, which normally expel organisms that reach the lower airways. Insults that interfere with respiratory defenses, including influenza, other viral respiratory illnesses, smoking and alcoholism, allow *S. pneumoniae* to reach the alveoli. Once there, the organisms proliferate and elicit an acute inflammatory response. As the bacteria multiply and fill alveoli, they spread to other alveoli. Their polysaccharide capsule prevents activation of the alternate complement pathway, thereby blocking production of the opsonin C3b. Consequently, the organism can proliferate and spread unimpeded by phagocytes until antibody is produced. In the lungs, *S. pneumoniae* spreads rapidly to involve an entire lobe or several lobes (lobar pneumonia).

PATHOLOGY: Alveoli fill with proteinaceous fluid, neutrophils and bacteria. Clinical features of pneumococcal infections are discussed in Chapter 18. Pneumonia caused by *S. pneumoniae* often resolves completely, unlike that caused by *S. aureus,* which can cause permanent lung damage. If there is an underlying problem such as chronic aspiration, diabetes or alcohol abuse, or if bacterial opsonization is compromised, as in multiple myeloma, hypogammaglobulinemia or sickle cell disease, pneumococcal disease may spread. Patients with prior splenectomies are at high risk of rapid, fulminant septic shock and death. Immunization for pneumococcal pneumonia, particularly among the elderly, is available.

Group B Streptococci Are the Leading Cause of Neonatal Pneumonia, Meningitis and Sepsis

Group B streptococci are gram-positive bacteria that grow in short chains. Several thousand neonatal infections with group B streptococci occur in the United States each year; 30% of infected infants die. Group B streptococci are part of the normal vaginal flora in 10%–30% of women. Most babies born to colonized women acquire the organisms as they pass through the birth canal. Group B streptococci infrequently cause pyogenic infections in adults.

PATHOPHYSIOLOGY AND PATHOLOGY: Particular risk factors associated with development of neonatal group B streptococcal infections include premature delivery and low levels of maternally derived IgG antibodies against the organism. Newborns have little functional reserve for granulocyte production, so once the bacterial infection is established, it rapidly overwhelms the body's defenses. Group B streptococcal infection may be limited to the lungs or CNS or may be widely disseminated. The involved tissues show a pyogenic response, often with overwhelming numbers of gram-positive cocci.

BACTERIAL INFECTIONS OF CHILDHOOD

Diphtheria Is a Necrotizing Upper Respiratory Tract Infection

Infection with *Corynebacterium diphtheriae*—an aerobic, pleomorphic, gram-positive rod—may lead to cardiac and neurologic disturbances due to toxin production. The disease is preventable by vaccination with inactivated *C. diphtheriae* toxin (toxoid).

EPIDEMIOLOGY: Humans are the only known reservoir for *C. diphtheriae,* and most people are asymptomatic carriers. The organism spreads from person to person in respiratory droplets or oral secretions. Diphtheria was once a leading cause of death in children 2–15 years of age. Immunization programs have largely eliminated the disease in the Western world, but diphtheria persists as a major health problem in less developed countries. A recent outbreak in Nigeria mainly affected children, with a case-fatality ratio of 20%.

MOLECULAR PATHOGENESIS: *C. diphtheriae* enters the pharynx and proliferates, often on the tonsils. Diphtheria toxin is absorbed systemically and acts on many tissues, with the heart, nerves and kidneys being most susceptible to damage. Diphtheria toxin is a protein composed of two peptide chains—the A and B subunits—held together by a disulfide bond. The B subunit binds glycolipid receptors on target cells, and the A subunit acts within the cytoplasm on elongation factor 2 to interrupt protein synthesis. The toxin is one of the most potent known: one molecule suffices to kill a cell. Not all strains of *C. diphtheriae* produce exotoxin. The exotoxin is encoded by a lysogenic β-bacteriophage.

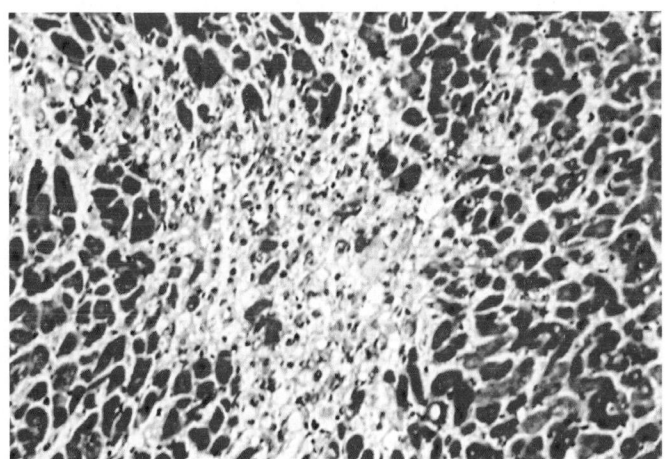

FIGURE 9-15. Diphtheric myocarditis. Focal degeneration of cardiac myocytes is evident.

PATHOLOGY: The characteristic lesions of diphtheria (from the Greek, *diphtheria*, "pair of leather scrolls") are the thick, gray, leathery membranes composed of sloughed epithelium, necrotic debris, neutrophils, fibrin and bacteria that line affected respiratory passages. The epithelial surface beneath the membranes is denuded, and the submucosa is acutely inflamed and hemorrhagic. The inflammation often causes swelling in surrounding soft tissues, which can be severe enough to cause respiratory compromise. When the heart is affected, the myocardium displays fat droplets in the myocytes and focal necrosis (Fig. 9-15). In the case of neural involvement, affected peripheral nerves show demyelination.

**CLINICAL FEATURES:** Diphtheria begins with fever, sore throat and malaise. The dirty gray membrane usually develops first on the tonsils and then spreads throughout the posterior oropharynx (Fig. 9-16). The membrane is firmly adherent, and an attempt to strip it from the underlying mucosa produces bleeding. Cardiac and neurologic symptoms develop in a minority of those infected, usually people with the most severe local disease.

Cutaneous diphtheria results from inoculation of the organism into a break in the skin and manifests as a pustule or ulcer; it rarely leads to cardiac or neurologic complications. Diphtheria is treated by prompt administration of antitoxin and antibiotics.

Pertussis Features Debilitating Paroxysmal Coughing

The paroxysm is followed by a long, high-pitched inspiration, the "whoop," which gives the disease its name, "whooping cough." The causative organism is *Bordetella pertussis*, a small, gram-negative coccobacillus.

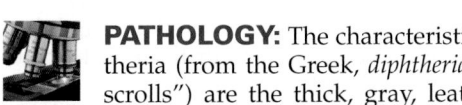**EPIDEMIOLOGY:** *B. pertussis* is highly contagious and spreads from person to person, primarily by respiratory aerosols. Humans are the only reservoir of infection. In susceptible populations, pertussis is primarily a disease of children under 5 years, but incidence is increasing among adults. Vaccination is protective, but there are 50 million cases of pertussis each year worldwide,

and almost 1 million deaths, particularly in infants. In 2012, the United States experienced the worst outbreak of pertussis in 50 years—over 40,000 new cases—highlighting a major public health problem in a vaccine-preventable disease.

MOLECULAR PATHOGENESIS: *B. pertussis* initiates infection by attaching to the cilia of respiratory epithelial cells. The organism then elaborates a cytotoxin that kills ciliated cells. Progressive destruction of ciliated respiratory epithelium and the ensuing inflammatory response cause the local respiratory symptoms. Several other toxins include "pertussis toxin," an agent that causes the pronounced lymphocytosis often associated with whooping cough. Another toxin inhibits adenylyl cyclase, an effect that blocks bacterial phagocytosis.

PATHOLOGY: *B. pertussis* causes an extensive tracheobronchitis, with necrosis of ciliated respiratory epithelium and an acute inflammatory response. With the loss of the protective mucociliary blanket, there is increased risk of pneumonia from aspirated oral bacteria. Coughing paroxysms and vomiting make aspiration likely. Secondary bacterial pneumonia is the most common cause of death.

CLINICAL FEATURES: Whooping cough is a prolonged upper respiratory tract illness, lasting 4–5 weeks and passing through three stages:

- The **catarrhal stage** resembles a common viral upper respiratory tract illness, with low-grade fever, runny nose, conjunctivitis and cough.
- The **paroxysmal stage** occurs 1 week into the illness. Cough worsens and becomes paroxysmal, with 5–15 consecutive coughs, often followed by an inspiratory whoop.

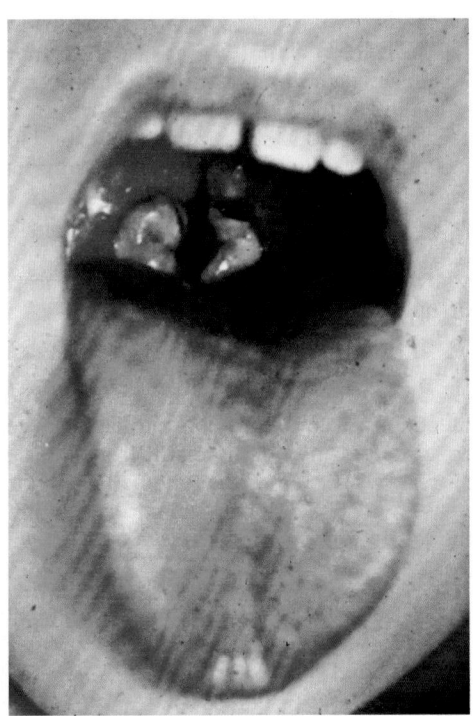

FIGURE 9-16. Child with characteristic diphtheric membrane in the oropharynx.

The patient develops a marked lymphocytosis; total leukocyte counts often exceed 40,000 cells/μL. The paroxysms persist for 2–3 weeks.

- The **convalescent phase** usually lasts for several weeks.

Haemophilus influenzae Causes Pyogenic Infections in Young Children

Haemophilus influenzae infections involve the middle ear, sinuses, facial skin, epiglottis, meninges, lungs and joints. The organism is a major pediatric pathogen and a leading cause of bacterial meningitis worldwide. It is an aerobic, pleomorphic gram-negative coccobacillus that may or may not be encapsulated. Nonencapsulated strains (type a) usually produce localized infections; encapsulated strains, type b, are more virulent and cause over 95% of the invasive bacteremic infections.

EPIDEMIOLOGY: *H. influenzae* only infects humans and spreads from person to person, mainly in respiratory droplets and secretions. It resides in the human nasopharynx of 20%–50% of healthy adults. Most colonizing strains are nonencapsulated, but 3%–5% are *H. influenzae* type b.

Most severe *H. influenzae* type b infections occur in children under the age of 6 years. The incidence of serious disease peaks at 6–18 months of age, corresponding to the period between the loss of maternally acquired immunity and the acquisition of native immunity. The *H. influenzae* type b vaccine has been credited with greatly reducing the complications of invasive *H. influenzae* type b disease, particularly meningitis, in children. However, as vaccination also reduces *H. influenzae* type b carriage and the repeated immunologic boosting effect that carriage provides, continued vigilance is important.

PATHOPHYSIOLOGY: Unencapsulated *H. influenzae* strains produce disease by spreading locally from their normal sites of residence to adjoining sterile locations, such as the sinuses or middle ear. This is facilitated by injury to normal defense mechanisms, as with a viral upper respiratory tract illness. At these previously sterile sites, unencapsulated organisms proliferate and elicit acute inflammatory responses, which injure local tissue but eventually contain the infection. Unencapsulated strains do not usually produce bacteremia.

By contrast, encapsulated H. influenzae type b is capable of tissue invasion. The capsular polysaccharide of type b organisms allows them to evade phagocytosis, and bacteremic infections are common. Epiglottitis, facial cellulitis, septic arthritis and meningitis result from invasive bacteremic infections. *H. influenzae* type b also elaborates an IgA protease, which facilitates local survival of the organism in the respiratory tract.

PATHOLOGY: *H. influenzae* elicits strong acute inflammatory responses. Specific pathologic features vary according to the sites affected. *H. influenzae* meningitis resembles other acute bacterial meningitides, with a predominantly acute inflammatory leptomeningeal infiltrate, sometimes involving the subarachnoid space.

H. influenzae pneumonia usually complicates chronic lung disease. In half of patients, it follows a viral infection of the respiratory tract. Alveoli are filled with neutrophils and macrophages, containing bacilli and fibrin. The bronchiolar epithelium is necrotic and infiltrated by macrophages.

Epiglottitis is swelling and acute inflammation of the epiglottis, aryepiglottic fold and pyriform sinuses. It may sometimes completely obstruct the upper airway. In **facial cellulitis,** the site of infection and inflammation is the dermis, usually of the cheek or periorbital region.

CLINICAL FEATURES: Most bacteremic *H. influenzae* infections afflict young children. **H. influenzae** *is the most common cause of meningitis in children under 2 years,* **although vaccination has reduced its frequency.** Onset is insidious and may follow an otherwise unremarkable upper respiratory tract infection or otitis media.

- **Bronchopneumonia and lobar pneumonia** are characterized by fever, cough, purulent sputum and dyspnea.
- **Epiglottitis** affects primarily children aged 2–7 years but also occurs in adults. Death may occur from obstruction of the upper respiratory tract.
- **Septic arthritis** is due to bacteremic seeding of large weight-bearing joints. Symptoms include fever, heat, erythema, swelling and pain on movement.
- **Facial cellulitis** or periorbital cellulitis is another severe bacteremic infection affecting primarily young children. Patients present with fever, profound malaise and a raised, hot, red-blue discolored area of the face, usually involving the cheek or an area about the eye. There is often concomitant meningitis or septic arthritis.

Neisseria meningitides Causes Pyogenic Meningitis and Overwhelming Shock

Neisseria meningitidis, or **meningococcus,** produces disseminated blood-borne infections, often accompanied by shock and profound disturbances in coagulation (Fig. 9-17). The organism is aerobic and appears as paired, bean-shaped, gram-negative cocci.

EPIDEMIOLOGY: Meningococci spread from person to person, primarily via respiratory droplets. About 5%–15% of the population carries them as commensals in the nasopharynx. Carriers develop antibodies to their colonizing strain and are not susceptible to disease caused by that strain.

Meningococcal diseases appear as sporadic cases, clusters of cases and epidemics. Most infections in industrialized countries are sporadic and afflict children under the age of 5 years. Epidemic disease occurs mostly in crowded quarters, such as among military recruits in barracks. There are over 6000 cases of meningococcal meningitis each year in the United States, and over 600 deaths. Fatal meningococcal disease is more common in less developed countries.

PATHOPHYSIOLOGY: Upon colonizing the upper respiratory tract, *N. meningitidis* attaches to nonciliated respiratory epithelium by means of its pili. Most exposed people then develop protective

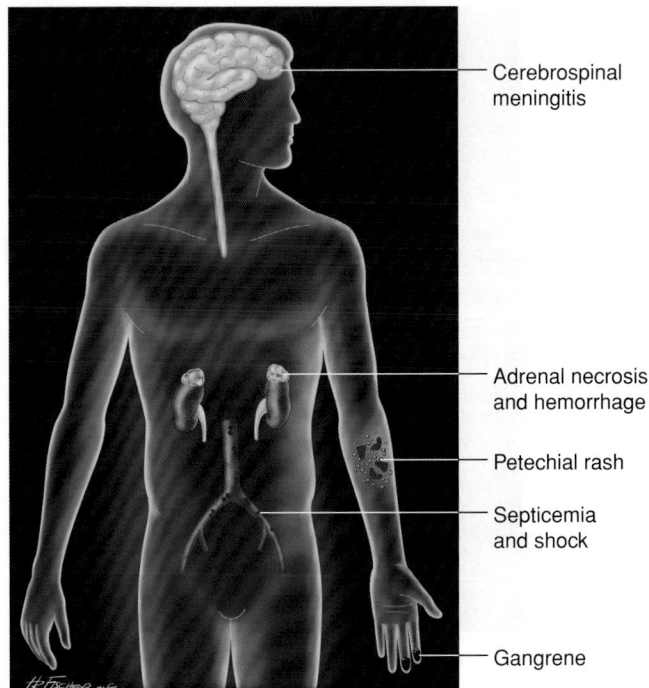

FIGURE 9-17. **Meningococcemia.** Meningococcal infections have a variety of clinical manifestations including meningitis, septicemia, shock and associated complications.

bactericidal antibodies over the following weeks, and some become carriers. If the organism spreads to the bloodstream before protective immunity develops, it can proliferate rapidly and cause fulminant meningococcal disease.

Many of the systemic effects of meningococcal disease are due to the endotoxin of the bacterial outer membrane lipopolysaccharide. Endotoxin promotes a conspicuous increase in TNF production and simultaneous activation of complement and coagulation cascades. Disseminated intravascular coagulation, fibrinolysis and shock follow.

PATHOLOGY: Meningococcal disease can be confined to the CNS or may be disseminated throughout the body in the form of septicemia. In the former case, the leptomeninges and subarachnoid space are infiltrated with neutrophils and the underlying brain parenchyma is swollen and congested. Meningococcal septicemia is characterized by diffuse damage to the endothelium of small blood vessels, with widespread petechiae and purpura in the skin and viscera.

Rarely (4% of cases), vasculitis and thrombosis produce hemorrhagic necrosis of both adrenals, **Waterhouse-Friderichsen syndrome**.

CLINICAL FEATURES: Meningitis begins with rapid onset of fever, stiff neck and headache. In meningococcal sepsis, fever, shock and mucocutaneous hemorrhages appear abruptly. Patients may progress to shock within minutes, and treatment requires blood

pressure support and antibiotics. Meningococcal disease was once almost invariably fatal, but antibiotic treatment has reduced mortality to less than 15%. Some patients who survive the early phase of meningococcemia develop late immunologic complications, such as polyarthritis, cutaneous vasculitis and pericarditis. Severe vasculitis may be associated with extensive cutaneous ulceration and even gangrene of the distal extremities.

SEXUALLY TRANSMITTED BACTERIAL DISEASES

Gonorrhea Remains a Common Infection That Causes Sterility

Neisseria gonorrhoeae, also called **gonococcus,** causes gonorrhea, an acute suppurative genital tract infection, which manifests as urethritis in men and endocervicitis in women. It is one of the oldest and still one of the most common sexually transmitted diseases. *N. gonorrhoeae* is an aerobic, bean-shaped, gram-negative diplococcus.

Gonococcal pharyngitis and proctitis are not uncommon and are also sexually transmitted. In women, infection often ascends the genital tract, producing endometritis, salpingitis and pelvic inflammatory disease. Ascending spread in men is less common, but if it occurs, epididymitis results. Gonococcal infection may rarely be bacteremic, in which case septic arthritis and skin lesions develop. Neonatal infections, derived from the birth canal of a mother with gonorrhea, usually manifest as conjunctivitis, although disseminated infections occur occasionally. Neonatal gonococcal conjunctivitis is still a major cause of blindness in much of Africa and Asia but has been largely eliminated in developed countries by routine instillation of antibiotics into the conjunctiva at birth.

EPIDEMIOLOGY: This common infection is spread directly from person to person. Except for perinatal transmission, spread is almost always by sexual intercourse. Infected people who are asymptomatic are a significant reservoir of infection.

PATHOPHYSIOLOGY: Gonorrhea begins in the mucous membranes of the urogenital tract (Fig. 9-18). Bacteria attach to surface cells, after which they invade superficially and provoke acute inflammation. Gonococcus lacks a true polysaccharide capsule, but hair-like extensions, termed "pili," project from the cell wall. The pili contain a protease that digests IgA on the mucous membrane, thereby facilitating bacterial attachment to the columnar and transitional epithelium of the urogenital tract.

PATHOLOGY: Gonorrhea is a suppurative infection, eliciting a vigorous acute inflammatory response, with copious pus, and often forming submucosal abscesses. Smears of pus reveal numerous neutrophils, often containing phagocytosed bacteria. If untreated, the inflammation becomes chronic, with macrophages and lymphocytes predominant.

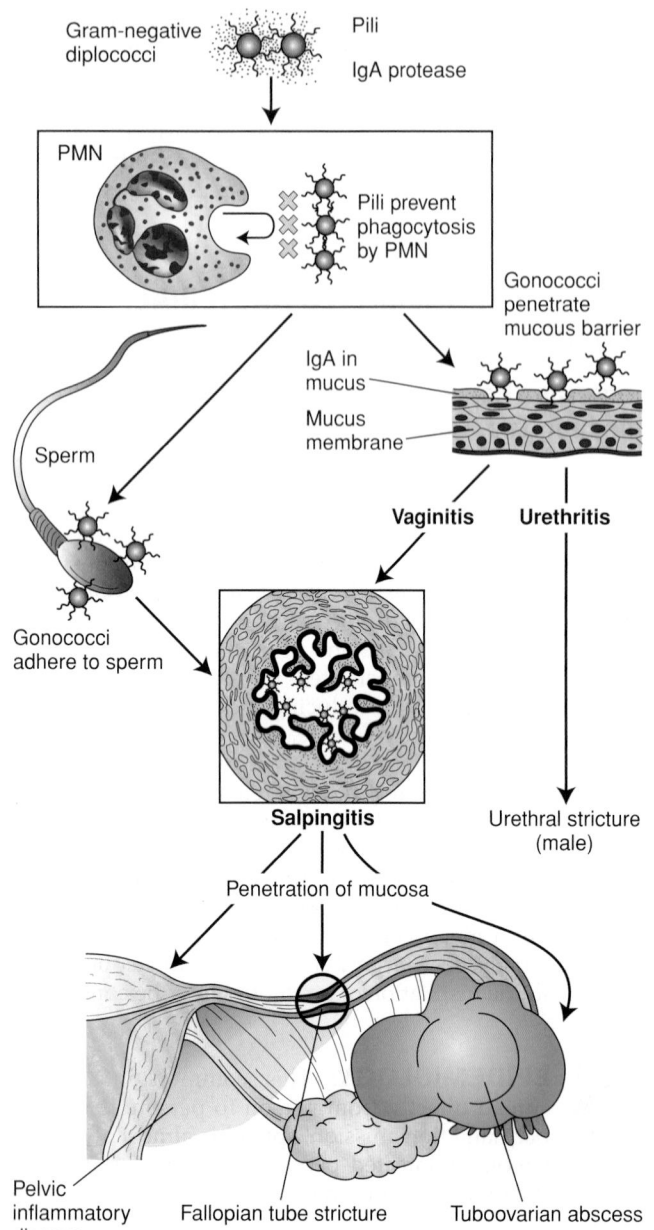

FIGURE 9-18. Pathogenesis of gonococcal infections. *Neisseria gonorrhoeae* is a gram-negative diplococcus whose surface pili form a barrier against phagocytosis by neutrophils. The pili contain an immunoglobulin A (IgA) protease that digests IgA on the luminal surface of the mucous membranes of the urethra, endocervix and fallopian tube, thereby facilitating attachment of gonococci. Gonococci cause endocervicitis, vaginitis and salpingitis. In men, gonococci attached to the mucous membrane of the urethra cause urethritis and, sometimes, urethral stricture. Gonococci may also attach to sperm heads and be carried into the fallopian tube. Penetration of the mucous membrane by gonococci leads to stricture of the fallopian tube, pelvic inflammatory disease (PID) or tuboovarian abscess.

 CLINICAL FEATURES: Men exposed to *N. gonorrhoeae* present with purulent urethral discharge and dysuria. If treatment is not instituted promptly, urethral stricture is a common complication. The organisms may also extend to the prostate, epididymis and accessory glands, where they cause epididymitis and orchitis, and may result in infertility.

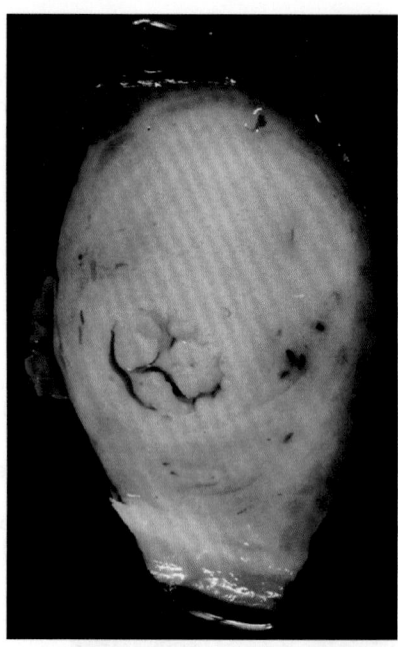

FIGURE 9-19. Gonorrhea of the fallopian tube. Cross-section of a "pus tube" shows thickening of the wall and a lumen swollen with pus.

In one half of infected women, gonorrhea remains asymptomatic. The other infected women initially exhibit endocervicitis, with vaginal discharge or bleeding. Urethritis presents as dysuria rather than as a urethral discharge. Infection often extends to the fallopian tubes, where it produces acute and chronic salpingitis and, eventually, pelvic inflammatory disease. Fallopian tubes swell with pus (Fig. 9-19), causing acute abdominal pain. Infertility occurs when inflammatory adhesions block the tubes.

From the fallopian tubes, gonorrhea spreads to the peritoneum, healing as fine "violin string" adhesions between the liver and the parietal peritoneum (Fitz-Hugh-Curtis syndrome). Chronic endometritis is a persistent complication of gonococcal infection and is usually the consequence of chronic gonococcal salpingitis.

Chancroid Causes Genital Ulcers in Less Developed Regions

Chancroid is an acute sexually transmitted infection caused by *Haemophilus ducreyi*. The organism is a small, gram-negative bacillus, which appears in tissue as clusters of parallel bacilli and as chains, resembling schools of fish. Infections lead to painful genital ulceration and lymphadenopathy. *Chancroid is the leading cause of genital ulcers in many less developed countries, especially in Africa and parts of Asia.* It has been suggested that these genital ulcers facilitate spread of HIV. In the United States, the incidence of chancroid has risen in the past decade; there are about 5000 cases annually.

PATHOLOGY: *H. ducreyi* enters through breaks in the skin, where it multiplies and produces a raised lesion, which then ulcerates. Ulcers vary from 0.1 to 2 cm in diameter. Organisms are carried within macrophages to regional lymph nodes, which may suppurate. Seven to 10 days after the primary lesion appears, half of patients develop unilateral, painful, suppurative, inguinal

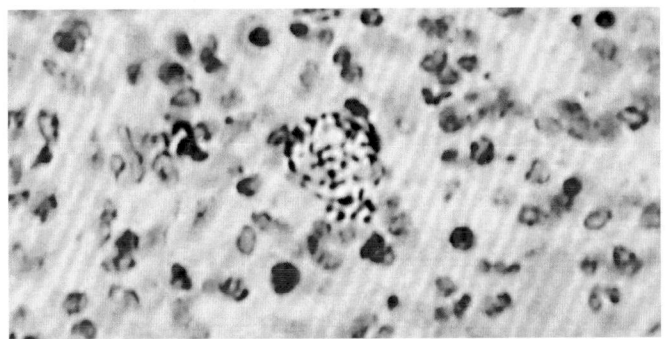

FIGURE 9-20. Granuloma inguinale. A photomicrograph of a skin lesion shows *Calymmatobacterium granulomatis* (Donovan bodies) clustered in a large macrophage. Intense silver staining by Warthin-Starry technique makes the organisms large, black and easily seen.

lymphadenitis **(bubo)**. Overlying skin becomes inflamed, breaks down and drains pus from the underlying node. The diagnosis is made by identifying the bacillus in tissue sections or Gram-stained smears from the ulcers. Treatment with erythromycin is usually effective.

Granuloma Inguinale Is a Tropical Ulcerating Disease

Granuloma inguinale is a sexually transmitted, chronic, superficial ulceration of the genitalia and inguinal and perianal regions. It is caused by *Calymmatobacterium granulomatis*, a small, encapsulated, nonmotile, gram-negative bacillus.

 **EPIDEMIOLOGY:** Humans are the only hosts of *C. granulomatis*. Granuloma inguinale is rare in temperate climates but is common in tropical and subtropical areas. Papua New Guinea, central Australia and India have the highest incidence. Most patients are 15–40 years old.

 PATHOLOGY: The characteristic lesion is a raised, soft, beefy-red, superficial ulcer. The exuberant granulation tissue resembles a fleshy mass herniating through the skin. Macrophages and plasma cells, and occasional neutrophils and lymphocytes, infiltrate the dermis and subcutis. Interspersed macrophages contain many bacteria, termed **Donovan bodies** (Fig. 9-20).

 CLINICAL FEATURES: Untreated granuloma inguinale follows an indolent, relapsing course, often healing with an atrophic scar. Secondary fusospirochetal infection may cause ulceration, mutilation or amputation of the genitalia. Massive scarring of the dermis and subcutis may obstruct lymphatics and cause genital **elephantiasis**. Antibiotic therapy is effective in early cases.

ENTEROPATHOGENIC BACTERIAL INFECTIONS

Escherichia coli Commonly Causes Diarrhea and Urinary Tract Infections

E. coli *is among the most frequent and important human bacterial pathogens, causing over 90% of all urinary tract infections and many cases of diarrheal illness worldwide.* It

is also a major opportunistic pathogen, frequently producing pneumonia and sepsis in immunocompromised hosts and meningitis and sepsis in newborns.

E. coli comprises a group of antigenically and biologically diverse, aerobic (facultatively anaerobic), gram-negative bacteria. Most strains are intestinal commensals, well adapted to growth in the human colon without harming the host. However, *E. coli* can be aggressive when it gains access to usually sterile body sites, such as the urinary tract, meninges or peritoneum. Strains of *E. coli* that produce diarrhea possess specialized virulence properties, usually plasmid-borne, that cause intestinal disease.

E. coli Diarrhea

There are four distinct strains of *E. coli* that cause diarrhea:

ENTEROTOXIGENIC E. coli: *Enterotoxigenic E. coli gives rise to diarrhea in poor tropical areas and probably causes most "traveler's diarrhea" among visitors to such regions.* It is acquired from contaminated water and food. Many people in Latin America, Africa and Asia are asymptomatic carriers of the infection.

 **MOLECULAR PATHOGENESIS:** Nonimmune people (local children or travelers from abroad) develop diarrhea when they encounter the organism. Enterotoxigenic strains produce diarrhea by adhering to the intestinal mucosa and elaborating one or more of at least three enterotoxins that cause secretory dysfunction of the small bowel. One of the enterotoxins is structurally and functionally similar to cholera toxin, and another acts on guanylyl cyclase. Enterotoxigenic *E. coli* produces no distinctive macroscopic or light-microscopic alterations in the intestine.

Enterotoxigenic *E. coli* causes an acute, self-limited diarrheal illness, with watery stools lacking neutrophils and erythrocytes. In severe cases, fluid and electrolyte loss can lead to extreme dehydration and even death.

ENTEROPATHOGENIC E. coli: Historically, enteropathogenic *E. coli* was the first group of this genus to be identified as a cause of diarrhea. The organism is responsible for diarrheal illness in poor tropical areas, especially in infants and young children. Although it has virtually disappeared from developed countries, it still produces sporadic outbreaks of diarrhea, particularly among hospitalized infants younger than 2 years. Enteropathogenic *E. coli* is acquired by ingesting contaminated food or water. The organism is not invasive and brings on disease by adhering to and deforming the microvilli of the intestinal epithelial cells (Fig. 9-21A). Enteropathogenic *E. coli* produces diarrhea, vomiting, fever and malaise.

ENTEROHEMORRHAGIC E. coli: Enterohemorrhagic *E. coli* (serotype 0157:H7) causes a bloody diarrhea, which may be followed by the **hemolytic–uremic syndrome** (see Chapter 16). The source of infection is usually ingestion of contaminated meat or milk. Bacteria adhere to colonic mucosa and elaborate an enterotoxin, virtually identical to Shigatoxin (see below), that destroys the epithelial cells. Patients infected with *E. coli* 0157:H7 present with cramping abdominal pain, low-grade fever and sometimes bloody diarrhea. Microscopic examination of stool shows both leukocytes and erythrocytes.

ENTEROINVASIVE E. coli: Enteroinvasive *E. coli* causes food-borne dysentery, which is clinically and pathologically

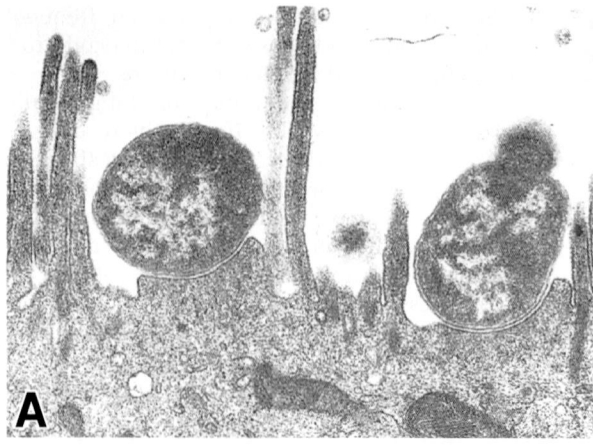
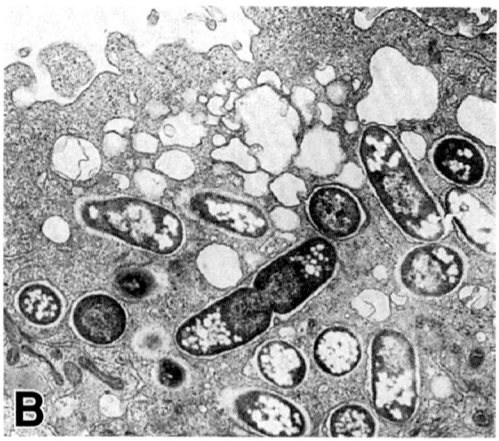

FIGURE 9-21. Enteric *Escherichia coli* infections. A. Enteropathogenic *E. coli* infection. An electron micrograph shows adherence of the bacteria to the intestinal mucosal cells and localized destruction of microvilli. **B.** Enteroinvasive *E. coli* infection. An electron micrograph shows organisms within a cell.

indistinguishable from that caused by *Shigella*. The agent shares extensive DNA homology and antigenic and biochemical characteristics with *Shigella*. It invades and destroys mucosal cells of the distal ileum and colon (Fig. 9-21B). As in shigellosis, the mucosa of the distal ileum and colon is acutely inflamed and focally eroded and is sometimes covered by an inflammatory pseudomembrane. Patients have abdominal pain, fever, tenesmus and bloody diarrhea, usually for about a week. Antibiotic treatment is similar to that for shigellosis.

E. coli Urinary Tract Infection

 **EPIDEMIOLOGY:** Urinary tract infections with *E. coli* are most common in sexually active women and in people of both sexes who have structural or functional abnormalities of the urinary tract. *Such infections afflict more than 10% of the human population, often repeatedly.* *E. coli* in the urinary tract usually derives from resident flora of the perineum and periurethral areas, reflecting fecal contamination of these regions.

PATHOPHYSIOLOGY: *E. coli* gains access to the sterile proximal urinary tract by ascending from the distal urethra. Because the shorter female urethra provides a less effective mechanical barrier to infection, women are much more prone to urinary tract infections. Sexual intercourse can suffice to propel organisms into the female urethra. Uropathogenic *E. coli* organisms have specialized adherence factors (Gal-Gal) on the pili, which enable them to bind to galactopyranosyl-galactopyranoside residues on the uroepithelium. Structural abnormalities of the urinary tract (e.g., congenital deformities, prostatic hyperplasia, strictures) and instrumentation (catheterization) overwhelm normal host defenses and facilitate the establishment of urinary tract infections. These conditions account for most urinary tract infections in men.

  PATHOLOGY AND CLINICAL FEATURES: *E. coli* urinary tract infections initially produce an acute inflammatory

infiltrate at the site of infection, usually the bladder mucosa. Infections involving the bladder or urethra manifest as urinary urgency, burning on urination **(dysuria)** and leukocytes in the urine. If infection ascends to involve the kidney **(pyelonephritis)**, patients develop acute flank pain, fever and elevated leukocyte counts. An infiltrate of neutrophils spills from the mucosa into the urine, and the blood vessels of the submucosa are dilated and congested. Chronic infections exhibit an inflammatory infiltrate of neutrophils and mononuclear cells. Chronic renal infection may lead to chronic pyelonephritis and renal failure (see Chapter 22).

E. coli Pneumonia

Pneumonia caused by enteric gram-negative bacteria is considered opportunistic, occurring mostly in debilitated persons. *E. coli* is the most common cause, but other normal bowel flora, such as *Klebsiella, Serratia* and *Enterobacter* species, produce similar disease. *The discussion below applies to all opportunistic gram-negative pneumonias.*

PATHOPHYSIOLOGY: Enteric gram-negative bacteria are transiently introduced into the oral cavity of healthy people but cannot compete successfully with the predominant gram-positive flora, which adhere to the fibronectin that coats mucosal cell surfaces. Chronically ill or severely stressed persons elaborate a salivary protease that degrades fibronectin, allowing gram-negative enteric bacteria to overcome the normal gram-positive flora and colonize the oropharynx.

Inevitably, droplets of the resident oral flora are aspirated into the respiratory tract. Debilitated patients often have weak local defenses and cannot destroy these organisms. Decreased gag and cough reflexes, abnormal neutrophil chemotaxis, injured respiratory epithelium and foreign bodies, such as endotracheal tubes, all facilitate entry and survival of the aspirated organisms.

 PATHOLOGY: *E. coli* pneumonia results from proliferation of aspirated organisms in terminal airways, usually at multiple sites in the lung.

Multifocal areas of consolidation result and terminal airways and alveoli are filled with proteinaceous fluid, fibrin, neutrophils and macrophages.

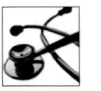 **CLINICAL FEATURES:** Because pneumonia caused by *E. coli* and other enteric gram-negative organisms afflicts patients who are often already severely ill, symptoms of pneumonia may be less obvious than in healthy persons. Increased malaise, fever and labored breathing are often the first signs of pneumonia. If *E. coli* pneumonia remains untreated, the organisms may invade the blood to produce fatal septicemia. Treatment requires parenteral antibiotics.

E. coli Sepsis (Gram-Negative Sepsis)

E. coli is the most common cause of enteric gram-negative sepsis, but other gram-negative rods, including *Pseudomonas*, *Klebsiella* and *Enterobacter* species, produce identical disease. The discussion below relates to gram-negative sepsis in general.

PATHOPHYSIOLOGY: *E. coli* sepsis is usually an opportunistic infection, occurring in people with predisposing conditions, such as neutropenia, pyelonephritis or cirrhosis, and in hospitalized patients. Together with other enteric gram-negative rods that normally reside in the human colon, *E. coli* occasionally seeds the bloodstream. In healthy individuals, macrophages and circulating neutrophils phagocytose these bacteria. Patients with neutropenia or cirrhosis develop *E. coli* sepsis because of impaired ability to eliminate even low-level bacteremias. People with ruptured abdominal organs or acute pyelonephritis suffer gram-negative sepsis because the large numbers of organisms that gain access to the circulation overwhelm the normal defenses.

The presence of *E. coli* in the bloodstream causes septic shock through the effects of TNF (among other factors), whose release from macrophages is stimulated by bacterial endotoxin. Septic shock is discussed in Chapters 7 and 26.

Neonatal *E. coli* Meningitis and Sepsis

E. coli and group B streptococci are the main causes of meningitis and sepsis in the first month after birth. Both colonize the vagina, and newborns acquire them on passage through the birth canal. *E. coli* then colonizes the infant's gastrointestinal tract. It is postulated that the organisms spread to the bloodstream from the gastrointestinal tract and then seed the meninges. The pathology of *E. coli* meningitis is identical to that of other bacterial meningitides. Although antibiotic treatment for neonatal *E. coli* meningitis and sepsis is often effective, the mortality rate is still up to 50%. Almost half of survivors suffer neurologic sequelae.

Salmonella Enterocolitis and Typhoid Fever Are Both Intestinal Infections

The bacterial genus *Salmonella* contains over 1500 antigenically distinct but biochemically and genetically related gram-negative rods. The agents cause two important human diseases, namely, *Salmonella* enterocolitis and typhoid fever.

Salmonella Enterocolitis

Salmonella enterocolitis is an acute, self-limited (1–3 days) gastrointestinal illness that presents as nausea, vomiting, diarrhea and fever. Infection is typically acquired by eating food containing nontyphoidal *Salmonella* strains and is commonly called ***Salmonella food poisoning***.

 EPIDEMIOLOGY: Nontyphoidal *Salmonella* infect diverse animal species, including amphibians, reptiles, birds and mammals. They also readily contaminate foodstuffs derived from infected animals (e.g., meat, poultry, eggs, dairy products). If these foods are not cooked, pasteurized or irradiated, the bacteria persist and proliferate, particularly at warm temperatures. Once someone is infected, the organism can spread from person to person by the fecal–oral route. Although such dissemination is infrequent among adults, it is common among small children in daycare settings or within families. *Salmonella* enterocolitis remains a major cause of childhood mortality in less developed countries.

 **PATHOPHYSIOLOGY:** *Salmonella* proliferate in the small intestine and invade enterocytes in the distal small bowel and colon. The nontyphoidal *Salmonella* species elaborate several toxins that injure intestinal cells. The mucosa of the ileum and colon is acutely inflamed and sometimes superficially ulcerated.

 CLINICAL FEATURES: *Salmonella* enterocolitis typically manifests as diarrhea, within 12–48 hours after consuming contaminated food. This contrasts with staphylococcal food poisoning, which is caused by a preformed toxin and begins 1–6 hours after eating. The diarrhea of *Salmonella* food poisoning is self-limited. It lasts 1–3 days and is often accompanied by nausea, vomiting, cramping abdominal pain and fever. Treatment is supportive and antibiotics rarely improve the clinical course.

Typhoid Fever

Typhoid fever is an acute systemic illness caused by infection with *Salmonella typhi*. **Paratyphoid fever** is a clinically similar but milder disease that results from infection with other species of *Salmonella*, including *Salmonella paratyphi*. The term **enteric fever** includes both typhoid and paratyphoid fever.

 **EPIDEMIOLOGY:** Humans are the only natural reservoir for *S. typhi*, and typhoid fever is acquired from infected patients or chronic carriers. The latter tend to be older women with gallstones or biliary scarring; *S. typhi* colonizes their gallbladder or biliary tree. The disease is spread primarily by ingestion of contaminated water and food, especially dairy products and shellfish. Less commonly, the organisms are disseminated by direct finger-to-mouth contact with feces, urine

or other secretions. Infected food handlers with poor personal hygiene and urine from patients with typhoid pyelonephritis can be a significant source of spread. Typhoid fever accounts for over 25,000 annual deaths worldwide but is uncommon in the United States.

 **MOLECULAR PATHOGENESIS:** *S. typhi* attaches to and invades the small bowel mucosa without causing clinical enterocolitis. Invasion tends to be most prominent in the ileum in areas overlying Peyer patches. The organisms are engulfed by macrophages, after which they block the respiratory burst of the phagocytes and multiply within these cells. Infected cells spread first to regional lymph nodes, then throughout the body via the lymphatics and bloodstream, affecting mononuclear macrophages in lymph nodes, bone marrow, liver and spleen. Infection of macrophages stimulates IL-1 and TNF production, thereby causing the prolonged fever, malaise and wasting characteristic of typhoid fever.

 PATHOLOGY: The earliest pathologic change in typhoid fever is degeneration of the intestinal epithelium brush border. As bacteria invade, Peyer patches become hypertrophic. In some cases, intestinal lymphoid hyperplasia progresses to capillary thrombosis, causing necrosis of overlying mucosa and the characteristic ulcers oriented along the long axis of the bowel (Fig. 9-22). These ulcers frequently bleed and occasionally perforate, producing infectious peritonitis. Systemic dissemination of the organisms leads to focal granulomas in the liver, spleen and other organs, termed **typhoid nodules**. These are composed of aggregates of macrophages ("typhoid cells") containing ingested bacteria, erythrocytes and degenerated lymphocytes.

 CLINICAL FEATURES: Untreated typhoid fever was classically divided into five stages (Fig. 9-23):

- **Incubation:** 10–14 days.
- **Active invasion/bacteremia:** The patient suffers for about a week with a variety of nonspecific symptoms, including daily stepwise elevation in temperature (up to 41°C [105.8°F]), malaise, headache, arthralgias and abdominal pain.

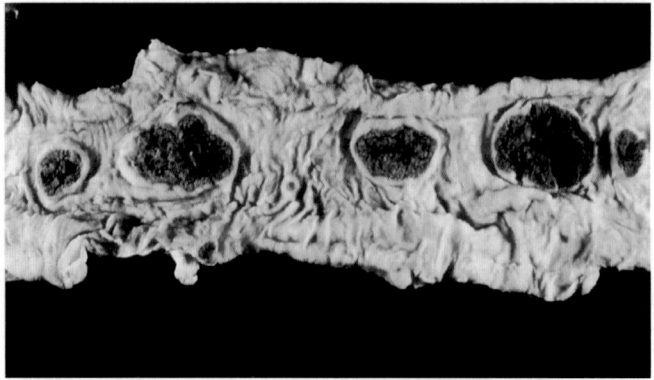

FIGURE 9-22. Ulcers of the terminal ileum in fatal typhoid fever. The ulcers have a longitudinal orientation because they are located over hyperplastic and necrotic Peyer patches.

- **Fastigium:** Fever and malaise increase over several days until the infected person is prostrate. Patients may become toxic from the release of endotoxins from dead bacteria. Hepatomegaly is accompanied by derangement in liver function. The spleen is conspicuously enlarged.
- **Lysis:** In patients destined to survive, fever and toxic symptoms gradually diminish. Gastrointestinal bleeding and intestinal perforation at sites of ulceration may occur in any stage but are most common during lysis, which commonly lasts a week.
- **Convalescence:** Fever abates and patients gradually recover over several weeks to months. Some relapse or have metastatic foci of infection.

The treatment of typhoid fever entails antibiotics and supportive care. Ten to 20% of untreated patients die, usually of secondary complications, such as pneumonia. However, treatment within 3 days of the onset of fever is generally curative.

Shigellosis Is a Necrotizing Infection of the Distal Small Bowel and Colon

It is caused by any of four species of *Shigella* (*Shigella boydii, Shigella dysenteriae, Shigella flexneri* and *Shigella sonnei*), which are aerobic, gram-negative rods. Of these species, *S. dysenteriae* is the most virulent. Shigellosis is a self-limited disease that typically presents with abdominal pain and bloody, mucoid stools.

 **EPIDEMIOLOGY:** *Shigella* organisms are spread from person to person by the fecal–oral route. They have no animal reservoir and do not survive well outside the stool. Infection usually occurs through ingestion of fecally contaminated food or water but can be acquired by oral contact with any contaminated surface (e.g., clothing, towels or skin surfaces). As a result, endemic shigellosis is more common in areas with poor hygiene and sanitation. It is also spread in closed communities, such as hospitals, barracks and households. In developed countries, *S. flexneri* and *S. sonnei* are more common, and infection tends to be sporadic.

In the United States, about 300,000 cases occur annually, but the incidence of the disease is much higher in countries lacking sanitary systems for human waste disposal. Like other diarrheal illnesses, shigellosis is a significant cause of childhood mortality in developing countries.

 **MOLECULAR PATHOGENESIS:** Shigellae are among the most virulent enteropathogens. Disease is produced by ingesting as few as 10–100 organisms, and there are few asymptomatic carriers. The agent proliferates rapidly in the small bowel and attaches to enterocytes, where it replicates within the cytoplasm. Endocytosis is essential for virulence, and the virulence factor is encoded by a plasmid. Replicating shigellae kill infected cells and then spread to adjacent cells.

Shigellae also produce a potent exotoxin, known as **Shiga toxin,** that is like the verotoxin of *E. coli* O157:H7. This toxin interferes with 60S ribosomal subunits and inhibits protein synthesis. It also causes watery diarrhea, probably by interfering with fluid absorption in the colon. Although shigellae extensively damage the epithelium of the ileum and colon, they rarely invade beyond the intestinal lamina propria, and bacteremia is uncommon.

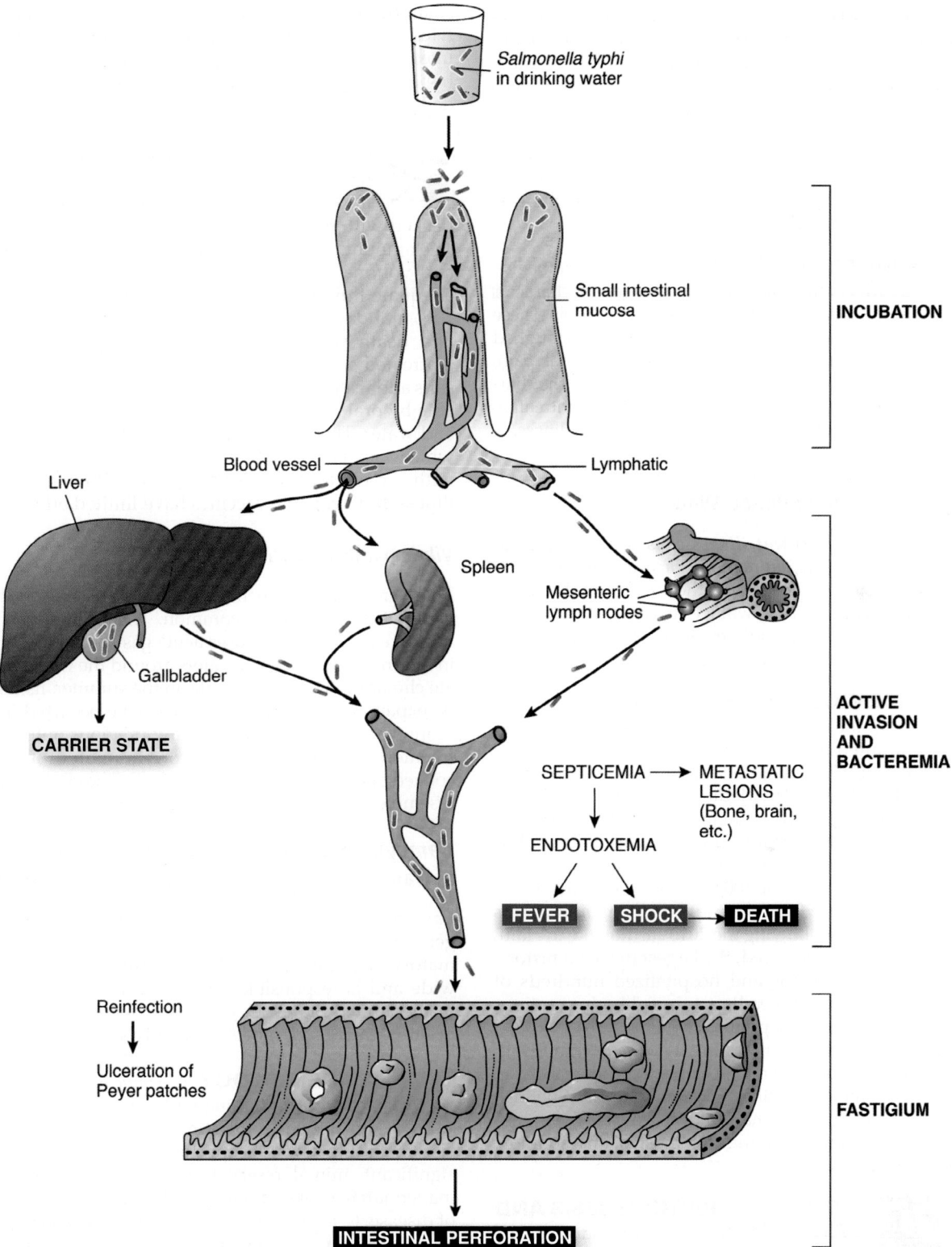

FIGURE 9-23. Stages of typhoid fever. Incubation (10–14 days). Water or food contaminated with *Salmonella typhi* is ingested. Bacilli attach to the villi in the small intestine, invade the mucosa and pass to the intestinal lymphoid follicles and draining mesenteric lymph nodes. The organisms proliferate further within mononuclear phagocytic cells of the lymphoid follicles, lymph nodes, liver and spleen. Bacilli are sequestered intracellularly in the intestinal and mesenteric lymphatic system. **Active invasion/bacteremia** (1 week). Organisms are released and produce a transient bacteremia. The intestinal mucosa becomes enlarged and necrotic, forming characteristic mucosal lesions. The intestinal lymphoid tissues become hyperplastic and contain "typhoid nodules"—aggregates of macrophages ("typhoid cells") that phagocytose bacteria, erythrocytes and degenerated lymphocytes. Bacilli proliferate in several organs, reappear in the intestine, are excreted in stool and may invade through the intestinal wall. **Fastigium** (1 week). Dying bacilli release endotoxins that cause systemic toxemia. **Lysis** (1 week). Necrotic intestinal mucosa sloughs, producing ulcers, which hemorrhage or perforate into the peritoneal cavity.

PATHOLOGY: The distal colon is almost always affected, although the entire colon and distal ileum can be involved. The mucosa is edematous, acutely inflamed and focally eroded. Ulcers appear first on the edges of mucosal folds, perpendicular to the long axis of the colon. A patchy inflammatory **pseudomembrane,** composed of neutrophils, fibrin and necrotic epithelium, is commonly found on the most severely affected areas. Regeneration of infected colonic epithelium occurs rapidly, and healing is usually complete within 10–14 days.

 CLINICAL FEATURES: Shigellosis often begins with watery diarrhea, which changes in character within 1–2 days to the classic dysenteric stools. These are small-volume stools that contain gross blood, sloughed pseudomembranes and mucus. Cramping abdominal pain, tenesmus and urgency at stool typically accompany the diarrhea. Symptoms persist for 3–8 days, if the disease is untreated. Treatment with antibiotics shortens the course of the illness.

Cholera Is an Epidemic Enteritis Usually Acquired from Contaminated Water

Cholera is a severe diarrheal illness caused by the enterotoxin of Vibrio cholerae, *an aerobic, curved gram-negative rod.* The organism proliferates in the lumen of the small intestine and causes profuse watery diarrhea, rapid dehydration and (if fluids are not restored) shock and death within 24 hours of the onset of symptoms.

 **EPIDEMIOLOGY:** Cholera is common in most parts of the world, but it periodically "disappears" spontaneously. A major pandemic occurred between 1961 and 1974, extending throughout Asia, the Middle East, southern Russia, the Mediterranean basin and parts of Africa. Cholera remains endemic in the river deltas of India and Bangladesh. This infection is a worldwide public health problem, affecting an estimated 3–5 million people per year. It is responsible for 100,000–130,000 deaths annually, a marked decrease from the estimated 3 million deaths per year in the 1980s. Following the 2010 earthquake in Haiti, an outbreak of cholera occurred, the largest in recent history, which killed 8000 Haitians and hospitalized hundreds of thousands more, while spreading to neighboring nations Cuba and the Dominican Republic.

Cholera is acquired by ingesting *V. cholerae,* mainly in contaminated food or water. Epidemics spread readily in areas where human feces pollute the water supply. Shellfish and plankton may serve as a natural reservoir for the organism. Shellfish ingestion accounts for most of the sporadic cases in the United States.

 **MOLECULAR PATHOGENESIS AND PATHOLOGY:** Bacteria that survive passage through the stomach thrive and multiply in the mucous layer of the small bowel. They do not invade the mucosa but cause diarrhea by elaborating a potent exotoxin, **cholera toxin,** which is composed of A and B subunits. The latter binds to GM_1 ganglioside in the enterocyte cell membrane. The A subunit then enters the cell, where it activates adenylyl cyclase. The consequent rise in cell cyclic adenosine 3′,5′-monophosphate (cAMP) content causes massive secretion of sodium and water by the enterocyte into the intestinal lumen (Fig. 9-24). Most fluid secretion occurs in the

small bowel, where there is a net loss of water and electrolytes. *V. cholerae* causes little visible alteration in the affected intestine, which appears grossly normal or only slightly hyperemic. The intestinal epithelium remains intact but depleted of mucus.

 CLINICAL FEATURES: Cholera begins with a few loose stools, usually evolving within hours into severe watery diarrhea. The stools are often flecked with mucus, imparting a "rice water" appearance. The amount of diarrhea is highly variable, but the rapidity and volume loss in severe cases can be staggering. With adequate fluid replacement, infected adults can lose up to 20 L in a day. Water and electrolyte loss can lead to shock and death within hours if the volume is not replaced. Untreated cholera has a 50% mortality rate. Replacing lost salts and water is a simple, effective treatment, often achievable by oral rehydration with preparations of salt, glucose and water. The illness subsides spontaneously in 3–6 days, which can be shortened by antibiotic therapy. Infection with *V. cholerae* confers long-term protection from recurrent illness, but available vaccines have limited effectiveness.

Vibrio parahaemolyticus

There are several "noncholera" vibrios, of which *Vibrio parahaemolyticus* is the most common. This organism is a gram-negative bacillus that causes acute gastroenteritis. It is found in marine life and coastal waters around the world in temperate climates, causing outbreaks in the summer. Its range may be expanding, as confirmed cases have occurred in Alaska, more than 1000 miles north of any previous outbreaks. Gastroenteritis is associated with consumption of inadequately cooked or poorly refrigerated seafood. The clinical syndrome resembles *Salmonella* enteritis. No deaths have been reported.

Campylobacter jejuni Is the Most Common Cause of Bacterial Diarrhea in the Developed World

Campylobacter jejuni is the major human pathogen in the genus *Campylobacter.* It causes an acute, self-limited, inflammatory diarrheal illness. The organism is distributed worldwide and is responsible for over 2 million cases annually in the United States. *C. jejuni* is a microaerophilic, curved gram-negative rod, morphologically similar to the vibrios.

 **EPIDEMIOLOGY:** *C. jejuni* infection is acquired through contaminated food or water. The bacteria inhabit gastrointestinal tracts of many animal species, including cows, sheep, chickens and dogs, which are a significant animal reservoir for infection. Raw milk and inadequately cooked poultry and meat are frequent sources of disease. *C. jejuni* can also spread from person to person by the fecal–oral route. The organism is a major cause of childhood mortality in developing countries and causes many cases of "travelers' diarrhea."

 **PATHOPHYSIOLOGY:** Ingested *C. jejuni* that survives gastric acidity multiplies in the alkaline environment of the upper small intestine. The agent elaborates several toxic proteins that correlate with the severity of the symptoms.

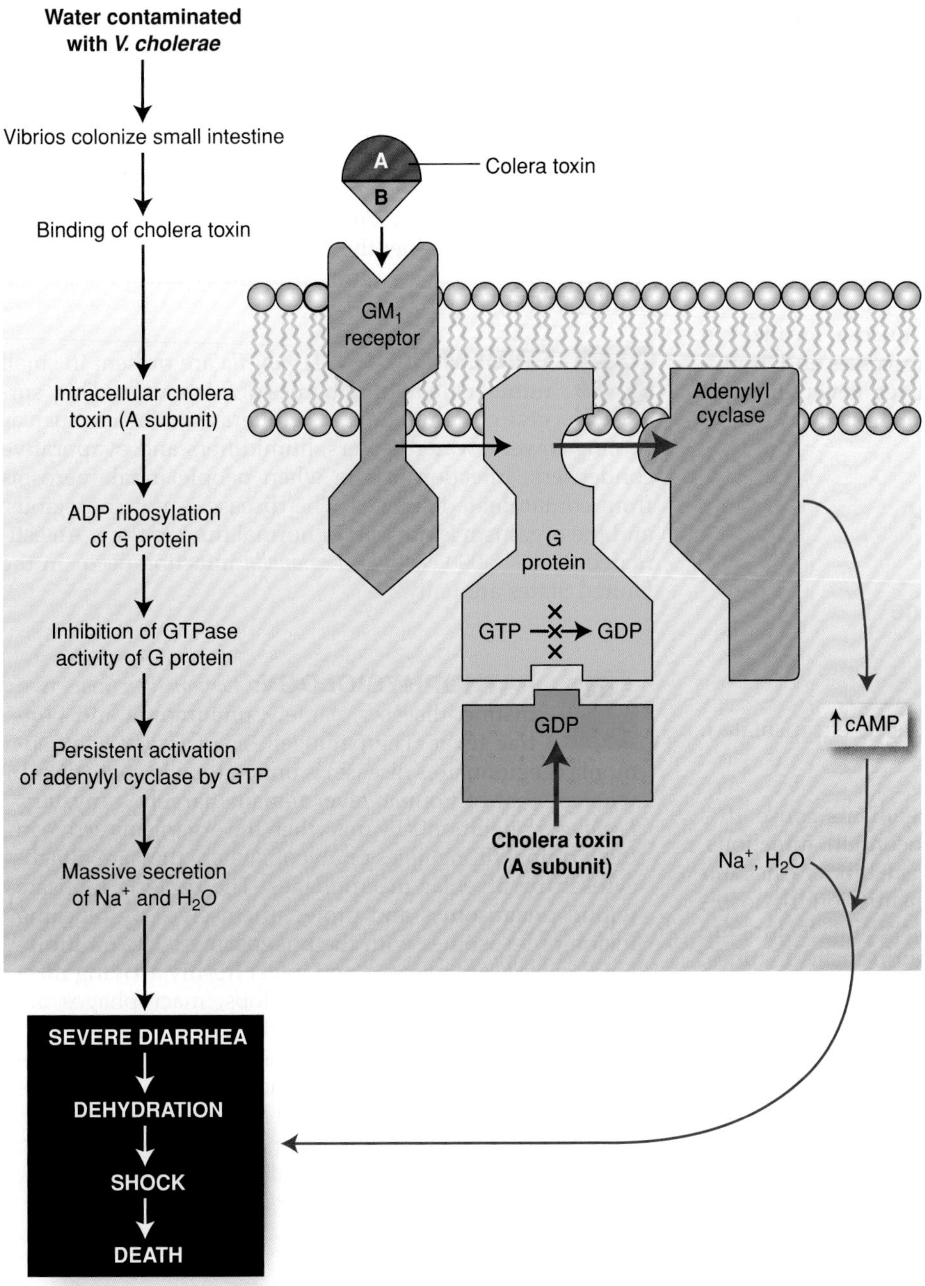

**Water contaminated
with *V. cholerae***

↓

Vibrios colonize small intestine

↓

Binding of cholera toxin

↓

Intracellular cholera
toxin (A subunit)

↓

ADP ribosylation
of G protein

↓

Inhibition of GTPase
activity of G protein

↓

Persistent activation
of adenylyl cyclase by GTP

↓

Massive secretion
of Na^+ and H_2O

↓

SEVERE DIARRHEA
↓
DEHYDRATION
↓
SHOCK
↓
DEATH

Colera toxin

GM₁
receptor

Adenylyl
cyclase

G
protein

GTP —×→ GDP

GDP

**Cholera toxin
(A subunit)**

↑cAMP

Na^+, H_2O

FIGURE 9-24. Cholera. Infection comes from water contaminated with *Vibrio cholerae* or food prepared with contaminated water. Vibrios traverse the stomach, enter the small intestine and propagate. Although they do not invade the intestinal mucosa, vibrios elaborate a potent toxin that induces a massive outpouring of water and electrolytes. Severe diarrhea ("rice water stool") leads to dehydration and hypovolemic shock.

 PATHOLOGY: *C. jejuni* causes a superficial enterocolitis, primarily involving the terminal ileum and colon, with focal necrosis of intestinal epithelium and acute inflammation. In severe cases, infection progresses to small ulcers and patchy inflammatory exudates (pseudomembranes) composed of necrotic cells, neutrophils, fibrin and debris. Epithelial crypts in the colon often fill with neutrophils, forming so-called crypt abscesses. These changes resolve in 7–14 days.

 CLINICAL FEATURES: Patients with *C. jejuni* usually produce more than 10 stools per day, varying from profuse watery stools to small-volume stools containing gross blood and mucus. Symptoms resolve in 5–7 days. Treatment with antibiotics is probably of marginal benefit. A few patients develop a more severe, protracted illness, resembling acute ulcerative colitis. Gastrointestinal infections with *C. jejuni* have been associated with Guillain-Barré syndrome.

Yersinia Infections Produce Painful Diarrhea

Yesinia enterocolitica and *Yersinia pseudotuberculosis* are gram-negative coccoid or rod-shaped bacteria.

 **EPIDEMIOLOGY:** These organisms are facultative anaerobes found in feces of wild and domestic animals, including rodents, sheep, cattle, dogs, cats and horses. *Y. pseudotuberculosis* is also often seen in domestic birds, including turkeys, ducks, geese and canaries. Both organisms have been isolated from drinking water and milk. *Y. enterocolitica* is more likely to be acquired from contaminated meat, and *Y. pseudotuberculosis* from contact with infected animals.

PATHOLOGY AND CLINICAL FEATURES: *Y. enterocolitica* proliferates in the ileum and invades the mucosa, causing ulceration and necrosis of Peyer patches. It migrates by way of lymphatics to mesenteric lymph nodes. Fever, diarrhea (sometimes bloody) and abdominal pain begin 4–10 days after mucosal penetration. Abdominal pain in the right lower quadrant has led to an incorrect diagnosis of appendicitis. Arthralgia, arthritis and erythema nodosum are complications. Septicemia is uncommon but kills about one half of those in whom it occurs.

Y. pseudotuberculosis penetrates ileal mucosa, localizes in ileal–cecal lymph nodes and produces abscesses and granulomas in the lymph nodes, spleen and liver. Fever, diarrhea and abdominal pain may also suggest appendicitis.

PULMONARY INFECTIONS WITH GRAM-NEGATIVE BACTERIA

Klebsiella and *Enterobacter* Produce Nosocomial Infections That Cause Necrotizing Lobar Pneumonia

Klebsiella and *Enterobacter* species are short, encapsulated, gram-negative bacilli.

 **EPIDEMIOLOGY:** These organisms cause 10% of all hospital-acquired (nosocomial) infections, involving the lungs, urinary tract, biliary tract and surgical wounds. Person-to-person transmission by hospital personnel is a special hazard. Predisposing factors are obstructive pulmonary disease in endotracheal tubes, indwelling catheters, debilitating conditions and immunosuppression. Secondary pneumonia caused by these bacteria may complicate influenza or other respiratory viral infections.

 PATHOLOGY: *Klebsiella* and *Enterobacter* are inhaled and multiply in the alveolar spaces. The pulmonary parenchyma becomes consolidated, and a mucoid exudate of macrophages, fibrin and edema fluid fills the alveoli. As the exudate accumulates, alveolar walls become compressed and then necrotic. Numerous small abscesses may coalesce and lead to cavitation.

 CLINICAL FEATURES: The onset of pneumonia is sudden, with fever, pleuritic pain, cough and a characteristic **thick mucoid sputum**. When infection is severe, these symptoms progress to dyspnea, cyanosis and death in 2–3 days. *Klebsiella* and *Enterobacter* infections may be complicated by fulminating, often fatal, septicemia, and aggressive antibiotic therapy is required. Recently, a group of highly drug-resistant members of the Enterobacteriaceae, including *Klebsiella* and *Enterobacter*, have emerged and are spreading throughout the world. These organisms, termed carbapenem-resistant Enterobacteriaceae (CRE), are resistant to the carbapenem class of antibiotics, considered the "drugs of last resort" for such infections. Carbapenem-resistant *Klebsiella pneumoniae* (CRKP) produces an enzyme, or a β-metallo-lactamase 1 (NDM-1), such that these strains are resistant to almost all available antibiotics.

Legionella Cause Mild to Life-threatening Pneumonia

Legionella pneumophila is a minute aerobic bacillus that has the cell wall structure of a gram-negative organism but reacts poorly with Gram stains. It was first identified 6 months after an outbreak of a severe respiratory disease of unknown cause at the 1976 American Legion convention in Philadelphia. Subsequently, retrospective studies demonstrated antibodies in sera from previously unexplained epidemics, dating to 1957.

 **EPIDEMIOLOGY:** *Legionella* are present in small numbers in natural bodies of fresh water. They survive chlorination and proliferate in devices such as cooling towers, water heaters, humidifiers and evaporative condensers. Infection occurs when people inhale aerosols from contaminated sources. The disease is not contagious, and the organism is not part of normal human flora. An estimated 8000–18,000 cases of *Legionella* infection occur in the United States annually.

 **PATHOPHYSIOLOGY:** *Legionella* cause two distinct diseases, namely, **pneumonia** and **Pontiac fever**. The pathogenesis of *Legionella* pneumonia (Legionnaires disease) is understood in some detail, whereas that of Pontiac fever remains largely a mystery. *Legionella* pneumonia begins when the organisms arrive in the terminal bronchioles or alveoli, where they are phagocytosed by alveolar macrophages. The bacteria replicate within phagosomes and protect themselves by blocking fusion of lysosomes with the phagosomes. The multiplying *Legionella* are released and infect freshly arriving macrophages. When immunity develops, macrophages are activated and cease to support such intracellular growth.

Native respiratory tract defenses, such as the mucociliary blanket of the airway, provide a first line of defense against *Legionella* infection in the lower respiratory tract. Conditions that interfere with respiratory defenses, such as smoking, alcoholism and chronic lung diseases, increase the risk of developing *Legionella* pneumonia.

 PATHOLOGY: Legionnaires disease is an acute bronchopneumonia. It is usually patchy but may show a lobar pattern of infiltration. Affected alveoli and bronchioles are filled with an exudate composed of proteinaceous fluid, fibrin, macrophages and neutrophils (Fig. 9-25) and microabscesses. Alveolar walls become necrotic and are destroyed. Many macrophages show eccentric nuclei, pushed aside by cytoplasmic vacuoles containing *L. pneumophila*. As the pneumonia resolves, the lungs heal with little permanent damage.

 CLINICAL FEATURES: After incubating 2–10 days, clinical onset is characterized by rapidly progressive pneumonia, fever, nonproductive cough and myalgia. Chest radiographs reveal unilateral, diffuse, patchy consolidation, progressing to widespread nodular consolidation. Toxic symptoms, hypoxia and obtundation may be prominent, and death may follow within a few days. In those who survive, convalescence is prolonged. Mortality

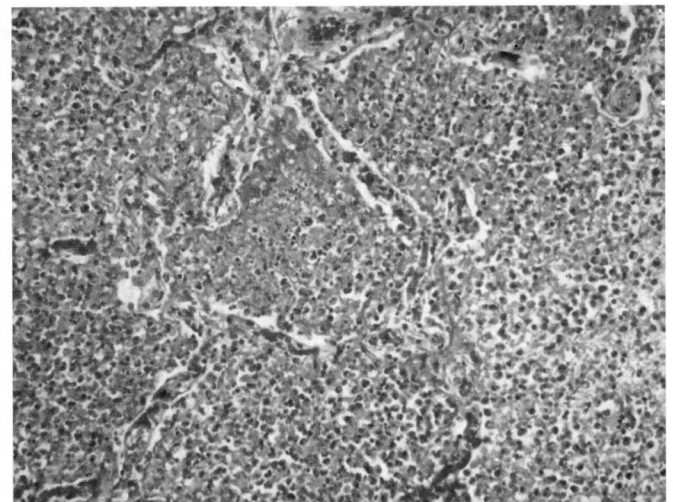

FIGURE 9-25. Legionnaires pneumonia. The alveoli are packed with an exudate composed of fibrin, macrophages and neutrophils.

among hospitalized patients averages 15% but is much greater if there is a serious underlying illness. Infection is amenable to treatment with macrolide antibiotics.

Pontiac fever is a self-limited, flu-like illness with fever, malaise, myalgias and headache. It differs from Legionnaires disease in that it lacks pulmonary consolidation and resolves spontaneously in 3–5 days.

Pseudomonas aeruginosa Is a Highly Antibiotic-Resistant Opportunistic Pathogen

The organism only infrequently infects humans. However, it causes disease, particularly in hospital environments, where it is associated with pneumonia, wound infections, urinary tract disease and sepsis in debilitated or immunosuppressed persons. Burns, urinary catheterization, cystic fibrosis, diabetes and neutropenia all predispose to infection with *Pseudomonas aeruginosa*.

The organism is a ubiquitous aerobic, gram-negative rod that requires moisture and only minimal nutrients. It thrives in soil and water, on animals and on moist environmental surfaces. Antibiotic use selects for *P. aeruginosa,* as it is resistant to most antibiotics.

  PATHOPHYSIOLOGY: *P. aeruginosa* elaborates an array of proteins that allow it to attach to, invade and destroy host tissues while avoiding host inflammatory and immune defenses. Injury to epithelial cells uncovers surface molecules that serve as binding sites for the pili of *P. aeruginosa.* Many strains of *P. aeruginosa* produce a proteoglycan that surrounds and protects them from mucociliary action, complement and phagocytes. The organism releases extracellular enzymes—including an elastase, an alkaline protease and a cytotoxin—which facilitate tissue invasion and are partially responsible for the necrotizing lesions of *Pseudomonas* infections. The elastase probably determines the distinctive ability of *P. aeruginosa* to invade blood vessel walls. The organism also causes systemic pathologic effects through endotoxin and several systemically active exotoxins.

 PATHOLOGY: *Pseudomonas* infection produces an acute inflammatory response. The bacterium often invades small arteries and veins, causing thrombosis and hemorrhagic necrosis, particularly in the lungs and skin. Blood vessel invasion predisposes to dissemination and sepsis and causes multiple nodular lesions in the lungs. Gram stains of necrotic tissue infected with *Pseudomonas* commonly show blood vessel walls densely infiltrated with organisms. Sometimes disseminated infection is marked by skin lesions called **ecthyma gangrenosum**. These nodular, necrotic lesions represent sites where the organism has disseminated to the skin, invaded blood vessels and produced localized hemorrhagic infarcts.

 CLINICAL FEATURES: These are among the most aggressive human bacterial diseases, often progressing rapidly to sepsis. They require immediate medical intervention and are associated with a high mortality.

Melioidosis Is Characterized by Abscesses in Many Organs

Melioidosis (Rangoon beggars disease) is an uncommon disease caused by *Burkholderia* (formerly *Pseudomonas*) *pseudomallei,* a small gram-negative bacillus in the soil and surface water of Southeast Asia and other tropical areas. During the Vietnam conflict, several hundred American servicemen acquired melioidosis. The organism flourishes in wet environments, such as rice paddies and marshes. The skin is the usual portal of entry; organisms enter preexisting lesions, including penetrating wounds and burns. Humans may also be infected by inhaling contaminated dust or aerosolized droplets. The incubation period may last months to years, and the clinical course is variable.

PATHOLOGY AND CLINICAL FEATURES: Acute melioidosis is a pulmonary infection, ranging from a mild tracheobronchitis to an overwhelming cavitary pneumonia (Fig. 9-26). Patients with severe cases present with the sudden onset of high fever, constitutional symptoms and a cough that may produce blood-stained sputum. Splenomegaly, hepatomegaly and jaundice are sometimes present. Diarrhea may be as severe as in cholera. Fulminating septicemia,

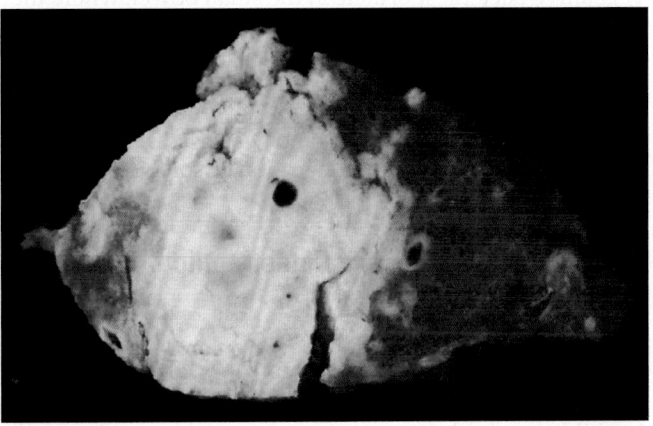

FIGURE 9-26. Acute melioidosis. The lung is consolidated and necrotic.

shock, coma and death may develop in spite of antibiotic therapy. Acute septicemic melioidosis causes discrete abscesses throughout the body, especially in the lungs, liver, spleen and lymph nodes.

Chronic melioidosis is a persistent localized infection of the lungs, skin, bones or other organs. Lesions are suppurative or granulomatous abscesses and in the lung may be mistaken for tuberculosis. In some cases, chronic melioidosis lies dormant for months or years, only to appear suddenly.

CLOSTRIDIAL DISEASES

Clostridia are gram-positive, spore-forming, obligate anaerobic bacilli. The vegetative bacilli are found in the gastrointestinal tract of herbivorous animals and humans. Anaerobic conditions promote vegetative division. Aerobic environments lead to sporulation. Spores pass in animal feces and contaminate soil and plants and survive well in unfavorable environments. Under anaerobic conditions, spores revert to vegetative cells, thus completing the cycle. During sporulation, vegetative cells degenerate, and their plasmids produce a variety of specific toxins that cause widely differing diseases, depending on the species (Fig. 9-27).

- **Food poisoning and necrotizing enteritis** are caused by enterotoxins of *Clostridium perfringens*.
- **Gas gangrene** is produced by myotoxins of *C. perfringens*, *Clostridium novyi*, *Clostridium septicum* and other species.
- **Tetanus** is due to *Clostridium tetani* neurotoxin.
- **Botulism** results from neurotoxins of *C. botulinum*.
- **Pseudomembranous enterocolitis** is caused by exotoxins made by *Clostridium difficile*.

Clostridial Food Poisoning Is Self-Limited

C. perfringens is one of the most common causes of bacterial food poisoning in the world, causing an acute, generally benign, diarrheal disease, usually lasting less than 24 hours. It is omnipresent in the environment, contaminating soil, water, air samples, clothing, dust and meat.

Its spores survive cooking and germinate to yield vegetative forms, which proliferate when food is allowed to stand without refrigeration. Cooking drives out enough air to make the food anaerobic, which is conducive to growth but not to sporulation. As a result, contaminated food contains vegetative clostridia but little preformed enterotoxin. The vegetative bacteria sporulate in the small bowel, where they elaborate several exotoxins, which are cytotoxic to enterocytes and cause loss of intracellular ions and fluid. Certain types of food, including meats, gravies and sauces, are ideal substrates for *C. perfringens*. Clostridial food poisoning presents as abdominal cramping and watery diarrhea. Symptoms begin 8–24 hours after ingestion of contaminated food and usually resolve within 24 hours.

Necrotizing Enteritis Is a Catastrophic Childhood Infection in New Guinea

C. perfringens type C also produces an enterotoxin that causes necrotizing enterocolitis. The illness is rare in the industrialized world but is endemic in parts of New Guinea, especially in children who have participated in pig feasts (hence the pidgin term, *pigbel*). Adults, because they have circulating

antibodies, tend not to develop the disease. Pigbel is segmental and may be restricted to a few centimeters or may involve the entire small intestine. Green, necrotic pseudomembranes are seen in areas of necrosis and peritonitis. More-advanced lesions perforate the bowel wall. Infarction of intestinal mucosa, with edema, hemorrhage and a suppurative transmural infiltrate, is characteristic. The mortality in children is high.

Gas Gangrene May Complicate Penetrating Wounds

Gas gangrene (clostridial myonecrosis) is a necrotizing, gasforming infection that begins in contaminated wounds and spreads rapidly to adjacent tissues. It can be fatal within hours of onset. *C. perfringens* is the most common cause of gas gangrene, but other clostridial species occasionally produce the disease.

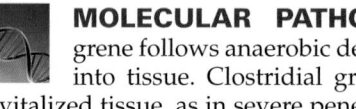 **MOLECULAR PATHOGENESIS:** Gas gangrene follows anaerobic deposition of *C. perfringens* into tissue. Clostridial growth requires extensive devitalized tissue, as in severe penetrating trauma, wartime injuries and septic abortions. Clostridial myonecrosis is rare if wounds are débrided promptly.

Necrosis of previously healthy muscle is caused by myotoxins elaborated by a few species of clostridia. *C. perfringens* type A is the source of the myotoxin in 80%–90% of cases, but *C. novyi* and *C. septicum* may also produce myotoxin. Clostridial myotoxin is a phospholipase that destroys the membranes of muscle cells, leukocytes and erythrocytes.

 PATHOLOGY: Affected tissues rapidly become mottled and then frankly necrotic. Muscle may even liquefy. Overlying skin becomes tense, as edema and gas expand underlying soft tissues. There is extensive tissue necrosis with dissolution of the cells. A striking feature is the paucity of neutrophils, which are destroyed by the myotoxin. Affected tissues often show typical, lozengeshaped, gram-positive rods.

 CLINICAL FEATURES: The incubation period of gas gangrene is 2–4 days after injury. Sudden, severe pain occurs at the wound site, which is tender and edematous. Skin darkens, because of hemorrhage and cutaneous necrosis. The lesion develops a thick, smelly serosanguineous discharge that may contain gas bubbles. Hemolytic anemia, hypotension and renal failure may develop; in the terminal stages, coma, jaundice and shock supervene.

Tetanus Is Spastic Skeletal Muscle Contractions Caused by *Clostridium tetani* Neurotoxin

It is also known as "lockjaw" because of early involvement of the muscles of mastication.

 **EPIDEMIOLOGY:** *C. tetani* is present in the soil and lower intestine of many animals. Tetanus occurs when the organism contaminates wounds and proliferates in tissue, releasing its exotoxin. A vaccine composed of inactivated tetanus toxin has largely eliminated the disease from developed countries. Nonetheless, tetanus is still a common and lethal disease in developing countries.

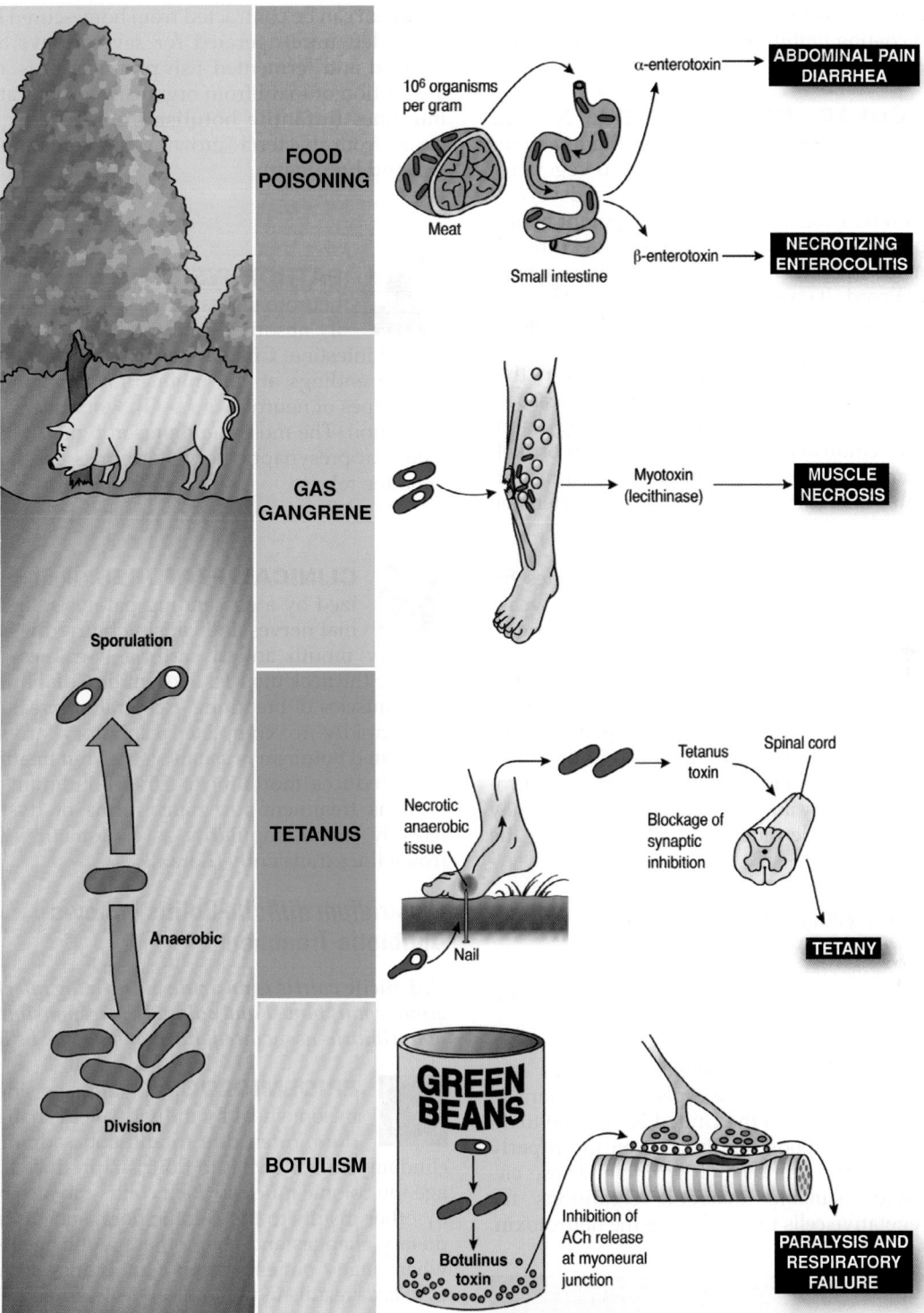

FIGURE 9-27. Clostridial diseases. Clostridia in the vegetative form (bacilli) inhabit the gastrointestinal tract of humans and animals. Spores pass in the feces, contaminate soil and plant materials and are ingested or enter sites of penetrating wounds. Under anaerobic conditions, they revert to vegetative forms. Plasmids in the vegetative forms elaborate toxins that cause several clostridial diseases. **Food poisoning and necrotizing enteritis.** Meat dishes left to cool at room temperature grow large numbers of clostridia (>10^6 organisms per gram). When contaminated meat is ingested, *Clostridium perfringens* types A and C produce α enterotoxin in the small intestine during sporulation, causing abdominal pain and diarrhea. Type C also produces β enterotoxin. **Gas gangrene.** Clostridia are widespread and may contaminate a traumatic wound or surgical operation. *C. perfringens* type A elaborates a myotoxin (α toxin), an α lecithinase that destroys cell membranes, alters capillary permeability and causes severe hemolysis following intravenous injection. The toxin causes necrosis of previously healthy skeletal muscle. **Tetanus.** Spores of *Clostridium tetani* are in soil and enter the site of an accidental wound. Necrotic tissue at the wound site causes spores to revert to the vegetative form (bacilli). Autolysis of vegetative forms releases tetanus toxin. The toxin is transported in peripheral nerves and (retrograde) through axons to the anterior horn cells of the spinal cord. The toxin blocks synaptic inhibition, and the accumulation of acetylcholine in damaged synapses leads to rigidity and spasms of the skeletal musculature (tetany). **Botulism.** Improperly canned food is contaminated by the vegetative form of *Clostridium botulinum,* which proliferates under aerobic conditions and elaborates a neurotoxin. After the food is ingested, the neurotoxin is absorbed from the small intestine and eventually reaches the myoneural junction, where it inhibits the release of acetylcholine (ACh). The result is a symmetric descending paralysis of cranial nerves, trunk and limbs, with eventual respiratory paralysis and death.

Many deaths occur in newborns in primitive societies owing to the custom of coating umbilical stumps with dirt or dung to prevent bleeding.

 **MOLECULAR PATHOGENESIS:** Necrotic tissue and suppuration create a fertile anaerobic environment for the spores to revert to vegetative bacteria. Tetanus toxin is released from autolyzed vegetative cells. Infection remains localized, but the potent neurotoxin **(tetanospasmin)** is transported retrograde through the ventral roots of peripheral nerves to the anterior horn cells of the spinal cord. It crosses the synapse and binds to ganglioside receptors on presynaptic terminals of motor neurons in the ventral horns. After it is internalized, its endopeptidase activity selectively cleaves a protein that mediates exocytosis of synaptic vesicles. Thus, release of inhibitory neurotransmitters is blocked, permitting unopposed neural stimulation and sustained contraction of skeletal muscles **(tetany)**. The loss of inhibitory neurotransmitters also accelerates the heart rate and leads to hypertension and cardiovascular instability.

 CLINICAL FEATURES: Tetanus incubates for 1–3 weeks, then begins subtly with fatigue, weakness and muscle cramping that progresses to rigidity. Spastic rigidity often begins in the muscles of the face, hence **"lockjaw,"** which extends to several facial muscles, causing a fixed grin **(risus sardonicus)**. Rigidity of the muscles of the back produces a backward arching **(opisthotonos)** (Fig. 9-28). Abrupt stimuli, including noise, light or touch, can precipitate painful generalized muscle spasms. Prolonged spasm of respiratory and laryngeal musculature may be fatal. Infants and people older than 50 years have the highest mortality.

Botulism Is a Paralyzing Disease Due to *Clostridium botulinum* Neurotoxin

The disease entails symmetric descending paralysis of cranial nerves, limbs and trunk.

 **EPIDEMIOLOGY:** *C. botulinum* spores are widely distributed and are especially resistant to drying and boiling. In the United States, the toxin is most often present in foods that have been improperly home canned and stored without refrigeration. These circumstances provide suitable anaerobic conditions for growth of the vegetative cells that elaborate the neurotoxin.

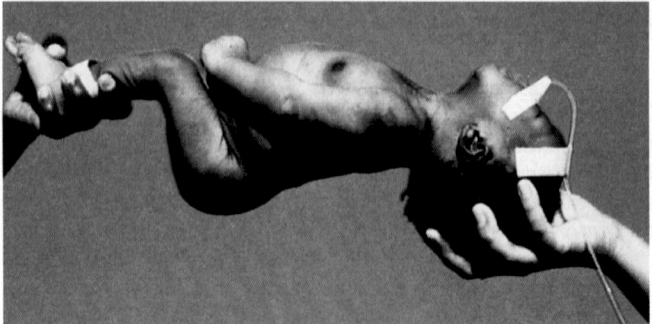

FIGURE 9-28. Tetanus. Opisthotonus (backward arching) in an infant due to intense contraction of the paravertebral muscles.

Botulism can be contracted from home-cured ham and other meats left unrefrigerated for several days and from raw, smoked and fermented fish products. It is also caused by absorption of toxin from organisms proliferating in infants' intestines **(infantile botulism)** or rarely by absorption of toxin from bacteria growing in contaminated wounds **(wound botulism)**.

 PATHOPHYSIOLOGY: Ingested botulinum neurotoxin resists gastric digestion and is readily absorbed into the blood from the proximal small intestine. Circulating toxin reaches the cholinergic nerve endings at the myoneural junction. There are 7 serotypes of neurotoxin (A–G), with diverse mechanisms of action. The most common serotype, A, binds gangliosides at presynaptic nerve terminals and inhibits acetylcholine release.

 CLINICAL FEATURES: Botulism is characterized by a descending paralysis, first affecting cranial nerves and causing blurred vision, photophobia, dry mouth and dysarthria. Weakness progresses to involve the neck muscles, extremities, diaphragm and accessory muscles of breathing. Respiratory weakness can progress rapidly to complete respiratory arrest and death. Untreated botulism is usually lethal, but treatment with antitoxin reduces mortality to 25%. Botulinum toxin is often used as treatment for many forms of dystonia and has recently found popularity as a cosmetic vehicle to erase frown lines transiently (Botox).

Clostridium difficile Colitis Follows Antibiotic Treatment

C. difficile colitis is an acute necrotizing infection of the terminal small bowel and colon. It is responsible for 25%–50% of antibiotic-associated diarrhea and can be lethal.

 **EPIDEMIOLOGY:** *C. difficile* resides in the colon in some healthy individuals. A change in intestinal flora, often due to antibiotic administration (e.g., clindamycin), allows it to flourish, produce toxin and damage the colonic mucosa. Such colitis can also be precipitated by other insults to the colonic flora, such as bowel surgery, dietary changes and chemotherapeutic agents. In hospitals where many patients receive antibiotics, fecal shedding of *C. difficile* results in person-to-person spread.

 MOLECULAR PATHOGENESIS: Commensal colonic bacteria normally limit growth of *C. difficile*, but when normal flora are disturbed (e.g., by antibiotic treatment), the organism can proliferate, elaborate toxins and destroy mucosal cells. *C. difficile* does not invade, but rather produces two exotoxins. Toxin A causes fluid secretion; toxin B is directly cytopathic.

PATHOLOGY: *C. difficile* destroys colonic mucosal cells and incites an acute inflammatory infiltrate. Lesions range from focal colitis limited to a few crypts and only detectable on biopsy, to massive confluent mucosal ulceration. Inflammation initially involves only the mucosa, but it can extend into the submucosa and muscularis propria. An inflammatory exudate, "pseudomembrane" of cellular debris, neutrophils and fibrin, often forms over affected areas of the colon. *C. difficile* colitis is often called **pseudomembranous colitis,** even though that condition may have many etiologies.

 CLINICAL FEATURES: *C. difficile* colitis may start with very mild symptoms or with diarrhea, fever and abdominal pain. Stools may be profuse and often contain neutrophils. The symptoms and signs are not specific and do not distinguish *C. difficile* colitis from other acute inflammatory diarrheal illnesses. Mild cases can often be treated simply by discontinuing the precipitating antibiotic. More-severe cases require an antibiotic effective against *C. difficile.*

BACTERIAL INFECTIONS WITH ANIMAL RESERVOIRS OR INSECT VECTORS

Brucellosis Is a Chronic Febrile Disease Acquired from Domestic Animals

Human brucellosis may manifest as an acute systemic disease or as a chronic infection with waxing and waning febrile episodes, weight loss and fatigue. *Brucella* are small, aerobic, gram-negative rods. In humans, they primarily infect monocytes/macrophages.

 **EPIDEMIOLOGY:** Brucellosis is a zoonotic disease caused by one of four *Brucella* species. Each species of *Brucella* has its own animal reservoir:

- *Brucella melitensis:* sheep and goats
- *Brucella abortus:* cattle
- *Brucella suis:* swine
- *Brucella canis:* dogs

Brucellosis occurs worldwide; virtually every type of domesticated animal and many wild ones are infected. The organisms reside in the animals' genitourinary systems, and infection is often endemic in animal herds. Humans acquire the bacteria by (1) contact with infected blood or tissue, (2) ingesting contaminated meat or milk or (3) inhaling contaminated aerosols. Brucellosis is an occupational hazard among ranchers, herders, veterinarians and slaughterhouse workers.

Elimination of infected animals and vaccination of herds have reduced the incidence of brucellosis in many countries, so that only about 200 cases are reported annually in the United States. Yet, the disease remains prevalent throughout Central and South America, Africa, Asia and Southern Europe, where unpasteurized milk and cheese are major sources of infection. In the arctic and subarctic regions, humans acquire brucellosis by eating raw bone marrow of infected reindeer.

 PATHOLOGY: Bacteria enter the circulation through skin abrasions, lungs, conjunctiva or oropharynx. They then spread in the bloodstream to the liver, spleen, lymph nodes and bone marrow, where they multiply in macrophages. Generalized hyperplasia of these cells may ensue, causing lymphadenopathy and hep-

atosplenomegaly in 15% of patients infected with *B. melitensis,* and in 40% of those infected with *B. abortus.* Patients infected with *B. abortus* develop conspicuous noncaseating granulomas in the liver, spleen, lymph nodes and bone marrow. By contrast, patients infected with *B. melitensis* do not develop classic granulomas, but may have only small aggregates of mononuclear inflammatory cells scattered throughout the liver. *B. suis* infection may cause suppurative liver abscesses. The organisms usually cannot be demonstrated histologically. Periodic release of organisms from infected phagocytic cells may be responsible for the febrile episodes of the illness.

 CLINICAL FEATURES: Brucellosis is a systemic infection that can involve any organ or organ system, with an insidious onset in half of cases. It is characterized by a multitude of somatic complaints, such as fever, sweats, anorexia, fatigue, weight loss and depression. Fever occurs in all patients at some time during the illness, but it can wax and wane (hence the term **undulant fever**) over weeks to months if untreated. Mortality from brucellosis is less than 1%; death is usually caused by endocarditis.

The most common complications of brucellosis involve the bones and joints and include spondylitis of the lumbar spine and suppuration in large joints. Peripheral neuritis, meningitis, orchitis, endocarditis, myocarditis and pulmonary lesions are described. Prolonged treatment with tetracycline is usually effective; the relapse rate is dramatically reduced if rifampin or an aminoglycoside antibiotic is used.

Yersinia pestis Causes Bubonic Plague

Plague is a bacteremic, often fatal, infection that is usually accompanied by enlarged, painful regional lymph nodes **(buboes)**. Historically, plague caused massive epidemics that killed much of the then-civilized world and has been credited with major impact on the course of history.

Major plague epidemics have occurred when *Yersinia pestis* was introduced into large urban rat populations in crowded, squalid cities. Infection spread first among rats; then, as they died, infected fleas fed on the human population, causing widespread disease. Plague has been a common cohabitant of war. An Athenian plague in the 5th century BC developed during the Peloponnesian wars. Two huge epidemics occurred in the Roman empire, one in the 2nd century AD and one in the 6th century AD, both involving either wars or trade routes. The latter may have killed as many as 100 million people. The Black Death pandemic in mid-14th-century (1347–1350) Europe killed 30%–60% of Europe's population. In the United States, 30–40 cases of plague occur annually, mostly in the desert Southwest. Between 2000 and 3000 cases of plague are reported worldwide each year, but the likely number of infections is considerably higher.

Y. pestis is a short gram-negative rod that stains more heavily at the ends (i.e., bipolar staining), particularly with Giemsa stains.

 **EPIDEMIOLOGY:** *Y. pestis* infection is an endemic zoonosis in many parts of the world, including the Americas, Africa and Asia. The organisms are found in wild rodents, such as rats, squirrels

and prairie dogs. Fleas transmit it from animal to animal, and most human infections result from bites of infected fleas. Some infected humans develop plague pneumonia and shed large numbers of organisms in aerosolized respiratory secretions, which allows person-to-person transmission.

 PATHOPHYSIOLOGY: After inoculation into the skin, *Y. pestis* is phagocytosed by neutrophils and macrophages. Organisms ingested by neutrophils are killed, but those engulfed by macrophages survive and replicate intracellularly. The bacteria are carried to regional lymph nodes, where they continue to multiply, producing extensive hemorrhagic necrosis. From regional lymph nodes, they disseminate via the bloodstream and lymphatics. In the lungs, *Y. pestis* produces a necrotizing pneumonitis that releases organisms into the alveoli and airways. These are expelled by coughing, enabling pneumonic spread of the disease. Affected lymph nodes, known as "buboes," are frequently enlarged and fluctuant, owing to extensive hemorrhagic necrosis. Infected patients often develop necrotic, hemorrhagic skin lesions, hence the name "black death" for this disease.

 **CLINICAL FEATURES:** The three clinical presentations of *Y. pestis* infection often overlap.

- **Bubonic plague** begins 2–8 days after the flea bite. Symptoms include headache, fever and myalgias and painful enlargement of regional lymph nodes, mostly in the groin, because flea bites usually occur in the lower extremities. Disease progresses to septic shock within hours to days after appearance of the bubo.
- **Septicemic plague** (10% of cases) occurs when bacteria enter directly into the blood and do not produce buboes. Patients die of overwhelming bacterial growth in the bloodstream. Fever, prostration and meningitis occur suddenly, and death ensues within 48 hours. All blood vessels contain bacilli, and fibrin casts surround the organisms in renal glomeruli and dermal vessels.
- **Pneumonic plague** results from inhalation of airborne particles from carcasses of animals or the cough of infected people. Within 2–5 days after infection, high fever, cough and dyspnea begin suddenly. The sputum teems with bacilli. Respiratory insufficiency and endotoxic shock kill patients within 1–2 days.

All types of plague carry a high mortality rate (50%–75%) if untreated. Tetracycline, combined with streptomycin, is the recommended therapy.

Tularemia Is a Febrile Disease Caused by *Francisella tularensis*

Francisella tularensis is a small, gram-negative coccobacillus.

 EPIDEMIOLOGY: Tularemia is a zoonosis whose most important reservoirs are rabbits and rodents, although other wild and domestic animals may harbor the organisms. Human infection results from contact with infected animals or from the bites of infected insects, including ticks, deerflies and mosquitoes.

Ticks and rabbits are responsible for most human cases. Bacteria enter the body when blood-sucking insects inoculate them through the skin or via unnoticed breaks in the skin if there is direct contact with an infected animal, ingestion of contaminated food and water or inoculation into the eye. Inhalational tularemia can also result from inhalation of infected aerosols. It is found in temperate zones. The incidence of tularemia has declined dramatically in the United States, to about 250 cases annually, probably owing to a decline in hunting and trapping.

 PATHOPHYSIOLOGY: *F. tularensis* multiplies at the site of inoculation, producing a focal ulcer. The bacteria then spread to regional lymph nodes. Dissemination in the bloodstream leads to metastatic infections that involve the monocyte/macrophage system and sometimes the lungs, heart and kidneys. *F. tularensis* survives within macrophages until these cells are activated by a cell-mediated immune response to the infection.

 PATHOLOGY: Lesions of tularemia occur at the inoculation site and in lymph nodes, spleen, liver, bone marrow, lungs (Fig. 9-29), heart and kidneys. Initial skin lesions are exudative, pyogenic ulcers. Later, disseminated lesions undergo central necrosis and are surrounded by a perimeter of granulomatous reaction resembling the lesions of tuberculosis. Hyperemia and abundant macrophages in the sinuses make lymph nodes large and firm; they later soften as necrosis and suppuration develop. Pulmonary lesions resemble those of primary tuberculosis.

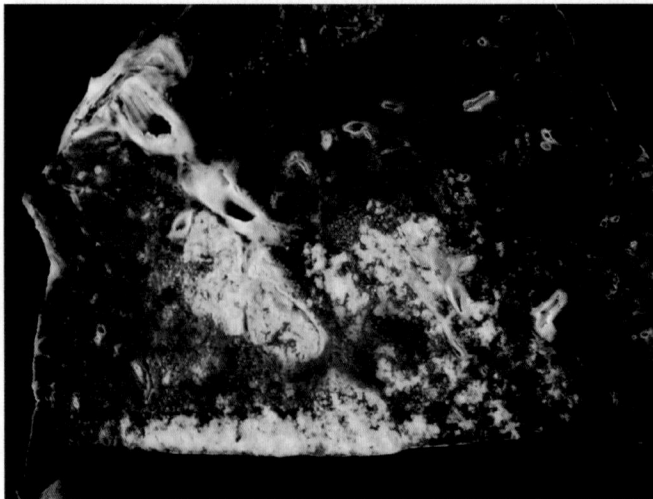 **CLINICAL FEATURES:** The incubation period of tularemia is 1–14 days, depending on the dose and route of transmission, with a mean of 3–4 days. There are four distinct clinical presentations:

- **Ulceroglandular tularemia** is the most common (80%–90% of cases). It begins as a tender, erythematous papule at the site of inoculation, usually on a limb. This develops

FIGURE 9-29. Tularemia. The lung shows firm, consolidated and necrotic areas.

into a pustule, which then ulcerates. Regional lymph nodes become large and tender and may suppurate and drain through sinus tracts. In some instances, generalized lymphadenopathy **(glandular tularemia)** is the first manifestation of infection.

Initial bacteremia is accompanied by fever, headache, myalgias and occasionally prostration. Within a week, generalized lymphadenopathy and splenomegaly develop. The most serious infections are complicated by secondary pneumonia and endotoxic shock, in which case the prognosis is grave. Some patients develop meningitis, endocarditis, pericarditis or osteomyelitis.

- **Oculoglandular tularemia** is rare (<2% of cases) and is characterized by a primary conjunctival papule, which forms a pustule and ulcerates. Lymphadenopathy develops in the head and neck. Severe ulceration may cause blindness if infection penetrates the sclera and reaches the optic nerve.
- **Typhoidal tularemia** is diagnosed when fever, hepatosplenomegaly and toxemia are the presenting signs and symptoms.
- **Pneumonic tularemia,** in which pneumonia is a major feature, may complicate any of the other types.

Tularemia lasts 1 week to 3 months, but this may be shortened by prompt treatment with streptomycin.

Anthrax is Rapidly Fatal When It Disseminates

Anthrax is a necrotizing disease caused by *Bacillus anthracis,* which is a large spore-forming, gram-positive rod.

 **EPIDEMIOLOGY:** Anthrax has been recognized for centuries, and descriptions of disease consistent with anthrax were reported in early Hebrew, Roman and Greek records. The major reservoirs are goats, sheep, cattle, horses, pigs and dogs. Spores form in the soil and dead animals, resisting heat, desiccation and chemical disinfection for years. Humans are infected when spores enter the body through breaks in the skin, by inhalation or by ingestion. Human disease may also result from exposure to contaminated animal byproducts, such as hides, wool, brushes or bone meal.

Anthrax has been a persistent problem in Iran, Turkey, Pakistan and Sudan. One of the largest recorded naturally occurring outbreaks of anthrax occurred in Zimbabwe, when an estimated 10,000 persons became infected in 1978–1980. In North America, human infection is extremely rare (one case per year for the past few years) and usually results from exposure to imported animal products. However, increased vigilance for anthrax has emerged following a recent bioterrorism episode involving transport of organisms by the postal system (see below).

PATHOPHYSIOLOGY: The spores of *B. anthracis* germinate in the human body to yield vegetative bacteria that multiply and release a potent necrotizing toxin. In 80% of cases of cutaneous anthrax, infection remains localized and host immune responses eventually eliminate the organism. If the infection disseminates, as occurs when the organisms are inhaled or ingested, the resulting widespread tissue destruction is usually fatal.

 PATHOLOGY: *B. anthracis* produces extensive tissue necrosis at the sites of infection, with only a mild infiltrate of neutrophils. Cutaneous lesions are ulcerated, contain numerous organisms and are covered by a black scab. Pulmonary infection produces a necrotizing, hemorrhagic pneumonia, associated with hemorrhagic necrosis of mediastinal lymph nodes and widespread dissemination of the organism.

 CLINICAL FEATURES: The mode of presentation of anthrax depends on the site of inoculation.

- **Malignant pustule,** the cutaneous form, accounts for 95% of all anthrax. The patient presents with an elevated skin papule that enlarges and erodes into an ulcer. Bloody purulent exudate accumulates and gradually darkens to purple or black. The ulcer is often surrounded by a zone of brawny edema, which is disproportionately large for the size of the ulcer. Regional lymphadenitis portends a poor prognosis, since lymphatic invasion precedes septicemia. If infection does not disseminate, cutaneous lesions heal without sequelae.
- **Pulmonary, or inhalational, anthrax,** sometimes called "woolsorters' disease," is a hazard of handling raw wool and develops after inhaling the spores of *B. anthracis*. It begins as a flu-like illness that rapidly progresses to respiratory failure and shock. Death often ensues within 24–48 hours. Inhalational anthrax is very rare in the United States. During a bioterror attack in the United States in 2001, 11 cases of inhalational anthrax occurred. The only hope is early antibiotic therapy.
- **Septicemic anthrax** more commonly follows pulmonary anthrax than malignant pustule. Disseminated intravascular coagulation is a common complication. Moreover, a bacterial toxin depresses the respiratory center, which explains why death can occur even when antibiotic therapy has cured the infection.
- **Gastrointestinal anthrax** is rare and is acquired by eating contaminated meat. Stomach or bowel ulceration and invasion of regional lymphatics are common. Death is caused by fulminant diarrhea and massive ascites.

Listeriosis Is a Systemic Multiorgan Infection with a High Mortality

Listeriosis is caused by *Listeria monocytogenes,* a small, motile, gram-positive coccobacillus. It is particularly important as a cause of perinatal disease in newborn babies.

 **EPIDEMIOLOGY:** Listeriosis is usually sporadic but may be epidemic. The organism has been isolated worldwide from surface water, soil, vegetation, feces of healthy persons, many species of wild and domestic mammals and several species of birds. However, spread of infection from animals to humans is rare. Most human infections occur in urban rather than rural environments, usually in the summer. *L. monocytogenes* grows at refrigerator temperatures, and outbreaks have been traced to unpasteurized milk, cheese and dairy products.

 **MOLECULAR PATHOGENESIS:** *L. monocytogenes* has an unusual life cycle, which accounts for its ability to evade intracellular and extracellular

host antibacterial defenses. After phagocytosis by host cells, the organisms enter phagolysosomes, where acidic pH activates *listeriolysin O*, an exotoxin that disrupts the vesicular membrane and allows bacteria to escape into the cytoplasm. After replicating, bacteria usurp host cytoskeleton contractile elements to form elongated protrusions that are engulfed by adjacent cells. Thus, *Listeria* spread from one cell to another without exposure to the extracellular environment.

 PATHOLOGY AND CLINICAL FEATURES: Listeriosis of pregnancy includes prenatal and postnatal infections. Listeriosis of the adult population is characterized by meningoencephalitis and septicemia but may be localized to the skin, eyes, lymph nodes, endocardium or bone.

Maternal infection early in pregnancy may lead to abortion or premature delivery. Infected infants rapidly develop respiratory distress, hepatosplenomegaly, cutaneous and mucosal papules, leukopenia and thrombocytopenia. Intrauterine infections involve many organs and tissues, including amniotic fluid, the placenta and the umbilical cord. Abscesses are found in many organs. Foci of necrosis and suppuration contain many bacteria. Older lesions tend to be granulomatous. Neurologic sequelae are common, and the mortality of neonatal listeriosis is high even with prompt antibiotic therapy. Neonatal listeriosis may also be acquired during delivery, in which case the onset of clinical disease is 3 days to 2 weeks after birth.

Chronic alcoholics, patients with cancer or receiving immunosuppressive therapy and those with AIDS are far more susceptible to infection than is the general population. Meningitis is the most common form of the disease in adults and resembles other bacterial meningitides.

Septicemic listeriosis is a severe febrile illness most common in immunodeficient patients. It may lead to shock and disseminated intravascular coagulation, accounting for misdiagnosis as gram-negative sepsis. Prolonged treatment with antimicrobials is usually required because patients tend to experience relapse if therapy is administered for less than 3 weeks. The mortality from systemic listeriosis remains at 25%.

Bartonella henselae Causes Cat-Scratch Disease

Cat-scratch disease is a self-limited infection usually caused by *Bartonella* strain *Bartonella henselae* and, more rarely, *Bartonella quintana*. The bacteria are small (0.2–0.6 μm) gram-negative rods. They are difficult to culture but are easily seen in tissue sections of the skin, lymph nodes and conjunctiva when stained with a silver impregnation technique (Fig. 9-30).

 **EPIDEMIOLOGY:** The animal reservoir is thought to be cats; surveys have shown that up to 30% of cats are bacteremic. Infection begins when the bacillus is inoculated into the skin by the claws of cats (or rarely other animals) or by thorns or splinters. Sometimes the conjunctiva is contaminated by close contact with a cat, possibly by licking around the eye. Infections are more common in children (80%) than in adults.

 PATHOLOGY AND CLINICAL FEATURES: Bacteria multiply in the walls of small vessels and about collagen fibers at

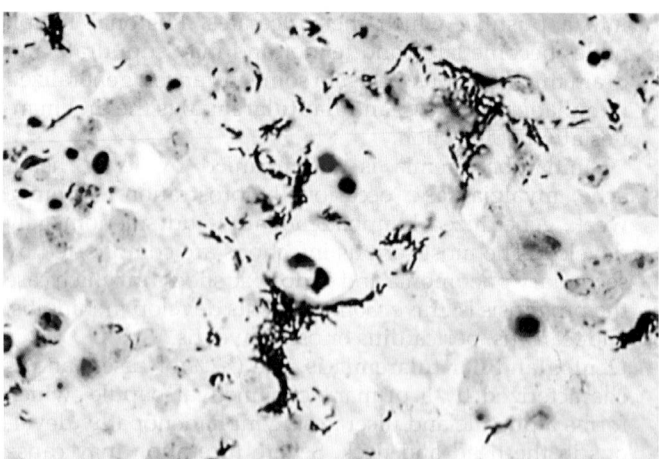
FIGURE 9-30. Cat-scratch disease. Section of a lymph node shows the bacilli, which are gram negative but difficult to visualize with tissue Gram stains. They are blackened by the Warthin-Starry silver impregnation technique.

the site of inoculation. The organisms are then carried to regional lymph nodes, where they cause a **suppurative** and **granulomatous lymphadenitis**. In early lesions, clusters of bacteria fill and expand lumina of small blood vessels. However, bacteria are rare in late lesions. A papule develops at the site of inoculation, followed by tenderness and enlargement of regional lymph nodes. Nodes remain enlarged for 3–4 months and may drain through the skin. About half of patients have other symptoms, including fever and malaise, rash, a brief encephalitis and erythema nodosum. There are other clinical presentations. **Parinaud oculoglandular syndrome** (preauricular adenopathy secondary to conjunctival infection) is common. **Bacillary angiomatosis** is a vascular skin disease that can extend to other organs—it is most commonly seen in immunocompromised persons. **Bacillary peliosis** affects the liver and spleen, causing blood-filled cystic spaces; it affects patients with severe immunologic compromise. Antibiotics are not known to help.

Glanders Is a Granulomatous Infection Acquired from Horses

Glanders is an infection of equine species (horses, mules, donkeys) that is only rarely transmitted to humans, in whom it causes acute or chronic granulomatous disease. It is caused by *Pseudomonas mallei*, a small gram-negative, nonmotile bacillus. Although uncommon, the infection remains endemic in South America, Asia and Africa. People acquire the disease by contact with infected equines through broken skin or inhalation of contaminated aerosols.

- **Acute glanders** is characterized by bacteremia, severe prostration and fever. Granulomatous abscesses may form in subcutaneous tissues and many other organs, including the lung, liver, spleen, muscles and joints. Acute glanders is almost always fatal.
- **Chronic glanders** features low-grade fever, draining abscesses of the skin, lymphadenopathy and hepatosplenomegaly. Granulomas in many organs mimic tuberculosis. The mortality in chronic glanders exceeds 50%.

Bartonellosis Causes Acute Anemia and Skin Disease

Bartonellosis is an infection by *Bartonella bacilliformis,* a small, multiflagellated, gram-negative coccobacillus.

 EPIDEMIOLOGY: Bartonellosis occurs only in Peru, Ecuador and Colombia, in river valleys of the Andes, and is transmitted by sandflies. Humans are the only reservoir and acquire the infection at sunrise and sunset, when sandflies are most active. In endemic areas, 10%–15% of the population have latent infections. Newcomers are susceptible, whereas the indigenous population tends to be resistant.

  PATHOLOGY AND CLINICAL FEATURES: Bartonellosis presents a biphasic pattern, with acute hemolytic anemia **(Oroya fever)** first, followed some months later by a chronic dermal phase **(verruga peruana)**. Either phase may occur by itself.

The most severe consequence of bartonellosis is hemolytic anemia. After *B. bacilliformis* is inoculated into the skin by a sandfly, bacteria proliferate in the vascular endothelium and then invade erythrocytes, leading to profound hemolysis.

The **acute anemic phase** follows 3 weeks of incubation and is characterized by abrupt onset of fever, skeletal pains and severe, hemolytic anemia. If untreated, 40% of patients in the anemic phase die. Secondary *Salmonella* sepsis is common and contributes to the high mortality.

The **dermal eruptive phase** may coexist with the anemic phase but usually appears 3–6 months later. Many small hemangioma-like lesions stud the dermis, and bacteria may be identified in endothelial cells. Nodular lesions may be prominent on extensor surfaces of the arms and legs. Large deep-seated lesions, which tend to ulcerate, develop near joints and limit motion. The dermal eruptive phase is often prolonged but eventually heals spontaneously. The mortality in this phase is less than 5%.

INFECTIONS CAUSED BY BRANCHING FILAMENTOUS ORGANISMS

Actinomycosis Features Abscesses and Sinus Tracts

Actinomycosis is a slowly progressive, suppurative, fibrosing infection involving the jaw, thorax or abdomen. It is caused by a number of anaerobic and microaerophilic bacteria termed *Actinomyces.* These are branching, filamentous, gram-positive rods that normally reside in the oropharynx, gastrointestinal tract and vagina. Several *Actinomyces* species cause human disease, the most common being *Actinomyces israelii.*

 PATHOPHYSIOLOGY: *Actinomyces* is not ordinarily virulent; the organisms reside as saprophytes in the body without producing disease. Two uncommon conditions must occur for *Actinomyces* to cause disease. First, it must be inoculated into deeper tissues, since it cannot invade. Second, an anaerobic atmosphere is necessary for bacterial proliferation. Trauma can produce tissue necrosis, providing an excellent anaerobic medium for growth of *Actinomyces* and inoculating the organism into normally sterile tissue. Actinomycosis occurs at four distinct sites:

- **Cervicofacial actinomycosis** results from jaw injury, dental extraction or dental manipulation.
- **Thoracic actinomycosis** is due to aspiration of organisms contaminating dental debris.
- **Abdominal actinomycosis** follows traumatic or surgical disruption of the bowel, especially the appendix.
- **Pelvic actinomycosis** is associated with the prolonged use of intrauterine devices (IUDs).

Actinomycosis begins as a nidus of proliferating organisms that attract an acute inflammatory infiltrate. The small abscess grows slowly, becoming a series of abscesses connected by sinus tracts. Tracts burrow, characteristically, across normal tissue boundaries and into adjacent organs. Eventually, a tract may reach an external surface or mucosal membrane and produce a draining sinus. The walls of abscesses and tracts are granulation tissue, often thick, densely fibrotic and chronically inflamed. Within abscesses and sinuses are pus and colonies of organisms.

Actinomyces colonies can grow to several millimeters and be visible to the naked eye. They appear as hard, yellow grains called **sulfur granules,** because they resemble elemental sulfur. These are tangled masses of narrow, branching filaments in a polysaccharide–protein matrix. Histologically, colonies are rounded, basophilic grains with scalloped eosinophilic borders (Fig. 9-31A). Individual filaments of *Actinomyces* cannot be discerned with hematoxylin and eosin stain but are readily visible on Gram staining or silver impregnation (Fig. 9-31B).

 CLINICAL FEATURES: The presentation of actinomycosis depends on the site of infection. If infection originates in a tooth socket or the tonsils, it is characterized by swelling of the jaw ("lumpy jaw"), face and neck, at first painless and fluctuant but later painful. In pulmonary infections, sinus tracts may penetrate from lobe to lobe, through the pleura and into ribs and vertebrae. Abdominal or pelvic disease may present as an expanding mass, suggesting an enlarging tumor. Actinomycosis responds to prolonged antibiotic therapy; penicillin is highly effective.

Nocardiosis Is a Suppurative Respiratory Infection in Immunocompromised Hosts

Nocardia are aerobic, gram-positive filamentous, branching bacteria. They are weakly acid-fast, as distinguished from the morphologically similar actinomycetes. From the lungs, infection often spreads to the brain and skin.

 **EPIDEMIOLOGY:** *Nocardia* species are widely distributed in soil, and human disease is caused by inhaling or inoculating soil-borne organisms. It is not transmitted from person to person. *Nocardia asteroides* is the species most often involved in human disease. Nocardiosis is most common in patients with impaired immunity, particularly cell-mediated immunity. Organ transplantation,

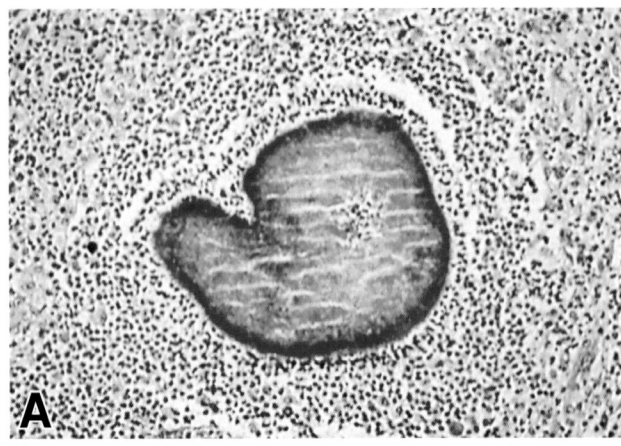
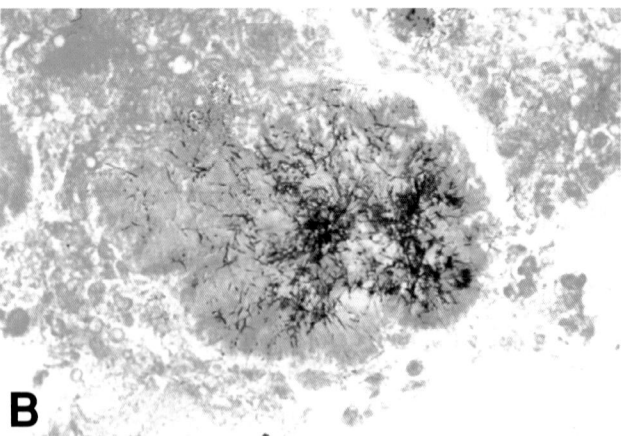

FIGURE 9-31. Actinomycosis. A. A typical sulfur granule lies within an abscess. **B.** The individual filaments of *Actinomyces israeli* are readily visible with the silver impregnation technique.

long-term corticosteroid therapy, lymphomas, leukemias and other debilitating diseases are predisposing factors.

Two other pathogenic species of *Nocardia*, *Nocardia brasiliensis* and *Nocardia caviae*, may cause pulmonary nocardiosis resembling that produced by *N. asteroides.* They are usually encountered in underdeveloped countries as a cause of mycetomas.

  PATHOLOGY AND CLINICAL FEATURES: The respiratory tract is the usual portal of entry. The organism elicits a brisk infiltrate of neutrophils, and disease begins as a slowly progressive, pyogenic pneumonia. If an infected person mounts a vigorous cell-mediated immune response, the infection may be eliminated. In immunocompromised people, however, *Nocardia* produces pulmonary abscesses, which are frequently multiple and confluent. Direct extension to the pleura, trachea and heart and blood-borne metastases to the brain or skin carry a grave prognosis. Nocardial abscesses are filled with neutrophils, necrotic debris and scattered organisms. Bacteria can be demonstrated by silver impregnation (Fig. 9-32). With the Gram

stain, they appear as beaded, filamentous, gram-positive rods. Untreated nocardiosis is usually fatal. Sulfonamides or related antibiotics for several months are often effective therapy.

Spirochetal Infections

Spirochetes are long, slender, helical bacteria with specialized cell envelopes that permit them to move by flexion and rotation. The thinner organisms are below the resolving power of routine light microscopy. Specialized techniques, such as darkfield microscopy or silver impregnation, are needed to visualize them. They have the basic cell wall structure of gram-negative bacteria but stain poorly with the Gram stain.

Three genera of spirochetes, *Treponema*, *Borrelia* and *Leptospira*, cause human disease (Table 9-5). They are adept at evading host inflammatory and immunologic defenses, and diseases caused by these organisms are all chronic or relapsing.

SYPHILIS

Syphilis (lues) is a chronic, sexually transmitted, systemic infection caused by *Treponema pallidum*, a thin, long spirochete (Fig. 9-33) that cannot be grown in artificial media. The disease was first recognized in Europe in the 1490s and has been related to Columbus's return from the New World. Urbanization and mass movements of people caused by war contributed to its rapid spread. Originally, syphilis was an acute disease that caused destructive skin lesions and early death, but it has become milder, with a more protracted and insidious clinical course.

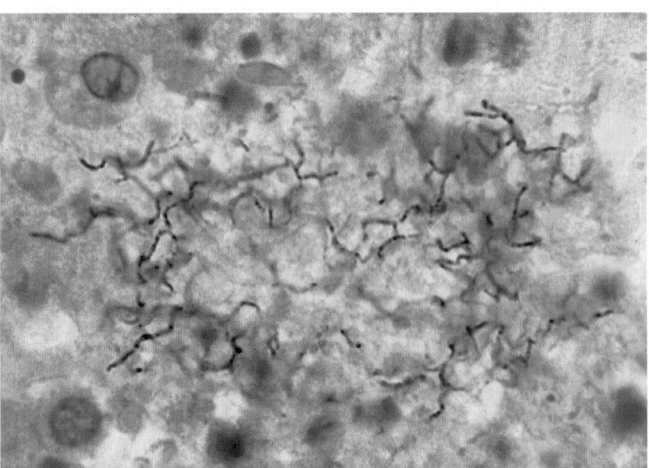

FIGURE 9-32. Nocardiosis. A silver stain of a necrotic exudate reveals the branching, filamentous rods of *Nocardia asteroides.*

 **EPIDEMIOLOGY:** Syphilis is a worldwide disease that is transmitted almost exclusively by sexual contact. Infection may also spread from an infected mother to her fetus (**congenital syphilis**). The incidence of primary and secondary syphilis has declined since the introduction of penicillin therapy at the end of World War II.

TABLE 9-5
SPIROCHETE INFECTIONS

Disease	Organism	Clinical Manifestation	Distribution	Mode of Transmission
Treponemes				
Syphilis	*Treponema pallidum*	See text	Common worldwide	Sexual contact, congenital
Bejel	*Treponema endemicum (Treponema pallidum,* subspecies *endemicum)*	Mucosal, skin and bone lesions	Middle East	Mouth-to-mouth contact
Yaws	*Treponema pertenue (Treponema pallidum* subspecies *pertenue)*	Skin and bone	Tropics	Skin-to-skin contact
Pinta	*Treponema carateum*	Skin lesions	Latin America	Skin-to-skin contact
Borrelia				
Lyme disease	*Borrelia burgdorferi*	See text	North America, Europe, Russia, Asia, Africa, Australia	Tick bite
Relapsing fever	*Borrelia recurrentis*	Relapsing flu-like illness	Worldwide	Tick bite, louse bite and related species
Leptospira				
Leptospirosis	*Leptospira interrogans*	Flu-like illness, meningitis	Worldwide	Contact with animal urine

 **ETIOLOGIC FACTORS AND PATHO-PHYSIOLOGY:** *T. pallidum* is very fragile and is killed by soap, antiseptics, drying and cold. Person-to-person transmission requires direct contact between a rich source of spirochetes (e.g., an open lesion) and mucous membranes or abraded skin of the genital organs, rectum, mouth, fingers or nipples. The organisms reproduce at the site of inoculation, pass to regional lymph nodes, gain access to systemic circulation and disseminate throughout the body. Although *T. pallidum* induces an inflammatory response and is taken up by phagocytic cells, it persists and proliferates. Chronic infection and inflammation cause tissue destruction, sometimes for decades. The course of syphilis is classically divided into three stages (Fig. 9-34).

The Classical Lesion of Primary Syphilis Is the Chancre

Chancres (Fig. 9-35) are characteristic ulcers at sites of *T. pallidum* entry, usually the penis, vulva, anus or mouth. They appear 1 week to 3 months after exposure, with an average of 3 weeks, and tend to be solitary, with firm raised borders. Spirochetes concentrate in vessel walls and in the epidermis around the ulcer. Chancres, as well as the lesions of the other stages of syphilis, show a characteristic **"luetic vasculitis,"** with endothelial cell proliferation and swelling and vessel walls thickened by lymphocytes and fibrosis.

Chancres quickly erode to characteristic ulcers. They are painless and may go unnoticed especially in the uterine cervix, anal canal and mouth. Chancres last 3–12 weeks, are frequently accompanied by inguinal lymphadenopathy and heal without scarring.

Secondary Syphilis Reflects Dissemination of Spirochetes

In secondary syphilis, *T. pallidum* spreads systemically and proliferates to cause lesions in the skin, mucous membranes, lymph nodes, meninges, stomach and liver. Lesions show

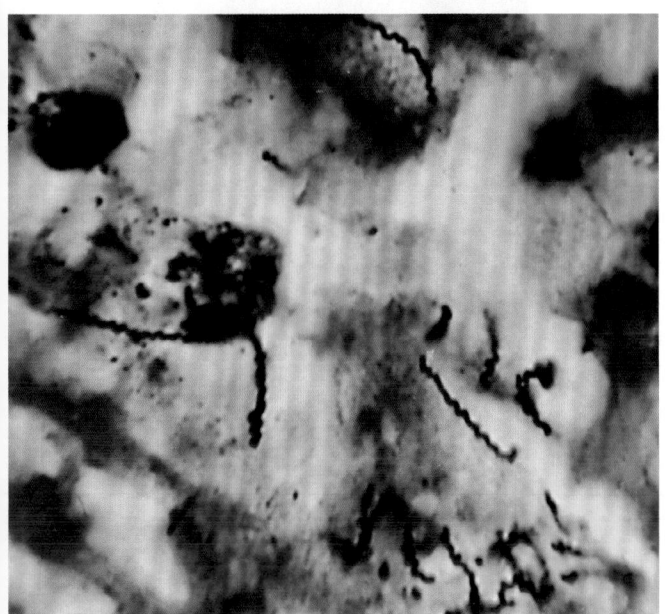
FIGURE 9-33. Syphilis. Spirochetes of *Treponema pallidum,* visualized by silver impregnation, in the eye of a child with congenital syphilis.

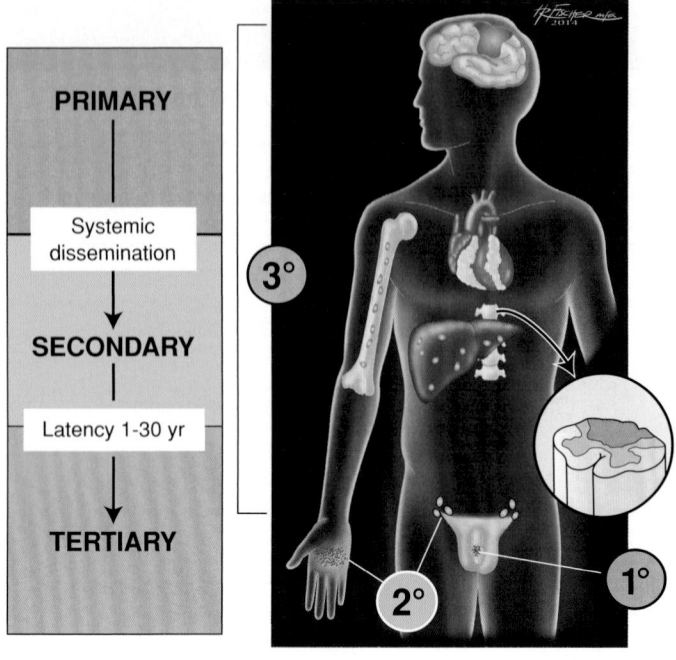

PRIMARY

Systemic
dissemination

SECONDARY

Latency 1-30 yr

TERTIARY

3°

2°

1°

Chancre
(male or female
genitalia)

Lymphadenopathy
Rash: palms, soles

Paralytic dementia
Aortic aneurysm
Aortic insufficiency
Tabes dorsalis
Gummas
(widespread)

FIGURE 9-34. Clinical characteristics of the various stages of syphilis.

perivascular lymphocytic infiltration and obliterative end-arteritis.

- **Skin:** Secondary syphilis most often appears as an erythematous and maculopapular rash of the trunk and extremities, often including the palms (Fig. 9-36) and soles. The rash appears 2 weeks to 3 months after the chancre heals. Other skin lesions in secondary syphilis include **condylomata lata** (exudative plaques in the perineum, vulva or scrotum, which abound in spirochetes) (Fig. 9-37), **follicular syphilids** (small papular lesions around hair follicles that cause loss of hair) and **nummular syphilids** (coin-like lesions of the face and perineum).
- **Mucous membranes:** Lesions on mucosal surfaces of the mouth and genital organs, called **mucous patches,** teem with organisms and are highly infectious.

- **Lymph nodes:** Characteristic changes in lymph nodes, especially epitrochlear nodes, include a thickened capsule, follicular hyperplasia, increased plasma cells and macrophages and luetic vasculitis. Spirochetes are numerous in the lymph nodes of secondary syphilis.
- **Meninges:** Although the meninges are commonly seeded with *T. pallidum,* the condition is frequently asymptomatic.

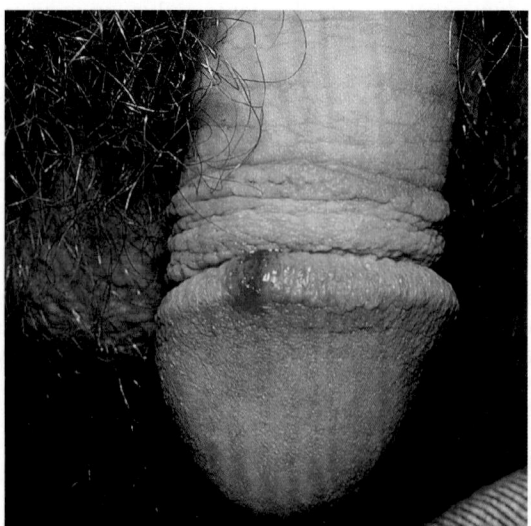

FIGURE 9-35. Syphilitic chancre. A patient with primary syphilis displays a raised, erythematous penile lesion.

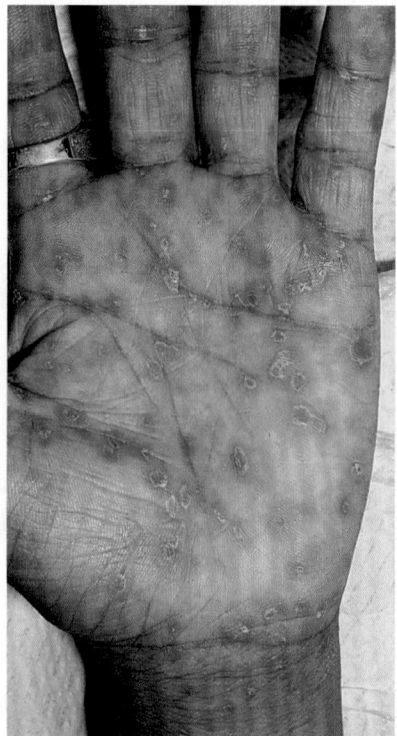

FIGURE 9-36. Secondary syphilis. A maculopapular rash is present on the palm.

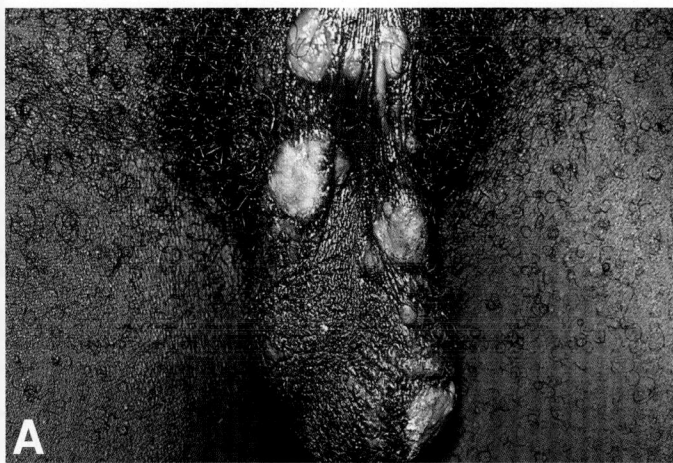
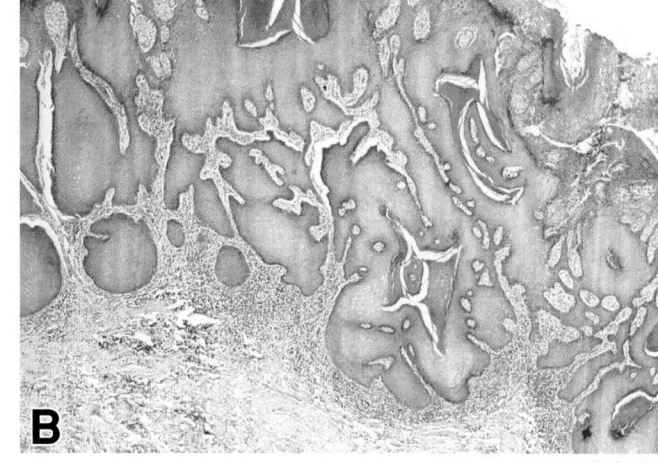

FIGURE 9-37. Condylomata lata in secondary syphilis. A. Whitish plaques are seen on the vulva and perineum. **B.** A photomicrograph shows papillomatous hyperplasia of the epidermis with underlying chronic inflammation.

Tertiary Syphilis Causes Neurologic and Vascular Diseases

After lesions of secondary syphilis subside, an asymptomatic period of years to decades follows. During this time, spirochetes continue to multiply, and the deep-seated lesions of tertiary syphilis gradually develop in one third of untreated patients. *Focal ischemic necrosis secondary to obliterative endarteritis is the underlying mechanism for many of the processes associated with tertiary syphilis.* T. pallidum elicits mononuclear inflammation, mainly of lymphocytes and plasma cells. These cells infiltrate small arteries and arterioles, producing a characteristic obstructive vascular lesion **(endarteritis obliterans)**. Small arteries are inflamed and their endothelial cells are swollen. They are surrounded by concentric layers of proliferating fibroblasts, giving the vascular lesions an "onion skin" appearance.

- **Syphilitic aortitis:** This disorder results from a slowly progressive endarteritis obliterans of vasa vasorum that eventually leads to necrosis of the aortic media, gradual weakening and stretching of the aortic wall and aortic aneurysm. Syphilitic aneurysms are saccular and involve the ascending aorta, which is an unusual site for the much more common atherosclerotic aneurysms. On gross examination, the aortic intima is rough and pitted **(tree-bark appearance;** Fig. 9-38) (see Chapter 16). The aortic media is gradually replaced by scar tissue, after which the aorta loses strength and resilience. The aorta stretches, becoming progressively thinner to the point of rupture, massive hemorrhage and sudden death. *Damage to, and scarring of, the ascending aorta also commonly leads to dilation of the aortic ring, separation of the valve cusps and regurgitation of blood through the aortic valve (aortic insufficiency).* Luetic vasculitis may narrow or occlude the coronary arteries and cause myocardial infarction.

- **Neurosyphilis:** The slowly progressive infection damages the meninges, cerebral cortex, spinal cord, cranial nerves or eyes. Tertiary syphilis of the CNS is subclassified according to the predominant tissue affected. Thus, there are **meningovascular syphilis** (meninges), **tabes dorsalis** (spinal cord) and **general paresis** (cerebral cortex) (see Chapter 32).

- **Benign tertiary syphilis:** The appearance of a gumma (Fig. 9-39) in any organ or tissue is the hallmark of benign

FIGURE 9-38. Syphilitic aortitis. The ascending aorta exhibits a roughened intima (*arrow*, "tree bark" appearance), owing to destruction of the media.

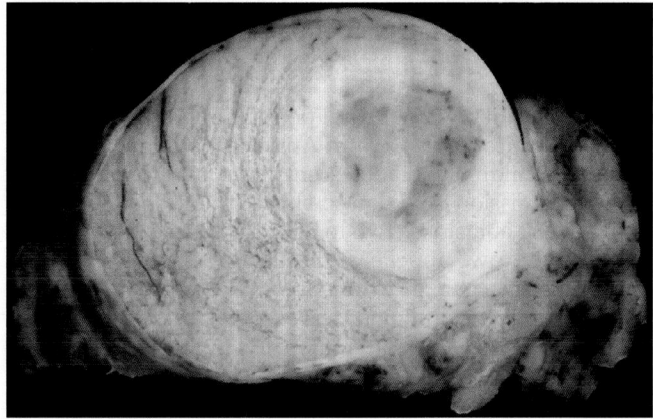

FIGURE 9-39. Syphilitic gumma. A patient with tertiary syphilis shows a sharply circumscribed gumma in the testis, characterized by a fibrogranulomatous wall and a necrotic center.

tertiary syphilis. Gummas are most common in the skin, bone and joints but can occur anywhere. These granulomatous lesions have a central area of coagulative necrosis, epithelioid macrophages, occasional giant cells and peripheral fibrous tissue. Gummas are usually localized lesions that do not significantly damage the patient.

Congenital Syphilis Is Transmitted from an Infected Mother to the Fetus

In this setting, the treponeme disseminates in fetal tissues, which are injured by the proliferating organisms and accompanying inflammatory response. Fetal infection produces stillbirth, neonatal illness or death or progressive postnatal disease.

 PATHOLOGY: Lesions of congenital syphilis are identical to those of adult disease. Infected tissues show a chronic inflammatory infiltrate of lymphocytes and plasma cells and endarteritis obliterans. Virtually any tissue can be affected, but the skin, bones, teeth, joints, liver and CNS are characteristically involved (see Chapter 6).

 CLINICAL FEATURES: Congenital syphilis presents variably. Infected newborns are often asymptomatic. Early signs of infection include rhinitis **(snuffles)** and a desquamative rash. Infections of periosteum, bone, cartilage and dental pulp produce deformities of bones and teeth, including **saddle nose,** anterior bowing of the legs **(saber shins)** and peg-shaped upper incisor teeth **(Hutchinson teeth)**. Disease progression can be arrested by penicillin.

NONVENEREAL TREPONEMATOSES

In tropical and subtropical climes, there are nonvenereal, chronic diseases caused by treponemes indistinguishable from *T. pallidum.* Like syphilis, they result from inoculation of the organism into mucocutaneous surfaces. They also pass through clearly defined clinical and pathologic stages, including a primary lesion at the site of inoculation, secondary skin eruptions, a latent period and a tertiary late stage.

Yaws Is a Tropical Disease Caused by *Treponema pertenue*

Yaws occurs among poor rural populations in warm, humid areas of tropical Africa, South America, Southeast Asia and Oceania. Children and adolescents in tropical regions are at risk. Transmission is by skin-to-skin contact and is facilitated by breaks or abrasions. Two to 5 weeks after exposure, a single "mother yaw" appears at the site of inoculation, usually on an exposed part. It evolves from a papule to a 2–5-cm "raspberry-like" papilloma. The secondary or disseminated stage begins with the eruption of similar, but smaller, yaws on other parts of the skin. The mother yaw and secondary lesions show hyperkeratosis, papillary acanthosis and an intense neutrophilic infiltrate of the epidermis. The epidermis at the apex of the papilloma lyses to form a shallow ulcer, and plasma cells invade the upper dermis. Spirochetes are numerous in the dermal papillae.

Painful papillomas on the soles of the feet lead patients to walk on the side of their feet like a crab, a condition called **"crab yaw."** Treponemes are borne by the blood to bones, lymph nodes and skin, where they grow during a latent period of 5 or more years. The lesions in the late stage include cutaneous gummas, which are destructive to the face and upper airway. Periostitis of the tibia causes "saber shins" or "boomerang legs." One dose of long-acting penicillin cures yaws.

Bejel Is Characterized by Gummas of the Skin, Airways and Bone

Bejel (also known as "endemic syphilis") has a focal distribution in Africa, western Asia and Australia. It is transmitted from an infected infant to the breast of the mother, from mouth to mouth or from utensils to the mouth. The causative agent, *T. pallidum* subspecies *endemicum,* is morphologically and serologically indistinguishable from the agent of syphilis. Other than on the nursing breast, primary lesions are rare. Secondary lesions in the mouth are identical to the mucosal lesions of syphilis and may spread from the upper airway to the larynx. Lesions of the perineum and bone are encountered, and gummas of the breast occur.

Pinta Is a Tropical Skin Disease

Pinta (from the Spanish for "painted" or "blemish") is a treponematosis (*Treponema carateum*) characterized by variably colored spots on the skin. It was first described in the 16th century in Aztec and Caribbean Amerindians. It is prevalent in remote, arid, inland regions and river valleys of the American tropics. The lesions of the three stages of pinta are limited to the skin and tend to merge. Transmission is by skin-to-skin inoculation, usually after long intimate contact with an infected person. Currently, there are only a few hundred new cases reported each year from endemic areas, but this is probably an underestimate.

LYME DISEASE

Lyme disease is a chronic systemic infection that begins with a characteristic skin lesion and later manifests as cardiac, neurologic or joint disturbances. The causative agents are large, microaerophilic spirochetes belonging to the genus *Borrelia.*

 **EPIDEMIOLOGY:** Lyme disease was first described in patients from Lyme, Connecticut, but has since been recognized in many other areas. *Borrelia burgdorferi* is the major cause of Lyme disease in the United States, while *Borrelia afzelii* and *Borrelia garinii* cause most cases in Europe. The spirochete is transmitted from its animal reservoir to humans by the bite of the minute *Ixodes* tick. This pinhead-sized insect is found in wooded areas, where it usually feeds on mice and deer. Transmission to humans is most likely from May through July, when nymph forms of the tick feed.

In the United States, Lyme disease is the most common tick-borne illness, causing an estimated 15,000–20,000 cases annually. It is concentrated along the eastern seaboard from Maryland to Massachusetts, in the Midwest in Minnesota and Wisconsin and in the West in California and Oregon. It also occurs in Europe, Australia and Asia.

  PATHOLOGY AND CLINICAL FEATURES: *B. burgdorferi* reproduces locally at the site of inoculation, spreads to regional lymph nodes and disseminates throughout the body via the bloodstream. Like other spirochetal diseases, Lyme disease is chronic, occurring in stages, with remissions and exacerbations. In patients who die of the disease, organisms are seen at autopsy in virtually every organ affected, including the skin, myocardium, liver, CNS and musculoskeletal system.

Three clinical stages are described:

- **Stage 1:** The characteristic skin lesion, **erythema chronicum migrans,** appears at the site of the tick bite. It begins 3–35 days after the bite as an erythematous macule or papule, which grows into an erythematous patch 3–7 cm in diameter. It often is intensely red at its periphery, with some central clearing, imparting an annular appearance. Studies of skin and synovium have shown that *B. burgdorferi* elicits a chronic inflammatory infiltrate, composed of lymphocytes and plasma cells. It is accompanied by fever, fatigue, headache, arthralgias and regional lymphadenopathy. Secondary annular skin lesions develop in about half of patients and may persist for long periods. During this phase, patients experience constant malaise and fatigue, headache and fever. Intermittent manifestations may also include meningeal irritation, migratory myalgia, cough, generalized lymphadenopathy and testicular swelling.
- **Stage 2:** The second stage begins weeks to months after the skin lesion and is characterized by exacerbation of migratory musculoskeletal pains and cardiac and neurologic abnormalities. In 10% of cases, conduction abnormalities, particularly atrioventricular block, result from myocarditis. Neurologic abnormalities, most commonly meningitis and facial nerve palsies, occur in 15% of patients.
- **Stage 3:** The third stage of Lyme disease begins months to years afterward, with joint, skin and neurologic abnormalities. Over half of these patients have arthralgia and severe arthritis of the large joints, especially the knee. The histopathology of affected joints is virtually indistinguishable from that of rheumatoid arthritis, including villous hypertrophy and a conspicuous mononuclear infiltrate in the subsynovial lining area.

Neurologic manifestations may begin months to years after disease begins. They range from intermittent tingling paresthesias without demonstrable neurologic deficits to slowly progressive encephalomyelitis, transverse myelitis, organic brain syndromes and dementia.

Distinctive late skin manifestations of Lyme disease include acrodermatitis chronica atrophicans. This occurs years after erythema chronicum migrans and presents as patchy atrophy and sclerosis of the skin.

Antibody titers (initially IgM, later IgG) against the organism are the most practical way to establish the diagnosis. Treatment with tetracycline or erythromycin is effective in eliminating early Lyme disease. In later stages, and when there are extensive extracutaneous manifestations, high doses of intravenous penicillin or other combinations of antibiotic regimens for long periods are necessary.

Leptospirosis

Leptospirosis is an infection with spirochetes of the genus *Leptospira.* Usually (90% of patients) leptospirosis is a mild, self-limited, febrile disease. More severe infections may entail hepatic and renal failure, which may prove fatal.

 **EPIDEMIOLOGY:** Leptospirosis is a worldwide zoonosis. Leptospires penetrate abraded skin or mucous membranes following contact with infected rats, contaminated water or mud. Since warm, moist environments favor survival of the spirochetes, the incidence is higher in the tropics. Between 30 and 100 cases are reported annually in the United States, some of them in slaughterhouse workers and trappers, but recently some cases occurred among destitute people in urban areas.

  PATHOLOGY AND CLINICAL FEATURES: The symptoms of leptospirosis begin 4 days to 3 weeks after exposure to *Leptospira interrogans.* In most cases, the disease resolves within a week without sequelae. In more severe infections, leptospirosis is a biphasic disease.

- In the **leptospiremic phase,** leptospires are present in the blood and cerebrospinal fluid. There is an abrupt onset of fever, shaking chills, headache and myalgias. Symptoms abate after 1–2 weeks, as the leptospires disappear from the blood and bodily fluids.
- The **immune phase** begins within 3 days of the end of the leptospiremic phase and is accompanied by the production of IgM antibodies. The earlier symptoms recur, and signs of meningeal irritation become apparent. At this time, the cerebrospinal fluid shows a prominent pleocytosis. In severe cases, jaundice appears and may be followed by hepatic and renal failure and the appearance of widespread hemorrhages and shock. This severe form of leptospirosis has historically been referred to as **Weil disease**.

Untreated Weil disease has a mortality rate of 5%–30%. At autopsy tissues are bile stained, and hemorrhages are seen in many organs. The principal lesion is a diffuse vasculitis with capillary injury. Livers show dissociation of liver cell plates, erythrophagocytosis by Kupffer cells, minimal necrosis of hepatocytes, neutrophils in the sinusoids and a mixed inflammatory cell infiltrate in portal tracts. Renal tubules are swollen and necrotic. Spirochetes are numerous in tubular lumina, and particularly in bile-stained casts (Fig. 9-40).

RELAPSING FEVER

Relapsing fever is an acute, febrile, septicemic illness caused by spirochetes of the genus *Borrelia.* There are two main types of relapsing fever:

- **Epidemic relapsing fever** is caused by *Borrelia recurrentis* and is transmitted by the bite of an infected louse. Humans are the only reservoir.
- **Endemic relapsing fever** is produced by a number of *Borrelia* species and is transferred from rodents and other animals by the bite of an infected tick.

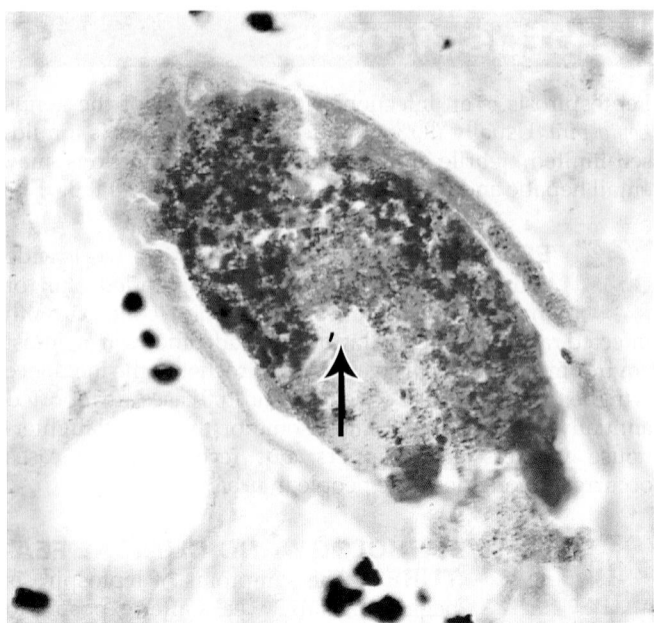

FIGURE 9-40. Leptospirosis. A distal renal tubule is obstructed by a bile-stained mass of hemoglobin and cellular debris. A leptospire (*arrow*) is in the center of this mass.

 **EPIDEMIOLOGY:** The human body louse, *Pediculus humanus humanus,* becomes infected with *B. recurrentis* when it feeds on an infected person. The spirochetes only enter a subsequent person if the louse is crushed when feeding. War, crowded migrant worker camps and heavy clothing during cold weather all favor mobilization of lice and the spread of relapsing fever. Lice also dislike the higher temperatures of feverish victims and seek new hosts, another factor in the rapid spread of relapsing fever during epidemics. Louse-borne relapsing fever is currently seen in several African countries, especially Ethiopia and Sudan, and also in the South American Andes.

In endemic, tick-borne relapsing fever, the insects are infected while biting rats and other hosts. Humans are infected by saliva or coxal fluid of the tick. Ticks live much longer than lice and may harbor spirochetes for 12–15 years without a blood meal. Tick-borne relapsing fever occurs sporadically worldwide.

 PATHOLOGY: In fatal infections, the spleen is enlarged and contains miliary microabscesses. Spirochetes form tangled aggregates around the necrotic centers. Lymphocytes and neutrophils infiltrate central and midzonal areas of the liver, where spirochetes lie free in the sinusoids. Focal hemorrhages involve many organs.

 CLINICAL FEATURES: Arthralgias, lethargy, fever, headache and myalgias appear within 1–2 weeks of a bite of an infected arthropod. The liver and spleen enlarge, and there are petechiae of the skin, conjunctival hemorrhages and abdominal tenderness. The fever ends abruptly within 3–9 days, only to begin anew 7–10 days later. During the afebrile period, spirochetes disappear from the blood and change their antigenic coats. With each relapse, symptoms are milder and the illness shorter. In severe cases,

the initial episode may be characterized by a rash, meningitis, myocarditis, liver failure and coma. Tetracycline is an effective treatment for both types of relapsing fever.

FUSOSPIROCHETAL INFECTIONS

Tropical Phagedenic Ulcer Is a Painful Lesion of the Leg

Tropical phagedenic (rapid spreading and sloughing) ulcer, also known as **tropical foot,** is a painful, necrotizing lesion of the skin and subcutaneous tissues of the leg that afflicts people in tropical climates. *Bacillus fusiformis* and *Treponema vincentii* are two causes. Malnutrition may predispose to infection.

 CLINICAL FEATURES: The lesion usually starts on the skin at a point of trauma and develops rapidly. The surface sloughs to form an ulcer with raised borders and a cup-shaped crater, which contains a gray, putrid exudate (Fig. 9-41). The ulcer may be so deep that the underlying bone and tendons are exposed. The margin becomes fibrotic, but complete healing may be delayed for years. In addition to secondary infection, tibial osteomyelitis and squamous cell carcinoma may be late complications. Antibiotics may be effective, but reconstructive plastic surgery is often necessary to close the defect.

Noma Is a Destructive Lesion of the Face

Noma (gangrenous stomatitis, cancrum oris) is a rapidly progressive necrosis of soft tissues and bones of the mouth and face. Less commonly, it involves other sites, such as the chest, limbs and genitalia. It afflicts malnourished children in the tropics, many of whom are further debilitated by recent infections (e.g., measles, malaria, leishmaniasis). *T. vincentii, B. fusiformis, Bacteroides* spp. and *Corynebacterium* spp. tend to predominate in these lesions.

 CLINICAL FEATURES: The ulcer is destructive, disfiguring and usually unilateral (Fig. 9-42). Initially it is a small papule, often on the cheek opposite the molars or premolars. Large malodorous defects quickly develop. The lesions are painful and advanced ulcers

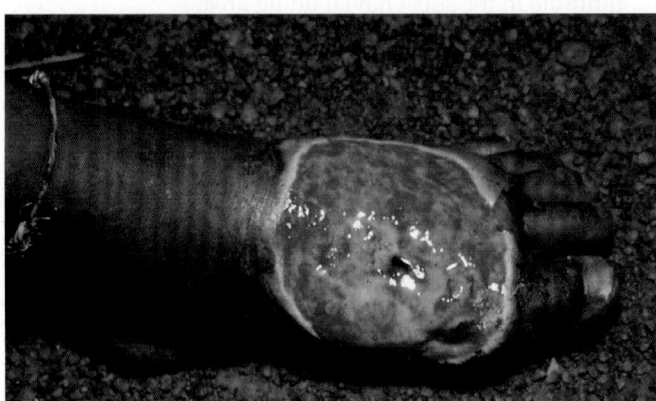

FIGURE 9-41. Tropical phagedenic ulcer caused by infection by fusospirochetal organisms, following penetrating trauma.

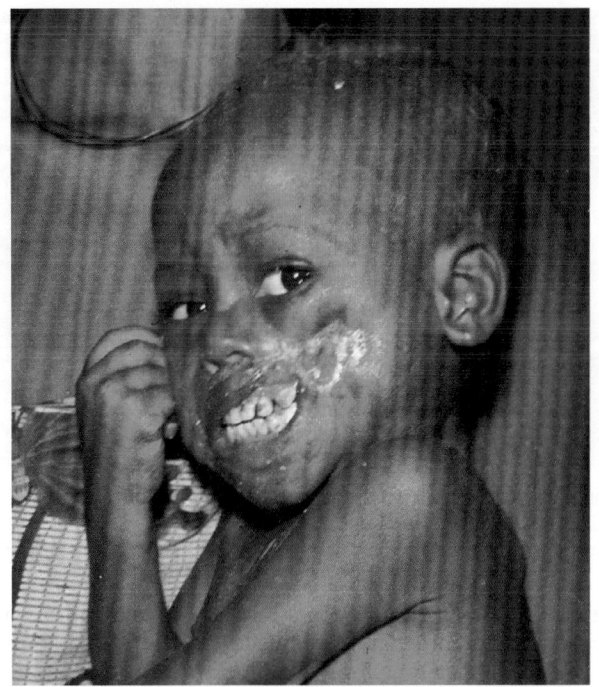

FIGURE 9-42. Noma. There is massive destruction of the soft tissues and bones of the mouth and cheek.

reveal necrosis of skin, muscle and adipose tissue, with exposure of underlying bone. Without treatment, patients usually die. Antibiotics are helpful, but reconstructive surgery is often required.

Chlamydial Infections

Chlamydiae are obligate intracellular parasites that are smaller than most other bacteria. They cannot make adenosine triphosphate (ATP), and so must parasitize the metabolic machinery of a host cell to reproduce. The life cycle involves two morphologic forms. The **elementary body** is the smaller, metabolically inactive form, which survives extracellularly. It attaches to the appropriate host cell and induces endocytosis, forming a vacuole. It then transforms into the larger, metabolically active form, the **reticulate body,** which commandeers host cell metabolism to fuel chlamydial replication. The reticulate body divides repeatedly, forming daughter elementary bodies and destroying the host cell. Necrotic debris elicits inflammatory and immunologic responses that further damage infected tissue.

Chlamydial infections are widespread among birds and mammals, and as many as 20% of humans are infected. Three species of chlamydiae (*Chlamydia trachomatis, Chlamydia psittaci* and *Chlamydia pneumoniae*) cause human infection.

CHLAMYDIA TRACHOMATIS INFECTION

C. trachomatis contains a variety of strains (serovars), which cause three distinct types of disease: (1) genital and neonatal disease, (2) lymphogranuloma venereum and (3) trachoma.

Infections with *Chlamydia trachomatis* Are among the Most Common Sexually Transmitted Diseases

C. trachomatis serovars D through K cause genital epithelial infections that are the most common sexually contracted disease in North America. In men, they produce urethritis and sometimes epididymitis or proctitis. In women, infection usually begins with cervicitis, which can progress to endometritis, salpingitis and generalized infection of the pelvic adnexal organs (pelvic inflammatory disease). Repeated episodes of salpingitis are associated with scarring, which can lead to infertility or ectopic pregnancy. Perinatal transmission of *C. trachomatis* causes neonatal conjunctivitis and pneumonia.

 EPIDEMIOLOGY: The organism spreads in genital secretions. Infection is chronic and frequently asymptomatic, providing an enormous reservoir for transmission. As with all sexually transmitted diseases, people with the largest number of sexual partners are at greatest risk of infection. Newborns acquire the organism by contact with infected endocervical secretions on passage through the birth canal. Two thirds of exposed newborns develop *C. trachomatis* conjunctivitis.

 PATHOLOGY: Chlamydial infection elicits an infiltrate of neutrophils and lymphocytes. Lymphoid aggregates, with or without germinal centers, may appear at the site of infection. In newborns, the conjunctival epithelium often contains characteristic vacuolar cytoplasmic inclusions and the disease is frequently called **inclusion conjunctivitis**.

 CLINICAL FEATURES: Most genital infections are asymptomatic. In men, clinically apparent infection presents as a purulent penile discharge, with dysuria and urinary urgency. Chlamydial cervicitis causes a mucopurulent drainage from the cervical os. Chlamydial disease in the newborn presents as reddened conjunctivae with a watery or purulent discharge. Untreated neonatal conjunctivitis is potentially serious, although it may resolve without sequelae. Chlamydial pneumonia manifests in the second or third month with tachypnea and paroxysmal cough, usually without fever. Inclusion conjunctivitis is treated with systemic or topical antibiotics.

Lymphogranuloma Venereum Is a Sexually Transmitted Disease That Causes Necrotizing Lymphadenitis

Lymphogranuloma venereum (LGV) begins as a genital ulcer, spreads to lymph nodes (Fig. 9-43A) and may cause local scarring. It is caused by *C. trachomatis* serovars L1 to L3.

 EPIDEMIOLOGY: LGV is uncommon in developed countries but is endemic in the tropics and subtropics. It accounts for 5% of sexually transmitted disease in Africa, India, parts of southeast Asia, South America and the Caribbean. Since 2003, LGV has been increasingly reported from developed countries. Large outbreaks, primarily in men who have sex with men, have occurred, especially in New York City and the United Kingdom. In these outbreaks the disease has presented

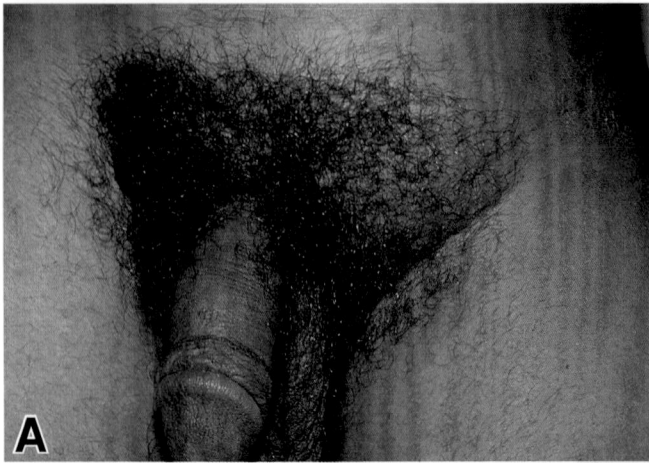
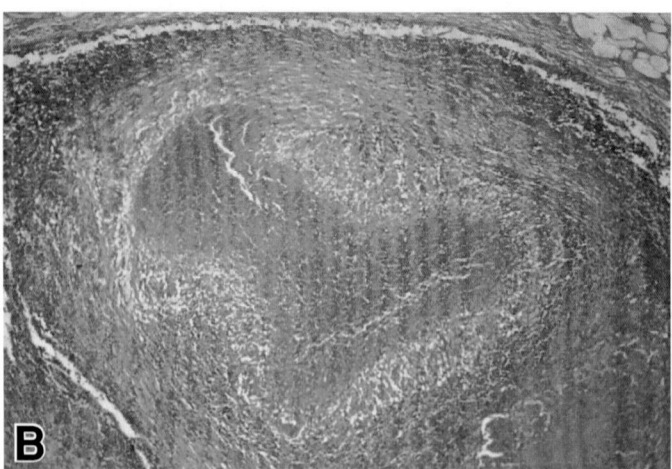

FIGURE 9-43. Lymphogranuloma venereum. A. Painful inguinal lymphadenopathy in a man infected with *Chlamydia trachomatis*. **B.** Microscopic section of a lymph node shows a necrotic central area surrounded by a granulomatous zone.

mostly as proctitis, and the majority of men were HIV coinfected (up to 75%).

 PATHOLOGY: The organism is introduced through a break in the skin. After incubation for 4–21 days, an ulcer appears, usually on the penis, vagina or cervix, although the lips, tongue and fingers may also be primary sites. The organisms are transported by lymphatics to regional lymph nodes, where a **necrotizing lymphadenitis** with abscesses erupts 1–3 weeks after the primary lesion. The nodes become tender and fluctuant and frequently ulcerate and discharge pus. The intense inflammation can cause severe scarring, leading to chronic lymphatic obstruction, ischemic necrosis of overlying structures or strictures and adhesions. Enlarged and matted lymph nodes result, containing multiple, coalescing abscesses, which often develop a stellate shape (Fig. 9-43B). Abscesses have neutrophils and necrotic debris in the center, surrounded by palisading epithelioid cells, macrophages and occasional giant cells. There is a rim of lymphocytes, plasma cells and fibrous tissue.

 CLINICAL FEATURES: Patients with lymphogranuloma venereum present with lymphadenopathy. Most infections resolve completely, even without antimicrobial therapy. However, progressive ulceration of the penis, urethra or scrotum, with fistulas and urethral stricture, develops in 5% of men. Women and men who have sex with men often present with hemorrhagic proctitis, and most late complications, such as rectal stricture, rectovaginal fistulas and genital elephantiasis, occur in women.

Trachoma Is a Leading Cause of Blindness in Many Developing Countries

Trachoma is a chronic infection that causes progressive scars of the conjunctiva and cornea. *C. trachomatis* serovars A, B, Ba and C cause the disease.

 **EPIDEMIOLOGY:** Trachoma is worldwide, associated with poverty and most prevalent in dry or sandy regions. Only humans are naturally infected, and poor personal hygiene and inadequate public sanitation

are common factors. Trachoma remains a major problem in parts of Africa, India and the Middle East. It is spread mostly by direct contact but may also be transmitted by fomites, contaminated water and probably flies. Subclinical infections are an important reservoir. In endemic areas, infection is acquired early in childhood, becomes chronic and eventually progresses to blindness.

 PATHOLOGY: When *C. trachomatis* is inoculated into the eye, it reproduces in the conjunctival epithelium, inciting a mixed acute and chronic inflammatory infiltrate. Histologic examination of early lesions shows chronic inflammation, lymphoid aggregates, focal degeneration and chlamydial inclusions in the conjunctiva. As trachoma progresses, lymphoid aggregates enlarge, and the conjunctiva becomes scarred and focally hypertrophic. The cornea is invaded by blood vessels and fibroblasts, forming a scar reminiscent of a cloth (*pannus* in Latin) and is eventually opacified (see Chapter 33).

 CLINICAL FEATURES: Early trachoma is characterized by the abrupt onset of palpebral and conjunctival inflammation, leading to tearing, purulent conjunctivitis and photophobia. The lymphoid aggregates appear as small yellow grains beneath the palpebral conjunctivae within 3–4 weeks. After months or years, eyelid deformities eventually interfere with normal ocular function, and secondary bacterial infections and corneal ulcers are common. Blindness is a common endpoint.

PSITTACOSIS (ORNITHOSIS)

Psittacosis is a self-limited pneumonia transmitted to humans from birds. The causative agent, *C. psittaci*, is spread by infected birds. The resulting disease is known as both psittacosis (association with parrots) and ornithosis (contact with birds in general).

 **EPIDEMIOLOGY:** *C. psittaci* is present in the blood, tissues, excreta and feathers of infected birds. Humans inhale infectious excreta or dust from feathers. Infection is endemic in tropical birds, but *C. psittaci* can

infect almost any species and can spread to humans from any bird. Use of tetracycline-containing bird feeds and quarantine of imported tropical birds limit the spread of disease, and fewer than 50 cases are reported annually in the United States.

 PATHOLOGY: *C. psittaci* first infects pulmonary macrophages, which carry the organism to the phagocytes of the liver and spleen, where it reproduces. It then spreads via the bloodstream, producing systemic infection, with particularly diffuse involvement of the lungs. *C. psittaci* reproduces in alveolar lining cells, whose destruction elicits an inflammatory response. The pneumonia is predominantly interstitial, with an interstitial lymphocytic inflammatory infiltrate. Dissemination of the infection is characterized by foci of necrosis in the liver and spleen and diffuse mononuclear cell infiltrates in the heart, kidneys and brain.

 CLINICAL FEATURES: The spectrum of clinical illness varies widely. There is usually a persistent dry cough, with constitutional symptoms of high fever, headache, malaise, myalgias and arthralgias. Untreated, fever persists for 2–3 weeks, then subsides as pulmonary disease regresses. With tetracycline therapy, the disease is rarely fatal.

CHLAMYDIA PNEUMONIAE

C. pneumoniae is a cause of acute, self-limited, usually mild respiratory tract infections, including pneumonia. It is transmitted from person to person, and infection appears to be very common. In the developed world, half of all adults show evidence of past exposure, but only 10% of infections cause clinical pneumonia. Symptoms include fever, sore throat and cough. Severe pneumonia occurs only if there is an underlying pulmonary condition. Untreated disease usually resolves in 2–4 weeks.

Rickettsial Infections

The rickettsiae are small, gram-negative coccobacillary bacteria that are obligate intracellular pathogens and cannot replicate outside a host. Unlike chlamydiae, rickettsiae replicate by binary fission. They synthesize their own ATP and can obtain ATP from the host. The organisms induce endocytosis by target cells and replicate in their cytoplasm. Rickettsiae have cell wall structures like gram-negative bacteria, but do not stain well with the Gram stain. They are best demonstrated by the Gimenez method or with acridine orange.

Humans are accidental hosts for most species of *Rickettsia*. The organisms reside in animals and insects and do not require humans for perpetuation. Human infections result from insect bites. Several species of *Rickettsia* cause different human diseases (Table 9-6) that share many common features. ***In humans, the target cells for all rickettsiae are capillary and small vessel endothelial cells.*** The organisms reproduce within these cells, killing them in the process and producing a necrotizing vasculitis. Human rickettsial infections are traditionally divided into the **"spotted fever group"** and the **"typhus group."**

ROCKY MOUNTAIN SPOTTED FEVER

Rocky Mountain spotted fever is an acute, potentially fatal, systemic vasculitis that is usually attended by headache, fever and rash. The causative organism, *Rickettsia rickettsii*, is transmitted to humans by tick bites.

TABLE 9-6

RICKETTSIAL INFECTIONS

Disease	Organism	Distribution	Transmission
Spotted-Fever Group (genus *Rickettsia*)			
Rocky Mountain spotted fever	*R. rickettsii*	Americas	Ticks
Queensland tick fever	*R. australis*	Australia	Ticks
Boutonneuse fever, Kenya tick fever	*R. conorii*	Mediterranean, Africa, India	Ticks
Siberian tick fever	*R. sibirica*	Siberia, Mongolia	Ticks
Rickettsialpox	*R. akari*	United States, Russia, Central Asia, Korea, Africa	Mites
Flea-borne spotted fever	*R. felis*	North and South America, Europe, Australia	Ticks
Typhus Group			
Louse-borne typhus (epidemic typhus)	*R. prowazekii*	Latin America, Africa, Asia	Lice
Murine typhus (endemic typhus)	*R. typhi*	Worldwide	Fleas
Scrub typhus	*Orientia tsutsugamushi*	South Pacific, Asia	Mites
Q fever	*Coxiella brunetti*	Worldwide	Inhalation

 **EPIDEMIOLOGY:** Rocky Mountain spotted fever is acquired by bites of infected ticks, which are the vectors for *R. rickettsii*. The organism is transmitted from mother to progeny ticks, thereby maintaining a natural reservoir for human infection. Rocky Mountain spotted fever occurs in various areas throughout North, Central and South America. About 500 cases occur annually in the eastern United States. Its name derives from its discovery in Idaho, but the disease is uncommon in the Rocky Mountain region.

 PATHOPHYSIOLOGY: *R. rickettsii* in salivary glands of ticks are introduced into the skin as the ticks feed. Organisms spread via lymphatics and small blood vessels to the systemic and pulmonary circulation. They enter vascular endothelial cells, reproduce in the cytoplasm and are then shed into the vascular and lymphatic systems. Further infection and destruction of vascular endothelium causes a systemic vasculitis. The rash, produced by inflammatory damage to cutaneous vessels, is the most visible manifestation of the generalized vascular injury. Other rickettsiae infect only capillary endothelial cells, but *R. rickettsii* spreads to vascular smooth muscle and endothelium of larger vessels. Extensive damage to blood vessel walls causes loss of vascular integrity, fluid exudation and disseminated intravascular coagulation. Fluid loss can be so extensive as to lead to shock. Damage to pulmonary capillaries can produce pulmonary edema and acute alveolar injury.

 PATHOLOGY: The vascular lesions of Rocky Mountain spotted fever are seen throughout the body, affecting capillaries, venules, arterioles and sometimes larger vessels. Necrosis and reactive hyperplasia of vascular endothelium are often associated with thrombosis of small-caliber vessels. Vessel walls are infiltrated, initially with neutrophils and macrophages and later by lymphocytes and plasma cells. Microscopic infarcts and extravasation of blood into surrounding tissues are common. The orientation of the intracellular bacilli in parallel rows and in an end-to-end pattern gives them the appearance of a "flotilla at anchor facing the wind."

 CLINICAL FEATURES: Rocky Mountain spotted fever manifests with fever, headache and myalgias, followed by a rash. Skin lesions begin as a maculopapular eruption but rapidly become petechial, spreading centripetally from the distal extremities to the trunk (Fig. 9-44). Cutaneous lesions usually appear on the palms and soles, a distinctive feature of the disease. If untreated, more than 20%–50% of infected people die within 8–15 days. Prompt diagnosis and antibiotic treatment (chloramphenicol and tetracycline) is life saving; mortality in the United States is less than 5%.

EPIDEMIC (LOUSE-BORNE) TYPHUS

Epidemic typhus is a severe systemic vasculitis transmitted by bites of infected lice. It is caused by *Rickettsia*

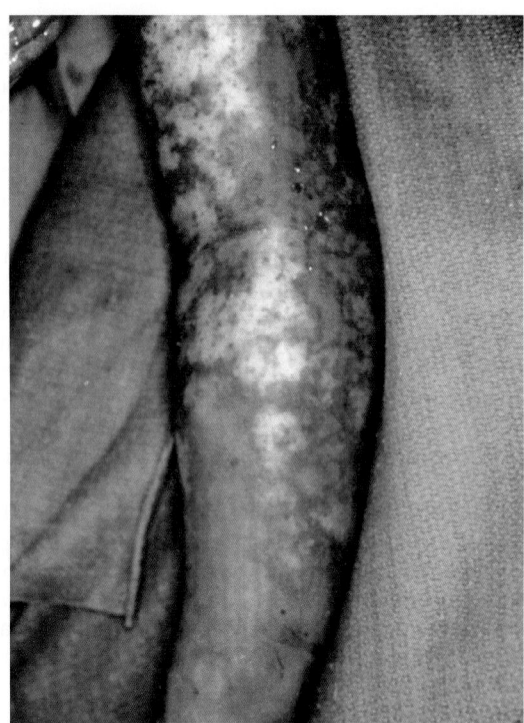

FIGURE 9-44. Rocky mountain spotted fever. A severe petechial and purpuric eruption is noted on the arm in this fatal case.

prowazekii, an organism that has a human–louse–human life cycle (Fig. 9-45).

EPIDEMIOLOGY: The disease is widely distributed in some regions of Africa, Asia, Europe and the Western Hemisphere. Devastating epidemics of typhus were associated with cold climates, poor sanitation and crowding during natural disasters, famine or war. Infrequent bathing and lack of changes of clothing lead to louse infestation of human populations and consequently epidemics of typhus. Mass displacements of populations in Eastern Europe in World War I led to epidemic typhus, which affected 30 million people and killed 3 million. Epidemic louse-borne typhus last occurred in the United States in 1921.

PATHOPHYSIOLOGY: After a louse takes blood from someone infected with *R. prowazekii,* large numbers of rickettsiae contaminate louse feces. These are deposited on the skin or clothing of a second host and may remain infectious for more than 3 months. Human infection begins when contaminated louse feces penetrate an abrasion or scratch, or when the person inhales airborne rickettsiae from clothing containing louse feces. Epidemic typhus begins as a localized infection of capillary endothelium and progresses to a systemic vasculitis. Louse-borne typhus differs from other rickettsial diseases in that *R. prowazekii* can establish latent infection and produce recrudescent disease (Brill-Zinsser disease) many years after primary infection.

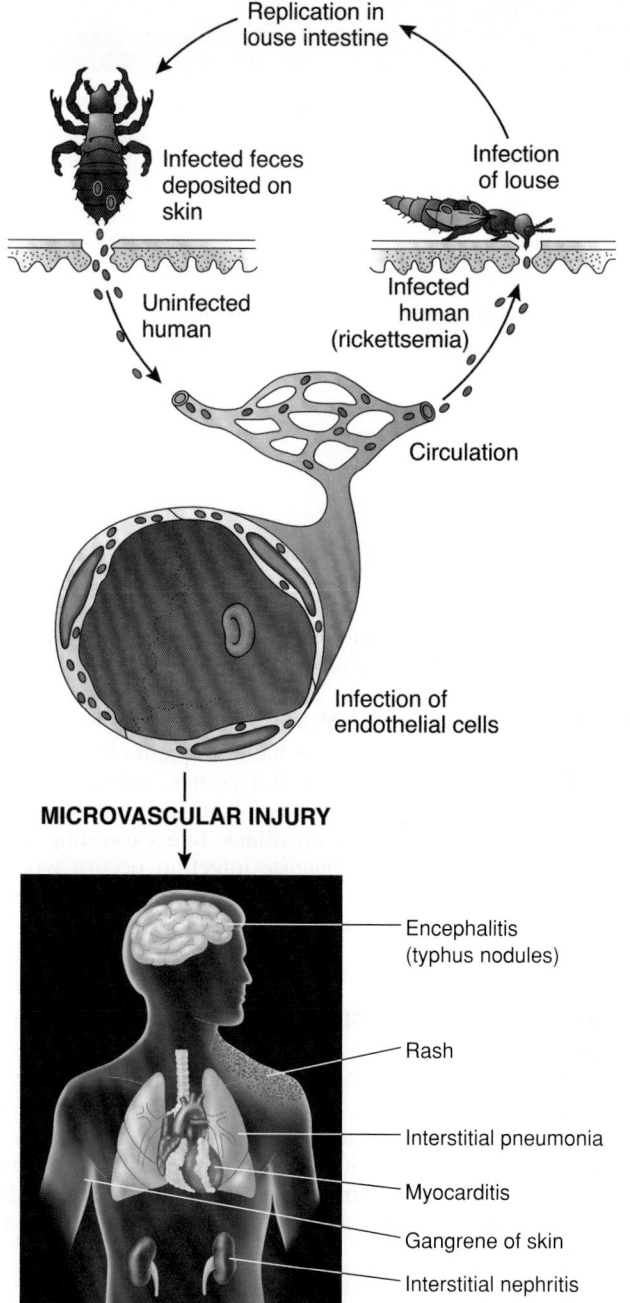

FIGURE 9-45. Epidemic typhus (louse-borne typhus). *Rickettsia prowazekii* has a man–louse–man life cycle. The organism multiplies in endothelial cells, which detach, rupture and release organisms into the circulation (rickettsemia). A louse taking a blood meal becomes infected with rickettsiae, which enter the epithelial cells of its midgut, multiply and rupture the cells, thereby releasing rickettsiae into the lumen of the louse intestine. Contaminated feces are deposited on the skin or clothing of a second host, penetrate an abrasion or are inhaled. The rickettsiae then enter endothelial cells, multiply and rupture the cells, thus completing the cycle.

 PATHOLOGY: The pathologic findings produced by *R. prowazekii* are similar to those in Rocky Mountain spotted fever and other rickettsial diseases. At autopsy, there are few gross findings except for splenomegaly and occasional areas of necrosis. Collections of

mononuclear cells are found in various organs (e.g., skin, brain and heart). The infiltrate includes mast cells, lymphocytes, plasma cells and macrophages, frequently arranged as **typhus nodules** around arterioles and capillaries. Throughout the body, the endothelium of small blood vessels is focally necrotic and hyperplastic, and the walls contain inflammatory cells. Rickettsiae can be demonstrated within the endothelial cells.

CLINICAL FEATURES: Symptoms of louse-borne typhus are fever, headache and myalgias, followed by a rash. Macular lesions, which become petechial, appear on the upper trunk and axillary folds and spread centrifugally to the extremities. In fatal cases, the rash commonly becomes confluent and purpuric. Mild rickettsial pneumonia may precede a bacterial pneumonia. Dying patients may exhibit the symptoms of encephalitis, myocarditis, interstitial pneumonia, interstitial nephritis and shock. Fatalities usually occur during the second or third week of illness. In patients who recover, the symptoms abate after about 3 weeks.

Epidemic typhus can be controlled by large-scale delousing of the population, steam sterilization of clothing and use of insecticides. Prompt treatment with azithromycin or other broad-spectrum antibiotics is curative.

ENDEMIC (MURINE) TYPHUS

Endemic typhus is similar to epidemic typhus but tends to be milder. Humans are infected with *Rickettsia typhi,* interrupting the rat–flea–rat cycle of transmission. Contaminated flea feces on the skin may enter the body via the small wound made by the bite. *R. typhi* may also contaminate clothes and become airborne. If inhaled, they cause pulmonary infection. Outbreaks of murine typhus are associated with an exploding population of rats, although sporadic infections occur in the southwestern United States. These are associated with rat-infested dwellings and with occupations that bring humans into contact with rats, such as the handling and storage of grain.

SCRUB TYPHUS

Scrub typhus **(Tsutsugamushi fever)** is an acute, febrile illness of humans caused by *Orientia tsutsugamushi,* the only member of its genus. It was previously designated *Rickettsia tsutsugamushi.* Rodents are the natural mammalian reservoir, from which the organism is passed to trombiculid mites known as chiggers. These insects transmit infection to their larvae, which crawl to the tips of vegetation and attach to passersby. While feeding, mites inoculate the organisms into the skin. Rickettsemia and lymphadenopathy follow shortly. Scrub typhus is widely distributed in eastern and southern Asia and the islands of the southern and western Pacific, including Japan. Endemic infection is unknown in the Western world.

A multiloculated vesicle forms at the inoculation site and ulcerates, followed by an eschar. As the lesion heals, headache and fever appear suddenly, followed by pneumonia, a macular rash, lymphadenopathy and hepatosplenomegaly. Severe infections are complicated by myocarditis, meningoencephalitis and shock. Mortality rates in untreated patients have ranged up to 30%.

Q FEVER

Q fever is a self-limited, systemic infection, usually manifesting as headache, fever and myalgias. The disease is caused by *Coxiella burnetii,* a small pleomorphic coccobacillus with a gram-negative cell wall. Unlike true rickettsiae, *C. burnetii* enters cells passively upon phagocytosis by macrophages. It does not produce a vasculitis, so there is no associated rash.

 **EPIDEMIOLOGY:** Humans acquire Q fever by exposure to infected animals or animal products. Infection is endemic in many wild and domesticated animals, but cattle, sheep and goats are the usual sources of human infection. These animals shed large numbers of organisms in urine, feces, milk, bodily fluids and birth products. Q fever is most often seen in herders, slaughterhouse workers, veterinarians, dairy workers and others with occupational exposure to infected domesticated animals. Aerosol droplets may spread infection from person to person. Q fever is rare in the United States.

 PATHOLOGY: Q fever begins with inhalation of organisms, which are phagocytosed by alveolar macrophages and replicate in phagolysosomes. Recruitment of neutrophils and macrophages produces a focal bronchopneumonia. The nonactivated phagocytes fail to kill *C. burnetii,* and the organism disseminates through the body, primarily infecting monocytes/macrophages. Most infections resolve with the onset of specific cell-mediated immunity, but occasional cases persist as chronic infections.

The lungs and liver are most prominently involved in Q fever. The lungs show single or multiple irregular areas of consolidation, in which the pulmonary parenchyma is infiltrated by neutrophils and macrophages. Organisms may be demonstrated in macrophages by the Giemsa stain. In the liver, Q fever is usually characterized by multiple microscopic granulomas with a distinctive "fibrin ring." In these granulomas epithelioid macrophages encircle a ring of fibrin, sometimes containing a lipid vacuole.

 CLINICAL FEATURES: Q fever is usually a self-limited mildly symptomatic febrile disease. More-severe cases may present with headache, fever, fatigue and myalgias, with no rash. Pulmonary infection is virtually always present, but it may appear as an atypical pneumonia with dry cough, a rapidly progressive pneumonia or chest roentgenographic abnormalities without significant respiratory symptoms. Many patients have some hepatosplenomegaly. Q fever usually resolves spontaneously in 2–14 days.

Mycoplasmal Infections

At less than 0.3 µm in greatest dimension, mycoplasmas are the smallest free-living **prokaryotes**. They lack the rigid cell walls of more complex bacteria. Mycoplasmas are widespread, geographically and ecologically, as saprophytes and as parasites of many animals and plants. Many *Mycoplasma* species inhabit the human body, but only three are pathogenic: *Mycoplasma pneumoniae, Mycoplasma hominis* and

TABLE 9-7
MYCOPLASMAL INFECTIONS

Organism	Disease
Mycoplasma pneumoniae	Tracheobronchitis
	Pneumonia
	Pharyngitis
	Otitis media
Ureaplasma urealyticum	Urethritis
	Chorioamnionitis
	Postpartum fever
Mycoplasma hominis	Postpartum fever

Ureaplasma urealyticum. The diseases associated with these organisms are shown in Table 9-7.

M. pneumoniae *produces acute, self-limited lower respiratory tract infections, affecting mostly children and young adults.* It can also cause pharyngitis and otitis media.

 **EPIDEMIOLOGY:** Most infections occur in small groups of people who have frequent close contact (e.g., families, college fraternities, military units). The organism is spread by aerosol from person to person over several months, with an attack rate exceeding 50% within the group. *M. pneumoniae* infection occurs worldwide, and in developed countries, the organism causes 15%–20% of all pneumonias.

 **PATHOPHYSIOLOGY:** *M. pneumoniae* initiates infection by attaching to a glycolipid on the surface of the respiratory epithelium. The agent remains outside the cells, where it reproduces and causes progressive dysfunction and eventual death of host cells. Because *M. pneumoniae* infection rarely produces symptomatic disease in children younger than the age of 5 years, it is thought that the host immune response plays a role in tissue injury.

 PATHOLOGY: Pneumonia caused by *M. pneumoniae* usually shows patchy consolidation of a single segment of a lower lung lobe, although the process can be more widespread. The mucosa of affected airways is edematous and infiltrated by a mostly mononuclear inflammatory infiltrate. Alveoli show a largely interstitial process, with reactive alveolar lining cells and mononuclear infiltration. Pulmonary changes are often complicated by bacterial superinfection. The organism itself is too small to be seen by routine light microscopy.

 CLINICAL FEATURES: *Mycoplasma* pneumonia tends to be milder than other bacterial pneumonias and is sometimes called "walking pneumonia." Fever rarely lasts more than 2 weeks, although cough may linger for 6 weeks or more. Death from *M. pneumoniae*

infection is rare. However, life-threatening cases of Stevens-Johnson syndrome have been linked to mycoplasma infection.

Mycobacterial Infections

Mycobacteria are distinctive organisms, 2–10 μm in length, with cell wall architecture like that of gram-positive bacteria, but also containing large amounts of lipid. The high lipid content interferes with staining by aniline dyes, including crystal violet used in the Gram stain. Thus, although mycobacteria are structurally gram-positive, this property is difficult to demonstrate by routine staining. *The waxy lipids of the cell wall make the mycobacteria "acid fast" (i.e., they retain carbolfuchsin after rinsing with acid alcohol).*

Mycobacteria grow more slowly than other pathogenic bacteria, and their diseases are chronic, slowly progressive illnesses. They produce no known toxins but damage human tissues by inducing inflammatory and immune responses. Most mycobacterial pathogens replicate within cells of the monocyte/macrophage lineage and elicit granulomatous inflammation. The outcome of mycobacterial infection is largely determined by the host's capacity to contain the organism through cell-mediated immune responses.

The two main mycobacterial pathogens, *Mycobacterium tuberculosis* and *Mycobacterium leprae*, only infect humans and have no environmental reservoir. Other pathogenic mycobacteria are environmental organisms that only occasionally cause human disease.

TUBERCULOSIS

Tuberculosis is a chronic, communicable disease in which the lungs are the prime target, although any organ may be infected. Disease is mainly caused by M. tuberculosis hominis *(Koch bacillus) but also occasionally by* M. tuberculosis bovis. *The characteristic lesion is a spherical granuloma with central caseous necrosis.*

M. tuberculosis is a slender, beaded, nonmotile, acid-fast bacillus, which is an obligate aerobe (Fig. 9-46). It grows

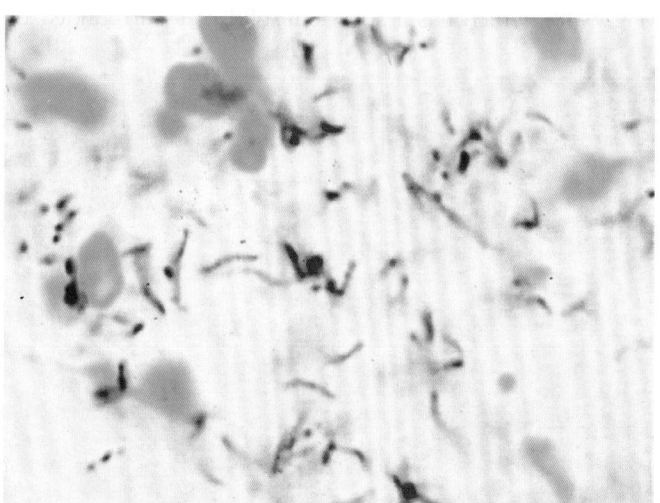

FIGURE 9-46. *Mycobacterium tuberculosis.* A smear of a pulmonary lesion shows slender, beaded, acid-fast bacilli.

slowly in culture, with a doubling time of 24 hours, and 3–6 weeks are commonly required to produce visible growth in culture.

 **EPIDEMIOLOGY:** Tuberculosis is one of the most important human bacterial diseases worldwide. Rates of infection are now low in developed countries. HIV-infected, homeless and malnourished people are highly susceptible, as are immigrants from areas where the disease is endemic. In the United States, the annual incidence is 12 per 100,000 and mortality is 1–2 per 100,000. In some developing countries, the incidence reaches 450 per 100,000, with a high fatality rate. There are also racial and ethnic differences—Africans, Native Americans and Eskimos are more susceptible than are white people. In the United States, tuberculosis is most common among the elderly, possibly reflecting reactivation of infections acquired early in life before the decline in the prevalence of the disease.

M. tuberculosis is transmitted from person to person by aerosol. Coughing, sneezing and talking all create aerosolized respiratory droplets. Droplets usually evaporate, leaving an organism (droplet nucleus) that is readily carried in the air. Tuberculosis can also be caused by the closely related *M. tuberculosis bovis,* which is acquired by drinking nonpasteurized milk from infected cows.

 **CLINICAL FEATURES:** The course of tuberculosis depends on age and immune competence, as well as total burden of organisms. Some patients have only an indolent, asymptomatic infection, while in others, tuberculosis is a destructive, disseminated disease. Many more people are infected with *M. tuberculosis* than develop clinical symptoms. Thus, one must distinguish between infection and active tuberculosis. **Tuberculous infection** means that the organism is growing in a person, whether or not there is symptomatic disease. **Active tuberculosis** denotes the subset of tuberculous infections manifested by destructive, symptomatic disease.

Primary tuberculosis occurs on first exposure to the organism and can pursue either an indolent or aggressive course (Fig. 9-47). **Secondary tuberculosis** develops long after a primary infection, mostly due to reactivation of a primary infection. Secondary tuberculosis can also be produced by exposure to exogenous organisms and is always an active disease.

Primary Tuberculosis Occurs upon First Exposure to the Tubercle Bacillus

 PATHOPHYSIOLOGY: Inhaled *M. tuberculosis* is deposited in alveoli, usually in the lower segments of lower and middle lobes and anterior segments of upper lobes. The organisms are phagocytosed by alveolar macrophages but resist killing; cell wall lipids of *M. tuberculosis* block fusion of phagosomes and lysosomes and allow the bacilli to proliferate within macrophages. As bacilli multiply, the macrophages degrade some organisms and present antigens to T lymphocytes. Some macrophages carry bacilli from the lung to regional (hilar and mediastinal) lymph nodes, from which they may disseminate by the bloodstream. Tubercle bacilli

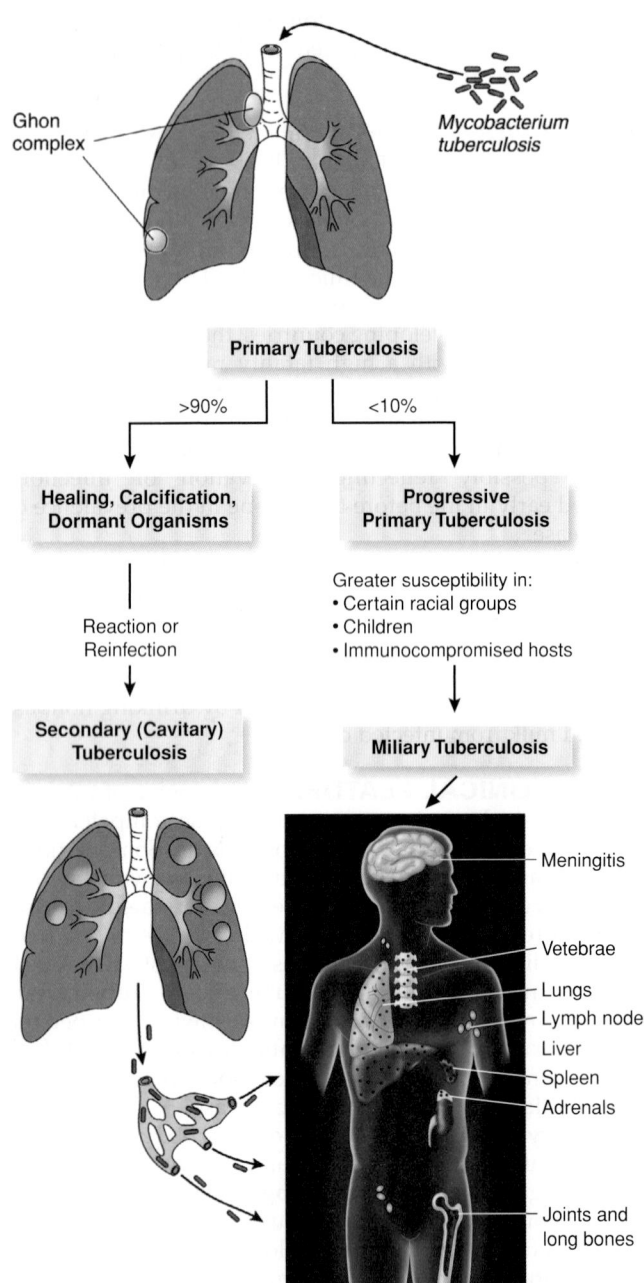

FIGURE 9-47. Stages of tuberculosis. Primary tuberculosis develops in a person lacking previous contact or immune responsiveness. **Progressive primary** tuberculosis develops in less than 10% of infected normal adults, but more frequently in children and immunosuppressed patients. **Secondary** (cavitary) tuberculosis results from reactivation of dormant endogenous bacilli or reinfection with exogenous bacilli. **Miliary** tuberculosis is caused by dissemination of tubercle bacilli to produce numerous, minute, yellow-white lesions (resembling millet seeds) in distant organs.

continue to proliferate at the primary site in the lungs and elsewhere, including lymph nodes, kidneys, meninges, epiphyseal plates of long bones and vertebrae and apical areas of the lungs.

Although the macrophages that first ingest *M. tuberculosis* cannot kill it, hypersensitivity and cell-mediated immunologic responses eventually contain the infection.

Infected macrophages present mycobacterial antigens to T cells. Clones of sensitized T cells proliferate, produce interferon-γ and activate macrophages, thereby increasing their concentrations of lytic enzymes and augmenting their capacity to kill mycobacteria. The lytic enzymes of these activated macrophages may, if released, also damage host tissues.

Development of activated lymphocytes responsive to *M. tuberculosis* antigen is the hypersensitivity response to the organism. The emergence of activated macrophages that can ingest and destroy the bacilli accounts for the cell-mediated immune response. These responses together combat the organisms, a process that requires 3–6 weeks to come into play.

If an infected person is immunologically competent and the burden of organisms is small, a vigorous granulomatous reaction is produced. Tubercle bacilli are ingested and killed by activated macrophages, surrounded by fibrous tissue and successfully contained. When the number of organisms is high, the hypersensitivity reaction produces significant tissue necrosis, which has a characteristic cheese-like (caseous) consistency. Although not invariably caused by *M. tuberculosis,* caseous necrosis is so strongly associated with tuberculosis that its discovery in tissue inevitably raises suspicion of this disease.

In immunologically immature or compromised subjects (young children or immunosuppressed patients), granulomas are poorly formed or not formed at all, and infection may progress at the primary site in the lung, in the regional lymph nodes or in multiple sites of dissemination. This process produces **progressive primary tuberculosis**.

PATHOLOGY: The lung lesion of primary tuberculosis is known as a **Ghon focus**. It is found in the subpleural area of the upper segments of the lower lobes or in the lower segments of the upper lobes. Initially, it is a small, ill-defined area of inflammatory consolidation, which then drains to hilar lymph nodes. The combination of a peripheral Ghon focus and involved mediastinal or hilar lymph nodes is called the **Ghon complex**.

The classic lesion of tuberculosis is a caseous granuloma (Fig. 9-48), which has a soft, semisolid core surrounded by

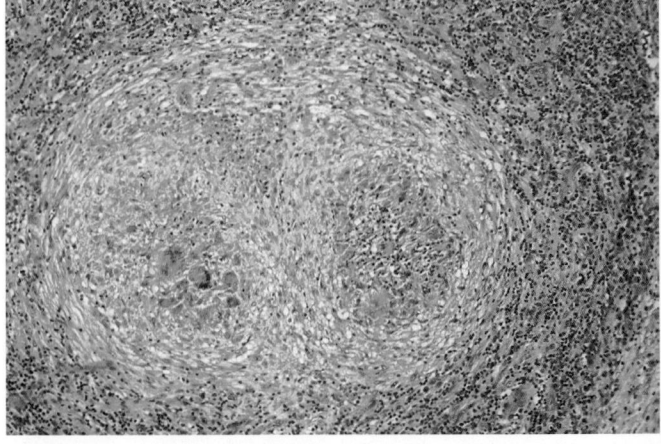

FIGURE 9-48. Primary tuberculosis. Photomicrograph of a hilar lymph node shows a tuberculous granuloma with central caseation.

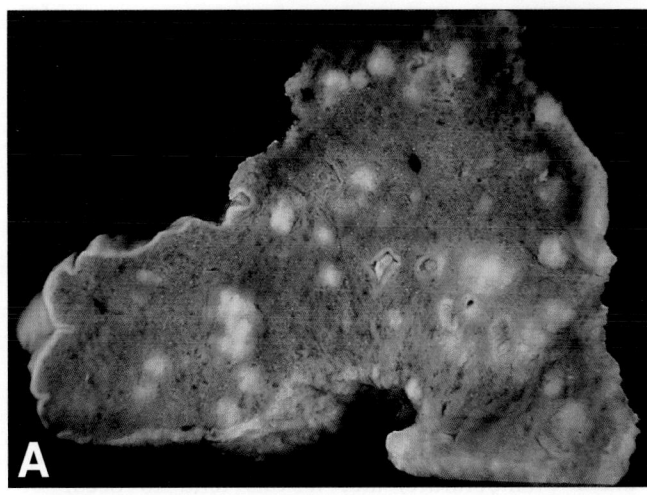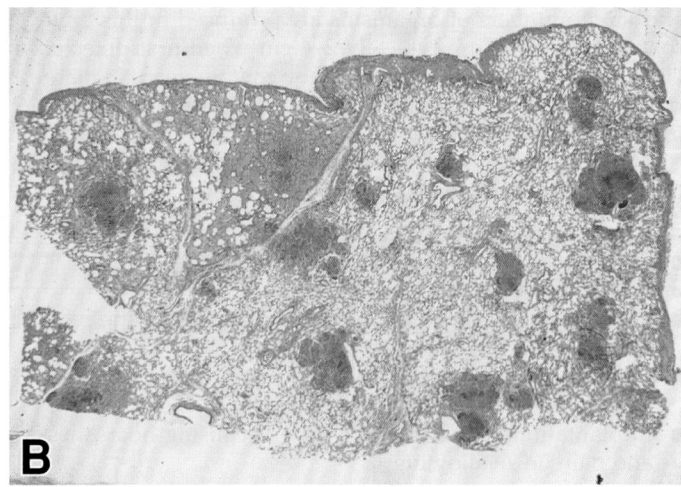

FIGURE 9-49. Miliary tuberculosis. A. The cut surface of the lung reveals numerous uniform, white nodules. **B.** A low-power photomicrograph discloses many foci of granulomatous inflammation.

epithelioid macrophages, Langhans giant cells, lymphocytes and peripheral fibrous tissue. If the host is immunocompromised, the granulomas elicited by *M. tuberculosis* may be less organized and consist of only aggregates of macrophages, without the architecture or Langhans giant cells of the classic granuloma.

In over 90% of normal adults, tuberculous infection is self-limited. In both lungs and lymph nodes, the Ghon complex heals, undergoing shrinkage, fibrous scarring and calcification, the latter visible radiographically. Small numbers of organisms may remain viable for years. Later, if immune mechanisms wane or fail, resting bacilli may proliferate and break out, causing serious secondary tuberculosis.

In **progressive primary tuberculosis,** the host immune response fails to control the tubercle bacilli. This happens in less than 10% of normal adults, but it is common in children younger than 5 years and in patients with suppressed or defective immunity. The Ghon focus enlarges and may even erode into the bronchial tree. Affected hilar and mediastinal lymph nodes also enlarge, sometimes compressing the bronchi to produce atelectasis of the distal lung; collapse of the middle lobe **(middle lobe syndrome)** is a common result of this compression. In some instances, the infected lymph nodes erode into an airway to spread organisms throughout the lungs.

Miliary tuberculosis occurs when infection disseminates to produce multiple, small, yellow, nodular lesions in several organs (Fig. 9-49). The term "miliary" refers to the resemblance of these lesions to millet seeds. The lungs, lymph nodes, kidneys, adrenals, bone marrow, spleen and liver are common sites of miliary lesions. Progressive disease may involve the meninges and cause tuberculous meningitis.

CLINICAL FEATURES: Most people contain primary infection successfully, and primary tuberculosis is generally asymptomatic. In those who develop progressive primary disease, symptoms are usually insidious and nonspecific, with fever, weight loss, fatigue and night sweats. Sometimes the onset of symptoms is abrupt, with high fever, pleurisy, pleural effusion and lymphadenitis. Cough and hemoptysis develop only when active pulmonary disease is well established. In miliary tuberculosis, symptoms vary according to the organs affected and tend to occur late in the course of disease.

Secondary (Cavitary) Tuberculosis Follows a Previously Contained Infection

The mycobacteria in secondary tuberculosis may be either dormant organisms from old granulomas (which is usually the case) or newly acquired bacilli. Various conditions, including cancer, antineoplastic chemotherapy, immunosuppressive therapy, AIDS and old age, predispose to reemergence of dormant *M. tuberculosis*. Secondary tuberculosis may develop even decades after primary infection.

 PATHOLOGY: Any location may be involved, but the lungs are by far the most common site for secondary tuberculosis. In the lungs, secondary tuberculosis usually begins in apical–posterior segments of the upper lobes, where organisms are commonly seeded during primary infection. There, the bacilli proliferate and elicit an inflammatory response, causing localized consolidation. *Ensuing T-cell–mediated immune responses to the now familiar tuberculous antigens lead to tissue necrosis and production of tuberculous cavities* (Fig. 9-50). Apical cavities are optimal sites for multiplication of *M. tuberculosis,*

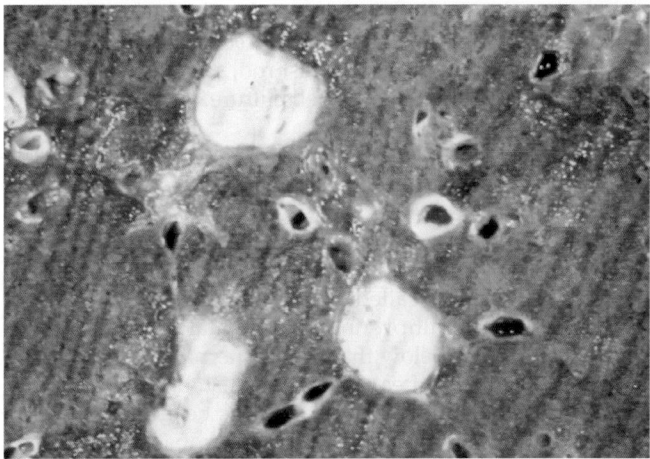

FIGURE 9-50. Secondary pulmonary tuberculosis. A cross-section of lung shows several tuberculous cavities filled with necrotic, caseous material.

and large numbers of organisms are produced in this environment. Cavities are typically 2–4 cm when first detected clinically but can exceed 10 cm. They contain necrotic material teeming with mycobacteria and are surrounded by a granulomatous response.

Lung lesions in secondary tuberculosis may be complicated by secondary effects:

- Scarring and calcification
- Spread to other areas
- Pleural fibrosis and adhesions
- Rupture of a caseous lesion, spilling bacilli into the pleural cavity
- Erosion into a bronchus, which seeds bronchioles, bronchi and trachea
- Implantation of bacilli in the larynx, causing hoarseness and pain on swallowing

Tubercle bacilli may also spread throughout the body through the lymphatics and bloodstream to cause miliary tuberculosis.

CLINICAL FEATURES: Cough (which may be mistakenly attributed to smoking or a cold), low-grade fever, general malaise, fatigue, anorexia, weight loss and often night sweats are the usual manifestations. Cavitation may be accompanied by hemoptysis, on occasion severe enough to cause exsanguination. Chest radiographs that show unilateral or bilateral apical cavities suggest the diagnosis of secondary tuberculosis. If disease is disseminated, the signs and symptoms reflect the particular organs involved.

Untreated secondary tuberculosis is a wasting disease that is eventually fatal, and at one time chronic cavitary tuberculosis was a common cause of secondary amyloidosis. Tuberculosis is now treated with prolonged courses of antituberculous antibiotics, including isoniazid, pyrazinamide, rifampin and ethambutol. Strains of *M. tuberculosis* resistant to these antibiotics have recently emerged, often as a consequence of poor compliance with the full regimen of antibiotic therapy.

LEPROSY

Leprosy (Hansen disease) is a chronic, slowly progressive, destructive process involving peripheral nerves, skin and mucous membranes, caused by *Mycobacterium leprae*. This agent is a slender, weakly acid-fast rod, which cannot be cultured on artificial media or in cell culture.

EPIDEMIOLOGY: Leprosy is one of the oldest recognized human diseases. Lepers were isolated from the community in the Old Testament. For centuries, leprosy was widespread in Europe, including England. In 1873, Hansen first documented the causative agent (leprosy is also called "Hansen disease").

Lepra bacilli multiply in experimental animals at sites with temperatures below that of the internal organs, such as foot pads of mice and ear lobes of hamsters, rats and other rodents. Naturally acquired leprosy has been recognized in armadillos in Louisiana and Texas. Lepra bacilli have been experimentally transmitted to armadillos, whose susceptibility is related, at least in part, to their low body temperature (32°C–35°C [89.6°F–95°F]).

Leprosy is transmitted from person to person, after years of intimate contact. *M. leprae* is present in nasal secretions or ulcerated lesions of infected persons. The mode of infection is unclear, but probably involves inoculation of bacilli into the respiratory tract or open wounds. Leprosy is now rare in developed countries, but worldwide 15 million people are infected, mainly in tropical areas such as India, Papua New Guinea, Southeast Asia and tropical Africa. Fewer than 400 cases are diagnosed yearly in the United States, mostly in immigrants from endemic areas. In total, there are approximately 6500 people with leprosy in the United States, of whom 3300 require active management.

PATHOPHYSIOLOGY: *M. leprae* multiplies best at temperatures below core human body temperature, and lesions tend to occur in cooler parts of the body (e.g., hands and face). Leprosy exhibits a bewildering variety of clinical and pathologic features. Lesions vary from the small, insignificant and self-healing macules of tuberculoid leprosy to the diffuse, disfiguring and sometimes fatal ones of lepromatous leprosy (Fig. 9-51). This extreme variation in disease presentation probably reflects differences in immune reactivity.

Most (95%) persons have a natural protective immunity to *M. leprae* and are not infected, despite intimate and prolonged exposure. Susceptible individuals (5%) span a broad spectrum of immune function, from anergy to hyperergy, and may develop symptomatic infection. At one end of the spectrum, anergic patients have little or no resistance and develop **lepromatous leprosy,** whereas hyperergic patients with high resistance manifest **tuberculoid leprosy**. Most patients, in between these extremes, have **borderline leprosy**.

TUBERCULOID LEPROSY: This condition is characterized by a single lesion or very few lesions of the skin, usually on the face, extremities or trunk. Microscopically, lesions show well-formed, circumscribed dermal granulomas, with epithelioid macrophages, Langhans giant cells and lymphocytes. Nerve fibers are almost invariably swollen and infiltrated with lymphocytes. Destruction of small dermal nerve twigs accounts for the sensory deficit associated with tuberculoid leprosy. Bacilli are rare and often not found with acid-fast stains. The term "tuberculoid leprosy" is used because the granulomas vaguely resemble those of tuberculosis. However, leprous granulomas lack caseation. The lesions of tuberculoid leprosy cause minimal disfigurement and are not infectious.

LEPROMATOUS LEPROSY: This form exhibits multiple, tumor-like lesions of the skin, eyes, testes, nerves, lymph nodes and spleen. Nodular or diffuse infiltrates of foamy macrophages contain myriad bacilli (Fig. 9-52). The epidermis is stretched thinly over the nodules, and beneath it is a narrow, uninvolved "clear zone" of the dermis. Rather than destroying the bacilli, macrophages seem to act as microincubators. When subjected to acid-fast stains, the numerous organisms within the foamy macrophages appear as aggregates of acid-fast material, called "globi." The dermal infiltrates expand slowly to distort and disfigure the face, ears and upper airway and to destroy the eyes, eyebrows and eyelashes, nerves

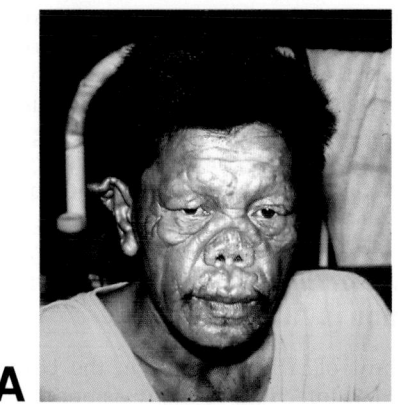

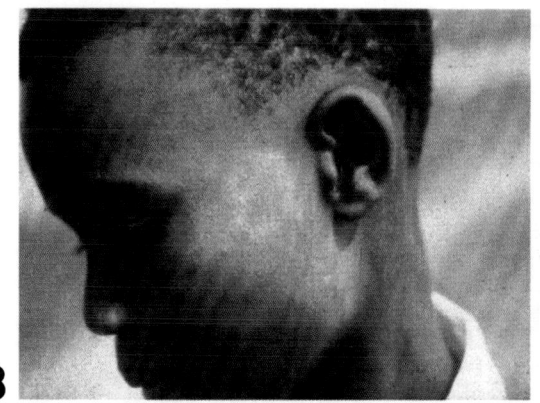

A

B

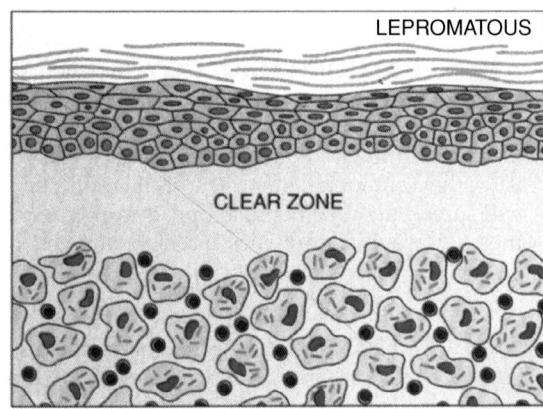

LEPROMATOUS

CLEAR ZONE

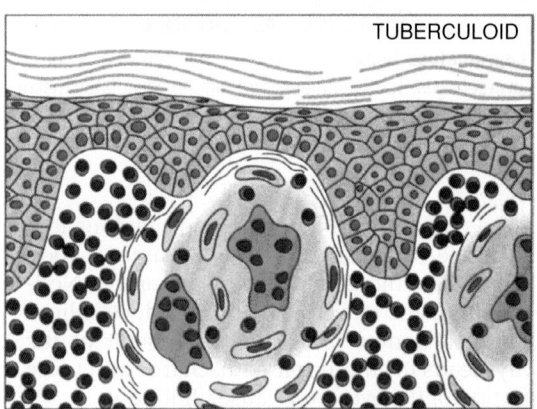

TUBERCULOID

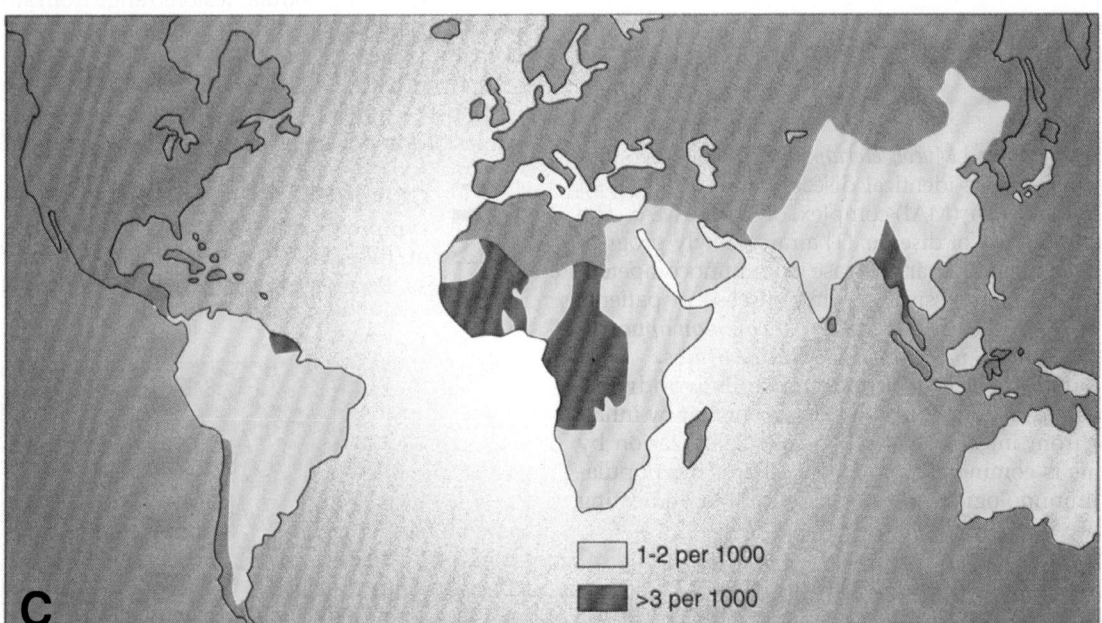

1-2 per 1000

>3 per 1000

C

FIGURE 9-51. A. (*Top*) **Leonine facies of lepromatous leprosy.** There is diffuse involvement, including a loss of eyebrows and eyelashes and nodular distortions of the face and ears, the exposed (cool) parts of the body. The septum and bone of the nose are damaged, producing "saddle nose" deformity. This Filipino patient also had deformities of the hands and feet. (*Bottom*) The nodular skin lesions of advanced lepromatous leprosy. Swelling has flattened the epidermis (loss of rete ridges). A characteristic "clear zone" of uninvolved dermis separates the epidermis from tumor-like accumulations of macrophages, each containing numerous lepra bacilli *(Mycobacterium leprae)*. **B.** (*Top*) **Tuberculoid leprosy** on the cheek, showing a hypopigmented macule with a raised, infiltrated border. The central portion may be hypesthetic or anesthetic. (*Bottom*) Macular skin lesion of tuberculoid leprosy. Skin from the raised "infiltrated" margin of the plaque contains discrete granulomas that extend to the basal layer of the epidermis (without a clear zone). The granulomas are composed of epithelioid cells and Langhans giant cells and are associated with lymphocytes and plasma cells. Lepra bacilli are rare. **C. Distribution of leprosy.** Prevalence is greatest in tropical regions of Africa, Asia and Latin America.

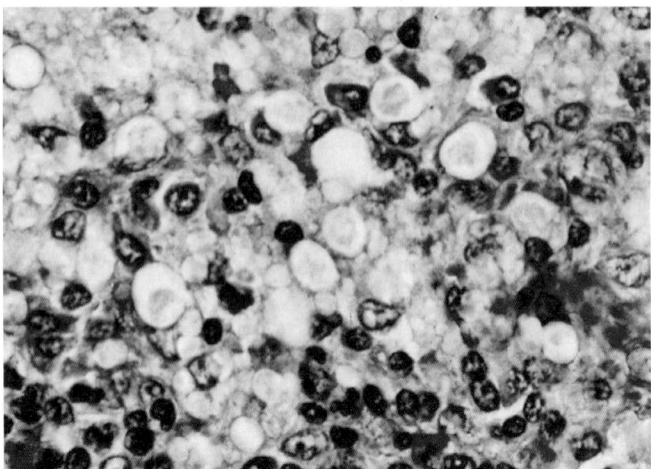

FIGURE 9-52. Lepromatous leprosy. A section of skin shows a tumor-like mass of foamy macrophages. The faint masses within the vacuolated macrophages are enormous numbers of lepra bacilli.

and testes. The nodular skin lesions of lepromatous leprosy may ulcerate. Claw-shaped hands, hammer toes, saddle nose and pendulous ear lobes are common. Nodular lesions of the face may coalesce to produce a lion-like appearance ("leonine facies"). Involvement of the upper airways leads to chronic nasal discharge and voice change. Infection of the eyes may cause blindness.

MYCOBACTERIUM AVIUM-INTRACELLULARE COMPLEX

Mycobacterium avium and *Mycobacterium intracellulare* are similar species, which cause identical diseases and are grouped as *M. avium-intracellulare* (MAI) complex, or simply MAI. The agents cause two types of disease: (1) a rare, slowly progressive granulomatous pulmonary disease in immunocompetent persons, and (2) a progressive systemic disease in patients with AIDS. *MAI infection is the third most common opportunistic infection in AIDS patients in the United States.*

MAI is found in soil, water and foodstuffs worldwide. Humans probably acquire it from the environment by inhaling aerosols from infected water sources. Colonization by the organisms is common. As much as 70% of the population shows immunologic responsiveness to MAI, indicating prior exposure.

Granulomatous MAI Disease Affects Some Immunocompetent Persons

Most immunocompetent persons with granulomatous pulmonary disease caused by MAI are older (50–70 years), and many suffer from preexisting pulmonary disease. *Clinically and pathologically, MAI disease resembles tuberculosis but progresses much more slowly. It causes pulmonary nodules and cavities and caseating granulomas.*

 CLINICAL FEATURES: The most common antecedent illnesses predisposing to pulmonary MAI infection in people with a normal immune system are chronic obstructive pulmonary disease, treated tuberculosis, pneumoconioses and bronchiectasis. Cough is a common symptom, but most symptoms that characterize tuberculosis are lacking. MAI lung disease is indolent or only slowly progressive, causing lung function to decline gradually over years or decades. The organism is resistant to first-line antituberculous drugs, and combination therapies often yield disappointing results.

M. Avium-Intracellulare Causes Disseminated Infection in AIDS

One third of AIDS patients in the United States develop overt MAI infection; as many as one half have evidence of infection at autopsy.

 **PATHOPHYSIOLOGY:** In patients with AIDS, progressive depletion of helper T cells cripples immune responses that normally prevent MAI disease. Although macrophages phagocytose the organisms, they cannot kill them. The bacilli replicate, fill the cells and spread first to other macrophages and then throughout the body via the lymphatics and bloodstream.

 PATHOLOGY: Infected macrophages are found in many organs, and proliferation of the organisms leads to recruitment of additional macrophages. As a result, expanding nodular lesions range from structured epithelioid granulomas with few organisms to loose aggregates of foamy macrophages packed with acid-fast bacilli (Fig. 9-53). Eventually, lymph nodes, spleen and bone marrow may be almost completely replaced by aggregates of macrophages, and lesions in the bowel erode into the lumen of the gut.

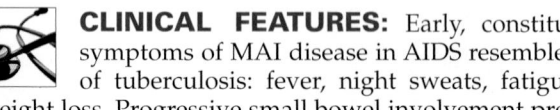 **CLINICAL FEATURES:** Early, constitutional symptoms of MAI disease in AIDS resemble those of tuberculosis: fever, night sweats, fatigue and weight loss. Progressive small bowel involvement produces

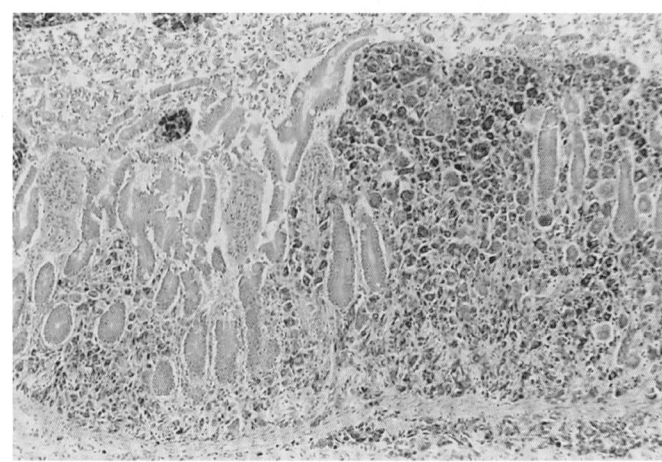

FIGURE 9-53. *Mycobacterium avium-intracellulare* (MAI). A section of small bowel from a patient with acquired immunodeficiency syndrome (AIDS) reveals the presence of numerous macrophages stuffed with acid-fast bacilli in the lamina propria.

malabsorption and diarrhea, often with abdominal pain. Pulmonary involvement is common but does not usually produce symptoms. Combinations of five or more different antibiotics, including clarithromycin, may control, but rarely cure, widespread MAI infection in AIDS patients.

ATYPICAL MYCOBACTERIA

Several other species of environmental mycobacteria occasionally produce human disease. These organisms are also present in surface waters, dust and dirt, and people acquire infection by inhalation, inoculation or ingestion of environmental material.

These bacteria, including MAI, are often lumped together as the "atypical mycobacteria" (in contrast to *M. tuberculosis*, regarded as the "typical" mycobacterium). The atypical mycobacteria are biologically diverse and the uncommon diseases that they produce in humans differ in circumstances of acquisition, pathology, clinical presentations and therapies. The features of these diseases are compared in Table 9-8.

- *Mycobacterium kansasii* causes a chronic, slowly progressive, granulomatous pulmonary disease in people over 50 years, similar to that produced by MAI in immunocompetent patients.
- *Mycobacterium scrofulaceum,* a common soil inhabitant, produces a draining, granulomatous, cervical lymphadenitis in young children (aged 1–5 years). The infection affects the submandibular lymph nodes and probably results from inoculation or ingestion of organisms by toddlers playing in soil. The disease is localized, and surgical excision of affected lymph nodes is curative.
- *Mycobacterium marinum,* commonly found on underwater surfaces, leads to a localized nodular skin lesion ("swimming pool granuloma"), sometimes with lymphatic involvement. Infection is acquired by traumatic inoculation, such as abrading an elbow on a swimming pool ladder or cutting a finger on a fish spine. Tissue reactions may be pyogenic or granulomatous.
- *Mycobacterium ulcerans* is associated with severe ulcerating skin disease in Australia, Africa and New Guinea. Infection presents as a solitary, undermining, deep ulcer of the skin and subcutaneous fat of the extremities.
- *Mycobacterium chelonae* and *Mycobacterium fortuitum* are closely related organisms that are ubiquitous in the environment. Infection follows traumatic or iatrogenic inoculation of material contaminated with organisms. Painless, fluctuant abscesses appear at the site of inoculation, ulcerate and gradually heal spontaneously. The tissue reaction can be pyogenic or granulomatous.

Fungal Infections

Of more than 100,000 known fungi, only a few cause human disease. Of these, most are "opportunists"; they only infect people with impaired defenses. ***Thus, corticosteroid administration, antineoplastic therapy and congenital or acquired T-cell deficiencies all predispose to mycotic infections.***

Fungi are larger and more complex than bacteria. They vary in size from 2 to 100 μm and are eukaryotes. Thus, they possess nuclear membranes and cytoplasmic organelles, such as mitochondria and endoplasmic reticulum.

There are two morphologic types of fungi: yeasts and molds.

- **Yeasts** are unicellular forms of fungi. They are round or oval cells that reproduce by budding, a process by which daughter organisms pinch off from a parent. Some yeasts produce buds that do not detach but instead create

TABLE 9-8

ATYPICAL MYCOBACTERIAL INFECTIONS

Organism	Disease	Ages Affected	Pathology	Source	Distribution
Mycobacterium kansasii	Chronic granulomatous pulmonary disease (similar to that caused by *Mycobacterium avium-intracellulare*)	50–70	Granulomatous inflammation	Inhaled organisms from soil, dust or water	Worldwide
Mycobacterium scrofulaceum	Cervical lymphadenitis	1–5	Granulomatous inflammation	Probably ingested organisms from soil or dust	Worldwide
Mycobacterium marinum	Localized skin lesions	All	Granulomatous inflammation	Direct inoculation of organisms from fish or underwater surfaces (swimming pools, fish tanks)	Worldwide
Mycobacterium ulcerans	Large, solitary, severe ulcer of skin and subcutaneous tissue	Usually 5–25	Coagulative necrosis	Probably inoculation of environmental organisms	Australia, Africa
Mycobacterium fortuitum and *Mycobacterium chelonae*	Infections associated with traumatic or iatrogenic inoculations	All	Pyogenic inflammation	Inoculation of environmental organisms	Worldwide

pseudohyphae (i.e., chains of elongated yeast cells that resemble hyphae).

- **Molds** are multicellular filamentous fungal colonies with branching tubules, or **hyphae,** 2–10 μm in diameter. The mass of tangled hyphae in the mold form is called a **mycelium.** Some hyphae are separated by septa that are located at regular intervals; others are nonseptate.
- **Dimorphic fungi** may grow as yeasts or molds, depending on their environment.

Most fungi are visible on tissue sections stained with hematoxylin and eosin. The periodic acid–Schiff (PAS) and Gomori methenamine silver (GMS) stains outline fungal cell walls and are commonly used to detect fungal infection in tissues.

PNEUMOCYSTIS JIROVECI PNEUMONIA

Pneumocystis jiroveci (formerly, carinii) *causes progressive, often fatal, pneumonia in people with impaired cell-mediated immunity. It is a common opportunistic pathogen in AIDS.* The organism has recently been reclassified with the fungi.

 **EPIDEMIOLOGY:** *P. jiroveci* is distributed worldwide. Since 75% of the population have antibodies by 5 years of age, it is likely that the organisms are inhaled by all. If cell-mediated immunity is intact, infection is rapidly contained without producing symptoms.

In the 1960s and 1970s, 100–200 cases of active *Pneumocystis* disease were reported annually in the United States, mainly in people with hematologic malignancies, transplant recipients or those treated with corticosteroids or cytotoxic therapy. Pneumocystis became a common pathogen with the AIDS pandemic. Before the use of highly active antiretroviral therapy (see Chapter 4), 80% of AIDS patients developed *Pneumocystis* pneumonia.

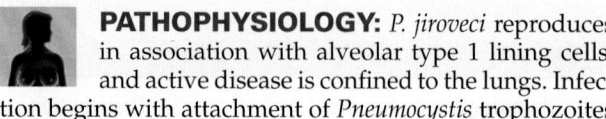 **PATHOPHYSIOLOGY:** *P. jiroveci* reproduces in association with alveolar type 1 lining cells, and active disease is confined to the lungs. Infection begins with attachment of *Pneumocystis* trophozoites

to alveolar lining cells. Trophozoites feed on host cells and enlarge and transform into the cyst form, which contains daughter organisms. The cyst ruptures to release new trophozoites, which attach to additional alveolar lining cells. If the process is not checked by the host immune system or antibiotics, infected alveoli eventually fill with organisms and proteinaceous fluid. The progressive filling of alveoli prevents adequate gas exchange and the patient slowly suffocates.

It is assumed, but not proved, that most cases of pneumocystosis derive from latent endogenous infection. Outbreaks of *Pneumocystis* pneumonia have also occurred among severely malnourished (and thus immunosuppressed) infants in nurseries; these represent primary infection with the organism.

 PATHOLOGY: *P. jiroveci* causes progressive consolidation of the lungs. Microscopically, alveoli contain a frothy eosinophilic material, composed of alveolar macrophages and cysts and *P. jiroveci* trophozoites (Fig. 9-54). Hyaline membranes and type 2 pneumocytes are prominent. In newborns, alveolar septa are thickened by lymphoid cells and macrophages. The prominent plasma cells in the infantile disease led to the now obsolete term *plasma cell pneumonia.*

The various forms of *P. jiroveci* are best visualized with methenamine silver stains. The cyst form measures about 60 μm in diameter (Fig. 9-54B); extracellular trophozoites and intracystic forms of the organism appear as irregularly shaped cells, 1–3 μm across, with punctate violet nuclei by Giemsa staining.

 CLINICAL FEATURES: *P. jiroveci* pneumonia features fever and progressive shortness of breath, often exacerbated by exertion and accompanied by a nonproductive cough. Dyspnea may be subtle in onset and slowly progressive over many weeks. Chest radiographs show a diffuse pulmonary process. The diagnosis requires recovery of alveolar material (by bronchoscopy, endobronchial washing or sputum induction) for staining. The disease

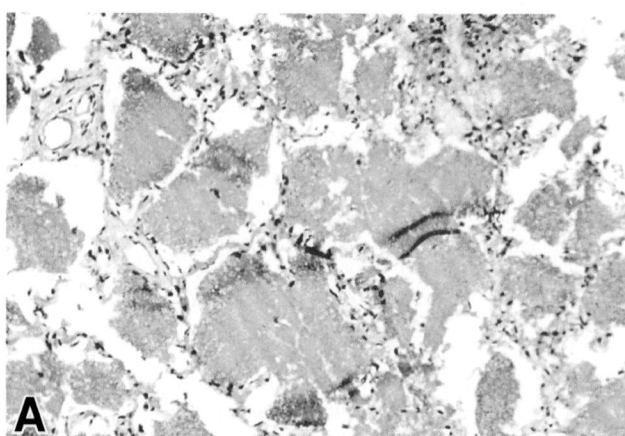
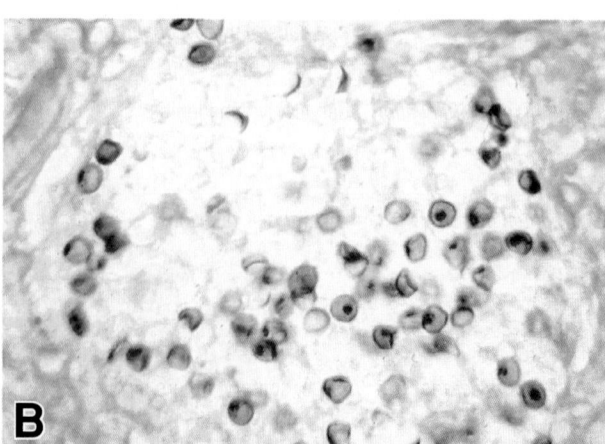

FIGURE 9-54. ***Pneumocystis jiroveci* pneumonia. A.** The alveoli contain a frothy eosinophilic material that is composed of alveolar macrophages and cysts and trophozoites of *P. jiroveci.* **B.** A silver stain shows crescent-shaped organisms, which are collapsed and degenerated. Some have a characteristic dark spot in their walls.

is fatal if untreated. Therapy is with trimethoprim-sulfamethoxazole or pentamidine.

CANDIDA

The genus *Candida,* comprising over 20 species of yeasts, includes the most common opportunistic pathogens. Many are endogenous human flora, well adapted to life on or in the human body. However, they can cause disease when host defenses are compromised. Although the various forms of candidiasis vary in clinical severity, most are localized, superficial diseases, limited to a particular mucocutaneous site, including:

- **Intertrigo:** infection of opposed skin surfaces
- **Paronychia:** infection of the nail bed
- **Diaper rash**
- **Vulvovaginitis**
- **Thrush:** oral infection
- **Esophagitis**

Candidal infections of deep tissues are much less common than superficial infections but can be life-threatening. The most common deep sites affected are the brain, eye, kidney and heart. Deep infections, with candidal sepsis and disseminated candidiasis, occur only in immunologically compromised people and are often fatal.

Most candidal infections derive from endogenous flora. *Candida albicans* resides in small numbers in the oropharynx, gastrointestinal tract and vagina and accounts for more than 95% of these infections.

PATHOPHYSIOLOGY: Mechanical barriers, inflammatory cells, humoral immunity and cell-mediated immunity relegate *Candida* to superficial, nonsterile sites. In turn, the resident bacterial flora normally limit the number of fungal organisms. Bacteria (1) block candidal attachment to epithelial cells, (2) compete with them for nutrients and (3) prevent conversion of the fungus to tissue-invasive forms. When any of these defenses is compromised, candidal infections can occur (Table 9-9). *Antibiotic use suppresses competing bacterial flora and is the most common precipitating factor for candidiasis.* Under conditions of unopposed growth, the yeast converts to its invasive form (hyphae or pseudohyphae), invades superficially and elicits an inflammatory or immunologic response.

Although *Candida* inhabits skin surfaces, it does not cause cutaneous disease without a predisposing skin lesion. The most common such factor is maceration, or softening and destruction of the skin. Chronically warm and moist areas, such as between fingers and toes, between skinfolds and under diapers, are prone to maceration and superficial candidal disease.

The incidence of invasive candidal infections is increasing. Frequent use of potent broad-spectrum antibiotics eliminates bacteria that otherwise limit *Candida* colonization. Expanded use of medical devices, such as intravascular catheters, monitoring devices, endotracheal tubes and urinary catheters, provides access to sterile sites. AIDS and iatrogenic neutropenias render individuals susceptible to even weak pathogens, such as *Candida*. Finally, intravenous drug users develop deep candidal infections because of inoculation of the fungi into the bloodstream.

TABLE 9-9
CANDIDAL INFECTIONS

Disease	Predisposing Conditions
Superficial Infections	
Intertrigo (opposed skin surfaces)	Maceration
Paronychia (nail beds)	Maceration
Diaper rash	Maceration
Vulvovaginitis	Alteration in normal flora
Thrush (oral)	Decreased cell-mediated immunity
Esophagitis	Decreased cell-mediated immunity
Deep Infections	
Urinary tract infections	Indwelling urinary catheters
Sepsis and disseminated infection	Neutropenia, indwelling vascular catheters and change in normal flora

PATHOLOGY AND CLINICAL FEATURES: Superficial infections of the skin, oropharynx (Fig. 9-55A) and esophagus feature invasive organisms in the most superficial epithelial layers and are associated with acute inflammatory infiltrates. Yeast, pseudohyphae and hyphae are present (Fig. 9-55B). The yeasts are round, are 3–4 μm in diameter and display septate hyphae. Candidal vaginitis is characterized by superficial invasion of the squamous epithelium, but inflammation is usually scanty. Deep infections consist of multiple microscopic abscesses, which contain yeast, hyphae, necrotic debris and neutrophils. Rarely, *Candida* elicit granulomatous responses.

The various superficial cutaneous infections manifest as tender, erythematous papules, which expand to form confluent erythematous areas:

- **Thrush:** This disorder involves the tongue and mucous membranes of the mouth. Early in life, it is the most common form of mucocutaneous candidiasis. Candidal vaginitis during pregnancy predisposes newborns to infection. Friable, white, curd-like membranes are adherent to affected surfaces. These patches contain fungi, necrotic debris, neutrophils and bacteria, and can be dislodged by scraping. Removal of the membranes leaves a painful, bleeding surface.
- **Candidal vulvovaginitis:** This condition causes a thick, white vaginal discharge, with vaginal and vulvar itching. Involved areas of the vulva are erythematous and tender. Candidal vaginitis is most intense when vaginal pH is low. Antibiotics, pregnancy, diabetes and corticosteroids predispose to this form of vaginitis.
- **Candidal sepsis and disseminated candidiasis:** Systemic candidiasis is rare and is ordinarily a terminal event in someone with altered immunity or neutropenia. Several candidal species can produce invasive disease in this context. Organisms may enter through ulcerated skin or

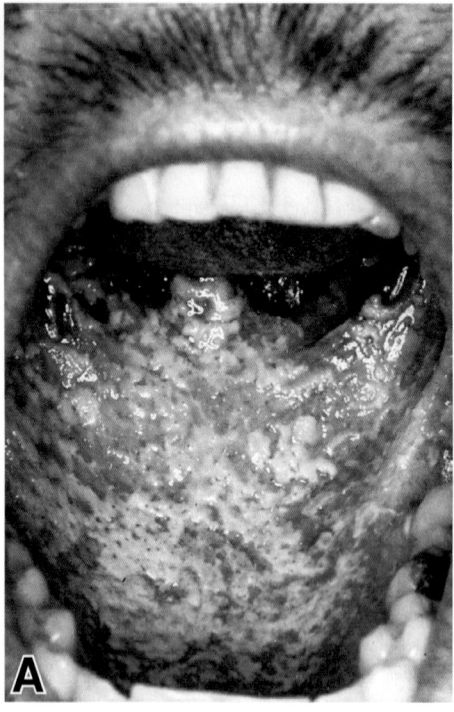
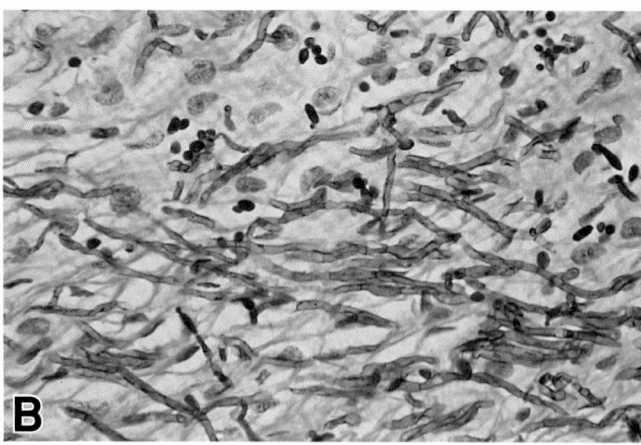

FIGURE 9-55. Candidiasis. A. The oral cavity of a patient with acquired immunodeficiency syndrome (AIDS) is covered by a white, curd-like exudate containing numerous fungal organisms. **B.** A periodic acid–Schiff (PAS) stain shows numerous septate hyphae and yeast forms.

mucous membrane lesions or may be introduced iatrogenically (e.g., peritoneal dialysis, intravenous lines or urinary catheters). The urinary tract is most commonly involved, and the incidence in women is four times that in men. Renal lesions may be blood-borne or may arise from an ascending pyelonephritis.

- **Candidal endocarditis:** This infection is characterized by large vegetations on the heart valves and a high incidence of embolization to large arteries. In most patients with candidal endocarditis, the cause is not immunosuppression but unusual vulnerability. Drug addicts who use unsterilized needles and persons with preexisting valvular disease who have had prolonged antibacterial therapy or indwelling vascular catheters are at risk for endocarditis. One of the most serious complications of invasive candidiasis is septic embolism to the brain.

ASPERGILLOSIS

Aspergillus species are common environmental fungi that cause opportunistic infections, usually involving the lungs. There are three types of pulmonary aspergillosis: (1) **allergic bronchopulmonary aspergillosis,** (2) **colonization of a preexisting pulmonary cavity (aspergilloma or fungus ball)** and (3) **invasive aspergillosis** (see Chapter 18). Of the over 200 identified species of *Aspergillus,* approximately 20 cause human disease. *Aspergillus fumigatus* is by far the most frequent human pathogen.

 **EPIDEMIOLOGY:** *Aspergillus* is a saprophyte found worldwide in soil, decaying plant matter and dung. Pulmonary aspergillosis is acquired by inhaling small (2–3 μm) spores, termed **conidia,** that are in the air in almost every human environment. The spores are small enough to reach the alveoli when inhaled. Exposure is

greatest when the habitat of the fungus is disturbed, as during soil excavations or handling decaying organic matter.

In tissues, *Aspergillus* spp. show septate hyphae, 2–7 μm in diameter, branching progressively at acute angles. The multiple dichotomous branching led to the name *Aspergillus,* which is derived from a fancied resemblance to the aspergillum, a device used to sprinkle holy water during Catholic religious ceremonies.

Allergic Bronchopulmonary Aspergillosis Complicates Asthma

Inhalation of *Aspergillus* spores delivers fungal antigens to airways and alveoli; contact subsequently initiates an allergic response in susceptible people. The situation is aggravated if spores can germinate and grow in the airways, thereby causing long-term exposure to the antigen. Allergic bronchopulmonary aspergillosis is virtually restricted to asthmatics, 20% of whom eventually develop this disorder (see Chapter 18).

Bronchi and bronchioles show infiltrates of lymphocytes, plasma cells and variable numbers of eosinophils. Sometimes airways are impacted with mucus and fungal hyphae. Patients experience exacerbations of asthma, often accompanied by pulmonary infiltrates and eosinophilia.

Aspergillomas Reside in Pulmonary Cavities or Bronchiectasis

Inhaled spores germinate in the warm humid atmosphere provided by these hollows and fill them with masses of hyphae (see Chapter 18).

 PATHOLOGY: An aspergilloma is a dense, roundish mass of tangled hyphae, 1–7 cm in diameter, within a fibrous cavity. The cavity wall is collagenous connective tissue, with lymphocytes and plasma cells. The hyphae do not invade adjacent tissues.

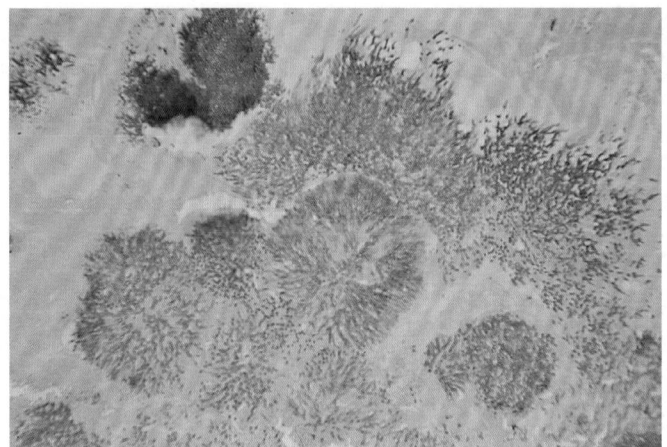

FIGURE 9-56. Invasive aspergillosis. A section of lung impregnated with silver shows branching fungal hyphae surrounding blood vessels and invading the adjacent parenchyma.

 CLINICAL FEATURES: Aspergillomas occur most commonly in old tuberculous cavities. Symptoms reflect the underlying disease. The radiologic appearance of a dense round ball in a cavity is characteristic. Aspergillomas are usually best left untreated, although surgical excision may be indicated in some cases.

Invasive Aspergillosis Generally Affects Neutropenic Patients

Whenever neutrophil number or activity is compromised, invasive aspergillosis may occur. The most common settings are high-dose steroid or cytotoxic therapy or acute leukemia. In profoundly neutropenic patients, inhaled spores germinate to produce hyphae, which invade through bronchi into the lung parenchyma, from where the fungi may spread widely.

 PATHOLOGY: *Aspergillus* readily invades blood vessels and produces thrombosis (Fig. 9-56). As a result, multiple nodular infarcts are seen throughout both lungs. Involvement of larger pulmonary arteries results in large, wedge-shaped, pleural-based infarcts. Vascular invasion also leads to fungus dissemination to other organs. *Aspergillus* hyphae are arranged radially around blood vessels and extend through their walls. Acute aspergillosis may also start in a nasal sinus and spread to the face, orbit and brain.

 CLINICAL FEATURES: Invasive aspergillosis presents as fever and multifocal pulmonary infiltrates in a compromised patient. Because of frequent thrombosis and bloodstream dissemination, the disease is often fatal. Antifungal therapy with amphotericin B may be successful but must be initiated early and given in high doses.

MUCORMYCOSIS (ZYGOMYCOSIS)

Several related environmental fungi, members of the class Zygomycetes (*Rhizopus, Mucor, Rhizomucor, Absidia*) produce severe, necrotizing, invasive, opportunistic infections that begin in the nasal sinuses or lungs. The infections they produce are usually called **mucormycoses** or **zygomycoses**.

In tissues, zygomycetes have large (8–15 μm across) hyphae that branch at right angles, have thin walls and lack septa. In tissue sections, they appear as hollow tubes. Since they lack cross-walls, their liquid contents flow, leaving long empty segments. They also may resemble "twisted ribbons," which represent collapsed hyphae.

 EPIDEMIOLOGY: Zygomycetes are ubiquitous, inhabiting soil, food and decaying vegetable matter. Their spores are inhaled, and in susceptible people, disease begins in the lungs. Mucormycosis occurs almost exclusively in the setting of compromised defenses. Common causes include severe neutropenia (e.g., after treatment for leukemia), high-dose glucocorticoid therapy and, particularly, severe diabetes.

  PATHOLOGY AND CLINICAL FEATURES: The three predominant forms of mucormycosis are rhinocerebral, pulmonary and subcutaneous.

■ **Rhinocerebral mucormycosis:** Fungi proliferate in nasal sinuses, invade surrounding tissues and extend into facial soft tissues, nerves, blood vessels and the brain. The palate or nasal turbinates are covered by a black crust, and underlying tissue is friable and hemorrhagic. Fungal hyphae grow into the arteries and cause devastating, rapidly progressive, septic infarction of affected tissues. Extension into the brain leads to fatal, necrotizing, hemorrhagic encephalitis. Therapy requires surgical excision of involved tissues, amphotericin B and correction of the predisposing abnormality.
■ **Pulmonary mucormycosis:** This infection resembles invasive pulmonary aspergillosis, including vascular invasion and multiple areas of septic infarction (Fig. 9-57). Both rhinocerebral and pulmonary mucormycosis are usually fatal.
■ **Subcutaneous zygomycosis:** This infection is limited to the tropics and is caused by *Basidiobolus haptosporus*. The fungus grows slowly in the panniculus, producing a gradually enlarging, hard inflammatory mass, usually on the shoulder, trunk, buttock or thigh.

CRYPTOCOCCOSIS

Cryptococcosis is a systemic mycosis caused by *Cryptococcus neoformans*, which principally affects the meninges and lungs (Fig. 9-58). *C. neoformans* has a worldwide distribution. Its main reservoir is pigeon droppings, which are alkaline and hyperosmolar. These conditions keep cryptococci small, allowing inhaled organisms to reach the terminal bronchioles. *C. neoformans* is unique among pathogenic fungi in having a proteoglycan capsule, which is essential for pathogenicity. The organisms appear as faintly basophilic yeasts with a clear, 3–5-μm-thick, mucinous capsule.

 **PATHOPHYSIOLOGY:** Cryptococcus *almost exclusively affects people with impaired cell-mediated immunity*. Although the organism is ubiquitous and exposure is common, cryptococcosis is rare in the absence of predisposing illness. Disease is

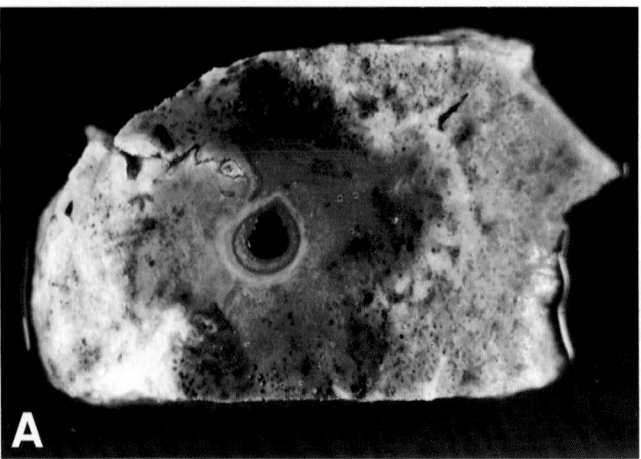
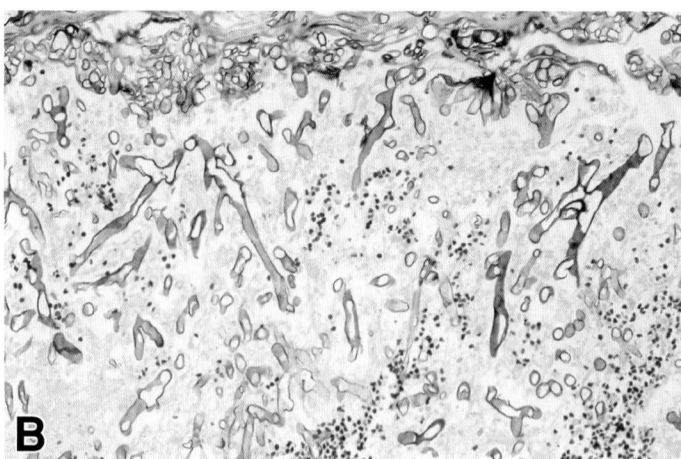

FIGURE 9-57. Pulmonary mucormycosis. A cross-section of the lung shows the vessel in the center of the field to be invaded by mucormycetes and occluded by a septic thrombus. The surrounding tissue is infarcted.

uncommon even among persons such as pigeon fanciers, who are exposed to high concentrations of the organism. Cryptococcosis occurs in patients with AIDS, lymphomas (particularly Hodgkin disease), leukemias and sarcoidosis, and in those treated with high doses of corticosteroids.

In immunologically intact individuals, neutrophils and alveolar macrophages kill *C. neoformans,* and no clinical disease develops. By contrast, in a patient with defective cell-mediated immunity, the cryptococci survive, reproduce locally and then disseminate. Although the lung is the portal of entry, the CNS is the most common site of disease, owing to the nourishing environment provided by the cerebrospinal fluid.

 PATHOLOGY: Over 95% of cryptococcal infections involve the meninges and brain. Lesions in the lungs can be demonstrated in half of patients. In a small minority, skin, liver and other involvement occurs. In cryptococcal meningoencephalitis, the entire brain is swollen and soft, and leptomeninges are thickened and gelatinous from infiltration by the thickly encapsulated organisms. Inflammatory responses are variable but are often minimal, with large numbers of cryptococci infiltrating tissue. When present, inflammation may be neutrophilic, lymphocytic or granulomatous.

Cryptococcosis in the lung may appear as diffuse disease or as isolated areas of consolidation. Affected alveoli are distended by clusters of organisms, usually with minimal inflammation.

Because of its thick capsule, *C. neoformans* stains poorly with the routine hematoxylin and eosin stain and appears as bubbles or holes in tissue sections (Fig. 9-59A). Fungal stains (PAS and GMS) demonstrate the yeasts well but do not stain the polysaccharide capsule. The organism thus appears to be surrounded by a halo. The capsule can be highlighted by the mucicarmine stain (Fig. 9-59B).

 CLINICAL FEATURES: Cryptococcal CNS disease often begins insidiously, with headache, dizziness, sleepiness and loss of coordination. Untreated

cryptococcal meningitis is invariably fatal. Therapy requires prolonged systemic administration of antifungal agents. Cryptococcal pneumonia presents as diffuse progressive pulmonary disease.

HISTOPLASMOSIS

Histoplasmosis reflects an infection with *Histoplasma capsulatum. **The disease is usually self-limited but may lead to a systemic granulomatous disease.*** Most cases of histoplasmosis are asymptomatic, although progressive disseminated infections occur in people with impaired cell-mediated immunity. *H. capsulatum* is a dimorphic fungus of worldwide distribution, which grows as a mold at ambient temperatures and as a yeast in the body (37°C [98.6°F]). The yeast cell is round and has a central basophilic body surrounded by a clear zone or halo, which in turn is encircled by a rigid cell wall. In caseous lesions, silver impregnation identifies the remains of degenerating yeast forms.

 EPIDEMIOLOGY: Histoplasmosis is acquired by inhalation of infectious spores of *H. capsulatum* (Fig. 9-55). The reservoir for the fungus is bird droppings and soil. In the Americas, hyperendemic areas are the eastern and central United States, western Mexico, Central America, the northern countries of South America and Argentina. In the tropics, bat nests, caves and soil beneath trees are foci of exposure.

PATHOPHYSIOLOGY: Histoplasmosis resembles tuberculosis in many ways. Primary infection begins with phagocytosis of microconidia by alveolar macrophages. Like *M. tuberculosis, H. capsulatum* reproduces in immunologically naive macrophages. As organisms grow, additional macrophages are recruited to the site of infection, producing an area of pulmonary consolidation. A few macrophages carry organisms first to hilar and mediastinal lymph nodes and then throughout the body, where fungi further infect monocytes/macrophages. The organisms proliferate within these cells

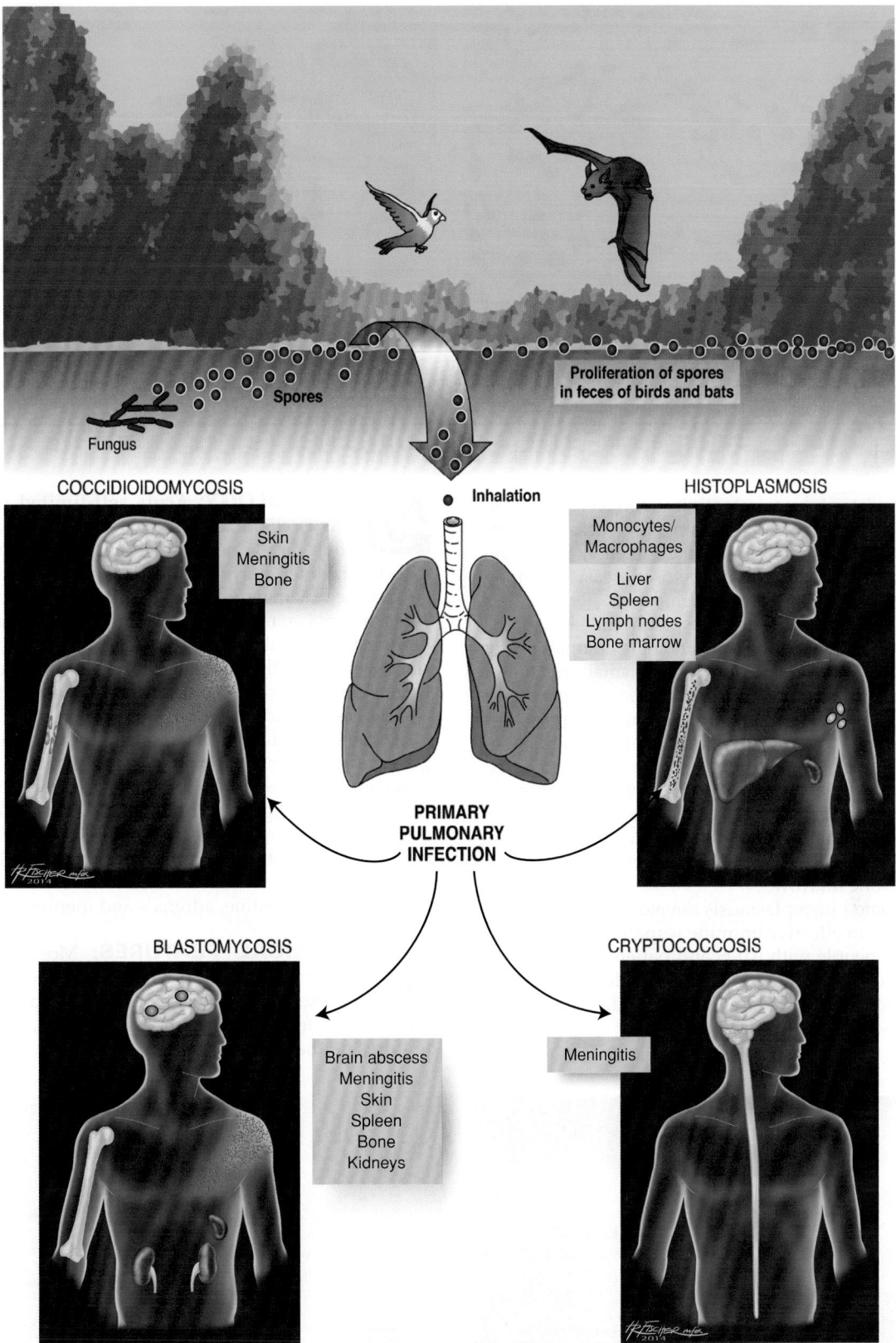

FIGURE 9-58. Pulmonary and disseminated fungal infection. Fungi grow in soil, air and the feces of birds and bats; they produce spores, some of which are infectious. When inhaled, spores cause primary pulmonary infection. In a few patients, the infection disseminates. **Histoplasmosis.** Primary infection is in the lung. In susceptible patients, the fungus disseminates to target organs, namely, the monocyte/macrophage system (liver, spleen, lymph nodes and bone marrow) and the tongue, mucous membranes of the mouth and the adrenals. **Cryptococcosis.** Primary infection of the lung disseminates to the meninges. **Blastomycosis.** Primary infection of the lung disseminates widely. The principal targets are the brain, meninges, skin, spleen, bone and kidney. **Coccidioidomycosis.** Primary infection of the lung may disseminate widely. The skin, meninges and bone are common targets.

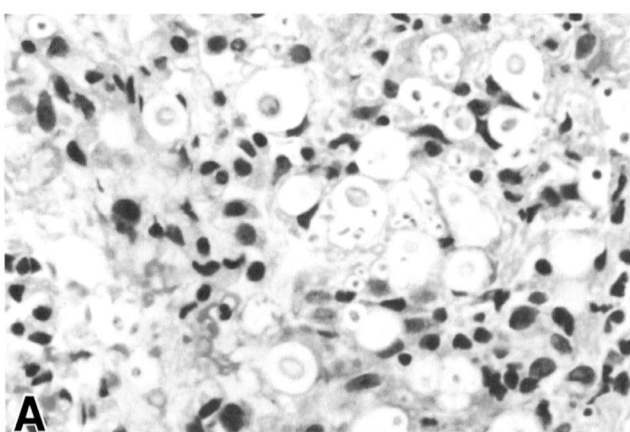 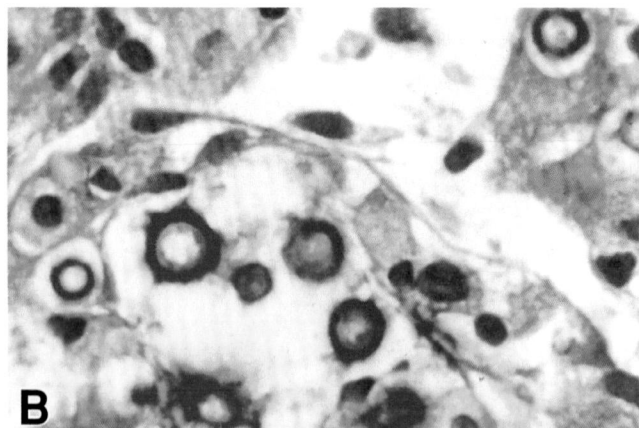

FIGURE 9-59. Cryptococcosis. A. In a section of the lung stained with hematoxylin and eosin, *Cryptococcus neoformans* appears as holes or bubbles. **B.** The same section stained with mucicarmine illustrates the capsule of the organism.

until the onset of hypersensitivity and cell-mediated immune responses, usually within 1–3 weeks. Normal immune responses usually limit the infection. Activated macrophages destroy the phagocytosed yeasts, forming necrotizing granulomas at sites of infection.

The course of infection varies with the size of the infecting inoculum and the immunologic competence of the host. Most infections (95%) involve small inocula of organisms in immunologically competent people. They affect small areas of the lung and regional lymph nodes and invariably remain unnoticed. On the other hand, exposure to a large inoculum, as occurs in an excavated bird roost, may lead to rapidly evolving pulmonary disease. Such cases feature large areas of pulmonary consolidation, prominent mediastinal and hilar nodal involvement and extension of the infection to the liver, spleen and bone marrow.

Disseminated histoplasmosis develops in people who do not mount an effective immune response to *H. capsulatum*. Infants, people with AIDS and patients treated with corticosteroids are at particular risk. In addition, on rare occasions individuals with no known underlying illness develop disseminated histoplasmosis.

 PATHOLOGY: Acute self-limited histoplasmosis is characterized by necrotizing granulomas in the lung, mediastinal and hilar lymph nodes, spleen and liver. Early in infection, the caseous material is surrounded by macrophages, Langhans giant cells, lymphocytes and plasma cells. Yeast forms of *H. capsulatum* can be demonstrated within macrophages and in the caseous material. Eventually, the cellular components of the granuloma largely disappear and the caseous material calcifies, forming a "fibrocaseous nodule" (Fig. 9-60A).

Disseminated histoplasmosis is characterized by progressive organ infiltration with macrophages carrying *H. capsulatum* (Fig. 9-60B). In mild cases, immune responses can control the organism, but not eliminate it. For long periods, disease is largely confined to macrophages in infected organs. If the patient is immunocompromised, clusters of macrophages filled with *H. capsulatum* infiltrate the liver, spleen, lungs, intestine, adrenals and meninges.

 CLINICAL FEATURES: Most infections are asymptomatic, but with extensive disease, patients present with fever, headache and cough. The symptoms persist for a few days to a few weeks, but the disease requires no therapy.

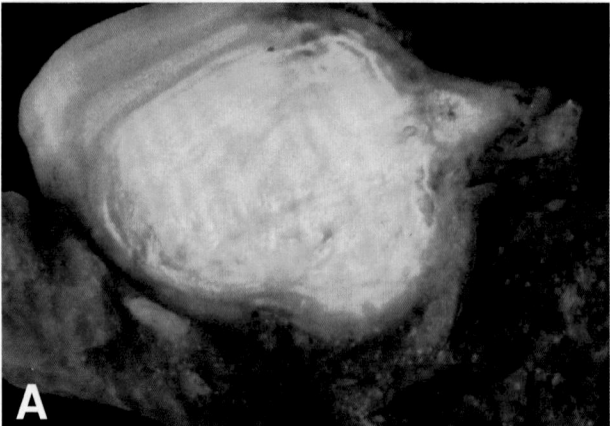 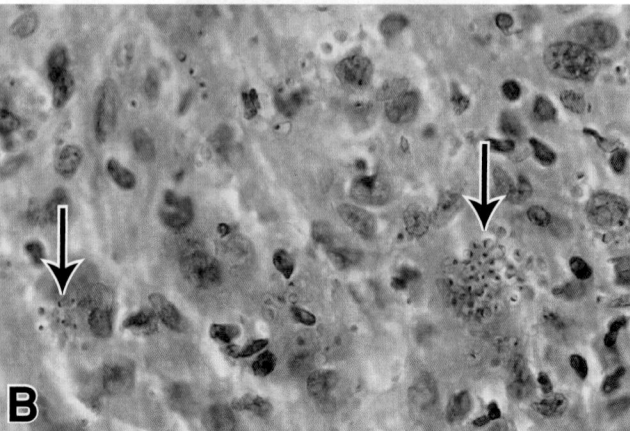

FIGURE 9-60. Histoplasmosis. A. A section of lung shows an encapsulated, subpleural, fibrocaseous nodule. **B.** A section of liver from a patient with disseminated histoplasmosis reveals Kupffer cells containing numerous yeasts of *Histoplasma capsulatum* (*arrows*) (periodic acid–Schiff [PAS] stain).

Disseminated histoplasmosis features weight loss, intermittent fever and weakness. In cases of subtle immunodeficiency, the disease may persist and progress for years, even decades. With more-profound immunodeficiency, dissemination progresses rapidly, often with high fever, cough, pancytopenia and changes in mental status. Disseminated histoplasmosis is treated with systemic antifungal agents.

COCCIDIOIDOMYCOSIS

Coccidioidomycosis is a chronic, necrotizing mycotic infection that clinically and pathologically resembles tuberculosis. The disease caused by *Coccidioides immitis* includes a spectrum of infections that begins as focal pneumonitis. Most cases are mild and asymptomatic and are limited to the lungs and regional lymph nodes. Occasionally, *C. immitis* infections spread outside the lungs to produce life-threatening disease.

  **EPIDEMIOLOGY AND ETIOLOGIC FACTORS:** *C. immitis* is a dimorphic fungus that grows as a mold in the soil, where it forms spores. Inhaled spores reach the alveoli and terminal bronchioles, enlarge into spherules and then mature to form sporangia (30–60 μm across). These gradually fill with 1–5-μm endospores, which accumulate by endosporulation, a process unique among pathogenic fungi. The sporangia eventually rupture and release endospores, which then repeat the cycle.

C. immitis is found in the soil in restricted climatic regions, particularly the Lower Sonoran life zones of the Western Hemisphere. These are areas with sparse rainfall, hot summers and mild winters. In the United States, large portions of California, Arizona, New Mexico and Texas are natural habitats for *C. immitis*. The disease is particularly common in California's San Joaquin Valley, where it is called **"valley fever."** It also occurs in Mexico and parts of South America.

Long-term residents of endemic regions are almost always infected with *C. immitis*. Even brief visits to these areas can cause infection (usually asymptomatic). Dry, windy weather, which lifts spores into the air, favors infection. The disease is not contagious.

 PATHOPHYSIOLOGY: Coccidioidomycosis begins with focal bronchopneumonia, where the spores are deposited. Mixed inflammatory infiltrates of neutrophils and macrophages follow, but the spores survive these immunologically naive inflammatory cells. As in tuberculosis and histoplasmosis, the host controls *C. immitis* infection only when inflammatory cells become immunologically activated. Necrotizing granulomas form with the onset of specific hypersensitivity and cell-mediated immune responses, which kills or contains the fungi.

The course of coccidioidomycosis varies from acute, self-limited disease to disseminated infection, depending on the size of the infecting dose and the immune status of the host. Coccidioidomycosis begins with focal bronchopneumonia. Most infections are produced by small inocula of organisms in immunologically competent hosts and are acute and self-limited. Extensive pulmonary involvement and fulminant disease may occur in persons from a nonendemic region exposed to large numbers of organisms.

Disseminated coccidioidomycosis occurs in immunocompromised people, from a primary infection or reactivation of old disease. Immunologically compromised patients are at greatest risk. Certain racial groups, including Filipinos, other Asians and blacks, are particularly susceptible to dissemination of coccidioidomycosis, probably because of a specific immunologic defect. For example, the risk of dissemination in Filipinos is 175 times that in whites. Pregnant women are also unusually susceptible to spread of the disease if they develop primary infection during the latter half of pregnancy.

PATHOLOGY: Acute self-limited coccidioidomycosis causes solitary lesions or patchy pulmonary consolidation, in which affected alveoli are infiltrated by neutrophils and macrophages. *C. immitis* spherules elicit an infiltrate of macrophages, whereas endospores predominantly attract neutrophils. Once an immune reaction begins, necrotizing, caseous granulomas develop. Successful immune responses cause the granuloma to heal, sometimes leaving a fibrocaseous nodule composed of caseous material and rimmed by residual macrophages and a thin capsule. In contrast to histoplasmosis, old granulomas of coccidioidomycosis rarely calcify.

The spherules and endospores of *C. immitis* stain with hematoxylin and eosin (Fig. 9-61). Spherules in various stages of development appear as basophilic rings. Mature spherules (sporangia) contain endospores that appear as smaller basophilic rings. As in other fungal infections, PAS and GMS stains can be used to enhance the staining of *C. immitis*.

Disseminated coccidioidomycosis may involve almost any body site and may manifest as a single extrathoracic site or as widespread disease, involving the skin (Fig. 9-62), bones, meninges, liver, spleen and genitourinary tract. Inflammatory responses at sites of dissemination are highly variable, ranging from infiltrates of neutrophils to granulomas.

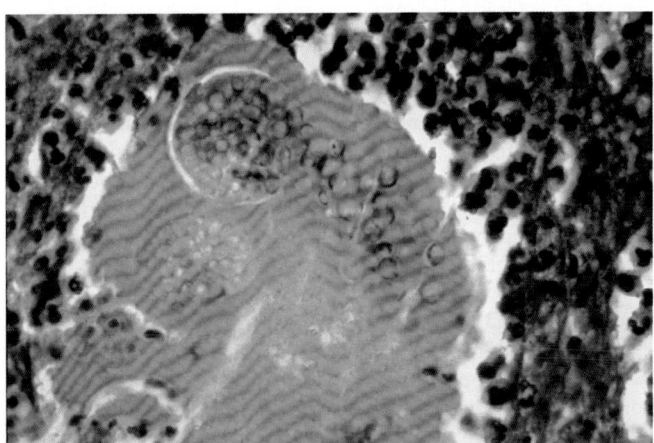

FIGURE 9-61. Coccidioidomycosis. A photomicrograph of the lung from a patient with acute coccidioidal pneumonia shows two spherules containing numerous endospores of *Coccidioides immitis.*

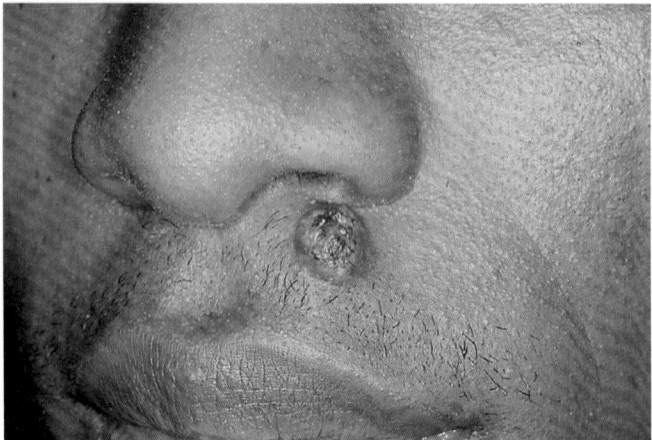

FIGURE 9-62. Disseminated coccidioidomycosis. A single raised, central ulcerated lesion is present on the face.

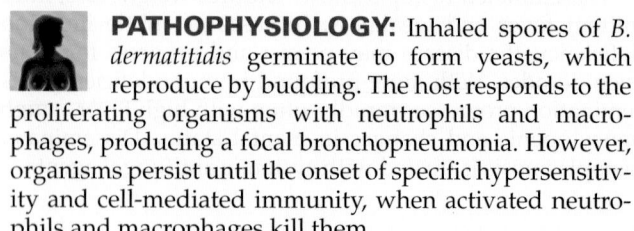

PATHOPHYSIOLOGY: Inhaled spores of *B. dermatitidis* germinate to form yeasts, which reproduce by budding. The host responds to the proliferating organisms with neutrophils and macrophages, producing a focal bronchopneumonia. However, organisms persist until the onset of specific hypersensitivity and cell-mediated immunity, when activated neutrophils and macrophages kill them.

PATHOLOGY: Blastomycosis is usually confined to the lungs, where infection mostly produces small areas of consolidation. *B. dermatitidis* incites a mixed suppurative and granulomatous inflammatory response and, even in the same patient, lesions range from neutrophilic abscesses to epithelioid granulomas. Pulmonary disease usually resolves by scarring, but some patients develop progressive miliary lesions or cavities. The skin (>50%) and bones (>10%) are the most common sites of extrapulmonary involvement. Skin infection often elicits marked pseudoepitheliomatous hyperplasia, imparting a warty appearance to the lesions.

Infected areas contain numerous yeasts of *B. dermatitidis*, which are spherical and 8–14 µm across, with broad-based buds and multiple nuclei in a central body (Fig. 9-63). With hematoxylin and eosin stains, the yeasts are rings with thick, sharply defined cell walls. They may be found in epithelioid cells, macrophages or giant cells, or they may lie free in microabscesses.

CLINICAL FEATURES: Coccidioidomycosis is a disease of protean manifestations, which vary from a subclinical respiratory infection to one that disseminates and is rapidly fatal. Like syphilis and typhoid fever, this disease is a great imitator; almost any complaint or syndrome may be its initial presentation.

Most people with coccidioidomycosis (>60%) are asymptomatic. The others develop a flu-like syndrome, with fever, cough, chest pain and malaise. Infection usually resolves spontaneously. Cavitation is the most frequent complication of pulmonary coccidioidomycosis, although it fortunately occurs in only few patients (<5%). The cavity, which may be mistaken for tuberculosis, is usually solitary and may persist for years. Progression or reactivation may lead to destructive lesions in the lungs or, more seriously, to disseminated lesions.

The signs and symptoms of disseminated coccidioidomycosis vary according to the site affected. Coccidioidal meningitis manifests with headache, fever, alteration in mental status or seizures and is fatal if untreated. Skin lesions in disseminated disease often have a warty appearance (Fig. 9-62). Even with prolonged amphotericin B therapy, the prognosis is poor in acute disseminated coccidioidomycosis, although the response rate has been improved with some of the newer azole antifungal agents.

BLASTOMYCOSIS

Blastomycosis is a chronic granulomatous and suppurative pulmonary disease, which is often followed by dissemination to other body sites, principally the skin and bone. The causative organism, *Blastomyces dermatitidis,* is a dimorphic fungus that grows as a mold in warm moist soil, rich in decaying vegetable matter.

EPIDEMIOLOGY: Blastomycosis is acquired by inhalation of infectious spores from the soil. The infection occurs within restricted geographic regions of the Americas, Africa and possibly the Middle East. In North America, the fungus is endemic along the distributions of the Mississippi and Ohio Rivers, the Great Lakes and the St. Lawrence River. Disturbance of the soil, either by construction or by leisure activities such as hunting or camping, leads to formation of aerosols containing fungal spores.

CLINICAL FEATURES: Pulmonary blastomycosis is self-limited in one third of cases. Symptomatic acute infection presents as a flu-like illness, with fever, arthralgias and myalgias. Progressive pulmonary disease is characterized by low-grade fever, weight loss, cough and predominantly upper lobe infiltrates on the chest radiograph. Skin lesions often resemble squamous cell carcinomas of the skin (Fig. 9-64) and are the most common signs of extrapulmonary dissemination. Although the lung infection may appear to resolve totally, in some patients blastomycosis may appear at distant sites months to years later.

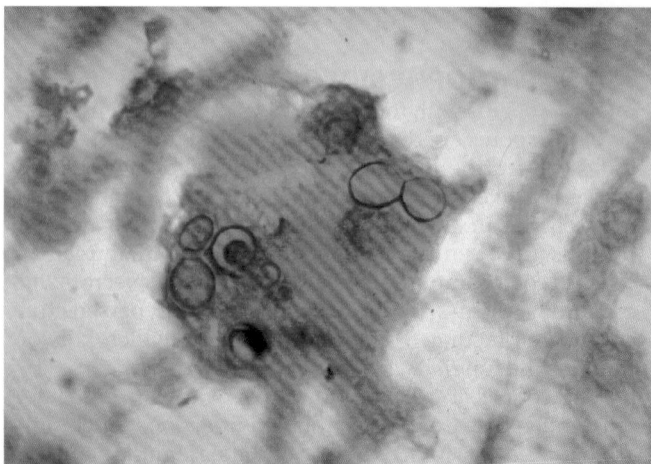

FIGURE 9-63. Blastomycosis. The yeasts of *Blastomyces dermatitidis* have a doubly contoured wall and nuclei in the central body. The buds have broad-based attachments.

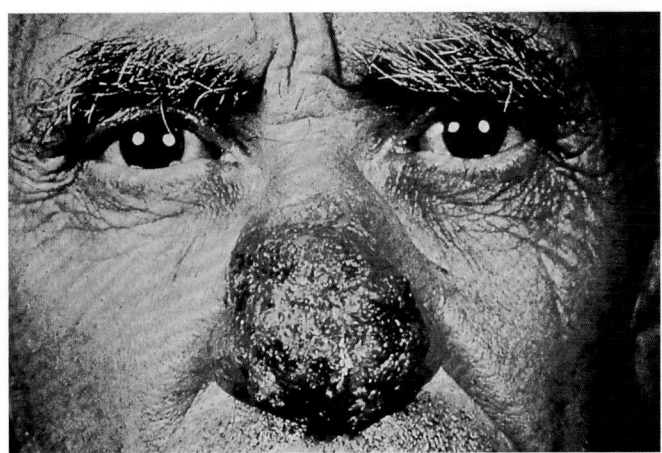

FIGURE 9-64. Cutaneous blastomycosis with ulceration.

PARACOCCIDIOIDOMYCOSIS (SOUTH AMERICAN BLASTOMYCOSIS)

Paracoccidioidomycosis is a chronic granulomatous infection that begins with lung involvement and disseminates to involve skin, oropharynx, adrenals and the macrophages of the liver, spleen and lymph nodes. The causative organism is *Paracoccidioides brasiliensis*, a dimorphic fungus, whose mold form resides in the soil.

 **EPIDEMIOLOGY:** Paracoccidioidomycosis is acquired by inhaling spores from the environment in restricted regions of Central and South America. Most infections are asymptomatic. Reactivation of latent infection occurs, and active disease can develop many years after someone leaves an endemic region. Interestingly, men develop symptomatic infections 15 times more often than women.

 PATHOLOGY: Paracoccidioidomycosis can involve the lungs alone (Fig. 9-65) or multiple extrapulmonary sites, most commonly skin, mucosal surfaces and lymph nodes. *P. brasiliensis* elicits a mixed suppurative and granulomatous response, producing lesions similar to those seen in blastomycosis and coccidioidomycosis.

 CLINICAL FEATURES: Paracoccidioidomycosis is usually an acute, self-limited and mild disease. Symptoms of progressive pulmonary

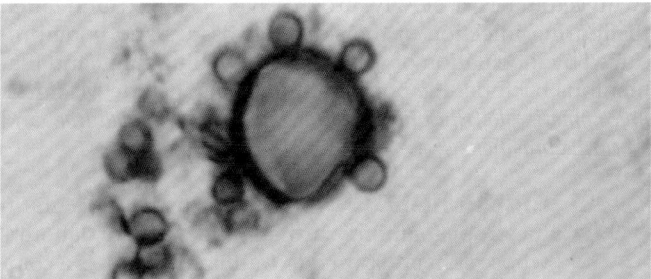

FIGURE 9-65. Paracoccidioidomycosis. The lung contains *Paracoccidioides braziliensis*, which displays many external buds arising circumferentially from the mother organism.

involvement resemble those of tuberculosis. Chronic mucocutaneous ulcers are a frequent manifestation of extrapulmonary disease.

SPOROTRICHOSIS

Sporotrichosis is a chronic infection of the skin, subcutaneous tissues and regional lymph nodes caused by *Sporothrix schenckii*. This dimorphic fungus grows as a mold in soil and decaying plant matter and as yeast in the body.

 EPIDEMIOLOGY: Sporotrichosis is endemic in parts of the Americas and southern Africa. Most cases are cutaneous, resulting from accidental inoculation of the fungus from thorns (especially rose thorns) or splinters, or by handling reeds or grasses. Cutaneous sporotrichosis is particularly common among gardeners, botanical nursery workers and others who suffer abrasions while working with soil, moss, hay or timbers. Infected animals, particularly cats, can also transmit the disease.

 PATHOLOGY: On entry into the skin, *S. schenckii* proliferates locally, eliciting an inflammatory response that produces an ulceronodular lesion. The infection frequently spreads along subcutaneous lymphatic channels, resulting in a chain of similar nodular skin lesions (Fig. 9-66A). Extracutaneous disease is much less common than skin disease. Joint and bone involvement is the commonest form of extracutaneous disease, and infections of the wrist, elbow, ankle or knee account for most (80%) of the cases.

The lesions of cutaneous sporotrichosis are usually in the dermis or subcutaneous tissue. The periphery of the nodules is granulomatous and the center is suppurative. Surrounding skin shows exuberant pseudoepitheliomatous hyperplasia. Some yeasts are surrounded by an eosinophilic, spiculated zone and are termed "asteroid bodies" (Fig. 9-66B). The material surrounding the yeasts ("Splendore-Hoeppli substance") probably consists of antigen–antibody complexes.

 CLINICAL FEATURES: Cutaneous sporotrichosis begins as a solitary nodular lesion at the site of inoculation, typically on a hand, arm or leg. Weeks afterward, additional nodules may appear along the lymphatic drainage of the primary lesion. Nodules often ulcerate and drain serosanguineous fluid. Joint involvement appears as pain and swelling of the affected joint, without involving overlying skin. Untreated cutaneous sporotrichosis continues to spread along the skin. The skin infection responds to systemic iodine therapy, but extracutaneous sporotrichosis requires systemic antifungal therapy.

CHROMOMYCOSIS

Chromomycosis is a chronic skin infection caused by several species of fungi that live as saprophytes in soil and decaying vegetable matter. The fungi are brown, round, thick walled and 8 μm across, and have been likened to "copper pennies" (Fig. 9-67). The infection is most common in barefooted agricultural workers in the tropics, in whom the fungus is implanted by trauma, usually below the knee. The lesions begin as papules and over the years become verrucous,

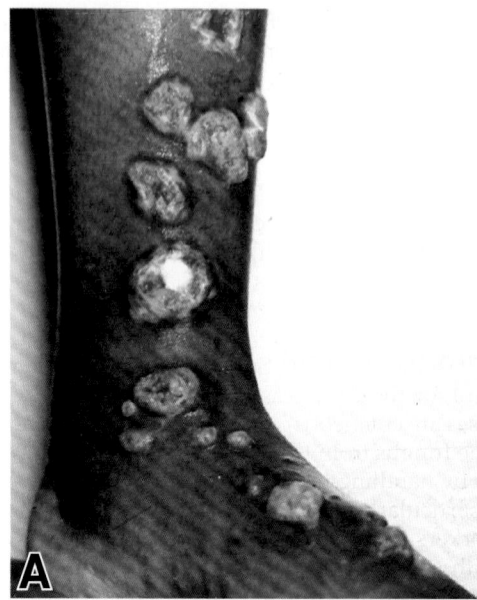
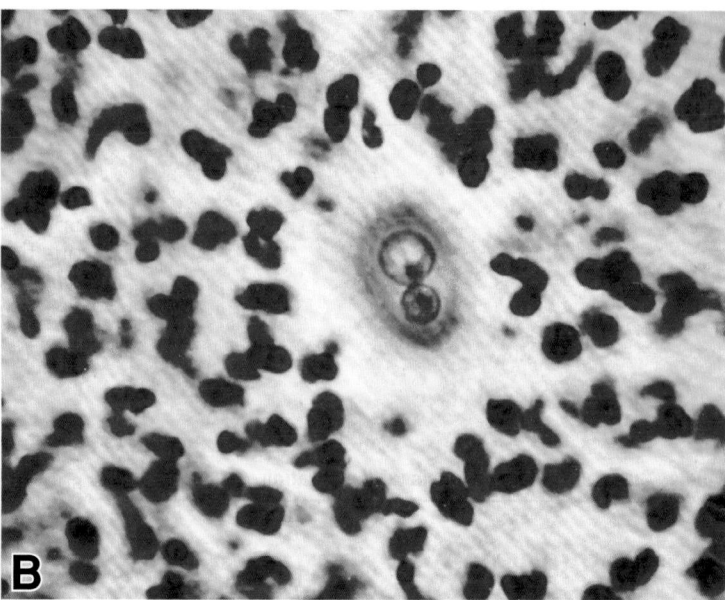

FIGURE 9-66. Sporotrichosis. A. The leg shows typical lymphocutaneous spread. **B.** A section of the lesion in **(A)** shows an asteroid body, composed of a pair of budding yeasts of *Sporothrix schenckii* surrounded by a layer of Splendore-Hoeppli substance, with radiating projections.

crusted and sometimes ulcerated. The infection spreads by contiguous growth and through lymphatics, and eventually may involve an entire limb.

DERMATOPHYTE INFECTIONS

Dermatophytes are fungi that cause localized superficial infections of keratinized tissues, including skin, hair and nails. There are about 40 species of dermatophytes in 3 genera: *Trichophyton*, *Microsporum* and *Epidermophyton*. *Dermatophyte infections are minor illnesses, but are among the most common skin diseases for which medical help is sought.* They are resident in soil, on animals and on humans. Most dermatophyte infections in temperate countries are acquired by direct contact with people who have infected hairs or skin scales.

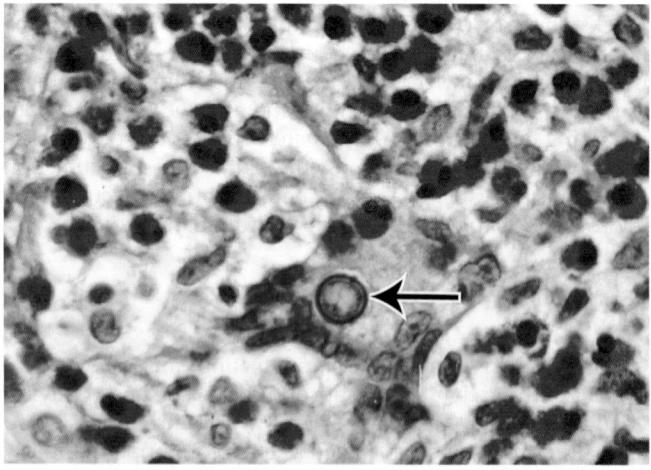

FIGURE 9-67. Chromomycosis. A section of skin shows a giant cell in the center, which contains a thick-walled, brown, sclerotic body (copper penny, *arrow*), representing the fungus.

 PATHOLOGY: Dermatophytes proliferate within the superficial keratinized tissues. They spread centrifugally from the initial site, producing round, expanding lesions with sharp margins. The appearance once suggested that a worm was responsible for the disease, hence the names **ringworm** and **tinea** (from the Latin *tinea*, "worm").

Dermatophyte infections produce thickening of the squamous epithelium, with increased numbers of keratinized cells. Lesions severe enough to be biopsied show a mild lymphocytic inflammatory infiltrate in the dermis. Hyphae and spores of the infecting dermatophytes are confined to the nonviable portions of skin, hair and nails.

 CLINICAL FEATURES: Dermatophyte infections are named according to the sites of involvement (e.g., scalp, tinea capitis; feet, tinea pedis, "athlete's foot"; nails, tinea unguium; intertriginous areas of the groin, tinea cruris, "jock itch"). These infections range from asymptomatic disease to chronic, fiercely pruritic eruptions and are treated with topical antifungal agents.

MYCETOMA

A mycetoma is a slowly progressive, localized and often disfiguring infection of the skin, soft tissues and bone produced by inoculation of various soil-dwelling fungi and filamentous bacteria. Responsible organisms include *Madurella mycetomatis*, *Petrilidium boydii*, *Actinomadura madurae* and *Nocardia brasiliensis*.

 **EPIDEMIOLOGY:** Mycetoma usually occurs in the tropics among farmers and outdoor laborers whose skin is exposed to trauma. The foot is a common site of infection in locales where persons walk barefoot on soggy ground, and the disease is also known as **Madura foot**. Frequent immersion of the foot macerates the skin and facilitates deep inoculation with soil organisms.

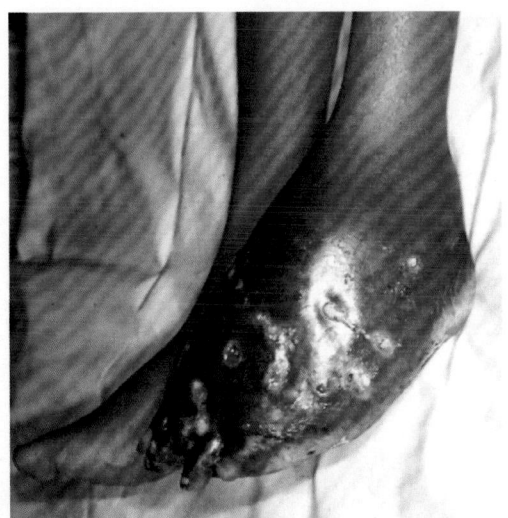

FIGURE 9-68. Mycetoma of the foot. The foot is swollen and painful and drains through the skin. The extremity was amputated.

 PATHOLOGY: The organisms proliferate in the subcutis and spread to adjacent tissues, including bone. This incites a mixed suppurative and granulomatous inflammatory infiltrate, which fails to eliminate the infecting organism. Surrounding granulation tissue and scarring produce progressive disfigurement of the affected sites.

A mycetoma begins as a solitary subcutaneous abscess and slowly expands to form multiple abscesses interconnected by sinus tracts (Fig. 9-68), which eventually drain to the skin surface. Abscesses contain colonies of compact bacteria or fungi, surrounded by neutrophils and an outer layer of granulomatous inflammation. The colonies of organisms, called "grains," resemble the "sulfur granules" of actinomycosis.

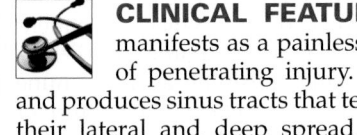 **CLINICAL FEATURES:** A mycetoma initially manifests as a painless, localized swelling at a site of penetrating injury. The lesion slowly expands and produces sinus tracts that tend to follow fascial planes in their lateral and deep spread through connective tissue, muscle and bone. Treatment is usually wide excision of the affected area.

Protozoal Infections

Protozoa are single-celled eukaryotes that fall into three general classes: **amebae, flagellates** and **sporozoites**. Amebae move by projection of cytoplasmic extensions termed **pseudopoda**. Flagellates move through thread-like structures, flagella, which extend out from the cell membrane. Sporozoites do not have organelles of locomotion and also differ from amebae and flagellates in their mode of replication.

Protozoa cause human disease by diverse mechanisms. Some, such as *Entamoeba histolytica,* are extracellular parasites that digest and invade human tissues. Others, such as plasmodia, are obligate intracellular parasites that replicate in, and kill, human cells. Still others, such as trypanosomes, damage human tissue largely by inflammatory and immunologic responses. Some protozoa (e.g., *Toxoplasma gondii*)

can establish latent infections and cause reactivation disease in immunocompromised hosts.

MALARIA

Malaria is a mosquito-borne, hemolytic, febrile illness. It affects over 200 million people worldwide and kills more than 1 million yearly. Four *Plasmodium* species cause malaria: *Plasmodium falciparum, Plasmodium vivax, Plasmodium ovale* and *Plasmodium malariae.* All infect and destroy human erythrocytes, producing chills, fever, anemia and splenomegaly. *P. falciparum* causes more severe disease than the others and accounts for most malarial deaths.

 EPIDEMIOLOGY: Although malaria has been eradicated in developed countries, it continues to afflict people in tropical and subtropical areas, especially Africa, South and Central America, India and Southeast Asia (Fig. 9-69). The rural poor, infants, children, malnourished people and pregnant women are especially susceptible to infection.

Malaria is transmitted by the bite of the female *Anopheles* mosquito. *P. falciparum* and *P. vivax* are the most common pathogens, but there is considerable geographic variation in species distribution. *P. vivax* is rare in Africa, where much of the black population lacks the erythrocyte cell surface receptors required for infection. *P. falciparum* and *P. ovale* are the predominant species in Africa. *P. malariae* is the least common and mildest form of malaria, although it has a broad geographic distribution.

 **ETIOLOGIC FACTORS:** The life cycle of the *Plasmodium* species responsible for human malaria requires both human and mosquito hosts (Fig. 9-70). Infected humans produce forms of the organism (gametocytes) that mosquitoes acquire upon feeding. Within these insects, the organism reproduces sexually, producing plasmodial forms (sporozoites), which the mosquito transmits to humans when it feeds.

The anopheline mosquito inoculates the sporozoites into the human bloodstream. There, they undergo asexual division ("schizogony"). Circulating sporozoites rapidly invade hepatocytes and reproduce in the liver, yielding numerous daughter organisms, termed "merozoites" (exoerythrocytic phase). Within 2–3 weeks of hepatic infection, these agents rupture host hepatocytes, exit into the bloodstream and invade erythrocytes.

Merozoites feed on hemoglobin and grow and reproduce inside erythrocytes. Within 2–4 days, mature progeny merozoites are produced. These daughter merozoites burst from infected erythrocytes, invade naive red cells and so initiate another cycle of erythrocytic parasitism. This cycle is repeated many times. Eventually, subpopulations of merozoites differentiate into sexual forms called gametocytes, which are ingested when a mosquito feeds on an infected host, thus completing the parasite's life cycle.

The rupture of infected erythrocytes releases pyrogens and causes the chills and fever of malaria. Anemia results both from loss of circulating infected erythrocytes and sequestration of cells in the enlarging spleen. The fixed mononuclear phagocytes of the liver and spleen respond to the infestation by proliferating and causing enlargement of the liver and spleen.

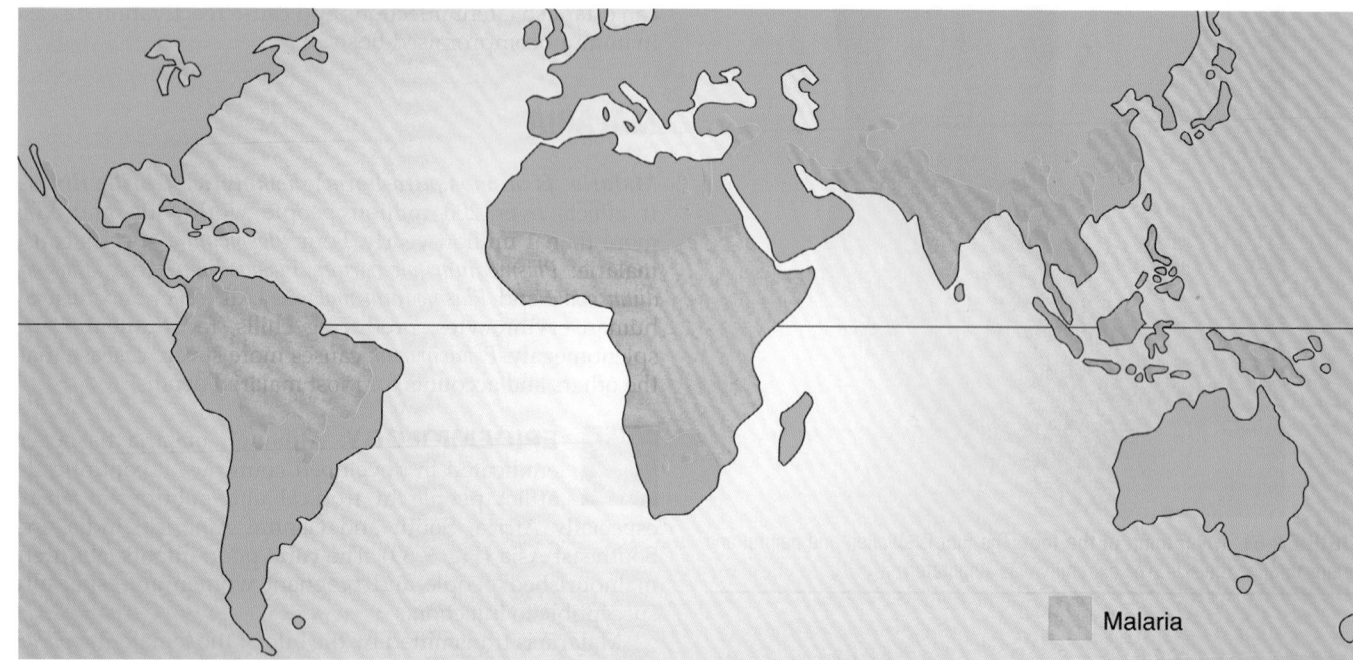

FIGURE 9-69. **The geographic distribution of malaria.**

P. falciparum infestation produces **malignant malaria,** a much more aggressive disease than the other plasmodia. It is distinguished from other malarial parasites in four respects:

- It has no secondary exoerythrocytic (hepatic) stage.
- It parasitizes erythrocytes of any age, causing marked parasitemia and anemia. In other types of malaria, only subpopulations of erythrocytes (e.g., only young or old forms) are parasitized, leading to lower-level parasitemias and more modest anemias.
- There may be several parasites in a single red cell.
- *P. falciparum* alters flow characteristics and adhesive properties of infected erythrocytes, so that they adhere to endothelial cells of small blood vessels. Obstruction of small blood vessels frequently produces severe tissue ischemia, which is probably the most important factor in the organism's virulence.

 PATHOLOGY: All forms of malaria show hepatosplenomegaly, as red blood cells are sequestered by fixed mononuclear phagocytes. The organs of this system (liver, spleen, lymph nodes) are darkened ("slate gray") by macrophages filled with hemosiderin and malarial pigment, the end-product of parasitic digestion of hemoglobin.

Adherence of infected red cells to microvascular endothelium in falciparum malaria has two consequences. First, parasitized erythrocytes attached to endothelial cells do not circulate, so patients with severe falciparum malaria have few circulating parasites. Second, capillaries of deep organs, especially the brain, become obstructed, leading to ischemia of the brain, kidneys and lungs. Brains of patients who die of cerebral malaria show congestion and thrombosis of small blood vessels in the white matter, which are rimmed with edema and hemorrhage ("ring hemorrhages") (Fig. 9-71). Obstruction of renal blood flow produces acute renal failure, while intravascular hemolysis results in hemoglobinuric nephrosis

(blackwater fever). In the lung, damage to alveolar capillaries generates pulmonary edema and acute alveolar damage.

CLINICAL FEATURES: Malaria is characterized by recurrent **paroxysms** of chills and high fever. They begin with chills and sometimes headache, followed by a high, spiking fever, with tachycardia, nausea, vomiting and abdominal pain. The high fever produces marked vasodilation and is often associated with orthostatic hypotension. The patient defervesces after several hours and is usually exhausted and drenched in sweat.

A period of 2–3 days follows, during which the patient feels well, only to be followed by a new paroxysm. Paroxysms recur for weeks, eventually subsiding as an immune response is mounted. Each paroxysm reflects the rupture of infected erythrocytes and release of daughter merozoites. As the mononuclear macrophage system responds to the infection, patients develop hepatosplenomegaly. Indeed, some of the largest spleens on record are the result of chronic malaria. Hypersplenism can exacerbate the anemia of malarial infection. As the level of parasitemia grows, fever may become virtually continuous. Ischemic brain injury causes symptoms from somnolence, hallucinations and behavioral changes to seizures and coma. CNS disease has a mortality of 20%–50%.

Malaria is diagnosed by demonstrating the organisms on Giemsa-stained blood smears. The several species are distinguished by their appearance in infected erythrocytes. Malarias other than falciparum malaria are treated with oral chloroquine, sometimes with primaquine. Therapy for falciparum malaria varies, as widespread chloroquine resistance requires new treatments.

BABESIOSIS

Babesiosis is a malaria-like infection caused by protozoa of the genus *Babesia,* which is transmitted by hard-bodied ticks.

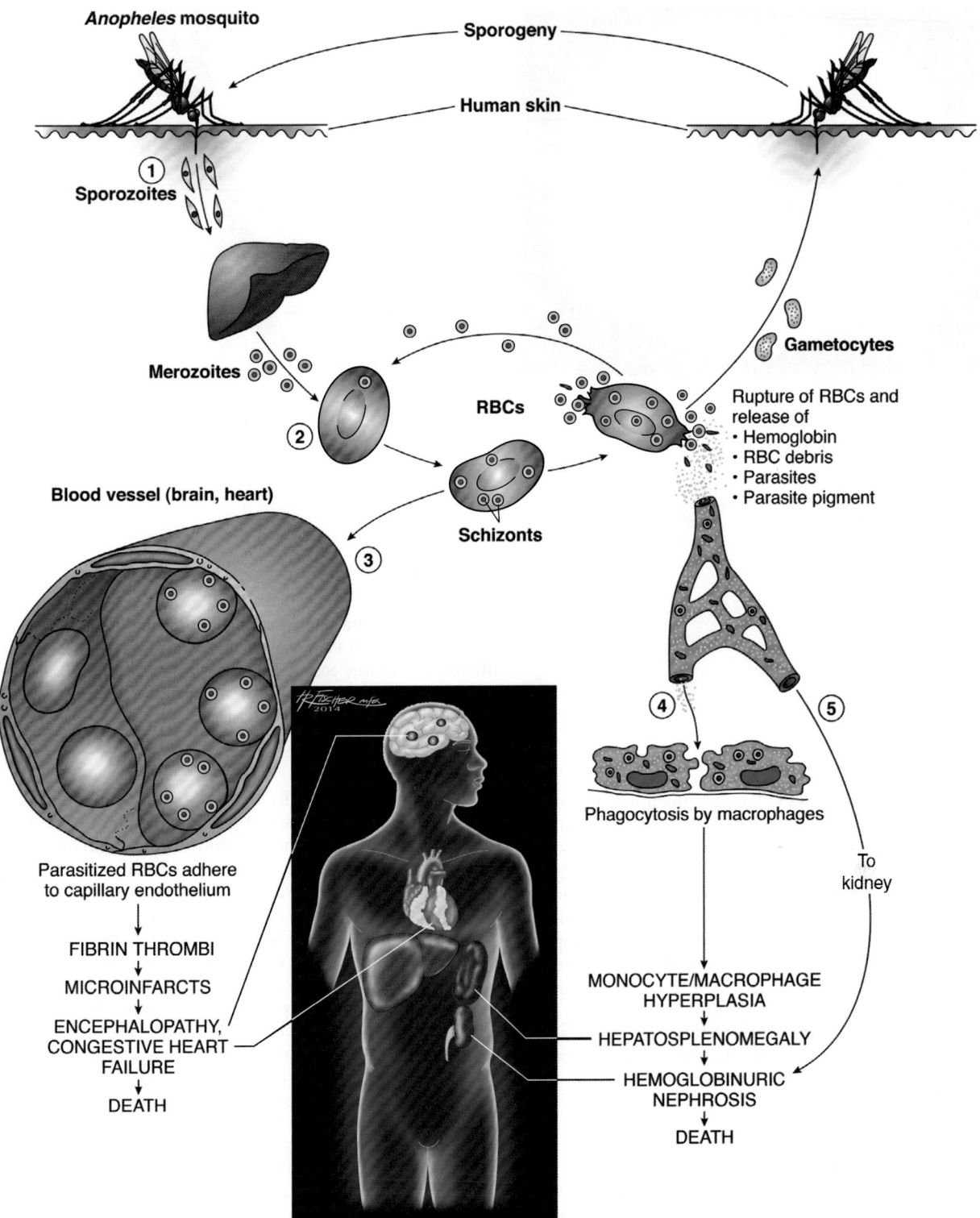

FIGURE 9-70. Life cycle of malaria. An *Anopheles* mosquito bites an infected person, taking blood that contains micro- and macrogametocytes (sexual forms). In the mosquito, sexual multiplication (sporogony) produces infective sporozoites in the salivary glands. **(1)** During the mosquito bite, sporozoites are inoculated into the bloodstream of the vertebrate host. Some sporozoites leave the blood and enter the hepatocytes, where they multiply asexually (exoerythrocytic schizogony) and form thousands of uninucleated merozoites. **(2)** Rupture of hepatocytes releases merozoites, which penetrate erythrocytes and become trophozoites, which then divide to form numerous schizonts (intraerythrocytic schizogony). Schizonts divide to form more merozoites, which are released on the rupture of erythrocytes and reenter other erythrocytes to begin a new cycle. After several cycles, subpopulations of merozoites develop into micro- and macrogametocytes, which are taken up by another mosquito to complete the cycle. **(3)** Parasitized erythrocytes obstruct capillaries of the brain, heart, kidney and other deep organs. Adherence of parasitized erythrocytes to capillary endothelial cells causes fibrin thrombi, which produce microinfarcts. These result in encephalopathy, congestive heart failure, pulmonary edema and frequently death. Ruptured erythrocytes release hemoglobin, erythrocyte debris and malarial pigment. **(4)** Phagocytosis leads to monocyte/macrophage hyperplasia and hepatosplenomegaly. **(5)** Released hemoglobin produces hemoglobinuric nephrosis, which may be fatal. *RBCs* = red blood cells.

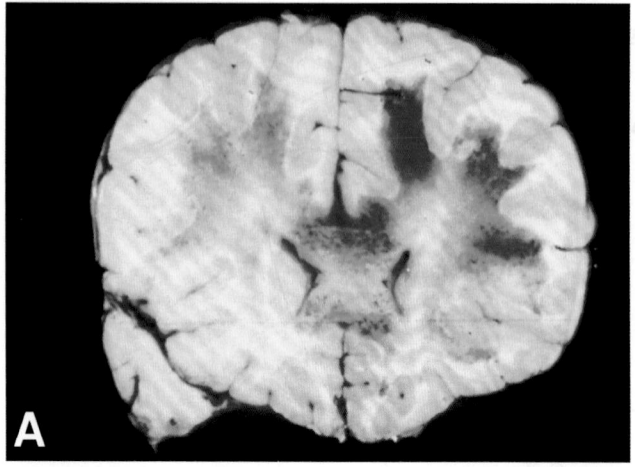

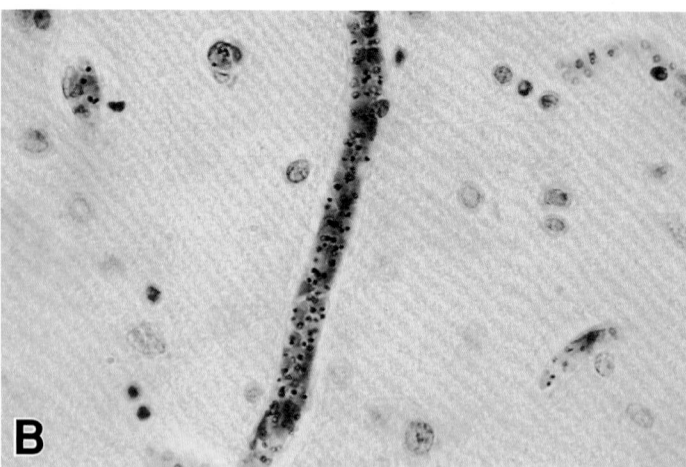

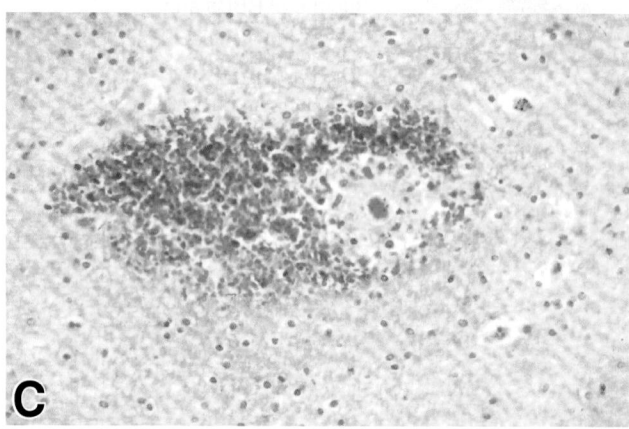

FIGURE 9-71. Acute falciparum malaria of the brain. A. There is severe diffuse congestion of the white matter and focal hemorrhages. **B.** A section of **(A)** shows a capillary packed with parasitized erythrocytes. **C.** Another section of **(A)** displays a ring hemorrhage around a thrombosed capillary, which contains parasitized erythrocytes in a fibrin thrombus.

 **EPIDEMIOLOGY:** *Babesia* infections are common in animals and in some locations are responsible for serious economic losses to the livestock industry. By contrast, human babesiosis is almost a medical curiosity, with the parasites infecting humans only when people intrude into the zoonotic cycle between the tick vector and its vertebrate host. Human babesiosis is reported only in Europe and North America. Infections in the United States have been concentrated in islands off the New England coast. The organisms invade and destroy erythrocytes, causing hemoglobinemia, hemoglobinuria and renal failure. The disease is usually self-limited, but uncontrolled infections can be fatal. *Babesia* spp. are resistant to most antiprotozoal drugs.

TOXOPLASMOSIS

Toxoplasmosis is a worldwide infectious disease caused by a protozoan, *Toxoplasma gondii*. Most infections are asymptomatic, but if they occur in a fetus or immunocompromised host, devastating necrotizing disease may result.

  **EPIDEMIOLOGY AND ETIOLOGIC FACTORS:** In some areas (e.g., France), the prevalence of *T. gondii* infection exceeds 80% of adults; in other regions (e.g., the southwestern United States), few people are affected. *T. gondii* infects many mammals and birds as intermediate hosts. The only final host is the cat, which becomes infected by ingesting toxoplasma cysts in tissues of an infected mouse or other intermediate host. In the cat's intestinal epithelium, five multiplicative stages end with shedding of oocysts. Oocysts sporulate in feces and soil and differentiate into sporocysts, which contain sporozoites. These are ingested by intermediate hosts, such as birds, mice or humans, and develop in the intermediate host to complete the life cycle.

T. gondii has two stages in tissue, tachyzoites and bradyzoites, both crescent shaped and 2×6 μm. In acute infection, tachyzoites multiply rapidly to form "groups" within intracellular vacuoles of parasitized cells, eventually causing the cells to rupture. Tachyzoites spread from the gut through lymphatics to regional lymph nodes, and through the blood to the liver, lungs, heart, brain and other organs. During chronic infection, the organisms, now called "bradyzoites," multiply slowly. The bradyzoites store PAS-positive material, and hundreds of organisms are tightly packed in "cysts." The cysts originate in intracellular vacuoles, enlarge beyond the usual size of the cell and push the nucleus to the periphery.

Except for congenital infection, toxoplasmosis is acquired by eating infectious forms of the organism. In the tropics, where infection is generally acquired in childhood, oocysts in contaminated soil are the main source of infection. In developed countries, the major mechanism of infection is eating incompletely cooked meat (lamb and pork) that carries *Toxoplasma* tissue cysts. Another source of infection is cat feces; oocysts contaminate the hands and food of people who live in close proximity to cats. **Congenital infection** is acquired by transplacental transmission of infectious forms from an acutely infected (usually asymptomatic) mother to the fetus.

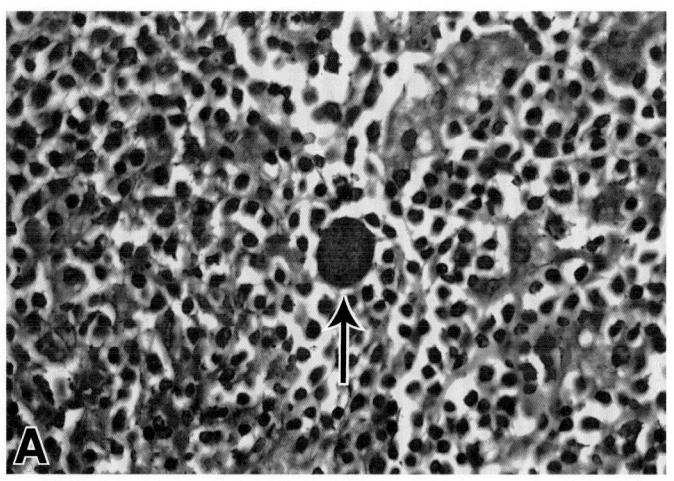
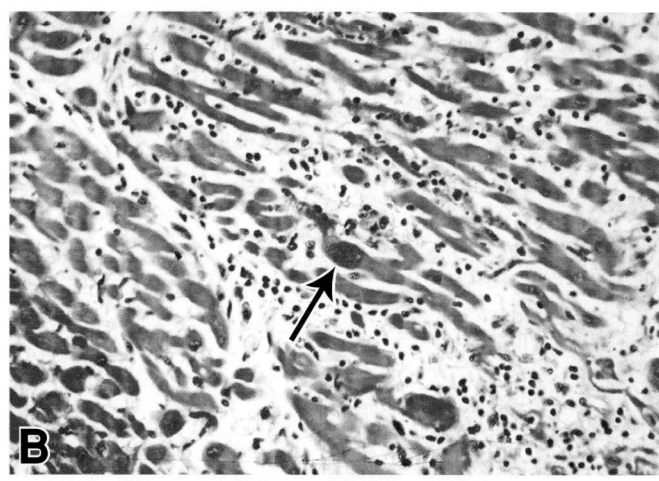

FIGURE 9-72. Toxoplasmosis. A. A photomicrograph of an enlarged lymph node reveals bradyzoites of *Toxoplasma gondii* within a cyst (*arrow*). **B.** A section of heart shows a cyst of bradyzoites of *T. gondii* within a myofiber (*arrow*), with edema and inflammatory cells in the adjacent tissue.

The active infection is usually terminated by the development of cell-mediated immune responses. In most *T. gondii* infections, little significant tissue destruction occurs before the immune response brings the active phase of the infection under control, and those infected suffer few clinical effects. *T. gondii* establishes latent infection, however, by forming dormant tissue cysts in some infected cells. These survive for decades in host cells. If an infected individual loses cell-mediated immunity, the organism can emerge from its encysted form and reestablish a destructive infection.

Toxoplasma Lymphadenopathy Occurs in Immunocompetent Persons

PATHOLOGY: The most common manifestation of *T. gondii* infection in immunocompetent hosts is lymphadenopathy (see Chapter 26). Virtually any lymph node group may be involved, but enlarged cervical nodes are most readily apparent. The histologic appearance of affected lymph nodes is distinctive, with numerous epithelioid macrophages surrounding and encroaching on reactive germinal centers.

CLINICAL FEATURES: In *Toxoplasma* lymphadenitis (Fig. 9-72A), patients present with nontender regional lymph node enlargement, sometimes accompanied by fever, sore throat, hepatosplenomegaly and circulating atypical lymphocytes. Hepatitis, myocarditis (Fig. 9-72B) and myositis have been documented. Lymphadenopathy usually resolves spontaneously in several weeks to several months, and therapy is seldom required.

Congenital *Toxoplasma* Infections Principally Affect the Brain

T. gondii infection in a fetus is far more destructive than is postnatal infection (see Chapter 6).

PATHOLOGY: The fetus lacks the immunologic capacity to contain *T. gondii* infection. The developing brain and eye are readily infected, leading to a necrotizing meningoencephalitis, which in the most severe cases causes loss of brain parenchyma, cerebral calcifications

(Fig. 9-73) and marked hydrocephalus. Ocular infection results in chorioretinitis (i.e., necrosis and inflammation of the choroid and retina).

CLINICAL FEATURES: The most severe fetal disease is associated with infection early in pregnancy and often terminates in spontaneous abortion. In infants born with congenital toxoplasmosis, the effects of brain involvement range from severe mental retardation and seizures to subtle psychomotor defects. Ocular involvement may cause congenital visual impairment. Latent ocular infection established in utero may also recrudesce later in life to produce visual loss. Some newborns have *Toxoplasma* hepatitis, with large areas of necrosis and giant cells. Adrenal necrosis is also occasionally observed. Congenital toxoplasmosis requires therapy with antiprotozoal agents.

Toxoplasmosis in Immunocompromised Hosts Produces Encephalitis

Devastating *T. gondii* infections occur in people with impaired cell-mediated immunity (e.g., patients with AIDS or receiving immunosuppressive therapy). In most cases, the

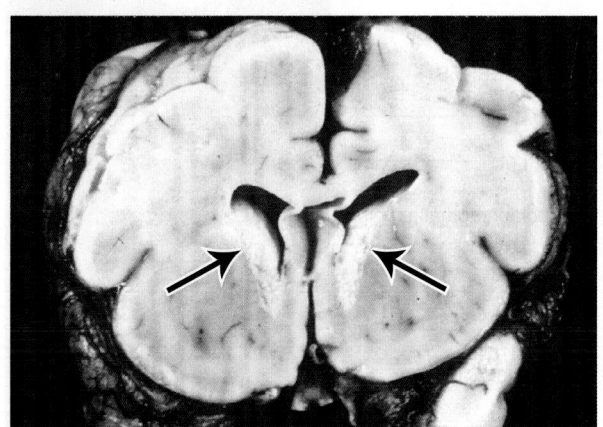

FIGURE 9-73. Congenital toxoplasmosis. The brain of a premature infant reveals subependymal necrosis with calcification appearing as bilaterally symmetric areas of whitish discoloration (*arrows*).

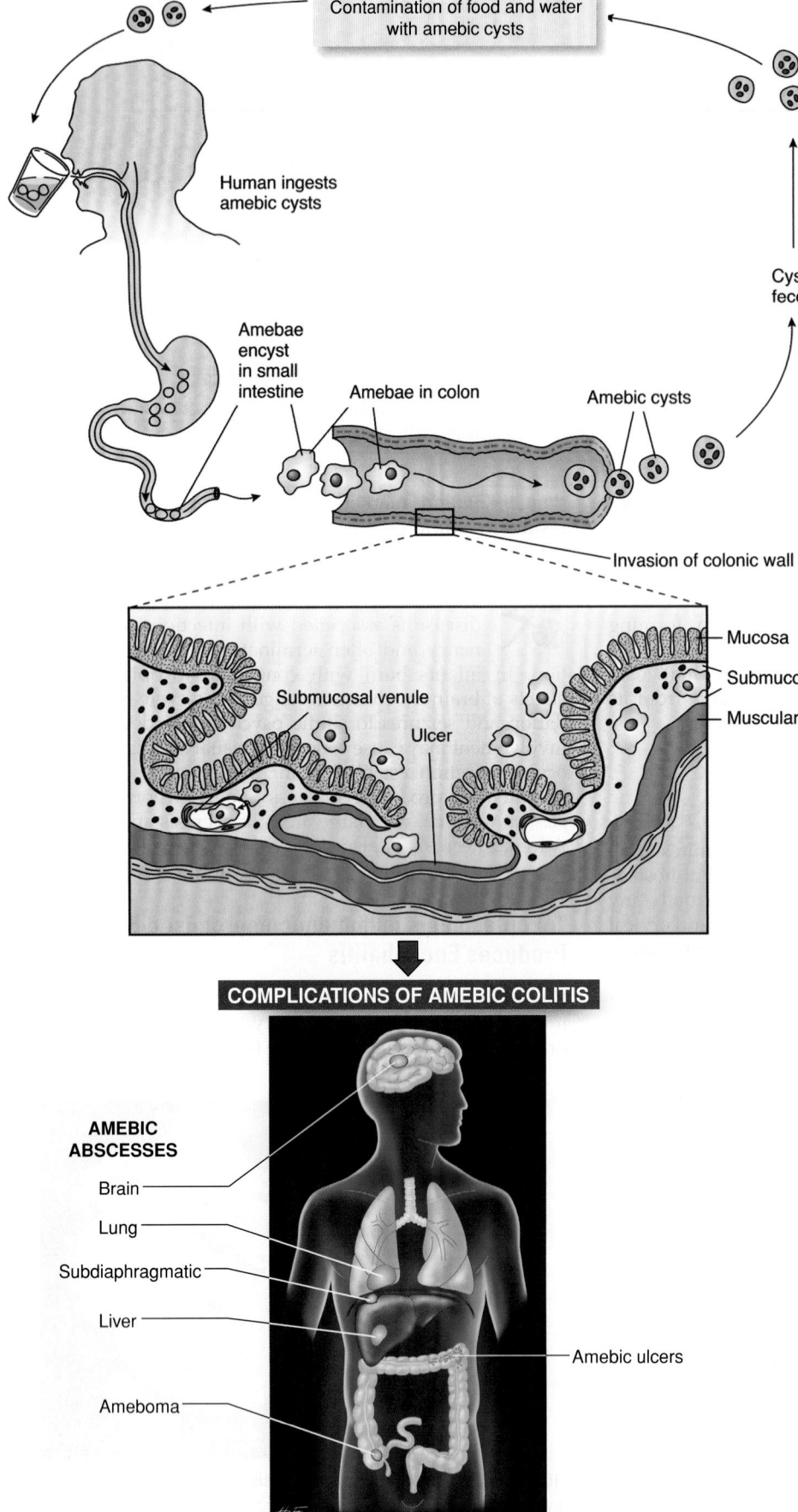

Contamination of food and water
with amebic cysts

Human ingests
amebic cysts

Cysts in
feces

Amebae
encyst
in small
intestine

Amebae in colon

Amebic cysts

Invasion of colonic wall

Mucosa

Submucosa

Muscularis

Submucosal venule

Ulcer

COMPLICATIONS OF AMEBIC COLITIS

**AMEBIC
ABSCESSES**

Brain

Lung

Subdiaphragmatic

Liver

Ameboma

Amebic ulcers

FIGURE 9-74. Amebic colitis and its complications. Amebiasis results from the ingestion of food or water contaminated with amebic cysts. In the colon, the amebae penetrate the mucosa and produce flask-shaped ulcers of the mucosa and submucosa. The organisms may invade submucosal venules, thereby disseminating the infection to the liver and other organs. The liver abscess can expand to involve adjacent structures.

disease reflects reactivation of a latent infection. The brain is most commonly affected, and infection with *T. gondii* produces a multifocal necrotizing encephalitis. Patients with encephalitis present with paresis, seizures, alterations in visual acuity and changes in mentation. *Toxoplasma* encephalitis in immunocompromised patients is fatal if not treated with antiprotozoal agents.

AMEBIASIS

Amebiasis is infection with *Entamoeba histolytica*, which principally involves the colon and occasionally refers to the liver. The parasite is named for its lytic actions on tissue. Intestinal infection ranges from asymptomatic colonization to severe invasive infection with bloody diarrhea. On occasion, the organisms spread beyond the colon to involve other organs. The most common site of extraintestinal disease is the liver, where *E. histolytica* causes slowly expanding, necrotizing abscesses.

 EPIDEMIOLOGY: Humans are the only known reservoir for *E. histolytica,* which reproduces in the colon and passes in the feces. Although amebiasis is found worldwide, it is more common and more severe in tropical and subtropical areas, where poor sanitation prevails. *Amebiasis is acquired by ingestion of materials contaminated with human feces.*

 **ETIOLOGIC FACTORS:** *E. histolytica* has three distinct stages: the trophozoite, the precyst and the cyst.

Amebic trophozoites, 10–60 μm across, are found in stools of patients with acute symptoms. They are spherical or oval and have a thin cell membrane, a single nucleus, condensed chromatin on the interior of the nuclear membrane and a central karyosome. The trophozoites sometimes contain phagocytosed erythrocytes. PAS stains the cytoplasm of the trophozoites and makes them stand out in tissue sections. In the colon, trophozoites develop into cysts through an intermediate form, the **precyst.** During this process, trophozoites stop feeding, become round and nonmotile, lose some digestive vacuoles and form glycogen masses and chromatoidal bodies.

Amebic cysts are the infecting stage and are found only in stools, since they do not invade tissue. They are spherical, have thick walls, measure 5–25 μm across and usually have four nuclei. From the stools, the cysts contaminate water, food or fingers (Fig. 9-74). On ingestion, cysts traverse the stomach and excyst in the lower ileum. A metacystic ameba containing four nuclei divides to form four small, immature trophozoites, which then grow to full size. These organisms thrive in the colon and feed on bacteria and human cells. They may colonize any part of the large bowel, but the cecum is most affected. Patients with symptomatic amebic colitis pass both cysts and trophozoites. The latter survive only briefly outside the body and are also destroyed by gastric secretions. Host factors, such as nutritional status, coexistent colonic flora and immunologic status, also affect the course of *E. histolytica* infection. Invasion begins with attachment of a trophozoite to a colonic epithelial cell. The parasite kills target cells by elaborating a lytic protein that breaches the cell membrane. Progressive death of mucosal cells produces a superficial ulcer.

Intestinal Amebiasis Is an Ulcerating Disease of the Colon

 PATHOLOGY: Amebic lesions begin as small foci of necrosis that progress to ulcers (Fig. 9-75A). Undermining of the ulcer margin and confluence of expanding ulcers lead to irregular sloughing of the mucosa. The ulcer bed is gray and necrotic, with fibrin and cellular debris. The exudate raises the undermined mucosa, producing chronic amebic ulcers, whose shape has been described as resembling a flask or a bottle neck.

Trophozoites are found on the ulcer surface, in the exudate and in the crater (Fig. 9-75B). They are also frequent in the submucosa, muscularis propria, serosa and small veins of the submucosa. There is little inflammatory response in early amebic ulcers. However, as the ulcers enlarge, acute and chronic inflammatory cells accumulate.

An **ameboma** is an infrequent complication of amebiasis, occurring when amebae invade through the intestinal wall. It is an inflammatory thickening of the bowel wall that resembles colon cancer and tends to form a "napkin-ring constriction." It consists of granulation tissue, fibrosis and clusters of trophozoites.

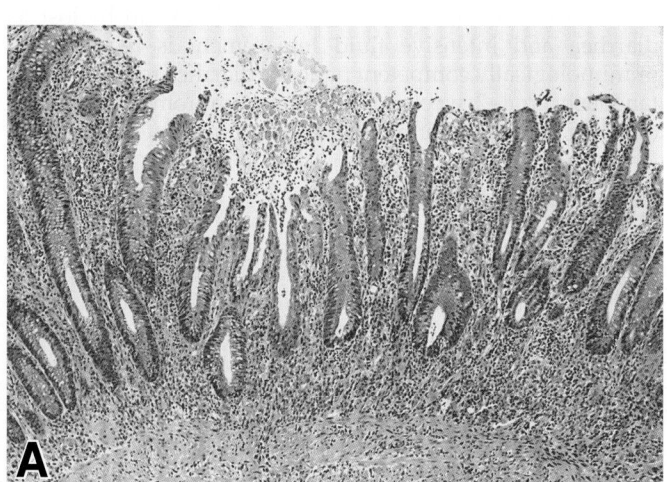

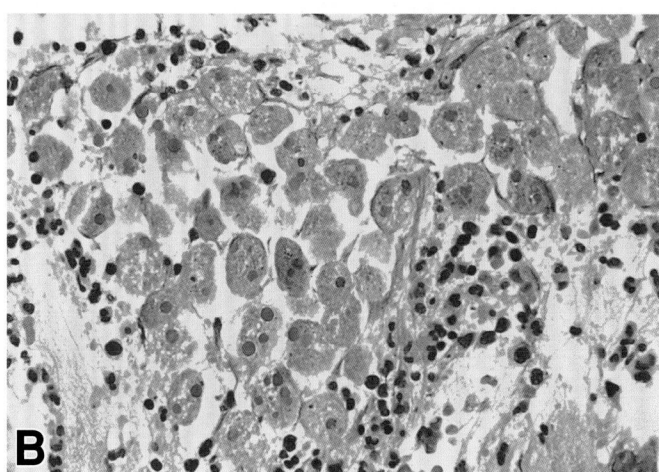

FIGURE 9-75. Intestinal amebiasis. A. The colonic mucosa shows superficial ulceration beneath a cluster of trophozoites of *Entamoeba histolytica.* The lamina propria contains excess acute and chronic inflammatory cells, including eosinophils. **B.** Higher-power view shows numerous trophozoites in the luminal exudate.

CLINICAL FEATURES: Intestinal amebiasis ranges from completely asymptomatic to a severe dysenteric disease. The incubation period for acute amebic colitis is 8–10 days. Gradually increasing abdominal discomfort, tenderness and cramps are accompanied by chills and fever. Nausea, vomiting, malodorous flatus and intermittent constipation are typical features. Liquid stools (up to 25 a day) contain bloody mucus, but diarrhea is rarely prolonged enough to cause dehydration. Amebic colitis often persists for months or years, and patients may become emaciated and anemic. Clinical features are often bizarre and sometimes must be differentiated from those of appendicitis, cholecystitis, intestinal obstruction or diverticulitis. In severe amebic colitis, massive destruction of colonic mucosa may lead to fatal hemorrhage, perforation or peritonitis. Therapy for intestinal amebiasis includes metronidazole, which acts against trophozoites, and diloxanide, which is effective against cysts.

Amebic Liver Abscess Is a Major Complication of Intestinal Amebiasis

 PATHOLOGY: E. histolytica trophozoites that have invaded submucosal veins of the colon enter the portal circulation and reach the liver. Here the organisms kill hepatocytes, producing a slowly expanding necrotic cavity, which is filled with a dark brown, odorless, semisolid material, reported to resemble "anchovy paste" in color and consistency (Fig. 9-76). Neutrophils are rare within the cavity and trophozoites are found along the edges adjacent to hepatocytes.

Amebic liver abscesses may expand or rupture through the capsule. In the latter case, infestation extends into the peritoneum, diaphragm, pleural cavity, lungs or pericardium. Rarely, a liver abscess, or even a lesion in the colon, may spread amebae to the brain by a hematogenous route to form large necrotic lesions.

 CLINICAL FEATURES: Patients with amebic liver abscess present with severe right upper quadrant pain, low-grade fever and weight loss. Only a minority of patients give a history of an antecedent diarrheal

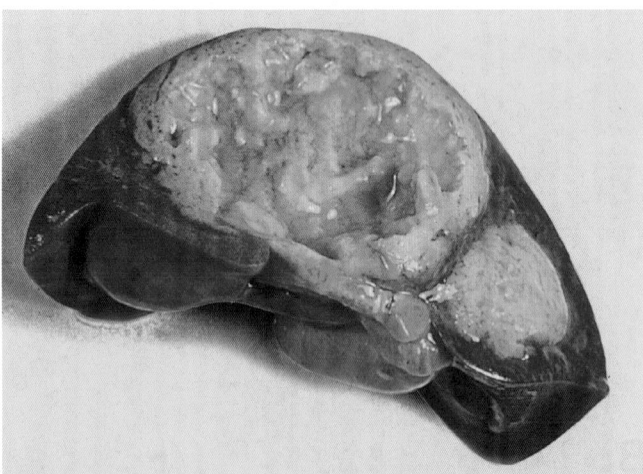

FIGURE 9-76. Amebic abscesses of the liver. The cut surface of the liver shows multiple abscesses containing "anchovy paste" material.

illness, and E. histolytica is demonstrated in the feces of less than one third of patients with extraintestinal disease. The diagnosis is usually made by radiologic or ultrasound demonstration of the abscess, in conjunction with serologic testing for antibodies to E. histolytica. Amebic abscess is treated by percutaneous or surgical drainage and antiamebic drugs.

CRYPTOSPORIDIOSIS

Cryptosporidiosis is an enteric infection with protozoa of the genus Cryptosporidium that cause diarrhea in persons with compromised immunity. The infection varies from a self-limited gastrointestinal infection to a potentially life-threatening illness. It is acquired by ingesting Cryptosporidium oocysts, which are shed in feces of infected humans and animals. Most infections probably result from person-to-person transmission, but many domesticated animals harbor the parasite and are a reservoir for human infection.

 **ETIOLOGIC FACTORS AND PATHOLOGY:** Cryptosporidium oocysts survive passage through the stomach and release forms that attach to the microvillous surface of the small bowel. Unlike Toxoplasma and other coccidia, Cryptosporidia remain extracellular. They reproduce on the luminal surface of the gut, from stomach to rectum, forming progeny that also attach to the epithelium.

In immunocompetent people, infection is terminated by immune responses. Patients with AIDS and some congenital immunodeficiencies cannot contain the parasite and develop chronic infections, which may spread from the bowel to involve the gallbladder and intrahepatic bile ducts.

Cryptosporidiosis produces no grossly visible alterations. The organisms are visible microscopically as round, 2–4-μm blebs attached to the luminal surface of the epithelium (Fig. 9-77). In the small intestine, moderate or severe chronic inflammation in the lamina propria and villous atrophy are directly related to the density of the parasites. The colon has a chronic active colitis, with minimal architectural disruption.

 CLINICAL FEATURES: Cryptosporidiosis presents as a profuse, watery diarrhea, sometimes accompanied by cramping abdominal pain or low-grade fever. Extraordinary volumes of fluid can be lost as diarrhea and intensive fluid replacement is required. In immunologically competent patients, diarrhea resolves spontaneously in 1–2 weeks. In immunocompromised persons, diarrhea persists indefinitely and may contribute to death.

GIARDIASIS

Giardiasis is an infection of the small intestine caused by the flagellated protozoan Giardia lamblia and is characterized by abdominal cramping and diarrhea.

 **EPIDEMIOLOGY:** G. lamblia has a worldwide distribution, with a prevalence of infection from less than 1% to more than 25% in some areas with warmer climates and crowded, unsanitary environments. Children are more susceptible than adults. Giardiasis is acquired by ingesting infectious cyst forms of the organism, which are shed in the feces of infected humans and animals.

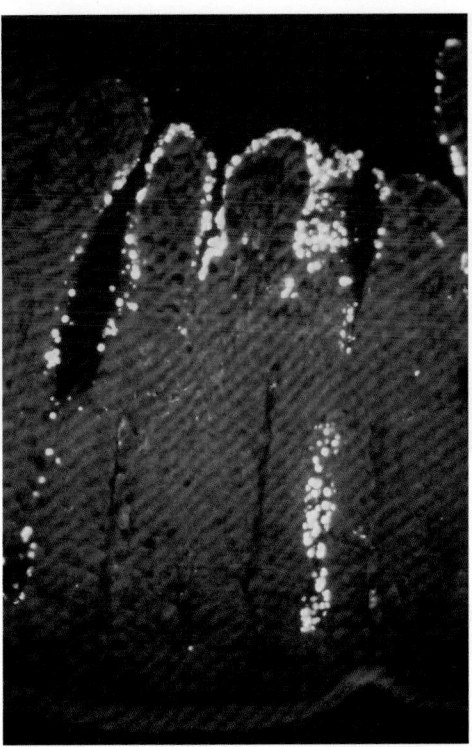

FIGURE 9-77. Cryptosporidiosis. A small intestinal biopsy stained with fluorescent antibody to *Cryptosporidium parvum* shows numerous sporozoites covering the villi and lining the crypts.

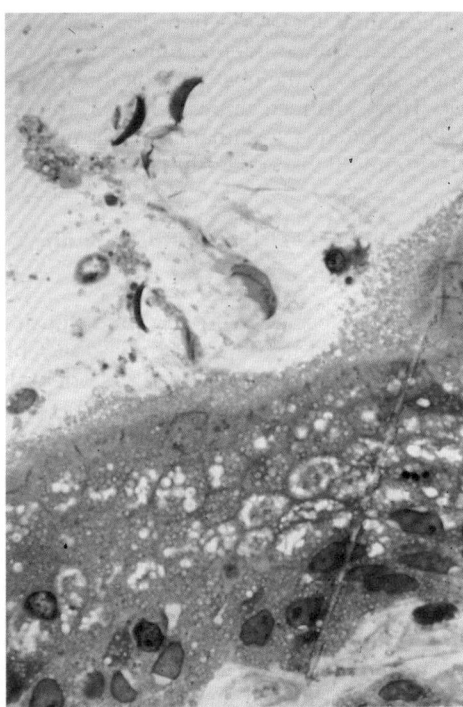

FIGURE 9-78. Giardiasis. Crescent-shaped trophozoites of *Giardia lamblia* are present overlying the small intestinal mucosa.

Infection spreads directly from person to person and also in contaminated water or food. *Giardia* can be acquired from wilderness water sources, where infected animals, such as beavers and bears, serve as the reservoir of infection. Infection may be epidemic, and outbreaks have occurred in orphanages and institutions.

 **ETIOLOGIC FACTORS AND PATHOLOGY:** *G. lamblia* has two stages: trophozoites and cysts. The former are flat, pear-shaped, binucleate organisms with 4 pairs of flagella. They are most numerous in the duodenum and proximal small intestine. A curved, disc-like "sucker plate" on their ventral surface aids mucosal attachment. Ingested cysts contain 2 or 4 nuclei and revert to trophozoites on reaching the intestine. The stools usually contain only cysts, but trophozoites may also be present in patients with diarrhea.

Giardia cysts survive gastric acidity and rupture in the duodenum and jejunum to release trophozoites. These attach to small bowel epithelial microvilli and reproduce. Giardiasis produces no grossly visible alterations. Microscopic examination shows minimal associated mucosal changes, with crescentic or semilunar-shaped *Giardia* trophozoites on villous surfaces and within crypts (Fig. 9-78).

 CLINICAL FEATURES: *G. lamblia* is usually a harmless commensal, but can cause acute or chronic symptoms. Acute giardiasis occurs with abrupt onset of abdominal cramping and frequent, foul-smelling stools. The infection is highly variable. In some patients, symptoms resolve spontaneously in 1–4 weeks. Others complain of persistent abdominal cramping and

poorly formed stools for months. In children, chronic giardiasis may cause malabsorption, weight loss and retarded growth. The infection is treated effectively with various antibiotics, including metronidazole.

LEISHMANIASIS

Leishmaniae are protozoans that are transmitted to humans by insect bites and cause a spectrum of clinical syndromes, from indolent, self-resolving cutaneous ulcers to fatal disseminated disease. There are numerous *Leishmania* species, which differ in their natural habitats and the types of disease that they produce.

 EPIDEMIOLOGY: Leishmaniasis is transmitted by *Phlebotomus* sandflies, which acquire the infection by feeding on infected animals. In many subtropical and tropical areas, leishmanial infection is endemic in animal populations; dogs, ground squirrels, foxes and jackals are reservoirs and potential sources for transmission to humans. It is mainly a disease of less developed countries where humans live in close proximity to animal hosts and the fly vector. There are estimated to be 20 million people infected worldwide.

 **ETIOLOGIC FACTORS:** Infection begins when the organisms are inoculated into human skin by a sandfly bite. Shortly thereafter, leishmaniae are phagocytosed by mononuclear phagocytes and transformed into amastigotes, which reproduce within the macrophage. Daughter amastigotes eventually rupture from the cell and spread to other macrophages. Reproduction continues in this way, and eventually a cluster of infected macrophages forms at the site of inoculation.

From this initial local infection, the disease may take widely divergent courses depending on two factors: the immunologic status of the host and the infecting species of *Leishmania*. Three distinct clinical entities are recognized: (1) localized cutaneous leishmaniasis, (2) mucocutaneous leishmaniasis and (3) visceral leishmaniasis.

Localized Cutaneous Leishmaniasis Is an Ulcerating Disorder

Several *Leishmania* species in Central and South America, Northern Africa, the Middle East, India and China cause a localized skin disease, also known as "oriental sore" or "tropical sore."

 PATHOLOGY: Localized cutaneous leishmaniasis begins as a collection of amastigote-filled macrophages that ulcerates the overlying epidermis. In tissue sections, the oval amastigotes measure 2 μm and contain two internal structures, a nucleus and a kinetoplast. Amastigotes in macrophages appear as multiple regular cytoplasmic dots, **Leishman-Donovan bodies**. With progressive development of cell-mediated immunity, macrophages are activated and kill the intracellular parasites. The lesion slowly becomes a more mature granuloma, with epithelioid macrophages, Langhans giant cells, plasma cells and lymphocytes. Over the course of months, the cutaneous ulcer heals spontaneously.

 CLINICAL FEATURES: Cutaneous leishmaniasis begins as an itching, solitary papule, which erodes to form a shallow ulcer with a sharp, raised border. This ulcer can grow to 6–8 cm in diameter. Satellite lesions develop along draining lymphatics. The ulcers begin to resolve at 3–6 months, but healing may take a year or longer.

Diffuse cutaneous leishmaniasis develops in some patients who lack specific cell-mediated immune responses to leishmaniae. The disease begins as a single nodule, but adjacent satellite nodules slowly form, eventually involving much of the skin. These lesions so closely resemble lepromatous leprosy that some patients have been cared for in leprosaria. The nodule of anergic leishmaniasis is caused by enormous numbers of macrophages replete with leishmaniae.

Mucocutaneous Leishmaniasis Is a Late Complication of Cutaneous Leishmaniasis

Mucocutaneous leishmaniasis is caused by infection with *Leishmania braziliensis*. Most cases occur in Central and South America, where rodents and sloths are reservoirs.

  PATHOLOGY AND CLINICAL FEATURES: The early course and pathologic changes of mucocutaneous leishmaniasis are like those of localized cutaneous leishmaniasis. A solitary ulcer appears, expands and resolves. Years afterward, an ulcer develops at a mucocutaneous junction, such as the larynx, nasal septum, anus or vulva. The mucosal lesion progresses slowly, is highly destructive and disfiguring and erodes mucosal surfaces and cartilage (Fig. 9-79). Destruction of the nasal septum sometimes produces a "tapir nose" deformity. The patient may die if the ulcers obstruct the airways. Mucocutaneous leishmaniasis requires treatment with systemic antiprotozoal agents.

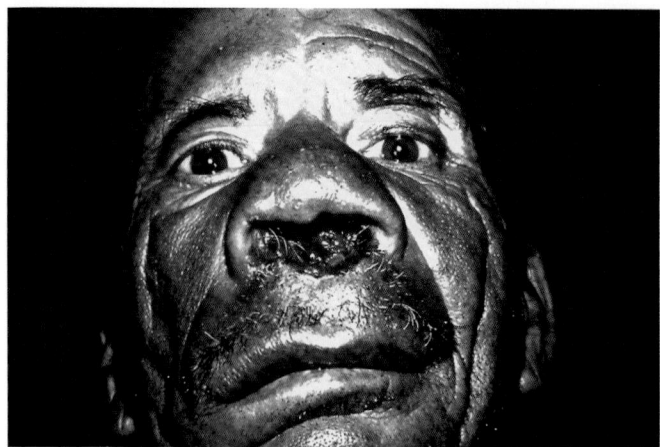

FIGURE 9-79. Mucocutaneous leishmaniasis. There is complete destruction of the basal septum and mucocutaneous ulceration.

Visceral Leishmaniasis (Kala Azar) Is a Potentially Fatal Infection

 **EPIDEMIOLOGY:** Kala azar is produced by several subspecies of *Leishmania donovani*. Reservoirs of the agent and susceptible age groups vary in different parts of the world. Humans are the reservoir in India, and foxes in southern France and central Italy. Other canine and rodent species are reservoirs elsewhere in the world.

 PATHOLOGY: Infection with *L. donovani* begins with localized collections of infected macrophages at the site of a sandfly bite (Fig. 9-80); these spread the organisms throughout the mononuclear phagocyte system. *L. donovani* are mostly destroyed by cell-mediated immune responses, but 5% of patients develop visceral leishmaniasis. Children and malnourished people are especially susceptible. The liver (Fig. 9-81A), spleen and lymph nodes become massively enlarged, as macrophages in these organs fill with proliferating leishmanial amastigotes (Fig. 9-81B). Normal organ architecture is gradually replaced by sheets of parasitized macrophages. Eventually, these cells accumulate in other organs, including the heart and kidney.

 CLINICAL FEATURES: Patients with visceral leishmaniasis have persistent fever, progressive weight loss, hepatosplenomegaly, anemia, thrombocytopenia and leukopenia. Light-skinned people develop darkening of the skin; the Hindi name for leishmaniasis, *kala azar*, means "black sickness." Over the course of months, a patient with visceral leishmaniasis becomes profoundly cachectic and exhibits massive splenomegaly. The untreated disease is invariably fatal. Treatment entails systemic antiprotozoal therapy.

CHAGAS DISEASE (AMERICAN TRYPANOSOMIASIS)

Chagas disease is an insect-borne, zoonotic infection by the protozoan *Trypanosoma cruzi*, which causes a systemic infection of humans. Acute manifestations and long-term sequelae occur in the heart and gastrointestinal tract.

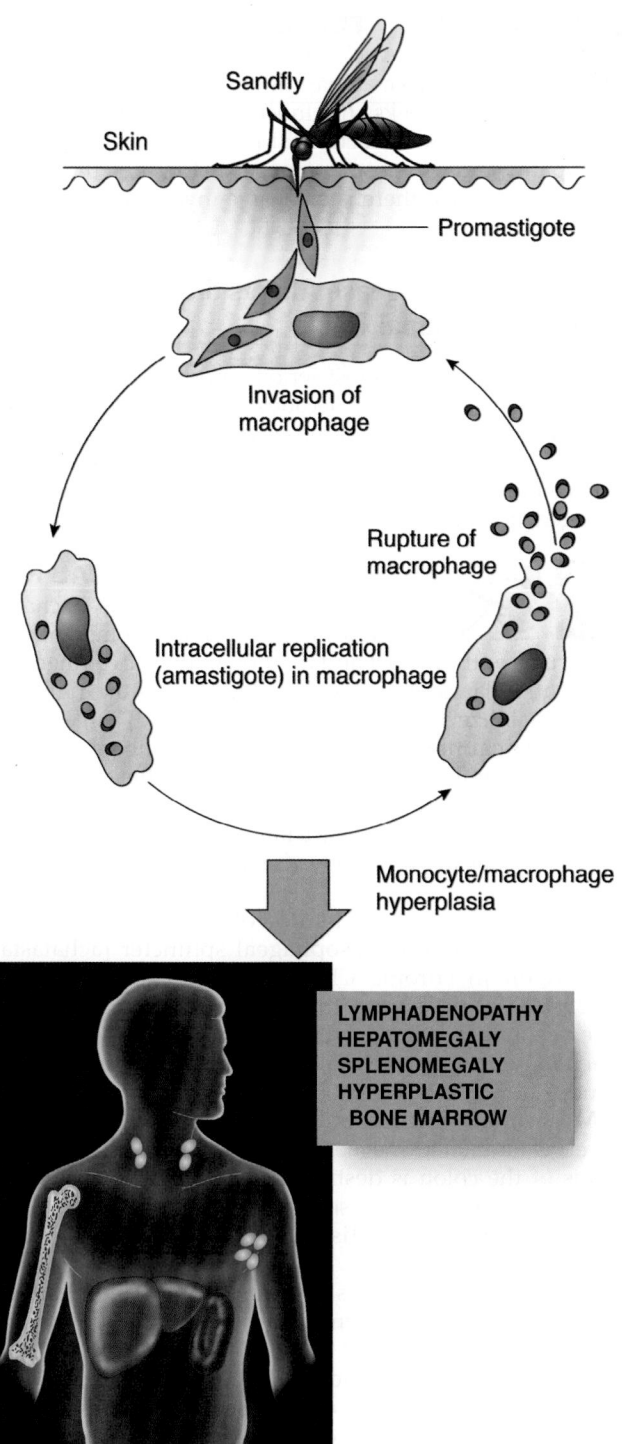

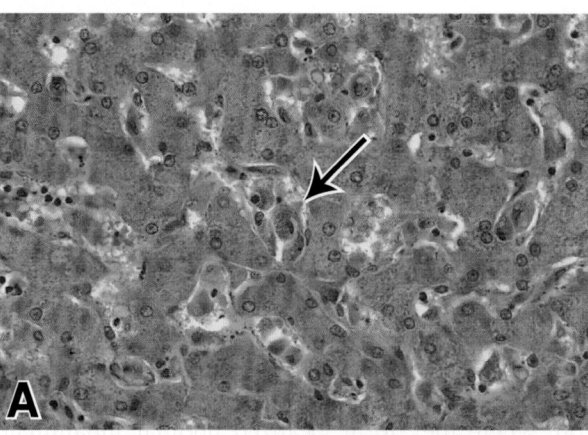

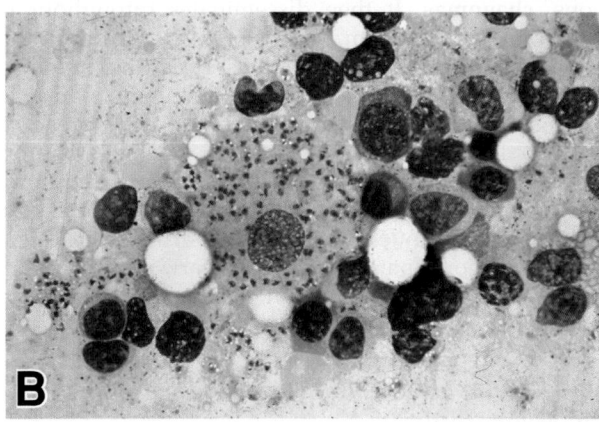

FIGURE 9-81. Visceral leishmaniasis. A. A photomicrograph of an enlarged liver shows prominent Kupffer cells distended by leishmanial amastigotes (*arrows*). **B.** A bone marrow aspirate from a patient with visceral leishmaniasis. Numerous leishmanial amastigotes are present, some of which are intracytoplasmic.

LYMPHADENOPATHY
HEPATOMEGALY
SPLENOMEGALY
HYPERPLASTIC
BONE MARROW

FIGURE 9-80. Leishmaniasis. Blood-sucking sandflies ingest amastigotes from an infected host. These are transformed in the sandfly gut into promastigotes, which multiply and are injected into the next vertebrate host. There they invade macrophages, revert to the amastigote form and multiply, eventually rupturing the cell. They then invade other macrophages, thus completing the cycle.

humans and infected bugs, usually in mud or thatched dwellings of the rural and suburban poor. The bugs emerge at night and feed on sleeping victims. Congenital infection occurs upon passage of the parasite from mother to fetus. It is estimated that some 20 million people are infected with *T. cruzi*, more than half of them in Brazil. It is present in 18 nations on the American continents, with an estimated 300,000 infected people residing in the United States. Although exact figures are not known, it is thought that up to 50,000 deaths are attributable to Chagas disease every year.

 ETIOLOGIC FACTORS: Infective forms of *T. cruzi* are discharged in the feces of the reduviid bug as it takes its blood meal. Itching and scratching promote contamination of the wound. The trypomastigotes penetrate at the site of the bite or at other abrasions, or may enter the mucosa of the eyes or lips. Once inside the body, they lose their flagella and undulating membranes, round up to become amastigotes and enter macrophages, where they undergo repeated divisions. Amastigotes also invade other sites, including cardiac myocytes and brain. Within host cells, amastigotes differentiate into trypomastigotes, which break out and enter the bloodstream (Fig. 9-82). Ingested in a subsequent bite of a reduviid bug, trypomastigotes multiply in the insect's alimentary tract and differentiate into metacyclic trypomastigotes, which congregate in the rectum of the bug and are discharged in the feces.

EPIDEMIOLOGY: *T. cruzi* infection is endemic in wild and domesticated animals (e.g., rats, dogs, goats, cats, armadillos) in Central and South America, where it is transmitted by the reduviid ("kissing") bug. Infection with *T. cruzi* is promoted by contact between

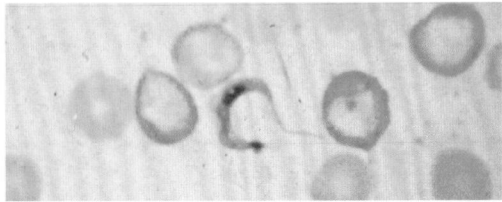

FIGURE 9-82. Chagas disease. A blood smear demonstrates a trypomastigote of *Trypanosoma cruzi* with its characteristic "C" shape, flagellum, nucleus and terminal kinetoplast.

T. cruzi infects and reproduces in cells at sites of inoculation, where they form localized nodular inflammatory lesions, **chagomas.** It then disseminates throughout the body via the bloodstream. Strains of *T. cruzi* differ in their predominant target cells; infections of cardiac myocytes, gastrointestinal ganglion cells and meninges cause the most significant disease. Parasitemia and widespread cellular infection are responsible for the systemic symptoms of acute Chagas disease. The onset of cell-mediated immunity eliminates the acute manifestations, but chronic tissue damage may continue. Progressive destruction of cells at sites of infection—particularly the heart, esophagus and colon—causes organ dysfunction, manifested decades after the acute infection.

Acute Chagas Disease May Cause Fatal Myocarditis

PATHOLOGY: *T. cruzi* circulates in the blood as a 20-μm long, curved flagellate that is easily recognized on blood films. Within infected cells, it reproduces as a nonflagellated amastigote, 2–4 μm in diameter. In fatal cases, the heart is enlarged and dilated, with a pale, focally hemorrhagic myocardium. Many parasites are seen in the heart, and amastigotes are evident within pseudocysts in myofibers (Fig. 9-83). There is extensive chronic inflammation and phagocytosis of parasites is conspicuous.

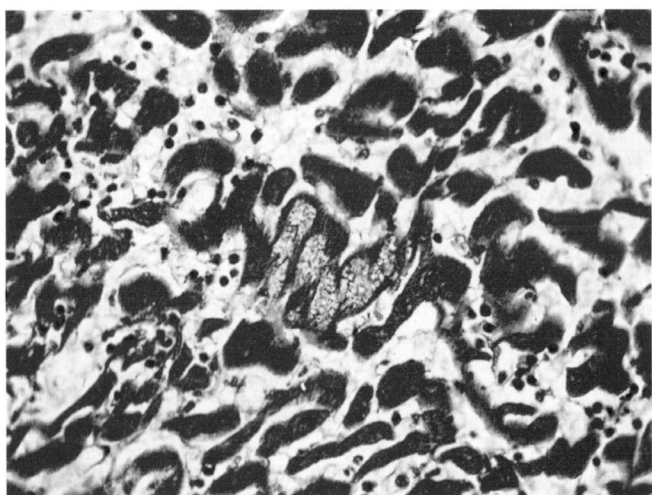

FIGURE 9-83. Acute Chagas myocarditis. The myofibers in the center contain numerous amastigotes of *Trypanosoma cruzi* and are surrounded by edema and chronic inflammation.

CLINICAL FEATURES: Acute symptoms develop 1–2 weeks after inoculation with *T. cruzi*. A chagoma (see above) develops at the site. Parasitemia appears 2–3 weeks after inoculation, usually associated with a mild illness characterized by fever, malaise, lymphadenopathy and hepatosplenomegaly. However, the disease can be lethal when there is extensive myocardial or meningeal involvement.

Chronic Chagas Disease Affects the Heart and Gastrointestinal Tract

The most frequent and most serious consequences of *T. cruzi* infection develop years or decades after acute infection. It is estimated that up to 40% of those acutely infected eventually develop chronic disease. In this phase of the illness, *T. cruzi* is no longer present in blood or tissue. Infected organs have been damaged, however, by chronic, progressive inflammation.

PATHOLOGY AND CLINICAL FEATURES: Chronic myocarditis is characterized by a dilated heart, prominent right ventricular outflow tract and dilation of the valve rings. The interventricular septum is often deviated to the right and may immobilize the adjacent tricuspid leaflet. There is extensive interstitial fibrosis, hypertrophied myofibers and focal lymphocytic inflammation, often involving the cardiac conduction system. Progressive cardiac fibrosis causes dysrhythmia or congestive heart failure. In endemic regions, chronic Chagas disease is a leading cause of heart failure in young adults.

Megaesophagus (i.e., dilation of the esophagus caused by failure of the lower esophageal sphincter [achalasia]) is common in chronic Chagas disease. It results from destruction of parasympathetic ganglia in the wall of the lower esophagus and leads to difficulty in swallowing, which may be so severe that the patient can consume only liquids.

Megacolon, which refers to massive dilation of the large bowel, is similar to megaesophagus in that the myenteric plexus of the colon is destroyed. The progressive aganglionosis of the colon causes severe constipation.

Congenital Chagas disease occurs in some pregnant women with parasitemia. Infection of the placenta and fetus leads to spontaneous abortion. In the infrequent live births, the infants die of encephalitis within a few days or weeks.

Antiprotozoal chemotherapy is effective for acute Chagas disease but not for its chronic sequelae. Cardiac transplantation has been effective in a number of patients.

AFRICAN TRYPANOSOMIASIS

African trypanosomiasis, popularly termed **sleeping sickness,** is an infection with *Trypanosoma brucei gambiense* or *Trypanosoma brucei rhodesiense* that leads to life-threatening meningoencephalitis. Gambian trypanosomiasis is a chronic infection often lasting more than a year. By contrast, East African (Rhodesian) trypanosomiasis is a rapidly progressive infection that kills the patient in 3–6 months. The organisms are curved flagellates, 15–30 μm in length. Although they can be demonstrated in blood or cerebrospinal fluid, they are difficult to find in infected tissues.

 **EPIDEMIOLOGY:** *T. brucei gambiense* and *T. brucei rhodesiense* are hemoflagellate protozoa that are transmitted by several species of blood-sucking tsetse flies of the genus *Glossina*. The patchy distribution of African trypanosomiasis is related to the habitats of these flies. In Gambian trypanosomiasis, *T. brucei gambiense* is transmitted by tsetse flies of the riverine bush, mainly in endemic pockets of West and Central Africa. ***Humans are the only important reservoir for this trypanosome.***

In East African trypanosomiasis, *T. brucei rhodesiense* is spread by tsetse flies of the woodland savanna of East Africa. Antelope, other game animals and domestic cattle are natural reservoirs of the parasite. Infection of humans is an occupational hazard of game wardens, fishermen and cattle herders.

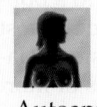 **ETIOLOGIC FACTORS:** While biting an infected animal or human, the tsetse fly ingests trypomastigotes with the blood (Fig. 9-84). These (1) lose their coat of surface antigen, (2) multiply in the midgut of the fly, (3) migrate to the salivary gland, (4) develop for 3 weeks through the epimastigote stage and (5) multiply in the fly's saliva as infective metacyclic trypomastigotes. During another bite, metacyclic trypomastigotes are injected into the lymphatics and blood vessels of a new host. They disseminate to the bone marrow and tissue fluids and some eventually invade the CNS. After replicating by binary fission in blood, lymph and spinal fluid, trypomastigotes are ingested by another fly to complete the cycle.

 PATHOPHYSIOLOGY: African trypanosomiasis involves immune complex formation by variable trypanosomal antigens and antibodies. Autoantibodies to antigens of erythrocytes, brain and heart may participate in the pathogenesis of this disease. The trypanosome evades immune attack in mammals by periodically altering its glycoprotein antigen coat, which occurs in a genetically determined pattern, not by mutation. Thus, each wave of circulating trypomastigotes includes different antigenic variants that are a step ahead of the immune response.

PATHOLOGY: *T. brucei* multiplies at sites of inoculation, occasionally producing localized nodular lesions, termed "primary chancres." Generalized involvement of lymph nodes and spleen is prominent early in the disease. Affected nodes and spleen show foci of lymphocyte and macrophage hyperplasia. Infection eventually localizes to small blood vessels of the CNS, where replicating organisms elicit a destructive vasculitis, producing the progressive decrease in mentation characteristic of sleeping sickness. In *T. brucei rhodesiense* infection, the organisms also localize to blood vessels in the heart, sometimes causing a fulminant myocarditis.

Lesions in the lymph nodes, brain, heart and various other sites (including the inoculation site) show vasculitis of small blood vessels, with endothelial cell hyperplasia and dense perivascular infiltrates of lymphocytes, macrophages and plasma cells. The CNS vasculitis causes destruction of neurons, demyelination and gliosis. The perivascular infiltrate thickens the leptomeninges and involves the Virchow-Robin spaces (Fig. 9-85).

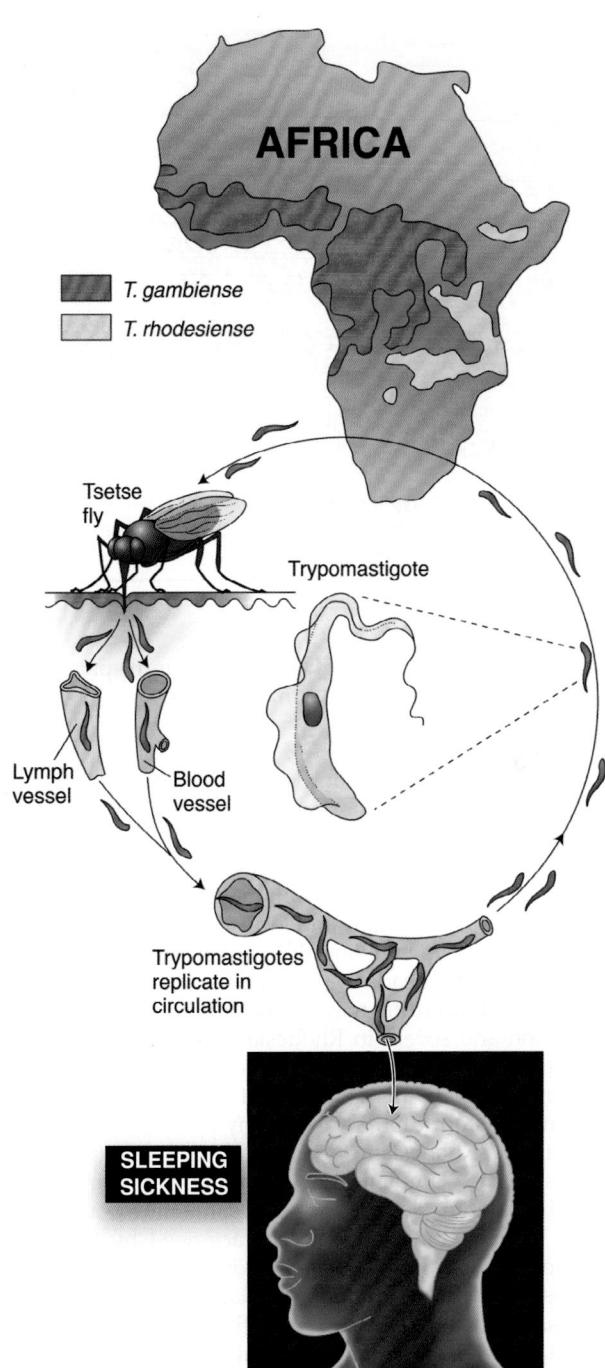

FIGURE 9-84. African trypanosomiasis (sleeping sickness). The distribution of Gambian and Rhodesian trypanosomiasis is related to the habitats of the vector tsetse flies (*Glossina* spp.). A tsetse fly bites an infected animal or human and ingests trypomastigotes, which multiply into infective, metacyclic trypomastigotes. During another fly bite, these are injected into lymphatic and blood vessels of a new host. A primary chancre develops at the site of the bite (stage 1a). Trypomastigotes replicate further in the blood and lymph, causing a systemic infection (stage 1b). Another fly ingests hypomastigotes to complete the cycle. In stage 2, invasion of the central nervous system by trypomastigotes leads to meningoencephalomyelitis and associated symptoms, including lethargy and daytime somnolence. Patients with Rhodesian trypanosomiasis may die within a few months. *T. gambiense* = *Trypanosoma brucei gambiense*; *T. rhodesiense* = *Trypanosoma brucei rhodesiense*.

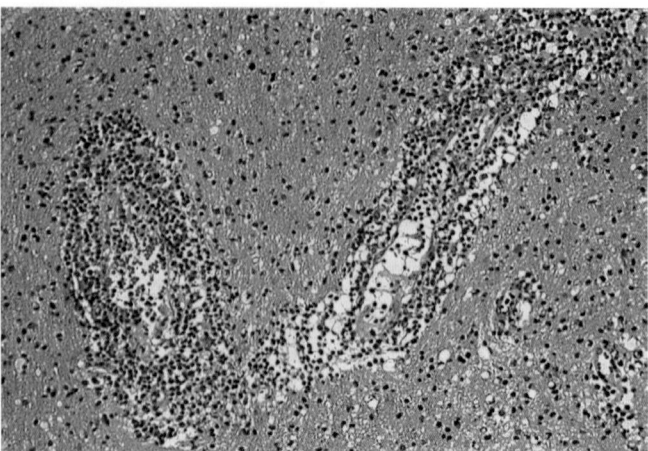

FIGURE 9-85. African trypanosomiasis. A section of brain from a patient who died from infection with *Trypanosoma brucei rhodesiense* shows a perivascular mononuclear cell infiltrate.

CLINICAL FEATURES: African trypanosomiasis is divided into 3 clinical stages:

1. **Primary chancre:** After 5–15 days, a 3–4-cm papillary swelling topped by a central red spot appears at the inoculation site. It subsides spontaneously within 3 weeks.
2. **Systemic infection:** Shortly after the appearance of the chancre (if any) and within 3 weeks of a bite, bloodstream invasion is marked by intermittent fever, for up to a week, often with splenomegaly and local and generalized lymphadenopathy. The evolving illness is marked by remitting irregular fevers, headache, joint pains, lethargy and muscle wasting. Myocarditis may be a complication and is more common and severe in Rhodesian trypanosomiasis. Dysfunction of the lungs, kidneys, liver and endocrine system occurs commonly in both forms of the disease.
3. **Brain invasion:** CNS invasion may occur early (weeks or months) in Rhodesian trypanosomiasis or late (months or years) in the Gambian form. Brain invasion is marked by apathy, daytime somnolence and sometimes coma. A diffuse meningoencephalitis is characterized by tremors of the tongue and fingers; fasciculations of the muscles of the limbs, face, lips and tongue; oscillatory movements of the arms, head, neck and trunk; indistinct speech; and cerebellar ataxia, causing problems in walking.

PRIMARY AMEBIC MENINGOENCEPHALITIS

Amebic meningoencephalitis, caused by *Naegleria fowleri,* is a fatal illness.

EPIDEMIOLOGY: *N. fowleri* is a free-living, soil ameba that inhabits ponds and lakes throughout tropical and subtropical regions but it is reported in temperate areas, including the United States. Primary amebic meningoencephalitis is rare (fewer than 300 reported cases), affecting people who swim or bathe in these waters.

ETIOLOGIC FACTORS AND PATHOLOGY: *N. fowleri* is inoculated into the nasal mucosa near the cribriform plate when a person swims in or dives into water containing high concentrations of the organism. Amebae invade the olfactory nerves, migrate into the olfactory bulbs and then proliferate in the meninges and brain.

The trophozoites are 8–15 μm across, with sharply outlined nuclei that stain deeply with hematoxylin. Grossly, the brain is swollen and soft, with vascular congestion and a purulent meningeal exudate, most prominent over the lateral and basal areas. The amebae invade the brain along the Virchow-Robin spaces and cause massive tissue damage. Thrombosis and destruction of blood vessels are associated with extensive hemorrhage. The olfactory tract and bulbs are enveloped and destroyed, and there is an exudate between the bulb and the inferior surface of the temporal lobe. Proliferation of *Naegleria* in the brain may produce solid masses of amebae (amebomas). Meningitis can extend the full length of the spinal cord.

CLINICAL FEATURES: Primary amebic meningoencephalitis due to *N. fowleri* begins suddenly with fever, nausea, vomiting and headache. Within hours, the patient suffers profound deterioration in mental status. Cerebrospinal fluid contains numerous neutrophils, blood and amebae. The disease is rapidly fatal.

Helminthic Infection

Helminths, or worms, are among the most common human pathogens. At any given time, 25%–50% of the world's population carries at least one helminth species. Although most do little harm, some cause significant disease. Schistosomiasis, for instance, is among the leading global causes of morbidity and mortality.

Helminths are the largest and most complex organisms capable of living within the human body. Their adult forms range from 0.5 mm to over 1 m in length. Most are visible to the naked eye. They are multicellular animals with differentiated tissues, including specialized nervous tissues, digestive tissues and reproductive systems. Their maturation from eggs or larvae to adult worms is complex, often involving multiple morphologic transformations (molts). Some undergo these metamorphoses in different hosts before attaining adulthood, and the human host may be only one in a series that supports this maturation process. Within the human body, the helminths frequently migrate from the port of entry through several organs to a site of final infection.

Most helminths that infect humans are well adapted to human parasitism, causing limited or no host tissue damage. They gain entry by ingestion, skin penetration or insect bites. With two exceptions, they do not multiply in the human body, so a single organism cannot become an overwhelming infection. The exceptions are *Strongyloides stercoralis* and *Capillaria philippinensis,* which can complete their life cycle and multiply within the human body.

Helminths cause disease in various ways. A few compete with their human host for certain nutrients. Some grow to block vital structures, producing disease by mass effect. Most, however, cause dysfunction through the destructive inflammatory and immunologic responses that they elicit. For example, morbidity in schistosomiasis, the most destructive helminthic infection, results from granulomatous responses to schistosome eggs deposited in tissue.

Eosinophils contain basic proteins toxic to some helminths and are a major component of inflammatory responses to these organisms. Parasitic helminths are categorized based on overall morphology and the structure of digestive tissues:

- **Roundworms (nematodes)** are elongate cylindrical organisms with tubular digestive tracts.
- **Flatworms (trematodes)** are dorsoventrally flattened organisms with digestive tracts that end in blind loops.
- **Tapeworms (cestodes)** are segmented organisms with separate head and body parts; they lack a digestive tract and absorb nutrients through their outer walls.

FILARIAL NEMATODES

Lymphatic Filariasis Results in Massive Lymphedema (Elephantiasis)

Lymphatic filariasis (bancroftian and Malayan filariasis) is an inflammatory parasitic infection of lymphatic vessels caused by the roundworms *Wuchereria bancrofti* and *Brugia malayi*. Adult worms inhabit the lymphatics, most frequently in inguinal, epitrochlear and axillary lymph nodes, testis and epididymis. There they cause acute lymphangitis and, in a minority of infected subjects, lymphatic obstruction, leading to severe lymphedema (Fig. 9-86). These and similar organisms are known as filarial worms, because of their thread-like appearance (from the Latin *filum*, meaning "thread").

 **EPIDEMIOLOGY:** The elephantiasis characteristic of lymphatic filariasis was familiar to Hindi and Persian physicians as early as 600 BC. Humans, the only definitive host of these filarial nematodes, acquire infection from the bites of at least 80 species of mosquitoes of the genera *Culex, Aedes, Anopheles* and *Mansonia*. *W. bancrofti* infection is widespread in southern Asia, the Pacific, Africa and parts of South America. *B. malayi* is localized to coastal southern Asia and western Pacific islands. Worldwide, 100–200 million people are estimated to be infected.

 **ETIOLOGIC FACTORS:** Mosquito bites transmit infectious larvae that migrate to lymphatics and lymph nodes. After maturing into adult forms over

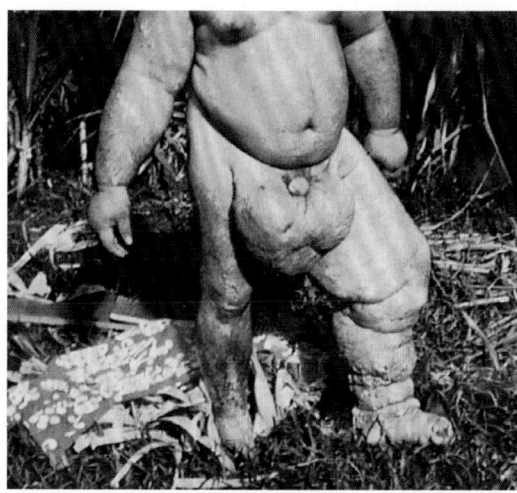

FIGURE 9-86. Bancroftian filariasis. Massive lymphedema (elephantiasis) of the scrotum and left lower extremity are present.

several months, worms mate and the female releases microfilariae into lymphatics and the bloodstream. The manifestations of filariasis result from inflammatory responses to degenerating adult worms in the lymphatics. Repeated infections are common in endemic regions and produce numerous bouts of lymphangitis (filarial fevers), which cause extensive scarring and obstruction of lymphatics over years. This blockage causes localized dependent edema, most commonly affecting legs, arms, genitalia and breasts. In its most severe form (<5% of the infected population), this is known as **elephantiasis**.

 PATHOLOGY: The adult nematode is a white, thread-like worm that is very convoluted within lymph nodes. Females are 80–100 mm in length and 0.20–0.3 mm in width, twice the size of males. In blood films stained with Giemsa, the microfilariae appear as curved worms.

Lymphatic vessels harboring adult worms are dilated, and their endothelial lining is thickened. In adjacent tissues, worms are surrounded by chronic inflammation, including eosinophils. A granulomatous reaction may develop, and degenerating worms can provoke acute inflammation. Microfilariae are seen in blood vessels and lymphatics, and degenerating microfilariae also provoke a chronic inflammatory reaction. After repeated bouts of lymphangitis, lymph nodes and lymphatics become densely fibrotic, often containing calcified remnants of the worms.

 CLINICAL FEATURES: In endemic areas, most of the infected population either has antifilarial antibodies with no detectable infection or asymptomatic microfilaremia. A smaller number develop recurrent episodes of filarial fevers, with malaise, lymphadenopathy and lymphangitis, which persist for 1–2 weeks and then resolve spontaneously. In a small subset, late manifestations of disease appear after two to three decades of recurrent bouts of filarial fevers. Lymphatic obstruction leads to chronic edema of dependent tissues. The overlying skin becomes thickened and warty. The diagnosis is made by identifying microfilariae in blood samples. Diethylcarbamazine and ivermectin are the agents effective against lymphatic filariasis.

Occult filariasis, characterized by indirect evidence of filarial infection (antifilarial antibodies), is the cause of **tropical pulmonary eosinophilia**. This condition is virtually restricted to southern India and some Pacific Islands. Patients present with cough, wheezing, diffuse pulmonary infiltrates and peripheral eosinophilia. The severity ranges from mild asthma to fatal pneumonia.

Onchocerciasis Causes Blindness

Onchocerciasis **("river blindness")** is a chronic inflammatory disease of the skin, eyes and lymphatics caused by the filarial nematode *Onchocerca volvulus*.

 **EPIDEMIOLOGY:** Onchocerciasis is one of the world's major endemic diseases, afflicting an estimated 40 million people, of whom 2 million are blind. The disease is transmitted by bites of *Simulium damnosum* blackflies, which transmit infectious larvae to humans, who are the only definitive hosts. The flies require rapidly running water for breeding. Onchocerciasis is thus endemic along rivers and streams (hence, "river blindness") in parts of tropical Africa, southern Mexico, Central America and South America.

 **PATHOPHYSIOLOGY:** Adult worms live as coiled tangled masses in deep fascia and subcutaneous tissues. They do not cause tissue damage or elicit inflammatory responses. However, gravid females release millions of microfilariae, which migrate into the skin, eyes, lymph nodes and deep organs, producing corresponding onchocercal lesions. Ocular onchocerciasis results from migration of microfilariae into all regions of the eye, from the cornea to the optic nerve head.

When microfilariae die, they incite vigorous inflammatory and immune responses. Inflammatory damage to the cornea, choroid or retina causes partial or total loss of vision. Cutaneous inflammation results in microabscess formation and chronic degenerative changes in the epidermis and dermis. In lymph nodes and lymphatics, responses to dying microfilariae produce chronic lymphatic obstruction and localized dependent edema.

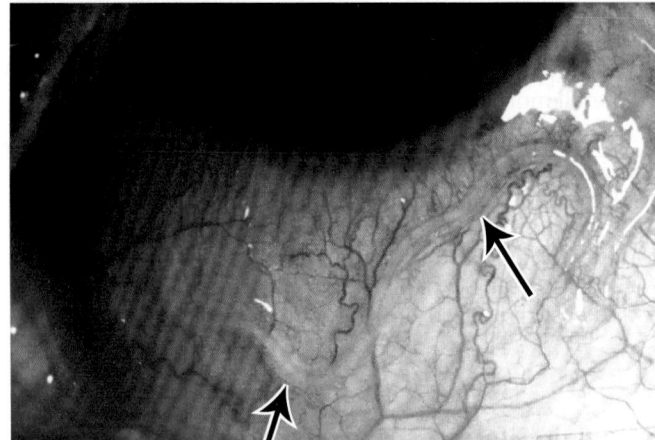

FIGURE 9-87. Loiasis. A thread-like *Loa loa* (*arrows*) is migrating in the subconjunctival tissues.

 PATHOLOGY: *Onchocerca volvulus* is a thin, very long nematode; the female is 400 × 0.3 mm and the male 30 × 0.2 mm. Masses of adult worms become encapsulated by a fibrous scar, forming discrete, 1–3-cm, **onchocercal nodules** in the deep dermis and subcutis. Nodules form over bony prominences of the skull, scapula, ribs, iliac crest, trochanter, sacrum and knee. Microscopically, these nodules have an outer fibrous layer and a central inflammatory infiltrate, which varies from suppurative to granulomatous. Active lesions in the eyes and lymphatics all show degenerating microfilariae surrounded by chronic inflammation, including eosinophils. Ocular involvement leads to sclerosing keratitis, iridocyclitis, chorioretinitis and optic atrophy. The femoral inguinal nodes become enlarged and then fibrotic.

 CLINICAL FEATURES: Symptoms of onchocerciasis result from inflammatory responses to degenerating microfilariae. Skin manifestations begin with generalized pruritus, which becomes so intense that it can interfere with sleeping. Continuing damage produces areas of depigmentation, hypertrophy or atrophy of the skin. Progressive destruction of the cornea, choroid or uvea results in loss of vision. Chronic lymphadenitis is followed by localized edema, which may cause chronic swelling (elephantiasis) of the legs, scrotum or other dependent portions of the body. Systemic antihelminthic therapy, particularly with ivermectin, is effective.

Loiasis Principally Affects the Eyes and Skin

Loiasis is infection by the filarial nematode *Loa loa,* the African "eyeworm."

 **EPIDEMIOLOGY AND PATHOPHYSIOLOGY:** Loiasis is prevalent in the rain forests of Central and West Africa. Humans and baboons are the definitive hosts, and infection is transmitted by mango flies. Adult worms (4 cm long) migrate in the skin and occasionally cross the eye beneath the conjunctiva, making the patient acutely aware of this infection (Fig. 9-87). Gravid worms discharge microfilariae, which circulate in the blood during the day but reside in capillaries of the skin, lungs and other organs at night.

 PATHOLOGY: Migrating worms cause no inflammation, but static ones are surrounded by eosinophils, other inflammatory cells and a foreign body giant cell reaction. Rarely, those infected may develop acute generalized loiasis, characterized by obstructive fibrin thrombi, containing degenerating microfilariae in small vessels of most organs. Brain involvement, with obstruction of vessels by filarial thrombi, may cause lethal and sudden diffuse cerebral ischemia.

 CLINICAL FEATURES: Most infections are asymptomatic but persist for years. Some patients have pruritic, red, subcutaneous "Calabar" swellings, which may be a reaction to migrating adult worms or to microfilariae in the skin. Ocular symptoms include swelling of the eyelids, itching and pain. Worms may be extracted during their migration beneath the conjunctiva. Systemic reactions include fever, pain, itching, urticaria and eosinophilia. Dead worms in or near major nerves may cause paresthesia or paralysis. Treatment with microfilariacides may initiate massive death of microfilariae and provoke fever, meningoencephalitis and death.

INTESTINAL NEMATODES

The adult forms of several nematode species (Table 9-10) reside in the human bowel but rarely cause symptomatic disease. Clinical symptoms occur almost exclusively in patients with very large numbers of worms or who are immunocompromised. Humans are the exclusive or primary hosts for all of intestinal nematodes. Infection spreads from person to person via eggs or larvae passed in the stool or deposited in the perianal region. Infection is most prevalent in settings where hand washing and hygienic disposal of feces are lacking (e.g., less developed countries). Warm, moist climates are required for the infectious forms of many intestinal nematodes to survive outside the body. These worms are, thus, endemic in tropical and subtropical climates.

Ascariasis Is an Infestation of the Small Bowel

Ascariasis refers to infection by the large roundworm *Ascaris lumbricoides.* It is the most common helminthic infection of

TABLE 9-10			
INTESTINAL NEMATODES			
Species	**Common Name**	**Site of Adult Worm**	**Clinical Manifestations**
Ascaris lumbricoides	Roundworm	Small bowel	Allergic reactions to lung migration; intestinal obstruction
Ancylostoma duodenale	Hookworm	Small bowel	Allergic reactions to cutaneous inoculation and lung migration; intestinal blood loss
Necator americanus	Hookworm	Small bowel	Allergic reactions to cutaneous inoculation and lung migration; intestinal blood loss
Trichuris trichiura	Whipworm	Large bowel	Abdominal pain and diarrhea; rectal prolapse (rare)
Strongyloides stercoralis	Threadworm	Small bowel	Abdominal pain and diarrhea; dissemination to extraintestinal sites in immunocompromised persons
Enterobius vermicularis	Pinworm	Cecum, appendix	Perianal and perineal itching

humans, affecting at least 1 billion people, usually without causing symptoms. Infection is worldwide but is most common in areas with warm climates and poor sanitation.

 PATHOPHYSIOLOGY: Adult worms live in the small intestine, where gravid females discharge eggs that pass in the feces. These eggs hatch when ingested. *Ascaris* larvae emerge in the small intestine, penetrate the bowel wall and reach the lungs through the venous circulation. They leave the pulmonary capillaries, enter the alveoli and then migrate up the trachea to the glottis, where they are swallowed and again reach the small bowel. There, they mature and live as adult worms within the lumen for 1–2 years.

 PATHOLOGY AND CLINICAL FEATURES: Adult worms (15–35 cm long) usually cause no pathologic changes. Heavy infections may be complicated by vomiting, malnutrition and sometimes intestinal obstruction (Fig. 9-88). On rare occasions, worms enter the ampulla of Vater or pancreatic or biliary ducts, where they may cause obstruction, acute pancreatitis, suppurative cholangitis and liver abscesses. Eggs deposited in the liver or other tissues produce necrosis, granulomatous inflammation and fibrosis. *Ascaris* pneumonia, which may be fatal, develops when large numbers of larvae migrate within the air spaces.

Ascariasis is diagnosed by identifying eggs in the feces. Occasionally, adult worms may pass with the stools or even emerge from the nose or mouth. Ascaricidal drugs are effective.

Trichuriasis Is an Infestation of the Large Bowel

Trichuriasis is caused by the intestinal nematode *Trichuris trichiura* (**"whipworm"**).

 EPIDEMIOLOGY: Whipworm infection is found worldwide, affecting over 800 million people. Parasitism is most common in warm, moist places with poor sanitation, but over 2 million persons in the United

States are infected. Children are especially susceptible. Adult worms live in the cecum and upper colon, where females produce eggs that pass in the feces. Eggs embryonate in moist soil and become infective in 3 weeks. Humans are infected by ingesting eggs in contaminated soil, food or drink.

PATHOPHYSIOLOGY: Larvae emerge from ingested eggs in the small bowel and migrate to the cecum and colon, where adult worms burrow their anterior portions into the superficial mucosa (Fig. 9-89). This invasion causes small erosions, focal active inflammation and continuous loss of small quantities of blood. *T. trichiura* measures 3–5 cm in length, with a long, slender anterior portion and a short, blunt posterior.

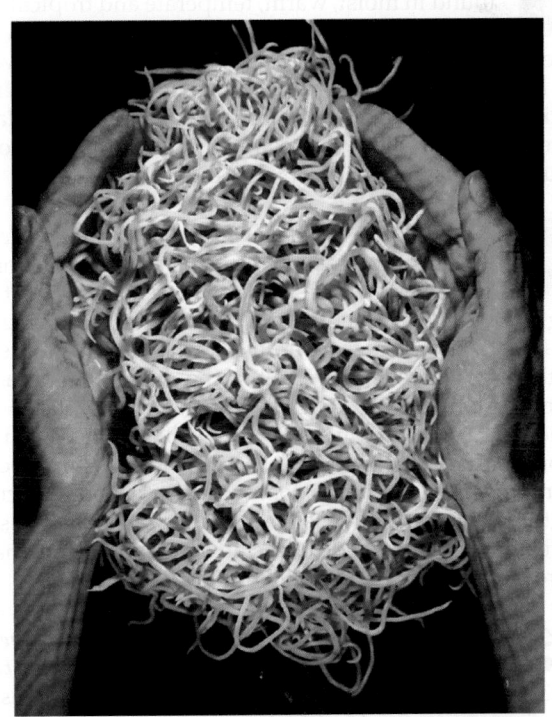

FIGURE 9-88. Ascariasis. This mass of over 800 worms of *Ascaris lumbricoides* obstructed and infarcted the ileum of a 2-year-old girl in South Africa.

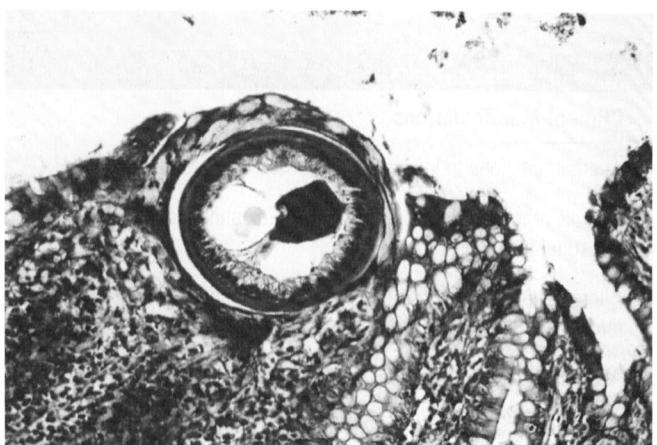

FIGURE 9-89. Trichuriasis. The anterior "whip" end of *Trichuris trichiura* is threaded into the mucosa of the colon.

 CLINICAL FEATURES: Most *T. trichiura* infections are asymptomatic. Heavy infestation produces cramping abdominal pain, bloody diarrhea, weight loss and anemia. The diagnosis is made by finding the characteristic eggs in the stool. Mebendazole is effective therapy.

Hookworms Cause Intestinal Blood Loss and Anemia

Necator americanus and *Ancylostoma duodenale* ("hookworms") are intestinal nematodes that infect the human small bowel. They produce intestinal blood loss by lacerating the bowel mucosa, thereby resulting in anemia.

 **EPIDEMIOLOGY:** Hookworm infections are found in moist, warm, temperate and tropical areas and cause serious public health problems worldwide. In fact, both *A. duodenale* ("Old World" hookworm) and *N. americanus* ("American" hookworm) prevail on most continents and have overlapping epidemiologic boundaries. More than 700 million people are infected with hookworms, including half a million people in the United States.

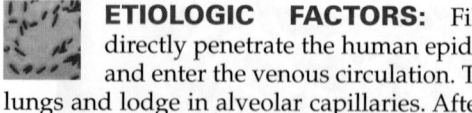 **ETIOLOGIC FACTORS:** Filariform larvae directly penetrate the human epidermis on contact and enter the venous circulation. They travel to the lungs and lodge in alveolar capillaries. After rupturing into the alveoli, larvae migrate up the trachea to the glottis and are then swallowed. They molt in the duodenum, attach to the mucosal wall with tooth-like buckle plates, clamp off a section of a villus and ingest it (Fig. 9-90). In extensive infestations, particularly with *A. duodenale*, blood loss can be sufficient to cause anemia. Hookworms are about 1 cm in length. They are grossly visible and are attached to the small bowel mucosa alongside punctate areas of hemorrhages. There is no attendant inflammation.

 CLINICAL FEATURES: *Although most people with hookworm infection have no symptoms, this parasite is the most important cause of chronic anemia worldwide.* In people with heavy worm burdens (particularly women who consume a diet low in

iron) and in populations with inadequate iron intake, chronic intestinal blood loss can produce severe iron-deficiency anemia. Skin penetration is sometimes associated with a pruritic eruption ("ground itch"), and the phase of larval migration through the lungs occasionally causes asthma-like symptoms.

Strongyloidiasis Is Disseminated in Immunocompromised Hosts

Strongyloidiasis is a small intestinal infection with a nematode, *Strongyloides stercoralis* ("threadworm"). *Although most cases are asymptomatic, the infection can progress to lethal disseminated disease in immunocompromised persons.* Infection is most frequent in areas with warm, moist climates and poor sanitation. Endemic pockets of strongyloidiasis still exist in the United States, particularly in the Appalachian region.

 **ETIOLOGIC FACTORS AND PATHOPHYSIOLOGY:** *S. stercoralis* is the smallest of the intestinal nematodes, measuring 0.2–0.3 cm in length. Adult females are buried in the crypts of the duodenum or jejunum but produce no visible alterations. Microscopically, the coiled females, along with eggs and developing larvae, lie within the mucosa, usually with no associated inflammation (Fig. 9-91).

Parasitic females survive in the mucosa of the small intestine, where they lay eggs that hatch quickly and release rhabditiform larvae. These are passed in the feces, and in the soil become filariform, the infective stage that penetrates human skin. On entering the skin, *S. stercoralis* larvae pass in the bloodstream to the lungs and then to the small bowel, similarly to hookworms. The worms mature in the small bowel. Unlike other intestinal nematodes, *S. stercoralis* may reproduce in human hosts by a mechanism known as **autoinfection**. This occurs when rhabditiform larvae become infective (filariform) within a host's intestine and repenetrate either the intestinal wall or the perianal skin, thereby starting a new parasitic cycle within a single host.

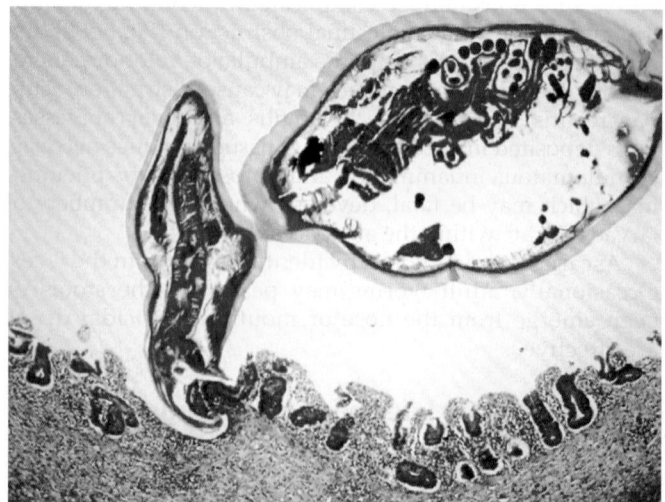

FIGURE 9-90. Ancylostomiasis. Section of the ileum shows two portions of a single adult worm, *Ancylostoma duodenale*. A plug of mucosa is in the buccal cavity of the hookworm.

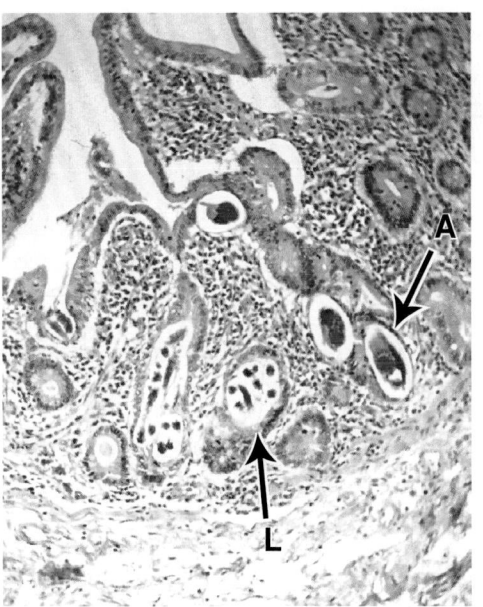

FIGURE 9-91. Strongyloidiasis. A section of jejunum shows adult worms, larvae and eggs of *Strongyloides stercoralis* in the mucosal crypts. The lamina propria is infiltrated with lymphocytes, plasma cells and eosinophils. The patient had a hyperinfected syndrome and presented with malabsorption.

 CLINICAL FEATURES: Most infected people are asymptomatic, but moderate eosinophilia is common. **Disseminated strongyloidiasis** or **hyperinfection syndrome** occurs in patients with suppressed immunity, particularly those receiving corticosteroids. In such individuals, internal autoinfection is greatly increased, and extraordinary numbers of filariform larvae penetrate intestinal walls and disseminate to distant organs. In disseminated strongyloidiasis, the gut may show ulceration, edema and severe inflammation. Sepsis, usually with gramnegative organisms, and infection of parenchymal organs eventuate. Untreated, disseminated strongyloidiasis is fatal; even with prompt treatment with thiabendazole or ivermectin, only one third of patients survive.

Pinworm Infection (Enterobiasis) Leads to Perianal Itching

Enterobius vermicularis ("pinworm") is a worldwide intestinal nematode, most often encountered in temperate zones. Although people can be infected at any age, parasitism is most common among young children. More than 200 million people are estimated to be infected with *E. vermicularis* worldwide, including some 5 million school-age children in the United States.

The adult female worm resides in the cecum and appendix but migrates to the perianal and perineal skin to deposit eggs. The eggs stick to fingers, bed linens, towels and clothing and are readily transmitted from person to person. Ingested eggs hatch in the small bowel to yield larvae that mature into adult worms. Some infected people are asymptomatic, but most complain of perineal pruritus, caused by migrating worms depositing eggs. Several agents, including mebendazole, are effective against pinworms.

TISSUE NEMATODES

Trichinosis Is Myositis Acquired by Eating Pork

Trichinosis is produced by the roundworm *Trichinella spiralis.*

 EPIDEMIOLOGY: Infection with *T. spiralis* occurs worldwide. Humans acquire trichinosis by eating inadequately cooked meat with encysted *T. spiralis* larvae. The larvae are found in the skeletal muscles of various carnivorous or omnivorous wild and domesticated animals, including pigs, rats, bears and walruses. Pork is the most common source of human trichinosis (Fig. 9-92).

Animals acquire trichinosis by feeding on the flesh of other infected animals. Infection is common among some wild animal populations and can be readily introduced into domesticated animals, such as pigs, when they feed on garbage or uncooked meat. Meat inspection programs and restriction of feeding practices have largely eliminated *T. spiralis* from domesticated pigs in many developed countries. Only about 100 cases of trichinosis are reported in the United States annually, but these represent only the most severely symptomatic cases, and infection is probably much more common.

 **ETIOLOGIC FACTORS:** In the small bowel, *T. spiralis* larvae emerge from the ingested tissue cysts and burrow into the intestinal mucosa, where they develop into adult worms. The adults mate, and the female liberates larvae that invade the intestinal wall and enter the circulation. Production of larvae may continue for 1–4 months, until the worms are finally expelled from the intestine. The larvae can invade nearly any tissue but can survive only in striated skeletal muscle, where they encyst and remain viable for years. The resulting myositis is especially prominent in the diaphragm, extrinsic ocular muscles, tongue, intercostal muscles, gastrocnemius and deltoids. Sometimes the CNS or heart is also inflamed, causing meningoencephalitis or myocarditis.

 PATHOLOGY: Skeletal muscle is the major site of tissue damage in trichinosis. When a larva infects a myocyte, the cell undergoes basophilic degeneration and swelling. Early myocyte infection elicits an intense inflammatory infiltrate rich in eosinophils and macrophages. Larvae grow to 10 times their initial size, fold on themselves and develop a capsule. With encapsulation, inflammation subsides. Several years later, the larvae die and the cysts calcify. The small bowel is grossly unremarkable but adult worms may be found on microscopic examination at the base of villi in heavy infestations, and may be associated with an inflammatory infiltrate.

 CLINICAL FEATURES: Most human infections with *T. spiralis* involve small numbers of cysts and are asymptomatic. Symptomatic trichinosis is usually self-limited and patients recover in a few months. If large numbers of cysts are eaten, abdominal pain and diarrhea may result from small bowel invasion by the worms. Major symptoms, in the form of fever, weakness and severe pain and tenderness of affected muscles, usually develop several days later. **Eosinophilia may be extreme (over 50% of all leukocytes).** Involvement of extraocular muscles produces periorbital edema. Infection of the brain or myocardium can

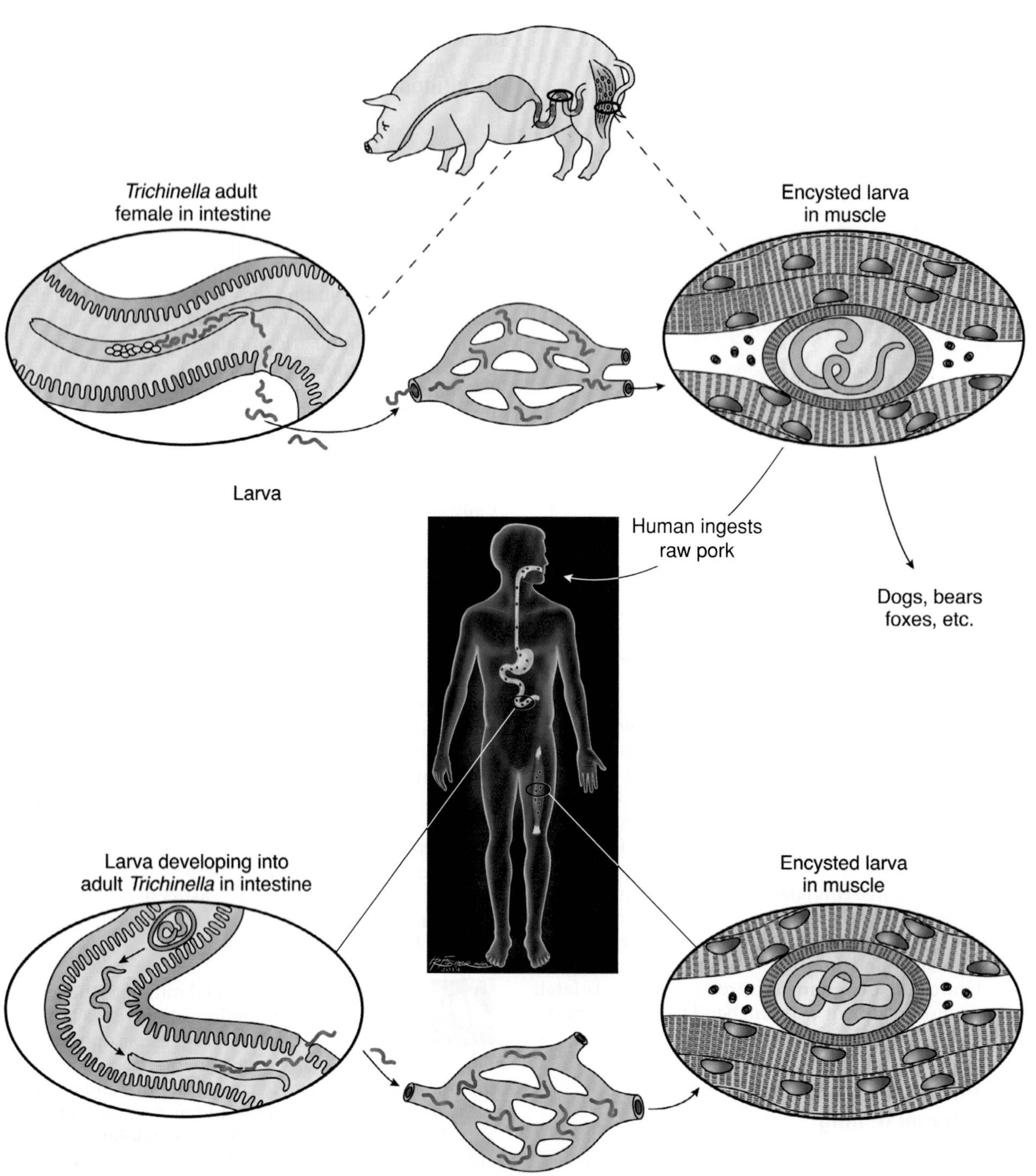

FIGURE 9-92. Trichinosis. After being ingested by the pig, cysts of *Trichinella* are digested in the gastrointestinal tract, liberating larvae that mature to adult worms. Female worms release larvae that penetrate the intestinal wall, enter the circulation and lodge in striated muscle, where they encyst. When humans ingest inadequately cooked pork, the cycle is repeated, resulting in the muscle disease characteristic of trichinosis.

be fatal. Severe trichinosis is treated with corticosteroids to attenuate the inflammation. Antihelminthic drugs are required to remove adult worms from the intestine.

Visceral Larva Migrans (Toxocariasis) Is Transmitted by Cats and Dogs

Toxocariasis is an infection of deep organs by helminthic larvae migrating in aberrant hosts.

 ETIOLOGIC FACTORS: The infestation is a sporadic disease, mainly of young children, typically in the setting of overcrowded dwellings, living with dogs and cats. The most common causes of visceral larva migrans are *Toxocara* species, especially *T. canis* and *T. cati*. These roundworms live in the intestines of dogs and cats, and infection is transmitted to humans by ingestion of embryonated ova. Eggs hatch and larvae invade the intestinal wall. They are carried to the liver, from where a few emerge to reach the systemic circulation and may be carried to any part of the body. In tissues, larvae die and elicit small granulomas, which eventually heal by scarring.

 CLINICAL FEATURES: Many cases of visceral larva migrans are asymptomatic, but any infection can potentially cause severe disease. The typical symptomatic patient is a child with hypereosinophilia, pneumonitis and hypergammaglobulinemia. In these patients, ocular manifestations are common, and the chief complaint is often loss of vision in one eye. In fact, eyes with toxocaral endophthalmitis have been mistakenly enucleated for retinoblastoma. The infection is generally self-limited and symptoms disappear within a year. It is treated with diethylcarbamazine and thiabendazole.

Cutaneous Larva Migrans Is a Pruritic Eruption

Cutaneous larva migrans is caused by larval nematodes migrating through the skin, where they provoke severe inflammation that appears as serpiginous urticarial trails (Fig. 9-93). The names applied to cutaneous larva migrans are as varied as the organisms that cause it and include creeping eruptions, sand worm, plumber's itch, duck hunter's itch and epidermis linearis migrans. The more common larval nematodes include *Strongyloides stercoralis*, *Ancylostoma braziliensis* and *Necator americanus*. Dogs and cats infected with hookworms are the major source of the disease. Outbreaks of cutaneous larva migrans occur at subtropical and tropical beaches. Plumbers who crawl under houses and animal caretakers are frequently infected. Thiabendazole is the treatment of choice.

Dracunculiasis Features Long Adult Worms beneath the Skin

Dracunculiasis (guinea worm) is an infection of connective and subcutaneous tissues with the guinea worm, *Dracunculus medinensis*.

 EPIDEMIOLOGY: Dracunculiasis is common in rural areas of sub-Saharan Africa, the Middle East, India and Pakistan, where it is estimated that

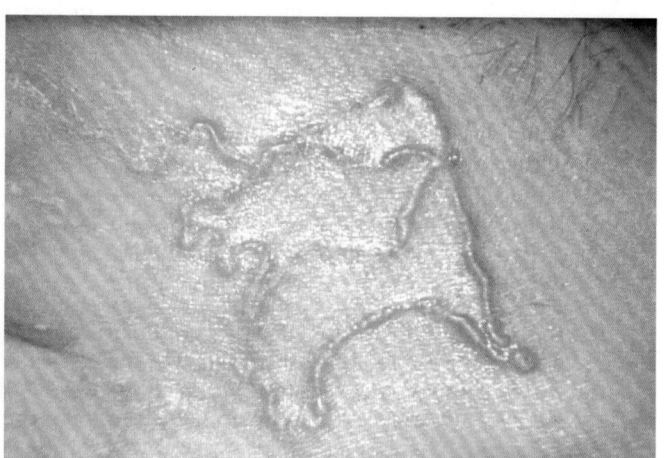

FIGURE 9-93. Cutaneous larva migrans. The skin shows a creeping eruption with the characteristic serpiginous, raised lesion.

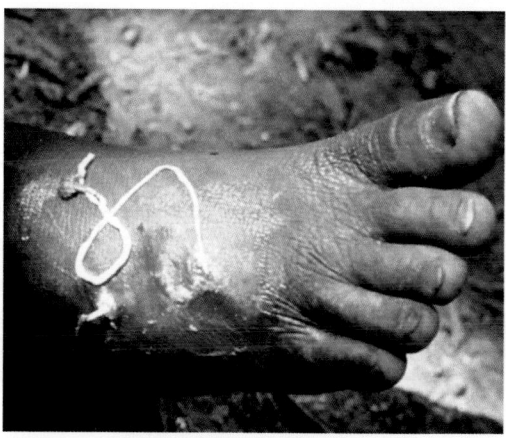

FIGURE 9-94. Dracunculiasis. A female guinea worm is seen emerging from the foot, which is swollen because of secondary bacterial infection.

10 million people are infected. The disease is transmitted in drinking water contaminated with the intermediate host, a microscopic aquatic crustacean of the genus *Cyclops*.

 **ETIOLOGIC FACTORS AND PATHOLOGY:** The adult female nematode resides in subcutaneous tissues and releases numerous larvae through an ulcerated blister. When the blister is immersed in water, larvae are ingested by the *Cyclops* crustaceans, which are in turn ingested by humans.

About a year after ingestion of infected crustaceans, systemic allergic symptoms appear, including a pruritic urticarial rash. A reddish papule, often around the ankles, develops and vesiculates. Beneath this sterile blister is the anterior end of the female worm. The blister bursts upon contact with water and the female worm, now measuring up to 120 cm and containing 3 million larvae, partially emerges (Fig. 9-94). The worm then spews myriad larvae into the water. Secondary infection of the blister, often with spreading cellulitis, is common. Dead worms provoke an intense inflammatory response, causing debilitation in many patients with dracunculosis. The worm is often extracted by local practitioners by progressively twisting it onto a small stick. Treatment also includes anthelminthic drugs.

TREMATODES (FLUKES)

Schistosomiasis Produces Diseases of the Liver and Bladder

Schistosomiasis (bilharziasis) is the most important human helminthic disease. Intense inflammatory and immune responses damage the liver, intestine or urinary bladder. Three species of schistosomes, *Schistosoma mansoni*, *Schistosoma haematobium* and *Schistosoma japonicum*, are the causative agents.

 **EPIDEMIOLOGY:** *Schistosomiasis causes greater morbidity and mortality than all other worm infections.* It affects about 10% of the world's population and is second only to malaria as a cause of disabling disease. The three schistosomal pathogens affect distinct geographic regions, as dictated by the distribution of

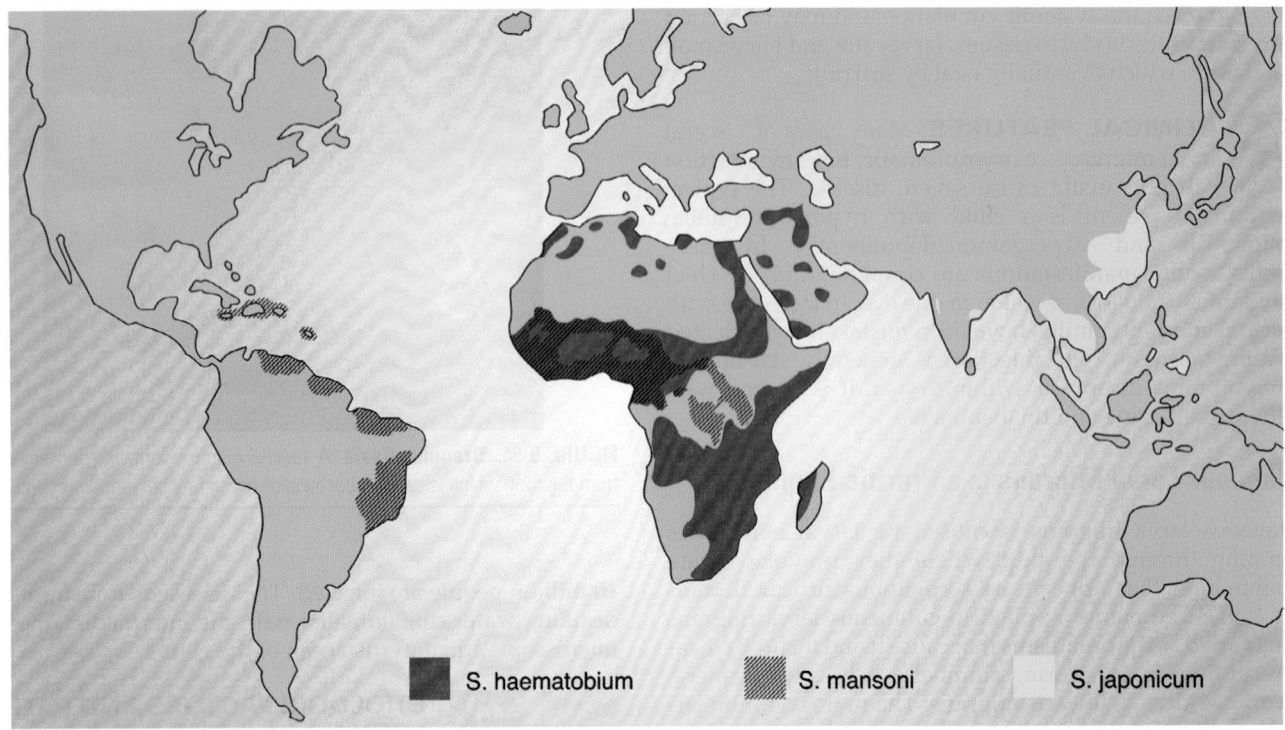

FIGURE 9-95. Distribution of schistosomiasis caused by *Schistosoma mansoni*, *Schistosoma haematobium* and *Schistosoma japonicum*.

their specific host snail species (Fig. 9-95). *S. mansoni* is found in much of tropical Africa, parts of southwest Asia, South America and the Caribbean islands. *S. haematobium* is endemic in large regions of tropical Africa and parts of the Middle East. *S. japonicum* occurs in parts of China, the Philippines, Southeast Asia and India.

 **ETIOLOGIC FACTORS:** Schistosomes have complicated life cycles, alternating between asexual generations in their invertebrate host (snail) and sexual generations in the vertebrate host (Fig. 9-96). A schistosome egg hatches in fresh water, liberating a motile **miracidium** that penetrates a snail, where it develops into the final larval stage, the **cercaria**. Cercariae escape into the water and penetrate human skin, during which process they lose their forked tails and become "schistosomula." These migrate through tissues, penetrate blood vessels and migrate to the lungs and liver. In intestinal venules of the portal drainage, schistosomula mature, forming pairs of male and female worms. Female *S. mansoni* and *S. japonicum* deposit eggs in intestinal venules, whereas *S. haematobium* lays eggs in those of the urinary bladder. Embryos develop as the eggs pass through these tissues. The larvae are mature when eggs pass through the wall of the intestine or the bladder and are discharged in feces or urine. They hatch in fresh water, liberating miracidia and completing the life cycle.

 PATHOLOGY: *The basic lesion is a circumscribed granuloma or a cellular infiltrate of eosinophils and neutrophils around an egg.* Adult schistosomes provoke no inflammation while alive in the veins. Granulomas that form about the eggs also obstruct microvascular blood flow and produce ischemic damage to adjacent tissue. The result is progressive scarring and dysfunction in affected organs.

Female worms deposit hundreds or thousands of eggs daily for 5–35 years. Most infected people harbor fewer than 10 adult females. However, if the worm burden is large, the granulomatous response to the enormous number of eggs poses significant problems. The site of involvement is determined by the tropism of the particular schistosome species.

- *S. mansoni* inhabits the branches of the inferior mesenteric vein, thereby affecting the distal colon and liver.
- *S. haematobium* winds its way to the veins serving the rectum, bladder and pelvic organs.
- *S. japonicum* deposits eggs predominantly in the branches of the superior mesenteric vein, thereby damaging the small bowel, ascending colon and liver.

Liver disease caused by *S. mansoni* or *S. japonicum* begins as periportal granulomatous inflammation (Fig. 9-97) and progresses to dense periportal fibrosis **(pipestem fibrosis)** (Fig. 9-98). In severe hepatic schistosomiasis, this causes obstruction of portal blood flow and portal hypertension. *S. mansoni* and *S. japonicum* also damage the intestine, where granulomatous responses produce inflammatory polyps and foci of mucosal and submucosal fibrosis.

In **urogenital schistosomiasis,** caused by *S. haematobium*, eggs are most numerous in the bladder, ureter and seminal vesicles, although they may also reach the lungs, colon and appendix. Eggs in the bladder and ureters provoke a granulomatous reaction, inflammatory protuberances and patches of mucosal and mural fibrosis. These may obstruct urine flow, and so cause secondary inflammatory damage to the bladder, ureters and kidneys. Bladder disease produced by *S. haematobium* may lead to **squamous cell carcinoma of the bladder**. In areas where *S. haematobium* is prevalent, this is the most common form of cancer.

The granulomas of schistosomiasis surround schistosome eggs. Eosinophils often predominate in early granulomas.

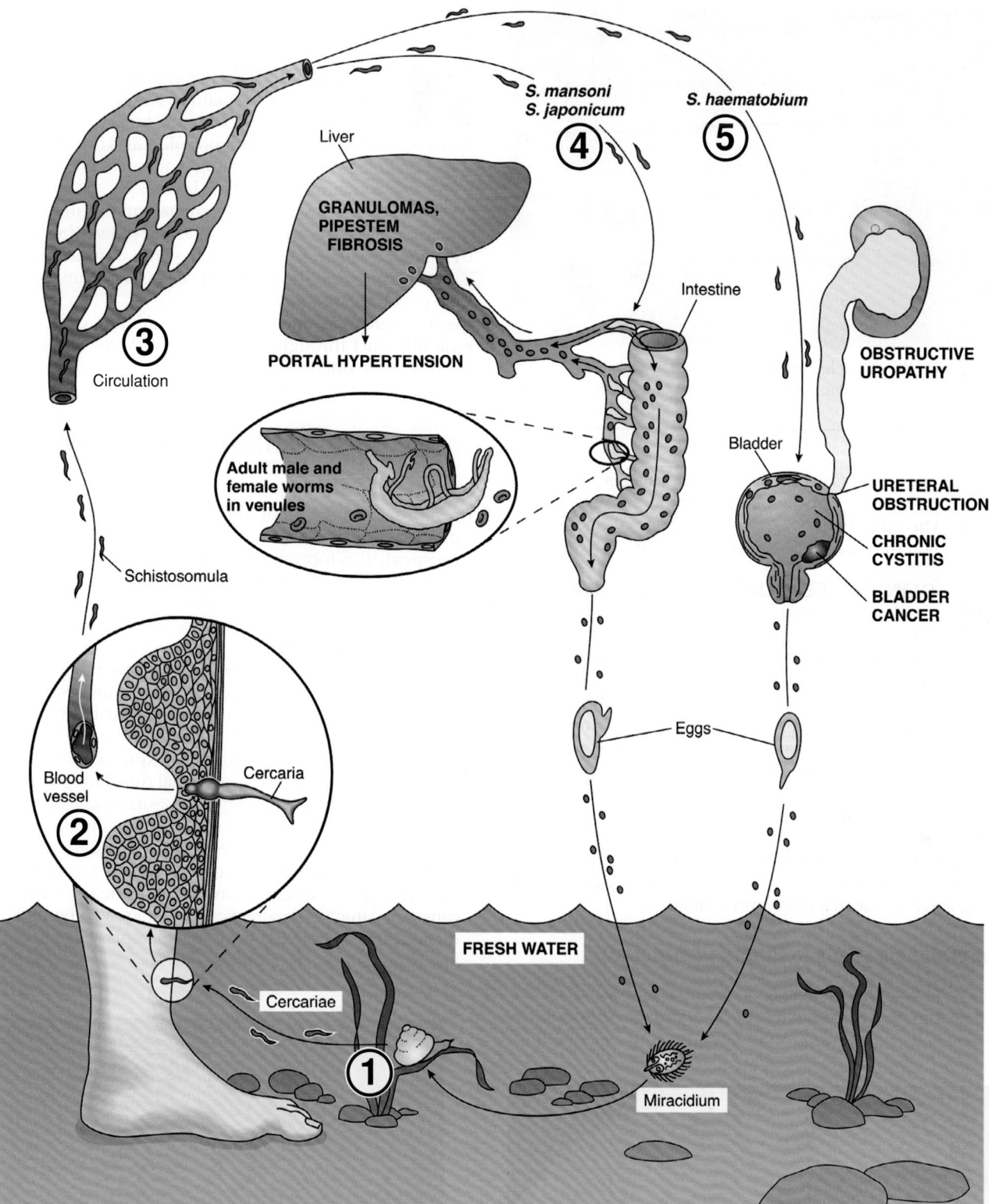

FIGURE 9-96. Life cycle of *Schistosoma* and clinical features of schistosomiasis. The schistosome egg hatches in water, liberates a miracidium that penetrates a snail and develops through two stages to a sporocyst to form the final larval stage, the cercaria. **(1)** The cercaria escapes from the snail into water, "swims" and penetrates the skin of a human host. **(2)** The cercaria loses its forked tail to become a schistosomulum, which migrates through tissues, penetrates a blood vessel and **(3)** is carried to the lung and later to the liver. In hepatic portal venules, the schistosomula become sexually mature and form pairs, each with a male and a female worm, the female worm lying in the gynecophoral canal of the male worm. The organism causes lesions in the liver, including granulomas, portal ("pipestem") fibrosis and portal hypertension. **(4)** The female worm deposits immature eggs in small venules of the intestine and rectum (*Schistosoma mansoni* and *Schistosoma japonicum*) or **(5)** of the urinary bladder (*Schistosoma haematobium*). The bladder infestation leads to obstructive uropathy, ureteral obstruction, chronic cystitis and bladder cancer. Embryos develop during passage of the eggs through tissues, and larvae are mature when eggs pass through the wall of the intestine or urinary bladder. Eggs hatch in water and liberate miracidia to complete the cycle.

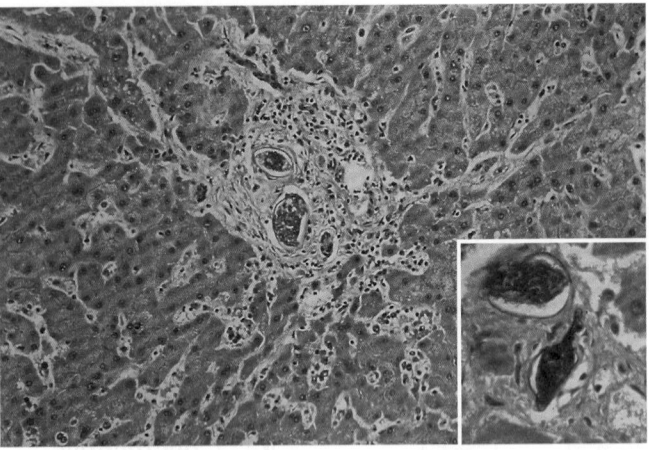

FIGURE 9-97. Hepatic schistosomiasis. A hepatic granuloma surrounds a degenerating egg of *Schistosoma mansoni*. A higher power of the organism is shown in the inset.

In older granulomas, epithelioid macrophages and giant cells are prominent and the oldest granulomas are densely fibrotic. The eggs of the various schistosomal species are identified on the basis of their size and shape.

 CLINICAL FEATURES: Skin penetration by the schistosome larvae is sometimes associated with a self-limited, intensely pruritic rash. Most cases are dominated by the manifestations of chronic granulomatous tissue damage. Hepatic involvement is accompanied by portal hypertension, splenomegaly, ascites and bleeding esophageal varices. Intestinal disease is usually only minimally symptomatic, but some patients have abdominal pain and bloody stools. Schistosomiasis of the bladder is complicated by hematuria, recurrent urinary tract infections and sometimes progressive urinary obstruction, leading to renal failure. Identification of schistosome eggs in the urine or feces establishes the diagnosis. Schistosomes are effectively killed by systemic antihelminthic agents, but structural changes due to extensive scarring are irreversible.

Clonorchiasis Leads to Biliary Obstruction

Clonorchiasis is an infection of the hepatic biliary system by the Chinese liver fluke, *Clonorchis sinensis*. Although the fluke usually causes only mild symptoms, it is sometimes associated with bile duct stones, cholangitis and bile duct cancer.

 **EPIDEMIOLOGY:** Clonorchiasis is endemic in east Asia, from Vietnam to Korea, where uncooked freshwater fish is common fare. In parts of these regions, over 50% of the adult population is infected. Human infection is acquired by ingesting inadequately cooked freshwater fish containing *C. sinensis* larvae.

Adult worms are flat and transparent, live in human bile ducts and pass eggs to the intestine and feces. After ingestion by a specific snail, the egg hatches into a miracidium. Cercariae escape from the snail and seek out certain fish, which they penetrate and in which they encyst. When humans eat the fish, cercariae emerge in the duodenum, enter the common bile duct through the ampulla of Vater and mature in the distal bile ducts to adult flukes.

 PATHOPHYSIOLOGY AND PATHOLOGY: The presence of *Clonorchis* in the bile ducts elicits an inflammatory response that does not eliminate the worm, but causes dilation and fibrosis of the ducts. Sometimes the worms cause calculus formation in the hepatic bile ducts, leading to ductal obstruction. The adult *Clonorchis* persists in the ducts for decades, and long-standing infection is associated with an increased incidence of bile duct carcinoma (**cholangiocarcinoma**).

In heavy *Clonorchis* infections, the liver may be up to three times normal size. Dilated bile ducts are seen through the capsule, and the cut surface is punctuated with thick-walled dilated bile ducts (Fig. 9-99). Flukes (up to 2.5 cm), sometimes in the thousands, can be expressed from the bile ducts. Microscopically, the epithelial duct lining is initially hyperplastic and then metaplastic. Surrounding stroma is fibrotic. Secondary bacterial infection is common and may be associated with suppurative cholangitis. Eggs deposited in the liver parenchyma elicit a fibrous and granulomatous reaction. Masses of eggs may lodge in the bile ducts and cause cholangitis. Pancreatic ducts may also be invaded, dilated and thickened; lined by metaplastic epithelium; and eventually surrounded by fibrosis.

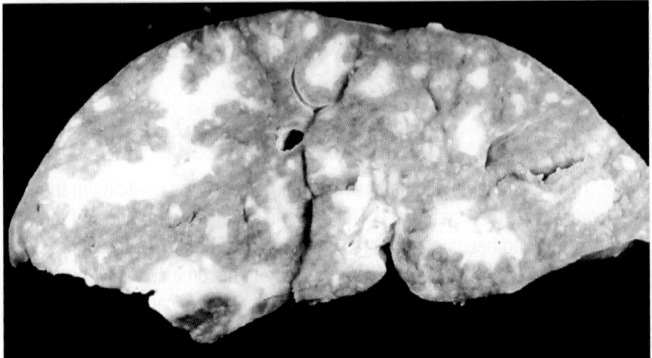

FIGURE 9-98. Hepatic schistosomiasis. Chronic infection of the liver with *Schistosoma japonicum* has led to the characteristic "pipestem" fibrosis.

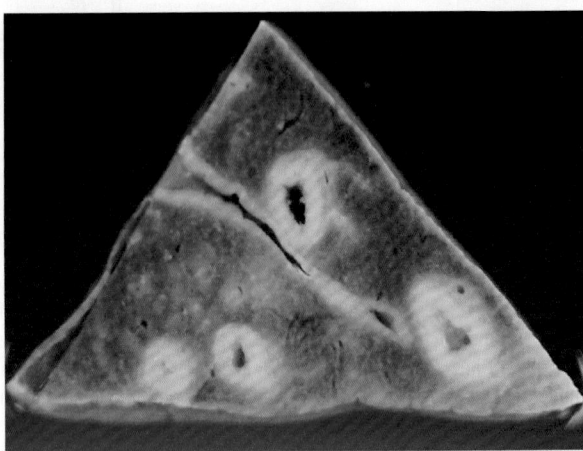

FIGURE 9-99. Clonorchiasis of the liver. The bile ducts are greatly thickened and dilated because of the presence of adult flukes (*Clonorchis sinensis*).

CLINICAL FEATURES: Migration of *C. sinensis* into the bile ducts causes transient fever and chills, but most infected persons are asymptomatic. Patients with clonorchiasis may die of a variety of complications, including biliary obstruction, bacterial cholangitis, pancreatitis and cholangiocarcinoma. The diagnosis is made by identifying eggs of *C. sinensis* in stools or duodenal aspirates. The infestation is treated effectively with systemic antihelminthic agents.

Paragonimiasis Is a Lung Disease

Paragonimiasis is a pulmonary infection by several species of the genus *Paragonimus,* the oriental lung fluke. The most common human pathogen is *Paragonimus westermani,* which is common in Asian countries (Korea, the Philippines, Taiwan and China), where uncooked, lightly salted or wine-soaked fresh crabs are delicacies. Use of raw crab juices as medicines or seasonings also has been associated with the infection.

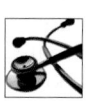 **CLINICAL FEATURES:** Pulmonary paragonimiasis is frequently misdiagnosed as tuberculosis. It manifests as fever, malaise, night sweats, chest pain and cough. However, unlike tuberculosis, peripheral eosinophilia is common. The sputum is sometimes blood tinged and chest radiographs reveal transient diffuse pulmonary infiltrates. The prognosis in pulmonary paragonimiasis is good, but ectopic lesions of the brain may be fatal. Eggs in the sputum or stools provide the definitive diagnosis.

Fascioliasis Is a Biliary Disease Acquired from Sheep

Fascioliasis is an infection of the liver by the sheep liver fluke, *Fasciola hepatica.* Humans may acquire the infection wherever sheep are raised. People become infected by eating vegetation, such as watercress, that is contaminated with the cysts passed by sheep.

 **ETIOLOGIC FACTORS:** After reaching the duodenum, cysts liberate metacercariae that pass into the peritoneal cavity, penetrate the liver and migrate through the hepatic parenchyma into the bile ducts. The larvae mature to adults and live in both the intrahepatic and extrahepatic bile ducts. Later, the adult flukes penetrate the wall of the bile ducts and wander back into the liver parenchyma, where they feed on liver cells and deposit their eggs.

  PATHOLOGY AND CLINICAL FEATURES: Eggs of *F. hepatica* lead to hepatic abscesses and granulomas. The worms induce hyperplasia of bile duct epithelium, portal and periductal fibrosis, proliferation of bile ductules and varying degrees of biliary obstruction. Eosinophilia, vomiting and acute gastric pain are characteristic. Severe untreated infections may be fatal. The diagnosis is made by recovering eggs from the stools or biliary tract.

Fasciolopsiasis Is an Infestation of the Small Intestine

Fasciolopsiasis is caused by the giant intestinal fluke, *Fasciolopsis buski.* The disease is common in the Orient. Humans are infected by eating aquatic vegetables contaminated with

encysted cercariae. The large worm (3 × 7 cm) attaches to the duodenal or jejunal wall, which may ulcerate, become infected and cause pain like that of a peptic ulcer. Acute symptoms may also be due to intestinal obstruction or by toxins released by large numbers of worms. The diagnosis is made by identifying *F. buski* eggs in the stool. Treatment is with systemic antihelminthic agents.

CESTODES: INTESTINAL TAPEWORMS

Taenia saginata, Taenia solium and *Diphyllobothrium latum* are tapeworms that infect humans, growing to their adult forms within the intestine (Table 9-11). Presence of these adult worms rarely damages the human host.

 **EPIDEMIOLOGY:** Intestinal tapeworm infections are acquired by eating inadequately cooked beef (*T. saginata*), pork (*T. solium*) or fish (*D. latum*) containing larvae. Tapeworm life cycles involve cystic larval stages in animals and worm stages in the human. The life cycles of beef and pork tapeworms require that the animals ingest material tainted with infected human feces. The cystic larval forms develop in the animals' muscles. Modern cattle and pig farming practices, plus meat inspection, have largely eliminated beef and pork tapeworms in industrialized countries, but infection remains common in the underdeveloped world. Fish tapeworm infection is prevalent in areas where raw, pickled or partly cooked freshwater fish are common fare. Tapeworm infections are usually asymptomatic, although it may be distressing when an infected person passes portions of the worm in the stool. The fish tapeworm (*D. latum*) takes up vitamin B_{12}, and a small number (<2%) of infected persons develop pernicious anemia (see Chapter 26).

Cysticercosis Is a Systemic Infection by the Larvae of the Pork Tapeworm

Adult *T. solium* is acquired by eating undercooked pork infected with cysticerci (measly pork).

 **PATHOPHYSIOLOGY:** Pigs acquire cysticerci by ingesting eggs of *T. solium* in human feces. This cycle, although a public health concern, is essentially benign for both humans and pigs.

	TABLE 9-11

TABLE 9-11
TAPEWORM INFECTIONS

Species	Human Disease	Source of Human Infection
Taenia saginata	Adult tapeworm in intestine	Beef
Taenia solium	Adult tapeworm in intestine; cysticercosis	Pork; human feces
Diphyllobothrium latum	Adult tapeworm in intestine	Fish
Echinococcus granulosus	Hydatid cyst disease	Dog feces

However, when humans accidentally ingest tapeworm eggs from human feces and become infected with cysticerci, the consequences may be catastrophic. The eggs release oncospheres, which penetrate the gut wall, enter the bloodstream, lodge in tissue, encyst and differentiate to cysticerci.

 PATHOLOGY: The cysticercus is a spherical, milky white cyst, about 1 cm in diameter, containing fluid and an invaginated scolex (head of the worm) with birefringent hooklets. Cysts can remain viable for an indefinite period and provoke no inflammation; rather, as they grow, they compress adjacent tissues. Degenerating cysts are the ones usually responsible for symptoms. They attach to tissue and are densely inflamed with eosinophils, neutrophils, lymphocytes and plasma cells. Multiple cysticerci in the brain may impart a "Swiss cheese" appearance to the tissue (Fig. 9-100).

 CLINICAL FEATURES: Cysticercosis of the brain manifests as headaches or seizures, and symptoms depend on the sites affected. Massive cerebral cysticercosis causes convulsions and death. Cysticerci in the retina blind the patient. In the heart, they may cause arrhythmias and sudden death. Depending on the site involved, cysticercosis is treated with surgery or antihelminthic therapy.

Echinococcosis Features Cysts of the Liver and Lungs

Echinococcosis (hydatid disease) is a zoonotic infection caused by larval cestodes of the genus *Echinococcus*. The most common offender is *Echinococcus granulosus*, which causes cystic hydatid disease. Rarely, *Echinococcus multilocularis* and *Echinococcus vogeli* infect humans.

 **EPIDEMIOLOGY:** Infestation with the tapeworm *E. granulosus* is endemic in sheep, goats and cattle, as well as their attendant dogs. Dogs contaminate their habitats (and their human keepers) with infectious eggs. Humans become infected when they inadvertently ingest the tapeworm eggs. The resulting hydatid disease is present worldwide among herding populations who live in close proximity to dogs and herd animals, especially Australia, New Zealand, Argentina, Greece and herding countries of Africa and the Middle East. In the United States, hydatid cyst disease is seen among immigrants and among the indigenous sheep-herding populations of the southwest.

E. multilocularis causes alveolar hydatid disease in humans. Dogs and cats are domestic definitive hosts; the domestic intermediate host is the house mouse. Rare infections by *E. multilocularis* have been reported in Germany, Switzerland, China and the republics of the former Soviet Union.

Dogs are definitive hosts for *E. vogeli*. Humans may become accidental intermediate hosts for *E. vogeli* by ingesting eggs shed by domestic dogs. Polycystic hydatid disease caused by *E. vogeli* has been reported in Central and South America.

 **ETIOLOGIC FACTORS:** The adult tapeworms (2–6 mm long) live in the small intestines of carnivorous hosts (e.g., wolves, foxes, etc.; Fig. 9-101). *E. granulosus* has a scolex with suckers and numerous hooklets to attach to intestinal mucosa. A short neck is followed by three segments (proglottids). The terminal gravid proglottid breaks off and releases eggs, which are eliminated in feces. Contaminated herbage is then eaten by herbivorous intermediate hosts, such as cattle and sheep. Humans are also infected by ingesting plant material contaminated by cestode eggs. Larvae released from the eggs penetrate the gut wall, enter the bloodstream and disseminate to deep organs, where they grow to form large cysts containing brood capsules and scolices. If the flesh of the herbivore is eaten by a carnivore, scolices develop into sexually mature worms in the latter, thereby completing the cycle.

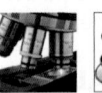 **PATHOLOGY AND CLINICAL FEATURES:** The slowly growing hydatid cyst is found by chance or becomes obvious when its size and position interfere with normal functions. A hepatic cyst may manifest as a palpable right upper quadrant mass. Compression of intrahepatic bile ducts by the cyst leads to obstructive jaundice. Pulmonary cysts (Fig. 9-102) are often asymptomatic and discovered incidentally on a chest radiograph.

A major complication of cyst rupture is seeding of adjacent tissues with brood capsules and scolices. When these "seeds" germinate, they produce many additional cysts, each with the growth potential of the original cyst. Traumatic rupture of a hydatid cyst of the liver or other abdominal organ results in severe diffuse pain, resembling that of peritonitis. Rupture of a pulmonary cyst may cause pneumothorax and empyema. Moreover, when a hydatid cyst ruptures into a body cavity, release of cyst contents can cause fatal allergic

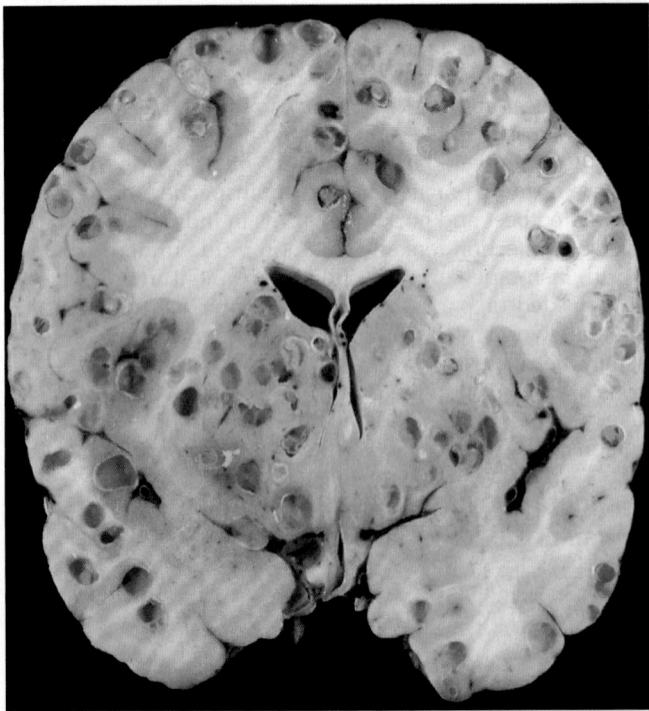

FIGURE 9-100. Cysticercosis. A cross-section of the brain from a patient infected with the larvae of *Taenia solium* shows many cysticerci in the gray matter, imparting a "Swiss cheese" appearance.

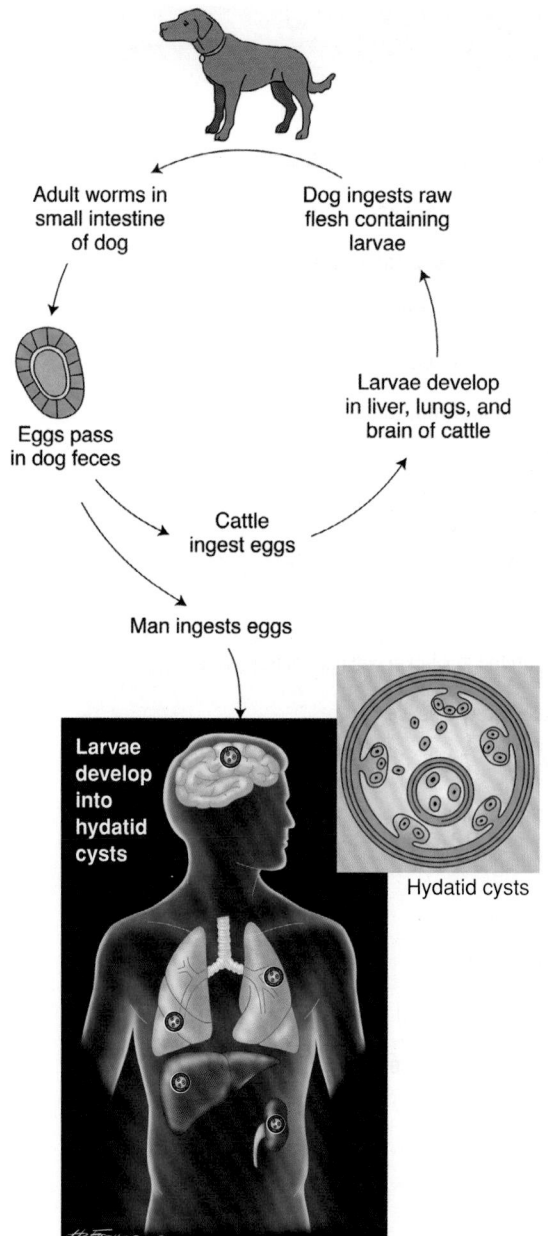

FIGURE 9-101. Life cycle of *Echinococcus granulosus* and cystic hydatid disease. The adult cestode lives in the small intestine of a dog (the definitive host). A gravid proglottid ruptures, releasing cestode eggs into the dog's feces. Cestode eggs are ingested by cattle or sheep (the intermediate hosts), hatch in the intestine and release oncospheres that penetrate the wall of the gut, enter the bloodstream, disseminate to various deep organs and grow to form hydatid cysts, containing brood capsules and scolices. When another dog ingests raw flesh from the cattle or sheep, the scolices are ingested and develop into mature worms in the dog's intestine to complete the cycle. A person who ingests cestode eggs in contaminated plant material becomes an accidental intermediate host. The larvae increase in size, but the parasite reaches a "dead end" without developing into an adult tapeworm. Hydatid cysts in humans occur predominantly in the liver but may also involve lung, kidney, brain and other organs.

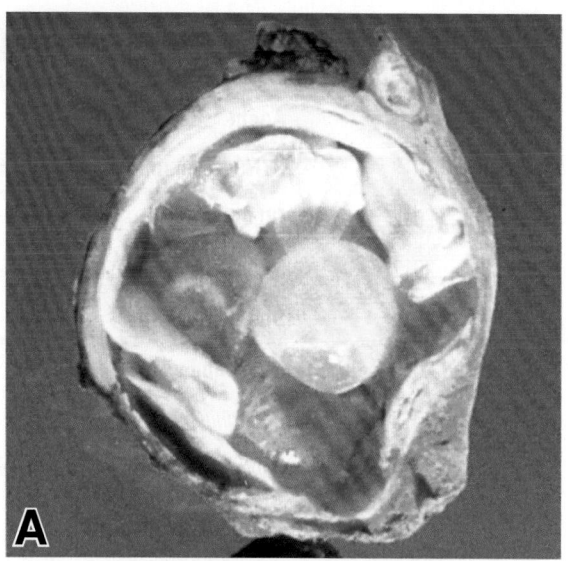

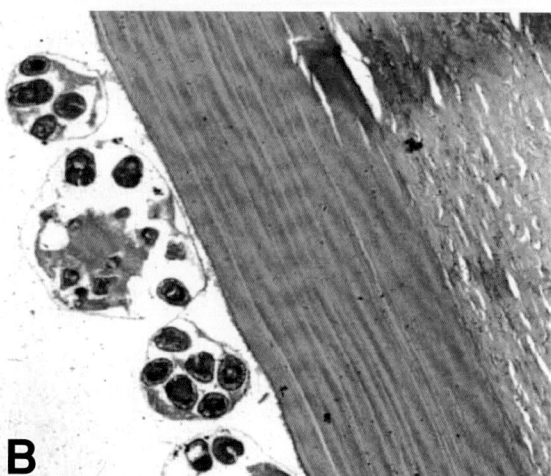

FIGURE 9-102. Echinococcal cyst. A. An echinococcal cyst showing daughter cysts was resected from the liver of a patient infected with *Echinococcus granulosus*. **B.** A photomicrograph of the cyst wall shows (*from right to left*) a laminated, nonnuclear layer, a nucleated germinal layer with brood capsules attached and numerous scolices in the cyst cavity.

Emerging and Reemerging Infections

Several decades ago, the antibiotic revolution, vaccinations and modern public health measures understandably led to the notion that the traditional global scourges of infectious diseases had been brought to bay. However, in the last few decades, we have witnessed the reemergence of microbial threats, including resurgent well-known agents (e.g., cholera, dengue fever, influenza, anthrax), as well as previously unknown pathogens. Antibiotic resistance among organisms, particularly communicable ones, such as tuberculosis, presents a new set of challenges.

Equally important has been the discovery of new pathogens belonging to all classes: viruses, bacteria, parasites and fungi. AIDS and hepatitis C were unknown in the 1970s and alone have caused many millions of deaths, despite

reactions. Treatment of echinococcal cysts requires careful surgical removal: cysts must be sterilized with formalin before drainage or extirpation to prevent intraoperative anaphylactic shock.

TABLE 9-12

EXAMPLES OF RECENTLY DISCOVERED AND EMERGING INFECTIONS

Year	Agent	Human Disease/Association
2013	**H7N9 avian influenza virus**	**Pneumonia**
2012	**GII.4 Sydney**	**Epidemic viral gastroenteritis**
2012	**Novel coronavirus 2012**	**SARS-like respiratory infection**
2012	**Bas Congo virus**	**Hemorrhagic fever**
2012	**Heartland virus**	**Systemic disease**
2012	*Exserohilum rostratum*	**Fungal meningitis outbreak**
2011	*Candidatus Neoehrlichia mikurensis*	**Sepsis**
2010	*Listeria ivanovii*	Gastroenteritis and bacteremia
2009	H1N1 "swine" influenza virus	Pneumonia
2008	Human parvovirus 4 (PARV4)	Viremia
2008	Merkel cell polyomavirus (MC PyV)	Identified in Merkel cell carcinoma tissue
2007	*Segniliparus rugosus*	Respiratory disease
2007	*Mycobacterium massiliense*	Sepsis
2007	*Schineria larvae*	Human myiasis
2007	Saffold virus	Acute gastroenteritis
2007	KI virus (KI PyV)	Respiratory
2007	WU virus (WU PyV)	Respiratory
2006	*Rickettsia massiliae*	Rickettsial spotted fever
2006	*Mycobacterium tilburgii*	Multiorgan disease
2005	Coronavirus HCoV-HKU-1	Pneumonia
2005	*Rickettsia mongolotimonae*	Lymphangitis
2004	H5N1 "avian" influenza	Pneumonia
2004	*Arcobacter* species	Intestinal infection
2004	*Rickettsia parkeri*	Rickettsial spotted fever
2002	SARS-associated coronavirus	Severe atypical pneumonia (SARS-CoV)
2002	*Rickettsia aeschlimannii*	Rickettsial spotted fever
2000	*Rickettsia felis*	Rickettsial spotted fever
2000	Human metapneumovirus (hMPV)	Respiratory tract infection
1999	Nipah virus	Acute respiratory syndrome
1997	Alkhurma hemorrhagic fever virus	Saudi Arabian hemorrhagic fever
1997	*Rickettsia slovaca* (tick-borne lymphade-nopathy); TIBOLA	Lymph node enlargement
1996	*Rickettsia africae*	African tick bite fever
1995	New variant Creutzfeldt-Jakob Disease	Spongiform encephalopathy ("mad cow")

TABLE 9-12

EXAMPLES OF RECENTLY DISCOVERED AND EMERGING INFECTIONS (*Continued*)

Year	Agent	Human Disease/Association
1994	Hendra virus	Acute respiratory syndrome
1994	Sabia virus	Brazilian hemorrhagic fever
1994	Human herpesvirus 8 (HHV8)	Kaposi sarcoma, body cavity lymphomas
1994	*Ehrlichia phagocytophilia*-like agent	Human granulocytic ehrlichiosis
1993	*Balamuthia mandrillaris*	Amebic meningoencephalitis
1993	*Cyclospora cayetanensis*	Coccidian diarrhea
1993	Sin nombre virus	Hantavirus pulmonary syndrome
1993	*Septata intestinalis* (now *Encephalitozoon intestinalis*)	Intestinal and disseminated microsporidiosis
1992	*Vibrio cholerae* O139	Epidemic cholera
1992	*Bartonella henselae*	Bacillary angiomatosis, cat-scratch fever
1991	*Ehrlichia chaffeensis*	Human ehrlichiosis
1991	Guanarito virus	Venezuelan hemorrhagic fever
1991	*Encephalitozoon hellem*	Disseminated microsporidiosis
1990	*Anaplasma phagocytophilum*	Human granulocytic anaplasmosis
1990	*Haemophilus influenzae* biotype *aegyptius*	Brazilian purpuric fever
1990	Human herpesvirus 7 (HHV7)	Aseptic meningitis
1989	*Pythium insidiosum*	Cutaneous and deep fungal infections
1989	*Chlamydia pneumoniae* (TWAR)	Respiratory infection
1989	Hepatitis C virus	Chronic hepatitis, cirrhosis, liver cancer
1989	Barmah Forest virus	Polyarthritis
1986	Human herpesvirus 6 (HHV6)	Roseola (Exanthema subitum)
1986	Porogia virus	Hemorrhagic fever/renal syndrome (HFRS)
1986	HIV-2	AIDS-like illness
1985	*Enterocytozoon bieneusi*	Intestinal and hepatobiliary microsporidiosis
1983	HIV-1	AIDS
1983	*Helicobacter pylori*	Gastric and duodenal infection, ulcers
1983	Hepatitis E virus	"Epidemic" non-A non-B hepatitis
1983	*Borrelia burgdorferi*	Lyme disease

SARS = severe acute respiratory syndrome; SARS-CoV = severe acute respiratory syndrome-associated corona virus.

therapeutic advances. The resilience of influenza virus as a pathogen is underscored by the global influenza pandemics (e.g., H1N1, H5N1).

Table 9-12 is a partial list of newly recognized human infections. It should serve as a reminder that the equilibrium between humans and the pathogens that confront them is a dynamic one: continuous vigilance is obligatory, and complacency invites disaster. The reader is referred to other sources for those infections not discussed above.

AGENTS OF BIOWARFARE

Biological agents have been used as weapons since ancient times. The earliest documentation of use of biological weapons is described in Hittite texts from 1500 to 2000 BC, in which victims of plague were driven into enemy lands. The great Carthaginian warrior, Hannibal, first delivered bioweapons in 184 BC when, in preparing for a naval battle against King Eumenes of Pergamum, his army filled earthenware pots with serpents and hurled them to the decks of the Pergamene ships. In 1346, the Tatars lay siege to the Genoese-controlled seaport of Caffa (modern-day Feodosiya, Ukraine). During the siege, the Tatars were ravaged by plague. The Tatar leader catapulted his own dead soldiers, victims of the disease, into the besieged town to spread the epidemic, and forced the Genoese army to flee to Italy. Similar tactics were used at Karlstein in Bohemia in 1422 and by Russian troops in fighting Swedish forces in Reval in 1710.

Smallpox was used as a biological weapon by Francisco Pizarro in his conquest of South America in the 15th century when he presented variola-contaminated clothing as gifts. The English used a similar tactic in the French-Indian War in 1763, when Sir Jeffrey Amherst presented smallpox-laden blankets to the Delaware Indians loyal to the French. During the Revolutionary War, there were accusations of the potential use of smallpox as a weapon of terror from both sides. There was a plan by the British and their colonial allies to spread smallpox among the revolutionary American colonists (Fig. 9-103). In addition, a smallpox outbreak was spreading through the Northern Continental Army. By 1777, General George Washington ordered mandatory smallpox inoculation of all military recruits who had not had the disease.

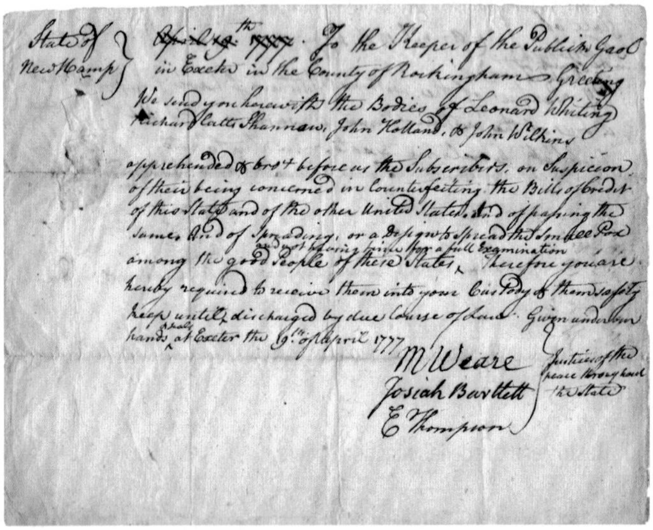

State of New Hamps. April 19th 1777. To the Keeper of the Publick Gaol in Exeter in the County of Rockingham Greeting

We send you herewith the Bodies of Leonard Whiting Richard Flatts Shannaw, John Holland, & John Wilkins apprehended & brot before us the Subscribers, on Suspicion of their being concerned in Counterfeiting the Bills of Credit of this State and of the other United States. And of passing the same, And of Spreading, or a Design to Spread the Small Pox among the good People of these States, Therefore you are hereby required to receive them into your Custody & them safely keep untill discharged by due Course of Law. Given under our hands at Exeter the 19th of April 1777

M Weare
Josiah Bartlett
E Thompson

FIGURE 9-103. American Revolutionary War handwritten document describing the arrest and transport of three men "*... on Suspicion of their being concerned in Counterfeiting the Bills of Credit of this State and of the other United States, and of passing the same* ***And of Spreading or a Design to spread the Small Pox among the good People of these States...,***" dated April 19, 1777 and signed by Josiah Bartlett, a famed New Hampshire physician and signer of the Declaration of Independence. This letter describes the threat of deliberate biowarfare by British sympathizers (Loyalists) in the War of Independence, and led to General George Washington's order for smallpox inoculation of the Continental Army.

TABLE 9-13

POTENTIAL BIOLOGICAL AGENTS OF WARFARE AND BIOTERROR

Bacteria
Bacillus anthracis
Brucella abortus, Brucella suis, Brucella melitensis
Listeria monocytogenes
Vibrio cholerae
Rickettsia prowazekii, Rickettsia rickettsii
Burkholderia mallei, Burkholderia pseudomallei
Coxiella burnetii, Francisella tularensis, Yersinia pestis
Clostridium botulinum and botulinum neurotoxin-producing species of *Clostridium*
Viruses
Arenaviruses—Lassa, Machupo, Sabia, Junin, Guanarito
Bunyaviruses—Rift Valley fever virus, Congo-Crimean hemorrhagic fever virus
Filoviruses—Ebolavirus, Marburg virus
Flaviviruses—Kyasanur Forest disease
Influenza
Kumlinge, Omsk hemorrhagic fever, Russian spring-summer encephalitis, tick-borne encephalitis
Poxviruses—smallpox (variola) and monkeypox
Togaviruses—eastern equine encephalitis virus
Venezuelan equine encephalitis virus
Biological Toxins
Botulinum, *Clostridium perfringens* ε toxin
Staphylococcal enterotoxin B
Shigatoxin
Conotoxins
Abrin
Ricin
Tetrodotoxin
Saxitoxin
T-2 toxin
Diacetoxyscirpenol
Microcystins
Aflatoxins
Satratoxin H
Palytoxin
Anatoxin A

Allegations of biowarfare surfaced in World War I. The Germans were reported to spread cholera to Italy, plague to St. Petersburg and anthrax and glanders to the United States and elsewhere. Although the League of Nations following the war found no definite proof of any of these actions by Germany, the psychological impact of the potential use of biological weaponry in inducing terror was firmly established in modern times. The United States established Camp Detrick in Maryland in 1942–1943 to investigate biological weapons.

The 20th century has unfortunately witnessed many national bioweapons programs, mainly covert, and a few notorious for human experimentation. During the Sino-Japanese War, 1937–1945, Japanese Army Unit 731 conducted bioweapons experimentation on many thousands of Chinese civilians, as well as Russian and American prisoners of war. The Japanese Army used bioweapons during military campaigns against Chinese soldiers and civilians. In 1940, Japanese planes bombed Ningbo with ceramic bombs containing plague-infested fleas. It is estimated that 400,000 Chinese died as a direct result of this use of biological weapons.

Accidental biological contamination has also occurred. In 1942, Gruinard Island off the northwest coast of Scotland was rendered uninhabitable for almost 50 years after British field trials of anthrax. In 1979, accidental release of anthrax from a Sverdlovsk (now Yekaterinburg) military facility, Compound 19, was perhaps the largest biological weapons accident known; sheep developed anthrax 200 kilometers from the release point and over 60 people died.

There is legitimate fear in modern times over the use of bioweapons as a terrorist tool. In September 1984, an outbreak of salmonella gastroenteritis was caused by followers of the Indian guru Bagwan Shree Rajneesh in Oregon, infecting over 700 people. In 1993, an apocalyptic Japanese cult group sprayed anthrax spores from a high-rise building in Tokyo, but no one was injured. The same cult group was found to be preparing vast quantities of C. difficile spores for terrorist use. In 1995, the American Type Culture Collection (ATCC), a nonprofit organization that supplies biological specimens to scientists, shipped a package containing three vials of Y. pestis to the home of a political extremist in Ohio. A search of his home revealed a variety of explosive devices, detonating fuses and triggers. Most recently, dried anthrax was mailed in letters through the U.S. postal system, causing five deaths.

Only a few biological agents have been considered or proven to be effective as weapons of biowarfare or bioterrorism (Table 9-13). Key factors that make an infectious agent suitable for large-scale biowarfare include (1) ease of large-scale production; (2) ability to cause death or incapacity of humans at doses that are deliverable; (3) appropriate particle size as an aerosol; (4) ease of dissemination; (5) stability during storage, in the environment or during placement into a delivery system; and (6) susceptibility of intended victims, but nonsusceptibility of friendly forces. Some biological weapons are potentially extremely lethal: 1 gram of purified botulinum toxin could kill 10 million people.

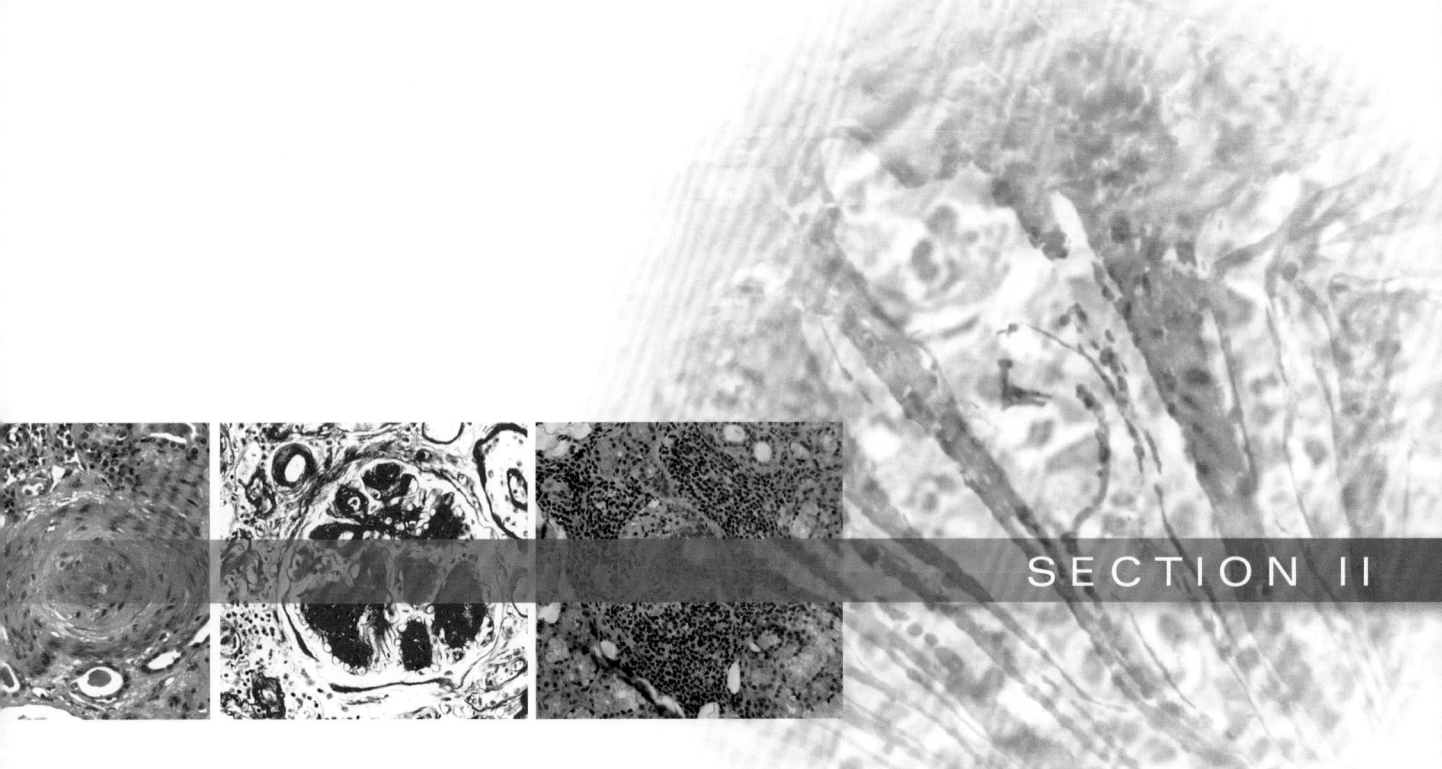

Pathogenesis of Systemic Conditions

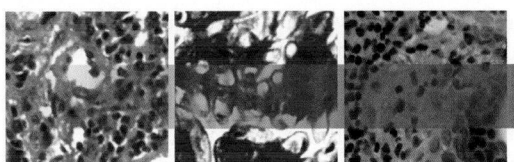

Aging

David Lombard

Biological Aging
Life Span
Model Systems

Cellular Senescence and Organismal Aging
Telomeres
Molecular Control of Aging

Reactive Oxygen Species
Proteostasis
Mitochondrial Dysfunction
Stem Cell Function

Genetic Diseases Resembling Premature Aging
Defects in DNA Repair

Reduced Caloric Intake and Longevity
Active Aspects of DR-Induced Longevity
Insulin and IGF-1 Signaling
Sirtuins

> Harsh old age (Geras) will soon enshroud you—ruthless age which stands someday at the side of every man, deadly, wearying, dreaded even by the gods.
>
> *Homeric Hymn V to Aphrodite 243-24*

BIOLOGICAL AGING

Questions related to aging and death have obsessed humanity since the dawn of recorded history. For example, after the debacle in the Garden of Eden, Adam and Eve were cursed with (among other problems) the certainty of mortality, implying predestined aging. *Aging can be defined as a process characterized by progressive dysfunction, frailty and increasing mortality.* Biological aging is distinct from disease, in that the latter represents an abnormal and unpredictable pathologic condition, whereas aging is both universal and inevitable. Yet, aging and disease are intimately related; aging represents a key risk factor—and in many cases the dominant risk factor—for many of the afflictions described elsewhere in this volume.

The insidious effects of aging can be detected in otherwise healthy persons. For example, in many sports, an athlete in his or her 30s is considered "old." Even in the absence of specific diseases or vascular abnormalities, beginning in the fourth decade of life, there is a progressive decline in many physiologic functions, including such measurable parameters as muscular strength, cardiac reserve, nerve conduction time, pulmonary vital capacity, glomerular filtration and vascular elasticity (Fig. 10-1). This functional deterioration is accompanied by structural changes. Lean body mass decreases and the proportion of fat rises. Connective tissue matrix constituents are increasingly cross-linked. Lipofuscin ("aging") pigment accumulates in organs such as the brain, heart and liver. At the cellular level, the challenges imposed by aging on postmitotic cells (e.g., neurons and cardiomyocytes) are likely quite different than those faced by rapidly dividing cells, such as those of the gut or skin.

Life Span Is Subject to Environmental and Genetic Influences

Considerable evidence shows that aging is subject to strong genetic and environmental influences. For example, it is now possible to achieve dramatic life span extension (up to 65%) in rodent models through single-gene mutations in specific signaling pathways, or even by administering certain small molecules. Reduced food intake without malnutrition (dietary restriction [DR]) promotes longevity in many species, from budding yeast to rodents and perhaps even nonhuman primates.

Those who live in advanced industrialized societies already benefit from a greatly increased life span, relative to our forebears. It is estimated that a typical age at death of Neolithic humans was 20–25 years, and the average life span today in some underdeveloped regions is often barely 10 years more. By contrast, female life expectancy at birth in industrialized countries over the past 160 years has risen

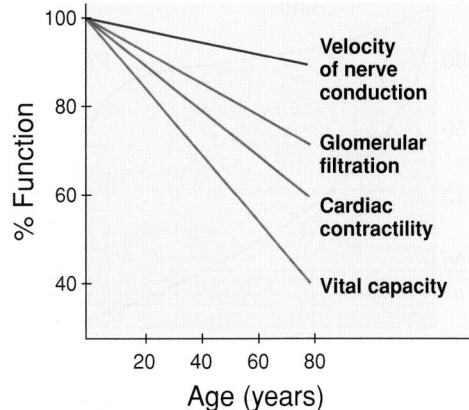

FIGURE 10-1. Decrease in human physiologic capacities as a function of age.

linearly by nearly 3 months a year, from about 45 years in the mid-19th century to nearly 85 years in the present day (women live 5–6 years longer than men, on average). This dramatic increase in life span stems mostly from reduced child mortality and improved public health measures, as well as advances in medical care. If current trends hold, life expectancy at birth in developed countries may reach 100 years by the mid-21st century. The **maximum** documented life span for any human is 122 years, and very few people live to be significantly older than 100.

Health Span

Health span is the *period of life spent free from major disease.* Remarkably, the prolongevity interventions described below not only extend life span but also delay or prevent many common diseases. For example, mice on a DR diet remain healthy into late old age, sometimes showing no evidence of clinically significant pathology at necropsy. By contrast, animals allowed to eat as much as they want typically show a diverse spectrum of advanced pathologies.

An Evolutionary Perspective on Aging

Why do we age at all? Once development has ceased, why do we not remain in good health and young perpetually? The notion that aging is programmed is an intuitively appealing explanation. That is to say, older individuals die to "make room" and free up resources for the next generation. However, from the standpoint of evolutionary biology, there are major conceptual problems with the notion of programmed aging. Among these is the issue of "cheating"—that is, if a gene existed whose sole purpose was to cause those possessing it to age and die, lucky individuals in whom that gene had been inactivated by chance would experience a selective breeding advantage and eventually take over the population. By similar reasoning, mutations that speed aging would confer selective disadvantages and so would not be maintained during evolution.

So if aging is not a strictly programmed process, akin to development, why does it occur? Evolutionary biology offers a conceptual answer to this question, if not a biological mechanism. We observe aging of organisms in the laboratory, or in other protected settings such as zoos. In this context, the maximal life span of animals in the wild is no different from the same animals in the zoo (Fig. 10-2).

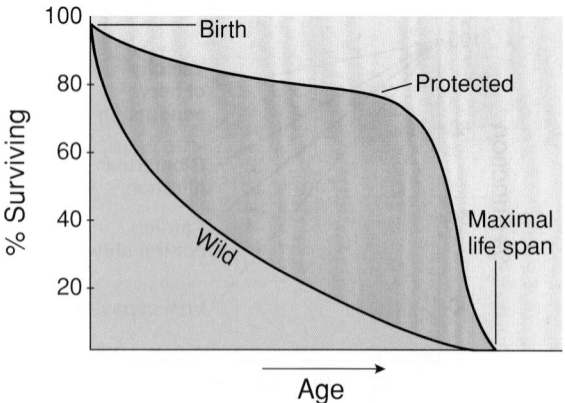

FIGURE 10-2. Life span of animals in their natural environment compared with that in a protected habitat. Note that both curves reach the same maximal life span.

In humans, aging is most evident in industrialized societies, where most people escape the ravages of infant mortality, infectious disease, trauma, starvation and other causes of early death. However, these sorts of protected environments differ greatly from those that occurred over the course of evolution. Most organisms evolved under conditions in which predation, infectious disease, competition for resources and environmental exposure eliminated most of the population early in life, independently of any effects of aging. For organisms evolving under such strong pressures, there was no evolutionary selective advantage in longevity, as most people died early from non-age-related causes. This idea generates several predictions that are borne out experimentally. For example, evolutionary biology predicts that species that evolve in relatively protected environments will inherently live longer than those evolving in less forgiving circumstances. In fact, this is the case. Birds, bats and flying squirrels, all of which can fly to escape from potential predators, are far longer lived than are mice. Other rodents that have evolved inherent protection against would-be predators (e.g., porcupines) or that live in safe environments underground (the naked mole rat) also live longer than their less fortunate exposed kin.

Antagonistic Pleiotropy

Evolutionary biology postulates **antagonistic pleiotropy,** that is, that *genes with deleterious effects at older ages may nevertheless be favorably selected if they confer some advantage early in life.* Thus, genes that improve reproductive efficiency, running speed or pathogen resistance in young adults would be greatly favored, even if they were associated with increases in the risks of cancer, neurodegeneration or other pathologies of old age.

Diverse Systems Exist to Study the Biology of Aging

Maximal life spans range from a few hours for adult forms of some insects, to a few weeks for the nematode *Caenorhabditis elegans* and fruitfly *Drosophila melanogaster,* to many decades for humans and other large mammals. At the upper end of longevity, there are clams that can live for centuries. A few species, such as hydra and lobster, may be entirely immune to aging. Key pathways that modulate longevity in invertebrates function similarly in rodents, and so potentially operate in the same way in humans.

Short-Lived Organisms and Mechanistic Insights into Aging

Model organisms have helped elucidate aging biology (Fig. 10-3). Brewer's yeast (*Saccharomyces cerevisiae*) reproduces by budding, producing a larger mother cell and a smaller daughter cell. Individual yeast cells can bud only a finite number of times before ceasing to divide, a point known as *senescence.* Several yeast genes (e.g., *mTOR* [mammalian target of rapamycin] and *SIR2*) influence this process and also play key roles in modulating longevity in mammals. The roundworm (*C. elegans*) and the fruitfly (*Drosophila*) are more complex organisms that possess tissue types seen in higher organisms, such as skeletal muscle and a nervous system. As they age, they show degenerative effects like those in higher organisms, including decreased movement and lipofuscin accumulation.

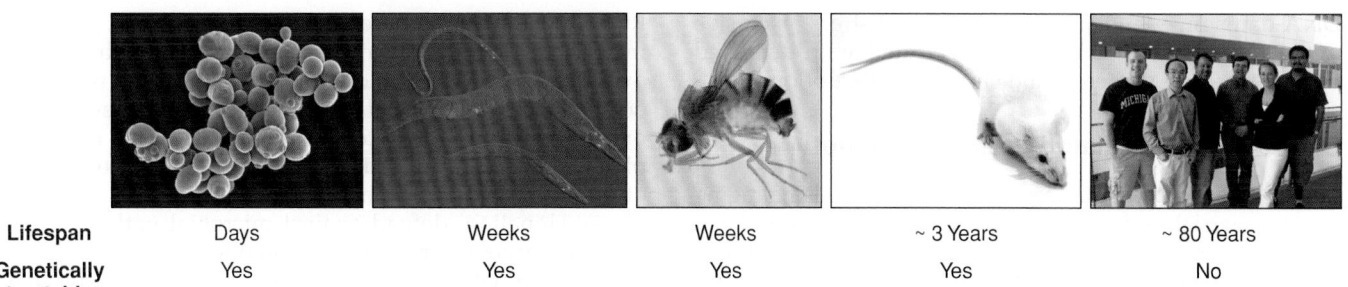

Lifespan	Days	Weeks	Weeks	~ 3 Years	~ 80 Years
Genetically tractable	Yes	Yes	Yes	Yes	No

FIGURE 10-3. Model organisms commonly used in aging research.

Among mammals, the laboratory mouse (*Mus musculus*) is by far the most common system used in life span studies. Aged mice show many of the same pathologies as older humans. Thus, their small size, rapid generation time of roughly 12 weeks, and short life span of 2–3 years, make mice the prime system for studying mammalian aging. The ease with which mouse strains with specific genomic alterations can be produced has facilitated dissection of mechanisms of mammalian aging. Many diverse pathologies of old age in humans are also manifest in aged mice.

Scaling

Conserved aging phenotypes show a phenomenon called **scaling**—that is, they manifest at proportionately the same point in the lifespan, irrespective of absolute chronological time. Thus, cancer incidence increases at roughly the midpoint of life span in both mice and humans. However, in mice, this phenomenon occurs at 1–1½ years, whereas in humans, it occurs in the 5th decade. Although the biological basis of scaling is not well understood, it implies that interventions that slow the aging rate in humans would probably also delay the onset of age-associated disease and dysfunction.

CELLULAR SENESCENCE AND ORGANISMAL AGING

When human fibroblasts are passaged serially in culture, they do not replicate forever. Instead (like yeast), after many passages, they enter a nondividing state called **replicative senescence**. During this time, they remain postmitotic but are viable for an extended period. Senescent cells are characterized by (1) an enlarged, flattened appearance; (2) absence of molecular markers of proliferation; (3) persistent foci of unrepaired DNA damage; and (4) expression of senescence-associated β-galactosidase and p16^{Ink4a} protein.

Telomere Shortening Promotes Replicative Senescence

In human cells, replicative senescence is largely due to attrition of **telomeres,** which are a series of short repetitive nucleotide sequences (TTAGGG in vertebrates) at the 3' ends of chromosomes (see Chapters 1 and 5). DNA polymerase, the enzyme that replicates DNA, begins at the 5' and works toward the 3' end. It cannot copy linear chromosomes all the way to their distal ends, so telomeres tend to shorten with each cell division. Telomeres protect the genes that are near chromosomal termini from being lost with repeated cell divisions. Certain crucial cell types, such as stem cell populations, express an enzyme, **telomerase,** that restores sequences lost during replication and thus stabilizes the length of their telomeres. By contrast, most human somatic cells, such as fibroblasts, do not express significant levels of telomerase. Consequently, their telomeres shorten with each cell division, thus representing a "mitotic clock" that counts DNA replication events. Some types of cellular injury, such as oxidative stress, can directly damage telomeres, independent of replication.

Telomeres are normally protected by a protein complex termed **shelterin**. When telomeres shorten beyond a critical point, shelterin is released and telomeres are exposed, triggering a DNA damage response that can cause irreversible cell cycle arrest or apoptosis (Fig. 10-4). Telomere attrition can also lead to end-to-end chromosomal fusions and other types of genomic instability via breakage–fusion–bridge cycles (see Chapter 5). Reintroduction of telomerase into human fibroblasts enables them to bypass senescence, showing that telomere attrition is limiting for their growth in culture.

In addition to telomere shortening, other types of cellular injury also induce cellular senescence. These include many

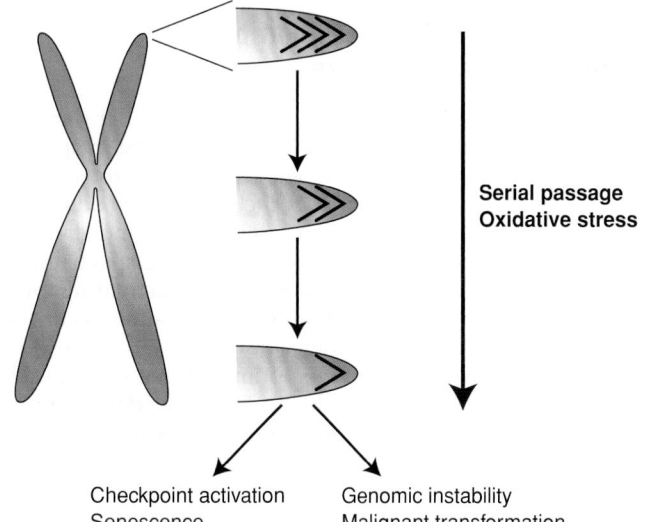

FIGURE 10-4. **Deleterious consequences of telomere shortening in mammalian cells.**

DNA-damaging agents, such as oxidative stress, excessive mitogenic stimulation like that associated with activated oncogenes (see Chapter 5), and chromatin disruption.

Senescence-Associated Secretory Phenotype

The link between cellular senescence and organismal aging is controversial and complex. There is solid evidence that senescence prevents replication of cells with potentially oncogenic mutations (oncogene-induced senescence; see Chapter 5), thereby helping protect from tumors. Senescent cells also secrete proinflammatory cytokines, proteases and other factors (the **senescence-associated secretory phenotype,** or **SASP**). Via SASP, senescent cells might potentially contribute to age-related pathologies, such as atherosclerosis, epidermal thinning, immune dysfunction and degenerative joint disease. Furthermore, it is possible that senescent cells create a microenvironment that promotes the growth of malignant cells, thus contributing to the increased rate of cancer observed in older people. Experimentally eliminating senescent cells can mitigate some effects of aging in mouse models.

Precise Molecular Mechanisms of Aging Remain Obscure

Many factors probably contribute to the degenerative manifestations of aging. Accumulated unrepaired macromolecular damage—to DNA, chromatin, proteins and lipids—eventually may induce cellular dysfunction, manifesting at the organismal level as aging. To counter the effects of such damage, cells have evolved elaborate, well-regulated mechanisms to repair many types of macromolecular lesions. Alternatively, cells with certain types of severe damage, such as to mitochondria and nuclear DNA, can also be removed by apoptosis (see Chapter 1). This damage-based model of aging predicts that mutant organisms with increased longevity should also show more robust resistance to damage-inducing stressors. This is in fact typically—though not always—observed. The model also predicts that cellular repair systems should be intimately related, genetically speaking, to prolongevity pathways. This is also observed empirically, as outlined in greater detail below.

Reactive Oxygen Species Contribute to Age-Associated Disease

A long-standing theory holds that macromolecular damage in the context of aging is caused by **reactive oxygen species (ROS),** generated mostly endogenously in mitochondria (see Chapter 1). Important ROS include superoxide, peroxide and nitric oxide. ROS can interact with and damage all cellular macromolecules, causing a diverse spectrum of lesions in nucleic acids, modifying and inactivating proteins and damaging lipids. Most ROS generation occurs in mitochondria, owing to "leakage" at complexes I and III of the electron transport chain. It is estimated that a single cell undergoes some 100,000 attacks on DNA per day by ROS, and that at any time 10% of protein molecules in the cell are modified by oxidative carbonyl adducts.

Antioxidants

To counter the potentially toxic consequences of ROS, cells possess a network of antioxidant defenses that detoxify ROS and repair ROS-related damage. These pathways include superoxide dismutase, catalase, glutathione peroxidase, thioredoxins, thioredoxin reductase and many others. An excess of ROS relative to cellular defenses is called **oxidative stress**. It is noteworthy that ROS play important physiologic roles, in addition to being a potential source of macromolecular damage. For example, ROS modulate kinase signaling, defend against microbial pathogens and regulate vascular tone. Thus, it is neither possible nor desirable to eliminate cellular ROS entirely. Yet most long-lived invertebrate mutants have enhanced antioxidant defenses. DR induces increased antioxidant defenses, concomitant with diminished ROS levels and reduced macromolecular oxidation products.

However, it is unlikely that ROS are the single major driver of age-associated damage. In many invertebrate models, *elevated* ROS levels are associated with *increased* longevity. Enhancement of ROS defenses in mouse models through genetic overexpression of antioxidant enzymes generally does not extend longevity. Studies in hundreds of thousands of people given supraphysiologic doses of antioxidant dietary supplements have not found any significant benefit on life span, disease development or health; indeed, adding certain antioxidants is associated with *increased* mortality.

A corollary to the free radical theory of aging, the **rate of living theory** aims to explain why larger species in general live longer and show a reduced metabolic rate than smaller ones. One current form of this idea postulates that each gram of tissue from any organism (shrew, human, elephant) can metabolize the same amount of total energy over the life span before losing function, presumably owing to accumulated ROS-related injury. Several observations have cast doubt on this theory: (1) some small creatures with high metabolic rates nevertheless live for a relatively long time (e.g., birds and bats); (2) *within* species, larger individuals tend to have a shorter life span than smaller ones (e.g., larger breeds of dogs are shorter lived than smaller ones); and (3) DR does not reduce overall metabolic rate but (counterintuitively) may actually *increase* it.

The Role of Telomere Maintenance in Longevity

The role of telomere erosion in aging is attributed to progressive cellular dysfunction and senescence, eventually leading to the overall phenomenon of organismal aging. However, laboratory mice have very long telomeres, and yet these animals age, so that (at least in mice) telomere attrition may not be needed for aging to occur. In humans, rare mutations in telomerase or shelterin components lead to shortened telomeres and aplastic anemia, skin and nail defects, infertility, pulmonary fibrosis and cancer. Even in people without such defects, shortened telomeres are also found in association with human diseases such as cirrhosis, atherosclerosis and ulcerative colitis, consistent with extended proliferative histories or high levels of oxidative stress in these conditions. Short telomere length in peripheral blood cells predicts susceptibility to coronary artery disease, neoplasia and overall mortality in older people. These findings suggest that eroded telomeres can indeed contribute to age-associated pathologies, if not necessarily to aging per se.

Genetically engineered mouse strains that cannot maintain telomeres show reduced longevity, as well as defects in tissues that require rapid cell proliferation and stem and progenitor cell activity, principally bone marrow, skin, gut and testes. Altogether, these studies demonstrate that telomere maintenance contributes to cellular and organismal homeostasis, but that its role in human longevity is less clear.

Maintenance of Proteostasis May Contribute to Longevity

Increasing evidence points to maintenance of cellular protein homeostasis (proteostasis) as an important factor in longevity (see Chapter 1). All cellular proteins, collectively called the proteome, are subject to diverse challenges. Translational errors, oxidative damage, mutations and polymorphisms can lead to protein misfolding and aggregation, which can cause cellular injury. All of these mechanisms can be regulated by interventions that also promote longevity, thus suggesting an important relationship between proteostasis and life span. Moreover, older cells and organisms accumulate oxidatively damaged and cross-linked proteins. Studies of invertebrates suggest that collapse of proteostasis is an early, and perhaps causative, event in organismal aging. One proteostatic mechanism that is closely linked to aging is autophagy, a regulated process by which cells degrade damaged proteins, and even whole organelles, in lysosomes (see Chapter 1). In model organisms, autophagy is required for longevity induced by many environmental or genetic manipulations. Autophagic function declines with age in mammals and lower organisms, and restoration of autophagy in older mice can improve tissue function.

Mitochondrial Function Declines with Aging

With age, mitochondria produce less adenosine triphosphate (ATP) and generate more ROS. It is thought that this mitochondrial energetic decline contributes to age-associated conditions such as sarcopenia, insulin resistance and type 2 diabetes, cardiac dysfunction, neurodegeneration and so forth. The molecular basis for mitochondrial functional decline during aging is unclear; damage to the mitochondrial genome may play a role. Since mitochondrial DNA lies in close proximity to components of the respiratory chain, the mitochondrial genome is highly susceptible to ROS-induced DNA damage. However, the role of mitochondria in longevity is not that straightforward. In *C. elegans, Drosophila* and even rodents, certain mitochondrial defects present during development actually *extend* longevity. Mitochondria thus help determine organismal longevity, but via complex and uncertain mechanisms.

Stem Cell Function Declines with Aging

Adult stem cells in mammalian tissues are critical for proper organ function and for repair following injury. These stem cells may lose functionality with age, thus impairing tissue homeostasis and contributing to degenerative disease. This notion has been best evaluated in the context of hematopoietic stem cells (HSCs), which give rise to all mature cell types in the blood. Aging is not characterized by fewer HSCs, but it is associated with impaired HSC function. Clinically, it has long been known that HSC transplants from young donors are more likely to be successful than those from older donors. In aged people, HSCs increasingly follow myeloid, rather than lymphoid, differentiation. There are progressive defects in HSC mobilization and homing, and aged HSCs also accumulate unrepaired ROS-induced DNA damage.

As mentioned previously expression of the tumor suppressor p16^{Ink4a} is induced in senescent cells. More generally, in aging tissues, p16^{Ink4a} and the related gene p19^{ARF} (the murine equivalent of human p14^{ARF}) are normally inhibited by Bmi-1, a protein required for renewal of all adult stem cell types. In aged mice, p16^{Ink4a} limits proliferative capacity in different types of stem cells. Increased p16^{Ink4a} in aging stem cells may be a defense against malignant transformation of these cells, at the expense of stem cell function, tissue repair and overall organismal homeostasis. Interestingly, genetic studies in humans have linked polymorphisms near the p16^{Ink4a} locus to diverse age-associated pathologies (e.g., coronary atherosclerosis, type 2 diabetes and frailty). These data suggest that p16^{Ink4a} or a closely linked gene product can regulate aging in humans in important ways, via effects on stem cells or other cell types.

In recent years, it has become possible to convert somatic cells into induced pluripotent stem cells (iPSCs). Remarkably, this process reverses many effects of aging, including senescence, telomere erosion and mitochondrial dysfunction. Although the mechanisms underlying these effects are poorly understood, it may eventually be possible to harness these processes to ameliorate the ravages of aging in differentiated cells.

Alternatives to the ROS-Centric Model of Aging

The free radical theory of aging dominated thinking in aging biology for decades, but aging is unlikely to have a single "root cause." As noted above, genetic data support the concept that protein quality control mechanisms are key to organismal longevity and health; hence, unrepaired damage to proteins may be a major cause of age-associated decline. As well, diverse chemicals (xenobiotics) in food and the environment may cause diverse types of macromolecular damage, thus contributing to the effects of aging. Xenobiotics are detoxified and chemically processed for eventual excretion by xenobiotic metabolizing enzymes. Intracellular signaling itself, in particular via mTOR kinase, may be central to organismal aging. Signaling through mTOR and its downstream targets significantly limits life span (see below). The mTOR-centric model postulates that this kinase drives inappropriate cellular hypertrophy and hyperplasia as organisms age, contributing to, or even causing, many of the manifestations of aging.

It seems likely that the protean effects of aging reflect multiple molecular causes, including diverse types of molecular damage and other phenomena, such as excess mTOR signaling. These effects may then converge to cause progressive dysfunction and eventual death. Processes underlying biological aging persist, since there has been little evolutionary pressure to weed them out. However, experimental biologists have now developed powerful means of extending life span; there is great promise that such tools will provide additional mechanistic insights into the aging process and eventually, perhaps, the means to extend healthy life spans in humans.

GENETIC DISEASES RESEMBLING PREMATURE AGING

There are rare diseases that seem to resemble accelerated aging (progerias). The two best-studied such conditions are Werner syndrome (WS) and Hutchinson-Guilford progeria syndrome (HGPS).

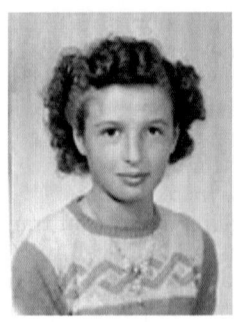 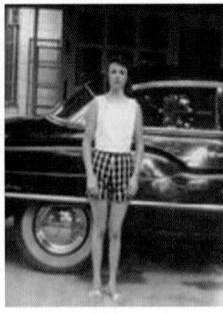 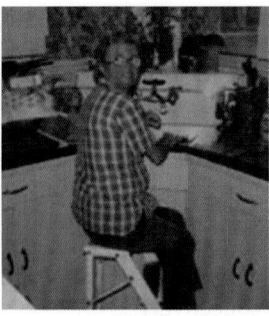 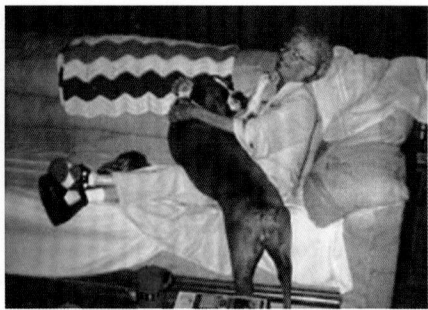

Age 8 Age 21 Age 36 Age 56

FIGURE 10-5. Werner syndrome. The premature appearance of aging phenotypes is evident.

Werner Syndrome

WS is caused by recessive mutations in the *WRN* gene, encoding a DNA helicase involved in many aspects of DNA metabolism, including replication, repair and telomere maintenance. Patients with mutations in *WRN* show poor growth in adolescence, premature hair graying, thinning of the skin, cataracts, diabetes and atherosclerosis (Fig. 10-5). They also have a tendency to develop cancer, specifically sarcomas, leukemias and other malignancies. WS patients typically succumb to myocardial infarction or cancer by their 40s or 50s.

Despite the apparent similarities of WS to normal aging, this disease is by no means a perfect mimic of the aging process. For example, some disorders commonly associated with physiologic aging, such as Alzheimer disease, are not observed in WS. Thus, WS is an example of a **segmental progeria**—that is, a syndrome that recapitulates some, but not all, aspects of accelerated aging. Cultured WS fibroblasts show chromosomal instability, sensitivity to DNA crosslinking agents and a reduced replicative life span. This last observation has been used to argue for the validity of cellular senescence as a model system to study aging.

Hutchinson-Guilford Progeria Syndrome

HGPS is caused by autosomal dominant mutations in the *LMNA* gene, whose product is a protein, **lamin A**. These children show reduced growth, hair loss, scleroderma-like skin changes and atherosclerosis (Fig. 10-6). Patients with HGPS die at an average age of 13 years, typically from myocardial infarction or stroke. The most common mutation associated with HGPS causes missplicing of the LMNA transcript, leading to accumulation of **progerin,** a defective precursor of lamin A protein. Normally, lamin A is a key part of the nuclear lamina that provides structural integrity to the nucleus in differentiated cells. By contrast, progerin accumulates in the nucleus, resulting in a distorted nuclear outline and nuclear blebbing. The buildup of progerin interferes with chromatin organization, impairing gene expression and DNA repair. HGPS is at the severe end of a spectrum of disorders associated with mutations in the *LMNA* gene, collectively termed "**laminopathies**." These diseases are associated with defects in muscle, adipose tissue and peripheral nerves.

It is unclear whether and to what extent the study of WS, HGPS and related disorders improves understanding of the biology of aging. These conditions may represent disease phenotypes whose pathogenesis is unrelated to physiologic aging.

Defects in DNA Repair Cause Degenerative Phenotypes

WS and HGPS are members of a larger group of progerias that show accelerated appearance of degenerative, aging-like (**progeroid**) phenotypes. Since most of these conditions have been produced in the mouse by inactivation of genes involved in nuclear DNA repair, a model holds that DNA is an important target, perhaps the principal target, of age-associated damage. In this respect ROS are thought to represent one major source of aging-associated DNA damage (see above). This is an intuitively appealing notion; unlike other cellular macromolecules such as proteins and lipids, nuclear DNA cannot simply be replaced, but instead must be repaired once damaged. Consistent with this notion, increased levels of chromosomal aberrations, as well as more

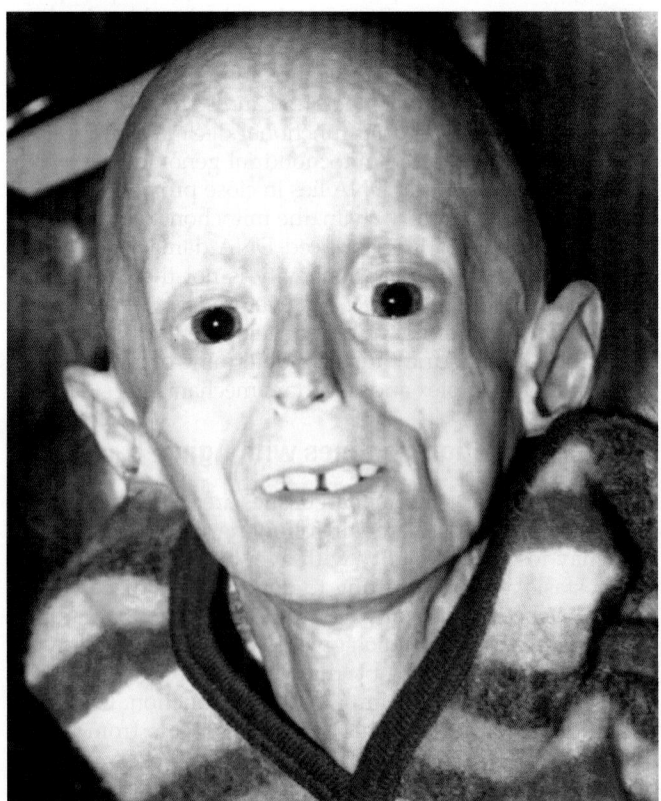

FIGURE 10-6. Hutchinson-Guilford progeria syndrome. A 10-year-old girl shows typical features of this disease.

subtle mutations, occur in peripheral blood leukocytes and other mammalian tissues with advancing age.

Cells have evolved numerous systems to repair distinct DNA lesions (see Chapter 5). Double-strand breaks are repaired through (1) homologous recombination, (2) non-homologous end-joining and (3) alternative end-joining. Single-strand lesions are mended via (1) nucleotide excision repair and its subsystems, (2) base excision repair and (3) mismatch repair. Unrepaired DNA damage activates cellular checkpoint responses, resulting in cell cycle arrest, apoptosis or senescence. Although defects in DNA repair systems cause dramatic harmful effects, that fact does not prove that DNA damage is at the root of physiologic aging. Thus, a connection between DNA repair and aging remains an attractive, but unproven hypothesis.

A related model implicates **epigenetic** alterations in aging. Gene expression is regulated by many mechanisms affecting DNA, histones, chromatin-binding factors, protein alterations and noncoding RNAs. DNA methylation and histone modifications change progressively with age, leading to less accurate regulation of gene expression. In invertebrate systems, genetic manipulations involving the epigenome can prolong life span. Increased cell-to-cell variation in gene expression has been observed with age in mammalian cardiomyocytes, arguing that age-associated epigenetic dysregulation may have deleterious consequences. Further studies are needed to elucidate the significance of epigenetic influences in mammalian aging.

REDUCED CALORIC INTAKE AND LONGEVITY

As noted above, DR promotes increased longevity in the vast majority of organisms in which it has been tested, from budding yeast to rodents. In mice, DR is typically achieved by reducing caloric intake by 30%–50%. This routinely extends life span by 25%–40%. Perhaps even more striking than its prolongevity effects, DR delays or prevents the onset of many age-associated conditions, including cancers, cardiovascular disease, neurodegeneration, diabetes, sarcopenia and many others. However, DR is not a "free ride"; in rodents, it impairs certain immune responses and delays wound healing. In humans, DR has been associated with reduced bone density and muscle mass, and with depression.

Prolonged Longevity with DR Is an Active Phenomenon

Longevity occurring in response to DR is not simply a passive consequence of reduced caloric intake. Even reduction of specific dietary constituents can dramatically prolong longevity. For example, in rodents, restriction of a particular amino acid, methionine, extends life span similarly to the prolongation that is seen with overall reduced caloric intake. Yet methionine-restricted animals actually consume *more* calories than do controls (Fig. 10-7).

In rodent models, DR initiated even in middle-aged adults has beneficial effects, although the increase in longevity is progressively less as DR is started later in life. Remarkably, in mice, DR imposed during the brief 3-week period from birth until weaning is sufficient to confer extended life span. This finding suggests that early DR may provoke long-lasting epigenetic changes that favor longevity.

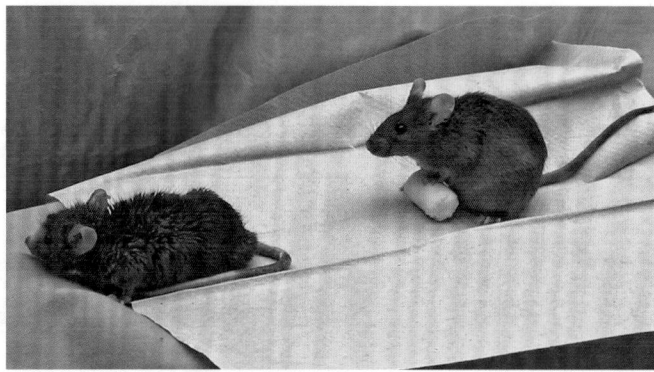

FIGURE 10-7. Methionine restriction extends mouse life span. Both mice are roughly 30 months old. The one in front is the last surviving member of a control group of mice fed regular chow. The one playing with the chalk was fed a low-methionine diet.

Can DR extend life span in humans? Studies of DR in our close cousins, rhesus monkeys, have so far yielded conflicting results as to its impact on longevity, though DR does have consistent health benefits in these animals. Until recently, residents of the Japanese island of Okinawa ate on average substantially fewer calories than did those on the Japanese mainland or the United States. This diet was associated with markedly reduced incidences of cardiac disease and cancer, and one of the world's largest populations of centenarians on a per capita basis. Members of the Calorie Restriction Society voluntarily limit their dietary intake and show improved serum lipid parameters, increased insulin sensitivity, reduced blood pressure and protection against obesity, type 2 diabetes, inflammation, carotid artery intimal hyperplasia and left ventricular diastolic dysfunction. Thus, DR in humans does confer dramatic protection against cardiovascular risk factors. Yet the overall lowest mortality rate in humans is associated with a body mass index (BMI) of roughly 25, corresponding to a normal to slightly overweight status; both lower and higher BMIs are associated with an increased risk of death. Thus, the low BMIs associated with DR in humans may have unforeseen negative consequences.

Hormesis

Conceptually, the longevity associated with DR represents an example of **hormesis:** a low-level stress such as reduced food intake may prime the organism to respond more effectively to other forms of stress, such as those linked to aging. As noted previously, DR is associated with reduced mitochondrial ROS production and decreased ROS-associated damage. It also reduces overall adiposity; visceral adiposity in particular has negative health effects. DR in rodents also increases insulin sensitivity in skeletal muscle and lowers serum levels of insulin and insulin-like growth factor-I (IGF-I). Genetic lesions in nutrient signaling pathways also extend longevity, providing a potential link between DR-induced and genetic longevity. DR modulates the activities of specific sirtuin proteins, NAD^+-dependent deacetylases that promote aspects of mammalian health span. DR also decreases inflammation and upregulates autophagy and DNA repair mechanisms. In sum, DR can extend health and life span. The molecular mechanisms underlying this effect are only beginning to be elucidated, but are likely to be complex.

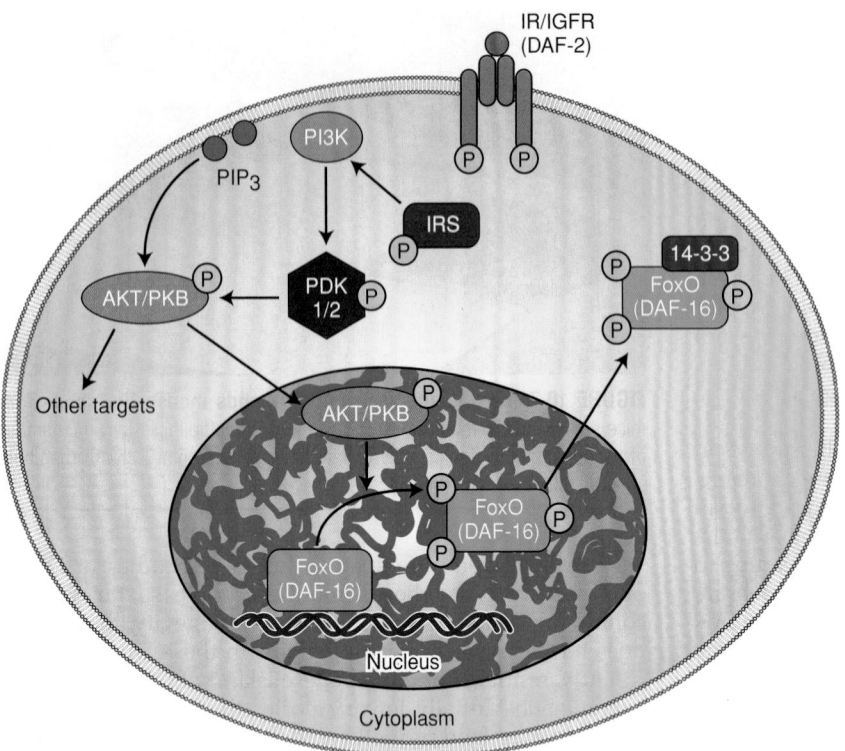

FIGURE 10-8. Insulin/insulin-like growth factor-I (IGF-I)-like signaling (IIS) pathway. IIS begins when insulin or IGF-I binds to its cell surface receptors, which are tyrosine kinases. This initiates an intracellular signaling cascade involving generation of phosphatidylinositol triphosphate by phosphatidylinositol-3-kinase (PI3K), in turn leading to activation of the downstream kinases PDK1 and Akt. FoxO transcription factors are key targets of this signaling pathway; in *C. elegans*, FoxO is termed DAF-16.

Insulin and IGF-I Signaling Shorten Life Span

Insulin/IGF-I-like signaling (IIS) negatively regulates longevity. IIS is initiated when insulin or IGF family members bind their cognate cell surface receptor tyrosine kinases (Fig. 10-8). These interactions activate the kinase Akt, which phosphorylates downstream proteins to regulate diverse processes, including cell survival, growth, cell cycle, metabolism and stress resistance. The FoxO transcription factors are key targets of Akt; when IIS is active, Akt phosphorylation sequesters FoxO factors in the cytoplasm, where they are transcriptionally inert.

In 1993, the first mutation that increased life span in any organism was characterized. Mutations in the *C. elegans* insulin receptor homolog *daf-2* were found to extend life span by more than twofold. This effect required the activity of a FoxO homolog. Subsequent work showed that genetic lesions that impair several IIS components also extend life span. Increased FoxO activity is a key element in longevity driven by reduced IIS. Surprisingly, detailed studies have revealed that increased FoxO activity in only a subset of tissues is sufficient to confer extended life span. These findings highlight the role of neuro endocrine signaling in controlling overall life span.

Two naturally occurring mouse mutants, the Snell and Ames dwarf lines, have pituitary defects that reduce growth hormone (GH) and IGF-I levels, along with greatly extended longevity and delayed onset of age-associated disease. Remarkably, these mice also show preserved cognition in old age. Although they have reduced levels of several pituitary-derived hormones, it is their GH deficiency that is critical for their long life span. Indeed, mutations in many genetically engineered strains of mice with increased longevity impinge upon IIS signaling. In dogs and horses, small breeds show low serum IGF-I levels and longer life spans, compared to their larger cousins. Collectively, these data point to a role for IIS in limiting mammalian life span.

Several mechanistic hypotheses have been proposed to explain how reduced IIS promotes longevity in mammals. In the Ames and Snell dwarf mice, as well as in some other long-lived mouse strains, cells show increased resistance to oxidative and other stressors. Insulin sensitivity is a feature of mice with reduced GH signaling, an improved metabolic profile that may contribute to their longevity, although some other IIS mutants paradoxically show insulin resistance. It has been proposed that reduced IIS contributes to the pro-longevity effects of DR, but mechanisms of longevity underlying DR and reduced GH–IGF-I–IIS overlap only partially.

Could reduced IIS contribute to longevity in humans as well? Since insulin *resistance* in humans is typically a pathologic condition associated with disease states (obesity, atherosclerosis, dyslipidemia, etc.; see Chapter 13), the intuitive response to this question might be no. Yet genetic studies in humans support the notion that under some circumstances, reduced IIS may provide health and even longevity benefits. Congenital mutations in the GH receptor and consequent low serum IGF-I levels are the basis of **Laron dwarfism**. Affected individuals show very short stature and striking protection from cancer and type 2 diabetes. In more typical populations, polymorphisms in the IGF-I receptor (IGFR), Akt and FoxO genes have been identified in centenarians. In the case of IGFR, these polymorphisms are associated with reduced IGF-I signaling. Overall, there is solid evidence that chronically reduced IGF-I signaling in humans protects against disease and potentially promotes longevity.

mTOR Signaling

mTOR is a protein kinase (see Chapters 1 and 5) with conserved roles in limiting longevity seen in widely divergent species. Through complex signaling pathways, mTOR phosphorylates many targets in the cell (Fig. 10-9). Genetic or pharmacologic inhibition of mTOR activity experimentally

Growth factors, amino acids, energy levels, oxygen, etc

FIGURE 10-9. mTOR signaling. The mTOR kinase participates in two major complexes, termed mTORC1 and mTORC2. mTORC1 has been most closely linked to longevity. Multiple stimuli activate mTORC1. Two key downstream targets of mTORC1 are S6K1 and 4EBP1, through which mTORC1 promotes protein synthesis. Rapamycin acutely inhibits mTORC1 in a substrate-specific manner, but chronically can also inhibit mTORC2.

extends longevity in invertebrate models. As with IIS, DR may work in part through reduction of mTOR signaling. Genetic disruption of mTOR signaling components extends longevity in invertebrate models of female mice. Remarkably, the mTOR inhibitor rapamycin robustly extends mouse life span, even when treatment is initiated in older adults. Rapamycin also suppresses neoplasia (see Chapter 5) and several other phenotypes of aging in treated animals. Overall, these data indicate that mTOR signaling limits longevity in a manner that is conserved in many different organisms.

Sirtuins Are Linked to Health Span and Life Span

Sirtuins are a family of enzymes whose best-characterized biochemical function is NAD$^+$-dependent **deacetylation** of target proteins. Intracellular NAD$^+$ levels rise with nutrient deprivation and stress; hence, sirtuin activity is a means by which cells sense and respond to their environments, akin to IIS and mTOR signaling.

Interest in the potential involvement of sirtuins in longevity began with the observation that the prototypical sirtuin, SIR2, extends life span when overexpressed in *S. cerevisiae*. One mechanism by which SIR2 promotes yeast longevity is by deacetylating histones in repetitive genomic regions, thereby suppressing recombination and enhancing genomic stability. These observations have led to investigation of SIR2 homologs (i.e., sirtuins) in mammals (which possess seven sirtuins). Sirtuin function helps promote mammalian health span (Fig. 10-10) and, in the case of at least two sirtuins (SIRT6), longevity.

Most research on mammalian sirtuins has focused on SIRT1, the closest homolog of yeast SIR2. This protein deacetylates dozens of cellular proteins, including histones, p53, FoxO transcription factors, PGC-1α and many others, thus regulating key aspects of cell biology. SIRT1 attenuates many diseases associated with aging, including cardiac hypertrophy, neoplasia, glucose intolerance, neurodegeneration and others. SIRT1 overexpression in the hypothalamus increases mouse life span.

Acetylation on mitochondrial proteins is particularly abundant, and the mitochondrial sirtuin SIRT3 deacetylates and regulates many protein targets in mitochondria. It influences core organelle processes, promoting electron transport and suppressing ROS generation. SIRT3 also plays a key role in promoting cardiac health and suppressing tumors. Interestingly, mice normally lose hearing acuity progressively with age, a change blocked by DR. DR-driven preservation of hearing requires SIRT3, likely due to the function of this sirtuin in lowering ROS. Overall, SIRT3 is strongly linked to health span, and potentially to the DR response.

Mammalian SIRT6 has also been connected to the biology of aging. SIRT6 maintains chromosomal stability and metabolic homeostasis. Mice lacking SIRT6 suffer from a degenerative metabolic disorder and typically die by 1 month of age. SIRT6 protein is a histone deacetylase that suppresses the transcriptional output of key signaling pathways, in particular nuclear factor-κB (NF-κB) and hypoxia-induced factor-1α (HIF-1α). It also facilitates DNA repair through several different mechanisms. In mice, SIRT6 promotes cardiac health and suppresses hypertrophy and is a potent tumor suppressor. Overexpression of SIRT6 extends mouse life span.

Perspective: The Biology of Aging and Longevity

Although in some respects aging remains an enigma, we now have important molecular insights into its mechanisms, as well as environmental and genetic interventions that can dramatically slow the rate of aging in invertebrates and in mammals. Eventually, these efforts are likely to yield large dividends in medicine. In industrialized societies, most elderly persons suffer from multiple diseases of old age. Consequently, disease-specific interventions, against heart disease or cancer for example, actually have fairly modest payoffs in terms of years of life gained. For example, based on demographic data, it has been estimated that for a 50-year-old woman, curing all forms of cancer would extend her life expectancy by less than 3 years. Even curing cancer, heart disease, stroke and diabetes all simultaneously would add only 14 years of life, on average. These gains are fairly modest because deaths due to all causes of mortality rise exponentially with age. Thus, as she ages, our hypothetical 50-year-old woman will likely succumb to some other age-associated disease anyway (i.e., soon after she would have otherwise died from cancer, heart disease, stroke or diabetes). On the other hand, life span extension proportional to that observed in a typical rodent DR study would increase the life expectancy of a 50-year-old woman by roughly 40%, from 80 to about 112 years. Moreover, based on animal studies, most of those added years would likely be spent in good health. These figures illustrate how a deep, mechanistic understanding of the biology of aging may offer a powerful means to improve human health.

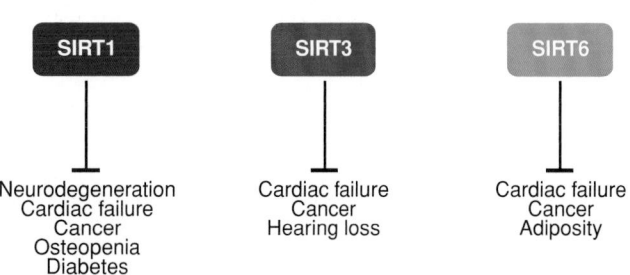

FIGURE 10-10. Mammalian sirtuins promote diverse aspects of health span.

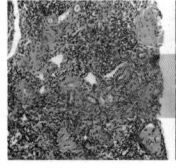
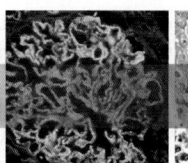
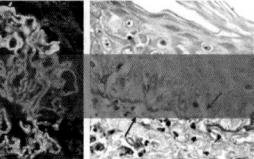

Systemic Autoimmune Diseases

Philip L. Cohen ■ Jeffrey Warren ■ Sergio A. Jimenez

MECHANISMS OF AUTOIMMUNITY Autoimmunity and the Adaptive Immune System Marker Autoantibodies **SYSTEMIC AUTOIMMUNE DISEASES** T- and B-Cell Autoreactivity Immune Function in Patients	Autoantibodies Predate Disease Onset Skewed Autoantibody Specificities **Systemic Lupus Erythematosus** SLE as a Multisystem Disease Variants of SLE **Rheumatoid Arthritis** **Vasculitides**	**Sjögren Syndrome** **Systemic Sclerosis (Scleroderma)** Abnormalities of Immune Function Vascular Dysfunction Myofibroblasts in Systemic Sclerosis **Mixed Connective Tissue Disease**

Mechanisms of Autoimmunity

Both the innate and adaptive immune systems have the capacity to injure host tissues. This process gives rise to a large number of human diseases, some entirely caused by self-reactivity, and others mediated secondarily by autoreactivity. Broadly speaking, human autoimmune diseases are divided into those affecting primarily one organ (e.g., myocarditis) and those whose effects extend to multiple body systems (e.g., systemic lupus). More recently, a third group of autoimmune illnesses caused by inappropriate activation of the innate immune system has been recognized.

Autoimmunity Is Specific Reactivity by the Adaptive Immune System against Self-Tissue

This includes recognition of self by autoantibodies and by self-reactive T cells. A broader definition of autoimmunity would include immune damage to tissues initiated by the innate immune system, for example, inflammation due to inappropriate activation of **inflammasomes** (see Chapter 2), key complexes of membrane-linked enzymes and adapter proteins that lead to generation of biologically active interleukin-1 (IL-1), with subsequent inflammation. Similar conditions of activation of innate immunity include activation of the complement system owing to faulty control proteins (such as factor H) or of the response to cytokines such as tumor necrosis factor-α (TNF-α) owing to an inappropriately sensitive receptor.

Autoimmunity is woven into the normal immune response. T cells normally recognize peptide antigens only when associated with self–major histocompatibility complex (MHC) molecules (see Chapter 4). Certain autoantibodies are present even in normal individuals (e.g., rheumatoid

factor; see below) and play a housekeeping role in removing superfluous antigens. B cells that make autoantibodies constitute a very large part of the fetal, and even neonatal, repertoire. Such cells are lost or inactivated as a normal part of development (Fig. 11-1).

Humoral Autoimmunity

Autoantibodies are generated normally as a consequence of random association of VH and VL gene segments. B cells

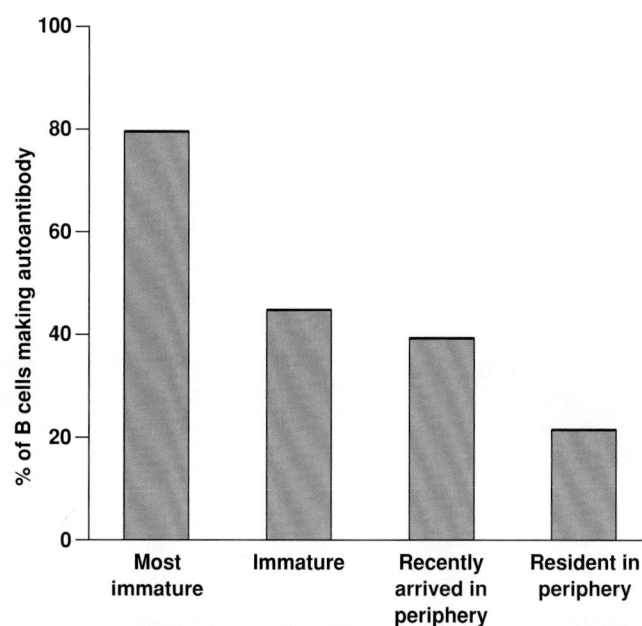

FIGURE 11-1. Autoantibody formation by normal B cells. Fractions of human B-cell lymphocytes produced autoantibodies, taken at different stages of development.

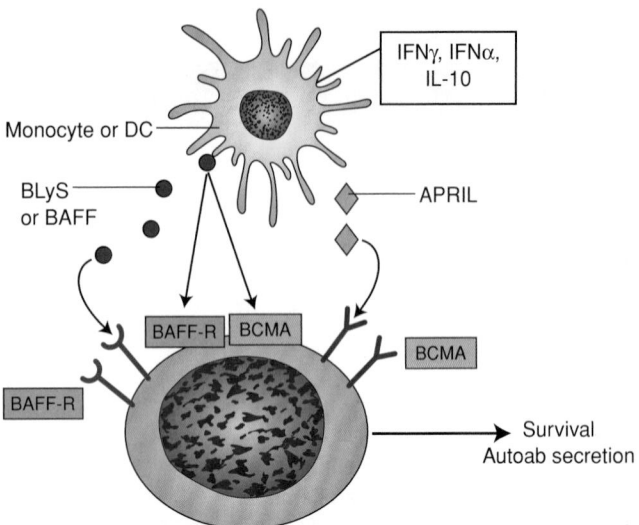

FIGURE 11-2. BAFF and APRIL binding to B lymphocytes. Monocytes and dendritic cells produce BAFF (BLys) and APRIL when driven by certain cytokines. These bind to receptors on B cells, promoting their survival.

that by chance are autoreactive must be eliminated or at least inactivated. Autoreactive B cells are vetted and removed or marginalized at multiple checkpoints in normal B-cell development. For example, heavy (H) or light (L) chains of autoreactive B cells are replaced by different H or L chains. This process, called **receptor editing,** changes the specificity of autoreactive B cells so that they are no longer autoreactive. Receptor editing is thought to be an important mechanism of avoiding autoreactivity. Another key mechanism is the action of BAFF (also known as BLyS), a cytokine derived mainly from monocytes, which regulates B-cell maturation (Fig. 11-2). Far more B cells are produced than are needed. BAFF (and a related molecule called APRIL) control the number of B cells that can mature by rescuing immature B cells from apoptosis. Overproduction of BAFF causes hypergammaglobulinemia and humoral autoimmunity.

T-Cell–Mediated Autoimmunity

Acquisition of a T-cell repertoire is a complex process involving both positive and negative selection in the thymus. The repertoire is further shaped by selection among peripheral T cells (i.e., mature T cells that have already exited the thymus). AIRE thymic transcription factor plays a crucial role in allowing many self-proteins to be expressed in the thymus so that potentially self-reactive T cells can be exposed to them and be eliminated (Fig. 11-3). Mutations in AIRE lead to a serious pediatric diffuse autoimmune disease (autoimmune polyendocrinopathy–candidiasis–ectodermal dystrophy [APECED]). T-cell autoreactivity is also controlled by regulatory T cells (T_{reg}), which dampen potentially harmful

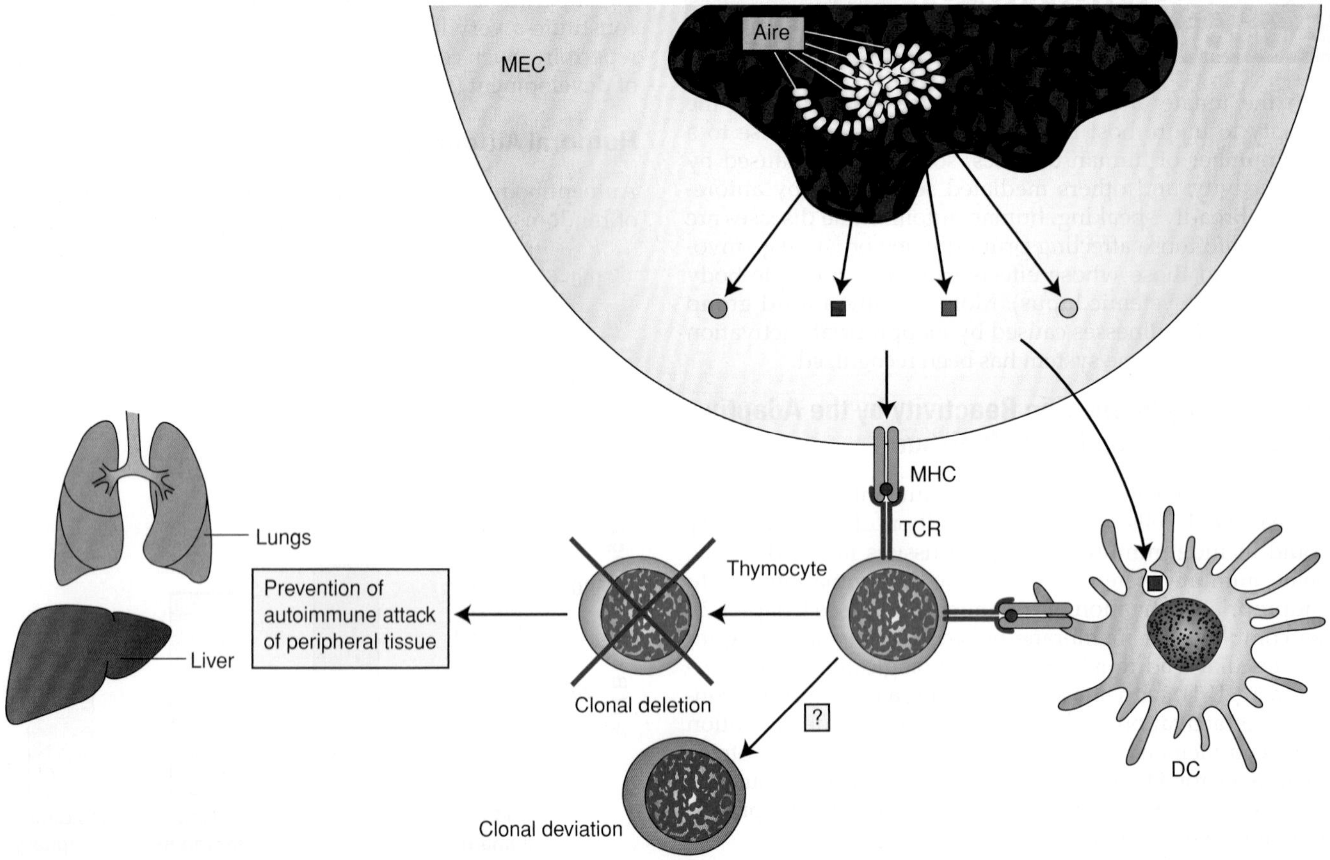

FIGURE 11-3. T-lymphocyte clonal deletion in tolerance. AIRE transcription factor activates expression of antigens normally expressed in peripheral tissues, so that they are expressed in thymic medulla epithelial cells (MEC). Antigens so regulated may include those of any tissue, the liver and lungs being shown here as representatives. Such self-antigens are presented to T lymphocytes developing in the thymus, directly by the MEC or by dendritic cells (DCs). The result is deletion of autoreactive T lymphocytes.

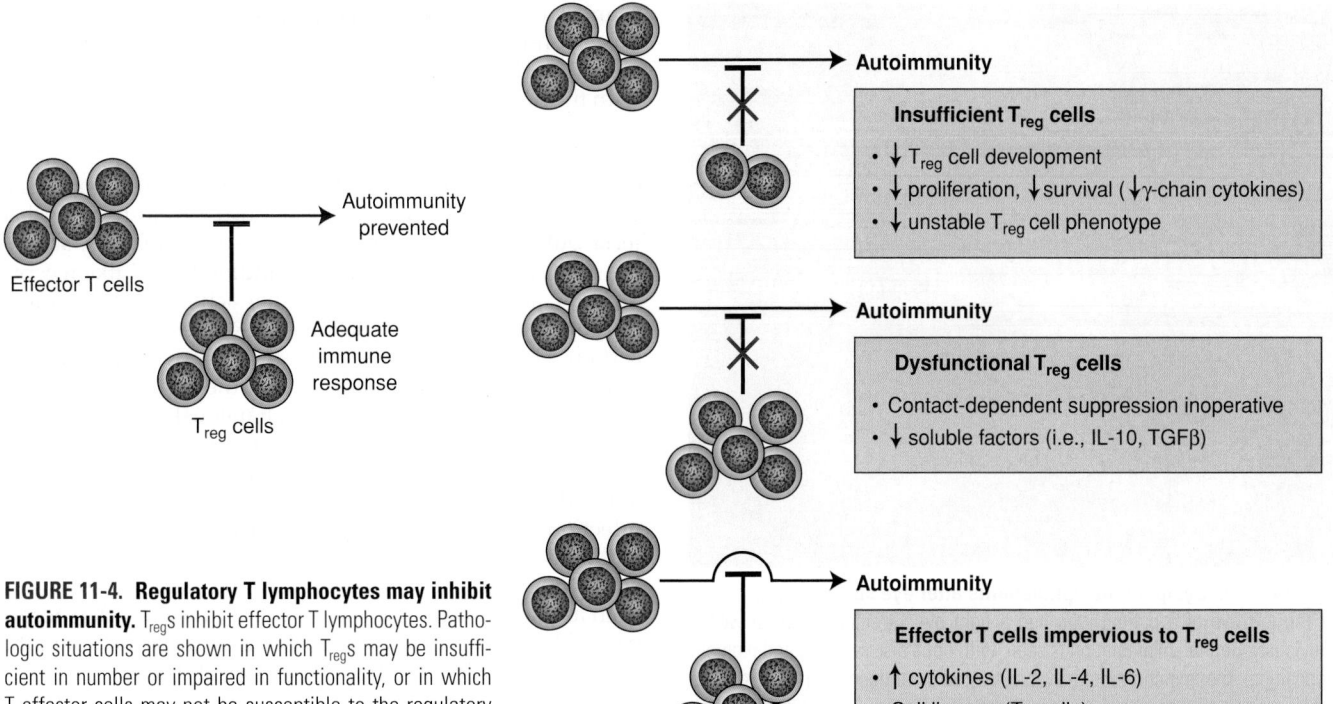

FIGURE 11-4. Regulatory T lymphocytes may inhibit autoimmunity. T_{reg}s inhibit effector T lymphocytes. Pathologic situations are shown in which T_{reg}s may be insufficient in number or impaired in functionality, or in which T effector cells may not be susceptible to the regulatory activities of T_{reg}s.

responses by other T cells. Mutations in FoxP3, a key transcription factor for regulatory T cells, lead to another serious autoimmune disease (immunodysregulation, polyendocrinopathy and enteropathy, X-linked [IPEX]) (Fig. 11-4).

Innate Immunity as a Form of Autoimmunity

Certain inflammatory diseases are caused by improper control of the innate immune system. The periodic fever syndromes, an important cause of morbidity in many parts of the world, are caused by genetic defects in the control of the **inflammasome** (see Chapter 2), a complex of proteins that regulates the conversion of prointerleukin-1 to interleukin-1 (Fig. 11-5). The "autoinflammatory" diseases also include several inherited disorders characterized by widespread inflammation, for example, neonatal onset multisystem inflammatory disease (NOMID), a condition in which a mutated cryopyrin protein (a key component of the inflammasome) is constitutively activated and leads to skin inflammation and arthritis. Mutations of TRAPS, a key intracellular protein involved in TNF signaling, also lead to inherited inflammatory conditions.

Inherited or acquired defects of complement control proteins (factor H and others) can result in severe microangiopathic disease (the hemolytic–uremic syndrome), and defects in red cell proteins that control complement activation can lead to paroxysmal nocturnal hemoglobulinuria, a serious form of anemia and hemolysis.

Causes of Autoimmunity

Thinking about autoimmunity is still influenced by a famous monograph by Paul Ehrlich, the father of modern immunology. He understood that animals generally did not make immune responses even when deliberately immunized with

their own tissues, and he coined the term *horror autotoxicus* to indicate the terrible consequences that might occur if autoimmunity were allowed to happen. Yet we now recognize that autoimmunity is a common feature of the immune system, and that there are many diseases that appear to be a result of abnormal autoimmunity.

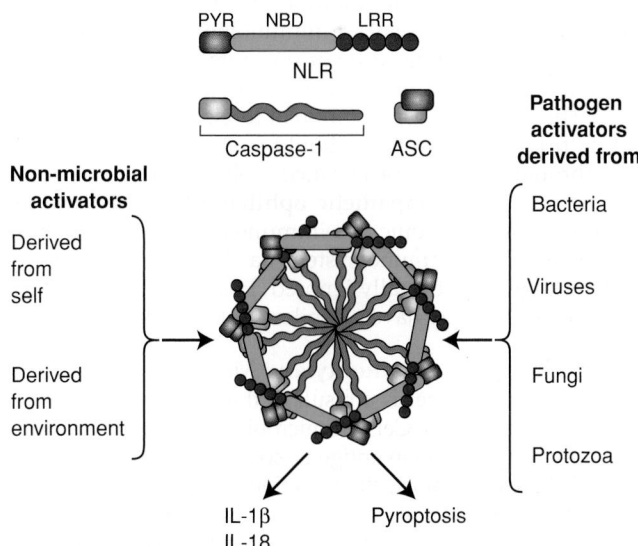

FIGURE 11-5. The inflammasome. The NLRP3 inflammasome, the best studied of these pro-inflammatory complexes, is a cluster of proteins (NLR, caspase 1, ASC) on macrophages and other innate immune cells. Several stimuli activate it to cause production of active interleukin-1 (IL-1) and IL-18 and to elicit cell death. *ASC* = apoptosis-associated speck-like protein containing a caspase recruitment domain; *CPPD* = calcium pyrophosphate dihydrate; *MDP* = muramyl dipeptide; *MSU* = monosodium urate; *NLR* = nucleotide-binding domain, leucine-rich repeat containing; *PAMP* = pathogen-associated molecule patterns.

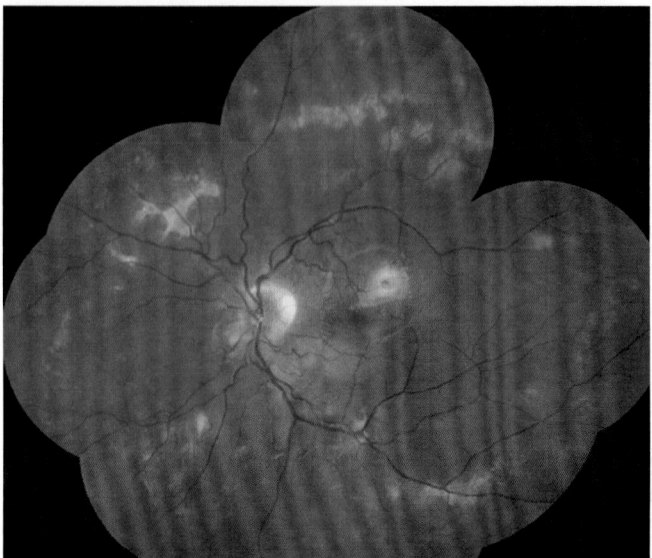

FIGURE 11-6. Sympathetic ophthalmitis after eye surgery. Optic fundus of the left eye of a patient who had a right eye vitrectomy several weeks previously. Retinal inflammation is seen, with optic disc swelling and pigment deposition. The immune system was activated by antigens from the left eye that were released as a consequence of the prior surgery. The result is damage in the previously normal right eye.

What are the causes of abnormal autoimmunity? In many cases, the answer is incompletely understood, but what follows are the principal views of scientists in this area of active investigation.

Breach of Immunologic Privilege

This is a rare cause of autoimmunity. Certain body areas (e.g., the anterior part of the eye) are immunologically "privileged": the immune system has little or no contact with these areas, and tolerance is not established to tissue-specific antigens there. This allows transplantation of foreign corneas, happily. But if "privileged" proteins should contact the immune system (through trauma, for instance), self-reactivity can occur. This accounts for **sympathetic ophthalmitis,** when trauma to one eye causes chronic autoimmune inflammation of both eyes because the immune system has become sensitized to ocular antigens it normally ignored. Post–myocardial infarction pericarditis may have a similar etiology (Fig. 11-6).

Postinfectious Autoimmunity and Molecular Mimicry

Acute rheumatic fever is a result of the immune response to group A *Streptococcus.* Certain microbial antigens share structural similarity to human antigens, so that immunity triggered by, and directed against, the infectious agent may elicit antibodies or T cells that react to self-tissues. In this vein, immunity that develops against certain streptococcal antigens is thought to stimulate antibodies that cross-react with tissue in joints, the nervous system and the heart. This causes an acute febrile illness with inflammation in and around the heart and in the joints, and sometimes in the brain (see Chapter 17). It may lead to scarring in heart valves and may recur with reinfection. Why some people are susceptible and others are not remains unclear (see below). **Guillain-Barré syndrome** is a postviral autoimmune neuropathy apparently resulting from immunity originally directed against viral products. A large

number of viral diseases have been associated with autoimmune consequences—for example, postmeasles encephalomyelopathy. The extent to which this represents cross-reactivity with the host or other mechanisms is unclear (Fig. 11-7).

Polyclonal Activation and Autoimmunity

Certain environmental agents—famously, the lipopolysaccharide (LPS) that is part of the coating of gram-negative bacteria, but also many other substances—may diffusely activate the immune system. LPS acts by binding to Toll-like receptor 4 (TLR4; see Chapter 2). Many other activators of the innate immune system can also activate TLRs. Because B cells have certain TLRs, they can be powerfully activated by ligands binding these receptors. For B cells, the result is that many different clones are activated simultaneously, causing a burst of antibody formation that represents all the specificities possessed by available B cells, including autoantibodies. Autoantibodies can thus be stimulated by certain viral or bacterial infections. For example, Epstein-Barr virus (EBV) binds to and activates B cells, and autoantibodies are regularly present during acute EBV infection. Chronic bacterial infections, such as endocarditis and osteomyelitis, are also often accompanied by autoantibodies. In most cases, these are not pathogenic, but occasionally they cause clinical disease.

Drugs and Toxins as Causes of Autoimmunity

Certain drugs can provoke autoantibodies and even clinical autoimmunity in ways that are still ill-defined but that

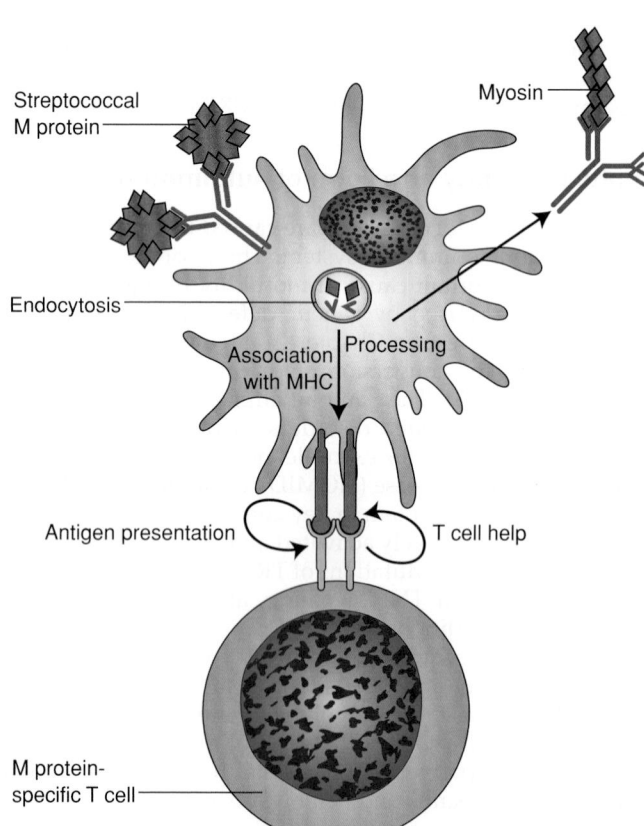

FIGURE 11-7. Molecular mimicry. In molecular mimicry, the immune system is sensitized by foreign proteins (here, *Streptococcus* M protein). M-protein–reactive T cells help B cells, which make antibody that cross-reacts with autologous cardiac myosin, to cause damage to the heart, as in rheumatic fever.

involve aberrations of tolerance. Well-known examples are antinuclear antibodies that follow treatment with hydralazine and procainamide, antierythrocyte autoantibodies from methyldopa and antiplatelet antibodies from quinine. Environmental toxins, notably mercury and other heavy metals, result in autoantibodies and immune-mediated renal and nervous system disease. There have been outbreaks of inflammatory connective tissue disease from contaminated tryptophan and other food supplements. Recently, it has been appreciated that cocaine, especially when taken with the antihelminth levamisole, may induce granulomatous vasculitis. Mechanisms are still obscure.

Genetics and Autoimmunity

Host genes profoundly affect susceptibility to autoimmune diseases. Concordance for certain autoimmune diseases among identical twins may reach 35%. As well, autoimmune disease patients frequently report that family members have or have had the same or similar autoimmune disorders. Except for rare inherited conditions (e.g., APECED), inheritance is complex and multiple genes are believed to conspire together with multiple environmental factors. Among the genetic links that influence development of autoimmune diseases are MHC alleles (mostly class II, but class I for the spondyloarthropathies), together with multiple genes involving the immune system, such as IL-7 and its receptor and IL-23. As well, TLR genes and other genes for cytokines, cytokine receptors and tyrosine kinases involved in immune cell activation are associated with development of immune responses to self-antigens.

Gender and Autoimmunity

Most autoimmune diseases occur more often in females. Female-to-male ratios range from up to 20:1 for autoimmune thyroiditis and lupus to perhaps 3:1 for rheumatoid arthritis and multiple sclerosis. The increased susceptibility of women to autoimmunity remains incompletely understood. A large but not conclusive body of evidence supports the notion that it is sex hormones, through their influence on the immune response, that account for the difference, but X-chromosome gene dosage effects are also possible.

Chance and Autoimmunity

Both B- and T-cell receptor formation involve random genetic recombination events. These are compounded by somatic mutation of receptors. The variability of autoimmunity—even in completely inbred susceptible animal strains—has led to the view that stochastic (random) events, probably in repertoire generation, may have a profound effect both on the normal immune repertoire and on the development of autoimmunity.

Apoptosis and Autoimmunity

Many autoantibodies—at least in systemic autoimmune diseases—recognize intracellular antigens, and in particular those that normally reside within the cell nucleus. Such intracellular antigens may gain access to the immune system during the process of cell death. Nuclear antigens can be demonstrated on the surfaces of dying cells and may be the source of immunization leading to autoantibodies. Apoptosis is characterized by cell death without inflammation (see Chapter 1). Apoptotic cells are phagocytosed whole, via a choreographed set of interactions with macrophages (Fig. 11-8). However, abnormalities of the mononuclear

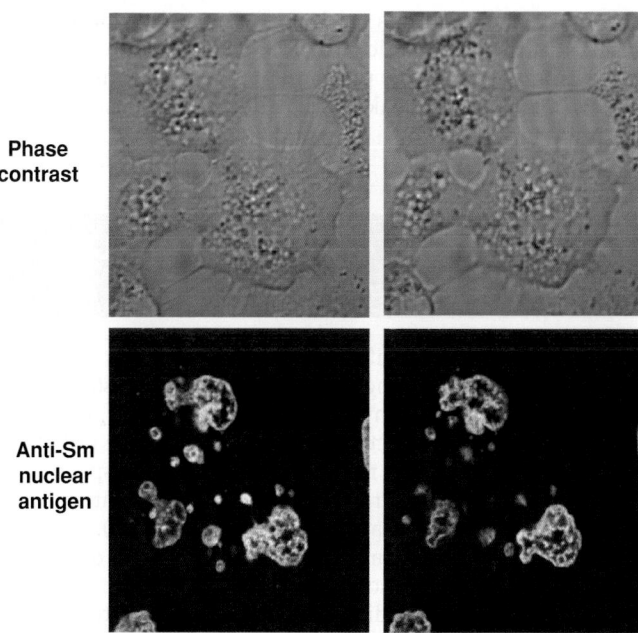

FIGURE 11-8. Expression and release of nuclear antigens by cells early (left) and late (right) in apoptosis. UV-irradiated skin cells became apoptotic, demonstrating the typical morphology (*upper panel*, phase contrast). Immunofluorescence staining was used to identify Sm nuclear antigen (*lower panel*). Sm was present on surface blebs. Such nuclear antigens may thus trigger autoimmune responses.

phagocyte system may lead to abnormal persistence of apoptotic cells and cause autoimmunity in experimental systems. Thus, mice lacking an apoptotic cell receptor–signaling intermediate develop a lupus-like syndrome (see below) because they cannot clear apoptotic debris. Along these lines, unengulfed apoptotic debris is detectable in human lupus and in other autoimmune diseases.

Graft-versus-Host Disease

Allogeneic T cells provoke inflammation when they recognize noncompatible tissue (as in recipients of allogeneic bone marrow; see Chapter 4). Autoantibodies may arise during chronic graft-versus-host disease (GVHD). This is believed to result in the abnormal interaction between the foreign T cells and host B cells, probably because the T cells have not been "educated" in the host thymus.

During Cycles of Remission and Exacerbation, Marker Autoantibodies May Provide Clues about Autoimmunity

Marker autoantibodies are disease-specific autoantibodies that are so tightly linked to certain diseases that their presence suffices to confirm the diagnosis. Some of these are very surprising; for instance, antibodies to transfer RNA (tRNA) synthetases (e.g., methionine tRNA synthetase) are virtually diagnostic of inflammatory myositis, and antibody to topoisomerase I (a DNA unwinding enzyme) is specific for scleroderma.

Remission–Exacerbation

Many autoimmune diseases, even if untreated, tend to flare and then to remit. Multiple sclerosis is especially prone to exacerbations and remissions, but other diseases (lupus, rheumatoid arthritis, etc.) can show marked regression (usually not permanent). The reasons for this pattern of episodic peaks and valleys of disease activity are uncertain.

Systemic Autoimmune Diseases

It is customary to classify autoimmune diseases as organ specific (affecting a single organ or organ system)—for example, autoimmune thyroiditis—or as systemic, in which multiple organs are affected. Such distinctions are not absolute, as some diseases may be mainly organ specific in most cases but demonstrate systemic involvement in some individuals (e.g., rheumatoid arthritis; see below). As well, organ-specific autoimmune symptomatologies are often part of systemic autoimmune disease. Manifestations of autoimmune diseases in individual organs (e.g., autoimmune hepatitis) are mainly described in the chapters that focus on organ-based pathology. We address below systemic autoimmune diseases as they affect the whole patient. It should be emphasized that almost every organ can be afflicted with autoimmune disease.

Autoantibodies

Autoantibodies can be detected in normal individuals and may not cause disease. Some autoantibodies clearly induce pathology if given to normal individuals. (This is not done anymore but was done in the past for several autoimmune diseases.) Such antibodies may also cross the placenta and be pathogenic for the fetus. Other autoantibodies can transfer disease manifestations when given to experimental animals. For most autoimmune diseases, the inference that autoantibodies or autoreactive T cells are the cause of pathology is made based on the presence of autoantibodies or T cells in affected tissue, often together with complement components.

Autoimmune Diseases May Reflect Both T- and B-Cell–Mediated Autoreactivity

Demonstrating that antibodies cause an autoimmune disease is technically much easier than doing so for T cells, and many autoimmune diseases do seem to be largely caused by antibody. Some autoimmune diseases (e.g., lupus; see below) seem to involve both autoreactive T and B cells. Even today, there is debate about the relative importance of humoral versus cellular immunity for many autoimmune diseases. The surprising effectiveness of B-cell depletion (using anti-CD20) has provoked a reevaluation of the relative role of T cells in certain autoimmune diseases, notably multiple sclerosis.

For some autoimmune diseases, the target antigens are few and are well defined (e.g., α-gliadin in celiac disease, although, strictly speaking, this is not autoimmune because the antigen is in food). For others, it has been difficult to incriminate specific antigens, or the antigenic spectrum of certain autoimmune diseases may be highly complex.

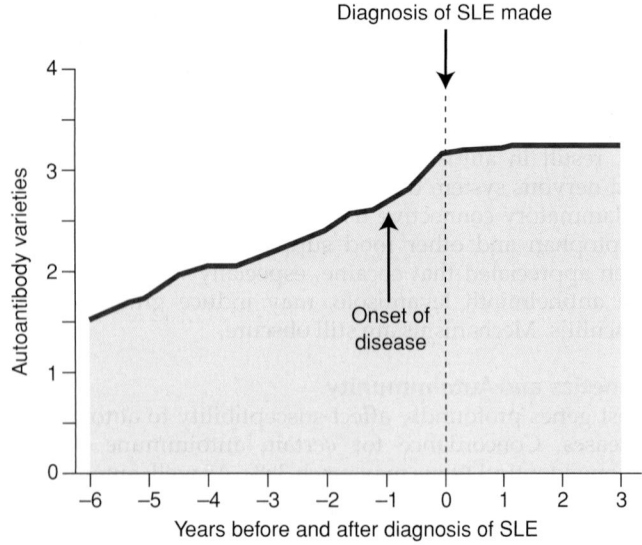

FIGURE 11-9. Time course of autoantibody formation in systemic lupus erythematosus (SLE). Average numbers of the different kinds of autoantibodies as a function of time of symptom onset and diagnosis in patients with SLE.

Immunity Is Usually Depressed in Patients with Autoimmune Diseases

People suffering from systemic autoimmune disorders have **reduced** immune responses to exogenous antigens (i.e., conventional antigens, such as in vaccines or natural infections). This observation is independent of immunosuppressive treatments they may be receiving. It is almost as if an immune system that is obsessed with responding to self cannot do its real job of defending against infection. This disease-associated reduction in immunocompetence has clinical implications.

The antibodies found in systemic autoimmune disease patients have all of the characteristics of mature, high-affinity immune responses. There are antibodies present against multiple epitopes on complex autoantigens, supporting the idea that the original autoantibody response was indeed antigen driven and not due to a fortuitous cross-reaction or an aberrancy in immune regulation (Fig. 11-9).

Autoantibodies Predate Disease Onset

Patients with systemic lupus and rheumatoid arthritis generally have significant levels of disease-specific autoantibodies in their sera years before the disease began to manifest clinically. Thus, at least in these instances, autoimmunity precedes disease, and autoantibodies most likely play causative roles in pathogenesis.

Autoantibody Specificities Are Skewed

The specificities of disease-related autoantibodies are not easily predictable. Of the thousands of proteins present in the nucleus, only a few are targets of autoantibodies. For example, the Smith (Sm) ribonuclear protein (RNP) complex, crucial to splicing of premessenger RNA (pre-mRNA), is a highly specific antibody for lupus, yet Sm RNP is not an abundant nuclear protein. Neither the amount nor the location of an individual self-protein determines whether it will be a disease-related autoantigen. There is some evidence that the degree of molecular disorder positively correlates with autoantigenicity.

SYSTEMIC LUPUS ERYTHEMATOSUS

Systemic Lupus Erythematosus Is a Multisystem Inflammatory Disease that May Involve Almost Any Organ

SLE characteristically affects the skin, joints, serous membranes, central nervous system and kidneys. Autoantibodies are formed against a variety of self-antigens, including plasma proteins (complement components, clotting factors) and protein–phospholipid complexes, cell surface antigens (lymphocytes, neutrophils, platelets, erythrocytes), intracellular cytoplasmic components (microfilaments, microtubules, lysosomes, ribosomes, RNA) and nuclear DNA, ribonucleoproteins and histones. The spectrum of intracellular autoantigens includes the proteins and DNA that make up chromatin, proteins of the spliceosome complex (small nuclear RNPs [snRNPs]) and the Ro/La small cytoplasmic ribonucleoprotein particle. The most important diagnostic autoantibodies are those against nuclear antigens—in particular, antibody to double-stranded DNA (dsDNA) and to a soluble nuclear antigen complex, Sm antigen, that is part of the spliceosome. In clinical context, high titers of these two **antinuclear antibodies** (ANAs) are very suggestive of SLE. Antigen–antibody complexes form or deposit in tissues, leading to characteristic vasculitis, synovitis and glomerulonephritis. SLE is a prototypical type III hypersensitivity reaction. Occasionally, directly cytotoxic antibodies are present, particularly antibodies against cell surface antigens of leukocytes and erythrocytes. There is also evidence that cell-mediated immune responses are involved.

EPIDEMIOLOGY: The prevalence of SLE varies worldwide. In North America and northern Europe, it is 40 in 100,000. In the United States, it appears to be more common and severe in blacks and Hispanics, although socioeconomic factors may in part be responsible. Nearly 90% of cases are in women of childbearing age, as many as 1 in 700 of whom may have this disease.

The etiology of SLE is unknown. Genetic, immunologic and environmental factors contribute (Fig. 11-10). The presence of numerous autoantibodies, particularly ANAs, suggests a loss of tolerance. Some manifestations of SLE result from tissue injury due to immune complex–mediated vasculitis, while other manifestations (e.g., thrombocytopenia or the secondary antiphospholipid syndrome) are caused by autoantibodies to cell membrane molecules or serum components. However, many diagnostically helpful ANAs are not incriminated in the pathogenesis of SLE.

MOLECULAR PATHOGENESIS: Unlike some other purely genetic diseases, the effects of a single gene do not dominate the genetics of lupus. Instead, susceptibility to lupus results from the sum of small effects of multiple genes. In the past two decades, at least 17 genetic linkages have been established and independently confirmed. For some of those linkages, the responsible gene within the specific chromosome interval has been also identified, for

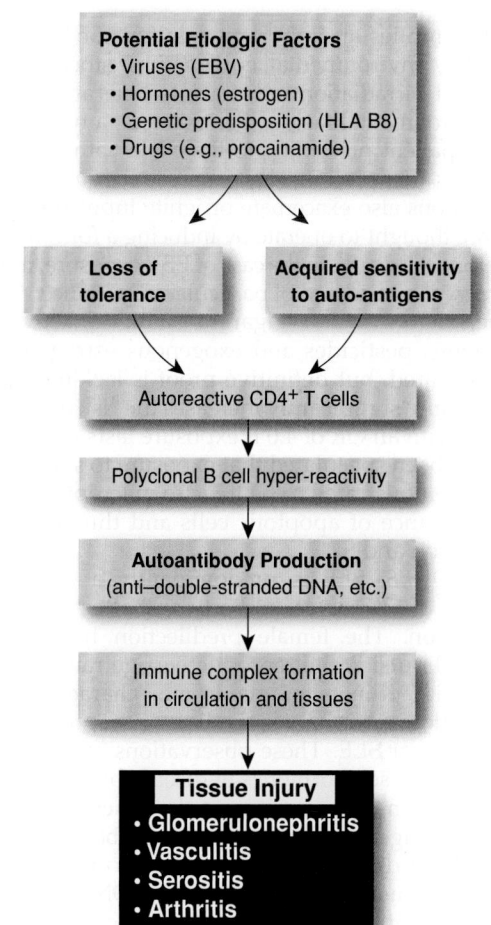

FIGURE 11-10. The pathogenesis of systemic lupus erythematosus is multifactorial. *EBV* = Epstein-Barr virus; *HLA* = human leukocyte antigen.

example, FcγRIIIA and FcγRIIA, PDCD1 and human leukocyte antigen-DR (HLA-DR). There are also at least 20 independent genetic effects (polymorphisms) identified and confirmed that are risk factors in lupus. Among those are HLA-DR2 (odds ratio [OR] 1.5–4), C2/C4 (OR 1.5–5), FcγRIIA (OR 1.3), PDCD1 (OR 2.6), PTPN22 (1.6), IRF5 (OR 1.3), TYK2 (1.6) and TNF-α (OR 4).

PATHOPHYSIOLOGY: Among the effector functions associated with these HLA haplotypes is a decrease in C3b receptors on cells that clear circulating immune complexes. A critical role for the D/DR region in the pathogenesis of SLE is supported by the observation that inherited deficiencies of certain complement components, particularly C2, C4 and C1q, are associated with an increased incidence of SLE and lupus-like disorders. The genes that encode C2 and C4 are within the MHC.

ENVIRONMENT. Lupus has an important genetic component as illustrated above and by the 20%–30% concordance of disease between monozygotic twins. In dizygotic twins, there is only 2% concordance. However, the observation that the second monozygotic twin does not develop lupus in three quarters of monozygotic twin pairs also implies an important role for nongenetic factors, be they environmental, epigenetic or stochastic.

Ultraviolet irradiation and viral infections are two established environmental factors. For example, a typical lupus onset is a patient presenting to the clinic with malar rash and arthritis after prolonged exposure to the sun. Common viral infections also exacerbate or ignite lupus onset. Both factors are thought to operate by inducing a form of proinflammatory cell death. In the case of EBV exposure, molecular mimicry is considered of particular importance.

Other factors such as cigarette smoking, heavy metals, solvents, pesticides and exogenous estrogens have been implicated, but definitive proof is lacking. Finally, silica exposure significantly increases the risk of developing lupus with an OR of 4.0 if exposure lasts more than 1 year. It has been speculated that exposure to silica, which has been demonstrated to be toxic to macrophages, may impair clearance of apoptotic cells and thus favor self-immunization and SLE.

HORMONES. SLE is predominantly a female disease. Onset of SLE before puberty and after menopause is uncommon. The female predilection becomes less pronounced outside the reproductive age range. Finally, patients with Klinefelter syndrome, characterized by hypergonadotrophic hypogonadism, are prone to the development of SLE. These observations suggest a role for endogenous sex hormones in disease predisposition.

Indeed, hormones can impact the function of T cells and macrophages, and estrogens have been shown to increase B-cell differentiation and in vitro immunoglobulin (Ig) production including anti-dsDNA. Yet other explanations for the female predominance in SLE have been proposed, including incomplete inactivation of the X chromosome in females with SLE, leading to increased dosage of genes affecting the immune system.

Immunologic Factors in the Pathogenesis of SLE

B Cells

Pathogenic autoantibodies produced by B cells are an important cause of tissue damage in SLE. B cells are also relevant as antigen-presenting cells (APCs) and contribute to lupus autoantigen presentation. Recently, lupus has been associated with abnormal early B-cell tolerance, resulting in the escape of autoreactive B cells to the periphery.

Recent studies suggest roles for TLR-driven and interferon-α (IFN-α)-driven B-cell responses. Evidence for specific antigen-driven responses comes from the observation that, with time, the antibodies of SLE demonstrate gene rearrangements and mutations that are typical of antigen-driven responses. Moreover, patients with SLE often have antibodies to more than one epitope on a single antigen, further suggesting a primary role for an antigen-driven process. Although inciting antigens have not been identified, a number of factors render normal body constituents more immunogenic, including infection, ultraviolet light exposure and other environmental agents that damage cells.

T Cells

Two important observations in humans suggest a role for T cells in the pathogenesis of lupus: (1) the association of SLE

with several MHC class II genes and (2) the autoantibodies found in lupus show features associated with T-cell–dependent responses such as isotype switching and somatic mutation.

CD4+ T cells become autoreactive following DNA hypomethylation and they overexpress the LFA (CD11a) cell adhesion molecules, which stabilize the interaction between T cells and APCs. Autoreactive CD4+ T cells have been best described in mouse models; no consistent defect in this regulatory T-cell population has been found in humans.

Dendritic Cells

The most potent APCs in our immune system have been shown to contribute to lupus autoimmunity by producing IFN-α, particularly plasmacytoid dendritic cells (DCs), and having a proinflammatory phenotype. Both characteristics predispose DCs to break tolerance, present autoantigens and sustain the ongoing autoimmunity.

Cytokines

The cytokine network is also abnormal in lupus and reflects (1) the systemic inflammatory status and (2) an ongoing antigen-driven autoimmune response. Some of the increased cytokines are IL-4, IL-6, IL-10 and IFN-α (Fig. 11-11).

Immune Complexes

A significant portion of injury in lupus is due to deposition of circulating immune complexes against self-antigens, particularly against DNA: the occurrence of circulating immune complexes that contain nuclear antigen; the presence of those

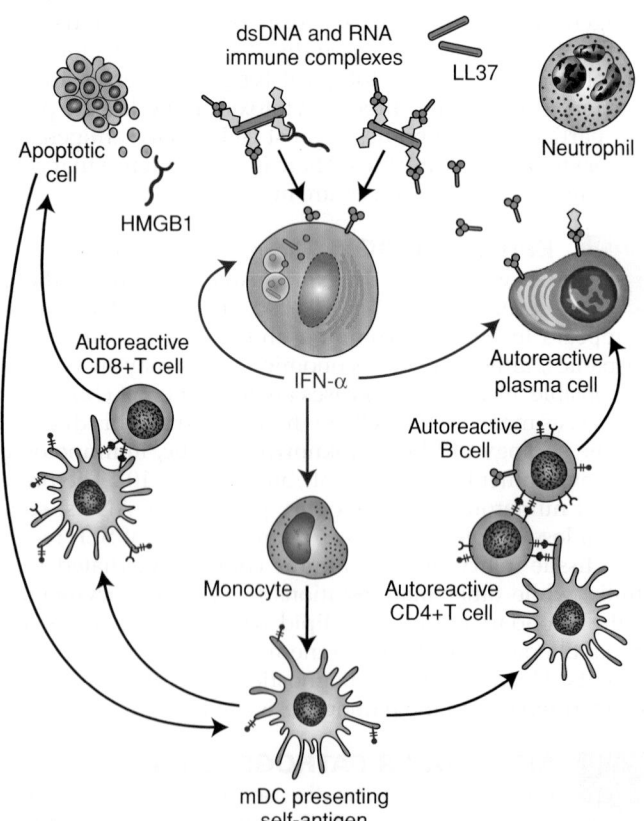

FIGURE 11-11. Immune pathogenesis of systemic lupus erythematosus (SLE). Nucleic acid complexes or Toll-like receptor (TLR) agonists elicit interferon-α (IFN-α) βψ dendritic cells (DCs). This, in turn, triggers autoantigen presentation and autoantibody production by plasma cells.

immune complexes in injured tissues, as identified by immunofluorescence; and the observation that immune complexes can be extracted from tissues that contain nuclear antigens. Additional evidence suggests that under certain conditions, immune complex formation also occurs in situ—that is, in tissues rather than in the circulation. Examples include antibodies against connective tissue components and perhaps the membranous form of lupus glomerulonephritis. Type II hypersensitivity reactions are also implicated in lupus, since cytotoxic antibodies against rbc and platelet membrane proteins can cause cytopenias (see Chapter 26).

Cell Death

Apoptosis (see Chapter 1) is characterized by nuclear condensation, membrane blebbing and subsequent cell shrinkage with preservation of an intact plasma membrane. The process culminates in the destruction of the nuclear components such as chromatin and snRNPs, incidentally the two major autoantigens in SLE.

Apoptosis avoids release of intracellular contents into the extracellular microenvironment, where they might have a powerful proinflammatory effect. Specifically, apoptosis would isolate intracellular autoantigens and render them inaccessible to the autoimmune system. Consequently, the body would be protected from developing responsiveness to such autoantigens. As mentioned above, impaired apoptotic mechanisms have led to development of experimental lupus-like disease, with production of lupus autoantibodies and glomerulonephritis. Such experimental lupus is greatly reduced in severity if release of intracellular material during cell death is prevented.

Along these lines, lupus patients have increased levels of circulating apoptotic debris and impaired capacity for uptake of dying cells. DNA/histones and RNA/proteins from apoptotic cells specifically bind to lupus autoantibodies and activate both DCs and autoreactive B cells via TLRs.

Toll-Like Receptors

TLRs recognize molecular microbial structures and constitute an important group of pattern recognition receptors of the innate immune system (see Chapter 2). Microbial TLR ligands include a wide range of molecules with strong adjuvant activity (such as lipopolysaccharide, lipopeptides, bacterial DNA and viral RNA and DNA). These ligands are powerful activators of DCs, macrophages and other APCs, and allow effective presentation of microbial antigens to cells of the adaptive immune system. However, endogenous ligands have also been identified for a substantial proportion of TLRs. In particular, in SLE, circulating DNA/histone and RNA/protein complexes from apoptotic debris (see above) become endogenous ligands, especially when complexed with autoantibodies. DNA/histone and RNA/protein, once taken up by DCs, engage TLR9 and TLR7 and stimulate DCs to produce large amounts of IFN-α. Indeed, studies from genetically modified mice show that the absence of TLR-9 or TLR-7 dramatically reduces the production of antichromatin or anti-snRNPs, respectively.

IFN-α

There are two major types of IFNs: type I (IFN-α, IFN-β) and type II (IFN-γ, which is secreted only by T cells). IFN-α is secreted by virally infected cells and by plasmacytoid DCs, whereas IFN-β is produced by many types of cells, such as myeloid DCs, following many—not necessarily infectious—stimuli. Type I IFNs share a ubiquitous heterodimeric receptor, mediate innate responses to viral infections and are also required for full DC response to TLRs and their stimulation of T and B cells.

IFN-α strongly stimulates both innate and adaptive immune responses. In lupus in particular, circulating DNA/histone and RNA/protein complexes from apoptotic debris chronically stimulate its production via engagement and activation of TLR7 and TLR9. Experimental manipulations confirm that IFN responsiveness correlates directly with severity of lupus: increased sensitivity to IFN magnifies the disease, while interventions that decrease IFN responses mitigate disease activity. Most lupus patients have increased circulating levels of IFN-α. Levels of expression of many genes that are upregulated by IFN-α are higher in patients with SLE than in normal patients.

 CLINICAL FEATURES: Because circulating immune complexes deposit in many tissues, virtually every organ in the body may be involved (Fig. 11-12).

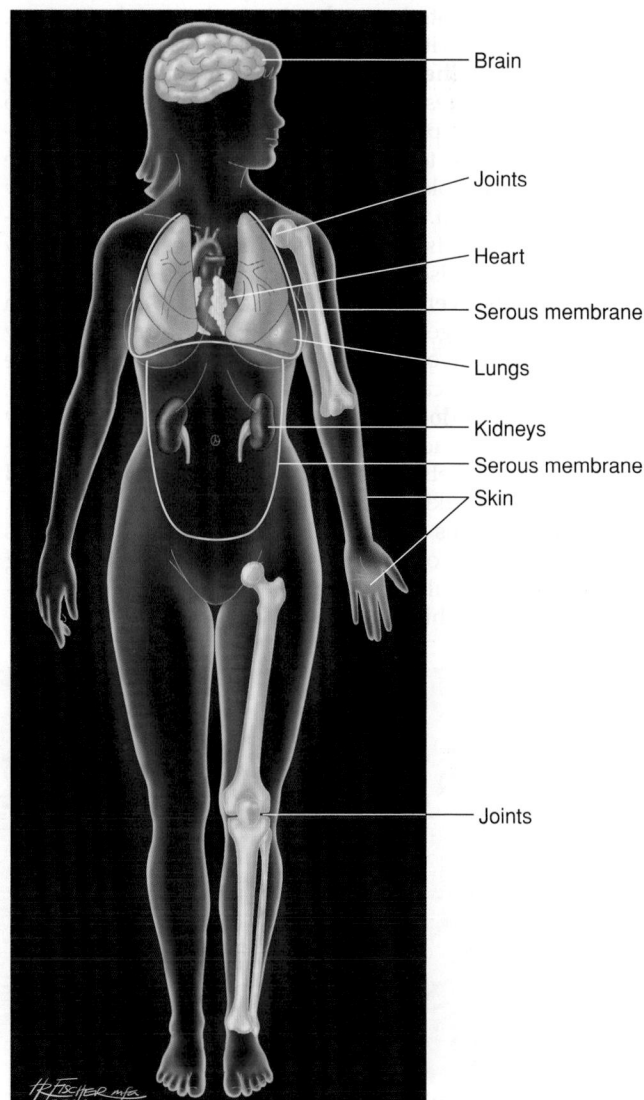

FIGURE 11-12. Organ involvement in systemic lupus erythematosus.

Joint disease is the most common manifestation of SLE; over 90% of patients have polyarthralgia. An inflammatory synovitis occurs, but unlike rheumatoid arthritis, joint destruction is unusual.

Skin involvement (see Chapter 28) is common. An erythematous rash in sun-exposed sites, a malar "butterfly" rash, is characteristic. Microscopically, perivascular lymphoid infiltrates and liquefactive degeneration of the basal cells are seen. Immunofluorescence studies reveal immunoglobulin and complement deposition along the dermal–epidermal junction ("lupus band").

Renal disease, especially glomerulonephritis, affects more than 50% of patients with SLE. Immune complexes that contain IgG antibodies to double-stranded DNA deposit in glomeruli and lead to various forms of glomerulonephritis including mesangial disease, focal proliferative nephritis, diffuse proliferative nephritis and membranous glomerulopathy (see Chapter 22). Although glomerulonephritis is the most common renal manifestation of SLE, interstitial nephritis or vasculitis (rarely) can also been seen. In many cases, immunoglobulins and complement are detectable in the interstitium and in renal blood vessels.

Serous membranes are commonly involved. More than one third of patients have pleuritis and pleural effusions. Pericarditis and peritonitis occur, but less frequently.

Disorders of the respiratory system occur frequently, with clinical manifestations ranging from pleural disease to upper airway and pulmonary parenchymal disease. Pneumonitis is thought to be caused by deposition of immune complexes in alveolar septa and is associated with patchy acute inflammation. Progressive interstitial fibrosis develops in some patients. An increased incidence of pulmonary hypertension has also been observed.

Cardiac involvement (see Chapter 17) is often seen in SLE, although congestive heart failure is rare and is usually associated with myocarditis. All layers of the heart may be involved, with pericarditis being the most common finding. **Libman-Sacks endocarditis,** which is usually not clinically significant, is characterized by small nonbacterial vegetations on valve leaflets. These lesions should be differentiated from the larger, bulkier vegetations of bacterial endocarditis.

Central nervous system (CNS) disease can manifest as psychiatric disease or vasculitis, the latter a life-threatening complication. Vasculitis can lead to hemorrhage and infarction of the brain, which may be fatal.

Antiphospholipid antibodies and antibodies directed against related protein–phospholipid complexes are identified in one third of SLE patients. These findings are associated with thromboembolic complications, including stroke, pulmonary embolism, deep venous thrombosis, portal vein thrombosis and spontaneous abortions.

Other organ involvement is less common and is often due to **vasculitis**. Lesions in the spleen are characterized by thickening and concentric fibrosis of the penicillary arteries, the so-called onion skin pattern.

The clinical course of SLE is extremely variable, typically with exacerbations and remissions. Because of immunosuppressive therapies, better recognition of mild forms of the disease and improved antihypertensive medication, overall 10-year survival approaches 90%. Patients with severe renal or CNS disease or with systolic hypertension have the worst prognosis.

 PATHOLOGY: The renal lesions of SLE are largely due to deposition of immune complexes, leading to glomerular inflammation (Fig. 11-13). There is deposition of IgG and complement components in a "lumpy bumpy" pattern, and electron-dense complexes can be visualized using electron microscopy (see Chapter 22). There is T-lymphocyte infiltration of kidneys as well, with a variable amount of interstitial nephritis. Skin lesions are characterized by lymphocytic infiltration and by hydropic degeneration of keratinocytes (see Chapter 30).

There Are Several Variants of Lupus Erythematosus

Drug-Induced Lupus

A lupus-like syndrome may be precipitated in some people by the use of certain medications, notably procainamide (for arrhythmias), hydralazine (for hypertension) and isoniazid (for tuberculosis). Drug-induced lupus ranges from asymptomatic laboratory abnormalities (positive ANA test) to a syndrome clinically similar to SLE. Unlike SLE, drug-induced lupus shows no gender predominance and most patients are over 50 years old. Factors that predispose include large daily doses of the offending drug, slow drug-acetylator status and (in hydralazine-induced lupus) HLA-DR4 genotype. As in SLE, deposition of immune complexes

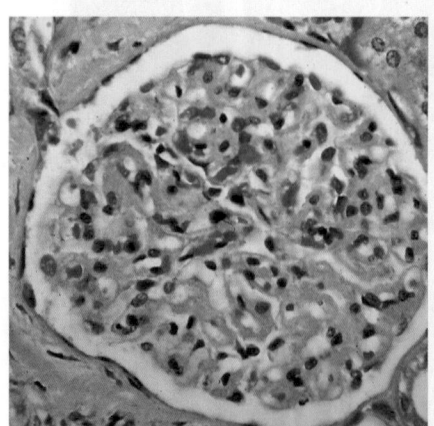
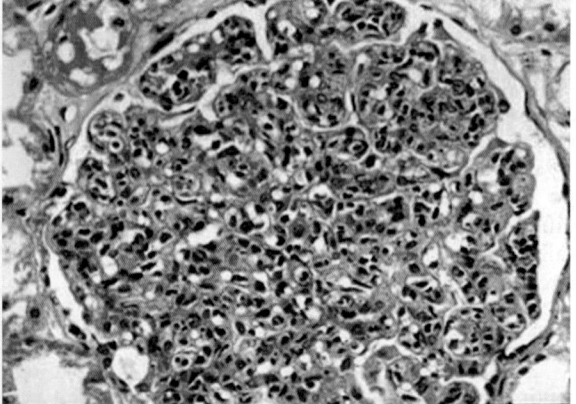

FIGURE 11-13. Glomerulonephritis in systemic lupus erythematosus (SLE). A normal glomerulus is shown at left, highlighting the inflammatory hypercellularity of the glomerulus from a patient with lupus, shown at right.

is a feature of drug-induced lupus. Patients typically exhibit constitutional signs, polyarthritis, pleuritis and antinuclear antibodies. Patients may develop rheumatoid factor, false-positive tests for syphilis and a positive direct antiglobulin (Coombs) test. Renal and CNS involvement rarely occur, and antibodies to double-stranded DNA and Sm antigen are distinctly uncommon. Autoantibodies to histones account for the positive ANA test result and are typical. As in idiopathic SLE, autoreactive CD4+ T cells have been implicated in polyclonal B-cell activation. The syndrome usually resolves when the offending drug is discontinued.

Chronic Discoid Lupus

The most common variety of localized lupus erythematosus is a skin disorder, although identical lesions can occur in some cases of SLE. Erythematous, depigmented and telangiectatic plaques occur most commonly on the face and scalp. Lesional deposition of immunoglobulins and complement at the dermal–epidermal interface is similar to that in SLE. However, unlike SLE, uninvolved skin contains no immune deposits. Although ANAs develop in about one third of the patients, antibodies to double-stranded DNA and Sm antigen are not seen. Most patients with discoid lupus are not otherwise ill, but up to 10% eventually exhibit features of systemic disease.

Subacute Cutaneous Lupus

Subacute cutaneous lupus is characterized by papular and annular lesions, typically on the trunk. The disorder is aggravated by exposure to ultraviolet light, although lesions usually eventually resolve without scarring. Antibodies to SS-A (Ro antigen) (ribonucleoprotein complex) and an association with HLA-DR3 genotype are characteristic.

RHEUMATOID ARTHRITIS

Rheumatoid arthritis (RA) is a systemic autoimmune disease, in which many organs are affected, in addition to the joints. As an inflammatory disorder of the joints, RA has a particular predilection for involvement of the hands and wrists. Patients are usually (3:1) women, with a peak incidence in early middle age. They usually complain of symmetric stiffness and pain in the joints, with swelling and warmth often noted by clinicians. Untreated, the disease can lead to destruction of cartilage and bone, with loss of joint function and considerable disability.

MOLECULAR PATHOGENESIS:
GENETIC FACTORS: A contribution of hereditary factors to RA susceptibility is suggested by the increased frequency of the disease in first-degree relatives of affected patients and by the concordance for the illness in monozygotic twins (15%). In addition, it is generally agreed that certain major histocompatibility genes are expressed in a nonrandom manner in patients with RA. An important genetic locus that predisposes to RA is present in HLA II genes, and a specific set of HLA-DR alleles (DR4, DR1, DR10, DR14) is consistently increased in these patients. These alleles share a pentapeptide sequence motif (shared epitope) in a hypervariable segment of the HLA-DRB1 gene, which forms the peptide-binding pocket on the HLA molecule. It is likely that the binding properties of this pocket influence the type of

peptides that can be bound by RA-associated HLA-DR molecules and so affect the immune response to these peptides. Interestingly, seropositive RA (poor prognosis) is associated with a high frequency of an arginine in the shared epitope, whereas seronegative disease (good prognosis) commonly exhibits a lysine in the same position, further suggesting that the physical characteristics of the rheumatoid pocket influence the immune response in RA. Several non-HLA loci have been linked to RA, including a region of chromosome 18q21 that encodes the receptor activator of NFκB, or RANK.

HUMORAL IMMUNITY: Immunologic mechanisms are important in the pathogenesis of RA. Lymphocytes and plasma cells accumulate in the synovium, where they produce immunoglobulins, mainly of the IgG class. In addition, immune complex deposits are present in the articular cartilage and the synovium. Increased serum levels of IgM, IgA and IgG are also seen.

Some 80% of patients with classic RA are positive for rheumatoid factor (RF). RF represents multiple antibodies, mostly IgM, but sometimes IgG or IgA, directed against the Fc fragment of IgG. Significant titers of RF are also found in patients with related collagen vascular diseases, such as systemic lupus erythematosus, progressive systemic sclerosis and dermatomyositis. RF also occurs in many nonrheumatic disorders, including pulmonary fibrosis, cirrhosis, sarcoidosis, Waldenström macroglobulinemia, tuberculosis, kala-azar, lepromatous leprosy and viral hepatitis. Even healthy elderly individuals, particularly women, occasionally test positive for RF.

Although patients with classic RA may be seronegative, the presence of RF in high titer is frequently associated with severe and unremitting disease, many systemic complications and a serious prognosis. The presence of IgG-type RF is sometimes associated with the development of systemic complications, such as necrotizing vasculitis.

Immune complexes (IgG RF + IgG) and complement components are found in the synovium, synovial fluid and extra-articular lesions of patients with RA. Furthermore, patients with seropositive RA have lower levels of complement in their synovial fluid than do those who are seronegative.

Anticitrullinated protein antibody (ACPA) is a recently developed serologic test that, like RF, is positive in 2/3 of cases of RA. The test may be positive even before the onset of clinical disease.

CELLULAR IMMUNITY: It has also been postulated that cell-mediated immunity contributes to RA. Abundant T lymphocytes in rheumatoid synovium are frequently Ia positive ("activated") and of the helper type (CD4+). They are often in close contact with HLA-DR–positive cells, which are either macrophages or dendritic Ia-positive cells.

T cells may directly or indirectly interact with macrophages through production of cytokines that inhibit migration and proliferation of the latter. Such substances have been found in rheumatoid synovial fluid and in supernatants from rheumatoid tissue explants. These studies provide strong evidence that joint destruction in RA reflects local production of cytokines, especially TNF-α and IL-1.

INFECTIOUS AGENTS: Infectious bacteria and viruses are not detected in joints of patients with RA, although structures resembling viruses have been reported early in the disease. Most patients with RA develop antibodies against a nuclear antigen in B cells infected with EBV. This antigen, RA-associated nuclear antigen (RANA), is closely related to the nuclear antigen encoded by EBV (EBNA). Moreover, EBV is a polyclonal B-cell activator that stimulates production of RF. Interestingly, the blood of many patients with RA has increased numbers of EBV-infected B cells.

LOCAL FACTORS: Synovial cells cultured from rheumatic joints exhibit a decreased response to glucocorticoids and increased production of hyaluronate. These cells release a peptide (connective tissue–activating peptide) that may influence the function of other cells, producing increased amounts of prostaglandins, particularly PGE2.

A hypothetical scenario consistent with the evidence presented earlier might be constructed as follows:

1. In a genetically susceptible person, an unknown agent (possibly a virus, such as EBV) infects a joint or some other tissue and stimulates antibody formation.
2. These immunoglobulins act as new antigens, triggering production of anti IgG antibodies (RF).
3. Immune complexes containing RF are deposited in the synovium and activate complement. This increases vascular permeability and uptake of immune complexes by leukocytes, which in turn release lysosomal enzymes, activated oxygen species and other injurious products.
4. Activated macrophages in the synovium present unknown antigens to T cells, thus stimulating production of cytokines, which amplify inflammation, tissue injury and synovial cell proliferation.

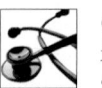 **CLINICAL FEATURES:** RA patients suffer from joint pain and stiffness. As the disease progresses, inflammation is accompanied by loss of bone and cartilage and with progressive loss of motion and instability in the joints. Involvement of weightbearing joints like the hips and knees may lead to difficulty with gait and to increased immobility. RA inflammation outside the joints can present as subcutaneous nodules and occasionally nodules in the lungs; to pericarditis and pleurisy; to inflammation of the conjunctivae and sclera, sometimes accompanied by diffuse eye inflammation; to skin vasculitis with troublesome ulcerations; to anemia and decreased numbers of circulating neutrophils; and to secondary Sjögren syndrome, with infiltration of salivary and lacrimal glands with lymphocytes leading to dry mouth and eyes (see below for primary Sjögren syndrome) (Fig. 11-14).

 PATHOLOGY: The synovium (see Chapter 30) is normally a delicate layer of just a few cells that lines the joints and secretes lubricating synovial fluid. In RA, dense infiltrates of inflammatory cells (lymphocytes, macrophages, DCs) cause dramatic enlargement of the synovium, and there is frequently production of large amounts of inflammatory joint fluid leading to joint effusions. Swelling and pain are noted by patients, together with stiffness, particularly upon arising. Along with activated immune cells, fibroblast-like synoviocytes contribute to the process through their secretion of proteolytic enzymes (matrix metalloproteinases, collagenases), which aid in cartilage destruction. Occasionally, leukocytoclastic vasculitis is seen in extra-articular sites, primarily skin.

VASCULITIDES

Vasculitis is a term for a broad category of diseases characterized by inflammation of blood vessels of different

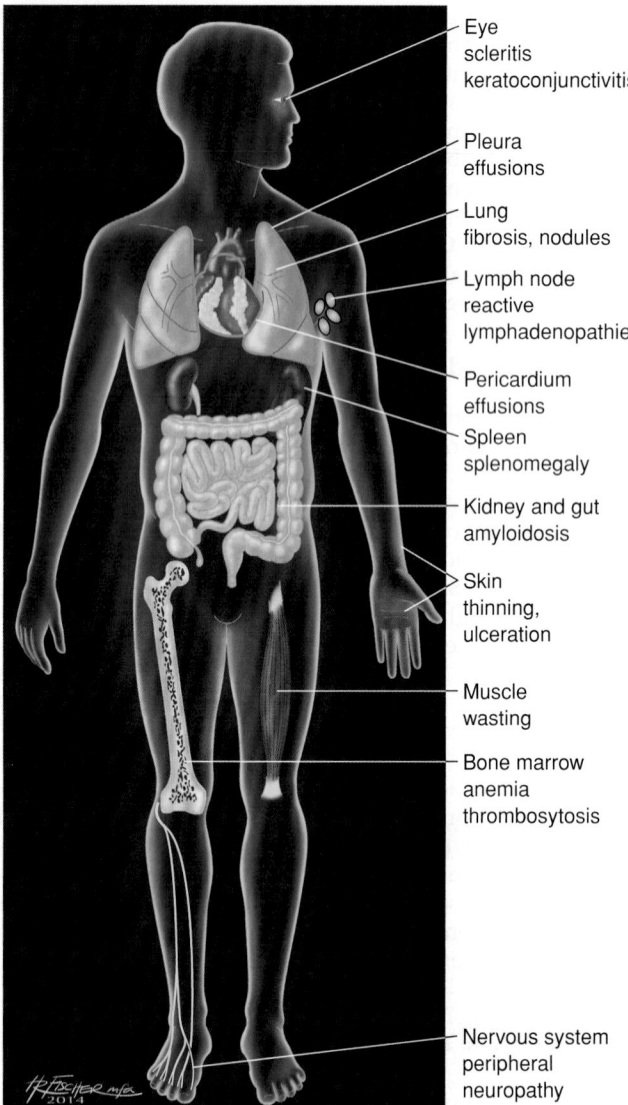

FIGURE 11-14. Organ involvement in rheumatoid arthritis.

types (see Chapter 16), leading to pathology because of the impairment of blood flow to tissues. This group of diseases is generally subdivided depending on the caliber of blood vessel involved and on whether there is an associated rheumatic disease. Thus, both SLE and RA can be associated with vasculitis, which is also seen in dermatomyositis (see below), especially in children. Vasculitis is seen in conjunction with a number of infections, particularly viral infections, and as a consequence of taking certain drugs. Vasculitides that are not associated with systemic autoimmune diseases are discussed in Chapter 16. Vasculitic processes that are part of a constellation of particular diseases are addressed in sections that cover those specific diseases.

SJÖGREN SYNDROME

This disease is marked by lymphocytic infiltration of exocrine glands, primarily salivary and lacrimal glands, leading to dry mouth (**xerostomia**) and dry eyes (**xerophthalmia** or **keratoconjunctivitis sicca**). It exists as a single entity (primary Sjögren syndrome [SS]) or together with other systemic

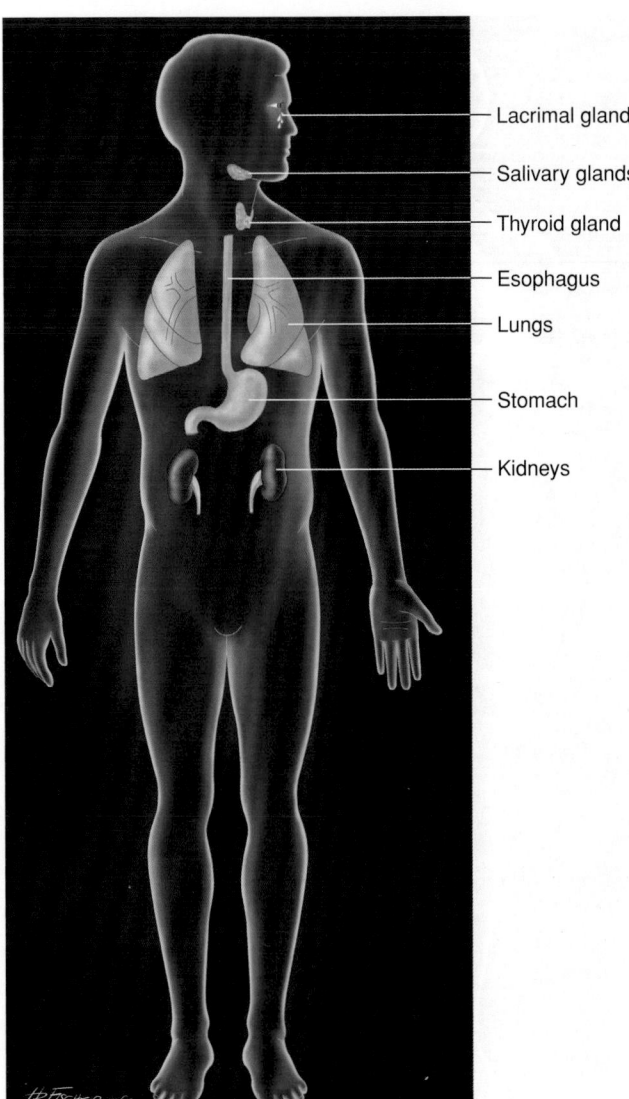

FIGURE 11-15. Organ involvement in Sjögren syndrome.

— Lacrimal glands

— Salivary glands

— Thyroid gland

— Esophagus

— Lungs

— Stomach

— Kidneys

autoimmune diseases such as SLE and RA. Primary SS is also frequently associated with involvement of other organs, including the thyroid, lungs and kidneys (Fig. 11-15). The primary form of the disease most commonly begins in late middle age and patients are overwhelmingly female.

 PATHOPHYSIOLOGY: The basis of lymphocyte accumulation in Sjögren disease is unknown. The majority of lymphocytes found in glands are CD4+, with a significant CD8+ minority. B cells are also present, with occasional germinal centers. It has been proposed that the primary abnormality is autoimmunity to salivary epithelial cells. Most patients with primary Sjögren disease produce antibodies to the cytoplasmic RNA-associated proteins SS-A (Ro) and SS-B (La). Antinuclear antibodies are frequently present, as is rheumatoid factor.

Autoantibodies to DNA or histones are rare; their presence suggests secondary SS associated with lupus. Organ-specific autoantibodies (e.g., against salivary

gland antigens) are quite uncommon. As in SLE, it is controversial whether autoantibodies in SS mainly reflect polyclonal B-cell activation or are chiefly antigen driven, although these processes are not mutually exclusive.

SS has become the focus for investigation of possible viral etiology for autoimmune disease. Particular attention has been paid to possible roles of EBV and human T-cell leukemia virus-1 (HTLV-1). Although difficult to assign a role for EBV in the pathogenesis of SS, there is evidence that reactivation of this virus may be involved in perpetuating SS, polyclonal B-cell activation and development of lymphoma. In Japan, seropositivity for HTLV-1 among patients with SS is 23%, compared with 3.4% among unselected blood donors. Conversely, more than three quarters of HTLV-1–seropositive people have evidence of SS.

PATHOLOGY: Sjögren syndrome is characterized by intense lymphocytic infiltrates in salivary and lacrimal glands (see Chapter 29 and Fig. 11-16). Lymphocytic infiltrates are initially periductal. Most lobules are affected, especially the centers. Well-defined germinal centers are rare. The lymphoid infiltrates destroy acini and ducts; the latter often become dilated and filled with cellular debris. Preservation of glandular stroma helps distinguish SS from lymphoma. The lymphocytic infiltrates are predominantly CD4+ T cells admixed with some B cells. Late in disease, affected glands atrophy and may be replaced by hyalinized fibrotic tissue. Owing to the absence of tears, corneas can become dry and fissured, and may ulcerate. Lack of saliva causes atrophy, inflammation and cracking of the oral mucosa. The pathology of the salivary and lacrimal glands is described in greater detail in Chapter 29.

Involvement of extraglandular sites is also common in SS. Pulmonary disease occurs in many patients, particularly

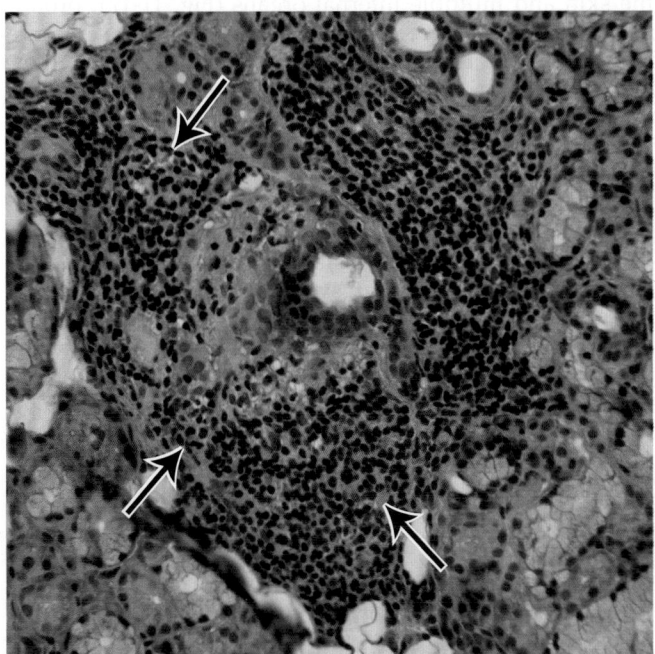

FIGURE 11-16. **Histologic appearance of salivary glands in Sjögren syndrome.** Note the infiltration of lymphocytes into the salivary gland tissue (*arrows*).

bronchial gland atrophy in association with lymphoid infiltration. Pulmonary SS is accompanied by thick tenacious secretions, focal atelectasis, bronchiectasis and recurrent infections. The gastrointestinal tract can be affected, and many patients have difficulty swallowing (dysphagia). Esophageal submucosal glands are infiltrated by lymphocytes. In addition, atrophic gastritis occurs secondary to lymphoid infiltration of the gastric mucosa. Liver disease, especially primary biliary cirrhosis, is present in 5%–10% of patients with SS and is associated with nodular lymphoid infiltrates and destruction of intrahepatic bile ducts (see Chapter 20). Interstitial nephritis and chronic thyroiditis occasionally accompany SS. SS is associated with a 40-fold increased risk of lymphoma, probably through B-cell clonal expansion.

CLINICAL FEATURES: Patients with Sjögren syndrome suffer the consequences of lack of tears and saliva. They complain of eye discomfort and can develop ulcerations and infections of the cornea and conjunctivae. Dry mouth symptoms are sometimes accompanied by increased dental caries and by thrush or other mouth infections. Lymphocytic infiltration of other glandular tissue can lead to dry skin and dryness in the female reproductive tract. Patients may develop extraglandular disease, with lymphocytic infiltration leading to impaired clearance of respiratory mucus and to interstitial lung and kidney disease. Hypergammaglobulinemia can lead to vasculitis, and some patients develop CNS involvement with transverse myelitis or cranial neuropathies. Patients are at a much greater risk of developing B-cell lymphomas.

SYSTEMIC SCLEROSIS (SCLERODERMA)

Systemic sclerosis is a systemic autoimmune disease of unknown origin characterized by excessive deposition of collagen and other connective tissue macromolecules in the skin and multiple internal organs (Fig. 11-17), prominent and often severe alterations in the microvasculature and humoral and cellular immunologic abnormalities. Systemic sclerosis is a complex and heterogeneous disease with clinical forms ranging from limited skin involvement with minimal systemic alterations (**limited cutaneous systemic sclerosis,** previously known as CREST syndrome; see below) to forms with diffuse skin sclerosis and severe and often progressive internal organ involvement (**diffuse cutaneous systemic sclerosis**), and occasionally a fulminant course (**fulminant systemic sclerosis**). Systemic sclerosis is the third most common systemic autoimmune disease (following rheumatoid arthritis and systemic lupus erythematosus) and is 3–8 times more frequent in women, with a peak occurrence from 40 to 50 years of age. Although systemic sclerosis is not inherited, it is accepted that genetic predisposition plays an important role in its development. Familial clusters have been reported, and there is an association between HLA-DQB1 and the characteristic autoantibodies.

Patients with Scleroderma Exhibit Abnormalities of Humoral and Cellular Immune Systems

There are normal numbers of circulating B lymphocytes, but hypergammaglobulinemia and cryoglobulinemia suggest

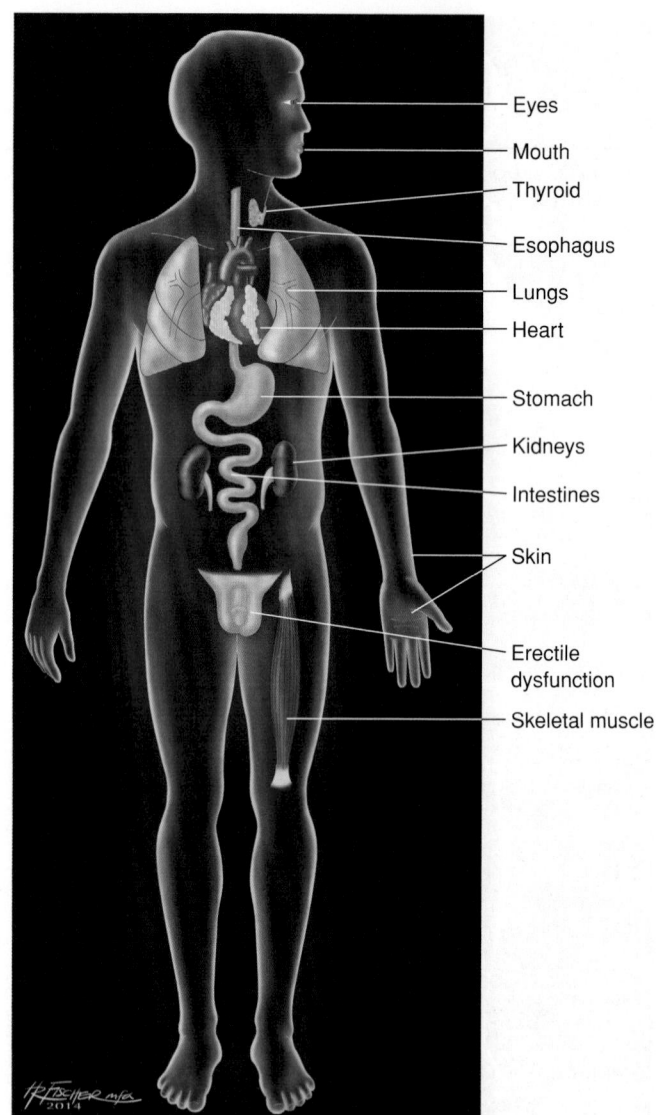

FIGURE 11-17. Organ involvement in systemic sclerosis.

that they may be hyperactive. The presence of specific antibodies is one of the most common manifestations of systemic sclerosis, and they are present in over 90% of patients. ANAs are common but usually at lower titers than in SLE. Commonly found antibodies include nucleolar autoantibodies (primarily against RNA polymerase). Antibodies to Scl-70, a nonhistone nuclear protein topoisomerase, are found in 30%–40% of patients with the diffuse form of systemic sclerosis. Anticentromere antibodies are associated with the CREST variant (see below). The Scl-70 autoantibody is the most common and specific for diffuse scleroderma, seen in 60% of patients. There is no correlation between ANA titer and disease severity. Rheumatoid factor is commonly present, as are autoantibodies against other tissues, such as smooth muscle, thyroid and salivary glands. Antibodies to collagen types I and IV have also been described.

Although autoantibodies are common in systemic sclerosis, they do not cause the clinical manifestations of the disease. However, owing to their high frequency and to their specificity for certain clinical subsets of the disease, their presence is very helpful to establish the diagnosis and to predict a likely pattern of organ involvement, severity and progression of systemic sclerosis.

Cellular immune derangements are also seen in patients with progressive systemic sclerosis. Reduced circulating CD8$^+$ T suppressor cells, evidence of T-cell activation, alterations in functions mediated by IL-1 and elevated IL-2 and soluble IL-2 receptor occur in active disease. Increased levels of IL-4 and IL-6 have also been described. Tissues show active mononuclear inflammation, which precedes development of the vasculopathy and fibrosis characteristic of this disease. The infiltrates contain increased numbers of CD4$^+$ and $\gamma\delta$-T cells (which adhere to fibroblasts), as well as macrophages. Mast cells (degranulated) are also present in the skin of scleroderma patients. The incidence of other autoimmune disorders, such as thyroiditis and primary biliary cirrhosis, is increased.

PATHOPHYSIOLOGY: The pathogenesis of systemic sclerosis is extremely complex and the exact mechanisms involved are not well understood. The clinical and pathologic manifestations of systemic sclerosis result from three distinct processes: (1) fibroproliferative vascular lesions of small arteries and arterioles, (2) excessive and often progressive deposition of collagen and other extracellular matrix macromolecules in skin and various internal organs and (3) alterations of humoral and cellular immunity. The immunologic alterations include innate immunity abnormalities, tissue infiltration with macrophages and T and B lymphocytes, production of numerous disease-specific autoantibodies and dysregulation of cytokine, chemokine and growth factor production. It is not clear which of these processes is of primary importance or how they are temporally related during the development and progression of the disease.

Unknown etiologic factors trigger a sequence of pathogenetic events initiated by a genetically receptive host. These entail microvascular injury, characterized by structural and functional endothelial cell abnormalities. The endothelial cell abnormalities result either in increased production and release of many potent mediators including cytokines, chemokines, polypeptide growth factors and various other substances such as prostaglandins, reactive oxygen species (ROS) and thrombogenic and procoagulant activities, or in the reduction of important compounds such as prostacyclin and nitric oxide. The endothelial cell dysfunction allows chemokine- and cytokine-mediated attraction of inflammatory cells and fibroblast precursors from the bloodstream and bone marrow. These cells transmigrate into the surrounding tissues to establish a chronic inflammatory process with participation of macrophages and T and B lymphocytes.

These cells produce and secrete additional cytokines and growth factors. As a result, resident fibroblasts, epithelial cells, endothelial cells and pericytes become activated and undergo a phenotypic conversion into myofibroblasts (Fig. 11-18). This sequence of events causes a severe and often progressive fibroproliferative vasculopathy, vessel rarefaction and exaggerated and widespread accumulation of fibrotic tissue, the hallmark of the fibrotic process characteristic of the disease.

Vascular Dysfunction Is One of the Earliest Manifestations of Systemic Sclerosis

This is heralded by Raynaud phenomenon. This episodic circulatory compromise in the distal extremities, particularly the hands, often triggered by exposure to cold, is accompanied by nailfold capillary microvascular alterations that often precede any clinical evidence of tissue fibrosis.

The initial events responsible for the vascular and endothelial cell injury and subsequent activation are not known. Numerous putative etiologic factors have been suggested, including vasculotropic viral pathogens, antiendothelial cell antibodies, cellular products from inflammatory cells

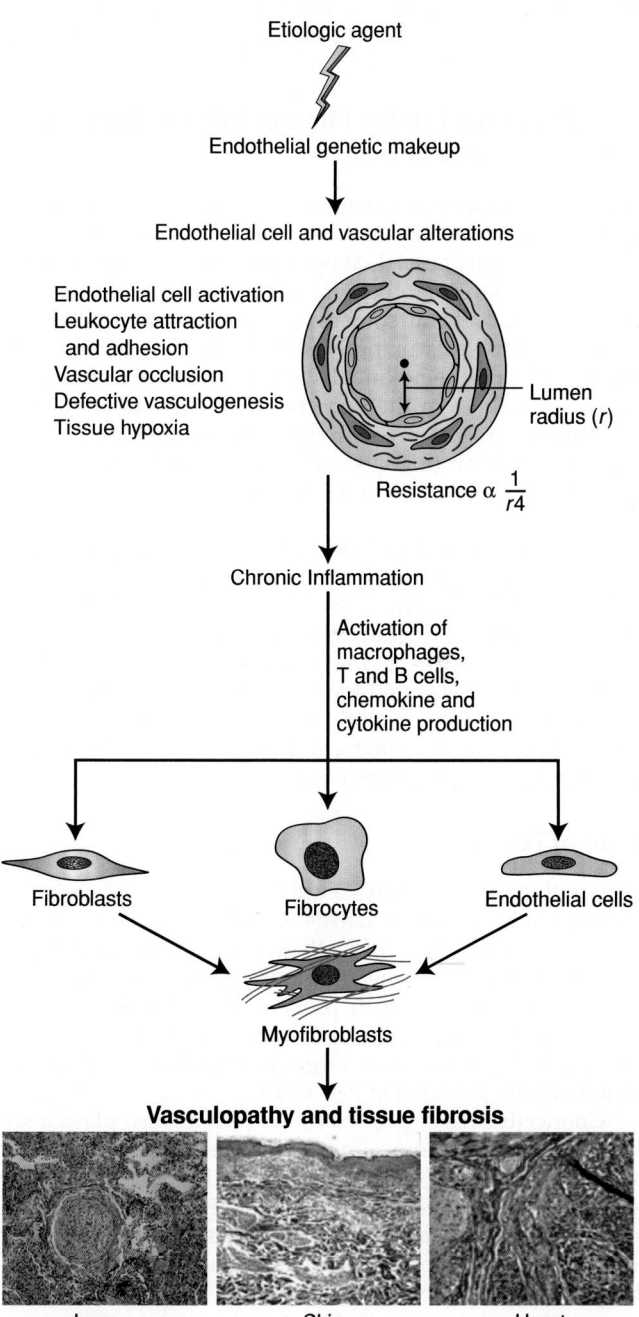

FIGURE 11-18. Involvement of endothelial cell and vascular alteration in the pathogenesis of systemic sclerosis.

or ROS generated during episodes of ischemia/reperfusion. Endothelial cell activation induces expression of chemokine and cell adhesion molecules, causes transendothelial cellular migration and leads to perivascular accumulation of immunologic/inflammatory cells. The latter include T and B lymphocytes and various macrophage populations. These produce and secrete diverse cytokines and/or growth factors, including transforming growth factor-β (TGF-β) and other profibrotic mediators such as endothelin-1, which stimulate smooth muscle cell proliferation and marked accumulation of subendothelial fibrotic tissue and initiation of platelet aggregation. They also trigger intravascular thrombosis, eventually leading to microvascular occlusion. The effects of vascular dysfunction in patients with systemic sclerosis are most dramatic when they involve the pulmonary and renal arterioles, causing renal crisis and pulmonary hypertension, respectively.

Myofibroblasts Are the Effector Cells in Systemic Sclerosis Tissue Fibrosis

The fibrotic process is the most notable characteristic of systemic sclerosis and causes most of its clinical manifestations (Fig. 11-17). This crucial component results from the accumulation in skin and other affected tissues of myofibroblasts derived from several sources: proliferation and activation of tissue fibroblasts or perivascular and vascular adventitial fibroblasts; chemokine-driven recruitment of fibroblast precursor cells from the bone marrow; transdifferentiation of epithelial cells to myofibroblasts via epithelial-to-mesenchymal transition (EMT; see Chapter 5); and other cellular transitions in which endothelial cells acquire mesenchymal phenotypes.

This increased population of myofibroblasts produces more fibrillar type I and type III collagens and expresses α-smooth muscle actin. They also produce less extracellular matrix (ECM)-degradative enzymes. Accumulation of myofibroblasts in affected tissues and the uncontrolled persistence of their elevated biosynthetic functions are crucial determinants of the extent and rate of progression of the fibrotic process in systemic sclerosis and of its clinical course, response to therapy, prognosis and mortality.

Role of TGF-β

A growth factor that plays a crucial role in the fibrosis that accompanies systemic sclerosis is TGF-β (Fig. 11-19). It also decreases production of collagen-degrading metalloproteinases while simultaneously upregulating production of protease inhibitors, which prevent ECM breakdown. The pathways involved in the activation of collagen genes following TGF-β binding to target cell surface receptors are schematically depicted in Fig. 11-19.

Connective tissue growth factor (CTGF) also plays a key role in systemic sclerosis–associated tissue fibrosis. TGF-β strongly stimulates CTGF synthesis in fibroblasts, vascular smooth muscle cells and endothelial cells. It magnifies the profibrotic phenotype and also enhances its own production via an autocrine loop. It thus maintains a continuous, prolonged cycle of excessive fibrosis.

 PATHOLOGY: Sclerodermatous skin initially reveals edema, then induration. The thickened skin exhibits a striking increase in collagen fibers in the

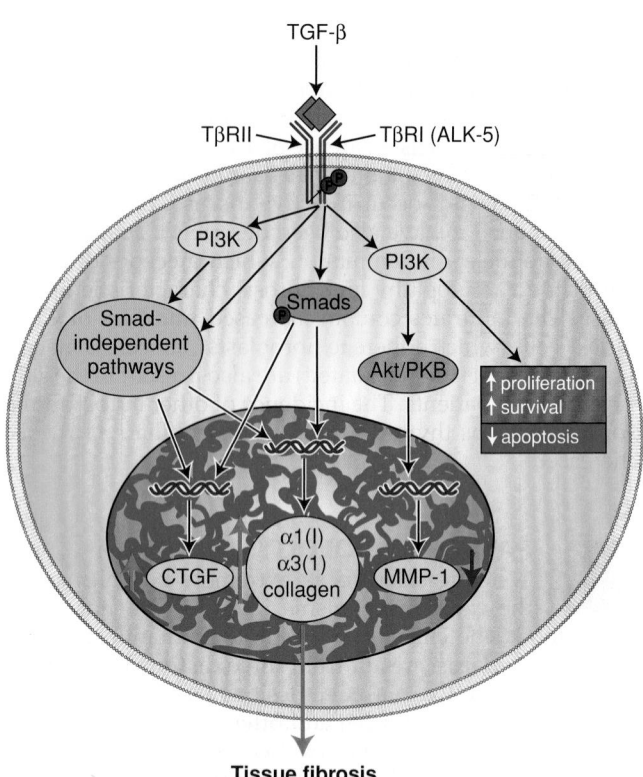

FIGURE 11-19. Involvement of transforming growth factor-β (TGF-β) in systemic sclerosis. Fibrogenic pathways are stimulated by TGF-β, and production of enzymes that degrade collagen is inhibited by TGF-β. Signaling pathways that are both independent of and that involve Smads may be involved in mediating these effects. *PI3K* = phosphoinositol-3-kinase; *CTGF* = connective tissue growth factor; *MMP-1* = matrix metalloproteinase-1.

reticular dermis; thinning of the epidermis with loss of rete pegs; atrophy of dermal appendages (Fig. 11-20A); hyalinization and obliteration of arterioles; and variable mononuclear infiltrates, primarily of T cells. The stage of induration may progress to atrophy or revert to normal. Increased collagen deposition can also occur in the synovia, lungs, gastrointestinal tract, heart and kidneys.

Lesions in arteries, arterioles and capillaries are typical, and in some cases may be the first demonstrable pathology. Initial subintimal edema with fibrin deposition is followed by thickening and fibrosis of the vessel wall and reduplication or fraying of the internal elastic lamina. Involved vessels may become severely narrowed or occluded by thrombi.

The kidneys, involved in more than half of patients, show marked vascular changes, often with focal hemorrhage and cortical infarcts (see Chapter 22). The interlobular arteries and afferent arterioles tend to be the most severely affected vessels. Early fibromuscular thickening of the subintima causes luminal narrowing, followed by fibrosis (Fig. 11-20B). Fibrinoid necrosis is commonly seen in afferent arterioles. Glomerular alterations are nonspecific, and focal changes range from necrosis extending from the afferent arterioles to fibrosis. Early in disease, there is diffuse deposition of immunoglobulin, complement and fibrin in affected vessels, probably because of increased vascular permeability.

Heightened pulmonary vascular reactivity ("pulmonary Raynaud phenomenon") and, later, hypertension and

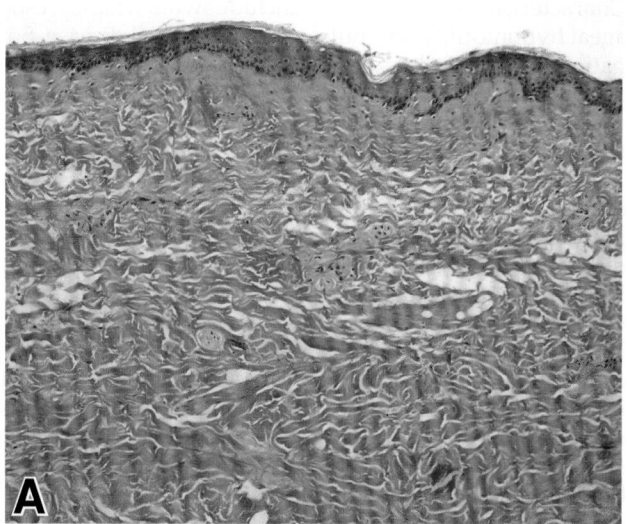 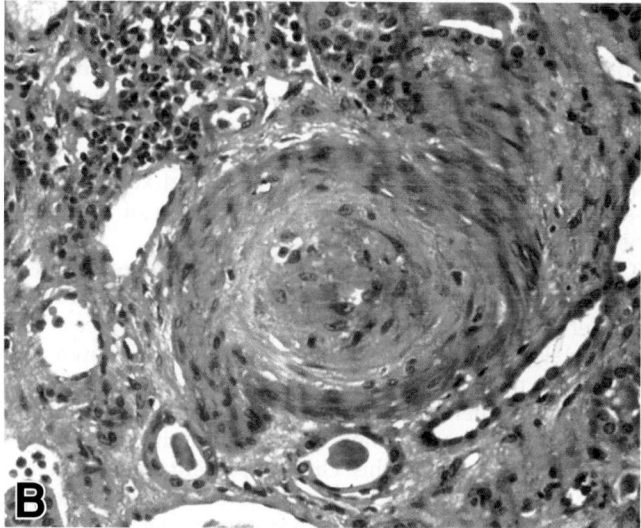

FIGURE 11-20. Histologic appearance of systemic sclerosis. A. Dermal fibrosis is characteristic of scleroderma. Dense collagen accumulation occurs beneath the epidermis. Note the absence of dermal appendages. **B.** Scleroderma that affects the kidney is manifested by vascular involvement. Here, the interlobular artery exhibits marked luminal narrowing due to pronounced intimal thickening.

diffuse interstitial fibrosis are the primary lung abnormalities. Pulmonary disease can progress to end-stage fibrosis, so-called honeycomb lung (see Chapter 18).

Most patients with scleroderma have patchy myocardial fibrosis, and in about one fourth of cases, more than 10% of the myocardium is involved. These lesions result from focal myocardial necrosis, which may reflect focal ischemia secondary to Raynaud-like reactivity of cardiac microvasculature.

Progressive systemic sclerosis can also involve any portion of the gastrointestinal tract. Esophageal dysfunction is the most common and troublesome gastrointestinal complication. Atrophy and fibrous replacement of smooth muscle are seen in the lower esophagus. The small bowel often exhibits patchy fibrosis of the muscular layers.

 CLINICAL FEATURES: The most apparent and almost universal clinical features of systemic sclerosis are related to the progressive thickening and fibrosis of the skin. Scleroderma manifests as two distinct clinical syndromes, a generalized or diffuse **(progressive systemic)** form and a **limited variant**. Progressive systemic sclerosis (diffuse scleroderma) is characterized by severe and progressive disease of skin and early onset of all or most of the associated abnormalities of visceral organs. Symptoms usually begin with Raynaud phenomenon, namely, intermittent episodes of ischemia of the fingers, marked by triphasic color changes, paresthesias and pain. Raynaud phenomenon is accompanied or followed by edema of the fingers and hands, thickening and tightening of the skin, polyarthralgia and involvement of specific internal organs. The affected skin is tight, indurated and firmly bound to the subcutaneous tissue. The skin over the hands and face is most frequently involved, and as the disease progresses, the sclerotic changes extend and may affect the entire body.

The typical patient with generalized scleroderma exhibits "stone facies," owing to tightening of facial skin and restricted motion of the mouth. Progression of vascular lesions in the fingers leads to ischemic ulceration of the fingertips, with subsequent shortening and atrophy of the digits. Many patients suffer from painful tendonitis and joint pain.

OTHER ORGAN INVOLVEMENT. Musculoskeletal symptoms are often the first manifestations of the disease. Severity may vary from mild polyarthralgias to more severe arthralgias, but synovitis and frank arthritis are rare. In more advanced stages, thickening and fibrosis of periarticular tissues result in severe joint flexion contractures and distal phalangeal resorption also known as **acroosteolysis**. Muscle infiltration with fibrotic tissue may lead to an inflammatory myopathy or a more indolent noninflammatory form.

The gastrointestinal tract is the internal organ system most commonly involved. Esophageal involvement is almost universal, with symptoms of gastroesophageal reflux, heartburn and dysphagia due to dysfunctional esophageal sphincter motility. In severe cases, stricture may result. Impaired gastric emptying and small intestine peristalsis may cause distention, bloating, nausea and pain. Bacterial overgrowth may lead to secondary malabsorption and diarrhea.

Pulmonary involvement frequently leads to severe respiratory disability and is the most common cause of death. Patients develop progressively worsening tachypnea and exertional dyspnea, secondary to pulmonary fibrosis and/or pulmonary hypertension. The former usually develops early in the disease, but pulmonary hypertension is most commonly a late complication.

Cardiac involvement is not uncommon and may manifest as chest pain, arrhythmias and conduction defects. Infiltrative cardiomyopathy may cause left ventricular or biventricular failure. Cor pulmonale can develop in patients with pulmonary hypertension.

"Scleroderma renal crisis," as the renal disease may be known, typically begins abruptly, with malignant hypertension and rapidly progressive renal insufficiency. It is often heralded by severe headache, hypertensive retinopathy, seizures and other central nervous system symptoms, and/or myocardial ischemia, infarction or left ventricular failure. Prompt aggressive treatment can usually reverse this process, which otherwise is often fatal or may cause renal failure.

Functional thyroid abnormalities including elevated levels of antithyroid autoantibodies and clinical and subclinical hypothyroidism are common. Impotence caused by erectile failure may be an early feature of systemic sclerosis, and some degree of erectile dysfunction ultimately develops in many systemic sclerosis patients. Patients may develop the sicca syndrome (keratoconjunctivitis sicca and xerostomia) caused by fibrosis and lymphocytic infiltration of the salivary and lacrimal glands.

CREST. In many cases, the cutaneous involvement is confined to the digits and the dorsum of the hands and feet (acrosclerosis), and progression of the sclerotic process is relatively slow. This form of disease, previously known as the CREST syndrome (acronym for calcinosis, long-standing Raynaud phenomenon, esophageal dysmotility, sclerodactyly and telangiectases) is now known as limited systemic sclerosis to differentiate this clinical presentation from a more severe form with extensive cutaneous involvement. This latter form is known as diffuse systemic sclerosis. Other cutaneous manifestations include skin ulcerations, usually localized to fingertips or knuckles, and peculiar pigmentary changes with hyper- and hypopigmentation. Calcinosis is most commonly found in the fingertips and periarticular tissues. Many patients with CREST have circulating anticentromere antibodies.

MIXED CONNECTIVE TISSUE DISEASE

As suggested by the name, mixed connective tissue disease (MCTD) patients exhibit features of several different collagen vascular diseases including SLE, scleroderma and polymyositis. The exact incidence of MCTD is unclear. Between 80% and 90% of patients are female, and most are adults (mean age, 37 years). Findings characteristic of SLE include rash, Raynaud phenomenon, arthralgias and arthritis.

Characteristics of scleroderma include swollen hands, esophageal hypomotility and pulmonary interstitial disease. Some patients also develop symptoms suggestive of rheumatoid arthritis. Patients with MCTD have been reported to respond well to corticosteroid therapy, although some studies have challenged this assertion.

The pathogenesis of MCTD is poorly understood. Patients often have evidence of B-cell activation with hypergammaglobulinemia and rheumatoid factor. ANAs are present but, differently from SLE, do not usually bind double-stranded DNA. The most distinctive ANA is directed against an extractable nuclear antigen. Specifically, patients with MCTD have high titers of antibody to uridine-rich ribonucleoprotein (anti-U1-RNP) in the absence of other extractable nuclear antigens, including PM-1 and Jo-1. Most diagnostic criteria for MCTD include high-titer anti-U1-RNP ANA as a sine qua non. Anti-RNP antibodies may be detected in SLE, but in much lower titers than in MCTD.

The cause of high titers of anti-U1-RNP antibody is unclear. However, there is an association with HLA-DR4 and HLA-DR2 genotypes, suggesting a role for T cells in autoantibody production. There is no direct evidence that these antibodies participate in the development of any of the characteristic lesions of MCTD.

There is controversy whether MCTD is a separate disease or a heterogeneous collection of patients with nonclassical presentations of SLE, scleroderma or polymyositis. For example, in some patients, MCTD seems to evolve into typical scleroderma; other patients develop renal disease similar to that seen in SLE; still others develop features of rheumatoid arthritis. Thus, MCTD may be an intermediate stage in the progression to another recognized autoimmune disease. Patients whose disease remains undifferentiated may constitute a distinct subset. Thus, it remains unclear whether MCTD is a distinct entity or simply an overlap of findings in patients with other types of collagen vascular disease.

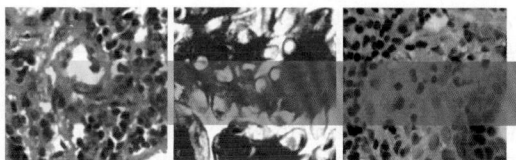

Sepsis

Kendra Iskander ▪ David S. Strayer ▪ Daniel Remick

Definitions Systemic Inflammatory Response Syndrome **Triggers of Sepsis** Infection	Age, Debility, Immune Status and Organ Function Diverse Organisms as Triggers Anti-Inflammatory Mediators	Balance of Pro- and Anti-Inflammatory Activities Abnormal Circulation and Coagulation **Physiologic Responses to SIRS/Sepsis**

DEFINITIONS

Systemic Inflammatory Response Syndrome Is a Bodily Reaction to a Broad Range of Insults

The insults that elicit systemic inflammatory response syndrome (SIRS) reactions include—but are not limited to—trauma, ischemia, inflammation and infection. Multiple insults may contribute simultaneously to the development of SIRS. Therefore, the triggering stimuli for the development of SIRS need not be specific and may represent combinations of multiple processes acting concurrently to initiate protective mechanisms for human self-defense. The American College of Chest Physicians and the Society of Critical Care Medicine Consensus Conference defined the terms "SIRS," "sepsis," "severe sepsis," "septic shock," and "multiple organ dysfunction syndrome (MODS)" in 1992 to standardize the classification of the human response to infection. The relationship between the conditions is represented in Fig. 12-1. The definition of SIRS requires that two or more of the abnormal findings described in Table 12-1 be present.

Should these criteria be met, and if an infection is documented in the patient, **sepsis** is the appropriate diagnosis. Sepsis represents the body's systemic inflammatory reaction to a documented or suspected infection. A patient's inability to eradicate pathogens can cause them to spread systemically and damage normal tissues and organ systems that are distant from the original insult.

Sepsis can progress to severe sepsis with clinical features of hypoperfusion including lactic acidosis, oliguria or acute change in mental status. If hypotension with perfusion abnormalities occurs despite adequate fluid replenishment, then septic shock develops along the continuum of worsening severity in sepsis. In a study of 3500 septic patients, mortality ranged from 25% in sepsis, to 40% in severe sepsis, to 60% in septic shock. MODS is defined as progressive organ dysfunction in critically ill patients with physiologic dysregulation leading to impaired homeostasis. Mortality strongly correlates with organ dysfunction, so that the more organs that fail, the greater the mortality. If five organs fail, mortality may exceed 80%.

 **EPIDEMIOLOGY:** The incidence of sepsis is increasing despite advances in intensive care management and significant resource utilization allocated to caring for septic patients. Hospitalizations for sepsis in the United States have more than doubled, to over 725,000 in an 8-year period. There are now more than 200,000 deaths from sepsis per year. Sepsis is the leading cause of mortality in noncoronary intensive care units (ICUs) and the 11th most common cause of death in the United States. It affects nearly 20 million people globally, and its incidence is anticipated to rise owing to a constellation of factors. These include increasing antimicrobial resistance to available antimicrobial therapies, an aging population, the prevalence and frequency of use of immunosuppressive medications, infectious diseases like HIV/AIDS that compromise the

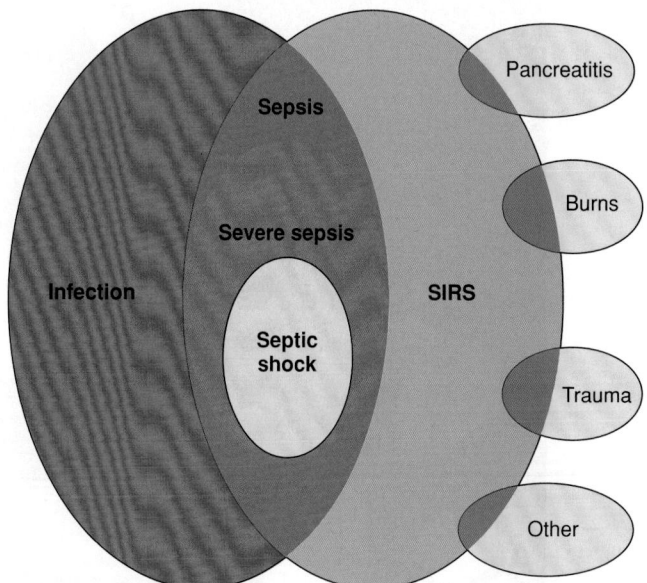

FIGURE 12-1. Venn diagram demonstrating the relationship between systemic inflammatory response syndrome (SIRS), sepsis, severe sepsis and septic shock. After Bone, et al., *Chest*, 1992;101(6):1644–1655.

TABLE 12-1

DIAGNOSTIC CRITERIA FOR SIRS, SEPSIS, SEVERE SEPSIS AND SEPTIC SHOCK

Systemic Inflammatory Response Syndrome (SIRS) (two or more of the following abnormalities)

Temperature >38.5°C or <35°C

Heart rate >90 beats per minute

Respiratory rate >20 breaths per minute or $PaCO_2$ <32 mm Hg

White blood cell count >12,000 cells/mm³ or <4,000 cells/mm³ or >10% bands

Sepsis

SIRS with a documented or suspected infection

Severe Sepsis

Sepsis with organ dysfunction, hypoperfusion or hypotension

Septic Shock

Sepsis-induced hypotension (systolic blood pressure <90 mm Hg or drop of ≥40 mm Hg from baseline) despite adequate fluid resuscitation with inadequate perfusion

Multiple Organ Dysfunction Syndrome (MODS)

Physiologic dysregulation in a critically ill patient in which impaired homeostasis manifests as organ dysfunction

immune system and more widely available health care technologies and interventions.

Even though there has been an overall reduction in the proportional mortality from sepsis, the total number of deaths from sepsis is greater than in the past as more individuals are affected. Survival studies in sepsis usually monitor patients for 28 days. This contrasts with, for example, most cancer trials, which evaluate 5-year survival. Such a juxtaposition underscores the acutely damaging and life-threatening nature of sepsis. A hospitalized patient with severe sepsis has a greater risk of death than a patient admitted for acute myocardial infarction or stroke. Advancements in supportive care for sepsis continue to reduce early deaths, but initial sepsis survivors often suffer from functional deficits and reduced quality of life, as well as being at risk for higher long-term mortality.

Severe sepsis most frequently occurs in children younger than 1 year and elderly patients who are older than 65 years. In this context, the elderly represent only 12% of the U.S. population but account for over 65% of sepsis cases. Older age is an independent predictor of mortality in sepsis. Compared to younger people, elderly patients are more likely to have medical comorbidities and earlier mortality during hospitalization for sepsis. The most common comorbidities seen in septic patients overall are diabetes mellitus, chronic obstructive pulmonary disease, cancer, end-stage renal disease, HIV/AIDS and cirrhosis. Sepsis survivors older than 65 years more often need considerable nursing and/or rehabilitative care upon discharge. With the average age of the U.S. population rising, the incidence of sepsis is predicted to increase.

TRIGGERS OF SEPSIS

Infection in Any Part of the Body May Lead to Sepsis

The most common site of sepsis-related infection is the lungs. Over 40% of septic patients have a respiratory source of infection such as pneumonia. Fig. 12-2 shows the typical histopathology of bacterial pneumonia. Abdominal infections are the second most frequent cause of sepsis. These occur in many circumstances, including ruptured appendicitis, penetrating injuries to the bowel and postsurgical

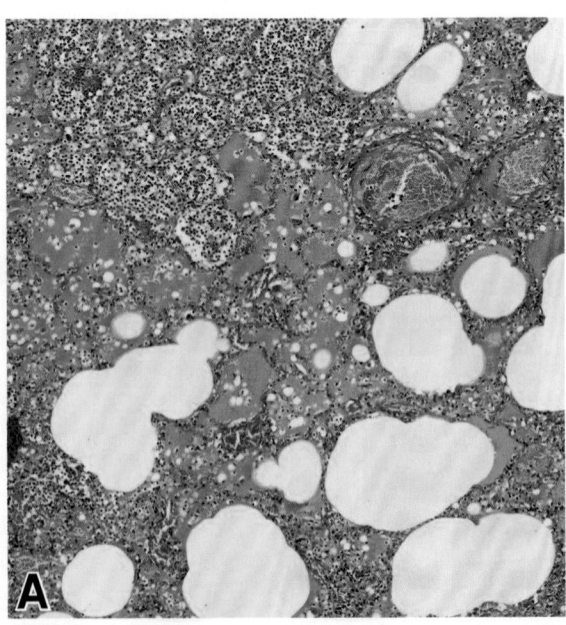
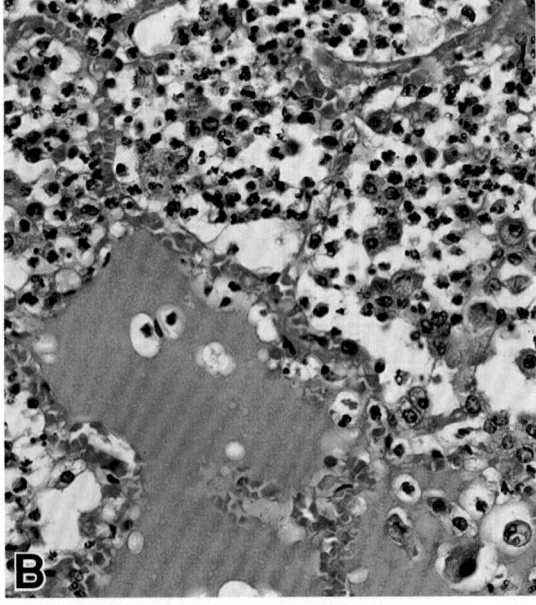

FIGURE 12-2. Histopathology of bacterial pneumonia. A. Some alveolar airspaces are filled with pink-stained protein-filled fluid. Numerous neutrophils have also infiltrated the alveolar space. The white spaces show alveoli where air was still exchanged through breathing. **B.** Higher power, showing intraalveolar fluid and many neutrophils.

anastomotic leaks. Urinary tract infections are the third most common starting point for sepsis. Additional causes of sepsis are attributable to soft tissue infections, primary bacteremia, meningitis, encephalitis, endocarditis and others. Infections that precipitate sepsis may be acquired in the community or during the course of hospitalization (i.e., nosocomial infections). Patients who develop sepsis as a result of nosocomial infections have higher mortality rates than those with community-acquired pathogens.

Age, Debility, Immune Status and Organ Function Help Determine the Risk of Sepsis

Sepsis occurs more often in those who are at the extremes of life: the aged and very young children. Males are more likely to develop sepsis than females, and blacks are more susceptible than whites. People with chronic illnesses, especially if their immune systems are compromised, are particularly at risk. AIDS, iatrogenic immunosuppression (e.g., postchemotherapy), long-standing respiratory or circulatory insufficiency and so forth predispose patients to sepsis.

Other, more poorly understood contributors relate to specific organ or organ system impairments and to the involvement of individual genetic, epigenetic and environmental factors. Many contributors participate in the pathophysiology of sepsis, including inflammatory mediators, clotting and complement systems and so forth (see below), and person-to-person variability in these systems undoubtedly affects susceptibility to development of sepsis in ways that are not yet quantified.

Infections with Many Different Organisms and Different Types of Organisms May Precipitate Sepsis

Infections with diverse types of pathogens may lead to sepsis, depending on the host response to the infectious insult. The nature of the infectious organisms that precipitate sepsis has shifted over time. Gram-positive bacteria are now responsible for more cases than are gram-negative organisms. A single bacterial species is responsible in over 85% of cases, with the remainder being due to polymicrobial bacterial infections or infections with fungi, anaerobes, viruses or parasites. The incidence of fungal sepsis has increased sharply in recent years, but fungi still provoke only about 5%–10% of cases overall.

Bacteremia (i.e., microbial infection of the bloodstream) may occur during sepsis, but it is not an essential component, because local infections can lead to distant tissue damage and organ dysfunction. Blood cultures are positive in only 20%–40% of patients with severe sepsis and 40%–70% of those with septic shock. Clinical suspicion for sepsis should remain high particularly if an infection is suspected but not detectable, and then empirical management should be initiated.

PATHOPHYSIOLOGY: Sepsis is part of a systemic overreaction that begins with inflammatory responses to infection (see Chapters 2 and 4). These responses reflect host recognition of pathogen-associated molecular patterns (PAMPs) that are present on invading microorganisms. PAMPs are perceived via pattern response receptors (PRRs), such as Toll-like

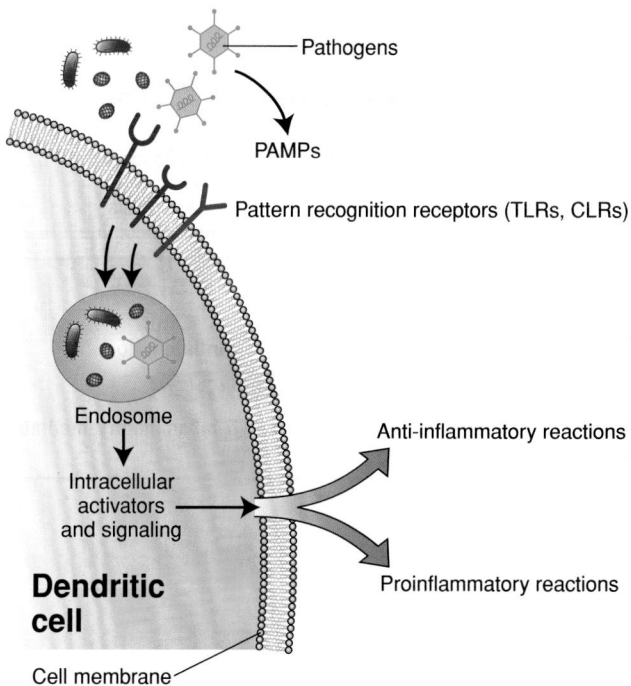

FIGURE 12-3. Mechanisms triggering soluble mediators in sepsis. Pathogen associated molecular pattern-containing molecules (PAMPs) are recognized by pattern recognition receptors (PRRs, mainly Toll-like receptors [TLRs] and C-type lectin receptors [CLRs]) on cells of the innate immune system, principally dendritic cells. Among other things, these interactions lead to endocytosis of the pathogens, which is in turn followed by activation of intracellular response systems. As a consequence, dendritic cells secrete a plethora of both proinflammatory and anti-inflammatory substances.

receptors (TLRs) and C-type lectin receptors (CLRs) on dendritic cells (Fig. 12-3). For example, the cells of the innate immune system bind the peptidoglycan of gram-positive bacteria to TLR2 and the lipopolysaccharide of gram-negative bacteria to TLR4, as well as to other fungal, viral and parasitic components.

Endocytosis of these pathogens triggers major intracellular receptors of several types. Transmembrane TLR receptor binding to these mediators also activates nuclear factor-κB (NFκB) within monocytes and stimulates production of proinflammatory cytokines such as tumor necrosis factor-α (TNF-α) and interleukin-6 (IL-6), chemokines like IL-8 and intracellular adhesion molecule-1 (ICAM-1) and nitric oxide (NO; see Chapter 1).

Simultaneously, anti-inflammatory pathways are activated (see below), which are important as mediators of downstream or secondary effects of sepsis. The interplay of the triggering pathogen with the cells of the innate immune helps to determine whether pro- or anti-inflammatory forces predominate. Additional factors that participate in the decision as to the outcome include influences described above. The timing of the outcome, and the diverse intra- and extra-cellular pathways triggered, hang in the balance (Fig. 12-4). The opening act may favor a proinflammatory situation (Fig. 12-5).

The initial sequence is but the beginning, however. Tissue necrosis releases damage-associated molecular pattern molecules (DAMPs, or alarmins; see Chapters 2 and 4).

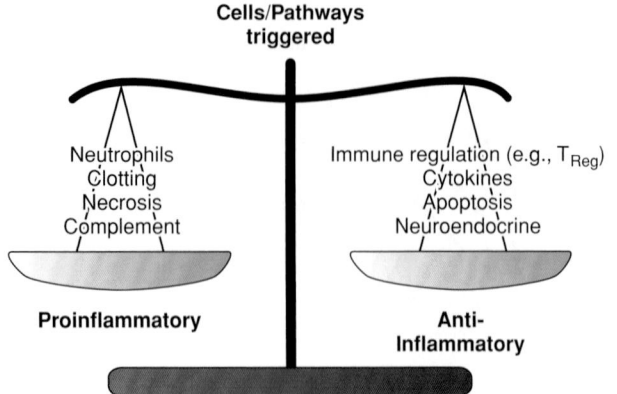

FIGURE 12-4. The balance of pro- and anti-inflammatory mediators that participate in sepsis.

DAMPs are recognized by pattern recognition receptors in cells of the innate immune system. Interaction between DAMPs and PRRs in turn drives those cells to produce more proinflammatory mediators. For reasons that are as yet unclear, and that probably reflect the interplay of host and environmental factors, this proinflammation stimulatory process spirals out of control and the body is flooded with inflammation-inducing, -potentiating and -sustaining factors that lead to uncontrolled inflammation.

Neutrophils are recruited to the site of injury and release mediators that lead to characteristic signs of local inflammation, such as protein-rich edema from microvascular leakage along with erythema and warmth from vasodilation (see below). A combination of proinflammatory and anti-inflammatory mediators is produced by macrophages in an effort to kill invading pathogens and to remove debris by phagocytosis of damaged tissue in a controlled approach. However, sepsis develops when the inflammatory response to infection cannot be contained in the local environment and becomes systemic.

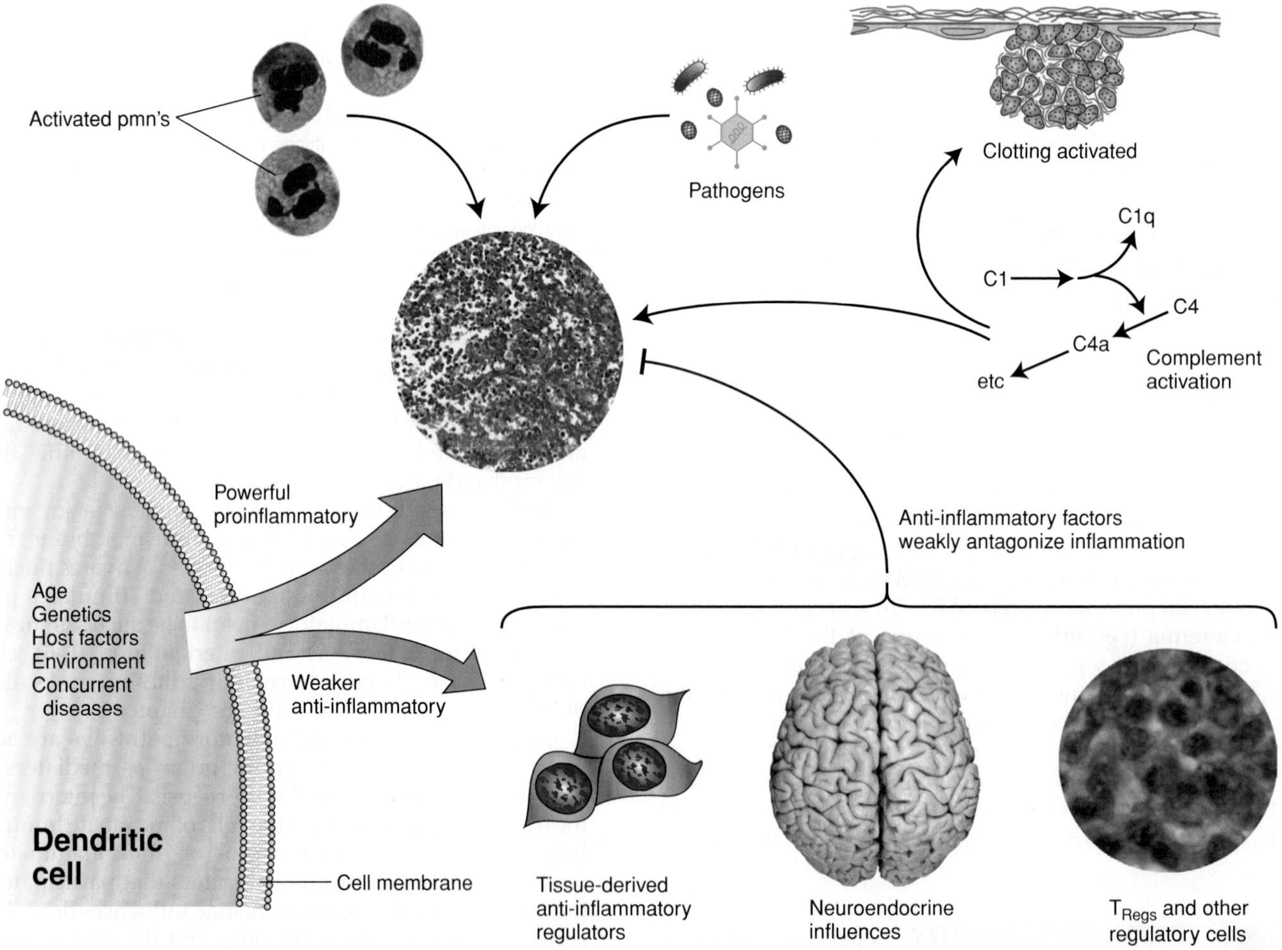

FIGURE 12-5. The elements of host responses favoring inflammatory activity during sepsis. Dendritic cell responses are determined, both quantitatively and qualitatively, by a combination of genetics, environment, age, other concurrent illnesses and other factors. When stimulated by an appropriate microbial trigger, whether bacterial, fungal or viral, pro- and anti-inflammatory substances are secreted by these dendritic cells. Here, the former (*upper*) predominate and are involved in a series of reactions. These include activation of neutrophils, blood-clotting elements and complement, all of which lead to tissue necrosis. This, in turn, magnifies the proinflammatory response. Anti-inflammatory elements (*lower*) include tissue-derived anti-inflammatory regulators, neuroendocrine influences and regulatory cells of different lineages, including T regulatory cells (T$_{reg}$s) and others.

Many Organ Systems Produce Anti-Inflammatory Mediators in Sepsis

Nervous System

Anti-inflammatory influences entail intricate regulatory pathways in which nervous system–derived mediators modulate inflammation. These mediators act in part via vagal stimulation, which triggers several intermediaries to stimulate acetylcholine (ACh) secretion by a subset of CD4$^+$ T cells. ACh directly downregulates macrophage production of proinflammatory cytokines. The neuroendocrine axis also acts through hypothalamic–pituitary intermediaries to increase corticosteroid production. The net effect of both ACh and cortisol secretion is to reduce inflammation.

Regulatory Cells

T-cell interactions with antigen-presenting cells (APCs; see Chapter 4) involve complex recognition processes, triggered by cell membrane molecules on each. In sepsis, these interactions are skewed, so that T regulatory cells (T$_{reg}$s, CD4$^+$/CD25$^+$) are activated. T$_{reg}$s act to dampen T-cell–mediated immune responses. Suppressor cells from other sources, such as bone marrow–derived suppressor cells (see Chapter 5), are also recruited and activated.

The Role of Apoptosis

An important feature of the pathogenesis of sepsis is the contribution of apoptosis to continued infection and the body's ongoing inability to handle it. This dysfunction of the programmed cell death (PCD) mechanism (see Chapter 1) has two features: excessive death among cell populations and insufficient elimination of others.

Excessive apoptosis occurs among lymphocytes and dendritic cells. Thus, in sepsis, both B lymphocytes and certain T-cell subsets are lost to PCD at a high rate. This is most pronounced among CD4$^+$ T lymphocytes, but CD8$^+$ T cells may also be affected. Certain populations of APCs, particularly interdigitating and follicular dendritic cells, undergo excessive PCD as well. Other types of macrophages are unaffected, or less dramatically impaired. Resulting decreases in total circulating lymphocyte counts (lymphopenia) impair immune responsiveness and are characteristic of people with sepsis. Lymphocyte apoptosis has been shown to be present in such patients. Apoptotic lymphocytes are found in the peripheral blood, bone marrow, spleen and even lymphoid aggregates such as the Peyer patches in the intestinal tract.

Circulating monocytes from patients with sepsis typically express less immune-stimulatory molecules on their cell membranes. However, monocytes expressing immunomodulatory molecules are not generally decreased. As a consequence of these diverse contributors, cells from patients with sepsis show impaired responsiveness to antigen stimulation.

Apoptosis of gastrointestinal epithelium also contributes to propagation of sepsis. Gut epithelial cells are lost to both PCD and ischemic necrosis as a result of circulatory impairment (see below). Intercellular tight junctions are loosened. Consequently, the epithelial barrier to gut flora becomes more porous. Bacteria from the gastrointestinal (GI) tract then enter the submucosal lymphoid tissue and then the general circulation, where they perpetuate the cycle of infection and inflammation.

Neutrophils are among the first line of antimicrobial defense (see Chapter 2). They are also programmed to undergo rapid PCD, the result being that the acute arm of the inflammatory response is, at least in part, self-limited by the cell death program of neutrophils. Altered apoptosis involving neutrophils also contributes to sepsis, but the alteration in cell death is in the opposite direction from that seen with lymphocytes and mononuclear phagocytes: PCD of polymorphonuclear leukocytes is markedly decreased. Impaired neutrophil apoptosis prolongs the acute inflammatory response, increases the release of degradative enzymes by these longer-lived neutrophils and so magnifies tissue injury.

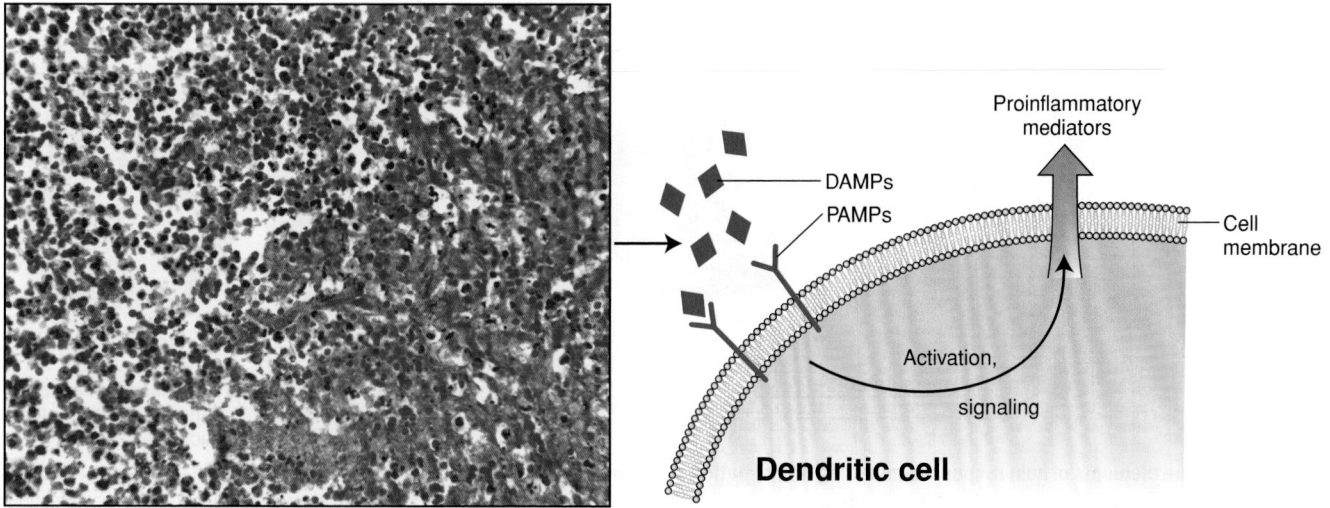

FIGURE 12-6. Tissue necrosis stimulates inflammation. Necrotic tissues, whether due to infections or other causes, release patterned molecules called damage-associated molecular patterns, or alarmins. These are similar to pathogen-associated molecular patterns (PAMPs) and bind to pattern recognition receptors (PRRs), in turn activating dendritic cells to release proinflammatory cytokines.

Alarmins and the Tissue Damage Response

Endogenous molecules released by damaged tissues also stimulate inflammatory responses. These molecules are DAMPs, also called alarmins. They are recognized by pattern recognition receptors similar to those that recognize PAMPs. Alarmins comprise nuclear, cytoplasmic and other cellular materials that are released by cells undergoing non-apoptotic cell death. Some types of cells may even produce and secrete alarmins despite the fact that they may not be dead or dying.

Alarmins bind specific receptors on innate immune system cells, such as dendritic cells, to activate innate immunity, inflammation (Fig. 12-6) and, subsequently, adoptive immunity. These pattern recognition receptors include TLRs as well as others. Alarmins may also engage and activate the IL-1 receptor.

As they are tissue derived, and not microbial in origin, alarmins signal tissue injury, not infection. They can trigger innate immune and inflammatory responses in settings of tissue death that occur in the absence of infectious agents, such as wounds or blunt trauma. They therefore represent the link between the pathogenesis of MODS in sepsis and MODS that occurs in settings that do not involve infection.

The Balance Between Pro- and Anti-Inflammatory Activities Helps to Determine the Course of Sepsis

Teleologically, proinflammatory influences protect the host against invading pathogens, and anti-inflammatory circuits should protect the host from potentially injurious overly exuberant inflammatory activity. In sepsis, however, it does not always work this way. Proinflammatory influences, for reasons that are still being studied, overwhelm counterregulatory braking mechanisms and engage in inflammatory excesses, which lead to tissue necrosis beyond what is elicited by pathogens or necessary to contain the infection.

Anti-inflammatory influences in sepsis may finally supervene, but when they do, they are too much and too late. That is, the net effect of anti-inflammatory activities is not so much to rein in inflammation that can damage tissues but rather to suppress immune responses and render the host susceptible to subsequent secondary or other infections (Fig. 12-7). In so doing, they magnify the impact of the initial infection and

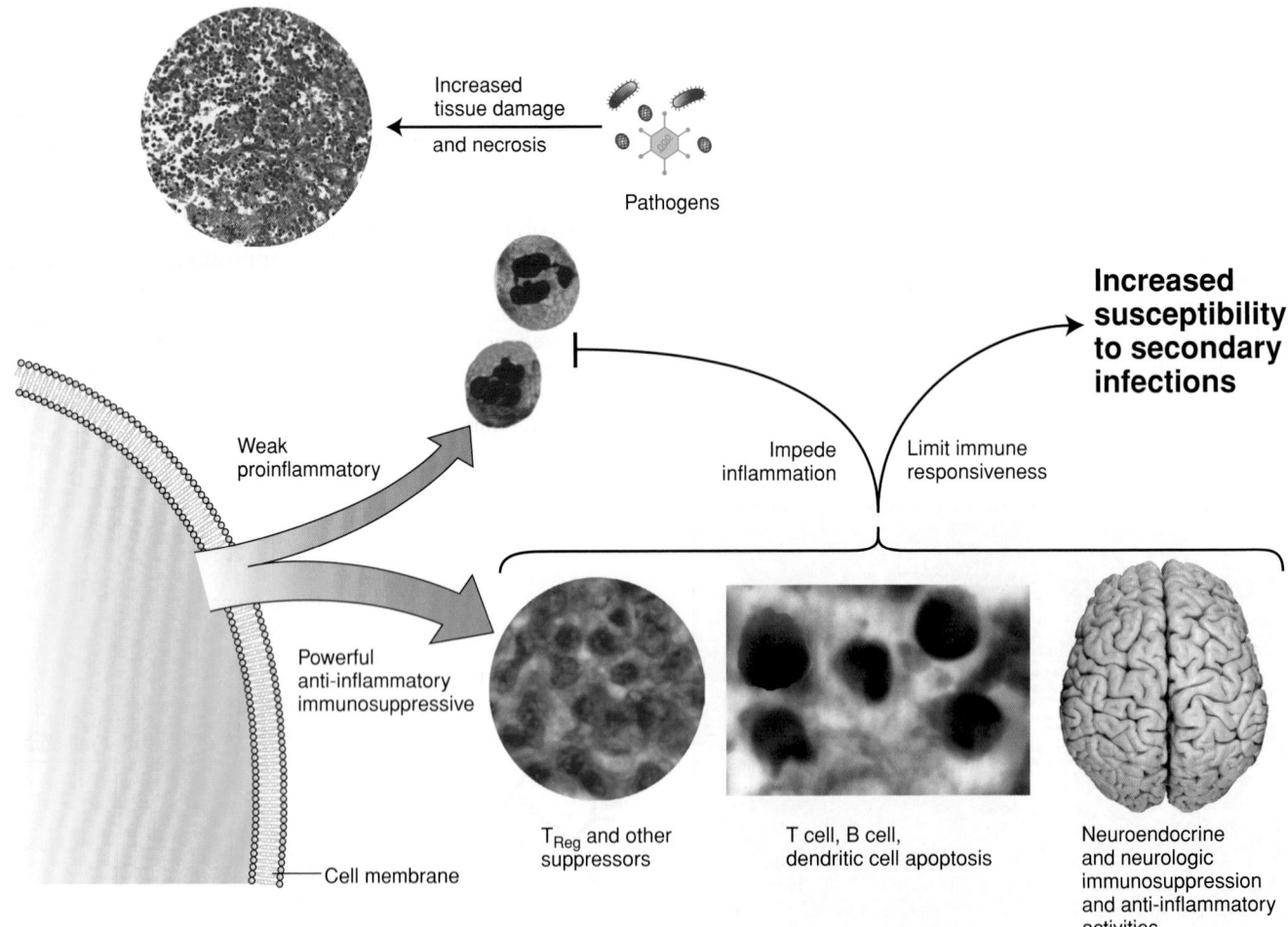

FIGURE 12-7. The elements of host responses impeding inflammation and immune responsiveness during sepsis. The same dendritic cell responses described in Fig. 12-5 may be balanced differently, either because of genetics, environment and so forth or as a function of timing following the initial infectious stimulus. In this setting, anti-inflammatory elements (*lower*) may predominate over proinflammatory agents (*upper*). Depending on when such anti-inflammatory responses predominate during sepsis, they may impair immune responsiveness and limit inflammatory responses to secondarily invading pathogens. This may magnify the tissue damage that was initially due to exaggerated proinflammatory responses.

simultaneously have the exact opposite of their seemingly intended purpose: they lead to more inflammation.

Circulation and Coagulation Are Abnormal in Sepsis

Disseminated intravascular coagulation (DIC) and dysfunctional patterns of circulation are characteristic of sepsis. PAMPs trigger expression of tissue factor (TF) by endothelial and other cells, particularly monocytes. TF activates the coagulation cascade (see Chapter 16) via factor VII. This leads to intravascular microthrombus formation. Pathogen-activated neutrophils release neutrophil extracellular traps (NETs; see Chapter 1), which also precipitate coagulation (Fig. 12-8).

Under normal circumstances, clot formation activates fibrinolytic pathways, which should limit the extent of clotting. However, in sepsis, mediators of fibrinolysis (tissue factor inhibitor, antithrombin, plasminogen activator and others) are impaired or inhibited. As a result, unimpeded formation of intravascular thrombi (DIC) limits blood flow and hence hampers adequate oxygen delivery to organs.

Simultaneously, additional factors magnify this vascular insufficiency. The ability of endothelial cells themselves to limit blood coagulation is impaired. Provoked by large amounts of thrombin (and freed of restraint normally exercised by protein C, which is decreased in sepsis), protease activated receptors (PARs) on endothelial cells downregulate endothelial anticoagulant activities.

At the same time, endothelial cells activate inducible nitric oxide synthase (iNOS). NO stimulates vasodilation,

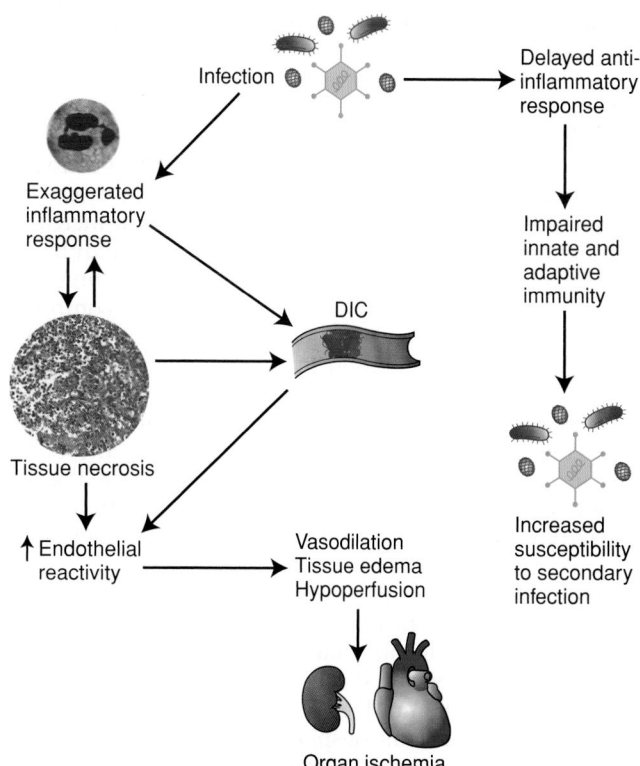

FIGURE 12-9. Sequence of events in many cases of sepsis. Following an infection as the initiating event, an exaggerated inflammatory response leads to excessive tissue necrosis (which, in turn, increases inflammation). Tissue necrosis and inflammation cause disseminated intravascular coagulation (DIC). Endothelial cell hyperreactivity results from all three of these stimuli and, together with DIC, provokes vasodilation and tissue edema and leads to hypoperfusion of tissues. This, in turn, causes organ dysfunction and failure. In parallel, delayed anti-inflammatory activities impair immune responses and render the patient more susceptible to secondary infection.

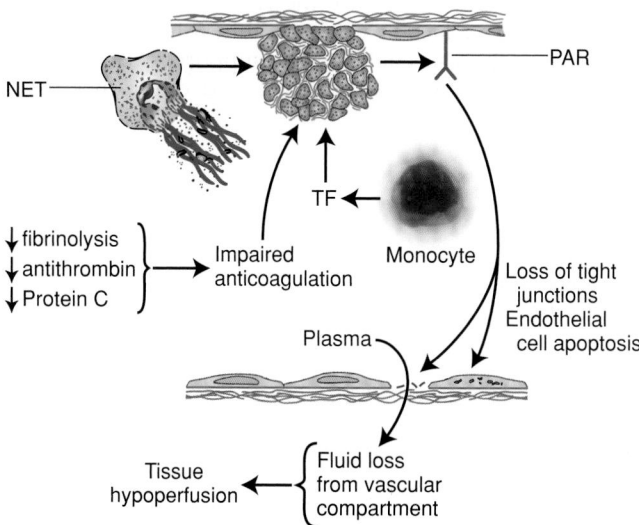

FIGURE 12-8. Pathogenesis of disseminated intravascular coagulation (DIC) and vascular insufficiency in sepsis. Several factors contribute to the development of DIC in patients with sepsis. These include the release of extracellular nets by neutrophils, trapping the microbial pathogens, and the production of tissue factor (TF) by activated monocytes and endothelial cells. TF both sets clotting in motion and inhibits fibrinolysis, the end result being excessive intravascular coagulation. At the same time, excessive thrombin activation in DIC triggers protease activated receptors (PARs) on endothelial cells. Endothelium undergoes apoptosis and intercellular tight junctions loosen, leading to vasodilation and fluid leakage from the circulation into extravascular spaces. Activated endothelial cells produce nitric oxide (NO), which causes vasodilation and vascular leakiness. Impaired red blood cell deformability adds to these factors to decrease the effectiveness of oxygen delivery to tissues.

increases vascular permeability and causes leakage of plasma from the vascular system into tissue spaces. In the setting of DIC (see Chapters 7 and 16), sepsis-related impairments in erythrocyte deformability further limit oxygenation of organs and peripheral tissues.

Mechanistically, then, these diverse dysfunctions play into each other to increase the severity of the resulting pathophysiology. Invading pathogens, in the context of host and environmental factors that limit host modulatory activities, trigger excessively exuberant inflammatory responses and DIC, both of which lead to a cycle of tissue death, circulatory insufficiency and poor oxygen delivery to tissues. When anti-inflammatory activities start to participate in the process, they make matters worse because their net effect is to limit the ability of the adaptive immune system to respond to invading pathogens. Anti-inflammatory regulators therefore set the stage for subsequent secondary infection with additional pathogens (Fig. 12-9).

PHYSIOLOGIC RESPONSES TO SIRS/SEPSIS

The patient's response to inflammation and systemic infection depends on the severity of the condition, ranging from SIRS to sepsis to severe sepsis to septic shock to MODS.

Physiologic alterations vary, depending on where an individual falls in that spectrum. The SIRS response includes the clinical signs of tachycardia, tachypnea and hyperthermia or hypothermia.

Tachycardia is an important compensatory mechanism to maintain adequate perfusion in order to offset intravascular volume loss, vasodilation and diminished cardiac contractility. Tachypnea in sepsis may be due to increased stimulation of the respiratory center in the medulla by inflammatory mediators or be a response to counterbalance metabolic acidosis. Body temperature is controlled by the hypothalamus, which may readjust to a higher set point owing to an alteration in heat equilibrium, leading to hyperthermia in sepsis. Rigors may also be present with fever as skeletal muscle contractions generate additional heat. However, some individuals do not show any of the typical signs of sepsis. Development of hypothermia occurs more frequently in patients who die from sepsis than those who survive. It is associated with other adverse effects, such as surgical wound infections.

Severe sepsis arises in the presence of hypoperfusion or organ dysfunction, which may appear physiologically as an acute alteration in mental status or oliguria. In the course of development of septic shock, hypotension (systolic blood pressure [SBP] < 90 mm Hg or a decrease of more than 40 mm Hg in SBP) occurs despite adequate fluid resuscitation, resulting in perfusion abnormalities. These individual clinical signs are not specific for sepsis and may develop in other settings. In contrast, classic indicators of systemic inflammation may be absent in severe sepsis, particularly in higher-risk patient populations such as elderly and immunosuppressed patients.

Virtually every organ in the body is susceptible to impairment during septic responses, and MODS is a particularly life-threatening complication of sepsis. The renal, pulmonary, hepatic, endocrine, cardiovascular and central nervous systems frequently sustain injury in septic patients (Fig. 12-10). Primary organ damage is difficult to distinguish from injury that results from inadequate perfusion caused by cardiovascular insufficiency. Frequent physiologic and laboratory measurements are necessary to monitor end-organ function and direct supportive interventions.

 PATHOLOGY: Laboratory pathology plays a central role in evaluating patients with possible sepsis and in following both their clinical course and the effectiveness of treatment (see below).

LABORATORY ABNORMALITIES IN SIRS/SEPSIS. One of the SIRS criteria is leukocytosis (white blood cell [WBC] count >12,000/mm^3), leukopenia (WBC count <4,000/mm^3) or greater than 10% bands. In a study of patients with gram-negative sepsis, leukopenia was more frequently seen among nonsurvivors of sepsis than among survivors, identifying it as a finding often related to more severe disease in sepsis. To facilitate the diagnosis and management of the septic patient, cultures should be obtained from all potentially infected sites including but not limited to blood, urine, sputum and indwelling catheters. Patients with positive cultures should receive appropriate antimicrobial therapy; however, a definitive site of infection may not be identified in a subset of patients and empiric broad-spectrum coverage is indicated for suspected infection.

Clinical measurements of poor perfusion in severe sepsis and septic shock include lactic acidosis, base deficit and decreased mixed central venous oxyhemoglobin saturation (ScvO$_2$). Significantly elevated lactate levels, greater than or equal to 4 mmol/L, increase the risk of mortality. Prompt normalization of lactate values within 6 hours of presentation through resuscitation and supportive care reflects resolution of global tissue hypoxia and diminishes organ

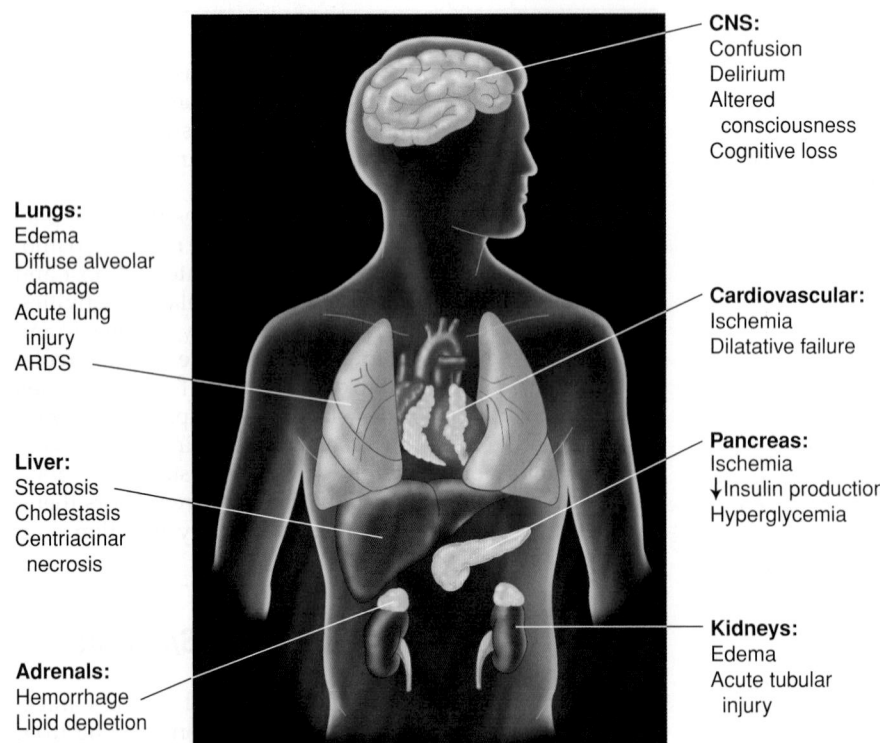

Lungs:
Edema
Diffuse alveolar
 damage
Acute lung
 injury
ARDS

Liver:
Steatosis
Cholestasis
Centriacinar
 necrosis

Adrenals:
Hemorrhage
Lipid depletion

CNS:
Confusion
Delirium
Altered
 consciousness
Cognitive loss

Cardiovascular:
Ischemia
Dilatative failure

Pancreas:
Ischemia
↓Insulin production
Hyperglycemia

Kidneys:
Edema
Acute tubular
 injury

FIGURE 12-10. End-organ damage in septic patients. Individual organ or multisystem organ failure may occur during the human response to sepsis.

dysfunction and mortality in sepsis. Improved mortality is also associated with rapidly achieving $ScvO_2$ greater than 70% to enhance tissue oxygenation.

Septic patients develop a range of coagulation abnormalities, from mildly prolonged bleeding time and thrombocytopenia to life-threatening DIC. Proinflammatory cytokine production upregulates TF (see above), suppresses antithrombin, interferes with protein C anticoagulation activity and impedes fibrinolysis. Systemic intravascular microthrombi occur and may lead to tissue ischemia, necrosis or MODS. Platelets and coagulation factors are consumed while activation of fibrinolysis contributes, leading to failed hemostasis. Elevations in bleeding time and impaired clotting are common. The latter is measured by international normalized ratio (INR, which is a value calculated from the ratio of a patient's prothrombin time to a normal prothrombin time) and partial thromboplastin time (PTT). Platelet levels and fibrinogen may also be decreased.

End-organ damage in sepsis also leads to laboratory abnormalities depending on which organs are involved. Kidney injury increases serum creatinine and may also alter blood electrolyte levels. Hepatic damage may lead to elevated transaminases, severe hypoglycemia and reduced synthesis of coagulation factors. The latter may further impair hemostasis that may already be problematic as a result of DIC. Decreased partial pressure of oxygen in the arterial blood (PaO_2) results from lung dysfunction. Impaired adrenal function in sepsis can markedly decrease blood cortisol levels, which may lead to hypotension in septic shock.

BIOMARKERS. Biomarker identification in sepsis is helpful to diagnose the condition better, detect which patients may benefit from immunomodulatory therapies and predict outcomes. C-reactive protein (CRP) is a well-known marker of inflammation, but it is not sufficiently specific to discriminate septic patients from those with noninfectious SIRS. Multiple cytokines such as IL-6 and TNF-α lack adequate prognostic value to be useful markers in sepsis.

Other potential biomarkers, particularly procalcitonin (PCT), have potential utility in diagnosis. PCT is made in the lungs and intestines in the context of bacterial infection. Normally, it is not detectable in the circulation, but high circulating PCT levels in septic patients help to identify sepsis. It does not generally become elevated in nonbacterial infections, so PCT is a useful clinical adjunct to help determine if infection is present in a critically ill patient who develops a new fever. Its measurement also appears to have a role in antibiotic management. Implementing a PCT-based algorithm to guide antimicrobial therapy has reduced days of antibiotic exposure and costs in septic patients.

CLINICAL FEATURES:

ORGAN SYSTEM MANIFESTATIONS OF SEPSIS.
Clearly, the clinical presentation of sepsis depends in part on the anatomic location(s) of the precipitating infection. However, some clinical features tend to be consistent regardless of the source of the infection. Respiratory compromise and cardiovascular dysfunction are most common. Pulmonary failure in the form of acute respiratory distress syndrome (ARDS; see Chapter 18), with impaired blood oxygenation and pulmonary infiltrates, is common. Circulatory insufficiency entails prolonged low blood pressure, which contributes to poor oxygen delivery to peripheral tissues, despite compensatory tachycardia.

Consequently, many other organ systems experience dysfunction relating to the effects of poor perfusion and inadequate oxygen delivery. Almost any organ system may be affected. Renal function often declines, as evidenced by oliguria (low urine output) and rising serum creatinine levels. Both central and peripheral nervous systems may evidence dysfunction: decreased cognition, impaired mental status and both myopathies and neuropathies. Sepsis has a substantial impact on endocrine homeostasis, as glycemic control and thyroid function are both compromised. Gut motility and liver function may decline.

CURRENT TREATMENT OF SEPSIS. Severe sepsis is a medical emergency and the first priority is to evaluate and maintain the "A, B, Cs:" airway, breathing and circulation. Mechanical ventilation may be needed to provide respiratory support for increased work of breathing or airway protection in septic patients. Blood pressure is assessed frequently to detect signs of hypoperfusion. Subsequent management continues after initial stabilization and evaluation of the septic patient.

Early goal-directed therapy (EGDT), antibiotics and source control of infection are effective in the management of human sepsis, but no targeted sepsis therapy exists; despite decades of intense research, treatment remains primarily supportive. EGDT is a valuable algorithm for initiating early, aggressive end-point–driven resuscitation, and it has been proven to improve survival in severe sepsis and septic shock. EGDT has been adapted into the Surviving Sepsis clinical practice guidelines, last revised in 2012. The international recommendations seek to minimize barotrauma from mechanical ventilation, maintain organ perfusion, control infection and reduce hyperglycemia. Additionally, corticosteroids may be useful if a patient's hemodynamic status does not stabilize with fluid resuscitation and vasopressors.

Hyperglycemia occurs with many nosocomial infections and correlates with decreased survival in sepsis. However, optimal blood glucose levels in sepsis remain controversial. Hypoglycemia is also detrimental and entails increased mortality. The Surviving Sepsis 2012 guidelines currently recommend maintaining glucose less than 180 mg/dL.

Multiple unsuccessful drug trials in sepsis underscore the difficulty in developing new therapies for patients. For many years, research efforts were focused on using anti-inflammatory agents to suppress hosts' robust inflammatory responses. These efforts have not borne fruit. The complex, simultaneous abnormalities of multiple pathways that likely drive sepsis present a significant challenge to developing efficacious therapeutics. Given the variability in the human response to sepsis, treatment targeted at specific patient populations or particular infectious sources may prove more successful than previous investigational therapies. Currently, no pharmacologic agent is approved in the United States for treatment of sepsis, and morbidity and mortality remain high.

SEPSIS

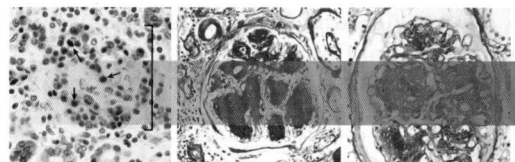

Obesity and Diabetes Mellitus

Kevin Jon Williams ▪ Elias S. Siraj

Obesity

Only three decades ago, obesity was relatively uncommon, but its prevalence has been increasing rapidly. Astonishingly, on a global scale, 1 billion adults might be classified as overweight, and at least 400 million meet established criteria for obesity. One third of American adults are overweight and 1/3 are obese. Although overall prevalence of obesity in the United States may be leveling off, extreme obesity continues to increase. That is, individuals already in the obese category are growing heavier. In the developed world, obesity is more common among women and the poor, while in developing countries, it affects primarily the well-to-do. The explosion in obesity rates indicates that the fundamental problem is a recent change in environment, not genetics. It is especially worrisome that at least one in seven children in the United States is obese; a recent longitudinal study showed that childhood obesity more than doubles the risk of death from endogenous causes before the age of 55 years.

Chronic, Positive Caloric Imbalances Cause Obesity, but Underlying Factors Are Complex

Obesity is rooted in complex interactions of genetic, metabolic, physiologic, social, behavioral, technologic, governmental and commercial influences that lead to overnutrition and underexertion. The imbalance in energy intake and expenditure may be quite small: just 35 kcal/day—merely 1% of the typical flux of 3500 kcal/day in the developed world—becomes a weight gain of 14 kg (~30 lbs) of adiposity in a decade. For comparison, there are 300 kcal in two cans of regular soda or three 8-ounce servings of fruit juice. Thus, a child who consumes high-calorie snacks on the way to and from school substantially increases his risk for obesity, if there are no compensatory changes in intake or expenditure.

As another way to illustrate the precision of energy balance required to defend body weight and adiposity over the long run, consider that we consume and expend roughly 10^6 kcal per year. Proportionately small cumulative errors on this scale add up quickly. Severe clinical obesity may rarely entail monogenic causes that impair satiety (see below), but most cases result from the combined effects of lifestyle and other environmental factors, superimposed on several traits that are partially heritable.

In the past, eating was a highly social and cultural endeavor, and vigorous physical activity was necessary for typical daily life. Several factors associated with rising rates of obesity disrupt long-standing patterns of dining and movement. Altered eating habits include rising consumption of sugar, particularly sugary beverages; replacement of regular, social meals with unscheduled snacking; agricultural and other subsidies that lower the cost of carbohydrate calories; and the growth of a sophisticated industry for manufacturing processed foods that are savory and calorically dense. Simultaneously, physical activity has declined because of labor-saving devices, such as washing machines and private cars; television and other electronic entertainment; and jobs that have become more sedentary. These factors, alone and in moderation, may be highly desirable (e.g., the availability of enough food to sustain a world population of 7 billion people). Yet in combination and in excess, these factors help disrupt the normal physiologic mechanisms that balance body weight and adiposity. The result is chronic positive caloric imbalance and hence the global growth of obesity.

ENERGY INTAKE AND EXPENDITURE

Weight increases when energy intake exceeds expenditure; you are what you eat, minus what you burn. The normal human gastrointestinal (GI) tract absorbs essentially all simple fuels that enter it. Many behaviors related to caloric intake and expenditure have a significant inherited component. For example, offspring of mothers with high prepregnancy body weights tend to eat in the absence of hunger (EAH) and to seek foods of high energy density (kcal/g).

Total daily energy expenditure (TDEE) consists of several regulated components:

1. **Basal metabolic rate (BMR):** BMR is the energy expended at complete rest, lying down, in the postabsorptive state. It includes maintenance levels of breathing, circulation of blood and essential metabolic functions. For people with sedentary occupations, BMR accounts for ~60% of TDEE. Over 75% of interindividual variation in BMR reflects differences in lean body mass.
2. **Calories spent to digest, absorb and store ingested calories** (6%–12% of TDEE).
3. **Energetic costs of emotion, medication and adaptive thermogenesis owing to the environment** (e.g., changes in temperature, exposure to infectious agents).
4. **Activity thermogenesis** generated by physical movement during purposeful exercise and nonexercise activity thermogenesis (NEAT). Purposeful exercise is a key element of successful weight loss programs. Except for high-level athletes, most people burn relatively few calories during purposeful exercise, but without compensatory increases in intake, even small shifts in overall energy balance add up. Levels of NEAT may vary substantially among apparently normal individuals, by up to 2000 calories/day, and lower NEAT correlates strongly with obesity. Obese people in sedentary occupations sit 2.5 hours more each day than their comparable lean counterparts. The cumulative impact of such inactivity on energy balance over the years can be substantial.

The Brain Is the Central Controller of Body Weight

The brain receives hormonal and neuronal signals about food deficits or surpluses and the rate of fuel utilization. To maintain homeostasis, it then coordinates responses, modulating behavior and the endocrine and autonomic nervous systems to adjust energy balance.

The **hypothalamus** is the main processor of signals from the periphery and is crucial to managing energy balance. Many hypothalamic nuclei regulate metabolism, but the arcuate nucleus plays a central role via two distinct populations of neurons, which generate opposing actions on food intake. One group makes **anorexigenic** (appetite-suppressing) peptides, including proopiomelanocortin (POMC) and cocaine- and amphetamine-regulated transcripts (CARTs). POMC is cleaved into α-melanocyte–stimulating hormone (α-MSH), which binds melanocortin receptors MC3R and MC4R to decrease appetite.

The other population of neurons produces two **orexigenic** (appetite-stimulating) neuropeptides: **neuropeptide Y** (NPY) and **agouti-related protein** (AgRP). NPY is among the most abundant neuropeptides in the mammalian brain and strongly stimulates feeding. It may bind any of six G-protein–coupled NPY receptor subtypes (Y1 through Y6), but Y1 and Y2 NPY receptors stimulate feeding most. AgRP antagonizes melanocortin receptors, thus blocking α-MSH anorexigenic effects and stimulating food intake.

The GI Tract, Adipocytes and Other Tissues Produce Hormones That Contribute to Regulation of Hunger and Satiety

Key systemic soluble mediators of these responses include:

- **Leptin:** The discovery of **leptin** revealed a key link between neural and nonneural systems in the control of appetite and energy expenditure. Leptin (from the Greek, "thin") is the protein product of the *LEP* gene, known historically as the *Ob* gene. It is produced mainly by adipocytes. Its serum concentration is proportional to body fat mass (i.e., it is lower in lean people and rises with obesity). Its chief physiologic role appears to be signaling to the brain that body adipose stores are sufficient. Low serum leptin levels increase appetite and decrease energy expenditure, in part by dampening the thyroidal axis. This effect impedes weight loss during caloric restriction. By contrast, normal leptin levels decrease appetite.

  In the brain, leptin interacts with leptin receptors on POMC/CART and NPY/AgRP neurons, regulating them in opposite ways. It directly activates anorexigenic POMC/CART neurons while blocking the activity of orexigenic NPY/AgRP neurons. The result is decreased food intake. Blood leptin levels are above normal in most obese people, but unfortunately, this increased leptin fails to suppress appetite and halt excessive fat accumulation. There is evidence to support several explanations, including an inability of leptin to reach its neuronal targets, a failure of intracellular signaling by the leptin receptor despite occupancy with leptin (desensitization) and psychological cues to overeat that overwhelm physiologic restraints. Leptin injections to treat obesity have to date not been successful.
- **Circadian rhythms** affect, and are affected by, caloric flux. Mice with genetic disruption of the circadian system develop obesity, hyperleptinemia, hyperlipidemia and hyperglycemia. In humans, shift workers, who must alter their sleep rhythms, exhibit increased prevalence of high body mass indices (BMIs), metabolic syndrome (see below) and cardiovascular events. Forced sleep restriction in humans disturbs appetite control and glucose tolerance. This effect is of particular concern, given the disturbances in sleep caused by obstructive apnea in people who are already obese.
- **Endocannabinoids** are endogenous lipids that bind to cannabinoid receptors 1 and 2 (CB1 and CB2). CB1 receptors are found in hypothalamic nuclei involved in control of energy balance and weight. They are also present in adipose tissue and the GI tract. Activated CB1 receptor stimulates food intake and may play a role in the development and maintenance of obesity. Rimonabant, a synthetic blocker of the CB1 receptor, suppresses appetite, decreases weight and improves metabolic parameters in obese subjects, but a major side effect of depression has stopped its use in the treatment of obesity.
- **The GI tract** contains a diverse group of mechanoreceptors and chemosensitive receptors that relay information via vagal afferent fibers that terminate in the nucleus tractus solitarii in the brainstem. For example, vagal activation due to gastric distension causes satiety and meal termination. Taste receptors for bitter, sweet and umami (savory flavor imparted by glutamate and nucleotides)

have been found in regions besides the tongue, particularly the stomach, small intestine and pancreas, where they may act as nutrient sensors and affect appetite and insulin release. As well, several hormones produced by the GI tract signal the central nervous system (CNS) to regulate energy intake. **Glucagon-like peptide 1** (GLP-1) is made by posttranslational processing of proglucagon by L cells located primarily in the mucosa of the distal ileum and colon. GLP-1 decreases food intake, slows gastric emptying, generates a feeling of satiety, augments postprandial glucose-stimulated insulin secretion and decreases secretion of glucagon, a hormone that opposes insulin action (see Chapter 27). These combined effects reduce the rate of caloric delivery to the intestines, and hence to the rest of the body, while enhancing insulin secretion and action. Long-acting GLP-1 analogs (exenatide and liraglutide) are used to treat type 2 diabetes mellitus and to induce weight reduction.

- **Ghrelin** is a hormone that stimulates hunger. It is produced primarily by endocrine cells in the stomach and, to a lesser extent, in the duodenum, ileum and colon. Ghrelin stimulates orexigenic NPY neurons in the arcuate nucleus of the hypothalamus. Circulating ghrelin levels increase during fasting, and its administration to normal subjects increases caloric intake. Patients with anorexia nervosa have high plasma concentrations of ghrelin; however, administration of exogenous ghrelin to treat this condition has not been successful. Plasma ghrelin declines after gastric bypass surgery, which may facilitate continued weight loss after the procedure. Patients with hyperphagia in Prader-Willi syndrome have very high plasma ghrelin levels. Moreover, serum ghrelin increases after diet-induced weight loss, which may contribute to poor long-term results of clinical weight loss programs.

- **Cholecystokinin (CCK)** is made mainly in duodenal and jejunal mucosa. It is released after fat and protein intake and acts on two distinct receptors. CCK stimulates release of enzymes from the pancreas and gallbladder to aid digestion, slows gastric emptying and reduces food intake. Regulation of food intake is mediated via vagal afferent signals to the brain.

- **Peptide YY** (PYY) is secreted along the entire GI tract, but mostly in the ileum and colon. Of its two forms, PYY(3-36) is the major circulating type. It is released in response to food intake, and its many actions include delaying pancreatic and gastric secretions, gallbladder emptying and gastric emptying. PYY(3-36) decreases appetite, duration of eating and total caloric intake.

- **Pancreatic polypeptide** (PP) is in the same peptide family as PYY. Although it is primarily produced in the pancreas, it is also found in the colon and rectum. The main stimulus to its release is food intake; PP reduces appetite and food intake.

- **Amylin** is a peptide mainly produced by pancreatic beta cells, but also found in gut endocrine cells, visceral sensory neurons and the hypothalamus. It is a potent inhibitor of gastric emptying and decreases food intake. An analog of amylin, pramlintide, is currently used to treat diabetes mellitus. It is associated with weight reduction in these patients and is in clinical trials for obesity.

- **Insulin** is best known for its role in peripheral glucose uptake, but it also affects appetite. Injection of insulin into the third cerebral ventricle of rats decreases food intake via insulin receptors in the arcuate nucleus of the hypothalamus, where it increases messenger RNA (mRNA) for POMC (anorexigenic) and suppresses mRNA for NPY (orexigenic). Clinically, however, insulin is administered peripherally and often increases appetite, which can cause already overweight patients to eat more. Part of the explanation may be hypoglycemia.

- **Other substances** regulate hunger, satiety, fat deposition and so forth in rodents, including galanin, adipocyte complement-related protein (ACRP), peroxisome proliferator-associated receptors (PPARs) and others.

- **Gut flora** affect body weight. Germ-free mice are protected from diet-induced obesity. Colonization of these mice with intestinal flora from conventionally raised mice enhances caloric uptake from complex dietary plant polysaccharides. These flora also modulate expression of specific host genes to increase caloric storage in adipose tissue. Distal gut flora from obese people contain different microbes from the flora of lean individuals. Gut bacteria from obese individuals may extract calories from complex components of the diet more efficiently than microbiota from their lean counterparts. Nevertheless, modern foods of high-caloric density contain mostly simple carbohydrates and oils, which are readily absorbed without microbial assistance. Regulatory effects on the host from variations in gut flora are still likely to be important, and gut flora "transplants" from lean to obese subjects have been proposed.

Known orexigenic and anorexigenic factors are illustrated in Fig. 13-1.

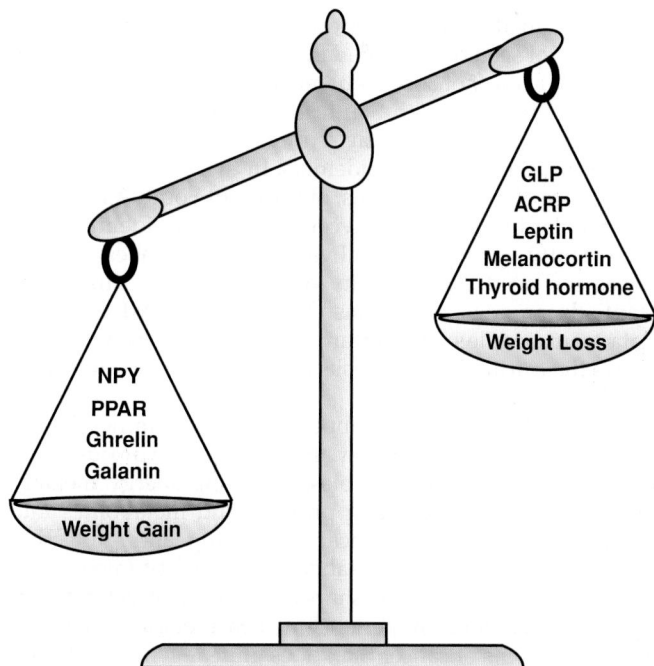

FIGURE 13-1. The balance of chemical mediators that promote fat accumulation (weight gain) and those that promote fat loss (weight loss). *ACRP* = adipocyte complement-related protein; *GLP* = glucagon-like peptide; *NPY* = neuropeptide Y; *PPAR* = peroxisome proliferator-activated receptor.

BODY MASS INDEX AND OBESITY

The standard most often used to define obesity is the BMI:

$$BMI = [weight (kg)] \div [height (m)]^2$$

Although BMI is an excellent indicator of obesity, it does not formally distinguish between fat mass and lean mass. A short, muscular person with little body fat may be misclassified as obese by BMI, while a person with excess adipose tissue and reduced muscle mass, such as an elderly or chronically ill individual, could have a normal BMI. There may also be ethnic variations in the amounts of adipose tissue, particularly visceral–abdominal adipose tissue, at a given BMI.

Obesity, Morbidity and Mortality in Multiethnic Populations

Most health organizations define overweight as a BMI between 25 and 29.9 kg/m². A BMI over 30 defines obesity, 30–35 class I obesity, 35–40 class II obesity and a BMI exceeding 40 extreme (class III) obesity. A high BMI correlates with excess morbidity, largely due to specific metabolic abnormalities like dyslipoproteinemia, hypertension, impaired regulation of plasma glucose concentrations, hypercoagulability and the risk of developing type 2 diabetes. A BMI above 35 (class II and class III obesity) is consistently associated with excess all-cause mortality, but BMIs of 25–30 (overweight) or 30–35 (class I obesity) are not. The correlation between obesity and mortality in Western countries has weakened over time, perhaps because of better treatments for cardiovascular risk factors and improved public health measures.

Various populations differ in susceptibility to metabolic abnormalities at similar BMIs. A multiethnic cross-sectional study in Canada found that the same degree of impaired glucose control seen on average in people of European descent with a BMI cutoff of 30—the barely obese—occurred at BMIs of only 21 in those with South Asian ancestry, 20.6 in Chinese people and 21.8 in Native Americans. Similar data were seen with respect to dyslipidemias. In this study, and in the experience of many clinicians, overweight South Asians face a particular burden of dysglycemia and dyslipidemia. Most importantly, appropriate BMI values to define obesity—and hence the need and intensity of intervention—differ substantially among populations. Thus, use of BMI based on data from people of European descent probably underestimates the cardiometabolic risks associated with weight gain in other ethnic groups.

Regional body fat distribution also determines health risks associated with obesity. Fat depots in various parts of the body play different roles, including energy metabolism, secretion of circulating proteins and metabolites into the bloodstream and physical cushioning and protection of internal organs. Visceral–abdominal obesity (also called central adiposity or "apple shaped") carries a greater risk of dyslipoproteinemia, hypertension, heart disease, diabetes and some forms of cancer than does gluteal–femoral obesity (lower-body obesity or "pear shaped"; Fig. 13-2).

BMI does not account for fat distribution, so abdominal obesity is better assessed by measuring waist circumference or the waist:hip ratio. Waist circumference above 102 cm (40 inches) and waist:hip ratio over 0.9 in men are associated with adverse outcomes. The same holds true for women

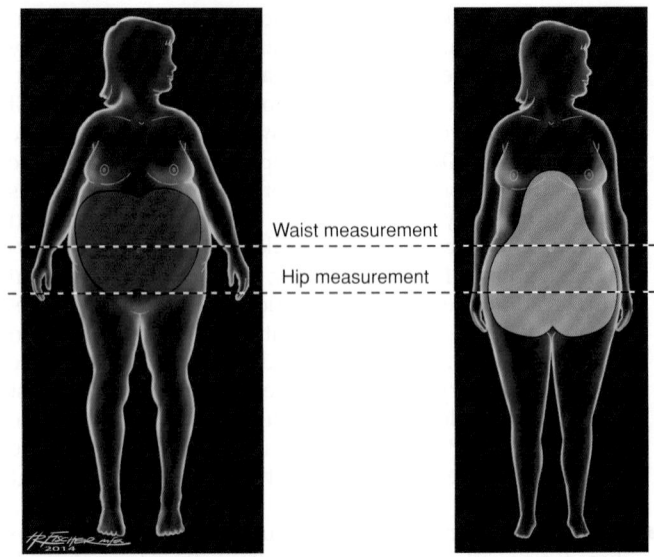

FIGURE 13-2. Regional adipose distribution and cardiometabolic risk. Individuals who accumulate adipose tissue in the abdomen ("apple shaped") exhibit increased risk of insulin resistance for glucose, type 2 diabetes mellitus and cardiovascular disease, compared to those with fat accumulations around the hips, buttocks and thighs ("pear shaped"). Standard methods to assess abdominal obesity include waist circumference and the waist:hip ratio.

with a waist circumference more than 88 cm (35 inches) or waist:hip ratio larger than 0.85. Thus, amounts of visceral fat and modifiable cardiovascular risk factors provide better guides to therapy than does BMI.

Studies of Heritable Causes and Molecular Mediators of Obesity

Nearly everyone living in developed countries is exposed to a calorie-rich, sedentary environment; yet BMIs vary considerably, from extremely thin to morbidly obese. An inherited propensity toward obesity is clear, based on comparisons of BMIs (1) between monozygotic and dizygotic twins, (2) between genetically full or half-siblings raised apart after adoption in infancy and (3) in multigenerational kindreds. These reports yield estimates of heritability for obesity ranging from 20% to 80%. Most of these studies were done on people born before the recent increase in obesity. Notably, a study of twin children growing up during the obesity epidemic found that BMI and waist circumference each showed 77% heritability. Behaviors linked to obesity all have substantial inherited components: eating in the absence of hunger, impaired responses to internal signals of satiety, exaggerated responses to external food cues, rapid eating and low levels of physical activity, including NEAT.

 MOLECULAR PATHOGENESIS: Many genetic studies have identified specific gene variants that, all together, contribute only slightly to the population-wide development of obesity:

- **Leptin gene mutations** have been linked to rare monogenic syndromes of severe obesity in humans. Homozygotes present with hyperphagia and severe, early-onset obesity. They die more readily after childhood infections and as adults develop hypothalamic hypogonadism, insulin resistance and diabetes. Heterozygotes have reduced blood levels of leptin and increased body weight compared with unaffected siblings. Replacement therapy with injections of recombinant leptin is effective.

- **Leptin receptor gene mutations** have been found in rare families with severe early-onset obesity. The phenotype is similar to that in patients with mutations in the leptin gene, except that people with receptor mutations have more elevated serum leptin levels. They also have hypogonadotropic hypogonadism, failure of pubertal development, growth delay and secondary hypothyroidism. As expected, leptin supplementation is ineffective in these individuals.
- **Melanocortin-4 receptor gene (*MC4R*) mutations,** both dominant and recessive, are the leading cause of severe, monogenic, childhood-onset obesity, accounting for 5% of such cases. Because this syndrome is rare, *MC4R* mutations have only a minor effect on population-wide prevalence of obesity. Patients tend to have no phenotype other than overeating, obesity and the well-known cardiometabolic sequelae of obesity.
- **Mutations or deficiencies in POMC/α-MSH,** prohormone convertase 1 and the hypothalamic transcription factor SIM1 may cause isolated cases of obesity.
- Genome-wide association studies have identified several genes that encode brain/hypothalamic proteins and are associated with variations in BMI. However, all specific gene polymorphisms identified to date account for under 1% of the genetic basis for obesity.
- **Epigenetic programming** during fetal or immediate postnatal life may influence adult physiology. Children born to obese mothers show high rates of obesity, but—remarkably—those born to the same woman who undergoes biliopancreatic bypass surgery and loses considerable weight before subsequent pregnancies tend not to be obese. It is not known if maternal weight loss from more widely used bariatric surgical methods, such as vertical sleeve gastrectomy or Roux-en-Y bypass, provides similar protection to children born postsurgery.

Body weight control mechanisms are believed to have evolved to protect from weight loss in times of scarcity, not obesity in times of plenty. Striking examples of environmental influence on genetic predisposition include the Pima Native Americans in Arizona and the Aboriginal population of northern Australia. Pimas are now largely sedentary and eat a diet in which 50% of energy derives from fat, unlike their traditional low-fat diets. They have experienced huge increases in obesity and diabetes. By contrast, the genetically related Pimas in the Sierra Madre Mountains of Northern Mexico are more physically active, maintain more traditional low-fat diets and have much lower rates of obesity and type 2 diabetes.

Urbanized Aboriginal people in Australia have a high prevalence of diabetes and hypertriglyceridemia, compared with their nonurbanized counterparts. As little as a 7-week reexposure of urbanized Aboriginals with diabetes and hypertriglyceridemia to traditional lifestyle—eating less and moving more—led to weight loss and improved glucose tolerance, blood glucose, insulin and triglycerides.

Regarding heritable predisposition, diabetes risk among the Pima community varies inversely with the extent of European ancestry in each. This is consistent with the 3-fold difference in disease prevalence between the two parental populations (i.e., Pima and European).

Overnutrition, Insulin Resistance and Responsiveness Syndromes

Imbalanced Insulin Action Often Follows Overnutrition and Obesity and Causes Metabolic Complications Including Type 2 Diabetes Mellitus

The **insulin receptor** is a tetrameric glycoprotein with two extracellular α-subunits that bind insulin and two transmembrane β-subunits with insulin-stimulated tyrosine kinase activity. Activation of the receptor kinase leads to tyrosine phosphorylation of several docking proteins, including **insulin receptor substrate** (IRS)-1, IRS2 and Src homologous and collagen-like protein (SHC) (Fig. 13-3). The newly phosphorylated sites on IRS1, IRS2 and SHC recruit other signal transduction kinases or adaptor proteins. These, in turn, activate downstream kinases. As a result, lipid and protein substrates are phosphorylated, leading to translocation of glucose transport proteins from the interior of the cell to the plasma membrane. This effect facilitates glucose entry, particularly into skeletal muscle and, to a lesser extent, adipocytes.

Insulin has several additional functions unrelated to importing glucose:

- Suppression of hepatic glycogenolysis and gluconeogenesis, thus inhibiting hepatic glucose production in the postprandial state.
- Induction of hepatic fatty acid and triglyceride biosynthesis (de novo lipogenesis) to export and store calories in a compact, osmotically inactive form.
- Activation of endothelial nitric oxide synthase (eNOS) to produce nitric oxide (NO), a vasodilator that increases blood flow and hence glucose availability to skeletal muscle.
- Activation of extracellular signal-regulated kinase (ERK), a mitogen-activated protein (MAP) kinase. This kinase drives protein synthesis and cell division and increases endothelial production of endothelin-1, a vasoconstrictor that may modulate eNOS-mediated vasodilation.

All of these effects are healthy responses to handle the caloric content of a normal meal.

Obesity is usually associated with resistance to insulin's glucose-lowering effects, or more simply, insulin resistance for glucose [IRg] (Fig. 13-4). However, many other actions of insulin remain fully intact in obese subjects. Hence, such people develop an imbalance among the actions of insulin. For example, the ability of insulin to increase blood flow into muscle, drive glucose uptake into skeletal myocytes and block postprandial glucose production from the liver is impaired in overnutrition. Paradoxically, insulin still stimulates hepatic triglyceride biosynthesis, which contributes to development of fatty liver and hypertriglyceridemia. Moreover, insulin-induced activation of ERK continues unimpaired, driving vasoconstriction through endothelin-1

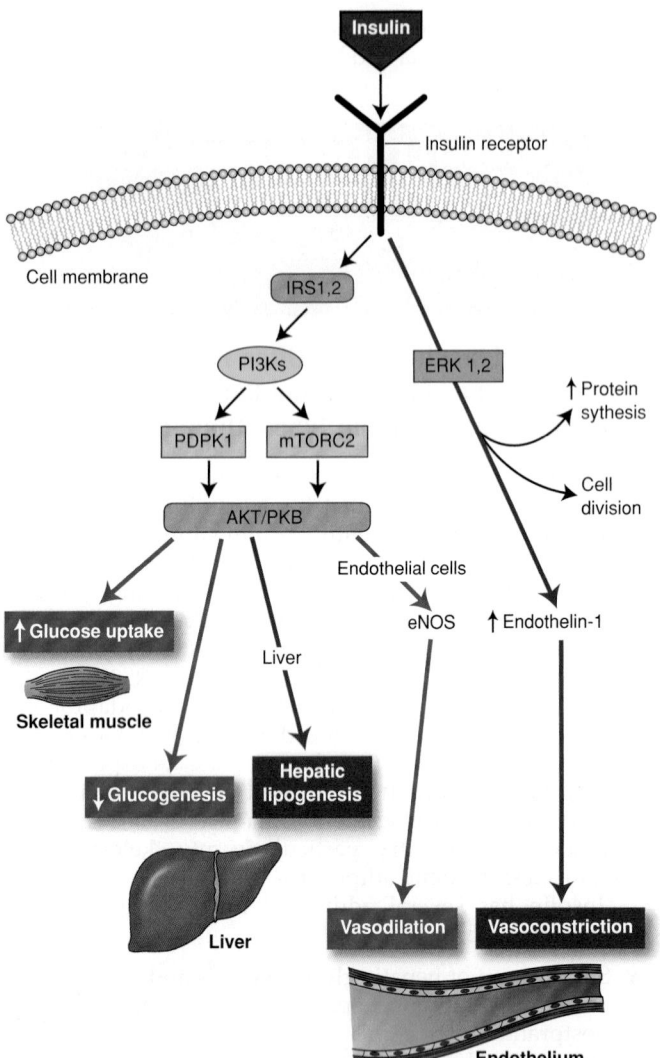

FIGURE 13-3. Key branches of insulin signaling and action. In normal physiology, insulin activates all pathways, but vasodilation produced by endothelial nitric oxide synthase (eNOS) dominates over vasoconstriction via ERK. Beneficial pathways when insulin is administered therapeutically are indicated in *blue* (glucose-lowering), while those that are potentially harmful are shown in *red* (hepatic lipogenesis and the ERK mitogen-activated protein [MAP] kinase). Strikingly, in obesity, type 2 diabetes and other conditions associated with pathway-selective insulin resistance and responsiveness (SEIRR), all pathways shown in blue become insulin resistant, while those in red remain insulin responsive. *From the standpoint of human health, it is the worst possible combination of effects.* Protein abbreviations: *AKT/PKB* = protein kinase B; *ERK* = extracellular signal-regulated kinase; *Gluc* = glucose; *IRS1,2* = insulin receptor substrates 1 and 2; *mTORC2* = mammalian target of rapamycin complex-2; *PDPK1* = 3′-phosphoinositide-dependent protein kinase-1; *PI3Ks* = isoforms of phosphatidylinositol 3′-kinases; *SHC* = Src homologous and collagen-like protein.

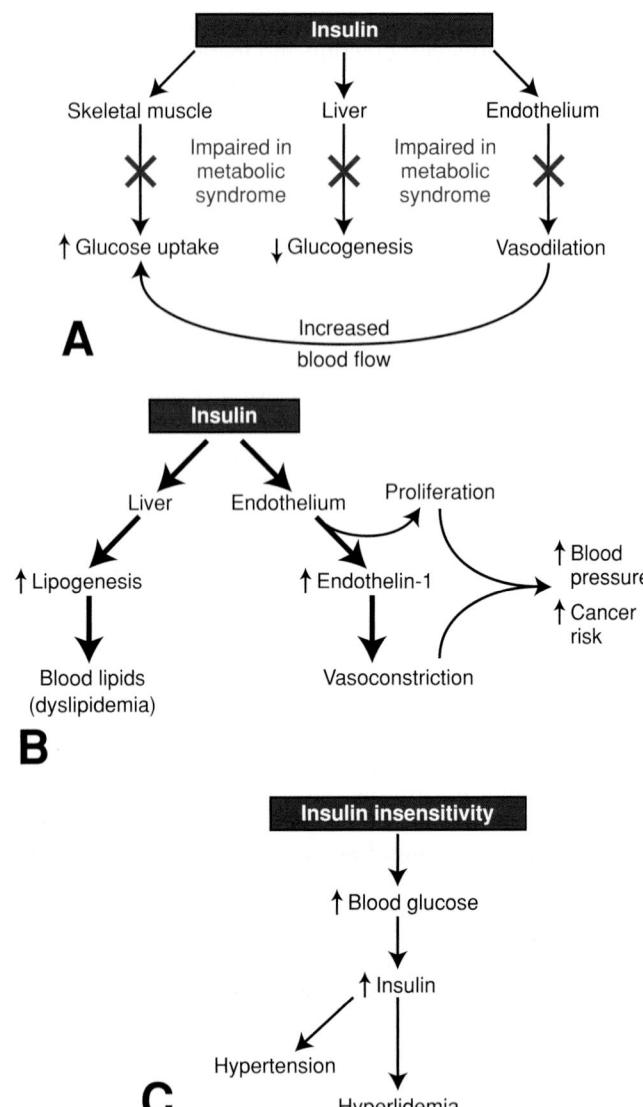

FIGURE 13-4. Mechanisms of insulin action that are impaired and that are intact in metabolic syndrome. A. Insulin activities that are impaired in metabolic syndrome. **B.** Insulin functions that remain intact in metabolic syndrome. **C.** Summary of insulin resistance for glucose and its consequences.

production and mitogenesis, possibly contributing to hypertension and cancer risk. This constellation of effects has been called pathway-selective insulin resistance and responsiveness (SEIRR). To control plasma concentrations of glucose, people with SEIRR become hyperinsulinemic, either from pancreatic overproduction of endogenous insulin or from therapeutic administration of exogenous insulin. Raising

insulin levels cannot make these individuals metabolically normal, *even if they achieve normoglycemia*, because hyperinsulinemia drives lipid synthesis in the liver and the ERK MAP kinase to become overactive.

Insulin Resistance for Glucose and SEIRR Are Not Understood

There are currently several suggested mechanisms to explain IRg and SEIRR. Each potential pathway explains some facets of these phenomena but leaves others unclear.

- **Lipotoxicity:** In obese people, plasma concentrations of nonesterified fatty acids (NEFAs) tend to be high, in part because the normal postprandial suppression of lipolysis of triglycerides in adipose tissue becomes insulin resistant. An excess of plasma nonesterified fatty acids can lead to ectopic accumulation of triglycerides, diacylglycerol and ceramide in liver and muscle cells. These molecules activate protein kinase C to induce insulin resistance for glucose by blocking the insulin receptor tyrosine kinase signal cascade (see above). Plasma levels of nonesterified fatty acids are preferentially increased in visceral–abdominal adiposity (Fig. 13-2). However, this hypothesis appears inconsistent with some newer information. For example, protein kinase C activation produces proximal blocks in insulin signaling, but such inhibition cannot explain ongoing insulin-dependent lipogenesis in the liver pathway–selective activation of ERK. Also, fatty liver in people with certain genetic defects in triglyceride disposal (and fatty liver in animals with analogous molecular manipulations) does not cause insulin resistance for glucose, even when the liver also shows remarkably high levels of diacylglycerol and ceramide.

- **Inflammation:** Adipose tissue in obesity often contains an inflammatory infiltrate, particularly of macrophages. Circulating levels of cytokines, particularly tumor necrosis factor-α (TNF-α) and interleukin-1β (IL-1β), are increased in visceral–abdominal obesity. These cytokines can also induce insulin resistance for glucose in experimental animals and cultured cells. However, in early stages of human overnutrition syndromes, TNF-α and other cytokines are not elevated; yet these people are already insulin resistant for glucose. A recent prospective clinical trial of high-dose salicylate as an anti-inflammatory agent produced only minor improvements in glycemic control. As well, TNF-α–induced blocks in insulin signaling may be too proximal to explain downstream pathway-selectivity.

- **Endoplasmic reticulum (ER) stress:** In animal models of obesity and insulin resistance for glucose, ER stress pathways are activated, as part of the unfolded protein response (see Chapter 1). Chemical induction of ER stress in cultured cells impairs insulin signaling, and relief of ER stress in obese animals improves their glucose handling. Evidence for this pathway in obese humans, however, has been mixed.

- **NAD(P)H oxidase-4 (NOX4):** NOX4, a molecule activated by insulin, affects the balance among other downstream limbs of the insulin signaling cascade. However, any role for NOX4 in SEIRR in people remains conjectural.

Imbalanced insulin action in target tissues and compensatory hyperinsulinemia are closely tied to a diverse set of cardiovascular risk factors that are prevalent in obese, sedentary people and patients with diabetes. These risk factors, together called the **metabolic syndrome,** include (1) abdominal adiposity with increased waist circumference, (2) mild hypertension (perhaps related to failure of endothelium-dependent vascular relaxation), (3) impaired fasting plasma glucose levels and (4) dyslipoproteinemia with elevated plasma triglycerides and low plasma high-density lipoprotein (HDL) cholesterol (Table 13-1).

The Complications of Overnutrition and Obesity Affect Most Organ Systems

Obesity and central adiposity are associated with increased morbidity and, for class II and III obesity, increased mortality as well (Fig. 13-5). Fat cells undergo both hyperplasia and hypertrophy. The excess from the imbalance between energy

TABLE 13-1
FREQUENTLY OBSERVED CONCOMITANTS OF THE METABOLIC SYNDROME

Clinical Signs

Central (upper body) obesity with increased waist circumference

Acanthosis nigricans (hypertrophic, hyperpigmented skin changes)

Laboratory Abnormalities

Elevated fasting and/or postprandial glucose

Insulin resistance for glucose, with hyperinsulinemia, but continued responsiveness—and hence overactivity—of other pathways downstream of the insulin receptor

Dyslipidemia characterized by increased triglycerides and low high-density lipoprotein cholesterol

Hypercoagulability and abnormal thrombolysis

Hyperuricemia

Endothelial and vascular smooth muscle dysfunction

Albuminuria

Comorbid Illnesses

Hypertension

Atherosclerosis

Hyperandrogenism with polycystic ovary syndrome

intake and energy expenditure is stored in adipocytes, which enlarge, increase in number or both. An extremely obese adult can have four times as many adipocytes as a lean one, each cell containing twice as much lipid.

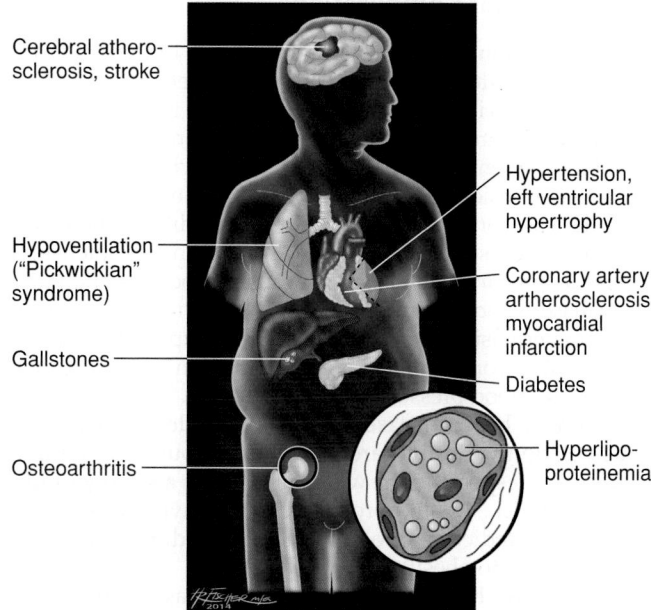

FIGURE 13-5. Medical complications of obesity.

Endocrine Complications

- **Type 2 diabetes mellitus (T2DM):** T2DM is strongly associated with obesity, and more than 80% of cases are attributed to obesity. The risk of diabetes increases linearly with BMI and with increments in abdominal fat, waist circumference or waist:hip ratio. Conversely, weight loss and exercise decrease risk of T2DM and can prevent progression of insulin resistance to diabetes. In a large American population with impaired glucose tolerance, simply engaging in brisk walking for 150 minutes per week and loss of 7% of body weight reduced the rate of progression of blood glucose levels to overt T2DM in 60% of subjects. More drastic measures for morbid obesity (e.g., weight loss after gastric bypass surgery) resulted in complete resolution of diabetes in almost 80% of patients. Thus, these harmful effects appear reversible.
- **Dyslipidemia and dyslipoproteinemia:** By far, the major killer in obesity and diabetes is atherosclerotic cardiovascular disease. Several deleterious plasma lipid and lipoprotein abnormalities often occur in obesity, including elevated fasting levels of triglyceride- and cholesterol-rich lipoproteins and nonesterified fatty acids and reduced HDLs. These abnormalities are strongly associated with an increased risk of cardiovascular disease, particularly in people with central adiposity. In addition, nonfasting plasma triglyceride concentrations independently predict subsequent heart attacks and strokes. They reflect the persistence of a particular class of harmful lipoproteins, called remnants, that appear in the circulation after each meal or snack. Like low-density lipoproteins (LDLs), these particles contain apolipoprotein B and cholesterol, and can be trapped within arterial walls, initiating and accelerating atherosclerotic vascular disease (see Chapter 16). As the prevalence of obesity rises, dyslipoproteinemias beyond simple elevations in plasma LDL cholesterol have contributed increasingly to cardiovascular risk.
- **Other endocrine complications:** Obesity is also associated with polycystic ovary syndrome, irregular menses, amenorrhea, infertility and hypogonadism.

Cardiovascular Complications

- **Hypertension:** Obesity entails a high risk of hypertension and is associated with heightened sympathetic activity. High insulin levels in obese patients with insulin resistance act on pathways unrelated to glucose importation. These include enhancing renal reabsorption of sodium, which contributes to hypertension, and stimulating endothelial production of the vasoconstrictor endothelin-1. In addition, obese adipose tissue also secretes substances including angiotensin II and its precursors that directly cause vasoconstriction and increase blood pressure. By interfering with the action of antihypertensive agents, obesity makes hypertension more difficult to control. Even a small reduction in weight may decrease blood pressure in this population.
- **Coronary heart disease:** BMI has a modest and graded association with myocardial infarction, but body fat distribution, especially the waist:hip ratio, is a stronger indicator of risk. Dyslipoproteinemia and hypertension are the best predictors of atherosclerotic cardiovascular disease linked to obesity.
- **Congestive heart failure:** Obesity is associated with increased risk of heart failure due to eccentric cardiac dilatation. Also, the combination of obesity and hypertension leads to ventricular wall thickening and larger heart volume. Obese patients are also at increased risk of atrial fibrillation and atrial flutter.
- **Thromboembolic disease:** Deep venous thromboses and pulmonary embolism are more common in obese patients. Thromboembolic disease of the lower extremities may be related to increased abdominal pressure, impaired fibrinolysis and increased circulating cytokines, particularly with abdominal obesity.

Additional Complications of Obesity

- **Neurologic:** Obesity increases risk of ischemic stroke as BMI increases.
- **Pulmonary:** Obesity may interfere mechanically with lung function. Increased weight, particularly excess abdominal obesity, decreases ventilatory drive, respiratory compliance and ventilation, particularly ventilation of lung bases. It thus adds to ventilation–perfusion mismatch. Obesity is a major risk factor for **obstructive sleep apnea,** which renders patients prone to breathing disorders during sleep. **Obesity-hypoventilation syndrome** refers to decreased ventilatory responsiveness to hypercapnia or hypoxia. This condition impairs responses to the increased ventilatory demands that are imposed by the mechanical effects of obesity. The severe form of this syndrome is **Pickwickian syndrome,** in which extreme obesity, irregular breathing, cyanosis, secondary polycythemia and right ventricular dysfunction all lead to fixed pulmonary hypertension.
- **Hepatobiliary:** Obese people, particularly women, suffer from an increased incidence of gallstones. Interestingly, weight loss may also precipitate gallstones, owing to increased cholesterol supersaturation in bile, enhanced cholesterol crystal nucleation and decreased gallbladder contractility. Many liver abnormalities, manifested by increased serum liver enzymes, hepatomegaly and altered liver histology, may also complicate obesity. These represent a spectrum of disease, **nonalcoholic fatty liver disease** (NAFLD), characterized by accumulation of fat within hepatocytes (see pathway-selective insulin resistance and responsiveness, above, and Chapter 20). A subset of patients with simple steatosis progress to nonalcoholic steatohepatitis (NASH), and inflammatory changes within the liver can cause fibrosis, cirrhosis and portal hypertension. NASH is the leading cause of so-called "idiopathic" cirrhosis.
- **Gastrointestinal:** Gastroesophageal reflux is more common in obese people.
- **Cancer:** Certain cancers occur with greater frequency in those who are obese. Specifically, risks for esophageal, gallbladder, pancreatic, breast, renal, uterine, cervical and prostate cancers are all increased. Once cancer is diagnosed, obesity is associated with a worse prognosis. Activation of ERK (see above) may provide a mitogenic stimulus that predisposes obese people to certain tumors. Obesity has also been associated with overexpression of aromatase in adipose tissue within the breast, local production of estrogen and increased breast cancer risk.
- **Musculoskeletal:** Hyperuricemia and gout are more common in obese people. Obesity increases the risk of osteoarthritis, particularly of weight-bearing joints such as the knees. However, non–weight-bearing joints can also be affected, suggesting mechanisms other than increased mechanical load. Weight loss decreases the risk of osteoarthritis.

- **Skin:** Obesity causes **striae,** stretching and thinning of the epidermis in a ribbon-like pattern. **Acanthosis nigricans** is a velvety, hypertrophic, hyperpigmented lesion, especially at skinfold areas (axillae, nape of the neck). It may be a response to high circulating insulin levels in patients with insulin resistance. Excessive hair growth **(hirsutism)** can result from increases in circulating androgens in susceptible women.
- **Psychological and social:** Obesity has also been associated with impaired quality of life, increased sick leave absences and disability claims and depression.

Diabetes Mellitus

Almost a century ago, Sir William Osler defined diabetes mellitus as "a syndrome due to a disturbance in carbohydrate metabolism from various causes, in which sugar appears in the urine, associated with thirst, polyuria, wasting and imperfect oxidation of fats." With the advent of insulin and other therapies, however, such extreme features are unusual in properly managed patients with diabetes.

Yet long-term consequences persist. Hence, diabetes mellitus in the modern setting is redefined as "a state of premature cardiovascular death that is associated with chronic hyperglycemia and may also be associated with blindness and renal failure." This emphasis reflects the fact that in industrialized countries, cardiovascular disease kills 70% of patients with diabetes, compared to 50% of the general population. It also affects them earlier in life, with greater morbidity. Adults with diabetes are two to four times more likely to have heart disease or stroke than those without diabetes.

Diabetes is a major health problem that affects increasing numbers of people throughout the world. Two major forms are recognized, distinguished by different underlying pathophysiologies. **Type 1 diabetes mellitus (T1DM),** formerly known as **insulin-dependent diabetes mellitus (IDDM) or juvenile-onset diabetes,** is caused by autoimmune destruction of insulin-producing beta cells in the pancreatic islets of Langerhans. It affects fewer than 10% of all patients with diabetes. By contrast, **T2DM,** formerly known as **non–insulin-dependent diabetes mellitus (NIDDM) or maturity-onset diabetes,** is usually associated with obesity. It results from a complex interrelationship between insulin resistance of target tissues and an oversecretion of insulin by the pancreas (see above). This balance may, or may not, be sufficient to control plasma glucose concentrations. Table 13-2 compares the key features of type 1 and type 2 diabetes.

Gestational diabetes develops in some pregnant women owing to resistance to the glucose-lowering actions of insulin in pregnancy, combined with a beta cell defect in the pancreas.

TABLE 13-2

COMPARISON OF TYPE 1 AND TYPE 2 DIABETES MELLITUS

	Type 1 Diabetes	Type 2 Diabetes
Age at onset	Usually before 20	Usually after 30
Type of onset	Abrupt; symptomatic (polyuria, polydipsia, dehydration); often severe with ketoacidosis	Gradual; usually subtle; often asymptomatic
Usual body weight	Normal; recent weight loss is common	Overweight
Family history	<20%	>60%
Monozygotic twins	50% concordant	90% concordant
HLA associations	+	No
Antibodies to islet cell antigens (insulin, glutamic acid decarboxylase [GAD-65], IA-2)	+	No
Islet lesions	Early—inflammation Late—atrophy and fibrosis	Late—fibrosis, amyloid
Beta cell mass	Markedly reduced	Normal or slightly reduced
Circulating insulin levels	Markedly reduced or absent	Elevated (early)
Insulin resistance for glucose (i.e., selective resistance to the glucose-lowering actions of insulin)	Normal sensitivity to glucose-lowering actions of insulin	Significant insulin resistance for glucose, but with continued insulin responsiveness of other pathways
Clinical management	Administration of exogenous insulin absolutely required	Exogenous insulin usually not needed initially; insulin supplementation may be needed at later stages; weight loss typically improves the condition

HLA = human leukocyte antigen; IA-2 = islet cell antigen-512.

TABLE 13-3
ETIOLOGIC CLASSIFICATION OF DIABETES MELLITUS

I. Type 1 diabetes (beta cell destruction, absolute insulin deficiency)
 – A. Immune mediated
 – B. Idiopathic

II. Type 2 diabetes (insulin resistance for glucose, with relative insulin deficiency)

III. Other specific types
 – Genetic defects of beta cell function (e.g., maturity-onset diabetes of the young)
 – Genetic defects in insulin action (e.g., type A insulin resistance, which can be caused by mutations in the insulin receptor)
 – Diseases of the exocrine pancreas
 – Endocrinopathies (e.g., Cushing disease, acromegaly, etc.)
 – Drug or chemical induced (e.g., glucocorticoids)
 – Infections (e.g., cytomegalovirus, rubella)
 – Uncommon forms of immune-mediated diabetes (e.g., "stiff-man syndrome")
 – Other genetic syndromes (e.g., Turner syndrome, Down syndrome)

IV. Gestational diabetes mellitus

Copyright 2013 American Diabetes Association. From *Diabetes Care,* Vol. 36, 2013. Modified with permission from the American Diabetes Association.

It almost always abates after delivery. Diabetes can also occur in other endocrine conditions or drug therapy, especially in Cushing syndrome or during treatment with glucocorticoids. Other rare clinical syndromes entail abnormal glucose metabolism or overt **hyperglycemia**. As these conditions are uncommon and have well-defined genetic etiologies that differ from the more common forms of diabetes, they will not be considered in detail. Table 13-3 shows the classification of diabetes as recommended by the American Diabetes Association (ADA).

Current criteria for the diagnosis of diabetes mellitus are based on abnormal threshold levels for glucose or

---

TABLE 13-4
CRITERIA FOR THE DIAGNOSIS OF DIABETES

1. HbA_{1c}[a] ≥6.5%

OR

2. FPG ≥126 mg/dL (7.0 mmol/L). Fasting is defined as no caloric intake for at least 8 h

OR

3. 2-h plasma glucose ≥200 mg/dL (11.1 mmol/L) during an OGTT

OR

4. In a patient with classic symptoms of hyperglycemia or hyperglycemic crisis, a random plasma glucose ≥200 mg/dL (11.1 mmol/L)

FPG = fasting plasma glucose; HbA_{1c} = hemoglobin A_{1c}; OGTT = oral glucose tolerance test.
[a]In the absence of unequivocal hyperglycemia, criteria 1–3 should be confirmed by repeat testing.
Copyright 2013 American Diabetes Association. From *Diabetes Care,* Vol. 36, 2013. Modified with permission from the American Diabetes Association.

TABLE 13-5
CATEGORIES OF INCREASED RISK FOR DIABETES (PREDIABETES)[a]

FPG 100 mg/dL (5.6 mmol/L) to 125 mg/dL (6.9 mmol/L) (IFG)

2-h PG in the 75-g OGTT 140 mg/dL (7.8 mmol/L) to 199 mg/dL (11.0 mmol/L) (IGT)

HbA_{1c} 5.7%–6.4%

FPG = fasting plasma glucose; HbA_{1c} = hemoglobin A_{1c}; IFG = impaired fasting glucose; IGT = impaired glucose tolerance; OGTT = oral glucose tolerance test; PG = plasma glucose.
[a]For all three tests, risk is continuous, extending below the lower limit of the range and becoming disproportionately greater at the higher ends of the range.
Copyright 2013 American Diabetes Association. From *Diabetes Care,* Vol. 36, 2013. Modified with permission from the American Diabetes Association.

hemoglobin A_{1c} that are closely associated with the chronic complications of this disorder. In particular, hyperglycemia causes the microvascular changes of diabetic retinopathy and renal glomerular damage. In a younger patient with abrupt onset of hyperglycemia and elevated plasma ketones or frank ketoacidosis, T1DM arises from absolute insulin deficiency. By contrast, T2DM typically develops gradually over years before it is recognized, most often in an overweight, middle-aged person with a genetic predisposition.

The ADA suggests any of four criteria to diagnose diabetes (Table 13-4). One of the four criteria has to be present for the diagnosis, but some criteria require repeat testing for confirmation. In addition, the ADA recognizes three categories of increased risk for diabetes (Table 13-5). Some of those are commonly referred to as "prediabetes," but the term should be used with caution, because only half of those patients will ultimately develop diabetes.

TYPE 2 DIABETES MELLITUS

T2DM is characterized by a combination of reduced tissue sensitivity to the glucose-lowering effects of insulin and oversecretion of insulin from the pancreas, which eventuates in an inadequate control of plasma glucose concentrations.

T2DM usually develops in adults, mostly in obese people and in the elderly. Recently, it has been appearing increasingly in younger adults and adolescents, as severe obesity and lack of exercise become more severe and common in this age group. Patients with T2DM exhibit hyperinsulinemia in terms of absolute concentrations, but these excessive insulin concentrations fail to control their blood sugar levels. When T2DM patients require administration of exogenous insulin, their total daily doses are much higher than in lean T1DM (insulin-deficient) patients. Because a number of insulin actions in obesity, prediabetes and T2DM still remain responsive, such as hepatic lipogenesis and ERK activation, some investigators attribute metabolic harm to hyperinsulinemia.

 **EPIDEMIOLOGY:** In 2010, about 8% of the American population and/or 11% of those older than 20 years had T2DM. More than a quarter were undiagnosed. Over 25% of people over 60 have diabetes, and 35% of adults are felt to have prediabetes. T2DM is most prevalent in women, especially of lower socioeconomic

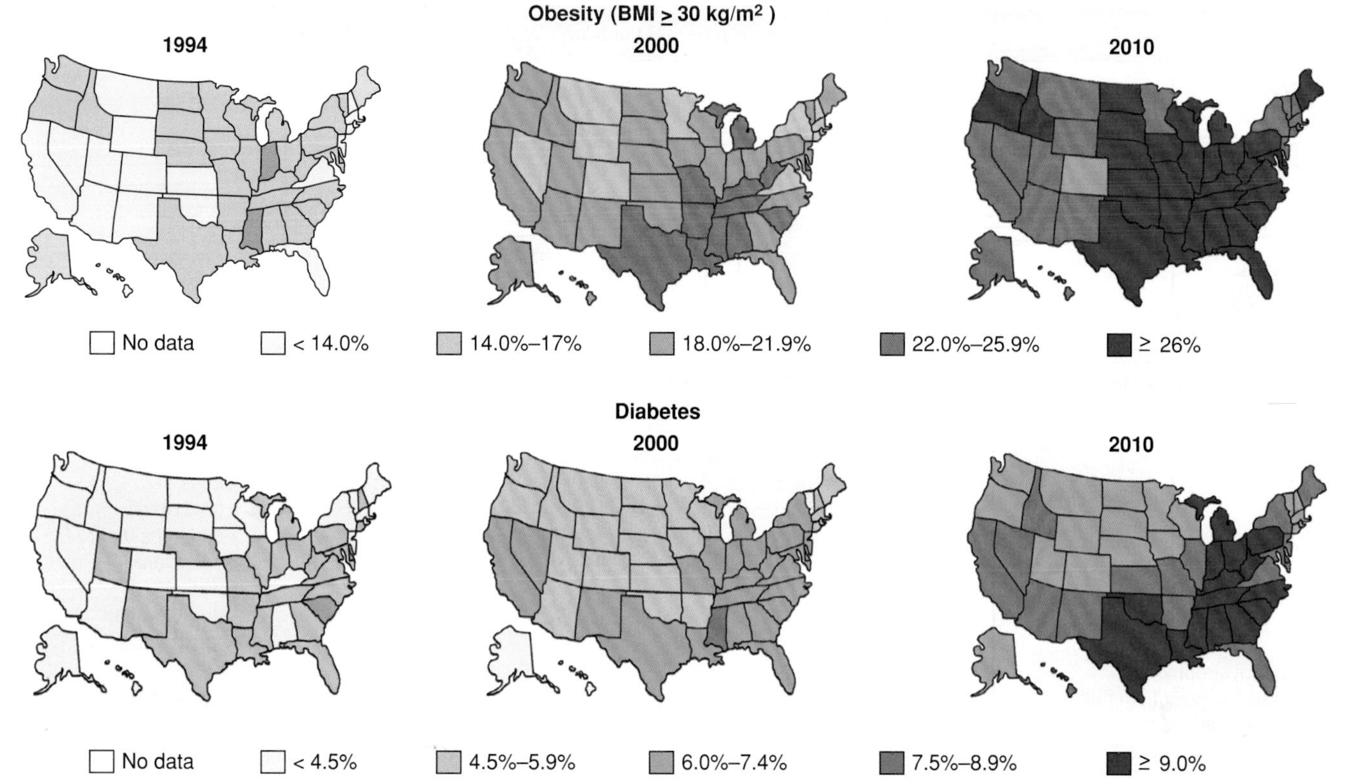

Obesity (BMI ≥ 30 kg/m²)

| 1994 | 2000 | 2010 |

☐ No data   ☐ < 14.0%   ◻ 14.0%–17%   ▨ 18.0%–21.9%   ▨ 22.0%–25.9%   ■ ≥ 26%

Diabetes

| 1994 | 2000 | 2010 |

☐ No data   ☐ < 4.5%   ◻ 4.5%–5.9%   ▨ 6.0%–7.4%   ▨ 7.5%–8.9%   ■ ≥ 9.0%

FIGURE 13-6. The increasing prevalence of obesity and diabetes in the United States.

strata. All nonwhite ethnic groups are more affected than white Americans. Diabetes is also increasing worldwide: in China, for example, it affects about 10% of adults.

Diabetes is the leading cause of kidney failure, nontraumatic lower limb amputations and new cases of blindness among American adults. It is also a major factor in heart disease and stroke, and is the 7th leading cause of death. Fig. 13-6 shows the dramatic increase in prevalence of diabetes in the United States from 1994 to 2010.

Type 2 Diabetes Mellitus Results from Insulin Resistance and Inability to Hypersecrete Insulin

T2DM is a two-hit disease. The first "hit" is resistance to the glucose-lowering actions of insulin in its target tissues (liver, skeletal muscle, adipose tissue). This defect alone provokes increased total pancreatic output of insulin and may later be followed by moderate defects in glucose handling, indicative of prediabetes. The second "hit" occurs when increased pancreatic insulin output can no longer compensate for the highly increased demand for insulin to control blood sugar levels. Pancreatic islets often show degenerative changes in these patients. Progression to overt diabetes occurs most commonly in patients with both of these hits (Fig. 13-7).

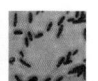 **ETIOLOGIC FACTORS:** Several risk factors are clearly associated with T2DM. The most important ones are **obesity, overnutrition and low levels of physical activity**. As noted above, the risk of T2DM increases linearly with BMI. More than 80% of cases of T2DM can be attributed to obesity. As noted above, visceral–abdominal obesity ("apple shaped") is more associated with insulin resistance for glucose and T2DM compared

to gluteal–femoral obesity ("pear shaped"). Accordingly, weight loss lowers the risk of T2DM and can prevent progression of high-risk individuals to frank diabetes.

 MOLECULAR PATHOGENESIS: *Multifactorial and multigenic inheritance is a key contributor to the development of T2DM.* Several observations demonstrate genetic influences in the development of T2DM:

■ More than 1/3 of patients with T2DM have at least one parent with the disease.
■ Among monozygotic twins, concordance for T2DM approaches 100%.
■ The prevalence of T2DM among different ethnic groups who are living in similar environments varies tremendously.
■ First-degree relatives of patients with T2DM have a significantly higher lifetime risk of T2DM compared with matched subjects without a family history.

Despite the high familial prevalence of the disease, inheritance is complex and involves multiple interacting susceptibility genes. As with obesity, monogenic causes of T2DM represent only a small fraction of cases, and commonly inherited polymorphisms contribute only small degrees of risk for, or protection from, T2DM. Factors such as obesity (which itself has strong genetic determinants; see above), hypertension and exercise influence phenotypic expression of T2DM and complicate genetic analysis.

A rare autosomal dominant form of inherited diabetes, known as **maturity-onset diabetes of the young (MODY),** is associated with gene defects that affect beta cell function, including the gene for glucokinase, a key sensor for glucose

OBESITY AND DIABETES MELLITUS

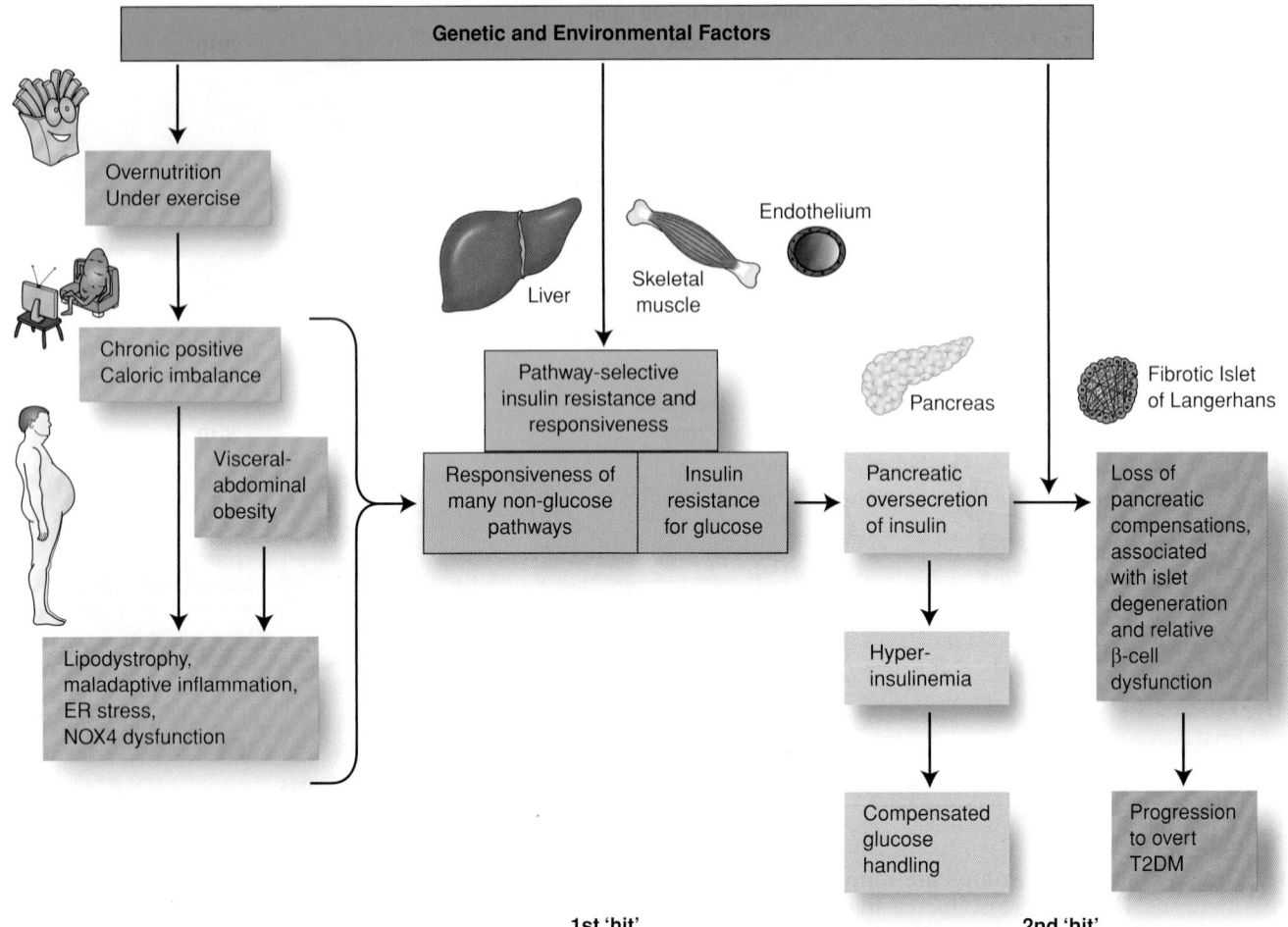

FIGURE 13-7. Pathogenesis of obesity-related type 2 diabetes mellitus (T2DM). The expanded visceral fat mass in upper body obesity elaborates several factors that may contribute to insulin resistance for glucose. These include an increase in circulating free (nonesterified) fatty acids (FFAs) and other cytokines and proteins that inhibit insulin action, as well as a decrease in factors that enhance insulin signaling, such as adiponectin. These changes result in impairments to insulin action in liver and skeletal muscle at the level of the insulin receptor and at postreceptor signaling sites, resulting in a failure of insulin to suppress hepatic glucose production and to promote glucose uptake into muscle. The resulting hyperglycemia is normally countered by increased insulin secretion by pancreatic beta cells. Continuing responsiveness of pathways downstream of the insulin receptor that are unrelated to glucose control, such as lipogenesis in the liver and activation of the extracellular signal-regulated kinase (ERK) mitogen-activated protein (MAP) kinase, may contribute to fatty liver, dyslipoproteinemia and hypertension. In many individuals, the combination of resistance to the glucose-lowering actions of insulin and a genetically determined impairment of the beta cell response to hyperglycemia eventually results in hyperglycemia, and T2DM ensues.

metabolism within the beta cell. Several mutations in genes that control beta cell development and function have been described. Mutations in these genes, however, do not account for typical T2DM.

Insulin Resistance for Glucose

After a carbohydrate-rich meal, the gut absorbs glucose. This increases blood glucose, which stimulates insulin secretion by pancreatic beta cells. In turn, insulin increases glucose uptake by skeletal muscle and adipose tissue (Fig. 13-4). At the same time, insulin suppresses hepatic glucose production by (1) inhibiting glycogenolysis and gluconeogenesis, (2) enhancing glycogen synthesis, (3) blocking the effects of glucagon on the liver and (4) antagonizing glucagon release from the pancreas.

All of these effects of insulin are impaired in IRg. Initially, compromised insulin action is subclinical. As the condition progresses, fasting glucose rises or impaired glucose tolerance develops. Eventually, the patient develops frank

hyperglycemia and overt T2DM (Fig. 13-8). IRg increases hepatic glucose output and reduces glucose uptake by peripheral tissues, primarily muscles and adipose tissue.

By itself, insulin resistance rarely causes T2DM: increased insulin secretion (hyperinsulinism) by beta cells compensates for these defects and prevents blood glucose levels from rising. Only when the pancreas can no longer keep up with this high demand do blood glucose levels start to increase (Fig. 13-8). In many obese and prediabetic patients, subclinical beta cell dysfunction exists before overt diabetes.

Beta Cell Dysfunction

At first, an impairment in the first phase of insulin secretion following glucose stimulation precedes glucose intolerance in T2DM (Fig. 13-9). Later in the second phase of the disease, release of newly synthesized insulin is faulty. This effect can be reversed, at least in some patients, by restoring good control of glycemia. This partially reversible reduction in

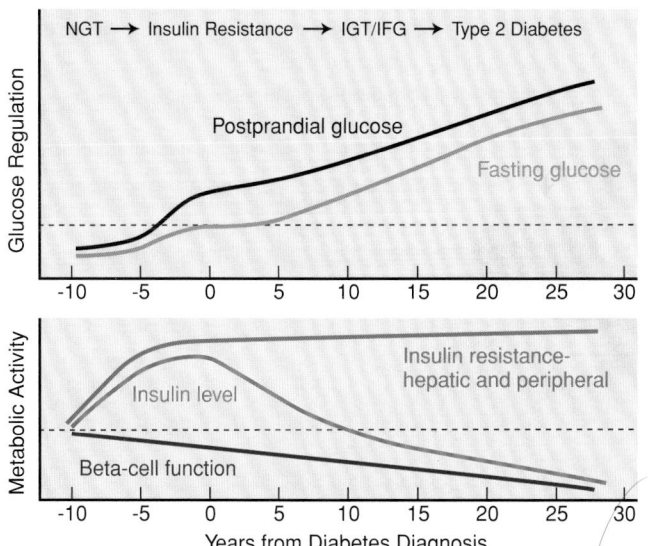

FIGURE 13-8. Glucose regulation and metabolic activity during the development of type 2 diabetes mellitus. *NGT* = normal glucose tolerance; *IGT* = impaired glucose tolerance; *IFG* = impaired fasting glucose.

insulin secretion results from a paradoxical inhibitory effect of glucose upon insulin release that may be seen at high blood glucose levels ("glucose toxicity").

Impaired first-phase insulin secretion can serve as a marker of risk for T2DM in family members of subjects with T2DM, and may be seen in patients with prior gestational diabetes. Over a long time, insulin secretion in T2DM gradually declines, together with beta cell mass.

The Role of Incretins

In the 1960s, it was discovered that the ability of an oral glucose load to stimulate insulin secretion was significantly

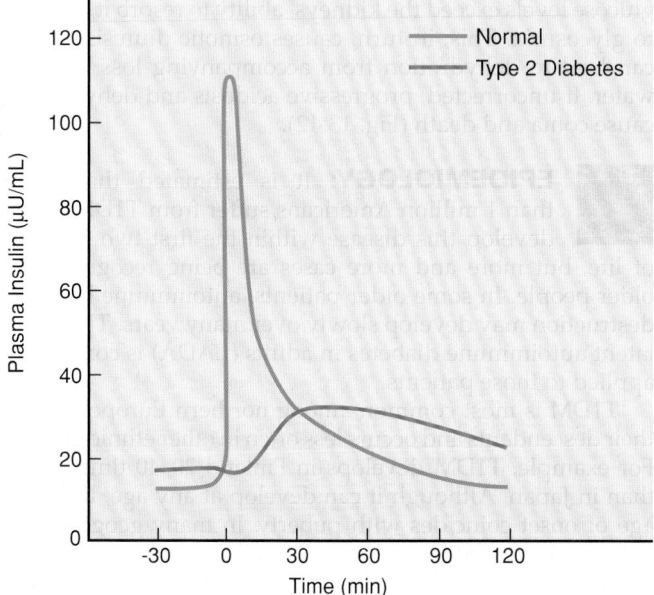

FIGURE 13-9. Insulin response in diabetes. Typical patterns of insulin production in response to glucose challenge in normal (*blue*) and type 2 diabetic (*red*) patients.

greater than that evoked from a comparable intravenous infusion of glucose. This discrepancy was named the **incretin effect** (Fig. 13-10A). Incretins are peptides secreted by the gut in response to meals that increase insulin secretion and decrease glucagon secretion. Most of this effect is now thought to be due to glucose-dependent insulinotropic peptide (GIP) and GLP-1. Incretins are rapidly inactivated by dipeptidyl peptidase 4 (DPP-4) in the circulation. Effects of incretins include (1) enhanced glucose-dependent stimulation of insulin secretion by beta cells, (2) inhibition of glucagon secretion by alpha cells, (3) inhibition of appetite and (4) slowed gastric emptying.

In patients with T2DM, the incretin effect is markedly reduced (Fig. 13-10B), an effect that has been attributed to defects in secretion of GLP-1 and GIP. The role, if any, of these changes in incretins in the pathogenesis of T2DM is unknown.

Therapeutic Implications

Early in T2DM, insulin resistance for glucose and hyperinsulinemia predominate. Both can improve dramatically with even modest weight loss and exercise, and lifestyle interventions are at the center of clinical management. In addition, insulin sensitizers are useful in those patients. Metformin is considered an "insulin sensitizer," because it improves glucose uptake by muscle and inhibits hepatic glucose production, although its mechanism of action at a molecular level remains in dispute. Thiazolidinediones, a class of PPAR-γ agonists, are also classified as insulin sensitizers because they lower insulin requirements and improve fatty liver. Some of their side effects, such as water retention, increased appetite and others, have limited their use.

Later in the course of diabetes, as beta cell dysfunction sets in, insulin sensitizers alone cannot control T2DM. Other agents (e.g., secretagogues such as sulfonylureas, incretin-based agents [GLP-1 analogs and DPP4 inhibitors] and, ultimately, exogenous insulin) are needed. Bariatric surgery has also become a therapeutic option, reducing caloric intake, BMI and the need for medications. Remarkably, some patients with T2DM before bariatric surgery require no medications after surgery.

 PATHOLOGY: Lesions may be found in the islets of Langerhans of many, but not all, patients with T2DM. Unlike T1DM (see below), the number of beta cells is not consistently reduced in T2DM, and no morphologic lesions of these cells have been found by light or electron microscopy.

In some islets, fibrous tissue accumulates, sometimes so much that islets are obliterated. Islet amyloid is often present (Fig. 13-11), particularly in patients older than 60 years. This type of amyloid is composed of a polypeptide molecule known as **amylin,** which is secreted with insulin by the beta cell. Importantly, as many as 20% of aged nondiabetics also have amyloid in their pancreatic islets, a finding that has been attributed to the aging process itself.

TYPE 1 DIABETES MELLITUS

T1DM is a lifelong disorder of glucose homeostasis that results from autoimmune destruction of beta cells in the islets of Langerhans. In contrast to T2DM, T1DM is a one-hit

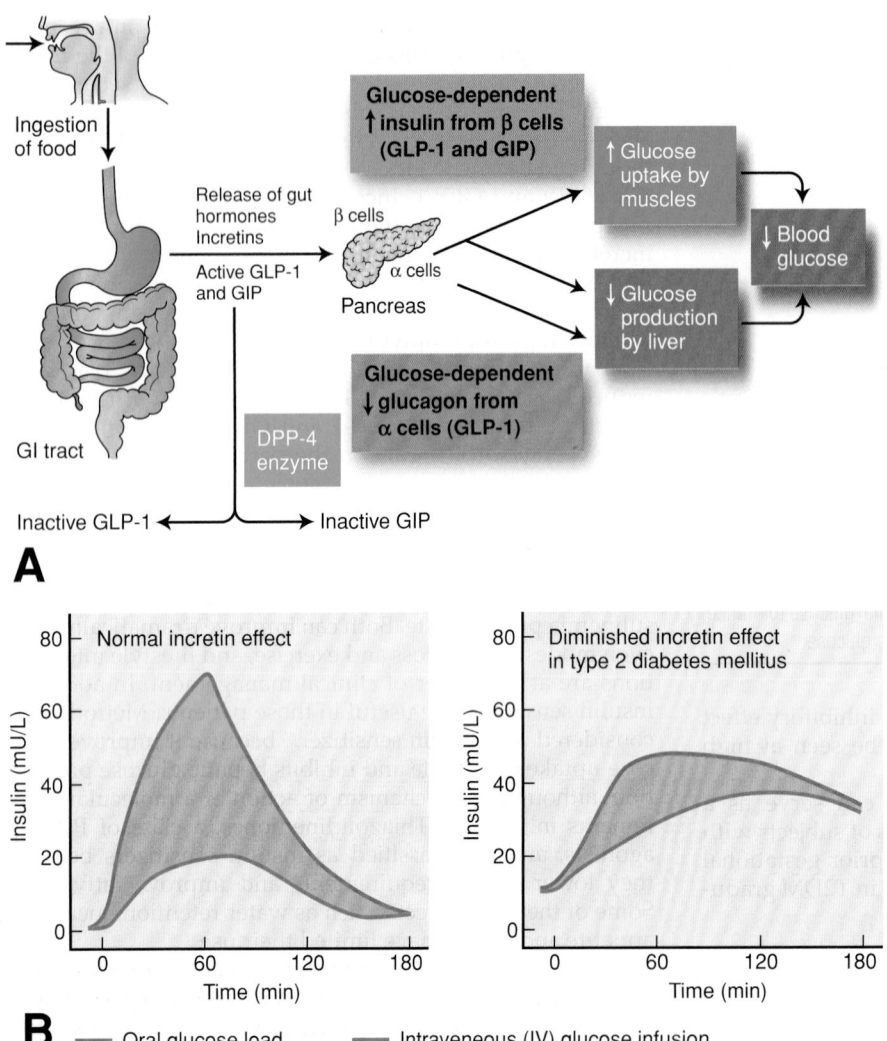

A

B

— Oral glucose load   — Intraveneous (IV) glucose infusion

FIGURE 13-10. Incretins. A. Physiologic roles of incretins in glucose metabolism. Involvement of incretins in regulating the responses of the body to a caloric load. *GIP* = glucose-dependent insulinotropic peptide; *GLP-1* = glucagon-like peptide-1. **B.** Diminished incretin responsiveness in type 2 diabetes mellitus.

disease that is caused by autoimmune destruction of pancreatic beta cells. Triggers for this autoimmune reaction remain unknown (see below). Because T1DM reflects absolute insulin deficiency, rather than complex defects in insulin action, these patients can be made almost metabolically normal by closely controlling the amounts, timing and preparations of exogenous insulin. Considerable research is being devoted to two independent approaches to supply insulin in a highly regulated fashion to T1DM patients—namely, islet cell transplantation and "closed loop" machines that simultaneously monitor glucose concentrations and administer exogenous insulin. Management of T1DM can be complicated if patients become obese; historically, T1DM patients were uniformly lean.

T1DM is characterized by few, if any, functional beta cells and extremely limited or nonexistent insulin secretion. Without insulin, the body switches energy use to a pattern that resembles starvation, regardless of the availability of food. Thus, adipose stores, rather than exogenous glucose, are preferentially metabolized for energy. Oxidation of fat overproduces **ketone bodies** (acetoacetic acid and β-hydroxybutyric acid), which are released into the blood from the liver and lead to metabolic ketoacidosis. Hyperglycemia results from unsuppressed hepatic glucose output and reduced glucose uptake into skeletal muscle and adipose tissue. Blood

glucose levels exceed the kidneys' ability to resorb it, leading to glycosuria. This, in turn, causes osmotic diuresis, which can lead to dehydration from accompanying loss of body water. If uncorrected, progressive acidosis and dehydration cause coma and death (Fig. 13-12).

EPIDEMIOLOGY: It is estimated that more than 1 million Americans suffer from T1DM. Most develop this disease within the first two decades of life, but more and more cases are being recognized in older people. In some older patients, autoimmune beta cell destruction may develop slowly over many years. The name latent autoimmune diabetes in adults (LADA) is commonly applied to those patients.

T1DM is most common among northern Europeans and their descendants and occurs less often in other ethnic groups. For example, T1DM develops in Finland 20–40 times more than in Japan. Although it can develop at any age, the peak age of onset coincides with puberty. In many geographical areas, an increased incidence in late fall and early winter suggests seasonal infections as autoimmune triggers (see below).

MOLECULAR PATHOGENESIS:
AUTOIMMUNITY: The concept of an autoimmune pathogenesis for T1DM is suggested by the

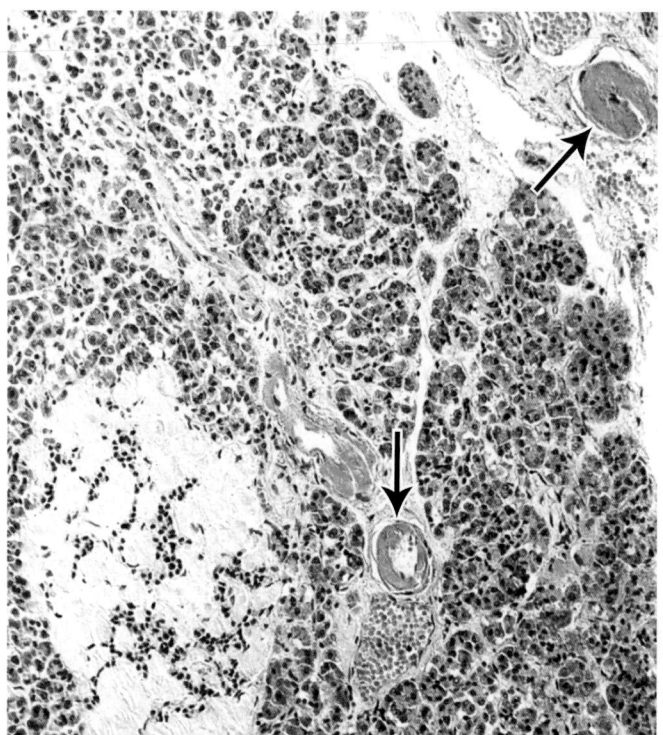

FIGURE 13-11. Amyloid deposition (hyalinization) of an islet in the pancreas of a patient with type 2 diabetes mellitus (*lower left*). Blood vessels adjacent to the islet show the advanced hyaline arteriolosclerosis (*arrows*) characteristic of diabetes.

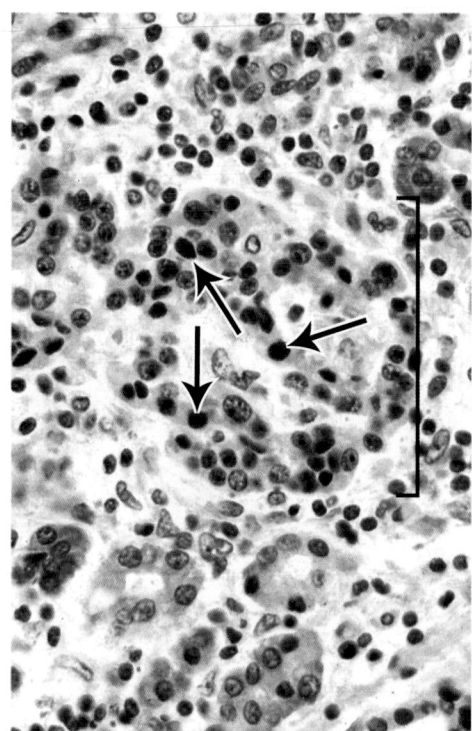

FIGURE 13-13. Insulitis in type 1 diabetes mellitus. A lymphocytic inflammatory infiltrate (*arrows*) is seen in and around the islet (*left of bracket*).

observation that pancreatic islets from patients who die shortly after the onset of the disease show mononuclear infiltrates, or **insulitis,** in their pancreatic islets (Fig. 13-13). CD8+ T lymphocytes predominate among these inflammatory cells. The infiltrating cells also elaborate proinflammatory cytokines, for example, IL-1, IL-6, interferon-α and nitric oxide, which may further contribute to beta cell injury.

Most newly diagnosed children with this disease have circulating antibodies against components of the beta cells. Major target antigens include insulin, glutamic acid

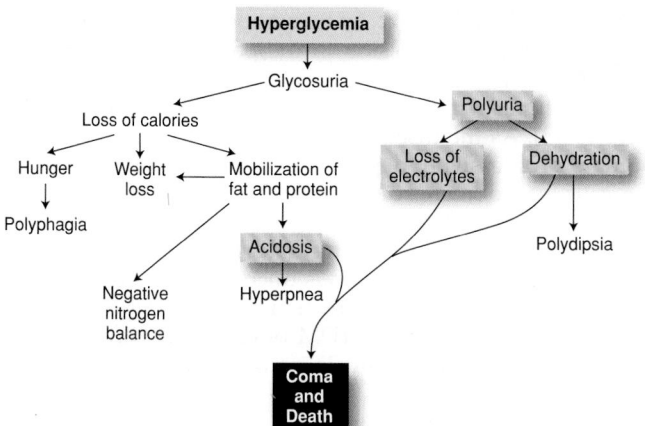

FIGURE 13-12. Symptoms and signs of uncontrolled hyperglycemia in diabetes mellitus.

decarboxylase (GAD) and insulinoma-associated protein 2 (IA-2), also known as islet cell antigen 512 (ICA-512). Many patients develop anti-islet cell antibodies months or years before insulin production decreases and clinical symptoms appear, a clinical state known as "pre-T1DM" (Fig. 13-14). However, these antibodies are now regarded as responses to beta cell antigens released during destruction of beta cells by cell-mediated immune mechanisms, rather than the cause of beta cell depletion. Nevertheless, detection of serum antibodies to islet cells and target islet antigens is a useful clinical tool for differentiating T1DM.

Cell-mediated immune mechanisms are fundamental to the pathogenesis of T1DM. Cytotoxic T lymphocytes sensitized to beta cells in T1DM persist indefinitely, possibly for a lifetime. Patients transplanted with a donor pancreas or a preparation of purified islets must be treated with immunosuppressive drugs. Ten percent of patients with T1DM develop at least one other organ-specific autoimmune disease, including Hashimoto thyroiditis, Graves disease, myasthenia gravis, Addison disease and pernicious anemia. Interestingly, most patients with polyendocrine immune syndromes (see Chapter 27) also exhibit human leukocyte antigen (HLA)-DR3 and -DR4.

Studies in first-degree relatives of subjects with T1DM have shown that antibodies against islet cells are present several years before the onset of the disease. Thus, beta cell destruction in T1DM generally develops slowly over years. Specific stages of the disease have been described (Fig. 13-14). Only when 80% or more of insulin-secreting cells are eliminated and insulin deprivation is severe is T1DM with hyperglycemia or ketoacidosis clinically evident.

OBESITY AND DIABETES MELLITUS

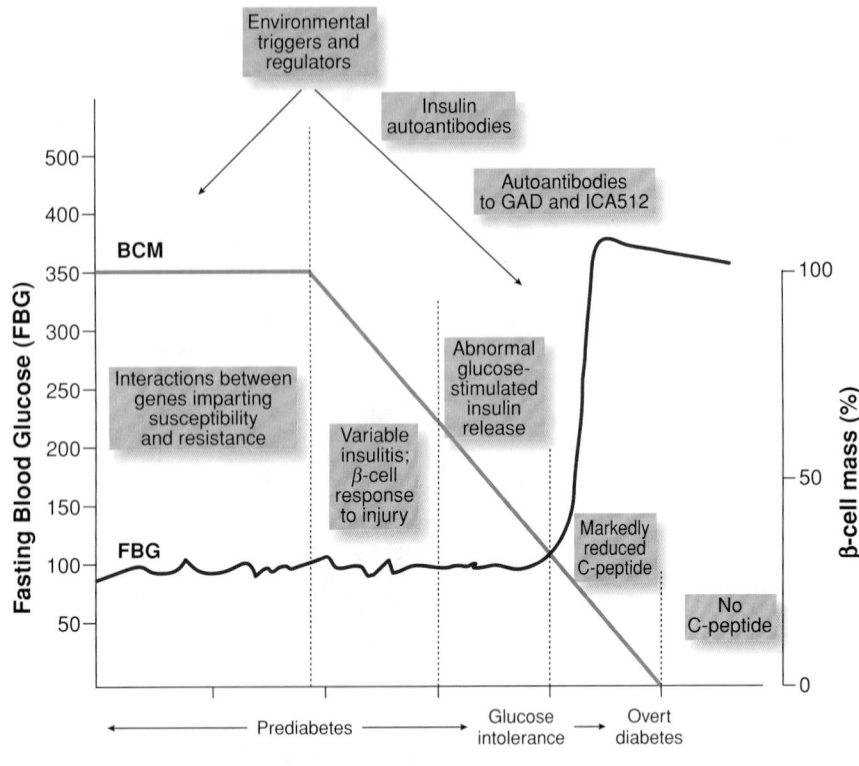

FIGURE 13-14. Pathogenetic stages in the development of type 1 diabetes (T1DM). The disease develops from an initial genetic susceptibility to defective recognition of beta cell epitopes and ends with essentially complete beta cell destruction in most patients. An environmental event is believed to trigger the immune attack, and people with certain genetic markers (human leukocyte antigen [HLA]-DR3 and -DR4) are particularly susceptible to the autoimmune disease. Patients with islet cell antibodies and normal blood glucose levels are considered to have a state of "pre–type 1 diabetes." The rate of decline in beta cell mass (*blue line*) determines the length of time between onset of beta cell destruction and eventual hyperglycemia (*red line,* fasting blood glucose) owing to loss of greater than 90% of functioning beta cells. In the serum, autoantibodies to insulin appear early, followed by antibodies to the beta cell antigen glutamic acid decarboxylase (GAD-65) and the islet cell antigen (ICA-512). *BCM* = beta cell mass.

GENETIC FACTORS: Evidence for the role of genetic factors in the pathogenesis of T1DM include the following:

1. Relatives of people with T1DM have an increased risk for development of T1DM. The lifetime risk of T1DM in the U.S. general population is 0.4%, but it is 3%–8% for first-degree relatives of people with T1DM. An identical twin of a T1DM patient has a 30%–50% risk of developing T1DM. Interestingly, children of fathers with T1DM are three times more likely to develop the disease than are children of mothers with T1DM. This suggests genetic imprinting involving paternal susceptibility genes or protective intrauterine or other maternal influences.
2. There are differences in risk among different ethnic groups who live in similar environments.
3. T1DM is strongly linked to the highly polymorphic HLA class II immune recognition molecules—DR and DQ—on chromosome 6. While only 45% of the population in the United States express DR3 or DR4, 95% of those who develop T1DM express these haplotypes. Because of the known role of HLA molecules in antigen presentation, the T1DM–HLA association is consistent with other evidence that T1DM has an autoimmune component.
4. Many other independent chromosomal regions (several of them non-HLA) are also associated with susceptibility to T1DM, but their contributions to the overall incidence of T1DM are small.

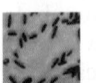

ETIOLOGIC FACTORS:

ENVIRONMENTAL FACTORS: Evidence for the role of environmental factors in the pathogenesis of T1DM includes the following:

■ Only 1/3 to 1/2 of monozygotic twins of T1DM patients develop T1DM.

■ Recent increases in T1DM incidence in some populations suggest a possible environmental role.
■ About 80% to 90% of patients with T1DM have no family history of the disease.
■ There are seasonal differences in the incidence of T1DM.

Viruses have been implicated in at least some cases. Thus, T1DM occasionally develops after infection with coxsackie B virus and, less often, mumps virus. Certain proteins may share antigenic determinants with human cell surface proteins and trigger autoreactivity by molecular mimicry. For example, a coxsackie B virus protein has close similarity to the human GAD-65 islet protein.

Dietary factors have been suggested as playing a role in the pathogenesis of T1DM. However, there is little to support this possibility.

 PATHOLOGY: As noted above, the most characteristic early lesion in the pancreas of T1DM is a chiefly lymphocytic infiltrate in the islets (insulitis), sometimes with scattered macrophages and neutrophils (Fig. 13-13). As the disease becomes chronic, islet beta cells become progressively depleted; eventually insulin-producing cells are no longer discernible. Loss of beta cells results in variably sized islets, many of which appear as ribbon-like cords that may be difficult to distinguish from surrounding acinar tissue. Islet fibrosis is uncommon. Unlike T2DM, amyloid is not seen in pancreatic islets in T1DM. The exocrine pancreas in chronic T1DM often shows diffuse interlobular and interacinar fibrosis, accompanied by atrophy of the acinar cells.

 CLINICAL FEATURES: The clinical picture of T1DM reflects lack of insulin, and insulin's unique role in energy metabolism in the body. The disease classically presents with acute metabolic decompensation, with hyperglycemia and ketoacidosis. Depending on the degree of absolute insulin deficiency, severe ketoacidosis may be preceded by weeks to months of increased urine output **(polyuria)** and increased thirst **(polydipsia).** Excessive diuresis results from the osmotic load from glucose in the urine. Weight loss in spite of increased appetite **(polyphagia)** results from unregulated catabolism of body stores of fat, protein and carbohydrate. Often the clinical onset of T1DM coincides with another acute illness, such as a febrile viral or bacterial infection (Fig. 13-12).

COMPLICATIONS OF DIABETES

The discovery of insulin in the early 20th century promised to cure diabetes, but as patients with diabetes lived longer, they began to develop complications. *The severity and chronicity of hyperglycemia in both T2DM and T1DM are the major pathogenetic factors leading to the "microvascular" complications of diabetes, including retinopathy, nephropathy and neuropathy. Thus, control of blood glucose remains the major means by which the development of microvascular diabetic complications can be minimized.* It has been more difficult to demonstrate that glucose control can prevent "macrovascular" (large-vessel) complications, meaning atherosclerosis and its sequelae (coronary artery disease, peripheral vascular disease and cerebrovascular disease). These macrovascular complications are especially common in patients with T2DM, in part since the patients tend to be older and frequently harbor additional cardiovascular risk factors, particularly dyslipoproteinemia, hypertension and hypercoagulability.

 **PATHOPHYSIOLOGY:** Several biochemical mechanisms have been proposed to account for the development of pathologic changes in diabetes.

ADVERSE EFFECTS ON KNOWN ATHEROSCLEROTIC CARDIOVASCULAR RISK FACTORS: In T2DM, the harmful pattern of pathway-selective insulin resistance and responsiveness promotes (1) fatty liver, (2) overproduction of triglyceride-rich apoB-lipoproteins, (3) impaired hepatic removal of atherogenic postprandial lipoproteins from the circulation, (4) vasoconstriction, (5) overexpression of tissue factor and (6) possibly salt retention. Enhanced production or action of angiotensin II may also play a role. Benefits have been shown from lipid-lowering agents (statins); treatment of hypertension, particularly with angiotensin-converting enzyme (ACE) inhibitors; and low daily doses of aspirin to inhibit platelet function. In T1DM, significant hypertriglyceridemia can develop in the context of poor glycemic control but usually corrects quickly once insulin doses and diet are properly managed.

EXCESSIVE REACTIVE OXYGEN SPECIES: In various cell types in culture, high concentrations of glucose increase production of reactive oxygen species (ROS) as byproducts of mitochondrial oxidative phosphorylation. Proposed mediators of glucose-induced oxidative damage include nitric oxide, superoxide anions and aldose reductase (see Chapter 1). Nevertheless, antioxidant supplementation does not affect the course of diabetes and atherosclerosis in people. Thus, there is no clinical evidence that ROS contribute to diabetes or its complications.

PROTEIN GLYCATION: Glucose covalently attaches to an assortment of proteins nonenzymatically, a process termed **glycation** (also termed **nonenzymatic glycosylation**). Glycation occurs roughly in proportion to the severity of hyperglycemia. Numerous cellular proteins are modified in this manner, including hemoglobin, components of the crystalline lens and cellular basement membrane proteins. A specific fraction of glycated hemoglobin in circulating red blood cells, hemoglobin A_{1c}, is used routinely to monitor the overall degree of hyperglycemia during the preceding 6–8 weeks. Because glycation of hemoglobin is irreversible, hemoglobin A_{1c} levels serve as a marker for glycemic control.

The initial glycation products (known chemically as Schiff bases) are labile and can dissociate rapidly. With time, these labile products undergo complex chemical rearrangements to form stable **advanced glycosylation end-products (AGEs),** which consist of glucose derivatives bound covalently to protein amino groups. AGE formation permanently alters protein structure and, possibly, function. For example, albumin and immunoglobulin G (IgG) do not normally bind to collagen, but they adhere to glycated collagen. Unstable chemical bonds in proteins containing AGEs can lead to physical cross-linking of nearby proteins, which may contribute to the characteristic thickening of vascular basement membranes in diabetes. Importantly, unlike the initial labile glycation products, AGEs can continue to cross-link proteins even if blood glucose returns to normal. Patients with diabetic retinopathy have higher levels of AGEs than do diabetics without retinopathy. Nevertheless, the role of AGEs in diabetic microvascular disease is uncertain. Compounds that inhibit AGE formation (e.g., aminoguanidine) do not protect people from diabetic complications, unlike experimental animals.

THE ALDOSE REDUCTASE PATHWAY: By mass action, hyperglycemia also increases glucose uptake by tissues that do not depend on insulin. Some of the increased flux of glucose is metabolized by aldose reductase, via the reaction:

$$\text{Glucose} + \text{NADPH} \rightarrow \text{Sorbitol} + \text{NADP}$$

This reaction depletes cellular reducing equivalents, which alters redox status and allows sorbitol to accumulate. Sorbitol's role, if any, in the complications of diabetes is undefined. Aldose reductase has a low affinity for glucose, but it generates considerable amounts of sorbitol in tissues when blood glucose is elevated. In the ocular lens, excess sorbitol may simply create an osmotic gradient that causes influx of fluid and consequent swelling. Increased intracellular sorbitol has been linked to decreased myo-inositol (a precursor of phosphoinositides), lower protein kinase C activity and inhibition of the plasma membrane sodium pump. However, inhibition of aldose reductase shows no benefit in human clinical trials, so the roles of aldose reductase and sorbitol in the complications of diabetes is unclear.

Atherosclerosis Is a Deadly Complication of Diabetes

Atherosclerotic heart disease and ischemic strokes account for over half of all deaths among adults with diabetes. The extent and severity of atherosclerotic lesions in medium-sized and large arteries are increased in patients with long-standing diabetes. Diabetes eliminates the usual protective effect of being female, and coronary artery disease develops at a younger age than in nondiabetic people. Moreover, mortality from myocardial infarction is higher in diabetics than in nondiabetics. As indicated above, patients with T2DM often have multiple risk factors of the metabolic syndrome that contribute to atherogenesis.

Atherosclerotic peripheral vascular disease, particularly of the lower extremities, commonly complicates diabetes. Vascular insufficiency may cause ulcers and gangrene of the toes and feet, ultimately necessitating amputation. *Diabetes accounts for more than 60% of nontraumatic limb amputations in the United States.*

Even though epidemiologic analyses suggest a correlation between chronic hyperglycemia and higher rates of cardiovascular disease, glucose levels per se are probably not the culprits. Most randomized clinical trials have failed to show that lower hemoglobin A_{1c} levels correlate with improved macrovascular outcomes in T2DM.

 **PATHOPHYSIOLOGY:** How diabetes promotes atherosclerosis is uncertain. There are at least three general schools of thought:

1. **Direct effects of diabetes or hyperglycemia on the arterial wall.** As noted above, however, none of the clinical therapies based on this idea (intensive glycemic control, aldose reductase inhibitors, antioxidants) reduces this type of complication of T2DM.
2. **Side effects of diabetic therapy,** such as high insulin concentrations associated with certain forms of treatment.
3. **Exacerbation of general risk factors for atherosclerosis** (e.g., hypertension, dyslipoproteinemia, hypercoagulability). Dyslipoproteinemia in T2DM is partly due to

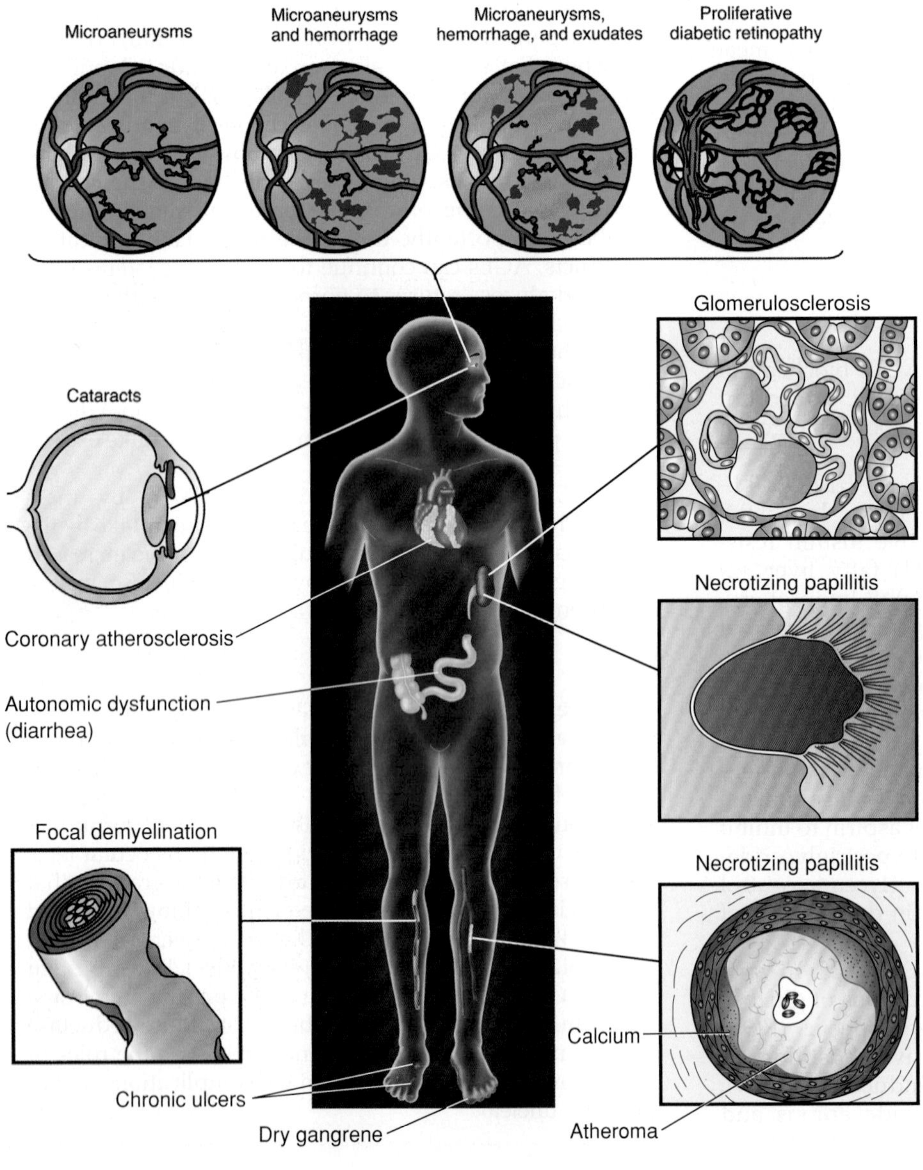

FIGURE 13-15. Secondary complications of diabetes. The effects of diabetes on a number of vital organs result in complications that may be incapacitating (cerebral and peripheral vascular disease), painful (neuropathy) or life-threatening (coronary artery disease, pyelonephritis with necrotizing papillitis).

Labels in figure: Microaneurysms; Microaneurysms and hemorrhage; Microaneurysms, hemorrhage, and exudates; Proliferative diabetic retinopathy; Glomerulosclerosis; Cataracts; Coronary atherosclerosis; Autonomic dysfunction (diarrhea); Focal demyelination; Necrotizing papillitis; Necrotizing papillitis; Chronic ulcers; Dry gangrene; Calcium; Atheroma

hepatic and intestinal overproduction of triglyceride-rich apoB-lipoproteins. A defect in lipoprotein lipase impairs clearance of chylomicrons and causes postprandial hypertriglyceridemia. In addition, the liver's uptake of atherogenic postprandial remnant lipoprotein particles is impaired. At this point, the most successful strategies to reduce cardiovascular events in T2DM involve management of these risk factors (e.g., administration of statins, antihypertensive agents and low-dose aspirin). Gastric bypass surgery for weight loss has been associated with substantial decreases in cardiovascular deaths.

Diabetic Microvascular Disease Is Responsible for Many of the Complications of Diabetes

Arteriolosclerosis and capillary basement membrane thickening are characteristic vascular changes in diabetes (see Chapter 16). The frequent occurrence of hypertension contributes to the development of the arteriolar lesions. Deposition of basement membrane proteins, which may also become glycated, increases in diabetes. Platelet aggregation in smaller blood vessels and impaired fibrinolysis may also contribute to diabetic microvascular disease.

However it develops, the effects of microvascular disease on tissue perfusion and wound healing are profound. Blood flow to the heart, already compromised by large-vessel disease (coronary atherosclerosis), is reduced. Chronic ulcers due to trauma and infection of the feet heal poorly in diabetic patients, in part because of microvascular disease. The major complications of diabetic microvascular disease involve the kidney and the retina (Fig. 13-15).

Diabetic Nephropathy

Diabetes is the leading cause of renal failure in the United States, accounting for almost half of new cases. One third of patients with T1DM ultimately develop renal failure, as do up to 20% of patients with T2DM. Some patients with T1DM may die from uremia, but most of those who develop nephropathy die of cardiovascular disease, which is 40 times more common in T1DM patients who have end-stage renal disease. The prevalence of diabetic nephropathy increases with the severity and duration of hyperglycemia. *Kidney disease due to diabetes is the most common reason for renal transplantation in adults.*

Initially, hyperglycemia leads to glomerular hypertension and renal hyperperfusion (Fig. 13-16). Increased glomerular pressure favors deposition of protein in the mesangium, resulting in glomerulosclerosis and, eventually, renal failure. AGEs and lipoprotein abnormalities may contribute to chemical changes in the glomerular basement membrane. The diabetic kidney produces growth factors, particularly transforming growth factor-β (TGF-β), that have been implicated in some of the cellular abnormalities. In animal models, inhibiting TGF-β attenuates renal disease. Whatever the underlying mechanism, strict control of blood glucose and blood pressure retards development of diabetic nephropathy. ACE inhibitors or angiotensin receptor blockers reduce systemic blood pressure, glomerular hypertension and renal perfusion, and thus retard progression of diabetic nephropathy.

Eventually, a unique lesion, **Kimmelstiel-Wilson disease or nodular glomerulosclerosis** (see Chapter 22), develops. It

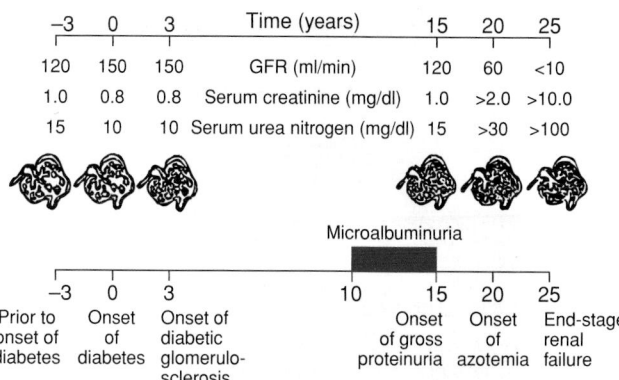

FIGURE 13-16. Natural history of diabetic nephropathy. Initially, renal hypertrophy and hyperfiltration lead to an increase in the glomerular filtration rate (GFR). Once the decline in renal function begins, on average at least 10 years after the onset of diabetes, leakage of a small amount of serum albumin into the urine (microalbuminuria) is the first abnormality that is easily and reliably measured. The elevation in serum creatinine and gross proteinuria occur much later.

assumes two microscopic patterns. Most commonly, spherical masses of basement membrane–like material accumulate in glomerular lobules (Fig. 13-17). Less often, this material deposits more diffusely and somewhat irregularly throughout the glomerulus. Clinically, the onset of glomerular disease is heralded by the appearance in the urine of small amounts of serum albumin, **microalbuminuria**. Proteinuria increases with time and with progressive decline in renal function.

Diabetic Retinopathy

Diabetic retinopathy is the leading cause of blindness in the Unites States in adults under 74. The risk is higher in T1DM than in T2DM. In fact, 10% of patients with T1DM of 30 years' duration become legally blind. Nevertheless, as there are many more patients with T2DM, they are the most

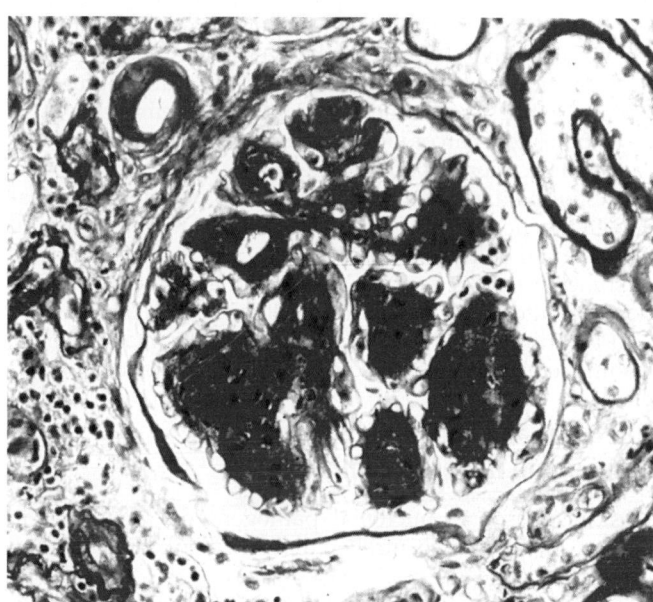

FIGURE 13-17. Diabetic glomerulosclerosis. A periodic acid–Schiff stain demonstrates nodular accumulations of basement membrane–like material in the glomerulus.

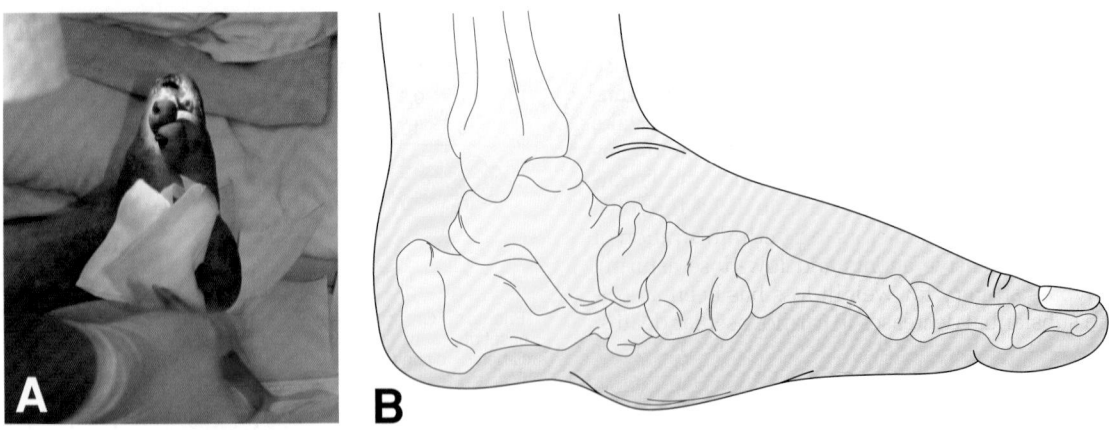

FIGURE 13-18. Foot complications of diabetes mellitus. A. Foot ulcer. **B.** Charcot foot.

numerous patients with diabetic retinopathy. Retinopathy is the most devastating ophthalmic complication of diabetes, although glaucoma, cataracts and corneal disease are also increased. Like nephropathy, the prevalence of diabetic retinopathy reflects the duration and degree of glycemic control (also see Chapter 33).

Diabetic Neuropathy Affects Sensory and Autonomic Innervation

Peripheral sensory impairment and autonomic nerve dysfunction are among the most common and distressing complications of diabetes. Changes in the nerves are complex, with abnormalities in axons, the myelin sheath and Schwann cells. Microvasculopathy involving the small blood vessels of nerves contributes to diabetic neuropathy. Hyperglycemia increases the perception of pain, independently of any structural lesions in the nerves.

Peripheral neuropathy is initially characterized by pain and abnormal sensations in the extremities. However, fine touch, pain detection and proprioception are ultimately lost. As a result, patients with diabetes tend to ignore irritation and minor trauma to the feet, joints and legs, and they develop foot ulcers (Fig. 13-18), which are common in patients with severe diabetes. Peripheral neuropathy also contributes to Charcot joint, a painless destructive joint disease that occasionally occurs (Fig. 13-18).

Abnormalities in autonomic regulation of cardiovascular and GI functions frequently lead to postural hypotension and altered gut motility (e.g., gastroparesis and diarrhea). Erectile dysfunction and retrograde ejaculation are other complications of autonomic dysfunction, although vascular disease also contributes. Hypotonic urinary bladder may develop, leading to urinary retention and predisposing to infection.

Bacterial and Fungal Infections Complicate Hyperglycemia

Host responses to microbial pathogens are abnormal in patients with poorly controlled diabetes. Leukocyte function

is compromised and immune responses are blunted. Before the use of insulin, tuberculosis and purulent infections were often life-threatening. Now, patients with well-controlled diabetes are much less susceptible to infections. However, **urinary tract infections** continue to be problematic because glucose makes the urine an enriched culture medium. Urinary retention from autonomic neuropathy may exacerbate this tendency. Infection ascending from the bladder to the kidney (i.e., **pyelonephritis**) is thus a constant concern. **Renal papillary necrosis** may be a devastating complication of urinary tract infection.

A dreaded infectious complication of poorly controlled diabetes is **mucormycosis**. This often fatal fungal infection tends to originate in the nasopharynx or paranasal sinuses and spreads rapidly to the orbit and brain (see Chapter 9).

Gestational Diabetes Puts Mother and Fetus at Risk

Gestational diabetes develops in only a few percent of seemingly healthy women during pregnancy. It may continue after parturition in a small proportion of these patients. Pregnancy is a state of IRg, but only pregnant women with impaired beta cell secretion of insulin become diabetic. Abnormalities in the amount and timing of pancreatic insulin secretion predispose these women to overt T2DM later in life.

Poor control of diabetes in pregnancy (either gestational diabetes or preexisting diabetes) may lead to the birth of large infants, complicate labor and delivery and necessitate a cesarean section. The fetal pancreas tries to compensate for poor maternal control of diabetes during gestation. Such fetuses develop beta cell hyperplasia, which may lead to hypoglycemia at birth and in the early postnatal period.

Infants of diabetic mothers have a 5% to 10% incidence of major developmental abnormalities, including anomalies of the heart and great vessels and neural tube defects, such as anencephaly and spina bifida. The frequency of these lesions is a function of the control of maternal diabetes during early gestation.

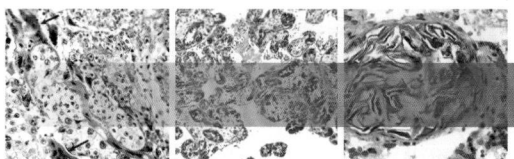

14

The Pathology of Pregnancy

David A. Schwartz

OBSTETRIC PATHOLOGY AND THE PATHOLOGY OF PREGNANCY

Normal pregnancy is characterized by profound changes in almost every maternal organ system in order to accommodate the demands of the fetoplacental unit. An important component of obstetric pathology is the study of the placenta, which has two separate vascular supplies from two genetically distinct individuals. It invades its host under normal circumstances, but can also result in potentially fatal cancer.

PLACENTA

Anatomy

The placenta includes the **placental disc, umbilical cord** and **extraplacental membranes** (Fig. 14-1). It is a flattened discoid organ with two surfaces. The fetus faces one aspect **(fetal** or **chorionic surface),** which is covered by membranes, the **amnion** and **chorion**. These contain the **amniotic fluid** that surrounds the fetus. The opposite surface is the **maternal surface** (or the **decidual surface,** since the endometrium becomes decidualized during pregnancy).

Fetal blood enters the placenta through two umbilical arteries that spiral around an umbilical vein. Each artery supplies half of the placenta. The umbilical cord inserts into the chorionic surface on the placenta. The major branches of the umbilical arteries and vein (chorionic plate blood vessels) then branch along the surface of the disc and penetrate into the placental disc to form the chorionic villous tree. Primary stem villi originate at the chorionic plate and contain the major branches of the umbilical arteries and veins. These villous trunks progressively subdivide into smaller branches, ending in the terminal (or, tertiary) villi, where oxygen and nutrient transport occurs. At term, the terminal villi constitute 40% of the villous volume and 60% of villous cross-sections.

The **decidua** forms the border between fetal tissue composing the villous trees and the underlying uterus. The decidua contains 80–100 small uterine arteries (**spiral**

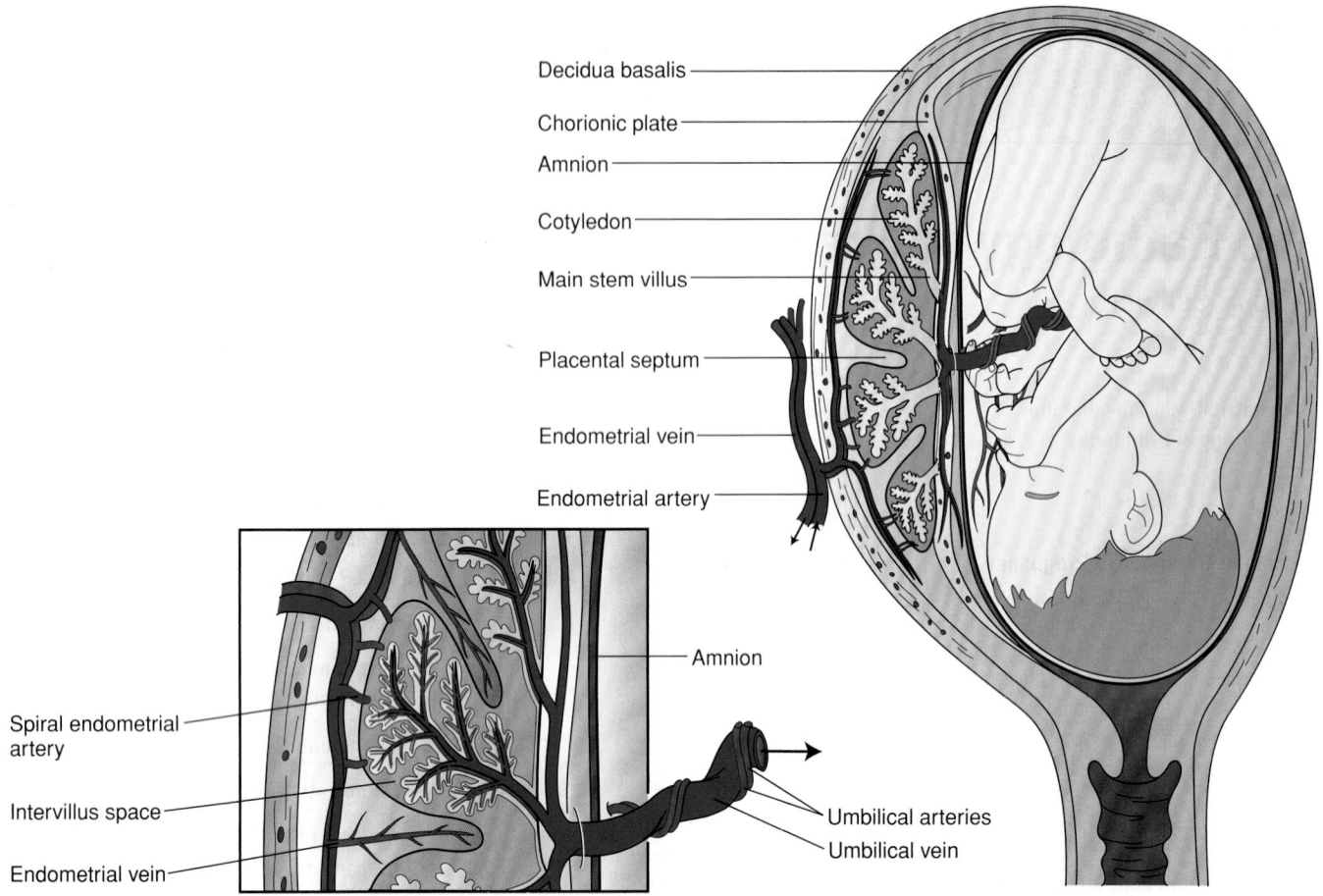

Decidua basalis

Chorionic plate

Amnion

Cotyledon

Main stem villus

Placental septum

Endometrial vein

Endometrial artery

Amnion

Spiral endometrial artery

Intervillus space

Endometrial vein

Umbilical arteries

Umbilical vein

FIGURE 14-1. **Modern diagram of the pregnant uterus including fetus, placenta and circulation.**

arterioles, branches of the myometrial arteries), which supply the placenta with maternal blood (Fig. 14-2). These arteries undergo a series of **remodeling** changes that decrease vascular resistance to uterine blood flow and support the developing placenta and fetus. Each spiral arteriole delivers maternal blood to the center of an anatomic subunit of the placenta, the **cotyledon.** Maternal blood entering the placental disc is no longer confined to a vessel, but instead occupies a cavity, the **intervillous space,** where it exchanges oxygen and nutrients. The maternal and fetal circulations in the placenta are entirely separate systems (Fig. 14-3).

The terminal villus is the placenta's functional unit of exchange. The chorionic villous tree is covered by the trophoblastic layer (Greek *trephein*: "to feed," *blastos:* "germinator"). It consists of an inner layer of **cytotrophoblast (Langhans cells),** a middle layer of **intermediate trophoblast** and an outer layer of **syncytiotrophoblast.** The villous stroma is loose mesenchyme containing embryonal macrophages, termed **Hofbauer cells.** In the third trimester, syncytiotrophoblast nuclei aggregate to form multinuclear protrusions **(syncytial knots).** In other areas along the villous surface, syncytium between the knots becomes markedly attenuated. At these points, the trophoblastic cytoplasm comes into direct contact with the endothelium of the fetal capillaries to form the **vasculosyncytial membrane.** These specialized zones facilitate gas and nutrient transfer across the placenta.

In addition to releasing waste and absorbing oxygen and nutrients, the villi are hormonally active. The syncytiotrophoblast secretes **human chorionic gonadotropin (hCG),** which prevents degeneration of the corpus luteum. It also secretes **progesterone** to maintain the integrity of the decidua and **human placental lactogen (HPL),** which raises maternal glucose levels and so assists in adequate fetal nutrition.

Placental Size

The placenta increases in size as gestation progresses. For example, the mean placental weight at 30 weeks' gestation is 316 grams, at 35 weeks 434 grams and at term (40 weeks) 537 grams. An abnormally small placenta (≤10th percentile for gestational age) is associated with maternal hypertensive disease of pregnancy and low birth weight. It can cause a poor fetal outcome, including neurologic abnormalities and perinatal death. Abnormally large placentas (≥90th percentile) also occur and can result from villous edema, fetal hydrops, placental hemorrhage, syphilis, placental tumors and maternal diabetes. At term, 1 gram of placenta can oxygenate 7 grams of fetal tissue. This relationship, called the **fetal–placental weight ratio,** determines how chronic uteroplacental malperfusion, or placental insufficiency, can occur. If the fetus is too large for its placenta, or the placenta is too small, the increased fetal–placental weight ratio can

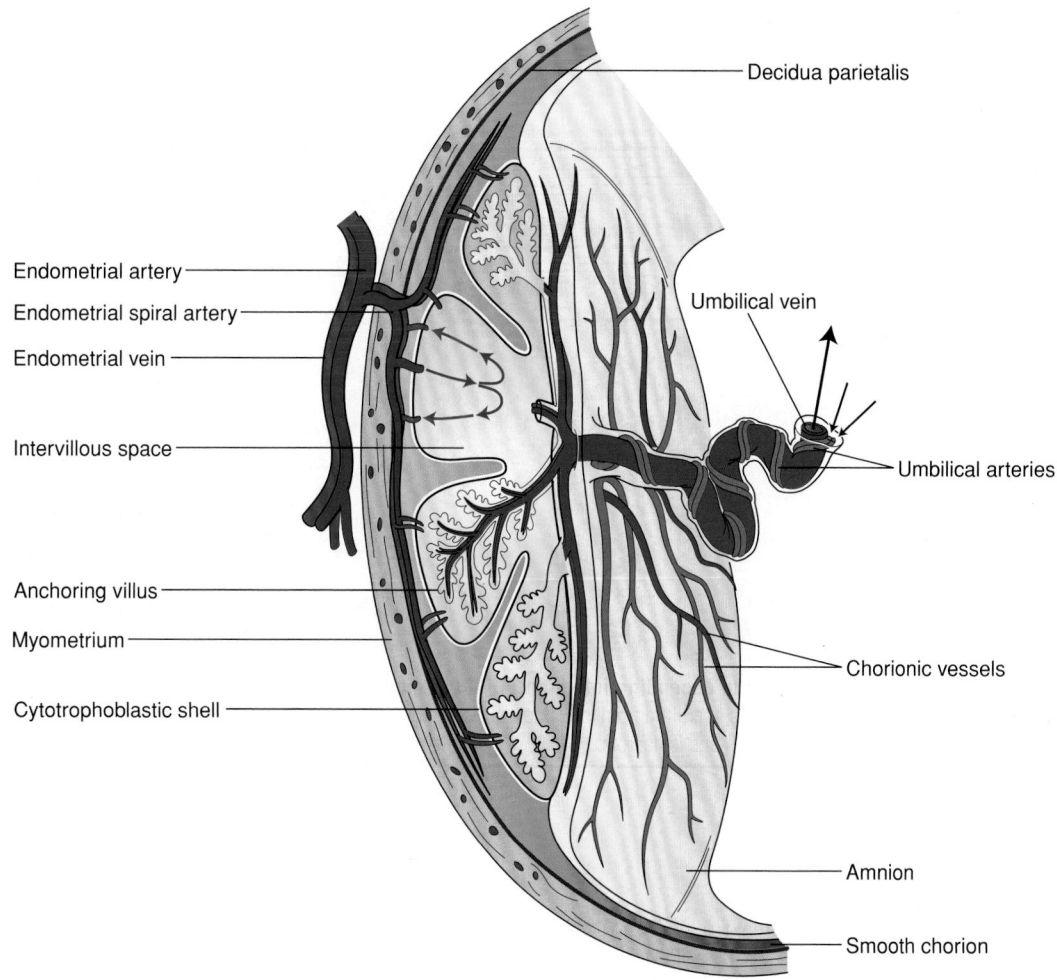

Decidua parietalis

Endometrial artery

Endometrial spiral artery

Endometrial vein

Umbilical vein

Intervillous space

Umbilical arteries

Anchoring villus

Myometrium

Chorionic vessels

Cytotrophoblastic shell

Amnion

Smooth chorion

FIGURE 14-2. Cross-sectional diagram of the placenta and its circulation.

contribute to a poor obstetric outcome. Abnormally thin placentas (<2 cm thickness at term) can also be associated with neonatal problems.

Placental Shape

A typical placental disc is round or ovoid.

- **Bilobed placenta** (2%–8%) appears as two equal-sized discs, separated by membranes.
- **Succenturiate placenta** (5%) is bilobed, with one lobe smaller than the other. Bilobed and succenturiate placentas have membranous blood vessels connecting each lobe, which can be susceptible to damage by compression, thrombosis or rupture.
- **Vasa previa** (1 in 2500) refers to membranous vessels situated between the fetus and the internal cervical os. Rupture of these vessels before or during delivery produces fetal bleeding and can rapidly result in fetal exsanguination.
- **Circumvallate placenta** (1%–6%) features membranes that extend away from the margin toward the center of the placental disc. The margin exhibits fibrin and clotted blood. It is thought to result from either marginal hemorrhage early in development or a deep implantation of the fetus into the decidua.

- **Circummarginate placenta** (4%) differs from circumvallate placenta by not having the reflected membranes fold back.

Placental Implantation

The placenta is normally implanted in the uterine wall above the internal cervical os. It may implant at the lower portion of the uterus and either partially or completely cover the internal os, a condition termed **placenta previa** (0.3%–1% of pregnancies). Risk factors include smoking, increased age, multiple prior pregnancies, previous cesarean sections and prior abortions. Placenta previa must be recognized before delivery to avoid the fetus being delivered through its own placenta, risking life-threatening hemorrhage. Placenta previa is one of the most frequent causes of 3rd-trimester bleeding and entails a high risk of abruption, postpartum hemorrhage, prolapsed umbilical cord, fetal malpresentation, intrauterine growth restriction and fetal and perinatal mortality. Placenta previa is often associated with another abnormal condition, placenta accreta (see below), in which case it is **placenta previa accreta**.

Ectopic pregnancy occurs when a placenta implants outside the uterine cavity. It usually occurs in the fallopian tube, but 2% of ectopic pregnancies occur in the ovary, cervix or abdomen. Unless removed surgically, abdominal pregnancy carries a high maternal mortality.

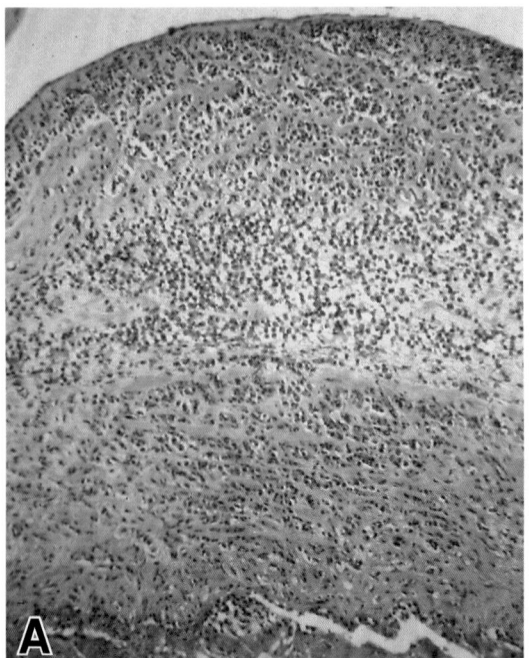
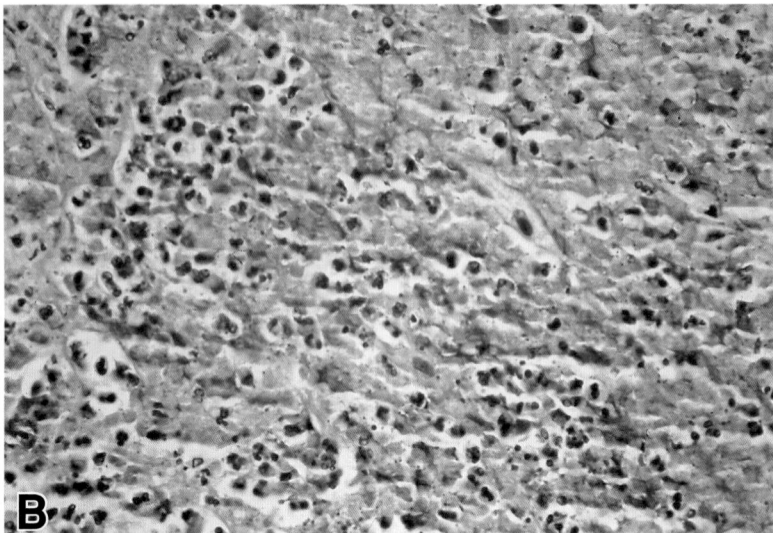

FIGURE 14-3. Maternal inflammatory responses to ascending infection. A. Acute chorioamnionitis (maternal inflammatory response [MIR]). The chorion contains numerous acute inflammatory cells, recruited from the maternal intervillous space. **B. Acute necrotizing deciduitis (MIR).** The decidua contains numerous inflammatory cells of maternal origin and is necrotic.

Abnormalities of the Umbilical Cord

At term, the umbilical cord normally measures 35–100 cm long. Abnormally short umbilical cords are associated with increased perinatal mortality, intrauterine fetal distress and intrauterine growth restriction. The point of insertion of the cord is usually at or near the center of the placental disc, but 7% show a **marginal insertion,** at the placenta's edge. About 1% of umbilical cords insert into the membranes, called a **velamentous** or **membranous insertion**. Velamentous and marginal cord insertions are often seen in spontaneous abortions and fetuses with congenital anomalies. A serious potential complication of velamentous vessels is **vasa previa** (see above).

IMMUNE TOLERANCE IN PREGNANCY

The Mother Tolerates the Fetus and Placenta as Allografts

The conceptus is genetically different from the mother and thus represents an allograft. Why, then, does the mother not reject her fetus as foreign tissue, as she would with transplantation of other genetically disparate tissues? **Immune tolerance in pregnancy** describes the absence of a maternal immune response against the fetus and its placenta.

PATHOPHYSIOLOGY: The placenta is the major immunologic barrier between the mother and the conceptus and creates an immunologically privileged site.

■ The placental trophoblast does not express major histocompatibility complex (MHC) class I isotypes human

leukocyte antigen (HLA)-A and HLA-B. The absence of these molecules prevents recognition of the fetus as "foreign tissue."
■ The trophoblast expresses atypical MHC class I isotypes HLA-E and HLA-G, which may prevent attack by maternal natural killer (NK) cells.
■ The trophoblast forms a continuous syncytium, lacking intercellular spaces or connections between cells. This situation serves to restrict passage of migratory immune cells between the maternal and fetal bloodstreams.
■ The placenta permits some maternal immunoglobulin G (IgG) antibody to cross the vasculosyncytial barrier and enter the fetal circulation to provide immune protection against infectious diseases.
■ Fetal cells that have entered the maternal circulation elicit antibodies targeting fetal antigens. If there are major blood group differences between mother and fetus, maternal antibodies against fetal ABO antigens can develop and cause antibody-mediated destruction of fetal erythrocytes, leading to **hemolytic disease of the newborn (HDN)**. However, ABO HDN is rare because maternal anti-A and anti-B antibodies are of the IgM class, which does not cross the placenta.
■ The placenta secretes **neurokinin B,** a peptide that binds the immune-cloaking molecule **phosphocholine**.
■ Regulatory T lymphocytes (T_{reg}; see Chapters 4 and 11) and NK cells are thought to play a role in avoidance of the maternal immunologic rejection by fetal tissues, but the mechanisms are uncertain.

PLACENTAL INFECTIONS

Chorioamnionitis Is the Hallmark of Ascending Infection

Infectious organisms, almost exclusively bacteria, can ascend from the maternal birth canal, pass through the cervical os and infect the decidua and placental tissues, the amniotic fluid and, potentially, the fetus.

 **ETIOLOGIC FACTORS:** Acute chorioamnionitis is usually caused by bacteria that are normally present in the maternal cervicovaginal canal. The most common bacterial causes of chorioamnionitis are group B *Streptococcus* sp., *Escherichia coli, Enterococcus,* other streptococcal species, *Staphylococcus* sp., Gram-negative bacilli, *Bacteroides, Mycoplasma hominis* and *Ureaplasma.*

 PATHOLOGY: Upon reaching the uterine cavity, bacteria elicit a maternal inflammatory response (MIR). Maternal neutrophils circulating in the intervillous space migrate upward toward the fetal surface, or chorionic plate, resulting in **acute subchorionitis.** The neutrophils then migrate up from the subchorion into the chorion. Maternal neutrophils are recruited from the decidual blood vessels and enter the chorion of the extraplacental membranes (Fig. 14-3A). Maternal neutrophil infiltration of either the chorion of the placenta or its membranes is termed **acute chorioamnionitis.** Maternal inflammatory cells can also migrate from the decidual and spiral arteries into the decidua underlying the extraplacental membranes or the placental disc to cause **acute deciduitis.** Deciduitis may be so

severe as to cause necrosis of the decidua **(necrotizing deciduitis)** (Fig. 14-3B), or it can form small collections of neutrophils, called **decidual microabscesses.** Because the maternal spiral arteries, which supply the placenta with oxygenated maternal blood, are in the decidua, decidual infection can threaten the pregnancy.

 PATHOLOGY: A fetal inflammatory response (FIR) may also develop. **Acute chorionic vasculitis,** a component of FIR, occurs when fetal neutrophils migrate from the fetal bloodstream into the walls of the large chorionic plate vessels (branches of the umbilical cord vessels) at the surface of the placental disc (Fig. 14-4A). Fetal neutrophils also migrate from the lumen of the umbilical cord blood vessels into the muscular vessel walls, resulting in a vasculitis of the cord vessels termed **acute funisitis** (Fig. 14-4B). Fetal neutrophils can migrate completely through umbilical vessel walls and infiltrate the mesenchyme (Wharton jelly). Cerebral palsy is statistically associated with severe FIR but not with mild to moderate MIR (see below).

 CLINICAL FEATURES: Acute chorioamnionitis (10% of placentas) can cause preterm labor, premature rupture of membranes, fetal and neonatal infections and intrauterine hypoxia. The mother may have fever, uterine tenderness and foul-smelling or cloudy amniotic fluid. Major risks are postpartum endometritis and pelvic sepsis with venous thrombosis.

In preterm, low–birth-weight (<2500 grams) infants, especially very low weight (<1500 grams), acute chorioamnionitis often leads to severe neurologic disease, stillbirth,

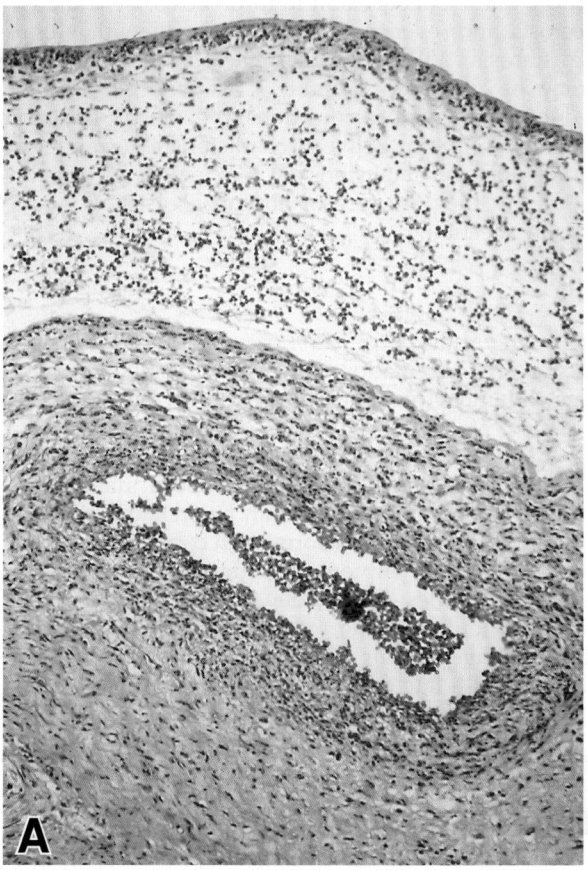

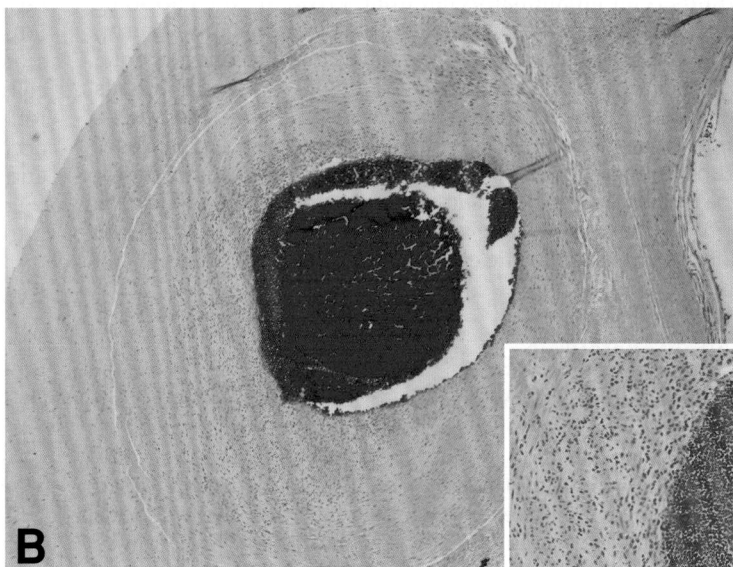

FIGURE 14-4. Fetal inflammatory responses to ascending infection. A. Acute chorionic vasculitis (fetal inflammatory response [FIR]). The wall of this large chorionic plate blood vessel is infiltrated by fetal neutrophils. The overlying chorion shows acute chorioamnionitis. **B. Acute funisitis (FIR).** The muscular wall of this umbilical vessel contains numerous fetal inflammatory cells (**inset:** higher magnification).

neonatal sepsis and death. However, it can also cause morbidity in full-term infants. The risks of chorioamnionitis to the fetus include (1) pneumonia after inhalation of infected amniotic fluid; (2) skin or eye infections from direct contact with organisms in the fluid; and (3) neonatal gastritis, enteritis or peritonitis from ingestion of infected fluid.

Amniotic Infection Syndrome Can Cause Intrauterine Fetal Infection

Amniotic Fluid

Amniotic fluid is initially formed as a transudate of maternal fluids, but later a combination of the amnion, fetal lungs and kidneys contributes to its formation. The fetus also inhales and exhales amniotic fluid during breathing movements before birth.

Intra-Amniotic Infection

Amniotic fluid is normally sterile, but in some cases it can be seeded with bacteria. Amniotic fluid infection gives microorganisms a portal of entry into the fetus, most frequently the respiratory tract, from which intrauterine infection can enter the bloodstream and disseminate to other fetal organs. These infants can be born with "congenital" or early-onset neonatal infections, including pneumonia, sepsis and meningitis. Placentas of these infants typically demonstrate acute chorioamnionitis, often with a component of FIR. Amniotic infections can portend a serious or fatal outcome for the neonate.

Villitis Can Indicate a Maternal Infection

Villitis is an inflammatory infiltrate involving the chorionic villi. Microorganisms in the maternal blood, usually viruses, or less commonly bacteria, can gain access to the placenta. Villitis can also be of unknown etiology. Potential agents include (1) bacteria (*Listeria*, *Treponema pallidum*, *Mycobacterium. tuberculosis*, *Mycoplasma* sp., *Chlamydia* sp.), (2) viruses (rubella, cytomegalovirus, herpes), (3) parasites and protozoa (*Toxoplasma* sp., *Trypanosoma cruzi*) and (4) fungi (*Candida* sp.). Villitis can interfere with oxygen transport to the fetus, and transmission of the etiologic agent through the villi can infect the fetus.

Cytomegalovirus

Cytomegalovirus (CMV) is one of the TORCH agents (see Chapter 6) that can cause congenital infection in a newborn. Intrauterine infection can occur when the mother acquires a primary (first-time) infection while pregnant—this form of transplacental infection is potentially the most serious to the fetus. Less dangerous to the infant is reactivation of latent maternal CMV infection during pregnancy. In Western nations, 8% of women develop primary infection during pregnancy, of which 1/2 will transmit the virus to their fetus. In developing nations and in poorer socioeconomic groups, congenital CMV infections are less common, because those women most likely were exposed to CMV previously.

 CLINICAL FEATURES: Among fetuses infected with CMV, 1/4 are born with clinical symptoms. Some 5%–10% of neonates will not have symptoms at birth but will subsequently develop hearing loss, visual

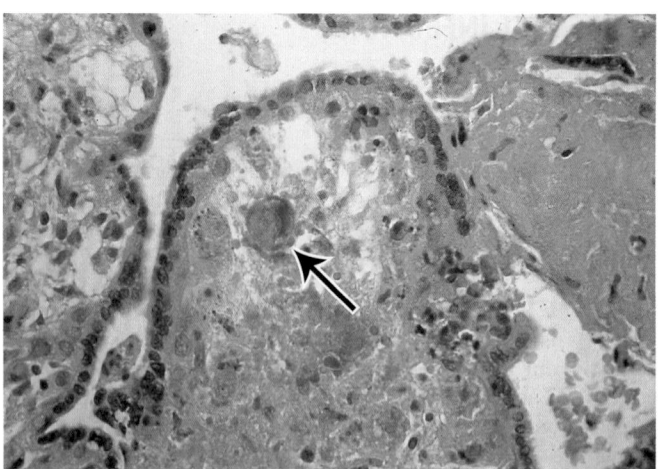

FIGURE 14-5. Chronic villitis caused by cytomegalovirus (CMV). The villi are infiltrated by chronic inflammatory cells. An enlarged cell with a CMV inclusion is present (*arrow*).

impairment and mental retardation. In more severe cases, generalized infections of the infant can occur, including low birth weight, microcephaly, seizures and skin manifestations. Multiorgan dissemination is characterized by cerebral abnormalities, splenomegaly and hepatitis. Occasionally, congenital CMV may be lethal for the infant.

 PATHOLOGY: CMV enters the placenta from maternal blood and results in chronic villitis. Endothelial infection causes cellular swelling, luminal occlusion, endothelial necrosis and eventual vascular destruction. These effects result in thrombosis, ischemic villous necrosis and, eventually, avascular villi with villous scarring (fibrosis). Villous stromal macrophages (Hofbauer cells) may be increased. Remote CMV infection can be reflected in villous microcalcifications. When CMV infection occurs near the time of delivery, characteristic intranuclear and intracytoplasmic inclusions of CMV may be identifiable (Fig. 14-5), but they are rare or absent in cases of remote intrauterine infection.

Syphilis

The agent of syphilis, *T. pallidum* (see Chapter 9), can pass from the maternal circulation to the fetal circulation through chorionic villi, most frequently during the secondary phase.

 CLINICAL FEATURES: Syphilis is an important cause of stillbirth, and liveborn infants with early congenital syphilis may be premature. Nevertheless, more than half of newborns with congenital syphilis are asymptomatic. Symptomatic infants suffer hepatosplenomegaly, snuffles, lymphadenopathy, mucocutaneous lesions, pneumonia, edema, rash, hemolytic anemia or thrombocytopenia at birth or within the first 4–8 weeks of age. Children with late congenital syphilis show numerous facial and other defects (see Chapter 6).

 PATHOLOGY: The placenta in infants with congenital syphilis can be unusually heavy, and may weigh 1000 or more grams. Villi appear hypercellular and enlarged, usually with Hofbauer cell hyperplasia

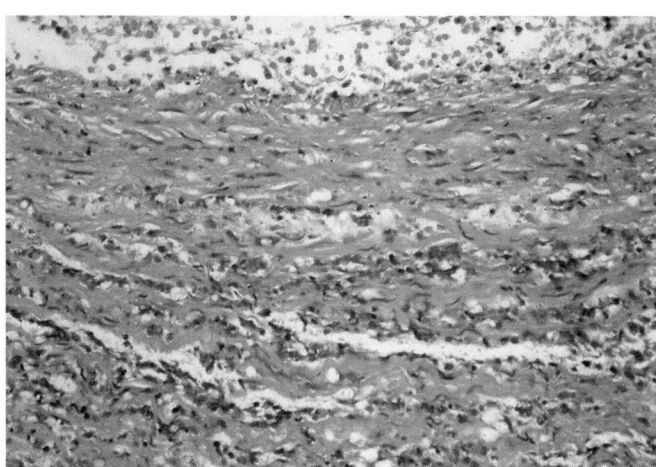

FIGURE 14-6. **Necrotizing funisitis due to syphilis.** The smooth muscle cells of the umbilical vessels are necrotic, and "smudgy" chronic inflammatory cells are causing a funisitis.

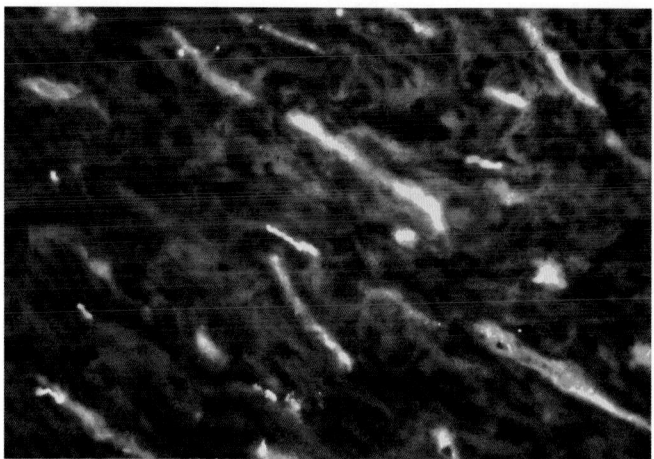

FIGURE 14-7. **Spirochetes of *Treponema pallidum* in the wall of an umbilical cord blood vessel with necrotizing funisitis.** The organisms are visible using a fluorescent antibody stain.

and stromal fibrosis. Chronic villitis is usually present and plasma cells may also be abundant in the decidua. The umbilical cord can demonstrate an unusual finding, termed **necrotizing funisitis**. This condition grossly resembles a "barber pole" and microscopically demonstrates smooth muscle necrosis of muscular walls of umbilical vessels and perivascular concentric rings of smudgy-appearing chronic inflammatory cells, necrotic debris or calcium deposits (Fig. 14-6). Spirochetes in placental tissues are visualized using the Warthin-Starry silver stain or fluorescent antibodies (Fig. 14-7).

Listeria

Listeriosis is a potentially serious infection most commonly acquired by eating food contaminated with the Gram-positive bacillus *Listeria monocytogenes*. Pregnant women and their infants are at increased risk for *listeriosis*. The bacteria can circulate in the maternal blood and infect the placenta and the fetus, causing miscarriage, stillbirth and premature delivery. In infants, *Listeria* infection is characterized by

granulomatous rash and pyogenic granulomas throughout the body. *Listeria* is also responsible for 5% of cases of neonatal meningitis.

 PATHOLOGY: Placentas infected with *Listeria* contain numerous microabscesses that destroy villi and produce an acute intervillositis (Fig. 14-8). Necrotizing chorioamnionitis and severe funisitis are frequent.

Toxoplasma

Toxoplasma gondii, a parasite in cats, is a protozoan that is a potential health problem in pregnancy. Infections acquired by the fetus early in pregnancy are more likely to be severe than those acquired later.

 CLINICAL FEATURES: The classical triad of congenital toxoplasmosis, namely, hydrocephalus, intracranial calcifications and chorioretinitis, is well known but does not occur in most infants infected in

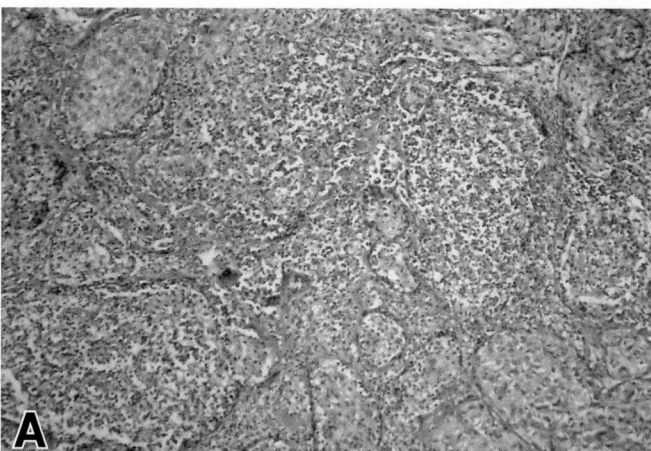

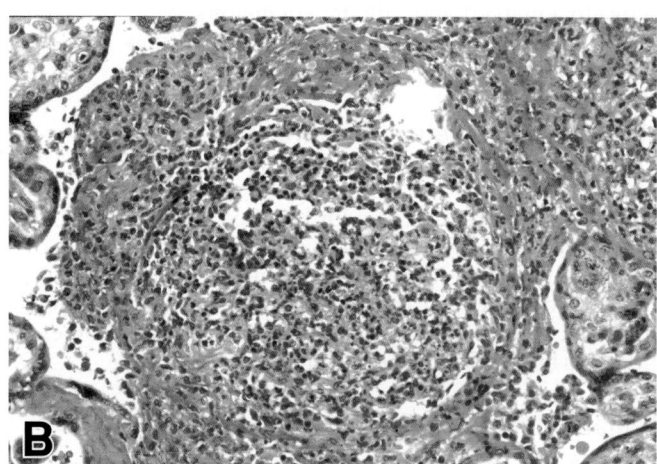

FIGURE 14-8. ***Listeria* infection. A. Necrotizing villitis and intervillositis with microabscesses caused by *Listeria monocytogenes*. B. Higher magnification of acute villitis caused *by L. monocytogenes*.** The central villus has been destroyed by acute inflammation and has the appearance of a microabscess. Neutrophils extend from the inflamed villus into the intervillous space and adjacent villi.

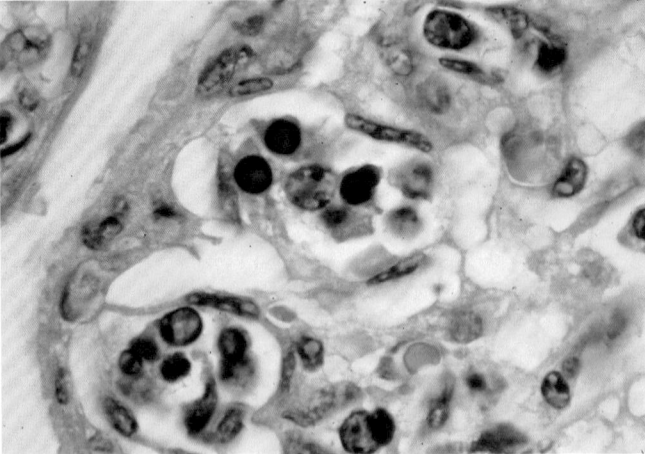

FIGURE 14-9. Intranuclear inclusions ("lantern cells") of erythrovirus (parvovirus) in nucleated fetal red blood cells in the placenta.

utero. Severe manifestations of congenital toxoplasmosis include encephalitis, multiple organ infection, epilepsy, mental retardation, blindness and stillbirth.

 PATHOLOGY: Characteristic cysts of *Toxoplasma* can be present in the subamnionic connective tissue, chorionic villi, trophoblast and umbilical cord. Like syphilis and CMV, Hofbauer cell hyperplasia can also occur in toxoplasmosis. In some cases, thrombosis of placental blood vessels occurs, with or without calcification.

Erythrovirus (Parvovirus B19) Causes Fetal Hydrops and Stillbirth

Erythrovirus, formerly called parvovirus B19, is a DNA virus that causes ecthyma infectiosum, a benign disease with fever and rash in children. When a pregnant woman becomes infected, the risk for stillbirth rises, especially if the infection occurs in the first and second trimester. Mothers transmit the agent to their fetus in 30% of cases of acute maternal infection. The virus produces distinctive ground-glass intranuclear inclusions, termed "lantern cells," which are most evident in nucleated fetal red blood (Fig. 14-9). Placentas are typically enlarged and villi are edematous. Newborns tend to be hydropic (Fig. 14-10) and anemic, and may have cardiac involvement.

Human Immunodeficiency Virus Can Be Transmitted from Mother to Fetus

When an woman infected with HIV becomes pregnant, her infant can become infected via 3 major routes. The virus can cross the placenta; it can infect the newborn at the time of delivery; or infection can be transmitted through breastfeeding. Risk factors for transmission of HIV from a mother to her fetus are shown in Table 14-1.

Malaria Remains a Perinatal Infection in Endemic Areas

Malaria occurring during pregnancy remains an important problem in parts of the world where *Plasmodium* infections are endemic. Pregnant women with no preexisting

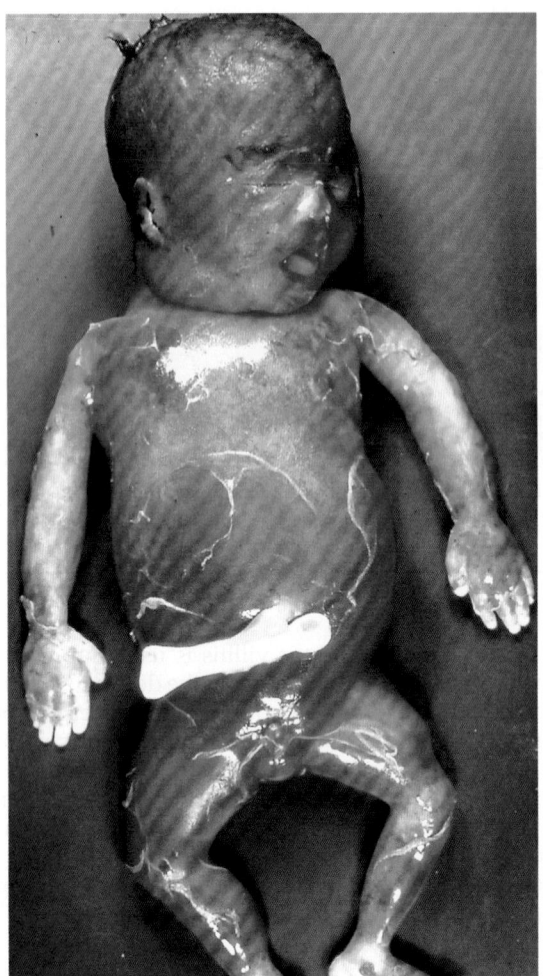

FIGURE 14-10. Stillbirth due to erythrovirus (parvovirus). The infant is hydropic (edematous).

TABLE 14-1
RISK FACTORS FOR PERINATAL TRANSMISSION OF HIV

Maternal Factors
Low CD4+ lymphocyte counts (T cells)
High HIV-1 RNA levels (viral load)
Acute retroviral syndrome during pregnancy
Presence of coinfections (hepatitis C, bacterial vaginosis, CMV)
Injection drug use
Absence of antiretroviral therapy or prophylaxis
Absence of prenatal care

Obstetric Factors
Duration of placental membrane rupture and/or chorioamnionitis
Invasive procedures
Vaginal delivery

Infant Factors
Premature delivery
Breastfeeding

CMV = cytomegalovirus.

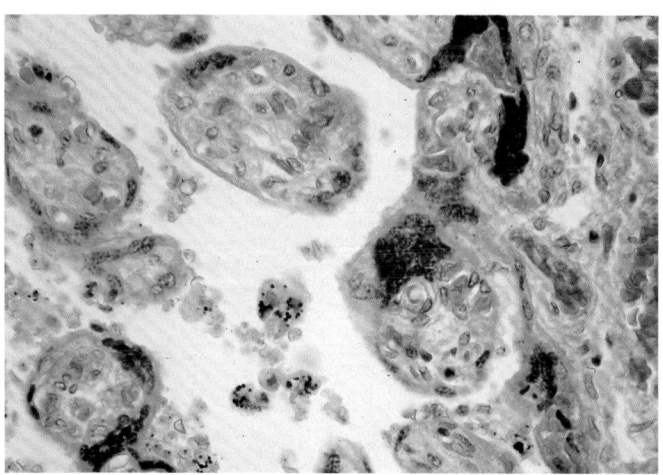

FIGURE 14-11. Placenta from mother with malaria. There is abundant intracellular brown pigment (hemosiderin) in the intervillous space.

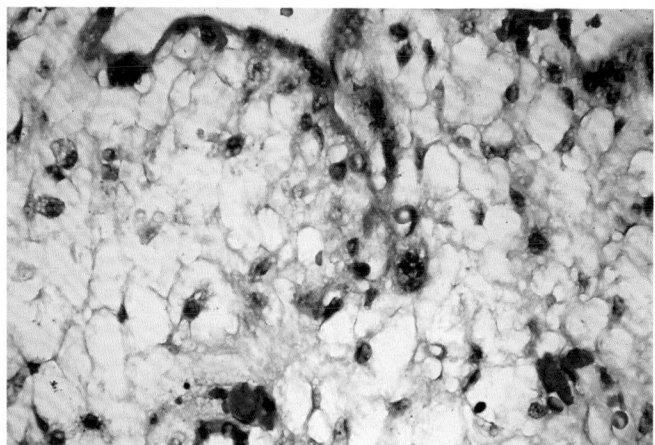

FIGURE 14-12. Villous edema. This villus is enlarged and hydropic, and the fetal capillaries appear compressed. Especially in premature infants, the stromal edema can inhibit oxygen transfer from maternal to fetal circulations.

immunity are at high risk for cerebral malaria, hypoglycemia, pulmonary edema, severe hemolytic anemia and death. Malaria infection can cause low birth weight, and possibly abortion and stillbirth. In malaria-endemic African countries, 15% of all infant deaths can be attributed to low birth weight.

 PATHOLOGY: Placentas of mothers with malaria may show maternal red blood cells infected with *Plasmodium* in the intervillous space. Malarial pigment may be abundant in the intervillous space, the villous stroma and fibrin deposits (Fig. 14-11). Chronic intervillositis is common.

NONINFECTIOUS CONDITIONS AFFECTING CHORIONIC VILLI

Villitis of Unknown Etiology Results in Reproductive Loss, Brain Damage and Recurrence in Subsequent Pregnancy

Villitis of unknown etiology (VUE) is an abnormal inflammatory process of chorionic villi in which no infectious agent is found. Severe cases of VUE are associated with a significant rate of recurrence and with poor obstetric outcomes. Pregnancy failures occur in about 60% of pregnancies complicated by recurrent VUE.

 PATHOLOGY: VUE may be focal or diffuse. If it destroys chorionic villi, it is called necrotizing villitis of unknown etiology. This is an ominous prognosis for the fetus. Chronic uteroplacental malperfusion and insufficiency often coexist with other pathologic findings, including fetal thrombotic vasculopathy and avascular chorionic villi.

Villous Edema Results from Fetal Stress

Villous edema, derived from the fetal chorionic circulation, is one of the most frequent causes of an enlarged placenta, especially in preterm deliveries.

 **ETIOLOGIC FACTORS:** Villous edema has many causes. When it accompanies immunologic reactions and certain infectious diseases, it is **villous hydrops** and is often associated with **hydrops fetalis** (see Chapter 6), such as occurs in maternal–fetal Rh incompatibility and intrauterine erythrovirus infection (see above). However, villous edema can also occur without an edematous fetus, in which case intrauterine fetal stress is usually the trigger. Other causes of villous edema include abruptio placentae, chorioamnionitis, umbilical cord accidents, fetal malformations and genetic disorders. If edema is severe, it can compress the fetal villous vessels, causing fetal hypoxia and stillbirth.

 PATHOLOGY: Terminal villi are enlarged and edematous (Fig. 14-12). Edema fluid may be phagocytized by villous Hofbauer cells, where it appears as intracellular microdroplets. As edema accumulates in the chorionic villi, it can cause clefts, or lacunae, in the villous interstitium, imparting a "bubbly" appearance. Villous edema tends to be most severe in immature placentas and in preterm infants.

VASCULAR DISORDERS OF THE PLACENTA

Fetal Thrombotic Vasculopathy Reflects Clotting in Placental Vessels

Thrombosis occurring anywhere in the circulation of the placenta is called fetal thrombotic vasculopathy (FTV) and indicates an unfavorable intrauterine environment for the fetus. Clots can develop in either the arterial or venous circulation of the placenta and umbilical cord, although the venous circulation is most often affected. Risk factors for development of FTV include villitis and disorders of coagulation, particularly hypercoagulable syndromes (see Chapter 26). A variety of poor outcomes are associated with FTV, including stillbirth, neonatal death, intrauterine growth restriction and, in surviving infants, neurologic injury. FTV may occur with similar clots in fetal organs.

 PATHOLOGY: Thrombi of varying ages are often seen in chorionic villous blood vessels. In cases of acute FTV, large thrombi may be present in the

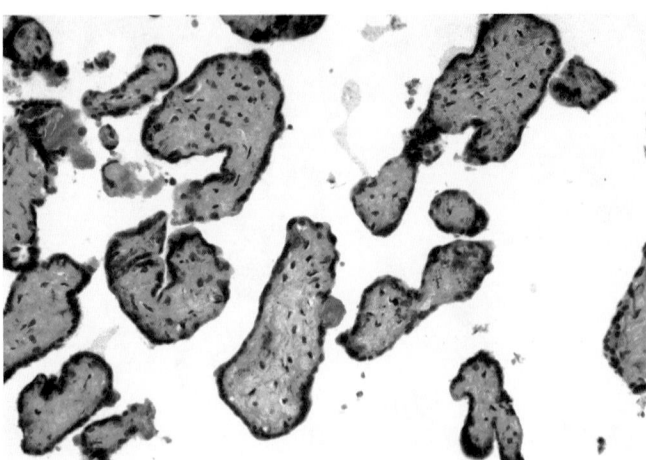

FIGURE 14-13. Avascular villi. The villous capillaries have been replaced by fibrous tissue as a result of a chronic thrombus in a larger upstream stem villus.

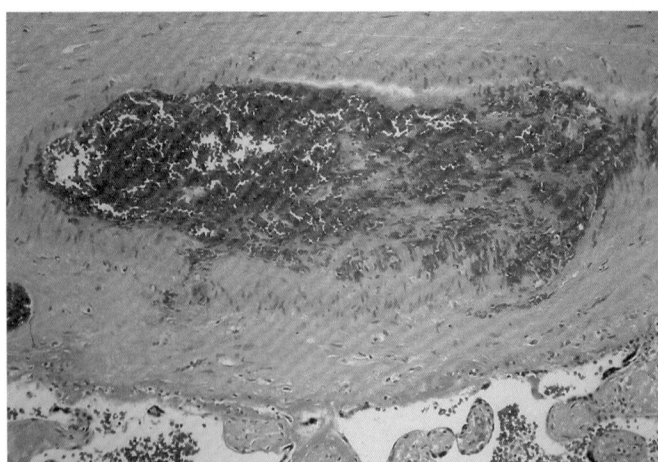

FIGURE 14-15. Hemorrhagic endovasculopathy (HEV). Fetal red blood cells in a large chorionic villus vessel extend from the lumen, through the ischemic endothelium and into the surrounding villous stroma.

umbilical cord vessels or in the large-sized vessels of the chorionic plate. Microscopically, acute thrombi may involve smaller fetal vessels, including the secondary and tertiary villi. In chronic FTV, chorionic villi downstream from thrombosed vessels undergo progressive fibrosis, giving a distinctive appearance to clusters of scarred, **avascular villi** (Fig. 14-13). A thrombus can be incorporated into the vessel wall to form a mural thrombus, or **cushion defect**. Microcalcifications, stromal fibrosis and deposition of hemosiderin result from degeneration of red blood cells.

FTV in the umbilical cord vessels (Fig. 14-14) can be catastrophic and can complicate abnormally long or excessively twisted cords, velamentous cord insertion, entanglement of the cord and cord knots.

Hemorrhagic Endovasculopathy Is Ischemic Injury to Chorionic Blood Vessels

Hemorrhagic endovasculopathy (HEV, formerly termed **hemorrhagic endovasculitis)** results from irreversible injury to the endothelial cells lining fetal blood vessels in the chorionic villi. It is associated with increased perinatal morbidity and mortality, neurologic impairment and abnormalities of fetal growth and development. HEV often occurs together

with other placental abnormalities, including fetal thrombotic vasculopathy, villitis of unknown etiology, villous fibrosis, infarcts, erythroblastosis and meconium staining. Hypertensive disease of pregnancy is the only known risk factor.

 PATHOLOGY: HEV can affect any vessel in the chorionic villous tree. Extravasated fetal red blood cells extend from the lumen through the intimal lining and into the surrounding blood vessel wall or stroma (Fig. 14-15). The vessel wall may be necrotic. Red blood cells can be fragmented, and karyorrhexis of endothelial and nucleated red blood cells is common. HEV may accompany inflammatory infiltrates in the villi, in which case it is called **hemorrhagic villitis**.

Abruptio Placentae Causes Retroplacental Hematoma

Retroplacental hematoma occurs between the basal plate of the placenta and the uterine wall and accounts for 8% of perinatal deaths. Hemorrhage derives from a ruptured maternal (spiral) artery or premature separation of the placenta. Retroplacental hemorrhage can be due to placental abruption **(abruptio placentae),** but in 1/3 of cases it occurs without clinical abruption, and the reverse is also true. Although abruptio placentae is often the final dramatic consequence of a chronic placental disorder, most cases result from maternal vascular disease. Key risk factors for retroplacental hematoma include maternal smoking, hypertensive disease of pregnancy, late maternal age, acute chorioamnionitis, uterine malformation, placenta previa, history of previous abruption, short umbilical cord, thrombophilia, multiparity and cocaine use.

 CLINICAL FEATURES: Abruptio placentae complicates 1% of pregnancies worldwide. Symptoms depend on the extent of abruption and include vaginal bleeding, uterine tenderness, abdominal or back pain, uterine tetanic contractions, fetal distress, maternal shock, hypofibrinogenemia, coagulopathy and maternal or fetal death.

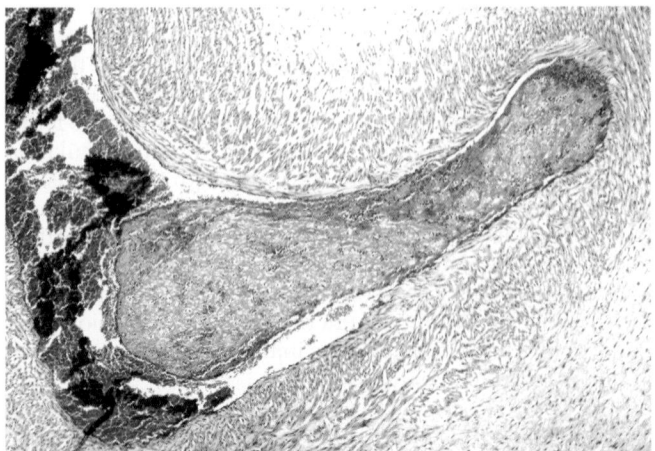

FIGURE 14-14. Thrombus within an umbilical cord blood vessel.

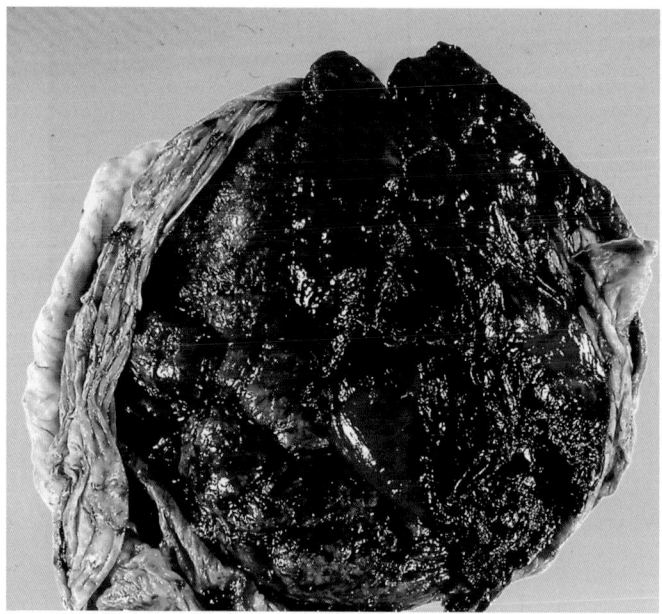

Figure 14-16. Retroplacental hematoma. The occurrence of a retroplacental hemorrhage such as this large hematoma may correlate with the presence of a clinical abruption.

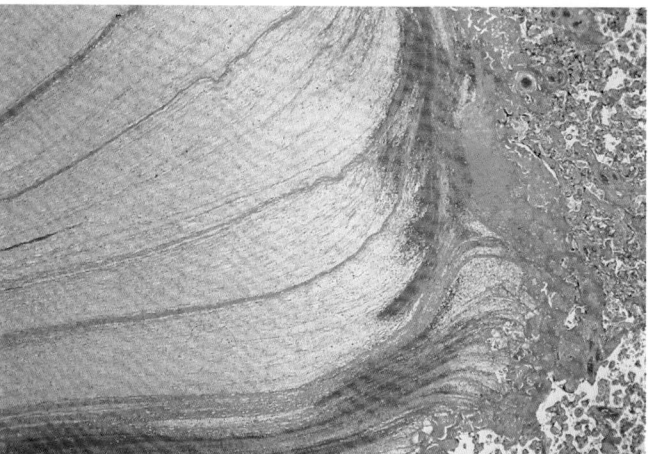

FIGURE 14-17. Intervillous thrombus (hematoma). This intraplacental hematoma represents an area of fetal–maternal hemorrhage. It is surrounded by a zone of fibrin and ischemic villi.

 PATHOLOGY: Premature detachment of the placenta or rupture of a uterine blood vessel causes blood to accumulate between the placenta and the decidua basalis, forming a hematoma (Fig. 14-16). When a retroplacental hematoma is present for some time, overlying villous tissue may show ischemic infarction.

In the half of placental abruptions that are mild, neither the fetus nor the mother suffers ill consequences. However, many abruptions result in poor fetal outcomes, including neonatal shock from hypoxia and anemia, irreversible neurologic injury and perinatal death.

In some cases, blood forces its way into the underlying myometrium, resulting in a **"Couvelaire uterus."** In such cases, mothers may develop anemia, coagulopathy, disseminated intravascular coagulation, adult respiratory distress syndrome (ARDS), shock and death. Maternal death due to abruptio placentae is rare in developed nations (0.4 per thousand cases of abruption), but it continues to be an important cause of maternal death in the resource-poor regions of the world.

Intervillous Thrombi Represent Fetomaternal Hemorrhage

Rupture of a chorionic villous blood vessel causes blood to accumulate in the placenta and to form an intervillous thrombus or hematoma. Since the pressure of the fetal circulation in the placenta is higher than that of the maternal circulation, this represents a **fetomaternal hemorrhage**. Entry of fetal blood into the maternal circulation can have clinical implications if there are blood group incompatibilities between the fetus and mother. Small intervillous thrombi occur in up to 20% of full-term-gestation placentas and are usually clinically insignificant. A larger thrombus or multiple thrombi cause fetal blood loss or hypoxia. Intervillous thrombi can develop as a result of preeclampsia or maternal thrombophilias, and when there is thrombosis in the maternal circulation.

PATHOLOGY: Intervillous thrombi appear as well-demarcated areas of red firm areas, much different from the surrounding spongy placental parenchyma. Hemorrhage compresses the surrounding villi (Fig. 14-17). When intervillous thrombi occur remotely from the time of delivery, the rim of surrounding compressed villi show infarction or avascular scarring.

If significant amounts of fetal blood enter the maternal bloodstream from an intervillous thrombus, the fetal red blood cells may be detected using the **Kleihauer-Betke (KB)** test, which utilizes the differing sensitivity of fetal and adult hemoglobin to acid.

Placenta Accreta Is Abnormal Adherence of the Placenta to the Uterus

Placenta accreta is caused by failure to form decidua. Normally, decidual endometrium separates the base of the placenta from the underlying uterine muscle. Placenta accreta occurs when the decidual layer is partially or totally absent, so that the villi are in direct contact with the underlying decidua or uterine muscle. In this case, the placenta does not separate normally from the uterine wall at the time of delivery, which may lead to life-threatening maternal hemorrhage. Risk factors for placenta accreta include placenta previa, prior cesarean sections, advanced maternal age, high parity and endometrial defects.

 PATHOLOGY: Placenta accreta is classified by the depth of myometrial invasion by the villi:

- **Placenta accreta** refers to attachment of villi to the surface of the uterine wall without further invasion (Fig. 14-18A).
- **Placenta increta** occurs when villi invade underlying myometrium, penetrating either superficially or deep into the myometrium (Fig. 14-18B).
- **Placenta percreta** describes villi penetrating the full thickness of the uterine wall. In some cases, placenta percreta penetrates through the uterine serosa and invades adjacent organs such as the colon or urinary bladder; it can also result in uterine rupture.

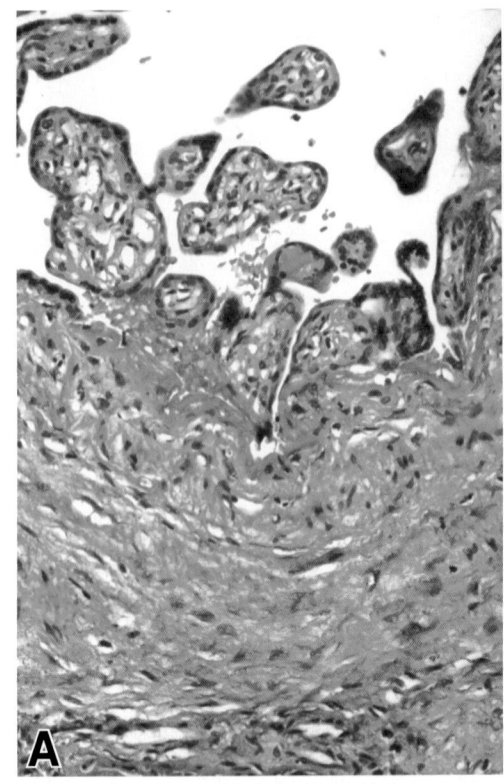

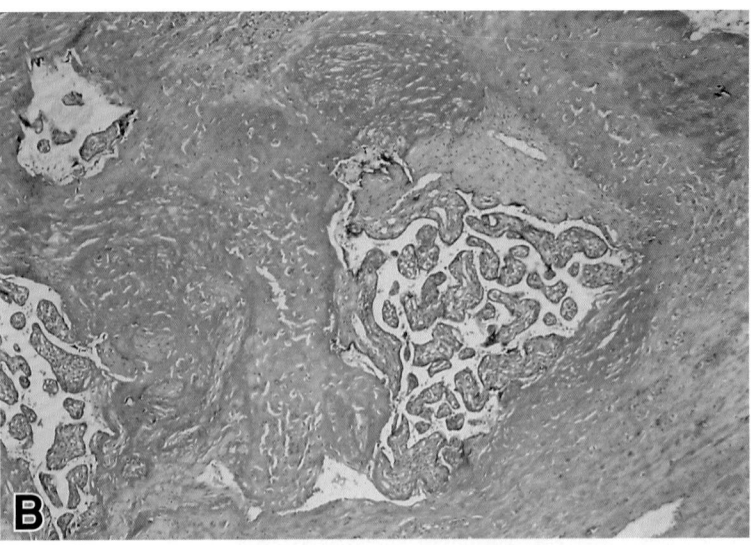

FIGURE 14-18. A. Placenta accreta. Some of the chorionic villi (*top*) are in contact with the underlying muscle. The decidua is absent. **B. Placenta increta.** The chorionic villi have invaded deeply into the uterine wall.

CLINICAL FEATURES: Patients with placenta accreta can have a normal pregnancy and delivery. However, complications may occur during pregnancy, during delivery or especially in the immediate postpartum period. Third-trimester bleeding is the most common presenting sign; substantial fragments of placenta may remain adherent after delivery and cause hemorrhage, endometritis and disseminated intravascular coagulation. Bleeding may threaten the lives of both mother and baby and necessitate emergency hysterectomy.

Chronic Uteroplacental Malperfusion Can Cause Poor Obstetric Outcomes

Adequate oxygenation of the fetus during pregnancy requires that both fetal and maternal circulations between the uteroplacental and fetal structures operate properly. Chronic uteroplacental malperfusion and insufficiency are important causes of perinatal morbidity and mortality. They can result in stillbirth, neonatal death, preterm birth, intrauterine growth restriction and, if the infant lives, neurologic damage. Some of the most frequent causes include villous hypoplasia, maternal floor infarction, massive perivillous fibrin deposition, diabetes, autoimmune diseases, villitis, placental infarcts, chronic abruption, fetal thrombotic vasculopathy, abnormally small or thin placentas, chorangiomas, large remote intervillous thrombi and chronic umbilical cord abnormalities.

Villous Hypoplasia Is Caused by Insufficient Maternal Blood Flow to the Placenta

Villous hypoplasia (also called uneven accelerated maturation) results from chronic underlying disease of the spiral arterioles, including stenosis, fluctuating vasoconstriction or, as occurs with preeclampsia, defective remodeling (see below). Decreased maternal perfusion of the intervillous space of the placenta leads to ischemic degeneration of chorionic villi (Fig. 14-19A, B). Resulting fetal hypoxia can produce stillbirth, neonatal death, intrauterine growth restriction, preterm birth and neurologic injury in infants who survive.

Increased Fibrin Results in a Spectrum of Placental Disorders

Small amounts of fibrin from the maternal circulation deposit in the placenta under normal conditions. **Rohr fibrin** is a necessary component of the basal plate of the placenta, where it faces the intervillous plate. **Nitabuch fibrin** deposits in the deep part of the basal plate. It is a deficiency of Nitabuch fibrin that causes placenta accreta.

Increased Perivillous Fibrin

Excess deposition of fibrin around villi can cause placental insufficiency by interfering with perfusion of the villi. Ischemic necrosis of the villi may eventuate (Fig. 14-20) and can cause placental insufficiency.

Massive perivillous fibrin deposition (MPFD) can cause perinatal death. The cause of MPFD is unknown. The fibrin extends from the basal (decidual) part of the placenta up to the fetal (chorionic) surface. Dense fibrin fills the intervillous space and results in villous ischemic necrosis (Fig. 14-21). MPFD often leads to poor pregnancy outcomes.

Maternal Floor Infarction

Maternal floor infarction (MFI) is not a true infarct but shares some morphologic features with MPFD. Excessive

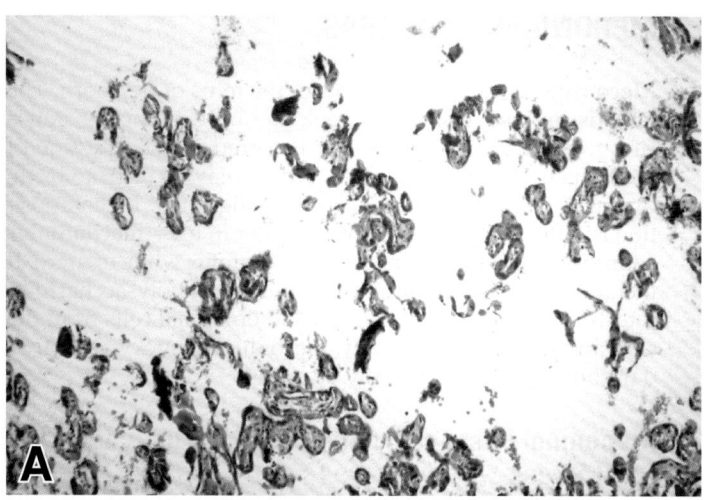
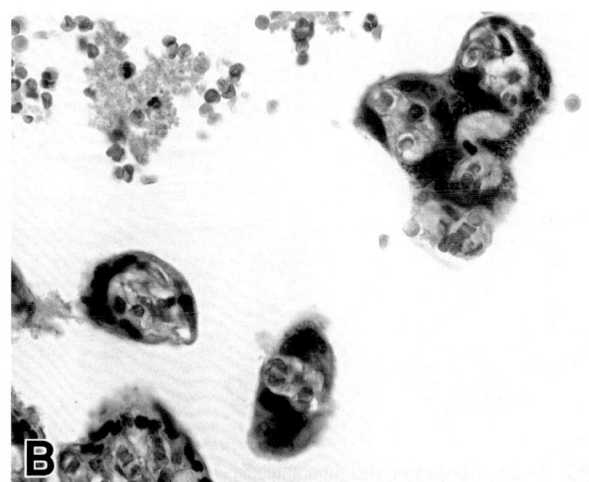

FIGURE 14-19. Villous hypoplasia. A. The diameter of the villi is decreased, resulting in an apparent increase in the intervillous space between villi. **B. High magnification of villous hypoplasia.** The characteristic features of chronic ischemia are present, including small, shrunken villi with stromal fibrosis and clumped trophoblast.

fibrin extends confluently across the width of the placenta. It mainly affects the basal surface and decidua and extends upward to involve the villi. The floor of the placenta is firm, thickened and often discolored tan-yellow. Like MPFD, villi involved with MFI are embedded in dense fibrin and are necrotic. MFI has the same perinatal outcomes as does MPFD.

Infarcts Are the Most Frequently Diagnosed Vascular Condition of the Placenta

Placental infarcts consist of an area of placental tissue that has undergone irreversible ischemic injury and death owing to complete interruption of maternal vascular supply to the infarcted area. The most frequent causes of placental infarction are hemorrhage between the base of the placenta and the uterine wall (retroplacental hemorrhage and abruptio placentae) and occlusion or thrombosis of the uterine spiral artery.

Placental infarcts often accompany hypertensive diseases of pregnancy, including preeclampsia, maternal thrombophilia and cigarette smoking. Multiple infarcts, especially if they are large or in the central part of the placenta, can result in placental insufficiency and give rise to intrauterine growth restriction, neurologic injury and perinatal death.

 PATHOLOGY: Infarcts are dark red areas that are firmer than surrounding placental tissue. With increasing age, they become firmer, change in color from dark red to yellow and then to tan, and finally become white and more sharply delineated from the adjacent tissue.

Chorangiosis Is Increased Chorionic Vasculature

Terminal chorionic villi have a markedly increased number of vessels. This endothelial proliferation increases the capillary surface area of the villi in the face of chronic intrauterine hypoxia. Chorangiosis does not cause fetal damage but is a microscopic marker of significant uteroplacental

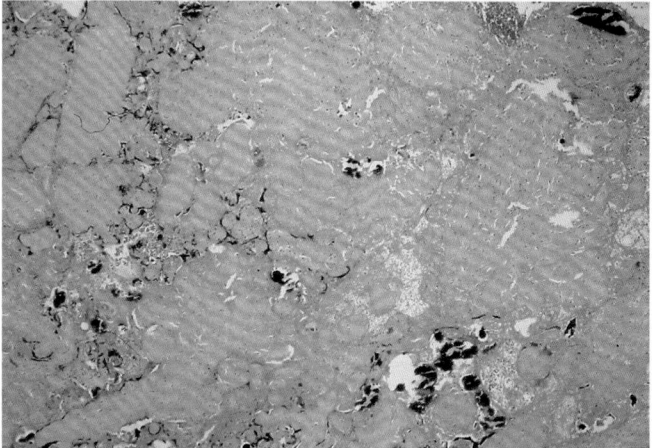

FIGURE 14-21. Massive perivillous fibrin deposition (MPFD). Low magnification showing confluent villous necrosis and fibrin deposition in the intervillous space. The small, dark purple microcalcifications attest to the chronicity of this process.

FIGURE 14-20. Increased villous fibrin. The fibrin has covered the chorionic villi, obstructed the intervillous space and resulted in villous necrosis.

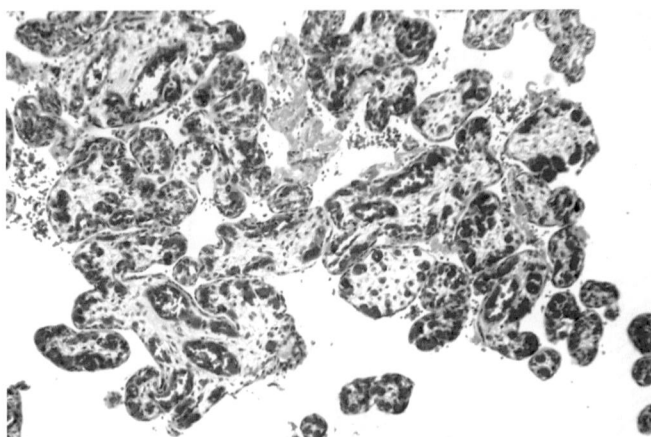

FIGURE 14-22. Chorangiosis. Chorangiosis results from chronic fetal hypoxia. Normal chorionic villi contain 5 or fewer capillaries. The chorionic villi in these villi are hypervascular—most contain greater than 10 capillary cross-sections, and a few villi contain 20 or more vessels.

insufficiency and fetal hypoxia that may arise from any variety of causes.

 PATHOLOGY: Chorangiotic villi contain 10 or more vessels, affecting numerous villi. The increased vascularity may be so marked that some villi have 30–40 or more fetal vessels (Fig. 14-22).

Increased Syncytial Knots Indicate Uteroplacental Malperfusion

Chorionic villi are covered by a layer of multinucleated cells, the syncytiotrophoblast (see above). In the face of chronic uteroplacental malperfusion, the syncytiotrophoblast forms prominent bulbous knots or folds, often bridging the intervillous space and touching the trophoblast of adjacent villi (Fig. 14-23). This abnormality, termed **syncytiotrophoblast hyperplasia**, often affects placentas with chronic malperfusion from all causes.

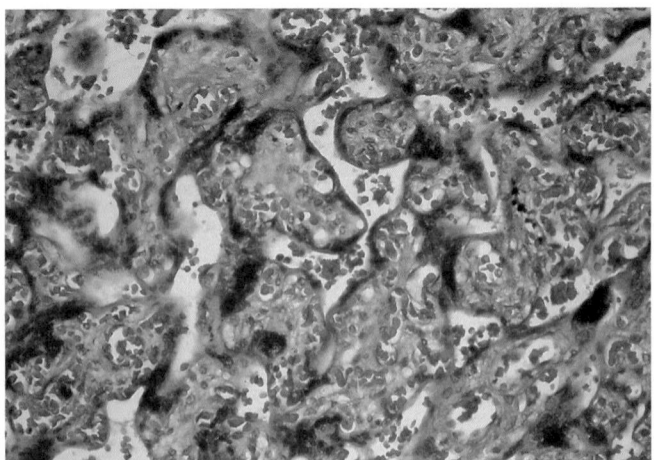

FIGURE 14-23. Tenney-Parker change (syncytiotrophoblast hyperplasia). The syncytiotrophoblast is knotted and hyperbasophilic and bridges the intervillous space to connect to adjacent villi. This is caused by chronic uteroplacental malperfusion of either maternal or fetal origin.

MECONIUM DISORDERS

Meconium is the earliest stools of the fetus or newborn. The term is derived from the Greek *mēkōn,* or "poppy," referring to its tarry appearance. It is stored in the intestine of the fetus until it is discharged, which may be prior to birth, during labor and delivery or following birth. Its composition is different from feces formed later in life—meconium is composed of materials ingested by the fetus while in utero. It includes water (80%), amniotic fluid, mucopolysaccharides, intestinal enzymes, bile, lanugo and epithelial cells from the skin and intestines. Typically, meconium is sticky and tarry, dark olive green and usually odorless.

Meconium Passage by the Fetus May Indicate Fetal Stress

Physiologic passage of meconium can be facilitated in full-term fetuses because of the maturity of the fetal gastrointestinal tract. It can also be released in the term fetus as a result of fetal hypoxia or fetal distress. Chorioamnionitis and amniotic infection syndrome, compression of the fetal head or umbilical cord, fetal asphyxia and acidosis and gestational cholestasis in the mother may all trigger meconium release. In preterm infants (<37 weeks), passage of meconium is always abnormal.

 PATHOLOGY: Following delivery, the fetal surfaces of the placenta, membranes or umbilical cord appear discolored, varying from brown to green to golden yellow. Within 1–3 hours after meconium passage, the amnion will be stained. Beyond 3 hours prior to delivery, intracellular meconium is evident within the resident macrophages in the membranes or chorionic surface of the placenta (Fig. 14-24). When meconium has been present for more than 24 hours, it may been seen in the umbilical cord mesenchyme (Wharton jelly) or in the trophoblast or decidual layers of the extraplacental membranes. In remote meconium passage, the amnionic epithelium is thickened or thrown up into finger-like projections owing to irritation, which is called **amnionic papillary hyperplasia**.

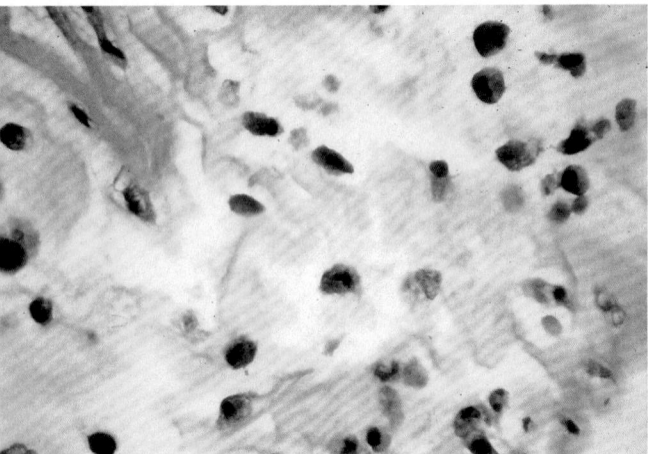

FIGURE 14-24. Abundant meconium present in chorionic macrophages in a premature infant. It takes a minimum of 3–4 hours for meconium to be absorbed into the chorion and macrophages from the amniotic fluid following its passage by the fetus.

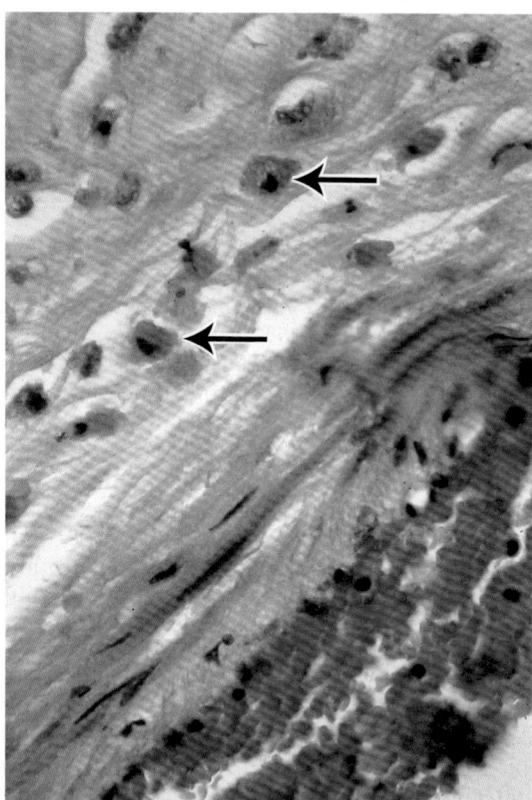

FIGURE 14-25. Meconium-induced vascular necrosis (MIVN). Smooth muscle cells of the fetal blood vessel have undergone ischemic degeneration and necrosis, and appear rounded and hyperchromatic (*arrows*).

Meconium-Induced Vascular Necrosis Can Threaten the Life of the Fetus or Cause Brain Damage

An important potential complication of meconium discharge is **meconium-induced vascular necrosis** (MIVN). In MIVN, meconium passed by the fetus long before delivery has sufficient time to penetrate the connective tissue of the umbilical cord or through the chorionic plate, to reach and permeate the muscular walls of the umbilical cord or large chorionic plate blood vessels. This causes necrosis of blood vessels, which compromises fetal blood flow and leads to poor obstetric outcomes.

 PATHOLOGY: The umbilical cord vessels and the large-sized chorionic plate blood vessels can be involved in MIVN (Fig. 14-25). In affected blood vessels, only eosinophilic remnants of the cytoplasm remain visible. In remote cases of MIVN, muscular walls of the affected vessel are thinned. Meconium is often identified within connective tissues near the injured vessels.

INTRAUTERINE GROWTH RESTRICTION AND LOW BIRTH WEIGHT

Intrauterine growth restriction (IUGR) is an abnormality of fetal growth and development that affects 3%–10% of deliveries and reflects chronic uteroplacental insufficiency. IUGR can be asymmetric (70%–80%) or symmetric (20%–30%). In the more common asymmetric form, head size, length and weight are often normal, but subcutaneous fat and muscle mass and abdominal circumference are decreased (see below).

The newborn with asymmetric IUGR has a 5–10-fold increased risk for perinatal mortality and morbidity. Asymmetric IUGR is also associated with neonatal hypoglycemia, meconium aspiration, persistent fetal circulation and neurologic injury due to chronic fetal hypoxia. Placentas from neonates with asymmetrical IUGR are almost always abnormal. *Maternal cigarette smoking is the most important preventable cause of asymmetric IUGR.* Symmetric IUGR results in an abnormally and proportionally small infant, with low birth weight, small head and short stature. It begins early in pregnancy and is usually due to genetic disorders, early fetal infections and chromosomal and congenital anomalies. Morbidity and mortality are increased in infants with symmetric IUGR, and 30% of infants who survive have neurodevelopmental problems.

Small- or Large-for-Gestational-Age Infants May Have Normal Development

Infants who are **small for gestational age,** or **SGA,** have birth weights below the 10th percentile for gestational age and gender. Similarly, **large-for-gestational-age,** or **LGA,** infants have birth weights above the 90th percentile. Average birth weights vary with geography, ethnicity and socioeconomic status. However, infants who are SGA or LGA may be so as a result of an abnormal intrauterine exposure or disease. Related terms for infant birth weight are as follows:

- **Low birth weight (LBW):** a newborn weighing less than 2500 grams regardless of gestational age
- **Very low birth weight (VLBW):** infants weighing less than 1500 grams
- **Extremely low birth weight (ELBW):** newborns weighing less than 1000 grams

Low Birth Weight Causes Neonatal Morbidity

LBW is a principal contributor to neonatal morbidity and mortality worldwide. In some countries, it accounts for up to 70% of neonatal deaths. LBW infants are 20 times more likely to die than are normal–birth-weight infants. They tend to remain malnourished and to have lower IQs and cognitive disabilities. More than 95% of LBW babies are born in developing countries. IUGR is the most common form of LBW in the developing world, whereas most LBW in developed countries is due to prematurity.

Extremely-Low-Birth-Weight Infants Have Perinatal Complications

Most **ELBW** infants are born at less than 27 weeks' gestation. ELBW infants represent less than 1% of all live births in Western nations. For infants with birth weights less than 500 grams, the first-year survival rate is 14%; between 500 and 749 grams, 51% survive the first year; infants weighing between 750 and 1000 grams at birth have a 1-year survival rate of 85%. In the resource-poor nations of the world, data for ELBW infants are scarce, and survival is most likely rare.

Macrosomia Can Be Constitutional or Caused by Intrauterine Disease

Depending on the criteria used, macrosomic newborns weigh greater than 4000 grams (8 lbs, 13 oz) or greater than 4500 grams (9 lbs, 15 oz), regardless of gestational age or gender. They differ from being large for gestational age, in that the classification LGA is based on a birth weight greater than the 90th percentile.

Fetal macrosomia presents problems for both the mother and infant. Potential maternal complications include difficulty in labor, genital tract lacerations, postpartum bleeding and uterine rupture. Complications affecting the infant include shoulder dystocia and brachial plexus injuries, impaired glucose tolerance and childhood obesity. The still-birth rate for macrosomic infants is twice as high as that for normal-sized infants, irrespective of maternal diabetes.

 **ETIOLOGIC FACTORS:** The most frequent cause of neonatal macrosomia is maternal diabetes. Gestational diabetes increases maternal serum glucose levels, leading to increased fetal insulin, which stimulates fetal growth. Male infants are at greater risk than females. Additional risk factors for macrosomia include maternal obesity, excessive maternal weight gain, a history of a previous macrosomic infant, prolonged pregnancy (>41 weeks) and advanced maternal age.

SPONTANEOUS ABORTION

A pregnancy that ends with expulsion of a conceptus before the 20th week of gestation is called a spontaneous abortion, or miscarriage. Some 15% of recognized pregnancies abort spontaneously. An additional 30% of women abort without being aware that they were pregnant. Thus, about half of all pregnancies miscarry, making it the most common complication of early pregnancy. The most common symptom of spontaneous abortion is bleeding.

 **ETIOLOGIC FACTORS:** Most spontaneous abortions occur before 12 weeks of gestation. Karyotypic anomalies are present in 50% of all spontaneous abortions, and in as many as 70% of those occurring before the 7th week of gestation. The principal factors responsible for spontaneous abortion are:

- Infection early in pregnancy (e.g., *Listeria*, CMV, *Toxoplasma*, coxsackievirus)
- Mechanical factors (e.g., uterine leiomyoma, septate uteri, cervical incompetence)
- Endocrine factors (e.g., maternal diabetes, polycystic ovary, luteal phase defects, progesterone deficiency, hypothyroidism)
- Immunologic factors
- Cigarette smoking
- Cocaine usage
- Congenital fetal malformations (e.g., neural tube defects)
- Chromosomal abnormalities
- Increasing maternal age
- Multiple gestation (e.g., twins, triplets, etc.)

 PATHOLOGY: An empty gestational sac with hydropic swelling of the chorionic villi (blighted ovum) suggests early fetal demise. The embryo may be grossly disorganized or show defects such as spina bifida, anencephaly or cleft palate. Chorionic villi may be histologically normal or show intravillous fibrosis or hydropic change. If infection preceded the miscarriage, there is often microscopic evidence of the infectious agent (see Chapter 9).

RECURRENT PREGNANCY LOSS

Pregnancy loss is the most common complication of human pregnancy, affecting 10%–15% of all human conceptions. For most fertile couples miscarriage is a sporadic event, but 1%–5% of fertile couples suffer from **recurrent pregnancy loss** (RPL; also termed **habitual abortion**).

 **ETIOLOGIC FACTORS:** The **antiphospholipid syndrome** accounts for 3%–15% of recurrent pregnancy loss. Another important cause of RPL is **thrombophilia**, mostly **factor V Leiden** and **prothrombin G20210A** (factor II) mutations. In 4% of couples with RPL, there are chromosomal aberrations in one or both partners. Diverse endocrine factors can cause RPL, including hypothyroidism, polycystic ovary disease, diabetes and inadequate production of progesterone. Anatomic conditions, such as cervical incompetence and uterine malformations, or immune factors including antithyroid autoantibodies and maternal immunization against male-specific minor histocompatibility (H-Y) antigens are also involved in some cases. Certain ovarian factors are risk factors for RPL. These include luteal phase defects and advanced maternal age, with decreased ovarian reserve and decreased egg quality.

MULTIPLE GESTATIONS

Slightly less than 1% of normal pregnancies yield dizygotic or monozygotic twins (Fig. 14-26).

DIZYGOTIC TWINS: Fertilization of two separate ova results in genetically different twins, of the same or opposite sex. Dizygotic twinning has a strong hereditary component, which is limited to the maternal side. Dizygotic twinning and multiple gestations occur more commonly in women who have used hormones to induce ovulation artificially or who have been impregnated after in vitro fertilization.

Separate placentas develop when two fertilized ova implant apart from one another. If they implant near each other, the two placentas show varying degrees of fusion, and may appear to be one. If the ova implant apart, there are discrete conceptuses, each placenta having its own amniotic sac. In cases when the placentas fuse, the membranes between the two fetuses show two amnions and two chorions (diamnionic, dichorionic gestation).

MONOZYGOTIC TWINS: Early division of a single fertilized ovum results in genetically identical twins of the same sex. If a fertilized ovum divides within 2 days of fertilization, before the trophoblast has differentiated, two separate embryos develop, each with its own placenta and amniotic sac (dichorionic, diamniotic twinning). Hence, dichorionic placentas may be either monozygotic or dizygotic, while monochorionic placentas are always monozygous. If division occurs from the third to eighth days after conception, the trophoblast (but not the amniotic cavity) has already differentiated. A single placenta with two amniotic sacs develops

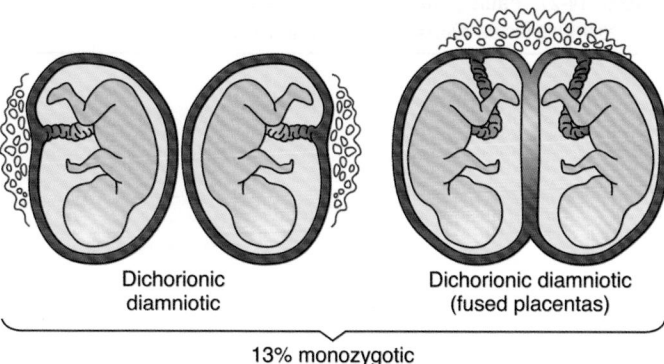

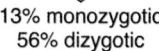

FIGURE 14-26. Placental structure in twin pregnancies. The percentages in the figure refer to the proportion of total twin pregnancies (100%) accounted for by each variant.

(monochorionic, diamniotic twinning). A monochorionic, monoamniotic placenta is formed if division occurs between the 8th and 13th day after conception, because the amniotic cavity has already developed. Incomplete separation of monozygous twins results in **conjoint (formerly Siamese) twins** within a monoamniotic, monochorionic placenta.

HYPERTENSIVE DISORDERS OF PREGNANCY

Preeclampsia and eclampsia define a syndrome of hypertension, proteinuria and edema and, most severely, convulsions. Preeclampsia occurs in 6% of pregnant women in their last trimester, especially with their first child. If convulsive seizures appear, the syndrome is called eclampsia. (The archaic term "toxemia" is rarely used anymore.) Preeclampsia causes some 50,000 maternal deaths worldwide each year.

 **ETIOLOGIC FACTORS:** Preeclampsia probably arises because of faulty remodeling of uterine spiral arteries that supply maternal blood to the placenta. Immunologic and genetic factors, as well as altered vascular reactivity, endothelial injury and coagulation abnormalities, may also contribute. The characteristics of preeclampsia are (Fig. 14-27):

- Maternal blood flow to the placenta is markedly reduced because of ineffective remodeling of maternal spiral arteries of the decidua.
- Renal involvement contributes to hypertension and proteinuria.
- Disseminated intravascular coagulation may occur in preeclampsia.
- The risk of preeclampsia in a first pregnancy is manyfold higher than in subsequent pregnancies.
- Rarely, preeclampsia may not occur until the time of labor and delivery, or shortly thereafter (postpartum preeclampsia).
- Eclampsia is a cerebrovascular disorder characterized by seizures, worsening hypertension and cerebral edema. It may precede other symptoms and does not necessarily evolve from preeclampsia.

 PATHOPHYSIOLOGY: Faulty cytotrophoblastic remodeling of the maternal uterine (spiral) arteries in early pregnancy (Fig. 14-27) is believed to result from abnormal expression of integrins by the fetal-derived cytotrophoblast, as well as generalized apoptosis of the cytotrophoblast. This situation leads to limited invasion of the decidua and spiral arteries, in which case, the spiral arteries cannot perfuse the growing fetus adequately. Resulting placental ischemia promotes release of cytokines such as tumor necrosis factor-α (TNF-α) and interleukin-6 (IL-6).

Upregulation and production of such placental antiangiogenic factors as vascular endothelial growth factor (VEGF) and soluble endoglin may play a role in the onset of the clinical features of preeclampsia, including hypertension and proteinuria. The roles, if any, of other factors are unclear.

The fundamental pathophysiology of preeclampsia reflects reduced maternal blood flow to the uteroplacental unit, as the spiral arteries of the uteroplacental bed never fully dilate.

Early in a normal pregnancy, fetal cytotrophoblast cells extend downward into the decidua and uterus. They invade the uterine spiral arteries and progressively replace the maternal-derived endothelium, medial elastic tissue, smooth muscle and neural tissue. By the end of the second trimester, the normally narrow spiral arteries are dilated tubes lined by fetal-derived cytotrophoblast. This low-resistance arterial circuit supplies the increasing oxygen and nutrient demands of the developing fetus.

In preeclampsia, many spiral arteries escape invasion by trophoblastic tissue and so never dilate. The combination of vasoconstriction and structural changes in spiral arteries contributes to inadequate blood flow, placental ischemia, villous hypoplasia and fetal hypoxia. The effectiveness of vasodilators in treating preeclampsia, including nitric oxide (NO•), prostacyclin (PGI₂) and endothelium-derived hyperpolarizing factor (EDHF), is further evidence for endothelial dysfunction in preeclampsia.

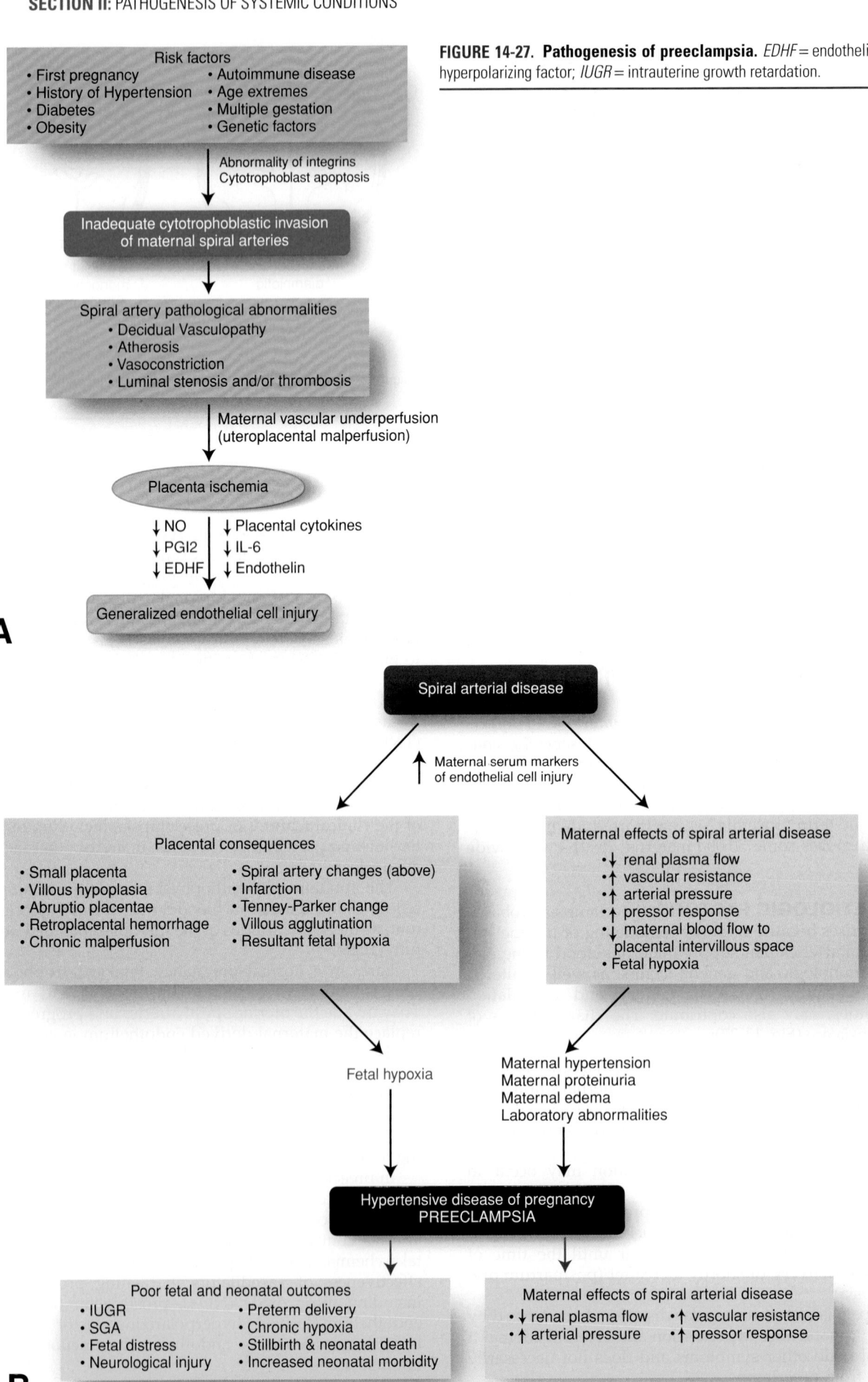

FIGURE 14-27. Pathogenesis of preeclampsia. *EDHF* = endothelium-derived hyperpolarizing factor; *IUGR* = intrauterine growth retardation.

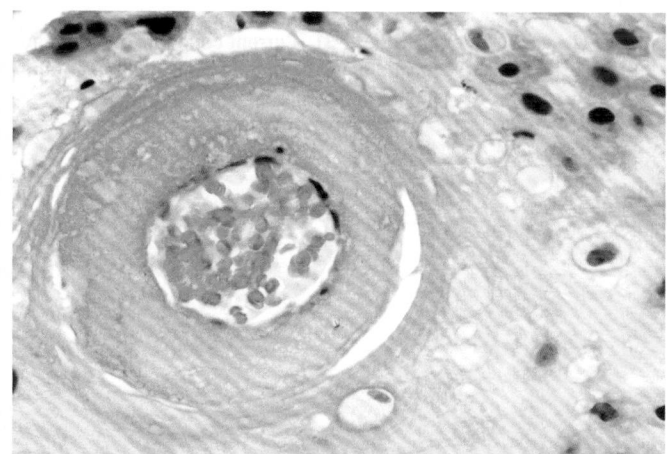

FIGURE 14-28. Decidual atherosis in preeclampsia. A small decidual artery shows fibrinoid thickening of the vessel wall.

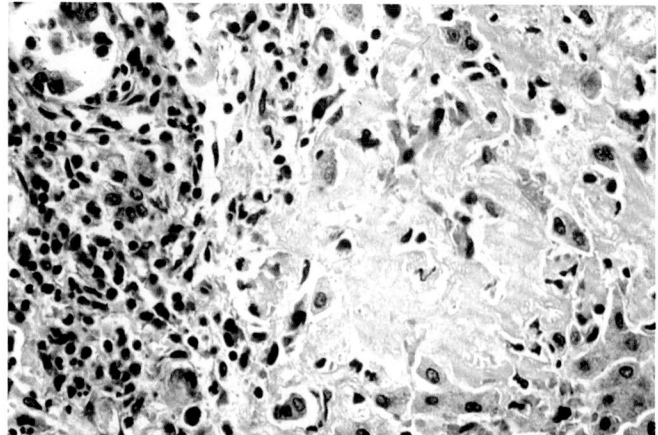

FIGURE 14-30. Liver of a woman with HELLP syndrome. The periportal area (zone 1) demonstrates fibrin deposition.

 PATHOLOGY: *Placental pathology usually precedes the clinical onset of maternal hypertension.* Extensive placental infarction is seen in 1/3 of women with severe preeclampsia, although it is often negligible in mild preeclampsia. Retroplacental hemorrhage or abruptio placentae occurs in 15% and abnormally small placentas (<10th percentile) in 10% of cases (Fig. 14-16). Chorionic villi show signs of chronic maternal underperfusion, consisting of ischemically degenerated chorionic villi (villous hypoplasia; Fig. 14-19), fibrin (Fig. 14-20), increased placental site giant cells, syncytiotrophoblastic hyperplasia (Tenney-Parker change) (Fig. 14-23) and mural hypertrophy of membrane arterioles. The spiral arteries commonly show fibrinoid necrosis, clusters of lipid-rich macrophages and a perivascular infiltrate of mononuclear cells; this constellation of findings is called **acute atherosis** (Fig. 14-28). These vessels are often thrombosed, causing focal placental infarcts.

Maternal kidneys always show glomerular changes. Glomeruli are enlarged and endothelial cells are swollen, forming classic "bloodless" glomeruli of preeclampsia (glomerular endotheliosis) (Fig. 14-29). Fibrin deposits between endothelial cells and the glomerular capillary basement membrane. Mesangial cell hyperplasia is the

rule. These maternal renal changes are reversible with therapy or after delivery.

Fatal cases of eclampsia often show cerebral hemorrhages, ranging from petechiae to large hematomas. *Liver abnormalities are present in 60% of women dying from preeclampsia,* including periportal fibrin deposits and necrosis (Fig. 14-30), lobular hemorrhage and hepatic infarction.

 CLINICAL FEATURES: Preeclampsia usually begins insidiously after the 20th week of pregnancy, with excessive weight gain due to fluid retention, increased maternal blood pressure and proteinuria. As preeclampsia progresses from mild to severe, diastolic pressure persistently exceeds 110 mm Hg, proteinuria is greater than 3 g/day and renal function declines. Disseminated intravascular coagulation (DIC) often supervenes. Preeclampsia is treated with antihypertensive and antiplatelet drugs, but definitive therapy requires removing the placenta. Eclampsia is treated with magnesium sulfate, which reduces cerebrovascular tone.

HELLP SYNDROME

HELLP syndrome is a potentially fatal condition of pregnant women and their infants that most often follows the diagnosis of preeclampsia in the third trimester. Its name is an acronym for its major findings—hemolytic anemia, elevated liver enzymes and low platelet count. It occurs in 0.2%–0.6% of all pregnancies, and in 4%–12% of women with preeclampsia or eclampsia. Some 70% of cases occur antepartum and 30% develop in the postpartum period.

 PATHOPHYSIOLOGY: The trigger for developing HELLP syndrome is unknown, but generalized activation of the coagulation cascade is thought to be the major problem. The syndrome is the final manifestation of an event that provokes microvascular endothelial damage and intravascular platelet activation. The latter causes vasospasm, platelet agglutination and aggregation and further endothelial damage. Excessive

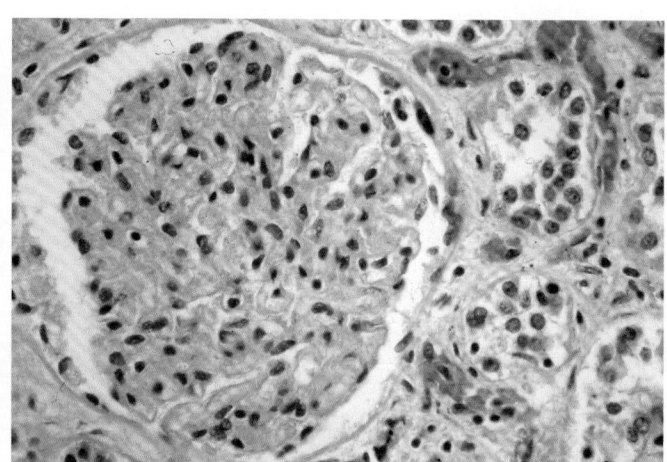

FIGURE 14-29. Glomerular endotheliosis. This is the "bloodless glomerulus" from a woman dying from preeclampsia.

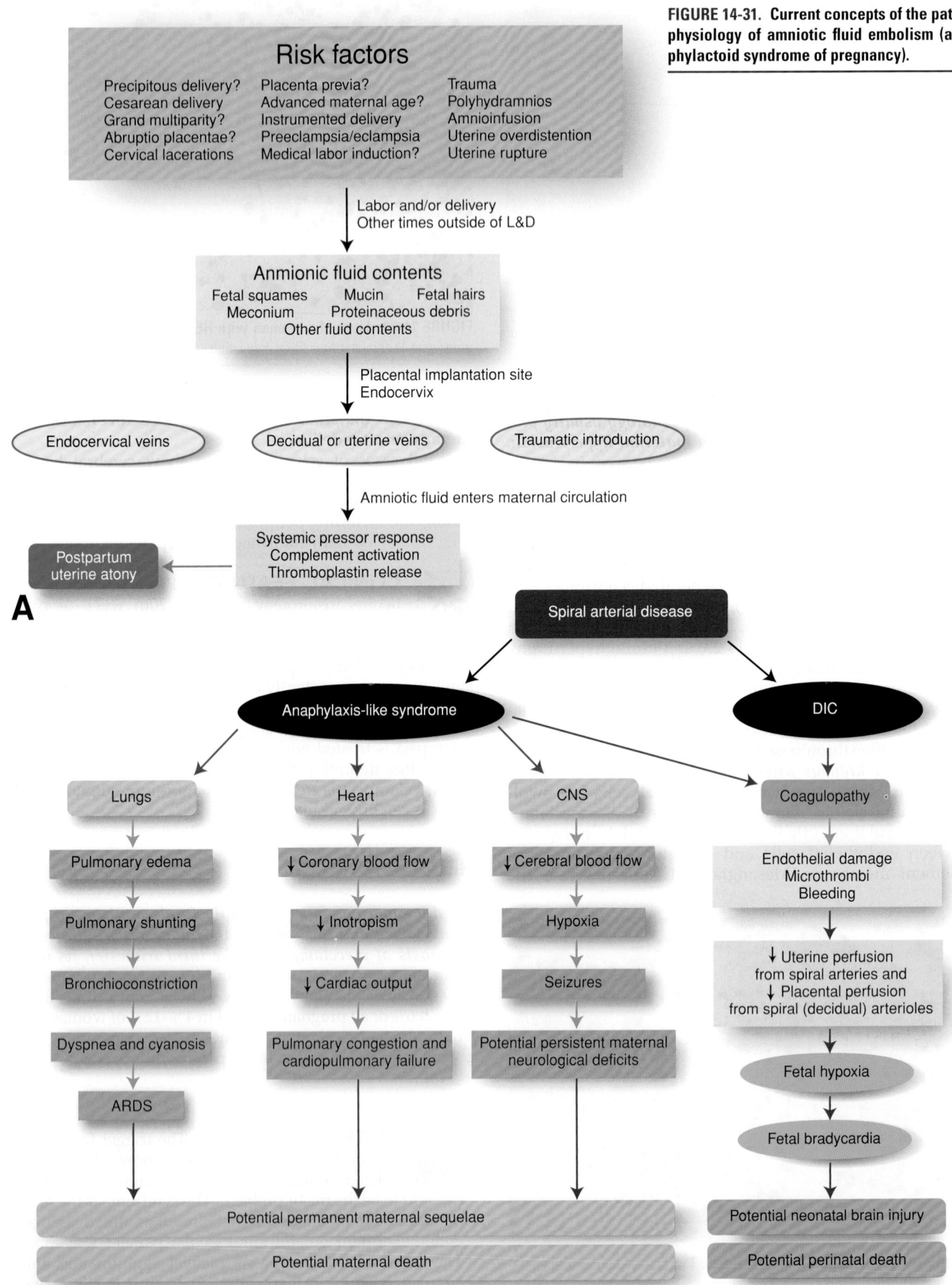

FIGURE 14-31. Current concepts of the pathophysiology of amniotic fluid embolism (anaphylactoid syndrome of pregnancy).

platelet consumption results in DIC and microangiopathic anemia in 20% of women with HELLP syndrome. Obstruction of hepatic blood flow by fibrin deposits in the sinusoids gives rise to liver ischemia, resulting in periportal necrosis, increased levels of liver enzymes and, in severe cases, intrahepatic hemorrhage, subcapsular hematoma formation or hepatic rupture. Additional complications include hemorrhage from DIC, pulmonary edema, placental abruption, ARDS, acute hepatorenal failure and fetal death. The maternal mortality rate is 1%. Infant morbidity and mortality rates vary from 10%–60%, depending on the severity of maternal disease.

AMNIOTIC FLUID EMBOLISM

Amniotic fluid embolism (AFE), also called anaphylactoid syndrome of pregnancy, is a rare, life-threatening obstetric emergency that results in an anaphylaxis-like syndrome. It occurs when amniotic fluid, fetal squamous cells, hair, vernix and other amniotic materials enter the maternal circulation through the uterine veins in the decidual bed at the base of the placenta. Maternal mortality has declined to 25%, but it accounts for 5%–10% of maternal deaths in the United States. About 20% of infants die after their mothers develop AFE.

 ETIOLOGIC FACTORS: The entry of amniotic fluid elements into the maternal bloodstream is thought to trigger the acute onset of symptoms of AFE. However, amniotic fluid cellular elements are not always identified in women with AFE, and they may be present in women who do not develop the disorder. Amniotic fluid materials that enter the maternal bloodstream at the time of labor and delivery trigger an anaphylactic reaction, complement activation or both. The pathophysiology of amniotic fluid embolism is summarized in Fig. 14-31.

PATHOLOGY: In fatal cases of AFE, the lungs show diffuse alveolar damage (see Chapter 18). Platelet–fibrin aggregates are present in pulmonary

vessels, and increased megakaryocytes are often seen in alveoli, indicative of the onset of DIC. Distinctive fetal squamous epithelial cells are often present in both alveolar capillaries and larger blood vessels (Fig. 14-32A). Rarely, other fetal elements are present, including fetal hair (Fig. 14-32B).

 CLINICAL FEATURES: Initially, pulmonary arterial vasospasm, pulmonary hypertension and elevation of right ventricular pressure cause hypoxia. Myocardial and pulmonary capillary damage ensue. Left heart failure and ARDS develop, further endangering the patient. Women surviving the first phase of AFE may develop a second phase, including uterine atony, hemorrhage and DIC. A fatal consumptive coagulopathy may be the initial presentation.

INTRAHEPATIC CHOLESTASIS OF PREGNANCY

Intrahepatic cholestasis of pregnancy (ICP) is the second leading cause of jaundice during pregnancy and may endanger the health of the fetus. ICP occurs in only 1 or 2 women per 1000 pregnancies. It typically presents as intense pruritus. ICP usually begins in the third trimester but can occur any time during pregnancy. It can result in fetal distress, spontaneous premature delivery, meconium aspiration syndrome, intrauterine fetal demise and neonatal death.

 **ETIOLOGIC FACTORS:** The etiology of ICP is not known, but pregnancy hormones and genetic factors are probably involved. ICP most commonly occurs in the third trimester, when maternal pregnancy hormone levels are at their highest, and it occurs more often in multifetal pregnancies, which are associated with higher levels of hormones. Estrogens and glucuronides can cause cholestasis, and high-dose estrogen oral contraceptives can result in features of ICP in nonpregnant women.

 CLINICAL FEATURES: The most common maternal complaint is intense itching without a rash, most often involving the palms and soles. Levels of liver enzymes and serum bile acids can be elevated.

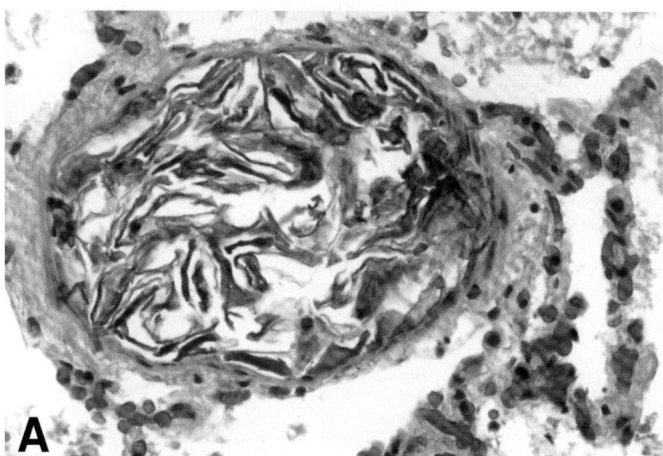
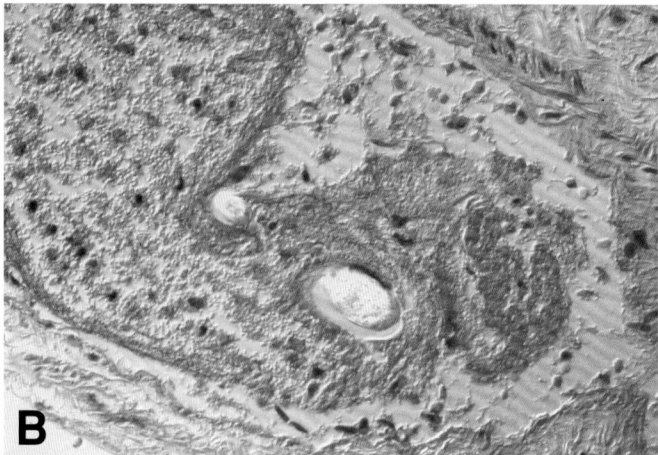

FIGURE 14-32. Amniotic fluid embolism. A. Lung from a woman who died from amniotic fluid embolism. Numerous tightly packed fetal squamous epithelial cells obstruct the lumen of this pulmonary blood vessel. **B.** Amniotic fluid embolism from another woman dying of this condition. Nomarski interference contrast highlights two golden brown cross-sections of a fetal hair in the maternal pulmonary circulation.

Less common symptoms include jaundice, dark urine, right upper quadrant pain and lighter stools. Risks of recurrence may be 90% in subsequent pregnancies.

GESTATIONAL DIABETES

In gestational diabetes, a pregnant woman without previous diabetes develops abnormally high blood glucose levels. The condition develops in 3%–10% of pregnancies. Gestational diabetes usually reverses after delivery, but entails an increased risk (30%–80%, depending on ethnicity) for recurring in future pregnancies. There is also a 50% risk

of diabetes within 6 years postpartum, which is highest in women who need insulin treatment during pregnancy, had antibodies (e.g., anti-islet cell antibodies) associated with diabetes, had more than two previous pregnancies and who are obese.

PATHOPHYSIOLOGY: The hallmark of gestational diabetes is resistance to maternal insulin (Fig. 14-33). Pregnancy hormones and other factors interfere with insulin binding to its receptor, leading to hyperglycemia.

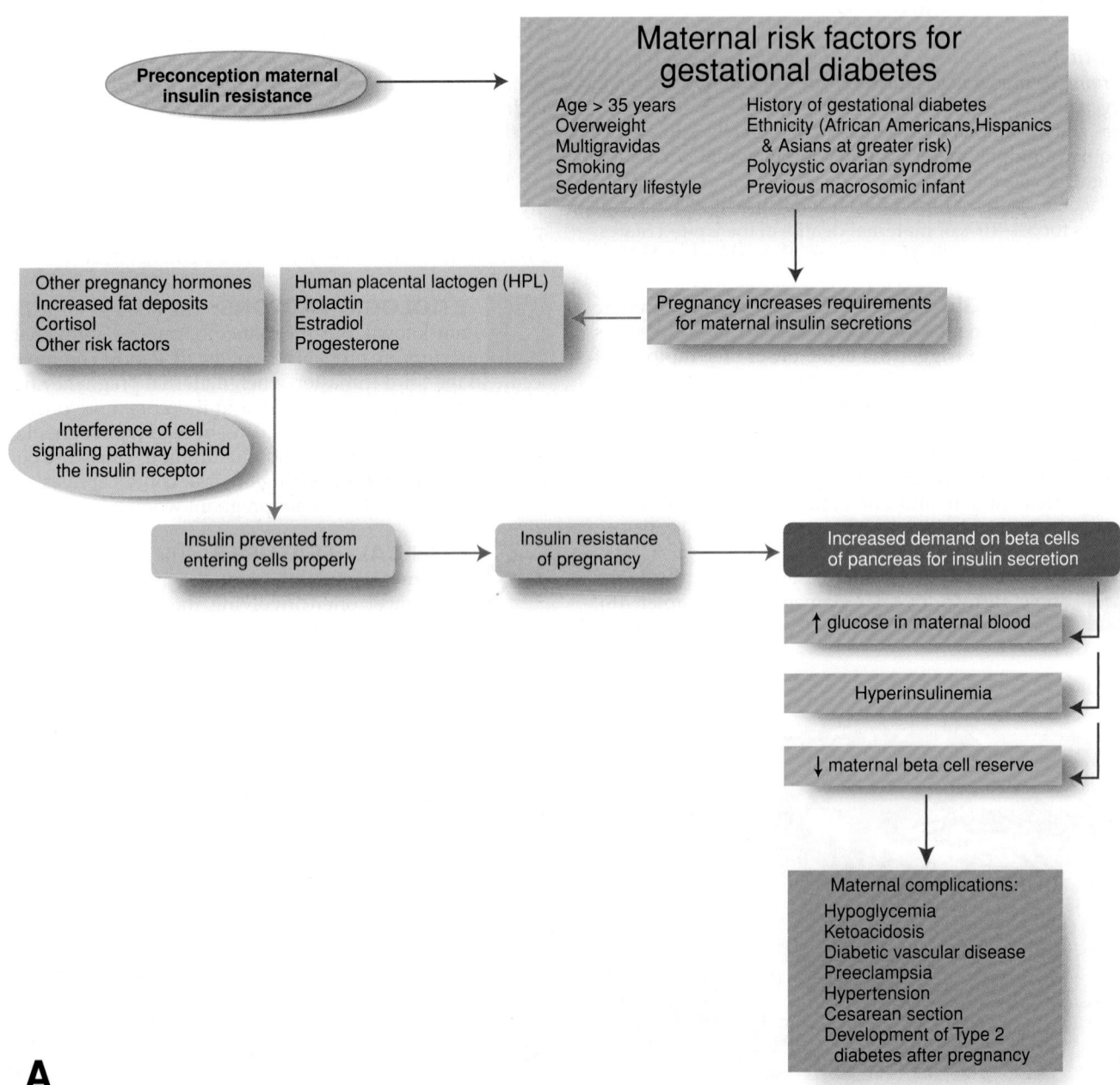

A

FIGURE 14-33. Current concepts of the pathophysiology of gestational diabetes.

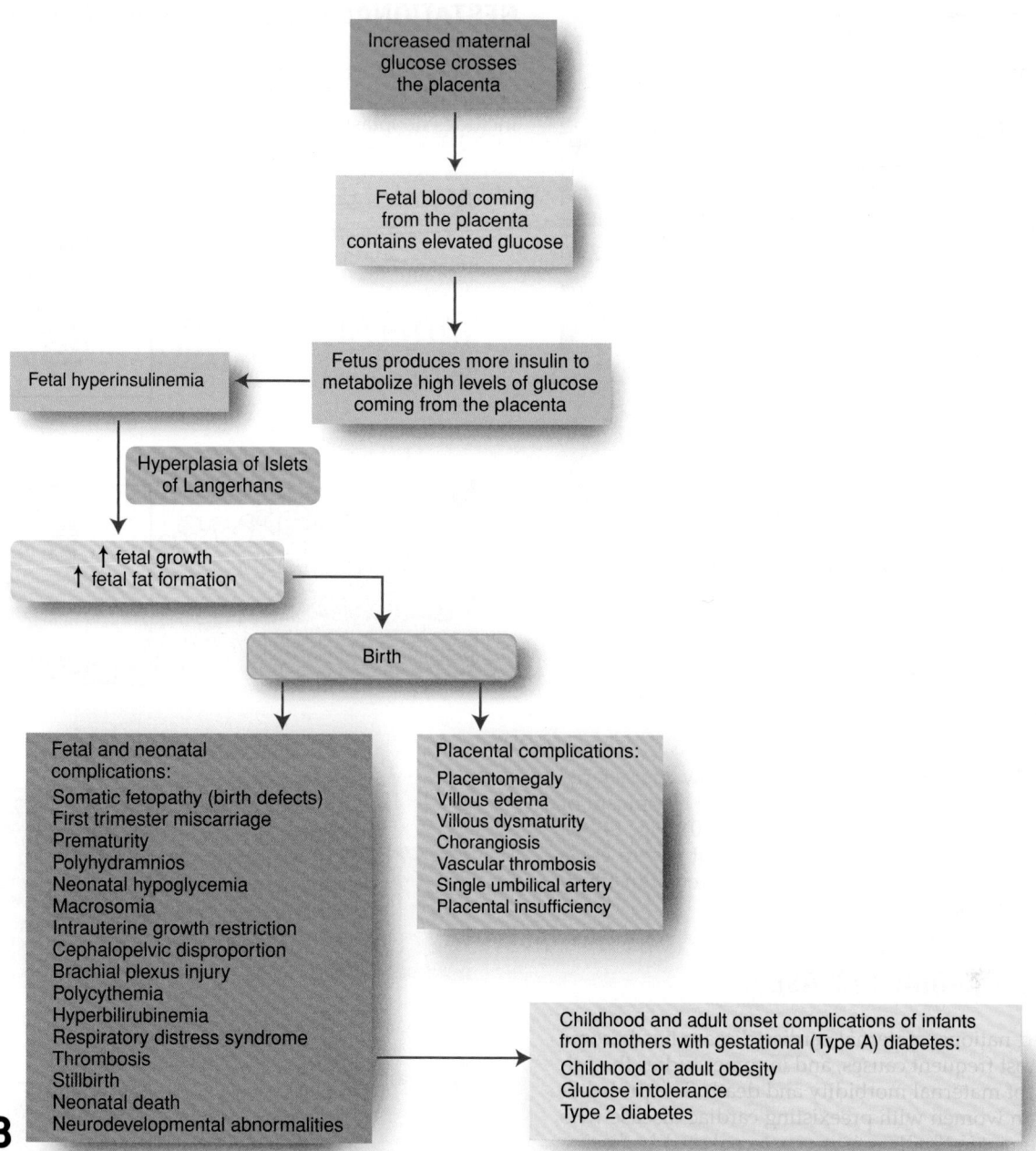

FIGURE 14-33. (*Continued*)

CLINICAL FEATURES: As mentioned above, infants of women with gestational diabetes may be abnormally large (macrosomia), unusually small or growth restricted. Congenital fetal malformations are increased with gestational diabetes, as are fetal and placental thrombosis. Neonates are at risk for a variety of metabolic abnormalities, including hypoglycemia, jaundice, polycythemia, hypocalcemia and hypomagnesemia.

ACUTE FATTY LIVER OF PREGNANCY

Acute fatty liver of pregnancy (AFLP) is a rare, lifethreatening complication of pregnancy caused by disordered metabolism of fatty acids by maternal mitochondria. It is commonly (50%–100%) associated with preeclampsia and can recur in subsequent pregnancies. AFLP occurs almost exclusively in the third trimester and is characterized by the onset of abdominal pain, jaundice and anorexia, with elevated levels of liver enzymes and bilirubin. DIC may occur in severe cases. Additional complications include pancreatitis and encephalopathy. AFLP is associated with 18% maternal mortality and 23% fetal mortality.

MOLECULAR PATHOGENESIS: Acute fatty liver of pregnancy is caused by a mitochondrial dysfunction, generally thought to be a deficiency in long-chain 3-hydroxyacyl-coenzyme A dehydrogenase (LCHAD). When fatty acid oxidation is deficient in the fetus, unmetabolized fatty acids reenter the maternal bloodstream

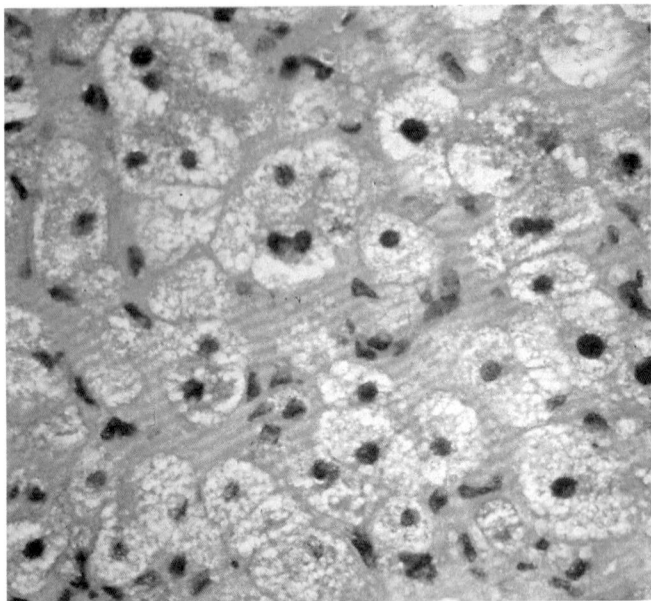

FIGURE 14-34. Acute fatty liver of pregnancy (AFLP). The hepatocytes contain microvesicular fat droplets.

through the placenta, overwhelming maternal β-oxidation enzymes. Microvesicular steatosis in the mothers' liver occurs as a result.

 PATHOLOGY: Livers in AFLP show characteristic microvesicular fat droplets in the cytoplasm of enlarged hepatocytes (see Chapter 20) (Fig. 14-34). Hepatocellular necrosis is usually absent, but severe cases may show hepatocyte dropout, collapse of reticulin fibers and portal tract inflammation.

MATERNAL CARDIAC DISEASE

In developed nations, maternal cardiac disease has become one of the most frequent causes, and in some studies the primary cause, of maternal morbidity and death. The probability of death in women with preexisting cardiac disease who become pregnant is 1%. Preexisting maternal cardiac disease also increases the risk of death of the infant 10-fold. Pregnancy is contraindicated in women with severe cardiac conditions, owing to a 25%–50% probability of maternal death.

Peripartum Cardiomyopathy Is Rarely Diagnosed before Delivery

This type of cardiomyopathy accounts for only 1% of cardiac events during pregnancy, but it is the cause of an increasing number of pregnancy-related maternal deaths. Only 10% of cases are diagnosed prior to delivery, with 75% detected in the postpartum period. Although the exact cause of peripartum cardiomyopathy is unknown, it is associated with increased maternal age, obesity, hypertension, multiparity, tocolysis with β-agonists, preeclampsia, low socioeconomic status and black race. Mortality is 25%–50%.

The large majority (65%) of pregnant women who die from preexisting heart conditions have congenital cardiac disease. The second leading cause of death is vascular heart disease (25%); 6% have cardiomyopathy.

GESTATIONAL TROPHOBLASTIC DISEASE

The spectrum of gestational trophoblastic disease reflects abnormal trophoblast proliferation and maturation and includes neoplasms derived from trophoblast (Fig. 14-35).

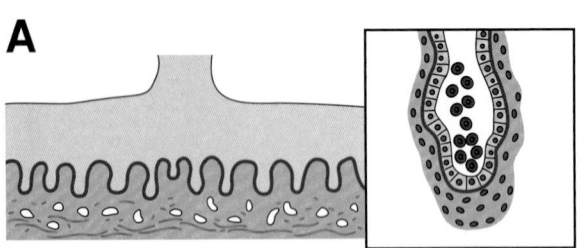

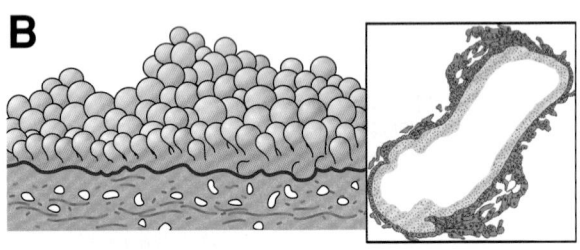

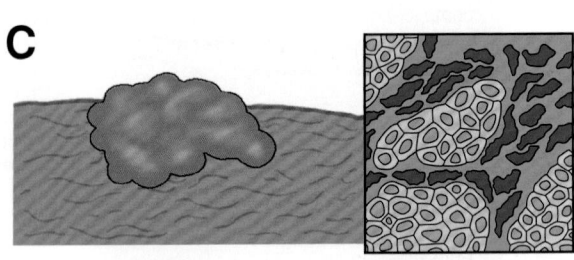

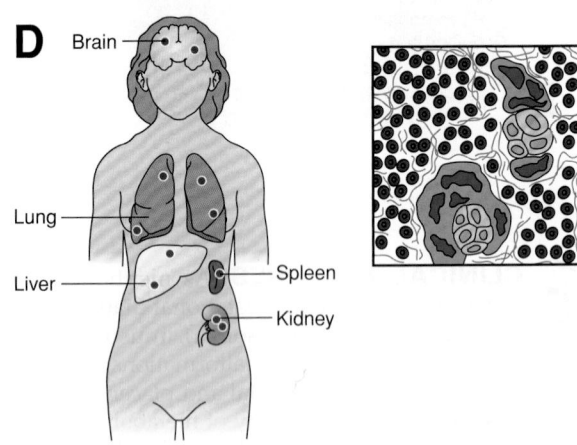

FIGURE 14-35. Proliferative disorders of the trophoblast. A. Normal chorionic villus of 8-week fetus, with blood vessel containing nucleated red blood cells. **B.** Complete hydatidiform mole with hydropic villi (also see Fig. 14-38). The villi are enlarged by an edematous stroma devoid of blood vessels. The trophoblastic epithelium is hyperplastic and exhibits variable atypia. **C.** Choriocarcinoma that has arisen in a molar pregnancy invades the myometrium and consists of admixed syncytiotrophoblastic and cytotrophoblastic elements. **D.** Common sites of metastasis from choriocarcinoma.

Complete Hydatidiform Mole Does Not Contain an Embryo

Complete hydatidiform mole is a placenta with grossly swollen chorionic villi, resembling bunches of grapes and showing varying degrees of trophoblastic proliferation. Villi are enlarged, often exceeding 5 mm in diameter (Fig. 14-36).

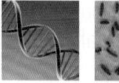 **MOLECULAR PATHOGENESIS AND ETIOLOGIC FACTORS:** Complete mole results from fertilization of an empty ovum that lacks functional maternal DNA. Most commonly, a haploid (23,X) set of paternal chromosomes introduced by monospermy duplicates to 46,XX, but dispermic 46,XX and 46,XY moles also occur. *Moles characteristically lack maternal chromosomes.* Paternally imprinted genes, such as *p57*, in which only the maternal allele is expressed, are not expressed in villous trophoblasts of androgenetic-derived complete moles. Since the embryo dies very early, before placental circulation has developed, few chorionic villi develop blood vessels, and fetal parts are absent.

 EPIDEMIOLOGY: The risk of hydatidiform mole relates to maternal age and has two peaks. Girls under 15 years of age have a 20-fold higher risk than women 20–35 years old. Risk increases progressively for women over 40 years. In fact, women older than 50 years of age have a 200-fold greater risk than those between 20 and 40 years. The incidence is manyfold higher in Asian women than in white women. In Taiwan, the risk is 25 times that in

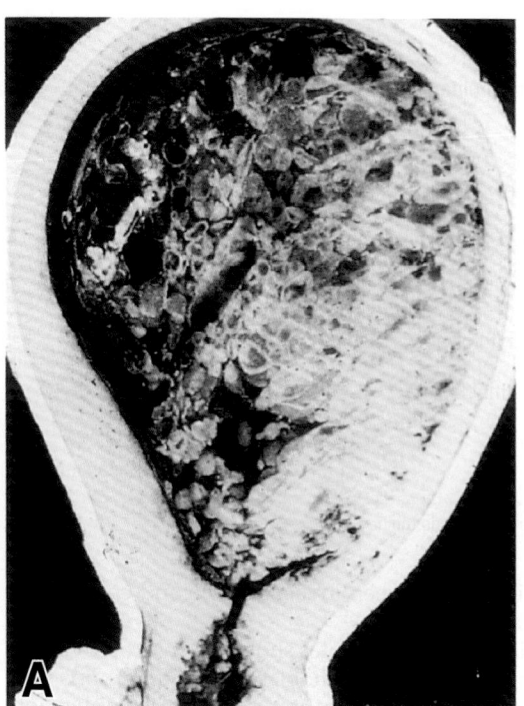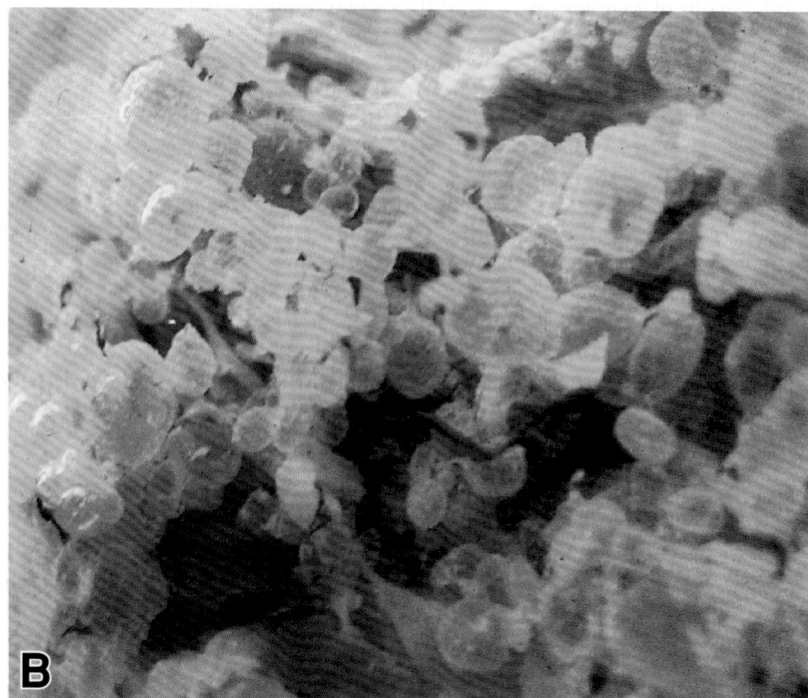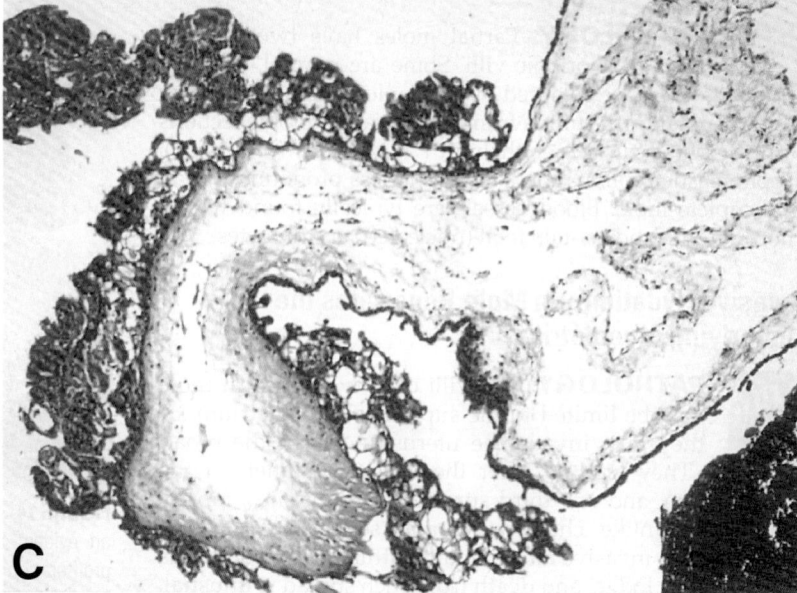

FIGURE 14-36. Complete hydatidiform mole. A. Complete mole in which the entire uterine cavity is filled with swollen villi. **B.** The villi are each 1–3 mm in diameter and appear grape-like. **C.** Individual molar villi, many of which have cavitated central cisterns, exhibit considerable trophoblastic hyperplasia and atypia. The blood vessels of the villi have atrophied and disappeared.

the United States. Women with a prior hydatidiform mole have a 20-fold greater risk of a subsequent molar pregnancy than does the general population.

 PATHOLOGY: Molar tissue is voluminous and consists of grossly visible villi that are obviously swollen (Fig. 14-36). Many individual villi have cisternae, which are central, acellular, fluid-filled spaces devoid of mesenchymal cells. Trophoblast is hyperplastic and composed of syncytiotrophoblast, cytotrophoblast and intermediate trophoblast. Considerable cellular atypia is present.

 CLINICAL FEATURES: Patients with complete moles commonly present between the 11th and 25th weeks of pregnancy with excessive uterine enlargement and often uterine bleeding. Passage of tissue fragments, which appear as small, grape-like masses, is common. Serum hCG levels are markedly elevated and increase rapidly.

Complications of complete mole include uterine hemorrhage, DIC, uterine perforation, trophoblastic embolism and infection. The most important complication is development of choriocarcinoma, which occurs in 2% of patients whose moles were evacuated.

Treatment consists of suction curettage of the uterus and subsequent monitoring of serum hCG levels. Up to 20% of patients require adjuvant chemotherapy for persistent disease, judging by stable or rising hCG levels. With such management, survival approaches 100%.

Partial Hydatidiform Mole Features Triploid Cells

Partial hydatidiform mole is a distinct entity that almost never evolves into choriocarcinoma (Table 14-2). Partial hydatidiform moles have 69 chromosomes (triploidy), of which one haploid set is maternal and two are paternal. This abnormal chromosomal complement results from fertilization of a normal ovum (23,X) by two spermatozoa, each with 23 chromosomes, or a single spermatozoon that failed meiotic reduction and has 46 chromosomes. Fetuses associated with a partial mole usually die after 10 weeks of gestation. Moles are aborted shortly thereafter. Thus, fetal parts may be present.

 PATHOLOGY: Partial moles have two populations of chorionic villi. Some are normal, whereas others are enlarged by hydropic swelling and show central cavitation, resulting from tangential histologic sections of invaginated surface epithelium ("fjord-like") (Fig. 14-37). Trophoblastic proliferation is focal and less pronounced than in complete mole. Blood vessels are typically found within chorionic villi and contain fetal (nucleated) erythrocytes.

Invasive Hydatidiform Mole Penetrates the Underlying Myometrium

 PATHOLOGY: The villi of a hydatidiform mole may be limited to the superficial myometrium, or they may invade the uterus and even the broad ligament. They tend to enter the venous channels of the myometrium, and one third spread to distant sites, mostly the lungs. Unlike choriocarcinoma (see below), distant deposits of an invasive mole remain within the blood vessels in which they lodge, and death from such spread is unusual.

TABLE 14-2

COMPARATIVE FEATURES OF COMPLETE AND PARTIAL HYDATIDIFORM MOLE

Features	Complete Mole	Partial Mole
Karyotype	46,XX	47,XXY or 47,XXX
Parental origin of haploid genome sets	Both paternal	1 maternal, 2 paternal
Preoperative diagnosis	Mole	Missed abortion
Marked vaginal bleeding	3+	1+
Uterus	Large	Small
Serum hCG	High	Less elevated
Hydropic villi	All	Some
Trophoblastic proliferation	Diffuse	Focal
Atypia	Diffuse	Minimal
hCG in tissue	3+	1+
Embryo present	No	Some
Blood vessels	No	Common
Nucleated erythrocytes	No	Sometimes
Persists after initial therapy	20%	7%
Choriocarcinoma	2% after mole	No choriocarcinoma

hCG = human chorionic gonadotropin.

Clinical distinction between invasive mole and choriocarcinoma is often difficult.

Histologically, invasive moles show less hydropic change than do complete moles. Trophoblastic proliferation is usually prominent. Uterine perforation is a major complication,

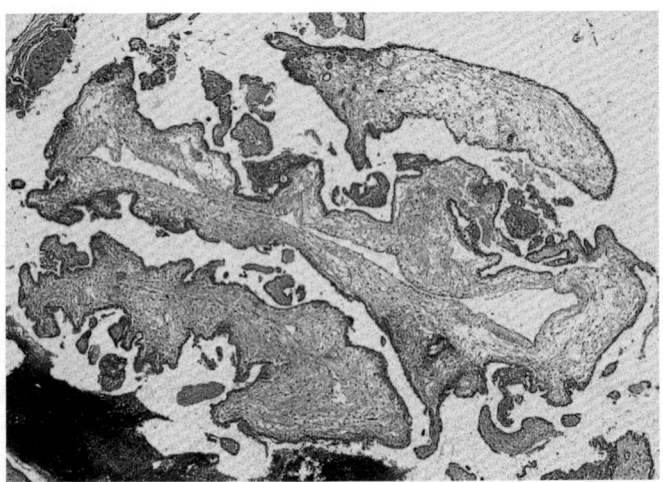

FIGURE 14-37. Partial hydatidiform mole. Two populations of chorionic villi are evident. Some are normal; others are conspicuously swollen. Trophoblastic proliferation is focal and less conspicuous than in a complete mole.

but occurs in only a minority of cases. Theca lutein cysts (see Chapter 24), which may occur with any form of trophoblastic disease as a result of hCG stimulation, are prominent with invasive moles.

Gestational Choriocarcinoma Is Derived from Trophoblast

 **EPIDEMIOLOGY:** Choriocarcinoma occurs in 1 in 30,000 pregnancies in the United States; in eastern Asia, the frequency is far greater. The incidence seems related to abnormalities of pregnancy. In whites, 25% arise from term deliveries, 25% from spontaneous abortions and 50% from complete hydatidiform moles. Although the risk that a complete hydatidiform mole will transform into choriocarcinoma is only 2%, it is still several orders of magnitude higher than if the pregnancy were normal.

 PATHOLOGY: Uterine lesions of choriocarcinoma range from microscopic foci to huge necrotic and hemorrhagic tumors. Viable tumor is usually confined to the rim of the neoplasm because, unlike most other cancers, choriocarcinomas lack intrinsic tumor vasculature. These tumors contain a dimorphic population of cytotrophoblast and syncytiotrophoblast, with varying degrees of intermediate trophoblast (Fig. 14-38). The tumor resembles the

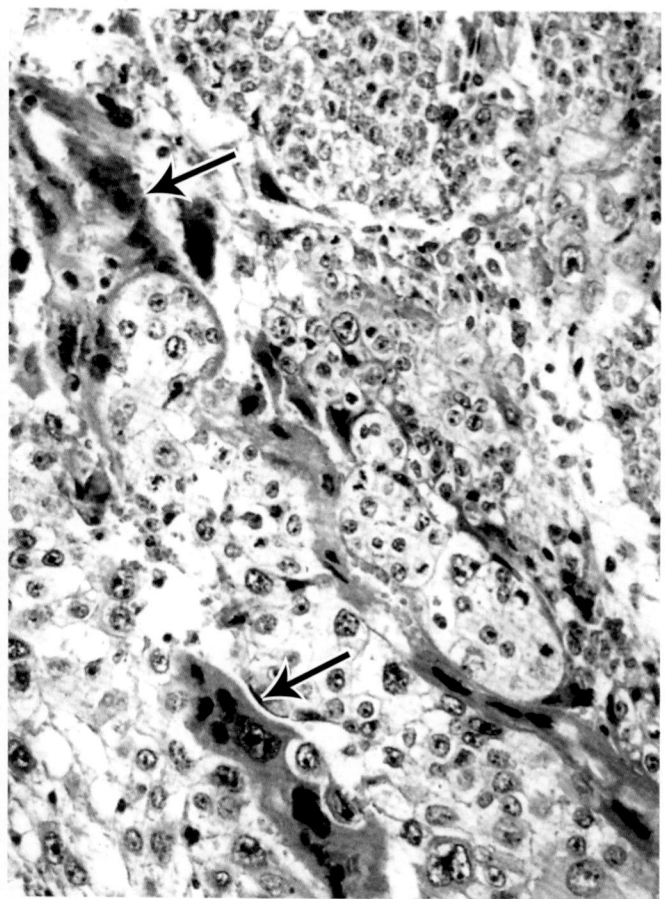

FIGURE 14-38. Choriocarcinoma. Malignant cytotrophoblast and syncytiotrophoblast (*arrows*) are present.

TABLE 14-3	
CLINICAL STAGING OF GESTATIONAL TROPHOBLASTIC TUMORS	
I	Confined to the uterus
Ia	0 risk factors
Ib	1 risk factor
Ic	2 risk factors
II	Extends outside of the uterus but limited to genital structures
III	Extends to lungs
IV	All other metastatic sites

Risk factors affecting stage include (1) human chorionic gonadotropin (hCG) >100,000 mIU/mL and (2) duration of disease >6 months from termination of antecedent pregnancy.

trophoblast of an early implanting blastocyst. Rims of syncytiotrophoblast surround central cytotrophoblastic cores, in addition to being arranged around maternal blood spaces, which resemble the intervillous space of normal placentation. hCG is localized to the syncytiotrophoblastic element. *By definition, tumors containing any villous structures, even if metastatic, are considered hydatidiform mole and not choriocarcinoma.*

Choriocarcinomas invade mainly via venous sinuses in the myometrium. They metastasize widely hematogenously, especially to lungs (>90%), brain, gastrointestinal tract, liver and vagina (Table 14-3).

 CLINICAL FEATURES: Abnormal uterine bleeding is the most common first symptom of choriocarcinoma. Occasionally, the tumor first presents with metastases to lungs or brain. In some cases, it may only become evident 10 or more years after the last pregnancy.

With current chemotherapy, survival rates exceed 70% even for tumors that have metastasized. Virtually 100% remission is expected if a tumor is localized. Serial serum hCG levels are used to monitor the effectiveness of treatment.

Placental Site Trophoblastic Tumor Outcomes Are Unpredictable

Placental site trophoblastic tumors are the least common trophoblastic tumors. They are mainly composed of intermediate trophoblastic cells.

 PATHOLOGY: The gross appearance of placental site trophoblastic tumor is more variable than that of choriocarcinoma. Often, the myometrium shows an ill-defined, yellowish tumor without conspicuous hemorrhage. The extent of myometrial invasion varies, and patterns of infiltration resemble that of normal trophoblast in the placental bed. Since intermediate trophoblast in a normal pregnancy anchors the pregnancy to the superficial myometrium, the microscopic appearance of these tumors is typically that of an exaggerated placental site. Mononuclear and multinuclear trophoblast may be present as single cells or as cords, islands and sheets of cells interspersed among myometrial cells. Neither necrosis nor chorionic villi are present. Placental site trophoblastic tumor is also distinguished from choriocarcinoma by its monomorphic (intermediate) trophoblastic proliferation, unlike the dimorphic pattern of trophoblast in choriocarcinoma. Most trophoblastic cells express human placental lactogen (hPL), but a few express hCG.

CLINICAL FEATURES: The age and parity of patients with placental site trophoblastic tumor are like those of patients with choriocarcinoma. Half of patients report amenorrhea, whereas vaginal bleeding usually occurs with choriocarcinoma. Past history of a molar pregnancy is much less common than in women with choriocarcinoma (5% vs. 50%).

Placental site trophoblastic tumors must be excised completely (hysterectomy) to prevent local recurrence. They sometimes metastasize and may be fatal. Large tumors and high mitotic indices are associated with a worse prognosis. Because of the short half-life of hPL, serum levels of hCG are more useful in monitoring response to treatment. Conservative management usually suffices. If hCG persists, even at low levels, or mitotic count is elevated, aggressive treatment with hysterectomy or chemotherapy is indicated.

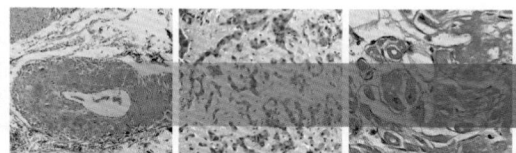

15

The Amyloidoses

Philip Hawkins

Constituents of Amyloid **Staining Properties of Amyloid Deposits**	**Clinical Classification of the Amyloidoses and Fibril Proteins** Acquired Amyloidosis Hereditary Amyloidosis	**Morphologic Features of Amyloidosis** **Clinical Features and Organ Involvement in Amyloidosis** **Treatment of Amyloidosis**

CONSTITUENTS OF AMYLOID

Amyloid refers to a group of diverse extracellular protein deposits that have (1) common morphologic properties, (2) affinities for specific dyes and (3) a characteristic appearance under polarized light. All proteins that form amyloid are folded so they share common ultrastructural and physical properties, despite different amino acid sequences. **Amyloidosis** encompasses the clinical disorders caused directly by localized or systemic amyloid deposition.

Diseases associated with amyloid deposition have been recognized for more than 300 years, but only in the mid-19th century were attempts made to define these tissue deposits by their staining properties. Amyloid stained blue with acidified iodine, a method that demonstrates cellulose or starch. Hence, the term **amyloid** (Greek for "starch-like") was coined, and has been retained, although the protein nature of these deposits has been recognized for over 100 years. Protein misfolding and aggregation are increasingly being recognized in various other diseases, but amyloidosis—the disease directly caused by extracellular amyloid deposition—is a precise term with critical implications for patients with a specific group of life-threatening disorders.

More than 25 different unrelated proteins can form amyloid in vivo, and clinical amyloidosis is classified by the identity of the fibril protein. Amyloid deposition is remarkably diverse: it can be systemic or localized, acquired or hereditary, life-threatening or merely incidental. Clinical consequences occur when amyloid accumulates sufficiently to disrupt the structure of tissues or organs and to impair function. Patterns of organ involvement vary among the amyloidoses, but clinical phenotypes overlap greatly. In **systemic amyloidosis,** virtually any tissue may be involved. This form of the disease is often fatal, although prognosis has improved due to better treatments for many of the underlying conditions. **Localized amyloid deposits** are confined to a particular organ or tissue and range from being clinically silent to life-threatening (e.g., cardiac amyloidosis).

In addition to clinical disorders classified as amyloidoses, local amyloid deposits are seen in other important disorders including Alzheimer disease (see Chapter 32), prion disorders and pancreatic islets in type 2 diabetes mellitus (see Chapter 13).

MOLECULAR PATHOGENESIS: Amyloidosis defies the dogma that tertiary structure of proteins is determined solely by primary amino acid sequence. Amyloid-forming proteins can exist in two completely different stable structures: (1) **a native form** and (2) transformation by massive refolding of the native form into predominantly **β-sheets** that can autoaggregate in a highly ordered manner to produce characteristic fibrils. Such amyloid fibrils are rigid, nonbranching, 10–15 nm in diameter and indeterminate in length. Acquired biophysical properties that are common to all amyloid fibrils include insolubility in physiologic solutions, relative resistance to proteolysis and the ability to bind **Congo red dye** in a spatially ordered manner to produce the diagnostic green birefringence under cross-polarized light (Fig. 15-1).

There are several circumstances in which amyloid deposition occurs (Fig. 15-2):

- *Sustained, abnormally high abundance of certain proteins that are normally present at low levels,* such as serum amyloid A protein (SAA) in chronic inflammation and β_2-microglobulin in renal failure, which underlie susceptibility to AA and $A\beta_2M$ amyloidosis, respectively (see below)
- *Normal concentrations of a normal, but to some extent inherently amyloidogenic, protein over a very prolonged period,* such as transthyretin in senile amyloidosis (ATTR) and β-protein in Alzheimer disease
- *Presence of an acquired or inherited variant protein with an abnormal, markedly amyloidogenic structure,* such as certain monoclonal immunoglobulin light chains in AL amyloidosis and the genetic amyloidogenic variants of transthyretin, lysozyme, apolipoprotein AI and fibrinogen Aα chain in hereditary amyloidosis

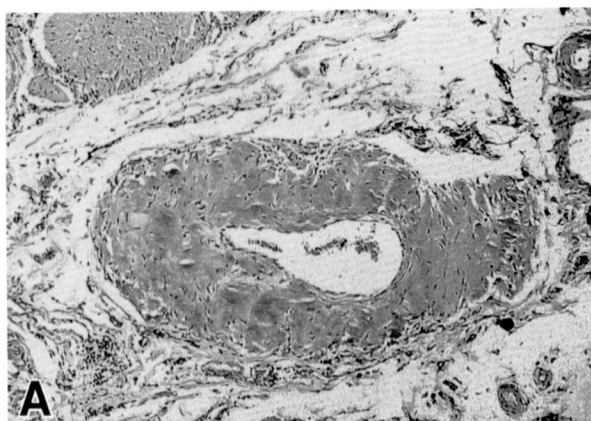
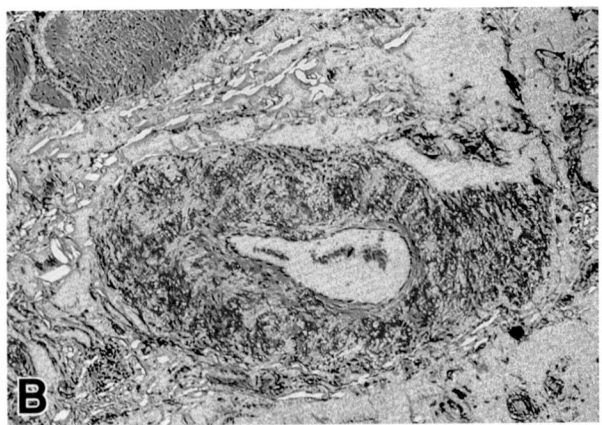

FIGURE 15-1. AL amyloid involving the wall of an artery stained with Congo red is shown under **(A)** ordinary light and **(B)** polarized light. Note the red-green birefringence of the amyloid. Collagen has a silvery appearance.

Although it is not clear why only the 20 or so known amyloidogenic proteins adopt the amyloid fold and persist as fibrils in vivo, a unifying theme is that amyloid precursors are relatively unstable. Even under normal physiologic conditions, these proteins can exist in partly unfolded states involving loss of tertiary structure but retention of β-sheet secondary structure, and which can autoaggregate into protofilaments and thence mature amyloid fibrils.

Amyloid deposits consist mainly of these protein fibrils but also contain some common minor constituents, including certain **glycosaminoglycans** (GAGs), the normal plasma protein **serum amyloid P component** (SAP) and various other trace proteins such as **apolipoprotein E** (apoE), **laminin** and **collagen IV** (Fig. 15-3).

- SAP binds in a specific calcium-dependent manner to a domain that is present on all amyloid fibrils but not on their respective precursor proteins. This phenomenon is the basis for the use of SAP scintigraphy for diagnostic imaging and quantitative monitoring of amyloid deposits. Animal studies indicate that SAP contributes to amyloidogenesis. SAP is also a minor, structural component of normal basement membranes.
- Amyloid fibril-associated GAGs are mainly heparan and dermatan sulphates. Their universal presence, restricted heterogeneity and intimate relationship with the fibrils are consistent with their contribution to the development or stability of amyloid deposits. This hypothesis has been supported by the inhibitory effect of low–molecular-weight GAG analogs on the experimental induction of AA amyloidosis in mice and people.

The genetic and/or environmental factors that determine the individual susceptibility and timing of amyloid deposition are unclear, although several factors may be at play:

- Once the process has begun, further accumulation of amyloid is unremitting so long as there is a continuous supply of the respective precursor protein. Initiation of amyloid accumulation may involve a "seeding" process, consistent with observations that amyloid deposition can be remarkably rapid following its initiation. Seeding may be a stochastic event. The notion of seeding is supported by observations in experimental murine AA amyloidosis, in which nanogram quantities of parenterally administered amyloid material result in massive amyloid deposition within 24 hours of developing an acute phase SAA response. The existence of an "amyloid-enhancing factor" (AEF) has been proposed.
- Both increasing age and male sex appear to be potent susceptibility factors in wild-type TTR amyloid deposition. Clinical sequelae of this kind of amyloid are almost unheard before age 60 years, and more than 90% of patients are male.
- The factors that influence the anatomic distribution of amyloid deposits are also unclear, but there is reasonable consistency among the organ involvement associated with AA and most hereditary types of amyloidosis in

Amyloid precursor proteins

Increased synthesis (e.g., SAA or L-chains)	Constitutive synthesis (e.g., TTR)	Mutant forms (e.g., TTR in FAP)

↓

Protein precursor pool

↓

Native protein conformation

Fibrillogenic microenvironment →

Amyloidogenic conformation

Tissue amyloid deposits →

Fibril formation

↓

Proteolysis and turnover of amyloid →

Pruning of amyloid proteins

FIGURE 15-2. General scheme for amyloidogenesis. *FAP* = familial amyloidotic polyneuropathy; *SAA* = serum amyloid A protein; *TTR* = transthyretin.

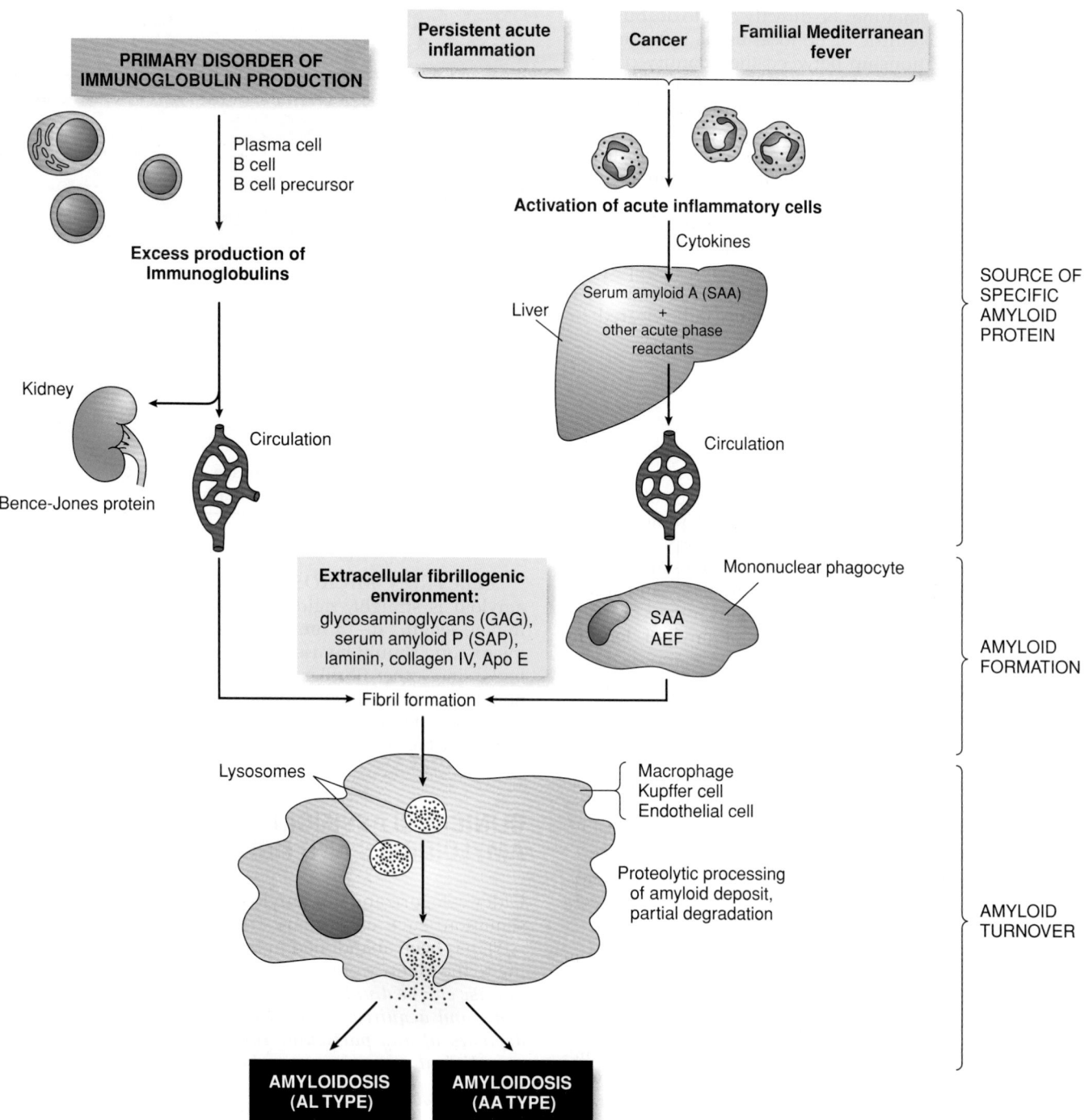

FIGURE 15-3. The mechanisms of amyloid deposition. For **AL amyloid:** Certain lymphocyte- and plasma cell–derived immunoglobulin light chains are amyloidogenic within a fibrillogenic environment. For **AA amyloid** deposition: A variety of diseases are associated with the activation of polymorphonuclear leukocytes and macrophages, which in turn leads to the synthesis and release of acute phase reactants by the liver, including serum amyloid A protein (SAA). SAA may undergo cleavage by macrophages, and its conversion into AA fibrils is promoted by amyloid-enhancing factor (AEF). In a fibrillogenic environment, the released products complex with glycosaminoglycans and serum amyloid P component (SAP). Macrophages are also involved in turnover of amyloid.

which the fibril protein has the same structure in all individuals. By contrast, the organ distribution in AL amyloidosis is extremely heterogeneous, probably reflecting the unique sequence of the respective monoclonal immunoglobulin light chain in each patient.

The pathologic effects of amyloid are due to its physical presence. Extensive deposits may total kilograms, are structurally disruptive and impair normal function, as do strategically located smaller deposits (e.g., in glomeruli or nerves). It is possible that amyloid fibrils or prefibrillar aggregates may sometimes be directly cytotoxic, but amyloid deposits evoke little or no local tissue inflammatory reaction. The relationship between the quantity of amyloid deposited and the degree of associated organ dysfunction differs greatly between individuals and between different organs, and there is a strong impression that the rate of new amyloid deposition may be as important a determinant of progressive organ failure as the absolute amyloid load.

Treatments that reduce the supply of amyloidogenic precursor proteins may result in stabilization or regression of existing amyloid deposits, preserving or improving the function of organs infiltrated by amyloid, although the mechanisms by which amyloid deposits can be cleared are poorly understood.

STAINING PROPERTIES OF AMYLOID DEPOSITS

The staining properties and general appearance of amyloid are governed primarily by its compact and proteinaceous nature. Because of this, amyloid has few morphologic features visible on light microscopy. With routine stains (hematoxylin and eosin), amyloid is amorphous, glassy and almost cartilage-like, appearing much like many other proteins. However, the nature and organization of amyloid deposits allow it to be stained in specific ways.

CONGO RED: All types of amyloid stain red with the Congo red dye but exhibit red-green birefringence when viewed under cross-polarized light (Fig. 15-1). The fibrillar deposits organized in one plane exhibit one color, and those opposite to that plane appear the other color. Congo red is the stain most commonly used for the diagnosis of amyloidosis, although published techniques vary in their sensitivity and specificity.

THIOFLAVIN T: Although not entirely specific for amyloid, staining with thioflavin T allows amyloid to fluoresce when viewed in ultraviolet light.

ALCIAN BLUE: The presence of glycosaminoglycans in all amyloid deposits is evident with a variety of Alcian blue stains, which cause GAGs to appear blue.

SPECIFIC ANTIBODIES: Immunohistochemistry is the best way to characterize amyloid, although its success varies with fibril protein type and depends on availability of a suitable tissue sample that contains neither too little nor too much amyloid. Antibodies to SAA virtually always stain AA deposits, as is the case with antibodies to β_2-microglobulin in hemodialysis-associated amyloid. In AL amyloid, deposits in fixed specimens are stained convincingly with antibodies to κ or λ immunoglobulin light chains in only about two thirds of cases, in part because AL fibrils are chiefly variable light-chain domains with unique sequences in each case. Immunohistochemical staining of TTR and other hereditary amyloid fibril proteins may require pretreatment of sections with formic acid, alkaline guanidine or deglycosylation, and even then, does not always yield definitive results. Demonstration of SAP, the most abundant nonfibrillar protein present in all types of amyloid, helps to corroborate that deposits are indeed amyloid and can be particularly useful in excluding light-chain deposition disease.

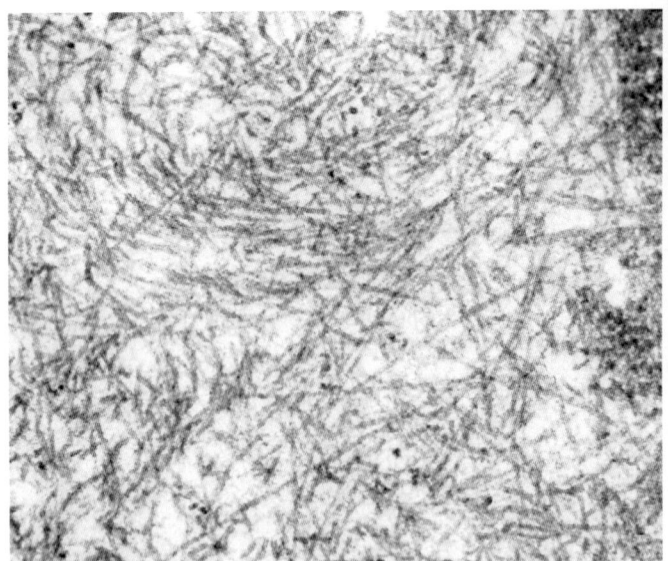

FIGURE 15-4. Amyloid deposits in tissue. Parallel and interlacing arrays of fibrils are evident in this electron micrograph.

ELECTRON MICROSCOPY: By electron microscopy, amyloid is straight, rigid nonbranching fibrils of indeterminate length, 10–15 nm in diameter (Fig. 15-4). Electron microscopy should be used to supplement other diagnostic tools, since other fibrillar deposition diseases occur. Immunogold staining of amyloidotic biopsies can sometimes be diagnostic of fibril protein type if light microscopic immunochemistry has not produced definitive results.

CLINICAL CLASSIFICATION OF THE AMYLOIDOSES AND FIBRIL PROTEINS

Older categorization of amyloidosis based on clinical presentation, such as primary (for AL) and secondary (for AA), has been abandoned in favor of classification according to the identity of the amyloid proteins (Table 15-1). *The disease can be divided into systemic or localized distributions and acquired or hereditary etiologies, but amyloid deposits of any particular type do not necessarily have any clinical consequences and can be merely an incidental finding.*

Acquired Amyloidosis Derives from Diverse Sources

Acquired systemic amyloidosis is thought to be the cause of death in about 1 in 1000 individuals in Western countries, and is probably underdiagnosed among the elderly, who are likely to be at greatest risk of developing it. Systemic AL amyloidosis is the most common and serious type, accounting for over 60% of cases. Although less serious, dialysis-related β_2-microglobulin amyloidosis affects about 1 million patients on long-term renal replacement therapy worldwide. Senile transthyretin amyloidosis, which predominantly involves the heart, occurs in about one quarter of individuals older than 80 years, a sector of the population that is ever rising.

TABLE 15-1
CLASSIFICATION OF HUMAN AMYLOIDS

Amyloid Protein	Protein Precursor	Clinical Setting
AL	k Or λ immunoglobulin light chain	Multiple myeloma, plasma cell dyscrasias and primary amyloid
AH	γ Immunoglobulin chain	Waldenström macroglobulinemia
A2M	β_2-Microglobulin	Hemodialysis related
ATTR	Transthyretin	Familial amyloidotic polyneuropathy (FAP), normal TTR in senile systemic amyloid
AA	Apo serum AA	Persistent acute inflammation; familial Mediterranean fever; certain malignancies
AApoAI	Apolipoprotein AI	FAP Iowa
AApoAII	Apolipoprotein AII	Familial
AApoAIV	Apolipoprotein AIV	Sporadic, age associated
Aβ	β-Protein precursor	Alzheimer disease, Down syndrome, hereditary cerebral hemorrhage with amyloid (HCHWA), Dutch
ABri	ABriPP	Familial dementia, British
ADan	ADanPP	Familial dementia, Danish
APrP	Prion protein	CJD, scrapie, BSE, GSS, Kuru
ACys	Cystatin C	HCHWA, Icelandic
ALys	Lysozyme	Hereditary systemic amyloidosis, Ostertag type
AFib	Fibrinogen	Hereditary renal amyloidosis
AGel	Gelsolin	Familial amyloidosis, Finnish
ACal	(Pro)calcitonin	Medullary carcinoma of the thyroid
AANF	Atrial natriuretic factor	Isolated atrial amyloid
AIAPP	Islet amyloid polypeptide	Type 2 diabetes, insulinomas
AIns	Insulin	Iatrogenic
APro	Prolactin	Pituitary, age associated
AMed	Lactadherin	Senile aortic, media
AKer	Keratoepithelin	Cornea, familial
ALac	Lactoferrin	Cornea

Apo = apolipoprotein; BSE = bovine spongiform encephalopathy; CJD = Creutzfeldt-Jakob disease; GSS = Gerstmann-Sträussler-Scheinker syndrome; TTR = transthyretin.

Reactive Systemic Amyloidosis, AA Amyloidosis

AA amyloidosis is a complication of chronic infections and inflammatory diseases, or any condition that leads to long-term overproduction of the acute phase reactant SAA. The amyloid fibrils are composed of an N-terminal cleavage fragment of SAA (i.e., AA protein). AA amyloidosis occurs in 1%–5% of patients with rheumatoid arthritis, juvenile idiopathic arthritis and Crohn disease, and is more common in those with untreated lifelong autoinflammatory diseases such as familial Mediterranean fever. Most patients present with proteinuria, and although liver and gastrointestinal involvement may occur later, clinically significant cardiac or neuropathic involvement is very rare.

 MOLECULAR PATHOGENESIS: *AA protein is a single nonglycosylated polypeptide chain usually of mass ~8 kd making up the 76-residue N-terminal portion of the 104-residue SAA.* Smaller and larger AA fragments occur. SAA is an apolipoprotein of high-density lipoprotein particles and is the polymorphic product of a set of genes located on chromosome 11. It is highly conserved in evolution and is a major acute phase reactant. Most SAA in plasma is produced by hepatocytes under transcriptional regulation by cytokines, especially interleukin 1 (IL-1), IL-6 and tumor necrosis factor-α (TNF-α). After secretion, SAA rapidly associates with high-density lipoproteins, from which it displaces apolipoprotein AI. Circulating SAA can rise from normal levels (≤3 mg/L) to over 2000 mg/L within 24–48 hours of an acute stimulus, and remains elevated indefinitely in the presence of chronic inflammation.

Cleavage of circulating SAA to AA can be done by macrophages and several proteinases, but it is not known whether cleavage of SAA occurs before and/or after aggregation of monomers during AA fibrillogenesis. Long-term overproduction of SAA is a prerequisite for deposition of AA amyloid, but it is not known why the latter occurs in only some individuals. SAA isoforms are complex, but homozygosity for particular types seems to favor amyloidogenesis, as may ethnic differences in susceptibility.

SAA function is not known, but it may modulate effects on reverse cholesterol transport and on lipid functions in the microenvironment of inflammatory foci. Regardless of its physiologic role, SAA as an exquisitely sensitive acute phase protein with enormous dynamic range, making it a very valuable empirical clinical marker. It can be used to monitor the extent and activity of many infective, inflammatory, necrotic and neoplastic diseases. Frequent long-term monitoring of SAA is vital in managing all patients with AA amyloidosis, as the primary inflammatory process must be controlled sufficiently to reduce SAA production if amyloid deposition is to be halted or enabled to regress. Automated immunoassays for SAA are available standardized on a World Health Organization International Reference Standard.

AA amyloidosis occurs in association with chronic inflammatory disorders, chronic local or systemic microbial infections and, occasionally, neoplasms. In the Western world, the most common predisposing conditions are chronic inflammatory diseases, particularly rheumatoid arthritis. Amyloidosis is exceptionally rare in ulcerative colitis or systemic lupus erythematosus and related connective tissue diseases, since these conditions provoke only modest acute phase responses. Tuberculosis and leprosy are important causes of AA amyloidosis in some parts of the world. Chronic osteomyelitis, bronchiectasis, chronically infected burns and decubitus ulcers and the chronic pyelonephritis of paraplegia are other well-recognized associations. Hodgkin disease and renal carcinoma often cause a major acute phase response and are the malignancies most commonly associated with systemic AA amyloid. The associated chronic inflammatory disease in about 7% of patients with AA amyloidosis may not be clinically evident, and these patients may be erroneously assumed to have AL amyloidosis.

AA amyloid deposits are widely distributed, and so random rectal and other biopsies are often used to make the diagnosis. However, clinically, AA amyloidosis is dominated by progressive proteinuria. Treatment entails measures to suppress the underlying inflammatory disorder. Prognosis is now often excellent among patients in whom the causative acute phase response can be substantially suppressed, but about 50% of patients with persistent uncontrolled inflammation die within 10 years of diagnosis.

Amyloidosis Associated with Monoclonal B-Cell Dyscrasias, AL Amyloidosis

Systemic AL, once known as "primary," amyloidosis occurs in about 2% of people with monoclonal B-cell dyscrasias.

AL fibrils are derived from monoclonal immunoglobulin light chains. These are unique in each patient, so that AL amyloidosis is highly heterogeneous in terms of organ involvement and overall clinical course. Virtually any organ other than the brain may be directly affected, but the kidneys, heart, liver and peripheral nerves bear the brunt of the clinical consequences. As the underlying monoclonal gammopathy is often missed by routine screening techniques, very sensitive methods, such as serum free light-chain analysis, may be needed to identify the causative subtle B-cell dyscrasias.

 **MOLECULAR PATHOGENESIS:** *AL amyloid fibrils are usually derived from the N-terminal region of monoclonal immunoglobulin light chains and consist of the whole or part of the variable (V$_L$) domain.* The molecular weight of the fibril subunit protein thus varies between 8 and 30 kd. Monoclonal light chains are unique to each individual, and only a small percentage are amyloidogenic, but it is not possible to predict which light chains will form AL amyloid.

The property of "amyloidogenicity" is inherent in certain monoclonal light chains. Thus, when purified human Bence Jones proteins (urinary light-chain proteins) were injected into mice, animals receiving light chains from patients with AL amyloid developed typical amyloid deposits, while mice given light chains from myeloma patients without amyloid did not. AL fibrils develop more commonly from λ than κ light chains, despite the fact that κ-chains are more common among normal immunoglobulins and monoclonal gammopathies. Compared to light chains that do not form amyloid, some amyloidogenic light chains have distinctive amino acid replacements or insertions that can promote aggregation and insolubility, including replacement of hydrophilic framework residues by hydrophobic ones. Certain light-chain types, notably Vλ$_{VI}$, are especially amyloidogenic, and some tend to be deposited as amyloid in particular organs. For example, Vλ$_{VI}$ light chains often deposit in the kidney, while Vλ$_{II}$ chains prefer the heart.

B-cell dyscrasias underlying systemic AL amyloidosis are also heterogeneous and include almost any clonal proliferation of differentiated B cells: multiple myeloma, Waldenström macroglobulinemia and occasionally other malignant lymphomas or leukemias. However, over 80% of cases are associated with low-grade and otherwise "benign" monoclonal gammopathies that may be difficult to detect. Histologically, minor and clinically insignificant amyloid deposits are seen in up to 10% of patients with myeloma, and similarly in a smaller proportion of patients with monoclonal gammopathy of undetermined significance (MGUS). Cytogenetic abnormalities common in multiple myeloma and MGUS, such as 14q translocations and 13q deletion, are also observed in AL amyloidosis, but their prognostic significance is not yet understood.

Localized AL Amyloidosis

A localized monoclonal B-cell dyscrasia may lead to AL deposits at the site of that B-cell lesion, almost anywhere in the body. Characteristic sites include the skin, airways, lungs, conjunctiva and urogenital tract. Deposits may be nodular or confluent, but the clonal B-cell infiltrate that is the culprit, producing the amyloidogenic light chains, may be inconspicuous. Lichenoid and macular forms of cutaneous amyloid are distinct and are thought to be derived from keratin or related proteins. Nodular cutaneous amyloid deposits are usually localized AL type but can also be part of systemic AL amyloidosis. Localized AL amyloid deposits can exert serious space-occupying effects or cause serious hemorrhage but otherwise are benign and enlarge slowly.

Dialysis-Related Amyloidosis, β₂-Microglobulin Amyloidosis

β₂-Microglobulin amyloid deposition occurs in patients with dialysis-dependent chronic renal failure, mainly affecting articular and periarticular structures, and typically causing arthralgia of the shoulders, knees, wrists and small joints of the hand, joint swelling and carpal tunnel syndrome. The amyloid fibril precursor protein is β₂-microglobulin, which is the invariant chain of the major histocompatibility complex (MHC) class I molecule, and is expressed by all nucleated cells. It is synthesized at an average rate of 150–200 mg/day and is normally filtered freely at the glomerulus, reabsorbed and catabolized by proximal tubular cells. Decreasing renal function causes a proportionate rise in concentration. β₂-Microglobulin amyloidosis was first described in 1980 and occurs in patients who have been on hemodialysis for several years and peritoneal dialysis for 5–10 years. Infrequently, it occurs in patients with long-term severe chronic renal impairment. Dialysis-related amyloidosis (DRA) is present in 20%–30% of patients within 3 years of starting dialysis for end-stage renal failure. Although it is a systemic disease, manifestations outside of the musculoskeletal system are unusual: there have been notable reports of DRA causing congestive cardiac failure and gastrointestinal bleeding, perforation and pseudo-obstruction.

Senile Transthyretin Amyloidosis, ATTR Amyloidosis

In the elderly, clinically silent systemic deposits of wild-type "senile" TTR amyloid are common, involving the heart and blood vessel walls, smooth and striated muscle, fat tissue, renal papillae and alveolar walls. Unlike most other forms of systemic amyloidosis, including hereditary transthyretin amyloid caused by point mutations in the transthyretin gene, the spleen and renal glomeruli are rarely affected. Neither is the brain involved, although symptomatic leptomeningeal deposits can occasionally occur in familial TTR amyloidosis. Senile transthyretin amyloidosis almost always presents with restrictive cardiomyopathy, and other than carpal tunnel syndrome, deposits elsewhere rarely ever attain clinical significance. About one quarter of patients can be demonstrated to have gastrointestinal amyloid deposits on rectal biopsy. Most patients are at least 70 years old, and there is a very strong male preponderance. Cardiac failure progresses and death usually occurs within about 5 years.

Endocrine Amyloidosis

Many hormone-producing tumors of APUD cells have amyloid deposits in their stroma (see Chapter 27). These are probably composed of the hormone peptides, and in the case of medullary carcinoma of the thyroid, fibril subunits are derived from procalcitonin.

In insulinomas, the amyloid fibril protein is called islet amyloid polypeptide (or **amylin**) and shows appreciable homology with calcitonin gene–related peptide. It has subsequently been shown to be the same protein as in the amyloid of the islets of Langerhans in type 2 diabetes. Islet polypeptide amyloid is almost always seen in the pancreatic islets in type 2 diabetes and becomes more extensive with increasing duration and severity of the disease. The amyloid itself probably does not initiate the metabolic defect in type 2 diabetes, but progressive amyloid deposition may facilitate islet destruction.

Amyloid and the Brain

The brain is a common and important site of amyloid deposition, although there are never any deposits in the cerebral parenchyma itself in any form of acquired systemic visceral amyloidosis. However, cerebrovascular and oculoleptomeningeal amyloid deposits that can be clinically significant do occasionally occur in hereditary TTR amyloidosis.

The common and major forms of brain amyloid are associated with Alzheimer disease, the most common type of dementia (see Chapter 33). In brief, intracerebral and cerebrovascular amyloid deposits derived from β-protein (Aβ), a 39- to 43-residue cleavage product of the large amyloid precursor protein, are neuropathologic hallmarks of Alzheimer disease. It is unclear whether or how Aβ per se, small prefibrillar aggregates or the amyloid fibrils that it forms contribute to the neuronal loss that underlies the dementia.

Intracerebral amyloid plaques derived from the normal physiologic cellular prion protein PrP^C are sometimes seen in acquired and hereditary spongiform encephalopathies. The pathogenetic significance of amyloid in these disorders is not clear. However, the amyloid-like proteinase-resistant conformational isoform of PrP^C, called PrP^Sc, is the transmissible agent of these spongiform encephalopathies. Neuron damage may be caused by cytotoxic interaction between prefibrillar PrP^Sc aggregates and normal PrP^C, or by other mechanisms entirely.

In Hereditary Amyloidosis Genetically Variant Proteins Accumulate as Amyloid

In hereditary systemic amyloidosis, mutations in the genes for transthyretin, cystatin C, gelsolin, lysozyme, fibrinogen A α-chain, apolipoprotein AI and, extremely rarely, apolipoprotein AII lead to deposition of these mutant proteins as amyloid. These diseases are all inherited dominantly with variable penetrance and present clinically from teenage to old age, though usually in midadult life. Hereditary transthyretin amyloidosis is by far the commonest, most often presenting as a syndrome of familial amyloid polyneuropathy with peripheral and autonomic neuropathy and/or cardiomyopathy. Cystatin C amyloidosis presents as cerebral amyloid angiopathy with recurrent cerebral hemorrhage and clinically silent systemic deposits, and has been reported only in Icelandic families. Gelsolin amyloidosis presents with cranial neuropathy but is also extremely rare. Apolipoprotein AI, lysozyme and fibrinogen A α-chain amyloidosis usually present as nonneuropathic systemic amyloidosis that can affect any or all major viscera, with renal involvement usually being prominent. Since a family history is often absent, these latter conditions are readily misdiagnosed as acquired "primary" AL amyloidosis and are much less rare than previously thought. *Of patients presenting with non-AA systemic amyloidosis, 5%–10% have hereditary forms of the disease.* It is imperative that hereditary amyloidosis is identified correctly, since prognosis, treatment and implications for family members differ substantially, compared to acquired amyloidosis.

Familial Amyloidotic Polyneuropathy, Variant Transthyretin (ATTR) Amyloidosis

Familial amyloidotic polyneuropathy (FAP) is associated with heterozygous point mutations in the TTR gene. It is an autosomal dominant syndrome with onset between the third and seventh decades. Over 100 TTR variants are associated with FAP, and amyloid fibrils are a mixture of variant and wild-type TTR protein. There are probably several thousand patients with FAP in the world. The disease is characterized by progressive and disabling peripheral and autonomic neuropathy and varying degrees of visceral amyloid involvement, prominently including cardiac amyloidosis, which can be the sole clinical feature in some cases. Deposits within the vitreous of the eye are well recognized and are pathognomonic, while deposits in the kidneys, thyroid, spleen and adrenals are usually asymptomatic. There is considerable phenotypic variation in age of onset, rate of progression, involvement of different systems and disease penetrance, even within one family. Typically the disease progresses inexorably, causing death within 5–15 years.

Familial Amyloid Polyneuropathy with Predominant Cranial Neuropathy

This is a very rare dominant form of hereditary amyloidosis that presents in mid- to late adult life with cranial neuropathy, lattice corneal dystrophy and mild distal peripheral neuropathy. It was first described in Finland but has since been reported in other ethnic groups. There may be skin, renal and cardiac manifestations, but these are usually covert and life expectancy approaches normal. There is no specific treatment and the disorder is progressively disfiguring and very distressing in its late stages. The responsible mutant gene encodes a variant form of gelsolin, which is an actin-modulating protein. The functional role of circulating gelsolin is unknown but may be related to clearance of actin filaments released by apoptotic cells.

Nonneuropathic Variants of Hereditary Systemic Amyloidosis

Hereditary lysozyme systemic amyloidosis has been ascribed to six lysozyme variants, all of which are very rare. Most patients present in middle age with proteinuria, sicca syndrome or upper gastrointestinal and liver involvement. Acute gastrointestinal hemorrhage or perforation and spontaneous liver rupture are well recognized and potentially fatal complications.

Apolipoprotein AI is a major constituent of high-density lipoprotein. Known amyloidogenic variants include single amino acid substitutions, deletions and a deletion/insertion. Associated clinical syndromes vary but often entail substantial amyloid deposits in the liver, spleen and kidneys; some mutations cause cardiomyopathy, and patients with the arginine 26 variant may develop polyneuropathy. In several C-terminal variants, laryngeal amyloid deposits lead to hoarseness. Other manifestations seen with particular mutations include male infertility and skin lesions. Many patients eventually develop renal failure, but liver function usually remains normal despite extensive hepatic amyloid deposits. Normal wild-type apolipoprotein AI amyloid is itself weakly amyloidogenic and is the precursor of small amyloid deposits that occur quite frequently in aortic atherosclerotic plaques.

Hereditary fibrinogen A α-chain amyloid is the commonest type of hereditary renal amyloidosis, caused by some 10 different mutations, the commonest being substitution of valine for glutamic acid at position 526. Penetrance in most families is low and a family history is often lacking. Most patients present in late middle age with proteinuria or hypertension and progress to end-stage renal failure during the next 5 years or so. Amyloid deposition occurs in the kidneys, spleen and sometimes the liver, but it is usually asymptomatic in the latter two sites.

MORPHOLOGIC FEATURES OF AMYLOIDOSIS

Amyloid fibrils are usually first deposited near subendothelial basement membranes (Fig. 15-5). Because amyloid accumulates along stromal networks, deposits take on the configurations of the organs involved. Morphologic differences in amyloid deposition among organs simply reflect organ-to-organ differences in stromal organization. For example, in the renal medulla, amyloid is laid down longitudinally, parallel to tubules and vasa recta, while in glomeruli amyloid (Fig. 15-6), it follows lobular glomerular architecture. In the spleen, amyloid may be mostly in the stroma of the red pulp or that of the white pulp. Grossly, amyloid in the

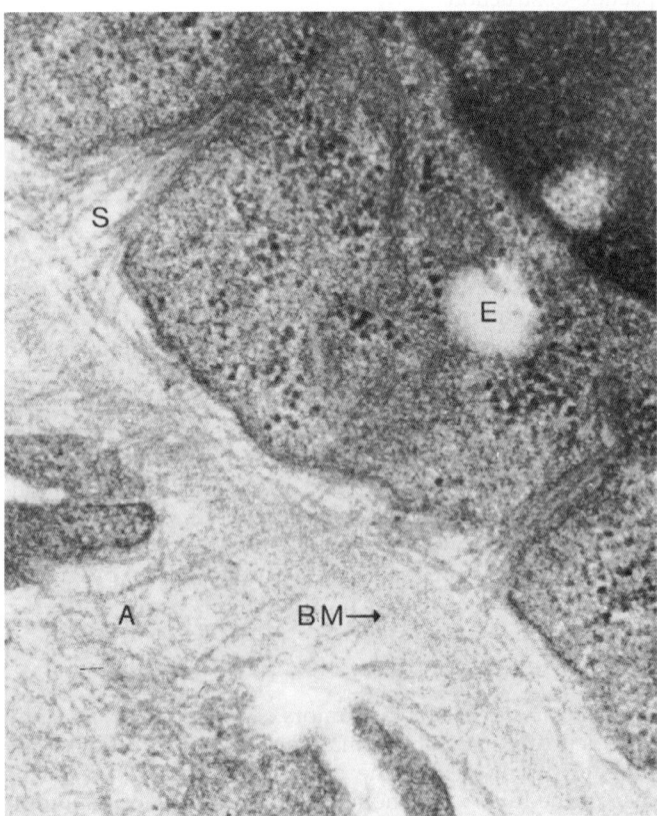

FIGURE 15-5. Electron micrograph of glomerular amyloid (*A*) illustrating its location relative to the basement membrane (*BM*). Amyloid spicules (*S*) extend into the cytoplasm of the glomerular epithelial cells (*E*).

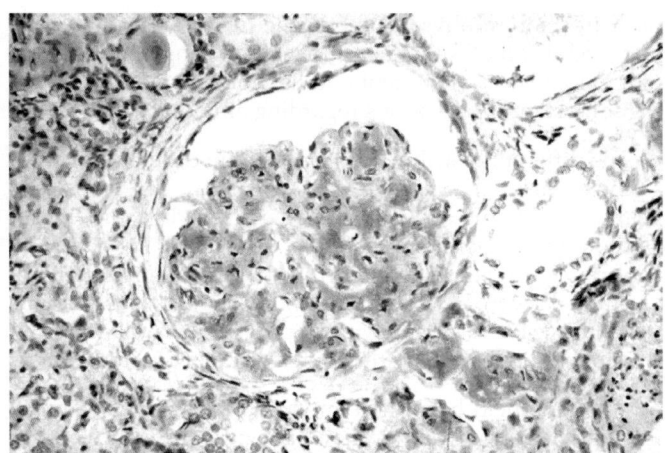

FIGURE 15-6. Microscopic appearance of AA amyloid in a glomerulus. Note the lobular pattern of the amyloid deposit and the involvement of the afferent arteriole.

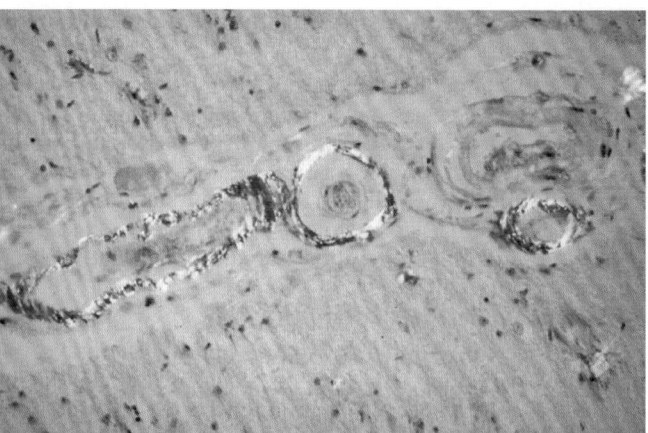

FIGURE 15-8. Cerebrovascular amyloid in a case of Alzheimer disease. The section was stained with Congo red and examined under polarized light.

red pulp imparts a diffusely pale and waxy appearance, the so-called lardaceous spleen. A spleen containing white pulp amyloid shows multiple pale foci scattered throughout the organ, which is called sago spleen. Deposits in the liver follow the arteries of the portal triads or are laid down along central veins and radiate into the parenchyma along liver cell plates (Fig. 15-7).

Amyloid adds interstitial material at sites of deposition, thus increasing the size of affected organs. This increase may be counterbalanced by the deposition of amyloid in blood vessels (Fig. 15-8), which might impair circulation and lead to organ atrophy. Affected organs may thus increase or decrease in size. Amyloid deposits are essentially avascular, so the involved organs are commonly pale and firm.

Regardless of whether amyloid is laid down in a systemic or local fashion, deposits tend to occur between parenchymal cells and their blood supply, interfering with normal nutrition and gas exchange. Amyloid may eventually entrap parenchymal cells. Alternatively, it may have an additional toxic effect on these cells through the interaction of protofibrils and cell membranes. In each case, amyloid deposits may lead to cell strangulation, atrophy and death (Fig. 15-9).

CLINICAL FEATURES AND ORGAN INVOLVEMENT IN AMYLOIDOSIS

No single set of symptoms points unequivocally to amyloidosis as a diagnosis. The symptoms of amyloidosis depend on the underlying disease and the type and organ locations of the amyloid deposits. Amyloidosis may also be diagnosed unexpectedly in the course of evaluation for something unrelated, with no clinical manifestations referable to the amyloidosis itself. In other cases, for example,

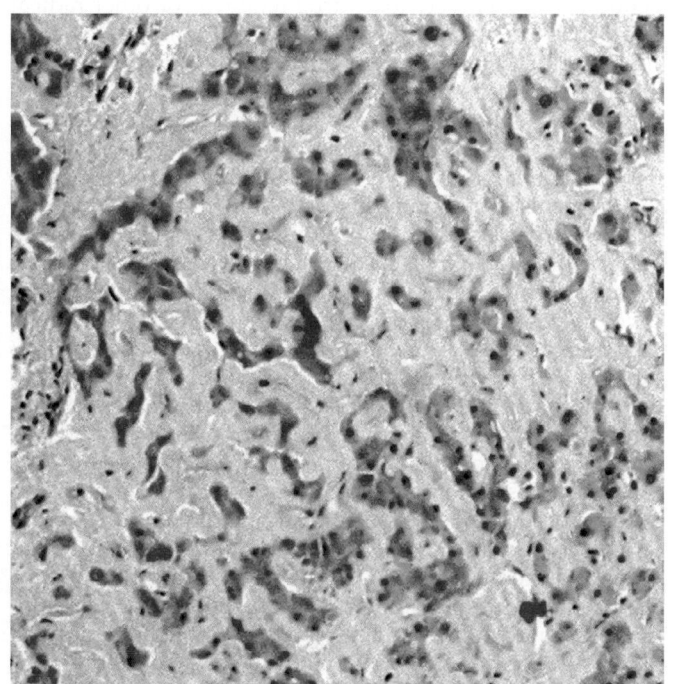

FIGURE 15-7. Hepatic amyloidosis. Amyloid is deposited along the sinusoids. Note the atrophic hepatocytes.

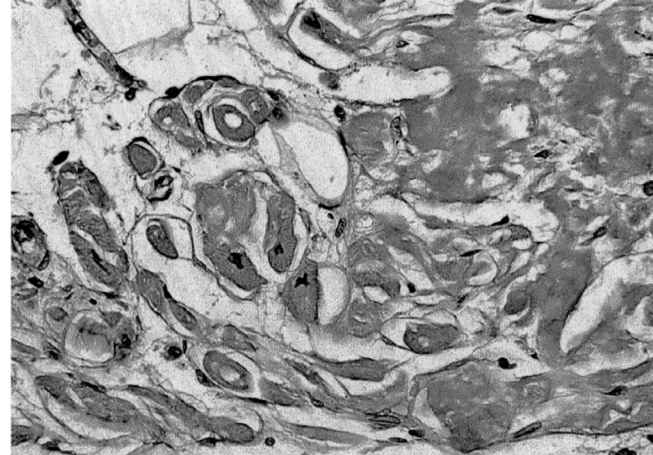

FIGURE 15-9. Myocardial amyloid (AL type), showing the encroachment upon, and strangulation of, individual myocardial fibers.

unexplained renal and cardiac dysfunction may be the presenting conditions.

KIDNEY: Patients with multiple myeloma and other clonal B-cell dyscrasias or long-standing inflammatory disorders who develop **nephrotic syndrome** should be suspected of having amyloidosis. Proteinuria, particularly in patients with plasma cell dyscrasias, may be overlooked if the patient is already excreting a Bence Jones protein. Progressive glomerular obliteration may ultimately lead to renal failure and uremia.

HEART: Amyloid involvement of the myocardium should be suspected in all patients with AL and TTR amyloidosis and in any patient with unexplained concentric thickening of the myocardium, especially if the latter is not associated with abnormally large voltage complexes on electrocardiography. Myocardial amyloid deposits cause **restrictive cardiomyopathy,** in which diastolic dysfunction is often associated with well-preserved systolic function. Short of biopsy, two-dimensional echocardiography and Doppler studies are helpful in suggesting the diagnosis. Cardiac magnetic resonance imaging with late gadolinium enhancement has been reported to be useful as well. Serum cardiac troponin and N-terminal pro-brain natriuretic peptide concentrations appear to be powerful predictors of cardiac involvement, as well as prognosis and survival after chemotherapy in AL amyloidosis. Cardiac amyloidosis is also associated with conduction abnormalities that cause arrhythmias and sudden death.

GASTROINTESTINAL TRACT: The ganglia, smooth muscle, vasculature and submucosa of the gastrointestinal tract may all be affected by amyloid. Deposits in these locations can alter gastrointestinal motility and absorption but are often clinically silent. Patients complain of either constipation or diarrhea, and insidious malnutrition is common. Enlargement of the tongue is virtually pathognomonic of AL amyloidosis, and interference with its motor function may be severe enough to affect speech and swallowing.

LIVER: AL, AA and familial forms of amyloidosis often cause amyloid deposits in the liver but rarely lead to clinically significant hepatic dysfunction. Substantial hepatomegaly may occur before any abnormalities in serum liver function tests are seen. Liver amyloidosis is typically associated with progressive elevation of serum alkaline phosphatase and γ-glutamyl transferase in these patients, but jaundice generally occurs late and is associated with frank liver failure and a very poor prognosis, particularly the AL type.

PERIPHERAL NERVES: The familial polyneuropathic forms of amyloid usually manifest as paresthesias, with loss in temperature and pain sensation of the extremities.

The diagnosis of amyloidosis generally requires histologic confirmation, although the mere demonstration of amyloid deposition does not by itself establish that it is clinically significant. While amyloidosis does not occur in the absence of amyloid deposits, the latter may be an incidental histologic finding, especially in older subjects. Immunohistochemical staining is the most accessible method for characterizing amyloid fibril protein type, but it does not always produce definitive results, especially in AL type. Amyloid deposits can be quite patchy and histology can never provide information about the overall whole body load or distribution of amyloid deposits, nor does it permit monitoring of the natural history of amyloidosis or its response to treatment. Radiolabeled human SAP is a specific, noninvasive, quantitative in vivo tracer for amyloid deposits and has been used in scintigraphy and metabolic turnover studies. This approach facilitates the diagnosis, monitoring and response of amyloidosis to treatment and has contributed the following important observations regarding amyloid:

- The different distribution of amyloid in different forms of the disease
- Major systemic deposits in forms of amyloid previously thought to be organ limited
- A poor correlation between the quantity of amyloid present in a given organ and the degree of organ dysfunction
- Evidence for surprisingly rapid progression and regression of amyloid deposits with different rates in different organs

The long-held belief that amyloid deposition is irreversible and inexorably progressive is evidently incorrect and simply reflects the usually persistent nature of the conditions that underlie it. Many case reports have described improvement in amyloidotic organ function when the underlying conditions have been controlled, suggesting that amyloid deposits may regress.

TREATMENT OF AMYLOIDOSIS

Systemic amyloidosis is a progressive disease that, without effective treatment, is ultimately fatal in most cases. Although no treatments yet exist that specifically promote the mobilization of amyloid, there have been substantial recent advances in the management of systemic amyloidosis, in particular active measures to support failing organ function while attempts are made to reduce the supply of the amyloid fibril precursor protein. Serial SAP scintigraphy has shown that control of the primary disease process, or removal of the source of the amyloidogenic precursor, often allows gradual regression of existing deposits and recovery or preservation of organ function. Thus, aggressive intervention, and relatively toxic drug regimens or other radical approaches, can be justified by the poor prognosis. However, clinical improvement is often delayed long after the underlying disorder has remitted, reflecting the very gradual regression of the deposits that is now recognized to occur in most patients. Continuing production of amyloid precursor protein should be monitored closely over time, to determine the requirement for, and intensity of, treatment for the underlying primary condition. In AA amyloidosis, this means frequent estimation of plasma SAA levels; in AL amyloidosis, it requires monitoring of serum free light chains or other markers of the underlying monoclonal plasma cell proliferation.

The treatment of AA amyloidosis ranges from potent anti-inflammatory, cytokine-inhibiting and immunosuppressive drugs in patients with rheumatoid arthritis to lifelong prophylactic colchicine in familial Mediterranean fever and surgery in conditions such as refractory osteomyelitis and the tumors of Castleman disease. Treatment of AL amyloidosis is based on that for myeloma, including oral administration of melphalan and dexamethasone, thalidomide-based regimens and the new agents such as the proteasome inhibitor bortezomib and the immunomodulatory agent lenalidomide. High-dose chemotherapy with autologous peripheral blood stem cell transplantation has high response rates but much toxicity and is restricted to selected patients. The disabling arthralgia of β_2-microglobulin amyloidosis usually responds dramatically to renal transplantation. The basis for this remarkable clinical response is unclear since although transplantation rapidly restores normal β_2-microglobulin metabolism, regression of β_2-microglobulin amyloid may not be evident for many years.

Liver transplantation is effective in familial amyloid polyneuropathy associated with transthyretin gene mutations since the variant amyloidogenic protein is produced mainly in the liver. Outcomes are best among younger patients with the methionine 30 variant, though even in this group the peripheral neuropathy usually only stabilizes. Unfortunately, paradoxical progression of established cardiac amyloidosis with wild-type transthyretin has been noted in many older patients. On a similar basis, hepatic transplantation has proven promising in some patients with hereditary fibrinogen A α-chain and apolipoprotein AI amyloidosis.

Supportive therapy remains critical in systemic amyloidosis, notably including attention to nutrition, rigorous control of hypertension in renal amyloidosis and diuretic and fluid balance management in cardiac amyloidosis. Dysrhythmias may respond to conventional pharmacologic therapy or to pacing. Replacement of vital organ function, notably dialysis, may be necessary, and cardiac and renal transplantation has been very successful in selected cases.

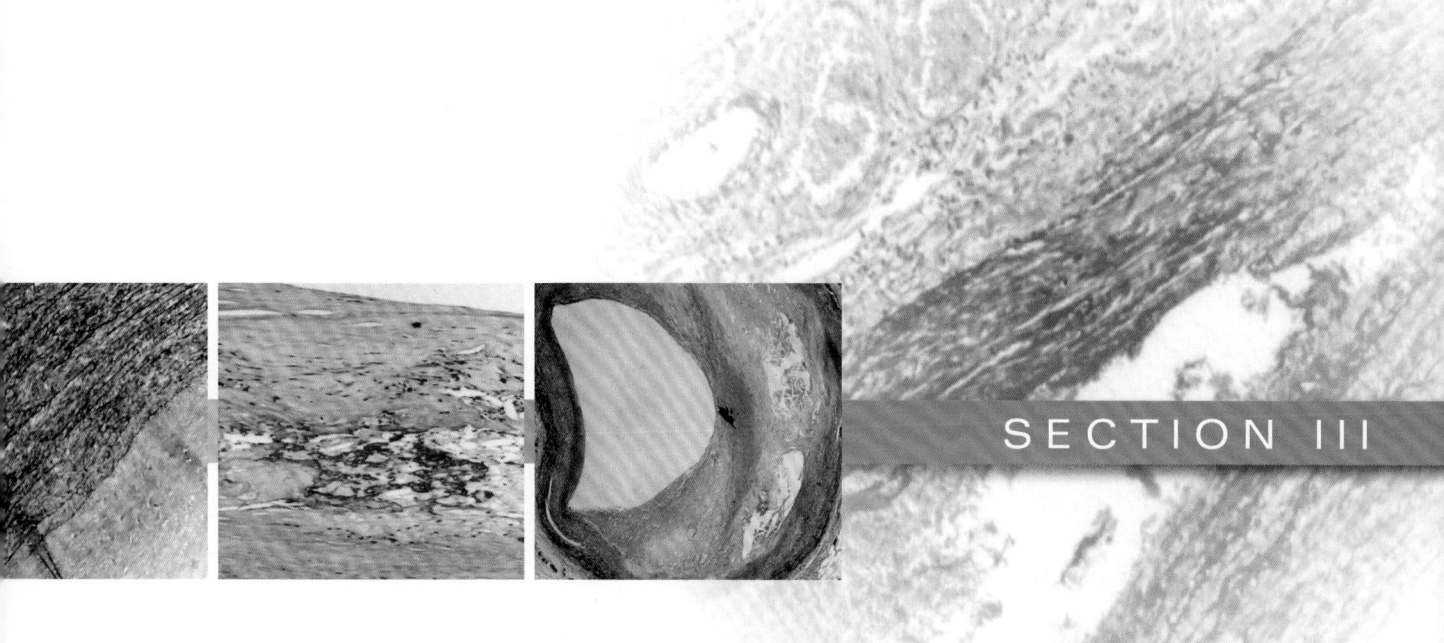

Diseases of Individual Organ Systems

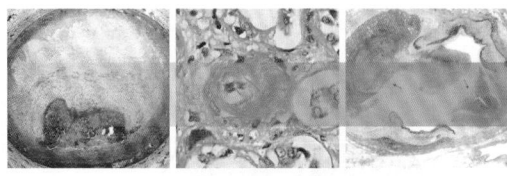

16

Blood Vessels

Avrum I. Gotlieb ■ Amber Liu

ANATOMY OF BLOOD VESSELS

Arteries Include Conducting and Resistance Vessels

The vascular portion of the circulatory system is composed of a variety of blood vessel compartments that are categorized by size, structure and function. These include arteries, which are conducting and resistance vessels; capillaries; and veins (Fig. 16-1).

Elastic Arteries

The largest blood vessels in the body, the aorta and the elastic arteries, are conduits for blood flow to smaller arterial branches and are composed of three layers:

■ **Tunica intima:** This consists of a single layer of endothelial cells, a subendothelial compartment containing a few smooth muscle cells and an extracellular matrix extending to the luminal side of the internal elastic lamina. The aortic intima is thicker than the other elastic arteries and contains matrix proteins including collagen, proteoglycans and small amounts of elastin. Occasional resident lymphocytes, macrophages, dendritic cells and other blood-derived inflammatory cells are also present.

■ **Tunica media:** The next layer outward is the tunica media, the thickest tunica. It is bounded by internal and external elastic laminae and itself displays numerous elastic laminae and smooth muscle cells within an extracellular connective tissue matrix. In the aorta, the media is organized into lamellar units, each consisting of two concentric elastic laminae, with smooth muscle cells and their associated matrix in between the laminae. The media of the thoracic aorta contains more elastin and the abdominal aorta contains more collagen. In elastic arteries, elastic fibers are interposed between smooth muscle cells and serve to minimize energy loss during the pressure changes between systole and diastole.

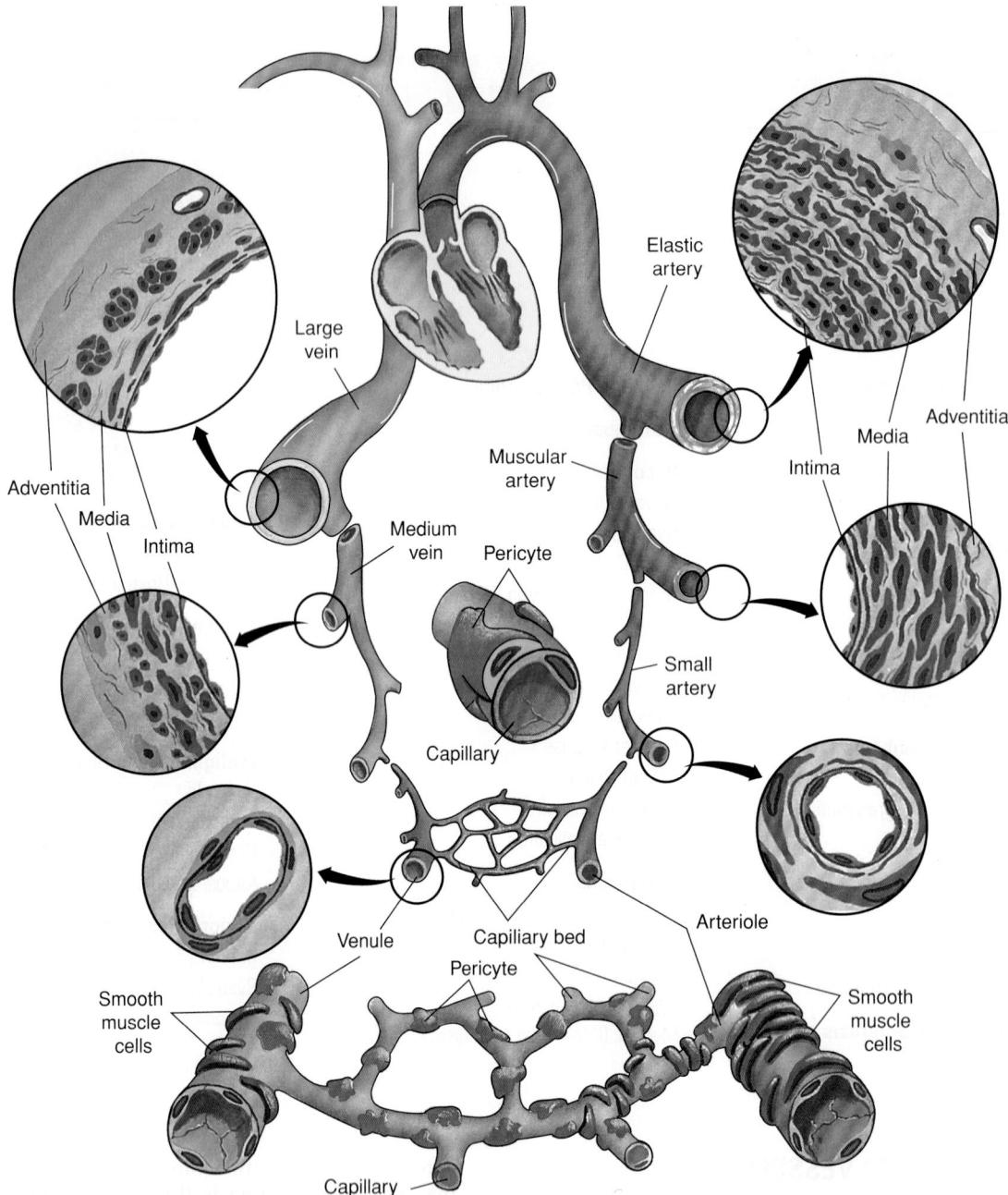

FIGURE 16-1. Subdivisions and histologic structure of the vascular system. Each subdivision is subject to a set of pathologic changes conditioned by the structure–function relationship of that part of the system. For example, the aorta, an elastic artery subject to great pressure, frequently shows a pathologic dilation (aneurysm) if the supporting elastic media is damaged. Muscular arteries are the most significant sites of atherosclerosis. Small arteries, particularly arterioles, are sites of hypertensive changes. Capillary beds, venules and veins each display their own types of pathologic changes.

In smaller elastic arteries, nutrition for the media is provided by diffusion from the blood vessel lumen through the endothelium and the layers of smooth muscle. However, blood vessels with more than 28 layers of smooth muscle cells have a vasculature of their own, the **vasa vasorum**. These small vessels arise from the visceral and parietal branches of the aorta, and both form a superficial plexus at the adventitia–media border, when they penetrate into the outer 2/3 of the media. The tunica media also contains autonomic nerve fibers that influence vascular contractility.

■ **Tunica adventitia:** The most external vessel wall layer contains fibroblasts, connective tissue, nerves and small vessels that give rise to the vasa vasorum. Occasional inflammatory cells, including collections of lymphocytes, may also be present in the adventitia.

Muscular Arteries

Blood conducted by the elastic arteries is distributed to individual organs through large muscular arteries (Figs. 16-1 and 16-2). The tunica media of a muscular artery consists of

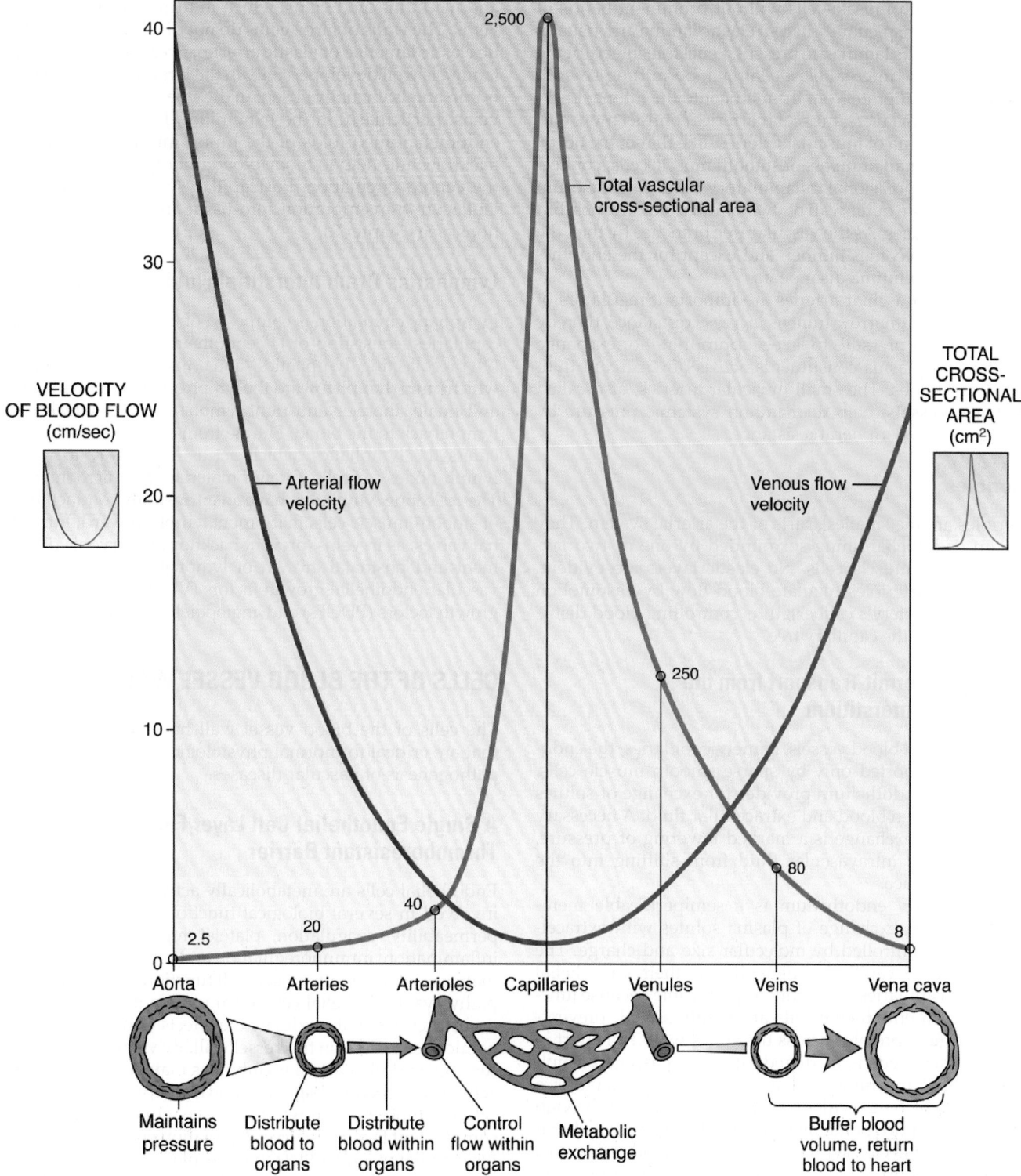

FIGURE 16-2. Relationship between velocity of blood flow and cross-sectional area in the vasculature. The vascular tree is a circuit that conducts blood from the heart through large-diameter, low-resistance conducting vessels to small arteries and arterioles, which lower blood pressure and protect the capillaries. The capillaries are thin walled and allow the exchange of nutrients and waste products between tissue and blood, a process that requires a very large surface area. The circuit back to the heart is completed by the veins, which are distensible and provide a volume buffer that acts as a capacitance for the vascular circuit.

layers of smooth muscle cells without prominent bands of elastin, but a conspicuous internal elastic lamina and usually an external elastic lamina are present. Fenestrae interrupt the continuity of the internal elastic lamina, permitting smooth muscle cells to migrate from the media into the intima. Lacking heavy elastin layers, muscular arteries contract more efficiently. The intima of muscular arteries, like that of the aorta, also contains small numbers of smooth muscle cells, connective tissue and occasional inflammatory cells. Vasa vasorum are present in the outer wall of thicker muscular arteries, but not in smaller ones. As the vascular tree branches further, the tunica media becomes thinner, and except for the endothelium, the tunica intima disappears.

The small muscular arteries are important regulators of blood flow. Their narrow lumens increase resistance, thereby reducing blood pressure to levels appropriate for exchange of water and plasma constituents across downstream thin-walled capillaries. The small muscular arteries, also called **resistance vessels,** help to maintain systemic pressure by regulating total peripheral resistance.

Arterioles

Arterioles are the smallest parts of the arterial system. They have an endothelial lining surrounded by one or two layers of smooth muscle cells. No elastic layers are evident. The smallest arterioles regulate blood flow by vasomotion (change in an artery's caliber), thus controlling blood distribution through the capillary tree.

Capillaries Permit Transport from the Blood to the Interstitium

In these smallest blood vessels, namely, capillaries, the endothelium is supported only by sparse smooth muscle cells. The capillary endothelium provides for exchange of solutes and cells between blood and extracellular fluid. A necessary feature of this exchange is a marked lowering of pressure, which prevents intravascular fluid from shifting into the extracellular space.

The capillary endothelium is a semipermeable membrane, in which exchange of plasma solutes with extracellular fluid is controlled by molecular size and charge. The permeability of capillaries depends on their endothelial cells. Brain capillaries are highly impermeable because junctions between endothelial cells are tightly sealed, preventing exchange of proteins across the vessel wall. Transport in other capillary beds is mediated either by passage of molecules through incomplete cell junctions or by pinocytosis, a process by which molecules traverse the cytoplasm through vesicular transport. Some investigators have suggested that vesicles are connected with each other to provide a channel for direct transport of plasma proteins across the cytoplasm. In some locations, the capillary endothelium itself may have permanent channels through discontinuous gaps between them. Fenestrated capillaries in renal glomeruli are specifically adapted to filter plasma. Liver sinusoids, which are not true capillaries, also show a fenestrated endothelium, which permits free access of plasma to liver cells.

Veins Return Blood to the Heart

Venules are the first vessels to collect blood from capillaries. Their thin media is appropriate for a vessel that does not face high intraluminal pressures. Venules merge into small and medium-sized veins, which in turn converge into large veins. The walls of large veins do not display the characteristic elastic lamellae of elastic arteries; even the internal elastic lamina is well developed only in the largest veins. The media is thin and is virtually absent in the smaller tributaries. Many veins, particularly in the extremities, have valves made of endothelial-lined folds of the tunica intima, which prevent backflow and help to move blood under the low pressure of the venous circulation. Postcapillary venules are the site of leukocyte transmigration into tissue in inflammatory reactions (see Chapter 2).

Lymphatics Drain Interstitial Fluid

Lymphatic circulation is composed of blind-ended lymphatic capillaries, consisting of (1) endothelium with no pericytes; (2) precollecting lymphatics; and (3) collecting lymphatics, which pump lymph toward the lymph nodes, lymphatic trunks and finally thoracic and right lymphatic ducts, which return lymph back to the blood. Filtrate from capillaries and venules enters the lymphatics, which act as a pathway to regional lymph nodes for cells, foreign material and microorganisms. The collecting lymphatics have an intrinsically contractile layer of smooth muscle cells that propel lymph forward. Intraluminal valves, as in veins, prevent backflow. Embryonic development and postnatal growth of lymphatics are regulated by vascular endothelial growth factors (VEGFs), platelet-derived growth factors (PDGFs) and angiopoietin 1 and 2.

CELLS OF THE BLOOD VESSEL WALL

The cells of the blood vessel wall have unique properties that are critical for normal physiologic functions and for the pathogenesis of vascular diseases.

A Single Endothelial Cell Layer Forms a Thromboresistant Barrier

Endothelial cells are metabolically active and are intimately involved in several biological functions, including vascular permeability, coagulation, platelet regulation, fibrinolysis, inflammation, immunoregulation and repair. They also modulate vascular smooth muscle cell function through paracrine pathways. Endothelial cells form unique mechanotransduction structures that modulate the effects of luminal hemodynamic shear stress on the vessel wall. By virtue of mechanical sensing, endothelial cell membranes may deform. This effect activates biochemical signaling and leads to expression of vasoactive compounds, growth factors, coagulation/fibrinolytic/complement factors, matrix degradation enzymes, inflammatory mediators and adhesion molecules.

Endothelial integrity depends on several types of adhesion complexes that promote cell–substratum and cell–cell adhesions (see Chapter 2).

- **Cell–substrate adhesion molecules** attach endothelial cells to their substratum (e.g., basal lamina). They complex with intracellular cytoskeleton, which participates in intracellular signal transduction. For example, integrins are transmembrane molecules that bind endothelial cells to extracellular matrix adhesive molecules, including laminin, fibronectin, fibrinogen, von Willebrand factor and thrombospondin. The cytoplasmic tails of the integrins bind the complex of proteins that regulate adhesion

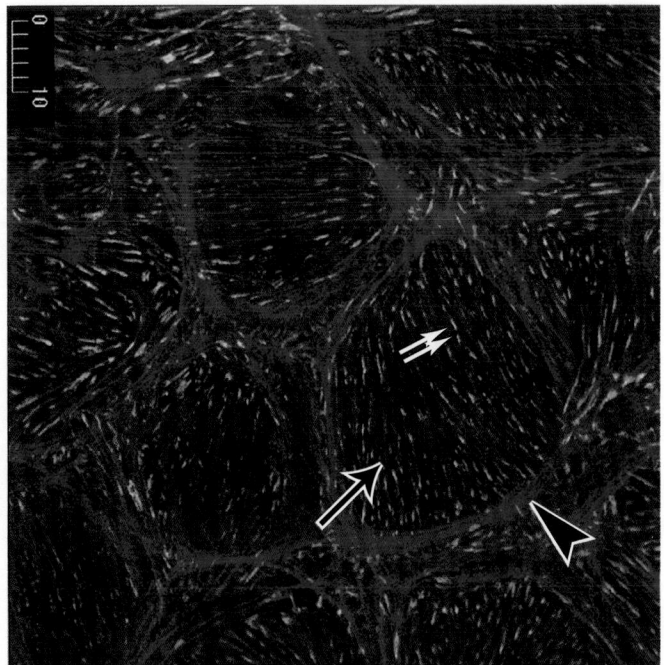

FIGURE 16-3. Focal adhesion protein, vinculin. Porcine aortic endothelial cells were grown to confluency and double-stained for actin/vinculin. Endothelial cells in confluent monolayers contain a dense peripheral band of actin microfilament bundles (*arrowhead*) and central microfilament or "stress fibers" (*single arrow*). Vinculin in confluent monolayer localizes to the tips of stress fibers (*double arrow*).

TABLE 16-1

FUNCTIONS OF ENDOTHELIAL CELLS OF THE BLOOD VESSELS

Permeability barrier

Vasoactive factors: Nitric oxide (EDRF), endothelin

Antithrombotic agent production: Prostacyclin (PGI$_2$), adenine metabolites

Anticoagulant production: Thrombomodulin, other proteins

Fibrinolytic agent production: Tissue plasminogen activator, urokinase-like factor, tissue factor pathway inhibitor

Procoagulant production: Tissue factor, plasminogen activator/inhibitor, factor V, factor VIIIa (von Willebrand factor)

Inflammatory mediator production: Interleukin-1, cell adhesion molecules

Receptors for factor IX, factor X, low-density lipoproteins, modified low-density lipoproteins, thrombin

Growth factor production: Blood cell colony-stimulating factors, insulin-like growth factors, fibroblast growth factor, platelet-derived growth factor

Growth inhibitor: Heparin

Replication

EDRF = endothelium-derived relaxing factor.

at focal contact sites and associate with actin microfilaments and microtubules of the cytoskeleton (Fig. 16-3).

- **Cell–cell adhesion molecules** attach one endothelial cell to its neighbors. Cadherin occurs at intercellular adhesion junctions and occludin at intercellular tight junctions. Cadherins bind to the actin cytoskeleton via catenins.

Endothelial cells carry out a large variety of important metabolic functions (Table 16-1). Many of these are regulated by serum and hemodynamic factors, which activate surface receptors and signal transduction pathways or regulate gene transcription. Endothelial cells do not normally proliferate, but after vascular injury and loss of endothelial cells, they spread, migrate and proliferate rapidly to reestablish the structural integrity of the endothelium and thus protect the wall (Fig. 16-4).

Endothelial cells release a number of biologically potent factors when they are activated. Some of these bioactive

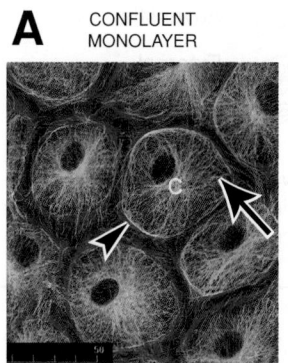 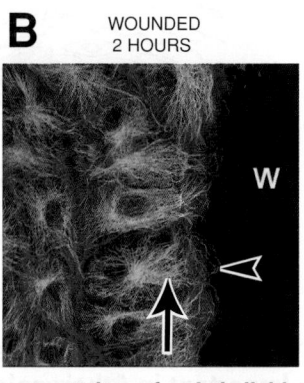 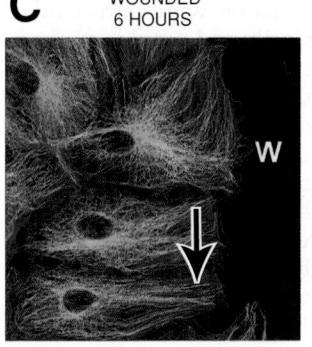 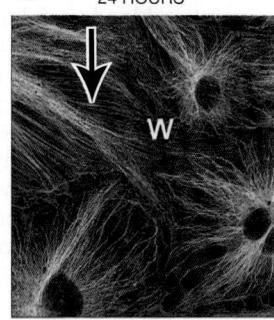

FIGURE 16-4. Remodeling in response to loss of endothelial integrity. Porcine aortic endothelial cells were grown to confluency, and a 1-mm wound was created using a scraper. Cells were fixed and double-stained for actin/tublin at 2, 6 and 24 hours after wounding. **A.** Endothelial cells in confluent monolayers contain a dense peripheral band (DPB) of actin microfilament bundles (*arrowhead*) and centrosomes (C) (*arrow*) toward the cell periphery. **B.** Two hours after wounding, there is formation of lamellipodia (*arrowhead*), and stress fibers (*arrow*) rearrange to become parallel to the wound edge (W). Centrosomes migrate around the nucleus toward the wound edge, and the microtubules begin emanating toward the wound (W). **C.** By 6 hours, changes in microtubules and microfilaments are more prominent, the microtubule/microfilaments are more prominent and the microtubule–microfilament networks (*arrow*) begin to reorganize perpendicular to the wound edge (W) as the cells begin to spread. **D.** Twenty-four hours after wounding, the microtubule–microfilament networks (*arrow*) are aligned perpendicular to the wound edge (W) as the cells migrate into the wound.

molecules are released locally, act at short distances and are rapidly inactivated. For example, prostacyclin (PGI₂), derived from the cyclooxygenase (COX) pathway, relaxes smooth muscle and inhibits platelet aggregation. Endothelial nitric oxide synthase (NOS) converts L-arginine and O_2 to L-citrulline and nitric oxide (NO•) (see below). It also modulates vascular tone and vascular smooth muscle cell proliferation by increasing cyclic guanosine monophosphate (cGMP), in turn activating cGMP-dependent protein kinase. NO• also helps to control the muscular tone of large arteries and resistance vessels. After stimulation of endothelial cell receptors by agonists, prostacyclin and NO• are released and together inhibit platelet aggregation. Compounds that promote NO• release include acetylcholine, bradykinin and adenosine diphosphate (ADP). NO• is even more labile than prostacyclin, with a half-life of 6 seconds.

Vascular tone is also affected by several bioactive peptides. **Endothelins** are a family of potent vasoconstrictive proteins made by endothelial cells. They bind two distinct receptors. Both are found on smooth muscle cells, but only one on endothelial cells. Angiotensin-converting enzyme (ACE), an endothelial product, converts angiotensin I to angiotensin II, a potent vasoconstrictor that is important in the pathogenesis of hypertension.

Endothelial cell–derived factors also control some immune responses. Like macrophages, when stimulated, endothelial cells express class II histocompatibility antigens. They may thus work with monocytes—or even replace them—in activating lymphocytes. Immune responses to endothelial cells are a major part of organ rejection following transplantation and play a role in the pathogenesis of graft arteriosclerosis.

Smooth Muscle Cells Maintain Blood Vessel Integrity

Vascular smooth muscle cells are derived from local mesoderm after endothelial tubes are formed (Fig. 16-5). However, the smooth muscle cells of major arteries in the upper part of the body are derived from neural crest. Thus, the structural and functional diversity of vascular smooth muscle cells has a developmental basis and may have pathogenetic implications for diseases of the adult vascular system.

Smooth muscle cells are in the contractile phenotype (differentiated state) and, in association with extracellular matrix, maintain blood vessel integrity and provide support for endothelium. They control blood flow by contracting or dilating in response to specific stimuli. Smooth muscle cells synthesize the connective tissue matrix of the vessel wall, which includes elastin; collagen, especially type I and III collagen; and proteoglycan. They also produce proteolytic enzymes and their inhibitors, which regulate tissue remodeling and repair. In normal arteries, smooth muscle cells rarely divide. Rather, like endothelial cells, they proliferate in response to injury and are important in the pathogenesis of atherosclerotic plaques. In the latter instance, they differentiate to a synthetic phenotype, expressing genes regulating secretion, migration and proliferation. Oxidized low-density lipoprotein (LDL) and platelet-derived growth factor (PDGF) are important stimuli in the switch of smooth muscle cells from a contractile to a synthetic phenotype. Vascular smooth muscle cell phenotype switching is also regulated by microRNA (miRNA). Smooth muscle cells are major producers of the growth factors, cytokines and chemokines involved in atherogenesis.

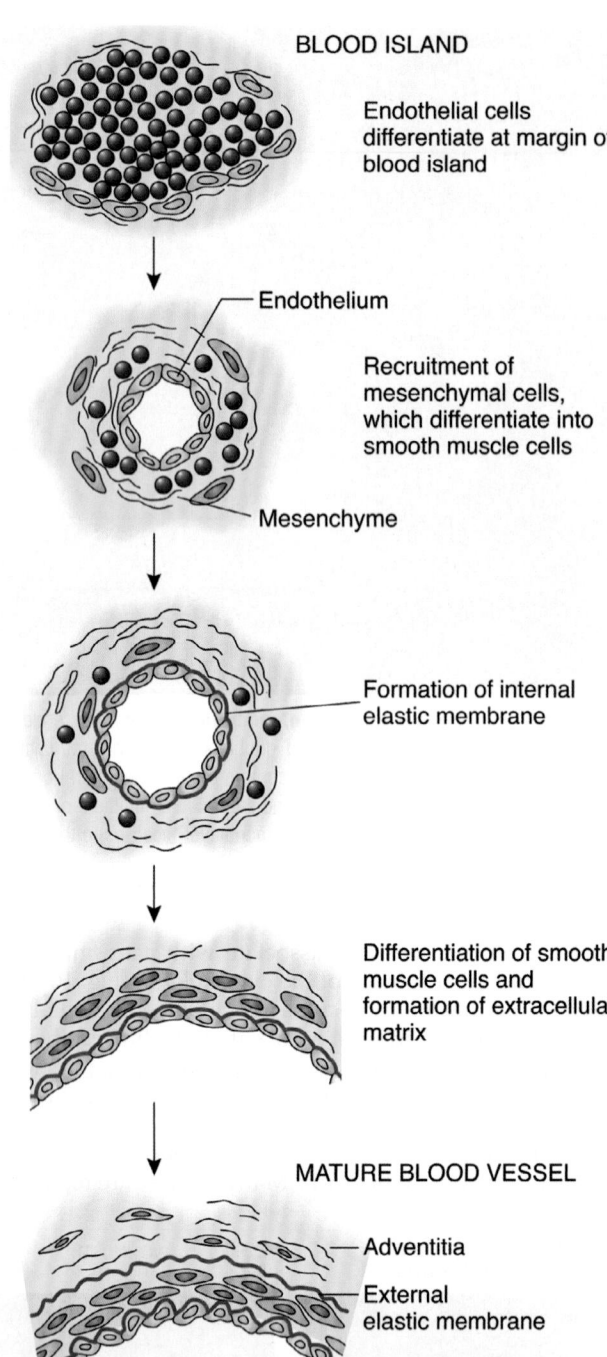

BLOOD ISLAND

Endothelial cells differentiate at margin of blood island

Endothelium

Recruitment of mesenchymal cells, which differentiate into smooth muscle cells

Mesenchyme

Formation of internal elastic membrane

Differentiation of smooth muscle cells and formation of extracellular matrix

MATURE BLOOD VESSEL

Adventitia

External elastic membrane

FIGURE 16-5. Differentiation of vessels in early embryos. The course of events from the development of blood islands on the chorioallantoic membrane starts with differentiation of endothelium and proceeds to fully developed arteries and veins.

Inflammatory Cells Enter Vessel Walls and Are Important in Atherosclerosis

Macrophages, dendritic cells and lymphocytes, in particular, promote vascular disease. Atherosclerosis (see below) may be viewed as an inflammatory disease in which monocyte-derived macrophages are very important. T lymphocytes are present in the adventitia in normal arteries and are increased in number in atherosclerotic plaques. Dendritic cells are found in intimal atherosclerotic lesions, and adventitial leukocytes are organized into clusters similar to lymphoid tissue in areas beneath plaques. Polymorphonuclear leukocytes are important in acute vasculitis, and T cells in acute and chronic vasculitis.

Pericytes Are Modified Smooth Muscle Cells around Capillaries

Pericytes are in close contact with endothelial cells. Both share the same basement membrane. The functions of pericytes are largely unknown. They may be contractile or regulate adjacent endothelial cells' activities and proliferation. The capillary adventitia merges with, and is indistinguishable from, the surrounding connective tissue.

Vascular Progenitor/Stem Cells Regulate Vasculogenesis

The discovery of vascular progenitor/stem cells has aided our understanding of blood vessel injury and repair. Several types of progenitor/stem cells have been identified. **Endothelial progenitor cells** (EPCs) are bone marrow–derived cells arising from perinatal hemangioblasts and are present in adult bone marrow and peripheral circulation. EPCs are identified by their expression of CD133, CD34, c-kit, VEGFR-2, CD144 and Sca-1. They are multipotent immature cells that can proliferate, migrate and differentiate into endothelial cells. Unlike mature endothelial cells, they express CD133, but not endothelial cadherin or von Willebrand factor. The presence of circulating EPCs in adults suggests that new blood vessel growth in adults occurs by **vasculogenesis,** not only by **angiogenesis** as previously thought. Angiogenesis refers to the sprouting of new capillaries from existing blood vessels, whereas vasculogenesis is the differentiation of angioblasts (precursor cells) into endothelial cells that form a vascular network de novo. Vasculogenesis, present in the developing embryo, reappears in adults when EPCs are mobilized and recruited to regions of new blood vessel formation. Embryonic and adult vasculogenesis show many similarities, suggesting that initiating stimuli and regulatory pathways for both are similar.

The number and migratory activity of circulating EPCs are decreased in patients with stable coronary artery disease and are inversely correlated with the number of risk factors in patients with coronary artery disease. EPC proliferation in people with type 2 diabetes mellitus is significantly less than in controls, and EPCs from subjects at high risk for cardiovascular events senesce in culture more readily than do cells from those at low risk. These findings suggest that EPCs may be sensitive indicators of increased risk of vascular disease, especially atherosclerosis.

EPCs have been the subject of intense experimental and clinical investigation, owing to their therapeutic potential in cardiovascular regeneration. EPC transplantation to promote collateral circulation is an innovative therapy to treat tissue ischemia. Blood EPCs from healthy humans can differentiate into endothelial cells and improve blood supply in experimentally injured limbs, and contribute to neovascularization following experimental myocardial infarction. EPC therapy also inhibits left ventricular fibrosis and preserves left ventricular function.

In addition, EPCs help to maintain blood vessel patency after therapeutic stenting. Technologies designed to capture EPCs, such as incorporating anti-CD34 antibody into stents, has shown promise in delaying or preventing restenosis of implanted stents. Therefore, the discovery of adult circulating EPCs may both improve our understanding and contribute to the treatment of vascular injury and repair.

HEMOSTASIS AND THROMBOSIS

Hemostasis is an exquisitely controlled physiologic process initiated to arrest hemorrhage by forming a blood clot. It is a response to vascular injury and involves local vasoconstriction, tissue swelling and platelet adhesion, aggregation and activation. These processes are followed by coagulation and fibrin formation, resulting in a hemostatic plug at sites of injury.

Thrombosis refers to the process that promotes the formation of a blood clot, or thrombus, within the circulation. A thrombus is an aggregate of coagulated blood that contains platelets, fibrin, leukocytes and red blood cells. Its formation involves a balance in favor of factors that promote clotting compared to those that inhibit it. *Thrombi are formed when antithrombotic systems fail to equal prothrombotic processes.* Thrombosis involves (1) activation of platelets, (2) activation of coagulation pathways, (3) participation of the monocyte/macrophage system and (4) active involvement of the endothelial cells of the vessel wall.

Coagulation can be induced in vitro in a test tube by activation of the coagulation cascade. In vivo hemostasis involves the coagulation network of activating and inactivating enzymes, and cofactors derived from different cells and tissues, some circulating and some locally produced (Table 16-2). Disorders of hemostasis are discussed in detail in Chapters 7 and 26.

TABLE 16-2	
COAGULATION FACTOR DESIGNATIONS	
Factor	**Standard Name**
I	Fibrinogen
II	Prothrombin
III	Tissue factor
IV	Calcium ions
V	Proaccelerin
VII	Proconvertin
VIII	Antihemophilic factor (AHF)
IX	Plasma thromboplastin (PTC)
X	Stuart factor
XI	Plasma thromboplastin antecedent (PTA)
XII	Hageman factor
XIII	Fibrin-stabilizing factor (FSF)
–	Prekallikrein
–	High–molecular-weight kininogen

Blood Coagulates When Fibrinogen Is Converted to Fibrin

The endpoint of blood coagulation is the conversion of soluble plasma fibrinogen to an insoluble fibrillar polymer–fibrin, a reaction catalyzed by the protease enzyme thrombin. This process must be carefully controlled to prevent a massive activation of the system and extensive clotting throughout the entire circulation. A series of finely tuned steps is mediated by a number of coagulation factors (Table 16-2), many of which are restricted by specific inhibitors. This coagulation cascade amplifies an initial signal into the eventual generation of thrombin, production of which is key to progression and stabilization of a thrombus. For example, one molecule of an upstream coagulation factor, factor Xa, generates about 1000 molecules of thrombin.

The coagulation cascade was once divided into the "intrinsic" and "extrinsic" pathways, now called the **contact activation pathway** and the **tissue factor pathway,** respectively. However, this dichotomy does not accurately reflect the main mechanisms of clotting, in which the contact activation pathway actually plays a minor role.

The current view of coagulation (Fig. 16-6) highlights the importance of **tissue factor** (TF), a membrane-bound glycoprotein. The dynamic association of factor VIIa–TF complexes with TF pathway inhibitor (TFPI) is crucial to thrombosis. TFPI inhibits initiation of coagulation by binding TF–FXa–FVIIa complex. A major pool of TFPI on the surface of endothelial cells thus probably regulates coagulation. Hemostasis starts when activated factor VII (VIIa) encounters TF at a site of injury, forming the TF–VIIa complex. This complex activates small amounts of factors IX and X to IXa

and Xa. Activation of larger amounts of X to Xa is promoted by factors VIIIa and IXa. Xa converts small amounts of prothrombin to thrombin, and these traces of thrombin catalyze activation of factor XI, which in turn augments conversion of factor IX to IXa. The IXa and VIIIa complex generates more factor Xa from X. In the presence of calcium, this Xa binds Va to form the **prothrombinase complex** on phospholipids from platelet membranes. This complex then catalyzes activation of the inactive zymogen prothrombin to thrombin. Thrombin converts fibrinogen to fibrin monomers, which then form polymers. Thrombin also activates factor XIII to factor XIIIa, forming cross-linked fibrin strands to stabilize the clot.

Besides its important role in coagulation and platelet aggregation, thrombin participates in production of fibrinolytic molecules and regulation of growth factors and leukocyte adhesion molecules. It also mediates the protein C anticoagulant pathway by binding thrombomodulin at the surface of endothelial cells. Factor V, an essential protein coagulation cofactor, also has anticoagulant activity by exerting a cofactor function in the activated protein C system, which then downregulates factor VIIIa activity. Thrombin also increases vessel permeability by promoting alterations in endothelial cell shape and disrupting endothelial cell–cell adhesion junctions.

Injury to Blood Vessels Causes Platelet Adhesion and Aggregation

Normally, circulating platelets are not adherent to each other and to the surface of the vessel wall. However, injury upregulates platelet adhesiveness, after which platelets interact with one another to form a platelet thrombus, that is, an aggregate of activated platelets (Fig. 16-7). This process requires changes in platelet shape that reflect reorganization of actin microfilaments. Several molecules may promote platelet aggregation including thrombin, collagen, ADP, epinephrine, thromboxane A_2, platelet-activating factor (PAF) and vasopressin. Platelet aggregates occlude injured small vessels and prevent leakage of blood.

Once platelets are stimulated to adhere to a vessel wall, their granular contents are released, in part by contraction of the platelet cytoskeleton. These granules promote aggregation of other platelets. Platelet adhesion is enhanced by release of subendothelial von Willebrand factor, which is adhesive for glycoprotein (Gp) Ib platelet membrane protein and for fibrinogen. Activated platelets also release ADP and thromboxane A_2, a product of arachidonic acid metabolism, which recruit additional platelets to the process. The platelet membrane protein complex GpIIb–IIIa binds fibrinogen to form fibrinogen bridges between platelets, enhance aggregation and stabilize the nascent thrombus. Activated platelets in turn release factors that initiate coagulation, thus forming a complex thrombus on the surface of the vessel wall. Thrombin itself stimulates further release of platelet granules and subsequent recruitment of new platelets.

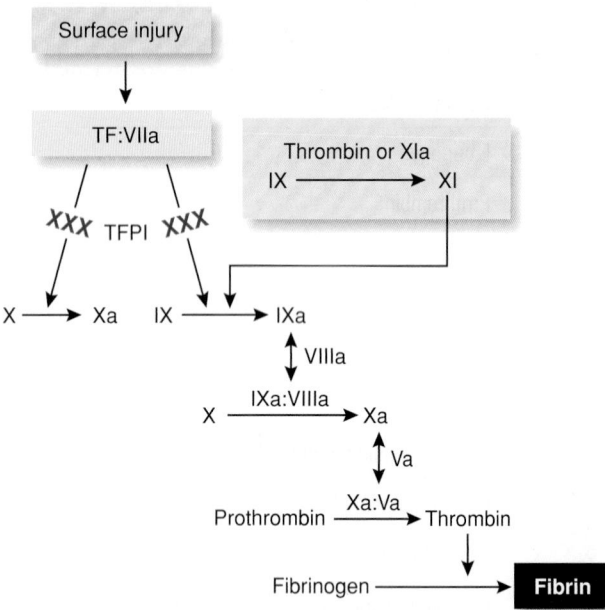

FIGURE 16-6. Coagulation cascade. The coagulation cascade is initiated by endothelial injury, which releases tissue factor (TF). The latter combines with activated factor VII (VIIa) to form a complex that activates small amounts of X to Xa and IX to IXa. The complex of IXa with VIIIa further activates X. The complex of Xa with Va then catalyzes the conversion of prothrombin to thrombin, after which fibrin is formed from fibrinogen. *TFPI* = tissue factor pathway inhibitor.

Endothelial Cells Regulate Clotting and Anticoagulation

Endothelium-derived modulators of coagulation are listed in Table 16-3. Endothelial cells synthesize a number of

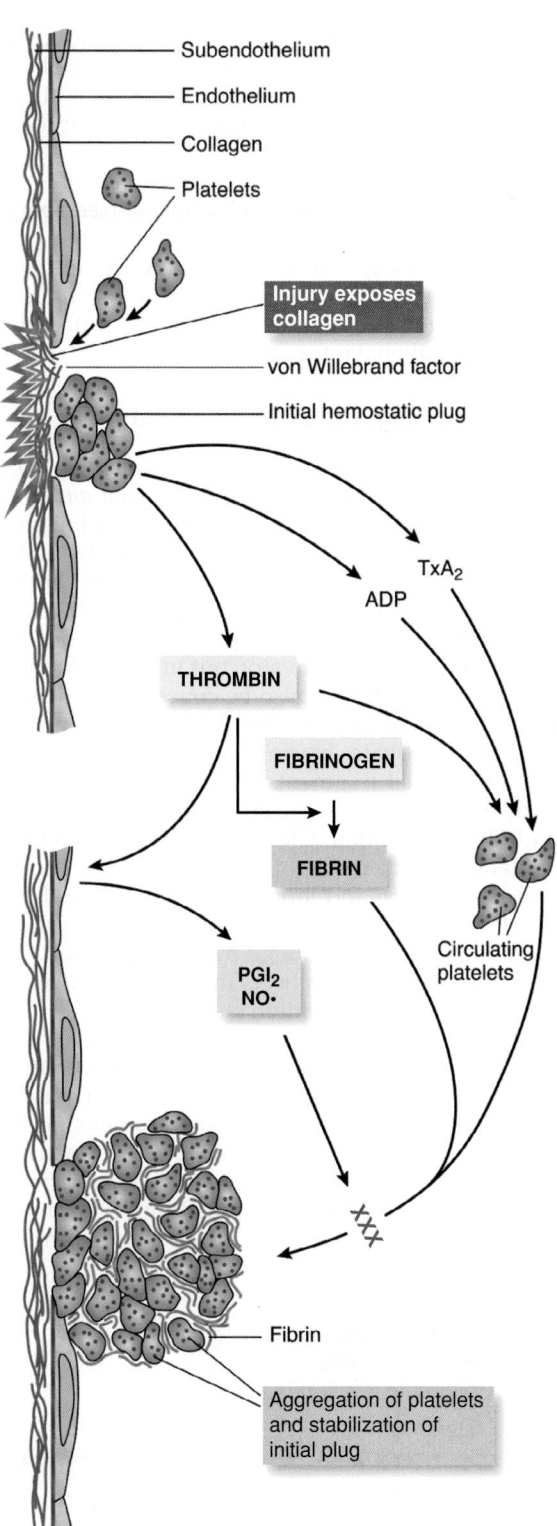

FIGURE 16-7. The role of platelets in thrombosis. Following vessel wall injury and alteration in flow, platelets adhere and then aggregate. Adenosine diphosphate (ADP) and thromboxane A_2 (TxA_2) are released and, along with locally generated thrombin, recruit additional platelets, causing the mass to enlarge. The growing platelet thrombus is stabilized by fibrin. Other elements, including leukocytes and red blood cells, are also incorporated into the thrombus. The release of prostacyclin (PGI_2) and nitric oxide (NO•) by endothelial cells regulates the process by inhibiting platelet aggregation.

TABLE 16-3
REGULATION OF COAGULATION AT THE ENDOTHELIAL CELL SURFACE

Downregulation

1. Thrombin inactivators
   a. Antithrombin III
   b. Thrombomodulin
2. Activated protein C pathway
   a. Synthesis and expression of thrombomodulin
   b. Synthesis and expression of protein S
   c. Thrombomodulin-mediated activation of protein C
   d. Inactivation of factor V_a and factor VIII_a by APC–protein S complex
3. Tissue factor pathway inhibition
4. Fibrinolysis
   a. Synthesis of tissue plasminogen activator, urokinase plasminogen activator and plasminogen activator inhibitor-1
   b. Conversion of Glu-plasminogen to Lys-plasminogen
   c. APC-mediated potentiation
5. Synthesis of unsaturated fatty acid metabolites
   a. Lipoxygenase metabolites—13-HODE
   b. Cyclooxygenase metabolites—PGI_2 and PGE_2

Procoagulant Pathways

1. Synthesis and expression of:
   a. Tissue factor (thromboplastin)
   b. Factor V
   c. Platelet-activating factor (PAF)
2. Binding of clotting factors IX/IX_a, X (prothrombinase complex)
3. Downregulation of APC pathway
4. Increased synthesis of plasminogen activator inhibitor
5. Synthesis of 15-HPETE

APC = adenomatous polyposis coli; 13-HODE = 13-hydroxy-octadeca-dienoic acid; 15-HPETE = 15-hydroperoxyeicosatetraenoic acid; PGE_2 = prostaglandin E_2; PGI_2 = prostacyclin.

anticoagulant factors. They produce and secrete **PGI_2,** which inhibits platelet aggregation. Endothelial NO• strongly inhibits platelet aggregation and adhesion to the vessel wall. Endothelial cells metabolize ADP, a strong promoter of thrombogenesis, to antithrombogenic metabolites. The luminal surface of the endothelium is coated with heparan sulfate, which binds a number of clotting factors, including the antiprotease β_2-macroglobulin. Endothelial heparan sulfate activates antithrombin, which binds to several coagulation factors, IIa, IXa, Xa, XIa and XIIa, which are free and not bound in complexes or in the clot. Endothelial cells may also lyse some clots as they form through the **plasminogen/ plasminogen activator/plasmin system**.

Endothelial cells have several other anticoagulant activities. A cofactor on the endothelial cell surface inactivates thrombin by forming a complex with thrombin and antithrombin III (a plasma antiprotease). Thrombin itself activates protein C by binding its receptor, **thrombomodulin,** at endothelial cell surfaces. Both protein C and thrombomodulin are synthesized by endothelial cells. Activated protein C destroys coagulation factors V and VIII. TFPI generated

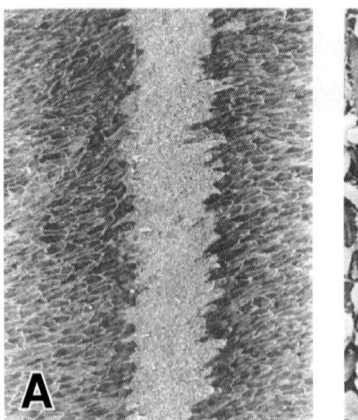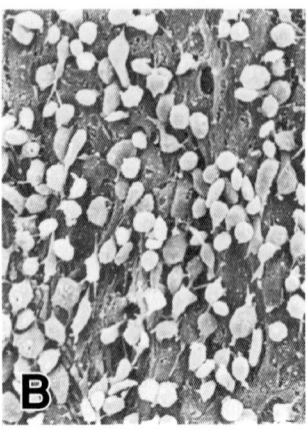

FIGURE 16-8. Scanning electron micrograph of the endothelial surface of a rat aorta 1 hour after the endothelial cells were removed by scraping with a nylon filament. A. Intact endothelium and scratched portion. **B.** Higher-power view of the scratched area shows a pavement of intact platelets that adheres to the underlying connective tissue in the high-velocity arterial stream.

during coagulation is bound to endothelium, where it inhibits the TF–VIIa complex (Fig. 16-6). TF and TFPI are synthesized and secreted by endothelial cells as well as other vascular cells.

In terms of balancing the system, the endothelium is also intimately involved in initiating and propagating thrombosis. The event that triggers most thrombosis is endothelial injury, which imparts a prothrombotic property to endothelium (Fig. 16-7). Endothelial cells synthesize von Willebrand factor, which promotes platelet adherence and activates clotting factor V. Endothelial cells also bind factors IX and X, a process that favors coagulation at the endothelial surface. Finally, inflammatory agents, including cytokines released from monocytes, activate procoagulants on the surface of intact endothelium. Interluekin-1 (IL-1) and tumor necrosis factor (TNF) cause endothelial cells to present thromboplastin to the plasma, thereby potentially triggering the extrinsic coagulation pathway.

Thus, thrombi may form when endothelial function is altered, when endothelial continuity is lost or when blood flow in a vessel becomes abnormal, such as turbulent or static. Simple loss of endothelial cells or injury to a vessel with good flow produces platelet pavementing but not thrombosis (Fig. 16-8).

Endothelial Cells Repair Defects in Damaged Areas

The most common denuding injury to endothelium is progressive disruption by atherosclerotic plaque. Denuding endothelial damage is also described in homocystinuria, hypoxia and endotoxemia, as well as during invasive therapeutic procedures such as harvesting and implantation of saphenous veins for bypass grafts, angioplasty, insertion of intravascular stents and atherectomy. Interactions of a thrombus with subjacent endothelial cells may further disturb endothelial integrity. Both fibrin and thrombin affect the endothelial cytoskeleton and initiate endothelial shape changes to form intercellular gaps that disrupt endothelial integrity.

In that setting, endothelial cells can spread rapidly and migrate into the denuded area to reestablish a thromboresistant barrier (Fig. 16-4). This is followed by endothelial cell proliferation to restore normal cell density. These mechanisms may become dysfunctional at sites of persistent endothelial cell damage and result in focal erosions, ulcers and fissures.

Another hypothesized mechanism of repair is migration of endothelial progenitor cells (EPCs) (see above and Chapter 3). EPCs are thought to proliferate after vascular injury and physiologic stress. They then are released into the peripheral circulation, where they target injured vessel walls, attach to the denuded surface and differentiate to reestablish endothelial integrity.

Clot Lysis Is a Regulatory Mechanism

A thrombus may undergo several fates, including (1) lysis, (2) growth and propagation, (3) embolization and (4) organization and canalization. The combination of aggregated platelets and clotted blood is made unstable by activation of the fibrinolytic enzyme plasmin (Fig. 16-9). During clot formation, plasminogen is bound to fibrin and therefore is an integral part of the forming platelet mass. Endothelial cells make plasminogen activator, but in larger thrombi, circulating plasminogen may also be converted to plasmin by products of the coagulation cascade. Plasminogen activator bound to fibrin activates plasmin. In turn, by digesting fibrin strands into smaller fragments, plasmin lyses clots and disrupts the thrombus. These smaller fragments inhibit thrombin and fibrin formation. Clearance of fibrin also limits its accumulation in atherosclerotic plaques, where it can promote plaque growth and attract inflammatory cells. Endothelial cells also synthesize plasminogen activator inhibitor-1 (PAI-1), and plasmin is inhibited by α_2-antiplasmin. Thus, a regional fibrinolytic state reflects the balance between plasminogen and plasmin activation and inhibition.

Thrombi may undergo organization and become incorporated into vessel walls. The fibrin meshwork contracts to reduce the size of the thrombus. Arterial smooth muscle cells or venous fibroblasts migrate into the thrombus meshwork of cross-linked fibrin and produce extracellular matrix.

Proteolytic enzymes and their inhibitors secreted by smooth muscle cells and macrophages remodel the thrombus, digest the fibrin and form a fibrous structure with its own

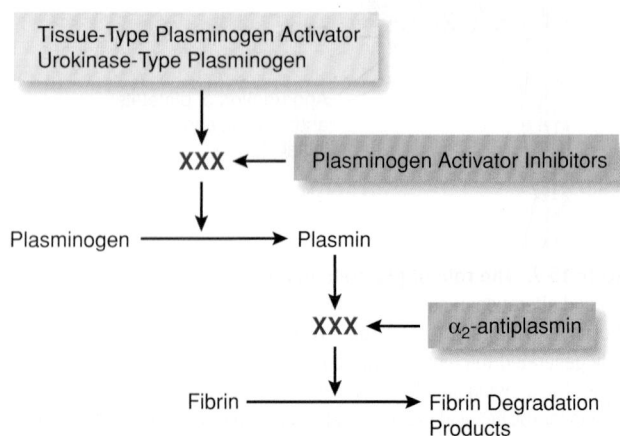

FIGURE 16-9. Mechanisms of fibrinolysis. Plasmin formed from plasminogen lyses fibrin. The conversion of plasminogen to plasmin and the activity of plasmin itself are suppressed by specific inhibitors.

TABLE 16-4
ATHEROGENESIS

- Initiation and growth of fibroinflammatory lipid atheroma is a slowly evolving dynamic process with superimposed acute events.

- Risk factors accelerate progression.

- The pathogenesis is multifactorial and thus the relative importance of specific genetic and environmental factors may vary in individuals.

- Interactions between cellular and matrix components of the vessel wall and serum constituents, leukocytes, platelets and physical forces regulate the formation of the fibroinflammatory lipid atheroma.

new blood vessels formed by angiogenic factors present in the thrombus. This revascularization is called **canalization**. However, blood flow through canalized thrombi is usually limited.

ATHEROSCLEROSIS

Atherosclerosis is characterized by progressive accumulation of inflammatory, immune and smooth muscle cells; lipids; and connective tissue in the intima of large and medium-sized elastic and muscular arteries. The classic atherosclerotic lesion is best described as a fibroinflammatory lipid plaque **(atheroma).** These plaques develop over several decades (Tables 16-4 and 16-5). Their continued growth encroaches on the media of the arterial wall and into the lumen of the vessel, narrowing its caliber. Atherosclerotic lesions are also called atherosclerotic plaques, atheromas, fibrous plaques or fibrofatty lesions.

 EPIDEMIOLOGY: The major complications of atherosclerosis, including ischemic heart disease (coronary artery disease), myocardial infarction, stroke and gangrene of the extremities, account for more than half of the annual mortality in the United States, with ischemic heart disease being the leading cause of death. The incidence of death from ischemic heart disease in Western countries peaked in the late 1960s, then declined by more than 30%. There are wide geographic and racial variations in the incidence of the disorder.

TABLE 16-5
IMPORTANT COMPONENTS OF FIBROINFLAMMATORY LIPID ATHEROMA

Cells		
	– Endothelial cells	Lipids and lipoproteins
	– Foam cells	Serum proteins
	– Giant cells	Platelet and leukocyte products
	– Lymphocytes	Necrotic debris
	– Mast cells	New microvessels
	– Macrophages	Hydroxyapatite crystals
Matrix		
	– Collagen	Growth factors
	– Elastin	Oxidants/antioxidants
	– Glycoproteins	Proteolytic enzymes
	– Proteoglycans	Procoagulant factors

 PATHOPHYSIOLOGY: Over the years, many theories have been proposed to explain the origins of atherosclerotic plaques. With the new knowledge from experimental and clinical observations, a comprehensive description of the pathogenesis of atherosclerosis is now possible, with the caveat that the formation, growth and clinical presentation of the plaques vary from patient to patient.

A Unifying Theory of Atherogenesis

The sequence of events in atherogenesis (Figs. 16-10 to 16-13) may begin in fetal life, with the formation of intimal cell masses, or perhaps shortly after birth, when fatty streaks begin to evolve. However, the typical atherosclerotic lesion, which is initially clinically insignificant, forms over 20–30 years. An exception is homozygous familial hypercholesterolemia, in which lesions develop in the first decade of life.

The life of a plaque can be divided into three stages: (1) initiation and formation, (2) adaptation and (3) clinical. Biologically active molecules regulate several dynamic cellular functions. Identification of a single "master" atherogenic gene responsible for most atherosclerosis is unlikely. Rather, it is probable that multiple gene polymorphisms interact with the environment and with each other.

Initiation and Formation Stage

1. Intimal lesions initially occur at sites that appear to be predisposed to lesion formation due to structural

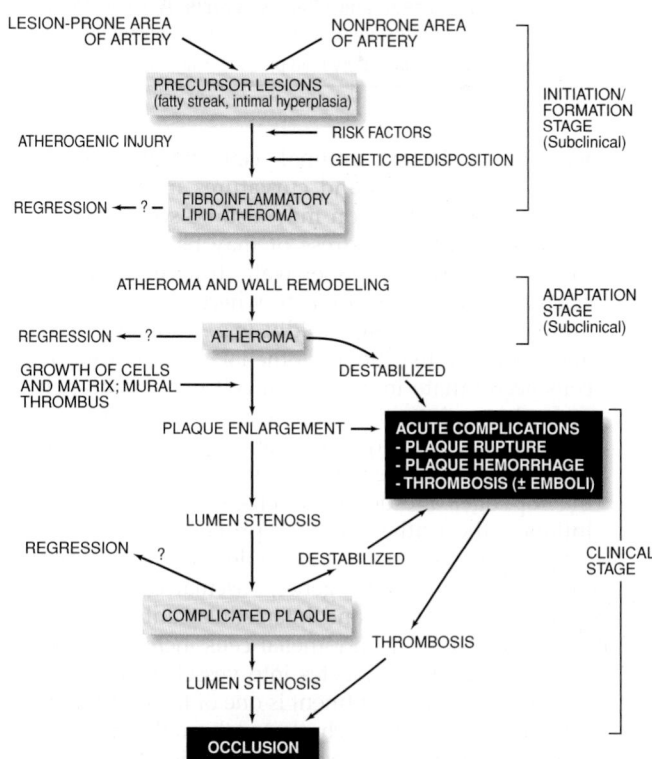

FIGURE 16-10. A unifying hypothesis for the pathogenesis of atherosclerosis.

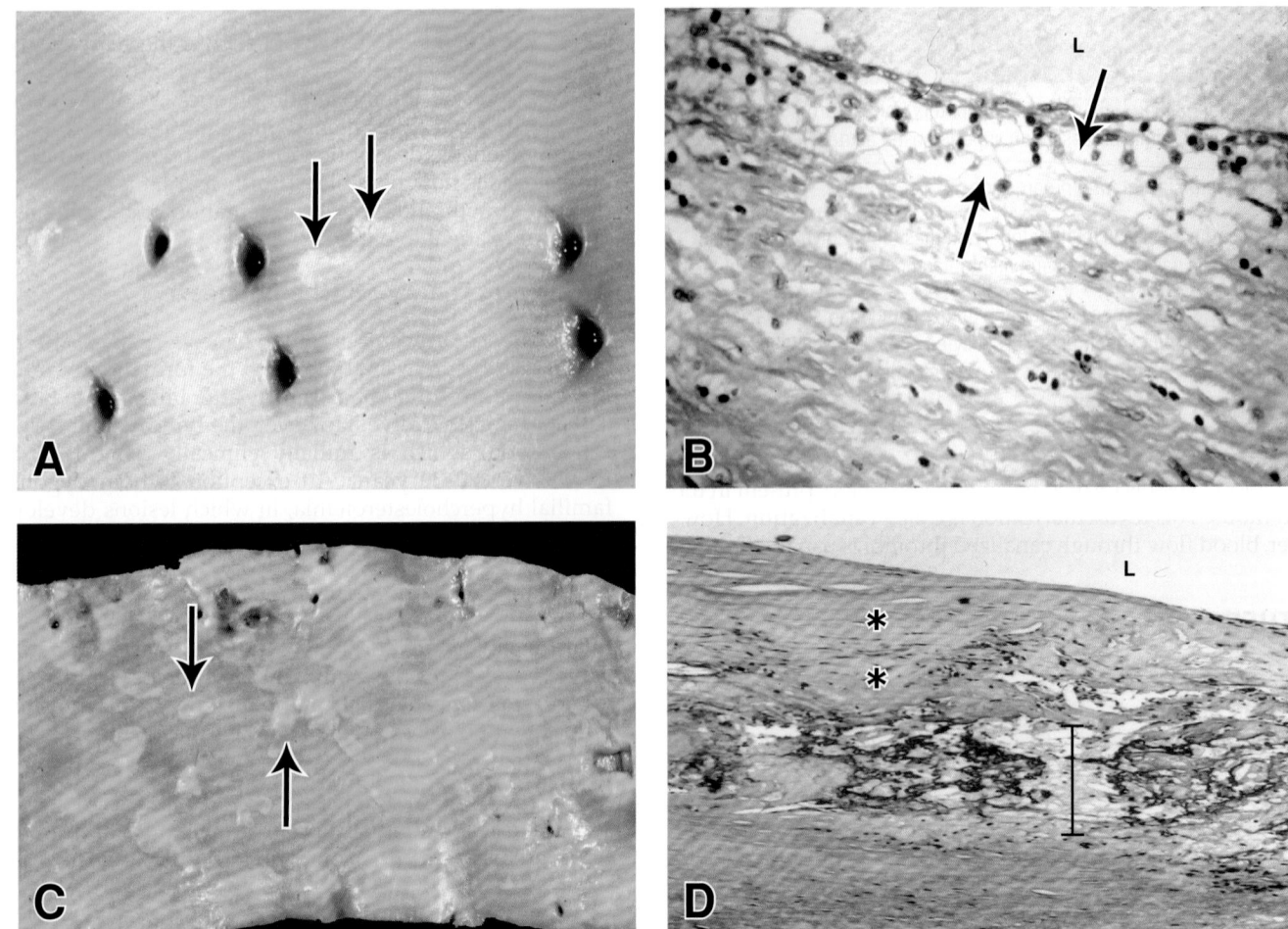

FIGURE 16-11. Fatty streak and atherosclerosis. A. Fatty streak. Gross photo of yellow fatty streaks (*arrows*) in the thoracic aorta. **B.** Fatty streak. Microscopic features of fatty streak in artery wall with intimal foam cells (*arrows*). *L* = lumen. **C.** Fibroinflammatory lipid plaques. Focal elevated plaques in thoracic aorta. **D.** Fibroinflammatory lipid plaques. Fibrous cap (*asterisks*) separating lumen (L) from central necrotic core (*bracket*).

features, including intimal cell mass, bifurcations, branch points and curvatures in the artery. Endothelial dysfunction may also be secondary to hemodynamic shear stress or may be constitutive in association with vessel wall structure. Atherosclerotic lesions tend to arise where shear stresses are low but fluctuate rapidly (e.g., branch points and bifurcations). Subendothelial smooth muscle cells accumulate in an intimal cell mass at branch and other points in certain vessels. This cell mass predisposes to plaque formation, particularly in the coronary arteries. Inflammatory cells, including macrophages and dendritic cells, are present in the intima of these atherosclerotic-prone areas.

At sites susceptible to plaque development, expression of proinflammatory genes, vascular cell adhesion molecule-1 (VCAM-1) and intercellular adhesion molecule-1 (ICAM-1) by endothelial cells increases. These molecules recruit monocytes into vessel walls. Monocyte/macrophage recruitment is one of the early events in atherogenesis and is orchestrated through a multistep process involving adhesion and transmigration. Adhesion is regulated by cell surface adhesion molecules including P-selectin, E-selectin, VCAM-1, ICAM-1 and

several chemokines. Transmigration involves platelet endothelial cell adhesion molecule-1 (PECAM-1).

The distribution of atherosclerotic lesions in large vessels and differences in location and frequency of lesions in different vascular beds encourage a belief in the role of hemodynamic factors. The fact that hypertension enhances the severity of atherosclerotic lesions further supports a role for hemodynamic factors in atherosclerogenesis. Hemodynamic forces induce unique gene expression patterns, including several factors in endothelial cells that are likely to promote atherosclerosis, for example, fibroblast growth factor 2 (FGF-2), TF, plasminogen activator, endothelin and PECAM. However, shear stress also induces gene expression of agents that may be antiatherogenic, including NOS and PAI-1. In people at increased risk of atherosclerosis, lesions also occur in areas that are not necessarily predisposed to the disease.

2. Lipid accumulation depends on disruption of the integrity of the endothelial barrier through gaps between cells, cell loss or endothelial cell dysfunction. This injury may be due to hypercholesterolemia, abnormal laminar flow, reactive oxygen species, cytokine- induced inflammation, advanced glycation end-products in

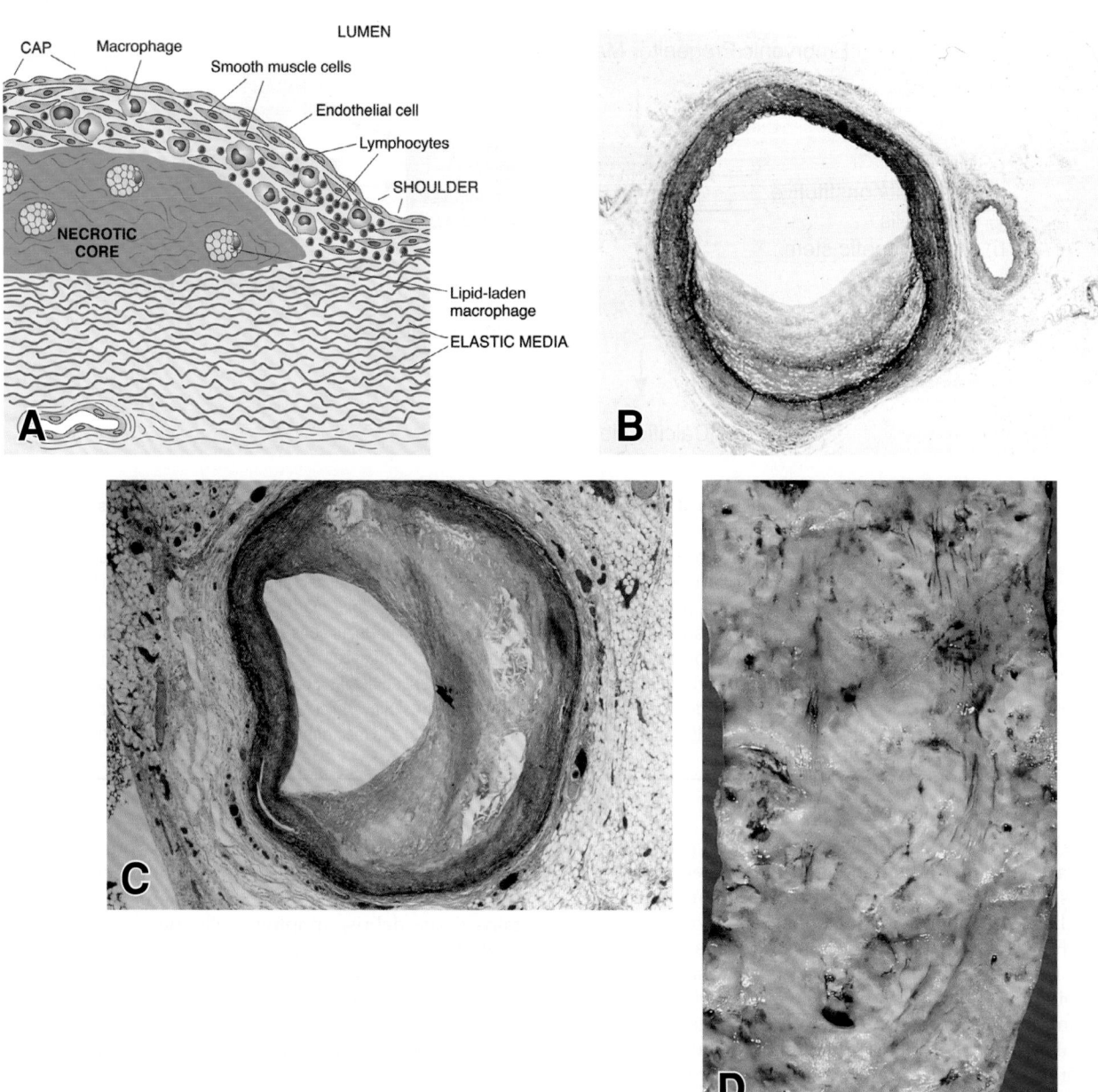

FIGURE 16-12. Fibrofatty plaque of atherosclerosis. A. In this fully developed fibrous plaque, the core contains lipid-filled macrophages and necrotic smooth muscle cell debris. The "fibrous" cap is composed largely of smooth muscle cells, which produce collagen, small amounts of elastin and glycosaminoglycans. Also shown are infiltrating macrophages and lymphocytes. Note that the endothelium over the surface of the fibrous cap frequently appears intact. **B.** Adaptive stage with atherosclerotic plaque and vessel wall dilatation to maintain the normal size of the lumen. Normal artery wall is at the top. **C.** Stenotic coronary artery with atherosclerotic plaque. **D.** The aorta shows discrete, raised, tan plaques. Focal plaque ulcerations are also evident.

diabetes and hyperhomocysteinemia. Hypertension also promotes endothelial dysfunction. Oxidative stress in endothelial cells and macrophages leads to cellular dysfunction and damage. LDLs carry lipids into the intima. Since oxidized LDL activates cell adhesion molecules, macrophages can adhere to activated endothelial cells and transmigrate between endothelial cells into the intima, bringing lipids with them. Some of these "foamy" macrophages undergo necrosis and release lipids. Alterations in types of matrix proteoglycans synthesized by the smooth muscle cells in the intima also render these sites prone to lipid accumulation by binding lipids and trapping them in the intima. *Reduced egress of lipids out of the artery wall also promotes lipid accumulation.*

3. Mononuclear macrophages, in addition to being central to atherogenesis by participating in lipid accumulation, also release growth factors that stimulate further accumulation of smooth muscle cells. **Oxidized LDL** induces tissue damage and recruits macrophages. It also promotes endothelial and smooth muscle cell release of chemokines, which regulate immune cell recruitment in the plaque. The nuclear factor-κB (NFκB) pathway is an important intracellular signal transduction system that

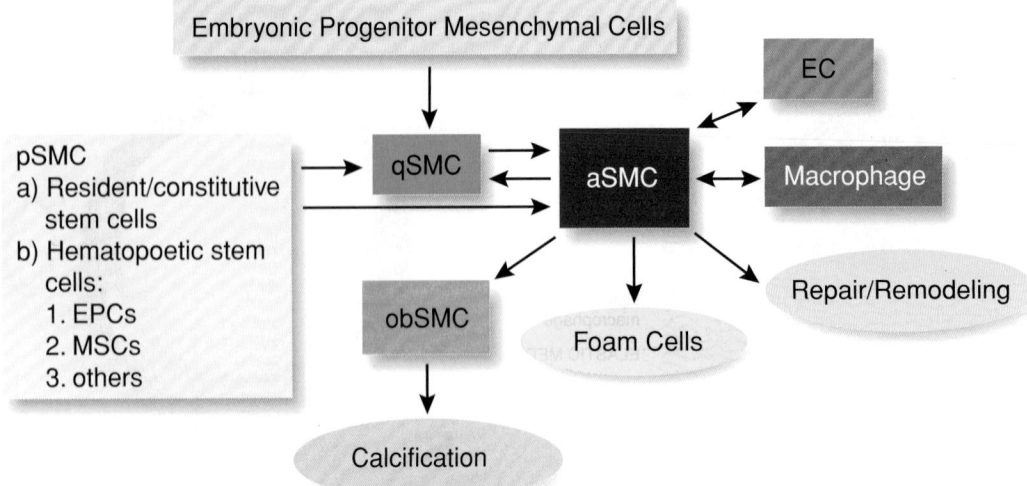

FIGURE 16-13. The hypothesized roles of smooth muscle cells (SMCs) in the pathogenesis of atherosclerosis. SMCs are quiescent (qSMC) in the normal artery wall and are derived embryonically from progenitor mesenchymal cells and neural crest cells. SMCs become activated (aSMC) by lipids and a variety of cytokines, chemokines, other mediators secreted by macrophages and endothelial cells through paracrine pathways in the lesion, and function in repair and remodeling of the lesion. aSMCs migrate, proliferate and secrete prominent extracellular matrix, while qSMCs exhibit a differentiated and contractile phenotype. aSMCs can accumulate lipids and become foam cells in the lesion. aSMCs can also undergo a change in phenotype to show osteoblastic functions (obSMC) promoting calcification in the atherosclerotic lesion. Progenitor SMCs (pSMCs) such as resident stem cells, bone marrow–derived hematopoietic stem cells, endothelial progenitor cells (EPCs) and bone marrow–derived mesenchymal stem cells (MSCs) may replenish SMCs in the vasculature, especially during a response to injury. aSMCs interact with endothelial cells (ECs) and macrophages directly or indirectly to regulate atherosclerotic plaque growth.

is active at several stages of plaque growth and progression. It activates recruitment of leukocytes by endothelial cells, cytokine expression and extracellular matrix remodeling. Monocytes/macrophages synthesize PDGF, FGF, TNF, IL-1, interferon-α and transforming growth factor-β (TGF-β), each of which can stimulate or inhibit growth of smooth muscle or endothelial cells. For example, interferon and TGF limit cell proliferation and could account for the failure of endothelial cells to maintain continuity over the lesion. Alternatively, they could inhibit growth-stimulatory peptides. IL-1 and TNF stimulate endothelial cells to produce PAF, TF and PAI. Thus, the combination of macrophages and endothelial cells may transform the normal anticoagulant vascular surface to a procoagulant one.

4. As a lesion progresses, mural thrombi often form on the damaged intimal surface. This stimulates PDGF release, accelerating smooth muscle proliferation and secretion of matrix components. The thrombus may grow, lyse or become organized and incorporated into the plaque.

5. The deeper parts of the thickened intima are poorly nourished because of a distance limitation for the diffusion of nutrients. This tissue undergoes ischemic necrosis, which is augmented by proteolytic enzymes released by macrophages (i.e., cathepsins) and tissue damage caused by oxidized LDL, reactive oxygen species and other agents. Thus, the central necrotic core is formed. Together with specific platelet- and macrophage-derived angiogenic factors, the necrotic core initiates angiogenesis, with new vasa vasorum forming in the plaque.

6. The fibroinflammatory lipid plaque is formed, with a central necrotic core and a fibrous cap, which separates the core from the blood in the lumen. The core contains tissue debris, apoptotic cells, necrotic foam cells, cholesterol crystals and focal calcification. Cholesterol clefts promote further inflammation. Inflammatory and immune cells infiltrate, mingling with smooth muscle cells, deposited lipids and variably organized matrix. TGF-β, a key regulator of extracellular matrix deposition, induces formation of several types of collagen, fibronectin and proteoglycans. It also enhances expression of proteolytic enzyme inhibitors that promote matrix degradation. TGF-β also has anti-inflammatory properties and has been reported to promote growth of smooth muscle cells. Since its effects depend on the environment, TGF-β may be both atherogenic and antiatherogenic.

7. The immune system participates in atherogenesis. Expression of human leukocyte antigen (HLA)-DR antigens on the endothelial and smooth muscle cells of plaques implies that these cells may have undergone immunologic activation, perhaps in response to interferon released by activated T cells in the plaque. In this scenario, the presence of T cells reflects an autoimmune response (e.g., against oxidized LDL). Dendritic cells are present in early lesions, and T lymphocytes also increase in the plaque.

Adaptation Stage
As the plaque protrudes into the lumen (e.g., in coronary arteries), the wall of the artery remodels to maintain lumen size. When a plaque occupies about half of the lumen, such remodeling can no longer compensate, and

the arterial lumen becomes narrowed (stenosis). Hemodynamic shear stress, an important regulator of vessel wall remodeling, acts through the mechanotransduction properties of endothelial cells. These include the cell cytoskeleton, ion channels in the cell membrane and the cell coat. Smooth muscle cell turnover, proliferation, apoptosis and matrix synthesis and degradation modulate remodeling of the vessel and the atherosclerotic plaque. Matrix metalloproteinases (MMPs) and their inhibitors (TIMPs) are important in this process (see Chapter 3). Just as remodeling maintains vessel patency, it also allows a plaque to be "clinically silent." Even a small plaque at this stage can rupture, with catastrophic results, as noted below.

Clinical Stage

1. As a plaque encroaches on the lumen, hemorrhage into it may increase its size without rupture. This hemorrhage occurs when fragile new vessels are formed in the plaques, which may rupture locally. Macrophages clean up the hemorrhagic material. Circulating blood may undermine the plaque, in which case the raised plaque, hemorrhage and thrombosis combine to obstruct the vessel.

2. Complications develop in the plaque, including surface ulceration, fissure formation, calcification and aneurysm formation. Activated mast cells at sites of erosion may release proinflammatory mediators and cytokines. Continued plaque growth leads to severe stenosis or occlusion of the lumen. Plaque rupture, involving the fibrous cap, and ensuing thrombosis and occlusion may precipitate catastrophic events in these advanced plaques (e.g., acute myocardial infarction). However, recent angiographic studies suggest that even plaques causing less than 50% stenosis may suddenly rupture. There are several conditions that appear to favor rupture, as noted in Fig. 16-10. These include hemodynamic shear stress, fissure formation, a thin fibrous cap, reduced number of smooth muscle cells, increased matrix metalloproteinase activity, inflammation, foam cell accumulation and focal nodular calcification.

Fig. 16-10 shows how these mechanisms may operate in atherogenesis.

The Initial Lesion of Atherosclerosis

PATHOLOGY: Two distinct lesions precede atherosclerotic plaques.

FATTY STREAK: Fatty streaks are flat or slightly elevated lesions in the intima in which intracellular and extracellular lipids accumulate. They are seen in young children as well as in adults. Cells filled with lipid droplets ("foam cells") congregate (Fig. 16-11). Macrophages contain the most lipid, but smooth muscle cells contain fat as well.

In children who die accidentally, significant fatty streaks may be evident in many parts of the arterial tree, but they do not reflect the distribution of atherosclerotic lesions in adults. Fatty streaks are common in the thoracic aorta in children, but atherosclerosis in adults is far more prominent in the abdominal aorta. Nonetheless, many believe that fatty infiltration is a precursor lesion of atherosclerosis and that other factors control the transition from fatty streak to clinically significant atherosclerotic plaque.

INTIMAL CELL MASS: The intimal cell mass is another candidate for a precursor lesion of atherosclerosis. Intimal cell masses are white, thickened areas at branch points in the arterial tree. Microscopically, they contain smooth muscle cells and connective tissue but no lipid. The location of these lesions, also known as "cushions," at arterial branch sites correlates well with the locations of later atherosclerotic lesions.

THE CHARACTERISTIC LESION OF ATHEROSCLEROSIS: The characteristic lesion of atherosclerosis is the fibroinflammatory lipid plaque. Simple plaques are focal, elevated, pale yellow, smooth-surfaced lesions, irregular in shape but with well-defined borders. Fibrofatty plaques (Fig. 16-12) represent more-advanced lesions and tend to be oval, with diameters of up to 12 cm. In smaller vessels, such as the coronary or cerebral arteries, a plaque is often eccentric; that is, it occupies only part of the circumference of the lumen. In later stages, fusion of plaques in muscular arteries can give rise to larger lesions, which occupy several square centimeters.

Atherosclerotic plaques are initially covered by endothelium and tend to involve the intima and very little of the upper media (Fig. 16-12B). The area between the lumen and the necrotic core—the **fibrous cap**—contains smooth muscle cells, macrophages, lymphocytes, lipid-laden cells (foam cells) and connective tissue components. The central core contains necrotic debris. Cholesterol crystals and foreign body giant cells may be present within the fibrous tissue and necrotic areas. Foam cells are both macrophages and smooth muscle cells that have taken up lipids. Numerous inflammatory and immune cells, especially T cells, are present within a plaque.

Neovascularization is an important contributor to plaque growth and its subsequent complications (Fig. 16-13). It is postulated that vessels grow inward from the vasa vasorum. They are rare in healthy coronary arteries but plentiful in atherosclerotic plaques.

COMPLICATED ATHEROSCLEROTIC PLAQUES: A **complicated** plaque may reflect erosion, ulceration or fissuring of the plaque surface; plaque hemorrhage; mural thrombosis; calcification; and aneurysm (Figs. 16-12C, D; 16-14; and 16-15). Progression from a simple fibrofatty atherosclerotic plaque to a complicated lesion may occur as early as the third decade of life, but most affected people are 50 or 60 years of age.

Cellular interactions in atherogenesis are summarized in Fig. 16-16.

- **Calcification** involving osteochondrocytic differentiation occurs in areas of necrosis and elsewhere in the plaque. Oxidized lipids and inflammatory cytokines promote vascular calcification. Calcification in the artery is thought to depend on mineral deposition and resorption, which are regulated by osteoblast-like and osteoclast-like cells in the vessel wall. These cells are considered to be rare precursor cells in the artery wall, derived from smooth muscle–type cells that have undergone a phenotypic transformation or possibly circulating stem/precursor cells derived from bone marrow. Several transcription factors (including Msx2, Runx2, Osterix and Sox9) promote cell osteoblast development. Calcification may also reflect changes in the physical-chemical properties of a diseased vessel wall that provoke formation of hydroxyapatite crystals.
- **Mural thrombosis** results from abnormal blood flow around the plaque, where it protrudes into the lumen

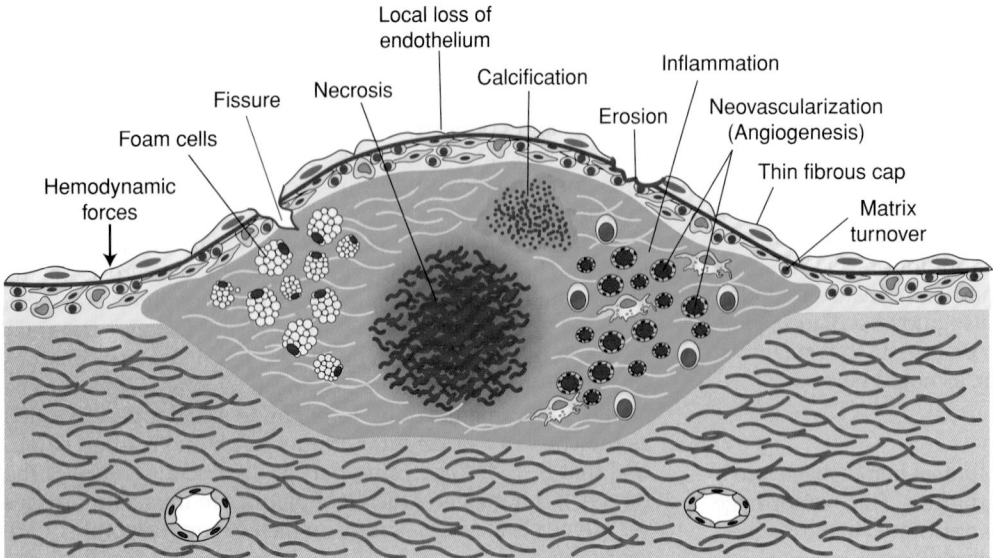

FIGURE 16-14. Complicated atherosclerotic plaque. The surface shows endothelial denudation, erosion and fissure formation. The plaque shows a thin fibrous cap, a central necrotic core, inflammation, lipids, calcification and neovascularization.

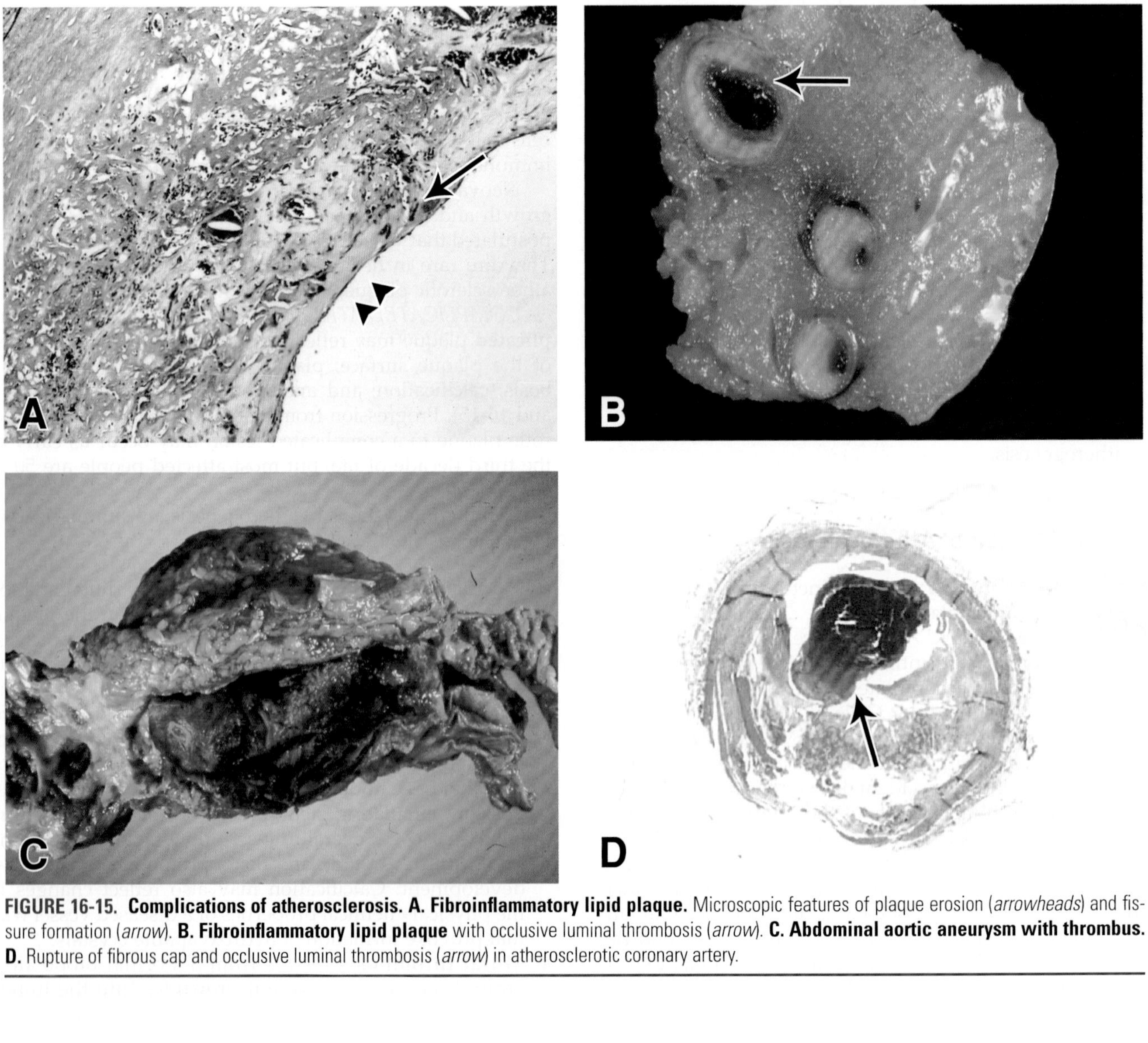

FIGURE 16-15. Complications of atherosclerosis. A. Fibroinflammatory lipid plaque. Microscopic features of plaque erosion (*arrowheads*) and fissure formation (*arrow*). **B. Fibroinflammatory lipid plaque** with occlusive luminal thrombosis (*arrow*). **C. Abdominal aortic aneurysm with thrombus. D.** Rupture of fibrous cap and occlusive luminal thrombosis (*arrow*) in atherosclerotic coronary artery.

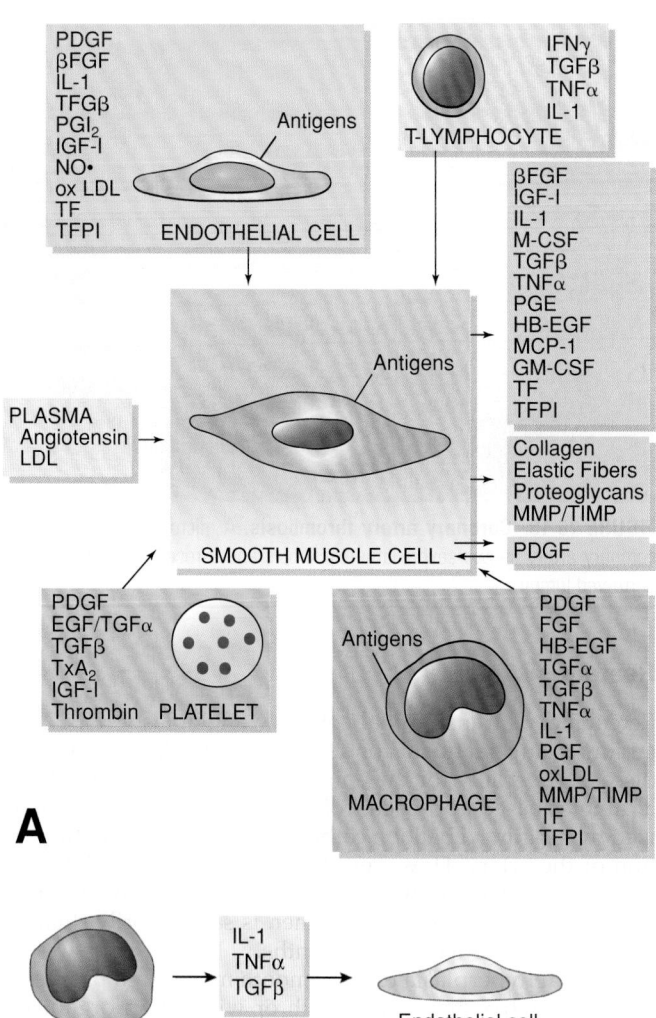

A

B

FIGURE 16-16. Cellular interactions in the progression of the athero-sclerotic plaque. A. Endothelium, platelets, macrophages, T lymphocytes and smooth muscle cells elaborate a variety of cytokines, growth factors and other substances. The scheme illustrated here emphasizes their influence on smooth muscle cells. **B.** The cellular interactions that promote the proliferation of smooth cells. *EGF* = endothelial growth factor; *FGF* = fibroblast growth factor; *HB-EGF* = heparin-binding epidermal growth factor; *IFN* = interferon; *IGF-I* = insulin-like growth factor I; *IL* = interleukin; *MCP-1* = monocyte chemotactic protein-1; *M-CSF* = macrophage colony-stimulating factor; *MMP* = matrix metalloproteinase; *NO•* = nitric oxide; *oxLDL* = oxidated low-density lipoprotein; *PDGF* = platelet-derived growth factor; *PGE* = prostaglandin; *PGI₂* = prostacyclin; *TF* = tissue factor; *TGF* = tumor growth factor; *TFPI* = tissue factor pathway inhibitor; *TNF* = tumor necrosis factor; *TIMP* = inhibitors of MMPs; *TxA₂* = thromboxane A₂.

and creates turbulence, reduced luminal flow or stasis. The disturbance in flow also causes damage to the endothelial lining, which may become dysfunctional or locally denuded, in which case it no longer presents a thromboresistant surface. Thrombi often form at sites

of erosion and fissuring on the surface of the fibrous cap. Mural thrombi in the proximal region of a coronary artery may embolize to more distal sites in the vessel.

- **The vulnerable atheroma** has structural and functional alterations that predispose to plaque destabilization.
- **Atheroma destabilization** often results in acute coronary syndromes. It may occur whenever the dynamic balance of opposing biological and physical processes is disrupted, leading to mural thrombosis, fibrous cap rupture or intraplaque hemorrhage. Some ruptures are clinically silent and can heal. In a ruptured plaque, the necrotic material that comes in contact with the blood contains TF and is highly thrombogenic. The adjacent endothelium has reduced inhibitor (TFPI) levels and lower antiplatelet and fibrinolytic activities, all favoring coagulation. The presence of circulating markers of inflammation suggests that procoagulant inflammatory mediators may also participate.

Once a plaque **ruptures,** the exposed thrombogenic material promotes clot formation in the lumen, causing an occlusive thrombus. Plaque hemorrhage due to rupture of thin, newly formed vessels may occur within a plaque, with or without a subsequent rupture of the fibrous cap. In the latter case, hemorrhage may expand the plaque and so narrow the lumen further. The hemorrhage will be resorbed over time within the plaque, leaving telltale residual hemosiderin-laden macrophages.

Most plaques that rupture show less than 50% luminal stenosis, and over 95% are less than 70% stenosed. Plaque rupture often occurs at the shoulder of the plaque, suggesting that hemodynamic shear stress weakens and tears the fibrous cap. If not repaired, endothelial loss leads to plaque erosion, weakening the fibrous cap and exposing the plaque to blood constituents. Plaque rupture has been associated with (1) areas of inflammation, (2) large lipid core size, (3) thin fibrous cap, (4) decreased smooth muscle cells owing to apoptosis, (5) imbalance of proteolytic enzymes and their inhibitors in the fibrous cap, (6) calcification in the plaque and (7) intraplaque hemorrhage, leading to inside-out rupture of the fibrous cap.

Several circulating markers have been associated with plaque burden, including C-reactive protein (CRP), fibrinogen, soluble VCAM, IL-1, IL-6 and TNF.

Complications of Atherosclerosis

The complications of atherosclerosis depend on the location and size of the affected vessel (Fig. 16-17) and the chronicity of the process.

- **Acute occlusion:** Thrombosis on an atherosclerotic plaque may abruptly occlude a muscular artery (Fig. 16-18). The result is ischemic necrosis (infarction) of the tissue supplied by that vessel, manifested clinically as myocardial infarction, stroke or gangrene of the intestine or lower extremities. Some occlusive thrombi can be dissolved therapeutically by enzymes that activate plasma fibrinolytic activity, including streptokinase and tissue plasminogen activator.
- **Chronic narrowing of the vessel lumen:** As an atherosclerotic plaque grows, it may narrow the lumen, progressively reducing blood flow to tissue served by that artery.

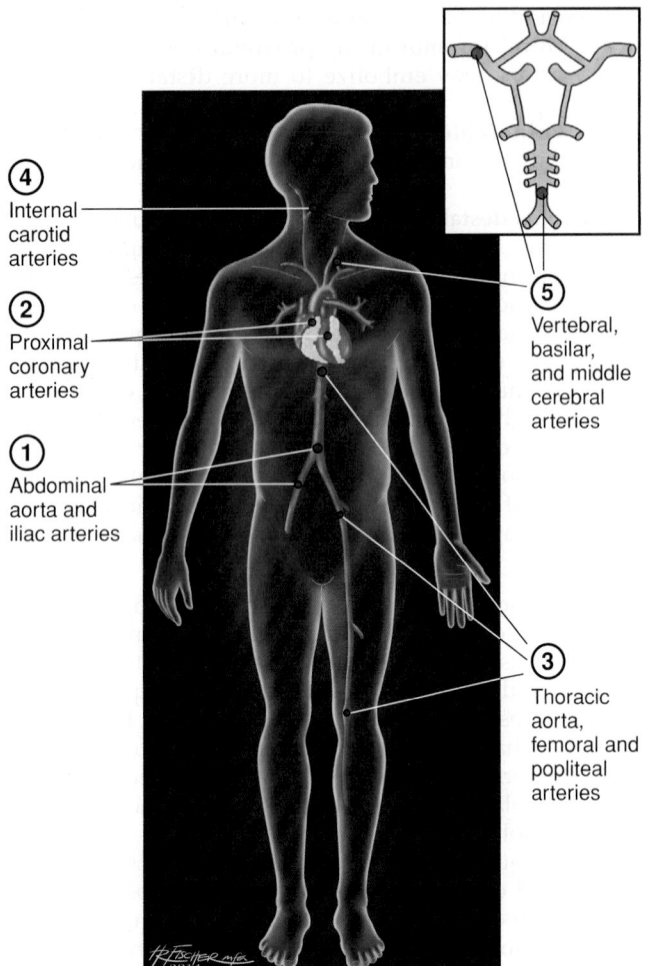

FIGURE 16-17. Sites of severe atherosclerosis in order of frequency.

Chronic ischemia of the affected tissue causes atrophy of the organ, for example, (1) unilateral renal artery stenosis giving rise to renal atrophy, (2) mesenteric artery atherosclerosis causing intestinal stricture or (3) ischemic atrophy of the skin occurring in a diabetic with severe peripheral vascular disease.

■ **Aneurysm formation:** The complicated lesions of atherosclerosis may extend into the media of elastic arteries and weaken their walls, so as to allow aneurysm formation, typically in the abdominal aorta. The reduced elastin promotes thinning and ballooning of the wall, while matrix metalloproteinases secreted by smooth muscle cells and macrophages break down collagen. Such aneurysms often contain thrombi, which may embolize. Sudden rupture of these aneurysms, especially in the aorta and cerebrum, may precipitate a vascular catastrophe.

■ **Embolism:** A thrombus formed over an atherosclerotic plaque may detach and lodge in a distal vessel. Thus, embolization from a thrombus in an abdominal aortic aneurysm may acutely occlude the popliteal artery, causing gangrene of the leg. Ulceration of an atherosclerotic plaque may also dislodge atheromatous debris and produce so-called cholesterol crystal emboli, which appear as needle-shaped spaces in affected tissues (Fig. 16-19), most often the kidney.

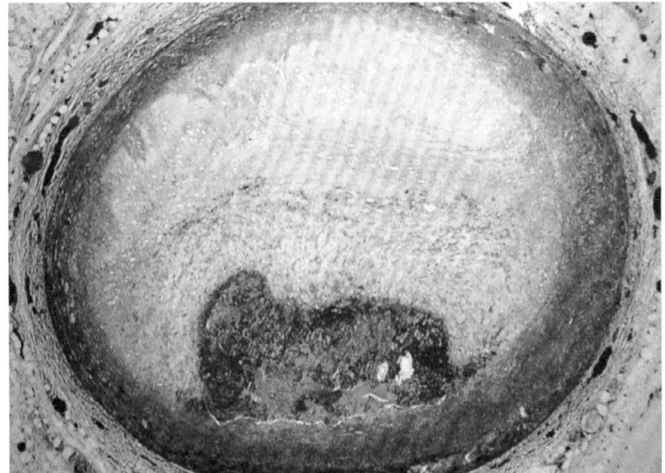

FIGURE 16-18. Coronary artery thrombosis. A microscopic section of a coronary artery shows severe atherosclerosis and a recent thrombus in the narrowed lumen.

Restenosis

Percutaneous transluminal coronary angioplasty (PTCA) is an important treatment for stenotic atherosclerotic vascular disease, especially for the epicardial coronary arteries. With a catheter-based approach, coronary arteries are revascularized by inflating a balloon catheter to dilate the stenotic portion of the artery. However, the balloon causes endothelial damage and tears in the plaque and the media. In 30%–40% of cases in which the vessel lumen is satisfactorily dilated, restenosis occurs within 3–6 months.

Intimal hyperplasia due to smooth muscle cell proliferation and matrix deposition, with or without an organized mural thrombus on the luminal surface, leads to restenosis. In addition, vascular wall remodeling, induced in part by trauma to the vessel wall and involving the adventitia, also results in luminal narrowing through contraction of the arterial wall.

Restenosis is reduced when a stent, a tubular scaffold device, is deployed by a catheter to keep the diseased

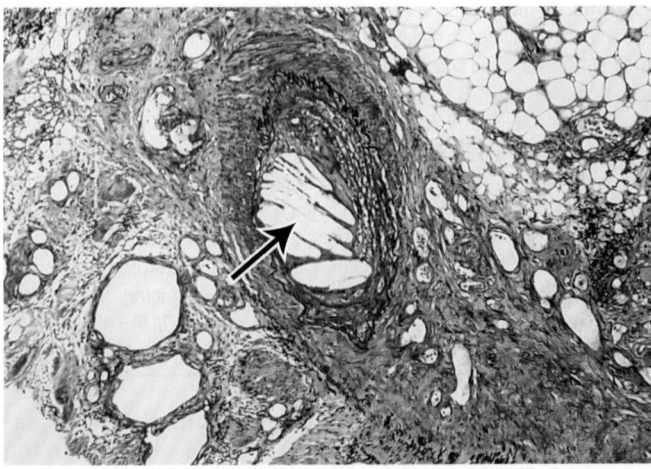

FIGURE 16-19. Cholesterol crystal embolus. Needle-shaped clefts (*arrow*) are seen in an atherosclerotic embolus that has occluded a small artery.

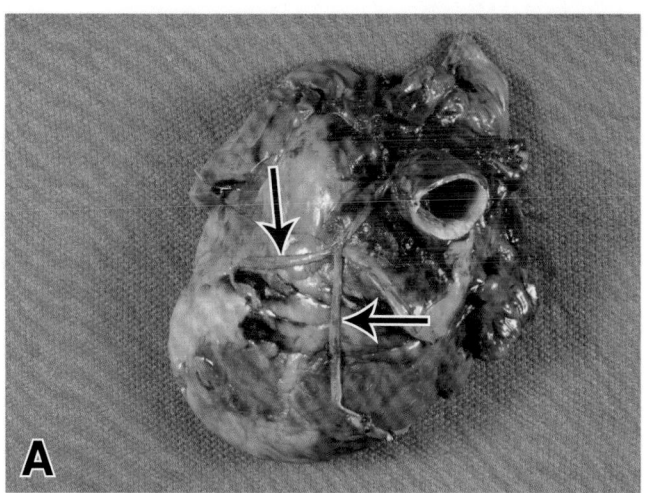
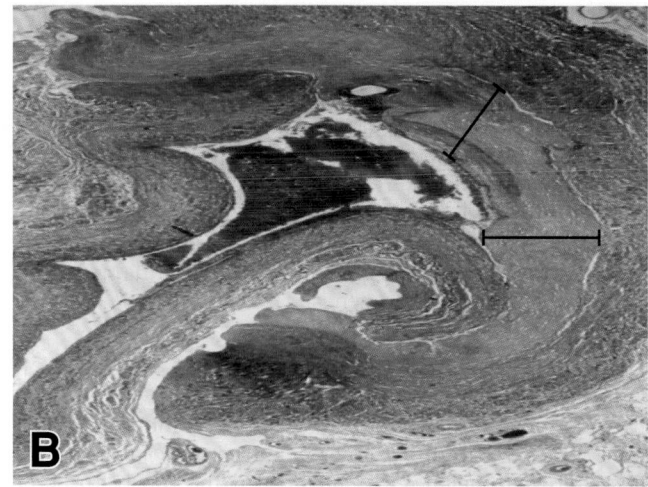

FIGURE 16-20. Saphenous vein aortocoronary bypass. A. Saphenous vein aortocoronary bypass on the surface of the heart (epicardium) (*arrows*). **B.** Distal anastomosis site with atherosclerotic coronary artery (*brackets*).

atherosclerotic artery open. Originally, bare metal stents were used, but because of frequent restenosis, these have been replaced by stents coated with biocompatible polymers and biologically active agents, with much less restenosis. For example, drug-eluting stents with antiproliferative agents block cell cycle progression and thus inhibit overgrowth of smooth muscle cells in the vessel wall. Although long-term complications are not fully known, especially as they relate to thrombosis, drug-eluting stents are used extensively.

Transplanted saphenous veins are used as autografts in coronary artery bypass operations and undergo a series of adaptive and reparative changes. These include (1) intimal thickening associated with phlebosclerosis, (2) occasional medial calcification, (3) focal muscle cell hypertrophy and, eventually, (4) adventitial scarring. Venous grafts in place for a few years develop atherosclerotic plaques indistinguishable from those found in native coronary arteries (Fig. 16-20). Half of bypass grafts occlude within 5–10 years as a result of neointimal hyperplasia and atherosclerosis.

Risk Factors for Atherosclerosis

Factors associated with a twofold or greater risk of ischemic heart disease include:

- **Hypertension:** High blood pressure increases the risk of myocardial infarction. Recent evidence indicates that both diastolic and systolic hypertension contribute equally to this increased risk. Men with systolic blood pressures over 160 mm Hg have almost triple the incidence of myocardial infarction compared to those with systolic pressures under 120 mm Hg. The use of antihypertensive drugs has significantly reduced myocardial infarction and stroke.
- **Blood cholesterol level:** Serum cholesterol levels correlate with development of ischemic heart disease and account for much of the geographic variation in the incidence of this condition. Absent genetic disorders of lipid metabolism (see below), blood cholesterol correlates strongly with dietary intake of saturated fat. Use of cholesterol-lowering drugs lowers the risk of myocardial infarction. Total serum cholesterol does not necessarily predict risk of ischemic heart disease, since cholesterol is transported by atherogenic and antiatherogenic lipoproteins. Thus, therapeutic decisions are mainly based on LDL cholesterol levels.
- **Cigarette smoking:** Coronary and aortic atherosclerosis are more severe and extensive in cigarette smokers than in nonsmokers, and the effect is dose related (see Chapter 8). Thus, smoking markedly increases the risk of myocardial infarction, ischemic stroke and abdominal aortic aneurysms.
- **Diabetes:** Diabetics are at increased risk for occlusive atherosclerotic vascular disease in many organs. However, the relative contribution of carbohydrate intolerance alone, as opposed to the hypertension and hyperlipidemias common in diabetics, is not well defined (see Chapter 13).
- **Increasing age and male sex:** Both correlate strongly with the risk of myocardial infarction, but probably as reflections of accumulated effects of other risk factors.
- **Physical inactivity and stressful life patterns:** These factors correlate with increased risk of ischemic heart disease, but their role in the evolution of atherosclerosis is not clear.
- **Homocysteine:** Homocystinuria is a rare autosomal recessive disease caused by mutations in the gene encoding cystathionine synthase. The disorder causes premature and severe atherosclerosis. Mild elevations of plasma homocysteine are common and are an independent risk factor for atherosclerosis of the coronary arteries and other large vessels. The increased risk is similar in magnitude to those of smoking and hyperlipidemia. Homocysteine is toxic to endothelial cells and impairs several anticoagulant mechanisms in endothelial cells. It inhibits thrombomodulin on the endothelial cell surface, antithrombin III–binding activity of heparan sulfate proteoglycan, binding of tissue plasminogen activator and ecto-ADPase activity on the endothelial cell surface, the last of which promotes platelet aggregation. In addition, oxidative interactions between homocysteine, lipoproteins and cholesterol further complicate the situation.

Low dietary folate intake may aggravate genetic predispositions to hyperhomocysteinemia, but it is not known whether folic acid treatment protects from atherosclerotic vascular disease.

- **C-reactive protein:** CRP is an acute phase reactant mainly produced by hepatocytes. It is a serum marker for systemic inflammation and has been linked to an increased risk of myocardial infarction and ischemic stroke. This observation, together with the presence of CRP in atherosclerotic plaques, suggests that systemic inflammation may contribute to atherogenesis.

Infection and Atherosclerosis

Seroepidemiologic studies suggest that some infectious agents may contribute to atherosclerosis. *Chlamydia pneumoniae* and cytomegalovirus have been the most studied, although there is also interest in *Helicobacter pylori,* herpesvirus and others. DNA from these agents has been found in human atherosclerotic lesions, but the nature of this association is obscure.

Lipid Metabolism

Since Rudolf Virchow in the 19th century first identified cholesterol crystals in atherosclerotic lesions, considerable information has accumulated on lipoproteins and their roles in lipid transport and metabolism in atherosclerosis. Cholesterol and other lipids (mainly triglycerides) are insoluble, and lipoprotein particles function as special transporters (Table 16-6; Fig. 16-21). These particles differ in protein and lipid composition, size and density. They are categorized according to density:

- Chylomicrons
- Very-low-density lipoproteins (VLDLs)
- LDLs
- High-density lipoproteins (HDLs)

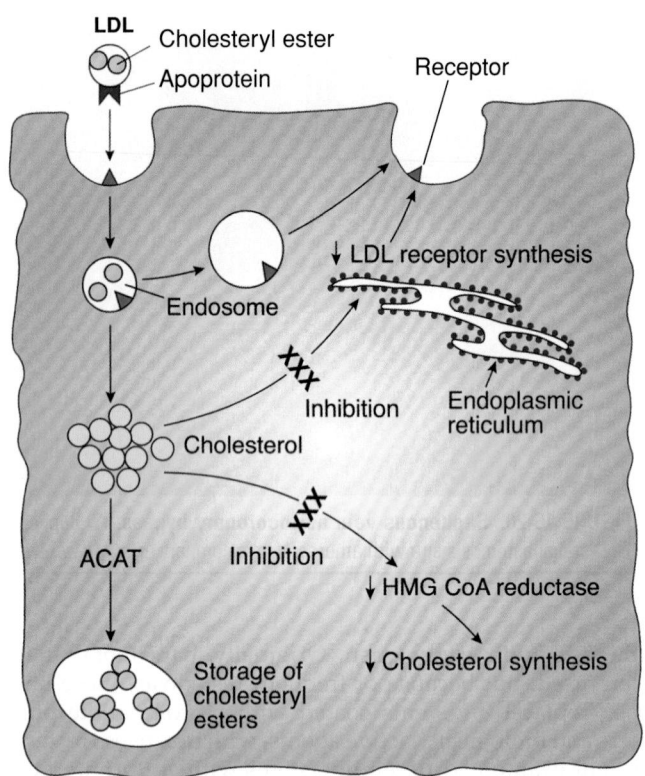

FIGURE 16-21. The relationship between circulating low-density lipoprotein (LDL) cholesterol, LDL receptors and the synthesis of cholesterol. LDL, which contains cholesteryl esters, is taken up by cells into vesicles by a receptor-mediated pathway to form an endosome. The receptor and lipids are dissociated, and the receptor is returned to the cell surface. The exogenous cholesterol, now in the cytoplasm, causes a reduction in receptor synthesis in the endoplasmic reticulum and inhibits the activity of hydroxymethylglutaryl–coenzyme A (HMG–CoA) reductase in the cholesterol-synthesizing pathway. Excess cholesterol in the cell is esterified to cholesteryl esters and stored in vacuoles. *ACAT* = acyl-CoA: cholesterol acyltransferase.

	TABLE 16-6

THE APOLIPOPROTEINS

Apolipoprotein	Approximate Molecular Weight	Major Density Class	Major Sites of Synthesis in Humans	Major Function in Lipoprotein Metabolism
AI	28,000	HDL	Liver, intestine	Activates lecithin:cholesterol acyltransferase
AII	18,000	HDL	Liver, intestine	
AIV	45,000	Chylomicrons	Intestine	
B-100	250,000	VLDL, IDL, LDL	Liver	Binds to LDL receptor
B-48	125,000	Chylomicrons, VLDL, IDL	Intestine	
CI	6500	Chylomicrons, VLDL, HDL	Liver	Activates lecithin:cholesterol acyltransferase
CII	10,000	Chylomicrons, VLDL, HDL	Liver	Activates lipoprotein lipase
CIII	10,000	Chylomicrons	Liver	Inhibits lipoprotein uptake by the liver
D	20,000	HDL		Cholesteryl ester exchange protein
E	40,000	Chylomicrons, VLDL, HDL	Liver, macrophage	Binds to E receptor system

HDL = high-density lipoprotein; IDL = intermediate-density lipoprotein; LDL = low-density lipoprotein; VLDL = very-low-density lipoprotein.

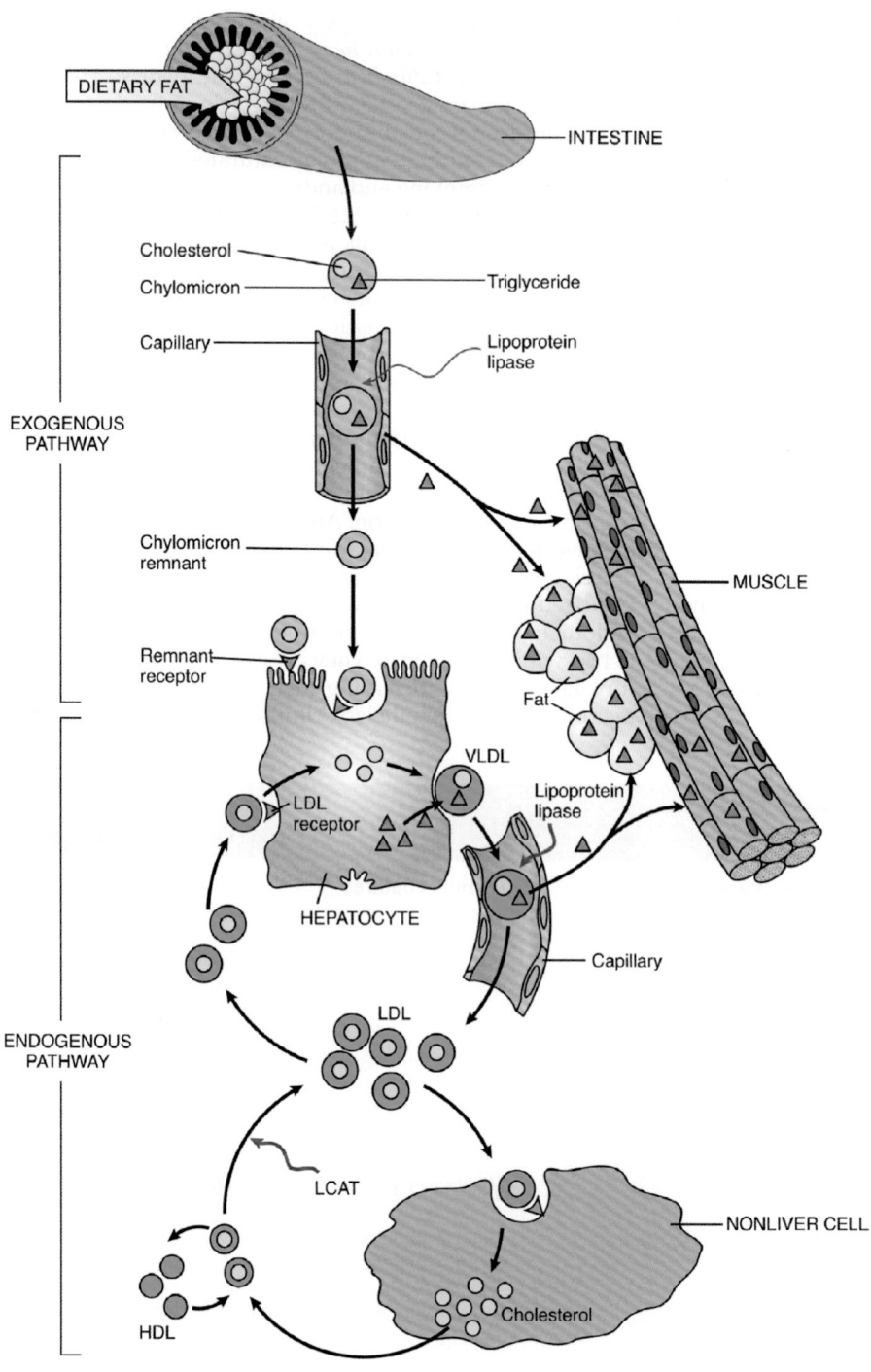

FIGURE 16-22. Exogenous and endogenous cholesterol transport pathway. In the exogenous pathway, cholesterol and fatty acids from food are absorbed through the intestinal mucosa. Fatty acid chains are linked to glycerol to form triglycerides. Triglycerides and cholesterol are packaged into chylomicrons that are returned via the lymph to the blood. The lipids are coupled to proteins by enzymes such as the microsomal transfer protein complex. In the capillaries (mainly of fat tissue and muscle, but also other tissues), the ester bonds holding the fatty acids in triglycerides are split by lipoprotein lipase. Fatty acids are removed, leaving cholesterol-rich lipoprotein remnants. These bind to special remnant receptors and are taken up by liver cells. The cholesterol of the remnant is either secreted into the intestine, largely as bile acids, or packaged as very-low-density lipoprotein (VLDL) particles, which are then secreted into the circulation. This is the first step in the endogenous cycle. In fat or muscle tissue, the triglyceride is removed from the VLDLs with the aid of lipoprotein lipase. The intermediate-density lipoprotein (IDL) particles (not shown) remain in the circulation. Some IDLs are immediately taken up by the liver via the mediation of low-density lipoprotein (LDL) receptors for apoB/E. The remaining IDLs in the circulation are either taken up by nonliver cells or converted to LDLs. Most of the LDLs in the circulation bind to hepatocytes or other cells and are removed from the circulation. High-density lipoproteins (HDLs) take up cholesterol from cells. This cholesterol is esterified by the enzyme lecithin:cholesterol acyltransferase (LCAT), after which the esters are transferred to LDLs and taken up by cells.

Each of these has a lipid core with associated proteins (apolipoproteins) (Table 16-6). The metabolic pathways for lipoproteins containing B apolipoproteins (apoB) are two major cascades, one from the intestine and the other from the liver (Fig. 16-22).

EXOGENOUS PATHWAY: This metabolic route involves chylomicrons containing the protein apoB-48, secreted by the intestine. After secretion, chylomicrons rapidly acquire apoCII and apoE from HDL. These triglyceride-rich lipoproteins mainly transport lipid from intestine to liver. The triglycerides in chylomicrons are hydrolyzed by lipoprotein lipase at the surface of capillary endothelial cells. ApoCII activates lipoprotein lipase, which removes triglycerides

and converts chylomicrons to "remnants," and finally to intermediate-density lipoproteins (IDLs). Hepatocytes take up chylomicron remnants through an apoE-mediated (remnant) receptor process.

ENDOGENOUS PATHWAY: This network of reactions involves triglyceride-rich lipoproteins containing apoB-100 secreted by the liver. Liver VLDL particles acquire apoCII and apoE from HDL shortly after their secretion. The triglycerides on VLDL are hydrolyzed by lipoprotein lipase. The particles containing apoB-100 are initially converted to IDLs, and then to LDLs. Hepatic lipoprotein lipase converts IDL to LDL, at least in part, at which point most apoCII and apoE dissociates from the particles and reassociates with HDL.

Lipoprotein lipase acts both as a triglyceride hydrolase and, more importantly, as a phospholipase. LDL, which contains apoB-100, interacts with high-affinity receptors on hepatocytes and other cells, including smooth muscle cells, fibroblasts and adrenal cells (Fig. 16-22). Interaction of LDL with its receptor initiates receptor-mediated endocytosis, leading to catabolism of LDL.

HIGH-DENSITY LIPOPROTEIN: HDL containing apoAI and apoAII is synthesized by several pathways. These include direct secretion of HDL by intestine and liver, and transfer of lipid and apolipoprotein constituents released during lipolysis of lipoproteins that contain apoB. Two major functions have been proposed for HDL: (1) a reservoir for apolipoproteins, mainly apoCII and apoE, and (2) interaction with cells in the transport system to carry extrahepatic cholesterol, including that in the arterial wall, to the liver for elimination. The latter function has been called **reverse cholesterol transport**. The cholesterol removed from cells is principally free cholesterol, which is rapidly esterified to cholesteryl esters. The latter are transferred to the cores of lipoprotein particles or are exchanged to VLDL and LDL. These transfers are mediated by specific transfer proteins (e.g., cholesterol ester transfer protein [CETP]). Defects in cholesteryl ester transfer and exchange lead to dyslipoproteinemia, increased intracellular cholesteryl ester concentrations and premature atherosclerosis.

HDL is referred to as "good" cholesterol. *An inverse correlation between ischemic heart disease and HDL cholesterol levels has been established.* Factors that increase HDL levels include female gender, estrogens, vigorous exercise and moderate alcohol consumption. Decreased HDL occurs with diets low in fat or high in polyunsaturated fats, truncal obesity, diabetes, smoking and androgen administration.

LOW-DENSITY LIPOPROTEIN: LDL contains apoB-100 and cholesterol esters as its main lipid entity. LDLs are heterogeneous in particle density, a characteristic that correlates with differences in atherogenicity. Macrophages, endothelial cells and smooth muscle cells in atherosclerotic lesions can oxidize LDL, thereby increasing LDL atherogenicity, facilitating LDL recognition by the macrophage scavenger receptor and leading to massive cholesterol uptake by macrophages. **Oxidized lipoproteins** also affect other processes that may contribute to atherogenesis, including regulation of vascular tone, activation of inflammatory and immune responses and coagulation. Autoantibodies to oxidized LDL are detected in both plasma and plaques in patients with atherosclerosis, and may be important in plaque development. Oxidized LDLs are toxic to vascular wall cells, may disrupt endothelial integrity and promote the accumulation of cell debris within atheromas. They are also chemotactic for macrophages, thereby increasing their accumulation in atheromas even more. Nonetheless, clinical trials of antioxidants to

TABLE 16-7

MOLECULAR DEFECTS IN DYSLIPOPROTEINEMIAS

Disease	Genetic Defect	Clinical Features
Apolipoprotein Defects		
ApoAI deficiency	ApoA1 truncations or rearrangements (11q23)	Absent HDL, severe atherosclerosis
ApoAI variants	ApoA1 point mutations (11q23)	Reduced HDL, variable atherosclerosis
Abetalipoproteinemia (absence of both apoB-100 defects, absence of atherosclerosis and apoB-48)	Microsomal triglyceride protein mutations (4q22–24)	Ataxia, malabsorption, hemolytic anemia, visual
ApoB-100 absence	Unknown (2p24)	Mild ataxia, malabsorption, absence of atherosclerosis
ApoCII deficiency	ApoCII mutations (19q13.2)	Type I hyperlipidemia: severe hypertriglyceridemia, variable atherosclerosis
ApoE variants	ApoE mutations (19q13.2)	Type III hyperlipidemia: elevated triglycerides, premature atherosclerosis
Enzyme Defects		
Lipoprotein lipase deficiency	Lipoprotein lipase mutations (8p22)	Type I hyperlipidemia: hypertriglyceridemia; minimal atherosclerosis
Hepatic lipase deficiency	Hepatic lipase mutations (15q21–23)	Elevations of IDL and HDL; severe atherosclerosis
Lecithin:cholesterol acyltransferase (LCAT) deficiency	LCAT mutations (16q22.1)	Mild hypertriglyceridemia; reduced HDL; corneal opacities; variable atherosclerosis
Receptor Defect		
Familial hypercholesterolemia	LDL receptor mutations (19p13.2)	Type II hyperlipidemia: severe elevation of LDL; premature atherosclerosis

Apo = apoprotein; HDL = high-density lipoprotein; IDL = intermediate-density lipoprotein; LDL = low-density lipoprotein.

prevent ischemic heart disease have not demonstrated any protection. An interesting therapeutic strategy is related to the inhibition of proprotein convertase subtilisin kexin type 9 (PCSK9), an enzyme that promotes degradation of the LDL receptor and thus impairs clearance of LDL.

Heritable Dyslipoproteinemias

Familial clustering of ischemic heart diseases is well documented (Table 16-7).

FAMILIAL HYPERCHOLESTEROLEMIA: The 1985 Nobel Prize was awarded to Brown and Goldstein for discovering the LDL receptor. They identified the pathways regulating cholesterol homeostasis (Fig. 16-21) and facilitated our understanding of receptor-mediated endocytosis and regulation of cell membrane receptors. The LDL receptor is a cell surface glycoprotein that regulates plasma cholesterol by mediating endocytosis and recycling of apoE, the major plasma cholesterol transport protein. Mutations in the LDL receptor gene, on the short arm of chromosome 19, give rise to familial hypercholesterolemia (FH), an autosomal dominant disease for which about 1 in 500 people are heterozygotes and 1 in a million are homozygotes.

Most untreated homozygotes die from coronary artery disease before the age of 20. Among people under 60 years of age who have suffered a myocardial infarction, 5% are heterozygous for familial hypercholesterolemia. Such heterozygotes have plasma LDL levels that are twice normal, whereas homozygotes exhibit a 6- to 10-fold increase in plasma LDL. Heterozygote patients also suffer from premature myocardial infarction but at a later age than do homozygotes (40–45 years of age in men).

More than 400 mutant alleles for familial hypercholesterolemia are known, including point mutations, insertions and deletions. These mutations fall into five main classes, based on their effects on receptor protein function (Fig. 16-23). Genetic issues in familial hypercholesterolemia are discussed more fully in Chapter 6.

In addition to accelerated accumulation of cholesterol in arteries (premature atherosclerosis), LDL cholesterol also deposits in skin and tendons to form xanthomas (Fig. 16-24). In some cases (before age 10 in homozygotes), an *arcus lipoides* is present in the cornea.

APOLIPOPROTEIN E: Genetic variations in various apoproteins are also accompanied by alterations in LDL levels. Polymorphisms in apoE and variants of apolipoprotein AI and AII have been observed. Apolipoprotein E is one of the main protein constituents of VLDL and of a subclass of HDL. The gene locus that codes for apoE is polymorphic; three common alleles, E2, E3 and E4, code for three major apoE isoforms and determine the six apoE phenotypes. Some 20% of the variability in serum cholesterol has been attributed to apoE polymorphism. In men, the apoE 3/2 phenotype is associated with a 20% lower LDL level than the most common phenotype, apoE 3/3. By contrast, the E4 allele is associated with elevated serum cholesterol. Interestingly, the E2 allele is increased and E4 decreased among male octogenarians. The E4 allele is also a major risk factor for late-onset Alzheimer disease. Patients who display E2/2 clear chylomicron remnants and IDLs poorly and have familial type III hyperlipoproteinemia, with premature atherosclerosis.

HIGH-DENSITY LIPOPROTEIN: The genes for apolipoproteins AI and CIII are on chromosome 11 and are physically linked, whereas the gene for AII is on chromosome 1.

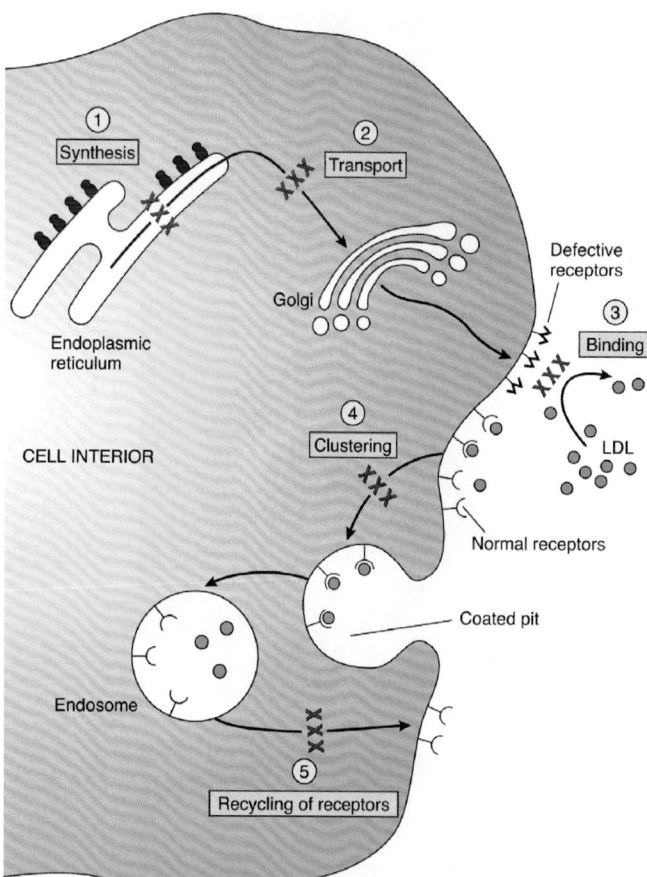

FIGURE 16-23. Mutations of the low-density lipoprotein (LDL) receptor in familial hypercholesterolemia.

Polymorphisms of apoAI are associated with premature atherosclerosis, as are rare cases of hereditary apoAI deficiency. Hypertriglyceridemia is often associated with low HDL cholesterol.

LIPOPROTEIN (a) (Lp[a]): Lp(a) is an LDL-like particle to which the glycoprotein apo(a) is attached through a disulfide bridge with apoB-100. High circulating levels of Lp(a) are associated with an increased risk of atherosclerosis of the coronary arteries and larger cerebral vessels in both sexes. Plasma levels of this cholesterol-rich lipoprotein vary greatly (<1 to >140 mg/dL) and appear to be independent of LDL levels. The Lp(a)-specific protein, apo(a), has been detected in atherosclerotic lesions, and high Lp(a) levels correlate with target organ damage in hypertensive patients.

Apo(a) is encoded by a gene on chromosome 6 (6q2.7), close to the gene for plasminogen, to which apo(a) is highly homologous. Apo(a) and plasminogen display similar domains that mediate interactions with fibrin and cell surface receptors. Lp(a) enhances cholesterol delivery to injured blood vessels, suppresses generation of plasmin and promotes smooth muscle proliferation. Thus, it may be an important link between atherosclerosis and thrombosis.

Lp(a) plasma levels are heritable and not altered by most cholesterol-lowering drugs, although they are reduced by nicotinic acid. Taken together, this information distinguishes a risk factor that appears superficially to be related to serum cholesterol but the effect of which may actually be linked to an alteration in clot lysis.

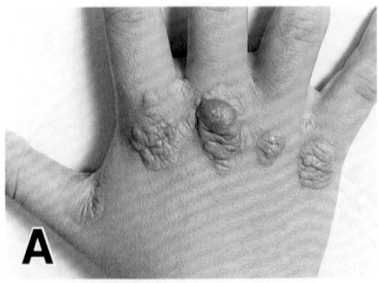
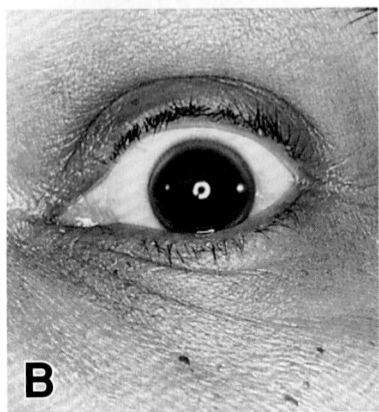
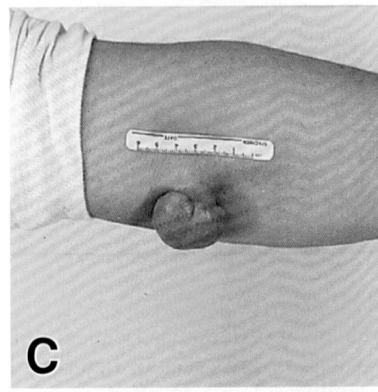
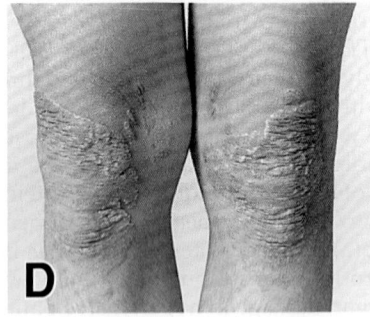

FIGURE 16-24. Xanthomas in familial hypercholesterolemia. A. Dorsum of the hand. **B.** Arcus lipoides represents the deposition of lipids in the peripheral cornea. **C.** Extensor surface of the elbow. **D.** Knees.

HYPERTENSIVE VASCULAR DISEASE

There has been a significant increase in the prevalence of hypertension worldwide, with dramatic increases since the beginning of the 20th century. Hypertension affects over 30% of the population of the United States. It is present in more than half of cases of myocardial infarction, stroke and chronic renal disease. It is included in the "metabolic syndrome"

(see Chapter 13), along with hyperglycemia, insulin resistance, dyslipidemia and obesity. Hypertension is present in 95% or greater of ascending aortic dissections or rupture. At least 3/4 of patients with dissecting aortic aneurysm, intracerebral hemorrhage or myocardial wall rupture also have elevated blood pressure. Blacks are particularly plagued by hypertension and are more likely than are whites to experience severe complications.

In 95% of patients, hypertension occurs without an identifiable cause, a condition referred to as **primary** hypertension. A number of diseases contribute to the development of hypertension, including renal artery stenosis, most forms of chronic renal disease, diabetes mellitus, primary elevation of aldosterone levels, Cushing syndrome, pheochromocytoma, hyperthyroidism, coarctation of the aorta and renin-secreting tumors. In addition, people with severe atherosclerosis may have high systolic pressure because a sclerotic aorta cannot properly absorb the kinetic energy of the pulse wave. Whatever the etiology, effective treatment of hypertension prolongs life.

The definition of hypertension depends on a statistical estimate of the distribution of systolic and diastolic blood pressures in the general population. Both systolic and diastolic pressures are important in determining the risk of cardiovascular disease, especially that due to atherosclerosis. Over the course of the day, blood pressure varies widely, depending on exertion, emotional state and other poorly understood factors. It also exhibits a circadian rhythm, falling at night or during sleep, as sympathetic nervous system tone declines. The mean systolic blood pressure in 20-year-old men is about 130 mm Hg, but 95% confidence limits range from 105 to 150 mm Hg. Average systolic blood pressure increases with age, so that in 80-year-olds, it reaches 170 mm Hg, with 95% confidence limits from 125 to 220. The World Health Organization (WHO) defines hypertension as systolic pressure above 160 mm Hg or diastolic pressure above 90.

 **ETIOLOGIC FACTORS:** Blood pressure is the product of cardiac output and systemic vascular resistance to blood flow. The most widespread hypothesis holds that primary hypertension results from an imbalance in the interactions between these mechanisms (Fig. 16-25). However, both of these functions are critically influenced by renal function and sodium homeostasis. Frequency of hypertension increases as the glomerular filtration rate (GFR) falls even with mild renal dysfunction. Reduced GFR causes sodium retention and volume expansion, which should be compensated by a decrease in tubular sodium reabsorption. Impaired renal tubular sodium handling and reduced GFR are likely to be important in hypertension that afflicts patients with chronic kidney disease due to diabetes or aging.

A complex endocrine axis centers on the renin–angiotensin system (RAS), which is both hormonal and tissue based, the latter present in many organs, including the brain. The RAS is important in regulation of normal blood pressure, and dysregulation of RAS is implicated in over 2/3 of the cases of hypertension. Renal artery occlusion or dietary salt restriction leads to increased renal secretion of renin. Renin is a protease that cleaves angiotensinogen to a decapeptide, angiotensin I. In turn, angiotensin I is converted to angiotensin II by ACE on the endothelial surface. Angiotensin II causes vasoconstriction and also affects centers in the brain

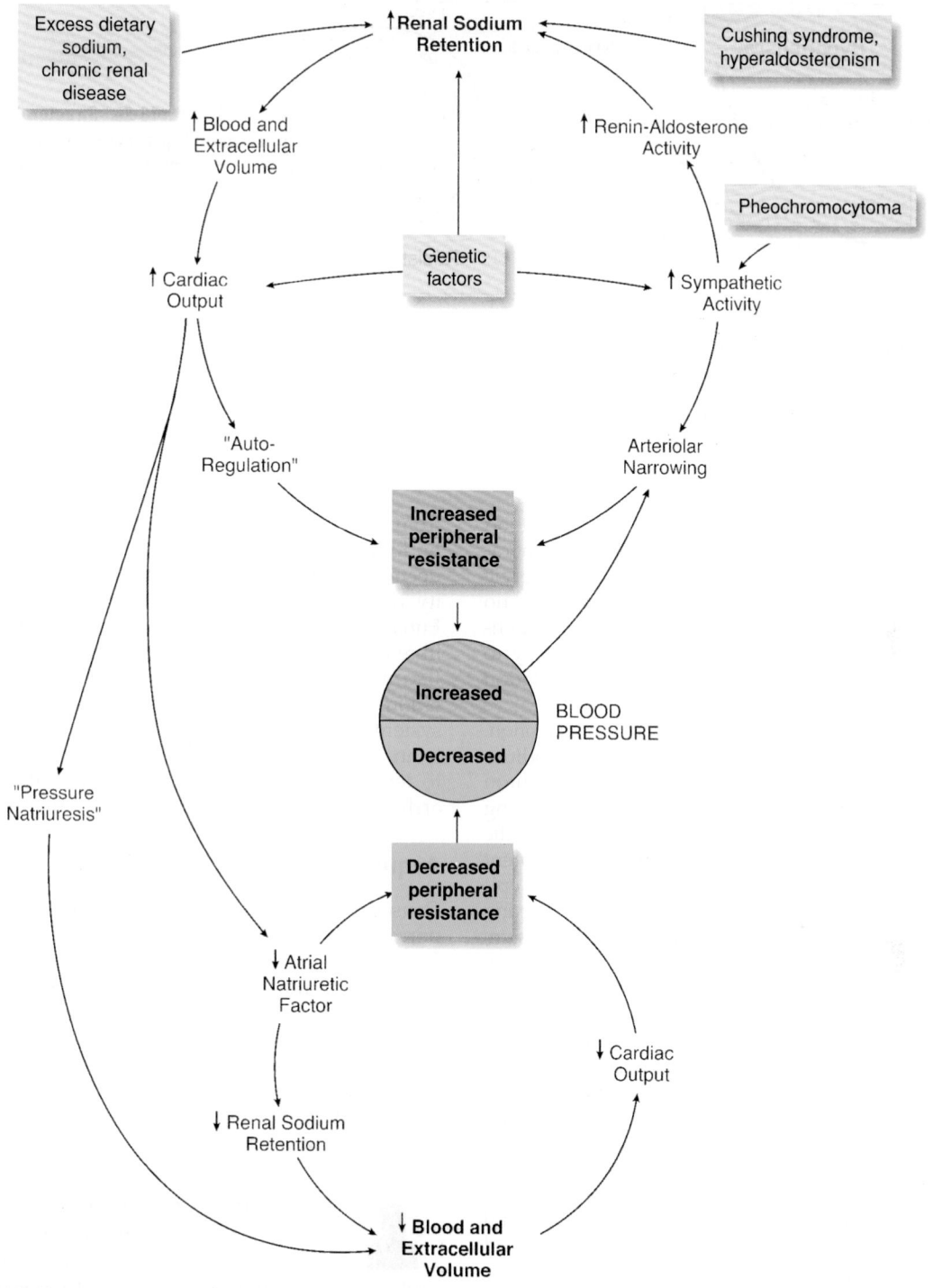

FIGURE 16-25. Factors contributing to hypertension and the counterregulatory factors that lower blood pressure. An imbalance in these factors results in the increased peripheral resistance that is responsible for most cases of essential (primary) hypertension. Note the central role of peripheral resistance.

that control sympathetic outflow and stimulate adrenal aldosterone release. Aldosterone increases sodium reabsorption by the renal tubules. The net effect of all these actions is increased total body fluid. Thus, the **renin–angiotensin** system elevates blood pressure by three mechanisms:

- Increased sympathetic output
- Increased mineralocorticoid secretion
- Direct vasoconstriction

This axis is antagonized by atrial natriuretic factor (ANF), a polypeptide hormone secreted by specialized cells in the cardiac atria. ANF binds specific receptors in the kidney and increases urinary sodium excretion, thereby opposing angiotensin II–induced vasoconstriction. Secretion of ANF may be controlled by stretch–secretion coupling after atrial distention, a consequence of increased volume, or by as-yet undefined endocrine interactions, possibly involving endothelin-1.

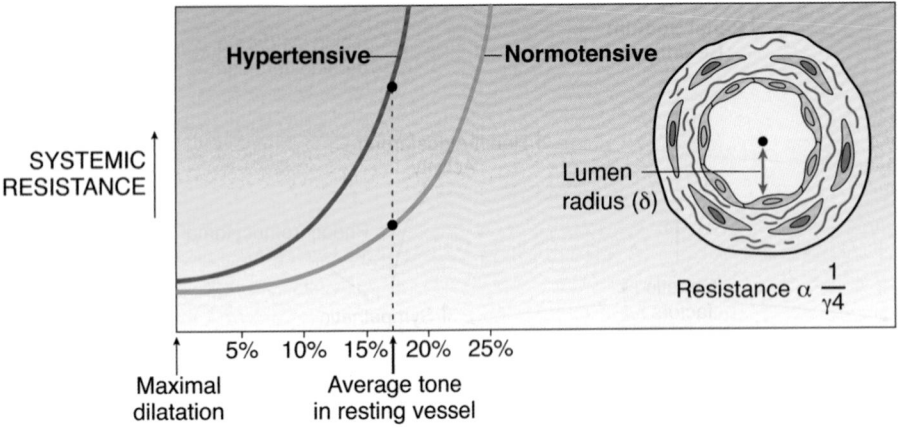

FIGURE 16-26. Structural autoregulation of blood pressure. Hypertension, regardless of its primary cause, increases the ability of the resistance vessel walls to respond to vasoactive stimuli. Resistance is increased even in maximally dilated vessels because the lumen size is decreased in the hypertensive vascular bed. As the smooth muscle cells contract, the increase in vessel wall thickness increases the resistance, which is inversely proportional to the fourth power of the radius of the lumen. Note that at the average resting muscular tone, the resistance in hypertensive patients is considerably higher than normal.

The importance of this hormonal axis in regulating blood pressure in hypertension is demonstrated by the therapeutic success of sympathetic antagonists (β-adrenergic blockers), diuretics and inhibitors of ACE. Nonetheless, no central defect in the renin–angiotensin axis has been identified, in part because the vasculature responds quickly to hemodynamic changes in the tissues by autoregulation (Fig. 16-26).

Extensive mechanisms regulate renal sodium excretion. Renal collecting ducts are important in maintaining sodium balance when alterations in more proximal parts of the nephron occur. Thus, dysregulation of sodium transport at the collecting duct can lead to the greatest deficit in sodium handling. Genetic mutations involving sodium reabsorption at this final segment are strongly associated with hypertension. Defects in the epithelial sodium channel in the renal distal tubule and collecting duct, or defects in signaling pathways regulating its expression, are responsible for several rare genetic forms of hypertension. These include mutations in WNK protein kinases and increased expression of epithelial sodium channels.

In the case of hypertension, the end result of autoregulation is always increased peripheral resistance. For example, hypertension can be induced experimentally by surgically removing large amounts of renal tissue, followed by administering excess sodium and water. Cardiac output, and therefore blood pressure, increases rapidly as a result of the rapid change in blood volume. However, within a few days, pressure-induced diuresis restores near-normal cardiac output and plasma volume. At that point, blood pressure is maintained by increased peripheral resistance. Thus, although the blood pressure elevation is initially due to increased volume, compensatory mechanisms successfully mask the volume changes and cause apparent primary hypertension. Many cases of human hypertension may also result from a process that begins with altered cardiac output, salt metabolism or ANF release.

The Prothrombotic Paradox

Hypertension exposes the arterial tree to increased pulsatile stress. Paradoxically, most major complications of chronic hypertension, such as myocardial infarction and stroke, are thrombotic, rather than hemorrhagic. This is known as the *prothrombotic paradox of hypertension.* This state can result

from chronic shear stress and low-grade inflammation. Endothelial dysfunction may be multifactorial and includes decreased activity of vasodilator agents and increased activity of, or increased sensitivity to, vasoconstrictor agents. Enhanced activity of the renin–angiotensin system and kallikrein–kinin system has opposite effects via angiotensin II–converting enzyme, causing vasoconstriction and vasodilation, respectively. Importantly, increased activity of these systems also leads to a hypercoagulable state. Thus, there is an increased load on the myocardium, which gives rise to left ventricular hypertrophy and ventricular and atrial arrhythmias and impairs coronary circulation.

Acquired Causes of Hypertension

Causes of hypertension are identifiable only in a small proportion of cases. These include renal artery stenosis, most forms of chronic renal disease, diabetes mellitus, primary elevation of aldosterone levels (Conn syndrome), Cushing syndrome, pheochromocytoma, hyperthyroidism, coarctation of the aorta and renin-secreting tumors. In addition, people with severe atherosclerosis may have high systolic pressure because a sclerotic aorta cannot properly absorb the kinetic energy of pulse waves, and because they often have renovascular hypertension.

PATHOPHYSIOLOGY: It is likely that many genes contribute small effects to individual cases of hypertension. Environmental factors play a role as well. However, a number of monogenic forms of hypertension have been defined:

- **Glucocorticoid-remediable aldosteronism (GRA):** GRA is an autosomal dominant trait, in which congenital hypertension is mediated by the renal mineralocorticoid receptor. Excess aldosterone production is caused by adrenocorticotropic hormone (ACTH) (see Chapter 27), rather than by the normal secretagogue for aldosterone, angiotensin II. The aldosterone synthase gene on chromosome 8 is normally expressed in the adrenal cortical zona glomerulosa, where the enzyme catalyzes aldosterone biosynthesis. This gene is 95% homologous with the steroid 11β-hydroxylase gene, which regulates adrenal cortisol biosynthesis. Nearby, on the same chromosome, mutations in aldosterone synthase and 11β-hydroxylase genes create a hybrid gene, with ectopic production of aldosterone in the zona fasciculate, under the control of ACTH. In turn, unrestrained secretion of mineralocorticoids leads to prolonged volume expansion and hypertension.

- **Syndrome of apparent mineralocorticoid excess (AME):** In this autosomal recessive form of early-onset hypertension, the mineralocorticoid receptor is stimulated, despite very low levels of aldosterone. Normally, the mineralocorticoid receptor responds both to aldosterone and to cortisol, albeit much more weakly to the latter. The aldosterone-like activity of cortisol is suppressed when 11β-hydroxysteroid dehydrogenase in renal tubular epithelial cells converts it to cortisone. In AME, inactivating mutations in the gene for this enzyme allow cortisol to accumulate and constitutively stimulate the mineralocorticoid receptor. Interestingly, consumption of large quantities of licorice can produce a similar syndrome, because glycyrrhetinic acid in licorice inhibits 11β-hydroxysteroid dehydrogenase.

- **Liddle syndrome:** This rare autosomal dominant form of hypertension stems from a gain-of-function mutation in a gene on chromosome 16 that codes for the amiloride-sensitive, epithelial sodium channel. Patients have constitutively activated renal tubule sodium channels but low mineralocorticoid levels. Sustained channel activation is due to lack of the repressor activity that normally promotes internalization and degradation of the cell surface channel. This effect causes kidneys to resorb too much salt and water, independently of mineralocorticoids, thereby leading to volume expansion and hypertension.

All mutations that cause hereditary hypertension constitutively increase renal sodium reabsorption. Conversely, diseases, such as pseudohypoaldosteronism type I and Gitelman syndrome (with inactivating mutations in *SLC12A3* encoding the thiazide-sensitive sodium chloride cotransporter), that result in sodium-losing syndromes are associated with profound hypotension. *Thus, these Mendelian disorders illustrate the central role of sodium homeostasis in determining blood pressure.*

Large genome-wide association studies have reported some loci associated with primary hypertension, including a susceptibility locus in the promoter region of endothelial NOS. Increasing evidence using targeted gene approaches indicates that common polymorphisms of the angiotensinogen gene contribute to primary hypertension: (1) the angiotensinogen locus is linked to elevated blood pressure in sibling pairs, (2) specific angiotensinogen variants have been tied to hypertension in case-control studies and (3) the same variants are associated with increased plasma angiotensinogen.

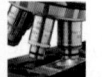 **PATHOLOGY:** In most cases of hypertension, the critical lesions are in resistance vessels that control blood flow through the capillary beds and in the kidney. The lumens of these small muscular arteries and arterioles may be restricted by active contraction of the vessel wall or increased vessel wall mass. Thicker vessel

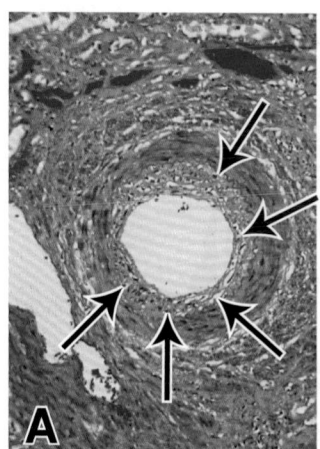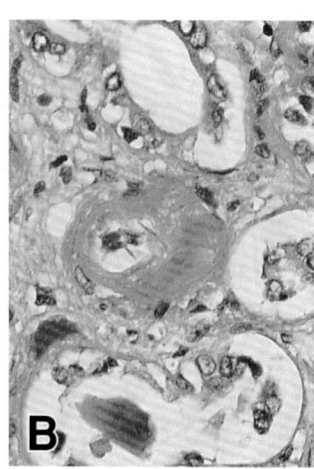

FIGURE 16-27. Benign arteriosclerosis. A. A cross-section of a renal intralobular artery shows irregular thickening of the intima (*arrows*). **B.** A renal arteriole exhibits hyaline arteriolosclerosis (*center*).

walls narrow vascular lumens more than do normal, thinner walls. Over time, chronic hypertension leads to reactive changes in smaller arteries (arteriosclerosis) and arterioles (arteriolosclerosis) throughout the body. Kidneys affected with chronic hypertension have a contracted and granular gross appearance, and microscopically often show tubular and glomerular changes.

Benign arteriosclerosis reflects mild chronic hypertension, the major change being a variable increase in arterial wall thickness (Fig. 16-27A). In the smallest arteries and arterioles, these lesions are referred to as **hyaline arteriosclerosis** and **arteriolosclerosis**. "Hyaline" refers to the glassy scarred appearance of the blood vessel walls by light microscopy. Thickened arterioles reflect deposition of basement membrane material and accumulation of plasma proteins (Fig. 16-27B). The small muscular arteries have new layers of elastin, which manifest as reduplication of the intimal elastic lamina and increased connective tissue. The vascular lesions of benign arteriosclerosis are particularly evident where they result in loss of renal parenchyma, termed **benign nephrosclerosis**. The presence of benign arteriosclerosis is not diagnostic of hypertension, since similar morphologic alterations are common with aging. Hyaline arteriosclerosis may also be present in diabetes.

In **malignant hypertension,** blood pressure is very high, leading to rapidly progressive vascular compromise with the onset of symptomatic disease of the brain, heart or kidney. Blood pressures usually exceed 160/110 mm Hg, but modern antihypertensive therapy has made malignant hypertension a rare disorder. Malignant hypertension produces dramatic microvascular pathologic changes. Segmental constriction and dilation of retinal arterioles in severely hypertensive patients are sufficiently prominent to allow one to make the diagnosis by ophthalmoscopy (see Chapter 33). If blood pressure rises rapidly, retinal arterioles show microaneurysms, focal hemorrhages and retinal scarring. Ischemic necrosis and edema of the retina appear as "cotton wool spots" with the ophthalmoscope. These retinal changes are typical of those in other resistance vessels when pressure rises rapidly.

In malignant hypertension, small muscular arteries show segmental dilation due to necrosis of smooth muscle

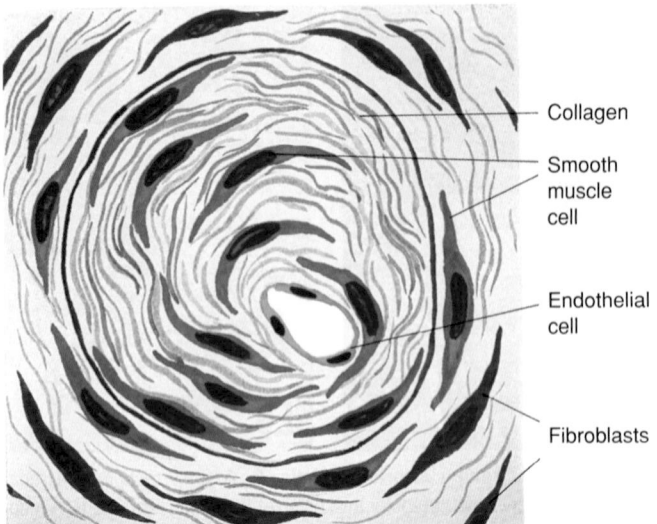

Collagen

Smooth
muscle
cell

Endothelial
cell

Fibroblasts

FIGURE 16-28. Arteriolosclerosis. In cases of hypertension, the arterioles exhibit smooth muscle cell proliferation and increased amounts of intercellular collagen and glycosaminoglycans, resulting in an "onion-skin" appearance. The mass of smooth muscle and associated elements tends to fix the size of the lumen and restrict the arteriole's capacity to dilate.

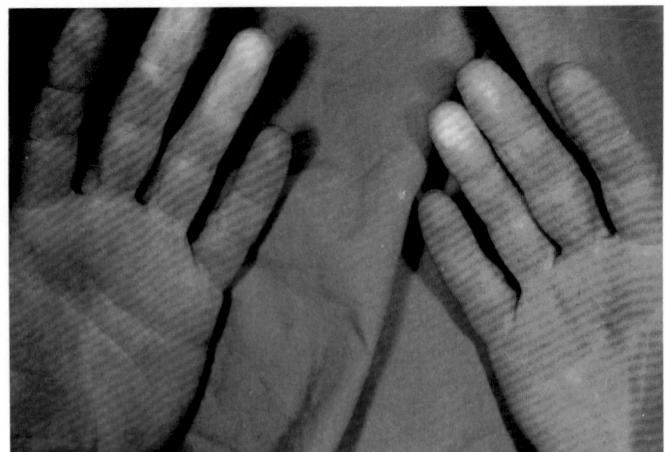

FIGURE 16-29. Raynaud phenomenon. The tips of the fingers show marked pallor.

cells. Endothelial integrity is lost in these regions, and increased vascular permeability leads to entry of plasma proteins into the vessel wall, deposition of fibrin and an appearance called **fibrinoid necrosis** (see Chapter 1). Acute injury is rapidly followed by smooth muscle proliferation and a striking concentric increase in the number of layers of smooth muscle cells, producing an "onion-skin" appearance (Fig. 16-28). This form of smooth muscle proliferation may be a response to release of growth factors from platelets and other cells at sites of vascular injury. Together, these changes are labeled **malignant arteriosclerosis** or **arteriolosclerosis,** depending on the size of the vessels affected. In the kidney, lesions of malignant hypertension are known as **malignant nephrosclerosis.**

MÖNCKEBERG MEDIAL SCLEROSIS

Mönckeberg medial sclerosis refers to degenerative calcification of the media of large and medium-sized muscular arteries. The disorder occurs principally in older people and most often involves arteries of the upper and lower extremities. It is also common in advanced chronic renal disease.

 PATHOLOGY: Involved arteries are hard and dilated. Microscopically, the smooth muscle of the media is focally replaced by pale-staining, acellular, hyalinized fibrous tissue, with concentric dystrophic calcification. In most cases the internal elastic lamina shows focal calcification. Osseous metaplasia in calcified areas is occasionally observed. Mönckeberg medial sclerosis is distinct from atherosclerosis and ordinarily does not entail any clinically significant impairment. Some assert that in patients with chronic renal disease, the features of Mönckeberg medial sclerosis in arteries should be considered a form of accelerated atherosclerosis.

RAYNAUD PHENOMENON

Raynaud phenomenon refers to intermittent bilateral attacks of ischemia of the fingers or toes, and sometimes the ears or nose. It is characterized by severe pallor (Fig. 16-29) and is often accompanied by paresthesias and pain. Symptoms are precipitated by cold or emotional stimuli and relieved by heat. Primary cold sensitivity of the Raynaud type is more common in women, and it often starts in the late teens. It is bilateral and symmetric and, on rare occasions, may lead to ulcers or gangrene of the tips of digits. The hands are more commonly affected than feet.

Raynaud phenomenon may occur as an isolated disorder or as part of systemic diseases of connective tissue (collagen vascular disorders), particularly scleroderma and systemic lupus erythematosus. It includes primary and secondary cold sensitivity, livedo reticularis and acrocyanosis. Whatever its cause, Raynaud phenomenon reflects vasospasm of the arteries and arterioles in the skin. Dysregulation of vascular tone by sympathetic nerve activity and by neurohumoral factors may play a role in its pathogenesis. Phosphodiesterase type 5 inhibitors induce vasodilation and have shown some therapeutic value.

FIBROMUSCULAR DYSPLASIA

Fibromuscular dysplasia is a rare noninflammatory thickening of large and medium-sized muscular arteries, which is distinct from atherosclerosis and arteriosclerosis. The cause is unknown; however, it may be developmental in nature. Renal artery stenosis due to this condition is an important cause of renovascular hypertension, although fibromuscular dysplasia may affect almost any other vessel, including carotid, vertebral and splanchnic arteries. It is typically a disease of women during their reproductive years but may appear at any age, even in childhood.

 PATHOLOGY: In most cases, the distal 2/3 of the renal artery and its primary branches have several segmental stenoses, which represent fibrous and muscular ridges that project into the lumen. Microscopically,

TABLE 16-8
INFLAMMATORY DISORDERS OF BLOOD VESSELS

Polyarteritis Nodosa Group of Systemic Necrotizing Vasculitis

Classic polyarteritis nodosa

Allergic angiitis and granulomatosis (Churg-Strauss variant)

"Overlap syndrome" of systemic angiitis

Hypersensitivity Vasculitis

Serum sickness and similar reactions

Henoch-Schönlein purpura

Vasculitis associated with connective tissue disorders

Vasculitis in cases of essential mixed cryoglobulinemia

Vasculitis associated with other primary disorders

Wegener Granulomatosis

Lymphomatoid Granulomatosis

Giant Cell Arteritis

Temporal arteritis

Takayasu arteritis

Central Nervous System Vasculitis

Vasculitis Associated with Cancer

Mucocutaneous Lymph Node Syndrome (Kawasaki Disease)

Thromboangiitis Obliterans (Buerger Disease)

Behçet Disease

Miscellaneous Vasculitis Syndromes

these segments show disorderly arrangement and proliferation of the cellular elements of the vessel wall, without necrosis or inflammation. Smooth muscle is replaced by fibrous tissue and myofibroblasts, and the media may be thinned. In some cases, intimal fibroplasia predominates, and in unusual instances, connective tissue encircles the adventitia. Other than renal hypertension, the major complication of fibromuscular dysplasia is dissecting aneurysm owing to thinning of the media of affected arteries.

VASCULITIS

Vasculitis is inflammation and necrosis of blood vessels. It may affect arteries, veins and capillaries (Table 16-8). Vessels may be damaged by immune mechanisms (see Chapter 4), infectious agents, mechanical trauma, radiation or toxins. However, in many cases, no specific cause is determined.

 **ETIOLOGIC FACTORS:** Vasculitic syndromes are thought to involve immune mechanisms, including (1) **deposition of immune complexes,** (2) **direct**

attack on vessels by circulating antibodies and (3) **various forms of cell-mediated immunity.** Agents that incite these reactions are largely unknown, although in some instances vasculitis is associated with viral infection.

Serum sickness was one of the first human immunologic disorders to be linked with vasculitis. In animal models of serum sickness, immune complexes and complement are found in local tissue reaction (see Chapter 4). However, in most human cases, immune complexes are only sometimes present, and firm evidence for them in most cases of vasculitis is lacking.

Viral antigens may cause vasculitis. Thus, chronic infection with hepatitis B virus is associated with some cases of polyarteritis nodosa (see below). In this case, viral antigen–antibody complexes circulate and are deposited in the vascular lesions. Human vasculitis has also been associated with other viral infections, including herpes simplex, cytomegalovirus and parvovirus, as well as with several bacterial antigens.

Small vessel vasculitides (e.g., polyangiitis with granulomatosis; see below) are associated with circulating **antineutrophil cytoplasmic antibodies (ANCAs),** but why these autoantibodies appear and how they lead to vasculitis are not known. Infection may play a role in the development of ANCAs. ANCA may cause endothelial damage by activating neutrophils, and antibody titers correlate with disease activity in some cases. ANCA is detected by indirect immunofluorescence assays using patients' sera and ethanol-fixed neutrophils. Common patterns include **perinuclear immunofluorescence (P-ANCA),** mostly against myeloperoxidase, and a more general **cytoplasmic immunofluorescence (C-ANCA),** mainly against proteinase 3.

Neutrophils activated by, for example, TNF degranulate and express myeloperoxidase and proteinase 3 at their surfaces. ANCA, which is present as a response to infection, can then bind and activate the neutrophils. Other autoantibodies that activate neutrophils and injure endothelial cells also occur in vasculitides (Fig. 16-30).

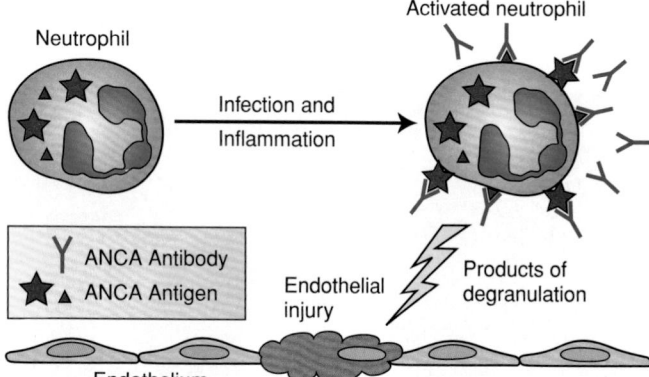

FIGURE 16-30. Model of the pathogenesis of antineutrophil cytoplasmic antibody (ANCA) vasculitis. ANCA antigens are normally found in the neutrophil cytoplasm with very little surface expression. In inflammation and infection, increased cell surface expression of ANCA antigens is induced in the neutrophils. ANCA present in the circulation owing to previous formation through unknown mechanisms binds to these ANCA antigens on the surface, leading to neutrophil activation and interaction with endothelial cells. Neutrophil degranulation releases toxic factors including reactive oxygen species, proteinase 3 (PR3) and myeloperoxidase, and other granule enzymes cause endothelial cell apoptosis and necrosis, leading to endothelial injury.

Polyarteritis Nodosa Is an Acute, Necrotizing Vasculitis

Polyarteritis nodosa affects medium-sized and smaller muscular arteries and, occasionally, larger arteries. It is more common in men than in women. The disease was rare until the 1940s, when there was a striking rise in its incidence. The increased frequency of polyarteritis nodosa at that time seemed to be associated with the widespread use of antisera to bacteria and toxins produced in animals, and with use of sulfonamides. The incidence of polyarteritis nodosa now seems to be subsiding.

 PATHOLOGY: The characteristic lesions of polyarteritis nodosa occur patchily in small to medium-sized muscular arteries. However, on occasion they extend into larger arteries, such as renal, splenic or coronary arteries. Each lesion is no more than 1 mm long and may involve part or all of the circumference of the vessel. Fibrinoid necrosis is the most prominent morphologic feature. The medial muscle and adjacent tissues are fused into a structureless eosinophilic mass that stains for fibrin. A vigorous acute inflammatory response envelops the area of necrosis, usually involving the entire adventitia (periarteritis), and extends through the other coats of the vessel (Fig. 16-31). Neutrophils, lymphocytes, plasma cells and macrophages are present in varying proportions, and eosinophils are often conspicuous.

Infarcts are common in involved organs and are caused by thrombosis in affected segments of arteries. Injury to larger arteries may cause small aneurysms (<0.5 cm), especially in branches of the renal, coronary and cerebral arteries. An aneurysm may rupture and, if located in a critical area, has resulted in fatal hemorrhage.

Over time, many vascular lesions start to heal, especially if corticosteroids have been given. Necrotic tissue and inflammatory exudate are resorbed, and the vessel is left with fibrosis of the media and conspicuous gaps in the elastic laminae.

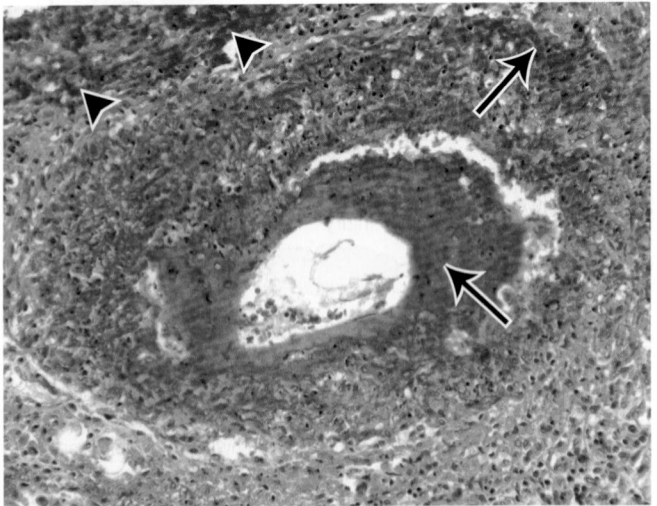

FIGURE 16-31. Polyarteritis nodosa. The intense inflammatory cell infiltrate in the arterial wall and surrounding connective tissue is associated with fibrinoid necrosis (*arrows*) and disruption of the vessel wall with hemorrhage into surrounding tissues (*arrowheads*).

 CLINICAL FEATURES: Clinical manifestations of polyarteritis nodosa are variable and depend on the organs affected by the lesions. Kidneys, heart, skeletal muscle, skin and mesentery are most often involved, but lesions may occur in almost any organ, including the bowel, pancreas, lungs, liver and brain. Constitutional symptoms such as fever and weight loss are common. Polyarteritis nodosa–like lesions may occur in viral infections including hepatitis B and C and HIV infection.

Without treatment, polyarteritis nodosa is usually fatal, but anti-inflammatory and immunosuppressive therapy, in the form of corticosteroids and cyclophosphamide, leads to remissions or cures in most patients.

Hypersensitivity Angiitis Is a Response to Exogenous Substances

Hypersensitivity angiitis refers to a broad category of inflammatory vascular lesions that are thought to represent a reaction to foreign materials (e.g., bacterial products or drugs). In the case of vascular lesions confined predominantly to skin, the terms **leukocytoclastic vasculitis** (referring to nuclear debris from disintegrating neutrophils), **cutaneous vasculitis** or **cutaneous necrotizing venulitis** (emphasizing the predominant involvement of the venules) are applied. **Systemic hypersensitivity angiitis,** also referred to as **microscopic polyangiitis,** affects many of the same organs as polyarteritis nodosa but is restricted to the smallest arteries and arterioles.

 CLINICAL FEATURES: Cutaneous vasculitis may follow administration of many drugs, including aspirin, penicillin and thiazide diuretics. It is also commonly related to such disparate infections as streptococcal and staphylococcal illnesses, viral hepatitis, tuberculosis and bacterial endocarditis. The disease typically presents as palpable purpura, principally on the lower extremities. Microscopically, superficial cutaneous venules show fibrinoid necrosis with acute inflammation. Cutaneous vasculitis is generally self-limited (see Chapter 28).

Systemic hypersensitivity angiitis may be an isolated entity or a feature of other conditions, including collagen vascular diseases (lupus erythematosus, rheumatoid arthritis, Sjögren syndrome), Henoch-Schönlein purpura, dysproteinemias and several malignancies. Patients with systemic hypersensitivity angiitis may also have cutaneous purpuric lesions. The most feared complication of microscopic polyangiitis is renal involvement, characterized by rapidly progressive glomerulonephritis and renal failure (see Chapter 22). *Microscopic polyarteritis is strongly associated with P-ANCA.*

Giant Cell Arteritis Mainly Affects the Temporal Arteries

Although it most often affects the temporal artery, granulomatous arteritis (temporal arteritis) may also involve other cranial arteries, the aorta (giant cell aortitis) and its branches and occasionally other arteries. Aortic aneurysms and dissection occur. The average age at onset is 70 years, and it is rare before age 50. Giant cell arteritis is the most common vasculitis; its incidence rises with age and may reach 1% by 80 years of age. Women are slightly more often affected than men. The age at onset helps differentiate it from other vasculitides that may involve the same vessels in younger people, such as Takayasu disease.

PATHOPHYSIOLOGY: The etiology of giant cell arteritis is obscure. Its association with HLA-DR4 and its occurrence in first-degree relatives support a genetic component in its pathogenesis. The morphologic alterations, including activated CD4⁺ T-helper cells and macrophages, and the association of the disease with a specific polymorphism of ICAM-1 suggest an immune reaction. B lymphocytes are lacking. Macrophages at the border of the intima and media produce matrix metalloproteinases that digest extracellular matrix. ANCA is absent in giant cell arteritis. Generalized muscle aching and widespread distribution of its manifestations are consistent with a relationship to rheumatoid diseases.

 PATHOLOGY: Affected vessels are cord-like with nodular thickening. Lumens are reduced to slits or may be obliterated by a thrombus (Fig. 16-32A). Microscopically, the media and intima show granulomatous inflammation; aggregates of macrophages, lymphocytes and plasma cells are admixed with variable numbers of eosinophils and neutrophils. Giant cells tend to be distributed at the internal elastic lamina (Fig. 16-32B) but vary widely in number. Foreign body giant cells and Langhans giant cells are both seen. Foci of necrosis are characterized by changes in the internal elastica, which becomes swollen, irregular and fragmented, and in advanced lesions may completely disappear. Fragments of the elastica occasionally appear in the giant cells. In the late stages, the intima is conspicuously thickened and the media is fibrotic. Thrombi may obliterate the lumen, after which organization and canalization occur.

 CLINICAL FEATURES: Giant cell arteritis tends to be benign and self-limited, and symptoms subside in 6–12 months. Patients present with headache and throbbing temporal pain. In some instances, there are early constitutional symptoms, including malaise, fever and weight loss, plus generalized muscular aching or stiffness in the shoulders and hips. Throbbing and pain over the temporal artery are accompanied by swelling, tenderness and redness in overlying skin. Almost half of patients have visual symptoms, which may proceed from transient to permanent blindness in one or both eyes, sometimes

rapidly. Occasionally, the disease causes myocardial, central nervous system (CNS) or gastrointestinal infarcts, which may be fatal. Because the inflammatory process is patchy, biopsy of the temporal artery may not be diagnostic in as many as 40% of patients with otherwise classic manifestations. Response to corticosteroids is usually dramatic, and symptoms subside within days.

Granulomatosis with Polyangiitis Is a Vasculitis That Affects the Respiratory Tract and Kidney

Granulomatosis with polyangiitis (GPA, formerly Wegener granulomatosis) is a systemic necrotizing vasculitis of unknown etiology, with granulomatous lesions of the nose, sinuses and lungs and renal glomerular disease. Men are affected more than women, usually in their fifth and sixth decades. Over 90% of patients with GPA are positive for ANCA, of whom 75% have C-ANCA. It has been suggested that these antibodies activate circulating neutrophils to attack blood vessels. The response to immunosuppressive therapy supports an immunologic basis for the disease.

PATHOLOGY: Lesions of GPA feature parenchymal necrosis, vasculitis and granulomatous inflammation composed of neutrophils, lymphocytes, plasma cells, macrophages and eosinophils. Individual lesions in the lung may be as large as 5 cm across and must be distinguished from tuberculosis. Vasculitis involving small arteries and veins may be seen anywhere but occurs most frequently in the respiratory tract (Fig. 16-33), kidney and spleen. Arteritis is characterized principally by chronic inflammation, although acute inflammation, necrotizing and nonnecrotizing granulomas and fibrinoid necrosis are often present. Medial thickening and intimal proliferation are common and often cause narrowing or obliteration of the lumen.

The most prominent pulmonary feature is persistent bilateral pneumonitis, with nodular infiltrates that undergo cavitation similar to tuberculous lesions (although the mechanisms are clearly different). Chronic sinusitis and nasopharyngeal mucosal ulcers are frequent. The kidney at first shows focal necrotizing glomerulonephritis, which progresses to crescentic glomerulonephritis (see Chapter 23).

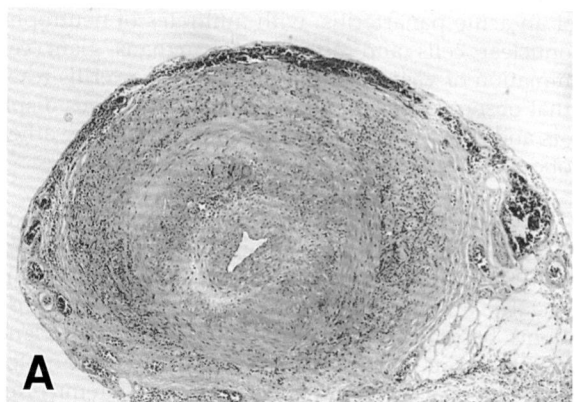 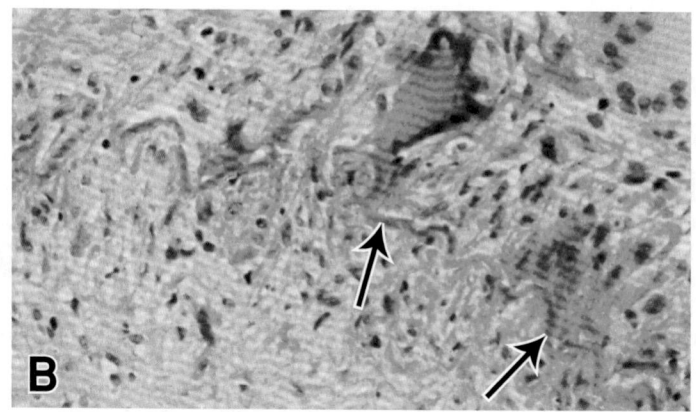

FIGURE 16-32. Temporal arteritis. A. A photomicrograph of a temporal artery shows chronic inflammation throughout the wall and a lumen severely narrowed by intimal thickening. **B.** A high-power view shows giant cells adjacent to the fragmented internal elastic lamina (*arrows*).

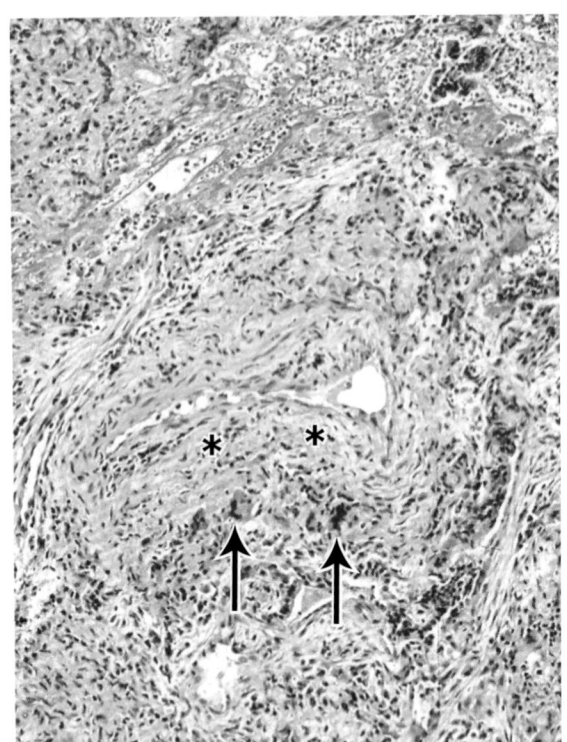

FIGURE 16-33. Granulomatosis with polyangiitis (GPA). A photomicrograph of the lung shows vasculitis of a pulmonary artery. There are chronic inflammatory cells and Langerhans giant cells (*arrows*) in the wall, together with thickening of the intima (*asterisks*).

 CLINICAL FEATURES: Most patients present with symptoms referable to the respiratory tract, particularly pneumonitis and sinusitis. In fact, the lung is eventually involved in over 90% of patients. Radiologically, multiple pulmonary infiltrates are prominent, which are often cavitary. Hematuria and proteinuria are common, and glomerular disease can progress to renal failure. Rash, muscular pains, joint involvement and neurologic symptoms occur. Most patients (80%) die within a year if untreated, with a mean survival of 5–6 months. Treatment with cyclophosphamide produces both complete remissions and substantial disease-free intervals in most patients. Interestingly, antimicrobial sulfa drugs significantly reduce the incidence of relapses, suggesting a relationship of the disease to bacterial infection.

Allergic Granulomatosis and Angiitis (Churg-Strauss Syndrome) Occurs in Young People with Asthma

PATHOLOGY: Two thirds of patients with Churg-Strauss syndrome have P-ANCA. Widespread necrotizing lesions of small and medium-sized arteries (Fig. 16-34), arterioles and veins are found in the lungs, spleen, kidney, heart, liver, CNS and other organs. These lesions are granulomas and intense eosinophilic infiltrates in and around blood vessels. The resulting fibrinoid necrosis, thrombosis and aneurysm formation may simulate polyarteritis nodosa, although Churg-Strauss syndrome seems to be a distinct entity. It must also be distinguished from other eosinophilic syndromes, such as parasitic and fungal infestations, polyangiitis with granulomatosis, eosinophilic pneumonia (Loeffler syndrome) and drug vasculitis.

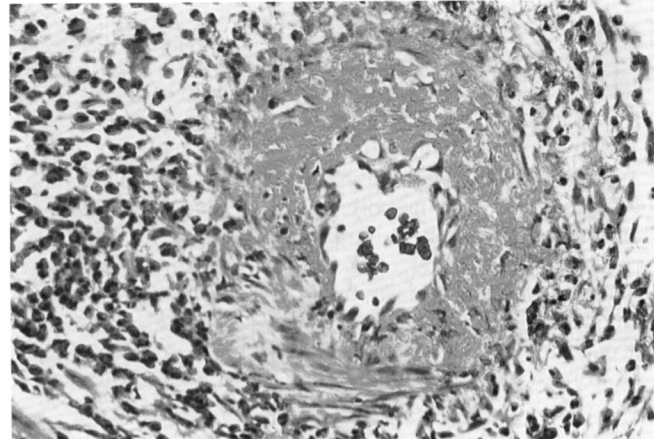

FIGURE 16-34. Churg-Strauss syndrome. A medium-sized artery shows fibrinoid necrosis and a surrounding eosinophilic infiltrate.

Untreated, these patients have a poor prognosis, but corticosteroid therapy is almost always effective.

Takayasu Arteritis Affects the Aorta and Its Branches

This form of arteritis is seen worldwide. It mainly affects women (90%), most of whom are under 30 years of age. The cause of Takayasu arteritis is unknown, but an autoimmune basis has been proposed.

 PATHOLOGY: Takayasu arteritis is classified according to the extent of aortic involvement: (1) disease restricted to the aortic arch and its branches, (2) arteritis only affecting the descending thoracic and abdominal aorta and its branches and (3) combined involvement of the arch and descending aorta. The pulmonary artery is also occasionally affected and the retinal vasculature is frequently involved.

The aorta wall is thickened, and the intima shows focal, raised plaques. Branches of the aorta often have localized stenosis or occlusion, which interferes with blood flow. If the subclavian arteries are affected, the synonym **pulseless disease** is used. The aorta, particularly the distal thoracic and abdominal segments, commonly shows variably sized aneurysms. Early lesions of the aorta and its main branches consist of an acute panarteritis, with infiltrates of neutrophils, mononuclear cells and occasional Langhans giant cells. Inflammation of vasa vasorum in Takayasu arteritis resembles that observed in syphilitic aortitis. Late lesions display fibrosis and severe intimal proliferation. Secondary atherosclerotic changes may obscure the basic disease.

 CLINICAL FEATURES: Patients with early Takayasu arteritis complain of constitutional symptoms, dizziness, visual disturbances, dyspnea and, occasionally, syncope. As the disease progresses, cardiac symptoms become more severe, with intermittent claudication of the arms or legs. Asymmetric differences in blood pressure may develop, and pulses in one extremity may sometimes actually disappear. Hypertension may reflect coarctation of the aorta or renal artery stenosis. Most patients eventually develop congestive heart failure. Loss of visual

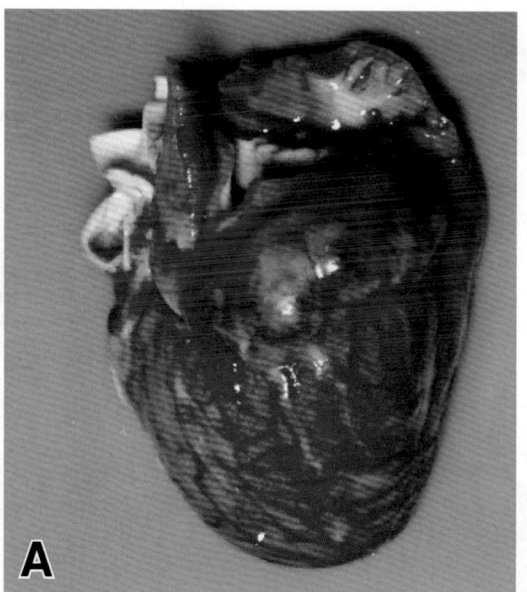
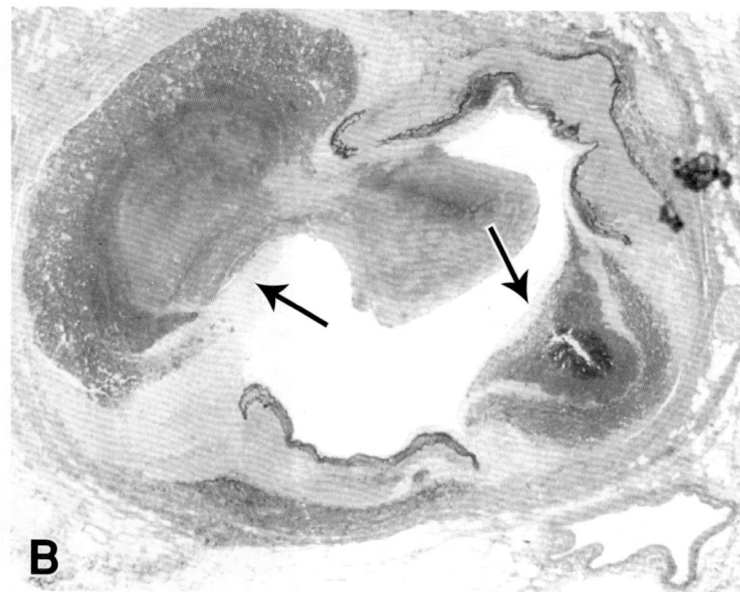

FIGURE 16-35. Kawasaki disease. A. The heart of a child who died from Kawasaki disease shows conspicuous coronary artery aneurysms. **B.** A microscopic section of a coronary artery from the same patient shows two large defects (*arrows*) in the internal elastic lamina, with two small aneurysms filled with thrombus.

acuity ranges from field defects to total blindness. Early Takayasu arteritis responds to corticosteroids, but the later lesions require surgical reconstruction.

Kawasaki Disease Mainly Targets Coronary Arteries in Children

Kawasaki disease (mucocutaneous lymph node syndrome) is an acute necrotizing vasculitis of infancy and early childhood, with high fever, rash, conjunctival and oral lesions and lymphadenitis. In 70% of patients, vasculitis of the coronary arteries leads to coronary artery aneurysms (Fig. 16-35), 1%–2% of which are lethal.

ETIOLOGIC FACTORS: Kawasaki disease is usually self-limited. Although an infectious cause has been sought, none has been conclusively demonstrated. Infection with *parvovirus B19* or with *New Haven coronavirus* has been implicated in some cases, and there is evidence for various bacterial infections, including *Staphylococcus, Streptococcus* and *Chlamydia* in others. The common theme seems to be viral or bacterial production of superantigens. These are molecules that bind to major histocompatibility complex (MHC) class II receptors and the V-beta region of the T-cell receptor, thereby massively activating immune responses. Autoantibodies to endothelial and smooth muscle cells have been identified in some patients.

Buerger Disease Is a Peripheral Vascular Disease of Smokers

Buerger disease (thromboangiitis obliterans) is an occlusive inflammatory disease of medium and small arteries in the distal arms and legs. It once occurred almost only in young and middle-aged men who smoked heavily, but it is now also described in women. It is more common in the Mediterranean area, Middle East and Asia.

ETIOLOGIC FACTORS: The etiologic role of smoking in Buerger disease is underscored by the fact that cessation of smoking may lead to remission, and resumption of smoking to exacerbation. Yet, how tobacco smoke produces the malady is obscure. Certain polyphenols from tobacco elicit antibodies and can induce inflammation. Smokers show a higher incidence of such sensitivity to tobacco than do nonsmokers. Cell-mediated hypersensitivity to collagen types II and III has also been observed. Endothelium-dependent vasodilatory responses in disease-free blood vessels are dysfunctional in some patients, suggesting that there may be a generalized impairment of endothelial function. HLA-A9 and HLA-B5 haplotypes are more common among Buerger patients, further suggesting that a genetically controlled hypersensitivity to tobacco is involved in the pathogenesis of disease.

PATHOLOGY: The earliest change in Buerger disease is acute inflammation of medium-sized and small arteries. Neutrophilic infiltrates extend to involve neighboring veins and nerves. Involvement of the endothelium in inflamed areas gives rise to thrombosis and obliteration of the lumen (Fig. 16-36A). Small microabscesses of the vessel wall, with a central area of neutrophils surrounded by fibroblasts and Langhans giant cells, distinguish this process from thrombosis associated with atherosclerosis. Early lesions often become severe enough to cause gangrene of the extremity, leading to amputation. Late in the course of the disease, thrombi are completely organized and partly canalized.

CLINICAL FEATURES: Symptoms of Buerger disease usually start between the ages of 25 and 40 years as intermittent claudication (cramping pains in muscles after exercise, quickly relieved by rest). Patients often present with painful ulceration of a digit, which progresses to destruction of the tips of the involved digits (Fig. 16-36B).

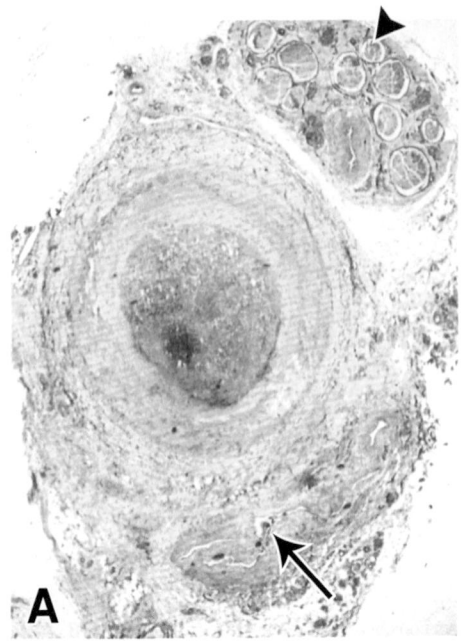
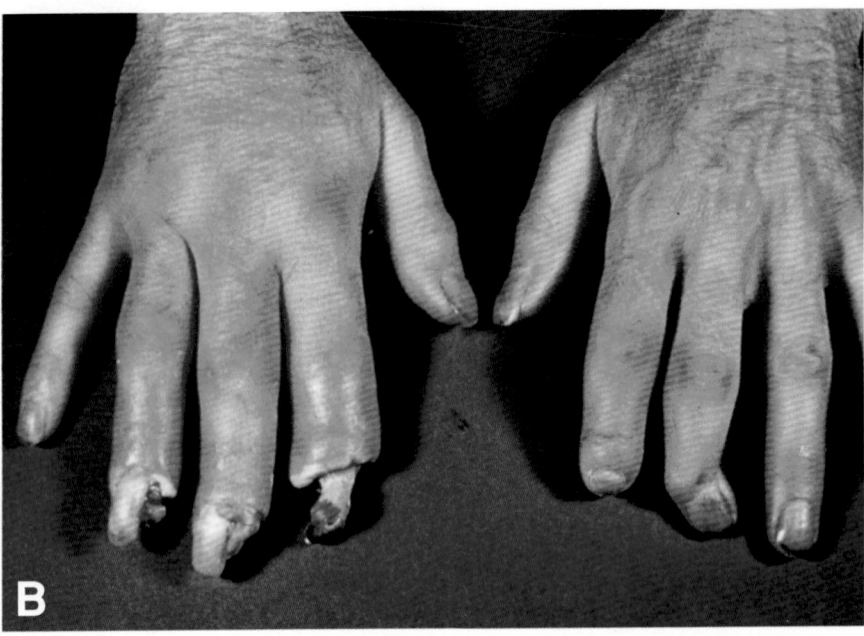

FIGURE 16-36. **Buerger disease. A.** Section of the upper extremity shows an organized arterial thrombus that has occluded the lumen. Some inflammatory cells are evident in the adventitial fat. In this instance, the vein (*arrow*) and the adjacent nerve (*arrowhead*) show foci of chronic inflammation. **B.** The hand shows necrosis of the tips of the fingers.

Those who continue to smoke may slowly lose both hands and feet.

Behçet Disease Is a Vasculitis of Many Mucous Membranes

Behçet disease is a systemic vasculitis characterized by oral aphthous ulcers, genital ulcers and ocular inflammation. Occasionally, there are lesions in the CNS, gastrointestinal tract and cardiovascular system. Both large and small vessels show vasculitis. The mucocutaneous lesions exhibit nonspecific vasculitis of arterioles, capillaries and venules, with infiltration of vessel walls and perivascular tissue by lymphocytes and plasma cells. Occasional endothelial cells are proliferated and swollen. Medium and large arteries show destructive arteritis, characterized by fibrinoid necrosis, mononuclear infiltration, thrombosis, aneurysms and hemorrhage. The cause is unknown, but the effectiveness of corticosteroid treatment and an association with specific HLA subtypes suggest an immune basis.

Radiation Vasculitis Has Acute and Chronic Phases

The acute phase of radiation vasculitis shows endothelial injury and denudation, ballooning degeneration of intimal smooth muscle cells, the presence of macrophages and smooth muscle cell necrosis of the media, which may appear fibrinoid. Thrombi may be seen in small arteries and arterioles. In the chronic phase, intimal hyperplasia and fibrosis of the vessel wall are noted. Occasionally, vessels display complete fibrous occlusion. Radiation damage predisposes to accelerated atherosclerosis.

Rickettsial Vasculitis Is Caused by Intracellular Parasites

Rickettsiae are obligate intracellular parasites that produce a characteristic vasculitis (see Chapter 9). Each different rickettsial disease affects different types of small vessels, and its extent and severity vary. The organisms usually disseminate from the entry site into the blood and invade endothelial cells, smooth muscle cells of the media of small vessels and capillaries.

ANEURYSMS

Arterial aneurysms are localized dilations of blood vessels caused by a congenital or acquired weakness of the media. They are not rare, and their incidence tends to rise with age. Aneurysms of the aorta and other arteries are found in as many as 10% of unselected autopsies. The wall of an aneurysm is formed by stretched remnants of the arterial wall.

Aneurysms are classified by location, configuration and etiology (Fig. 16-37). The location refers to the type of vessel involved—artery or vein—and the specific vessel affected, such as the aorta or popliteal artery. There are several categories of aneurysms:

- **Fusiform aneurysms** are ovoid swellings parallel to the long axis of the vessel.
- **Saccular aneurysms** are bubble-like arterial wall outpouchings at a site of weakened media.
- **Dissecting aneurysms** are actually dissecting hematomas, in which blood from hemorrhage into the media separates the layers of the vascular wall.
- **Arteriovenous aneurysms** are direct conduits between an artery and a vein.

Abdominal Aortic Aneurysms Complicate Atherosclerosis

Abdominal aortic aneurysms are dilations that increase vessel wall diameter by at least 50%. They are the most frequent aneurysms, usually developing after the age of

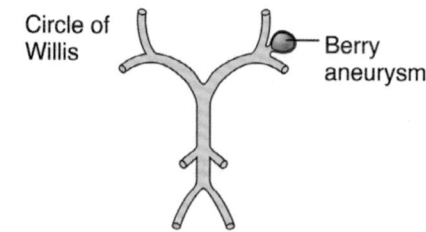

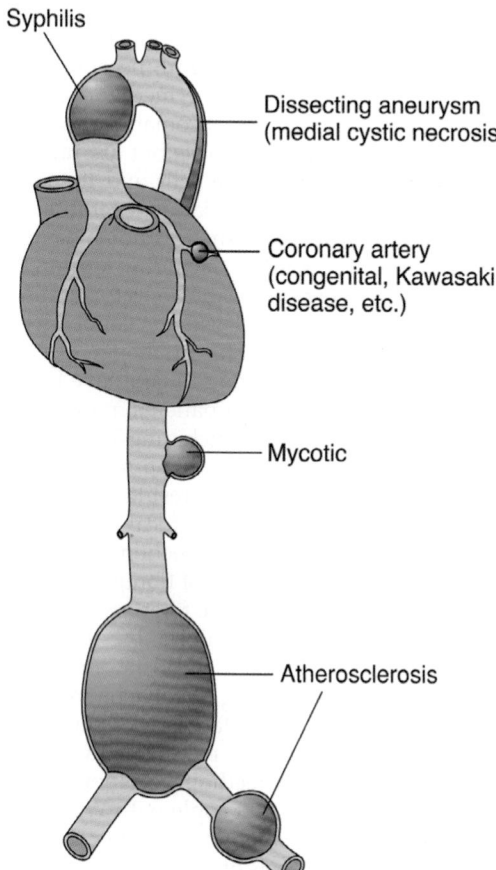

FIGURE 16-37. The locations of aneurysms. Syphilitic aneurysms are the common variety in the ascending aorta, which is usually spared by the atherosclerotic process. Atherosclerotic aneurysms can occur in the abdominal aorta or muscular arteries, including the coronary and popliteal arteries and other vessels. Berry aneurysms are seen in the circle of Willis, mainly at branch points; their rupture leads to subarachnoid hemorrhage. Mycotic aneurysms occur almost anywhere that bacteria can deposit on vessel walls.

50 years, and are associated with severe atherosclerosis of the artery. The prevalence rises to 6% after age 80. They occur much more often in men than in women, and half of patients are hypertensive. Occasionally, aneurysms may be found in all parts of the thoracic aorta and in iliac and popliteal arteries.

PATHOPHYSIOLOGY: Abdominal aortic aneurysms (AAAs) invariably occur in the context of atherosclerosis. However, it is thought that the disease is actually multifactorial, involving inflammation and dysregulation of matrix remodeling and repair.

The growth of the aneurysm is regulated in part by hemodynamic forces that occur in the aneurysm; as the radius of the vessel increases, so does the circumferential wall stress. Enzymes important in the proteolysis of medial and adventitial type I/III fibrillar collagen promote the growth of abdominal aneurysms. These include matrix metalloproteinases; cysteine protease cathepsins K, L and S; and osteoclastic proton pump vH^+-adenosine triphosphatase (ATPase). Proinflammatory cytokines, such as IL-1β, TNF-α, monocyte chemotactin protein-1 (MCP-1) and IL-8, have also been linked to the pathogenesis of abdominal aneurysms. The walls of AAAs contain chemokines and growth factors that regulate remodeling. Examples are granulocyte colony-stimulating factor (G-CSF), macrophage colony-stimulating factor (M-CSF), IL-13, IGF-1, TGF-β and macrophage inflammatory protein (MIP)-1α and -1β. Familial clustering suggests a genetic predisposition, although this is poorly understood.

PATHOLOGY: Most abdominal aortic aneurysms occur distal to the renal arteries and proximal to the aortic bifurcation (Fig. 16-38). They are usually fusiform, but saccular varieties are occasionally seen. Although most of the symptomatic lesions are over 5–6 cm in diameter, they may be of almost any size. Some extend into the iliac arteries, which occasionally exhibit distinct

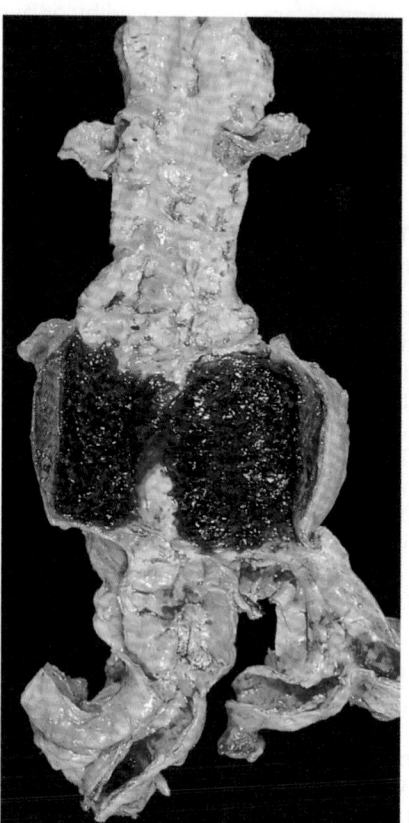

FIGURE 16-38. Atherosclerotic aneurysm of the abdominal aorta. The aneurysm has been opened longitudinally to reveal a large mural thrombus in the lumen. The aorta and common iliac arteries display complicated lesions of atherosclerosis.

aneurysms distal to the one in the aorta. Aneurysms that extend above the renal arteries may occlude the origin of the superior mesenteric artery and the celiac axis.

Most abdominal aortic aneurysms are lined by raised, ulcerated and calcified (complicated) atherosclerotic lesions. The majority contain mural thrombi of varying degrees of organization, portions of which may embolize to peripheral arteries. Infrequently, a thrombus itself enlarges enough to compromise the lumen of the aorta.

Microscopically, walls of AAAs complicated by atherosclerotic lesions are destroyed and replaced by fibrous tissue. Remnants of normal media are seen focally, and atheromatous lesions extend to variable depths. The adventitia is thickened and focally inflamed as a response to severe atherosclerosis.

 CLINICAL FEATURES: Many abdominal aortic aneurysms are asymptomatic and are discovered only after palpation of a mass in the abdomen or on radiologic examination for some other reason. In some cases the condition is brought to medical attention by the onset of abdominal pain, which often reflects expansion of the aneurysm. Abrupt occlusion of a peripheral artery by an embolus from a mural thrombus presents as sudden ischemia of a lower limb. The most dreaded complication of aortic aneurysms is rupture and exsanguination into the retroperitoneum (or chest), in which case the patient presents with pain, shock and a pulsatile mass in the abdomen. This is an acute emergency, and half of patients die, even with prompt surgical intervention. Therefore, even asymptomatic large aneurysms are often replaced by or bypassed with prosthetic grafts.

The risk of rupture of an abdominal aortic aneurysm is a function of its size. Aneurysms under 4 cm in diameter rarely rupture (2%), and 25%–40% of those larger than 5 cm rupture within 5 years of their discovery.

Aneurysms of Cerebral Arteries Cause Subarachnoid Hemorrhage

The most common type of cerebral aneurysm is a saccular structure known as **berry aneurysm,** because it resembles a berry attached to a twig of the arterial tree. Berry aneurysms occur due to congenital defects in arterial walls and tend to arise at branches in the circle of Willis or one of the arterial junctions. The most common sites are between the anterior cerebral and anterior communicating arteries; the internal carotid and posterior communicating arteries; and the first main divisions of the middle cerebral artery and the bifurcation of the internal carotid artery. These aneurysms are also discussed Chapter 32.

Dissecting Aneurysm Features Blood in the Arterial Wall

The dissection occurs on a path along the length of the vessel (Fig. 16-39) and essentially represents a false lumen within the wall of the artery. Although the lesion is usually designated an aneurysm, it is actually a form of hematoma. Dissecting aneurysms most often affect the aorta, especially the ascending portion, and its major branches. Thoracic dissections may involve the ascending aorta alone (type A) or only the distal aorta (type B). Their frequency has been estimated

to be as high as 1 in 400 autopsies, with men affected three times as frequently as women. They may occur at almost any age but are most common in the sixth and seventh decades. Almost all patients have a history of hypertension, and associated conditions include atherosclerosis, bicuspid aortic valve and idiopathic aortic root dilation.

 **PATHOPHYSIOLOGY:** The basis of dissecting aneurysms is usually weakening of the aortic media. The changes were originally described as **cystic medial necrosis (of Erdheim),** because focal loss of elastic and muscle fibers in the media leads to "cystic" spaces filled with a metachromatic myxoid material. These spaces are not true cysts but are rather pools of matrix collected between the cells and tissues of the media. The mechanisms of medial degeneration are not well understood. However, genetic studies have linked some cases to specific disorders, including Marfan, Ehlers-Danlos and Loeys-Dietz syndromes, and to filamin mutations. In Marfan syndrome, a systemic connective tissue abnormality, specific mutations in the gene encoding fibrillin (an extracellular matrix protein) have been identified (see Chapter 6). In some patients, mutations have been identified in other genes, including TGF-β receptors 1 and 2, smooth muscle cell–specific β-myosin (MYH11) and α-actin (ACTA2). Aging also results in mild degenerative changes in the aorta, with focal elastin loss and medial fibrosis. Patients with dissection of the thoracic aorta show decreased expression of fibulin-5, an extracellular protein that regulates elastic fiber assembly. Abnormal release of MMP-2 and its inhibitor by smooth muscle cells has also been implicated in aortic aneurysms. In animals, defective cross-linking of collagen induced by a copper-deficient diet (lysyl oxidase is a copper-dependent enzyme) causes dissecting aneurysm of the aorta. The same lesion is produced by feeding β-aminopropionitrile, an inhibitor of lysyl oxidase. People with Wilson disease who are treated with penicillamine, a copper chelator, also may develop medial necrosis of the aorta. Taken together, these data suggest that the common factor in these several situations is a molecular defect that brings on weakness of aortic connective tissue.

 PATHOLOGY: The initial event that triggers medial dissection is controversial. Over 95% of cases have a transverse tear in the intima and internal media, and it is widely held that spontaneous laceration of the intima allows blood from the lumen to enter and dissect the media. Alternatively, it has been proposed that hemorrhage from vasa vasorum into a media weakened by cystic medial necrosis initiates stress on the intima, which in turn leads to the ubiquitous intimal tear.

Most intimal tears are in the ascending aorta, 1 or 2 cm above the aortic ring. Dissection in the media occurs within seconds and separates the inner 2/3 of the aorta from the outer third. It can also involve coronary arteries, great vessels of the neck and renal, mesenteric or iliac arteries. Since the outer wall of the false channel of the dissecting aneurysm is thin, hemorrhage into the extravascular space—including the pericardium, mediastinum, pleural space and

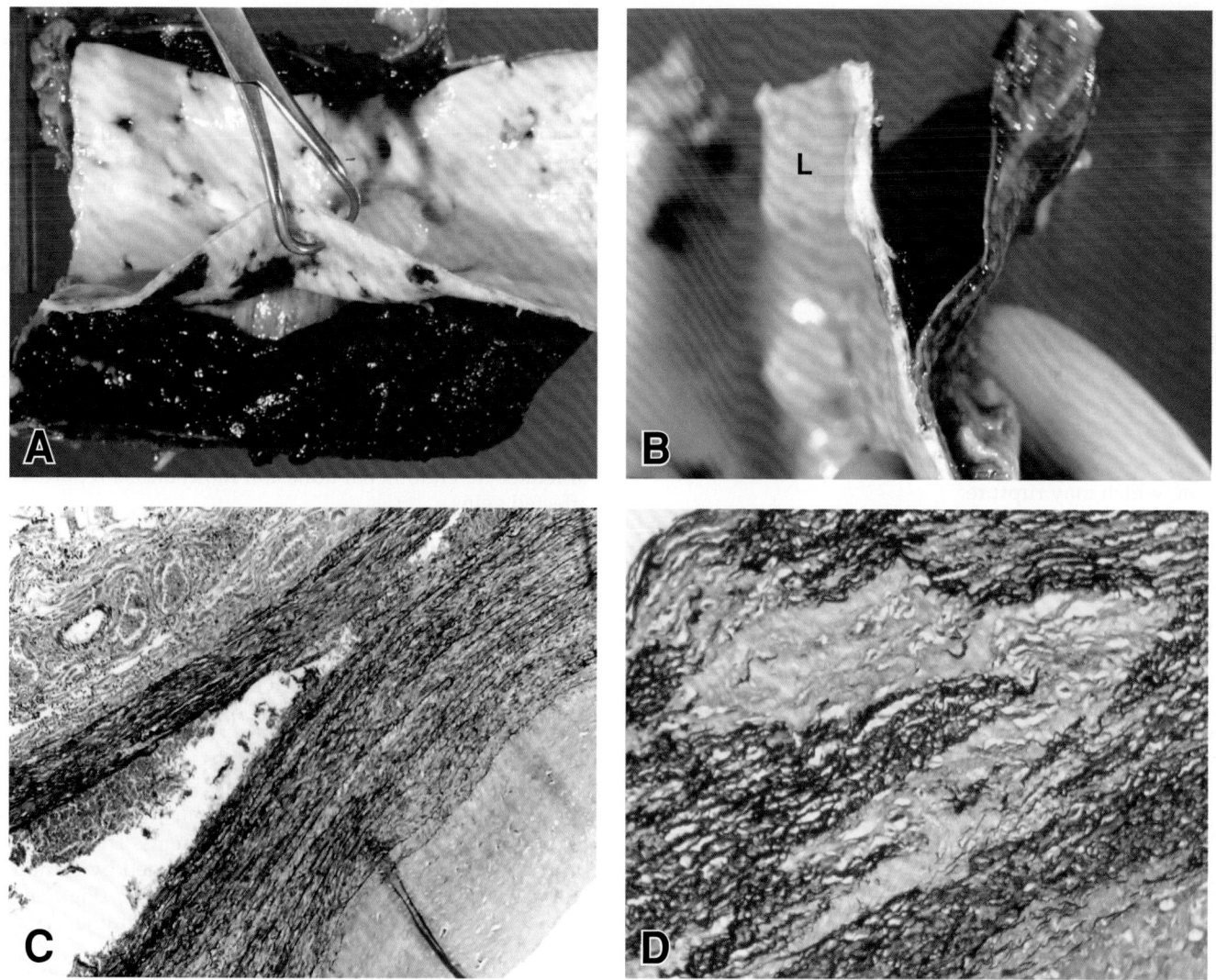

FIGURE 16-39. Dissecting aortic aneurysm. A. Thoracic aorta with metal clamps revealing the dissection and hematoma in the wall with old blood clot. **B.** The thoracic aorta has been opened longitudinally and reveals clotted blood dissecting the media of the vessel. *L* = lumen. **C.** Atherosclerotic aorta with dissection along the outer third of the media (elastic stain). **D.** A section of the aortic wall stained with aldehyde fuchsin shows pools of metachromatic material characteristic of the degenerative process known as cystic medial necrosis.

retroperitoneum—frequently causes death. In 5%–10% of cases, the blood within the dissection reenters the lumen via a second distal tear to form a "double-barreled aorta." In a comparable proportion, a reentry site produces communication of the aorta with a major artery, most often the iliac artery.

CLINICAL FEATURES: Patients typically present with acute onset of severe, "tearing" pain in the anterior chest, which is sometimes misdiagnosed as myocardial infarction. Loss of one or more arterial pulses is common, as is a murmur of aortic regurgitation. Whereas hypertension is a frequent finding in patients with dissecting aneurysms, hypotension is an ominous sign and suggests aortic rupture. Cardiac tamponade or congestive heart failure is diagnosed by the usual criteria.

Before antihypertensive and surgical treatment became available, more than a third of patients with aortic dissection died within 24 hours, and 80% succumbed by 2 weeks. Of the survivors, half died within 3 months. Prompt surgical

intervention and control of hypertension have reduced overall mortality to less than 20%.

Inflammation of Aortic Vasa Vasorum Causes Syphilitic Aneurysms

Syphilis was once the most common cause of aortic aneurysms, but as the infection has become less common, so has syphilitic vascular disease, including aortitis and aneurysms. Syphilitic aneurysms mainly affect the ascending aorta, which shows endarteritis and periarteritis of vasa vasorum. These vessels ramify in the adventitia and penetrate the outer and middle thirds of the aorta, where they become encircled by lymphocytes, plasma cells and macrophages. Obliterative changes in the vasa vasorum cause focal medial necrosis and scarring, and disruption and disorganization of elastic lamellae. The depressed medial scars create a roughened intimal surface, a "tree bark" appearance (Fig. 16-40). The relentless pressure of the blood eventually forces the weakened wall of the

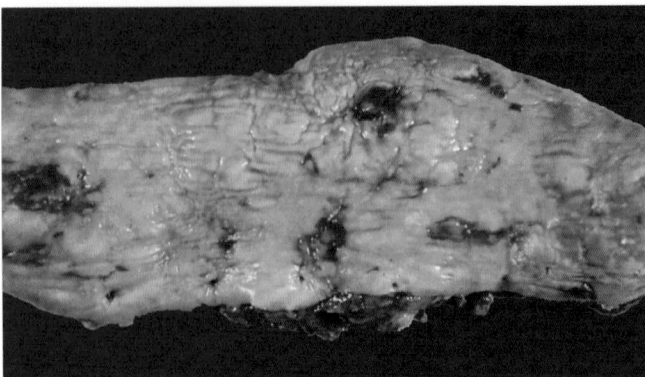

FIGURE 16-40. Syphilitic aortitis. The thoracic aorta is dilated, and its inner surface shows the typical "tree bark" appearance.

ascending aorta and aortic arch to form a fusiform aneurysm, which may rupture.

Mycotic Aneurysms Are Microbial Infections of a Vessel Wall

Mycotic (infectious) aneurysms tend to rupture and bleed. They may develop in the aortic wall or in cerebral vessels during septicemia, most commonly due to bacterial endocarditis. Mesenteric, splenic or renal arteries are also commonly affected. Mycotic aneurysms may also occur adjacent to a focus of tuberculous or a bacterial abscess.

VEINS

Varicose Veins Are Enlarged and Tortuous

Superficial varicosities of leg veins, usually in the saphenous system, are very common. They vary from a trivial knot of dilated veins to painful and disabling distention of the whole venous system of the leg, with secondary trophic disturbances. It is estimated that as much as 10%–20% of the population has some varicosities in the leg veins, but only a fraction of these develop symptoms.

 **ETIOLOGIC FACTORS:** There are several risk factors for varicose veins:

- **Age:** Varicose veins increase in frequency with age and may reach 50% in people over 50 years. This increased incidence may reflect age-related degenerative changes in connective tissues of venous walls, loss of supporting fat and connective tissues, more flaccid muscle tone and inactivity.
- **Sex:** Among 30- to 50-year-olds, women are more often affected by varicose veins than men, particularly those who have experienced increased venous pressure on the iliac veins from a pregnant uterus.
- **Heredity:** There is a strong familial predisposition to varicose veins, possibly owing to inherited configurations or structural weaknesses of the walls or valves of these vessels.
- **Posture:** Leg vein pressure is 5–10 times higher when a person is erect rather than recumbent. As a result, the incidence of varicose veins and its complications are greater in those whose occupations require them to stand in one place for long periods.

- **Obesity:** Excessive body weight increases the incidence of varicose veins, possibly because of increased intraabdominal pressure or poor support to vessel walls provided by subcutaneous fat.

Other factors that raise venous pressure in the legs can cause varicose veins, including pelvic tumors, congestive heart failure and thrombotic obstruction of the main venous trunks of the thigh or pelvis.

In the pathogenesis of varicose veins, it is not clear whether incompetence of the valves or dilation of the vessels comes first. Whatever the case, the two reinforce each other. As the vein increases in length and diameter, tortuousities develop. Once the process begins, the varicosity extends progressively throughout the length of the affected vein. As each valve becomes incompetent, increasing strain is put on the vessel and valve below. The role of inflammation is not well studied, although elevated expression of leukocyte-endothelial adhesion molecules is reported in affected veins.

 PATHOLOGY: Microscopically, varicose veins show variations in wall thickness. Some areas are thin, owing to dilation, while others are thickened by smooth muscle hypertrophy, subintimal fibrosis and incorporation of mural thrombi into the wall. Patchy calcification is frequently seen. Valvular deformities consist of thickening, shortening and rolling of the cusps.

 CLINICAL FEATURES: Visual inspection makes the diagnosis of varicose veins of the leg. Most affected vessels and veins have little clinical effect and are mainly cosmetic problems. The principal symptoms are aching in the legs, aggravated by standing and relieved by elevation. Severe varicosities (Fig. 16-41) may give rise to trophic changes in the skin drained by the

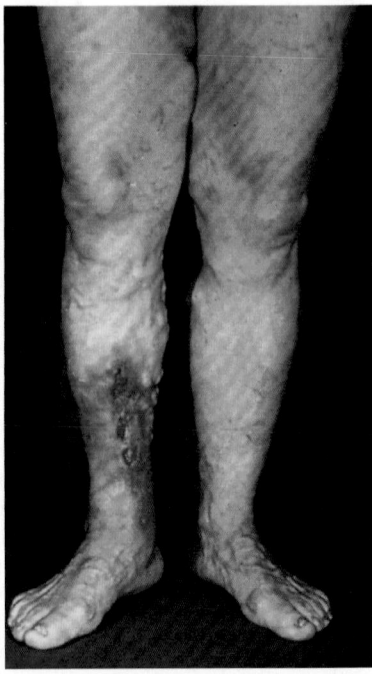

FIGURE 16-41. Varicose veins of the legs. Severe varicosities of the superficial leg veins have led to stasis dermatitis and secondary ulcerations.

affected veins, called **stasis dermatitis**. Surgery is mandated if the overlying skin has ulcerated or if spontaneous bleeding or extensive thrombosis (which may lead to pulmonary embolism) occurs.

Varicose Veins also Occur at Other Sites

HEMORRHOIDS: These are dilations of the veins of the rectum and anal canal and may occur inside or outside the anal sphincter (see Chapter 19). Although there may be a hereditary predisposition, the condition is aggravated by factors that increase intra-abdominal pressure. These include constipation, pregnancy and venous obstruction by rectal tumors. Hemorrhoids often bleed, an occurrence that may be confused with bleeding rectal cancers. Thrombosed hemorrhoids are exquisitely painful.

ESOPHAGEAL VARICES: This complication of portal hypertension is caused mainly by cirrhosis of the liver (see Chapter 20). High portal pressure distends the anastomoses between portal and systemic venous circulations at the lower end of the esophagus. Although they may be prominent radiologically, esophageal varices are usually unimpressive at autopsy. After their collapse at death, bluish streaks in the esophageal mucosa may be all that is evident. Hemorrhage from esophageal varices is a common cause of death in patients with cirrhosis.

VARICOCELE: This palpable scrotal mass represents varicosities of the pampiniform plexus (see Chapter 23).

Deep Venous Thrombosis Principally Affects Leg Veins

- **Thrombophlebitis** is inflammation and secondary thrombosis of small veins and sometimes larger ones, commonly as part of a local reaction to bacterial infection.
- **Phlebothrombosis** is the term for venous thrombosis that occurs without an initiating infection or inflammation.
- **Deep venous thrombosis** now refers to both phlebothrombosis and thrombophlebitis. Since most cases of venous thrombosis are not associated with inflammation or infection, the condition is currently associated with prolonged bed rest or reduced cardiac output. It is most frequent in deep leg veins and can be a major threat to life because of pulmonary embolization (witness the well-known phenomenon of sudden death with ambulation after surgery). Deficiencies of anticoagulants, such as protein C and antithrombin, increase the incidence of venous thromboembolism. Deep venous thrombosis is discussed more fully in Chapter 7.

LYMPHATIC VESSELS

Lymphatic vessels are thin-walled low-pressure channels. They are important for normal tissue fluid balance, providing drainage of plasma filtrates, cells and foreign material from the interstitial spaces. They are also important in fat digestion, through lacteals in the intestinal villi, and in immune surveillance. Lymphatic vessels are more permeable than blood vessels, in part because the former have fewer tight junctions. NO• may act as a mediator of several growth factors that are lymphangiogenic and may be important in lymphatic function. For example, NO• may inhibit

pumping in collecting lymphatics. Inflammation and tumors frequently spread via lymphatics.

 MOLECULAR PATHOGENESIS: Fox2, the forkhead transcription factor, regulates lymphatic valve morphogenesis and maintains the lymphatic capillary phenotype late in development. The VEGF-C/VEGFR-3 pathway mediates lymphatic endothelial cell migration, proliferation and survival. Missense mutations in VEGFR-3 result in lymphedema and lymphatic hypoplasia. PROX-1 is essential for early steps in lymphatic formation, such as budding from the anterior cardinal vein and forming lymph sacs. Along with podoplanin, VEGFR-3 and neuropilin-2, it also contributes to primary lymphatic plexus development. In inflammatory conditions, VEGF-C is upregulated by cytokines, and macrophages express VEGFR-3 and secrete VEGF-C. In experimental studies, tumor metastasis and lymphangiogenesis can be blocked by inhibiting VEGF-C/VEGFR-3. In some patients, primary lymphedema is associated with mutations in VEGFR-3, FOXC2, SOX18 and germline GATA2.

Lymphangitis Reflects Infection in Lymphatic Vessels

Transport of infectious material to regional lymph nodes incites **lymphadenitis**. The periphery of a focus of inflammation reveals dilated lymphatics filled with fluid exudate, cells, cellular debris and bacteria. When tissues are expanded by exudate, there is comparable distention of lymphatic channels and an opening of intercellular channels between endothelial cells.

Almost any pathogen can cause acute lymphangitis, but β-hemolytic streptococci (pyogenes) are particularly notorious offenders. The process may extend beyond these channels into surrounding tissues. Draining lymph nodes are regularly enlarged and inflamed. Painful subcutaneous red streaks, often accompanied by similarly painful regional lymph nodes, characterize acute lymphangitis.

Lymphatic Obstruction Causes Lymphedema

Lymphatics may be obstructed by scar tissue, intraluminal tumor cells, pressure from surrounding tumor tissue or plugging with parasites. As collateral lymphatic routes are abundant, lymphedema (distention of tissue by lymph) usually occurs only when major trunks are obstructed, especially in the axilla or groin. For example, when radical mastectomy for breast cancer was routine, axillary lymph node dissection frequently disrupted lymphatic channels and led to lymphedema of the arm. Prolonged lymphatic obstruction causes progressive dilation of lymphatic vessels, or **lymphangiectasia,** and overgrowth of fibrous tissue. The term **elephantiasis** describes a lymphedematous limb that is grossly enlarged. In the tropics, filariasis, in which a parasitic worm invades lymphatics, is a common cause of elephantiasis (see Chapter 9).

Milroy disease is an inherited type of lymphedema that is present at birth. It is associated with mutations in VEGF3 receptor, which is normally activated by VEGF-C and VEGF-D in lymphatic embryogenesis. It usually affects only one limb, but it may be more extensive and involve the eyelids and lips. Affected tissues show hugely dilated lymphatic channels, and the entire area appears honeycombed or spongy. This lesion is more properly considered lymphangiectasia rather than simply lymphedema.

BENIGN TUMORS OF BLOOD VESSELS

Tumors of the vascular system are common. Many are hamartomas rather than true neoplasms. Some mutations have been linked to vascular anomalies. For example, endoglin and ALK-1 mutations have been identified in hereditary hemorrhagic telangiectasia, and several gene mutations have been identified in familial cerebral cavernous malformation.

Hemangiomas Are Common Benign Tumors of Vascular Channels

Hemangiomas usually occur in the skin but may also be found in internal organs.

PATHOLOGY:

CAPILLARY HEMANGIOMA: This lesion is composed of vascular channels with the size and structure of normal capillaries. Capillary hemangiomas may occur in any tissue. The most common sites are skin; subcutaneous tissues; mucous membranes of the lips and mouth; and internal viscera, including spleen, kidneys and liver. Capillary hemangiomas vary from a few millimeters to several centimeters in diameter. They are bright red to blue, depending on the degree of oxygenation of the blood. In the skin, capillary hemangiomas are known as **birthmarks** or **ruby spots**. The only disability is cosmetic disfiguration.

JUVENILE HEMANGIOMA: Also called **strawberry hemangiomas,** these lesions are found on the skin of newborns. They grow rapidly in the first months of life, begin to fade at 1–3 years of age and completely regress in most (80%) cases by 5 years of age. Juvenile hemangiomas contain packed masses of capillaries separated by connective tissue stroma (Fig. 16-42). The endothelial-lined channels are usually filled with blood. Thromboses, sometimes organized, are common. Occasionally, the vascular channels rupture, causing scarring and accumulation of hemosiderin. Juvenile hemangiomas are usually well demarcated despite lacking capsules. Although finger-like projections of the vascular tissue may give the impression of invasion, these growths are benign; they do not invade or metastasize.

CAVERNOUS HEMANGIOMA: This term is reserved for lesions made of large vascular channels, often interspersed with small, capillary-type vessels. When cavernous hemangiomas occur in the skin (Fig. 16-43), they are called **port wine stains**. They also appear on mucosal surfaces and visceral organs, including the spleen, liver and pancreas. If they occur in the brain, they may enlarge slowly and cause neurologic symptoms after long quiescent periods.

A cavernous hemangioma is a red-blue, soft, spongy mass, with a diameter of up to several centimeters. Unlike capillary hemangiomas, cavernous hemangiomas do not regress spontaneously. Although the lesion is demarcated by a sharp border, it is not encapsulated. Large endothelial-lined, blood-containing spaces are separated by sparse connective tissue. Cavernous hemangiomas can undergo a variety of changes, including thrombosis, fibrosis, cystic cavitation and intracystic hemorrhage.

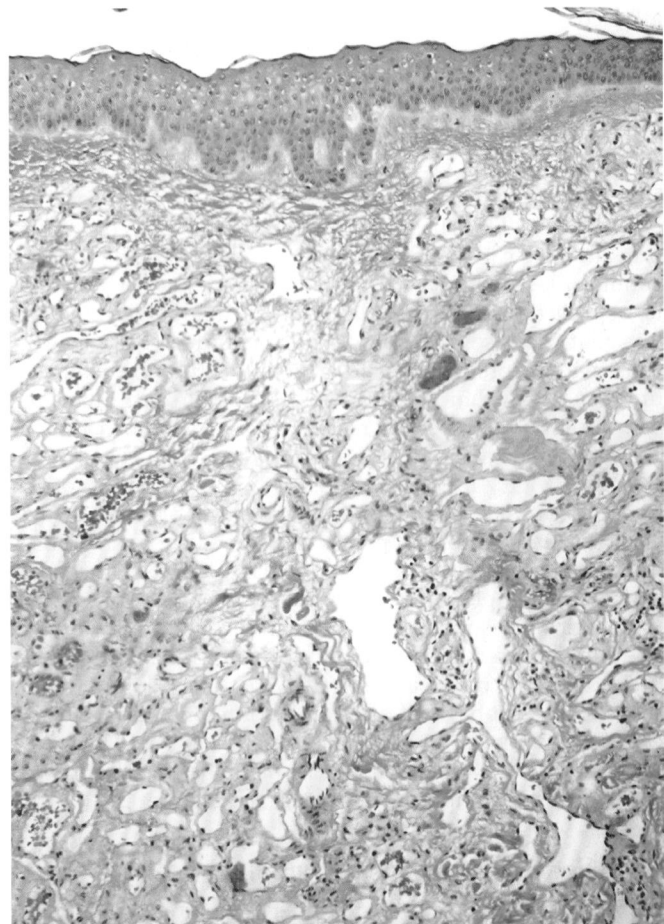

FIGURE 16-42. Juvenile hemangioma. A network of delicate, anastomosing vessels is present subcutaneously.

MULTIPLE HEMANGIOMATOUS SYNDROMES: More than one hemangioma may occur in a single tissue. Two or more tissues may be involved, such as skin and nervous system or spleen and liver. **von Hippel-Lindau syndrome** is a rare entity in which cavernous hemangiomas occur in the cerebellum or brainstem and the retina. **Sturge-Weber**

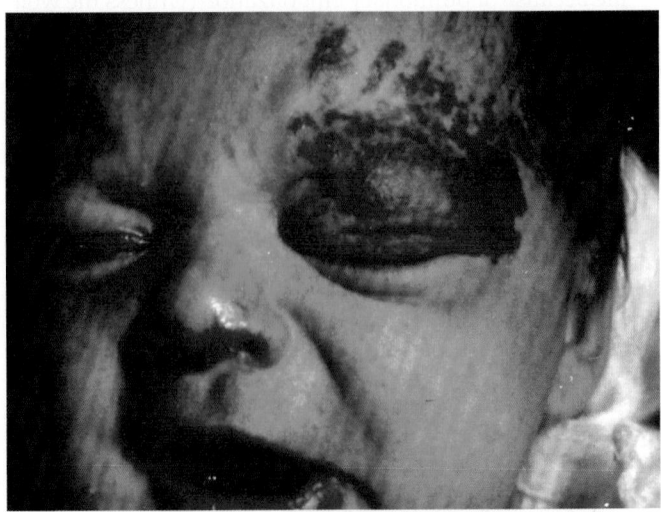

FIGURE 16-43. Congenital cavernous hemangioma of the skin.

syndrome involves a developmental disturbance of blood vessels in the brain and skin. Other closely related lesions are plexiform or racemose angiomas, cirsoid aneurysms and angiomatous dilation of vessels of the brain and elsewhere.

 **ETIOLOGIC FACTORS:** Although hemangiomas are clearly benign, their origin is uncertain; they may be true neoplasms or they may be hamartomas. The evidence favoring hamartoma includes (1) the lesion is present at birth; (2) it grows only as the rest of the body grows and remains limited in size; and (3) after growth ceases, it usually remains unchanged indefinitely absent trauma, thrombosis or hemorrhage.

The development of these vascular malformations recalls the embryology of the vascular system. A network of endothelial channels undergoes remodeling, acquiring a muscular coat and adventitia. In this view, vascular malformations reflect the persistence of the original or modified channels and mixtures of connective tissue elements derived from the mesenchyme. At present, hemangiomas are classified by histologic type and location, although molecular characterization will likely lead to new classifications and better understanding of the prognosis of given lesions.

Glomus Tumor Is a Painful Tumor of the Glomus Body

Glomus bodies are normal neuromyoarterial receptors that are sensitive to temperature and regulate arteriolar flow. Glomus bodies are widely distributed in the skin, mostly in distal parts of fingers and toes. This parallels the sites of glomus tumors (glomangiomas), typically under the nails. The lesions tend to be unusually painful.

 PATHOLOGY: Glomus tumors are usually under 1 cm in diameter; many are smaller than a few millimeters. In the skin, they are slightly elevated, rounded, red-blue and firm (Fig. 16-44). The two main histologic components are branching vascular channels in a connective tissue stroma and aggregates or nests of specialized glomus cells. The latter are regular, round to cuboidal cells that reveal typical smooth muscle cell features by electron microscopy.

Hemangioendothelioma Is Intermediate between Hemangiomas and Angiosarcomas

The epithelioid or histiocytoid hemangioendothelioma displays endothelial cells with considerable eosinophilic, often vacuolated, cytoplasm. Vascular lumina are evident, as are a few mitoses. These tumors occur in almost all locations. Although the lesion may recur locally, surgical removal is generally curative. However, about 1/5 of patients develop metastases.

Spindle cell hemangioendothelioma occurs principally in males of any age, usually in the dermis and subcutaneous tissue of distal extremities. It features vascular, endothelial-lined spaces into which papillary projections extend.

MALIGNANT TUMORS OF BLOOD VESSELS

Malignant vascular neoplasms are rare, and only rarely do they arise in preexisting benign tumors.

Angiosarcoma Is a Rare Malignant Tumor of Endothelial Cells

These tumors occur in either sex and at any age. They begin as small, painless, sharply demarcated, red nodules. The most common locations are skin, soft tissue, breast, bone, liver and spleen. Eventually, most enlarge to become pale gray, fleshy masses without a capsule. These tumors often undergo central necrosis, with softening and hemorrhage.

 PATHOLOGY: Angiosarcomas exhibit varying degrees of differentiation, ranging from those composed mainly of distinct vascular elements to undifferentiated tumors with few recognizable blood channels (Fig. 16-45). The latter display frequent mitoses, pleomorphism and giant cells and tend to be more malignant. Almost half of patients with angiosarcoma die of the disease.

Angiosarcoma of the liver is of special interest; it is associated with environmental carcinogens, particularly arsenic (a component of pesticides) and vinyl chloride (used in production of plastics). Hepatic angiosarcoma was observed after administration of thorium dioxide, a radioactive contrast

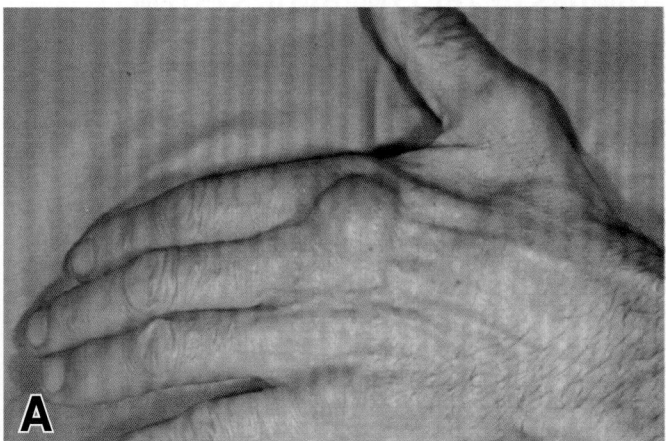
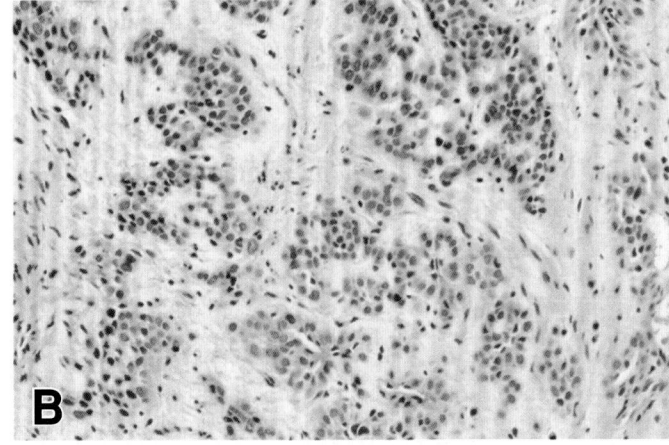

FIGURE 16-44. Glomus tumor. A. The dorsal surface of the hand displays a prominent tumor nodule on the proximal third finger. **B.** A photomicrograph of (A) reveals nests of glomus tumor cells embedded in a fibrovascular stroma.

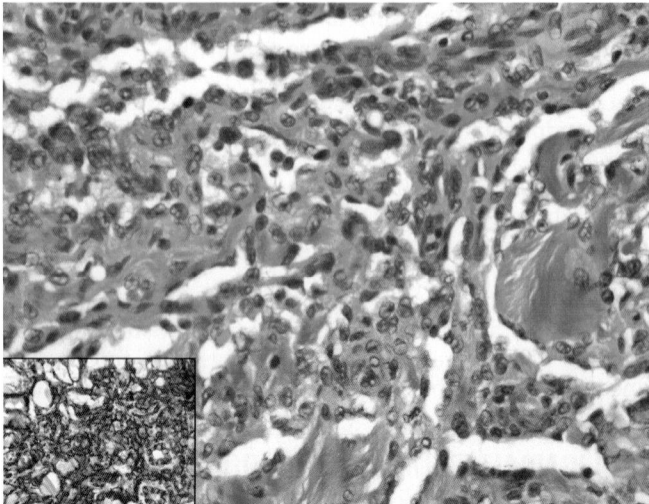

FIGURE 16-45. **Angiosarcoma.** Malignant spindly cells line vague channels. **Inset.** Immunostain for CD31, an endothelial marker.

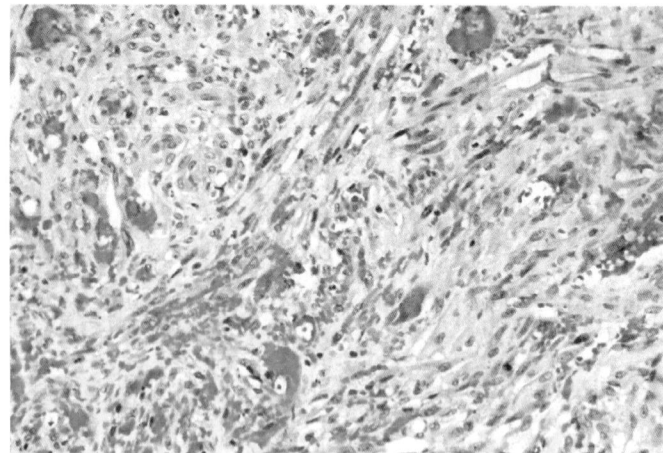

FIGURE 16-46. **Kaposi sarcoma.** A photomicrograph of a vascular lesion from a patient with acquired immune deficiency syndrome shows numerous poorly differentiated, spindle-shaped neoplastic cells and a vascular lesion filled with red blood cells.

medium (Thorotrast) used by radiologists prior to 1950. Thorotrast is engulfed by macrophages of the liver sinusoids, where it remains for life.

There is a long latent period between exposure to the chemicals or radionuclide and development of hepatic angiosarcoma. The earliest detectable changes are atypia and diffuse hyperplasia of the cells lining the hepatic sinusoids. The tumors are frequently multicentric and may arise in the spleen as well. Hepatic angiosarcomas are highly malignant and spread by both local invasion and metastasis.

Hemangiopericytoma

Hemangiopericytoma is a rare neoplasm previously thought to arise from pericytes, which are modified smooth muscle cells outside the walls of capillaries and arterioles. However, it is not clear that the neoplasm actually derives from these cells. These tumors present as small masses of capillary-like channels surrounded by, and frequently enclosed within, nests and masses of round to spindle-shaped cells. The tumor cells are characteristically invested by a basement membrane.

Hemangiopericytomas can occur anywhere but are most common in the retroperitoneum and lower extremities. Most are removed surgically without having invaded or metastasized. Malignant hemangiopericytomas metastasize to lungs, bone, liver and lymph nodes.

Kaposi Sarcoma Is Caused by Human Herpesvirus 8

Kaposi sarcoma is a malignant angioproliferative tumor derived from endothelial cells.

 **EPIDEMIOLOGY:** Kaposi sarcoma was originally described in the 19th century by Moritz Kaposi in Vienna. It also occurred as a sporadic tumor endemic in parts of central Africa, but was otherwise an oddity that mainly afflicted older men. Kaposi sarcoma is now seen in epidemic form in immunosuppressed patients, especially those with AIDS. Human herpesvirus 8 (HHV8), also called Kaposi sarcoma–associated herpes virus (KSHV),

is responsible for this tumor, which arises in endothelial cells. Only a small fraction of HHV8-infected people develop Kaposi sarcoma. VEGF and hypoxia-inducible factor (HIF) seem to play important roles in pathogenesis of the tumor, as does the PI3K/Akt/mTOR pathway. Cofactors that determine the occurrence of Kaposi sarcoma in individuals who are at risk are not well understood.

 PATHOLOGY: Kaposi sarcoma begins as painful purple or brown 1-mm to 1-cm cutaneous nodules. They appear most often on the hands or feet but may occur anywhere. Their microscopic appearance is highly variable. One form resembles a simple hemangioma, with tightly packed clusters of capillaries and scattered hemosiderin-laden macrophages. Other types are highly cellular with less prominent vascular spaces (Fig. 16-46). They may be difficult to distinguish from fibrosarcomas, but their endothelial origin is demonstrable by immunochemistry and by electron microscopy. Although Kaposi sarcoma is considered a malignant lesion and may be widely disseminated in the body, it rarely causes death.

TUMORS OF THE LYMPHATIC SYSTEM

Many histologic and clinical variants of local enlargements of the lymphatics have been described. It is difficult to distinguish among anomalies, proliferations due to stasis and true neoplasms. In general, lymphatic tumors are distinguished by their size and location. The spaces may be small, as in capillary lymphangiomas, or large and dilated, as in cystic or cavernous lesions. Lymphangiomatous lesions can arise at almost any site, including skin, mediastinum, retroperitoneum, spleen and elsewhere.

Capillary Lymphangioma

Sometimes called "simple lymphangiomas," these benign tumors are small, circumscribed, grayish pink, fleshy nodules, which can be single or multiple. They are subcutaneous and occur on the skin of the face, lips, chest, genitalia or extremities. Capillary lymphangiomas are composed of variably sized, thin-walled spaces lined by endothelial cells and contain lymph and occasional leukocytes.

Cystic Lymphangiomas Are Often Congenital Lesions

These benign lesions (also called cystic hygromas) are most common in the neck and axilla but also occur in the mediastinum and sometimes in the retroperitoneum. They may reach 10–15 cm or more in diameter and fill the axilla or distort the neck.

 PATHOLOGY: Cystic lymphangiomas are soft, spongy and pink. Watery fluid exudes from their cut surfaces. Microscopically, they contain endothelial-lined spaces with a protein-rich fluid. These spaces are distinguished from blood vessels because they lack erythrocytes and leukocytes. Abundant irregularly distributed smooth muscle and connective tissue cells may be present.

Lymphangiosarcoma May Occur after Lymphedema or Radiation

These are rare malignant tumors that develop in 0.1%–0.5% of patients with lymphedema of the arm after radical mastectomy. Distinction between this tumor and angiosarcoma is difficult, and some authors equate the two. Lymphangiosarcoma may also occur in other regions, for example, in the leg following radiation therapy for uterine cervical carcinoma.

 PATHOLOGY: Lymphangiosarcomas are purplish, frequently multiple, nodules in edematous skin. They are composed of cells resembling capillary endothelial cells and showing zonulae adherentes between cells. The walls of tumor vessels have a rudimentary form of basal basement membrane. Lymphangiosarcomas are highly malignant and, despite radical surgery, have a poor prognosis.

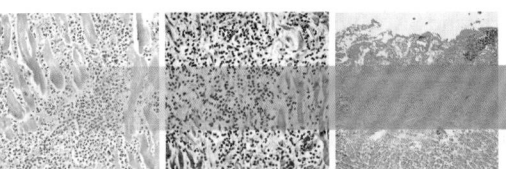

17

The Heart

Jeffrey E. Saffitz

Anatomy of the Heart
The Cardiac Myocyte
The Conduction System
The Coronary Arteries

Myocardial Hypertrophy and Heart Failure

Congenital Heart Disease
Classifications of Congenital Heart Disease
Initial Left-to-Right Shunt
Right-to-Left Shunt
Congenital Heart Diseases without Shunts

Ischemic Heart Disease
Conditions That Limit the Supply of Blood to the Heart
Conditions That Limit Oxygen Availability
Increased Oxygen Demand
Myocardial Infarcts
Therapeutic Interventions
Chronic Ischemic Heart Disease

Hypertensive Heart Disease
Effects of Hypertension on the Heart
Cause of Death in Patients with Hypertension

Cor Pulmonale

Acquired Valvular and Endocardial Diseases
Rheumatic Heart Disease
Collagen Vascular Diseases
Bacterial Endocarditis
Nonbacterial Thrombotic Endocarditis
Calcific Aortic Stenosis
Calcification of the Mitral Valve Annulus
Mitral Valve Prolapse
Papillary Muscle Dysfunction
Carcinoid Heart Disease

Myocarditis
Viral Myocarditis
Other Forms of Infectious Myocarditis
Granulomatous Myocarditis
Hypersensitivity Myocarditis
Giant Cell Myocarditis

Metabolic Diseases of the Heart
Hyperthyroid Heart Disease
Hypothyroid Heart Disease
Thiamine Deficiency (Beriberi) Heart Disease

Cardiomyopathy
Idiopathic Dilated Cardiomyopathy
Secondary Dilated Cardiomyopathy

Hypertrophic Cardiomyopathy
Arrhythmogenic Cardiomyopathy
Restrictive Cardiomyopathy

Sudden Cardiac Death
Sudden Death in Patients with Structurally Normal Hearts

Cardiac Tumors
Cardiac Myxoma
Rhabdomyoma
Papillary Fibroelastoma
Other Tumors

Diseases of the Pericardium
Pericardial Effusion
Acute Pericarditis
Constrictive Pericarditis

Pathology of Interventional Therapies
Coronary Angioplasty and Stenting
Coronary Bypass Grafts
Prosthetic Valves
Cardiovascular Complications in Cancer Survivors
Heart Transplantation

The heart is a fist-sized muscular pump that has the remarkable capacity to work unceasingly for the 90 or more years of a human lifetime. As demand requires, it can increase its output manyfold, in part because the coronary circulation can augment its blood flow to over 10 times normal. The ventricles also respond to short-term increases in workload by increasing heart rate and contractility, the latter in accordance with Starling's law of the heart. When an increased workload is imposed for longer periods (e.g., systemic hypertension), the left ventricle hypertrophies, an adaptation that increases its work capacity. However, this compensatory mechanism has its limits: a point is reached when the heart can no longer supply blood adequately to peripheral tissues; the result is congestive heart failure. Damage to the myocardium, caused most commonly by coronary artery

disease, also limits left ventricular capacity to pump blood and similarly results in heart failure.

ANATOMY OF THE HEART

The heart of a normal adult man weighs 280–340 g, and that of a normal adult woman, 230–280 g. It is a two-sided pump. Blood enters each side through a thin-walled **atrium,** from which it is propelled forward by thicker muscular **ventricles.** The right ventricle is considerably thinner (<0.5 cm) than the left ventricle (1.3–1.5 cm) owing to the low venous pressure and relatively low afterload on the right side. Blood enters the ventricles across atrioventricular valves, the mitral valve on the left and the tricuspid valve on the right. These valves'

621

leaflets are held in place by chordae tendineae, strong fibrous cords attached to the inner surface of the ventricular wall via papillary muscles. The entrances to the aorta and pulmonary arteries are guarded respectively by the aortic and pulmonary valves, each with three semilunar cusps.

The heart wall has three layers: outer epicardium, middle myocardium and inner endocardium. The heart is surrounded and enclosed by visceral and parietal pericardia, which are separated by the pericardial cavity.

Cardiac Myocytes Generate Contractile Force

The myocardium is a network of individual myocytes, most of which normally have a single nucleus. They are separated from each other by intercalated disks that contain cell–cell adhesion and electrical junctions. Electron microscopy reveals the structure and distribution of the sarcolemma, **sarcoplasmic reticulum** (SR), T system of tubules, nucleus and many mitochondria (Fig. 17-1A). The contractile elements of the myocyte, the **myofilaments,** are arranged in bundles called **myofibrils**. These are separated by mitochondria and SR. Myofibrils are organized into repeating units termed **sarcomeres**.

The sarcomere is the basic functional unit of the contractile apparatus. It consists of a Z disk on each end and interdigitated thick and thin filaments, oriented perpendicular to the Z disk (Fig. 17-1). The thick filaments contain myosin heavy chains, myosin-binding protein C and myosin light chains. The thick filaments are limited to the A band and interact with the giant sarcomeric protein, titin (~27,000 amino acids), which spans from the Z disk to the M line, to form a third sarcomere filament system. Titin helps maintain precise assembly of myofibrillar proteins and contributes to the viscoelastic properties of cardiac muscle. The thin filaments contain actin and regulatory proteins, including **α-tropomyosin-1** and the **troponin complex** (cardiac troponins I, C and T), and extend from the Z disk through the I band and into the A band. Interaction of these myofilaments generates the force for contraction. The amount of force that can be produced is proportional to the overlap between adjoining thick and thin filaments and is maximum when sarcomeres are 2.0–2.2 μm in length.

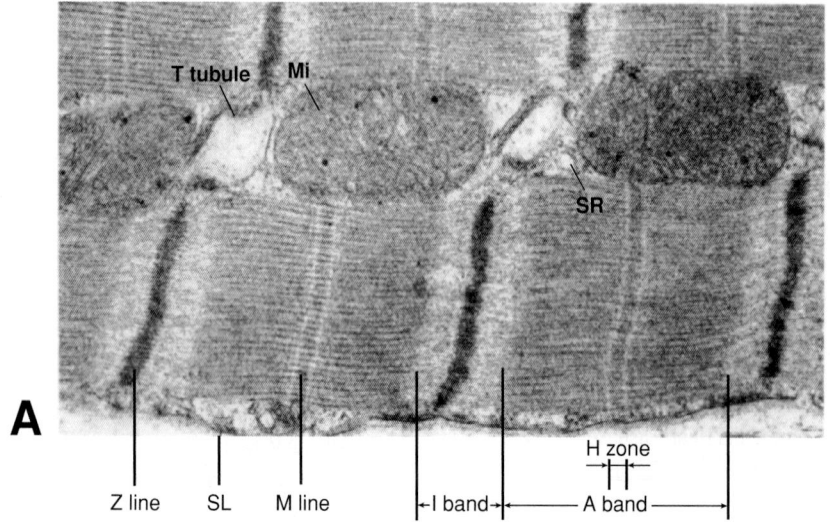

A

Z line   SL   M line   ⊢I band⊣   ⊢ A band ⊣   H zone

T tubule   Mi   SR

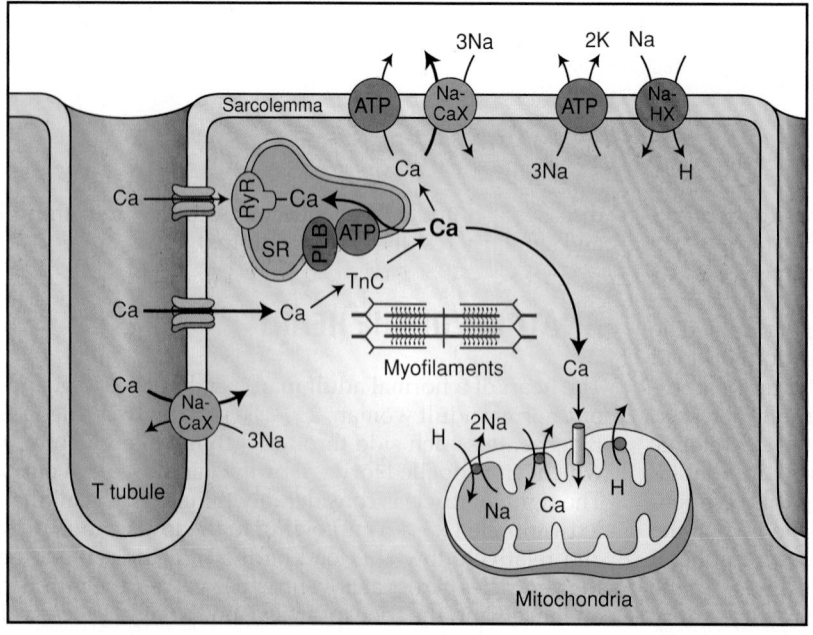

B

FIGURE 17-1. Ultrastructure of the myocardium. A. Electron micrograph of left ventricle in the longitudinal plane, showing the sarcolemma (SL); the sarcomeres of the myofibrils, delimited by Z lines; A bands; I bands; H zones; and M lines. Also present are mitochondria (Mi), sarcoplasmic reticulum (SR) and T tubules. The I bands and H zones are absent when the myofibrils are shortened. The structural basis for the banding is shown in the electron micrograph. The fine threads that extend at right angles to the thick (myosin) filaments are the cross-bridges that form the force-generating cross-links with actin. The amount of force that can be generated is proportional to the length of the adjoining myofilaments and is at a maximum when the sarcomeres are between 2 and 2.2 μm in length. When the sarcomeres are less than 2 μm in length, the thin filaments slide across each other and overlap, decreasing the potential for force-generating cross-links; similarly, when the sarcomeres are stretched beyond 2.2 μm, there is a decrease in force that is proportional to the widening of the H zone. This mechanism can be invoked as the basis for Starling's law of the heart. **B.** Pathways regulating Ca^{2+} homeostasis and excitation–contraction coupling in cardiac myocytes. The cardiac action potential brings depolarizing current into T tubules where voltage-gated L-type Ca^{2+} channels reside in high concentrations (green channel structures). Influx of Ca^{2+} through these channels (ICa) stimulates release of Ca^{2+} from the SR (located in immediate proximity to the T tubule) via RyR2. The transient increase in cytosolic Ca^{2+} promotes contraction through interactions with cardiac troponin T (TnC). Resting diastolic Ca^{2+} levels are restored by reuptake into the SR and extrusion via sodium–calcium exchange (Na-CaX) and an adenosine triphosphate (ATP) pump.

When sarcomere length is under 2 μm, the thin filaments slide across each other and overlap, decreasing the potential for force-generating cross-links. If it is stretched over 2.2 μm, force decreases in proportion to the widening of the H zone. *This is the basis for Starling law of the heart, which states that cardiac contractile force is a function of fiber length during diastole.* Average sarcomere length is about 2.2 μm when left ventricular end-diastolic pressure is at the upper limit of normal.

Contraction of cardiac muscle is initiated by increases in cytosolic free calcium. In a normal myocyte, an action potential triggers entry of calcium ions into the myocyte through voltage-gated L-type Ca^{2+} channels in T tubules. These invaginations of the sarcolemma bring depolarizing current and resultant voltage-gated Ca^{2+} entry into intimate proximity to intracellular organelles regulating calcium homeostasis (lateral cisterns of the SR) and the contractile apparatus itself (Fig. 17-1B). The entering calcium stimulates release of Ca^{2+} sequestered in the SR (Ca^{2+}-induced Ca^{2+} release) via cardiac ryanodine receptors (RyR2). Increased cytosolic Ca^{2+} produces a conformational change in the regulatory myofilament proteins, in particular troponin, allowing cross-bridges between actin and myosin to break and reform repeatedly. As a result, the filaments slide over one another, causing myocardial contraction. *The number of contractile sites activated and the resulting force generated are directly proportional to the concentration of Ca^{2+} near the myofibrils.*

The myocardium relaxes when cytosolic Ca^{2+} returns to its normal low (diastolic) concentration of 10^{-7} M. This process depends on calcium adenosine triphosphatase (ATPase) of the SR, which pumps Ca^{2+} from the cytosol into the SR. Cytosolic Ca^{2+} also returns to the normal resting diastolic concentration by its outward transport through $Na^+–Ca^{2+}$ exchange and sarcolemmal calcium pumps (Fig. 17-1B). *Thus, myocardial relaxation is an active, energy-requiring event.*

The Conduction System Consists of Specialized Myocytes

These myocytes have two major functions: (1) they initiate heartbeats by generating electrical current through their automatic rhythmicity, which is more rapid in the sinoatrial (SA) node than more distally in the system; and (2) they distribute this current to activate atrial and ventricular myocardium in an appropriate temporal–spatial pattern. Fibers of the atrioventricular conduction system generally conduct impulses faster (~1–2 m/sec) than do working (contractile) atrial and ventricular fibers (~0.5–1 m/sec). By contrast, conduction through the atrioventricular node is exceptionally slow (~0.1 m/sec). Slow conduction at the atrioventricular junction delays ventricular activation and facilitates ventricular filling.

Heartbeats normally originate in the SA node, which is near the junction of the superior vena cava and the roof of the right atrium. If the node is diseased or otherwise prevented from functioning as the pacemaker, more distal components of the conduction system or even ventricular muscle itself assume the role of pacemaker. *As a rule, the more distal the pacemaker site, the slower the heart rate.* On leaving the SA node, an electrical impulse activates the atria. Atrial wavefronts converge on the atrioventricular (AV) node, which conducts the impulse through the common bundle (bundle of His) to the left and right bundle branches of the Purkinje system. Purkinje fibers run within the endocardium on both sides of the interventricular septum and distribute current to overlying ventricular muscles. Each cycle, ventricular contraction begins along the interventricular septum and at the apex. It progresses from apex to base, resulting in smooth and efficient ejection of blood into the great vessels.

The His bundle in normal adult hearts is the only electrical connection between atria and ventricles. Additional abnormal connections may occasionally arise as small bundles or tracts of cardiac myocytes. Such "bypass tracts" can activate ventricular muscle before the normal impulse arrives via the conduction system. They are found in patients with the **Wolff-Parkinson-White syndrome** and can establish circuits that promote **supraventricular tachycardia**. Congenital conduction system discontinuities may be caused by placentally transmitted autoantibodies in mothers with diseases such as systemic lupus erythematosus (SLE). Acquired defects may arise due to infarction, inflammatory or infiltrative disease, cardiac surgery or cardiac catheterization.

Coronary Arteries Supply Blood to the Heart

The right and left main coronary arteries originate in, or immediately above, the sinuses of Valsalva of the aortic valve. The left main coronary artery bifurcates within 1 cm of its origin into the left anterior descending (LAD) and left circumflex coronary arteries. The latter rests in the left atrioventricular groove and supplies the lateral wall of the left ventricle (Fig. 17-2). The LAD coronary artery lies in the anterior interventricular groove and provides blood to the (1) anterior left ventricle, (2) adjacent anterior right ventricle and (3) anterior 1/2 to 2/3 of the interventricular septum. In the apical region, the LAD artery supplies the ventricles circumferentially (Fig. 17-2).

The right coronary artery travels along the right atrioventricular groove and feeds most of the right ventricle and posteroseptal left ventricle (Fig. 17-2), including the posterior third to half of the interventricular septum at the base of the heart (also referred to as the "inferior" or "diaphragmatic" wall). Thus, one can predict locations of infarcts that result from occlusion of any of these major epicardial coronary arteries.

The epicardial coronary arteries are usually arranged in a so-called right coronary–dominant distribution. The pattern of dominance is defined by the coronary artery that contributes the most blood to the posterior descending coronary artery. In 5–10% of human hearts, the left circumflex coronary artery supplies the posterior descending coronary artery (left dominant).

Blood flows in the myocardium inward from epicardium to endocardium. Thus, as a general rule, endocardium is most vulnerable to ischemia when flow through a major epicardial coronary artery is compromised. Some of the small intramyocardial coronary arteries branch as they traverse the ventricular wall; others maintain a large diameter and pass to the endocardial surface without branching (Fig. 17-3). Because capillary networks arising from penetrating arteries do not interconnect, the borders between viable and infarcted myocardium after coronary artery occlusion are distinct.

The epicardial portion of each coronary artery fills and expands during systole and empties and narrows during diastole. Intramyocardial arteries do the opposite and are

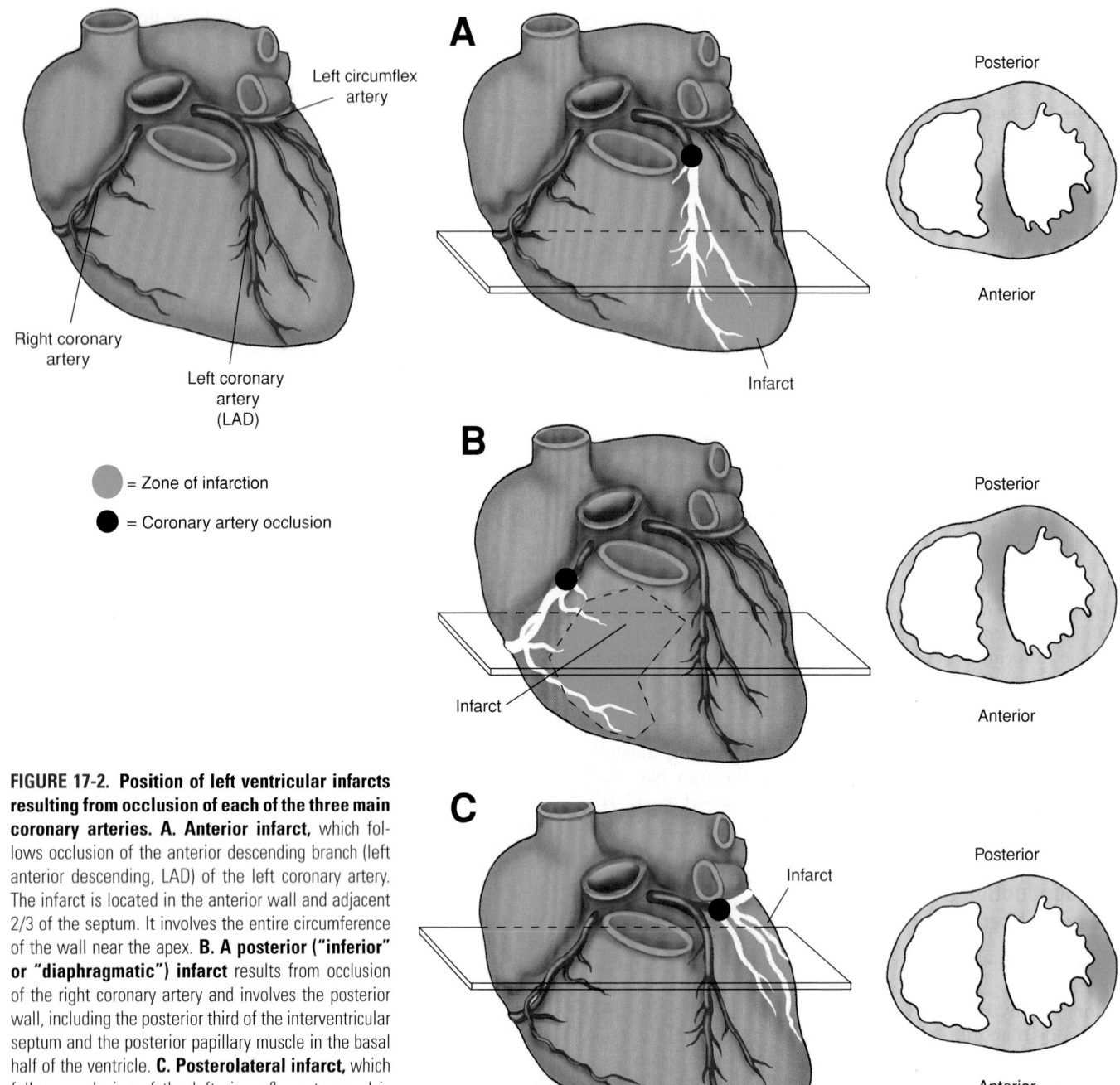

FIGURE 17-2. Position of left ventricular infarcts resulting from occlusion of each of the three main coronary arteries. A. Anterior infarct, which follows occlusion of the anterior descending branch (left anterior descending, LAD) of the left coronary artery. The infarct is located in the anterior wall and adjacent 2/3 of the septum. It involves the entire circumference of the wall near the apex. **B. A posterior ("inferior" or "diaphragmatic") infarct** results from occlusion of the right coronary artery and involves the posterior wall, including the posterior third of the interventricular septum and the posterior papillary muscle in the basal half of the ventricle. **C. Posterolateral infarct,** which follows occlusion of the left circumflex artery and is present in the posterolateral wall.

compressed by systolic muscular pressure. Thus, blood flow in the myocardium, especially in subendocardial ventricular regions, is lower or absent in systole. Autoregulation of blood flow roughly equalizes the myocardial supply, however.

MYOCARDIAL HYPERTROPHY AND HEART FAILURE

The ventricles are compliant in a normal heart, and diastolic filling occurs at low atrial pressures. During systole, ventricles contract vigorously and eject about 60% of the blood in them at the end of diastole **(ejection fraction)**. If a heart is injured, the clinical consequences are similar, regardless of the cause of cardiac dysfunction. *When initial impairment is severe, cardiac output is not maintained despite compensatory changes and the result is acute, life-threatening, cardiogenic shock.* For a lesser impairment, compensatory mechanisms (see below) maintain cardiac output by increasing diastolic ventricular filling pressure and end-diastolic volume. This results in the characteristic signs and symptoms of congestive heart failure. Because of the heart's capacity to compensate, congestive heart failure is often tolerated for years.

The heart's ability to adapt to injury is based on the same mechanisms that allow cardiac output to rise in response to stress. *Compensation reflects the Frank-Starling law: cardiac stroke volume is a function of diastolic fiber length;*

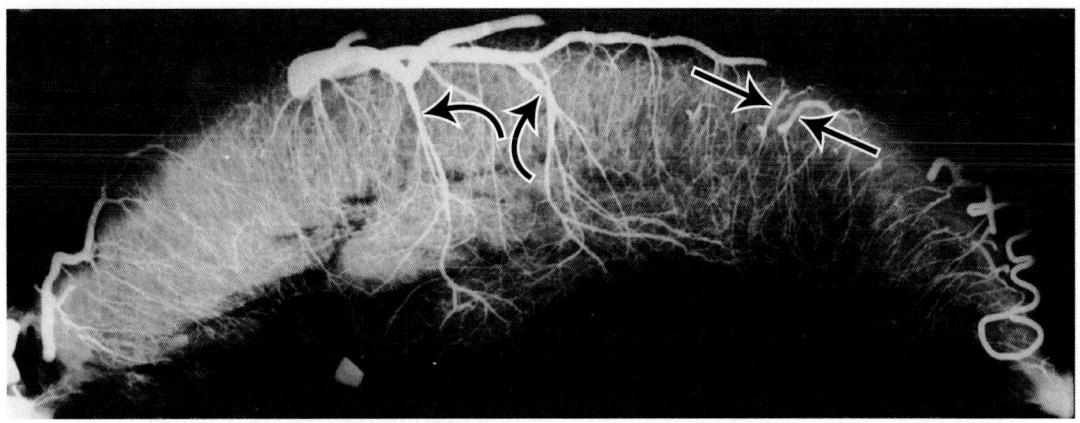

FIGURE 17-3. Arteriogram of a longitudinal segment of the posterior wall of the left ventricle including the posterior papillary muscle. Note the two types of branches passing into the myocardium at right angles to the epicardial artery (*top*): class A, which quickly divide into a fine network (*straight arrows*), and class B, which maintain a large diameter and pass with little branching into the subendocardial region and the papillary muscle (*curved arrows*).

within certain limits, a normal heart will pump whatever volume the venous circulation brings to it (Fig. 17-4). Stroke volume, a measure of ventricular function, increases with greater ventricular end-diastolic volume owing to increased atrial filling pressure.

Increased contractile force in response to ventricular dilation is a result of myofibrillar organization: stretching of sarcomeres allows greater potential overlap of thick and thin filaments during contraction. This permits enhanced force generation, as long as the sarcomere is not stretched

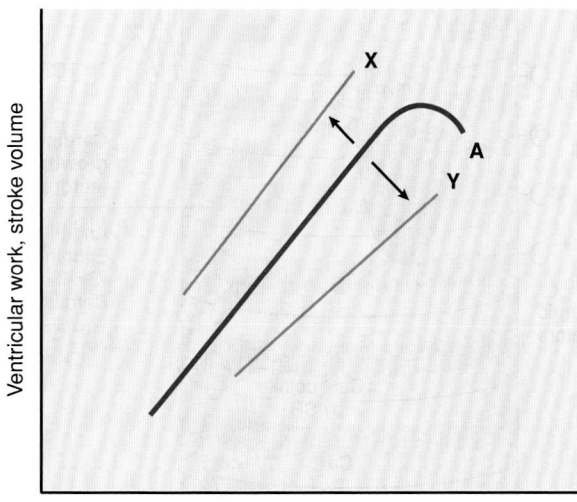

FIGURE 17-4. Relation between the work of the heart (or stroke volume) and the level of venous inflow, as measured by atrial pressure, ventricular end-diastolic volume (EDV) or end-diastolic pressure (EDP). *Curve A* indicates that as ventricular EDV, EDP or left atrial pressure increases, the amount of work done by the heart increases linearly up to a point. Beyond this point, the work done decreases, and the heart fails. However, the downslope of this curve is reached only at very high left atrial pressures. The curve may shift upward to position *X* or downward to position *Y,* depending on whether contractility has increased (e.g., because of the action of norepinephrine) or decreased (i.e., in failure), respectively. The failing heart usually functions on the ascending limb of a depressed curve.

beyond 2.2 µm. When there is a sudden need to increase cardiac output in a normal heart, as during exercise, catecholamine stimulation increases both heart rate and contractility. The latter is mainly mediated by modulating the activities of key proteins that regulate Ca^{2+} transients during excitation–contraction coupling. Thus, the normal relationship between end-diastolic volume and stroke volume is shifted upward (from curve A to curve X in Fig. 17-4). End-diastolic volume may also increase, causing a large increase in cardiac output.

If a heart is injured, overall cardiac function tends to be depressed in the basal state. Higher than normal filling pressures are then required to maintain cardiac output (curve Y in Fig. 17-4). Moreover, in cardiac failure, catecholamine stimulation is often present in the basal state. Comparable increases in cardiac output thus require greater increases in atrial pressure in failing hearts than in normal ones. *The most prominent feature of heart failure is abnormally high atrial filling pressure relative to stroke volume.* However, the absolute values of stroke volume and cardiac output are generally well maintained.

PATHOPHYSIOLOGY: Myocardial hypertrophy is an adaptive response that augments myocyte contractile strength. There is a distinction between **physiologic hypertrophy,** which develops in highly trained athletes, and **pathologic hypertrophy,** which occurs because of injury or disease. While there is considerable overlap in the molecular mechanisms leading to these different forms of hypertrophy, there must also be important differences, since the athlete's enlarged heart is highly efficient while a diseased heart of similar mass is structurally and functionally deficient. These disparities are not well understood but may reflect the fact that the demands of exercise are intermittent, while those of disease (e.g., chronic hypertension) are unceasing. Differences in angiogenesis may also play a role.

Pathologic hypertrophy is a compensatory response to hemodynamic overload, which occurs in association with chronic hypertension or valvular stenosis **(pressure overload),** myocardial injury, valvular insufficiency

(volume overload) and other stresses that increase the heart's workload. It also develops as a response to primary injury of cardiac myocytes as in cardiomyopathies (see below). It results in enlargement of cardiac myocytes by assembly of new sarcomeres. Until recently, this had been thought to occur without an increase in the number of cardiac myocytes, but it is now known that cardiac progenitor cells exist with at least the potential to contribute to hyperplastic growth (see below).

Hypertrophy at first entails compensatory and possibly reversible mechanisms, but with persistent stress, the myocardium becomes irreversibly enlarged and dilated.

MOLECULAR PATHOGENESIS: *Receptor-mediated myocardial events that are triggered by a stimulus promote the hypertrophic response by autocrine and paracrine mechanisms.* Contractile cells respond to mechanical stimuli, such as stretching or pressure overload, by releasing ligands that activate receptor-mediated signaling pathways to produce hypertrophy (Fig. 17-5). Among the most important ligands are (1) angiotensin II (AngII), (2) endothelin-1 (ET-1), (3) norepinephrine (NE) and (4) various growth factors, including insulin-like growth factor-I (IGF-I) and transforming growth factor-I (TGF-I). Some of these mediators may also act on interstitial

fibroblasts in the heart to promote synthesis and deposition of extracellular matrix. These ligands bind to and activate G-protein–coupled receptors and receptor tyrosine kinases to initiate intracellular signaling cascades, the most important of which include (1) mitogen-activated protein kinases (MAPKs), phosphoinositide-3-kinases (PI3Ks) and β-adrenergic (protein kinase A) and protein kinase C (PKC) pathways, which are all activated by G-protein–coupled receptors; and (2) Ca^{2+}/calmodulin-dependent protein kinase (CaMK) pathways, which are regulated by Ca^{2+}. Events mediated by β-adrenergic receptors are implicated in the transition from compensatory hypertrophy to heart failure. Ligands, signaling cascades, downstream targets and mechanisms mediating the hypertrophic response are described below (see also Chapter 1).

ANGIOTENSIN II: Cardiac myocytes and fibroblasts both contain all components of the renin–angiotensin system (renin, angiotensinogen, angiotensin-converting enzyme [ACE] and AngII receptors). AngII is released locally in response to load or stress stimuli and acts by autocrine and paracrine mechanisms to promote myocyte protein synthesis and hypertrophy and stimulate fibroblast proliferation and secretion of extracellular matrix. AngII interacts with two different classes of receptors to activate, directly or indirectly, multiple signaling cascades including those involving MAPKs and CaMK. Use of ACE inhibitors tends to reverse cardiac hypertrophy and to normalize heart size.

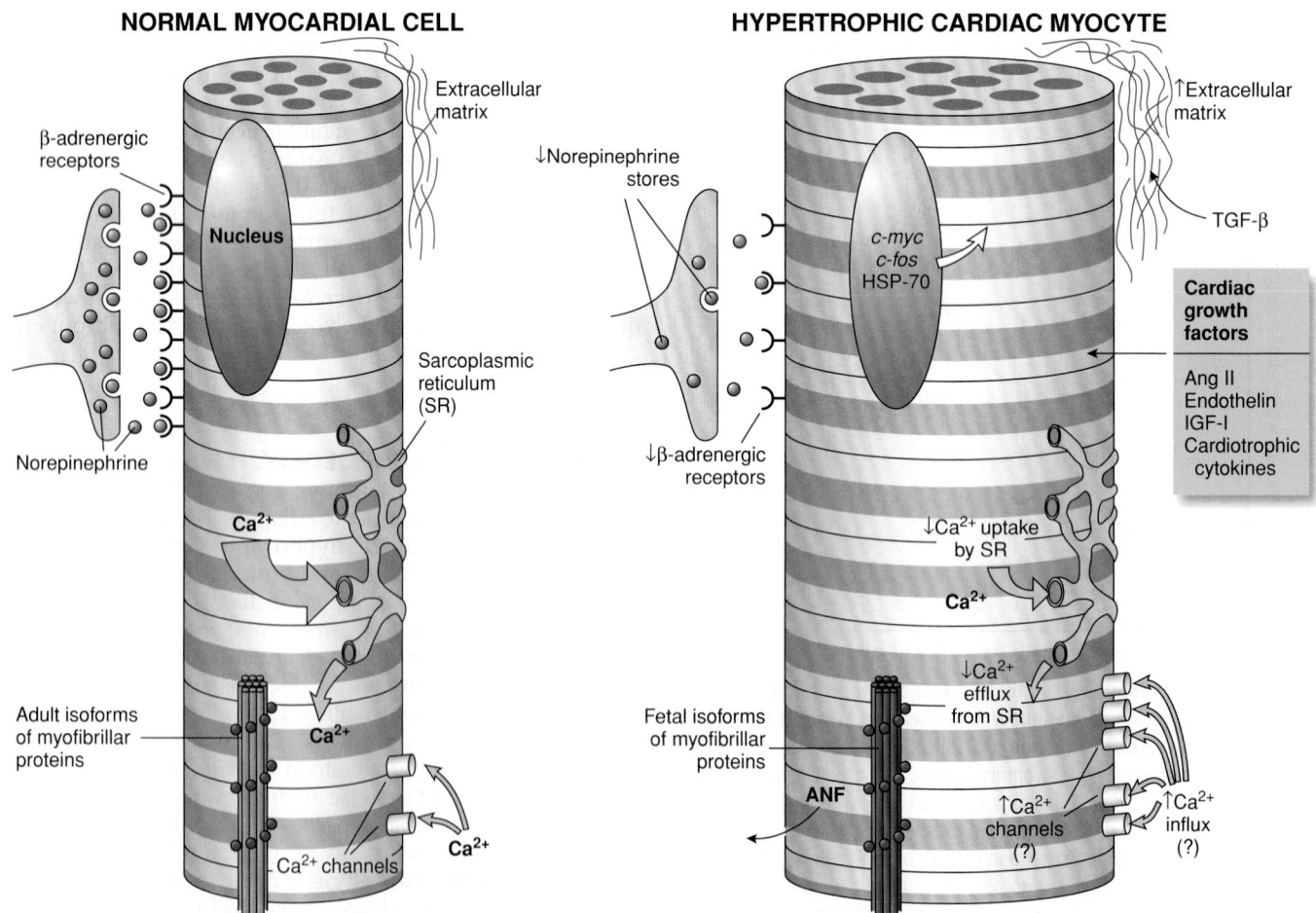

FIGURE 17-5. Biochemical characteristics of myocardial hypertrophy and congestive heart failure. *ANF* = atrial natriuretic factor; *Ang II* = angiotensin II; *HSP-70* = heat shock protein 70; *IGF* = insulin-like growth factor; *TGF* = transforming growth factor.

ACE inhibitors also prevent cardiac hypertrophy induced by experimental hypertension, without reducing the elevated arterial pressure.

ENDOTHELIN-1: ET-1 is a powerful vasoconstrictor produced by many cells, including endothelial cells and cardiac myocytes. It is also a potent growth factor for cardiac myocytes. Like AngII, ET-1 activates MAPK cascades upon binding to its receptor, to promote cardiac hypertrophy.

INSULIN-LIKE GROWTH FACTOR-I: IGF-I is a growth-promoting peptide synthesized in most tissues. As a growth factor for cardiac myocytes, IGF-I acts through PI3K pathways to promote cardiac hypertrophy.

EXTRACELLULAR MATRIX: Short-term heart overload leads to a prompt increase in collagen synthesis. Interstitial fibrosis, which occurs in virtually all forms of heart failure, is an obligatory feature of the hypertrophic response. Deposition of matrix proteins results, at least in part, from stimulation of cardiac fibroblasts by TGF-β and AngII. After myocardial infarction, fibrosis is important in replacing necrotic myocytes and preventing cardiac rupture. However, when it occurs diffusely, myocardial fibrosis can interfere with diastolic relaxation and impair diffusion of oxygen and nutrients. It can also lead to remodeling of electrical conduction pathways, and so is a major factor in the pathogenesis of atrial fibrillation and ventricular tachycardia.

MITOGEN-ACTIVATED PROTEIN KINASE PATHWAYS: MAPK cascades modulate hypertrophic responses to pressure overload. Activation of ERK1/2 (extracellular receptor kinase 1/2) signaling stimulates growth and survival of cardiac myocytes, while activation of JNK (c-Jun N-terminal kinase) and p38 MAPK cascades is involved in pathologic remodeling and apoptosis of cardiac myocytes.

PI3K PATHWAYS: Activation of PI3K leads to phosphorylation of membrane lipids and generation of second messengers such as phosphatidylinositol-3,4,5-trisphosphate. Receptor tyrosine kinases like IGF-I receptor activate the p110α isoform of PI3K. This isoform helps mediate physiologic hypertrophy in response to exercise training, promotes cell survival, inhibits cardiac fibrosis and attenuates pathologic hypertrophy. By contrast, activation of the p110α isoform of PI3K is detrimental as it promotes internalization of β-adrenergic receptors and inhibits sarco/endoplasmic reticulum Ca^{2+}-ATPase (SERCA) activity.

β-ADRENERGIC SIGNALING AND DESENSITIZATION: Stimulation of β-adrenergic receptors by norepinephrine (NE) turns on the stimulatory G protein G_S and activates adenylyl cyclase. The latter produces cyclic adenosine monophosphate (cAMP) as a second messenger, activating protein kinase A to enhance contractility. Poor responses to catecholamines by chronically failing hearts likely reflect adaptive responses to increases in circulating NE in heart failure. Desensitization of β-adrenergic receptors contributes to sluggish responses of a failing heart to exercise. Chronic overstimulation leads to decreased numbers and responsiveness of β-adrenergic receptors and a defect in coupling to adenylyl cyclase. Failing hearts also store less norepinephrine in autonomic nerve endings. Although $β_1$-adrenergic receptors are desensitized in heart failure, treatment to block this receptor class reduces mortality and improves contractile function in patients with advanced heart failure. Seemingly paradoxically, this response is consistent with abundant evidence that $β_1$-adrenergic receptors mediate cardiotoxic effects of NE in the failing heart including maladaptive cardiac myocyte hypertrophy and

apoptosis, interstitial fibrosis, contractile dysfunction and sudden death.

CALCIUM HOMEOSTASIS: Defects in Ca^{2+} homeostasis occur in hypertrophy and heart failure. Expression and function of key Ca^{2+}-regulating proteins in cardiac myocytes are altered (see Fig. 17-1B):

- **Ryanodine receptor-2 (RyR2),** the major Ca^{2+} release channel in the SR, is activated during the action potential by influx of extracellular Ca^{2+} through voltage-gated channels in T tubules. Decreased numbers of RyR2 channels impair contractile function by reducing the rate of Ca^{2+} release from SR.
- **SERCA** is the pump responsible for Ca^{2+} reuptake into SR after contraction. Lower SR Ca^{2+} uptake is caused by fewer and abnormal regulation of SERCA. As a result, impaired Ca^{2+} sequestration in diastole leads to impaired relaxation.
- **Phospholamban** is a key regulator of cardiac contractility that inhibits SERCA. Enhanced phospholamban–SERCA interactions lead to chronically elevated Ca^{2+} levels during diastole, which is considered to play a critical role in chronic heart failure and arrhythmias.
- **CaMK pathways** are important in excitation–contraction coupling. CaMKII, the main cardiac isoform, modulates actions of Ca^{2+} handling proteins such as SERCA, phospholamban, RyR2 and the voltage-gated L-type Ca^{2+} channel. Myocardial CaMKII is increased in heart failure, contributing to abnormal Ca^{2+} homeostasis.

PROTO-ONCOGENES AND MYOCARDIAL HYPERTROPHY: Cardiac myocytes respond to acute pressure overload within an hour of its onset, by expressing proto-oncogenes c-*jun* and c-*fos* and heat shock protein 70 (Hsp70). These effects are mediated by AngII signaling and other pathways. Transcription of proto-oncogenes helps to reexpress fetal protein isoforms in the hypertrophic heart.

EXPRESSION OF FETAL GENES: Several protein isoforms are expressed in fetal hearts, but not after birth. In cardiac hypertrophy induced by hemodynamic overload, many of these genes are reexpressed. For example, atrial natriuretic factor (ANF) is made in the fetal ventricle and atrium, but its production is restricted to the atrium after birth. In hypertrophic ventricles, however, ANF and brain natriuretic protein (now called B-type natriuretic protein or BNP) are abundantly reexpressed and reduce hemodynamic overload via effects on salt and water metabolism (see Chapter 7). Blood BNP levels are a useful biomarker of the severity of heart failure.

Cardiac hypertrophy also elicits reexpression of fetal isoforms of several contractile proteins. In the rat, the normal adult isoform is a β-myosin with high ATPase activity and a rapid shortening velocity. By contrast, the fetal β-myosin has less ATPase activity and a slower shortening velocity. In experimental cardiac hypertrophy, "fast" β-myosin is replaced by "slow" β-myosin, leading to impaired myocardial contractility. However, this change in myosin gene expression is also adaptive, as it increases the tension generated during systole and improves contraction efficiency, thus conserving energy. Hypertrophied hearts exhibit similar, but not identical, changes in myosin isoforms. Ventricles contain only slow myosin, and hypertrophic hearts change from fast to slow myosin only in the atrium. However, fetal isoforms of other myofibrillar proteins appear in ventricular myocardium, including fetal forms of actin and tropomyosin. Hypertrophied hearts also contain abnormal varieties of lactic dehydrogenase (LDH), creatine kinase (CK) and the sarcolemmal sodium pump.

Another adaptive gene switch occurs in energy metabolism. Fetal hearts rely mainly on maternally derived glucose for ATP production. After birth, however, the heart downregulates glycolytic enzymes and increases expression of genes that encode proteins mediating β-oxidation of fatty acids derived from breast milk. The failing heart reverts to using glucose by reexpressing fetal patterns of genes for energy generation. Although a mole of glucose yields less ATP than a mole of fatty acid, glycolytic metabolism uses less oxygen. For a failing heart, this switch is therefore advantageous.

Recent advances in understanding the molecular pathogenesis of heart failure have identified a role for histone acetylases and deacetylases in stress-activated myocyte signaling pathways. DNA-binding histone proteins control gene expression by modulating chromatin structure and controlling access of transcriptional activators and repressors to critical regulatory DNA sequences. Activation of stress-related signaling pathways involving G-protein–coupled receptors for NE, ET-1, AngII and others ultimately shifts patterns of histone acetylation and gene expression patterns. This switch entails changes in subcellular localization and activities of histone acetylases and deacetylases, suggesting that manipulation of histone-modifying enzymes may be useful in preventing heart failure.

Another emerging regulatory network in cardiac myocytes involves microRNAs (miRNAs; see Chapter 5), hundreds of species of which are expressed in the heart, where they may help to orchestrate expression of large groups of genes important in development and phenotypic specification. miRNAs do not encode proteins but rather bind target mRNAs in a sequence-specific manner, to promote their degradation or inhibit their translation. Specific patterns of miRNAs are upregulated in response to stress and have been implicated in mediating the hypertrophic response.

Apoptosis of cardiac myocytes may be important in heart failure. Apoptosis of cardiac myocytes increases 5-fold in animal models of heart disease, and senescent rats have 30% fewer cardiac myocytes than do young ones. Pathologic hypertrophy is generally associated with greater cardiac myocyte apoptosis, which may help transition from compensated hypertrophy to heart failure. Signaling by agonists such as AngII and ET-1 increases expression of proapoptotic genes via JNK and p38 MAPK pathways, and signaling by adrenergic agonists increases cardiac myocyte sensitivity to apoptotic stimuli. In contrast, p110α PI3K signaling via the IGF-I receptor enhances survival. Thus, diverse signaling pathways in cardiac hypertrophy may exert both proapoptotic and antiapoptotic influences, the final outcome depending on the balance between them.

CARDIAC STEM CELLS AND MYOCARDIAL REGENERATION: The heart has traditionally been thought of as a static organ incapable of growing new myocytes to regenerate or repair damage owing to a lack of cardiac stem cells. A few binucleated cardiac myocytes occur in normal hearts. These increase in number with age or in disease, indicating a capacity for nuclear division. However, it is clear that cardiac stem cells exist in adults and that during a lifetime, the heart continuously replaces myocytes, endothelial cells and fibroblasts at a slow rate (see Chapter 1). Increasing evidence also indicates that new cardiac myocytes can also arise directly from existing myocytes, and this process is increased

in response to stress or disease. Still, the heart's regenerative capacity is quite limited. Current research focuses on strategies to exploit this capacity in order to replace damaged or necrotic muscle.

 PATHOLOGY: Anything that increases cardiac workload for a prolonged period or produces structural damage may lead to myocardial failure. *Ischemic heart disease is by far the most common cause of cardiac failure, accounting for more than 80% of deaths from heart disease.* Most of the rest are caused by nonischemic heart muscle disease (cardiomyopathies) and congenital heart diseases. Virtually all body organs suffer when the heart fails (see Chapter 7).

Other than changes characteristic of specific diseases (e.g., ischemic heart disease or cardiac amyloidosis), the morphology of failing hearts is nonspecific. *Ventricular hypertrophy is seen in virtually all conditions associated with chronic heart failure.* Initially, only the left ventricle may be hypertrophied, as in compensated hypertensive heart disease. But when the left ventricle fails, some right ventricular hypertrophy usually follows, as the increased workload is imposed on the right ventricle by the failing left ventricle. *In most cases of clinically apparent systolic heart failure, the ventricles are conspicuously dilated.* The distribution of end-organ involvement depends on whether the heart failure is predominantly left sided or right sided.

Left-sided heart failure is more common, as the most common causes of cardiac injury (e.g., ischemic heart disease and hypertension) primarily affect the left ventricle. To compensate for left ventricular failure, left atrial and pulmonary venous pressures rise, resulting in passive pulmonary congestion. Alveolar septal capillaries fill with blood and small ruptures allow erythrocytes to escape. As a result, alveoli contain many hemosiderin-laden macrophages (so-called heart failure cells). If capillary hydrostatic pressure exceeds plasma osmotic pressure, fluid leaks from capillaries into alveoli. Resultant **pulmonary edema** (see Chapters 16 and 18) may be massive, with alveoli being "drowned" in a transudate. Interstitial pulmonary fibrosis results when congestion is present over an extended period.

Right-sided heart failure most commonly complicates left-sided failure, but it can develop independently due to intrinsic lung disease or pulmonary hypertension. The latter creates resistance to blood flow through the lung, causing right atrial pressure and systemic venous pressure to increase. Jugular veins become distended, edema accumulates in the legs and the liver and spleen become congested. Hepatic congestion in heart failure is characterized by distended central veins, which stand out on the cut surface of the liver as dark red foci against the yellow of cells in the lobular periphery. This gives the liver a gross appearance that has been compared to the cut surface of a nutmeg (hence, "nutmeg liver"; see Chapter 20).

Chronically injured cardiac myocytes lose myofibrils. Regardless of the type of injury, dysfunctional myocytes lose sarcomeres and correspondingly increase cytosol and glycogen. This process (**myocytolysis**) makes cells appear vacuolated (Fig. 17-6 shows a dramatic example). These changes likely result from reversible perturbations in myocyte metabolism. Myocytolysis may be an adaptive response to keep myocytes alive in the face of chronic injury and is quite prominent in "hibernating myocardium," in which contractile function is impaired at rest owing to reduced coronary blood flow.

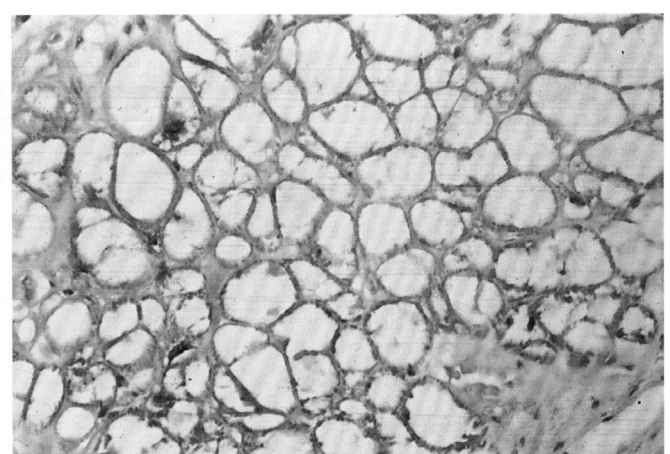

FIGURE 17-6. Severe myocytolysis in a patient with end-stage heart failure. Chronically injured myocytes show dramatic loss of myofibrils, giving the cells a marked vacuolated appearance. Only a thin rim of contractile cytoplasm is present, immediately beneath the sarcolemma.

TABLE 17-1

RELATIVE INCIDENCE OF SPECIFIC ANOMALIES IN PATIENTS WITH CONGENITAL HEART DISEASE

Ventricular septal defects: 25%–30%
Atrial septal defects: 10%–15%
Patent ductus arteriosus: 10%–20%
Tetralogy of Fallot: 4%–9%
Pulmonary stenosis: 5%–7%
Coarctation of the aorta: 5%–7%
Aortic stenosis: 4%–6%
Complete transposition of the great arteries: 4%–10%
Truncus arteriosus: 2%
Tricuspid atresia: 1%

Diastolic heart failure, often seen in elderly patients, has become an important clinical problem as life expectancy has increased. Ventricles become progressively stiffer with advancing age and require greater filling (diastolic) pressures. Some patients exhibit signs and symptoms of heart failure even though their hearts are normal in size and have normal systolic contractile function. These patients do not tolerate increases in blood volume well and are susceptible to developing pulmonary edema in response to a fluid challenge. These hearts typically show interstitial fibrosis, which may contribute to the decreased compliance of ventricular myocardium. Still, mechanisms responsible for diastolic heart failure are poorly understood.

 CLINICAL FEATURES: Symptoms of left-sided failure include respiratory distress with exercise **(dyspnea on exertion), orthopnea** (dyspnea when lying down) and **paroxysmal nocturnal dyspnea** (dyspnea that awakens patients from sleep). Dyspnea on exertion reflects the increasing pulmonary congestion that accompanies a higher end-diastolic pressure in the left atrium and ventricle. Orthopnea and paroxysmal nocturnal dyspnea result when lung blood volume increases, owing to reduced blood volume in the legs during recumbency.

Although much of the clinical presentation of heart failure can be explained by venous congestion **(backward failure),** important aspects of congestive failure involve inadequate perfusion of vital organs **(forward failure).** Most patients with left-sided heart failure retain sodium and water (edema) owing to poor renal perfusion, decreased glomerular filtration rate and renin–angiotensin–aldosterone system activation (see Chapter 7). Inadequate cerebral perfusion can lead to confusion, memory loss and disorientation. Reduced perfusion of skeletal muscle leads to fatigue and weakness.

CONGENITAL HEART DISEASE

Congenital heart disease (CHD) results from faulty embryonic development, expressed either as misplaced structures (e.g., transposition of the great vessels) or arrested progression of a normal structure from an early stage to a more advanced one (e.g., atrial septal defect).

Significant CHD occurs in almost 1% of live births. This does not include certain common defects that are not functionally important, such as an anatomically patent foramen ovale that is functionally closed by the left atrial flap that covers it. In this case, the foramen ovale remains closed as long as left atrial pressure exceeds that in the right atrium. Bicuspid aortic valves are also common and are usually asymptomatic until adulthood. Estimates of the incidence of specific cardiovascular anomalies depend on many factors. A range derived from several sources is shown in Table 17-1.

 ETIOLOGIC FACTORS: The best evidence for a role of intrauterine influence in congenital cardiac defects is maternal rubella infection during the first trimester, especially during the first 4 weeks of gestation. Associations with other viral infections are suspected but are not as well documented. Maternal use of certain drugs in early pregnancy is also associated with increased cardiac defects in offspring. For example, 10% of babies with thalidomide syndrome (phocomelia) had CHD (see Chapter 6). Other drugs implicated in CHD include alcohol, amphetamines, phenytoin, lithium and estrogens. Maternal diabetes is also associated with increased incidence of CHD.

 MOLECULAR PATHOGENESIS: Causes of CHD are not usually clear. However, it is worthwhile to determine whether a defect in any one case is most likely to be of genetic origin or probably acquired, as this issue is important to parents in planning future pregnancies. Most congenital heart defects reflect multifactorial genetic, epigenetic and environmental influences. As in other diseases with complex inheritance (see Chapter 6), risk of recurrence is greater among siblings of an affected child: CHD occurs in 1% of the general population; this increases to 2–15% for pregnancies after the birth of a child with a heart defect. The risk of a third affected child may reach 30%. Also, infants born to mothers with CHD have increased risk for CHD.

Chromosomal abnormalities may cause CHD, most prominently Down syndrome (trisomy 21), other trisomies, Turner syndrome and DiGeorge syndrome. Together, these account for no more than 5% of cases of CHD.

Much has been learned recently about genes encoding transcription factors that regulate cardiogenesis. The best studied is *Csx/NKX2.5*, a member of the evolutionarily conserved *NK* homeobox gene family. *Csx/NKX2.5* is a mammalian homolog of the *Drosophila* gene *NK4*, also known as *tinman* (from the *Wizard of Oz*) because deletion of this gene leads to failure of cardiac myocyte fate specification and lack of formation of a heart. Cardiac myocytes are formed when *Csx/NKX2.5* is deleted in mammals, but certain features of morphogenesis are arrested and growth of the heart tube is retarded. Expression of several cardiac genes is also reduced, including genes encoding myosin light chain 2v, ANF, cardiac ankyrin repeat protein and various transcription factors such as dHAND and eHAND, which are expressed in chamber-specific patterns and exert important regulatory influences over the development of the right and left ventricles. Various mutations in *Csx/NKX2.5* in humans have been associated with a spectrum of congenital cardiac malformations including atrial and ventricular septal defects, tetralogy of Fallot, double-outlet right ventricle, tricuspid valve abnormalities and hypoplastic left heart syndrome. Mutations in other transcription factors have been linked to congenital heart disease (*GATA4* and atrial and ventricular septal defects; *TBX1* and malformations of outflow septation such as tetralogy of Fallot and persistent truncus arteriosus), and mutations in *NOTCH1* (see Chapter 5) are linked to congenital malformations of the aortic valve. Increasing evidence also implicates alterations in histone methylation, an epigenetic mechanism that regulates expression of many genes during ontogeny and afterward. As many as 10% of patients with severe congenital cardiac malformations may harbor somatic mutations that arose during development in genes regulating histone methylation in the heart.

Classifications of Congenital Heart Disease Reflect Cyanosis and Shunting

There are several ways to categorize congenital heart defects. One clinically useful approach puts cases into three groups based on the presence or absence of cyanosis:

- The **acyanotic group** does not have an abnormal communication between systemic and pulmonary circuits. Examples of the acyanotic group include coarctation of the aorta, right-sided aortic arch and Ebstein malformation.
- The **cyanose tardive group** is defined as an initial left-to-right shunt with late reversal of flow, including patent ductus arteriosus (PDA), patent foramen ovale and ventricular septal defect. In patients with these anomalies, cyanosis supervenes later (i.e., tardive). Although the shunt is initially left to right, it later becomes right to left (**Eisenmenger complex**) because progressive increases in pulmonary vascular resistance cause the right ventricular pressure to rise to the point where it exceeds that in the left ventricle (see below).
- The **cyanotic group** entails a permanent right-to-left shunt. These CHDs include tetralogy of Fallot, truncus arteriosus, tricuspid atresia and complete transposition of the great vessels.

TABLE 17-2
CLASSIFICATION OF CONGENITAL HEART DISEASE
Initial Left-to-Right Shunt
Ventricular septal defect
Atrial septal defect
Patent ductus arteriosus
Persistent truncus arteriosus
Anomalous pulmonary venous drainage
Hypoplastic left heart syndrome
Right-to-Left Shunt
Tetralogy of Fallot
Tricuspid atresia
No Shunt
Complete transposition of the great vessels
Coarctation of the aorta
Pulmonary stenosis
Aortic stenosis
Coronary artery origin from pulmonary artery
Ebstein malformation
Complete heart block
Endocardial fibroelastosis

Additional classification schemes have been developed to provide the detail necessary to meet clinical requirements, especially those of the cardiac surgeon. **A more contemporary classification divides cases into the groups shown in Table 17-2.**

Early Left-to-Right Shunt Reflects the Higher Pressure on the Left Side of the Heart

Ventricular Septal Defect

Ventricular septal defects (VSDs) are among the most common congenital heart lesions (Table 17-1). They occur as isolated lesions or in combination with other malformations.

 **ETIOLOGIC FACTORS:** The fetal heart consists of a single chamber until the fifth week of gestation, after which development of interatrial and interventricular septa and formation of atrioventricular valves from endocardial cushions divide it. A muscular interventricular septum grows upward from the apex toward the base of the heart (Fig. 17-7). It is joined by the downward-growing membranous septum, separating right and left ventricles. *The most common VSD is related to partial or incomplete formation of the membranous portion of the septum.*

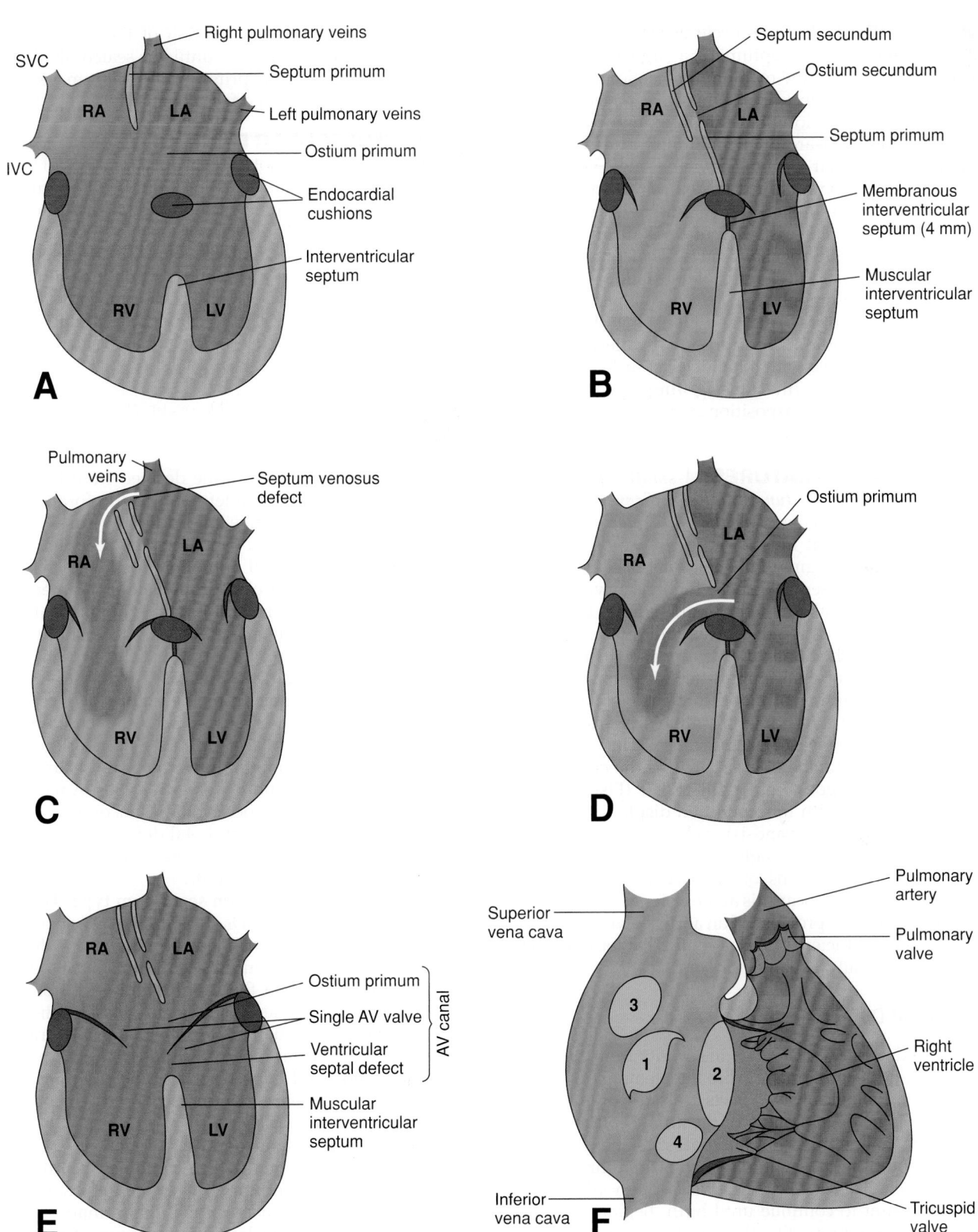

FIGURE 17-7. Pathogenesis of ventricular and atrial septal defects. A. The common atrial chamber is being separated into the right and left atria (RA and LA) by the septum primum. Because the septum primum has not yet joined the endocardial cushions, there is an open ostium primum. The ventricular cavity is being divided by a muscular interventricular septum into right and left chambers (right and left ventricles, RV and LV). *IVC* = inferior vena cava; *SVC* = superior vena cava. **B.** The septum primum has joined the endocardial cushions but at the same time has developed an opening in its midportion (the ostium secundum). This opening is partly overlaid by the septum secundum, which has grown down to cover, in part, the foramen ovale. Simultaneously, the membranous septum joins the muscular interventricular septum to the base of the heart, completely separating the ventricles. **C.** The **sinus venosus type of atrial septal** defect is located in the most cephalad region and is adjacent to the inflow of the right pulmonary veins, which thus tend to open into the RA. **D.** The **ostium primum defect** occurs just above the atrioventricular (AV) valve ring, sometimes in the presence of an intact valve ring. It may also, in conjunction with a defect of the valve ring and ventricular septum, form an AV canal, as shown in panel **E.** This common opening allows free communication between the atria and the ventricles. **F. Location of atrial septal defects.** In decreasing order of frequency: 1. Ostium secundum. 2. Ostium primum. 3. Sinus venosus. 4. Coronary sinus type.

PATHOLOGY: VSDs occur as (1) a small hole in the membranous septum; (2) a large defect involving more than the membranous region (perimembranous defects); (3) defects in the muscular portion, which are more common anteriorly but can occur anywhere in the muscular septum and are often multiple; or (4) complete absence of the muscular septum (leaving a single ventricle).

VSDs are most common in the superior portion of the septum below the pulmonary artery outflow tract (below the crista supraventricularis, i.e., infracristal) and behind the septal leaflet of the tricuspid valve. The common bundle (bundle of His) is located immediately below the defect (inlet type). Less commonly, the defect is above the crista supraventricularis (supracristal) and just below the pulmonary valve (infra-arterial). The supracristal variety of septal defect is often associated with other defects, such as an overriding pulmonary artery (the **Taussig-Bing** type of double-outlet right ventricle), transposition of the great vessels or persistent truncus arteriosus.

CLINICAL FEATURES: *A small septal defect may have little functional significance and may close spontaneously as the child matures.* Either hypertrophy of adjacent muscle or adherence of tricuspid valve leaflets to the margins of the hole may close the defect. In infants with large septal defects, higher left ventricular pressure creates initially a left-to-right shunt. Left ventricular dilation and congestive heart failure are common complications of such shunts. If a defect is small enough to permit prolonged survival, augmented pulmonary blood flow caused by shunting of blood into the right ventricle eventually results in thickening of pulmonary arteries and increased pulmonary vascular resistance. This increased vascular resistance may be so great that the direction of the shunt reverses, and goes from right to left **(Eisenmenger complex)**. A patient with this condition displays late onset of cyanosis (i.e., tardive cyanosis), right ventricular hypertrophy and right-sided heart failure.

Additional complications of ventricular septal defects include (1) infective endocarditis at the lesional site, (2) paradoxical emboli and (3) prolapse of an aortic valve cusp (with resulting aortic insufficiency). Large ventricular septal defects are repaired surgically, usually in infancy.

Atrial Septal Defects

Atrial septal defects (ASDs) range in severity from clinically insignificant and asymptomatic to life-threatening conditions. They arise embryologically by defects in atrial septum formation. Embryologic development of the atrial septum occurs in a sequence that permits continued passage of oxygenated placental blood from the right to the left atrium through the patent foramen. The developing atrial septum allows this right-to-left shunt to continue until birth. Beginning at the fifth week of intrauterine life, the septum primum extends downward from the roof of the common atrium to join to the endocardial cushions, thus closing the incomplete segment, or "ostium primum" (Fig. 17-7A). Before this closure is complete, the midportion of the septum primum develops a defect, or "ostium secundum," so that right-to-left flow continues. During the sixth week, a second septum (septum secundum) develops to the right of the septum primum, passing from the roof of the atrium toward the endocardial cushions (Fig. 17-7B). This process leaves a patent foramen,

the **foramen ovale,** in the position of the original ostium secundum. The defect persists until it is sealed off after birth by fusion of the septum primum and septum secundum, whereupon it is termed the **fossa ovalis**.

MOLECULAR PATHOGENESIS: The cause of most ASDs is not known, but a minority of them are parts of certain genetic syndromes. About 15% of familial ASDs and 3% of sporadic ASDs are associated with coding errors in *NKX2.5*. Deletion of the T-box gene *TBX1* in DiGeorge syndrome (chromosome 22Q11 deletion) has been implicated in ASD formation. Mutations in a related T-box gene, *TBX5*, cause Holt-Oram syndrome in which large secundum-type ASDs typically occur. Mutations in the cardiac transcription factor *GATA4* are associated with both ASDs and VSDs.

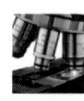

PATHOLOGY: ASDs occur at a number of sites (Fig. 17-7).

- **Patent foramen ovale:** Tissue derived from the septum primum situated on the left side of the foramen ovale functions as a flap valve that normally fuses with the margins of the foramen ovale, thereby sealing the opening. An incomplete seal of the foramen ovale, which can be traversed with a probe **(probe patent foramen ovale),** occurs in 25% of normal adults and is not normally problematic. However, it may become a true shunt if right atrial pressure increases (e.g., with recurrent pulmonary thromboemboli). In this case, a right-to-left shunt develops, and emboli from the right-sided circulation pass directly into the systemic circuit. Such **paradoxical emboli** may cause infarcts in many parts of the arterial circulation, most commonly in the brain, heart, spleen, intestines, kidneys and lower extremities. A widely patent foramen ovale is occasionally encountered and is actually an acquired atrial septal defect caused by a disproportion between the size of the foramen ovale and the length of the valve covering it.
- **Atrial septal defect, ostium secundum type:** This defect accounts for 90% of ASDs. It is a true deficiency of the atrial septum and should not be confused with a patent foramen ovale. Ostium secundum defects occur in the middle portion of the septum and vary from trivial openings to large defects of the entire fossa ovalis region. Small defects are usually not problematic, but larger ones may allow sufficient blood to shunt from left to right to cause dilation and hypertrophy of the right atrium and ventricle. In this setting, pulmonary artery diameter may exceed that of the aorta.

  Lutembacher syndrome, a variant of the ostium secundum atrial septal defect, combines mitral stenosis and an ostium secundum atrial septal defect. Mitral stenosis may be due to a congenital malformation or rheumatic fever. Increased left atrial pressure due to mitral valve obstruction keeps the atrial septum patent.
- **Sinus venosus defect:** This anomaly, accounting for 5% of ASDs, occurs in the upper portion of the atrial septum, above the fossa ovalis, near the entry of the superior vena cava (Fig. 17-7C). It is usually accompanied by drainage of right pulmonary veins into the right atrium or superior vena cava.
- **Atrial septal defect, ostium primum type:** This condition involves the region adjacent to the endocardial cushions

(Fig. 17-7D) and makes up 7% of atrial septal defects. There are usually clefts in the anterior mitral valve leaflet and the septal leaflet of the tricuspid valve, which may be accompanied by a defect in the adjacent interventricular septum.

- **Atrioventricular canal:**
    - **Persistent common atrioventricular canal** represents fully developed combined atrial and ventricular septal defects (Fig. 17-7E). Although quite uncommon, this defect occurs often in patients with Down syndrome.
    - **Complete atrioventricular canal** occurs when atrioventricular endocardial cushions fail to fuse. As a result, the defect includes (1) an enlarged ostium primum atrial septal defect, (2) an inlet ventricular septal defect and (3) clefts in the mitral valve anterior leaflet and the tricuspid valve septal leaflet.
    - **Incomplete (partial) atrioventricular canal** is a situation in which an ostium primum atrial septal defect is adjacent to the atrioventricular valves, which are often abnormal.
- **Coronary sinus atrial septal defect:** This is the rarest of atrial septal defects. It is situated in the posteroinferior part of the interatrial septum by the coronary sinus ostium and is associated with a persistent left superior vena cava, which drains into the roof of the left atrium.

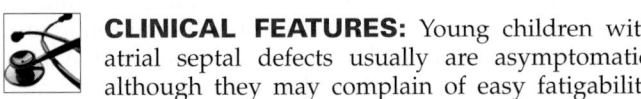 **CLINICAL FEATURES:** Young children with atrial septal defects usually are asymptomatic, although they may complain of easy fatigability and dyspnea on exertion. Later in life, usually in adulthood, changes in the pulmonary vasculature may reverse blood flow through the defect and create a right-to-left shunt. Then, cyanosis and clubbing of the fingers ensue. Complications of atrial septal defects include atrial arrhythmias, pulmonary hypertension, right ventricular hypertrophy, heart failure, paradoxical emboli and bacterial endocarditis. Symptomatic cases are treated surgically or with new closure devices, which can be delivered and placed percutaneously.

Patent Ductus Arteriosus

The early embryo supposedly recapitulates an ancestral evolutionary stage, with six aortic arches connecting ventral and dorsal aortas as part of the branchial cleft system (Fig. 17-8A). The left sixth aortic arch is partly preserved as the pulmonary arteries, and the arterial continuation on the left to the descending thoracic aorta becomes the **ductus arteriosus**. The ductus conveys most of the pulmonary outflow into the aorta. It constricts after birth in response to increased arterial oxygen content and becomes occluded by fibrosis **(ligamentum arteriosus)** (Fig. 17-8B).

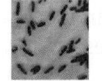 **ETIOLOGIC FACTORS:** Persistent PDA is one of the most common congenital cardiac defects, especially in infants whose mothers were infected with rubella virus early in pregnancy. It is also common in premature infants, in whom prematurity precluded closure. In these patients, the ductus usually closes spontaneously. In full-term infants with PDA, however, the ductus has an abnormal endothelium and media, and only rarely closes spontaneously. PDAs occur in some patients with Down and DiGeorge syndromes.

PRIMITIVE AORTIC ARCHES

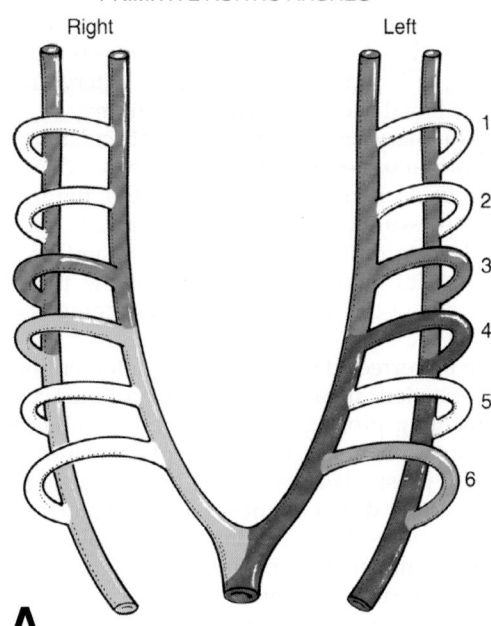

A

NORMAL ADULT

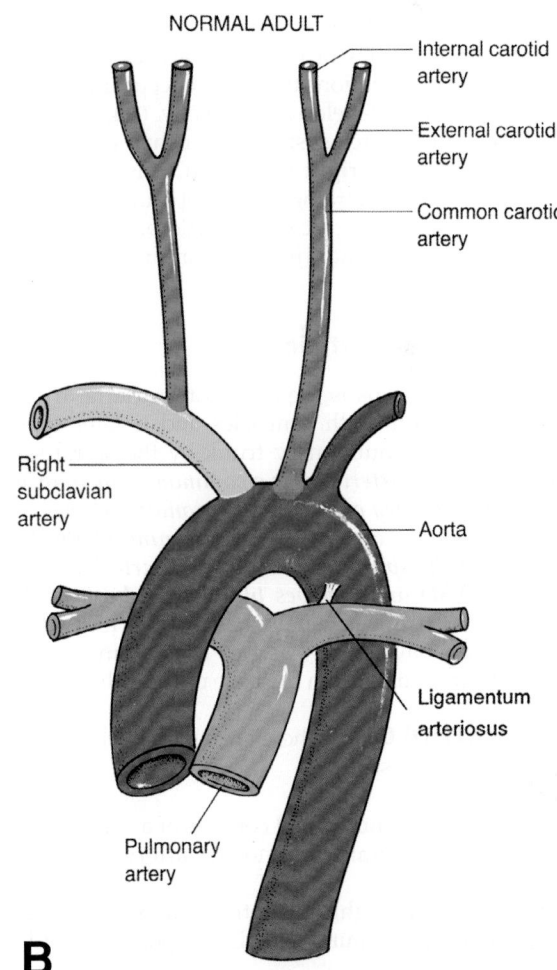

B

FIGURE 17-8. Derivatives of the aortic arches. A. Complete primitive aortic arch system. **B.** In the normal adult, the left fourth aortic arch is preserved as the arch of the adult aorta, and the left sixth arch gives rise to the pulmonary artery and ligamentum arteriosus (closed ductus arteriosus).

CLINICAL FEATURES: Luminal diameters of PDAs vary greatly. A small shunt has little effect on the heart, but a large one may divert blood from the aorta to the low-pressure pulmonary artery. In severe cases, over half of the left ventricular output may be shunted into the pulmonary circulation. Left ventricular hypertrophy and heart failure ensue owing to increased demand for cardiac output. In patients with large PDAs, the increased volume and pressure of blood in the pulmonary circulation eventually lead to pulmonary hypertension and its cardiac complications. Infective endarteritis involving the pulmonary artery side of the ductus is a frequent complication of untreated PDA.

PDA can be corrected surgically or by interventional cardiac catheterization. It can be caused to contract and then close by instilling prostaglandin synthesis inhibitors (e.g., indomethacin). Conversely, it can be kept open after birth by administering prostaglandins (PGE₂) if survival of patients born with a cardiac defect requires a left-to-right or right-to-left shunt. Examples include patients with isolated pulmonary stenosis, complete transposition of the great vessels or hypoplastic left heart syndrome.

Aortopulmonary window is a defect between the base of the aorta and the pulmonary artery. It is a rare condition that is functionally similar to PDA and is clinically difficult to differentiate from it.

Other abnormalities of the aortic arches can be understood in terms of variations that could occur if the complete aortic arch system develops incorrectly (Fig. 17-8). Thus, the right side of the arch system rather than the left may be retained, resulting in a **right aortic arch**. This is seen in about 25% of patients with tetralogy of Fallot and 50% of patients with truncus arteriosus. A right aortic arch is innocuous unless it creates a vascular ring that compresses the esophagus and trachea.

Persistent Truncus Arteriosus

The truncus arteriosus is the embryonic arterial trunk that initially opens from both ventricles and is later separated into the aorta and pulmonary trunk by the spiral septum. *Persistent truncus arteriosus is a common trunk of origin for the aorta, pulmonary arteries and coronary arteries, resulting from absent or incomplete partitioning of the truncus arteriosus by the spiral septum. Truncus arteriosus always overrides a VSD and receives blood from both ventricles.* The valve of the truncus usually has three or four semilunar cusps but may have as few as two or as many as six. The coronary arteries arise from the base of the valve.

PATHOLOGY: There are several variants of truncus arteriosus:

- **Type 1** is most common and consists of a single trunk that gives rise to a common pulmonary artery and ascending aorta.
- **Type 2** displays right and left pulmonary arteries that originate from a common site in the posterior midline of the truncus.
- **Type 3** has separate pulmonary arteries arising laterally from a common trunk.
- **Type 4** covers other rare variants in which there is no pulmonary trunk at all and in which the pulmonary circulation is supplied from the aorta by enlarged bronchial

arteries. This type is difficult to differentiate from tetralogy of Fallot with pulmonary artery atresia.

CLINICAL FEATURES: Most infants with truncus arteriosus have torrential pulmonary blood flow, causing heart failure, recurrent respiratory infections and often early death. Pulmonary vascular disease develops if children survive, in which case cyanosis, polycythemia and clubbing of the fingers appear. Open-heart surgery before significant pulmonary vascular changes develop is effective treatment.

Hypoplastic Left Heart Syndrome

PATHOLOGY: This usually profound malformation features hypoplasia of the left ventricle and ascending aorta and hypoplasia or atresia of the left-sided valves. Severe aortic valvular stenosis or aortic atresia is often the main defect. Some mitral valve structures are usually present, but the mitral valve may also be atretic. If the mitral valve is atretic rather than hypoplastic, the left ventricle may only be a thin slit lined by endocardium.

MOLECULAR PATHOGENESIS: No specific mutations are implicated in this complex malformation, but there is a 2–4% risk of recurrence in future pregnancies. In families with two affected children, the risk increases to 25%. Maternal chromosome abnormalities have been implicated in about 10% of cases, the most common being terminal 11q deletion (Jacobsen syndrome), in which 10% of children have hypoplastic left heart syndrome.

CLINICAL FEATURES: Aortic valve atresia precludes left ventricular outflow into the aorta. There is an obligate left-to-right shunt through a patent foramen ovale. Cardiac output is entirely via the right ventricle and pulmonary artery. Systemic blood flow depends on flow from the pulmonary trunk to the aorta through a PDA. Coronary blood flow depends on retrograde flow from a hypoplastic ascending aorta to the sinuses of Valsalva. Because pulmonary vascular resistance is high at birth and both the foramen ovale and ductus arteriosus are patent, newborns with hypoplastic left heart syndrome may appear well initially. As pulmonary vascular resistance falls and systemic (and especially coronary) blood flow decreases, infants become symptomatic. Without surgical correction or transplantation, over 95% die within their first month.

Anomalous Pulmonary Vein Drainage

The pulmonary veins form a network in the dorsal mesoderm. A bud from the region of the atrium joins the pulmonary venous confluence, and eventually all four pulmonary veins drain into the left atrium. Failure of these tissues to join correctly results in various venous anomalies.

PATHOLOGY: Total anomalous pulmonary vein drainage may occur as an isolated defect or as part of the asplenia syndrome (splenic agenesis, congenital heart defects and situs inversus of abdominal organs). Most commonly, the pulmonary veins drain into a common pulmonary venous chamber and then via a persistent left superior vena cava (persistent left pericardial vein) into the innominate vein or right superior vena cava. Alternate routes for common pulmonary vein drainage may lead into the coronary sinus or entail persistent posterior and subcardinal veins. The latter form a middorsal trunk that crosses the diaphragm and enters the portal vein or ductus venosus, and may be associated with some pulmonary venous obstruction.

 CLINICAL FEATURES: In total anomalous pulmonary drainage, there is no direct venous return to the left side of the heart. Life is sustained only by an atrial septal defect or patent foramen ovale. Heart failure, severe hypoxemia and pulmonary venous obstruction result from total anomalous pulmonary vein drainage. Good results have been obtained with surgical correction.

Partial anomalous pulmonary venous drainage may result from less severe circulatory impairment. This anomaly may involve one or two pulmonary veins, especially in association with a sinus venosus type of atrial septal defect. The prognosis is excellent, similar to that for atrial septal defects.

Right-to-Left Shunt Is the Most Common Cyanotic Congenital Heart Disease

Tetralogy of Fallot

Tetralogy of Fallot represents 10% of CHD. It has a familial recurrence rate of 2–3%, but little is known of its potential genetic and epigenetic causes.

 PATHOLOGY: Four changes define the tetralogy of Fallot (Fig. 17-9):

- **Pulmonary stenosis**
- **Ventricular septal defect**
- **Dextroposition of the aorta so that it overrides the ventricular septal defect**
- **Right ventricular hypertrophy**

The VSD, which may be as large as the aortic orifice, results from incomplete closure of the membranous septum and affects both the muscular septum and the endocardial cushions. In addition, development of the spiral septum, which normally divides the common truncus region into an aorta and a pulmonary artery, is abnormal. As a result, the aorta is displaced to the right and overlies the septal defect. The ventricular septal defect is immediately below the overriding aorta. Pulmonary stenosis is often due to subpulmonary muscular hypertrophy, with an enlarged infundibular muscle obstructing blood flow into the pulmonary artery. In about 1/3 of these hearts, the valve itself is the main cause of stenosis; in such cases, the valve is usually funnel shaped, with the narrow part more distal.

The heart is hypertrophied so as to give it a boot shape. Almost half of patients with tetralogy of Fallot have other cardiac anomalies, including ostium secundum atrial septal defects, PDA, left superior vena cava and endocardial cushion defects. The aortic arch is on the right side in about 25% of cases of tetralogy of Fallot. The surgeon must remember that a large branch of the right coronary artery may cross the pulmonary conus region, which is the site of the cardiotomy made to enlarge the outflow tract. Patency of the ductus arteriosus is actually protective, because it provides

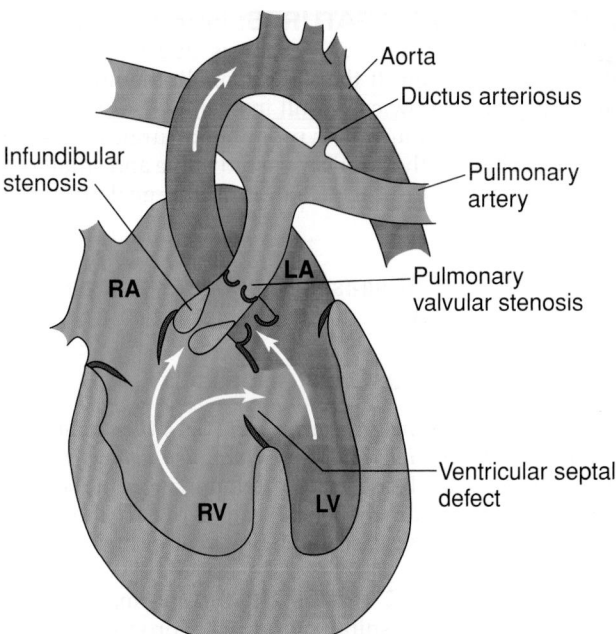

FIGURE 17-9. Tetralogy of Fallot. Note the pulmonary stenosis, which is due to infundibular hypertrophy as well as pulmonary valvular stenosis. The ventricular septal defect involves the membranous septum region. Dextroposition of the aorta and right ventricular hypertrophy are shown. Because of the pulmonary obstruction, the shunt is from right to left, and the patient is cyanotic. *LA* = left atrium; *LV* = left ventricle; *RA* = right atrium; *RV* = right ventricle.

a source of blood to the otherwise deprived pulmonary vascular bed.

 CLINICAL FEATURES: In the face of severe pulmonary stenosis, right ventricular blood is shunted through the ventricular septal defect into the aorta, causing arterial desaturation and cyanosis. Surgical correction is typically done in the first 2 years of life. Otherwise, the affected child complains of dyspnea on exertion and often assumes a squatting position to relieve the shortness of breath. Physical development is characteristically slow. Cerebral thromboses due to marked polycythemia may occur. Patients are also at risk for bacterial endocarditis and brain abscesses. Increasing cyanosis and shortness of breath may indicate that a beneficial PDA has closed spontaneously. Left-sided heart failure is not common.

Without treatment, the prognosis of tetralogy of Fallot is dismal. However, total correction is possible with surgery, which has less than 10% mortality. After successful surgery, patients become asymptomatic and have excellent long-term prognoses.

Tricuspid Atresia

 PATHOLOGY: *Tricuspid atresia, a congenital absence of the tricuspid valve, causes obligate right-to-left shunting through the patent foramen ovale.* This defect usually occurs with a VSD through which blood gains access to the pulmonary artery. In **type I** tricuspid atresia (75% of patients), the great arteries are normal, while in **type II** D-transposition of the great arteries occurs. The rare **type III** has L-malposition (see below).

THE HEART

CLINICAL FEATURES: Infants with tricuspid atresia present with cyanosis due to atrial right-to-left shunt. If the VSD is small, the limitation of pulmonary blood flow can result in even worse cyanosis. In that case, a cardiac murmur is prominent. Surgical intervention tries to bypass the atretic tricuspid valve and small right ventricle. Staged surgical palliation is the goal of current therapy.

Congenital Heart Diseases May Occur without Shunting of Blood

Transposition of the Great Arteries

In transposition of the great arteries (TGA), the aorta arises from the right ventricle and the pulmonary artery from the left ventricle. TGA has a male predominance and is more common if mothers are diabetic. It causes over half of deaths from cyanotic heart disease in the first year of life.

 **ETIOLOGIC FACTORS:** Abnormal development of the spiral septum can produce aberrant positioning of the great arteries, such that the aorta is anterior to the pulmonary artery and connects to the right ventricle. Then, the pulmonary artery receives the left ventricular outflow (Fig. 17-10). Because the venous blood from the right side of the heart flows to the aorta and the oxygenated blood from the lungs returns to the pulmonary

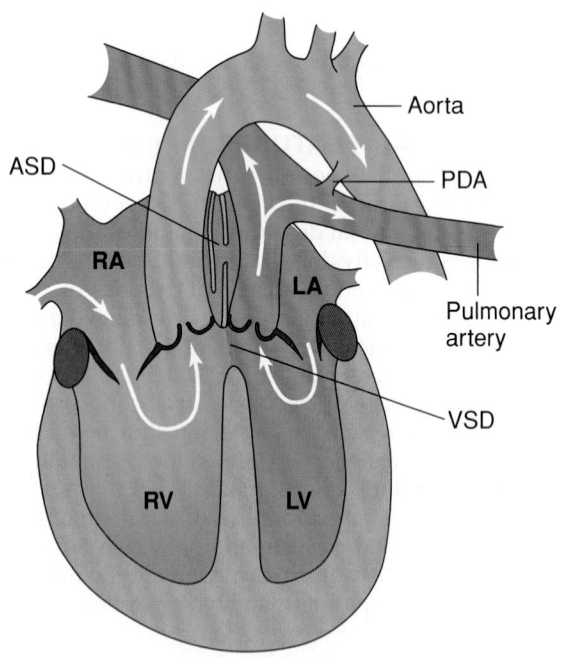

FIGURE 17-10. Complete transposition of great arteries, regular type. The aorta is anterior to, and to the right of, the pulmonary artery ("D-transposition") and arises from the right ventricle. In the absence of interatrial or interventricular connections or patent ductus arteriosus, this anomaly is incompatible with life. The volume and direction of blood flow through intracardiac communications and patent ductus arteriosus, if present, depend on pressure gradients across the communications, which can vary during early stages of extrauterine life. *ASD* = atrial septal defect; *LA* = left atrium; *LV* = left ventricle; *RA* = right atrium; *RV* = right ventricle; *PDA* = patent ductus arteriosus; *VSD* = ventricular septal defect.

artery, there are in effect two independent and parallel blood circuits for systemic and pulmonary circulations. Survival requires a communication between the circuits. Virtually all such infants have an ASD, 1/2 have a VSD and 2/3 have a PDA.

 PATHOLOGY: The aorta normally arises posterior and left of the pulmonary artery and ascends behind and right of it. In TGA, the aorta is anterior and right of the pulmonary artery **("D" or dextrotransposition)** all the way from its origin.

 CLINICAL FEATURES: It is possible to correct the malformation within the first 2 weeks of life using an arterial-switch operation, with overall survival of 90%.

Congenitally corrected transposition is a condition in which the aorta is anterior to, but passes to the left of, the pulmonary artery **("L" transposition)**. Although the great arteries are thus abnormally related to each other and arise from discordant ventricles, the circulatory pattern is functionally corrected because of coexistent atrioventricular discordance. Patients in whom corrected TGA is the only malformation are clinically entirely normal. Unfortunately, many cases are complicated by other anomalies that require their own specific interventions.

Taussig-Bing malformation is a double-outlet right ventricle (both great vessels arise from the right ventricle) in which a VSD is above the crista supraventricularis and directly beneath an overriding pulmonary artery. This condition is functionally and clinically similar to TGA with a VSD and pulmonary hypertension.

 **MOLECULAR PATHOGENESIS:** Various types of double-outlet right ventricle occur in patients with autosomal trisomies (13, 18, 21) and 22q11 deletions. Mutations in *NKX2.5* and maternal exposure to teratogens that influence neural crest development have also been implicated in a few cases.

Coarctation of the Aorta

Coarctation of the aorta is a local constriction that almost always occurs immediately below the origin of the left subclavian artery at the site of the ductus arteriosus. Rare coarctations may occur at any point from the aortic arch to the abdominal bifurcation. The condition is two to five times more common in males than females and is associated with a bicuspid aortic valve in 2/3 of cases. Mitral valve malformations, VSDs and subaortic stenosis may also be present. Turner syndrome, in particular, is associated with coarctation, and berry aneurysms in the brain are also more common.

 **ETIOLOGIC FACTORS AND PATHOGENESIS:** The pathogenesis of coarctation of the aorta reflects the pattern of flow in the ductus arteriosus in fetal life (Fig. 17-11). In utero, considerably more blood flows through the ductus than across the aortic valve. The blood leaving the ductus is diverted into two streams by a posterior aortic shelf opposite the orifice of the ductus. One stream passes cephalad into a relatively hypoplastic aortic isthmus to supply the head and arms; the other enters the descending thoracic aorta. In late

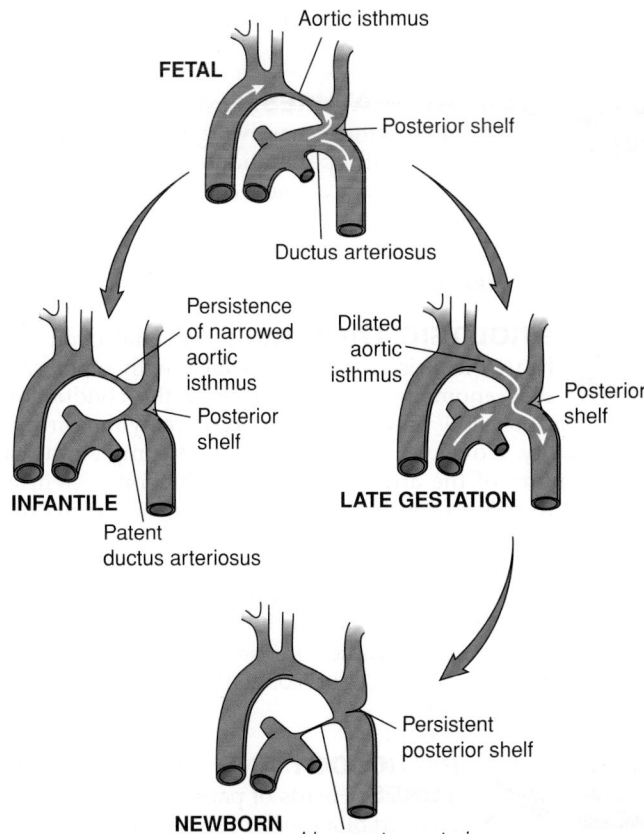

Aortic isthmus

FETAL

Posterior shelf

Ductus arteriosus

Persistence of narrowed aortic isthmus

Dilated aortic isthmus

Posterior shelf

Posterior shelf

INFANTILE

Patent ductus arteriosus

LATE GESTATION

Persistent posterior shelf

NEWBORN Ligamentum arteriosus

FIGURE 17-11. Pathogenesis of coarctation of the aorta. In the fetus, ductal blood is diverted into cephalad and descending streams by the posterior aortic shelf. In late fetal life, the isthmus dilates and the increased descending blood flow is accommodated by the ductal orifice. After birth, if the shelf does not undergo the normal involution, obliteration of the ductal orifice does not permit free flow around the persistent posterior shelf, thereby creating a juxtaductal obstruction of blood flow to the distal aorta. If the aortic isthmus does not dilate during late fetal life, it remains narrow, resulting in an infantile or preductal coarctation. In this circumstance, the ductus arteriosus usually remains patent.

fetal life, increasing left ventricular output dilates the isthmus and bypasses the obstruction (represented by the posterior shelf) through the wide ductal orifice. After birth, the ductal orifice is obliterated and the posterior shelf normally involutes, removing the obstruction. The shelf may not involute because of inadequate antegrade flow in the aortic arch in utero due to anomalies that limit left ventricular output (e.g., bicuspid aortic valve). Often the obstructing shelf fails to involute for unknown reasons. In any event, the result is the most common type of coarctation of the aorta, a **juxtaductal constriction**.

The **infantile (preductal) type of coarctation** occurs when the aortic isthmus remains narrow (hypoplastic) into late fetal life and after birth. This lesion is usually accompanied by a PDA and a right-to-left shunt through a VSD.

 **CLINICAL FEATURES:** *The clinical hallmark of coarctation of the aorta is a discrepancy in blood pressure between the upper and lower extremities.* The pressure gradient produced by the coarctation causes hypertension proximal to the narrowed segment and, occasionally, dilation of that portion of the aorta.

Hypertension in the upper part of the body results in left ventricular hypertrophy and may produce dizziness, headaches and nosebleeds. The increased pressure may also increase the risk of rupture of a berry aneurysm and consequent subarachnoid hemorrhage (see Chapter 32). Hypotension below the coarctation leads to weakness, pallor and coldness of the lower extremities. In an attempt to bridge the obstruction between the upper and lower aortic segments, collateral vessels enlarge. Chest radiography shows notching of the inner surfaces of the ribs, caused by increased pressure in markedly dilated intercostal arteries.

Most patients with coarctation of the aorta die by age 40 unless they are treated. Complications include (1) heart failure, (2) rupture of a dissecting aneurysm (secondary to cystic medial necrosis of the aorta), (3) infective endarteritis at the point of narrowing or at the site of jet-stream impingement on the wall immediately distal to the coarctation, (4) cerebral hemorrhage and (5) stenosis or infective endocarditis of a bicuspid aortic valve. Surgical excision of the narrowed segment, preferably between 1 and 2 years of age for asymptomatic patients, is effective treatment. Balloon dilation of the narrowed area by cardiac catheterization has also been performed.

Pulmonary Stenosis

Pulmonary stenosis results from (1) developmental deformities from the endocardial cushion region (with involvement of the pulmonary valves), (2) an abnormality of the right ventricular infundibular muscle (subvalvular or infundibular stenosis, especially as part of tetralogy of Fallot) or (3) abnormal development of the more distal parts of the pulmonary artery tree (peripheral pulmonary stenosis). Peripheral pulmonary stenosis, which is much less common than the other two, may cause pulmonary artery "coarctation" at one or more sites. This anomaly is more common in newborns with **Williams syndrome,** in which there are deletion mutations in the gene encoding elastin.

Isolated pulmonary stenosis ordinarily involves the valve cusps, which are fused to form an inverted cone or funnel type of constriction. The artery distal to the valve may develop poststenotic dilation after several years. In severe cases, infants have right ventricular and atrial hypertrophy. If the foramen ovale is patent, there is a right-to-left shunt with cyanosis, secondary polycythemia and clubbing of the fingers. Balloon dilation of the stenotic valve by cardiac catheterization can be effective.

Congenital Aortic Stenosis

The types of congenital aortic stenosis are valvular, subvalvular and supravalvular.

VALVULAR AORTIC STENOSIS: The most common congenital aortic stenosis, bicuspid valve, arises through abnormal development of the endocardial cushions. A congenitally bicuspid aortic valve is much more frequent (4:1) in males than females and is associated with other cardiac anomalies (e.g., coarctation of the aorta) in 20% of cases. Typically, two of the three semilunar cusps (the right coronary cusp with one of the adjacent two cusps) are fused.

 CLINICAL FEATURES: Many children with bicuspid aortic stenosis are asymptomatic. Over the years, the resulting bicuspid valve tends to become thickened and calcified, generally causing symptoms in adulthood. More severe forms of congenital aortic stenosis result in a unicommissural valve or one without any commissures. These malformations cause symptoms in early life. Exertional dyspnea and angina pectoris may be prominent. Sudden death, principally due to ventricular arrhythmias, is a distinct threat for patients with severe obstruction. Bacterial endocarditis sometimes complicates the disease. Valve replacement may be indicated.

SUBVALVULAR AORTIC STENOSIS: This defect accounts for 10% of cases of congenital aortic stenosis and is caused by abnormal development of a band of subvalvular fibroelastic tissue or a muscular ridge. Stenosis results from a membranous diaphragm or fibrous ring that surrounds the left ventricular outflow tract immediately below the aortic valve. It is twice as common in males as in females.

Many people with subvalvular aortic stenosis develop thickening and immobility of the aortic cusps, with mild aortic regurgitation. Bacterial endocarditis carries its own risks and may also aggravate the regurgitation. Surgical treatment of subvalvular aortic stenosis involves excising the membrane or fibrous ridge.

SUPRAVALVULAR AORTIC STENOSIS: This type of stenosis is much less common than the other two, and is often associated with idiopathic infantile hypercalcemia **(Williams syndrome)** characterized by mental retardation and multiple system disorders.

Origin of a Coronary Artery from the Pulmonary Artery

A single coronary artery or, rarely, both may originate from the pulmonary artery rather than the aorta. When one coronary artery has an anomalous origin (most often the left coronary), anastomoses develop between right and left coronary arteries. This produces an arterial–arterial shunt through which blood flows from the artery originating from the aorta to that arising from the pulmonary artery. The myocardium supplied by the anomalous artery is vulnerable to episodes of ischemia. The result may be myocardial infarction, fibrosis and calcification and endocardial fibroelastosis.

Ebstein Malformation

Ebstein malformation results from downward displacement of an abnormal tricuspid valve into an underdeveloped right ventricle. One or more tricuspid valve leaflets are plastered to the right ventricular wall for a variable distance below the right atrioventricular annulus.

 PATHOLOGY: Septal and posterior tricuspid valve leaflets are usually affected. They are irregularly elongated and adherent to the right ventricular wall, so that the upper part of the right ventricular cavity (inflow region) functions separately from the distal chamber. The anterior leaflet is usually the least involved, and may be normal. The valve ring may or may not be displaced downward from its usual position. In any event, the effective tricuspid valve orifice is displaced downward into the ventricle, thus dividing it into two separate parts: the "atrialized" (proximal) ventricle and the functional right (distal) ventricle. In 2/3 of cases, conspicuous dilation of the functional ventricle hinders its ability to pump blood efficiently via the pulmonary arteries. The degree of tricuspid valve

insufficiency depends on the severity and configuration of the defect in the leaflets.

 CLINICAL FEATURES: Ebstein malformation leads to heart failure, massive right atrial dilation, arrhythmias with palpitations and tachycardia and sudden death. Surgical treatment has met with variable success.

Congenital Heart Block

 **ETIOLOGIC FACTORS:** Congenital complete heart block is usually associated with other cardiac anomalies. Discontinuity of the conduction system is probably caused by the accompanying cardiac abnormality. However, in cases of isolated complete heart block, failure of the atrioventricular conduction system is believed to result from lack of regression of the sulcus tissue, which entirely encloses the conducting tissue during early development. Congenital heart block without structural heart disease has been linked to maternal connective tissue disease, especially systemic lupus. If maternal SS-A/Ro or SS-B/La autoantibodies are transmitted to the fetus transplacentally, incidence of congenital complete heart block approaches 100%.

 PATHOLOGY AND CLINICAL FEATURES: Hearts of patients with congenital heart block tend to show a discontinuity between the atrial myocardium and the AV node. Alternatively, the defect may be a fibrous separation of the AV node from the ventricular conducting tissue. The heart rate is abnormally slow, but patients with isolated heart block rarely have functional difficulty. Later in life, cardiac hypertrophy, attacks of Stokes–Adams syncope (dizziness and unexpected fainting), arrhythmias and heart failure may develop.

Endocardial Fibroelastosis

Endocardial fibroelastosis (EFE) is a fibroelastotic thickening of left ventricular endocardium. It may also affect the valves. This condition may be primary or, more often, secondary.

SECONDARY ENDOCARDIAL FIBROELASTOSIS: This occurs in association with underlying cardiovascular anomalies that lead to left ventricular hypertrophy in the face of inability to meet the increased myocardial oxygen demands. Thus, secondary EFE is a common complication of congenital aortic stenosis (including hypoplastic left ventricle syndrome) and coarctation of the aorta. Some type of endocardial injury is likely involved in its pathogenesis.

 PATHOLOGY: On gross examination, the left ventricle endocardium has irregular, opaque, gray-white patches, which may also affect the cardiac valves. These plaques are areas of endocardial fibroelastotic thickening, often with degeneration of adjacent subendocardial myocytes. Valves may show collagenous thickening.

PRIMARY ENDOCARDIAL FIBROELASTOSIS: Defined as fibroelastosis without any associated lesion, this disorder is now quite rare. It afflicts infants, usually 4–10 months old. Although it has occurred in siblings, no specific mode of inheritance has been established. Some evidence links primary EFE to mumps infection, which may explain why this condition is now seen so infrequently.

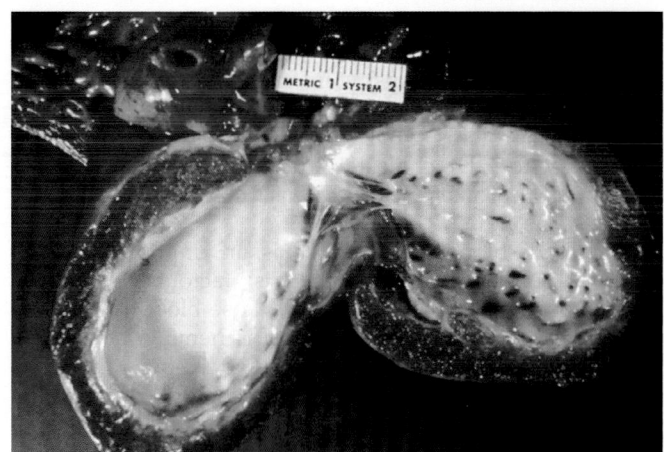

FIGURE 17-12. Endocardial fibroelastosis. The left ventricle of an infant who died of endocardial fibroelastosis has been opened to reveal a thickened endocardium lining most of the cavity and virtually obliterating the trabeculae carneae.

 PATHOLOGY: The left ventricle is usually conspicuously dilated but may be contracted and hypertrophic. Diffuse endocardial thickening involves most of the left ventricle (Fig. 17-12) and aortic and mitral valve leaflets. The thickened endocardium tends to obscure the trabecular pattern of the underlying myocardium, and papillary muscles and chordae tendineae are thick and short. Mural thrombi may be present.

Infants with primary EFE develop progressive heart failure. The prognosis is dismal, and cardiac transplantation offers the only hope for a cure.

Dextrocardia

Dextrocardia is rightward orientation of the base–apex axis of the heart. It is often associated with a mirror image of the normal left-sided location and configuration. The position of the ventricles is determined by the direction of the embryonic cardiac loop. If the loop protrudes to the right, the future right ventricle develops on the right, and the left ventricle comes to occupy its proper position. If the loop protrudes to the left, the opposite occurs.

 PATHOLOGY: Dextrocardia without abnormal positioning of the visceral organs **(situs inversus)** is invariably associated with severe cardiovascular anomalies. These include transposition of the great arteries, several atrial and ventricular septal defects, anomalous pulmonary venous drainage and others. If dextrocardia occurs with situs inversus, the heart is functionally normal, but minor anomalies may be seen.

ISCHEMIC HEART DISEASE

Ischemic heart disease is usually due to coronary artery atherosclerosis. It develops when blood flow is inadequate to meet the heart's oxygen needs. Ischemic heart disease is by far the most common type of heart disease in the United States and other industrialized nations, where it is the leading cause of death and is responsible for at least 80% of all deaths from heart disease. By contrast, atherosclerotic heart disease is far less frequent in underdeveloped countries. The principal effects of ischemic heart disease are angina pectoris, myocardial infarction, chronic congestive heart failure and sudden death.

ANGINA PECTORIS: This is the pain of myocardial ischemia. It typically feels like severe crushing or burning in the substernal portion of the chest, which may radiate to the left arm, jaw or epigastrium. It is the most common symptom of ischemic heart disease. Coronary atherosclerosis usually becomes symptomatic only when the luminal cross-sectional area of the affected vessel is reduced by more than 75%. A patient with angina pectoris typically has recurrent episodes of chest pain, usually brought on by physical or emotional stress. The pain is of limited duration (1–15 minutes) and is relieved by rest or treatment with sublingual nitroglycerin (a potent vasodilator).

Although the most common cause of angina pectoris is severe coronary atherosclerosis, decreased coronary blood flow can result from other conditions, including coronary vasospasm, aortic stenosis or aortic insufficiency. Angina pectoris is not usually associated with myocardial pathology as long as the duration and severity of the episodes do not cause myocardial necrosis. However, repetitive bouts of angina may eventually contribute to myocytolytic degeneration of the myocardium (Fig. 17-6).

Prinzmetal angina (variant angina) *is an atypical form of angina that occurs at rest and is caused by coronary artery spasm.* The mechanisms responsible are not fully understood, but endothelial dysfunction plays a major role. Patients typically show vasoconstrictor responses to acetylcholine, reflecting abnormal nitric oxide production. Thromboxane, derived from platelet activation, may also be involved. Spasm in structurally normal coronary arteries may be part of a systemic syndrome of abnormal arterial vasomotor reactivity, which includes migraine headache and Raynaud phenomenon. Usually, though, it develops in atherosclerotic coronary arteries, often in a portion of a vessel near an atherosclerotic plaque. In this case, coronary artery spasm may contribute to acute myocardial infarction or affect the size of an infarct but is generally not the principal cause of infarction.

In **unstable angina,** *chest pain has a less predictable relationship to exercise than does stable angina, may occur during rest or sleep and is often associated with nonocclusive thrombi over atherosclerotic plaques.* In some cases of unstable angina, episodes of chest pain become progressively more frequent and longer over a 3- to 4-day period. Electrocardiographic (ECG) changes are not characteristic of infarction and serum levels of cardiac-specific intracellular proteins, such as the MB isoform of CK (MB-CK) or cardiac troponins T or I (evidence of myocardial necrosis), remain normal. Unstable angina is also called **preinfarction angina, accelerated angina** or **"crescendo" angina.** Without pharmacologic or mechanical intervention to treat the coronary narrowing, many such patients progress to myocardial infarction.

MYOCARDIAL INFARCTION: A myocardial infarct is a discrete focus of ischemic muscle necrosis in the heart. This definition excludes patchy foci of necrosis caused by drugs, toxins or viruses. Development of an infarct is related to the duration of ischemia and the metabolic demands of the ischemic tissue. In experimental coronary artery ligation, foci of necrosis form after 20 minutes of ischemia and become more extensive as the period of ischemia lengthens.

CHRONIC CONGESTIVE HEART FAILURE: Early mortality associated with acute myocardial infarction is now less than 5%. Many patients with ischemic heart disease survive longer and develop chronic congestive heart failure. Coronary artery disease is responsible for over 75% of heart failure in patients. Contractile impairment in these people is due to irreversible loss of myocardium (previous infarcts) and hypoperfusion of surviving muscle, which leads to chronic ventricular dysfunction ("hibernating" myocardium; Fig. 17-6). Some of these patients die suddenly, especially those in whom contractile impairment is not severe. Others develop progressive pump failure and die of multiorgan failure. Because their coronary artery disease is often so extensive and many have already had coronary artery bypass surgery, the only treatments available for end-stage disease in these patients are heart transplantation or the use of artificial pumps (ventricular assist devices).

SUDDEN DEATH: In some patients, the first and only clinical manifestation of ischemic heart disease is sudden death due to spontaneous ventricular tachycardia that degenerates into ventricular fibrillation. Diagnoses of sudden death vary. Some authorities only consider death to be sudden if it occurs within 1 hour of the onset of symptoms. Others regard death within 24 hours after the onset of symptoms to be sudden or require that sudden death be diagnosed only if it is unexpected. *In any event, coronary atherosclerosis underlies most cases of cardiac death occurring during the first hour after the onset of symptoms.*

Experimental animals subjected to acute coronary occlusion show a high incidence of ventricular fibrillation within 1 hour. Sudden cardiac death due to ventricular fibrillation also occurs in humans as a result of acute coronary artery thrombosis. On the other hand, such an arrhythmia also appears in patients with marked coronary artery disease and no detectable thrombosis. Most patients who have been defibrillated and survived an arrhythmia have not suffered acute myocardial infarction: serum markers and ECG changes characteristic of infarction do not develop. *Thus, in many cases, lethal arrhythmia is likely triggered by acute ischemia without overt myocardial infarction.* The presence of a healed infarct or ventricular hypertrophy increases the risk that an episode of acute ischemia will initiate life-threatening ventricular arrhythmia.

 **EPIDEMIOLOGY:** *The major risk factors predisposing to coronary artery disease are (1) systemic hypertension, (2) cigarette smoking, (3) diabetes mellitus and (4) elevated blood cholesterol.* Any one of these factors significantly increases the risk of myocardial infarction, but a combination of multiple factors increases that risk by over 7-fold (see Chapter 8).

During the 20th century, the United States first experienced a dramatic increase and then a marked decrease in mortality from ischemic heart disease. In 1950, the age-adjusted death rate from myocardial infarction was 226 per 100,000 cases; 40 years later it was 108. This shift reflects many factors, including reduced smoking, lower dietary saturated fat and new drugs that control hypertension, reduce cholesterol and dissolve coronary thrombi. Important advances in medical technology include construction of coronary care units, coronary revascularization procedures and use of defibrillators and ventricular assist devices. Concurrently, the role of hyperlipidemia in the pathogenesis of coronary artery atherosclerosis attracted much more attention. This was driven initially by epidemiologic evidence showing that populations in which men have high mean serum cholesterol values had higher rates of coronary artery disease. Since then, multiple studies established that elevated serum low-density lipoproteins (LDLs) increase risk of myocardial infarction, but that high levels of high-density lipoproteins (HDLs) decrease that risk. The total cholesterol–to–HDL cholesterol ratio appears to be a better predictor of coronary artery disease than is serum cholesterol level alone.

Although blood lipid profile is an important indicator of risk of atherogenesis, other risk factors exert powerful independent effects. Someone whose blood pressure is 160/95 mm Hg has twice the risk of ischemic heart disease as someone whose blood pressure is 140/75 mm Hg or less. Risk of ischemic heart disease increases in proportion to the numbers of cigarettes smoked. Serum factors involved in thrombosis or thrombolysis or that contribute to endothelial injury have also been implicated in atherogenesis. For example, plasma fibrinogen levels directly correlate with risk of ischemic heart disease, presumably because of the role of fibrinogen in atherogenesis and coronary artery thrombosis. Other factors that increase risk of myocardial infarction include factor VII, plasminogen activator inhibitor-1 (PAI-1), homocysteine and low fibrinolytic activity. Levels of selected serum markers of inflammation such as C-reactive protein also predict greater ischemic heart disease risk.

In recent years, there has been a remarkable increase in the incidence of type 2 diabetes in the United States, which mirrors a similar increase in obesity (see Chapter 13). Ischemic heart disease is a complication of both type 1 and type 2 diabetes, the risk being 2- to 3-fold greater than in nondiabetic people. Conversely, atherosclerotic cardiovascular disease (myocardial infarction, stroke, peripheral vascular disease) accounts for 80% of all deaths in diabetics.

Other risk factors for ischemic heart disease include:

- **Obesity:** In a major, longitudinal study of one population (Framingham Heart Study), obesity was an independent risk factor for cardiovascular disease, with an increased risk for obese people over lean ones of 2–2.5.
- **Age:** Risk of infarction increases with increasing age, up to 80 years.
- **Sex:** Sixty percent of coronary events occur in men. Angina pectoris is more common in men than women; the ratio at ages under 50 years is 4:1, and is 2:1 after age 60.
- **Family history:** In one study that controlled for other risk factors, relatives of patients with ischemic heart disease had 2- to 4-fold higher risk for coronary artery disease. The genetics of familial risk may interact with other risk factors.
- **Use of oral contraceptives:** Women over 35 years of age who smoke cigarettes and use oral contraceptives have modestly increased chances of myocardial infarction.
- **Sedentary life:** Regular exercise reduces risk of myocardial infarction, perhaps by increasing HDL. In one study, people in the least-fit quartile had six times the risk of myocardial infarction of those in the fittest quartile.
- **Personality features:** Early studies suggested that aggressive, time-conscious, executive-type individuals ("type A" personality) have more heart disease than do easygoing, relaxed people ("type B" personality). "Coronary-prone" subjects, with type A behaviors, differ from type B individuals in having higher plasma triglyceride and cholesterol levels and greater urinary catecholamine excretion. Yet, the link between coronary

artery disease and personality is controversial. Recent studies have not shown the strong association previously reported.

Many Conditions Limit Blood Supply to the Heart

The heart is an aerobic organ, using oxidative phosphorylation to generate energy for contraction. The anaerobic glycolysis used by skeletal muscle under conditions of extreme physical exertion is insufficient to sustain the heart. Ischemic heart disease is caused by an imbalance between myocardial oxygen requirements and the supply of oxygenated blood (Table 17-3).

Atherosclerosis and Thrombosis

The pathogenesis of atherosclerosis is detailed in Chapter 16. Here we discuss only briefly the features of special importance to ischemic heart disease. Coronary arteries are conductance vessels—small muscular arteries with a prominent internal elastic lamina. Their main role is to deliver blood

TABLE 17-3
CAUSES OF ISCHEMIC HEART DISEASE
Decreased Supply of Oxygen
Conditions that influence the supply of blood
Atherosclerosis and thrombosis
Thromboemboli
Coronary artery spasm
Collateral blood vessels
Blood pressure, cardiac output, and heart rate
Miscellaneous: arteritis (e.g., periarteritis nodosa), dissecting aneurysm, luetic aortitis, anomalous origin of coronary artery, muscular bridging of coronary artery
Conditions that influence the availability of oxygen in the blood
Anemia
Shift in the hemoglobin–oxygen dissociation curve
Carbon monoxide
Cyanide
Increased Oxygen Demand (i.e., Increased Cardiac Work)
Hypertension
Valvular stenosis or insufficiency
Hyperthyroidism
Fever
Thiamine deficiency
Catecholamines

to the regulatory vasculature (small intramural arteries and arterioles), which controls nutritive myocardial blood flow. A healthy person has substantial coronary flow reserve and myocardial perfusion can increase to four to eight times the resting blood flow. In a normal heart, the large coronary arteries provide almost no resistance to blood flow and myocardial circulation is mainly controlled by constriction and dilation of small, intramyocardial branches less than 400 μm in diameter. In advanced atherosclerosis of the main epicardial coronary arteries, luminal stenosis decreases blood pressure distal to the narrowed zone. To compensate for reduced perfusion pressure, microvessels dilate, thus maintaining normal resting blood flow. Most patients with coronary atherosclerosis do not, as a result, have ischemia or angina at rest. However, the capacity of the microcirculation to dilate further is limited, so if myocardial oxygen demand with exercise exceeds the supply, the result is ischemia and angina.

Maximal blood flow to the myocardium is not impaired until about 75% of the cross-sectional area of an epicardial coronary artery (~50% of the diameter as assessed during coronary angiography) is compromised by atherosclerosis. Resting blood flow is not reduced until over 90% of the lumen is occluded. In patients with long-standing angina pectoris, the extent and distribution of collateral circulation exerts an important influence on the risk of acute myocardial infarction. In some settings (e.g., hypotension or tachycardia), demand for oxygen and perfusion pressure may be so out of balance that myocardial infarction ensues even when a coronary artery is not ordinarily sufficiently narrowed to produce ischemia.

Although myocardial infarction often occurs during physically demanding activities such as running or shoveling snow, many infarcts occur at rest or even while asleep. Thus, for most people, conversion of clinically silent coronary atherosclerosis to a catastrophic myocardial infarction involves a sudden, marked decrease in myocardial blood flow, with or without increased myocardial oxygen demand. *Coronary artery thrombosis is the event that usually precipitates acute myocardial infarction. Thrombosis typically results from spontaneous rupture of an atherosclerotic plaque, usually in a region with numerous inflammatory cells and a thin fibrous cap.* The initiating event may be hemorrhage into or beneath the plaque.

Thromboemboli

Thromboembolism is a rare cause of myocardial infarction. The coronary embolus often comes from the heart itself, usually valvular vegetations due to infective or nonbacterial endocarditis. Coronary emboli occur in patients with atrial fibrillation and mitral valve disease who have mural thrombi in the left atrial appendage (Fig. 17-13). Thromboembolic occlusion of a coronary artery is also seen in patients with left ventricular mural thrombi due to infarction, aneurysm or dilated cardiomyopathy.

Coronary Collateral Circulation

Normal coronary arteries act as endarteries. Most normal hearts have anastomoses 20–200 μm in diameter between coronary vessels. Collateral vessels do not function under normal circumstances as there is no pressure gradient between the arteries that they connect. However, a pressure differential resulting from abrupt occlusion of a coronary artery allows blood to flow from the patent artery to

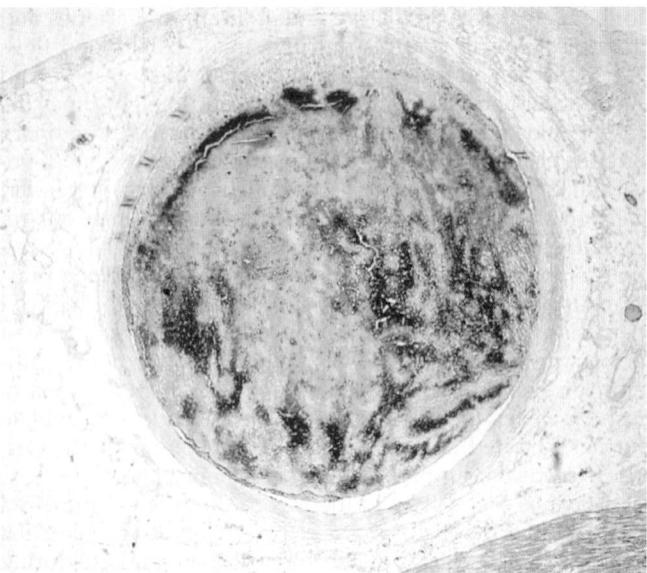

FIGURE 17-13. Thromboembolus in the left anterior descending coronary artery of a man who had old rheumatic heart disease, mitral stenosis and a mural thrombus in the left atrial appendage.

the ischemic area. Extensive collateral connections develop in hearts with severe coronary atherosclerosis. These collaterals may actually provide enough arterial flow to prevent infarction completely or to limit infarct size when a major epicardial coronary artery is acutely occluded.

Well-developed coronary collaterals can explain certain unusual situations, such as anterior infarction after recent thrombotic occlusion of the right coronary artery (so-called *infarction at a distance*). This reflects the opening of collaterals between the LAD and right coronary arteries (formed, e.g., in response to gradual atherosclerotic narrowing of the LAD). As a result, myocardium normally supplied by the LAD distal to the occlusion now depends on blood flow from the right coronary artery via collaterals. Acute thrombosis of the right coronary artery may then cause paradoxical infarction of the anterior left ventricular wall.

Other Conditions That Limit Coronary Blood Flow

- **Coronary arteritis** occurs in various vasculitides, such as polyarteritis nodosa or Kawasaki disease. It may cause luminal narrowing from vessel wall thickening. It can also create local aneurysms that may become occluded by thrombus.
- **Dissecting aortic aneurysms** may involve and obstruct coronary arteries. Rarely, medial necrosis and dissecting aneurysms are limited to a coronary artery.
- **Syphilitic aortitis** characteristically affects the ascending aorta, where it may obliterate a coronary artery orifice.
- **Congenital anomalous origin of a coronary artery** (origin of a coronary artery from the pulmonary trunk or passage of an anomalous coronary artery between the aorta and pulmonary artery) may cause sudden death in young, otherwise healthy individuals.
- **An intramural course of the LAD coronary artery** may cause myocardial ischemia and sudden death. The artery normally runs in the epicardial fat, but in some hearts, it dips into the myocardium for a short distance. The muscular bridge may compress the artery during systole or predispose to coronary spasm.

If the Blood Cannot Deliver Enough Oxygen, the Myocardium Is at Risk for Ischemia

Anemia is a common cause of decreased myocardial oxygen delivery. Although a heart with normal circulation can survive severe anemia, severe coronary atherosclerosis may limit the effectiveness of compensatory increases in coronary blood flow so severely that cardiac necrosis results. Anemia also increases cardiac workload because increased output is required to oxygenate vital organs adequately.

Carbon monoxide (CO) poisoning (see Chapter 8) decreases oxygen delivery to tissues. The high affinity of hemoglobin for CO displaces oxygen, thus depriving tissues of oxygen. It should be noted that cigarette smoking generates significant levels of carboxyhemoglobin (a measure of CO) in the blood.

Increased Oxygen Demand May Cause Cardiac Ischemia

Any increase in cardiac workload increases the heart's need for oxygen. Conditions that raise blood pressure or cardiac output, such as exercise or pregnancy, increase myocardial demand, which may lead to angina pectoris or infarction. Disorders in this category include valvular disease (mitral or aortic insufficiency, aortic stenosis), infection and conditions such as hypertension, coarctation of the aorta and hypertrophic cardiomyopathy (HCM) (Table 17-3).

Hyperthyroid patients have increased metabolic rates and tachycardia, leading to increased oxygen demand and greater cardiac workload. Treatment of the underlying thyroid disease is the best therapy for a hyperthyroid patient with symptoms of cardiac ischemia. Fever also increases basal metabolic rate, cardiac output and heart rate.

Myocardial Infarcts Are Mainly Subendocardial or Transmural

 PATHOLOGY:
Location of Infarcts

There are important differences between these two types of infarction (Table 17-4).

A **subendocardial infarct** affects the inner 1/3 to 1/2 of the left ventricle. It may arise within the territory of one of the major epicardial coronary arteries or it may be circumferential, involving subendocardial distributions of multiple coronary arteries. *Subendocardial infarction generally results from hypoperfusion.* It may be due to atherosclerosis in one coronary artery or due to diseases that limit myocardial blood flow globally, such as aortic stenosis, hemorrhagic shock or hypoperfusion during cardiopulmonary bypass. Most subendocardial infarcts are not consequences of occlusive coronary thrombi, although small particles of platelet–fibrin thrombus may be seen in the epicardial coronary artery that supplies the affected region. Circumferential subendocardial infarction caused by global hypoperfusion of the myocardium does not require that coronary artery stenosis to be present. Because necrosis is limited to the inner layers of the heart, complications arising in transmural infarcts (e.g., pericarditis and ventricular rupture) do not follow subendocardial infarction.

TABLE 17-4

DIFFERENCES BETWEEN SUBENDOCARDIAL AND TRANSMURAL INFARCTS

Subendocardial Infarcts	Transmural Infarcts
Multifocal	Unifocal
Patchy	Solid
May be circumferential	In distribution of a specific coronary artery
Coronary thrombosis rare	Coronary thrombosis common
Often result from hypotension or shock	Often cause shock
No epicarditis	Epicarditis common
Do not form aneurysms or lead to ventricular rupture	May result in aneurysm or ventricular rupture

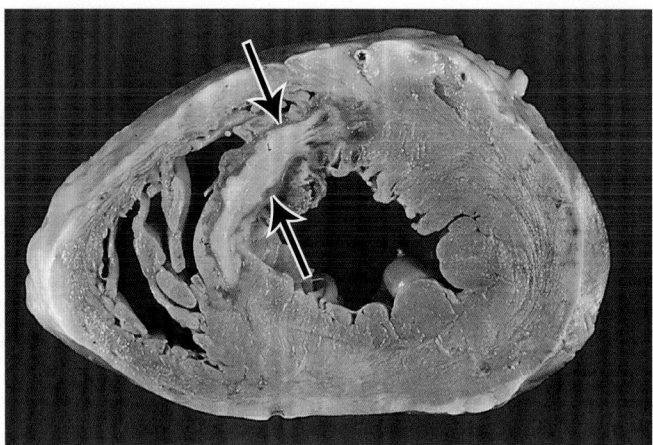

FIGURE 17-14. Acute myocardial infarct. A transverse section of the heart of a patient who died a few days after the onset of severe chest pain shows a transmural infarct in the anteroseptal region of the left ventricle (left anterior descending [LAD] coronary artery territory). The necrotic myocardium is soft, yellowish and sharply demarcated (*arrows*).

A **transmural infarct** involves the full left ventricular wall thickness, usually after occlusion of a coronary artery. As a result, transmural infarcts typically conform to the distribution of one of the three major coronary arteries (Fig. 17-2).

- **Right coronary artery:** Occlusion of this vessel's proximal portion results in an infarct of the posterior basal region of the left ventricle and the posterior third to half of the interventricular septum ("inferior" infarct).
- **LAD coronary artery:** Blockage of the LAD produces an infarct of the apical, anterior and anteroseptal walls of the left ventricle.
- **Left circumflex coronary artery:** Obstruction of this vessel is the least common cause of myocardial infarction, causing infarcts of the lateral left ventricle wall.

Myocardial infarction does not occur instantaneously. Rather, it first develops in the subendocardium and progresses as a wavefront of necrosis from subendocardium to subepicardium over several hours. Transient coronary occlusion may cause only subendocardial necrosis, but persistent occlusion eventually leads to transmural necrosis. The goal of acute coronary interventions (pharmacologic or mechanical thrombolysis) is to interrupt this wavefront and limit myocardial necrosis.

The volume of arterial collateral flow is the chief determinant of transmural progression of an infarct. In chronic cardiac hypoperfusion, extensive collaterals, which preferentially supply the outer or subepicardial layer, often limit infarction to the subendocardial myocardium. However, in fatal cases, acute transmural infarcts are more common than those restricted to the subendocardium.

Infarcts involve the left ventricle much more often and extensively than the right ventricle. This difference may be partly explained by the greater workload imposed on the left ventricle by systemic vascular resistance and the greater thickness of the left ventricular wall. Right ventricular hypertrophy (e.g., in pulmonary hypertension) increases the incidence of right ventricular infarction. Infarction of the posterior right ventricle occurs in about a third of left ventricular posteroseptal infarcts (right coronary artery territory), but infarcts limited to the right ventricle are rare.

Macroscopic Characteristics of Myocardial Infarcts

The early stages of myocardial infarction have been characterized most thoroughly in experimental animals. Within 10 seconds after ligation of a coronary artery, the affected myocardium becomes cyanotic and, rather than contracting, bulges outward during systole. If the obstruction is promptly relieved, myocardial contractions resume and there is no anatomic damage, although contractility may be depressed in the affected area for many hours **(stunned myocardium)** owing to the effects of oxygen radicals formed by reperfusion of acutely ischemic myocardium (see below). This reversible stage lasts for 20–30 minutes of total ischemia, after which damaged myocytes progressively die.

Acute myocardial infarcts are not grossly identifiable within the first 12 hours. By 24 hours, they are recognized by pallor on cut surfaces of the involved ventricle. After 3–5 days, they become mottled and more sharply outlined, with a central pale, yellowish, necrotic region bordered by a hyperemic zone (Fig. 17-14). By 2–3 weeks, the infarcted region is depressed and soft, with a refractile, gelatinous appearance. Older, healed infarcts are firm and contracted, with pale gray scar tissue (Fig. 17-15).

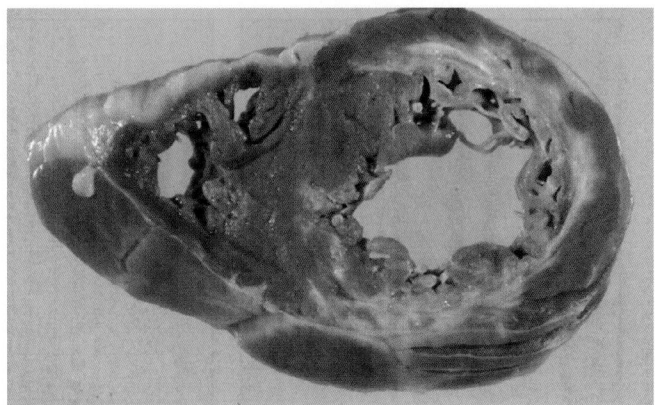

FIGURE 17-15. Healed myocardial infarct. A cross-section of the heart from a man who died after a long history of angina pectoris and several myocardial infarctions shows near-circumferential scarring of the left ventricle.

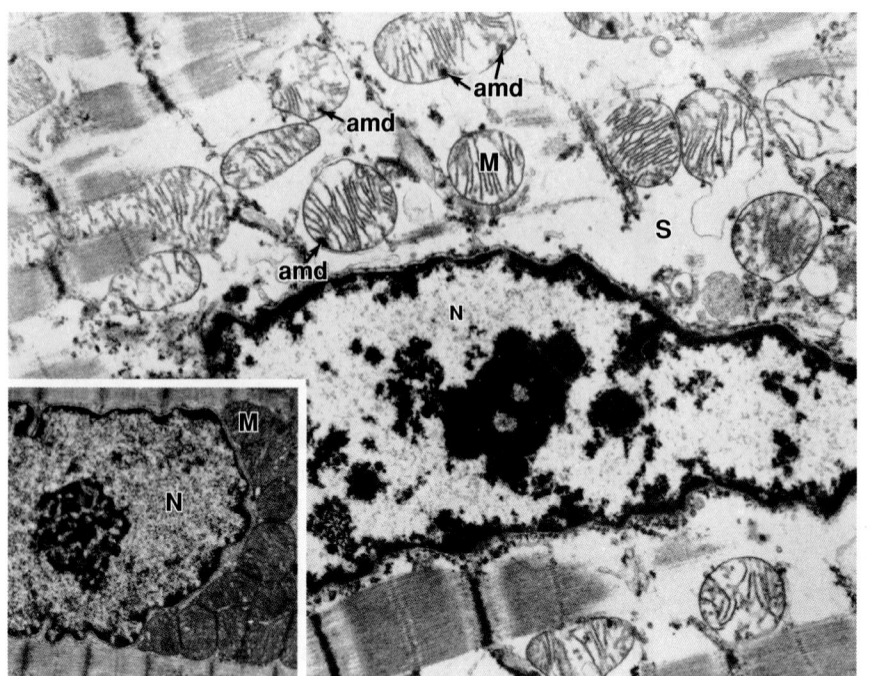

FIGURE 17-16. Ultrastructure of myocardial ischemia. Electron micrograph of an irreversibly injured myocyte from a canine heart subjected to 40 minutes of low-flow ischemia induced by proximal occlusion of the circumflex branch of the left coronary artery. (**Inset** shows a nonischemic control myocyte from the same heart. N = nucleus.) The affected myocyte is swollen and has abundant clear sarcoplasm (S). The mitochondria (M) are also swollen and contain amorphous matrix densities (amd), which are characteristic of lethal cell injury. The sarcolemma of this myocyte (*not shown*) exhibited small areas of disruption. The chromatin of the nucleus (N) is aggregated peripherally, in contrast to the uniformly distributed chromatin in normal tissue.

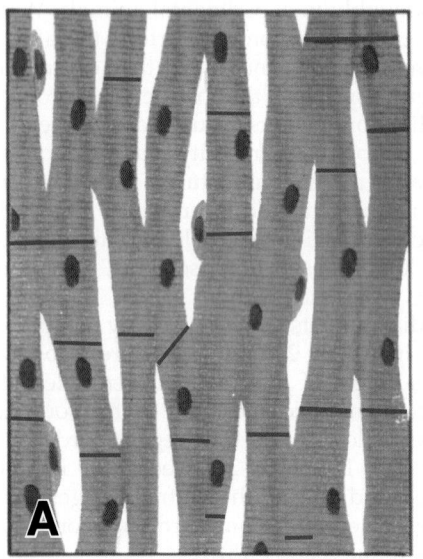

Normal

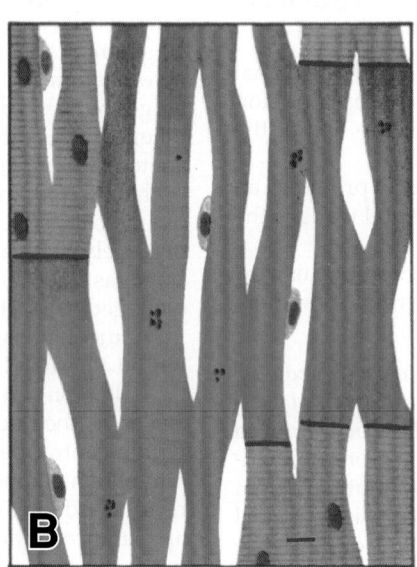

12–18 hours

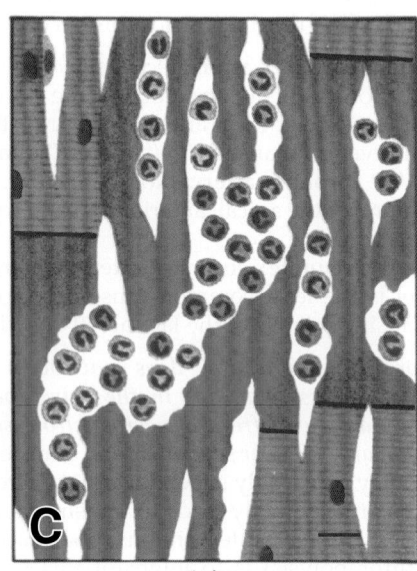

1 day

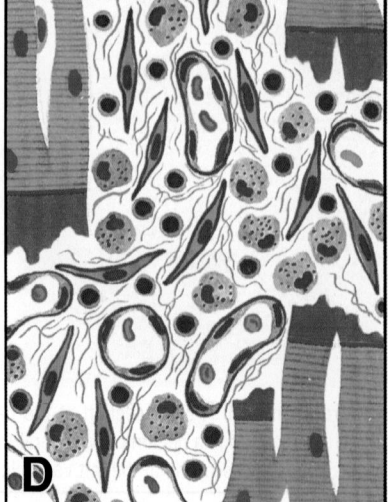

3 weeks

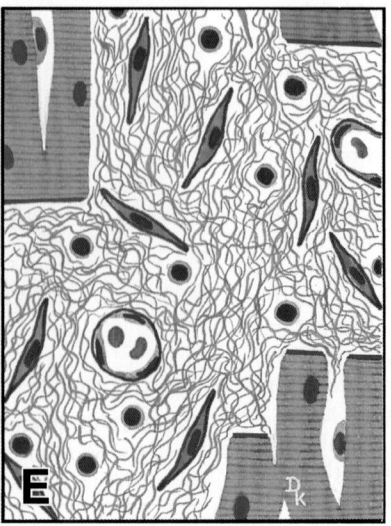

3 months

FIGURE 17-17. Development of a myocardial infarct. A. Normal myocardium. **B.** After about 12–18 hours, the infarcted myocardium shows eosinophilia (*red staining*) in sections of the heart stained with hematoxylin and eosin. **C.** About 24 hours after the onset of infarction, polymorphonuclear neutrophils infiltrate necrotic myocytes at the periphery of the infarct. **D.** After about 3 weeks, peripheral portions of the infarct are composed of granulation tissue with prominent capillaries, fibroblasts, lymphoid cells and macrophages. The necrotic debris has been largely removed from this area, and a small amount of collagen has been laid down. **E.** After 3 months or more, the infarcted region has been replaced by scar tissue.

Microscopic Characteristics of Myocardial Infarcts

THE FIRST 24 HOURS: Electron microscopy is required to discern the earliest morphologic features of ischemic injury (Fig. 17-16). Reversibly injured myocytes show subtle changes of sarcoplasmic edema, mild mitochondrial swelling and loss of glycogen (the ultrastructural correlates of stunned myocardium). After 30–60 minutes of ischemia, when myocyte injury has become irreversible, mitochondria are greatly swollen with disorganized cristae and amorphous matrix densities made of calcium phosphate salts formed by massive Ca^{2+} overload in severely injured cells. Nuclei show clumping and margination of chromatin and the sarcolemma is focally disrupted.

Loss of sarcolemmal integrity leads to release of intracellular proteins, such as myoglobin, LDH, CK and troponins I and T. Ion gradients are also dissipated, and tissue potassium decreases as sodium, chloride and calcium increase.

The noncontractile ischemic myocytes are stretched with each systole and become **"wavy fibers."** By 24 hours, they are deeply eosinophilic (Fig. 17-17) with the characteristic changes of coagulative necrosis (see Chapter 1). However, it takes several days for myocyte nuclei to disappear totally.

TWO TO 3 DAYS: Polymorphonuclear leukocytes are attracted to necrotic myocytes, but they gain access only at the edge of the infarct, where blood flow is intact. They accumulate at infarct borders and reach peak concentrations at 2–3 days (Figs. 17-17 and 17-18). Interstitial edema and microscopic areas of hemorrhage may also appear. By 2–3 days, muscle cells are more clearly necrotic, nuclei disappear and striations become less prominent. Some of the neutrophils begin to undergo karyorrhexis.

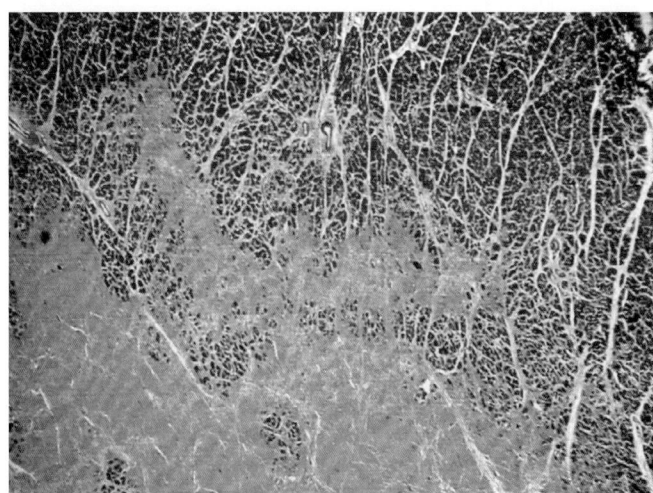

FIGURE 17-19. Healed myocardial infarct. A section at the edge of a healed infarct stained for collagen, which appears blue-green here, shows dense, acellular regions of collagenous matrix sharply demarcated from the adjacent viable myocardium.

FIVE TO 7 DAYS: By this time, few, if any, neutrophils remain. The periphery of the infarcted region shows phagocytosis of dead muscle by macrophages. Fibroblasts begin to proliferate. New collagen is deposited. Lymphocytes and pigment-laden macrophages are prominent. The process of replacing necrotic muscle with scar tissue starts at about 5 days, first at the edge of the infarct, gradually moving inward.

ONE TO 3 WEEKS: Collagen deposition proceeds, inflammation gradually recedes and the newly sprouted capillaries are progressively obliterated.

MORE THAN 4 WEEKS: Considerable dense fibrous tissue is present. The debris is slowly removed, and the scar is more solid and less cellular as it matures (Fig. 17-19).

This sequence of inflammatory and reparative events can be altered by local or systemic factors. For example, immediate extension of an infarct into a region that previously had patchy necrosis may not show expected changes. A large infarct tends not to mature at its center as rapidly as a smaller one. In estimating the age of a large infarct, it is more accurate to base interpretation on the outer border where repair begins, rather than on the central region. In fact, in some large infarcts, dead myocytes are not removed but rather remain indefinitely "mummified."

Reperfusion and Ischemic Myocardium

The above descriptions pertain to healing of infarcts caused by persistent coronary occlusion, such as those arising from thrombotic occlusion of an epicardial coronary artery. However, blood flow may be restored to regions of evolving infarcts either because of spontaneous thrombolysis or in response to therapeutic opening of occluded coronary arteries. When that happens, the infarct's gross and microscopic appearances change. Reperfused infarcts are typically hemorrhagic, from blood flow through damaged microvasculature. Thus, infarcts after persistent occlusion are only grossly apparent after about 12 hours and are pale, but hemorrhage immediately highlights reperfused infarcts. Reperfusion also accelerates acute inflammation: neutrophils gain access throughout

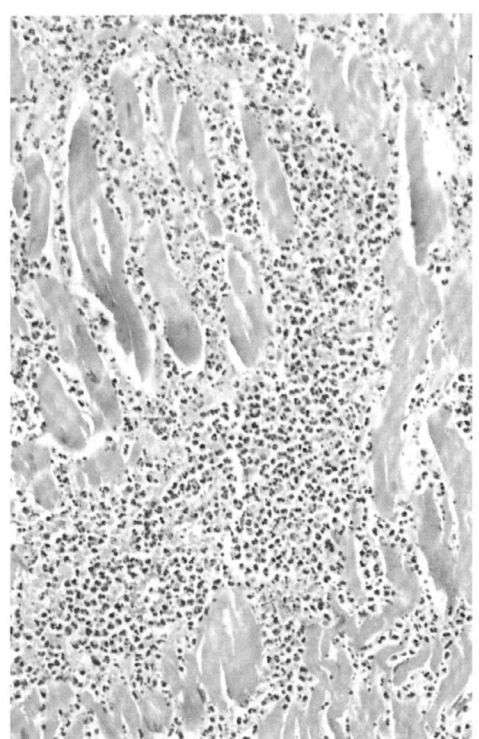

FIGURE 17-18. Acute myocardial infarct. The necrotic myocardial fibers, which are eosinophilic and devoid of cross-striations and nuclei, are immersed in a sea of acute inflammatory cells.

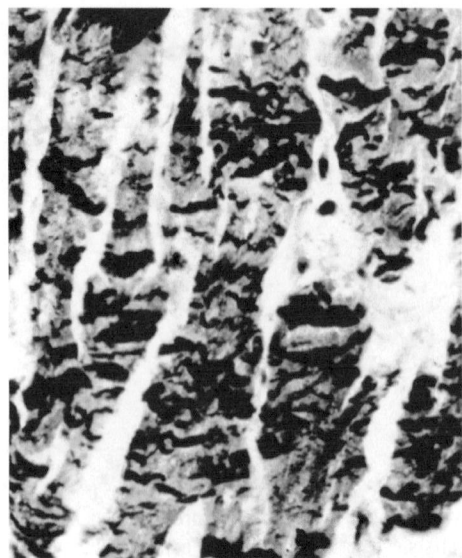

FIGURE 17-20. Contraction band necrosis. A section of infarcted myocardium shows prominent, thick, wavy, transverse bands in myofibers.

the infarct, rather than only at the periphery. They accumulate more rapidly, then also disappear more rapidly. Replacement of necrotic muscle by fibrous scar also occurs more quickly, at least in areas of the infarct in which perfusion persists.

One of the most characteristic features of reperfused infarcts is **contraction band necrosis**. Contraction bands are thick, irregular, transverse eosinophilic bands in necrotic myocytes (Fig. 17-20). By electron microscopy, these bands are small groups of hypercontracted and disorganized sarcomeres with thickened Z disks. The sarcolemma is disrupted and mitochondria located between the contraction bands swell. They may contain deposits of calcium phosphate in the matrix and amorphous matrix densities. Contraction bands occur whenever there is a massive influx of Ca^{2+} into cardiac myocytes. Reperfusion of ischemic myocardium causes extensive sarcolemmal damage mediated largely by reactive oxygen species (ROS), which permits unrestrained entry of extracellular Ca^{2+} into myocytes. This massive Ca^{2+} influx leads to hypercontraction in cells still able to contract. Ca^{2+} flow into more severely injured cells that can no longer contract but still produces dense deposits in mitochondria as in Fig. 17-16. Contraction band necrosis is most prominent when ischemic myocardium is reperfused (e.g., after thrombolytic therapy or with prolonged cardiopulmonary bypass during which the myocardium has sustained irreversible injury). In infarcts arising from persistent coronary occlusion, microscopic foci of contraction band necrosis are often seen at the margins, where dynamic ebb and flow of blood creates conditions that favor Ca^{2+} influx. Other conditions associated with contraction bands include massive catecholamine release in patients with pheochromocytoma or head injuries, or patients in shock treated with large doses of pressors.

 ## CLINICAL FEATURES:

Clinical Diagnosis

The onset of acute myocardial infarction is often sudden, with severe, crushing substernal or precordial pain. The pain may be felt as epigastric burning (simulating indigestion) or it may extend into the jaw or down the inside of either arm. It is often accompanied by sweating, nausea, vomiting and shortness of breath. In some cases an acute myocardial infarction is preceded by unstable angina of several days' duration. *One fourth to 1/2 of nonfatal myocardial infarctions occur without symptoms and are identified only later by ECG changes or at autopsy.* These "clinically silent" infarcts are particularly common among diabetics with autonomic dysfunction and in cardiac transplant patients whose hearts are denervated.

The diagnosis of acute myocardial infarction is confirmed by ECG and by increased serum levels of certain enzymes or proteins. The electrocardiogram shows new Q waves, ST-segment changes and altered conformation of T waves. There is a reasonable correlation between the pathologic distinction of transmural versus subendocardial infarcts and ECG distinction of STEMI (ST elevation myocardial infarction) versus non-STEMI events. Identification in serum of cardiac proteins such as MB-CK or cardiac troponins T and I is evidence of myocardial necrosis.

Complications of Myocardial Infarction

Early mortality in acute myocardial infarction (within 30 days) has dropped from 30% in the 1950s to less than 5% today. Nevertheless, the clinical course after acute infarction may be dominated by functional or mechanical complications of the infarct.

ARRHYTHMIAS: Virtually all patients who have a myocardial infarct have abnormal cardiac rhythm at some time during their illness. Arrhythmias still account for half of deaths caused by ischemic heart disease, but the advent of coronary care units and defibrillators has greatly reduced early mortality. Acute infarction is often associated with premature ventricular beats, sinus bradycardia, ventricular tachycardia, ventricular fibrillation and paroxysmal atrial tachycardia. Partial or complete heart block can also occur. The causes of these arrhythmias are often multifactorial. Acute ischemia alters conduction, increases automaticity and promotes triggered activity related to after-depolarizations. Enhanced sympathetic activity mediated by increased levels of local or circulating catecholamines plays an important role.

LEFT VENTRICULAR FAILURE AND CARDIOGENIC SHOCK: Development of left ventricular failure soon after myocardial infarction is an ominous sign that generally indicates massive loss of muscle. Fortunately, cardiogenic shock occurs in fewer than 5% of cases, owing to the development of techniques that limit the extent of infarction (thrombolytic therapy, angioplasty) or assist damaged myocardium (intra-aortic balloon pump). Cardiogenic shock tends to develop early after infarction when 40% or more of the left ventricle has been lost; mortality is as high as 90%.

EXTENSION OF THE INFARCT: Clinically recognizable extension of an acute infarct occurs in the first 1–2 weeks in up to 10% of patients. In careful echocardiographic studies, half of all patients with anterior myocardial infarction showed some infarct extension during the first 2 weeks, indicating that many episodes of infarct extension are not recognized. Clinically significant infarct extension is associated with a doubling of mortality.

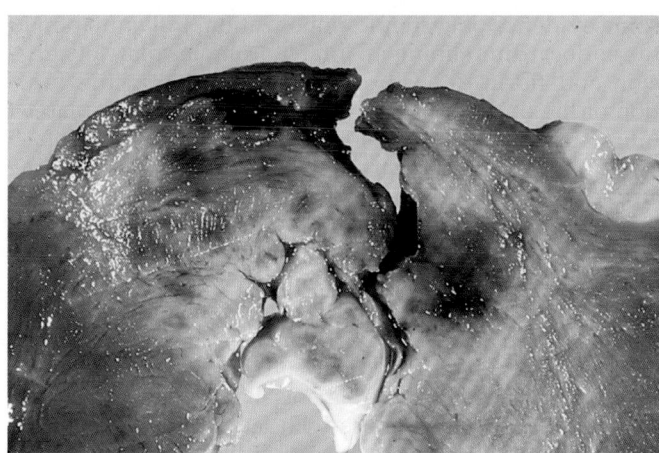

FIGURE 17-21. Rupture of an acute myocardial infarct. An elderly woman with a recent myocardial infarct died of cardiac tamponade. The pericardium was filled with blood, and the cut surface of the left ventricle shows a linear rupture of the necrotic myocardium.

RUPTURE OF THE FREE WALL OF THE MYOCARDIUM: Myocardial rupture (Fig. 17-21) may occur at almost any time in the 3 weeks after acute infarction but is most common between days 1 and 4, when the infarcted wall is weakest. During this vulnerable period, the infarct is composed of soft, necrotic tissue in which the extracellular matrix has been degraded by proteases released by inflammatory cells but new matrix deposition has not yet occurred. Once scars begin to form, rupture is less likely. Rupture of the free wall is a complication of transmural infarcts; surviving muscle overlying subendocardial infarcts prevents rupture. However, rupture usually occurs in relatively small transmural infarcts. The remaining viable, contractile myocardium produces mechanical forces that may initiate and propagate tearing along the infarct's edge, where neutrophils accumulate.

Rupture of the left ventricular free wall most often leads to hemopericardium and death from pericardial tamponade.

Myocardial rupture accounts for 10% of deaths after acute myocardial infarction among hospitalized patients. It is more common in elderly people having a first infarct (most often women). Rarely, a ruptured ventricle may become walled off and the patient survives with a false aneurysm (Fig. 17-22).

OTHER FORMS OF MYOCARDIAL RUPTURE: A few patients in whom a myocardial infarct involves the interventricular septum develop **septal perforations,** 1 cm or longer. The magnitude of the resulting left-to-right shunt and, therefore, the prognosis depend on the size of the rupture.

Rupture of a portion of a papillary muscle results in mitral regurgitation. In some cases, an entire papillary muscle is transected, in which case, massive mitral valve incompetence may be fatal.

ANEURYSMS: Left ventricular aneurysms complicate 10%–15% of transmural myocardial infarcts. After acute transmural infarction, the affected ventricular wall tends to bulge outward during systole in 1/3 of patients. As the infarct heals, the newly deposited collagenous matrix is susceptible to further stretching, although eventually the scar tissue becomes nondistensible. Localized thinning and stretching of the ventricular wall in the region of a healing infarct is called "infarct expansion" but is actually an early aneurysm. Such an aneurysm is composed of a thin layer of necrotic myocardium and collagenous tissue, which expands with each contraction of the heart. As evolving aneurysms become more fibrotic, their tensile strength increases. However, the aneurysms continue to dilate with each beat, thus "stealing" some left ventricular output and increasing the workload of the heart. Patients with left ventricular aneurysms are at increased risk for ventricular tachycardia owing to increased opportunities for electrical current reentry at the periphery of the aneurysm. Mural thrombi often develop within aneurysms and can be sources of systemic emboli.

A distinction should be made between "**true**" and "**false**" **aneurysms** (Fig. 17-22). True aneurysms are much more common than false ones, and are caused by bulging

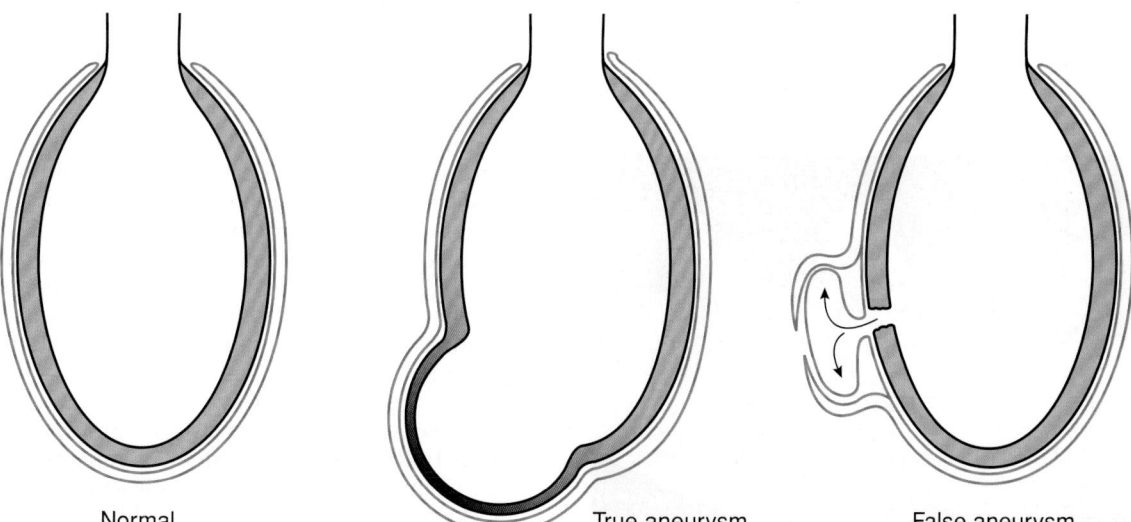

FIGURE 17-22. True and false aneurysms of the left ventricle. Left. Normal heart. The left ventricular wall (*shaded*) is enclosed by the pericardial sac. **Center.** True aneurysm shows an intact wall (*black*), which bulges outward. **Right.** False aneurysm shows a ruptured infarct that is walled off externally by adherent pericardium. Note that the mouth of the true aneurysm is wider than that of the false aneurysm.

Normal   True aneurysm   False aneurysm

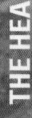

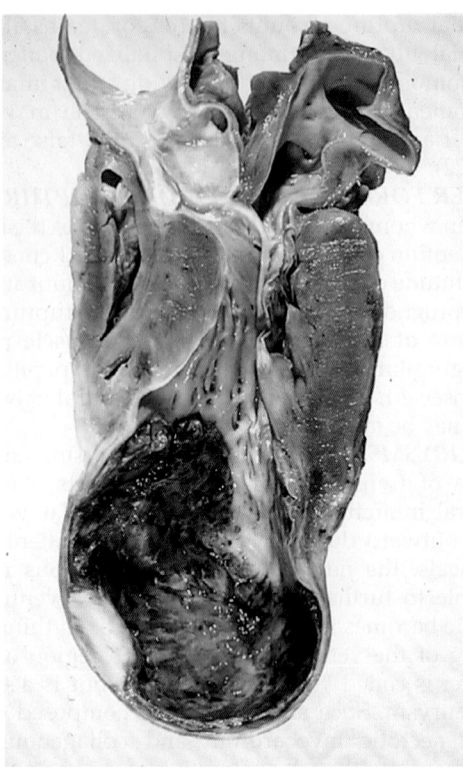

FIGURE 17-23. Ventricular aneurysm. The heart of a patient with a history of an anteroapical myocardial infarct who developed a massive ventricular aneurysm. The apex of the heart shows marked thinning and aneurysmal dilation.

of an intact, but weakened, left ventricular wall (Fig. 17-23). By contrast, false aneurysms result from rupture of a portion of the left ventricle that has been walled off by pericardial scar tissue. Thus, the wall of a false aneurysm is composed of pericardium and scar tissue, not left ventricular myocardium.

MURAL THROMBOSIS AND EMBOLISM: One third to 1/2 of patients who die after myocardial infarction have mural thrombi overlying the infarct at autopsy (Fig. 17-24). This occurs particularly often when the infarct involves the apex of the heart. In turn, half of these patients have

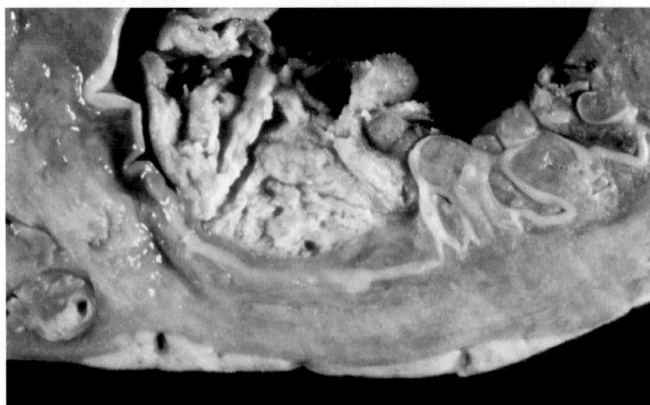

FIGURE 17-24. Mural thrombus overlying a healed myocardial infarct. In this cross-section of a fixed heart, an organized, friable, grayish white mural thrombus overlies a thickened endocardium situated over scarred myocardium.

some evidence of systemic embolization. Inflammation of the endocardium lining an infarct promotes platelet adhesion and fibrin deposition. Also, poor contractile function of the underlying myocardium allows fibrin–platelet mural thrombi to grow. Pieces of thrombus can detach and be swept with the arterial blood, potentially causing strokes or myocardial or visceral infarcts. Documented mural thrombosis justifies anticoagulant and antiplatelet therapy.

PERICARDITIS: A transmural myocardial infarct involves the epicardium and leads to inflammation of the pericardium in 10%–20% of patients. Pericarditis manifests clinically as chest pain and may produce a pericardial friction rub. One quarter of patients with acute myocardial infarction, particularly those with larger infarcts and congestive heart failure, develop pericardial effusions, with or without pericarditis. Less often, anticoagulant therapy may lead to hemorrhagic pericardial effusions and even cardiac tamponade.

Postmyocardial infarction syndrome (Dressler syndrome) is a delayed form of pericarditis that develops 2–10 weeks after infarction. A similar disorder may occur after cardiac surgery. Patients develop antibodies to heart muscle and improve with corticosteroid therapy, suggesting that the syndrome may have an immunologic basis.

Therapeutic Interventions Can Limit Infarct Size

Because the amount of myocardium that undergoes necrosis is an important predictor of morbidity and mortality, any therapy that limits infarct size should be beneficial. By definition, such therapy is directed at preventing reversibly injured, ischemic myocytes from dying and limiting infarct extension. Damaged myocytes can be salvaged for some time after the onset of ischemia if arterial blood flow resumes.

- **Restoration of arterial blood flow** is the only way to salvage ischemic myocytes permanently, although other interventions can slow ischemic injury. The most notable is hypothermia, which is used to minimize myocardial damage during cardiopulmonary bypass. Several methods have been developed to restore blood flow to myocardium supplied by an obstructed coronary artery.
- **Thrombolytic enzymes** such as tissue plasminogen activator or streptokinase can be infused intravenously to dissolve a clot causing vascular obstruction.
- **Percutaneous coronary intervention (PCI)** is dilation of a narrowed coronary artery by inflation with a balloon catheter. PCI can be applied as a primary procedure immediately after onset of ischemia or as a rescue procedure if thrombolytic agents fail to restore arterial blood flow. It nearly always includes placement of a drug-eluting stent in the coronary artery to maintain its patency. The slow release of drugs such as everolimus, an inhibitor of the mTOR (mammalian target of rapamycin) pathway (see Chapters 1 and 5), limits subsequent restenosis by blocking smooth muscle cell proliferative responses to local injury caused by inflation of the balloon catheter and deployment of the stent.
- **Coronary artery bypass grafting** can restore blood flow to the coronary artery segment beyond a proximal occlusion.

Procedures that restore blood flow must be performed as quickly as possible, preferably within the first few hours after symptoms begin. Beyond 12 hours, it is unlikely that much salvageable ischemic myocardium remains, although reperfusion at this point may aid infarct healing and limit maladaptive postinfarct remodeling.

Chronic Ischemic Heart Disease Can Lead to Cardiomyopathy

In a minority of patients with severe coronary atherosclerosis, myocardial contractility is impaired globally without discrete infarcts, as in dilated cardiomyopathy. This situation usually reflects a combination of ischemic myocardial dysfunction, diffuse fibrosis and multiple small healed infarcts. However, there is a group of patients with left ventricular failure in whom cardiac dysfunction occurs without obvious infarction. These patients are said to have **ischemic cardiomyopathy**. In some, the dysfunctional myocardium has experienced repetitive episodes of ischemic injury, which causes degenerative changes in myocytes, with loss of myofibrils (hibernating myocardium) (Fig. 17-6). Contractile function of hibernating myocardium is restored when affected tissue is revascularized. Thus, to the extent that hibernation plays a role in ischemic cardiomyopathy, surgical revascularization may be beneficial.

HYPERTENSIVE HEART DISEASE

Effects of Hypertension on the Heart

The World Health Organization defines hypertension as persistent increase of systemic blood pressure above 140 mm Hg systolic or 90 mm Hg diastolic, or both (see Chapter 16). Chronic hypertension is one of the most prevalent and serious causes of coronary artery and myocardial disease in the United States. It leads to pressure overload resulting first in compensatory left ventricular hypertrophy and, eventually, cardiac failure. The term **hypertensive heart disease** is used when the heart is enlarged in the absence of a cause other than hypertension.

 PATHOLOGY: The increased workload caused by hypertension leads to compensatory left ventricular hypertrophy. The left ventricular free walls and interventricular septum become thickened uniformly and concentrically (Fig. 17-25), and heart weight increases, exceeding 375 g in men and 350 g in women. Hypertrophic myocardial cells are thicker, with enlarged, hyperchromatic, and rectangular ("boxcar") nuclei (Fig. 17-26).

 CLINICAL FEATURES: Myocardial hypertrophy clearly allows the heart to handle increased workload. However, there is a limit beyond which additional hypertrophy no longer compensates. This upper limit to useful hypertrophy may reflect increasing diffusion distance between the interstitium and the center of each myofiber; if that distance is too great, oxygen supply to the myofiber will be impaired.

Diastolic dysfunction is the most common operative abnormality caused by hypertension and by itself can lead to congestive heart failure. Hypertrophy causes some interstitial fibrosis, which makes the left ventricle stiffer.

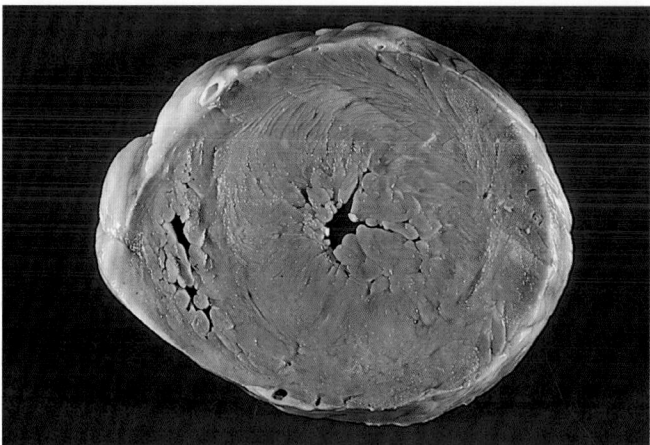

FIGURE 17-25. Hypertensive heart disease. A transverse section of the heart shows marked hypertrophy of the left ventricular myocardium without dilation of the chamber. The right ventricle is of normal dimensions.

Hypertension also is associated with more severe coronary artery atherosclerosis. *The combination of greater cardiac workload (systolic dysfunction), diastolic dysfunction and narrowed coronary arteries leads to greater risk of myocardial ischemia, infarction and heart failure.*

Congestive Heart Failure Is the Major Cause of Death in Patients with Untreated Hypertension

Fatal intracerebral hemorrhage is common as well. Death may also result from coronary atherosclerosis and myocardial infarction, dissecting aortic aneurysm or ruptured cerebral berry aneurysm. Renal failure may supervene when nephrosclerosis induced by hypertension becomes severe.

COR PULMONALE

Cor pulmonale is right ventricular hypertrophy and dilation due to pulmonary hypertension. Increased pulmonary

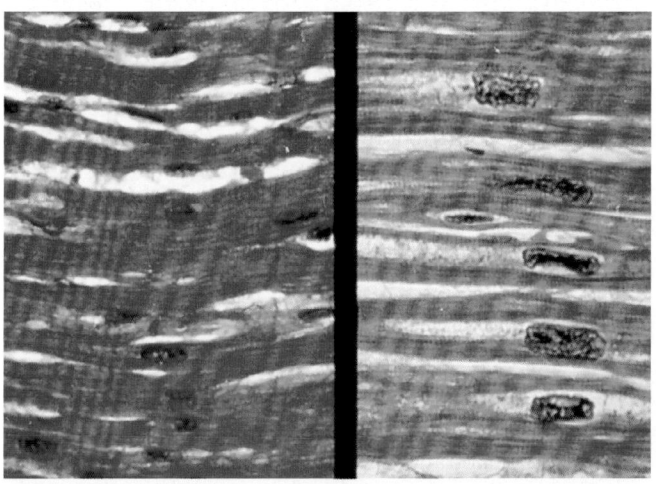

FIGURE 17-26. Hypertensive heart disease with myocardial hypertrophy. Left. Normal myocardium. Right. Hypertrophic myocardium (same magnification) shows thicker fibers and enlarged, hyperchromatic, rectangular nuclei.

arterial pressure may reflect a disorder of lung parenchyma or, more rarely, a primary vascular disease (e.g., primary pulmonary hypertension, recurrent small pulmonary emboli).

Acute cor pulmonale is an abrupt occurrence of pulmonary hypertension, most commonly due to sudden, massive pulmonary embolization. This condition causes acute right-sided heart failure and is a medical emergency. At autopsy, the only cardiac findings are severe right ventricular, and sometimes right atrial, dilation.

Chronic cor pulmonale is a common heart disease, accounting for 30%–40% of heart failure in an English study and 10%–30% in the United States. This frequency reflects the prevalence of lung disease in these countries, especially chronic bronchitis and emphysema. Often, in chronic lung disease, the degree of pulmonary hypertension correlates more closely with survival than any other variable: fewer than 10% of patients with pulmonary artery pressures over 45 mm Hg survive 5 years.

 **ETIOLOGIC FACTORS:** Chronic cor pulmonale may be caused by any pulmonary disease that interferes with ventilatory mechanics or gas exchange or obstructs the pulmonary vasculature (Table 17-5). *The most common causes of chronic cor pulmonale are chronic obstructive pulmonary disease and pulmonary fibrosis.* Severe kyphoscoliosis may deform the chest wall and impede its function as a bellows, leading to hypoxemia and pulmonary vasoconstriction. **Primary pulmonary hypertension** is a rare disorder that may also cause cor pulmonale. Some congenital heart diseases associated with increased pulmonary blood flow (see above) are complicated by pulmonary hypertension and cor pulmonale.

PATHOPHYSIOLOGY: The pathogenesis of pulmonary hypertension due to recurrent pulmonary emboli is related clearly to progressive mechanical obstruction of blood flow. However, mechanisms of pulmonary hypertension in chronic parenchymal diseases of the lungs are more complicated. In addition to obliteration of blood vessels in the lung, these disorders also lead to pulmonary arteriolar vasoconstriction, which reduces the effective cross-sectional area of the pulmonary vascular bed without destroying vessels. Hypoxia, acidosis and hypercapnia directly cause pulmonary vasoconstriction. Hypoxia also raises pulmonary vascular resistance indirectly by leading to polycythemia, which increases blood viscosity. People living at very high altitude (e.g., natives of the Andes mountain range) often develop cor pulmonale because of the effects of chronic hypoxemia.

MOLECULAR PATHOGENESIS: Some people with primary pulmonary hypertension have a familial disease with dominant inheritance and incomplete penetrance. Many of these individuals have mutations in the gene encoding bone morphogenic protein receptor type 2 (*BMPR2*). BMPR2 participates in signaling pathways that regulate gene expression and intersect with other signaling cascades (e.g., MAPK pathway). A

TABLE 17-5
CAUSES OF COR PULMONALE
Parenchymal Diseases of the Lung
Chronic bronchitis and emphysema
Pulmonary fibrosis (from any cause)
Cystic fibrosis
Pulmonary Vascular Diseases
Recurrent pulmonary emboli
Primary pulmonary hypertension
Peripheral pulmonary stenosis
Intravenous drug abuse
Residence at high altitude
Schistosomiasis
Congenital Heart Diseases
Impaired Movement of the Thoracic Cage
Kyphoscoliosis
Pickwickian syndrome
Pleural fibrosis
Neuromuscular disorders
Idiopathic hypoventilation

consequence of this aberrant signaling is endothelial dysfunction with insufficient production of vasodilators such as NO and prostacyclin and overexpression of vasoconstrictors such as thromboxane. Resulting imbalances promote vasoconstriction, which leads to smooth muscle hyperplasia and thickening of small pulmonary arteries, which is typically seen in pulmonary arterial hypertension.

 PATHOLOGY: Chronic cor pulmonale is characterized by conspicuous right ventricular hypertrophy (Fig. 17-27), which may exceed 1.0 cm in thickness (normal, 0.3–0.5 cm). Right ventricular and right atrial dilatation are often present. Normally, the interventricular septum is concave to the left (i.e., it is part of the left ventricle). When right ventricular hypertrophy is severe, the interventricular septum remodels by straightening or even becoming concave to the right.

ACQUIRED VALVULAR AND ENDOCARDIAL DISEASES

Many inflammatory, infectious and degenerative diseases damage heart valves and impair their function. Valves normally are thin flexible membranes that close tightly to prevent backward blood flow. The semilunar valves are

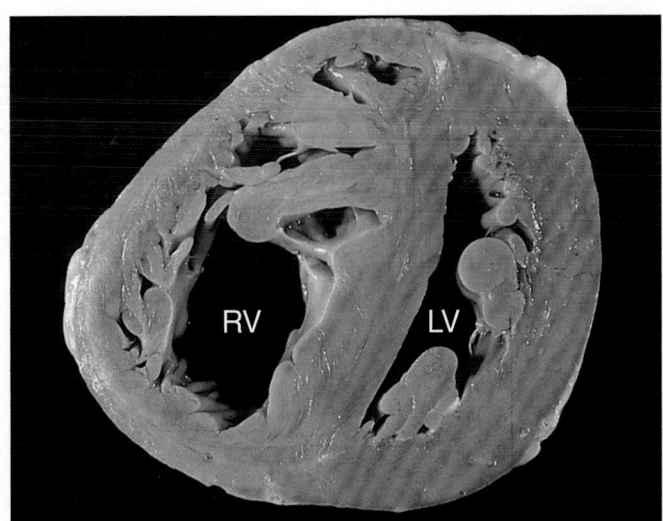

FIGURE 17-27. Cor pulmonale. A transverse section of the heart from a patient with primary (idiopathic) pulmonary hypertension shows a markedly hypertrophied right ventricle (on the left in this image). The right ventricular free wall has a thickness nearly equal to the left ventricular wall. The right ventricle is dilated. The straightened interventricular septum has lost its normal curvature toward the left ventricle as part of the remodeling process in cor pulmonale.

structurally and functionally simple compared with atrioventricular valves. The latter consist of the valve leaflets, muscular valve annuli and subvalvular apparatus (chordae tendineae and papillary muscles). In general, valvular stenosis involves pathologic changes of leaflets themselves, but regurgitation can be caused by abnormalities of valve leaflets, annulus or subvalvular apparatus.

When they become damaged, leaflets or cusps may be thickened and fused sufficiently to narrow the aperture and obstruct blood flow. This is called **valvular stenosis**. Diseases that destroy valve tissue may also allow retrograde blood flow into the atria during systole—**valvular regurgitation** or **insufficiency**. Diseases of the cardiac valves may produce both stenosis and insufficiency, but one or the other generally predominates.

Stenosis of a cardiac valve results in **pressure overload** hypertrophy of the myocardium proximal (i.e., upstream, in terms of blood flow) to the obstruction. Once compensatory mechanisms are exhausted, dilation and failure of the chamber proximal to the valve eventually occur. Thus, mitral stenosis leads to left atrial hypertrophy and dilation. As the left atrium decompensates and can no longer propel the pulmonary venous return through the stenotic mitral valve, blood backs up into the pulmonary venous circuit and signs of pulmonary congestion develop. This is followed by right ventricular hypertrophy and may even lead to cor pulmonale. Similarly, aortic stenosis causes left ventricular hypertrophy and eventually left heart failure.

Valvular regurgitation or insufficiency also results in hypertrophy and dilation of the chamber proximal to the valve, owing to **volume overload**. In aortic insufficiency, the left ventricle first hypertrophies, then, when it can no longer accommodate the regurgitant volume and maintain adequate cardiac output, it dilates. An incompetent mitral valve leads to hypertrophy and dilation of both the left atrium and left ventricle, as both experience volume overload.

Marked left ventricular dilation from any cause that limits cardiac contractility (e.g., congestive failure after a large myocardial infarct) may also widen the mitral valve ring and splay the left ventricular papillary muscles. These effects may be so severe that the valve leaflets do not close properly, leading to mitral regurgitation.

Rheumatic Heart Disease Encompasses Acute Myocarditis and Residual Valvular Deformities

Acute Rheumatic Fever

Rheumatic fever (RF) is a multisystem childhood disease that follows streptococcal infection. It entails an inflammatory reaction involving the heart, joints and central nervous system.

 **EPIDEMIOLOGY:** RF is a complication of acute streptococcal infection, almost always pharyngitis (i.e., "strep" throat; see Chapter 9). The cause is *Streptococcus pyogenes*, also known as group A β-hemolytic *Streptococcus*. In some epidemics of streptococcal pharyngitis, incidence of RF may be as high as 3%. RF is mainly a disease of children, the median age being 9 to 11 years, although it can occur in adults.

In the first half of the 20th century, RF reached almost epidemic proportions in the United States, but its incidence has decreased dramatically. Between 1950 and 1972, the death rate fell from 14.5 to 6.8 per 100,000, and has decreased further since then. This decline in part reflects widespread antibiotic treatment, but that therapy cannot explain the entire reduction, because the death rate had begun to decrease well before antibiotics were generally available. Better socioeconomic conditions, particularly less crowded living circumstances, probably also contributed. *RF, though less common in developed countries, is still a leading cause of cardiac deaths in young people elsewhere.*

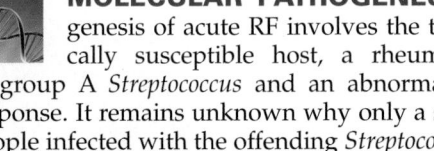 **MOLECULAR PATHOGENESIS:** The pathogenesis of acute RF involves the triad of a genetically susceptible host, a rheumatogenic strain of group A *Streptococcus* and an abnormal host immune response. It remains unknown why only a small number of people infected with the offending *Streptococcus* develop RF. Human leukocyte antigen (HLA) class II molecules appear to play a role in disease susceptibility; exactly how is unclear. The specific HLA molecules may present the bacterial antigens differently from other HLA molecules; there are similarities between some HLA class II alleles and streptococcal antigens. This may lead to aberrant cytokine production, causing antibodies to be directed against proteins on valves and other host tissues. Alternatively, bacterial antigens may mimic HLA molecules, and so initiate an aberrant immune response. These mechanisms suggest the possibility of an autoimmune etiology (Fig. 17-28).

Streptococcal antigens structurally akin to those in the heart include hyaluronate in the bacterial capsule, cell wall polysaccharides like to carbohydrates of heart valve glycoproteins and bacterial membrane antigens that share epitopes with sarcolemma and smooth muscle constituents.

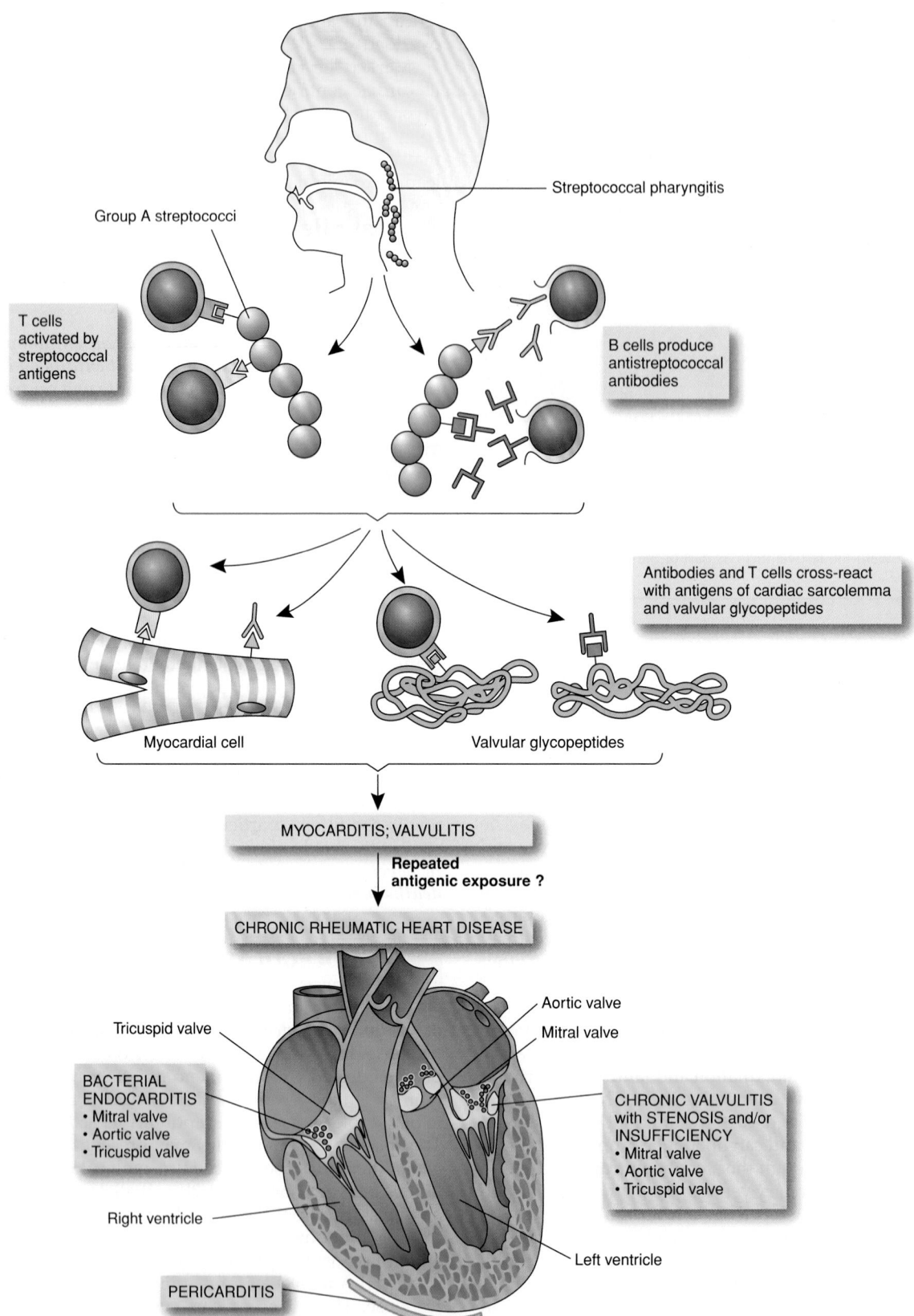

FIGURE 17-28. Biological factors in rheumatic heart disease. The upper portion illustrates the initiating β-hemolytic streptococcal infection of the throat, which introduces the streptococcal antigens into the body and may also activate cytotoxic T cells. These antigens lead to the production of antibodies against various antigenic components of the streptococcus, which can cross-react with certain cardiac antigens, including those from the myocyte sarcolemma and glycoproteins of the valves. This may be the mechanism for inflammation of the heart in acute rheumatic fever, which involves all cardiac layers (endocarditis, myocarditis and pericarditis). This inflammation becomes apparent after a latent period of 2–3 weeks. Active inflammation of the valves may eventually lead to chronic valvular stenosis or insufficiency. These lesions involve the mitral, aortic and tricuspid valves, in that order of frequency.

Although antibodies to these antigens are found in patients with RF, it has not been proved that they are cytotoxic or even that they are directly involved in the pathogenesis of the disease. A direct toxic effect of some streptococcal product on the myocardium has not yet been excluded.

 PATHOLOGY: Acute rheumatic heart disease is a pancarditis; that is, it affects all three layers of the heart (endocardium, myocardium, pericardium).

MYOCARDITIS: In severe cases of RF, a few patients may die during the earliest acute phase of the illness before the typical granulomatous inflammation develops. At this early stage, the heart tends to be dilated and shows a nonspecific myocarditis, with lymphocytes and macrophages predominating, although a few neutrophils and eosinophils may be present. Fibrinoid degeneration of collagen, in which fibers become swollen, fragmented and eosinophilic, is characteristic of this early phase.

The **Aschoff body** is the characteristic granulomatous lesion of rheumatic myocarditis (Fig. 17-29). It develops several weeks after symptoms begin. At first, it consists of a perivascular focus of swollen eosinophilic collagen surrounded by lymphocytes, plasma cells and macrophages. With time, the Aschoff body assumes a granulomatous appearance, with a fibrinoid central and a perimeter of lymphocytes, plasma cells, macrophages and giant cells. In time, it is replaced by a scarred nodule.

Anitschkow cells are unusual cells within Aschoff bodies, whose nuclei contain a central band of chromatin. These nuclei have an "owl eye" appearance in cross-section, and they resemble a caterpillar when cut longitudinally (Fig. 17-29). These cells are macrophages that are normally

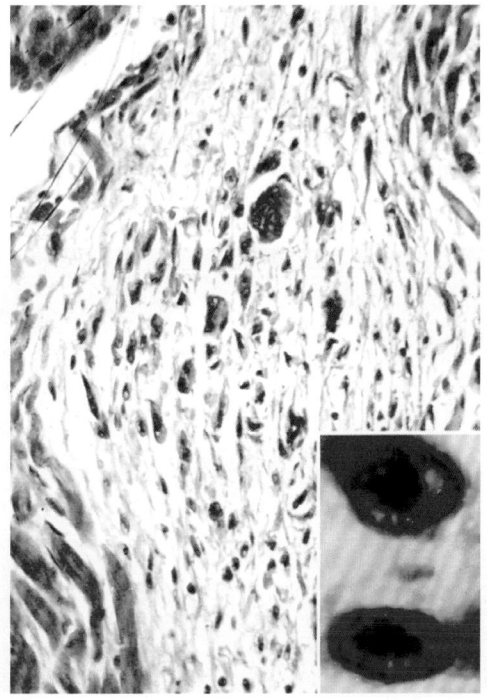

FIGURE 17-29. Acute rheumatic heart disease. An Aschoff body in the myocardial interstitium. Note collagen degeneration, lymphocytes and a multinucleated Aschoff giant cell. **Inset.** Nuclei of Anitschkow myocytes, showing "owl-eye" appearance in cross-section and "caterpillar" shape longitudinally.

present in small numbers but accumulate and are prominent in certain types of inflammatory diseases of the heart. Anitschkow cells may become multinucleated, in which case they are termed **Aschoff giant cells**.

PERICARDITIS: Tenacious irregular fibrin deposits are found on visceral and parietal pericardial surfaces during the acute inflammatory phase of RF. These exudates resemble the shaggy surfaces of two slices of buttered bread that have been pulled apart ("bread-and-butter pericarditis"). This pericarditis may manifest clinically as a friction rub, but it is functionally minor and only infrequently leads to constrictive pericarditis.

ENDOCARDITIS: During the acute stage of rheumatic carditis, valve leaflets become inflamed and edematous. All four valves are affected, but left-sided valves are most injured because they close under greater pressures than right-sided valves. The result is damage and focal loss of endothelium along valve leaflet closure lines. This leads to deposition of tiny nodules of fibrin, which can be recognized grossly as "verrucae" along the leaflets (so-called verrucous endocarditis of acute RF).

 CLINICAL FEATURES: There is no specific test for RF. Clinically, the diagnosis is made if two major—or one major and two minor—criteria **(Jones criteria)** are met. Evidence of recent streptococcal infection increases the probability of RF.

The **major criteria** of acute RF include carditis (murmurs, cardiomegaly, pericarditis and congestive heart failure), polyarthritis, chorea, erythema marginatum and subcutaneous nodules.

The **minor criteria** are previous history of RF, arthralgia, fever, certain laboratory tests indicating an inflammatory process (e.g., increased sedimentation rate, positive test result for C-reactive protein, leukocytosis) and ECG changes.

Symptoms of RF begin 2–3 weeks after an infection with *S. pyogenes.* By then, throat cultures are usually negative. Increasing serum antibodies to group A streptococcal antigens, such as antistreptolysin O, anti-DNAase B and antihyaluronidase, provide concrete evidence of a recent infection with group A *Streptococcus.* Acute symptoms of RF usually subside within 3 months, but with severe carditis, clinical activity may continue for 6 months or more. Mortality in acute rheumatic carditis is low. The main cause of death is heart failure due to myocarditis, although valvular dysfunction may also play a role.

Recurrent attacks of RF are associated with types of group A β-hemolytic streptococci to which the patient has not been exposed previously and, thus, to which immunity has not developed. The rate of RF recurrence is related to the time between the initial episode and a subsequent streptococcal infection. In patients with a history of a recent attack of RF, recurrence rates may reach 65%, while recurrence after 10 years affects only 5% of patients.

Prompt treatment of streptococcal pharyngitis with antibiotics prevents a first attack of RF and, less often, recurrences. There is no specific treatment for acute RF, but corticosteroids and salicylates are helpful in managing the symptoms.

Chronic Rheumatic Heart Disease

 PATHOLOGY: The myocardial and pericardial components of rheumatic pancarditis typically resolve without permanent sequelae. By contrast,

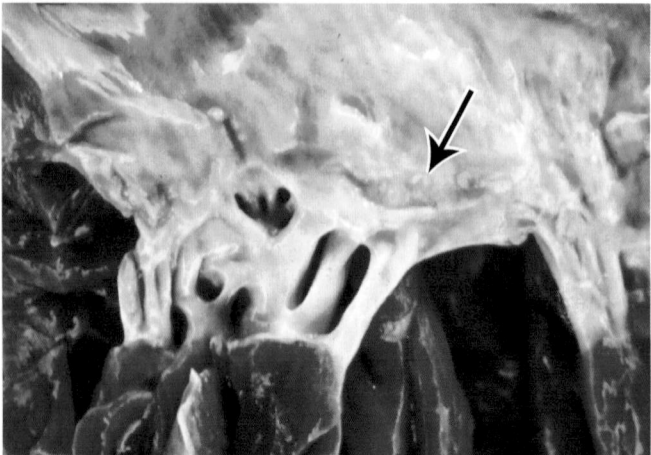

FIGURE 17-30. Chronic rheumatic valvulitis. The mitral valve leaflets are thickened and focally calcified (*arrow*), and the commissures are partially fused. The chordae tendineae are also short, thick and fused.

valvulitis due to RF often leads to long-term structural and functional changes. During the healing phase, valve leaflets develop diffuse fibrosis and become thickened, shrunken and less pliable. At the same time, healing of the verrucous lesions along the lines of closure often generates fibrous "adhesions" between leaflets, especially at the commissures (commissural fusion). The result is a stenotic valve that does not open freely because its leaflets are rigid and partially fused. Blood flow across such a valve is turbulent, which can cause even more scarring and deformation of leaflets because of chronic "wear and tear" on the valve. Severe valvular scarring may develop months or years after a single bout of acute RF. On the other hand, recurrent episodes of acute RF are common and result in repeated and progressively increasing damage to the heart valves.

The mitral valve is the most commonly and severely affected valve in chronic rheumatic disease. It snaps shut under systolic pressure and, thus, bears the greatest mechanical burden of all the valves. In chronic mitral valvulitis, valve leaflets become conspicuous, irregularly thickened and calcified, often with fusion of commissures and chordae tendineae (Fig. 17-30). In severe chronic rheumatic mitral valvular disease, valve orifices become reduced to fixed narrow slits resembling "fish mouths" when viewed from the ventricular aspect (Fig. 17-31). Stenosis is dominant functionally, but mitral valves are also regurgitant. Chronic regurgitation produces a "jet" of blood directed at the posterior aspect of the left atrium, damaging atrial endocardium and producing focal rough, wrinkled endocardium called "MacCallum patches."

The aortic valve, which snaps shut under diastolic pressure, is the second most commonly involved valve in rheumatic heart disease. Diffuse fibrous thickening of the cusps and fusion of the commissures cause aortic stenosis, which may be mild initially but which progresses because of the chronic effects of turbulent blood flow across the valve. Often, cusps become rigidly calcified as the patient ages, resulting in stenosis and insufficiency, although either lesion may predominate (Fig. 17-32). The lower pressures experienced by the right-sided valves are usually protective. In recurrent RF, however, tricuspid valves may become deformed, virtually always in association with mitral and aortic lesions. Pulmonic valves are rarely affected.

Complications of Chronic Rheumatic Heart Disease

- **Bacterial endocarditis** follows episodes of bacteremia (e.g., during dental procedures). The scarred valves of rheumatic heart disease provide an attractive environment for bacteria that would bypass a normal valve.
- **Mural thrombi** form in atrial or ventricular chambers in 40% of patients with rheumatic valvular disease. They give rise to thromboemboli, which can produce infarcts in various organs. Rarely, a large thrombus in the left atrial appendage develops a stalk and acts as a ball valve to obstruct the mitral valve orifice.
- **Congestive heart failure** complicates rheumatic disease of both mitral and aortic valves.

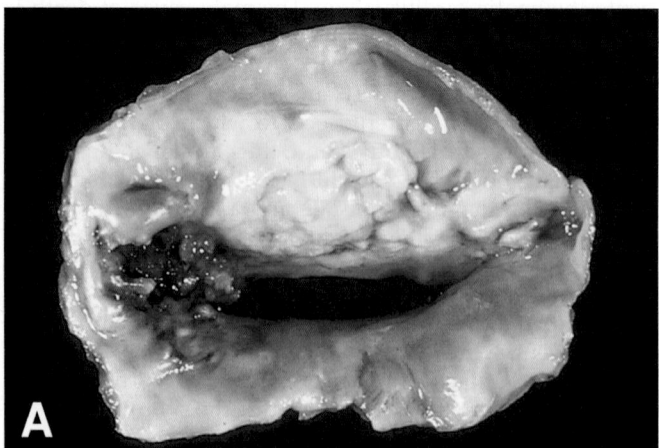
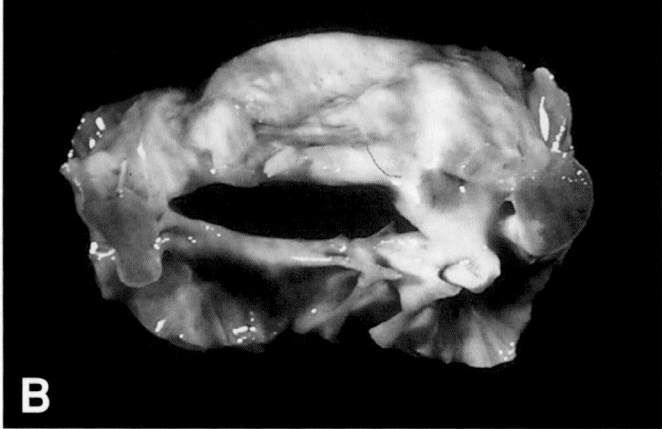

FIGURE 17-31. Chronic rheumatic valvulitis. A view of a surgically excised rheumatic mitral valve from the left atrium **(A)** and left ventricle **(B)** shows rigid, thickened and fused leaflets with a narrow orifice, creating the characteristic "fish mouth" appearance of rheumatic mitral stenosis. Note that the tips of the papillary muscles (shown in B) are directly attached to the underside of the valve leaflets, reflecting marked shortening and fusion of the chordae tendineae.

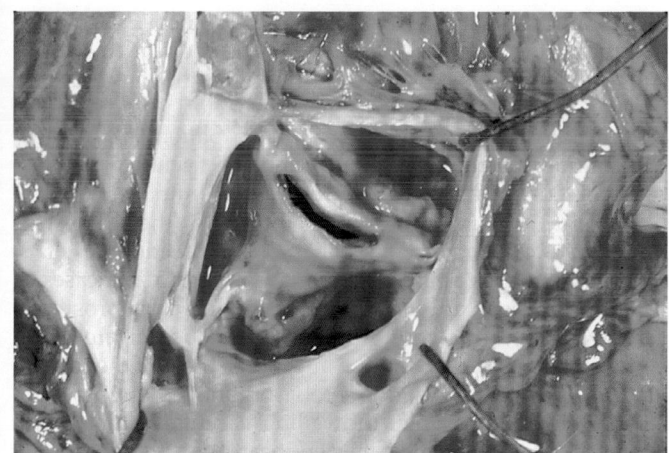

FIGURE 17-32. Chronic rheumatic aortic valvulitis. An example of severe rheumatic aortic stenosis. Three sinuses of Valsalva are recognizable, but the cusps are rigidly fibrotic and calcified, and extensive fusion of the commissures has narrowed the orifice into a fixed slit-like configuration that does not change during the cardiac cycle.

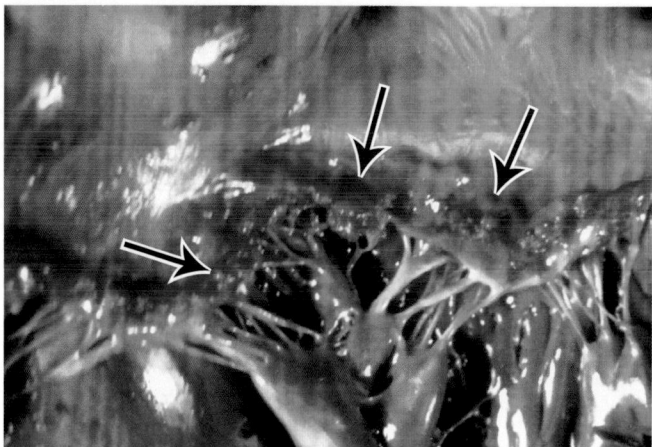

FIGURE 17-33. Libman-Sacks endocarditis. The heart of a patient who died of complications of systemic lupus erythematosus displays verrucous vegetations (*arrows*) on the leaflets of the mitral valve.

- **Adhesive pericarditis** often follows the fibrinous pericarditis of acute attacks, but rarely causes constrictive pericarditis.

Autoimmune Diseases Affect Cardiac Valves and Myocardium

Systemic Lupus Erythematosus

The heart is often involved in SLE, but cardiac symptoms are usually less prominent than other manifestations of the disease.

 PATHOLOGY: The most common cardiac lesion is **fibrinous pericarditis,** usually with an effusion. **Myocarditis** in SLE, manifesting as subclinical left ventricular dysfunction, is also common and reflects the severity of the disease in other organs. Fibrinoid necrosis of small vessels and focal degeneration of interstitial tissue are seen.

Endocarditis is the most striking cardiac lesion of SLE. Verrucous vegetations, up to 4 mm, occur on endocardial surfaces and are called **Libman-Sacks endocarditis.** They occur most often on the mitral valve (Fig. 17-33), usually on atrial surfaces, close to the origin of the leaflets from the valve ring. They may also extend onto chordae tendineae and papillary muscles. Aortic valve involvement is rare. Ordinarily, *Libman-Sacks endocarditis heals without scarring and does not produce a functional deficit.*

Rheumatoid Arthritis

The heart is rarely involved in patients with rheumatoid arthritis. Characteristic rheumatoid granulomatous inflammation, with fibrinoid necrosis and palisaded lymphocytes and macrophages, may occur in the pericardium, myocardium or valves. Cardiac function remains intact.

Ankylosing Spondylitis

A characteristic aortic valve lesion develops in up to 10% of patients with long-standing ankylosing spondylitis. The aortic valve ring is dilated and its cusps are scarred and shortened. Focal inflammatory lesions occur in all layers of the aortic wall, particularly near the valve ring. Aortic regurgitation is the principal functional consequence.

Scleroderma (Progressive Systemic Sclerosis)

Cardiac involvement is second only to renal disease as a cause of death in scleroderma. The myocardium shows intimal sclerosis of small arteries, which leads to small infarcts and patchy fibrosis. As a result, congestive heart failure and arrhythmias are common. In fact, ECGs show ventricular ectopy in up to 2/3 of patients with scleroderma, and serious arrhythmias in 1/4. Cor pulmonale (due to pulmonary interstitial fibrosis) and hypertensive heart disease (caused by renal involvement) are also seen.

Polyarteritis Nodosa

The heart is affected in up to 75% of patients with polyarteritis nodosa. Necrotizing lesions in branches of the coronary arteries cause myocardial infarction, arrhythmias or heart block. Cardiac hypertrophy and failure due to renal vascular hypertension are common.

Bacterial Endocarditis Is Infection of the Cardiac Valves

Fungi, chlamydia and rickettsiae may also cause infective endocarditis, but do so uncommonly. Before the antibiotic era, bacterial endocarditis was untreatable and almost invariably fatal. The infection was classified according to its clinical course as acute or subacute endocarditis. **Acute bacterial endocarditis** was infection of normal cardiac valves by highly virulent suppurative organisms, typically *Staphylococcus aureus* and *S. pyogenes.* Affected valves were rapidly destroyed, and patients usually died within 6 weeks from acute heart failure or overwhelming sepsis.

Subacute bacterial endocarditis was less fulminant, with less virulent organisms (e.g., *Streptococcus viridans* or *Staphylococcus epidermidis*) infecting structurally abnormal valves, which typically had been deformed by rheumatic

TABLE 17-6

ETIOLOGIC FACTORS IN BACTERIAL ENDOCARDITIS

	Children (%)		Adults (%)	
	Newborns	<15 y	15–60 y	>60 y
Underlying Disease				
Congenital heart disease	30	80	10	2
Rheumatic heart disease	—	5	25	8
Mitral valve prolapse	—	10	10	10
Valvular calcification	—	—	5	30
Intravenous drug abuse	—	—	15	10
Other	—	—	10	10
None	70	5	25	30
Microorganisms[a]				
Staphylococcus aureus	45	25	35	30
Coagulase-negative staphylococci	10	5	5	10
Streptococci	15	45	45	35
Enterococci	—	5	5	15
Gram-negative bacteria	10	5	5	5
Fungi	10	Rare	Rare	Rare
Negative culture	5	10	5	5

[a]Five percent of neonatal infections are polymicrobial.

heart disease. These patients usually survived for 6 months or more, and infectious complications were uncommon.

Antimicrobial therapy changed clinical patterns of bacterial endocarditis, and the above classical presentations are now unusual. The disease is now classified by the anatomic location and the offending organism (Table 17-6).

 **EPIDEMIOLOGY:** Most children with bacterial endocarditis have an underlying cardiac lesion. In the past, rheumatic heart disease accounted for 1/3 of such cases. However, as incidence of RF has declined, RF is responsible for fewer than 10% of children with bacterial endocarditis. *The most common predisposing condition for bacterial endocarditis in children currently is congenital cardiac malformations.*

Epidemiology of bacterial endocarditis has also changed in adults. Rheumatic heart disease once made up 75% of cases, but now underlies only a few. Most adults with bacterial endocarditis have no predisposing cardiac lesion. *Mitral valve prolapse (MVP) and congenital heart disease are now the most frequent bases for bacterial endocarditis in adults.*

- In patients in whom bacterial endocarditis is superimposed on **rheumatic heart disease,** mitral valves are affected in over 85%, and aortic valves in 50%. A lone mitral valve is affected more often in women (2:1), but the ratio is reversed, 4:1, in isolated aortic endocarditis.

- **Intravenous drug abusers** inject pathogenic organisms along with illicit drugs, and bacterial endocarditis is a notorious complication. In such patients, 80% have no underlying cardiac lesion, and the tricuspid valve is involved in half of cases. The most common source of bacteria in intravenous drug abusers is the skin, with *S. aureus* causing more than half of the infections.

- **Prosthetic valves** are sites of infection in 15% of cases of endocarditis in adults, and 4% of patients with prosthetic valves have this complication. Staphylococci are again responsible for half of these infections. Most of the rest are caused by gram-negative aerobic organisms, streptococci, enterococci and fungi. Indwelling vascular catheters are another source of iatrogenic endocarditis.

- **Transient bacteremia** from any procedure may lead to infective endocarditis. Examples include dental procedures, urinary catheterization, gastrointestinal endoscopy and obstetric procedures. Antibiotic prophylaxis is recommended during such maneuvers for patients at increased risk for bacterial endocarditis (e.g., those with a history of RF or a cardiac murmur).

- **The elderly** are increasingly prone to developing endocarditis. Degenerative changes in heart valves, including calcific aortic stenosis and calcification of mitral annuli, predispose to endocarditis.

- **Diabetes** and **pregnancy** may also increase the incidence of bacterial endocarditis.

  **ETIOLOGIC FACTORS AND MOLECULAR PATHOGENESIS:** Virulent organisms, such as *S. aureus*, can infect apparently normal valves, but the mechanism of such bacterial colonization is poorly understood. Infection of previously damaged valves by less virulent organisms has been tied to (1) hemodynamic factors, (2) formation of an initially sterile platelet–fibrin thrombus and (3) adherence properties of the microorganisms. A key feature is abnormal blood flow across a damaged valve. Lesions form on the inflow portions of valves, where high pulsatile shear stresses occur. The pressure gradient across a narrow orifice (valve or congenital defect) produces turbulent flow at the periphery and a high-velocity jet at the center, both of which tend to denude valve endothelial surfaces. This leads to focal deposition of platelets and fibrin, creating small sterile vegetations that are hospitable sites for bacterial colonization and growth. Indeed, platelet adhesion is enhanced at high shear rates, which occur at leaflet free edges. Surrounding endothelium becomes activated by the presence of platelet–fibrin thrombi and upregulates expression of adhesion molecules (vascular cell adhesion molecule-1 [VCAM-1], intracellular adhesion molecule-1 [ICAM-1] and E-selectin). These, in turn, attract inflammatory cells. Microorganisms that gain access to the circulation, as a result of dental manipulation for example, can be deposited within the vegetations. In this protected environment, there may be 10^{10} organisms per gram of tissue. Matrix metalloproteinases made by bacteria begin to destroy valves, facilitating formation of adjacent vegetations.

Factors that promote bacterial adherence to sterile vegetations are believed to be important in the pathogenesis of endocarditis. Cell-associated and circulating fibronectin both bind to surface molecules of the bacteria, facilitating

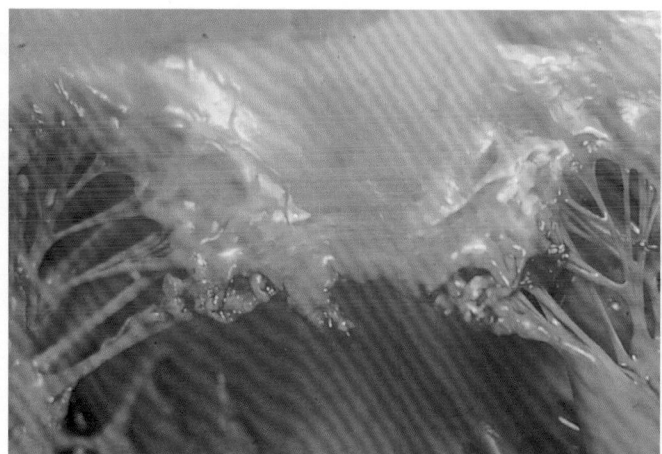

FIGURE 17-34. Bacterial endocarditis. The mitral valve shows destructive vegetations, which have eroded through the free margins of the valve leaflets.

adhesion of fibrin, collagen and cells. Some microorganisms produce extracellular polysaccharides, which also function as adhesion factors.

PATHOLOGY: Bacterial endocarditis most commonly involves the left-sided heart valves (mitral, aortic or both). The most common congenital heart lesions that underlie bacterial endocarditis are PDA, tetralogy of Fallot, VSD and bicuspid aortic valve, which is an increasingly recognized risk factor, especially in men over 60. *As a rule, the vegetations form on the upstream sides of the valves (i.e., the atrial side of atrioventricular valves and the ventricular side of semilunar valves), often at points where leaflets or cusps close* (Fig. 17-34). Vegetations consist of platelets, fibrin, cell debris and masses of organisms. Underlying valve tissue is edematous and inflamed, and may eventually become so damaged that a leaflet perforates, causing regurgitation. Lesions vary from small, superficial deposits to bulky, exuberant vegetations. The infective process may spread locally to involve valve rings or adjacent mural endocardium and chordae tendineae.

Infected thromboemboli travel to multiple systemic sites, causing infarcts or abscesses in many organs, including the brain, kidneys, intestine and spleen.

Focal segmental glomerulonephritis may complicate infective endocarditis (see Chapter 22). It results from immune complex deposition in glomeruli, producing a patchy hemorrhagic appearance—so-called flea-bitten kidneys.

CLINICAL FEATURES: Many patients show early symptoms of bacterial endocarditis within a week of the bacteremic episode, and almost all are symptomatic within 2 weeks. Nonspecific symptoms—low-grade fever, fatigue, anorexia, weight loss—predominate at first. Heart murmurs develop almost invariably and often change during the course of the disease. In cases lasting more than 6 weeks, splenomegaly, petechiae and clubbing of the fingers are frequent. In 1/3 of patients, systemic emboli are recognized at some time during the illness. One third of patients show some neurologic dysfunction, owing to the frequency of cerebral emboli. Mycotic aneurysms of cerebral vessels, brain abscesses and intracerebral bleeding

are observed. Pulmonary emboli typify tricuspid valve endocarditis in drug addicts.

Antibacterial therapy is effective in limiting the morbidity and mortality of bacterial endocarditis. Most patients defervesce within a week of instituting such therapy. However, prognosis depends to some extent on the offending organism and the stage at which infection is treated. *A third of cases of* **S. aureus** *endocarditis are still fatal.* Surgical replacement of a valve destroyed by endocarditis is risky and carries high surgical mortality as long as infection is active. *The most common serious complication of bacterial endocarditis is congestive heart failure, usually due to valvular destruction, and portending a grim prognosis.* Myocardial abscesses and infarction due to coronary artery emboli may contribute to heart failure.

Nonbacterial Thrombotic Endocarditis Is a Complication of Wasting Diseases

Nonbacterial thrombotic endocarditis (NBTE), also known as marantic endocarditis, entails sterile vegetations on apparently normal cardiac valves, almost always in association with cancer or some other wasting disease. It affects mitral (Fig. 17-35) and aortic valves equally often. NBTE resembles infective endocarditis grossly, but it does not destroy affected valves and lacks both inflammation and microorganisms.

The cause of NBTE is poorly understood. It is seen commonly as a paraneoplastic condition, usually complicating adenocarcinomas (particularly of pancreas and lung) and hematologic malignancies. NBTE may also occur in disseminated intravascular coagulation or accompany debilitating nonneoplastic diseases, accounting for the term "marantic endocarditis" (from the Greek, *marantikos,* "wasting away"). It may reflect increased blood coagulability or immune complex deposition. Lacking bacteria, the vegetations remain small and there is no valve destruction. The main danger posed by NBTE is distant embolization, clinically presenting as infarcts of many organs, but this is unusual and NBTE is often an incidental finding at autopsy.

Calcific Aortic Stenosis Reflects Chronic Damage to the Valve

Calcific aortic stenosis is narrowing of the aortic valve orifice due to calcium deposition in the valve cusps and ring.

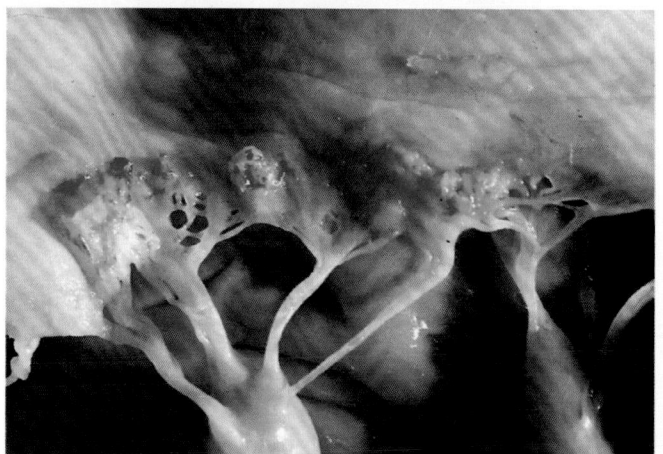

FIGURE 17-35. Marantic endocarditis. Sterile platelet–fibrin vegetations are seen on the leaflets of a structurally normal mitral valve.

 **ETIOLOGIC FACTORS AND PATHOLOGY:** Calcific aortic stenosis has three main causes.

- **Rheumatic aortic valve disease** is characterized by diffuse fibrous thickening and scarring of aortic cusps, commissural fusion and calcium deposition, all of which reduce the valve orifice and limit valve mobility (Fig. 17-32). Rheumatic aortic stenosis almost never occurs in isolation; it accompanies rheumatic mitral valve disease. Now that acute RF has become so rare in the United States and most elderly patients with rheumatic valve disease have either undergone valve replacement or died, calcific aortic stenosis is usually attributed to other causes.
- **Degenerative (senile) calcific stenosis** develops in the elderly as a degenerative process in a tricuspid aortic valve. Valve cusps become rigidly calcified, but commissural fusion (Fig. 17-36), which is a hallmark of rheumatic aortic valves, is not seen. The mitral valve is usually normal in patients with senile calcific aortic stenosis, although the mitral annulus may also be calcified.
- **Congenital bicuspid aortic stenosis** often develops with age (Fig. 17-37).
- **Calcific aortic stenosis** in both congenitally malformed valves and normal ones is probably related to cumulative effects of years of turbulent blood flow around the valve. Thus, although a bicuspid valve is not inherently stenotic, its orifice is elliptical rather than round, and flow across the valve is more turbulent than with a tricuspid aortic valve. Increasing cusp rigidity eventually produces functional derangements, typically in patients over age 60.

In any form of calcific aortic stenosis, calcification produces nodules restricted to the base and lower half of the cusps, and rarely involves the free margins. Without rheumatic scarring, commissures are not fused and three distinct cusps are evident.

Aortic valve calcification is not a purely passive process in which devitalized tissue becomes mineralized, as the term "dystrophic calcification" seems to imply. In fact, valvular calcification is an active process involving modulation of valvular interstitial cells to an osteoblastic phenotype and new gene expression resulting in cell-mediated mineralization of the extracellular matrix. Many of the mechanisms and

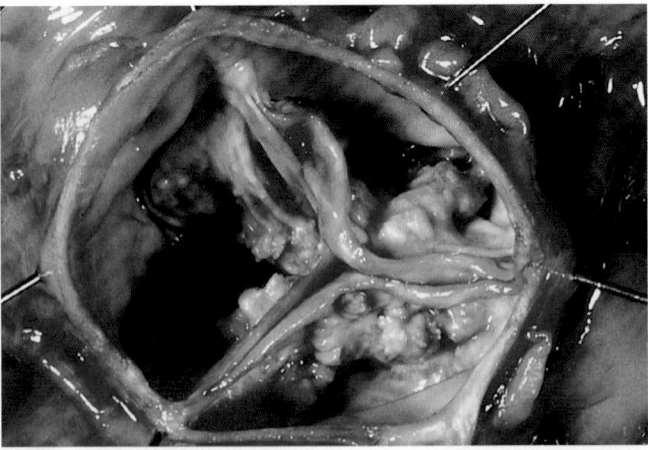

FIGURE 17-36. Calcific aortic stenosis in a three-cuspid aortic valve in an elderly person. The leaflets are heavily calcified, but there is no commissural fusion (compare with Fig. 17-32).

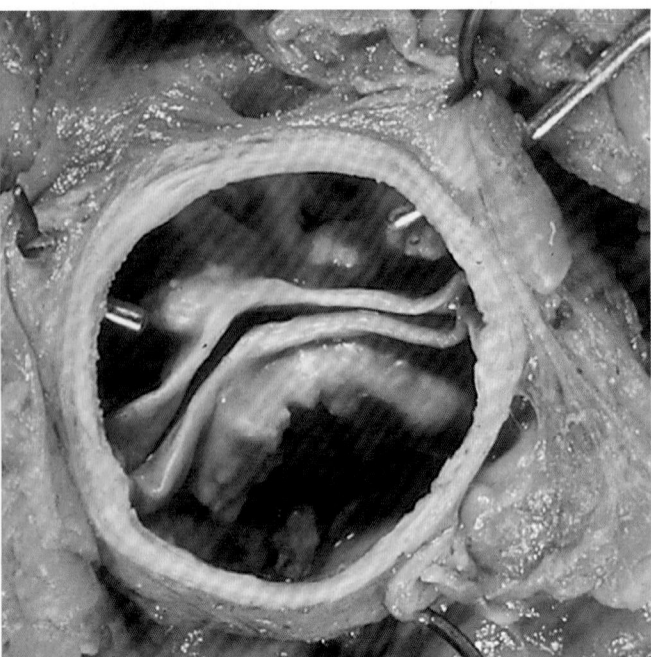

FIGURE 17-37. Calcific aortic stenosis of a congenitally bicuspid aortic valve. The two leaflets are heavily calcified, but there is no commissural fusion. Probes show the openings of the coronary ostia.

risk factors associated with valvular calcification are similar to those for atherosclerosis. Mechanical forces promote accumulation of LDL particles and other factors, leading to inflammation, activation and transformation of valvular interstitial cells, remodeling of extracellular matrix and secretion of osteogenic proteins such as bone morphogenic protein-2 and other noncollagenous matrix proteins. Despite these pathogenetic similarities to atherosclerosis, effective prevention of the latter, as with statins, does not prevent the development of calcific aortic stenosis.

 CLINICAL FEATURES: Severe aortic stenosis causes striking concentric left ventricular hypertrophy. Eventually, the ventricle dilates and fails. Surgical valve replacement is highly successful (5-year survival rate of 85%), if done before ventricular dysfunction is irreversible. The hypertrophic left ventricle then returns to normal size.

Mitral Valve Annulus Calcification Is Usually Asymptomatic

Calcification of the mitral valve annulus occurs commonly in the elderly and is usually without functional significance, although it often produces a murmur. However, if it is severe enough to interfere with posterior mitral leaflet excursion during systole, mitral regurgitation occurs. Unlike calcification in RF-damaged valves, valve leaflets are not deformed in mitral valve annulus calcification in the elderly, and calcification affects the annulus most, rather than the leaflets. About 40% of women older than 90 have this lesion, compared to only 15% of men. Calcification of the mitral valve annulus is aggravated if the patient has aortic stenosis, hypertension or diabetes.

Calcific deposits transform the mitral ring into a rigid, curved bar up to 2 cm in diameter, which may be evident

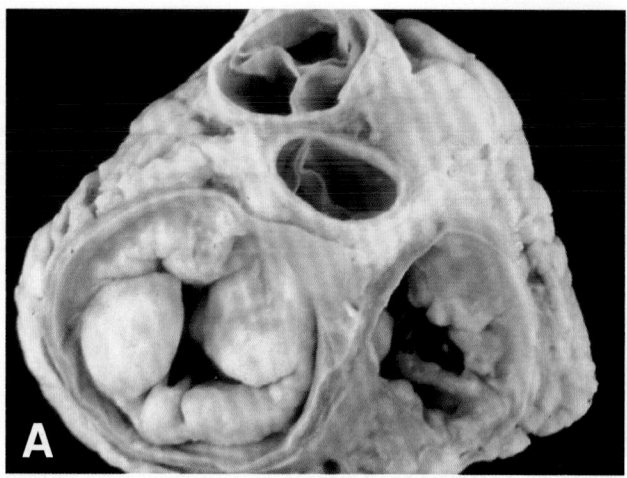
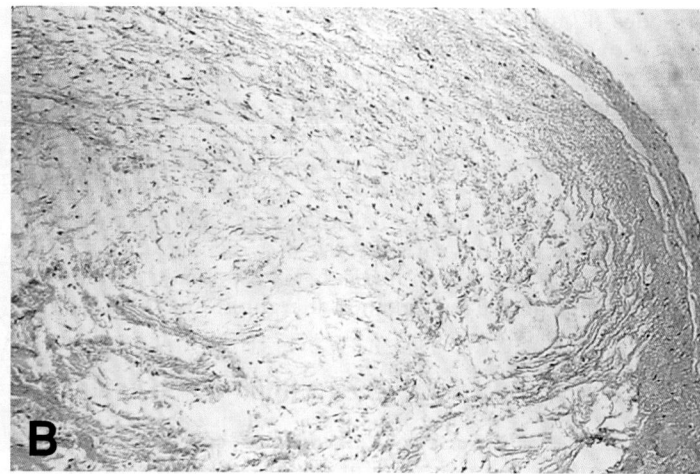

FIGURE 17-38. Mitral valve prolapse. A. A view of the mitral valve (*left*) from the left atrium shows redundant and deformed leaflets, which billow into the left atrial cavity. **B.** A microscopic section of one of the mitral valve leaflets reveals conspicuous myxomatous connective tissue in the center of the leaflet.

radiologically. Amorphous masses of calcified material first develop in the connective tissue of the valve ring, but, with time, extend into the base of the leaflets and eventually to the ventricular septum.

Mitral Valve Prolapse Is the Most Common Indication for Valve Repair or Replacement

In MVP, mitral valve leaflets become enlarged and redundant. Chordae tendineae are thinned and elongated, so that the leaflets billow and prolapse into the left atrium during systole (Fig. 17-38A). Also called "floppy mitral valve syndrome," MVP is the most common cause of mitral regurgitation that requires surgical valve repair or replacement. Up to 5% of adults may show echocardiographic evidence of MVP, although most will not have severe enough regurgitation to require surgery.

 MOLECULAR PATHOGENESIS: Many cases of MVP appear to be transmitted as an autosomal dominant trait. Three different loci on chromosomes 16, 11 and 13 are associated with MVP, but no specific gene mutations have been identified. Prolapsed mitral valves accumulate striking amounts of myxomatous connective tissue in the center of the valve leaflet (Fig. 17-38B). Proteoglycans in the valve are increased, and electron microscopy shows fragmentation of collagen fibrils. Presumably, these changes reflect a molecular defect in the extracellular matrix that allows leaflets and chordae to enlarge and stretch under the high-pressure conditions they experience during the cardiac cycle. MVP is usually an isolated finding, but is particularly prevalent in patients with Marfan syndrome, Ehlers-Danlos syndrome, osteogenic imperfecta and other collagen-related disorders. This association with inherited connective tissue disorders suggests an abnormality of connective tissue in the pathogenesis of myxomatous degeneration, but thus far, no abnormalities in fibrillar collagen genes or TGF-β signaling have been identified. Pectus excavatum, scoliosis and loss of kyphosis of the thoracic spine are common in patients with MVP, but it is not known how or if these bony abnormalities are genetically linked to MVP.

The risk of sudden death in patients with MVP, presumably due to ventricular tachyarrhythmias, is twice that in the general population. Repair of a regurgitant floppy mitral valve lowers this risk. The mechanisms are not well understood, but the risk appears to depend primarily on the degree of mitral regurgitation, perhaps related to ventricular remodeling associated with volume overload.

 PATHOLOGY: Mitral valve leaflets are redundant and deformed (Fig. 17-38A). On cross-section they have a gelatinous appearance and slippery texture, owing to accumulation of acid mucopolysaccharides (proteoglycans). Myxomatous degeneration also affects the annulus and chordae tendineae, increasing prolapse and regurgitation. Damage to chordae may be so severe that they break. Rupture of multiple chordae can yield a flail mitral valve that is totally incompetent. Although the mitral valve is usually the only valve affected, myxomatous degeneration can occur in other valves, especially in patients with Marfan syndrome, 90% of whom have clinical evidence of MVP.

CLINICAL FEATURES: Most patients with MVP are asymptomatic. Clinical recognition of MVP is based on classical auscultatory findings: a mid- to late systolic click, caused by the snap of the redundant leaflets as they prolapse into the left atrium. A late systolic murmur is present if regurgitation is significant. Endocarditis, both infective and nonbacterial, may develop as a serious complication, and cerebral emboli are common. Significant mitral regurgitation develops in 15% of patients after 10–15 years of MVP, after which mitral valve repair or replacement is indicated.

Papillary Muscle Dysfunction May Cause Mitral Regurgitation

Left ventricular papillary muscle dysfunction is usually due to ischemia. These muscles are especially vulnerable to ischemic injury as they are supplied by terminal branches of intramyocardial coronary arteries. Any reduction in coronary blood flow thus preferentially interferes with papillary muscle function. Brief periods of ischemia (e.g., during episodes of angina pectoris) can cause transient papillary muscle dysfunction (stunning) and temporary mitral regurgitation. Permanent mitral regurgitation may be due to myocardial infarction and subsequent scarring of papillary muscles. One third of patients being evaluated for coronary artery bypass surgery show evidence of "ischemic mitral regurgitation." Papillary muscle dysfunction may also be associated with a healed myocardial infarct, in which impaired myocardial contractility at the base of a papillary muscle impedes its function. Rarely, patients may suddenly develop life-threatening mitral regurgitation after rupture of an acutely infarcted papillary muscle.

Carcinoid Heart Disease Affects Right-Sided Valves

Carcinoid heart disease is an unusual condition that uniquely affects the right side of the heart, leading to tricuspid regurgitation and pulmonary stenosis. It occurs in people with carcinoid tumors, usually of the small intestine, after they have spread to the liver.

 **PATHOPHYSIOLOGY:** The pathogenesis of carcinoid heart disease is not fully understood, but the valvular and endocardial lesions are thought to be caused by high concentrations of serotonin or other vasoactive amines and peptides secreted by the tumor in the liver. These moieties are metabolized in the lung, so carcinoid heart disease affects the right side of the heart almost exclusively. There are reports of left-sided involvement in patients with atrial or ventricular septal defects.

During the 1990s, reports surfaced of mitral and aortic valve disease in patients taking the appetite-suppressing drugs fenfluramine-phentermine ("fen-phen"). Pathologic features of those valve lesions were strikingly similar to those seen in carcinoid heart disease, except that they developed on left-sided valves. Since then, other anorexigenic drugs and ergot alkaloid drugs such as methysergide and ergotamine used to treat migraine headaches have also been linked to this type of valve disease. Since these drugs interfere with serotonin metabolism and signaling, the pathogenesis of drug-related and carcinoid valve disease is similar.

 PATHOLOGY: The cardiac lesions are plaque-like deposits of dense, pearly gray, fibrous tissue on the tricuspid (Fig. 17-39) and pulmonary valves and on the endocardial surface of the right ventricle. These patches appear "tacked on" to valve leaflets, without associated inflammation or apparent damage to underlying valve structures. However, leaflets become deformed, and their surface area reduced. As a result, tricuspid leaflets become "stuck down" onto adjacent right ventricular mural endocardium, resulting in tricuspid insufficiency or stenosis. Shrinkage of the pulmonary valve and its annulus leads to pulmonary stenosis.

MYOCARDITIS

Myocarditis is inflammation of the myocardium associated with myocyte necrosis and degeneration. This definition specifically excludes ischemic heart disease. The true incidence of myocarditis is difficult to establish because many cases are asymptomatic. It can occur at any age but is most common

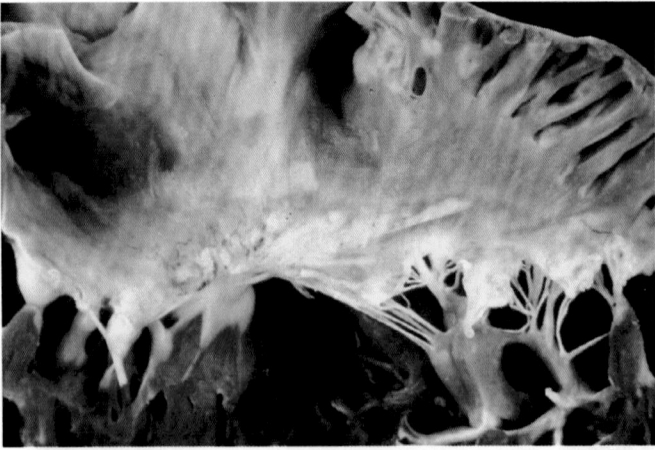

FIGURE 17-39. Carcinoid heart disease. Pearly white deposits are seen on the tricuspid valve leaflets and adjacent endocardium. Although the valve leaflets have not been destroyed, they have become deformed and "stuck down" on the ventricular endocardium, which usually produces tricuspid regurgitation.

in children 1–10 years old. It is one of the few heart diseases that can cause acute heart failure in previously healthy children, adolescents or young adults. Severe myocarditis can cause arrhythmias and even sudden cardiac death.

Most Cases of Viral Myocarditis Have No Demonstrable Cause

Viral etiology is generally suspected, but the evidence is usually circumstantial unless polymerase chain reaction (PCR) studies identify viral genomes in heart biopsies. The most common viral causes of myocarditis are listed in Table 17-7.

TABLE 17-7
CAUSES OF MYOCARDITIS
Idiopathic
Infectious
• Viral: Coxsackievirus, adenovirus, echovirus, influenza virus, human immunodeficiency virus and many others
• Rickettsial: Typhus, Rocky Mountain spotted fever
• Bacterial: Diphtheria, staphylococcal, streptococcal, meningococcal, *Borrelia* (Lyme disease) and leptospiral infection
• Fungi and protozoan parasites: Chagas disease, toxoplasmosis, aspergillosis, cryptococcal and candidal infection
• Metazoan parasites: *Echinococcus, Trichina*
Noninfectious
• Hypersensitivity and immunologically related diseases: Rheumatic fever, systemic lupus erythematosus, scleroderma, drug reaction (e.g., to penicillin or sulfonamide) and rheumatoid arthritis
• Radiation
• Miscellaneous: Sarcoidosis, uremia

MOLECULAR PATHOGENESIS: The pathogenesis of viral myocarditis involves direct viral cytotoxicity and cell-mediated immune reactions against infected myocytes. In animal models, inoculation of a cardiotropic virus is followed shortly by viral replication in the myocardium. There are only scattered foci of acute myocyte necrosis with little, if any, inflammation, and there is little evidence of functional impairment. Over the next few days, mononuclear cells, principally T lymphocytes and macrophages, infiltrate the myocardium extensively. At the point of maximum inflammation, signs of heart failure develop, although viral cultures of blood and myocardium are negative. This finding is consistent with the observation that patients with symptomatic myocarditis generally have negative viral cultures, although viral nucleic acid sequences can still be detected by PCR.

The most common viruses to infect the heart, coxsackievirus and adenovirus, both enter cardiac myocytes after binding the same cell surface receptor, the coxsackie-adenovirus receptor (CAR). Deletion of this molecule in mice prevents viral infection. CAR belongs to the family of intercellular adhesion molecules. It is especially abundant in children, which may explain why viral myocarditis is so common in childhood. Once inside a myocyte, coxsackieviruses produce proteases, such as protease 2A, which play a role in viral replication. These proteases may impede myocardial function. They also cleave myocyte proteins such as dystrophin, which may be involved in virus exiting from myocytes (intracellular viral load is higher if dystrophin is absent).

Cardiac myocytes contain powerful innate antiviral defenses mediated by Janus kinase (JAK) and STAT pathways activated by interferon (IFN)-α/β, IFN-γ and interleukin-6 (IL-6). However, these actions can be inhibited by suppressors of cytokine signaling (SOCS), proteins that limit potentially deleterious actions of cytokine signaling in cardiac myocytes. Levels of SOCS profoundly affect susceptibility to coxsackievirus infection. Thus, the highly variable clinical and pathologic manifestations of viral myocarditis depend on the dynamic interplay between mechanisms that determine viral entry, replication and release, and immune mechanisms (innate and T-cell mediated) of host responsiveness.

PATHOLOGY: The hearts of patients with myocarditis who develop clinical heart failure during the active inflammatory phase show biventricular dilation and generalized myocardial hypokinesis. At autopsy, such hearts are flabby and dilated. Histologic features of viral myocarditis vary with the clinical disease severity, but with few exceptions, microscopic features are nonspecific and indistinguishable from toxic myocarditis. Most cases show patchy or diffuse interstitial, predominantly mononuclear, inflammatory infiltrates, mainly of T lymphocytes and macrophages (Fig. 17-40). Multinucleated giant cells may also be present. The inflammatory cells often surround individual myocytes, and focal myocyte necrosis is seen. During the resolving phase, fibroblasts proliferate and interstitial collagen is deposited. Neutrophils are uncommon in viral myocarditis. However, if necrosis is extensive, the histology may resemble that of an infarct—a neutrophilic infiltrate followed by organization and repair. Most viruses that cause myocarditis also cause pericarditis.

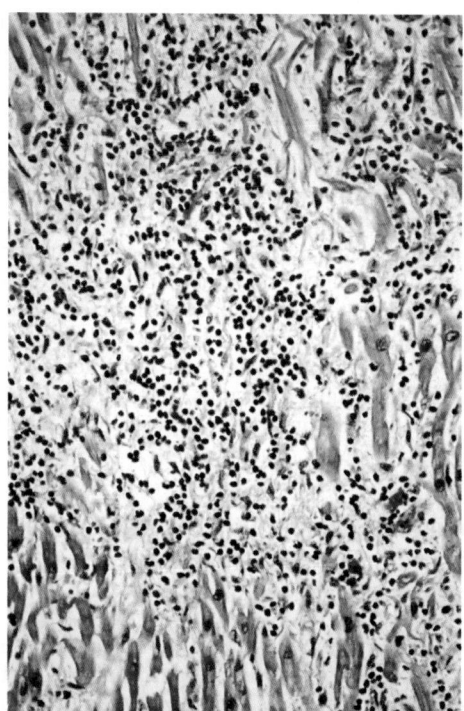

FIGURE 17-40. Viral myocarditis. The myocardial fibers are disrupted by a prominent interstitial infiltrate of lymphocytes and macrophages.

CLINICAL FEATURES: Many people with viral myocarditis have no symptoms. When symptoms do occur, they usually start a few weeks after infection. Most patients recover from acute myocarditis, although a few die of congestive heart failure or arrhythmias. The disease may be unusually severe in infants and pregnant women. Despite resolution of the active inflammatory phase of viral myocarditis, subtle functional impairment may persist for years and progression to overt cardiomyopathy is well documented. There is no specific treatment for viral myocarditis; supportive measures are the rule. Antiviral and immunomodulatory therapies are not useful.

MYOCARDITIS IN ACQUIRED IMMUNODEFICIENCY SYNDROME: A significant number of patients with AIDS have clinical or pathologic evidence of cardiac disease (pericardial effusions, myocarditis, endocarditis or cardiomyopathy). They are prone to an unusually high incidence of viral myocarditis, which largely reflects cardiotropic viruses, such as coxsackievirus and adenovirus. Human immunodeficiency virus type 1 (HIV-1) infection of cardiac myocytes appears to play a minor role.

Nonviral Transmissible Agents May Cause Myocarditis

Other microorganisms that gain access to the bloodstream can infect the heart. Among these, brucellosis, meningococcemia and psittacosis (see Chapter 9) often lead to infectious myocarditis. Some bacteria (e.g., diphtheria) produce cardiotoxins, which may cause fatal myocarditis. The most common cause of myocarditis in South America is a protozoan, *Trypanosoma cruzi,* the agent of Chagas disease (see below, Chapter 9).

- **Bacterial infection** of the myocardium is characterized by multiple foci of a mixed inflammatory infiltrate, with neutrophils predominant. Microabscesses occur when septic emboli lodge in the coronary circulation, often secondary to infective endocarditis.

- **Rickettsial diseases** often cause widespread vasculitis, which affects small coronary blood vessels.
- **Fungal infection** of the myocardium typically occurs in immunocompromised patients, although the heart is relatively resistant to fungal infection.
- **Toxoplasmosis** can involve the myocardium in immunosuppressed patients; these intracellular parasites proliferate in cardiac myocytes and elicit a focal mixed inflammatory response, with neutrophils and eosinophils.
- **Chagas disease** is associated with proliferation of parasites within cardiac myocytes and a mixed inflammatory cell infiltrate, composed principally of lymphocytes, plasma cells and macrophages.

Granulomatous Myocarditis May Be Caused by Microorganisms or Immunologically Mediated Injury

Granulomatous myocarditis, with myocyte necrosis, occurs in a variety of diseases. Microorganisms associated with granulomatous myocarditis include *Mycobacteria* and some types of fungi. Immunologically mediated injury of the myocardium, for example, rheumatic myocarditis (Fig. 17-29) and sarcoidosis (see Fig. 17-46), may also cause granulomatous myocarditis.

Hypersensitivity Myocarditis Is a Reaction to Drugs

 PATHOLOGY: In hypersensitivity myocarditis, the inflammation is interstitial and perivascular and is often confined to the myocardium without affecting other organs. The inflammatory infiltrate in hypersensitivity myocarditis resembles that in viral myocarditis but tends to have numerous eosinophils, in addition to lymphocytes and plasma cells. Another typical feature is the virtual absence of myocyte necrosis, even when the infiltrate is intense.

 CLINICAL FEATURES: Hypersensitivity myocarditis is usually clinically silent. The diagnosis is often made as an incidental finding at autopsy. However, it may produce chest pain and ECG changes resembling acute myocardial ischemia. Occasionally, hypersensitivity myocarditis causes fatal ventricular arrhythmias. When the disease causes symptoms, treatment consists of discontinuing the offending drug and administering corticosteroids or immunosuppressive agents.

Giant Cell Myocarditis Is Usually Fatal

Giant cell myocarditis is a rare, highly aggressive disease characterized by intense inflammation, extensive areas of myocyte necrosis and many multinucleated giant cells derived from macrophages. Its cause is unknown, but it sometimes occurs in patients with SLE, hyperthyroidism or thymoma. An autoimmune etiology has been suggested, but there is no persuasive evidence for this theory.

Giant cell myocarditis is usually a rapidly fatal disease of adults in the third to fifth decades, although it also occurs in adolescents. Patients die of congestive heart failure or suddenly from arrhythmias. At autopsy, the heart is flabby

and dilated and may contain mural thrombi. Prominent giant cells, lymphoid cells and macrophages are present at the margins of serpiginous areas of myocardial necrosis. Although giant cells are many, there are no granulomas. A few patients may recover, but the only effective treatment for most is cardiac transplantation. However, giant cell myocarditis may recur in transplanted hearts in 1/4 of cases.

METABOLIC DISEASES OF THE HEART

Hyperthyroidism Causes High-Output Failure

Thyroid hormone has direct inotropic and chronotropic effects on the heart: (1) it increases activity of the sarcolemmal sodium-potassium pump (Na^+/K^+-adenosine triphosphatase [ATPase]); (2) it enhances synthesis of a myosin isoform with rapid ATPase activity and reduces production of a slower isoform; and (3) it upregulates expression of SERCA and exerts direct effects on voltage-gated Ca^{2+} channels in the sarcolemma, thus facilitating contractility. Hyperthyroidism therefore causes tachycardia and increases cardiac workload, owing to decreased peripheral resistance and increased cardiac output. It may eventually lead to angina pectoris, high-output failure and/or arrhythmias (atrial fibrillation, most commonly).

Hypothyroid Heart Disease Diminishes Cardiac Output

Patients with severe hypothyroidism (**myxedema**) have low cardiac output, reduced heart rate and poor myocardial contractility—the opposite changes of those seen in hyperthyroidism. There may be a pericardial effusion created by increased capillary permeability and leakage of fluid and protein into the pericardial cavity. Pulse pressure is low because of higher peripheral resistance and lower blood volume.

The hearts of patients with myxedema are flabby and dilated, and the myocardium shows myofiber swelling. Basophilic (mucinous) degeneration is common. Interstitial fibrosis may also be present. Despite these changes, myxedema does not cause congestive heart failure in the absence of other cardiac disorders.

Thiamine Deficiency (Beriberi) Heart Disease Resembles Hyperthyroidism

Beriberi heart disease develops in people who eat insufficient vitamin B_1 (thiamine) for at least 3 months (see Chapter 8). It is seen in parts of Asia where the diet consists largely of shelled rice. In the United States, thiamine deficiency is occasionally seen in alcoholics or neglected people. Beriberi heart disease results in decreased peripheral vascular resistance and increased cardiac output, thus resembling hyperthyroidism with high-output failure. Interestingly, heart failure may develop so abruptly that patients die within 2 days of the onset of symptoms. At autopsy, the heart is dilated and shows only nonspecific microscopic changes.

CARDIOMYOPATHY

Cardiomyopathies are primary diseases of the myocardium exclusive of damage caused by extrinsic factors. Usually, primary cardiomyopathies are divided into the major clinicopathologic groups of **dilated cardiomyopathy (DCM)**, **hypertrophic cardiomyopathy (HCM)**, **arrhythmogenic cardiomyopathy (AC)** and **restrictive cardiomyopathy (RCM)**. DCM is most common and is a leading indication for heart transplantation. It is characterized by biventricular dilation, impaired contractility and eventually congestive heart failure. DCM can develop after a large number of known insults that injure cardiac myocytes directly **(secondary DCM),** or it may be idiopathic **(primary DCM)**.

In Idiopathic Dilated Cardiomyopathy Contractility Is Impaired

MOLECULAR PATHOGENESIS: Many etiologies have been implicated in idiopathic DCM. Most cases probably represent interplay between genetic, epigenetic and environmental factors.

Genetic factors play an important role in the pathogenesis of DCM. At least 1/3 of DCM patients inherited the disease as a single-gene disorder in a Mendelian pattern. The proportion may be even greater, as incomplete penetrance often makes it difficult to identify early or latent disease in family members. Most familial cases seem to be transmitted as autosomal dominant traits, but autosomal recessive, X-linked recessive and mitochondrial inheritance patterns have all been described (Table 17-8).

Mutations in more than 50 genes have been linked to DCM. Several occur in genes encoding cytoskeletal proteins such as lamin A/C, desmin and metavinculin. Others occur in genes such as δ-sarcoglycan and dystrophin, which are involved in anchoring the cytoskeleton and the sarcolemma to the extracellular matrix (Table 17-8). *This has led to the hypothesis that defects in force transmission lead to development of a dilated, poorly contracting heart* (Fig. 17-41). However, 35%–45% of genetic causes of DCM may be related to mutations in genes encoding sarcomeric proteins such as

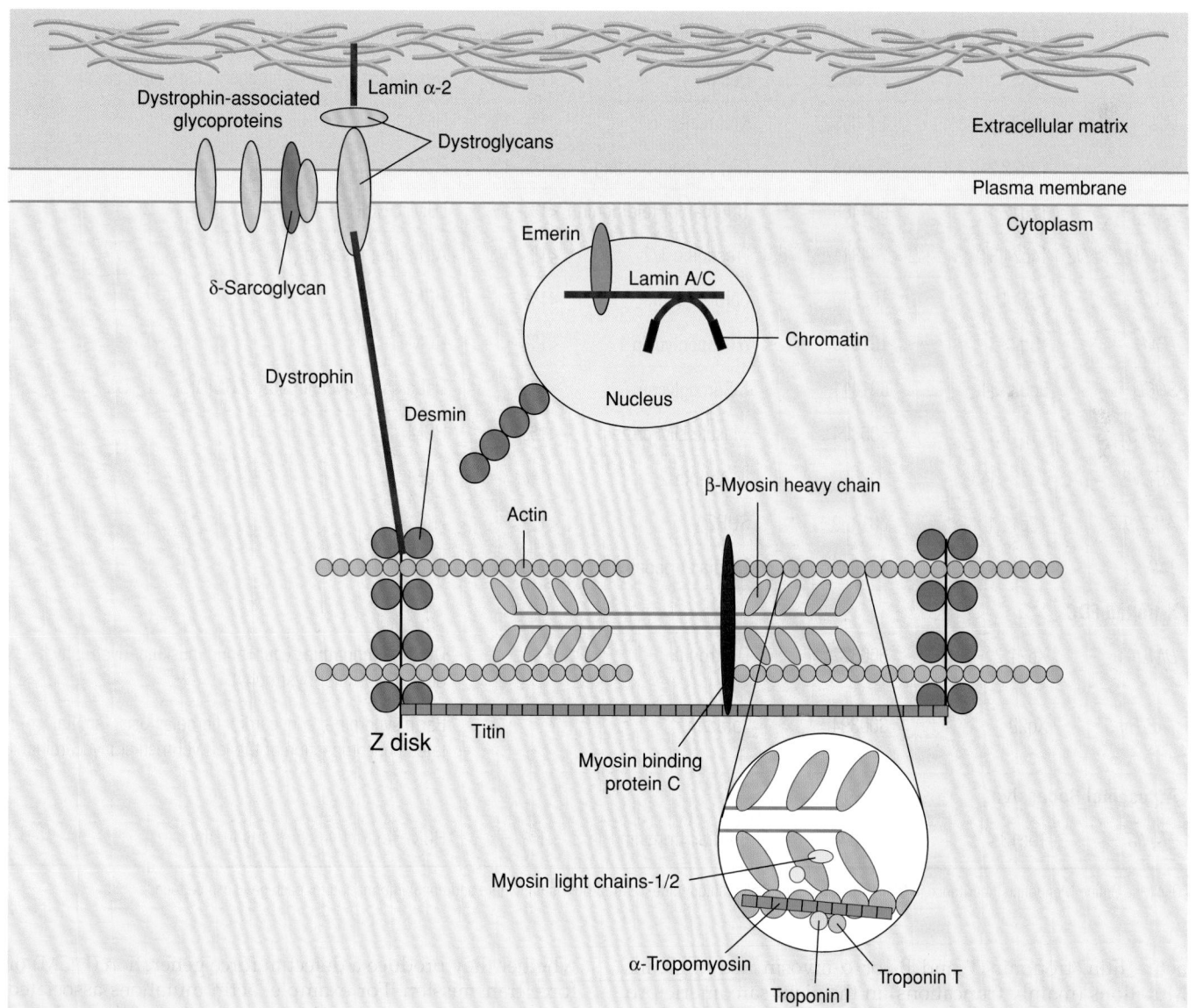

FIGURE 17-41. **Subcellular distribution and molecular interactions of mutant proteins implicated in the pathogenesis of dilated and hypertrophic cardiomyopathy.** The specific mutations responsible for each type are provided in Tables 17-8 and 17-9.

TABLE 17-8

GENE DEFECTS ASSOCIATED WITH DILATED CARDIOMYOPATHY (DCM)

Gene	Chromosome Locus	OMIM[a]	Gene Product	Frequency	Related Disorders
Autosomal Dominant					
TTN	2q31	188840	Titin	20%–25%	Hypertrophic cardiomyopathy (HCM)
LMNA	1q21.2	150330	Lamin A/C	4%–8%	Lipodystrophy, Charcot-Marie-Tooth, Emery-Dreifuss muscular dystrophy, Hutchinson-Gilford progeria syndrome, limb girdle muscular dystrophy (LGMD)
MYH7	14q12	160760	β-Myosin heavy chain	4%–6%	Laing distal myopathy, HCM
TNNT2	1q32	191045	Cardiac troponin T	3%	HCM
SCN5A	3p21	600163	Sodium channel	2%–3%	Long QT syndrome, Brugada syndrome, idiopathic ventricular fibrillation, sick sinus syndrome, cardiac conduction system disease
MYH6	14q12	160710	α-Myosin heavy chain	? 2%–3%	HCM, dominantly inherited atrial septal defect
DES	2q35	125660	Desmin	<1%–1%	Desminopathy, arrhythmogenic cardiomyopathy
VCL	10q22.1–23	193065	Metavinculin	<1%–1%	HCM
LDB3	10q22.2–23.3	605906	LIM domain-binding 3	<1%–1%	HCM
TCAP	17q12	604488	Titin-cap or telethonin	<1%–1%	LGMD, HCM
PSEN1/PSEN2	14q24.3/1q31–q42	104311/600759	Presenilin 1/2	<1%–1%	Alzheimer disease
ACTC	15q14	102540	Cardiac actin	<1%	HCM
TPM1	15q22.1	191010	α-Tropomyosin 1	<1%	HCM
SGCD	5q33–34	601411	δ-Sarcoglycan	<1%	Delta sarcoglycanopathy (LGMD)
CSRP3	11p15.1	600824	Muscle LIM protein	<1%	HCM
ACTN2	1q42–q43	102573	α-Actinin-2	<1%	HCM
ABCC9	12p12.1	601439	SUR2A	<1%	NA
TNNC1	3p21.3–p14.3	191040	Cardiac troponin C	<1%	NA
X-linked FDC					
DMD	Xp21.2	300377	Dystrophin	?	Dystrophinopathies (Duchenne muscular dystrophy, Becker muscular dystrophy)
TAZ/G4.5	Xq28	300394	Tafazzin	?	Barth syndrome, endocardial fibroelastosis, familial isolated noncompaction of the left ventricular myocardium
Autosomal Recessive					
TNNI3	19q13.4	191044	Cardiac troponin I	<1%	HCM, restrictive cardiomyopathy

[a]OMIM is Online Mendelian Inheritance in Man, http://www.ncbi.nlm.nih.gov/sites/entrez?db=omim, where additional information for each gene can be found.

actin, titin, troponin T and β- or α-myosin heavy chains. Mutations (mainly truncations) in the giant sarcomeric protein titin, which has 35,000 amino acids, may alone account for up to 25% of genetic causes.

Interestingly, some sarcomeric protein mutations may produce either DCM or HCM phenotypes, perhaps depending on whether they produce a defect in force generation (HCM) or force transmission. For example, actin mutations associated with HCM have been localized to a portion of the molecule near a myosin-binding site, which could impair sarcomeric function. By contrast, DCM-associated mutations in actin are within the region that binds to the dystrophin–sarcoglycan complex (Fig. 17-41). While the force transmission hypothesis is appealing, it may not account for other mutations linked to DCM such as those involving the cardiac sodium channel or presenilin, both of which have also been implicated in other types of diseases (Table 17-8). As the list of genetic factors expands, so too does the breadth of potential molecular mechanisms and insights into genotype–phenotype relationships. For example, mutations in genes encoding proteins of the cytoskeleton and sarcomere tend to produce phenotypes dominated by contractile dysfunction and heart failure, while mutations in genes for desmosomal proteins, lamin A/C and the cardiac sodium channel protein Nav1.5 lead to a more arrhythmogenic DCM picture.

Viral myocarditis may eventually lead to DCM, but how this would develop is not clear. Once they have infected cardiac myocytes, viruses can harness the host ubiquitin/proteasomal system and autophagy machinery to facilitate their replication. Ongoing interactions between viruses and these host systems can impair normal host protein turnover kinetics and promote oxidative stress. This could, in turn, lead to abnormal regulation of contractile proteins and promote apoptosis and autophagic cell death with the eventual emergence of a clinical phenotype of ventricular remodeling and failure. Indeed, persistence of viral genomes in the heart detected by PCR is associated with progressive impairment of left ventricular function, whereas spontaneous viral elimination is associated with improved function.

Immunologic abnormalities, both cellular and humoral, have been recognized in both myocarditis and idiopathic DCM. Autoantibodies have been identified against several cardiac antigens, including a variety of mitochondrial antigens, cardiac myosin and β-adrenergic receptors. However, as in many cases of autoimmune disease, a pathogenic role for immune mechanisms remains to be proven: circulating autoantibodies may be the result of myocardial injury, rather than its cause.

 PATHOLOGY: The pathology of DCM is generally nonspecific, and is similar whatever its genesis. At autopsy, the heart is invariably enlarged, with conspicuous left and right ventricular hypertrophy. Heart weight may be tripled (>900 g). As a rule, all chambers of the heart are dilated, though the ventricles are more severely affected than are the atria (Fig. 17-42). At end stage, left ventricular dilation is usually so severe that the left ventricle wall appears to be of normal thickness or even thinned. The myocardium is flabby and pale, sometimes with small subendocardial scars. The left ventricle endocardium tends to be thickened, especially at the apex. Adherent mural thrombi are often present in this area.

DCM is characterized by atrophic and hypertrophic myocardial fibers. Cardiac myocytes, especially in the subendocardium, often show advanced degenerative changes characterized by myofibrillar loss (myocytolysis), an effect that gives cells a vacant, vacuolated appearance. Interstitial and perivascular fibrosis of myocardium is evident, also most prominently in the subendocardial zone. Scattered chronic inflammatory cells may be present, but are not conspicuous. Electron microscopy typically shows loss of sarcomeres and an apparent increase in mitochondria.

CLINICAL FEATURES: The clinical courses of idiopathic and secondary DCM are comparable. Both begin insidiously with compensatory

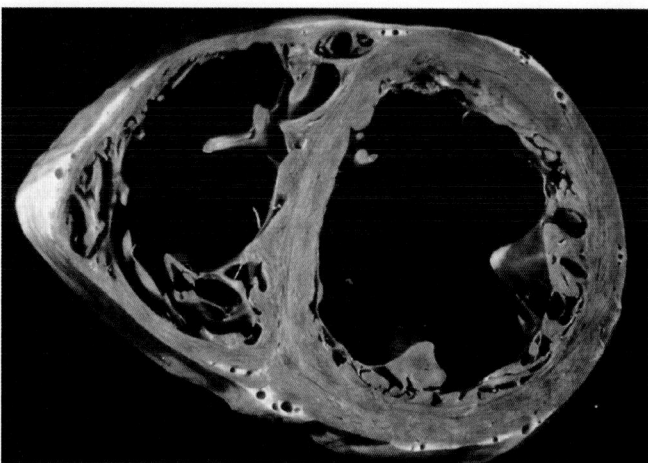

FIGURE 17-42. Idiopathic dilated cardiomyopathy. A transverse section of the enlarged heart reveals conspicuous dilation of both ventricles. Although the ventricular wall appears thinned, the increased mass of the heart indicates considerable hypertrophy.

ventricular hypertrophy and asymptomatic left ventricular dilation. Exercise intolerance usually progresses relentlessly to frank congestive heart failure and 75% of patients die within 5 years of the onset of symptoms. Half of all deaths in DCM patients are sudden and are attributed to ventricular arrhythmias. Abnormalities in intracellular Ca^{2+} handling and certain repolarizing (K^+) currents are common features in all forms of heart failure. They tend to prolong QT intervals and increase the likelihood of arrhythmias initiated by triggered activity. Supportive treatment is useful, but cardiac transplantation or a ventricular assist device is eventually necessary.

Over 100 Diseases May Cause Clinical Features of Secondary Dilated Cardiomyopathy

Thus, secondary DCM is best viewed as a final common pathway for virtually any toxic, metabolic or infectious disorder that directly injures cardiac myocytes. In this context, alcohol abuse, hypertension, pregnancy and viral myocarditis predispose to secondary DCM. Diabetes mellitus and cigarette smoking are also associated with an increased incidence of DCM.

Toxic Cardiomyopathy

Many chemicals and drugs cause myocardial injury, but only a few of the more important chemicals are discussed here.

ETHANOL: Alcohol is the single most common identifiable cause of DCM in the United States and Europe. Ethanol abuse can lead to chronic, progressive cardiac dysfunction, which may be fatal. The disorder is more common in men, because alcoholism is more frequent in men. The typical patient is between 30 and 55 years old and has been drinking heavily for at least 10 years.

MOLECULAR PATHOGENESIS: The pathogenesis of alcoholic cardiomyopathy is obscure. In experimental animals, the presence of ethanol exerts a negative inotropic effect (decreased contractile strength) on cardiac muscle, impairs calcium flux, inhibits protein synthesis and produces oxidative stress. Moreover, adducts of ethanol, metabolic products such as acetaldehyde and fatty acid ethyl esters impair cardiac myocyte function. Yet all of these effects are entirely reversible if ethanol is discontinued. Since the development of human alcoholic cardiomyopathy requires more than 10 years of alcohol abuse and is related to the total lifetime dose of alcohol, the role of reversible changes is questionable. Alcohol abuse increases the rate of apoptosis in human cardiac myocytes, and inhibitory effects on certain types of progenitor cells have been shown. Whether alcoholic cardiomyopathy represents an imbalance between apoptosis and replacement of cardiac myocytes, as has been claimed for biological aging (see Chapter 10), is a subject for further study.

COBALT: The cardiac toxicity of cobalt is discussed in Chapter 8.

CATECHOLAMINES: In high concentrations, catecholamines can cause focal myocyte necrosis (contraction band necrosis). Toxic myocarditis may occur in patients with pheochromocytomas or who require high doses of inotropic drugs to maintain blood pressure and in accident victims who sustain massive head trauma. Multiple mechanisms contribute to myocardial injury, but the most important is enhanced calcium flux into myocytes. Focal ischemia caused by platelet aggregation and microvascular constriction may also contribute. Catecholamine toxicity has been implicated in Takotsubo cardiomyopathy, also known as apical ballooning cardiomyopathy or stress-induced cardiomyopathy, which is characterized by the abrupt onset of transient left ventricular dysfunction with apical dilation, often brought on by severe emotional or physical stress.

ANTHRACYCLINES: Doxorubicin (Adriamycin) and other anthracycline drugs are potent chemotherapeutic agents whose usefulness is limited by cumulative, dose-dependent, cardiac toxicity. The clinical major effect is poor myocyte contractility due to chronic, irreversible degeneration of cardiac myocytes. The histopathology of this disorder includes vacuolization and loss of myofibrils. Myocyte necrosis is rare, but once severe degeneration occurs, intractable congestive heart failure develops and the prognosis is grim.

PATHOPHYSIOLOGY: DCM begins to appear in patients who receive a cumulative dose of more than 500 mg doxorubicin per m^2, and 35% of those receiving more than 550 mg/m^2 develop cardiomyopathy. The mechanism by which anthracyclines damage the heart appears related mainly to formation of ROS through redox cycling of aglycone metabolites and anthracycline–iron complexes. Although the heart is relatively resistant to radiation injury, anthracyclines and radiation act synergistically. Thus, a patient who has received radiotherapy to the mediastinum is likely to develop anthracycline toxicity at a lower dose than someone who was never irradiated. As detailed below, DCM due to anthracyclines is only one example of long-term cardiovascular complications in patients who have survived cancer therapies.

CYCLOPHOSPHAMIDE: This alkylating agent is often used in high doses before bone marrow transplantation. It does not cause classical DCM but can cause pericarditis and occasionally massive hemorrhagic myocarditis. The latter is thought to be secondary to endothelial injury and thrombocytopenia.

COCAINE: Cocaine use is often associated with chest pain and palpitations. True DCM is an unusual complication of cocaine abuse, but myocarditis, focal necrosis and thickening of intramyocardial coronary arteries have been reported. Myocardial ischemia or infarction associated with cocaine use has been attributed to coronary vasoconstriction in the face of increased myocardial oxygen demand. Sudden death due to spontaneous ventricular tachyarrhythmias is well documented. Cocaine-induced arrhythmias may be due to drug-related vasoconstriction, sympathomimetic activity, hypersensitivity responses and direct toxicity.

Cardiomyopathy of Pregnancy

A unique form of DCM develops in the last trimester of pregnancy or the first 6 months after delivery. The disorder is relatively uncommon in the United States, but in some areas in Africa, it occurs in as many as 1% of pregnant women. Risk of cardiomyopathy of pregnancy is greatest in black, multiparous women older than 30 years. Some patients exhibit inflammatory cells in heart biopsies taken during the symptomatic phase of the illness, consistent with the hypothesis that disordered immunity may underlie development of DCM in this setting.

Unlike most other varieties of DCM, half of women with cardiomyopathy of pregnancy spontaneously recover normal cardiac function. In the other half, left ventricular dysfunction persists or becomes overt congestive heart failure, leading to early death. In patients who survive, subsequent pregnancies pose a high risk of recurrence and maternal mortality.

PATHOPHYSIOLOGY: Overproduction of prolactin has been implicated in cardiomyopathy of pregnancy. In normal pregnancy, prolactin increases blood volume, decreases blood pressure and diminishes renal excretion of water and salts. Patients with peripartum cardiomyopathy have increased blood levels of a biologically active proteolytic fragment of prolactin. Small clinical studies using the prolactin secretion inhibitor bromocriptine have shown promising results.

In Hypertrophic Cardiomyopathy Cardiac Hypertrophy Is Out of Proportion to Hemodynamic Load

HCM develops for no apparent physiologic reason, is probably genetically determined in most patients and is an autosomal dominant trait in half of patients. Many people with no family history probably have spontaneous mutations or a mild form of disease that is hard to detect. The prevalence of HCM in the United States is about 1 in 500.

MOLECULAR PATHOGENESIS: The clinical picture of HCM is typically caused by dominant mutations in genes encoding proteins of the sarcomere (Table 17-9). Roughly 80% of HCM cases for which a genetic basis is identified involve mutations in one of two

TABLE 17-9

GENETIC CAUSES OF HYPERTROPHIC CARDIOMYOPATHY

Gene	Locus	OMIM[a]	Gene Product	Frequency	Related Disorders
Autosomal Dominant					
MYH7	14q12	160760	β-Myosin heavy chain	45%	Dilated cardiomyopathy (DCM)
MYBPC3	11p11.2	600958	Myosin-binding protein C	35%	DCM
TNNT2	1q32	191045	Cardiac troponin T	5%	DCM
TNNI3	19q13.4	191044	Cardiac troponin I	5%	DCM, restrictive cardiomyopathy
TPM1	15q22.1	191010	α-Tropomyosin 1	≈1%–2%	DCM
MYL2	12q23–q24.3	160781	Cardiac myosin light chain 2	?	
MYL3	3p	160790	Myosin light chain 3	≈1%	
ACTC	15q14	102540	Cardiac actin	≈1%	DCM
TTN	2q31	188840	Titin	Rare	DCM
MYH6	14q12	160710	α-Myosin heavy chain	<1%	DCM, dominantly inherited atrial septal defect
TCAP	17q12	604488	Titin cap or telethonin	<1%	DCM, limb girdle muscular dystrophy (LGMD)
MYOZ2	4q26–q27	605602	Myozenin 2	<1%	
CSRP3	11p15.1	600824	Muscle LIM protein	Rare	DCM
MYLK2	20q13.3	606566	Myosin light chain kinase 2	Rare	
LDB3	10q22.2–q23.3	605906	LIM domain-binding 3	Rare	DCM
VCL	10q22.1–q23	193065	Metavinculin	Rare	DCM
ACTN2	1q42-q43	102573	α-Actinin 2	Rare	DCM
PLN	6q22.1	172405	Phospholamban	Rare	DCM
JPH2	20q12	605267	Junctophilin 2	Rare	
CAV3	3p25	601253	Caveolin 3	Rare	Long QT syndrome, LGMD
CALR3	19p13.12	611414	Calreticulin 3	Rare	

[a]OMIM is Online Mendelian Inheritance in Man, http://www.ncbi.nlm.nih.gov/sites/entrez?db=omim.

genes: those encoding β-myosin heavy chain and myosin-binding protein C. Mutations in genes for cardiac troponin T, cardiac troponin I and α-tropomyosin-1 (components of the troponin complex) account for most remaining cases. However, like DCM, there is marked allelic heterogeneity in HCM such that most mutations occur "privately" or at frequencies of less than 1%. Thus, hundreds of different mutations, mostly missense, have been identified. In addition, mutations in several nonsarcomeric protein genes have rarely been linked to the clinical phenotype of HCM. As noted in the discussion of DCM, different mutations in the same gene can give rise to diverse clinical phenotypes of DCM or HCM.

The mechanistic link between the mutations and the resultant clinical and pathologic phenotypes of HCM is poorly understood. In general, it is thought that the mutant protein is incorporated into the sarcomere, where it acts in a dominant-negative fashion to cause a loss of sarcomeric function. *This proposed mechanism has led to the hypothesis that HCM is related to defects in force generation due to altered sarcomeric function.* Hypertrophy may then be a compensatory response. Other mutations (e.g., involving myosin light-chain or α-tropomyosin-1 genes) may actually enhance contractility and thus lead to hypertrophy. Still others (e.g., mutations in the myosin-binding protein C gene) may produce proteins that do not become incorporated into sarcomeres. These might lead to hypertrophy because a functional protein is missing, rather than by a dominant-negative effect.

Because of the risk of sudden death in HCM, there have been many attempts to use genetics to help stratify risk. Overall, results have been disappointing, although some correlations have been recognized. For example, selected mutations in β-myosin heavy-chain and troponin T genes involve a high likelihood of sudden death. In the case of the β-myosin heavy-chain mutations, the risk of sudden death correlates with the amount of hypertrophy, whereas troponin T mutations, which are also linked to sudden death, produce minimal or no hypertrophy. HCM in patients with myosin-binding protein C mutations is usually benign clinically, and is associated with slowly progressive hypertrophy developing late in life. A few patients (2%–5%) have mutations in two genes and generally show earlier onset and a more severe clinical phenotype.

 PATHOLOGY: The heart in HCM is always enlarged, but the extent of hypertrophy varies in different genetic forms. The left ventricular wall is thick, and its cavity is small, sometimes only a slit. Papillary muscles and trabeculae carneae are prominent and encroach on the lumen. More than half of cases exhibit asymmetric hypertrophy of the interventricular septum, with a ratio of septum to left ventricular free wall thickness greater than 1.5 (Fig. 17-43A). In some rare genetic forms of HCM, only the apical portion of the left ventricle or the papillary muscles may be selectively hypertrophied. Often, the thickened, hypertrophied interventricular septum bulges into the left ventricular outflow tract early in ventricular systole, obstructing the aortic outflow tract. In this situation, an endocardial mural plaque is typically seen in the outflow tract, corresponding to the contact point where the anterior mitral valve leaflet impinges on the septal wall of the outflow tract during systole. Both atria are commonly dilated.

The most notable histologic feature of HCM is **myofiber disarray,** which is most extensive in the interventricular septum. Instead of the usual parallel arrangement of myocytes into muscle bundles, myofiber disarray is characterized by oblique and often perpendicular orientations of adjacent hypertrophic myocytes (Fig. 17-43B). By electron microscopy, myofibrils and myofilaments within individual myocytes are also disorganized. Such structural disarrangements may be present in infants with congenital heart defects and in several other settings, but they are always extensive in HCM and are not as widespread in other situations. Interstitial cells are usually hyperplastic, and intramural coronary arteries may be thick and cellular (Fig. 17-43C).

 CLINICAL FEATURES: Many patients with HCM have few, if any, symptoms, and the diagnosis is commonly made during screening of the family with an affected member. Despite a lack of symptoms, such people may be at risk for sudden death, particularly during severe exertion. In fact, unsuspected HCM is commonly found at autopsy in young competitive athletes who die suddenly (see Fig. 17-47). Clinical recognition of HCM can occur at any age, often in the third to fifth decades of life, but it also is encountered in the elderly (mainly in people with myosin-binding protein C mutations). Some patients with HCM are incapacitated by cardiac symptoms, of which dyspnea, angina pectoris and syncope are most common. The clinical course tends to remain stable for many years, although eventually the disease can progress to congestive heart failure. In 10% of patients, DCM supervenes.

Despite the fact that mutant proteins impair the sarcomere, contractile function in HCM tends to be hyperdynamic.

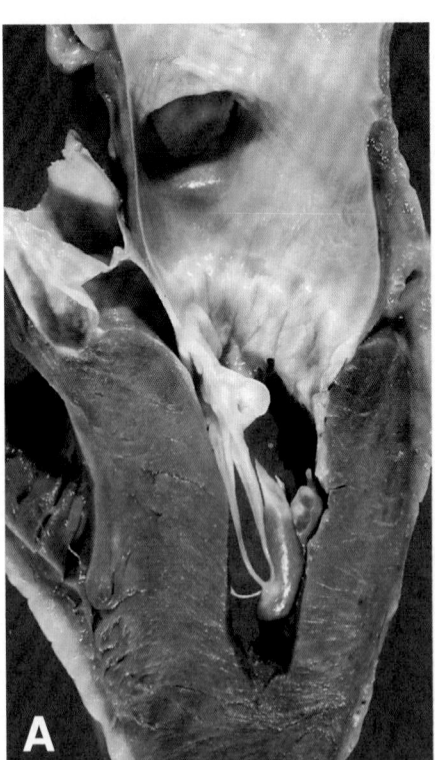 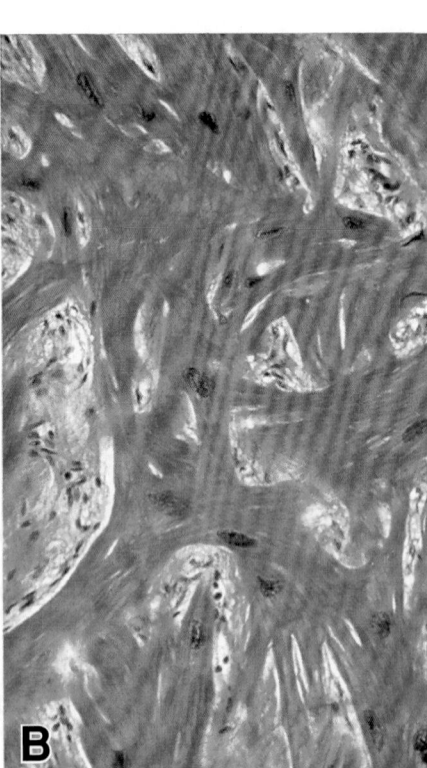 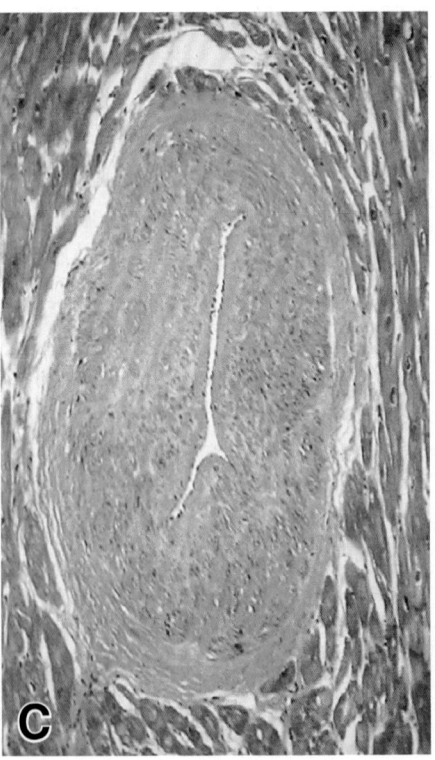

FIGURE 17-43. Hypertrophic cardiomyopathy (HCM). A. The heart has been opened to show striking asymmetric left ventricular hypertrophy. The interventricular septum is thicker than the free wall of the left ventricle and impinges on the outflow tract such that it contacts the underside of the anterior mitral valve leaflet. The left atrium is markedly enlarged. **B.** A section of the myocardium shows the characteristic myofiber disarray and hyperplasia of interstitial cells. **C.** A small intramural coronary artery shows a thickened, hypercellular media. This type of remodeling of coronary vessels could contribute to development of angina-like symptoms in some patients with HCM.

Ejection fractions are typically very high and most of the stroke volume is ejected during early systole. The most prominent dysfunctional aspect of HCM is decreased left ventricular compliance (diastolic dysfunction), which results in increased end-diastolic pressure. Mitral regurgitation is also seen in many such patients, leading to the atrial dilation commonly seen in HCM (note the enlarged left atrium in Fig. 17-43). In 1/4 of patients, functional obstruction of the left ventricular outflow tract occurs near the end of systole, resulting in a pressure gradient between the apex and the subvalvular region of the left ventricle.

HCM responds paradoxically to pharmacologic interventions. Heart failure from other causes is typically treated with cardiac glycosides to increase myocardial contractility and with diuretics to reduce intravascular volume. These drugs aggravate symptoms of HCM. Rather, HCM is treated with β-adrenergic blockers and Ca^{2+} channel blockers, which reduce contractility, decrease outflow tract obstruction and may improve left ventricular relaxation during diastole. Surgical removal of part of the hypertrophic septum or injection of ethanol into a septal artery to cause localized infarction may relieve symptoms of obstruction, but the risk of sudden death remains.

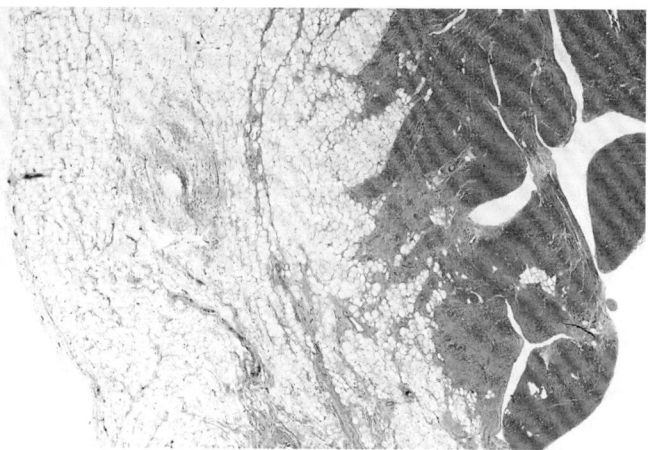

FIGURE 17-44. Arrhythmogenic cardiomyopathy. This section of the right ventricular free wall from a patient with classical arrhythmogenic right ventricular cardiomyopathy shows that much of the myocardium has been replaced by mature adipose tissue and fibrosis such that only subendocardial muscle bundles remain.

Arrhythmogenic Cardiomyopathy Is a Disease of the Desmosome with a High Risk of Sudden Death

Arrhythmogenic cardiomyopathy (AC) is a highly arrhythmogenic form of human heart disease. First described as a right ventricular disease (arrhythmogenic right ventricular cardiomyopathy, or ARVC), AC is now recognized to include biventricular and left dominant forms, which may be misdiagnosed as dilated cardiomyopathy or myocarditis. It affects roughly 1 in 5000 individuals and occurs most commonly in Mediterranean countries where it is a leading cause of sudden death in young people (under 35 years of age).

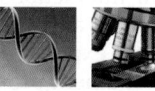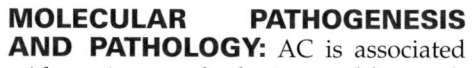 **MOLECULAR PATHOGENESIS AND PATHOLOGY:** AC is associated with serious arrhythmias and/or sudden death, which may occur early in the disease before significant structural remodeling and contractile dysfunction develop. The classical form (ARVC) affects the right ventricular free wall. The characteristic pathologic features are degeneration of cardiac myocytes and replacement by fat and fibrous tissue (Fig. 17-44), but the extent of this change can be quite variable and it is not necessarily conspicuous in patients who die suddenly.

AC is a familial disease, usually inherited in an autosomal dominant pattern. Its true incidence is probably underestimated because of variable penetrance, age-related progression and large phenotypic variation. The diagnosis can be difficult to make and requires analysis of various clinical criteria, which, although relatively specific, are not very sensitive. Mutations in genes encoding proteins in desmosomes, cell–cell adhesion organelles, can be identified in more than half of individuals who fulfill these criteria. These include genes for desmosomal adhesion molecules such as desmoglein-2 and intracellular desmosomal proteins including plakoglobin, desmoplakin and plakophilin-2, which form a complex that links the adhesion molecules to the desmin cytoskeleton in cardiac myocytes. Mutations in the gene for plakophilin-2 are most commonly seen in classical

ARVC, whereas mutations in the gene for desmoplakin are often associated with biventricular or left-sided forms of AC. Desmosomes are particularly abundant in heart and skin, two organs that experience the greatest mechanical burden, and mutations in desmosomal genes generally give rise to cutaneous and/or cardiac disease depending on the tissue-specific expression pattern of the mutant isoform. The mechanism by which desmosome mutations cause AC is unresolved, but increasing evidence implicates deranged Wnt signaling pathways and abnormal responses to mechanical stimulation of the heart during exercise.

Restrictive Cardiomyopathy Impairs Diastolic Function

Restrictive cardiomyopathy describes a group of diseases in which myocardial or endocardial abnormalities limit diastolic filling while contractile function is normal. It is the least common category of cardiomyopathy in Western countries, but in some less developed areas (e.g., equatorial Africa, South America and Asia), endomyocardial diseases due to parasitic infections lead to many cases of restrictive cardiomyopathy.

 ETIOLOGIC FACTORS AND PATHOLOGY: Restrictive cardiomyopathy is caused by (1) interstitial infiltration of amyloid, metastatic carcinoma or sarcoid granulomas; (2) endomyocardial disease characterized by marked fibrotic thickening of the endocardium; (3) genetic and storage diseases, including hemochromatosis and desmin-related cardiomyopathies; and (4) markedly increased interstitial fibrous tissue. The pathophysiologic consequence is a preload-dependent state, characterized by defective diastolic compliance, restricted ventricular filling, increased end-diastolic pressure, atrial dilation and venous congestion. In many respects, these hemodynamic changes are similar to the consequences of constrictive pericarditis. Many cases of restrictive cardiomyopathy are classified as idiopathic, with interstitial fibrosis as the only histologic abnormality.

The disease almost invariably progresses to congestive heart failure, and only 10% of the patients survive for 10 years.

Amyloidosis

The heart is affected in most forms of generalized amyloidosis (see Chapter 15). In fact, restrictive cardiomyopathy is the most common cause of death in the AL amyloidosis of plasma cell dyscrasias.

 PATHOLOGY: Amyloid infiltration of the heart results in cardiac enlargement without ventricular dilation. The gross appearance of the heart may resemble that seen in hypertrophic cardiomyopathy. Ventricular walls are typically thickened, firm and rubbery. Amyloid accumulation is most prominent in interstitial, perivascular and endocardial regions (Fig. 17-45). Endocardial involvement is common in the atria, where nodular endocardial deposits often impart a granular appearance and gritty texture to the endocardial surface. Amyloid deposits also can thicken cardiac valves. In rare cases, amyloid in the walls of intramural coronary arteries narrows their lumens and causes ischemic injury.

 CLINICAL FEATURES: Cardiac amyloidosis is most often a restrictive cardiomyopathy, with progressive diastolic and eventually systolic dysfunction. Infiltration of the conduction system can result in varying degrees of heart block and ventricular tachyarrhythmias. Echocardiography shows concentric ventricular thickening with right ventricular involvement and, usually, near-normal ejection fraction. Atrial enlargement, due to the noncompliant ventricular walls, is often seen. Low voltage of the QRS complex is a characteristic feature of the electrocardiogram.

The outlook for patients with symptomatic cardiac amyloidosis is grim: most survive less than 1 year. However, some patients have experienced more prolonged survival following successful treatment of their underlying plasma cell dyscrasia with chemotherapy or bone marrow transplantation. Durable remissions with bortezomib, a proteasome inhibitor used in multiple myeloma, have also been reported.

SENILE CARDIAC AMYLOIDOSIS: In senile cardiac amyloidosis, a protein related to prealbumin (transthyretin) is deposited in the hearts of elderly people (see Chapter 15). The disorder may be present to some extent in up to 25% of patients 80 years old or older. It involves not only the heart (atria and ventricles) but also, in many cases, the lungs and rectum as well. Amyloid deposits also may be found in blood vessel walls in many organs, but virtually never in renal glomeruli. Senile cardiac amyloidosis is usually an incidental finding at autopsy, and rarely is functionally significant. Even if amyloid deposits are extensive and there is symptomatic congestive heart failure, progression of the disease is much slower than that in AL amyloidosis.

Two additional forms of isolated cardiovascular amyloidosis are common in the elderly: **senile aortic amyloidosis** and **isolated atrial amyloidosis**. Neither of these forms of amyloid contains prealbumin or closely related proteins.

Desmin-Related Cardiomyopathies

Desmin is the intermediate filament protein in cardiac, striated and smooth muscle. Desmin filaments bind to desmosomes at intercalated disks and span the length of the cardiac myocyte by binding to Z disks of sarcomeres and other intracellular organelles.

 **MOLECULAR PATHOGENESIS AND PATHOLOGY:** Many mutations in desmin are known in patients with skeletal and cardiomyopathies; most are inherited as autosomal dominant traits. The heart disease usually manifests as a restrictive cardiomyopathy, with ventricular wall thickening, loss of ventricular compliance and diastolic dysfunction. Yet, some desmin-related cardiomyopathies resemble AC or DCM, presumably related to altered molecular interactions between desmin and components of desmosomes and the cytoskeleton, In many forms, the mutant protein is expressed and apparently interferes with normal desmin filament production. Large intracellular aggregates of refractile material can be seen by light microscopy, which are tangled masses of misfolded desmin filaments.

Endomyocardial Disease

Endomyocardial disease (EMD) consists of two geographically separate disorders.

ENDOMYOCARDIAL FIBROSIS: This disorder is particularly common in equatorial Africa, where it accounts for 10%–20% of deaths from heart disease. It also occurs occasionally in other tropical and subtropical regions of the world. While it is most common in children and young adults, endomyocardial fibrosis may occur in people up to age 70. It leads to progressive myocardial failure and has a poor prognosis, although some patients survive for as long as 12 years.

EOSINOPHILIC ENDOMYOCARDIAL DISEASE (LÖFFLER ENDOCARDITIS): This is a cardiac disorder of temperate regions characterized by hypereosinophilia (up to 50,000/μL). It usually occurs in men in the fifth decade and is often accompanied by rash. Löffler endocarditis typically progresses to congestive heart failure and death, although corticosteroids may improve survival.

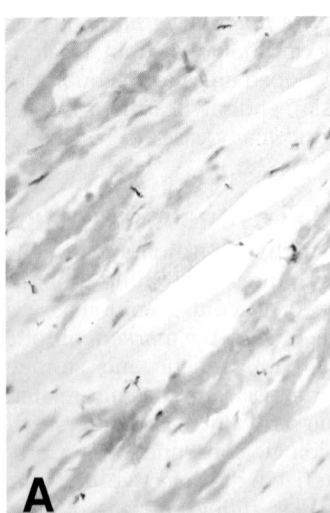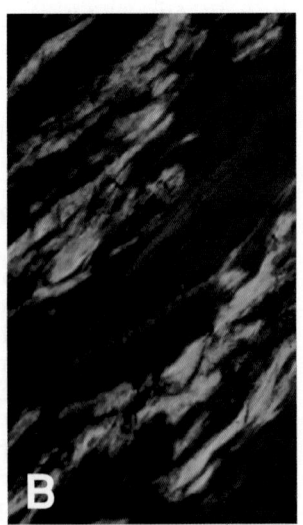

FIGURE 17-45. Cardiac amyloidosis. A. A section of myocardium stained with Congo red shows interstitial, pink-staining deposits of amyloid. **B.** Under polarized light, the same section displays the characteristic green birefringence of amyloid fibrils.

 **ETIOLOGIC FACTORS:** Endomyocardial fibrosis and Löffler endocarditis are variants of the same basic disease. *EMD probably results from myocardial injury caused by eosinophils, possibly mediated by cardiotoxic granule components.* In the tropics, transient high blood eosinophil counts often result from parasitic infestations; in temperate climates, idiopathic hypereosinophilia is often persistent.

EMD can be divided into three stages:

1. The necrotic stage occurs within the first few months of the illness and is characterized by an intense eosinophilic infiltrate of the inner myocardial layers, usually of both ventricles. The infiltrate is perivascular and interstitial, and there is evidence of vascular injury and myocyte necrosis. This stage lasts for several months, usually without significant functional impairment.
2. The thrombotic stage develops about a year later. Mural thrombi attach to injured, slightly thickened endocardium. At this time, the myocardium is no longer inflamed but shows early hypertrophy. Emboli may occur at this time.
3. The fibrotic stage is the chronic phase of EMD, with conspicuous fibrotic endocardial thickening and marked fibrosis. This decreases compliance and causes diastolic dysfunction. Posterior valve leaflets may adhere to the endocardium, causing mitral—or on the right side, tricuspid—regurgitation.

 PATHOLOGY: At autopsy, a grayish white thickened endocardium extends from the apex of the left ventricle over the posterior papillary muscle to the posterior leaflet of the mitral valve and for a short distance into the left outflow tract. Endocardial fibrosis involves the inner 1/3 to 1/2 of the ventricle wall. Mural thrombi in various stages of organization may be present. When the right ventricle is involved, the entire cavity may show endocardial thickening, which may extend to the epicardium. The fibrotic endocardium contains only a few elastic fibers. Myofibers trapped within the collagenous tissue display nonspecific degenerative changes.

Storage Diseases

Lysosomal storage diseases are detailed in Chapter 6. Only the cardiac manifestations are reviewed here.

GLYCOGEN STORAGE DISEASES: Of the various forms of glycogen storage disease, types II (Pompe disease), III (Cori disease) and IV (Andersen disease) affect the heart. Pompe disease is the most common and severe. Infants with this condition have markedly enlarged hearts (up to seven times normal), and 20% have endocardial fibroelastosis. Myocytes are vacuolated owing to large amounts of stored glycogen. These patients show a restrictive type of cardiomyopathy and usually die of cardiac failure.

MUCOPOLYSACCHARIDOSES: Several of the mucopolysaccharidoses involve the heart. Cardiac disease results from lysosomal accumulation of mucopolysaccharides (glycosaminoglycans) in various cells. In general, pseudohypertrophy of the ventricles develops and contractility gradually diminishes. The coronary arteries may be narrowed by intimal and medial thickening. In Hurler and Hunter syndromes, myocardial infarction is common. Valve leaflets may be thickened, thus causing progressive valvular dysfunction, manifested as aortic stenosis (Scheie syndrome) or mitral regurgitation (Hurler, Morquio syndromes). Cor pulmonale may result from pulmonary hypertension related to narrowing of the airways.

SPHINGOLIPIDOSES: In **Fabry disease,** glycosphingolipid accumulation in the heart may cause functional and pathologic changes like those in the mucopolysaccharidoses. Fabry disease produces gross and microscopic changes that mimic HCM, but the characteristic vacuolated appearance of cardiac myocytes is an important clue of an underlying storage disease. **Gaucher disease** only rarely involves the heart but may feature left ventricular interstitial infiltration by cerebroside-laden macrophages, impaired left ventricular compliance and cardiac output.

HEMOCHROMATOSIS: This multiorgan disease is associated with excessive iron deposition in many tissues (see Chapter 20). The degree of iron deposition in the heart varies and only roughly correlates with that in other organs. Cardiac involvement has features of both dilated and restrictive cardiomyopathy, with systolic and diastolic impairment. *Congestive heart failure occurs in up to 1/3 of patients.*

At autopsy, the heart is dilated; ventricular walls are thickened. The myocardium reflects iron deposition in cardiac myocytes. Interstitial fibrosis is invariable, but its extent does not correlate well with the extent of iron accumulation. The severity of myocardial dysfunction seems to be proportional to the quantity of iron deposited.

Sarcoidosis

Sarcoidosis is a generalized granulomatous disease that may involve the heart (see Chapter 18). One quarter of cases show some granulomas in the heart at autopsy, but fewer than 5% of patients with this condition have cardiac symptoms. Sarcoid heart disease is seen clinically as a mixed pattern of dilated and restrictive cardiomyopathy. Sarcoid granulomas often cause extensive myocardial damage, preferentially involving the base of the interventricular septum. Because this region contains major components of the atrioventricular conduction system, bundle branch blocks or complete heart block is common. More serious life-threatening arrhythmias and sudden death are frequent. Microscopic examination of the heart in severe cases of sarcoid heart disease reveals infiltration of the myocardium by noncaseating granulomas, massive destruction of myocytes and replacement by interstitial fibrosis (Fig. 17-46).

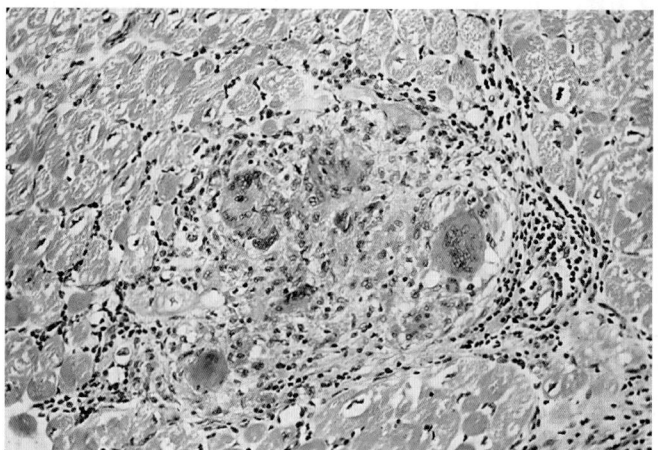

FIGURE 17-46. Cardiac sarcoidosis. The myocardium is infiltrated by noncaseating granulomas, with prominent giant cells. There is considerable destruction of cardiac myocytes with fibrosis.

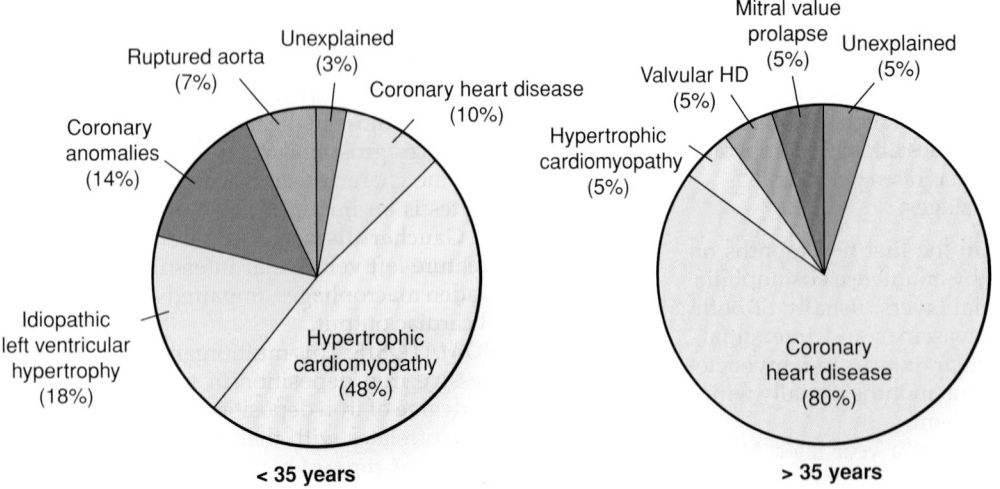

FIGURE 17-47. Different causes of sudden cardiac death in young and older adult competitive athletes. *HD* = heart disease.

SUDDEN CARDIAC DEATH

Over 300,000 people in the United States die suddenly each year. Most of these deaths are caused by spontaneous lethal ventricular tachyarrhythmias—ventricular tachycardia and ventricular fibrillation—in patients with some type of heart disease. Many sudden deaths occur out of the hospital in apparently healthy individuals who have coronary artery disease at autopsy but may have had little clinical evidence of it during life.

Common causes of sudden cardiac death differ in young and old individuals. This has been studied most thoroughly in competitive athletes (Fig. 17-47). In subjects younger than 35, HCM, idiopathic left ventricular hypertrophy (presumably reflecting genetic forms of heart muscle disease in at least some) and congenital coronary anomalies account for over 75% of sudden deaths. In Italy and other Mediterranean countries, arrhythmogenic cardiomyopathy is a leading cause of sudden death in young people. *However, in economically developed nations, coronary artery disease is responsible for most sudden deaths in middle-aged and older adults.*

PATHOLOGY: The surface ECG may occasionally indicate a specific pathologic structure that can be implicated in causing sudden death, such as an accessory atrioventricular connection in Wolff-Parkinson-White syndrome or a lesion that disrupts a discrete component of the ventricular conduction system causing new bundle branch block. *However, lethal arrhythmias usually arise from pathologic changes affecting conduction in the working ventricular myocardium.* At autopsy, hearts of sudden death victims typically exhibit myocardial alterations that create "anatomic substrates of arrhythmias." These changes may be localized (e.g., healed myocardial infarcts or left ventricular aneurysms) or diffuse (e.g., variable degrees of cardiac myocyte hypertrophy and interstitial fibrosis). Spontaneous development of a lethal cardiac arrhythmia may be regarded as a stochastic event arising from complex interactions between relatively fixed anatomic substrates and acute, transient triggering events such as acute ischemia, neurohormonal activation, changes in electrolytes or other stresses. Many patients have potential arrhythmia substrates in their hearts. In most cases, they may be necessary but they are not

sufficient for arrhythmogenesis. Arrhythmias are most likely when acute electrophysiologic changes (triggers) are superimposed on an existing substrate of remodeled myocardium with characteristic conduction abnormalities. Indeed, most often sudden death involves acute ischemia (a transient triggering event) in an area of the heart containing a healed infarct (a common anatomic substrate).

Sudden Cardiac Death Occurs in Patients with Structurally Normal Hearts, but This Is Rare

Some (perhaps many) of such patients have "channelopathies," genetic diseases in which mutations in genes for Na^+, K^+ and Ca^{2+} channel proteins are responsible for sudden death syndromes (see Chapter 1). Although these syndromes are rare, they have provided valuable insights into molecular mechanisms of lethal arrhythmias.

MOLECULAR PATHOGENESIS:
LONG QT SYNDROME: This condition is defined by prolonged QT intervals and T-wave abnormalities on the surface ECG and a history of syncope, ventricular arrhythmias or sudden, unexpected death. More than 10 different types of congenital long QT syndrome have been defined. Most are caused by loss-of-function mutations in genes encoding proteins that form various K^+ channels. The loss of function prolongs repolarization of the cardiac action potential (thus increasing QT intervals on surface ECGs) and promotes arrhythmias by increasing the likelihood of after-depolarizations. Long QT syndrome can also be caused by gain-of-function mutations in *SCN5A*, the gene encoding the cardiac Na^+ channel protein. These mutations prolong QT intervals by allowing leakage of depolarizing current during repolarization. Mutations in proteins responsible for ion channel trafficking or scaffolding, such as ankyrin B and caveolin-3, are also implicated in long QT syndrome. Arrhythmias occur in long QT syndrome because the mutated ion channels are normally distributed in the heart in a spatially heterogeneous fashion. The functional defect caused by the mutation creates ionic gradients that promote abnormal electrical impulse formation (after-depolarizations) and abnormal impulse conduction, conditions conducive to development of ventricular tachycardias.

BRUGADA SYNDROME: This is an autosomal dominant disease in a structurally normal heart with characteristic ST-segment elevation in right precordial leads, right bundle branch block and susceptibility to life-threatening arrhythmias. Loss-of-function mutations in *SCN5A* are identified in approximately 25% of cases.

CATECHOLAMINERGIC POLYMORPHIC VENTRICULAR TACHYCARDIA: In this condition, arrhythmias and sudden death occur in response to catecholamine surges associated with exercise or emotional stress. Mutations in genes encoding proteins that regulate intracellular Ca^{2+} homeostasis and excitation–contraction coupling, such as RyR2 and calsequestrin, are typical. These mutations promote leakage of Ca^{2+} from the SR and resultant arrhythmias triggered by after-depolarizations.

CARDIAC TUMORS

Primary cardiac tumors are rare, but can cause serious problems when they occur.

Myxomas Are the Most Common Primary Cardiac Tumors

These tumors account for 30%–50% of all primary cardiac tumors.

 MOLECULAR PATHOGENESIS: Most cardiac myxomas are sporadic, but about 7% are part of a familial autosomal dominant syndrome that also includes pigmented lesions of the skin and adrenocortical hyperplasia. These cases have been linked to mutations in the gene encoding a regulatory subunit of cyclic adenosine monophosphate (cAMP)-dependent protein kinase (protein kinase A), which, among other actions, appears to be a tumor suppressor gene that controls cell proliferation.

 PATHOLOGY: Myxomas can occur in any cardiac chamber or on a valve, but most (75%) arise in the left atrium. The tumors appear as glistening, gelatinous, polypoid masses, usually 5–6 cm, with a short stalk (Fig. 17-48), and may be sufficiently mobile to obstruct the mitral valve orifice. They show loose myxoid stroma containing abundant proteoglycans. Polygonal stellate cells are found within the matrix, singly or in small clusters.

CLINICAL FEATURES: More than half of patients with left atrial myxomas have clinical evidence of mitral valve dysfunction. The tumor does not metastasize in the usual sense, but it often embolizes. Some patients with myxomas of the left heart die from tumor emboli to the brain. Surgical tumor removal is usually curative.

Rhabdomyomas Are the Most Common Primary Childhood Cardiac Tumors

They form nodular myocardial masses. These lesions may really be hamartomas (see below) rather than true neoplasms, but the issue is still debated. Almost all are multiple and involve both ventricles and, in 1/3 of cases, the atria as well. In half of cases, the tumors project into a cardiac chamber and obstruct the lumen or valve orifices.

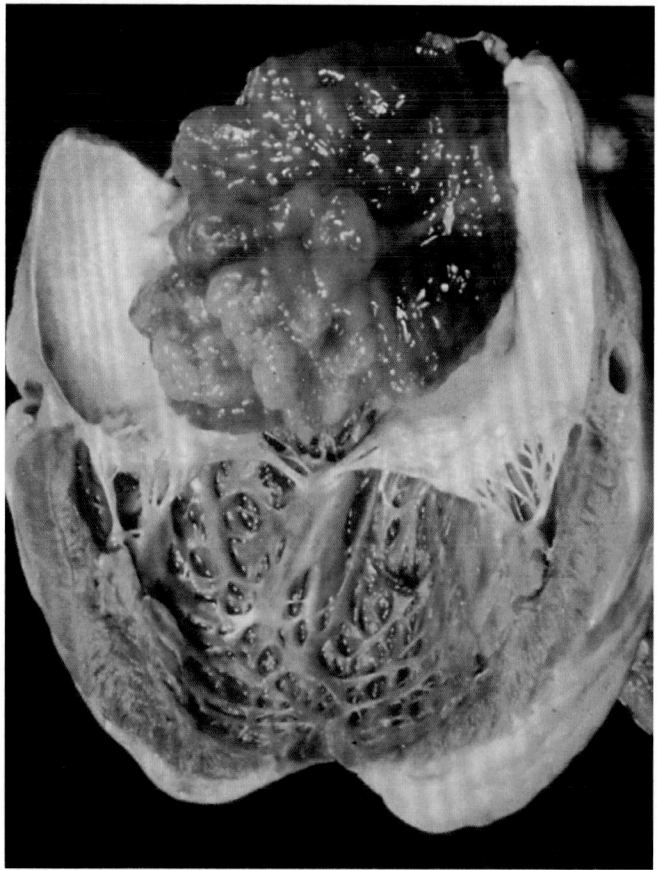
FIGURE 17-48. Cardiac myxoma. The left atrium contains a large, polypoid tumor that protrudes into the mitral valve orifice.

 **MOLECULAR PATHOGENESIS:** Rhabdomyomas occur in 1/3 of patients with tuberous sclerosis, the familial form of which is caused by mutations in *TSC1* and *TSC2*, genes that encode hamartin and tuberin, respectively. Both genes are tumor suppressors (see Chapter 5) and regulate embryonic and neonatal growth and differentiation of cardiac myocytes.

 PATHOLOGY: Cardiac rhabdomyomas are pale masses, 1 mm to several centimeters. Tumor cells show small central nuclei and abundant glycogen-rich clear cytoplasm, in which fibrillar processes containing sarcomeres radiate to the margin of the cell ("spider cell"). About 1/3 to 1/2 of these tumors occur in association with tuberous sclerosis. A few cardiac rhabdomyomas have been successfully excised.

Papillary Fibroelastoma Involves the Valves

Papillary fronds resembling a sea anemone and measuring up to 3–4 cm may grow on the heart valves. These are not neoplasms, and are more appropriately termed **hamartomas**. The fronds have central dense cores of collagen and elastic fibers surrounded by looser connective tissue. They are covered by a continuation of valvular endothelium on which the tumor originates. In most instances, papillary fibroelastomas are not clinical problems, but they can fragment and embolize to other organs or occlude a coronary artery orifice and produce myocardial ischemia.

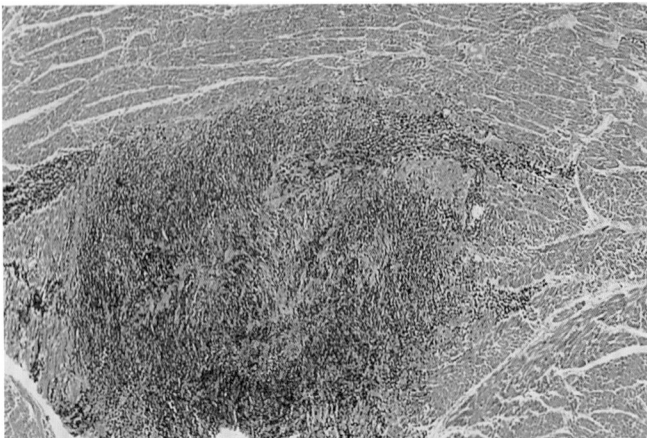

FIGURE 17-49. Malignant melanoma metastatic to the heart. The myocardium contains a heavily pigmented tumor metastasis.

Other Tumors in the Heart Are Rare

Other primary tumors of the heart include angiomas, fibromas, lymphangiomas, neurofibromas and their sarcomatous counterparts. Lipomatous hypertrophy of the interatrial septum and encapsulated lipomas have been reported.

Metastatic tumors to the heart are seen most often in patients with the most common carcinomas—that is, lung, breast and gastrointestinal tract. Still, only a minority of patients with these tumors develop cardiac metastases. Lymphomas and leukemia also may involve the heart. Of all tumors, the one most likely to metastasize to the heart is malignant melanoma (Fig. 17-49). Metastatic cancer involving the myocardium can result in clinical manifestations of restrictive cardiomyopathy, particularly if the cardiac tumors are associated with extensive fibrosis. Occasionally, metastatic tumors may disrupt components of the atrioventricular conduction system, giving rise to heart block or bundle branch block patterns on the surface electrocardiogram.

DISEASES OF THE PERICARDIUM

Pericardial Effusions Can Cause Cardiac Tamponade

Pericardial effusions are accumulations of excess fluid within the pericardial cavity, as either a transudate or an exudate. The pericardial sac normally contains no more than 50 mL of lubricating fluid. If the pericardium is slowly distended, it can accommodate up to 2 L of fluid without notable hemodynamic consequences. However, rapid accumulation of as little as 150–200 mL of pericardial fluid or blood may significantly increase intrapericardial pressure and restrict diastolic filling, especially of the right atrium and ventricle.

- **Serous pericardial effusion** often complicates an increase in extracellular fluid volume, as occurs in congestive heart failure or nephrotic syndrome. The fluid has a low protein content and few cellular elements.
- **Chylous effusion** (fluid containing chylomicrons) results from a communication of the thoracic duct with the pericardial space due to lymphatic obstruction by tumor or infection.

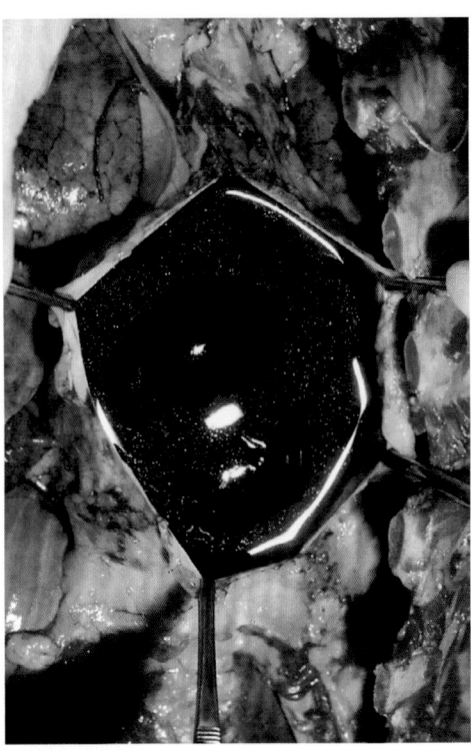

FIGURE 17-50. Hemopericardium. The parietal pericardium has been opened to reveal the pericardial cavity distended with fresh blood. The patient sustained a rupture of a myocardial infarct.

- **Serosanguineous pericardial effusion** may develop after chest trauma, either accidentally or after cardiopulmonary resuscitation.
- **Hemopericardium** is bleeding directly into the pericardial cavity (Fig. 17-50). The most common cause is ventricular free wall rupture at a myocardial infarct. Less frequent causes are penetrating cardiac trauma, rupture of a dissecting aneurysm of the aorta, infiltration of a vessel by tumor or a bleeding diathesis.

Cardiac tamponade *is the syndrome caused by rapid accumulation of pericardial fluid, restricting the filling of the heart.* Hemodynamic consequences range from a minimally symptomatic condition to abrupt cardiovascular collapse and death. As pericardial pressure increases, it reaches and then exceeds central venous pressure, thus limiting blood return to the heart. Cardiac output and blood pressure decrease, and **pulsus paradoxus** (an abnormal decrease in systolic pressure with inspiration) occurs in almost all patients. Acute cardiac tamponade is almost always fatal unless the pressure is relieved by removing pericardial fluid, via needle pericardiocentesis or surgery.

Acute Pericarditis May Follow Viral Infections

Pericarditis is inflammation of the visceral or parietal pericardium.

 **ETIOLOGIC FACTORS:** The causes of pericarditis are similar to those for myocarditis (Table 17-7). In most cases, the cause of acute pericarditis is obscure and (as in myocarditis) is attributed to undiagnosed

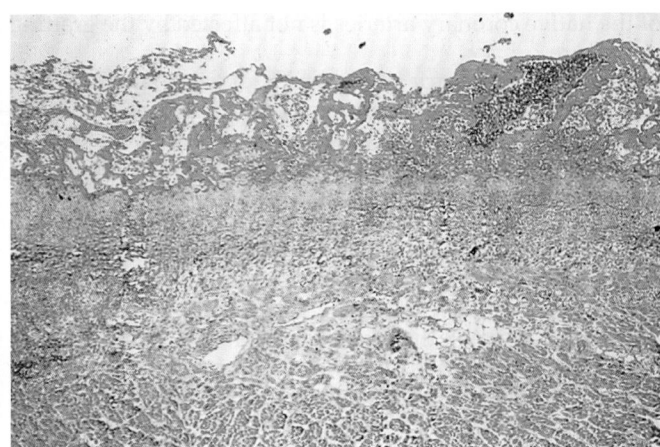

FIGURE 17-51. Fibrinous pericardial exudate. The epicardial surface is edematous, inflamed and covered with tentacles of fibrin.

viral infection. Bacterial pericarditis is unusual in the antibiotic era. Metastatic tumors may induce serofibrinous or hemorrhagic exudative and inflammatory reactions when they involve the pericardium. The most common tumors to involve the pericardium and cause malignant pericardial effusions are breast and lung carcinomas. Pericarditis associated with myocardial infarction and rheumatic fever is discussed above.

 PATHOLOGY: Acute pericarditis can be **fibrinous, purulent** or **hemorrhagic,** depending on gross and microscopic characteristics of the pericardial surfaces and fluid. The most common form is fibrinous pericarditis, in which the normal smooth, glistening pericardial surfaces are replaced by a dull, granular fibrin-rich exudate (Fig. 17-51). The rough texture of inflamed pericardial surfaces produces a characteristic friction rub on auscultation. Effusion fluid in fibrinous pericarditis is usually rich in protein, and the pericardium contains mainly mononuclear inflammatory cells. Uremia can cause fibrinous pericarditis (Fig. 17-52), but with the widespread availability of renal dialysis, uremic pericarditis is now unusual in the United States. The most common causes are viral infection and pericarditis after myocardial infarcts.

Bacterial infection leads to a purulent pericarditis, in which the pericardial exudate resembles pus and is full of neutrophils. Bleeding into the pericardial space caused by aggressive infectious or neoplastic processes or coagulation defects leads to hemorrhagic pericarditis.

 CLINICAL FEATURES: Initial manifestations of acute pericarditis are sudden, severe, substernal chest pain, sometimes referred to the back, shoulder or neck. These differ from the pain of angina pectoris or myocardial infarction by their failure to radiate down the left arm. A characteristic pericardial friction rub is easily heard. Electrocardiographic changes reflect repolarization abnormalities of the myocardium.

Idiopathic or viral pericarditis is a self-limited disorder, but it may infrequently lead to constrictive pericarditis. Corticosteroids are the treatment of choice. Therapy for other specific forms of acute pericarditis varies with the cause.

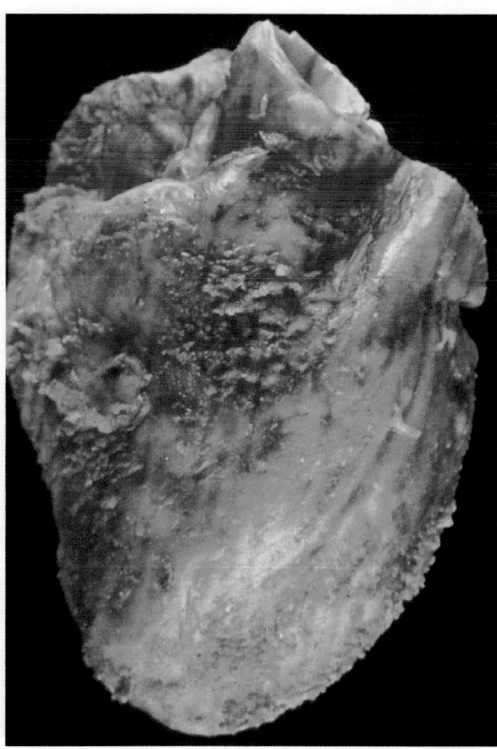

FIGURE 17-52. Fibrinous pericarditis. The heart of a patient who died in uremia displays a shaggy, fibrinous exudate covering the visceral pericardium.

Constrictive Pericarditis May Mimic Right Heart Failure

Constrictive pericarditis is a chronic fibrosing disease of the pericardium that compresses the heart and restricts inflow.

 **ETIOLOGIC FACTORS AND PATHOLOGY:** Constrictive pericarditis is not an active inflammatory condition. Rather, it reflects exuberant healing after acute pericardial injury. The pericardial space becomes obliterated, and visceral and parietal layers become fused in a dense, rigid mass of fibrous tissue. The scarred pericardium may be so thick (up to 3 cm) that it narrows the orifices of the venae cavae (Fig. 17-53). The fibrous envelope may contain calcium. The condition is uncommon today and, in developed countries, is predominantly idiopathic. Prior radiation therapy to the mediastinum and cardiac surgery account for more than 1/3 of cases. In others, it follows a purulent or tuberculous infection. Tuberculosis today accounts for fewer than 15% of cases of constrictive pericarditis in industrialized countries, but it is still the major cause in underdeveloped regions.

 CLINICAL FEATURES: Patients with constrictive pericarditis have small, quiet hearts in which venous inflow is restricted, as the rigid pericardium limits the diastolic volume of the heart. These patients have high venous pressure, low cardiac output, small pulse pressure and fluid retention with ascites and peripheral edema. Total pericardiectomy is the treatment of choice.

Adhesive pericarditis is a much milder form of healing of an inflamed pericardium. Commonly seen as an incidental

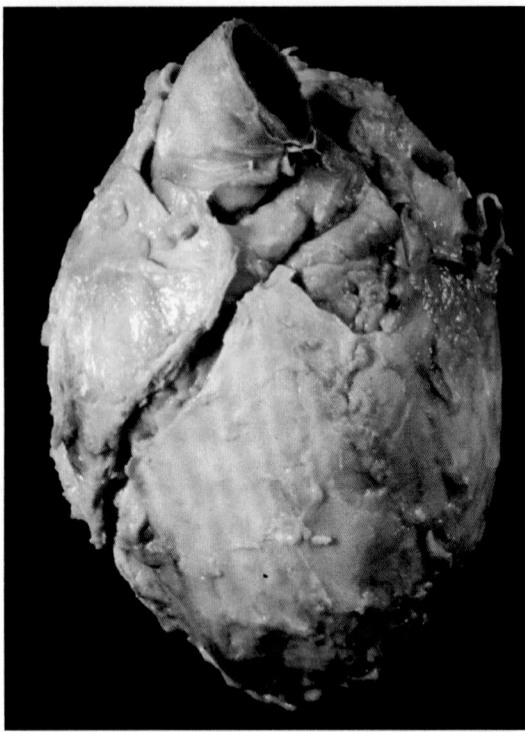

FIGURE 17-53. Constrictive pericarditis. The pericardial space has been obliterated, and the heart is encased in a fibrotic, thickened pericardium.

finding at autopsy, it is the outcome of many different types of pericarditis that have healed and left only minor fibrous adhesions between the visceral and parietal surfaces.

PATHOLOGY OF INTERVENTIONAL THERAPIES

Percutaneous Coronary Interventions Are Used to Treat Atherosclerotic Coronary Arterial Disease

PCI is used to mechanically dilate an artery narrowed by atherosclerosis and keep the lumen open. A catheter with a deflated balloon covered by a collapsed cylindrical metallic mesh **(stent)** is positioned in the stenotic segment. Inflating the balloon fractures the plaque and stretches the vessel wall. As the stent deploys, it holds the fragmented wall open and keeps the vessel lumen patent. Acute complications of PCI such as coronary artery dissection, acute thrombotic occlusion and perforation are uncommon. Most patients receive drug-eluting stents, which slowly release antiproliferative agents such as everolimus or paclitaxel. Their use has dramatically reduced the incidence of restenosis.

Coronary Bypass Grafts Circumvent Obstructed Segments

Coronary bypass grafting, using a saphenous vein or left internal mammary artery to redirect blood around a blockage, is common treatment for proximal coronary stenosis. Although operative mortality is low and early symptomatic relief occurs in most patients, myocardial perfusion is not permanently improved, owing to several complications: (1) early thrombosis, (2) intimal hyperplasia and (3) atherosclerosis of vein grafts. Moreover, progressive atherosclerosis

of the native coronary arteries is not affected by the grafting procedure.

Internal mammary artery grafts develop fewer pathologic changes and so last longer than vein grafts. Excised saphenous vein segments used as grafts are subjected to unavoidable surgical manipulation and an interval of ischemia during harvesting, which injures endothelial cells. Grafted veins are also exposed to arterial pressures that are much higher than those in their native location. Finally, the caliber of the vein, which is expanded by arterial blood pressure, is usually much greater than that of the distal coronary artery at the graft anastomosis, and this mismatch promotes blood stasis. In the immediate postoperative period, these factors enhance the chance of thrombosis and probably eventually lead to intimal hyperplasia. Intimal hyperplasia is a concentric increase of smooth muscle cells, fibroblasts and collagen in the intima of the vein. After several years, lipids may deposit and atherosclerotic plaques may form in the thickened intima of vein grafts. Atherosclerosis is the most frequent cause of vein graft failure in patients who have had good graft function for several years after surgery.

Since arteries are better aortocoronary bypass conduits than veins, some surgeons have developed total arterial bypass procedures that use internal mammary, radial and selected abdominal arteries that can be taken without endorgan damage.

Tissue Xenografts and Mechanical Valves Typically Are Used to Replace Damaged Cardiac Valves

In most patients with severe valve dysfunction, valve replacement is the best prospect for long-term symptomatic improvement. Operative mortality is low, especially for patients with good preoperative myocardial function. Half of all patients with prosthetic valves are free of complications after 10 years.

TISSUE VALVES: The most commonly used tissue-valve prostheses use a mechanical frame to which glutaraldehyde-fixed porcine aortic valve cusps or pieces of bovine pericardium are attached. These valves have good hemodynamic characteristics, cause little obstruction and resist thromboembolic complications. Unfortunately, they are not very durable. The most common cause of failure of tissue-valve prostheses is tissue degeneration with calcification and fragmentation of prosthetic valve cusps. This developed within 5 years of implantation in virtually all early-generation porcine aortic valves and led to valve failure in 20%–30% of patients within 10 years. Improved understanding of prosthetic tissue-valve calcification has led to development of anticalcification treatments that improve valve longevity and performance. Tissue-valve calcification occurs mainly within residual cells killed by glutaraldehyde treatment. Strategies to prevent or delay such calcification include removal of residual cells, binding of calcification inhibitors to the glutaraldehyde-fixed tissue and use of other tissue cross-linking and preservation reagents.

MECHANICAL VALVES: The most widely used mechanical prostheses involve single or bileaflet tilting disk designs that do not obstruct blood flow across the valve and have excellent durability. However, the risk of thromboembolism makes long-term anticoagulant therapy imperative.

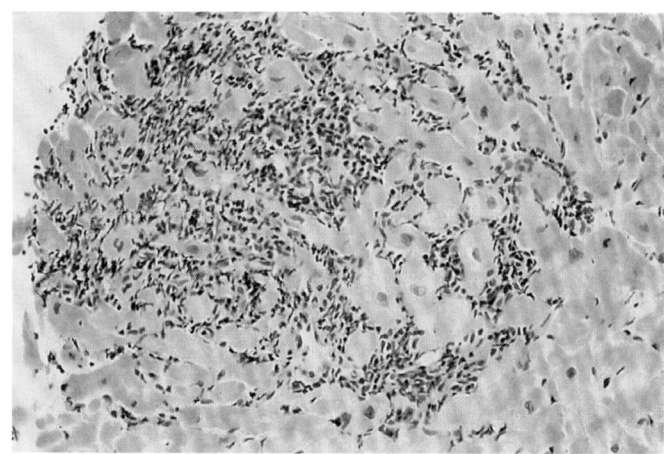

FIGURE 17-54. Cardiac transplant rejection. An endomyocardial biopsy shows lymphocytes surrounding individual myocytes and expanding the interstitium.

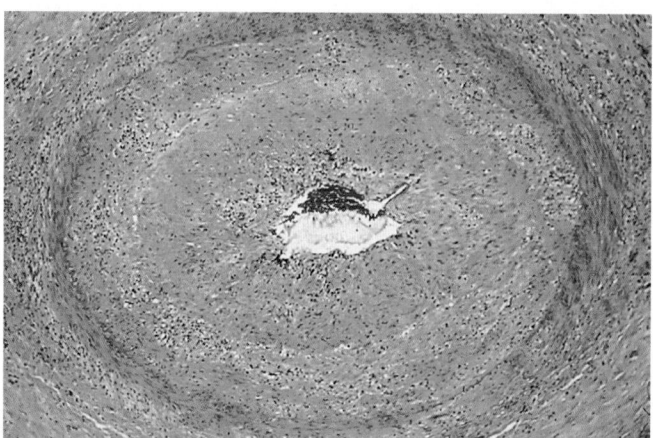

FIGURE 17-55. Chronic cardiac transplant rejection. An intramyocardial branch of a coronary artery shows prominent intimal proliferation and inflammation with concentric narrowing of the lumen.

Cancer Survivors May Experience Long-Term Cardiovascular Complications

As more patients survive cancer chemotherapy and/or radiation therapy, increased rates of cardiovascular disease attributable to their therapy are becoming recognized. Exposing the heart to radiation increases the rate of ischemic heart disease. Each gray of radiation (see Chapter 8) is associated with an estimated 7.4% increase in risk of a major coronary event, which apparently persists for at least two decades after the radiation ends. Radiation also contributes to pericardial disease, cardiomyopathy and valvular dysfunction. Breast cancer patients treated with drugs that target HER2/neu experience greater risk of both coronary events and ventricular dysfunction.

Heart Transplantation May Cure Many End-Stage Heart Diseases but Is Subject to Host Rejection Processes

The development of effective immunosuppressive regimens and surveillance endomyocardial biopsy protocols has made cardiac transplantation an effective treatment for end-stage heart disease. Allograft rejection (see Chapter 4), however, is a major complication of cardiac transplantation.

Hyperacute rejection occurs if there are blood-group incompatibility or major histocompatibility differences. In these situations, preformed antibodies cause immediate vascular injury to the donor heart, with diffuse hemorrhage, edema, intracapillary platelet–fibrin thrombi, vascular necrosis and infiltration of neutrophils. Screening for blood-group incompatibility has rendered this complication rare.

Acute humoral rejection is characterized by vascular deposition of antibody and complement, endothelial cell swelling and edema. This unusual form of rejection has a worse prognosis than acute cellular rejection.

Acute cellular rejection, the most common form of allograft rejection, usually occurs in the first few months after transplantation. It begins as perivascular T-cell infiltration, which is focal and is not associated with acute myocyte necrosis. This reaction often resolves spontaneously and, therefore, does not necessitate a change in the immunosuppressive regimen. Moderate cellular rejection is characterized by T-cell infiltration into adjacent interstitial spaces, where lymphocytes surround individual myocytes and expand the interstitium (Fig. 17-54). In this instance, focal acute myocyte necrosis is also present. Moderate cellular rejection usually does not produce detectable functional impairment and tends to resolve within a few days to a week after treatment. However, additional immunosuppressive therapy is instituted because moderate cellular rejection can progress to severe rejection. The latter is characterized by vascular damage, widespread myocyte necrosis, neutrophil infiltration, interstitial hemorrhage and functional impairment, which is difficult to reverse.

The early stage of cellular allograft rejection is often asymptomatic. Once symptoms develop, rejection is usually advanced and has caused irrecoverable loss of cardiac myocytes. The most reliable screening procedure is endomyocardial biopsy of the right side of the interventricular septum, via cardiac catheterization.

Chronic vascular rejection, also referred to as **accelerated coronary artery disease,** is the most common cause of death in heart transplant patients beyond the first year after transplantation. It affects proximal and distal epicardial coronary arteries, the penetrating coronary artery branches and even arterioles. Accelerated coronary artery disease is characterized by concentric intimal proliferation (Fig. 17-55), which can lead to coronary occlusion and myocardial infarction. This complication is silent because the transplanted heart is denervated. Thus, extensive myocardial damage can develop before a transplant patient is aware that ischemic injury has occurred.

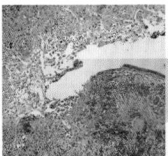
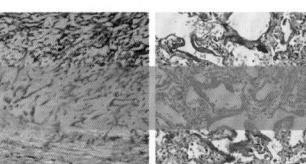
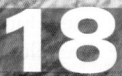

The Respiratory System
Mary Beth Beasley ▪ William D. Travis

The Normal Respiratory System

EMBRYOLOGY

The respiratory system includes the larynx, trachea, bronchi, bronchioles and alveoli. During the fourth week of gestation, the laryngotracheal groove develops as a ventral outpouching of the foregut.

1. **Embryonic period:** Between 4 and 6 weeks' gestation, the tracheobronchial bud divides to form proximal airways to the level of segmental bronchi.
2. **Pseudoglandular period:** From 6 to 16 weeks' gestation, the distal airways are formed to the level of the terminal bronchioles.

3. **Acinar or canalicular development:** During weeks 17–28, (a) the framework of the gas-exchanging unit of the lung develops, (b) acini are formed, (c) the vascular system develops, (d) capillaries reach the epithelium and (e) gas exchange can occur. At this point extrauterine life becomes possible.

4. **Saccular period:** At 28–34 weeks of gestation, primary saccules become subdivided by secondary crests, resulting in greater complexity of the gas-exchanging surface and thinning of airspace walls.

5. **Alveolar period:** The last step is alveolar development during weeks 34–36. At birth, the number of alveoli is highly variable, ranging from 20 to 150 million. Most alveoli develop in the first 2 years of life.

ANATOMY

TRACHEA AND BRONCHI: The trachea is a hollow tube up to 25 cm in length and 2.5 cm in diameter. The right bronchus diverges at a lesser angle from the trachea than does the left, which is why foreign material is more frequently aspirated on the right side. On entering the lung, the main bronchi divide into lobar bronchi, then into segmental bronchi, which supply the 19 lung segments. Since segments are individual units with their own bronchovascular supply, they can be resected individually.

The tracheobronchial tree contains cartilage and submucosal mucous glands in the wall (Fig. 18-1). The latter are compound tubular glands, which contain **mucous cells** (pale) and **serous cells** (granular, more basophilic). The pseudostratified epithelium appears as layers, but all cells reach the basement membrane. Most cells are ciliated, but there are also mucus-secreting **(goblet)** cells and basal cells. The **basal cells,** which do not reach the surface, are precursors that differentiate into more specialized tracheobronchial epithelial cells. There are also nonciliated columnar cells, or **club cells** (formerly **Clara cells**), which accumulate and detoxify many inhaled toxic agents (e.g., nitrogen dioxide [NO_2]). **Neuroendocrine cells** are scattered in the tracheobronchial mucosa and contain a variety of hormonally active polypeptides and vasoactive amines.

BRONCHIOLES: Distal to the bronchi are the bronchioles, which differ from bronchi in that they lack cartilage and mucus-secreting glands (Fig. 18-1). Bronchiolar epithelium becomes thinner with progressive branching, until only one cell layer is present. The last purely conducting structure free of alveoli is the **terminal bronchiole,** which exhibits pseudostratified ciliated respiratory epithelium and a smooth muscle wall. Mucous cells gradually disappear from the lining of the bronchioles until they are entirely replaced in the small bronchioles by nonciliated, columnar club cells (formerly Clara cells). Terminal bronchioles divide into **respiratory bronchioles,** which merge into **alveolar ducts** and **alveoli.** The gas exchange units of the lung are called **acini** and consist of respiratory bronchioles, alveolar ducts and alveoli.

ALVEOLI: Alveoli are lined by two types of epithelium (Fig. 18-1). **Type I cells** cover 95% of the alveolar surface but constitute only 40% of alveolar epithelial cells. They are thin and have a large surface area, a combination that facilitates gas exchange. **Type II cells** produce surfactant and make up 60% of the alveolar lining cells. As they are more cuboidal than type I cells, they cover only 5% of the alveolar surface. Type I cells are highly vulnerable to injury. When they are lost, type II pneumocytes multiply and differentiate to form new type I cells, restoring the integrity of the alveolar surface.

Alveolar epithelial and endothelial cells are ideally arranged for gas exchange. The cytoplasm of epithelial and endothelial cells is spread very thinly on either side of a fused basement membrane, allowing efficient exchange of oxygen and carbon dioxide. An extensive capillary network supplies 85%–95% of the alveolar surface. Away from the site of gas exchange, interstitial connective tissue is more abundant, consisting of collagen, elastin and proteoglycans. Fibroblasts and myofibroblasts may also be present. This expanded region forms the interstitial space of the alveolar wall, where significant fluid and molecular exchange occurs.

PULMONARY VASCULATURE: The lung has a **dual blood supply** from the pulmonary and the bronchial systems. Pulmonary arteries accompany airways in a sheath of connective tissue, the **bronchovascular bundle**. The more proximal arteries are elastic and are succeeded by muscular arteries, pulmonary arterioles and eventually pulmonary capillaries.

The smallest veins, which resemble the smallest arteries, join other veins and drain into lobular septa, connective tissue partitions that subdivide the lung into small respiratory units. In these septa, the veins form a network separate from the bronchovascular bundles.

Bronchial arteries arise from the thoracic aorta and nourish the bronchial tree as far as the respiratory bronchioles. These arteries are accompanied by their respective veins, which drain into the azygous or hemiazygous veins.

There are no lymphatics in most alveolar walls. These vessels begin in alveoli at the periphery of acini, which lie along lobular septa, bronchovascular bundles or the pleura. The lymphatics of the lobular septa and bronchovascular bundle accompany these structures, and the pleural lymphatics drain toward the hilus through the bronchovascular lymphatics.

DEFENSE MECHANISMS

The respiratory system has effective defense mechanisms to cope with the numerous particulates and infectious agents inhaled on inspiration.

The **nose and trachea** warm and humidify air entering the lung. The nose traps almost all particles over 10 μm in diameter and about half of all particles of 3 μm aerodynamic diameter (Fig. 18-2, see also Chapter 8). (Aerodynamic diameter refers to the way particles behave in air rather than to their actual size.)

The **mucociliary blanket** of the airway epithelium disposes of particles 2–10 μm in diameter. The ciliary beat drives the mucous blanket toward the trachea. Particles that land on it are thus removed from the lungs and swallowed or coughed up.

Alveolar macrophages protect the alveolar space. These cells are derived from the bone marrow, probably undergo a maturation division in the interstitium of the lung and then enter the alveolar space. They are particularly effective in dealing with particles with aerodynamic diameters under 2 μm. Very small particles are not phagocytosed and are exhaled.

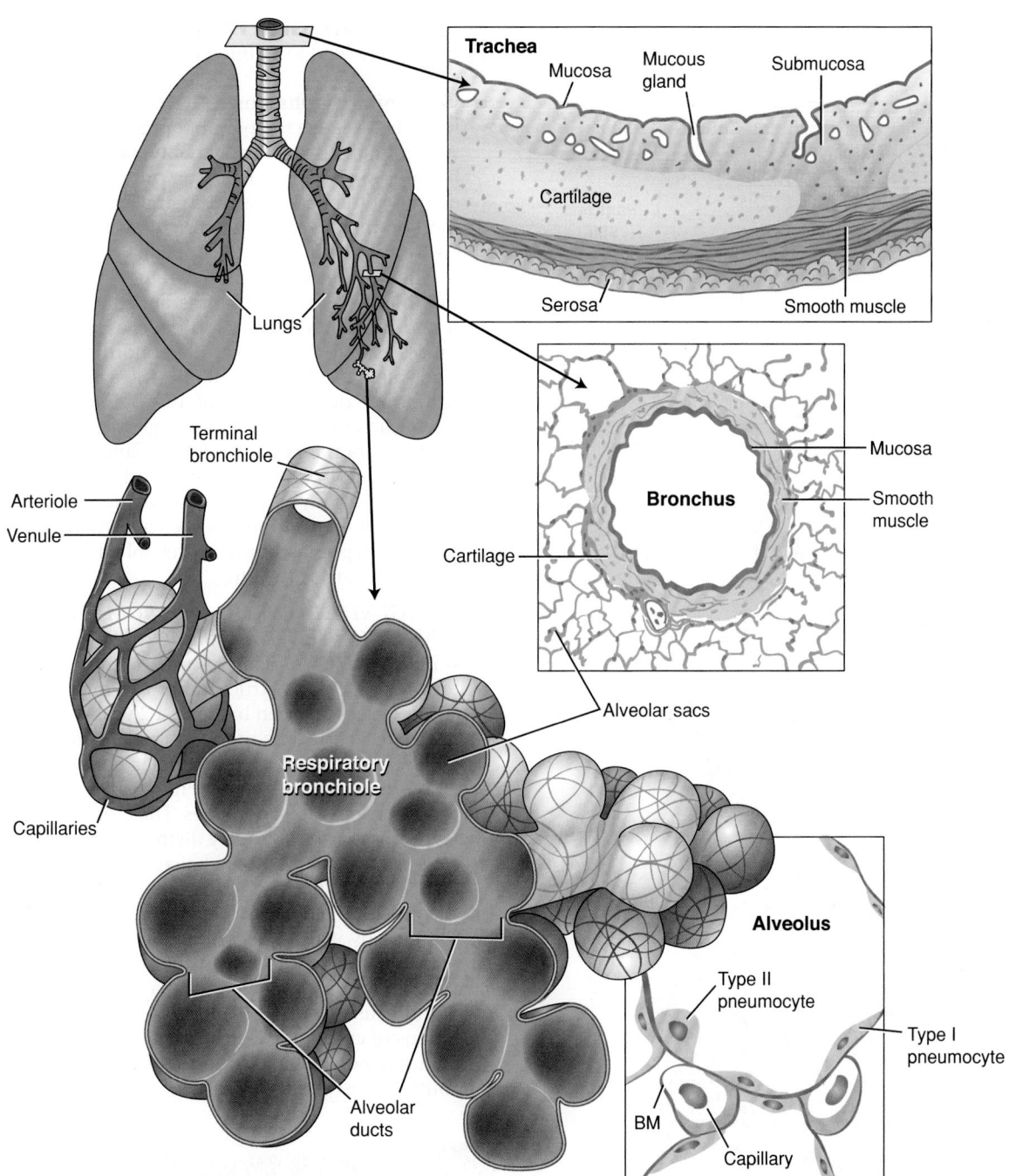

FIGURE 18-1. Anatomy of the lung. The conducting structures of the lung include (1) the trachea, which has horseshoe-shaped cartilages; (2) the bronchi, which have plates of cartilage in their walls (both the trachea and bronchi have mucus-secreting glands in their walls); and (3) the bronchioles, which do not have cartilage in their walls and terminate in the terminal bronchioles. The gas-exchanging components compose the unit distal to the terminal bronchiole, namely, the acinus. Alveoli are lined by type I cells, which are large, flat cells that cover most of the alveolar wall, and by type II cells, which secrete surfactant and are the progenitor cells of the alveolar epithelium. Gas exchange occurs at the level of the alveolar wall.

The Lungs

CONGENITAL ANOMALIES

BRONCHIAL ATRESIA: This abnormality most often involves the bronchus to the apical posterior segment of the left upper lobe. In infants, the lesion may result in an overexpanded part of the lung. In later life, the overexpanded lobe may also be emphysematous. Bronchial mucus accumulating distal to the atretic region may appear on radiologic examination as a mass.

PULMONARY HYPOPLASIA: This condition reflects incomplete or defective lung development. The lung is smaller than normal, with fewer and smaller acini. This is the most common congenital lesion of the lung, found in 10% of

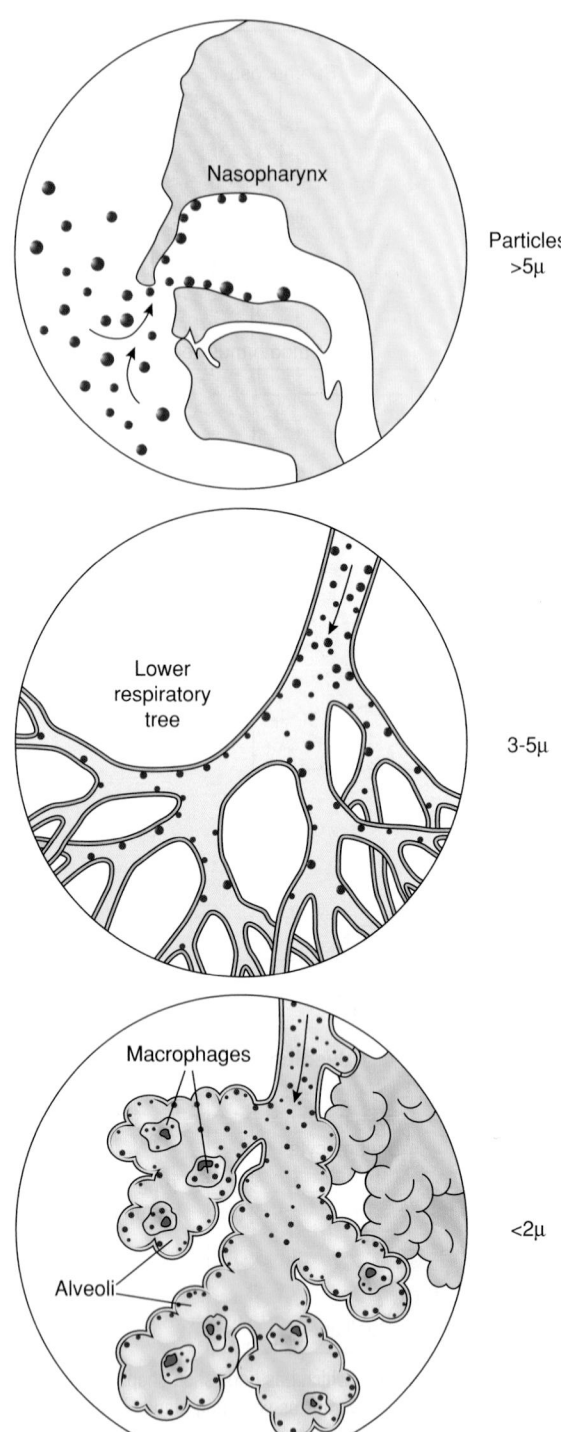

FIGURE 18-2. Deposition of particles in the respiratory tract. Large particles are trapped in the nose. Intermediate-sized particles deposit on the bronchi and bronchioles and are removed by the mucociliary blanket. Smaller particles terminate in the airspaces and are removed by macrophages. Very small particles behave as a gas and are breathed out.

neonatal autopsies. In most cases (90%), it occurs in association with other congenital anomalies, most of which involve the thorax. The lesion may be accompanied by hypoplasia of bronchi and pulmonary vessels if the insult occurs early in gestation, as in congenital diaphragmatic hernia. Pulmonary hypoplasia also is seen in trisomies 13, 18 and 21.

 **ETIOLOGIC FACTORS:** Three major factors may lead to pulmonary hypoplasia:

- **Congenital diaphragmatic hernia** typically occurs on the left side, because the pleuroperitoneal canal fails to close. Abdominal viscera are variably present in the affected hemithorax and result in compression of the lung. The degree of hypoplasia is thus variable. At one extreme, the lung on the affected side is reduced to a small nubbin of tissue and the lung on the opposite side is severely hypoplastic. At the other extreme, hypoplasia is so slight that the infant has no symptoms and the abnormalities are found incidentally on a routine chest radiograph. Other causes of hypoplasia include abnormalities of the chest wall, pleural effusions and ascites, as in hydrops fetalis. Abnormal development of the pulmonary vasculature often leads to persistent pulmonary hypertension.
- **Oligohydramnios** (low amniotic fluid volume) is usually due to genitourinary anomalies and is an important cause of pulmonary hypoplasia (see Chapter 6).
- **Decreased respiration** has been shown experimentally to produce hypoplastic lungs, probably due to lack of repetitive stretching of the lung.

CONGENITAL CYSTIC ADENOMATOID MALFORMATION (CONGENITAL PULMONARY ADENOMATOID MALFORMATION): This common anomaly consists of abnormal bronchiolar structures of varying sizes or distribution. Most cases are seen in the first 2 years of life. The lesion usually affects one lobe of the lung and consists of multiple cyst-like spaces lined by bronchiolar epithelium and separated by loose fibrous tissue (Fig. 18-3). Some patients will have other congenital anomalies. The most common presenting symptoms are respiratory distress and cyanosis. Surgical resection is the treatment of choice.

BRONCHOGENIC CYSTS: These are discrete, extrapulmonary, fluid-filled masses lined by respiratory epithelium and limited by walls that contain muscle and cartilage. They are most commonly found in the middle mediastinum. In newborns, a bronchogenic cyst may compress a major airway and cause respiratory distress. Later in life, secondary infections of cysts may lead to hemorrhage and perforation. Many bronchogenic cysts are asymptomatic and are found on routine chest radiographs.

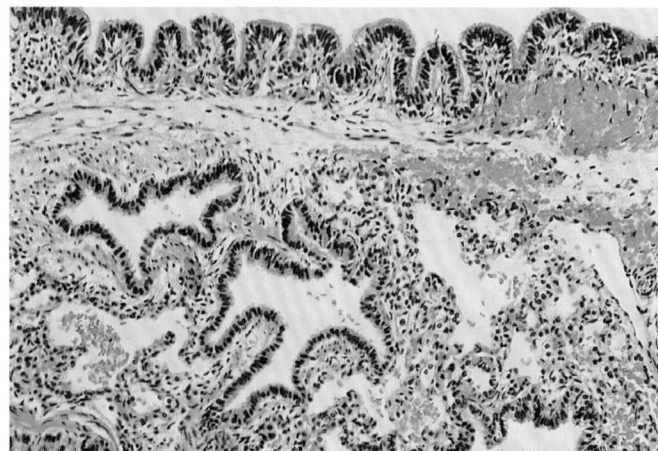

FIGURE 18-3. Congenital cystic adenomatoid malformation. Multiple gland-like spaces are lined by bronchiolar epithelium.

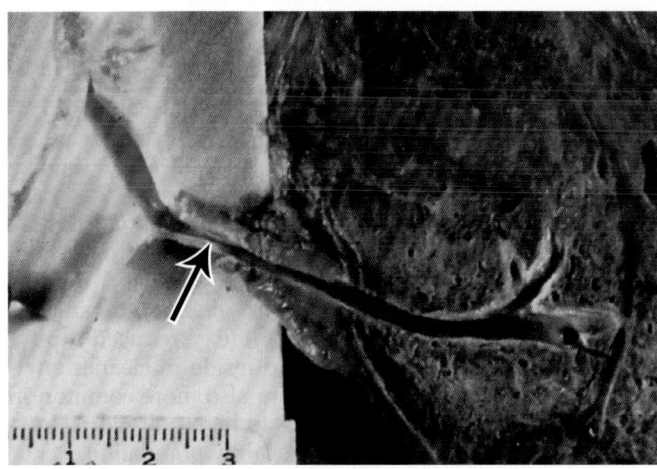

FIGURE 18-4. Extralobar sequestration. The sequestered pulmonary tissue is situated outside the lung parenchyma. It is supplied by an aberrant artery (*arrow*) from the aorta and is not connected to the bronchial tree.

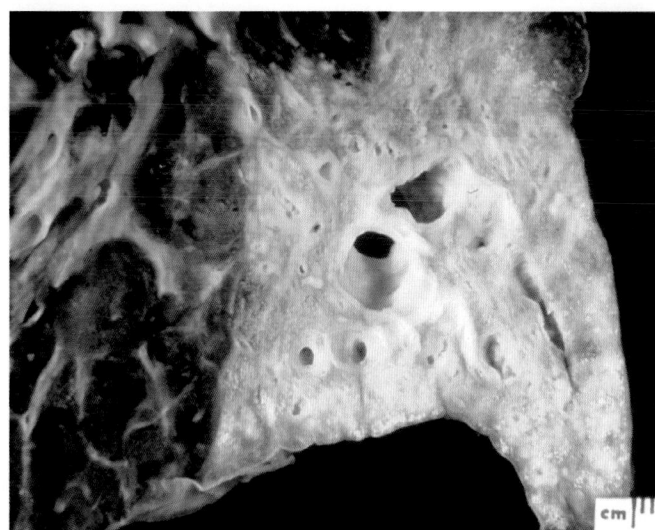

FIGURE 18-5. Intralobar sequestration. The sequestered tissue lies within the visceral pleura and exhibits cystic change and dense fibrosis. An aberrant arterial supply to this lesion was identified (not shown).

EXTRALOBAR SEQUESTRATION: Extralobar sequestration is a mass of lung tissue that is not connected to the bronchial tree and is located outside the visceral pleura. An abnormal artery, usually arising from the aorta, supplies the sequestered tissue (Fig. 18-4).

 **ETIOLOGIC FACTORS:** This lesion is thought to originate from an outpouching of the foregut, distinct from the pulmonary anlage, but later loses its connection to the original foregut. It occurs three to four times more often in males than in females and is associated with other anomalies in two thirds of patients.

 PATHOLOGY: Extralobar sequestrations are 1–15-cm pyramidal or round masses, covered by pleura. Microscopically, dilated bronchioles, alveolar ducts and alveoli are noted. Infection or infarction may alter the histologic appearance.

 CLINICAL FEATURES: In half of cases, extralobar sequestration is detected before 1 month of age, and is recognized by 2 years of age in 75% of patients. The condition is often associated with congenital cystic adenomatoid malformation. In the neonatal period, extralobar sequestration may cause dyspnea and cyanosis, often in the first day of life. In older children, recurrent bronchopulmonary infections may bring it to medical attention. Surgical excision is curative.

INTRALOBAR SEQUESTRATION: Intralobar sequestrations are masses of lung tissue in the visceral pleura, isolated from the tracheobronchial tree and supplied by a systemic artery (Fig. 18-5). These are felt to be acquired abnormalities.

 PATHOLOGY: Intralobar sequestrations are almost always found in a lower lobe. Bilateral involvement is distinctly unusual. On gross examination, the sequestered tissue shows the result of chronic recurrent pneumonia, with end-stage fibrosis and honeycomb cystic changes. These cysts range up to 5 cm in diameter and lie in a dense fibrous stroma. Microscopically, the cystic spaces are mostly lined by cuboidal or columnar epithelium and the lumen contains foamy macrophages and eosinophilic material. Interstitial chronic inflammation and follicular lymphoid hyperplasia are often prominent. Acute and organizing pneumonia may be seen.

 CLINICAL FEATURES: Cough, sputum production and recurrent pneumonia are seen in almost all patients. Most cases are discovered in adolescents or young adults. Only one fourth of patients are in the first decade of life, and the lesion is rarely identified in infants. Surgical resection is often indicated.

DISEASES OF THE BRONCHI AND BRONCHIOLES

Most bronchial and bronchiolar diseases are acute conditions and their sequelae. Chronic bronchitis is discussed later.

Airway Infections Are Caused by Diverse Organisms

Here, we distinguish between airway and parenchyma infections for convenience and for reasons of classification, but this division should not be thought of as rigid. Causative agents are discussed in Chapter 9.

Many infectious agents that involve the intrapulmonary airways tend to affect the more peripheral airways (**bronchiolitis**), for example, adenovirus, respiratory syncytial virus (RSV) and measles. All are more serious in malnourished children and in populations not ordinarily exposed to these agents. Severe symptomatic infections occur more often in infants and children, and recovery is the rule. Symptoms include cough, a feeling of tightness in the chest and, in extreme cases, shortness of breath and even cyanosis.

INFLUENZA: This is a characteristic example of tracheobronchitis, and in the occasional patient who dies with this infection, the appearance of the bronchi is dramatic. The surface of the airway is fiery red, reflecting acute inflammation and congestion of the mucosa.

ADENOVIRUS: Infection with adenovirus causes the most serious sequelae, with extensive bronchiolitis (Fig. 18-6) and then healing by fibrosis. Bronchioles may become

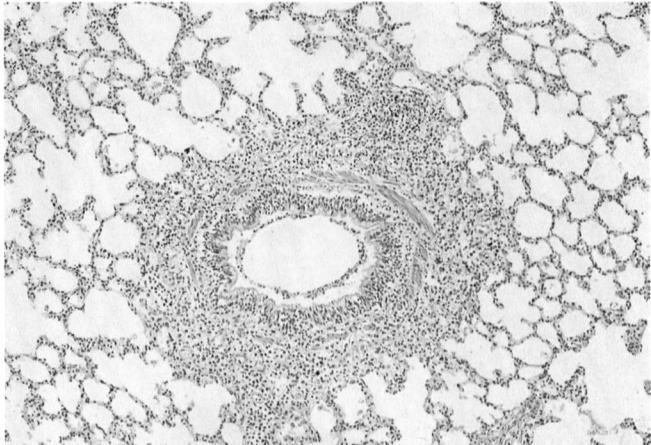

FIGURE 18-6. Bronchiolitis due to adenovirus. The wall of this bronchiole shows an intense chronic inflammatory infiltrate with local extension into the surrounding peribronchial tissue.

obliterated or occluded by loose fibrous tissue **(obliterative bronchiolitis).**

RESPIRATORY SYNCYTIAL VIRUS (RSV): RSV infection often occurs in epidemics in nurseries. It is usually self-limited, but rare fatal cases do occur. It can cause nosocomial infection in children and (rarely) in adults. Histologically, peribronchiolar inflammation and disorganization of the epithelium are evident. Severe overdistention may be found without obvious bronchiolar obstruction, possibly due to displacement of surfactant from the bronchiolar surface.

MEASLES: At one time a major cause of bronchiolitis, measles is rarely a problem in developed countries since the advent of the measles vaccine. However, measles-induced bronchiolitis remains a serious problem particularly in populations seldom exposed to the virus. Similar to adenovirus, it may cause bronchiolar obliteration and bronchiectasis.

BORDETELLA PERTUSSIS: This bacterium commonly infects the airways and is the cause of whooping cough. With widespread use of a pertussis vaccine, the disease became rare in the United States. Unfortunately, vaccination is no longer compulsory in England, and the incidence of pertussis is rising. Clinically, whooping cough is typified by fever and severe prolonged bouts of coughing, followed by a characteristic deep whooping inspiration. Severe bronchial and bronchiolar inflammation are found in fatal cases. Before immunization was available, whooping cough commonly led to the development of bronchiectasis.

HAEMOPHILUS INFLUENZAE AND STREPTOCOCCUS PNEUMONIAE: In addition to causing pneumonia, these organisms have been implicated in exacerbations of chronic bronchitis. Such episodes contribute to the morbidity of chronic bronchitis and are treated with antibiotics.

CANDIDA ALBICANS: This fungus is a normal commensal organism in the oral cavity, gut and vagina and is best known for infections in those regions. It may also affect the lungs, usually as a noninvasive growth on airway surface epithelium, where it may produce mucosal ulceration. Predisposing factors for invasive growth include trauma, burns, gastrointestinal surgery, indwelling catheters and neutropenia, such as may be associated with cytotoxic chemotherapy for acute leukemia.

Irritants Derive from Air Pollution and Industrial Accidents

The most important irritant gases in the atmosphere are oxidants (ozone, nitrogen oxides) and sulfur dioxide (SO_2). Oxidants derive from the action of sunlight on automobile exhaust and are important in major urban areas (see Chapter 8). SO_2 is produced mainly by burning fossil fuels. These gases, plus particulate carbon carrying toxins from diesel exhaust, may also compound adverse effects of tobacco smoke. Indeed, inhabitants of urban and more polluted areas have worse pulmonary function (e.g., reduced expiratory flow rates) than do those who reside in cleaner environments. Respiratory infections are also more common in young children who live in regions of high pollution. However, these effects are small in the healthy population.

In people with chronic pulmonary disease, the situation is different: experimentally, ozone makes airways more reactive, an effect related to airway inflammation. *Thus, air pollution may exacerbate symptoms in asthmatic people and in those with established respiratory disease. In high concentrations, irritant gases produce serious morphologic and functional effects.*

NO_2: NO_2 is often encountered in industrial settings, including welding, electroplating, metal cleaning and blasting. It is also produced by decaying grain stored in silos. As NO_2 is heavier than air, it accumulates immediately above the surface of the grain. A worker entering the silo inhales it in high concentrations, resulting in lung injury known as **silo-filler disease.** Respiratory symptoms in such cases may be delayed for up to 30 hours, after which cough and dyspnea develop. Most patients recover, but some develop progressive bronchiolitis obliterans and may die of respiratory failure.

SO_2: This highly soluble gas, when inhaled chronically by experimental animals, produces lesions in the more central airways that resemble chronic bronchitis and that may progress to squamous metaplasia. In humans, exposure to very high concentrations of SO_2 has been associated with severe inflammation and bronchiolitis.

CHLORINE AND AMMONIA: These gases may be released in high concentrations in industrial accidents. If inhaled, they produce extensive bronchial and bronchiolar mucosal injury. Secondary inflammation may cause bronchiectasis, owing partly to bronchiolar obliteration and partly to direct bronchial damage.

Bronchocentric Granulomatosis Is Usually a Response to Infection

Bronchocentric granulomatosis is a nonspecific granulomatous inflammation centered on bronchi or bronchioles (Fig. 18-7). *This histologic pattern can be seen in a number of clinical settings and is not a distinct clinical entity.*

Asthmatic patients, for the most part, have allergic bronchopulmonary aspergillosis (see below). In addition to having bronchocentric granulomatosis, they have bronchial mucous plugs, bronchiectasis and bronchiolectasis and eosinophilic pneumonia. Irregular, fragmented *Aspergillus* hyphae may be seen in the mucous plugs. A nonspecific secondary vasculitis is centered on airways rather than vessels.

Nonasthmatic patients with bronchocentric granulomatosis are likely to have an infection, especially tuberculosis or fungi such as *Histoplasma capsulatum.* The disorder can also

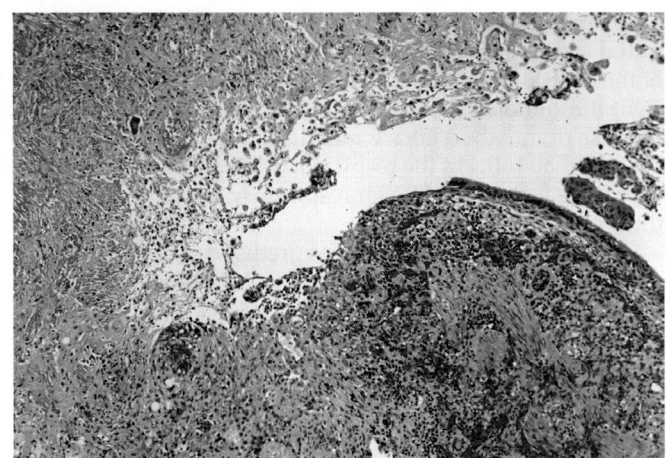

FIGURE 18-7. Bronchocentric granulomatosis. This bronchiole shows ulceration and necrosis of the mucosa and submucosa with granulomatous inflammation. The patient had granulomatosis polyangiitis (formerly Wegener granulomatosis) with lung involvement in the pattern of bronchocentric granulomatosis.

be a manifestation of immune problems, such as rheumatoid arthritis, ankylosing spondylitis and granulomatosis with polyangiitis (formerly Wegener granulomatosis). Patients with bronchocentric granulomatosis of either allergic or nonallergic type generally respond well to corticosteroid therapy.

Constrictive Bronchiolitis May Obliterate an Airway

In constrictive bronchiolitis, an initial inflammatory bronchiolitis is followed by bronchiolar scarring and fibrosis, with progressive narrowing and, eventually, complete destruction of the airway lumen (Fig. 18-8). **Obliterative bronchiolitis** is a synonym.

 PATHOLOGY: Bronchioles show chronic mural inflammation and varying amounts of fibrosis between the epithelium and smooth muscle, with resultant narrowing of the lumen. These lesions are often

focal and may be difficult to identify. Elastic stains may help in recognizing the scarred bronchioles. Bronchiolectasis and mucous plugs may be seen in adjacent airways. The surrounding lung is usually normal.

 CLINICAL FEATURES: Patients may have dyspnea and wheezing due to severe obstructive pulmonary function. Chest radiographs and computed tomography (CT) scans may be normal or show overinflation caused by air trapping distal to the obliterated bronchioles. This pattern of fibrosis is seen in several situations, including (1) bone marrow transplantation (graft-versus-host disease), (2) lung transplantation (chronic rejection), (3) collagen vascular diseases (especially rheumatoid arthritis), (4) postinfectious disorders (especially viral infections), (5) after inhalation of toxins (SO_2, ammonia, phosgene) and (6) ingestion of certain drugs (penicillamine). It may also be idiopathic. Most patients have a relentless progressive clinical course. Although many patients are treated with steroids, no therapy is effective for this disease.

Bronchial Obstruction Leads to Atelectasis

Bronchial obstruction in adults occurs mostly because of endobronchial extension of primary lung tumors, although mucous plugs, aspirated gastric contents or foreign bodies may also be responsible, especially in children. If obstruction is partial, trapped air may cause overdistention of the distal affected segment; complete obstruction results in atelectasis. Areas distal to the obstruction may also develop pneumonia, abscesses and bronchiectasis (see below).

Atelectasis is the collapse of expanded lung tissue (Fig. 18-9). If the air supply is obstructed, gas transfers from the alveoli to the blood, causing the affected region to collapse. Atelectasis occurs as an important postoperative complication of abdominal surgery, because of mucous

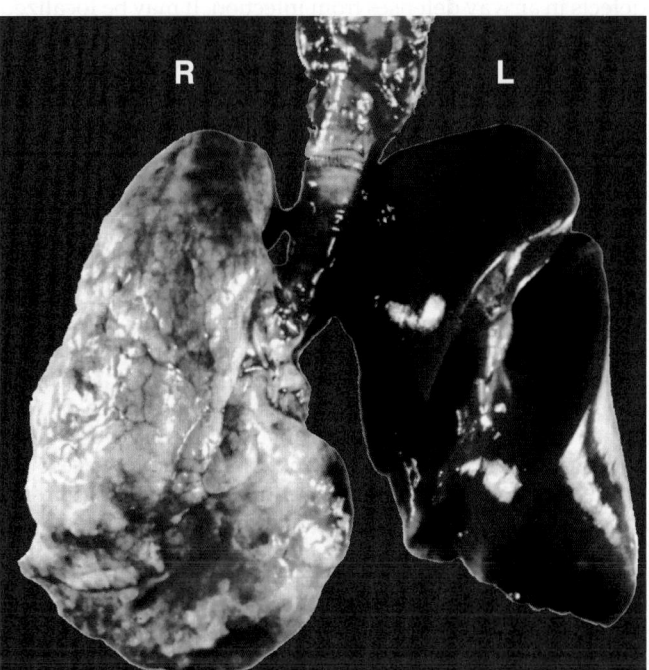

FIGURE 18-9. Atelectasis. The right lung (R) of an infant is pale and expanded by air; the left lung (L) is collapsed.

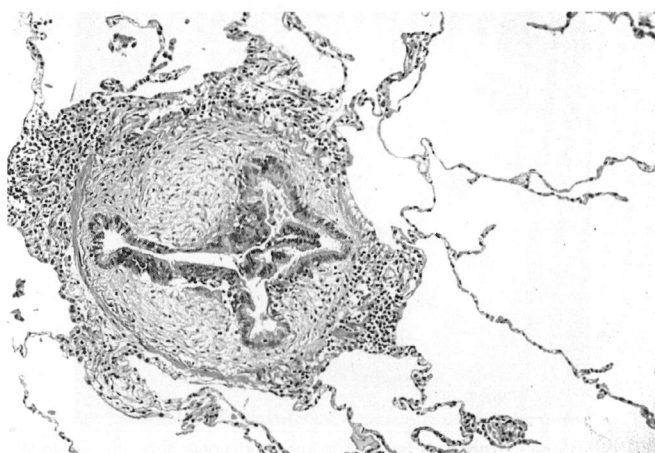

FIGURE 18-8. Constrictive bronchiolitis. The lumen of a bronchiole is markedly narrowed, owing to marked submucosal fibrosis.

obstruction of a bronchus and/or diminished respiratory movement resulting from postoperative pain. It is often asymptomatic, but when severe, it results in hypoxemia and a shift of the mediastinum *toward* the affected side.

Atelectasis is usually caused by bronchial obstruction but may also result from direct compression of the lung (e.g., hydrothorax or pneumothorax). If the compression is severe enough, the function of the affected lung may be jeopardized and the mediastinum may shift *away* from the affected side.

In long-standing atelectasis, the area of collapsed lung becomes fibrotic and bronchi dilate, in part owing to infection distal to the obstruction. Permanent bronchial dilation (bronchiectasis) results.

Right middle lobe syndrome refers to atelectasis due to obstruction of the bronchus to the right middle lobe, usually from external compression by hilar lymph nodes. This bronchus is particularly susceptible to external compression because it is long and slender and surrounded by lymph nodes. Histologically, the lung shows bronchiectasis, chronic bronchitis and bronchiolitis, lymphoid hyperplasia, abscess formation and dense fibrosis. Acute and organizing pneumonia may both be present. Tuberculous lymphadenitis or metastatic lung cancer may cause the lymph node enlargement, but the cause of the obstruction is often undetermined.

Bronchiectasis Is Irreversible Bronchial Dilation Caused by Destruction of Bronchial Wall Muscle and Elastic Elements

 ETIOLOGIC FACTORS: Bronchiectasis may be obstructive or nonobstructive.

Obstructive bronchiectasis is localized and occurs distal to a mechanical obstruction of a central bronchus by, for example, tumors, inhaled foreign bodies, mucous plugs in asthma or lymph node enlargement. **Nonobstructive bronchiectasis** usually follows respiratory infections or defects in airway defenses from infection. It may be localized or generalized.

Localized nonobstructive bronchiectasis was once common, usually after childhood bronchopulmonary infections with measles, pertussis or other bacteria. Vaccines and antibiotics have reduced the incidence of bronchiectasis, but most cases still follow bronchopulmonary infection, usually with adenovirus or RSV. Childhood respiratory infections still cause bronchiectasis in less developed parts of the world.

Generalized bronchiectasis is, for the most part, secondary to inherited impairment in host defense mechanisms or acquired conditions that permit introduction of infectious organisms into the airways. Acquired disorders that predispose to bronchiectasis include (1) neurologic diseases that impair consciousness, swallowing, respiratory excursions and the cough reflex; (2) incompetence of the lower esophageal sphincter; (3) nasogastric intubation; and (4) chronic bronchitis. The main **inherited conditions** associated with generalized bronchiectasis are cystic fibrosis, dyskinetic ciliary syndromes, hypogammaglobulinemias and deficiencies of specific immunoglobulin (Ig) G subclasses.

Kartagener syndrome is one of the immotile cilia syndromes (ciliary dyskinesia) and consists of the triad of dextrocardia (with or without situs inversus), bronchiectasis and sinusitis. It is caused by defects in the outer or inner dynein arms of cilia, which generate or regulate cilia beats,

respectively. Other dyskinetic ciliary syndromes include **radial spoke deficiency** ("Sturgess syndrome") and absence of the central doublet of cilia. In these diseases, cilia are deficient throughout the body. Both men and women are sterile, because of impaired ciliary mobility in the vas deferens and the fallopian tube. In the respiratory tract, ciliary defects lead to repeated upper and lower respiratory tract infections and, thus, to bronchiectasis.

Immunodeficiencies may also predispose to repeated pulmonary infection and bronchiectasis. In hypogammaglobulinemias, lack of IgAs or IgGs that protect against viruses or bacteria can lead to recurrent lung infections. Acquired and inherited defects of neutrophils also increase the risk of respiratory infections and bronchiectasis.

PATHOLOGY: Bronchial dilation is saccular, varicose or cylindrical.

- **Saccular bronchiectasis** affects the proximal third to fourth bronchial branches (Fig. 18-10). These bronchi are severely dilated and end blindly in dilated sacs, associated with collapse and fibrosis of the distal lung parenchyma.
- **Cylindrical bronchiectasis** involves the sixth to eighth bronchial branchings, which show uniform, moderate dilation. It is a milder disease than saccular bronchiectasis and leads to fewer clinical symptoms.
- **Varicose bronchiectasis** results in bronchi that resemble varicose veins on bronchographic examination, with irregular dilations and constrictions. Two to eight branchings of bronchi are recognized grossly. Bronchiolar obliteration is not as severe, and parenchymal abnormalities are variable.

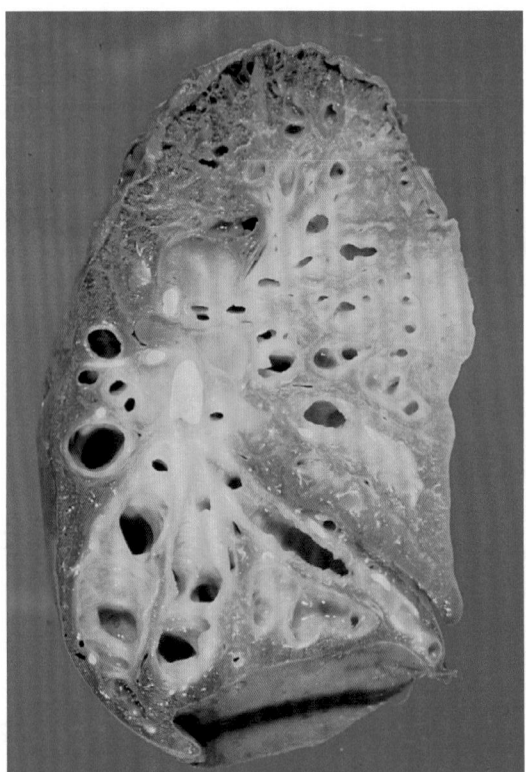

FIGURE 18-10. Bronchiectasis. The resected upper lobe shows widely dilated bronchi, with thickening of the bronchial walls and collapse and fibrosis of the pulmonary parenchyma.

Generalized bronchiectasis is usually bilateral and is most common in the lower lobes, the left more than the right. Localized bronchiectasis may occur wherever there was obstruction or infection. Bronchi are dilated, with thick, white or yellow walls. Bronchial lumens often contain dense, mucopurulent secretions. Severe inflammation of bronchi and bronchioles results in destruction of all components of the bronchial wall. Collapse of distal lung parenchyma causes damaged bronchi to dilate. Inflammation of central airways leads to mucus hypersecretion and abnormalities of the surface epithelium, including squamous metaplasia and increased goblet cells. Lymphoid follicles are often seen in bronchial walls, and distal bronchi and bronchioles are scarred and often obliterated. Bronchial arteries enlarge to supply the inflamed bronchial wall and fibrous tissue. A vicious circle may be established in which pools of mucus become infected, which further promotes destruction of the bronchial walls.

 CLINICAL FEATURES: Patients with bronchiectasis have chronic cough, often producing several hundred milliliters of mucopurulent sputum a day. Hemoptysis is common, as bronchial inflammation erodes the walls of adjacent bronchial arteries. Dyspnea and wheezing are variable, depending on the extent of the disease. Pneumonia is common, and patients with longstanding cases are at risk of chronic hypoxia and pulmonary hypertension. Radiologically, the bronchi appear dilated and have thickened walls. Definitive diagnosis is made by CT scan of the lung. Surgical resection of localized bronchiectasis may be necessary, especially if complications such as severe hemoptysis or pneumonia arise. However, in the generalized disease, surgical resection is more palliative than curative.

Acute, reversible bronchial dilation may follow bacterial or viral respiratory infections; it may take months before the bronchi return to normal size.

INFECTIONS

Pulmonary infections are discussed in detail in Chapter 9. The major pulmonary entities are described below, with particular emphasis on pathologic features.

Bacterial Pneumonia Is Inflammation and Consolidation of Lung Parenchyma

Bacterial pneumonia was once divided into lobar pneumonia or bronchopneumonia, but these terms have little clinical relevance today. In **lobar pneumonia,** an entire lobe is consolidated (Fig. 18-11), whereas **bronchopneumonia** refers to scattered solid foci in the same or several lobes (Fig. 18-12).

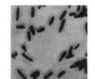 **ETIOLOGIC FACTORS:** *Streptococcus pneumoniae* (pneumococcus) was the classic cause of lobar pneumonia, but with antibiotic therapy, involvement of a lobe tends to be incomplete, and more than one lobe is usually affected. By contrast, bronchopneumonia is still a common cause of death. It typically develops in terminally ill patients, usually in dependent and posterior portions of the lung. Scattered irregular foci of pneumonia are centered on terminal bronchioles and respiratory bronchioles. Bronchiolitis is seen, with polymorphonuclear exudates

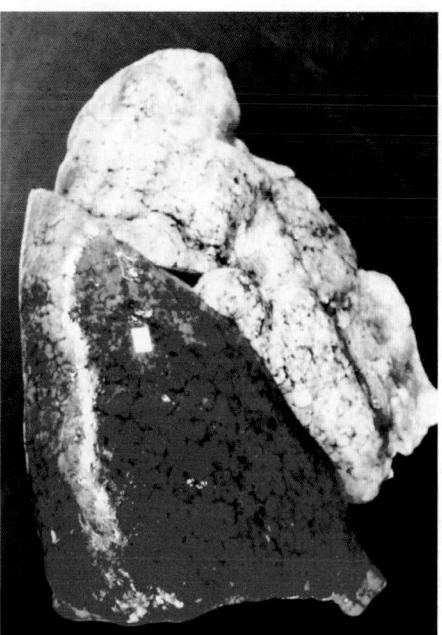

FIGURE 18-11. Lobar pneumonia. The entire left lower lobe is consolidated and in the stage of red hepatization. The upper lobe is normally expanded.

in adjacent alveoli. Large contiguous areas of alveolar involvement do not occur in bronchopneumonia.

Bacterial pneumonias occur in three settings:

■ **Community-acquired pneumonia** arises outside the hospital in people with no primary disorder of the immune system. The term is also used loosely to denote lobar pneumonia.

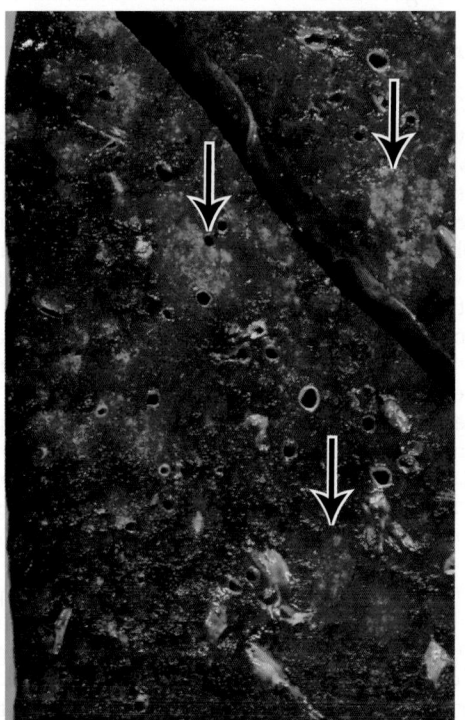

FIGURE 18-12. Bronchopneumonia. Scattered foci of consolidation (*arrows*) are centered on bronchi and bronchioles.

- **Nosocomial pneumonia** is infection that develops in hospital environments and tends to affect compromised patients.
- **Opportunistic pneumonia** afflicts people whose immune status is defective.

Bacterial pneumonias are best classified by etiologic agent, as clinical and morphologic features, and thus therapies, often vary with the causative organism.

Most bacteria that cause pneumonia are normal inhabitants of the oropharynx and nasopharynx that reach alveoli by aspiration of secretions. Other routes of infection include inhalation from the environment, hematogenous dissemination from an infectious focus elsewhere and (rarely) spread of bacteria from an adjacent site. Emergence of a virulent organism in the oropharyngeal flora often precedes the development of pneumonia. Predisposing conditions usually entail depressed host defenses related to cigarette smoking, chronic bronchitis, alcoholism, severe malnutrition, wasting diseases and poorly controlled diabetes. Debilitated or immunosuppressed patients in the hospital often have altered oropharyngeal flora, and as many as 25% may develop nosocomial pneumonia.

Pneumococcal Pneumonia

Antibiotic therapy notwithstanding, *S. pneumoniae* (pneumococcus) pneumonia remains a significant problem. It is mainly a disease of young to middle-aged adults. It is rare in infants, less common in the elderly and much more frequent in men than women.

 **ETIOLOGIC FACTORS:** Pneumococcal pneumonia is mostly a result of altered respiratory tract defenses. For example, a viral upper respiratory infection (e.g., influenza) stimulates bronchial secretions. These provide a hospitable environment for *S. pneumoniae*, which are normal flora of the nasopharynx, to proliferate. The thin, watery secretions carry the organisms into the alveoli, thus initiating an inflammatory response. The remarkably severe acute inflammation with spreading edema suggests that immunologic mechanisms may be involved. Aspiration of pneumococci may also follow impaired epiglottic reflexes, as occurs with exposure to cold, anesthesia and alcohol intoxication. Lung injury caused, for example, by congestive heart failure or irritant gases also increases susceptibility to pneumococcal pneumonia.

The pneumococcal capsule protects the bacteria against phagocytosis by alveolar macrophages. The organisms must therefore be opsonized before they can be ingested and killed. In an immune-competent person, antipneumococcal antibodies act as opsonins, but a host not previously exposed to the specific infecting strain of *S. pneumoniae* must use the alternative complement pathway to opsonize the bacteria.

 PATHOLOGY: In the earliest stage of pneumococcal pneumonia, protein-rich edema fluid with abundant organisms fills the alveoli (Fig. 18-13). Marked capillary congestion leads to massive outpouring of polymorphonuclear leukocytes and intra-alveolar hemorrhage (Fig. 18-14). Because the color and firm consistency of the affected lung are reminiscent of the liver, this stage has been aptly named **"red hepatization"** (Fig. 18-13).

The next phase, 2 or more days later (depending on the success of treatment), involves lysis of neutrophils and appearance of macrophages, which phagocytose the fragmented leukocytes and other inflammatory debris. At this stage, the congestion has diminished, but the lung is still firm **("gray hepatization")** (Fig. 18-13). The alveolar exudate is then removed and the lung gradually returns to normal.

A number of complications may follow pneumococcal pneumonia:

- **Pleuritis (inflammation of the pleura),** often painful, is common, because the pneumonia readily extends to the pleura.
- **Pleural effusion** (fluid in the pleural space) is common but usually resolves.
- Empyema/**pyothorax (pus in the pleural space)** results from infection of a pleural effusion and may heal with extensive fibrosis.
- **Bacteremia** occurs during the early stages of pneumococcal pneumonia in more than 25% of patients and may lead to endocarditis or meningitis. Patients whose spleens have been removed often die of this bacteremia.
- **Pulmonary fibrosis** is a rare complication of pneumococcal pneumonia. The intra-alveolar exudate organizes to form intra-alveolar plugs of granulation tissue, known as **organizing pneumonia**. Gradually, increasing alveolar fibrosis leads to a shrunken and firm lobe, a rare complication known as **carnification**.
- **Lung abscess (localized collection of pus)** is an unusual complication of pneumococcal pneumonia.

 CLINICAL FEATURES: Pneumococcal pneumonia begins abruptly, with fever and chills. Chest pain due to pleural involvement is common. Sputum is characteristically "rusty," because it is derived from altered blood in alveolar spaces. Radiologic studies show alveolar filling in large areas of lung, producing a solid appearance that extends to entire lobes or segments. Before antibiotic therapy, severe fever, dyspnea, debility and even loss of consciousness were common. Such symptoms were followed by **"crisis"** after 5–10 days, when a moribund patient would suddenly become afebrile and return from death's door. Satisfactory resolution of a crisis reflected effective immune responses to the infection. Nevertheless, about 1/3 of patients died. Current treatment for pneumococcal pneumonia is effective, and although symptoms resolve rapidly, radiographic lesions still take several days to clear.

Klebsiella Pneumonia

Other than *S. pneumoniae*, *Klebsiella pneumoniae* is the only organism that causes lobar pneumonia with any frequency. However, *K. pneumoniae* accounts for only about 1% of community-acquired pneumonias. *Klebsiella* pneumonia occurs mostly in middle-aged, often alcoholic, men. Diabetes and chronic lung disease also increase the risk.

 PATHOLOGY: The pathologic stages of *Klebsiella* pneumonia are not as distinctly defined as those in pneumococcal pneumonia, but acute phase congestion and hemorrhage are less pronounced. *K. pneumoniae* has a thick, gelatinous capsule, giving the cut lung surface a characteristic mucoid appearance. Another distinctive feature of *Klebsiella* pneumonia is increased size of the affected

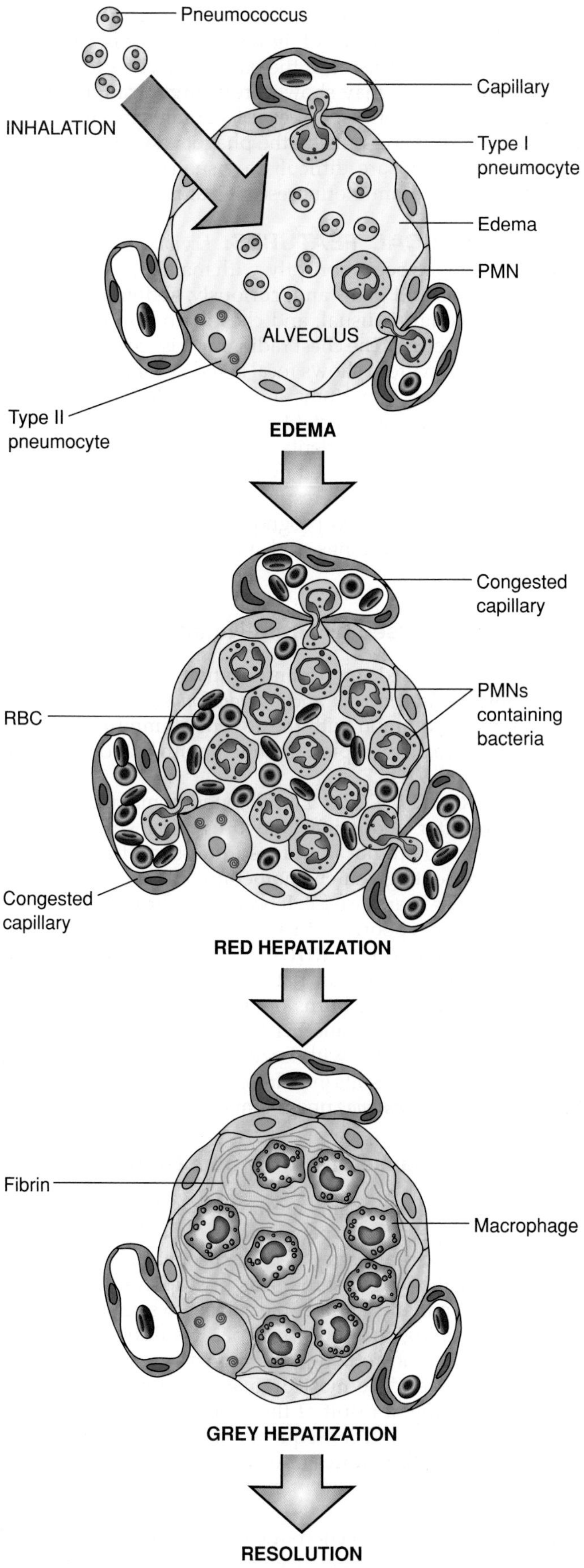

Pneumococcus

Capillary

Type I pneumocyte

INHALATION

Edema

PMN

ALVEOLUS

Type II pneumocyte

EDEMA

Congested capillary

PMNs containing bacteria

RBC

Congested capillary

RED HEPATIZATION

Fibrin

Macrophage

GREY HEPATIZATION

RESOLUTION

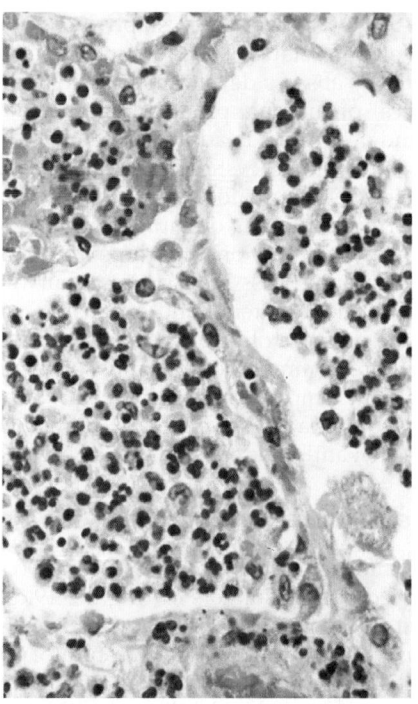

FIGURE 18-14. Pneumococcal pneumonia. Alveoli are packed with an exudate composed of polymorphonuclear leukocytes and occasional macrophages.

lobe, causing the fissure to "bulge" toward the unaffected region. There is a tendency toward tissue necrosis and abscess formation. A serious complication is **bronchopleural fistula** (i.e., a communication between the bronchial airway and the pleural space).

The onset of *Klebsiella* pneumonia is less dramatic than that of pneumococcal pneumonia, but the disease may be more dangerous. Before antibiotics, mortality from *Klebsiella* pneumonia was 50%–80%. Even with prompt antibiotic treatment, mortality remains considerable.

Staphylococcal Pneumonia

Staphylococci account for only 1% of community-acquired bacterial pneumonias. However, *S. aureus* is a common pulmonary superinfection after influenza and other viral respiratory tract infections. Repeated episodes of staphylococcal pneumonia are seen in patients with cystic fibrosis, owing to colonization of bronchiectatic airways. Nosocomial staphylococcal pneumonia typically occurs in chronically ill people who are prone to aspiration and in intubated patients.

FIGURE 18-13. Pathogenesis of pneumococcal lobar pneumonia. Pneumococci, characteristically in pairs (diplococci), multiply rapidly in alveolar spaces and produce extensive edema. They incite an acute inflammatory response in which polymorphonuclear leukocytes and congestion are prominent (red hepatization). As the inflammatory process progresses, macrophages replace the polymorphonuclear leukocytes and ingest debris (gray hepatization). The process usually resolves, but complications may ensue. *PMN* = polymorphonuclear neutrophil; *RBC* = red blood cell.

PATHOLOGY: Like staphylococcal infections elsewhere, staphylococcal pneumonia is characterized by abscess development. The multiple foci of staphylococcal pneumonia produce many small abscesses. In infants and, less often, in adults, these may lead to **pneumatoceles,** thin-walled cystic spaces lined primarily by respiratory tissue. Pneumatoceles may enlarge rapidly and compress surrounding lung or rupture into the pleural cavity and cause a tension pneumothorax. A pneumatocele develops when an abscess breaks into an airway, allowing drainage of purulent material and expansion of the former abscess by the pressure of inspired air. Cavitation and pleural effusions are common complications of staphylococcal pneumonia, but empyema is infrequent. Staphylococcal pneumonia requires aggressive therapy, particularly because *S. aureus* is often antibiotic resistant.

Other Streptococcal Pneumonias

Pulmonary infections with group A *Streptococcus pyogenes* were identified among soldiers during the 19th century. Its features were described during World War I. Streptococcal pneumonia typically follows viral respiratory tract infections. It is distinctly unusual in a community setting but is occasionally encountered in debilitated patients.

 PATHOLOGY: On gross examination, the lungs of patients who die of streptococcal pneumonia are heavy, with bloody edema. Dry consolidation (hepatization) is not a feature of this disease. Microscopically, alveoli are filled with fibrin-containing fluid, but neutrophils are few. Alveolar necrosis may follow prolonged pneumonia. Empyema is a common complication.

 CLINICAL FEATURES: Patients with streptococcal pneumonia have abrupt fever, dyspnea, cough, chest pain, hemoptysis and often cyanosis. Radiographically, a bronchopneumonia pattern is observed; lobar consolidation is not seen. Intensive antibiotic therapy is indicated.

Streptococcal pneumonia in the newborn is usually caused by group B streptococci (*Streptococcus agalactiae*), a normal resident of the female genital tract. Symptoms are similar to those of the infantile respiratory distress syndrome. The infants, however, are often full term, have severe toxemia and may die within a few hours.

Legionella Pneumonia

In 1976, a mysterious respiratory disease with high mortality broke out at an American Legion convention in Philadelphia. The responsible organism, *Legionella pneumophila*, is a fastidious bacterium that is difficult to grow in culture. Serologic and histologic studies showed that several previously unrecognized epidemics of the same disease had occurred. *Legionella* organisms thrive in aquatic environments, and outbreaks of pneumonia have been traced to contaminated water in air-conditioning cooling towers, evaporative condensers and construction sites. Person-to-person spread does not occur, and there is no animal or human reservoir.

 PATHOLOGY: In fatal *Legionella* pneumonia, multiple lobes show bronchopneumonia, with large confluent areas. Alveoli contain fibrin and inflammatory cells, with either neutrophils or macrophages predominating. Necrosis of inflammatory cells (leukocytoclasis) may be extensive. If the patient survives for several weeks, the exudate may show fibrous organization. Empyema occurs in 1/3 of cases. *Legionella* organisms are usually abundant within and outside the phagocytic cells. They are gram-negative but are difficult to visualize without silver impregnation or immunofluorescent stains.

 CLINICAL FEATURES: *Legionella* pneumonia tends to begin abruptly, with malaise, fever, muscle aches and pains and, curiously, abdominal pain. A productive cough is usual, and chest pain due to pleuritis occasionally occurs. The chest radiograph is variable, but the most common pattern shows focal alveolar infiltrates, which may be bilateral. Symptoms are usually less severe than radiographs suggest. Mortality is 10%–20%, especially in immunocompromised patients.

Pontiac fever, also caused by *Legionella* species, is mainly a febrile illness with slight respiratory symptoms, radiologic abnormalities and a good prognosis. It has occurred in epidemics in office buildings and affects apparently healthy individuals.

Pneumonia Caused by Gram-Negative Bacteria

Pneumonias caused by gram-negative organisms, most commonly *Escherichia coli* and *Pseudomonas aeruginosa,* have become more common with the advent of immunosuppressive and cytotoxic therapies, treatment with broad-spectrum antibiotics and AIDS.

ESCHERICHIA COLI: E. coli pneumonia may follow bacteremia after abdominal and urogenital surgery, even in patients who are not immunosuppressed. It also is seen in cancer patients given chemotherapy and in people with chronic lung or heart disease. It occurs as a bronchopneumonia and responds poorly to treatment.

PSEUDOMONAS AERUGINOSA: Pseudomonas pneumonia is most common in patients who are immunocompromised or who have burns or cystic fibrosis. A history of antibiotic treatment for another infection is common. Often an infectious vasculitis, with large numbers of organisms in blood vessel walls, results in pulmonary infarction. Antibiotic treatment of *Pseudomonas* pneumonia is often unsatisfactory.

Pneumonias Caused by Anaerobic Organisms

Many anaerobic organisms are normal commensals of the oral cavity, especially in people with poor dental hygiene. These include certain streptococci, fusobacteria and *Bacteroides* sp. Swallowing disorders, as in stuporous alcoholics, anesthetized patients and people subject to seizures, predispose to aspirating anaerobic bacteria. Resulting pulmonary infections cause necrotizing pneumonias, which often lead to lung abscesses. The most dramatic complication is gangrene of the lung, a result of thrombosis of a branch of the pulmonary artery and consequent infarction. This is a medical emergency and requires resection of the affected lung.

Psittacosis

Psittacosis is a lung infection due to inhalation of *Chlamydia psittaci* in dust contaminated with excreta from birds, usually pets and often parrots. It is characterized by severe systemic symptoms, with fever, malaise and muscle aches, but surprisingly few respiratory symptoms other than cough. Chest radiographs may be negative, and when abnormal, they show irregular consolidation and an interstitial pattern. The morphologic patterns in most cases are unknown, but the disease is likely to be an interstitial pneumonia. In fatal cases, varying degrees of diffuse alveolar damage are present, together with edema, intra-alveolar pneumonia and necrosis.

Anthrax Pneumonia and Pneumonic Plague

Recent world events have focused attention on infectious agents that could be used as weapons of bioterrorism. Chief among these are **Bacillus anthracis** and **Yersinia pestis**.

B. anthracis, a gram-positive, spore-forming bacillus, is the causative agent of anthrax. Anthrax occurs in many species of domestic animals, but human infection occurs rarely, or in sporadic outbreaks. Transmission is via direct contact with the spores; person-to-person transmission is uncommon. Cutaneous anthrax is rarely fatal, but inhalational anthrax has a high mortality. Anthrax spores are extremely resistant to drying. When inhaled, they are transported to mediastinal lymph nodes where bacilli emerge and disseminate rapidly through the bloodstream to other organs, including the lungs. Hemorrhagic necrosis of infected organs ensues along with severe hemorrhagic mediastinitis related to local lymphadenopathy. In the lungs, the disease is manifested by hemorrhagic bronchitis and confluent areas of hemorrhagic pneumonia.

Y. pestis, the causative agent of **plague,** produces two main forms of infection, a bubonic form and a pneumonic form. In pneumonic plague, the organisms are inhaled directly without an intermediary arthropod vector, and disease may be spread from person to person. The lungs typically show extensive hemorrhagic bronchopneumonia, pleuritis and mediastinal lymph node enlargement. Untreated disease progresses rapidly and is highly fatal.

Mycoplasma Pneumoniae Causes "Atypical Pneumonia"

Unlike lobar pneumonia, atypical pneumonia begins insidiously. Leukocytosis is absent or slight and the course is prolonged. Respiratory symptoms may be minimal or severe, and chest radiography shows patchy intra-alveolar pneumonia or interstitial infiltrates. Infection characteristically causes a bronchiolitis with a neutrophilic intraluminal exudate and intense lymphoplasmacytic infiltration in bronchiolar walls (Fig. 18-15). *Mycoplasma* lack rigid cell walls that most bacteria possess. They grow slowly and are difficult to culture by traditional methods. Diagnosis is usually established by serologic detection of *Mycoplasma pneumoniae* antibodies or cold agglutinins. Erythromycin is effective, and the infection is only rarely fatal.

Tuberculosis Is the Classic Granulomatous Infection

Known since ancient Egypt, tuberculosis was the scourge of the industrialized world in the 19th and early 20th centuries. It declined quickly as living and working conditions improved during the 20th century, and the introduction of antituberculosis drugs further decreased its impact. However, tuberculosis has recently reemerged, particularly drug-resistant strains and among patients with AIDS (see Chapter 9).

Tuberculosis mostly represents infection with *tuberculosis,* although atypical mycobacterial infections may cause

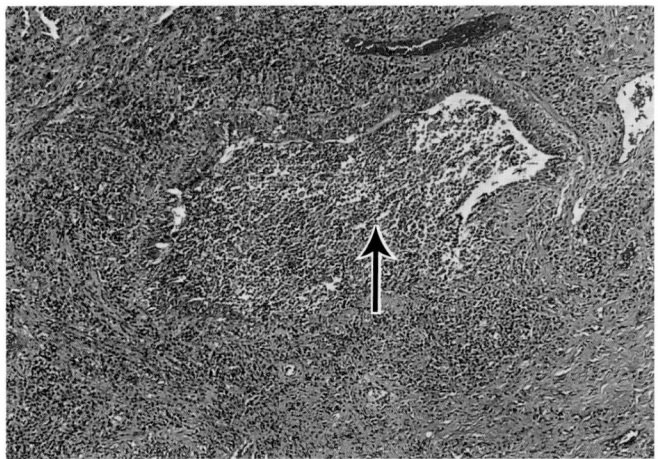

FIGURE 18-15. Mycoplasma pneumonia. Chronic bronchiolitis with a neutrophilic luminal exudate (*arrow*).

similar manifestations. The disease is divided into primary and secondary (or reactivation) tuberculosis.

PRIMARY TUBERCULOSIS: The disease is acquired after initial exposure to *Mycobacterium tuberculosis,* most commonly from inhaling infected aerosols generated when a person with cavitary tuberculosis coughs. Inhaled organisms multiply in the alveoli because alveolar macrophages cannot readily kill them.

 PATHOLOGY: The **Ghon lesion** is the first lesion of primary tuberculosis and consists of a peripheral parenchymal granuloma, often in the upper lobes. When this lesion is associated with an enlarged mediastinal lymph node, a **Ghon complex** is formed (Fig. 18-16). On gross examination, the healed, subpleural Ghon nodule is

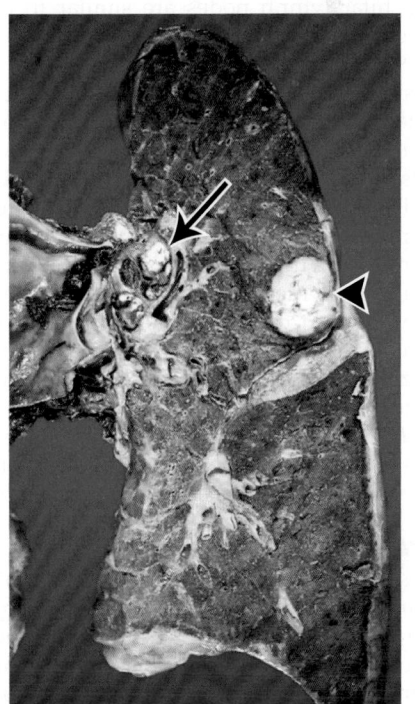

FIGURE 18-16. Primary tuberculosis. A healed Ghon complex is represented by a subpleural nodule (*arrowhead*) and involved hilar lymph nodes (*arrow*).

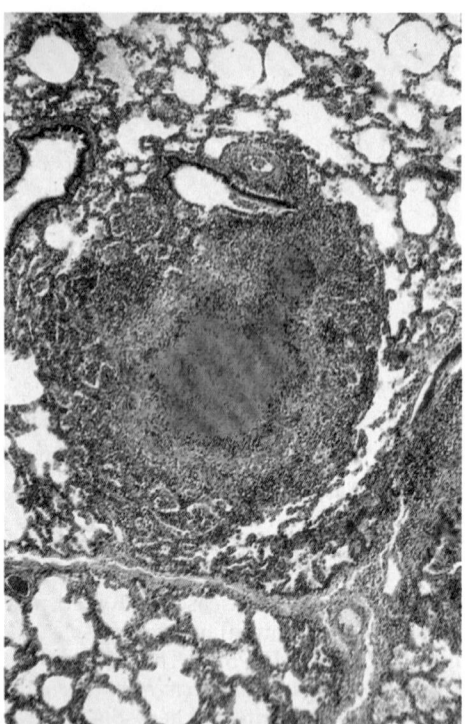

FIGURE 18-17. Necrotizing granuloma due to *Mycobacterium tuberculosis*. A small tuberculous granuloma with conspicuous central caseation is present in the pulmonary parenchyma. The necrotic center is surrounded by histiocytes, giant cells and fibrous tissue.

1–2 cm in diameter, well circumscribed and centrally necrotic. In later stages, it is fibrotic and calcified. Microscopically, a granuloma with central caseous necrosis (Fig. 18-17) shows varying degrees of fibrosis. The microscopic features of draining hilar lymph nodes are similar to those of the peripheral parenchymal lesion.

Most (>90%) primary tuberculous infections are asymptomatic; lesions remain localized and heal. Sometimes there is self-limited extension to the pleura, with secondary pleural effusion. Less often, primary tuberculosis is not limited but spreads to other parts of the lung **(progressive primary tuberculosis)**. This usually occurs in young children or immunosuppressed adults. In this situation, the initial lesion enlarges, producing necrotic areas up to 6 cm. Central liquefaction results in cavities, which may expand to occupy most of the lower lobe. At the same time, draining lymph nodes display similar histologic changes. Erosion of a bronchus by the necrotizing process leads to further pulmonary dissemination of the disease.

SECONDARY TUBERCULOSIS: This stage represents reactivation of primary pulmonary tuberculosis or new infection in someone previously sensitized by primary tuberculosis.

PATHOLOGY: The initial reaction to *M. tuberculosis* is different in secondary tuberculosis. A cellular immune response occurs after a latent interval and leads to formation of many granulomas and extensive tissue necrosis. Apical and posterior segments of the upper lobes are most commonly involved, but the superior segment of the lower lobe is also often affected, and no part of the lung can be excluded. A diffuse, fibrotic, poorly defined lesion develops, with focal areas of caseous necrosis. Often

these foci heal and calcify, but some may erode into bronchi, after which drainage of infectious material creates a tuberculous cavity.

Tuberculous cavities range from under 1 cm to large, cystic areas occupying almost the entire lung. Most measure 3–10 cm. They prefer the apices of the upper lobes (Fig. 18-18) but may occur anywhere in the lung. The cavity wall is composed of an inner, thin, gray membrane encompassing soft necrotic nodules; a middle zone of granulation tissue; and an outer collagenous border. The lumen is filled with caseous material containing acid-fast bacilli. Cavities often communicate with a bronchus, and the release of infectious material into airways spreads infection within the lung. The walls of healed tuberculous cavities eventually become fibrotic and calcified.

Secondary tuberculosis is associated with a number of complications:

- **Miliary tuberculosis** is the presence of multiple, small (size of millet seeds), tuberculous granulomas (Fig. 18-19) in many organs. The organisms disseminate from the lung or other sites via the blood, usually during secondary tuberculosis, but occasionally in primary disease.
- **Hemoptysis** is caused by erosion into small pulmonary arteries adjacent to the cavity wall. It may be severe enough to drown patients in their own blood.
- **Bronchopleural fistula** occurs when a subpleural cavity ruptures into the pleural space. In turn, tuberculous empyema and pneumothorax result.
- **Tuberculous laryngitis** is a consequence of coughing up infectious material.
- **Intestinal tuberculosis** may follow swallowing of the same tuberculous material.
- **Aspergilloma** is a fungal mass arising by superinfection of a persistent open cavity with *Aspergillus;* the fungi may fill the entire cavity.

MYCOBACTERIUM AVIUM-INTRACELLULARE (MAI): In immunodeficient patients, whose ability to mount a granulomatous reaction may be impaired, MAI pneumonia is characterized by an extensive infiltrate of macrophages and innumerable acid-fast organisms (Fig. 18-20). MAI may colonize airways of older, immunocompetent individuals with underlying pulmonary disorders such as bronchiectasis, or it may produce granulomatous inflammation with or without

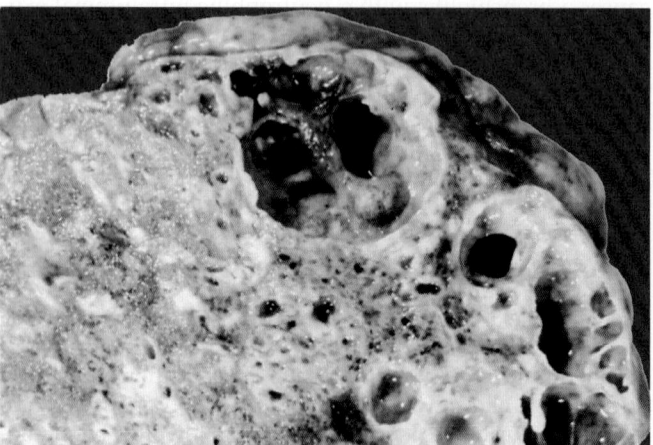

FIGURE 18-18. Cavitary tuberculosis. The apex of the left upper lobe shows tuberculous cavities surrounded by consolidated and fibrotic pulmonary parenchyma that contains small tubercles.

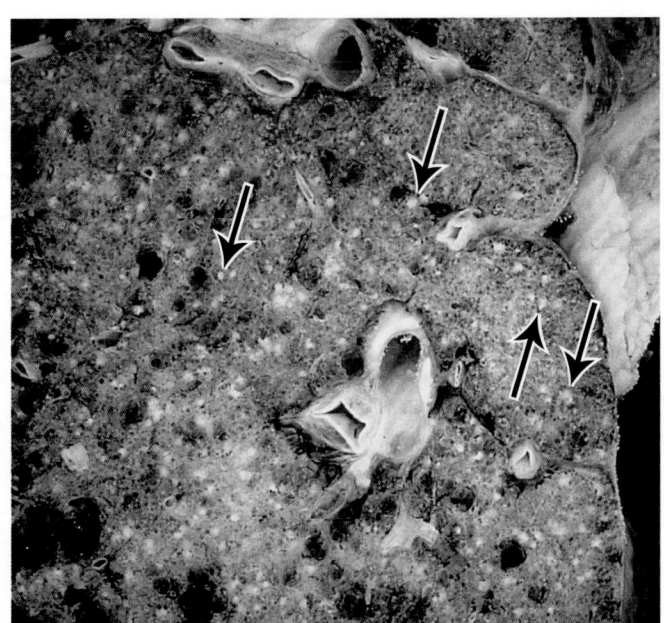

FIGURE 18-19. Miliary tuberculosis. Multiple millimeter-sized nodules (*arrows*) are scattered throughout the lung parenchyma.

cavitation. *Mycobacterium kansasii* produces a spectrum of disease similar to that of MAI but is not as frequently encountered, owing to a more restricted geographic distribution.

Actinomycosis Features Multiple Lung Abscesses

Actinomycosis is caused by infection with actinomycetes, and the usual pulmonary organism is *Actinomyces israelii*. Although actinomycetes resemble fungi in appearance, they are anaerobic, gram-positive, filamentous bacteria. They normally inhabit the mouth and nose and infect the lung by aspiration of oropharyngeal contents or by extension from an actinomycotic subdiaphragmatic abscess or liver abscess.

 PATHOLOGY: Lung lesions of actinomycosis consist of multiple, interconnecting, small lung abscesses. The abscess margins are granulomatous,

but central necrotic areas are purulent and contain colonies of thin, branching, filamentous, gram-positive bacteria. Clubbed basophilic filaments, noted at the colony margins, are visible to the naked eye as small yellow particles (**"sulfur granules"**). The abscesses may extend to the pleura and produce bronchopulmonary fistulas and empyema. They may also invade the chest wall.

Nocardia Is Usually an Opportunistic Organism

Nocardia is a gram-positive filamentous bacterium that causes an acute progressive or chronic bacterial pneumonia. Infection is mostly seen in immunocompromised patients, particularly those with lymphomas, neutropenia, chronic granulomatous disease of childhood and pulmonary alveolar proteinosis. *Nocardia asteroides* is the most common *Nocardia* sp. to cause pneumonia.

 PATHOLOGY: Histologically, lungs show abscesses (Fig. 18-21A), which may have granulomatous features in chronic infections. The organisms are delicate, beaded, thin filaments, which branch mostly at right angles (Fig. 18-21B). They are best seen with Gram or Gomori methenamine silver stains (Fig. 18-21B) and are also weakly acid fast.

Fungal Infections May Be Geographic or Opportunistic

Histoplasmosis

Histoplasmosis is a disease of the midwestern and southeastern United States, particularly the Mississippi and Ohio river valleys. It is caused by inhalation of *Histoplasma capsulatum* in infected dust, commonly from bird droppings.

 PATHOLOGY: Histoplasmosis resembles tuberculosis clinically and pathologically. Most infections are asymptomatic and result in lesions like Ghon complexes, including a parenchymal granuloma and similar lesions in the draining lymph nodes. The granulomas are particularly prone to calcify, often with a concentric laminar pattern. In the acute phase, numerous organisms

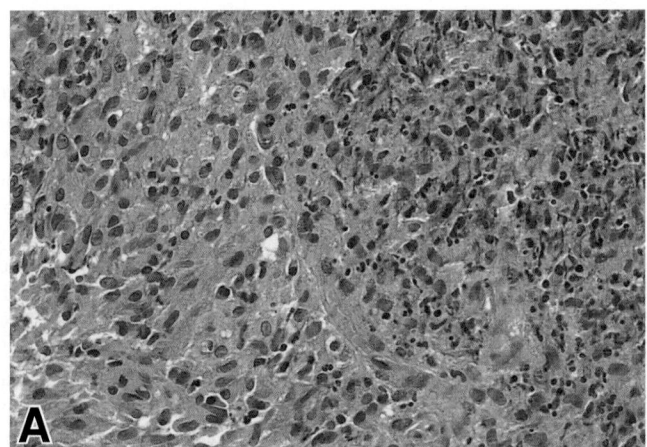
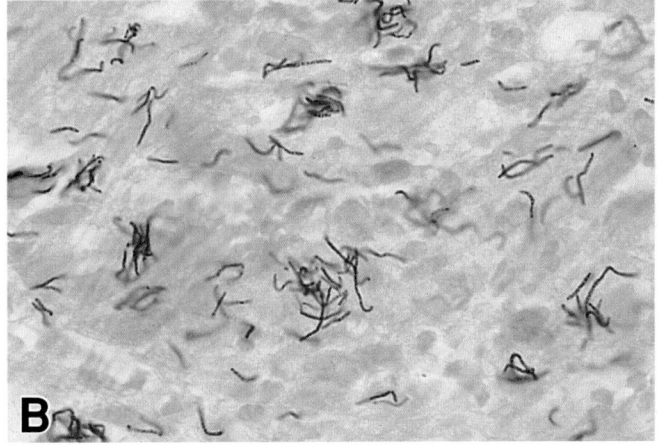

FIGURE 18-20. *Mycobacterium avium-intracellulare* pneumonia in AIDS. **A.** The pneumonia is characterized by an extensive infiltrate of macrophages. **B.** The Ziehl-Neelsen stain shows numerous acid-fast organisms.

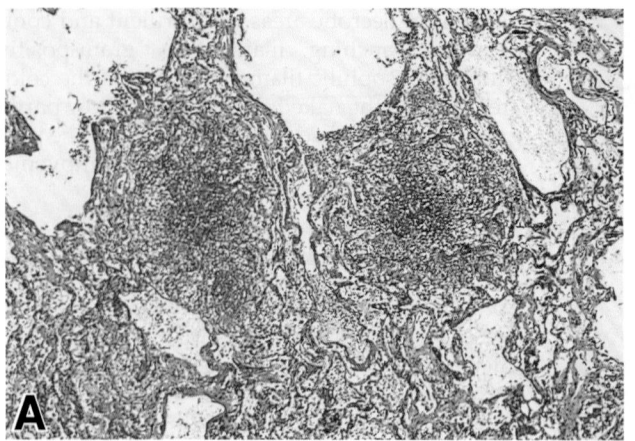
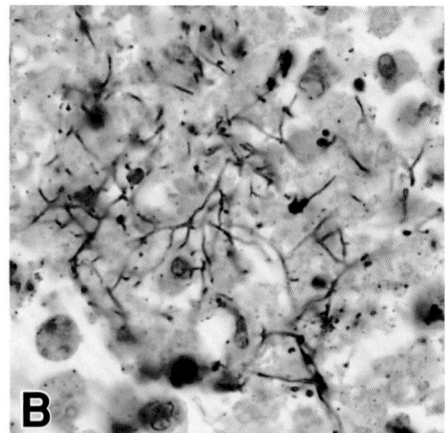

FIGURE 18-21. Nocardiosis. A. This lung shows abscesses consisting of focal collections of acute inflammation. **B.** The organisms are thin, filamentous, branching bacteria (Gomori methenamine silver stain).

are seen within macrophages. Granulomatous inflammation follows, often with central areas of necrosis. The granulomas heal by fibrosis and calcification, but central necrotic areas may persist. The spherical organisms are best seen with a silver stain as 2–4 μm in diameter with narrow-based budding.

In a few cases, pulmonary lesions progress or reactivate, leading to a progressive fibrotic and necrotic lesion that closely resembles that of reactivation tuberculosis. However, histoplasmosis lesions are more fibrotic than those of tuberculosis, and cavitation is less common. The reason for progression is not known, although large infective doses and poor host responses are usually considered to be responsible. Immunocompromised patients are at particular risk for the dissemination of *Histoplasma* within the lungs and spread to other organs.

Coccidioidomycosis

Coccidioidomycosis, caused by inhalation of spores of *Coccidioides immitis*, was originally known as San Joaquin Valley fever, after the location where the disease has been endemic for many years. However, the infection is widespread throughout the southwestern part of the United States and shares many of the clinical and pathologic features of histoplasmosis and tuberculosis. In histologic sections, the organism is a spherule, 30–100 μm, with a thick refractile wall. Spherules contain innumerable 2–5-μm endospores. Empty spherules or endospores that have been released into the tissue may also be visible.

 PATHOLOGY: In most instances, lesions are limited to a peripheral parenchymal granuloma, with or without lymph node granulomas. Sometimes, the lesion may be slowly progressive. In immunocompromised hosts, the disease may progress rapidly, with release of endospores into the lung, in which case the tissue reaction may be purulent as well as granulomatous.

Cryptococcosis

Cryptococcosis results from the inhalation of spores of *Cryptococcus neoformans*, which are often found in pigeon droppings. Lung lesions range from small parenchymal granulomas to several large granulomatous nodules, pneumonic consolidation and even cavitation. Most serious cases of pulmonary cryptococcosis occur in immunocompromised patients, in whom the organisms proliferate extensively within alveolar spaces, with little tissue reaction. The organisms are 4–6 μm, but may be larger, with narrow-based budding and a thick mucoid capsule.

North American Blastomycosis

Blastomycosis is an uncommon condition caused by *Blastomyces dermatitidis*. It is concentrated in the Missouri, Mississippi and Ohio river basins in the United States, and in southern Manitoba and northwestern Ontario in Canada. Clinical and pathologic features resemble those of the fungi mentioned above. Initial infection produces a lesion resembling a Ghon complex or progressive pneumonitis. Unlike tuberculous Ghon complexes, the focal lesions of blastomycosis show central necrosis with a purulent reaction, surrounded by granulomatous inflammation. The organisms are 8–15 μm, have a thick refractile wall and exhibit broad-based budding.

Aspergillosis

Lung infections by *Aspergillus* spp., usually *Aspergillus niger* or *Aspergillus fumigatus*, may occur as:

- **Invasive aspergillosis:** This is the most serious form of *Aspergillus* infection, occurring almost exclusively as an opportunistic infection in people with compromised immunity, usually due to cytotoxic therapy or AIDS. The lungs show patchy, multifocal consolidation and, occasionally, cavities. Extensive blood vessel invasion (usually arterial [Fig. 18-22]) results in occlusion, thrombosis and infarction of lung tissue. Invasive aspergillosis is a fulminant pulmonary infection that is not amenable to therapy.
- **Aspergilloma ("fungus ball" or mycetoma):** *Aspergillus* spp. may grow in preexisting cavities, such as those caused by tuberculosis or bronchiectasis, where they proliferate to form fungus balls (Fig. 18-23). Radiographs show a large mass within an air-filled cavity. Fungus balls are usually clinically silent and merely represent interesting radiologic findings. However, if they become

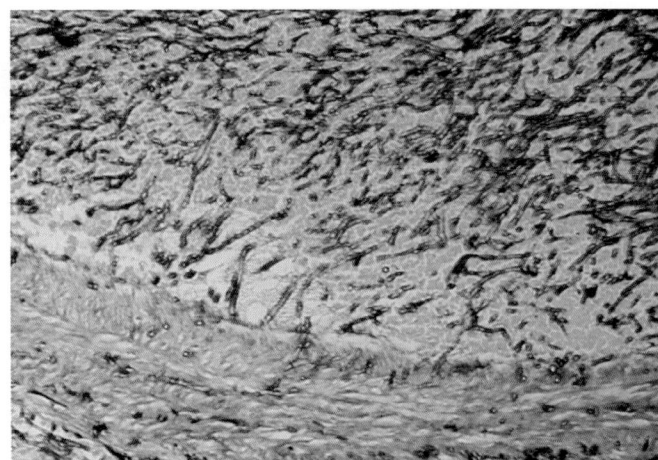

FIGURE 18-22. **Invasive pulmonary aspergillosis.** A branch of the pulmonary artery shows fungal hyphae in the wall and within the lumen (Gomori methenamine silver stain).

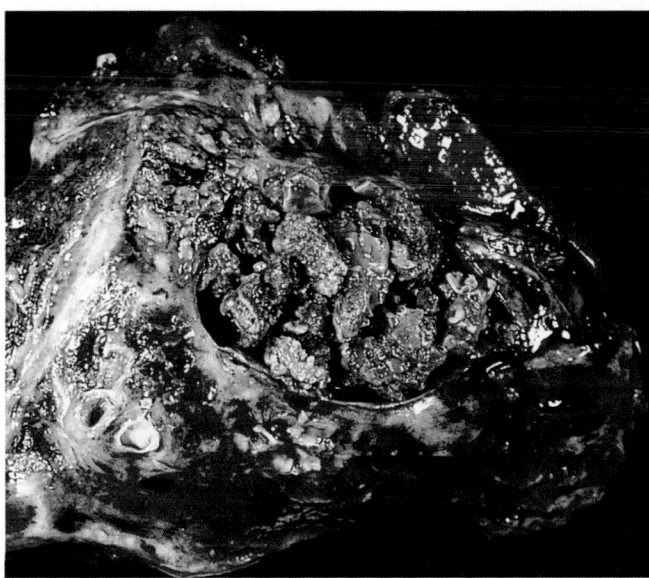

FIGURE 18-23. *Aspergillus* **fungus ball.** The lung contains a cavity filled with a fungus ball.

clinically evident, they most often present with hemoptysis, arising either from the underlying condition or, less commonly, fungal infection of the cavity wall.

■ **Allergic bronchopulmonary aspergillosis (ABPA):** Certain asthmatics have an unusual immunologic reaction to *Aspergillus* that is characterized by (1) transient pulmonary infiltrates on chest radiographs, (2) eosinophilia of blood and sputum, (3) skin sensitivity and serum precipitins to *A. fumigatus* antigens and (4) increased serum IgE. Computed tomography shows thickened bronchial walls and mucous plugs in the bronchi.

 PATHOLOGY: ABPA is invariably associated with proximal (central) bronchiectasis, involving segmental bronchi and the next 2–4 orders of subsegmental bronchi. There are bronchial and bronchiolar mucous plugs, eosinophilic infiltrates and Charcot-Leyden crystals (Fig. 18-24A,B). Bronchocentric granulomatosis and eosinophilic pneumonia may be present. The bronchial mucus may contain septate, fungal hyphae, with 45-degree branching. Interestingly, the peripheral bronchial tree is spared.

 CLINICAL FEATURES: Patients with ABPA wheeze, with chest pain and cough, and often have thick mucous plugs. Systemic corticosteroids usually control acute episodes.

Pneumocystis jiroveci

First described as "plasma cell pneumonia" in malnourished infants at the end of World War II, pulmonary infections with *Pneumocystis jiroveci* (formerly *Pneumocystis carinii*) most often cause pneumonia in immunosuppressed patients or those with immunodeficiencies such as HIV/AIDS. Patients receiving immunosuppressive drugs after organ transplantation or chemotherapy for malignant disease are particularly at risk. Once considered a protozoan, *Pneumocystis* is now recognized as a fungus.

 PATHOLOGY: The classic lesions of *Pneumocystis* pneumonia are interstitial infiltrates of plasma cells and lymphocytes and hyperplasia of type II

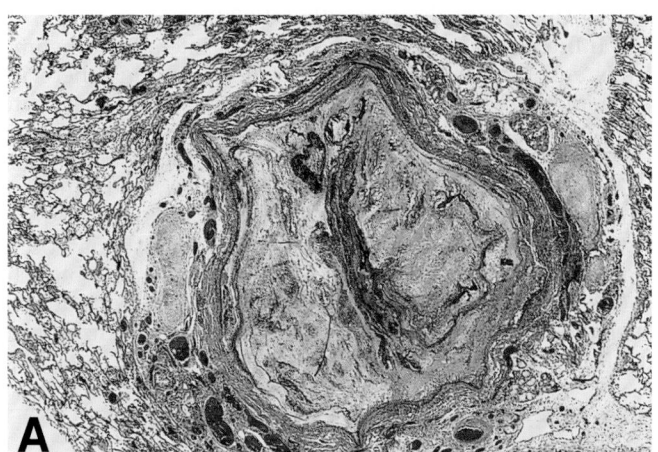
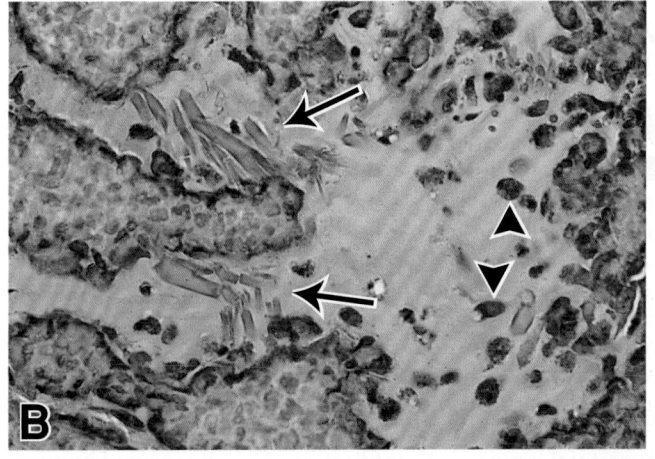

FIGURE 18-24. **Allergic bronchopulmonary aspergillosis. A.** A dilated bronchus is filled with a mucous plug that has dense layers of eosinophilic infiltrates. **B.** Higher magnification shows numerous eosinophils (*arrowheads*) and Charcot-Leyden crystals (*arrows*).

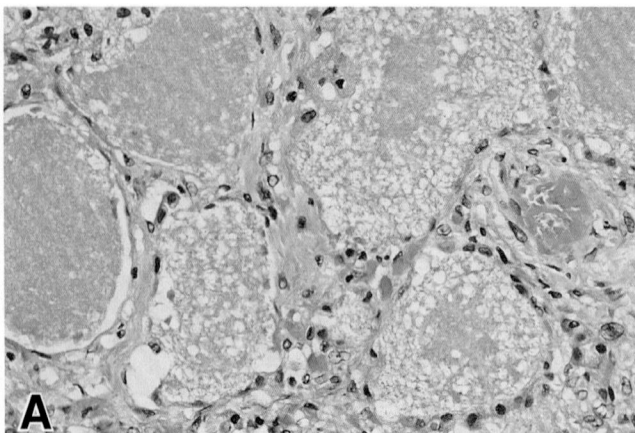
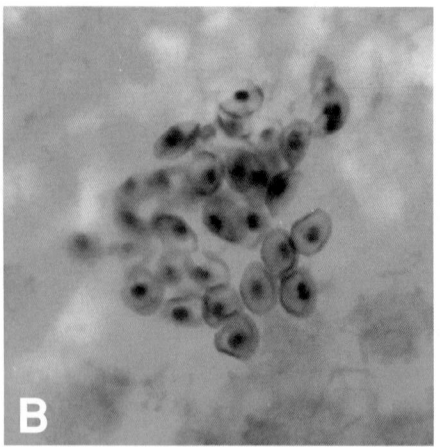

FIGURE 18-25. *Pneumocystis jiroveci* **pneumonia. A.** The alveoli are filled with a foamy exudate, and the interstitium is thickened and contains a chronic inflammatory infiltrate. **B.** A centrifuged bronchoalveolar lavage specimen impregnated with silver shows a cluster of *Pneumocystis* cysts.

pneumocytes. Alveoli are filled with a characteristic foamy exudate, in which the organisms appear as small bubbles in a background of proteinaceous exudate (Fig. 18-25A). With silver impregnation, cysts appear as round or indented ("crescent moon") bodies, 5 μm in diameter (Fig. 18-25B). After sporozoites develop within the cyst, it ruptures and assumes an indented shape. Sporozoites develop into trophozoites, which may be seen with stains such as Giemsa in cytology specimens but are very difficult to see in routine histologic sections. Granulomatous inflammation in *Pneumocystis* pneumonia is rare but occurs in up to 5% of lung biopsies from HIV-infected patients. In some cases, *Pneumocystis* also produces diffuse alveolar damage (see below).

 CLINICAL FEATURES: Clinically and radiologically, *Pneumocystis* pneumonia presents a variable picture. At one extreme, symptoms may be minimal, while at the other, there is rapidly progressive respiratory failure. In AIDS patients, thin-walled parenchymal cysts may develop and predispose to pneumothorax. The diagnosis is made by identifying the organism by sputum examination, bronchoalveolar lavage, transbronchial biopsy, needle aspiration of the lung or open lung biopsy. Treatment is with trimethoprim–sulfamethoxazole or pentamidine.

Viral Pneumonitides Cause Diffuse Alveolar Damage or Interstitial Pneumonia

 PATHOLOGY: Viral infections initially affect the alveolar epithelium and elicit interstitial mononuclear infiltrates (Fig. 18-26). Hyaline membranes and necrosis of type I epithelial cells lead to an appearance indistinguishable from diffuse alveolar damage from other causes. Sometimes, alveolar damage is indolent, and disease is characterized by type II pneumocyte hyperplasia and chronic interstitial inflammation. This is unlike most bacterial infections, in which intra-alveolar neutrophilic exudates predominate and the interstitium is only incidentally involved (Fig. 18-27).

Cytomegalovirus (CMV) pneumonia entails intense interstitial lymphocytic infiltration. Alveoli are lined by type II cells that have regenerated to cover the epithelial defect left by necrosis of type I cells. The infected alveolar cells are very large (cytomegaly) with a single, dark, basophilic

nuclear inclusion with a peripheral halo and multiple, indistinct cytoplasmic, basophilic inclusions (Fig. 18-28).

Measles infection involves both the airways and the parenchyma. It is characterized by very large (100 μm across) multinucleated giant cells with nuclear inclusions and large eosinophilic cytoplasmic inclusions (Fig. 18-29). Interstitial pneumonia, a well-characterized complication of measles, is rarely fatal, except in immunocompromised, previously unexposed individuals.

Varicella infection (chickenpox and herpes zoster) produces disseminated, focally necrotic lung lesions and interstitial pneumonia. Pulmonary involvement is usually asymptomatic, except in immunocompromised hosts, in whom it may be fatal. The viral inclusions are nuclear, eosinophilic and refractile and are surrounded by a clear halo. Multinucleation can occur.

Herpes simplex can cause a necrotizing tracheobronchitis as well as diffuse alveolar damage. Viral inclusions are identical to those seen in varicella infection.

Adenovirus causes necrotizing bronchiolitis and bronchopneumonia. Two types of nuclear inclusions are seen: eosinophilic nuclear inclusions surrounded by a clear halo and "smudge cells," with indistinct, basophilic, nuclear inclusions that fill the entire nucleus and are surrounded by only a thin rim of chromatin (Fig. 18-30).

Influenza virus typically produces interstitial pneumonitis and bronchiolitis similar to those seen in other viral pneumonias. It does not produce characteristic viral cytopathic changes in histologic sections. A recent pandemic of H1N1 influenza drew attention to the pathology of influenza pneumonia. Most cases of H1N1 infection are fortunately mild and self-limited. But in some patients, mainly those with underlying health problems, fatal disease may occur. Pathologies vary from interstitial pneumonia and bronchiolitis to diffuse alveolar damage. In some cases, extensive hemorrhage is present. With most strains of influenza, bacterial superinfection is not uncommon.

The Most Common Cause of Lung Abscess Is Aspiration

Lung abscesses are localized accumulations of pus, with destruction of pulmonary parenchyma, including alveoli, airways and blood vessels.

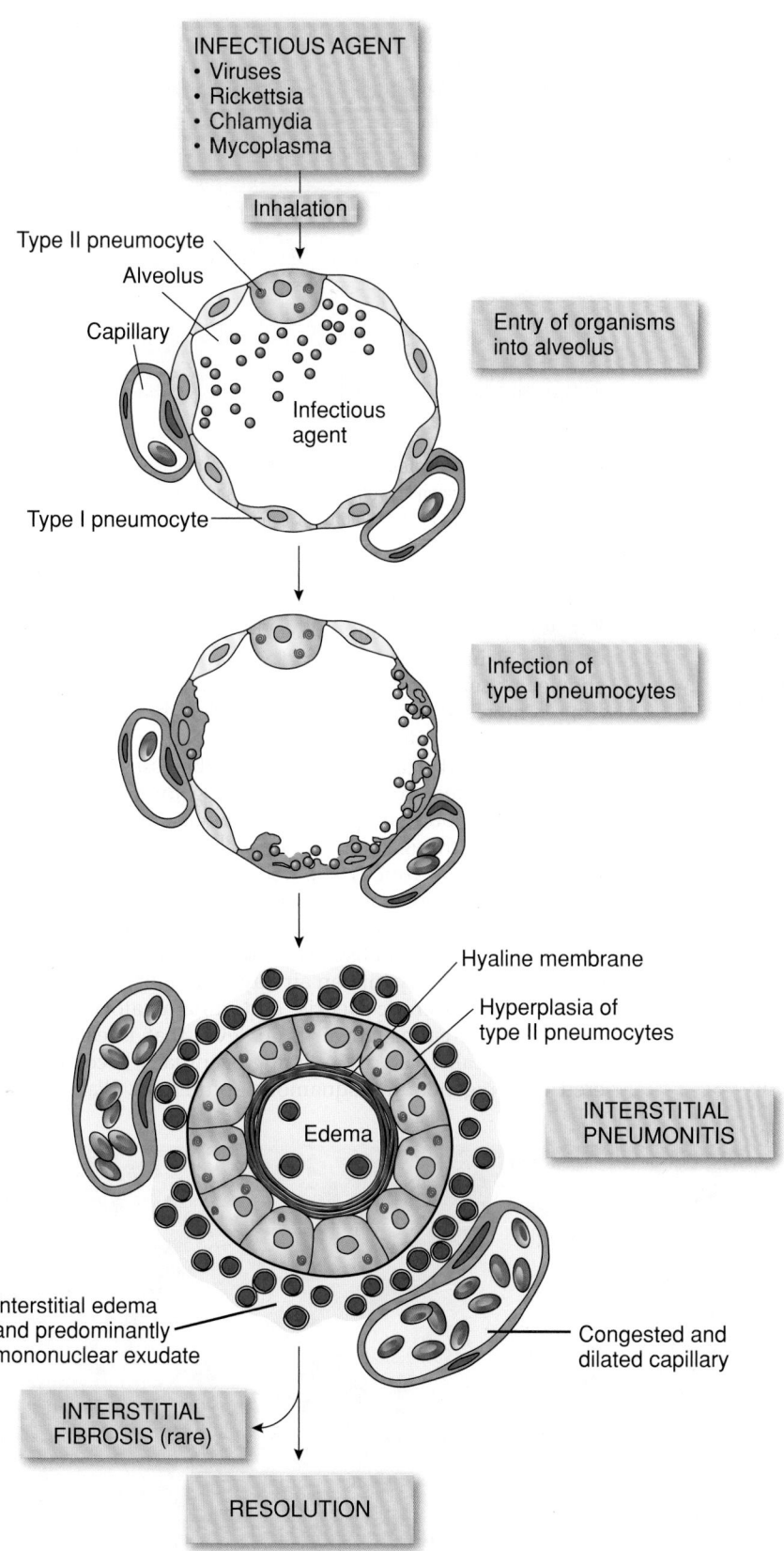

INFECTIOUS AGENT
- Viruses
- Rickettsia
- Chlamydia
- Mycoplasma

Inhalation

Type II pneumocyte

Alveolus

Capillary

Entry of organisms
into alveolus

Infectious
agent

Type I pneumocyte

Infection of
type I pneumocytes

Hyaline membrane

Hyperplasia of
type II pneumocytes

Edema

**INTERSTITIAL
PNEUMONITIS**

Interstitial edema
and predominantly
mononuclear exudate

Congested and
dilated capillary

**INTERSTITIAL
FIBROSIS (rare)**

RESOLUTION

FIGURE 18-26. Pathogenesis of interstitial pneumonia. Although interstitial pneumonia is most commonly caused by viruses, other organisms also may cause significant interstitial inflammation. Type I cells are the most sensitive to damage, and loss of their integrity leads to intra-alveolar edema. The proteinaceous exudate and cell debris form hyaline membranes, and type II cells multiply to line the alveoli. Interstitial inflammation is characterized mainly by mononuclear cells. The disease usually resolves completely but occasionally progresses to interstitial fibrosis.

States of depressed consciousness often predispose to the aspiration that causes lung abscesses, and aspirated oropharyngeal anaerobic bacteria are responsible in over 90% of cases. Infections are typically polymicrobial, often with fusiform bacteria and *Bacteroides* spp. Other organisms encountered in lung abscesses caused by aspiration include *S. aureus, K. pneumoniae, S. pneumoniae* and *Nocardia*.

Development of lung abscess after aspiration requires a large number of anaerobic bacteria in the oral flora, as in people with poor oral hygiene or periodontal disease. The cough

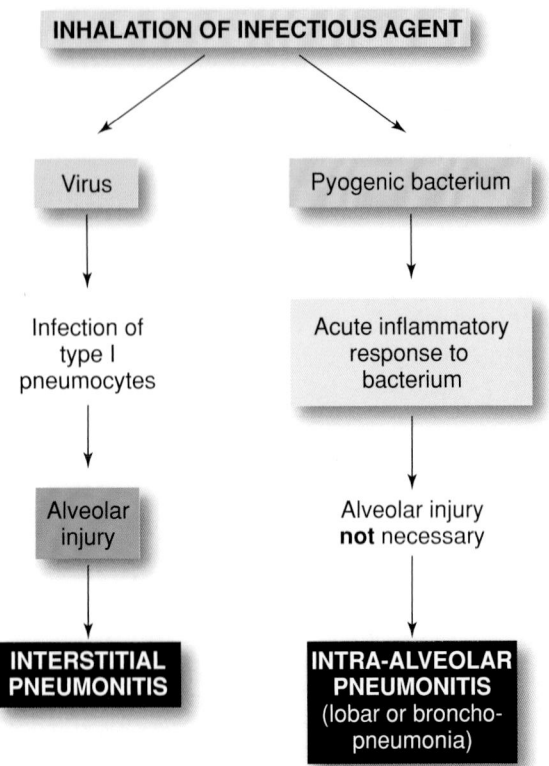

INHALATION OF INFECTIOUS AGENT

Virus

Pyogenic bacterium

Infection of type I pneumocytes

Acute inflammatory response to bacterium

Alveolar injury

Alveolar injury **not** necessary

INTERSTITIAL PNEUMONITIS

INTRA-ALVEOLAR PNEUMONITIS (lobar or broncho-pneumonia)

FIGURE 18-27. Pathogenesis of interstitial and intra-alveolar pneumonitis.

reflex or tracheobronchial clearance must also be impaired. Not surprisingly, alcoholism is the most common condition predisposing to lung abscess. Drug overdoses, epilepsy and neurologic impairment also increase the risk. Other causes of lung abscess include necrotizing pneumonias, bronchial obstruction, infected pulmonary emboli, penetrating trauma and extension of infection from adjacent tissues.

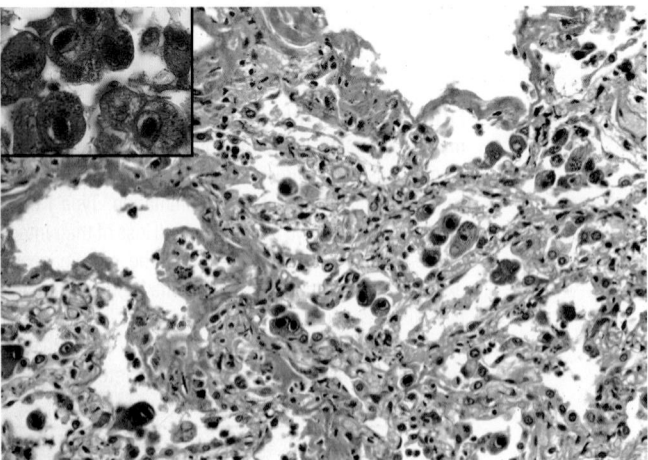

FIGURE 18-28. Cytomegalovirus pneumonitis. Infected alveolar cells are enlarged and display the typical dark blue nuclear inclusions. *Inset.* A higher-power view shows infected alveolar cells that display a single basophilic nuclear inclusion with a perinuclear halo and multiple, indistinct, basophilic, cytoplasmic inclusions.

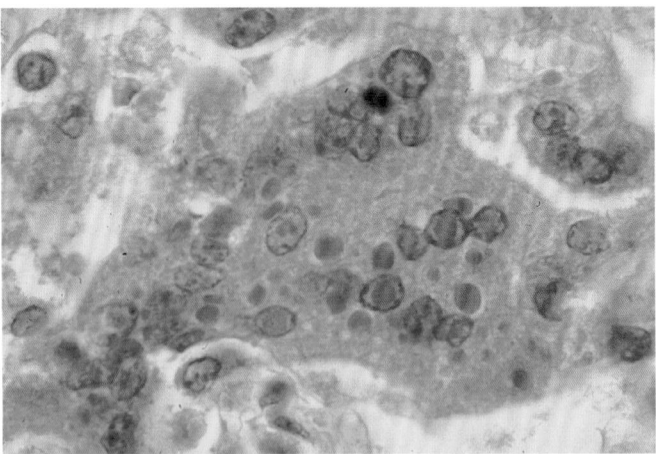

FIGURE 18-29. Measles pneumonitis. This multinucleated giant cell shows single, eosinophilic, refractile inclusions within each of the nuclei, as well as multiple, irregular, eosinophilic, cytoplasmic inclusions.

PATHOLOGY: Lung abscesses typically range from 2 to 6 cm; 10%–20% have multiple cavities, usually arising after a necrotizing pneumonia or a shower of septic pulmonary emboli. The right side of the lung is more often involved than the left, because the right main bronchus follows the direction of the trachea more closely at its bifurcation. Acute lung abscesses are not distinctly separated from the surrounding lung parenchyma. They contain abundant polymorphonuclear leukocytes and, depending on the age of the lesion, variable numbers of macrophages and necrotic tissue debris. Initially, they are surrounded by hemorrhage, fibrin and inflammation, but as they age, a fibrous wall forms around the margin. Lung abscesses differ from abscesses elsewhere in that they may drain spontaneously into an airway. The cavity thus formed contains air, necrotic debris and inflammatory exudate (Fig. 18-31), creating an air-fluid level that is easily seen radiographically. The cavity lining eventually becomes covered with regenerating squamous epithelium. Walls of old

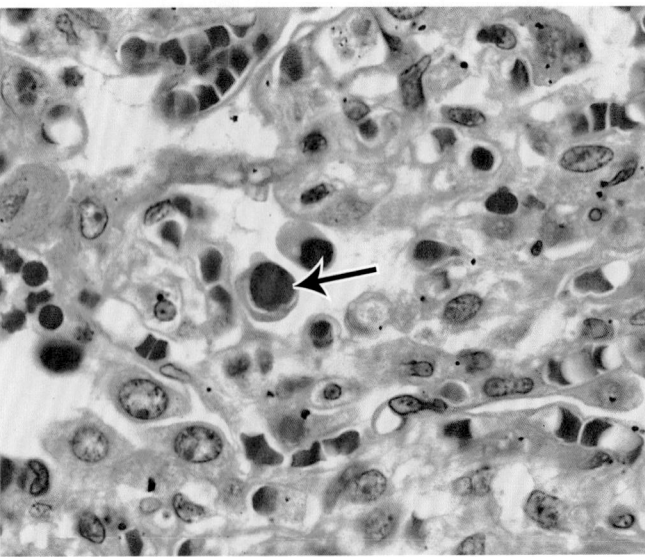

FIGURE 18-30. Adenovirus pneumonia. The "smudge" cell in the center (*arrow*) contains a smudgy basophilic nuclear inclusion.

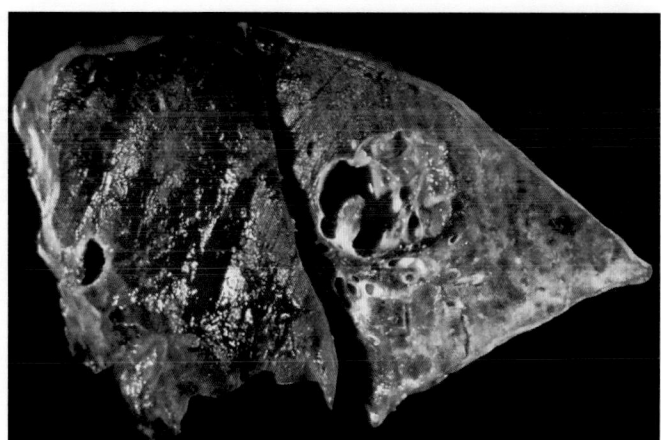

FIGURE 18-31. Pulmonary abscess. A large cystic abscess contains a purulent exudate and is lined by a fibrous wall. Pneumonia is present in the surrounding pulmonary parenchyma.

abscesses may be lined by ciliated respiratory epithelium, making them difficult to distinguish from bronchiectasis.

CLINICAL FEATURES: Almost all patients with lung abscess present with fever and cough, characteristically producing large amounts of foul-smelling sputum. Many patients complain of pleuritic chest pain, and 20% develop hemoptysis.

The differential diagnosis of lung abscess includes lung cancer and cavitary tuberculosis. Indeed, cancer is a more common cause of cavitation than lung abscess. Cavitation due to cancer arises from tumor necrosis half the time, with the other half following bronchial obstruction with subsequent infection. Tuberculous cavities only rarely show the air-fluid levels characteristic of lung abscesses.

Complications of lung abscess include rupture into the pleural space, which causes empyema, and severe hemoptysis. Abscess drainage into a bronchus may spread infection to other parts of the lung. Despite vigorous antimicrobial therapy, principally directed against anaerobic bacteria, the mortality of lung abscess remains 5%–10%.

DIFFUSE ALVEOLAR DAMAGE

Diffuse alveolar damage (DAD) is a pattern of reaction of alveolar epithelial and endothelial cells to a variety of acute insults (Table 18-1). The clinical expression of severe DAD

is **acute respiratory distress syndrome** (ARDS). In ARDS, apparently normal lungs sustain damage that progresses rapidly to respiratory failure. Lung compliance is impaired (usually requiring mechanical ventilation), with hypoxemia and extensive bilateral radiologic opacities ("white-out"). ARDS mortality exceeds 50%, and in patients over 60, it is as high as 90%.

 ETIOLOGIC FACTORS: DAD is a final common pathologic pathway triggered by a large variety of insults (Table 18-1), including infections, sepsis, shock, aspiration of gastric contents, inhalation of toxic gases, near-drowning, radiation pneumonitis and many drugs and other chemicals. The common pathogenic link is acute alveolar epithelial and endothelial cell injury, thus producing DAD. *Unless a specific infectious agent is identified, the trigger for DAD is not evident from the lung histology alone.* In some patients, no cause is found. Such idiopathic DAD, referred to clinically as **acute interstitial pneumonia** (AIP), also includes cases historically called **Hamman-Rich disease (see below)**.

 **MOLECULAR PATHOGENESIS:** Endothelial cell injury allows protein-rich fluid to leak from alveolar capillaries into the interstitial space (Fig. 18-32). Loss of type I pneumocytes permits fluid to enter alveolar spaces, where plasma proteins form fibrin-containing precipitates (hyaline membranes) on the injured alveolar walls (Fig. 18-33). In response to cell injury in DAD, inflammatory cells accumulate in the interstitium. Although lacking type I pneumocytes, alveolar basement membranes remain intact and act as scaffolds for type II pneumocytes, which proliferate to replace the normal alveolar epithelial lining.

If the patient survives the acute phase of ARDS, fibroblasts proliferate in the interstitial space and deposit collagen in the alveolar walls (Fig. 18-34). With complete recovery, the alveolar exudate and hyaline membranes are resorbed and normal alveolar epithelium is restored. Fibroblast proliferation ceases, the extra collagen is metabolized and patients regain normal lung function. In patients who do not recover, DAD can progress to end-stage fibrosis: remodeling of lung architecture produces many cyst-like spaces throughout the lung **(honeycomb lung)**. These spaces are separated by thick fibrous walls lined by type II pneumocytes, bronchiolar epithelium or squamous cells.

Mechanisms of acute injury in DAD are not entirely clear. It is thought that activation of complement (e.g., by endotoxin in the case of gram-negative septicemia) leads to

TABLE 18-1			
IMPORTANT CAUSES OF ACUTE RESPIRATORY DISTRESS SYNDROME			
Nonthoracic Trauma	**Infection**	**Aspiration**	**Drugs and Therapeutic Agents**
Shock due to any cause	Gram-negative septicemia	Near-drowning	Heroin
Fat embolism	Other bacterial infections	Aspiration of gastric contents	Oxygen
	Viral infections		Radiation
			Paraquat
			Cytotoxic drugs

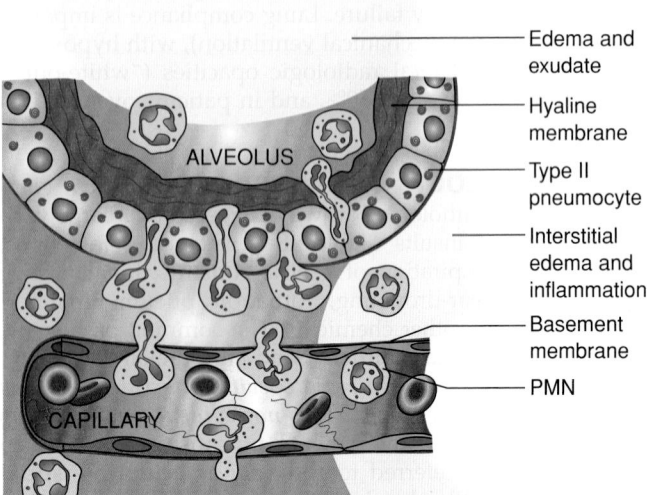

- Edema and exudate
- Hyaline membrane
- Type II pneumocyte
- Interstitial edema and inflammation
- Basement membrane
- PMN

FIGURE 18-32. Diffuse alveolar damage (acute respiratory distress syndrome [ARDS]). In ARDS, type I cells die as a result of diffuse alveolar damage. Intra-alveolar edema follows, after which there is formation of hyaline membranes composed of proteinaceous exudate and cell debris. In the acute phase, the lungs are markedly congested and heavy. Type II cells multiply to line the alveolar surface. Interstitial inflammation is characteristic. The lesion may heal completely or progress to interstitial fibrosis. *PMN =* polymorphonuclear neutrophil.

sequestration of neutrophils in the marginating pool. Only a small proportion, perhaps 1/3, of neutrophils actively circulate in the blood; most of the rest are in the lung. Normally, they cause no damage there, but after activation by complement, they release oxygen radicals and hydrolytic enzymes, which damage pulmonary capillary endothelium. However, neutrophils cannot be obligatory for DAD, because ARDS can develop in severely neutropenic patients.

In DAD following toxic gas inhalation or near-drowning, the damage is mostly at the alveolar epithelial surface. Normal alveolar epithelial junctions are very tight, but epithelial injury disrupts these junctions, permitting exudation of fluid and proteins from the interstitium into alveolar spaces.

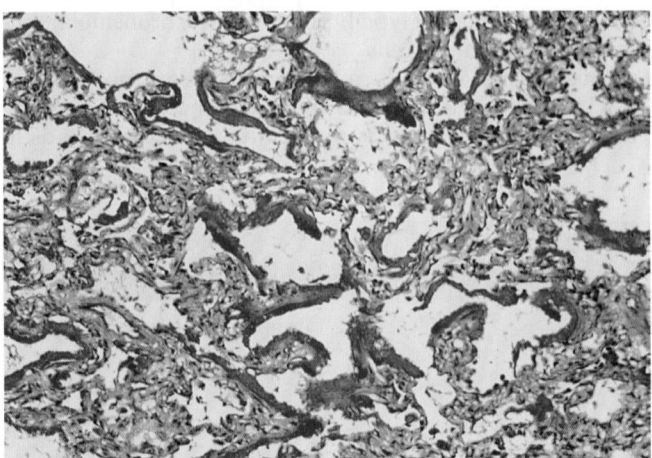

FIGURE 18-33. Diffuse alveolar damage, acute (exudative) phase. Alveolar septa are thickened by edema and a sparse inflammatory infiltrate. Alveoli are lined by eosinophilic hyaline membranes.

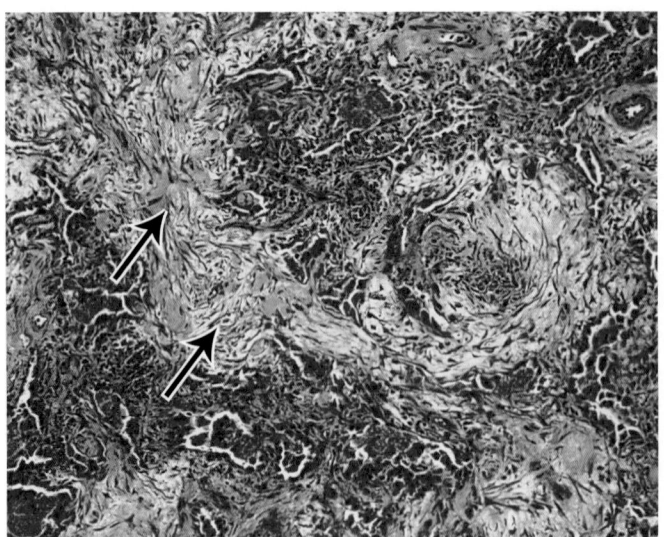

FIGURE 18-34. Diffuse alveolar damage, acute and organizing phase. The alveolar walls are thickened by fibroblasts and loose connective tissue (*arrows*).

PATHOLOGY: The first step is the **exudative phase of DAD,** which develops within a week after pulmonary insult. Edema, hyaline membranes and leakage of plasma proteins are evident, as is accumulation of inflammatory cells (Fig. 18-33). The earliest evidence of alveolar injury is seen by electron microscopy as degenerative changes in endothelial cells and type I pneumocytes. This is followed by sloughing of type I cells, thus denuding basement membranes. Interstitial and alveolar edema is prominent by the first day but soon recedes. **"Hyaline membranes"** appear by the second day and are the most conspicuous morphologic feature of the exudative phase after 4–5 days. They are eosinophilic and glassy, consisting of precipitated plasma proteins and cytoplasmic and nuclear debris from sloughed epithelial cells. Interstitial inflammation, with lymphocytes, plasma cells and macrophages, develops early and peaks in about a week. Toward the end of the first week and persisting during the subsequent **organizing stage,** regularly spaced, cuboidal type II pneumocytes become arrayed along the denuded alveolar septa. Alveolar capillaries and pulmonary arterioles may contain fibrin thrombi. If DAD is fatal, the lungs are heavy, edematous and virtually airless.

The organizing phase of DAD starts about a week after the initial injury and is marked by fibroblast proliferation within alveolar walls (Fig. 18-34). Interstitial inflammation and proliferated type II pneumocytes persist, but hyaline membranes are no longer formed. Alveolar macrophages digest the remnants of hyaline membranes and other debris. Loose fibrosis expands alveolar septa but resolves in mild cases. In severe DAD, fibrosis progresses to restructuring of the pulmonary parenchyma.

CLINICAL FEATURES: Patients destined to develop ARDS have a symptom-free interval for a few hours after the initial insult. Tachypnea and dyspnea mark the onset of ARDS. Blood gas analyses show arterial hypoxemia and decreased pCO_2. As ARDS progresses, dyspnea worsens and the patient becomes cyanotic.

Diffuse, bilateral, interstitial and alveolar infiltrates are noted radiologically. Increasing inspired oxygen concentrations does not restore adequate blood oxygenation, necessitating mechanical ventilation. In fatal cases, the combination of increasing tachypnea and decreasing tidal volume causes alveolar hypoventilation, progressive hypoxemia and increasing pCO_2.

Patients who survive ARDS may recover normal pulmonary function, but in severe cases, they are left with scarred lungs, respiratory dysfunction and, in some instances, pulmonary hypertension.

Diffuse Alveolar Damage Has Diverse Causes

Oxygen Toxicity

Patients who receive high oxygen levels for respiratory problems can develop DAD. Lung lesions may rarely follow long-term exposure to as little as 28% oxygen, but it is usually safe to breathe 40%–60% oxygen for long periods. Oxygen toxicity is thought to be caused by increased production of reactive oxygen species in the lung (see Chapter 1).

Shock

ARDS often follows shock from any cause, including sepsis (see Chapter 12), trauma or blood loss, the pulmonary consequences of which are often called "shock lung." The pathogenesis of DAD associated with shock is poorly understood but is likely multifactorial. Tissue necrosis in organs damaged by trauma or ischemia may lead to release of vasoactive peptides into the circulation. These enhance vascular permeability in the lung. Disseminated intravascular coagulation may damage alveolar capillaries, and fat emboli from bone fractures may obstruct the distal capillary bed of the lung. The pathogenesis of endothelial cell injury in endotoxic shock is discussed in Chapter 7.

Aspiration

Aspiration of gastric contents introduces acid with a pH less than 3.0 into the alveoli. The severe chemical injury to the alveolar lining cells leads to DAD. In near-drowning, aspiration of water produces pulmonary injury and ARDS.

Drug-Induced DAD

Many drugs cause DAD, especially cytotoxic chemotherapeutic agents. The best known is bleomycin, but others include 1,3-bis-(2-chloroethyl)-1-nitrosourea (BCNU), methotrexate, 5-fluorouracil, busulfan and cyclophosphamide. With bleomycin, an imprecise dose-dependent relation has been demonstrated, but such an effect is not apparent with most other drugs.

Bizarre, atypical, hyperchromatic nuclei in type II cells are particularly common when alveolar damage is due to chemotherapy (Fig. 18-35). Damage progresses even when the offending agent is discontinued, but corticosteroid treatment may be helpful. Progressive interstitial fibrosis occurs, usually with retention of lung structure. Methotrexate differs from other chemotherapeutic agents in that it may sometimes cause a hypersensitivity reaction in the lung, in which case the DAD is reversible after the drug is discontinued. Hypersensitivity lesions are characterized by

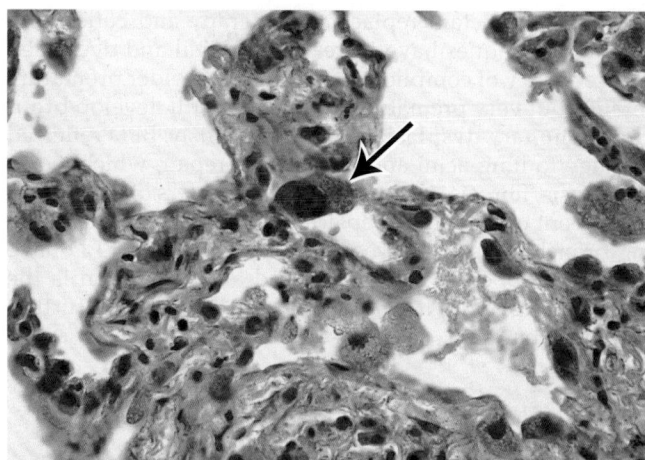

FIGURE 18-35. Diffuse alveolar damage (DAD) associated with busulfan treatment. An atypical pneumocyte (*arrow*) is seen in a case of organizing DAD associated with busulfan therapy.

granulomatous inflammation and occasionally vasculitis. Drugs other than chemotherapeutic agents that may cause DAD include nitrofurantoin, amiodarone and penicillamine.

Radiation Pneumonitis

There are two forms of radiation pneumonitis: acute DAD and chronic pulmonary fibrosis. Alveolar injury is believed to be caused by oxygen radicals generated by the radiolysis of water (see Chapter 1).

Acute radiation pneumonitis occurs in as many as 10% of patients irradiated for lung or breast cancer or for mediastinal lymphoma. DAD caused by radiation is mostly dose related and appears 1–6 months after radiation therapy, when patients develop fever, cough and dyspnea. Pathologically, the lungs show atypical alveolar lining cells, with enlarged hyperchromatic nuclei and multinucleated cells. Most patients recover from acute radiation pneumonitis.

In **chronic radiation pneumonitis,** interstitial fibrosis may follow acute DAD or develop insidiously. Lung biopsy demonstrates interstitial fibrosis, radiation-induced vascular changes and atypical type II pneumocytes. The disease is asymptomatic unless it affects a substantial volume of the lung.

Paraquat

Exposure to paraquat, a common herbicide, may cause DAD. Pulmonary disease becomes apparent 4–7 days after ingestion, as ARDS develops. Patients rarely recover once pulmonary complications have evolved. A curious intra-alveolar exudate and organization occur, as well as the more usual interstitial fibrosis. The intra-alveolar exudate organizes in such a way that the alveolar framework persists and the airspaces are filled with loose granulation tissue.

Neonatal Respiratory Distress Syndrome Resembles ARDS

Neonatal respiratory distress syndrome (NRDS) (see Chapter 6) results from immaturity of the surfactant system at birth, usually because of severe prematurity. The advent of surfactant replacement therapy and better ventilatory techniques have increased survival and decreased the frequency of complications of NRDS in older premature infants, but very premature infants may still develop **bronchopulmonary dysplasia (BPD)**. Previously, BPD reflected damage to lung acini and subsequent repair, which led to atelectasis, fibrosis and destruction of clusters of acini. With the advent of surfactant replacement therapy, the necrotizing bronchiolitis and alveolar septal fibrosis of BPD have largely disappeared, and decreased alveolarization is the main finding now. NRDS and BPD are discussed in further detail in Chapter 6.

RARE ALVEOLAR DISEASES

Alveolar Proteinosis Features Excess Intra-Alveolar Lipid-Rich Material

Alveolar proteinosis, also called **lipoproteinosis,** is a rare condition in which alveoli are filled with a granular eosinophilic material rich in surfactant. Initially considered idiopathic, alveolar proteinosis is now known to be associated with compromised immunity; various cancers, particularly leukemia and lymphoma; respiratory infections; and exposure to environmental inorganic dusts. There is also a rare congenital form caused by a point mutation in the gene for the granulocyte-macrophage colony-stimulating factor (GM-CSF) receptor.

 PATHOPHYSIOLOGY: Alveolar proteinosis is thought to be related to defective surfactant clearance by macrophages. It has recently been attributed to defective activity, or deficiency, of GM-CSF. Anti–GM-CSF autoantibodies are detected in most patients with the idiopathic form of the disease, suggesting an autoimmune etiology. The pathogenesis of secondary alveolar proteinosis is less clear, but appears related to defective macrophage function via altered GM-CSF activity.

 PATHOLOGY: The lungs are very heavy and viscid, and yellow fluid leaks from cut surfaces. They contain scattered, firm, yellow-white nodules that vary in diameter from a few millimeters to 2 cm. Granular material composed of surfactant, cell debris, foamy macrophages and detached type II pneumocytes is seen in alveoli, respiratory bronchioles and alveolar ducts (Fig. 18-36). Electron microscopy shows characteristic surfactant tubular myelin structures. Importantly, the interstitial architecture of the lung is intact, and little inflammation is present.

CLINICAL FEATURES: A few cases have been reported in infants and children, but alveolar proteinosis is a disease of adults. Patients have fever, productive cough and dyspnea. Chest radiographs show diffuse, bilateral, symmetric, alveolar infiltrates, which may radiate from the hilar regions. Repeated respiratory tract infections, often with fungi or *Nocardia*, are common, perhaps due to altered neutrophil and macrophage activity. Infections occur at both pulmonary and extrapulmonary

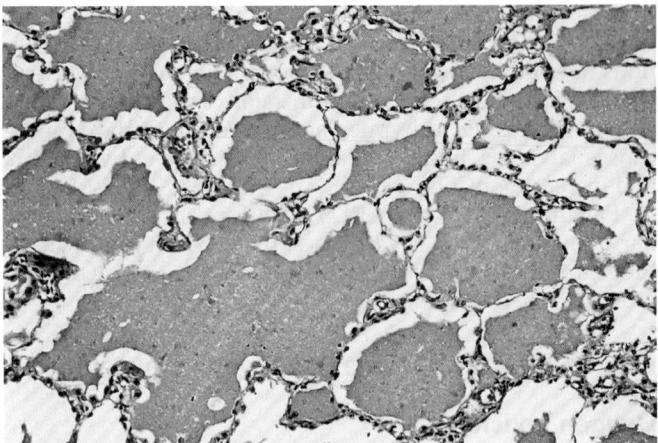

FIGURE 18-36. Alveolar proteinosis. Alveoli and alveolar ducts contain abundant granular, eosinophilic material.

sites, suggesting a systemic predisposition to infections. Before treatment became available, alveolar proteinosis often progressed gradually to respiratory failure. Today, bronchoalveolar lavage can remove the alveolar material, and repeated lavage (sometimes for years) cures or arrests the disease. GM-CSF reconstitution is being investigated.

Diffuse Pulmonary Hemorrhage Syndromes Are Immunologic Disorders

Diffuse alveolar hemorrhage can occur in diverse clinical settings (Table 18-2). These diseases are characterized by acute hemorrhage (numerous intra-alveolar red blood cells) or chronic hemorrhage (hemosiderosis). In virtually all of these disorders, neutrophils infiltrate the alveolar capillary walls **(neutrophilic capillaritis),** reminiscent of leukocytoclastic vasculitis seen in other organs such as the skin. This finding tends to be most prominent in hemorrhagic syndromes associated with polyangiitis with granulomatosis (formerly Wegener granulomatosis) or systemic lupus erythematosus.

Some diffuse pulmonary hemorrhage syndromes are associated with characteristic immunofluorescence patterns. Linear fluorescence along alveolar walls is seen in antibasement membrane antibody disease, or Goodpasture syndrome. A granular pattern occurs in immune complex–associated diseases, such as systemic lupus erythematosus. Pauci-immune disorders consist of antineutrophil cytoplasm antibody (ANCA)-associated diseases (e.g., polyangiitis with granulomatosis, microscopic polyangiitis or idiopathic pulmonary hemorrhage syndromes), in which no etiology or immunologic mechanism can be determined (Table 18-2).

Goodpasture Syndrome

Goodpasture syndrome entails a triad: diffuse alveolar hemorrhage, glomerulonephritis and circulating cytotoxic autoantibody to a component of basement membranes. Cross-reactivity between alveolar and glomerular basement membranes accounts for the simultaneous attack on the lung and kidney (see Chapter 22 for pathogenetic details).

 PATHOLOGY: Patients with Goodpasture syndrome have extensive intra-alveolar hemorrhage (Fig. 18-37A). Their lungs are dark red and heavy

TABLE 18-2

CONDITIONS OF PULMONARY HEMORRHAGE

Disease	Immunologic Mechanism	Immunofluorescence Pattern
Goodpasture syndrome	Antibasement membrane antibody	Linear
Microscopic polyangiitis	Antineutrophilic cytoplasmic antibody (ANCA)	Negative/pauci-immune
Systemic lupus erythematosus	Immune complexes	Granular
Mixed cryoglobulinemia		
Henoch-Schönlein purpura		
Immunoglobulin A (IgA) disease		
Granulomatosis with polyangiitis (formerly Wegener granulomatosis)	ANCA	Negative or pauci-immune
Idiopathic glomerulonephritis		
Idiopathic pulmonary hemorrhage	No immunologic marker	

in the acute phase and rusty brown later, when the erythrocytes have been phagocytosed. Red blood cells and hemosiderin-laden macrophages fill airspaces. The presence of neutrophils in and around alveolar capillaries may suggest an "alveolitis," but this reaction may be transient. Alveolar septa are mildly thickened by interstitial fibrosis and type II pneumocyte hyperplasia is seen. By immunofluorescence, IgG and complement are deposited in the basement membranes of alveoli and glomeruli (Fig. 18-37B).

CLINICAL FEATURES: Goodpasture syndrome may affect adults of either sex and any age, but it occurs mostly in young men. Most (95%) patients present with hemoptysis, often accompanied by dyspnea, weakness and mild anemia. Evidence of glomerulonephritis follows pulmonary manifestations within about 3 months (1 week to 1 year), although some patients do not develop renal disease. Radiography reveals diffuse, bilateral alveolar infiltrates, which may resolve rapidly in a

matter of days as erythrocytes lyse and are phagocytosed. Hypoxemia and respiratory alkalosis are common, but respiratory function returns to normal as the hemorrhage resolves. The diagnosis is made on the basis of a renal or pulmonary biopsy.

Goodpasture syndrome is treated with corticosteroids, cytotoxic drugs and plasmapheresis. Before such aggressive treatment was used, the mortality of Goodpasture syndrome was 80%. Even with current therapy, 2-year survival is now only 50%, and the outlook is worse if renal failure develops.

Idiopathic Pulmonary Hemorrhage

This rare disease (also called **idiopathic pulmonary hemosiderosis**) is characterized by diffuse alveolar bleeding similar to that of Goodpasture syndrome but without renal involvement or antibasement membrane antibodies. It is microscopically indistinguishable from the lung of Goodpasture syndrome.

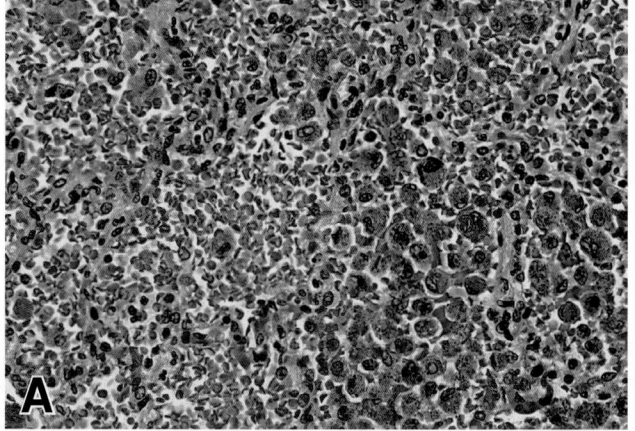
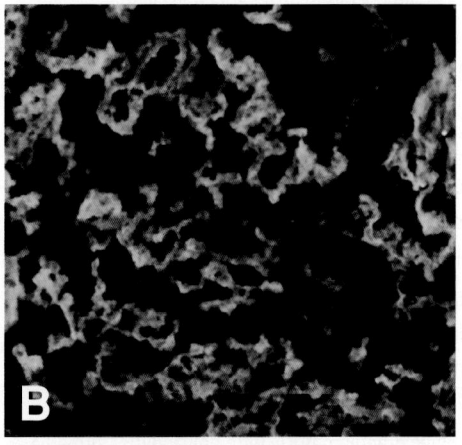

FIGURE 18-37. Goodpasture syndrome. A. A section of lung shows extensive intra-alveolar hemorrhage (*left*) and collections of hemosiderin-laden macrophages (*right*). Alveolar septa are thickened, and alveoli are lined by hyperplastic type II pneumocytes. **B.** Linear deposition of immunoglobulin G (IgG) within the alveolar septa is demonstrated by immunofluorescence.

CLINICAL FEATURES: Idiopathic pulmonary hemosiderosis affects mainly children, but 20% of patients are adults, usually younger than 30. Males predominate, 2:1, among adults, but sex distribution is equal in children. Patients complain of cough (with or without hemoptysis), dyspnea, substernal chest pain, fatigue and iron-deficiency anemia. Pulmonary hemorrhages are recurrent and intermittent. The course is more protracted than that of Goodpasture syndrome.

The response to corticosteroids is variable, and mean survival is 3–5 years. One fourth of patients die rapidly of massive hemorrhage. Another 25% have persistent, active disease; repeated episodes of hemoptysis result in interstitial fibrosis and cor pulmonale. In another 1/4 of patients, the disease remains inactive, but dyspnea and anemia may persist. The remaining patients recover completely without recurrence.

Hypersensitivity to cow's milk in infants and children generally younger than 2 years can result in diffuse pulmonary hemorrhage similar to that seen in idiopathic pulmonary hemorrhage. Removal of milk from the diet ameliorates the condition.

Eosinophilic Pneumonia Is Largely a Hypersensitivity Reaction

Eosinophilic pneumonia entails accumulation of eosinophils in alveolar spaces. The disease is classified as **idiopathic** or **secondary** to an underlying illness (Table 18-3).

TABLE 18-3
TYPES OF EOSINOPHILIC PNEUMONIA
Idiopathic
Chronic eosinophilic pneumonia
Acute eosinophilic pneumonia
Simple eosinophilic pneumonia (Löffler syndrome)
Secondary Eosinophilic Pneumonia
Infection
Parasitic
Tropical eosinophilic pneumonia
Ascaris lumbricoides, Toxocara canis, filaria
Dirofilaria
Fungal
Aspergillus
Drug induced
Antibiotics
Cytotoxic drugs
Anti-inflammatory agents
Antihypertensive drugs
L-Tryptophan (eosinophilic fasciitis)
Immunologic or systemic diseases
Allergic bronchopulmonary aspergillosis
Eosinophilic granulomatosis with polyangiitis (formerly Churg-Strauss syndrome)
Hypereosinophilic syndrome

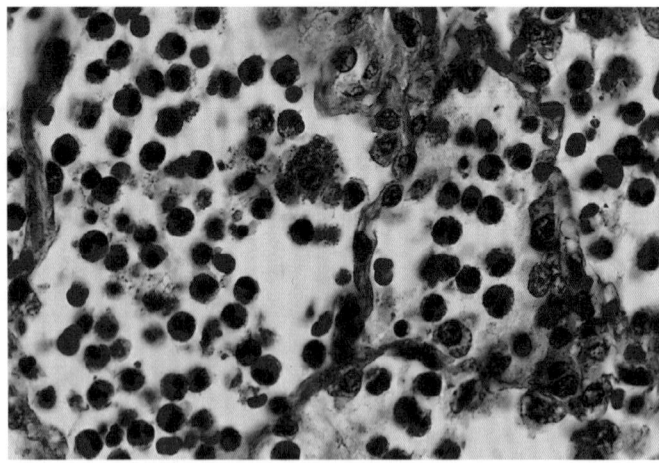

FIGURE 18-38. Eosinophilic pneumonia. Alveolar spaces are filled with an inflammatory exudate composed of eosinophils and macrophages. Alveolar septa are thickened by the presence of numerous eosinophils.

Idiopathic Eosinophilic Pneumonia

SIMPLE EOSINOPHILIC PNEUMONIA: Simple eosinophilic pneumonia (Löffler syndrome) is a mild condition characterized by fleeting pulmonary infiltrates, which usually resolve within a month. Patients typically have peripheral blood eosinophilia but are often asymptomatic. Histologically, the lung shows eosinophilic pneumonia, but the diagnosis is usually established clinically, and lung biopsy is rarely performed.

ACUTE EOSINOPHILIC PNEUMONIA: Patients present with acute (<7 days) symptoms, including fever, hypoxemia and diffuse interstitial and alveolar infiltrates on chest radiograph. The etiology is not known but is thought to be a hypersensitivity reaction. Peripheral blood eosinophilia is often absent, but bronchoalveolar lavage consistently contains increased eosinophils. Histologically, the lung shows eosinophilic pneumonia accompanied by features of diffuse alveolar damage (i.e., hyaline membranes). Patients respond dramatically to corticosteroids, and unlike chronic eosinophilic pneumonia, acute eosinophilic pneumonia does not recur.

CHRONIC EOSINOPHILIC PNEUMONIA: The etiology of chronic eosinophilic pneumonia is unknown, but an allergic diathesis is noted in some patients.

PATHOLOGY: Alveolar spaces are flooded with eosinophils, alveolar macrophages and a proteinaceous exudate (Fig. 18-38). Some cases may also show an eosinophilic interstitial pneumonia. Hyperplasia of type II pneumocytes may be prominent. Eosinophilic abscesses, with central masses of necrotic eosinophils surrounded by palisaded macrophages, are sometimes found. A mild eosinophilic vasculitis may be seen. An organizing pneumonia pattern is also occasionally described (see below).

CLINICAL FEATURES: Patients have fever, night sweats, weight loss, cough productive of eosinophils and dyspnea. Asthma is present in many patients, and circulating eosinophilia may be conspicuous. The chest radiograph is diagnostic and has been described as "the photographic negative of pulmonary edema," characterized by peripheral alveolar infiltrates with sparing of the hilum. The response to corticosteroids is dramatic and helps confirm the diagnosis.

Secondary Eosinophilic Pneumonia

Eosinophilic pneumonia can occur in a variety of clinical settings, including parasitic or fungal infection, drug toxicity and systemic disorders such as Churg-Strauss syndrome (Table 18-3). In industrialized countries, the most frequent cause of eosinophilic pneumonia is drug hypersensitivity, including reactions to antibiotics, anti-inflammatory agents, cytotoxic drugs and antihypertensive agents. The pulmonary disease resolves without long-term sequelae. The clinical presentations and histologic findings are the same as described above.

The classic form of **infectious eosinophilic pneumonia** associated with parasitic infection is **tropical eosinophilic pneumonia**. Migration of parasites through the lung elicits an acute, self-limited, respiratory illness, characterized clinically by fever, a cough productive of sputum containing eosinophils and transient pulmonary infiltrates.

In temperate zones, *Ascaris lumbricoides* is the usual culprit, but *Toxocara canis* also occasionally is involved. However, the most distinctive infection associated with eosinophilic pneumonia is allergic bronchopulmonary aspergillosis (see above).

In tropical regions, eosinophilic pneumonia is most commonly a response to infestation with the filarial nematodes *Wuchereria bancrofti* and *Brugia malayi*, although other parasites may also be responsible.

Endogenous Lipid Pneumonia Reflects Bronchial Obstruction

This disease, also called "golden pneumonia," is a localized condition distal to an obstructed airway, which is characterized by lipid-laden macrophages in alveolar spaces. The size of the affected area corresponds to the caliber of the involved bronchus. Bronchial obstruction leads to retention of secretions and breakdown products of inflammatory and epithelial cells. Although the protein component is readily digested, lipids are phagocytosed by macrophages, which fill alveoli distal to the obstruction.

 PATHOLOGY: Endogenous lipid pneumonia has a characteristic golden-yellow color, from lipid accumulation within alveolar macrophages. Alveoli are flooded by foamy macrophages with needle-shaped clefts characteristic of cholesterol crystals, with mild chronic inflammation and fibrosis. Alveolar walls are intact. If the obstruction is relieved, the affected lung can return to its normal state unless bronchiectasis and chronic recurrent bronchopneumonia have caused irreversible damage.

Exogenous Lipid Pneumonia Is a Response to Aspirated Oils

Causes of exogenous pneumonia include mineral oil (a laxative and a carrier for medications in nose drops), vegetable oils used in cooking and animal oils ingested in the form of cod-liver oil and other vitamin preparations. Oil-based contrast media used for radiologic bronchography have also been associated with the disorder. Exogenous lipid pneumonia is most common in older individuals, who take nose

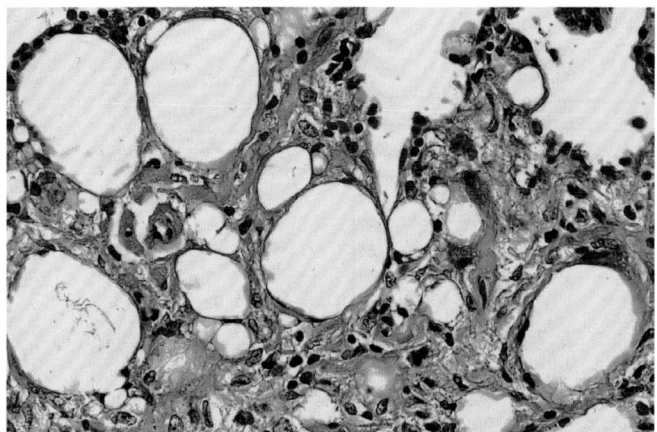

FIGURE 18-39. Exogenous lipoid pneumonia (mineral oil aspiration). The cystic spaces are empty because the lipid was washed out during tissue processing. A giant cell reaction is also present.

drops or laxatives at bedtime and aspirate during sleep. Computed tomography may reveal a spiculated mass that appears worrisome for malignancy. Children may aspirate oily medications while vigorously resisting the dosing.

 PATHOLOGY: Exogenous lipid pneumonia is gray, greasy and poorly demarcated. Foamy macrophages are seen in alveolar and interstitial spaces (Fig. 18-39). Large oil droplets in both locations are surrounded by foreign body granulomas. As processing for paraffin embedding removes most of the oil, there are empty vacuolar spaces in histologic sections. In chronic cases, affected areas may become densely fibrotic.

Patients with exogenous lipid pneumonia are usually asymptomatic; the condition comes to medical attention when a mass simulating an infection or a tumor is seen on a chest radiograph.

OBSTRUCTIVE PULMONARY DISEASES

Several diseases, including chronic bronchitis, emphysema, asthma and in some classifications bronchiectasis and cystic fibrosis, are grouped because they all entail obstruction to airflow in the lungs.

Chronic obstructive pulmonary disease (COPD) includes chronic bronchitis and emphysema, in which forced expiratory volume, measured by spirometry, is decreased.

Airflow can be reduced by increasing resistance to airflow or by reducing outflow pressure. In the lung, narrowed airways produce increased resistance, whereas loss of elastic recoil results in diminished pressure. Airway narrowing occurs in chronic bronchitis or asthma, and emphysema causes loss of recoil.

In Chronic Bronchitis Patients Have a Chronic Productive Cough without a Discernible Cause for 50% or More Days during 2 or More Years

The pathologic definition of the disease is less satisfactory, as its morphologic alterations are a continuum; mild chronic bronchitis may show normal histology.

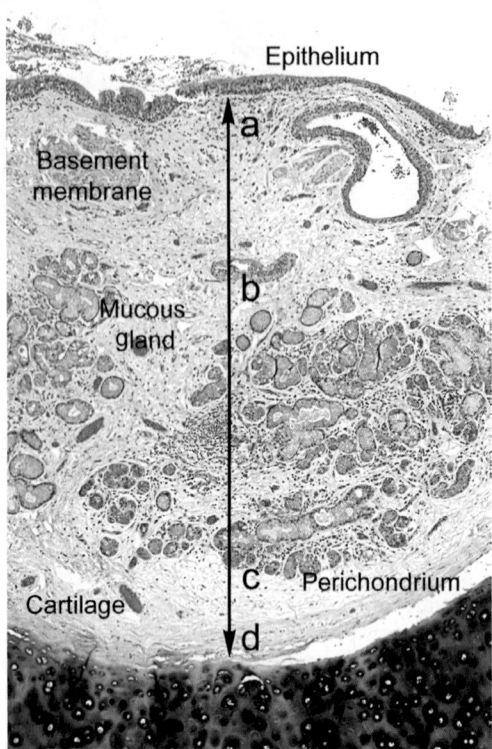

FIGURE 18-40. **Chronic bronchitis.** The bronchial submucosa is greatly expanded by hyperplastic submucosal glands that compose well over 50% of the thickness of the bronchial wall. The Reid index equals the maximum thickness of the bronchial mucous glands internal to the cartilage (*b* to *c*) divided by the bronchial wall thickness (*a* to *d*).

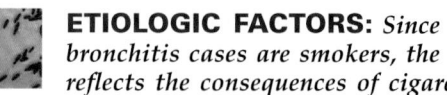

ETIOLOGIC FACTORS: *Since 90% of chronic bronchitis cases are smokers, the disease mainly reflects the consequences of cigarette smoke (see Chapter 8).* Chronic bronchitis occurs in less than 5% of nonsmokers, 10%–15% of moderate smokers and over 25% of heavy smokers. The frequency and severity of acute respiratory tract infections are increased in patients with chronic bronchitis; conversely, infections have been incriminated in its etiology and progression. Chronic bronchitis occurs more often in people in areas of substantial air pollution and in workers exposed to toxic industrial inhalants, but the effects of cigarette smoking far outweigh other contributing factors.

How cigarette smoke and other pollutants injure bronchi is not well understood. Experimentally, rodents that inhale cigarette smoke or SO_2, or are given dilute acids by instillation, exhibit squamous metaplasia of the bronchial epithelium. A similar change occurs when certain proteases are introduced into the bronchi, and this effect can be prevented by pretreating with antiproteases. Bronchial epithelial metaplasia also occurs in rodents given adrenergic and cholinergic agonists, suggesting that autonomic stimulation may play a role in the pathogenesis of chronic bronchitis.

PATHOLOGY: The main pathology in chronic bronchitis is increased bronchial mucus-secreting tissue (Fig. 18-40). Two types of cells line bronchial mucous glands: the more abundant pale mucous cells, and basophilic, granular serous cells. In *chronic bronchitis, mucous cells undergo hyperplasia and hypertrophy and are increased relative to serous cells.* Thus, both individual acini and glands enlarge (Fig. 18-41).

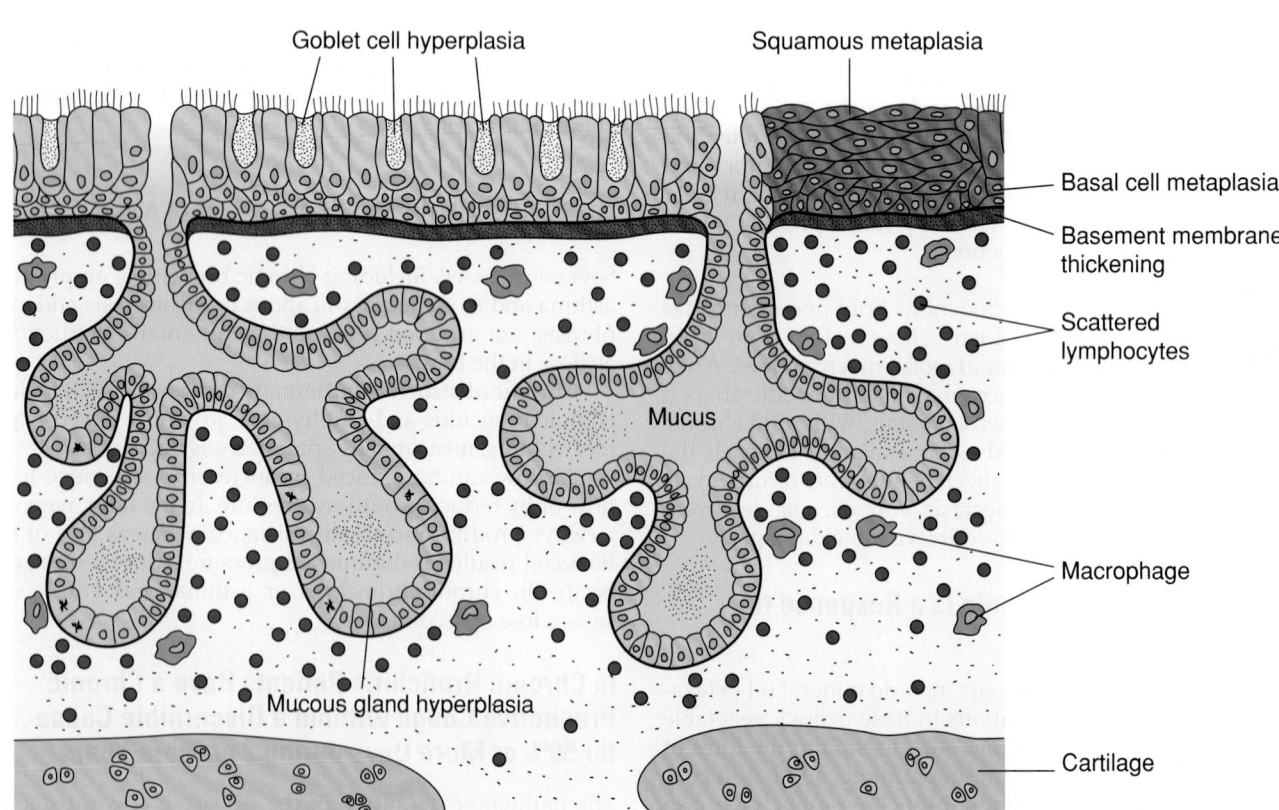

FIGURE 18-41. **Chronic bronchitis.** Morphologic changes in chronic bronchitis.

The Reid index measures the size of the mucous glands (Fig. 18-40): the area occupied by the glands in the plane vertical to the epithelium as a proportion of the thickness of the entire bronchial wall (basement membrane to inner perichondrium). A normal Reid index is 0.4 or less; in chronic bronchitis, it is more than 0.5.

Other morphologic changes in chronic bronchitis are variable and include:

- Excess mucus in central and peripheral airways
- "Pits" on the surface of the bronchial epithelium, which represent dilated ducts into which several bronchial glands open
- Thickening of the bronchial wall by mucous gland enlargement and edema, encroaching on the bronchial lumen
- Increased numbers of goblet cells (hyperplasia) in the bronchial epithelium
- Increased smooth muscle, which may indicate bronchial hyperreactivity
- Squamous metaplasia of the bronchial epithelium, reflecting epithelial damage from tobacco smoke, an effect that is probably independent of the other changes seen in chronic bronchitis

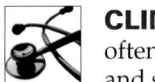 **CLINICAL FEATURES:** Chronic bronchitis is often accompanied by emphysema (see below), and separating the contributions of each in an individual patient may be difficult. In general, patients with mainly chronic bronchitis have had a productive cough for many years. Cough and sputum production are initially more severe in the winter but progress over time from hibernal to perennial. Exertional dyspnea and cyanosis supervene, and cor pulmonale may ensue. The combination of cyanosis and edema due to cor pulmonale has led to the label "blue bloater" for such patients.

In patients with advanced chronic bronchitis, multiple factors such as pulmonary infections, thromboembolism, left ventricular failure and major episodes of air pollution may precipitate acute respiratory failure, with progressive hypoxemia and hypercapnia. Because of retained mucous secretions, people with chronic bronchitis are prone to bacterial lung infections, particularly with *Haemophilus influenzae* and *S. pneumoniae*.

People with chronic bronchitis must be warned to stop smoking. Prompt antibiotic treatment of pulmonary infections, use of bronchodilator drugs and occasionally bronchopulmonary drainage are mainstays of treatment.

Emphysema Causes Overinflation of the Lungs in Smokers

Emphysema is a chronic lung disease in which airspaces distal to terminal bronchioles are enlarged owing to destruction of their walls, without fibrosis. Although it is classified in anatomic terms, the severity of emphysema is more important than the anatomic type. In practical terms, as emphysema becomes more severe, it becomes more difficult to classify. Moreover, several anatomic patterns may be present in the same lung.

 **ETIOLOGIC FACTORS AND PATHOPHYSIOLOGY:** The major cause of emphysema is cigarette smoking. Moderate to severe emphysema is rare in nonsmokers (see Chapter 8). In considering the pathogenesis of emphysema, it is thought that a balance exists between elastin synthesis and catabolism in the normal lung. Emphysema results when elastolytic activity increases or antielastolytic activity is reduced (Fig. 18-42).

Increased numbers of neutrophils, which contain serine elastase and other proteases, are found in the bronchoalveolar lavage fluid of smokers. Smoking also interferes with α_1-antitrypsin (α_1-AT) activity, by oxidizing methionine residues in α_1-antitrypsin. In this way, unopposed and increased elastolytic activity leads to destruction of elastic tissue in the walls of distal airspaces, impairing elastic recoil. At the same time, other cellular proteases may be involved in injury to the airspace walls. This theory, although attractive, awaits further confirmation.

α_1-*ANTITRYPSIN* (α_1-*AT*) *DEFICIENCY:* Hereditary lack of α_1-AT accounts for about 1% of patients with COPD and is much more common in young people with severe emphysema. α_1-AT is a circulating inhibitor of serine proteases, including elastase, trypsin, chymotrypsin, thrombin and bacterial proteases. Made in the liver, it accounts for 90% of blood antiproteinase activity. In the lung, it inhibits neutrophil elastase, an enzyme that digests elastin and other alveolar wall components.

 **MOLECULAR PATHOGENESIS:** The amount and type of α_1-AT is determined by a pair of codominant *Pi* (protease inhibitor) alleles. The most common allele is *PiM and the most common genotype is PiMM*, but more than 100 variants are known. The amount of α_1-AT in the blood depends on the genotype. Some mutant forms fail to fold properly and are thus targeted for proteasomal degradation in liver cells. Other mutant forms may polymerize and accumulate within hepatocytes. The most serious abnormality involves the *PiZ* allele, which occurs in 5% of the population. It is more common in people of Scandinavian origin and is rare in Jews, blacks and Japanese. Because the abnormal protein is poorly secreted by the liver, plasma α_1-AT in *PiZZ* homozygotes is only 15%–20% of normal. These people are at risk for cirrhosis of the liver (see Chapter 20) and emphysema. **Most patients with clinically diagnosed emphysema under age 40 have α_1-AT deficiency (PiZ).** In *PiZZ* homozygotes who do not smoke, emphysema begins between ages 45 and 50; those who smoke develop it 5–10 years earlier. Most nonsmoking *PiZZ* homozygotes show no evidence of emphysema. The association of α_1-AT deficiency with emphysema supports the concept that cigarette smoking by itself causes emphysema by altering the balance of proteases and antiproteases in the lung.

 PATHOLOGY: Emphysema is morphologically classified according to the location of the lesions within the pulmonary acinus (Fig. 18-43). Only the proximal acinus (the respiratory bronchiole) is affected in centrilobular emphysema, whereas the entire acinus is destroyed in panacinar emphysema.

CENTRILOBULAR EMPHYSEMA: This form of emphysema is most common. It usually accompanies cigarette smoking and is symptomatic. The clusters of terminal bronchioles near the end of the bronchiolar tree in the central part of the pulmonary lobule are destroyed (Fig. 18-44A). These are the smallest portion of the lung bounded by septa and

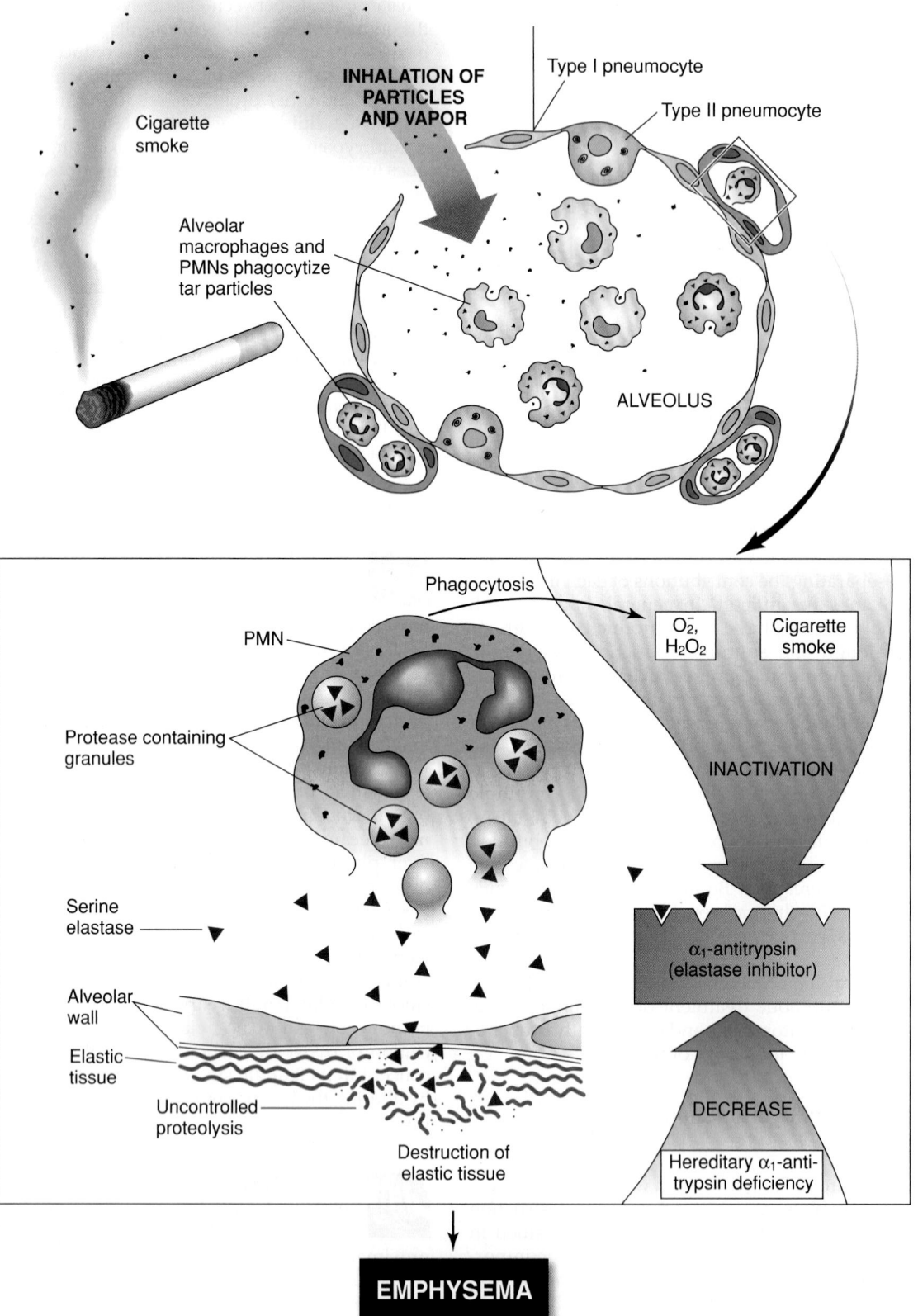

FIGURE 18-42. The proteolysis–antiproteolysis theory of the pathogenesis of emphysema. Cigarette (tobacco) smoking is closely related to the development of emphysema. Some products in tobacco smoke induce an inflammatory reaction. The serine elastase in polymorphonuclear leukocytes, a particularly potent elastolytic agent, injures the elastic tissue of the lung. Normally, this enzyme activity is inhibited by α_1-antitrypsin, but tobacco smoke, directly or through the generation of free radicals, inactivates α_1-antitrypsin (protease inhibitor). H_2O_2 = hydrogen peroxide; O_2^- = superoxide ion; *PMN* = polymorphonuclear neutrophil.

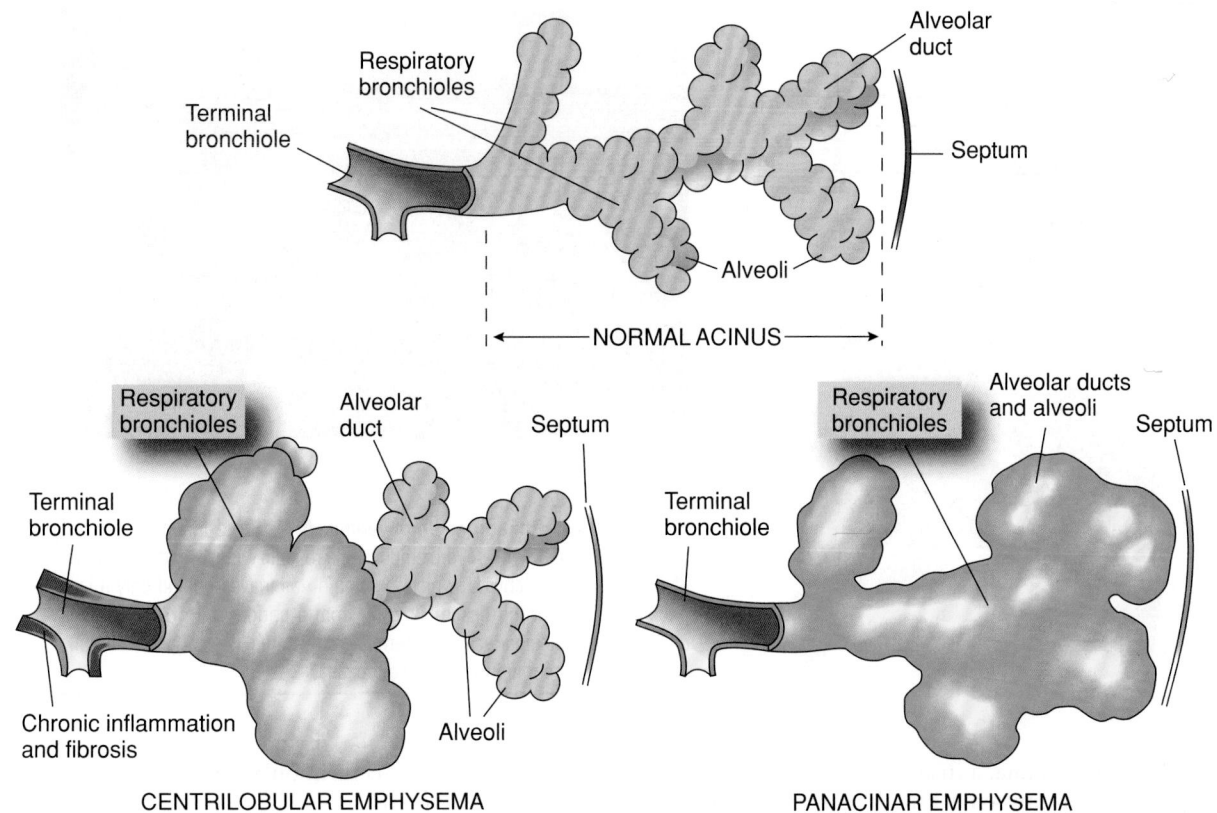

FIGURE 18-43. Types of emphysema. The acinus is the gas-exchanging structural unit of the lung distal to the terminal bronchiole. It consists of (from proximal to distal) respiratory bronchioles, alveolar ducts, alveolar sacs and alveoli. In centrilobular (proximal acinar) emphysema, the respiratory bronchioles are predominantly involved. In paraseptal (distal acinar) emphysema, the alveolar ducts are particularly affected. In panacinar (panlobular) emphysema, the acinus is uniformly damaged.

include several acini. Dilated respiratory bronchioles form enlarged airspaces separated from each other and from lobular septa by normal alveolar ducts and alveoli. As centrilobular emphysema progresses, these distal structures may also be involved (Fig. 18-44B). Bronchioles proximal to emphysematous spaces are inflamed and narrowed. Centrilobular emphysema is most severe in the upper lobes and in superior segments of the lower lobes.

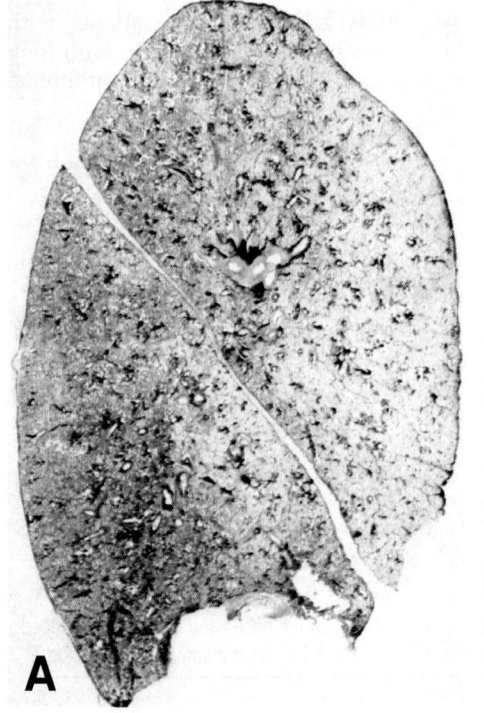

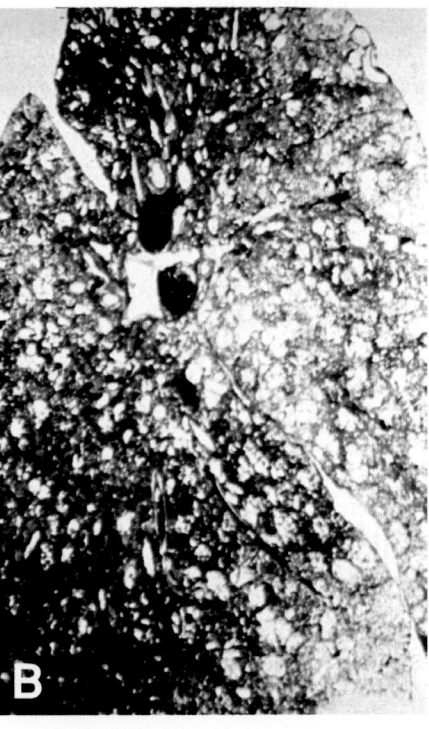

FIGURE 18-44. Centrilobular emphysema. A. A whole mount of the left lung of a smoker with mild emphysema shows enlarged airspaces scattered throughout both lobes, which represent destruction of the terminal bronchioles in the central part of the pulmonary lobule. These abnormal spaces are surrounded by intact pulmonary parenchyma. **B.** In a more advanced case of centrilobular emphysema, destruction of the lung has progressed to produce large, irregular airspaces.

THE RESPIRATORY SYSTEM

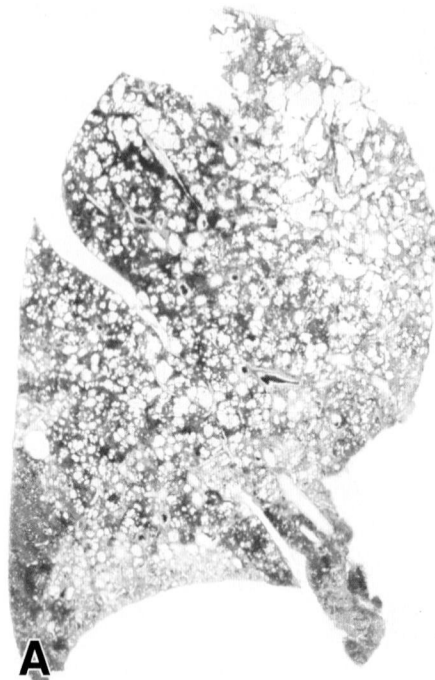

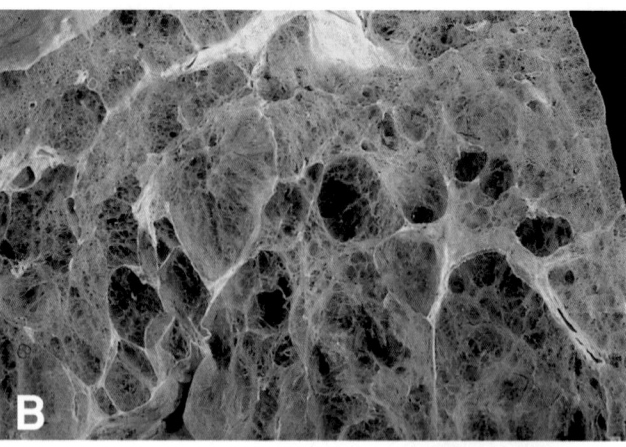

FIGURE 18-45. Panacinar emphysema. A. A whole mount of the left lung from a patient with severe emphysema reveals widespread destruction of pulmonary parenchyma, which in some areas leaves behind only a lacy network of supporting tissue. **B.** Lung from a patient with α_1-antitrypsin deficiency shows a panacinar pattern of emphysema. Loss of alveolar walls has resulted in markedly enlarged airspaces.

Focal dust emphysema, a disease of coal miners, resembles centrilobular emphysema but differs in that affected spaces are smaller and more regular and lack inflammation of the bronchioles. The lesions mainly distend, rather than destroy, alveolar walls. This disease is discussed below with coal workers' pneumoconiosis.

PANACINAR EMPHYSEMA: In panacinar emphysema, acini are uniformly involved, with destruction of alveolar septa from the center to the periphery of acini (Fig. 18-45). Loss of alveolar septa is illustrated by histologic comparison of normal lungs with those affected by α_1-AT deficiency (Fig. 18-46). In its final stage, panacinar emphysema leaves behind a lacy network of supporting tissue ("cotton-candy lung"). This type of emphysema is typically associated with α_1-AT deficiency. But it may also occur in cigarette smokers in association with centrilobular emphysema, in which cases the panacinar pattern tends to occur in more basal lung zones, while centrilobular emphysema prefers upper regions (see above).

LOCALIZED EMPHYSEMA: This disease, once called "paraseptal emphysema," entails alveolar destruction and leads to emphysema at only one or at most a few locations. The remainder of the lungs is normal. The lesion is usually found at the apex of an upper lobe in a subpleural location but may occur anywhere (Fig. 18-47). It is not clinically significant itself, but a focus of localized emphysema may rupture and cause spontaneous pneumothorax (see below). Localized emphysema can also progress to large areas of destruction, or **bullae,** which can be as small as 2 cm or can occupy an entire hemithorax.

 CLINICAL FEATURES: Most patients with emphysema present at age 60 or older, with long histories of exertional dyspnea but minimal,

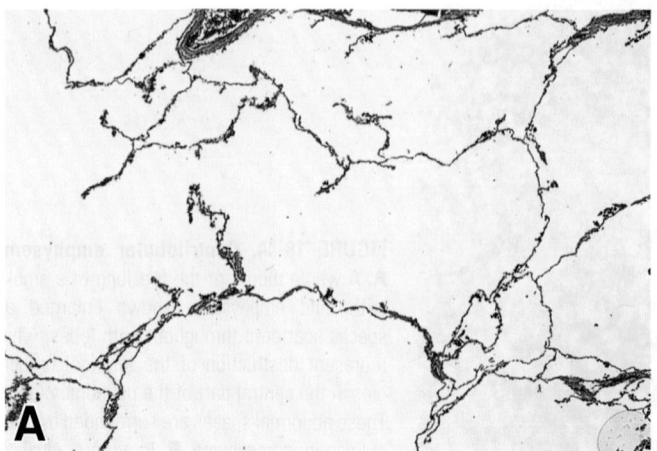

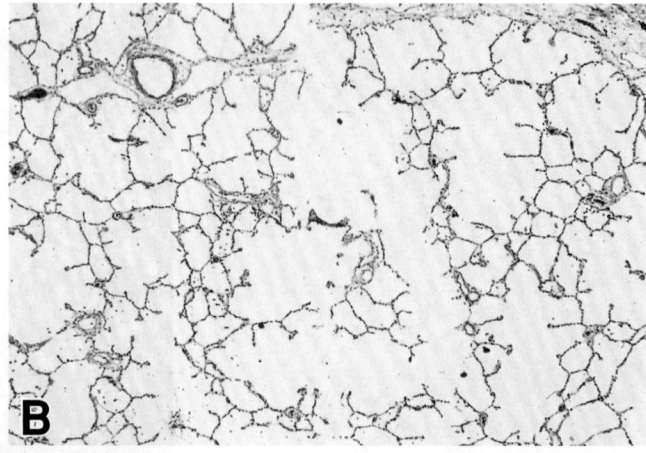

FIGURE 18-46. Panacinar emphysema. A. This lung, from a patient with α_1-antitrypsin deficiency, shows large, irregular airspaces and a markedly reduced number of alveolar walls. **B.** Extensive loss of alveolar walls in **A** is emphasized by comparison with this section of normal lung at the same magnification.

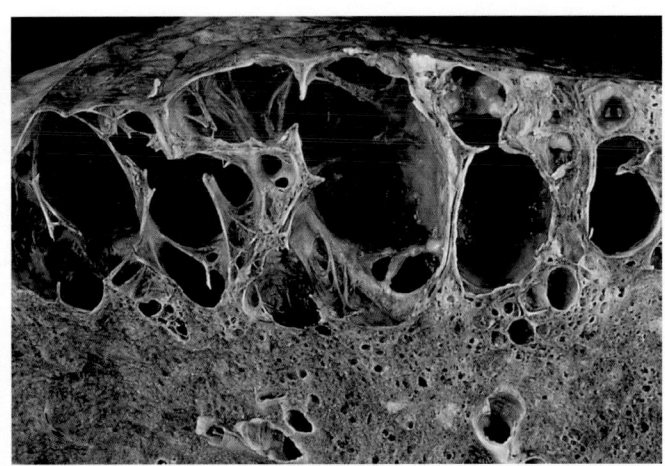

FIGURE 18-47. Localized emphysema. The subpleural parenchyma shows markedly enlarged airspaces owing to the loss of alveolar tissue.

nonproductive cough. They have lost weight and use accessory muscles of respiration to breathe. Weight loss is probably due less to lack of calories than to the increased work of breathing. Tachypnea and a prolonged expiratory phase are typical. Radiologically, the lungs are overinflated: they are enlarged, diaphragms are depressed and the posteroanterior diameter is increased (barrel chest). Bronchovascular markings do not reach the peripheral lung fields. Since these patients have increased respiratory rates and minute volumes, they can maintain arterial hemoglobin saturation at near-normal levels and so are called "pink puffers." Unlike patients with predominantly chronic bronchitis, those with emphysema are not at higher risk for recurrent pulmonary infections and are not so prone to develop cor pulmonale. Emphysema entails an inexorable decline in respiratory function and progressive dyspnea, for which no treatment is adequate.

In Asthma a Number of Stimuli Trigger Episodic Airflow Obstruction

Asthmatic patients typically have paroxysms of wheezing, dyspnea and cough. Attacks may alternate with asymptomatic periods or be superimposed on a background of chronic airway obstruction. Severe acute asthma that is unresponsive to therapy is **status asthmaticus**. Most asthmatic patients, even when apparently well, have some persistent airflow obstruction and morphologic lesions.

In the United States, bronchial asthma affects up to 10% of children and 5% of adults. The prevalence of asthma in the United States has doubled since 1980. Initial asthma attacks may occur at any age, but half of cases begin in patients under age 10, and they are twice as common in boys as in girls. By age 30, both sexes are affected equally.

ETIOLOGIC FACTORS: Asthma was once divided into **extrinsic (allergic)** and **intrinsic (idiosyncratic)** forms, depending on inciting factors. Asthma is now described in terms of the different inciting factors and the common effector pathways.

Bronchial hyperresponsiveness in asthma generally reflects inflammatory reactions to diverse stimuli. After exposure to an inciting factor (e.g., allergens, drugs, cold, exercise), inflammatory mediators released by activated macrophages, mast cells, eosinophils and basophils trigger bronchoconstriction, increased vascular permeability and mucous secretion. Resident inflammatory cells release chemotactic factors, which in turn recruit more effector cells and amplify the response of the airways. Inflammation of bronchial walls also may injure the epithelium, stimulating nerve endings and initiating neural reflexes that further aggravate and propagate the bronchospasm.

Many inflammatory mediators and chemotactic factors may participate in the bronchospasm and mucous hypersecretion of asthma. The relative contributions of the different substances probably vary with the inciting stimulus. The best-studied situation associated with the induction of asthma is inhaled allergens.

In a sensitized person, an inhaled allergen interacts with T_H2 cells and IgE antibody bound to the surface of mast cells, which are interspersed among the bronchial epithelial cells (Fig. 18-48). The T_H2 cells and mast cells release mediators of type I (immediate) hypersensitivity, including histamine, bradykinin, leukotrienes, prostaglandins, thromboxane A_2 and platelet-activating factor (PAF), as well as cytokines such as interleukin (IL)-4 and IL-5. These inflammatory mediators lead to (1) **smooth muscle contraction,** (2) **mucous secretion** and (3) **increased vascular permeability and edema.** Each of these effects is a potent, albeit reversible, cause of airway obstruction. IL-5 causes terminal differentiation of eosinophils in the bone marrow. Chemotactic factors, including leukotriene B_4 and neutrophil and eosinophil chemotactic factors, attract neutrophils, eosinophils and platelets to the bronchial wall. Eosinophils then release leukotriene B_4 and PAF, aggravating bronchoconstriction and edema. Discharge of eosinophil granules containing eosinophil cationic protein and major basic protein into the bronchial lumen further impairs mucociliary function and damages epithelial cells. Epithelial cell injury is suspected to stimulate nerve endings in the mucosa, initiating autonomic discharge that contributes to airway narrowing and mucus secretion. Leukotriene B_4 and PAF recruit more eosinophils and other effector cells, and thus act to prolong and amplify the attack.

Bronchial epithelium also plays a role in the pathogenesis of various asthma phenotypes. The barrier function of the bronchial epithelium is impaired, with disruption of tight junctions and increased permeability. The mucosal epithelium itself also secretes various cytokines and chemokines that participate in regulating cells of the immune system. Since the bronchial mucosa is the first structure to come into contact with inhaled allergens and infectious agents, the importance of epithelial cells in the pathogenesis of asthma has recently been emphasized.

ALLERGIC ASTHMA: This is the most common form of asthma and is usually seen in children. One third to one half of all patients with asthma have known or suspected reactions to such allergens as pollens, animal hair or fur and house dust contaminated with mites. Allergic asthma correlates strongly with skin-test reactivity. Half of children with asthma have substantial or complete remission of symptoms by age 20, but in many, asthma may recur after age 30.

INFECTIOUS ASTHMA: A common precipitating factor in childhood asthma is a viral respiratory tract infection rather than an allergic stimulus. In children under 2 years of age, RSV is the usual agent; in older children, rhinovirus,

A IMMEDIATE RESPONSE

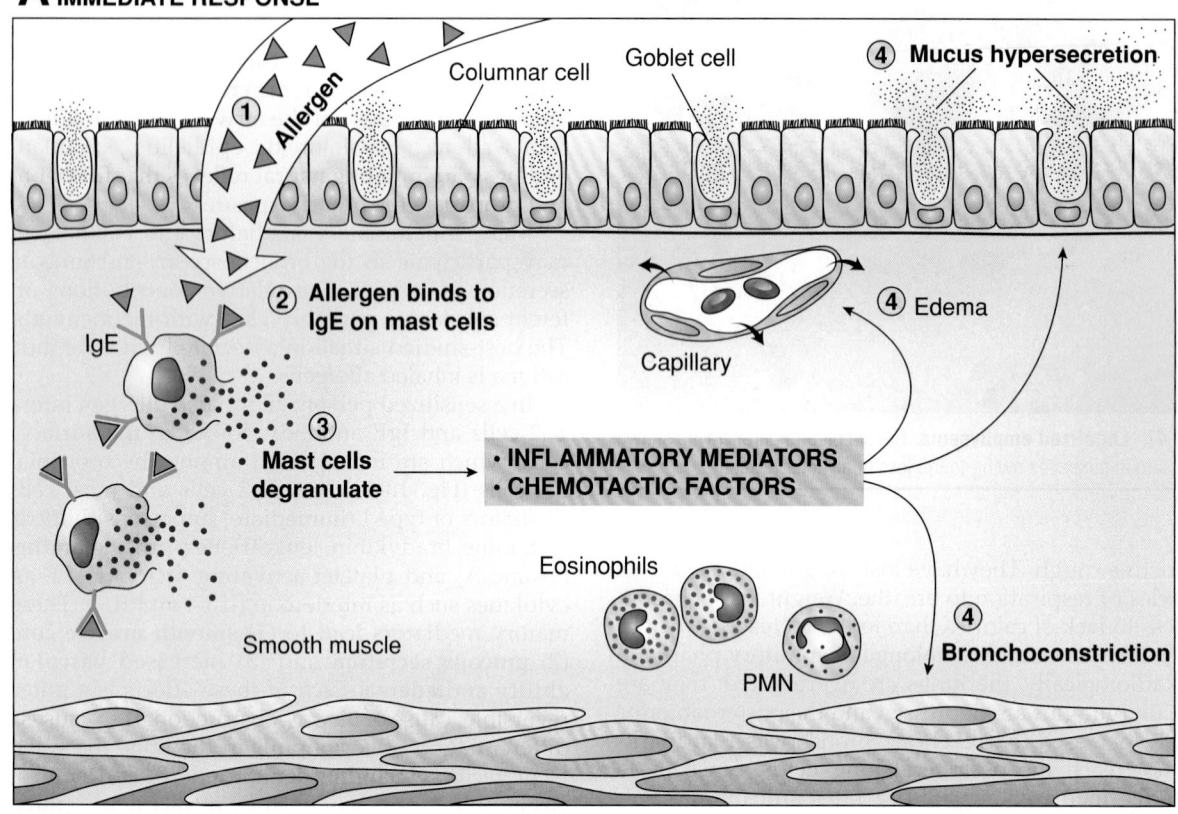

B DELAYED RESPONSE

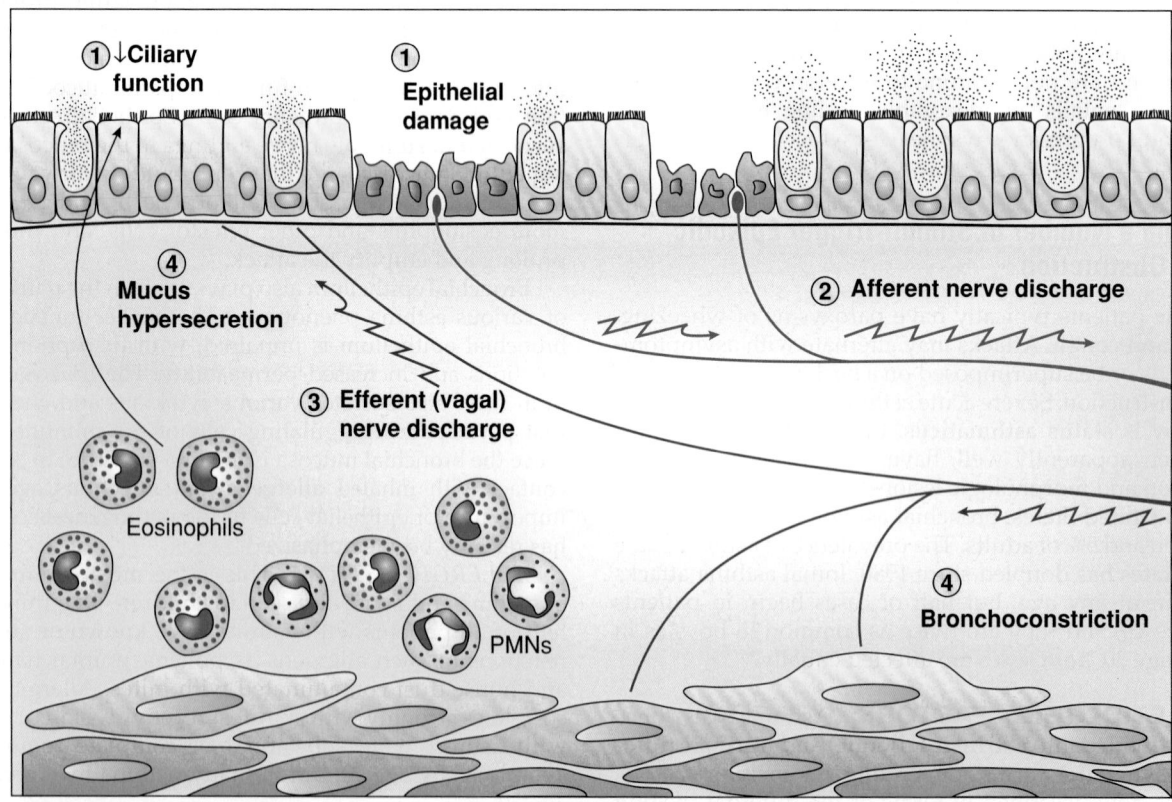

FIGURE 18-48. Pathogenesis of asthma. A. Immunologically mediated asthma. Allergens interact with immunoglobulin E (IgE) on mast cells, either on the surface of the epithelium or, when there is abnormal permeability of the epithelium, in the submucosa. Released mediators may react locally or by vagal reflexes. **B.** Discharge of eosinophilic granules further impairs mucociliary function and damages epithelial cells. Epithelial cell injury stimulates nerve endings (*in red*) in the mucosa, initiating an autonomic discharge that contributes to airway narrowing and mucus secretion. *PMNs* = polymorphonuclear neutrophils.

influenza and parainfluenza are common inciting organisms. Inflammatory responses to viral infection in susceptible people may trigger the episode of bronchoconstriction. In support of this hypothesis, bronchial hyperreactivity may persist for as long as 2 months after a viral infection in non-asthmatics.

EXERCISE-INDUCED ASTHMA: Exercise can precipitate bronchospasm in more than half of all asthmatics. In some patients, it may be the only inciting factor. Exercise-induced asthma is related to the magnitude of heat or water loss from airway epithelium. The more rapid the ventilation (severity of exercise) and the colder and drier the air breathed, the more likely is an attack of asthma. Thus, an asthmatic playing hockey on an outdoor rink in Canada in winter is more likely to have an attack than one swimming slowly in Texas during the summer. The mechanisms underlying exercise-induced asthma are unclear. It may be related to mediator release or vascular congestion secondary to rewarming of bronchi after the exertion.

OCCUPATIONAL ASTHMA: More than 80 different occupational exposures have been linked to asthma. Some substances may provoke allergic asthma via IgE-related hypersensitivity (e.g., in animal handlers, bakers and workers exposed to wood and vegetable dusts, metal salts, pharmaceutical agents and industrial chemicals). Occupational asthma may also result from direct release of mediators of smooth muscle contraction after contact with an offending agent, as is postulated in byssinosis ("brown lung"), an occupational lung disease of cotton workers. Some occupational exposures affect the autonomic nervous system directly. For instance, organic phosphorus insecticides act as anticholinesterases and produce overactivity of the parasympathetic nervous system. Substances such as toluene diisocyanate and western red cedar dust are thought to operate through hypersensitivity mechanisms, although specific IgE antibodies to these substances have not been identified.

DRUG-INDUCED ASTHMA: Drug-induced bronchospasm occurs mostly in patients with known asthma. The best-known offender is aspirin, but other nonsteroidal anti-inflammatory agents also have been implicated. Up to 10% of adult asthmatics may be sensitive to aspirin. Immediate hypersensitivity does not seem to be involved, and these patients can be desensitized by daily administrations of small doses of aspirin. Rhinitis and nasal polyps are also common in these individuals. β-Adrenergic antagonists consistently induce bronchoconstriction in asthmatics and are contraindicated in such patients.

AIR POLLUTION: Massive air pollution, usually occurring during temperature inversions, may cause bronchospasm in patients with asthma and other preexisting lung diseases. Gasses such as SO_2, nitrogen oxides and ozone are commonly implicated, but particulate carbon, carrying toxic chemicals in diesel exhaust, may also participate.

EMOTIONAL FACTORS: Psychological stress can aggravate or precipitate attacks of bronchospasm in as many as half of asthmatics. Vagal efferent stimulation is thought to be the underlying mechanism.

 PATHOLOGY: The pathology of asthma has been studied in autopsies of patients who died in status asthmaticus, where the most severe lesions are described. Grossly, the lungs are highly distended with air, and airways are filled with thick, tenacious, adherent mucous plugs. Microscopically, these plugs (Fig. 18-49A) contain strips of epithelium and many eosinophils. Charcot-Leyden crystals, derived from phospholipids of the eosinophil cell membrane, are also seen (Fig. 18-24B). In some

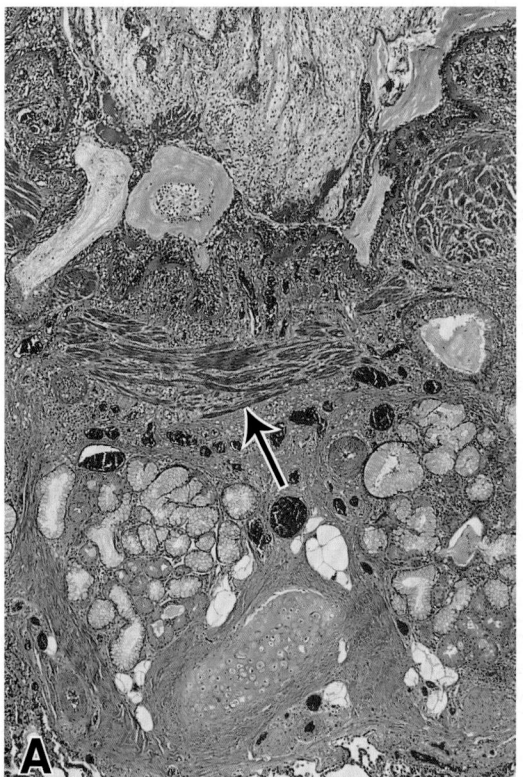

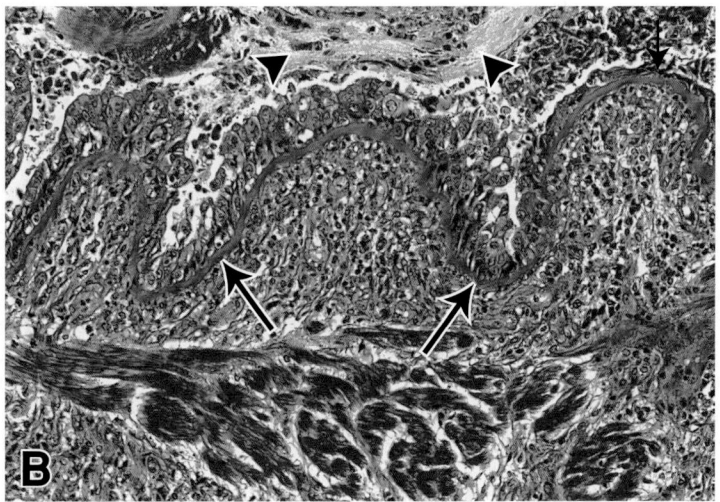

FIGURE 18-49. Asthma. A. A section of lung from a patient who died in status asthmaticus reveals a bronchus containing a luminal mucous plug, submucosal gland hyperplasia and smooth muscle hyperplasia (*arrow*). **B.** Higher magnification shows hyaline thickening of the subepithelial basement membrane (*long arrows*) and marked inflammation of the bronchiolar wall, with numerous eosinophils. The mucosa exhibits an inflamed and metaplastic epithelium (*arrowheads*). The epithelium is focally denuded (*short arrow*).

cases, mucoid casts of the airways (Curschmann spirals) may be expelled with coughing, as may compact clusters of epithelial cells (Creola bodies).

One of the most characteristic features of status asthmaticus is hyperplasia of bronchial smooth muscle. Bronchial submucosal mucous glands are also hyperplastic (Fig. 18-49A). The submucosa is edematous, with a mixed inflammatory infiltrate containing variable numbers of eosinophils. The epithelium does not show the normal pseudostratified appearance and may be denuded, with only basal cells remaining (Fig. 18-49B). The basal cells are hyperplastic, and squamous metaplasia and goblet cell hyperplasia are seen. Bronchial epithelial basement membranes are thickened, owing to an increase in collagen deep to the true basal lamina.

 CLINICAL FEATURES: A typical attack of asthma begins with tightness in the chest and nonproductive cough. Inspiratory *and* expiratory wheezes appear, respiratory rate increases and the patient becomes dyspneic. The expiratory phase is particularly prolonged. The attack often ends with fits of severe coughing and expectoration of thick, mucus-containing Curschmann spirals, eosinophils and Charcot-Leyden crystals.

Status asthmaticus is severe bronchoconstriction that does not respond to drugs that usually abort the acute attack. It is serious and requires hospitalization. Patients in status asthmaticus have hypoxemia and often hypercapnia. They require oxygen and other pharmacologic interventions. Severe episodes may be fatal. The cornerstone of asthma treatment includes administration of β-adrenergic agonists, inhaled corticosteroids, cromolyn sodium, methylxanthines and anticholinergic agents. Systemic corticosteroids are reserved for status asthmaticus or resistant chronic asthma. The inhalation of bronchodilators often provides dramatic relief.

PNEUMOCONIOSES

Pneumoconioses are pulmonary diseases caused by mineral dust inhalation. Over 40 inhaled minerals cause lung lesions and radiographic abnormalities. Most, like tin, barium and iron, are innocuous and simply accumulate in the lung. However, some lead to crippling lung diseases. The specific types of pneumoconioses are named by the substance inhaled (e.g., silicosis, asbestosis, talcosis). Sometimes, the offending agent is uncertain, and the occupation is simply cited (e.g., "arc welder's lung"), as before etiologies were identified, some occupations were known to predispose to lung disease. Thus, "knife grinder's lung" was used before the disease was recognized as silicosis.

 **ETIOLOGIC FACTORS:** *The key factor in the genesis of symptomatic pneumoconioses is the capacity of inhaled dusts to stimulate fibrosis* (Fig. 18-50). Thus, small amounts of silica produce extensive fibrosis, whereas coal and iron are only weakly fibrogenic.

In general, lung lesions produced by inorganic dusts reflect the dose and size of inhaled particles. The dose is a function of the concentration of dust in the air and the duration of exposure. As inhaled particles are often irregular, their size should be expressed as aerodynamic particle diameter, a parameter that describes the particle's motion in inspired air and that determines where inhaled dusts deposit in the lung (Fig. 18-2, Chapter 8). The most dangerous particles are those that reach the farthest periphery (i.e., the smallest bronchioles and acini). Particles 2.5–10 μm in diameter deposit on bronchi and bronchioles and are removed by mucociliary action. Smaller particles (<2.5 μm) reach acini, and the tiniest ones (<100 nm) may penetrate alveolar walls and enter the bloodstream.

Alveolar macrophages ingest inhaled particles and are the main defenders of the alveolar space. Most phagocytosed particles ascend to the mucociliary carpet, to be coughed up or swallowed. Others migrate into the lung interstitium, and thence into lymphatics. Many ingested particles accumulate in and about respiratory bronchioles and terminal bronchioles. Others are not phagocytosed but migrate through epithelial cells into the interstitium.

Silicosis Is Caused by Inhaled Silicon Dioxide (Silica)

The earth's crust is composed largely of silicon and its oxides, and silicosis is one of the oldest recorded diseases, possibly having begun in the Paleolithic period when humans began to fashion flint instruments. Dyspnea in metal diggers was reported by Hippocrates, and early Dutch pathologists wrote that the lungs of stone cutters sectioned like a mass of sand. The 19th-century English literature provided numerous descriptions of silicosis, and the disease remained the major cause of death in workers exposed to silica dust for the first half of the 20th century.

Silicosis was first described as a disease of sandblasters, but exposure to silica occurs in many occupations, including mining, stone cutting, polishing and sharpening of metals, ceramic manufacturing, foundry work and cleaning of boilers. The use of air-handling equipment and face masks has substantially reduced the incidence of silicosis.

 **ETIOLOGIC FACTORS:** The biological effects of silica particles depend on a number of factors, some involving the particle itself and others related to the host response. Crystalline silica (quartz) is more toxic than amorphous forms, and its biological activity is related to its surface properties. Particles of 0.2–2.0 μm are the most dangerous. Removal of the soluble surface layer by acid washing or creation of new surfaces by sandblasting enhances the biological activity of silica particles.

After their inhalation, silica particles are ingested by alveolar macrophages. Silicon hydroxide groups on the particles' surface form hydrogen bonds with phospholipids and proteins. This interaction damages cellular membranes and so kills the macrophages. The dead cells release free silica particles and fibrogenic factors. The released silica is then reingested by macrophages and the process is amplified.

 PATHOLOGY:
SIMPLE NODULAR SILICOSIS: This is the most common form of silicosis and is almost inevitable in any worker with long-term exposure to silica. Twenty to 40 years (but sometimes only 10 years) after initial exposure to silica, the lungs contain silicotic nodules less than 1 cm in diameter (usually 2–4 mm). Histologically, they have

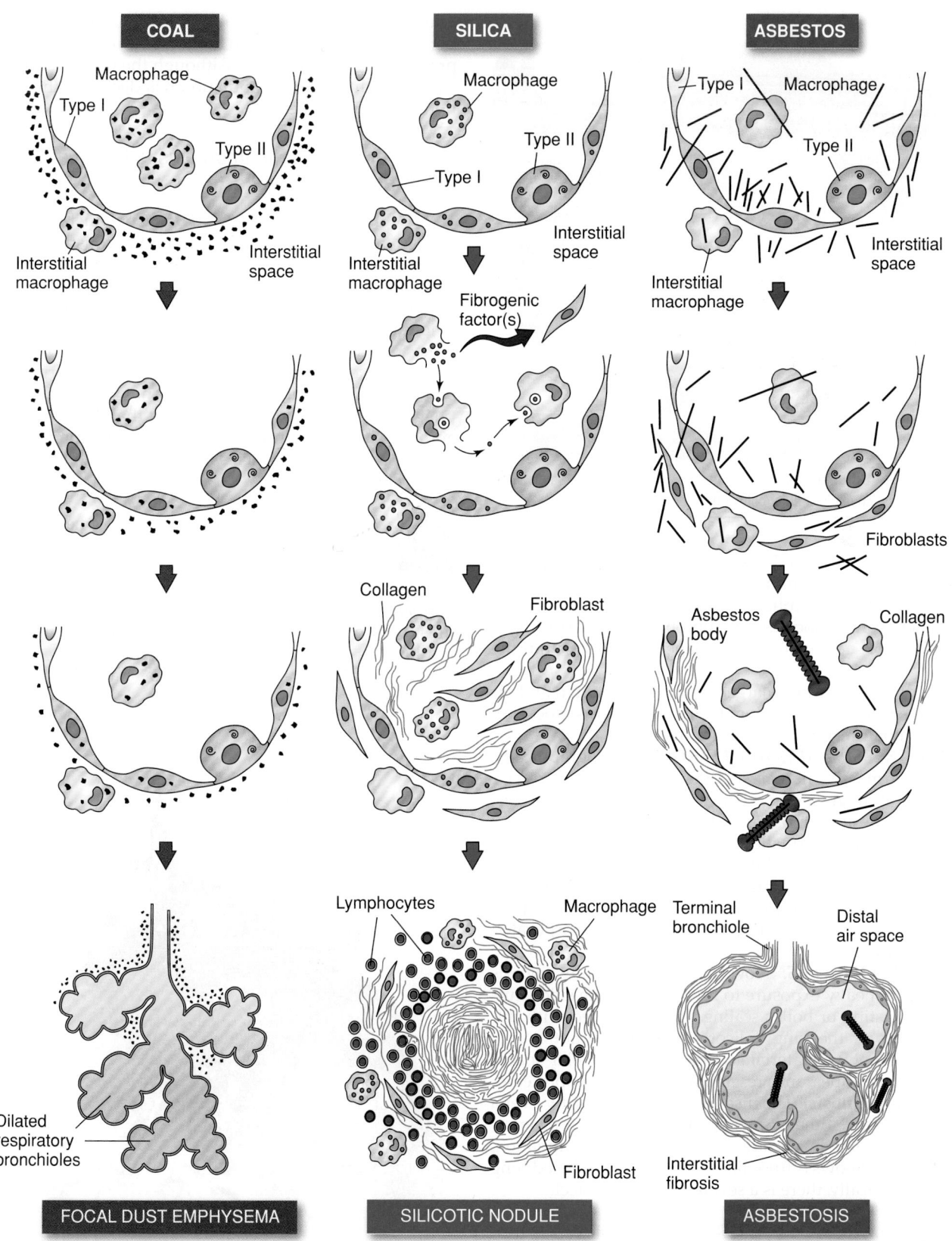

FIGURE 18-50. Pathogenesis of pneumoconioses. The three most important pneumoconioses are illustrated. In simple coal workers' pneumoconi-osis, massive amounts of dust are inhaled and engulfed by macrophages. The macrophages pass into the interstitium of the lung and aggregate around respiratory bronchioles, which subsequently dilate. In silicosis, silica particles are toxic to macrophages, causing them to die and release a fibrogenic factor. In turn, the released silica is again phagocytosed by other macrophages. The result is a dense fibrotic nodule, the silicotic nodule. Asbestosis is characterized by considerable interstitial fibrosis. Asbestos bodies are the classic features.

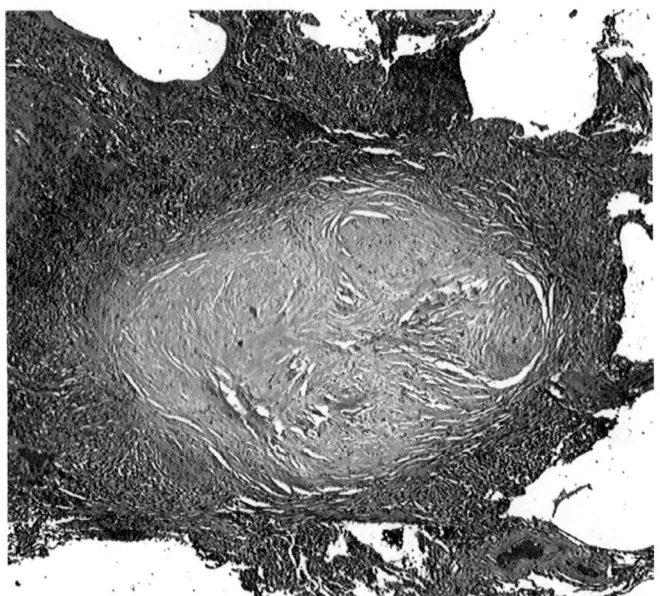

FIGURE 18-51. Silicosis. A silicotic nodule is composed of concentric whorls of dense, sparsely cellular collagen.

a characteristic whorled appearance, with concentrically arranged collagen forming the largest part of the nodule (Fig. 18-51). At the periphery are aggregates of mononuclear cells, mostly lymphocytes and fibroblasts. Polarized light reveals doubly refractile needle-shaped silicates within the nodule.

Hilar nodes may be enlarged and calcified, often at their edges ("eggshell calcification"). Simple silicosis does not usually impair respiration significantly.

PROGRESSIVE MASSIVE FIBROSIS: Radiographically, progressive massive fibrosis signifies nodular masses greater than 2 cm in diameter, in a background of simple silicosis. These larger lesions, most of which are 5–10 cm across, represent coalescence of smaller nodules and are usually in the upper zones of the lungs bilaterally (Fig. 18-52). The lesions often exhibit central cavitation. Progressive massive fibrosis is related to the amount of silica in the lung. Disability is caused by destruction of lung tissue that was incorporated into the nodules.

ACUTE SILICOSIS: Now uncommon, acute silicosis results from heavy exposure to finely particulate silica during sandblasting or boiler scaling. It is associated with diffuse fibrosis of the lung. Silicotic nodules are not found. Dense eosinophilic material accumulates in alveolar spaces to produce an appearance resembling alveolar lipoproteinosis **(silicoproteinosis)**. The disease progresses rapidly over a few years, unlike other forms of silicosis in which progression is measured in decades. On radiologic examination, acute silicosis shows diffuse linear fibrosis and reduced lung volume. Clinically, there is a severe restrictive defect.

 CLINICAL FEATURES: Simple silicosis is usually a radiologic diagnosis without significant symptoms. Dyspnea on exertion and later at rest suggests progressive massive fibrosis or other complications of silicosis. In acute silicosis, dyspnea may become rapidly disabling, after which respiratory failure ensues.

It is well recognized that **tuberculosis** is much more common in patients with silicosis than in the general population.

The incidence of tuberculosis in patients with silicosis is higher in acute silicosis and among populations with a high prevalence of tuberculosis. Although the incidence of tuberculosis in the general population has declined, the association with silicosis persists.

Coal Workers' Pneumoconiosis Is Due to Inhalation of Carbon Particles

 **ETIOLOGIC FACTORS:** Coal dust is composed of amorphous carbon and other constituents of the earth's surface, including variable amounts of silica. Anthracite (hard) coal contains significantly more quartz than does bituminous (soft) coal. Workers who inhale large amounts of quartz particles, such as those who work within mines, are at greater risk than those working above ground or loading coal for transport. In this context, amorphous carbon by itself is not fibrogenic. It does not kill alveolar macrophages, but is simply a nuisance dust that causes innocuous anthracosis. By contrast, silica is highly fibrogenic, and inhaled anthracotic particles may thus lead to **anthracosilicosis** (Fig. 18-53).

 PATHOLOGY: Coal workers' pneumoconiosis (CWP) is typically divided into **simple CWP** and **complicated CWP** (a.k.a. progressive massive fibrosis). The typical lung lesions of simple CWP include nonpalpable **coal-dust macules** and palpable **coal-dust nodules,** both of which are multiple and scattered throughout the lung as 1–4-mm black foci. Microscopically, coal-dust macules contain many carbon-laden macrophages, which

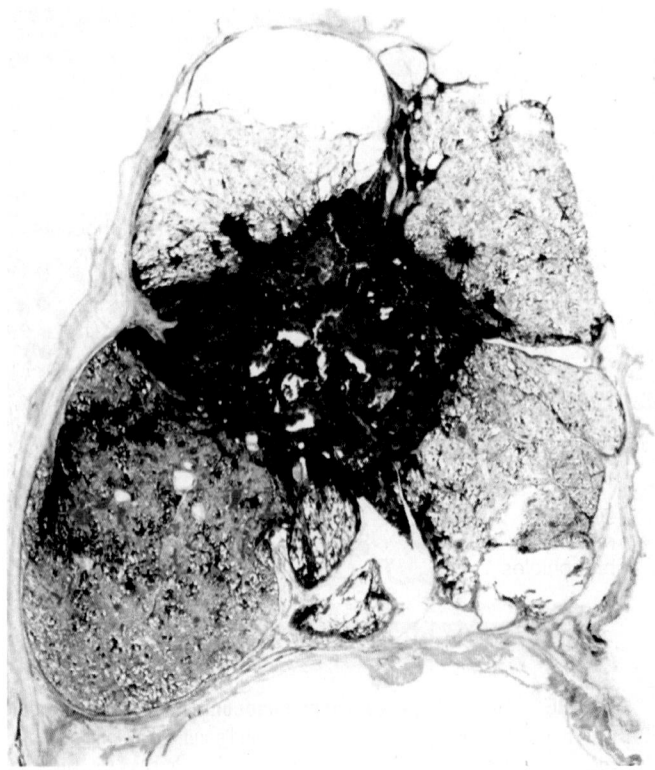

FIGURE 18-52. Progressive massive fibrosis. A whole mount of a silicotic lung from a coal miner shows a large area of dense fibrosis containing entrapped carbon particles.

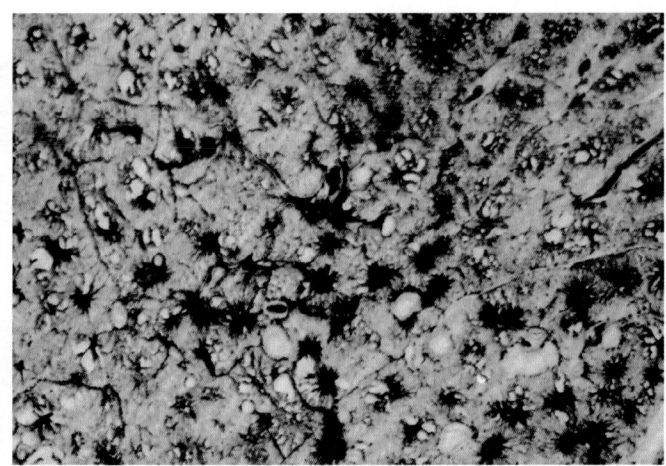

FIGURE 18-53. Anthracosilicosis. A whole mount of the lung of a coal miner demonstrates scattered, irregular, pigmented nodules throughout the parenchyma.

surround distal respiratory bronchioles, extend to fill adjacent alveolar spaces and infiltrate peribronchiolar interstitial spaces. Respiratory bronchioles may be mildly dilated (focal dust emphysema), probably owing to atrophy of smooth muscle.

Nodules are round or irregular, may or may not be associated with bronchioles and consist of dust-laden macrophages associated with a fibrotic stroma. They occur when coal is admixed with fibrogenic dusts such as silica, and are more properly classified as anthracosilicosis (Fig. 18-53). Coal-dust macules and nodules appear on chest radiographs as small nodular densities. Simple CWP was once thought to cause severe disability, but it is now clear that at worst it causes minor impairment of lung function. If coal miners have severe airflow obstruction, it is usually due to smoking. **Complicated CWP** occurs on a background of simple CWP and is defined as a lesion 2.0 cm or greater in size. It may cause significant respiratory impairment.

Caplan syndrome was first described as rheumatoid nodules **(Caplan nodules)** in the lungs of coal miners with rheumatoid arthritis. However, it now also refers to the association of pulmonary rheumatoid nodules with other pneumoconioses, such as silicosis or asbestosis. The nodular lesions are large (1–10 cm), multiple, bilateral and usually peripheral. Microscopically, they resemble rheumatoid nodules associated with inhaled dust deposits. Rheumatoid nodules are large, central, necrotic areas with a border of chronic inflammation and palisading macrophages (see Chapters 11 and 30). Caplan nodules are not identical to rheumatoid nodules and may represent a combination of silicotic and rheumatoid nodules.

Asbestos-Related Diseases May Be Reactive or Neoplastic

Asbestos (Greek, "unquenchable") includes a group of fibrous silicate minerals that occur as thin fibers. It has been used for diverse purposes for over 4000 years, since early Finns fashioned pottery from it. Roman vestal virgins used it to manufacture oil-lamp wicks, and Marco Polo remarked that asbestos-containing Chinese cloth resisted fire. More recently, asbestos has been used in insulation, construction materials and automative brake linings. Asbestos mining proceeded exponentially in the 20th century until its deleterious effects eventually elicited alarm.

There are six natural types of asbestos, which can be divided into two mineralogic groups. **Chrysotile** accounts for the bulk of commercially used asbestos. The **amphiboles** include amosite, crocidolite, tremolite, actinolite and anthophyllite. Of the amphiboles, only amosite and crocidolite have been used commercially to any significant extent. Erionite, a fibrous zeolite, is found in Turkey and adjacent areas. It has pathogenic properties similar to the amphiboles. Exposure to asbestos can cause asbestosis, benign pleural effusion, pleural plaques, diffuse pleural fibrosis, rounded atelectasis and mesothelioma (Table 18-4). All commercially used forms of asbestos are associated with lung diseases, but the amphiboles, and crocidolite in particular, have a much greater propensity to produce disease than does chrysotile.

ASBESTOSIS: Asbestosis is diffuse interstitial fibrosis resulting from inhalation of asbestos fibers. Development of asbestosis requires heavy exposure to asbestos of the type historically seen in asbestos miners, millers and insulators.

 **ETIOLOGIC FACTORS:** Asbestos fibers may be long (up to 100 μm) but thin (0.5–1 μm), so their aerodynamic particle diameter is small. They deposit in distal airways and alveoli, particularly at bifurcations of alveolar ducts. The smallest particles are engulfed by macrophages, but many larger fibers penetrate into the interstitial space. The first lesion is an alveolitis that is directly related to asbestos exposure. Release of inflammatory mediators by activated macrophages and the fibrogenic character of the free asbestos fibers in the interstitium promote interstitial pulmonary fibrosis.

 PATHOLOGY: Asbestosis is characterized by bilateral, diffuse interstitial fibrosis and asbestos bodies in the lung (Figs. 18-54 and 18-55). In early stages, fibrosis occurs in and around alveolar ducts and respiratory bronchioles, and in the periphery of the acinus. When the fibers deposit in bronchioles and respiratory bronchioles, they incite a fibrogenic response that leads to mild chronic airflow obstruction. Thus, asbestos may produce obstructive as well as restrictive defects. As the disease progresses, fibrosis spreads beyond the peribronchiolar location and eventually results in an end-stage or "honeycomb" lung. Asbestosis is usually more severe in the lower zones of the lung.

TABLE 18-4
ASBESTOS-RELATED LUNG DISEASE
Pleural Lesions
Benign pleural effusion
Parietal pleural plaques
Diffuse pleural fibrosis
Rounded atelectasis
Interstitial Lung Disease
Asbestosis
Malignant Mesothelioma
Carcinoma of the lung (in smokers)

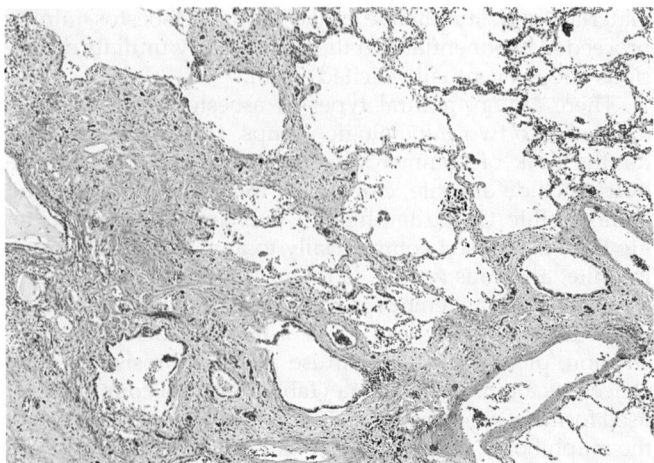

FIGURE 18-54. Asbestosis. The lung shows patchy, dense, interstitial fibrosis.

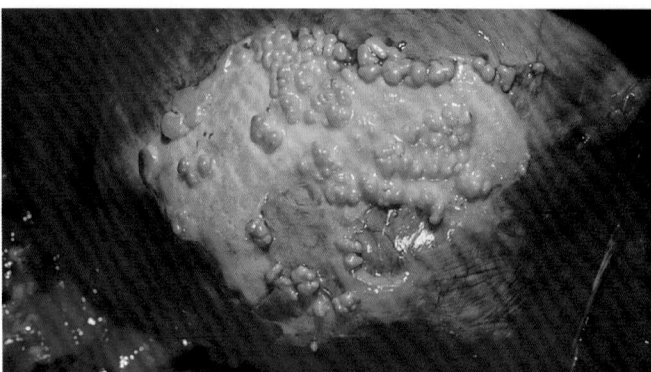

FIGURE 18-56. Pleural plaque. The dome of the diaphragm is covered by a pearly white, nodular plaque.

Asbestos bodies are found in the walls of bronchioles or within alveolar spaces, often engulfed by alveolar macrophages. The particles have a distinctive morphology, consisting of a clear, thin asbestos fiber (10–50 μm long) surrounded by a beaded iron–protein coat. By light microscopy, they are golden brown (Fig. 18-55) and react strongly with the Prussian blue stain for iron. The fibers are only partly engulfed by macrophages because they are too large for a single cell. The macrophages coat the asbestos fiber with protein, proteoglycans and ferritin.

Finding asbestos bodies incidentally at autopsy does not warrant a diagnosis of asbestosis; the lungs must also show diffuse interstitial fibrosis. Digests and concentrates of autopsy lungs demonstrate asbestos bodies to varying degrees in the lungs of virtually all adults.

BENIGN PLEURAL EFFUSION: Benign pleural effusion associated with asbestos inhalation is diagnosed by (1) a history of asbestos exposure, (2) identification of a pleural effusion with radiographs or thoracentesis, (3) absence of other diseases that could cause effusion and (4) no malignant tumor after 3 years of follow-up. Pleural effusions often occur within 10 years of initial exposure and are seen in about 3% of workers exposed to asbestos.

PLEURAL PLAQUES: Pleural plaques, mainly on parietal and diaphragmatic pleura, occur 10–20 years after exposure to asbestos. They may be found in up to 15% of the general population, and half of all patients with plaques at autopsy may not have a known history of asbestos exposure. Plaques occur most often on the parietal pleura, in the posterolateral regions of the lower thorax and on the domes of the diaphragm.

Grossly, pleural plaques are pearly white and have a smooth or nodular surface (Fig. 18-56). They are usually bilateral, but not necessarily symmetric. Plaques may measure over 10 cm in diameter and become calcified. Histologically, they consist of acellular, dense, hyalinized fibrous tissue, with numerous slit-like spaces in a parallel fashion ("basket-weave pattern"). Pleural plaques are not predictors of asbestosis, nor do they evolve into mesotheliomas.

DIFFUSE PLEURAL FIBROSIS: Fibrosis limited to the pleura is usually detected at least 10 years after the initial exposure and should be distinguished from asbestosis, in which fibrosis affects the interstitium of the underlying lung diffusely.

ROUNDED ATELECTASIS: Asbestosis exposure occasionally leads to pleural fibrosis and adhesions associated with atelectasis, which has a rounded appearance on chest radiograph. Radiographically, rounded atelectasis is characterized by a pleural-based, rounded or oval, 2.5–5-cm shadow, which usually lies along the posterior surface of a lower lobe. Pathologically, the lung shows pleural fibrosis or plaques, with curved pleural invaginations extending several centimeters into the underlying parenchyma. The condition is clinically benign.

MESOTHELIOMA: *The relation between asbestos exposure and malignant mesothelioma is firmly established.* Sometimes exposure is indirect and slight (e.g., wives of asbestos workers who wash their husbands' clothes). More often, mesothelioma is seen in workers with heavy occupational exposure to asbestos, mainly crocidolite and amosite. This malignancy is discussed below with diseases of the pleura.

CARCINOMA OF THE LUNG: There are reports that lung cancer is more common in nonsmoking asbestos workers than in similar workers not exposed to asbestos, but data are limited and no firm conclusion is possible at this point. However, in asbestos workers who smoke, the incidence of carcinoma of the lung is vastly increased: up to 40–60 times that of the general nonsmoking population. The link between asbestos and lung cancer is most convincingly supported in the presence of asbestosis (diffuse interstitial fibrosis).

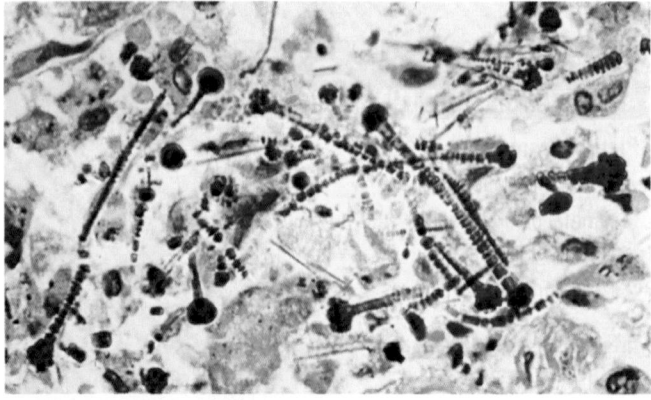

FIGURE 18-55. Asbestos bodies. These ferruginous bodies are golden brown and beaded, with a central, colorless, nonbirefringent core fiber. Asbestos bodies are encrusted with protein and iron.

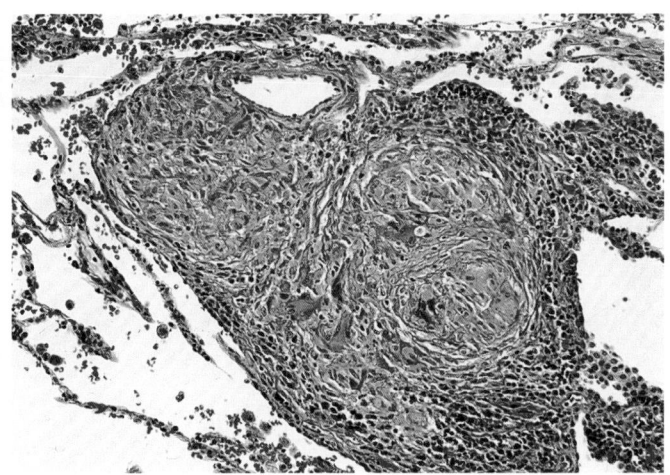

FIGURE 18-57. Berylliosis. A noncaseating granuloma consists of a nodular collection of epithelioid macrophages and multinucleated giant cells.

Berylliosis Is Characterized by Noncaseating Granulomas

Berylliosis refers to the pulmonary disease that follows the inhalation of beryllium. Today this metal is used principally in structural materials in aerospace, industrial ceramics and nuclear industries. Exposure to beryllium may also occur in those who mine and extract beryllium ores.

 PATHOLOGY: Berylliosis may occur as an acute chemical pneumonitis or a chronic pneumoconiosis. In the acute form, symptoms begin within hours or days after inhalation of metal particles and manifest pathologically as diffuse alveolar damage. Of all patients with acute beryllium pneumonitis, 10% progress to chronic disease, although chronic berylliosis is often observed in workers without any history of an acute illness.

Chronic berylliosis differs from other pneumoconioses in that exposure may be brief and minimal. The lesion is thus suspected to be a hypersensitivity reaction. Pulmonary lesions are indistinguishable from those of sarcoidosis (see below). Multiple noncaseating granulomas are distributed along the pleura, septa and bronchovascular bundles (Fig. 18-57). The beryllium lymphocyte proliferation test (demonstration of beryllium sensitization by proliferation of isolated peripheral blood lymphocytes incubated with beryllium) may aid in separating these two entities. The disease may progress to end-stage fibrosis and **honeycomb lung** (see below). Patients with chronic berylliosis have an insidious onset of dyspnea 15 or more years after the initial exposure. The disease appears to be associated with an increased risk of lung cancer.

Talcosis Results from Prolonged and Heavy Exposure to Talc Dust

Talc consists of magnesium silicates that are used in several industries as lubricants, and in cosmetics and pharmaceuticals. Occupational exposure to talc occurs among workers engaged in mining and milling the mineral and in the leather, rubber, paper and textile industries. Industrial talcs may include other minerals such as tremolite

or silica. Cosmetic talc is more than 90% pure and rarely causes lung disease.

 PATHOLOGY: Talcosis lesions vary from tiny nodules to severe fibrosis. Foreign body granulomas associated with birefringent plate-like talc particles are scattered throughout the parenchyma, which displays fibrotic nodules and interstitial fibrosis. Associated minerals such as silica may contribute to the fibrotic changes.

People who inject illicit drugs that include talc as a carrier may develop vascular and interstitial granulomas in the lung and variable fibrosis. Arterial changes of pulmonary hypertension are common and may be associated with cor pulmonale.

INTERSTITIAL LUNG DISEASE

Many pulmonary disorders are characterized by interstitial inflammatory infiltrates and have similar clinical and radiologic presentations, and so are grouped as interstitial, infiltrative or restrictive diseases. These may be acute or chronic and of known or unknown etiology and vary from minimally symptomatic to severely incapacitating and lethal interstitial fibrosis. Restrictive lung diseases are characterized by decreased lung volume and decreased oxygen-diffusing capacity on pulmonary function studies.

Hypersensitivity Pneumonitis Is a Response to Inhaled Antigens

Inhalation of many antigens leads to hypersensitivity pneumonitis (also called extrinsic allergic alveolitis), with acute or chronic interstitial inflammation in the lung. Most such antigens are encountered in occupational settings, and resulting diseases are labeled accordingly: **farmer's lung** occurs in people exposed to *Micropolyspora faeni* from moldy hay; **bagassosis** results from exposure to *Thermoactinomyces sacchari* in moldy sugar cane; **maple bark–stripper's disease** follows exposure to the fungus *Cryptostroma corticale* in moldy maple bark; and **bird fancier's lung** affects bird keepers with long-term exposure to proteins from bird feathers, blood and excrement. Other causes of hypersensitivity pneumonitis include inhalation of pituitary snuff **(pituitary snuff taker's disease),** moldy cork **(suberosis)** and moldy compost **(mushroom worker's disease)**. Hypersensitivity pneumonitis may also be caused by fungi that grow in stagnant water in air conditioners, swimming pools, hot tubs and central heating units. Skin tests and serum precipitating antibodies are often used to confirm the diagnosis. Often, especially in chronic hypersensitivity pneumonitis, an inciting antigen is never identified. In acute cases, the diagnosis is usually established clinically, so lung biopsies are performed only in chronic cases.

 **PATHOPHYSIOLOGY:** Acute hypersensitivity pneumonitis is characterized by neutrophilic infiltrates in alveoli and respiratory bronchioles; chronic lesions show mononuclear cells and granulomas, typical of delayed hypersensitivity. Most cases have serum IgG precipitating antibodies against the offending

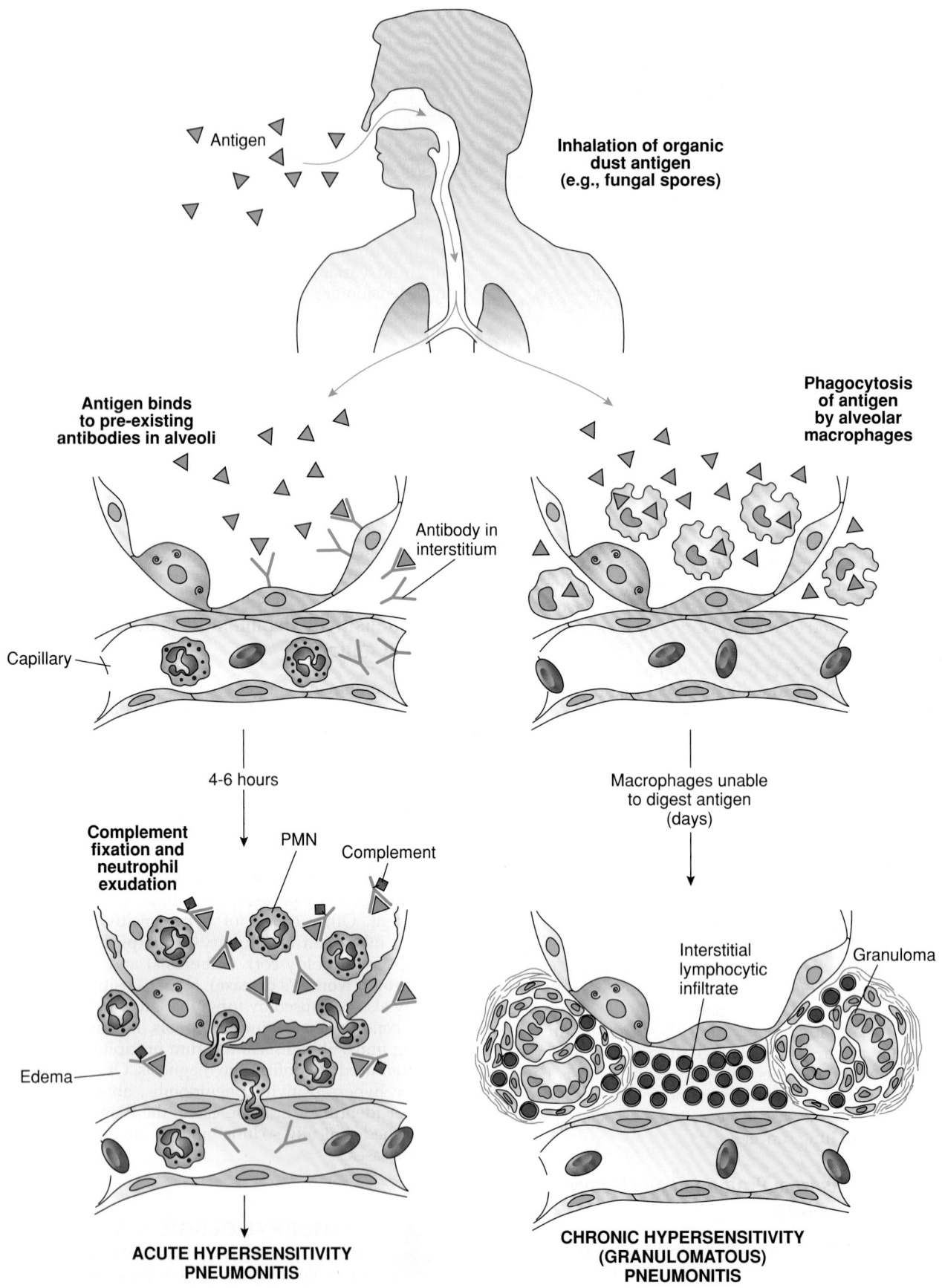

FIGURE 18-58. Hypersensitivity pneumonitis. An antigen–antibody reaction occurs in the acute phase and leads to acute hypersensitivity pneumonitis. If exposure is continued, this is followed by a cellular or subacute phase, with formation of granulomas and chronic interstitial pneumonitis. *PMN* = polymorphonuclear neutrophil.

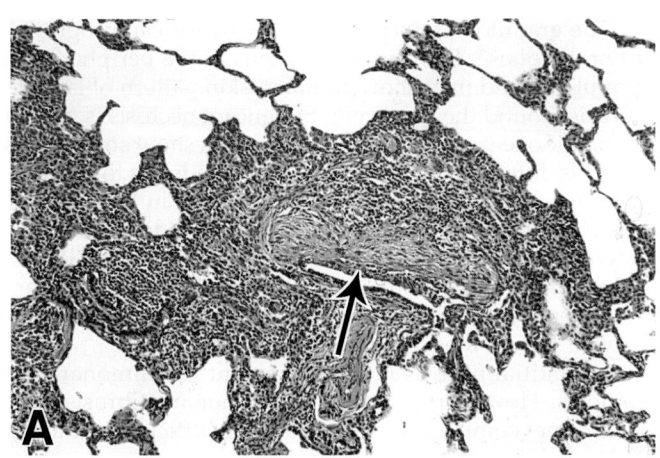 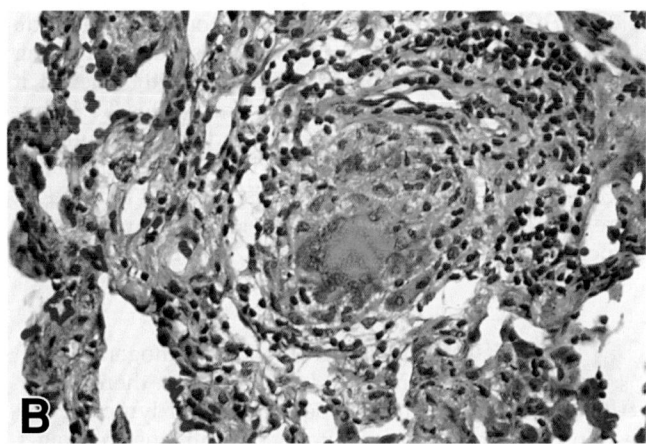

FIGURE 18-59. Hypersensitivity pneumonitis. A. A lung biopsy specimen shows a mild peribronchiolar chronic inflammatory interstitial infiltrate, with a focus of intraluminal organizing fibrosis (*arrow*). **B.** Focal poorly formed granulomas were scattered in the lung biopsy specimen.

agent. Hypersensitivity pneumonitis represents a combination of immune complex–mediated (type III) and cell-mediated (type IV) hypersensitivity reactions, although the precise contribution of each is still debated (Fig. 18-58). Importantly, most people who have serum precipitins to inhaled antigens do not develop hypersensitivity pneumonitis, suggesting a genetic component in host susceptibility.

 PATHOLOGY: The histology in florid cases of chronic hypersensitivity pneumonitis is virtually diagnostic. However, in subtle cases, the diagnosis may require careful clinical and radiologic correlation, and even then it may remain tentative. Microscopic features of chronic hypersensitivity pneumonitis are bronchiolocentric cellular interstitial pneumonia, noncaseating granulomas and organizing pneumonia (Fig. 18-59A,B). The bronchiolocentric cellular interstitial infiltrate consists of lymphocytes, plasma cells and macrophages and varies from severe to subtle; eosinophils are uncommon. Poorly formed noncaseating granulomas are seen in two thirds of cases (Fig. 18-59B), as is organizing pneumonia (Fig. 18-59A). In the end stage, interstitial inflammation recedes, leaving pulmonary fibrosis, which may resemble usual interstitial pneumonia.

 CLINICAL FEATURES: Hypersensitivity pneumonitis may present as acute, subacute or chronic pulmonary disease, depending on the frequency and intensity of exposure to the offending antigen. Farmer's lung is the prototype of hypersensitivity pneumonitis, caused by inhaling thermophilic actinomycetes from moldy hay. Typically, a farm worker enters a barn where hay has been stored for winter feeding. After a lag period of 4–6 hours, he or she rapidly develops dyspnea, cough and mild fever. Symptoms remit within 24–48 hours but return on reexposure; with time, the disorder becomes chronic. Patients with chronic hypersensitivity pneumonitis have a more nonspecific presentation, with a gradual onset of dyspnea and cor pulmonale.

Pulmonary function studies show a restrictive pattern, with decreased compliance, reduced diffusion capacity

and hypoxemia. In the chronic stage, airway obstruction may be troublesome. Bronchoalveolar fluid has increased T lymphocytes, mostly CD8+ suppressor/cytotoxic cells. Removing the offending antigen is the only adequate treatment for hypersensitivity pneumonitis. Steroid therapy may be effective in acute forms and for some chronically affected patients.

Sarcoidosis Is a Granulomatous Disease of Unknown Etiology

In sarcoidosis, the lung is the organ most often involved, but lymph nodes, skin, eye and other organs are also common targets (Fig. 18-60).

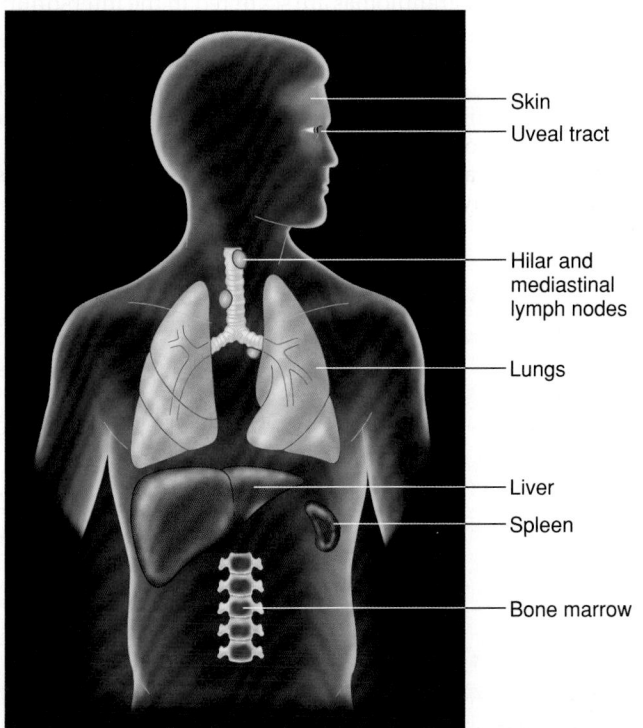

FIGURE 18-60. Organs commonly affected by sarcoidosis. Sarcoidosis involves many organs, most commonly the lymph nodes and lung.

 **EPIDEMIOLOGY:** Sarcoidosis occurs worldwide and affects all races and both sexes, but with strong racial and ethnic predilections. In North America, it is much more common among blacks than whites (15:1), but it is uncommon in tropical Africa. In Scandinavian countries, its prevalence is 64 in 100,000, but is 10 in 100,000 in France and 3 in 100,000 in Poland; among Irish women in London, its prevalence is an astonishing 200 in 100,000. Sarcoidosis is distinctly uncommon in China.

 **PATHOPHYSIOLOGY:** The pathogenesis of sarcoidosis remains obscure, but there is a consensus that helper/inducer T-lymphocyte responses to exogenous or autologous antigens are exaggerated. These cells accumulate in affected organs, where they secrete lymphokines and recruit macrophages, which help form noncaseating granulomas. $CD4^+:CD8^+$ T-cell ratios are 10:1 in organs with sarcoid granulomas, but are 2:1 in uninvolved tissues. Why helper/inducer T lymphocytes accumulate is unclear. A defect in suppressor cell function may permit unopposed helper cell proliferation. Inherited or acquired differences in immune response genes may favor one type of T-cell response over another. Nonspecific polyclonal activation of B cells by T-helper cells leads to hyperglobulinemia, a characteristic feature of active sarcoidosis.

 PATHOLOGY: Pulmonary sarcoidosis most often affects the lungs and hilar lymph nodes, although either involvement may occur separately. Radiologically, a diffuse reticulonodular infiltrate is typical, but occasional cases may show larger nodules. Histologically, multiple sarcoid granulomas are scattered in the interstitium of the lung (Fig. 18-61). The distribution is distinctive—along the pleura and interlobular septa and around bronchovascular bundles (Fig. 18-61A). Frequent bronchial or bronchiolar submucosal infiltration by sarcoid granulomas accounts for the high diagnostic yield ($\cong$90%) on bronchoscopic biopsy. Granulomas in airways may occasionally be so prominent as to lead to airway obstruction (endobronchial sarcoid).

The granulomatous phase of sarcoidosis can progress to a fibrotic phase. Fibrosis often begins at the periphery of a granuloma and may show an onion-skin pattern of lamellar fibrosis around the giant cells. Significant necrosis is uncommon, but one third of open lung biopsies show small foci of necrosis. Interstitial chronic inflammation tends to be inconspicuous. Granulomatous vasculitis is seen in two thirds of open lung biopsies from patients with sarcoidosis. Although **asteroid bodies** (star-shaped crystals) (Fig. 18-61B) and **Schaumann bodies** (small lamellar calcifications) are commonly encountered, they are not specific for sarcoidosis and may be seen in most granulomatous processes.

Interstitial fibrosis is not prominent in pulmonary sarcoidosis. However, progressive pulmonary fibrosis leads to a honeycomb lung, respiratory insufficiency and cor pulmonale.

 CLINICAL FEATURES: Sarcoidosis is most common in young adults of both sexes. **Acute sarcoidosis** has an abrupt onset, usually followed by spontaneous remission within 2 years and an excellent response to steroids. **Chronic sarcoidosis** begins insidiously, and patients are more likely to have persistent or progressive disease. Sarcoidosis causes several chest radiographic patterns, the most classic of which is bilateral hilar adenopathy, with or without interstitial pulmonary infiltrates. It may also affect the skin (erythema nodosum), mostly in women. Black patients tend to have more severe uveitis, skin disease and lacrimal gland involvement. Cough and dyspnea are the major respiratory complaints. However, the disease can be mild and may be discovered as an incidental finding on a chest radiograph in an asymptomatic patient.

No laboratory test is specific for the diagnosis of sarcoidosis. Transbronchial lung biopsy via a fiberoptic bronchoscope often reveals granulomas. Occasionally, the diagnosis is made by mediastinoscopy, identifying multiple noncaseating granulomas in a mediastinal lymph node. Bronchoalveolar lavage often shows an increase in the proportion of $CD4^+$ T lymphocytes. Increased uptake of gallium-67, a material phagocytosed by activated macrophages, can demonstrate granulomatous areas. Serum angiotensin-converting enzyme (ACE) levels are elevated in two thirds of patients with active sarcoidosis, and 24-hour urine calcium

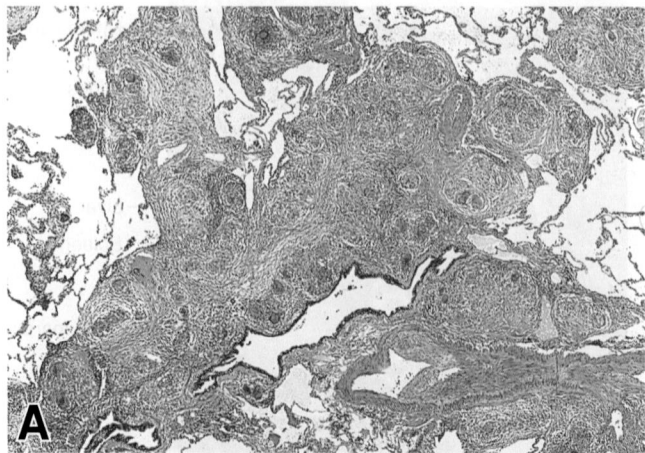
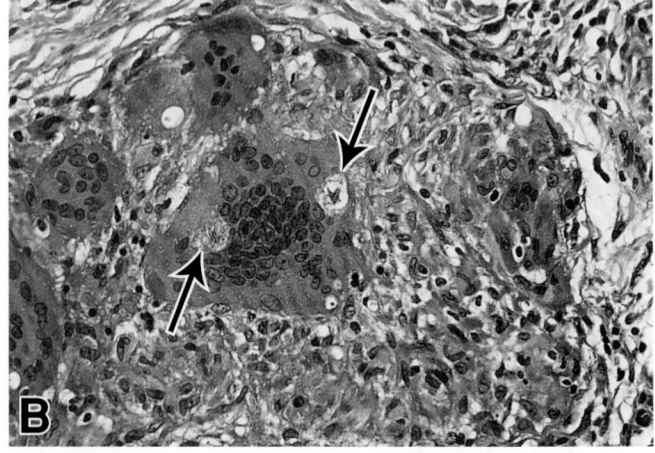

FIGURE 18-61. Sarcoidosis. A. Multiple noncaseating granulomas are present along the bronchovascular interstitium. **B.** Noncaseating granulomas consist of tight clusters of epithelioid macrophages and multinucleated giant cells. Several asteroid bodies are present (*arrows*).

is frequently increased. These laboratory data, together with supportive clinical and radiologic findings, allow the diagnosis of sarcoidosis to be made with a high probability.

Other organs commonly involved include the skin, eye (uveal tract), heart, central nervous system, extrathoracic lymph nodes, spleen and liver (Fig. 18-60). These are discussed separately in individual chapters.

The prognosis in pulmonary sarcoidosis is favorable; most patients do not develop clinically significant sequelae. In 60% of patients, pulmonary sarcoidosis resolves, but this is less likely in older patients and those with extrathoracic disease, particularly in the bone and skin. In up to 20% of cases, sarcoidosis does not remit or recurs at intervals, but it leads to death in only 10% of cases. Corticosteroid therapy is effective for active sarcoidosis.

Usual Interstitial Pneumonia Is the Most Common Histology Seen in Clinical Idiopathic Pulmonary Fibrosis

Usual interstitial pneumonia (UIP) is one of the most common types of interstitial pneumonia, with an annual incidence of 6–14 cases per 100,000 people. It has a slight male predominance and a mean age at onset of 50–60 years. UIP is the histologic pattern present on biopsy, and the clinical term **idiopathic pulmonary fibrosis** (IPF) is applied when the disease is determined to be of unknown origin.

 **ETIOLOGIC FACTORS:** The etiology of IPF is unknown, but immunologic, viral and genetic factors probably contribute. Some patients have histories of flu-like illnesses, suggesting viral involvement. Familial clusters of IPF, and association of UIP-like diseases in patients with inherited disorders such as neurofibromatosis and Hermansky-Pudlak syndrome, indicate that genetic factors contribute. Mutations in telomerase genes, particularly telomerase reverse transcriptase (TERT), surfactant protein C and MUC5B, are common in familial IPF but involve less than 1/3 of cases; the genetic abnormality is unknown in most patients.

UIP histology accompanies autoimmune diseases, including rheumatoid arthritis, systemic lupus erythematosus and progressive systemic sclerosis, in 20% of cases, suggesting impaired immunity. It also occurs with autoimmune disorders like Hashimoto thyroiditis, primary biliary cirrhosis, autoimmune hepatitis, idiopathic thrombocytopenic purpura and myasthenia gravis. Autoantibodies (e.g., antinuclear antibodies and rheumatoid factor) and immune complexes are often found in blood, inflamed alveolar walls and bronchoalveolar lavage fluids. No antigen has yet been identified. Activated alveolar macrophages may release cytokines, which recruit neutrophils. These in turn damage alveolar walls, stimulating a series of events that culminates in interstitial fibrosis.

 PATHOLOGY: UIP is a histologic pattern that occurs in several clinical settings (e.g., collagen vascular disease, chronic hypersensitivity pneumonitis, drug toxicity and asbestosis). Many cases have no identifiable etiology and are so considered idiopathic (IPF). The lungs are small in UIP, and fibrosis tends to be worse in the lower lobes, in the subpleural regions and along interlobular septa. Retraction of the scars, especially of lobular septa, gives the pleural surface of the lung a hobnail appearance, reminiscent of cirrhosis of the liver. Fibrosis is often patchy, with areas of dense scarring and honeycomb cystic change (Fig. 18-62A).

The histologic hallmark of UIP is patchy interstitial fibrosis, with areas of normal lung adjacent to fibrotic areas (Fig. 18-62B). The fibrosis is of different ages, which has been called **"temporal heterogeneity."** Areas of loose fibroblastic tissue **(fibroblast foci)** may be adjacent to dense collagen (Fig. 18-62C). The fibrosis is most pronounced beneath the pleura and adjacent to interlobular septa (Fig. 18-62B).

Bronchiolar epithelium grows into the dilated airspaces, which may be damaged but unrecognizable proximal respiratory bronchioles (Fig. 18-63). The areas of dense scarring fibrosis cause remodeling of the lung architecture, leading to alveolar wall collapse and formation of cystic spaces (Fig. 18-62A). These spaces are typically lined by bronchiolar or cuboidal epithelium and contain mucus, macrophages or neutrophils. If such changes are extensive, the term **"honeycomb lung"** may be used to describe the gross cystic changes. Interstitial chronic inflammation is mild or moderate. Lymphoid aggregates, sometimes containing germinal centers, are occasionally noted, particularly in UIP associated with a collagen vascular disease such as rheumatoid arthritis. Extensive vascular changes of intimal fibrosis and medial thickening may be associated with pulmonary hypertension.

 CLINICAL FEATURES: UIP begins insidiously, with gradual onset of dyspnea on exertion and dry cough, usually for 1–3 years. Patients have restrictive lung disease by pulmonary function testing. Finger clubbing is common, especially late in the disease. In half of patients, CT scans show distinctive peripheral, subpleural reticular opacities, traction bronchiectasis and honeycombing, mostly in posterior lower lobes.

The classic auscultatory finding is late inspiratory crackles and fine ("Velcro") rales at the lung bases. Tachypnea at rest, cyanosis and cor pulmonale eventually follow. The prognosis is bleak, with a mean survival of 4–6 years. Patients are treated with corticosteroids and sometimes cyclophosphamide, but lung transplantation generally offers the only hope of survival.

Nonspecific Interstitial Pneumonia Has Multiple Etiologies

Nonspecific interstitial pneumonia (NSIP) is a histologic pattern that reflects diverse potential etiologies (infection, collagen vascular disease, hypersensitivity pneumonitis, drug reaction) or it may be idiopathic.

 PATHOLOGY: NSIP shows a spectrum of **cellular** and **fibrosing patterns**. Unlike the patchy distribution and temporal heterogeneity of UIP, lung changes in NSIP are diffuse and uniform. In the **cellular form,** alveolar septa are diffusely involved by a mild to moderate lymphocytic infiltrate. In the **fibrosing form,** septa show diffuse fibrosis, with or without significant associated inflammation. Honeycombing and fibroblastic foci are inconspicuous or absent.

 CLINICAL FEATURES: In NSIP, shortness of breath and cough develop over months to years. Computed tomography is variable but mostly

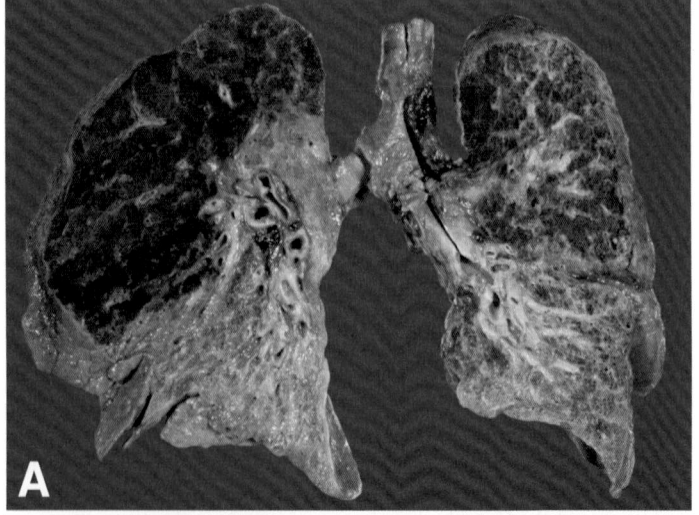

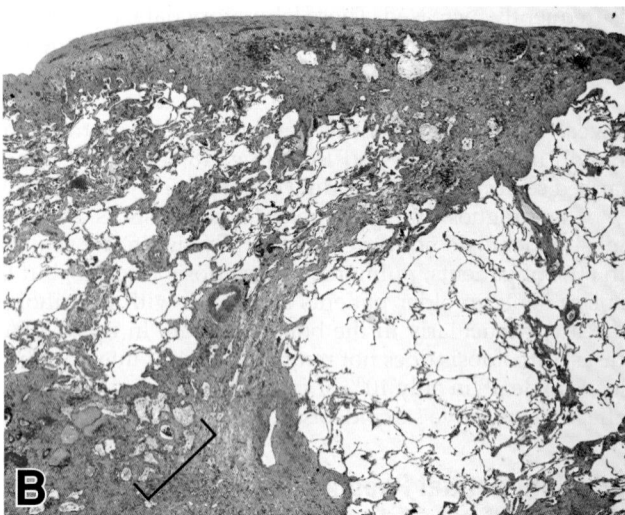

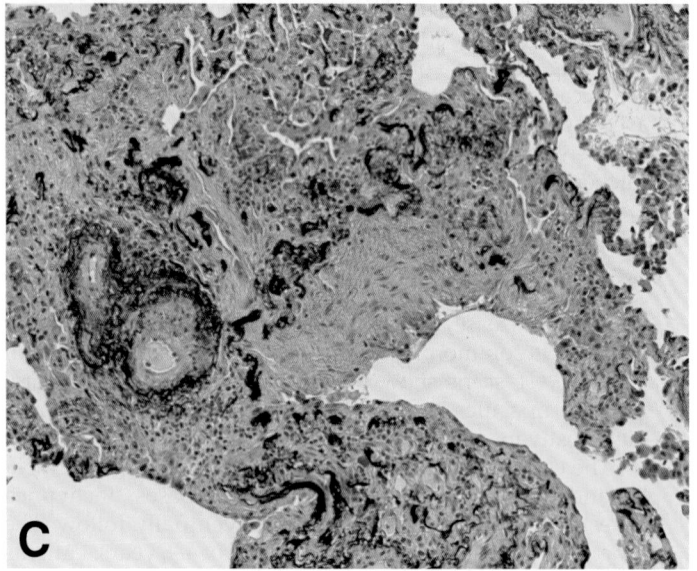

FIGURE 18-62. Usual interstitial pneumonitis. A. A gross specimen of the lung shows patchy dense scarring with extensive areas of honeycomb cystic change, predominantly affecting the lower lobes. This patient also had polymyositis. **B.** A microscopic view shows patchy subpleural fibrosis with microscopic honeycomb fibrosis (*bracket*). The areas of dense fibrosis display remodeling, with loss of the normal lung architecture. **C.** Elastin stain highlights the fibroblastic focus in green, which contrasts with the adjacent area of yellow staining of dense collagen and black staining of collapsed elastic fibers.

shows bilateral lower lobe "ground glass" changes or reticulation with traction bronchiectasis. The prognosis of idiopathic NSIP is favorable compared to IPF; 5-year survival is 80%.

Desquamative Interstitial Pneumonia Is a Diffuse Lung Disease Seen Mostly in Smokers

Interstitial fibrosis is minimal in desquamative interstitial pneumonia (DIP) (Fig. 18-64A,B). The term "desquamative" reflected the misconception that the intra-alveolar cells were desquamated epithelial cells, but they are now recognized as macrophages. In DIP, unlike UIP, alveolar architecture is preserved, and the disorder lacks the patchy scarring and remodeling of lung parenchyma of UIP. The macrophages contain a fine golden-brown pigment. Alveolar walls in DIP may, however, be mildly thickened by chronic inflammation and interstitial fibrosis (Fig. 18-64B). Scattered lymphoid aggregates also may be present. Hyperplasia of type II pneumocytes is often prominent.

DIP occurs almost exclusively in cigarette smokers, typically in the fourth or fifth decade, and is twice as common in men as in women. Probably, DIP and respiratory

bronchiolitis–interstitial lung disease (see below) are a spectrum of disease related to cigarette smoking, although the mechanism is unclear. The radiographic picture of DIP is not specific but is most often bilateral lower lobe ground glass infiltrates. DIP has a much better prognosis than UIP, with an overall 10-year survival between 70% and 100%. Most patients respond well to steroid therapy and smoking cessation.

Respiratory Bronchiolitis–Interstitial Lung Disease Occurs in Smokers

Respiratory bronchiolitis (RB) is a histologic lesion that occurs in cigarette smokers. It is most often an incidental histologic finding, but it may rarely be the sole cause of interstitial lung disease (ILD), and the clinical term **respiratory bronchiolitis–interstitial lung disease** (RB-ILD) is appropriate in this setting.

 PATHOLOGY: RB is a patchy accumulation of pigmented macrophages in airspaces, centered on bronchioles (Fig. 18-65). These macrophages are

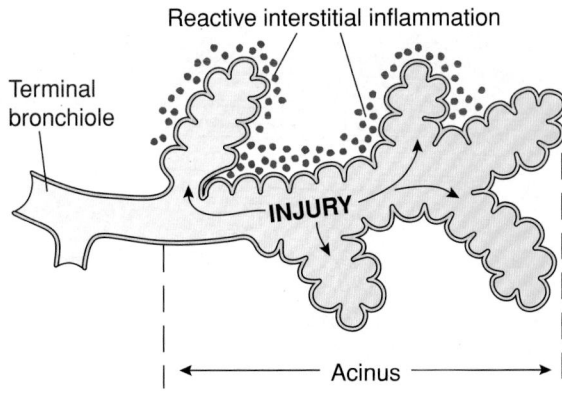

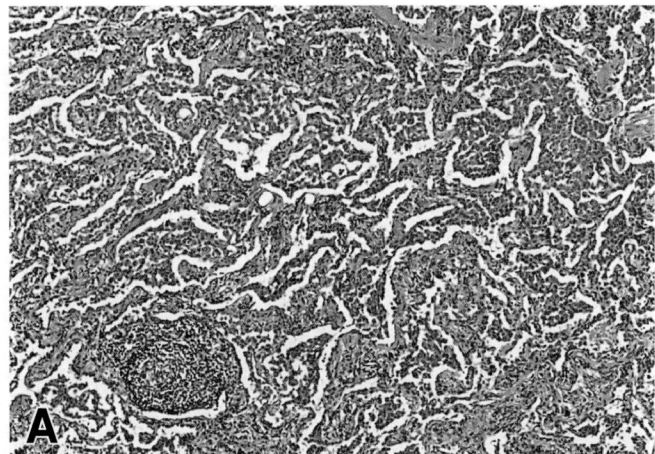

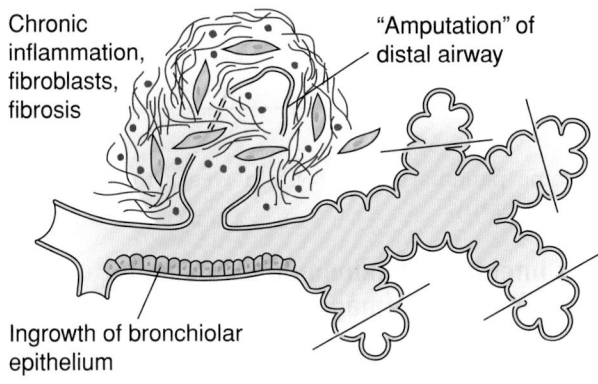

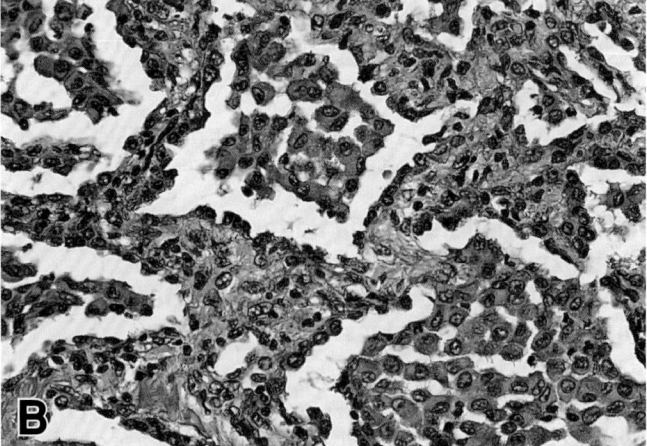

FIGURE 18-64. Desquamative interstitial pneumonia (DIP). A. A diffuse process in the lungs is characterized by accumulation of alveolar macrophages, preservation of alveolar architecture and lymphoid aggregates. **B.** In addition to alveolar macrophage accumulation, there is mild alveolar septal fibrosis, type II pneumocyte hyperplasia and mild interstitial chronic inflammation.

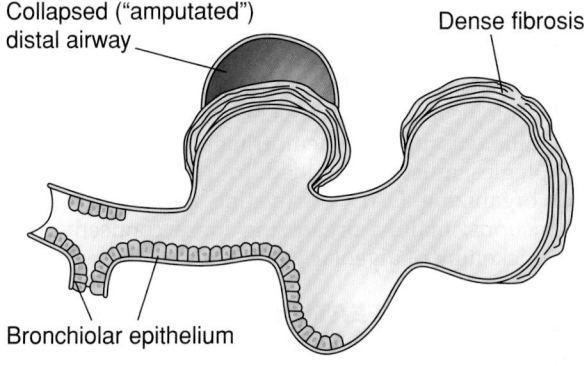

FIGURE 18-63. Pathogenesis of honeycomb lung. Honeycomb lung is the result of a variety of injuries. Interstitial and alveolar inflammation destroys ("amputates") the distal part of the acinus. The proximal parts dilate and become lined by bronchiolar epithelium.

present in bronchiolar lumens and adjacent alveoli. Bronchiolar walls show mild chronic inflammation and fibrosis. However, interstitial fibrosis does not extend into the surrounding lung. Macrophages usually contain finely granular, brown pigment. The lesions in RB are bronchiolocentric and patchy.

 CLINICAL FEATURES: Patients have mild respiratory dysfunction. Upper lobes are most affected, with thickening of peripheral bronchioles.

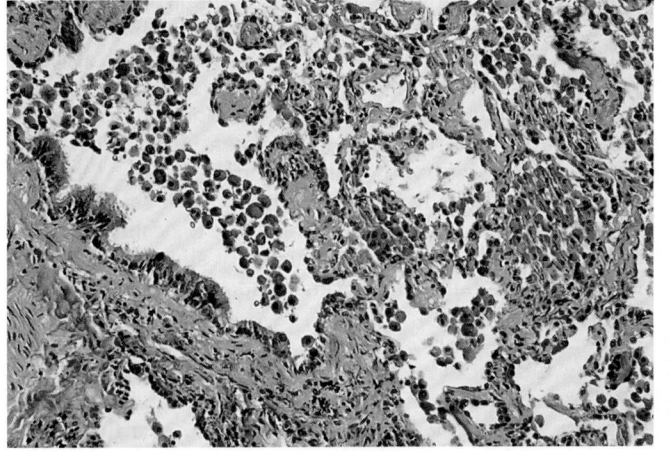

FIGURE 18-65. Respiratory bronchiolitis. There is marked accumulation of macrophages within bronchioles and surrounding airspaces. Mild fibrotic thickening and chronic inflammation of the bronchiolar wall are present.

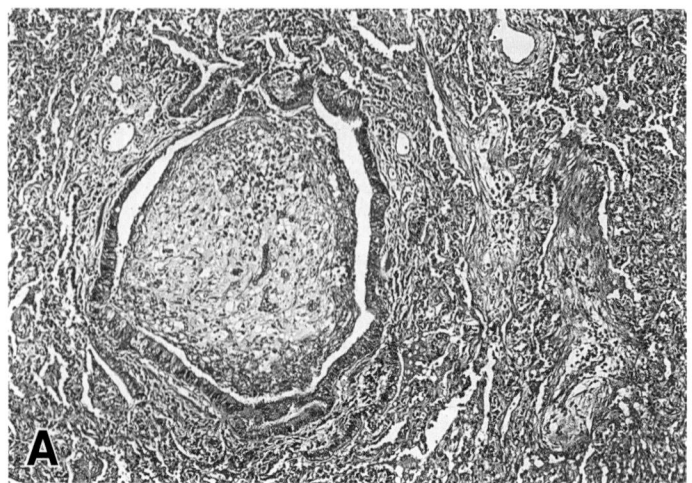
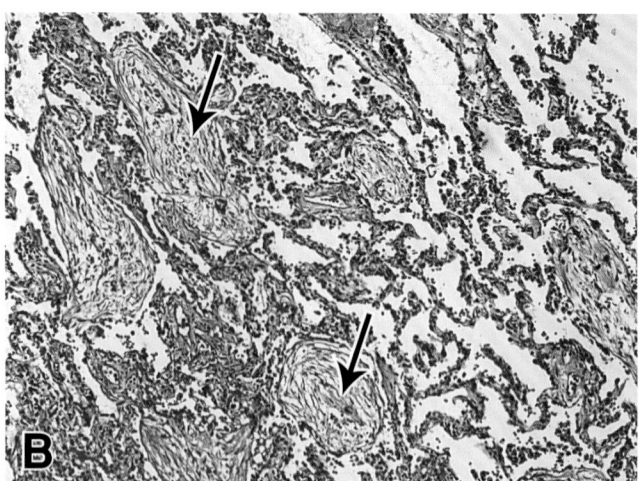

FIGURE 18-66. Organizing pneumonia pattern. A. Polypoid plugs of loose fibrous tissue are present in a bronchiole and adjacent alveolar ducts and alveoli. **B.** Alveolar spaces contain similar plugs of loose organizing connective tissue (*arrows*).

Patients with RB-ILD have an excellent prognosis, and the symptoms usually resolve after smoking cessation.

In Organizing Pneumonia Pattern (Cryptogenic Organizing Pneumonia) Polypoid Plugs of Tissue Fill Alveolar Spaces, Alveolar Ducts and Bronchiolar Lumens

Organizing pneumonia pattern, previously called "bronchiolitis obliterans–organizing pneumonia" (BOOP), is not specific for any etiologic agent, and its cause cannot be determined from the histopathology. Thus, it is seen in many settings, including respiratory tract infections (particularly viral bronchiolitis), inhalation of toxic materials, after administration of a number of drugs and various inflammatory processes (e.g., collagen vascular diseases). *A substantial number of cases are idiopathic and are called cryptogenic organizing pneumonia (or idiopathic BOOP).*

 PATHOLOGY: Organizing pneumonia pattern has patchy areas of loose organizing fibrosis and chronic inflammatory cells in distal airways, adjacent to normal lung. Plugs of organizing fibroblastic tissue occlude bronchioles (bronchiolitis obliterans), alveolar ducts and surrounding alveoli (organizing pneumonia; Fig. 18-66). Alveolar organizing pneumonia predominates; bronchiolitis obliterans may not be seen in all cases. Lung architecture is preserved, without honeycombing. Obstructive or endogenous lipid pneumonia may develop if there is significant bronchiolitis obliterans due to occlusion of the distal airways. Alveolar septa are only slightly thickened with chronic inflammatory cells, and type II pneumocyte hyperplasia is mild.

 **CLINICAL FEATURES:** The average age at presentation is 55. The onset is acute, with fever, cough and dyspnea, often with a history of a flu-like illness 4–6 weeks previously. Some patients may have predisposing conditions. Chest radiographs reveal localized opacities or bilateral interstitial infiltrates, which may migrate over time. Pulmonary function studies demonstrate a restrictive ventilatory pattern. Corticosteroid therapy is effective, and some patients recover within weeks to months even without therapy.

Acute Interstitial Pneumonia Is Idiopathic Diffuse Alveolar Damage

Acute interstitial pneumonia (AIP) is a clinical term for diffuse alveolar damage of unknown cause. The diagnosis requires exclusion of clinical and pathologic causes such as infection, collagen vascular disease and drug toxicity.

 PATHOLOGY: The pathology is identical to DAD associated with known causes (see above), but histologic features such as necrosis, acute pneumonia, eosinophilia, vasculitis or hemorrhage, which suggest specific etiologies, must be excluded. In AIP, the pattern is usually of organizing DAD, so hyaline membranes may be inconspicuous; mainly, organizing loose connective tissue causes thickening of alveolar walls.

 CLINICAL FEATURES: AIP has a mean age at onset of 50 with a wide range and no sex predominance. It usually begins after an illness that resembles an upper respiratory tract infection with myalgias, arthralgias, fever, chills and malaise. Patients develop severe exertional dyspnea over several days and usually present less than 3 weeks after experiencing the first symptoms. CT scan shows widespread consolidation. Mortality is approximately 50%, and those who survive may either recover completely or follow a course with recurrences and progressive interstitial lung disease.

Lymphoid Interstitial Pneumonia Often Accompanies Autoimmune Diseases

Lymphoid interstitial pneumonia (LIP) is a rare disease with lymphoid infiltrates distributed diffusely in interstitial spaces.

 PATHOLOGY: The hallmark of LIP is diffuse lymphocytic infiltration of alveolar septa and peribronchiolar spaces, with plasma cells and macrophages

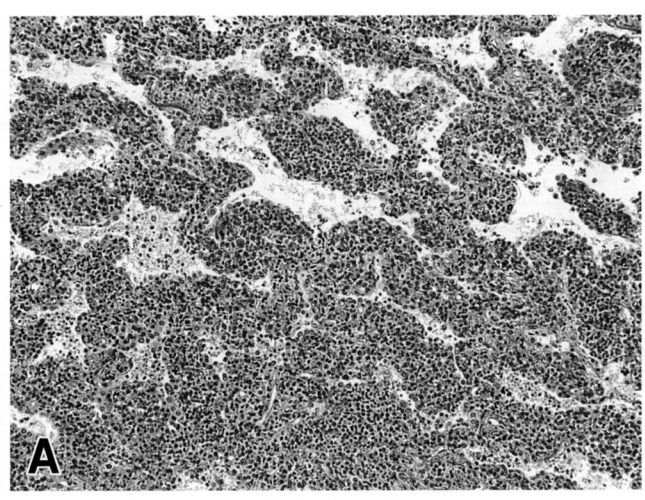
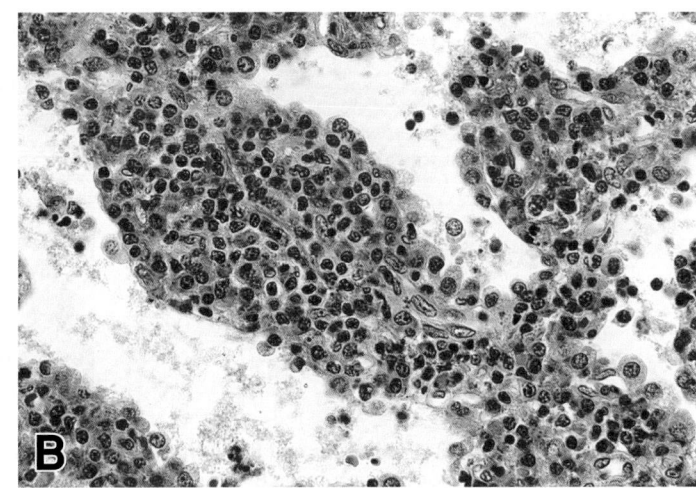

FIGURE 18-67. Lymphocytic interstitial pneumonia (LIP). A. The walls of the alveolar septa are diffusely infiltrated by chronic inflammation. **B.** The inflammatory infiltrate is composed of lymphocytes and plasma cells.

(Fig. 18-67). Alveolar architecture is preserved without scarring or remodeling. Marked type II pneumocyte hyperplasia may be seen, and inconspicuous foci of organizing interstitial fibrosis are occasionally present. Noncaseating sarcoid-like granulomas are often seen. Alveolar spaces tend to contain a proteinaceous exudate. Occasionally, scattered lymphoid aggregates are present, some containing germinal centers. Hyperplasia of peribronchiolar lymphoid tissue may be prominent.

CLINICAL FEATURES: LIP may be idiopathic but often occurs in patients with collagen vascular disease (especially Sjögren syndrome), dysproteinemia or HIV infection (Table 18-5). It is largely a disease of adults, but pediatric cases are recorded. In children, LIP is a defining criterion for the diagnosis of AIDS. Associated autoimmune manifestations include increased or reduced serum γ-globulins, various dysproteinemias and increased circulating autoantibodies, such as rheumatoid factor and antinuclear antibodies. Lymphoma may rarely develop in patients with LIP, particularly in patients with Sjögren syndrome and AIDS.

Symptoms of LIP include cough and progressive dyspnea. The disease varies from an indolent condition to one that progresses to end-stage lung and respiratory failure. Corticosteroids and cytotoxic agents have been of some benefit.

Langerhans Cell Histiocytosis Entails Diverse Histiocyte Proliferations

Different presentations of Langerhans cell histiocytosis (LCH) have been called **eosinophilic granuloma, Hand-Schüller-Christian disease** and **Letterer-Siwe disease** (see Chapter 26). LCH can affect the lung as a distinctive form of interstitial lung disease. In adults, LCH is *primarily seen in cigarette smokers* and may occur as an isolated lesion (previously **pulmonary eosinophilic granuloma**) or as diffuse cystic lung disease. Extrapulmonary manifestations such as bone lesions or diabetes insipidus occur in 10%–15% of cases. In children, lung involvement may occur in association with the multisystemic Letterer-Siwe disease or Hand-Schüller-Christian disease.

PATHOLOGY: Histologically, pulmonary LCH appears as scattered nodular infiltrates with a stellate border extending into the surrounding interstitium (Fig. 18-68A). These lesions are frequently subpleural or centered on bronchioles. They contain varying proportions of Langerhans cells admixed with lymphocytes, eosinophils and macrophages. Langerhans cells are round to oval,

TABLE 18-5
CONDITIONS ASSOCIATED WITH LYMPHOCYTIC INTERSTITIAL PNEUMONIA
Idiopathic
Dysproteinemia
Polyclonal gammopathy
Macroglobulinemia
Hypogammaglobulinemia
Pernicious anemia
Collagen Vascular Disease
Sjögren syndrome
Systemic lupus erythematosus
Rheumatoid arthritis
Immunodeficiency
HIV infection
Severe combined immunodeficiency syndrome
Infection
Pneumocystis jiroveci pneumonia
Epstein-Barr virus (lymphoproliferative disorder)
Chronic hepatitis
Iatrogenic
Bone marrow transplantation
Phenytoin (Dilantin)

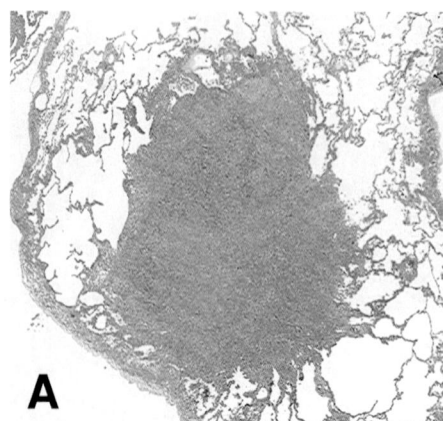
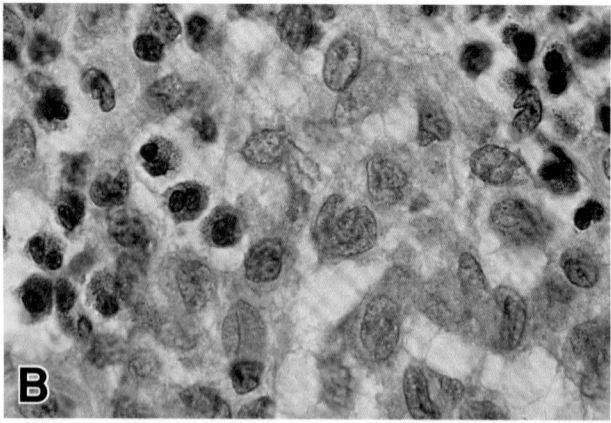

FIGURE 18-68. Langerhans cell histiocytosis. A. The nodular interstitial infiltrate has a stellate shape, with extension of cells into adjacent alveolar septa. **B.** Higher-power view shows Langerhans cells with moderate amount of eosinophilic cytoplasm and prominently grooved nuclei. Eosinophils are present.

with a moderate amount of eosinophilic cytoplasm and prominently grooved nuclei with small inconspicuous nucleoli (Fig. 18-68B). As the disease progresses, lesions cavitate and become fibrotic, and honeycomb fibrosis may result. Parenchyma adjacent to the nodular lesions may show marked accumulation of intra-alveolar macrophages, owing to respiratory bronchiolitis caused by smoking.

Langerhans cells are distinctive: they show cytoplasmic Birbeck granules (on electron microscopy), C3, IgG-F$_c$ receptors, CD1a and human leukocyte antigen (HLA)-DR and S-100 protein expression. Whether pulmonary LCH is a neoplastic proliferation or an abnormal immunologic response to antigens within cigarette smoke is unclear. Recently, BRAF mutations have been reported in a subset of pulmonary LCH.

 CLINICAL FEATURES: Pulmonary LCH usually affects patients in their third and fourth decades. The most common presenting symptoms are nonproductive cough, dyspnea on exertion and spontaneous pneumothorax, but 25% of patients are asymptomatic at the time of diagnosis. Chest radiographs show diffuse, bilateral, reticulonodular lesions, usually in the upper lobes. The lesions frequently undergo cavitation. Although most patients have a good prognosis, some develop chronic pulmonary dysfunction. In a few cases, progressive pulmonary fibrosis can lead to death. Cessation of smoking is beneficial in early stages of the disease.

In Lymphangioleiomyomatosis Abnormal Smooth Muscle Proliferates in the Lung and Lymphatics

Lymphangioleiomyomatosis (LAM) is a rare interstitial lung disease that occurs almost exclusively in women of child-bearing age and is characterized by widespread abnormal proliferation of smooth muscle in the lung, mediastinal and retroperitoneal lymph nodes and major lymphatic ducts. Its etiology is unknown, but clinical responses to oophorectomy and progesterone therapy suggest that the smooth muscle proliferation is under hormonal control. Its occurrence in patients with tuberous sclerosis and its association with renal angiomyolipomas suggest that LAM may be a forme fruste of **tuberous sclerosis**. LAM is

also associated with tuberous sclerosis gene complex (TSC) mutations, whether or not the patient has fully developed tuberous sclerosis. LAM cells are thought to be derived from perivascular epithelioid cells similar to other lesions associated with tuberous sclerosis, such as angiomyolipoma and clear cell tumor.

 PATHOLOGY: The lungs show bilateral, diffuse enlargement, with extensive cystic changes as in emphysema (Fig. 18-69A). Many cystic spaces are lined by focal nodules or bundles of abnormal smooth muscle cells. These round or spindle-shaped cells (LAM cells) resemble immature smooth muscle cells but lack the parallel orientation of normal smooth muscle around airways and blood vessels (Fig. 18-69B). This proliferation typically follows a lymphatic distribution in the lung, around blood vessels and bronchioles and along pleura and interlobular septa. Blood vessel walls, especially in small pulmonary veins, may also be infiltrated, causing microscopic hemorrhage and hemosiderin accumulation in alveolar macrophages. Immunostaining for HMB-45 (a melanoma antigen) specifically identifies LAM cells and distinguishes them from other lung smooth muscle cells. They usually also express estrogen or progesterone receptors.

 CLINICAL FEATURES: Patients with LAM have shortness of breath, spontaneous pneumothorax, hemoptysis, cough and chylous effusions. In early stages, the chest radiograph may be normal, but may show a diffuse interstitial reticular or cystic pattern as the disease progresses. Pleural effusions, marked hyperinflation of the lungs and pneumothorax may ensue. Pulmonary function tests show markedly increased total lung capacity, decreased diffusing capacity and obstructive or restrictive features. Some patients have an indolent clinical course, but many die of progressive respiratory failure. Hormonal ablation through oophorectomy, as well as antiestrogen (tamoxifen) and progesterone therapy, showed initial promise but has not proven to be effective therapy over time. Mutations of the TSC genes lead to activation of the mammalian target of rapamycin (mTOR) pathway, and as such, sirolimus is currently under investigation as a potential therapy.

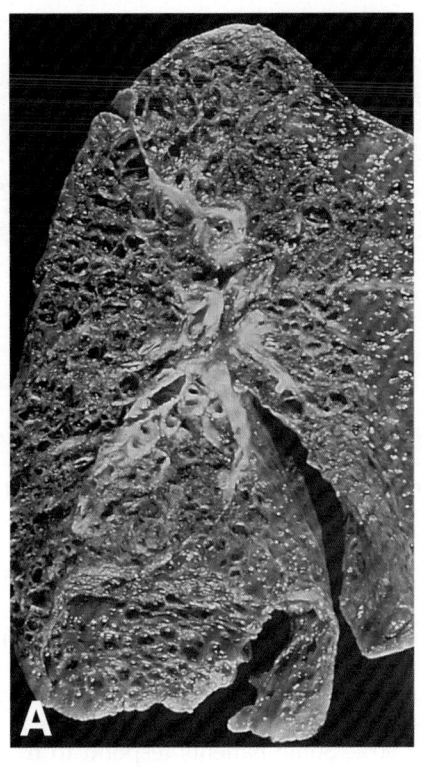
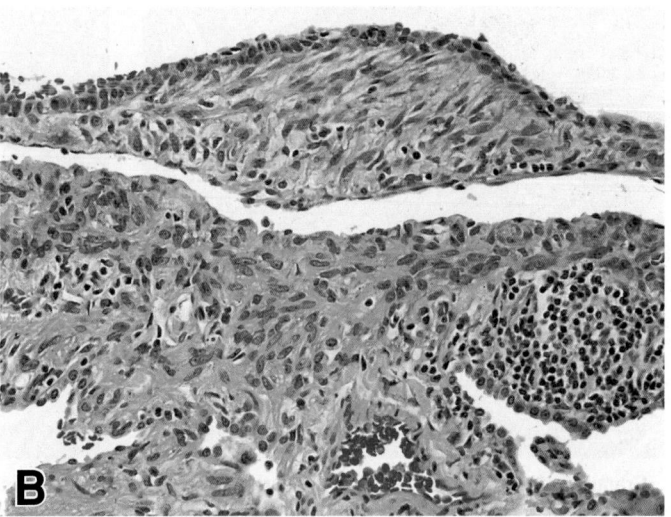

FIGURE 18-69. Lymphangioleiomyomatosis. A. The cut surface of the lung displays extensive cystic change. **B.** Abnormal cystic spaces are lined by smooth muscle bundles in which myocytes are haphazardly arranged.

LUNG TRANSPLANTATION

Patients who undergo lung transplantation are prone to acute and chronic rejection and infection. The histology of acute rejection includes perivascular infiltrates of small round lymphocytes, plasmacytoid lymphocytes, macrophages and eosinophils. In severe cases, inflammation may involve adjacent alveoli, and hyaline membranes may be seen. The major pattern of chronic rejection is bronchiolitis obliterans, characterized by bronchiolar inflammation and varying degrees of fibrosis. The latter can take the form of polypoid plugs of intraluminal granulation tissue or concentric mural fibrosis, with the pattern of constrictive bronchiolitis (Fig. 18-70). Bronchiectasis is common in

long-term survivors of lung transplants, perhaps related to poor perfusion of the airways, denervation and/or recurrent airway infection.

Opportunistic infections, including bacteria, fungi, viruses and *Pneumocystis,* are common in transplant patients. The most common fungal pathogens are *Candida* and *Aspergillus* spp. CMV is the most common cause of viral pneumonia. Of lung transplant patients who survive more than 30 days, 3%–8% develop **lymphoproliferative disorders,** owing to uncontrolled proliferation of Epstein-Barr virus (EBV)–infected B lymphocytes as a result of immunosuppression by cyclosporine.

VASCULITIS AND GRANULOMATOSIS

Many pulmonary conditions result in vasculitis, most of which are secondary to other inflammatory processes, such as necrotizing granulomatous infections. Only a few primary idiopathic vasculitis syndromes affect the lung, the most important of which are granulomatosis with polyangiitis (GPA, formerly Wegener granulomatosis), microscopic polyangiitis, eosinophilic granulomatosis with polyangiitis (EGPA, formerly Churg-Strauss granulomatosis) and necrotizing sarcoid granulomatosis.

Granulomatosis with Polyangiitis Has Aseptic, Necrotizing Granulomas and Vasculitis

GPA (formerly called Wegener granulomatosis) is a disease of unknown cause. Blood vessels affected by the disease are small and medium sized. It chiefly affects upper and lower respiratory tracts and the kidneys (see Chapters 16, 22 and 29), but many cases also involve the eyes, joints, skin and peripheral nerves. Here, we deal only with pulmonary manifestations of GPA.

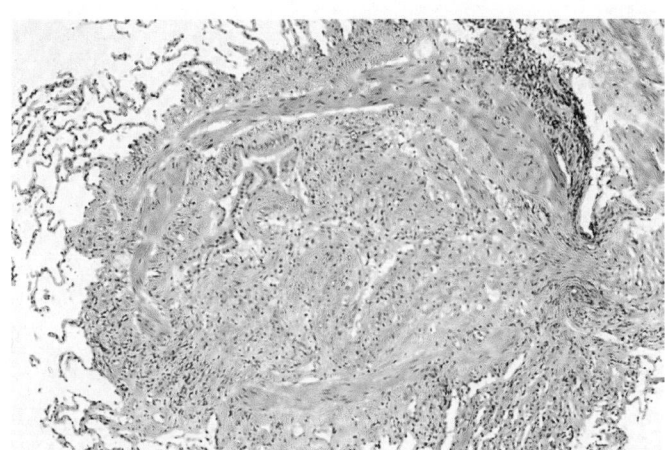

FIGURE 18-70. Obliterative bronchiolitis, chronic rejection in lung transplantation. The lumen of this bronchiole is virtually obliterated by concentric fibrosis.

THE RESPIRATORY SYSTEM

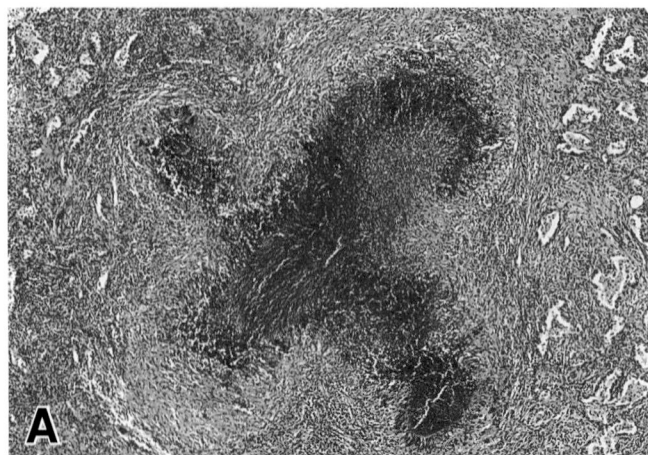
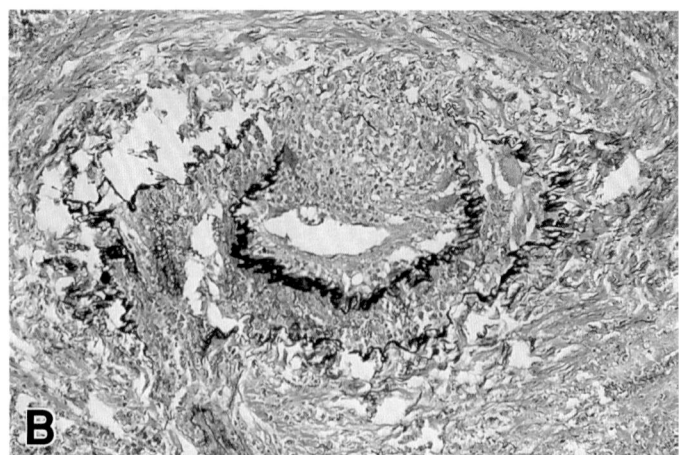

FIGURE 18-71. Granulomatosis with polyangiitis (formerly Wegener granulomatosis). A. This large area of necrosis has a "geographical" pattern with serpiginous borders and a basophilic center. **B.** Vasculitis in this artery is characterized by a focal, eccentric, transmural chronic inflammatory infiltrate that destroys the inner and outer elastic laminae (elastic stain).

PATHOLOGY: GPA in the lung is characterized by necrotizing granulomatous inflammation, parenchymal necrosis and vasculitis. Most cases show multiple bilateral nodules, averaging 2–3 cm, with irregular edges, tan-brown or hemorrhagic cut surfaces and frequent central cavitation.

Nodules of parenchymal consolidation show (1) tissue necrosis; (2) granulomatous inflammation with a mixture of lymphocytes, plasma cells, neutrophils, eosinophils, macrophages and giant cells; and (3) fibrosis. Necrosis may feature neutrophilic microabscesses or large basophilic zones of "geographical" necrosis with irregular serpiginous borders (Fig. 18-71A). Patterns of GPA granulomas include palisading macrophages along the border of the large necrotic zones, loosely clustered multinucleated giant cells and scattered giant cells. Vasculitis may affect arteries (Fig. 18-71B), veins or capillaries and may show acute, chronic or granulomatous inflammation. Organizing pneumonia is common at the edges of the nodules of inflammatory consolidation. The lungs often show acute or chronic alveolar hemorrhage. "Neutrophilic capillaritis," with neutrophils in alveolar walls, is common.

CLINICAL FEATURES: GPA mostly affects the head and neck, then the lung, kidney and eye. Respiratory manifestations include cough, hemoptysis and pleuritis. Chest radiographs often show multiple intrapulmonary nodules, although single nodules may also be seen. Head and neck manifestations include sinusitis, nasal disease, otitis media, hearing loss, subglottic stenosis, ear pain, cough and oral lesions. Systemic symptoms include arthralgias, fever, skin lesions, weight loss, peripheral neuropathy, central nervous system abnormalities and pericarditis.

Diffuse pulmonary hemorrhage, an important complication of GPA, is a fulminant life-threatening crisis with severe respiratory failure. It is usually accompanied by acute renal failure.

It is currently thought that ANCAs are responsible for the inflammation in GPA. Serum ANCAs are a useful marker for GPA and other vasculitis syndromes. This test yields two major immunofluorescence patterns: cytoplasmic (C-ANCA) and perinuclear (P-ANCA). C-ANCAs reacting with proteinase 3 occur in more than 85% of patients with active generalized GPA. Most P-ANCAs are specific for myeloperoxidase and are seen with idiopathic necrotizing and crescentic

glomerulonephritis, polyarteritis nodosa or Churg-Strauss syndrome.

Most patients with GPA are treated effectively with corticosteroids and cyclophosphamide, and 5-year survival is now almost 90%. Some patients respond to trimethoprim-sulfamethoxazole, suggesting a possible bacterial infection.

Microscopic Polyangiitis

Microscopic polyangiitis is a pauci-immune vasculitis involving arterioles, venules and capillaries. Almost all patients also show evidence of glomerulonephritis, and microscopic polyangiitis has emerged as one of the more common causes of "pulmonary-renal syndrome." Joints and muscle, upper respiratory tract and skin may also be involved. Over 80% of patients have a positive ANCA, most often of the "perinuclear" type (P-ANCA), directed against myeloperoxidase. Microscopic polyangiitis may occur at any age and is of equal incidence in both males and females. Lung biopsies show alveolar hemorrhage with neutrophilic capillaritis (Fig. 18-72). Immunoglobulin deposition is not seen.

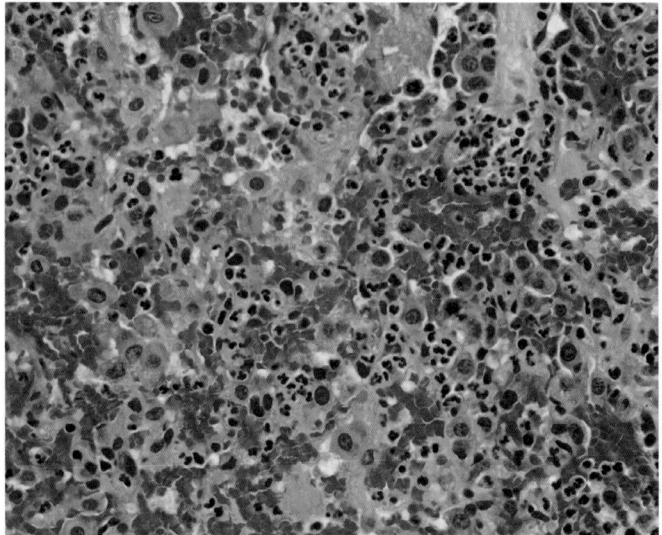

FIGURE 18-72. Microscopic polyangiitis. Alveolar walls are thickened owing to prominent infiltration by neutrophils.

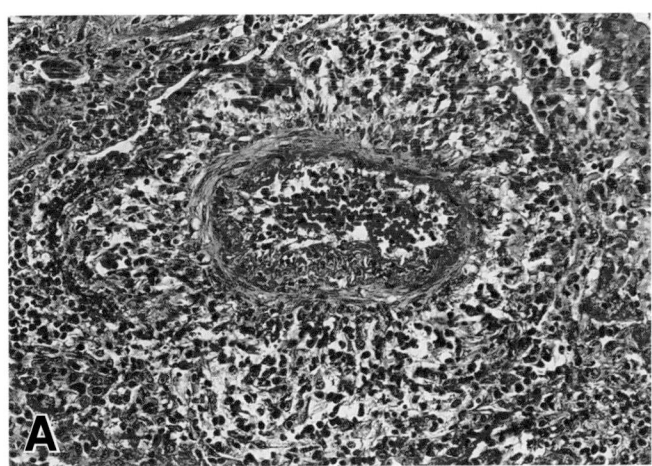
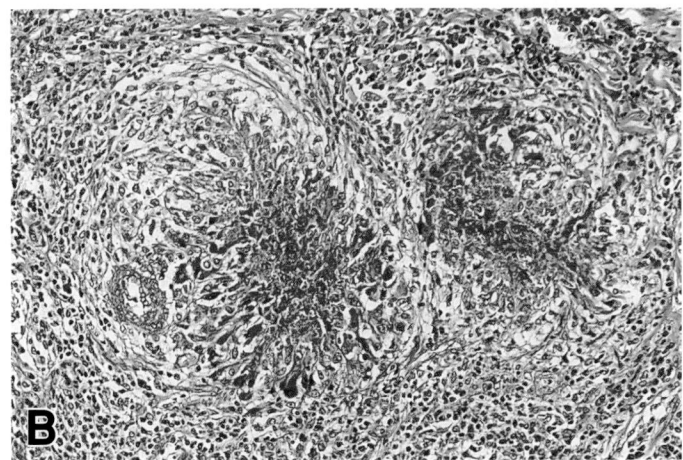

FIGURE 18-73. **Allergic granulomatosis with polyangiitis (formerly Churg-Strauss syndrome). A.** An artery shows severe vasculitis consisting of a dense infiltrate of chronic inflammatory cells and eosinophils. **B.** A necrotic ("allergic") granuloma has a central eosinophilic area of necrosis surrounded by palisading macrophages and giant cells.

Eosinophilic Granulomatosis with Polyangiitis Is a Disorder of Unknown Etiology, Defined by Asthma, Eosinophilia and Vasculitis

 PATHOLOGY: The lungs of patients with EGPA (formerly Churg-Strauss syndrome or allergic angiitis and granulomatosis) show changes of asthmatic bronchitis or bronchiolitis (see above), including eosinophilic pneumonia, vasculitis (Fig. 18-73A), parenchymal necrosis (Fig. 18-73B) and granulomatous inflammation. Infiltrates of eosinophils may be seen in any anatomic compartment of the lung. Involvement of blood vessel walls causes vasculitis and damage to airway walls and results in bronchitis or bronchiolitis. The vasculitis includes eosinophils, lymphocytes, plasma cells, macrophages, giant cells and neutrophils (Fig. 18-73A). Necrotic foci have eosinophilic centers owing to accumulation of dead eosinophils (Fig. 18-73B).

CLINICAL FEATURES: EGPA has 3 clinical phases.

- **Prodrome:** Patients have one or more of the following: allergic rhinitis, asthma, peripheral eosinophilia and eosinophilic infiltrative disease (eosinophilic pneumonia or eosinophilic enteritis).
- **Systemic vasculitic phase:** Extrapulmonary vasculitic manifestations are present, such as cutaneous leukocytoclastic vasculitis or peripheral neuropathy.
- **Postvasculitic phase:** Asthma, allergic rhinitis and complications of neuropathy and hypertension may persist. Cardiovascular manifestations are common and include pericarditis, hypertension and cardiac failure. Renal disease and sinus involvement are usually less severe than those in GPA.

The cause of EGPA is obscure. An autoimmune mechanism is likely, in view of the hypergammaglobulinemia, increased IgE, rheumatoid factor and ANCA.

Patients with EGPA usually are positive for P-ANCA in the vasculitic phase. Most patients respond to corticosteroid therapy, but cyclophosphamide may be needed in severe cases. With treatment, the 5-year survival is 60%.

Necrotizing Sarcoid Granulomatosis Shows Large Zones of Necrosis and Vasculitis

Necrotizing sarcoid granulomatosis is a rare condition featuring nodular confluent sarcoidal granulomas (Fig. 18-74).

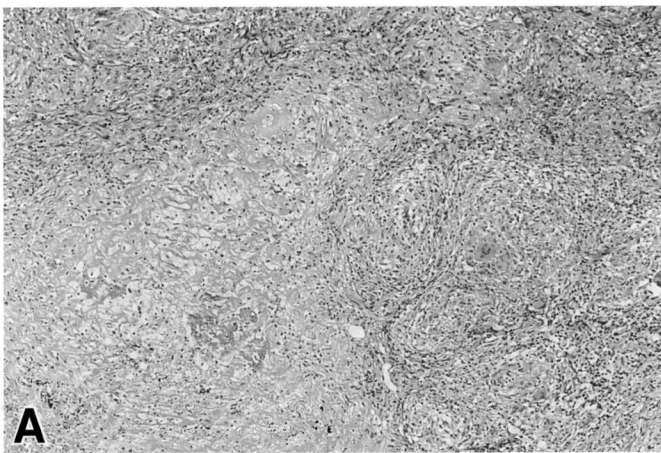
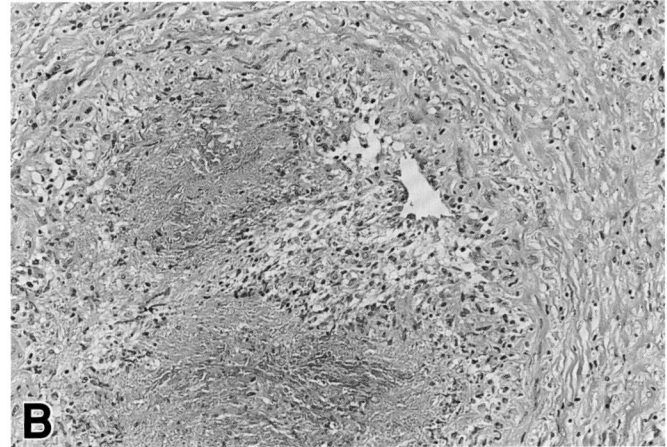

FIGURE 18-74. **Necrotizing sarcoid granulomatosis. A.** A large area of necrosis is surrounded by confluent sarcoid granulomas. **B.** The vasculitis consists of a necrotizing granuloma in the wall of an artery.

It is not a systemic vasculitis, but is usually limited to the lung. Giant cells and necrotizing granulomas (Fig. 18-74B) are seen, as is chronic inflammation with lymphocytes and plasma cells. Most patients are asymptomatic, and chest radiographs typically show multiple, well-circumscribed, pulmonary nodules. Extrapulmonary disease is uncommon, and localized lesions may be treated effectively by surgical removal. Corticosteroids are usually effective for patients with multiple lesions. The prognosis is excellent.

PULMONARY HYPERTENSION

In fetal life, pulmonary arterial walls are thick, as pulmonary arterial pressure is high. Blood is oxygenated through the placenta, not the lungs, and high fetal pulmonary arterial resistance helps to shunt right ventricular output through the ductus arteriosus into the systemic circulation. After birth, the ductus arteriosus closes and the lungs must oxygenate venous blood. The lungs must therefore adapt to accept the entire cardiac output, which demands the high-volume and low-pressure system of the mature lung. By the third day of life, pulmonary arteries dilate, their walls become thin and pulmonary arterial pressure declines.

Elevated pulmonary arterial pressure is defined as a mean pressure over 25 mm Hg at rest. Increased pulmonary blood flow or vascular resistance may lead to higher pulmonary arterial pressure. Whatever the cause, increased pulmonary artery pressure alters pulmonary artery histology (Fig. 18-75). The Heath and Edwards grading system was devised to determine if the arterial changes of pulmonary hypertension could be reversed with corrective cardiac surgery. Grades 1, 2 and 3 are generally reversible; grades 4 and above are generally not.

- **Grade 1:** Medial hypertrophy of muscular pulmonary arteries and appearance of smooth muscle in pulmonary arterioles.
- **Grade 2:** Intimal proliferation with increasing medial hypertrophy.
- **Grade 3:** Intimal fibrosis of muscular pulmonary arteries and arterioles, which may be occlusive (Fig. 18-76A).
- **Grade 4:** Plexiform lesions, dilation and thinning of pulmonary arteries. These nodular lesions are composed of

irregular interlacing blood channels and further obstruct pulmonary blood flow (Fig. 18-76B).
- **Grade 5:** Plexiform lesions in combination with dilation or angiomatoid lesions. Rupture of dilated thin-walled vessel, with parenchymal hemorrhage and hemosiderosis, is also present.
- **Grade 6:** Fibrinoid necrosis of arteries and arterioles.

Even mild pulmonary atherosclerosis is uncommon if pulmonary arterial pressure is normal. However, atherosclerosis is seen in the largest pulmonary arteries with all grades of pulmonary hypertension. Increased pressure in the lesser circulation leads to hypertrophy of the right ventricle (**cor pulmonale**).

Pulmonary Hypertension May Be Precapillary or Postcapillary in Origin

Whether the primary source of increased flow or resistance is proximal or distal to the pulmonary capillary bed may be used to understand the pathophysiology of pulmonary hypertension. Precapillary hypertension includes left-to-right cardiac shunts, primary pulmonary hypertension, thromboembolic pulmonary hypertension and hypertension due to fibrotic lung disease and hypoxia. Postcapillary hypertension includes pulmonary veno-occlusive disease and hypertension secondary to left-sided cardiac disorders, such as mitral stenosis and aortic coarctation.

Left-to-Right Shunts

Shunts from the systemic to the pulmonary circuit increase blood flow to the lungs. Most cases represent congenital left-to-right shunts (see Chapter 17). At birth, the pulmonary artery and the aorta have about the same number of elastic lamellae in their media. Normally, elastic lamellae in the pulmonary artery are lost after birth, but if pulmonary hypertension is present, the fetal pattern of elastic lamellation persists.

Primary Pulmonary Hypertension

Primary pulmonary hypertension is a rare precapillary disorder caused by increased pulmonary arterial tone. The

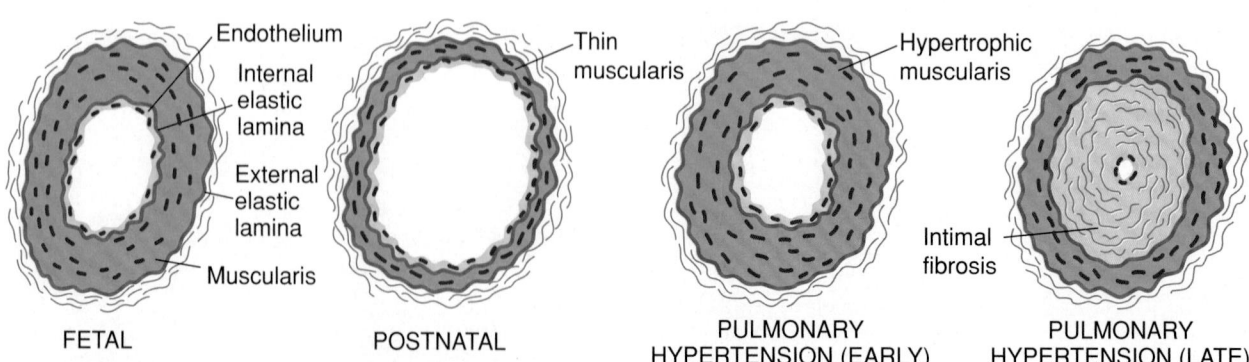

SMALL PULMONARY ARTERIES

FETAL — Endothelium, Internal elastic lamina, External elastic lamina, Muscularis

POSTNATAL — Thin muscularis

PULMONARY HYPERTENSION (EARLY) — Hypertrophic muscularis

PULMONARY HYPERTENSION (LATE) — Intimal fibrosis

FIGURE 18-75. Histopathology of pulmonary hypertension. In late gestation, the pulmonary arteries have thick walls. After birth, the vessels dilate, and the walls become thin. Mild pulmonary hypertension is characterized by thickening of the media. As pulmonary hypertension becomes more severe, there is extensive intimal fibrosis and muscle thickening.

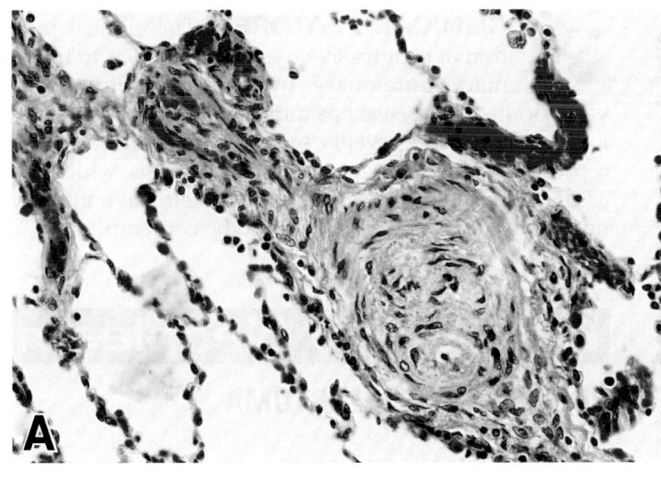

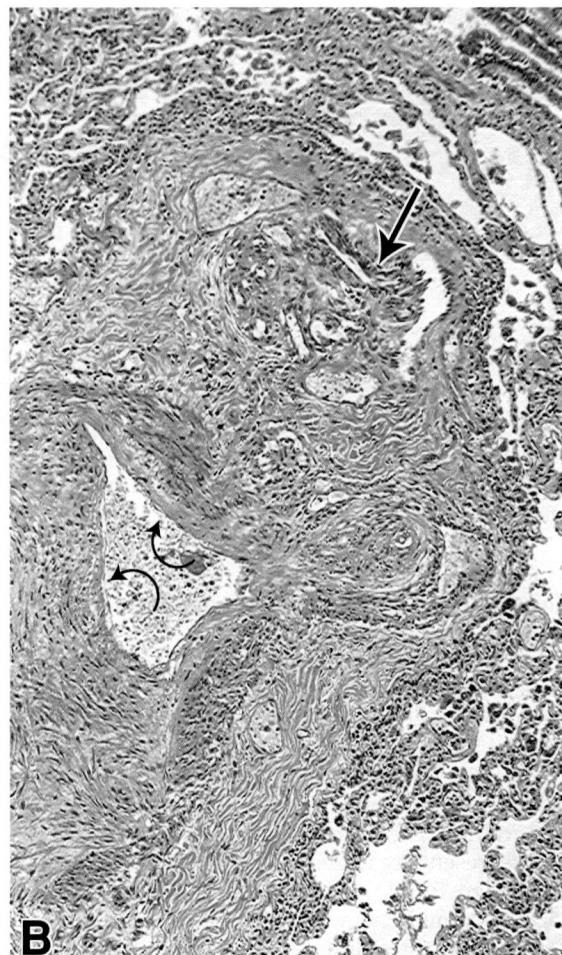

FIGURE 18-76. Pulmonary arterial hypertension. A. A small pulmonary artery is virtually occluded by concentric intimal fibrosis and thickening of the media. **B.** A plexiform lesion (*arrow*) is characterized by a glomeruloid proliferation of thin-walled vessels adjacent to a parent artery, which shows marked hypertensive changes of intimal fibrosis and medial thickening (*curved arrows*).

condition may be idiopathic, but some cases are hereditary and have been associated with mutations of bone morphogenetic protein receptor type 2 (*BMPR2*), activin receptor-like kinase 1 (*ALK1*) and endoglein. Pulmonary arterial hypertension may also be encountered in association with underlying collagen vascular diseases or may be induced by drugs or toxins (an example being the diet drug "phen-phen"). Pulmonary arterial hypertension occurs at all ages but is most common in young women in their 20s and 30s. It presents with insidious onset of dyspnea. Physical signs and radiologic abnormalities are initially slight but become more apparent with time. Severe pulmonary hypertension, typically associated with plexiform lesions histologically, eventually ensues, and patients die of cor pulmonale. Although medical treatment is mostly ineffective, recent use of prostacyclin analogs, endothelin receptor antagonists and phosphodiesterase-5 inhibitors have led to a 5-year survival of about 30%. Heart–lung transplantation is often indicated.

Recurrent Pulmonary Emboli

Multiple thromboemboli in smaller pulmonary vessels often result from asymptomatic, episodic showers of small emboli from the periphery. They gradually limit pulmonary circulation and lead to pulmonary hypertension. Some patients have peripheral venous thromboses, usually in leg veins, or a history of circumstances predisposing to

venous thrombosis. In addition to the vascular lesions of pulmonary hypertension, organized thromboemboli are evidenced by fibrous bands ("webs") that extend across the lumina of small pulmonary arteries. If the condition is diagnosed during life, placement of a filter in the inferior vena cava usually prevents further embolization.

Any Disorder That Produces Hypoxemia Can Constrict Small Pulmonary Arteries and Lead to Pulmonary Hypertension

Predisposing conditions include chronic airflow obstruction (chronic bronchitis), interstitial lung disease and living at high altitude. Severe kyphoscoliosis or extreme obesity **(Pickwickian syndrome)** may impede ventilation and lead to hypoxemia and pulmonary hypertension.

Left Ventricular Failure Increases Pulmonary Venous Pressure and Secondarily Pulmonary Arterial Pressure

Both mitral stenosis and insufficiency can produce severe venous hypertension and significant pulmonary artery hypertension. In such cases, the lungs exhibit lesions of both pulmonary hypertension and chronic passive congestion (see Chapter 7).

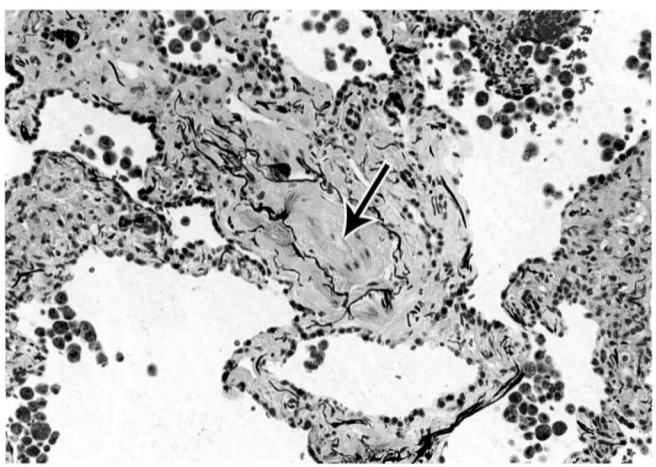

FIGURE 18-77. Veno-occlusive disease of the lung. This pulmonary vein is occluded by intimal fibrosis (*arrow;* Movat stain).

Pulmonary Veno-Occlusive Disease Involves Fibrotic Obstruction of Small Veins

Pulmonary veno-occlusive disease (PVOD) is a rare condition of uncertain etiology in which small pulmonary veins and venules are occluded by loose, sparsely cellular, intimal fibrosis (Fig. 18-77). Some large veins may also be involved, and in half of cases, similar but less severe lesions affect pulmonary arteries. The obstructive lesions may canalize, and so could represent organized thrombi, possibly due to endothelial damage. PVOD may follow viral infections, exposure to toxic agents and chemotherapy. More than half of cases occur in the first three decades of life. In children, girls and boys are affected similarly, but after age 15, it is more common in men.

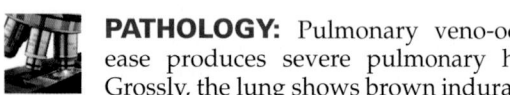 **PATHOLOGY:** Pulmonary veno-occlusive disease produces severe pulmonary hypertension. Grossly, the lung shows brown induration and atherosclerosis of large pulmonary arteries. Microscopically, small veins and venules are partly or totally occluded and larger veins show eccentric intimal thickening. Moderate alveolar wall fibrosis and foci of hemosiderosis are common. Pulmonary arteries show recent thrombi and lesions of severe pulmonary hypertension.

 CLINICAL FEATURES: The clinical presentation of progressive dyspnea is similar to that of primary pulmonary hypertension, but pulmonary veno-occlusive disease has a more fulminant course. Radiologic examination reveals scattered infiltrates in the lung, representing hemorrhage and hemosiderosis, which increase as the disease progresses. There is no effective therapy, and heart–lung transplantation should be contemplated.

Pulmonary Neoplasms

PULMONARY HAMARTOMA

The term "hamartoma" implies a malformation, but hamartomas are true tumors. They typically occur in adults, with a peak in the sixth decade of life, and account for 10% of "coin" lesions discovered incidentally on chest radiographs. A characteristic ("popcorn") pattern of calcification is often seen by x-ray.

 PATHOLOGY: Grossly, pulmonary hamartomas are solitary, circumscribed, lobulated masses, averaging 2 cm in diameter, with a white or gray, cartilaginous cut surface (Fig. 18-78A). The tumor has elements usually present in the lung: cartilage, fibromyxoid connective tissue, fat, bone and occasionally smooth muscle (Fig. 18-78B), interspersed with clefts lined by respiratory epithelium. Hamartomas are benign and well circumscribed and shell out from the surrounding lung parenchyma. Most are seen in the periphery, but 10% occur in a central endobronchial location. The latter may cause symptoms due to bronchial obstruction.

CARCINOMA OF THE LUNG

 **EPIDEMIOLOGY:** Regarded as a rare tumor as recently as 1945, lung cancer is the most common cause of cancer mortality worldwide. In the United States, where it is the leading cause of cancer death in both men and women, 85%–90% of lung cancers occur in cigarette smokers (see Chapter 8); conversely, the lifetime risk of developing lung cancer in smokers is 12%–17%. Smokers are

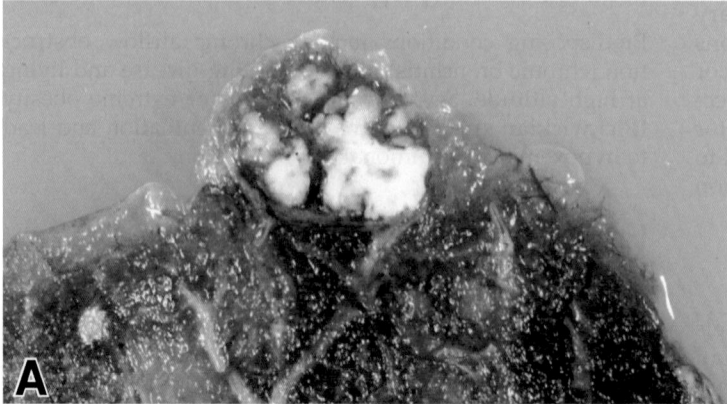
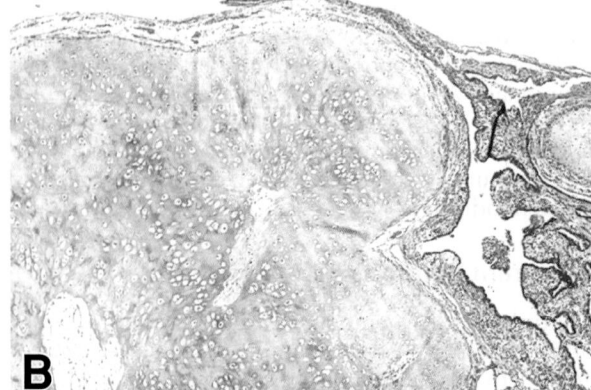

FIGURE 18-78. Pulmonary hamartoma. A. The cut surface of a sharply circumscribed, peripheral pulmonary nodule shows a lobulated structure. **B.** A photomicrograph reveals nodules of hyaline cartilage separated by connective tissue lined by respiratory epithelium.

TABLE 18-6

FREQUENCY OF LUNG CARCINOMA HISTOLOGIC TYPES BY GENDER (NCI SEER DATA, HISTOLOGICALLY CONFIRMED, 2006–2010)

Subtype	Males	Females	Males and Females
Adenocarcinoma	32.9	40.5	36.4
Squamous cell carcinoma	23.8	15.6	20
Small cell carcinoma	13.0	14.7	13.8
Large cell carcinoma	3.6	2.9	3.3
Other carcinomas	23.7	21.8	22.8
Carcinoid	2.0	3.5	2.7
Adenosquamous carcinoma	1.0	1.0	1.0

at risk for "non–small cell lung carcinomas" (NSCLCs)—encompassing squamous cell carcinoma, adenocarcinoma and large cell carcinoma (see also Pathology paragraph below)—and for small cell lung carcinoma (SCLC). Most of the never-smokers who develop lung cancer have an adenocarcinoma. In general, 80% of lung cancers are NSCLC and 17% are SCLC. The distribution of histologic subtypes of NSCLC according to gender is shown in Table 18-6. The peak age for lung cancer is between 60 and 70 years, with most patients between 50 and 80 years. The former male predominance is decreasing as smoking increases among women.

General Features of Lung Cancer

 CLINICAL FEATURES: Lung cancer presents in early stages in 30% of patients where the primary treatment approach is surgical resection and pathology assessment is based on evaluation of the entire tumor. However, the remaining 70% of lung cancers present as advanced, unresectable disease. Then, diagnosis is based on nonresection specimens (small biopsies and cytology) and treatment is mostly chemotherapy and/or radiation.

Lung cancers were categorized as SCLCs and NSCLCs, with the latter encompassing squamous cell carcinoma, adenocarcinoma and large cell carcinoma. The reason for this was that small cell carcinomas responded to specific chemotherapies, but non–small cell tumors did not. Now, some NSCLCs can be treated with chemotherapy: lung adenocarcinoma patients whose tumors express endothelial growth factor receptor (*EGFR*) mutations or rearrangements involving the anaplastic lymphoma kinase gene (ALK, or CD246, not to be confused with ALK1, see above) show better progression-free survival if treated with tyrosine kinase inhibitors or crizotinib, respectively. Patients with advanced-stage adenocarcinoma—but not squamous cell carcinoma—respond to a folate antimetabolite, pemetrexed. Furthermore, patients with advanced squamous carcinoma are at risk for life-threatening hemorrhage.

Overall survival for all patients with NSCLC was 15% for the past few decades. However, advanced lung cancer patients with *EGFR* mutations or ALK rearrangements show improved 2-year progression-free survival, from 20%

to 60%, with tyrosine kinase inhibitor and ALK therapy, respectively. The molecular landscape of lung cancer is evolving rapidly.

Small cell carcinomas have a dismal prognosis: 5-year survival of 5% or less. *Tumor stage is the single most important predictor of prognosis.* The staging system for lung carcinoma is based primarily on tumor size, extent of spread in the lung and chest, lymph node involvement and distant metastases or malignancy involving the pleural fluid. The staging system for lung cancer is summarized in Table 18-7.

LOCAL EFFECTS: Lung cancer can produce cough, dyspnea, hemoptysis, chest pain, obstructive pneumonia and pleural effusion. A lung cancer (usually squamous) in the apex of the lung **(Pancoast tumor)** may extend to involve the eighth cervical and first and second thoracic nerves, leading to shoulder pain that radiates down the arm in an ulnar distribution **(Pancoast syndrome)**. A Pancoast tumor also may paralyze cervical sympathetic nerves and cause **Horner syndrome** on the affected side with (1) depression of the eyeball (enophthalmos), (2) ptosis of the upper eyelid, (3) constriction of the pupil (miosis) and (4) absence of sweating (anhidrosis).

Most central endobronchial tumors produce symptoms related to bronchial obstruction: persistent cough, hemoptysis and obstructive pneumonia, or atelectasis. Effusions can result from tumor extension into the pleura or pericardium. Lymphangitic spread of the tumor within the lung may interfere with oxygenation. Tumors arising peripherally are more likely to be discovered on routine chest radiographs or after they have become advanced. The latter circumstance features invasion of the chest wall with resulting chest pain, superior vena cava syndrome and nerve entrapment syndromes.

MEDIASTINAL SPREAD: Tumor growth within the mediastinum can cause superior vena cava syndrome (owing to tumorous obstruction of this vein) and nerve entrapment syndromes.

METASTASES: Lung cancers metastasize most often to regional lymph nodes, particularly hilar and mediastinal nodes, and to the brain, bone and liver. Extranodal metastases often involve the adrenal gland, but adrenal insufficiency is uncommon.

PARANEOPLASTIC SYNDROMES: Disorders associated with lung cancer include acanthosis nigricans, dermatomyositis/polymyositis, clubbing of the fingers and myasthenic syndromes, such as Eaton-Lambert syndrome and progressive multifocal encephalopathy. Endocrine syndromes are also seen, for example, Cushing syndrome or the syndrome of inappropriate release of antidiuretic hormone (SIADH) in small cell carcinomas, and hypercalcemia (secretion of a parathormone-like substance) in squamous cell carcinomas. Small cell carcinomas may also be associated with a syndrome of paraneoplastic encephalomyelitis and sensory neuropathy associated with circulating anti-Hu antibodies.

 **MOLECULAR PATHOGENESIS:** No single mutation determines the development of lung cancer, but some are common and may allow for targeted chemotherapy.

- *EGFR:* Activating mutations in the tyrosine kinase domain of this gene are of particular interest in lung adenocarcinomas,

TABLE 18-7

AMERICAN JOINT COMMISSION ON CANCER LUNG CANCER STAGING SYSTEM

T1   Tumor <3 cm surrounded by lung or visceral pleura and not involving the mainstem bronchus

   T1a: <2 cm

   T1b: 2–3 cm

T2   Tumor >3 cm but ≤7 cm OR tumor with any of the following features:

   Involves main bronchus, ≥2 cm distal to the carina

   Invades visceral pleura

   Associated with atelectasis or obstructive pneumonitis that extends to the hilar region but does not involve the entire lung

   T2a: >3 cm but ≤5 cm

   T2b: >5 cm but ≤7 cm

T3   Tumor >7 cm OR a tumor with involvement of any of the following: chest wall (including superior sulcus tumors), diaphragm, mediastinal pleura, pericardium or main stem bronchus 2 cm from carina OR entire lung atelectasis OR separate tumor nodules in the same lobe

T4   Tumor with invasion of mediastinum, heart, great vessels, trachea, esophagus, vertebral body or carina OR separate tumor nodules in a different ipsilateral lobe

N0   No demonstrable metastasis to regional lymph nodes

N1   Ipsilateral hilar or peribronchial nodal involvement

N2   Metastasis to ipsilateral mediastinal or subcarinal lymph nodes

N3   Metastasis to contralateral mediastinal or hilar lymph nodes, ipsilateral or contralateral scalene or supraclavicular lymph nodes

M0   No distant metastasis

M1   Distant metastasis

   M1a: separate tumor nodule in contralateral lobe or separate pleural nodules or malignant pleural effusion

   M1b: distant metastasis

Lung Cancer Stage Groupings

Stage Ia	T1	N0	M0
Stage Ib	T2	N0	M0
Stage IIa	T1	N1	M0
Stage IIb	T2	N1	M0
	T3	N0	M0
Stage IIIa	T1–3	N2	M0
	T3	N1	M0
Stage IIIb	Any T	N3	M0
	T3	N2	M0
	T4	Any N	M0
Stage IV	Any T	Any N	M1

Data from Edge SB, Byrd DR, Compton CC, et al., eds. AJCC Cancer Staging Manual. 7th Ed. New York: Springer, 2010.

owing to the responsiveness of mutated tumors to tyrosine kinase inhibitor drugs targeted against this receptor, such as erlotinib and gefitinib. *EGFR* mutations are more common in adenocarcinomas in nonsmokers, Asians and women. These mutations occur in 10%–15% of lung adenocarcinomas in the United States, with higher percentages in nonsmokers and women, but 40%–60% of East Asians have *EGFR* mutations.

- **K-ras:** Mutations in this oncogene, particularly codons 12 and 13, occur in 25% of adenocarcinomas, 20% of large cell carcinomas and 5% of squamous carcinomas, but rarely in SCLCs. These mutations correlate with cigarette smoking and with a poor prognosis in patients with adenocarcinoma. No effective targeted molecular therapy is available for *K-ras* mutations.

- **EML4-ALK translocations:** Fusion between echinoderm microtubule-associated protein-like 4 (*EML4*) and anaplastic lymphoma kinase (*ALK*) is encountered in approximately 5% of advanced pulmonary adenocarcinomas, most frequently in nonsmokers. Adenocarcinomas harboring this translocation are responsive to targeted therapy with crizotinib.

- **Myc:** Overexpression of this oncogene occurs in 10%–40% of small cell carcinomas but is rare in other types.

- **p53:** Mutations of *p53* are identified in more than 80% of small cell carcinomas and 50% of non–small cell tumors.

- **Rb:** Mutations in the retinoblastoma (*Rb*) gene occur in over 80% of small cell cancers and 25% of non–small cell carcinomas.

- **Chromosome 3 (3p):** Deletions in the short arm of this chromosome are frequently found in all types of lung cancers.

- **bcl-2:** This protooncogene encodes a protein that inhibits apoptosis (see Chapter 1). It is expressed in 25% of squamous cell carcinomas and 10% of adenocarcinomas.

- **PTEN:** This tumor suppressor gene regulates cell survival signaling and is deficient by one of a number of mechanisms (loss of heterozygosity, mutation, promoter methylation, etc.) in many non–small cell lung cancers. Loss of PTEN is associated with poor prognosis and drug resistance.

- **FGFR1** (fibroblast growth factor receptor 1): Amplification of FGFR1 has been reported in 20% of squamous cell carcinoma, and FGFR inhibitors are currently the subject of clinical testing.

- **Other mutations:** Abnormalities of *BRAF, PIK3CA, ERBB2, ROS-1, RET* and others have been reported in small percentages of lung carcinoma and are the focus of ongoing efforts to identify effective targeted therapies.

 PATHOLOGY: Squamous cell carcinoma, adenocarcinoma, large cell carcinoma and small cell carcinoma are the major forms of lung cancer. Although the term **bronchogenic** carcinoma was once used, about one fourth of primary lung cancers do not have an obvious bronchial origin, so this term is no longer recommended. Squamous cell carcinoma, adenocarcinoma and large cell carcinoma have traditionally been lumped together from a clinical standpoint as "non–small cell carcinoma" because of historically similar treatment; however, advances in chemotherapy and targeted therapies in particular have made subtyping of critical importance, and the usage of "non–small cell carcinoma" is discouraged.

Histologic subtyping of lung cancer is based on the best-differentiated component, unless an area of small cell carcinoma is present. However, the degree of differentiation is graded according to the worst-differentiated component. If a tumor is mostly poorly differentiated large cells but has foci of squamous cells or adenocarcinoma, it is classified as a poorly differentiated squamous cell carcinoma or adenocarcinoma, respectively. Any cancer with a component of small cell carcinoma is regarded as a subtype of that tumor (see below).

Histologic Subtypes of Lung Carcinoma

Squamous Cell Carcinoma

Squamous cell carcinoma is the second most common histologic type of lung cancer, accounting for 20% of all lung cancers in the United States, and is more common in men than in women (Table 18-6). After injury to the bronchial epithelium, such as occurs with cigarette smoking, regeneration from the pluripotent basal layer commonly entails squamous metaplasia. The metaplastic squamous mucosa follows the same sequence of dysplasia, carcinoma in situ and invasive tumor seen in other sites normally lined by squamous epithelium, such as the cervix or skin.

Most squamous cell carcinomas arise centrally in the lung, from major or segmental bronchi, although 10% originate in the periphery. They tend to be firm, gray-white, 3–5-cm ulcerated lesions that extend through the bronchial wall into the adjacent lung parenchyma (Fig. 18-79A). Central cavitation is frequent. On occasion, a central squamous carcinoma occurs as an endobronchial tumor.

These tumors vary widely in degrees of squamous differentiation. Many show overt keratinization or intercellular bridges. Well-differentiated tumors have keratin "pearls," small round nests of brightly eosinophilic aggregates of keratin surrounded by concentric ("onion skin") layers of squamous cells (Fig. 18-79B). Individual cell keratinization also occurs, in which the cytoplasm becomes glassy and intensely eosinophilic. Intercellular bridges in some well-differentiated squamous cancers are slender gaps between adjacent cells, traversed by fine strands of cytoplasm. By

contrast, some squamous tumors are very poorly differentiated: they lack keratinization and are difficult to distinguish from large cell, small cell or spindle cell carcinomas.

Adenocarcinoma

Worldwide, adenocarcinoma has overtaken squamous cell carcinoma as the most common subtype of lung cancer in most countries, and it is the most common type in nonsmokers. In the United States, it accounts for 36% of all invasive lung malignancies and is more common in women (41% of all lung cancers) than in men (33% of all lung cancers) (Table 18-6). It tends to arise in the periphery and is often associated with pleural fibrosis and subpleural scars, which can lead to pleural puckering (Fig. 18-80). These cancers were once thought to arise in scars left by old tuberculosis or healed infarcts, but it is now recognized that such scars represent a desmoplastic response to the tumor. Adenocarcinoma classification has recently been revised. The term "bronchioloalveolar carcinoma" has been dropped because it was found to represent 5 different entities. Also, the term "mixed subtype adenocarcinoma" is no longer used.

Atypical adenomatous hyperplasia (AAH) is recognized as a putative precursor lesion for adenocarcinomas. AAH is a well-demarcated lesion, usually less than 5 mm, with atypical proliferation of epithelial cells along alveolar septa (Fig. 18-81). In a sequence similar to the "adenoma–carcinoma" sequence in colon cancers, lung adenocarcinomas are thought potentially to originate as AAH and progress to adenocarcinoma in situ and then to more aggressive invasive adenocarcinomas. The finding of progressive accumulation of mutations as the lesions advance supports this hypothesis. It remains unclear whether all foci of AAH will progress to carcinoma or if all adenocarcinomas arise via this sequence of events.

Adenocarcinoma in Situ

Adenocarcinoma in situ (AIS), once called bronchioloalveolar carcinoma, is a preinvasive form of adenocarcinoma in which tumor cells grow only along preexisting alveolar

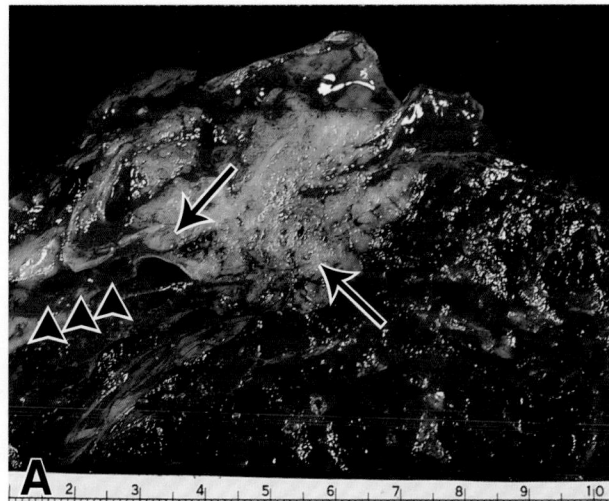
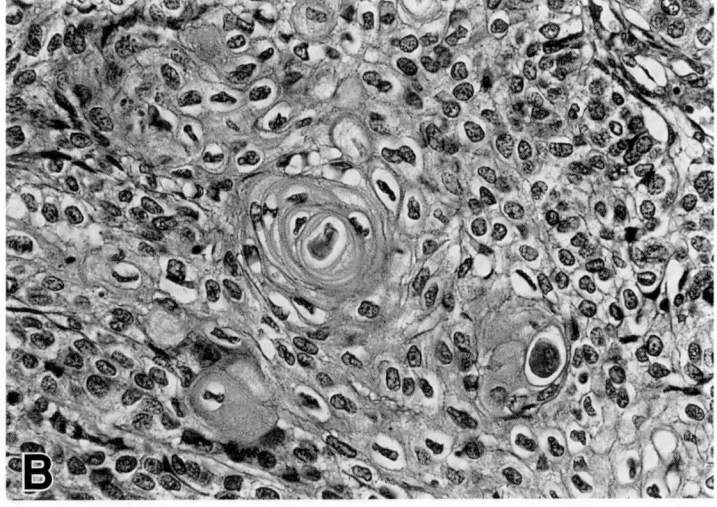

FIGURE 18-79. Squamous cell carcinoma of the lung. A. The tumor (*large arrow*) grows within the lumen of a bronchus (*arrowheads* highlight the course of the bronchus) and invades the adjacent intrapulmonary lymph node (*small arrow*). **B.** A photomicrograph shows well-differentiated squamous cell carcinoma with a keratin pearl composed of cells with brightly eosinophilic cytoplasm.

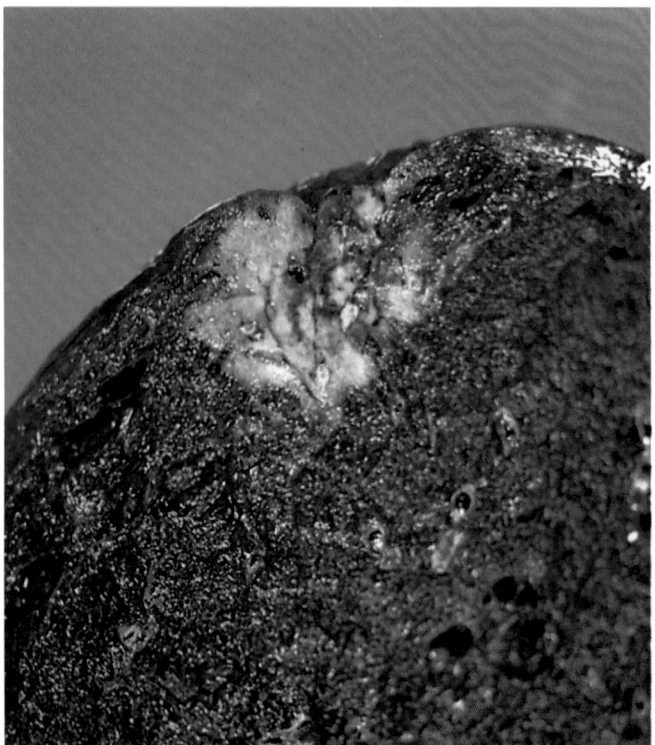

FIGURE 18-80. Invasive adenocarcinoma of the lung. A peripheral tumor of the right upper lobe has an irregular border and a tan or gray cut surface and causes puckering of the overlying pleura.

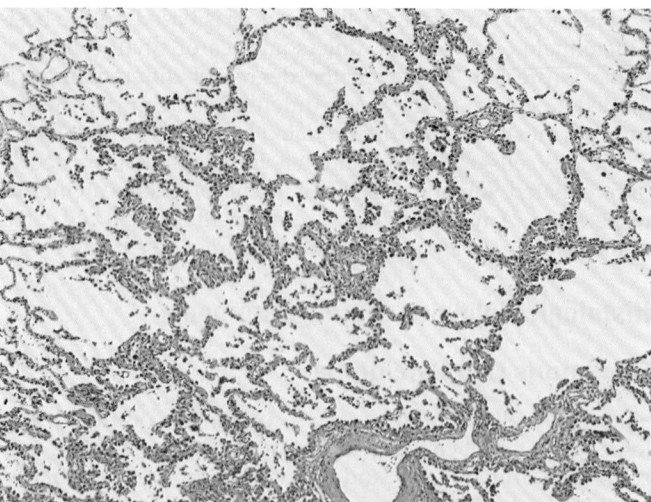

FIGURE 18-81. Atypical adenomatous hyperplasia. This millimeter-sized bronchioloalveolar proliferation is ill-defined with mild thickening of alveolar walls lined by hyperplastic pneumocytes that show minimal atypia.

walls (lepidic growth). It accounts for 1%–5% of lung adenocarcinomas. Patients with tumors meeting criteria for AIS have a 100% 5-year survival rate after resection.

Minimally Invasive Adenocarcinoma

For adenocarcinomas, a small amount of invasion in a tumor otherwise showing lepidic growth does not adversely affect prognosis. This has led to the introduction

of a category of adenocarcinoma called minimally invasive adenocarcinoma (MIA, formerly bronchioloalveolar carcinoma), which has the same favorable prognosis as AIS. MIA is defined as a tumor with lepidic growth as seen in AIS, but with foci of invasive tumor measuring 5 mm or less in maximal diameter and lacking pleural or lymphovascular invasion and necrosis.

Both AIS and MIA may be seen radiographically as single peripheral nodules with a "ground glass" appearance or as multiple nodules. AIS shows pure ground glass changes radiographically, while MIA may show a small solid component. Grossly, both tumors should measure less than or equal to 3 cm and typically appear as ill-defined tan lesions, which may be difficult to distinguish from surrounding normal tissue.

Most AIS and MIA are nonmucinous, with club cells (formerly Clara cells) and/or type II pneumocytes. Only rarely

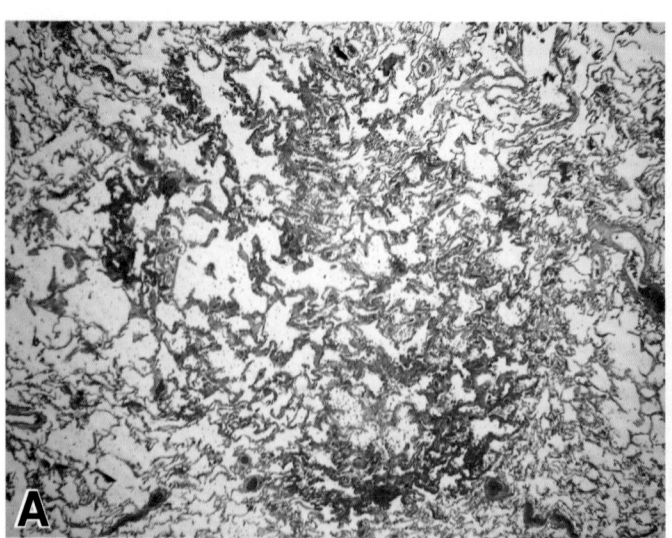

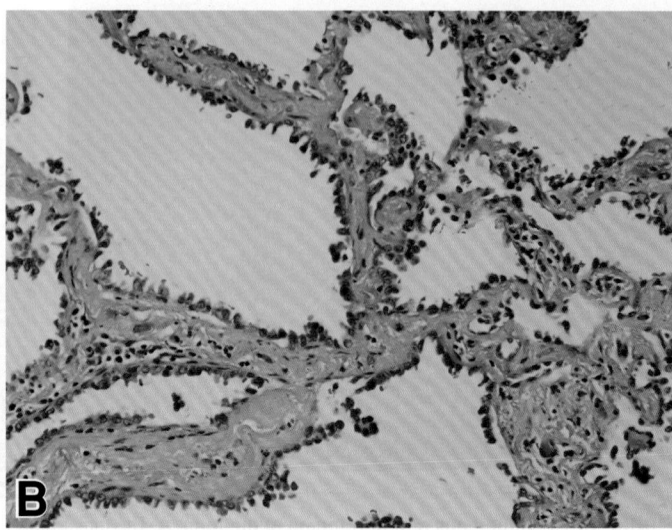

FIGURE 18-82. Adenocarcinoma in situ. A. This circumscribed nonmucinous tumor grows purely with a lepidic pattern. No foci of invasion or scarring are seen. **B.** A layer of atypical pneumocytes lines the alveolar walls.

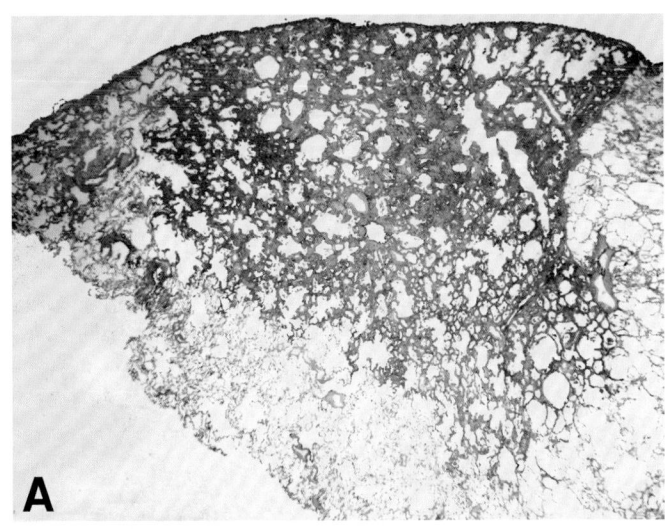

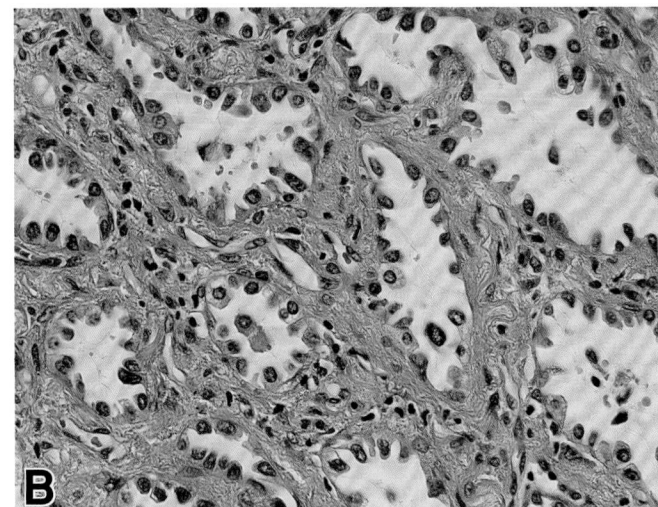

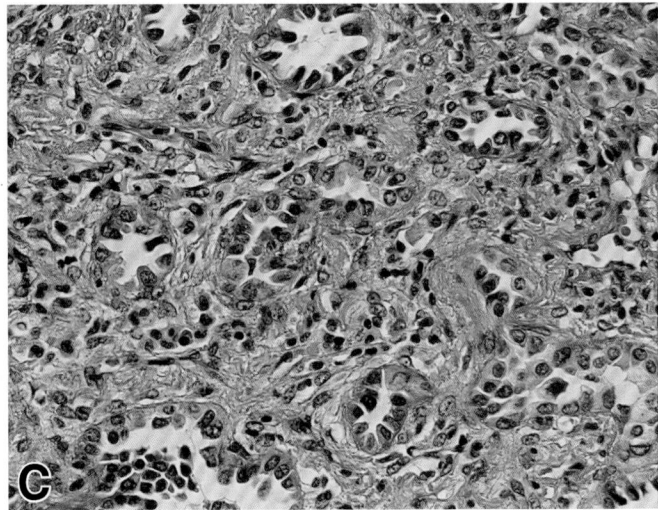

FIGURE 18-83. Minimally invasive adenocarcinoma. A. This nonmucinous adenocarcinoma consists primarily of lepidic growth with a small (<0.5 cm) area of invasion. **B.** The lepidic component shows alveolar walls lined by atypical pneumocytes. **C.** From the area of invasion, these acinar glands are invading in the fibrous stroma.

are they mucinous. AIS has a pure lepidic pattern without invasion. (Fig. 18-82A,B). MIA is lepidic-predominant adenocarcinoma with an invasive component less than or equal to 5 mm in maximal dimension (Fig. 18-83). In nonmucinous tumors, cuboidal cells grow along alveolar walls. Mucinous tumors contain columnar cells with abundant apical cytoplasm filled with mucus, sometimes with a goblet cell appearance. Particularly for mucinous tumors, the possibility that the tumor is metastatic from another site must be excluded.

Invasive Adenocarcinomas

AIS and MIA account for only 5% of adenocarcinomas. Most lung adenocarcinomas are more invasive. They are typically very heterogeneous and consist of a mixture of growth patterns. Invasive tumors are now classified based on the predominant growth pattern. Such patterns include lepidic, acinar, papillary, solid and micropapillary. Rarely, tumors will contain only a single growth pattern. For completely resected tumors, the predominant histologic subtype has prognostic significance. AIS and MIA have 100% 5-year disease-free survival. For stage I invasive adenocarcinomas, lepidic-predominant adenocarcinoma has excellent 5-year

disease-free survival (>90%), with an intermediate survival for acinar and papillary types (80%–90%). The worst disease-free survival is for solid and micropapillary adenocarcinoma (60%–80%).

 PATHOLOGY: Invasive lung adenocarcinomas appear mostly as irregular 2–5-cm masses but may be so large as to replace an entire lobe. On cut section, nonmucinous tumors are grayish white. Mucinous tumors may be glistening or gelatinous depending on the amount of mucin production. Central adenocarcinomas may grow mainly endobronchially and invade bronchial cartilage.

Most invasive adenocarcinomas contain heterogeneous mixtures of lepidic, acinar, papillary, micropapillary and solid patterns. Lepidic-predominant tumors are invasive lung adenocarcinomas in which lepidic growth is the most prominent pattern (Fig. 18-84A,B). The acinar pattern is distinguished by regular glands lined by cuboidal or columnar cells (Fig. 18-85A). Acinar-predominant adenocarcinomas are the most common category of invasive adenocarcinomas. Papillary adenocarcinomas exhibit a single cell layer on a core of fibrovascular connective tissue (Fig. 18-85B).

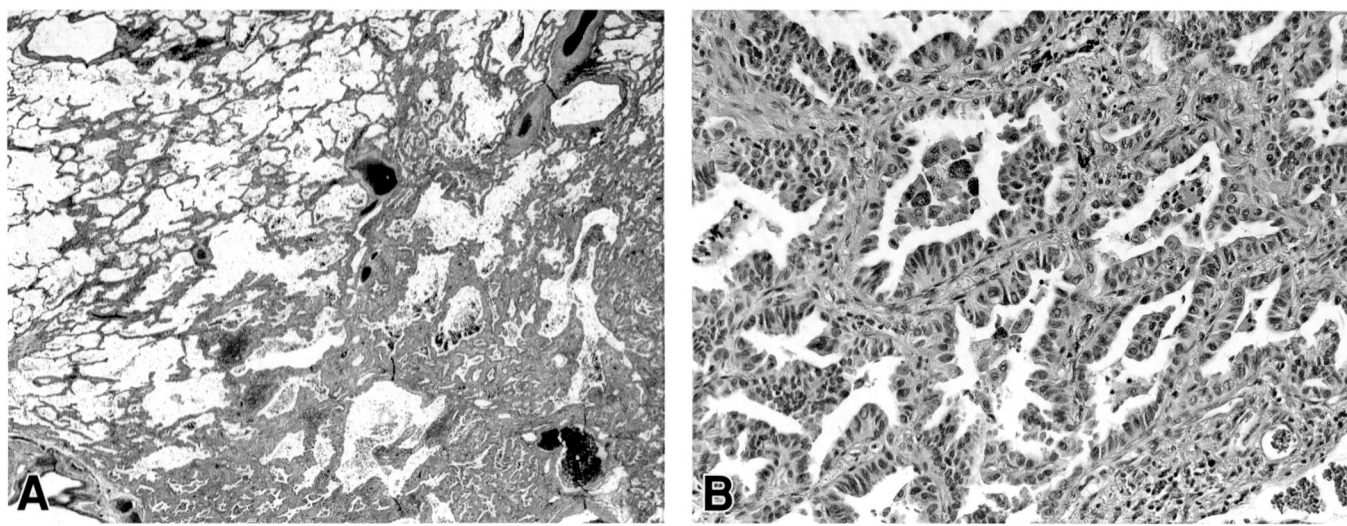

FIGURE 18-84. Adenocarcinoma with lepidic-predominant *pattern*. A. The tumor shows mostly lepidic growth and an area of invasive acinar adenocarcinoma. **B.** Lepidic pattern consists of a proliferation of type II pneumocytes and Clara cells along the surface alveolar walls.

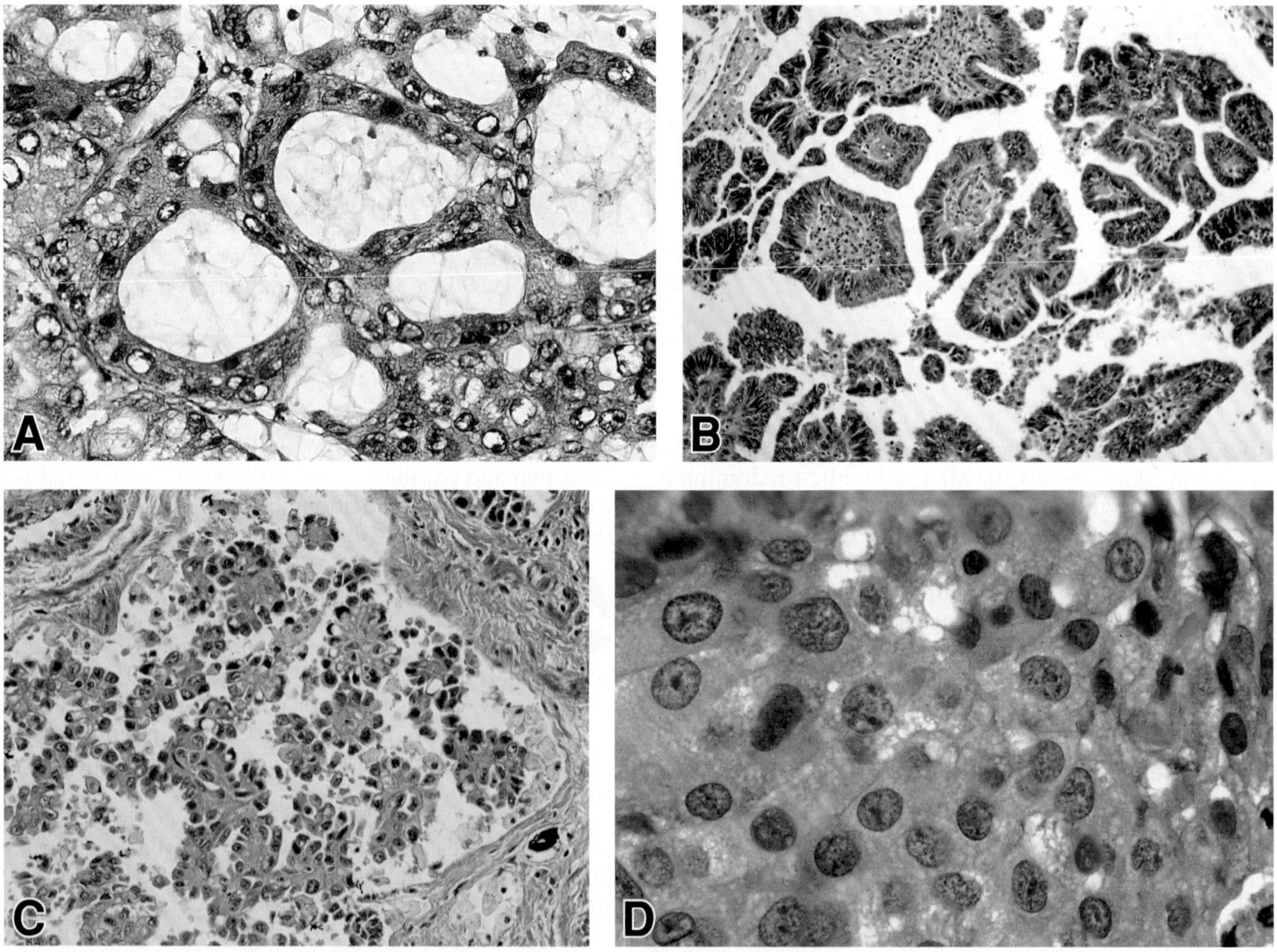

FIGURE 18-85. Invasive adenocarcinoma of the lung. A. Acinar adenocarcinoma composed of round to oval-shaped malignant glands. **B. Papillary adenocarcinoma** consists of malignant cuboidal to columnar tumor cells growing on the surface of fibrovascular cores. **C. Micropapillary adenocarcinoma** consists of small papillary clusters of glandular cells growing within this airspace, most of which do not show fibrovascular cores. **D.** Solid adenocarcinoma with mucin formation consists of solid sheets of tumor cells with several red intracytoplasmic mucin droplets that stain positively with the mucicarmine stain.

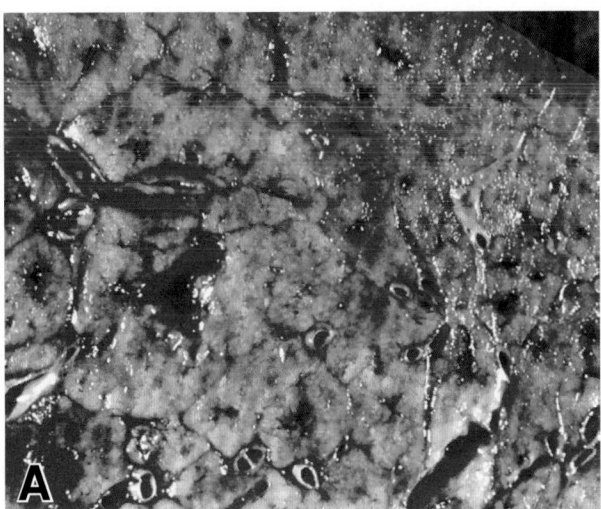
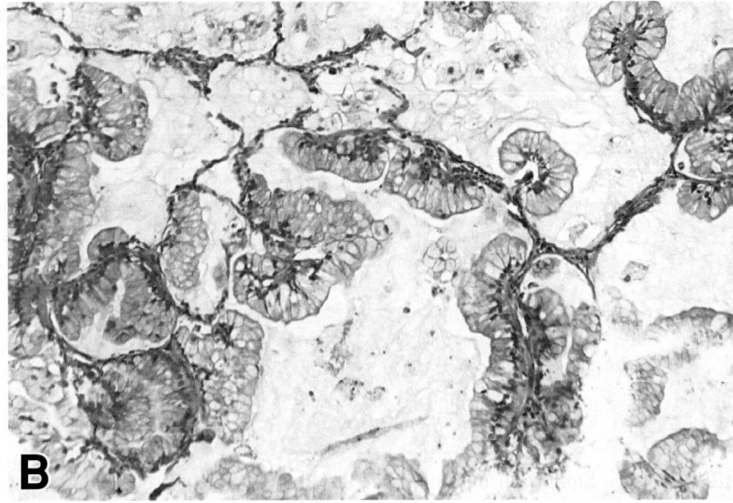

FIGURE 18-86. Invasive mucinous adenocarcinoma. A. The cut surface of the lung is solid, glistening and mucoid, an appearance that reflects a diffusely infiltrating tumor. **B.** Mucinous bronchioloalveolar carcinoma consists of tall columnar cells filled with apical cytoplasmic mucin that grow along existing alveolar walls.

Micropapillary carcinomas show small papillary tufts of tumor cells with no fibrovascular core. The cells may appear to float in alveolar spaces, glands or spaces in fibrous stroma (Fig. 18-85C). Solid adenocarcinomas with mucus formation are poorly differentiated tumors. They are different from large cell carcinomas by having mucin detected with mucicarmine or periodic acid–Schiff (with diastase digestion) stains (Fig. 18-85D). Invasive mucinous adenocarcinomas show solid mucoid cut surfaces (Fig. 18-86A) and have tall columnar cells with apical cytoplasmic mucin (Fig. 18-86B).

Large Cell Carcinoma

Large cell carcinoma is a diagnosis of exclusion: a poorly differentiated tumor lacking squamous or glandular differentiation that is not a small cell carcinoma (Fig. 18-87). This tumor type accounts for 30% of invasive lung tumors in the United States (Table 18-6). The cells are large and exhibit ample cytoplasm. Nuclei frequently show prominent nucleoli and vesicular chromatin.

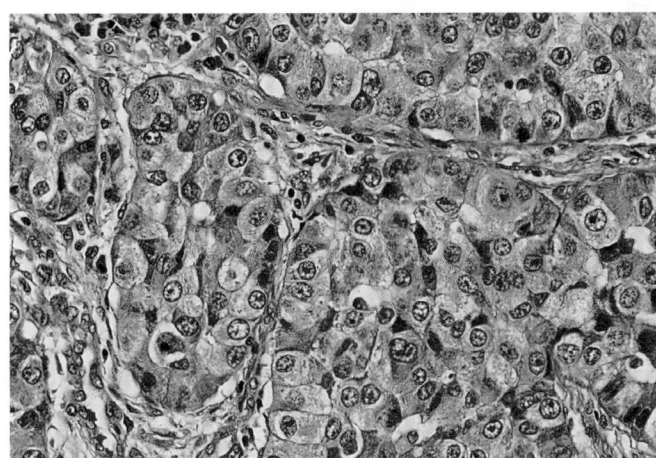

FIGURE 18-87. Large cell carcinoma of the lung. This poorly differentiated tumor is growing in sheets. Tumor cells are large and contain ample cytoplasm and prominent nucleoli.

Some large cell carcinomas called **large cell neuroendocrine carcinoma** grow like carcinoid tumors (see below), with an organoid pattern, trabecular growth, peripheral palisading of cells and rosette formation, and show evidence of neuroendocrine differentiation by immunohistochemistry or ultrastructure. Mitotic rates are high and necrosis is common. These are aggressive tumors with 5-year survival rates similar to small cell carcinoma.

Small Cell Carcinoma

Small cell carcinoma (formerly "oat cell" carcinoma) is a highly malignant epithelial tumor of the lung with neuroendocrine features. It accounts for 14% of all lung cancers in the United States (Table 18-6) and is strongly associated with cigarette smoking. SCLCs grow and metastasize rapidly: 70% of patients are first seen at advanced stages. These tumors often cause paraneoplastic syndromes, including **diabetes insipidus, ectopic adrenocorticotropic hormone (ACTH; corticotropin) syndrome** and **Eaton-Lambert syndrome**.

 PATHOLOGY: SCLCs are usually perihilar masses, with extensive lymph node metastases. They are soft and white, often with extensive hemorrhage and necrosis. The tumor typically spreads along bronchi in a submucosal and circumferential fashion.

Small cell carcinomas have sheets of small, round, oval or spindle-shaped cells with scant cytoplasm. Their nuclei are distinctive, with finely granular nuclear chromatin and absent or inconspicuous nucleoli (Fig. 18-88). Most tumors express detectable neuroendocrine markers such as CD56, chromogranin or synaptophysin. Mitotic rates are very high, with 60–70 mitoses per 2-mm^2 area of tumor (10 high-power fields). Necrosis is frequent and extensive. Although there is no absolute measure for the size of the tumor cells, a useful rule of thumb in small cell carcinoma is the diameter of three small resting lymphocytes. Rarely, a small cell carcinoma may occur with a "non–small cell carcinoma." In such cases, tumor behavior and clinical outcome reflect the small cell component, so they are classified as combined small

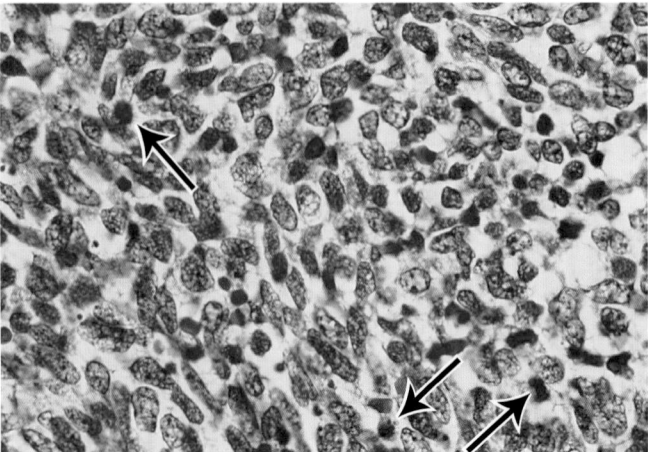

FIGURE 18-88. Small cell carcinoma of the lung. This tumor consists of small oval to spindle-shaped cells with scant cytoplasm, finely granular nuclear chromatin and conspicuous mitoses (*arrows*).

cell carcinoma plus the non–small cell type (e.g., combined small cell carcinoma and adenocarcinoma). Unlike other lung cancers, small cell tumors, at least initially, are very sensitive to chemotherapy, which is the mainstay of treatment for this tumor type.

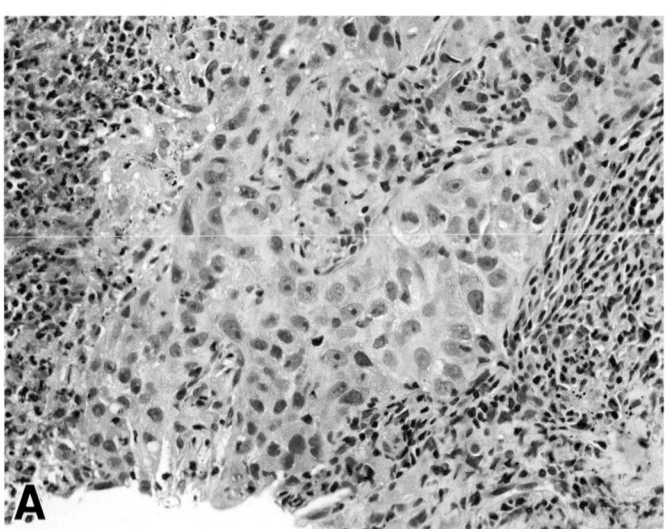

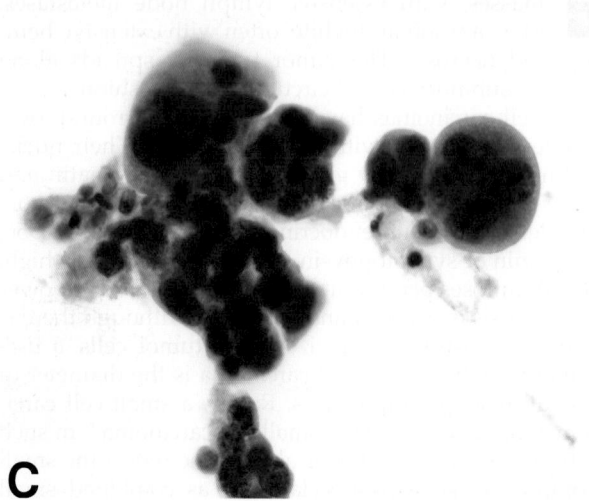

Lung Carcinomas with Combined Histology

Lung carcinomas may contain a combination of histologic subtypes within one tumor: small cell carcinomas may occur in combination with components of non–small cell carcinomas (known as "combined small cell carcinoma"), or different non–small cell subtypes may also occur in the same tumor, primarily exemplified by adenosquamous carcinomas. Combined small cell carcinomas are treated as small cell carcinomas.

Sarcomatoid tumors make up less than 1% of lung cancers. Most are pleomorphic carcinomas with at least 10% spindle and/or giant cell carcinoma in addition to other non–small cell carcinoma patterns such as adenocarcinoma or squamous cell carcinoma. If true sarcomatous components are present such as osteosarcoma, chondrosarcoma or rhabdomyosarcoma, these tumors are classified as carcinosarcomas. Their prognosis is poor, with a median survival of 9–12 months.

DIAGNOSIS OF LUNG CANCER IN SMALL BIOPSIES AND CYTOLOGY SPECIMENS: The diagnosis of small cell carcinoma is reliably made based on small biopsy and cytology specimens. However, in 20%–40% of advanced NSCLCs where the diagnosis is based on small biopsies or cytology, tumors may be difficult to further reclassify as adenocarcinoma or squamous cell carcinoma because they lack clear

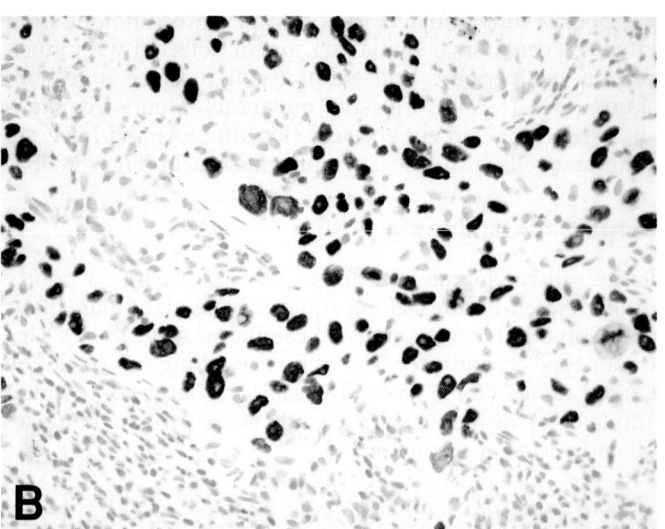

FIGURE 18-89. Non–small cell carcinoma, favor adenocarcinoma. A. This tumor shows features of a non–small cell carcinoma with large cell size, abundant cytoplasm and prominent nucleoli. **B.** Tumor cells show strong nuclear staining for the immunohistochemical marker thyroid transcription factor-1 (TTF-1), a marker not only for adenocarcinoma differentiation but also for lung origin. Staining for p40 was negative (not shown). **C.** Papanicolaou stain of fine needle aspiration shows malignant cells in clusters with glandular structures and large hyperchromatic nuclei with some nucleoli.

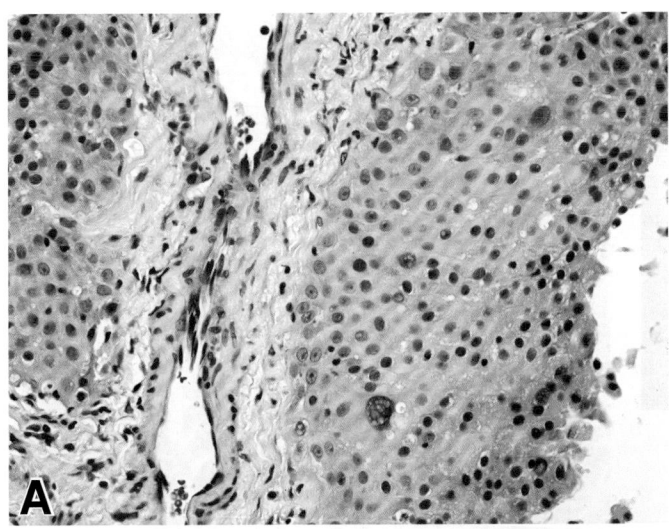

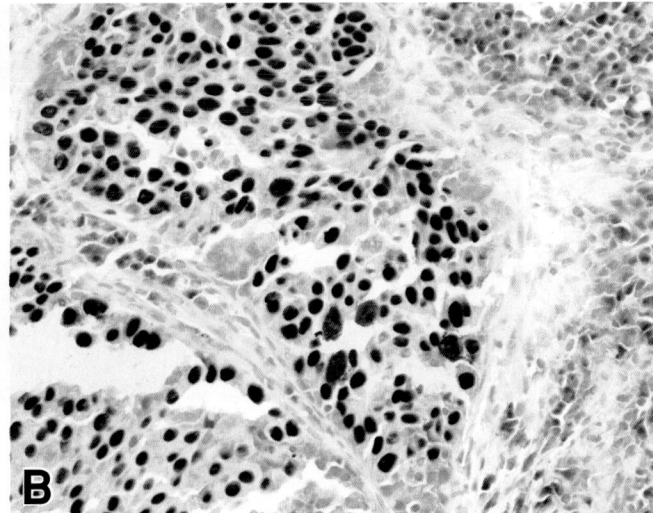

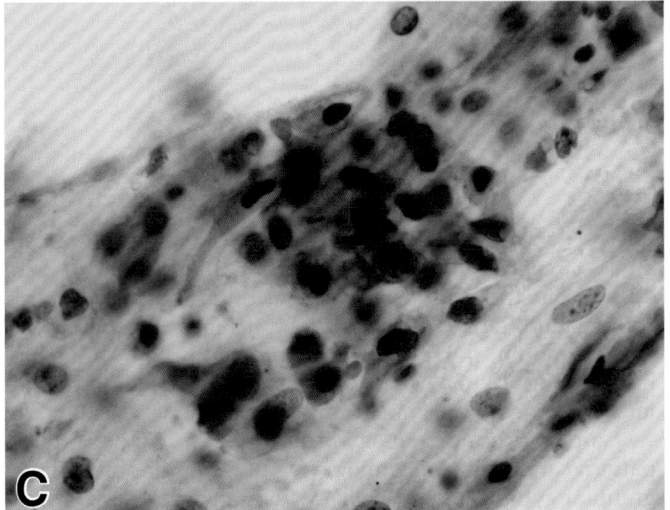

FIGURE 18-90. Non–small cell carcinoma, favor squamous cell carcinoma. A. This tumor shows features of a non–small cell carcinoma consisting of sheets of malignant cells with abundant eosinophilic cytoplasm, hyperchromatic nuclei and some prominent nucleoli. **B.** The tumor cells show strong nuclear staining for p40, a marker of squamous differentiation. Staining for thyroid transcription factor-1 (TTF-1) was negative (not shown). **C.** Papanicolaou stain of fine needle aspiration biopsy shows clusters of cells with dense eosinophilic cytoplasm, hyperchromatic nuclei with sharply angulated shapes. Some cells are elongated with pointed ends. All of these are features of squamous cell carcinoma.

patterns of differentiation. In such cases, the term "non–small cell carcinoma, not otherwise specified (NSCC-NOS)" has been used. As noted above, because targeted chemotherapy for advanced lung cancer patients is dependent on accurate histologic classification and knowledge of *EGFR* mutation or *ALK* rearrangement status, an initial NSCC-NOS pattern in small biopsies and cytology specimens prompts immunohistochemical analyses using a single adenocarcinoma marker such as thyroid transcription factor-1 (TTF-1) and a single squamous marker such as p40 to further classify these tumors. A histochemical stain for mucin may also be helpful. The recommended terminology and criteria for these tumors are summarized below:

- **Non–small cell carcinoma, favor adenocarcinoma:** An NSCC-NOS by light microscopy that is positive for adenocarcinoma markers (TTF-1 or mucin) and negative for squamous markers (Fig. 18-89)
- **Non–small cell carcinoma, favor squamous carcinoma:** An NSCC-NOS by light microscopy that is positive for squamous markers (p40 or p63) but negative for adenocarcinoma markers (Fig. 18-90)
- **Non–small cell carcinoma, not otherwise specified:** An NSCC-NOS by light microscopy either that is negative for adenocarcinoma and squamous markers or where the staining pattern is not clear (Fig. 18-91)

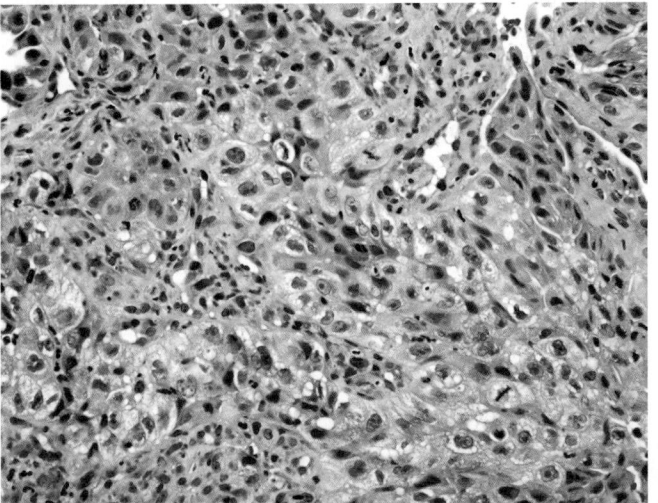

FIGURE 18-91. Non–small cell carcinoma, not otherwise specified. This tumor consists of sheets of large malignant cells with abundant eosinophilic cytoplasm and hyperchromatic and vesicular nuclei, many of which show prominent nucleoli.

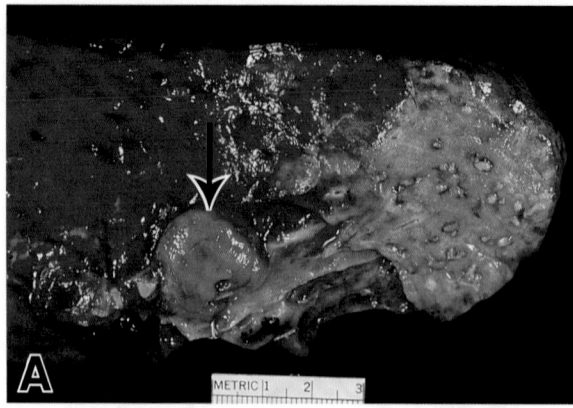

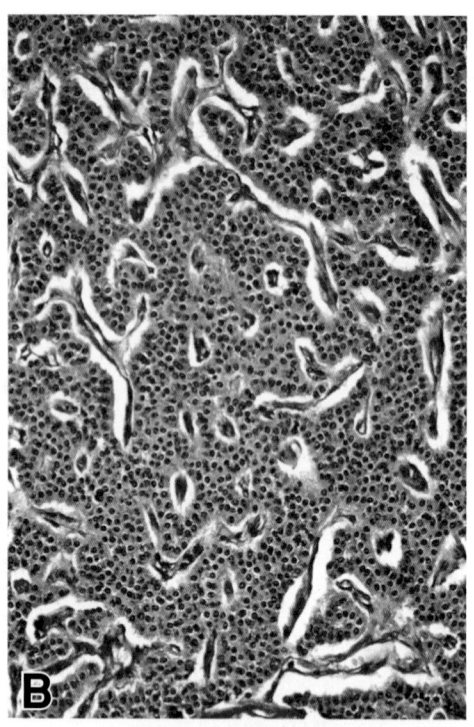

FIGURE 18-92. Carcinoid tumor of the lung. A. A central carcinoid tumor (*arrow*) is circumscribed and protrudes into the lumen of the main bronchus. Compression of the bronchus by the tumor caused the postobstructive pneumonia seen in the distal lung parenchyma (*right*). **B.** A microscopic view shows ribbons of tumor cells embedded in a vascular stroma.

This approach can reduce the percentage of NSCC-NOS from 20%–40% to less than 5%, allowing many patients to get a clear histologic diagnosis that defines eligibility for molecular testing for *EGFR* mutation and *ALK* rearrangement. It emphasizes the need to minimize use of special stains to further classify the tumor in small specimens and preserves tissue for molecular testing. All tumors classified as adenocarcinoma, NSCC-NOS and NSCC-NOS must be tested for *EGFR* mutation and *ALK* rearrangement. Treatments are given accordingly. If the tumor is negative for both, or if mutation status is unknown, patients are eligible for pemetrexed or bevacizumab-based regiments.

Evidence-based molecular targeted therapies are not yet established for squamous cell carcinomas. Thus, routine molecular testing for squamous cell carcinomas is not currently recommended.

Carcinoid Tumors

There are two subtypes of carcinoid tumors of the lung **(typical carcinoid and atypical carcinoid)**, which are thought to arise from the resident neuroendocrine cells normally in the bronchial epithelium. Carcinoid tumors account for 2%–32% of all primary lung cancers in the United States (Table 18-6), show no sex predilection and are not related to cigarette smoking. Although neuropeptides are readily demonstrated in the tumor cells, most are endocrinologically silent. A small subset of cases is associated with an endocrinopathy, such as Cushing syndrome with ectopic ACTH production by tumor cells. The carcinoid syndrome (see Chapter 19) occurs in 1% of cases, usually in the setting of hepatic metastases. Nodular neuroendocrine proliferations less than 0.5 cm are called tumorlets. They may arise in the setting of interstitial fibrosis or small airway disorders and usually represent incidental findings of no clinical significance.

 PATHOLOGY: One third of carcinoid tumors are central, 1/3 are peripheral (subpleural) and 1/3 are in the midportion of the lung. Central carcinoid tumors tend to have a large endobronchial component, with fleshy, smooth, polypoid masses protruding into bronchial lumens (Fig. 18-92A). The tumors average 3.0 cm in diameter, but range from 0.5 to 10 cm.

Carcinoid tumors are characterized by organoid growth patterns and uniform cytologic features: eosinophilic, finely granular cytoplasm and nuclei with finely granular chromatin (Fig. 18-92B). A variety of neuroendocrine patterns may be seen, including trabecular growth, peripheral palisading and rosettes.

Atypical carcinoid tumors differ from typical carcinoids by (1) increased mitoses, with 2–10 mitoses per 2 mm^2 of tumor; (2) tumor necrosis (Fig. 18-93); (3) areas of

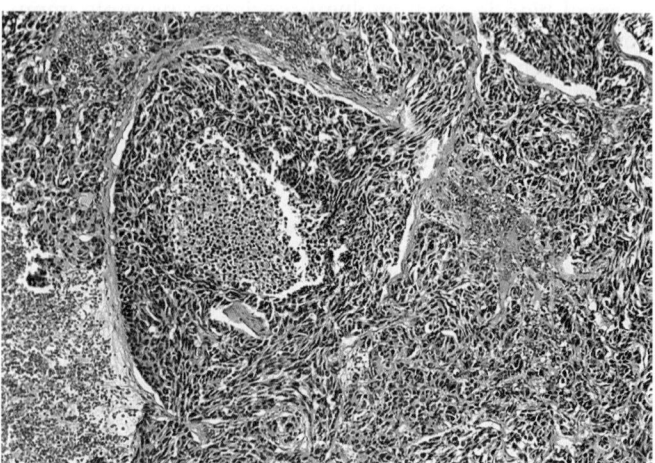

FIGURE 18-93. Atypical carcinoid tumor of the lung. A cellular tumor shows central necrosis and a disorganized architecture.

increased cellularity and architectural disorganization; and (4) nuclear pleomorphism, hyperchromatism and a high nuclear:cytoplasmic ratio.

 CLINICAL FEATURES: Carcinoid tumors grow slowly, so half of patients are asymptomatic at presentation. They are often discovered incidentally as a mass in a chest radiograph. If a patient is symptomatic, the most common pulmonary manifestations are hemoptysis, postobstructive pneumonitis and dyspnea. There is a slight female predominance. The mean age at diagnosis is 55, but these tumors can occur at any age. In fact, bronchial carcinoids are the most common lung tumor in childhood. Atypical carcinoid tumors tend to be more aggressive than typical ones. Regional lymph node metastases occur in 15% of patients with typical carcinoids and 50% of those with atypical carcinoids. Patients with typical carcinoids have 90% 5-year survival after surgery, compared with 60% for atypical carcinoids.

Rare Pulmonary Tumors

INFLAMMATORY MYOFIBROBLASTIC TUMOR/INFLAMMATORY PSEUDOTUMOR: Inflammatory myofibroblastic tumor of the lung is an uncommon lesion that consists of variable amounts of inflammatory cells, foamy macrophages and fibroblasts. Most of these masses are within the lung, although the pleura may be involved. In 5% of cases, tumors invade structures outside the lung, such as the esophagus, mediastinum, chest wall, diaphragm or pericardium.

Inflammatory myofibroblastic tumors encompass a spectrum of lesions with a range of histologic findings as described below; as knowledge expands, some of these lesions may be better classified as other entities. Some thought previously to be a nonneoplastic inflammatory process are now known to be inflammatory myofibroblastic tumors, a lesion originally described in soft tissue. Identification of *ALK* gene mutations provides additional evidence that at least some are true neoplasms. Other lesions previously categorized as so-called plasma cell granuloma variants of inflammatory myofibroblastic tumor may be pulmonary manifestations of immune-related processes such as IgG4-related systemic sclerosing disease.

 PATHOLOGY: The tumors are solitary circumscribed, with a mean size of 4 cm. Virtually any type of inflammatory cell may be present, including lymphocytes, plasma cells, macrophages, giant cells, mast cells and eosinophils. Inflammatory myofibroblastic tumor causes consolidation of the lung parenchyma and loss of architecture. Two major histologic patterns are fibrohistiocytic (Fig. 18-94) and plasma cell granuloma, depending on the predominant component. In some cases, foamy macrophages impart a xanthomatous picture.

 CLINICAL FEATURES: Most patients are under 40, but inflammatory myofibroblastic tumor can occur at any age and is one of the most common lung tumors of childhood. Half of patients are asymptomatic at presentation. A previous history of a pulmonary infection can be elicited in one third of patients. Most inflammatory myofibroblastic tumors are cured by surgical excision, but 5% recur within the chest.

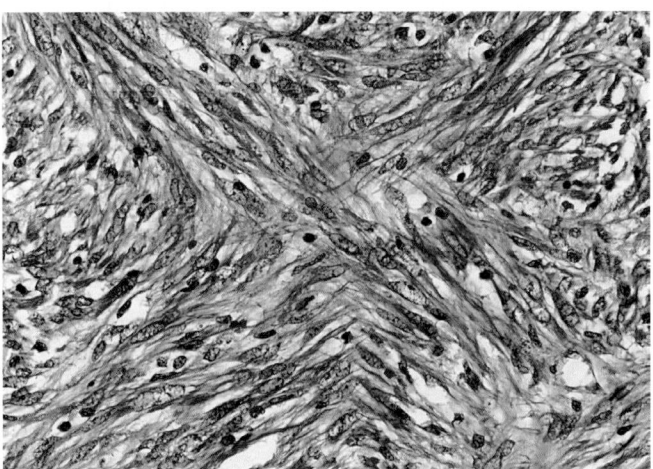

FIGURE 18-94. Inflammatory pseudotumor. A photomicrograph shows intersecting spindle cells and scattered lymphocytes and macrophages.

PULMONARY EPITHELIOID HEMANGIOENDOTHELIOMA: Pulmonary epithelioid hemangioendotheliomas are rare low- to intermediate-grade vascular sarcomas. Most patients are young adults; 80% are women. Half are asymptomatic.

 PATHOLOGY: Most patients are first seen with multiple pulmonary nodules. Histologically, the tumor consists of oval-shaped nodules with central, sclerotic, hypocellular zones and cellular peripheral zones. The tumors spread within alveolar spaces (Fig. 18-95). Tumor cells have abundant cytoplasm, with frequent intracytoplasmic vascular lumens, which may contain red blood cells. The tumor matrix is abundant and eosinophilic. The tumors express vascular markers, such as factor VIII, CD34 or CD31. Epithelioid hemangioendotheliomas with a histologic pattern similar to that seen in the lung may occur in the liver, bone and soft tissue. Pulmonary epithelioid hemangioendothelioma has a variable clinical course, with a mean survival of 5 years.

PULMONARY BLASTOMA: This malignant tumor resembles embryonal lung, with a glandular component

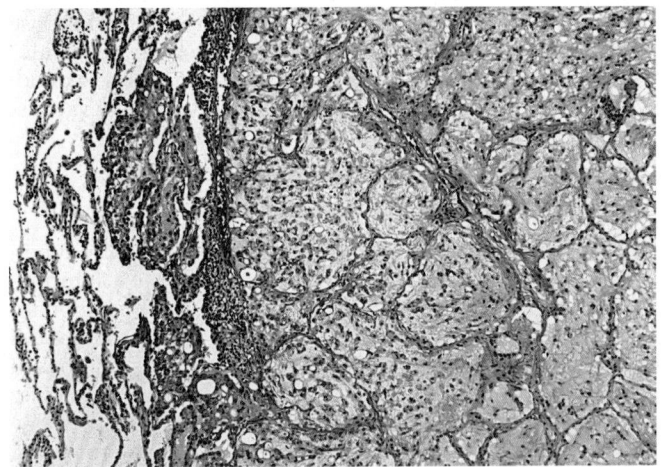

FIGURE 18-95. Epithelioid hemangioendothelioma. A nodule of tumor has spread within alveolar spaces.

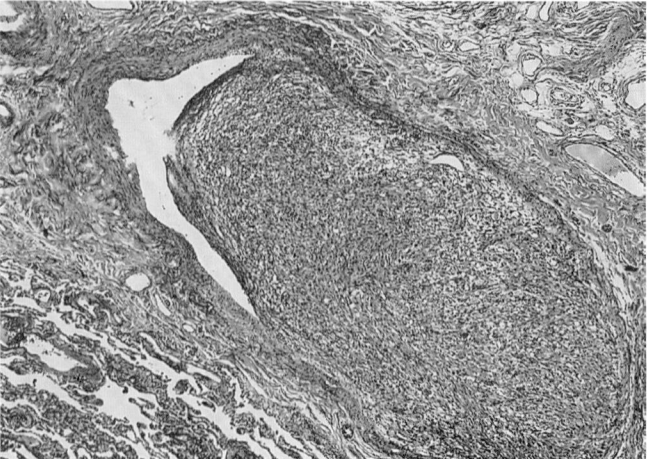

FIGURE 18-96. Pulmonary artery sarcoma. A polypoid mass of malignant spindle cells is spreading within the lumen of this pulmonary artery.

of poorly differentiated columnar cells in tubules, lacking mucus secretion. The intervening tumor contains spindle cells that resemble embryonal mesoderm. There is histologic overlap between pulmonary blastoma and carcinosarcoma, including heterologous elements. The clinical features are also similar.

Despite its embryonal appearance, pulmonary blastomas occur mainly in adults (median age range, 35–43), and most patients are cigarette smokers. The prognosis for patients with biphasic tumors is poor and comparable to that for carcinoma of the lung. Pulmonary blastomas are often associated with β-catenin mutations.

MUCOEPIDERMOID CARCINOMA AND ADENOID CYSTIC CARCINOMA: These neoplasms resemble their namesakes in the salivary glands. They are derived from tracheobronchial mucous glands and are seen in the trachea or proximal bronchus as a luminal mass, often associated with obstructive symptoms. Adenoid cystic carcinomas are difficult to resect locally and often metastasize.

PULMONARY ARTERY SARCOMA: Pulmonary artery sarcoma is a rare tumor of connective tissue (Fig. 18-96), which has a broad histologic spectrum, including fibrosarcoma, leiomyosarcoma, osteosarcoma, rhabdomyosarcoma, angiosarcoma or unclassifiable sarcoma. These tumors are rarely diagnosed during life and may be discovered because of pulmonary hypertension. They often grow in an intraluminal fashion, within proximal arteries, and may extend, worm-like, to peripheral pulmonary artery branches, causing peripheral infarcts.

Pulmonary Lymphomas

All lymphomas, both Hodgkin and non-Hodgkin types, may involve the lung (see also Chapter 26). Most lymphomas involving the lung are metastatic. Primary pulmonary lymphomas are rare, the most common being **extranodal marginal zone B-cell lymphoma.** These tumors are thought to arise from *mucosa-associated lymphoid tissue* of the lung and are sometimes designated "MALT" lymphomas. They are low-grade tumors, generally with a favorable prognosis.

Diffuse large B-cell lymphoma may also arise as a primary pulmonary lymphoma (see Chapter 26). **Lymphomatoid granulomatosis,** a subtype of diffuse large B-cell lymphoma, is characterized by nodular pulmonary lymphoid infiltrates with frequent central necrosis and vascular permeation (Fig. 18-97). It affects middle-aged people and is more common in immunosuppressed individuals. The lung is the major location, but the kidney, skin and upper respiratory tract may also be involved. The lymphoid infiltrate is angiocentric and angioinvasive, with polymorphous, small to medium-sized lymphocytes, mainly T cells, admixed with variable numbers of large atypical B cells. The latter typically express EBV, which is thought to drive the proliferation. Lymphomatoid granulomatosis is typically divided into grades depending on the percentage of atypical B cells present. Previously, only the highest grade was considered a "true" lymphoma, the lower grades being considered as less aggressive lesions; however, all grades are now considered to be subtypes of diffuse large B-cell lymphoma for treatment purposes. Despite remissions with chemotherapy, half of all patients eventually develop large cell lymphoma.

Extrapulmonary Tumors Often Metastasize to the Lung

In 1/3 of all fatal cancers, there are lung metastases at autopsy. In fact, metastatic tumors are the most common malignancies in the lung. They are typically multiple and circumscribed. Large metastatic nodules in the lungs seen radiologically are called "cannon ball" metastases (Fig. 18-98). Most metastases resemble their primary tumors. Rarely, metastatic tumors show lepidic growth, particularly mucinous types, in which cases the usual primary site is the pancreas or stomach.

In **lymphangitic carcinoma,** metastatic tumor spreads widely through pulmonary lymphatic channels to form a sheath of tumor around the bronchovascular tree and veins. Clinically, patients suffer from cough and shortness of breath and display a diffuse reticulonodular pattern on the chest radiograph. The common primary sites are the breast, stomach, pancreas and colon.

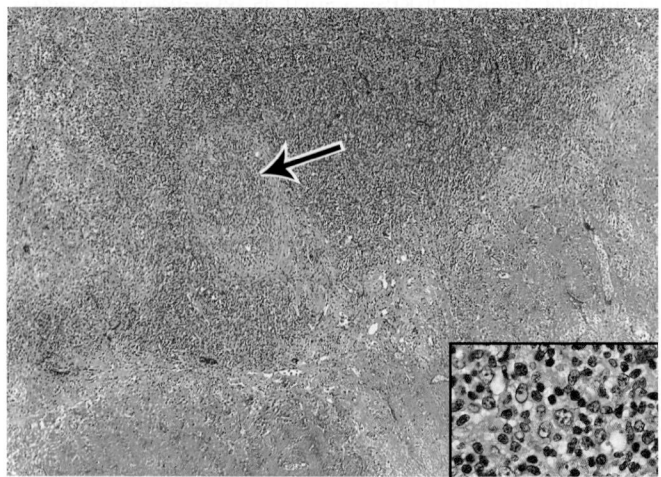

FIGURE 18-97. Lymphomatoid granulomatosis. This extensively necrotic nodular mass consists of a cellular lymphoid infiltrate that penetrates a blood vessel (*arrow*) at the edge of the lesion. *Inset.* The lymphoid infiltrate is composed of a polymorphous population of small, medium-sized and large atypical lymphoid cells.

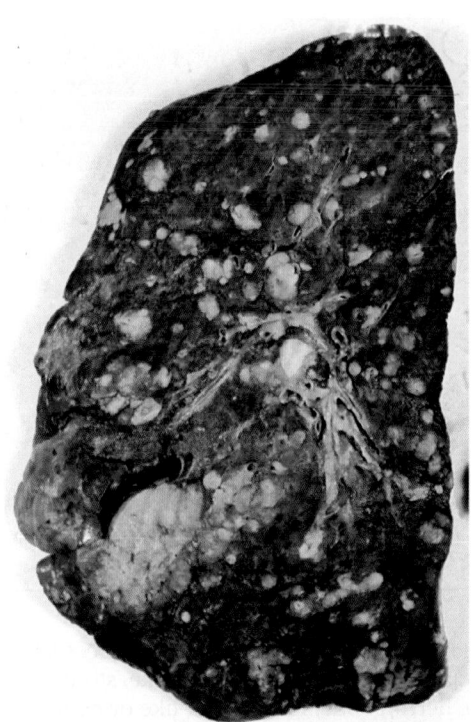

FIGURE 18-98. Metastatic carcinoma of the lung. A section through the lung shows numerous nodules of metastatic carcinoma corresponding to "cannon ball" metastases seen radiologically.

The Pleura

PNEUMOTHORAX

Pneumothorax is the presence of air in the pleural cavity. It may occur with traumatic perforation of the pleura or may be "spontaneous." Traumatic causes include penetrating wounds of the chest wall (e.g., a stab wound or a rib fracture). Traumatic pneumothorax is most commonly iatrogenic and is seen after therapeutic aspiration of fluid from the pleura (thoracentesis), pleural or lung biopsies, transbronchial biopsies and positive pressure–assisted ventilation.

Spontaneous pneumothorax is typically seen in young adults. For example, a young man may develop acute chest pain and shortness of breath during vigorous exercise. A chest radiograph shows collapse of the lung on the side of the pain and a large collection of air in the pleural space. The cause is rupture, usually of a subpleural emphysematous bleb. In most cases, spontaneous pneumothorax resolves by itself, but some patients require withdrawal of the air.

Tension pneumothorax refers to unilateral pneumothorax extensive enough to shift the mediastinum to the opposite side, with compression of the opposite lung. The condition may be life-threatening and must be relieved by immediate drainage.

Bronchopleural fistula is a serious condition in which there is free communication between an airway and the pleura. It is usually iatrogenic, caused by the interruption of bronchial continuity by biopsy or surgery. It may also be due to extensive infection and necrosis of lung tissue, in which case the infection is more important than the air.

PLEURAL EFFUSION

Pleural effusion is accumulation of excess fluid in the pleural cavity. Normally, only a small amount of fluid in the pleural cavity lubricates the space between the lungs and chest wall. Fluid is secreted into the pleural space by the parietal pleura and absorbed by the visceral pleura. Effusions vary from a few milliliters, detectable only radiologically as blunting of the costophrenic angle, to massive accumulations that shift the mediastinum and the trachea to the opposite side.

HYDROTHORAX: Hydrothorax is an effusion that resembles water and would be regarded as edema elsewhere. It may be due to increased capillary hydrostatic pressure, as occurs in patients with heart failure or in any condition that produces systemic or pulmonary edema. Hydrothorax also occurs in patients with low serum osmotic pressure, as in nephrotic syndrome, cirrhosis of the liver or severe starvation. Other important causes of hydrothorax are collagen vascular diseases (notably systemic lupus erythematosus and rheumatoid arthritis) and asbestos exposure.

PYOTHORAX: A turbid effusion full of polymorphonuclear leukocytes (pyothorax) results from infections of the pleura. It may occasionally be caused by an external penetrating wound that introduces pyogenic organisms into the pleural space but more commonly is a complication of bacterial pneumonia that extends to the pleural surface, the classic example of which is pneumococcal pneumonia. Pyothorax is a rare complication of medical procedures involving the pleural cavity.

EMPYEMA: This disorder is a variant of pyothorax in which thick pus accumulates within the pleural cavity, often with loculation and fibrosis.

HEMOTHORAX: Blood in the pleural cavity as a result of trauma or rupture of a vessel (e.g., dissecting aneurysm of the aorta) is hemothorax. A pleural effusion may be blood stained in tuberculosis, cancers involving the pleura and pulmonary infarction.

CHYLOTHORAX: Chylothorax is accumulation of milky, lipid-rich fluid (chyle) in the pleural cavity due to lymphatic obstruction. It has an ominous portent, because lymphatic obstruction suggests disease of the lymph nodes in the posterior mediastinum. Chylothorax is thus a rare complication of mediastinal tumors, such as lymphoma. In tropical countries, it may result from nematode infestations. It can also be seen in pulmonary lymphangioleiomyomatosis.

PLEURITIS

Pleuritis, or inflammation of the pleura, may result from extension of any pulmonary infection to the visceral pleura, bacterial infections within the pleural cavity, viral infections, collagen vascular disease or pulmonary infarction that involves the lung surface. The most striking symptom is sharp, stabbing chest pain on inspiration. It is often associated with pleural effusions.

TUMORS OF THE PLEURA

Localized (Solitary) Fibrous Tumors of the Pleura Are Usually Benign

Solitary fibrous tumor of the pleura is an uncommon localized neoplasm arising in the pleura. Most are benign, but a

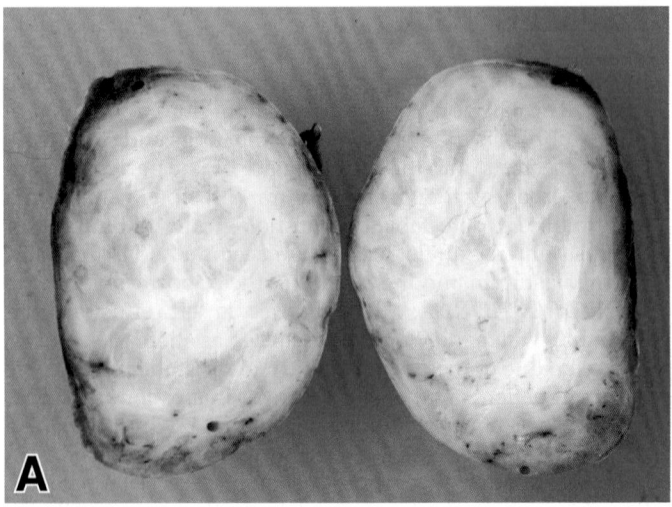
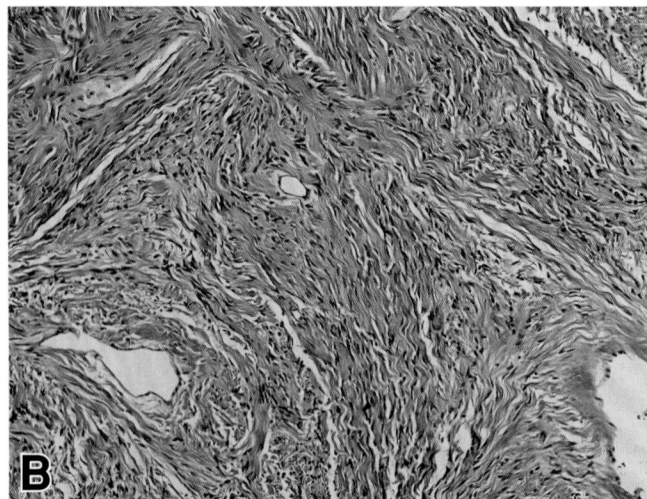

FIGURE 18-99. Pleural localized (solitary) fibrous tumor. A. The tumor is circumscribed with a whorled, tan cut surface. **B.** Tumor cells are round to oval and spindle shaped, with a dense eosinophilic or "ropy" collagen stroma and slit-like blood vessels.

small percentage are malignant. Some 80% arise on the visceral pleura, the remainder being from the parietal pleura. Similar tumors can develop on any mesothelial surface, including the mediastinum, peritoneum, pericardium, liver and tunica vaginalis. They arise from submesothelial connective tissue, not mesothelium, and are unrelated to asbestos.

 PATHOLOGY: The tumors are usually pedunculated. More than 60% are over 10 cm in diameter and some reach 40 cm and may weigh up to 3800 g. The cut surface is gray-white, with a nodular, whorled or lobulated appearance (Fig. 18-99A). Cysts are occasionally present, especially at the base near the pleural attachment.

The most common histologic appearance is the "patternless pattern" of disorderly or randomly arranged mixtures of fibroblast-like cells and connective tissue. Other arrangements include hemangiopericytoma-like, storiform (star-like, or spiral), herringbone, leiomyoma-like or neurofibroma-like arrangements (Fig. 18-99B). The tumor cells are spindle to oval shaped, often with a fibroblast-like appearance. The collagen is compressed between the cells in a lacy network or it may form dense, wire-like bands. Histologic features suggesting malignancy include increased cellularity, pleomorphism, necrosis and more than four mitoses per 10 high-power fields. Most tumors are immunopositive for CD34 and *bcl*-2.

 CLINICAL FEATURES: The median age of patients diagnosed with localized fibrous tumor of the pleura is 55 years (range, 9–86 years) without any sex predominance. They present most often with chest

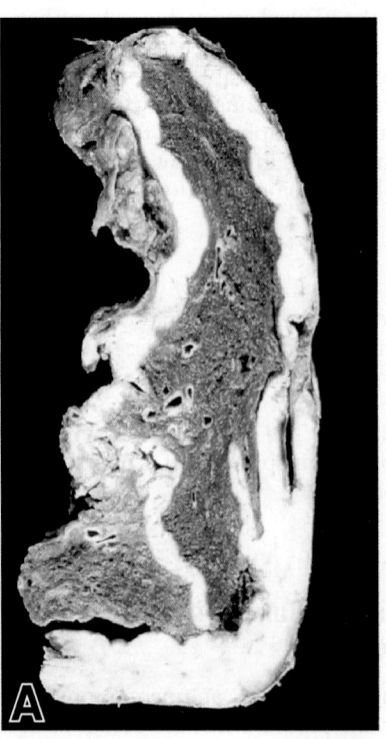
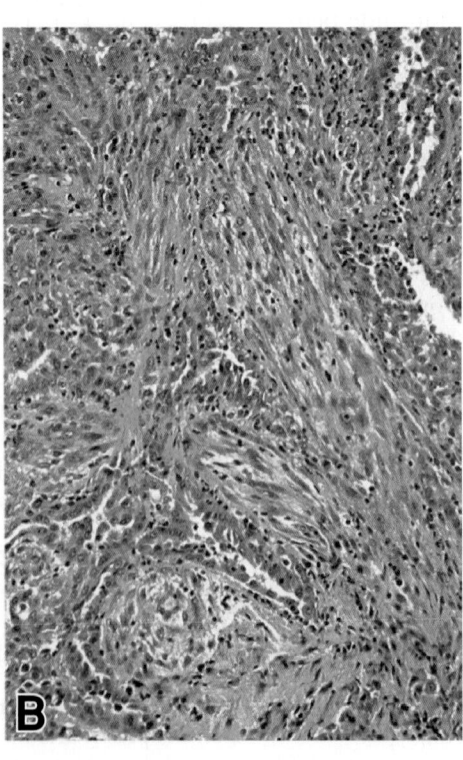

FIGURE 18-100. Pleural malignant mesothelioma. A. The lung is encased by a dense pleural tumor that extends along the interlobar fissures but does not involve the underlying lung parenchyma. **B.** This mesothelioma is composed of a biphasic pattern of epithelial and sarcomatous elements.

pain, followed by shortness of breath, cough, hypoglycemia, weight loss, hemoptysis, fever and night sweats. Patients with benign fibrous tumors of pleura have an excellent prognosis. Half of histologically malignant tumors are cured if resected completely.

Malignant Mesothelioma Usually Reflects Asbestos Exposure

Malignant mesothelioma is a neoplasm of mesothelial cells. It is most common in the pleura but also occurs in the peritoneum, pericardium and tunica vaginalis of the testis.

EPIDEMIOLOGY: Some 2000 new cases of malignant mesothelioma develop yearly in the United States. In the United States, Great Britain and South Africa, 80% of patients report exposure to asbestos. Mesothelioma typically develops after a long latency period, which averages 30–40 years.

PATHOLOGY: Grossly, pleural mesotheliomas often encase and compress the lung, extending into fissures and interlobar septa, a distribution often referred to as a "pleural rind" (Fig. 18-100A). Invasion of pulmonary parenchyma is generally limited to the periphery adjacent to the tumor. Lymph nodes tend to be spared. Microscopically, classic mesotheliomas show both epithelial and sarcomatous patterns (Fig. 18-100B). Glands and tubules that resemble adenocarcinoma are admixed with sheets of

spindle cells similar in appearance to a fibrosarcoma. In some instances, only one or the other component is present: if it is epithelial, the tumor may be difficult to distinguish from adenocarcinoma. Less commonly, only a sarcomatous component is present.

Immunohistochemistry is essential for differentiating mesothelioma from adenocarcinoma (see Chapter 5). Both are positive for cytokeratins; however, adenocarcinomas often, but not always, express carcinoembryonic antigen, Leu-M1, B72.3 and BER-EP4, but mesotheliomas are negative for these markers. In contrast, mesotheliomas are typically positive for calretinin, WT-1 and D2-40 (podoplanin), for which adenocarcinomas are typically negative. Other criteria supportive of a diagnosis of mesothelioma include absence of mucin, presence of hyaluronic acid (positive Alcian blue staining) and long, slender microvilli seen by electron microscopy.

CLINICAL FEATURES: The average age of patients with mesothelioma is 60 years. Patients first present with a pleural effusion or a pleural mass, chest pain and nonspecific symptoms, such as weight loss and malaise. Pleural mesotheliomas tend to spread locally within the chest cavity, invading and compressing major structures. Metastases can occur to the lung parenchyma and mediastinal lymph nodes, as well as to extrathoracic sites such as liver, bones, peritoneum and adrenals. Treatment is largely ineffective and prognosis is poor: few patients survive longer than 18 months after diagnosis.

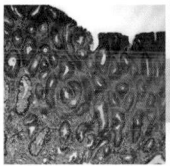
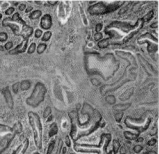
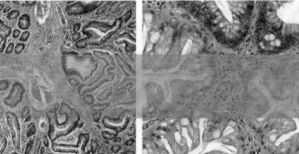

19

The Gastrointestinal Tract

Leana Guerin ■ Frank Mitros

The Esophagus

ANATOMY

The gut and respiratory tract arise embryologically from the foregut, which then divides into two separate tubes, the dorsal esophagus and the ventral trachea. The adult esophagus is a 23–25-cm conduit for food and liquid into the stomach. During upper endoscopy, the esophagus is measured from the incisor teeth with a range of 38 to 43 (average 40) cm from teeth to gastroesophageal junction. The esophagus contains striated and smooth muscle in its upper portion and smooth muscle alone in its lower portion. It is fixed superiorly at the cricopharyngeal and inferior pharyngeal constrictor muscles, which together form the upper esophageal sphincter. It courses inferiorly through the posterior mediastinum behind the trachea and heart and exits the thorax through the diaphragm. Tonic muscular contraction at its lower end creates the **lower esophageal sphincter,** which is a functional sphincter, rather than a true anatomic one.

The esophagus has a mucosa, muscularis mucosae, submucosa, muscularis propria and adventitia. The former is lined by a nonkeratinizing, stratified squamous epithelium. A transition to gastric mucosa at the **gastroesophageal (GE) junction** occurs abruptly at the level of the diaphragm. The esophageal submucosa contains mucous glands, a rich lymphatic plexus and nerve fibers. Lymphatics of the upper third of the esophagus drain to cervical lymph nodes, those of the middle third to mediastinal nodes and those of the lower third to celiac and gastric lymph nodes. These anatomic features are significant in the spread of esophageal cancer.

Venous drainage of the esophagus is important, because the veins can form varices if there is portal hypertension. Varices occur invariably in the lower third of the esophagus, as the veins of the upper third drain into the superior vena cava and those of the middle third drain into the azygous system. Only the veins of the lower third drain into the portal vein via the gastric veins.

CONGENITAL DISORDERS

Tracheoesophageal Fistula Leads to Aspiration Pneumonia

Congenital **atresias** and **stenoses** may occur at any site in the gastrointestinal (GI) tract. Esophageal atresia occurs in 1 in 3500 births and stenosis in 1 in 50,000 births. Atresia may be present alone or, more often, with an associated tracheoesophageal fistula. Stenoses are usually acquired but can be congenital, are usually in the distal esophagus and reflect abnormal wall architecture.

Esophageal atresia with or without tracheoesophageal fistula is the most common esophageal congenital anomaly (Fig. 19-1). Esophageal atresia without a fistula appears in only about 8% of cases. Half of patients have other congenital anomalies, 25% being other gastrointestinal malformations. One fifth have VACTERL syndrome (vertebral defects, anal atresia, cardiac defects, tracheoesophageal fistula, renal dysplasia and limb abnormalities). The etiology of esophageal atresias and fistulas is unknown, but genetic and environmental factors are felt to contribute. Prenatal diagnosis is suggested by polyhydramnios, prominent esophageal pouch and small or absent stomach bubble with fluid-filled loops of bowel on ultrasonography. Polyhydramnios develops because amniotic fluid cannot reach the stomach.

 PATHOLOGY: In about 85% of tracheoesophageal fistulas, the upper portion of the esophagus ends in a blind pouch and the superior end of the lower segment communicates with the trachea (Fig. 19-1). *In this type of atresia, the upper blind sac soon fills with mucus, which the infant then aspirates.* Surgical correction is feasible but difficult.

Another type of fistula is a communication between the proximal esophagus and the trachea; the lower esophageal pouch communicates with the stomach. *Infants with this condition aspirate shortly after birth.* In an **H-type fistula,** there is a communication between an intact esophagus and

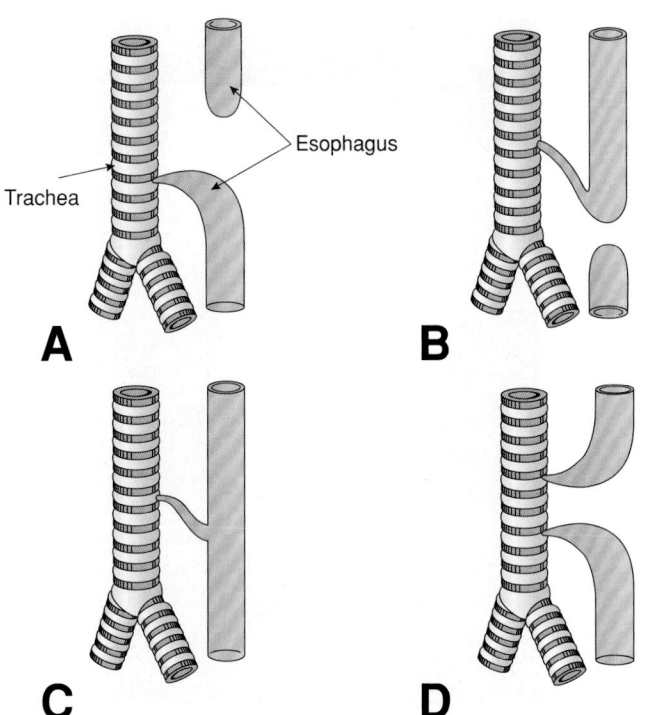

FIGURE 19-1. Congenital tracheoesophageal fistulas. A. The most common type (85% of cases) is a communication between the trachea and the lower portion of the esophagus. The upper segment of the esophagus ends in a blind sac. **B.** In a few cases, the proximal esophagus communicates with the trachea. **C.** H-type fistula without esophageal atresia. **D.** Tracheal fistulas to both a proximal esophageal pouch and distal esophagus.

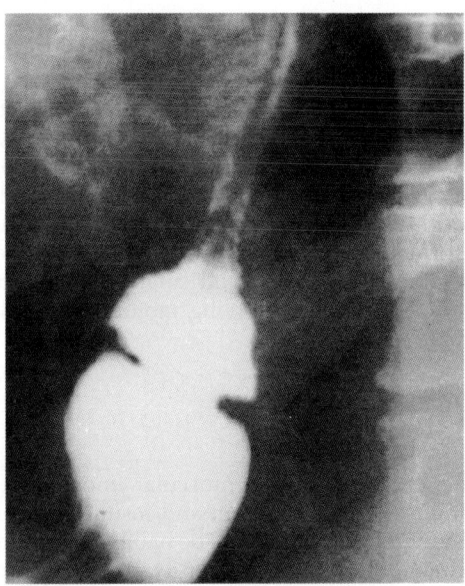

FIGURE 19-2. Schatzki mucosal ring. A contrast radiograph illustrates the lower esophageal narrowing.

an intact trachea. In some cases, this lesion is first symptomatic in adulthood, presenting with repeated pulmonary infections.

Duplication Cysts Replicate the Normal Anatomy of the Affected Bowel

Cystic or tubular remnants of a segment of the gut are duplications. These may occur anywhere in the gut but affect the small bowel most often (50%), followed by the esophagus (15%). Duplications are usually continuous with the segment of bowel from which they arise, although ectopic sites may occur. They may form expanding, intramural masses, which may cause partial or complete bowel obstruction.

Rings and Webs Cause Dysphagia

ESOPHAGEAL WEBS: Occasionally, a thin mucosal membrane projects into the esophageal lumen. Webs are usually single and thin (2 mm) and occur anywhere in the esophagus. They have a core of fibrovascular tissue lined by normal mucosa and submucosa. Middle-aged women are most affected and present with difficulty swallowing (dysphagia). They are often successfully treated by dilation with large rubber bougies; if needed, webs can be excised with biopsy forceps via endoscopy.

PLUMMER-VINSON (PATERSON-KELLY) SYNDROME: This exceedingly rare disorder is characterized by (1) a cervical esophageal web, (2) mucosal lesions of the mouth and pharynx and (3) iron-deficiency anemia. Dysphagia, often

associated with aspiration of swallowed food, is the most common clinical manifestation. Ninety percent of cases occur in women. *Carcinoma of the oropharynx and upper esophagus is a possible complication.*

SCHATZKI RING: This lower esophageal narrowing is usually seen at the GE junction (Fig. 19-2). The upper surface of the mucosal ring has stratified squamous epithelium; the lower, columnar epithelium. Although they are seen in up to 14% of barium examinations, Schatzki rings are usually asymptomatic. Patients with narrow Schatzki rings, however, may complain of intermittent dysphagia. Often dietary and lifestyle changes improve symptoms. If these interventions are ineffective, dilation with bougies can also be done.

Esophageal Diverticula Often Reflect Motor Dysfunction

A **true diverticulum** is an outpouching of the wall that contains all layers of the wall. If a sac has no muscular layer, it is a **false diverticulum** (or pseudodiverticulum). Esophageal diverticula occur in the hypopharyngeal area above the upper esophageal sphincter, in the middle esophagus and just proximal to the lower esophageal sphincter.

ZENKER DIVERTICULUM: Zenker diverticula are uncommon lesions that appear high in the esophagus and affect men more than women. These false diverticula probably reflect disordered function of cricopharyngeal musculature. Most affected people who come to medical attention are older than 60, suggesting that Zenker diverticula are acquired.

These diverticula can enlarge conspicuously and accumulate a large amount of food. The typical symptom is regurgitation of food eaten some time previously (occasionally days), without dysphagia. Patients may develop recurrent aspiration pneumonia. When symptomatic, these lesions are surgically removed or treated endoscopically.

MIDESOPHAGEAL (TRACTION) DIVERTICULA: Diverticula in the middle of the esophagus often reflect a disturbance in esophageal motor function but may also be due to adhesions. They ordinarily have wide stomas and the pouches are usually higher than their orifices. Thus, these diverticula do not retain food or secretions and remain asymptomatic, with only rare complications.

EPIPHRENIC DIVERTICULA: These diverticula are located in the distalmost 10 cm of the esophagus, usually immediately above the diaphragm. Motor disturbances of the esophagus (e.g., achalasia, diffuse esophageal spasm) are found in two thirds of patients with this true diverticulum. Abnormalities of the lower esophageal sphincter may also lead to an epiphrenic diverticula. When symptomatic, surgery to correct the underlying motor abnormality (e.g., myotomy) is appropriate.

MOTOR DISORDERS

Automatic coordination of muscular movement during swallowing is a **motor function** and results in free passage of food through the esophagus. The hallmark of motor disorders is difficulty in swallowing, or **dysphagia**. Dysphagia is often an awareness that food is not moving downward and in itself is not painful. Pain on swallowing is **odynophagia**. Motor disorders can be caused by:

- **Systemic diseases of skeletal muscle** (in the upper esophagus) such as myasthenia gravis, dermatomyositis, amyloidosis, hypothyroidism and myxedema
- **Neurologic diseases** affecting nerves to skeletal or smooth muscle (e.g., cerebrovascular accidents, amyotrophic lateral sclerosis)
- **Peripheral neuropathy** associated with diabetes or alcoholism

In Achalasia Lower Esophageal Sphincter Function Is Abnormal

Achalasia, once called cardiospasm, involves failure of the lower esophageal sphincter to relax with swallowing and poor peristalsis in the body of the esophagus. As a result of these defects in both the outflow tract and esophageal pumping mechanisms, food is retained in the esophagus, and the organ hypertrophies and dilates (Fig. 19-3).

Achalasia is an inflammatory disease that causes loss of inhibitory neurons in the esophageal myenteric plexus. Chronic inflammation (mainly T cells) in the myenteric plexus leads to neuritis and ganglionitis, and eventually to ganglion cell loss and fibrosis. The cause of the inflammation is unknown, but genetic, viral and autoimmune factors have been suggested. Degenerative changes in the dorsal motor nucleus of the vagus and extraesophageal vagus nerves may also contribute. In Latin America, secondary achalasia is a common complication of **Chagas disease** (see Chapter 9), in which ganglion cells are destroyed by the protozoan *Trypanosoma cruzi.* Amyloidosis, sarcoidosis and infiltrative malignancies may also cause achalasia.

Dysphagia (to both solids and liquids), occasionally odynophagia and regurgitation of material retained in the esophagus are common symptoms of achalasia. Squamous cell carcinoma may develop in long-standing cases. Radiography may show a "bird-beak" gastroesophageal junction, but manometry is the standard diagnostic test for confirming achalasia. Treatment may include endoscopic balloon dilation, botulinum toxin injection of the lower esophageal sphincter, endoscopic myotomy or surgical myotomy of the

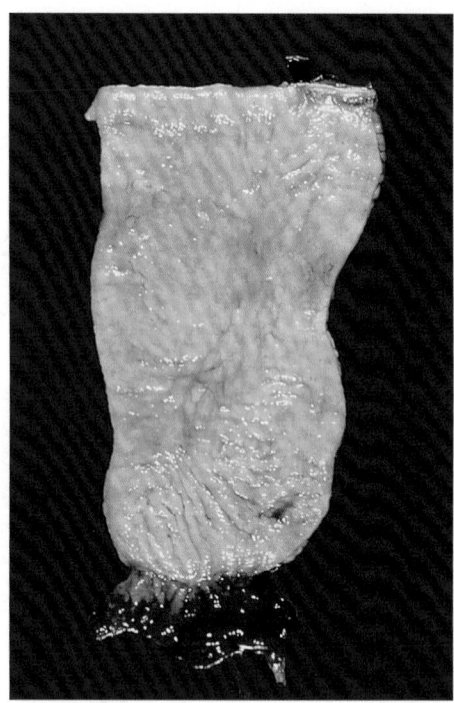

FIGURE 19-3. Esophagus and upper stomach of a patient with advanced achalasia. The esophagus is markedly dilated above the esophagogastric junction, where the lower esophageal sphincter is located. The esophageal mucosa is redundant and has hyperplastic squamous epithelium.

lower esophageal sphincter. Patients may develop GE reflux after treatment.

Systemic Sclerosis Causes Fibrosis of the Esophageal Wall

Systemic sclerosis (scleroderma) causes fibrosis in many organs and involves the GI tract 80% of the time (see Chapter 11). Any segment of the tubal gut may be affected. The esophagus is most frequently impacted, often with severely abnormal esophageal muscle function. The lower esophageal sphincter may be so impaired that the lower esophagus and upper stomach are no longer distinct functional entities and are visualized as a common cavity. Peristalsis may be impaired throughout the esophagus.

 PATHOLOGY: Fibrosis is present in the esophageal smooth muscle (especially the inner muscularis propria). Nonspecific inflammation is also evident. Small arteries and arterioles show intimal fibrosis, which may contribute to the fibrosis.

 CLINICAL FEATURES: Patients have dysphagia, regurgitation and heartburn caused by peptic esophagitis, owing to reflux of acid from the stomach. Severe reflux changes may occur (see below).

HIATAL HERNIA

Hiatal hernia is a protrusion of the stomach into the chest, through an enlarged diaphragmatic opening. There are two basic types of hiatal hernia (Fig. 19-4).

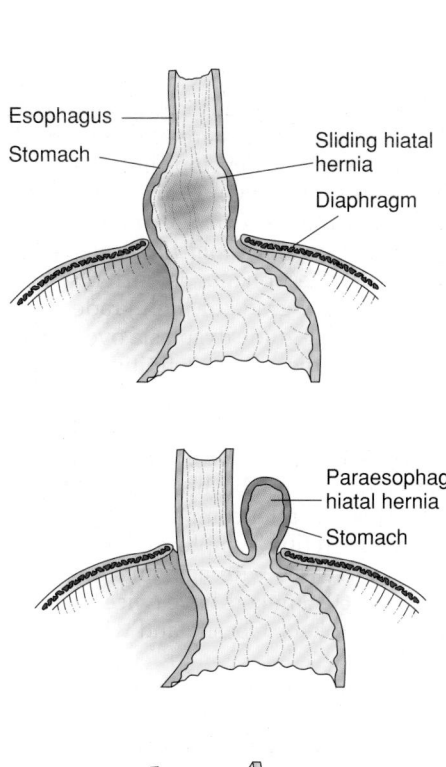

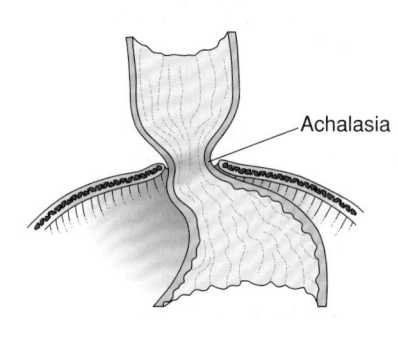

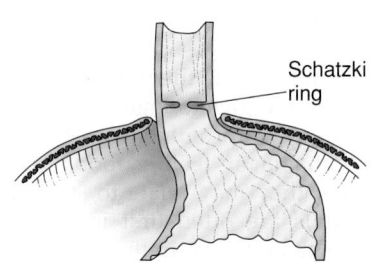

FIGURE 19-4. Disorders of the esophageal outlet.

SLIDING HERNIA: Enlargement of the diaphragmatic hiatus and laxity of the circumferential connective tissue allow a cap of gastric mucosa to move upward, above the diaphragm. This common condition accounts for 85% of hiatal hernias and is usually asymptomatic. The most commonly associated symptom is GE reflux, although it is unclear whether hernias are the causes or results of reflux.

PARAESOPHAGEAL HERNIA: In this uncommon form of hiatal hernia, a portion of gastric fundus herniates through a defect in the diaphragmatic connective tissue that defines the esophageal hiatus and lies beside the esophagus. The hernia progressively enlarges and the hiatus grows increasingly wide, which can compress the esophagus, leading to decrease in reflux of gastric contents. In extreme cases, the entire stomach and other abdominal organs can herniate into the thorax.

 CLINICAL FEATURES: Symptoms of sliding hiatal hernia, mostly heartburn and regurgitation, reflect reflux of gastric contents into the esophagus, primarily due to incompetence of the lower esophageal sphincter. Classically, symptoms are worse when subjects recline, as this position facilitates acid reflux. Dysphagia, fullness after meals, shortness of breath, painful swallowing and occasionally bleeding peptic ulcers may be seen in paraesophageal hernias. Large hernias carry a risk of gastric volvulus or intrathoracic gastric dilation.

Sliding hiatal hernias generally do not require surgery and symptoms are treated medically. An enlarging paraesophageal hernia should be corrected surgically, even if it is asymptomatic.

ESOPHAGITIS

Reflux Esophagitis Is Caused by Reflux of Gastric Contents (Gastroesophageal Reflux Disease)

This is by far the most common type of esophagitis. It often occurs together with sliding hiatal hernias but may develop as the result of an incompetent lower esophageal sphincter with no anatomic lesion.

 **ETIOLOGIC FACTORS:** The main barrier to reflux of gastric contents into the esophagus is the lower esophageal sphincter. Episodic reflux is normal, particularly after a meal. The mucosa is partially protected by the alkaline secretions of submucosal glands. Esophagitis results when episodes are frequent and prolonged. Agents that decrease lower esophageal sphincter pressure (e.g., alcohol, chocolate, fatty foods, cigarette smoking) also cause reflux, as may certain central nervous system (CNS) depressants (e.g., morphine, diazepam), abdominal obesity, pregnancy, estrogen therapy and the presence of a nasogastric tube. Acid damages the esophageal mucosa, but the combination of acid plus pepsin is particularly injurious. Moreover, gastric fluid often contains refluxed bile from the duodenum, which magnifies injury to the esophageal mucosa. Alcohol, hot beverages and spicy foods may also injure the mucosa directly.

 PATHOLOGY: The first grossly evident effect of GE reflux is hyperemia. Affected areas are susceptible to superficial mucosal erosions and ulcers, which often appear as vertical linear streaks. Mild injury to the squamous epithelium appears as cell swelling (hydropic change; see Chapter 1). With continued injury, hyperplasia develops: the basal epithelium is thickened and the papillae of the lamina propria are elongated and approach the surface (Fig. 19-5). Capillary vessels in the papillae are often dilated. Lymphocytes, neutrophils and eosinophils infiltrate the epithelium. Mucosal ulceration develops in severe cases. Esophageal stricture may occur if the ulcer persists and damages the esophageal wall deep to the lamina propria. In this circumstance, reactive fibrosis can narrow the esophageal lumen.

 CLINICAL FEATURES: Gastroesophageal reflux disease (GERD) can occur at any age and can be nonerosive, erosive or involved by Barrett esophagus

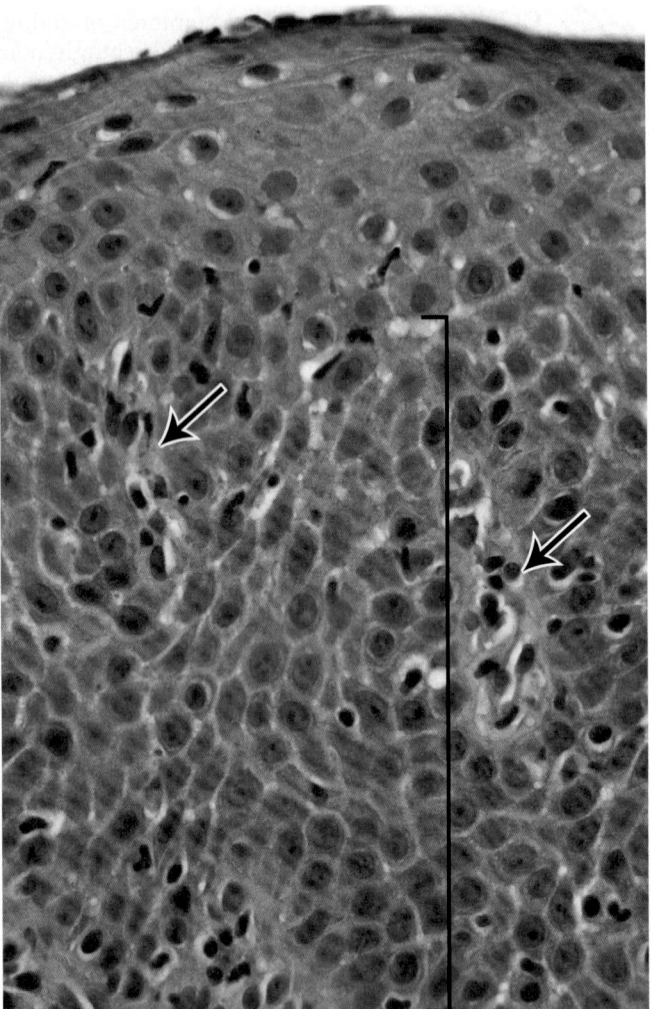

FIGURE 19-5. Reflux esophagitis. Biopsy from a patient with long-standing heartburn. Note the basal hyperplasia (*bracket*) and papillae, squamous hyperplasia and inflammation.

(see below). Heartburn and dysphagia are the usual presenting symptoms and generally respond to agents that reduce gastric acidity, in particular proton pump inhibitors. In cases of erosive GERD, ulceration, hematemesis and stricture may occur.

Barrett Esophagus Is Replacement of Esophageal Squamous Epithelium by Columnar Epithelium (Intestinal Metaplasia)

Barrett esophagus is a result of chronic GERD. For reasons unknown, its incidence has been increasing in recent years, particularly among white men. This disorder occurs in the lower third of the esophagus but may extend higher.

PATHOLOGY: Metaplastic Barrett epithelium may partially involve the circumference of short segments or may line the entire lower esophagus (Fig. 19-6A). The sine qua non of Barrett esophagus is a distinctive "specialized epithelium." By endoscopy, it has a typical salmon-pink color and is an admixture of intestine-like epithelium with well-formed goblet cells, mixed with

gastric foveolar cells (Fig. 19-6B). Complete intestinal metaplasia, with Paneth cells and absorptive cells, occurs occasionally. Inflammatory changes are often superimposed on these alterations. Dysplasia develops in this epithelium in a minority of patients (Fig. 19-6C). *The risk of Barrett esophagus transforming into adenocarcinoma correlates with the length of esophagus involved and the degree of dysplasia.* Dysplasia in a Barrett esophagus is currently classified as negative, indefinite, low grade or high grade. The cytology and architecture of high-grade dysplasia overlap intramucosal adenocarcinoma, the latter definitively identified by invasion into the lamina propria (Fig. 19-6D).

CLINICAL FEATURES: The diagnosis of Barrett esophagus is established by endoscopy with biopsy, usually after complaints of GERD, although many do not report reflux symptoms. Males predominate (3:1). Prevalence increases with age, and most patients are diagnosed after age 60. Smokers have twice the risk of Barrett esophagus as nonsmokers. Obesity and white race are other risk factors.

Patients with Barrett esophagus are followed closely to detect early microscopic evidence of dysplastic mucosa. Many cases, particularly low-grade dysplasia (or even microscopic foci of high-grade dysplasia), regress after pharmacologic reduction in gastric acidity. However, high-grade dysplasia and intramucosal carcinoma require intervention. Techniques used to ablate these lesions (short of esophagectomy) include endoscopic mucosectomy, laser treatment and photodynamic therapy. Standards of care for high-grade dysplasia/intramucosal adenocarcinoma are evolving.

Eosinophilic Esophagitis Is Increasing in Incidence

A diagnosis of eosinophilic esophagitis requires clinical–pathologic correlation. While the pathogenesis is not completely understood, allergies to ingested food and inhaled allergens likely play a prominent role. Patients often complain of dysphagia or feeling food "sticking" upon swallowing, which they may relate to specific foodstuffs. Affected individuals are often first identified after they fail to improve on standard antireflux therapy. It is important to rule out GERD with several weeks of proton pump inhibitor therapy before biopsy or with pH monitoring. The incidence of eosinophilic esophagitis is increasing, likely from a combination of increasing disease prevalence and increasing awareness of the entity and thus more frequent diagnosis.

PATHOLOGY: On endoscopy, eosinophilic esophagitis shows concentric mucosal rings (called trachealization or felinization because it resembles the trachea or cat esophagus), vertical linear furrows, narrow esophagus, strictures and small white plaques/exudates (Fig. 19-7A). Some patients have a normal-appearing esophagus at endoscopy. Since the disease can be quite patchy, multiple biopsies from various levels of esophagus should be assessed. The epithelium shows hyperplasia (papillary and basal layer hyperplasia), intercellular edema, increased intraepithelial eosinophils (≥15 per high-power field), superficial layering of eosinophils, eosinophilic microabscesses

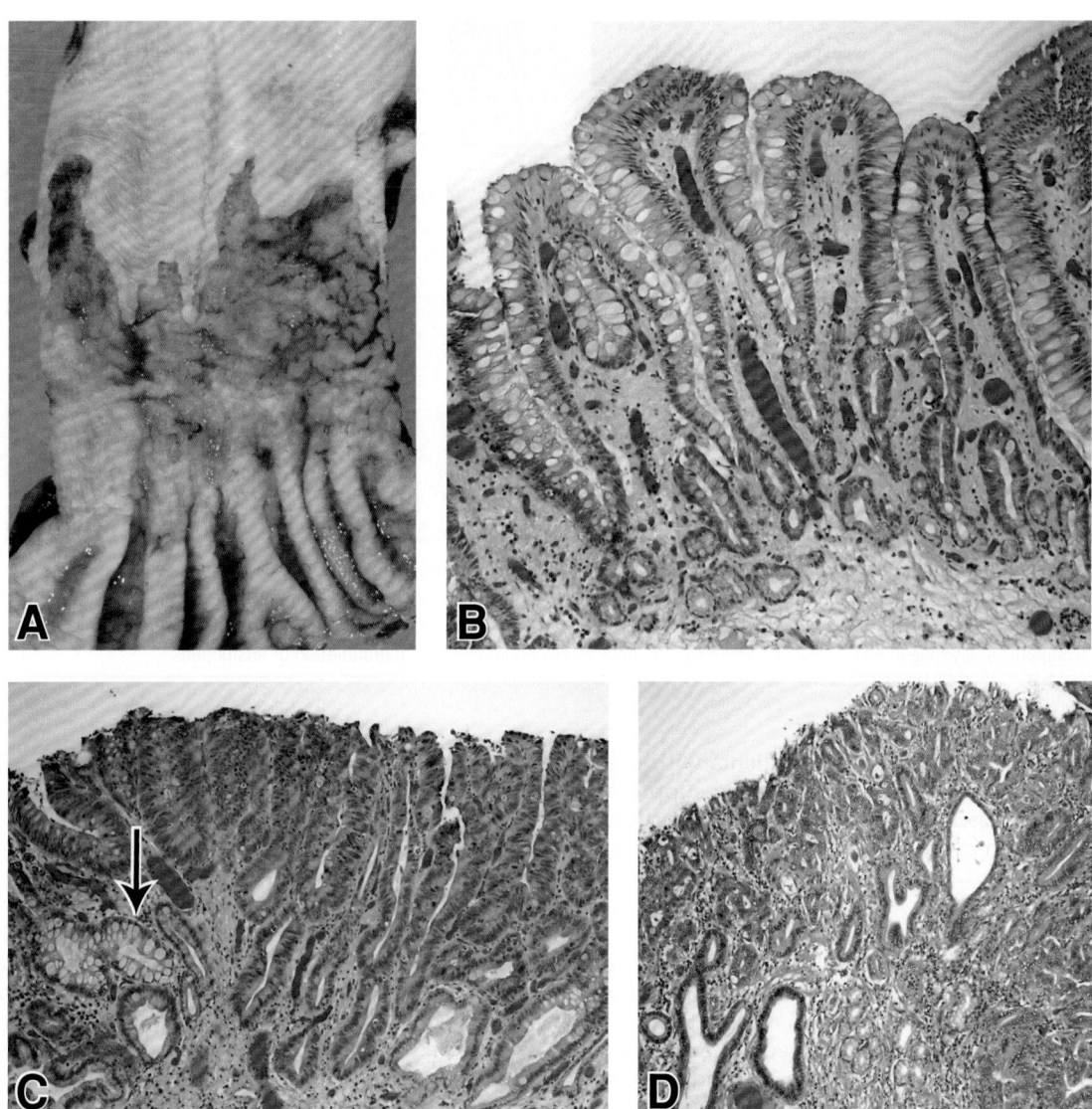

FIGURE 19-6. Barrett esophagus. A. The presence of the tan tongues of epithelium interdigitating with the more proximal squamous epithelium is typical of Barrett esophagus. **B.** The specialized epithelium has a villiform architecture and is lined by cells that are foveolar gastric-type cells and intestinal goblet-type cells. **C. High-grade dysplasia.** Markedly dysplastic glands predominate with hyperchromatic nuclei and early architectural distortion. Intestinalized, nondysplastic glands persist (*arrow*). **D. Intramucosal adenocarcinoma.** Malignant glands are restricted to the mucosa.

and prominent degranulation of eosinophils (Fig. 19-7B). Deeper samples may show subepithelial fibrosis and eosinophils in the lamina propria.

CLINICAL FEATURES: Eosinophilic esophagitis can present at any age and is more common in males. Adults typically complain of dysphagia to solids or food impaction, while young children may show food intolerance, vomiting, feeding difficulties or failure to thrive. Many patients have a personal or family history of atopy (asthma, allergic rhinitis, eczema, atopic dermatitis), and some may have mildly increased blood eosinophils. Eliminating inciting food from the diet can lead to remission in many patients. Swallowed corticosteroids, leukotriene inhibitors and other immunomodulators can also be used to treat eosinophilic esophagitis.

Lymphocytic Esophagitis Is an Emerging Form of Esophagitis

This rare entity is defined by marked esophageal lymphocytosis in peripapillary zones, with rare or absent granulocytes. Intercellular edema is frequent. Patients present with a variety of clinical symptoms, and no specific underlying etiology is known.

Infective Esophagitis Is Associated with Immunosuppression

CANDIDA ESOPHAGITIS: This fungal infection became common as increasing numbers of patients are immunocompromised owing to chemotherapy for malignant disease, immunosuppression after organ transplantation or AIDS.

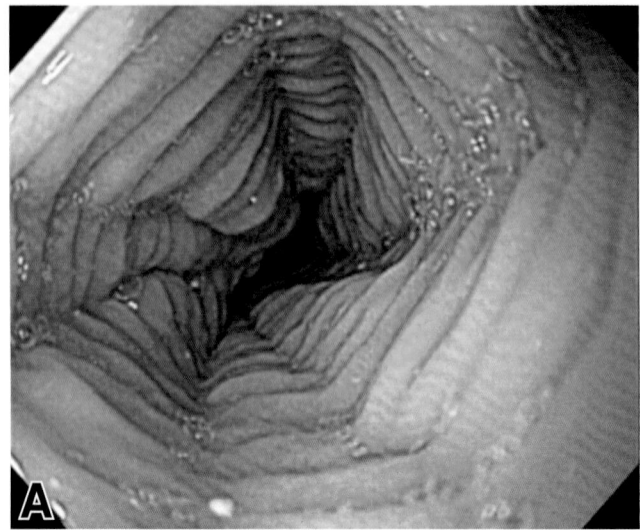
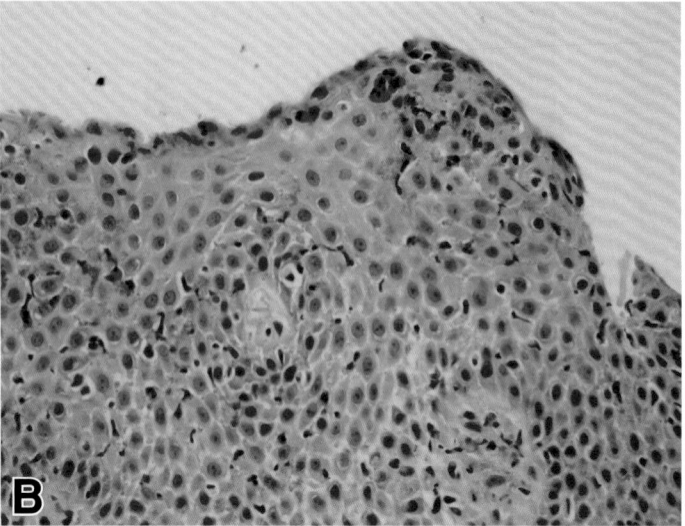

FIGURE 19-7. Eosinophilic esophagitis. A. Endoscopic view of an esophagus from a patient with eosinophilic esophagitis showing concentric mucosal rings (called trachealization or felinization because of its resemblance to the trachea or cat esophagus), vertical linear furrows and small white plaques/exudates. **B.** Microscopic image showing epithelial hyperplasia (papillary and basal layer hyperplasia), intercellular edema, increased intraepithelial eosinophils (≥15 per high-power field), superficial layering of eosinophils, eosinophilic microabscesses and prominent degranulation of eosinophils.

Esophageal candidiasis also occurs in patients with diabetes, in those receiving antibiotic therapy or acid-suppressive therapy or in people using inhaled or swallowed corticosteroids. It is uncommon in the absence of known predisposing factors. Dysphagia and severe pain on swallowing are the usual symptoms.

 PATHOLOGY: In mild cases, a few small, elevated white mucosal plaques are surrounded by a hyperemic zone in the middle or lower third of the esophagus. In severe cases, confluent pseudomembranes lie on a hyperemic and edematous mucosa. Candidal pseudomembranes contain fungal forms, necrotic debris and fibrin. *Candida* may involve only the superficial epithelium, but invasion deeper into the esophageal wall can lead to disseminated candidiasis or fibrosis, sometimes severe enough to create a stricture.

HERPETIC ESOPHAGITIS: Esophageal infection with herpesvirus type I most commonly follows solid organ or bone marrow transplantation. Patients complain of odynophagia. Herpetic esophagitis may occur on occasion in otherwise healthy people.

 PATHOLOGY: Well-developed lesions of herpetic esophagitis grossly resemble those of candidiasis. Early cases show vesicles, small erosions or plaques; as infection progresses, these coalesce into larger lesions. Epithelial cells show typical nuclear herpetic inclusions and occasional multinucleation. Necrosis of infected cells leads to ulceration. Candidal or bacterial superinfection may cause pseudomembranes.

CYTOMEGALOVIRUS (CMV) ESOPHAGITIS: Involvement of the esophagus, or other segments of the GI tract, with CMV usually reflects systemic viral disease in severely immunosuppressed patients (e.g., those with AIDS, transplant recipients, etc.). Mucosal ulceration, as in herpetic esophagitis, is common. Characteristic CMV inclusion bodies are seen in endothelial cells and granulation tissue fibroblasts.

Chemical Esophagitis Results from Ingestion of Corrosive Agents

Chemical injury to the esophagus usually reflects accidental poisoning in children, attempted suicide in adults or contact with medication ("pill esophagitis"). Strong alkaline agents (e.g., lye) or strong acids (e.g., sulfuric or hydrochloric acid), which are used in various cleaning solutions, can produce chemical esophagitis. The former are particularly insidious, since they are generally odorless and tasteless and so easily swallowed before protective reflexes come into play.

 PATHOLOGY: Alkaline agents cause liquefactive necrosis with conspicuous inflammation and saponification of membrane lipids of all layers of the esophagus and stomach. Small vessel thrombosis adds ischemic necrosis to the injury. Severe damage is the rule with liquid alkali, but less than 25% of those who ingest granular preparations have severe complications.

Strong acids produce immediate coagulative necrosis. Resultant protective eschars limit injury and penetration. Still, half of patients who ingest concentrated hydrochloric or sulfuric acid develop severe esophageal injury.

Drug-related esophagitis is most often caused by direct chemical effects on the squamous-lined mucosa, especially with capsules; esophageal dysmotility and cardiac enlargement (which impinges on the esophagus) may be contributing factors.

Esophagitis May Complicate Systemic Illnesses

Esophageal squamous mucosa resembles, and shares some reactions with, the skin.

The **dermolytic (dystrophic) form of epidermolysis bullosa** (see Chapter 28) involves all organs lined by, or derived from, squamous epithelium, including skin, nails, teeth and esophagus. Bullae occur episodically and evolve from fluid-filled vesicles to weeping ulcers. Dysphagia and painful swallowing are common. Stricture, usually in the upper esophagus, may occur.

Bullous pemphigoid causes subepithelial bullae in the skin and esophagus without scarring. Other dermatologic disorders associated with esophagitis include pemphigus vulgaris, dermatitis herpetiformis, Behçet syndrome and erythema multiforme.

Graft-versus-host disease (GVHD; see Chapter 4) in recipients of bone marrow transplants can cause esophageal lesions and dysphagia, odynophagia and GE reflux.

Esophagitis May Be Iatrogenic

External irradiation for treatment of thoracic cancers may affect parts of the esophagus and lead to esophagitis and stricture. **Nasogastric tubes** may cause pressure ulcers if they are in place for prolonged periods, but acid reflux also plays a role in these cases.

ESOPHAGEAL VARICES

Esophageal varices are dilated veins just beneath the mucosa (Fig. 19-8) *that are prone to rupture and hemorrhage* (also see Chapter 20). They arise in the lower third of the esophagus, virtually always in patients with hepatic cirrhosis and portal hypertension. GE anastomoses link lower esophageal veins to the portal system. If portal pressure exceeds a critical level, these anastomoses dilate in the upper stomach and lower esophagus. Without treatment, varices rupture in approximately 1/3 of patients, leading to life-threatening hemorrhage. Reflux injury or infective esophagitis can contribute to variceal bleeding. Esophageal banding and a variety of medications are used to prevent esophageal varices from rupturing.

LACERATIONS AND PERFORATIONS

Lacerations of the esophagus result from external trauma, such as automobile accidents or medical instrumentation,

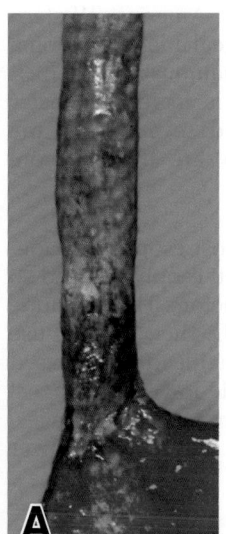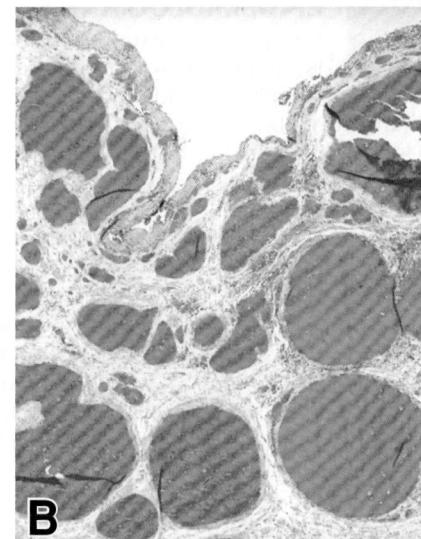

FIGURE 19-8. Esophageal varices. A. Numerous prominent blue venous channels are seen beneath the mucosa of the everted esophagus, particularly above the gastroesophageal junction. **B.** Section of the esophagus reveals numerous dilated submucosal veins.

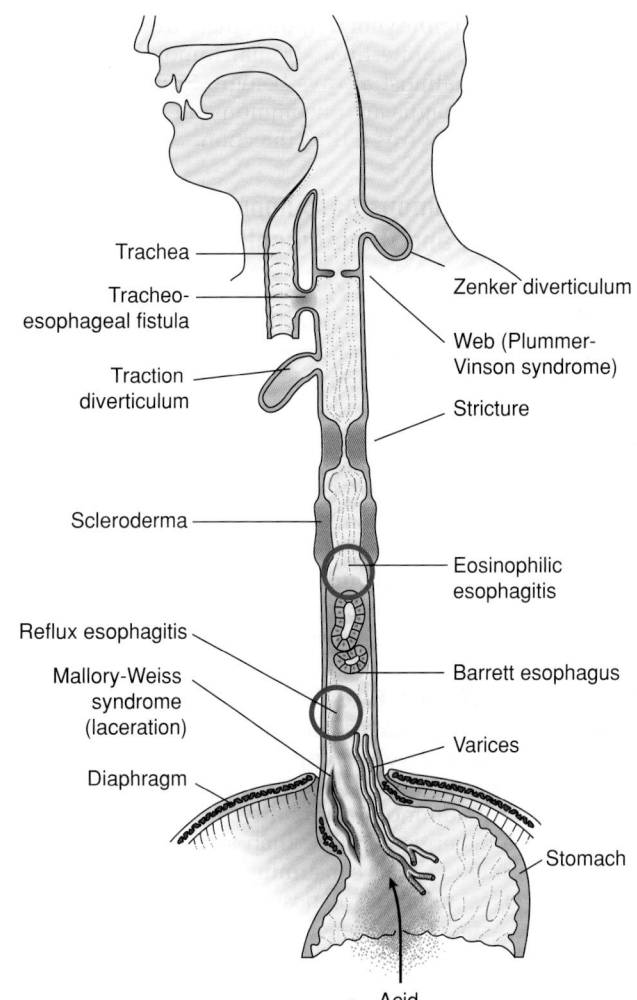

FIGURE 19-9. Nonneoplastic disorders of the esophagus.

or from severe vomiting, during which intraesophageal pressure may reach 300 mm Hg. Forceful retching may cause mucosal tears, first in the gastric epithelium and then extending into the esophagus.

Mallory-Weiss syndrome refers to severe retching, often associated with alcoholism. It leads to mucosal lacerations of the upper stomach and lower esophagus. These tears cause patients to vomit bright red blood. Bleeding may be so severe as to require transfusion of many units of blood. Perforation into the mediastinum, called **Boerhaave syndrome,** may result.

Esophageal perforation, whether from trauma, from vomiting or iatrogenic, can be catastrophic. It is a well-known occurrence in newborns, in whom it is caused occasionally by suctioning or feeding with a nasogastric tube. However, it may also occur spontaneously.

The major nonneoplastic esophageal disorders are summarized in Fig. 19-9.

NEOPLASMS OF THE ESOPHAGUS

Benign Tumors of the Esophagus Are Uncommon

Unlike other parts of the gastrointestinal tract, most spindle cell submucosal tumors of the esophagus derive from smooth muscle (**leiomyoma**) rather than from interstitial cells of Cajal (gastrointestinal stromal tumors [GISTs]; see below). They are almost always benign. **Squamous papillomas** of the esophagus are uncommon and may be related to human papillomavirus (HPV) infection.

Esophageal Squamous Carcinomas Vary Geographically and Histologically

 **EPIDEMIOLOGY:** Worldwide, most esophageal cancers are squamous cell carcinomas. Esophageal cancer is the eighth most common cancer. In the United States, adenocarcinoma is now more common (see below).

Global geographic variations in the incidence of esophageal squamous carcinomas are striking: areas of high incidence often abut areas of low incidence. The greatest frequency is in China, Iran, South America and South Africa. In the United States, black men have a much higher incidence than whites, and American urban dwellers are at greater risk than those in rural areas. Esophageal squamous cell carcinoma is more common in older males.

 **ETIOLOGIC FACTORS:** The variable distribution of esophageal squamous carcinomas, even among relatively homogeneous populations, suggests that environmental factors strongly affect its development. The most common factors are smoking and alcohol, which have a synergistic rather than additive effect. Other contributors include diet, consuming large amounts of hot beverages, HPV, radiation exposure, dietary nitrates and nitrosamines, vitamin deficiencies, genetic factors, Plummer-Vinson syndrome, achalasia and prior caustic injury.

 PATHOLOGY: About half of cases of esophageal squamous cell carcinoma involve the middle and upper thirds of the esophagus. Tumors may be endophytic or exophytic (Fig. 19-10). They can also be infiltrating, growing mainly in the wall. Bulky polypoid tumors tend to obstruct early, but ulcerated ones are more likely to bleed. Infiltrating tumors gradually narrow the lumen by circumferential compression. Extension of tumor into mediastinal structures is often a major problem.

Neoplastic squamous cells range from well differentiated, with squamous "pearls," to poorly differentiated, without evident squamous differentiation. Some tumors have a predominant spindle cell population of tumor cells.

The rich lymphatic drainage of the esophagus provides a route for most metastases. Tumors of the upper third spread to cervical, internal jugular and supraclavicular nodes. Those of the middle third metastasize to paratracheal and hilar lymph nodes and to nodes in the aortic, cardiac and paraesophageal regions. Since the lower third of the esophagus is supplied by the left gastric artery, lower esophageal tumors spread via accompanying lymphatics to retroperitoneal, celiac and left gastric nodes. Metastases to liver and lung are common, but almost any organ may be affected.

 CLINICAL FEATURES: Dysphagia is the most common presenting complaint, but by the time this occurs, most tumors are inoperable. Patients may become cachectic from anorexia, difficulty in swallowing and the remote effects of a cancer. Odynophagia occurs in

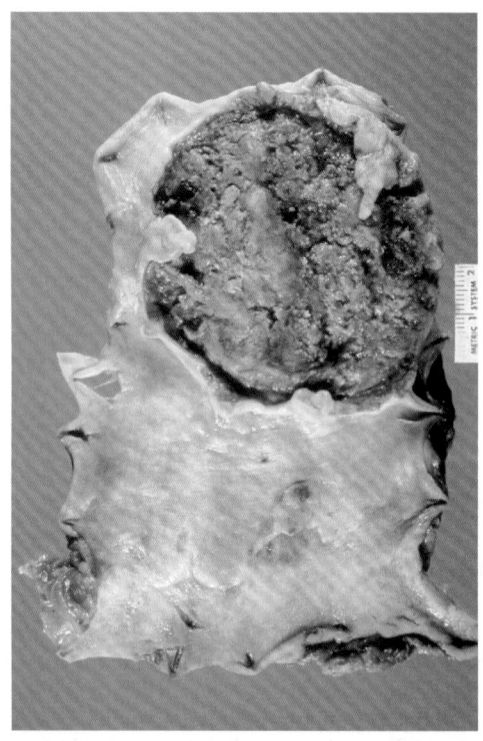

FIGURE 19-10. Esophageal squamous cell carcinoma. There is a large ulcerated mass present in the squamous mucosa with normal squamous mucosa intervening between the carcinoma and the stomach.

half of patients. Persistent pain suggests extension to the mediastinum or to spinal nerves. Compression of the recurrent laryngeal nerve causes hoarseness, and tracheoesophageal fistula presents clinically as a chronic cough. Treatment is similar to esophageal adenocarcinoma (see below).

Adenocarcinoma of the Esophagus Often Arises in a Background of Barrett Esophagus

 **EPIDEMIOLOGY:** In North America, Western Europe and Australia, esophageal adenocarcinoma is far more common than squamous cancer. Incidence of esophageal adenocarcinoma is increasing faster than any solid tumor: it has increased sevenfold in the United States in the last 30 years. Men are affected more often than women.

 **ETIOLOGIC FACTORS:** Most esophageal adenocarcinomas arise from Barrett esophagus and so have similar underlying risk factors. These include white race, male gender, obesity, GERD, diet, tobacco use and genetic factors. Other risk factors that lead to increased gastric acid production or reflux include lower esophageal sphincter dilation or myotomy, scleroderma, Zollinger-Ellison syndrome or use of medications that relax the lower esophageal sphincter.

 PATHOLOGY: The majority of esophageal adenocarcinomas involve the distal esophagus or GE junction, and can extend into the proximal stomach. Tumors may be flat, ulcerated, polypoid or fungating. Often there is surrounding nonneoplastic Barrett mucosa that can be seen grossly or microscopically (Fig. 19-11).

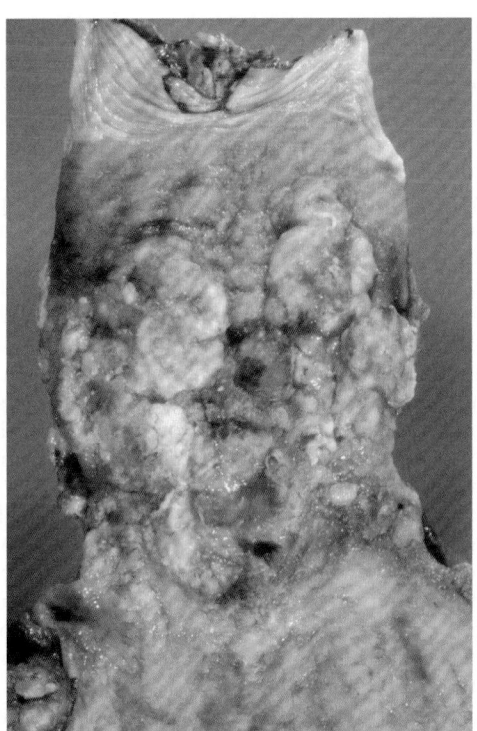

FIGURE 19-11. Esophageal adenocarcinoma. There is a large exophytic ulcerated mass lesion just proximal to the gastroesophageal junction. This well-differentiated adenocarcinoma was separated from the most proximal squamous epithelium by a tan area representing Barrett esophagus.

These tumors may be well differentiated, with well-developed glands, ranging to poorly differentiated tumors with essentially no glandular differentiation. Some poorly differentiated adenocarcinomas have signet ring cellular morphology.

 CLINICAL FEATURES: The symptoms and clinical course of esophageal adenocarcinoma are like those of squamous carcinoma. Symptoms

generally appear in white, obese men with histories of GERD. Diagnosis and staging are typically done using endoscopy with ultrasound. Early invasive cancers (T1) can be treated with endoscopic mucosal resection. Patients with T2 cancers (invading into the submucosa) usually undergo primary esophagectomy. More advanced disease requires neoadjuvant chemotherapy and radiation treatment, which can then be followed by surgical resection in patients who have a good clinical response.

It is controversial as to whether there is an improvement in survival for esophageal adenocarcinoma, but endoscopic surveillance is commonly done in the United States for people with Barrett esophagus. Patients with dysplasia undergo more frequent screening endoscopies. The goal is to identify and treat precursor lesions and early cancers.

The Stomach

ANATOMY

The stomach arises as a dilatation of the embryonic foregut. In adult life, it assumes a J configuration with its convexity (the greater curvature) extending leftward from the GE junction. The concave aspect (lesser curvature) extends from the GE junction to the right. The whole stomach is covered by peritoneum; the omentum extends downward from the greater curvature.

The stomach is commonly divided into four regions: the cardia, fundus, body (corpus) and antrum (Fig. 19-12A,B). The **cardia** separates the esophagus from the rest of the stomach; in many ways it mirrors more the problems of the distal esophagus than of the rest of the stomach. Its exact proximal and distal limits are controversial. Most would consider its distal margin to be where gastric rugal folds begin. The proximal margin is more difficult to define as columnar metaplasia in the distal esophagus may blur the border between esophagus and stomach. The cardia is said

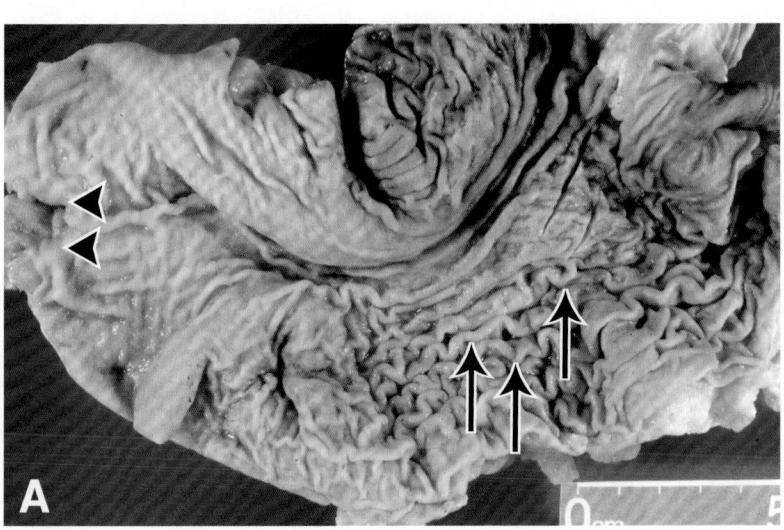

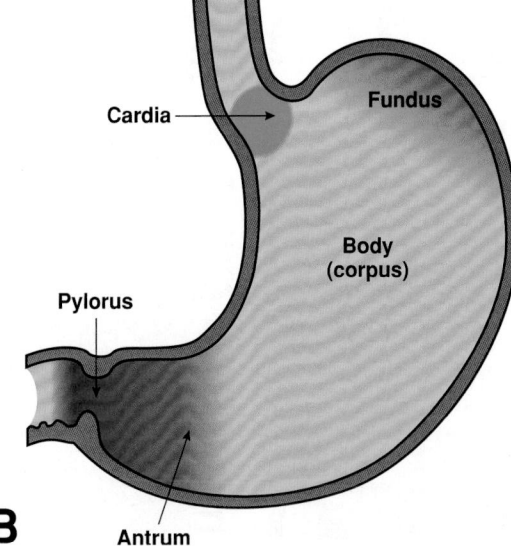

FIGURE 19-12. A. A **normal stomach** from an autopsy. The rugal folds are readily seen in the body (*arrows*). The sweep of the lesser curvature leads into the V-shaped antrum (*arrowheads*). **B.** Anatomic regions of the stomach.

to range between 0.5 and 3 cm in length, although some concern has been raised that the longer cardias (over 2 cm) may represent metaplasia responding to reflux.

The **fundus** and **body** are basically identical except that the fundus is that part of the stomach which bulges above the GE junction. Acid and intrinsic factor are produced in these regions. The boundary between the body and antrum is usually taken to be the incisura angularis, a notch in the lesser curvature.

The **antrum** is the distal stomach, ending in the duodenum, from which it is separated by the pyloric sphincter. The hormone gastrin is made here, eliciting acid production in the gastric body.

In addition to the inner circular and outer longitudinal layers of the muscularis propria seen elsewhere in the gut, there is an oblique layer that aids in the mixing necessary in early phases of digestion.

The histology of the stomach is quite distinct in the cardia, fundus/body and antrum. However, the top mucosal layer of the entire stomach is a characteristic foveolar epithelium (Fig. 19-13A); the term "foveolar" refers to the shallow pits covering the entire gastric surface. The neutral pink mucin in these epithelial cells is periodic acid–Schiff (PAS) positive and Alcian blue negative; it provides a safe haven for *Helicobacter pylori*. The foveolae are separated from underlying glands by a small neck region. This is important since it is the proliferative region and differs from the rest of the gastrointestinal tract where cell division occurs in the base of the glands.

In the glands underlying the foveolae, the main regions of the stomach take on their characteristic features.

The glands of the cardia (Fig. 19-13B) are loosely packed and lined by cells containing neutral mucous. They somewhat resemble the antral glands but do not produce gastrin cells. They often show a slight degree of cystic dilatation.

The gastric fundus and body glands (Fig. 19-13C) are where the acid-producing parietal cells (Fig. 19-13D) are located. These cells also produce intrinsic factor. They are large and polygonal, with slightly granular pink cytoplasm. Deeply in these glands, chief cells predominate; they have a granular blue cytoplasm marking production of pepsinogen. The deepest aspect of the glands is also home to neuroendocrine cells: the enterochromaffin-like (ECL) cells.

The antral (or pyloric) mucosa (Fig. 19-13E) also contains loosely packed glands lined by cells that make neutral mucous. However, it is by the neuroendocrine cells that the antrum differs from the cardia. Gastrin-producing G cells (Fig. 19-13F) are numerous here. There are also enterochromaffin cells (ECs) that produce serotonin and some somatostatin-producing D cells.

The cardia, body and antrum are distinct in their anatomy and function. Thus, it is important to keep track of landmarks during endoscopic examination and biopsy of

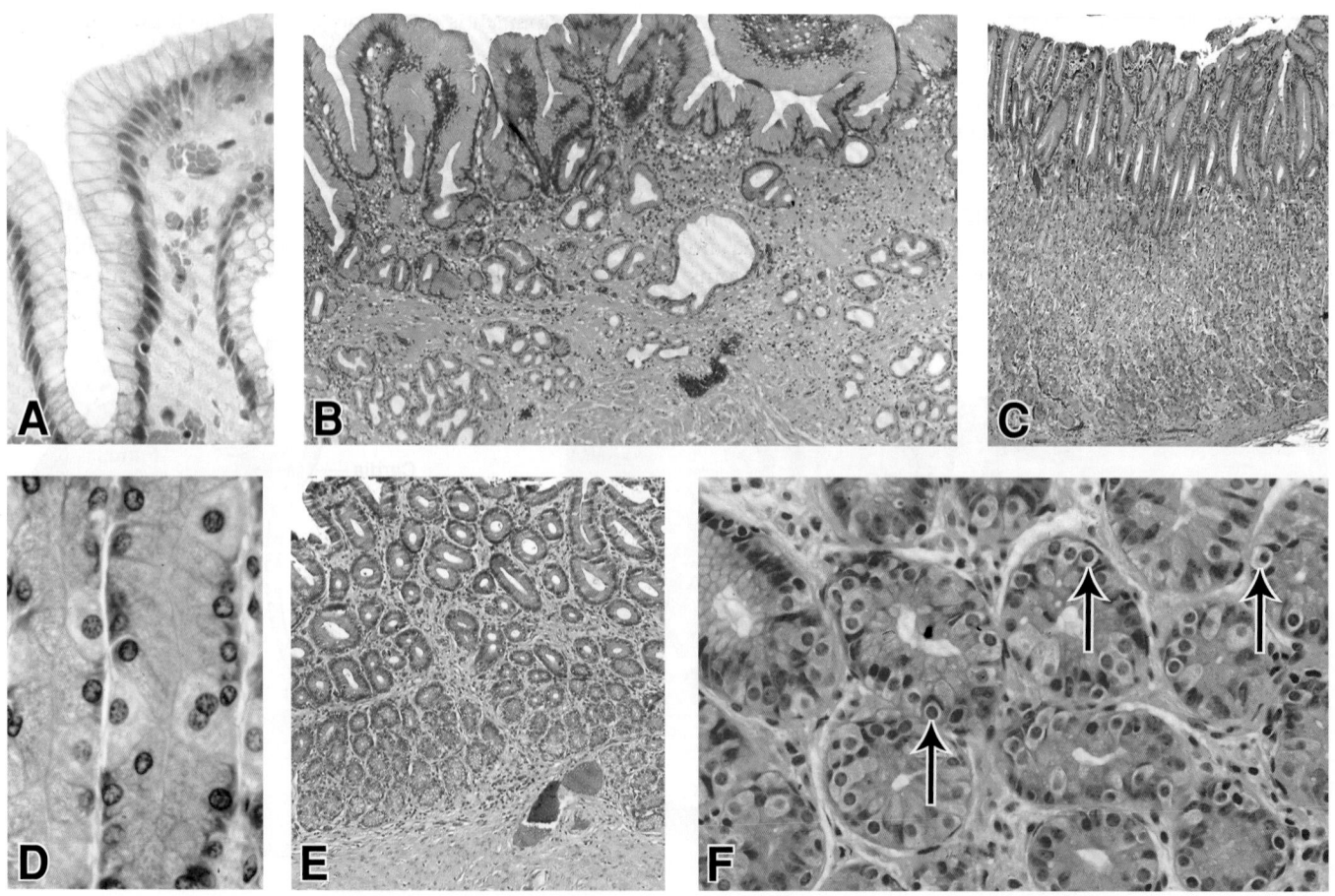

FIGURE 19-13. Histology of the stomach. A. The **foveolar epithelium. B.** The gastric **cardia. C.** The gastric **body. D. Parietal** cells (pink) and **chief cells** (granular blue). **E.** The gastric **antrum. F. Gastrin**-producing cells in antrum; they resemble fried eggs (*arrows*). See text for further description.

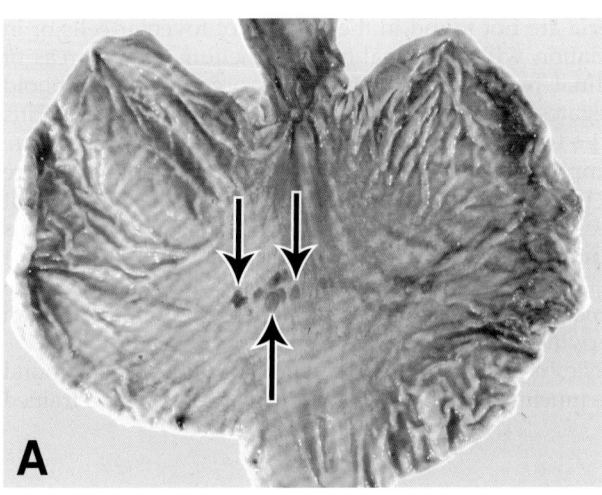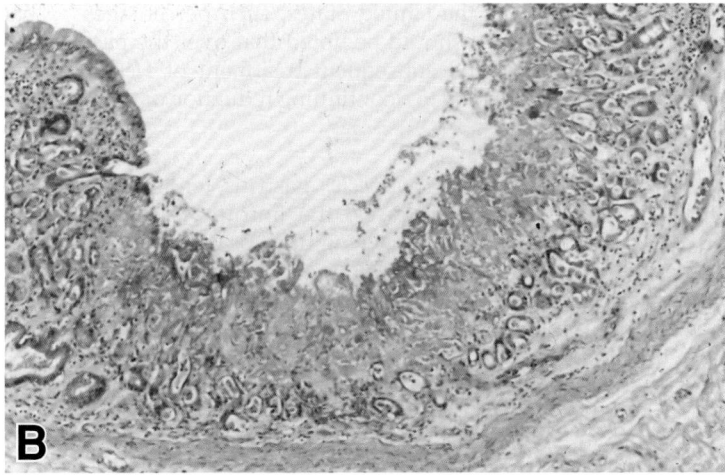

FIGURE 19-14. A. Several shallow erosions/ulcers are scattered in the gastric body (*arrows*). **B.** There is an area of erosion with hemorrhage.

the stomach. It should also be noted that the transition from each of these areas to the other is not very sharp and they may intermingle somewhat in areas of transition.

CONGENITAL DISORDERS

Congenital disorders of the stomach are uncommon. Of these, the most common is **congenital pyloric stenosis**. This condition presents with projectile vomiting during the first 6 months of life. It is more common in boys than girls and may have a genetic basis.

ACUTE GASTRITIS

Acute Gastritis/Acute Gastric Ulceration

These conditions usually occur in specific clinical situations: severe physiologic stress such as trauma, severe burns, increased intracranial pressure or sepsis. At times, acute gastritis may be related to back-diffusion of hydrogen ions related to ingestion of alcohol or aspirin or other nonsteroidal anti-inflammatory drugs (NSAIDs). Superficial ulcers related to burns are called Curling ulcers; if such ulcers are related to increased intracranial pressure, they are Cushing ulcers. Unlike chronic peptic ulcers, which are usually in the antrum or the junction of the body and antrum, these ulcers are usually shallow and multiple and found in the acid-producing mucosa of the body (Fig. 19-14A,B). The gastritis itself (Fig. 19-15) is usually hemorrhagic (acute hemorrhagic gastritis) but can show a significant fibroinflammatory reaction (acute erosive gastritis). These processes can be life-threatening and patients with predisposing conditions may be treated prophylactically.

CHRONIC GASTRITIS

Chronic gastritis is an increase in lamina propria inflammatory cells and is very common worldwide. It may be asymptomatic, or it may present with vague dyspeptic symptoms. Endoscopic examination is less accurate in assessing gastritis

than similar examinations are for esophagitis and colitis. In part for this reason, and partly because of the heterogeneity of this disorder, there has been a profusion of classifications of gastritis and subsequent variable nomenclature.

Helicobacter pylori Infection Is the Major Cause of Gastritis Worldwide

Helicobacter are short rod-shaped bacteria with a unique habitat: the surface of foveolar cells. The presence and significance of these bacteria went unnoticed for many years, until the astute observations of Warren and Marshall in 1984, for which they were awarded the Nobel Prize, explained the mystery of chronic gastritis. In some countries, over 80% of

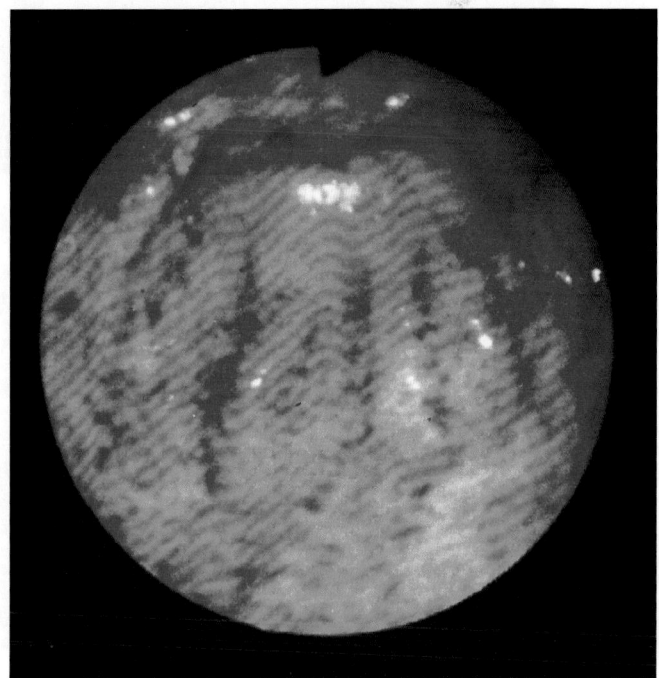

FIGURE 19-15. Endoscopic view of erosive gastritis from a patient who had ingested aspirin. Note the hemorrhagic lesions.

people are affected. In the United States, such percentages vary from 4% to 30%. It should be noted that over the past 30 years, recognition and subsequent treatment of *Helicobacter pylori* gastritis has led to a continuing reduction of these percentages.

PATHOLOGY: *Helicobacter* gastritis tends to be localized. In most cases, the antrum is mostly affected. But with advancing time, or with therapy with proton pump inhibitors (PPIs), the more proximal stomach may become involved. Inflammation in involved areas starts in the superficial lamina propria (Fig. 19-16A), since the organisms are in a thin layer of mucus adherent to the surface foveolar cells. *Helicobacter* do not invade. The

bacteria are not found in the absence of foveolar cells or in association with intestinal-type epithelium. Thus, areas of intestinal metaplasia are devoid of organisms. Lymphoid aggregates are often present in *Helicobacter* gastritis (Fig. 19-16B). The inflammatory infiltrate is largely a mixture of lymphocytes and plasma cells, although neutrophils are often present. They can accumulate in foveolae to form "pit abscesses" (Fig. 19-16C). The presence of such neutrophils does not denote acute gastritis, which is an entirely different process (see above). Rather, neutrophils indicate an active chronic gastritis, with ongoing flares of inflammation in an underlying chronic gastritis.

Helicobacter (Fig. 19-16D) are small curvilinear bacilli found in the mucin-covered surface of foveolar cells. With a trained

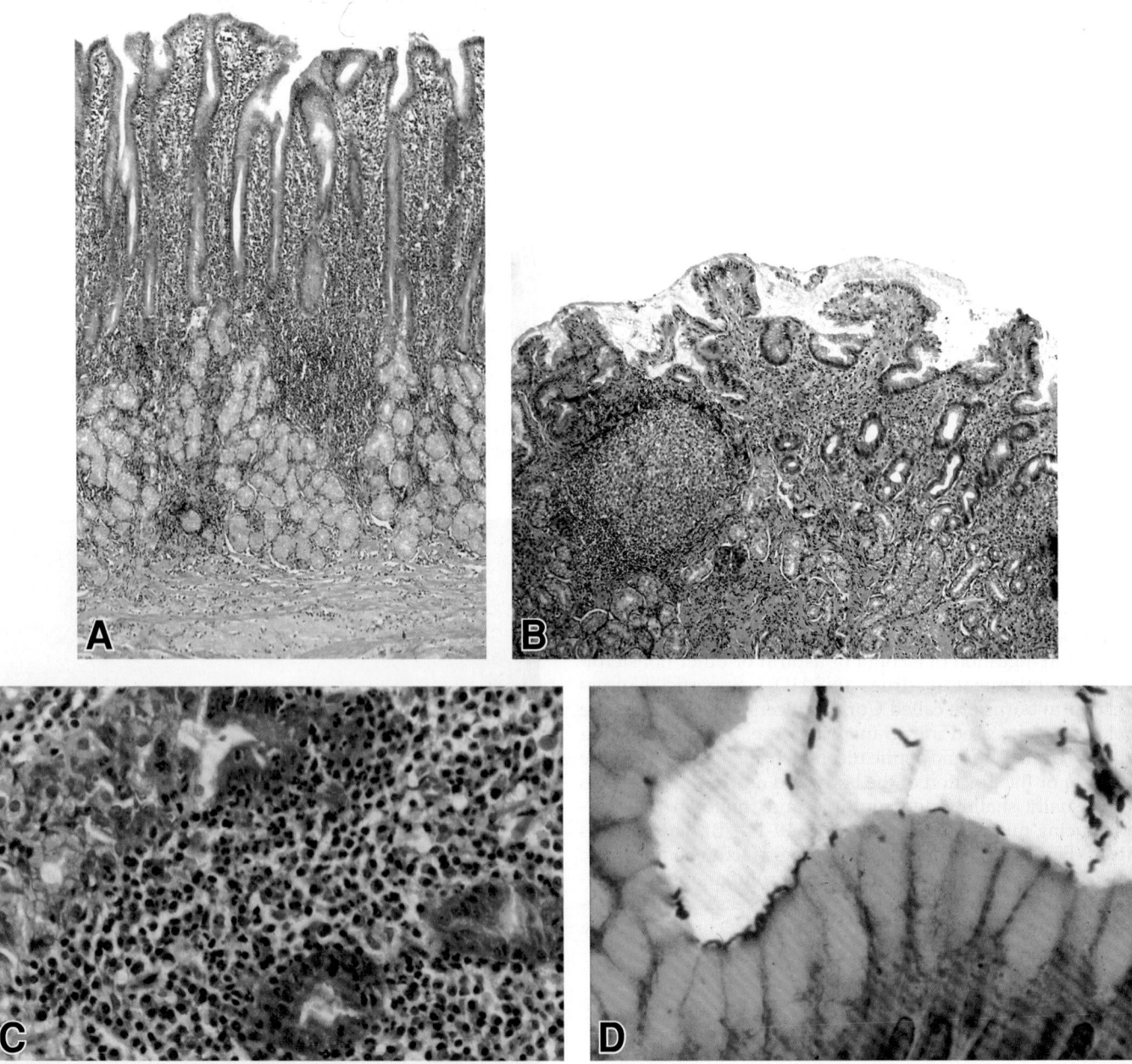

FIGURE 19-16. A. There is a superficial dense lymphoplasmacytic infiltrate in the lamina propria. **B.** A lymphoid aggregate; when present, these are highly suggestive of *Helicobacter*. **C.** Neutrophils are scattered in the lamina propria infiltrate and can penetrate the glandular epithelium. **D.** The Warthin-Starry stain highlights the small curvilinear organisms at the foveolar surface.

eye (and mind), they are usually visible with hematoxylin and eosin stains, but several special stains enhance their recognition: silver impregnation, as in the Warthin-Starry stain, is most often used; immunostaining is also effective.

Gastritis Caused by Non–*Helicobacter pylori* *Helicobacter* Species

Several other species of *Helicobacter,* often collectively called *Helicobacter heilmannii,* can cause human disease. These species are commonly found in the stomachs of domestic animals such as cats, dogs and pigs. They are longer and thicker than *H. pylori* and have several tight spirals. Gastritis caused by these organisms is quite similar to that seen with *H. pylori.* Like *H. pylori,* they produce urease and respond to the same treatment regimens.

Significance of *Helicobacter* Infections

The most common serious problem related to chronic *Helicobacter* gastritis is peptic ulcer disease. Duodenal ulcers occur in 10%–20% of patients with antral-predominant gastritis. This is the main pattern in Western countries, where for years duodenal ulcer disease had been epidemic. Such ulcer disease was often refractory to medical therapy, resulting in a large number of gastrectomies. Recognition of the role of *Helicobacter* has greatly lessened the incidence of duodenal ulcers and their complications. The disease is now largely treated medically and surgical intervention is rarely necessary.

H. pylori infection involving the gastric body increases the risk for gastric cancer. The magnitude of this risk is difficult to ascertain as the involved stomach often shows intestinal metaplasia and *H. pylori* may no longer be readily identifiable. Still, it is widely held that *H. pylori* infection is the most common known cause of gastric cancer. Countries with a high incidence of *H. pylori* carriage have a high gastric cancer risk.

Active Chronic Gastritis without Identified *Helicobacter*

In many cases, this likely represents prior therapy with antibiotics and PPIs, which partly or totally eradicated the organisms. Other infections (e.g., CMV), or adverse drug effects, may also be responsible. Similar gastric inflammation occurs with some frequency in patients with idiopathic inflammatory bowel disease, particularly Crohn disease.

Causes of Chronic Gastritis with Atrophy and Metaplasia Are Controversial

Save for that associated with pernicious anemia (see below), the etiology of chronic gastritis (Fig. 19-17) with atrophy (loss of glands) and metaplasia is uncertain. Still, this condition is felt to predispose to gastric carcinoma. It occurs in multiple scattered foci, though the antrum is usually most affected. At least some cases probably result from long-standing *Helicobacter* infection, and the possibility of other as yet unidentified exposures has led to the use of the noncommittal term "environmental."

Identification of atrophy is difficult in less severe cases. Intestinal metaplasia may be complete (faithfully replicating

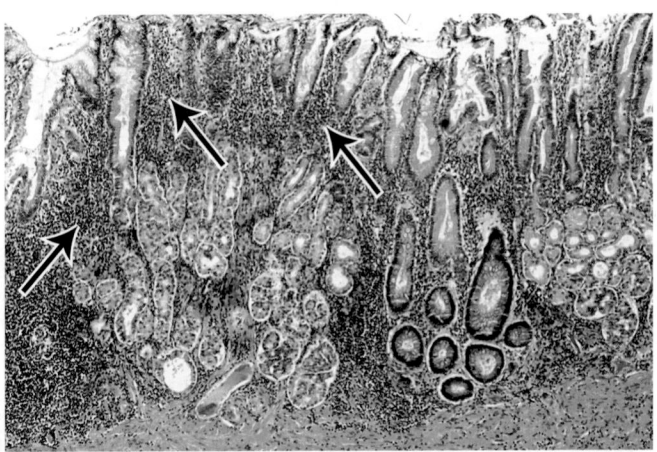

FIGURE 19-17. The inflammatory infiltrate fills the lamin propria (*arrows*). There is loss of gland volume, and a patch of intestinal metaplasia (*arrows*) has replaced the gastric epithelium.

all aspects of small intestine epithelium) or incomplete. The latter is felt to be the major type predisposing to carcinoma. Pyloric (pseudopyloric) metaplasia is more difficult to recognize; it mimics the glands of the antrum but lacks G cells. It is recognized by its presence outside the antral area.

Autoimmune Gastritis Is Limited to the Gastric Antrum

Autoimmune gastritis is often unrecognized, and its overall significance is often not appreciated. The target of the autoimmune reaction is gastric parietal cells, hence its limitation to the gastric antrum. Without parietal cells, the stomach does not produce acid, and clinical achlorhydria results. Also lost is the other product of the parietal cells, intrinsic factor, which mediates absorption of vitamin B_{12} in the distal small intestine.

Immunologically mediated destruction of parietal cells leads to production of antiparietal cell and anti-intrinsic factor antibodies. These antibodies are the basis of diagnostically useful serum tests. With careful sampling from the proximal (body) and distal (antrum) stomach, the diagnosis can be established long before loss of B_{12} results in clinical anemia, known as pernicious anemia (see Chapter 26). Unlike other forms of chronic gastritis, the antrum is spared from inflammation and metaplasia. Hyperplasia of antral G cells occurs because there is no feedback inhibition, as there is no acid production. These G cells consequently produce large amounts of gastrin, which exerts a trophic effect on neuroendocrine ECL cells of the proximal stomach. Hyperplasia of these ECL cells predisposes to development of neoplasms (neuroendocrine tumors or gastric carcinoids; see below).

These conditions lead to a characteristic histology of autoimmune gastritis (Fig. 19-18A,B). Parietal cells are gone and there is significant mononuclear inflammation and intestinal and pseudopyloric metaplasia. In time, neuroendocrine hyperplasia may become prominent. Autoimmune gastritis indicates a significant predisposition to other autoimmune diseases (see Chapter 11) in both the patient and family members. These diseases include type I diabetes, hypothyroidism and Addison disease.

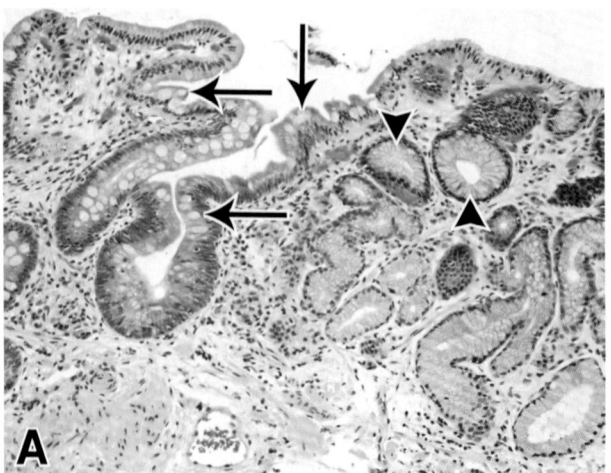
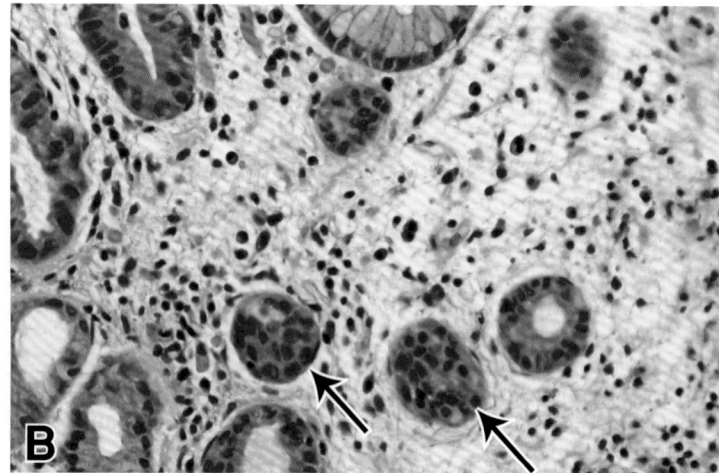

FIGURE 19-18. A. The gastric body is atrophic and devoid of parietal cells. There is intestinal metaplasia (goblet cells, *arrows*) and pseudopyloric metaplasia (*arrowhead*). **B.** Elsewhere in the body there are micronodules composed of enterochromaffin-like (ECL) cells (*arrows*). Note: these biopsies were from the stomach of one of the authors (FAM).

Lymphocytic Gastritis

As the name suggests, this process is characterized by increased numbers of lymphocytes. These occur both in the lamina propria and, importantly, in the surface epithelium (Fig. 19-19). A characteristic "varioliform" endoscopic appearance describes the mucosal lesion's resemblance to poxvirus infection. Several clinical associations account for the importance of this entity. The most important of these is its relationship to celiac disease. Some 10% of patients with celiac disease have lymphocytic gastritis. Diagnostic confusion with *Helicobacter* gastritis may occur as occasional patients with *Helicobacter* have increased lymphocytes at the gastric surface; organisms are usually sparse in these cases, and serology may be needed to confirm this relationship. Lymphocytic gastritis may also be seen together with Menetrier disease (see below).

Focal Enhanced Gastritis

In this process, there are foci of inflammation centered on small portions or groups of glands, which are surrounded by normal mucosa. The inflammation consists of a mixture of lymphocytes and histiocytes, often admixed with neutrophils. Some reports suggest a close relationship to Crohn disease or ulcerative colitis, but this pattern can occur in patients without idiopathic inflammatory bowel disease. Still, its presence, particularly in children, should raise awareness of the possibility of Crohn disease.

Portal Hypertensive Gastropathy

This lesion is seen in patients with portal hypertension, typically from cirrhosis. A typical endoscopic appearance ("mosaic" or "snakeskin") is due to abnormal dilatation of submucosal vasculature. As these vessels are not usually included in endoscopic biopsies, mucosal biopsies often are bland, belying the endoscopic appearance.

Granulomas in Gastric Mucosa

There are multiple causes of gastric granulomas. Finding granulomas in the gastric mucosa should prompt a search for responsible processes (e.g., sarcoidosis or Crohn disease). Typical findings elsewhere (lung, ileum, etc.) are necessary to establish such diagnoses. Infections (fungal and mycobacterial) must also be excluded.

Reactive (Chemical) Gastropathy Is Most Often Due to NSAIDs

While it is clear that exposure to NSAIDs or bile can alter the gastric mucosa, it is not clear when these changes represent a clinically significant condition. These agents lead to hyperplasia of foveolar cells, resulting in loss of the normal nearly flat surface. Resulting short abortive villus-like structures impart a villiform appearance. These structures may become irregular, resulting in a "corkscrew" appearance (Fig. 19-20A). Additional changes may include reactive hyperplasia of foveolar cells and proliferation of lamina propria smooth muscle (Fig. 19-20B). Inflammation is infrequent unless there has been an ulcer or erosion with a subsequent localized inflammatory response.

Much confusion and controversy continue to surround this entity. This is not surprising, given the facts that the

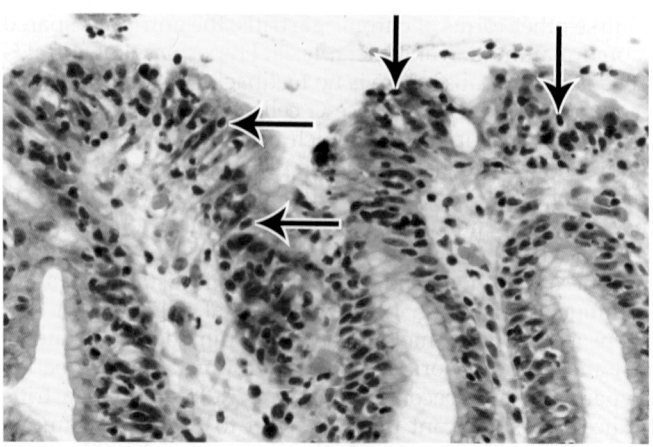

FIGURE 19-19. There is a dense infiltrate of T lymphocytes (*arrows*) in the surface, and here extending into the rest of the gland.

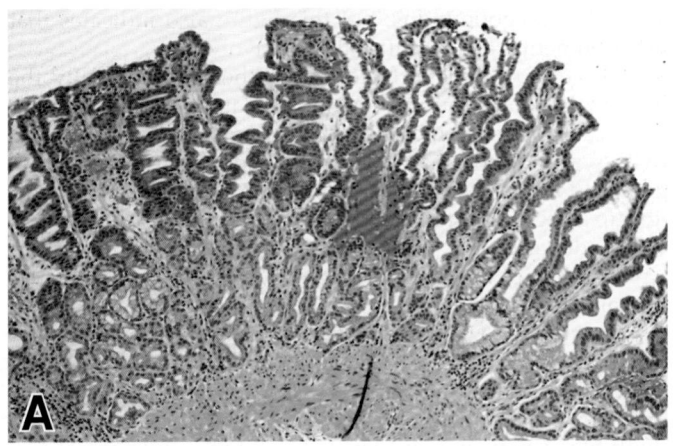
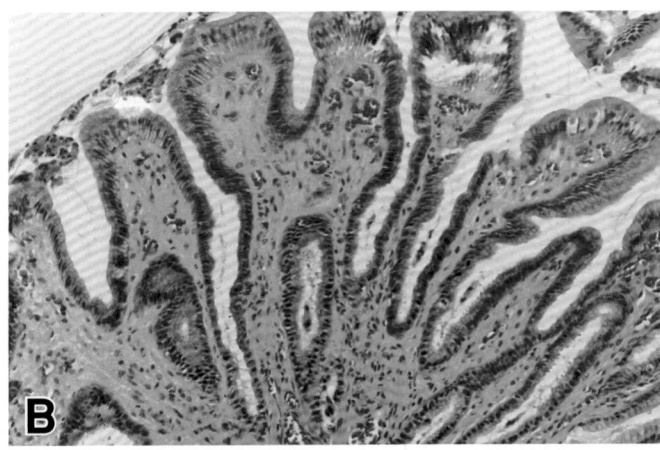

FIGURE 19-20. **A.** The corkscrew contour of the antral glands deviates from normal architecture in this patient with bile reflux. **B.** There is increased smooth muscle in the villiform structures in the antrum of a patient with chronic use of nonsteroidal anti-inflammatory drugs (NSAIDs).

symptoms of gastric mucosal disease are usually vague and that endoscopic appearances are neither specific nor particularly sensitive. A practical approach is helpful. A patient with dyspepsia or ulcer who shows these changes instead of the previously described changes of *Helicobacter* likely has a clinically significant condition, and any NSAID ingestion should be curtailed.

Drug Effects

The most common drug effect is caused by PPIs, which is not surprising given their widespread use. In the gastric body, glands lined by parietal cells show luminal dilatation and some protrusion into these lumens by parietal cells' cytoplasm. Many patients develop fundic gland polyps (see below). Since acid production is blocked, antral G cells visibly multiply in compensation and produce excess gastrin. This causes ECL cell proliferation in the gastric body, though less so than in autoimmune gastritis.

Reactions to NSAIDs are also very common and may result in the reactive or chemical gastropathy described above. Ulceration may occur.

Iron sulfate tablets may cause surface encrustation by the mineral and its congeners. Colchicine and mycophenolate may produce changes mimicking gastritis.

PEPTIC ULCER DISEASE

"Peptic ulcer disease" is focal destruction of the mucosa of the stomach and small intestine, mainly the proximal duodenum. It is caused by gastric secretions. Duodenal ulcers have declined greatly in frequency over the past 30 years.

Peptic ulceration may occur as far proximally as the esophagus and as far distally as the Meckel diverticulum with gastric heterotopia, but the disease mostly affects the distal stomach and proximal duodenum. Many clinical and epidemiologic features distinguish gastric from duodenal ulcers; the common factors that unite them are gastric hydrochloric acid secretion and *H. pylori* infection.

 **EPIDEMIOLOGY:** Peptic ulcers may occur at any age (including infancy), but the peak incidence has progressively changed, so that it is now

between age 30 and 60. Gastric ulcers usually afflict the middle-aged and elderly and affect both sexes equally. Duodenal ulcers are more common in males.

Racial differences have been postulated, but most data suggest that all ethnic groups are susceptible in an urban Western setting. Surveys in the United States and Great Britain show a trend toward an inverse relation between duodenal ulcers and socioeconomic status and education.

 **ETIOLOGIC FACTORS:** No single agent seems to be responsible, although many etiologies have been proffered.

H. PYLORI: H. pylori is isolated from the gastric antrum of virtually all patients with duodenal ulcers. The converse is not true; that is, only a small minority of those carrying the bacterium have duodenal ulcer disease. Thus, *H. pylori* infection may be necessary, but is not sufficient, for peptic duodenal ulcers to develop. Such ulcers heal more quickly after treatment for *H. pylori* infection, and recur less.

Just how *H. pylori* infection predisposes to duodenal ulcers is not completely clear, but several mechanisms have been proposed. Cytokines produced by inflammatory cells in response to the infection stimulate gastrin release and suppress somatostatin secretion. Interleukin-1β (IL-1β), an acid inhibitor, is a key mediator of inflammation in *H. pylori*–infected gastric mucosa. These effects, plus release of histamine metabolites from the organism itself, may stimulate basal gastric acid secretion. In addition, luminal cytokines from the stomach may enter and injure duodenal epithelium.

H. pylori infection may also block inhibitory signals from the antrum to G cells and the parietal cell region, thus increasing gastrin release and impairing inhibition of gastric acid secretion. Such an effect might increase acid load in the duodenum, contributing to duodenal ulceration. Acidification of the duodenal bulb leads to islands of metaplastic gastric mucosa in the duodenum in many patients with peptic ulcers. Such gastric epithelium in the duodenum is sometimes colonized with *H. pylori*, like the gastric mucosa, and infection of the metaplastic epithelium by *H. pylori* may render the mucosa more susceptible to peptic injury (Fig. 19-21).

H. pylori infection is probably also important in the pathogenesis of gastric ulcers, because the organism causes most of the chronic gastritis that underlies this disease. About 75% of patients with gastric ulcers harbor *H. pylori*. The other 25%

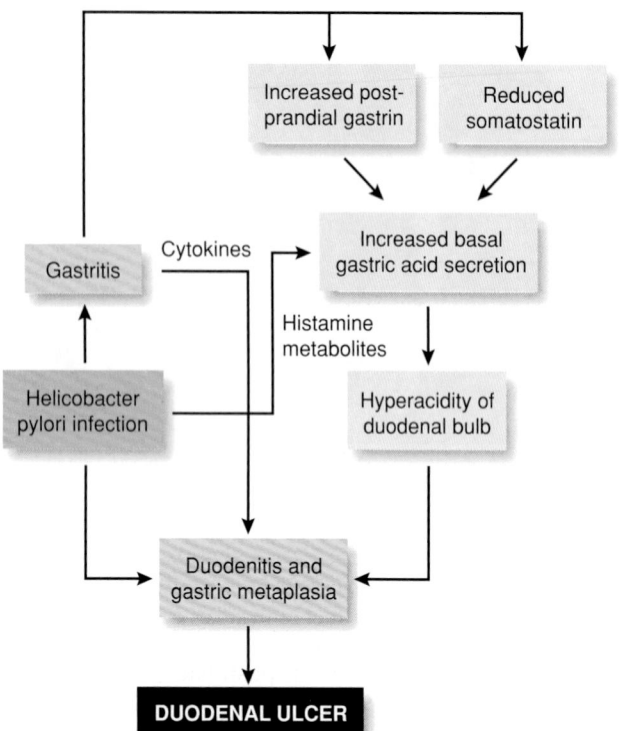

FIGURE 19-21. Possible mechanisms in the pathogenesis of duodenal ulcer disease associated with *Helicobacter pylori* infection.

than do dizygotic twins, but this figure also indicates that environmental factors must also be involved.

The role of genetic factors is further supported by the fact that blood-group antigens correlate with peptic ulcer disease. Duodenal ulcers occur 30% more often in people with type O blood than in those with other types. This does not hold for gastric ulcers. People who do not secrete blood-group antigens in saliva or gastric juice have 50% higher risk of duodenal ulcers. Those who are both type O and nonsecretors (10% of white people) have a 2.5-fold increase in duodenal ulcers.

Pepsinogen I is secreted by gastric chief and mucous neck cells and appears in gastric juice, blood and urine. Serum levels of this proenzyme correlate with the capacity for gastric acid secretion and reflect parietal cell mass. Someone with high blood pepsinogen I levels has 5 times the normal risk of developing a duodenal ulcer. Hyperpepsinogenemia has been attributed to autosomal dominant inheritance and may reflect an inherited tendency to increased parietal cell mass. Half of children of ulcer patients with hyperpepsinogenemia have hyperpepsinogenemia themselves.

Familial tendencies for other features are reported in ulcer patients. Many such patients have normal pepsinogen I levels and still show familial aggregation. Family clustering of duodenal ulcers and rapid gastric emptying have been noted, as has familial hyperfunction of antral G cells. Patients with a childhood duodenal ulcer are much more likely to have a family history of ulcers than people in whom the disease begins when they are adults.

of cases may reflect the influences of other types of chronic gastritis. The gastric and duodenal factors that have been implicated as possible mechanisms in the pathogenesis of duodenal ulcers are summarized in Fig. 19-22.

HCl SECRETION: Hyperacidity due to increased hydrochloric acid secretion is necessary for peptic ulcers to form and persist in the stomach and duodenum. This is evidenced principally by the following: (1) all patients with duodenal ulcers and almost all with gastric ulcers are gastric acid secretors; (2) experimental ulcer production in animals requires acid; (3) hypersecretion of acid is present in many, but not all, patients with duodenal ulcers (there is no evidence that acid overproduction alone explains duodenal ulceration); and (4) surgical and medical treatment that reduces acid production results in the healing of peptic ulcers. Gastric secretion of pepsin, which may also play a role in peptic ulceration, parallels that of hydrochloric acid.

DIET: Despite the folk wisdom that spicy food and caffeine are ulcerogenic, there is little evidence that any food or beverage, including coffee and alcohol, leads to the development or persistence of peptic ulcers.

DRUGS: Aspirin is an important contributor to duodenal, and especially gastric, ulcers. Other nonsteroidal anti-inflammatory agents and analgesics have been incriminated in peptic ulcerogenesis. Prolonged treatment with high doses of corticosteroids may also increase the risk of peptic ulceration slightly.

CIGARETTE SMOKING: Smoking is a definite risk factor for duodenal and gastric ulcers, particularly gastric ulcers.

GENETIC FACTORS: First-degree relatives of people with duodenal or gastric ulcers have a 3-fold higher risk of developing an ulcer—but only at the same site. Monozygotic twins show much higher (50%) concordance for these ulcers

PATHOPHYSIOLOGY:
DUODENAL ULCERS: Maximal capacity for gastric acid production is a function of total parietal cell mass. Patients with duodenal ulcers may have up to double the normal parietal cell mass and maximal acid secretion. However, there is a large overlap with normal values, and only one third of ulcer patients secrete excess acid. Increased chief cell mass often accompanies increased parietal cells, reflecting the prevalence of hyperpepsinogenemia in patients with ulcers.

Food-stimulated gastric acid secretion is increased in magnitude and duration in people with duodenal ulcers, but here, too, there is significant overlap with normal values. This may involve, at least in part, altered G-cell responses to meals. Such patients show postprandial hypergastrinemia and increased antral G cells. Most people with duodenal ulcers, however, show no G-cell hyperfunction. Acid secretion in people with duodenal ulcers may also be more sensitive than normal to gastric secretagogues such as gastrin, possibly owing to increased vagal tone or increased affinity of parietal cells for gastrin. Brisk secretion of acid after a meal may reflect increased vagal tone.

Patients with duodenal ulcers show accelerated gastric emptying. This might lead to excessive duodenal acidification. However, as with other factors, there is overlap with normal rates. Duodenal bulb acidification normally inhibits further gastric emptying, but not in most people with duodenal ulcers. In them, duodenal acidification leads to continued, rather than delayed, gastric emptying. Rapid gastric emptying may in some cases be an inherited trait.

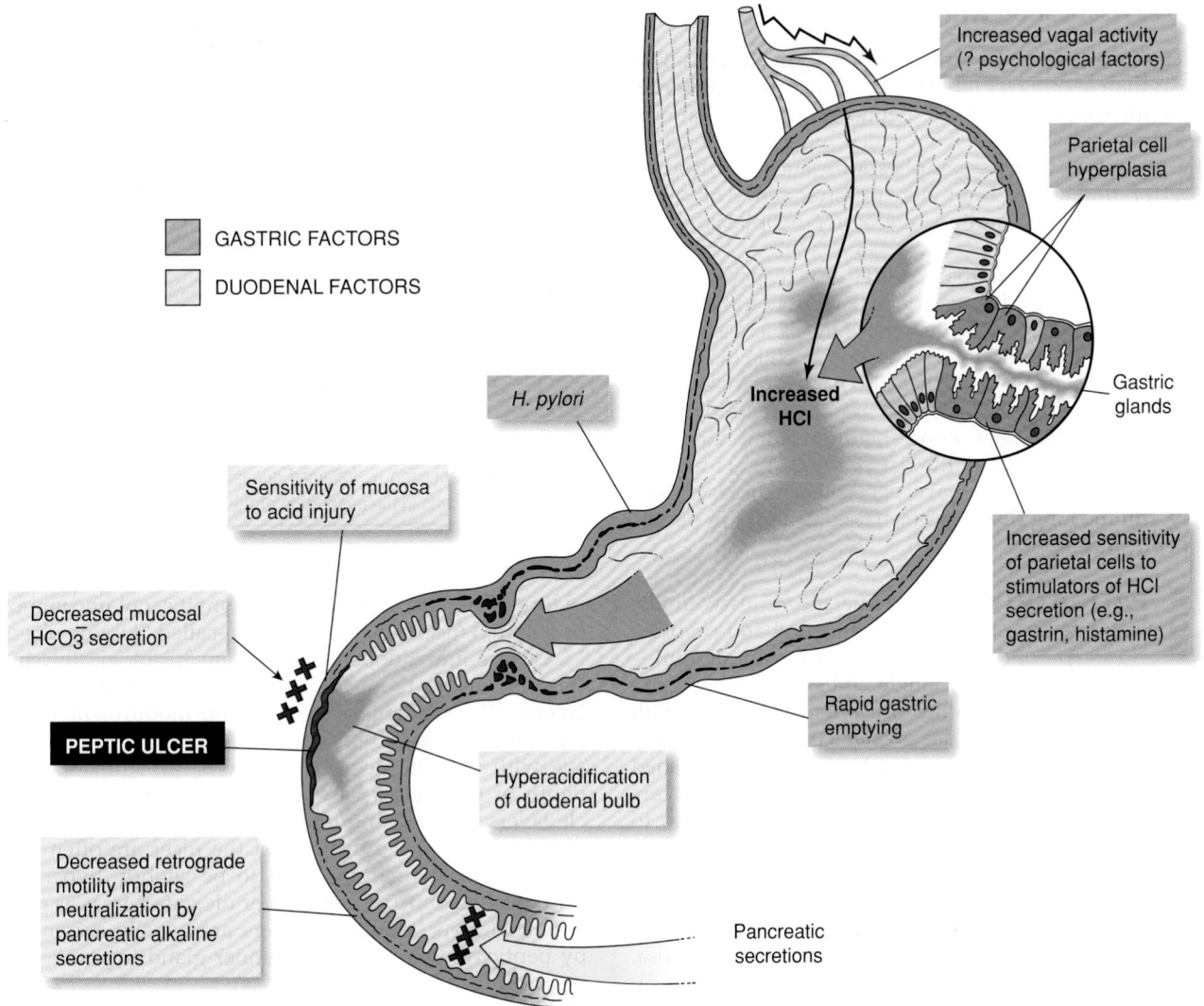

GASTRIC FACTORS

DUODENAL FACTORS

Increased vagal activity
(? psychological factors)

Parietal cell
hyperplasia

H. pylori

Sensitivity of mucosa
to acid injury

Increased
HCl

Gastric
glands

Decreased mucosal
HCO_3^- secretion

Increased sensitivity
of parietal cells to
stimulators of HCl
secretion (e.g.,
gastrin, histamine)

PEPTIC ULCER

Rapid gastric
emptying

Hyperacidification
of duodenal bulb

Decreased retrograde
motility impairs
neutralization by
pancreatic alkaline
secretions

Pancreatic
secretions

FIGURE 19-22. Gastric and duodenal factors in the pathogenesis of duodenal peptic ulcers.

The pH of the duodenal bulb reflects a balance between delivery of gastric juice and its neutralization by biliary, pancreatic and duodenal secretions. Duodenal ulceration requires an acidic pH in the bulb. In ulcer patients, duodenal pH after a meal decreases to a lower level and remains depressed longer than in normal people. Such duodenal hyperacidity certainly reflects the gastric factors discussed above. The role of neutralizing factors, particularly bicarbonate secretion by the duodenal mucosa or by the pancreas in response to secretin, is uncertain.

Impaired mucosal defenses may also contribute to peptic ulceration. Factors such as prostaglandins may or may not protect the duodenum as they do the gastric mucosa (see above).

GASTRIC ULCERS: Gastric ulcers almost invariably arise in the setting of epithelial injury by *H. pylori* or chemical gastritis. Just how chronic gastritis predisposes to gastric ulceration is obscure. Most patients with gastric ulcers secrete less acid than do those with duodenal ulcers and even less than normal people. Factors implicated include (1) back-diffusion of acid into the mucosa,

(2) decreased parietal cell mass and (3) abnormalities of parietal cells themselves. A few gastric ulcer patients produce excess acid. Their ulcers are usually near the pylorus and are considered variants of duodenal ulcers. Interestingly, intense gastric hypersecretion such as occurs in the Zollinger-Ellison syndrome (see below) is associated with severe ulceration of the duodenum and even the jejunum, but rarely of the stomach.

The concurrence of gastric ulcers and gastric hyposecretion implies that (1) the gastric mucosa may in some way be particularly sensitive to low concentrations of acid; (2) something other than acid may damage the mucosa (e.g., NSAIDs); or (3) the gastric mucosa may be exposed to potentially injurious agents for unusually long periods. As discussed above, the mucosal barrier to the action of acid and perhaps to other contents of the stomach may be impaired in some patients with gastric ulcers, although evidence is not conclusive. Bile reflux (particularly deoxycholic acid and lysolecithin) and pancreatic secretions may contribute to the development of gastric ulcers.

Diseases Associated with Peptic Ulcers

Duodenal ulcers occur 10 times more often in patients with cirrhosis than in others. End-stage renal disease with hemodialysis increases the risk of peptic ulceration. Patients with kidney transplants have a much higher incidence of peptic ulceration and its complications, such as bleeding and perforation. There is an increased frequency of peptic ulcers in people with multiple endocrine neoplasia type 1 (see Chapter 27).

Zollinger-Ellison syndrome causes severe peptic ulceration. It is characterized by gastric hypersecretion, caused by a gastric-producing islet cell adenoma of the pancreas. Almost one third of patients with this disease have peptic ulcers, and the incidence is even higher if they also have lung disease.

Peptic ulcers are also increased in people heterozygous for mutant α_1-antitrypsin. Long-standing pulmonary dysfunction significantly raises the risk of ulcers. One fourth of those with such disorders have peptic ulcer disease. Conversely, chronic lung disease is increased 2–3-fold in people with peptic ulcers.

 PATHOLOGY: Most peptic ulcers arise in the lesser gastric curvature, in the antral and prepyloric regions and in the first part of the duodenum.

Gastric ulcers are usually single and smaller than 2 cm. Ulcers on the lesser curvature are often associated with chronic gastritis; those on the greater curvature are commonly related to NSAIDs. Edges tend to be sharply punched out, with overhanging margins. Deeply penetrating ulcers produce a serosal exudate that may cause the stomach to adhere to nearby structures. Scarring of ulcers in the prepyloric region may be severe enough to cause pyloric stenosis. Grossly, chronic peptic ulcers may resemble ulcerated gastric carcinomas. They differ from the latter by their tendency to produce radiating folds in the surrounding mucosa, their lack of a raised border and a "clean" (fibrin-covered)-appearing base (Fig. 19-23). Endoscopists must biopsy the edges and bed of gastric ulcers multiply, as ulcer centers tend to show only necrotic tissue.

Duodenal ulcers (Fig. 19-24) are ordinarily on the anterior or posterior wall of the first part of the duodenum, near the

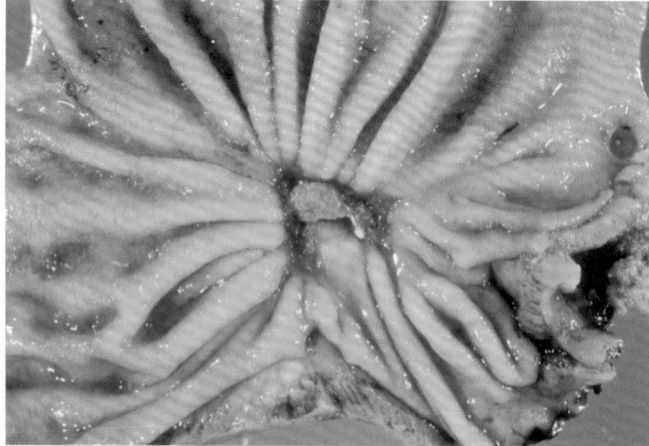

FIGURE 19-23. Gastric ulcer. There is a characteristic sharp demarcation from the surrounding mucosa, which has prominent radiating folds. The base of the ulcer is covered with fibrin, giving it a gray color.

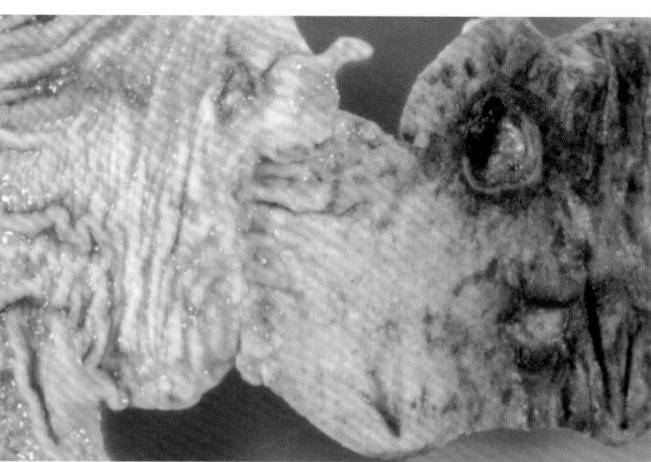

FIGURE 19-24. Duodenal ulcers. There are two sharply demarcated duodenal ulcers surrounded by inflamed duodenal mucosa. The gastroduodenal junction can be seen in the midportion of the photograph.

pylorus. They are usually solitary, but it is not uncommon to find paired ulcers on both walls, so-called "kissing ulcers."

Gastric and duodenal ulcers are histologically similar (Fig. 19-25A,B). From the lumen inward, there are several layers: (1) a superficial zone of fibrinopurulent exudate, (2) necrotic tissue, (3) granulation tissue and (4) fibrotic tissue with variable degrees of chronic inflammation at the depth of the ulcer's base. Ulceration may penetrate muscle layers, interrupting them with scar tissue after healing. Blood vessels at the margins of the ulcer are often thrombosed. Mucosal margins tend to be slightly hyperplastic. With healing, mucosa grows over ulcerated areas as a single epithelial layer. Duodenal ulcers are usually accompanied by peptic duodenitis, with Brunner gland hyperplasia and gastric mucin cell metaplasia.

 CLINICAL FEATURES: The symptoms of gastric and duodenal ulcers are generally not distinguishable by history or physical examination. Classic duodenal ulcers are characterized by epigastric pain 1–3 hours after a meal or that awakens a patient at night. Alkali and food relieve these symptoms. Dyspeptic symptoms often associated with gallbladder disease, such as fatty food intolerance, distention and belching, occur in half of patients with peptic ulcers.

The major complications of peptic ulcer disease are hemorrhage, obstruction and perforation with peritonitis. Of these, the most common is bleeding, which occurs in up to 20% of patients. It is often occult. If there are no other symptoms, it may manifest as iron-deficiency anemia or occult blood in stools. Massive life-threatening bleeding is a well-known complication of active peptic ulcers.

Perforation is a serious complication that occurs in 5% of patients. In 1/3 of these, there are no antecedent symptoms of a peptic ulcer. Duodenal ulcers perforate more often than do gastric ulcers, mostly on the anterior wall of the duodenum. As the anterior gastric and duodenal walls are undefended by contiguous tissue, perforations there are more likely to lead to generalized peritonitis and to air in the abdominal cavity, called **pneumoperitoneum**. Posterior gastric ulcers perforate into the lesser peritoneal sac, where inflammation may be contained. An ulcer that penetrates the

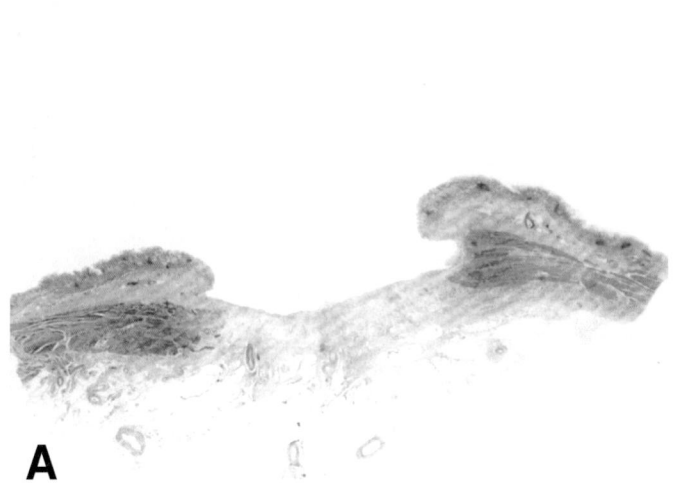
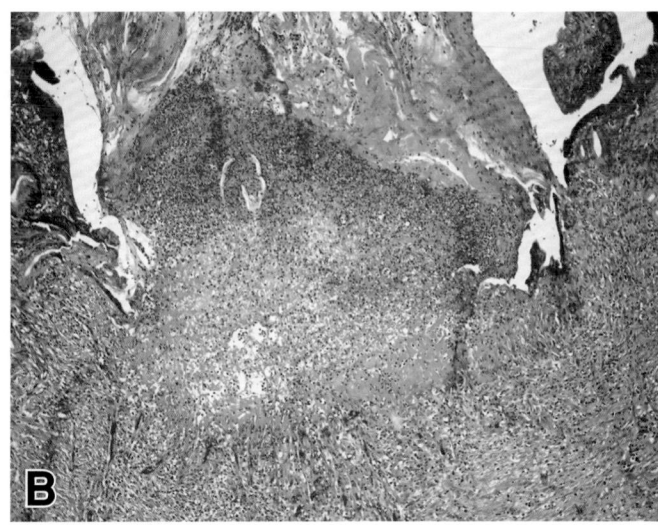

FIGURE 19-25. A. Gastric ulcer: The destructive nature of this lesion is shown by the loss of the underlying muscle in the muscularis propria with replacement by fibrous tissue. **B.** Classic appearance of peptic ulcer with superficial fibrin exudate over necrosis, followed by granulation tissue and fibrosis in the deep aspect.

pancreas, liver or greater omentum can cause severe intractable pain. Ulcers may also penetrate the biliary tract and fill it with air, a condition known as **pneumobilia**.

Perforation carries a high mortality rate, which is 10%–40% for gastric ulcers, 2–4 times more than for duodenal ulcers (10%). Perforations may be complicated by hemorrhage. Shock, abdominal distension and pain are common symptoms, but perforations are occasionally diagnosed for the first time at autopsy, particularly in institutionalized, elderly patients.

Pyloric obstruction occurs in up to 10% of ulcer patients, and peptic ulcer disease is its most common cause in adults. Narrowing with eventual obstruction of the pyloric lumen by an adjacent peptic ulcer may be caused by muscular spasm, edema, muscular hypertrophy or contraction of scar tissue, or, most commonly, a combination of these.

Gastric and duodenal ulcers may occur together in the same patient far more often than can be accounted for by chance alone. Patients with either one have a much greater risk of developing the other later.

ENLARGED RUGAL FOLDS USUALLY REFLECT MÉNÉTRIER OR ZOLLINGER-ELLISON DISEASES

In Ménétrier disease (Fig. 19-26), there is massive foveolar hyperplasia with no increase in underlying glands. This is due to overexpression of transforming growth factor-α (TGF-α) and may cause intramucosal cysts lined by foveolar epithelium. There is often adherent surface mucin or proteinaceous material. Lymphocytic gastritis may be present and may cause a varioliform appearance (see above). The process is more common in men. There is postprandial pain. Protein loss from the mucosa results in hypoalbuminemia and subsequent peripheral edema. Patients with Ménétrier disease have a predisposition to develop gastric carcinoma.

The other prominent condition causing enlarged rugal folds is due to a proliferation of parietal cells rather than foveolar cells (Zollinger-Ellison [Z-E] syndrome). The cause is gastrin production by a neuroendocrine tumor (gastrinoma). Most cases are sporadic, in which case the gastrinomas are more commonly duodenal than pancreatic. A minority of cases are related to multiple endocrine neoplasia syndrome type 1 (MEN1). Gastrinomas in Z-E patients may occur in the duodenum, pancreas or gastric antrum, and they may be multiple and exceedingly small. Rugal folds are enlarged owing to increased numbers of hypertrophied parietal cells; the rugae consequently have a characteristic bumpy appearance (Fig. 19-27). These patients have intractable peptic ulcer disease, with the ulcers often being multiple and in unusual locations.

BENIGN NEOPLASMS

Polyps are endoscopically or grossly identifiable elevations of the mucosa. In the stomach, unlike the colon, the vast majority are not true neoplasms.

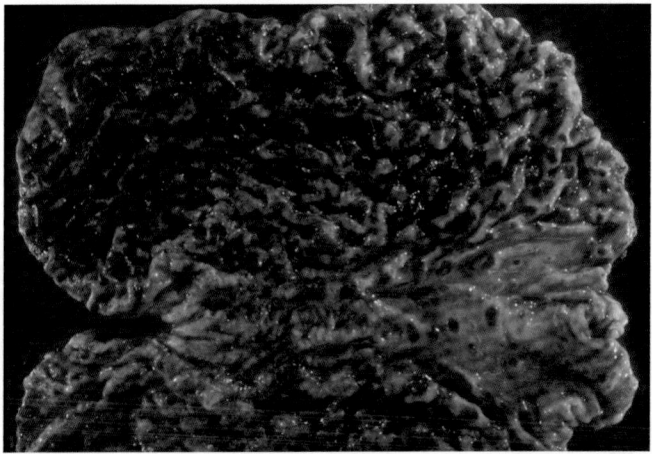

FIGURE 19-26. Menetrier disease. The rugal folds are diffusely enlarged. They appear to be hemorrhagic because of the accompanying lymphocytic gastritis.

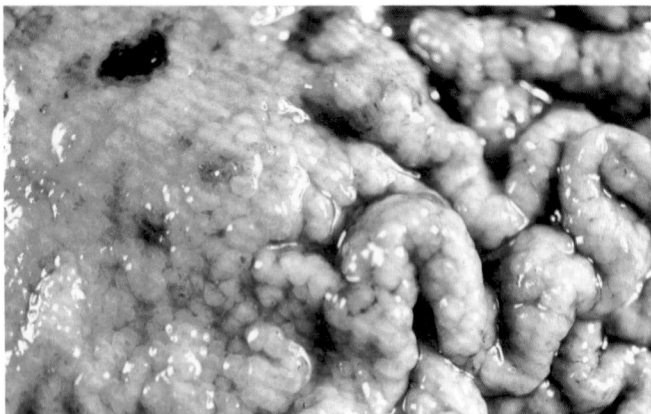

FIGURE 19-27. Zollinger Ellison syndrome. The rugal folds are convoluted and thickened. They appear bumpy owing to hyperplasia of the parietal cells occurring in groups.

Fundic Gland Polyps Occur Only in the Body and Fundus

They are mucosal elevations composed of cystically dilated glands lined by a mixture of parietal cells, chief cells and neutral mucous cells (Fig. 19-28A,B). They were first described in patients with familial adenomatous polyposis (FAP; see below); in affected patients, a myriad of such polyps carpet the proximal gastric mucosa. Rarely, fundic gland polyps in these patients show focal dysplasia. Far more common are isolated or small numbers of fundic polyps in patients taking PPIs.

The mechanism for their formation is unknown. Polyps related to PPI use appear to be innocuous. Because of the ever-increasing use of PPIs in recent years, fundic gland polyps are now the most common form of polyp seen in the stomach.

Hyperplastic Polyps

This term is something of a misnomer, and these polyps have nothing but the name in common with polyps of the colon that bear the same name (see below). They occur in the setting of chronic gastritis or reactive gastropathy, may be single or multiple and are exaggerated focal responses to mucosal injury. Gastric hyperplastic polyps consist of

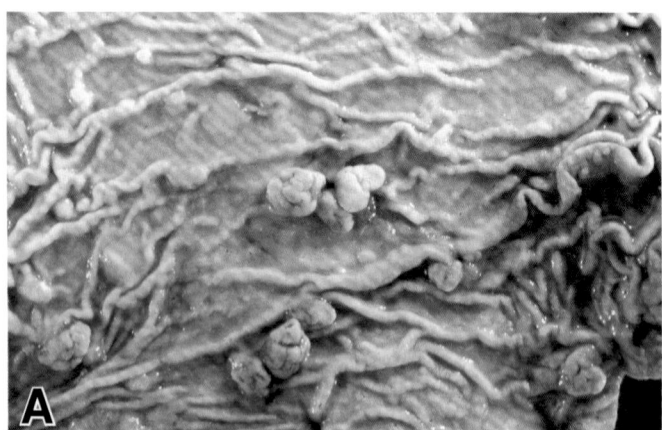

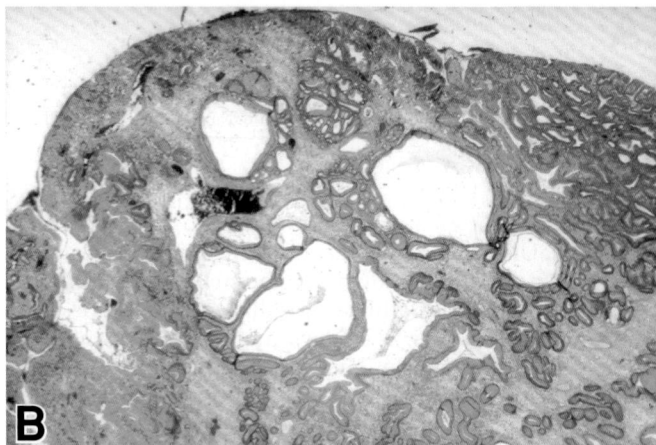

FIGURE 19-29. Hyperplastic polyp. A. Multiple mucosal elevations are seen in this resected stomach. **B.** The polyp is a mound of inflamed lamina propria. The cystically dilated glands are lined by foveolar epithelium.

hyperplastic foveolar cells sometimes forming small cysts, and an inflamed lamina propria (Fig. 19-29A,B). Reactive atypia may be present, particularly if there are surface erosions. They are sometimes called "hyperplastic/inflammatory" polyps, reflecting the manner in which they arose. Their malignant potential is that of the background mucosa from which they arose.

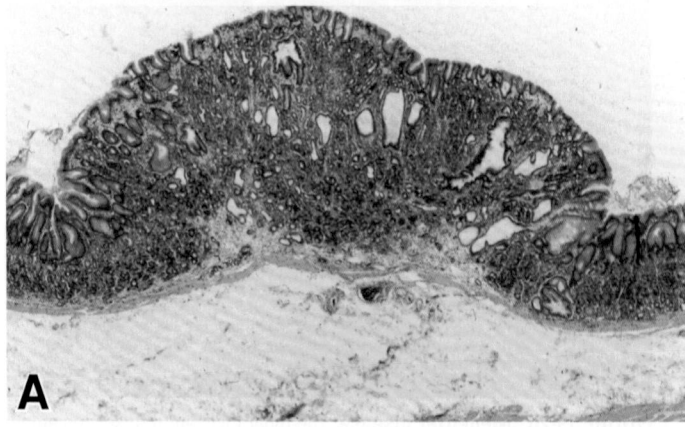

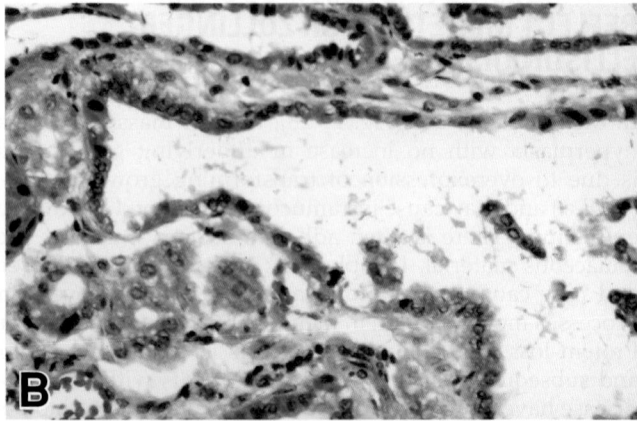

FIGURE 19-28. Fundic gland polyp. A. Low-power view shows the polyp as a slight elevation above the surrounding body-type mucosa. **B.** The cystically dilated glands contain parietal and chief cells.

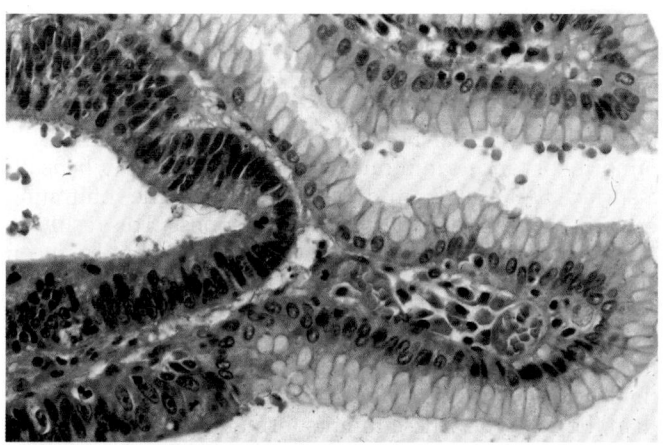

FIGURE 19-30. Gastric adenoma. There is sharp demarcation between the glandular epithelium with enlarged, hyperchromatic pencil-shaped nuclei (*left*) and adjacent normal foveolar epithelium (*right*).

Gastric Adenomas Are Relatively Uncommon

True adenomas of the stomach occur far less often than adenomas of the colon. They are usually single except in FAP, and can be of foveolar- or intestinal-type mucosa. By definition, dysplastic changes are present (Fig. 19-30). Intestinal-type adenomas are far more common and usually arise in stomachs with intestinal metaplasia. Nuclei tend to be enlarged, elongated and hyperchromatic, like their intestinal counterparts.

In contrast, foveolar-type adenomas have no relationship to intestinal metaplasia; there does appear to be a relationship to FAP.

Although gastric adenomas can be related to gastric carcinoma, the very close relationship of adenoma to carcinoma seen in the colon is not present.

Gastric Polyposis Syndromes

Multiple gastric polyps can be seen in FAP and in several distinct syndromes. These include generalized familial juvenile polyposis (Fig. 19-31A–C) and Peutz-Jeghers, Cronkhite-Canada and Cowden syndromes. The polyps in these syndromes are usually bland in appearance, often somewhat resembling large hyperplastic polyps. Their true nature is established by identifying other features of the respective syndrome.

MALIGNANT NEOPLASMS

Adenocarcinoma Is the Most Common Gastric Malignancy

 **EPIDEMIOLOGY:** There are striking geographical differences in its incidence. Gastric adenocarcinoma has declined markedly in incidence in Western countries over the past century. Many Eastern countries have a far higher incidence. There are a number of factors involved, but the most important appears to

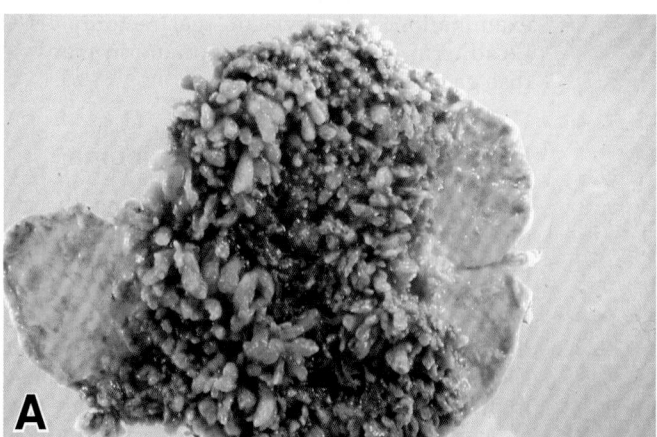

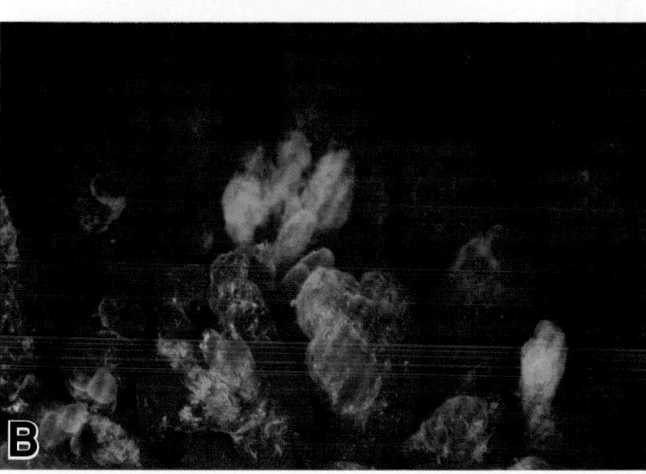

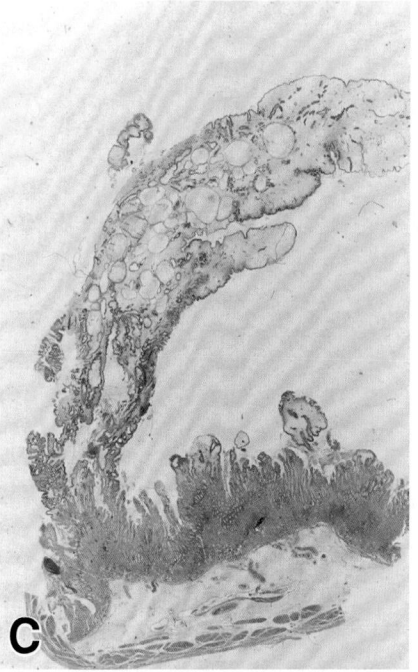

FIGURE 19-31. Familial juvenile polyposis. A, B. While the colon is the main target organ in this syndrome, the stomach can be involved and carpeted by polyps. **C.** Histologically, they are innocuous and somewhat resemble hyperplastic polyps.

reflect differences in the prevalence of *Helicobacter* and chronic gastritis. With improved recognition and treatment of *Helicobacter* infections, gaps between the West and East are narrowing. Other environmental factors also contribute, especially food. Diets high in smoked or pickled foods are associated with a higher cancer rate, while consumption of fresh vegetables and leafy greens has the opposite effect. Genetic factors also play a significant role, particularly with some types of gastric cancer.

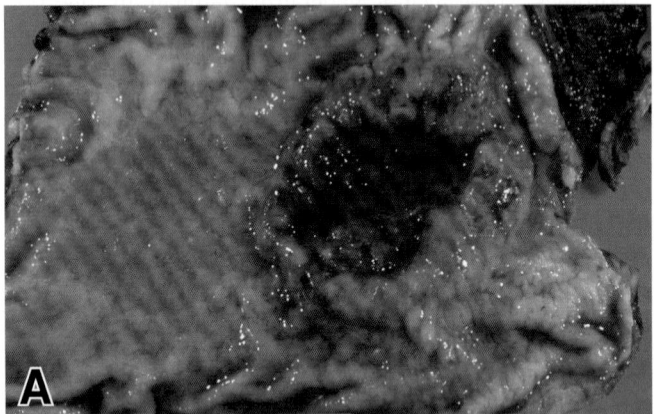

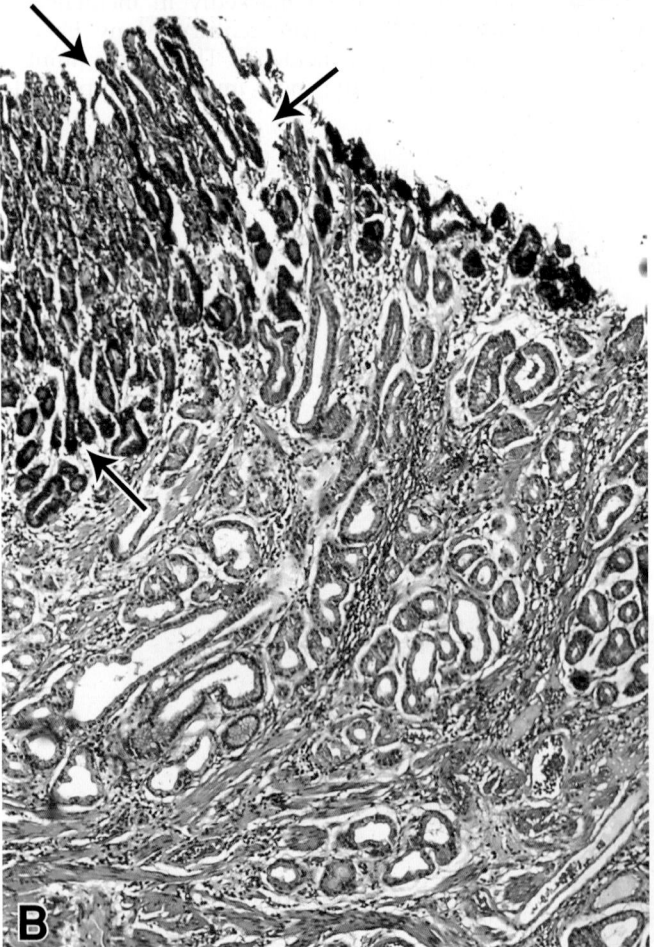

FIGURE 19-32. Gastric carcinoma. A. This large antral lesion is clearly distinguished from a benign ulcer by its raised firm edges and necrotic base. **B.** Microscopically, there are innumerable poorly formed glands (*arrows*) replacing mucosa in this intestinal-type carcinoma.

PATHOLOGY: Gross appearance is variable. Most carcinomas form large polypoid masses or growths with significant ulceration (Fig. 19-32A,B). The latter differ from benign peptic ulcers by their large size, raised firm irregular borders and ragged ulcer surfaces. A minority of cancers infiltrate the gastric wall deeply, beneath a surface that may seem deceptively intact. The infiltrating cells elicit a prominent desmoplastic response. This results in a rigid thick-walled stomach, an appearance that has been classically described as **linitis plastica** (Fig. 19-33A–C).

Gastric carcinoma has traditionally been separated into two categories, intestinal and diffuse, with some cases showing overlap; this is the Lauren classification. The term "intestinal" in this context mainly describes the architecture, rather than the cell type. These tumors form glands or papillae, as well as some solid areas; mucin production may occur. This is the more common pattern and is the one associated with chronic gastritis. It is declining in incidence because of its relationship to *Helicobacter.*

Diffuse-type carcinoma contains poorly cohesive cells, widely infiltrating the gastric wall, often with striking desmoplasia. Although the diffusely infiltrating cells may have a signet ring appearance, other cells may more mimic histiocytes or even lymphocytes. The incidence of this tumor has been more stable in all countries. It has a clearer genetic component. In fact, a hereditary diffuse gastric cancer exists as an uncommon autosomal dominant condition due to germline mutations in *CDH1,* the gene that encodes E-cadherin. These patients may develop cancer at an early age and often have multiple small foci of signet ring carcinoma in situ detectable only by thorough microscopic examination. Prophylactic gastrectomy is considered. E-cadherin inactivation also occurs in many sporadic diffuse gastric carcinomas.

Early versus Late Gastric Carcinoma

There are complex systems describing the character and depth of gastric carcinomas, but there is one simple fact of paramount importance: *patients with early gastric cancer (i.e., tumors confined to the mucosa and submucosa) are very likely to survive. Patients with late cancers (i.e., lesions that extend beyond the submucosa into the muscularis propria or beyond) are likely doomed.* The significance of this fact is that most carcinomas in the lower-incidence Western countries are diagnosed only at later stages.

The Stomach Is a Common Site of Extranodal Lymphomas

The gastrointestinal tract is the most common location for extranodal lymphomas, and the stomach is the most common portion of the GI tract affected. Most gastric lymphomas are either extranodal marginal zone lymphomas of mucosa-associated lymphoid tissue (MALT lymphoma; see Chapter 26) or diffuse large B-cell lymphomas. Both are associated with *Helicobacter* infection; eradication of the organisms leads to remission in the striking majority of cases. MALT lymphoma is difficult to distinguish from chronic gastritis with lymphoid hyperplasia. The presence of gastric glands infiltrated by lymphocytes (lymphoepithelial lesions) and a uniform monocytoid morphology of the cells infiltrating the lamina propria are distinguishing features (Fig. 19-34). Diffuse large

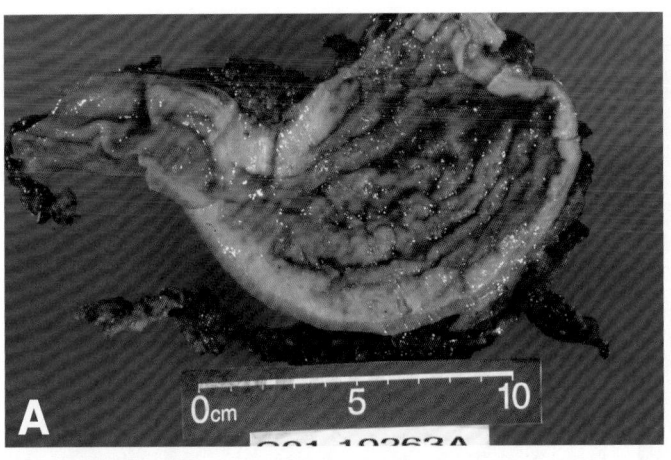

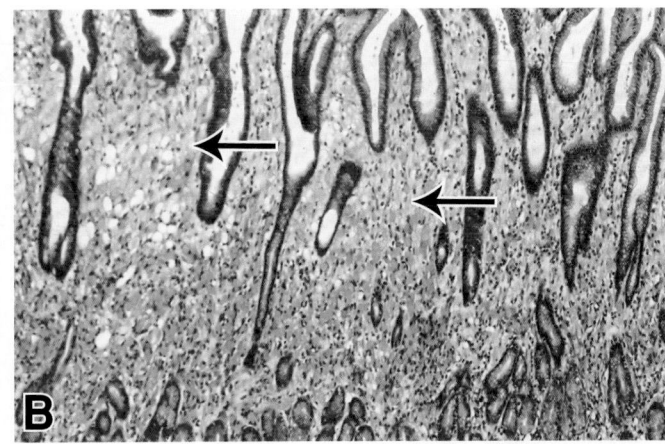

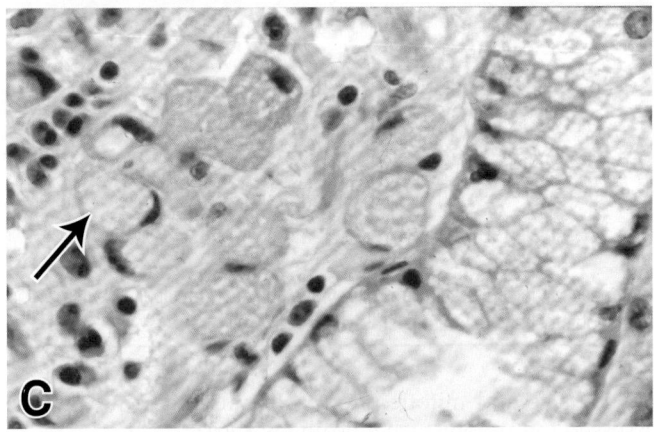

FIGURE 19-33. Gastric carcinoma. A. The wall is white and thickened owing to the diffuse infiltrate of tumor cells. The mucosal surface is deceptively free of mass lesions. **B.** The infiltrate fills and expands the lamina propria (*arrows*) but leaves glands and surface epithelium intact. **C.** The tumor cells in this diffuse-type cancer are present next to an intact gland. Note the signet ring appearance (*arrow*).

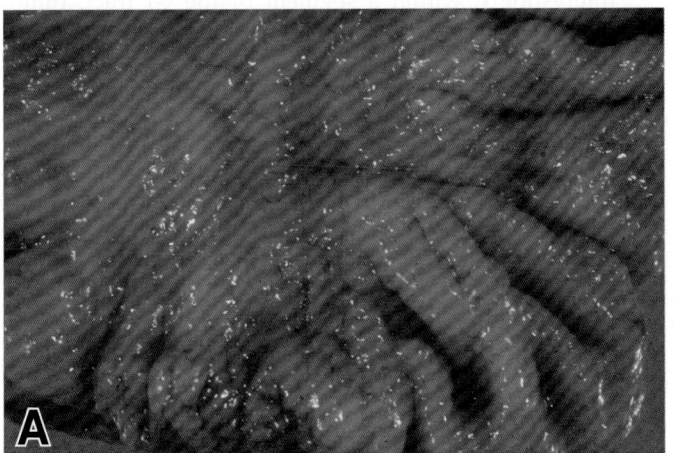

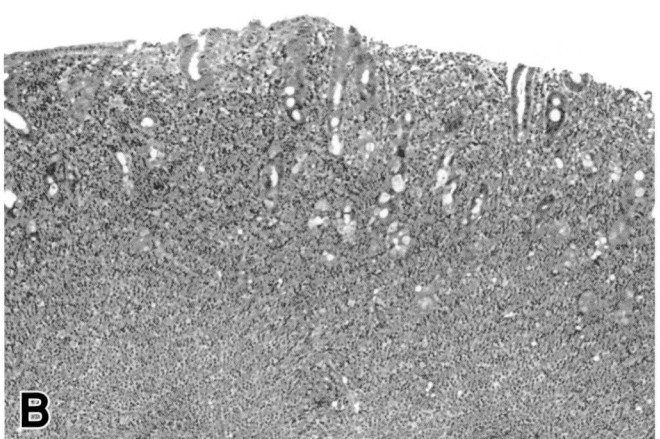

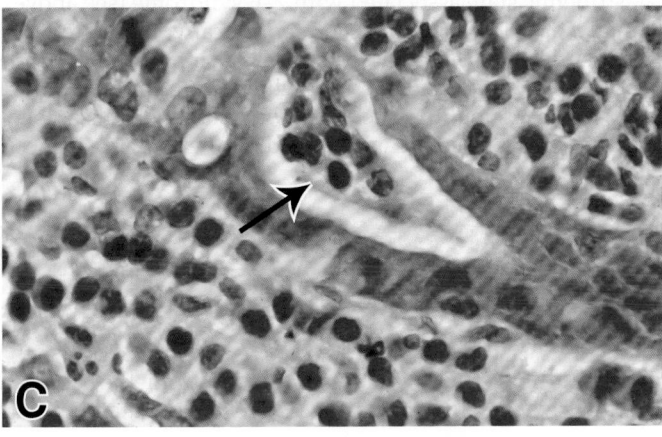

FIGURE 19-34. Gastric lymphoma, mucosa-associated lymphoid tissue (MALT) type. A. There is loss of detail within the gastric mucosa as a MALT lymphoma infiltrates the mucosa over a large surface area, although a discrete mass was not formed. **B.** Microscopically, a monotonous population of lymphoid cells greatly expands the lamina propria. **C.** A **lymphoepithelial lesion,** with tumor lymphocytes penetrating into a gland (*arrows*).

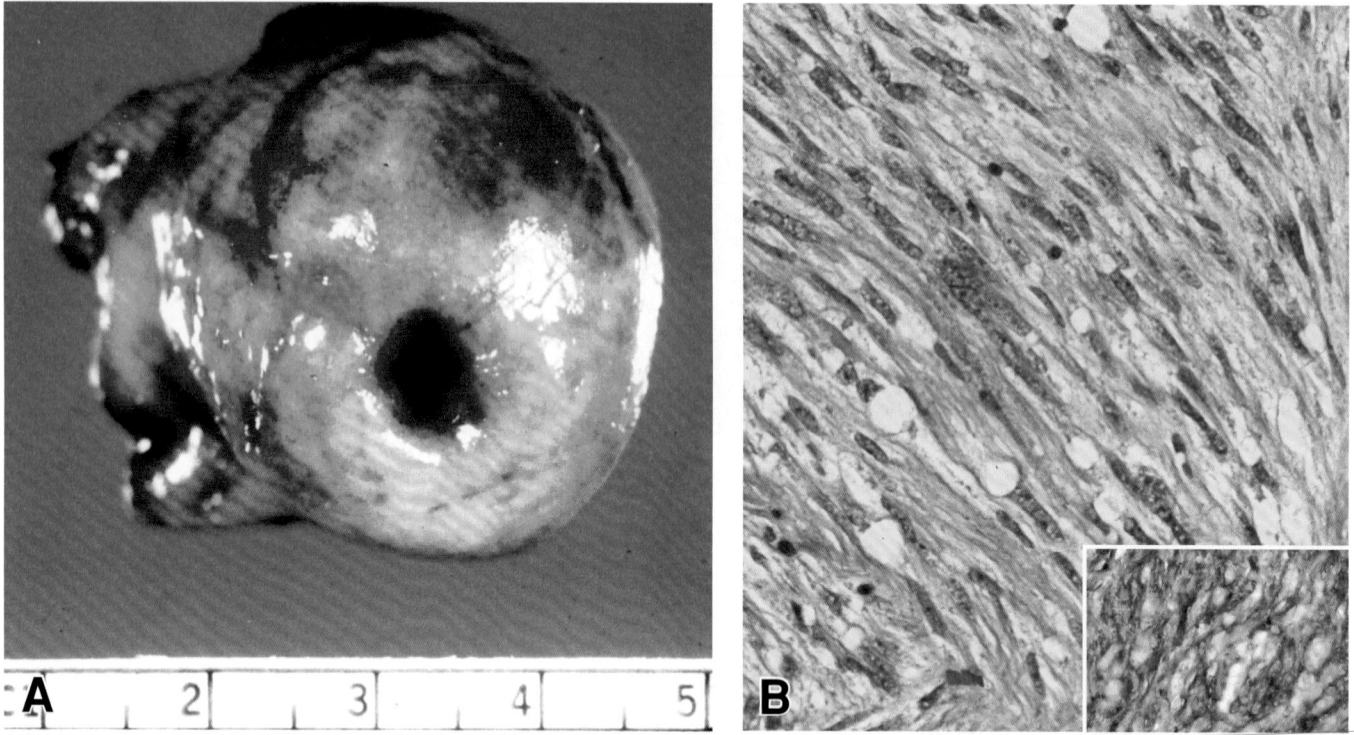

FIGURE 19-35. Gastrointestinal stromal tumor (GIST). A. The resected tumor is submucosal and covered by mucosa with a deep central ulcer. **B.** Microscopic appearance of tumor cells that are spindled and have cytoplasmic vacuoles. **Inset:** Immunohistochemical stain positive for c-kit.

B-cell lymphomas are more easily recognized because of their more pleomorphic appearance.

GI Stromal Tumors Derive from the Interstitial Cells of Cajal

For years these tumors, which contain elongate spindly cells, were felt to be of smooth muscle origin and were called leiomyomas and leiomyosarcomas. In fact, true smooth muscle gastric tumors are very uncommon. The interstitial cells of Cajal, from which these tumors derive, normally reside in the muscularis propria and are pacemakers.

The tumors are usually large and bulky, arising in the muscularis propria (Fig. 19-35A,B). They may show central ulceration in the overlying mucosa, and so present with bleeding. Most stain positively for CD117, although not all. CD117-negative GISTS are often immunopositive with another antibody, DOG1.

GISTs occur throughout the GI tract but are particularly common in the stomach. It is not possible to distinguish clearly between benign and malignant GISTs. Rather, criteria predicting progressively more aggressive behavior are being established for each site in the gut, since behavior varies in this regard. More distal lesions show a greater tendency toward malignant behavior. In addition to site, tumor size and mitotic rate are reliable discriminators. Fortunately, most gastric GISTs are less likely to show aggressive behavior.

Neuroendocrine Tumors

These tumors were once called "carcinoids," but that term is being replaced by "neuroendocrine tumor" (NET). As for GISTs, the site of origin is the major determinant of likely behavior. The best predictive features within a given site are the size and mitotic rate (proliferative activity may be assessed immunohistochemically by Ki67).

Interestingly, within a segment of the GI tract, tumor behavior depends on the conditions under which the neoplasms arise. This is especially so for gastric NETs. There are three major clinical scenarios in which such tumors are found. The first of these is autoimmune gastritis. As described previously, the profound activity of antral G cells results in a proliferation of ECL cells in the body and fundus. An identifiable sequence of proliferation has been identified. At first there are merely increased numbers of these cells. Then, strings of such cells form linear arrays, which later coalesce to form micronodules, which separate from the bases of gastric glands. As time progresses, propelled by prominent hypergastrinemia, these micronodules coalesce into larger and larger structures until a clinically evident neoplasm is formed. Patients with NETs arising in autoimmune gastritis often have multiple visible tumors (Fig. 19-36).

Gastric neuroendocrine tumors also arise in the hypergastrinemic state associated with Z-E syndrome (see above). Finally, gastric NETs can occur sporadically; these are more frequently antral. Of interest, tumors arising in autoimmune gastritis are rarely aggressive, while sporadic NETs often are. Those arising in association with Zollinger-Ellison syndrome are intermediate with regards to their aggressiveness.

The Small Intestine

ANATOMY

The intestinal tract develops as a tube from the stomach to the cloaca. This tube progressively elongates, and its

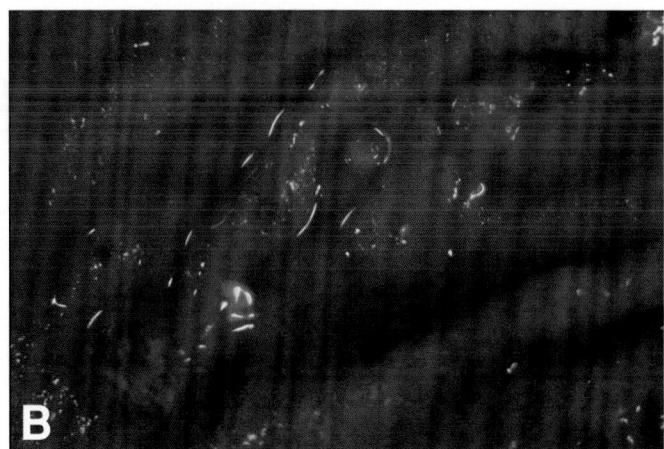

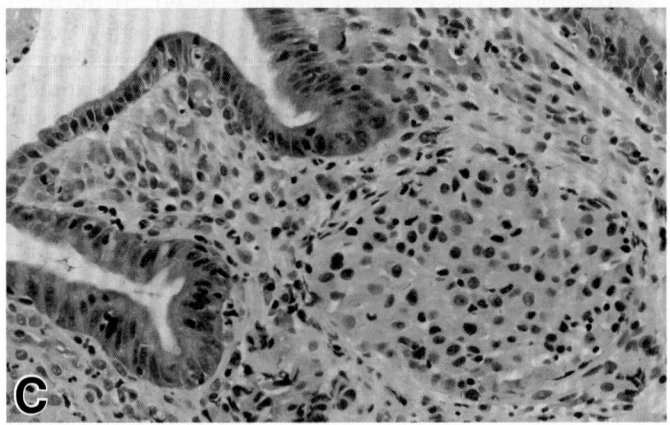

FIGURE 19-36. Neuroendocrine tumor (NET) of stomach. A, B. Multiple small elevated mucosal nodules dot the severely atrophic mucosa in this patient with autoimmune gastritis and pernicious anemia. C. Microscopically, the bland-appearing neuroendocrine tumor cells (*arrows*) push aside the atrophic mucosa.

cephalic part becomes the segment that extends from the distal duodenum to the proximal ileum. The more caudal portion develops into distal ileum and the proximal 2/3 of transverse colon. The vitelline duct, which connects the primitive duct to the yolk sac, may persist as a Meckel diverticulum (see below). To reach its final position, the fetal gut undergoes a complex series of rotations.

The small intestine extends from the pylorus to the ileocecal valve and, depending on its muscle tone, is from 3.5 to 6.5 m long. It is divided into three regions:

1. **The duodenum** extends to the ligament of Treitz.
2. **The jejunum** is the proximal 40% of the remainder of the small intestine.
3. **The ileum** is the distal 60%.

The duodenum is almost entirely retroperitoneal and thus fixed. The remainder of small intestine, which is disposed in redundant loops, is movable.

The C-shaped duodenum surrounds the head of the pancreas. It receives biliary drainage of the liver and pancreatic secretions through the common bile duct at the ampulla of Vater. The distal duodenum becomes invested by mesentery and merges with the jejunum at the ligament of Treitz. There is no demarcation between jejunum and ileum, which merge gradually. The wall of the jejunum is thicker and its lumen wider than those of the ileum.

The plicae circularis, spiral folds of mucosa and submucosa, are most prominent in the distal duodenum and proximal jejunum, usually disappearing in the terminal ileum. Peyer patches are submucosal lymphoid aggregates up to 3 cm in diameter, in the antimesenteric aspect of the distal

half of the ileum. The ileocecal valve is a muscular sphincter that regulates flow of intestinal contents into the cecum.

The duodenum is served by the pancreaticoduodenal branch of the hepatic artery, which arises from the celiac artery. The jejunum and ileum are supplied by the superior mesenteric artery (a branch of the aorta), which is arranged in arcades in the mesentery, thus providing abundant collateral circulation in its distal reaches. Venous flow from the small intestine empties into the portal venous system. The small intestinal wall has four layers: mucosa, submucosa, muscularis and serosa. In the retroperitoneal duodenum, however, only the anterior wall is covered by a serosa.

The serosa contains loose connective tissue bounded by a single layer of mesothelium. The muscularis propria has an outer longitudinal layer and an inner circular layer, which act together to propel intestinal contents by peristalsis.

The submucosa consists of vascularized connective tissue and scattered lymphocytes, plasma cells and macrophages, occasional mast cells and eosinophils. In the proximal duodenum, the submucosa is occupied by Brunner glands, branched structures with mucous and serous cells. These secrete mucus and bicarbonate, which protect the duodenal mucosa from peptic ulceration. Mucosal lymphatics and venous capillaries drain into a highly developed system of lymphatic and venous plexuses in the submucosa.

The distinctive feature of intestinal mucosa is its unique villi (Fig. 19-37), 0.5–1-mm-long finger-like projections that expand the absorptive area enormously. Villi in the proximal duodenum tend to be broad and blunted, but in the distal duodenum and proximal jejunum they are more slender. Shorter, finger-shaped villi are the rule in the distal jejunum and ileum.

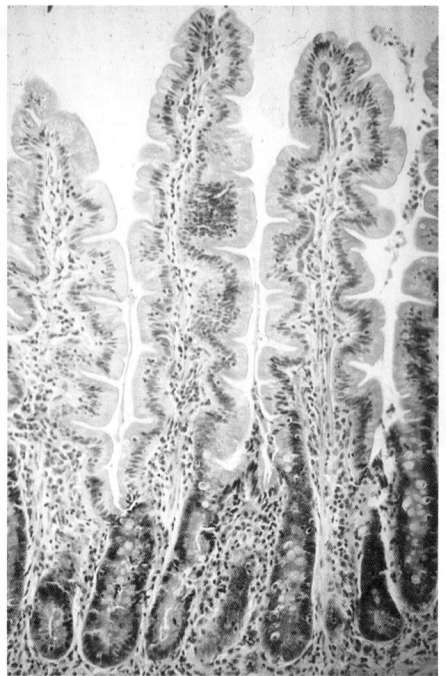

FIGURE 19-37. Intestinal villi from the proximal jejunum. The villi are several times longer than the crypts that gave rise to them. The lamina propria normally contains a mixture of lymphocytes and plasma cells with some scattered eosinophils.

In villi, the columnar epithelium sits on a basement membrane. A lamina propria and muscularis mucosae separate the mucosa from the submucosa. The connective tissue of the lamina propria forms the core of the villus and surrounds the crypts of Lieberkühn at the base of the villi. The normal lamina propria contains lymphocytes, plasma cells and macrophages. Plasma cells here mainly secrete immunoglobulin A (IgA) into the intestinal lumen or the lamina propria itself. Scattered eosinophils and mast cells and a few smooth muscle cells and fibroblasts are present. This cellular composition reflects the roles of the lamina propria: preventing bacteria from penetrating the mucosa and segregating foreign material that breaches the mucosa.

Some IgA made by lamina propria plasma cells is dimeric. It diffuses through the basement membrane of the crypt, then reaches the basal or lateral surfaces of epithelial cells, where it combines with a secretory component produced by that cell. Resulting secretory IgA is taken up by epithelial cells and secreted into the lumen. Secretory IgA is more resistant to proteolysis than is serum IgA. It binds food antigens and prevents bacterial adherence to intestinal epithelium. Moreover, it can neutralize bacterial toxins and inhibit viral replication and mucosal penetration.

Lymphoid nodules are scattered throughout the mucosa and aggregate into visible Peyer patches (Fig. 19-38A,B). The villous columnar epithelial cells are mainly absorptive, while those lining the crypts are the source of cell renewal and secretion. There are normally a moderate number of intraepithelial T lymphocytes.

Absorptive cells, or enterocytes (Fig. 19-39), are the main lining cells of intestinal villi, which also contain a few goblet and endocrine cells. Enterocytes are tall, with basal nuclei and microvilli extending from their surfaces into the lumen, thus hugely increasing the absorptive area. The plasma membrane of the microvilli is covered by a glycocalyx (fuzzy coat), wherein reside disaccharidases and peptidases. In the ileum, the glycocalyx also contains receptors for the intrinsic factor–vitamin B_{12} complex.

The cytosol just under the microvilli has a network of actin microfilaments, the terminal web. These also associate with myosin and other contractile proteins, insert into the core of the microvilli and likely serve as a contractile apparatus. The plasma membranes of adjacent cells form tight junctions that permit passive paracellular transport of small molecules but are impermeable to macromolecules. Absorbed material moves from epithelial cells to intercellular spaces between absorptive cells, via lateral or basal plasma membranes. It then penetrates the basement membrane, traverses the lamina propria and enters capillaries or lymphatic channels.

There are four cell types in the crypts:

■ **Paneth cells** at crypt bases resemble pancreatic or salivary zymogen cells and are active in exocrine secretion. Their eosinophilic secretory granules fill a basophilic cytoplasm. Paneth cells function in mucosal defense, as evidenced by the presence of lysozyme; antimicrobial products,

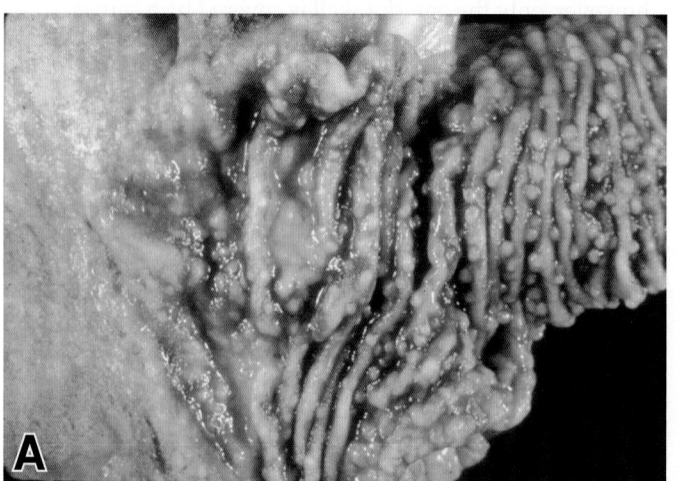
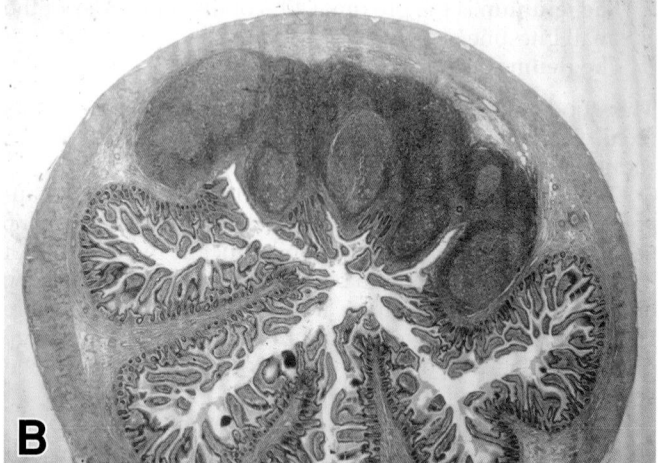

FIGURE 19-38. A. Peyer patches are particularly prominent in the terminal ileum; they are small dome-shaped mucosal mounds. **B.** The Peyer patch is composed of lymphoid tissue, often with prominent germinal centers, displacing the epithelial structures.

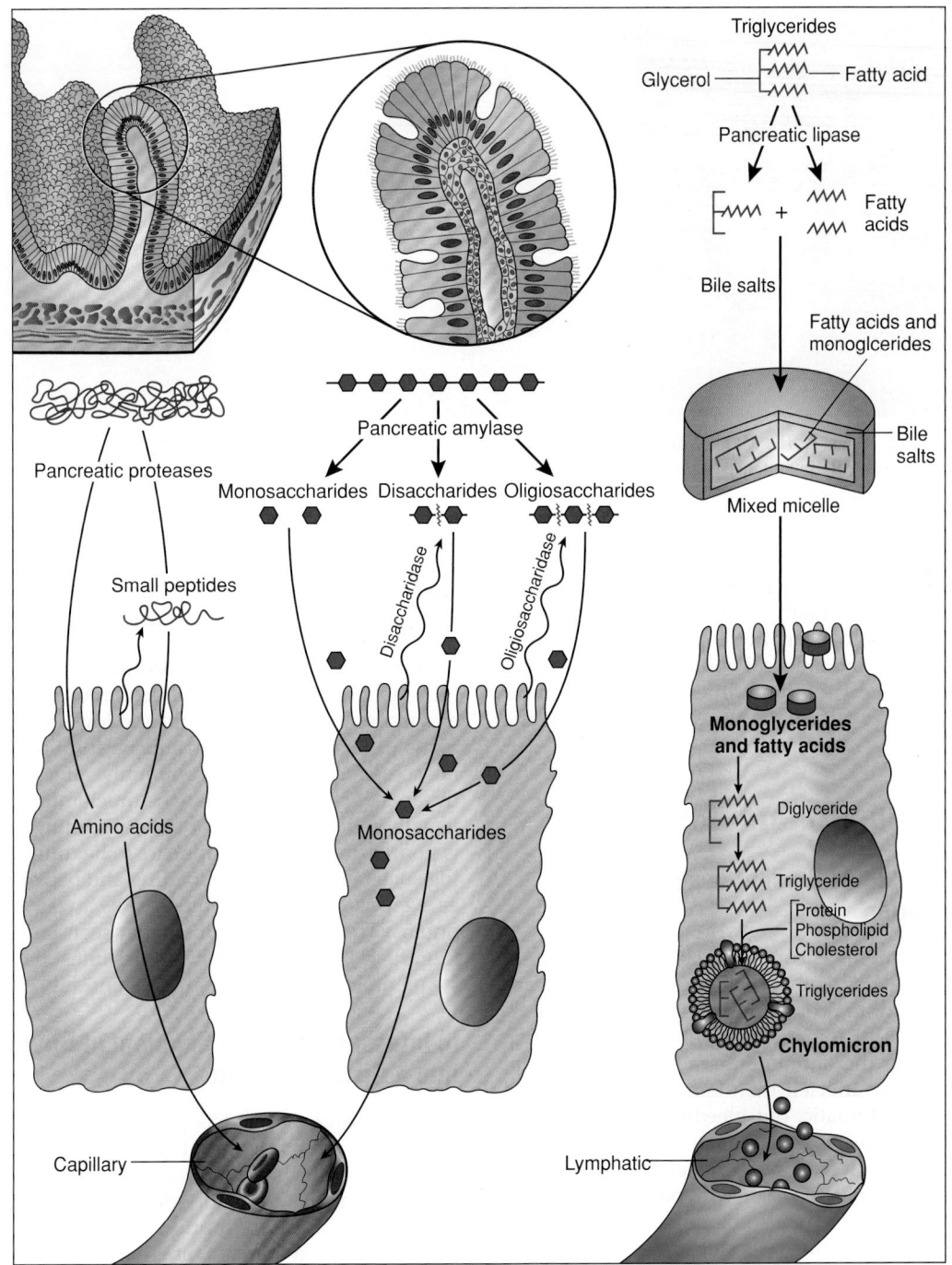

FIGURE 19-39. Mechanisms of nutrient absorption in the small intestine.

including peptides called crypt defensins (cryptdins); and CD95 ligand, a member of the tumor necrosis factor (TNF) family of cytokines.

■ **Goblet cells** of the lateral walls of the crypts are flask shaped and filled with mucous granules. They resemble goblet cells elsewhere both structurally and functionally, with neutral and acid mucins.

■ **Endocrine cells** have apical nuclei and basal eosinophilic granules. These cells make several gastrointestinal hormones and peptides, including gastrin, secretin, cholecystokinin, glucagon, vasoactive intestinal peptide (VIP) and serotonin. These hormones regulate many gastrointestinal functions, and tumors derived from these cells often exhibit striking hormone secretion.

■ **Undifferentiated cells** in the lateral crypt walls and interspersed between Paneth cells at their bases are the most abundant cells in the crypts. Small glycoprotein secretory granules may be grouped in their apical cytoplasm. These cells act as reserve cells, from which all other mucosal cell populations are renewed, and thus they show abundant mitotic activity.

Cell renewal in the small intestine is limited to the crypts, where undifferentiated cells divide. Resulting cells migrate

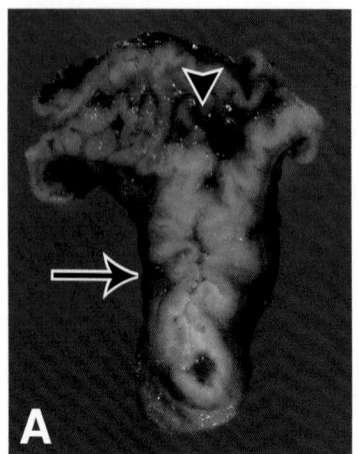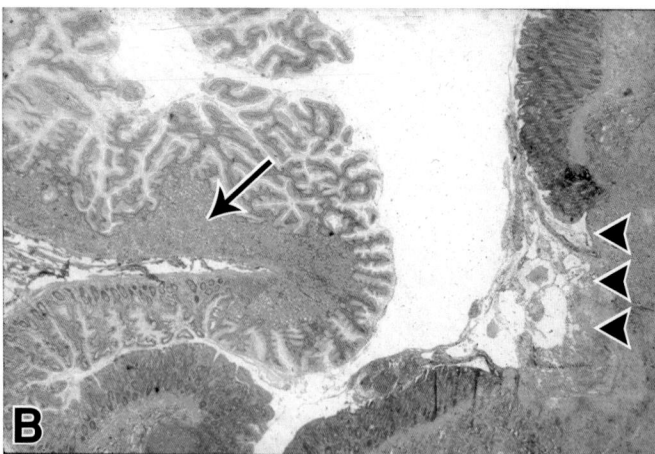

FIGURE 19-40. **A.** The **Meckel diverticulum** (*arrow*) here is seen extending downward from the lumen of the ileum (*arrowhead*). **B.** Heterotopic gastric mucosa with parietal cells (*arrow*) sits opposite the peptic ulcer (*arrowheads*) in the intestinal mucosa.

up the villus, where they differentiate into goblet cells and absorptive cells, and eventually slough into the lumen at the tip of the villus. Their absorptive capacity is maximal in the upper 1/3 of villi. The mucosal epithelium of the small intestine is replaced every 4–7 days. Intestinal epithelium is therefore very sensitive to radiation and chemotherapeutic agents.

CONGENITAL AND NEONATAL DISORDERS

Meckel Diverticulum Is Present in about 2% of the Population

This is the most commonly encountered clinically significant congenital disorder affecting the small intestine. It is solitary and is a true diverticulum, containing all layers of the intestinal wall (Fig. 19-40A,B). It is a remnant of the vitelline duct, and so extends from the antimesenteric side of the distal ileum. Males are more affected than females. Most Meckel diverticula are asymptomatic, but bleeding, perforation or obstruction due to intussusception may occur. The bleeding and perforation result from peptic ulceration, due to the presence of heterotopic gastric tissue with parietal cells. Heterotopic pancreatic tissue may also be present. Rarely, neoplasms develop, usually neuroendocrine tumors.

Meconium Ileus May Be an Early Complication of Cystic Fibrosis

In the neonatal period, infants with cystic fibrosis may develop intestinal obstruction owing to the thick viscid mucus characteristic of that condition plugging the lumen of the distal ileum. Perforation and peritonitis due to the meconium may occur.

Other Congenital Conditions

Atresia and stenosis are uncommon but can cause obstruction in the newborn. Duplications or enteric cysts are spherical or tubular structures adjacent to the long axis of the intestine; they too are rare.

Necrotizing Enterocolitis Is the Most Serious Acquired Neonatal GI Disorder

Neonatal necrotizing enterocolitis, commonly known as NEC, is, unfortunately, not uncommon. It is more common and more severe in premature and low–birth-weight infants. Signs of obstruction occur and perforation may occur. The ileocecal region is most commonly affected; in fatal cases, the area of involvement may be much more extensive. Onset usually follows the start of enteral feeding. Its pathogenesis is poorly understood; it appears to be multifactorial, involving such factors as solute loading and bacterial proliferation, as well as diversion of blood flow away from abdominal organs. The bowel resembles that seen in ischemic damage (Fig. 19-41). Pneumatosis cystoides intestinales (see below) is frequent. Healing may result in stenosis.

In Intussusception, a Segment of Bowel Is Drawn into a Distal Segment

In this setting, peristalsis pushes a part of bowel distally, causing it to telescope (Fig. 19-42A,B). The mesentery and blood vessels accompany the bowel and can become compressed, leading to edema, ischemic damage and entrapment. Intussusception can reverse spontaneously, or sometimes a barium enema may reduce it. Surgical

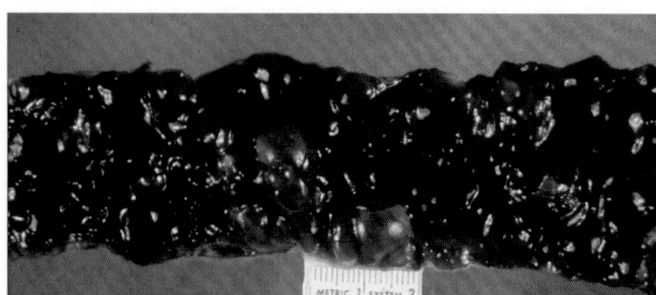

FIGURE 19-41. A segment of necrotic ileum with hemorrhage and pneumatosis from a premature infarct with **Neonatal necrotizing enterocolitis (NEC).**

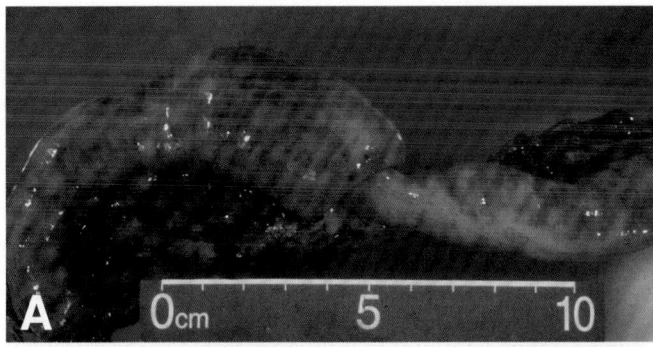

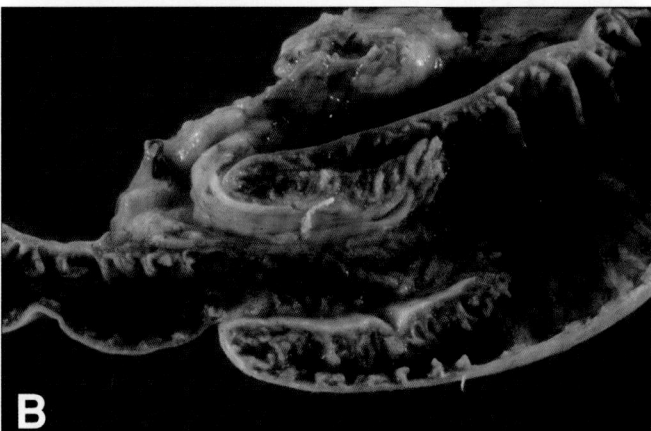

FIGURE 19-42. A, B. The proximal ileum has telescoped into the distal ileum in this case of **intussusception;** the anatomy is well seen in the cut section.

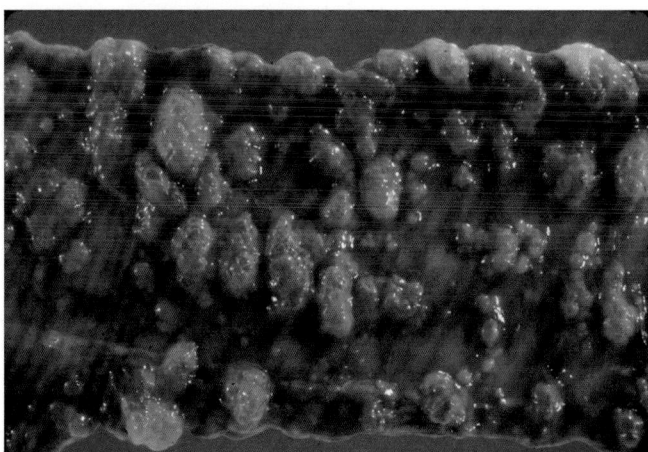

FIGURE 19-43. Multiple gas-filled blebs protrude into the lumen in this case of **pneumatosis cystoides intestinales.**

removal may be necessary. In children, there is usually no causative anatomic defect, other than lymphoid hyperplasia. This may be physiologic for age, but in some, rotavirus or adenovirus may be implicated in causing the hyperplasia. In adults, there is often a neoplastic luminal process, with the mass serving as a point of traction.

Pneumatosis Cystoides Intestinales Is Gas Bubbles in the Bowel Wall

The small intestine and colon are most commonly affected (Fig. 19-43). Pneumatosis almost always complicates another condition, such as NEC. In adults, it may be seen in pulmonary disease such as emphysema or complicating such processes as endoscopic polypectomy, ischemia, *Clostridium difficile* colitis or AIDS. Entrapped gas may cause a mass effect that can be mistaken for a neoplastic process.

Gas may enter the bowel by several routes. In pulmonary disease, air from ruptured blebs may track through the retroperitoneum and follow vascular adventitia into the bowel wall. Increased intra-abdominal pressure may force gas through minute mucosal defects. Finally, some cases result from gas formed by luminal anaerobic organisms. Prognosis is related to the underlying condition.

MALABSORPTION

Malabsorption is a general term that covers diverse clinical conditions in which important nutrients are inadequately absorbed by the gut. Some nutrient absorption occurs in the stomach and colon, but only absorption from the small intestine, mainly in the proximal portion, is clinically important. Two substances are preferentially absorbed by the distal small intestine: bile salts and vitamin B_{12}.

In normal intestinal absorption, there is a luminal phase and an intestinal phase. In the luminal phase (i.e., those processes that occur within the small intestine lumen), the physicochemical state of nutrients is altered so they can be taken up by absorptive cells. **The intestinal phase** includes processes occurring in cells and transport channels of the intestinal wall. Each phase has several critical components; derangement of any one or more of these components can impair absorption.

In the luminal phase, adequate amounts of pancreatic enzymes and bile acids are secreted into the duodenum in normal physicochemical conditions. Also, normal, regulated flow of gastric contents into the duodenum and a sufficiently high duodenal pH are needed. Normal pancreatic enzyme excretion into the duodenum requires adequate pancreatic exocrine function and unobstructed flow of pancreatic juice.

Supplying bile in normal quantity and quality to the duodenum requires (1) adequate liver function, (2) unobstructed bile flow and (3) intact enterohepatic bile salt circulation. Enterohepatic circulation of bile begins with absorption of most intestinal bile salts from the distal ileum and ends with their excretion into the duodenum through the bile ducts. Normally, 95% of intestinal bile salts are recycled via this circuit; 5% are excreted in the stool. Normal functioning of the enterohepatic circulation requires (1) normal intestinal microflora, (2) normal ileal absorptive function and (3) an unobstructed biliary system.

Intestinal-Phase Malabsorption Frequently Reflects Specific Enzyme Defects or Impaired Transport

Abnormalities in any of the four parts of the intestinal phase may cause malabsorption, but some diseases affect more than one of these components.

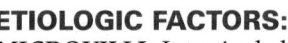 **ETIOLOGIC FACTORS:**
MICROVILLI: Intestinal disaccharidases and oligopeptidases are integrally bound to microvillous membranes. Disaccharidases are essential for sugar

absorption, since only monosaccharides can be absorbed by intestinal epithelial cells. Oligopeptides and dipeptides may be absorbed by alternate routes that do not require peptidases. Abnormal microvillous function may be primary—as in primary disaccharidase deficiencies—or secondary, if there is damage to villi, as in celiac disease (see below). Enzyme deficiencies (e.g., of lactase) entail intolerance to the respective disaccharides.

ABSORPTIVE AREA: The considerable length of the small bowel and the amplification of its surface by the intestinal folds (valves of Kerckring) provide a large absorptive surface. Severe diminution in this area may cause malabsorption. Surface area may be decreased by (1) small bowel resection (short bowel syndrome), (2) gastrocolic fistula (bypassing the small intestine) or (3) mucosal damage due to various small intestinal diseases (celiac disease, tropical sprue, Whipple disease).

METABOLIC FUNCTION OF ABSORPTIVE CELLS: For their subsequent transport to the circulation, nutrients in absorptive cells must be metabolized within these cells. Monoglycerides and free fatty acids are reassembled into triglycerides and coated with proteins (apoproteins) to make chylomicrons and lipoprotein particles. Specific metabolic dysfunction occurs in abetalipoproteinemia (associated with erythrocyte acanthocytosis; see Chapter 26), in which absorptive cells cannot synthesize the apoprotein required for assembling lipoproteins and chylomicrons. Nonspecific damage to small intestinal epithelial cells occurs in celiac disease, tropical sprue, Whipple disease and hyperacidity due to gastrinoma.

TRANSPORT: Nutrients are moved from the intestinal epithelium through the intestinal wall via blood capillaries and lymphatic vessels. Impaired transport of nutrients through these conduits is probably important in malabsorption due to Whipple disease, intestinal lymphoma and congenital lymphangiectasia.

CLINICAL FEATURES: Malabsorption may be specific or generalized:

- **Specific or isolated malabsorption** reflects an identifiable molecular defect that leads to malabsorption of one nutrient. Examples are disaccharidase deficiencies (e.g., lactase deficiency) and vitamin B_{12} insufficiency (pernicious anemia) from lack of intrinsic factor. Anemias may be caused by deficiencies of iron, folic acid, vitamin B_{12} or a combination of these. A bleeding diathesis may be due to vitamin K deficiency; malabsorption of vitamin D and calcium may lead to tetany, osteomalacia (in adults) or rickets (in children) (also see Chapter 8).
- **Generalized malabsorption** occurs when absorption of several or all major nutrient classes is impaired. It leads to generalized malnutrition. In adults, this appears as weight loss and sometimes cachexia; in children, it is "failure to thrive" with poor growth and weight gain.

Diverse Laboratory Studies May Detect Specific Forms of Malabsorption

Thus, disaccharidase deficiency is diagnosed by measuring blood sugar after ingestion of a standard amount of disaccharide, as in a lactose tolerance test, or by measuring enzyme activity in small bowel biopsies.

In generalized malabsorption, absorption of dietary fat is almost always impaired. Quantitative fecal fat analysis is the most reliable and sensitive test of overall digestive and absorptive function and is a standard for all other tests for malabsorption. **Steatorrhea** (fat in the stools) is a hallmark of generalized malabsorption.

Several key tests are often used to assess causes of malabsorption.

- **D-xylose absorption:** Xylose is a 5-carbon sugar whose absorption does not require any component of the luminal phase. Blood levels and urinary excretion after eating a defined amount of it thus are tested in the intestinal phase of absorption.
- **$^{14}CO_2$-cholyl-glycine breath test:** Measuring $^{14}CO_2$ in exhaled air after oral administration of $^{14}CO_2$-cholylglycine tests bile salt absorption by the ileum. It is used to diagnose blind- or stagnant-loop syndrome (due to bacterial overgrowth) and to assess ileal absorptive function. A ^{14}C-xylose breath test detects bacterial overgrowth.

Lactase Deficiency Causes Intolerance to Milk Products

The intestinal brush border contains disaccharidases that are important for absorption of carbohydrates. Lactose is present in milk and other dairy products and is one of the most common disaccharides in the diet. Before domestication of milk-producing animals about 9000 years ago, human milk was probably the only milk consumed by babies and young children. Dairy products were nonexistent. The availability of nonhuman milk favored lactase production, perhaps leading cattle-herding societies (e.g., Europeans) to be lactose tolerant, while non–cattle herders (e.g., Native Americans, Asians) are lactose intolerant.

Acquired lactase deficiency is widespread. Symptoms typically begin in adolescence, with abdominal distention, flatulence and diarrhea after consuming dairy products. Removing milk and dairy products from the diet provides relief. Diseases that injure the intestinal mucosa (e.g., celiac disease) may also cause acquired lactase deficiency. Congenital lactase deficiency is rare but may be lethal if recognized.

Celiac Disease Is Due to Sensitivity to Gluten

PATHOPHYSIOLOGY: Gluten is found in wheat, rye and barley; the main culprit appears to be a peptide fraction of gluten, namely, **gliadin**. Other environmental factors may be operative. Many patients have evidence of previous infection with adenovirus 12; a protein component of this virus shows homology with α-gliadin. Gluten-sensitive enteropathy (GSE) is an immunologic disorder that occurs in genetically susceptible individuals. The genetic nature was first established by family studies; the fact that a significant percentage of people with type 1 diabetes, another immunologic disorder (see Chapter 13), have GSE is further confirmation. It appears that two separate genes involved in the major histocompatibility complex, namely, class I human leukocyte antigen (HLA)-B8 and class II HLA-DR3 and DQW2, are present in almost all patients (Fig. 19-44).

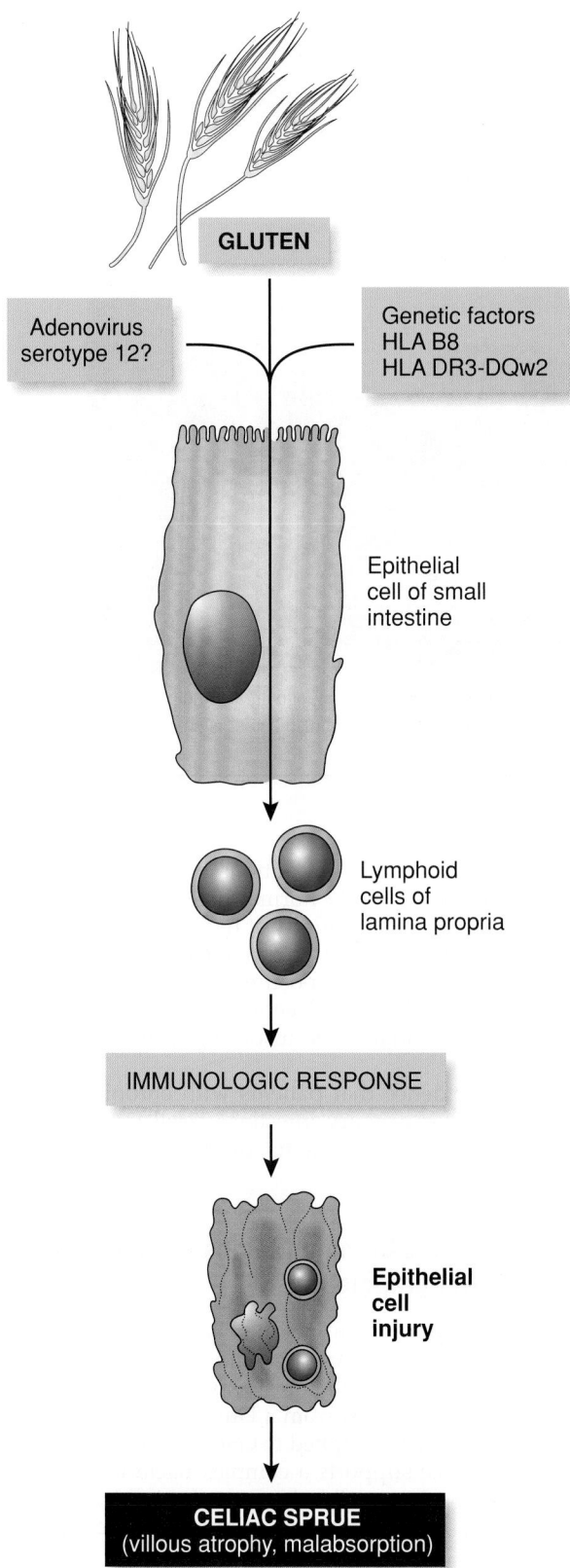

FIGURE 19-44. Proposed mechanism of the pathogenesis of celiac disease. HLA = human leukocyte antigen.

Although many patients with these genes do not have celiac disease, it is thought that absence of these genes virtually excludes the diagnosis.

Both cellular immunity and antibodies are involved. Activated mucosal T lymphocytes cause mucosal injury via release of cytokines; antigen–antibody complex deposition with complement activation may also lead to injury. Because of this, a number of serologic tests are useful in diagnosing GSE. The most important of these are **tissue transglutaminase (tTG)** and **antiendomysial antibody;** the former is now the test of choice. Testing for antigliadin antibody has a much lower sensitivity than these two tests.

 CLINICAL FEATURES: The classic symptoms are abdominal discomfort and diarrhea. With more advanced disease and consequent increased difficulty in absorbing fat, steatorrhea develops. Because of its high fat content, the stool tends to float and develops a particularly offensive odor owing to the action of intestinal bacteria on lipid. Eventually there can be severe malnutrition with weight loss, muscle wasting and hypoalbuminemia with edema. Other findings reported are osteoporosis and short stature compared to siblings.

These "classic" findings in GSE are becoming increasingly rare with better means of diagnosis and subsequent treatment. However, improved understanding of the pathogenesis of GSE and better means of recognizing the process serologically and morphologically has led to the concept of a much broader spectrum of the disease. Patients may even be asymptomatic, only to be discovered after a proband in their family has been identified. More importantly, it is now recognized that patients with GSE commonly present with iron-deficiency anemia resistant to oral therapy.

The last several decades have seen a particularly wide swing of the pendulum. Early on GSE was very much underdiagnosed, since the process was not considered unless the patient had several classic findings. With the current realization that GSE can manifest much more subtly than previously believed, many symptoms or conditions are attributed to GSE without unequivocal evidence. Care must be taken, as the diagnosis requires strong clinical, serologic or histologic evidence.

Treatment is exclusion of gluten from the diet and is usually quite effective. However, gluten is ubiquitous and adhering to the diet can be difficult. As well, diet change has been known to lead to a placebo effect, underscoring the need for concrete evidence before diagnosing GSE.

 PATHOLOGY: The histologic hallmark of GSE is both increased inflammation and architectural derangement in the small intestinal villi. The previously accepted classic histology of the disease included total or near-total loss of villi, resulting in a flat mucosa, plus an increase in lamina propria inflammation, including lymphocytes, plasma cells and some eosinophils.

In recent years there has been an increased emphasis on the character of the inflammation, in particular, the increase in intraepithelial lymphocytes (IELs). T lymphocytes are normally present in the surface epithelium (Fig. 19-45A,B), but in the GSE these T cells may increase to the point where

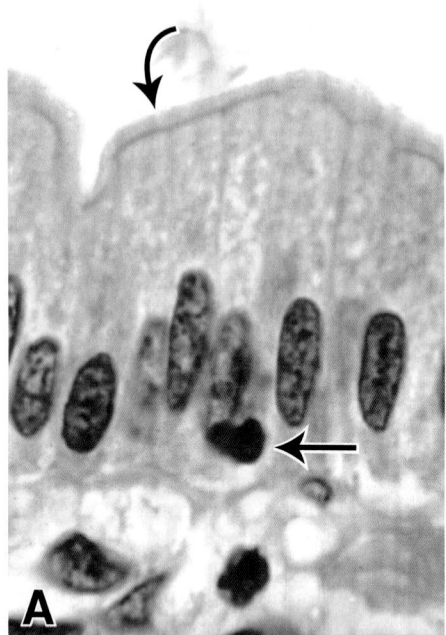
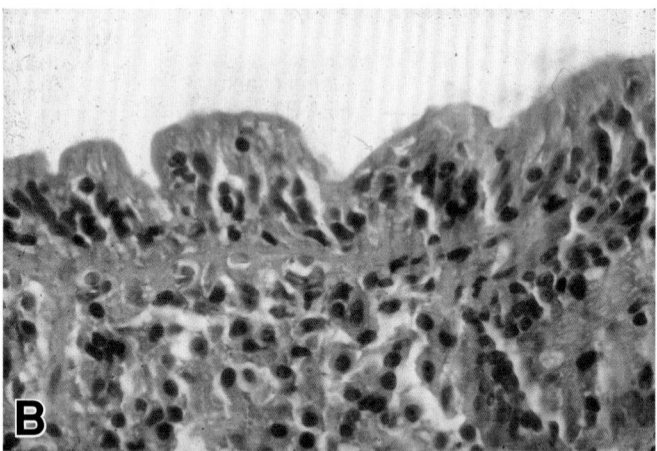

FIGURE 19-45. A. High-power view of small intestine surface epithelium; note the **brush border** (*arrow*) and intraepithelial lymphocyte (*curved arrow*). **B.** The surface epithelium in **celiac disease:** the epithelial height is reduced, the brush border is destroyed and intraepithelial lymphocytes are numerous.

they outnumber the surface epithelial cells. The exact number necessary to diagnose GSE is controversial, as is the best method for enumerating them. Increased T cells are not specific for GSE (they may be seen in, e.g., NSAID exposure and *H. pylori* gastritis), but IELs are essentially always increased in patients with GSE, as would be expected from the pathophysiology of that process.

Surface epithelial cells are damaged and lose their brush border. This damage shortens their life span, so that mitotic activity in the crypts increases to compensate for the increased cell loss. As a result, there is hyperplasia of the crypts. This leads to deeper crypts, even as villi decrease in height (Fig. 19-46). Eventually a flat mucosa may result,

but there are a series of gradations between total loss of villi and villi of relatively normal height notable only for an increase in IELs, particularly at their tips. These changes are most prominent in the proximal small intestine where the most intense gluten exposure occurs; the distal ileum is only rarely involved. In severe cases, the surface area of small intestine available for absorbing nutrients is greatly reduced.

There is evidence that patients with chronic GSE have increased risk for primary intestinal T-cell lymphoma and small intestinal adenocarcinoma, but the magnitude of this risk is unclear.

Tropical Sprue Is Chronic Malabsorption That Is Restricted Geographically

Affected locations are the Indian subcontinent, portions of Southeast Asia, Central America and the Caribbean. Tropical sprue can develop both in residents and in visitors to the area. The term "sprue" is from a Dutch term meaning diarrhea and has also been applied to GSE at times ("nontropical sprue"). Evidence supports a complex bacterial etiology in that broad-spectrum antibiotics are effective in alleviating the condition. The exact nature of the causative agent(s) is uncertain.

The entire small intestine including ileum is involved. The histologic appearance is very similar to that of GSE; however, IELs are more prominent in the crypts than in the villus tips. Completely flat mucosa is less common than in GSE.

Severe folate and B_{12} deficiency may occur, the latter reflecting ileal involvement; this may lead to megaloblastic change.

FIGURE 19-46. Classic advanced **celiac disease:** villi are no longer visible, crypts are taller than normal and a lymphoplasmacytic infiltrate expands the lamina propria. Even at low power, damage to the surface epithelium is evident.

Autoimmune Enteritis Is a Rare Disease but Is Increasing in Frequency

It is characterized by severe diarrhea. Small intestinal biopsies are similar in appearance to those in GSE. Antibodies are present, but these are directed against the intestinal epithelial cells themselves. Severe villous atrophy may be present, but IELs are not as prominent as in GSE. Also, there is usually loss of goblet and Paneth cells. Importantly, the stomach and colon are often involved in addition to the small intestine. Likewise, extraintestinal involvement, such as the pancreas and lung, may also be present. Treatment differs radically from that for GSE; potent immunosuppressives are needed and gluten restriction has no effect.

Whipple Disease Is Caused by *Tropheryma whippelii*

While this disease is uncommon, it is important to recognize this process, which also presents as malabsorption. The causative bacterium is an actinobacterium and was identified only many years after the disease was first described. Villi are enlarged and bulbous owing to massive numbers of bacteria within macrophages, which are unable to degrade

the organisms; these macrophages take on a foamy appearance (Fig. 19-47A–D). Defective T-cell function may also be present. Because of their polysaccharide content, the bacteria impact striking positivity to the foamy macrophages when the PAS stain is employed. This time-honored method of establishing the diagnosis of the disease is being replaced by specific polymerase chain reaction (PCR) testing for the causative organism. Extraintestinal manifestations are very common and affect the heart, joints, lymph nodes and brain. Because of the CNS involvement, these patients may first present with neuropsychiatric symptoms. This disease responds dramatically to antibiotic therapy.

Giardiasis Is the Leading Gastrointestinal Protozoal Infection in the United States

The causative agent is *Giardia lamblia*. Symptoms may include severe watery diarrhea as well as abdominal discomfort with nausea and vomiting. Malabsorption can occur. Infection usually occurs after drinking from unprotected water sources. *Giardia* spores are extremely hardy; person-to-person transmission can occur, particularly among children in day care centers. The trophozoites can be identified in duodenal fluid or stool, but they are often

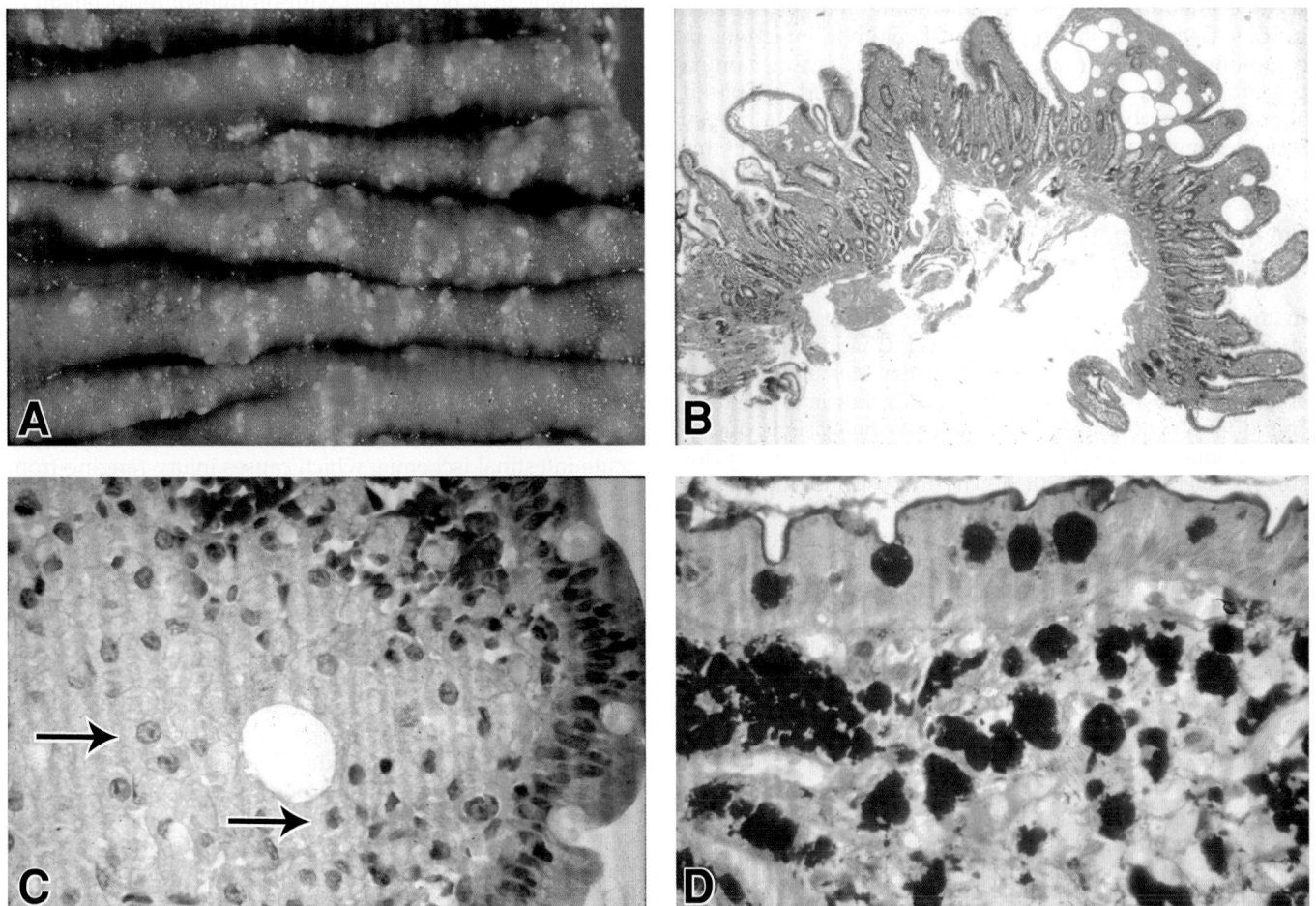

FIGURE 19-47. Whipple disease. A. The gross specimen shows white elevated areas; these are due to lipid collecting in the damaged mucosa. **B.** At low power the villi are short and club shaped; the large cystic-appearing areas represent fat trapped owing to compression of mucosal lymphocytes. **C.** The lamina propria contains abundant foamy macrophages (*arrows*). **D.** The partially digested bacteria in these macrophages impart strong periodic acid–Schiff (PAS) positivity.

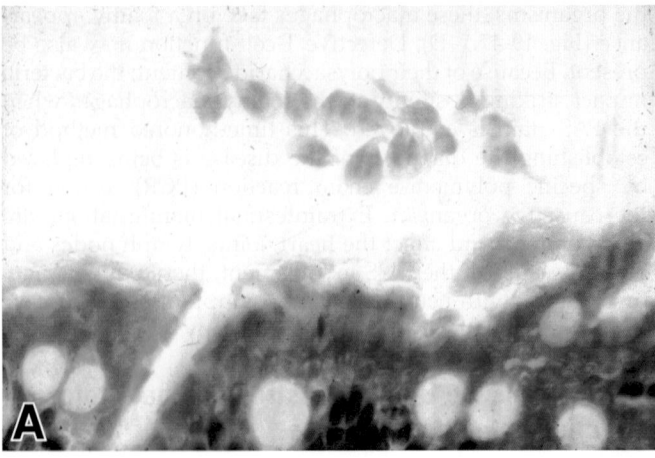 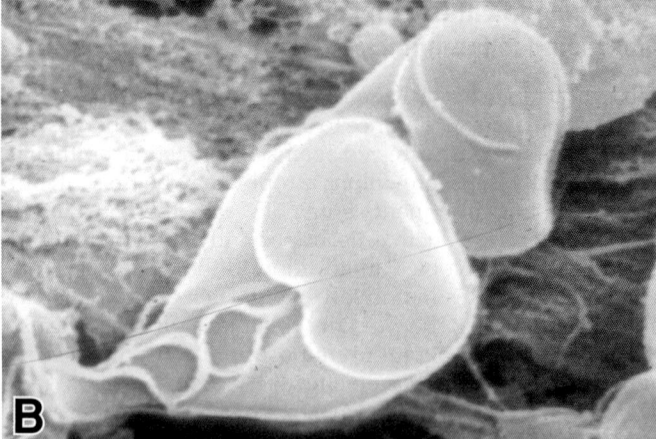

FIGURE 19-48. A. A group of **_Giardia_** is seen just above the surface epithelium in this jejunal biopsy. **B.** A single trophozoite from this area is seen here by scanning electron microscopy.

first identified in a duodenal biopsy. While they have a characteristic pear shape when seen in fluids, they tend to be seen in profile as sickle or triangular shapes in biopsies (Fig. 19-48A,B). They are usually very numerous, adhere to the epithelial surface and do not invade. The underlying mucosa is often completely normal or may show mild nonspecific inflammatory changes including a slight increase in IELs. _Giardia_ are among the most common infections in common variable immunodeficiency. In such cases, lamina propria plasma cells are sparse to absent and lymphoid aggregate may be present. Identifying _Giardia_ in a biopsy should trigger a search for plasma cells to exclude this possibility.

Small Bowel Bacterial Overgrowth Usually Results from Disordered Motility

In this condition, there is an overgrowth of colonic-type anaerobic bacteria in the small bowel. Conditions interfering with overall gut motility, such as diabetes, scleroderma, and pseudo-obstruction, can lead to the syndrome. The term "blind loop syndrome" may be used if the stasis is due to an anatomic defect such as small bowel diverticula or prior surgery such as a Billroth II. The mucosa may appear to be normal or show varying degrees of patchy nonspecific inflammation. It is thought that deconjugation of bile salts by the bacteria or their use of micronutrients is the major contributing pathogenic factor. Diagnosis is by breath test and cultures of intestinal fluid; antibiotic therapy usually results in symptomatic improvement. This and the other multiple causes of malabsorption are depicted in Fig. 19-49.

OBSTRUCTION

Mechanical obstruction can affect any segment of the gastrointestinal tract; the small bowel is frequently involved. The common causes include entrapment of bowel in hernias, intussusception (see above), adhesions from prior surgery or peritoneal infection, and volvulus. In volvulus, a segment of the intestinal tract twists on its mesentery, causing obstruction and ischemic damage. Neoplasms can also cause luminal obstruction with or without intussusception.

Pseudo-Obstruction

In pseudo-obstruction, symptoms and signs of obstruction are present but without any of the mechanical lesions previously discussed. There are both primary and secondary causes for this phenomenon. In primary pseudo-obstruction, the muscle may be affected with prominent replacement of smooth muscle with fibrous tissue leading to profoundly altered motility. Some of these cases are familial. Muscular abnormalities are more common than neural defects, which are often difficult to identify morphologically. Secondary forms of pseudo-obstruction complicate well-defined systemic diseases. Chief among these is scleroderma; amyloidosis and endometriosis affecting the muscularis are other causes of secondary damage.

INTESTINAL ISCHEMIA

Impaired intestinal blood flow for any reason can cause ischemic bowel disease. Manifestations of intestinal ischemia are diverse. The most common type of ischemic bowel disease is acute intestinal ischemia, which causes injury ranging from mucosal necrosis to transmural bowel infarction. Chronic intestinal ischemia syndromes are less common and generally require severe compromise of two or more major arteries, usually by atherosclerosis.

Superior Mesenteric Artery Occlusion

This is the most common cause of acute intestinal ischemia. Sudden occlusion of a large artery by thrombosis or embolization leads to small bowel infarction before collateral circulation can compensate. Depending on the size of the artery, infarction may be segmental or may lead to gangrene of virtually the entire small bowel. Occlusive intestinal infarction is most often caused by embolic or thrombotic occlusion of the superior mesenteric artery. A lesser number are the result of vasculitis, which often involves small arteries. In addition to intrinsic vascular lesions, volvulus, intussusception and incarceration of the intestine in a hernial sac may all lead to arterial as well as venous occlusion.

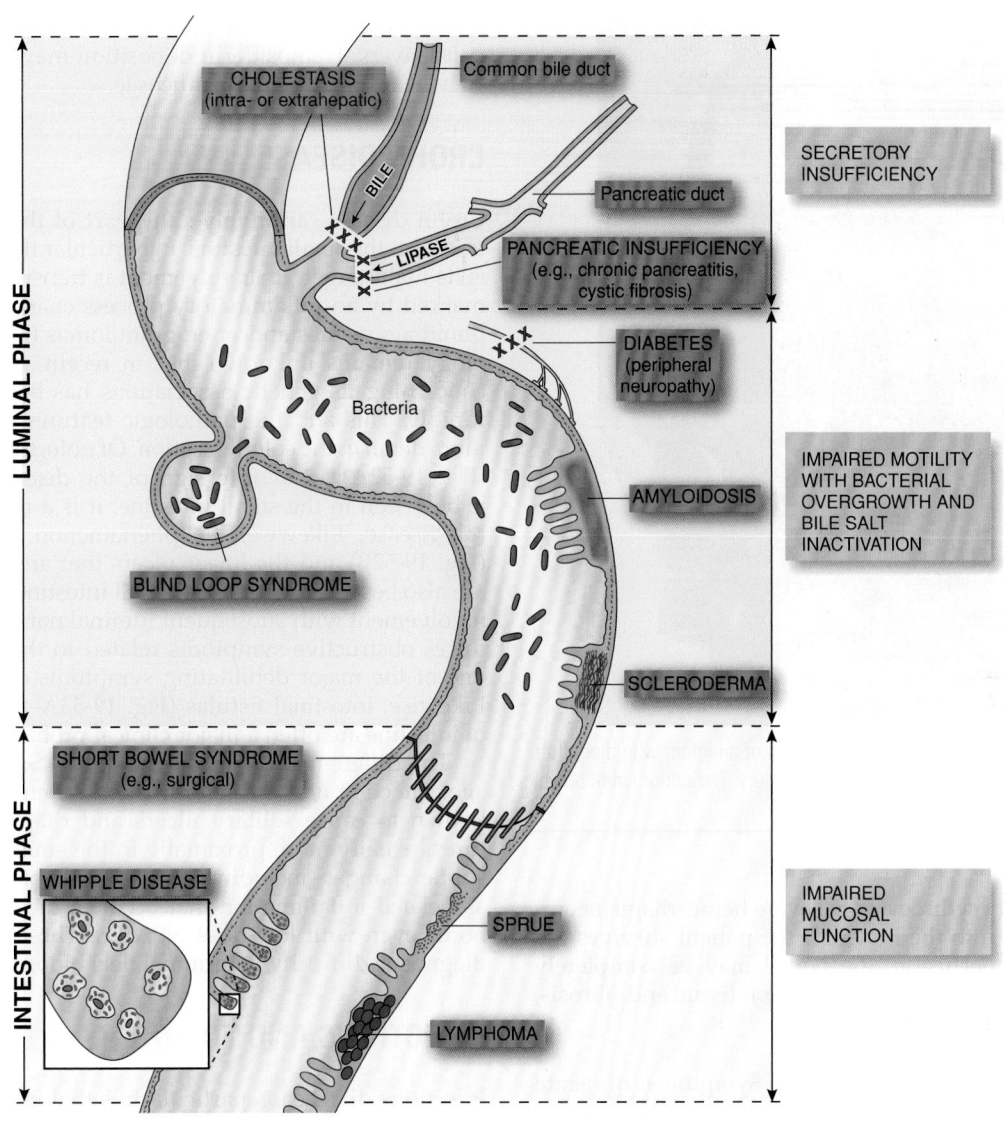

FIGURE 19-49. The causes of malabsorption.

Intestinal Ischemic Necrosis without Acute Vascular Occlusion

This type of vascular insufficiency is more common than the occlusive variety and may be just as extensive. It is seen in hypoxic patients with reduced cardiac output from shock of a variety of causes including hemorrhage, sepsis and acute myocardial infarction. In shock, blood flow redistributes to favor the brain and other vital organs, and patients often received α-adrenergic agents, which further shunt blood away from the intestine. Drastically lowered perfusion pressure leads to arteriolar collapse, aggravating the ischemia.

Mesenteric Vein Thrombosis

Mesenteric vein thrombosis is also a common cause of ischemic damage. Causes of mesenteric vein thrombosis include hypercoagulable states, stasis and inflammation (pylephlebitis). Almost all thromboses affect the superior mesenteric vein; only 5% involve the inferior mesenteric vein. The collateral flow in the distribution of the superior mesenteric vein usually suffices to preclude infarction of the intestine.

Infarcted bowel is edematous and diffusely purple (Fig. 19-50). The demarcation between the infarcted bowel and normal tissue is usually sharp, although venous occlusion may lead to a more diffuse appearance. Hemorrhage is prominent in the mucosa and submucosa, especially in venous occlusion (e.g., mesenteric vein thrombosis). The mucosal surface shows irregular wide areas of sloughing, and the wall becomes thin and distended. Bubbles of gas (pneumatosis) may be present in the bowel wall and mesenteric veins. The serosal surface is cloudy and covered by an inflammatory exudate.

Other Causes of Intestinal Ischemia

SMOOTH MUSCLE DYSFUNCTION: Dysfunctional smooth muscle interferes with peristalsis and leads to adynamic ileus, in which the bowel proximal to the lesion is dilated and filled with fluid. Intestinal organisms may pass through the damaged wall and cause peritonitis or septicemia.

NONOCCLUSIVE INTESTINAL ISCHEMIA: In this setting, the principal lesion is restricted initially to the mucosa. Mucosal changes range from foci of dilated capillaries with a

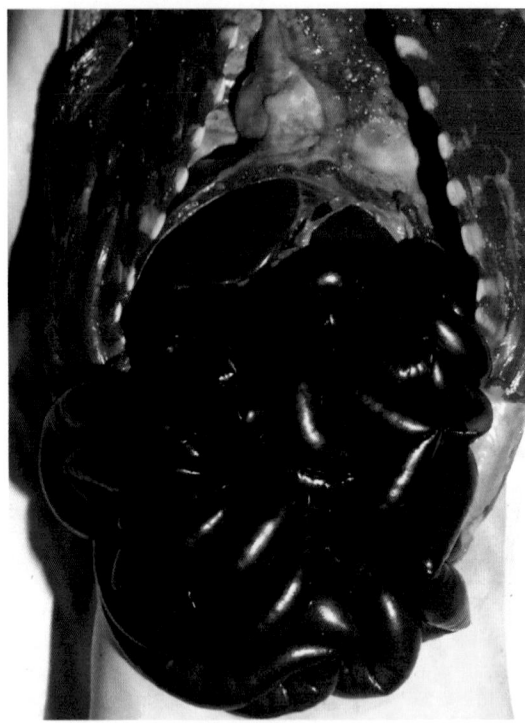

FIGURE 19-50. Infarcted small bowel at autopsy of an infant who died after volvulus had occluded the superior mesenteric artery. The entire small bowel is dilated, hemorrhagic and necrotic.

few extravasated erythrocytes to severe hemorrhagic necrosis and bleeding into the lumen. If the patient survives the episode of hypoperfusion, the bowel may be completely repaired, or it may heal with granulation tissue and fibrosis, with eventual **stricture formation**.

CLINICAL FEATURES: Symptoms of acute ischemia include abdominal pain, which begins abruptly, often with bloody diarrhea, hematemesis and shock. In untreated cases, perforation is frequent. As infarction progresses, systemic symptoms become more severe (multiple organ dysfunction syndrome). In extensive infarction that is a result of occlusion in the proximal superior mesenteric artery, almost the entire small bowel must be resected, a situation not compatible with ultimate survival.

Atherosclerotic narrowing of major splanchnic arteries leads to chronic intestinal ischemia. As in the heart, it causes intermittent abdominal pain, called intestinal (abdominal) angina. The pain usually starts within a half hour of eating and lasts for a few hours. Frank intestinal infarction may be heralded by abdominal angina. Recurrent abdominal pain may also reflect pressure on the celiac axis from surrounding structures, called the celiac compression syndrome.

Chronic Small Bowel Ischemia

Chronic vascular insufficiency of the small intestine may lead to fibrosis and stricture formation. Ischemic strictures of the small bowel may be single or multiple and produce intestinal obstruction or, occasionally, malabsorption owing to stasis and bacterial overgrowth. These strictures are concentric, and the mucosa of this region is atrophic, often with one or more small ulcers. The submucosa is thickened and

fibrotic with granulation tissue, which may involve the muscular layers. Hemosiderin deposition may be seen, particularly near the muscularis mucosae.

CROHN DISEASE

Crohn disease can involve any part of the gastrointestinal tract, but the small intestine, in particular the terminal ileum, is its main target. Its involvement is transmural and patchy, marked by an inflammatory process characterized by lymphoid aggregates and often granulomas (Fig. 19-51). Its etiology remains unknown, but in recent years information concerning its genetic associations has been accumulating rapidly. This and the pathologic features are described in more detail in the colonic section. Of note, the "fat wrapping" (Fig. 19-52A), a favorite sign of the disease for surgeons, is best seen in the small intestine; it is a result of transmural disease. Likewise, the phenomenon of cobblestoning (Fig. 19-52B) and the linear ulcers that are so characteristic are also best seen within the small intestine. The transmural involvement with subsequent luminal narrowing often produces obstructive symptoms related to the small intestine, one of the major debilitating symptoms of Crohn disease. Likewise, intestinal fistulas (Fig. 19-53A–C) between loops of intestine are often a major clinical problem.

The differential diagnosis includes NSAID-related damage, infection and radiation-related strictures. NSAIDs are known to cause solitary ulcers and diaphragm-like strictures, usually more proximally in the small intestine. More subtle changes, including erosive and shallow ulcers with associated inflammation that occur in the distal ileum, can occur even with low-dose NSAIDs. These can cause great diagnostic difficulty in terminal ileal biopsies.

INFECTIONS AND TOXINS

Infectious diarrhea is particularly lethal in underdeveloped countries and in infants. In countries with poor sanitation,

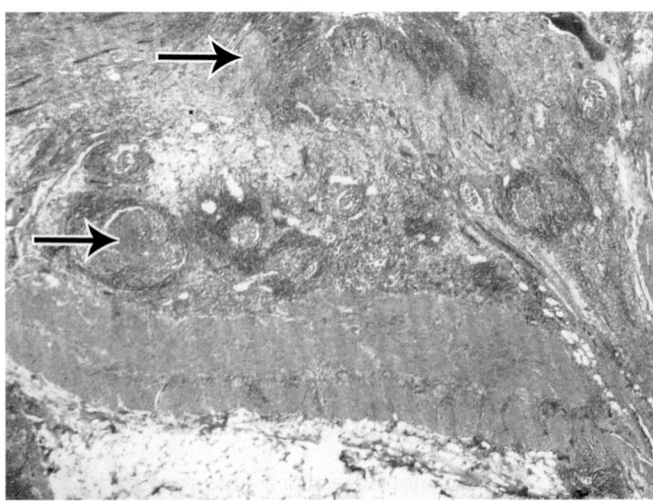

FIGURE 19-51. This full-thickness histologic section shows transmural involvement by lymphoid aggregates and granulomas. The mucosa and submucosa (*arrows*) are most severely affected, but the infiltrate also involves muscle and mesentery. Note the tendency to be more severe in perivascular areas. See also Figure 19-72.

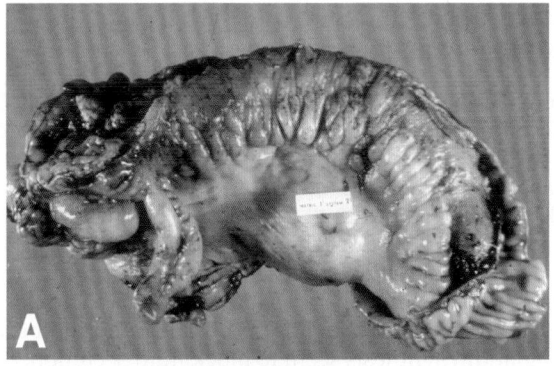

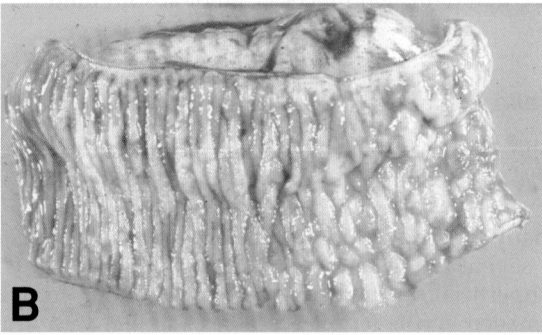

FIGURE 19-52. **A.** Fat wrapping is a manifestation of transmural involvement but is not always evident. **B.** The cobblestoning is a result of the patchy nature of **Crohn** disease. See also Figure 19-71 for a linear ulcer.

the death toll from childhood diarrhea is staggering: 1.5 million children under 5 years die annually of diarrhea, over 80% of them in Africa and south Asia.

The small bowel normally has few bacteria (usually <10^4/mL), mostly such bacilli as lactobacilli. These organisms travel in the food stream and ordinarily do not colonize the small intestine. Infectious diarrhea is caused by bacterial colonization (e.g., with toxigenic strains of *Escherichia coli* and *Vibrio cholerae*). The most significant factor in infectious diarrhea is increased intestinal secretion, stimulated by bacterial toxins and enteric hormones. Decreased absorption and increased peristaltic activity contribute less to the diarrhea.

The colon harbors abundant bacteria, at concentrations seven orders of magnitude greater than in the small intestine. Anaerobic bacteria in the colon (e.g., *Bacteroides* and *Clostridium* species) outnumber aerobic organisms 1000-fold. With the more rapid transit of intestinal contents during diarrhea, flora are shifted to more aerobic populations, including *E. coli, Klebsiella* and *Proteus.* Moreover, offending organisms themselves become conspicuous and pathogens of the small intestine such as *V. cholerae* may be the major isolate in the stool.

Several factors limit the numbers of bacteria in the stomach and small bowel: (1) gastric acid inhibits bacterial growth, which explains bacterial overgrowth in the stomach in achlorhydria; (2) bile has an antimicrobial activity; (3) peristalsis propels intestinal contents, limiting bacterial accumulation; (4) normal flora secrete their own antimicrobial

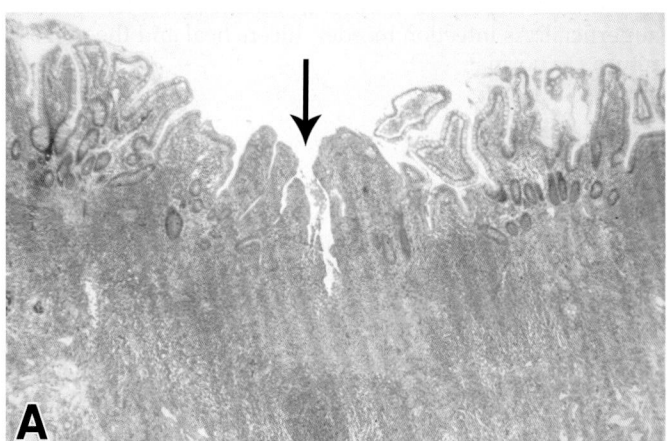

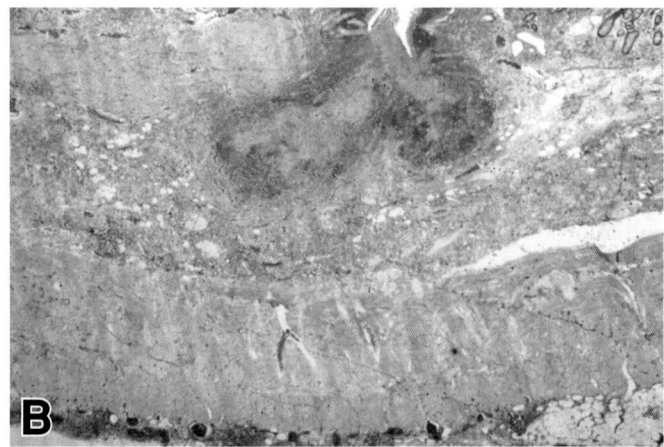

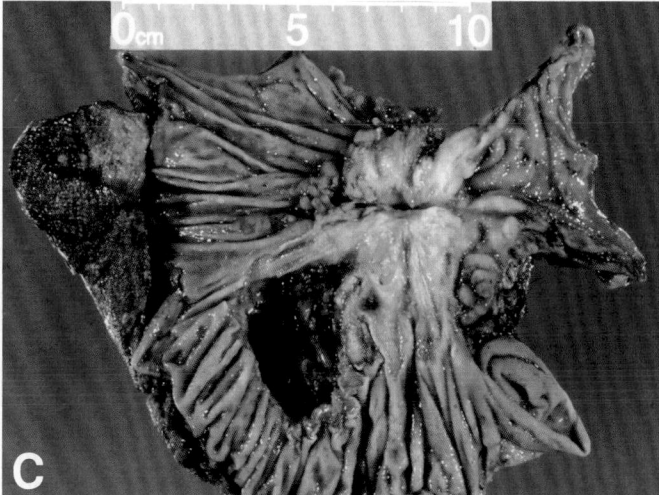

FIGURE 19-53. **A.** A small **fissure ulcer,** here knife-like (*arrow*), often starts over a lymphoid aggregate. **B.** The process continues, causing a fissure extending into the submucosa and beyond, ultimately penetrating the bowel wall. **C.** A **fistula** may result from such transmural involvement. Here an ileocolonic fistula has resulted.

TABLE 19-1

HISTOLOGIC PATTERNS OF BACTERIAL INFECTIONS OF THE GASTROINTESTINAL TRACT

Minimal inflammatory changes	*Vibrio cholerae*
	Toxigenic *Escherichia coli*
	Neisseria sp.
Acute self-limited colitis	*Shigella*
	Campylobacter jejuni
	Aeromonas
	Salmonella
	Clostridium difficile
Pseudomembranous pattern	*C. difficile*
	Shigella
	Enterohemorrhagic *E. coli*
Granulomas	*Yersinia* sp.
	Mycobacterium bovis
	Mycobacterium avium-intracellulare
	Actinomycosis
Histiocytic	Whipple disease (*Tropheryma whippelii*)
	M. avium-intracellulare
Lymphohistiocytic	*Lymphogranuloma venereum*
Architectural distortion	*Salmonella typhimurium*
	Shigella

substances to maintain an ecologic balance (indeed, treatment with broad-spectrum antibiotics alters the natural flora and allows overgrowth of ordinarily harmless organisms); and (5) plasma cells of the lamina propria secrete IgA into the intestinal lumen.

Individual agents responsible for infectious diarrhea are discussed in Chapter 9. Here we review the major entities only briefly. Agents of infectious diarrhea are classified into **toxigenic** (i.e., producing diarrhea by elaborating toxins) or as adherent or invasive bacteria (Table 19-1 lists reaction patterns).

Toxigenic Diarrhea Is Most Often Due to *Escherichia coli*

The prototypical organisms that cause diarrhea by secreting toxins are *V. cholerae* and toxigenic strains of *E. coli.*

The characteristics of toxigenic diarrhea are:

- Damage to the intestinal mucosal is minimal or absent.
- The organism remains on the mucosal surface, where it secretes its toxin.
- Fluid secreted into the small intestine causes watery diarrhea, which can lead to dehydration, particularly in the case of cholera.

Many organisms have been isolated in so-called travelers' diarrhea, but toxigenic *E. coli* is the most common in almost all studies.

Invasive Bacteria Cause Diarrhea by Direct Mucosal Injury

Among these invasive organisms, *Shigella, Salmonella,* and certain strains of *E. coli, Yersinia* and *Campylobacter* are the most widely recognized. Invasive organisms tend to infect the distal ileum and colon, while toxigenic bacteria mainly involve the upper intestinal tract. The mechanisms by which invasive bacteria produce diarrhea are uncertain. Enterotoxins have been identified, but their role in causing diarrhea is not established. Mucosal invasion by bacteria increases synthesis of prostaglandins in affected tissues, and inhibitors of prostaglandin synthesis seem to block fluid secretion. It also may be that damaged mucosa cannot absorb fluid from the lumen.

Shigella

Shigellosis, caused by any of the four species of the genus *Shigella,* mainly affects the colon, but the terminal ileum is occasionally involved. A granular and hemorrhagic mucosa has many shallow serpiginous ulcers. Inflammation is especially severe in the sigmoid colon and rectum, but is usually superficial. In the early stage, neutrophils accumulate in damaged crypts (crypt abscesses), similarly to in ulcerative colitis (see below), and the lymphoid follicles of the mucosa break down to form ulcers. Unlike ulcerative colitis (see below), signs of chronicity are not present. There is no crypt branching, and the dense lymphoplasmacytic infiltrate in the lamina propria is absent; inflammation tends to be superficial. As infection recedes, ulcers heal and the mucosa returns to normal.

Typhoid Fever

Typhoid fever (*Salmonella typhi* enteritis) is uncommon in the industrialized world but is still a problem in underdeveloped countries. Necrosis of lymphoid tissue, mainly in the terminal ileum, leads to scattered ulcers. Infection of Peyer patches results in oval ulcers, in which the longer dimension is in the long axis of the intestine. Occasionally, lymphoid follicles in the large bowel or the appendix are ulcerated. The base of the ulcer contains black necrotic tissue mixed with fibrin.

Early lesions of typhoid fever show large basophilic macrophages filled with typhoid bacilli, erythrocytes and necrotic debris. Necrosis of lymphoid follicles becomes confluent and mucosal ulceration follows. Similar lymphoid hyperplasia and necrosis are seen in regional lymph nodes. Within a week of the acute symptoms, ulcers heal completely, leaving little fibrosis or other sequelae. Intestinal hemorrhage and perforation, principally in the ileum, are the most feared complications of typhoid fever and tend to occur in the third week and during convalescence.

Nontyphoidal Salmonellosis

Formerly known as **paratyphoid fever,** enteritis caused by *Salmonella* strains other than *S. typhi* is generally far less serious than typhoid fever. The principal target is the ileum, but minor involvement of the colon may also occur. Organisms invade the mucosa, which shows mild ulceration, edema and infiltration with neutrophils. Hematogenous dissemination from the intestine may carry infection to bones, joints and meninges. People with sickle cell disease tend to develop *Salmonella* osteomyelitis, possibly because phagocytosis of products of hemolysis prevents further cellular ingestion of the organisms and allows their dissemination through the bloodstream.

Escherichia coli

Enteroinvasive, enteroadherent and enterohemorrhagic strains of *E. coli* may uncommonly cause bloody diarrhea similar to shigellosis and are a prominent cause of traveler's diarrhea. Certain strains of *E. coli*, particularly serotype 0157:H7, produce *Shigella*-like toxins, but the role of these proteins in the pathogenesis of the enterocolitis is not understood. Serotype 0157:H7 has also been implicated in the hemolytic–uremic syndrome in children.

Yersinia

Yersinia enterocolitica and *Yersinia pseudotuberculosis* are transmitted by pets or contaminated food, and infection is most common in young children. *Yersinia* infection causes diarrhea, cramps and fever and lasts 1–3 weeks. Peyer patches are hyperplastic, with acute ulceration of overlying mucosa. A fibrinopurulent exudate covering the ulcers often contains many organisms.

In addition to causing enterocolitis, *Yersinia* causes acute mesenteric adenitis and right lower quadrant pain. It may so resemble appendicitis that infected children have mistakenly been taken to laparotomy for *Yersinia* infection. Lymph nodes show epithelioid granulomas with central necrosis in the case of *Y. pseudotuberculosis*. The ileum and appendix may contain similar granulomas, imparting an appearance that resembles that of Crohn disease.

Adults, who are less susceptible to *Yersinia* infection than are children, have acute diarrhea, often followed within a few weeks by erythema nodosum, erythema multiforme or polyarthritis. Patients with chronic debilitating diseases may develop *Yersinia* bacteremia, resistant to antibiotic treatment. Interestingly, people with thalassemia are particularly susceptible to *Y. enterocolitica* infection. Identification by culture can be difficult; PCR analysis is effective.

Campylobacter jejuni

Campylobacter jejuni is one of the most common causes of bacterial diarrhea, with a higher incidence than nontyphoidal *Salmonella* and *Shigella* in some U.S. studies. In a report from Great Britain, *Campylobacter* caused half of bacterial diarrhea. Humans contract the disease mainly by contact with infected domestic animals or by eating poorly cooked or contaminated food. The histology is similar to that of *Shigella*. Adults usually recover in less than 1 week.

Food Poisoning Reflects Bacterial Toxins in Contaminated Food

STAPHYLOCOCCUS AUREUS: *S. aureus* is a common cause of food poisoning. Symptoms result from eating food contaminated with *Staphylococcus* strains that make an exotoxin that damages gastrointestinal epithelium. Severe vomiting and abdominal cramps occur within 6 hours, often followed by diarrhea. Most patients recover in 1–2 days.

CLOSTRIDIUM PERFRINGENS: This bacterium produces an enterotoxin that causes vomiting and diarrhea. The organism is anaerobic but tolerates exposure to air for up to 3 days. Enterotoxin activity is maximal in the ileum. In most cases, watery diarrhea and severe abdominal pain begin 8–24 hours after ingestion of contaminated food and last about 1 day.

Rotavirus and Norwalk Virus Are the Most Common Causes of Viral Gastroenteritis in the United States

ROTAVIRUS: Rotavirus infection is a common cause of infantile diarrhea. It accounts for about half of acute diarrhea in hospitalized children younger than 2 years. Rotavirus has been demonstrated in duodenal biopsy specimens. It is associated with injury to the surface epithelium and impaired intestinal absorption for periods of up to 2 months.

NORWALK VIRUSES: These highly infectious agents account for one third of the epidemics of viral gastroenteritis in the United States. There have been a number of notorious outbreaks on cruise ships of late. The virus targets the upper small intestine, causing patchy mucosal lesions and malabsorption. Vomiting and diarrhea are usual, but symptoms resolve within 2 days.

Other viruses implicated as etiologic agents of infective diarrhea include echovirus, coxsackievirus, cytomegalovirus, adenovirus and coronavirus.

Intestinal Tuberculosis Is Mostly Caused by Ingesting Bacteria in Food or Swallowing Infectious Sputum

The tubercle bacillus (either *Mycobacterium tuberculosis* or *Mycobacterium bovis*) is protected from gastric acid by its waxy capsule and passes into the small bowel. There, it establishes a locus of infection, usually (90% of patients) in the ileocecal region, where lymphoid tissue is abundant. Infection also occurs in the colon, jejunum, appendix, rectum and duodenum, in that order of frequency.

 PATHOLOGY: Intestinal tuberculosis may present with ulcers of varying size in the transverse plane of the bowel. As these ulcers heal, reactive fibrosis may cause a circumferential ("napkin ring") stricture of the bowel lumen. Mesenteric lymph nodes are typically enlarged, with caseous necrosis.

Granulomas occur in all layers of the bowel wall, particularly Peyer patches and lymphoid follicles. Tuberculous strictures are difficult to distinguish from other causes of stricture, such as ischemic enterocolitis or Crohn disease.

 CLINICAL FEATURES: Almost all patients with intestinal tuberculosis complain of chronic abdominal pain and 2/3 have a palpable abdominal mass, usually in the right lower quadrant. Malnutrition, weight loss, fever and weakness are common. Complications include obstruction, fistulas, perforation and abscess.

NEOPLASMS

Despite the length and large surface area of the small intestine, primary small intestinal neoplasms occur less commonly than do those in the esophagus, stomach or colon.

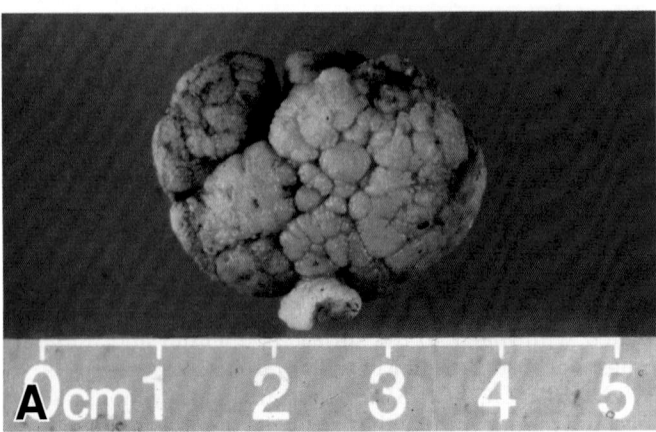

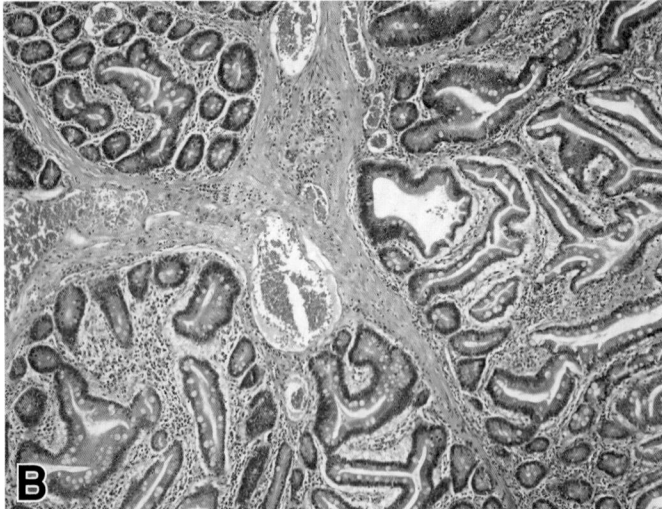

FIGURE 19-54. A. This **Peutz-Jeghers polyp** has a characteristic striking bosselated appearance. **B.** The histology is characterized by arborizing bundles of smooth muscle. The epithelium and glands between closely resemble the bland appearance of their normal counterparts but form an unusual architectural configuration.

Benign Neoplasms

Small Bowel Adenomas Resemble Those in the Colon

They are, however, far less common. Also, unlike the colon, they are not known to be frequent precursors to adenocarcinoma. They occur sporadically and are also seen commonly in FAP.

Peutz-Jeghers Polyps Are Hamartomas

Polyps in this syndrome may occur anywhere in the GI tract but are most common in the small intestine. They have a characteristic gross and microscopic (Fig. 19-54A,B) appearance. Bland-appearing small intestinal epithelium, often with an unusual architectural arrangement, is intermixed with large arborizing branches of smooth muscle. This autosomal dominant disorder is characterized by buccal pigmentation and macular lesions on the lips, hands, feet and genitals. Most patients have mutations in the *LKB1* tumor suppressor gene (on chromosome 19p13.3; see Chapter 5). There is an increased risk for cancer, largely outside the gastrointestinal tract, involving the testis, ovary, uterus or pancreas.

Malignant Tumors Are Far Less Common in the Small Intestine Than Elsewhere in the GI Tract

Adenocarcinoma

These tumors resemble their colonic counterparts but are much less frequent. They occur more often proximally, particularly in the duodenum. They can be polypoid or ulcerated or have a peculiar constricted napkin ring appearance (Fig. 19-55A,B). There is a much greater (80-fold) risk of small bowel adenocarcinoma in patients with Crohn disease or celiac disease. In the former, the tumors arise distally, in inflamed intestine. These tumors are also increased in FAP and Peutz-Jeghers syndrome.

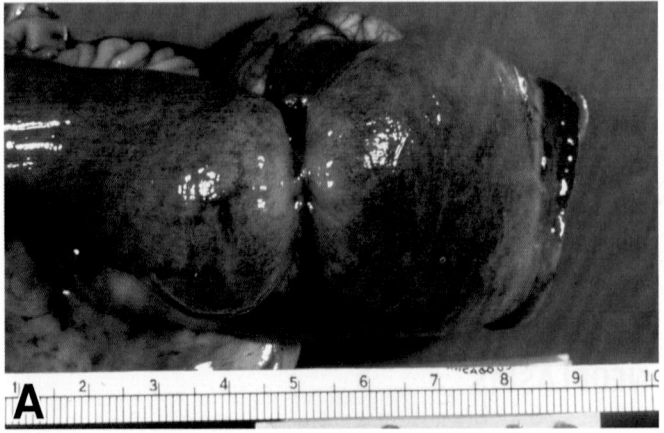

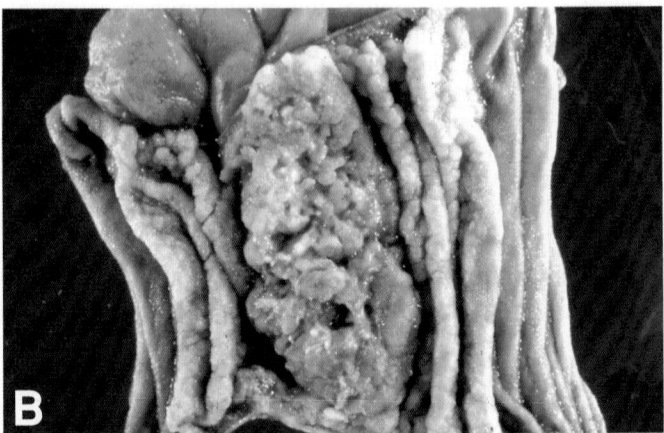

FIGURE 19-55. A. The external aspect of a small intestinal **adenocarcinoma** often has this peculiar constricted appearance. **B.** The luminal tumor is usually raised and often ulcerated, resembling its colonic counterpart.

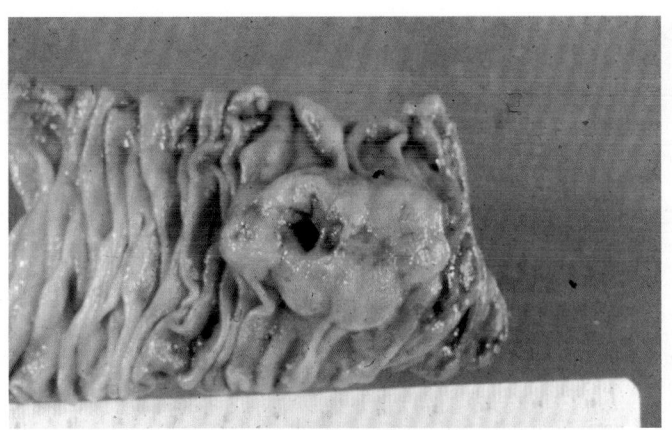

FIGURE 19-56. This mucosal-covered **gastrointestinal stromal tumor (GIST)** has a striking area of deep central ulceration.

Metastases

Secondary carcinomas are about as common as are primary adenocarcinomas in the small intestine. The primary tumor may be of any origin, but melanomas and tumors of the lung, breast, colon and kidney are the most common. Careful attention to historical and histologic detail is necessary to establish the diagnosis.

Gastrointestinal Stromal Tumors

The small intestine is second to the stomach in the incidence of these tumors. Those arising in the small intestine are more likely to behave aggressively. They frequently have a deep central ulceration, which can cause severe bleeding (Fig. 19-56). These GISTs tend more to be composed of spindled cells than gastric GISTs, which often have areas with an epithelioid appearance.

Neuroendocrine Tumors (Carcinoid Tumors)

As noted above, the term **neuroendocrine tumors** has largely replaced "carcinoid" in designating these tumors. All NETs are considered malignant, but they vary greatly in their metastatic potential. The GI tract is the most common

site for NETs (the bronchus being the next most common site). In addition to the site of origin, the size, depth of invasion, hormonal responsiveness and presence or absence of function are major indicators of likely aggressiveness.

The appendix is the most common gastrointestinal site of origin, followed by the rectum; these tumors are usually innocuous. Tumors of the ileum are usually small but are often quite aggressive.

 PATHOLOGY: Small NETs usually present as submucosal nodules covered by intact mucosa. Larger tumors may grow in polypoid, intramural or annular patterns and often undergo secondary ulceration. Cut surfaces are firm and white to yellow. As they enlarge, the tumors invade the muscular coat and penetrate the serosa, often causing a conspicuous desmoplasia, which can lead to peritoneal adhesions, kinking of the bowel and possible intestinal obstruction. Ileal NETs are multiple in about 40% of cases (Fig. 19-57A,B).

Small, round cells in NETs form nests, cords and rosettes. Occasional gland-like structures are also seen (hence the term "carcinoid"). Nuclei are remarkably regular and mitoses are rare. The abundant eosinophilic cytoplasm contains neurosecretory-type granules. Despite their bland appearance, jejunal and ileal tumors behave more aggressively than do similar-appearing NETs originating at other sites.

When these tumors metastasize to regional lymph nodes, they may produce a bulky mass far larger than the primary tumor. Subsequent hematogenous spread causes metastases at distant sites, particularly the liver. Patients occasionally present with a huge amount of metastatic NETs in the liver, all due to a small, clinically silent primary tumor in the ileum.

 CLINICAL FEATURES: Carcinoid syndrome occurs in a small percentage of patients with NETs. It is a unique but uncommon clinical condition caused by release of active tumor products. Most NETs are somewhat functional, but carcinoid syndrome mainly occurs in patients with extensive hepatic metastases. *Classic symptoms include diarrhea (often the most distressing symptom), episodic flushing, bronchospasm, cyanosis, telangiectasia and skin lesions.* Half of patients also have right-sided cardiac valvular disease (see Chapter 17). Diarrhea is thought to be caused by serotonin.

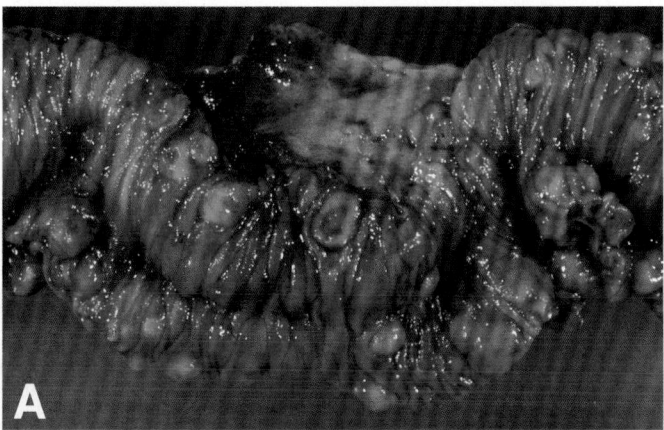

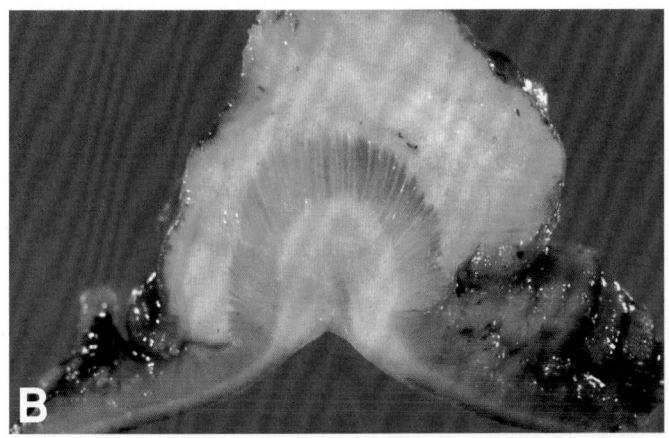

FIGURE 19-57. A. Ileal neuroendocrine tumors (NETs) are frequently multiple, here producing several mucosal-covered pale yellow tumors. **B.** The frequent characteristic "knuckling" of the intestinal wall is due to the brisk fibrous response to the invading tumor.

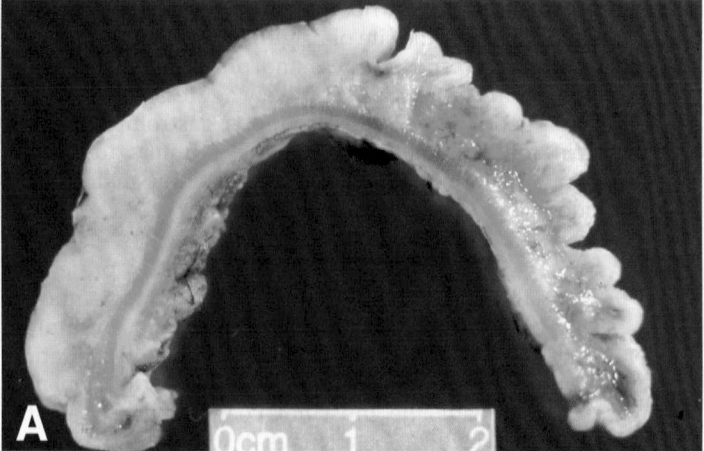

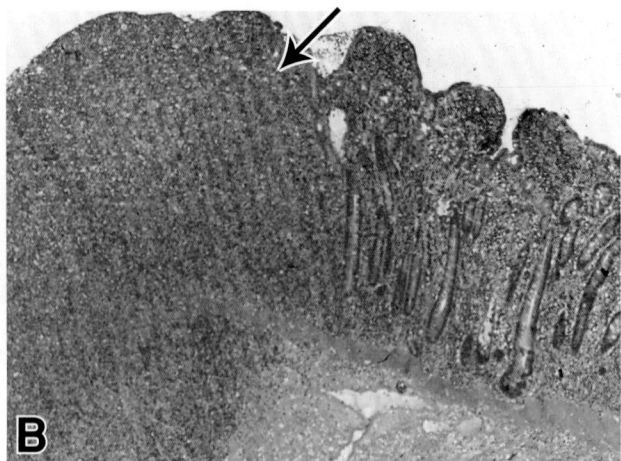

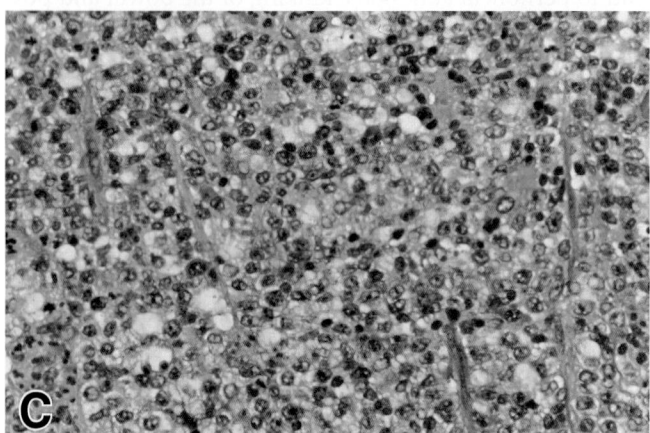

FIGURE 19-58. A. The **lymphoma** diffusely penetrating the bowel wall has given it a peculiar pale white color often referred to as "fish flesh." **B.** The infiltrate in this enteropathy-associated T-cell lymphoma (EATL) (*arrow*) is adjacent to the flat mucosa (*arrowhead*) in this patient with celiac disease. **C.** The lymphomatous infiltrate pushes aside the epithelial and muscular structures.

After its release into the blood, serotonin is metabolized to 5-hydroxyindoleacetic acid (5-HIAA) by monoamine oxidase (MAO) in the liver or other tissues. Urine 5-HIAA is a diagnostic test for carcinoid syndrome. Liver, lung and brain all have high levels of MAO activity, but the right side of the heart is affected mainly when there are metastases in the liver, allowing secreted serotonin to bypass hepatic detoxification. Fibrous plaques form on tricuspid and pulmonic valves, the endocardium of the right-sided cardiac chambers, the vena cava, the coronary sinus and the pulmonary artery. Valvular distortion leads to pulmonic stenosis and tricuspid regurgitation.

Lymphoma

Four major types of lymphoma occur in the small intestine (see Chapter 26): Burkitt lymphoma, immunoproliferative small intestinal disease (Mediterranean lymphoma), diffuse large B-cell lymphoma ("Western" lymphoma) and enteropathy-associated intestinal T-cell lymphoma (EATL).

Burkitt lymphoma develops mainly in the terminal ileum of children, with males predominating. The tumors form bulky masses. The B cells composing the tumor may have a plasmacytoid appearance. Many cases are EBV positive. The process can be seen in young adults who have some immunodeficiency; some are HIV positive.

Patients with immunoproliferative small intestinal disease (IPSID) are most commonly young adults of a lower socioeconomic status living in the Middle East. It appears to be a distinctive type of extranodal marginal B-cell lymphoma. Environmental factors are thought to play a role, and there is evidence implicating *C. jejuni*. Abdominal pain, malabsorption, diarrhea and weight loss dominate the clinical picture. Diffuse mural thickening with luminal dilatation is often present. Free α–heavy chains are often found in the serum. An extensive mucosal lymphoid infiltrate may distort small intestinal villi.

Diffuse large B-cell lymphoma often presents as a large luminal mass in an older adult. It tends to be quite aggressive.

EATL complicates celiac disease, which may be longstanding but can be of short duration (Fig. 19-58A–C). Severe malnutrition despite adherence to a gluten-free diet often heralds its onset. It has the worst prognosis of the intestinal lymphomas.

The Ampulla

ANATOMY

The ampulla is unique and of great importance since it is the confluence of three major organs, the liver, pancreas and small intestine. In most individuals, the common bile duct and the main pancreatic duct meet to form a common chamber, the ampulla (Fig. 19-59). There are several variations in anatomy, the most common being that the two ducts empty

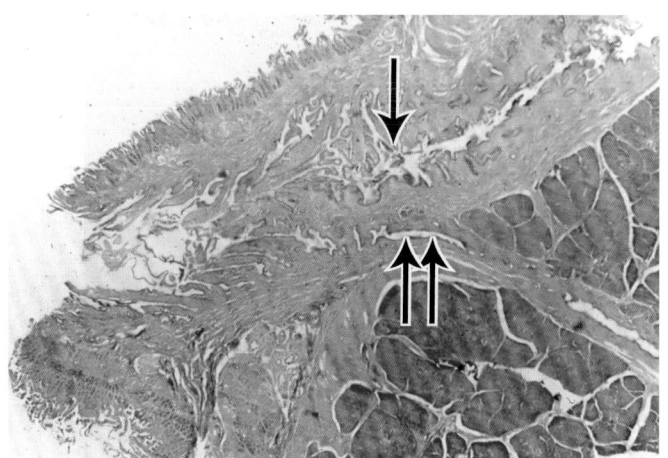

FIGURE 19-59. Small intestinal mucosa covers the protruding **papilla of Vater.** There is a common chamber, the **ampulla** (*arrowhead*), where the common bile duct (*arrow*) and the pancreatic duct (*double arrow*) meet.

separately into the duodenum, separated by a thin septum. Regardless, this meeting of the ducts projects into the duodenal lumen as the papilla of Vater.

The well-known relationship of gallstones to pancreatitis reflects the intimate proximity of the related ducts. Inflammatory processes can affect the periampullary area, causing clinical symptoms, and potentially mimicking neoplasia. The inflammation may be nonspecific or related to infection, such as involvement by *Cryptosporidia* or CMV in immunosuppressed individuals. Significant ampullitis may be a major feature of IgG4-related autoimmune pancreatitis.

NEOPLASMS

The ampulla and periampullary area is a common site for small intestinal neoplasms. There are occasional benign proliferations of smooth muscle and epithelium, so-called adenomyomatous hyperplasia. Adenomas may also occur here. They can be sporadic but are particularly frequent in individuals with familial adenomatous polyposis.

NETs also tend to arise in this location. Some develop as part of neurofibromatosis, produce somatostatin and are known as somatostatinomas.

Adenocarcinoma involving the ampulla may arise from the duct in the head of the pancreas, from the distal common bile duct, from the ampullary epithelial lining itself (Fig. 19-60A,B) or from the duodenal mucosa of the surface of the papilla or periampullary area.

Adenocarcinomas are by far the most common malignancy in the area. Most probably arise from preexisting adenomas. Because of their crucial anatomic location, tumors may present clinically with jaundice even when relatively small. Tumors may have an intestinal or a pancreaticobiliary phenotype. The former tend to have a somewhat better prognosis.

The Appendix

The appendix is a true diverticulum of the cecum. Its histology is the same as that of the colon from which it arises, although the submucosal lymphoid tissue is particularly robust, especially in childhood.

APPENDICITIS

The most important disease of the appendix is acute appendicitis (Fig. 19-61). This may occur at any age, but children and adults over 60 are most affected. The familiar presenting sign is right lower quadrant pain, which, if not treated, is followed by signs of peritoneal inflammation. Treatment is surgical removal. It must be admitted that the genesis of appendicitis remains largely mysterious. In many there appears to be some component of luminal obstruction by lumps of fecal concretions known as fecaliths. However, these are often not present. On occasion, a specific infectious agent is identified, such *Yersinia, Actinomyces* or *Campylobacter*. In some children, a tangle of pinworms (*Enterobius vermicularis*) may contribute to luminal obstruction.

However, in most cases, there is no apparent specific infectious agent. There is often a mucosal erosion or ulceration,

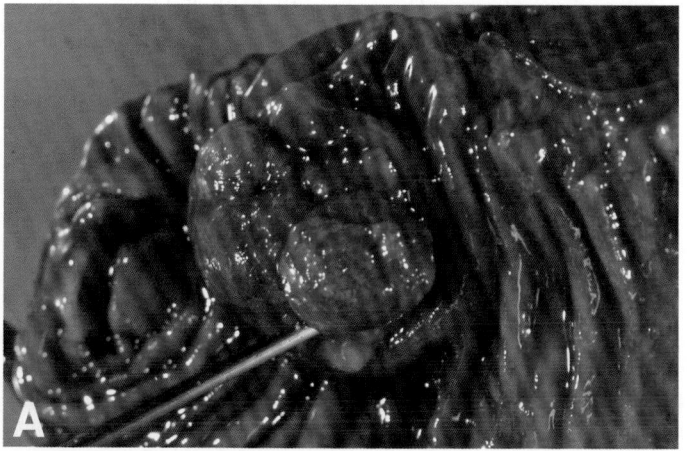

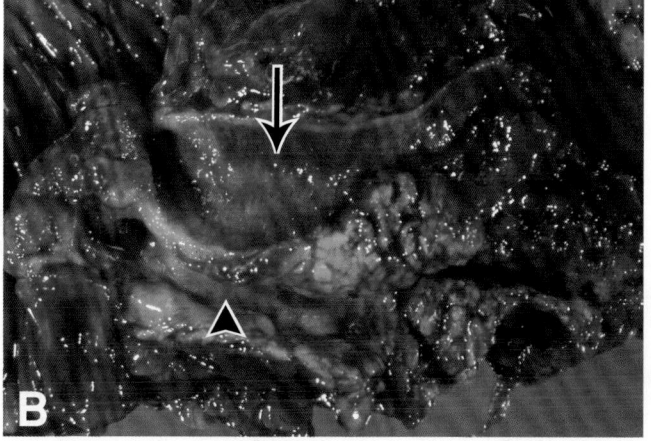

FIGURE 19-60.   A. A probe was placed into the ampulla and common bile duct in this carcinoma of the ampulla. **B.** Upon dissection, both the common bile duct (*arrow*) and the pancreatic duct (*arrowhead*) are dilated owing to obstruction by the tumor.

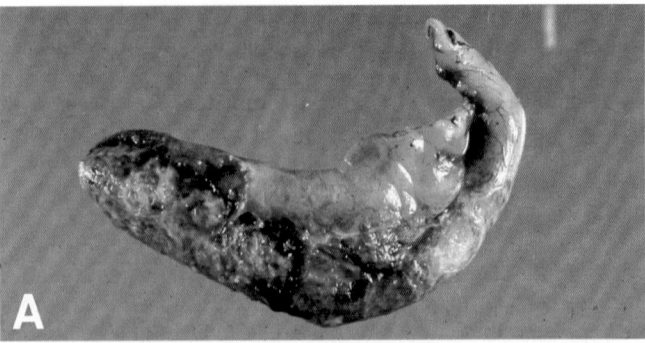

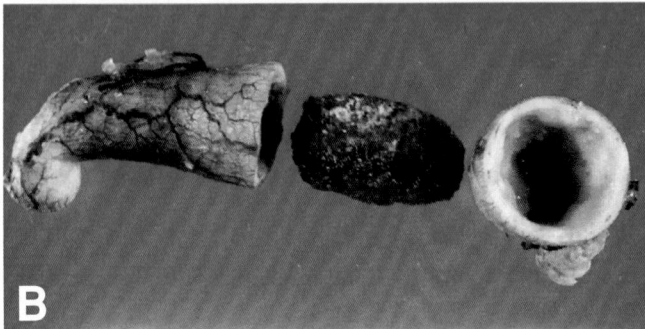

FIGURE 19-61. A. The distal appendix is dilated, congested and partly covered by fibrin (*arrow*) in this case of **appendicitis. B.** The lumen in this case of appendicitis was dilated owing to a large **fecalith.**

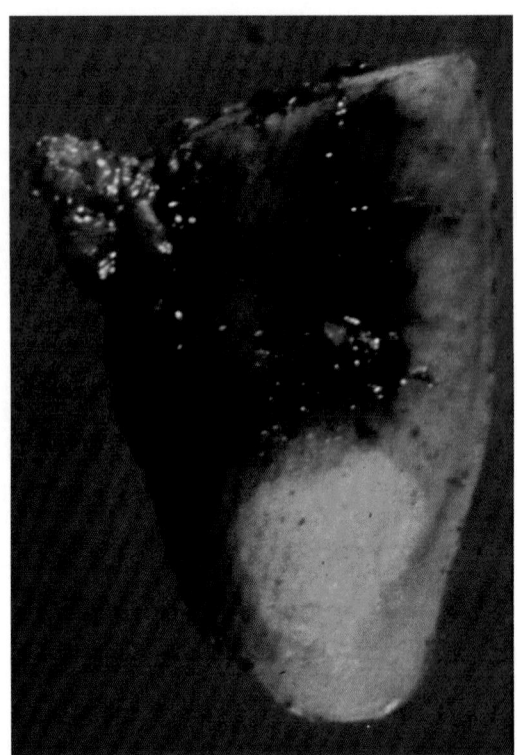

FIGURE 19-62. An oval yellow 1.1-cm **neuroendocrine tumor** was found incidentally in this appendix removed for appendicitis.

followed by a transmural infiltrate of neutrophils. Care must be taken not to confuse an acute inflammatory process centered in the subserosal area with acute appendicitis. Such periappendicitis reflects secondary involvement of the appendix from an external source, such as pelvic inflammatory disease involving the ovary or fallopian tube.

Granulomatous appendicitis may represent involvement by Crohn disease (see above) or an infectious agent. However, most granulomas involving the appendix involve neither of these entities and are of unknown cause and significance.

A **mucocele** is a distended appendix filled with mucinous material. Rarely these are due to inflammation causing focal luminal obstruction; these lesions rarely exceed 2 cm in diameter. More commonly, a dilated mucin-filled appendix reflects a neoplastic process (see below).

APPENDICEAL NEOPLASMS

Appendiceal NETs Are Generally Benign

Neuroendocrine tumors are very common in the appendix. Most such tumors are quite small and benign and are found incidentally at the time of appendectomy. Large amounts of empirical data show that small (<1.5 cm) NETs of the appendix are of no clinical significance.

Most NETs of the appendix arise from ECs. These tumors are almost always under 1 cm in diameter. At this size, the behavior of these tumors is invariably clinically benign. They tend to be oval and located at the tip of the appendix (Fig. 19-62). Tumors between 1 and 2 cm in diameter show a low rate of metastasis (about 1%). Larger lesions are increasingly aggressive.

Epithelial Tumors Are the Most Clinically Important Appendiceal Neoplasms

The nomenclature and classification of appendiceal tumors is controversial and unsettled. Some lesions resemble hyperplastic polyps, adenomas or the serrated lesions of the colon (see below). When these become larger, they tend to resemble hybrids of these forms, accounting for the difficulty in classification.

Regardless of the precise nomenclature, it is important to realize that these are the most clinically important neoplasms of the appendix. They dilate the lumen and expand its length. Resulting structures have been called mucoceles, but these differ radically from the banal lesions described above. A better descriptive term is **cystadenoma** (Fig. 19-63) or **mucinous tumor**. The neoplastic epithelial lining of these

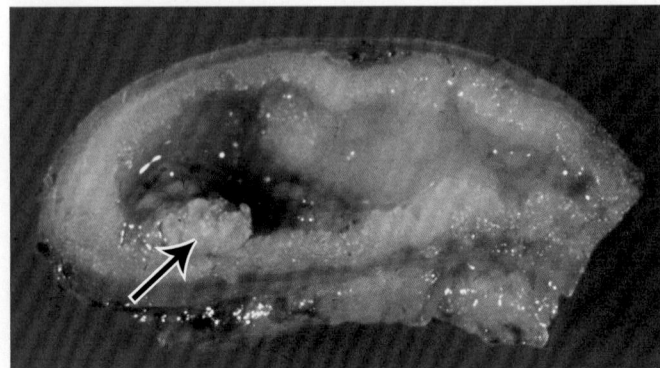

FIGURE 19-63. This **mucinous neoplasm** (*arrow*) has led to the dilatation of the appendix by massive mucin production producing a **cystadenoma.**

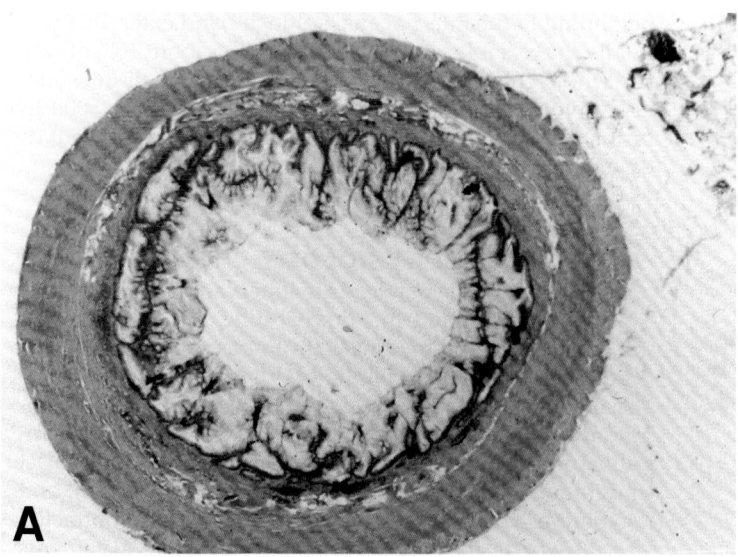
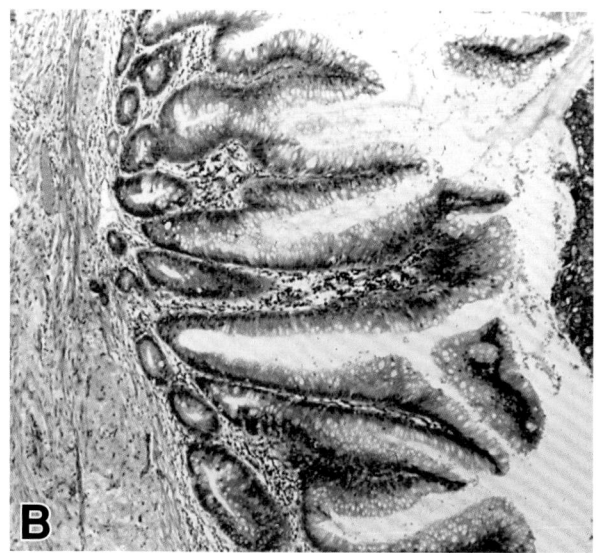

FIGURE 19-64. **A.** The mucinous neoplasm here encircles the entire lumen. **B.** At higher power its peculiar villous configuration is appreciated.

lesions is usually well differentiated (Fig. 19-64A,B) but can invade and penetrate the wall of the appendix. When this happens, abundant mucin may fill the peritoneal cavity, causing a lesion known as **pseudomyxoma peritonei** (Fig. 19-65). Rarely, neoplasms of the pancreas, gallbladder or stomach may cause a similar lesion. Some consider ovary to be another such organ of origin, but these cases usually prove to be appendiceal in origin.

Rarely, frank adenocarcinomas like their colonic counterparts are described.

The Large Intestine

ANATOMY

The large intestine is that portion of the gut from the ileocecal valve to the anus. It is 90–125 cm long in adults and includes the colon and rectum. The proximal colon derives

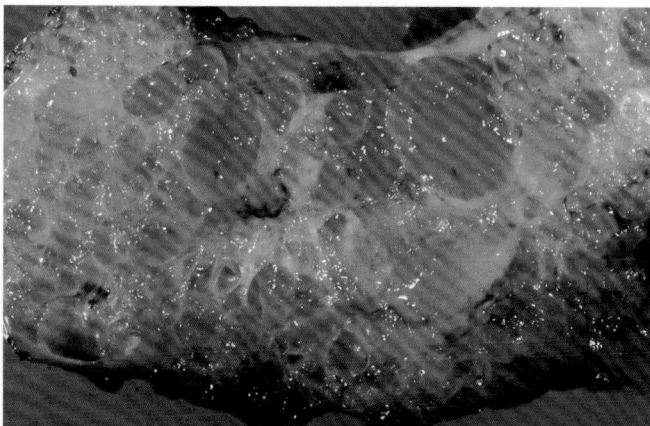

FIGURE 19-65. This large mass of mucin was removed from the abdomen of a patient with **pseudomyxoma peritonei** due to a mucinous tumor of the appendix.

from the embryonic midgut and is supplied by the superior mesenteric artery. The distal large intestine is of embryonic hindgut origin and is supplied by the inferior mesenteric artery. Its main function is to conserve water and salt and to store and dispose of waste material in the form of feces.

MACROSCOPIC FEATURES: The large intestine has six regions, distally from the ileocecal valve: (1) cecum, (2) ascending colon, (3) transverse colon, (4) descending colon, (5) sigmoid colon and (6) rectum. The bend between the ascending and transverse colon in the right upper quadrant is the **hepatic flexure,** and that between the transverse and descending segments in the left upper quadrant is the **splenic flexure**. The lumen progressively narrows from the cecum to the sigmoid colon.

Like the small intestine, the colon has outer longitudinal and inner circular muscle coats. However, in the colon, the longitudinal muscle has three separate bundles, the **taeniae coli**. Evaginations of the colonic wall between taeniae, the **haustra,** appear as external sacculations. The appendices epiploicae are small serosal masses of fat, invested by peritoneum.

The ileocecal valve is a sphincter that regulates the flow of intestinal contents into the cecum. However, it is an incompetent sphincter, and reflux of cecal contents into the ileum is usual. The internal sphincter of the anal canal is continuous with colonic smooth muscle. The external anal sphincter is the major mechanism by which bowel continence is maintained. It surrounds the anal canal with a layer of skeletal muscle. The mucosal surface of the large bowel has prominent folds, which are less pronounced in the rectum.

MICROSCOPIC FEATURES: Colonic mucosa is flat and punctuated by numerous pits, the **crypts of Lieberkühn**. The surface epithelium is primarily simple columnar cells with occasional goblet cells. The crypts mostly contain goblet cells, except at their bases, where a few undifferentiated cells and a variety of neuroendocrine cells are located. The basal undifferentiated cells are the mucosa reserve cells and divide continuously. Mucosal cells migrate from crypt bases toward the luminal surface. Mucosal cells are sloughed, balancing proliferation and maintaining an equilibrium in the crypt epithelial cell population.

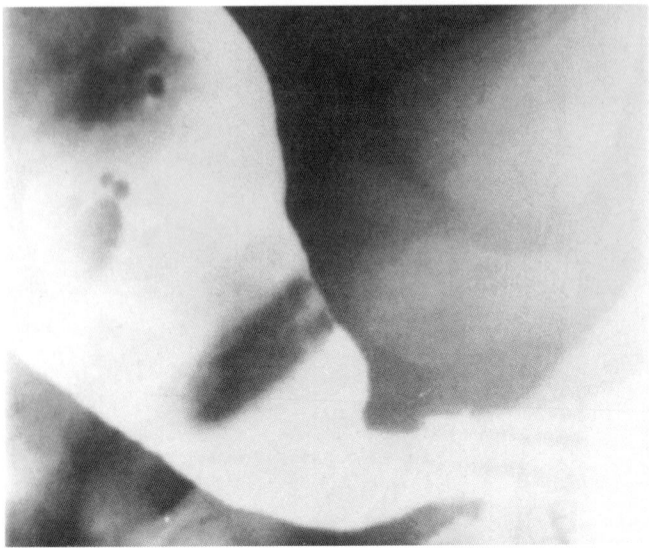

FIGURE 19-66. Hirschsprung disease. A contrast radiograph shows marked dilation of the rectosigmoid colon proximal to the narrowed rectum.

The lamina propria contains lymphocytes, plasma cells, macrophages and fibroblasts, plus occasional eosinophils. Lymphoid aggregates traverse the muscularis mucosae and extend into the submucosa. The submucosa is like that in the small intestine, but lymphatic channels are far less prominent. Colonic lymphatics drain into paracolic nodes in the mesenteric fat, intermediate nodes along the colic blood vessels and central nodes near the aorta. Parasympathetic and sympathetic innervations terminate in Meissner submucosal and Auerbach myenteric plexuses.

CONGENITAL DISORDERS

Hirschsprung Disease Is Due to Segmental Absence of Ganglion Cells

In Hirschsprung disease, colon dilation (Fig. 19-66) is due to defective colorectal innervation: ganglion cells are absent beginning in the internal anal sphincter and extending proximally for variable lengths (Fig. 19-67). In about 10% of cases, the whole colon is aganglionic; rarely, the small intestine is also involved. Hirschsprung disease affects 1 in 5000 live births; 80% of patients are male except in long segment disease where the male:female ratio is equal.

 PATHOPHYSIOLOGY: The developmental sequence that leads to innervation of the colon is interrupted in Hirschsprung disease. The normal caudal migration of cells from the neural crest to the intramural ganglion cells is aborted. Since the internal anal sphincter is at the far end of this migration, the aganglionic segment always starts there. It may extend variably proximally, depending on where primitive neuroblast migration halts. Given that the aganglionic rectum, and sometimes the adjacent colon, are permanently contracted because of the absence of relaxation stimuli, fecal contents cannot readily enter the stenotic area. The proximal bowel becomes dilated because of functional distal obstruction.

MOLECULAR PATHOGENESIS: Most cases of Hirschsprung disease are sporadic, but 10% are familial. Half of familial cases, and 15% of sporadic ones, reflect inactivating mutations of the RET receptor tyrosine kinase gene on chromosome 10q (see MEN2 syndrome, Chapter 27). Some cases involve mutations in the endothelin-B receptor or genes that encode ligands of these two receptors.

The incidence of Hirschsprung disease is 1 in 300 in infants with Down syndrome, and Down syndrome is found in approximately 4% of all patients with Hirschsprung disease. Most cases are solitary lesions, but congenital anomalies of the kidneys and lower urinary tract, as well as imperforate anus and ventricular septal defects, are reported.

PATHOLOGY: The large intestine in Hirschsprung disease has a constricted and spastic aganglionic segment. Proximal to this, the bowel is very dilated. Definitive diagnosis requires demonstrating the

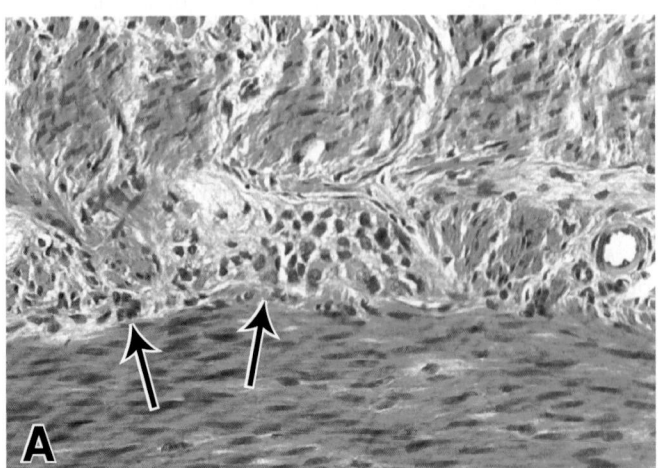
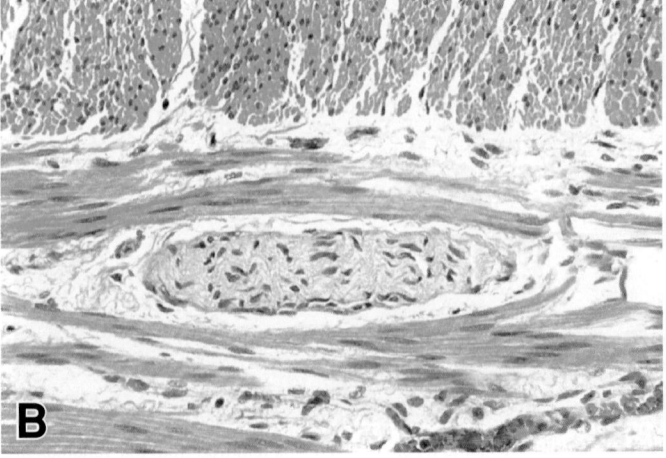

FIGURE 19-67. Hirschsprung disease. A. A photomicrograph of ganglion cells in the wall of a normal rectum (*arrows*). **B.** A rectal biopsy specimen from a patient with Hirschsprung disease shows a nonmyelinated nerve in the mesenteric plexus and an absence of ganglion cells.

absence of ganglion cells on rectal biopsy (Fig. 19-67B). There is also a striking increase in nonmyelinated cholinergic nerve fibers in the submucosa and between muscle coats (neural hyperplasia). The lack of ganglion cells leads to accumulation of acetylcholine and acetylcholinesterase, which are evident using histochemical staining. Calretinin immunohistochemistry aids in diagnosing Hirschsprung disease in rectal suction biopsies. Interestingly, like achalasia, which is caused by destruction of esophageal ganglion cells, Chagas disease may also cause aganglionic megacolon.

 CLINICAL FEATURES: *Hirschsprung disease is the most common cause of congenital intestinal obstruction.* Typically, newborns show delayed passage of meconium and vomiting in the first few days of life. In some cases, complete intestinal obstruction may require immediate surgical relief. Children whose involved rectal segments are short may experience only partial obstruction, constipation, abdominal distention and recurrent fecal impactions.

The most serious complication is enterocolitis, in which necrosis and ulceration affect the dilated proximal segment of the colon and may extend into the small intestine. Hirschsprung disease is treated by surgical removal of the aganglionic segment and reconstruction.

Acquired Megacolon Is Any Cause of Constipation with Colonic Dilatation

Acquired megacolon sometimes occurs in children and often has a psychogenic component. In adults, acquired megacolon can result from disorders that interfere with bowel innervation or smooth muscle function, such as Chagas disease, diabetic neuropathy, Parkinsonism, myotonic dystrophy, scleroderma, amyloidosis and hypothyroidism.

Anorectal Malformations Often Accompany Other Developmental Defects

These malformations vary from minor narrowing to serious and complex defects. They result from arrested development of the caudal region of the gut in the first 6 months of fetal life. These anomalies are now categorized by their precise anatomic anatomy:

- **Anorectal agenesis and rectal atresia.**
- **Anal agenesis and anorectal stenosis.**
- **Imperforate anus** is a deformity in which the anal opening is covered by a cutaneous membrane behind which meconium is visible. **Anal stenosis** is a variant of imperforate anus.
- **Fistulas** between the rectum and perineum, bladder, urethra or vagina may occur alone or in association with other anorectal anomalies.

INFECTIONS OF THE LARGE INTESTINE

The principal infections of the colon, including tuberculosis and amebiasis, are discussed in Chapter 9 or above, in the context of small intestine infectious diarrhea. Most remaining infectious diseases are sexually transmitted and involve the anorectal region, often in men who have sex with men (MSM). These include gonorrhea, syphilis, lymphogranuloma venereum, anorectal herpes and HPV infections (venereal warts or condylomata acuminata). Immunosuppressed people have a high incidence of colonic infections (e.g., amebiasis, shigellosis). Bone marrow transplant recipients are at high risk for contracting CMV and herpesvirus infections involving the colon.

Pseudomembranous Colitis Usually Follows Antibiotic Treatment

Pseudomembranous colitis is a generic term for an inflammatory disease of the colon that is characterized by **exudative mucosal plaques**. It is most often caused by *C. difficile.*

 **ETIOLOGIC FACTORS:** The major risk factor for developing *C. difficile* infection is antibiotic therapy. Virtually all antibiotics have been implicated, although some have been associated with a higher risk. Hospitalization is another major risk factor. About 1%–5% of adults are *C. difficile* carriers, but 30% of hospitalized patients become carriers. In elderly hospitalized patients, *C. difficile* carriage may approach 70%. Immunosuppression and underlying inflammatory bowel disease are also risk factors.

C. difficile is transmitted via the fecal–oral route and is ingested in vegetative form or as spores. When normal protective gut flora are killed by antibiotics, the more resistant *C. difficile* can gain a foothold and begin producing its toxins: toxins A and B. Toxin A activates and recruits inflammatory mediators, and toxin B is directly cytotoxic. *It is important to note that* **C. difficile** *is not invasive and mediates damage via production of toxins.*

Other conditions that can produce pseudomembranes include various diseases of the colon, shock, burns, uremia and chemotherapy.

 PATHOLOGY: The characteristic gross feature is raised yellowish plaques up to 2 cm that adhere to the underlying mucosa (Fig. 19-68). The intervening mucosa is congested and edematous, but not ulcerated. In severe cases, plaques coalesce into extensive pseudomembranes. Superficial epithelial necrosis is believed to be the initial pathologic event. Colonic crypts then become disrupted and expanded by mucin and neutrophils. The pseudomembrane consists of debris from necrotic epithelial cells, mucus, fibrin and neutrophils. In milder cases, well-formed pseudomembranes may be absent and the pathology is more subtle, with focal damage to the surface epithelium.

The entire colon is often involved and sometimes the small intestine is as well. If both small and large bowel are affected, the condition is called **pseudomembranous enterocolitis**. Pseudomembranes occur occasionally in ischemic colitis and in other enteric infections, most notably verotoxin-producing *E. coli.*

 CLINICAL FEATURES: Antibiotic-associated *C. difficile* infections are virtually always accompanied by mild to moderate watery diarrhea, but the disorder does not usually progress to colitis. In patients with pseudomembranous colitis, fever, leukocytosis and abdominal cramps are superimposed on a severe diarrhea that can be bloody. In some cases, the disease can progress to fulminant colitis, which can lead to serious complications such as colonic perforation, toxic megacolon and death.

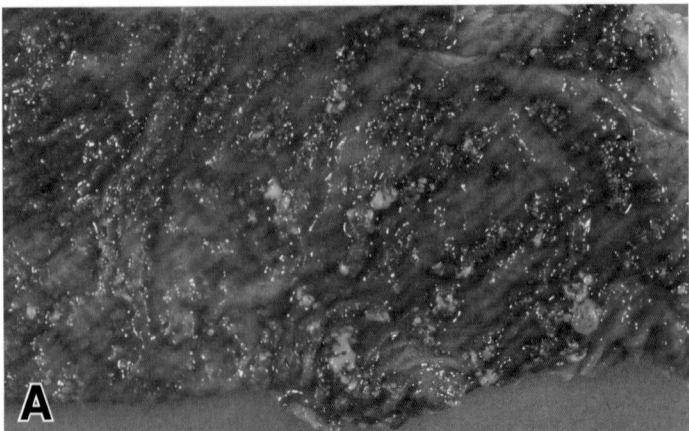
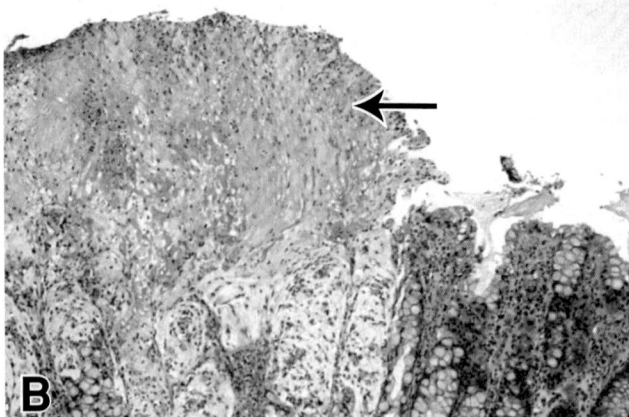

FIGURE 19-68. Pseudomembranous colitis. A. The colon shows variable involvement ranging from erythema to yellow-green areas of pseudomembrane. **B.** Microscopically, the pseudomembrane consists of fibrin, mucin and inflammatory cells (largely neutrophils).

The diagnosis is usually made by identifying toxins in stool by cytotoxin assay, enzyme-linked immunosorbent assay (ELISA) or molecular methods. *C. difficile* infections are treated with antibiotics (metronidazole or vancomycin) and supportive fluid and electrolyte therapy. It is important to withdraw the inciting antibiotic as soon as possible. In cases of fulminant colitis, colectomy may be necessary. *C. difficile* infection recurs in 1/5 of patients. Treatment for patients with multiple recurrences is replenishment of normal gut flora with a **"fecal transplant."** Preventing *C. difficile* transmission in hospitals is critically important in reducing the incidence of the disease.

Neonatal Necrotizing Enterocolitis Complicates Prematurity

Necrotizing enterocolitis is one of the most common acquired surgical emergencies in newborns. It is particularly common in premature infants after oral feeding and is likely related to an ischemic event involving the intestinal mucosa. This event is followed by bacterial colonization, usually with *C. difficile*, which is found in the stool of up to 50% of neonates. Lesions vary from those of typical pseudomembranous enterocolitis to gangrene and perforation of the bowel.

Gastrointestinal Infections Are Common Complications of AIDS

The AIDS epidemic has resulted in many gastrointestinal infections that were once considered rare. Most AIDS patients have chronic diarrhea. Virtually all forms of infectious agents—bacteria, fungi, protozoa and viruses—afflict these patients (Table 19-2).

Kaposi sarcoma in the gut is almost exclusively seen in AIDS patients, and up to half of such patients who have cutaneous Kaposi sarcoma also show digestive tract involvement. In most, intestinal Kaposi sarcoma does produce symptoms, although bleeding, obstruction and malabsorption have been reported.

A common presentation of lymphoma in AIDS patients is involvement of the gastrointestinal tract. Any portion of the gut may be affected. The histology and prognosis of these tumors in AIDS patients are similar to those elsewhere.

DIVERTICULAR DISEASE

Diverticular disease covers two entities: **diverticulosis** and its inflammatory complication, **diverticulitis**.

Diverticulosis Reflects Environmental and Structural Factors

Diverticulosis entails acquired herniation of the mucosa and submucosa through the muscularis propria.

TABLE 19-2
GASTROINTESTINAL PATHOGENS ASSOCIATED WITH AIDS

Bacteria
Mycobacterium avium-intracellulare
Shigella
Salmonella
Clostridium difficile

Viruses
Cytomegalovirus
Herpes simplex

Fungi
Candida
Aspergillus

Protozoa
Cryptosporidium
Toxoplasma
Giardia
Entameba histolytica
Microsporidia
Isospora belli

Helminths
Strongyloides
Enterobius

 **EPIDEMIOLOGY:** Diverticulosis shows striking geographic variability: it is common in Western societies but not in Asia, Africa and underdeveloped countries. Diverticulosis increases in frequency with age and is increasing worldwide.

 **ETIOLOGIC FACTORS:** Because of the striking predominance in developed countries and rising incidence throughout the world, diet and lifestyle changes are thought to play a prominent role in the development of diverticulosis. People who consume a vegetarian diet and/or a diet rich in fiber are at lower risk for diverticular disease than those whose diet is rich in refined carbohydrates and meat.

INCREASED INTRALUMINAL PRESSURE: According to the fiber theory, Western diets lack dietary residue, leading to sustained bowel contraction and thus increased intraluminal pressure. Such prolonged increased pressure may lead to herniation of the mucosa and submucosa of the colon.

DEFECTS IN THE WALL OF THE COLON: In addition to pressure, defects in the colon wall are required. The circular muscle of the colon is interrupted by connective tissue clefts at the sites of penetration by the nutrient vessels that supply the submucosa and mucosa. In older people, this connective tissue loses its resilience and thus its resistance to the effects of increased intraluminal pressure. This concept is supported by the fact that people with heritable connective tissue disorders (e.g., Marfan syndrome, Ehlers-Danlos syndrome) acquire precocious diverticulosis, primarily of the small bowel.

 PATHOLOGY: True diverticula involve all layers of the intestinal wall. In diverticulosis, the structures are actually pseudodiverticula, in which only the mucosa and submucosa are herniated through the muscle layers. The sigmoid colon is affected in 95% of cases, but diverticulosis can affect any segment of the colon, including the cecum. Diverticula vary in number from a few to hundreds. They measure up to 1 cm and are connected to the intestinal lumen by necks of varying length and caliber. The muscular wall of the affected colon is often thickened.

Diverticula are characteristically seen as flask-like structures that extend from the lumen through the muscle layers (Fig. 19-69). Their walls are continuous with the surface mucosa and thus have epithelium *and* submucosa. The outer base is formed by serosal connective tissue.

 CLINICAL FEATURES: *At least 80% of affected individuals are symptom free.* Symptomatic patients complain of episodic colicky abdominal pain. Both constipation and diarrhea, sometimes alternating, may occur, and flatulence is common. Sudden, painless and severe bleeding from colonic diverticula is a cause of serious lower gastrointestinal hemorrhage in the elderly, occurring in as many as 5% of patients with diverticulosis. Chronic blood loss may lead to anemia.

Diverticulitis Is Inflammation at the Base of a Diverticulum

Of patients with diverticulosis, 10%–20% will develop diverticulitis at some point. Acute diverticulitis is believed to be precipitated by irritation due to retained fecal material. This irritation and obstruction lead to inflammation of the diverticulum, which can eventually rupture. Beyond this acute episode, chronic diverticular disease may develop from a combination of abnormal colonic motility, visceral hypersensitivity, imbalance among intestinal flora (called dysbiosis) and chronic inflammation leading to an irritable bowel–like syndrome.

 PATHOLOGY: Diverticulitis produces inflammation of the wall of the diverticulum, which may lead to perforation and release of fecal bacteria into peridiverticular tissues. The resulting abscess is usually contained by the appendices epiploicae and pericolonic adipose tissue. Infrequently, free perforation leads to generalized peritonitis. Fibrosis in response to repeated episodes of diverticulitis may constrict the bowel lumen, causing obstruction. Fistulas may form between the colon and adjacent organs, including the bladder, vagina, small intestine and skin of the abdomen. Additional complications include pylephlebitis and liver abscesses.

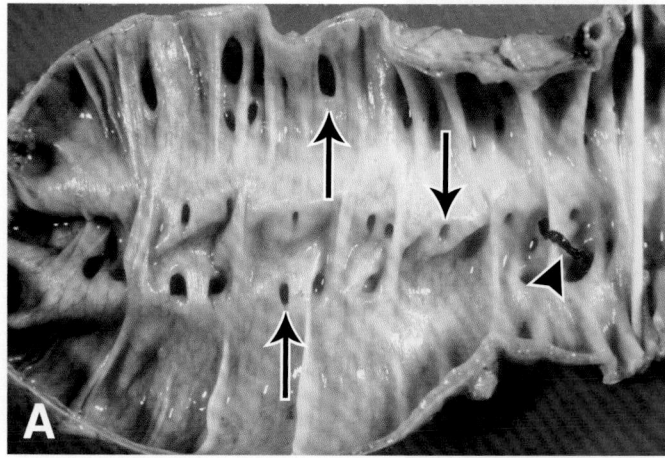 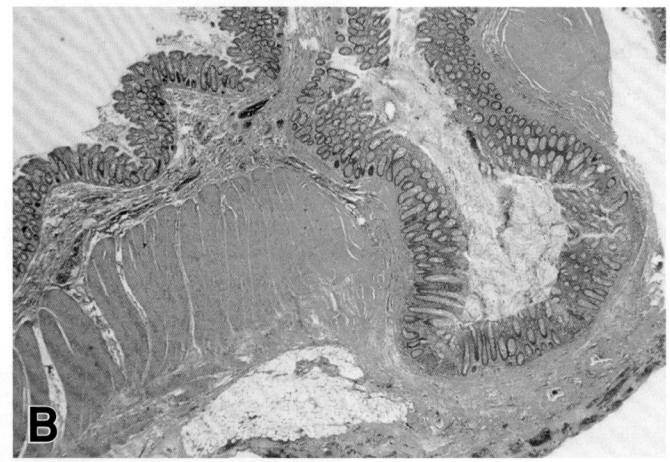

FIGURE 19-69. Diverticulosis of the colon. A. The mouths of numerous diverticula are seen between the taenia (*arrows*). There is a blood clot seen protruding from the mouth of one of the diverticula (*arrowhead*). This was the source of massive gastrointestinal bleeding. **B.** Sections show mucosa including muscularis mucosa and submucosa, which has herniated through a defect in the bowel wall, producing a diverticulum.

CLINICAL FEATURES: The most common symptoms of acute diverticulitis, which usually occur after perforation, are persistent lower abdominal pain and fever. Changes in bowel habits, from diarrhea to constipation, are frequent. Dysuria indicates bladder irritation. Most patients have left lower quadrant tenderness and, often, a palpable mass in that area. Leukocytosis is the rule. Antibiotics and supportive measures usually alleviate acute diverticulitis, but about 20% of patients eventually require surgery. Medical management to prevent subsequent attacks and chronic diverticular disease includes high-fiber diet; long-term, cyclical antibiotic therapy; anti-inflammatory medication (mesalamine); and, potentially, probiotics.

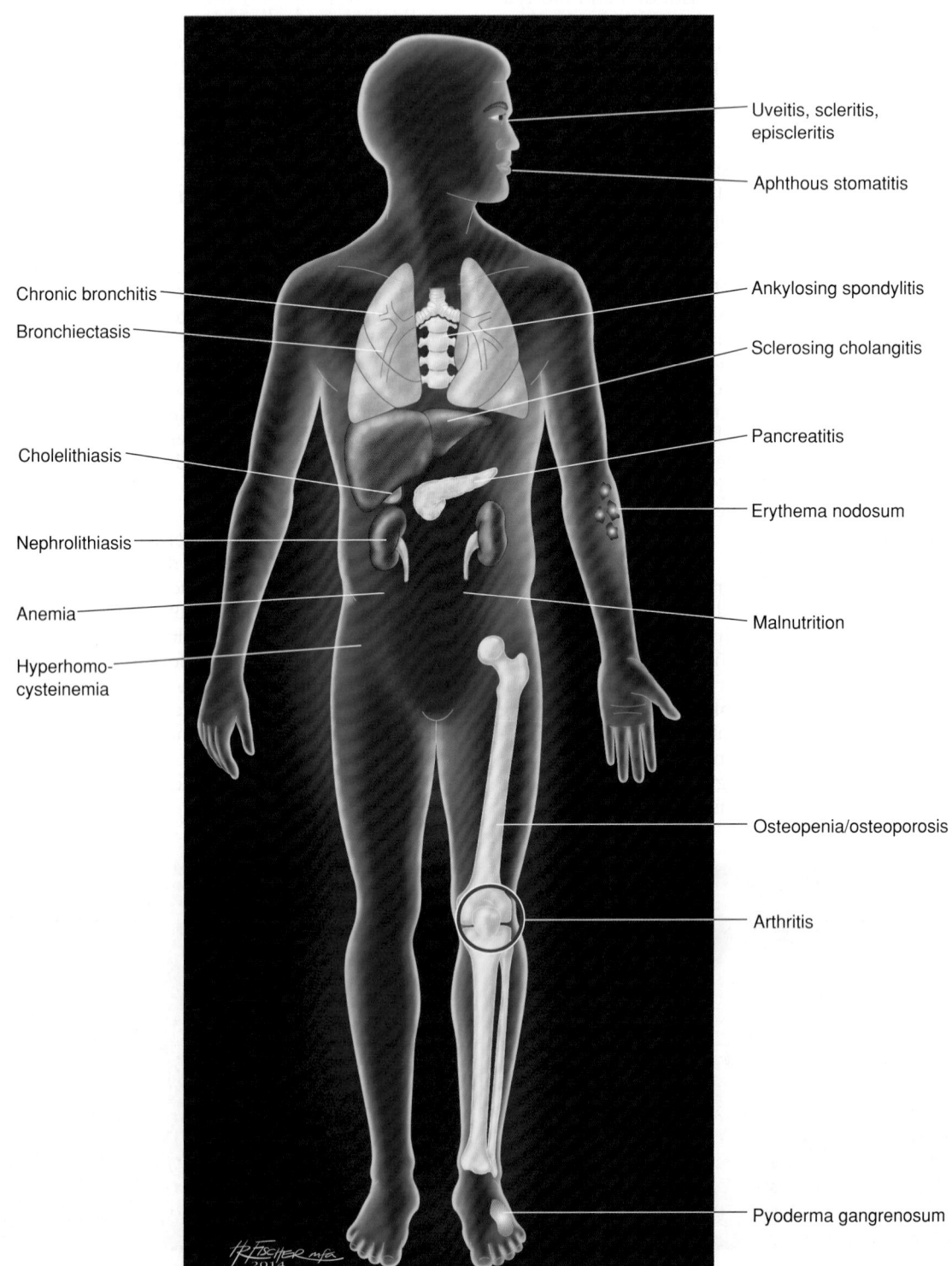

FIGURE 19-70. Systemic complications of inflammatory bowel disease. These conditions are more common with Crohn disease but may also be seen in ulcerative colitis.

INFLAMMATORY BOWEL DISEASE

The term **inflammatory bowel disease** (IBD) encompasses **Crohn disease** and **ulcerative colitis**. These two disorders have certain common features but usually differ enough to be clearly distinguishable. Cases that cannot be distinguished are labeled **indeterminate colitis**.

Both Crohn and ulcerative colitis show histologic features of chronicity including architectural glandular distortion, increased chronic inflammation with or without active neutrophilic inflammation and metaplasia. Extraintestinal complications of IBD are more common with Crohn disease but also occur in ulcerative colitis (Fig. 19-70). While their precise causes are unknown, epidemiologic, clinical and animal studies suggest that mucosal injury accrues from altered immune responses and abnormal interactions of bacteria with intestinal epithelia. The differences between the two diseases are described below.

Crohn Disease Is Chronic Segmental Transmural Intestinal Inflammation

Crohn disease mainly affects the distal small intestine but may involve any part of the digestive tract and even extraintestinal tissues. The colon, particularly the right colon, is often affected.

 **EPIDEMIOLOGY:** Crohn disease has a worldwide incidence of 0.7–14.6 per 100,000 but is more common in developed countries. Its incidence has increased dramatically in the past 30 years, probably owing to a combination of factors related to adoption of a "Western lifestyle." Age distribution is bimodal, with a peak in adolescents or young adults and a second smaller peak in the 50s and 60s. It is most common in people of European origin, with a considerably higher frequency among Ashkenazi Jews. Males predominate among children, but in adults there is a slight female predominance. Smokers are at an increased risk of developing Crohn disease and of having more severe disease, compared with nonsmokers.

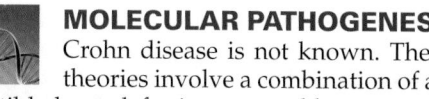 **MOLECULAR PATHOGENESIS:** The cause of Crohn disease is not known. The current leading theories involve a combination of a genetically susceptible host, defective mucosal barrier, intestinal dysbiosis (altered intestinal flora) and inadequate/inappropriate immune response. Genome-wide association studies have identified more than 30 loci that confer susceptibility for Crohn disease, although these account for a minority of cases. Some genetic associations involve genes controlling innate and adaptive immunity. Polymorphisms identified in the innate system are in *NOD2 (CARD15)* and in two genes related to autophagy (*ATG16L1, IRGM*). These defects imply problems in recognition and handling of intracellular bacteria. The T-cell response (adaptive immune system) in Crohn disease involves T_H1 (see Chapter 4), which is mediated by interleukin-12, interferon-γ (IFN-γ) and TNF.

PATHOLOGY: Two key features of Crohn disease differentiate it from other GI inflammatory diseases. First, inflammation usually involves all layers of the bowel wall and is thus referred to as **transmural**. Second, intestinal involvement is discontinuous: areas of inflammation are separated by apparently normal intestine.

Crohn disease may involve different parts of the bowel singly or in combination. It affects the ileum and cecum in half of cases, only the small intestine in 30% and only the colon in 20%. Ileal and cecal disease is more common in younger patients; colitis is common among older patients. Crohn disease sometimes affects the duodenum, stomach and esophagus as focal acute inflammation with or without granulomas. In women with anorectal disease, inflammation may spread to the external genitalia.

The pathology of Crohn disease is highly variable. The bowel and adjacent mesentery are thickened and edematous. Mesenteric fat often surrounds the bowel (so-called creeping fat). Mesenteric lymph nodes are frequently enlarged, firm and matted together. The intestinal lumen is narrowed by edema in early cases and by a combination of edema and fibrosis in long-standing disease. Nodular swelling, fibrosis and mucosal ulceration lead to a "cobblestone" appearance (Fig. 19-71). In early cases, ulcers have either an aphthous or a serpiginous appearance; later they become deeper and appear as linear clefts or fissures (Fig. 19-71B).

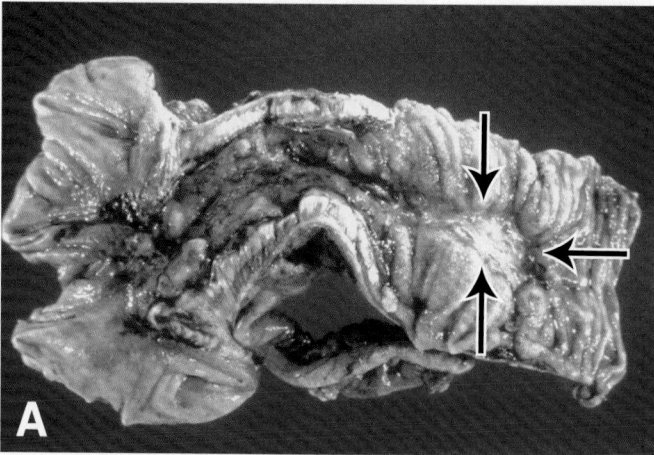
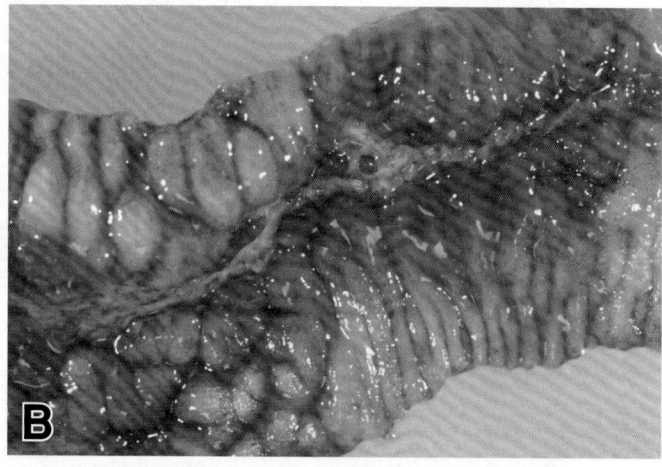

FIGURE 19-71. Crohn disease. A. The terminal ileum shows striking thickening of the wall of the distal portion with distortion of the ileocecal valve. A longitudinal ulcer is present (*arrows*). **B.** Another longitudinal ulcer is seen in this segment of ileum. The large rounded areas of edematous damaged mucosa give a "cobblestone" appearance to the involved mucosa. A portion of the mucosa to the lower right is uninvolved.

The appearance of the bowel wall underscores the fact that the process affects the entire thickness of the bowel wall: there are thickening, edema and fibrosis of all layers. Involved loops of bowel are often adherent. Fistulas may form between such segments. These are late results of deep mural ulcers and may also penetrate from the bowel into, for example, the bladder, uterus, vagina and skin. Most fistulas end blindly, to form abscess cavities in the peritoneum, mesentery or retroperitoneal structures. Lesions in the distal rectum and anus may create perianal fistulas, a well-known presenting feature.

Crohn disease is mainly a chronic inflammatory process. Early in the disease, inflammation may be confined to the mucosa and submucosa. Small, superficial mucosal ulcers (aphthous ulcers) are seen, as are mucosal and submucosal edema and infiltrates of lymphocytes, plasma cells, eosinophils and macrophages. Mucosal architecture is abnormal, often showing regenerative changes in crypts and villous distortion. Pyloric metaplasia and Paneth cell hyperplasia and/or metaplasia are common in the small and large intestines. Later, long, deep, fissure-like ulcers; vascular hyalinization; and fibrosis appear.

Lymphocytes form aggregates throughout the wall and the muscularis mucosae and nerves of the submucosal and myenteric plexuses all proliferate (Fig. 19-72). Discrete, non-caseating granulomas may be present, mostly in the submucosa (Fig. 19-72B). These resemble those of sarcoidosis, with focal aggregates of epithelioid cells, surrounded by a rim of lymphocytes. Multinucleated giant cells may be present. The centers of the granulomas usually have hyaline material but only very rarely necrosis.

Such discrete granulomas strongly suggest Crohn disease. However, their absence does not exclude the diagnosis, as they are present in less than half of cases.

The pathologic features of Crohn disease are summarized in Fig. 19-73.

CLINICAL FEATURES: The clinical manifestations and natural history of Crohn disease are highly variable and reflect the diversity of anatomic sites affected. The most common symptoms are abdominal pain and diarrhea, with passage of blood and/or mucus. Recurrent fever is frequent. If it mainly involves the ileum and cecum, its sudden onset may mimic appendicitis, with right lower quadrant pain, intermittent diarrhea, fever and a tender right lower quadrant mass. When the small intestine is diffusely involved, malabsorption and malnutrition may be major features. Lipid malabsorption may also result from interruption of the enterohepatic cycle of bile salts secondary to ileal disease. Colonic involvement leads to **diarrhea** and sometimes **colonic bleeding**. In a few patients, the major site of involvement may be the anorectal region and recurrent anorectal fistulas may be the presenting sign.

Intestinal obstruction and fistulas are the most common intestinal complications of Crohn disease. Occasionally, free perforation of the bowel occurs. When it begins in childhood, it may slow growth and physical development.

There are many extraintestinal manifestations and associated disorders (Fig. 19-70). Small bowel cancer occurs at least 3-fold more commonly in patients with Crohn disease. Risk of colorectal cancer is also higher, more in patients with more extensive involvement of the colon, a family history of colorectal cancer and/or sclerosing cholangitis.

There is no known cure. Corticosteroids, sulfasalazine, metronidazole, azathioprine, 6-mercaptopurine, methotrexate and anti–TNF-α antibodies such as infliximab may suppress the inflammatory reaction. However, these medications put patients at increased risk for opportunistic infections.

Surgical resection of obstructed or severely involved portions of intestine and drainage of abscesses caused by fistulas are required in some cases. Unfortunately, preanastomotic or prestomal recurrences after an enterostomy is constructed occur often and make clinical management difficult. The

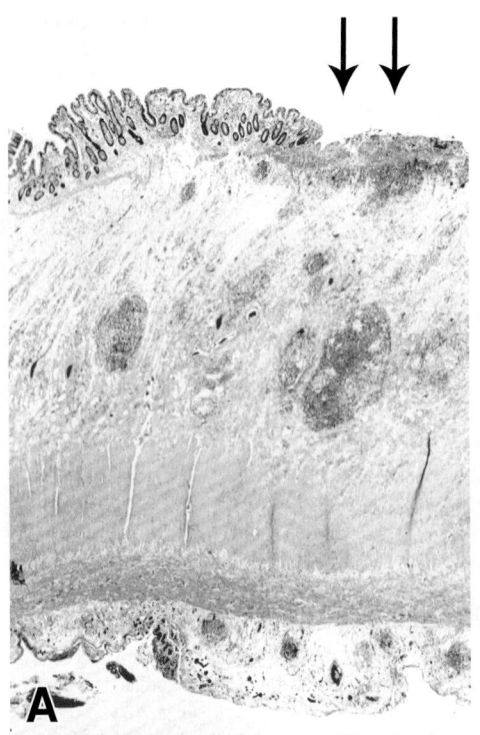

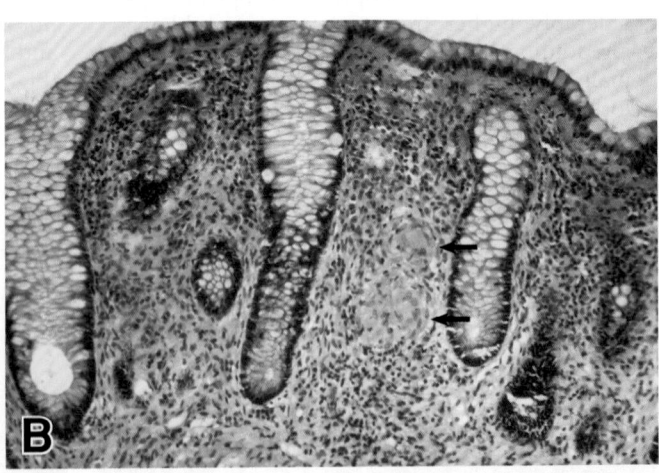

FIGURE 19-72. Crohn disease. A. The colon involved with Crohn disease shows an area of mucosal ulceration, an expanded submucosa with lymphoid aggregates and numerous lymphoid aggregates in the subserosal tissues immediately adjacent to the muscularis propria. **B.** This mucosal biopsy in Crohn disease shows a small epithelioid granuloma (*arrows*) between two intact crypts.

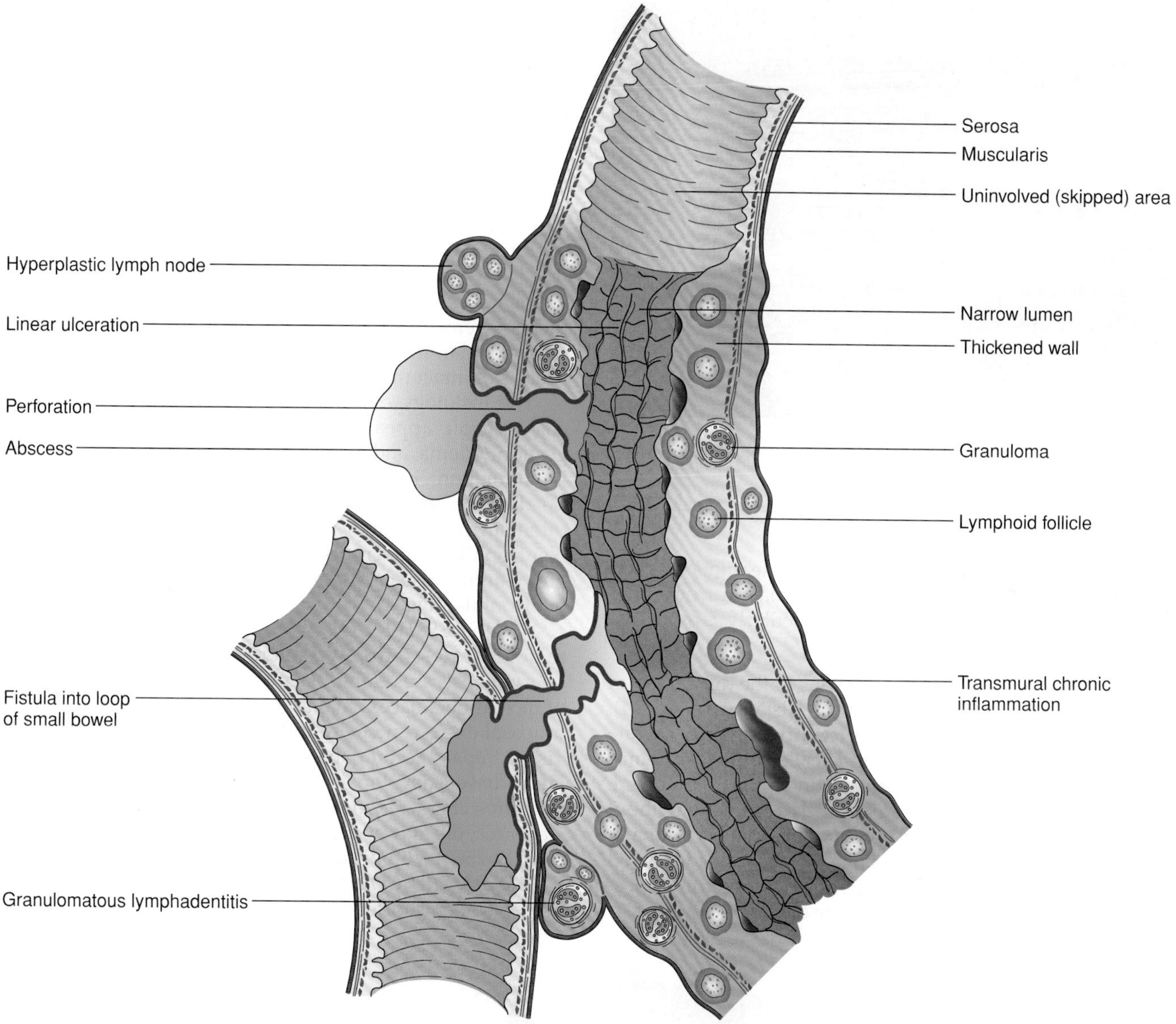

Hyperplastic lymph node

Linear ulceration

Perforation

Abscess

Fistula into loop
of small bowel

Granulomatous lymphadentitis

Serosa

Muscularis

Uninvolved (skipped) area

Narrow lumen

Thickened wall

Granuloma

Lymphoid follicle

Transmural chronic
inflammation

FIGURE 19-73. Crohn disease. A schematic representation of the major features of Crohn disease in the small intestine.

need for repeated resections can lead to short-bowel syndrome in some patients.

Additional adjunct therapies that show possible benefit in small series include dietary modifications, antibiotics, probiotics and fecal transplant.

Ulcerative Colitis Is Chronic, Superficial Inflammation of the Colon and Rectum

It is characterized by chronic diarrhea and rectal bleeding, with episodic exacerbations and remissions.

 **EPIDEMIOLOGY:** Worldwide, ulcerative colitis incidence ranges from 1.5 to 24.5 per 100,000 and occurs more often in developed countries. Like Crohn disease, its incidence is increasing in countries that adopt "Western" lifestyles, suggesting that environmental factors may contribute to the pathogenesis of the disease. It also has a bimodal age distribution, with a peak from 15 to 30 years and another between 50 and 70. In the United States,

whites are affected more than blacks. Smoking seems to inhibit development of ulcerative colitis, but ex-smokers are at an increased risk. People with a family history of IBD have a higher risk of developing ulcerative colitis, although this relationship is not as strong as that in Crohn disease.

MOLECULAR PATHOGENESIS: *The cause of ulcerative colitis is unknown.* Leading theories suggest that genetically predisposed individuals develop dysregulated mucosal immune responses to gut flora, leading to bowel inflammation. Over 40 susceptibility loci are associated with ulcerative colitis. Of these, 20 overlap with Crohn disease. Some encode proteins involved in epithelial cell adhesion and so perhaps contribute to mucosal barrier dysfunction. The T-cell response in ulcerative colitis is T_H2 dominant and mediated by natural killer T cells. This combination of factors leads to mucosal hyperresponsiveness to commensal bacteria and an exaggerated immune response causing chronic inflammation and damage.

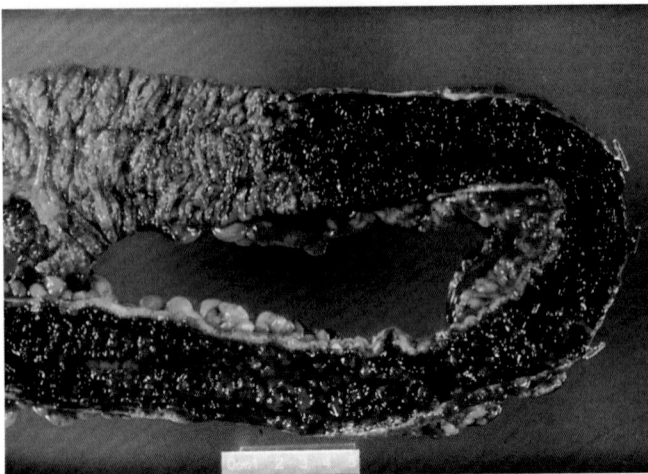

FIGURE 19-74. Ulcerative colitis. Prominent erythema and ulceration of the colon begins in and are most severe in the rectosigmoid area and extend into the ascending colon.

 PATHOLOGY: Major pathologic features of ulcerative colitis that help to differentiate it from other inflammatory conditions, particularly Crohn disease, are:

- **Ulcerative colitis is diffuse.** It begins in the distal rectum and extends proximally for a variable distance (Fig. 19-74). Isolated rectal involvement is **ulcerative proctitis,** while extension to the splenic flexure is called **proctosigmoiditis** or **left-sided colitis.** If the entire colon is involved, it is called **pancolitis.** The disease is confluent without skip lesions. The exception to this rule is that occasionally patients with left-sided colitis may have an area involved in the cecum, a "cecal patch." Sparing of the rectum is possible but should raise the possibility of Crohn disease.

- **Inflammation in ulcerative colitis is limited to the colon and rectum.** If the cecum is affected, the disease ends at the ileocecal valve, although minor inflammation of the adjacent ileum **(backwash ileitis)** may sometimes occur.
- **Ulcerative colitis is a mucosal disease.** Deeper layers are involved mainly in infrequent fulminant cases and are usually associated with toxic megacolon.

This morphologic sequence may develop rapidly or it may take years.

EARLY COLITIS: Early in the disease, the mucosal surface is raw, red and granular. It is frequently covered with a yellowish exudate and bleeds easily. Later, small superficial ulcers or erosions may appear. These occasionally coalesce into irregular, shallow, ulcerated areas that seem to surround islands of intact mucosa.

The histology of early ulcerative colitis correlates with colonoscopic appearances and includes (1) mucosal congestion, edema and tiny hemorrhages; (2) diffuse chronic inflammation in the lamina propria (Fig. 19-75); and (3) damage and distortion of colorectal crypts, which are often surrounded and infiltrated by neutrophils (cryptitis). Neutrophils in the crypts and suppurative necrosis of crypt epithelium cause crypt abscesses (dilated crypts filled with neutrophils) (Fig. 19-75B).

PROGRESSIVE COLITIS: As disease progresses, mucosal folds are lost (atrophy). Lateral extension and coalescence of crypt abscesses can undermine the mucosa, leaving areas of ulceration adjacent to hanging fragments of mucosa. Such mucosal excrescences are inflammatory polyps (Fig. 19-76). Tissue repair accompanies tissue destruction, and granulation tissue develops in denuded areas. Importantly, the strictures characteristic of Crohn disease are absent. In late stages, crypts may appear tortuous, branched and shortened (Fig. 19-75C), with diffuse mucosal atrophy.

ADVANCED COLITIS: In long-standing cases, the large bowel is often shortened, especially on the left side. Mucosal

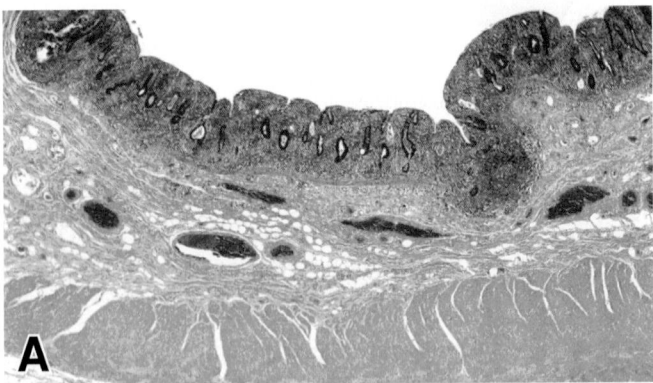

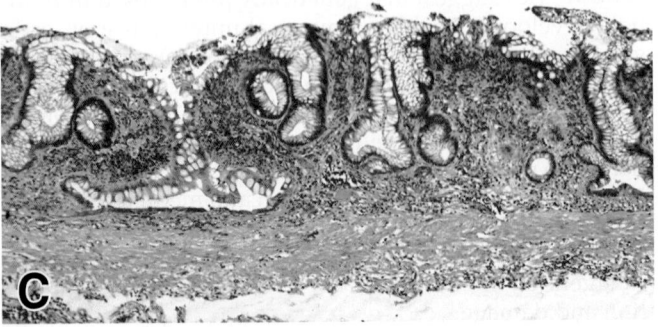

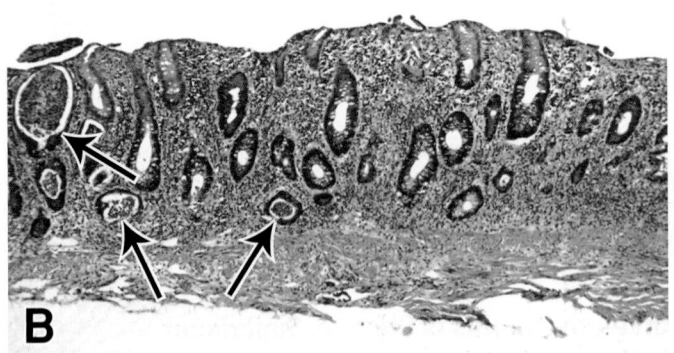

FIGURE 19-75. Ulcerative colitis. A. A full-thickness section of colon resected for ulcerative colitis shows inflammation affecting the mucosa with sparing of the submucosa and muscularis propria. **B.** A mucosal biopsy from a patient with active ulcerative colitis shows expansion of the lamina propria and several crypt abscesses (*arrows*). **C.** Chronic ulcerative colitis shows significant crypt distortion and atrophy.

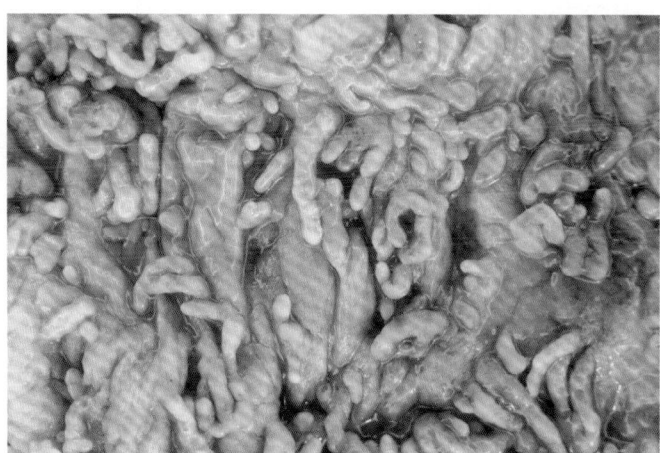

FIGURE 19-76. Inflammatory polyps of the colon in ulcerative colitis. Nodules of regenerative mucosa and inflammation surrounded by denuded areas provide a diffuse polypoid appearance of the mucosa.

folds are indistinct and are replaced by a granular or smooth mucosal pattern. In advanced ulcerative colitis, mucosal atrophy and chronic inflammation are present in the mucosa and superficial submucosa. Paneth cell metaplasia is common.

The pathologic features of ulcerative colitis are summarized in Fig. 19-77B.

CLINICAL FEATURES: The clinical course and manifestations are quite variable. Most patients have intermittent attacks, with partial or complete remissions in between. A few (<10%) have a very long remission (several years) after their first attack. About 20% have continuous symptoms without remission.

MILD COLITIS: Half of patients with ulcerative colitis have mild disease. Their major symptom is rectal bleeding, sometimes with **tenesmus** (rectal pressure and discomfort). In these patients, disease is usually limited to the rectum but may extend to the distal sigmoid colon. Extraintestinal complications are uncommon. In most patients in this category, the disease remains mild throughout their lives.

MODERATE COLITIS: About 40% of patients have moderate disease. They usually have episodic loose bloody stools, crampy abdominal pain and often low-grade fever, lasting days or weeks. Anemia is commonly due to chronic fecal blood loss.

SEVERE COLITIS: About 10% of patients have severe or fulminant disease. The disease may start out this way, but more often severe colitis supervenes during a flare of activity. They have many (sometimes >20) bloody bowel movements daily, often with fever and other systemic symptoms. Blood and fluid loss rapidly lead to anemia, dehydration and electrolyte depletion. Massive hemorrhage may be life-threatening. Toxic megacolon—extreme dilation of the colon that carries a high risk for perforation—is particularly dangerous. Fulminant ulcerative colitis is a medical emergency. It requires immediate, intensive medical therapy and, sometimes, prompt colectomy. Despite aggressive management, some patients with fulminant disease die.

The medical treatment of ulcerative colitis depends on the sites involved and the severity of the inflammation. The 5-aminosalicylate–based compounds (e.g., mesalazine) are mainstays of treatment for patients with mild to moderate disease. Corticosteroids and immunosuppressive/immunoregulatory agents (azathioprine, ciclosporin or anti–TNF-α agents) are used in patients with severe and refractory disease. Because infection with *C. difficile* or CMV can precipitate or exacerbate an attack of ulcerative colitis, these should be ruled out and treated if identified. There may be some benefit of fecal transplant in patients with refractory disease.

Differential Diagnosis

The most important conditions to be distinguished from ulcerative colitis are other forms of chronic colitis due to specifically treatable causes, and Crohn disease. Other conditions in the differential diagnosis of ulcerative colitis are bacterial infections and amebic colitis, especially in areas where it is endemic. If inflammation is limited to the rectum, other infectious agents, including viruses, chlamydia, fungi and other parasites, merit consideration. Proctitis due to these agents is common in MSM and a variety of opportunistic bowel infections occur in patients with AIDS (see above). Other conditions that may mimic ulcerative colitis are ischemic colitis, antibiotic-associated colitis, radiation injury and solitary rectal ulcer syndrome.

The distinction between ulcerative colitis and Crohn colitis is based on different anatomic localization and histopathology (Table 19-3). Ulcerative colitis is a diffuse process, usually more severe distally, while Crohn colitis is patchy or segmental and often spares the rectum. Inflammation in ulcerative colitis is superficial (i.e., usually limited to the mucosa), but that in Crohn colitis is transmural and involves all layers, with granulomas in some of the specimens.

If disease stops at the ileocecal valve or is limited to the distal colon, ulcerative colitis is more likely. Involvement of the terminal ileum suggests Crohn colitis, unless there is pancolitis with backwash ileitis.

In 10% of cases, definitive discrimination is impossible and the disease is denoted as indeterminate colitis. This occurs mostly in fulminant colitis.

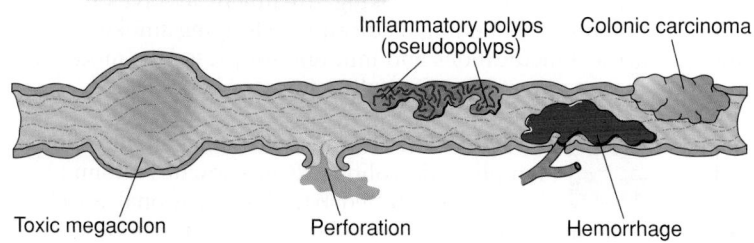

LOCAL COMPLICATIONS

Inflammatory polyps (pseudopolyps)

Colonic carcinoma

Toxic megacolon

Perforation

Hemorrhage

FIGURE 19-77. Ulcerative colitis. A schematic representation of the major features of ulcerative colitis in the colon.

TABLE 19-3

COMPARISON OF THE PATHOLOGIC FEATURES IN THE COLON OF CROHN DISEASE AND ULCERATIVE COLITIS

Lesion	Crohn Disease	Ulcerative Colitis
Macroscopic		
Thickened bowel wall	Typical	Uncommon
Luminal narrowing	Typical	Uncommon
"Skip" lesions	Common	Absent
Right colon predominance	Typical	Absent
Fissures and fistulas	Common	Absent
Circumscribed ulcers	Common	Absent
Confluent linear ulcers	Common	Absent
Inflammatory polyps	Absent	Common
Microscopic		
Transmural inflammation	Typical	Rare
Submucosal fibrosis	Typical	Absent
Fissures	Typical	Rare
Granulomas	Common	Absent
Crypt abscesses	Typical	Typical

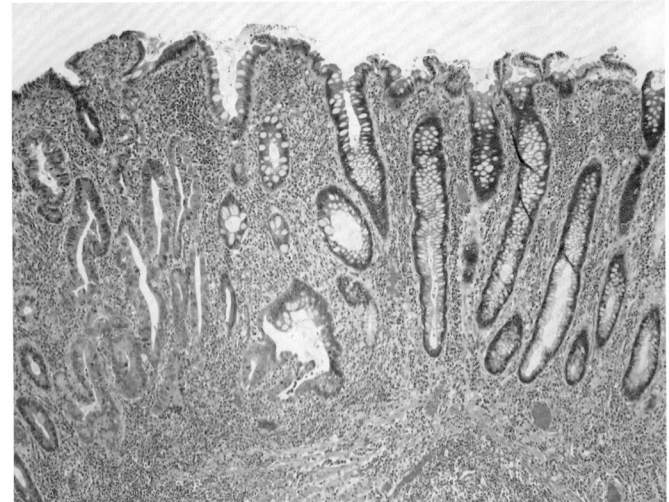

FIGURE 19-78. Dysplasia in ulcerative colitis. The colonic mucosa shows the chronic changes of ulcerative colitis (see Fig. 19-53C). The crypts to the left are dysplastic, showing architectural distortion, hyperchromatic nuclei and lack of glandular maturation.

Distinguishing between ulcerative colitis and Crohn colitis is important because (1) surgical approaches are different (Crohn disease often recurs, so continent ileostomy and ileoanal pouches may be contraindicated), (2) ulcerative colitis carries a higher risk of cancer and (3) medical treatments differ.

Ulcerative Colitis and Colorectal Cancer

Patients with long-standing ulcerative colitis have a much higher risk of colorectal cancer than does the general population. The magnitude of this increased risk is related to the extent and duration of the disease. It is greater if the entire colon is involved. If inflammation is limited to the rectum, the risk of colorectal cancer is like that of the general population. After 10 years with ulcerative colitis, chances for colorectal cancer are estimated to be 2% after 10 years of disease, 8% after 20 years and 18% after 30 years. Patients with ulcerative colitis who develop primary sclerosing cholangitis are at a higher risk of dysplasia and colorectal cancer.

Colorectal epithelial dysplasia is a neoplastic epithelial proliferation and precursor to colorectal carcinoma (Fig. 19-78). The dysplasia can be flat, adenoma-like or a non–adenoma-like lesion called dysplasia-associated lesion or mass (DALM), based on its endoscopic appearance. Epithelial dysplasia entails variation in nuclear size, shape and staining qualities and may be low grade or high grade, depending on the degree of cytologic organd architectural atypia. Extensive inflammation may preclude a definitive

diagnosis of dysplasia, in which case the term "indefinite for dysplasia" is used. High-grade dysplasia has a high risk for eventual colorectal cancer. When identified in a biopsy, it is a strong indication for colectomy.

The appropriate follow-up for low-grade dysplasia is controversial. Routine colonoscopy and biopsy of all patients with ulcerative colitis are recommended after 8–10 years of pancolitis, after 15 years of left-sided colitis or immediately in patients with primary sclerosing cholangitis. Newer technologies such as chromoendoscopy (applying a topical dye to the mucosa during endoscopy) or confocal laser endomicroscopy (enhancing magnification of the endoscopic picture down to the cellular level) may increase biopsy yields of dysplastic lesions via colonoscopy. With surveillance endoscopy with routine biopsies and chemoprevention to reduce inflammation, dysplasia and cancer risk can be reduced.

Microscopic Colitis Causes Chronic Diarrhea

This entity encompasses lymphocytic colitis and collagenous colitis, which can be distinguished histologically. The incidence of microscopic colitis has been increasing over the past 20 years. At least part of this increase reflects greater awareness of the disease. The main presenting symptom is chronic watery diarrhea. Patients may also have abdominal pain and weight loss, which are typically mild.

Microscopic colitis is so named because the colon appears grossly normal and only microscopic evaluation reveals an abnormality. The disease increases with age, is more common in women and is associated with some medications, autoimmune diseases and smoking. Treatment involves removing potentially offending medications, stopping smoking, antidiarrheal medications and immune suppressants/modulators. In rare refractory cases, colectomy may be indicated.

 ETIOLOGY: The causes for collagenous colitis and lymphocytic colitis are unknown. Autoimmunity has been suggested, based on occasional association with autoimmune diseases such as rheumatoid arthritis,

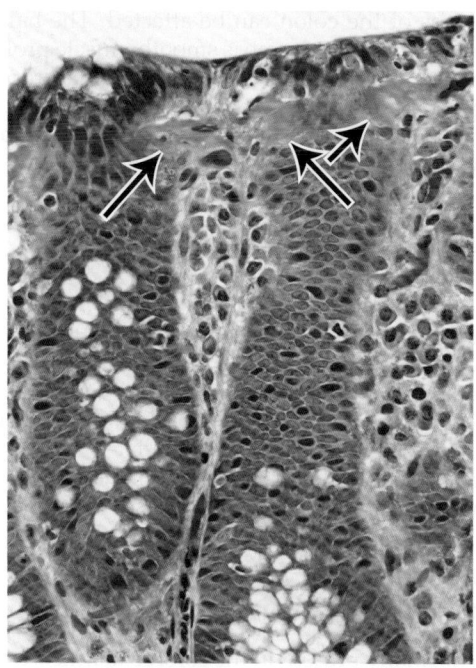

FIGURE 19-79. Collagenous colitis. A trichrome stain highlights the characteristic thickening of the collagen table (*blue*, note *arrows*) with entrapment of capillaries. The intercryptal surface epithelium is flattened and contains an increased number of intraepithelial lymphocytes.

thyroid dysfunction and psoriasis. Microscopic colitis is also frequently associated with celiac disease. Several medications are associated with both diseases; most are NSAIDs, but whether this association is causal or incidental is unclear, as many of these patients use NSAIDs for arthralgias.

 PATHOLOGY: Lymphocytic colitis has surface damage with increased intraepithelial lymphocytes (>20 per 100 epithelial cells). Chronic inflammation of the lamina propria is increased, and typically more prominent more superficially. Mild acute inflammation may also be present. Gland architecture is normal, unlike IBD, as is the collagen table. Changes may be more pronounced in the right colon, so random biopsies of the whole colon are useful in evaluating microscopic colitis.

Collagenous colitis typically shows similar changes to the colonic mucosa as lymphocytic colitis (normal architecture, surface damage, increased lamina propria inflammation, intraepithelial lymphocytosis), plus an irregularly thickened subepithelial collagen band, usually greater than 10 μm, which entraps capillaries (Fig. 19-79). The collagen table is usually thickened irregularly, and thus multiple biopsies may be needed to make this diagnosis (Fig. 19-79).

VASCULAR DISEASES

Extensive Infarction of the Colon is Uncommon

Segmental, and sometimes chronic, ischemic disease is the rule. *The parts of the colon most vulnerable to nonocclusive ischemia (usually due to hypotension) are areas between adjacent arterial distributions, so-called watershed areas.* For example, the splenic flexure is between the

regions supplied by the superior and inferior mesenteric arteries. Also, the rectosigmoid area shares blood from the inferior mesenteric and internal iliac arteries. The rectum itself, however, is usually spared because it has a dual blood supply, from the splanchnic and systemic arterial systems. Most cases of ischemic colitis are caused by atherosclerosis of major intestinal arteries, and recurrent bouts of abdominal pain due to ischemic colitis are called **intestinal angina**. Increasing age, especially older than 65 years, and female gender are risk factors. Patients with IBD may have reduced bowel perfusion and thus develop ischemic injury.

Infections with *E. coli* O157:H7 and *Shigella* spp. can cause ischemic injury via direct toxin damage to vascular endothelium. Thrombophilic states, several prescription medications and the illicit drug cocaine also increase the risk of ischemic bowel disease.

PATHOLOGY: On endoscopy, multiple ulcers, hemorrhagic nodular lesions or a pseudomembrane may be seen. Biopsy shows ischemic necrosis: coagulative necrosis of surface epithelium with ghost cells, mucosal ulceration, crypt abscesses, edema and hemorrhage (Fig. 19-80). In more severe cases, necrosis affects deeper layers of bowel and can evolve to full-thickness necrosis. Patients may recover completely or develop a stricture, in which case surgical removal of the obstructed segment may be necessary. Segments of ischemic stricture show variable mucosal ulceration and inflammation, submucosal granulation tissue, fibrosis and hemosiderin-laden macrophages.

CLINICAL FEATURES: Acute bowel ischemia usually presents with bright red blood in stools or with maroon stools, depending on the location of the bleeding. Patients without bleeding may have a worse prognosis. Ischemic colitis may be indistinguishable clinically from other forms of colitis (infectious, IBD). Prognosis and treatment depend on the primary cause and extent of involvement. The goal is to improve blood supply to the colon by treating patients' overall cardiovascular status and providing bowel rest. There may also be a role for antibiotics. In severe cases, mortality exceeds 50%, and urgent removal of the involved bowel may be necessary.

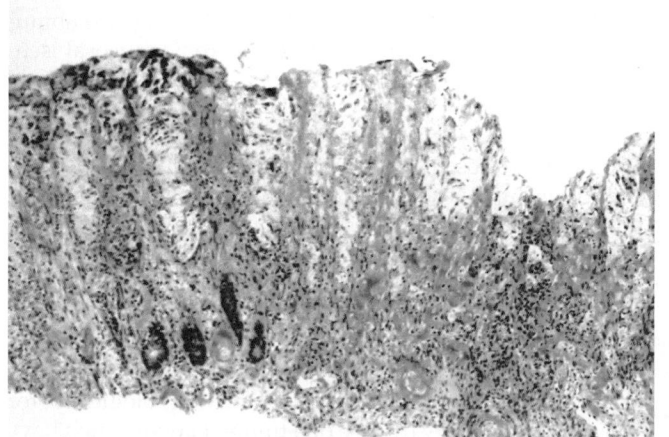

FIGURE 19-80. Ischemic colitis. A mucosal biopsy shows coagulative necrosis with "ghostly" outlines of the preexisting crypts. Only a small portion of the base of several crypts remains.

Angiodysplasia (Vascular Ectasia) May Cause Intestinal Bleeding

Angiodysplasia (vascular ectasia) is localized arteriovenous malformations, mainly in the cecum and ascending colon. These may cause lower intestinal bleeding, especially in people over 60. Younger people may have lesions at other sites, including the rectum, stomach and small bowel. Aortic valvular disease may be associated in some cases.

It has been suggested that angiodysplasia results from chronic intestinal circulatory insufficiency, intestinal muscle hypertrophy and consequent venous obstruction. Patients complain of multiple bleeding episodes, but chronic bleeding may also be occult. Radiologic studies and examination at laparotomy are usually negative. Thus, the diagnosis is difficult and often requires selective mesenteric arteriography or colonoscopy. Colonoscopic interventions are usually sufficient to stop the bleeding, but surgical removal of the affected segment may be necessary in some cases.

 PATHOLOGY: The resected specimen often has multiple vascular lesions, usually less than 0.5 cm. Submucosal veins and capillaries are tortuous, thin walled and dilated. These vessels have attenuated walls, presumably accounting for their propensity to bleed.

RADIATION ENTEROCOLITIS

Radiation therapy for malignancies in the pelvis or abdomen may be complicated by injury to the small intestine (radiation enteritis) and colon (radiation colitis).

 PATHOLOGY: Clinically significant radiation colitis occurs most often in the rectum (radiation proctitis). Lesions vary from reversible intestinal mucosal injury to chronic inflammation, ulceration and fibrosis of the intestine. In the short term, radiation damages epithelium and endothelium, impairs normal bowel mucosal renewal and, in the small bowel, leads to villous shortening. Mucosal inflammation is conspicuous and abscesses may be seen in colonic crypts. Failure of epithelial renewal may lead to ulceration. Chronic changes occur 9–14 months after radiation therapy, after the mucosa has healed. Damage to submucosal vessels leads to thrombosis and chronic mucosal ischemia. The submucosa becomes fibrotic and often has bizarre fibroblasts.

Complications of radiation enterocolitis include perforation and subsequent development of internal fistulas, hemorrhage and strictures. These may be severe enough to obstruct the intestines.

SOLITARY RECTAL ULCER SYNDROME

Internal rectal mucosal prolapse can cause mucosal changes that are easily mistaken clinically and pathologically for chronic inflammatory disease or a tumor. Patients often have a history of severe straining during defecation. Despite the name, some patients have no ulcers, while others have multiple erosions, ulcers or even polypoid lesions/masses that can simulate a neoplasm. While often found in the rectum, other regions of the colon can be affected. The hallmark of solitary rectal ulcer syndrome is smooth muscle proliferation from the muscularis mucosae into the lamina propria often with accompanying mucosal hyperplastic changes. Dilated glands can be trapped in the rectal wall, a condition called **colitis cystica profunda**.

POLYPS OF THE COLON AND RECTUM

A gastrointestinal polyp is a mass that protrudes into the gut lumen. Polyps are classified by their attachment to the bowel wall (e.g., sessile, or pedunculated with a discrete stalk), their histology (e.g., hyperplastic or adenomatous) and their neoplastic potential (i.e., benign or malignant). By themselves, polyps are not usually symptomatic and their clinical importance lies in their potential for malignant transformation.

Lymphoid Polyps Are Solitary Submucosal Lymphoid Accumulations

They are normally present in the colorectal mucosa and vary in size from pinpoint to up to 5 cm. On occasion, multiple lesions impart a cobblestone appearance to the mucosa. They are covered by intact mucosa and contain prominent lymphoid follicles with germinal centers. Lymphoid polyps are benign and usually asymptomatic.

Nodular lymphoid hyperplasia occurs mainly in children or patients with **common variable immunodeficiency syndrome** (see Chapter 4) and is characterized by excessive accumulation of normal colonic lymphoid follicles. The condition is rarely related to malignant lymphoma, but its radiologic appearance can be mistaken for FAP.

Inflammatory Polyps Are Elevated Areas of Inflamed, Regenerating Epithelium

They are commonly found in patients with ulcerative colitis and Crohn disease but may result from any cause of colitis. They also occur without demonstrable colonic disease and may be related to prior, resolved acute/infectious colitis. These polyps have variable components of distorted and inflamed mucosal glands, often intermixed with granulation tissue. They are not precancerous but must thus be distinguished from adenomatous polyps, which are potentially precancerous (see below).

Hamartomatous Polyps Typically Have Both Stromal and Epithelial Elements

They are composed of an overgrowth of cells and tissue native to the anatomic location. They occur sporadically and may also be associated with a variety of syndromes.

Juvenile Polyps (Retention Polyps)

Juvenile polyps occur most commonly in children younger than 10 years, although 1/3 may be in adults. They develop sporadically or may be part of a polyposis syndrome. When sporadic, they typically arise in the rectum and present with rectal bleeding or with the polyp prolapsing through the rectum.

A juvenile polyposis syndrome can be diagnosed if there are:

1. Five or more juvenile polyps in the colorectum
2. Juvenile polyps occurring outside the colon
3. Any number of juvenile polyps, plus a family history of juvenile polyposis

 **MOLECULAR PATHOGENESIS:** Mutations of *SMAD4* or *BMPR1A*, which affect the TGF-β pathway, have been identified in some families with this syndrome. However, 30%–40% of patients do not have an identified mutation. Patients with juvenile polyposis syndrome have an increased risk for gastrointestinal and pancreatic carcinomas. By contrast, people who present with sporadic juvenile polyps do not have an increased risk of malignancy.

 PATHOLOGY: Juvenile polyps are single or (rarely) multiple. They occur mostly in the rectum but may be anywhere in the small or large bowel. Most are pedunculated lesions up to 2 cm, with smooth, rounded surfaces. Dilated and cystic epithelial tubules are filled with mucus and inflammatory cells and are embedded in a fibrovascular lamina propria (Fig. 19-81). Surface epithelial erosion with underlying granulation tissue is common, as is reactive epithelial proliferation. But the epithelium usually lacks dysplasia.

Peutz-Jeghers Syndrome

This is a rare, autosomal dominant syndrome with variable penetrance. It may entail polyps anywhere in the GI tract and has been described above.

Cowden Syndrome

This syndrome is associated with germline *PTEN* mutations (see Chapter 5), is rare and is inherited as an autosomal dominant trait, with near-complete penetrance. These patients develop hamartomas of the skin, intestine, breast and thyroid gland. Gastrointestinal polyps in these patients are indistinguishable in appearance from juvenile polyps. Thus, the diagnosis of Cowden syndrome is made clinically and by identifying extraintestinal manifestations. Patients with Cowden syndrome are at increased risk of developing breast, thyroid, ovarian, cervical, uterine and bladder cancers as well as meningiomas (see Chapter 32). They do not appear to be at increased risk of gastrointestinal cancers.

Cronkhite-Canada Syndrome

Cronkhite-Canada syndrome is characterized by hamartomatous polyps of the GI tract, indistinguishable from juvenile polyps. However, unlike juvenile polyposis or Cowden syndrome, these polyps show changes in the mucosa between polyps (edema, cystically dilated glands, increased inflammatory cells). Such patients can develop a protein-losing enteropathy, anemia and electrolyte disturbances. They also present with scalp and body alopecia, nail dystrophy and skin hyperpigmentation. It is not entirely clear, but these patients may be at an increased risk for gastric and colorectal cancers.

Hyperplastic Polyps Are Benign Serrated Lesions

Hyperplastic polyps are small, sessile mucosal protrusions with exaggerated crypt architecture. They are the most common polyps of the colon, especially in the rectum. Hyperplastic polyps are present in 40% of rectal specimens in

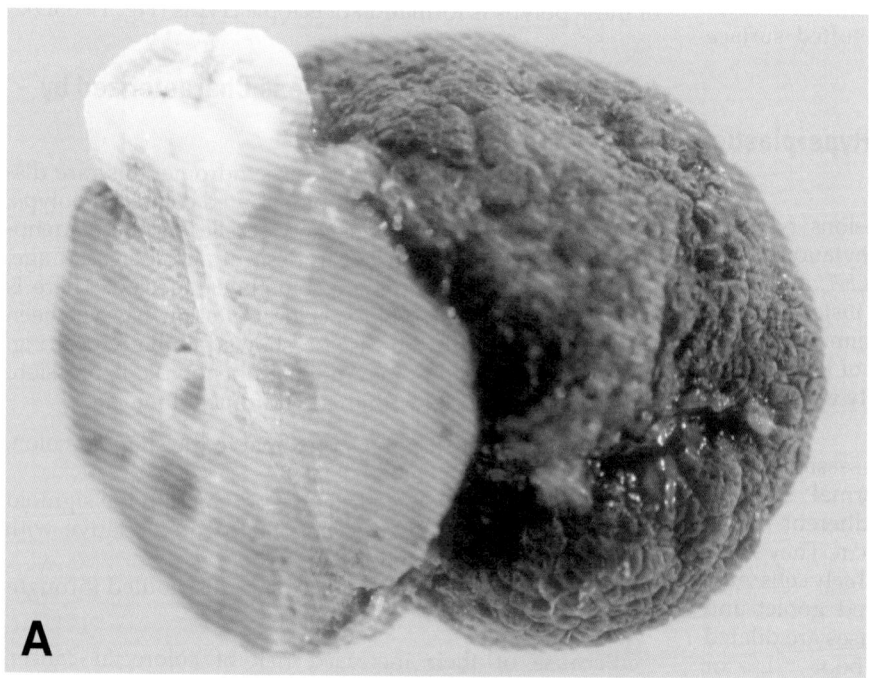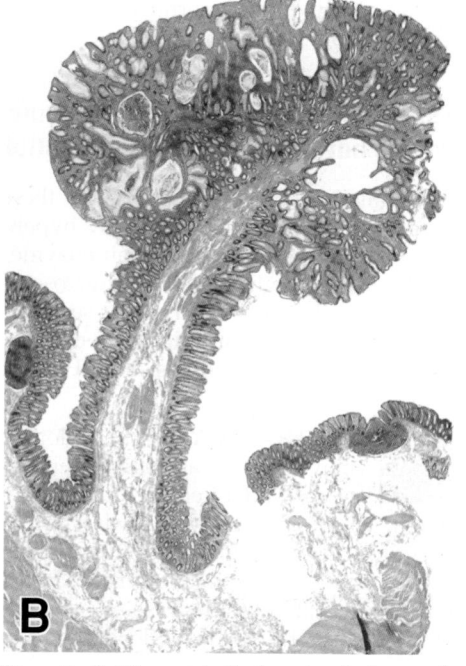

FIGURE 19-81. Juvenile polyp. A. The resected specimen shows a rounded surface. The cut surface (*left*) is cystic. **B.** Microscopically, the polyp displays cystically dilated glands.

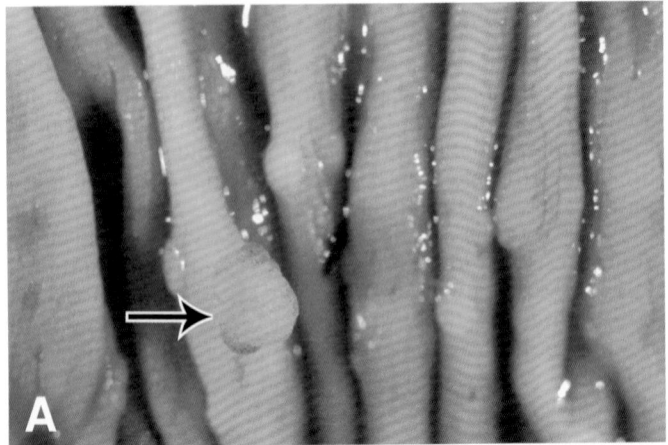
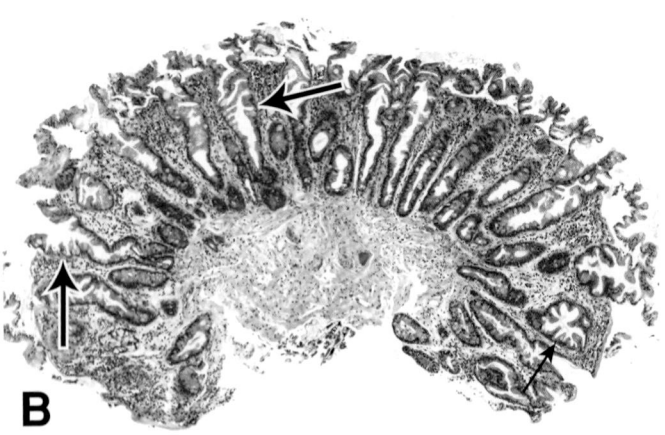

FIGURE 19-82. Hyperplastic polyp. A. This hyperplastic polyp is small, sessile and pale (*black arrow*). The larger adjacent polyp (*white arrow*) is an adenoma. **B.** Microscopically, there is a "sawtooth" appearance to the surface (*arrows*) with relatively normal-appearing crypt bases.

people younger than 40 and in 75% of older people. They are more common in colons with adenomatous polyps and in populations with higher rates of colorectal cancer. Hyperplastic polyps are felt to be due to defective proliferation and maturation of normal epithelium. Thus, cell proliferation occurs at the base of the crypt, and upward migration of the cells is slowed. The epithelial cells differentiate and acquire absorptive characteristics lower in the crypts and persist at the surface longer than do normal cells.

 PATHOLOGY: Hyperplastic polyps are small, sessile, raised mucosal nodules, up to 0.5 cm, but occasionally larger (Fig. 19-82A). They are almost always multiple. The crypts of hyperplastic polyps are elongated and show relatively normal crypt bases. The epithelium in the upper third of the crypts contains hyperplastic goblet and mucinous cells and absorptive cells, with no dysplasia, giving them a serrated contour and tufted surface (Fig. 19-82B).

Sessile Serrated Adenomas Resemble Hyperplastic Polyps but Have Malignant Potential

Also called sessile serrated polyps, these lesions typically arise in the right colon and show hypermethylation of the promoter for the mismatch-repair enzyme, *MLH1;* mutations in *BRAF;* and a high incidence of microsatellite instability. **The carcinomas that arise from sessile serrated adenomas tend to be bulky, mucinous and right sided. Because of their malignant potential, these polyps should be entirely resected.**

 PATHOLOGY: These lesions are sessile or flat; may appear as misshapen, abnormal mucosal folds; and often have abundant adherent mucin (Fig. 19-83A). They are typically larger than 1 cm. They show irregular, asymmetric cell proliferation in which cells may divide anywhere along the crypt. Intermixed goblet and mucin cells extend to the base. Some crypt bases are dilated with abundant mucin, while others show boot-, "L"- or inverted "T"-shaped crypts (Fig. 19-83B). These lesions may develop low- to high-grade dysplasia (Fig. 19-83C) and eventually invasive carcinoma.

Traditional Serrated Adenomas Occur Mainly in the Distal Colon and May Be Premalignant

These polyps are much less common than hyperplastic polyps or sessile serrated adenomas. They show diverse molecular abnormalities: some have *BRAF* mutations, some have *KRAS* mutations and some show a CpG island methylator phenotype that involves methylation of the promoter for *MGMT* (see Chapter 5). Like sessile serrated adenomas, these polyps should be entirely removed.

 PATHOLOGY: Traditional serrated adenomas typically show tubulovillous or villous architecture. Lining epithelial cells have abundant eosinophilic cytoplasm with an elongated nucleus and open or hyperchromatic chromatin. The most characteristic feature of these polyps is formation of ectopic crypts (Fig. 19-83D).

Serrated Polyposis Syndrome Is Characterized by Multiple Serrated Polyps

Also called hyperplastic polyposis syndrome, this rare disorder is characterized by multiple serrated colorectal polyps, usually hyperplastic polyps and sessile serrated adenomas. Risk factors are European descent and increased age, although younger people are sometimes affected. There is no gender preference. No specific mutation has yet been identified, although the disease shows familial clustering. Environmental factors may impact phenotypic expression. People are diagnosed with this syndrome if there are:

1. At least 5 serrated polyps proximal to the sigmoid colon, and 2 or more >1 cm
2. Any number of serrated polyps proximal to the sigmoid colon in an individual with a first-degree relative with serrated polyposis syndrome
3. Over 20 serrated polyps of any size, distributed throughout the colon

Because of their increased risk of colorectal cancer, patients with a first-degree relative with serrated polyposis syndrome should begin screening colonoscopy at age 40, or 10 years younger than age at diagnosis of the youngest

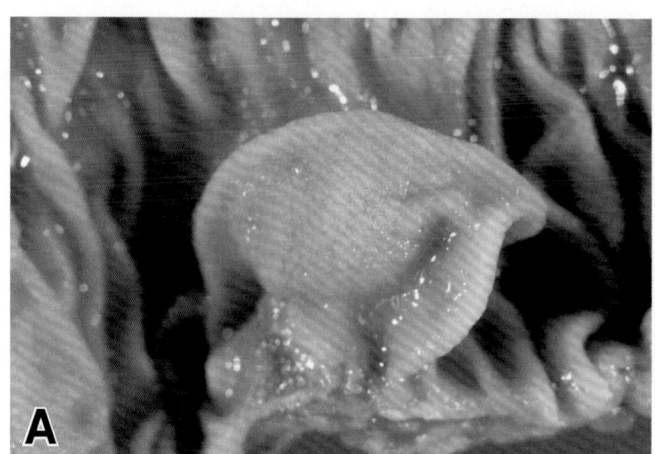
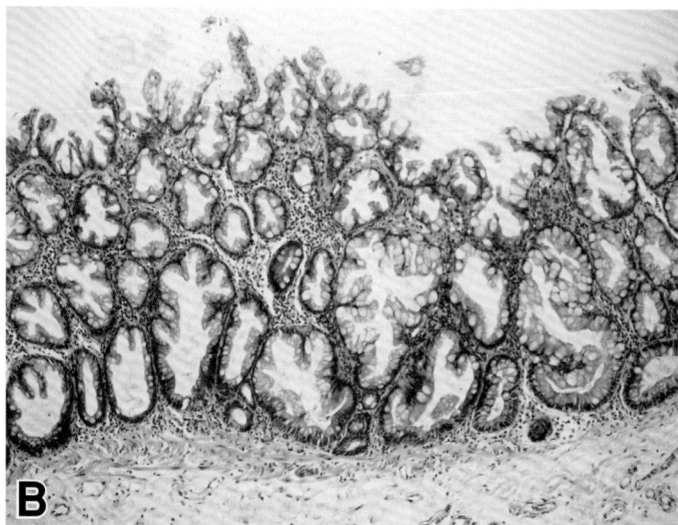
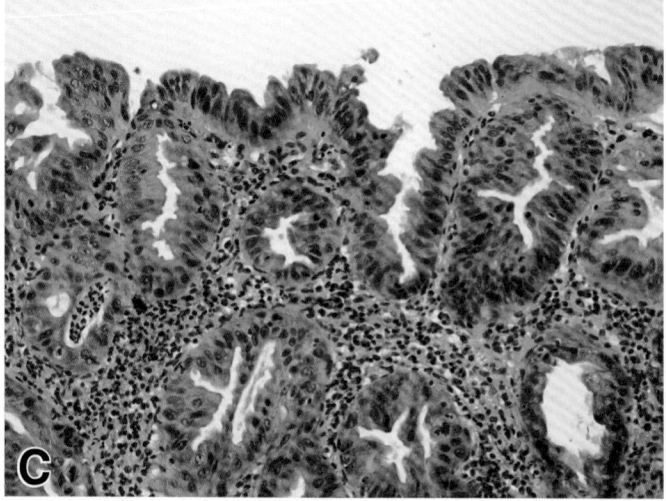
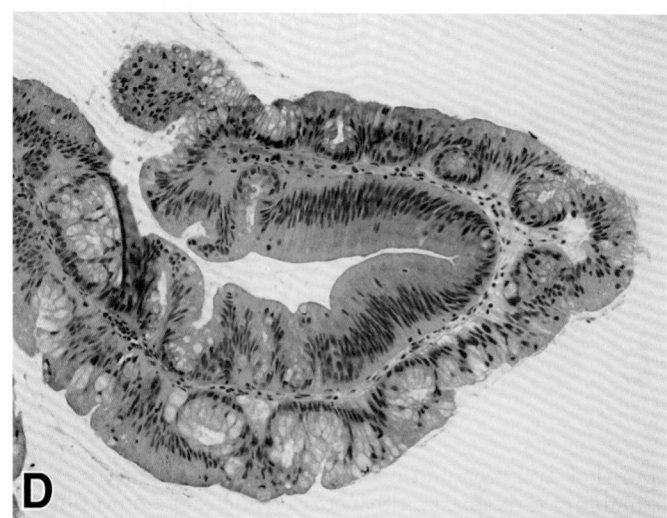

FIGURE 19-83. Premalignant serrated polyps. A. Sessile serrated adenoma. The gross appearance is often that of an enlarged flattened mucosal fold. **B. Sessile serrated adenoma.** Microscopically, the abnormal proliferation of goblet cells gives the crypts a serrated appearance down to the bases, causing the bases to become dilated with abundant mucin and the characteristic formation of boot-, "L"- or inverted "T"-shaped crypts. **C. Sessile serrated adenoma** with cytologic high-grade dysplasia. **D. Traditional serrated adenoma.** The most characteristic feature of this polyp type is formation of ectopic crypts, often with a villous architecture and lining epithelial cells with abundant eosinophilic cytoplasm.

affected relative. All lesions greater than 5 mm, especially if right sided, should be removed.

Adenomatous Polyps Are Premalignant

Adenomatous polyps (tubular adenomas) are neoplasms of colonic epithelium. They are composed of neoplastic epithelial cells that migrated to the surface and accumulated beyond the needs for replacement of the cells sloughed into the lumen.

 **EPIDEMIOLOGY:** These polyps occur most in industrialized countries. As with diverticular disease, the only known consistent environmental difference between high-risk and low-risk populations is a "Western" diet. After age 50, the incidence of adenomas rises rapidly such that in the United States, at least one adenomatous polyp is present in half of the adult population. This proportion reaches greater than 2/3 among those older than

65. Smoking, obesity and a family history of colon adenomas or carcinoma increase the risk of having adenomas.

 PATHOLOGY: Almost half of adenomatous polyps of the colon in the United States are in the rectosigmoid. The remaining half are evenly distributed throughout the rest of the colon. Adenomas vary from barely visible nodules or small, pedunculated adenomas to large, sessile (flat) lesions. They are classified by architecture into tubular, villous and tubulovillous types. These polyps are the usual precursors to colon carcinoma, and their epithelium is by definition dysplastic.

TUBULAR ADENOMAS: These represent 2/3 of large bowel adenomas. They are typically smooth-surfaced lesions, less than 2 cm, often with a stalk (Fig. 19-84). Some tubular adenomas, particularly the smaller ones, may be sessile.

Tubular adenomas show closely packed epithelial tubules, which may be uniform or irregular and excessively branched (Fig. 19-84C). Tubular adenomas show at least low-grade

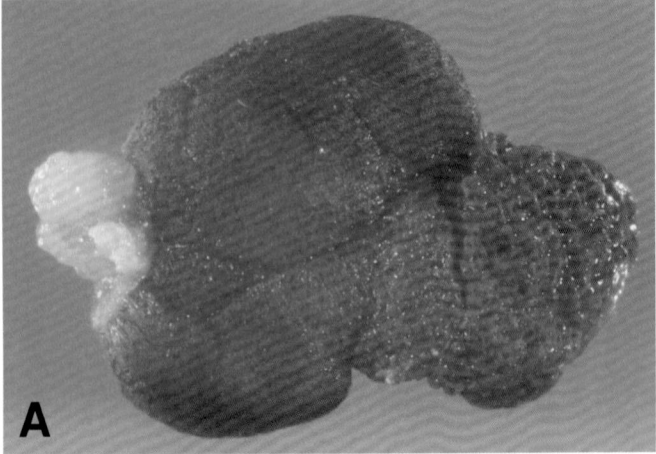

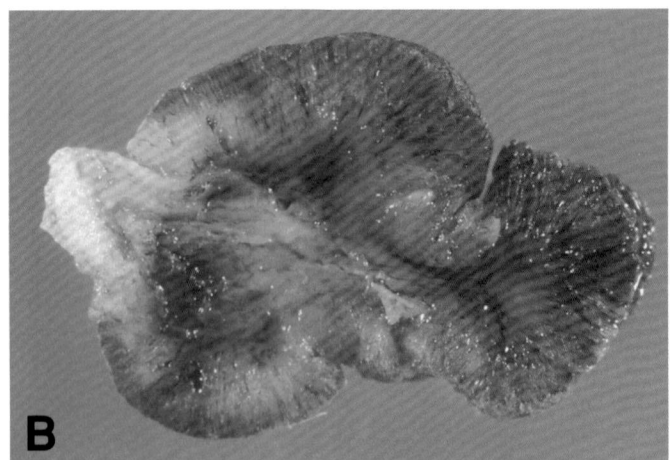

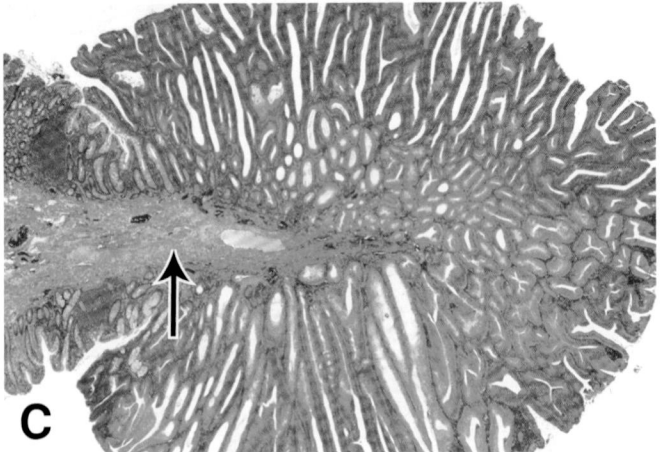

FIGURE 19-84. Tubular adenoma of the colon. A. The adenoma shows a characteristic stalk and bosselated surface. **B.** The bisected adenoma shows the stalk covered by the adenomatous epithelium. The ashen white color is cautery at the polypectomy resection margin from the polypectomy. **C.** Microscopically, the adenoma shows a repetitive pattern that is largely tubular. The stalk, which is in continuity with the submucosa of the colon, is not involved and is lined by normal colonic epithelium.

epithelial dysplasia and may occasionally show progression to high-grade dysplasia with increased nuclear pleomorphism and complex architecture. High-grade dysplasia can progress to invasive adenocarcinoma, the diagnosis of which requires neoplastic glands below the muscularis mucosae (Fig. 19-85). As long as dysplasia is confined to the mucosa, the lesion is cured by complete polypectomy. Invasive adenocarcinoma may be cured by polypectomy alone if the tumor shows low-risk features and there is an adequate margin of resection at the base.

The risk of invasive carcinoma correlates with the size of the adenoma. Only 1% of tubular adenomas less than 1 cm

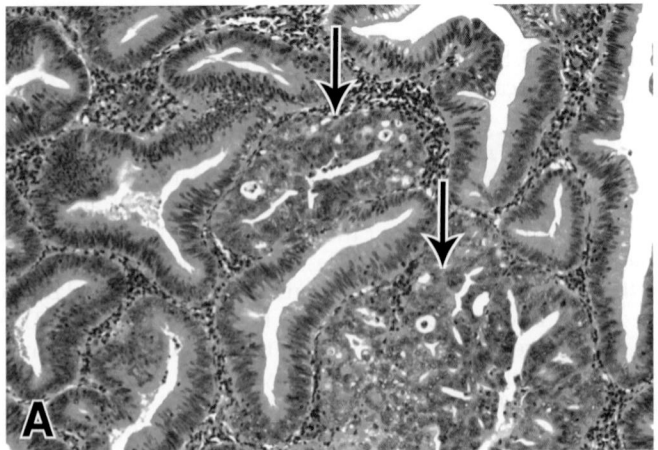

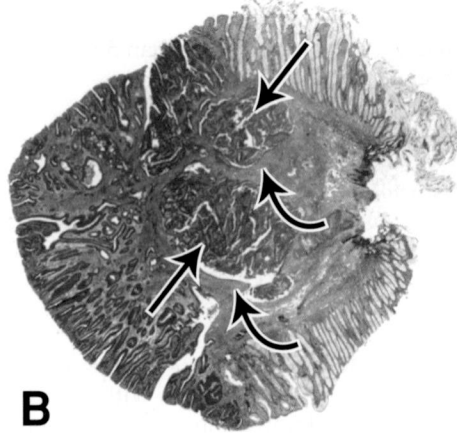

FIGURE 19-85. Adenocarcinoma arising in a pedunculated adenomatous polyp. A. Both low-grade dysplasia and high-grade dysplasia are present. The former is characterized by elongated, hyperchromatic, pseudostratified nuclei. The latter is characterized by a cribriform pattern and increased nuclear pleomorphism (*arrows*). **B.** Trichrome stain showing tumor invading the stalk (*blue*). Since there was a margin of resection of over 1 mm, polypectomy was sufficient therapy.

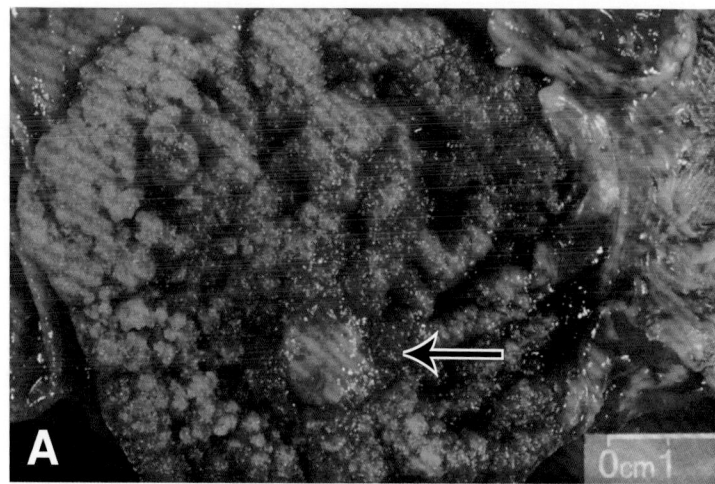

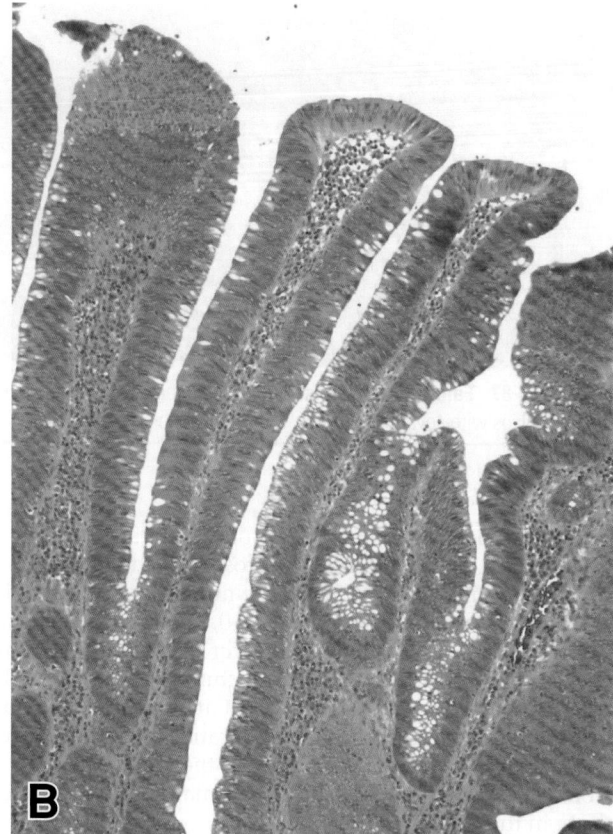

FIGURE 19-86. Villous adenoma of the colon. A. The colon contains a large, broad-based, elevated lesion that has a cauliflower-like surface. A firm area near the center of the lesion proved on histologic examination to be an adenocarcinoma. **B.** Microscopic examination shows finger-like processes with fibrovascular cores lined by low-grade dysplastic epithelium.

have invasive cancer at the time of resection; of those 1–2 cm, 10% harbor malignancy; and of those greater than 2 cm, 35% are malignant. Small flat adenomas may be missed during conventional endoscopy and thus have a high risk of progression to cancer.

VILLOUS ADENOMAS: These polyps constitute 1/10 of colonic adenomas and are found mainly in the rectosigmoid region. They are typically large, broad-based, elevated lesions with shaggy, cauliflower-like surfaces (Fig. 19-86A), but they can be small and pedunculated. Most exceed 2 cm, and they may reach 10–15 cm. Villous adenomas are composed of thin, tall, finger-like processes that resemble the villi of the small intestine. They are lined externally by neoplastic epithelial cells and are supported by a core of normal lamina propria (Fig. 19-86B).

Dysplasia in villous adenomas resembles that in tubular adenomas. However, villous adenomas contain foci of carcinoma more often than do tubular adenomas. In villous adenomas under 1 cm, the risk of cancer is 10 times higher than that for tubular adenomas of comparable size. Half of villous adenomas greater than 2 cm harbor invasive carcinoma. Since most villous adenomas exceed 2 cm, more than 1/3 of all resected villous adenomas contain invasive cancer.

TUBULOVILLOUS ADENOMAS: Many adenomatous polyps have both tubular and villous features. Polyps with 25%–75% villous architecture are **"tubulovillous."** These tend to be intermediate in distribution and size between tubular and villous forms, with 1/3 being greater than 2 cm. Tubulovillous polyps are also intermediate between tubular and villous adenomas in the risk of invasive carcinoma.

PATHOPHYSIOLOGY: The precursor to colorectal carcinoma is dysplasia, usually in the form of an adenoma. The pathogenesis of adenomas of the colon and rectum involves neoplastic alteration of crypt epithelial homeostasis with (1) diminished apoptosis, (2) persistent cell replication and (3) failure of epithelial cells to mature and differentiate as they migrate toward crypt surfaces. Normally, DNA synthesis stops when cells reach the upper 1/3 of crypts, after which they mature, migrate to the surface and then are sloughed into the lumen. Adenomas represent focal disruption of this orderly sequence, in that epithelial cells may proliferate throughout the entire depth of the crypt: mitotic figures are present along the entire length of the crypt and on the mucosal surface. As the lesion evolves, the proliferation rate exceeds that of sloughing, and cells accumulate in upper crypts and on the surface.

Familial Adenomatous Polyposis Is an Autosomal Dominant Trait That Invariably Leads to Cancer

Also called adenomatous polyposis coli (APC), FAP accounts for less than 1% of colorectal cancers. It is caused by a heritable, germline mutation in the APC gene on the long arm of chromosome 5 (5q21-22) (see below). Most cases are familial, but 30%–50% reflect new mutations. In FAP, there are hundreds to thousands of adenomas carpeting the colorectal mucosa, sometimes throughout its entire length, but particularly in the rectosigmoid region (Fig. 19-87). These are

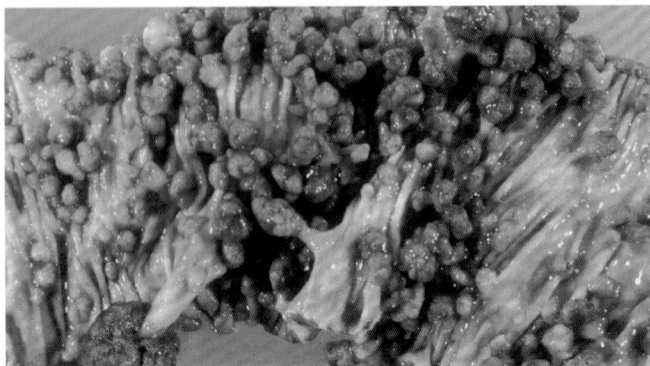

FIGURE 19-87. Familial polyposis. The colon contains thousands of adenomatous polyps with several exceeding 1 cm in diameter.

mostly tubular adenomas, but tubulovillous and villous adenomas may also be present. Microscopic adenomas, sometimes involving a single crypt, are numerous. A few polyps are usually already present by age 10, but symptoms usually begin by age 36. By this time cancer is often already present. Carcinoma of the colon and rectum is inevitable in FAP patients, with the mean age of onset at 40 years. Total colectomy before the onset of cancer is curative, but some patients may also have tubular adenomas in the small intestine and stomach, and these have the same malignant potential as those in the colon.

FAP mutations are found in only 3/4 of familial cases. Some APC mutation-negative patients have mutations in MYH (a distinct, rare, autosomal recessive, polyposis syndrome that clinically overlaps FAP). Subtypes of FAP include:

- **Attenuated FAP:** In this condition there are fewer than 100 adenomas in the colon. Colorectal cancer develops an average of 15 years later than in classical FAP and carries a 70% risk of invasive cancer by age 80.
- **Gardner syndrome:** In this variant, extracolonic lesions include osteomas of the skull, mandible and long bones; epidermoid cysts; desmoid tumors; and congenital hypertrophy of retinal pigment epithelium. *APC* mutations do not predict this phenotype.
- **Turcot syndrome:** This rare disorder combines FAP with malignant CNS tumors. Many cases, especially those with medulloblastoma, are due to germline mutations of the *APC* gene.

Colorectal Adenocarcinomas Mostly Arise in Adenomatous Polyps

In Western societies, colorectal cancer is the third most common cause of cancer and the second leading cause of cancer death. There is a marked geographic difference in the incidence of this cancer, with rates differing by 10-fold between developing and developed countries. This difference is largely attributed to environmental factors since countries that more recently adopted "Western" diets and lifestyles have seen marked increases in colorectal cancer rates, and people who migrate from low-incidence regions to high-incidence regions develop these cancers at rates similar to the high-incidence region. The term "colorectal" is used because cancers of the colon and rectum share certain biological features, but there are also differences between colonic and rectal cancers. For instance, colon cancer rates are about equal between men and women, but rectal cancer shows a slight male predominance. The two tumors are also treated differently.

 **ETIOLOGIC FACTORS:** Most colorectal cancers arise in adenomatous polyps; thus, factors that lead to the development of such polyps favor colorectal cancer as well. There are several modifiable and nonmodifiable risk factors (see below). While no one feature of a "Western" lifestyle is identified as causative, multiple factors contribute to higher incidence, and diet seems to have the greatest impact—either via a direct effect or because of its effect on altering gut flora.

Risk Factors for Colorectal Carcinoma

AGE: Increasing age is probably the single most important risk factor for colorectal cancer in the general population. The risk is low (but not zero) before age 40. It then increases steadily to age 50, after which it doubles each decade.

PRIOR COLORECTAL CANCER: Patients with one colorectal cancer are at increased risk for a subsequent tumor. In fact, 5%–10% of patients treated for colorectal cancer develop a second such malignancy. Moreover, 2%–5% of those with a new colorectal cancer have a simultaneous (synchronous) colorectal primary cancer.

ULCERATIVE COLITIS AND CROHN DISEASE: These chronic inflammatory diseases increase colorectal cancer risk in proportion to their duration and extent of large bowel involvement.

GENETIC FACTORS: Risk of colorectal cancer is increased in relatives of patients with the disease, suggesting a genetic contribution to tumorigenesis. People with two or more first- or second-degree relatives with colorectal cancer constitute 20% of all patients with this tumor. Some 5%–10% of colorectal cancers are inherited as autosomal dominant traits, the most common syndrome being hereditary nonpolyposis colorectal carcinoma (HNPCC, Lynch syndrome [see below]).

DIET: Consumption of animal products including fat, cholesterol and protein parallels incidence of colorectal cancer. Moreover, certain ethnic and religious groups in the United States whose diets are lower in animal products have less colorectal cancer. Possibly, ingestion of animal products favors bacterial flora that degrade bile salts to N-nitroso compounds, which may contribute to tumorigenesis.

Diets low in fruits, vegetables and whole grains (fiber) have also been implicated in colorectal carcinogenesis. Reasons for this are not entirely clear but may be related to an effect on gut flora and stool transit time.

PHYSICAL ACTIVITY AND OBESITY: These factors combined are thought to account for up to 1/3 of colorectal cancers. While not well understood, physical inactivity decreases gut motility. Obesity increases circulating estrogens and decreases insulin resistance, factors that are believed to influence cancer risk.

CIGARETTE SMOKING AND ALCOHOL: Cigarette smoking and heavy alcohol consumption are independent risk factors for colon cancer. If present together, they may act synergistically. DNA mutations induced by smoking are repaired less efficiently in the presence of alcohol. Nutritional deficiencies may also play a role in heavy alcohol users.

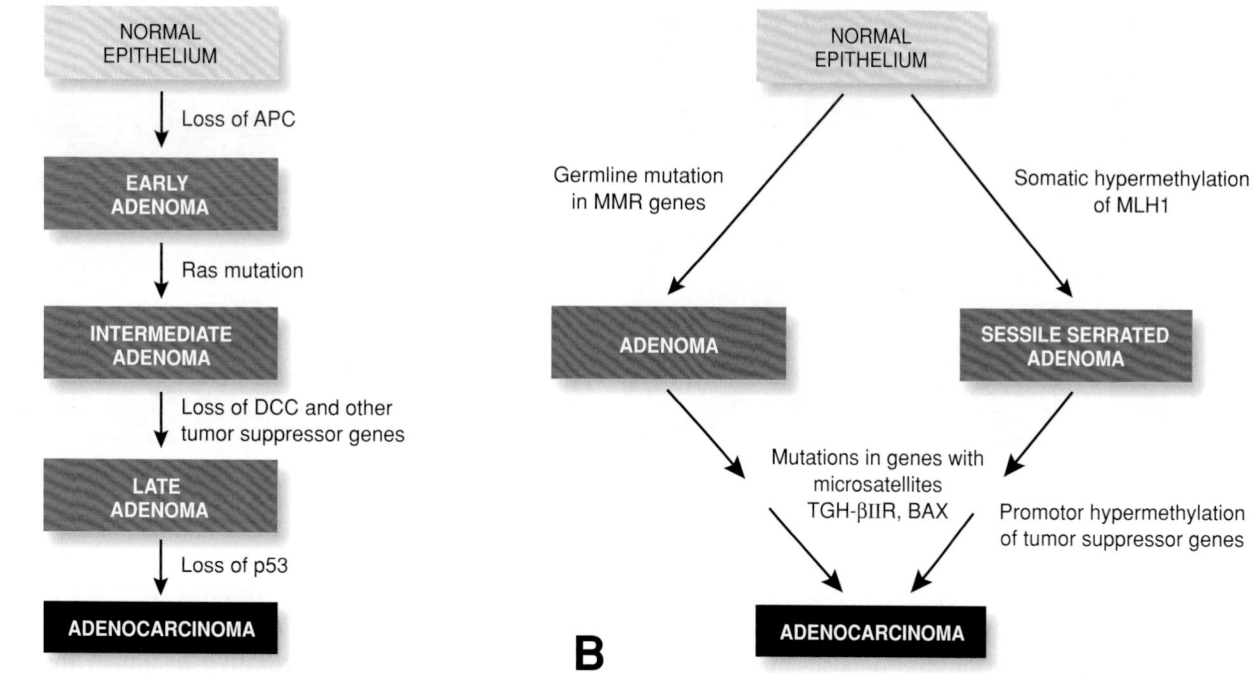

FIGURE 19-88. Model of some of the genetic alterations involved in colonic carcinogenesis. A. The tumor suppressor pathway. **B.** The mismatch repair (MMR) defect pathway. *APC* = adenomatous polyposis coli; *DCC* = deleted in colon cancer; *MLH1* = MutL homolog 1; *TGF-βIIR* = transforming growth factor-β2 receptor; *BAX* = BCL2 associated X protein.

 MOLECULAR PATHOGENESIS: In 85% of cases of colorectal carcinoma, it is estimated that at least 8–10 mutational events must accumulate before an invasive cancer with metastatic potential develops. This process is initiated in histologically normal mucosa, proceeds through an adenomatous precursor stage and ends as invasive adenocarcinoma (see Chapter 5).

The most important mutational events involve (Fig. 19-88A):

- **APC gene:** As noted above, germline mutations in the *APC* (adenomatous polyposis coli) tumor suppressor gene lead to familial adenomatous polyposis. Normal APC is a negative regulator of β-catenin: it binds β-catenin and causes its phosphorylation, followed by ubiquitination and proteasomal degradation. Mutant APC allows β-catenin to accumulate in the nucleus, where it is a transcriptional activator of key proliferation genes (e.g., *cyclin D1* and *MYC*). *APC is somatically mutated in 70%–80% of sporadic colorectal cancers.* Some tumors with normal *APC* have mutations in the β**-catenin gene** itself. A specific *APC* mutation (isoleucine → lysine at codon 1307) occurs in 6% of Ashkenazi Jews, renders surrounding regions of the gene susceptible to inactivating frame-shift mutations and increases risk of colon cancer. *APC* mutations in normal colonic mucosa precede development of sporadic adenomas. Thus, *APC* is central to the early development of most colorectal neoplasms.
- **KRAS:** Activating mutations of the *KRAS* proto-oncogene occur early in tubular adenomas of the colon.
- **DCC** gene: A putative tumor suppressor gene, *DCC* ("deleted in colon cancer") is located on chromosome 18 and is often missing in colorectal cancers.

- **TP53:** Mutations in p53 facilitate the transition from adenoma to the most common type of adenocarcinoma and are late events in colon carcinogenesis.

In 15% of colorectal cancers, the process of **DNA mismatch repair** (MMR; see Chapter 5) is impaired, leading to deficient repair of spontaneous replication errors, particularly in regions with simple repetitive sequences (microsatellites). MMR deficiencies occur via two mechanisms. In a hereditary form (HNPCC; see below), a germline mutation in one of the MMR genes is followed by somatic mutation of the other allele ("second hit"; see Chapter 5) later in life. In sporadic tumors, hypermethylation of an MMR promoter, usually for the *MLH1* gene, inactivates transcription of the gene (Fig. 19-88B).

PATHOLOGY: Grossly, colorectal cancers resemble adenocarcinomas elsewhere in the gut. They tend to be polypoid and ulcerating or infiltrative, and may be annular and constrictive (Fig. 19-89). Polypoid cancers are more common in the right colon, particularly the cecum, where the large lumen allows unimpeded intraluminal growth. Annular constricting tumors occur more often in the distal colon. Tumors often ulcerate, regardless of growth pattern.

The vast majority of colorectal cancers are adenocarcinomas that resemble their counterparts elsewhere in the digestive tract (Fig. 19-89B). About 15% secrete abundant mucin and are called **mucinous** adenocarcinomas. Degree of differentiation influences prognosis; better-differentiated tumors tend to have a more favorable outlook.

Colon cancers spread by direct extension or vascular invasion. The former is common in resected specimens. Serosal connective tissue offers little resistance to tumor spread, and

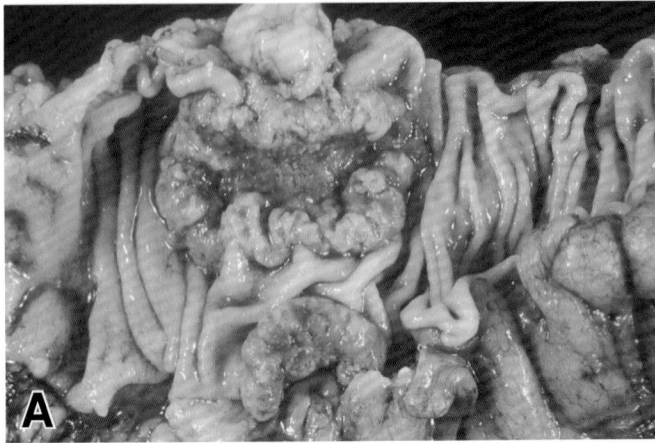
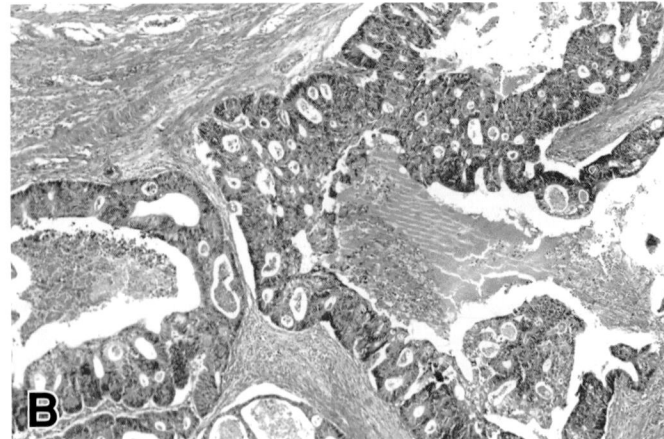

FIGURE 19-89. Adenocarcinoma of the colon. A. A resected colon shows an ulcerated mass with enlarged, firm, rolled borders. **B.** Microscopically, this colon adenocarcinoma consists of moderately differentiated glands with a prominent cribriform pattern and frequent central necrosis.

cancer cells are often seen in the pericolorectal fat far from the primary site. The peritoneum is occasionally involved, in which case there may be multiple deposits throughout the abdomen.

Colorectal cancer invades lymphatic channels and initially involves lymph nodes just below the tumor. The liver is the most common metastatic organ site, but the tumor may spread widely. The prognosis of colorectal cancer is more closely related to tumor extension through the large bowel wall than to its size or histopathology.

Staging of these tumors uses the TNM system (tumor, lymph nodes, metastasis; see Chapter 5). T1 tumors invade the submucosa; T2 tumors infiltrate into, but not through, the muscularis propria; T3 tumors invade pericolorectal soft tissue; and T4 tumors penetrate the serosa (T4a) or involve adjacent organs (T4b). N reflects the presence or absence of lymph node metastases, and M the presence or absence of distant metastases.

CLINICAL FEATURES: Initially, colorectal cancer is clinically silent. As the tumor grows, the most common sign is **fecal occult blood** when the tumor is in the proximal colon. Both occult blood and **bright red blood** in the feces may occur if a lesion is in the distal colorectum.

Cancers on the left side of the colon, where the lumen is narrow and feces are more solid, often constrict the lumen and produce **obstructive symptoms**. These include changes in bowel habits and abdominal pain. Colorectal cancers may **perforate** early and cause peritonitis. By contrast, right-sided cancers may grow large without causing obstruction, especially in the cecum where the lumen is large and fecal contents are liquid. As a result, right-sided tumors can lead to asymptomatic chronic bleeding. **Iron-deficiency anemia** may be the first indication of colorectal cancer. A tumor that spreads beyond the colorectum may cause enterocutaneous and rectovaginal **fistulas,** tumor masses in the abdominal wall, bladder symptoms and sciatic nerve pain. Spread within the abdomen may cause **small intestinal obstruction** and malignant **ascites**.

A positive test for fecal occult blood predicts the presence of a cancer or an adenoma in 50% of cases. Periodic fiberoptic colonoscopy and testing for occult blood in feces can detect tumors at early stages and have improved survival in colorectal cancer.

Resection is the only curative treatment for colorectal cancer. Small polyps are easily removed endoscopically; large lesions require segmental resection. Tumors near the anal verge often necessitate abdominal–perineal resection and colostomy, although newer surgical techniques may preserve sphincter function. Preoperative (neoadjuvant) chemotherapy and radiotherapy are typically used in all but very early rectal cancers.

Hereditary Nonpolyposis Colorectal Cancer (Lynch Syndrome)

HNPCC is an autosomal dominant inherited disease that accounts for 3%–5% of colorectal cancers.

MOLECULAR PATHOGENESIS: Lynch syndrome is caused by germline mutations in a DNA MMR gene. Usually, *hMSH2* (human MutS homolog 2) on chromosome 2p and *hMLH1* (human MutL homolog 1) on chromosome 3p are affected. Less common mutations involve *hMSH6* (human MutS homolog 6) or *hPMS2* (human postmeiotic segregation 2) on chromosomes 2p and 7p, respectively. In HNPCC, there is a germline mutation in one allele of one MMR gene. The fact that one allele is mutated hinders repair of any second sporadic mutation in the other (formerly) wild-type allele: a somatic "second hit" (see Chapter 5). Thereafter, repair of spontaneous replication errors is ineffective. Widespread genomic instability results, particularly in simple repetitive sequences (microsatellites), which are particularly prone to replication errors. Thus, genes that regulate growth and differentiation, and other mismatch repair genes, are disabled by unrepaired mutations.

Mismatch repair deficiency can be identified by sequencing MMR genes, testing for microsatellite instability and immunostaining to assess levels of MMR proteins in a tumor. A specific mutation can be used to evaluate other family members.

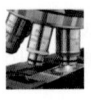 **PATHOLOGY AND CLINICAL FEATURES:** Lynch syndrome tumors more often show mucinous, signet ring cell and

<table>
<tr><td colspan="1">

TABLE 19-4

LYNCH SYNDROME/HEREDITARY NONPOLYPOSIS COLORECTAL CANCER (HNPCC)

Amsterdam II Criteria (must meet all criteria)

At least three relatives must have histologically verified HNPCC-associated cancer

One must be a first-degree relative of the other two

At least two successive generations must be affected

At least one of the relatives with colorectal cancer must have received the diagnosis before the age of 50 years

Familial adenomatous polyposis must have been excluded

Revised Bethesda Guidelines (only one criterion needs to be met)

Diagnosed with colorectal cancer (CRC) before the age of 50 years

Individuals with more than one CRC or other HNPCC-related tumor

CRC with high-microsatellite instability morphology, diagnosed before the age of 60 years

CRC and a first-degree relative with CRC or other HNPCC-related tumor. One cancer must have been diagnosed at younger than age 50 years or one adenoma at younger than age 40 years

CRC with at least two relatives with CRC or other HNPCC-related tumor, regardless of age

</td></tr>
</table>

solid (medullary) histologies than sporadic tumors, with many intratumor lymphocytes and Crohn-like lymphocytic reactions. HNPCC patients tend to (1) present with cancer at a young age; (2) have few adenomas (hence "nonpolyposis"); (3) develop tumors proximal to the splenic flexure (70%); (4) have multiple synchronous or metachronous colorectal cancers; and (5) develop extracolonic cancers, especially of the endometrium, ovary, stomach, small intestine, urinary tract, pancreas, hepatobiliary tract, skin and CNS. Patients with Lynch syndrome who have skin involvement (sebaceous adenomas and carcinomas) are said to have **Muir-Torre syndrome** (see Chapter 28). Specific criteria for the diagnosis of Lynch syndrome are listed in Table 19-4.

OTHER TUMORS OF THE LARGE INTESTINE

Colonic Mesenchymal Tumors Encompass the Range of Benign and Malignant Soft Tissue Tumors

Mesenchymal tumors arising from tissues normally in the colon include lipoma, liposarcoma, neurofibroma, ganglioneuroma, peripheral nerve sheath tumors, leiomyoma, leiomyosarcoma, vascular tumors and GISTs (see above). Of these, the most common are submucosal lipomas and leiomyomas.

Colonic Neuroendocrine Tumors Resemble NETs of the Small Intestine

These tumors were also called carcinoid tumors (see above). Half of colorectal NETs have metastasized by the time they are discovered.

Large Bowel Lymphomas Are Usually B-Cell Tumors

Primary lymphoma of the colorectum is uncommon. It may be seen with (1) segmental mucosal involvement, (2) diffuse polypoid lesions or (3) a mass extending beyond the colorectum. Symptoms are like those of other intestinal cancers, but the diffuse polypoid form may resemble inflammatory or adenomatous polyps. Most colonic lymphomas are tumors of B cells.

Endometriosis Involving the Colon Can Mimic Colorectal Cancer

Colorectal endometriosis is mostly asymptomatic and is discovered incidentally during laparotomy for other reasons. If symptoms occur (abdominal pain, constipation, intestinal obstruction), they may be mistaken for those of colorectal cancer. As a result of repeated hemorrhage, the lesions are surrounded by reactive fibrosis, which, when severe, can lead to a classic "apple core" appearance to the colon or rectum and grossly mimic a primary colorectal carcinoma (see Chapter 24).

The Anus

The anal canal extends from the level of the pelvic floor to the proximal margin of the anal verge. It is about 4 cm long and is divided into 3 parts, based on its lining epithelium: the colorectal zone (lined by glandular mucosa), the transition zone (varying, transitional mucosa) and the distal, squamous zone (lined by squamous mucosa). The dentate (pectinate) line (formed by the anal valves, roughly midway through the anal canal) is easily identified, and the superior border of the anal canal may be defined as 2 cm above this line.

BENIGN LESIONS OF THE ANAL CANAL

Hemorrhoids Are Dilated Venous Channels of the Hemorrhoidal Plexuses

They result from downward displacement of the anal cushions. Internal hemorrhoids arise from the superior hemorrhoidal plexus above the dentate (pectinate) line. They are covered by rectal or transitional mucosa. External hemorrhoids originate from the inferior hemorrhoidal plexus, below that line, and are covered by squamous mucosa. *Hemorrhoids affect at least 5% of people in Western countries (likely a gross underestimate since most people treat themselves for this condition).* They are most common in whites between 45 and 65 years old. Pregnancy is another risk factor, presumably related to increased abdominal pressure.

 PATHOLOGY: Hemorrhoids are dilated vascular spaces with excess smooth muscle in their walls. Hemorrhage and thrombosis are common.

 **CLINICAL FEATURES:** Hemorrhoids cause painless rectal bleeding associated with bowel movements. While chronic blood loss may lead to **iron-deficiency anemia,** other causes must be ruled out before

it is attributed to hemorrhoidal bleeding. **Rectal prolapse** is common and may cause perineal irritation or anal itching. Prolapsed hemorrhoids may become irreducible and lead to painful, strangulated hemorrhoids. **Thrombosed** external hemorrhoids are exquisitely painful and require evacuation of the offending clots. Hemorrhoids are treated with dietary and lifestyle modifications aimed at improving the quality of stools and reducing straining on the toilet. Medical and surgical interventions are also available.

Anal Condylomata Acuminata (Anal Warts) Are Related to HPV Infection

These lesions are typically benign but may potentially develop into squamous cancers.

 PATHOLOGY: Condylomata have a cauliflower-like growth pattern of papillary excrescences lined by squamous epithelium that is often hyperkeratotic. The squamous cells show characteristic koilocytic change, having enlarged nuclei with irregular nuclear contours, often binucleated, with perinuclear cytoplasmic clearing. These can develop dysplasia—graded mild, moderate or severe, similarly to the grading scheme in the cervix (see Chapter 24).

MALIGNANT TUMORS OF THE ANAL CANAL

Anal Canal Cancers Are Mostly Squamous Cell Carcinomas

These cancers, while increasing in frequency, are relatively uncommon. They are more common in women than in men, and their incidence is 1.4 per 100,000. In the highest-risk group, people who practice anal-receptive intercourse, incidence approaches 35 per 100,000.

 PATHOLOGY: Anal cancers have various histologic patterns (e.g., squamous or basaloid [cloacogenic]). But all tumor types tend to behave similarly

and so are simply classified as **squamous cell carcinomas. Bowen disease of the anus** is squamous carcinoma in situ. Anal carcinomas spread directly into surrounding tissues, including internal and external sphincters, perianal soft tissues, the prostate and the vagina.

 CLINICAL FEATURES: The major risk factor for anal squamous cell carcinoma is infection with HPV. Other risk factors include HIV infection, immunosuppression in organ transplantation, presence of an immune disorder and smoking.

The usual symptom of anal cancers is bleeding, but pain and/or a palpable mass are also possible. Often a tumor is not first recognized as malignant and may be discovered only in a hemorrhoidectomy specimen. Combined chemotherapy and radiation therapy is the customary treatment, although abdominal–perineal resection is sometimes used. The 5-year survival rate averages 75%, but patients with more advanced tumors (greater size, lymph node and/or distant metastases) do worse.

Extramammary Paget Disease May Involve the Anus

Paget disease is classically described in the breast (Chapter 25) but also occurs elsewhere, including the anogenital region. It can be primary when it arises from the epidermis or secondary if it is associated with an underlying adenocarcinoma.

 PATHOLOGY: Grossly involved areas may appear normal or be erythematous, scaly or ulcerated. The epidermis often shows reactive changes including hyperplasia and hyperkeratosis. The hallmark finding is malignant cells with pale, granular or vacuolated cytoplasm scattered throughout the epidermis (Fig. 19-90).

Figs. 19-91 through 19-94 summarize the causes of gastrointestinal bleeding and obstruction and the major benign and malignant tumors of the GI tract.

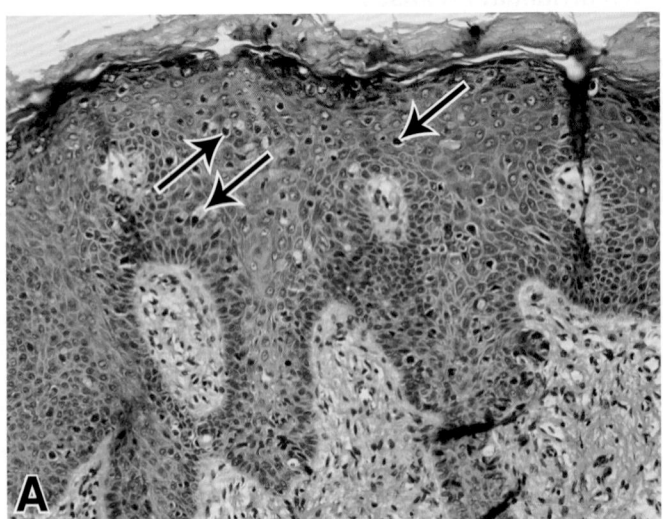
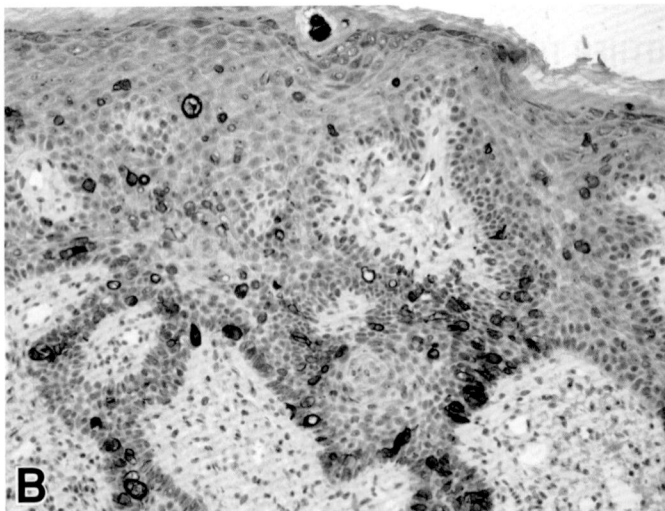

FIGURE 19-90. Paget disease of the anal canal. A. Microscopic image showing squamous epithelium with scattered malignant cells with pale or vacuolated cytoplasm seen throughout the epidermis (*arrows*). **B.** Immunohistochemical stain for CK20 highlights the malignant cells.

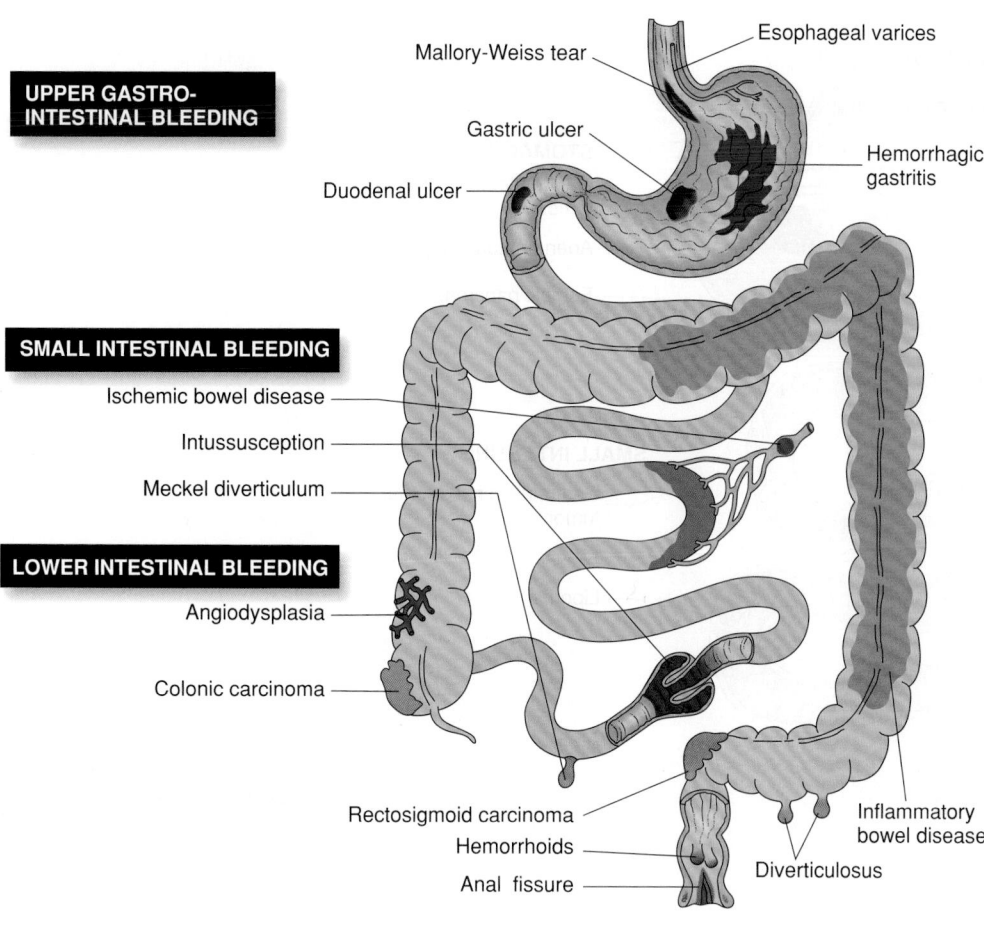

FIGURE 19-91. Causes of gastrointestinal bleeding.

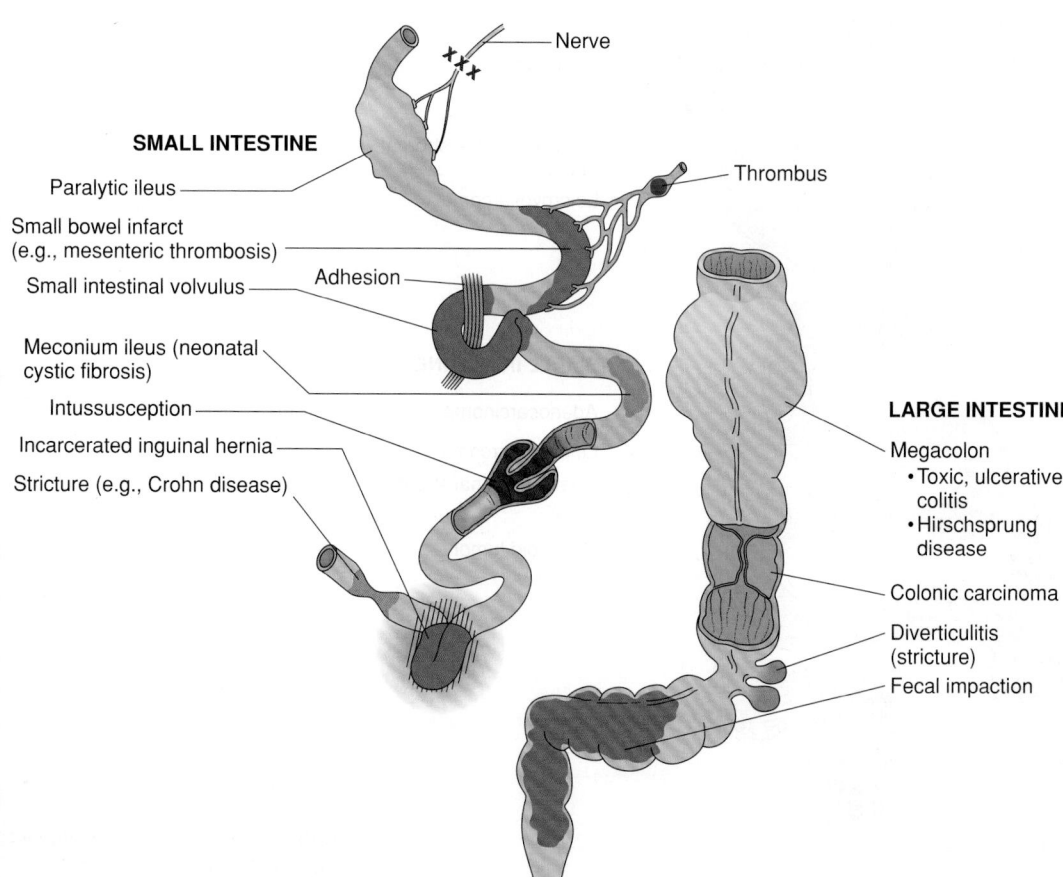

FIGURE 19-92. Causes of gastrointestinal obstruction.

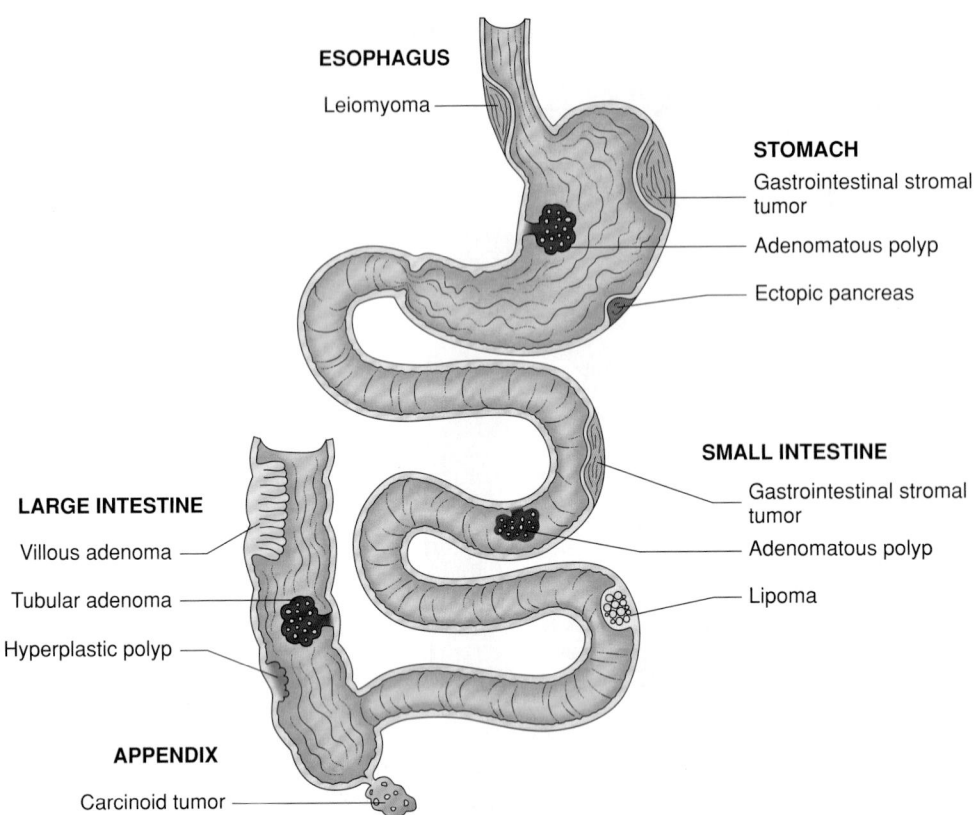

FIGURE 19-93. Major benign tumors of the gastrointestinal tract.

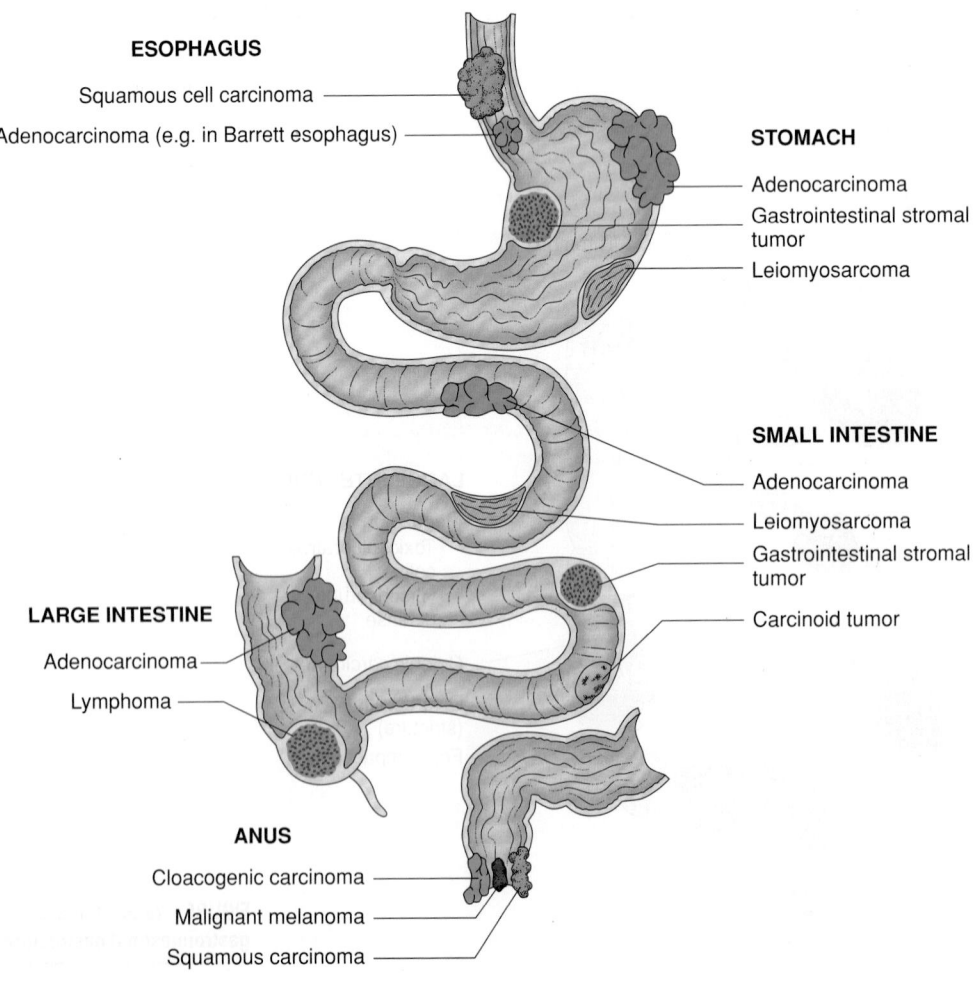

FIGURE 19-94. Major malignant tumors of the gastrointestinal tract.

The Peritoneum

The peritoneum is the mesothelial lining of the abdominal cavity and its viscera. The visceral peritoneum invests the gastrointestinal tract from stomach to rectum and encircles the liver. The parietal peritoneum lines the abdominal wall and retroperitoneal space. The omentum, which has a double layer of peritoneum, encloses blood vessels and a variable amount of fat.

PERITONITIS

Bacterial Peritonitis Is Usually Caused by Intestinal Organisms

 **ETIOLOGIC FACTORS:**
PERFORATION: The most common cause of bacterial peritonitis is perforation of an abdominal viscus (e.g., an inflamed appendix, peptic ulcer or colon diverticulum). Peritonitis results in an acute abdomen, with severe abdominal pain and tenderness. Nausea, vomiting and a high fever are usual. In severe cases, generalized peritonitis, paralytic ileus and septic shock (see Chapter 12) ensue. Often the perforation is "walled off," in which case a peritoneal abscess results.

The bacteria released into the peritoneal cavity from the gastrointestinal tract vary according to the site of perforation and the duration of the peritonitis. Diverse aerobic and anaerobic species usually participate, including *E. coli, Bacteroides* sp., various *Streptococcus* spp. and *Clostridium.* Despite antibiotic treatment, surgical drainage and supportive measures, generalized peritonitis still carries substantial mortality and is especially dangerous in the elderly.

PERITONEAL DIALYSIS: Chronic peritoneal dialysis is a frequent cause of bacterial peritonitis, due to contamination of instruments or dialysate. The clinical course is usually milder than with a perforated viscus; *Staphylococcus* and *Streptococcus* spp. are most often responsible. Chronic dialysis can also cause aseptic peritonitis, presumably due to a chemical in the dialysate to which the peritoneum is sensitive.

SPONTANEOUS BACTERIAL PERITONITIS: Sometimes, peritoneal infection lacks a clear cause. *Such spontaneous bacterial peritonitis occurs most often in adults with cirrhosis complicated by portal hypertension and ascites* (see Chapter 20). Enteric organisms, mainly gram-negative bacilli, appear to move from the gut to mesenteric lymph nodes. From there, they seed the ascitic fluid, where phagocytic and antibacterial activities are low.

In children, spontaneous bacterial peritonitis can complicate the **nephrotic syndrome** (see Chapter 22). Spontaneous peritonitis in children is mostly due to gram-negative organisms, usually from urinary tract infections. The disease causes symptoms of an acute abdomen and usually leads to surgical intervention, unless the child is known to have nephrotic syndrome. Even with antibiotic treatment, mortality is 5%–10%.

TUBERCULOUS PERITONITIS: Tuberculous peritonitis is rare in industrialized countries, but it may occur in developing countries. Many patients with tuberculous peritonitis do not have apparent pulmonary or miliary disease, which suggests that it represents activation of latent tuberculous foci in the peritoneum derived from previous hematogenous dissemination.

 PATHOLOGY: Grossly, bacterial peritonitis resembles purulent infection elsewhere. A fibrinopurulent exudate covers the surface of the intestines. When it organizes, fibrinous and fibrous adhesions form between loops of bowel, which then adhere to each other. Such adhesions may eventually be lysed, or they may lead to **volvulus** and **intestinal obstruction**. Bacterial salpingitis, usually due to gonococcus, may lead to pelvic peritonitis and adhesions. This occurrence defines **pelvic inflammatory disease** (see Chapter 24).

Chemical Peritonitis Usually Results from Endogenous Sources

- **Bile peritonitis** occurs when bile enters the peritoneum, usually from a perforated gallbladder but sometimes from needle biopsy of the liver. This abrupt insult may lead to shock.
- **Hydrochloric acid or hemorrhage** from a perforated peptic ulcer of the stomach or duodenum may elicit an inflammatory reaction in the peritoneum.
- In **acute pancreatitis,** activated lipolytic and proteolytic enzymes are released into the peritoneum, where they cause severe peritonitis with fat necrosis. Shock is common and may be lethal unless it is adequately treated.
- **Foreign materials** introduced by surgery (e.g., talc) or by trauma are unusual causes of chemical peritonitis.
- **Leakage of urine** can produce ascites.

NEOPLASMS OF THE PERITONEUM

Mesenteric and Omental Cysts Are Usually of Lymphatic Origin

They may also derive from other embryonic tissues. Usually a slowly enlarging, painless mass is discovered in a child older than 10 years. The cyst may come to medical attention because of rupture, bleeding, torsion or intestinal obstruction. Surgical excision is curative.

Malignant Peritoneal Mesotheliomas Are Rare, Aggressive Tumors

One quarter of mesotheliomas arise in the peritoneum. *Like pleural mesotheliomas, most of these malignant tumors are associated with exposure to asbestos.* Pathologic characteristics of peritoneal mesotheliomas are identical to those of their pleural counterparts (see Chapter 18).

Primary Peritoneal Carcinomas Resemble Ovarian Carcinoma

Primary peritoneal carcinomas present as tumor masses involving the omentum and peritoneum. They are morphologically identical to serous carcinomas of the ovary, except that in primary peritoneal carcinomas, the ovaries are normal (see Chapter 24).

The Most Common Malignancies of the Peritoneum Are Metastatic Carcinomas

Ovarian, gastric and pancreatic carcinomas are particularly likely to seed the peritoneum, but any intra-abdominal malignancy can spread to the peritoneum.

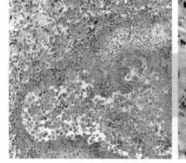
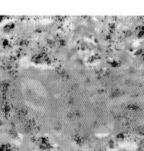
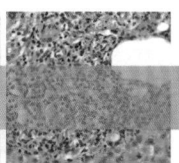

20

The Liver and Biliary System

Arief A. Suriawinata ▪ Swan N. Thung

The Liver

ANATOMY

The liver arises from the embryonic foregut as an endodermal bud that differentiates into the hepatic diverticulum. Strands of endodermal cells mingle with proliferating mesenchymal cells to form the adult liver, gallbladder and extrahepatic bile ducts.

The liver weighs about 1500 g in an average adult man and is in the right upper quadrant of the abdomen, just below the diaphragm. It has two lobes, a larger **right lobe** and a smaller **left lobe,** which meet at the level of the gallbladder bed. Inferiorly, the right lobe has lesser segments, the **caudate** and **quadrate lobes.** The **gallbladder** lies inferiorly, in a fossa of the right hepatic lobe, and extends a little below the inferior margin of the liver.

The liver has a dual blood supply: (1) the **hepatic artery,** a branch of the celiac axis, and (2) the **hepatic portal vein,** formed when the splenic and superior mesenteric veins join. The **hepatic veins** empty into the inferior vena cava, which is partly surrounded by the posterior surface of the liver. Hepatic lymphatics drain mainly into porta hepatis and celiac lymph nodes.

The right and left hepatic ducts merge to form the **hepatic duct,** which joins the cystic duct from the gallbladder to make the **common bile duct.** The latter meets the pancreatic duct just before emptying into the duodenum. It terminates in the ampulla of Vater, where its lumen is guarded by the sphincter of Oddi.

The Lobule Is the Basic Unit of the Liver

Liver lobules are polyhedral (Figs. 20-1 and 20-2), classically depicted as hexagons. **Portal triads** (or portal tracts) are

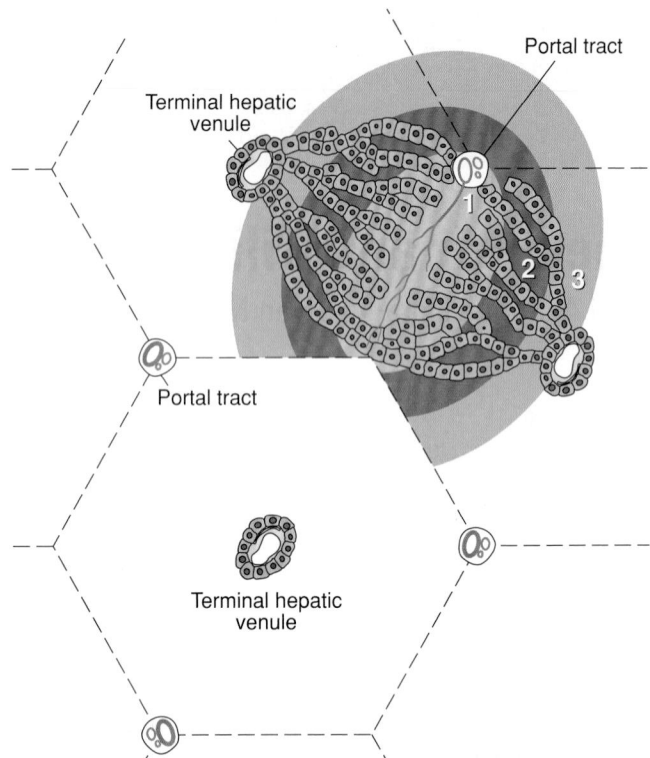

FIGURE 20-2. Morphologic and functional concepts of the liver lobule. In the classic *morphologic* liver lobule, the periphery of the hexagonal lobule is anchored in the portal tracts, and the terminal hepatic venule is in the center. The *functional* liver lobule is an acinus derived from the gradients of oxygen and nutrients in the sinusoidal blood. In this scheme, the portal tract, with the richest content of oxygen and nutrients, is in the center (zone 1). The region most distant from the portal tract (zone 3) is poor in oxygen and nutrients and surrounds the terminal hepatic venule.

peripheral, at the angles of the polygon, and contain intrahepatic branches of the (1) **bile ducts,** (2) **hepatic artery** and (3) **portal vein.** Portal tracts are invested by the **limiting plate,** a layer of adjacent hepatocytes. The **central venule** (or, **terminal hepatic venule**) is at the center of the lobule. Radiating from it are **one-cell-thick plates of hepatocytes,** which extend to the edge of the lobule, where they are continuous with plates of other lobules. Between plates of hepatocytes are **hepatic sinusoids,** which are lined by endothelial cells, Kupffer cells and stellate cells.

The hepatic artery and portal vein enter the liver at the porta hepatis and eventually divide into the small interlobular branches in the portal triads. From there, interlobular vessels distribute blood into hepatic sinusoids, where it flows centripetally toward the central venule. Central venules coalesce into sublobular veins, which eventually merge into the hepatic veins.

Bile is secreted by hepatocytes into **bile canaliculi.** These are formed by apposed lateral surfaces of contiguous hepatocytes. Bile flows in a direction opposite to that of the blood. Contraction of the bile canaliculus by the hepatocyte pericanalicular cytoskeleton propels bile toward the portal tract. From canaliculi, bile flows into canals of Hering, to **bile ductules,** or **cholangioles,** at the border of portal tracts. It then enters a branch of the **intrahepatic bile ducts.** Within each liver lobe, smaller bile ducts progressively merge, eventually forming right and left hepatic ducts.

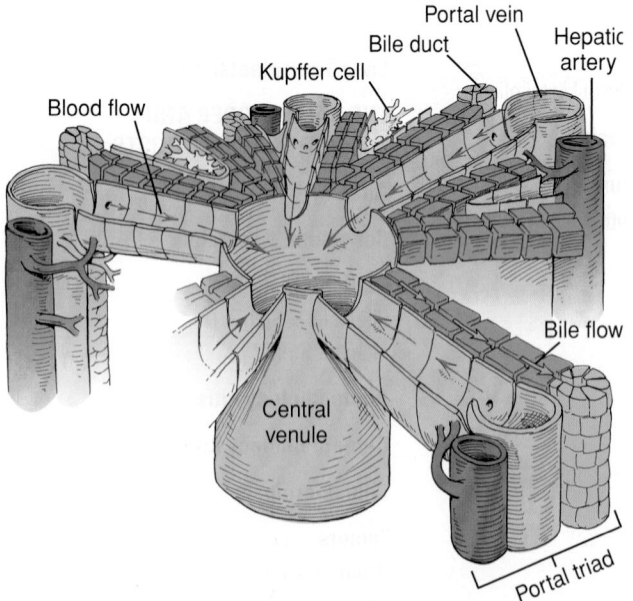

FIGURE 20-1. Microanatomy of the liver. The classic lobule is composed of portal triads, hepatic sinuses, a terminal hepatic venule (central venule) and associated plates of hepatocytes. *Red arrows* indicate the direction of sinusoidal blood flow. *Green arrows* show the direction of bile flow.

The Liver Acinus Is the Functional Interpretation of the Lobule

The structural lobule described above is arranged around a central venule and reflects the liver's histologic appearance. *However, a functional unit can be conceptualized with the portal tract* at the center (Fig. 20-2). Such a construct reflects the functional gradients within lobules. That is, oxygen, nutrients, etc., delivered by the blood are most concentrated near the portal tracts, then progressively decline as hepatocytes extract these materials from the blood going through the sinusoids toward the central venule. Such a construct allows for concentric functional zones. **Zone 1** is the most highly oxygenated zone, around portal tracts. **Zone 3** surrounds central venules and is oxygen-poor. **Zone 2** is intermediate and midlobular. Ischemic injury usually affects zone 3 first. Differences between hepatocytes are not limited to blood flow. The acinus is also heterogeneous with respect to metabolism, independent of oxygenation. In particular, toxic injury is often prominent in zone 3, which is enriched in hepatocyte enzymes that perform drug detoxification and biotransformation. For convenience, pathologic changes in the liver are usually designated in relation to the classic histologic lobule. For example, centrilobular necrosis describes a lesion around central venules, and periportal fibrosis occurs at the periphery of the classic lobule.

Hepatocytes Carry Out the Major Functions of the Liver

Hepatocytes comprise 60% of liver cells and about 90% of the organ's volume. They are roughly 30 μm across and have three specialized surfaces: **sinusoidal, lateral and canalicular.** Each cell has two sinusoidal surfaces, with numerous slender microvilli. Hepatocyte sinusoidal surfaces are separated from the endothelial cells that line sinusoids by the **space of Disse** (Fig. 20-3). Canalicular surfaces of adjacent hepatocytes form the **bile canaliculus,** which is actually an intercellular space without a separate wall. Along this surface, microvilli extend into the lumen. Tight junctions between adjacent hepatocytes prevent bile leakage from canaliculi. Lateral, or intercellular, surfaces of adjacent hepatocytes are in close contact and contain gap junctions.

Centrally placed, occasionally multiple, hepatocyte nuclei are spherical, with one or more nucleoli. Most are diploid, but tetraploid and octaploid nuclei are common. The cytoplasm is rich in organelles, with prominent rough and smooth endoplasmic reticulum (SER), Golgi complexes,

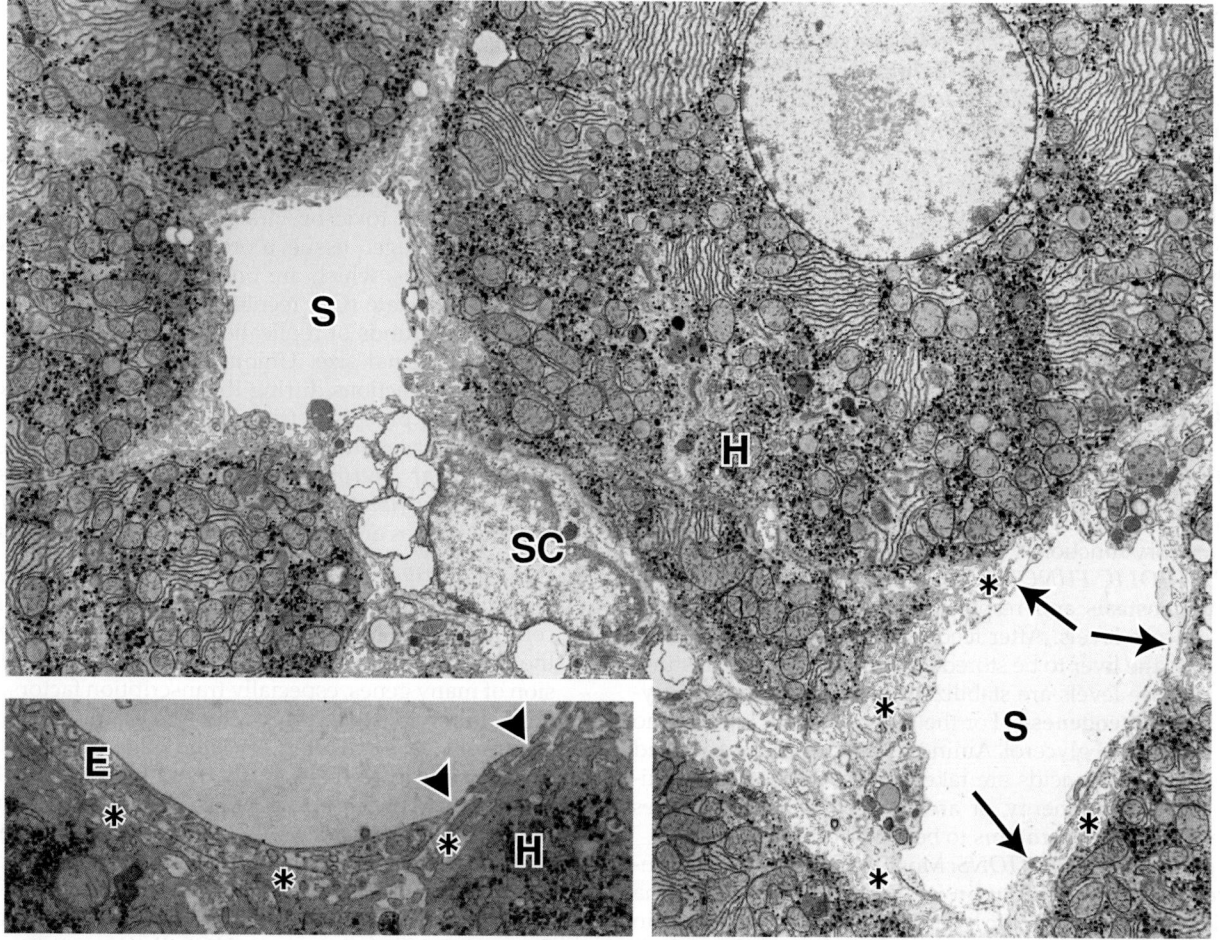

FIGURE 20-3. Hepatic sinusoids and space of Disse. An electron micrograph illustrates the relationship between hepatocytes, sinusoids, the space of Disse and hepatic stellate cells (Ito cells, fat-storing cells). The *arrow* indicates the endothelial cell, and the *asterisk* indicates the space of Disse. H = hepatocyte; S = sinusoid; SC = stellate cell. *Inset.* The relationship between hepatocytes (*H*) and endothelial cells (*E*). The *arrowheads* indicate fenestrae in the endothelial cells; the *asterisks* are in the space of Disse.

mitochondria, lysosomes and peroxisomes. In addition, in the fed state, abundant glycogen and occasional fat droplets are evident.

Blood Traverses the Liver through Hepatic Sinusoids

Sinusoids contain three cell types: endothelial, Kupffer and stellate cells.

ENDOTHELIAL CELLS: Endothelial cells line sinusoids and are penetrated by many holes, or **fenestrae** (Fig. 20-3). Adjacent endothelial cells do not form junctions in the liver, and there are many gaps between them. The result is a sieve-like structure that provides free communication between the sinusoidal lumen and the space of Disse. There is no basement membrane between endothelial cells and hepatocytes, further facilitating access of sinusoidal plasma to hepatocytes.

KUPFFER CELLS: Kupffer cells are macrophages, found in gaps between adjacent endothelial cells or on their surfaces (Fig. 20-1). Because they derive from bone marrow, the Kupffer cells that repopulate transplanted livers are from the recipient, not the donor. Like other macrophages, they protect against infection and circulating toxins (e.g., endotoxin), but with higher efficiency. Activated Kupffer cells also release cytokines, such as TNF-α, interleukins, interferons and TGFs α and β.

STELLATE CELLS: Stellate cells (also known as Ito cells) are occasionally seen beneath endothelial cells in the space of Disse and have specialized storage capacities. They contain fat, vitamin A and other lipid-soluble vitamins. Stellate cells also secrete extracellular matrix components, including collagens, laminin and proteoglycans. In some diseases, they make these species in great excess, leading to hepatic fibrosis and eventually cirrhosis.

The most abundant extracellular matrix component in the space of Disse is fibronectin. Bundles of type I collagen fibers provide a scaffold for liver lobules.

FUNCTIONS OF THE LIVER

Hepatocytes Serve Myriad Functions

Hepatocytes perform metabolic, synthetic, storage, catabolic and excretory functions.

METABOLIC FUNCTIONS: The liver is a center of **glucose homeostasis** and responds rapidly to fluctuations in blood glucose levels. After feeding, excess blood glucose is shunted to the liver to be stored as glycogen. During fasting, blood glucose levels are stabilized by hepatic **glycogenolysis** and **gluconeogenesis**. For the latter, the liver uses amino acids, lactate and glycerol. Amino acid nitrogen is converted to urea. Free fatty acids are taken up by the liver and oxidized to produce energy, or are converted to triglycerides and secreted as **lipoproteins** to be used elsewhere.

SYNTHETIC FUNCTIONS: Most serum proteins are synthesized in the liver. **Albumin** is the main source of plasma oncotic pressure; in chronic liver disease, decreased albumin causes edema and ascites. Blood **clotting factors,** including prothrombin and fibrinogen, are produced by hepatocytes. Severe and often life-threatening bleeding may thus complicate liver failure. Hepatic endothelial cells manufacture **factors V and VIII;** thus, hemophilia can be treated by

liver transplantation. **Complement** and other "acute-phase reactants" (e.g., ferritin, C-reactive protein, serum amyloid A) are also secreted by the liver. Numerous specific **binding proteins** (such as those for iron, copper and vitamin A) are also made by the liver.

STORAGE FUNCTIONS: The liver stores glycogen, triglycerides, iron, copper and lipid-soluble vitamins. Severe liver disease can result from excessive storage—for example, abnormal glycogen deposition in type IV glycogenosis, excess iron in hemochromatosis and copper in Wilson disease (WD).

CATABOLIC FUNCTIONS: The liver catabolizes many endogenous substances, such as hormones and serum proteins. As a result, in chronic liver disease, impaired elimination of estrogens causes feminization in men. The liver is also the principal **detoxifier of foreign compounds** such as drugs, industrial chemicals, environmental contaminants and, perhaps, products of intestinal bacterial metabolism.

Ammonia from amino acid metabolism is mainly removed by the liver. Serum ammonia increases in liver failure and is used as a marker for this condition.

EXCRETORY FUNCTIONS: The principal excretory product of the liver is **bile,** an aqueous mixture of conjugated bilirubin, bile acids, phospholipids, cholesterol and electrolytes. Bile is a repository for the products of heme catabolism and is vital for fat absorption in the small intestine. Normal bile production is critical for eliminating environmental toxins, carcinogens and drugs and their metabolites.

Regeneration Is a Unique Characteristic of the Liver

Liver size is normally maintained within narrow limits, relative to body size. If there is substantial loss of liver tissue (e.g., after mechanical, toxic or viral insult), the organ regrows from the undamaged tissue, a process called **liver regeneration**. Hepatocytes, which are normally in a fully differentiated, quiescent state (G_0), reenter the cell cycle for as many synchronized rounds of replication as are needed to recover the organ's original size. Uniquely, the liver maintains its differentiated functions during this process. Little is known about how this process is triggered or how the liver recognizes when it has reattained its normal size and architecture. *Conditions that interfere with regeneration may cause permanent liver dysfunction and may bring about liver failure.*

Several phases are distinguished in liver regeneration:

- **Priming:** Liver tissue recognizes that damage has occurred and that remaining functional parenchymal cells must transition from their peaceful G_0 state to enter the cell cycle. This process, called *priming*, entails expression of many genes, especially transcription factors. These are required to drive cell cycling (see Chapter 5). Priming requires release of TNF-α, IL-6 and other cytokines.
- **Progression to mitosis:** In the next phase, the cell progresses through G_1 into S phase, where DNA synthesis occurs. This is followed by G_2 and M phases, where cell division occurs. Several growth factors drive this part of the process, including hepatocyte growth factor (HGF/SF), epidermal growth factor (EGF), TGF-α and others. Several growth factors (e.g., HGF, IL-6) promote protection of the liver and survival in various models of hepatic injury. After one or two rounds (depending on need) of mitosis, hepatocytes become quiescent again and resume normal function.

■ **Nonparenchymal and progenitor cells:** In the final phase, nonparenchymal cells (sinusoidal endothelium, Kupffer cells, stellate cells and biliary epithelium) replicate. The tissue remodels to recover the original structure of liver cell plates.

Hepatic progenitor cells ("oval cells"), which lie within the terminal branches of bile ductules and canals of Hering, contribute to ductular proliferation after extensive hepatic necrosis. However, the role of these cells in hepatic regeneration is unclear, as is any involvement of bone marrow–derived stem cells (see Chapter 3).

BILIRUBIN METABOLISM AND MECHANISMS OF JAUNDICE

Bilirubin Is the End-Product of Heme Catabolism

About 80% of this heme comes from senescent erythrocytes, removed by mononuclear phagocytes of the spleen, bone marrow and liver from the circulation. The remainder of the heme comes from other sources, including cytochrome P450 isoenzymes, myoglobin and premature breakdown of erythroid progenitors in the bone marrow. Beyond this, no specific physiologic role for bilirubin is known.

Bilirubin dissolves poorly in water but is quite miscible with fat. Thus, in the circulation, it is transported bound to albumin. The albumin in the blood and extracellular space is a large reservoir for binding bilirubin, ensuring a low extracellular concentration of free (unbound) bilirubin. Bilirubin that is not bound to albumin or conjugated to glucuronic acid easily enters the lipid-rich brain. There, it is very toxic, and high concentrations of it in newborns causes irreversible brain injury, **kernicterus**.

Transfer of bilirubin from blood to the bile involves four steps:

1. **Uptake:** The albumin–bilirubin complex is dissociated when it reaches hepatocytes, and the bilirubin is transported across the plasma membrane. Transporter proteins facilitate mostly passive uptake by hepatocytes.
2. **Binding:** Once inside hepatocytes, bilirubin binds to cytosolic proteins, known collectively as **glutathione S-transferases** (also termed *ligandin*).
3. **Conjugation:** Bilirubin is converted to a water-soluble glucuronic acid conjugate for excretion. This is done in the endoplasmic reticulum (ER), where the uridine diphosphate-glucuronyl transferase (UGT) system attaches glucuronic acid to bilirubin. The process yields mostly water-soluble bilirubin diglucuronide and a small amount (<10%) of monoglucuronide.
4. **Excretion:** Conjugated bilirubin diffuses through the cytosol to bile canaliculi and is excreted into the bile by an energy-dependent carrier-mediated process. This is the rate-limiting step in the transhepatic transport of bilirubin.

Conjugated bilirubin enters the small intestine as part of mixed micelles but is not absorbed there. It remains intact until it reaches the distal small bowel and colon, where it is hydrolyzed by bacterial flora into free (unconjugated) bilirubin, which is reduced to a mixture of pyrroles, collectively called **urobilinogen**. Most urobilinogen is excreted in feces, but a small amount is absorbed in the terminal ileum and colon, returned to the liver and reexcreted into the bile. Bile acids are also reabsorbed in the terminal ileum and salvaged

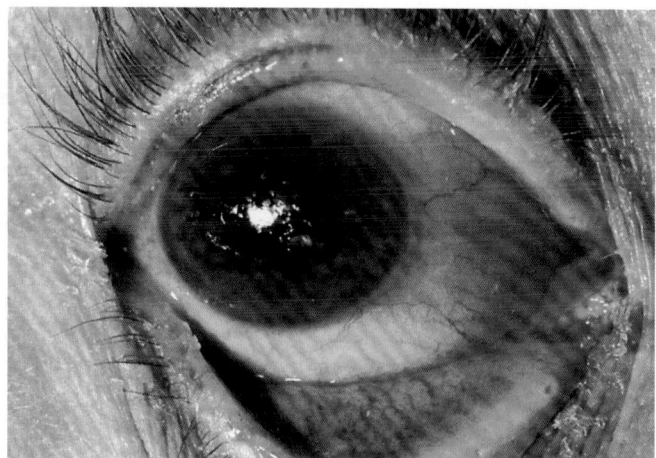

FIGURE 20-4. Jaundice. A patient in hepatic failure displays yellow sclera.

by the liver. This recycling process is the **enterohepatic circulation of bile**. Some urobilinogen escapes reabsorption by the liver, reaches the systemic circulation and is excreted in the urine.

■ **Hyperbilirubinemia** means increased blood levels of bilirubin (>1.0 mg/dL).
■ **Jaundice** or **icterus** is yellow skin and sclerae (Fig. 20-4), the color becoming apparent when circulating bilirubin concentrations exceed 2.5–3.0 mg/dL.
■ **Cholestasis** is pathological plugging of dilated bile canaliculi by inspissated bile. Bile pigment, which is normally invisible, is seen in hepatocytes.
■ **Cholestatic jaundice** is histologic cholestasis and hyperbilirubinemia. Many conditions are associated with hyperbilirubinemia (Fig. 20-5).

Overproduction of bilirubin, interference with its hepatic uptake or intracellular metabolism and impaired bile excretion and flow may all cause jaundice (Fig. 20-5).

Bilirubin Overproduction Can Lead to Unconjugated Hyperbilirubinemia

Increased production of free bilirubin results from enhanced destruction of erythrocytes (e.g., hemolytic anemia) or ineffective erythropoiesis. Rarely, erythrocyte breakdown in a large hematoma (e.g., after trauma) may also generate excess unconjugated bilirubin.

In adults, even severe hemolytic anemia does not lead to sustained increases in serum bilirubin above 4.0 mg/dL as long as hepatic bilirubin clearance is normal. However, prolonged hemolysis, as in sickle cell anemia, in the context of intrinsic liver disease, such as viral hepatitis, may cause extremely high blood bilirubin levels (up to 100 mg/dL) and pronounced jaundice.

Hyperbilirubinemia from uncomplicated hemolysis is mainly unconjugated bilirubin, whereas parenchymal liver disease causes elevation of both conjugated and unconjugated bilirubin. Unconjugated hyperbilirubinemia is of little clinical significance in adults but can cause kernicterus with catastrophic brain damage in newborns (see Chapter 6). This occurs if bilirubin concentrations exceed 20 mg/dL, but subtle psychomotor retardation may follow considerably lower bilirubin concentrations.

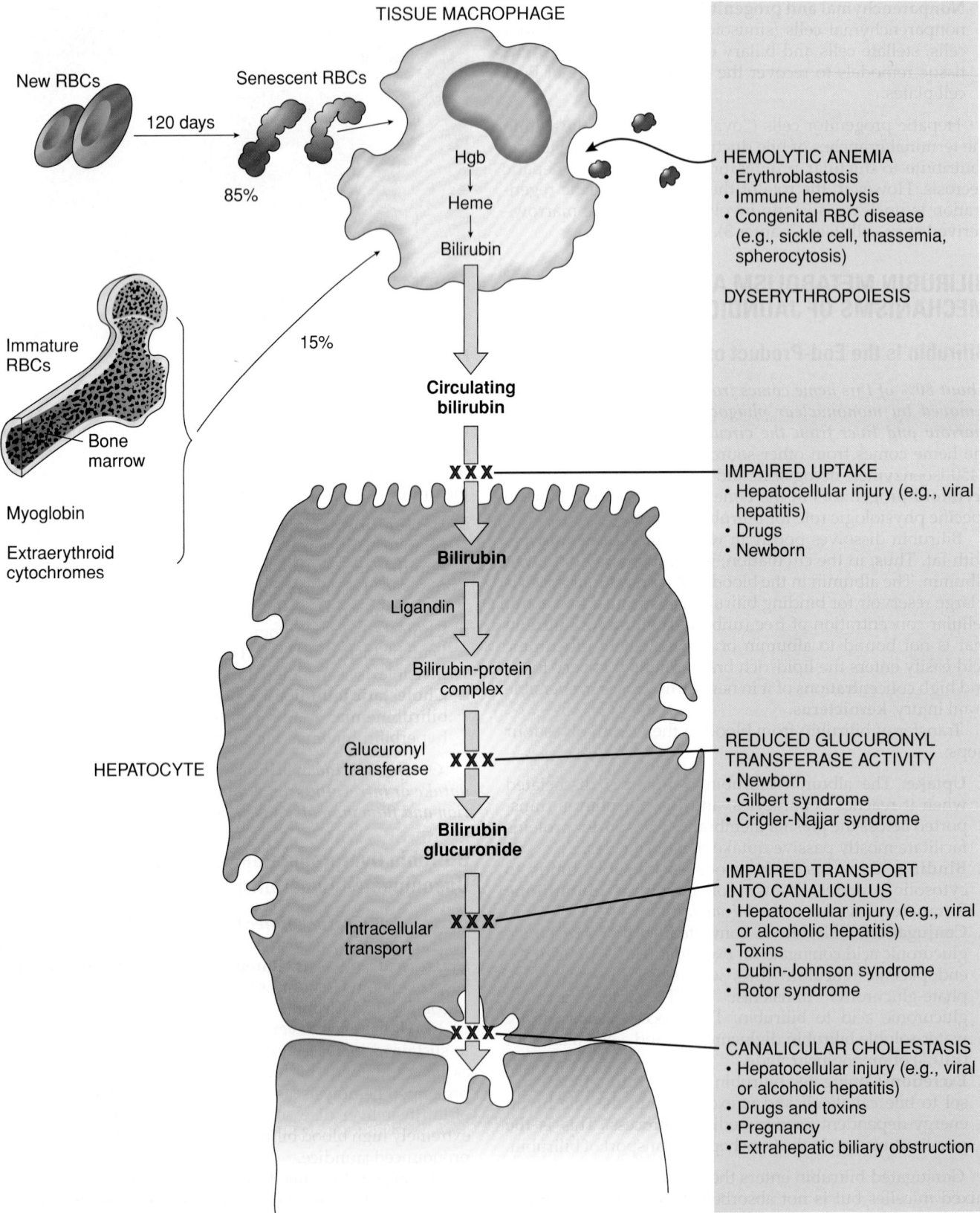

FIGURE 20-5. Mechanisms of hyperbilirubinemia at the level of the hepatocyte. Bilirubin is derived principally from the senescence of circulating red blood cells (RBCs), with a smaller contribution from the degradation of erythropoietic elements in the bone marrow, myoglobin and extraerythroid cytochromes. Hyperbilirubinemia and jaundice result from overproduction of bilirubin (hemolytic anemia), dyserythropoiesis, impaired bilirubin uptake or defects in its hepatic metabolism. The locations of specific blocks in the metabolic pathway of bilirubin in the hepatocyte are illustrated. Hgb = hemoglobin.

In disorders of ineffective erythropoiesis (e.g., megaloblastic or sideroblastic anemias; see Chapter 20), increased bone marrow–derived bilirubin may cause hyperbilirubinemia. In a rare hereditary disease of unknown etiology, "primary shunt hyperbilirubinemia" or "idiopathic dyserythropoietic jaundice," massive overproduction of bone marrow–derived bilirubin is associated with chronic unconjugated hyperbilirubinemia.

Decreased Hepatic Uptake of Bilirubin Is a Common Cause of Jaundice

Generalized liver cell injury (e.g., due to viral hepatitis or certain drugs, such as rifampin or probenecid) may interfere with net uptake of bilirubin by liver cells. This can cause mild unconjugated hyperbilirubinemia.

Decreased Bilirubin Conjugation Occurs in Several Hereditary Syndromes

Crigler-Najjar Syndrome

Crigler-Najjar syndrome type I is a rare, recessively inherited disease due to a complete lack of hepatic UGT activity. Affected patients show chronic, severe, unconjugated hyperbilirubinemia beginning in early childhood.

The appearance of the liver is normal. Crigler-Najjar syndrome type I was invariably lethal before the advent of phototherapy and liver transplantation.

Crigler-Najjar syndrome type II is similar to type I but is less severe and entails only a partial decrease in UGT activity. Almost all patients with type II syndrome develop normally, but some show neurologic changes resembling kernicterus.

Gilbert Syndrome

Gilbert syndrome is an inherited, mild, chronic unconjugated hyperbilirubinemia (<6 mg/dL). Bilirubin clearance is impaired, without functional or structural liver disease. The mode of inheritance is unclear, but autosomal recessive inheritance is most likely. Mutations in the *UGT* gene promotor region lead to reduced transcription of the *UGT* gene and, thus, inadequate synthesis of UGT. In a few patients the *UGT* promotor is normal, and missense mutations in the coding region are responsible for the disorder. Factors that elevate serum bilirubin concentrations in normal persons, such as fasting or an intercurrent illness, produce exaggerated increases in people with Gilbert syndrome. Mild hemolysis, which also tends to increase bilirubin levels, occurs in more than 1/2 of persons with Gilbert syndrome, but the mechanism is unclear.

Gilbert syndrome is exceptionally common, occurring in 5%–10% of the population. It occurs more often in men than in women and is usually recognized after puberty. Differences and the age at onset and patient gender suggest that hormones influence hepatic bilirubin metabolism. Gilbert syndrome is generally without clinical import, except for the possibility that drug metabolism may be altered.

Mutations in the Multidrug Resistance Protein Gene Family Often Alter Transport of Conjugated Bilirubin

Multidrug resistance proteins (MRPs) mediate transmembrane transport of organic ions, including conjugated bilirubin, bile acids and phospholipids. Mutations in genes encoding these proteins, or in other canalicular transporters, impair hepatocellular secretion of bilirubin glucuronides and other organic anions into canaliculi. The spectrum of resultant diseases varies from innocuous to lethal.

Dubin-Johnson Syndrome

This syndrome is caused by mutations in the *ABCC2/MRP2* gene. It is a benign, autosomal recessive disease with chronic conjugated hyperbilirubinemia and conspicuous deposition of melanin-like pigment in the liver.

Dubin-Johnson syndrome can be distinguished from other conditions with conjugated hyperbilirubinemia by testing **urinary coproporphyrin excretion**. There are two forms of human coproporphyrins, **isomer I** and **isomer III**. A shift in the ratio of urinary coproporphyrin isomer I and III from 1:3 (normal) to 4:1 (abnormal) is diagnostic of Dubin-Johnson syndrome.

 PATHOLOGY: Liver histology is entirely normal, except for coarse, iron-free, **dark-brown granules** in hepatocytes and Kupffer cells, mainly in the centrilobular zone (Fig. 20-6). By electron microscopy, the pigment is in enlarged lysosomes. As liver cells do not synthesize melanin, the pigment may reflect auto-oxidation of anionic metabolites (e.g., tyrosine, phenylalanine, tryptophan), and possibly of epinephrine. Accumulation of this pigment causes the liver to be grossly pigmented, or "black."

 CLINICAL FEATURES: Symptoms are mild: slight intermittent jaundice and vague nonspecific complaints. Dark urine is present in 1/2 of those affected. In women, the disease may be diagnosed when

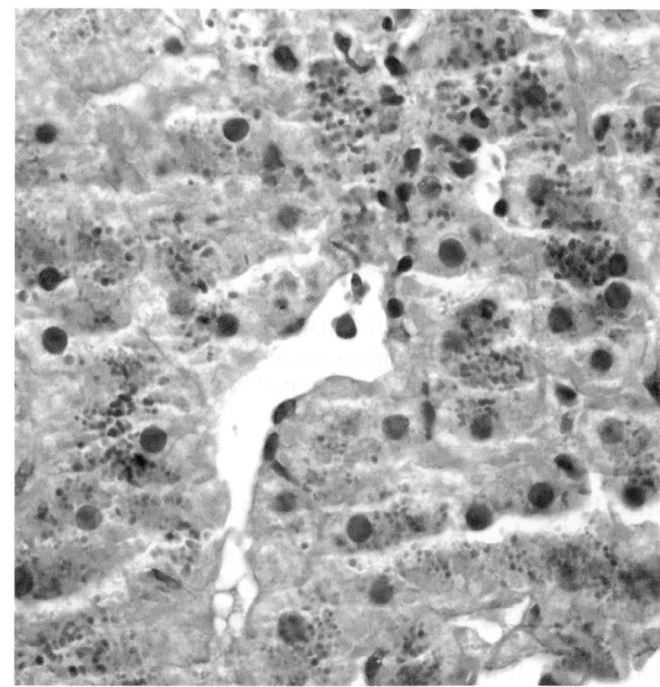

FIGURE 20-6. Dubin-Johnson syndrome. The hepatocytes contain coarse, iron-free, dark-brown granules.

jaundice appears with use of oral contraceptives or during pregnancy. Serum bilirubin is 2–5 mg/dL but may transiently be much higher.

Rotor Syndrome

Rotor syndrome is an autosomal recessive, familial conjugated hyperbilirubinemia, clinically similar to Dubin-Johnson syndrome but without liver pigmentation. Defective hepatic uptake or intracellular binding of organic ions has been blamed. The pattern of urinary coproporphyrins is like that of most hepatobiliary disorders with conjugated hyperbilirubinemia (i.e., increased total urinary coproporphyrins, 65% of which are isomer I). Patients with Rotor syndrome have few symptoms and lead normal lives.

Progressive Familial Intrahepatic Cholestasis

Progressive familial intrahepatic cholestases (PFICs) are a heterogeneous group of rare, inherited, autosomal recessive disorders of infancy or early childhood in which intrahepatic cholestasis progresses relentlessly to cirrhosis. PFIC1, PFIC2 and PFIC3 are due to mutations of different genes. In PFIC1, mutant *ATP8B1* causes deficiency in FIC1 protein. PFIC2 is a defect in a bile salt export pump (BSEP) encoded by the *ABCB11* gene. PFIC3 is caused by multidrug resistant 3 (MDR3) protein deficiency, encoded by the *ABCB4* gene. Both benign recurrent intrahepatic cholestasis and intrahepatic cholestasis of pregnancy (ICP; see below) are milder forms of PFIC that do not progress to cirrhosis.

The first patients with PFIC1 were descendents of an Amish man, Jacob Byler (Byler syndrome), but PFIC is not limited to that ethnic group. There is an associated high incidence of retinitis pigmentosa. The children are often mentally retarded. Most affected children die within the first 2 years of life.

Benign Recurrent Intrahepatic Cholestasis

In benign recurrent intrahepatic cholestasis, self-limited, episodic intrahepatic cholestasis may be preceded by malaise and itching. The occurrence of familial cases suggests a genetic origin. Symptoms tend to last several weeks to several months. Patients usually have 3–5 episodes in their lives, but some may have as many as 10. Recurrences may be separated by weeks to years. Serum bilirubin during the acute episodes ranges from 10 to 20 mg/dL, mostly conjugated.

The liver shows centrilobular cholestasis (bile plugs in bile canaliculi) and a few mononuclear inflammatory cells in portal tracts. All structural and functional alterations disappear during remissions. No permanent sequelae have been reported.

Intrahepatic Cholestasis of Pregnancy

ICP is a rare disease marked by pruritus and cholestasis, usually in the last trimester of each pregnancy. These promptly disappear after delivery. Women with ICP fare well, but fetal morbidity and mortality are increased, as are premature labor, fetal distress and placental insufficiency. Mutations in the ATP-cassette transporter B4 (*ABCB4*) and the multidrug resistance protein-3 (MDR3) have been described in women with ICP. Increased gonadal and placental hormones during pregnancy most likely cause cholestasis in susceptible women. Mothers' livers show mainly centrilobular cholestasis. The diagnosis is generally made by clinical observation and is confirmed by the markedly increased maternal total bile acid levels. Therapy with ursodeoxycholic acid (UDCA) provides some relief of pruritus.

Sepsis Can Cause Jaundice

Severe conjugated hyperbilirubinemia may occur in sepsis involving either gram-positive or gram-negative bacteria. In such situations, serum alkaline phosphatase and cholesterol levels are usually low, suggesting a defect in excretion of conjugated bilirubin. Liver pathology is nonspecific and includes mild canalicular cholestasis and slight fat accumulation. Portal tracts may contain excess inflammatory cells and variable bile ductule proliferation. Occasionally, dilated ductules are filled with inspissated bile.

Neonatal (Physiologic) Jaundice Occurs in Most Newborns

Neonatal hyperbilirubinemia occurs in the absence of any specific disorder. Hepatic clearance of bilirubin in the fetus is minimal; hepatic uptake, conjugation and biliary excretion are all much lower than in children and adults. Liver UGT activity is less than 1% of that in adults, and ligandin levels are low. Fetal bilirubin levels are low because bilirubin crosses the placenta and is conjugated and excreted by the mother's liver.

The livers of newborns thus become responsible for clearing bilirubin before the conjugation and excretion are fully developed. Moreover, increased erythrocyte destruction in the postnatal period adds to the liver's duties in the newborn. ***Thus, 70% of normal infants have transient unconjugated hyperbilirubinemia.*** Such physiologic jaundice is more pronounced in premature infants, because liver clearance of bilirubin is less developed and red blood cell turnover is greater than in term infants. When hepatic bilirubin-conjugating capacity reaches adult levels, about 2 weeks after birth (ligandin takes somewhat longer), serum bilirubin levels rapidly decline to adult values. Absorption of light by unconjugated bilirubin generates water-soluble bilirubin isomers. ***Thus, phototherapy is now routinely used to treat neonatal jaundice.***

Maternal–fetal blood group incompatibilities may lead to **erythroblastosis fetalis** (see Chapter 6), in which striking bilirubin overproduction in the fetus is due to immune-mediated hemolysis. Newborns with erythroblastosis fetalis show increased cord blood bilirubin. However, jaundice becomes severe only after birth, since the mother's liver no longer compensates for the immaturity of the neonatal liver.

Cholestasis Reflects Extra- or Intrahepatic Biliary Obstruction

Functionally, cholestasis represents decreased bile flow through the canaliculus and reduced secretion of water, bilirubin and bile acids by hepatocytes. Clinical diagnosis depends on the accumulation in the blood of materials that are normally transferred to the bile, including bilirubin, cholesterol and bile acids, and elevated blood activities of

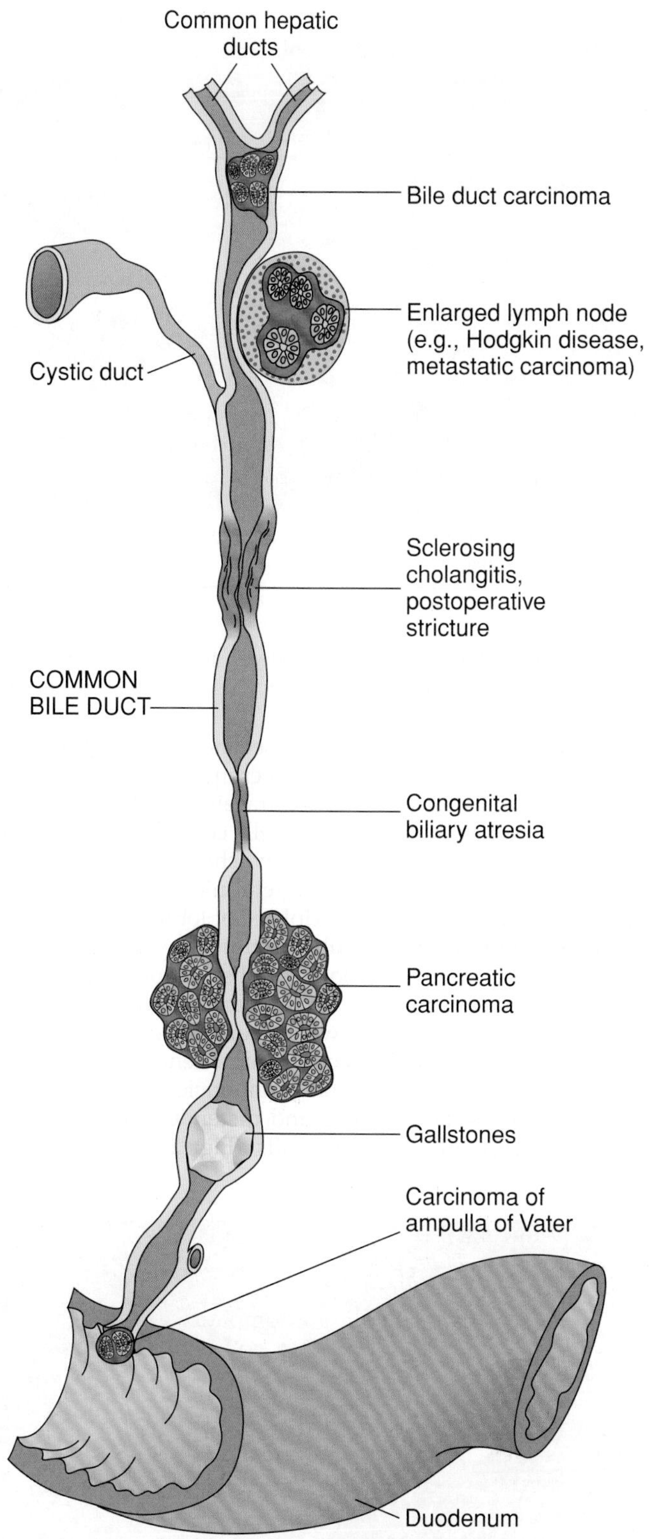
Common hepatic ducts
Bile duct carcinoma
Enlarged lymph node (e.g., Hodgkin disease, metastatic carcinoma)
Cystic duct
Sclerosing cholangitis, postoperative stricture
COMMON BILE DUCT
Congenital biliary atresia
Pancreatic carcinoma
Gallstones
Carcinoma of ampulla of Vater
Duodenum

FIGURE 20-7. Major causes of extrahepatic biliary obstruction.

certain enzymes, typically alkaline phosphatase. Cholestasis due to intrinsic liver disease is **intrahepatic cholestasis** (Fig. 20-5), whereas that caused by obstruction of large bile ducts is extrahepatic cholestasis. ***In any event, it reflects a defect in bile transport across the canalicular membrane.***

The inability to excrete bile acids into canaliculi raises serum and hepatocellular bile acid levels. As detergents, bile acids injure cells by both detergent action and direct activation of apoptosis. They are thus potent hepatotoxins, and their accumulation within hepatocytes causes much of the hepatic injury and progression to cirrhosis associated with cholestasis. Elevation of serum bile acids is the likely cause of severe itching **(pruritus)**.

The extrahepatic biliary system may be obstructed by gallstones lodged in the common bile duct, cancers of the bile duct or surrounding tissues (pancreas or ampulla of Vater), external compression by enlarged neoplastic lymph nodes in the porta hepatis (as in lymphoma), benign strictures (postoperative scarring or primary sclerosing cholangitis [PSC]) and congenital extrahepatic biliary atresia (EHBA) (Fig. 20-7).

PATHOPHYSIOLOGY: Bile secretion into canaliculi and passage into the biliary collecting system depend on (1) functional and structural characteristics of canalicular microvilli, (2) permeability of canalicular plasma membranes, (3) intracellular contractile systems around canaliculi (microfilaments, microtubules) and (4) interactions of bile acids with the secretory apparatus.

The biochemical basis of cholestasis is unclear, but several abnormalities in bile formation and movement of bile are described. For extrahepatic biliary obstruction, the effects clearly begin with increased pressure within bile ducts. However, in the early stages, the biochemistry and morphology at the canalicular level resemble those in intrahepatic cholestasis, including initial centrilobular canalicular bile plugs (Fig. 20-8).

The invariable presence of bile constituents in the blood of people with cholestasis implies regurgitation of conjugated bilirubin from hepatocytes into the blood. Hepatic clearance of unconjugated bilirubin in cholestasis is normal. Even if bile duct obstruction is complete, serum bilirubin levels only reach 30–35 mg/dL because renal excretion of bilirubin prevents further accumulation.

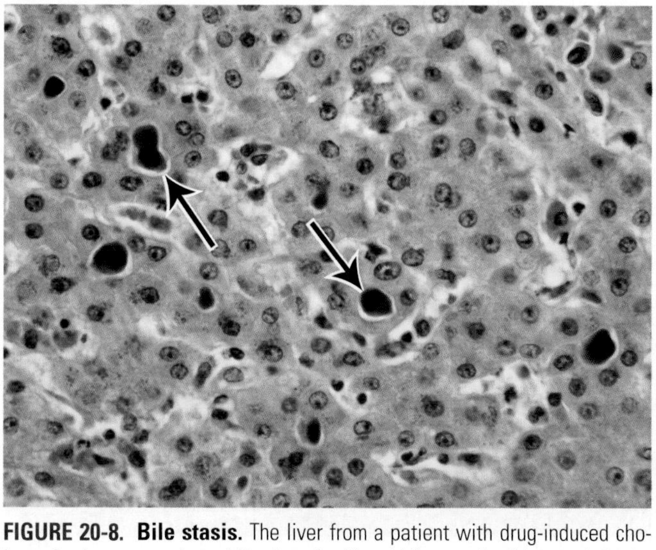

FIGURE 20-8. Bile stasis. The liver from a patient with drug-induced cholestasis shows prominent bile plugs in dilated bile canaliculi (*arrows*). In the absence of inflammation, this lesion may be termed *pure cholestasis.*

In both intrahepatic and extrahepatic cholestasis, bile pigment initially is centrilobular. Fluid secretion into the canalicular bile has two components: one that is dependent on bile acid secretion and the other that is not. Since periportal hepatocytes secrete most of the bile acids, the fluid content in the periportal zone of the canaliculus exceeds that in the central zone, thus keeping bilirubin in solution. In addition, the bile acids themselves act as detergents in the intestine and solubilize aggregates of bilirubin in the periportal areas. As well, the higher activity of microsomal mixed-function oxidases in the central zone predisposes central hepatocytes to injury by a variety of drugs and toxins. Such an effect may favor bile deposition in centrilobular areas in cholestasis.

Several mechanisms of cholestasis have been proposed.

DAMAGE TO CANALICULAR PLASMA MEMBRANES: The canalicular plasma membrane is the site of sodium (and therefore fluid) secretion into the bile. This membrane also participates in bile acid and bilirubin secretion. Fluid secretion is controlled by the Na$^+$/K$^+$-ATPase of the canalicular membrane. Alterations in the canalicular membrane by drugs and other agents that can perturb its structure inhibit the Na$^+$/K$^+$-ATPase, decrease bile flow or produce morphologic alterations.

ALTERED CONTRACTILE PROPERTIES OF THE CANALICULUS: Bile is propelled along the canaliculus by a peristalsis-like contractile activity of hepatocytes. Agents that interact with the pericanalicular actin microfilaments (e.g., cytochalasin and phalloidin) inhibit this peristalsis and may cause cholestasis.

ALTERATIONS IN CANALICULAR MEMBRANE PERMEABILITY: Agents that cause cholestasis, including estrogens and taurolithocholate, may allow back-diffusion of bile components by making canalicular membranes more permeable, or "leaky."

PATHOLOGY: *Cholestasis is characterized by the presence of brownish bile pigment within dilated canaliculi and in hepatocytes* (Figs. 20-8, 20-9 and 20-10). Canaliculi are enlarged. By electron microscopy,

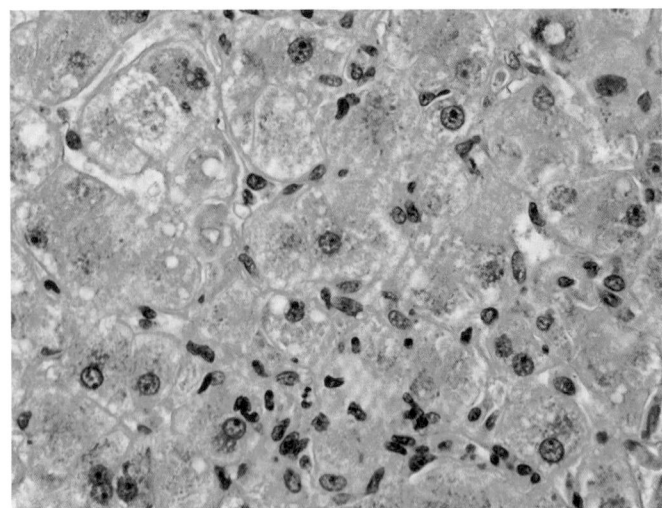

FIGURE 20-10. Cholestasis. Hepatocytes are swollen and bile stained (feathery degeneration).

the microvilli are blunted and fewer in number or even absent. Bile accumulates in hepatocytes in large, bile-laden lysosomes.

When cholestasis persists, secondary morphologic abnormalities develop. Scattered necrotic hepatocytes probably reflect the toxicity of excess intracellular bile. Intrasinusoidal macrophages and Kupffer cells contain bile pigment and cellular debris. Whereas early cholestasis is limited almost entirely to the central zone, chronic cholestasis is also marked by bile plugs at the periphery of lobules.

In **extrahepatic biliary obstruction,** the liver is swollen and bile stained. Prolonged obstruction suppresses bile secretion, causing the bile to become almost colorless ("white bile"). The liver, however, remains green. At first, edema in portal tracts accompanies centrilobular cholestasis, progressing to portal mononuclear infiltrates as obstruction persists. Tortuous and distended bile ductules proliferate and attract neutrophils (Fig. 20-9). Damaged

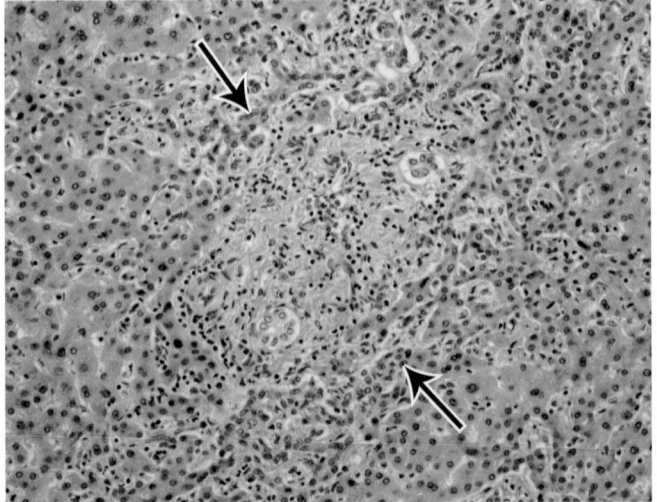

FIGURE 20-9. Extrahepatic biliary obstruction. A portal tract is expanded by ductular reaction (*arrows*) and acute and chronic inflammation.

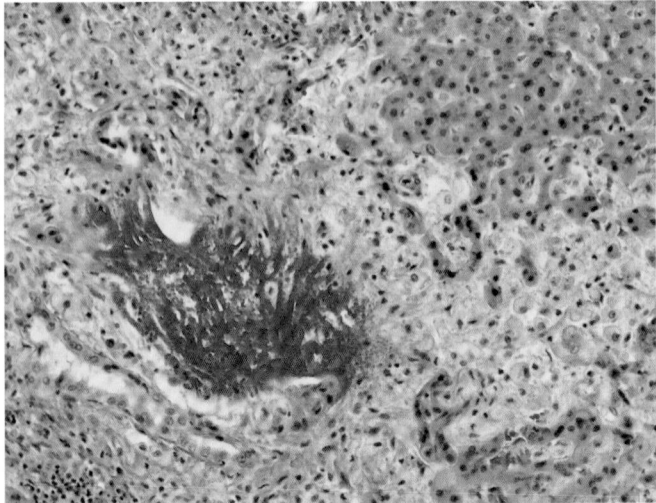

FIGURE 20-11. Bile infarct (bile lake). The liver in a patient with extrahepatic biliary obstruction, showing an area of necrosis and accumulation of extravasated bile.

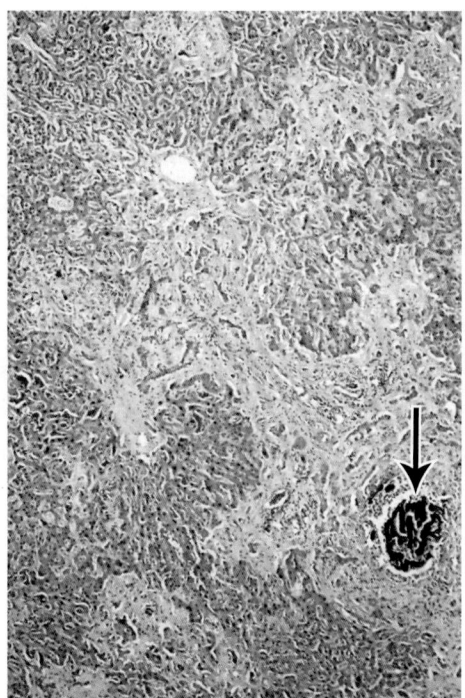

FIGURE 20-12. Secondary biliary cirrhosis. Liver from a patient with a carcinoma of the pancreas that obstructed the common bile duct. Irregular fibrous septa extend from enlarged portal tracts containing a dilated interlobular bile duct that encloses a dense bile concretion (*arrow*). Ductular reaction are seen within the septa.

hepatocytes swollen with bile show (1) hydropic swelling, (2) diffuse impregnation with bile pigment and (3) a reticulated appearance. This triad is **feathery degeneration** (Fig. 20-10). Cholestasis eventually reaches the periphery of the lobule. Dilated bile ducts may rupture, leading to **bile lakes** (Fig. 20-11)—focal, golden-yellow deposits surrounded by degenerating hepatocytes. Infection of obstructed biliary passages often leads to superimposed suppurative cholangitis, intraluminal pus and even intrahepatic abscesses. Within bile ducts and ductules, biliary concretions may be conspicuous.

In time, portal tracts become enlarged and fibrotic (Fig. 20-12). If extrahepatic biliary obstruction is untreated, septa eventually extend between portal tracts of contiguous lobules to form **micronodular cirrhosis** (see below).

CLINICAL FEATURES: Whatever the cause, cholestasis usually presents with jaundice. **Pruritus** (itching) is common and can be severe and intractable. It may be caused by deposition of bile acids in the skin, but other bile components may play a role. Cholesterol accumulates in the skin to form **xanthomas**. **Malabsorption** may develop in cases of protracted cholestasis (see Chapter 13).

CIRRHOSIS

Cirrhosis is destruction of normal liver architecture by fibrous bands around regenerative nodules of hepatocytes. This pattern invariably results from persistent liver cell necrosis. Advanced cases of cirrhosis all tend to have a similar appearance, and the cause often can no longer be

ascertained by morphologic examination alone. In earlier stages, on the other hand, features characteristic of an inciting pathogenic insult may be evident. For example, fat and Mallory bodies are typical of alcoholic liver injury, whereas chronic inflammation and periportal necrosis are prominent in chronic hepatitis.

The pathogenesis of cirrhosis involves death and regeneration of hepatocytes, extracellular matrix deposition by activated hepatic stellate cells and resulting alterations in hepatic vascular architecture.

Many terms are applied to the different forms of cirrhosis, rivaling the number of etiologies incriminated in chronic liver disease, but some patterns emerge. At one end of this spectrum, usually early in the evolution of cirrhosis, is the **micronodular** type (Fig. 20-13), characterized by small, uniform nodules separated by thin fibrous septa. At the other end, ordinarily late in the disease, is **macronodular cirrhosis** (Fig. 20-14), with grossly visible, coarse, irregular nodules, mirrored histologically by large nodules that vary in size and shape and are encircled by similarly variably broad bands of connective tissue. *Between these extremes are many cases with features of both. In practice, the different appearances of cirrhosis are less important than their etiologies.*

Once considered to be irreversible, cirrhotic livers may undergo collagen resorption, hepatic regeneration and remodeling over years to decades—if the underlying cause of cirrhosis is removed. However, even as functional and structural improvement may occur, complete regression is unlikely.

MICRONODULAR CIRRHOSIS: This form of liver disease was previously termed **Laennec cirrhosis,** to honor the early 19th-century French physician who first described it accurately. (He also invented the stethoscope.) Nodules in micronodular cirrhosis are usually less than 3 mm, scarcely larger than a lobule (Fig. 20-13). They show no landmarks of lobular architecture, such as portal tracts or central venules. Connective tissue septa separating nodules are usually thin, but irregular focal collapse of parenchyma may lead to wider septa. In its active stages, mononuclear inflammatory cells and proliferated bile ductules inhabit the septa. *The prototypical cause of micronodular cirrhosis is alcoholic injury, but other etiologies may also be responsible.*

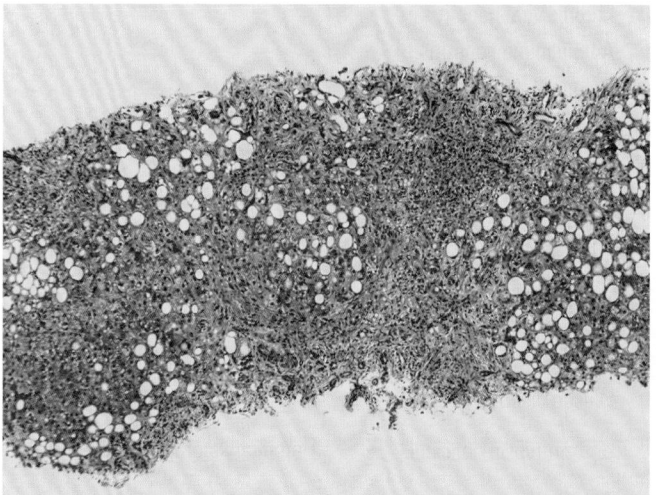

FIGURE 20-13. Micronodular cirrhosis. Cirrhotic liver from a chronic alcoholic. Note the small, regenerative nodules of parenchyma and fatty change.

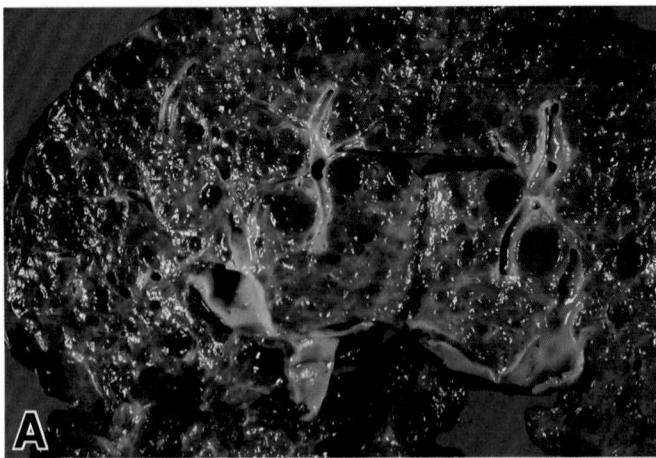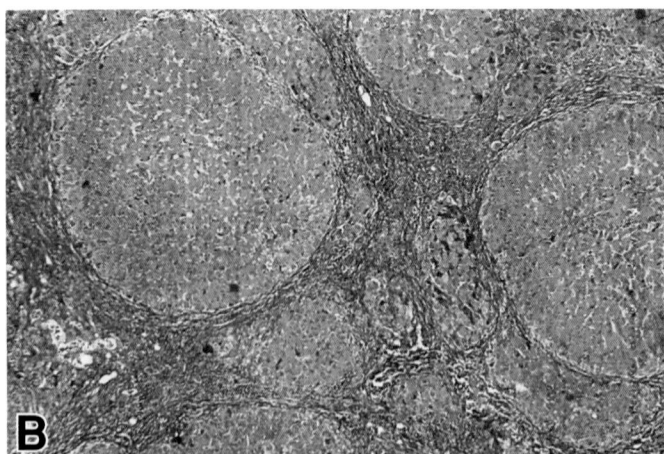

FIGURE 20-14. Macronodular cirrhosis. A. The liver is misshapen, and the cut surface reveals irregular nodules and connective tissue septa of varying width. **B.** Nodules of varying size and irregular fibrous septa.

MACRONODULAR CIRRHOSIS: Macronodular cirrhosis is classically due to chronic hepatitis. Broad connective tissue septa (Fig. 20-14) show elements of preexisting portal tracts, mononuclear inflammatory cells and proliferated bile ductules. Micronodular cirrhosis can become macronodular with continued regeneration and expansion of existing nodules, especially in alcoholics who stop drinking.

The diseases associated with cirrhosis are listed in Table 20-1. They have little in common except that they all entail persistent liver cell necrosis. Most cases of cirrhosis are attributable to alcoholism and chronic viral hepatitis. And for 15% of cases, etiologies remain unknown. These are labeled **cryptogenic cirrhosis**. Nonalcoholic steatohepatitis

(NASH) is now felt to account for a significant proportion of cryptogenic cirrhosis.

HEPATIC FAILURE

Hepatic failure is the clinical syndrome that occurs when the liver cannot sustain its vital activities. It may develop acutely, mostly due to viral hepatitis or toxic exposure. Or, chronic liver diseases, such as chronic viral hepatitis or cirrhosis, may lead to insidious onset of hepatic failure. Advances in supportive care have improved survival in acute hepatic failure, but mortality for this condition without liver transplantation exceeds 50%. The consequences of hepatic failure are depicted in Figure 20-15.

Jaundice Reflects Inadequate Clearance of Bilirubin by the Liver

Hyperbilirubinemia in hepatic failure is mostly conjugated, although unconjugated bilirubin levels also tend to increase. On occasion, increased erythrocyte turnover may add to unconjugated hyperbilirubinemia, thus aggravating the jaundice.

The Effect of Liver Failure on the CNS Is Hepatic Encephalopathy

Altered mental status is common in patients with acute liver failure and portal hypertension (see below).

TABLE 20-1	
MAJOR CAUSES OF CIRRHOSIS	
Alcoholic Liver Disease	
Nonalcoholic Fatty Liver Disease	
Chronic Hepatitis	
Chronic viral hepatitis	
Autoimmune hepatitis	
Drugs	
Biliary Disease	
Extrahepatic biliary obstruction	
Primary biliary cirrhosis	
Primary sclerosing cholangitis	
Metabolic Disease	
Hemochromatosis	Glycogen storage disease
Wilson disease	Hereditary fructose intolerance
α_1-Antitrypsin deficiency	Hereditary storage diseases
Tyrosinemia	Galactosemia
Cryptogenic	

PATHOPHYSIOLOGY: No one factor explains the clinical syndrome of hepatic encephalopathy. Because of hepatocyte dysfunction and/or structural or functional vascular shunts, harmful compounds absorbed from the intestine escape hepatic detoxification. This is particularly evident after surgical construction of a portal–systemic anastomosis (portal vein to inferior vena cava or its equivalent) to relieve portal hypertension (see below). Hence, the term

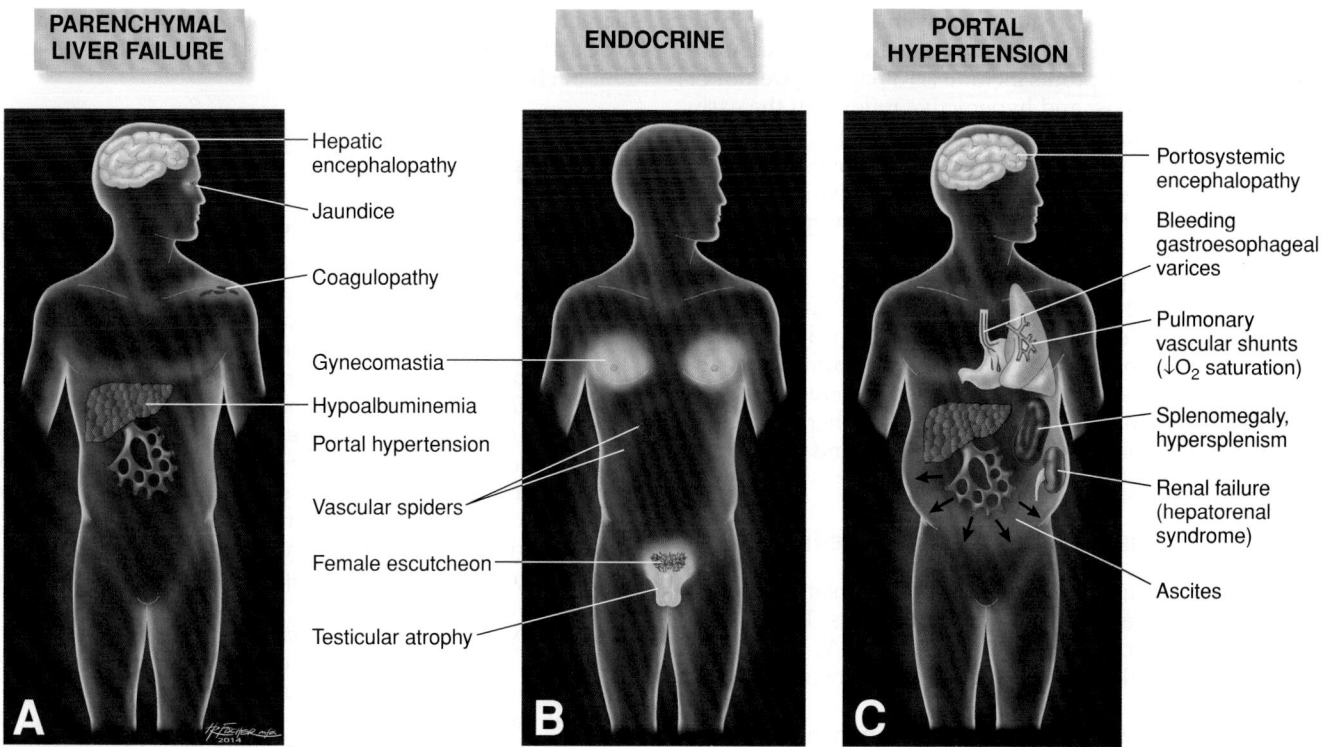

FIGURE 20-15. Complications of cirrhosis and hepatic failure. Clinical features related to **(A) parenchymal liver failure, (B) endocrine distur-bances** and **(C) portal hypertension.** There is considerable overlap of these clinical features with regard to their pathogeneses.

portal–systemic encephalopathy is used to describe post-shunt encephalopathy.

AMMONIA: Ammonia levels are usually increased in the blood and brain of patients with hepatic encephalopathy. Most of the body's ammonia is derived from ingestion of ammonia in foods, digestion of proteins in the small intestine and bacterial catabolism of dietary protein and urea secreted into the intestine. Ammonia is produced in the small bowel when glutamine is deaminated by glutaminase, an enzyme that is more active in cirrhosis than normally. Ammonia is detoxified by the liver. However, in patients with acute liver failure or cirrhosis, reduced hepatocyte mass or portal–systemic shunts, respectively, an excess of ammonia escapes into the systemic circulation.

Ammonia has several harmful effects. The brain detoxifies ammonia by synthesizing glutamate and glutamine. Excess levels of these molecules may alter neurotransmission and brain osmolality. However, correlation between blood ammonia levels and the severity of hepatic encephalopathy is inexact, thus the neurotoxicity of ammonia remains only partly understood.

γ-AMINOBUTYRIC ACID: Neural inhibition, mediated by the γ-aminobutyric acid (GABA)–benzodiazepine receptor complex, is accentuated in hepatic encephalopathy by increased levels of benzodiazepine-like molecules.

OTHER SUBSTANCES: Other compounds that may contribute to hepatic encephalopathy include **mercaptans** from the breakdown of sulfur-containing amino acids in the colon. A characteristic breath odor of patients with hepatic failure, **fetor hepaticus,** is due to these mercaptans in saliva. Blood levels of aromatic amino acids are increased in hepatic failure. They impair synthesis of normal neurotransmitters such as norepinephrine but increase production of **false neurotransmitters** (e.g., octopamine). Toxicity of **phenols** and **short-chain fatty acids** on the brain has also been postulated. Finally, the blood-brain barrier may be impaired in patients with hepatic failure.

 PATHOLOGY: Cerebral edema is the major cause of death in most patients with acute hepatic failure. It often coincides with uncal and cerebellar herniation. This edema is a specific lesion associated with hepatic coma, although the precise mechanism is obscure.

In brains of patients who died with chronic liver disease and hepatic coma, the most striking changes are in astrocytes. Termed **Alzheimer type II astrocytes** (see Chapter 28), these cells are swollen, increased in number and size and show nuclear enlargement and nuclear inclusions. Deep layers of the cerebral cortex and subcortical white matter, the basal ganglia and the cerebellum show laminar necrosis and a spongiform appearance.

 CLINICAL FEATURES: Hepatic encephalopathy traverses four stages:

- **Stage I:** Sleep disturbance, irritability and personality changes
- **Stage II:** Lethargy and disorientation
- **Stage III:** Deep somnolence
- **Stage IV:** Coma

This sequence may require many months, or it may evolve in days or weeks in cases of acute liver failure. Associated neurologic symptoms include (1) a flapping tremor of the hands, or **asterixis,** and hyperactive reflexes in the early stages; (2) extensor toe responses (Babinski reflex) later; and (3) a decerebrate posture in terminal stages. Intensive supportive measures may suffice early in hepatic encephalopathy, but patients with stages III and IV encephalopathy usually require liver transplantation.

Treatment of hepatic encephalopathy hinges on reversal of the underlying hepatic disease and reduction in ammonia levels. The latter requires purgatives (to rid the bowel of protein, the substrate for ammonia formation), nonabsorbable antibiotics (to reduce the urease-producing bacteria that make ammonia) and correction of other sources of ammonia production, including infections and electrolyte disturbances.

Defects of Coagulation Often Cause Bleeding

In liver failure, impaired synthesis of coagulation factors and thrombocytopenia lead to poor hemostasis. The clotting factors—fibrinogen, prothrombin, and factors V, VII, IX and X—are reduced, reflecting generalized impairment of hepatic protein synthesis.

Thrombocytopenia ($<80,000/\mu L$) is common in hepatic failure, as are qualitative defects in platelet function. Hypersplenism, bone marrow depression and platelet loss due to **disseminated intravascular coagulation** (DIC) decrease circulating platelets.

DIC occurs frequently in liver failure. It may be stimulated by liver cell necrosis, activation of factor XII (Hageman factor; see Chapter 4) by endotoxin or inadequate hepatic clearance of activated clotting factors from the circulation.

Hypoalbuminemia Complicates Hepatic Failure

Impaired hepatic albumin synthesis causes hypoalbuminemia. This is an important factor in the pathogenesis of the edema that often complicates chronic liver disease.

Liver Failure Causes Imbalances in Steroid Hormones

Hyperestrogenism in chronic liver failure in men leads to **gynecomastia,** a female body habitus and female distribution of pubic hair (female escutcheon). Vascular effects of hyperestrogenism are common and include **spider angiomas** in the drainage territory of the superior vena cava (upper trunk and face) and **palmar erythema**.

Feminization reflects reduced catabolism of estrogens and weak androgens by a dysfunctional liver. Weak androgens (androstenedione and dehydroepiandrosterone) are converted to estrogens in peripheral tissues, thus increasing circulating estrogen levels. Extrahepatic portal–systemic shunts due to portal hypertension in cirrhosis (see below) permit these hormones to bypass the liver.

Men with alcoholic liver disease are more likely to be feminized than those with liver disease from other causes, and the feminization is usually more severe. Chronic alcoholics also suffer hypogonadism, with testicular atrophy, impotence and loss of libido. Alcoholic women also have gonadal failure, which presents as oligomenorrhea, amenorrhea, infertility, ovarian atrophy and loss of secondary sex characteristics. These effects in both sexes reflect a direct toxic action of alcohol on gonadal function and are independent of chronic liver disease.

PORTAL HYPERTENSION

The superior mesenteric and splenic vein meet to make the hepatic portal vein. This vessel carries the major venous drainage from the gastrointestinal tract, pancreas and spleen to the liver. It accounts for 2/3 of the liver's blood flow but less than 1/2 of its total oxygen supply. The remainder is supplied by the hepatic artery. *Portal hypertension is either an absolute increase in portal venous pressure, usually above 8 mm Hg, or an increase in the pressure gradient between the portal vein and the hepatic vein of 5 mm Hg or more.* Obstruction to blood flow somewhere in the portal circuit is responsible. Increased portal pressure causes opening of **portal–systemic collateral channels,** bleeding from gastroesophageal varices, ascites, splenomegaly and renal and pulmonary disease (Fig. 20-15).

Portal hypertension is most accurately assessed by directly measuring hepatic vein pressure: a balloon-tipped catheter is inserted into the internal jugular vein and advanced to a terminal hepatic vein to obtain the **free hepatic vein pressure** (FHVP). The **wedged hepatic vein pressure** (WHVP) is determined after balloon inflation and is an indirect measure of the portal vein pressure. The difference between WHVP and FHVP is the **hepatic vein pressure gradient** (HVPG); that is, WHVP – FHVP = HVPG.

Increased resistance to portal blood outflow is the basis for diagnosing portal hypertension (Fig. 20-16). This increase in resistance can originate in one of three areas:

1. **Sinusoidal (intrahepatic):** Injury to sinusoids leads to sinusoidal, or intrahepatic, portal hypertension. In the Western world, cirrhosis is the most common cause of all forms of portal hypertension. In cirrhosis, fibrosis leads to obstruction of intrahepatic sinusoids. This, in turn, impedes the inflow of portal blood. The result is increased pressure in the portal vein, relative to the hepatic vein. In sinusoidal portal hypertension, the pressure difference between the WHVP and FHVP (HVPG) is usually 5 mm Hg or more.
2. **Presinusoidal:** Resistance to blood flow in the extrahepatic portal vein or intrahepatic portal veins or venules (e.g., thrombotic occlusion) is known as **presinusoidal portal hypertension**. If the point of resistance is within portal venules (i.e., within the liver), the HVPG may be increased. However, if the point of resistance is more distal, allowing for a zone of normal pressure in the portal vein, between the occlusion and the sinusoids, the HVPG can be normal.
3. **Postsinusoidal:** If the point of resistance is in the hepatic veins, venules or cardiac circulation, **postsinusoidal portal hypertension** may result. This can occur if blood flow in the hepatic veins is impeded, as in Budd-Chiari syndrome or congestive heart failure. The HVPG usually is normal in this situation. That is, if the hepatic vein pressure is measured distal to the point of postsinusoidal obstruction, the FHVP will be increased, and the HVPG can be expected to be normal, as the sinusoids are normal and pose no significant resistance to the flow of blood into the liver. However, if high pressure due to outflow resistance is constant, the sinusoids may become progressively injured, leading to eventual elevation in the HVPG.

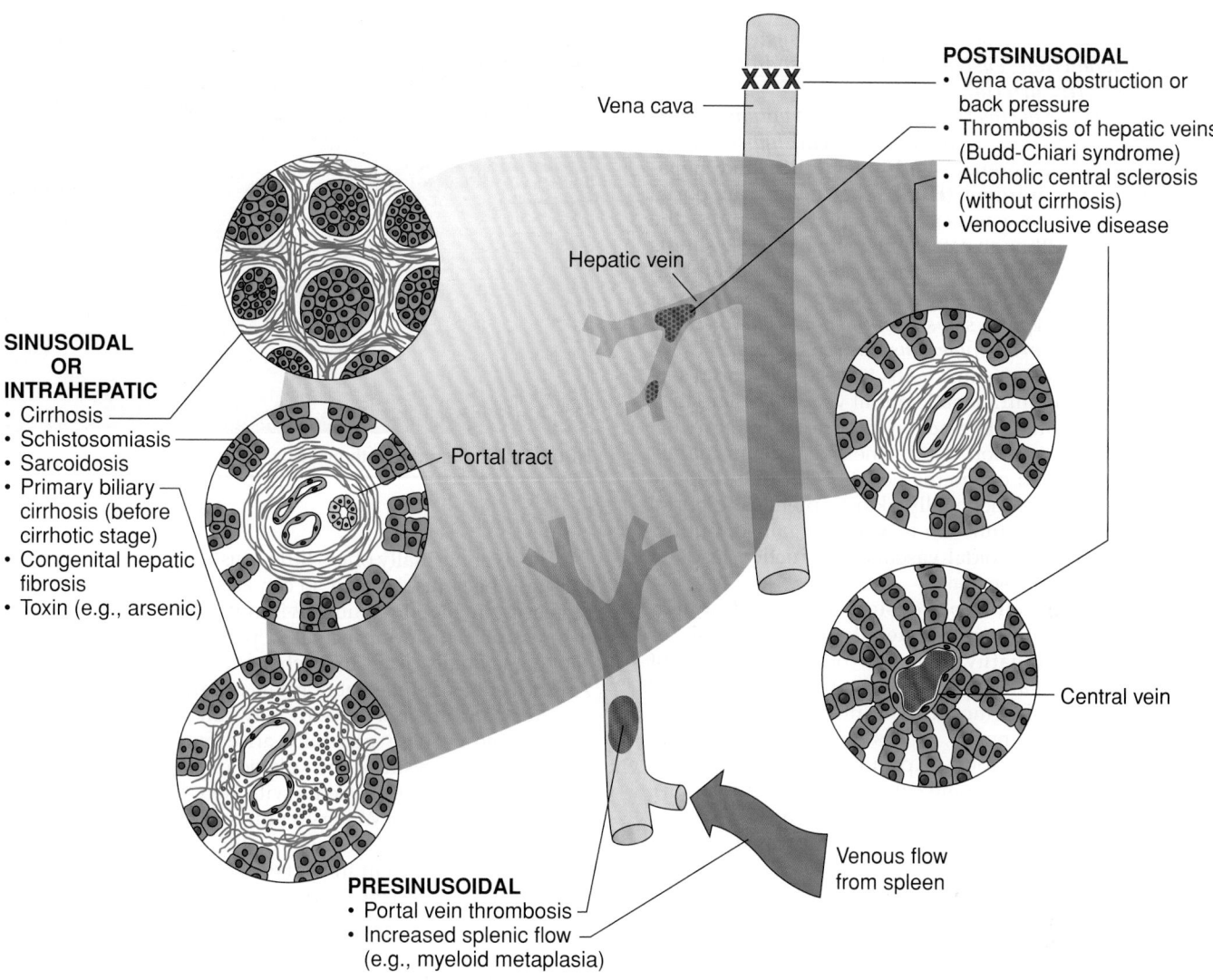

**SINUSOIDAL
OR
INTRAHEPATIC**
- Cirrhosis
- Schistosomiasis
- Sarcoidosis
- Primary biliary
  cirrhosis (before
  cirrhotic stage)
- Congenital hepatic
  fibrosis
- Toxin (e.g., arsenic)

Vena cava

Hepatic vein

Portal tract

POSTSINUSOIDAL
- Vena cava obstruction or
  back pressure
- Thrombosis of hepatic veins
  (Budd-Chiari syndrome)
- Alcoholic central sclerosis
  (without cirrhosis)
- Venoocclusive disease

Central vein

Venous flow
from spleen

PRESINUSOIDAL
- Portal vein thrombosis
- Increased splenic flow
  (e.g., myeloid metaplasia)

FIGURE 20-16. Causes of portal hypertension.

Intrahepatic Portal Hypertension Is Usually Caused by Cirrhosis

PATHOPHYSIOLOGY: Intrahepatic portal hypertension, such as occurs in cirrhosis, offers the best paradigm for understanding the pathogenesis of portal hypertension. Even before fibrosis distorts sinusoidal architecture, active contraction of vascular smooth muscle and stellate cells initiates resistance to the flow of blood into the liver from the portal vein. The trigger for this is not clear but is probably related to factors that incite inflammation, such as alcoholic hepatitis and viral hepatitis. As fibrosis develops, sinusoids become increasingly disordered. Regenerative nodules in the cirrhotic liver impinge on the hepatic veins, obstructing blood flow beyond the lobules. The small portal veins and venules are trapped, narrowed and often obliterated by scarring of the portal tracts. Blood flow through the hepatic artery is increased and small arteriovenous communications open. In this way, arterial blood flow increases and adds to portal

hypertension due to obstruction of blood flow distal to the sinusoid.

In cirrhosis, **endothelial cell dysfunction** occurs in the liver and in the systemic circulation. Hepatic vascular tone increases, and intrahepatic vessels constrict. Impaired endothelial nitric oxide sythetase (eNOS) phosphorylation, reduced nitric oxide (NO) availability due to oxidative stress and excess vasoconstrictive factors (e.g., angiotensinogen, endothelin and eicosanoids) all reduce eNOS activity. This decreases hepatic NO production. Ensuing vasoconstriction increases resistance to portal blood flow into the liver.

Progressive portal hypertension parallels mesenteric arterial vasodilation. That is, to make matters worse, **mesenteric arterial vasodilation** increases blood flow into the portal vein just when portal vein resistance is going up. This vasodilation reflects increased NO caused by greater sheer forces upon the mesenteric vessels, owing to increased resistance to portal blood flow into the liver, increased vascular endothelial growth factor (VEGF) and inflammatory mediators such as TNF-α.

Mesenteric artery vasodilation provokes systemic circulatory dysfunction, systemic arterial vasodilation and reduced effective arterial blood volume.

This decrease in effective arterial blood volume causes the clinical syndrome of advanced portal hypertension: ascites, and **hepatorenal syndrome (HRS)** and **hepatopulmonary syndrome (HPS)**. The increase in portal pressure also opens vascular shunts that decompress the portal circuit. Although ostensibly valuable, these shunts are a mixed blessing, as they may cause such complications as bleeding varices and encephalopathy (see above).

Worldwide, hepatic schistosomiasis is a major cause of intrahepatic portal hypertension (see Chapter 9). Ova released from the intestinal veins traverse the portal system and lodge in intrahepatic portal venules, where they elicit a granulomatous reaction that heals by scarring. Because the obstruction within the liver occurs mainly before portal blood enters the hepatic sinusoids, hepatic schistosomiasis is functionally akin to prehepatic portal hypertension. Liver function is well maintained, but the intrahepatic presinusoidal vascular obstruction leads to severe portal hypertension.

Idiopathic portal hypertension, also called **noncirrhotic portal hypertension, hepatoportal sclerosis or obliterative venopathy,** refers to occasional cases of intrahepatic portal hypertension with splenomegaly in the absence of demonstrable intrahepatic or extrahepatic disease. Known causes of idiopathic portal hypertension are chronic exposure to copper, arsenic and vinyl chloride. In some countries (England, Japan), idiopathic portal hypertension accounts for 15%–35% of all cases that require surgery to decompress the portal circulation.

Intrahepatic portal hypertension can be caused by other conditions that interfere with blood flow through the liver, including cystic disease of the liver (see Chapter 16), partial nodular transformation of the liver in the region of the porta hepatis and nodular regenerative hyperplasia (small regenerative nodules without fibrosis that compress the intervening hepatic parenchyma).

Portal Vein Thrombosis Often Causes Presinusoidal Portal Hypertension

 **ETIOLOGIC FACTORS:** Portal vein thrombosis occurs most often in the setting of cirrhosis. Other causes include tumors, infections, hypercoagulability states, pancreatitis and surgical trauma. Some cases are of unknown etiology. Primary hepatocellular carcinoma (HCC) may invade branches of the portal vein and occlude the main portal vein. When the portal vein is obstructed by a septic thrombus, bacteria may seed the intrahepatic branches of the portal vein (suppurative pylephlebitis) and cause multiple hepatic abscesses.

Portal vein occlusion (Fig. 20-17) may occur in the neonatal period or in early childhood. In some cases, umbilical sepsis is an important cause, but other local and systemic infections may also play a role. Sometimes the thrombosed portal or splenic vein is replaced by a fibrous cord or interlacing vascular channels, a condition termed **cavernous transformation.**

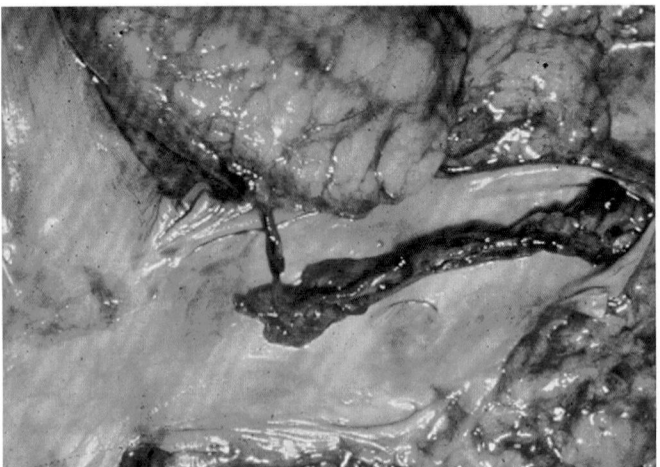

FIGURE 20-17. Portal vein thrombosis.

The liver normally offers little resistance to blood outflow through the sinusoids and so can accommodate substantial increases in blood volume without a secondary increase in pressure. However, increased portal venous blood flow can occasionally lead to prehepatic portal hypertension. Arteriovenous fistulas (abnormal communications between an artery and the portal vein) may cause prehepatic portal hypertension. These generally arise from trauma or rupture of an aneurysm of the splenic or hepatic artery. They may also develop in patients with hereditary hemorrhagic telangiectasia (Osler-Weber-Rendu syndrome). Splenomegaly due, for example, to myeloproliferative neoplasms (see Chapter 20) may result in portal hypertension. The splenomegaly that accompanies cirrhosis tends to aggravate portal hypertension.

Postsinusoidal Portal Hypertension Is Obstruction to Blood Flow beyond Liver Lobules

Budd-Chiari Syndrome

Budd-Chiari syndrome is a congestive disease of the liver caused by occlusion of the hepatic veins and their tributaries.

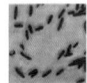 **ETIOLOGIC FACTORS:** Hepatic vein thrombosis is the main cause of Budd-Chiari syndrome, and it may occur in such diverse diseases as myeloproliferative neoplasms (especially polycythemia vera), hypercoagulable states associated with malignancies, use of oral contraceptives, pregnancy, bacterial infections, paroxysmal nocturnal hemoglobinuria, metastatic and primary tumors in the liver and surgical trauma. In 20% of cases, there is no clear cause. Thrombi form most often in the large hepatic veins, near their exit from the liver, and in the intrahepatic part of the inferior vena cava. In parts of Africa and Asia, membranous webs of unknown cause can compromise the vena cava above the orifices of the hepatic veins and lead to Budd-Chiari syndrome. Increased venous backpressure from severe congestive heart failure, tricuspid stenosis or regurgitation or constrictive pericarditis may mimic the syndrome.

Hepatic veno-occlusive disease is a variant of Budd-Chiari syndrome, caused by hepatic sinusoidal injury

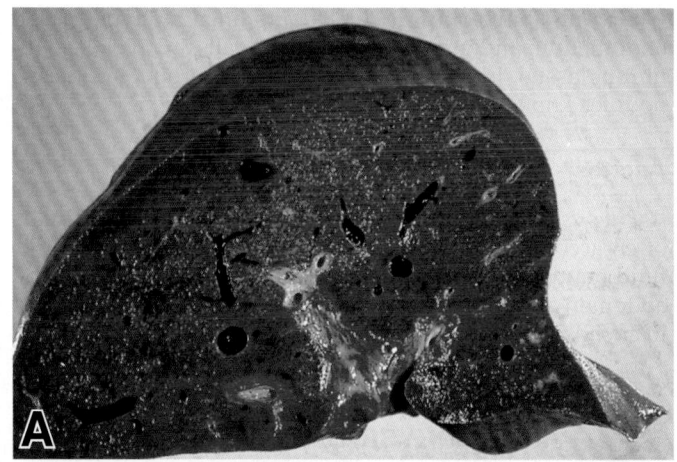

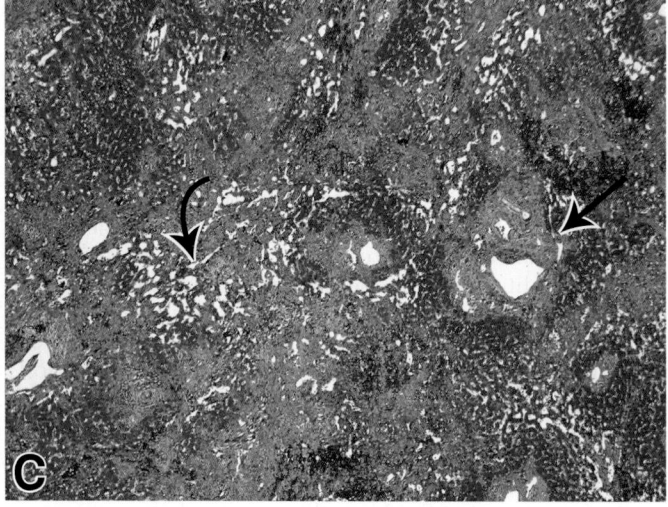

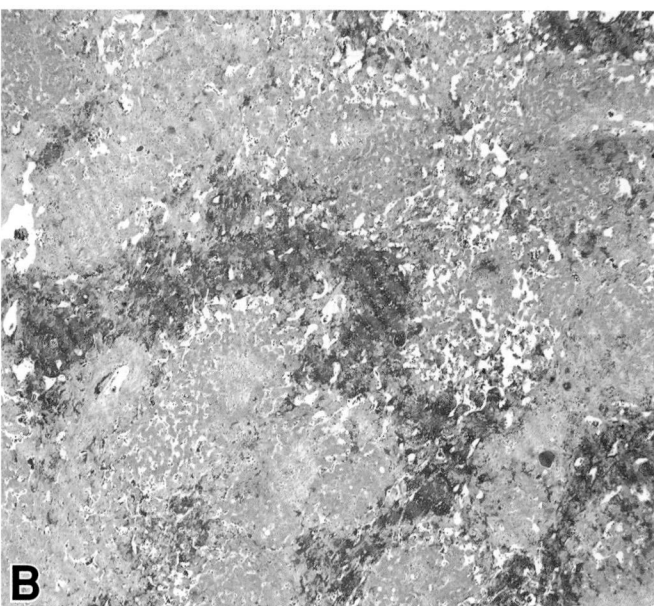

FIGURE 20-18. Budd-Chiari syndrome. A. The cut surface of the liver from a patient who died of Budd-Chiari syndrome shows thrombosis of the hepatic veins and diffuse congestion of the parenchyma. **B.** Liver parenchyma from a patient with **acute Budd-Chiari syndrome** reveals centrilobular necrosis and hemorrhage. **C. Chronic Budd-Chiari syndrome.** Cirrhosis has developed with bridging fibrosis emanating from the central venules rather than the portal tracts. Note the dilated sinusoids (*curved arrow*) and intact portal tract (*arrow*).

resulting in occlusion of the centrilobular hepatic sinusoids, central venules and small branches of the hepatic veins. This disorder is most often traced to ingestion of toxic pyrrolizidine alkaloids in plants of the *Crotalaria* and *Senecio* genera, which are used in "bush teas." It is also seen in patients given certain antineoplastic agents, after hepatic irradiation and after bone marrow transplantation, possibly as a manifestation of graft-versus-host disease.

 PATHOLOGY: In the acute stage of **hepatic vein thrombosis,** the liver is swollen and tense. Its cut surface is mottled and oozes blood (Fig. 20-18A). In the chronic stage, the cut surface is paler, and the liver is firm, owing to an increase in connective tissue. The hepatic veins have thrombi in varying stages of evolution, from recent clots to well-organized thrombi that have been rcanalized.

In the acute stage of both Budd-Chiari syndrome and veno-occlusive disease, the sinusoids of the central zone are dilated and packed with erythrocytes (Fig. 20-18B). Liver cell plates are compressed, with hemorrhage and necrosis of centrilobular hepatocytes. In long-standing venous congestion, fibrosis of the central zone may radiate to more peripheral portions of the lobules (Fig. 20-18C). Sinusoids are dilated, and central to midzonal hepatocytes show pressure atrophy. Eventually, **reverse lobulation** occurs, with connective tissue septa linking adjacent central zones to form nodules with a single central portal

tract. This fibrosis is usually not severe enough to justify a label of cirrhosis.

CLINICAL FEATURES: Complete thrombosis of the hepatic veins presents as an acute illness with abdominal pain, enlargement of the liver, ascites and mild jaundice. Acute hepatic failure and death often follow quickly. Most often, the obstruction of the hepatic venous circulation is incomplete, and similar symptoms persist for periods from a month to a few years. More than 90% of patients with Budd-Chiari syndrome develop ascites, usually severe, and splenomegaly is common. Typically, serum bilirubin and aminotransferase activities increase only modestly. Most patients eventually die in hepatic failure or from complications of portal hypertension. Liver transplantation may be curative.

Portal Hypertension Affects Many Organ Systems

Esophageal Varices

Esophageal varices are the most important complication of portal hypertension. They arise when collateral portal–systemic vascular channels open to relieve pressure in the portal circuit. One of the most common causes of death in patients with disorders associated with portal hypertension is exsanguinating upper gastrointestinal hemorrhage from **bleeding esophageal varices** (see Chapter 13).

PATHOPHYSIOLOGY: The collaterals of most clinical significance are in the submucosa of the lower esophagus and upper stomach, which communicate between the portal vein and the gastric coronary vein. Normally, these collaterals are closed. However, when the portal circulation sustains increased blood flow and higher pressures that follow, these collaterals open. They are submucosal veins near the esophagogastric junction, and they become dilated and protrude into the lumen. There is no simple correlation between the magnitude of the portal venous pressure and the risk of variceal bleeding, but that risk does rise with increasing size of the varices.

CLINICAL FEATURES: Bleeding esophageal varices portend a poor prognosis: acute mortality may be as high as 40%. In patients with cirrhosis who have survived one episode of variceal bleeding, long-term survival is unlikely because the chances of rebleeding or worsening liver failure are high. By contrast, patients in whom portal hypertension is caused by a presinusoidal block without underlying hepatic dysfunction, as in schistosomiasis, have a much better prognosis than those with cirrhosis. Death from bleeding esophageal varices is usually due to hepatic failure precipitated by stress, ischemic necrosis of the liver and the encephalopathy caused by the nitrogenous load imposed by blood in the intestinal tract. Exsanguination and shock are only infrequently the direct causes of death.

Initial treatment of acute variceal hemorrhage focuses on stopping the bleeding, by endoscopic variceal ligation, injection of varices with a sclerosing agent during endoscopy or direct tamponade with an inflatable balloon. In addition, intravenous administration of a somatostatin analog, octreotide, inhibits splanchnic vasodilation. This, in turn, reduces splanchnic blood flow and portal venous pressure. If these measures fail and varices rebleed, permanent portal circulation decompression may be needed. Angiographically a small stent, or shunt, is placed into the liver to join the portal and systemic circulations (transjugular intrahepatic portal–systemic shunt [TIPS]). This procedure, in addition to surgically constructed portal–systemic shunts, diverts blood from the high-pressure portal circulation to the lower-pressure systemic venous circulation. In some cases, liver transplantation is an alternative to shunt surgery.

Back-pressure in the portal vein also dilates its tributaries, including the inferior hemorrhoidal veins, which become dilated and tortuous **(anorectal varices)**. Collateral veins radiating about the umbilicus produce a pattern known as **caput medusae**.

Splenomegaly

The spleen in portal hypertension enlarges progressively and often causes **hypersplenism,** leading to decreased life spans and consequent reduced levels in the circulation of all formed elements of the blood (pancytopenia). Hypersplenism is attributed to a prolonged transit time through the hyperplastic spleen.

The spleen is firm and weighs up to 1000 g (normal, <180 g). Its cut surface is uniformly deep red, with inapparent white pulp. Sinusoids are dilated and lined by hyperplastic endothelium and macrophages. Their walls are thickened by fibrous tissue. Focal hemorrhages cause fibrotic, iron-laden nodules known as **Gamna-Gandy bodies**.

Ascites

Ascites is accumulation of fluid in the peritoneal cavity. It often accompanies portal hypertension, and the amount of fluid may be so great (often many liters) that it distends the abdomen and interferes with breathing. The onset of ascites in cirrhosis is associated with a poor prognosis.

PATHOPHYSIOLOGY: Reduced effective arterial blood volume and mean arterial pressure lead to predictable homeostatic responses. Early in portal hypertension, heart rate and cardiac output increase, thus preserving arterial pressure. However, as peripheral arterial vasodilation worsens, circulatory dysfunction worsens; cardiac output cannot keep pace with homeostatic demand, and endogenous vasoactive mechanisms become engaged. To preserve arterial pressure, the activities of the renin–angiotensin system and sympathetic nervous system increase. These effects raise renal sodium and water resorption. Vasodilation also activates antidiuretic hormone secretion, promoting to additional water retention and dilutional hyponatremia.

Increased liver sinusoidal pressure results in hydrostatic movement of fluid and lymph from the sinusoids into the space of Disse. This compounds the effects of greater sodium and water retention. These fluids spill into the peritoneal cavity as ascites. Decreased albumin synthesis lowers intravascular oncotic pressure and facilitates movement of fluid into the peritoneal space.

Accumulation of fibrous tissue makes the sinusoidal endothelium less and less permeable. Decreased permeability lowers the amounts of protein and albumin that spill into the ascites fluid. This effect increases the serum:ascites albumin gradient (SAAG). A SAAG exceeding 1.1 is associated with ascites due to portal hypertension from cirrhosis.

The pathogenesis of ascites is illustrated in Figure 20-19.

Spontaneous Bacterial Peritonitis

Spontaneous bacterial peritonitis (SBP) is an important complication in patients with both cirrhosis and ascites.

ETIOLOGIC FACTORS: SBP is due to translocation of intestinal bacteria into the systemic circulation, with secondary infection of ascitic fluid. The most common bacteria are the gram negatives of the gut (*E. coli, Klebsiella*); *Strep. pneumoniae* is also a common cause of SBP. Patients with low complement levels in ascitic fluid, reflected as low protein levels (<1 g/dL), are at particular risk for SBP.

CLINICAL FEATURES: Patients with SBP typically present with ascites and abdominal pain, or other signs of infection such as fever or leukocytosis. Up to 20% of patients are asymptomatic. A finding of

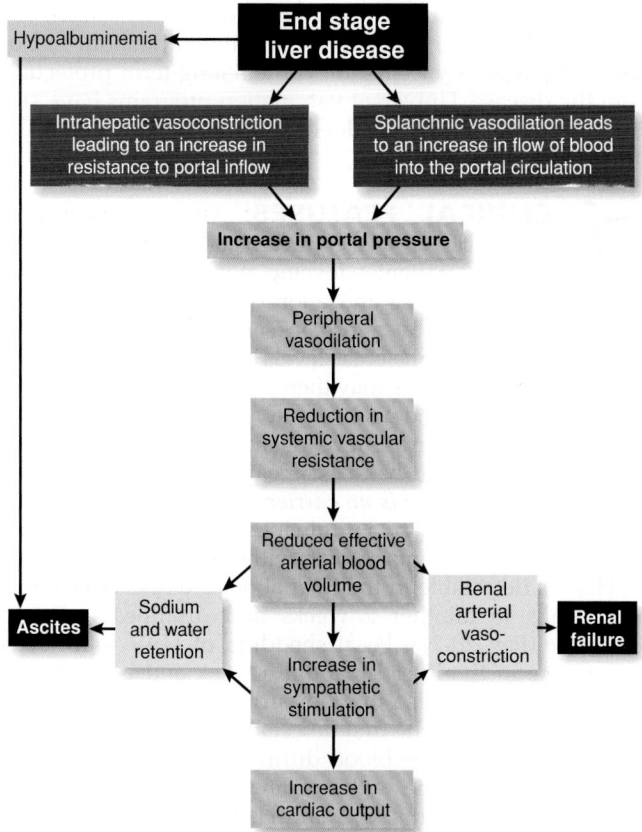

FIGURE 20-19. Pathogenesis of ascites.

more than 250 neutrophils/µL in ascitic fluid establishes the diagnosis of SBP. *Without appropriate therapy, SBP mortality exceeds 80%.* Even if it is treated with resolution of the acute infection, an episode of SBP is associated with a 70% 1-year mortality. Therefore, SBP is often an indication for liver transplantation.

Hepatorenal Syndrome

HRS is characterized by renal hypoperfusion, with oliguria, azotemia and increased plasma creatinine. It usually occurs in the setting of cirrhosis and indicates a poor prognosis. Oddly, the kidneys can still function normally, as kidneys from patients who died with HRS function well when transplanted into recipients with chronic renal failure. Conversely, in patients with HRS, liver transplantation can restore renal function.

PATHOPHYSIOLOGY: In the early stages of portal hypertension, glomerular filtration pressure is protected from systemic arteriolar vasodilation by intrarenal prostaglandins. As vasodilation worsens, these intrarenal factors become ineffective; renal vasoconstriction intensifies and glomerular perfusion and filtration decline. Eventually, this leads to clinically evident renal dysfunction, or HRS. A diagnosis of HRS also requires that serum creatinine exceeds 1.5 mg/dL and does not improve after diuretic withdrawal and volume expansion.

There are two types of HRS. Type I HRS is rapidly and inexorably progressive. Liver transplantation is the only definitive therapy. Type II HRS progresses more slowly and usually occurs in the setting of severe ascites unresponsive to conventional therapies with salt restriction and diuretics. This form of HRS may be mitigated by volume expansion or diuretic withdrawal. However, type II ultimately progresses to type I HRS if portal hypertension is not reversed.

Pulmonary Complications of Portal Hypertension

Cirrhosis and portal hypertension can lead to hepatopulmonary syndrome (HPS), **portopulmonary hypertension** (PPHTN) and **hepatic hydrothorax**. Directly or indirectly, these are due to the circulatory and vascular disturbances of advanced liver disease.

Up to 1/3 of patients with cirrhosis show signs of HPS, which results from shunts in the pulmonary vascular bed due to portal hypertension. These patients present with progressive shortness of breath, although chest radiography and pulmonary hemodynamics are typically normal. Treatment with supplemental oxygen may be useful, but liver transplantation is the only effective therapy because it reverses the intrapulmonary shunting. HPS is associated with reduced survival, particularly if arterial oxygen is less than 50 mm Hg.

PPHTN is increased pulmonary vascular resistance in the setting of portal hypertension. Usually, it is associated with increased mean pulmonary arterial pressure, to more than 25 mm Hg, and occurs in 2% of those with portal hypertension. The pathophysiology of the disorder is unclear. It may reflect aspects of the hyperdynamic circulation of portal hypertension: shear stress, endothelial injury, vasoconstriction and liberation of vasoactive factors. Proliferative pulmonary arteriopathy develops. PPHTN is inexorably progressive and usually does not reverse following liver transplantation. In fact, severe PPHTN it is a risk factor for intraoperative death due to acute heart failure and represents a contraindication to liver transplantation.

Hepatic hydrothorax is a pleural effusion attributed to portal hypertension. Most such effusions occur in the right chest and are caused by ascitic fluid moving through the diaphragm into the pleural space. Thus, the fluid has the same composition and protein content as ascites and, like ascites, is prone to spontaneous infection.

VIRAL HEPATITIS

Viral hepatitis is infection of hepatocytes that causes liver necrosis and inflammation. It was known as "epidemic jaundice" for millennia. Worldwide, more than 500 million people are infected with hepatotropic viruses and are at great risk for HCC. Many viruses and other infectious agents can produce hepatitis and jaundice (Table 20-2), but in the industrialized world, more than 95% of cases of viral hepatitis are caused by hepatitis A, B, C, D and E viruses (HAV, HBV, etc.). HGV is 25% homologous with HCV but does not lead to acute or chronic hepatitis.

The following discussion emphasizes the illnesses commonly termed **viral hepatitis**. The reader is referred to Chapter 9 for consideration of the other agents.

TABLE 20-2

INFECTIOUS AGENTS THAT CAUSE HEPATITIS

Hepatitis A virus (HAV)	Herpes simplex virus
Hepatitis B virus (HBV)+/− HDV	Cytomegalovirus
Hepatitis C virus (HCV)	Enteroviruses other than HAV
Hepatitis E virus (HEV)	
Yellow fever virus	Leptospires (leptospirosis)
Epstein-Barr virus (infectious mononucleosis)	*Entamoeba histolytica* (amebic hepatitis)
Lassa, Marburg and Ebola viruses	

Hepatitis A Virus Is the Most Common Cause of Acute Hepatitis

Hepatitis A virus (HAV) is a small RNA-containing enterovirus of the picornavirus family (which includes polio virus) (Fig. 20-20). It mainly replicates in hepatocytes, but gastrointestinal epithelial cells may also be infected. Infectious virus progeny are shed into the bile and present in the feces. HAV is not directly cytopathic, and hepatic injury has been attributed to the immunologic reaction against virally infected hepatocytes.

 **EPIDEMIOLOGY:** The only reservoir for HAV is acutely infected people, so transmission is mostly from person to person by the fecal–oral route. Epidemics of hepatitis A occur in crowded and unsanitary conditions, such as exist in warfare, or by fecal contamination of water and food. Edible shellfish in contaminated waters concentrate the virus and may transmit infection if they are not adequately cooked.

In industrialized countries, which have low rates of infection, most cases of hepatitis A are seen in older children and adults. By contrast, in less developed regions, where the disease is endemic, most of the population is infected before 10 years of age.

In the United States, about 10% of the population younger than 20 years show serologic evidence of previous HAV infection, indicating that *most HAV infections are anicteric*. Hepatitis A is common in day care centers and among international travelers and men who have sex with men. However, no source is identified in about 1/2 of cases. Hepatitis A vaccination confers long-term protection from the disease. Universal vaccination programs have significantly reduced the incidence of acute hepatitis A in the United States.

 CLINICAL FEATURES: After an incubation period of 3–6 weeks (mean, about 4 weeks), HAV-infected patients develop nonspecific symptoms, including fever, malaise and anorexia. Concomitantly, liver injury is evidenced by a rise in serum aminotransferases (Fig. 20-21). Aminotransferase levels begin to decline, usually 5–10 days later. Jaundice may then appear. It remains evident for an average of 10 days but may persist for more than a month. Aminotransferase levels generally return to normal by the time jaundice has disappeared. *Hepatitis A never becomes chronic. There is no carrier state, and infection provides lifelong immunity.* Fulminant hepatitis is rarely seen, and virtually all patients recover without sequelae.

HAV is detectable in the liver about 2 weeks after infection, peaks in another 2 weeks and disappears shortly thereafter (Fig. 20-21). Fecal shedding of HAV follows its appearance in the liver by about a week and is brief. The period of viremia is also short, occurring early in the disease.

IgM anti-HAV is the first detectable immune response to HAV. It appears in the blood during the acute illness. IgM titers begin to decline within a few weeks and are undetectable by 3–5 months. IgG anti-HAV appears as patients recover and persists for life. Serum IgM anti-HAV in a patient with acute hepatitis confirms HAV as the cause.

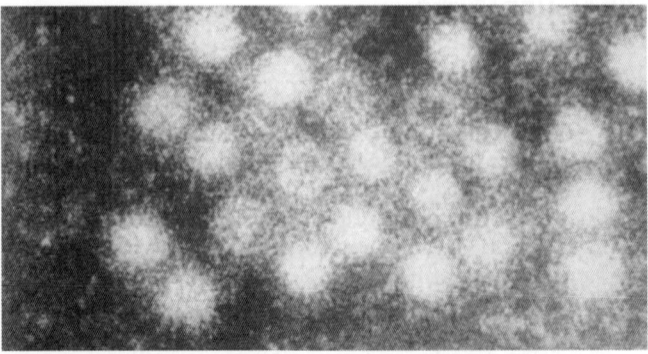

FIGURE 20-20. Electron micrograph of hepatitis A virus (HAV). A fecal extract was treated with convalescent serum containing anti-HAV.

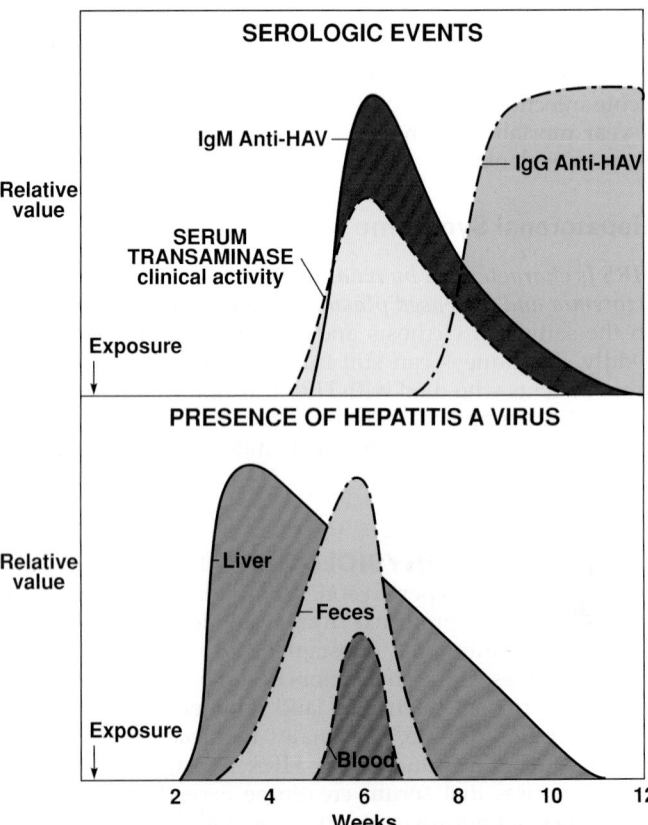

FIGURE 20-21. Typical serologic events associated with hepatitis A (HAV).

Hepatitis B Is a Major Cause of Acute and Chronic Liver Disease

 **ETIOLOGIC AGENT:** Hepatitis B virus (HBV) is a hepatotropic DNA virus of the **hepadnavirus** group, whose genomes are among the smallest of all known viruses. The HBV genome is circular and predominantly double-stranded DNA with the entire genome, plus a shorter complementary strand that varies from 50% to 85% of the length of the longer strand (Fig. 20-22). The viral particle is a 42-nm sphere (*Dane particle*) that contains the viral DNA. The HBV genome has four genes:

- **Core (*C*) gene:** The core of the virus contains the **core antigen (HBcAg)** and the **e antigen (HBeAg),** both of which are products of the *C* gene. The *C* gene includes two consecutive open reading frames: the precore and core regions. Transcription of the core frame alone yields

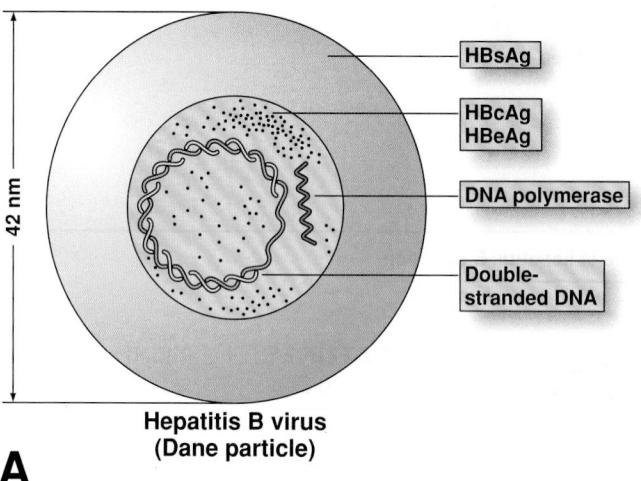

Hepatitis B virus (Dane particle)

A

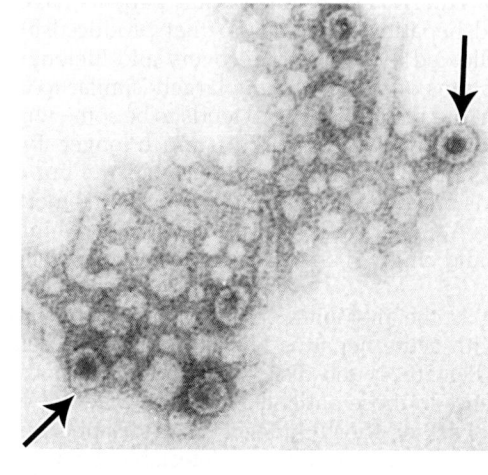

B

FIGURE 20-22. Hepatitis B virus (HBV). A. Schematic representation of HBV and serum particles associated with HBV infection. (Antigens [Ag] for hepatitis B are indicated by their letters: c = core, e, and s = surface.) **B.** Electron micrograph of particles from centrifuged serum in a case of hepatitis B. Rod-like and spherical particles containing HBsAg are evident. The complete virion, composed of the viral core and its surrounding envelope, is represented by Dane particles (*arrows*).

HBcAg. HBeAg is derived from the translation product of the entire *C* gene by proteolysis.

- **Surface gene:** The outer viral coat contains **hepatitis B surface antigen (HBsAg).** HBsAg is synthesized by infected hepatocytes independently of the viral core, and vast amounts are secreted into the blood. Electron microscopy of centrifuged serum identifies two distinct HBsAg particles (Fig. 20-22): a 22-nm sphere and a tubular structure 22 nm in diameter and 40–400 nm in length. These particles are immunogenic but not infectious.
- **Polymerase gene:** The *P* gene encodes viral DNA polymerase.
- **X gene:** The small X protein activates viral transcription and probably plays a role in HBV-related hepatocarcinogenesis associated with chronic HBV infection.

HBV attaches to host hepatocytes and then enters the cell, where it uncoats. Its genome then goes into the nucleus, where it is converted into a covalently closed circular DNA (cccDNA) that is the template for transcription of viral mRNA. Persistence of cccDNA prevents HBV clearance from the host, even with potent antiviral pharmacotherapy.

There are six distinct HBV serotypes (A through F). Mutations are common, both in unmolested infection and under the influence of pharmacotherapy. *Precore mutant HBV DNA-containing viruses do not express HBeAg,* and their function is unclear. Antiviral treatment selects for HBV mutants at high (50%) rates after years of therapy. Newer nucleoside and nucleotide analogs cause lower rates of HBV mutation.

 **EPIDEMIOLOGY:** It is estimated that there are more than 350 million chronic carriers of HBV in the world, constituting an enormous reservoir of infection (Fig. 20-23). Depending on the rate of primary infection with HBV, carrier rates of chronic infection vary from 0.3% (United States, Western Europe) to 20% (Southeast Asia, sub-Saharan Africa, Oceania and the Pacific and Amazon basins). In endemic areas, high carrier rates are sustained by vertical transmission from carrier mothers to newborns.

In the United States, between 500,000 and 1.5 million people are chronically infected HBV carriers. Between 200,000 and 300,000 new cases of HBV occur annually. The use of a protective vaccine lowered the incidence of HBV in the United States from 10.7/100,000 in 1983 to 1.6/100,000 in 2006. Only 1/4 of new cases present with jaundice. Fulminant hepatitis B causes 250–300 deaths annually in the United States. Posttransfusion hepatitis, once common, is now a memory due to routine blood screening for HBsAg.

The incidence of HBV chronicity is inversely proportional to the age at viral acquisition. In countries with high endemicity, the high chronicity rate is due to vertical transmission and unsafe injection practices. In areas with lower rates of infection, HBV transmission is most frequently horizontal. No more than 10% of people infected with HBV as adults become carriers, but neonatal hepatitis B generally leads to persistent infection. Males become carriers more often than females. In the United States, chronic HBV carriers are common among male homosexuals and IV drug users.

Humans are the only significant reservoir of HBV. Unlike hepatitis A, HBV is not transmitted by the fecal–oral route, nor does it contaminate food and water supplies. *HBsAg is found in most secretions, but infectious virus is only present*

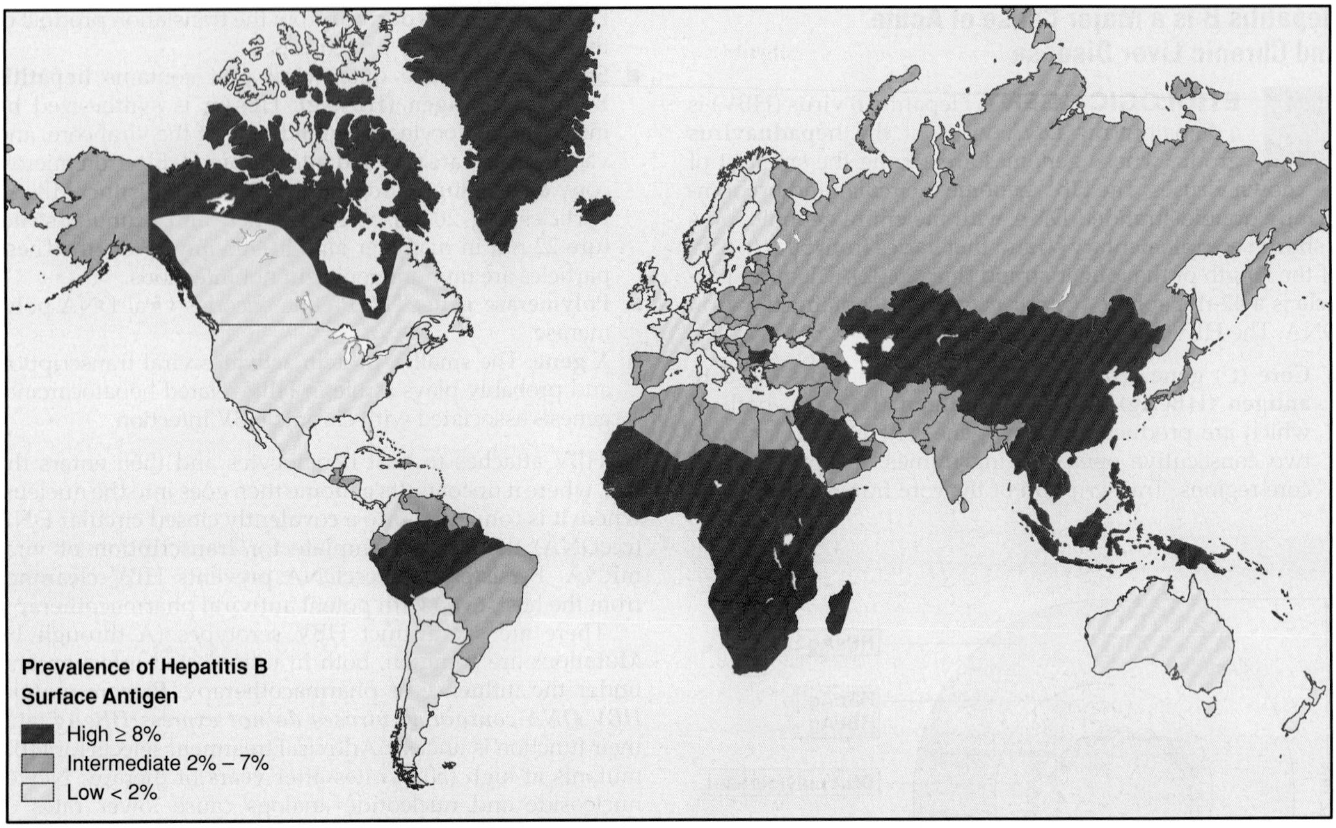

Prevalence of Hepatitis B Surface Antigen

■ High ≥ 8%
■ Intermediate 2% – 7%
□ Low < 2%

FIGURE 20-23. Geographic prevalence of hepatitis B infection.

in blood, saliva and semen. Most cases of hepatitis B are now transmitted by intimate contact. Such contact transmission largely involves direct transfer of virus through breaks in the skin or mucous membranes. Anal sexual contact is thus an important mode of transmission.

Synthetic hepatitis B vaccines, containing recombinant HBsAg or its immunogenic epitopes, are highly effective and confer lifelong immunity. In some regions where hepatitis B is endemic, vaccination has significantly reduced the prevalence of the disease. In the United States, it is now routine to administer the vaccine. Vaccination of infants is common in most nations (currently 177 of 193 countries).

PATHOPHYSIOLOGY: HBV is not directly cytopathic, as asymptomatic chronic carriers of the virus have a large load of infectious virus in the liver for years without functional or biochemical evidence of liver cell injury. Cytotoxic (CD8$^+$) T lymphocytes (CTLs) that target multiple HBV epitopes cause most of the destruction of hepatocytes and consequent clinical liver disease. Target viral antigens are expressed on the surface of infected hepatocytes, where they are recognized by CD8$^+$ cells. These CTLs, in turn, kill infected hepatocytes.

The infectivity of blood from patients with chronic hepatitis B declines with the duration of the disease. This is largely due to decreased episomal (extrachromosomal) replication of infectious virions. The intact viral genome does not integrate into host DNA. However, genomic fragments are progressively integrated, after which they produce several viral antigens, contributing to viral persistence.

CLINICAL FEATURES: Hepatitis B may follow three courses (Fig. 20-24):

■ Acute hepatitis
■ Fulminant hepatitis
■ Chronic hepatitis

ACUTE HEPATITIS B: Most adult patients have acute, self-limited hepatitis B, similar to that produced by HAV, usually followed by complete recovery and lifelong immunity. Symptoms of hepatitis B are largely similar to those of hepatitis A, but acute hepatitis B tends to be somewhat more severe, and its incubation period is much longer. Typically, symptoms appear 2–3 months after exposure, but incubation periods may vary from under 6 weeks to 6 months. As in hepatitis A, many cases, including virtually all infections in infants and children, are anicteric and thus not clinically apparent.

HBsAg is the first marker to appear in the serum of patients with acute hepatitis B. It appears 1–8 weeks after exposure (Fig. 20-24) and disappears from the blood during convalescence in those patients who recover rapidly. Simultaneously with, or shortly after, HBsAg disappears, serum antibody to HBsAg (anti-HBs) is detectable. Its appearance heralds complete recovery, and it provides lifelong immunity.

HBcAg (core antigen) is not seen in blood of persons with acute hepatitis B, but antibody to HBcAg (anti-HBc) appears shortly after HBsAg. Antibody to HBcAg is a marker of a prior HBV infection but does not clear the virus or protect from reinfection.

HBeAg circulates before the onset of clinical disease and after the appearance of HBsAg. It generally disappears within

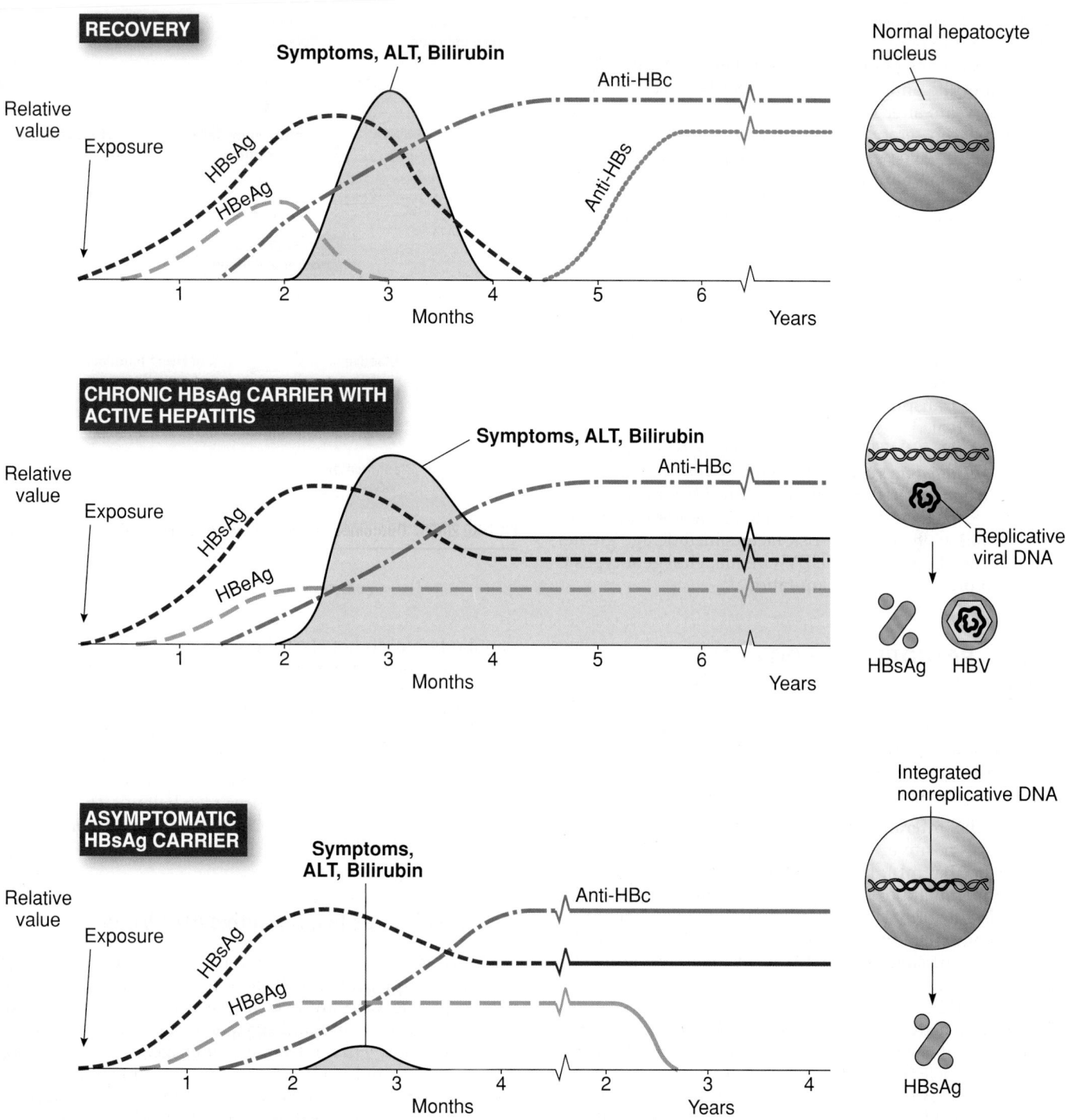

FIGURE 20-24. Typical serologic events in three distinct outcomes of hepatitis B. Top panel. In most cases, the appearance of antibody to hepatitis B surface antigen (HBsAg; anti-HBs) ensures complete recovery. Viral DNA disappears from the nucleus of the hepatocyte. **Middle panel.** In about 10% of cases of hepatitis B, HBs antigenemia is sustained for longer than 6 months, owing to the absence of anti-HBs. Patients in whom viral replication remains active, as evidenced by sustained high levels of HBeAg in the blood, develop active hepatitis. In such cases, the viral genome persists in the nucleus but is not integrated into host DNA. **Lower panel.** Patients in whom active viral replication ceases or is attenuated, as reflected in the disappearance of HBeAg from the blood, become asymptomatic carriers. In these individuals, fragments of the hepatitis B virus (HBV) genome are integrated into the host DNA, but episomal DNA is absent.

about 2 weeks, whereas HBsAg is still present. Serum HBeAg correlates with a period of intense viral replication and, hence, maximal infectivity of the patient. Anti-HBe antibody appears shortly after the antigen disappears and is detectable up to 2 or more years after the hepatitis resolves. A minor subset of patients who seroconvert to anti-HBe antibody and lose serum HBeAg have persistent HBV replication. HBV viruses in these cases are replication competent but do not produce HBeAg because of mutations in the HBV genome.

FULMINANT HEPATITIS B: More often than hepatitis A, but still only rarely, acute hepatitis B can be a fulminant disease, with massive liver cell necrosis, hepatic failure and high mortality. Nucleoside and nucleotide analogs have improved outcomes for patients with fulminant hepatitis B compared to historical controls. Patients with fulminant acute hepatitis B can decompensate rapidly. Death is primarily caused by cerebral edema, cardiopulmonary collapse or sepsis. Liver transplantation, when available, gives excellent patient survival.

CHRONIC HEPATITIS B: Chronic hepatitis is characterized by continued necrosis and inflammation in the liver for more than 6 months. People with chronic HBV infection are at increased risk for cirrhosis and HCC. Men are more susceptible than women. Other risk factors include age greater than 40 years, high levels of HBV viremia, viral genotypes C and F or a precore promoter mutation.

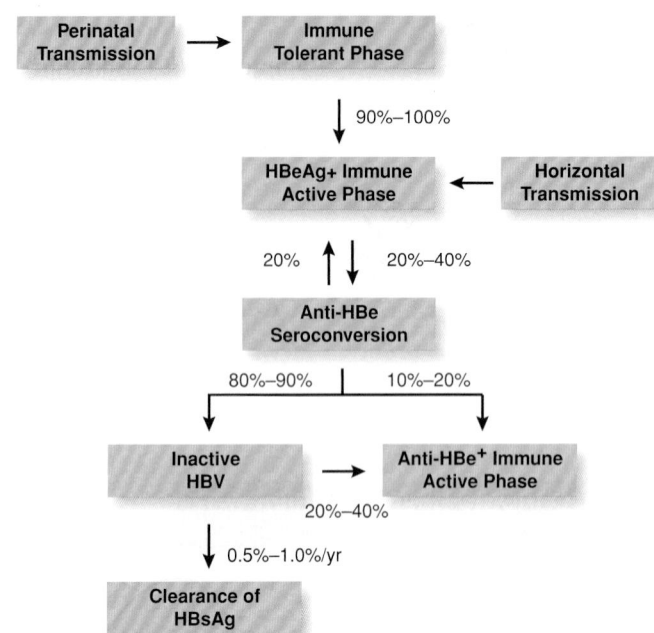

FIGURE 20-25. Outcomes of infection with the hepatitis B virus (HBV).

PATHOPHYSIOLOGY: Three phases of chronic hepatitis B are recognized: (1) immune tolerant phase, (2) immune active phase and (3) inactive phase. A fourth phase, recovery, is not yet generally accepted. People chronically infected with HBV often progress temporally through these phases but can also revert backward.

1. **Immune tolerant phase:** Patients in this phase are HBeAg positive, with very high HBV DNA levels (>20,000 IU/mL). There is little significant hepatocellular inflammation or necrosis: serum aminotransferase levels are normal. This phase may last for decades and is common among those who acquired HBV by vertical transmission. Since HBV DNA integrates into cellular DNA, even patients in this phase are at increased risk for HCC.

2. **Immune active phase:** This phase is characterized by HBV viremia and liver cell necrosis (i.e., elevated serum aminotransferases). Portal-based inflammatory infiltrates and hepatocyte necrosis are seen. Patients with detectable HBe tend to have greater viremia than those who are HBe negative/anti-HBe positive. Significant liver injury, cirrhosis and HCC tend to develop in this phase. Antiviral therapy is often initiated in the immune active phase.

3. **Inactive phase:** In the inactive phase, anti-HBe antibody circulates and HBeAg does not, serum aminotransferases are normal and blood HBV DNA is low (<2000 IU/mL). These people are "asymptomatic carriers" and are at very low risk of progression to cirrhosis or HCC. However, these people may revert to immune active disease and thus require long-term follow-up.

In some chronic HBV carriers, HBsAg–anti-HBs complexes circulate in the blood. Thus, these patients produce antibody but do not clear the virus antigen from the circulation. Such circulating immune complexes may lead to **extrahepatic** complications, including a serum sickness–like syndrome (fever, rash, urticaria, acute arthritis), polyarteritis, glomerulonephritis and cryoglobulinemia. In fact, 1/3 to 1/2 of patients with polyarteritis nodosa are HBV carriers. Chronic hepatitis B is associated with a significant risk of liver cancer (see below). *The possible outcomes of infection with HBV are summarized in Figures 20-24 and 20-25.*

Hepatitis D Virus Is a Defective RNA Virus

Assembly of hepatitis D virus (HDV) in the liver requires HBsAg to be present. Therefore, infection with HDV is limited to people who are also infected with HBV. The two infections may be simultaneous (coinfection), or HDV infection may follow HBV infection (superinfection). HDV and HBsAg are cleared together, and the clinical course is usually similar to that for the usual acute hepatitis B. However, in some patients, coinfection with HDV leads to severe, fulminant and often fatal hepatitis, particularly in intravenous drug abusers. *Superinfection of an HBV carrier with HDV typically increases the severity of an existing chronic hepatitis.* In fact, 70%–80% of HBsAg carriers superinfected with HDV develop chronic hepatitis. Since the discovery of HDV in 1979, recognition of its natural history has led to a significant drop in HDV transmission. The virus remains a clinical problem especially in developing nations endemic for HBV.

Hepatitis C Virus Commonly Causes Chronic Hepatitis and Cirrhosis

Hepatitis C virus (HCV) is an enveloped flavivirus. Its single-stranded RNA genome of 9600 bases encodes one transcript. This mRNA is translated into a polyprotein of about 3000 amino acids, which is cleaved into three structural proteins (one core and two envelope proteins) and six nonstructural proteins. Short untranslated regions at the end of the genome are required for replication.

The virus is genetically unstable, which leads to the existence of multiple genotypes and subtypes. Six different but related HCV genotypes are known. Types 1, 2 and 3 are most common (about 75% in the United States and Western Europe). Genotypes 2 and 3 respond better to antiviral therapy than does type 1. In an individual patient, many mutant HCVs arise, which likely accounts for several features of infection, including (1) the inability of anti-HCV antibodies to clear the infection, (2) persistent and relapsing infection in the chronic hepatitis phase and (3) lack of progress in developing a vaccine.

 **EPIDEMIOLOGY:** The prevalence of HCV ranges from under 1% in Canada and Scandinavia to 1.8% in the United States to as high as 22% in Egypt. It is estimated that some 170 million people (3% overall prevalence) are infected worldwide. HCV accounts for the majority of patients waiting for liver transplants.

HCV infection is transmitted by contact with infected blood through direct percutaneous exposure to blood or unsafe injection practices. Less efficient transmission occurs via smaller percutaneous exposures (needlestick injuries) or mucosal routes such as vertical and sexual transmission. Intravenous drug abuse (especially with unsafe injection practices), high-risk sexual behavior (particularly male homosexuals) and alcoholism place individuals at high risk for contracting infection with HCV. Screening of the blood supply for anti-HCV antibodies has virtually eliminated transfusions as a source of HCV infection. Transmission from infected mothers to newborn babies is infrequent (2.7%–8.4%) but is four to five times more common in women coinfected with HIV. In a minority of cases, there are no known risk factors. The incidence of new cases of acute HCV infection in the United States has fallen from 230,000 annually in the 1980s to 16,000 now, a drop of 93%. Much of this decrease probably reflects declining use of injectable illicit drugs. Mortality due to hepatitis C is increasing, as people infected long ago are aging. This aging population will likely be increasingly susceptible to decompensated cirrhosis and HCC over the next 20 years.

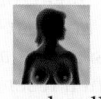 **PATHOPHYSIOLOGY:** HCV is not directly cytopathic, and many chronic HCV carriers have no liver cell injury. Despite active humoral and cellular immune responses against all viral proteins, most patients have persistent viremia. *Liver cell injury probably reflects CTL killing of virus-infected hepatocytes.* HCV persistence is not well understood. The high level of virus genome mutation (see above) and defects in HCV-specific cellular immunity probably contribute.

 CLINICAL FEATURES: The incubation period of hepatitis C is similar to that of hepatitis B. Serum aminotransferases (Fig. 20-26) usually rise

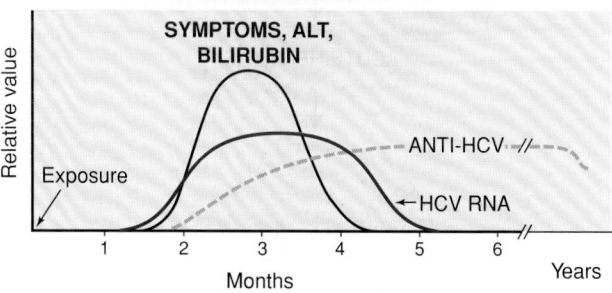

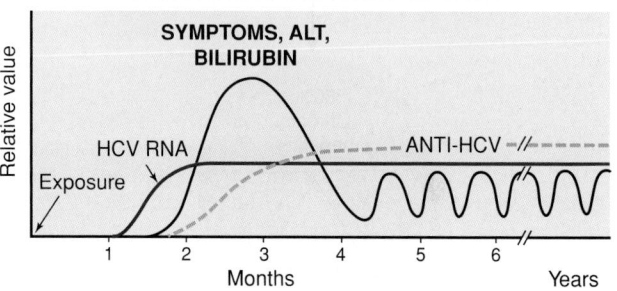

FIGURE 20-26. Clinical course of hepatitis C virus (HCV). Typical serologic events in two distinct outcomes. **Top panel.** About 20% of the patients with acute hepatitis C have a self-limited infection that resolves in a few months. Anti-HCV appears at the end of the clinical course and persists. **Bottom panel.** The remaining patients with hepatitis C develop chronic illness, with exacerbations and remissions of clinical symptoms. The development of anti-HCV does not affect the clinical outcome. Chronic hepatitis often eventuates in cirrhosis. ALT = alanine aminotransferase.

in 4–12 weeks after exposure (range, 2–26 weeks). Within 1–3 weeks of infection, HCV RNA circulates in the blood. Anti-HCV antibodies usually appear 7–8 weeks after infection and persist during the chronic phase. Acute hepatitis C is quite mild, or asymptomatic, in most people: only 10%–20% develop jaundice. About 20% of HCV patients spontaneously clear the virus. Persistent viremia is milder in patients who develop jaundice and greater in those who acquire HCV via IV drug use. Fulminant hepatitis, if it occurs at all, is rare.

The most important consequences of HCV infection relate to chronic disease. Despite complete recovery from clinical and biochemical acute liver disease, 85% of patients develop chronic disease (Fig. 20-27). Cirrhosis develops in 15%–20% of people chronically infected with HCV for 10–30 years. The risk of cirrhosis is greater in men, older people, alcoholics and those who are also infected with HIV or HBV. Even in the absence of elevated aminotransferases or significant risk factors for progression, patients can present with significant fibrosis and even cirrhosis. Liver biopsy is vital to estimating the risk of clinical progression.

Chronic hepatitis is mild in most patients for at least 10 years and often for 20 or more years. Some 20% of patients with chronic hepatitis C eventually develop cirrhosis. *Of patients with cirrhosis, up to 5% per year develop HCC.*

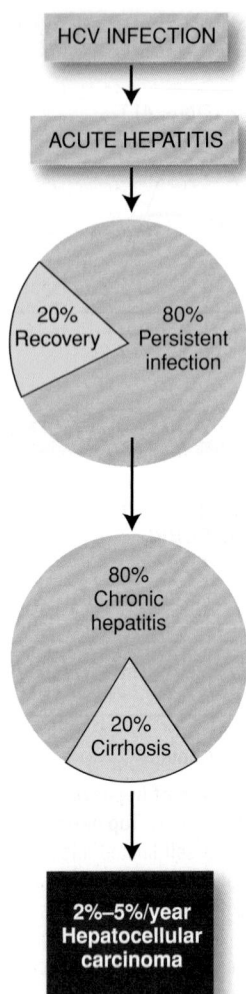

FIGURE 20-27. Outcomes of infection with the hepatitis C virus (HCV).

TABLE 20-3			
COMPARATIVE FEATURES OF THE COMMON FORMS OF VIRAL HEPATITIS			
	Hepatitis A	**Hepatitis B**	**Hepatitis C**
Genome	RNA	DNA	RNA
Incubation period	3–6 weeks	6 weeks–6 months	7–8 weeks
Transmission	Oral	Parenteral	Parenteral
Blood	No	Yes	Yes
Feces	Yes	No	No
Vertical	No	Yes	5%
Fulminant	Very rare	Yes	Rare hepatic necrosis
Chronic hepatitis	No	10%	80%
Carrier state	No	Yes	Yes
Liver cancer	No	Yes	Yes

protease and polymerase inhibitors offer even greater promise of effective control of HCV. A sustained virologic response (i.e., no detectable HCV RNA) is associated with a conspicuous decrease in the risk of HCC.

Table 20-3 compares the major features of the common forms of viral hepatitis.

Hepatitis E Virus Is a Major Cause of Epidemic Hepatitis

Hepatitis E is a self-limited, acute, icteric disease similar to hepatitis A. Hepatitis E virus (HEV) is an enteric RNA virus of the Hepeviridae family, four genotypes of which are now known. It accounts for more than 1/2 of cases of acute viral hepatitis in young to middle-aged people in the poorer regions of the world. Large outbreaks have been reported in India, Nepal, Burma, Pakistan, the former Soviet Union, Africa and Mexico. Most of these epidemics have followed heavy rains in areas with inadequate sewage disposal. HEV infection may be transmitted via several routes: waterborne, zoonotic (especially eating raw or undercooked meat of infected wild animals such as pig, boar or deer) and parenteral and vertical transmission. HEV closely resembles a swine virus, suggesting that the latter may represent a reservoir of infection.

The incubation period for HEV is 35–40 days. Jaundice, hepatomegaly, fever and arthralgias are common and usually resolve within 6 weeks, with 1%–12% mortality. Like hepatitis A, clinical illness from hepatitis E is far more common in adults than in children; in the latter, infection may often be subclinical. The disease is very dangerous in pregnant women, in whom mortality may reach 20%–40%. Chronic disease and carrier states are unknown in immunocompetent patients, but immunocompromised people may develop chronic hepatitis E. A successful vaccine against HEV infection has been developed and tested in Nepal but is not yet licensed in the United States.

Liver disease in patients with chronic HCV infection tends to be more severe in the face of concurrent hepatitis B, alcoholic liver disease, hemochromatosis or α_1-antitrypsin (α_1-AT) deficiency. About 25% of patients with advanced alcoholic liver disease have antibodies to HCV, although rates vary in different locales. The relationship is unexplained, and some cases classified as alcoholic cirrhosis may really be due to HCV.

Extrahepatic manifestations of hepatitis C are common and include mixed cryoglobulinemia (see Chapter 20), a systemic vasculitis due to deposition of circulating immune complexes in the microvasculature. The skin (leukocytoclastic vasculitis), salivary glands (sicca syndrome), nervous system (mononeuritis multiplex) and kidney (membranoproliferative glomerulonephritis) may be affected. Non-Hodgkin B-cell lymphomas are more common in patients with chronic hepatitis C.

Since it is largely asymptomatic, acute HCV rarely comes to medical attention. For patients who are treated for acute HCV, success rates are higher than in chronic cases. Chronic hepatitis C is generally treated with a combination of injected interferon-α and oral ribavirin. With genotype 1, 40%–50% of patients eliminate circulating HCV genomes; 75%–80% with genotypes 2 or 3 do the same. Newer therapies including

Other Human Hepatitis Viruses Remain Conjectural

Hepatitis F virus was a hypothetical virus linked to hepatitis, but reports of it in the 1990s were never substantiated. It was consequently disregarded as a cause of viral hepatitis.

Hepatitis G virus (HGV), now more commonly referred as GB virus C (GBV-C), is a lymphotropic flavivirus discovered in 1995 in relation to HCV infection. HGV infection by itself does not cause any known disease; however, several studies found an association between persistent GBV-C infection and improved survival in HIV-positive patients. GBV-C infection may alter T-cell function by modulating chemokine and cytokine release and by reducing T-cell activation, proliferation and apoptosis.

PATHOLOGY OF VIRAL HEPATITIS

All Forms of Acute Viral Hepatitis Are Pathologically Similar

PATHOLOGY: The hallmark of acute viral hepatitis is liver cell death (Fig. 20-28). Within the hepatic lobule, scattered single cell necrosis or death of small clusters of hepatocytes is seen. A few apoptotic liver cells appear as small, deeply eosinophilic bodies **(acidophilic bodies),** sometimes with pyknotic nuclei. Acidophilic bodies are characteristic of viral hepatitis but are also seen in many other liver diseases. In acute viral hepatitis, many liver cells show varying degrees of hydropic swelling and differences in size, shape and staining properties. Concomitantly, regenerative liver cells may have larger nuclei and basophilic cytoplasm. Resulting irregular liver cell plates are described as **lobular disarray.**

Mononuclear cells, mostly lymphocytes, infiltrate lobules diffusely, surround individual necrotic liver cells and accumulate in areas of focal necrosis. Macrophages may be prominent, whereas eosinophils and polymorphonuclear

leukocytes are not uncommon. Characteristically, lymphocytes infiltrate between the wall of the central vein and the liver cell plates, an appearance termed **central phlebitis.** Swelling and proliferation of the endothelium of central veins **(endophlebitis)** may develop. Kupffer cells are enlarged, project into sinusoid lumens and contain lipofuscin pigment and phagocytosed debris. Cholestasis is common. If severe, it is called **cholestatic hepatitis,** in which many liver cells are arrayed around dilated bile canaliculi, giving an acinar or glandular appearance. Lumens of dilated canaliculi may contain large bile plugs.

Mononuclear inflammatory cells accumulate within portal tracts. Lymphocytes in portal tracts may form follicles, particularly in hepatitis C. The limiting plate of hepatocytes around the portal tracts is usually intact. These changes are gradually reversed during recovery, and normal hepatic architecture is completely restored.

Confluent Hepatic Necrosis Affects Whole Regions of the Lobule

Confluent hepatic necrosis reflects particularly severe forms of acute viral hepatitis, characterized by death of many hepatocytes in a geographical distribution. In extreme cases, almost all liver cells in a lobule die **(massive hepatic necrosis).** The most common viral cause is acute hepatitis B; only rarely does confluent hepatic necrosis result from infection with other hepatotropic viruses. The lesions are not unique to viral hepatitis but may also occur after exposure to hepatotoxic chemicals and in autoimmune hepatitis (see below). Unlike most common forms of acute viral hepatitis, in which liver cell necrosis appears to be random and patchy, confluent hepatic necrosis typically affects whole regions of lobules. The lesions of confluent hepatic necrosis, in order of increasing severity, are bridging necrosis, submassive necrosis and massive necrosis.

BRIDGING NECROSIS: At the milder end of the spectrum of lesions that make up confluent hepatic necrosis are bands of necrosis (bridging necrosis) between adjacent portal tracts, between adjacent central veins and from portal tracts to central veins (Fig. 20-29). Adjacent plates of

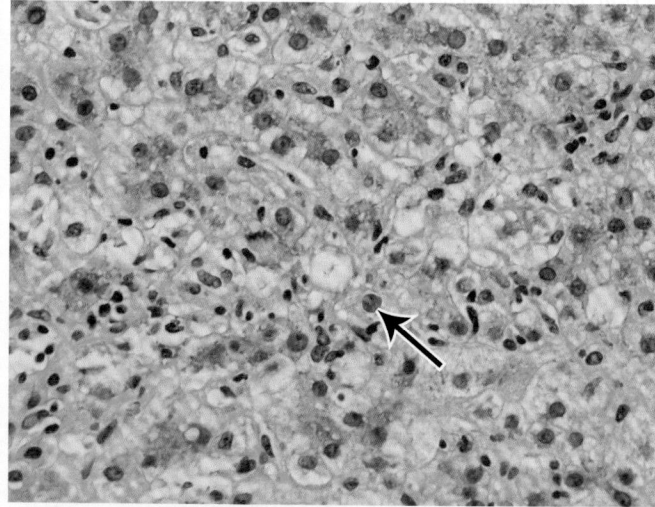

FIGURE 20-28. Acute viral hepatitis. Disarray of liver cell plates, swollen (ballooned) hepatocytes and an infiltrate of lymphocytes and scattered mononuclear inflammatory cells. The remnants of apoptotic hepatocytes have been extruded into the sinusoids, where they appear as acidophilic bodies (*arrow*).

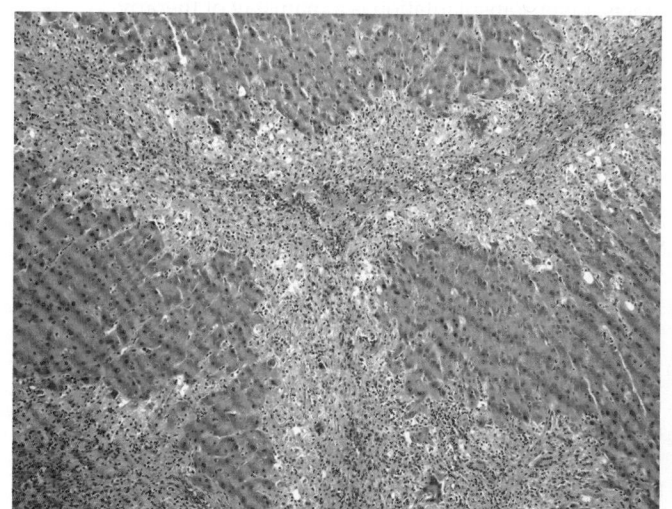

FIGURE 20-29. Confluent hepatic necrosis. Hemorrhagic zones of necrosis bridge adjacent central veins and portal tracts (bridging necrosis).

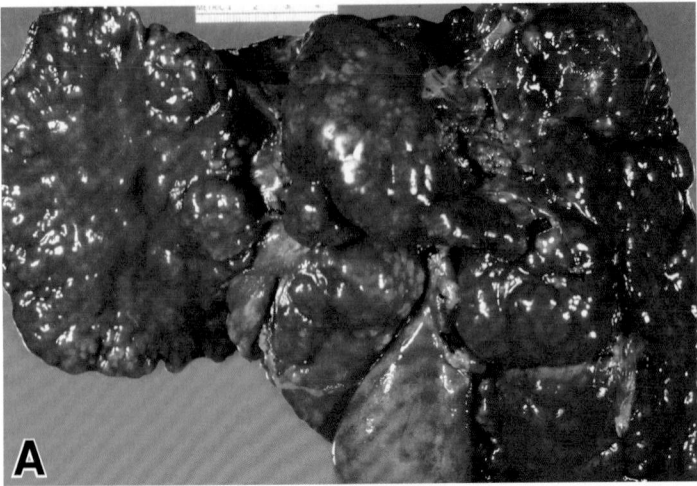

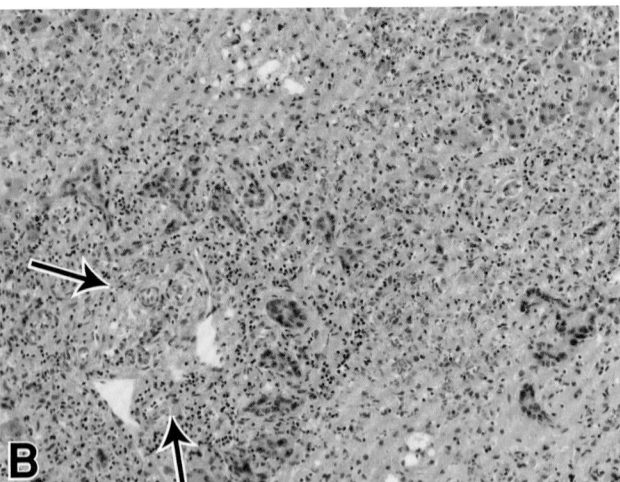

FIGURE 20-30. Massive hepatic necrosis. A. The liver is soft and reduced in size and shows a mottled, yellowish surface ("acute yellow atrophy"). **B.** Complete loss of the hepatocytes. The framework of the lobule has collapsed. The portal tracts (*arrows*) are expanded and contain ductular reaction.

hepatocytes die, causing collapse of the collagenous stroma to form bands of connective tissue. These are best seen with a reticulin stain. If such bands encircle an area of liver cells, they may impart a nodular appearance, as in cirrhosis.

SUBMASSIVE HEPATIC NECROSIS: This form of acute hepatitis defines an even more severe injury in which entire lobules or groups of adjacent lobules die. Clinically, these patients manifest severe hepatitis, which may rapidly proceed to hepatic failure, in which case the disease is classed clinically as **fulminant hepatitis**.

MASSIVE HEPATIC NECROSIS (ACUTE YELLOW ATROPHY): Massive hepatic necrosis, the most feared form of acute viral hepatitis, is fortunately rare. It is almost invariably fatal. Grossly, the liver is shrunken to as little as 500 g (1/3 of normal weight). The capsule is wrinkled, with mottled, soft and flabby red-tan parenchyma. Virtually all hepatocytes are dead (Fig. 20-30), and only the collagenous frameworks remain as epitaphs of liver lobules that collapsed and perished. Macrophages, erythrocytes and necrotic debris fill sinusoids. For unknown reasons, the massive necrosis does not elicit a vigorous inflammatory response in either the parenchyma or portal tracts. Liver transplantation is a mainstay of therapy.

Chronic Hepatitis May Complicate Hepatitis B and C, Metabolic Diseases and Immune Disorders

The morphologic spectrum of chronic hepatitis ranges from mild portal inflammation with little or no liver cell necrosis (Fig. 20-31) to widespread inflammation, necrosis and fibrosis eventuating in cirrhosis (Fig. 20-32).

PORTAL TRACT LESIONS: In chronic hepatitis, portal tracts are variably infiltrated by lymphocytes, plasma cells and macrophages (Figs. 20-31 and 20-32). These expanded portal tracts often show mild to severe proliferation of bile ductules, which is a nonspecific response to chronic liver injury. In the case of chronic hepatitis C, lymphoid aggregates or follicles with reactive centers are often present.

PIECEMEAL NECROSIS: Piecemeal necrosis is focal inflammatory destruction of the limiting plate of hepatocytes. A periportal chronic inflammatory infiltrate creates an irregular border between portal tracts and the lobular parenchyma (Fig. 20-32A).

INTRALOBULAR LESIONS: Focal necrosis and parenchymal inflammation typify chronic hepatitis. Scattered acidophilic bodies and enlarged Kupffer cells are common (Fig. 20-28). In chronic hepatitis B, scattered hepatocytes may show large granular cytoplasm with abundant HBsAg **(ground-glass hepatocytes)** (Fig. 20-33).

PERIPORTAL FIBROSIS: Progressive loss of periportal hepatocytes by piecemeal necrosis leads to deposition of collagen, giving portal tracts a stellate (star-shaped) appearance. In time, fibrosis may join adjacent portal tracts or approach the central vein, ultimately developing into cirrhosis (Fig. 20-32B).

AUTOIMMUNE HEPATITIS

Autoimmune hepatitis is a severe type of chronic hepatitis associated with circulating autoantibodies and elevated serum immunoglobulins. The disorder may appear at any

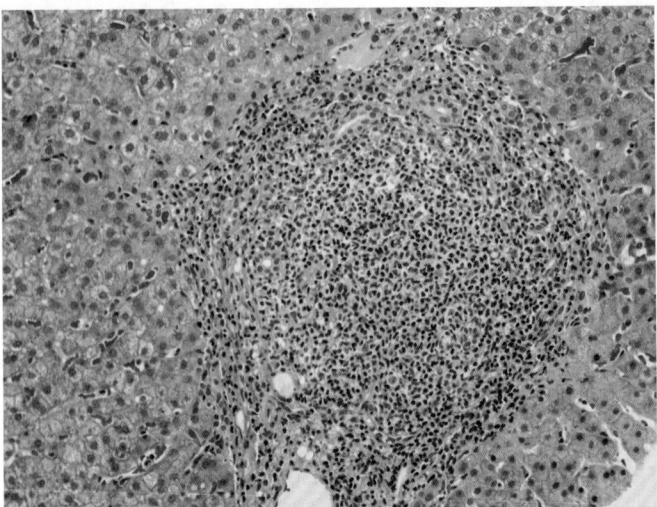

FIGURE 20-31. Mild chronic hepatitis. A portal tract infiltrated by mononuclear inflammatory cells. The lobular parenchyma is intact. Nonzonal or periportal mild fatty change often accompanies hepatitis C.

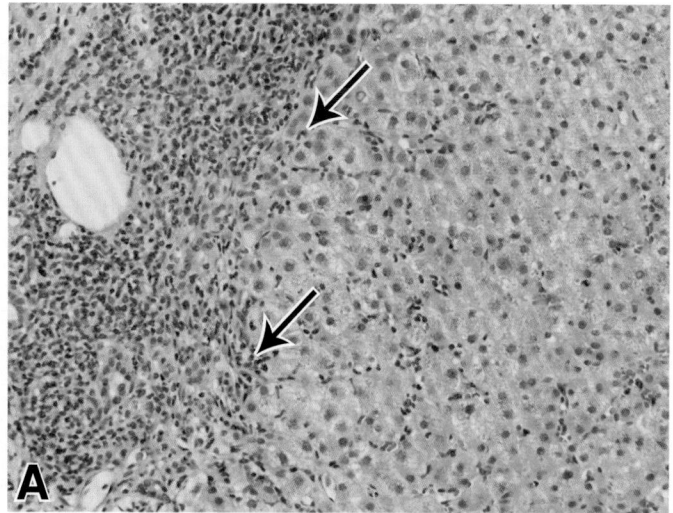
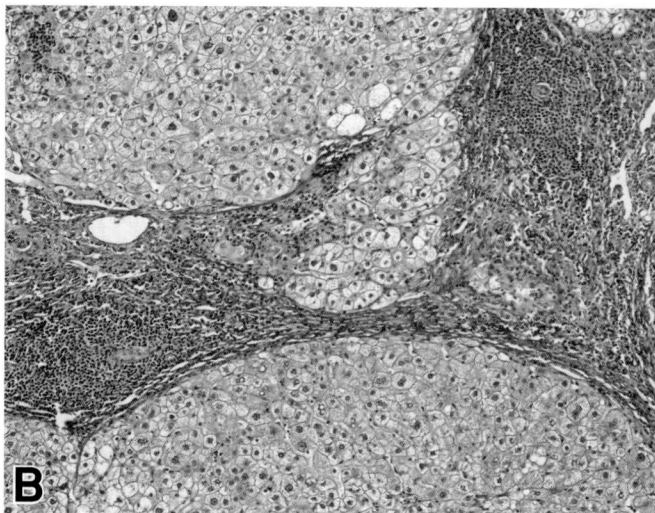

FIGURE 20-32. Severe chronic hepatitis. A. Mononuclear inflammatory infiltration in an expanded portal tract (*left*). Interface hepatitis is penetration of inflammation to the limiting plate and surrounds groups of hepatocytes at the border of the portal tract (*arrows*). **B. Chronic hepatitis with cirrhosis.** A liver from a patient with long-standing chronic hepatitis C shows lymphocytic aggregates, bridging fibrosis and nodular transformation.

age; 70% of cases occur in women. In the United States, auto-immune hepatitis affects up to 200,000 people and accounts for 6% of liver transplants.

PATHOPHYSIOLOGY: There are two types of autoimmune hepatitis:

- **Type I** disease is more common (80% of cases). It features antinuclear and anti–smooth muscle antibodies. Some 70% of cases occur in women younger than 40 years, among whom 1/3 have other autoimmune diseases, including thyroiditis, rheumatoid arthritis and ulcerative colitis. Of those patients with type I autoimmune hepatitis, 1/4 present with cirrhosis, indicating that the disease usually has a prolonged asymptomatic course. There are antibodies against many cytosolic

enzymes, but the hepatocyte membrane asialoglyco-protein receptor is the main candidate target for anti-body-dependent cell-mediated cytotoxicity (ADCC). The HLA-*DRB1* gene confers particular susceptibility to type I autoimmune hepatitis. Some patients may present with a poorly characterized "overlap syndrome" with mixed clinical and histologic features of autoimmune hepatitis and either primary biliary cirrhosis (PBC) or PSC.

- **Type II** autoimmune hepatitis occurs mainly in children who are 2–14 years old. Antibodies against liver and kidney microsomes (anti-LKM) are characteristic. However, the key autoantigen is a P450-type drug-metabolizing enzyme (CYP 2D6). These patients often have other autoimmune diseases (i.e., type I diabetes and thyroiditis). Genetic determinants of type II disease are not defined.

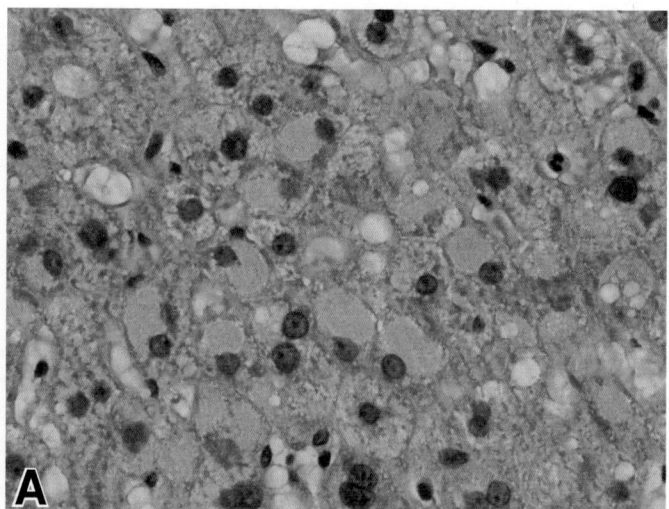
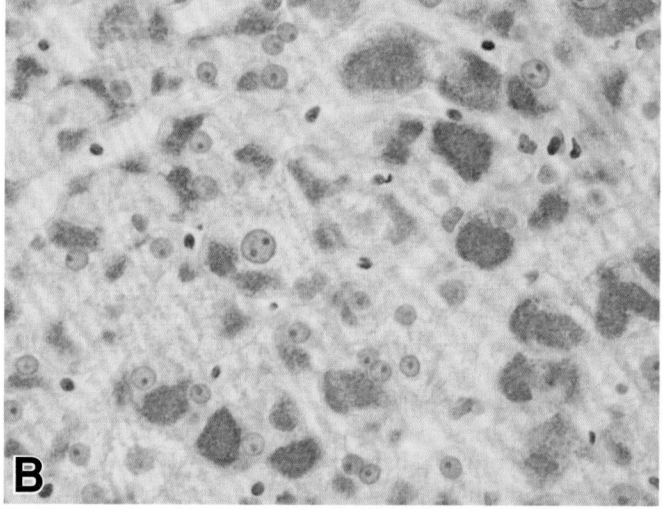

FIGURE 20-33. "Ground-glass" hepatocytes. A. Liver from a patient with chronic hepatitis B shows scattered hepatocytes (*arrow*) with an abundant granular cytoplasm containing hepatitis B surface antigen (HBsAg). **B.** The same specimen has been stained for HBsAg by the immunoperoxidase method. The abundant cytoplasmic HBsAg appears brown.

PATHOLOGY: Autoimmune hepatitis basically resembles acute and chronic viral hepatitis histologically, but lobular inflammation and necrosis are more pronounced. The inflammatory infiltrate is rich in plasma cells, an important diagnostic feature. Confluent hepatic necrosis may be seen in severe acute cases.

CLINICAL FEATURES: Autoimmune hepatitis can arise insidiously, with fatigue and mild right upper quadrant discomfort. Often, there is a personal or family history of autoimmunity. With time, aminotransferase levels rise markedly and may exceed 1000 IU/mL. Marked hyperglobulinemia is common. In severe cases, jaundice, hepatic synthetic dysfunction and even liver failure ensue, but it rarely presents as fulminant disese. Untreated, autoimmune hepatitis often progresses to cirrhosis.

Autoimmune hepatitis usually responds to combinations of corticosteroids and immunosuppressants such as azathioprine. Patients whose disease progresses to cirrhosis may receive liver transplants. Autoimmune hepatitis recurs in up to 20% of patients after liver transplantation.

ALCOHOLIC LIVER DISEASE

The harmful effects of excess alcohol (ethanol, ethyl alcohol) consumption have been recognized almost since the dawn of recorded history. The prophet Isaiah warned, "Woe to him that is mighty to drink wine." Ethanol is now seen as a hepatotoxin that acts both directly and indirectly.

EPIDEMIOLOGY: *Alcoholic cirrhosis is most common in countries where people consume the most alcohol,* regardless of the specific alcoholic beverage (e.g., wine in France, beer in Australia, spirits in Scandinavia). Only a minority of chronic alcoholics develop cirrhosis, but there is a dose-response relationship between lifetime dose of alcohol (duration of exposure and daily amount of alcohol consumed) and the appearance of cirrhosis.

About 10% of men and 5% of women in the United States abuse alcohol. In some other countries, this figure is much higher. *Some 15% of alcoholics develop cirrhosis; many of them die in hepatic failure or from extrahepatic complications of cirrhosis.* In many urban areas of the United States with high alcoholism rates, cirrhosis of the liver is the third or fourth leading cause of death in men younger than 45 years.

The amount of alcohol required to produce chronic liver disease depends on body size, age, gender and ethnicity, but the lower range seems to be about 20 g/day (about 2 ounces of 86 proof [43%] whiskey, two glasses of wine or two 12-ounce bottles of beer daily) for women and 40 g/day in men. In general, more than 10 years of alcohol use at this level is needed to produce cirrhosis, although a few cirrhotic patients give shorter histories of heavy alcohol use.

Women are more predisposed to the harmful effects of alcohol, for unknown reasons. However, women metabolize alcohol differently and have lower body masses.

The epidemiology of alcoholic liver disease is complicated by its association with the hepatotropic viruses. HBV seropositivity is two- to fourfold more common in alcoholics than in control populations. The prevalence of anti-HCV antibodies is up to 10% among alcoholics and is even higher among alcoholics with chronic liver disease. As noted above, people who abuse alcohol and also have hepatitis C are more likely to develop liver disease than their counterparts not so infected.

Ethanol Is Mainly Metabolized in the Liver

Ethanol is rapidly absorbed from the stomach and eventually distributed in body water space. Between 5% and 10% is excreted unchanged, mostly in the urine and expired breath. The remaining 90% is metabolized by the liver to acetaldehyde and acetate, largely by cytosolic **alcohol dehydrogenase (ADH)**. The mixed-function oxidases in the **microsomal ethanol-oxidizing system** in the SER are a minor metabolic pathway for alcohol. Clearance of alcohol from the body, unlike most drugs, is linear—that is, a fixed quantity is metabolized per unit time. Roughly, for the average man, 7–10 g of alcohol is eliminated per hour. However, since the microsomal pathway (see above) is upregulated in chronic alcoholics, they metabolize ethanol more rapidly, as long as they do not suffer from active liver disease.

Alcohol Consumption Causes a Spectrum of Liver Diseases

Alcoholic liver disease spans three major morphologic and clinical entities: **fatty liver, acute alcoholic hepatitis** and **cirrhosis**. These lesions usually occur in sequence, but they may coexist in any combination and may actually be independent entities.

Fatty Liver

MOLECULAR PATHOGENESIS: Virtually all chronic alcoholics, regardless of their pattern of drinking, accumulate fat in hepatocytes **(steatosis)**. The relative contributions of different metabolic pathways to steatosis may depend on the amount of alcohol consumed, dietary lipid content, body stores of fat, hormonal status and other variables. *Still, accumulation of fat clearly depends on alcohol intake, as it is fully and rapidly reversible if alcohol ingestion stops.*

Dietary fat, as chylomicrons and free fatty acids, is transported to the liver, where it is taken up by hepatocytes. Triglycerides are then hydrolyzed to free fatty acids. These, in turn, undergo β-oxidation in mitochondria or are converted by the ER to triglycerides. These newly synthesized triglycerides are secreted as lipoproteins or are retained for storage.

Most of the fat deposited in the liver after chronic alcohol consumption is from the diet. Ethanol increases lipolysis and thus delivery of free fatty acids to the liver. Within hepatocytes, ethanol (1) increases fatty acid synthesis, (2) decreases mitochondrial oxidation of fatty acids, (3) raises triglyceride production and (4) impairs release of lipoproteins. Collectively, these metabolic consequences produce a fatty liver.

PATHOLOGY: In the setting of high alcohol intake, the liver becomes yellow and enlarged, sometimes to as much as three times its normal weight. This increased weight does not only reflect fat accumulation; protein and water content also increase. The extent of visible fat accumulation varies from minute droplets scattered in the cytoplasm of a few hepatocytes to distention of

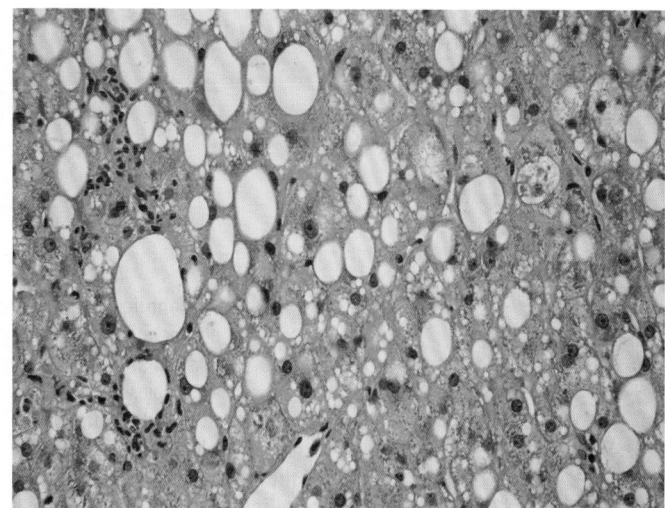

FIGURE 20-34. Alcoholic fatty liver. The cytoplasm of almost all of the hepatocytes distended by fat that displaces the nucleus to the periphery.

the entire cytoplasm of most cells by coalesced droplets (Fig. 20-34). In the latter case, liver cells may be barely recognizable as such and resemble adipocytes, with their cytoplasm distended by a clear area and their nuclei flattened and displaced to the periphery of the cell.

Ultrastructurally, hepatocytes in alcohol-induced fatty livers reflect the cytotoxicity of ethanol rather than an effect of fat. Mitochondria are enlarged, with occasional bizarre giant forms. The SER is hyperplastic, resembling that produced by other inducers of microsomal drug-metabolizing enzymes (see Chapter 1).

Chronic ethanol ingestion elicits pronounced hepatic functional alterations. Liver mitochondria show decreased rates of substrate oxidation (e.g., of fatty acids) and impaired ATP formation. SER hyperplasia is accompanied by increased activity of the cytochrome P450–dependent mixed-function oxidases. Not only is the microsomal ethanol-oxidizing system induced, but metabolism of a variety of drugs is also enhanced. *This increased microsomal function also augments metabolism of hepatic toxins, thus exaggerating the danger of agents such as acetaminophen, in which it is the drug's metabolic products that are most toxic.* Whereas chronic alcohol consumption promotes microsomal functions, acute alcohol ingestion inhibits mixed-function oxidases and acutely reduces the rate of clearance of drugs from the body.

 CLINICAL FEATURES: Patients with uncomplicated alcoholic fatty liver have surprisingly few symptoms of liver disease. Despite the striking morphologic change in the liver, alcoholic fatty liver is fully reversible and does not by itself progress to more severe disease. The best treatment for fatty liver due to alcohol is abstinence. Fatty liver, although characteristic of alcoholism, is not limited to it. Fatty liver may also be seen in nonalcoholic fatty liver disease (NAFLD; see below), hepatitis C, after certain drugs and in many other conditions.

Alcoholic Hepatitis

Alcoholic hepatitis is characterized by (1) hepatocyte necrosis, mainly in the central zone; (2) cytoplasmic hyaline inclusions within hepatocytes (Mallory bodies); (3) an acute inflammatory infiltrate in the lobule and (4) perivenular fibrosis (Fig. 20-35). **The pathogenesis of alcoholic hepatitis is a mystery.** Alcoholics may have mild fatty liver for many years and, without any change in drinking habits, suddenly develop acute alcoholic hepatitis. It may be that long-standing, subclinical alcoholic hepatitis precedes clinically overt hepatitis. Nevertheless, the often explosive presentation of alcoholic hepatitis suggests that some environmental or physiologic cofactor is involved, although none has been identified.

 PATHOLOGY: Typically, hepatic architecture is intact. Hepatocytes show variable hydropic swelling, giving them a heterogeneous appearance. Isolated necrotic liver cells or clusters of them have pyknotic nuclei and show karyorrhexis. Scattered hepatocytes contain **Mallory bodies (alcoholic hyaline)** (Fig. 20-35). These cytoplasmic inclusions are more common in visibly damaged, swollen hepatocytes and appear as irregular skeins of eosinophilic material or as solid eosinophilic masses, often perinuclearly. They are aggregates of intermediate (cytokeratin) filaments (Fig. 20-35C). The damaged, ballooned hepatocytes, particularly those with Mallory bodies, are surrounded by neutrophils. A more diffuse, intralobular inflammatory infiltrate is also present. Mallory bodies are characteristic of, but not specific for, alcoholic liver disease, as they may also be present in NASH, chronic cholestatic syndromes, WD and HCC. Mild to severe cholestasis is seen in up to 1/3 of cases. Alcoholic hepatitis is usually superimposed on an existing fatty liver, but there is no evidence that fat accumulation predisposes or contributes to development of alcoholic hepatitis.

Collagen deposition is always seen in alcoholic hepatitis, especially around central veins (terminal hepatic venules). Chronic alcohol exposure activates hepatic stellate cells to deposit intrasinusoidal collagen. In severe cases, venules and perivenular sinusoids are obliterated and surrounded by dense fibrous tissue to yield **central hyaline sclerosis** (Figs. 20-35 and 20-36). This condition is often associated with noncirrhotic portal hypertension.

Portal tracts in alcoholic hepatitis are highly variable. Some are virtually normal, whereas others are enlarged, with a mononuclear infiltrate and proliferated bile ductules. The altered portal tracts often show spurs of fibrous tissue that penetrate the lobules.

 CLINICAL FEATURES: Patients with alcoholic hepatitis have malaise and anorexia, fever, right upper quadrant abdominal pain and jaundice. Leukocytosis is common. Serum aminotransferases, particularly AST, are moderately elevated but not as high as in viral hepatitis: AST usually remains under 400. The AST:ALT ratio is typically 2:1. Serum alkaline phosphatase is usually increased. In severe cases, a prolonged prothrombin time often portends an ominous prognosis.

The outlook in patients with alcoholic hepatitis reflects the severity of liver cell injury. In some patients, the disease progresses rapidly to hepatic failure and death. Mortality in the acute stage of alcoholic hepatitis is about 10%. Most of those who abstain from alcohol after recovery from acute alcoholic hepatitis recover. However, of those who continue to drink, up to 70% ultimately develop cirrhosis.

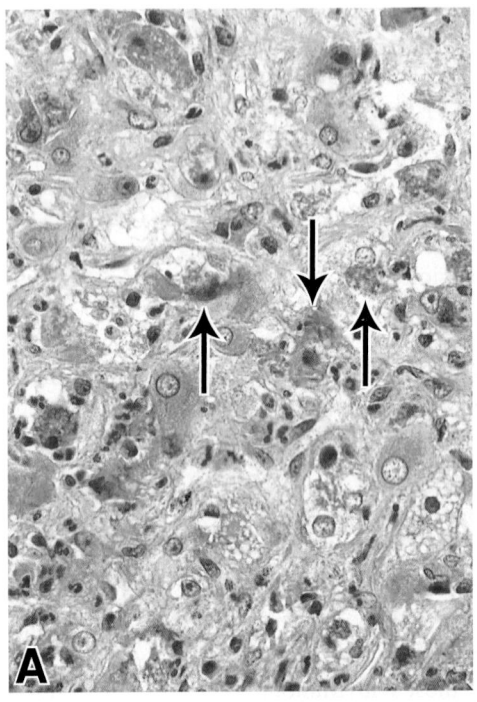

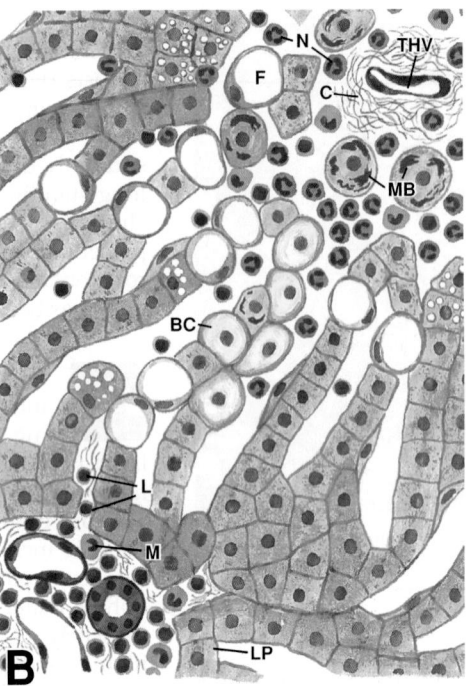

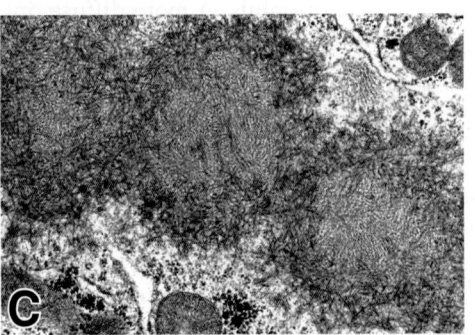

FIGURE 20-35. Alcoholic hepatitis. A. Necrosis and degeneration of hepatocytes, Mallory-Denk bodies (eosinophilic inclusions) in the cytoplasm of injured hepatocytes (*arrows*) and infiltration by neutrophils. **B. Schematic representation of the major pathologic features of alcoholic hepatitis.** The lesions are predominantly centrilobular and include necrosis and loss of hepatocytes, ballooned cells (*BC*) and Mallory-Denk bodies (*MB*) in the cytoplasm of damaged hepatocytes. The inflammatory infiltrate consists predominantly of neutrophils (*N*), although a few lymphocytes (*L*) and macrophages (*M*) are also present. The central venule, or terminal hepatic venule (*THV*), is encased in connective tissue (*C*) (central hyaline sclerosis; also see Fig. 14–36). Fat-laden hepatocytes (*F*) are evident in the lobule. The portal tract displays moderate chronic inflammation, and the limiting plate (*LP*) is focally breached. **C. Ultrastructure of Mallory-Denk bodies.** Dense, interwoven bundles of cytokeratin filaments are in the cytoplasm of hepatocytes.

There is no specific treatment for acute alcoholic hepatitis. Corticosteroids improve short-term mortality and thus are often given if there is no infection or renal failure. Nutritional therapy can be beneficial.

Alcoholic Cirrhosis

In about 15% of alcoholics, hepatocellular necrosis, fibrosis and regeneration eventually lead to formation of fibrous septa around hepatocellular nodules (Fig. 20-13). The other lesions of alcoholic liver disease—fatty liver and acute or persistent alcoholic hepatitis—are often seen in conjunction with cirrhosis. Some assert that progression to alcoholic cirrhosis requires at least subclinical alcoholic hepatitis. Activated hepatic stellate cells, which produce perisinusoidal collagen, probably contribute to the development of cirrhosis. The prognosis in cases of established alcoholic cirrhosis is much better in those who abstain from alcohol. Nevertheless, many patients progress to end-stage liver disease, and alcoholic liver disease is a common indication for liver transplantation.

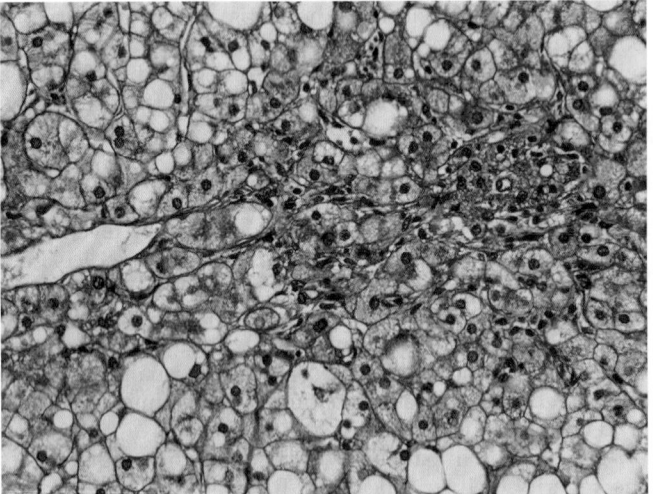

FIGURE 20-36. Pericellular fibrosis in nonalcoholic steatohepatitis (NASH). This trichrome stained liver from a patient with NASH shows pericellular fibrosis around the central venule (*blue*). Note the macrovesicular fat. This lesion mimics that seen in alcoholic liver disease.

NONALCOHOLIC FATTY LIVER DISEASE

NAFLD is so named because of its close resemblance to alcoholic liver disease. It represents diverse liver injuries from simple steatosis, with or without associated hepatitis (NASH) to bridging fibrosis and cirrhosis. Risk factors for NAFLD include obesity, type 2 diabetes mellitus, hyperlipidemia and metabolic syndrome (see Chapter 22). About 1/2 of people with both severe obesity and diabetes have NASH, of whom up to 1/5 develop cirrhosis.

NAFLD overlaps alcoholic liver disease histologically, with steatosis, lobular and portal inflammation, hepatocyte necrosis, Mallory-Denk bodies and fibrosis. As in alcoholic liver disease, centrilobular fibrosis is common (Fig. 20-36). If cirrhosis develops, steatosis often disappears. *Thus, NAFLD is the likely cause of many cases of so-called cryptogenic cirrhosis.*

 PATHOPHYSIOLOGY: The pathogenesis of NAFLD and NASH may overlap that of alcoholic hepatitis. Insulin resistance is associated with increased hepatic mitochondrial oxidation of free fatty acids, increased oxidative stress and lipid peroxidation, and it appears to be the strongest risk factor for NAFLD and NASH. Progression to cirrhosis in NAFLD is often insidious, and many patients remain asymptomatic, with only moderate increases in serum liver enzyme activities.

NAFLD is considered the hepatic manifestation of the metabolic syndrome, which consists of abdominal obesity, dyslipidemia, insulin resistance and hypertension (see Chapter 13). Weight reduction, including that via bariatric surgery, tends to improve NAFLD and NASH, but no definitive treatment is yet available.

PRIMARY BILIARY CIRRHOSIS

PBC is an immune-mediated, chronic, progressive cholestatic disease in which intrahepatic bile ducts are destroyed **(nonsuppurative destructive cholangitis)**. Loss of bile ducts leads to impaired bile secretion, cholestasis and hepatic damage. PBC occurs mainly in middle-aged women (10:1 female predominance). The term *cirrhosis* in this context is somewhat misleading, as it is actually a late complication of the disease.

PBC accounts for up to 2% of deaths from cirrhosis. Cases are sporadic, although the prevalence of PBC in families of patients with PBC is considerably higher than that in the general population, suggesting a hereditary predisposition.

 MOLECULAR PATHOGENESIS: PBC is associated with many immune abnormalities and thus is widely held to be an autoimmune disease. Most (85%) patients have at least one other autoimmune disease (chronic thyroiditis, rheumatoid arthritis, scleroderma, Sjögren syndrome, systemic lupus erythematosus), and almost 1/2 (40%) have two or more such diseases.

The *DRB1*008* family of major histocompatibility complex–encoded genes is associated with PBC, whereas the disease is less common in people carrying *DRB1*11* and *DRB1*13*. Polymorphisms of key immune regulatory genes, such as those encoding TNF-α and the CTL antigen 4 (CTLA4), are reported in patients with several autoimmune diseases, including PBC. Increased X chromosome monosomy may explain the strong female predominance of PBC.

PATHOPHYSIOLOGY: Humoral and cellular immunity are both impaired. Serum immunoglobulin levels are increased, especially IgM. *More than 95% of patients have circulating antimitochondrial antibodies (AMAs), a finding of which is commonly used to diagnose PBC.* Autoantibodies bind epitopes associated with the mitochondrial pyruvate dehydrogenase complex. Despite their specificity, AMAs do not affect mitochondrial function and play no known role in the pathogenesis or progression of the disease. Other circulating autoantibodies are antinuclear, antithyroid, antiplatelet, antiacetylcholine receptor and antiribonucleoprotein antibodies. The complement system is also chronically activated.

The cells surrounding and infiltrating the sites of bile duct damage are mostly suppressor/cytotoxic (CD8+) lymphocytes, suggesting that they mediate the destruction of the ductal epithelium.

PATHOLOGY: Pathologic stages of PBC are portal stage, periportal stage, septal stage and biliary cirrhosis.

- **STAGE 1: FLORID DUCT LESION OR PORTAL STAGE:** Early PBC features a unique lesion, a **chronic destructive cholangitis** involving small and medium-sized intrahepatic bile ducts. Injury to the ducts is segmental and thus appears focal in tissue sections. Lymphocytes, plasma cells and macrophages surround the ducts, disrupting the basement membrane (Fig. 20-37). Bile duct epithelium is irregular and hyperplastic, with stratification and occasional papillary ingrowths of epithelial cells. Epithelioid granulomas often occur in portal tracts and may impinge on the bile ducts.
- **STAGE 2: PERIPORTAL STAGE:** Bile ducts are reduced in number and ductular proliferation is evident in periportal areas. Inflammation is less than in stage 1.
- **STAGE 3: SEPTAL STAGE:** As a result of the destructive inflammation in stages 1 and 2 PBC, small bile ducts virtually disappear. Scarring of medium-sized bile ducts is

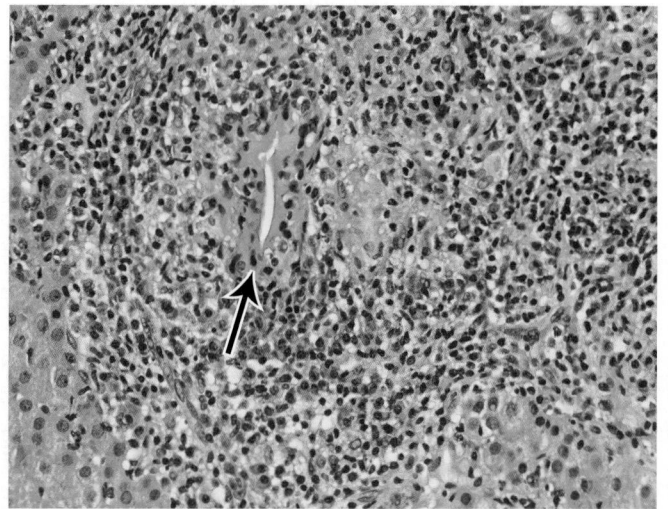

FIGURE 20-37. Florid duct lesion in primary biliary cirrhosis (PBC), stage I. A portal tract expanded by an inflammatory infiltrate consisting of lymphocytes, plasma cells, eosinophils and macrophages. Florid duct lesion represents a damaged bile duct (*arrow*) by the inflammation.

common. Collagenous septa extend from the portal tracts into the lobular parenchyma and begin to encircle some lobules.

- *STAGE 4: CIRRHOSIS:* The end stage of PBC is cirrhosis, with a dark-green bile-stained nodular liver with mainly portal-to-portal bridging fibrous septa. This fibrosis gives a "jigsaw puzzle" appearance to the cirrhotic nodules. Small bile ducts are scarce, and medium-sized ducts are conspicuously fewer in number. There is little inflammation within either the fibrous septa or the parenchymal nodules.

 CLINICAL FEATURES: *Some 90%–95% of those afflicted with PBC are women, usually those who are 30–65 years old.* Fatigue and pruritus are the most common initial symptoms, but many patients have no symptoms during the early stage of PBC. Some remain asymptomatic and appear to have an excellent prognosis; others ultimately develop advanced cirrhosis and its complications. The diagnosis of PBC is confirmed when a patient meets two of three criteria: (1) AMA titer of 1:40 or higher; (2) biochemical cholestasis, as indicated by elevated serum alkaline phosphatase for at least 6 months and (3) typical liver histology. The unusual diagnosis of so-called AMA-negative PBC rests on characteristic histologic and clinical findings (criteria 2 and 3).

Early in PBC, serum alkaline phosphatase is usually high, but bilirubin is normal or slightly elevated. The patient may complain of severe pruritus. As the disease advances, serum bilirubin progressively increases in most patients. Serum AST and ALT are only moderately elevated. Blood cholesterol levels increase strikingly, and an abnormal lipoprotein (lipoprotein-X) appears, a finding in many forms of chronic cholestasis. Cholesterol-laden macrophages accumulate in subcutaneous tissues, where they form localized lesions termed **xanthomas**. Impaired bile excretion into the intestine often leads to severe **steatorrhea** due to fat malabsorption. Associated malabsorption of vitamin D and calcium leads to **osteomalacia** and **osteoporosis,** two important complications of PBC. About 1/3 of patients develop gallstones. Those patients who eventually develop cirrhosis die of liver failure or complications of portal hypertension.

PBC is treated with UDCA, which increases transplant-free survival and leads to biochemical remission in about 40% of patients. The course of PBC is usually indolent and may be as long as 20–30 years. Liver transplantation is highly effective in end-stage PBC.

PRIMARY SCLEROSING CHOLANGITIS

PSC is a chronic cholestatic liver disease of unknown etiology, in which inflammation and fibrosis narrow and then obstruct intrahepatic and extrahepatic bile ducts. It usually occurs in men (70%), with a mean age of 40 years. PSC prevalence is 14 cases per 100,000 population. Progressive biliary obstruction typically leads to persistent obstructive jaundice, recurrent cholangitis and eventually to secondary biliary cirrhosis.

 PATHOPHYSIOLOGY: *The cause of PSC is unknown, but 2/3 of patients also have ulcerative colitis.* A few cases have been described in patients with Crohn disease of the colon. Associations with retroperitoneal fibrosis, lymphoma and the fibrosing variant of chronic thyroiditis (Riedel struma) are also reported. In 1/4 of cases, no other disease is present. Increased colonic permeability to bacteria has been suggested as a factor, but this possibility remains speculative.

Genetic and immunologic factors are implicated in the pathogenesis of PSC. PSC can occur in families, sometimes associated with certain HLA haplotypes, including HLA B8. Hypergammaglobulinemia is common, as are circulating immune complexes and antineutrophil cytoplasmic antibodies (perinuclear or P-ANCAs), and complement activation by the classic pathway. Portal tracts contain an increased number of T cells.

 PATHOLOGY: The pathology of PSC liver disease has four stages:

- *STAGE 1: PORTAL STAGE:* At first, there is periductal inflammation and "concentric, onion skin" fibrosis in the portal tracts (Fig. 20-38A).

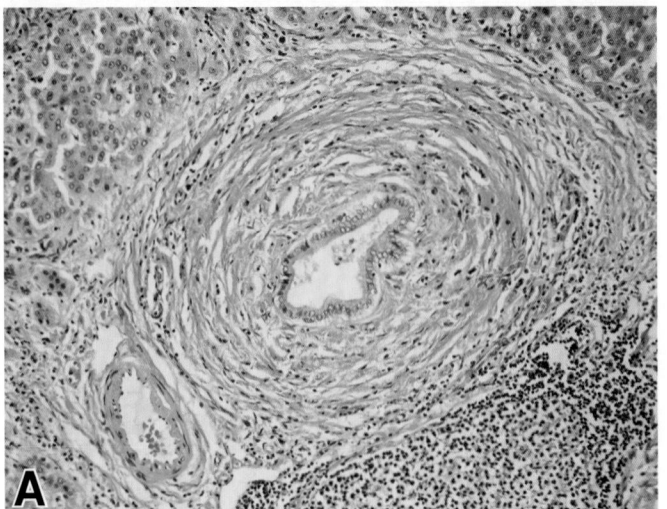
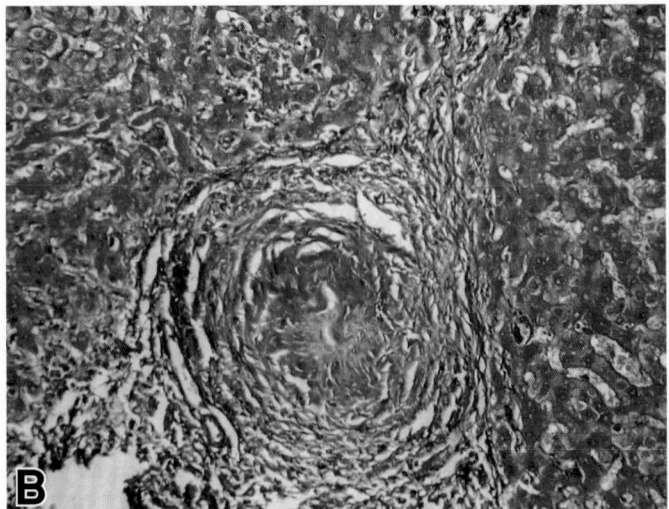

FIGURE 20-38. Primary sclerosing cholangitis (PSC). A. An inflammed portal tract with a dilated bile duct and "onion skin" periductal fibrosis. **B.** A bile duct scar represents a destroyed bile duct in PSC (trichrome stain).

- **STAGE 2: PERIPORTAL STAGE:** Many bile ducts become obliterated (Fig. 20-38B), portal fibrosis with fibrous septa extends into the parenchyma.
- **STAGE 3: SEPTAL STAGE:** Bridging fibrosis.
- **STAGE 4: CIRRHOSIS:** Secondary biliary cirrhosis eventuates (Fig. 20-38B).

Similar inflammatory and fibrotic changes may be seen in large intrahepatic and extrahepatic bile ducts, and these changes can obstruct both. The disease tends to be segmental; thus, the intrahepatic biliary tree shows a characteristic beaded appearance with contrast radiography. The same inflammatory process affects the gallbladder wall. Some patients with typical clinical features of PSC have normal-appearing bile ducts on cholangiography, in which case the condition is termed *small duct PSC.*

 CLINICAL FEATURES: The median survival in symptomatic patients with PSC is 8–9 years. Asymptomatic patients have a better prognosis. Clinical presentations vary from asymptomatic elevations in cholestatic liver tests to symptoms of biliary obstruction, recurrent cholangitis and evidence of end-stage liver disease. Infection may lead to abscess formation. *Cholangiocarcinoma develops in up to 20% of patients with PSC.* Liver transplantation may be curative; however, PSC often recurs in the transplanted liver.

IRON OVERLOAD SYNDROMES

In several conditions, excessive iron accumulates in the body (siderosis). There are two major groups of iron overload syndromes, divided on the basis of etiology. **Hereditary hemochromatosis (HH)** is caused by a common genetic alteration in control of intestinal iron absorption. **Secondary iron overload** complicates certain hematologic disorders. It entails parenteral iron overload, in which the iron accrues due to multiple blood transfusions or parenteral administration of iron itself, or is caused by huge dietary intake of iron. Secondary iron overload alone rarely causes liver disease.

Body Iron Stores Are Tightly Regulated

An understanding of normal iron metabolism is central to an appreciation of the pathophysiology of diseases of iron overload, such as HH. The normal total body content of iron is 3–4 g. Most of this (about 2.5 g) is bound up in hemoglobin. Iron normally enters the body by being absorbed through the duodenal mucosa. There is no mechanism for iron excretion: men and postmenopausal women eliminate 1–2 mg daily in desquamated cells. Therefore, keeping body iron within acceptable limits requires strict control of intestinal iron uptake (Fig. 20-39).

Several principal proteins control this process:

- **Hepcidin:** This 25 amino acid peptide is manufactured and exported by the liver and is the key to iron regulation. Hepcidin blocks transit of iron through enterocytes to the blood and inhibits its secretion from stores in hepatocytes and macrophages. It does this by binding the main iron export channel in these cells, **ferroportin,** and promoting its degradation.

  Control of hepcidin levels is thus central to iron homeostasis. Hepcidin synthesis is stimulated when

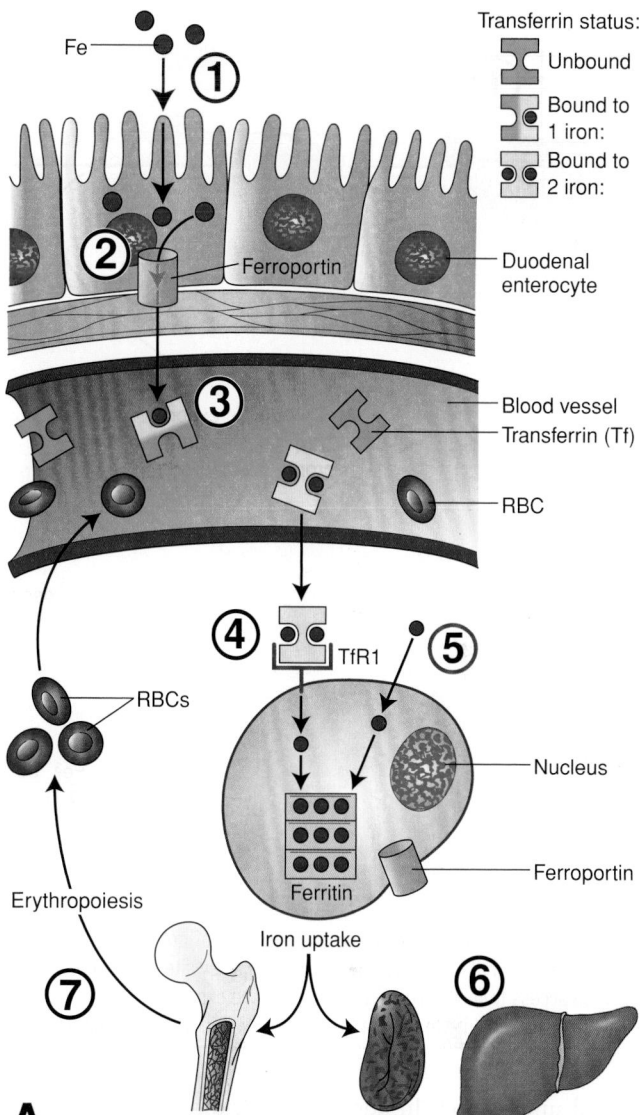

FIGURE 20-39. Normal iron metabolism and the role of hepcidin in its regulation. A. Iron absorption and utilization. 1. Iron enters duodenal enterocytes. These cells have a specific transporter that mediates iron entry. 2. Iron traverses enterocytes on its way to the circulation. Once in enterocyte cytosol, iron is exported by a specific channel, ferroportin, which mediates iron export in enterocytes and other cells. 3. Having traversed the enterocytes, Fe^{3+} binds to Tf, the principal means by which iron circulates. (Some free iron, i.e., iron not bound to Tf, circulates in normal circumstances.) 4. Tf is recognized by a receptor (TfR1) on cells that are engaged in iron uptake. It is stored bound to ferritin. 5. A small amount of iron enters cells as free iron, unbound to Tf. It, too, is stored as ferritin. 6. Excess iron supplies are stored in macrophages and hepatocytes. 7. Cells in the bone marrow incorporate iron into hemoglobin for use in erythrocytes. (*continued*)

body iron stores are sufficient and is downregulated when the body needs more iron. Upregulation of hepcidin requires several important proteins. This group of proteins—transferrin receptor 2 (TfR2), hemojuvelin and HFE—are all necessary to stimulate hepcidin production. Interestingly, hepcidin is also an acute phase reactant and is upregulated by the pro-inflammatory cytokine, IL-6 (see below). Other factors, such as bone morphogenesis proteins, increase hepcidin levels in ways that are not

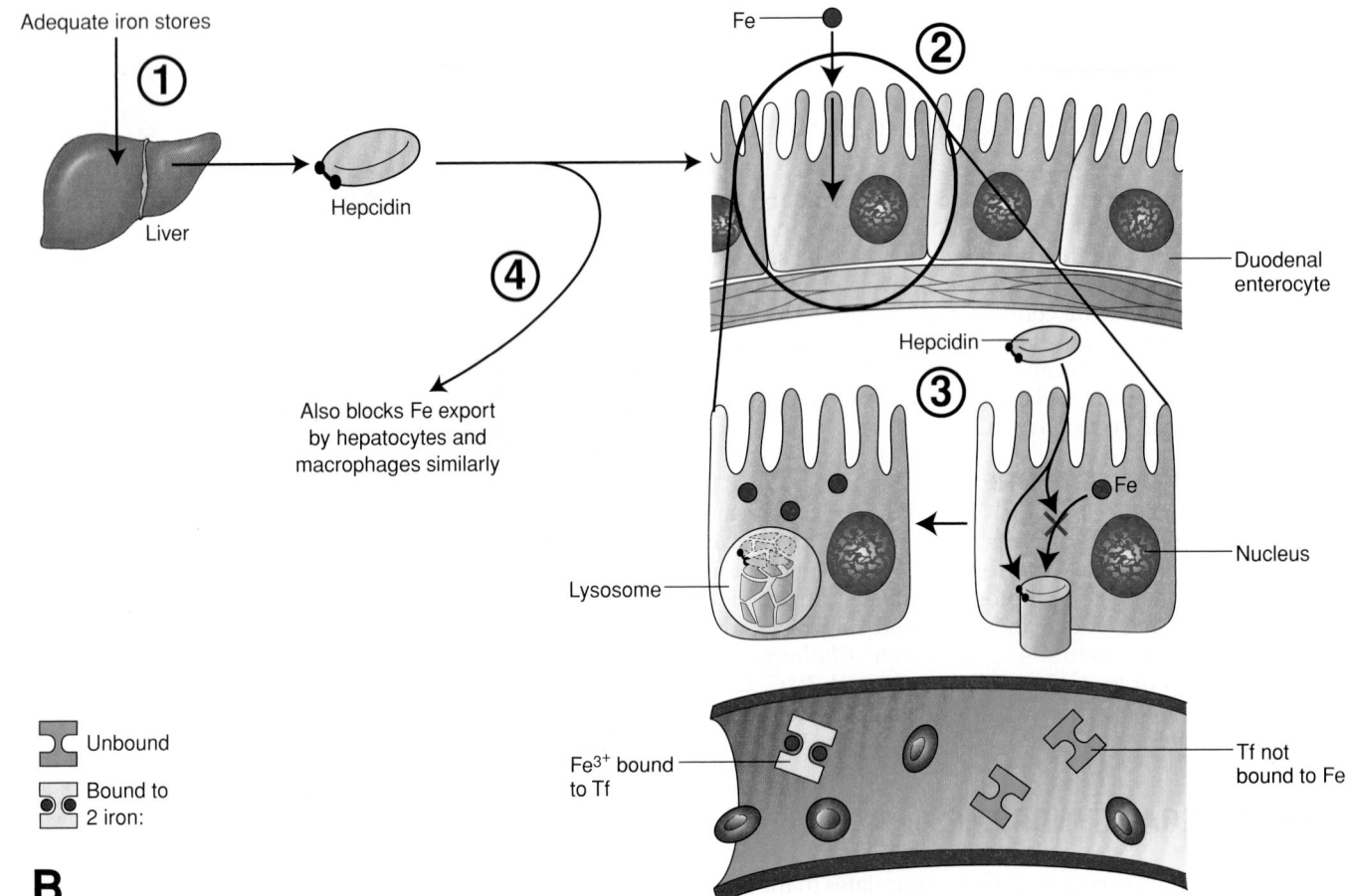

B

FIGURE 20-39. (*Continued*) **B.** Hepcidin regulation of iron uptake. 1. Hepcidin is produced by hepatocytes and exported into the circulation. 2. The duodenum, the principal portal of iron entry into the body, is a key site of hepcidin action. 3. If hepcidin is present, it binds ferroportin. This has two consequences. First, iron is denied access to ferroportin and thus cannot be exported. Second, hepcidin binding causes the hepcidin–ferroportin complex to be internalized and degraded. 4. The sequence is illustrated here for enterocytes but applies comparably to the other cells that store and export iron, such as macrophages and hepatocytes.

well understood. In addition, hepcidin, as a small peptide, passes through glomeruli. It is degraded in proximal tubules. As a consequence, in renal failure, hepcidin is not eliminated efficiently and its levels are generally elevated.

- **Ferroportin:** This protein is the obligatory iron channel in cells. It is required for cells (mainly enterocytes, hepatocytes and macrophages) to export iron or to transport it through the cell. Hepcidin inhibits ferroportin function by displacing iron from it, then causing the hepcidin–ferroportin complex to be internalized and degraded.
- **Transferrin (Tf):** There is more than one form of this molecule. However, the principal form of the Tf molecule is the main iron carrier in the blood. One Tf molecule binds two Fe^{3+} ions. Tf also mediates iron uptake by cells via its main receptor (TfR1). Normal plasma iron ranges from 80 to 100 mg/dL, and Tf is ordinarily about 33% saturated. A small amount of free iron—not bound by Tf—also circulates normally. In times of huge iron excess, free iron may be the predominant form of iron in the blood.
- **Ferritin:** This multimeric protein is responsible for storing iron within cells and is present in every cell type. It binds the ferric (Fe^{3+}) form of iron to form a complex called **hemosiderin,** and in so doing prevents the stored iron from generating free radical species via the Fenton reaction (see Chapter 1). Every ferritin complex (molecular size, 450 kDa) can store up to 4500 Fe^{3+} ions. Blood

ferritin levels generally reflect the status of the body's iron stores: low serum ferritin generally reflects iron deficiency. High ferritin levels occur when the body has large amounts of stored iron or, as well, during acute inflammatory reactions.

Iron Entry into Cells

Under normal circumstances, the main iron portal of entry into enterocytes is a cell membrane channel referred to as divalent metal transporter 1 (DMT-1). Other cells generally admit iron via a different receptor-mediated pathway: Tf-bound iron is recognized by TfR1 and internalized. Free iron (not bound by Tf) enters cells differently, via poorly understood mechanisms. It is this pathway, by which unbound iron enters cells, that allows intracellular iron accumulation when regulatory mechanisms malfunction (see below). Generally, iron is stored in macrophages and hepatocytes bound to **ferritin**.

Hereditary Hemochromatosis Is a Systemic Disease Caused by Excessive Iron Absorption

Toxic iron accumulation in HH is harmful to parenchymal cells, particularly of the liver, heart and pancreas. Up to 20–40 g of iron may accumulate, only within body storage

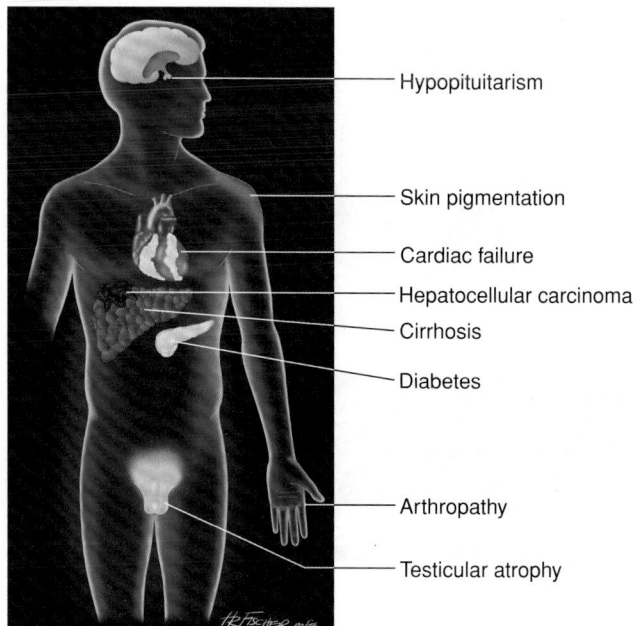

FIGURE 20-40. Complications of hemochromatosis.

compartments. *The clinical hallmarks of advanced HH are cirrhosis, diabetes, skin pigmentation and cardiac failure* (Fig. 20-40). HH is the most common inherited metabolic disorder in whites. It manifests most often in patients 40–60 years of age. Men are affected 10 times as often as women, probably because women lose iron by menstruation. However, postmenopausal women may also develop HH. As maximum daily iron absorption is about 4 mg, hemochromatosis develops over years.

Iron Metabolism in Hereditary Hemochromatosis

MOLECULAR PATHOGENESIS: There are several different known forms of HH. In most, it is the *HFE* gene, on the short arm of chromosome 6, that is mutated. Mutations in other genes that control iron metabolism less commonly lead to iron overload and syndromes like hemochromatosis. A particular mutation (C282Y), when present in both alleles of the *HFE* gene, is responsible for HH in 90% of patients. A less common HFE mutation is H63D. Among Europeans, 10% are heterozygous for C282Y, and 1 of 200–400 is homozygous. Oddly, some homozygotes do not develop HH or iron overload, and clinically apparent hemochromatosis only occurs 1 in 400 of the general population. Rarer forms of hemochromatosis are caused by mutations in other genes that control hepcidin expression, such as TfR2 and hemojuvelin. Rarely, the hepcidin gene itself (*HAMP*) is mutated.

PATHOPHYSIOLOGY: At the center of HH is hepcidin. Mutations that decrease hepcidin production mimic a situation in which there is insufficient iron. Iron uptake by enterocytes thus increases (Fig. 20-41). As well, iron transit through enterocytes, and iron export from macrophages and hepatocytes, into the circulation is increased because hepcidin is not present to

mediate downregulation of the ferroportin exporter. The exporter thus operates unchecked.

The combination of enhanced iron absorption through the gut and increased export from storage sites overwhelms the Tf system and results in very high circulating free iron levels. Massive influx of iron into many cells ensues. In hepatocytes, this flood of free iron exceeds even the accelerated iron export (see above) that occurs in the absence of hepcidin-mediated inhibition of ferroportin. Hepatocytes thus accumulate iron.

As noted in Chapter 1, iron is a key factor in cell injury mediated by reactive oxygen species (ROS). Excess cellular iron probably renders HH patients more susceptible to oxidative injury. Serum iron levels in HH patients exceed twice the normal, with 100% saturation of Tf. Blood ferritin, which parallels the amount of stored iron, is greatly increased.

The causes of iron overload are summarized in Table 20-4.

 PATHOLOGY: In HH, large amounts of iron accumulate in parenchymal cells of a variety of organs and tissues.

LIVER: The liver is always affected in HH and has more than 0.5 g iron per 100 g wet weight in the late stages. It is enlarged and red-brown with micronodular cirrhosis. Hepatocytes and bile duct epithelium are filled with iron granules (Fig. 20-42). Excess cellular iron is mostly stored in lysosomes as ferric iron. Late in the disease, iron is conspicuous in Kupffer cells due to phagocytosis of necrotic hepatocytes. Within the fibrous septa, iron is prominent in bile ductules and macrophages. Eventually, as with other forms of micronodular cirrhosis, macronodular cirrhosis supervenes.

SKIN: In HH, the skin is pigmented, but iron deposits in the skin in only 1/2 of patients. Most patients have increased melanin in the basal melanocytes.

PANCREAS: Diabetes due to deposition of iron in the pancreas is common in HH. The organ is rust colored and

TABLE 20-4
CAUSES OF IRON OVERLOAD
Increased Iron Absorption
Hereditary hemochromatosis
HFE associated: C282Y and H63D homozygotes and C282/H63D heterozygotes
Hemochromatosis associated with mutations in transferrin receptor 2 (TfR2) and ferroportin
Juvenile hemochromatosis: mutations in hemojuvelin and hepcidin
Chronic liver disease (e.g., alcoholic liver disease)
Iron-loading anemias
Porphyria cutanea tarda
Dietary iron overload; excess medicinal iron
Parenteral Iron Overload
Multiple blood transfusions
Injectable medicinal iron

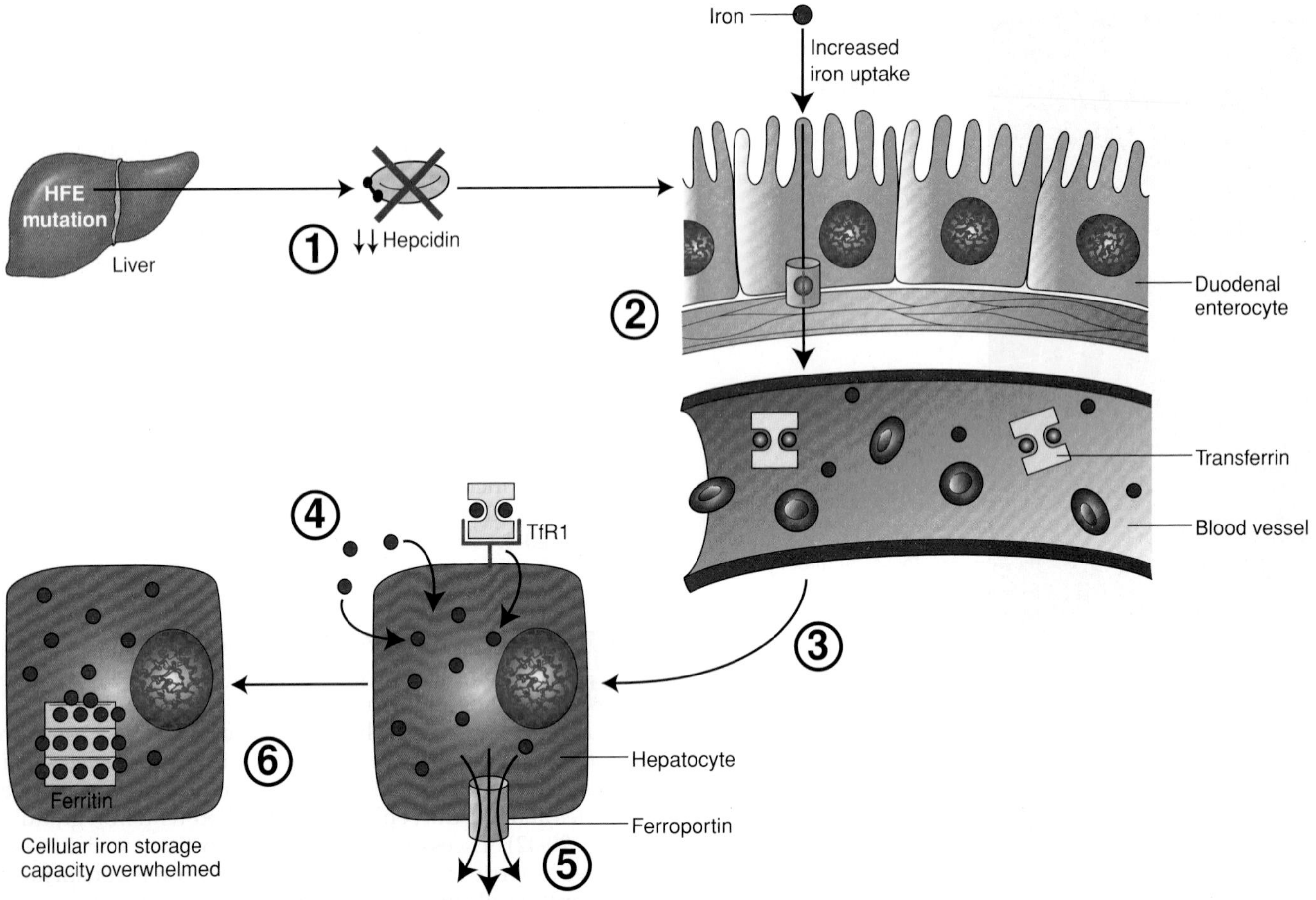

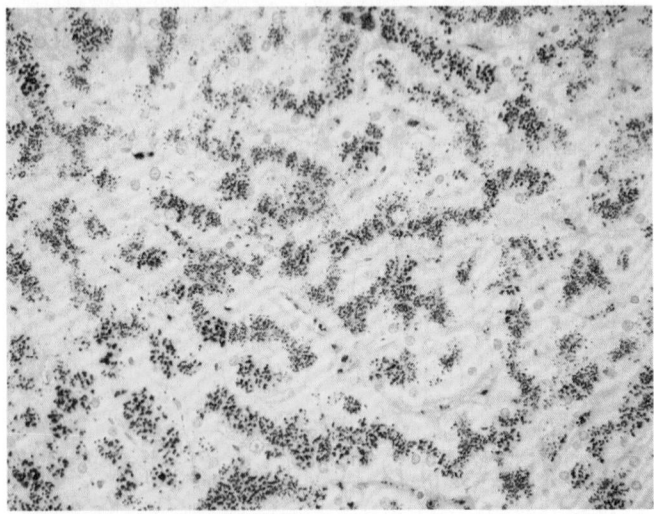

FIGURE 20-41. The fate of iron in the absence of hepcidin in hereditary hemochromatosis (HH). 1. The genetic defect in HH leads to decreased hepatic production of hepcidin. 2. As a consequence, when iron in the duodenal lumen enters enterocytes, its export through ferroportin is not regulated appropriately. The situation mimics that which occurs in iron deficiency (when hepcidin production is suppressed because of the need for increased iron uptake), even though there is abundant iron. Too much iron is absorbed and transported through the enterocytes into the blood. 3. Normally, iron is transported in the blood bound to Tf, and Tf is usually about 1/3 saturated with iron. In HH, not only is Tf iron-carrying capacity saturated (100%), but free iron (i.e., unbound to Tf) is also abundant in the blood. 4. Iron enters hepatocytes both as Tf-bound iron and as free iron. Tf-bound iron enters via the TfR1 pathway. Free iron enters via a different, poorly understood pathway. 5. Lacking inhibition by hepcidin, ferroportin export of iron is very active. 6. However, probably because of overwhelming entry of free iron into hepatocytes, iron storage and export capacities are overwhelmed. Therefore, the excess iron accumulates.

FIGURE 20-42. Hemochromatosis. Perl iron stain demonstrates marked iron (blue) in hepatocytes along the bile canaliculi.

fibrotic. Exocrine and endocrine cells have excess iron, and there is cell loss both in acini and islets of Langerhans. The combination of pigmented skin and glucose intolerance in HH is called **bronze diabetes**.

HEART: Congestive heart failure is a frequent cause of death in HH. Myocardial fibers contain iron pigment, more extensively in ventricles than in atria. Cardiac myocyte necrosis and resulting interstitial fibrosis are common.

ENDOCRINE SYSTEM: Many endocrine glands are affected in HH, including the pituitary, adrenal, thyroid and parathyroid glands. Except for the pituitary, in which release of gonadotropins is impaired, tissue damage does not occur in these organs. As a result, testicular atrophy is seen in 1/4 of male patients, even without iron deposition in the testes. Altered pituitary–gonadal axis function presents as loss of libido and amenorrhea in women, and impotence and sparse body hair in men.

JOINTS: About 1/2 of patients with HH show arthropathy, which is worst in the fingers and hands. HH arthritis affecting larger joints, like the knee, can be disabling.

CLINICAL FEATURES: HH generally becomes symptomatic in midlife. The liver disease usually progresses slowly, but 1/4 of untreated patients eventually die in hepatic coma or from gastrointestinal hemorrhage. Cirrhosis may lead to HCC; the 10-year cumulative chance of liver cancer may reach 30%.

Treatment of HH involves removal of iron from the body, most effectively by repeated phlebotomy. Weekly phlebotomies for 2–3 years can remove 20–40 g of iron, after which phlebotomies every 2–3 months maintain iron balance. In homozygotes without cirrhosis or diabetes, iron depletion allows a life expectancy identical to that of the general population. Without treatment, 10-year survival with HH is only 6%.

Secondary Iron Overload Occurs in People without HH Mutations

PATHOPHYSIOLOGY: Within certain limits, the amount of iron absorbed is a function of the amount ingested. For example, hemochromatosis is unlikely to develop in someone with a diet low in iron. Many patients (up to 40%) with secondary iron overload have a long history of alcohol abuse; it is thought that alcohol increases both iron storage and associated cell injury.

Iron accumulation among blacks of sub-Saharan Africa, commonly misnamed "Bantu siderosis," is an example of secondary iron overload. This disorder occurs because these populations consume large amounts of iron-containing alcoholic beverages. As "home-brewed" beverages (low alcohol, high iron) have been replaced by Western spirits (high alcohol, low iron), the incidence of siderosis has declined, whereas alcoholic cirrhosis has increased.

Massive iron overload occurs in patients with certain diseases with ineffective erythropoiesis, such as sickle cell anemia, thalassemia major and other anemias. The excess iron derives from hemolysis or transfused blood. Increased iron absorption also occurs despite Tf saturation. Multiple blood transfusions alone are generally insufficient to produce secondary iron overload, even in patients with hypoplastic anemia given many transfusions (250 mg iron/500 mL unit of blood). In these patients, iron is concentrated principally in mononuclear phagocytes, and cirrhosis is rare.

PATHOLOGY: In transfusion-related and other types of siderosis, there is uniform, initial iron deposition in Kupffer cells, eventually spilling over into hepatocytes. Cirrhosis associated with secondary iron overload shows varying degrees of iron accumulation, but hepatic iron deposition is generally less than that in HH and is often restricted to the periphery of the nodules.

A Footnote to Hepcidin-Regulated Iron Metabolism

The centrality of hepcidin to iron metabolism may have implications far beyond hereditary iron storage disorders. As mentioned above, in chronic renal failure, the inability of the kidneys to eliminate hepcidin may lead to its accumulation.

Excess hepcidin production, such as is stimulated by IL-6 in settings of chronic infection and inflammation, and in some malignancies, may also lead to excessively high levels of hepcidin.

In this setting, elevated hepcidin concentrations may severely restrict ferroportin function. This could impair iron absorption in the gut and lead to excessive iron retention in stores due to inadequate release from macrophages and hepatocytes. If hepcidin remains elevated for prolonged periods of time, iron deficiency anemia may develop. Thus, anemia in some chronic inflammatory diseases, such as Crohn disease and rheumatoid arthritis, or in some tumors, such as certain lymphomas, may be associated with anemia and high circulating hepcidin levels. Such anemias, although they show low blood iron levels, are not amenable to treatment with dietary iron, as high hepcidin levels impede enteric iron absorption.

HERITABLE DISORDERS ASSOCIATED WITH CIRRHOSIS

Wilson Disease Is an Inherited Disorder of Copper Metabolism

WD is an autosomal recessive disease in which excess copper is deposited in the liver and brain (Fig. 20-43). One in 150–180 people is a carrier, and 1 in 30,000 children develop clinical disease.

MOLECULAR PATHOGENESIS: Dietary copper intake usually exceeds the body's needs. The excess is excreted by the liver into the bile. Copper is normally bound to ceruloplasmin in hepatocytes and then secreted into the blood. The gene for WD, namely *ATP7B* on chromosome 13, codes for an ATP-dependent, transmembrane cation channel, which transports copper

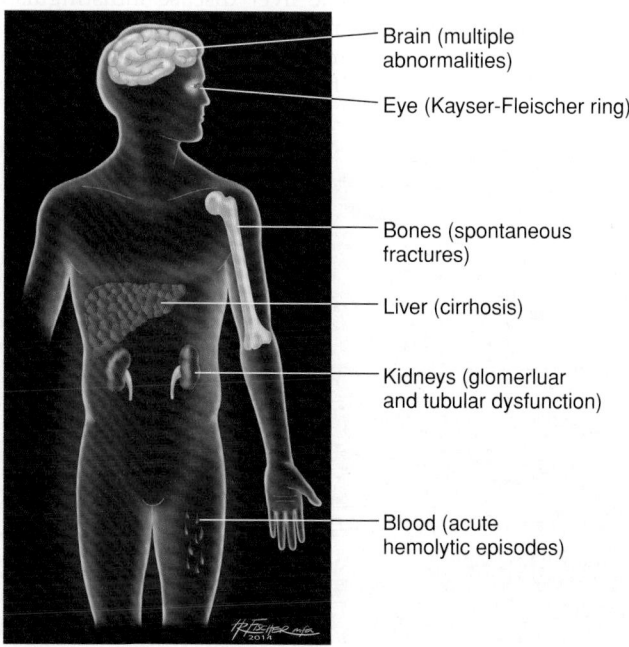

FIGURE 20-43. Wilson disease. The organs principally affected in Wilson disease.

within hepatocytes before it is excreted. *Mutations in ATP7B impair copper transport. Both biliary copper excretion and incorporation into ceruloplasmin are deficient.* Some 200 different mutations in the WD gene are known. In European and North American populations, a single mutation, H1069Q, accounts for 70% of WD, but this mutation is rare in India and Asia. Most patients are compound heterozygotes and possess two different mutant alleles.

In WD, serum ceruloplasmin levels are very low, a deficiency thought to be due to hepatic copper overload. Excess copper is toxic to hepatocytes, which die and release their copper into the blood, to then deposit in extrahepatic tissues. The central role of the liver in WD is underscored by the fact that liver transplantation is curative.

Just how excess copper injures cells is unclear. Copper can replace iron in the Fenton reaction to convert hydrogen peroxide into hydroxyl radicals (see Chapter 1).

 PATHOLOGY: *In WD, the liver progresses from mild to severe chronic hepatitis. Cirrhosis may develop rapidly, even in childhood (Fig. 20-44).* Features of severe hepatocyte injury and steatosis may be seen. Hepatocytes often contain Mallory bodies, and cholestasis is common. Initially, cirrhosis is micronodular, but in time, it becomes macronodular. Chemical measurement of liver copper in unfixed tissue from livers of patients with WD reveals more than 250 μg of copper per gram of dry weight.

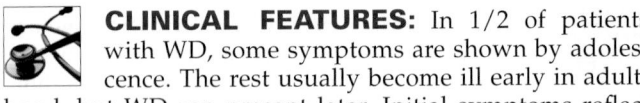 **CLINICAL FEATURES:** In 1/2 of patients with WD, some symptoms are shown by adolescence. The rest usually become ill early in adulthood, but WD can present later. Initial symptoms reflect chronic liver disease in about 1/2 of patients, 1/3 are first seen with neurologic complaints and about 1/10 have psychiatric illnesses.

LIVER: Liver-related symptoms are nonspecific at first and may progress to chronic liver disease indistinguishable from that of other forms of chronic hepatitis. Eventually, chronic hepatitis and cirrhosis result in jaundice, portal hypertension and hepatic failure. WD presents rarely as

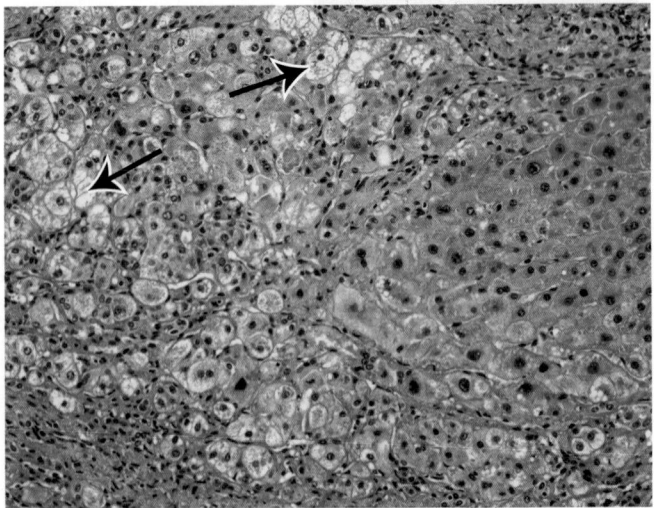

FIGURE 20-44. Wilson disease. The liver shows cirrhosis. There is severe hepatocyte injury with hydropic change (*arrows*).

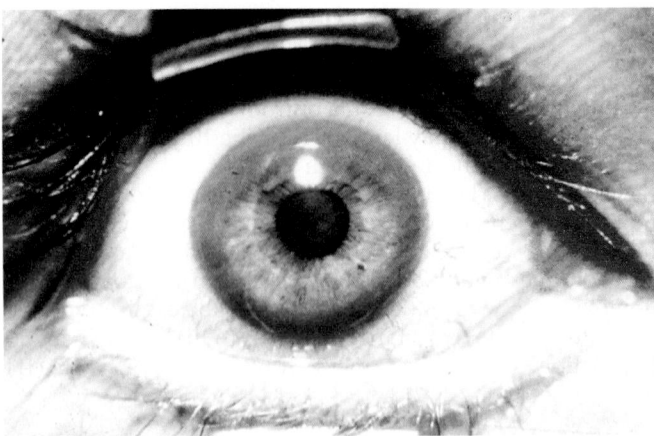

FIGURE 20-45. Kayser-Fleischer ring. The deposition of copper in the Descemet membrane is reflected in a peripheral brown color, which obstructs the view of the underlying iris.

acute liver failure. Unlike hemochromatosis, there is no increased risk of liver cancer.

BRAIN: Neurologic disease begins with mild incoordination and tremors. If untreated, dysarthria and dysphagia appear, then disabling dystonia and spasticity.

EYE: Ocular manifestations invariably accompany neurologic disease. **Kayser-Fleischer rings** are golden-brown, bilateral corneal discolorations around the edge of the iris that obscure its muscular pattern (Fig. 20-45). They represent copper deposited in Descemet membrane. In some patients, these rings are accompanied by "sunflower cataracts," which are green copper discs in the anterior capsule of the lens.

BONES: Skeletal lesions are common and include osteomalacia, osteoporosis, spontaneous fractures and various arthropathies.

KIDNEY: Renal glomerular and tubular dysfunction is common in WD and is manifested by proteinuria, lowered glomerular filtration, aminoaciduria and phosphaturia. These abnormalities are due to copper deposition in renal tubules.

BLOOD: Transient acute hemolytic episodes, presumably related to a sudden release of free copper from the liver, occur in 15% of patients with WD.

Treatment of WD prevents copper accumulation in tissues and removes copper already deposited. Copper-chelating agents, trientine and d-penicillamine, augment urinary copper excretion. Treatment often reverses central nervous system (CNS) dysfunction and liver disease. Presymptomatic patients are maintained with zinc, which blocks intestinal absorption of copper. Liver transplantation is curative for WD.

Cystic Fibrosis May Cause Biliary Obstruction

The cystic fibrosis transmembrane regulator (CFTR; see Chapter 6) is expressed in biliary epithelial cells. In cystic fibrosis (CF), tenacious mucus plugs obstruct intrahepatic biliary channels, sometimes as early as the first few weeks of life. Some infants die in hepatic failure. The most common hepatic lesion is focal or diffuse biliary cirrhosis. In patients who survive to adolescence, liver involvement becomes clinically symptomatic in 15%. Secondary biliary cirrhosis occurs in 10% of those who survive beyond 25 years. Liver disease accounts for 2.5% of deaths in CF, making it the most common nonpulmonary cause of death in this disease. UDCA therapy improves liver function, chemistry and histology, but not survival.

α₁-Antitrypsin Deficiency Leads to Cirrhosis

α₁-AT deficiency is an autosomal recessive disease that was initially described as a cause of emphysema (see Chapter 12). Later, cases of liver disease without lung involvement were reported. Diseases involving both organs are recognized. α₁-AT deficiency is the most common genetic liver disease and the most common genetic disease treated by liver transplantation. Although it occurs in 1 of 2000 live births, only 10%–15% of those affected develop liver disease.

 **MOLECULAR PATHOGENESIS:** α₁-AT is a serine protease inhibitor (serpin) made largely in the liver. It inactivates neutrophil elastase. Both pulmonary and hepatic disorders are due to inadequate α₁-AT secretion by the liver. The α₁-AT gene locus, *Pi*, has more than 75 known isoforms. PiZ is the most common (95% of cases) mutant α₁-AT protein, substituting a lysine for a glutamate at position 342. The mutant protein is retained within the hepatocyte ER, where it folds abnormally. Insoluble aggregates of the mutant protein cannot be exported and accumulate, thereby damaging the cell.

 PATHOLOGY: Hepatocytes in patients with α₁-AT deficiency contain faintly eosinophilic, PAS-positive cytoplasmic droplets (Fig. 20-46), which contain amorphous material within dilated ER cisternae. The disease often presents with chronic hepatitis, which terminates in cirrhosis.

α₁-AT deficiency may cause hepatitis in the newborn (see below). Micronodular cirrhosis develops by the age of 2–3 years in these children and may ultimately become macronodular.

 CLINICAL FEATURES: Liver disease in α₁-AT deficiency varies from rapidly fatal neonatal hepatitis to no hepatic dysfunction at all. *Of infants with*

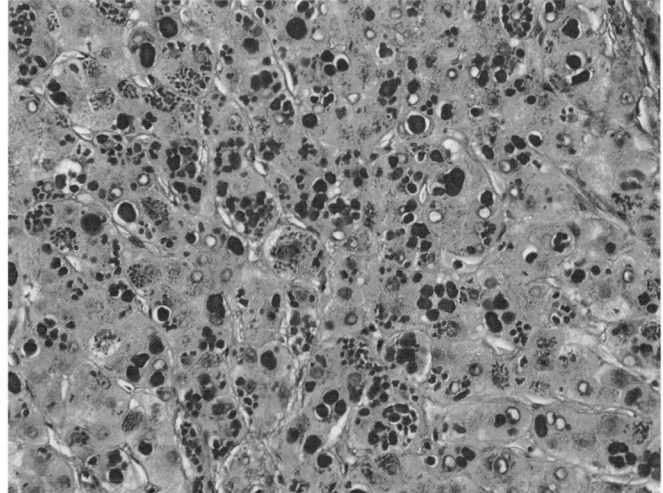

FIGURE 20-46. α₁-Antitrypsin deficiency. A cirrhotic liver stained by the periodic acid–Schiff (PAS) reaction with diastase digestion to remove glycogen reveals numerous cytoplasmic globules in the hepatocytes.

the ZZ genotype—who are susceptible to development of clinical disease—10% have neonatal cholestatic jaundice (conjugated hyperbilirubinemia). In fact, α₁-AT deficiency accounts for 30% of cases of neonatal conjugated hyperbilirubinemia. Most infants recover within 6 months, but 10%–20% develop permanent liver disease. Children with cirrhosis usually die before 10 years of age from hepatic failure or other complications of the disease. However, liver transplantation is curative.

Some patients are asymptomatic until early adulthood, when symptoms of cirrhosis may be the initial complaint. *Cirrhosis in α₁-AT deficiency is prone to a high incidence of HCC.*

Inborn Errors of Carbohydrate Metabolism Affect the Liver

Glycogen Storage Diseases

The biochemical basis of glycogen storage diseases is discussed in Chapter 6. *Only glycogenosis type IV (brancher deficiency, Andersen disease) is usually complicated by cirrhosis.* A slowly developing cirrhosis may also occur in glycogenosis type III (debrancher deficiency, Cori disease) but is not inevitable. Glycogenosis type I (glucose-6-phosphatase deficiency, von Gierke disease) is associated with striking hepatomegaly, and type II (acid-glucosidase deficiency, Pompe disease) features mild hepatomegaly. Neither type I nor type II is complicated by cirrhosis.

GLYCOGENOSIS TYPE I: Hepatocytes are distended by large amounts of glycogen, which appears pale in sections stained with hematoxylin and eosin and red with PAS. Fat accumulation varies from mild to severe, but fibrosis is usually absent. Hepatic adenomas often develop in adolescence but regress with dietary therapy.

GLYCOGENOSIS TYPE II: Infants with Pompe disease typically present with muscle weakness (myopathy), poor muscle tone (hypotonia), hepatomegaly, and cardiomegaly. The hepatocyte appearance with abundant glycogen is similar to glycogenosis type I.

GLYCOGENOSIS TYPE III: Infants with Cori disease show severe hepatomegaly, and the liver morphologically resembles that seen in type I. Fat is less conspicuous, but fibrosis is present and may progress to cirrhosis.

GLYCOGENOSIS TYPE IV: Infants present with severe hepatomegaly and usually succumb to cirrhosis by 4 years of age. Sharply circumscribed, PAS-positive inclusions are seen in enlarged hepatocytes. These inclusions are fibrillar and represent abnormal glycogen. Deposits of mutant glycogen are also found in the heart, skeletal muscle and brain. Liver transplantation is curative for glycogenosis type IV.

Galactosemia

Galactosemia is an autosomal recessive trait in which galactose-1-phosphate uridyl transferase is lacking. This enzyme catalyzes the second step in the conversion of galactose to glucose. Thus, galactose and its metabolites accumulate in the liver and other organs. Affected infants who are fed milk rapidly develop hepatosplenomegaly, jaundice and hypoglycemia. Cataracts and mental retardation are common.

Within 2 weeks of birth, the liver shows extensive and uniform fat accumulation and striking bile ductule proliferation in and around portal tracts. Cholestasis is often seen in canaliculi and bile ductules. Bile plugs fill many of these pseudoacini. At about 6 weeks of age, fibrosis begins to extend from portal tracts into the lobules and progresses to cirrhosis by 6 months. Institution of a galactose-free diet improves the disease and reverses many of the morphologic alterations.

Hereditary Fructose Intolerance

This disease is an autosomal recessive deficiency of fructose-1-phosphate aldolase. Fructose feeding early in infancy causes hepatomegaly, jaundice and ascites. However, if initial exposure to fructose occurs after 6 months, resulting disease is far milder; the only clinical impairment is spontaneous hypoglycemia. Infants with liver disease show many of the changes of neonatal hepatitis. Fat accumulation may be marked, resembling that in galactosemia. Progressive fibrosis culminates in cirrhosis.

Tyrosinemia

Tyrosinemia is an autosomal recessive trait in which tyrosine catabolism to fumarate and acetoacetate is impaired. The missing enzyme is fumarylacetoacetate hydrolase (FAH). More than 30 different mutations in the *FAH* gene are known. Succinyl acetone and succinyl acetoacetate accumulate. Both are potent electrophiles that can react with the sulfhydryl groups of glutathione and proteins, and damage the liver and kidneys.

Acute tyrosinemia begins within a few weeks or months of birth with hepatosplenomegaly. Liver failure and death are usual before 1 year of age. The liver is remarkably like that in galactosemia, and progression to cirrhosis is the rule.

Chronic tyrosinemia begins in the first year of life, manifesting as growth retardation, renal disease and hepatic failure. Death usually supervenes before 10 years of age. Tyrosinemia is treated by liver transplantation. *The incidence of HCC in untreated chronic tyrosinemia is extremely high.*

Miscellaneous Inherited Causes of Cirrhosis

Several inborn errors of metabolism are associated with cirrhosis, including storage diseases such as Gaucher disease, Niemann-Pick disease, mucopolysaccharidoses, neonatal adrenoleukodystrophy, Wolman disease and Zellweger syndrome.

INDIAN CHILDHOOD CIRRHOSIS

Indian childhood cirrhosis (ICC) is a fatal disorder mainly, but not only, affecting preschool children in India. ICC predominantly affects boys 1–4 years old. The liver shows micronodular cirrhosis and many Mallory bodies, as in alcoholic liver disease.

The etiology and pathogenesis of ICC are not well understood. Familial cases are reported, but no hereditary pattern is established. Interestingly, children with this disease have a marked excess of copper and copper-binding protein in the liver, but the significance of these findings remains obscure.

DRUG-INDUCED LIVER INJURY

Drug-induced liver injury can mimic nearly any type of liver disease, with severity ranging from asymptomatic elevations of transaminases to acute liver failure. *In fact, drugs are the most common cause of acute liver failure in the United States.* Chapter 1 includes a discussion of mechanisms by which toxins may produce liver necrosis. Chapter 4 reviews immune-mediated mechanisms of injury.

Drugs cause injury in either **predictable** or **unpredictable** patterns. The former refers to drugs that cause liver injury in a dose-dependent manner (e.g., carbon tetrachloride, the mushroom poison phalloidin, the analgesic acetaminophen). The latter reflects injury that can occur with low frequency, irrespective of dose and without obvious predisposition (**idiosyncratic reaction**).

The defining characteristics of predictable drug-induced hepatoxicity are:

- The agent, in sufficiently high doses, always produces liver cell damage.
- The extent of hepatic injury is dose dependent.
- The same lesions are seen in different animal species.
- Liver necrosis is zonal and often, but not always, centrilobular.
- The time between exposure and development of liver cell necrosis is short.

Most drug reactions are unpredictable and seem to represent idiosyncratic events. This type of hepatotoxicity occurs in people with metabolic or genetic predispositions. In them, injury usually reflects unusual sensitivity to a dose-related side effect. Thus, individuals may be predisposed to idiosyncratic reactions because their metabolic pathways differ from those of the general population (*metabolic idiosyncrasy*) or because they possess genetic variations in systems of biotransformation or detoxification of reactive metabolites. As well, some drugs or their metabolites may trigger immunologic reactions in the liver (autoimmune hepatitis).

There is no specific test to predict or diagnose drug-induced hepatotoxicity. A close history of medications, drugs and dietary supplements must be elicited from patients with elevated liver enzymes or jaundice. Other liver diseases must be ruled out (e.g., viral hepatitis, genetic disease, autoimmune hepatitis, alcoholic hepatitis). Liver biopsy is often of limited value in diagnosing drug injury, as histologic patterns of acute or chronic drug-induced liver disease overlap with non–drug-related diseases.

Histologic Patterns of Drug-Induced Liver Disease Are Diverse

Drug toxicities can span nearly the whole gamut of pathologies seen in non–drug-induced liver diseases. However, individual drugs usually have characteristic patterns of liver toxicity.

Zonal Hepatocellular Necrosis

Toxic doses of acetaminophen *predictably* cause centrilobular necrosis (Fig. 20-47A), but very high doses can cause panlobular necrosis (see Chapter 1). This zonal pattern probably reflects the greater activity of drug-metabolizing enzymes in the central zones. Classic agents that produce such injury are carbon tetrachloride and the toxin of the mushroom *Amanita phalloides.* In affected zones, hepatocytes show coagulative necrosis, hydropic swelling and variable small droplet fat. Inflammation is sparse. Patients either die in acute hepatic failure or recover without sequelae. *Acetaminophen-induced*

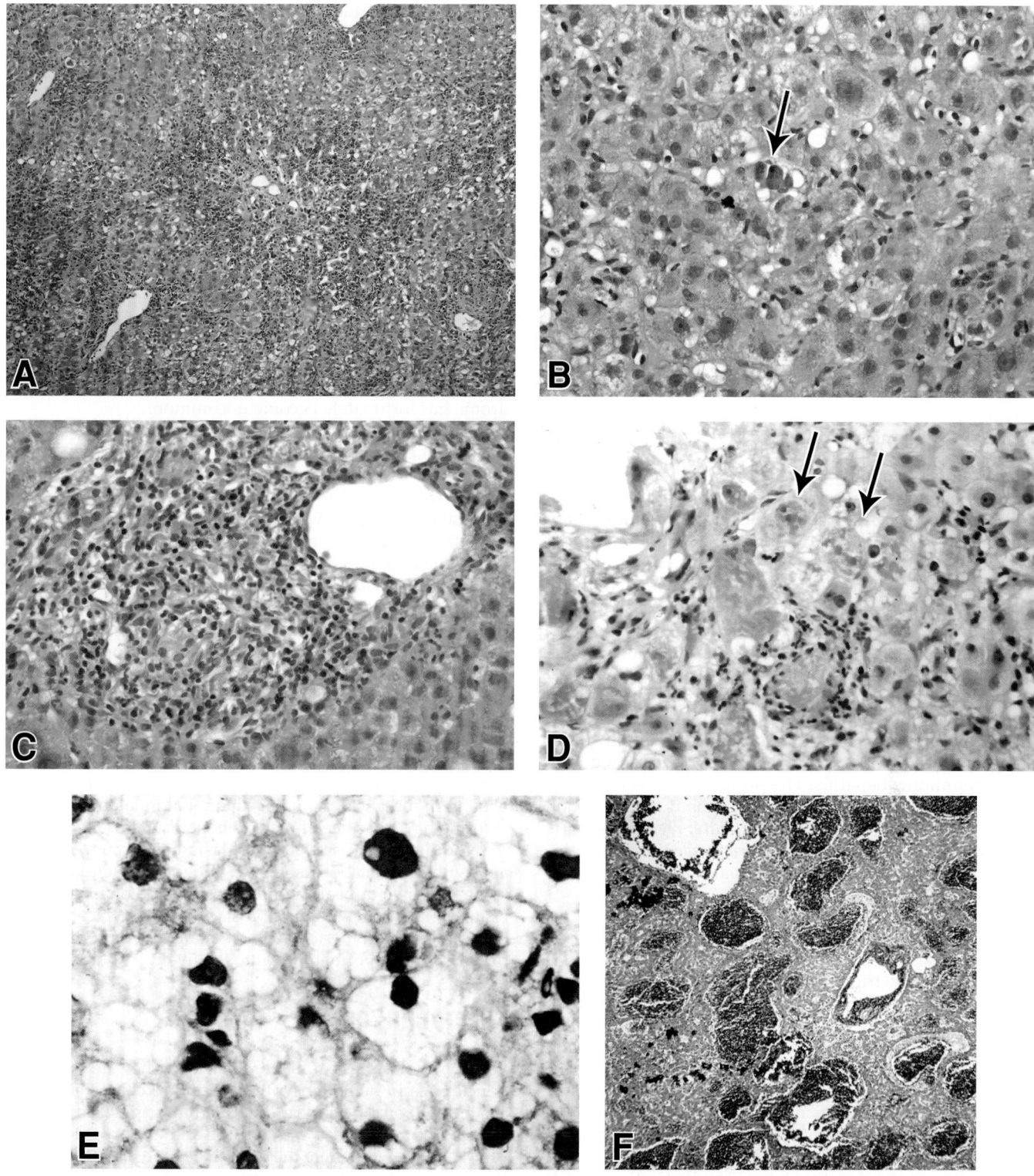

FIGURE 20-47. Drug-induced hepatotoxicity. A. Toxic centrilobular necrosis. This liver biopsy was from a 20-year-old man who attempted suicide with an overdose of acetaminophen. There is centrilobular hemorrhagic necrosis. Note that the surviving hepatocytes are markedly swollen. **B. Acute hepatitis.** The patient was started on isoniazid for treatment of tuberculosis. After 3 weeks, the aspartate aminotransferase (AST) and alanine aminotransferase (ALT) were elevated. The liver biopsy shows features of acute hepatitis including lobular disarray, inflammation, acidophilic bodies (*arrow*) and focal necrosis. **C. Eosinophilic portal inflammatory infiltrate.** A 33-year-old woman developed fatigue 2 weeks after initiating therapy with a nonsteroidal anti-inflammatory agent. The AST was 250 U/L. Portal tracts show expansion by acute and chronic inflammation with eosinophils. **D. Phospholipidosis.** Liver biopsy from a patient treated with amiodarone. The hepatocytes are swollen and display ample Mallory-Denk bodies (*arrows*). **E. Reye syndrome.** A liver biopsy specimen shows small-droplet fat in hepatocytes and centrally located nuclei. **F. Peliosis hepatis.** The patient was a 44-year-old weight lifter who used anabolic steroids. The liver contains numerous large, irregular, blood-filled spaces.

hepatotoxicity is the most common cause of acute liver failure in the United States and is frequently seen in suicidal gestures. Patients usually present soon after an ingestion.

Chronic exposure to some hepatotoxins that cause zonal necrosis (e.g., carbon tetrachloride) is not generally a problem: once acute toxic injury is recognized, reexposure to the offending agent is rare.

Cholestasis

Injury to intralobular and interlobular bile ducts is a common, unpredictable reaction to drugs. When it occurs, bile accumulates in hepatocytes and canaliculi. It is called *pure cholestasis* (Fig. 20-8) if there is no inflammation. Drugs that cause pure cholestasis include estrogens, androgens and several antibiotics (e.g., sulfamethoxazole). If cholestasis is accompanied by inflammation, the term **cholestatic hepatitis** is used.

Acute and Chronic Hepatitis

Inflammatory reactions are common in many *unpredictable* hepatotoxic drug reactions. All of the features of acute viral hepatitis can occur after exposure to a wide variety of drugs (e.g., isoniazid, antibiotics). The inflammation is a general response to cell injury and necrosis, such as in viral or autoimmune hepatitis (Fig. 20-47B). *The entire range of acute liver injury, from mild anicteric hepatitis to rapidly fatal massive hepatic necrosis, is encountered.* Typically, drug-induced hepatitis and liver enzyme elevations associated with it resolve when the offending drug is withdrawn. If exposure continues, chronic hepatitis and even cirrhosis may develop. Sometimes, inflammation may reflect **drug-induced autoimmune hepatitis** (e.g., nitrofurantoin) either as an immune response to the drug or by unmasking classical autoimmune hepatitis. The presence of eosinophils in the inflammatory infiltrate suggests such a drug reaction (Fig. 20-47C). *An inflammatory infiltrate, regardless of its composition, is not specific for drug-associated hepatotoxicity.* Granulomatous hepatitis is also a rare reaction to drugs.

Fatty Liver

Accumulation of triglycerides within hepatocytes (i.e., hepatic steatosis or fatty liver) generally occurs in a predictable fashion. Although there may be substantial overlap, two morphologic patterns are recognized: macrovesicular and microvesicular steatosis.

Macrovesicular Steatosis

In addition to its association with chronic ethanol ingestion, macrovesicular fat results from accidental exposure to direct hepatotoxins, such as carbon tetrachloride. Corticosteroids and some antimetabolites, such as methotrexate, may also cause macrovesicular steatosis. Fat per se does not injure hepatocytes (see above). A variant of toxic macrovesicular steatosis that resembles alcoholic hepatitis **(steatohepatitis)** occurs after administration of certain drugs (e.g., the antiarrhythmic agent amiodarone). Both hepatocytes and Kupffer cells are enlarged, with foamy cytoplasm that represents accumulation of **phospholipids**. Mallory bodies are abundant (Fig. 20-47D). Macrovesicular steatosis is itself clinically inconsequential.

Microvesicular Steatosis

Unlike macrovesicular steatosis, microvesicular fatty liver is often associated with severe, and sometimes fatal, liver disease. Small fat vacuoles are dispersed throughout the cytoplasm of hepatocytes, and the nucleus retains its central position (Fig. 20-47E). The microvesicular fat is important, not in and of itself but as a manifestation of metabolic severe injury to subcellular structures, mainly mitochondria.

REYE SYNDROME: This rare acute disease of children is characterized by microvesicular steatosis, hepatic failure and encephalopathy. Edema and fat accumulation are reported in the brain. Symptoms usually begin after a febrile illness, such as influenza or varicella infection, and may correlate with aspirin administration. However, in some cases, the doses of aspirin involved were far too low to cause liver injury, and Reye syndrome is more complex than simple aspirin toxicity. In any event, as the use of aspirin and the incidence of influenza has declined in children, Reye syndrome has fortunately become uncommon.

Vascular Lesions

Occlusion of hepatic veins **(Budd-Chiari syndrome; Fig. 20-18)** may follow use of oral contraceptives, perhaps because they induce hypercoagulability in some people.

Peliosis hepatis is a peculiar hepatic lesion with cystic, blood-filled cavities that are not lined by endothelial cells (Fig. 20-47F). Anabolic sex steroids, contraceptive steroids and the antiestrogen tamoxifen sometimes produce this lesion.

Mass Lesions and Altered Hepatic Morphology

Hepatocellular adenoma, induced by exogenous steroids (estrogens and anabolic steroids), and **hemangiosarcoma,** caused by intravenous administration of the radioactive contrast agent thorium dioxide (Thorotrast; see Chapter 8) dye (no longer used), are among the very few mass lesions caused by drugs. Chronic exposure to inorganic arsenic, usually in insecticides, and occupational inhalation of vinyl chloride have also been linked to hepatic angiosarcomas.

Nodular regenerative hyperplasia may occur after therapy with antimetabolites (e.g., 6-thioguanine) and azathioprine. The liver appears nodular, grossly and on microscopic examination, but without fibrosis. Patients typically present with portal hypertension as the architectural distortion impairs flow of portal blood into the liver.

THE PORPHYRIAS

Porphyrias may be acquired or inherited. They are caused by deficiencies in heme biosynthesis and are characterized by accumulation of porphyrin intermediates (see Chapter 20). Porphyrias are divided into hepatic and erythropoietic porphyrias, based on where the defective heme metabolism and the accumulation of porphyrins and their precursors occur. Genetic porphyrias are heterogeneous, usually with unique mutations in individual families.

Hepatic porphyrias are inherited as autosomal dominant traits and are often precipitated by administration of drugs, sex hormones, starvation, hepatitis C, HIV infection and alcohol. The liver shows variable steatosis, hemosiderosis, fibrosis and cirrhosis. Needle-shaped cytoplasmic inclusions may be present.

ACUTE INTERMITTENT PORPHYRIA: This is the most common genetic porphyria and reflects a deficiency of porphobilinogen deaminase activity in the liver. Only 10% of gene carriers show clinical symptoms, which generally affect young adults. Colicky abdominal pain and neuropsychiatric symptoms predominate.

PORPHYRIA CUTANEA TARDA: This chronic hepatic porphyria is the most frequent porphyria. It may be acquired or inherited as an autosomal dominant trait and is characterized by deficient uroporphyrinogen decarboxylase activity. Typical patients are of middle age or elderly, with cutaneous photosensitivity and liver disease with hepatic iron overload.

Other inherited porphyrias, termed **erythropoietic porphyrias** and **congenital erythropoietic porphyrias,** are caused by enzyme deficiencies in erythrocytes. They are characterized by cutaneous photosensitivity and occasionally liver disease.

VASCULAR DISORDERS

Congestive Heart Failure Is the Major Cause of Liver Congestion

Acute Passive Congestion

At autopsy, the liver is often acutely congested, presumably because of a terminal failing heart (see Chapter 7). On cut section, the liver is diffusely speckled with small red foci, which represent centrilobular zones with dilated and congested sinusoids and terminal venules. These changes are not clinically significant.

Chronic Passive Congestion

Chronic passive liver congestion occurs when congestive heart failure increases the back-pressure in the peripheral venous circulation, impeding venous outflow from the liver. Chronically congested livers are often small with an accentuated lobular pattern of alternating light and dark areas (Fig. 20-48A), called **nutmeg liver.** In severe cases, centrilobular terminal venules and adjacent sinusoids are greatly dilated and filled with blood (Fig. 20-48B). Liver cell plates in this zone are thinned by pressure atrophy.

If **right-sided heart failure** is severe and long-standing (e.g., tricuspid valvular disease or constrictive pericarditis), chronic passive congestion may progress to hepatic fibrosis (Fig. 20-48C). Delicate fibrous strands envelop terminal venules, and septa radiate from centrilobular zones. Fibrous septa may link adjacent central veins, producing a "reverse lobulation." Pressure atrophy of centrilobular hepatocytes is prominent. This is not "cardiac cirrhosis": complete septa and regenerative nodules, as are seen in true cirrhosis, are rarely encountered.

Chronic passive liver congestion rarely affects hepatic function. Infrequently, features of portal hypertension, such as splenomegaly and ascites, may develop.

Shock Results in Decreased Liver Perfusion

Shock from any cause may cause ischemic necrosis of centrilobular hepatocytes and hemorrhage. The centrilobular zone—that is, zone 3 (Fig. 20-2)—is farthest from the blood that originates in the portal tracts and thus is the area most vulnerable to ischemic insult.

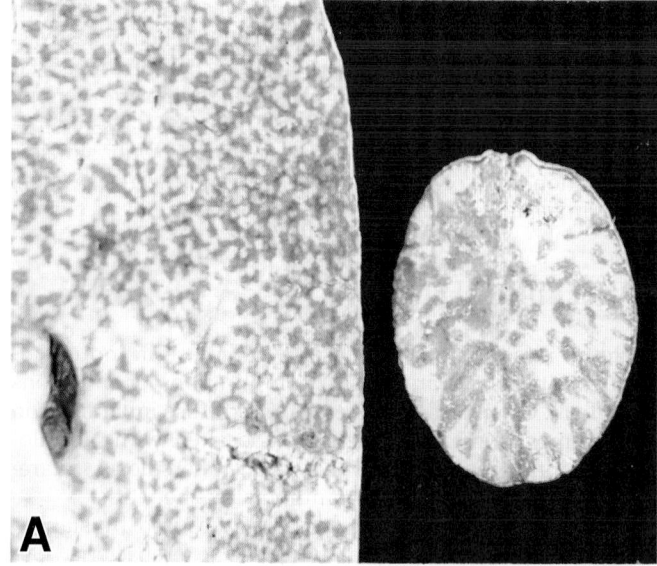

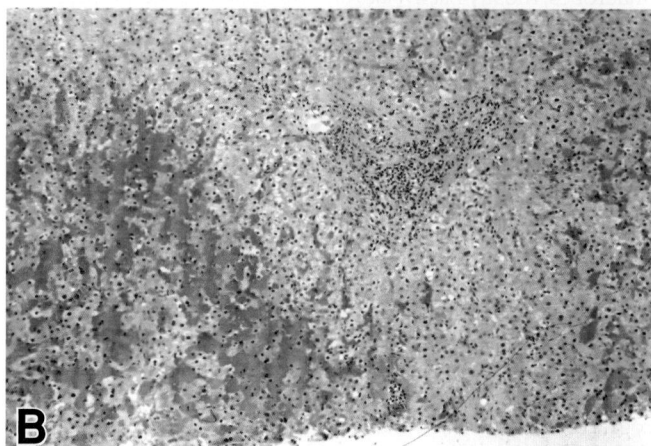

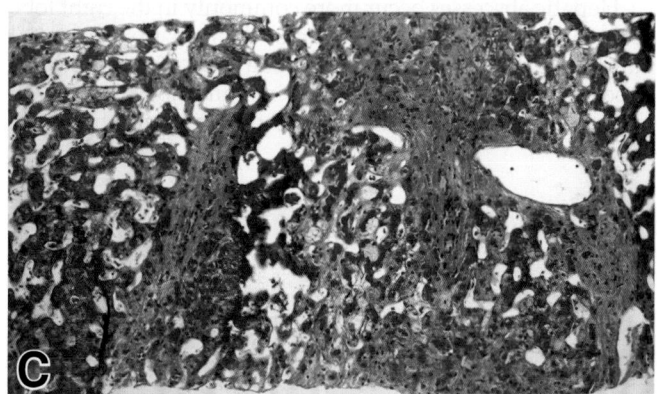

FIGURE 20-48. Chronic passive congestion of the liver. A. The surface of this fixed liver exhibits an accentuated lobular pattern, an appearance resembling that of a nutmeg (*right*). **B.** There is congestion and widening of central sinusoids. **C.** A Masson-trichrome stain shows fibrosis (*blue*) emanating out of central veins.

Liver Infarction Is Uncommon Because of Its Dual Blood Supply

Acute occlusion of the hepatic artery or its branches is rare and due to embolism, polyarteritis nodosa or accidental ligation during surgery. In such an event, irregular pale areas, often surrounded by a hyperemic zone, reflect the ischemic necrosis.

Acute occlusion of intrahepatic branches of the portal vein, generally in the setting of elevated hepatic venous pressure, classically produces a **Zahn infarct,** a dark-red, triangular area with its base at the liver surface. Only sinusoidal dilation and congestion are present, not necrosis. Thus, the term *infarct* is actually a misnomer.

BACTERIAL INFECTIONS

Bacterial infections rarely cause liver disease in industrialized countries and are mostly complications of infections elsewhere. Granulomas, abscesses and diffuse inflammation are the most common. Infections associated with granulomatous inflammation elsewhere (e.g., tuberculosis, tularemia, brucellosis) also cause granulomatous hepatitis.

Pyogenic liver abscesses are usually caused by staphylococci, streptococci and gram-negative enterobacteria. Gut anaerobes, mostly *Bacteroides* and microaerophilic streptococci, commonly cause liver abscesses. These resemble abscesses in other sites. Organisms reach the liver in arterial or portal blood, or via the biliary tract. In sepsis, the liver is seeded with organisms from distant sites through the arterial blood.

Pylephlebitic abscesses (Fig. 20-49) result from intra-abdominal suppuration, as in peritonitis or diverticulitis, with the organisms entering the liver in the portal blood. Pylephlebitis was once the most common cause of hepatic abscesses, but with antibiotic control of abdominal sepsis, this has become an uncommon route of infection.

Cholangitic abscesses in the liver are the most common form of hepatic abscess in Western countries today. Biliary obstruction from any cause is often complicated by bacterial infection of the biliary tree, called **ascending cholangitis.** Retrograde biliary dissemination of organisms (usually *E. coli*) then leads to cholangitic abscesses.

Hepatic abscesses occur more commonly in the right lobe of the liver. Diffuse inflammation of the liver from bacterial infection is distinctly uncommon today but may be encountered in septicemia, particularly in immunocompromised patients. The source of infection is unknown in about 1/2 of cases.

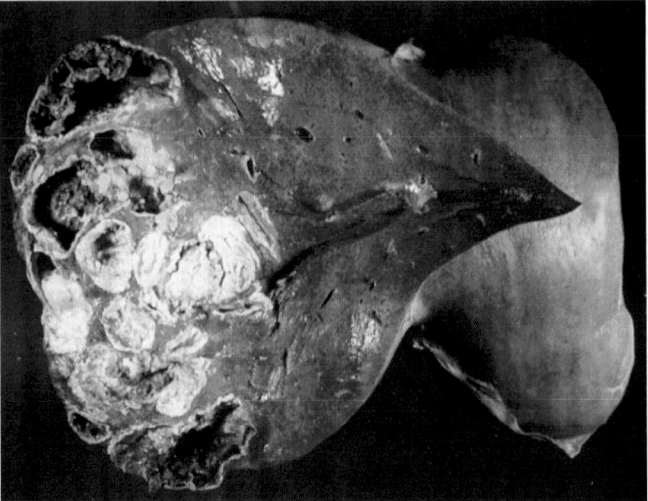

FIGURE 20-49. Pylephlebitic abscesses of the liver. The cut surface of the liver shows large, confluent, irregular abscess cavities.

 CLINICAL FEATURES: A patient with a hepatic abscess typically presents with high fever, rapid weight loss, right upper quadrant abdominal pain and hepatomegaly. Jaundice occurs in 1/4 of cases; serum alkaline phosphatase is almost always elevated. Solitary abscesses are treated with percutaneous or surgical drainage and antibiotics, but if abscesses are multiple, treatment is more problematic. The main complications are rupture and direct spread of infection. Pleuropulmonary fistulas, from rupture of an abscess through the diaphragm, and peritonitis, from leakage into the abdominal cavity, occur. Dissemination of organisms in the blood may promote septicemia and metastatic abscesses elsewhere in the body. The mortality from hepatic abscess, even when treated, is high, ranging from 40% to 80%.

PARASITIC INFESTATIONS

Parasitic disease in the liver is a serious public health problem worldwide but is rare in industrialized countries (for details, see Chapter 9). We summarize these diseases here.

Protozoal Diseases Frequently Involve the Liver

AMEBIASIS: In the United States, the carrier rate for *Entamoeba histolytica* in the colon is probably less than 5%, but rates approaching 35% are reported in homosexual men. Amebiasis of the liver, the most common extraintestinal site, causes amebic abscesses, which are multiple in about 1/2 of cases (Fig. 20-50). Amebic abscesses are 8–12 cm, well circumscribed and filled with thick, dark pasty material. Trophozoites are usually seen by the edge of the necrotic debris.

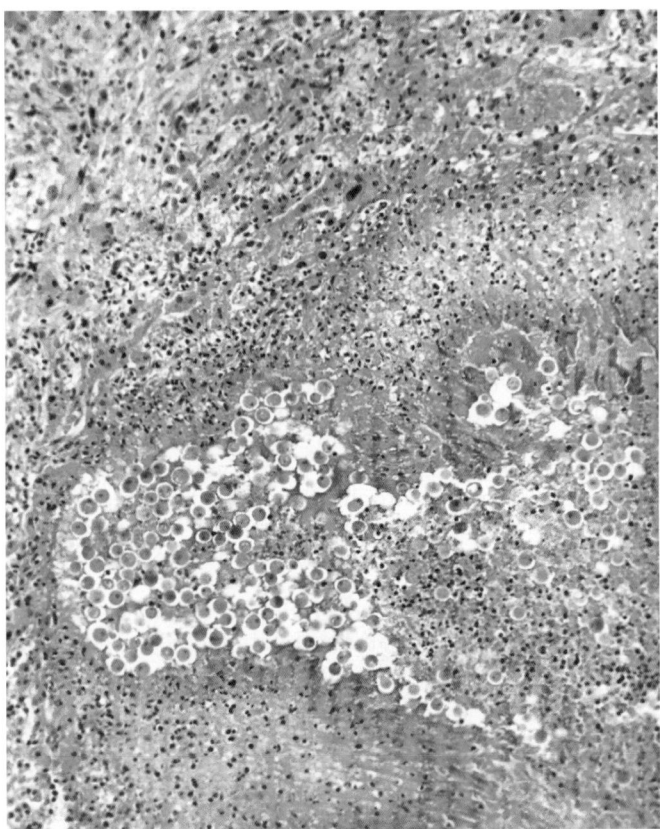

FIGURE 20-50. Amebic abscess of the liver. An amebic abscess shows fibroblastic proliferation surrounding the cavity and amebic trophozoites in the lumen.

The symptoms associated with amebic abscesses are similar to those of pyogenic abscesses. With appropriate treatment (tissue amebicides), the abscess may heal with only a residual scar remaining. Percutaneous or surgical drainage of large abscesses is important. If an amebic abscess continues to grow, it may rupture into the peritoneum and produce peritonitis, which carries a mortality rate as high as 40%. Amebae may also invade the blood and cause abscesses of the brain and lung.

MALARIA: Hepatic involvement in malaria is a common cause of hepatomegaly in endemic areas (see Chapter 9). It reflects Kupffer cell hypertrophy and hyperplasia owing to phagocytosis of debris from the rupture of parasitized erythrocytes. Liver function is intact.

VISCERAL LEISHMANIASIS (KALA-AZAR): As in malaria, chronic visceral leishmaniasis causes hyperplasia of mononuclear phagocytes in the liver. Unlike malaria, however, the Kupffer cells ingest the parasitic organisms themselves, which appear as **Donovan bodies.** Clinically, there is little evidence of hepatic dysfunction.

Helminthic Diseases Are Problems of Underdeveloped Areas

Diseases caused by helminths are described in Chapter 9, and **hepatic schistosomiasis** is discussed above in the context of portal hypertension.

ASCARIASIS: From the duodenum, *Ascaris lumbricoides* worms enter the biliary tree, where they may cause acute biliary colic. They lodge in intrahepatic biliary passages, where they disintegrate, liberating innumerable eggs that cause severe, suppurative cholangitis. Cholangitic abscesses may rupture into the peritoneum or pleural space. Spread into the hepatic or portal veins causes pylephlebitis, a highly dangerous complication. The liver is enlarged, with many irregular cavities full of foul-smelling material containing remnants of degenerated parasites.

LIVER FLUKES: The major parasitic flukes of the human liver are *Clonorchis sinensis* and *Fasciola hepatica.* Humans are the definitive host for *C. sinensis,* but sheep and cattle are the main reservoir of *F. hepatica.* Both parasites lodge in the intrahepatic biliary tree, where they provoke hyperplasia of the biliary epithelium, particularly severely in clonorchiasis (Fig. 20-51). In high-grade infestations with *C.*

sinensis, degenerated worms, parasite eggs and viscid mucus (secreted by metaplastic goblet cells in the biliary epithelium) accumulate and obstruct intrahepatic bile flow. This leads to intrahepatic pigment gallstones. Secondary infection of the bile with *E. coli* causes cholangitis and cholangitic abscesses, which are common causes of surgical emergencies in some Asian countries. **Biliary C. sinensis infestation is associated with the development of cholangiocarcinoma.**

ECHINOCOCCOSIS (CYSTIC HYDATID DISEASE): Hepatic infection with tapeworms of the genus *Echinococcus,* principally *E. granulosus,* is an important zoonosis affecting humans. Echinococcal cysts expand slowly and produce symptoms only after many years. The cysts behave as space-occupying lesions. Systemic manifestations reflect toxic or allergic reactions to the absorption of constituents of the organisms.

Leptospirosis Is an Accidental Human Infection from a Zoonosis

Leptospira spirochetes infect many animal species. Despite the large animal reservoir, fewer than 1/5 of patients who develop leptospirosis give a history of direct contact with animals. **Weil syndrome** is leptospirosis that is complicated by prolonged fever and jaundice, and, in severe cases, azotemia, hemorrhages and altered consciousness. Weil syndrome occurs in only 1%–6% of cases of leptospirosis. Liver pathology in fatal cases is nonspecific and includes focal necrosis, enlarged Kupffer cells and centrilobular cholestasis. The organisms are generally not demonstrable in the liver.

Liver Lesions May Occur in Congenital or Tertiary Syphilis

Congenital syphilis causes neonatal hepatitis, with diffuse fibrosis in portal tracts and around individual liver cells or groups of hepatocytes. In **tertiary syphilis,** hepatic gummas (i.e., focal lesions resembling granulomas) develop, which heal with dense scars. Retraction produces deep clefts and a gross pseudolobation of the liver called **hepar lobatum,** a condition that should not be confused with cirrhosis.

CHOLESTATIC SYNDROMES OF INFANCY

Diseases characterized by prolonged cholestasis and jaundice in infants either primarily affect hepatocytes or cause biliary obstruction.

Neonatal Hepatitis Entails Prolonged Cholestasis, Inflammation and Liver Cell Injury

 ETIOLOGIC FACTORS: In about 1/2 of cases of neonatal hepatitis, the cause is known (Table 20-5). About 30% are due to α_1-AT deficiency. Most other cases of known etiology are due to congenital infections with HBV, toxoplasma, rubella, cytomegalovirus, herpes simplex virus or other agents. Hepatic injury caused by metabolic defects (e.g., galactosemia or fructose intolerance) account for some cases, and neonatal hepatitis occurs occasionally in patients with Down syndrome and other chromosomal disorders. The other 1/2 of cases of neonatal hepatitis are unexplained.

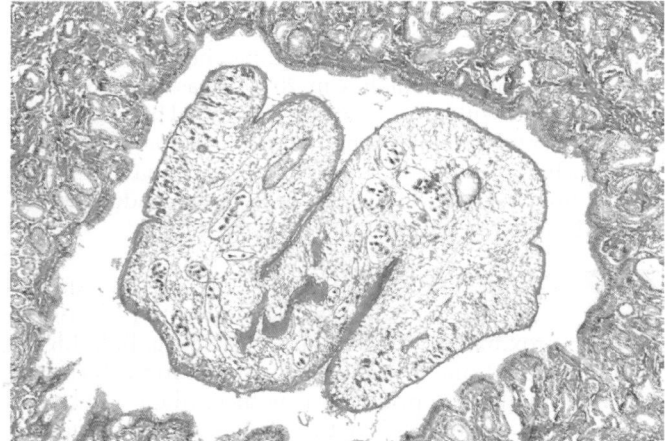

FIGURE 20-51. Infection of the liver by *Clonorchis sinensis.* The lumen of a bile duct contains an adult liver fluke, and the mucosa is hyperplastic.

TABLE 20-5
CAUSES OF NEONATAL HEPATITIS

Idiopathic

Idiopathic neonatal hepatitis

Prolonged intrahepatic cholestasis

    Arteriohepatic dysplasia (Alagille syndrome)

    Paucity of intrahepatic bile ducts not associated with specific syndromes

    Zellweger syndrome (cerebrohepatorenal syndrome)

    Byler disease

Mechanical Obstruction of the Intrahepatic Bile Ducts

Congenital hepatic fibrosis

Caroli disease (cystic dilation of intrahepatic ducts)

Metabolic Disorders

Defects of carbohydrate metabolism

    Galactosemia

    Hereditary fructose intolerance

    Glycogenosis type IV

Defects in lipid metabolism

    Gaucher disease

    Niemann-Pick disease

    Wolman disease

Tyrosinemia (defect of amino acid metabolism)

α_1-Antitrypsin deficiency

Cystic fibrosis

Parenteral nutrition

Hepatitis

Hepatitis B

TORCH agents (toxoplasmosis, "other," rubella, cytomegalovirus and herpes simplex)

Varicella

Syphilis

ECHO (enteric cytopathic human orphan) viruses

Neonatal sepsis

Chromosomal Abnormalities

Down syndrome

Trisomy 18

Extrahepatic Biliary Obstruction

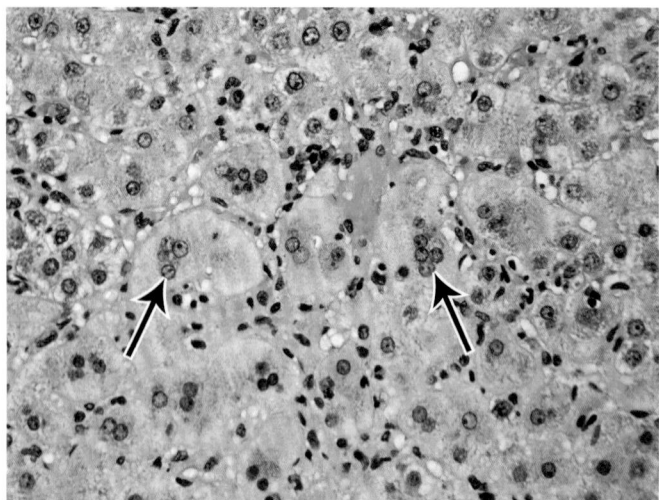

FIGURE 20-52. Neonatal hepatitis. Severe hepatocyte swelling (hydropic change), multinucleated giant hepatocytes (*arrows*), a mild chronic inflammatory infiltrate and fibrosis.

hepatocytes, acinar transformation of hepatocytes and acidophilic bodies are also typical of neonatal hepatitis. Extramedullary hematopoiesis is often conspicuous. Chronic inflammatory infiltrates are seen in the portal tracts as well as in the lobular parenchyma. Pericellular fibrosis around degenerating hepatocytes, singly or in groups, is common, and fibrous tissue septa extend from the portal tracts.

Part of the Biliary Tree Has No Lumen in Biliary Atresia

Extra- and intrahepatic biliary atresias may resemble neonatal hepatitis pathologically.

Extrahepatic Biliary Atresia

EHBA is a cholestatic disease in which inflammation obliterates the lumen of all or part of the biliary tree outside the liver, in the absence of calculi, tumor or rupture. EHBA is rare. Its estimated incidence is 1 in 5000–19,000 live births, with higher frequency being in East Asia. Biliary atresia is the most common indication for liver transplantation in children. EHBA is thought to represent the end result of heterogeneous conditions during gestational and perinatal development. Other organs, including the heart, intestine and spleen, show anomalies in 20% of cases. EHBA may occur together with known causes of neonatal hepatitis, such as a number of viral infections and chromosomal abnormalities (e.g., trisomy 18 and 21). Cholangiograms in EHBA show no bile flow into the duodenum or liver, depending on the site of the affected segment of the biliary tract.

 PATHOLOGY: The characteristic lesion of neonatal hepatitis is giant cell transformation of hepatocytes, hence the older term **giant cell hepatitis** (Fig. 20-52). These giant cells may contain up to 40 nuclei and may appear detached from other cells in the liver plate. Their pale, distended cytoplasm contains large amounts of glycogen and iron. Numbers of these cells decline with time, and they are rare in children older than 1 year. Bile pigment is prominent within canaliculi and hepatocytes. Ballooned

 PATHOLOGY: EHBA may involve all extrahepatic bile ducts or may be limited to parts of the proximal or distal biliary tree. The gallbladder is often atretic. At one extreme, acute and chronic periluminal inflammation is prominent, with epithelial necrosis, and cellular debris within the obstructed or narrowed lumen. At the other extreme, the original lumen is completely replaced by mature connective tissue, and little or no inflammation is seen. Histologically, cholestasis and periportal bile ductular proliferation in the liver are evident. Some cases have multinucleated giant hepatocytes, like those in neonatal hepatitis. Although the intrahepatic bile ducts may initially appear normal, they are gradually obliterated with the persistence of cholestasis. Eventually, secondary biliary cirrhosis supervenes.

Intrahepatic Biliary Atresia

In intrahepatic biliary atresia, there are few bile ducts within the liver. This occurs under three circumstances:

- In association with known causes of neonatal hepatitis (e.g., α_1-AT deficiency, various chromosomal anomalies and metabolic derangements).
- **Alagille syndrome** (syndromic bile duct paucity), an autosomal dominant disease, also characterized by congenital abnormalities of the heart, eye, skeleton, kidneys and CNS. This syndrome involves mutations in the Notch signaling pathway. Affected patients show five major features: chronic cholestasis, peripheral pulmonary artery stenosis, butterfly-like vertebral arch, hypertelic facies and eye abnormality known as posterior embryotoxon. The liver pathology is characterized by the absence of bile ducts in portal tracts.
- Unassociated with other conditions (idiopathic).

Neonatal hepatitis, intrahepatic biliary atresia, EHBA and possibly choledochal cyst all probably result from infantile obstructive cholangiopathy, a common inflammatory process.

 PATHOLOGY: In intrahepatic biliary atresia, there are very few bile ducts in the liver. Giant cell transformation, cholestasis and bile ductular proliferation are common; cirrhosis is not.

 CLINICAL FEATURES: Most patients with uncomplicated neonatal hepatitis recover without sequelae, but if it is associated with intrahepatic biliary atresia, the prognosis is poor. Many such children develop biliary cirrhosis. By contrast, the outlook in Alagille syndrome is good. If uncorrected, EHBA invariably leads to progressive secondary biliary cirrhosis and death. Surgical correction may be curative in some anatomically favorable cases, but transplantation is the best treatment for both extra- and intrahepatic biliary atresia.

BENIGN TUMORS AND TUMOR-LIKE LESIONS

Liver Adenomas Are Benign Tumors That Occur Mainly in Women

Once rare, these tumors became more common with oral contraceptive use. Lower-dose estrogen and progesterone combinations have reduced the incidence of liver adenomas.

 PATHOLOGY: Hepatocellular adenomas are usually solitary, sharply demarcated masses measuring up to 40 cm and weighing 3 kg (Fig. 20-53A). Multiple smaller adenomas are present in 1/4 of cases. If a liver has more than 10 adenomas, it is diagnosed as hepatocellular adenomatosis. These tumors are encapsulated and paler than nearby liver parenchyma. *The neoplastic hepatocytes resemble normal hepatocytes but are not arrayed in a lobular architecture.* Portal tracts and central venules are absent (Fig. 20-53B). The cells of adenomas may be very large and eosinophilic, or filled with glycogen or fat, which makes the cytoplasm appear clear or vacuolated. The presence of small arteries within the parenchyma suggests an adenoma as opposed to normal liver.

 CLINICAL FEATURES: In about 1/3 of patients with hepatic adenomas (particularly pregnant women who have used oral contraceptives), these tumors bleed into the peritoneal cavity and require immediate surgery. Even large adenomas may disappear if oral contraceptives are discontinued. Occasional liver adenomas have been reported in men who use anabolic steroids.

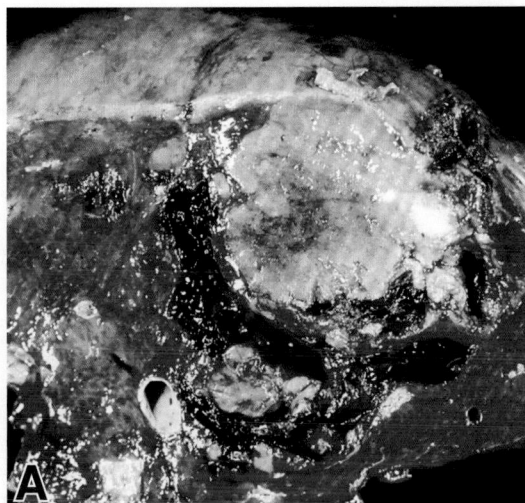
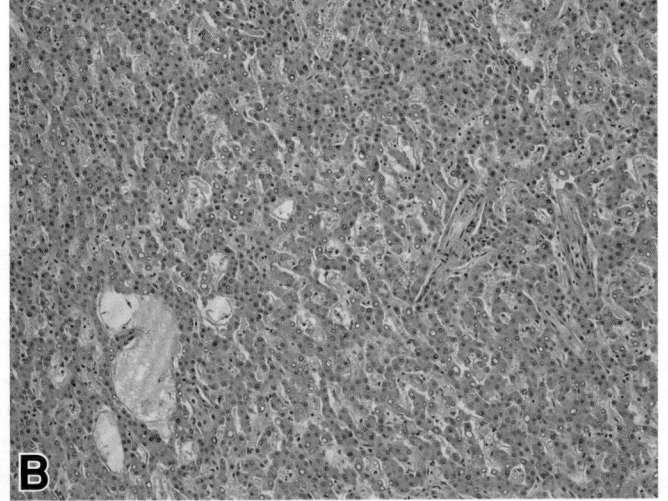

FIGURE 20-53. Hepatocellular adenoma. A. A surgically resected portion of liver shows a tan, lobulated mass beneath the liver capsule. The tumor has ruptured, resulting in intraparenchymal and intraperitoneal hemorrhage. The patient was a woman who had taken birth control pills for a number of years and presented with sudden intraperitoneal bleeding. **B.** The adenomatous hepatocytes do not differ from normal hepatocytes and are arranged without discernible lobular architecture. Note the absence of portal tracts.

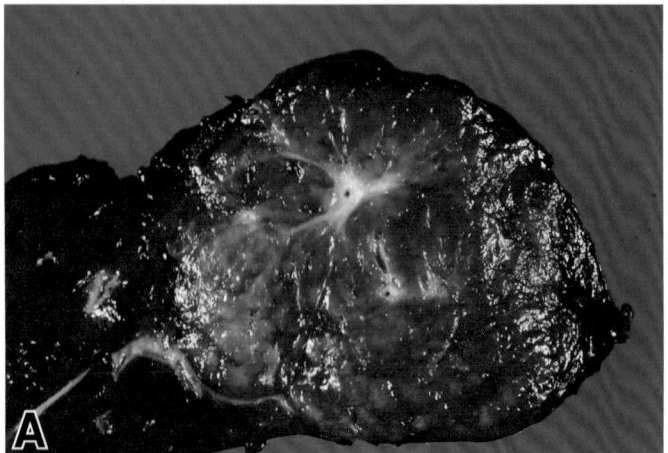
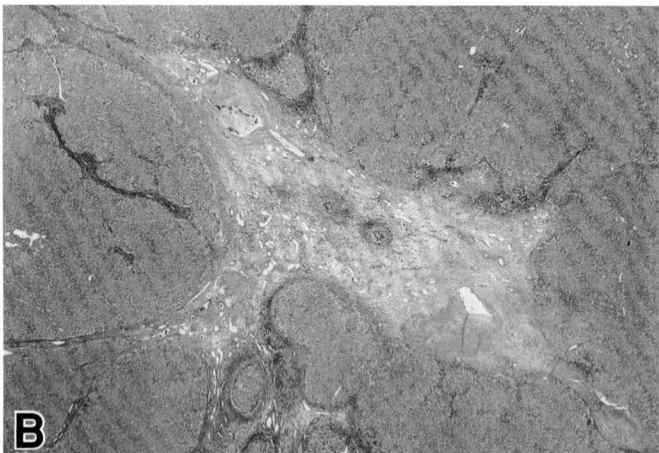

FIGURE 20-54. Focal nodular hyperplasia. A. A resected mass shows nodules with central scarring. **B.** This surgically resected mass from the liver shows a vascular central scar and irregular fibrous septa dissecting hepatic parenchyma, accounting for the resemblance to cirrhosis.

Focal Nodular Hyperplasia Resembles Cirrhosis

Focal nodular hyperplasia (FNH) is characterized by multiple fibrous septa and regenerative nodules (Fig. 20-54A). It measures up to 15 cm and weighs as much as 700 g. On occasion, FNH protrudes from the surface of the liver, and it may even be pedunculated. The cut surface has a central scar from which fibrous septa radiate. Hepatocytic nodules are circumscribed by fibrous septa (Fig. 20-54B), with many tortuous bile ductules and mononuclear inflammatory cells. Lobular architecture is absent within nodules. Septa contain large dystrophic arteries and veins, but little hemorrhage. These abnormal vessels suggest that FNH forms as a result of localized vascular malformation.

FNH occurs in both sexes and at all ages. It is not a neoplasm, is not associated with use of oral contraceptives, and rarely bleeds.

Nodular Regenerative Hyperplasia Causes Portal Hypertension

Nodular regenerative hyperplasia is also called *nodular transformation of the liver* or *partial nodular transformation*. It is neither neoplastic nor preneoplastic and is characterized by small, hyperplastic nodules without fibrosis in an otherwise normal liver. The lesion may be partial and located predominantly in the perihilar region, or it may be diffuse throughout the liver. Nodules are composed of liver cells in plates two and three cells thick, compressing the surrounding parenchyma.

Nodular regenerative hyperplasia is associated with portal hypertension and was once called **noncirrhotic portal hypertension**. Its etiology is unknown, but it has been associated with use of oral contraceptives or anabolic steroids, extrahepatic infections, tumors and chronic inflammatory and autoimmune diseases.

Hemangiomas Are the Most Common Tumors of the Liver

Benign hemangiomas in the liver occur at all ages and in both sexes. They are common, being present in up to 7% of autopsy livers (Fig. 20-55). They are normally small and asymptomatic, although larger tumors may cause abdominal symptoms and even hemorrhage into the peritoneum. Grossly, hemangiomas are usually solitary and under 5 cm, but multiple hemangiomas and giant forms (>15 cm) have been described. They resemble cavernous hemangiomas found elsewhere (see Chapter 10).

Cystic Disease of the Liver Represents a Spectrum of Lesions

BILE DUCT MICROHAMARTOMAS: These clinically inapparent lesions (also called *von Meyenburg complexes*) have anomalous, small cystic bile ducts in a fibrous stroma. They are usually multiple and vary from pinpoint grayish white foci to nodules up to 1 cm. Cysts are lined by bile duct epithelium and may have inspissated bile (Fig. 20-56).

SOLITARY AND MULTIPLE SIMPLE CYSTS: Simple liver cysts are lined by cuboidal to columnar epithelium and may be associated with adult polycystic kidney disease (see Chapter 16). They may be seen in livers with von Meyenburg complexes.

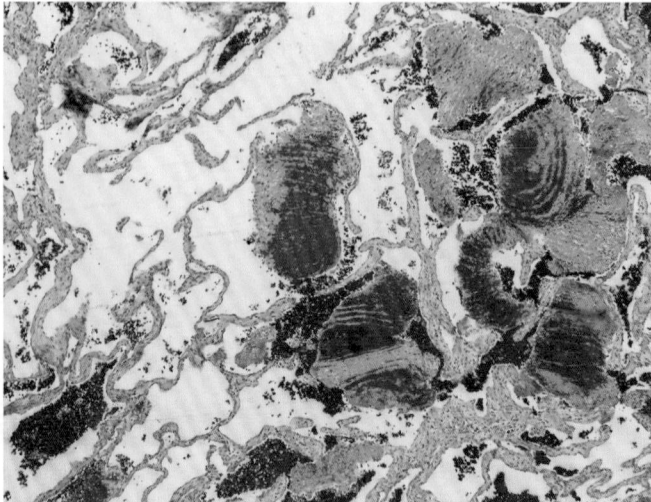

FIGURE 20-55. Cavernous hemangioma. A benign vascular tumor composed of blood-filled cavernous spaces.

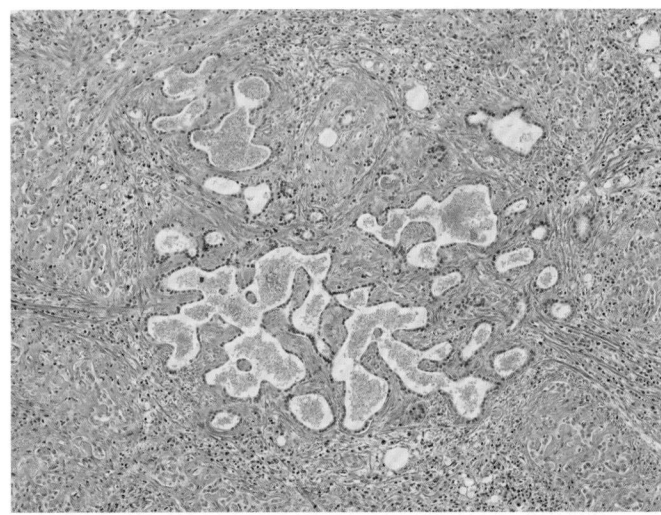

FIGURE 20-56. Bile duct microhamartoma (von Meyenburg complex). A photomicrograph of bile duct microhamartoma composed of cystically dilated spaces lined by a single layer of duct epithelium and containing inspissated bile.

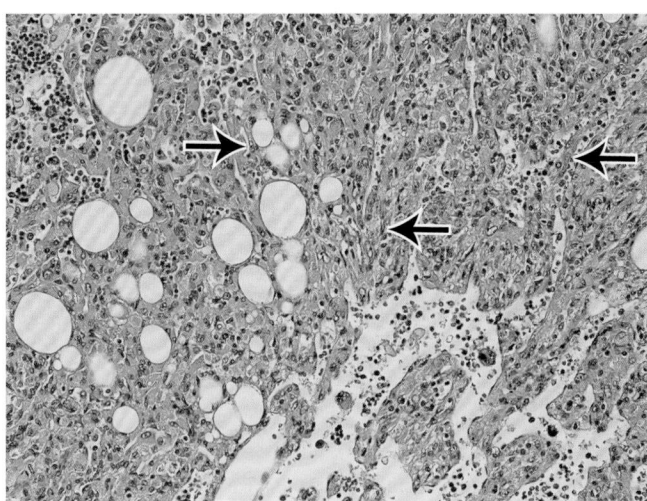

FIGURE 20-58. Angiomyolipoma. An angiomyolipoma composed of mixtures of epithelioid and spindle-shaped smooth muscle (*arrows*), vascular spaces and round fat cells.

CONGENITAL HEPATIC FIBROSIS: This recessively inherited disorder is marked by enlarged portal tracts with extensive fibrosis and many well-formed bile ductules (Fig. 20-57). It is seen mainly in children and adolescents. Bile ducts may be so dilated that they resemble microcysts, but they still communicate with the biliary system. Regenerative nodules are absent, distinguishing this condition from cirrhosis. The origin of the lesion is unknown. The main complication of congenital hepatic fibrosis is severe portal hypertension with recurrent bleeding from esophageal varices. **Infantile polycystic disease** of the liver resembles congenital hepatic fibrosis and is also inherited as an autosomal recessive trait.

Angiomyolipoma Is a Benign Tumor of Stromal Elements

Angiomyolipoma is a rare tumor composed of varying proportions of blood vessels, smooth muscle and mature fatty tissue (Fig. 20-58). It is derived from perivascular epithelial cells (PECs) and thus belongs to a group of tumors usually associated with tuberous sclerosis, referred as PEC-omas. Hepatic angiomyolipomas resemble the more common angiomyolipoma of the kidney (see Chapter 16).

Infantile Hemangioendothelioma Is a Type of Hemangioma That Occurs in Infants

Infantile hemangioendothelioma is a benign vascular tumor of intercommunicating vascular channels lined by a single layer of plump endothelial cells in a fibrous stroma (Fig. 20-59). It is mostly found in infants, usually females. Spontaneous involution is common. A large tumor may cause high-output cardiac or liver failure.

Mesenchymal Hamartoma Is a Developmental Malformation

Mesenchymal hamartoma is a benign liver tumor formed as a developmental malformation of liver mesenchyme. It

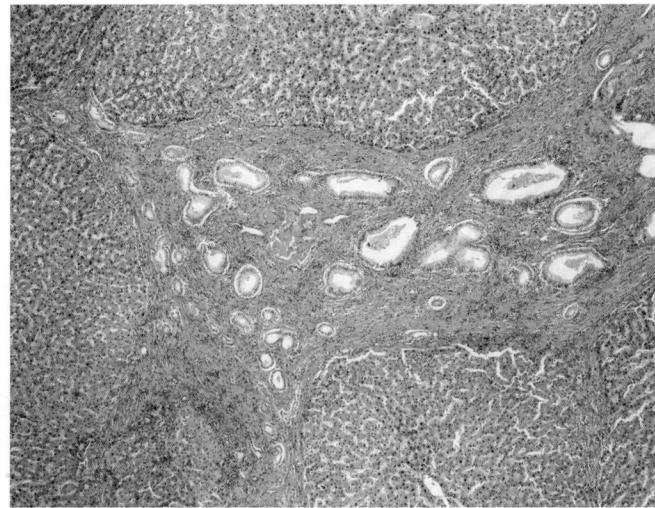

FIGURE 20-57. Congenital hepatic fibrosis. Enlarged and fibrotic portal tract containing ductal plate remnant microcysts.

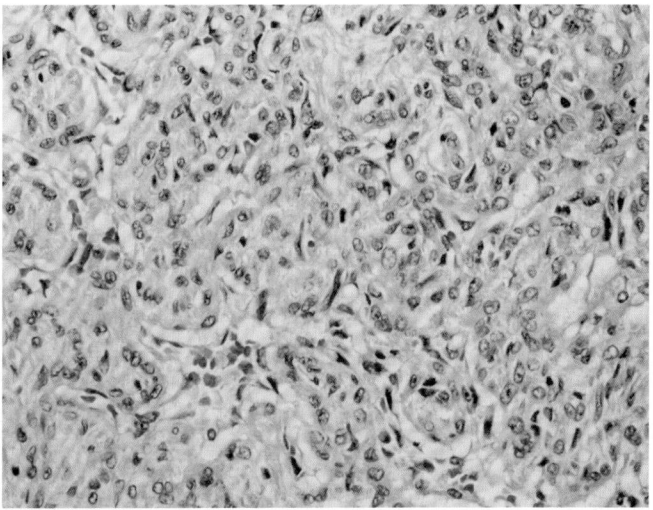

FIGURE 20-59. Infantile hemangioendothelioma. Plump endothelial cells lining anastomosing slit-like vascular spaces.

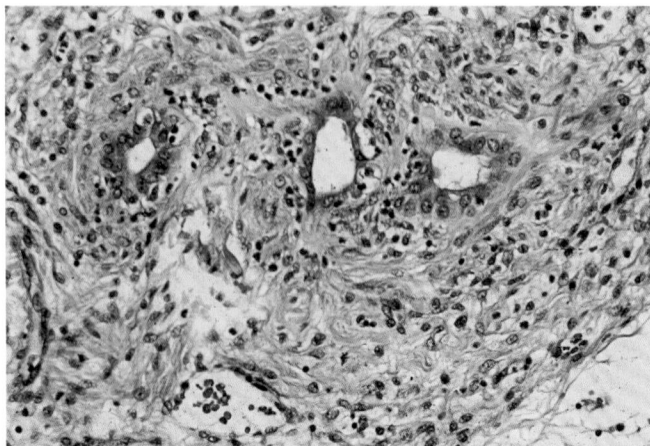

FIGURE 20-60. **Mesenchymal hamartoma.** Bile ducts in loose mesenchymal tissue stroma.

shows large, serous fluid cysts surrounded by loose mesenchyme containing a mixture of bile ducts, hepatocyte cords and clusters of vessels (Fig. 20-60). The mesenchymal tissue consists of scattered stellate-shaped cells in a loose matrix. Complete surgical excision is curative.

MALIGNANT TUMORS OF THE LIVER

Hepatocellular Carcinoma Is a Malignant Tumor of Hepatocytes

 **EPIDEMIOLOGY:** HCC is probably the most common human cancer. It occurs all over the world but shows a striking geographical variability. In Western industrialized countries, HCC is uncommon, but its incidence has nearly doubled in the past 20 years, mostly in patients with chronic hepatitis C. In sub-Saharan Africa, Southeast Asia and Japan, HCC may occur up to 50 times more often. For example, in Mozambique, which has the highest incidence in the world, 2/3 of all cancers in men and 1/3 in women are HCC.

 PATHOPHYSIOLOGY:
HEPATITIS B: More than 85% of cases of HCC occur in countries with a high prevalence of chronic HBV infection. Most patients have had chronic hepatitis B for years, often after perinatal transmission from an infected mother to her newborn child. Persistent HBV infection is very dangerous, with up to 200-fold increased risk for HCC. Of people with chronic hepatitis B acquired at or near birth, 1/4 will ultimately develop HCC. Risk of this cancer in men who are positive for HBsAg and HBeAg is about four times as great as in those only positive for HBsAg. Most (>80%) cases of HCC associated with HBV infection occur in patients with cirrhosis.

Cirrhosis has been blamed for the development of HCC in HBV-infected livers, but many HBV-associated HCCs occur in patients without cirrhosis. It is likely that integration of the HBV genome into cell DNA and expression of HBV genes are the key factors. Thus, the *X* gene of HBV encodes a viral protein (HBxAg) that inactivates tumor suppressor proteins and transactivates certain oncogenes.

HEPATITIS C: HCV is less common than HBV worldwide, but most cases of HCC in Europe, North America and Japan are associated with hepatitis C. In the United States, HCV infection is present in about 50% of HCC. As with HCC in hepatitis B, most patients with HCV who develop HCC have underlying cirrhosis, and the cumulative occurrence of HCC in HCV-induced cirrhosis is as high as 70% after 15 years.

Coinfection with HBV and HCV increases the risk of liver cancer threefold, relative to infection with either virus alone. Carcinogenesis by HCV is poorly understood, but interactions between virus proteins and cellular constituents is likely involved.

OTHER CAUSES OF HEPATOCELLULAR CARCINOMA: Alcoholic cirrhosis predisposes to HCC, but the risk is not large, and the mechanism is unknown. Because many alcoholics are infected with HBV and HCV, the role of alcohol alone in HCC is difficult to determine. Alcoholics with chronic hepatitis C have double the risk for HCC compared with HCV infection alone.

Hemochromatosis and α_1**-AT deficiency** carry a substantial risk of HCC: about 10% of patients with hemochromatosis may be expected to develop the tumor. On the other hand, HCC is not increased in patients with "autoimmune" chronic hepatitis and cirrhosis, WD or PBC. *As with HCC in patients with chronic hepatitis B without cirrhosis, this suggests that cirrhosis itself is not sufficient to cause liver cancer but that it may magnify HCC risk due to other etiologies.*

Aflatoxin B_1 is a fungal contaminant of many foods, mostly in less developed countries. It causes HCC in a number of animal species. The incidence of liver cancer in humans correlates roughly with dietary content of aflatoxin. The presence of urinary aflatoxin B_1 metabolites is associated with a 3-fold increased risk of HCC. Aflatoxin and HBV infection are synergistic; combined exposure increases the risk of HCC 60-fold.

Mutations in the *TP53* gene are present in 1/2 of DNA samples from HCCs occurring in areas endemic for aflatoxin. Most of these mutations are G-to-T substitutions at codon 249, a change that is produced experimentally by aflatoxin B_1.

PATHOLOGY: HCCs are solitary or multiple soft, hemorrhagic tan masses (Fig. 20-61A). Occasionally, a green color indicates bile production. HCCs tend to grow into portal and hepatic veins, and they may extend from the latter into the vena cava and even the right atrium. The tumor may spread widely, but metastases favor the lungs and portal lymph nodes.

HCCs range from so well differentiated as to be hard to distinguish from normal liver to anaplastic or undifferentiated neoplasms. In most, tumor cells are arranged in trabeculae or plates as in normal liver ("trabecular pattern"). These plates are separated by endothelium-lined sinusoids. In a "pseudoglandular (adenoid, acinar) pattern," malignant hepatocytes are arranged around a lumen, which may contain

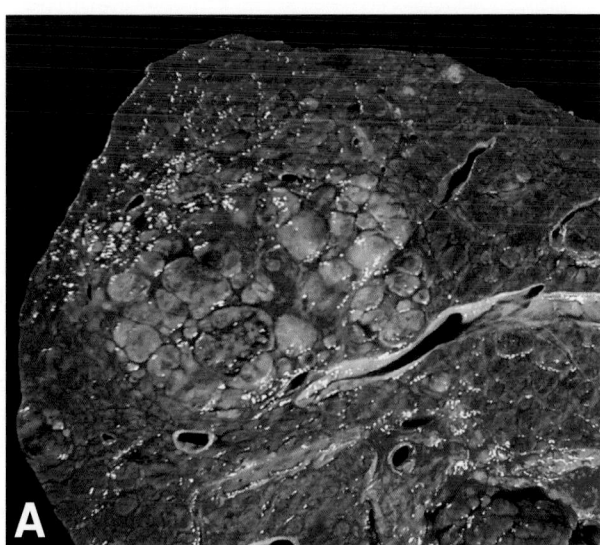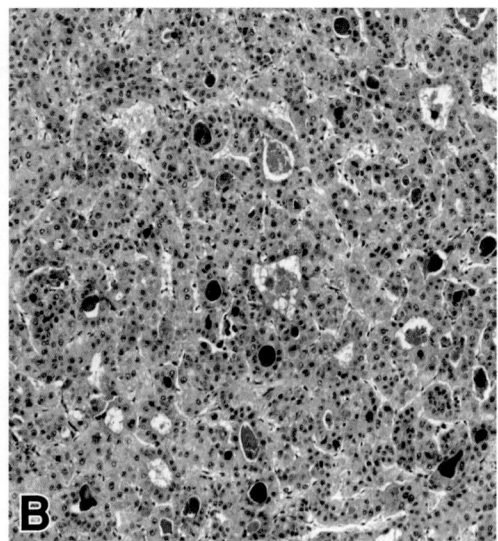

FIGURE 20-61. Hepatocellular carcinoma (HCC). A. Cross-section of a cirrhotic liver shows a poorly circumscribed, nodular area of yellow, partially hemorrhagic HCC. **B.** In this moderately differentiated tumor, HCC cells are arranged in an acinar pattern and surround concretions of inspissated bile.

bile (Fig. 20-61B). Despite their resemblance to glands, these are not true glands, and the lesion should not be confused with cholangiocarcinoma or other adenocarcinomas. Neither histologic pattern carries a particular prognostic significance.

Fibrolamellar HCC is an uncommon variant with a distinctive histology. It arises in apparently normal livers, mostly in adolescents and young adults, and is composed of clusters of large, eosinophilic, neoplastic hepatocytes surrounded by delicate collagen fibers (Fig. 20-62). The prognosis of fibrolamellar HCC is similar to that of other types of HCC.

 CLINICAL FEATURES: HCC usually presents as a painful and enlarging mass. If discovered at an advanced stage, the prognosis is dismal. Patients die of malignant cachexia, rupture of the tumor

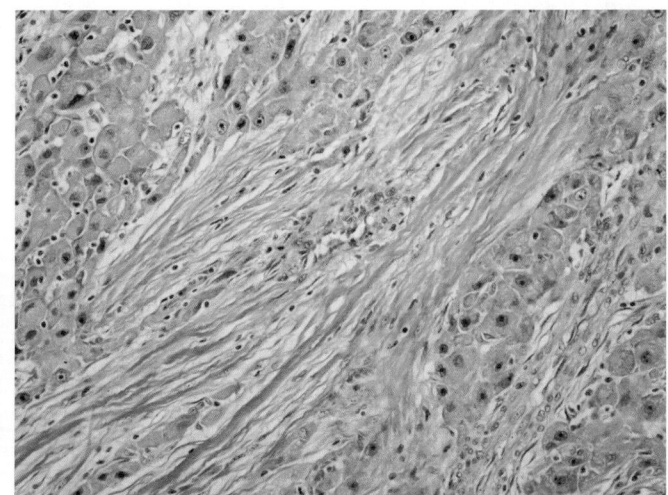

FIGURE 20-62. Fibrolamellar hepatocellular carcinoma. Clusters of eosinophilic tumor cells with abundant cytoplasm are separated by a lamellated fibrous band.

with catastrophic bleeding into the peritoneal cavity or complications of cirrhosis.

HCC may cause paraneoplastic syndromes (e.g., polycythemia, hypoglycemia, hypercalcemia) due to ectopic hormone production by the tumor. α-Fetoprotein (AFP) levels are often elevated, as in other benign and malignant liver diseases and some extrahepatic disorders.

If a small tumor is confined to one hepatic lobe, segmental resection can provide acceptable tumor-free survival rates. Ablative therapies (e.g., absolute alcohol injection, radiofrequency ablation, cryotherapy and transarterial embolization) can slow tumor progression. In patients with cirrhosis and limited tumor burden, liver transplantation gives the best tumor-free survival.

Cholangiocarcinomas Arise from Biliary Epithelium

Cholangiocarcinoma is a bile duct carcinoma that originates anywhere in the biliary tree, from large intrahepatic bile ducts at the porta hepatis to the smallest ducts at the edges of hepatic lobules, and peribiliary glands. It occurs mainly in older people of both sexes, with an average age at presentation of 60 years. It may occur anywhere but is particularly common in parts of Asia where the liver fluke (*C. sinensis*, see above) is endemic. In fact, the incidence of cholangiocarcinoma is also increasing in association with hepatitis C. PSC predisposes strongly to cholangiocarcinoma. Of livers with PSC removed for transplantation, 1/4 have cholangiocarcinoma. Choledochal cysts and Caroli disease (see below) are also risk factors.

 PATHOLOGY: Peripheral tumors or intrahepatic cholangiocarcinomas contain small cuboidal cells in ductular or glandular patterns (Fig. 20-63). They often show substantial fibrosis and thus may be confused with metastatic breast or pancreas carcinomas on liver biopsy. Tumors with both HCC and intrahepatic cholangiocarcinoma morphology are **combined hepatocellular-cholangiocarcinoma**.

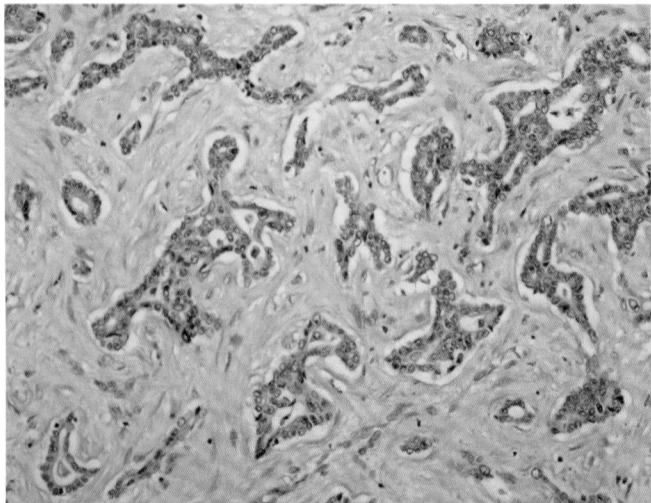

FIGURE 20-63. Cholangiocarcinoma. Well-differentiated neoplastic glands are embedded in a dense fibrous stroma.

Hilar cholangiocarcinomas are bile duct carcinomas that arise around the convergence of the right and left hepatic ducts. They present as (1) small sclerosing tumors that obliterate the duct, (2) tumors that spread within the duct wall or (3) a rare intraductal papillary variant. They may grow to "mass-forming" tumors. All produce symptoms of extrahepatic biliary obstruction.

Cholangiocarcinomas invade portal and hepatic veins less than do HCCs. They spread locally along nerves and metastasize throughout the body, particularly to portal lymph nodes. Liver transplantation is rarely successful in eradicating the tumor.

Hepatoblastoma Is a Rare Malignant Tumor of Children

Hepatoblastomas are usually discovered at birth or before the age of 3 years.

PATHOLOGY: Hepatoblastomas are circumscribed masses up to 25 cm that are partially necrotic and hemorrhagic, with epithelial- and mesenchymal-appearing cells. Occasionally, the latter are not seen. The epithelial component resembles embryonic and fetal cells. "Embryonal" cells are small and fusiform, arranged in ribbons or rosettes. The "fetal" cells resemble hepatocytes, contain glycogen and fat and form trabeculae with intervening sinusoids. The mesenchymal elements include connective tissue, cartilage and osteoid. Foci of squamous epithelium are occasionally encountered.

CLINICAL FEATURES: Abdominal enlargement, vomiting and failure to thrive are common presenting symptoms. Serum AFP is almost always elevated, and occasionally secretion of ectopic gonadotropin leads to sexual precocity. Congenital anomalies, including cardiac and renal malformations, hemihypertrophy and macroglossia, may be present. Untreated, these tumors are fatal, but liver transplantation or partial hepatectomy is often curative.

Epithelioid Hemangioendothelioma Is a Low-Grade Malignancy

This type of vascular tumor occurs predominantly in middle-aged women.

PATHOLOGY: Epithelioid hemangioendotheliomas typically may be single or multiple firm, gray tumors. They have a zonal pattern of cellularity with a hypocellular central area and a hypercellular periphery, the latter corresponding to its advancing front. The central zone is often sclerotic or calcified. Tumor cells, which are endothelial in origin, are spindle shaped, dendritic patterned or epithelioid (Fig. 20-64). The latter commonly form lumina, which may contain red blood cells.

CLINICAL FEATURES: Patients present with abdominal pain, enlarging mass, weight loss or malaise. Imaging studies show single or multiple avascular or calcified tumors. Treatment includes surgical resection for localized tumor or liver transplantation for patients with multiple tumors.

Hemangiosarcoma May Result from Chemical Exposures

Hemangiosarcoma is the only significant sarcoma of the liver. It is linked to thorium dioxide, vinyl chloride or inorganic arsenic and is now distinctly uncommon.

PATHOLOGY: These are mostly multicentric tumors, starting as multiple hemorrhagic nodules that may coalesce. Spindle-shaped, neoplastic, endothelial cells line sinusoids and compress liver cell plates (Fig. 20-65). Cavernous blood spaces and solid masses of neoplastic cells are common. Widespread metastases are usual.

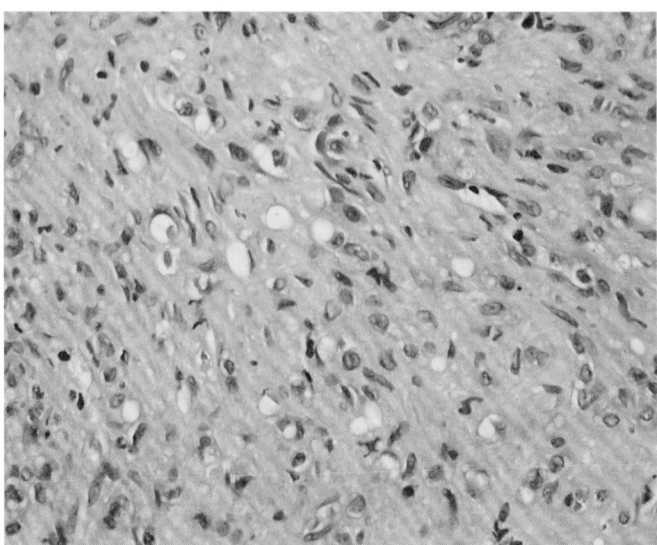

FIGURE 20-64. Epithelioid hemangioendothelioma. The tumor cells are scattered in a fibrous stroma. Some of them resemble a signet ring with intracellular lumen containing red blood cells.

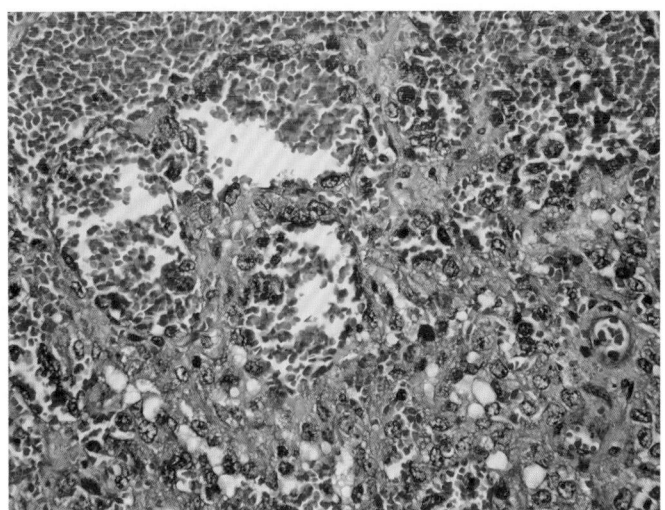

FIGURE 20-65. Hemangiosarcoma. Tumor cells with bizarre nuclei line the vascular spaces.

 CLINICAL FEATURES: Patients present with hepatomegaly, jaundice and ascites. Hematologic abnormalities, including pancytopenia and hemolytic anemia, are often prominent and in many cases due to splenomegaly from noncirrhotic portal hypertension. Tumor rupture with vigorous intra-abdominal hemorrhage is common. The prognosis is dismal.

Metastatic Cancer Is the Most Common Malignancy in the Liver

Of all metastatic cancers, 1/3 affect the liver, including 1/2 of cancers of the gastrointestinal tract, breast and lung. Pancreatic carcinoma, malignant melanoma and hematologic malignancies also often metastasize the liver, but any tumor may do so.

PATHOLOGY: The liver may have a single metastatic nodule or be almost replaced by metastases (Fig. 20-66). The organ may exceed 5 kg. *Such*

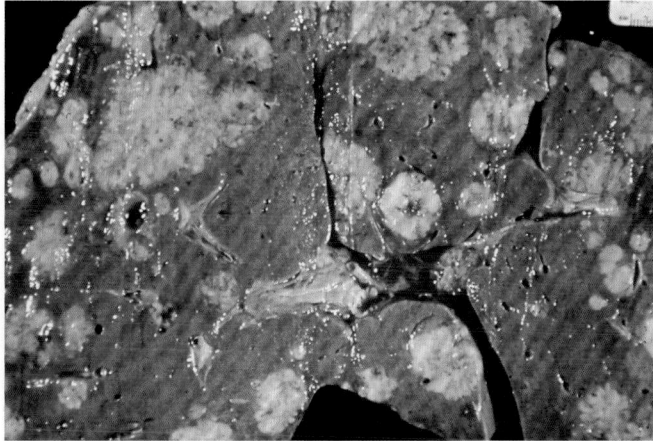

FIGURE 20-66. Metastatic carcinoma in the liver. The cut surface of the liver shows many firm, pale masses of metastatic colon cancer.

metastases are the most common cause of massive hepatomegaly. Metastatic tumors can appear on the liver surface as umbilicated masses. Hepatic metastases tend to resemble their primary tumors but may be so poorly differentiated that a primary site cannot be determined.

 CLINICAL FEATURES: Metastatic cancers to the liver often present with weight loss. Portal hypertension and its complications may occur. Bile duct obstruction or replacement of most of the liver parenchyma may cause jaundice. If the patient lives long enough, hepatic failure may ensue. Often the first indication of a metastatic tumor is an unexplained increase in serum alkaline phosphatase. Most patients die within a year of diagnosis, but surgical resection of a solitary metastasis may be curative.

LIVER TRANSPLANTATION

The increasing use of hepatic transplantation and the diagnosis and treatment of allograft rejection require useful pathologic criteria by which outcome can be assessed and therapy recommended.

 PATHOLOGY: In acute rejection, bile ducts are distorted by mixed cellular portal inflammation that may involve the ductal epithelium itself. Eosinophils are almost always present. Epithelial atypia may be seen (Fig. 20-67). Lymphocytes often adhere to the endothelium of terminal venules and small branches of the portal veins, with or without subendothelial inflammation (endothelialitis).

In allograft rejection lasting more than 2 months, there is damage to interlobular bile ducts. These small bile ducts are progressively destroyed, causing persistent cholestasis, the end stage of which is **chronic ductopenic rejection** or

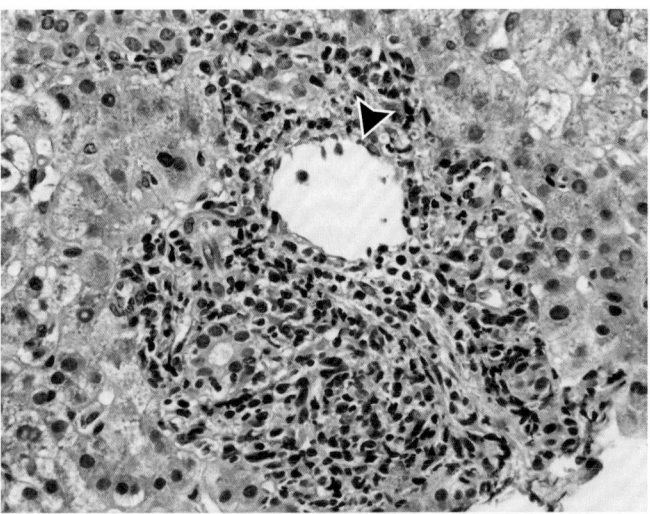

FIGURE 20-67. Acute rejection of a liver allograft. A portal tract is expanded by a polymorphous inflammatory infiltrate consisting of large and small lymphocytes, plasma cells, macrophages, neutrophils and eosinophils. The bile ducts (*arrows*) are damaged. A vein (*arrowhead*) is also inflamed (endophlebitis).

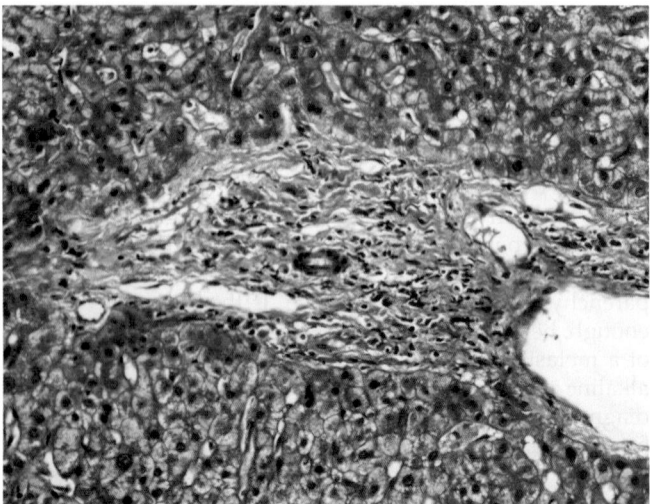

FIGURE 20-68. Chronic ductopenic rejection (vanishing bile duct syndrome). A portal tract shows mild chronic inflammation and absence of the bile duct.

vanishing bile duct syndrome (Fig. 20-68). Subintimal foam cells, intimal sclerosis and myointimal hyperplasia may cause arterial narrowing or occlusion (Fig. 20-69).

The Gallbladder and Extrahepatic Bile Ducts

ANATOMY

The gallbladder is a thin, elongated sac about 8 cm long and about 50 mL in volume, which occupies a fossa on the inferior surface of the liver between the right and quadrate lobes. It originates from the same foregut diverticulum that gives rise to the liver. Its primary function is storage, concentration and release of bile. The cystic duct is about 3 cm long and drains the gallbladder into the hepatic duct. It conducts

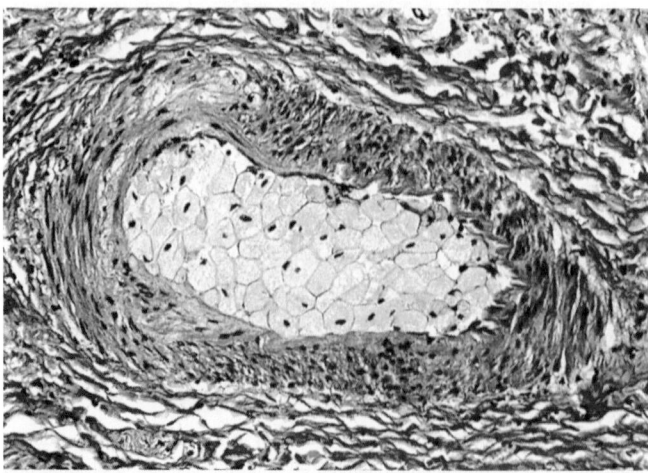

FIGURE 20-69. Arterial lesions in chronic rejection of a liver transplant. Subintimal foam cells, intimal sclerosis and myointimal hyperplasia virtually obliterate the lumen of a hepatic artery.

dilute bile from the hepatic duct into the gallbladder, where it is concentrated and subsequently discharged into the common bile duct.

The gallbladder wall is composed of a mucous membrane, a muscularis and an adventitia. It is covered by a reflection of visceral peritoneum. The mucosa is thrown into folds and consists of columnar epithelium and a lamina propria of loose connective tissue. **Rokitansky-Aschoff sinuses** are mucosal diverticula that dip into the gallbladder wall.

CONGENITAL ANOMALIES

Developmental anomalies of the gallbladder are rare and of little clinical significance except for surgeons. Bile duct anomalies include **duplication** and **accessory bile ducts.** Congenital bile duct dilations are **choledochal cysts** (85% of all cases), **choledochal diverticula** or **choledochoceles** (Fig. 20-70). Multiple cysts may occur as segmental dilations in the entire extrahepatic biliary tree. Similar multiple dilations in the intrahepatic biliary tree, called **Caroli disease,** predispose to bacterial cholangitis.

CHOLELITHIASIS

Cholelithiasis means stones in the gallbladder lumen or in the extrahepatic biliary tree. In the industrialized countries, 3/4 of gallstones are mainly **cholesterol;** the rest are **calcium bilirubinate** and **other calcium salts (pigment gallstones).**

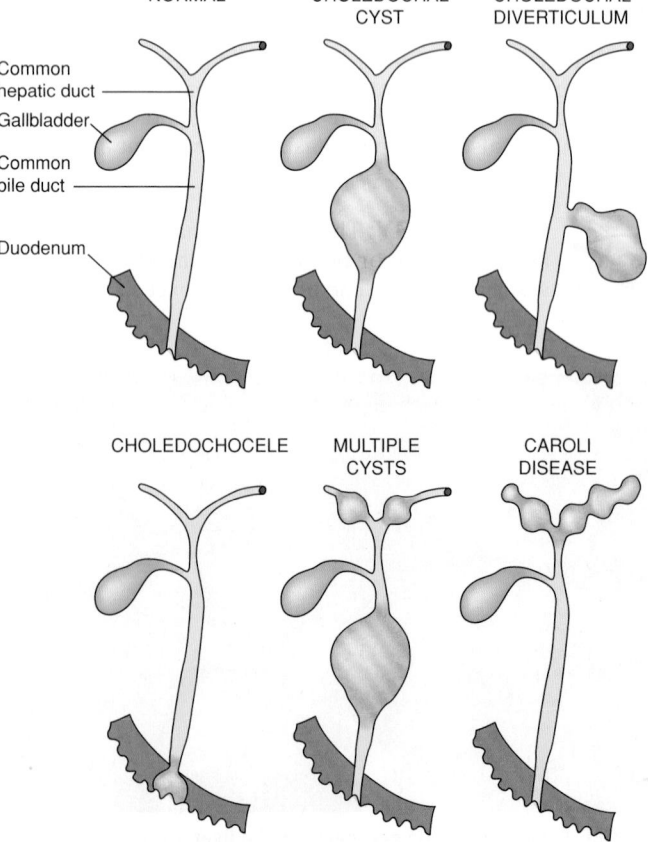

FIGURE 20-70. Congenital dilations of the bile ducts.

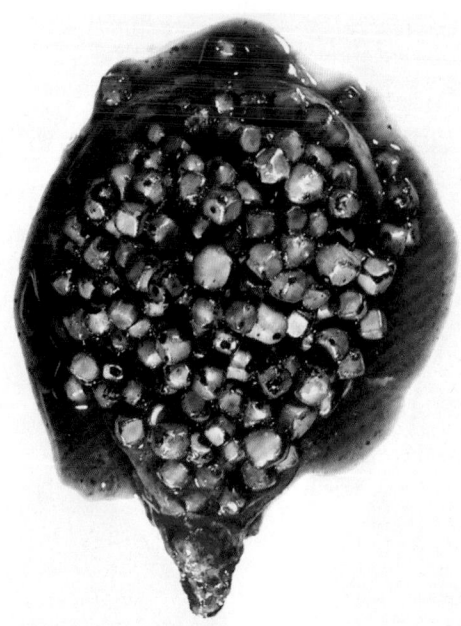

FIGURE 20-71. Cholesterol gallstones. The gallbladder has been opened to reveal numerous yellow cholesterol gallstones.

Pigment stones are more common in the tropics and Asia. Most gallstones are not radiopaque but are readily detected by ultrasonography. They are often asymptomatic but cause mild to severe pain **(biliary colic)** if they lodge in the cystic or common bile ducts.

Cholesterol Stones Are the Most Common Gallstones

Cholesterol stones measure up to 4 cm and may be round or faceted, yellow to tan, single or multiple (Fig. 20-71). They are mostly cholesterol, plus some calcium salts and mucin.

 **EPIDEMIOLOGY:** Some 20% of American men and 35% of women older than 75 years have gallstones at autopsy. *Premenopausal women develop cholesterol gallstones three times more often than do men. The incidence is highest in users of oral contraceptives and women with several pregnancies.* Cholesterol gallstones are very common in Pima Indian women of the American Southwest; 75% are affected by age 25 years and 90% by age 60.

 **PATHOPHYSIOLOGY:** Formation of cholesterol gallstones reflects the physicochemical qualities of bile and local factors in the gallbladder (Fig. 20-72):

■ **Bile formation in the liver:** Cholesterol is insoluble in water. When secreted by hepatocytes into the bile, it is held in solution by the combined action of bile acids and lecithin and is carried as mixed lipid micelles. Bile containing too much cholesterol or that is deficient in bile acids becomes supersaturated in cholesterol. Cholesterol then precipitates as solid crystals to form stones **(lithogenic bile)**. Bile from people who have cholesterol gallstones contains more cholesterol and less bile salts as it leaves the liver than does bile of normal people. Obesity increases hepatic cholesterol secretion even more, further supersaturating the bile with cholesterol.

■ **Local factors in the gallbladder:** Bile in the gallbladder from patients with gallstones crystallizes more easily than normal. Biliary proteins can function as nuclei of crystallization, and hypersecretion of gallbladder mucus accelerates cholesterol precipitation from gallbladder bile.

■ **Gallbladder motility:** Impaired gallbladder motor function leads to stasis causing bile sludging, which progresses to macroscopic stones.

Estrogens increase hepatic secretion of cholesterol and decrease secretion of bile acids, perhaps explaining why women form cholesterol gallstones more often. Pregnancy magnifies these effects. Progesterone, the main hormone of pregnancy, inhibits discharge of bile from the gallbladder. The gallbladder empties more slowly, and the resulting stasis increases the opportunity for cholesterol crystals to precipitate. Similar mechanisms may also explain the increase in gallstones with oral contraceptive use.

Other major risk factors for cholesterol gallstones include increased biliary cholesterol secretion, decreased secretion of bile salts and lecithin or both.

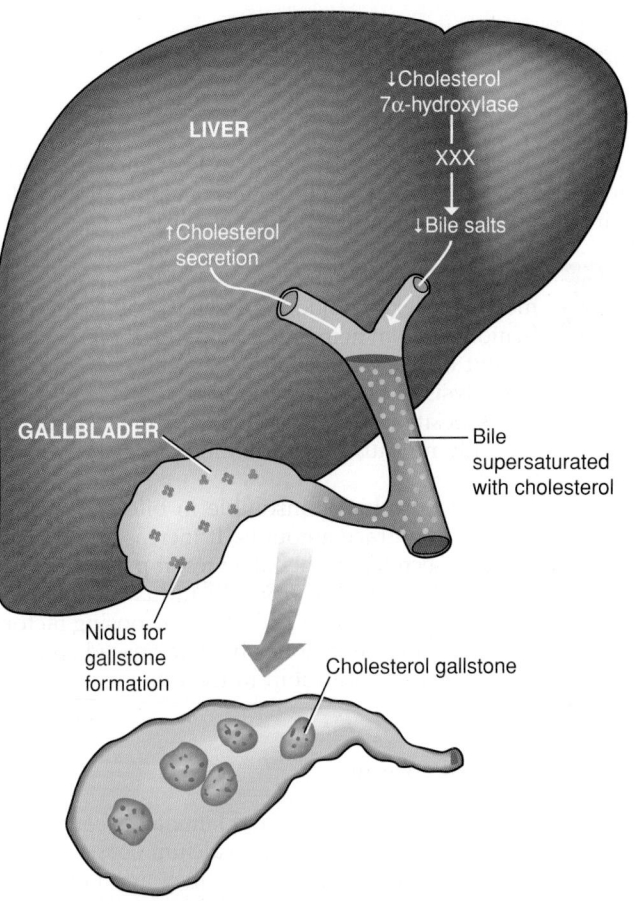

FIGURE 20-72. Pathogenesis of cholesterol gallstones.

Factors associated with **increased biliary cholesterol secretion** include:

- Increasing age
- Obesity
- Ethnicity (e.g., Native Americans, Chilean women, some northern Europeans)
- Familial predisposition
- Diet high in calories and cholesterol
- Certain metabolic abnormalities associated with high blood cholesterol levels (e.g., diabetes, some genetic hyperlipoproteinemias, PBC)

The risk of symptomatic gallstones is a direct function of body weight. In people who are obese, the relative risk of gallstones may be fivefold above normal. Hepatic cholesterol synthesis is stimulated by insulin, and the hyperinsulinism that accompanies increased body fat may explain why biliary excretion of cholesterol increases with obesity.

Decreased secretion of bile salts and lecithin occurs in nonobese whites who develop gallstones. Disorders that interfere with enterohepatic circulation of bile acids (e.g., pancreatic insufficiency in CF or Crohn disease) also decrease bile acid secretion and favor gallstone formation.

Cholesterol synthesis is elevated and bile salts and lecithin are lower in Pima Indians and in people taking certain drugs (e.g., clofibrate). Moderate alcohol intake lowers biliary cholesterol concentration and decreases the risk of gallstones.

Pigment Stones May Be Black or Brown

Black Pigment Stones

Black pigment stones measure less than 1 cm and are irregular and glassy (Fig. 20-73). They contain calcium bilirubinate, bilirubin polymers, calcium salts and mucin.

PATHOGENESIS: Black stones are more common in older or undernourished people. Chronic hemolysis, as in hemoglobionopathies, predisposes to development of black pigment stones. Either because it increases hemolysis or because of damage to liver cells, cirrhosis is also associated with a high incidence of black stones. However, usually no cause for formation of black pigment stones is found.

Unconjugated bilirubin is insoluble in bile and is normally present in only trace amounts. If increased unconjugated bilirubin is secreted by hepatocytes, it precipitates as calcium bilirubinate, probably around a nidus of mucinous glycoproteins. Patients without known predisposing factors who develop black pigment stones have increased concentrations of unconjugated bilirubin in the bile for unknown reasons.

Brown Pigment Stones

Brown pigment stones are spongy and laminated, containing calcium bilirubinate, cholesterol and calcium soaps of fatty acids. Unlike other types of gallstones, they are more common in intrahepatic and extrahepatic bile ducts than in the gallbladder.

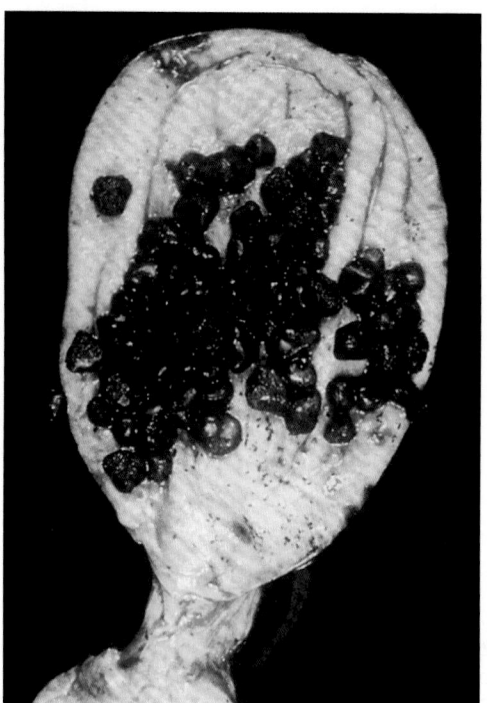

FIGURE 20-73. Pigment gallstones. The gallbladder has been opened to reveal numerous small, dark stones composed of calcium bilirubinate.

ETIOLOGIC FACTORS: *Brown stones are almost always associated with bacterial cholangitis, for which E. coli is the main cause.* They are uncommon in Western countries but are not infrequent in Asia, where they are almost entirely seen in people infested with *A. lumbricoides* or *C. sinensis,* helminths that may invade the biliary tract. The rare cases in Western countries are seen in patients with chronic mechanical obstruction to bile flow, as in sclerosing cholangitis, or the presence of a catheter in the common bile duct after common bile duct surgery. Bacterial β-glucuronidase or other hydrolytic enzymes hydrolyze conjugated bilirubin to its unconjugated form, which favors formation of brown stones.

CLINICAL FEATURES: Gallstones in the gallbladder may remain "silent" for many years, and few patients die as a result of cholelithiasis itself. The 15-year cumulative probability that asymptomatic stones will lead to biliary pain or other complications is less than 20%. Laparoscopic cholecystectomy is the treatment of choice.

Most complications of cholelithiasis relate to gallstones obstructing the cystic or common bile ducts. Passage of a stone into the cystic duct often, but not always, causes severe biliary colic and may lead to acute cholecystitis. Repeated bouts of acute cholecystitis give rise to chronic cholecystitis, which may also result from the presence of stones alone. Gallstones entering the common duct **(choledocholithiasis)** may cause obstructive jaundice, cholangitis and pancreatitis. They are the most common cause of acute pancreatitis in people who do not drink alcohol. Passage of a large gallstone into the small intestine can even cause intestinal obstruction, known as **gallstone ileus.** In cystic duct obstruction, with or without acute cholecystitis, bile in

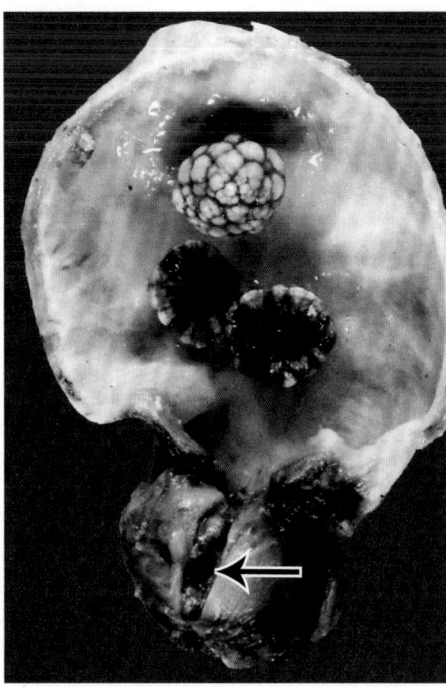

FIGURE 20-74. Hydrops of the gallbladder. The lumen of the dilated gall-bladder is filled with clear mucus and contains cholesterol stones. Note the stone (*arrow*) obstructing the cystic duct.

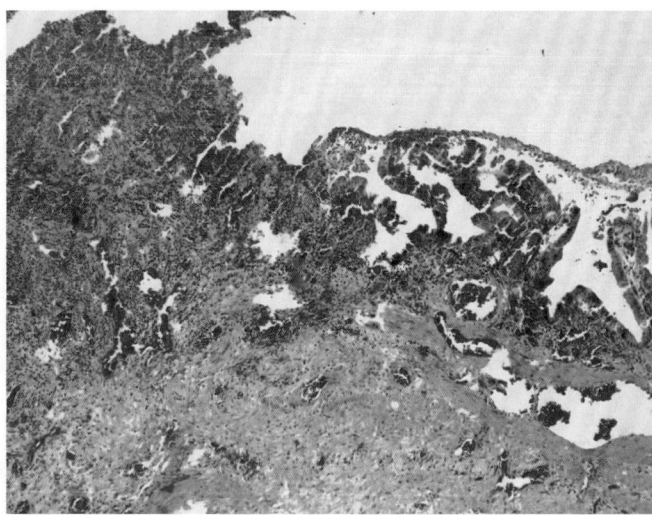

FIGURE 20-75. Acute cholecystitis. Gallbladder removed from a patient with acute cholecystitis demonstrates ulceration of the mucosa (*left*) and acute and chronic inflammation.

the gallbladder is reabsorbed and replaced by a clear muci-nous fluid secreted by gallbladder epithelium. **Hydrops of the gallbladder (mucocele)** (Fig. 20-74) entails a distended and palpable gallbladder, which may become secondarily infected.

ACUTE CHOLECYSTITIS

Acute cholecystitis is diffuse inflammation of the gallbladder, usually secondary to obstruction of the gallbladder outlet.

PATHOPHYSIOLOGY: *People with gall-stones account for 90% of cases of acute cho-lecystitis.* The remaining cases **(acalculous cholecystitis)** are linked to sepsis, severe trauma, infec-tion of the gallbladder with *Salmonella typhosa* and polyar-teritis nodosa. Bacterial infection is usually a consequence of biliary obstruction rather than a primary event.

Obstruction of the cystic duct by a gallstone may lead to release of phospholipase by the gallbladder epithe-lium. This enzyme hydrolyzes lecithin to lysolecithin, a membrane-active toxin. The mucous coat of the epithe-lium is disrupted, exposing mucosal cells to the detergent action of concentrated bile salts. Bile supersaturated with cholesterol may be toxic to the epithelium.

PATHOLOGY: In acute cholecystitis, the external surface of the gallbladder is congested and layered with a fibrinous exudate. The wall is thickened by edema, and the mucosa is fiery red or purple. Gallstones are

usually found in the lumen, and one is often seen obstructing the cystic duct. Rarely, in **empyema of the gallbladder,** the cystic duct is completely obstructed, allowing bacteria to invade the gallbladder and distending the organ with cloudy, purulent fluid.

In the gallbladder wall, edema and hemorrhage are strik-ing, with accompanying acute and chronic inflammation (Fig. 20-75). Suppuration in the wall often follows bacterial invasion. The mucosa shows focal ulcers or, in severe cases, widespread necrosis **(gangrenous cholecystitis)**.

Perforation is a dreaded complication of bacterial infection. Bile leakage into the peritoneum can cause **bile peritonitis**. More often, inflammatory adhesions form a **pericholecystic abscess** and limit spread of gallbladder contents after perfora-tion. Erosion of gallbladder contents into a viscus may create a **cholecystenteric fistula**.

CLINICAL FEATURES: Right upper quadrant abdominal pain is usually the presenting symptom. Most patients have already had episodes of biliary colic. Mild jaundice, caused by stones in, or edema of, the com-mon bile duct, is seen in 20% of patients. The acute illness gen-erally subsides within a week, but persistent pain, fever, leuko-cytosis and shaking chills herald progression of the disease and the need for cholecystectomy. As inflammation resolves, the gallbladder wall becomes fibrotic and the mucosa heals. However, the function of the gallbladder remains impaired.

CHRONIC CHOLECYSTITIS

Chronic cholecystitis (i.e., persistent chronic inflammation) is the most common disease of the gallbladder. It is almost always associated with gallstones but may also result from repeated attacks of acute cholecystitis. In the latter case, the pathogenesis probably relates to chronic irritation and chemical injury to the gallbladder epithelium.

PATHOLOGY: The wall of a chronically inflamed gallbladder is thickened and firm (Fig. 20-76A), and its serosal surface commonly shows fibrous

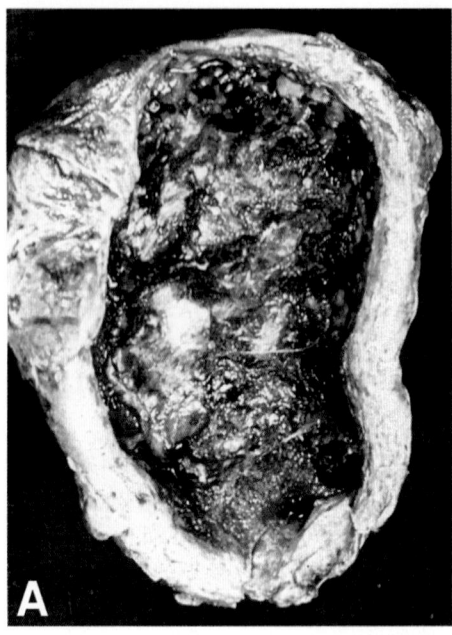
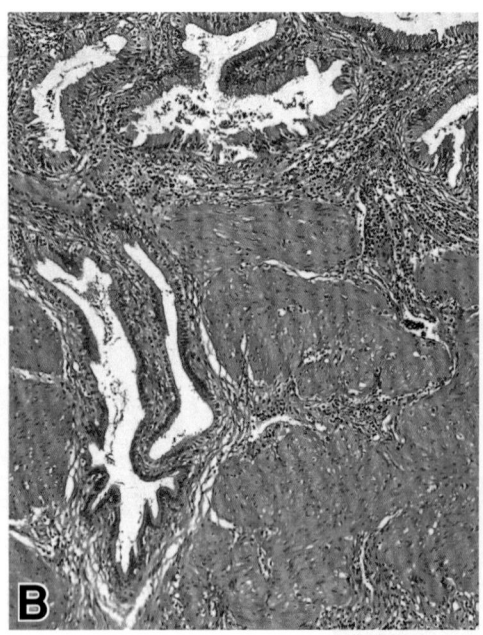

FIGURE 20-76. Chronic cholecystitis.
A. The gallbladder is thickened and fibrotic. The lumen had contained several gallstones. **B.** The same specimen as in A shows chronic inflammation of the gallbladder and a sinus of Rokitansky-Aschoff extending into the muscularis.

adhesions to surrounding structures, which are residues of previous episodes of acute cholecystitis. Gallstones are usually found within the lumen. The bile frequently contains gravel or sludge (i.e., fine precipitates of calculous material) with coliform organisms in about 1/2 of cases. The mucosa tends to be focally ulcerated and atrophic but may be intact. The fibrotic wall is chronically inflamed throughout and penetrated by Rokitansky-Aschoff sinuses (Fig. 20-76B). Long-standing inflammation may lead to calcification of the gallbladder wall **(porcelain gallbladder).**

 CLINICAL FEATURES: Many patients with chronic cholecystitis complain of nonspecific abdominal symptoms, but it is not at all clear that these are related to the gallbladder disease. On the other hand, pain in the right hypochondrium is typical and often episodic. The diagnosis is best made by ultrasound examination, which shows gallstones in a thick, contracted gallbladder. Cholecystectomy is the final treatment.

CHOLESTEROLOSIS

Cholesterolosis of the gallbladder is accumulation of cho-lesterol-laden macrophages in the submucosa. It reflects supersaturation of bile with cholesterol and does not ordinarily cause symptoms. The mucosa shows scattered, yellow flecks (strawberry gallbladder), and mucosal folds are swollen with large, foamy macrophages, in which a small nucleus is displaced to the periphery.

TUMORS

Benign Tumors of the Gallbladder and Extrahepatic Biliary Ducts Are Rare

Papillomas are the most common benign tumors of the gallbladder and may be single or multiple. They are associated

with gallstones in 75% of cases. A combined proliferation of smooth muscle and Rokitansky-Aschoff sinuses is an **adenomyoma and is adenomyomatus hyperplasia when it diffusely involves the gallbladder.** Fibromas, lipomas, leiomyomas and myxomas have also been recorded. Similar benign tumors may occur in the bile ducts, where they may obstruct biliary flow and cause jaundice and thus come to clinical attention.

Adenocarcinoma Is the Most Common Tumor of the Gallbladder

Adenocarcinoma of the gallbladder is not rare. It is found incidentally in 2% of patients who undergo cholecystectomy. Because this cancer is usually associated with cholelithiasis and chronic cholecystitis, it is much more common in women and in populations with a high incidence of cholelithiasis, such as Native Americans. Calcified (porcelain) gallbladders (see above) are particularly prone to developing gallbladder cancer.

 PATHOLOGY: Gallbladder carcinoma may occur anywhere in the gallbladder but most often involves the fundus. The tumor is usually an infiltrative, well-differentiated adenocarcinoma. It is usually desmoplastic, and thus the gallbladder wall becomes thickened and leathery (Fig. 20-77). Anaplastic, giant cell and spindle cell forms, as well as adenosquamous carcinoma of the gallbladder, have been reported. Metastases occur via both lymphatic spread and direct extension into the liver, contiguous structures and peritoneum.

 CLINICAL FEATURES: The symptoms of gallbladder carcinoma are like those of gallstone disease. However, by the time these tumors are symptomatic, they are almost always incurable; 5-year survival is less than 3%. For practical purposes, only those patients whose tumors are discovered incidentally during cholecystectomy are cured.

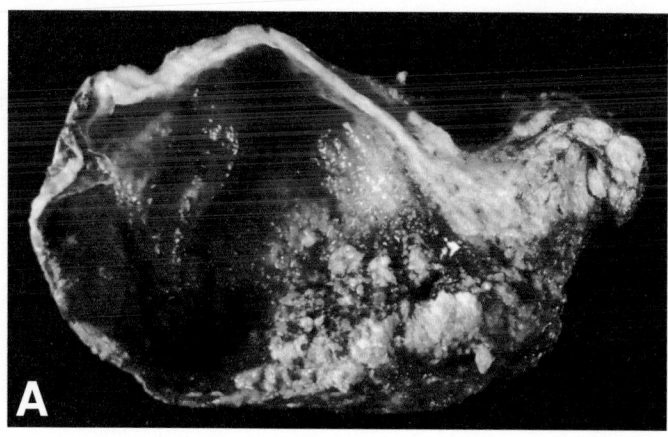

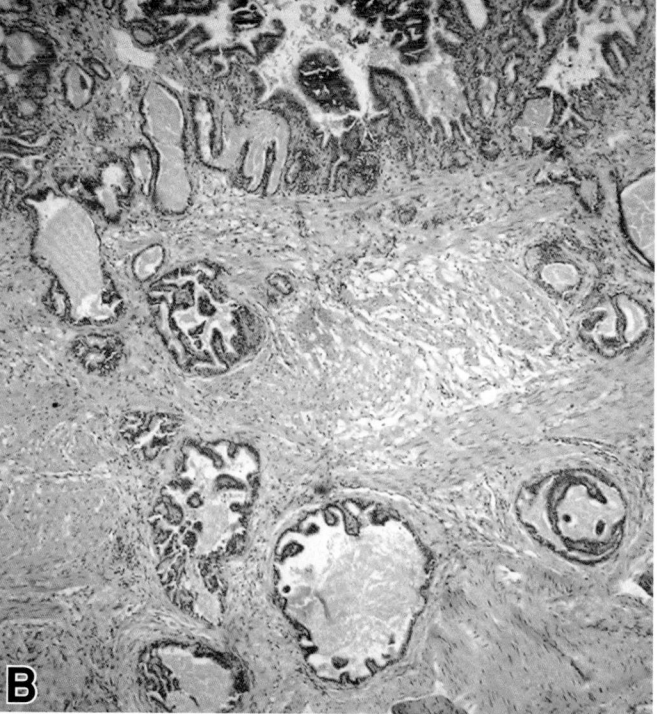

FIGURE 20-77. Carcinoma of the gallbladder. A. A surgically resected gallbladder has been opened to reveal a thickened wall infiltrated by adenocarcinoma, which also demonstrates exophytic growth into the lumen. **B.** The gallbladder wall is infiltrated by adenocarcinoma.

Carcinomas of the Bile Duct and Ampulla of Vater Present as Obstructive Jaundice

Cancer of the extrahepatic bile ducts (extrahepatic cholangiocarcinoma; see above) is almost always adenocarcinoma. It may occur anywhere along the duct, including the point where the right and left hepatic ducts join to form the common hepatic duct (hilar cholangiocarcinoma).

These tumors are less common than gallbladder cancer and affect both sexes comparably. Gallstones are often found in those affected, and there is an association with inflammatory diseases of the colon. The tumor may occur in choledochal cysts and in Caroli disease. In Asia, bile duct carcinoma is associated with biliary infestation by the fluke *C. sinensis*. As in carcinoma of the gallbladder, growth may be endophytic (into the lumen) or diffusely infiltrative. The prognosis is poor, but as symptoms arise early in the disease, the outcome is somewhat better than for gallbladder carcinoma.

Adenocarcinomas of the ampulla of Vater may also obstruct bile flow. They usually present as obstructive jaundice but occasionally as pancreatitis. Surgical treatment of cancer of the ampulla of Vater gives a 5-year survival rate of about 35%.

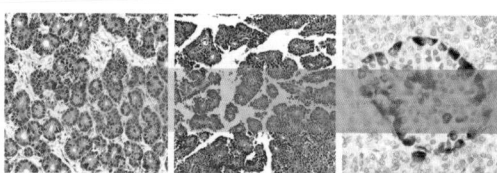

21

The Pancreas

David S. Klimstra ▪ Edward B. Stelow

ANATOMY AND PHYSIOLOGY

Pancreatic development begins at 4 weeks as two endodermal outpouchings on the dorsal and ventral sides of the embryonic duodenal tube. The ventral pancreas and the common bile duct migrate posteriorly around the duodenum. The ductal systems of the two embryonic pancreatic anlagen merge at 7 weeks, to form a main pancreatic duct (**duct of Wirsung**). This duct derives from the ventral pancreatic duct that extends from the ampulla of Vater at the duodenum into the distal portion of the dorsal pancreatic duct. The proximal dorsal duct remnant becomes the **duct of Santorini**, which may remain patent through the minor papilla into the duodenum, but this connection usually obliterates. The ducts branch progressively into smaller ducts and ductules that extend into the pancreatic lobules. Acinar cells arise from ductules and acquire their distinctive zymogen granules. The enzymatic secretions of the acinar cells drain into the smallest ductules between centroacinar cells, which bridge the acinar lumina into the ductal system. Islet cells are also derived from ducts and acquire several types of small, dense, secretory granules, corresponding to the various peptides they produce.

The pancreas is a mixed exocrine and endocrine gland, 10–15 cm long and weighing 60–150 g, that lies transversely in the upper abdomen, cradled between the loop of the duodenum and the hilum of the spleen. It is retroperitoneal, behind the lesser omental sac and the stomach, although the anterior surface is covered by peritoneum. It is thus inaccessible to physical examination. It has three anatomic subdivisions: (1) the **head** is in the concavity of the duodenum and extends to the superior mesenteric vessels, which pass through a groove immediately behind the organ; (2) the **neck** connects the head to the distal portion of the gland; and (3) the **tail** constitutes the distal two thirds of the pancreas and extends to the hilum of the spleen.

Exocrine pancreatic secretions drain into the major ducts of Wirsung and Santorini, which join the common bile duct and empty into the duodenum through the papilla of Vater. These pancreatic and biliary ducts usually merge a variable distance (1–5 mm) below the duodenal mucosa in a common channel that is the prototypical ampulla of Vater. In a significant minority of individuals, these ducts remain separated by a septum and enter the duodenum independently. The ampulla is surrounded by a circular complex of smooth muscle fibers, the **sphincter of Oddi,** that controls passage of pancreatic juice and bile into the duodenum.

Exocrine tissue makes up 80%–85% of the pancreas and contains acini with a single layer of pyramidal cells, whose basal cytoplasm is basophilic owing to abundant rough endoplasmic reticulum. The apical cytoplasm contains eosinophilic zymogen granules. Acinar cells synthesize some 20 different digestive enzymes, mostly in the form of inactive proenzymes. These enzymes include trypsin, chymotrypsin, amylase, lipase and elastase, which are secreted upon neural and hormonal stimulation and are subsequently activated in the duodenum. Amylase and lipase are secreted in their active forms. The daily secretion of 1.5–3 liters of pancreatic juice attests to the remarkable synthetic and secretory capacity of the exocrine pancreas.

The endocrine pancreas is organized into **islets of Langerhans**. These are present throughout the organ but account for only 1%–2% of the total pancreatic mass. Most islets consist of circumscribed lobules of cells derived from the dorsal embryonic pancreas. These *compact islets* contain several cell types, principally alpha and beta cells that produce glucagon and insulin, respectively; somatostatin-producing delta cells and pancreatic polypeptide cells are present in small numbers. Islets derived from the ventral embryonic pancreas are present in the head of the pancreas and mainly contain beta and pancreatic polypeptide cells. These *diffuse islets* are arranged in cords interspersed between acinar cells. Each islet cell makes only one peptide hormone, which is secreted directly into the blood (see below). The major endocrine disease of the pancreas, diabetes mellitus, is discussed in Chapter 22.

CONGENITAL ANOMALIES

There are many anatomic variations in the major pancreatic ducts and their relationship to the common bile duct, most of which are considered normal and are rarely of clinical significance. Other developmental variations have clinical consequences and are therefore regarded as developmental defects.

PANCREAS DIVISUM: Pancreas divisum, the most common congenital anomaly, results from failure of the two embryonic pancreatic ducts to fuse, leading to retention of two separate ductal systems, each draining into the duodenum through the major and minor papillae, respectively. Thus, the major portion of the pancreas is drained by the duct of Santorini through the minor papilla. Usually the two lobes of the organ do fuse, so the abnormality is not evident unless the course of the pancreatic ducts is specifically defined; sometimes the ventral and dorsal lobes fail to fuse entirely. Chronic pancreatitis develops in up to 25% of people with pancreas divisum.

HETEROTOPIC PANCREAS: Pancreatic tissue occurring outside its normal location, mostly in the walls of the duodenum, stomach and jejunum, is an incidental finding in 2%–15% of autopsies. Such heterotopic tissue may contain all components of normal pancreas, but some cases contain only ducts, and coexisting acini and islets are not always found. Smooth muscle is usually abundant in pancreatic heterotopia involving the tubular gastrointestinal tract. Pancreatic neoplasms of various types may arise in heterotopic tissue, most often infiltrating ductal adenocarcinoma.

ANNULAR PANCREAS: In this uncommon condition, the pancreatic head partly or completely surrounds the second portion of the duodenum. Infants with annular pancreas often have other congenital anomalies, including trisomy 21 (Down syndrome). Some affected patients also have duodenal atresia, which requires surgery immediately after birth. Half of patients with annular pancreas only develop symptoms in their 60s or 70s.

CYSTS: True nonneoplastic cysts of the pancreas are believed to arise from faulty development of pancreatic ducts. There is an association with other anatomic anomalies, including renal tubular dysplasia, anorectal malformations, polydactyly and thoracic dystrophy.

PARTIAL OR COMPLETE PANCREATIC AGENESIS: Homozygous mutations of homeodomain transcription factor IPF1 (PDX1) are reported in these rare conditions.

ACUTE PANCREATITIS

Acute Pancreatitis Results from Aberrant Release of Pancreatic Enzymes

It is not truly an inflammatory condition, but instead reflects myriad local, regional and systemic changes seen with release of these enzymes. The devastation of acute pancreatitis was described by Lord Moynihan in 1925 as the "most terrible of all calamities [of] the abdominal viscera. The suddenness of its onset, the illimitable agony which accompanies it and the mortality attendant upon it render it a formidable disease." For unknown reasons, the incidence of acute pancreatitis has increased in the past few decades.

The severity of acute pancreatitis varies greatly from case to case. At one end of the spectrum, it is a mild, self-limited disease, with acute inflammation and stromal edema, and little or no acinar cell necrosis. This is usually not associated with systemic manifestations of disease. At the other extreme is a severe, sometimes fatal, acute hemorrhagic pancreatitis with massive necrosis. In these cases, systemic manifestations such as shock, acute respiratory distress, acute renal failure and disseminated intravascular coagulation may develop in the face of massive enzymatic leak from the gland, reflected in extremely high serum levels of amylase and lipase.

Repeated bouts of acute pancreatitis may lead to chronic pancreatitis, which is characterized by recurrent attacks of severe abdominal pain and progressive fibrosis and atrophy of the gland, culminating in pancreatic insufficiency. However, antecedent acute episodes are only appreciated clinically in half of cases of chronic pancreatitis.

ETIOLOGIC FACTORS: **Acinar cell injury** and **duct obstruction** are the major causes of acute pancreatitis. These processes progress to inappropriate extracellular leakage of activated digestive enzymes and consequent autodigestion of pancreatic and extrapancreatic tissues. There may be some genetic predispositions to the development of acute pancreatitis; however, since the same molecular pathogenetic factors are generally associated with the development of chronic pancreatitis, they are discussed in that section.

ACTIVATED PANCREATIC ENZYMES: Inappropriate activation of pancreatic proenzymes occurs in all forms of pancreatitis. Acinar cells are shielded from the potentially destructive action of their digestive enzymes (proteases, nucleases, amylase, lipase and phospholipase A) by three mechanisms:

1. Enzymes are physically isolated from the cytosol by an intricate, intracellular, cavitary system of endoplasmic reticulum, Golgi complex and zymogen granule membranes.
2. Many digestive enzymes are synthesized as inactive forms (e.g., chymotrypsinogen, proelastase, prophospholipase and trypsinogen).
3. Specific enzyme inhibitors tend to protect the pancreas.

Inhibitors of proteolytic enzymes defend against inappropriate activation of pancreatic proenzymes and are present in many body fluids and tissues. The plasma protease inhibitors are α_1-antitrypsin, α_2-macroglobulin, C_1 esterase inhibitor and pancreatic secretory trypsin inhibitor. Several trypsin inhibitors are described in different body compartments, but they protect only incompletely from trypsin activation. Trypsin itself does not produce cell necrosis. Rather, it activates other pancreatic proenzymes, such as prophospholipase A_2 and proelastase, and so is central to the pathogenesis of acute pancreatitis.

SECRETION AGAINST OBSTRUCTION AND DUCT INSUFFICIENCY: Most enzymes secreted by acinar cells are discharged into the ductal system and enter the duodenum. A small amount diffuses back into periductular extracellular fluid and eventually into plasma. Whenever lumina of pancreatic ducts are narrowed or easy outflow of exocrine secretions is impaired, intraductal pressure and back-diffusion across the ducts increase. This is suspected to cause inappropriate activation of digestive proenzymes. Heavy meals may induce release of pancreatic secretagogues, and so augment production of pancreatic enzymes.

Gallstones sometimes obstruct pancreatic ducts, and 45% of patients with acute pancreatitis also have cholelithiasis.

Conversely, the risk of acute pancreatitis in patients with gallstones is 25 times higher than in the general population, and 5% of patients with gallstones develop acute pancreatitis. Also, if gallstones are not eliminated after one attack, pancreatitis recurs in half the cases. The reason for the association between pancreatitis and cholelithiasis is obscure. Under 5% of patients with acute pancreatitis have impacted stones at the ampulla of Vater. Neither ligation of the pancreatic duct nor its occlusion by tumor generally produces severe acute pancreatitis. Reflux of bile or duodenal contents into the pancreatic duct may cause pancreatitis, but there is little evidence to support this theory.

Anatomic anomalies (e.g., pancreas divisum) and **neoplasms** (ampullary and pancreatic neoplasms, including intraductal processes) can also lead to acute pancreatitis due to duct insufficiency or obstruction, respectively.

ETHANOL: Chronic alcohol abuse accounts for a third of cases of acute pancreatitis, although only 5%–10% of chronic alcoholics develop this complication. The pathogenesis of ethanol-induced pancreatitis (acute and chronic) is not well understood (see below). Ethanol does not cause significant injury to pancreatic acinar or duct cells.

Alcohol consumption may cause spasm or acute edema of the sphincter of Oddi, especially after an alcoholic binge. It also stimulates secretion from the small intestine, which triggers the exocrine pancreas to release pancreatic juice.

OTHER CAUSES OF ACUTE PANCREATITIS: Rare causes include:

- **Viruses,** such as mumps, coxsackievirus and cytomegalovirus. The incidence of acute pancreatitis is particularly high in patients with AIDS due to HIV-1 itself or, most commonly, cytomegalovirus (CMV) infection.
- **Therapeutic drugs.** These include immunosuppressive drugs (e.g., azathioprine), antineoplastic agents, estrogens, sulfonamides and diuretics. The mechanisms of pancreatic injury by these compounds are unclear.
- **Blunt trauma** to the upper abdomen with contusive injury to the pancreas and leakage of digestive enzymes into the pancreas and peripancreatic tissues. Patients undergoing endoscopic retrograde cholangiopancreatography (ERCP), fine needle aspiration biopsy and surgical manipulation occasionally develop acute pancreatitis.
- **Acute ischemia** due to shock, vasculitis and thrombosis.
- **Hyperlipidemia:** Hydrolysis of triglycerides in the extracellular space by inappropriate leakage of pancreatic lipase may be responsible. Released free fatty acids are cytotoxic.
- **Hypercalcemia.**
- **Obesity:** Obese people are at greater risk for severe pancreatitis. Increased peripancreatic fat may predispose them to greater fat necrosis after local release of pancreatic lipase.
- **Idiopathic pancreatitis:** This is the third most common form of the disease and accounts for 10%–20% of cases.
- **Parasites** (e.g., *Ascariasis*), bacteria (e.g., *Mycoplasma* species) and **pregnancy.**

Factors implicated in acute hemorrhagic pancreatitis are shown in Fig. 21-1.

 **PATHOLOGY:** In acute hemorrhagic pancreatitis, the pancreas is initially edematous and hyperemic. Within a day, pale, gray foci appear, rapidly becoming friable and hemorrhagic (Fig. 21-2A). In severe cases,

these foci enlarge so that most of the pancreas is converted into a large retroperitoneal hematoma, in which pancreatic tissue is barely recognizable. Yellow-white areas of fat necrosis appear around the pancreas, including in the adjacent mesentery (Fig. 21-2B). These nodules of necrotic fat have a pasty consistency that becomes firmer and chalk-like as more calcium and magnesium soaps are produced. Saponification reflects the interaction of cations with free fatty acids released by the action of activated lipase on triglycerides in fat cells. As a result, blood calcium may be depressed, sometimes to the point of causing neuromuscular irritability.

The most prominent microscopic findings in acute pancreatitis are acinar cell and fat necrosis, often with some degree of acute inflammation (Fig. 21-3). Necrosis is usually patchy and rarely involves the entire gland. Irregular fibrosis of the pancreas and occasionally calcification (i.e., chronic pancreatitis) result from healed acute pancreatitis.

PANCREATIC PSEUDOCYST: Half of patients surviving acute pancreatitis may develop pancreatic pseudocysts, which are usually centered in peripancreatic tissues (Fig. 21-4). Pseudocysts are surrounded by connective tissue, with no epithelial lining, and contain degraded blood, inflammatory cells, debris and fluid rich in pancreatic enzymes. Pseudocysts may enlarge to compress and even obstruct the duodenum or other structures. They may become secondarily infected and form abscesses. Rupture is a rare complication that may lead to chemical or septic peritonitis, or both.

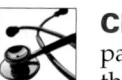 **CLINICAL FEATURES:** Patients with acute pancreatitis present with severe epigastric pain that is referred to the upper back, nausea and vomiting. Within hours, catastrophic peripheral vascular collapse and shock may ensue. With sustained, profound shock, **acute respiratory distress syndrome** and **acute renal failure** may occur within the first week. Early in the disease, pancreatic digestive enzymes from injured acinar cells enter the blood and retroperitoneal area. *Elevated serum amylase and lipase within 24–72 hours is diagnostic for acute pancreatitis.* Infection of the pancreas with gram-negative bacteria from the intestinal tract greatly increases mortality.

CHRONIC PANCREATITIS

Chronic Pancreatitis Results from Progressive Destruction of Pancreatic Parenchyma and Its Replacement by Fibrosis

Since its original description and its association with stones two centuries ago, the pathogenesis, clinical course and treatment of chronic pancreatitis remain enigmatic. Its symptoms include recurrent or persisting abdominal pain or simply evidence of pancreatic exocrine or endocrine insufficiency.

ETIOLOGIC FACTORS: Most factors that cause acute pancreatitis also cause chronic pancreatitis. The fact that chronic pancreatitis is often characterized by intermittent "acute" attacks with periods of quiescence suggests that it may evolve from repeated episodes of acute pancreatitis, with scarring. However, half of patients give no history of acute pancreatitis.

- **Chronic alcoholism** is the major cause of chronic pancreatitis, accounting for nearly 80% of adult cases. Even

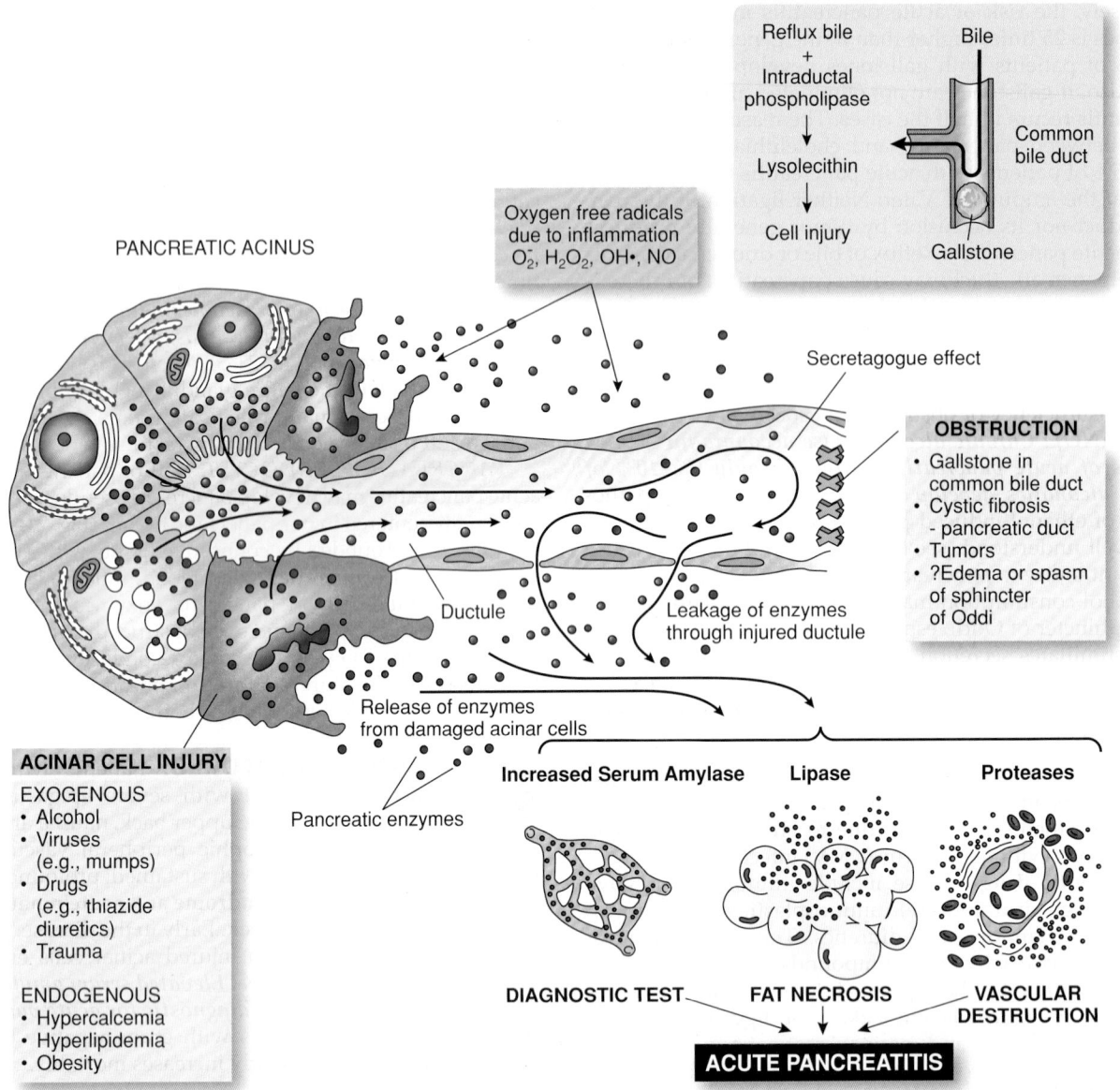

FIGURE 21-1. The pathogenesis of acute pancreatitis. Injury to the ductules or the acinar cells leads to the release of pancreatic enzymes. Lipase and proteases destroy tissue, thus causing acute pancreatitis. The release of amylase is the basis of a test for acute pancreatitis. H_2O_2 = hydrogen peroxide; $NO\bullet$ = nitric acid; O_2^- = superoxide ion; $OH\bullet$ = hydroxyl radical.

among alcoholics without symptoms of chronic pancreatitis, autopsy reveals evidence of this disease in about half. A comparable proportion of asymptomatic alcoholics show abnormal results for pancreatic exocrine function tests. The role of alcohol is undisputed, but the mechanism by which it causes chronic pancreatitis is still debated.

PATHOPHYSIOLOGY: The link between alcohol and pancreatitis may rest on the fact that alcohol is a pancreatic secretagogue. Hypersecretion of enzymes by acinar cells without increased fluid leads to precipitation of "protein plugs" in small pancreatic ducts. These deposits obstruct the small ducts, at first

causing only mild acute pancreatitis. Resolution with fibrosis facilitates development of more plugs (that grow and become the nidus for calcium carbonate stones), causing a vicious cycle that increases the risk of developing more and worse acute pancreatitis. Since only a minority of severe alcoholics develop clinical chronic pancreatitis, other factors may also play a role. Malformations (e.g., pancreatic divisum) or mutations (e.g., cystic fibrosis) may predispose some alcoholics to developing chronic pancreatitis.

■ **Obstruction or insufficiency of the pancreatic duct** sometimes causes chronic pancreatitis. However, acute obstruction by gallstones may cause acute pancreatitis but not progression to chronic pancreatitis.

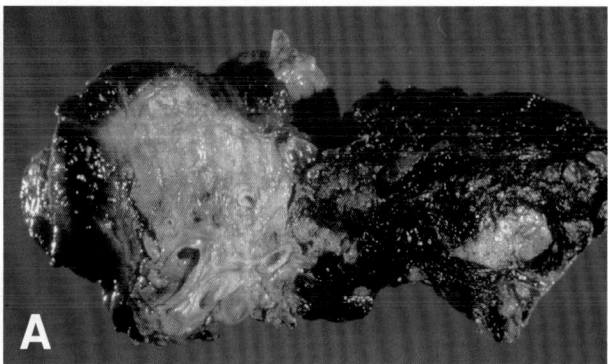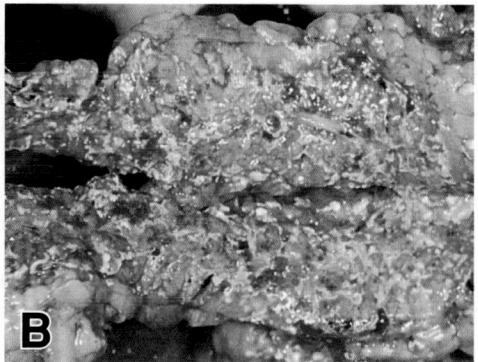

FIGURE 21-2. Acute hemorrhagic pancreatitis. A. Large areas of the pancreas are intensely hemorrhagic. **B.** The cut surface of the pancreas in a less severe case of acute pancreatitis, and at a somewhat later stage than in (A), shows numerous yellow-white foci of fat necrosis.

■ **Groove** or **paraduodenal pancreatitis** is a particular form of chronic pancreatitis that develops within the "groove" between the head of the pancreas, the common bile duct and the duodenum. Its etiology is not entirely clear. But since it usually develops in alcoholics, some have suggested that certain anatomic variations in the region of the minor papilla predispose these people to develop disease in the underlying portion of the pancreas. Because of the location of the disease, patients frequently develop jaundice (secondary to bile duct obstruction) or duodenal obstruction.

Cystic changes are also common in this condition. Because the process only focally affects the pancreas, patients are often brought to surgery for a suspected pancreatic neoplasm.

■ **Chronic injury to acinar cells** (e.g., in hemochromatosis) is associated with pancreatic fibrosis and atrophy.

■ **Chronic renal failure** increases the incidence of acute and chronic pancreatitis.

■ **Autoimmune chronic pancreatitis (lymphoplasmacytic sclerosing pancreatitis, duct-destructive chronic pancreatitis, etc.)** often occurs in association with other autoimmune and sclerosing disorders (e.g., chronic sclerosing sialadenitis and retroperitoneal fibrosis). The disorder affects both sexes, often in early adulthood. Symptoms vary from abdominal pain to painless jaundice. Imaging studies may suggest a mass-like lesion (mimicking carcinoma) or irregular beading of the pancreatic or bile ducts.

PATHOPHYSIOLOGY: The pathogenesis of autoimmune pancreatitis is unknown, and two forms of the disease appear to exist. In the most classic form of autoimmune pancreatitis (type I), serum immunoglobulin G4 (IgG4) is often elevated and plasma cells immunolabeled for IgG4 are numerous in the

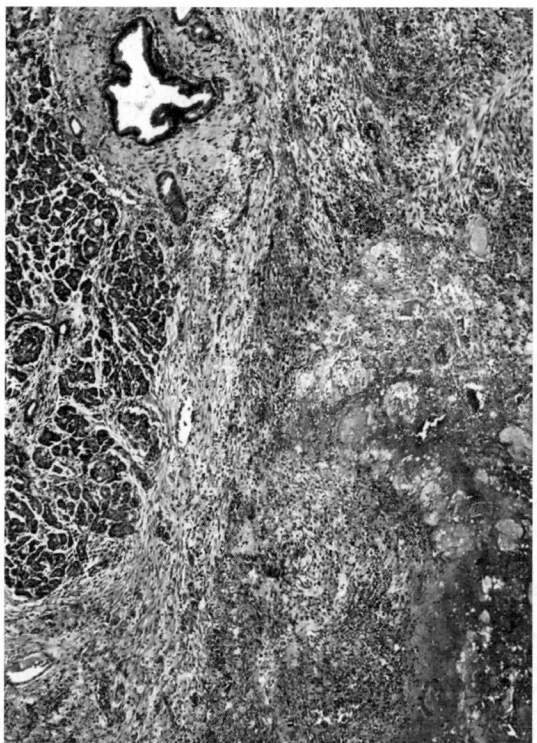

FIGURE 21-3. Acute hemorrhagic pancreatitis. A photomicrograph of the pancreas shows areas of acinar cell necrosis, hemorrhage and fat necrosis (*lower right*). An intact lobule is seen on the left.

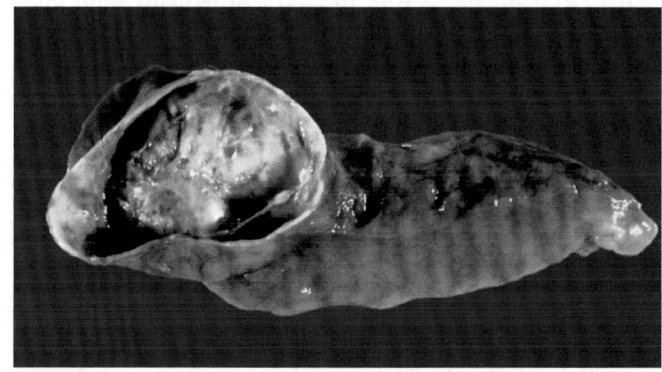

FIGURE 21-4. Pancreatic pseudocyst. A cystic cavity arises from the head of the pancreas.

parenchyma. Immunoglobulin deposits within basement membranes are described. The presence of hypergammaglobulinemia and autoantibodies, including antinuclear antibody (ANA), rheumatoid factor, antilactoferrin and anticarbonic anhydrase, support the suggestions of an autoimmune etiology.

- **Cystic fibrosis** (CF; see Chapters 6 and 22) may manifest as chronic pancreatitis. In patients with CF, intraductal secretions are abnormally viscid, accounting for the older name, **mucoviscidosis**. Plugs of inspissated mucus obstruct cystically distended pancreatic ducts, causing chronic pancreatitis and eventually exocrine pancreatic insufficiency. In late stages of CF, the entire organ is replaced by adipose tissue. Malabsorption is common in CF, causing bulky, fatty stools (steatorrhea). Death in CF is usually due to pulmonary disease.

- **Hereditary pancreatitis** is a rare autosomal dominant disease with 80% penetrance. It is characterized by recurring severe abdominal pain that often manifests in childhood.

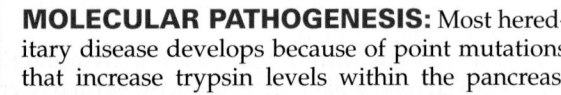

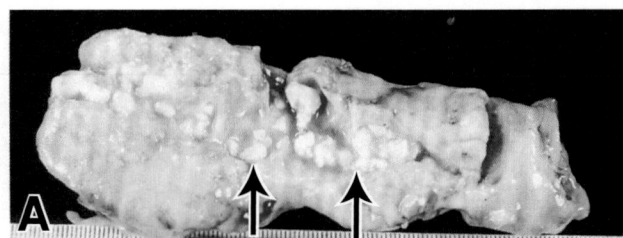

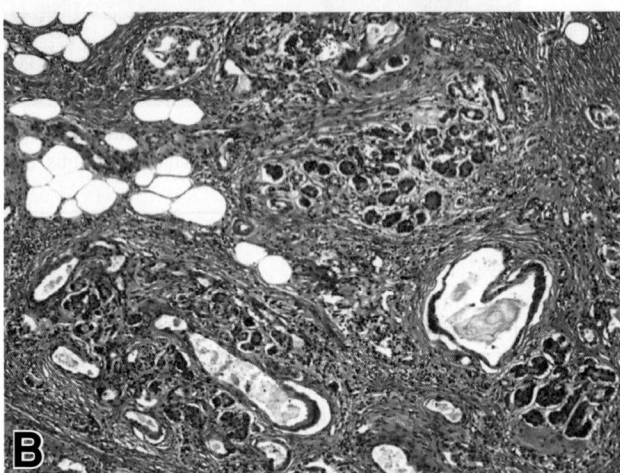

FIGURE 21-5. Chronic calcifying pancreatitis. A. The pancreas is shrunken and fibrotic, and the dilated duct contains numerous stones (*arrows*). **B.** Atrophic lobules of acinar cells are surrounded by dense fibrous tissue infiltrated by lymphocytes. The pancreatic ducts are dilated and contain inspissated proteinaceous material.

MOLECULAR PATHOGENESIS: Most hereditary disease develops because of point mutations that increase trypsin levels within the pancreas, largely due to autoactivation of trypsinogen. Point mutations in the **cationic trypsinogen gene** (**protease serine 1,** *PRSS1*; chromosome 7q) and in the **serine protease inhibitor gene** (*SPINK1*) are associated with the disease, and most forms of hereditary pancreatitis are caused by one of three point mutations in the **cationic trypsinogen** gene.

Hereditary pancreatitis is occasionally accompanied by aminoaciduria, although the two conditions are not necessarily linked etiologically. Some patients exhibit hypercalcemia secondary to parathyroid hyperplasia or adenomas. *About 40% of patients with hereditary pancreatitis later develop pancreatic ductal carcinomas.* Clinically and pathologically, the features of hereditary pancreatitis are indistinguishable from those of other forms of chronic pancreatitis, including ductal stones and the late complications.

- **Idiopathic chronic pancreatitis** has a bimodal distribution: a juvenile form with a mean age of 25 years, and a second form in older patients with a peak at age 60. Mutations in the cystic fibrosis transmembrane conductance regulator *(CFTR)* gene are seen in 10%–30% of patients with idiopathic chronic pancreatitis. Somatic mutations in the gene for pancreatic secretory trypsin inhibitor *(SPINK1)* are also associated with this disease. Thus, many cases of chronic idiopathic pancreatitis may be related to CF or hereditary pancreatitis but lack other signs of the diseases.

PATHOLOGY: By the time chronic pancreatitis is clinically evident, it is usually advanced. The pathology may vary somewhat, based on the etiology. Chronic calcifying pancreatitis is the most common type of the disease and is associated with chronic alcoholism in over 90% of cases. The pancreas can be affected focally, segmentally or diffusely. The parenchyma is firm, and the cut surface lacks the usual lobular appearance (Fig. 21-5A). The main pancreatic duct and its tributaries are commonly dilated, owing to obstruction by thick proteinaceous plugs, intraductal stones or strictures. Pseudocysts or abscess formation are common.

Microscopically, large regions of the gland show irregular areas of fibrosis with loss of acinar, then ductal and, eventually, endocrine parenchyma (Fig. 21-5B). Remaining pancreatic islets are embedded in the sclerotic tissue and may appear fused and enlarged until they, too, disappear. Some cases exhibit significant infiltration of adipose tissue into the gland, and the remaining islets may become suspended in the fat. Fibrotic areas show myofibroblasts and variable amounts of lymphocytes, plasma cells and macrophages. Pancreatic ducts of all sizes contain variably calcified proteinaceous material, a finding more commonly associated with alcoholism. Ductal epithelium may be atrophic or hyperplastic and may show squamous metaplasia.

In autoimmune pancreatitis, a dense lymphoplasmacytic inflammatory infiltrate and fibrosis surround the ductal epithelium (Fig. 21-6). Intraepithelial acute inflammation and obliterative venulitis may be seen with some forms of the disease.

CLINICAL FEATURES: Half of patients with chronic pancreatitis suffer repeated episodes of acute pancreatitis. One third of cases present with gradual onset of continuous or intermittent pain, with no acute attacks (Fig. 21-7). In some patients, chronic pancreatitis is initially painless but presents with diabetes or malabsorption. Once pancreatic calcifications are visible radiologically, most patients have diabetes, malabsorption or both.

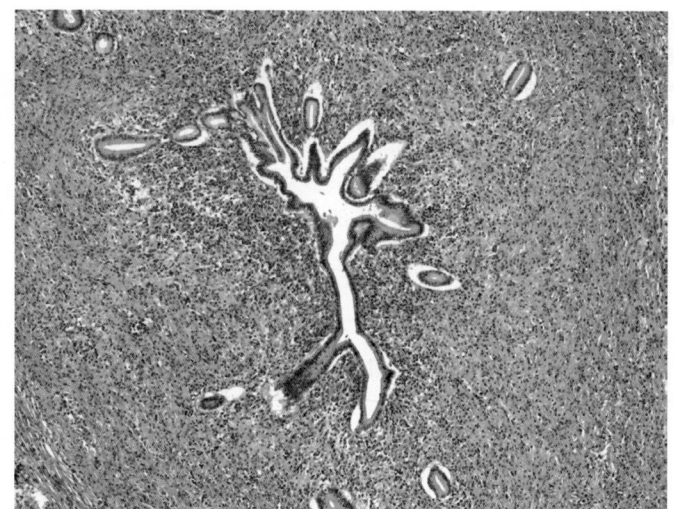

FIGURE 21-6. Autoimmune pancreatitis. There is loss of acinar tissue and the pancreatic duct is surrounded by a dense lymphoplasmacytic inflammatory infiltrate.

Conspicuous weight loss is common, and unrelenting epigastric pain, radiating to the back, may cripple the patient. Mortality is 3%–4% per year, approaching 50% within 20–25 years. One fifth of patients die of complications of attacks of acute pancreatitis. The other deaths are from other causes, particularly alcohol-related disorders. Autoimmune pancreatitis often responds favorably to steroid therapy, and a dramatic resolution of a mass lesion in response to steroids can be helpful in confirming the diagnosis in patients who have not had surgical resection.

PANCREATIC EXOCRINE NEOPLASIA

Most (~85%) Pancreatic Tumors in Adults Are Infiltrating Ductal Adenocarcinomas

Adenocarcinoma is the most common pancreatic malignancy and is often synonymous with "pancreatic cancer." It

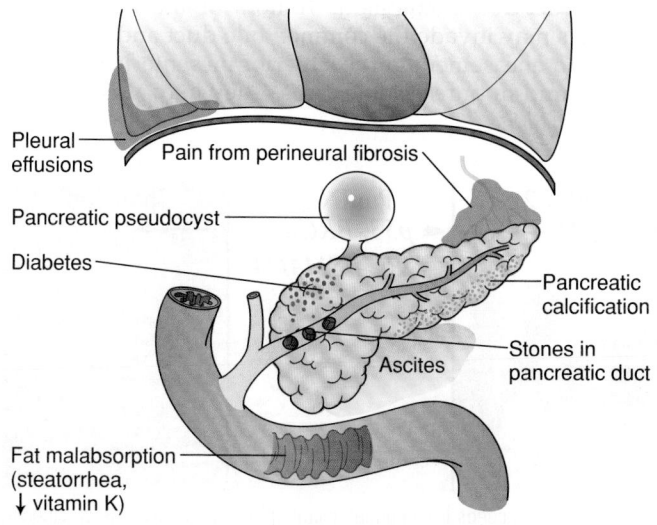

FIGURE 21-7. Complications of chronic pancreatitis.

is the 4th most common cause of cancer death in American men and the 5th in women. The prognosis is dismal: 5-year survival is less than 5%, and even the 20% of patients who can undergo surgical resection are rarely cured—the 5-year survival is less than 20% even when lymph nodes are uninvolved. Pancreatic cancer is increasing in many countries and has tripled in the United States over the past 50 years.

 **EPIDEMIOLOGY:** Pancreatic cancer occurs worldwide. The highest incidence (twice that in the United States) is among male Maoris, Polynesian aborigines of New Zealand and female natives of Hawaii. Over 45,000 new cases occur yearly in the United States, where it occurs 50% more often in Native Americans and blacks than in whites. Pancreatic cancer is a disease of late life, with peak incidence in people over 60 years old, although it may occur as early as the third decade. Males predominate (up to 3:1) at younger ages, but sex distribution equalizes in old age.

 ETIOLOGIC FACTORS: The pathogenesis of pancreatic cancer is obscure. Epidemiologic studies implicate hereditary and environmental factors.

SMOKING: About 25% of pancreatic cancers are attributable to cigarette smoking; cigarette smoking increases pancreatic cancer risk 2–3-fold, proportionate to the number of cigarettes smoked per day. Smokers may show proliferative lesions (pancreatic intraepithelial neoplasia; see below) in the pancreatic ducts at autopsy. However, as only a small fraction of smokers develop pancreatic cancer, additional genetic and environmental factors are undoubtedly important.

BODY MASS INDEX (BMI) AND DIETARY FACTORS: Diets high in meat, fat and nitrates may increase the risk of pancreatic cancer. However, confounding factors such as methods of cooking (e.g., frying, boiling, barbecuing, etc.) may play a role. Increased BMI raises the risk of pancreatic cancer. Diets high in fruits, vegetables, fiber and vitamin C seem to protect against pancreatic cancer. There is no clear link to coffee or alcohol consumption.

DIABETES MELLITUS: Diabetics have greater risk for carcinoma of the pancreas. Up to 80% of patients with pancreatic cancer have evidence of diabetes mellitus at the time of cancer diagnosis. In some patients, the diabetes may be caused by the pancreatic cancer, rather than the reverse. However, patients with diabetes mellitus for 5 or more years have double the risk for pancreatic cancer.

CHRONIC PANCREATITIS: Chronic pancreatitis is a risk factor for pancreatic cancer, although conventional types (such as alcoholic pancreatitis) likely account for few cases. Hereditary pancreatitis is more clearly linked to cancer. Since chronic pancreatitis is often mild and clinically silent, its role in development of pancreatic carcinoma may be underestimated. On the other hand, pancreatic cancers may cause obstructive chronic pancreatitis since they invade pancreatic ducts and obstruct the distal gland. Thus, the relationship of pancreatitis and cancer has been difficult to unravel.

ADDITIONAL FACTORS: Other environmental factors are suggested by increased risk linked to specific occupations. Workers exposed to coal gas, metal, dry cleaning agents and leather tanning have a higher incidence of pancreatic cancer.

FAMILIAL PANCREATIC CANCER: Hereditary factors play a role in pancreatic cancer risk, and several hereditary

TABLE 21-1

FAMILIAL CANCER SYNDROMES AND RELATIVE RISK FOR PANCREATIC CANCER

Syndrome	Chromosome	Gene Mutation	Relative Risk of Pancreatic Cancer
Peutz-Jeghers syndrome	19p13	STK11/LKB1	132-fold
Hereditary pancreatitis	7q35	PRSS1	50–80-fold
Familial atypical multiple mole melanoma syndrome (FAMMM)	9p21	P16 (CDKN2A)	9–38-fold
Hereditary breast-ovarian cancer syndrome (HBOC)	13q12–13	BRCA2	3.5–10-fold
Hereditary nonpolyposis cancer syndrome (HNPCC)	3p21, 2p22	hMLH1, hMSH2	Unknown

diseases are implicated (Table 21-1; also see Chapter 5). However, cases associated with known germline mutations represent only a small fraction of all pancreatic cancers, and even families with multiple affected members usually do not have a known hereditary syndrome. Increased risk may be linked to specific ABO blood types, but genetic bases for familial pancreatic cancers are largely unknown.

 MOLECULAR PATHOGENESIS: Infiltrating ductal cancers exhibit a number of genetic alterations. Some of these occur in most cases; others are infrequent. A genetic tumor progression model is supported by morphologic findings of preneoplastic ductal proliferative lesions, called **pancreatic intraductal neoplasia (PanIN),** the more recent nomenclature for dysplasia of the ducts. PanINs are characterized by mucinous epithelium replacing the normal lining of the ducts. PanINs are separated into 3 grades with increasing cytoarchitectural and genetic abnormalities. Early events, found in PanIN1, include telomere shortening and mutational activation of the *KRAS* oncogene, which is mutated in up to 95% of ductal adenocarcinomas. Later in the sequence of neoplastic progression, there is mutational inactivation or deletion of tumor suppressor genes, including *TP53* (50%–75%), *p16/CDKN2A* (95%) and *SMAD4/DPC4* (deleted in pancreatic cancer, locus 4) (55%). Interestingly, deletions in chromosome 18 are present in 90% of pancreatic cancers. Although *SMAD4* is on chromosome 18, only half of all pancreatic cancers show loss or inactivation of this gene, suggesting that other nearby tumor suppressors contribute to tumor development in the remaining 40%. Overactivity or inappropriate expression of several

growth factors and their receptors has been described, including epidermal growth factor (EGF) and its receptor (EGFR), transforming growth factor-β (TGF-β), fibroblast growth factor (FGF) and its receptor (FGFR) and HER2/neu. BRCA2 is inactivated in 7% of pancreatic carcinomas, and a similar fraction lose DNA mismatch repair genes. Many other genes involved in ductal adenocarcinoma are being identified, but most are implicated in only a small proportion of cases. The timing of abnormalities of the most common involved genes in the progression of PanIN to invasive carcinoma is shown in Fig. 21-8.

 PATHOLOGY: Ductal adenocarcinoma may arise anywhere in the pancreas but is most common in the head (60%–70%), followed by the body (10%) and tail (10%–15%). Sometimes, the pancreas is diffusely involved. Tumors of the pancreatic head may cause biliary obstruction by compressing the intrapancreatic common bile duct or ampulla of Vater. Classically, both the bile and pancreatic ducts are dilated ("double duct sign"). Carcinomas of the head tend to be smaller at the time of diagnosis than those elsewhere, with less spread to regional lymph nodes or distant sites.

Ductal adenocarcinomas are usually firm, gray, poorly demarcated masses (Fig. 21-9A) that can be difficult to distinguish from surrounding areas of fibrosing chronic pancreatitis. Invasion of peripancreatic tissues and other local structures is common. Tumors of the head of the pancreas may invade the common bile duct and duodenal wall, and encasement of the superior mesenteric vessels is often found in unresectable cases. They may also obstruct

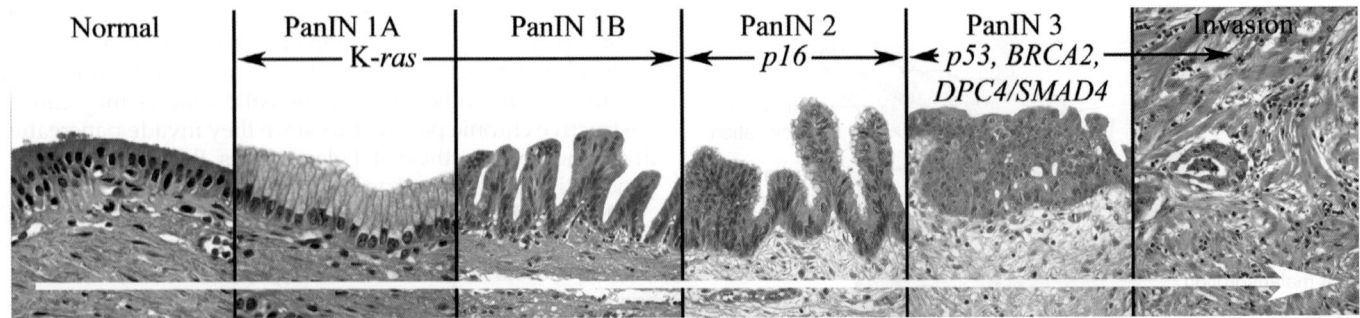

FIGURE 21-8. Pancreatic intraepithelial neoplasia (PanIN). From the left to the right, one proceeds from normal ductal epithelium to invasive carcinoma. Frequently mutated genes are shown when they are typically mutated within the spectrum of PanIN.

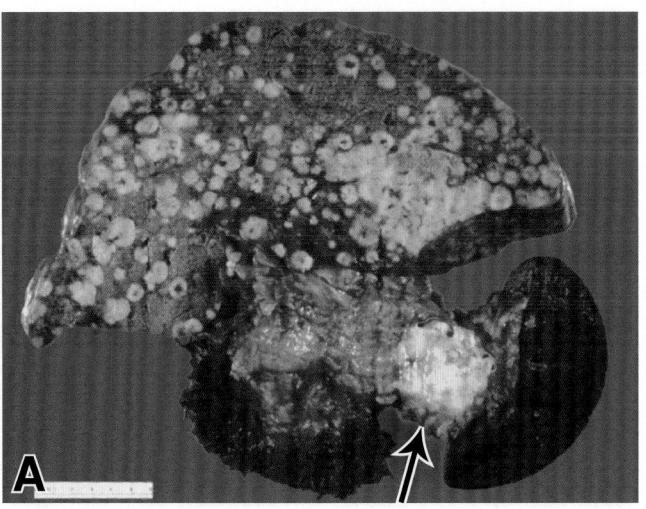
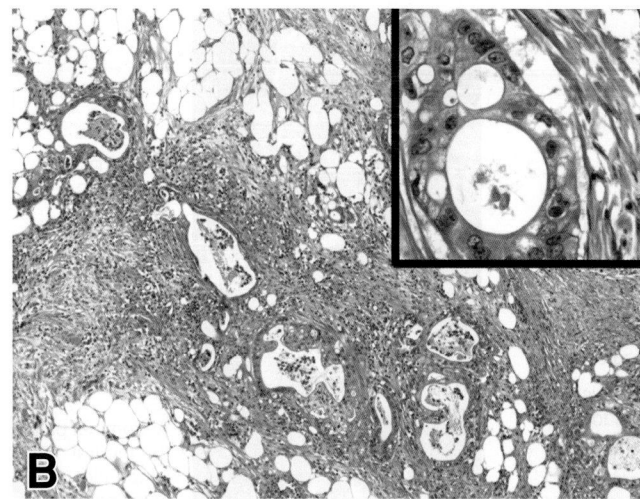

FIGURE 21-9. Infiltrating ductal adenocarcinoma of the pancreas. A. An autopsy specimen shows a large tumor in the tail of the pancreas (*arrow*) and extensive metastases in the liver. **B.** A section of the tumor reveals malignant glands infiltrating into adipose tissue with surrounding fibrous stroma. *Inset:* High-power image of a malignant gland.

the main pancreatic duct and cause atrophy of the body and tail. Carcinomas of the tail of the gland may extend into the spleen, transverse colon or stomach. Metastases in regional lymph nodes and liver are common. Other frequent metastatic sites include peritoneum, lungs, adrenals and bones; distant metastases and local spread render most cases unresectable.

Over 75% of infiltrating ductal adenocarcinomas are well to moderately differentiated (Fig. 21-9B), with well-formed individual tubular glands containing mucin-producing epithelial cells. Nuclear atypia may be focally marked, but some malignant glands may be so bland as to be difficult to distinguish from nonneoplastic ducts. Striking stromal desmoplasia around the neoplastic glands is the rule. The tumors are highly infiltrative and poorly circumscribed. Microscopic extension well beyond the gross limits of the tumor is common. Perineural invasion is a characteristic of these tumors and accounts for the early and persistent pain associated with them. Of the 25% of ductal adenocarcinomas that are poorly differentiated, sheets of cells or individual cells are seen. Additional variants include colloid carcinoma, medullary carcinoma, adenosquamous carcinoma and various undifferentiated carcinomas, including undifferentiated carcinoma with osteoclast-like giant cells.

Some ductal adenocarcinomas and variants arise in association with preinvasive cystic neoplasms such as mucinous cystic neoplasms and intraductal papillary mucinous neoplasms (see below).

CLINICAL FEATURES: Patients with pancreatic cancer present with anorexia, conspicuous weight loss and gnawing epigastric pain that often radiates to the back. Painless jaundice is seen in half of patients with cancer localized to the head of the pancreas but is uncommon in tumors of the body or tail. Depression may also be a presenting symptom. Serum levels of cancer antigen (CA) 19-9, a Lewis blood group antigen, are usually increased, but this finding is not specific. Early diagnosis of pancreatic cancer is unusual because the tumor is rarely symptomatic until it is advanced. Most have already metastasized at the time of diagnosis, and curative surgery is uncommon. Progressive

deterioration almost invariably ensues, with intractable pain, cachexia and death. Half of patients die within a year of diagnosis, and overall 5-year survival is less than 5%.

Courvoisier sign is acute, painless gallbladder dilation accompanied by jaundice, due to common bile duct obstruction by tumor. In about one third of patients, it may be the first sign of pancreatic cancer, but it does not identify potentially curable tumors.

Migratory thrombophlebitis (Trousseau syndrome, deep venous thrombosis) develops in 10% of patients with pancreatic cancer, especially when the tumor involves the body and tail of the pancreas. It is not uncommon for migratory thrombophlebitis to be the first evidence of an underlying pancreatic malignancy, and it is also seen with other cancers. Unexplained thrombophlebitis in an otherwise healthy person demands a careful search for occult malignancy. The mechanisms underlying the hypercoagulable state that leads to migratory thrombophlebitis are not completely understood, but (1) a serine protease synthesized and released by malignant tumor cells directly activates plasma factor X, and (2) tumor cells shed plasma membrane vesicles, tissue factor and mucins, which have procoagulant activity.

The complications of pancreatic ductal carcinoma are shown in Fig. 21-10.

Acinar Cell Carcinoma Is an Uncommon Tumor of Older Adults

Acinar cell carcinomas are rare (1%–2% of pancreatic carcinomas) and recapitulate normal pancreatic acinar tissue, including production of exocrine enzymes. These tumors usually develop in people in their 60s but may rarely also occur in children. Some patients show a characteristic paraneoplastic syndrome of subcutaneous fat necrosis, polyarthralgia and peripheral eosinophilia, due to hypersecretion of massive amounts of lipase into the serum. The prognosis of acinar cell carcinoma is poor, but they are less rapidly fatal than are ductal adenocarcinomas. Acinar cell carcinomas are large and circumscribed and lack the desmoplastic stroma of ductal cancers. Microscopically, they

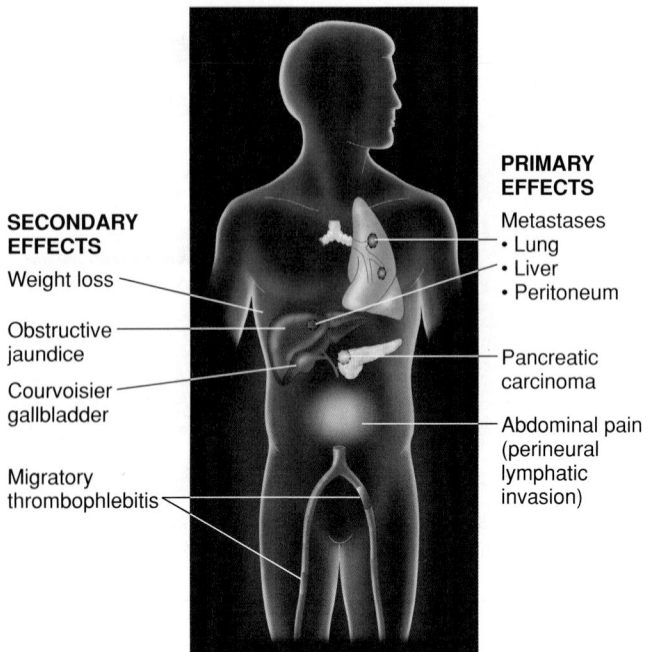

SECONDARY EFFECTS

Weight loss

Obstructive jaundice

Courvoisier gallbladder

Migratory thrombophlebitis

PRIMARY EFFECTS

Metastases
• Lung
• Liver
• Peritoneum

Pancreatic carcinoma

Abdominal pain (perineural lymphatic invasion)

FIGURE 21-10. Complications of pancreatic ductal adenocarcinoma.

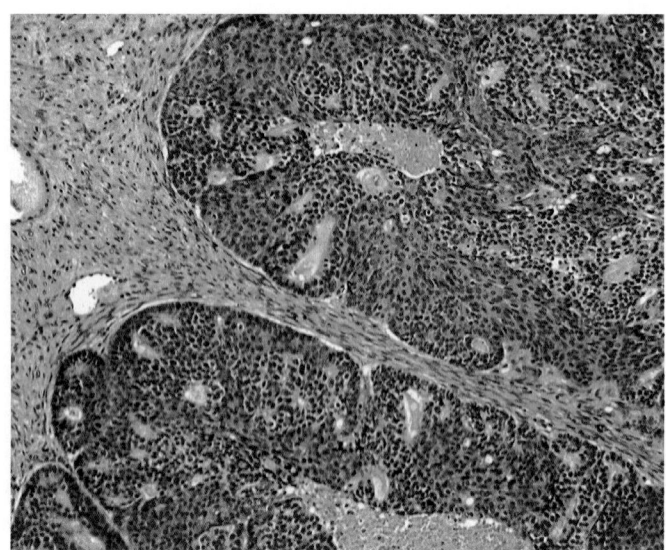

FIGURE 21-12. Pancreatoblastoma. There are spindle cell areas with scattered acinar structures.

are composed of uniform cells arranged in small acini and nests (Fig. 21-11). Immunohistochemistry demonstrates production of exocrine enzymes such as trypsin and chymotrypsin. The molecular pathogenesis of acinar cell carcinoma differs from that of ductal adenocarcinoma. Some cases have abnormalities in the APC/β-catenin pathway, but the genes typically abnormal in ductal adenocarcinoma are not altered.

Pancreatoblastoma Is a Childhood Tumor

These tumors are usually seen in the first decade of life and may occur in the setting of Beckwith-Wiedemann syndrome. Serum α-fetoprotein levels may be elevated.

Microscopically, tumors are composed of polygonal cells in solid islands and acinar structures, with interspersed squamoid nests (Fig. 21-12). Acinar differentiation, with production of exocrine enzymes, is consistently present, and some cases also have ductal or neuroendocrine differentiation. Lymph node or hepatic metastases occur in 1/3 of patients and are associated with a poor prognosis. Surgery and chemotherapy can be curative in patients without metastatic disease.

Serous Cystic Neoplasms of the Pancreas Are Nearly Always Benign

Serous cystic neoplasms are composed of numerous small cystic structures uniformly lined by glycogen-rich cuboidal epithelium with marked cytoplasmic clearing (Fig. 21-13).

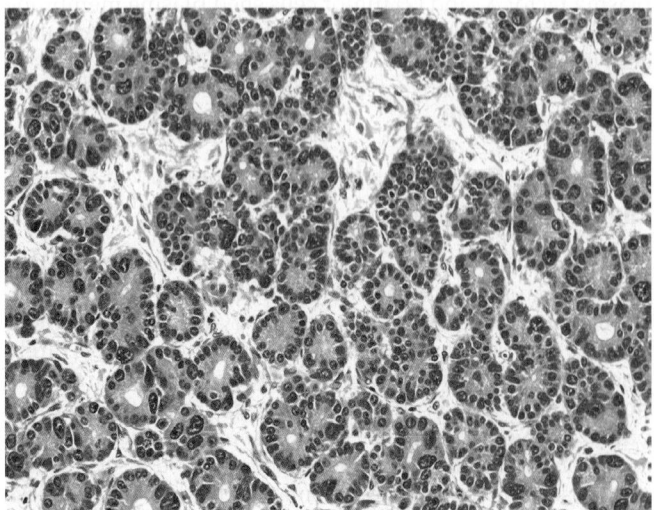

FIGURE 21-11. Acinar cell carcinoma. This malignant tumor is characterized by acinar formations reminiscent of normal pancreatic parenchyma.

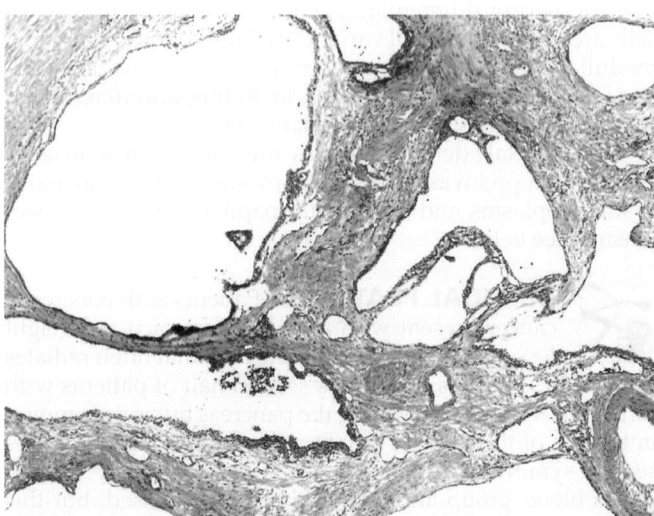

FIGURE 21-13. Serous cystadenoma. Cysts are embedded in a dense, fibrous stroma. The epithelial lining is composed of a single layer of glycogen-rich clear cells.

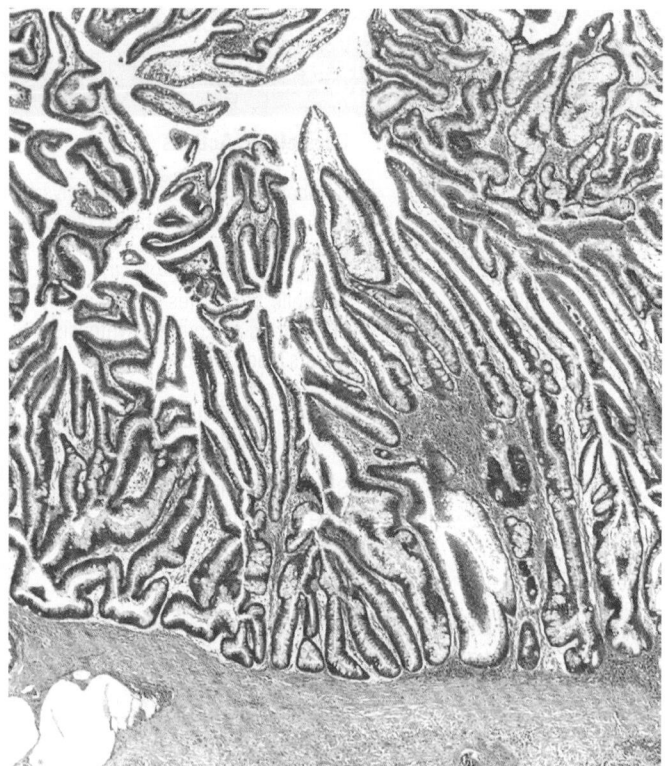

FIGURE 21-14. Intraductal papillary mucinous neoplasm. An exuberant papillary proliferation of tall mucin-secreting epithelium fills the pancreatic duct.

They usually occur in adults, in the pancreatic body or tail. Females predominate (3:1). Patients with von Hippel-Lindau syndrome are at increased risk for its development. It is not surprising, then, that these tumors are often associated with inactivation of the *VHL* gene. Serous cystadenomas range from 1 to 25 cm. Most patients present with nonspecific symptoms related to local mass effects, but many are asymptomatic. There is often a large, stellate central scar, sometimes with microcalcifications, giving a "sunburst" pattern on imaging studies. The tumors are sometimes removed owing to clinical concern for malignancy or because of symptoms.

Intraductal Papillary Mucinous Tumors May Be Associated with Invasive Carcinoma

Intraductal papillary mucin-producing neoplasms (IPMNs) are composed of dilated pancreatic ducts (>5 mm) lined by neoplastic mucinous epithelium and filled with mucus. Numerous papillary projections extend into the duct lumen (Fig. 21-14). IPMNs most often arise in the head of the pancreas and are usually diagnosed in late adulthood, after being found incidentally or in patients with symptoms of chronic pancreatitis. Duct involvement may be unifocal, multifocal or diffuse. Some IPMNs involve the main pancreatic ducts, while others are in peripheral (branch) ducts and mimic other cystic lesions on imaging studies. IPMNs exhibit varying degrees of epithelial dysplasia, similar to PanINs, and are graded in a similar fashion. Morphologically different types of epithelium occur in IPMNs, including gastric, intestinal, pancreatobiliary and oncocytic; each is associated with different immunohistochemical phenotypes and

spectra of mutational changes. A focus of invasive adenocarcinoma is found in up to one third of larger cases. Because they may harbor invasive carcinomas, larger tumors or those with atypical radiographic features are often resected. The molecular pathogenesis of IPMNs involves many of the same genes altered in PanIN and pancreatic ductal adenocarcinoma. However, some develop via alternative molecular pathways, perhaps explaining the diverse phenotypes of these tumors compared to PanIN. Additionally, mutations in *GNAS*, *RNF43* and *APC* occur in 60%, 75% and 25% of IPMNs, respectively; these genes are not mutated in most conventional ductal adenocarcinomas.

Mucinous Cystic Neoplasms Occur Most Often in the Pancreatic Tails of Middle-Aged Women

Mucinous cystic neoplasm (MCN) is usually a multilocular cystic neoplasm lined by mucin-secreting epithelium with underlying cellular stroma (ovarian-like stroma) (Fig. 21-15). MCNs occur almost exclusively in middle-aged women. Tumors may reach 10 cm and do not communicate with the pancreatic duct system. They have a predilection for the pancreatic body and tail. Like IPMNs, these tumors may have varying degrees of epithelial atypia and are sometimes associated with invasive carcinoma. The prognosis of MCN (noninvasive) is excellent if it is completely removed. Molecular changes in MCNs are similar to those in PanIN and invasive pancreatic ductal adenocarcinoma, and like IPMNs, MCNs have mutations in *RNF43* in 1/2 of cases.

Solid Pseudopapillary Neoplasms Are Very-Low-Grade Tumors of Young Women

Solid pseudopapillary neoplasms (SPNs) are solid and circumscribed, often with large cystically degenerated areas filled with blood and necrotic debris. The tumors are composed of monomorphic cells forming loose solid sheets and pseudopapillary structures (Fig. 21-16). These result from degeneration of the cells distant from the numerous small vessels that traverse the neoplasm. The cell lineage of SPN is

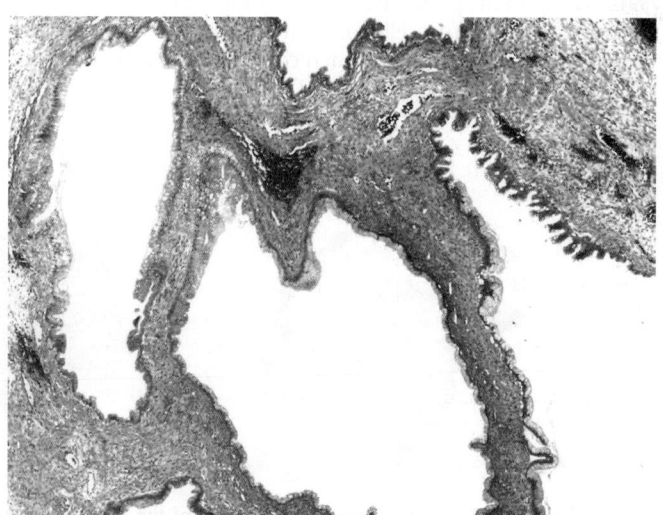

FIGURE 21-15. Mucinous cystic neoplasm. A mucin-rich epithelial lining of this cystic lesion rests on hypercellular, ovarian-like stroma.

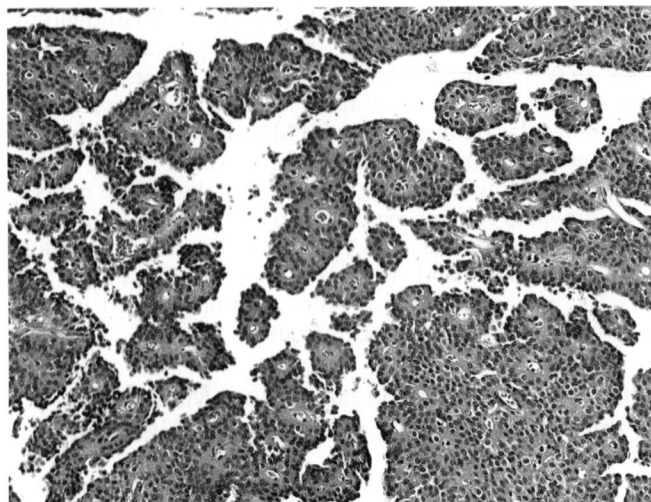

FIGURE 21-16. Solid pseudopapillary neoplasm. The tumor is composed of pseudopapillae with vascular cores.

TABLE 21-2		
SECRETORY PRODUCTS OF ISLET CELLS AND THEIR PHYSIOLOGIC ACTIONS		
Cell	**Secretory Product**	**Physiologic Actions**
Alpha	Glucagon	Catabolic; stimulates glycogenolysis and gluconeogenesis; raises blood glucose
Beta	Insulin	Anabolic; stimulates glycogenesis, lipogenesis and protein synthesis; lowers blood glucose
Delta	Somatostatin	Inhibits secretion of alpha, beta, D_1 and acinar cells
D_1	Vasoactive intestinal polypeptide (VIP)	Same as glucagon; also regulates tone and motility of the GI tract and activates cAMP of intestinal epithelium
PP	Human pancreatic polypeptide (hpp)	Stimulates gastric enzyme secretion; inhibits intestinal motility and bile secretion

cAMP = cyclic adenosine 3′,5′-monophosphate; GI = gastrointestinal.

unclear, and most cases fail to express any of the characteristic immunohistochemical markers of ductal, acinar or neuroendocrine differentiation. Most SPNs are very indolent and curable by complete surgical resection. Metastases, usually to the liver, occur in 10% of cases, and even those patients usually live for many years, underscoring the slow-growing nature of this neoplasm. Clinically, SPNs may mimic other malignancies of the pancreas. Most SPNs have mutations of the *β-catenin* gene, which results in abnormal nuclear localization of the protein—a useful diagnostic feature when detected using immunohistochemistry.

THE ENDOCRINE PANCREAS

The Islets of Langerhans Form the Endocrine Pancreas

The islets are irregularly scattered throughout the pancreas and consist of richly vascularized aggregates of endocrine cells arranged in spherical clusters (compact islets) or irregular trabeculae (diffuse islets). Four major distinct cell types are present in the islets, and each cell produces only one specific peptide hormone (Table 21-2).

- **Alpha cells** synthesize glucagon and are found at the periphery of islet lobules. They make up 15%–20% of the total islet cell population (Fig. 21-17A). Glucagon induces glycogenolysis and gluconeogenesis in the liver, thus raising blood glucose. Its secretion is stimulated by hypoglycemia and by ingestion of a low-carbohydrate, high-protein meal. By virtue of these responses, glucagon, together with insulin, serves to maintain glucose homeostasis.
- **Beta cells** make up 60%–70% of islet cells and produce insulin (Fig. 21-17B). They are found toward the centers of islets. By electron microscopy, beta cells contain characteristic polygonal and rhomboidal crystals enclosed in secretory vesicles. Insulin secretion is activated when glucose binds to receptors on the beta cell surface.
- **Delta cells** secrete somatostatin. They are few in number (5%–10%) and, like alpha cells, tend to be at the periphery of islets (Fig. 21-17C). Pancreatic somatostatin inhibits pituitary release of growth hormone and secretion by

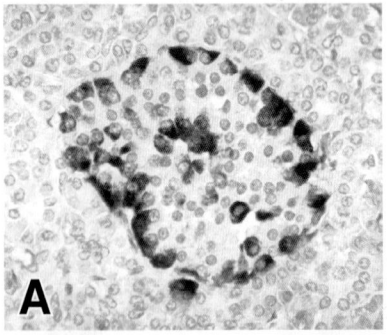
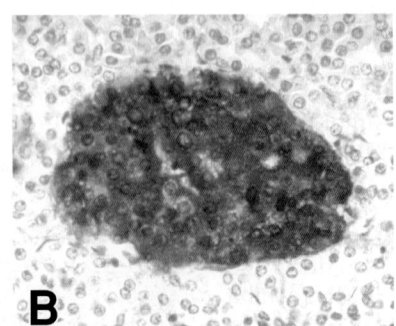
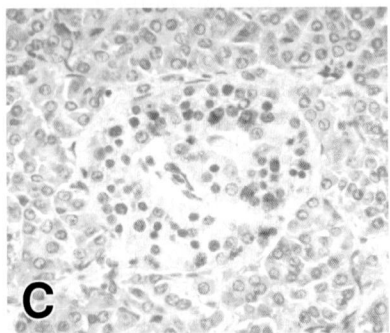

FIGURE 21-17. Localization of hormones of the pancreatic islet by specific antibodies. The immunoperoxidase technique reveals **(A)** glucagon in alpha cells at the periphery of the islet, **(B)** insulin in beta cells distributed throughout the islet and **(C)** somatostatin in sparsely distributed delta cells.

pancreatic alpha, beta and acinar cells and certain hormone-secreting cells in the gastrointestinal tract. These hormonal interactions suggest that somatostatin plays a regulatory role in glucose homeostasis.

- **Pancreatic polypeptide-secreting cells** are primarily in the diffuse islets within the part of the head of the pancreas derived from the embryonic ventral pancreas. They synthesize a polypeptide that appears to have diverse functions, including stimulation of enzyme secretion by the gastric mucosa, inhibition of smooth muscle contraction in the intestine and gallbladder, production of gastric acid and secretion by the exocrine pancreas and biliary system.

Well-Differentiated Pancreatic Neuroendocrine Tumors Make Up about 5% of Pancreatic Neoplasms

Pancreatic neuroendocrine tumors (PanNETs) are distinctive: they resemble normal islet cells and other well-differentiated endocrine (or neuroendocrine) tumors of the body, such as carcinoid tumors. Previously called "islet cell tumors," PanNETs may secrete hormones that cause dramatic paraneoplastic syndromes, or they may be nonfunctioning. Functioning varieties include insulinoma, glucagonoma, somatostatinoma, gastrinoma, VIPoma and other rare types.

These tumors show a range of clinical aggressiveness. If small, they can be cured by surgical resection, but larger tumors may develop incurable metastases. Predicting their likely clinical behavior is difficult, but features such as large size, high proliferative activity and more extensive invasion increase the chance of recurrence. Even in the presence of distant metastases, PanNETs often grow relatively slowly, and survival for years can occur. If functioning PanNETs cannot be completely removed by surgery, the hormonal syndromes they cause may be debilitating. Very small PanNETs (<0.5 cm), called pancreatic neuroendocrine microadenomas, are common incidental findings.

Most PanNETs are nonfunctioning, but among functioning PanNETs, insulinomas are most common. PanNETs occur at any age but are most common between 40 and 60 years, affecting men and women equally. The distinctive clinical syndromes of the more common functioning types are shown in Fig. 21-18 and discussed further below. Nonfunctioning PanNETs are detected incidentally by imaging studies and attract attention by local effects or metastases (e.g., in the liver).

MOLECULAR PATHOGENESIS: PanNETs are a component of multiple endocrine neoplasia syndrome type 1 (MEN1), which also involves pituitary and parathyroid adenomas, and less commonly endocrine tumors of other organs. Affected patients usually have multiple pancreatic neuroendocrine microadenomas and PanNETs, at least one of which is functioning. Patients with von Hippel-Lindau (VHL) syndrome also develop nonfunctioning PanNETs that may be histologically distinguished by their clear cytoplasm.

The genes involved in MEN1 and VHL syndromes (*MEN1* and *VHL* tumor suppressors, respectively) show biallelic inactivation in the hereditary PanNETs in these patients. Sporadic PanNETs also show mutations in the *MEN1* gene in 45% of cases. Other genes involved include members of the mammalian target of rapamycin (mTOR) pathway (e.g., *TSC1, PTEN, PIK3CA*) in 14% and a pair of genes involved in telomere maintenance, *DAXX* (death domain–associated protein) and *ATRX* (α-thalassemia/mental retardation syndrome X-linked), which are mutually exclusively lost in 43% of cases. PanNETs do not usually have mutations in the genes commonly mutated in ductal adenocarcinomas (see above).

Functioning PanNETs Produce Dramatic Paraneoplastic Syndromes

- **Insulinomas,** the most common functioning PanNETs, secrete sufficient insulin to cause hypoglycemia. Insulin secretion by the tumor cells is not regulated by blood glucose levels, so the tumors secrete insulin continuously. Although these tumors are usually small (75% are <2 cm), the symptoms may be profound and include both the direct central nervous system effects of hypoglycemia and the secondary effects of the resulting catecholamine response. Patients complain of sweating, visual changes, nervousness and hunger, which may progress to confusion, lethargy and even seizures or coma. Their abnormal behavior may falsely suggest a psychiatric disorder. Insulinomas occur somewhat more often in the tail of the pancreas (Fig. 21-19). Although 30% of the functioning PanNETs in patients with MEN1 are insulinomas, only 5% of insulinomas arise in the setting of MEN1. Compared to other PanNETs, insulinomas have a benign clinical course, perhaps because they are usually very small when detected. Surgical removal, even by enucleation, is usually curative.

- **Glucagonomas** are associated with a syndrome of (1) mild diabetes; (2) a necrotizing, migratory, erythematous rash; (3) anemia; (4) diarrhea; and (5) deep vein thromboses. Psychiatric disturbances also occur. Glucagonomas constitute 8%–13% of functioning PanNETs and occur between the ages of 40 and 70 years, with a slight female predominance. In patients with alpha cell tumors, plasma glucagon levels may be up to 30 times above normal. Like other functioning PanNETs (except insulinomas) and nonfunctioning PanNETs, glucagonomas exhibit malignant behavior in 50%–70% of cases.

- **Somatostatinomas** are rare and produce a syndrome of mild diabetes, gallstones, steatorrhea, hypochlorhydria, anemia and weight loss, due to the inhibitory actions of somatostatin on other cells of the pancreatic islets and on neuroendocrine cells of the gastrointestinal tract. Consequently, blood levels of insulin and glucagon are low.

- **Pancreatic gastrinoma** is a functioning PanNET composed of so-called G cells, which produce gastrin, a potent hormonal stimulus for gastric acid secretion. The location of this tumor in the pancreas is curious, because gastrin-producing cells do not normally occur in the islets. Pancreatic gastrinoma causes Zollinger-Ellison syndrome, a disorder showing (1) intractable gastric hypersecretion, (2) severe peptic ulceration of the duodenum and jejunum and (3) high blood gastrin levels. Among functioning PanNETs, gastrinomas are second in frequency to insulinomas, and they are the most common functioning tumor in MEN1 patients. However, the pancreas is a less common location for gastrinomas than is the duodenum, especially in cases not associated with MEN1. Gastrinomas of the pancreas are usually over 2 cm, but duodenal gastrinomas can measure only a few millimeters. Sometimes only lymph node metastases are found, with no

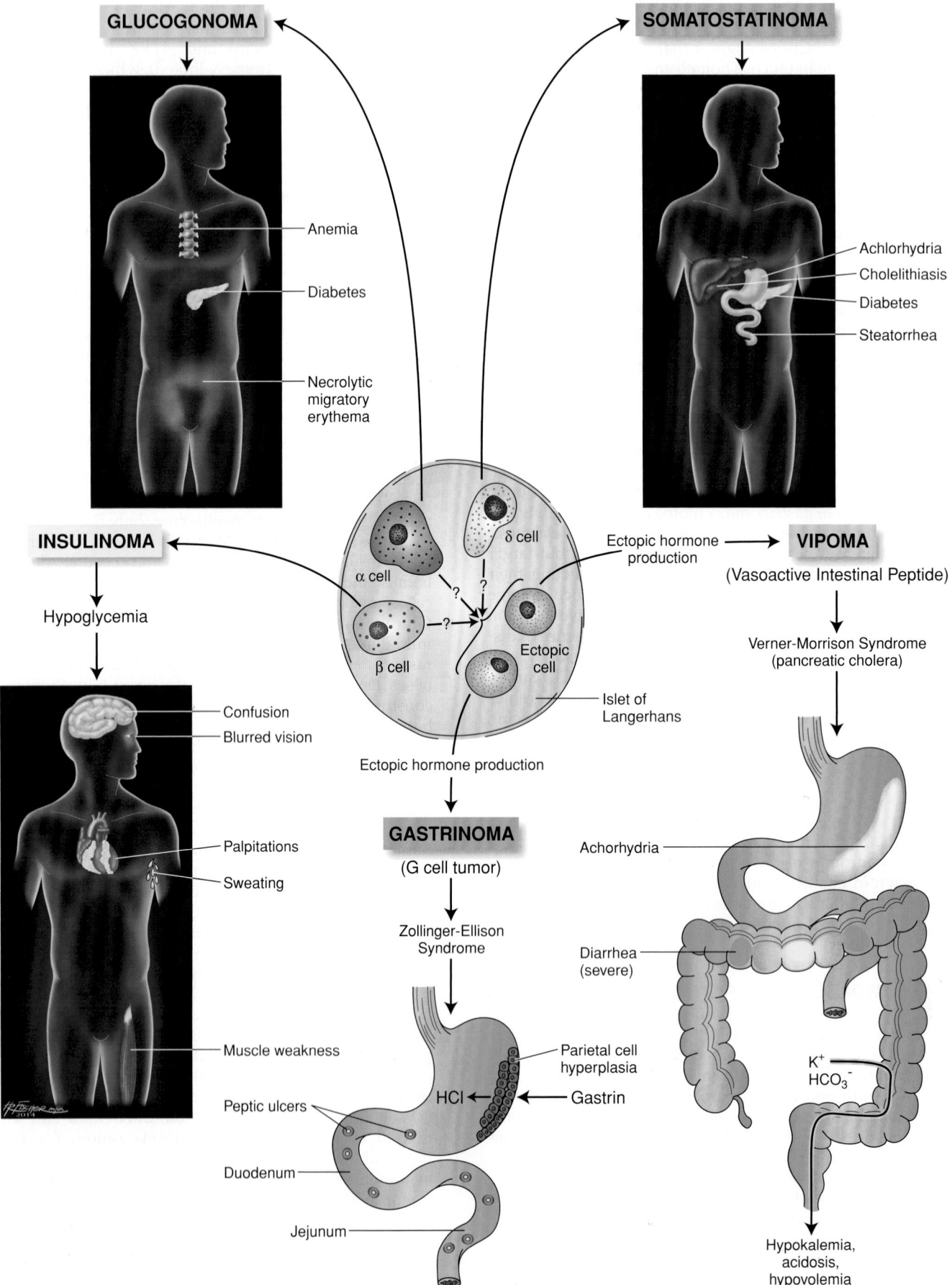

FIGURE 21-18. Syndromes associated with well-differentiated pancreatic neuroendocrine tumors.

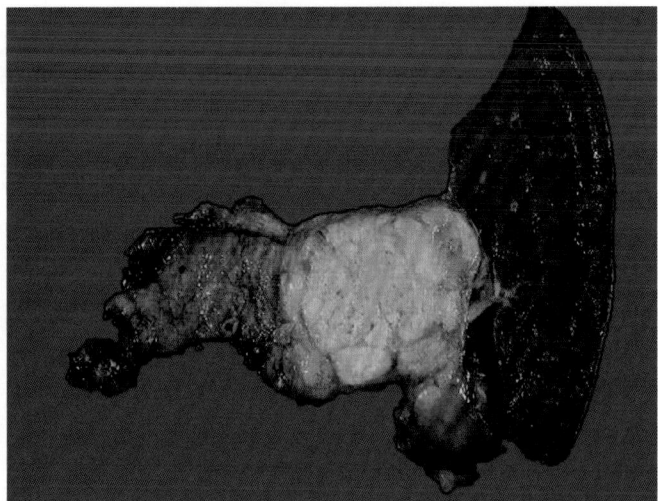

FIGURE 21-19. Well-differentiated pancreatic neuroendocrine tumor. This well-circumscribed somewhat nodular tumor was located in the tail of the pancreas near the spleen.

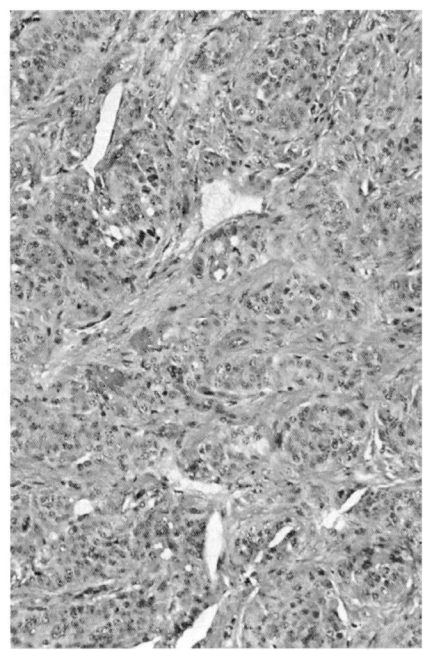

FIGURE 21-21. Insulinoma. Nests of tumor cells are surrounded by numerous capillaries.

evidence of a primary gastrinoma. Gastrinomas are most common between the ages of 30 and 50, with a slight male predominance. Most pancreatic examples arise in the head of the gland. Pancreatic gastrinomas are aggressive, although those arising in the duodenum usually remain localized, even when lymph node metastases are present.

- **VIPomas** are functioning PanNETs that produce vasoactive intestinal polypeptide (VIP). Like gastrin, VIP is not normally found in nonneoplastic islet cells but rather is made in ganglion cells and nerve fibers of the pancreas, gut and brain. VIP induces glycogenolysis and hyperglycemia and regulates ion and water secretion by the gastrointestinal epithelium. VIPomas induce Verner-Morrison syndrome, which is characterized by explosive and profuse watery diarrhea, hypokalemia and achlorhydria (also known as WDHA syndrome or pancreatic cholera). VIPomas are rare (3%–8% of all PanNETs and 10% of functioning PanNETs) and are usually large and solitary.

- PanNETs may rarely secrete **other hormones not ordinarily produced by the pancreas (ectopic hormones),** including adrenocorticotropic hormone (ACTH), parathyroid hormone, calcitonin and vasopressin. These ectopic hormones may be produced either alone or in combination

with normally occurring pancreatic hormones. Pancreatic polypeptide can also be secreted by some PanNETs, dubbed "PPomas," but no specific clinical syndrome is attributed to this hormone, so technically PPomas are clinically nonfunctioning.

PATHOLOGY: Other than the smaller size for insulinomas, functioning and nonfunctioning PanNETs appear similar. They are usually solitary, circumscribed masses of pink to tan, soft tissue (Fig. 21-19). Larger tumors are multinodular and have areas of hemorrhage. Cystic degeneration can occur, or some cases are firm and fibrotic. They have uniform cells, arranged in so-called organoid patterns, including nests, ribbons, glands and festoons (Figs. 21-20 and 21-21). Nuclei are uniform and the chromatin is coarsely stippled. The proliferative rate is low; by definition, there should be fewer than 20 mitotic figures in 10 high-power microscopic fields, and under 20% of nuclei should be positive for the immunohistochemical proliferation

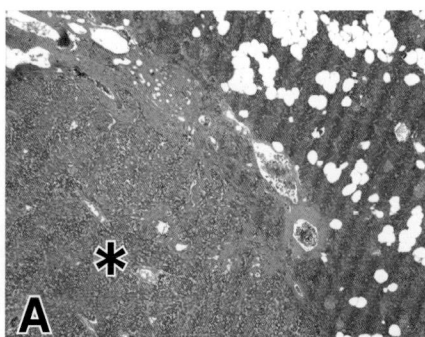
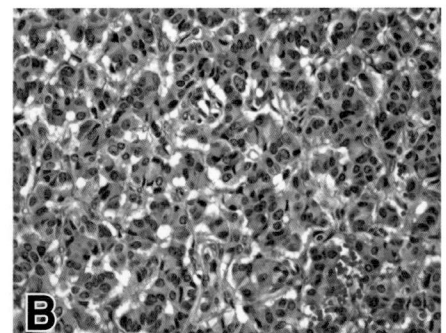
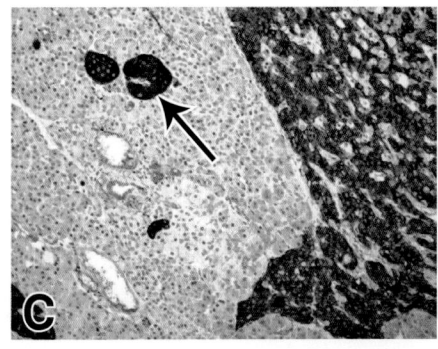

FIGURE 21-20. Well-differentiated pancreatic neuroendocrine tumor. A. The well-circumscribed nature of the tumor (*) can be appreciated at low power. **B.** A higher-power image showed the uniform neoplastic epithelioid cells to be arranged in cords. **C.** An immunohistochemical stain for chromogranin highlights tumor and the islets (*arrow*) within the adjacent pancreas.

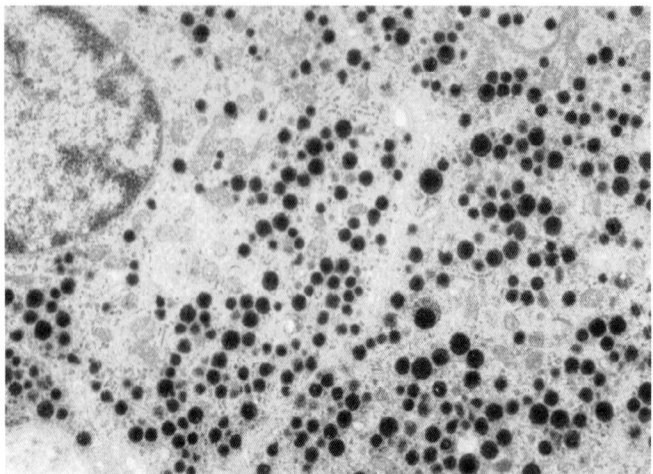

FIGURE 21-22. Alpha cells in a functional glucagonoma. The granules are indistinguishable from those of normal alpha cells (electron micrograph).

marker Ki67. Low- and intermediate-grade groups of Pan-NETs can be further defined based on these measures of proliferation, and the grade correlates well with prognosis. Sometimes the stroma contains amyloid, or it may be sclerotic.

Certain histologic patterns have been attributed to the various functioning types of PanNETs, but this relationship is loose at best and cannot be used to determine the cell type of the PanNET. The neuroendocrine nature of the tumor is demonstrated using immunohistochemistry with antibodies against chromogranin A (Fig. 21-20) and synaptophysin. Often, functioning PanNETs can be shown to produce the hormone responsible for the clinical syndrome using immunohistochemistry, but production of a number of different hormones in minor cell populations is not uncommon, even in clinically nonfunctioning PanNETs. Electron microscopy also shows characteristic neurosecretory granules (Fig. 21-22), and in some functioning PanNETs, granule morphology matches that of the specific granules in the nonneoplastic islet cell counterparts.

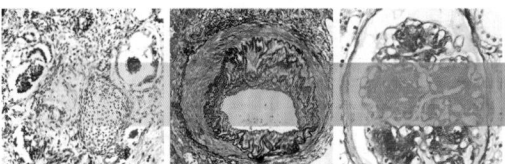

The Kidney

J. Charles Jennette

Anatomy

The kidneys are paired, bean-shaped organs located on both sides of the vertebral column in the retroperitoneal space. Adult kidneys average 150 g and are approximately 11 cm long, 6 cm wide and 3 cm thick. Each kidney consists of an outer cortex and an inner medulla (Fig. 22-1). When a kidney is bisected, the medulla has approximately 12 pyramids, with their bases at the corticomedullary junction. A medullary pyramid and its overlying cortex constitute a renal lobe. A pyramid has an inner and an outer zone.

The inner zone, the **papilla,** empties into a calyx, a funnel-shaped structure that conducts urine into the renal pelvis, which empties into the ureter.

BLOOD VESSELS

The kidney is one of the most vascular organs in the body and receives about 20%–25% of the cardiac output. The blood supply to each kidney usually derives from a single main renal artery, although 1/4 of kidneys have one or more

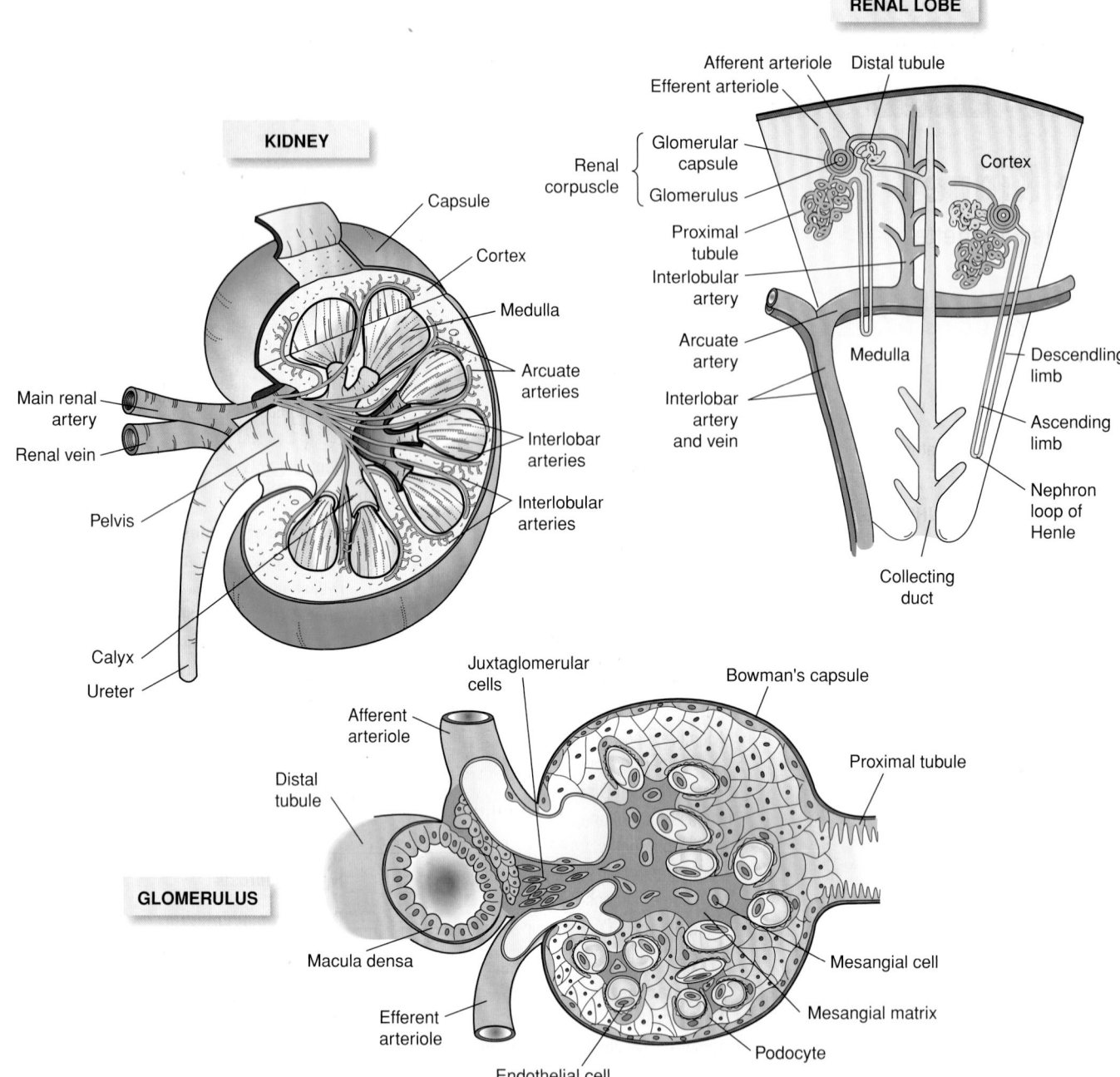

FIGURE 22-1. The gross and microscopic anatomy of the kidney.

accessory renal arteries. Before entering the renal parenchyma, the renal artery divides into anterior and posterior branches, which in turn give rise to interlobar arteries (Fig. 22-1). The latter branch into arcuate arteries, which run parallel to the renal surface near the corticomedullary junction. Interlobular arteries arise from the arcuate arteries and extend toward the renal surface, giving off afferent arterioles, each of which supplies a single glomerulus. Efferent arterioles drain the glomeruli and then branch into capillaries. Those in the outer cortex give rise to capillaries that supply blood to the cortical parenchyma, and those in the deep cortex, adjacent to the medulla, provide vessels that extend into the medulla to become the medullary peritubular vessels, the **vasa recta**.

The Glomerulus Is the Renal Filter

The **nephron** is the functional unit of the kidney and includes the glomerulus and its tubule, the latter terminating at a common collecting system (Fig. 22-1). The glomerulus is a specialized network of capillaries covered by epithelial cells called **podocytes** and supported by modified smooth muscle cells called **mesangial cells** (Figs. 22-1, 22-2, 22-3, 22-4). As it enters the glomerulus, the afferent arteriole branches into capillaries, which form the convoluted glomerular tuft and eventually coalesce into the efferent arteriole that exits the glomerulus. Glomerular capillaries are lined by fenestrated endothelial cells lying on a basement membrane. The outer surface of this basement membrane is covered by podocytes.

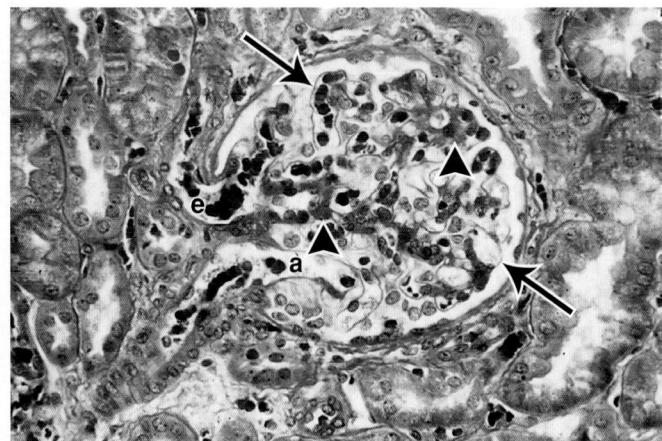

FIGURE 22-2. Normal glomerulus, light microscopy. The Masson trichrome stain shows a glomerular tuft with delicate blue capillary wall basement membranes (*arrows*), small amounts of blue matrix (*arrowheads*) surrounding mesangial cells and the hilum on the left. The afferent arteriole (*a*) enters below, and the efferent arteriole (*e*) exits above.

The Bowman space lies between the podocytes and the epithelial cells that line the Bowman capsule.

Glomerular Basement Membrane

The glomerular basement membrane (GBM) (Figs. 22-3, 22-4, 22-5) separates endothelial cells from podocytes in peripheral

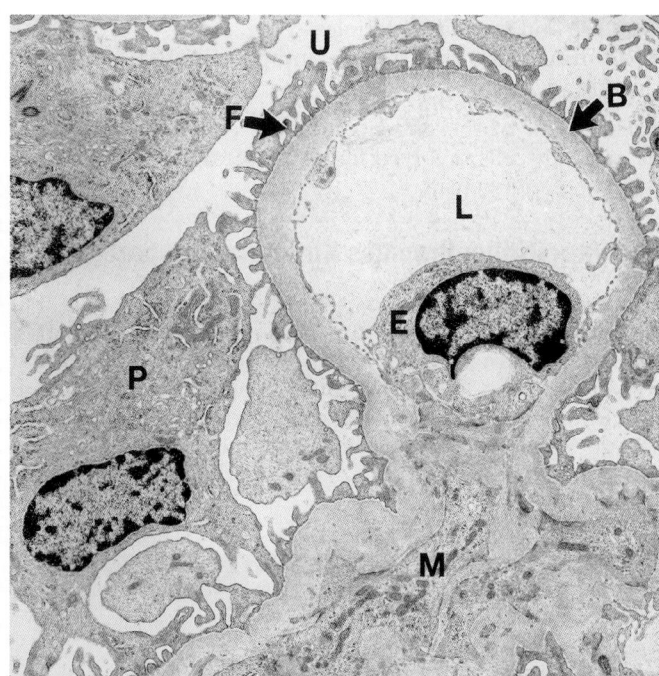

FIGURE 22-3. Normal glomerular capillary. In this electron micrograph of a single capillary loop and adjacent mesangium, the capillary wall portion of the lumen (L) is lined by a thin layer of fenestrated endothelial cytoplasm (shown at higher magnification in Fig. 22-5) that extends out from the endothelial cell body (E). The endothelial cell body is in direct contact with the mesangium, which includes the mesangial cell (M) and adjacent matrix. The outer aspect of the basement membrane (B) is covered by foot processes (F) from the podocyte (P) that line the urinary space (U). Compare this figure with Figs. 22-4 and 22-5.

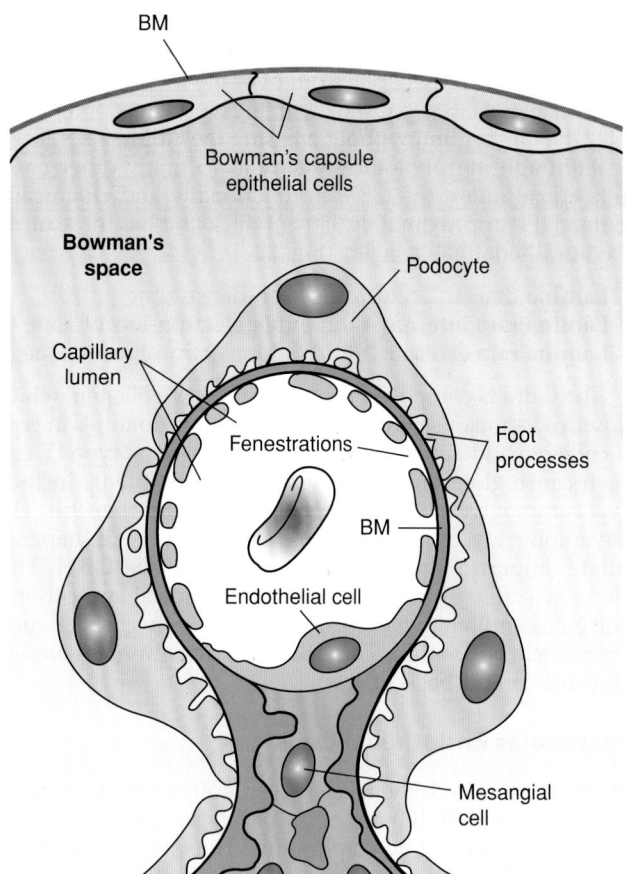

FIGURE 22-4. Normal glomerulus. The relationship of the different glomerular cell types to the basement membrane and mesangial matrix is illustrated using a single glomerular loop. The entire outer aspect of the glomerular basement membrane (peripheral loop and stalk) is covered by the visceral epithelial cell (podocyte) foot processes. The outer portions of the fenestrated endothelial cell are in contact with the inner surface of the basement membrane, whereas the central part is in contact with the mesangial cell and adjacent mesangial matrix. Compare with Fig. 22-3.

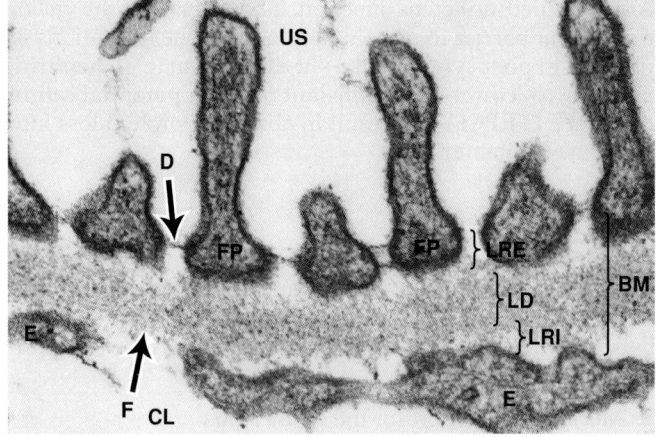

FIGURE 22-5. The glomerular filter. An electron micrograph illustrates the structures of the glomerular filter. Molecules that pass from the capillary lumen (CL) to the urinary space (US) traverse the fenestrations (F) of the endothelial cell (E), the trilaminar basement membrane (BM) (lamina rara interna [LRI], lamina densa [LD] and lamina rara externa [LRE]) and the slit pore diaphragm (D) that connects podocyte foot processes (FP).

capillary walls and also podocytes from the mesangium. Since the GBM does not completely surround each capillary lumen, but rather splays out over the mesangium as the paramesangial GBM, substances in the blood may potentially enter the mesangium without crossing the GBM.

Although morphologically similar to many other basement membranes, the GBM is functionally and chemically distinct. It is approximately 350 nm thick and has three ultrastructurally definable layers (Fig. 22-5):

- **Lamina densa:** A central electron-dense zone
- **Lamina rara interna:** A thin inner electron-lucent zone
- **Lamina rara externa:** A thin outer electron-lucent zone

The GBM is composed mainly of type IV collagen, which provides its major scaffolding. Genetic abnormalities in type IV collagen and autoantibodies directed against type IV collagen cause glomerular disease. Other constituents include glycosaminoglycans, laminin, entactin and fibronectin. The polyanionic glycosaminoglycans, which are rich in heparan sulfate, impart a strong negative charge to the GBM. This allows selective filtration of electrically neutral and cationic molecules and relative exclusion of negatively charged molecules such as albumin. The GBM also discriminates among molecules on the basis of size.

Glomerular Endothelial Cells

The glomerular endothelial cell layer is 50 nm thick and contains numerous 60–100-nm pores or fenestrations (Fig. 22-5) that are not spanned by diaphragms. Thus, they permit passage of fluid, ions and proteins (Fig. 22-4). Endothelial surface membrane proteins (e.g., adhesion molecules) and endothelial secretory products (e.g., prostaglandins and nitric oxide) play important roles in the pathogenesis of inflammatory and thrombotic glomerular diseases (Figs. 22-4, 22-5).

Podocytes

Podocytes rest on the outer aspect of the GBM and send cytoplasmic projections, **foot processes,** onto the lamina rara externa of the GBM (Fig. 22-5). Between adjacent foot processes is a thin membrane called the **slit diaphragm,** which is a modified adherens junction. Podocytes are the major glomerular barrier to protein loss in the urine. Mutations in proteins in podocytes and the slit diaphragm (e.g., **nephrin, podocin, α-actinin-4** and **transient receptor potential cation channel 6 [TRPC6]**) can result in abnormal protein loss into the urine (proteinuria).

Mesangium

The mesangium is a cellular and matrix network that supports the glomerulus. Mesangial cells are modified smooth muscle cells situated in the center of the glomerular tuft between capillary loops. Important functions of the mesangium are:

- Mechanical support for the glomerulus
- Endocytosis and processing of plasma proteins, including immune complexes
- Maintenance of basement membrane and matrix elements
- Modulation of glomerular filtration by mesangial cell contractility
- Generation of molecular mediators (e.g., prostaglandins and cytokines)

Tubules Comprise Most of the Nephron

The major segments of the tubule that arise from each glomerulus are the proximal tubule, loop of Henle and distal tubule, which empties into the collecting duct. At the origin of the proximal tubule from the glomerulus, the flat epithelium of the Bowman capsule abruptly transforms into tall columnar cells of the **proximal tubule,** which have numerous tall microvilli that form a brush border. The initial segment is very tortuous and is called the **proximal convoluted tubule.** As it descends into the medulla, the proximal tubule straightens into the thick **descending limb of the loop of Henle.** Further into the medulla, the thick descending limb thins into the **thin limb of the loop of Henle,** which eventually loops back toward the cortex.

Approaching the cortex, the thin limb becomes the **thick ascending limb.** This abuts the glomerulus from which it arose, contributes to that glomerulus' juxtaglomerular apparatus and then becomes the **distal convoluted tubule.** Several distal tubules unite to form a **collecting duct,** which ultimately empties into the ducts of Bellini, which discharge urine through the papillae into the calyces.

The Juxtaglomerular Apparatus Secretes Renin and Angiotensin

The juxtaglomerular apparatus is at the hilus of the glomerulus and consists of:

- **Macula densa,** a region of the thick ascending limb of the loop of Henle that has closely packed nuclei
- **Extraglomerular mesangial cells,** between the macula densa and the hilar arterioles
- **Terminal afferent arteriole** and **proximal efferent arteriole**

The wall of the afferent arteriole contains characteristic granular cells involved in the synthesis and secretion of renin and angiotensin.

The Interstitium Provides Structural Support

The renal interstitium is composed of interstitial cells that resemble fibroblasts and surrounding collagenous matrix. The interstitium occupies only 10% of cortical volume but constitutes 20%–30% of medullary volume. In addition to providing structural support, some cortical interstitial cells secrete erythropoietin and some medullary cells elaborate prostaglandins.

Congenital and Inherited Renal Diseases

CONGENITAL ANOMALIES

Potter Sequence Results from Insufficient Amniotic Fluid

Potter sequence (oligohydramnios sequence) is a syndrome of pathologic abnormalities that are caused by markedly

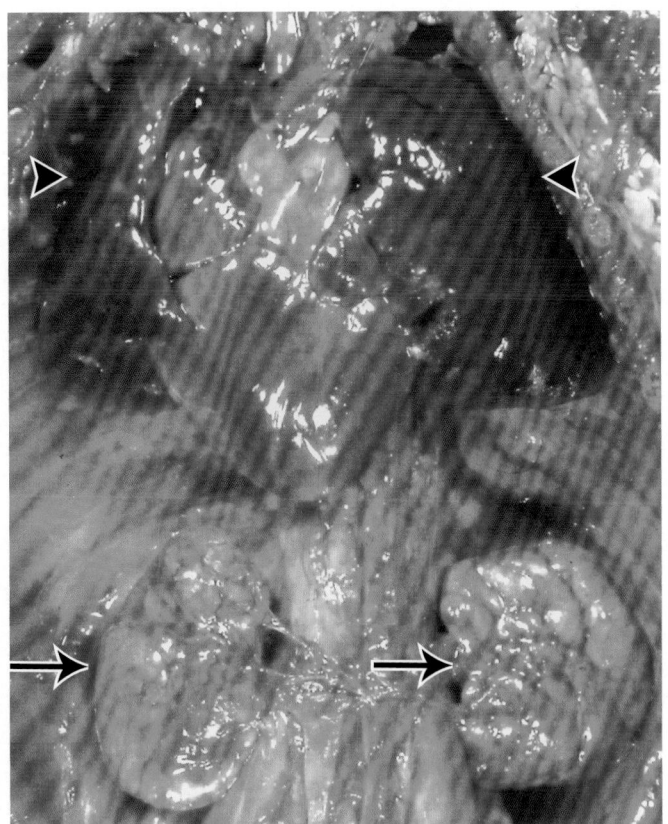

FIGURE 22-6. Bilateral renal agenesis. The Potter sequence includes congenitally nonfunctional kidneys, pulmonary hypoplasia and many other anomalies. In this case, there was bilateral renal agenesis, with only mesenchymal elements in the renal rudiments (*arrows*). Consequently, the lungs were hypoplastic (*arrowheads*). This infant was stillborn.

reduced intrauterine urine production (also see Chapter 6). Reduced urine production due, for example, to bilateral renal agenesis (Fig. 22-6) results in less amniotic fluid (oligohydramnios). The amniotic fluid normally cushions the fetus. With less fluid, the fetus is compressed by the uterus. This compression causes flattening of the face with low-set ears, a small receding chin and a beak-like nose; it also restricts movement of the arms and legs, often leading to abnormally bent lower extremities. The most life-threatening component of Potter sequence is pulmonary hypoplasia (Fig. 22-6), which is caused by inadequate maturational stimuli from amniotic fluid and by compression of the chest wall by the uterus. Because even neonates can be dialyzed, severe respiratory insufficiency due to Potter sequence (rather than renal insufficiency) may be the cause of death in infants with severe congenital renal anomalies.

Renal Agenesis Is the Complete Absence of Renal Tissue

Most infants born with bilateral renal agenesis (Fig. 22-6) are stillborn and have Potter sequence. Bilateral agenesis is often associated with other anomalies, especially elsewhere in the urinary tract or lower extremities. Unilateral renal agenesis is not serious if there are no associated anomalies, as the contralateral kidney hypertrophies sufficiently to maintain

normal renal function. If unilateral renal agenesis is accompanied by hypoplasia of the contralateral kidney, there is an increased risk for developing progressive glomerular sclerosis (secondary focal segmental glomerulosclerosis [FSGS]) due to overwork of nephrons.

In Renal Hypoplasia, Kidneys Are Histologically Normal but Smaller

Congenital hypoplastic kidneys are formed by six or fewer renal lobes (medullary pyramids with overlying cortex). Hypoplasia must be differentiated from small kidneys due to atrophy or scarring. A frequent variant of hypoplasia features enlargement of the too few glomeruli and thus is called **oligomeganephronia**. This enlargement indicates overwork of too few nephrons and predisposes to developing FSGS.

Renal Ectopia Is a Normal Kidney in an Abnormal Location

The misplaced kidney is usually in the pelvis, due to failure of the fetal kidney to migrate from the pelvis to the flank. One or both kidneys may be affected. In **simple ectopia,** the ureters drain into the appropriate side of the bladder. In **crossed ectopia,** the ectopic kidney is on the same side as its normal mate; the ectopic ureter crosses the midline and drains into the contralateral side of the bladder.

Horseshoe Kidney Is a Single, Large, Midline Organ

The kidneys are fused, usually at the lower poles (Fig. 22-7). This anomaly increases the risk for obstruction and renal

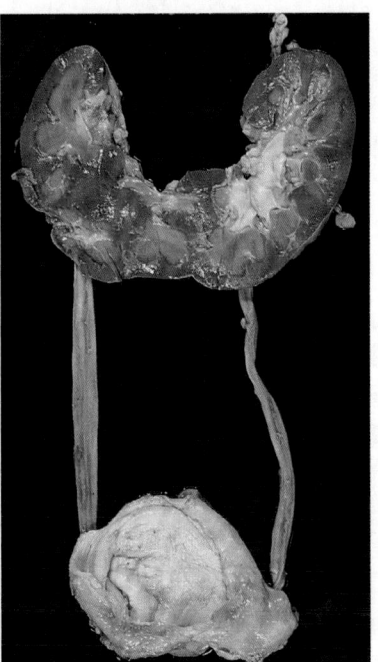

FIGURE 22-7. Horseshoe kidney. The kidneys are fused at the lower pole.

infection (pyelonephritis) because the ureters are compressed as they cross over the junction between the two kidneys when the organ is fused at the lower pole.

In Renal Dysplasia, Primitive Mesenchyme Surrounds Undifferentiated Tubules

This mesenchyme sometimes contains heterotopic tissue such as cartilage. Cysts often form from the abnormal tubules.

PATHOPHYSIOLOGY: Renal dysplasia results from abnormal metanephric differentiation and has multiple genetic and somatic causes. Some familial forms of dysplasia probably result from abnormal differentiation signals that affect the inductive interactions between the ureteric bud and the metanephric blastema. Many forms of dysplasia are accompanied by other urinary tract abnormalities, especially ones that cause obstruction of urine flow. This association suggests that obstruction to urine flow in utero can cause dysplasia. Frequent associated anomalies include:

- Ureteral agenesis
- Ureteral atresia
- Ureteropelvic junction obstruction
- Ureterovesical stenosis or posterior urethral valves

PATHOLOGY: The histologic hallmark of renal dysplasia is undifferentiated tubules and ducts lined by cuboidal or columnar epithelium. These

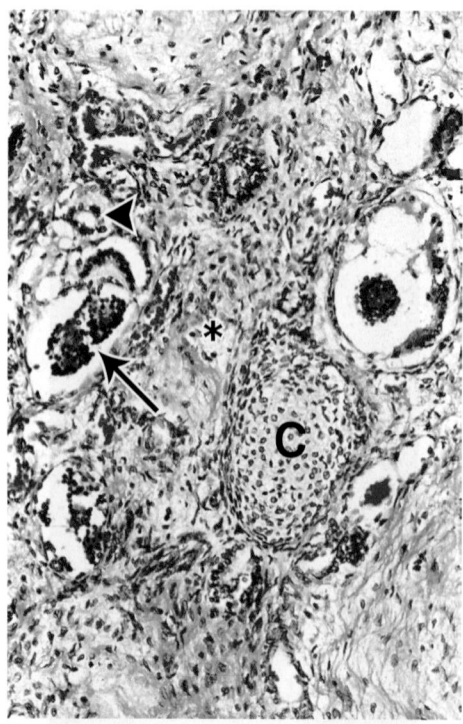

FIGURE 22-8. Renal dysplasia. Immature glomeruli (*arrow*), tubules (*arrowhead*) and cartilage (*C*) are surrounded by loose, undifferentiated mesenchymal tissue (*).

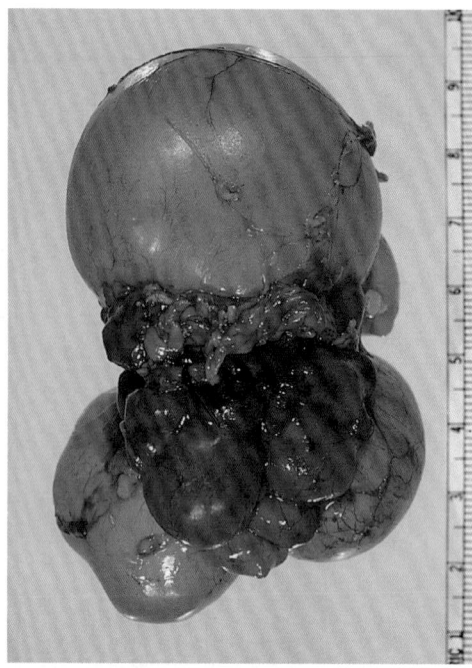

FIGURE 22-9. Multicystic renal dysplasia. An irregular mass of variably sized cysts does not have a reniform shape.

structures are surrounded by mantles of undifferentiated mesenchyme that may contain smooth muscle and islands of cartilage (Fig. 22-8). Rudimentary glomeruli may be seen, and tubules and ducts may be cystically dilated. Renal dysplasia can be unilateral or bilateral, and the affected kidney may be quite large or very small:

- **Aplastic renal dysplasia** results in very small misshapen dysplastic kidneys, which may be difficult to identify by gross examination.
- **Multicystic renal dysplasia** is usually unilateral and is characterized by renal enlargement by multiple cysts, ranging from microscopic to several centimeters in diameter. The kidney does not have the usual kidney shape but is rather an irregular mass of cysts (Fig. 22-9).
- **Diffuse cystic renal dysplasia** features more uniformly sized cysts and preservation of a kidney shape.
- **Obstructive renal dysplasia,** focal or diffuse, unilateral or bilateral, is caused by intrauterine obstruction to urine flow, such as posterior urethral valves or ureteropelvic junction stenosis.

CLINICAL FEATURES: In most patients with multicystic renal dysplasia, a palpable flank mass is discovered shortly after birth, although small multicystic kidneys may not be apparent until years later. *Unilateral multicystic renal dysplasia is the most common cause of an abdominal mass in newborns* and is adequately treated by removing the affected kidney. Bilateral aplastic dysplasia and diffuse cystic dysplasia cause oligohydramnios and the resultant Potter sequence and life-threatening pulmonary hypoplasia. Aplastic renal dysplasia and diffuse cystic dysplasia are more often hereditary than multicystic dysplasia, especially if they are associated with multiple anomalies in other organs, as in Meckel-Gruber syndrome.

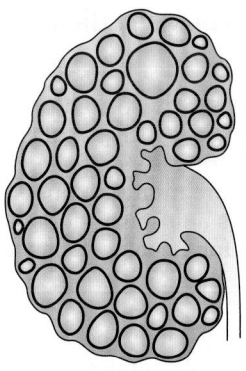
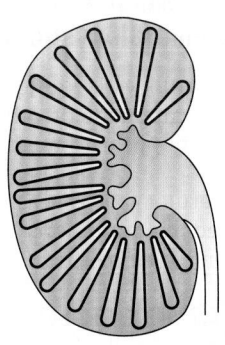

Autosomal dominant
polycystic disease

Autosomal recessive
polycystic disease

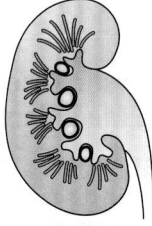
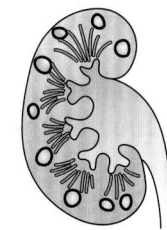

Medullary
sponge kidney

Medullary cystic
disease

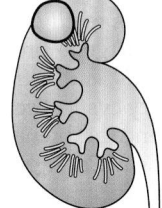

Simple cyst

FIGURE 22-10. Cystic diseases of the kidney.

In Autosomal Dominant Polycystic Kidney Disease, Kidneys Are Enlarged and Multicystic

Autosomal dominant polycystic kidney disease (ADPKD) is the most common of a group of congenital diseases in which the renal parenchyma contains many cysts (Fig. 22-10). It affects 1:400–1:1000 people in the United States, 1/2 of whom eventually develop end-stage renal failure. ADPKD is responsible for 5% of end-stage renal disease (ESRD) requiring dialysis or transplantation. Only diabetes and hypertension cause more ESRD than does ADPKD.

 MOLECULAR PATHOGENESIS: Some 85% of ADPKD is caused by mutations in polycystic kidney disease 1 gene (*PKD1*) and 15% by mutations in *PKD2*. The products of these genes, polycystin-1 and polycystin-2, are in the primary cilia of tubular epithelial cells and in cell–cell adhesion complexes. These structures sense the extracellular environment including urine flow, resulting in regulation of intracellular calcium and of tubule epithelial proliferation, cell polarity and apoptosis. Defects in these proteins result in dysfunction of primary cilia (ciliopathy) that disrupt calcium signaling, cause disturbed cell polarity and induce tubular epithelial cell proliferation.

Although the precise pathogenesis of ADPKD remains unclear, it is held that cysts arise in segments of renal tubules from a few cells that proliferate abnormally. The tubule wall becomes covered by undifferentiated cells with large nuclei and only few microvilli. Concomitantly, a defective basement membrane just below the abnormal epithelium allows the affected tubule to dilate. Cyst fluid is initially derived from the glomerular filtrate, but eventually most cysts lose connection with the tubules, in which case fluid accumulates by transepithelial secretion. The cysts in ADPKD originate in fewer than 2% of nephrons. Thus, factors other than crowding of normal tissue by expanding cysts likely impair functional renal tissue. Apoptotic loss of renal tubules and accumulation of inflammatory mediators have been incriminated in the destruction of normal renal mass.

 PATHOLOGY: The kidneys in ADPKD both are markedly enlarged and weigh up to 4500 g (Fig. 22-11). The external contours are distorted by numerous cysts, as large as 5 cm, filled with a straw-colored fluid. These cysts are lined by cuboidal and columnar epithelium. Cysts arise from any point along the nephron, including glomeruli, proximal tubules, distal tubules and collecting ducts. Areas of normal renal parenchyma between the cysts undergo progressive atrophy and fibrosis as the disease advances with age.

Of patients with ADPKD, 1/3 also have **hepatic cysts,** whose lining resembles bile duct epithelium. Cysts occur in the spleen (10% of patients) and pancreas (5%) as well. **Cerebral aneurysms** occur in 1/5 of patients, and intracranial hemorrhage is the cause of death in 15% of patients with ADPKD. Interestingly, many patients with ADPKD also develop colonic diverticula.

CLINICAL FEATURES: Most patients with ADPKD do not manifest clinically until the fourth decade of life, which is why this condition was once

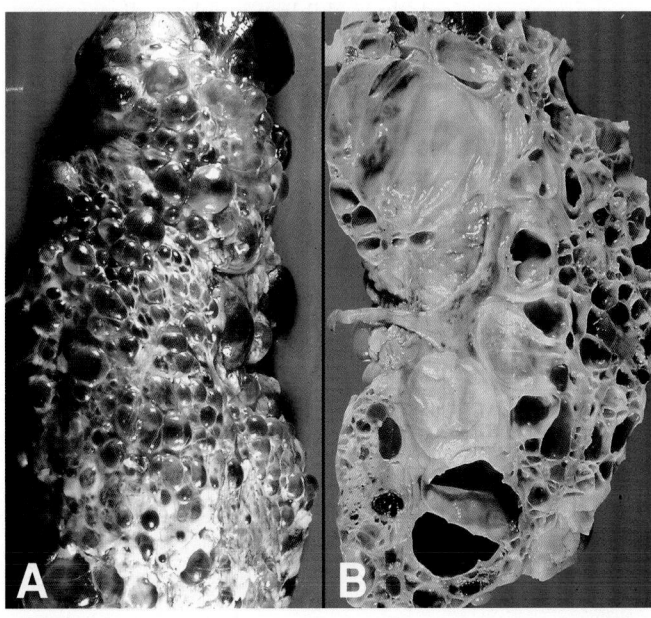

FIGURE 22-11. Autosomal dominant polycystic kidney disease. A. The kidneys are enlarged and studded with multiple fluid-filled structures. **B.** The parenchyma is almost entirely replaced by cysts of varying size.

called *adult* polycystic kidney disease. A small minority of patients develop symptoms during childhood, and rarely are they symptomatic at birth. Symptoms include a sense of heaviness in the loins, bilateral flank and abdominal pain, and abdominal masses. Hypertension is one of the earliest and most common manifestations. Eventually, hematuria, low-level proteinuria and progressive renal insufficiency develop.

Collecting Ducts Are Cystically Dilated in Infants with Autosomal Recessive Polycystic Kidney Disease

Compared with ADPKD, autosomal recessive polycystic kidney disease (ARPKD) is rare, occurring in about 1 in 6000–140,000 live births. In the neonatal period, 1/4 of these infants die, often because of pulmonary hypoplasia caused by oligohydramnios (Potter sequence) and because the large size of the kidneys impairs lung development and function. Children who survive the neonatal period have varying onset and rate of progression of renal insufficiency as well as hepatic fibrosis with portal hypertension.

 MOLECULAR PATHOGENESIS: ARPKD is caused by mutations in the *PKHD1* gene. The gene product, **fibrocystin,** is found in the primary cilia of the collecting ducts of the kidney, biliary ducts of the liver and exocrine ducts of the pancreas, and it appears to be involved in regulation of cell differentiation, proliferation and adhesion. Mutations of *PKHD1* also cause pancreatic cysts and hepatic biliary dysgenesis and fibrosis.

PATHOLOGY: Unlike ADPKD, the external kidney surface in ARPKD is smooth. The disease is invariably bilateral. The kidneys are often so large that delivery of the infant is impeded. The cysts are fusiform dilations of cortical and medullary collecting ducts and have a striking radial arrangement, perpendicular to the renal capsule (Fig. 22-12). Interstitial fibrosis and tubular atrophy are common, particularly in children in whom disease presents later. As in ADPKD, the calyceal system is normal. The liver is usually affected by **congenital hepatic fibrosis,** with fibrous expansion of portal tracts with bile duct proliferation (see Chapter 20).

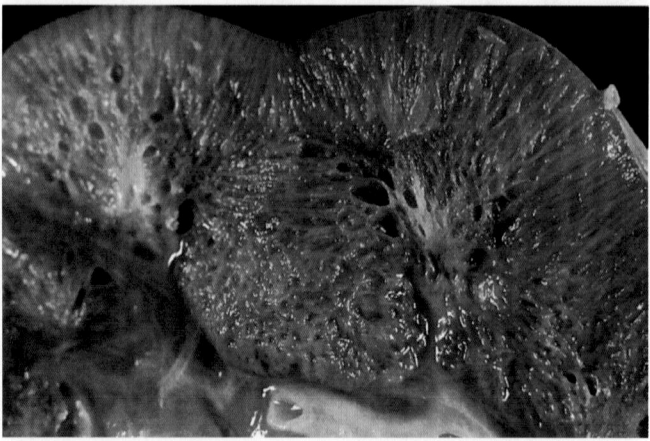

FIGURE 22-12. Autosomal recessive polycystic kidney disease. The dilated cortical and medullary collecting ducts are arranged radially, and the external surface is smooth.

The Bowman Capsule Is Dilated in Many Glomeruli in Glomerulocystic Disease

Glomerulocystic kidney disease may be an isolated process or a component of other cystic disease, such as ADPKD, nephronophthisis–medullary cystic disease complex and diffuse cystic dysplasia. Thus, there are multiple causes for glomerulocystic disease. One form is autosomal dominant, caused by mutations in the gene for hepatocyte nuclear factor-1β (HNF-1β).

 PATHOLOGY: The kidneys may be large or small. The cut surface reveals numerous small round cysts rarely of more than 1 cm. Light microscopy shows dilation of the Bowman capsule in many glomeruli. The residual glomerular tuft is often distorted or appears immature.

Nephronophthisis and Medullary Cystic Disease Cause Tubulointerstitial Injury and Medullary Cysts

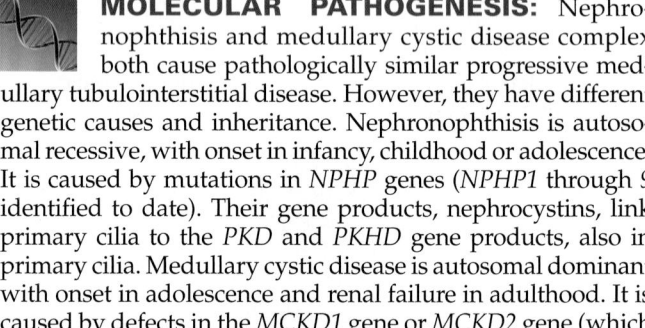 **MOLECULAR PATHOGENESIS:** Nephronophthisis and medullary cystic disease complex both cause pathologically similar progressive medullary tubulointerstitial disease. However, they have different genetic causes and inheritance. Nephronophthisis is autosomal recessive, with onset in infancy, childhood or adolescence. It is caused by mutations in *NPHP* genes (*NPHP1* through *9* identified to date). Their gene products, nephrocystins, link primary cilia to the *PKD* and *PKHD* gene products, also in primary cilia. Medullary cystic disease is autosomal dominant with onset in adolescence and renal failure in adulthood. It is caused by defects in the *MCKD1* gene or *MCKD2* gene (which codes for uromodulin).

 PATHOLOGY: The kidneys often, but not always, have multiple, variably sized cysts (up to 1 cm) at the corticomedullary junction (Fig. 22-10). These cysts arise from distal portions of the nephron. Atrophic tubules with markedly thickened and laminated basement membranes and loss of tubules out of proportion to glomerular loss are early histologic features of the disease. Eventually, corticomedullary cysts may develop, and the rest of the parenchyma becomes increasingly atrophic. Secondary glomerular sclerosis, interstitial fibrosis and nonspecific inflammatory infiltrates dominate the late histologic picture.

CLINICAL FEATURES: Patients present initially with deteriorating tubular function, such as impaired concentrating ability and sodium wasting, manifested as polyuria, polydipsia and enuresis (bedwetting). Progressive azotemia and renal failure follow. Nephronophthisis is seen in three clinical variants: infantile, juvenile and adolescent. The juvenile form is most common and accounts for 5%–10% of ESRD in children. Symptoms begin between 4 and 6 years, and ESRD usually develops within 10 years. The onset and progression to ESRD of adolescent nephronophthisis overlap with the juvenile form, but the adolescent form results from defects in *NEPH3* and more often causes ESRD at 10–20 years. Defects in *NPHP2* are most common in the infantile form, which progresses to ESRD before 2 years. Among all patients with nephronophthisis, the *NEPH1* mutation is most common.

Medullary cystic disease is characterized by onset of renal failure after the fourth decade and usually presents with polyuria. Hyperuricemia and gout may be accompanying findings.

Medullary Sponge Kidney Is Distinguished by Cysts in the Papillae

The papillary cysts are multiple and small (<5 mm in diameter) (Fig. 22-10), arise from collecting ducts in the renal papillae and are lined by cuboidal or columnar epithelium. The disease is bilateral in 75% of patients. A few familial cases have been described.

Medullary sponge kidney is asymptomatic in young adults. Symptomatic cases are usually discovered between the ages of 30 and 60 years, presenting with flank pain, dysuria, hematuria or "gravel" in the urine caused by stone formation in the cysts. Although the disease itself does not pose a threat to health, the cysts may predispose to secondary pyelonephritis.

ACQUIRED CYSTIC KIDNEY DISEASE

Simple Renal Cysts Occur in Half of People Older Than 50 Years

Simple cysts are usually incidental findings at autopsy and are rarely clinically symptomatic unless they are very large. They may be solitary or multiple and are usually found in the outer cortex, where they bulge the capsule. Simple cysts occur less commonly in the medulla. Microscopically, they are lined by flat epithelium.

Long-Term Dialysis Leads to Acquired Cystic Disease

Multiple cortical and medullary cysts may form in kidneys of patients with ESRD who are maintained on dialysis. After 5 years of dialysis, more than 75% of patients show bilateral cystic kidneys. The cysts are initially lined by flat-to-cuboidal epithelium, but hyperplastic and neoplastic epithelial proliferation may develop within 10 years of initiating dialysis. **Renal cell carcinoma (RCC)** develops in approximately 5% of patients with acquired cystic disease.

Acquired Nonneoplastic Diseases of the Kidney

GLOMERULAR DISEASES

Many renal disorders are caused by injury to the glomerulus. Glomeruli may be the only major site of disease (primary glomerular disease; e.g., immunoglobulin [Ig]A nephropathy) or part of a disease affecting several organs (secondary glomerular disease; e.g., lupus glomerulonephritis). Signs and symptoms of glomerular disease fall into one of the following categories:

- Asymptomatic proteinuria
- Nephrotic syndrome
- Asymptomatic hematuria
- Acute nephritic syndrome
- Rapidly progressive nephritic syndrome
- Chronic kidney injury
- ESRD

Proteinuria Exceeds 3.5 g/day in Nephrotic Syndrome

It is also characterized by hypoalbuminemia, edema, hyperlipidemia and lipiduria. Increased glomerular capillary permeability allows loss of protein from plasma into the urine (proteinuria). Proteinuria is caused by many different glomerular diseases and by a variety of mechanisms.

Severe proteinuria causes the nephrotic syndrome (Fig. 22-13), but lower levels of proteinuria may be asymptomatic. Nephrotic syndrome results from **primary** glomerular diseases unrelated to a systemic disease, or they may be **secondary** to a systemic disease that affects other organs as well as the kidneys. Diabetic glomerulosclerosis is the most common cause of secondary nephrotic syndrome in adults. Table 22-1 lists the major causes and approximate frequency of the primary nephrotic syndrome in adults and children. Table 22-2 details selected pathologic features of some of these diseases (discussed below).

There are important differences in the rates of specific glomerular diseases that cause nephrotic syndrome in adults versus those in children. For example, minimal-change disease is responsible for most (70%) cases of primary nephrotic syndrome in children, but only 15% in adults. The primary glomerular diseases that most often cause primary nephrotic syndrome in adults are membranous glomerulonephritis and FSGS. The most common cause of secondary nephrotic syndrome is diabetes. Membranous glomerulonephritis is the most frequent cause in whites and Asians, whereas FSGS is the most common etiology in American blacks. The incidence

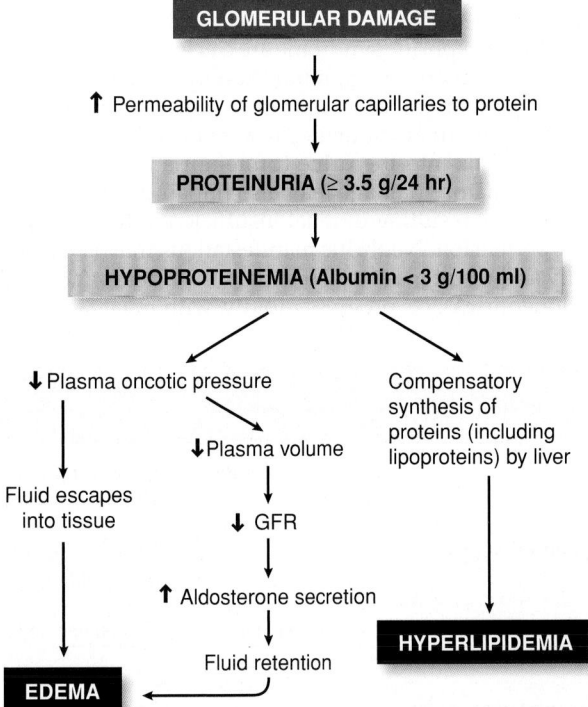

FIGURE 22-13. Pathophysiology of the nephrotic syndrome. GFR = glomerular filtration rate.

TABLE 22-1

FREQUENCY OF CAUSES FOR THE NEPHROTIC SYNDROME INDUCED BY PRIMARY GLOMERULAR DISEASES IN CHILDREN AND ADULTS

Cause	Children (%)	Adults (%)
Minimal-change disease	75	10
Membranous glomerulonephritis	5	30
Focal segmental glomerulosclerosis	10	35
Membranoproliferative glomerulone-phritis	5	5
Other glomerular diseases*	5	20

*Includes many forms of mesangioproliferative and proliferative glomerulonephritis, such as immunoglobulin A nephropathy, which may cause nephritic and nephrotic features.

TABLE 22-3

TENDENCIES OF GLOMERULAR DISEASES TO MANIFEST NEPHROTIC AND NEPHRITIC FEATURES

Disease	Nephrotic	Nephritic
Minimal-change disease	++++	–
Membranous glomerulonephritis	+++	++
Focal segmental glomerulosclerosis	+++	++
Mesangioproliferative glomerulonephritis*	++	++
Membranoproliferative glomerulonephritis	++	++
Proliferative glomerulonephritis*	+	+++
Crescentic glomerulonephritis*	+	++++

*These histologic phenotypes can be caused by many categories of glomerular disease, including immunoglobulin A nephropathy, postinfectious glomerulonephritis, lupus glomerulonephritis, antineutrophil cytoplasmic autoantibody glomerulonephritis, anti–glomerular basement membrane glomerulonephritis and C3 glomerulopathy.

of FSGS has been increasing over the past decade. Systemic diseases that involve the kidney, such as diabetes, amyloidosis and systemic lupus erythematosus (SLE), account for many cases of nephrotic syndrome in adults. In third world countries, where chronic infectious diseases are common, immune complex membranoproliferative glomerulonephritis (MPGN) is a much more frequent reason for nephrotic syndrome.

Nephritic (Glomerulonephritis) Syndrome Is an Inflammatory Disease with Hematuria, Proteinuria and Decreased Glomerular Filtration Rate

Hematuria may be microscopic or grossly visible, and proteinuria varies. Decreased GFR causes elevated blood urea nitrogen and serum creatinine, oliguria, salt and water retention, hypertension and edema. Glomerular diseases associated with the nephritic syndrome are caused by inflammatory changes in glomeruli (e.g., infiltration by leukocytes, hyperplasia of glomerular cells and, in severe lesions, necrosis). Injury to glomerular capillaries results in spillage of protein and blood cells into the urine (proteinuria and hematuria). The inflammatory damage may also impair glomerular flow and filtration, resulting in renal insufficiency, fluid retention and hypertension. Nephritic manifestations may (1) develop rapidly and result in reversible renal insufficiency (acute glomerulonephritis); (2) progress rapidly, with renal failure that

resolves only with aggressive treatment (rapidly progressive glomerulonephritis); or (3) persist for years continuously or intermittently and proceed slowly to renal failure (chronic glomerulonephritis).

Some glomerular diseases tend to cause the nephrotic syndrome, but others lead to the nephritic syndrome (Table 22-3). However, except for minimal-change disease (which almost always causes nephrotic syndrome), all glomerular diseases may occasionally cause mixed nephritic and nephrotic manifestations that confound clinical diagnosis. *Renal biopsy evaluation is the only means of definitive diagnosis for most glomerular diseases, although clinical and laboratory data may provide presumptive evidence for a specific disease.*

PATHOPHYSIOLOGY: Glomerulonephritis is often caused by immunologic mechanisms. Antibody- and cell-mediated immunity may both lead to glomerular inflammation, but three types of antibody-induced inflammation have been incriminated as the major pathogenetic processes in most forms of glomerulonephritis (Fig. 22-14). A less frequent cause of

TABLE 22-2

PATHOLOGIC FEATURES OF IMPORTANT CAUSES OF THE NEPHROTIC SYNDROME

	Minimal-Change Disease	Focal Segmental Glomerulosclerosis	Membranous Glomerulnephritis	Membranoproliferative Glomerulonephritis
Light microscopy	No lesion	Focal and segmental glomerular consolidation	Diffuse global capillary wall thickening	Capillary wall thickening and endo-capillary hypercellularity
Immunofluorescence microscopy	No immune deposits	No immune deposits	Diffuse capillary wall immunoglobulin	Diffuse capillary wall complement with or without immunoglobulin
Electron microscopy	No immune deposits	No immune deposits	Diffuse subepithelial deposits	Subendothelial dense deposits; intramembranous dense deposits (dense deposit disease)

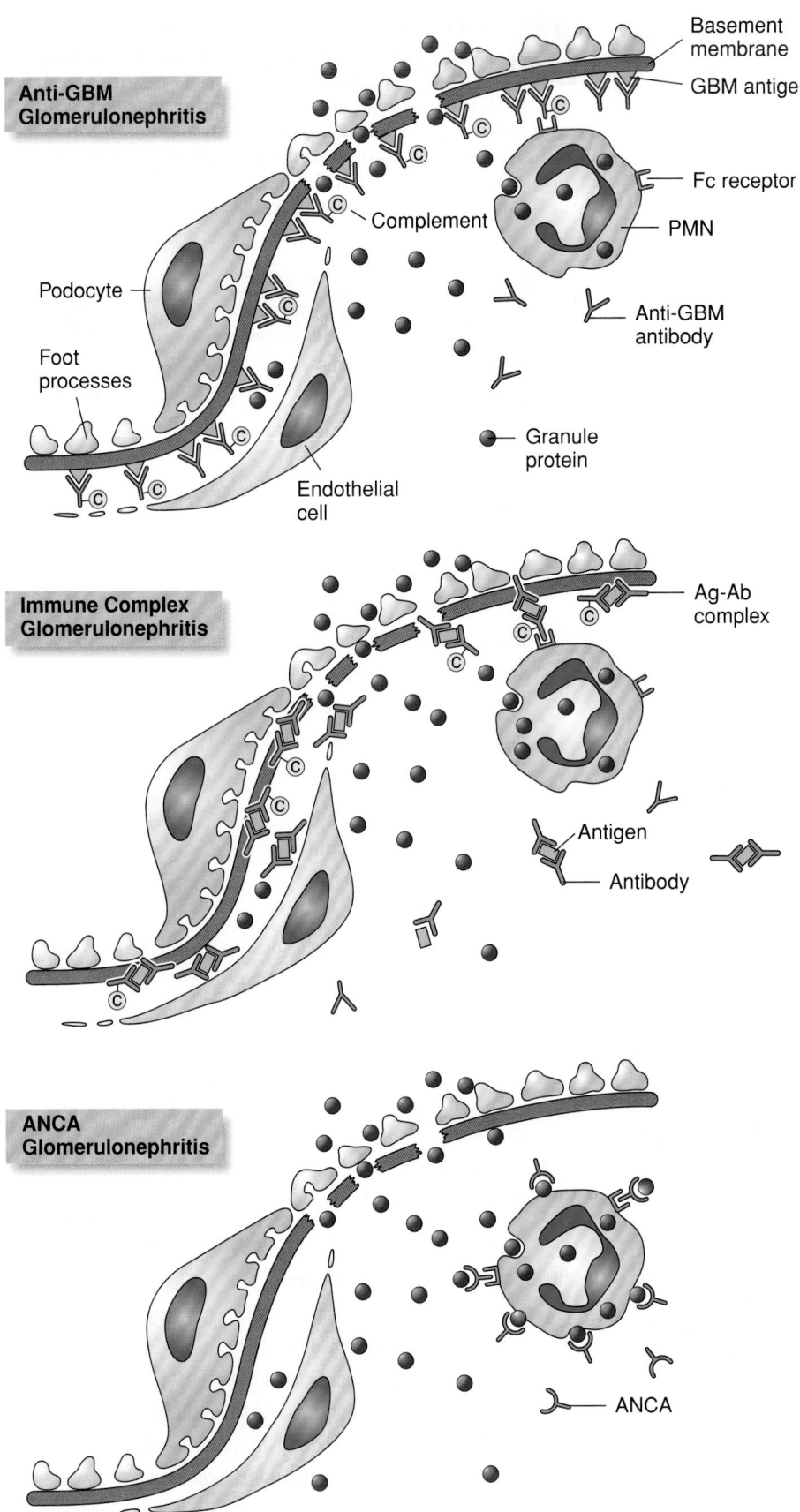

Anti-GBM Glomerulonephritis

- Basement membrane
- GBM antigen
- Fc receptor
- PMN
- Complement
- Anti-GBM antibody
- Podocyte
- Foot processes
- Granule protein
- Endothelial cell

Immune Complex Glomerulonephritis

- Ag-Ab complex
- Antigen
- Antibody

ANCA Glomerulonephritis

- ANCA

FIGURE 22-14. Antibody-mediated glomerulonephritis. Top panel. Anti–glomerular basement membrane (GBM) antibodies cause glomerulonephritis by binding in situ to basement membrane antigens. This activates complement and recruits inflammatory cells. PMN = polymorphonuclear neutrophil. **Middle panel.** Immune complexes that deposit from the circulation also activate complement and recruit inflammatory cells. Ag-Ab complex = antigen–antibody complex. **Bottom panel.** Antineutrophil cytoplasmic antibodies (ANCAs) cause inflammation by activating leukocytes by direct binding of the antibodies to the leukocytes and by Fc receptor engagement of ANCA bound to antigen.

THE KIDNEY

glomerulonephritis is dysregulation and uncontrolled activation of the alternative complement pathway.

- In situ immune complex formation
- Deposition of circulating immune complexes
- Antineutrophil cytoplasmic autoantibodies (ANCAs)
- Alternative pathway complement dysregulation

Immune complex formation in situ involves circulating antibodies binding to intrinsic antigens or foreign antigens within glomeruli. For example, anti-GBM autoantibodies bind a very specific epitope on the α4 chain of type IV collagen in GBMs. Resultant immune complexes in glomerular capillary walls attract leukocytes and activate complement and other humoral inflammatory mediators, resulting in inflammatory injury. In the most common form of primary membranous glomerulonephritis, immune complexes form in situ between an antigen produced by podocytes, phospholipase A_2 receptor (PLA$_2$R) and anti-PLA$_2$R antibodies from the circulation.

Circulating immune complexes may deposit in glomeruli and incite inflammation like that produced when immune complexes form in situ. For example, circulating antibodies can bind to antigens released into the blood by bacterial or viral infection to produce immune complexes. If these complexes escape phagocytosis, they can deposit in glomeruli and incite inflammation. Immunofluorescence microscopy detects such immune complexes in glomeruli. Anti-GBM antibodies produce linear staining of GBMs, but other immune complexes produce granular staining in capillary walls, mesangium or both.

Antineutrophil cytoplasmic autoantibodies cause severe glomerulonephritis with little or no glomerular immunoglobulin deposition. Such patients often have circulating autoantibodies specific for antigens in the cytoplasm of neutrophils, which activate them and so mediate glomerular inflammation. Most ANCAs are directed against myeloperoxidase (MPO-ANCA) or proteinase-3 (PR3-ANCA). Even minor stimulation of neutrophils and monocytes, such as by increased circulating levels of cytokines during viral infection, causes them to express surface MPO and PR3, which then can interact with ANCAs. This interaction activates neutrophils and causes them to adhere to microvascular endothelial cells, especially glomerular capillaries. There, they release products that promote vascular inflammation, including glomerulonephritis, arteritis and venulitis. This inflammation is amplified by release of factors from ANCA-activated neutrophils that activate the alternative complement pathway.

Formation of glomerular immune complexes in situ, deposition of immune complexes and interaction of ANCAs with leukocytes all initiate glomerular inflammatory injury, with attraction and activation of leukocytes (Fig. 22-14).

A fourth immunopathology category of glomerulonephritis **(C3 glomerulopathy)** is mediated by dysregulation of the alternative complement pathway caused either by the genetic absence or dysfunction of complement regulatory proteins (e.g., complement factor H, complement factor I), autoantibodies that inhibit complement regulatory proteins or autoantibodies that stabilize the alternative pathway C3 convertase (C3 nephritis factor).

PATHOLOGY: Specific glomerular diseases have distinctive pathologic features, as well as different natural histories and appropriate treatments. *Accurate pathologic diagnosis of glomerular diseases requires examination of renal tissue by light, immunofluorescence and electron microscopy, and integration of these findings with clinical information.* Table 22-4 lists pathologic features useful in diagnosing glomerular diseases (see Table 22-2 for a

---

TABLE 22-4

DIAGNOSTIC FEATURES OF GLOMERULAR DISEASES

I. Light microscopic features

  A. Increased cellularity

    Infiltration by leukocytes (e.g., neutrophils, monocytes, macrophages)

    Proliferation of "endocapillary" cells (i.e., endothelial and mesangial cells)

    Proliferation of "extracapillary" cells (i.e., epithelial cells) (crescent formation)

  B. Increased extracellular material

    Localization of immune complexes

    Thickening or replication of GBM

    Increases in collagenous matrix (sclerosis)

    Insudation of plasma proteins (hyalinosis)

    Fibrinoid necrosis

    Deposition of amyloid

II. Immunofluorescence features

  A. Linear staining of GBM

    Anti-GBM antibodies

    Multiple plasma proteins (e.g., diabetic glomerulosclerosis)

    Monoclonal immunoglobulin chains

  B. Granular immune complex staining or complement staining alone

    Mesangium (e.g., IgA nephropathy)

    Capillary wall (e.g., membranous glomerulonephritis)

    Mesangium and capillary wall (e.g., lupus glomerulonephritis, C3 glomerulopathy)

  C. Irregular (fluffy) staining

    Monoclonal light chains (AL amyloidosis)

    AA protein (AA amyloidosis)

III. Electron microscopic features

  A. Electron-dense immune complex deposits or complement deposits

    Mesangial (e.g., IgA nephropathy)

    Subendothelial (e.g., lupus glomerulonephritis)

    Subepithelial (e.g., membranous glomerulonephritis)

  B. GBM thickening (e.g., diabetic glomerulosclerosis)

  C. GBM remodeling (e.g., membranoproliferative glomerulonephritis)

  D. Collagenous matrix expansion (e.g., focal segmental glomerulosclerosis)

  E. Fibrillary deposits (e.g., amyloidosis)

GBM = glomerular basement membrane; IgA = immunoglobulin A.

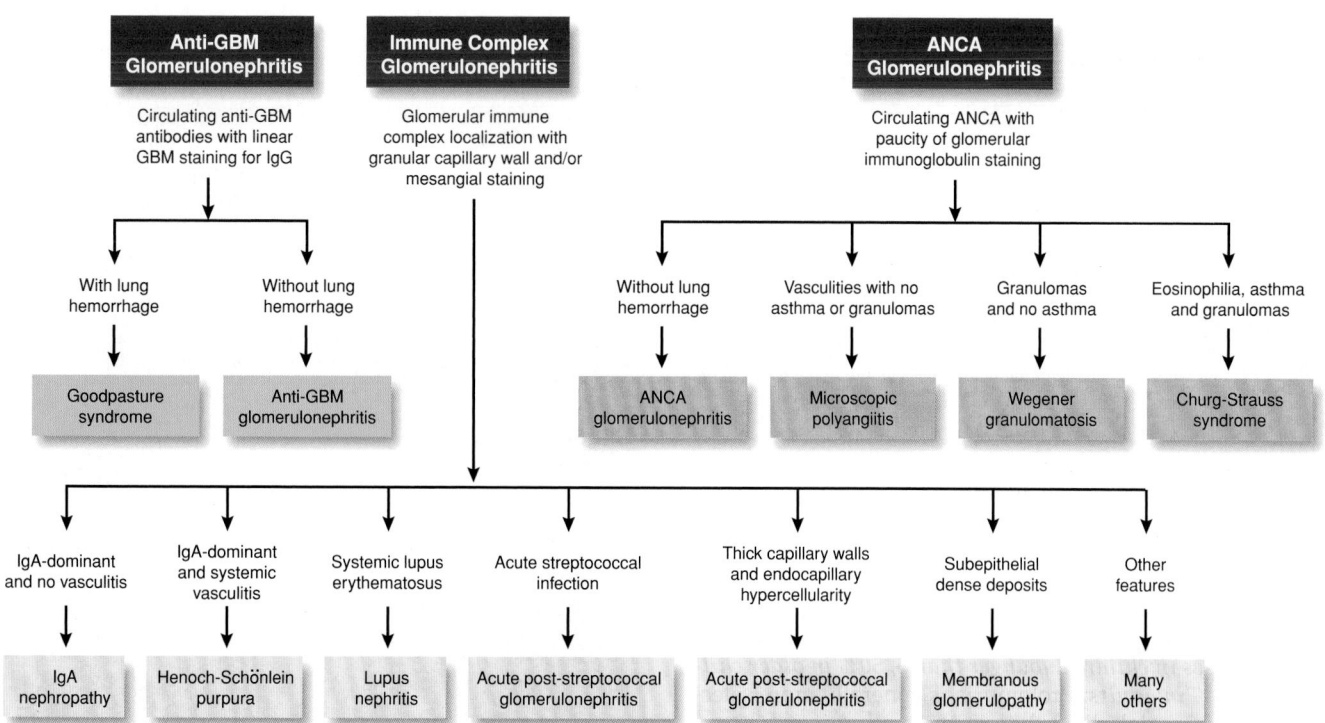

FIGURE 22-15. Algorithm demonstrating the integration of pathologic findings with clinical data to diagnose specific forms of primary or secondary glomerulonephritis. Note that an important initial categorization is as immune complex, anti–glomerular basement membrane (GBM), C3 or antineutrophil cytoplasmic autoantibody (ANCA) glomerulonephritis. Once this determination is made, more specific diagnoses depend on additional clinical or pathologic observations.

summary of pathologic features of important causes of the nephrotic syndrome). The algorithm in Fig. 22-15 shows how pathologic and clinical data mesh to diagnose specific glomerular diseases.

In general, pathologic features of acute inflammation, such as endocapillary and extracapillary hypercellularity, leukocyte infiltration and necrosis, are more common in disorders characterized mainly as nephritic than in those that are more typically nephrotic. **Glomerular crescent formation** (extracapillary proliferation) correlates with a more rapidly progressive course. Crescents are not specific for a particular cause of glomerular inflammation. They are, rather, markers of severe injury causing extensive rupture of capillary walls, which allows inflammatory mediators to enter the Bowman space, where they stimulate macrophage infiltration and epithelial proliferation.

Minimal-Change Disease Causes Nephrotic Syndrome

Pathologically, this disease entails effacement of podocyte foot processes.

PATHOPHYSIOLOGY: The pathogenesis of minimal-change disease is unknown. The immune system may be involved: the disease may remit with corticosteroid treatment, and it may occur in association with an allergic disease or a lymphoid neoplasm. Occasional associations with Hodgkin disease (in which there is T-cell dysfunction) and with thymomas and

T-cell lymphomas has led to speculation that minimal-change disease may reflect a disorder of T lymphocytes, possibly involving production of a cytokine that increases glomerular permeability via effects on podocytes. The heavy proteinuria of minimal-change disease is accompanied by loss of GBM and podocyte polyanionic sites. This allows anionic proteins, especially albumin, to pass more easily across capillary walls. There may be a pathogenic relationship between minimal-change disease and some forms of FSGS, with the potential for the former to evolve into the latter in some patients, but this has not been confirmed.

PATHOLOGY: *Glomeruli in minimal-change disease appear essentially normal on light microscopy* (Fig. 22-16). Proteinuria leads to hypoalbuminemia, and a compensatory increase in lipoprotein secretion by the liver results in hyperlipidemia. Loss of lipoproteins through glomeruli causes lipids to accumulate in proximal tubular cells, reflected histologically as glassy (hyaline) droplets in tubular epithelial cytoplasm. Such droplets are not specific for minimal-change disease but are seen in any glomerular disease causing nephrotic syndrome.

Electron microscopy shows extensive **fusion of podocyte cell foot processes** (Figs. 22-17, 22-18). This occurs in almost all cases of nephrotic range proteinuria; it is not specific for minimal-change disease. Immunofluorescence studies for immunoglobulin and complement deposition are most often negative, but there is occasional weak mesangial staining for IgM and the complement component C3.

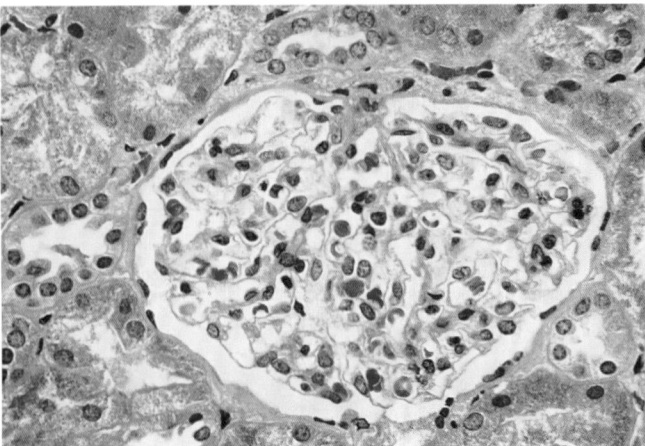

FIGURE 22-16. Minimal-change disease. A light micrograph shows no abnormality.

CLINICAL FEATURES: *Minimal-change disease causes 90% of primary nephrotic syndrome cases in children younger than 5, 50% in older children and 15% in adults.* Proteinuria is generally more selective (albumin > globulins) than in the nephrotic syndrome caused by other diseases, but there is too much overlap for this to be used as a diagnostic criterion. In more than 90% of

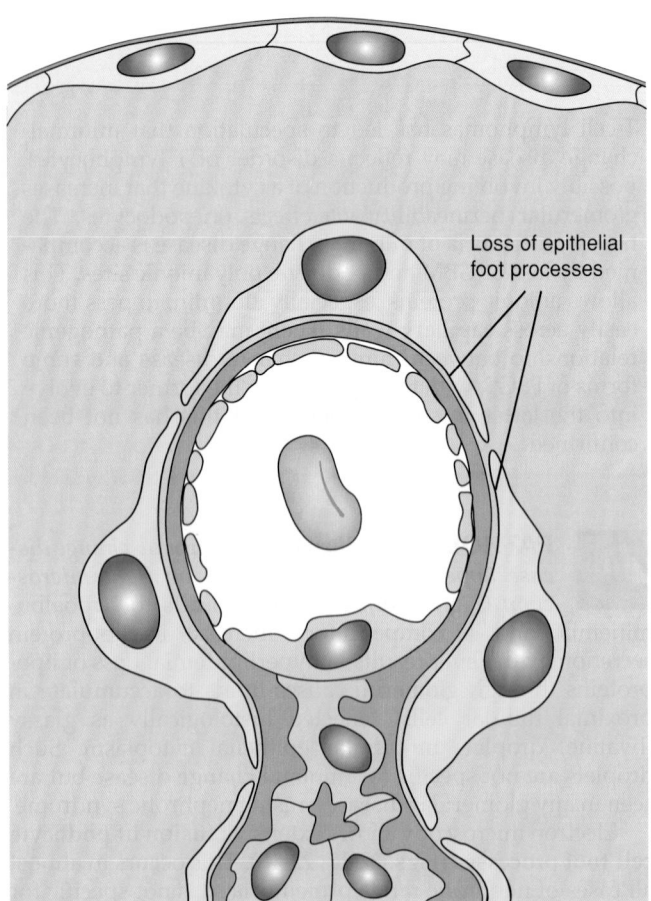

FIGURE 22-17. Minimal-change disease. This condition is characterized predominantly by epithelial cell changes, particularly effacement of foot processes. All other glomerular structures appear intact.

Loss of epithelial foot processes

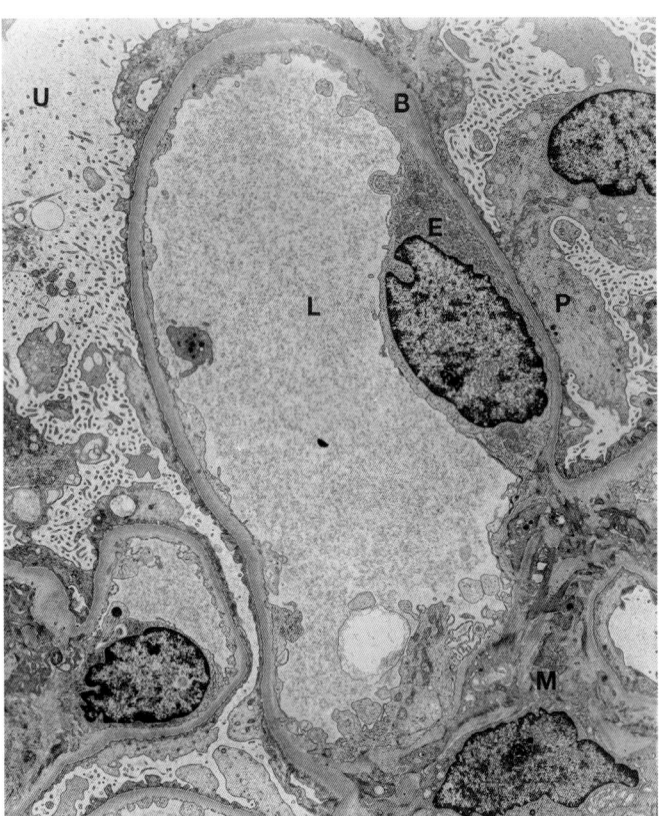

FIGURE 22-18. Minimal-change disease. In this electron micrograph, the podocyte (P) displays extensive effacement of foot processes and numerous microvilli projecting into the urinary space (U). B = basement membrane; E = endothelial cell; L = lumen; M = mesangial cell. Compare with Figure 22-3.

children and in fewer adults with minimal-change disease, proteinuria remits completely within 8 weeks of initiating corticosteroid therapy. Adults often require a longer course of steroids for remission. If corticosteroids are withdrawn, most patients have intermittent relapses for up to 10 years. A small subgroup of patients has only partial remission with corticosteroid therapy and continues to lose protein in the urine. An even smaller group is totally resistant to corticosteroid therapy. In such cases, the diagnosis of minimal-change disease may not be accurate, and FSGS that was not sampled in the initial biopsy specimen may be present.

In the absence of complications, the long-term outlook for patients with minimal-change disease is no different from that of the general population. Development of azotemia in a patient previously diagnosed as having minimal-change disease should suggest failure to sample FSGS in the original biopsy. It may also reflect evolution into FSGS or perhaps a complication such as drug-induced interstitial nephritis.

Focal Segmental Glomerulosclerosis May Reflect Diverse Etiologies and Pathogenetic Mechanisms

In FSGS, glomerular consolidation affects some (focal), but not all, glomeruli and initially involves only part of an affected glomerular tuft (segmental). Consolidated segments often show increased collagenous matrix (sclerosis; Fig. 22-19). There are primary (idiopathic) and secondary forms of FSGS.

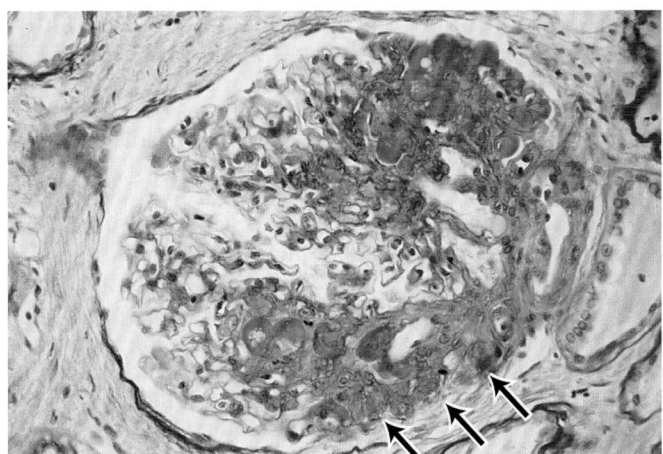

FIGURE 22-19. Focal segmental glomerulosclerosis. Periodic acid–Schiff (PAS) staining shows perihilar areas of segmental sclerosis and adjacent adhesions to the Bowman capsule (*arrows*).

  **MOLECULAR PATHOGENESIS AND ETIOLOGIC FACTORS:** The term **FSGS** describes a heterogeneous group of glomerular diseases with different causes, pathologies, responses to treatment and outcomes. It may be idiopathic (primary) or secondary to several conditions (Table 22-5). Multiple factors probably lead to a final common pathway of injury. Pathologic features and genetic evidence suggest that injury to podocytes may be common to all types of FSGS.

Several hereditary forms of FSGS reflect genetic abnormalities in podocyte proteins (e.g., podocin, nephrin, α-actinin-4 and TRPC6). This implicates injury to, or dysfunction of, podocytes in FSGS.

Congenital (e.g., unilateral agenesis with contralateral hypoplasia) and acquired (e.g., reflux nephropathy) reductions in renal mass place adaptive stress on the reduced number of nephrons. In turn, this strain appears to cause FSGS from overwork, with increased glomerular capillary pressure and filtration, and glomerular enlargement. A normal amount of renal tissue can also be stressed by excessive body mass (obesity), resulting in FSGS. Reduced blood oxygen (e.g., as in sickle cell disease or cyanotic congenital heart disease) also causes a similar pattern of glomerular injury. In all of these settings, glomerular enlargement reflects functional overwork, placing undue stress on podocytes because of their limited proliferative capacity.

Viruses, drugs and serum factors are implicated as causes of FSGS. Infection with HIV, especially in blacks, is associated with a variant of FSGS with a collapsing pattern of sclerosis (Fig. 22-20). Such an appearance may also occur in idiopathic FSGS. Collapsing FSGS may also be caused by viral infection of podocytes. Pamidronate, a drug used to treat osteolytic bone disease in patients with cancer, causes collapsing FSGS in some patients. The drug probably causes FSGS by injuring podocytes. A serum permeability factor has been detected in some patients with FSGS, which suggests a systemic cause for the glomerular injury. This is further supported by the recurrence of FSGS in renal transplants, especially in patients who have the permeability factor. Sequence variants in the gene encoding apolipoprotein 1 (*APOL1*) have been linked to FSGS in blacks, who are known to have a high incidence of FSGS and hypertension-related ESRD. Apparently, these variants provide protection against African sleeping sickness (trypanosomiasis), which may explain their prevalence in blacks. As in sickle cell disease, this is an example of how a genetic variant can cause a common disease while providing protection against a major infectious disease.

 PATHOLOGY: Varying numbers of glomeruli show segmental obliteration of capillary loops by increased matrix or accumulation of cells, or both. Insudation of plasma proteins and lipid gives lesions a glassy appearance, called **hyalinosis**. Adhesions to the Bowman

TABLE 22-5
CATEGORIES OF FOCAL SEGMENTAL GLOMERULOSCLEROSIS
Primary (idiopathic) focal segmental glomerulosclerosis (FSGS)
Secondary FSGS
Hereditary/genetic (e.g., mutations in podocyte genes)
Obesity (perihilar variant)
Reduced renal mass (perihilar variant)
Cyanotic congenital heart disease (usually perihilar variant)
Sickle cell nephropathy (usually perihilar variant)
Infection induced (e.g., HIV; collapsing variant)
Drug induced (e.g., pamidronate; collapsing variant)

Note: Primary and secondary FSGS can have various histologic patterns of injury: perihilar, tip lesion, cellular, collapsing, not otherwise specified (NOS).

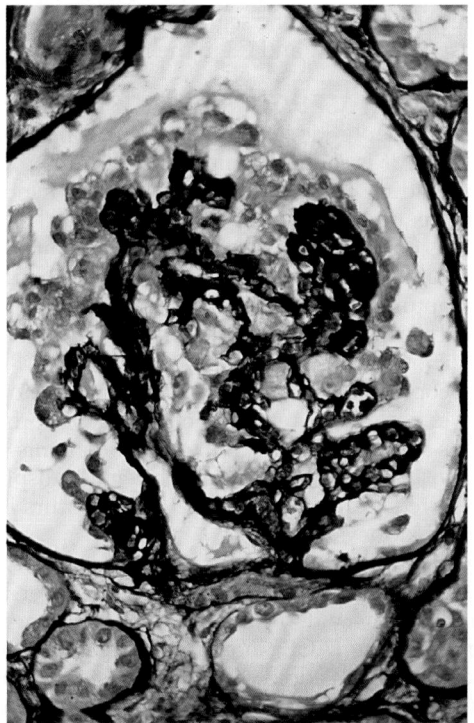

FIGURE 22-20. HIV-associated nephropathy. Silver staining shows a collapsing pattern of focal segmental glomerulosclerosis (FSGS), with collapse of glomerular capillaries, increased matrix material (sclerosis) and hypertrophy of podocytes.

capsule occur adjacent to sclerotic lesions. Uninvolved glomeruli may look entirely normal, although mild mesangial hypercellularity is occasionally present. Because uninvolved glomeruli usually appear normal, FSGS can be mistaken for minimal-change disease in small biopsy specimens that contain only nonsclerotic glomeruli.

Several histologic variants of FSGS are recognized. Particularly in patients with reduced renal mass or obesity, the sclerosis localizes in **perihilar** segments within glomeruli and in deep cortical (juxtamedullary) glomeruli (Fig. 22-19). A **collapsing** pattern of sclerosis with hypertrophied and hyperplastic podocytes adjacent to sclerotic segments is typical of HIV-associated nephropathy and also occurs with intravenous drug abuse, with pamidronate-induced disease and as an idiopathic process. This collapsing variant has a poor prognosis, and 1/2 of patients reach end-stage disease within 2 years. Sclerosis limited to glomerular segments adjacent to the origin of the proximal tubule has been designated **tip lesion** and is more likely to respond to steroid therapy than other forms of FSGS. A **cellular variant** of FSGS has prominent lipid-laden cells within the sites of glomerular consolidation.

By electron microscopy, epithelial cell foot processes are diffusely effaced in FSGS, with occasional focal detachment or loss of podocytes from the GBM. Sclerotic segments show increased matrix material, wrinkling and thickening of basement membranes and capillary collapse. Accumulation of electron-dense material in sclerotic segments represents insudative trapping of plasma proteins and corresponds to hyalinosis seen by light microscopy. *Immune complexes are absent.*

Immunofluorescence microscopy shows irregular trapping of IgM and C3 in the segmental areas of sclerosis and hyalinosis. IgG, C4 and C1q are less often found in sclerotic segments. Nonsclerotic segments do not stain or do so weakly, usually for IgM and C3 in the mesangium.

 CLINICAL FEATURES: FSGS causes 1/3 of primary nephrotic syndrome in adults and 10% in children. It is more common in blacks than in whites and is the leading cause of primary nephrotic syndrome in blacks. Its frequency has been increasing over the past few decades for unknown reasons. Clinical presentations and outcomes vary among the different patterns of injury. Most often, asymptomatic proteinuria begins insidiously and progresses to the nephrotic syndrome. Many patients are hypertensive. Microscopic hematuria is frequent.

Most people with FSGS show persistent proteinuria and progressive decline in renal function. Many progress to ESRD after 5–20 years. Some, but not all, patients improve with corticosteroid therapy. Although renal transplantation is the preferred treatment for ESRD, FSGS recurs in 1/2 of transplanted kidneys.

Patients with FSGS due to obesity or reduced renal mass usually have a more indolent course with lower levels of proteinuria that benefits from treatment with angiotensin-converting enzyme (ACE) inhibitors or angiotensin receptor blockers (ARBs). People with the tip lesion variant often present with severe nephrotic syndrome. This variant resembles minimal-change disease and responds better to corticosteroids than do other forms of FSGS. HIV-associated and idiopathic collapsing FSGS have the worst prognoses. They typically have severe nephrotic syndrome and renal failure, often progressing to ESRD within a year.

HIV-1–Associated Nephropathy Is a Severe, Rapidly Progressive Collapsing Form of FSGS

 ETIOLOGIC FACTORS: The occurrence of nephropathy in patients with HIV-1 infection has raised the possibility that it is caused by HIV-1 within the renal parenchyma. A different hypothesis proposes that the nephropathy is caused by another virus that has infected the kidney of an immunocompromised person.

 PATHOLOGY: HIV-1–associated nephropathy shows a segmental or global collapsing pattern of focal sclerosis (Fig. 22-20). Capillaries in sclerotic segments collapse, often with adjacent swollen podocytes that have numerous protein droplets. Interstitial fibrosis and infiltration by mononuclear leukocytes are common. Tubular epithelial atrophy and degeneration are conspicuous; cystically dilated tubules contain proteinaceous casts. By electron microscopy, many tubuloreticular inclusions are seen in endothelial cells, similar to those in lupus nephritis.

 CLINICAL FEATURES: Some 5% of HIV-positive patients, of whom more than 90% are black, develop collapsing FSGS. Idiopathic collapsing FSGS also occurs mainly in blacks. It presents with severe proteinuria (often >10 g/day) and renal insufficiency. More than 1/2 of patients progress to ESRD in less than 2 years.

Membranous Glomerulonephritis Is a Disease of Immune Complex Deposition

Membranous glomerulonephritis is a common cause of nephrotic syndrome in adults. It reflects subepithelial immune complex accumulation in glomerular capillaries.

PATHOPHYSIOLOGY: Immune complexes localize in the **subepithelial zone** (between podocytes and the GBM) as a result of immune complex formation in situ or deposition of circulating immune complexes. Formation in situ occurs in the animal model of membranous glomerulonephritis called **Heymann nephritis,** in which rats are immunized with a renal epithelial antigen and develop autoantibodies. The antibodies cross GBMs and bind antigens on podocytes. Resultant immune complexes are shed into the adjacent subepithelial zone to cause membranous glomerulonephritis. A rare form of neonatal membranous glomerulonephritis is caused by transplacental passage of antibodies that react with an alloantigen on neonatal podocytes (neutral endopeptidase) that is not shared by the mother. Most patients with primary membranous glomerulonephritis have circulating autoantibodies against a podocyte transmembrane receptor, PLA$_2$R. PLA$_2$R and anti-PLA$_2$R can be isolated from the immune complexes, supporting in situ subepithelial immune complex formation.

Repeated experimental exposure to foreign proteins elicits antibodies, which form circulating immune complexes. A subpopulation of these complexes deposits in glomerular capillary walls. Sometimes, free antigens and antibodies cross the GBM independently and form subepithelial immune complexes in situ.

General causes of membranous glomerulonephritis are:

- Primary membranous glomerulonephritis
  - Anti-PLA$_2$R autoantibodies
  - Anti–neutral endopeptidase alloantibodies
- Secondary membranous glomerulonephritis
  - Autoimmune disease (SLE, autoimmune thyroid disease)
  - Infectious disease (hepatitis B, malaria, syphilis, schistosomiasis)
  - Therapeutic agents (penicillamine)
  - Neoplasms (lung, prostate and gastrointestinal cancers)

 PATHOLOGY: Glomeruli are usually normocellular. Depending on the duration of the disease, capillary walls may be normal or thickened (Fig. 22-21). In intermediate disease stages, silver stains (which highlight basement membranes) reveal multiple "spikes" of argyrophilic material on the epithelial side of the basement membrane (Fig. 22-22). These spikes are projections of basement membrane material around subepithelial immune complexes (which do not stain with silver). As disease progresses, capillary lumens narrow, and glomerular sclerosis eventually ensues. Advanced membranous glomerulonephritis cannot be distinguished from other forms of chronic glomerular disease. Atrophy of tubules and interstitial fibrosis parallel the degree of glomerular sclerosis.

By electron microscopy, immune complexes appear in capillary walls as electron-dense deposits (Figs. 22-23, 22-24). The progressive ultrastructural changes caused by subepithelial immune complexes are divided into stages:

- **Stage I:** Subepithelial dense deposits without adjacent projections of GBM material
- **Stage II:** Projections of GBM material adjacent to dense deposits (Fig. 22-24)
- **Stage III:** Enclosure of dense deposits within GBM material
- **Stage IV:** Rarefaction of deposits within a thickened GBM

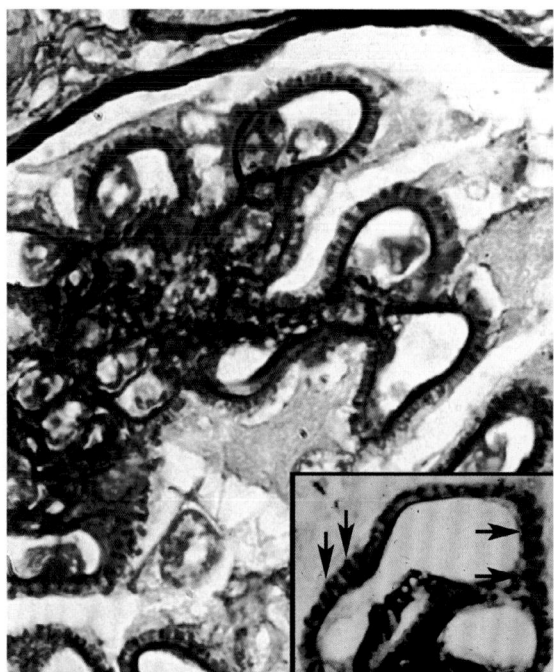

FIGURE 22-22. Membranous glomerulonephritis. Silver staining reveals multiple "spikes" diffusely distributed in the glomerular capillary basement membranes. This pattern corresponds to the stage II lesion illustrated in Figs. 22-23 and 22-24. The appearance is produced by the deposition of silver-positive basement membrane material around silver-negative immune complex deposits.

Mesangial electron-dense deposits are rare in primary membranous glomerulonephritis but are more common in secondary disease (e.g., in lupus nephropathy). This difference may reflect the fact that primary disease is caused by antigens normally present in the subepithelial zone (e.g., podocyte PLA$_2$R and neutral endopeptidase), but the secondary type is produced by circulating antigens (e.g., hepatitis B virus antigens) in complexes with circulating antibodies that can localize in mesangial as well as subepithelial locations.

Immunofluorescence reveals diffuse granular staining of capillary walls for IgG and C3 (Fig. 22-25). There is intense staining for terminal complement components, including the membrane attack complex, which participate in inducing glomerular injury, especially to podocytes.

CLINICAL FEATURES: Membranous glomerulonephritis is the most common primary glomerular cause of nephrotic syndrome in white and Asian adults in the United States (the most common secondary glomerular cause is diabetic glomerulosclerosis). The course of membranous glomerulonephritis is highly variable. Spontaneous remission occurs in 1/4 of patients within 20 years, and 10-year renal survival rate is greater than 65%. Lower survival correlates with male gender, age above 50, proteinuria of more than 6 g/day, extensive glomerular sclerosis and chronic tubulointerstitial disease. Patients with progressive renal failure receive corticosteroids and/or immunosuppressive drugs. The prognosis is better in children because of a higher rate of permanent spontaneous remission.

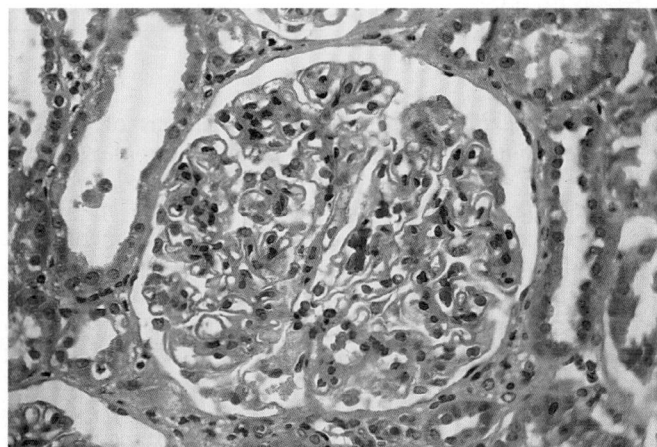

FIGURE 22-21. Membranous glomerulonephritis. The glomerulus is slightly enlarged and shows diffuse thickening of the capillary walls. There is no hypercellularity. Compare capillary walls to those shown in Fig. 22-15.

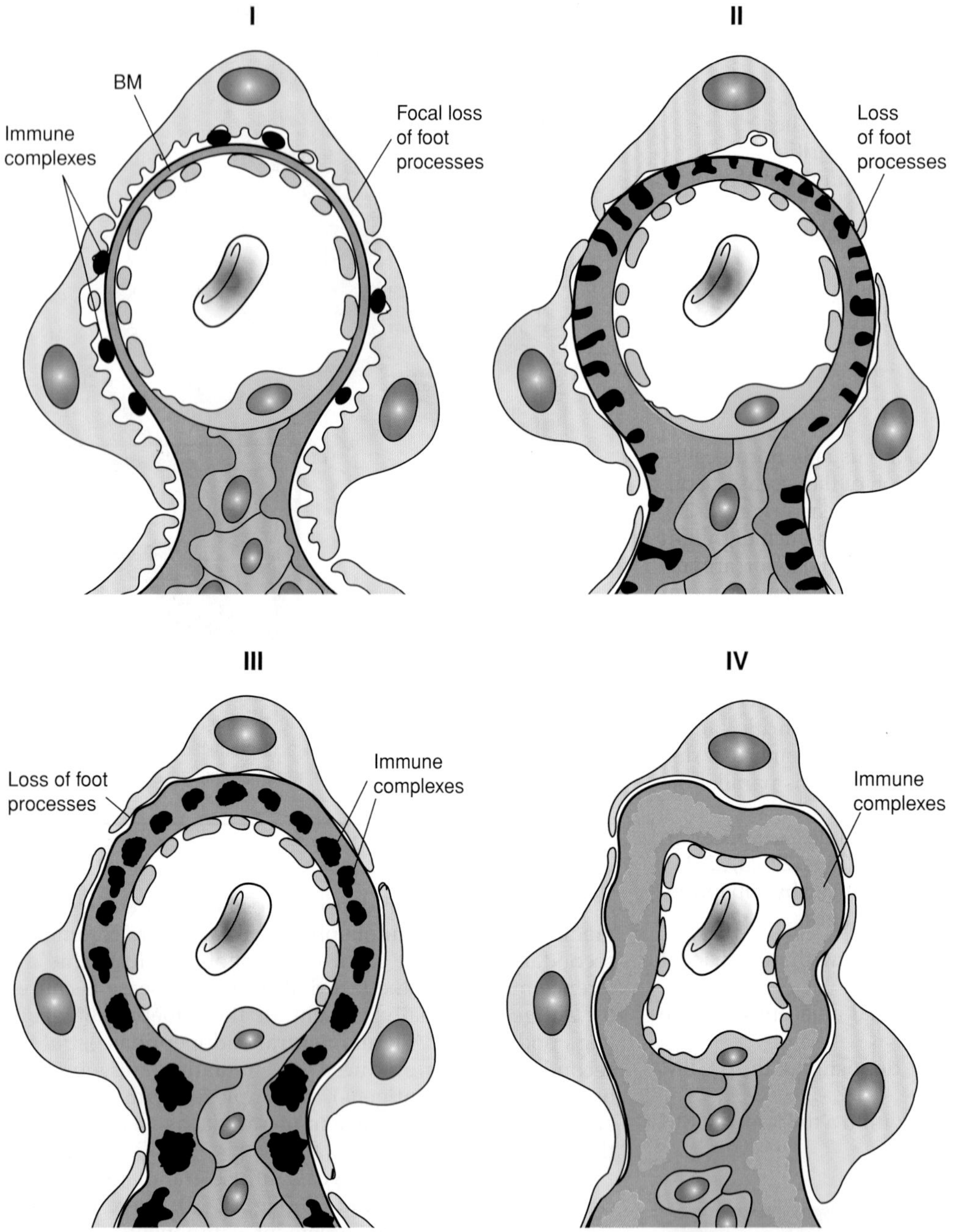

I

Immune complexes

BM

Focal loss of foot processes

II

Loss of foot processes

III

Loss of foot processes

Immune complexes

IV

Immune complexes

FIGURE 22-23. Membranous glomerulonephritis. This disease is caused by the subepithelial accumulation of immune complexes and the accompanying changes in the basement membrane (BM). Stage I exhibits scattered subepithelial deposits. The outer contour of the basement membrane remains smooth. Stage II disease has projections (spikes) of basement membrane material adjacent to the deposits. In stage III disease, newly formed basement membrane has surrounded the deposits. With stage IV disease, the immune complex deposits lose their electron density, resulting in an irregularly thickened basement membrane with irregular electron-lucent areas.

Diabetic Glomerulosclerosis Causes Proteinuria and Progressive Renal Failure

PATHOPHYSIOLOGY: Glomerulosclerosis is a part of vasculopathy that affects small vessels throughout the body in diabetic patients (see Chapter 13). The abnormal metabolic state leads to a general increase in synthesis of basement membrane material in the microvasculature. One hypothesis proposes that increased **oxidative injury** and abnormal **nonenzymatic glycosylation** of plasma proteins (e.g., immunoglobulins) and matrix proteins (including those of the GBM and mesangial matrix) induce excessive matrix production and podocyte injury.

PATHOLOGY: The earliest lesions of diabetic glomerulosclerosis are glomerular enlargement, GBM thickening and mesangial matrix expansion (Fig. 22-26). Numbers of podocytes decline. Mild mesangial hypercellularity may be present along with the increase in mesangial matrix. In patients who develop symptomatic disease, GBM thickening and especially mesangial matrix expansion result in changes visible on light microscopy. In diabetic glomerulosclerosis, diffuse global GBM thickening and diffuse mesangial matrix expansion are accompanied by sclerotic **Kimmelstiel-Wilson nodules** (Fig. 22-27). Insudated proteins form rounded nodules between the Bowman capsule and the parietal epithelium ("capsular drops") or subendothelial accumulations along capillary loops ("hyaline caps"). Tubular basement membranes are thickened. Sclerosing and insudative changes in afferent and efferent

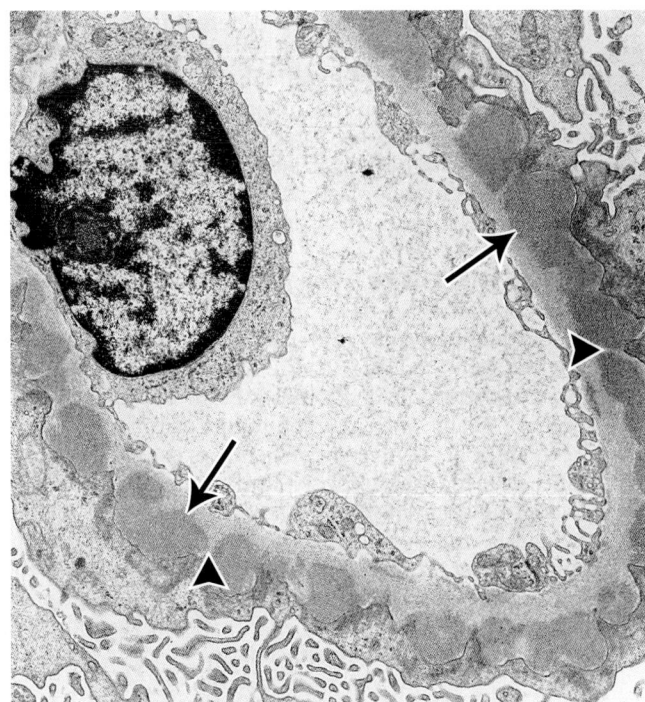

FIGURE 22-24. Stage II membranous glomerulonephritis. An electron micrograph shows deposits of electron-dense material (*arrows*), with intervening delicate projections of basement membrane material (*arrowheads*).

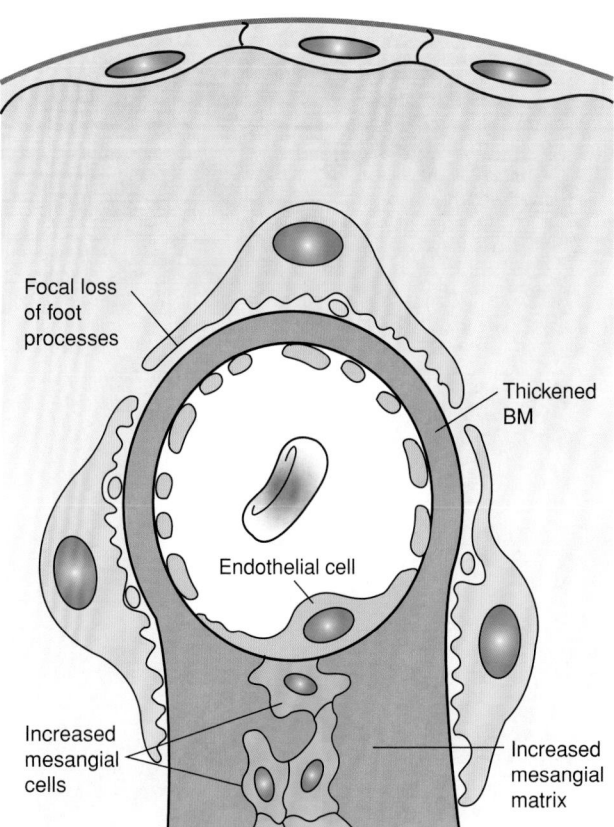

FIGURE 22-26. Diabetic glomerulosclerosis. The lamina densa of the glomerular basement membrane is thickened, and there is an increase in mesangial matrix material.

arterioles cause hyaline arteriolosclerosis. Generalized renal arteriosclerosis is usually present. Vascular narrowing and reduced blood flow to the medulla predispose to papillary necrosis and pyelonephritis.

By electron microscopy, the basement membrane lamina densa may be thicker by 5–10-fold. Mesangial matrix is increased, particularly in nodular lesions (Fig. 22-28). The hyaline insudative lesions appear as electron-dense masses that contain lipid debris. By immunofluorescence, there is diffuse linear trapping of IgG, albumin, fibrinogen and other plasma proteins in the GBM. This reflects nonimmunologic adsorption of these proteins to the thickened GBM, possibly due to nonenzymatic glycosylation of GBM and plasma proteins.

CLINICAL FEATURES: *Diabetic glomerulosclerosis accounts for 40% of ESRD and thus is the leading cause of ESRD in the United States.* It occurs in type 1 and type 2 diabetes mellitus. Approximately 25% of patients with diabetes develop diabetic glomerulosclerosis.

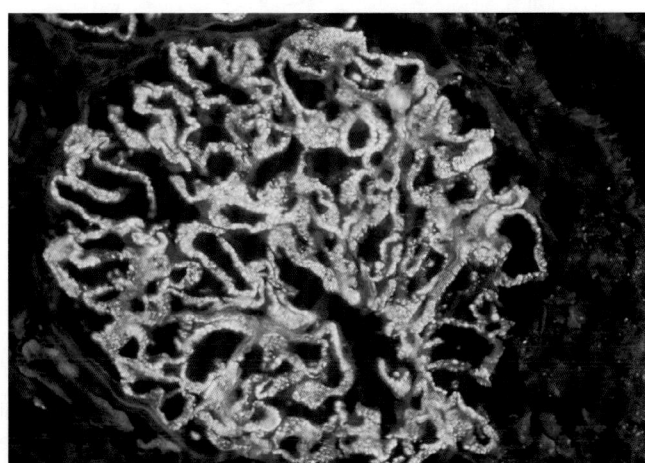

FIGURE 22-25. Membranous glomerulonephritis. Immunofluorescence microscopy shows granular deposits of immunoglobulin G (IgG) outlining the glomerular capillary loops.

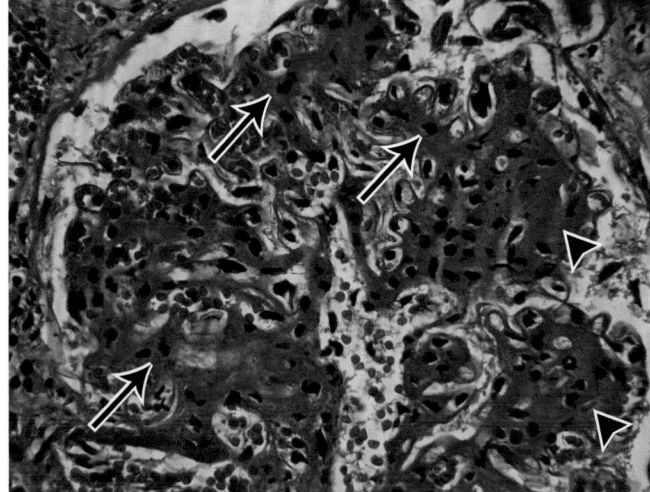

FIGURE 22-27. Diabetic glomerulosclerosis. There is a prominent increase in the mesangial matrix (*arrows*), forming several nodular lesions (*arrowheads*). Dilation of glomerular capillaries is evident, and some capillary basement membranes are thickened.

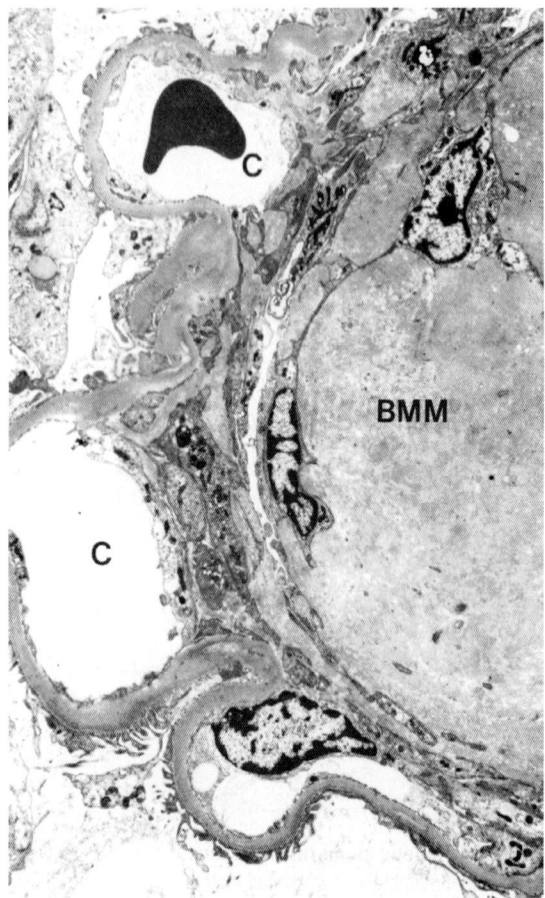

FIGURE 22-28. Advanced diabetic glomerulosclerosis. An electron micrograph shows a nodular aggregate of basement membrane–like material (BMM). The peripheral capillary (C) demonstrates diffuse basement membrane widening but a normal texture.

The earliest manifestation is microalbuminuria (slightly increased proteinuria). Overt proteinuria occurs between 10 and 15 years after the onset of diabetes and often becomes severe enough to cause the nephrotic syndrome. In time, diabetic glomerulosclerosis progresses to renal failure. Strict control of blood glucose reduces the incidence of diabetic glomerulosclerosis and retards progression once it develops. Control of hypertension and dietary protein restriction also slow progression of the disease.

Amyloidosis Leads to Nephrotic Syndrome and Renal Failure

Renal disease is a frequent complication of AA and AL amyloidosis (see Chapter 15).

MOLECULAR PATHOGENESIS: Amyloid may be formed from a number of different polypeptides. In North America, AL amyloidosis accounts for 80% of renal amyloidosis, 10% of AA amyloidosis and 10% of all other types of amyloidosis (e.g., composed of fibrinogen, leukocyte chemotactic factor 2, apolipoprotein). AA is more common is areas with high rates of endemic infections. All forms of amyloidosis appear similar histologically and ultrastructurally. Immunohistochemical tests are

required to differentiate among the different types. **AA amyloid** is derived from serum amyloid A (SAA) protein, which increases markedly during inflammation. Thus, AA amyloid is often associated with chronic inflammatory disorders (e.g., rheumatoid arthritis, chronic infections, familial Mediterranean fever). **AL amyloid** is derived from immunoglobulin light chains made by neoplastic clones of B cells or plasma cells. Thus, it often occurs in, or presages, multiple myeloma.

PATHOLOGY: Amyloid is an eosinophilic, amorphous material (Fig. 22-29) with a characteristic apple-green color under polarized light in sections stained with Congo red (Fig. 22-30). Acidophilic deposits are initially most apparent in the mesangium but later extend into capillary walls and may obliterate capillary lumens (Figs. 22-29, 22-31). Glomerular structure is completely obliterated in advanced amyloidosis, and glomeruli appear as large eosinophilic spheres.

Amyloid is composed of nonbranching fibrils, about 10 nm in diameter. These are initially most abundant in the mesangium but often extend into capillary walls, especially in advanced cases (Figs. 22-31, 22-32). Podocyte foot processes overlying the GBM are effaced.

CLINICAL FEATURES: Renal involvement is prominent in most cases of systemic AL and AA amyloidosis. Proteinuria is often the initial manifestation. Proteinuria is nonselective (i.e., albumin and globulins are in the urine) and nephrotic syndrome occurs in 60% of patients. Eventually, severe infiltration of glomeruli and

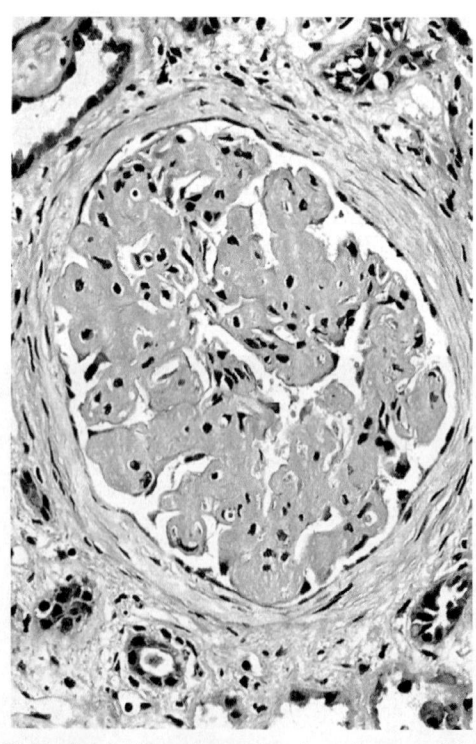

FIGURE 22-29. Amyloid nephropathy. Amorphous acellular material expands the mesangial areas and obstructs the glomerular capillaries. The deposits of amyloid may take on a nodular appearance, somewhat resembling those of diabetic glomerulosclerosis (see Fig. 22-27). However, amyloid deposits are not periodic acid–Schiff positive and are identifiable by Congo red staining.

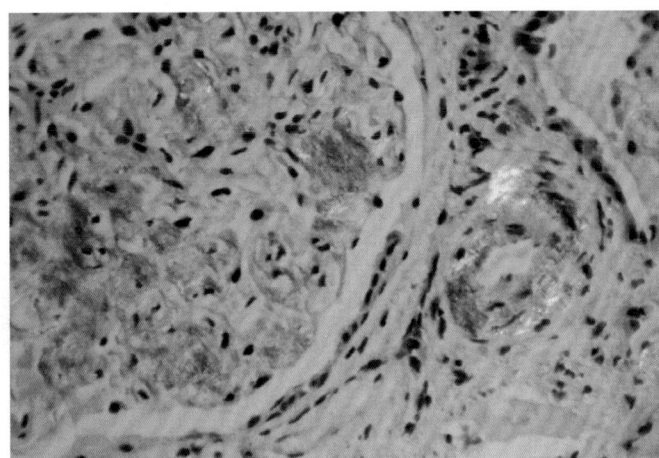

FIGURE 22-30. Amyloid nephropathy. In a section stained with Congo red and examined under polarized light, the amyloid deposits in the glomerulus and the adjacent arteriole show a characteristic apple-green birefringence.

blood vessels by amyloid results in renal failure. AL amyloidosis is treated with chemotherapy for multiple myeloma. AA amyloidosis, especially when caused by familial Mediterranean fever, is ameliorated by colchicine therapy.

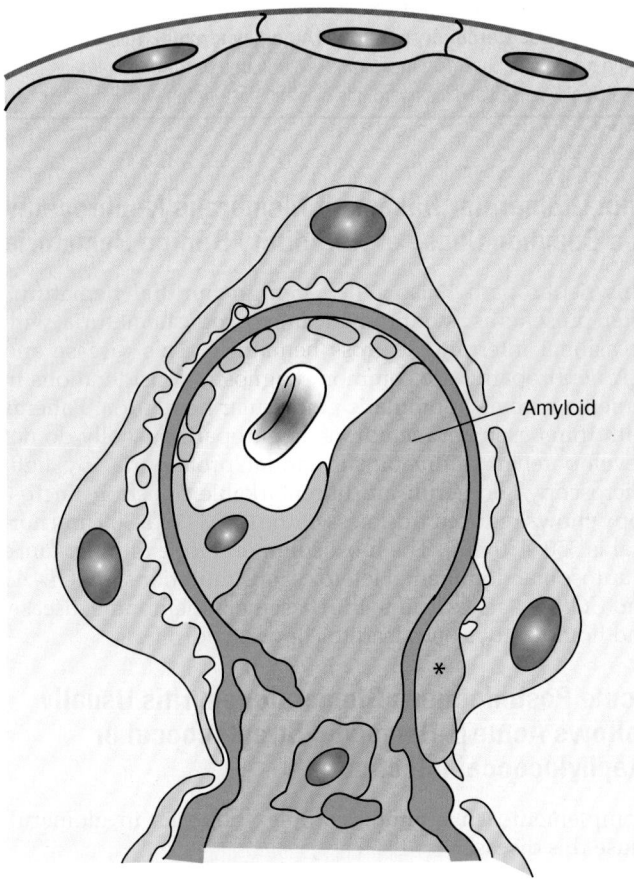

Amyloid

FIGURE 22-31. Amyloid nephropathy. This disorder is initially associated with the accumulation of characteristic fibrillar deposits in the mesangium. These inert masses, which are fibrillar by electron microscopy, extend along the inner surface of the basement membrane, frequently obstructing the capillary lumen. Focal extension of amyloid through the basement membrane (*) may elevate the epithelial cell.

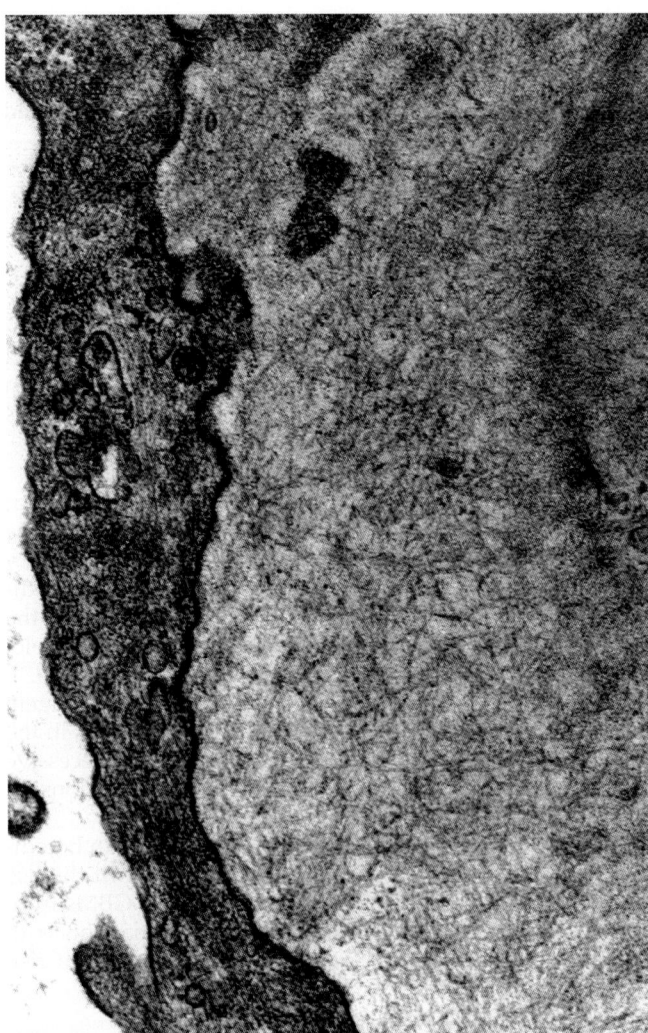

FIGURE 22-32. Amyloid nephropathy. Deposits of fibrils (10 nm in diameter) in a glomerulus adjacent to podocyte cytoplasm with effaced foot processes.

Nonfibrillary Monoclonal Immunoglobulin Deposition in Kidneys Can Cause Disease

Such deposition may be in GBMs, glomerular mesangial matrix, capillary walls and tubular basement membranes. Unlike the deposits of AL amyloid, these do not form fibrils. The two major phenotypes are nodular sclerosing glomerular disease with granular deposits by electron microscopy and proliferative (or membranoproliferative) glomerulonephritis with homogenous dense deposits by electron microscopy.

PATHOLOGY: The underlying B-cell dyscrasia may be occult, or there may be overt multiple myeloma or lymphoma. Monoclonal immunoglobulin deposition stimulates increased glomerular matrix production and/or mesangial hyperplasia. Nodular expansion of mesangial regions resembles diabetic glomerulosclerosis. The increased extracellular material does not stain with Congo red, which distinguishes monoclonal immunoglobulin deposition disease from amyloidosis. Immunofluorescence microscopy demonstrates staining for monoclonal immunoglobulin chains. Monoclonal immunoglobulin deposition disease with nodular sclerosis usually manifests clinically as nephrotic syndrome, whereas proliferative glomerulonephritis with monoclonal immunoglobulin often manifests as mixed nephritic and nephrotic syndrome.

Hereditary Nephritis (Alport Syndrome) Reflects Abnormal Glomerular Basement Membrane Type IV Collagen

Hereditary nephritis is a proliferative and sclerosing glomerular disease, often accompanied by defects of the ears or the eyes. It is caused by mutations in type IV collagen. In Alport syndrome, a hereditary hearing deficit accompanies nephritis.

 MOLECULAR PATHOGENESIS: Several genetic mutations cause molecular defects in the GBM that lead to the renal lesions of hereditary nephritis. The most common, accounting for 85% of hereditary nephritis, is X-linked and is caused by a mutation in the gene for the α5 chain of type IV collagen (*COL4A5*). A deletion at the 5′ end of *COL4A5* that extends into the *COL4A6* gene, which codes for the α6 chain of type IV collagen, causes hereditary nephritis and multiple leiomyomas in the gastrointestinal and genital tracts. An autosomal recessive form of hereditary nephritis is caused by mutations in *COL4A3* and *COL4A4*.

As basement membrane structure is disturbed in hereditary nephritis, serum from patients with anti-GBM disease (e.g., Goodpasture syndrome) fails to react with GBMs from patients with hereditary nephritis. Conversely, patients with hereditary nephritis who have renal transplants are at risk for developing antibodies to allograft GBMs.

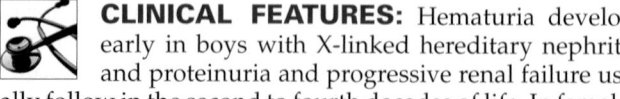 **PATHOLOGY:** Early glomerular lesions of hereditary nephritis show mild mesangial hypercellularity and matrix expansion. Renal disease progression is associated with increasing focal and eventually diffuse glomerular sclerosis. Tubular atrophy, interstitial fibrosis and foam cells in tubules and interstitium accompany advanced glomerular lesions. Electron microscopy makes the diagnosis, demonstrating an irregularly thickened GBM with splitting of the lamina densa into interlacing lamellae that surround electron-lucent areas (Fig. 22-33).

CLINICAL FEATURES: Hematuria develops early in boys with X-linked hereditary nephritis, and proteinuria and progressive renal failure usually follow in the second to fourth decades of life. In females, the X-linked disease is generally milder, with the rate of progression varying substantially among patients, possibly due to the degree of random inactivation (lyonization) of the mutated X chromosome. Autosomal recessive hereditary nephritis resembles X-linked disease except that males and females are affected equally. Autosomal dominant hereditary nephritis with progressive renal failure is rare and difficult to distinguish from severe thin basement membrane disease (see below). Sensorineural, high-frequency hearing loss affects 1/2 of males with X-linked disease and a higher proportion of males and females with autosomal disease. Ocular defects, largely of the lens, occur in 1/4 to 1/3 of patients.

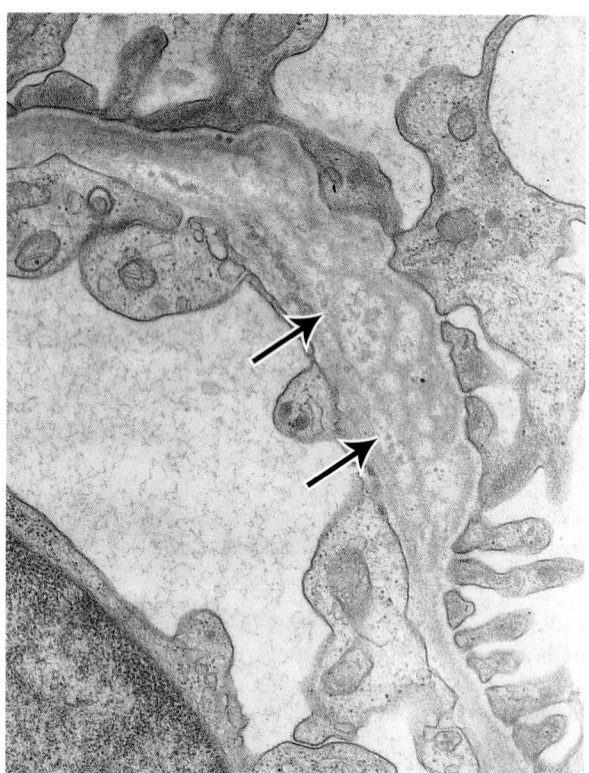

FIGURE 22-33. Hereditary nephritis (Alport syndrome). The lamina densa of the glomerular basement membrane is laminated (*arrows*) rather than forming a single dense band (compare this electron micrograph with Fig. 22-5).

Thin Glomerular Basement Membrane Nephropathy Is a Common Cause of Hereditary Benign Hematuria

This nephropathy, also called **benign familial hematuria**, often presents as asymptomatic microscopic hematuria, with occasional intermittent gross hematuria. This disease and IgA nephropathy are common diagnostic considerations in patients with asymptomatic glomerular hematuria. Patients with thin basement membrane nephropathy usually do not develop renal failure or substantial proteinuria. By light microscopy, glomeruli are unremarkable. Electron microscopy shows reduced thickness of the GBM (150–300 nm; normal is 350–450 nm). The most common mode of inheritance is autosomal dominant. Heterozygous mutations in *COL4A3* and *COL4A4* genes lead to thin basement membrane disease, and homozygous ones lead to Alport syndrome.

Acute Postinfectious Glomerulonephritis Usually Follows Acute β-Hemolytic Streptococcal or Staphylococcal Infection

Complement-rich immune complex deposits in glomeruli cause this disease.

 **PATHOPHYSIOLOGY:** Nephritogenic strains of group A streptococci or staphylococci usually cause acute postinfectious glomerulonephritis. Rare cases result from viral (e.g., hepatitis B) or parasitic (e.g., malaria) infections. The mechanism by which

infection causes the characteristic glomerular inflammation is not completely understood. Similarities to experimental acute serum sickness suggest that postinfectious glomerulonephritis reflects deposition in glomeruli of immune complexes containing antibody plus bacterial antigens. Poststreptococcal glomerulonephritis in patients and experimental acute serum sickness have 9–14-day latent periods between antigen exposure and glomerulonephritis. Both show granular immune complex deposits with similar ultrastructural appearance (dense deposits) (see below). Immune complexes could form in the circulation and deposit in glomeruli, or they may form in situ when bacterial antigens trapped in glomeruli bind to circulating antibodies. Potentially culpable (but not yet convicted) streptococcal antigens include glyceraldehyde phosphate dehydrogenase and cationic proteinase exotoxin B. Both can localize in glomerular capillary walls and activate complement even without antibodies. Alternatively, nephritogenic bacteria may release factors that activate complement without requiring immune complex formation. This would explain why complement—but not immunoglobulin—is sometimes present in glomerular deposits.

Complement activation, as well as activation of other humoral and cellular inflammatory mediators, causes glomerular inflammation. Complement activation is so extensive that more than 90% of patients develop hypocomplementemia. The inflammatory mediators attract and activate neutrophils and monocytes, and stimulate mesangial and endothelial cell proliferation. These effects result in marked glomerular hypercellularity, which defines acute diffuse proliferative glomerulonephritis.

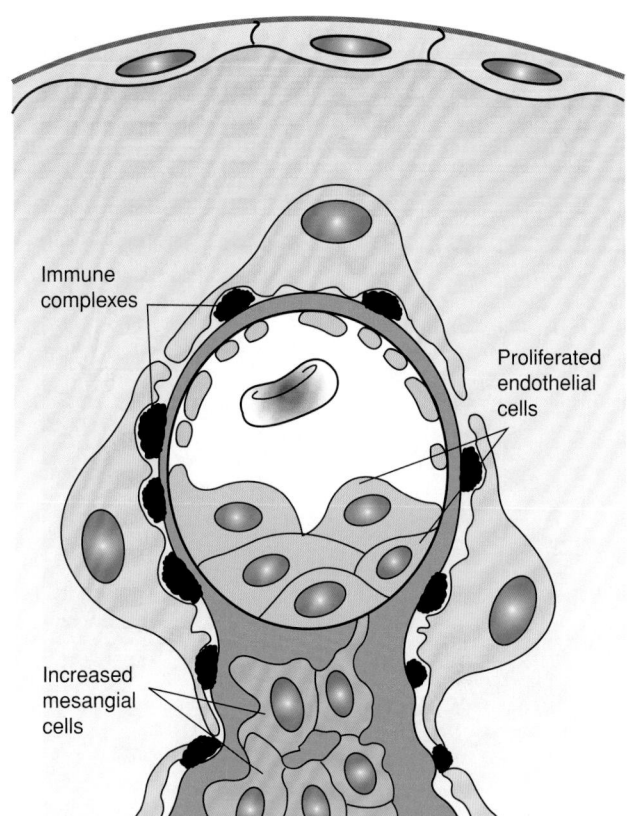

FIGURE 22-35. Postinfectious glomerulonephritis. Accumulation of numerous subepithelial immune complexes as hump-like structures is a characteristic feature. Less prominent subendothelial immune complexes are associated with endothelial cell proliferation and are related to increased capillary permeability and narrowing of the lumen. Frequently, proliferation of mesangial cells and a thickened mesangial matrix (BM) result in widening of the stalk and conspicuous trapping of immune complexes.

PATHOLOGY: In the acute phase, glomeruli are diffusely enlarged and hypercellular (Fig. 22-34). The latter reflects proliferation of endothelial and mesangial cells (Fig. 22-35), and infiltration by neutrophils and monocytes. Crescents are uncommon. Interstitial edema and mild mononuclear infiltration parallel the glomerular changes.

The acute phase begins 1–2 weeks after the onset of the nephritogenic infection and resolves in more than 90% of patients after several weeks. Neutrophils and endothelial hypercellularity disappear first. Mesangial hypercellularity and matrix expansion remain, but all of these changes resolve completely in most patients after several months.

Ultrastructurally, acute postinfectious glomerulonephritis shows distinctive **subepithelial dense deposits** shaped like **"humps"** (Figs. 22-35, 22-36). These are invariably accompanied by mesangial and subendothelial deposits, which may be more difficult to find but are probably more important in pathogenesis by virtue of their proximity to inflammatory mediator systems in the blood. The variably sized, dome-shaped humps are on the epithelial side of the GBM. They are not as widely distributed as the deposits of membranous glomerulonephritis (compare Figs. 22-23 and 22-35). Granular deposits of C3 with or without immunoglobulin are observed by immunofluorescence microscopy in capillary walls, corresponding to the humps (Fig. 22-37). A rare variant of postinfectious glomerulonephritis, usually caused by methicillin-resistant staphylococcus, has conspicuous IgA in the immune deposits.

CLINICAL FEATURES: The incidence of acute postinfectious glomerulonephritis is declining in most developed countries but remains high because of higher rates of nephritogenic infections. It is still

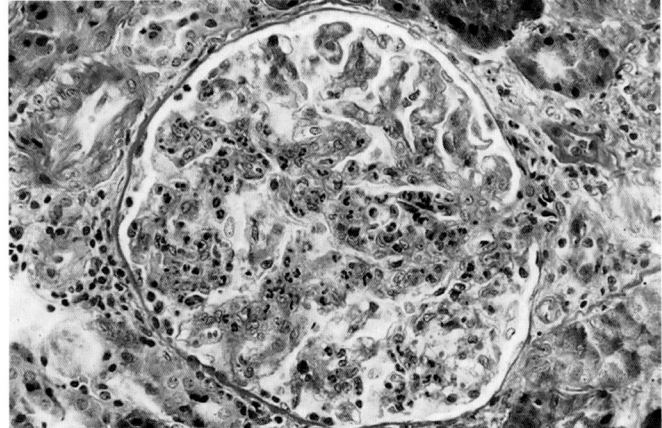

FIGURE 22-34. Acute poststreptococcal glomerulonephritis. A glomerulus of a patient who developed glomerulonephritis after a streptococcal infection contains many neutrophils (Masson trichrome stain).

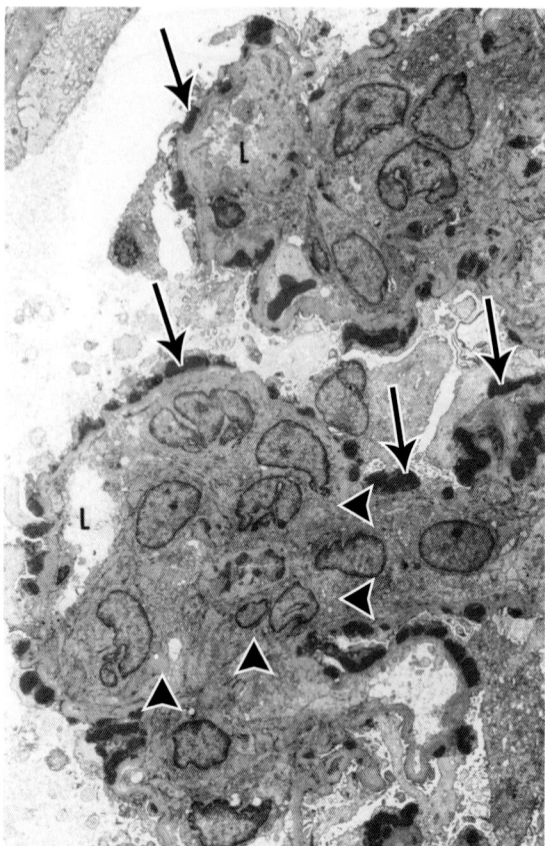

FIGURE 22-36. Acute postinfectious glomerulonephritis. An electron micrograph demonstrates numerous subepithelial humps (*arrows*) and mesangial hypercellularity (*arrowheads*). The capillary lumina (L) are markedly narrowed.

one of the most common childhood renal diseases. Primary infection involves the pharynx (pharyngitis) or, especially in hot and humid environments, the skin (pyoderma). In recent years, the proportion of cases following staphylococcal infection has been increasing. Because organisms may not be present at the time nephritis develops, the diagnosis may

depend on serologic evidence of increasing antibody titers to streptococcal antigens. The nephritic syndrome begins abruptly with oliguria, hematuria, facial edema and hypertension. Serum C3 levels are lower during the acute syndrome but return to normal within 1–2 weeks. Overt nephritis resolves after several weeks, but hematuria and especially proteinuria may persist for several months. A few patients have abnormal urinary sediment for years after the acute episode, and rare patients (particularly adults) develop progressive renal failure.

Immune Complex Membranoproliferative Glomerulonephritis Has Multiple Causes

MPGN is a pattern of glomerular inflammation with hypercellularity and capillary wall thickening caused by multiple different etiologies.

PATHOPHYSIOLOGY: MPGN is caused by deposits in the mesangium and subendothelial zone of capillary walls containing immune complexes or activated complement without immunoglobulin. Subepithelial deposits may also occur. The two major immunopathologic categories are immune complex MPGN and C3 glomerulopathy MPGN (Table 22-6). The nephritogenic antigens in immune complex MPGN are usually unknown. However, the apparent sources of the antigens may be infectious or autoimmune conditions (Table 22-6). C3 glomerulopathy MPGN is caused by genetic or autoimmune disruption of regulatory mechanisms that normally hold the alternative complement pathway in check. C3 glomerulopathy is discussed in the next section.

Eliminating the associated condition (e.g., bacterial endocarditis or osteomyelitis) may be followed by resolution of immune complex MPGN, thus suggesting a causal relationship between the two. Unlike the pathogens of

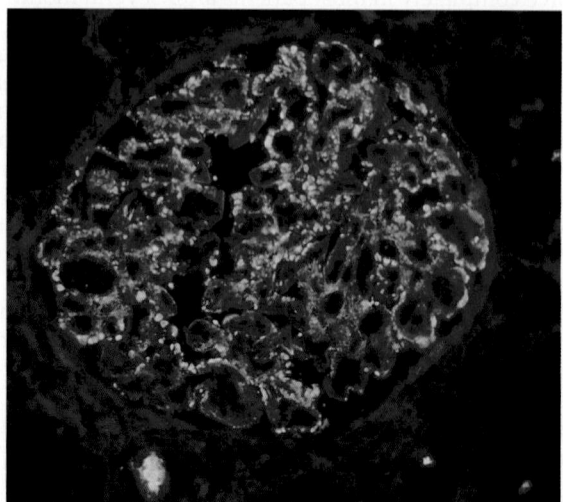

FIGURE 22-37. Acute postinfectious glomerulonephritis. An immunofluorescence micrograph demonstrates granular staining for C3 in capillary walls and the mesangium.

TABLE 22-6

CLASSIFICATION OF MEMBRANOPROLIFERATIVE GLOMERULONEPHRITIS

Primary Immune Complex (idiopathic) Membranoproliferative Glomerulonephritis (MPGN)

Secondary Immune Complex MPGN caused by:

    Subacute bacterial endocarditis

    Infected ventriculoatrial shunt

    Osteomyelitis

    Hepatitis C virus infection

    Cryoglobulinemia

    Monoclonal immunoglobulins

    Neoplasia

C3 Glomerulopathy

    Dense deposit disease

    C3 glomerulonephritis

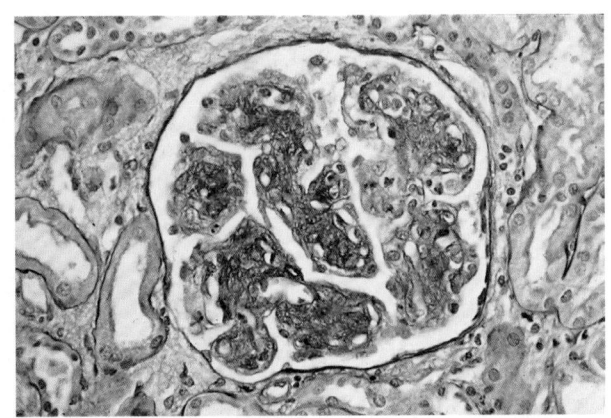

FIGURE 22-38. Type I membranoproliferative glomerulonephritis. The glomerular lobulation is accentuated. Increased cells and matrix in the mesangium and thickening of capillary walls are noted.

acute postinfectious glomerulonephritis, those associated with immune complex MPGN cause persistent, indolent infections with chronic antigenemia. This condition leads to chronic localization of immune complexes in glomeruli and resultant hypercellularity and matrix remodeling.

 PATHOLOGY: Glomeruli in MPGN are diffusely enlarged, with florid mesangial cell proliferation and infiltration of monocytes/macrophages. The resultant glomerular lobular distortion ("hypersegmentation"; Fig. 22-38) was once called **lobular glomerulonephritis**. Of these patients, 20% have crescents, usually involving only a minority of glomeruli. Capillary walls are thickened, and silver stains show a doubling or complex replication of GBMs.

Electron microscopy reveals thickening and replication of GBMs probably caused by endothelial cell activation as well as extension of mesangial cytoplasm into the subendothelial zone and deposition of new basement membrane material between the mesangial cytoplasm and endothelial cell (Figs. 22-39, 22-40). Subendothelial and mesangial electron-dense deposits, corresponding to immune complexes or complement deposits, are the likely stimuli for the endothelial and mesangial response. Variable numbers of subepithelial dense deposits may also be seen. Immunofluorescence microscopy shows granular deposition of immunoglobulins

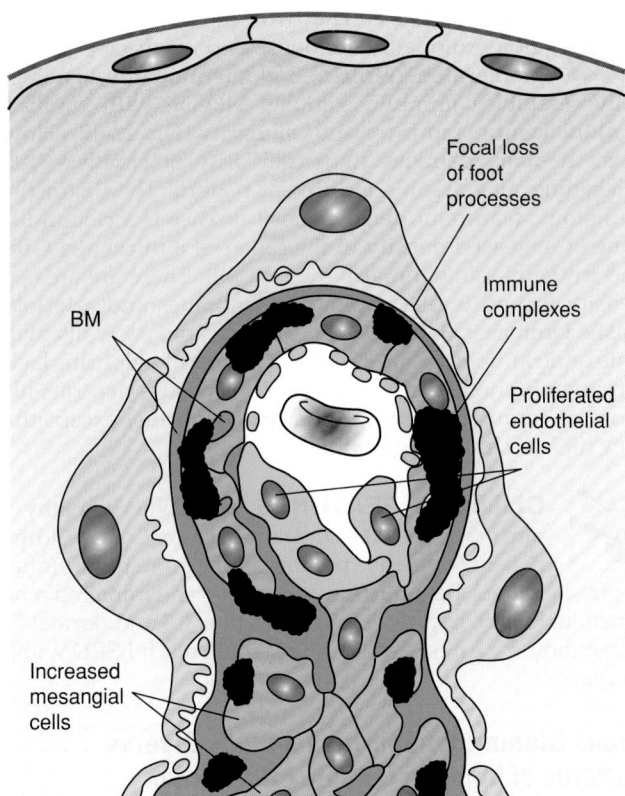

FIGURE 22-39. Type I membranoproliferative glomerulonephritis. In this disease, the glomeruli are enlarged. Hypercellular tufts and narrowing or obstruction of the capillary lumens are seen. Large subendothelial deposits of immune complexes extend along the inner border of the basement membrane (BM). The mesangial cells proliferate and migrate peripherally into the capillary. Basement membrane material accumulates in a linear fashion parallel to the basement membrane in a subendothelial position. The interposition of mesangial cells and basement membrane between the endothelial cells and the original basement membrane creates a double-contour effect. The accumulation of mesangial cells and stroma in the tufts narrows the capillary lumen. The proliferation of mesangial cells and the accumulation of basement membrane material also widen the mesangium. The entire process leads progressively to lobulation of the glomerulus. Note the proliferation of endothelial cells and focal effacement of foot processes.

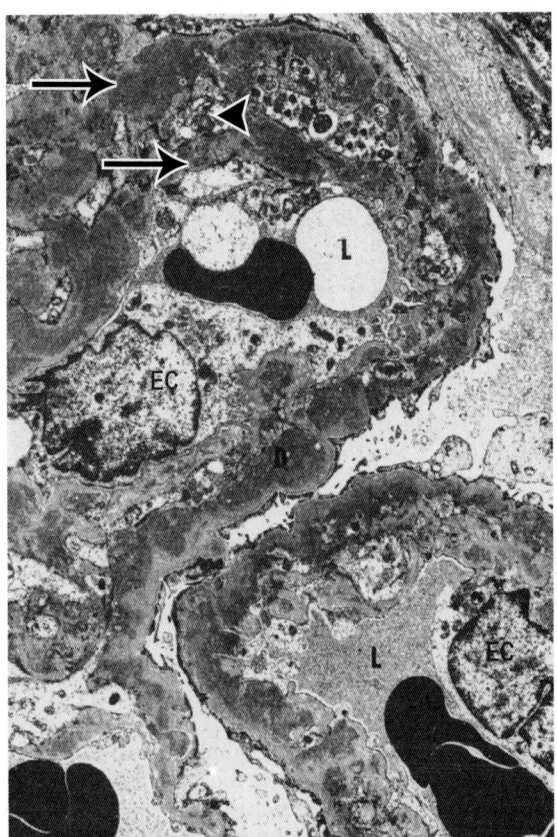

FIGURE 22-40. Type I membranoproliferative glomerulonephritis. An electron micrograph demonstrates a double-contour basement membrane (*arrows*), with mesangial interposition (*arrowhead*) and prominent subendothelial deposits. EC = endothelial cell; L = capillary lumen.

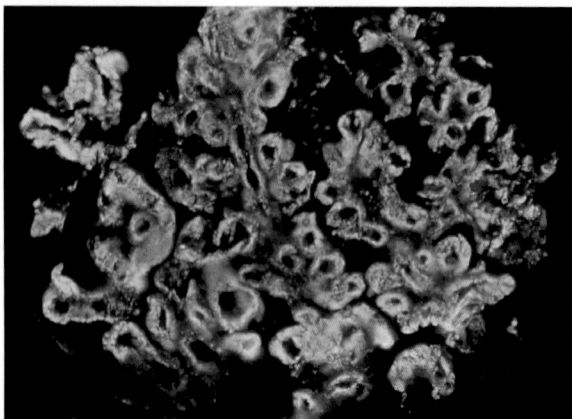

FIGURE 22-41. Type I membranoproliferative glomerulonephritis. An immunofluorescence micrograph demonstrates granular to band-like staining for C3 in the capillary walls and mesangium.

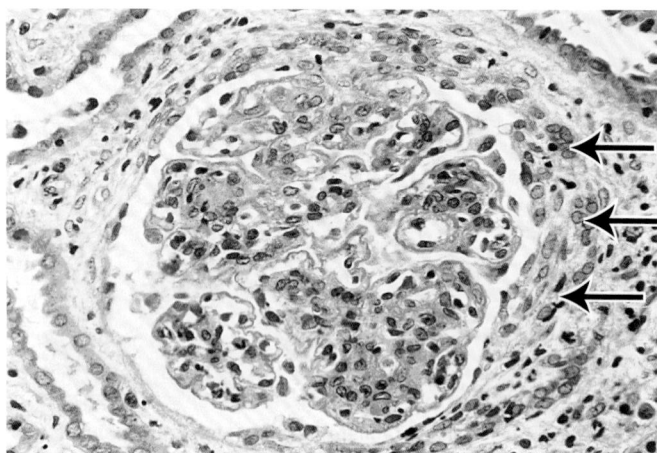

FIGURE 22-42. C3 glomerulopathy (dense deposit disease). Capillary wall thickening, hypercellularity and a small crescent (*arrows*) are evident.

and complement in glomerular capillary loops and mesangium in immune complex MPGN and complement alone in C3 glomerulopathy (Fig. 22-41).

CLINICAL FEATURES: Immune complex MPGN can occur at any age but is most frequent in older children and young adults. It may manifest as nephrotic or nephritic syndromes, or a combination of both. MPGN accounts for 5% of primary nephrotic syndrome in children and adults in the United States. Immune complex MPGN occurs much more commonly in countries where chronic infections are more prevalent. Patients often have low C3 levels. The differential diagnosis includes acute postinfectious glomerulonephritis and lupus glomerulonephritis, both of which can cause nephritis with hypocomplementemia. MPGN is usually a persistent, slowly progressive disease. After 10 years, 1/2 of patients reach ESRD.

C3 Glomerulopathy Is Caused by Dysregulation of the Alternative Complement Pathway

C3 glomerulopathy is a rare glomerulonephritis caused by complement dysregulation that includes **dense deposit disease** (formerly called *type II MPGN*) and **C3 glomerulonephritis** (including a variant with an MPGN pattern).

PATHOPHYSIOLOGY: The extensive glomerular localization of complement *without* immunoglobulin indicates that complement activation is a major mediator of the structural and functional abnormalities. Deficient or ineffective alternative pathway complement regulatory factors (e.g., complement factor H, complement factor I) cause C3 glomerulopathy. Complement activation abnormality results from genetic mutations or autoantibodies that impair alternative pathway regulatory mechanisms. Some patients have a serum IgG autoantibody, **C3 nephritic factor,** which stabilizes activated C3 convertase (C3bBb) of the alternative complement pathway and prolongs C3 activation. C3 glomerulopathy often recurs in renal transplants because the defect in complement regulation is in the recipient.

PATHOLOGY: The two pathologic types of C3 glomerulopathy are dense deposit disease and C3 glomerulonephritis. C3 glomerulopathy histologically resembles immune complex MPGN, with capillary wall thickening and increased cellularity (Fig. 22-42). However, in many patients, hypercellularity or capillary wall thickening may assume a different pattern. The distinctive pathologic feature of dense deposit disease is a ribbon-like zone of increased density in the center of a thickened GBM and in the mesangial matrix (Fig. 22-43). There are areas of density in peritubular capillary membranes and arteriolar elastic laminae. C3 deposits linearly in capillary walls, with little or no antibody (Fig. 22-44). C3 glomerulonephritis lacks intramembranous dense deposits. It has dense deposits like those of immune complex glomerulonephritis, except that they have no immunoglobulin.

CLINICAL FEATURES: C3 glomerulopathy is rare (<5/1,000,000), and 80% of patients are children. Patients usually present with proteinuria (often nephrotic range), hematuria, hypertension and impaired renal function. Hypocomplementemia with low C3 and normal C4 is common. Prognosis is sobering, as 40% reach ESRD within 10 years.

Lupus Glomerulonephritis Includes Diverse Patterns of Immune Complex Deposition

SLE (see Chapter 11) is an autoimmune disease with generalized B-cell dysregulation and hyperactivity, and production of autoantibodies to many nuclear and nonnuclear antigens, including DNA, RNA, nucleoproteins and phospholipids. SLE is most common in women, especially of child-bearing age. Blacks, Asians and Hispanics generally have more severe disease than do whites. Nephritis is one of the most common complications of SLE.

Immune complexes in the mesangium cause less inflammation than subendothelial immune complexes. The latter are more exposed to cellular and humoral inflammatory mediator systems in blood and are, therefore, more likely to initiate inflammation. Subepithelial localization of immune complexes causes proteinuria but does not stimulate overt glomerular inflammation.

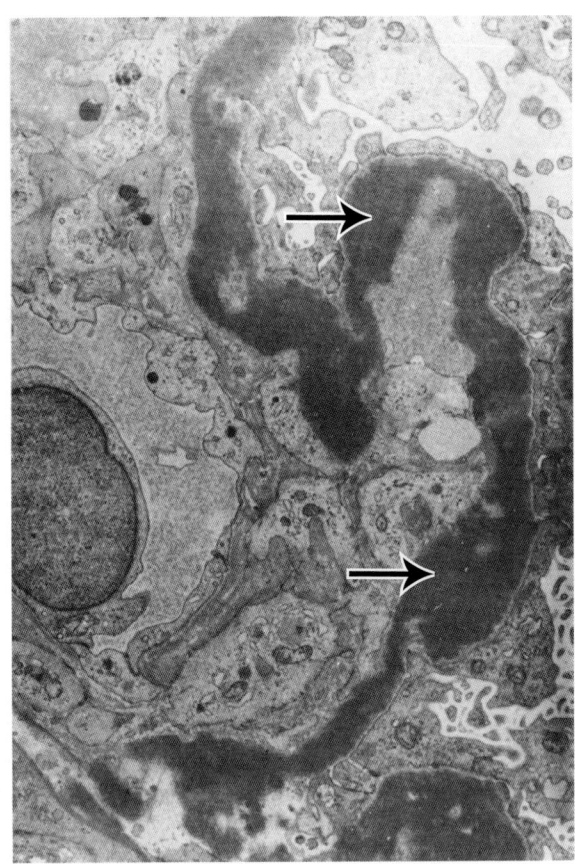

FIGURE 22-43. C3 glomerulopathy (dense deposit disease). An electron micrograph demonstrates thickening of the basement membrane with intramembranous dense deposits (*arrows*).

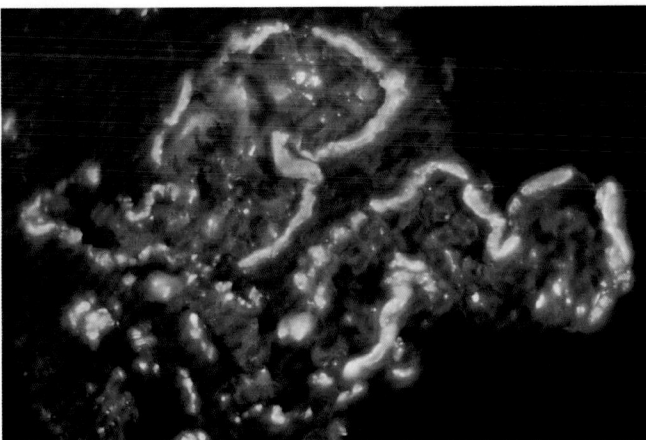

FIGURE 22-44. C3 glomerulopathy (dense deposit disease). An immunofluorescence micrograph demonstrates bands of capillary wall staining and coarsely granular mesangial staining for C3.

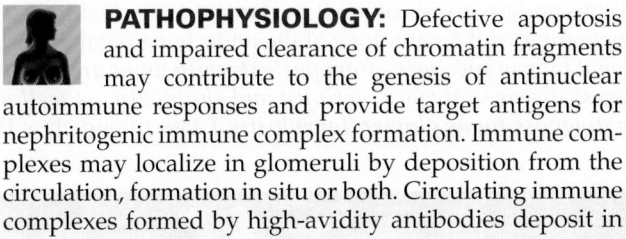

PATHOPHYSIOLOGY: Defective apoptosis and impaired clearance of chromatin fragments may contribute to the genesis of antinuclear autoimmune responses and provide target antigens for nephritogenic immune complex formation. Immune complexes may localize in glomeruli by deposition from the circulation, formation in situ or both. Circulating immune complexes formed by high-avidity antibodies deposit in subendothelial and mesangial zones; low-affinity antibodies form immune complexes in situ in the subepithelial zone. Immune complexes formed in situ may involve antigens such as double-stranded DNA and nucleosomes that accumulate on GBMs or in mesangial matrix due to charge interactions. Glomerular immune complexes activate complement and initiate inflammation. Complement activation often causes hypocomplementemia. Immune complexes also localize in the renal interstitium, walls of interstitial vessels and tubular basement membranes, where they may activate the tubulointerstitial inflammation seen in patients with lupus nephritis.

PATHOLOGY: The pathologic and clinical manifestations of lupus nephritis vary with the diverse patterns of immune complex accumulation in different patients (Table 22-7) and in the same patient over time.

- **Class I (minimal mesangial lupus glomerulonephritis):** Immune complexes are confined to mesangium and cause no changes by light microscopy.
- **Class II (mesangial proliferative lupus glomerulonephritis):** Immune complexes are confined to mesangium

Location of Immune Lupus Nephritis Class	Location of Immune Complexes	Clinical Manifestations
I: Minimal mesangial	Mesangial	Mild hematuria and proteinuria
II: Mesangial proliferative	Mesangial	Mild hematuria and proteinuria
III: Focal	Mesangial and subendothelial	Moderate nephritis
IV: Diffuse	Mesangial and subendothelial	Severe nephritis
V: Membranous	Subepithelial and mesangial	Nephrotic syndrome
VI: Chronic sclerosing	Variable	Chronic renal failure

TABLE 22-7

PATHOLOGIC AND CLINICAL FEATURES OF LUPUS NEPHRITIS

THE KIDNEY

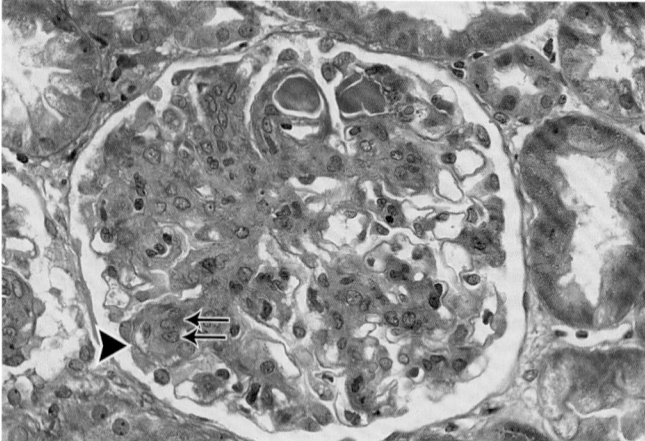

FIGURE 22-45. Proliferative lupus glomerulonephritis. Segmental endocapillary hypercellularity (*arrows*) and thickening of capillary walls (*arrowhead*) are present.

and cause varying degrees of mesangial hypercellularity and matrix expansion (Fig. 22-45).

■ **Class III (focal lupus glomerulonephritis):** Subendothelial immune complexes accumulate, together with mesangial immune complexes. These trigger mesangial and endothelial cell proliferation, inflammation and influx of neutrophils and monocytes. This overt glomerular inflammation is called **focal proliferative lupus glomerulonephritis** if it involves less than 50% of glomeruli.

■ **Class IV (diffuse lupus glomerulonephritis):** This type is similar to class III but involves more than 50% of glomeruli. Glomerular involvement may be predominantly global (IV-G) or predominantly segmental (IV-S).

■ **Class V (membranous lupus glomerulonephritis):** Immune complexes are mostly in the subepithelial zone. Some patients have a background of class V injury and a concurrent class III or IV injury. Even pure class V lupus nephritis has mesangial immune complexes that can be detected by electron microscopy.

■ **Class VI (advanced sclerosing lupus glomerulonephritis):** Advanced chronic disease.

Immune complex dense deposits occur in mesangial, subendothelial and subepithelial locations. Class I and II lesions have mainly mesangial deposits. Classes III and IV-G have mesangial and subendothelial deposits, and usually scattered subepithelial deposits (Fig. 22-46). Class IV-S tends to show fewer glomerular immune complexes and more segmental necrosis. Class V lesions contain many subepithelial dense deposits. In 80% of cases, endothelial cells have **tubuloreticular inclusions** (Fig. 22-46). These reflect high levels of interferon. Lupus nephritis and HIV-associated nephropathy are the only renal diseases that feature such inclusions.

By immunofluorescence, subepithelial complexes are granular; subendothelial deposits may be granular or band-like (Fig. 22-47). The immune complexes often stain most intensely for IgG, but IgA and IgM are also almost always present, as are C3, C1q and other complement components. Granular staining along tubular basement membranes and interstitial vessels occurs in more than 1/2 of patients.

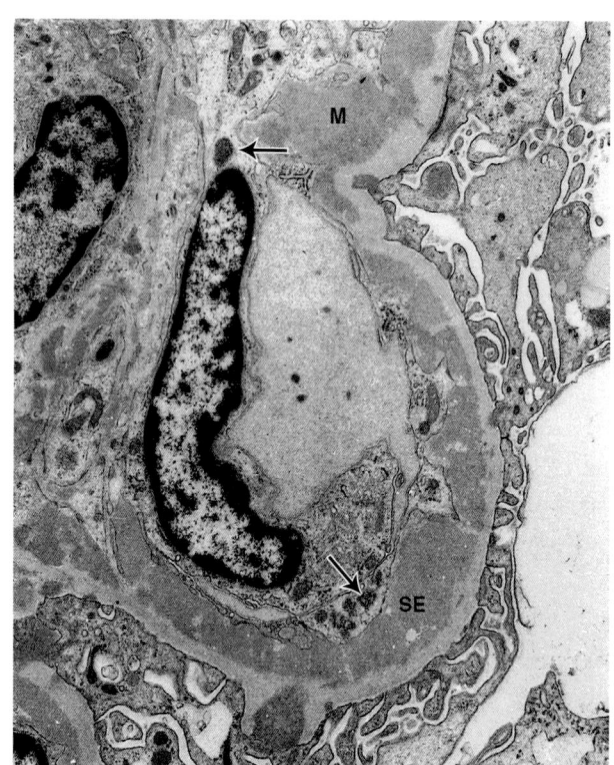

FIGURE 22-46. Diffuse proliferative class IV-G lupus glomerulonephritis. An electron micrograph reveals large subendothelial and mesangial dense deposits (*M*) and a few subepithelial (*SE*) deposits. Endothelial tubuloreticular inclusions (*arrows*) are present.

CLINICAL FEATURES: Renal disease develops in 70% of patients with SLE and is often the major cause of morbidity and mortality. Clinical manifestations and prognosis of renal dysfunction vary (Table 22-7), depending on the pathology of the underlying renal disease. *Renal biopsy specimens from patients with lupus are used to assess disease category, activity and chronicity, as well as to diagnose lupus glomerulonephritis.* Class III and class IV

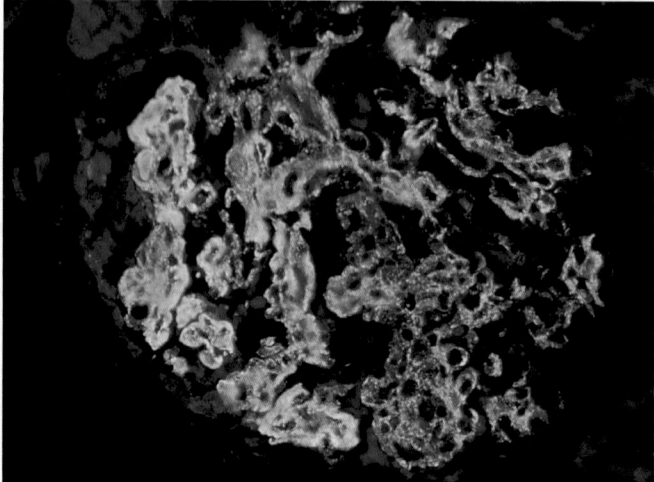

FIGURE 22-47. Diffuse proliferative lupus glomerulonephritis. An immunofluorescence micrograph demonstrates segmental staining for immunoglobulin G in the capillary walls and mesangium.

lupus nephritis have the poorest prognosis and are treated most aggressively, usually with high doses of corticosteroids and immunosuppressive drugs. Over time, sometimes due to treatment, lupus nephritis may change from one type to another, with parallel changes in clinical manifestations. Fewer than 20% of patients with class IV disease reach ESRD within 5 years.

IgA Nephropathy Is Caused by IgA1 Immune Complexes

PATHOPHYSIOLOGY: Deposition of IgA-dominant immune complexes is the cause of IgA nephropathy, but what the constituent antigens are and how they accumulate (deposition vs. formation in situ) are uncertain. Patients with IgA nephropathy often have aberrant IgA1 molecules, elevated blood levels of IgA1 and circulating IgA1-containing immune complexes or aggregated IgA1. Mesangial accumulation of IgA-dominant immune complexes may entail several mechanisms.

Respiratory or gastrointestinal infections often trigger exacerbations of IgA nephropathy. Mucosal exposure to viral, bacterial or dietary antigens stimulates IgA-dominant immune responses, leading to glomerular immune complex accumulation. Abnormal glycosylation of the IgA1 hinge region appears to be an important factor in many patients with IgA nephropathy. The immune deposits contain mainly IgA1 rather than IgA2. IgA1, but not IgA2, has a hinge region with O-linked glycan chains. In IgA nephropathy, serum IgA1 has less terminal galactosylation and sialylation of these chains. Autoantibodies against these abnormal chains may develop.

As well, the abnormal IgA1 galactosylation may lead to lack of receptor engagement of the abnormal IgA1, reducing clearance of immune complexes containing IgA1 from the blood. As a result, IgA forms aggregates in the circulation. The mesangium traps these aggregates. Immune complexes form between the abnormal IgA1 and IgG antibodies against the abnormal IgA1.

IgA-containing immune complexes in the mesangium most likely activate complement by the alternative pathway. The demonstration of C3 and properdin, but not C1q and C4, in the IgA deposits supports this hypothesis.

PATHOLOGY: Immunofluorescence microscopy is essential for diagnosis of IgA nephropathy. The diagnostic finding is mesangial immunostaining for IgA more intense than, or equivalent to, staining for IgG or IgM (Fig. 22-48). This is almost always accompanied by staining for C3. IgA deposited in the glomerular capillary wall (in addition to the mesangium) may be present in more severe cases and suggests a less favorable prognosis.

Depending on the severity and duration of the disease, a continuum of histologic findings is seen in IgA nephropathy, from (1) no discernible light microscopic changes to (2) focal or diffuse mesangial hypercellularity to (3) focal or diffuse proliferative glomerulonephritis (Fig. 22-49) to (4) chronic sclerosing glomerulonephritis. At the time of initial renal biopsy diagnosis, focal proliferative glomerulonephritis is the most frequent manifestation. Crescents are not common,

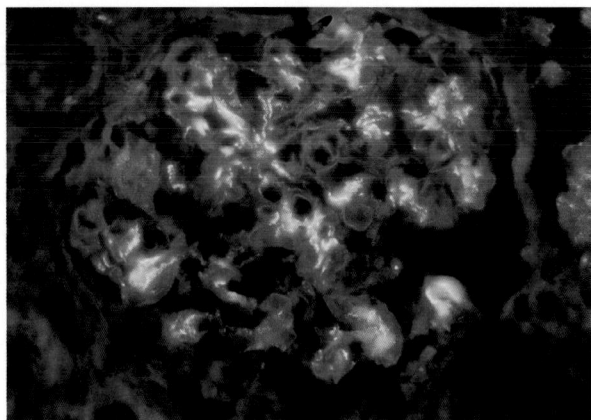

FIGURE 22-48. Immunoglobulin A (IgA) nephropathy. An immunofluorescence micrograph shows deposits of IgA in the mesangial areas.

except in unusually severe cases. This spectrum of pathologic changes is analogous to that seen with lupus nephritis but tends to be less severe.

Ultrastructural examination reveals mesangial electron-dense deposits (Figs. 22-50, 22-51). Dense deposits in capillary walls are usually seen in patients with severe disease.

CLINICAL FEATURES: *IgA nephropathy is the most common form of glomerulonephritis in developed countries.* It accounts for 10% of cases in the United States, 20% in Europe and 40% in Asia. IgA nephropathy is common in Native Americans and rare in blacks. It occurs most often in young men, with a peak age of 15–30 years at diagnosis. Clinical presentations vary, which reflects the varied pathologic severity: 40% of patients have asymptomatic microscopic hematuria, 40% have intermittent gross hematuria, 10% have nephrotic syndrome and 10% have renal failure. The disease rarely resolves completely but may follow an episodic course, with exacerbations often coinciding with upper respiratory tract infections. IgA nephropathy is slowly progressive, with 20% of patients reaching end-stage renal failure after 10 years. In systemic IgA vasculitis (Henoch-Schönlein purpura), the IgA deposits and resultant

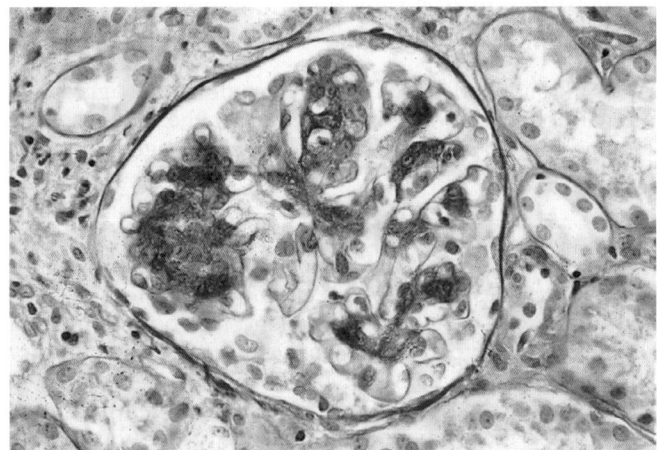

FIGURE 22-49. Immunoglobulin A nephropathy. Segmental mesangial hypercellularity and matrix expansion caused by the mesangial immune deposits (periodic acid–Schiff stain).

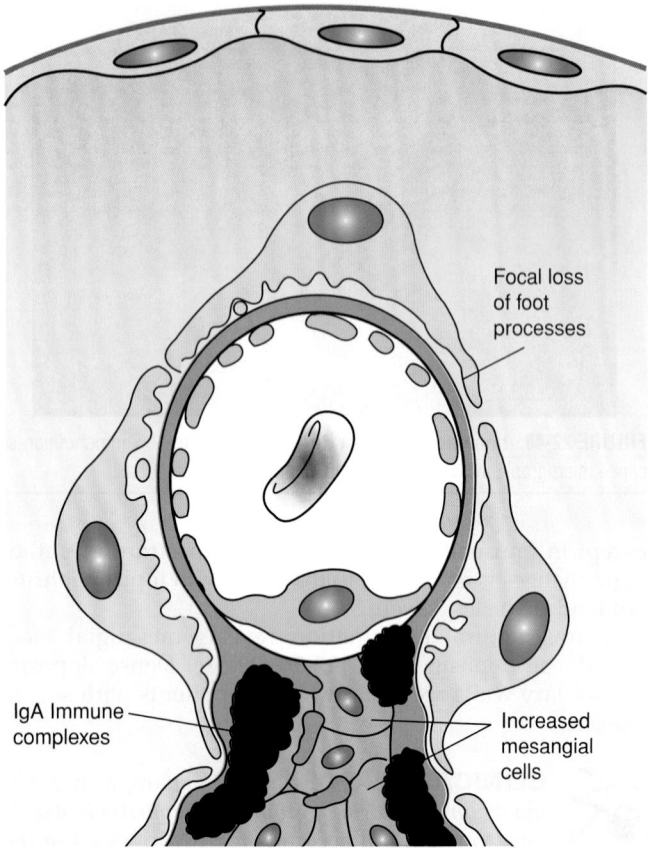

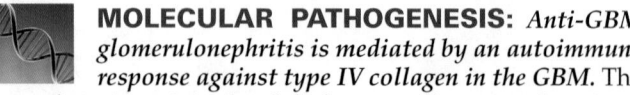

FIGURE 22-50. Immunoglobulin A (IgA) nephropathy. Significant accumulation of IgA is seen in the mesangium, most commonly between the mesangial cells and the basement membrane.

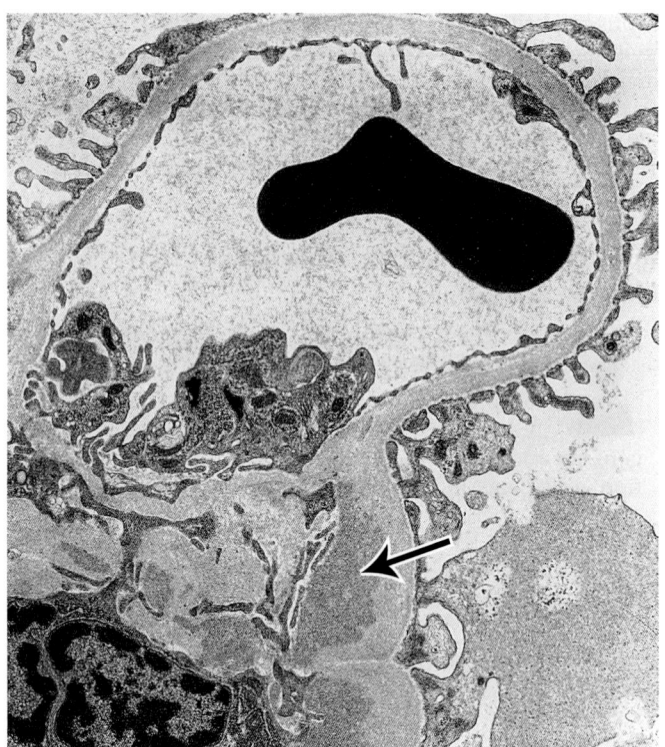

FIGURE 22-51. Immunoglobulin A nephropathy. An electron micrograph demonstrates prominent dense deposits in the mesangial matrix (*arrow*).

inflammation affect small vessels throughout the body including the skin (causing purpura) and gut (causing abdominal pain). When patients with IgA nephropathy are treated by renal transplantation, IgA deposits may recur in the allograft, although graft function is usually not impaired.

Anti–Glomerular Basement Membrane Glomerulonephritis May Be Accompanied by Pulmonary Hemorrhage

Anti-GBM antibody disease is an uncommon but aggressive glomerulonephritis that may only affect the kidneys, or it may be combined with pulmonary hemorrhage (Goodpasture syndrome).

MOLECULAR PATHOGENESIS: *Anti-GBM glomerulonephritis is mediated by an autoimmune response against type IV collagen in the GBM.* The specific epitope is in the globular noncollagenous domain of the α3 chain of type IV collagen. Disturbance of the tertiary structural conformation of type IV collagen is required to expose the epitopes that are targeted by anti-GBM antibodies. Because the target antigen is also expressed on pulmonary alveolar capillary basement membranes, 1/2 of patients also have pulmonary hemorrhages and hemoptysis, sometimes severe enough to be life-threatening. If lungs and kidneys are both involved, the eponym **Goodpasture syndrome**

is used (Fig. 22-15). Anti-GBM antibodies, anti-GBM T cells or both may mediate the injury. The antibodies bind the autoantigens in situ, initiating acute inflammation by activating mediator systems, such as complement. Experimental studies suggest that T cells specific for GBM antigens may also mediate vascular injury. Genetic susceptibility to anti-GBM disease is strongly associated with human leukocyte antigen (HLA)-DRB1. Disease onset often follows viral upper respiratory tract infections, and pulmonary involvement appears to require synergistic injurious agents, such as cigarette smoke.

PATHOLOGY: *The pathologic hallmark of anti-GBM glomerulonephritis is diffuse linear GBM immunostaining for IgG, indicating autoantibodies bound to the basement membrane* (Fig. 22-52). This finding is not, however, entirely specific. For example, binding of IgG to basement membranes occurs in diabetic glomerulosclerosis and monoclonal immunoglobulin deposition disease based on mechanisms other than antigen recognition. More than 90% of patients with anti-GBM glomerulonephritis have glomerular crescents **(crescentic glomerulonephritis)** (Figs. 22-53, 22-54), usually involving more than 50% of glomeruli. Focal glomerular fibrinoid necrosis is common. Involved lungs have marked intra-alveolar hemorrhage. By electron microscopy, GBMs show focal breaks, but no immune complex–type electron-dense deposits.

CLINICAL FEATURES: Anti-GBM glomerulonephritis typically presents with rapidly progressive renal failure and nephritic signs and symptoms. *It accounts for 10%–20% of rapidly progressive (crescentic) glomerulonephritis* (Table 22-8). Anti-GBM

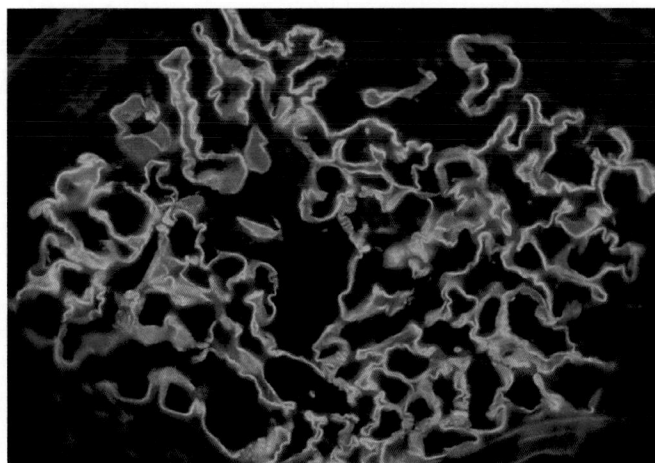

FIGURE 22-52. Anti–glomerular basement membrane (GBM) glomeru-lonephritis. Linear immunofluorescence for immunoglobulin G is seen along the GBM. Contrast this linear pattern of staining with the granular pattern of immunofluorescence typical for most types of immune complex deposition within capillary walls (see Fig. 22-36).

antibodies are detectable in approximately 90% of patients. Treatment consists of high-dose immunosuppressive therapy and plasma exchange, which are most effective at an early stage of the disease, before severe renal failure supervenes. If end-stage renal failure develops, renal transplantation is successful with little risk of losing the allograft to recurrent glomerulonephritis if transplantation is done after anti-GBM antibodies have disappeared.

Antineutrophil Cytoplasmic Autoantibody Glomerulonephritis Is an Aggressive Disease Mediated by Neutrophils

ANCA glomerulonephritis is characterized by glomerular necrosis and crescents.

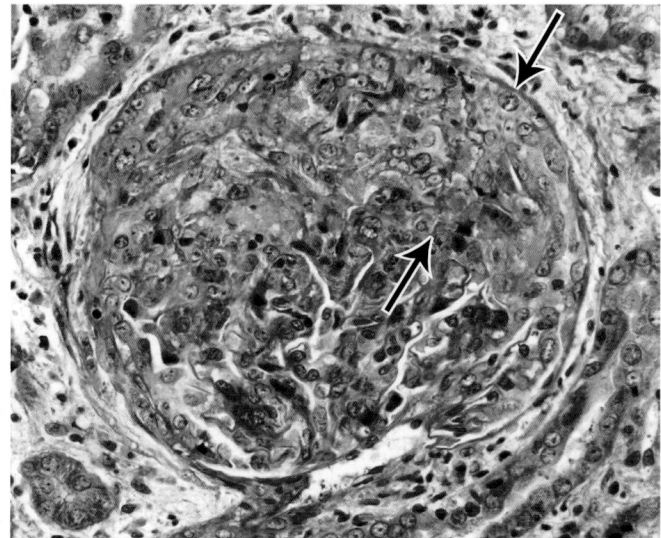

FIGURE 22-53. Crescentic anti–glomerular basement membrane glomerulonephritis. The Bowman space is filled by a cellular crescent (*between arrows*). The injured glomerular tuft is at the bottom (Masson trichrome stain).

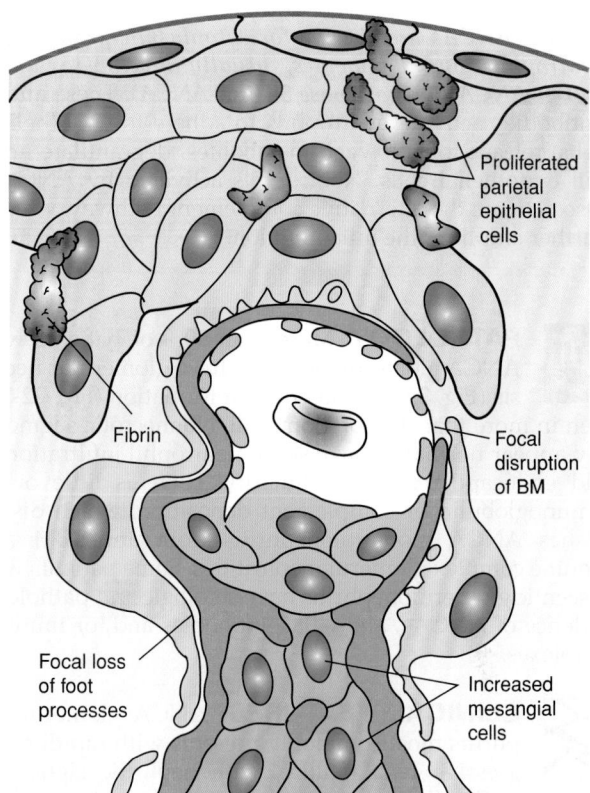

FIGURE 22-54. Crescentic (rapidly progressive) glomerulonephritis. A variety of different pathogenic mechanisms cause crescent formation by disrupting glomerular capillary walls. This allows plasma constituents into the Bowman space, including coagulation factors and inflammatory mediators. Fibrin forms, and there is proliferation of parietal epithelial cells and influx of macrophages (not shown), resulting in crescent formation.

PATHOPHYSIOLOGY: ANCA glomerulonephritis was once called *idiopathic crescentic glomerulonephritis* because there was no evidence of glomerular deposition of anti-GBM antibodies or immune complexes. The discovery that 90% of patients with this pattern of glomerular injury have circulating ANCAs led to the demonstration that these autoantibodies cause the

TABLE 22-8

FREQUENCY (%) OF IMMUNOPATHOLOGIC CATEGORIES OF CRESCENTIC GLOMERULONEPHRITIS* IN DIFFERENT AGE GROUPS

Category	Age (years)		
	<20	20–64	>65
Anti–glomerular basement membrane	10	10	10
Immune complex	55	40	10
Antineutrophil cytoplasmic autoantibody	30	45	75
No evidence for the three categories above	5	5	5

*Glomerulonephritis with crescents in more than 50% of glomeruli.

disease. *ANCAs are specific for cytoplasmic proteins in neutrophils and monocytes, usually myeloperoxidase (MPO-ANCA) or proteinase 3 (PR3-ANCA).* These autoantibodies activate neutrophils to adhere to endothelial cells, release toxic oxygen metabolites, degranulate and kill endothelial cells. Neutrophils activated by ANCAs also activate the alternative complement pathway, which further amplifies the inflammation.

 PATHOLOGY: More than 90% of patients with ANCA glomerulonephritis have glomerular necrosis (Fig. 22-55) and crescent formation (Fig. 22-56), often in more than 1/2 of glomeruli. Nonnecrotic segments may appear normal or have slight neutrophil infiltration or mild endocapillary hypercellularity. There is little or no immunoglobulin or complement deposition, which distinguishes ANCA glomerulonephritis from anti-GBM and immune complex glomerulonephritides. Some patients with crescentic glomerulonephritis have serologic and pathologic evidence of ANCAs, anti-GBM antibodies and/or immune complexes.

 CLINICAL FEATURES: ANCA glomerulonephritis most commonly presents with rapidly progressive renal failure, with nephritic signs and symptoms. The disease accounts for 75% of rapidly progressive (crescentic) glomerulonephritis in patients older than 60, 45% in middle-aged adults and 30% in young adults and children (Table 22-8). *In 3/4 of patients with ANCA glomerulonephritis, systemic small vessel vasculitis is present (see below), which has many systemic manifestations, including pulmonary hemorrhage.* ANCA glomerulonephritis with pulmonary vasculitis causes **pulmonary–renal vasculitic syndrome** much more often than does Goodpasture syndrome. More than 80% of patients with ANCA glomerulonephritis develop ESRD within 5 years if untreated. Immunosuppressive therapy reduces this to less than 20%. Once remission is induced with high-dose immunosuppression, patients are at risk for recurrent disease. The disease recurs in 15% of renal transplant recipients.

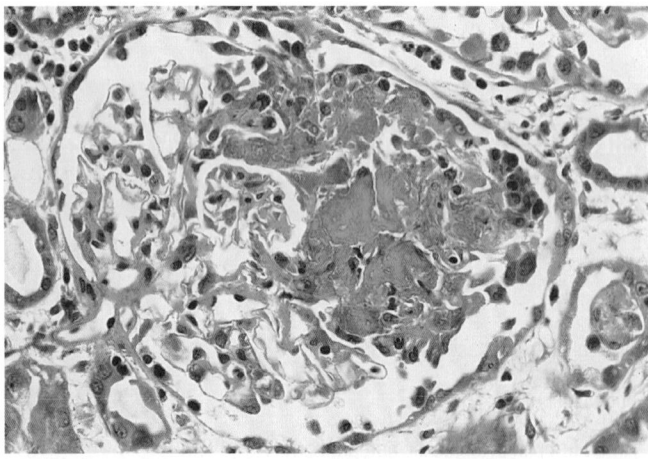

FIGURE 22-55. Antineutrophil cytoplasmic autoantibody glomerulonephritis. Segmental fibrinoid necrosis is illustrated. In time, this lesion stimulates crescent formation.

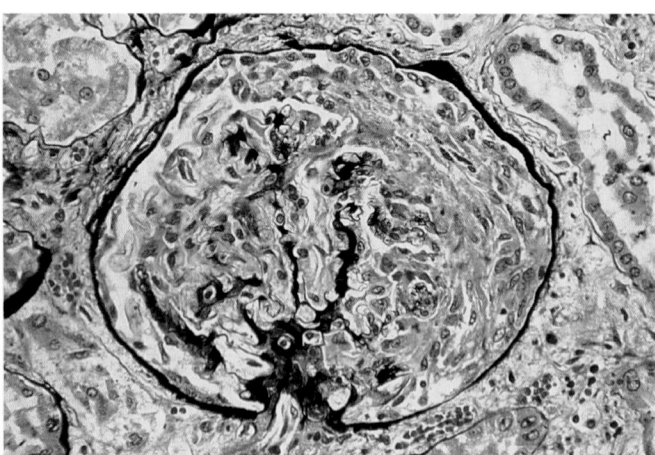

FIGURE 22-56. Antineutrophil cytoplasmic autoantibody glomerulonephritis. Silver staining shows focal disruption of glomerular basement membranes and crescent formation within the Bowman space.

VASCULAR DISEASES

Renal Vasculitis May Affect Vessels of All Sizes

Many types of systemic vasculitis affect the kidney (Table 22-9). *In a sense, glomerulonephritis is a local form of vasculitis that involves glomerular capillaries.* Glomeruli may be the only site of vascular inflammation, or the renal disease may be a component of a systemic vasculitis.

Small Vessel Vasculitides

Small vessel vasculitis affects small arteries, arterioles, capillaries and venules. Involvement of any of these can lead to glomerulonephritis. Other common manifestations include purpura, arthralgias, myalgias, peripheral neuropathy and pulmonary hemorrhage. Immune complexes, anti–basement membrane antibodies or ANCAs (Table 22-9) can cause small vessel vasculitides.

IgA vasculitis (Henoch-Schönlein purpura) is the most common childhood vasculitis. It is caused by vascular localization of immune complexes containing mostly IgA. The glomerular lesion is identical to that of IgA nephropathy.

Cryoglobulinemic vasculitis causes proliferative glomerulonephritis, usually type I MPGN. By light microscopy, aggregates of cryoglobulins ("hyaline thrombi") are often seen within capillary lumens (Fig. 22-57).

ANCA vasculitis involves vessels outside the kidneys in 75% of patients with ANCA glomerulonephritis. Based on clinical and pathologic features, patients with systemic ANCA vasculitis are classified as follows (Fig. 22-15):

- **Microscopic polyangiitis,** if there is pauci-immune vasculitis with no asthma or granulomatous inflammation
- **Granulomatosis with polyangiitis (formerly Wegener granulomatosis),** if there is necrotizing granulomatous inflammation, usually in the respiratory tract
- **Eosinophilic granulomatosis with polyangiitis (Churg-Strauss syndrome),** if there is eosinophilia and asthma

In addition to causing necrotizing and crescentic glomerulonephritis, ANCA vasculitides often entail necrotizing inflammation in other renal vessels, such as arteries (Fig. 22-58), arterioles and medullary peritubular capillaries.

TABLE 22-9

TYPES OF VASCULITIS THAT INVOLVE THE KIDNEYS

Type of Vasculitis	Major Target Vessels in Kidney	Major Renal Manifestations
Small Vessel Vasculitis		
Immune complex vasculitis		
IgA vasculitis (Henoch-Schönlein purpura)	Glomeruli	Nephritis
Cryoglobulinemic vasculitis	Glomeruli	Nephritis
Anti-GBM vasculitis		
Goodpasture syndrome	Glomeruli	Nephritis
ANCA vasculitis		
Granulomatosis with polyangiitis (Wegener granulomatosis)	Glomeruli, arterioles, interlobular arteries	Nephritis
Microscopic polyangiitis	Glomeruli, arterioles, interlobular arteries	Nephritis
Eosinophilic granulomatosis with polyangiitis (Churg-Strauss syndrome)	Glomeruli, arterioles, interlobular arteries	Nephritis
Medium-Sized Vessel Vasculitis		
Polyarteritis nodosa	Interlobar and arcuate arteries	Infarcts and hemorrhage
Kawasaki disease	Interlobar and arcuate arteries	Infarcts and hemorrhage
Large Vessel Vasculitis		
Giant cell arteritis	Main renal artery	Renovascular hypertension
Takayasu arteritis	Main renal artery	Renovascular hypertension

ANCA = antineutrophil cytoplasmic autoantibody; GBM = glomerular basement membrane.

Medium-Sized Vessel Vasculitis

Medium-sized vessel vasculitides affect arteries, but not arterioles, capillaries or venules (see Chapter 16). The necrotizing arteritides, such as **polyarteritis nodosa,** which occurs mainly in adults, and **Kawasaki disease,** which principally afflicts young children, rarely cause renal dysfunction. However, they may involve renal arteries and cause pseudoaneurysm formation and renal thrombosis, infarction and hemorrhage.

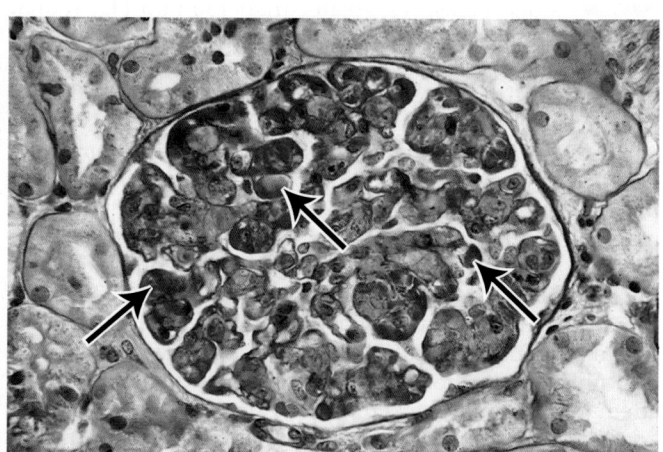

FIGURE 22-57. Cryoglobulinemic glomerulonephritis. The pattern of glomerular inflammation is similar to that of type I membranoproliferative glomerulonephritis. However, as in this specimen, there typically are conspicuous glassy aggregates ("hyaline thrombi," *arrows*) in the capillary lumina and subendothelial spaces. These are not true thrombi but rather are large aggregates of cryoglobulins (periodic acid–Schiff stain).

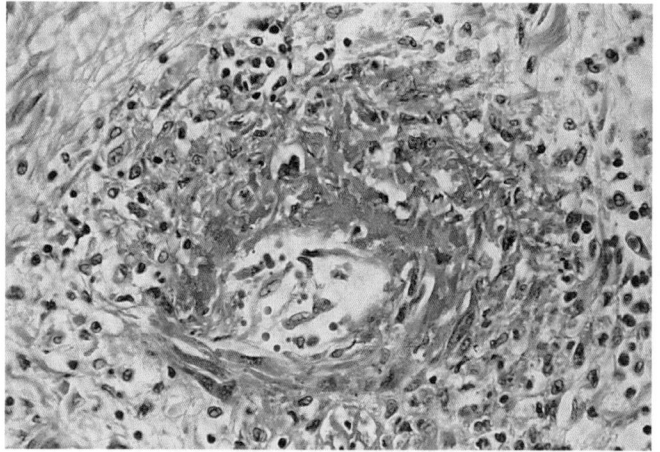

FIGURE 22-58. Antineutrophil cytoplasmic autoantibody necrotizing arteritis. Fibrinoid necrosis and inflammation involve an interlobular artery in the renal cortex.

Large Vessel Vasculitis

Large vessel vasculitides, such as **giant cell arteritis** and **Takayasu arteritis,** affect the aorta and its major branches. These disorders may cause renovascular hypertension by involving the main renal arteries or the aorta at the origin of the renal arteries (see Chapter 16). Narrowing or obstruction of these vessels results in renal ischemia, which stimulates increased renin production and consequent hypertension (Table 22-9).

Hypertensive Nephrosclerosis May Obliterate Glomeruli

 **ETIOLOGIC FACTORS:** Sustained systolic pressures greater than 140 mm Hg and diastolic pressures higher than 90 mm Hg define hypertension (see Chapter 16). Mild to moderate hypertension causes typical hypertensive nephrosclerosis, thus belying the previous term, *benign nephrosclerosis.* In fact, hypertensive nephrosclerosis is identified in about 15% of patients with "benign hypertension." Changes like those in hypertensive nephrosclerosis may occur in older individuals who have never had hypertension and are attributed to aging itself.

 PATHOLOGY: The kidneys are smaller than normal (atrophic) and are usually affected bilaterally. Renal cortical surfaces are finely granular (Fig. 22-59), but coarser scars are occasionally present. On cut section, the cortex is thinned. Many glomeruli appear normal; others show varying degrees of ischemic change. Initially, glomerular capillaries are broader because of thickening, wrinkling and collapse of GBMs. Cells of the glomerular tuft are progressively lost, and collagen and matrix material are deposited within the Bowman space. Eventually, glomerular tufts are obliterated by a dense, eosinophilic globular scar, all inside the Bowman capsule. Tubular atrophy, due to glomerular obsolescence, is associated with interstitial fibrosis and chronic inflammation. Globally, sclerotic glomeruli and surrounding atrophic tubules are often clustered in focal subcapsular zones, with adjacent areas of preserved glomeruli and tubules (Fig. 22-60), which accounts for the granular surfaces of nephrosclerotic kidneys.

The pattern of change in renal blood vessels depends on vessel size. Intimas of arteries as small as arcuate arteries have fibrotic thickening, replication of the elastica-like lamina and partial replacement of the muscularis with fibrous tissue. Interlobular arteries and arterioles may develop medial hyperplasia. Arterioles show concentric hyaline thickening of the wall, often with smooth muscle cell loss or displacement to the periphery. This arteriolar change is called **hyaline arteriolosclerosis**.

 CLINICAL FEATURES: Although hypertensive nephrosclerosis does not usually impair renal function, some people with hypertension develop progressive renal failure, which may lead to ESRD. Since hypertension is so common, the relatively small percentage of hypertensive patients who develop renal insufficiency amounts to 1/3 of patients with ESRD. *Hypertensive nephrosclerosis is most prevalent and aggressive in blacks, among whom hypertension is the leading cause of ESRD.*

Malignant Hypertensive Nephropathy Causes Rapid Loss of Renal Function

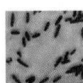 **ETIOLOGIC FACTORS:** No specific blood pressure defines malignant hypertension, but diastolic pressures greater than 130 mm Hg, retinal vascular changes, papilledema and renal functional impairment are usual criteria. There are prior histories of benign hypertension in 1/2 of patients, and many others have a background of chronic renal injury caused by many different diseases. Occasionally, malignant hypertension arises de novo in apparently healthy people, particularly young black men. The pathogenesis of the vascular injury in malignant hypertension is not entirely clear. One hypothesis proposes that very high blood pressure, combined with microvascular vasoconstriction, causes endothelial injury as blood slams into narrowed small vessels. At such sites, plasma constituents leak into injured arteriolar walls (causing fibrinoid necrosis), into arterial intimas (inducing edematous intimal thickening) and into the subendothelial zone of glomerular capillaries (consolidating glomeruli). At these sites of vascular injury, thrombosis can result in focal renal cortical necrosis (infarcts).

 PATHOLOGY: Renal sizes in malignant hypertensive nephropathy vary from small to enlarged, depending on the duration of preexisting benign hypertension. The cut surface is mottled red and yellow,

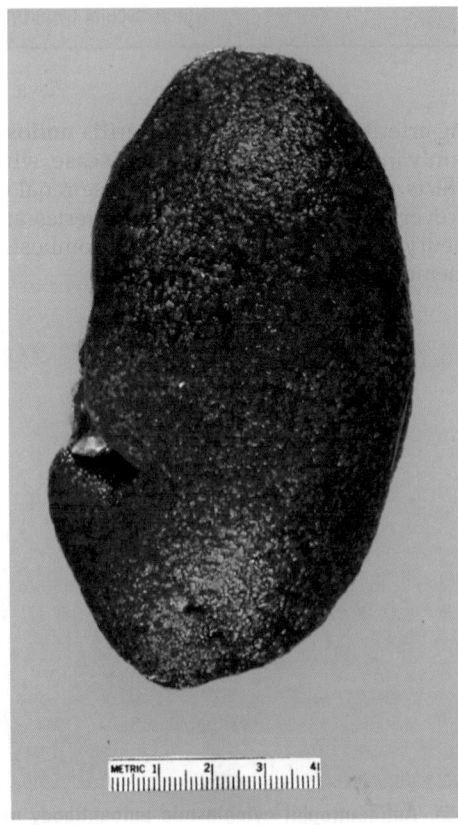

FIGURE 22-59. Hypertensive nephrosclerosis. The kidney is reduced in size, and the cortical surface exhibits fine granularity.

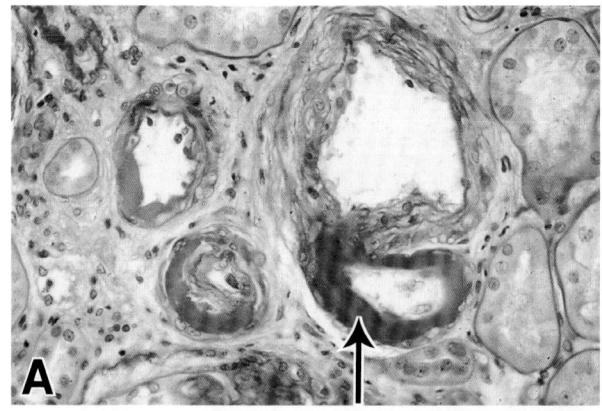

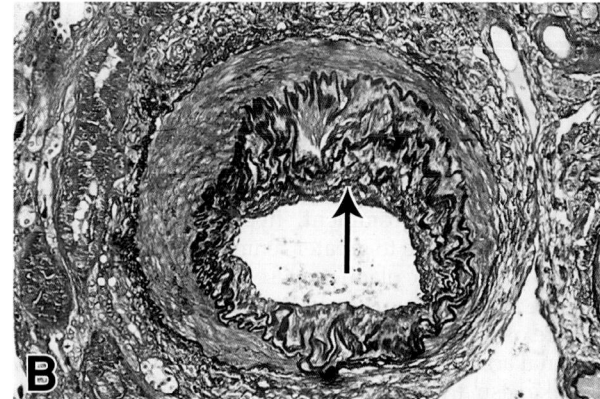

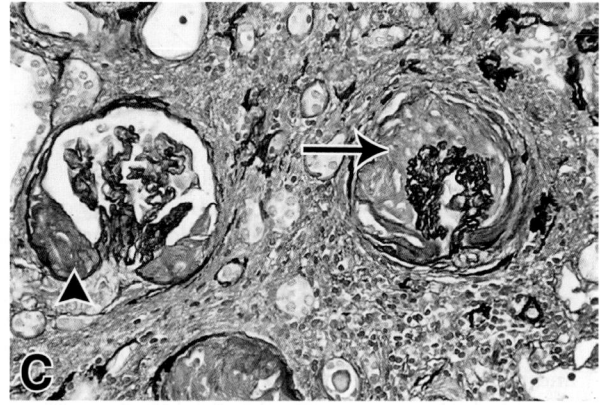

FIGURE 22-60. Hypertensive nephrosclerosis. A. Three arterioles with hyaline sclerosis (*arrow*) (periodic acid–Schiff stain). **B.** Arcuate artery with fibrotic intimal thickening causing narrowing of the lumen (*arrow*) (silver stain). **C.** One glomerulus with global sclerosis (*arrow*) and one with segmental sclerosis (*arrowhead*). Note also tubular atrophy, interstitial fibrosis and chronic inflammation (silver stain).

with occasional small cortical infarcts. Malignant hypertensive nephropathy is often superimposed on hypertensive nephrosclerosis, with edematous (myxoid, mucoid) intimal expansion in arteries and fibrinoid necrosis of arterioles. Glomerular changes vary from capillary congestion to consolidation to necrosis (Fig. 22-61). Severe cases show thrombosis and focal ischemic cortical necrosis (infarction). By electron microscopy, electron-lucent material expands glomerular subendothelial zones. There may be focal insudation of plasma proteins into injured vessel walls. These changes are identical to those seen in other forms of thrombotic microangiopathy (see below).

 CLINICAL FEATURES: Malignant hypertension is more common in men than in women, typically around the age of 40. Patients suffer headache, dizziness and visual disturbances and may develop overt encephalopathy. Hematuria and proteinuria are frequent. Progressive renal deterioration develops if the condition persists. Aggressive antihypertensive therapy often controls the disease.

Renovascular Hypertension Follows Narrowing of a Major Renal Artery

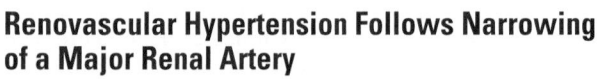 **PATHOPHYSIOLOGY:** Stenosis or total occlusion of a main renal artery produces hypertension that is potentially curable if the arterial lumen is restored. Harry Goldblatt carried out the initial studies of this syndrome in dogs in 1934. Since then, a kidney deprived of vascular supply has been known as a **Goldblatt kidney**. In patients with renal artery stenosis, hypertension reflects increased production of renin, angiotensin II and aldosterone. Renal vein renin from an ischemic kidney is elevated, but it is normal in the contralateral kidney. Most (95%) cases are caused by atherosclerosis, which explains why this disorder is twice as common in men as in women, and mainly at older ages (average age, 55). Fibromuscular dysplasia and vasculitis are less common causes overall but are the most frequent causes in children.

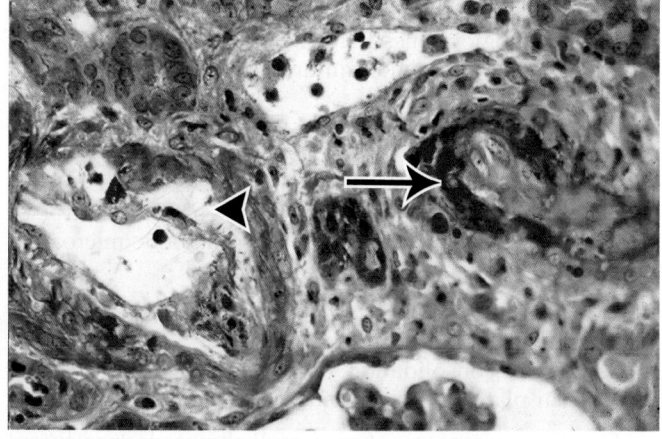

FIGURE 22-61. Malignant hypertensive nephropathy. Red fibrinoid necrosis (*arrow*) in the wall of the arteriole on the right and clear edematous expansion (*arrowhead*) in the intima of the interlobular artery on the left from a patient with malignant hypertension (Masson trichrome stain).

THE KIDNEY

PATHOLOGY: Regardless of the cause of renal artery stenosis, renal parenchymal changes are the same. The size of the involved kidney is reduced. Glomeruli appear normal but are closer to each other than normal, because intervening tubules show marked ischemic atrophy without extensive interstitial fibrosis. Many glomeruli lose their attachments to the proximal tubule. Juxtaglomerular apparati are prominent, hyperplastic and more granular than usual, due to greater renin production.

When atherosclerotic plaques cause the vascular stenosis, they impinge on the aortic ostium or narrow the renal artery lumen, more often on the left than on the right. Occasionally, an abdominal aortic aneurysm affects the origin of the renal arteries. Takayasu arteritis and giant cell arteritis cause renal artery stenosis by inflammatory and sclerotic thickening of the artery wall with resultant narrowing of the lumen.

In **fibromuscular dysplasia,** the renal artery becomes fibrous and shows stenosis due to muscular hyperplasia. There are several patterns of renal artery involvement: intimal fibroplasia, medial fibroplasia, perimedial fibroplasia and periarterial fibroplasia. As the names imply, these disorders affect different layers of the artery, from the intima to the adventitia. Medial fibroplasia is the most common and accounts for 2/3 of cases. This process creates areas of medial thickening alternating with areas of atrophy, producing a "string of beads" pattern in angiograms.

CLINICAL FEATURES: Renovascular hypertension is characterized by mild to moderate blood pressure elevations. A bruit may be heard over the renal artery. Diagnosis requires imaging studies, such as angiography. In more than 1/2 of patients, surgical revascularization, angioplasty or nephrectomy cures the hypertension. If the renovascular hypertension is long-standing, the uninvolved kidney may develop hypertensive nephrosclerosis.

Renal Atheroembolism May Complicate Aortic Atherosclerosis

In patients with severe aortic atherosclerosis, atheromatous debris may embolize into the renal arteries and vascular tree as far as glomerular capillaries and cause acute renal failure. This may occur spontaneously or be initiated by trauma, such as angiographic procedures. **Cholesterol clefts** are seen in vessel lumens (Fig. 22-62). Early lesions are surrounded by atheromatous material or thrombus. They may later elicit a foreign body reaction and may stimulate fibrosis in the adjacent vessel wall.

Thrombotic Microangiopathies Cause Microangiopathic Hemolytic Anemia and Renal Failure

**PATHOPHYSIOLOGY:** Thrombotic microangiopathy has a variety of causes and at least two distinct pathogenic pathways. One pathogenic pathway that causes typical and atypical **hemolytic–uremic syndrome (HUS)** produces endothelial damage that allows plasma constituents to enter the intima of arteries, walls of arterioles and subendothelial zone of glomerular capillaries, narrowing vessel lumens and causing

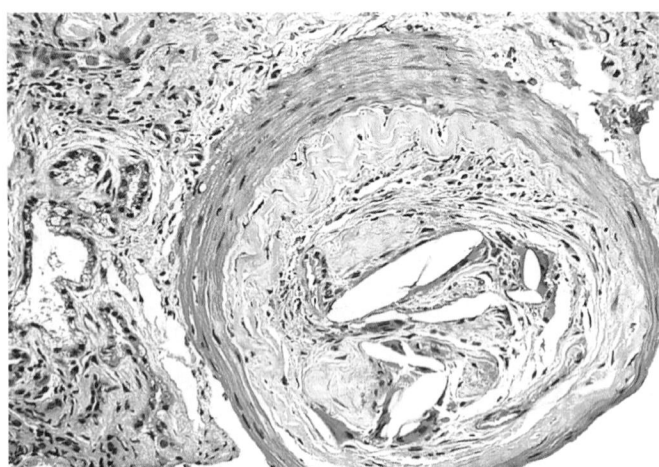

FIGURE 22-62. Atheroembolus. An atheroembolus obstructs an arcuate artery. Note the cholesterol clefts.

ischemia. The injured endothelial surfaces promote thrombosis, which worsens ischemia and may cause focal ischemic necrosis. **Typical HUS** follows diarrhea due to toxin-producing bacteria, most often *E. coli* (usually the O157:H7 strain), in contaminated food. The toxin injures glomerular endothelial cells, initiating the sequence described above. **Atypical HUS** is unrelated to diarrhea and is caused by different mechanisms, including genetic abnormalities in complement regulatory proteins (mostly factor H but also factor I and membrane cofactor protein), autoantibodies to complement regulatory proteins (anti–factor H) or both.

Thrombotic thrombocytopenic purpura (TTP) is caused by a genetic or acquired deficiency of a protease that cleaves multimers of von Willebrand factor on the surface of endothelial cells (see Chapter 26). The large uncleaved multimers promote platelet aggregation and microvascular thrombosis. Passage of blood through vessels injured by HUS or TTP leads to a nonimmune (Coombs-negative) hemolytic anemia, with misshapen and disrupted erythrocytes (schistocytes) and thrombocytopenia. This syndrome is **microangiopathic hemolytic anemia (MAHA).** Thus, because both HUS and TTP present with MAHA, they can be very difficult to distinguish clinically. Thrombotic microangiopathies that resemble HUS and TTP can also be due to drugs, autoimmune diseases and malignant hypertension (Table 22-10).

PATHOLOGY: The renal pathology of HUS is like that of malignant hypertensive nephropathy (see above), which is a form of thrombotic microangiopathy. The basic renal lesions are:

- Arteriolar fibrinoid necrosis
- Arterial edematous intimal expansion
- Glomerular consolidation, necrosis or congestion
- Vascular platelet-rich thrombosis

Electron microscopy of glomeruli shows electron-lucent expansion of the subendothelial zone (Figs. 22-63, 22-64), due to insudation of plasma proteins under injured endothelial cells. By fluorescence microscopy, fibrin and insudated plasma proteins are seen in injured vessel walls.

TABLE 22-10

CATEGORIES OF THROMBOTIC MICROANGIOPATHY

Thrombotic thrombocytopenic purpura

    Autoantibodies against ADAMTS13

    Inherited deficiency in ADAMTS13

Typical hemolytic–uremic syndrome

    E. coli

    Shigella spp.

    Pseudomonas spp.

Atypical hemolytic–uremic syndrome

    Genetic mutation (e.g., factor H, factor I, membrane cofactor protein)

    Autoantibodies to complement regulatory proteins (e.g., anti–factor H)

Drug-induced thrombotic microangiopathies

    Mitomycin

    Cisplatin

    Cyclosporin

    Tacrolimus

    Anti-VEGF therapy

Autoimmune diseases

    Systemic sclerosis (scleroderma)

    Systemic lupus erythematosus

    Antiphospholipid antibody syndrome

Malignant hypertension

Pregnancy and postpartum factors

VEGF = vascular endothelial growth factor.

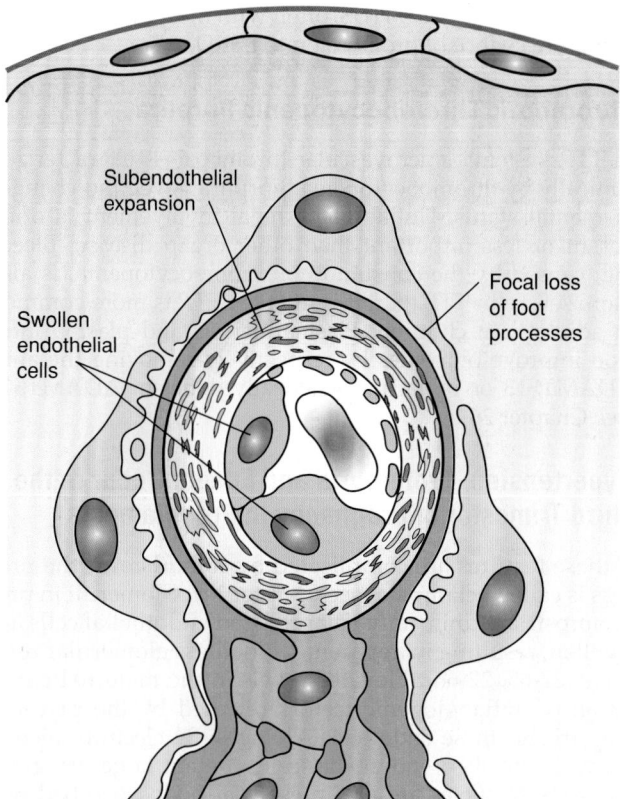

FIGURE 22-63. Hemolytic–uremic syndrome. A wide band of subendothelial expansion due to insudation of plasma proteins causes narrowing of the capillary lumen. Endothelial cell swelling also contributes to narrowing of the lumen.

TTP may have vascular lesions that resemble HUS, but TTP is characterized by more numerous platelet-rich thrombi in glomerular capillaries as well as in capillaries, arterioles and small arteries in many tissues of the body.

 CLINICAL FEATURES: Their clinical presentations and causes allow discrimination among the different categories of thrombotic microangiopathy. The MAHAs all have in common microangiopathic hemolytic anemia, thrombocytopenia, hypertension and renal failure, but to different degrees. In a patient with thrombotic microangiopathy, an accompanying diseases process (e.g., bloody diarrhea, SLE, systemic sclerosis) or treatment (e.g., mitomycin, cisplatin, vascular endothelial growth factor [VEGF] inhibitor) may point to the cause of the MAHA.

Hemolytic–Uremic Syndrome

Typical postdiarrheal HUS features MAHA and acute renal failure, with little or no significant vascular disease outside the kidneys. *Typical HUS is among the most common causes of acute renal failure in children.* It is less common in adults. HUS occurs as isolated cases or in epidemics caused by food contaminated with enterohemorrhagic *E. coli*. Patients present with hemorrhagic diarrhea and rapidly progressive renal failure. Even when dialysis is required, normal renal function usually returns within several weeks. However, impaired renal function may eventually reemerge after 15–25 years in in more than 1/2 of patients. Atypical HUS is more frequent in adults and is not preceded by diarrhea. Its prognosis is

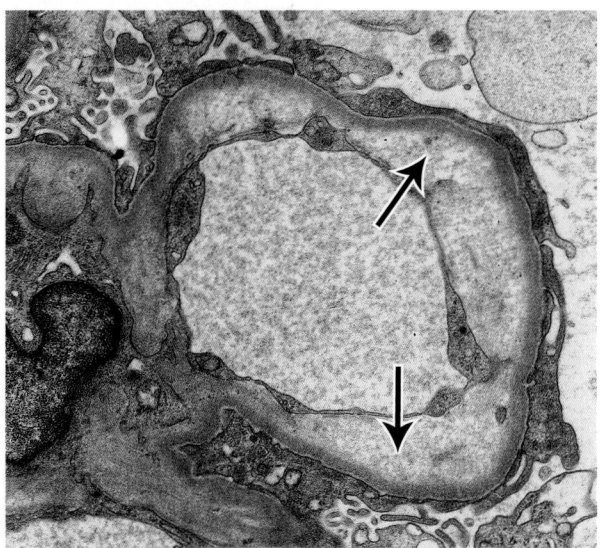

FIGURE 22-64. Thrombotic microangiopathy. An electron micrograph shows a wide band of lucent material in the subendothelial zone (*arrows*) corresponding to the subendothelial expansion shown in Fig. 22-62, which causes marked narrowing of the lumen.

worse than for typical HUS, often with multiple recurrences and more chance of progression to ESRD.

Thrombotic Thrombocytopenic Purpura

In TTP, systemic microvascular thrombosis is characterized clinically by thrombocytopenia, purpura, fever and changes in mental status. Unlike HUS, renal involvement is often absent or less important than other organ disease. Bleeding, caused by the consumptive thrombocytopenia, is also more severe in TTP than it is in HUS. TTP is more common in adults than children. Plasmapheresis and plasma infusion improve outcomes by respectively removing the anti-ADAMTS13 or replacing genetically deficient ADAMTS13 (see Chapter 26).

Hypertension, Proteinuria and Edema Occur in the Third Trimester of Pregnancy in Preeclampsia

If these features are complicated by **convulsions,** the process is called **eclampsia** (see Chapter 14). Glomeruli in preeclampsia are uniformly enlarged and endothelial cells are swollen, resulting in apparently bloodless glomerular tufts (Figs. 22-65, 22-66). Elevated levels in the maternal circulation of antiangiogenic factors released by the placenta may trigger these endothelial changes. By electron microscopy, the swollen endothelial cells contain large, irregular vacuoles. Vacuoles are also present in podocytes. Bed rest

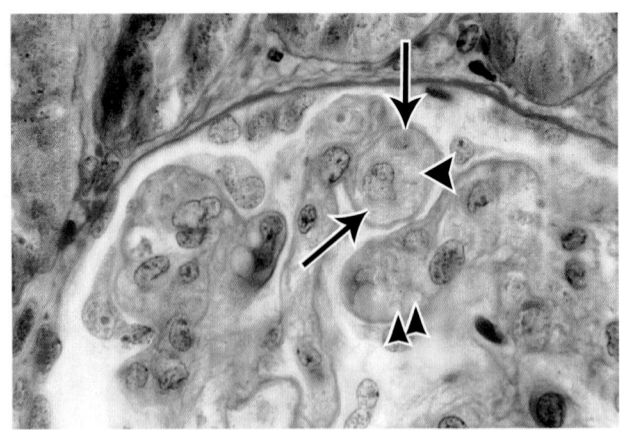

FIGURE 22-66. Preeclampsia. Capillary lumens (*large arrowhead*) are obliterated by swollen endothelial cells (*arrows*). Mesangial vacuolization is shown (*small double arrowheads*) (Masson trichrome stain).

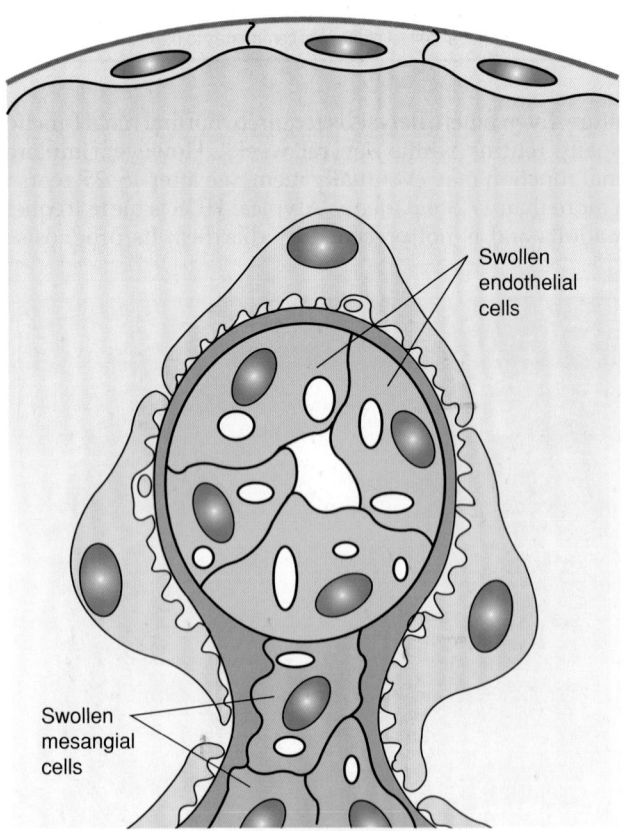

FIGURE 22-65. Preeclamptic nephropathy. Preeclamptic nephropathy, or pregnancy-induced nephropathy, exhibits marked swelling of endothelial cells with narrowing of the lumens. Both endothelial and mesangial cells are enlarged and have multiple vacuoles and vesicular structures.

and antihypertensive agents suffice to control mild to moderate disease. More severe cases may require induction of delivery. Hypertension and proteinuria typically disappear 1–2 weeks after delivery.

Nephropathy Is the Most Common Organ Manifestation of Sickle Cell Disease

The interstitial tissue in which the vasa recta course is hypertonic and has a low oxygen tension. As a result, in sickle cell patients, erythrocytes tend to sickle as they go through the vasa recta. In so doing, they occlude the vascular lumens and cause infarcts in the medulla and papilla. The latter may be severe enough to cause papillary necrosis. Ischemic scarring of the medulla leads to focal tubular loss and atrophy. Glomeruli are conspicuously congested with sickled cells. FSGS or, less often, MPGN occurs in a minority of patients and may cause nephrotic syndrome.

Renal Infarcts Are Mostly Due to Embolic Arterial Obstruction

Such emboli most often involve interlobar or arcuate arteries.

 ETIOLOGIC FACTORS: The size of the infarct varies with the size of the occluded vessel. Common sources of emboli include:

- **Mural thrombi** overlying myocardial infarcts or caused by atrial fibrillation
- **Infected valves** in bacterial endocarditis
- **Complicated atherosclerotic plaques** in the aorta

Occasionally, a branch of the renal artery is occluded by thrombosis superimposed on underlying atherosclerosis or arteritis. Lumens of the small branches of the renal artery may be so severely compromised in malignant hypertension, scleroderma or HUS that blood supply is insufficient to maintain tissue viability. Sickled erythrocytes in sickle cell anemia may cause renal infarcts, especially in the papillae, as noted above. Hemorrhagic renal infarction due to renal vein thrombosis may complicate severe dehydration, particularly in small infants, but also occurs in adults with septic thrombophlebitis and conditions associated with

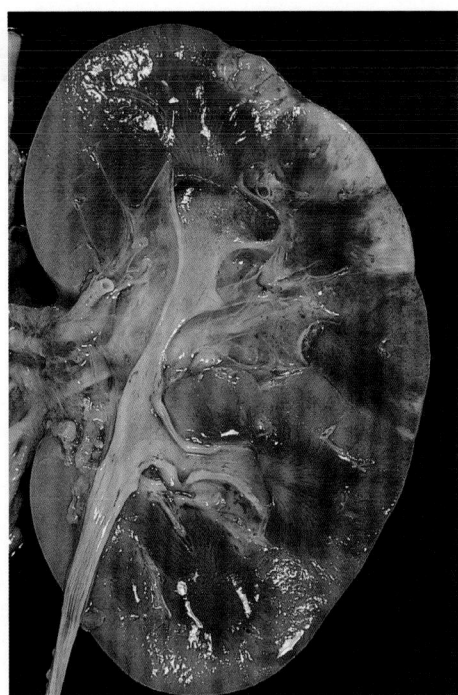

FIGURE 22-67. Renal infarcts. A bisected kidney shows three discrete areas of infarction characterized by marked pallor, which extends to the subcapsular surface.

hypercoagulability. Typically, an acute infarct causes sharp flank or abdominal pain and hematuria.

Infarction of an entire kidney by occlusion of the main renal artery is rare because collateral circulation generally maintains organ viability. Clearly, in such a circumstance, renal function ceases in that kidney.

 PATHOLOGY: Variably sized, wedge-shaped areas of pale ischemic necrosis, with the base on the capsular surface, are typical (Fig. 22-67). All structures in affected zones show coagulative necrosis. A hemorrhagic zone borders acute infarcts. As in other tissues, the histologic response to the infarct progresses through phases of acute inflammation, granulation tissue and fibrosis. Healed infarcts are sharply circumscribed and depressed cortical scars containing ghosts of obliterated glomeruli, atrophic tubules, interstitial fibrosis and a mild chronic inflammatory infiltrate. Old infarcts may undergo dystrophic calcification. At the margins of a healed infarct, the viable tissue resembles that seen in chronic ischemia, with tubular atrophy, interstitial fibrosis and infiltration by chronic inflammatory cells.

Cortical Necrosis Is Due to Severe Ischemia

Cortical necrosis affects all or part of the renal cortex. The term **infarct** applies if there is one area (or a few areas) of necrosis caused by arterial occlusion, but **cortical necrosis** implies more-widespread ischemic necrosis.

 **ETIOLOGIC FACTORS:** Renal cortical necrosis can complicate any condition associated with hypovolemic or endotoxic shock, the classical situation

being premature placental separation late in pregnancy (see Chapter 12). All forms of shock can result in reversible prerenal or intrarenal ischemia, which can precede irreversible cortical necrosis.

Vasa recta that supply arterial blood to the medulla arise from juxtamedullary efferent arterioles, proximal to vessels supplying the outer cortex. Thus, occlusion of outer cortical vessels (e.g., by vasospasm, thrombi or thrombotic microangiopathy) leads to cortical necrosis and spares the medulla. Experimentally, renal cortical necrosis may be caused by vasoconstrictors such as vasopressin and serotonin, or by eliciting disseminated intravascular coagulation (see Chapter 26).

 PATHOLOGY: Cortical necrosis may vary from patchy to confluent (Fig. 22-68). In the most severely involved areas, all parenchymal elements exhibit coagulative necrosis. The proximal convoluted tubules are invariably necrotic, as are most of the distal tubules. In adjacent viable portions of the cortex, glomeruli and distal convoluted tubules are usually unaffected, but many proximal convoluted tubules may show ischemic injury, such as epithelial flattening or necrosis.

With extensive necrosis, the cortex is pale and diffusely necrotic, except for thin rims of viable tissue just beneath the capsule and at the corticomedullary junction. These are supplied by capsular and medullary collateral blood vessels, respectively. Patients who survive cortical necrosis may develop dystrophic calcification of the necrotic areas.

 CLINICAL FEATURES: Severe cortical necrosis manifests as acute renal failure, which initially may be indistinguishable from that produced by acute

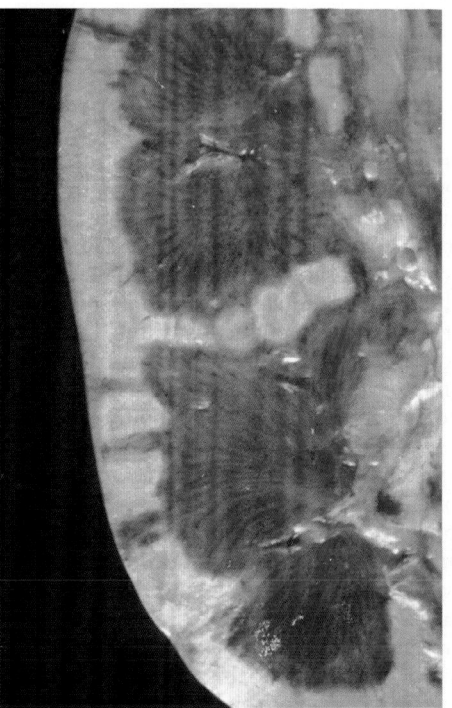

FIGURE 22-68. Renal cortical necrosis. The cortex of the kidney is pale yellow and soft owing to diffuse cortical necrosis.

tubular necrosis (ATN). However, the former is more often irreversible. A renal arteriogram or biopsy may be required for diagnosis. Recovery is determined by the extent of the disease, but hypertension is common among survivors.

DISEASES OF TUBULES AND INTERSTITIUM

Acute kidney injury (AKI) is an acute rise in serum creatinine. It is classified as **prerenal** if caused by reduced blood flow to the kidneys, **intrarenal** if due to injury to the renal parenchyma and **postrenal** if caused by urinary tract obstruction. Intrarenal AKI is further categorized by the portion of the kidney that is mainly injured: **glomeruli** (e.g., acute glomerulonephritis), **vessels** (e.g., thrombotic microangiopathy), **tubules** (e.g., ischemic acute tubular injury) or **interstitium** (acute tubulointerstitial nephritis). *The most common cause for intrarenal AKI is ischemic acute tubular injury.*

Acute Ischemic and Nephrotoxic Acute Tubular Injury Commonly Cause AKI

Ischemic AKI is severe, but potentially reversible, renal failure due to impaired tubular epithelial function caused by ischemia or toxic injury. Ischemic prerenal AKI is reversible pathophysiologic AKI with no structural tubular epithelial changes. *If ischemia is severe enough to cause histologic tubular epithelial injury, it is considered intrarenal ischemic AKI.* Extensive ischemia can cause overt necrosis of tubular epithelium, or **ATN**. However, most ischemic acute tubular injury does not produce widespread tubular epithelial necrosis, and thus in this setting, the term *ATN* would be a misnomer.

 **PATHOPHYSIOLOGY AND ETIO-LOGIC FACTORS:** Table 22-11 lists some causes of AKI due to acute tubular injury.

Ischemic acute tubular injury results from reduced renal perfusion, usually associated with hypotension. Tubular epithelial cells have a high metabolic rate and thus are particularly sensitive to oxygen deprivation, which rapidly depletes intracellular ATP. The most frequent histologic abnormality is flattening (simplification) of tubular epithelial cells due to sloughing of the apical cytoplasm into the urine. This generates granular pigmented casts that can be seen in the urine and detected by urinalysis. Tubular epithelial cells may be simplified (flattened) but not necrotic in some patients with typical clinical ischemic AKI. Overt necrosis is less common.

Nephrotoxic acute tubular injury is caused by chemical injury to epithelial cells. In addition to their sensitivity to ischemia, tubular epithelial cells' high needs makes them susceptible to injury by toxins that perturb oxidative or other metabolic pathways. At the same time, these cells absorb and concentrate toxins. Hemoglobin and myoglobin act as endogenous toxins that can induce acute tubular injury **(pigment nephropathy)** if they are present at high concentrations in the urine.

TABLE 22-11
CAUSES OF ACUTE ACUTE TUBULAR INJURY

Ischemic Prerenal Acute Renal Failure or Ischemic Acute Kidney Injury

Massive hemorrhage

Septic shock

Severe burns

Dehydration

Prolonged diarrhea

Congestive heart failure

Volume redistribution (e.g., pancreatitis, peritonitis)

Nephrotoxin Acute Tubular Injury

Antibiotics (e.g., aminoglycosides, amphotericin B)

Radiographic contrast agents

Heavy metals (e.g., mercury, lead, cisplatin)

Organic solvents (e.g., ethylene glycol, carbon tetrachloride)

Poisons (e.g., paraquat)

Heme Protein Cast Nephropathies

Myoglobin (from rhabdomyolysis, e.g., with crush injury)

Hemoglobin (from hemolysis, e.g., with transfusion reaction)

The pathophysiology of ischemic AKI involves decreased glomerular filtration and tubular epithelial dysfunction due to some or all of the following (Fig. 22-69):

- Intrarenal vasoconstriction
- Alteration of arteriolar tone by tubuloglomerular feedback
- Decreased glomerular hydrostatic pressure
- Decreased glomerular capillary permeability (K_f)
- Tubular obstruction by cellular debris, with increased hydrostatic pressure
- Back-leakage of glomerular filtrate into the interstitium through damaged tubular epithelium

 PATHOLOGY: In ischemic AKI, kidneys are swollen, with a pale cortex and a congested medulla. Glomeruli and blood vessels are normal. Tubule injury is focal and is most pronounced in the proximal tubules and thick ascending limb of the loop of Henle of the outer medulla. The epithelium is flattened, lumens are dilated and brush borders are lost (epithelial simplification), due in part to sloughing of apical cytoplasm, which appears in distal tubular lumens and urine as brown granular casts. (The color reflects renal cytochrome pigments.) Electron microscopy shows decreased basolateral membrane infoldings of proximal tubular epithelial cells. Widespread necrosis of tubular epithelial cells is uncommon, but simplification may be evident. Instead, "necrosis" is subtle and appears as individual necrotic cells in some proximal or distal tubules. These single necrotic cells, plus a few viable cells, are shed into the tubular lumen, thus focally denuding the tubular basement membrane (Fig. 22-70). Interstitial edema is common. The vasa recta of the outer medulla are congested and

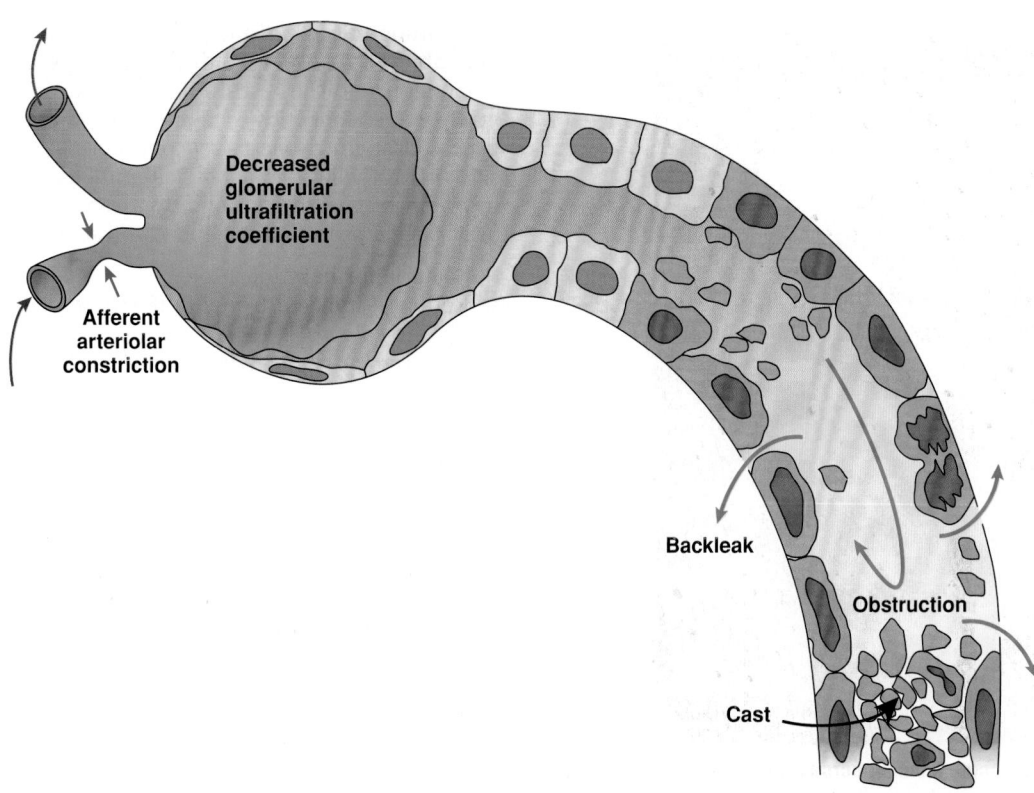

FIGURE 22-69. Pathogenesis of acute renal failure caused by acute tubular injury (acute tubular necrosis). Sloughing and necrosis of epithelial cells result in cast formation. Casts lead to obstruction and increased intraluminal pressure, which reduces glomerular filtration. Afferent arteriolar vasoconstriction, caused in part by tubuloglomerular feedback, results in decreased glomerular capillary filtration pressure. Tubular injury and increased intraluminal pressure cause fluid back-leakage from the lumen into the interstitium.

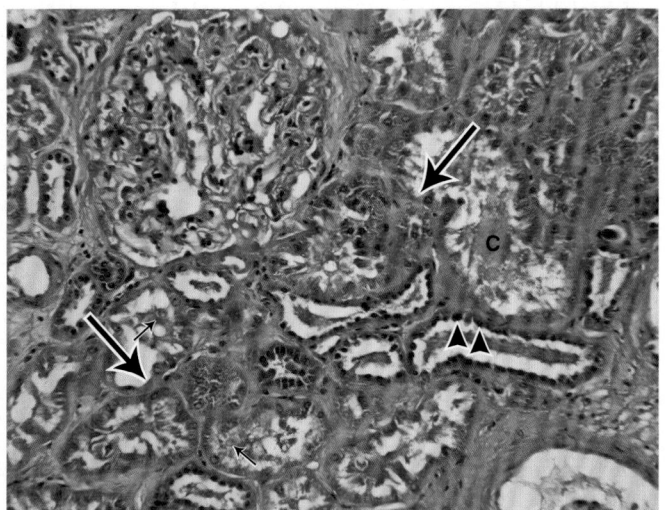

FIGURE 22-70. Ischemic acute tubular injury (ischemic acute kidney injury). Necrosis of individual tubular epithelial cells is evident both from focal denudation of the tubular basement membrane (*thick arrows*) and from the individual necrotic epithelial cells (*thin arrows*) present in some tubular lumina. Casts, the debris of dead tubular epithelium, fill many tubules (*C*). Some enlarged, regenerative-appearing epithelial cells are also present (*arrowheads*). Note the lack of significant glomerular or interstitial inflammation.

often contain nucleated cells, which are predominantly mononuclear leukocytes.

Toxic acute tubular injury shows more-extensive tubular epithelial necrosis than is typical for ischemic acute tubular injury (compare Figs. 22-70 and 22-71). However, toxic necrosis is largely limited to those tubular segments that are most sensitive to a particular toxin, usually the proximal tubule. In acute tubular injury due to hemoglobinuria or myoglobinuria, there are, as well, many red-brown tubular casts that are colored by heme pigments.

During the recovery phase of acute tubular injury, tubular epithelium regenerates, with mitoses, increased size of cells and nuclei, and cell crowding. Survivors eventually display complete restoration of normal renal architecture.

CLINICAL FEATURES: *Ischemia is the leading cause of AKI.* Rapidly rising serum creatinine, usually with decreased urine output **(oliguria),** is characteristic. **Nonoliguric** AKI is less common. Urinalysis shows degenerating epithelial cells and **"dirty brown" granular casts** (acute renal failure casts) with cell debris rich in cytochrome pigments. Urinalysis may help to differentiate among the three major intrinsic renal diseases that cause acute renal failure (Table 22-12). Prerenal ischemic acute tubular injury typically has a less than 1% fractional excretion of sodium, but intrarenal acute tubular injury has a fractional excretion of sodium greater than 2%, which is a marker of overt tubular epithelial damage.

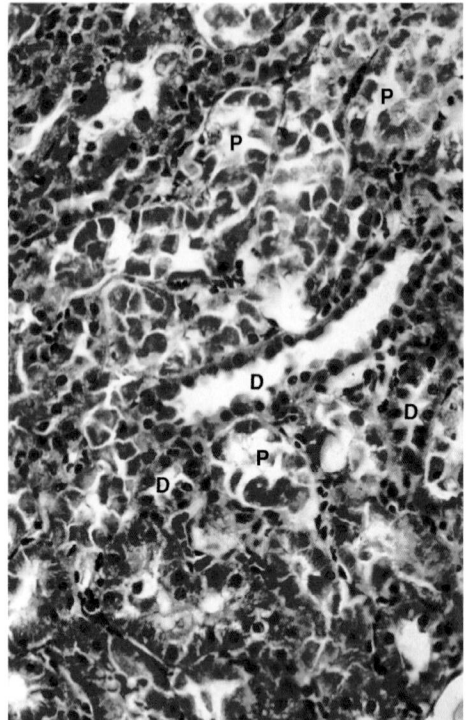

FIGURE 22-71. Toxic acute tubular necrosis due to mercury poisoning. There is widespread necrosis of proximal tubular (P) epithelial cells, with sparing of distal and collecting tubules (D). Interstitial inflammation is minimal.

The duration of renal failure in patients with ischemic acute tubular injury depends on many factors, especially the nature and reversibility of the cause. Many patients develop uremia (azotemia, fluid retention, metabolic acidosis, hyperkalemia), at least transiently, and may require dialysis. If the insult is removed right after injury begins, renal function may return within 1–2 weeks. However, recovery may take months. Increased urine output and decreased serum creatinine herald the recovery phase.

Pyelonephritis Usually Reflects Bacterial Infection of the Kidney

Acute Pyelonephritis

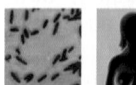 **ETIOLOGIC FACTORS AND PATHOPHYSIOLOGY:** Gram-negative bacteria from feces, mostly *E. coli*, cause 80% of acute pyelonephritis. *E. coli* that cause urinary tract infections

TABLE 22-12

URINALYSIS IN ACUTE KIDNEY INJURY

Causes of Acute Kidney Injury	Urinalysis Sediment Findings
Acute tubular injury	Dirty brown casts and epithelial cells
Acute glomerulonephritis	Red blood cell casts and proteinuria
Acute tubulointerstitial nephritis	White blood cell casts and pyuria

(uropathogenic *E. coli*) have virulence factors that enhance their ability to cause not only urinary tract infections but also pyelonephritis. The best studied of these are adhesins on fimbria (pili) encoded by pyelonephritis-associated pili (*PAP*) genes. Uropathogenic *E. coli* pili attach to adhesin-binding sites on urothelial cells as well as epithelial cells of the kidney. Infection reaches the kidney by ascending through the urinary tract, a process that depends on several factors:

- Bacterial urinary infection
- Reflux of infected urine up the ureters into the renal pelvis and calyces
- Bacterial entry through the papillae into the renal parenchyma

Bladder infections (cystitis) usually precede acute pyelonephritis. These occur more commonly in females because they have short urethras, they lack antibacterial prostatic secretions and sexual intercourse facilitates bacterial migration. Normal urethral commensal flora are replaced by fecal organisms in women who are unusually prone to recurrent urinary tract infections. Many factors may contribute to this change in flora, including hygiene, hormonal effects and genetic predisposition (e.g., increased receptors for *E. coli* on urothelial cells).

Pregnancy predisposes to acute pyelonephritis for several reasons, including a high frequency of asymptomatic bacteriuria (10%), of which 1/4 develops into acute pyelonephritis. Other causes include increased residual urine volume because high levels of progesterone make bladder musculature flaccid and less able to expel urine.

The bladder normally empties all but 2–3 mL of residual urine. Subsequent addition of sterile urine from the kidneys dilutes any bacteria that may have gained access to the bladder. However, if residual urine volume is increased (e.g., with prostatic obstruction or bladder atony due to neurogenic disorders such as paraplegia or diabetic neuropathy), sterile urine from the kidneys may be insufficient to dilute residual bladder urine to prevent bacterial accumulation. Diabetic glycosuria also facilitates infection by providing a rich bacterial growth medium.

Bacteria in bladder urine usually do not ascend to infect the kidneys. The ureter commonly inserts into the bladder wall at a steep angle (Fig. 22-72), and its most distal portion courses parallel to the bladder wall, between the mucosa and muscularis. Increased intravesicular pressure during micturition occludes the distal ureteral lumen and prevents urinary reflux. An anatomic abnormality, a short passage of the ureter within the bladder wall, causes the ureter to insert more perpendicularly to the bladder mucosal surface. As a result, rather than occluding the lumen, micturition increases intravesicular pressure and pushes urine into the patent ureter. This reflux can force the urine into the renal pelvis and calyces.

Even if reflux pressure delivers bacteria to the calyces, the renal parenchyma is not necessarily contaminated. The convexity of the simple papillae of central calyces blocks reflux urine from entering (Fig. 22-72), but the concavity of peripheral compound papillae allows easier access to the collecting system. *However, if pressure is prolonged, as in obstructive uropathy, even simple papillae are eventually vulnerable to retrograde entry of urine.* From the collecting tubules, bacteria access the renal interstitium and tubules.

In addition to ascending through urine, bacteria and other pathogens can gain access to renal parenchyma through the

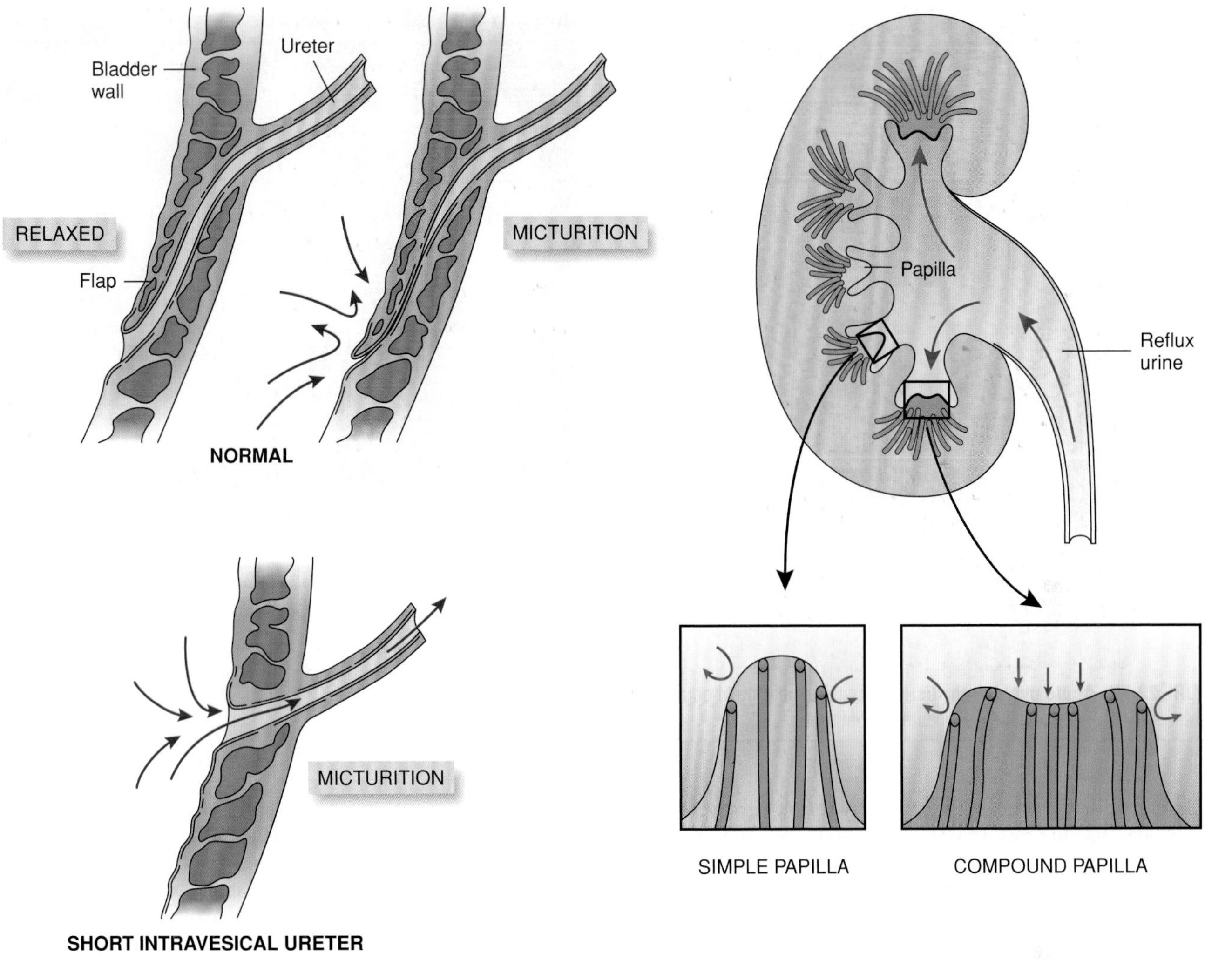

FIGURE 22-72. Anatomic features of the bladder and kidney in pyelonephritis caused by ureterovesical reflux. In the normal bladder, the distal portion of the intravesical ureter courses between the mucosa and the muscularis, forming a mucosal flap. On micturition, the elevated intravesicular pressure compresses the flap against the bladder wall, occluding the lumen. People with a congenitally short intravesical ureter have no mucosal flap, because the angle of entry of the ureter into the bladder approaches a right angle. Thus, micturition forces urine into the ureter. In the renal pelvis, simple papillae of the central calyces are convex and do not readily allow reflux of urine. By contrast, the peripheral compound papillae are concave and permit entry of refluxed urine.

bloodstream, causing **hematogenous pyelonephritis**. For example, in bacterial endocarditis, gram-positive organisms, such as staphylococci, can spread from an infected valve and establish infection in the kidney. The kidney is commonly involved in miliary tuberculosis. Fungi, such as *Aspergillus*, can seed kidneys in immunosuppressed hosts. Hematogenous infections preferentially affect the cortex.

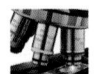 **PATHOLOGY:** The kidneys in acute pyelonephritis are swollen and may have abscesses in the medulla, if infection is ascending, and in the cortex, when it is hematogenous. Pelvic and calyceal urothelium may be hyperemic and covered by purulent exudate. The disease is often focal, and much of the kidney may be normal.

Most infections involve only a few papillary systems. Renal parenchyma, particularly the cortex, typically shows extensive focal destruction by inflammation, although vessels and glomeruli often are preferentially preserved. Infiltrates mainly contain neutrophils, which often fill tubules

and especially collecting ducts (Fig. 22-73). In severe cases of acute pyelonephritis, necrosis of the papillary tips may occur (Fig. 22-74) or infection may extend beyond the renal capsule to cause a perinephric abscess.

 CLINICAL FEATURES: Symptoms of acute pyelonephritis include fever, chills, sweats, malaise, flank pain and costovertebral angle tenderness. Blood neutrophilia is common. Differentiating upper from lower urinary tract infections clinically is often difficult, but **leukocyte casts** in the urine suggest pyelonephritis.

Chronic Pyelonephritis

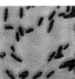 **ETIOLOGIC FACTORS:** Chronic pyelonephritis is caused by recurrent and persistent bacterial infection due to urinary tract obstruction, urine reflux or both (Fig. 22-75). Whether reflux without infection can produce chronic pyelonephritis is controversial.

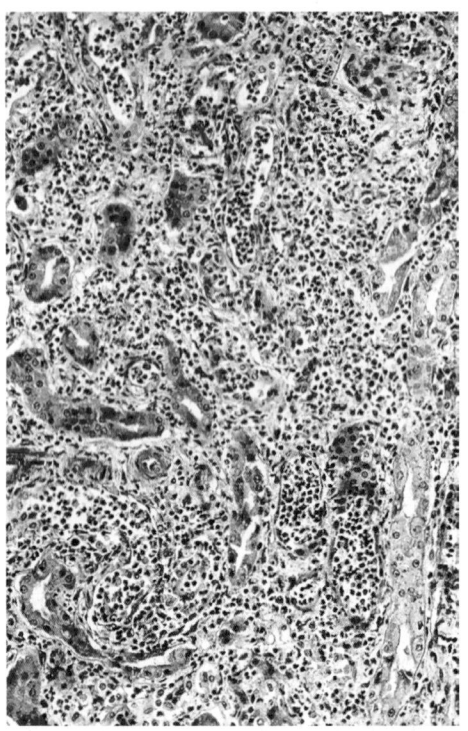

FIGURE 22-73. Acute pyelonephritis. An extensive infiltrate of neutrophils is present in the collecting tubules and interstitial tissue.

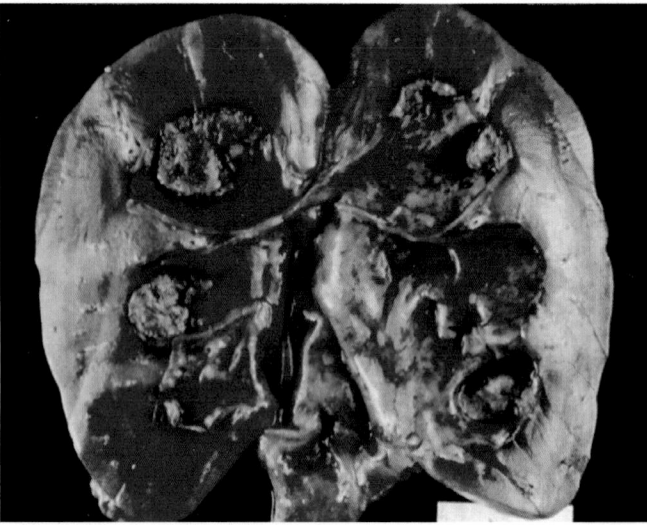

FIGURE 22-74. Papillary necrosis. The bisected kidney shows a dilated renal pelvis and dilated calyces secondary to urinary tract obstruction. The papillae are all necrotic and appear as sharply demarcated, ragged, yellowish areas.

In chronic pyelonephritis caused by reflux or obstruction, medullary tissue and overlying cortex are preferentially injured by recurrent acute and chronic inflammation. Progressive atrophy and scarring ensue, leading to contraction of involved papillary tips (or sloughing if there is papillary necrosis) and thinning of the overlying cortex. This process causes a distinctive gross appearance of broad depressed areas of cortical fibrosis and atrophy overlying a dilated calyx **(caliectasis)** (Fig. 22-76).

 PATHOLOGY: The histology of chronic pyelonephritis is nonspecific. Many diseases cause chronic injury to the tubulointerstitial compartment and induce chronic interstitial inflammation, interstitial fibrosis and tubular atrophy. Thus, chronic pyelonephritis is one of many causes of a pattern of injury called **chronic tubulointerstitial nephritis.** The gross appearance of chronic pyelonephritis is distinctive. Only chronic pyelonephritis and analgesic

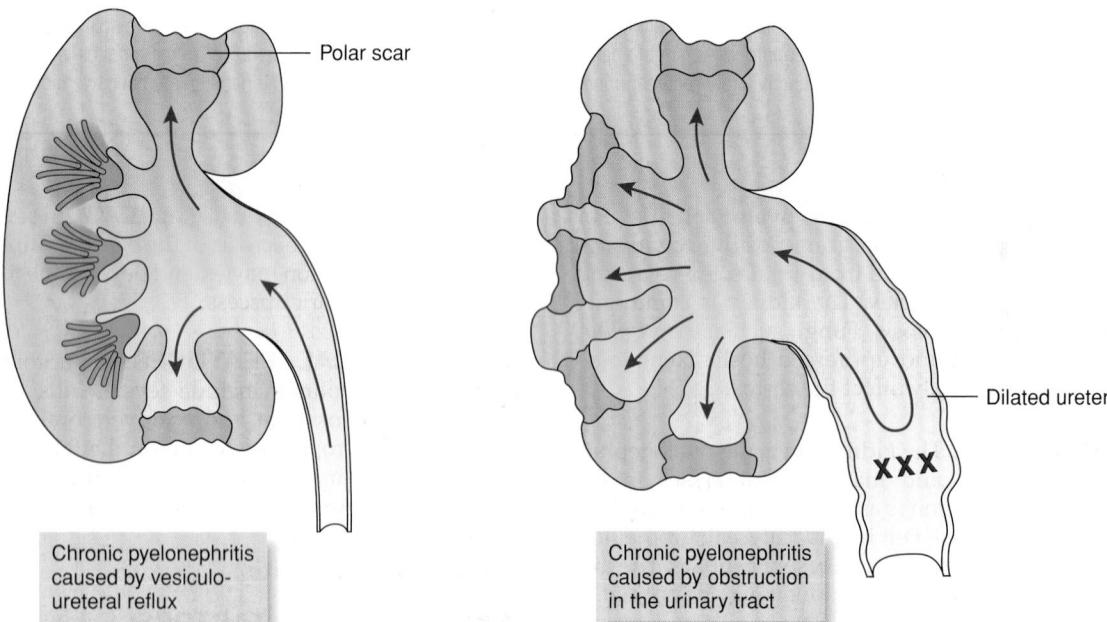

FIGURE 22-75. The two major types of chronic pyelonephritis. Left. Vesicoureteral reflux causes infection of the peripheral compound papillae and, therefore, scars in the poles of the kidney. **Right.** Obstruction of the urinary tract leads to high-pressure backflow of urine, which causes infection of all papillae, diffuse scarring of the kidney and thinning of the cortex.

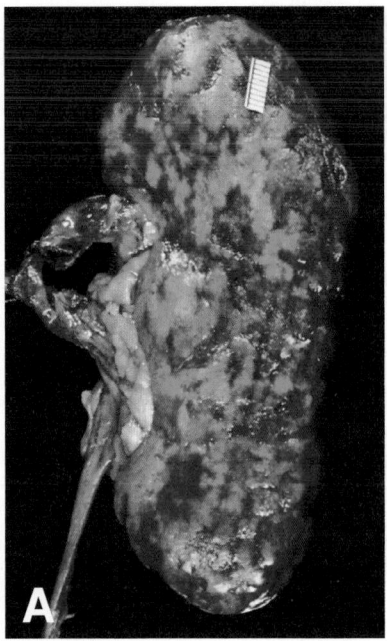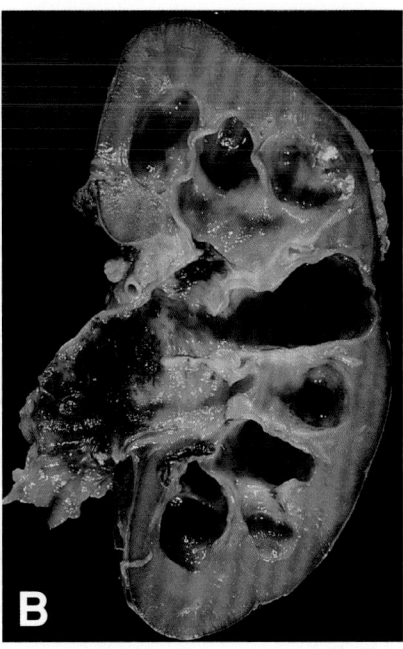

FIGURE 22-76. Chronic pyelonephritis. A. The cortical surface contains many irregular, depressed scars (reddish areas). **B.** There is marked dilation of calyces (caliectasis) caused by inflammatory destruction of papillae, with atrophy and scarring of the overlying cortex.

nephropathy produce both caliectasis and overlying corticomedullary scarring. In obstructive uropathy, all of the calyces and the renal pelvis are dilated, and the parenchyma is uniformly thinned (Fig. 22-76). In cases associated with vesicoureteral reflux, the calyces at the poles of the kidney are preferentially expanded and are associated with overlying discrete, coarse scars that indent the renal surface. The scars have atrophic dilated tubules surrounded by interstitial fibrosis and chronic inflammatory infiltrates (Fig. 22-77). The most characteristic (but not specific) tubular change is severe epithelial atrophy, with diffuse, eosinophilic, hyaline casts. Such tubules are "pinched-off" spherical segments, resembling colloid-containing thyroid follicles. This pattern, called **thyroidization,** results from breakup of tubules and residual segments forming spherules. Glomeruli may be uninvolved, show periglomerular fibrosis or be sclerotic. Loss of most functioning nephrons may lead to secondary FSGS. Fibrosis in arterial and arteriolar walls is common.

There is marked scarring and chronic inflammation of the calyceal mucosa.

Xanthogranulomatous pyelonephritis is an uncommon form of chronic pyelonephritis that is often caused by diverse pathogens, such as *Proteus, E. coli, Klebsiella* and *Pseudomonas.* Its name derives from the yellow gross appearance of nodular renal lesions, caused by numerous lipid-laden foamy macrophages **(xanthoma cells)** (Fig. 22-78A). The disease is usually unilateral. Because this form of inflammation often presents as a mass lesion (Fig. 22-78B), it can be confused with RCC.

CLINICAL FEATURES: Most patients with chronic pyelonephritis have episodic symptoms of urinary tract infection or acute pyelonephritis, such as recurrent fever and flank pain. Some have a silent course until ESRD develops. Urinalysis shows leukocytes, and imaging studies reveal caliectasis and cortical scarring.

Analgesic Nephropathy Results from Chronic Overconsumption of Phenacetin

Patients with analgesic nephropathy typically have taken more than 2 kg of analgesics, often in combinations, such as aspirin and phenacetin, or aspirin and acetaminophen. Phenacetin most often leads to nephropathy and is banned in many countries, including the United States. The pathogenesis of analgesic nephropathy is not clear. Possibilities include direct nephrotoxicity, ischemic damage due to drug-induced vascular changes or both. Analgesic nephropathy is distinct from AKI caused by analgesic-induced acute tubulointerstitial nephritis (e.g., caused by NSAIDs).

PATHOLOGY: Medullary injury with papillary necrosis occurs early in analgesic nephropathy. Atrophy, chronic inflammation and scarring of the overlying cortex follow. The earliest histologic abnormality is a distinctive homogeneous thickening of capillary walls just beneath the transitional epithelium of the urinary tract.

FIGURE 22-77. A light micrograph showing tubular dilation and atrophy. Many tubules contain eosinophilic hyaline casts resembling the colloid of thyroid follicles (so-called thyroidization). The interstitium is scarred and contains a chronic inflammatory cell infiltrate.

THE KIDNEY

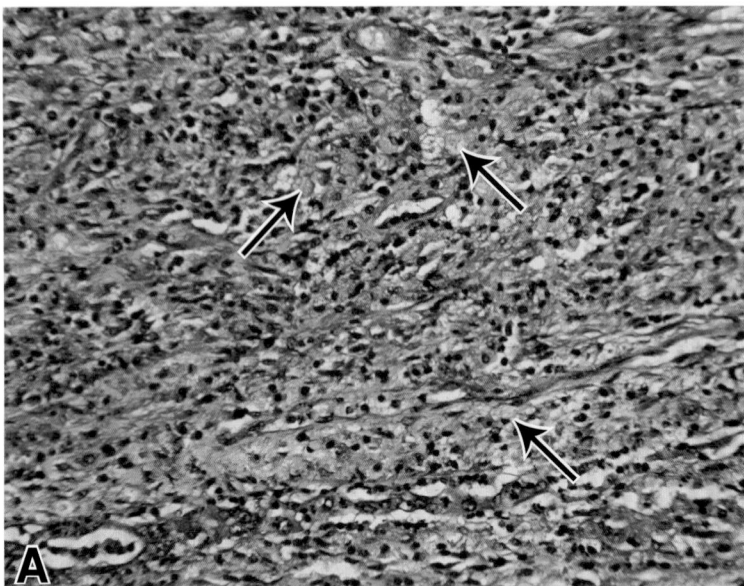
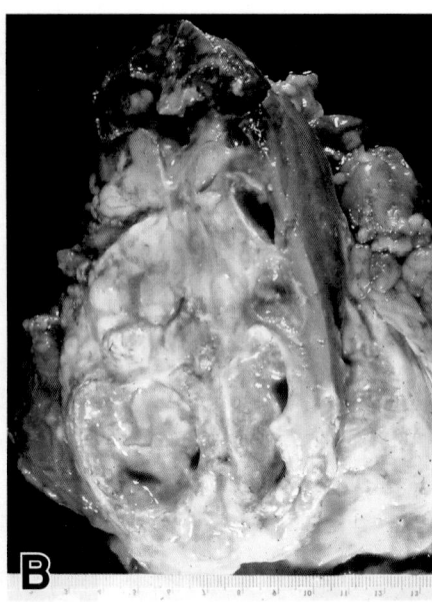

FIGURE 22-78. Xanthogranulomatous pyelonephritis. A. The lesion is characterized by a granulomatous reaction, full of foamy histiocytes (e.g., *arrows*), admixed with other types of inflammatory cells. **B.** This type of pyelonephritis can present as a mass lesion, simulating a tumor.

Early parenchymal changes are confined to papillae and the inner medulla, and they consist of focal basement membrane thickening of tubules and capillaries, interstitial fibrosis and focal coagulative necrosis. Necrotic areas eventually become confluent, first affecting the corticomedullary junction and then the collecting ducts. The necrotic foci contain few inflammatory cells. Eventually, the entire papilla becomes necrotic **(papillary necrosis),** often remaining in place as an amorphous mass. Dystrophic calcification of such necrotic papillae is common. Papillae may remain partly attached at the demarcation zone or be completely sloughed. There is secondary tubular atrophy, interstitial fibrosis and chronic inflammation in the overlying cortex.

 CLINICAL FEATURES: Signs and symptoms occur only late in analgesic nephropathy and include an inability to concentrate the urine, distal tubular acidosis, hematuria, hypertension and anemia. Sloughing of necrotic papillary tips into the renal pelvis may result in colic as they pass through the ureters. Progressive renal failure often develops and leads to ESRD.

Drug-Induced (Hypersensitivity) Acute Tubulointerstitial Nephritis Is a Cell-Mediated Immune Response

PATHOPHYSIOLOGY: Acute drug-induced tubulointerstitial nephritis causes AKI. It entails infiltration by activated T cells and eosinophils, indicating a type IV cell-mediated immune reaction. The immunogen could be the drug itself, the drug bound to certain tissue components, a drug metabolite or a tissue component altered by the drug. Drugs most commonly implicated include NSAIDs, diuretics and certain antibiotics, especially β-lactam antibiotics (e.g., synthetic penicillins, cephalosporins).

 PATHOLOGY: There is patchy cortical infiltration by lymphocytes and occasional eosinophils (5%–10% of the total leukocytes in the tissue) (Fig. 22-79). The medulla is usually less involved. Eosinophils tend to cluster, especially in tubular lumina and in the urine. Neutrophils are rare; their presence should raise suspicion of pyelonephritis or hematogenous bacterial infection. There may be

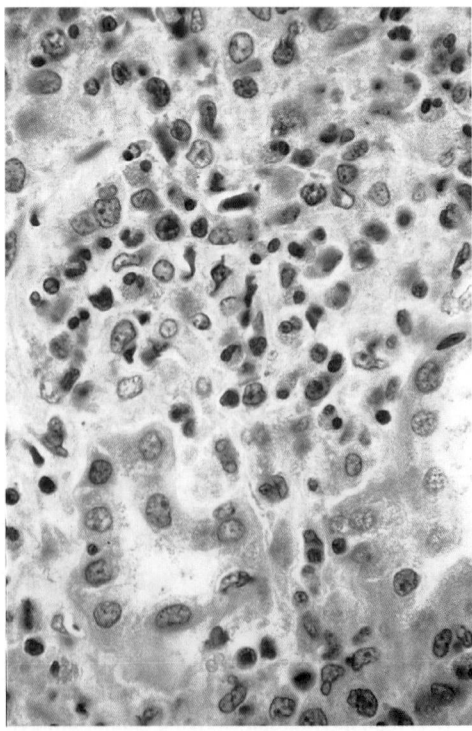

FIGURE 22-79. Hypersensitivity tubulointerstitial nephritis. There is interstitial edema and infiltration by mononuclear leukocytes, with admixed eosinophils.

granulomatous foci, especially later in the disease. Proximal and distal tubules are focally invaded by white blood cells ("tubulitis"). Glomeruli and vessels are not inflamed, but features of minimal-change disease may occur if drug-induced tubulointerstitial nephritis is caused by NSAIDs.

 CLINICAL FEATURES: Acute tubulointerstitial nephritis usually presents as acute renal failure, typically about 2 weeks after a drug is started. Urinalysis shows erythrocytes, leukocytes (including eosinophils) and sometimes leukocyte casts. Tubular defects are common, including sodium wasting, glucosuria, aminoaciduria and renal tubular acidosis. Systemic allergic symptoms, such as fever and rash, may also be present. Most patients recover fully within several weeks or months if the offending drug is discontinued.

Light-Chain Cast Nephropathy May Complicate Multiple Myeloma

Light-chain cast nephropathy is renal injury caused by monoclonal immunoglobulin light chains in the urine. These cause tubular epithelial injury and tubular casts.

PATHOPHYSIOLOGY: As discussed above, multiple myeloma may produce AL amyloidosis, light-chain deposition disease, heavy-chain deposition disease and light-chain cast nephropathy. The latter is the most common kidney disease in patients with multiple myeloma. Glomeruli filter circulating light chains. However, at the acidic pH typical of urine, these light chains form casts by binding to Tamm-Horsfall glycoproteins that are secreted by distal tubular epithelial cells. Renal dysfunction results from both the toxicity of free light chains for tubular epithelium and obstruction by the casts. Light chain structure determines whether they will induce light-chain cast nephropathy, AL amyloidosis or light-chain deposition disease. Occasional patients show several of these renal diseases.

 PATHOLOGY: Tubular lesions show many dense, brightly eosinophilic and glassy (hyaline) casts in distal renal tubules and collecting ducts (Fig. 22-80). Casts appear crystalline, often with fractures and angular borders. They may elicit foreign body reactions, with macrophages and multinucleated giant cells. Interstitial chronic inflammation and edema typically accompany the tubular lesions. More chronic lesions show interstitial fibrosis and tubular atrophy. Focal calcium deposits **(nephrocalcinosis)** often occur in the fibrotic tubular interstitium. Immunostaining visualizes antibody light chains and Tamm-Horsfall proteins.

 CLINICAL FEATURES: Light-chain cast nephropathy may manifest as acute or chronic renal failure. Proteinuria, predominantly of immunoglobulin light chains, is usually present, although not necessarily in the nephrotic range. Nephrotic-range proteinuria in patients with multiple myeloma suggests AL amyloidosis or light-chain deposition disease rather than light-chain cast nephropathy.

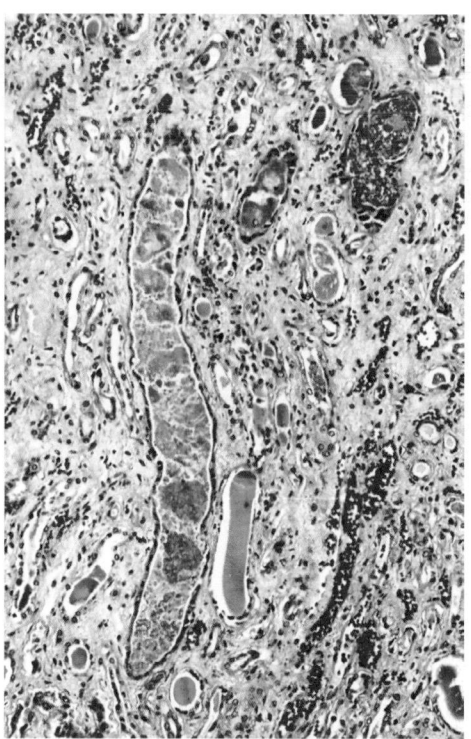

FIGURE 22-80. Light-chain cast nephropathy. A light micrograph shows numerous casts within tubular lumina.

Urate Crystals Deposit in the Tubules and Interstitium in Urate Nephropathy

Any condition with elevated blood levels of uric acid may cause urate nephropathy. The classic chronic disease in this category is primary gout (see Chapter 30).

 **PATHOPHYSIOLOGY:** In **chronic urate nephropathy** due to gout, crystalline monosodium urate deposits in the tubules and interstitium. **Acute urate nephropathy** can be due to increased cell turnover. For example, chemotherapy for malignant neoplasms may cause tumor cell death. In **tumor lysis syndrome,** blood uric acid suddenly increases as massive numbers of tumor cells die. Catabolism of huge amounts of purines from DNA released by dying tumor cells leads to hyperuricemia. Uric acid crystals precipitate in the acidic pH of collecting ducts, obstruction them and causing acute renal failure. Interference with uric acid excretion (e.g., chronic intake of certain diuretics) can also cause hyperuricemia. Chronic lead intoxication interferes with uric acid secretion by proximal tubules and leads to **saturnine gout**.

 PATHOLOGY: In acute urate nephropathy, uric acid precipitated in collecting ducts appears as yellow streaks in the papillae (Fig. 22-81A). The tubular deposits are amorphous after tissue processing, but birefringent crystals are visible in frozen sections (Fig. 22-81B). Tubules are dilated upstream of the obstruction. Uric acid crystals in collecting ducts may also elicit foreign body reactions.

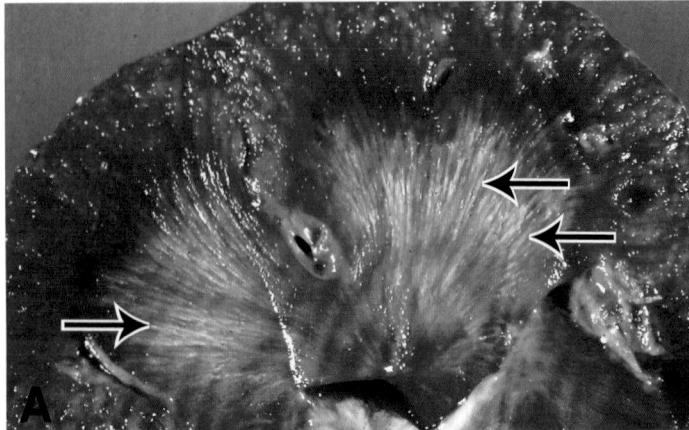
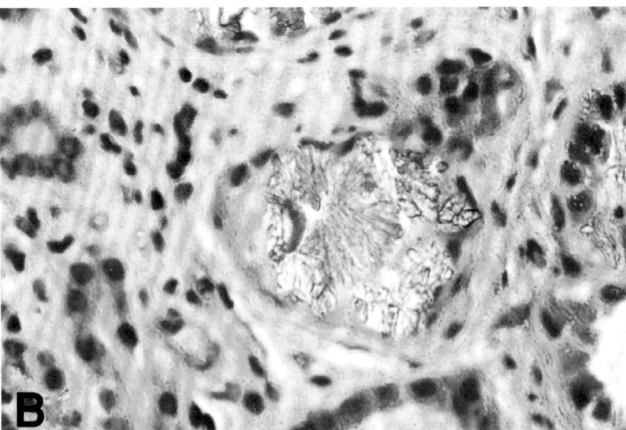

FIGURE 22-81. Urate nephropathy. A. Urate deposits appear as golden streaks in the medulla (*arrows*). **B.** A frozen section demonstrates tubular deposits of uric acid crystals.

The pathogenesis of chronic urate nephropathy is similar to that of the acute form, but because the course is prolonged, more urate deposits in the interstitium, causing interstitial fibrosis and cortical atrophy. The **gouty tophus** is diagnostic. It is a focal accumulation of urate crystals surrounded by inflammatory cells, which may appear granulomatous and include multinucleated giant cells. Uric acid stones account for 10% of **urolithiasis** and occur in 20% of patients with chronic gout and 40% of those with acute hyperuricemia.

 **CLINICAL FEATURES:** Acute urate nephropathy presents as acute renal failure; chronic urate nephropathy causes chronic renal tubular defects. Although histologic renal lesions occur in most patients with chronic gout, less than 1/2 have significant renal functional impairment.

Nephrocalcinosis Is Deposition of Calcium in the Renal Parenchyma

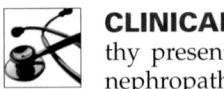 **PATHOPHYSIOLOGY:** Hypercalciuria may lead to **nephrocalcinosis** (Table 22-13), formation of calcium-containing stones **(nephrolithiasis)** or both. Nephrocalcinosis may impair renal function, especially tubular defects such as poor concentrating ability, salt wasting and renal tubular acidosis. If nephrocalcinosis is caused by hypercalcemia, it is **metastatic calcification,** whereas calcification at sites of renal parenchymal injury (e.g., infarcts or cortical necrosis) is representative of **dystrophic calcification.**

Acute phosphate nephropathy is a form of nephrocalcinosis that is an uncommon complication of phosphate bowel-cleansing preparations used in patients about to undergo colonoscopy. Risk factors for this complication include older age, renal insufficiency and use of ACE inhibitors or ARBs. Risk is reduced by avoiding excessive dehydration during bowel cleansing. In acute phosphate nephropathy, AKI occurs several weeks after use of phosphate bowel-cleansing preparations. Pathologically, calcium phosphate deposits in injured distal tubules and collecting ducts, usually accompanied by interstitial fibrosis and chronic inflammation.

 PATHOLOGY: At autopsy, 20% of kidneys have small calcium deposits that have no functional significance or recognized association with hypercalcemia. In patients with nephrocalcinosis caused by hypercalcemia, calcification varies from tiny deposits to grossly and radiologically visible calcium aggregates. If hypercalcemia is severe (e.g., as in primary hyperparathyroidism), kidneys may contain wedge-shaped scars interspersed with relatively normal renal tissue. These scars reflect parenchymal atrophy and interstitial fibrosis caused by the calcification. Renal tubular basement membrane calcification may be striking, particularly in proximal convoluted tubules. Interstitial tissues also contain calcium precipitates. Such deposits also accumulate in the cytoplasm of tubular epithelial cells, which eventually degenerate and are sloughed into the lumens to aggregate as calcified casts. Scattered glomeruli show calcification of the Bowman capsule. Intrarenal arteries may also be calcified. Calcium deposits stain deeply blue with hematoxylin. They are black with the more specific von Kossa stain. By electron microscopy, the mitochondria of renal tubular epithelial cells contain abundant calcium deposits.

TABLE 22-13
CAUSES OF HYPERCALCEMIA THAT LEAD TO NEPHROCALCINOSIS
Increased Resorption of Calcium from Bone
Renal osteodystrophy
Primary hyperparathyroidism
Neoplasms producing parathormone or parathormone-like protein
Osteolytic neoplasms and metastases
Increased Intestinal Absorption of Calcium
Idiopathic hypercalcemia
Vitamin D excess
Milk-alkali syndrome
Sarcoidosis

RENAL STONES (NEPHROLITHIASIS AND UROLITHIASIS)

Nephrolithiasis is stones within the renal collecting system and **urolithiasis** is stones elsewhere in the collecting system of the urinary tract. Calculi often form and accumulate in the renal pelvis and calyces. Stones vary in composition, depending on geography, metabolic alterations and the presence of infection.

For unknown reasons, renal stones are more common in men than in women. They vary in size from gravel (<1 mm) to large stones that dilate the entire renal pelvis. Although they may be well tolerated, in some cases they lead to severe hydronephrosis and pyelonephritis. They can also erode the mucosa and cause hematuria. Passage of a stone into the ureter causes excruciating flank pain, **renal colic**. Larger kidney stones required surgical removal in the past, but ultrasonic disintegration (lithotripsy) and endoscopic removal are now effective.

A urinary stone is usually associated with increased blood levels and urinary excretion of its principal component. This is the case with uric acid and cystine stones. However, many patients with calcium stones have hypercalciuria without hypercalcemia. Mixed urate and calcium stones are common with hyperuricemia, as urate crystals act as a nidus for calcium salts to precipitate.

- **Calcium stones:** Most (75%) renal stones are calcium complexed with oxalate or phosphate, or a mixture of these anions. Calcium oxalate is more common in the United States, whereas in England, calcium phosphate predominates. Calcium oxalate stones are hard and occasionally dark, because they are covered by hemorrhage from the mucosa of the renal pelvis injured by the sharp calcium oxalate crystals. Calcium phosphate stones tend to be softer and paler.
- **Infection stones:** Infection, often with urea-splitting bacteria like *Proteus* or *Providencia* spp., causes 15% of stones. Resulting alkaline urine favors magnesium ammonium phosphate **(struvite)** and calcium phosphate **(apatite)** precipitation. Such stones may be hard, or soft and friable. Infection stones occasionally fill the pelvis and calyces to form a cast of these spaces, a **staghorn calculus** (Fig. 22-82). Infection stones cause frequent complications, such as intractable urinary tract infection, pain, bleeding, perinephric abscess and urosepsis.
- **Uric acid stones:** These stones occur in 25% of patients with hyperuricemia and gout, but most patients with uric acid stones have neither **(idiopathic urate lithiasis)**. Urate stones are smooth, hard and yellow, and are usually less than 2 cm. Unlike calcium-containing stones, pure uric acid stones are radiolucent.
- **Cystine stones:** These account for only 1% of renal stones overall but are a significant fraction of childhood calculi. They occur only in hereditary cystinuria. Although composed only of cystine, they may be enveloped by a layer of calcium phosphate.

OBSTRUCTIVE UROPATHY AND HYDRONEPHROSIS

Obstructive uropathy is caused by structural or functional abnormalities in the urinary tract that impede urine flow,

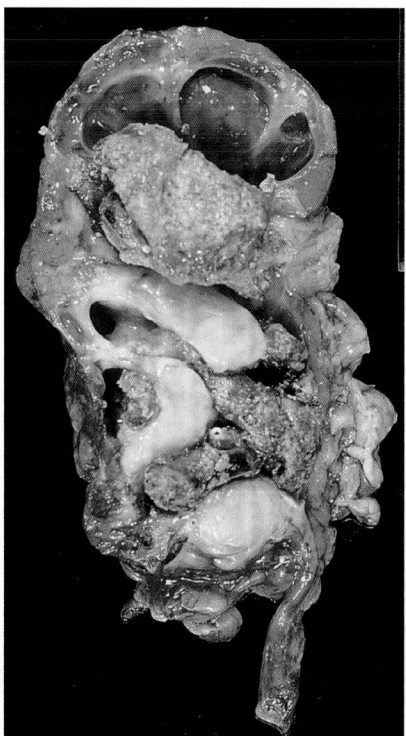

FIGURE 22-82. Staghorn calculi. The kidney shows hydronephrosis and stones that are casts of the dilated calyces.

which may cause renal dysfunction (obstructive nephropathy) and dilation of the collecting system (hydronephrosis). Urinary tract obstruction is detailed in Chapter 23.

 PATHOLOGY: The most prominent microscopic finding in early hydronephrosis is dilation of collecting ducts. This is followed by dilation of proximal and distal convoluted tubules. Eventually, the proximal tubules become widely dilated and are lost. Glomeruli are usually spared. Progressive dilation of the renal pelvis and calyces leads to renal parenchymal atrophy (Fig. 22-83). Hydronephrotic kidneys are more susceptible to pyelonephritis, adding injury to insult.

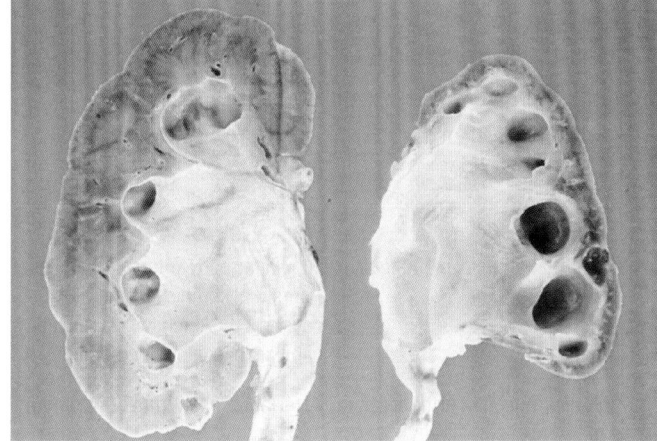

FIGURE 22-83. Hydronephrosis. Bilateral urinary tract obstruction has led to conspicuous dilation of the ureters, pelves and calyces. The kidney on the right shows severe parenchymal atrophy.

CLINICAL FEATURES: Bilateral acute urinary tract obstruction causes acute renal failure **(postrenal acute renal failure)**. Unilateral obstruction is often asymptomatic. Many causes of acute obstruction are reversible; thus, prompt recognition is important. Left untreated, an obstructed kidney undergoes atrophy. If obstruction is bilateral, chronic renal failure ensues.

RENAL TRANSPLANTATION

Kidney transplantation is the treatment of choice for most patients with ESRD. The major obstacle is allograft rejection. However, the transplanted organ is also susceptible to recurrence of the disease that destroyed the native kidneys and to nephrotoxicity from immunosuppressive drugs. Table 22-14 lists distinct, but often coexisting, patterns of antibody-mediated and cellular renal allograft rejection.

ABO blood group antigens and **HLA antigens** are the main antigenic targets on transplanted kidneys. ABO antigens

are expressed on endothelial cells and red blood cells, and are the most problematic barriers to transplantation. Because anti-ABO antibodies are preformed, they bind to graft endothelial cells and cause immediate (hyperacute) rejection (see below). *More common (and more gradual) patterns of acute and chronic rejection are mainly due to recipient reactivity against donor HLA antigens (see Chapter 4).* HLA antigens are expressed on most cells, including endothelial cells, but not erythrocytes. Development of donor-specific HLA immunity in allograft recipients causes cell-mediated and antibody-mediated reactions (see Chapter 4). Renal allograft rejection can be classified on the basis of its clinical course, pathologic features and presumed pathogenesis (Table 22-14). However, an allograft may undergo more than one type of rejection at the same time.

HYPERACUTE ANTIBODY-MEDIATED REJECTION: Hyperacute rejection is rare (<0.5% of grafts). If recipient blood contains antibodies to major graft alloantigens (usually ABO or class I HLA), those antibodies immediately bind endothelial cells in the transplanted organ and cause irreversible injury within minutes. The graft may become mottled, cyanotic and flaccid intraoperatively. Antibody binds endothelial cell antigens, activates complement and thus attracts neutrophils. The cytotoxic effects of complement and neutrophils cause endothelial cells to swell, become vacuolated and lyse. Accumulation of neutrophils in glomerular capillaries portends impending rejection. Endothelial cell changes are followed by platelet thrombi and later by fibrin thrombi (Fig. 22-84). Interstitial edema, hemorrhage (Fig. 22-84) and cortical necrosis develop over the next 12–24 hours.

ACUTE ANTIBODY-MEDIATED REJECTION: The most common type of acute antibody-mediated rejection is directed primarily at capillaries and may cause only subtle or no pathologic changes by light microscopy. Neutrophils or mononuclear leukocytes are increased in peritubular and glomerular capillaries, and in tubules. Complement activation products, especially C4d, localize consistently to the walls of peritubular and glomerular capillaries (Fig. 22-85A). The most severe, but least common, pattern of acute antibody-mediated rejection involves **necrotizing arteritis** with fibrinoid necrosis of the media (Fig. 22-85B). It occurs in less than 1% of allografts in patients whose immunosuppression includes a calcineurin inhibitor, although before these agents

TABLE 22-14
CATEGORIES OF RENAL ALLOGRAFT REJECTION

Category	Most Characteristic Lesion
Hyperacute antibody-mediated rejection	Neutrophils in peritubular capillaries, hemorrhage and necrosis
Acute antibody-mediated rejection	
Acute antibody-mediated capillary rejection	Leukocytes and C4d in peritubular capillaries
Acute necrotizing transplant arteritis	Arterial fibrinoid necrosis
Acute T-cell–mediated rejection	
Acute tubulointerstitial rejection	Tubulitis (mononuclear leukocytes between epithelial cells of tubules) and interstitial activated lymphocytes
Acute endarteritis	Mononuclear leukocytes in arterial intima
Acute transplant glomerulitis	Mononuclear leukocytes in glomerular capillaries
Acute transplant arteritis	Acute transmural inflammation or necrosis
Chronic rejection	
Interstitial fibrosis and tubular atrophy	Tubular atrophy, interstitial fibrosis, interstitial chronic inflammatory cells and thickening of peritubular capillary basement membranes
Chronic transplant arteriopathy	Arterial fibrotic intimal thickening
Chronic transplant glomerulopathy	Glomerular capillary wall thickening and glomerular basement membrane remodeling

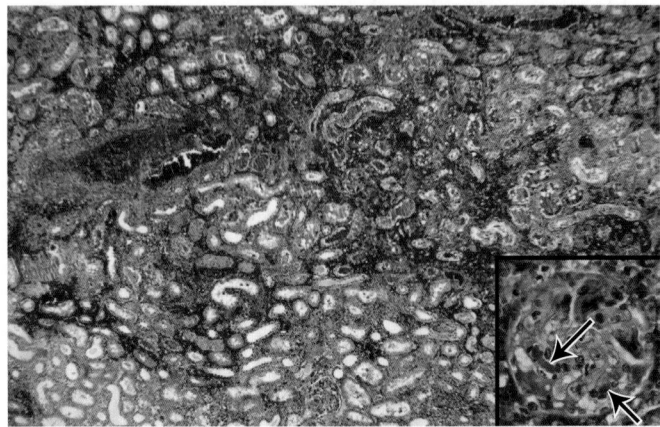
FIGURE 22-84. Hyperacute rejection. Preformed antibody against recipient antigens causes an immediate in situ reaction, with hemorrhage developing due to vascular necrosis. Fibrin thrombi (*inset*) are abundant in glomeruli.

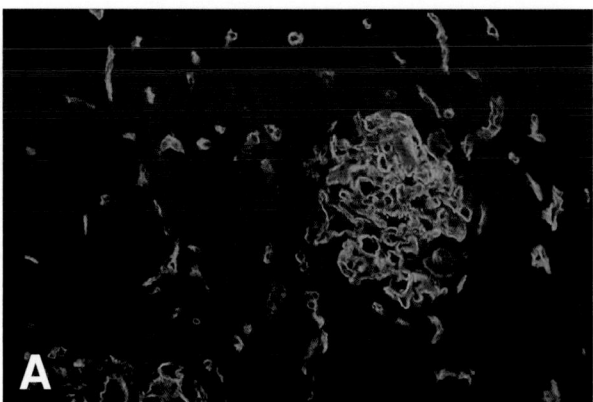
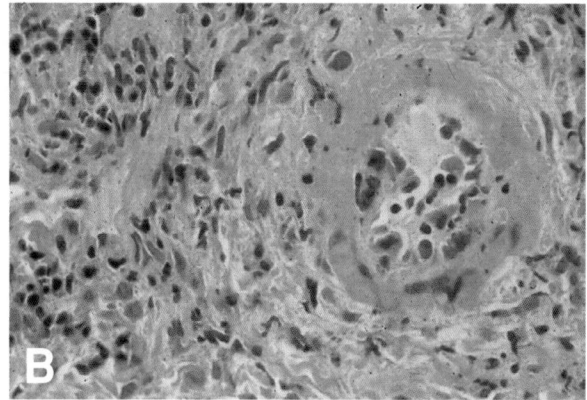

FIGURE 22-85. Acute antibody-mediated allograft rejection. A. Staining of peritubular and glomerular capillaries with an anti-C4d antibody showing evidence of complement activation by antibodies directed against donor antigens on endothelial cells. **B.** Acute antibody-mediated necrotizing acute vasculitis in an interlobular artery with extensive fibrinoid necrosis of the muscularis. The vascular and interstitial infiltrates of mononuclear leukocytes indicate concurrent acute cellular rejection.

were introduced it occurred in 5% of renal allografts. If necrotizing arteritis develops, fewer than 30% of grafts survive 1 year, even with aggressive immunosuppression.

ACUTE CELLULAR REJECTION: This is the most common form of acute rejection. It is characterized by infiltration of the interstitium, tubules, arteries, arterioles or glomeruli by T lymphocytes and macrophages. Nuclei of infiltrating lymphocytes vary in size and shape because the cells are at various stages of activation and include immunoblasts (see Chapter 26). Usually, interstitial infiltrates are patchy rather than diffuse. Involvement of tubules **(tubulitis)** is manifested by lymphocytes crossing tubular basement membranes and lying between tubular epithelial cells (Fig. 22-86A). Arterial involvement by cellular rejection involves T lymphocytes and monocytes traversing the endothelium, expanding the intima with mononuclear leukocytes **(endarteritis)** (Fig. 22-86B). Arterioles may be similarly affected. Glomerular infiltration by mononuclear leukocytes with obliteration of capillary lumens causes **acute transplant glomerulitis)**. Renal transplants with tubulitis but not endarteritis have an 80% chance of 1-year graft survival, compared with 60% for allografts with endarteritis.

CHRONIC REJECTION: Chronic rejection features interstitial fibrosis and tubular atrophy, interstitial mononuclear infiltrates, thickening (multilamination) of peritubular capillary basement membranes, **chronic transplant arteriopathy** and **chronic transplant glomerulopathy** (see below) (Table 22-14).

Chronic transplant arteriopathy affects arteries of all sizes, including the main renal artery. The intima is thickened by stromal cell proliferation and matrix deposition (Fig. 22-87), but without the dense fibrosis and elastic lamination seen in nonspecific arteriosclerosis. Inflammation is absent—or is much less prominent than in active acute cell-mediated intimal arteritis (compare to Fig. 22-83). Foam cells may be conspicuous, and the internal elastic lamina may be interrupted. Peritubular capillaries show basement membrane thickening and replication.

In chronic transplant glomerulopathy, glomerular capillary walls are thickened, due to expansion of the glomerular capillary subendothelial zone and GBM replication. This also occurs in peritubular capillaries. The mesangium is widened. Ischemia due to arterial and capillary narrowing may lead to tubular atrophy and interstitial fibrosis.

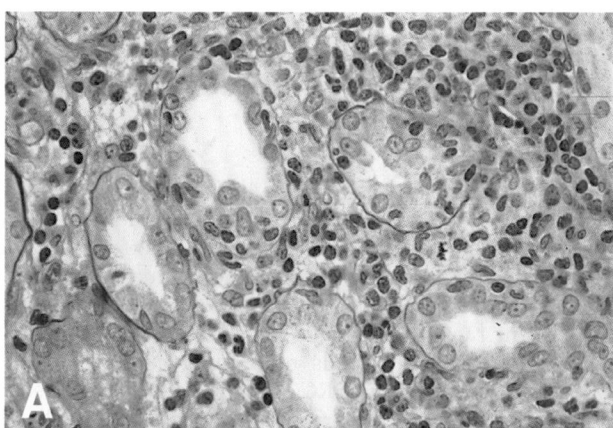
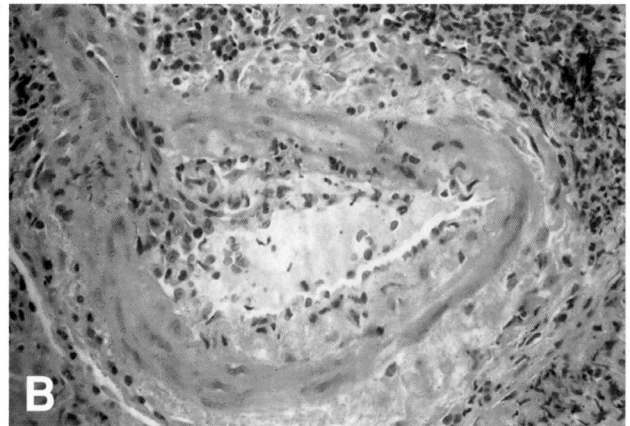

FIGURE 22-86. Acute cellular allograft rejection. A. Acute tubulointerstitial cellular rejection with tubulitis indicated by lymphocytes on the epithelial side of the basement membrane (periodic acid–Schiff stain). **B.** Acute cellular vascular rejection with endarteritis indicated by mononuclear leukocytes infiltrating the intima of an arcuate artery.

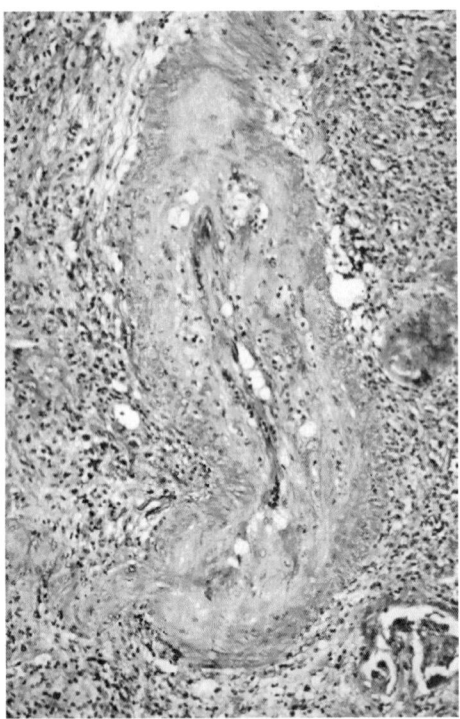

FIGURE 22-87. Chronic allograft rejection. The lumen of this medium-sized artery is occluded by a thickened intima, which contains a few inflammatory cells.

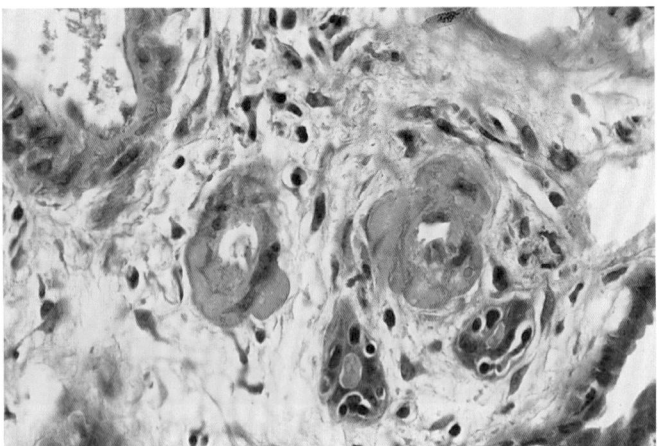

FIGURE 22-88. Cyclosporine nephrotoxicity with arteriolopathy. Marked destructive hyalinosis of arterioles is present.

Tubulointerstitial injury may also result from indolent tubulitis.

RECURRENCE OF KIDNEY DISEASE: The same disease that caused the native kidneys to fail may recur in a transplanted kidney. The frequency and significance of recurrence vary among different types of glomerular disease (Table 22-15).

TABLE 22-15
RECURRENCE OF DISEASE IN RENAL ALLOGRAFTS

Disease	Recurrence Rate (%)	Rate of Graft Loss (%)
C3 glomerulopathy (dense deposit disease)	>90	15
Diabetic glomerulosclerosis	>90	<5
IgA nephropathy	40	<10
Focal segmental glomerulosclerosis	35	30
Type I membranoproliferative glomerulonephritis	30	<10
Membranous glomerulonephritis	20	<5
ANCA glomerulonephritis	15	<5
Anti-GBM glomerulonephritis	5	<5
Lupus glomerulonephritis	5	<5

ANCA = antineutrophil cytoplasmic autoantibody; GBM = glomerular basement membrane; IgA = immunoglobulin A.

CALCINEURIN INHIBITOR NEPHROTOXICITY OF CYCLOSPORINE AND TACROLIMUS: Cyclosporine and tacrolimus are immunosuppressive inhibitors of calcineurin that have dramatically improved allograft survival for kidneys and other organs (e.g., liver, heart, lungs). Unfortunately, both drugs are nephrotoxic and can injure both kidney allografts and native kidneys of patients given these drugs for other reasons. Acute or chronic renal failure can result.

The most characteristic renal lesion is an **arteriolopathy** that begins with smooth muscle cell degeneration and necrosis. The destroyed arteriolar muscle cells are replaced by acidophilic hyaline material (Fig. 22-88). In fulminant cases, vascular lesions resemble full-blown thrombotic microangiopathy, with circumferential fibrinoid arteriolar necrosis. In chronic toxicity, there are zones of interstitial fibrosis and tubular atrophy ("striped fibrosis").

BK POLYOMAVIRUS INFECTION: Immunosuppression can reactivate latent BK virus infection in a transplanted kidney and can lead to acute tubular injury and tubulointerstitial nephritis. Intranuclear viral inclusions in tubular cells may suggest this possibility, and immunochemical staining can confirm the diagnosis.

Tumors of the Kidney

BENIGN RENAL TUMORS

PAPILLARY RENAL ADENOMA: There is controversy as to whether any epithelial renal cell tumor should be considered benign. Tumor size, which has been used to separate adenomas from carcinomas, is problematic because all carcinomas start out as small lesions. Renal epithelial neoplasms smaller than 3 cm rarely metastasize, but "rarely" is not "never." Tumors composed of cells resembling clear cell, chromophobe or collecting duct RCCs should not be referred to as adenomas even if they are small. Neoplasms smaller than 5 mm with papillary or tubulopapillary growth patterns can be considered adenomas. Papillary renal adenomas occur more often with advancing age and are incidental autopsy findings in 40% of patients older than 70.

RENAL ONCOCYTOMA: This benign neoplasm accounts for 5%–10% of primary renal tumors removed surgically. It derives from collecting duct intercalated cells. They are plump, with abundant, finely granular, acidophilic cytoplasm and round nuclei that lack atypia. The distinctive appearance of the tumor is due to abundant mitochondria in the cytoplasm. Oncocytomas are typically mahogany-brown due to mitochondrial lipochrome pigments. These tumors rarely metastasize.

MEDULLARY FIBROMA: Medullary fibromas (renomedullary interstitial cell tumors) are typically small (<0.5 cm in diameter), pale gray, well-circumscribed tumors, usually in the midportion of medullary pyramids. They are composed of small stellate to polygonal cells in a loose stroma. Renal medullary fibromas are incidental findings in as many as 1/2 of all adult autopsies (Fig. 22-89).

ANGIOMYOLIPOMA: These tumors are strongly associated with tuberous sclerosis. Of patients with tuberous sclerosis, 80% have angiomyolipomas, but most patients with angiomyolipomas do not have tuberous sclerosis. These lesions are mixtures of well-differentiated adipose tissue, smooth muscle and thick-walled vessels. Grossly, they are yellow and bosselated, and may resemble RCC. However, they are always well encapsulated and lack necrosis.

MESOBLASTIC NEPHROMA: Mesoblastic nephromas are benign congenital neoplasms or hamartomas usually found in the first 3 months of life. They must be differentiated from Wilms tumors. The lesions range from smaller than 1 cm to larger than 15 cm and are composed of spindle cells of fibroblastic or myofibroblastic lineage. Tumor margins are usually irregular, with bands of cells interdigitating with adjacent renal parenchyma. Mesoblastic nephromas may recur if some of these tongues of tumor tissue are left behind after surgical resection.

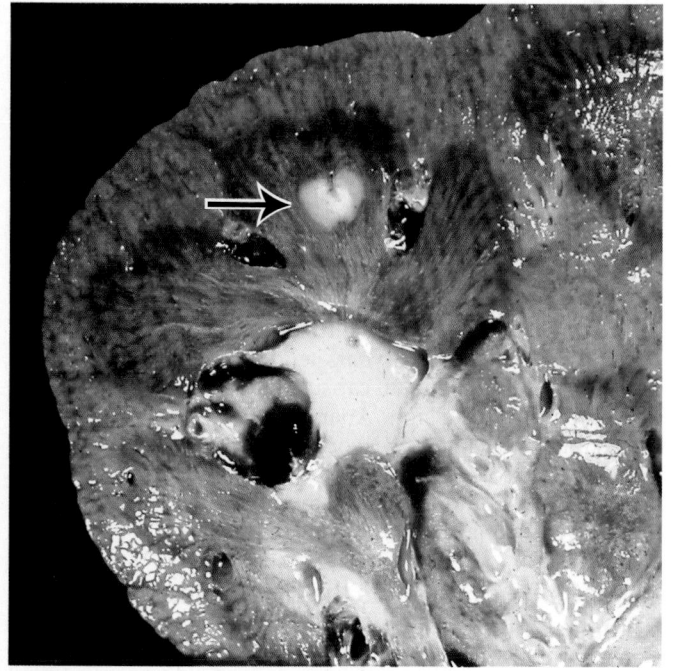

FIGURE 22-89. Medullary fibroma (*arrow*).

MALIGNANT TUMORS OF THE KIDNEY

Wilms Tumor (Nephroblastoma) Is a Malignancy of Embryonal Renal Elements

Component nephrogenic elements include admixed blastema, stroma and epithelium. Its incidence is 1 in 10,000, making it the most common abdominal solid tumor in children.

 **MOLECULAR PATHOGENESIS:** In most (90%) cases, the Wilms tumor is sporadic and unilateral. In 5% of cases, however, it arises as part of three different congenital syndromes, all of which increase the risk of developing Wilms tumors at an early age and often bilaterally:

- **WAGR syndrome:** **W**ilms tumor, **a**niridia, **g**enitourinary anomalies, mental **r**etardation
- **Denys-Drash syndrome (DDS):** Wilms tumor, intersexual disorders, glomerular mesangial sclerosis
- **Beckwith-Wiedemann syndrome (BWS):** Wilms tumor, overgrowth ranging from gigantism to hemihypertrophy, visceromegaly and macroglossia

Approximately 6% of Wilms tumors are familial, have an early onset and are bilateral but are not associated with any other syndrome.

WAGR syndrome is caused by a deletion in the short arm of chromosome 11 (11p13). Affected genes include the aniridia gene (*PAX6*) and **Wilms tumor gene 1 (*WT1*)**. WT1 protein (see below) is expressed in kidneys, thymus, spleen and gonads. Loss or mutation of one *WT1* allele leads to genitourinary anomalies. A defect in *PAX6* causes aniridia. Of children with WAGR syndrome, 1/3 develop Wilms tumors. The presence of a germline mutation in one *WT1* allele and loss of heterozygosity (LOH) at this locus in the tumors of WAGR syndrome implies that acquired somatic mutation in the remaining *WT1* allele is needed for Wilms tumor to occur (as in retinoblastomas; see Chapter 5). Unlike deletions in WAGR syndrome, mutations in the *WT1* gene in DDS are considered dominant negative mutations, possibly accounting for the fact that the DDS phenotype is far more severe than that of WAGR syndrome. *WT1* mutations also occur in Frasier syndrome, but affected patients develop gonadoblastomas, not Wilms tumors.

WT1 is a tumor-suppressor protein that regulates transcription of several other genes, including insulin-like growth factor-II (*IGF-II*), *Snail*, E-cadherin (*Cdh1*) and platelet-derived growth factor (*PDGF*). Wilms tumors arising in the context of WAGR syndrome all have *WT1* mutations, but only 10%–20% of sporadic Wilms tumors do. Thus, other genes besides *WT1* must contribute to the genesis of sporadic Wilms tumors. Among sporadic Wilms tumors, 10% have a gain-of-function mutation in β-catenin (*CTNNB1*), a part of the developmentally important WNT signaling pathway. An additional 5% have mutations in the p53 gene (*TP53*; see Chapter 5).

Approximately 70% of Wilms tumors show LOH or loss of imprinting (LOI) at a second locus on chromosome 11 (11p15.5). This site, also linked to BWS, is distinct from, but close to, the *WT1* gene. Interestingly, LOH at this locus in sporadic Wilms tumors invariably results in loss of the maternal allele. In addition, some BWS patients have germline duplications of the paternal locus, whereas others have two copies of chromosome 11 with the same imprinting pattern at this locus as the father (*paternal uniparental isodisomy*). Because *IGF-II 2* maps to chromosome 11p15 and has paternal imprinting, an increased dose of *IGF-II 2* might contribute to BWS and to tumorigenesis. Another possibility is that another closely linked gene, such as the *H19* gene, expressed only by the maternal allele, is a tumor suppressor or regulates imprinting in the region.

The *WTX* gene on the X chromosome is mutated in 20%–30% of Wilms tumors with about 2/3 of these carrying deletions of the entire gene. WTX may act as a tumor suppressor by downregulating WNT/β-catenin signaling by causing degradation of β-catenin. Mutations in *CTNNB1* that increase WNT /β-catenin stability occur in approximately 15% of Wilms tumors. Thus, constitutive activation of WNT/β-catenin signaling may be important in Wilms tumorigenesis. About 3/4 of Wilms tumors with mutant *WT1* also have *CTNNB1* mutations, suggesting that WT1 loss does not fully activate WNT/β-catenin signaling.

Nephrogenic rests (small foci of persistent primitive blastemal cells) are found in the kidneys of all children with syndromic Wilms tumors and in 1/3 of sporadic cases. Given that such rests in the nontumorous kidney have the same somatic *WT1* mutations as are present in the tumors, these rests may represent clonal precursor lesions one or more steps along the pathway to tumor formation.

PATHOLOGY: Wilms tumors tend to be large when detected, with bulging, pale tan, cut surfaces enclosed by a thin rim of renal cortex and capsule (Fig. 22-90). Wilms tumors resemble normal fetal renal tissue (Fig. 22-91), including metanephric blastema, immature stroma (mesenchymal tissue) and immature epithelial elements.

Most Wilms tumors contain all three elements in varying proportions, but only two elements or even only one may be present on occasion. The blastema-like component contains small ovoid cells with scanty cytoplasm, in nests and

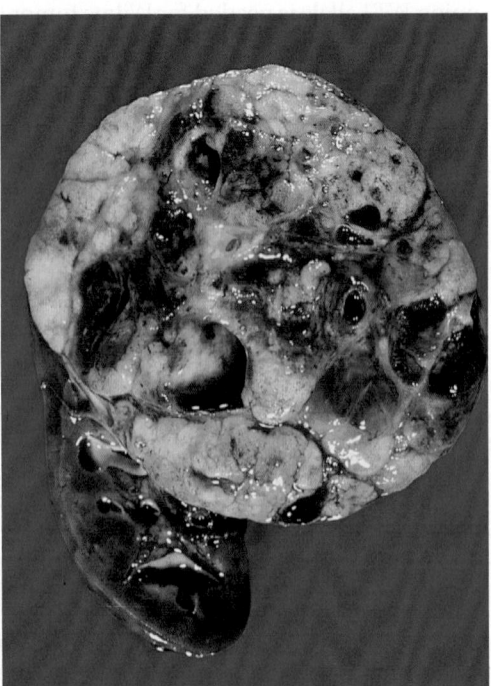

FIGURE 22-90. Wilms tumor. A cross-section of a pale tan neoplasm attached to a residual portion of the kidney.

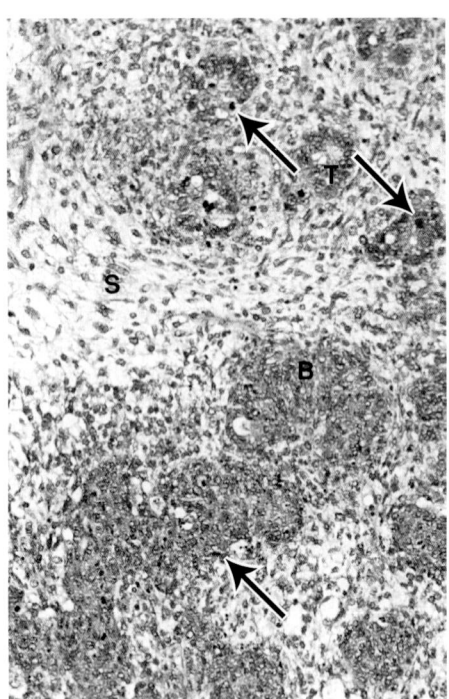

FIGURE 22-91. Wilms tumor (nephroblastoma). This Wilms tumor shows highly cellular areas composed of undifferentiated blastema (*B*), loose stroma (*S*) containing undifferentiated mesenchymal cells and immature tubules (*T*). Note the many mitotic figures (*arrows*).

trabeculae. The epithelial component appears as small tubular structures. Structures resembling immature glomeruli may sometimes be seen. The tumor stroma contains spindle cells, which are mostly undifferentiated but may show smooth muscle or fibroblast differentiation. Skeletal muscle is the most common heterotopic stromal element, although bone, cartilage, fat or neural tissue may rarely be encountered.

CLINICAL FEATURES: Wilms tumors represent 85% of pediatric renal neoplasms. They occur in 1 in 10,000 children, usually 1–3 years old, and 98% present before age 10. Familial cases usually show autosomal dominant inheritance. Only 5% of sporadic cases are bilateral, in contrast to 20% of familial cases. Most often, diagnosis is made after recognition of an abdominal mass. Additional manifestations include abdominal pain, intestinal obstruction, hypertension, hematuria and symptoms of traumatic tumor rupture.

Several histologic and clinical parameters are used to predict the behavior of these tumors, with varying success. Patients younger than 2 years tend to fare better. Presence of tumor outside the renal capsule at the time of surgery is a negative prognostic sign. Anaplasia (large, hyperchromatic nuclei and atypical mitoses) occurs more commonly in older patients and correlates with their overall worse prognosis. Chemotherapy and radiation therapy, plus surgical resection, provide long-term survival rates of 90%.

Renal Cell Carcinoma Is the Most Common Primary Cancer of the Kidney

RCC is a malignant neoplasm of renal tubular or ductal epithelial cells. It accounts for 80%–90% of primary renal cancers. More than 30,000 cases occur each year in the United States.

MOLECULAR PATHOGENESIS: Most RCCs are sporadic, but about 5% are inherited. Hereditary RCCs occur in the context of three distinct syndromes:

- **von Hippel-Lindau (VHL) syndrome,** an autosomal dominant cancer syndrome (see Chapter 5), with cerebellar hemangioblastomas, retinal angiomas, clear cell RCC (40% of cases of VHL disease), pheochromocytoma and cysts in various organs
- **Autosomal dominant RCC,** in which a clear cell tumor is the main manifestation and occurs in 1/2 of at-risk patients with genetic abnormalities like those in VHL syndrome
- **Hereditary papillary RCC,** an autosomal dominant inherited cancer characterized by multiple bilateral papillary tumors
- **Birt-Hogg-Dube (BHD) syndrome,** a hereditary disease with risk for bilateral, multifocal chromophobe RCC

Hereditary RCCs tend to be multifocal and bilateral, and appear in younger patients than do sporadic RCCs. A family history of RCC increases the risk for RCC four- to fivefold.

Several translocations involving a breakpoint on chromosome 3 contribute to VHL and autosomal dominant RCC syndromes. Patients with sporadic RCC may have deletions and LOH in the short arm of chromosome 3 (3p) in the tumor tissue. Finally, the *VHL* tumor suppressor gene is at 3p25. *In virtually all (98%) sporadic clear cell RCCs, one VHL allele is lost; VHL mutations occur in more than 50% of these tumors.* Thus, loss of *VHL* tumor-suppressor function plays a key role in clear cell RCC tumorigenesis.

Abnormal *VHL* gene function causes the transcriptional regulatory molecule, hypoxia-inducible factor-α (HIF-α), to accumulate. In turn, genes that make proteins that activate kinase-dependent signaling pathways are transcriptionally upregulated. Components of these pathways are targets for kinase inhibitors and mTOR (see Chapter 5) inhibitors that have proven useful for treating RCC.

Unlike clear cell RCC, hereditary papillary RCC is not linked to *VHL*. Trisomies or tetrasomies of chromosomes 7, 16 and 17, and loss of the Y chromosome, occur in many cases. Mutations in c-*met* proto-oncogene (*MET*) at 7q31 are implicated in the development of hereditary papillary RCC.

Chromophobe RCCs derive from intercalated cells of renal collecting ducts, and collecting duct RCCs originate in the ducts of Bellini of the medullary pyramids. Patients with BDH have germline inactivating mutations in the *BHD* gene, which produces folliculin (FLCN). These patients are at risk for developing bilateral, multifocal chromophobe RCCs.

Tobacco, whether smoked or chewed, increases the risk of RCC: 1/3 of RCCs are linked to tobacco use. Inherited and acquired renal cystic diseases may lead to RCC, especially papillary RCC. The cancer has also been tied to analgesic nephropathy.

PATHOLOGY: The pathologic variants of RCC reflect differences in histogenesis and predict different outcomes. The most common histologic categories of RCC are shown in Table 22-16.

TABLE 22-16

CATEGORIES OF RENAL CELL CARCINOMA

Category	Frequency (%)
Clear cell type	70–80
Papillary type	10–15
Chromophobe type	5
Collecting duct type	1

- **Clear cell RCC** is the most common type. It arises from proximal tubular epithelial cells. It is typically yellow-orange, solid or focally cystic, and focal hemorrhage and necrosis are common (Fig. 22-92). The removal of abundant cytoplasmic lipids and glycogen in tissue preparation accounts for the tumor cells' clear cytoplasm (Fig. 22-93). The cells are often arranged in round or elongated collections demarcated by a network of delicate vessels. Little cellular or nuclear pleomorphism is present.
- **Papillary RCC** contains tumor cells on fibrovascular stalks. Type 1 papillary RCC has small basophilic cells, and type 2 has large acidophilic cells. The latter is more aggressive, with a worse prognosis. Cytoplasm may be eosinophilic or basophilic. These tumors arise from proximal tubular epithelial cells (Fig. 22-94).
- **Chromophobe RCC** has a mixture of acidophilic granular cells and pale transparent cells with prominent cell borders, which impart a plant cell–like appearance (Fig. 22-95). Many cytoplasmic vesicles are filled with a distinctive mucopolysaccharide that stains with the Hale colloidal iron technique. These vesicles displace other organelles to the periphery, causing central cytoplasmic pallor. Chromophobe RCCs appear to arise from intercalated cells of the renal collecting ducts.

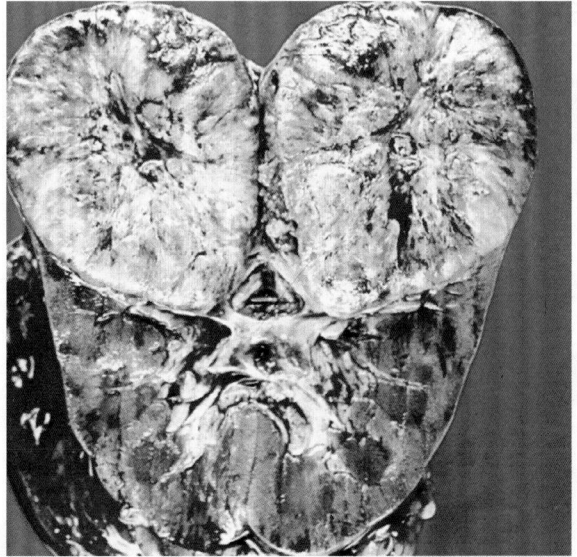

FIGURE 22-92. Clear cell renal cell carcinoma. The kidney contains a large irregular neoplasm with a variegated cut surface. Yellow areas correspond to lipid-containing cells.

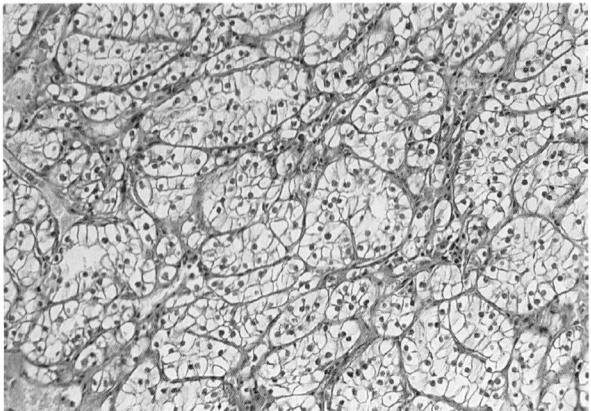

FIGURE 22-93. Clear cell renal cell carcinoma. Photomicrograph showing islands of neoplastic cells with abundant clear cytoplasm.

- **Collecting duct RCC** is a rare variety that originates in medullary collecting ducts (ducts of Bellini) but may extend into the cortex. It contains tubular and papillary structures lined by a single layer of cuboidal cells with a hobnail appearance. Renal medullary carcinomas are variants of collecting duct carcinomas that develop almost exclusively in blacks who have sickle cell trait or disease.
- **"Sarcomatoid" changes** may occur in any RCC and carry a worse prognosis.

Recommended histologic grading for RCC applies the Fuhrman system:

- **Grade I:** Nuclei round, uniform, 10 µm; nucleoli inconspicuous or absent
- **Grade II:** Nuclei irregular, 15 µm; nucleoli evident
- **Grade III:** Nuclei very irregular, 20 µm; nucleoli large and prominent
- **Grade IV:** Nuclei bizarre and multilobated, 20 µm or more; nucleoli prominent

 CLINICAL FEATURES: RCC incidence of peaks in the sixth decade, and the tumor occurs twice as often in men as in women. *Hematuria is*

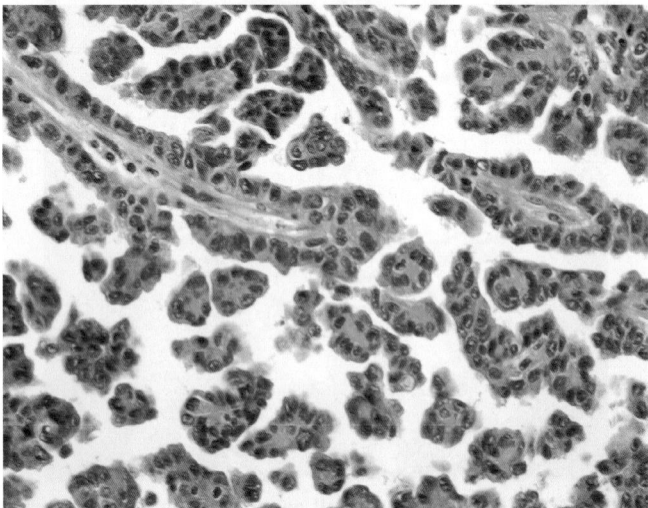

FIGURE 22-94. Papillary renal cell carcinoma. Photomicrograph showing papillary fronds covered by neoplastic cells.

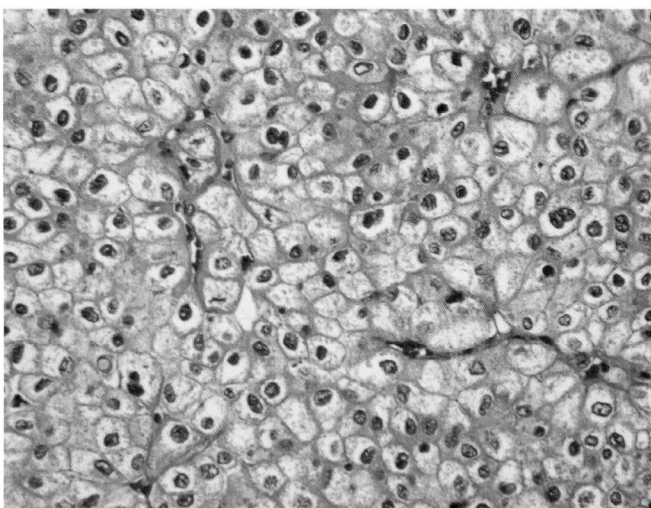

FIGURE 22-95. Chromophobe renal cell carcinoma. Photomicrograph showing pale acidophilic granular cells with prominent cell borders.

the most common presenting sign, but incidental discoveries are common, in imaging studies of the abdomen done for other reasons. The classic clinical triad of hematuria, flank pain and a palpable abdominal mass occurs in fewer than 10% of patients. RCC is known as a "great mimic," and it produces ectopic hormones that may cause fever and paraneoplastic syndromes. For example, secretion of a PTH-like substance leads to symptoms of hyperparathyroidism, production of erythropoietin causes erythrocytosis and RCC secretion of renin results in hypertension. Patients with RCC often come to medical attention because of symptoms from a metastasis. A sudden convulsion or a cough in a previously healthy person leads to discovery of an unsuspected tumor in the brain or lung, which on further examination proves to be RCC.

Prognosis for RCC reflects tumor size, extent of invasion and metastasis, histologic type and nuclear grade. Patients whose tumors show prominent sarcomatoid features rarely survive more than 1 year. By contrast, 1-year survival after nephrectomy for clear cell RCC is 50%. Papillary and chromophobe types have better prognoses than clear cell tumors, whereas collecting duct tumors have a worse prognosis. *Tumor stage is the single most important prognostic factor.* If RCC remains inside the renal capsule, 5-year survival is 90%. This drops to 30% if there are distant metastases. The tumor spreads most frequently to the lungs and bones.

Renal medullary carcinomas are rapidly growing neoplasms that are almost always associated with sickle cell disease.

Transitional Cell Carcinoma

Between 5% and 10% of primary kidney cancers are transitional cell carcinomas of the pelvis or calyces (see Chapter 23). These are morphologically identical to the more common transitional cell carcinomas of the urinary bladder and associated with them in 1/2 of cases. Fewer than 5% of transitional cell carcinomas occur in the collecting system proximal to the bladder.

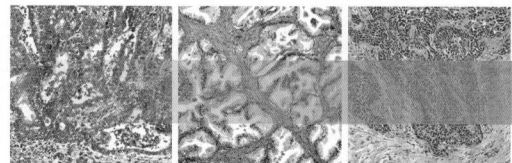

The Lower Urinary Tract and Male Reproductive System

Ivan Damjanov ■ Peter A. McCue

Anatomy and Embryology

LOWER URINARY TRACT

The ureters, urinary bladder and urethra—collectively known as the lower urinary tract—are the outflow part of the urinary system (Fig. 23-1). In males, the lower urinary tract is closely related to the reproductive system.

The Urinary Bladder Is in the Retroperitoneal Space of the Lower Abdomen

In males, the urinary bladder is anterior to the rectum and superior to the prostate. In females, it is anterior to the lower uterine corpus and anterior vaginal fornix.

The bladder is subdivided anatomically into the apex (dome), midportion and base, the last comprising the trigone and bladder neck. The apex is located behind the symphysis pubis and is linked in the midline to the umbilicus by the umbilical ligament, a fibrous remnant of the fetal **urachus**. The bladder neck in males rests on the upper surface of the prostate, where the smooth muscle fibers of the two organs intertwine. Inside the bladder, the **trigone** is the triangular area at the posterior aspect of the bladder base. It lacks mucosal folds and appears flattened. Superiorly, the trigone is bound by a muscular ridge joining the laterally placed orifices of the ureters. The inferior tip of the trigone is formed by the funnel-shaped internal orifice of the urethra.

The Ureters Are in the Posterior Retroperitoneal Space, Lateral to the Vertebrae

The ureters are paired organs linking each renal pelvis to the bladder. The lowermost part of the ureters is obliquely embedded in the smooth muscular wall of the urinary bladder, which acts as sphincters known as the **ureterovesical**

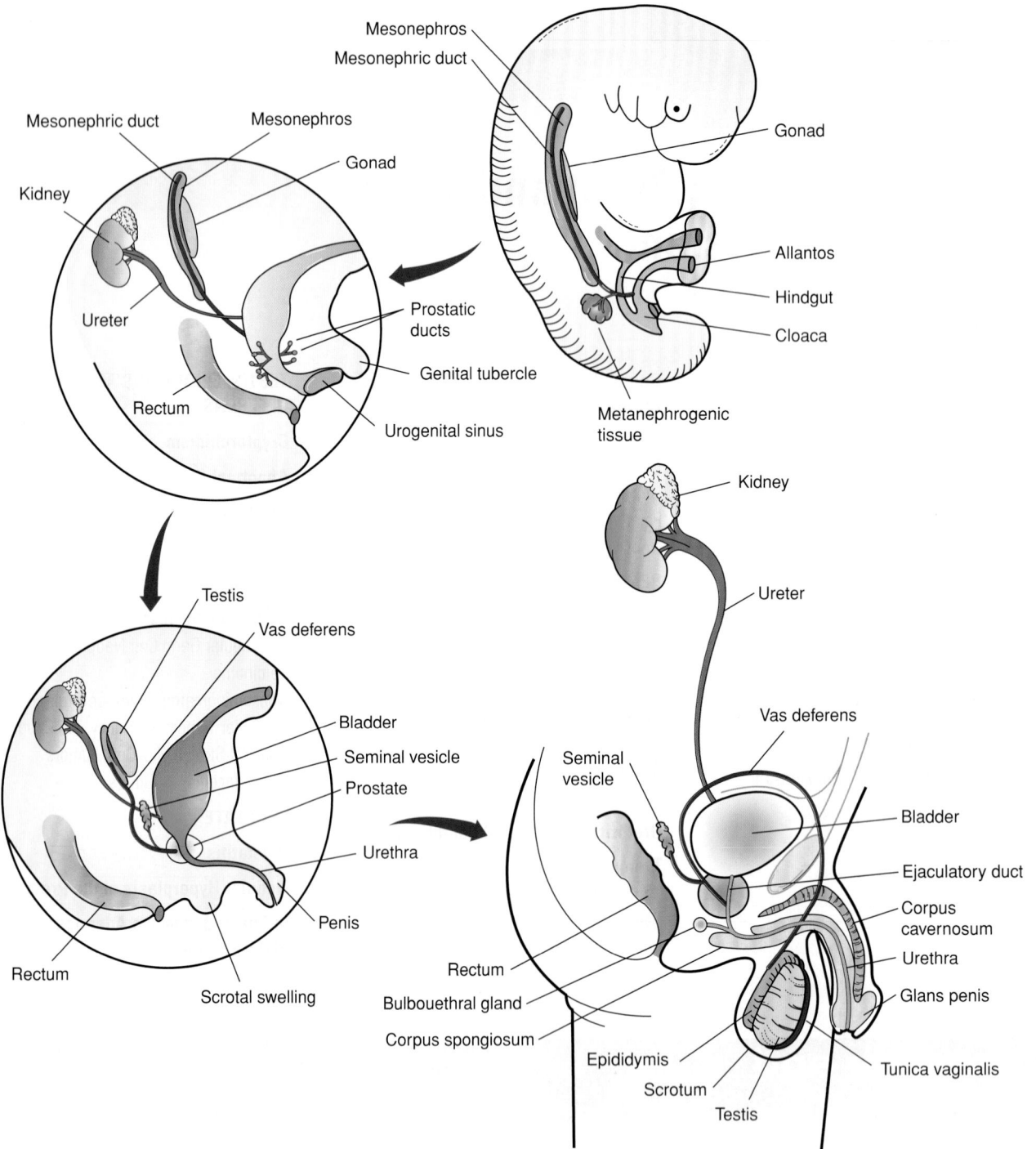

FIGURE 23-1. Embryologic development of the urinary tract and male reproductive system.

valves. These valves let urine pass downward into the bladder but not in the opposite direction.

The Urethra Is the Terminal Outflow Conduit of the Urinary Tract

The male urethra averages 20 cm long and has three parts: (1) **prostatic urethra,** traversing the prostate; (2) **membranous urethra,** penetrating the pelvic floor; and (3) **spongy or penile urethra,** in the central portion of the penis. The prostatic urethra contains ostia of the ejaculatory and prostatic

ducts. The posterior part of the penile urethra, also called the **bulbous urethra,** receives secretions from the mucous bulbourethral (Cowper) glands. The anterior part of the penile urethra contains scattered mucus-secreting glands of Littré. The penile urethra terminates in the fossa navicularis, just proximal to the external orifice, or meatus, on the tip of the penis.

The female urethra is shorter, only 3–4 cm in length. It extends from its internal orifice at the urinary bladder to its external orifice in the vulva, immediately below the clitoris. The wall of the female urethra also contains mucous glands.

Transitional Epithelium (Urothelium) Lines the Ureters, Bladder and Posterior Urethra

The urothelium has three epithelial zones. The **basal layer** lies on a basement membrane and contains cells that can divide and replace damaged superficial cells. Above the basal layer is the **intermediate zone,** 3–4 layers of polygonal cells. Both basal and polygonal cells can flatten when the bladder dilates. The **superficial layer** consists of "umbrella cells," which are resistant to the urine that constantly bathes them.

Under the epithelium, the lamina propria contains mainly loose connective tissue, smooth muscle cells and blood vessels. The muscularis mucosa is poorly developed and consists of thin discontinuous wisps of smooth muscle cells. Beyond the lamina propria lies a thick smooth muscle layer, covered by adventitia. Since the bladder, ureters and urethra are retroperitoneal, they do not have an external serosa. Only part of the bladder dome has a serosal covering.

The Lower Urinary Tract Develops Mostly from the Cloaca

The **cloaca** is a fetal structure that is partitioned early in ontogenesis into an anterior part, the **urogenital sinus,** and a posterior part, which is the primordium of the rectum (Fig. 23-1). The urogenital sinus is the anlage of the urinary bladder, proximal urethra and **urachus,** the latter being a temporary fetal structure that connects the urinary tract and umbilicus. Caudally, the urogenital sinus makes contact with an invagination of the urogenital membrane, to form the urethra. The urachus gradually involutes into the umbilical ligament. The fetal urinary bladder forms symmetrical lateral **ureteric buds** that grow cranially. When these epithelial buds reach the nephrogenic zone, they induce formation of the metanephros, the kidney primordium.

MALE REPRODUCTIVE SYSTEM

The male reproductive system includes the testis, epididymis, ductus (vas) deferens, seminal vesicles, prostate and penis (Fig. 23-1).

Testes Are Linked to the Epididymis and are Located in the Scrotum

Testes are paired oval organs measuring 4 × 3 × 3 cm. Each is invested with a **tunica vaginalis,** a layer of mesothelial cells that covers the outer fibrous capsule of the testis, which is called the **tunica albuginea.** This capsule has internal septal ramifications that divide the testis into about 250 **lobules.** Each lobule consists of coiled seminiferous tubules and loose interstitial tissue containing blood vessels and Leydig interstitial cells.

Testicular arteries originate from the abdominal aorta and nourish the testes. The right internal spermatic vein empties into the inferior vena cava, while the left drains into the left renal vein. This anatomic difference has several clinical implications discussed below.

Spermatogenesis Occurs in the Seminiferous Tubules

These tubules are the principal functional unit of the testes. They contain seminiferous epithelium and **Sertoli cells,** which support spermatogenesis. Sertoli cells also secrete **inhibin,** which communicates with the pituitary to regulate secretion of **gonadotropins** (i.e., follicle-stimulating hormone [FSH] and luteinizing hormone [LH]). The interstitial spaces of the testis contain **Leydig cells,** the primary source of testosterone.

In prepubertal testes, seminiferous tubules contain primitive **germ cells** (spermatogonia) and Sertoli cells. At puberty, LH stimulates testosterone production by Leydig cells to initiate spermatogenesis, and FSH acts on germ cells and Sertoli cells to drive spermatogenesis.

Hormonal stimuli increase numbers of germ cells, primarily **spermatogonia,** which also begin differentiating into **primary spermatocytes.** Meiotic division of the diploid primary spermatocytes produces **secondary spermatocytes,** which carry a haploid number (23) of chromosomes. Secondary spermatocytes mature to **spermatids,** and then to **spermatozoa,** which are discharged through the channels of rete testis into the epididymal ducts.

The **epididymis** lies along the lateral–posterior aspect of the testis and extends into the ductus deferens. In the epididymis, spermatozoa are admixed with fluid secreted by epididymal lining cells and travel through the **vas deferens,** which empties its contents into the urethra. Finally, semen is ejaculated through the penile urethra as a mixture of spermatozoa in epididymal secretions and fluids made by **accessory glands,** namely, the seminal vesicles, prostate, Cowper bulbourethral glands and urethral glands.

The Prostate Is an Accessory Gland Located in the Pelvis

It contacts the posterior and inferior external layers of the urinary bladder, close to the rectum. Posteriorly it is attached to **seminal vesicles.** Microscopically it is a tubuloalveolar gland with a rich fibromuscular stroma. It develops under the influence of testosterone, which is essential for maintaining its production of seminal fluid.

Functionally, the prostate is organized into three distinct zones. The **transition zone** is around the prostatic urethra. The **central zone** sits slightly posterior and extends toward the seminal vesicles. The **peripheral zone** envelops the other zones and defines the boundaries of the gland. Precise anatomic boundaries of the zones may be inapparent by light microscopy. However, the biological discrimination between the zones is important, as most cancers arise in the peripheral zone, while hyperplasias generally originate in the transition zone.

The gland lacks a true **capsule.** In some areas, there is a concentric band of fibromuscular tissue that blends into the adjacent glandular stroma. In the apex of the prostate, the capsular plane of dissection is essentially inseparable from the adjacent soft tissue. Thus, what constitutes capsular invasion by tumor is somewhat arbitrary, which carries important implications in cancer staging for the surgeon who removes the organ and for the pathologist assessing the extent of disease.

The Male Genital System Develops from Several Primordia

The testes develop from **genital ridges,** which occur on the posterior surface of the celomic cavity. These ridges are populated by migratory **primordial germ cells** (initially formed in the yolk sac) that enter the fetal body through the midline, then migrate laterally into the right and left genital ridges. Complex interactions of germ cells and stromal cells in the genital ridges lead to formation of the fetal testes on the posterior wall of the midabdomen. At the same time, the testes connect with the future epididymis and vas deferens, which develop from the **wolffian ducts**. At that point the testes begin a gradual descent into the inguinal canal to the scrotum.

The scrotum and penis develop simultaneously with the testes but from a different anlage that corresponds mostly to the genital tubercle and partly to the anterior urogenital sinus. These primordia of the external genital organs are initially identical in both sexes. In a male fetus, testosterone drives their development into penis, penile urethra and scrotum; in a female fetus, they become clitoris, labia minora and labia majora.

Renal Pelvis and Ureter

CONGENITAL DISORDERS

Developmental anomalies of the renal pelvis and ureters occur in 2%–3% of all people. They do not usually cause clinical problems, but on occasion may predispose to obstruction and urinary tract infections. The most important developmental anomalies include agenesis, ectopia, duplications, obstructions and dilations (Fig. 23-2).

AGENESIS OF THE RENAL PELVIS AND URETERS: This rare anomaly always entails agenesis of the corresponding kidney. Unilateral agenesis is usually asymptomatic. Bilateral agenesis of ureters and kidneys, a feature of **Potter syndrome,** is incompatible with extrauterine life (see Chapter 22).

ECTOPIC URETERS: Ureteric buds may develop at the wrong anatomic site during embryogenesis. The lower orifices of ectopic ureters can be found in many anomalous places, such as the midportion of the urinary bladder, seminal vesicles, urethra or vas deferens.

DUPLICATIONS: Ureteral duplication is the most common congenital abnormality of the urinary system. Duplicate or multiple ureteric buds may originate on the side of the fetal bladder and may be unilateral or bilateral, complete or partial. Usually there are two parallel ureters, each with its own renal pelvis and separate vesical orifice. **Bifid ureters** (subdivided by a septum), **bifurcate ureters** and many variations thereof may be encountered, but most are of no clinical significance.

URETERAL OBSTRUCTION: Obstructions can be traced to congenital **atresia** or abnormal **ureteral valves**. However, congenital **obstruction of the ureteropelvic junction (UPJ),** which is the most common form of hydronephrosis in infants and children, is thought to be related to abnormal layering of smooth muscle cells and/or fibrous tissue replacing the smooth muscle cells at the UPJ. Urinary obstruction in these children is usually unilateral but is bilateral in 20% of cases. Obstruction is more common in boys than girls and is usually diagnosed during the first 6 months of life. Congenital UPJ obstruction is often associated with other urinary tract anomalies, including, in some cases, agenesis of the contralateral kidney.

DILATIONS OF THE RENAL PELVIS OR URETERS: If dilations of the renal pelvis or ureters are localized, they are called **diverticula**. Generalized dilation of the entire ureter, **congenital megaureter,** may be unilateral or bilateral. Affected ureters are tortuous and lack peristalsis. Resulting stagnation of urine **(hydroureter)** is typically associated with progressive hydronephrosis, ultimately leading to renal failure.

URETERITIS AND URETERAL OBSTRUCTION

Ureteritis, or inflammation of the ureters, is a complication of descending infections from the kidneys or ascending infections due to vesicoureteric reflux. Ureteritis is often associated with ureteral obstruction, which may be intrinsic or extrinsic (Fig. 23-3).

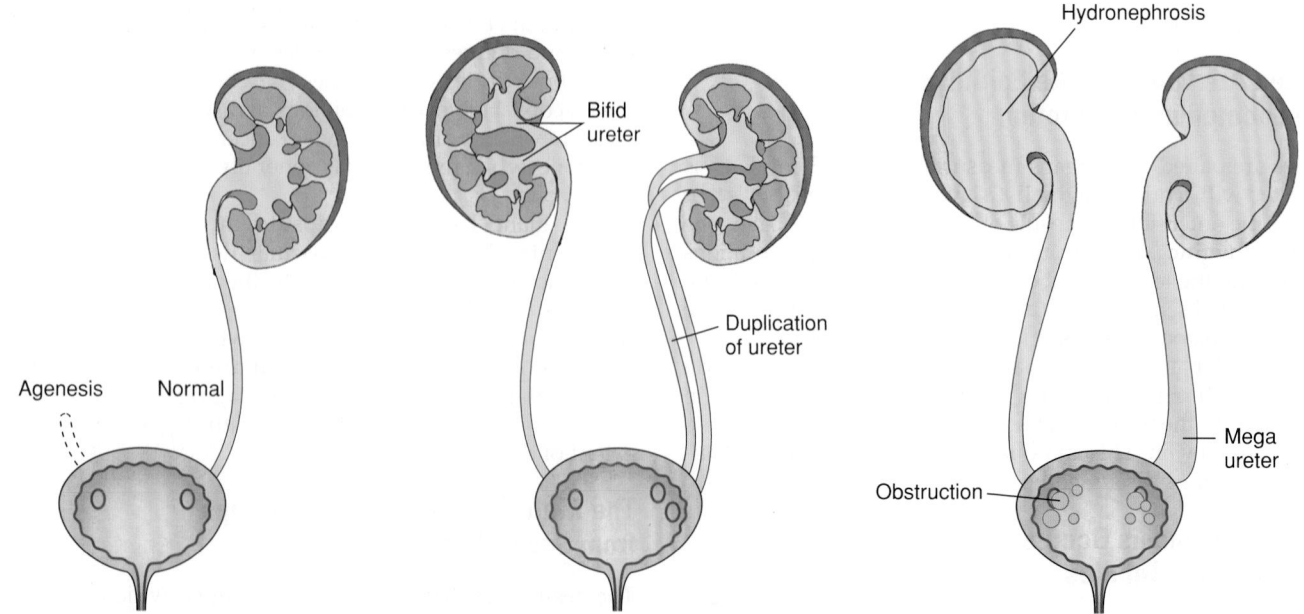

FIGURE 23-2. Anomalies of the renal pelvis and ureters.

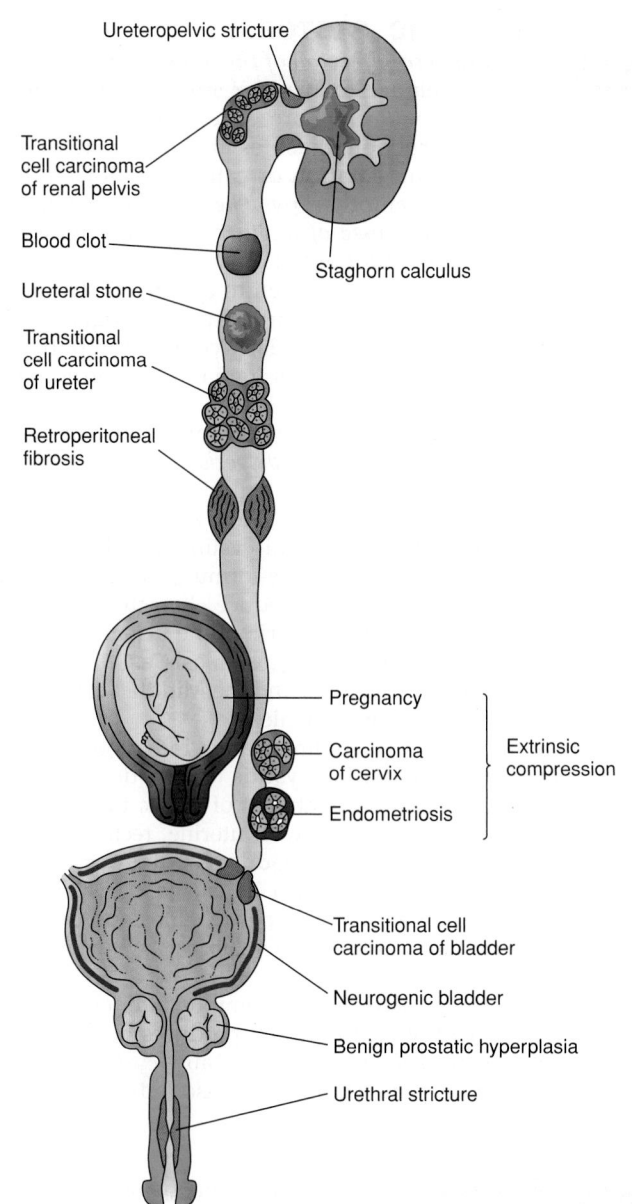

FIGURE 23-3. **Most common causes of ureteral obstruction.**

of retroperitoneal soft tissues and modest, nonspecific, chronic inflammation. On occasion, idiopathic retroperitoneal fibrosis is accompanied by inflammatory fibrosis in other areas, including Riedel struma (thyroid), primary sclerosing cholangitis (liver) and mediastinal fibrosis. Some of these multisystemic cases are associated with elevated serum immunoglobulin G4 (IgG4), and thus belong to the group of **IgG4-related diseases**. The fibrotic lesions are infiltrated with IgG4-positive plasma cells, which play an undefined pathogenetic role in the genesis of fibrosis. The disease may respond to treatment with corticosteroids or immunosuppression. **Secondary retroperitoneal fibrosis** resembles the idiopathic form of the disease clinically and pathologically and may evolve as a complication of surgery or radiation therapy, or as an adverse reaction to certain drugs such as methysergide or β-adrenergic blockers.

TUMORS OF THE RENAL PELVIS AND URETER

Tumors of the renal pelvis and ureter resemble those of urinary bladder (see below) except that they are 1/10 as common. Most (>90%) are **urothelial (transitional) cell carcinomas**. Etiologies associated with such tumors of the renal pelvis and ureter are similar to those found in bladder cancer, suggesting a "field effect" in which the entire urothelial mucosa is a continuous "target organ." About 2%–4% of tumors are bilateral, and almost half of treated patients develop subsequent urothelial bladder tumors.

CLINICAL FEATURES: Patients most often present in their sixth and seventh decades with hematuria (80%) and flank pain (25%). Urothelial cell carcinoma of the ureter or renal pelvis requires radical nephroureterectomy. The entire ureter must be removed because of the high frequency of concurrent and subsequent urothelial carcinomas. Prognosis reflects tumor stage at the time of diagnosis.

Urinary Bladder

CONGENITAL DISORDERS

Congenital developmental malformations of the urinary bladder include (1) bladder exstrophy, (2) diverticula, (3) urachal remnants and (4) congenital vesicoureteral valve incompetence.

EXSTROPHY OF THE BLADDER: This malformation is characterized by absence of the anterior bladder wall and part of the anterior abdominal wall. It occurs in 1 in 50,000 births. In some boys it is associated with **epispadias** (i.e., incomplete formation of the penile urethra).

Bladder exstrophy results from incomplete resorption of the anterior cloacal membrane. In normal embryogenesis, this membrane is replaced by smooth muscle, but if it persists, it forms the anterior vesical wall. As the membrane is thin, it ultimately ruptures to leave a large defect that is accompanied by defective closure of the anterior abdominal muscular wall. These two defects expose the posterior bladder wall to the exterior and transform the bladder into a cup-like organ that cannot hold urine (Fig. 23-4). The posterior wall of the exstrophic bladder is exposed to mechanical

Intrinsic ureteral obstruction may be caused by calculi, intraluminal blood clots, fibroepithelial polyps, inflammatory strictures, amyloidosis or tumors of the ureter.

Extrinsic causes of ureteral obstruction include the enlarged uterus during pregnancy, aberrant renal vessels to the lower pole of the kidney that cross the ureter or endometriosis. Tumors that compress the ureters usually originate from the digestive and female genital tracts, and may compress the ureters by direct extension or through metastases to retroperitoneal lymph nodes.

Ureteral obstruction can also result from diseases of the urinary bladder, prostate and urethra (e.g., bladder cancer near a ureteral orifice or bladder neck, neurogenic bladder and prostatic hyperplasia or cancer). Proximal causes of ureteral obstruction tend to be unilateral, while more distal ones, such as prostatic diseases, lead to bilateral hydronephrosis, with the possibility of renal failure in untreated cases.

Idiopathic retroperitoneal fibrosis (Ordmond disease) is a rare cause of ureteral obstruction, with dense fibrosis

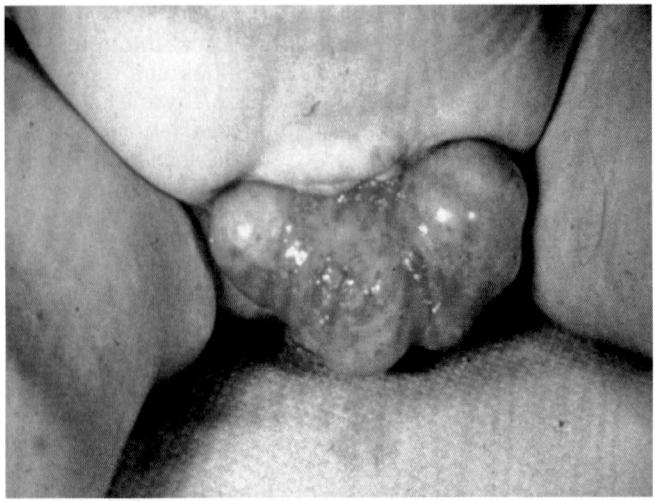

FIGURE 23-4. Exstrophy of the urinary bladder.

injury and prone to frequent infection, causing squamous or glandular metaplasia. Exstrophy can be surgically repaired, but the metaplastic mucosa is at increased risk of bladder cancer, even 50 to 60 years after surgical repair of exstrophy.

DIVERTICULA: These sac-like outpouchings of bladder wall are related to incomplete formation of muscular layers. They can be solitary or multiple. Urine retained inside such diverticula is commonly infected, which may lead to urinary stone formation. Congenital diverticula must be distinguished from **acquired vesical diverticula,** which typically occur in long-standing urinary tract obstruction due to prostatic hyperplasia in adults.

URACHAL REMNANTS: The urachus is the fetal allantoic stalk connecting the bladder and umbilicus. If it persists and remains patent throughout, it forms a vesical–umbilical fistula. Incomplete regression of the urinary end, midportion or umbilical end of the urachus leads to a **urachal diverticulum, umbilical–urachal sinus** or **urachal cyst,** respectively. The columnar epithelium of urachal remnants may give rise to **adenocarcinoma.** Only 0.2% of bladder cancers—but one third of bladder adenocarcinomas—arise in such remnants.

CONGENITAL VESICOURETERAL VALVE INCOMPETENCE: This anomaly results from an abnormal junction between the ureters and the urinary bladder. The ureters normally enter the bladder wall obliquely and have a long intravesical portion. The muscular layer of the bladder compresses the ureters and acts as a sphincter, to prevent backflow of urine into ureters. However, if ureters enter the bladder at right angles, they have a short intravesical segment that does not adequately prevent urine backflow during micturition. **Vesicoureteric reflux** (VUR) is more common in young girls than boys and is often familial. In 75% of cases, VUR is asymptomatic, but it may lead to reflux pyelonephritis. Congenital VUR is distinguished from acquired VUR that occurs during pregnancy or with bladder hypertrophy.

CYSTITIS

Cystitis is inflammation of the bladder. It may be acute or chronic. It is the most common urinary tract infection. Cystitis often occurs in hospitalized patients, especially those who have had indwelling bladder catheters.

 **ETIOLOGIC FACTORS:** *Cystitis is usually secondary to infection of the lower urinary tract.* Factors related to bladder infection include a patient's age and gender, the presence of bladder calculi, bladder outlet obstruction, diabetes mellitus, immunodeficiency, prior instrumentation or catheterization, radiation therapy and chemotherapy. *The risk of cystitis is greater in females because of a short urethra, especially during pregnancy.* Bladder outlet obstruction due to prostatic hyperplasia predisposes men to cystitis. Instrumentation (cystoscopy) may also introduce pathogens into the bladder, and cystitis is especially common in patients in whom indwelling catheters remain for prolonged periods.

Coliform bacteria are the most common cause of cystitis, mostly *Escherichia coli, Proteus vulgaris, Pseudomonas aeruginosa* and *Enterobacter* spp. Tuberculosis of the bladder is rarely seen in the Western world today and almost always follows renal tuberculosis. Fungal cystitis may be seen in immunosuppressed patients. Gas-forming bacilli, usually in people with diabetes, may produce characteristic interstitial bubbles in the lamina propria of the urinary bladder **(emphysematous cystitis).** Schistosomiasis as a common cause of cystitis in North Africa and the Middle East, where *Schistosoma haematobium* is endemic.

Iatrogenic cystitis is common after radiation therapy and chemotherapy. **Radiation cystitis** usually develops 4–6 weeks following radiation treatment of pelvic tumors, and is most often seen in patients with uterine, rectal or bladder cancer. Inflammation of the bladder is usually associated with epithelial cell atypia, which is usually transient and should not be mistaken for malignancy. Late consequences of radiation cystitis include extensive fibrosis, which may be transmural and incapacitating.

Drug-induced cystitis is most common after cyclophosphamide treatment, which typically produces hemorrhagic cystitis. Other cytotoxic drugs can also cause cystitis, but the injury is less prominent. These drugs also induce cytologic atypia, which is usually transient.

 PATHOLOGY: Stromal edema, hemorrhage and a neutrophilic infiltrate of variable intensity are typical of acute cystitis (Fig. 23-5). Focal petechial mucosal hemorrhages **(hemorrhagic cystitis)** are often seen in acute bacterial cystitis. Bleeding diatheses (e.g., leukemia or treatment with cytotoxic drugs) and disseminated intravascular coagulation often cause extensive hemorrhagic cystitis. *Acute cystitis that does not resolve is associated with chronic cystitis, including an infiltrate mainly of lymphocytes and plasma cells (Fig. 23-6), and fibrosis of the lamina propria.* Occasionally, an inflamed bladder mucosa may contain lymphocytic follicles **(follicular cystitis)** or dense infiltrates of eosinophils **(eosinophilic cystitis).** Granulomatous cystitis is characteristic of tuberculosis, but may also be seen in patients with bladder cancer treated with intravesical instillation of attenuated *Mycobacterium tuberculosis,* bacillus Calmette-Guerin (BCG). Ova of *Schistosoma hematobium* can cause simultaneous granulomatous reactions and eosinophilic infiltrates. Specific forms of chronic cystitis include:

- **Ulcerative cystitis:** Chronic irritation caused, for example, by indwelling catheters or traumatic cystoscopy may lead to ulceration and focal mucosal hemorrhage.

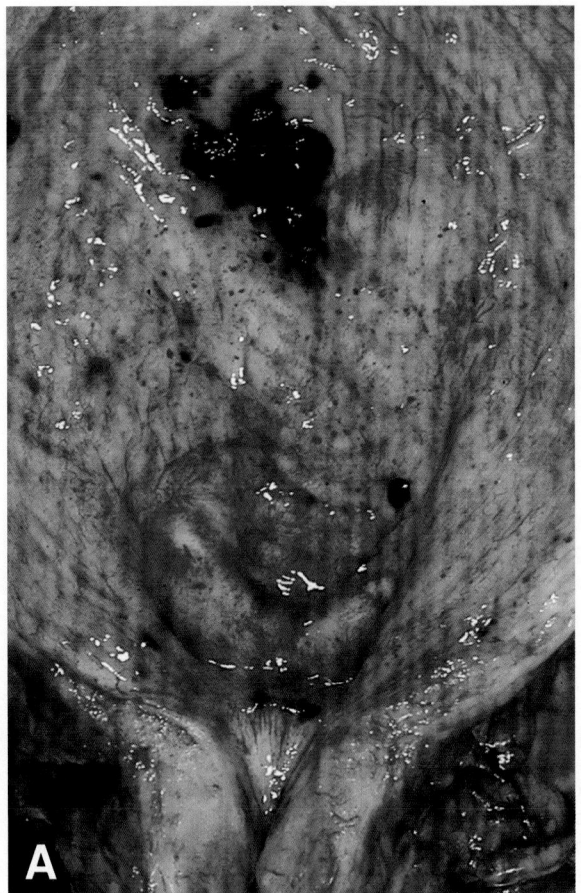

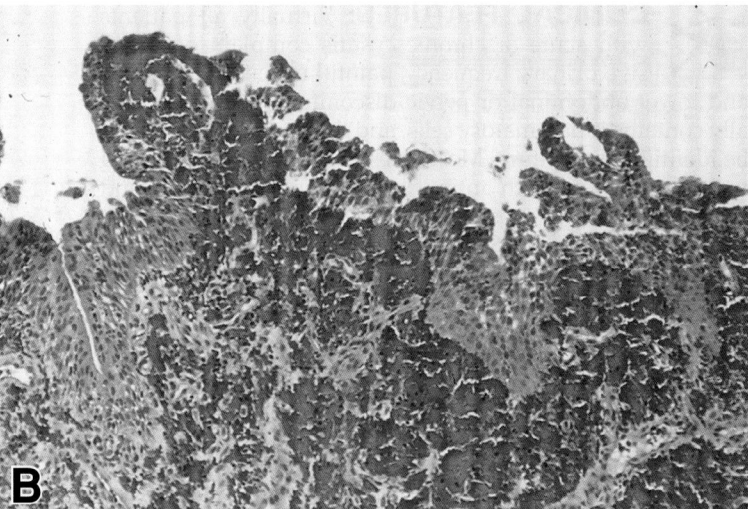

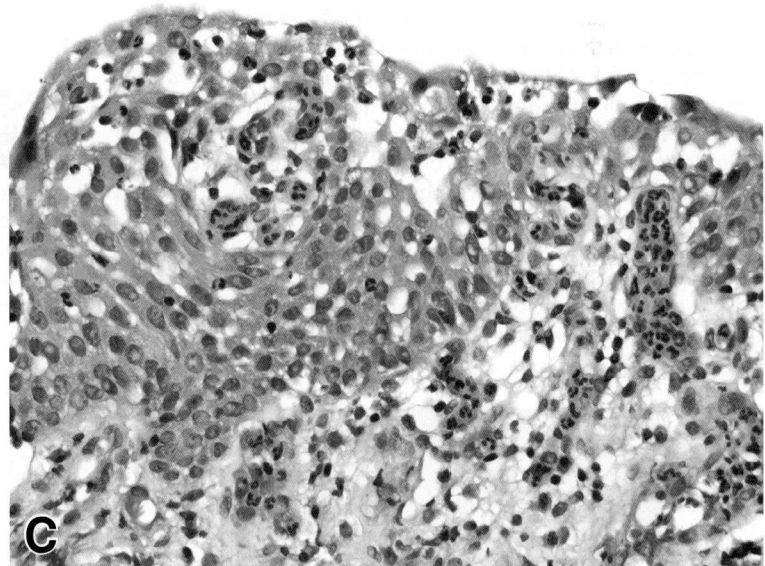

FIGURE 23-5. Acute cystitis. Cystitis was caused by an indwelling catheter. **A.** Several foci of hemorrhage are seen on the hyperemic bladder mucosa. **B.** Microscopic foci of mucosal hemorrhage. **C.** Acute cystitis. Polymorphonuclear leukocytes infiltrate the mucosa.

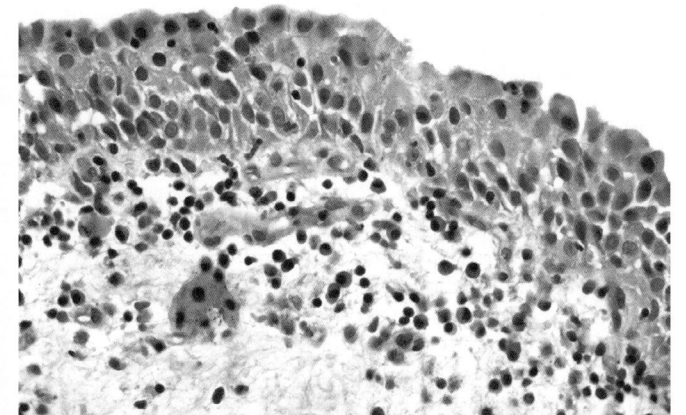

FIGURE 23-6. Chronic cystitis. A chronic inflammatory infiltrate of lymphocytes and plasma cells is present in the edematous lamina propria.

Solitary mucosal ulcer is also found in interstitial cystitis (see below).

- **Suppurative cystitis:** Pus may cover the bladder mucosa, fill the lumen or permeate the bladder wall. Suppurative cystitis may develop during local infection but more often is a complication of sepsis, pyelonephritis or purulent infections after bladder surgery.
- **Pseudomembranous cystitis:** Pseudomembranes—shaggy layers of necrotic, gray or yellow cell detritus; fibrin; inflammatory cells; and blood—sometimes cover the bladder mucosa. Underlying mucosa is hemorrhagic and ulcerated. Pseudomembranous cystitis typically complicates infections that follow treatment with cytotoxic drugs, such as cyclophosphamide.
- **Calcific cystitis:** This form of chronic inflammation is typically found in schistosomiasis. Calcification of ova produces bladder wall encrustations resembling grains of sand. These gradually coalesce, to transform the entire urinary bladder into a calcified rigid vessel.

THE LOWER URINARY TRACT

CLINICAL FEATURES: Virtually all patients with acute or chronic cystitis complain of excessive urinary frequency, painful urination **(dysuria)** and lower abdominal or pelvic discomfort. The urine usually contains inflammatory cells, and the causative agent can be identified by culture. Most cases of acute cystitis respond well to treatment with antimicrobial agents. Recurrent and chronic cystitis may pose therapeutic problems.

CHRONIC INTERSTITIAL CYSTITIS: This persistent painful inflammation of the bladder affects over 100,000 middle-aged women in the United States. It is has no known cause, and presents with suprapubic pain, an urge for frequent urination, hematuria and dysuria. During cystoscopic dilatation of the bladder, the mucosa typically develops hemorrhagic cracks and petechial hemorrhages. Urine cultures are almost always negative. In chronic stages of the disease, transmural inflammation of the bladder wall is occasionally associated with mucosal ulceration **(Hunner ulcer)** (Fig. 23-7). Chronic inflammation, including fibrosis and increased mast cells, is common in the mucosa and muscularis. Hunner ulcers contain intense acute inflammation. The disease is typically persistent and refractory to therapy.

MALAKOPLAKIA (from the Greek, **malakos,** *"soft";* **plax,** *"plaque"): This is an uncommon inflammatory disorder of unknown etiology.* Originally described in the bladder, malakoplakia may be seen in many other sites, within and outside the urinary tract. It occurs at all ages, with peak incidence in the fifth to seventh decades, and has a marked female preponderance.

Malakoplakia is often associated with urinary tract infection by *E. coli*, although a direct causal relationship is dubious. A clinical background of immunosuppression, chronic infections or cancer is common.

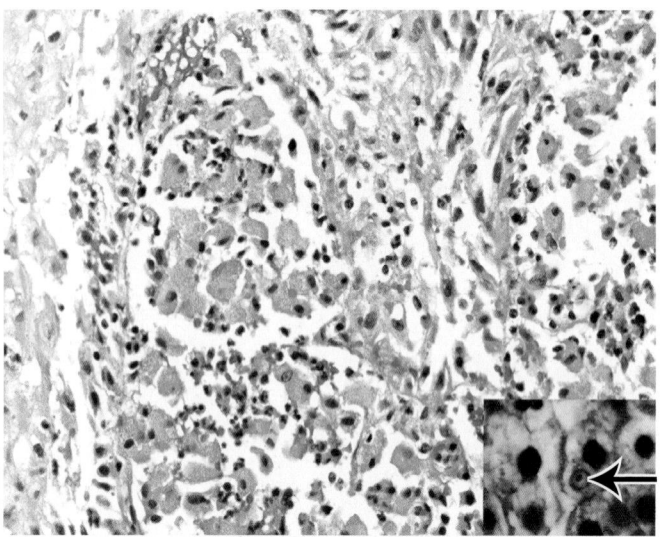

FIGURE 23-8. Malakoplakia. Inflammatory cells are mainly macrophages, with fewer lymphocytes. **Inset.** A Michaelis-Gutmann body (*arrow*) is seen at high magnification.

PATHOLOGY: Malakoplakia is characterized by soft, yellow plaques on the mucosal surface of the bladder. There is a striking chronic inflammatory cell infiltrate mainly of large macrophages with abundant, eosinophilic cytoplasm containing periodic acid–Schiff (PAS)-positive granules (Fig. 23-8). Ultrastructurally, these granules are engorged lysosomes that contain fragments of bacteria, suggesting that malakoplakia may reflect an acquired defect in lysosomal degradation. Some of these macrophages have laminated, basophilic calcospherites, called **Michaelis-Gutmann bodies,** caused by calcium salt deposition in the enlarged lysosomes.

The clinical symptoms of malakoplakia of the bladder are indistinguishable from those of other forms of chronic cystitis. Treatment is ineffective.

BENIGN PROLIFERATIVE AND METAPLASTIC UROTHELIAL LESIONS

Benign proliferative and metaplastic lesions of urothelium occur mostly in the urinary bladder but may be found anywhere in the urinary tract. These nonneoplastic lesions are characterized by hyperplasia (Fig. 23-9B) or combined hyperplasia and metaplasia, mostly in association with chronic inflammation due to urinary tract infections, calculi, neurogenic bladder and (rarely) bladder exstrophy. They may also occur without a known preexisting inflammatory condition.

- **Brunn buds** are bulbous invaginations of the surface urothelium into the lamina propria (Fig. 23-9C). They are found in over 85% of bladders and are considered normal variants of the urothelium. **Brunn nests** are similar to Brunn buds, but the urothelial cells are seen within the lamina propria, detached from the surface.
- **Cystic lesions of the urinary bladder (cystitis cystica)** appear as fluid-filled groups of cysts. Similar cysts can be seen in the urethra or ureter **(urethritis cystica, ureteritis cystica)** (Fig. 23-10). Cystitis cystica is found in 60% of otherwise normal bladders. Histologically, all these

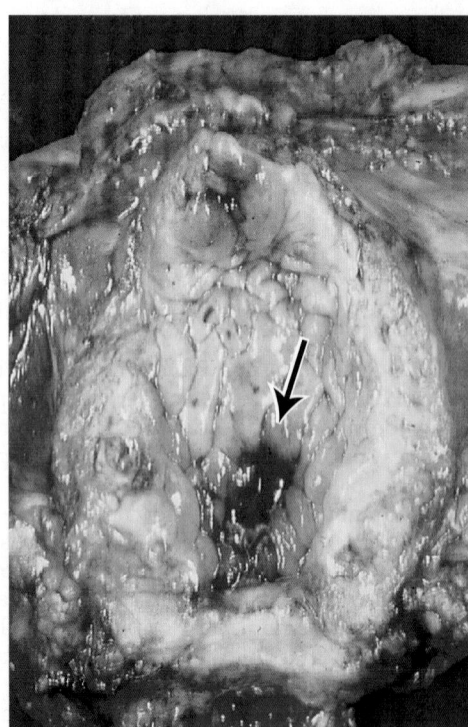

FIGURE 23-7. Interstitial cystitis. The hemorrhagic defect (*arrow*) in the edematous mucosa of the posterior wall of the bladder is clinically known as Hunner ulcer.

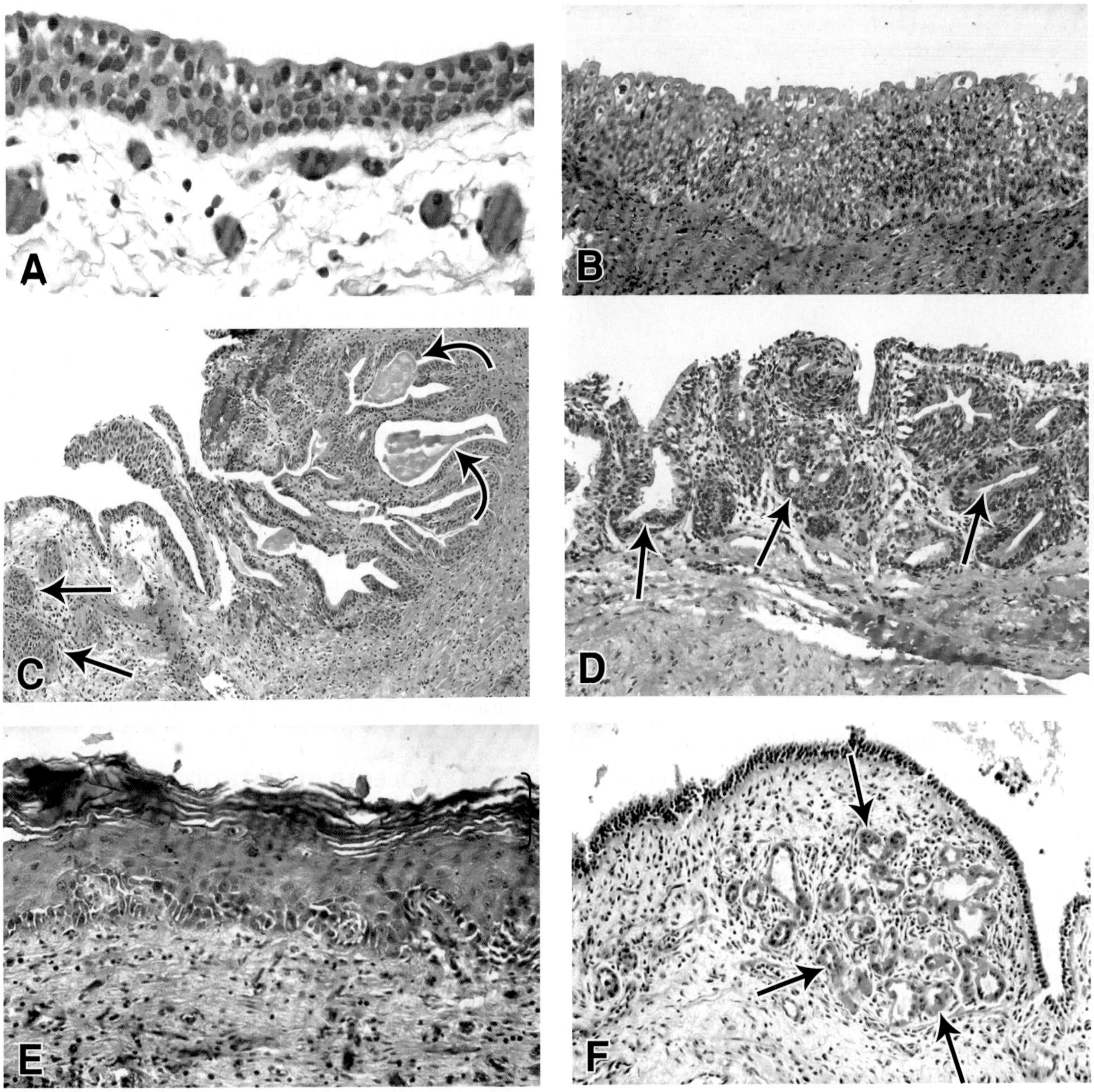

FIGURE 23-9. Proliferative and metaplastic changes of the urinary bladder. A. Normal bladder mucosa. B. Hyperplasia. Note the expansion of the normal 6–7 layers of urothelial cells. **C. Cystitis cystica.** Brunn nests (*straight arrows*) and cysts (*curved arrow*) protrude into the lamina propria. **D. Cystitis glandularis.** Metaplastic glandular mucosa is highlighted by the arrows. **E. Squamous metaplasia.** Note the keratinizing layer on the superficial epithelium (*bracket*). **F. Nephrogenic metaplasia** (*arrows*).

lesions correspond to cystic Brunn nests, lined by normal urothelium. Transitional epithelium may undergo metaplasia into mucus-secreting epithelium, which is then diagnosed as **cystitis glandularis** (Fig. 23-9D).

- **Squamous metaplasia** (Fig. 23-9E) is a reaction to chronic injury and inflammation and is particularly associated with calculi. It is seen in up to half of normal women and 10% of men.
- **Nephrogenic metaplasia** is a lesion caused by transformation of transitional epithelium to resemble renal tubules (Fig. 23-9F). It is most common in the urinary bladder but is also seen in the urethra and ureter. Many small tubules clustered in the lamina propria make a papillary exophytic

nodule. The histogenesis is unclear, but some cases seem to result from implants of detached renal tubular cells carried downstream by urine. The lesion may produce tumor-like protrusions in the bladder, which may obstruct the ureters and require surgical treatment.

 CLINICAL FEATURES: These proliferative and metaplastic urothelial lesions should not be confused with cancer. However, patients with such changes have higher risk of urothelial bladder carcinoma and, in the case of cystitis glandularis, of **adenocarcinoma** as well. Yet there is no evidence to suggest that these lesions themselves are preneoplastic.

THE LOWER URINARY TRACT

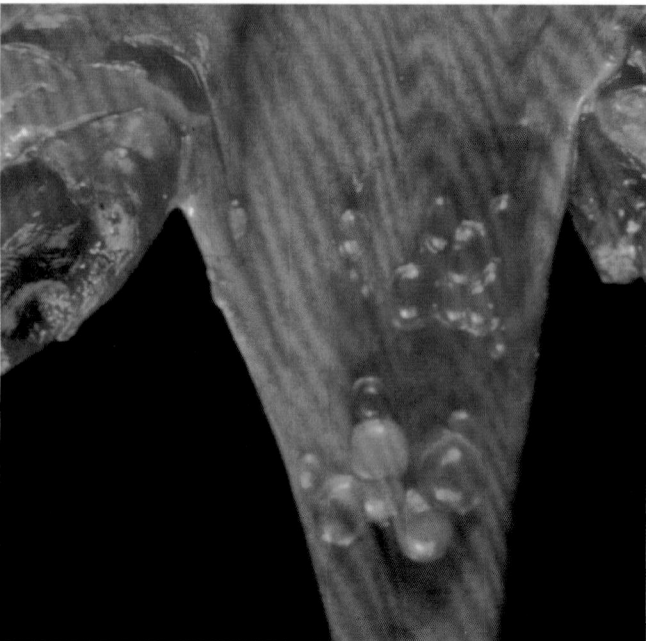

FIGURE 23-10. Ureteritis cystica. The mucosa of the proximal ureter exhibits small cystic structures.

TUMORS OF THE URINARY BLADDER

The most important facts about bladder cancer are:

- The urinary bladder is the most common site of urinary tract tumors.
- They mostly occur in older patients (median, 65 years) and are rare in patients under age 50.
- Tumors are much more common in men than in women.
- Most tumors (90%) are urothelial malignant neoplasms (formerly, "transitional cell" neoplasms). Squamous cell cancers, adenocarcinomas, neuroendocrine malignancies and sarcomas are rare.
- Tumors are often multifocal and can occur in any part of the urinary tract lined by transitional epithelium, from the renal pelvis to the posterior urethra.
- Local treatment is often followed by tumor recurrence.
- Tumor invasion into the muscularis propria markedly decreases the 5-year survival rate.

 **EPIDEMIOLOGY:** Bladder cancer represents 7% of all new cancers in men and 2% in women. It accounts for 3% of all cancer-related deaths in men and less than 1% in women. Bladder cancer shows significant geographic and sex differences throughout the world. The highest frequencies are among urban whites in the United States and western Europe. It is less common in Japan and among American blacks.

A high incidence of bladder cancer in Egypt, Sudan and some other African countries is due to endemic schistosomiasis. Most schistosomiasis-related cases are squamous cell carcinomas.

Bladder cancer may occur at any age, but most patients (80%) are 50–80 years old. Men are affected three times as often as women. There is no genetic predisposition to bladder cancer and no hereditary factors have been identified in the vast majority of cases.

The most important risk factors are:

- Cigarette smoking (4-fold increased risk)
- Industrial exposure to azo dyes
- Infection with *S. haematobium* (in endemic regions)
- Drugs, such as cyclophosphamide and analgesics
- Radiation therapy (following cervical, prostate or rectal cancer)

 **ETIOLOGIC FACTORS:** Bladder cancer following occupational exposure to certain organic chemicals was described in 1895 among workers in the German aniline dye industry and was subsequently confirmed in similar workers in the United States. This was one of the first occupational cancers known. Increased risk of bladder cancer was later noted in the leather, rubber, paint and organic chemical industries. Improved industrial hygiene has reduced this risk. *Today, polycyclic hydrocarbons from cigarette smoke are the most important risk factor for bladder carcinoma.*

A role for chemicals in bladder cancer has been strengthened by the demonstration that β-naphthylamine, to which the dye industry workers were exposed, produces bladder cancer in dogs. The metabolism of naphthylamines explains their organ specificity. Arylamines are conjugated to glucuronic acid in the liver, and the conjugates are excreted in the urine. In the bladder, β-glucuronidase in acidic urine hydrolyzes the glucuronic acid conjugate, producing reactive arylnitrenium ions that act as mutagens by binding guanines in DNA.

 **MOLECULAR PATHOGENESIS:** *Specific cytogenetic abnormalities occur in 50% of bladder cancers.* These often include deletion of chromosome 9 or its short (p) or long arm (q) (thus, 9p- or 9q-) and deletions of 11p, 13p, 14q or 17p, as well as aneuploidy of chromosomes 3, 7 and 17. Deletions within 9p, which contains the tumor suppressor gene *p16*, are the consistent findings in low-grade papillary tumors and flat carcinomas in situ. Deletions in 17p, the site of the tumor suppressor gene *TP53*, are often identified in invasive bladder cancers.

These genetic abnormalities suggest that cell cycle dysregulation due to mutated *p53* allows propagation of genetically abnormal urothelial cells. Unregulated proliferation reflects accumulated mutations in cyclin-dependent kinase inhibitors (e.g., p16/INK4a) or deletion of the tumor suppressor gene *RB1* (Fig. 23-11).

 PATHOLOGY: Over 90% of all primary bladder tumors are epithelial tumors, mostly urothelial carcinomas. Neoplastic urothelial lesions arising from the bladder mucosa make up a spectrum. One end includes benign papillomas and low-grade exophytic papillary carcinomas and the other end is invasive transitional cell carcinomas and highly malignant tumors (Fig. 23-12). Other tumors (Table 23-1) are considerably less common.

Urothelial Papilloma Is a Rare Benign Tumor

These papillomas are usually discovered incidentally in men aged 50 or older, during cystoscopy for an unrelated condition or for painless hematuria. They represent less than 1% of bladder tumors and have two forms: classical exophytic papilloma and inverted papilloma.

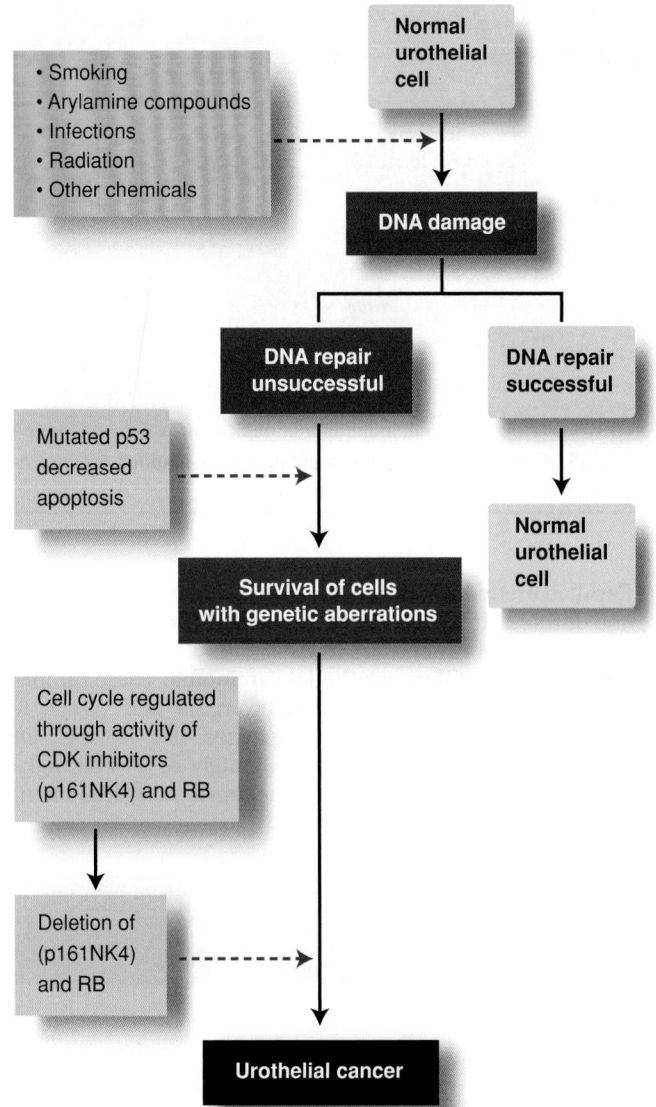

FIGURE 23-11. Hypothetical molecular model of urothelial neoplasms. The transition from normal urothelium to carcinoma occurs gradually in several steps.

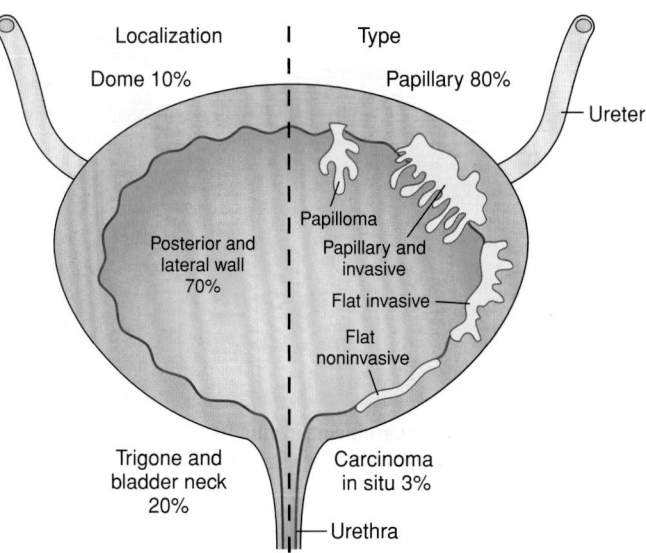

FIGURE 23-12. Urothelial neoplasms. Most tumors localize to the posterior and lateral walls; trigone and bladder neck are involved less often and the dome least. Malignant tumors may be papillary or flat. Both flat and papillary tumors may be invasive or noninvasive. Benign transitional cell papillomas are rare.

Urothelial Carcinoma In Situ Is a Flat, Full-Thickness Intraepithelial Lesion

This term is reserved for full-thickness lesions in which malignant changes are confined to nonpapillary bladder mucosa. The involved urothelium is of variable thickness, with cellular atypia from the basal layer to the surface (Fig. 23-13).

TABLE 23-1
TUMORS OF URINARY BLADDER
Urothelial Tumors
Urothelial cell papilloma
Exophytic papilloma
Inverted papilloma
Urothelial carcinoma in situ
Papillary urothelial neoplasm of low malignant potential (PUNLMP)
Papillary urothelial carcinoma, low grade[a]
Papillary urothelial carcinoma, high grade[a]
Invasive urothelial carcinoma
Other Malignant Tumors
Squamous cell carcinoma
Adenocarcinoma
Neuroendocrine (small cell) carcinoma
Carcinosarcoma
Sarcomas

[a]Papillary carcinomas may be invasive or noninvasive.

Exophytic papilloma features papillary fronds lined by transitional epithelium, virtually indistinguishable from normal urothelium. On cystoscopy, most patients show single lesions 2–5 cm in diameter, but some tumors may be multiple. Although considered benign, some recur or progress to carcinoma, mandating regular follow-up. Most "recurrences" are new tumors that develop elsewhere in the urinary bladder.

Inverted papillomas are rare and typically present as nodular mucosal lesions, usually in the trigone area. They have also been observed in the renal pelvis, ureter and urethra. Inverted papillomas are covered by normal urothelium, from which cords of transitional epithelium descend into the lamina propria. These lesions are most common in men in their sixth and seventh decades. Hematuria of recent onset is the usual clinical presentation. Inverted papillomas are benign tumors and are usually cured by simple excision.

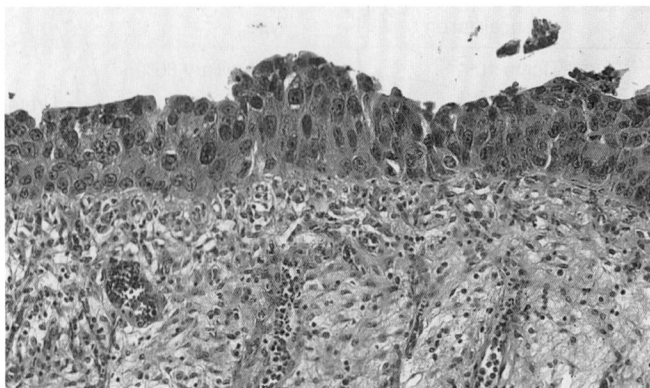

FIGURE 23-13. Urothelial carcinoma in situ. The urothelial mucosa shows nuclear pleomorphism and lack of polarity from the basal layer to the surface, without evidence of maturation.

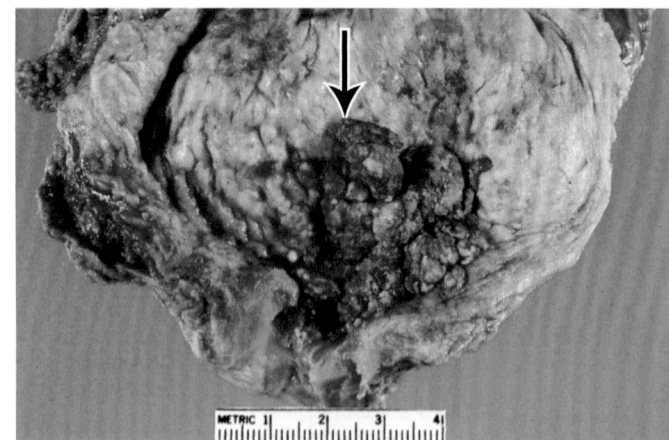

FIGURE 23-14. Urothelial carcinoma of the urinary bladder. A large exophytic tumor (*arrow*) is situated above the bladder neck.

Atypia entails loss of nuclear polarity, nuclear irregularity, enlargement, hyperchromatism and prominent nucleoli. *The basement membrane is intact and there is no invasion into underlying stroma.*

One third of carcinomas in situ of the bladder are associated with subsequent invasive carcinoma. In turn, most invasive transitional cell carcinomas arise from carcinoma in situ rather than from papillary transitional cell cancers. Confined to the mucosal surface, in situ lesions most often appear as multiple, red, velvety, flat patches that often are near exophytic papillary transitional cell carcinomas (see below). Concurrent in situ cancers elsewhere in the bladder or ureters, urethra and prostatic ducts are common. Carcinoma in situ is often multifocal at the time of discovery, or similar lesions may develop shortly thereafter. Lesions involving the bladder neck or the urethra may extend into the periurethral prostatic ducts.

Urothelial Carcinomas Vary from Superficial and Papillary to Deeply Invasive

PATHOLOGY: Papillary cancers arise most frequently in the lateral or posterior bladder walls. Grossly, tumors may be small, delicate, low-grade papillary lesions limited to the mucosal surface or larger, high-grade, solid masses that are invasive and ulcerated (Fig. 23-14).

They are graded as papillary urothelial neoplasms of low malignant potential (PUNLMP) and papillary urothelial carcinomas, low grade and high grade. The latter may be invasive.

- **Papillary urothelial neoplasms of low malignant potential:** These papillary tumors resemble urothelial papillomas but show increased cellularity. They are considered intermediate between benign papillomas and low-grade papillary urothelial carcinomas. These lesions are usually larger than papillomas but lack architectural and cytologic atypia that are characteristic of low-grade carcinomas. PUNLMP may recur or occasionally progress to higher-grade tumors.
- **Low-grade papillary urothelial carcinoma:** Low-grade tumors have fronds lined by neoplastic urothelial epithelium with minimal architectural and cytologic atypia (Fig. 23-15A, B). The cells are moderately hyperchromatic with little nuclear pleomorphism and low mitotic activity.

Papillae are long and delicate. Fusion of papillae is focal and limited. Invasion of the lamina propria or the deep muscularis propria occurs in 10%.

- **High-grade papillary urothelial carcinoma:** These tumors show significant nuclear hyperchromasia and pleomorphism. The epithelium is disorganized (Fig. 23-15C, D) with mitoses in all layers. Approximately 80% of all high-grade tumors invade the lamina propria and, less often,

TABLE 23-2
TNM STAGING OF UROTHELIAL CARCINOMA OF URINARY BLADDER

T—Primary Tumor

T0 No grossly visible tumor

Ta Noninvasive papillary carcinoma

Tis Carcinoma in situ

T1 Invasion of the lamina propria

T2 Invasion of the muscularis propria
    T2a Superficial invasion of the muscularis (inner half)
    T2b Invasion of deep muscle (outer half)

T3 Invasion of the perivesical tissue

T4 Extravesical spread into adjacent organs or distant metastases

N—Regional Lymph Nodes

N0 No lymph node involvement

N1 Single lymph node metastasis

N2, N3 More lymph nodes involved

M—Distant Metastases

M0 No metastases

M1 Distant metastases

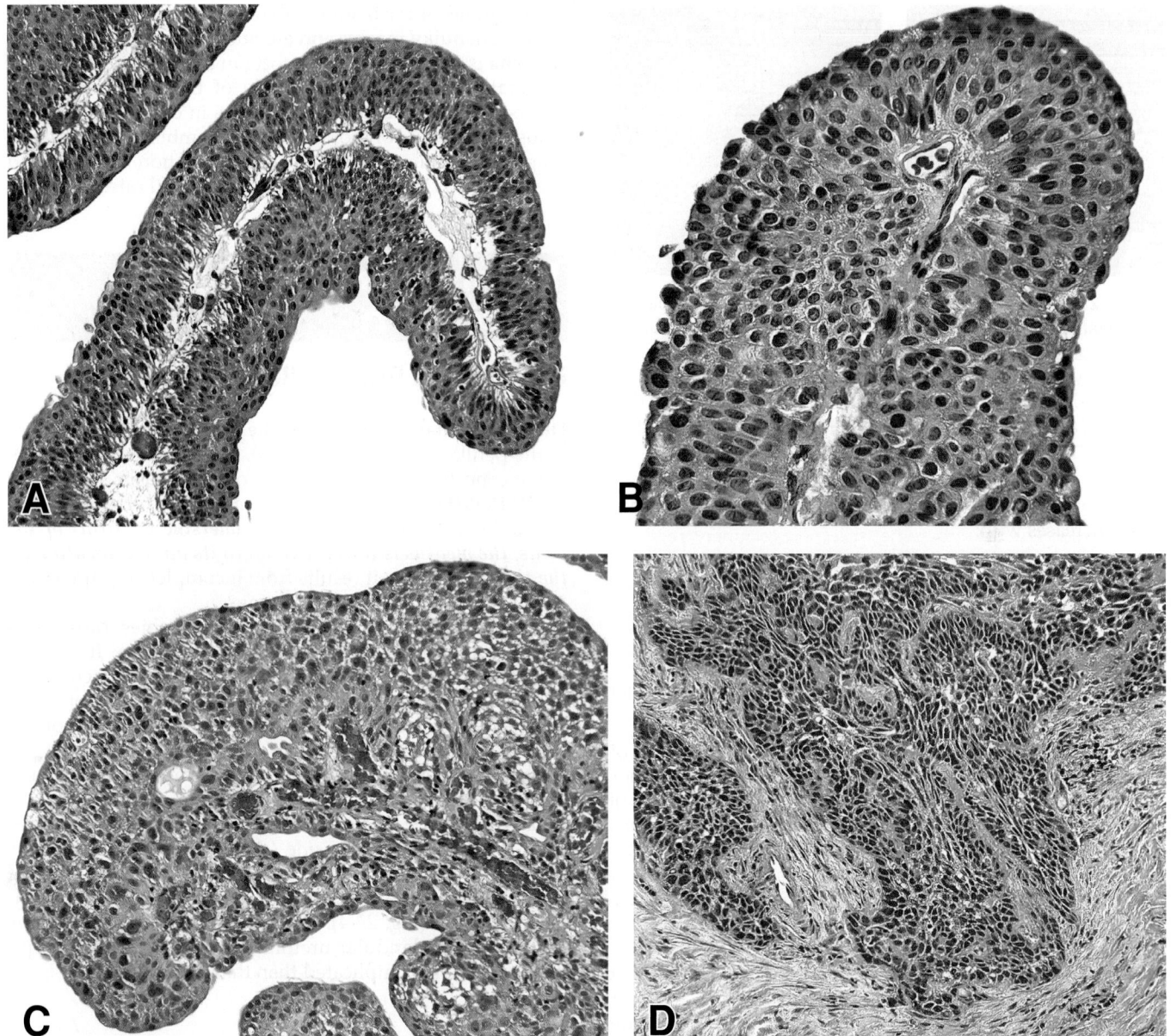

FIGURE 23-15. Urothelial tumors of the urinary bladder. A. Low-grade papillary urothelial carcinoma consists of exophytic papillae that have a central connective tissue core and are lined by slightly disorganized transitional epithelium. **B.** Low-grade papillary urothelial carcinoma at higher magnification shows mild architectural and cytologic atypia. **C.** High-grade papillary urothelial carcinoma displays prominent architectural disorganization of the epithelium, which contains cells with pleomorphic hyperchromatic nuclei. **D.** Invasive high-grade papillary urothelial carcinoma consists of irregular nests of hyperchromatic cells invading into the muscularis.

the muscularis propria or through the entire thickness of the bladder wall. Regional lymph nodes contain metastatic tumor in half of patients with these invasive tumors.

- **Invasive urothelial carcinoma:** These highly malignant tumors may evolve from papillary lesions or flat carcinomas in situ. In many cases the nature of the initial lesion is unknown. Most, if not all, invasive carcinomas are high-grade tumors. Depth of invasion into the bladder wall, or beyond, determines the prognosis.

Bladder cancers are staged according to the tumor–node–metastasis (TNM) system (Table 23-2). In order of decreasing frequency, metastases involve the regional and periaortic lymph nodes, liver, lung and bone.

CLINICAL FEATURES: Urothelial carcinoma of the bladder typically manifests as sudden **hematuria** and, less often, **dysuria**. Cystoscopy reveals one or more tumors. At the time of presentation, 85% of tumors are confined to the urinary bladder; 15% show regional or distant metastases. Papillary lesions limited to the mucosa or lamina propria (stage T1) are commonly treated conservatively by transurethral resection. Radical cystectomy is done for patients whose tumors show muscle invasion, and occasionally for advanced-stage tumors. In bladder cancer patients, the most common causes of death are uremia (from urinary outflow tract obstruction), extension into adjacent organs and effects of distant metastases.

THE LOWER URINARY TRACT

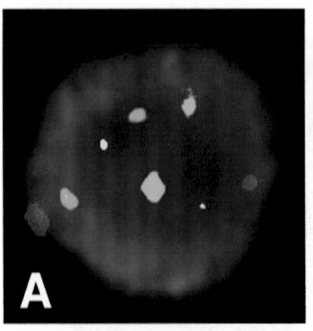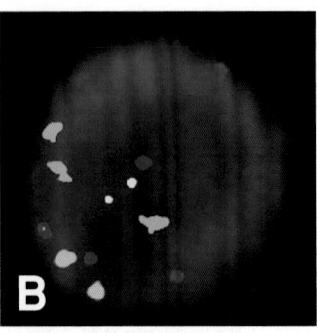

FIGURE 23-16. Fluorescence in situ hybridization of bladder cancer. A. Normal. Single urothelial cell collected from urine of normal person. Red fluorescence represents chromosome 3, green is chromosome 7, aqua is chromosome 17 and gold represents 9p21. The probe signals are present in two copies. **B.** Urothelial carcinoma of the bladder. There is aneuploidy of chromosomes 3 and chromosome 7. Chromosome 17 and 9p21 locus are euploid.

The probability of tumor extension and subsequent recurrence increases with:

- Increased tumor size
- High stage
- High grade
- Presence of multiple tumors
- Vascular or lymphatic invasion
- Urothelial dysplasia (including carcinoma in situ) at other sites in the bladder

The overall 10-year survival rate with noninvasive or superficially invasive low-grade urothelial tumors exceeds 95% irrespective of the number of recurrences. Only 10% of low-grade tumors progress to higher-grade tumors, and thus there is a worse prognosis. Conservative treatment includes fulguration, intravesicular immunotherapy with BCG or instillation of conventional chemotherapeutic agents. Invasive tumors or those refractory to conservative therapy are treated by cystectomy, possibly with adjuvant systemic chemotherapy. Tumors invading the bladder muscle bladder have 25%–30% overall mortality.

Recurrent or progressive disease is detected by cystoscopy and biopsy, or by less invasive techniques such as urinalysis for tumor markers, urine cytology and cytogenic analysis of desquamated cells. The latter analyzes cells from the patient's urine for ploidy values of specific chromosomal regions (see above) by fluorescence in situ hybridization (FISH) (Fig. 23-16; see Chapter 6). Currently, aneuploidy for chromosomes 3, 7 and 17 and loss of 9p21 are detected.

Nonurothelial Bladder Cancers Are Rare

Squamous cell bladder carcinomas develop in foci of squamous metaplasia, usually due to schistosomiasis. Bladder wall invasion is common by initial presentation and prognosis is poor.

Adenocarcinomas are 1% of malignant bladder tumors. They derive from urachal epithelial remnants, foci of cystitis glandularis or intestinal metaplasia. Most bladder adenocarcinomas are deeply invasive when they initially present and are not curable.

Neuroendocrine carcinoma, resembling small cell lung carcinoma, occurs uncommonly in the urinary bladder. It is highly malignant and has a poor prognosis.

Sarcomas of the bladder are rare. They are highly malignant, form bulky masses and are often inoperable. **Leiomyosarcoma** is the most common form in adults.

Rhabdomyosarcoma, typically of the embryonal type, occurs mostly as **sarcoma botryoides** in children, as edematous, mucosal, polypoid masses resembling a cluster of grapes. Combined treatment with radiation therapy and chemotherapy has greatly increased survival rates.

Penis, Urethra and Scrotum

CONGENITAL DISORDERS OF THE PENIS

Developmental anomalies of the penis include anomalies of the penile urethra and prepuce, as well as rare and infrequent conditions such as agenesis or hypoplasia.

HYPOSPADIAS: This term is a congenital anomaly in which the urethra opens on the underside (ventral) of the penis; the meatus is thus proximal to its normal location on the tip of the penis. It results from incomplete closure of the urethral folds of the urogenital sinus.

Hypospadias occurs in 1 in 350 male babies. Most cases are sporadic but familial occurrence is known. It may be associated with other urogenital anomalies and complex, multisystemic, developmental syndromes. In 90% of cases, the meatus is located on the underside of the glans, or the corona (Fig. 23-17). Less often, it occurs midshaft, in the scrotum or even in the perineum. Surgical repair is usually uncomplicated.

EPISPADIAS: In this rare congenital anomaly, the urethra opens on the upper side (dorsum) of the penis. In its most common form, all the penile urethra is open along the whole shaft. Severe epispadias may be associated with bladder exstrophy (Fig. 23-4). In its mildest form, the defect is limited to the glandular urethra. Surgical treatment of epispadias is more complicated than that of hypospadias.

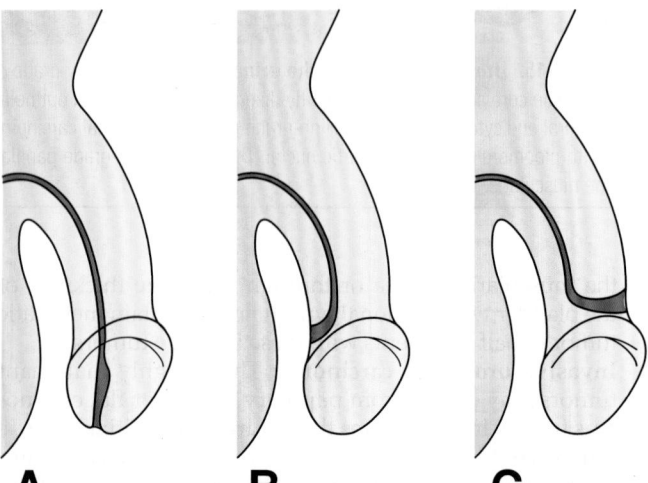

A. Normal **B.** Hypospadia **C.** Epispadia

FIGURE 23-17. Congenital anomalies of the penis. A. Normal penis has the urethral opening on the tip of the glans. **B.** Hypospadias is characterized by a urethral opening on the ventral side of the penis. **C.** Epispadias is characterized by a urethral opening on the dorsal side of the penis.

PHIMOSIS: *The orifice of the prepuce may be too narrow to allow retraction over the glans penis.* Phimosis may be congenital or acquired. The latter is usually a consequence of recurrent infections or trauma of the prepuce in uncircumcised men. Phimosis predisposes to penile infections. A narrow prepuce, if forcefully retracted, may strangulate the glans and impede the outflow of venous blood, a condition called **paraphimosis.** Circumcision is curative.

SCROTAL MASSES

Scrotal masses and conditions that lead to scrotal swelling or enlargement often reflect abnormalities of testicular, epididymal and scrotal development. Clinical problems related to these conditions are most often seen in children but may be found in adults (Fig. 23-18A–D).

HYDROCELE: This is a collection of serous fluid in the mesothelially lined scrotal sac between the two layers of the tunica vaginalis. Hydroceles may be congenital or acquired.

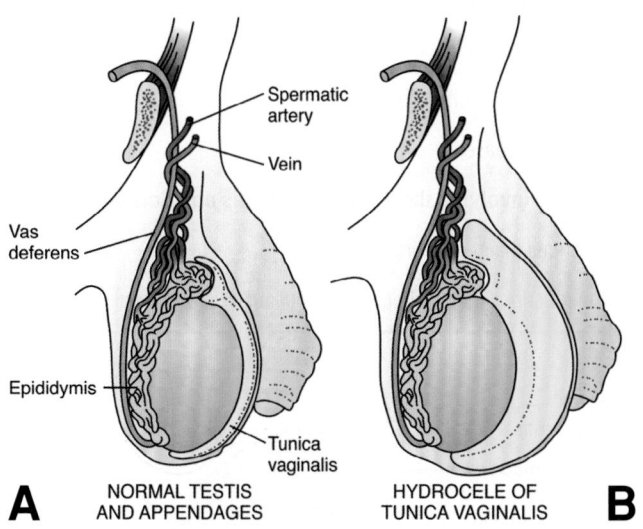

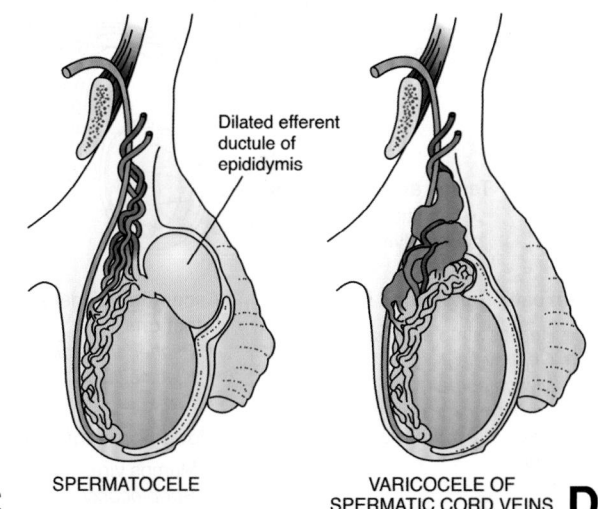

FIGURE 23-18. Scrotal masses. A. Normal testis. **B.** Hydrocele. **C.** Spermatocele. **D.** Varicocele.

Congenital hydrocele reflects patency or incomplete obliteration of the processus vaginalis testis. It is the most common cause of scrotal swelling in infants and is often associated with inguinal hernia.

Acquired hydrocele in adults is due to some other disease affecting the scrotum, such as infection, tumor or trauma. The diagnosis is made by ultrasound or by transluminating the fluid in the cavity. Hydrocele is a benign condition that disappears once the cause has been addressed. However, long-standing hydrocele may cause testicular atrophy or compress the epididymis, or the fluid may become infected and lead to **periorchitis.**

HEMATOCELE: *Blood may accumulate between the layers of tunica vaginalis after trauma or hemorrhage into a hydrocele,* or as a result of testicular tumors and infections.

SPERMATOCELE: *This mass is a cyst formed from protrusions of widened efferent ducts of the rete testis or epididymis.* It manifests as a hilar paratesticular nodule or a fluctuating mass filled with milky fluid. The cyst is lined by cuboidal epithelium that contains spermatozoa in various stages of degeneration.

VARICOCELE: *This dilation of testicular veins appears as a nodularity on the lateral side of the scrotum.* Most are asymptomatic and are discovered during physical examination of infertile men. Massive varicocele is described as resembling a "bag of worms." Varicoceles are considered a common cause of infertility and oligospermia, although it is unclear why dilation of veins should have such effects. Testicular atrophy occurs only rarely and only in long-standing cases. Surgical ligation of the internal spermatic vein often improves reproductive function.

SCROTAL INGUINAL HERNIA: *Intestinal protrusion into the scrotum through the inguinal canal is a scrotal hernia.* The bowel may be repositioned, but if it remains untreated, such a hernia may cause adhesions or testicular atrophy. Hernias can only be repaired surgically.

CIRCULATORY DISTURBANCES

SCROTAL EDEMA: *Lymph or serous fluid may accumulate in the scrotum from obstruction to lymphatic or venous drainage.* Lymphedema from lymphatic obstruction can be caused by pelvic or abdominal tumors, surgical scars or infections such as filariasis. **Transudation** of plasma is common in patients with heart failure, anasarca due to cirrhosis or nephrotic syndrome. Fluid accumulates in the loose connective tissue and the cavity lined by the tunica vaginalis testis.

ERECTILE DYSFUNCTION: This condition, also known as impotence, is *inability to achieve or maintain an erection sufficient for satisfactory sexual performance.* Its prevalence increases with age, from 20% at age 40 years to 50% by age 70.

Erection requires adequate filling of the penile corpora cavernosa and spongiosa with blood. Penile tumescence is the result of a complex interaction of mental, neural, hormonal and vascular factors. Filling of these vascular spaces depends on nitric oxide (NO•)-mediated relaxation of vascular smooth muscle cells in the erectile cylinders. NO• release is related to cyclic guanosine monophosphate (cGMP), so drugs that inhibit the phosphodiesterase that degrades cGMP (e.g., sildenafil [Viagra], vardenafil hydrochloride [Levitra], tadalafil [Cialis]) are used to treat erectile dysfunction. Disorders associated with erectile dysfunction are listed in Table 23-3.

TABLE 23-3
ERECTILE DYSFUNCTIONS

Neuropsychiatric

Psychiatric disorders (e.g., depression)

Spinal cord injury

Nerve injury during surgery (e.g., pelvic or perineal surgery)

Endocrine

Hypogonadism

Pituitary diseases (e.g., hyperprolactinemia)

Hypothyroidism, Cushing syndrome, Addison disease

Vascular

Diabetic microangiopathy

Hypertension

Atherosclerosis

Drugs

Antihypertensives

Psychotropic drugs

Estrogens, anticancer drugs, etc.

Idiopathic

"Performance anxiety"

Age-related "impotence"

TABLE 23-4
INFLAMMATORY LESIONS OF THE PENIS

Sexually Transmitted Diseases

Herpes genitalis

Syphilis

Chancroid

Granuloma inguinale

Lymphogranuloma venereum

Human papillomavirus infections

Nonspecific Infectious Balanoposthitis

Bacterial, fungal, viral

Diseases of Unknown Etiology

Balanitis xerotica obliterans

Circinate balanitis

Plasma cell balanitis (Zoon balanitis)

Peyronie disease

Dermatitis Involving the Shaft of the Penis and Scrotum

Infectious (bacterial, viral, fungal)

Noninfectious (e.g., lichen planus, bullous skin diseases)

PRIAPISM: Priapism is *continuous penile erection unrelated to sexual excitation.* It may be primary or secondary. Primary priapism is idiopathic and painful. Treatment is usually ineffective. Secondary priapism may occur in (1) pelvic diseases that impede outflow of blood from the penis (e.g., pelvic tumors or hematomas, thrombosis of pelvic veins, infections); (2) hematologic disorders (e.g., sickle cell anemia, polycythemia vera, leukemia); and (3) brain and spinal cord diseases (e.g., tumors, syphilis).

INFLAMMATORY DISORDERS

The most important inflammatory diseases of the penis are (1) sexually transmitted diseases (STDs); (2) nonspecific infections; (3) diseases of unknown etiology, such as balanitis xerotica obliterans; (4) dermatoses; and (5) dermatitis of the penile shaft and scrotum (Table 23-4).

Sexually Transmitted Diseases Cause Discrete Penile Lesions

STDs (see Chapter 9) as lower urinary tract infections (Fig. 23-19) include the following:

■ **Genital herpes** is most often caused by herpes simplex virus (HSV)-2 or, less commonly, by HSV-1. It is the most

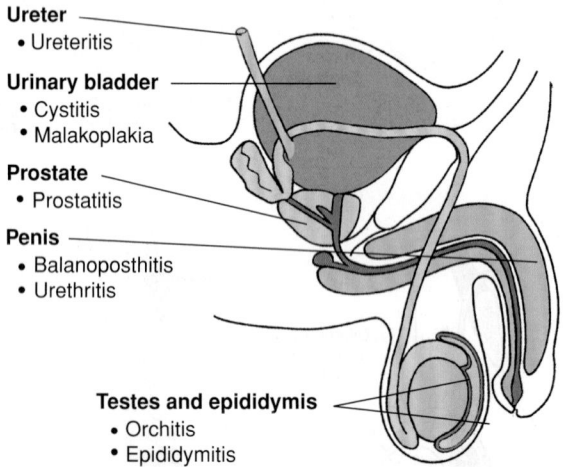

Ureter
• Ureteritis

Urinary bladder
• Cystitis
• Malakoplakia

Prostate
• Prostatitis

Penis
• Balanoposthitis
• Urethritis

Testes and epididymis
• Orchitis
• Epididymitis

Sexually transmitted infections
• Herpes simplex virus
• *Chlamydia*
• *Mycoplasma*
• *Treponema pallidum*
• *Neisseria gonorrhoeae*
• HIV

Ascending urinary tract infections
• *Escherichia coli*
• *Klebsiella*
• *Proteus*

Blood-borne infections
• Mumps virus
• *Streptococcus*
• *Staphylococcus*

FIGURE 23-19. Infections of the lower urinary tract and male reproductive system.

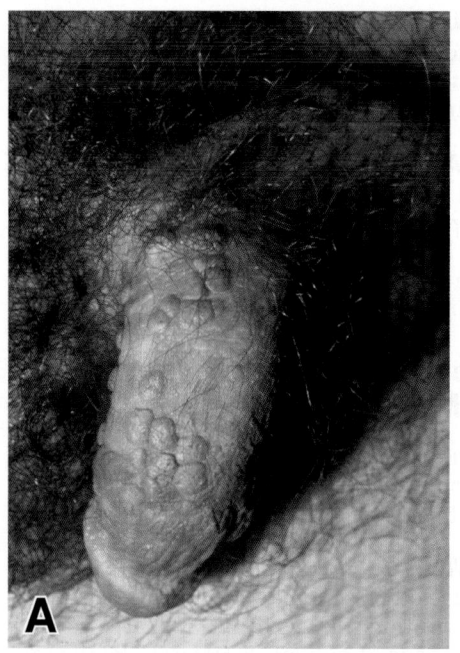
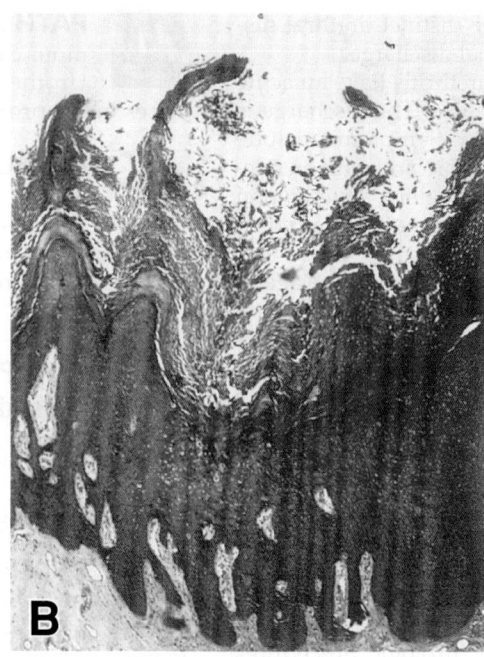

FIGURE 23-20. Condylomata acuminata of the penis. A. Raised, circumscribed lesions are seen on the shaft of the penis. **B.** Section of a lesion shows epidermal hyperkeratosis, parakeratosis, acanthosis and papillomatosis.

common STD affecting the glans and manifests typically as grouped vesicles that ulcerate and transform into crusts.

- **Primary syphilis,** caused by a spirochete, *Treponema pallidum,* may manifest as a solitary, soft ulcer **(chancre)** accompanied by palpable inguinal lymphadenopathy.
- **Chancroid** is caused by *Haemophilus ducreyi* and presents as a papule that transforms into a pustule and finally ulcerates. Shallow ulcers on the glans or the skin of the shaft are often associated with painful suppurative inguinal lymphadenitis.
- **Granuloma inguinale** is a tropical disease caused by *Calymmatobacterium granulomatis.* It appears as a raised ulcer with a copious chronic inflammatory exudate and granulation tissue. Such ulcers tend to enlarge and heal very slowly.
- **Lymphogranuloma venereum** is caused by *Chlamydia trachomatis.* It starts as a small, often innocuous, vesicle that ulcerates, typically accompanied by tender enlargement of inguinal lymph nodes that adhere to the skin and form sinuses draining pus and serosanguineous fluid.
- **Condyloma acuminatum** is caused by human papillomavirus type 6 or, less often, 11. It appears as flat-topped warts on the shaft (Fig. 23-20), small polyps on the glans and urethral meatus or larger cauliflower-like tumors that may be confused with verrucous carcinoma.

Balanitis Is Inflammation of the Glans Penis

In uncircumcised men, balanitis usually extends from the glans to the foreskin and is called **balanoposthitis.** Mostly it is caused by bacteria, but it may also be caused by fungi in diabetics or immunosuppressed people. Balanitis typically reflects poor hygiene. Significant complications of chronic balanoposthitis are meatal stricture, phimosis and paraphimosis.

BALANITIS XEROTICA OBLITERANS: This idiopathic chronic inflammatory condition is equivalent to lichen sclerosus of the vulva (see Chapter 24) and is characterized by fibrosis and sclerosis of subepithelial connective tissue. The affected portion of the glans is white and indurated. Fibrosis may constrict the urethral meatus or cause phimosis.

CIRCINATE BALANITIS: During oculo-urethro-synovial syndrome (OUS) (see below), the glans may show circular, linear or confluent plaque-like discolorations, occasionally associated with superficial ulcers.

PLASMA CELL BALANITIS: This chronic, innocuous disease of unknown origin (also called Zoon balanitis) causes macular discoloration or painless papules on the glans. Plasma cell and lymphocytic infiltrates are seen beneath a thickened overlying epithelium.

DERMATOSES: Many inflammatory skin diseases may involve the penis. Such conditions are discussed in Chapter 28.

Peyronie Disease Is an Idiopathic Fibrous Induration of the Penis

It is characterized by focal, asymmetric fibrosis of the penile shaft. During erections, the penis becomes curved and painful. Typically, it presents as an ill-defined induration of the penile shaft in a young or middle-aged man, with no change in the overlying skin. Microscopically, dense fibrosis is associated with sparse, nonspecific, chronic inflammatory infiltration. Collagen focally replaces muscle in the septum of the corpus cavernosum.

Peyronie disease affects 1% of men over age 40. In most instances, it is mild and does not interfere with sexual function. Severe cases may be so incapacitating as to require surgery, but the outcome is not always satisfactory.

URETHRITIS AND RELATED CONDITIONS

Urethritis is acute or chronic inflammation of the urethra.

SEXUALLY TRANSMITTED URETHRITIS: Urethritis presenting as urethral discharge is the most common sign of STDs in men. Women rarely notice distinct urethral discharge and usually complain of vaginal discharge.

Gonococcal and nongonococcal urethritis have an acute onset, related to recent sexual intercourse. The discharge is typically purulent and greenish yellow. Symptoms include pain or tingling at the meatus of the urethra and pain on micturition **(dysuria)**. Meatal redness and swelling are common in both sexes. Acute gonococcal and nongonococcal urethritis can both become chronic.

The diagnosis is made by identifying the causative agent. In gonococcal urethritis, the discharge contains *Neisseria gonorrhoeae,* which can be identified microscopically in smears of urethral exudates. Nongonococcal urethritis is mostly caused by *C. trachomatis* or *Ureaplasma urealyticum* but may be related to a variety of other pathogens.

NONSPECIFIC INFECTIOUS URETHRITIS: Uropathogens such as **E. coli** *and* **P. aeruginosa** *can cause urethritis.* Typically infection is associated with cystitis but may be caused by other diseases (e.g., prostatic hyperplasia or urinary stones). In men, infectious urethritis may be the only sign of prostatitis; in women, it may be a complication of vaginitis and vulvitis. In hospitalized patients, it commonly follows cystoscopy and other urologic procedures and is almost inevitable in patients with indwelling urethral catheters.

Nonspecific infectious urethritis manifests clinically with urgency and a burning sensation during urination. Usually there is no discharge, but men may express some milky fluid by "stripping" or "milking" the urethra.

URETHRAL CARUNCLES: Polypoid inflammatory lesions near the female urethral meatus cause pain and bleeding. They are idiopathic and occur only in women, mostly after menopause. Urethral mucosal prolapse and attendant chronic inflammation may be implicated.

Urethral caruncles present as 1- to 2-cm exophytic, often ulcerated, polypoid masses, at or near the urethral meatus. They show acutely and chronically inflamed granulation tissue and ulceration and hyperplasia of transitional cell or squamous epithelium. Complex patterns of papillomatosis and occasional dysplastic epithelium may suggest a superficial resemblance to carcinoma, but this inflammatory lesion does not lead to cancer. Treatment is surgical excision.

REACTIVE ARTHRITIS (PREVIOUSLY REITER SYNDROME): Reactive arthritis is a triad of urethritis, conjunctivitis and arthritis of weight-bearing joints (e.g., knee, intervertebral joints). Other findings may include circinate balanitis, cervicitis and skin eruptions. It tends to affect young adults with the human leukocyte antigen (HLA)-B27 haplotype, usually a few weeks after chlamydial urethritis or enteric infection with (e.g.) *Shigella, Salmonella or Campylobacter.* The disease may thus be an aberrant immune reaction to unknown microbial antigen(s). Symptoms usually disappear spontaneously in 3–6 months, but arthritis recurs in half of patients.

TUMORS

Urethral Cancers May Arise from Squamous or Transitional Epithelia

These uncommon tumors usually occur in elderly women. Some penile cancers arise in the terminal part of the penile urethra.

 PATHOLOGY: Most urethral cancers are squamous carcinomas originating in the distal urethra. Urothelial carcinoma, like that in the bladder, arises in the proximal urethra.

 CLINICAL FEATURES: Urethral cancer develops most often in the sixth and seventh decades. Patients present with urethral bleeding and dysuria. Most tumors have spread to adjacent tissues or lymph nodes at the time of presentation. Radical surgery is the main therapy.

Cancer of the Penis Occurs Mostly in Uncircumcised Men

Cancer of the penis originates from the squamous mucosa of the glans and contiguous urethral meatus or the prepuce and skin covering the penile shaft.

 **EPIDEMIOLOGY:** In the United States, invasive squamous cell carcinoma of the penis is uncommon, accounting for less than 0.5% of all cancers in men. The average age of patients is 60 years. Penile cancer is much more common in less developed countries: in some parts of Africa and Asia and South America, it constitutes 10% of cancers in men. It is virtually unknown in men circumcised at birth.

ETIOLOGIC FACTORS: No single agent has been identified as the cause of penile cancer. Current interest centers on the possible influence of smegma, the whitish material composed of accumulated keratin debris and secretion of the preputial (Tyson) glands that accumulates beneath the prepuce. Human papillomavirus (HPV) DNA has been found in 50% of all invasive carcinomas of the penis, suggesting that HPV types 16 and 18 play a role in some penile cancers. Cigarette smoking is also associated with a higher risk of penile cancer.

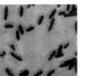 **PATHOLOGY:** Penile carcinoma may be preinvasive (in situ) or invasive.

SQUAMOUS CELL CARCINOMA IN SITU: Carcinoma in situ of the penis is similar to that in other sites (see Chapter 28). Grossly, it may present as Bowen disease or erythroplasia of Queyrat. **Bowen disease** is a sharply demarcated, erythematous or grayish white plaque on the shaft. **Erythroplasia of Queyrat** appears as solitary or multiple, shiny, soft, erythematous plaques on the glans and foreskin. Both of these resemble **squamous cell carcinoma in situ** elsewhere. They show cytologic atypia among keratinocytes of all layers of the epidermis, parakeratosis or hyperkeratosis; papillomatosis with broad epidermal papillae; and thinning of the granular layer. By definition, there is no invasion of the underlying dermis. Progression to invasive squamous cell carcinoma is estimated to occur in less than 10% of cases.

Bowenoid papulosis of the penis is caused by HPV and affects young, sexually active men. In contrast to the solitary lesion of Bowen disease, Bowenoid papulosis appears as multiple brownish or violaceous papules. Microscopically, it resembles other squamous carcinomas in situ, but there may be some differences. Most carcinoma in situ slowly merges at the margins with normal epithelium, but Bowenoid papulosis is sharply demarcated from normal epidermis, like HPV-induced warts. The altered epidermis

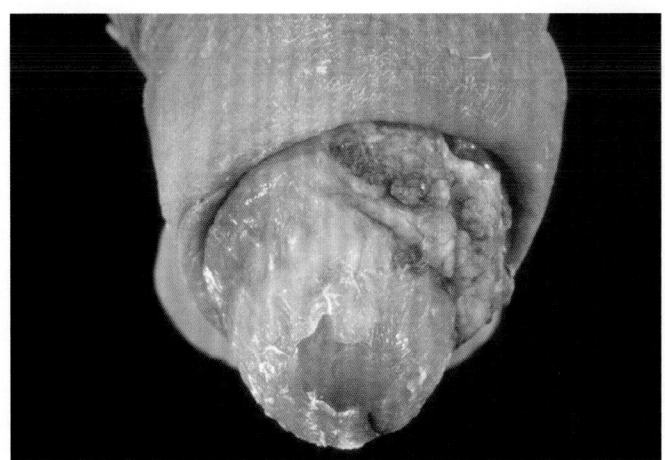

FIGURE 23-21. Carcinoma of the penis. This verrucous carcinoma arises on the glans and appears as an exophytic mass.

shows some superficial stratification and maturation and may contain giant keratinocytes with multinucleated atypical nuclei. HPV type 16 can be demonstrated in 80% of patients, and type 18 is occasionally implicated. Virtually all these lesions regress spontaneously and do not progress to invasive carcinoma.

INVASIVE SQUAMOUS CELL CARCINOMA: The tumor presents as (1) an ulcer; (2) an indurated crater; (3) a friable hemorrhagic mass; or (4) an exophytic, fungating, papillary tumor. It usually involves the glans or prepuce and less commonly the penile shaft. Extensive destruction of penile tissue, including the urethral meatus, is seen when the tumor has been neglected. Microscopically, these are typically well-differentiated, focally keratinizing, squamous cell carcinomas. Invasive tumors usually have underlying dense, chronic inflammation. The adjacent epidermis often shows dysplastic changes. The tumor may invade deeply along the shaft and spread to inguinal lymph nodes, then to iliac nodes and ultimately to distant organs.

VERRUCOUS CARCINOMA: This tumor is separated from other penile cancers because it is a cytologically benign but clinically malignant exophytic squamous cell carcinoma (Fig. 23-21). Grossly and cytologically, it resembles **condyloma acuminatum,** but it shows local invasion, unlike the latter. Verrucous carcinoma rarely metastasizes. Surgery is curative.

 CLINICAL FEATURES: Most squamous cell cancers are confined to the penis at the time of presentation. Occult metastases to inguinal lymph nodes are not uncommon, but half of patients with enlarged regional lymph nodes do not have nodal metastases, only reactive changes due to tumor-associated inflammation.

Survival of patients with penile cancer is related to the clinical stage and, to a lesser degree, histologic grade of the tumor. Amputation of the penis is usually necessary. Patients with superficially invasive cancer have 90% 5-year survival; inguinal lymph node metastases reduce 5-year survival to 20%–50%, depending on the extent of spread. HPV infection is seen in at least half of cases.

Cancer of the Scrotum Is Quite Uncommon

In 1775, Sir Percival Pott introduced the idea of chemical carcinogenesis by reporting scrotal cancer as an occupational disease of chimney sweeps (see Chapter 8). Many industrial chemicals were found to be causative. Improved industrial hygiene has made this a rare tumor.

Squamous carcinoma of the scrotum typically affects men mostly in their 50s and 60s. At presentation, many show invasion of the scrotal contents and metastases to regional nodes. Therapy is surgical excision. As in penile cancer, HPV has been often implicated.

Testis, Epididymis and Vas Deferens

CRYPTORCHIDISM

Cryptorchidism, clinically known as undesended testis, *is a congenital abnormality in which one or both testes are not in the scrotum.* It is the most common urologic condition requiring surgical treatment in infants. The testes are not in the scrotum or are easily retracted in 5% of term male infants and 30% of those born prematurely. In the large majority of these, testes descend into the scrotum in the first year of life. Thus, the prevalence of cryptorchidism from the end of the first year of life into adulthood is about 1%. It is bilateral in 30% of affected men.

 **ETIOLOGIC FACTORS:** Testicular maldescent is usually an idiopathic isolated developmental disorder. It may rarely be associated with other congenital anomalies.

 PATHOLOGY: Testicular descent may be arrested at any point from the abdominal cavity to the upper scrotum (Fig. 23-22). Cryptorchid testes are classified by their location as **abdominal, inguinal or upper scrotal**. Rarely, the testes are located in unusual locations, such as the perineum or calf.

Cryptorchid testes are smaller than normal even at an early age, and differences between the affected and unaffected testes increase with age. The testes are firm and show fibrosis.

The histology of cryptorchid testes varies with age. In infancy and early childhood, the seminiferous tubules in

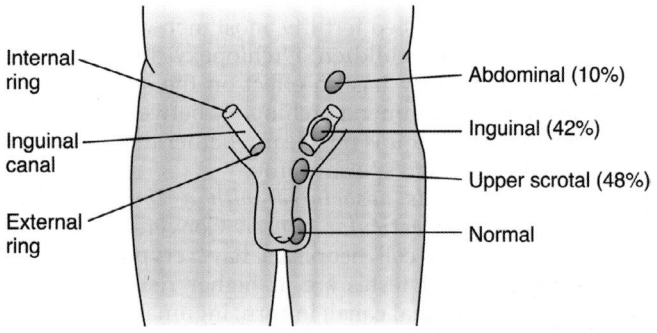

FIGURE 23-22. Cryptorchidism. In most instances, the testis has an upper scrotal location. It may also be retained in the inguinal canal and rarely in the abdominal cavity.

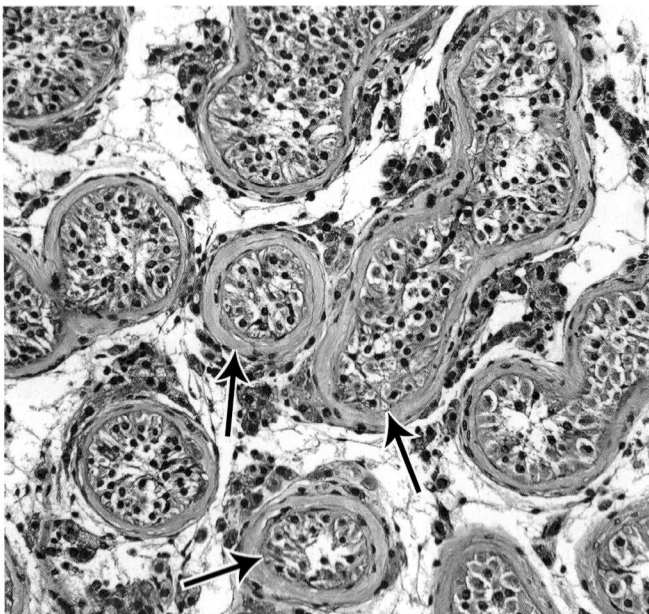

FIGURE 23-23. Cryptorchidism. This testis removed from a postpubertal man shows a markedly thickened hyalinized basement membrane (*arrows*) of seminiferous tubules, which show no signs of spermatogenesis.

affected testes are smaller, with fewer than normal germ cells. Postpubertal testes also show decreased germ cells, and spermatogenesis is limited to a minority of tubules. Hyaline thickening of tubular basement membranes and prominent stromal fibrosis are observed (Fig. 23-23). Eventually, tubules lose all spermatogenic cells and are entirely hyalinized. **Orchiopexy** (surgical placement of a testis into the scrotum) done either in childhood or after puberty does not prevent loss of seminiferous epithelium and tubules; both untreated and repositioned testes lack all spermatogenesis in half of the cases. A few adult cryptorchid testes (2%) contain atypical germ cells corresponding to carcinoma in situ.

CLINICAL FEATURES: The clinical significance of undescended testes is that they entail increased incidences of **infertility** and **germ cell neoplasia**. All men with bilateral cryptorchid testes have **azoospermia** and are infertile. Unilateral cryptorchidism is associated with **oligospermia,** defined as a sperm count below 20 million/mL, in 40% of cases. Although oligospermia is a cause of reduced fertility, most men with one normal testis can father children. Orchiopexy done in childhood or after puberty has no effect on the sperm count. Most urologists recommend orchiopexy between 6 months and 1 year of age, but it is not clear whether this treatment improves the eventual sperm count.

Cryptorchidism is associated with a 20- to 40-fold increased risk for testicular cancer. Conversely, 10% of patients with germ cell neoplasia have cryptorchid testes. Intra-abdominal testes are at higher risk than those retained in the inguinal canal; in turn, inguinal testes are at higher risk than those high in the scrotum. A contralateral, normally descended testis is also at risk, about 4 times that in normal men. Unfortunately, orchiopexy does not reduce cancer risk.

ABNORMALITIES OF SEXUAL DIFFERENTIATION

Disorders of gonadogenesis and formation of external genital organs, as well as development of secondary sex characteristics, can pertain to:

■ Genetic sex; the presence or absence of X and Y chromosomes
■ Gonadal sex; the presence or absence of testes or ovaries
■ Genital sex; the appearance of external genital organs
■ Psychosocial sexual orientation

Various conditions are listed in Table 23-5. Some of these, such as Klinefelter and Turner syndromes, are discussed in Chapter 6.

HERMAPHRODITISM: This rare developmental disorder is characterized by ambiguous genitalia in someone who has both male and female gonads. Gonads may become ovotestes (combination of ovary and testis) or one gonad may be testis and the other ovary. Half of these patients have a female karyotype (46,XX). The others are genetic males (46,XY) or mosaics or have a missing sex chromosome (45,X).

FEMALE PSEUDOHERMAPHRODITISM: Virilization of external genitalia may occur in genetic females (46,XX) who have normal ovaries and internal female genital organs. The vulva may fuse into scrotal folds and clitoromegaly is common. This phenotype is most often seen in the adrenogenital syndrome caused by 21-hydroxylase deficiency (see Chapter 27). Lack of this enzyme leads to excess androgen production in the adrenal gland during fetal life, and the ambiguous genitalia are seen at birth. Excess androgens in a pregnant woman can have the same effects on the external genitalia of the female baby in utero.

TABLE 23-5
DISORDERS OF SEXUAL DIFFERENTIATION
Sex Chromosomal Abnormalities
Klinefelter syndrome and its variants
Turner syndrome 46,XX males
Single-Gene Defects
Adrenogenital syndromes
Androgen insensitivity syndromes
Müllerian inhibitory substance deficiency
Prenatal Hormonal Effects
Exogenous hormones during pregnancy
Maternal hormone-producing tumors
Idiopathic Conditions
Hermaphroditism
Gonadal dysgenesis

A 46,XX karyotype is found in 1 of 25 patients with classical signs of Klinefelter syndrome. These 46,XX males carry the locus for the sex-determining region of chromosome Y (SRY) on one of their X chromosomes. It is not known how this translocation occurs.

MALE PSEUDOHERMAPHRODITISM: A spectrum of congenital disorders affects genetic males who have a normal 46,XY karyotype. The gonads are cryptorchid testes, but external genitalia appear feminine or ambiguously female with some virilization. Male pseudohermaphroditism occurs most often in **androgen insensitivity syndromes** due to deficiency of the androgen receptor, also known as **testicular feminization syndrome.**

MALE INFERTILITY

Infertility is empirically defined as inability to conceive after 1 year of coital activity with the same sexual partner without contraception. Some 15% of couples are childless in the United States, but the true prevalence of infertility is difficult to assess because it is confounded by cultural and social issues. The male is infertile in 20% of couples, the female in 40%, and both partners in 20%. In the remaining 20% of infertile couples, no cause can be identified. The

TABLE 23-6
CAUSES OF MALE INFERTILITY
Supratesticular Causes
Disorders of the hypothalamic–pituitary–gonadal axis
Endocrine disease of the adrenal, thyroid; diabetes
Metabolic disorders
Major organ diseases (e.g., renal, hepatic, cardiopulmonary diseases)
Chronic infectious and debilitating diseases (e.g., tuberculosis, AIDS)
Drugs and substance abuse
Testicular Causes
Idiopathic: hypospermatogenesis or azoospermia
Developmental (cryptorchidism, gonadal dysgenesis)
Genetic disorders (e.g., Klinefelter syndrome)
Orchitis (immune and infectious)
Iatrogenic testicular injury (radiation, cytotoxic drugs)
Trauma of the testis and surgical injury
Environmental (? phytoestrogens)
Posttesticular Causes
Congenital anomalies of the excretory ducts
Inflammation and scarring of excretory ducts
Iatrogenic or posttraumatic lesions of excretory ducts

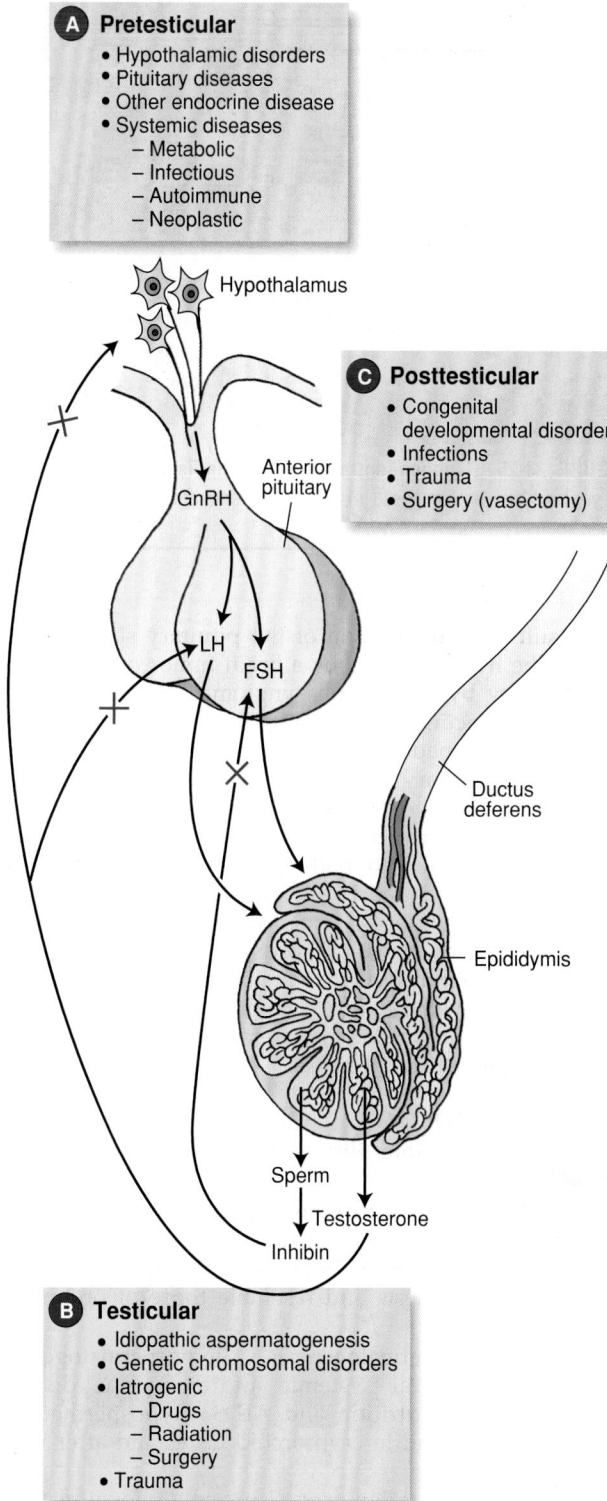

FIGURE 23-24. Causes of male infertility. A. Pretesticular infertility. *FSH* = follicle-stimulating hormone; *LH* = luteinizing hormone; *GnRH* = gonadotropin-releasing hormone. **B.** Testicular infertility. **C.** Posttesticular (obstructive) infertility.

causes of male infertility are listed in Table 23-6 and illustrated in Fig. 23-24.

Supratesticular causes of infertility affect hormonal and metabolic aspects of spermatogenesis. The best examples are injuries of the hypothalamic–pituitary area. Infertility

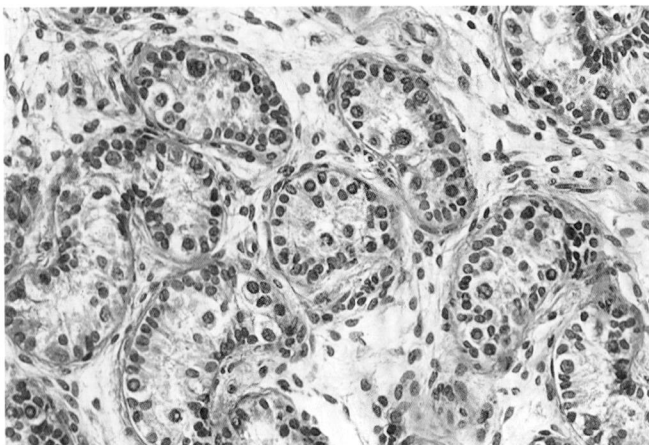

FIGURE 23-25. Hypogonadotropic hypogonadism. The testis of this 25-year-old man is composed of immature seminiferous tubules similar to those seen in prepubertal boys.

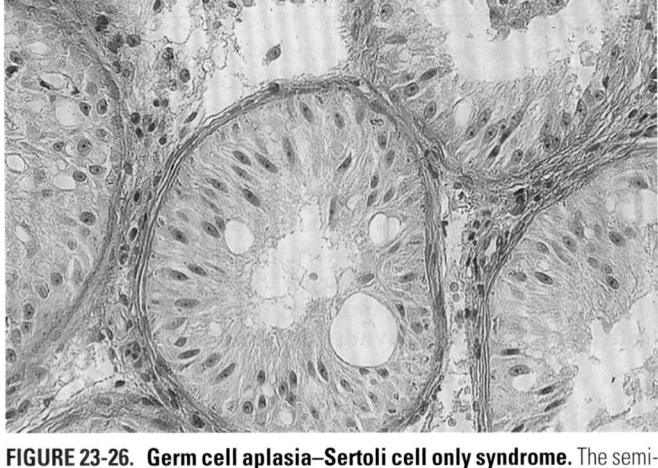

FIGURE 23-26. Germ cell aplasia–Sertoli cell only syndrome. The seminiferous tubules are lined by Sertoli cells and do not contain germ cells.

can result from transection of the pituitary stalk, destruction of the hypothalamus by a brain tumor or pressure on the pituitary by a craniopharyngioma. A pituitary tumor secreting prolactin (prolactinoma) may act as a mass lesion that destroys gonadotropin-secreting pituitary cells or compresses the pituitary stalk. It also secretes prolactin, which suppresses spermatogenesis.

Testicular infertility, the most common variety of male infertility, is related to pathologic changes in the testis. A male infertility (andrologic) workup includes urologic examination, sonography, semen analysis, hormonal studies and in some cases testicular biopsy.

Posttesticular infertility entails blockage of excretory ducts through which sperm reach the urethra. Chronic infections of the epididymis or vas deferens, previous trauma and congenital atresia are the causes.

 PATHOLOGY: Testicular biopsy may identify causes of infertility, such as the following:

- **Immaturity of seminiferous tubules** is seen in hypogonadotropic hypogonadism caused by pituitary or hypothalamic diseases (Fig. 23-25). Seminiferous tubules show no spermatogenesis and resemble those of prepubertal testes.
- **Decreased spermatogenesis (hypospermatogenesis)** occurs in several systemic and endocrine diseases, including malnutrition and AIDS. Hypospermatogenesis is also found in cryptorchid testes and after vasectomy.
- **Germ cell maturation arrest** is usually idiopathic. It can occur at any stage of maturation.
- **Germ cell aplasia** ("Sertoli cells only" syndrome) is mostly idiopathic (Fig. 23-26). An underlying genetic mutation has been identified in some patients. It can be seen in drug-induced and toxic injury of the seminiferous epithelium.
- **Orchitis** is caused by viruses (e.g., mumps) or autoimmune diseases.
- **Peritubular and tubular fibrosis** may be related to congenital disorders such as cryptorchidism or to previous infection, ischemia or radiation (Fig. 23-27).

EPIDIDYMITIS

Epididymitis is acute or chronic inflammation of the epididymis, usually caused by bacteria.

Bacterial epididymitis in young men most often occurs in an acute form as a complication of gonorrhea or a sexually acquired *Chlamydia* infection. It is characterized by suppurative inflammation (Fig. 23-28). In older men, *E. coli* from associated urinary tract infections is a more common culprit. Patients present with intrascrotal pain and tenderness, with or without associated fever. Epididymitis of recent origin shows the hallmarks of acute inflammation. Persistent chronic epididymitis is associated with accumulation of plasma cells, macrophages and lymphocytes and, ultimately, with fibrotic obstruction of infected ducts. Gonorrheal epididymitis is a common cause of acquired male infertility.

Tuberculous epididymitis is now uncommon and is usually associated with established pulmonary and renal tuberculosis. It manifests as palpable enlargement of the epididymis and beading of the vas deferens, with confluent caseating granulomas.

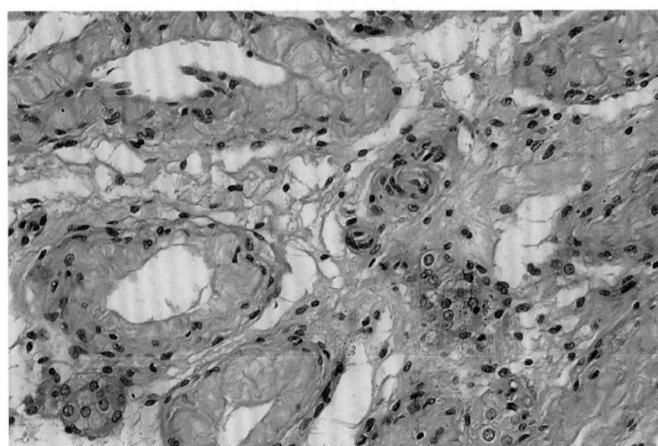

FIGURE 23-27. Postirradiation tubular atrophy of the testis. Seminiferous tubules are hyalinized, and there is no evidence of spermatogenesis.

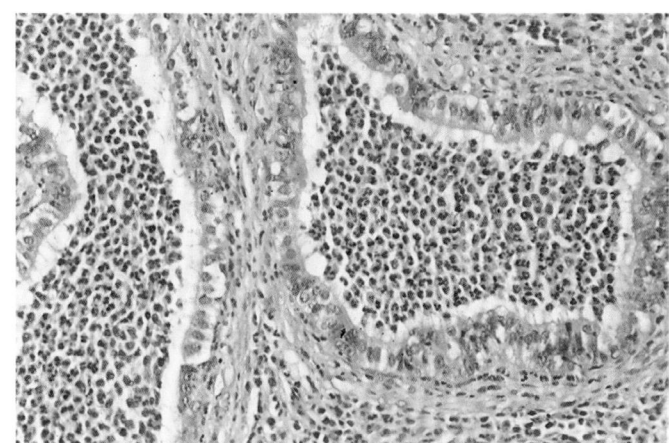

FIGURE 23-28. Bacterial epididymitis. The epididymal ducts contain numerous polymorphonuclear leukocytes.

Spermatic granulomas result from intense inflammatory responses to sperm outside of their usual channels. Traumatic rupture of epididymal ducts may play a role. Patients present with scrotal pain and swelling, frequently for weeks or months. The epididymis contains a mixed inflammatory cell infiltrate with many sperm fragments and macrophages phagocytosing sperm. Ultimately, inflammation results in interstitial fibrosis, ductal obstruction and infertility.

ORCHITIS

Orchitis is acute or chronic inflammation of the testis. It may occur as part of epididymo-orchitis, usually caused by ascending infection, or as isolated testicular inflammation. The latter is usually due to hematogenous spread of pathogens, but may be of autoimmune origin.

- **Gram-negative bacterial orchitis** is the most common form of the disease. It is often secondary to urinary tract infection and is typically associated with epididymitis. Infection may also manifest as intratesticular abscess or peritesticular suppuration and fibrosis.
- **Syphilitic orchitis** has two forms: (1) interstitial perivascular inflammation, with plasma cells, lymphocytes and macrophages; or (2) granulomatous inflammation (gummas).
- **Mumps orchitis** occurs in 20% of men who develop mumps but is uncommon because of widespread immunization against mumps. Viral infection is characterized by testicular pain and gonadal swelling, most often unilateral. Interstitial inflammation leads to destruction and loss of seminiferous epithelium (Fig. 23-29).
- **Granulomatous orchitis** of unknown cause is an uncommon disorder of middle-aged men that presents acutely as painful testicular enlargement or insidiously as induration. It shows noncaseating granulomas with neither organisms nor sperm remnants that might act as inciting agents. Variable numbers of seminiferous tubules are destroyed by the inflammatory process, which is considered to be a type IV (cell-mediated) hypersensitivity reaction.
- **Malakoplakia** of the testis has the same microscopic features and presumably the same histogenesis as malakoplakia elsewhere. It is typically related to *E. coli* infection.

TUMORS OF THE TESTIS

Tumors of the testis account for less than 1% of all cancers in men. More than 90% of these tumors are characterized by:

- Diagnosis between 25 and 45 years of age
- Germ cell origin
- Malignancy
- Curable by a combination of surgery and chemotherapy
- Cytogenetic marker, namely, isochromosome p12
- Metastasis first to periaortic abdominal lymph nodes

MOLECULAR PATHOGENESIS: The etiology of these tumors is not known. There is a geographic variation in the incidence of testicular cancer. The incidence is highest in Denmark, Sweden and Norway, but is low in Finland and southern European countries. The tumors are 5 times more common among Americans of European descent than in those of African heritage. Familial testicular cancers have been recorded but are rare. The only consistent cytogenetic abnormality is an additional fragment of chromosome 12 (isochromosome p12), found in 80% of germ cell tumors. As noted above, the only known risk factors are **cryptorchidism and gonadal dysgenesis**.

Malignant transformation of germ cells may occur during fetal development and involve (1) migrating primordial germ cells, (2) fetal germ cells interacting with stromal cells in the genital ridge or (3) early fetal spermatogonia. Since germ cell tumors rarely occur before puberty, some investigators believe that malignant transformation occurs in the peripubertal period and involves spermatogonia that are stimulated to proliferate and differentiate into spermatocytes. Although the initial events in testicular neoplasia are uncertain, a consensus holds that germ cell tumors progress through two pathways (Fig. 23-30). A carcinoma in situ stage, **intratubular testicular germ cell neoplasia** (ITGCN), precedes and progresses to invasive carcinoma (see below). This pathway accounts for most adult germ cell tumors. However, ITGCN is not found in testes harboring spermatocytic seminomas, teratomas of prepubertal testes or yolk sac tumors of infancy, which apparently develop directly from

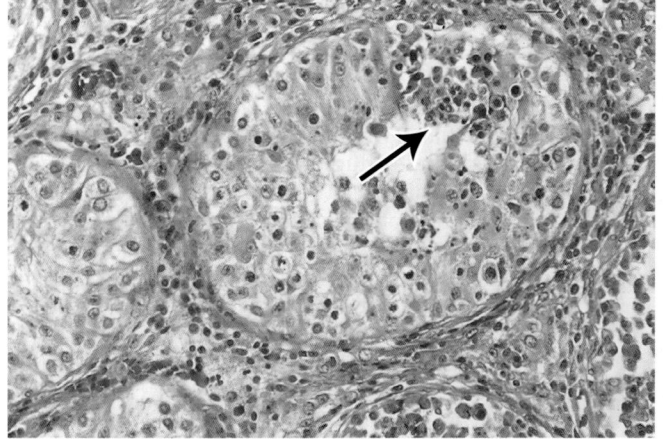

FIGURE 23-29. Viral orchitis. The interstitial spaces are infiltrated with mononuclear cells that spill focally into the lumen of seminiferous tubules (*arrow*). Note that the inflammation has interrupted normal spermatogenesis and that the seminiferous tubules do not contain sperm.

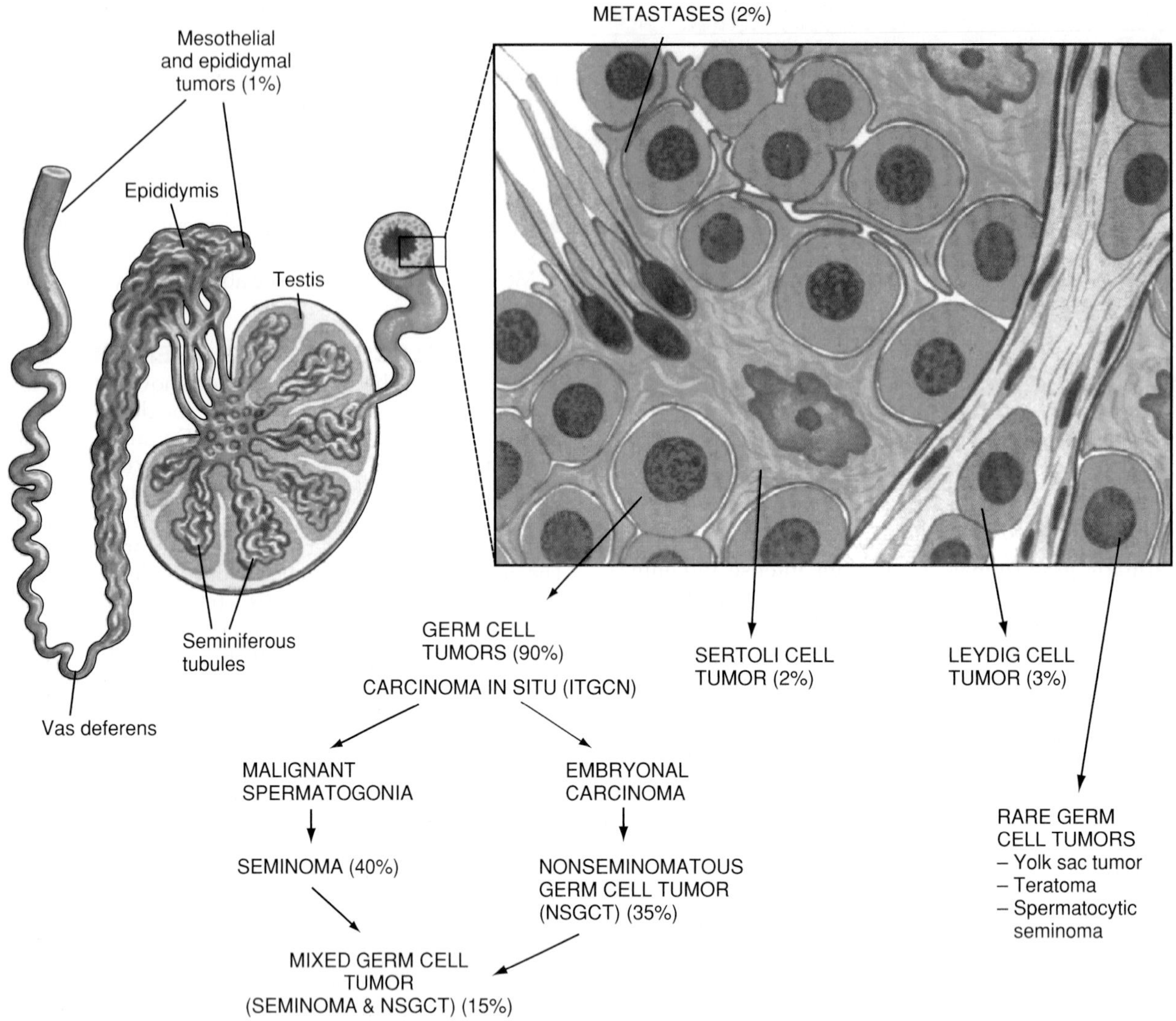

METASTASES (2%)

Mesothelial
and epididymal
tumors (1%)

Epididymis

Testis

Seminiferous
tubules

Vas deferens

GERM CELL
TUMORS (90%)
CARCINOMA IN SITU (ITGCN)

SERTOLI CELL
TUMOR (2%)

LEYDIG CELL
TUMOR (3%)

MALIGNANT
SPERMATOGONIA

EMBRYONAL
CARCINOMA

RARE GERM
CELL TUMORS
– Yolk sac tumor
– Teratoma
– Spermatocytic
  seminoma

SEMINOMA (40%)

NONSEMINOMATOUS
GERM CELL TUMOR
(NSGCT) (35%)

MIXED GERM CELL
TUMOR
(SEMINOMA & NSGCT) (15%)

FIGURE 23-30. Tumors of the testis, epididymis and related structures. Most testicular tumors originate from germ cells and are preceded by a carcinoma in situ stage known as intratubular germ cell neoplasia (ITGCN). Germ cell tumors of adult testes can be classified as seminomas (40%) or nonseminomatous germ cell tumors (NSGCTs) (35%). In 15% of cases, seminomatous elements are intermixed with NSGCT, forming mixed germ cell tumors. Some germ cell tumors (yolk sac tumor of childhood, childhood teratomas and spermatocytic seminomas) develop without passing through a preinvasive ITGCN stage. Tumors originating from sex cord stromal cells (Leydig and Sertoli cell tumors) account for 5% of testicular tumors. Epididymal tumors, tumors of the mesothelial lining of the tunica vaginalis (adenomatoid tumors) and metastases are rare.

germ cells without an in situ phase. It is possible that some migratory primordial germ cells may not find their way into the seminiferous tubules during fetal testicular organogenesis and that such "misplaced" cells become progenitors of yolk sac tumors and teratomas. Such cells may also give rise to midline extragonadal germ cell tumors in the retroperitoneum, sacral region, anterior mediastinum and area of the pineal gland.

 PATHOLOGY: Testicular tumors are classified histogenetically on the basis of their cell of origin into several groups (Table 23-7).

Tumor cells of ITGCN resemble spermatogonia or fetal germ cells but have much larger polyploid nuclei (Fig. 23-30). Like fetal germ cells, these cells express placental-like alkaline phosphatase (PlAP) on their surface. In infertile men with a history of cryptorchid testes, ITGCN

can persist unchanged for 5–10 years, after which the neoplastic cells acquire invasive properties, penetrate tubular basement membranes and give rise to infiltrating malignant tumors.

Malignant cells that retain the phenotype of spermatogonia give rise to **seminomas**. Alternatively, neoplastic germ cells can resemble malignant embryonic cells **(embryonal carcinoma)** by a process like **parthenogenetic activation** of oocytes in the female gonads of amphibians and reptiles.

In some cases, embryonal carcinoma cells proliferate in an undifferentiated form. Thus, the term "embryonal carcinoma" is used to designate undifferentiated embryonic cells and for tumors composed of these cells. In other cases, embryonal carcinoma cells differentiate into the three embryonic germ layers (ectoderm, mesoderm, endoderm) or extraembryonic tissues that form the fetal membranes and

TABLE 23-7		
TESTICULAR TUMORS		
Germ cell tumors—90%		
Seminoma (40%)		
Nonseminomatous germ cell tumors (NSGCTs)		
Embryonal carcinoma (5%)		
Teratocarcinoma (35%)		
Choriocarcinoma (<1%)		
Mixed germ cell tumors (15%)		
Teratoma (1%)		
Spermatocytic seminoma (1%)		
Yolk sac tumor of infancy (2%)		
Sex Cord Cell Tumors—5%		
Leydig cell tumors (60%)		
Sertoli cell tumors (40%)		
Metastases—2%		
Other Rare Tumors—3%		

placenta. Further differentiation of germ layer cells leads to formation of various somatic tissues. Ectoderm differentiates into skin, central nervous system, retinal pigment and other related tissues. Mesoderm gives rise to smooth and striated muscle, cartilage and bone. Endoderm forms intestinal tissue, bronchial epithelium, salivary glands and so forth. The extraembryonic derivatives of embryonal carcinoma cells give rise to chorionic epithelium (cytotrophoblast and syncytiotrophoblast) and yolk sac–like epithelium. These complex tumors composed of malignant undifferentiated embryonal cells and their somatic and extraembryonic derivatives are **teratocarcinomas** or **malignant teratomas**. Rarely, extraembryonic components of teratocarcinomas overgrow and destroy all other components. Such tumors are composed of a single tumor type and are classified as **yolk sac carcinoma** or **choriocarcinoma**.

For clinical purposes, all germ cell tumors with embryonal carcinoma as their malignant stem cells are termed **nonseminomatous germ cell tumors (NSGCTs),** to distinguish them from seminomas. Pure yolk sac carcinomas of the adult testis and choriocarcinomas are also included in this group because it is assumed that these tumors originated from embryonal carcinoma cells and still may contain a few such cells that are not readily recognizable.

In 15% of cases, germ cell tumors have both seminoma and nonseminomatous elements. Such **mixed germ cell tumors** are treated clinically as nonseminomatous neoplasms.

Intratubular Germ Cell Neoplasia Is Testicular Carcinoma in Situ

ITGCN represents a preinvasive form of germ cell tumors.

 EPIDEMIOLOGY: ITGCN can be seen as (1) an isolated focal histologic change in 2% of cryptorchid testes or testicular biopsies performed for infertility, (2) widespread carcinoma in situ adjacent to almost all invasive germ cell tumors and (3) lesions in 5% of contralateral testes in patients who had an orchiectomy for a testicular germ cell tumor.

 PATHOLOGY: ITGCN involves testes patchily, usually affecting less than 10%–30% of tubules. Seminiferous tubules harboring this lesion have thick basement membranes and no sperm. The normal germ cells are replaced by neoplastic ones that are broadly attached to the basal lamina (Fig. 23-31). The tumor cells are larger than normal spermatogonia and have large central nuclei with finely dispersed chromatin and prominent nucleoli. Their cytoplasm is abundant and clear, with abundant glycogen. Nuclear DNA content is increased, suggesting that the cells are triploid. Plasma membranes are distinct and stain with antibodies to PlAP. The transcription factor OCT3/4 is a reliable marker for nuclei of ITGCN cells.

 CLINICAL FEATURES: ITGCN is a precursor of invasive carcinoma, but the invasive tumor develops at an unpredictable pace. Half of men with ITGCN develop invasive cancer within 5 years and 70% in 7 years. Diagnosis of ITGCN on testicular biopsy is an indication for prophylactic orchiectomy.

Seminomas Contain Monomorphous Cells that Resemble Spermatogonia

 **EPIDEMIOLOGY:** Seminomas are the most common testicular cancer, making up 40% of all germ cell tumors. Peak incidence is 30–40 years, and they are not found before prepuberty, except in those who have dysgenetic gonads.

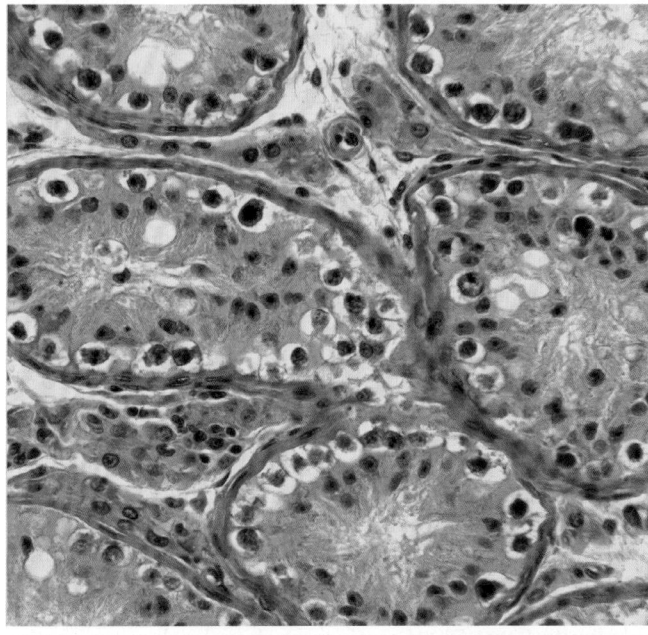

FIGURE 23-31. Intratubular germ cell neoplasia (ITGCN). The seminiferous tubules show no signs of spermatogenesis but instead contain large atypical cells corresponding to intratubular carcinoma in situ.

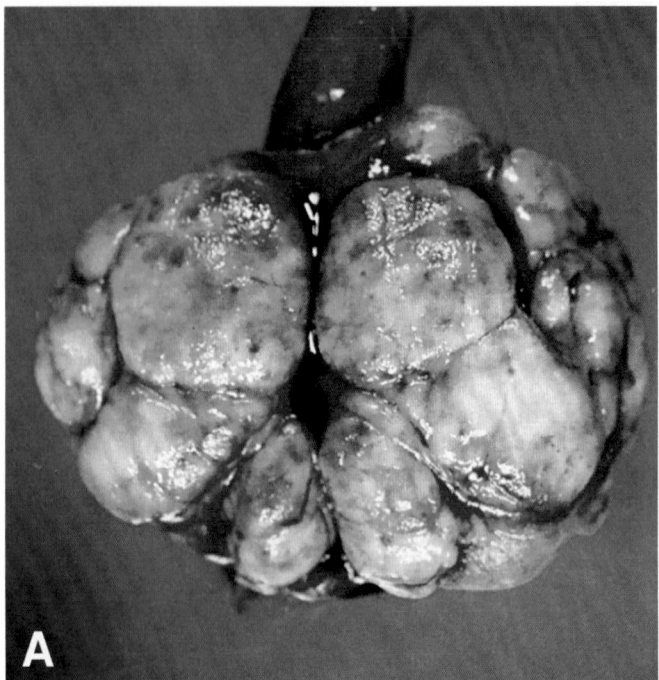

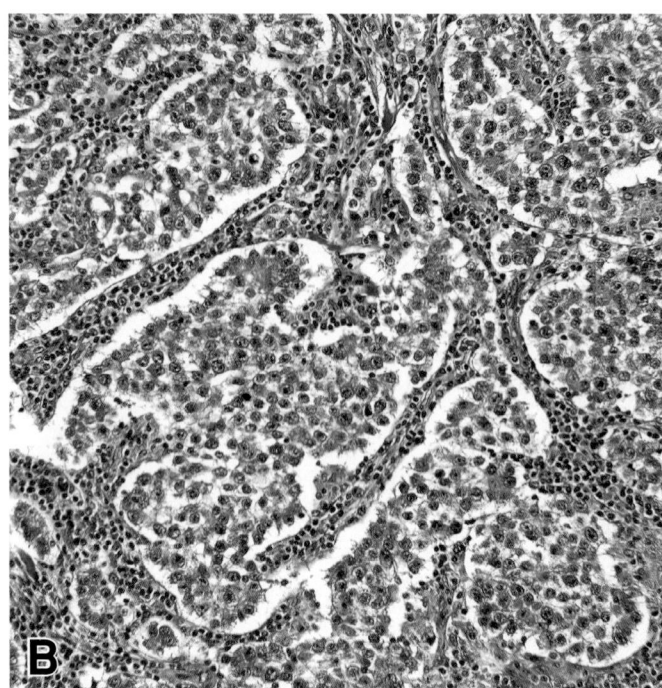

FIGURE 23-32. Seminoma. A. The cut surface of this nodular tumor is tan and bulging, suggesting that the tumor is firm and rubbery. **B.** Groups of tumor cells are surrounded by fibrous septa infiltrated with lymphocytes. Tumor cells have vesicular nuclei, which are much larger than the small round nuclei of the lymphocytes.

 **PATHOLOGY:** Seminomas are solid, rubbery-firm, bosselated masses that are usually sharply demarcated from normal tissue, which may be compressed, atrophic and fibrotic. On cross-section the tumors look lobulated and homogeneous tan or grayish yellow (Fig. 23-32). Areas of necrosis or hemorrhage are infrequent but may be seen in larger tumors.

Seminomas resemble **ovarian dysgerminoma** (see Chapter 24) microscopically. They feature a single population of uniform polygonal cells with central vesicular nuclei. Their ample cytoplasm may be pale and eosinophilic or clear, since it has considerable glycogen and some lipid. Cells grow in nests or sheets separated by fibrous septa infiltrated with lymphocytes, plasma cells and macrophages. Septa may contain granulomas with giant cells. Tumor cells invade the testicular parenchyma and spread through seminiferous tubules into rete testis. The epididymis is involved later in the disease, usually before spread to abdominal lymph nodes.

Seminoma cells resemble immature spermatogonia. Like fetal spermatogonia and primordial germ cells in the fetus, they express PlAP on the plasma membrane. Seminoma cells also react with antibodies to c-Kit (CD117) and OCT3/4, which are reliable markers for this tumor.

Pathologists recognize two subtypes of seminoma: (1) **seminoma with syncytiotrophoblastic giant cells** and (2) **anaplastic seminoma**. The first subgroup includes the 20% of tumors that contain syncytiotrophoblastic cells. These multinucleated giant cells are best demonstrated with antibodies to human chorionic gonadotropin (hCG). Although they secrete hCG, blood hCG levels are usually below detectable limits. Some 5% of seminomas show brisk mitotic activity and nuclear pleomorphism and are classified as **anaplastic seminoma**. There are no clinical differences between classical seminomas and these two microscopic tumor variants.

CLINICAL FEATURES: Seminomas are usually progressively growing scrotal masses that are often diagnosed while still curable by orchiectomy, with or without abdominal lymph node dissection. They are highly radiosensitive, and radiotherapy is important in treating tumors that are cured by surgery alone. Even in advanced stages of dissemination, chemotherapy can be curative. *The cure rate for all histologic subtypes of seminoma is now over 90%.*

Spermatocytic seminoma is a rare tumor, which, despite its name, is unrelated to classical seminoma. These are benign tumors of men over age 40. They are not associated with ITGCN and do not elicit lymphocytic reactions. Spermatocytic seminomas contain three cell types: large, small and intermediate cells. Immunohistochemically, the cells of these tumors do not express typical seminoma markers. Orchiectomy is curative.

Nonseminomatous Germ Cell Tumors Derive from Embryonal Cells

NSGCTs of the testis include several entities, two of which account for most of the cases: (1) pure embryonal carcinoma and (2) teratocarcinoma, also known as **malignant teratoma** or **mixed germ cell tumor**. **Pure choriocarcinoma, pure yolk sac carcinoma of the adult testis** and the so-called **growing benign teratoma** are rare NSGCTs. Mixed germ cell tumors are NSGCTs combined with seminomas.

EPIDEMIOLOGY: NSGCTs constitute 55% of all testicular germ cell tumors, of which 2/3 are teratocarcinomas, followed by mixed germ cell tumors and pure embryonal carcinomas. All other tumors of this group are extremely rare. Like seminomas, NSGCTs have a peak incidence in the third to fourth decades. At diagnosis, these patients are usually somewhat younger than those with seminomas.

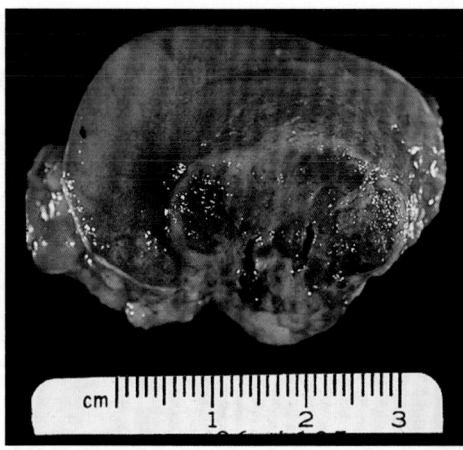

FIGURE 23-33. Nonseminomatous germ cell tumor (NSGCT) of the testis. The cut surface of this small testicular tumor shows considerable heterogeneity, varying in color from white to dark red.

PATHOLOGY: NSGCTs vary in size and shape. They may be solid or partially cystic. Solid areas vary from white to yellow to red, indicating that they are composed of viable tumor cells, foci of necrosis and hemorrhage, respectively (Fig. 23-33).

The histology of NSGCTs is highly variable. Pure embryonal carcinomas exclusively contain undifferentiated embryonal carcinoma cells like cells from preimplantation-stage embryos (Fig. 23-34). Because the tumor cells have little cytoplasm, their hyperchromatic, disproportionately large nuclei seem to overlap. Embryonal carcinoma cells may grow as broad solid sheets, cords, gland-like tubules and acini, and sometimes even line papillary structures. Mitoses and apoptotic cells are common. Embryonal carcinomas invade the testis, epididymis and blood vessels and metastasize to abdominal lymph nodes, lungs and other organs.

Embryonal carcinomas, like seminomas, react with antibodies to PlAP and OCT 3/4. Unlike seminomas and other tumors, they express cytokeratins and CD30, but not c-KIT (CD117).

Embryonal carcinoma cells are the stem cells of **teratocarcinomas (malignant teratomas),** which feature differentiated somatic elements (i.e., tissues normally found in various organs, and extraembryonic elements, including yolk sac cells and trophoblastic cells). Thus, such nonseminomatous tumors have foci of embryonal carcinoma and of other tissues (Fig. 23-35). Such a tumor might, for example, contain components of embryonal carcinoma, yolk sac and trophoblast. However, a similar tumor that also contains seminoma cells would be called a **mixed germ cell tumor.** In most tumors, the malignancy resides in the embryonal carcinoma cells. Interestingly, when these cells metastasize, they can differentiate into somatic or extraembryonic tissues, in which case the metastatic tumor can resemble the original one.

NSGCTs can give rise to clones of highly malignant cytotrophoblast and syncytiotrophoblast cells that overgrow other elements. Tumors composed exclusively of malignant chorionic epithelium are termed **choriocarcinomas.** Likewise, clones of malignant yolk sac epithelium produce **yolk sac carcinoma.**

Some histologically benign teratomas of postpubertal young men may have a malignant clinical course, even though they appear to be only mature, nonproliferating somatic tissues, without embryonal elements (Fig. 23-36). In some instances, it is assumed that the tumor was actually a teratocarcinoma in which almost all embryonal cells differentiated into mature somatic tissues but that a few remaining malignant cells were unnoticed, or had metastasized before resection. These tumors are clinically known as the **growing teratoma syndrome.** In other cases, teratoma tissues remain undifferentiated and resemble embryonic organs or embryonic tumors such as neuroblastoma. These **immature teratomas** are also potentially malignant.

CLINICAL FEATURES: Most NSGCTs present as testicular masses. They tend to grow faster than seminomas and metastasize more readily and more widely. Hence, for some NSGCTs, metastases may be the first sign of the neoplasm.

Unlike seminomas, NSGCTs often contain yolk sac and syncytiotrophoblastic components. Yolk sac cells secrete α-fetoprotein (AFP), a fetal protein not normally found in the blood. Syncytiotrophoblast cells release hCG, a hormone of pregnancy, that is also not found in males. *Elevated serum AFP or hCG is found in 70% of patients with NSGCTs and is thus a useful tumor marker.* Serum AFP, hCG and lactate dehydrogenase (a nonspecific tumor marker that reflects the extent of the total tumor mass) must be measured in all patients before orchiectomy and are included in the clinical staging of the tumor. These antigens are most useful to follow postoperative patients who have been treated for NSGCT. Persistently elevated AFP and/or hCG indicates that a patient is not tumor free. If initially high levels of AFP and hCG normalize after treatment but later rise again, metastatic spread is likely. AFP is a relatively insensitive marker of recurrence as elevated serum AFP is found only in 70% patients with recurrent cancer.

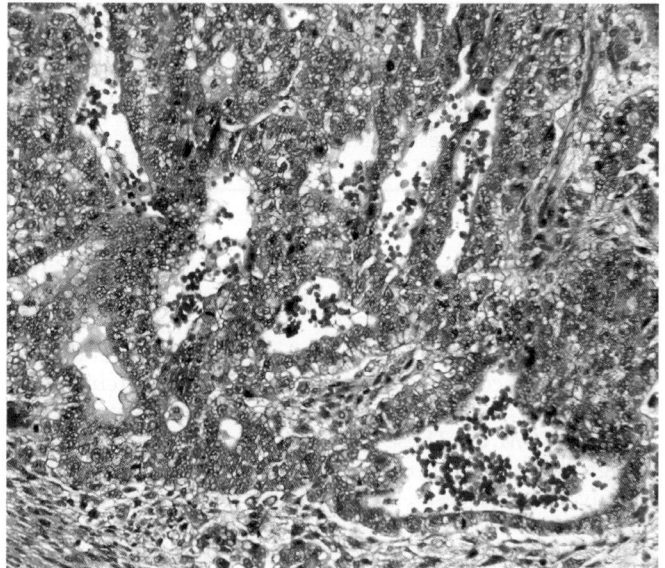

FIGURE 23-34. Embryonal carcinoma component of a nonseminomatous germ cell tumor (NSGCT). Because these undifferentiated cells have scant cytoplasm, their hyperchromatic nuclei impart a bluish color to the tumor. The nuclei appear crowded and seem to overlap each other. The cells form cords and sheets surrounding dilated vascular channels filled with red blood cells.

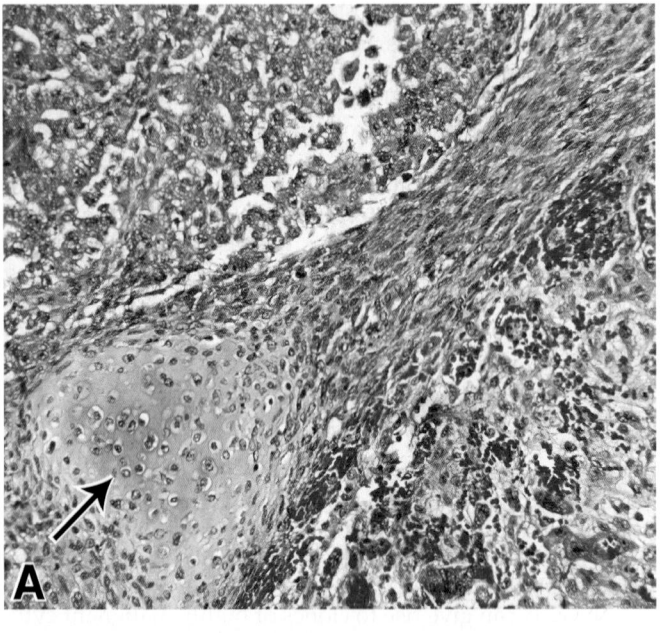

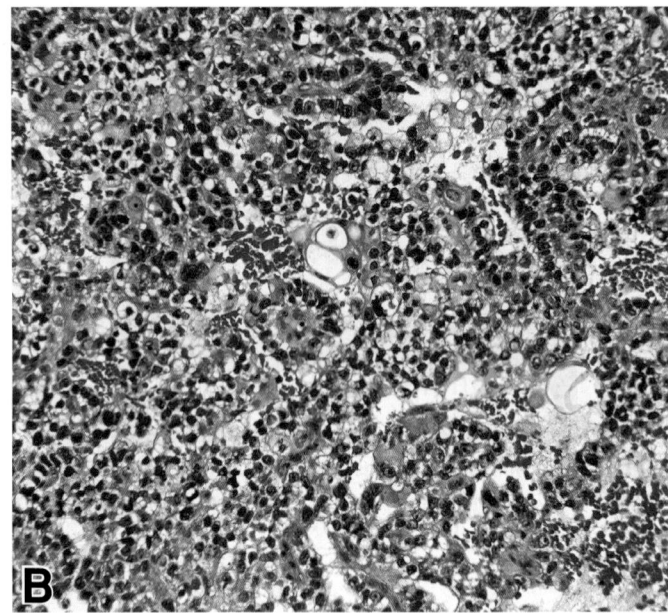

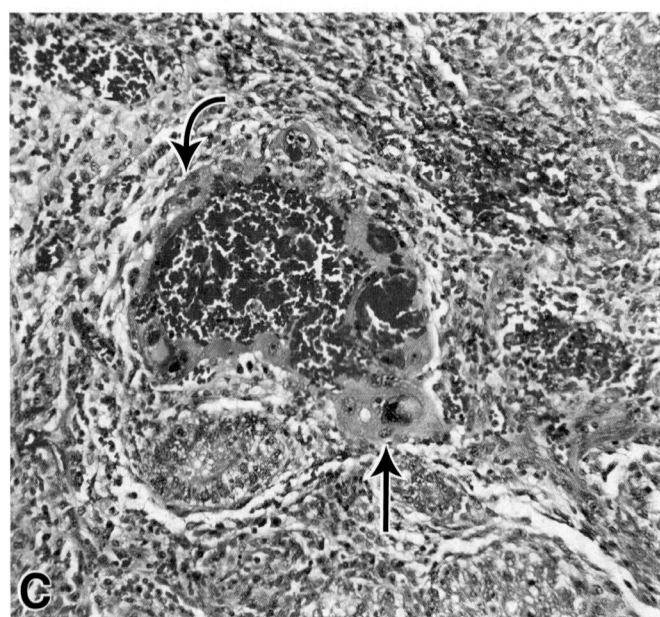

FIGURE 23-35. Nonseminomatous germ cell tumor (NSGCT). A. Somatic tissue of this tumor includes well-differentiated cartilage and nondescript connective tissue separating the embryonal carcinoma (*upper left corner*) from the hemorrhagic choriocarcinoma (*right lower corner*). **B.** Yolk sac component consists of interlacing cords of epithelial cells surrounded by loose stroma resembling the early yolk sac. **C.** Choriocarcinoma component of the NSGCT consists of multinucleated syncytiotrophoblastic giant cells and mononuclear cytotrophoblastic cells. Invasive growth of trophoblasts is usually associated with hemorrhage.

Treatment of NSGCT includes orchiectomy to remove the primary tumor, then platinum-based chemotherapy and, if indicated, surgical dissection of abdominal lymph nodes. Chemotherapy usually eliminates metastatic embryonal carcinoma cells, but differentiated tissues originating from them are resistant. Such tissues do not grow and are not likely to endanger the patient. Nevertheless, it is better to remove any residual tumor than to take a chance that a few malignant tumor cells might be lurking in residual tumors. *Complete cures of NSGCTs are now common in over 90% of cases.*

Testicular Tumors Are Rare in Prepubertal Boys

In the first 4 years of life, most testicular neoplasms are yolk sac tumors. Benign teratomas are the most common testicular tumor between ages 4 and 12 years.

YOLK SAC TUMORS: These neoplasms are composed of cells arranged into structures reminiscent of parts of fetal yolk sac. Diagnosis is based on recognizing multiple microscopic tumor patterns and glomeruloid **Schiller-Duval bodies** (Fig. 23-37). These neonatal tumors resemble those of the yolk sac elements in NSGCTs. All such tumors secrete AFP into the serum. Yolk sac tumors of infancy and early childhood are considered malignant, but timely orchiectomy and removal of the tumor cure over 95% of patients.

TERATOMAS: These tumors of prepubertal testes are benign and are composed of mature somatic tissues. Orchiectomy and even testis-sparing surgery are curative.

Gonadal Stromal/Sex Cord Tumors Are Composed of Cells that Resemble Sertoli or Leydig Cells

Gonadal stromal/sex cord tumors make up 5% of testicular tumors.

LEYDIG CELL TUMORS: These are rare neoplasms composed of cells resembling interstitial (Leydig) cells of the testis. They can be hormonally active and secrete androgens, estrogens or both. Leydig cell tumors occur at any age, with

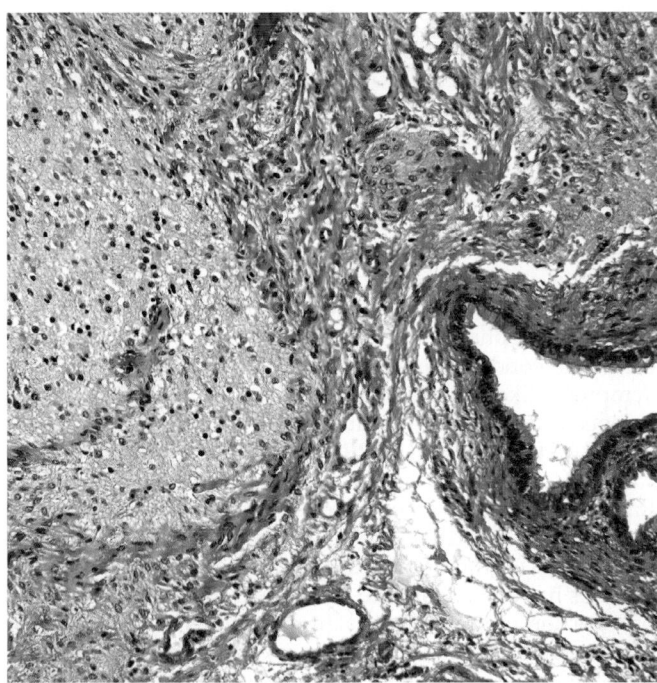

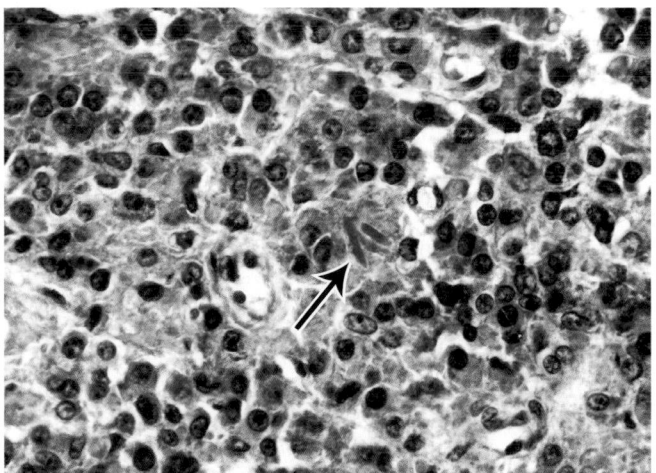

FIGURE 23-38. Leydig cell tumor. The tumor cells have uniform round nuclei and well-developed eosinophilic cytoplasm. Three cytoplasmic Reinke crystals are seen in the center of the field (*arrow*).

FIGURE 23-36. Teratoma. The tumor consists of neural tissue (*left*) connective tissue and smooth muscle cells (*midportion*) and glands lined by columnar epithelium (*right side of the picture*).

distinct peaks in childhood and then in adults from the third to the sixth decade.

PATHOLOGY: Leydig cell tumors vary from 1 to 10 cm and are circumscribed; some appear encapsulated. The cut surface is yellow to brown, and larger tumors have fibrous trabeculae, giving them a lobular appearance. Leydig tumor cells are uniform, with round nuclei and well-developed eosinophilic or vacuolated cytoplasm (Fig. 23-38). **Reinke crystals**—rectangular,

eosinophilic, cytoplasmic inclusions—are characteristic of normal Leydig cells and are seen in 30% of tumors. Most (90%) Leydig cell tumors are benign, but it is difficult to predict their biological behavior on histologic grounds.

CLINICAL FEATURES: Androgenic effects of testicular Leydig cell tumors in prepubertal boys lead to precocious physical and sexual development. By contrast, feminization and gynecomastia are seen in some adults with this tumor. Either estrogen or testosterone levels may be elevated, but there is no characteristic pattern. All Leydig cell tumors in children and almost all tumors in adults are cured by orchiectomy.

SERTOLI CELL TUMORS: Some testicular sex cord stromal cell tumors contain neoplastic Sertoli cells. Most (90%) are benign and produce few if any hormonal symptoms.

PATHOLOGY: Sertoli cell tumors are small (1–3 cm), solid, yellow-gray, well-circumscribed nodules. They contain columnar tumor cells arranged into tubules or cords in a fibrous trabecular framework (Fig. 23-39). The rare malignant variant shows greater

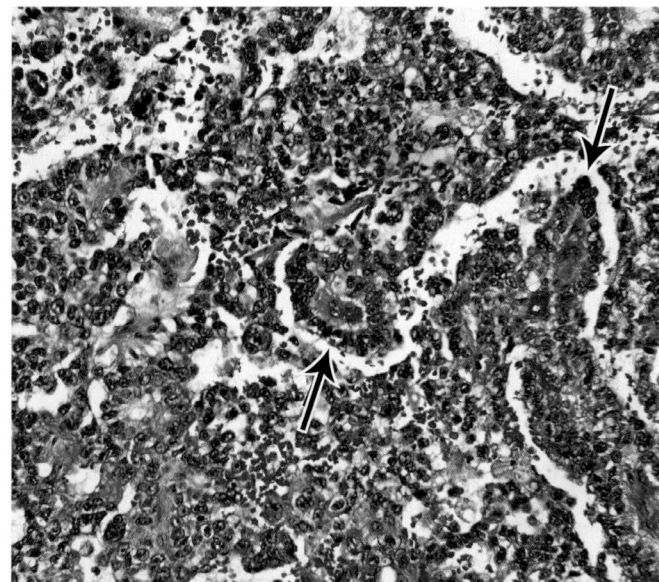

FIGURE 23-37. Yolk sac tumor. This childhood tumor is composed of interlacing strands of epithelial cells surrounded by loose connective stroma. The glomeruloid structures (Schiller-Duval bodies) are marked by arrows.

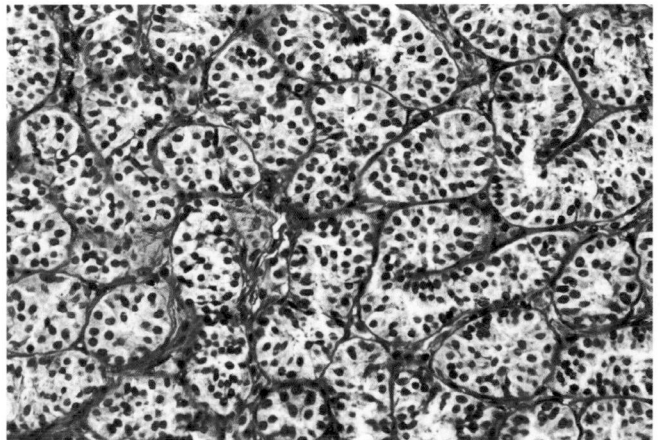

FIGURE 23-39. Sertoli cell tumor. The neoplastic cells are arranged in tubules surrounded by a basement membrane. These structures are reminiscent of seminiferous tubules devoid of germ cells.

cellular pleomorphism, focal necrosis and few cords and tubules. Most patients with Sertoli cell tumors are younger than age 40 and come to medical attention because of a scrotal mass. Endocrine effects are uncommon and, if present, are vague. Orchiectomy is curative.

All Other Germ Cell Tumors are Rare

Tumors may originate from the epithelium of the epididymis, connective tissue stroma, mesothelium and tunica vaginalis testis. All these tumors are rare. Metastatic tumors, including lymphomas, are also uncommon. All these tumors together account for less than 5% of all scrotal masses.

ADENOMATOID TUMOR: Adenomatoid tumor (benign mesothelioma) is a benign tumor that originates from the mesothelium of the testicular tunica vaginalis. These neoplasms usually occur in the upper pole of the epididymis, with fewer involving the tunica vaginalis or spermatic cord. They are well-demarcated nodules found by palpating the testis or epididymis. Microscopically, they contain mesothelial cells in cords or small duct-like structures embedded in dense fibrous stroma. Malignant mesotheliomas of tunica vaginalis testis are very rare.

METASTASES: Most of these spread from primary cancers of the prostate, large intestine or bladder (i.e., organs that are located in the pelvis and close to the testes).

MALIGNANT LYMPHOMA: This cancer is the most common neoplasm in the testes of men older than 60 years. It may be primary in the testis. More often, it reflects seeding of lymphoma from other sites or occurs in patients with leukemia. Diffuse large B-cell lymphoma is the most common form of lymphoma involving the testis. Most patients with lymphomatous involvement of the testis have a poor prognosis.

Prostate

The pathologic processes affecting the prostate can be simplified by considering just three processes: (1) inflammation, (2) hyperplasia and (3) neoplasia.

PROSTATITIS

Prostatitis is inflammation of the prostate. There are acute and chronic forms. Prostatitis is usually caused by coliform uropathogens, but often no etiology is found.

ACUTE PROSTATITIS: Typically a complication of other urinary tract infections, acute prostatitis results from reflux of infected urine into the prostate. An acute inflammatory infiltrate is seen in prostatic acini and stroma. It causes intense discomfort on urination and is often associated with fever, chills and perineal pain. Most patients respond well to antibiotics.

CHRONIC BACTERIAL PROSTATITIS: This infection is of longer duration that may or may not be preceded by an episode of acute prostatitis. Most patients complain of dysuria and burning at the urethral meatus. Suprapubic, perineal and low back pain or discomfort and nocturia may be also present. The urine usually contains bacteria. In addition to reflux of urine, prostatic calculi and local prostatic duct obstruction may contribute to development of chronic bacterial prostatitis. Infiltrates of lymphocytes, plasma cells

and macrophages are the rule. Prolonged antibiotic therapy is often, but not always, curative.

NONBACTERIAL PROSTATITIS: Sometimes in chronic prostatitis, no causative organism is identified. It is the most common form of inflammation in prostatic biopsies, in prostatectomy specimens or at autopsy. Nonbacterial prostatitis typically affects men older than 50 years but can be seen at any age. Some cases may be due to *C. trachomatis, Mycoplasma* or *U. urealyticum.* However, in practice, nonbacterial prostatitis is a diagnosis of exclusion. The most common histology shows dilated glands filled with neutrophils and foamy macrophages surrounded by chronic inflammatory cells. The condition may be asymptomatic or it may cause symptoms like those of chronic bacterial prostatitis. Usually, no specific therapy is available.

GRANULOMATOUS PROSTATITIS: In most cases, the cause of granulomatous prostatitis cannot be established. Rarely, this disease can be traced to specific causative agents, including *M. tuberculosis,* BCG or fungi such as *Histoplasma capsulatum.* A granulomatous lesion resembling rheumatoid nodules has been related to previous transurethral resection of a portion of the prostate. The symptoms of chronic granulomatous prostatitis are vague and the diagnosis is made histologically. Caseating or noncaseating granulomas are associated with localized destruction of prostatic ducts and acini and, in later stages, with fibrosis.

 CLINICAL FEATURES: As indicated above, symptoms of chronic prostatitis are highly variable and treatment may be ineffective. Most importantly, it may cause elevated serum prostate-specific antigen (PSA), a worrisome suggestion of prostatic malignancy (see below). Thus, the diagnosis is often made by biopsy done to exclude carcinoma.

NODULAR HYPERPLASIA OF THE PROSTATE

Nodular prostatic hyperplasia, also called benign prostatic hyperplasia *(BPH), is a common disorder characterized clinically by obstruction of urinary outflow and pathologically by proliferation of glands and stroma.*

 **EPIDEMIOLOGY:** BPH is most common in western Europe and the United States and least common in Asia. Its prevalence in the United States is higher among blacks than among whites. Clinical prostatism (i.e., BPH severe enough to interfere with urination) peaks in the seventh decade. However, prevalence of BPH is far greater at autopsy than is suggested by clinically apparent prostatism. In fact, 75% of men over age 80 have some degree of prostatic hyperplasia. The disorder is rare in men younger than 40 years of age.

 **MOLECULAR PATHOGENESIS:** The earliest histogenetic events in BPH remain unclear. Testosterone is necessary for prostatic development and to maintain secretory function. The active androgen form is dihydrotestosterone (DHT), a product of the enzyme 5α-reductase. DHT binds nuclear receptors in glandular and stromal cells. In men, exogenous testosterone does not induce hyperplasia and does not even stimulate atrophic glands. With aging, circulating testosterone levels decline in men with and without BPH. As well, no change in serum

DHT is seen in men with BPH, although the ratio of circulating testosterone to DHT may be low. Conversely, drugs that block 5α-reductase (e.g., finasteride or dutasteride) reduce the size of the prostate in men with BPH. Prepubertal castration prevents the development of age-related BPH and completely protects against prostate cancer.

 PATHOLOGY: Early nodular hyperplasia begins in the submucosa of the proximal urethra **(the transitional zone)**. Enlarging nodules compress the centrally located urethral lumen and the more peripherally located normal prostate (Fig. 23-40). In well-developed BPH, the normal gland is actually limited to an attenuated rim of tissue beneath the capsule. Individual nodules are demarcated by enveloping fibrous pseudocapsules (Fig. 23-41B). Larger nodules may show focal hemorrhage or infarction. Small stones may be seen as well.

In BPH, proliferation of epithelial cells of acini and ductules, smooth muscle cells and stromal fibroblasts are all

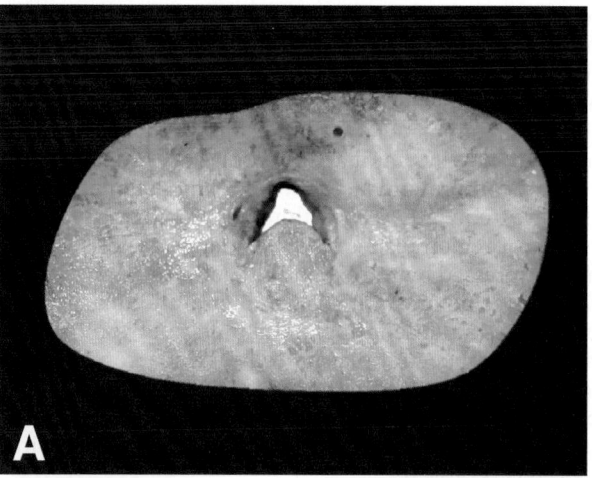

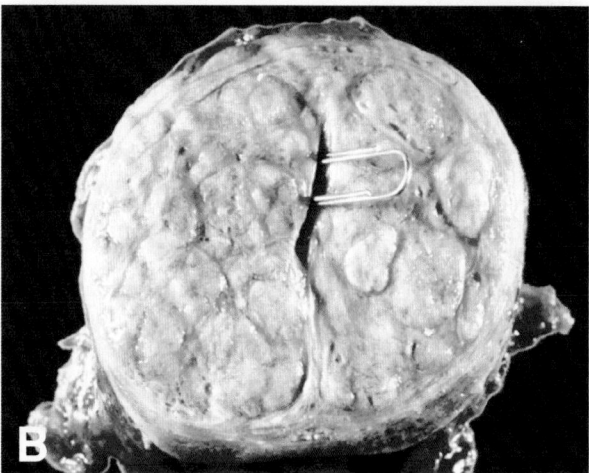

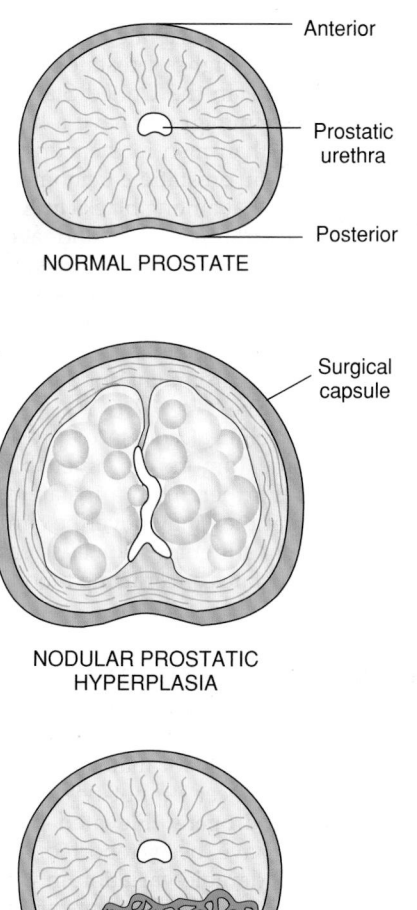

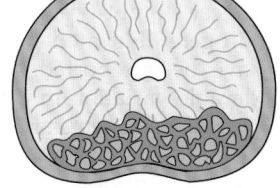

FIGURE 23-40. Normal prostate, nodular hyperplasia and adenocarcinoma. In prostatic hyperplasia, which involves predominantly the periurethral part of the gland, the nodules compress and distort the urethra. The expansion of the central prostatic glands leads to compression of the peripheral parts and fibrosis, resulting in the formation of a so-called surgical capsule. Prostatic carcinoma usually arises from the peripheral glands, and compression of the urethra is a late clinical event.

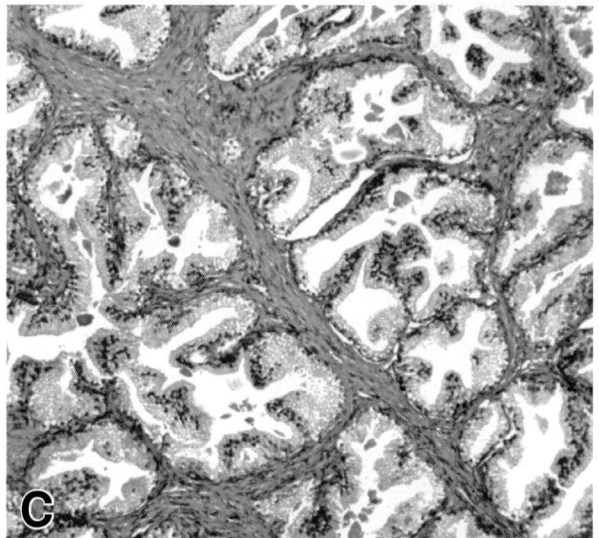

FIGURE 23-41. Nodular hyperplasia of the prostate. A. The cut surface of a prostate enlarged by nodular hyperplasia shows numerous well-circumscribed nodules of prostatic tissue surrounded by pseudocapsules. The prostatic urethra (*paper clip*) has been compressed to a narrow slit. **B.** Normal prostate. **C.** Hyperplastic prostate glands in nodular hyperplasia. The columnar epithelium lining the acini is composed of two cell layers: polarized clear cuboidal cells lining the acinar lumen and flattened basal cells interposed between the cuboidal acinar cells and the stroma. Hyperplastic cells line papillary projections protruding into the lumina of the acini.

seen in variable proportions. Typical fibromyoadenomatous nodules contain variably sized hyperplastic prostatic acini randomly scattered throughout their stroma. The epithelial (adenomatous) component contains a double layer of cells, with tall columnar cells overlying a basal layer (Fig. 23-41C) and often showing papillary hyperplasia. Chronic inflammation and corpora amylacea (eosinophilic laminated concretions) are frequently seen within the acini. In the uninvolved peripheral region of the prostate, glands are often atrophic and compressed by the expanding nodules.

Nonspecific prostatitis is common in nodular hyperplasia. There is a dense intraglandular and periglandular infiltrate of lymphocytes, plasma cells and macrophages, often with acute inflammatory cells and focal gland destruction. Focal infarcts of varying age are present in 20% of cases. Squamous metaplasia of ductal epithelium at the periphery of infarcts is typical.

CLINICAL FEATURES: The symptoms of nodular hyperplasia result from compression of the prostatic urethra and consequent bladder outlet obstruction (Fig. 23-42). A history of decreased vigor of the urinary stream and increasing urinary frequency is typical. Rectal examination reveals a firm, enlarged, nodular prostate. If severe obstruction is prolonged, back-pressure results in hydroureter, hydronephrosis and ultimately renal failure and death.

Treatment of BPH is either surgical or pharmacologic with drugs that block 5α-redutase. In addition, some patients receive α$_1$-adrenergic blockers to enhance urine flow. Transurethral radiofrequency ablation and cryotherapy are the surgical treatments of choice.

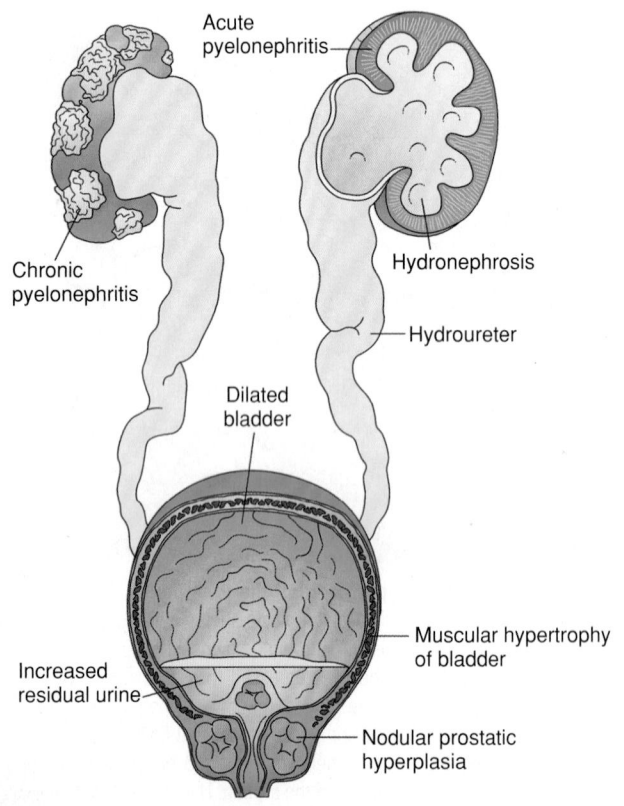

FIGURE 23-42. Complications of nodular prostatic hyperplasia.

IN SITU AND INVASIVE ADENOCARCINOMA OF THE PROSTATE

EPIDEMIOLOGY: *In 1990, prostatic adenocarcinoma surpassed lung cancer to become the cancer most frequently diagnosed in American men.* An estimated 220,000 new cases are diagnosed yearly in the United States. About 30,000 American men die annually from it, a figure equivalent to that of colorectal carcinoma. Prostate cancer is largely a disease of elderly men: 75% of patients are 60–80 years of age. Autopsy studies confirm that the tumor is more common with advancing age. Prostate cancer is diagnosed at autopsy in 20% of men in their 40s, and in 70% of men over age 70. The cumulative lifetime probability of being diagnosed with latent or symptomatic prostatic carcinoma is one in six for American men. There is considerable variation in age-related death rates for adenocarcinoma of the prostate throughout the world, the highest being in the United States and Scandinavian countries and the lowest in Mexico, Greece and Japan. Most western European countries have intermediate rates. American blacks, with a rate twice as high as that of white Americans, have the highest prostate carcinoma–related death rates in the world. In the United States, descendants of Polish and Japanese immigrants have a higher incidence of prostatic carcinoma than men in their original countries. Similarly, mortality from prostatic carcinoma among black American men exceeds that among blacks in Africa.

In addition to geography, racial and age differences, heredity and possibly diet influence prostate cancer risk. One tenth of cases have familial tendencies, so risk is significantly increased in persons with first-degree relatives with prostate cancer. Dietary fat content may increase risk of prostate cancer, but neither environment nor dietary factors have been found to be causative.

Unfortunately, the clinical course of prostate cancer is often capricious. Some tumors are amenable to therapy, while others are not. Further, many prostate cancers are so indolent (or latent) that they may never be clinically significant during the patient's lifetime. For this reason, the utility of screening for prostate cancer using blood PSA levels is controversial.

MOLECULAR PATHOGENESIS: Androgenic control of normal prostatic growth and the responsiveness of prostate cancer to castration and exogenous estrogens indicate a role for male hormones. However, patients with prostate cancer do not typically have higher levels of circulating androgens. Elevated urinary estrone-to-testosterone ratios have been reported. The androgen (AR) gene shows considerable variation in CAG repeats in exon 1. Men with fewer AR CAG repeats are at greater risk for developing prostate cancer. Some tumors show somatic mutations that place the transcription factor gene ETV1 under the control of the androgen-regulated TMPRSS2 promoter. Other cases show hypermethylation of the gene for the antioxidant enzyme glutathione S-transferase. Altered regulation of STAT transcription factors and dysregulation of the PTEN tumor suppressor are also documented.

There is consensus that intraductal dysplastic epithelial proliferation, termed **prostatic intraepithelial neoplasia (PIN)**, is a precursor lesion of prostatic adenocarcinoma. *PIN describes prostatic ducts lined by cytologically atypical luminal cells and a concomitant decrease in basal cells.*

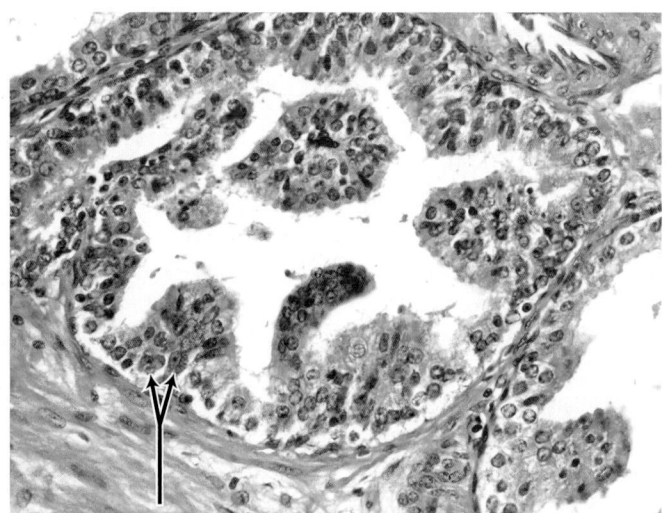

FIGURE 23-43. High-grade prostatic intraepithelial neoplasia (PIN). The large duct in the center is lined by atypical cells with enlarged nuclei and prominent nucleoli (*arrows*).

Nuclei of high-grade PIN are enlarged and show nucleoli and marked crowding (Fig. 23-43). Substantial data indicate that PIN lesions are premalignant and progress to adenocarcinoma. High-grade PIN may precede invasive cancer by up to two decades, and their severity increases with increasing age.

Morphologic evidence linking PIN to invasive prostate cancer includes (1) both lesions are mainly peripheral, (2) cytologic similarity of high-grade PIN to invasive cancer and (3) close topographic proximity of high-grade PIN to invasive cancer. Finally, PIN lesions are more frequent in prostates with cancer than in those without tumors. Certain indicators in high-grade PIN resemble those of invasive cancer (e.g., aneuploidy, transforming growth factor [TGF]-α, type IV collagenase, expression of *bcl-2* and *c-erb-2* oncogenes). Recognition of high-grade PIN on needle biopsy is important because many patients with high-grade PIN on initial biopsy have invasive carcinoma on follow-up biopsy.

 PATHOLOGY: Adenocarcinomas account for the vast majority of all primary prostatic tumors. They are commonly multicentric and located in the peripheral zones in over 70% of cases. The cut surface of a carcinomatous prostate shows irregular, yellow-white, indurated subcapsular nodules.

HISTOLOGIC FEATURES OF INVASIVE CARCINOMA: Most prostatic adenocarcinomas are of acinar origin and feature small to medium-sized glands that lack organization and infiltrate the stroma. Well-differentiated tumors show uniform medium-sized or small glands (Fig. 23-44) lined by

GLANDS

	Differentiation	Distribution
1	'Round,' lined by single layer of cuboidal cells	Close packed in rounded masses; definite edge
2	More variable in size and shape	Separated up to one gland diameter; 'loose' edge
3a	Irregular shape; medium to large size	Irregularly spaced apart; poorly defined 'edge'; surround normal strucutres
3b	Small to minute glands, not fused or 'chained'	
3c	Masses of cribriform or papillary epithelium with smooth outer surfaces	Very irregular spacing and distribution; no 'edge'; surround normal structures
4a	Ragged masses of fused glandular epithelium; bare tumor cells in stroma	Ragged infiltrating masses that overrun normal structures; No smooth surfaces against stroma
4b	Same as 4a; large clear cells	
5a	Smooth, cribriform to solid masses; often central necrosis 'comedocarcinoma'	Ragged infiltrating masses that infiltrate stromal fibers
5b	Anaplastic carcinoma with vacuoles and glands that suggest adenocarcinoma	

FIGURE 23-44. Prostatic carcinoma. Gleason grading system.

THE LOWER URINARY TRACT

a single layer of neoplastic epithelial cells. Malignant acini have no basal cells and no longer grow in lobular patterns. Progressive loss of differentiation of prostatic adenocarcinomas is characterized by:

- Increasing variability of gland size and configuration.
- Papillary and cribriform patterns.
- Rudimentary (or no) gland formation, with only solid cords of infiltrating tumor cells. Uncommonly, a prostate cancer is composed of small undifferentiated cells growing individually or in sheets, without evidence of any structural organization.

CYTOLOGIC FEATURES: The prominence of pleomorphic and hyperchromatic nuclei is highly variable. One or two conspicuous nucleoli in a background of chromatin clumped near the nuclear membrane is the most frequent nuclear feature. The cytoplasm stains slightly eosinophilic or may be so vacuolated that it simulates clear cells of renal cell carcinoma. Cell borders are distinct in better-differentiated tumors but are not well demarcated in poorly differentiated ones.

GRADING: Prostatic adenocarcinoma is most commonly classified according to the **Gleason grading system** (Figs. 23-44 and 23-45), which is based on five histologic patterns of tumor gland formation and infiltration. Recognizing the high frequency of mixed tumor patterns, the Gleason score is the sum of the grades (1 through 5) attributed to the most prominent pattern and that of the minority pattern. The best-differentiated tumors have Gleason scores of 2 (1 + 1), while the most poorly differentiated cancers score 10 (5 + 5). Gleason patterns 1 and 2 are rare. The most commonly diagnosed Gleason pattern is 3. Combined with tumor stage, Gleason grading has prognostic value: lower scores correlate with better prognoses.

INVASION AND METASTASIS: The high frequency of invasion of the prostatic capsule by adenocarcinoma reflects the tumor's subcapsular site of origin. Perineural tumor invasion within the prostate and in adjacent tissues is usual. Since peripheral nerves are devoid of perineural lymphatic channels, this mode of invasion represents contiguous spread of the tumor along a tissue space that offers a plane of low resistance.

The seminal vesicles are almost always involved by direct extension of prostate cancer. Invasion of the urinary bladder tends to occur later in the clinical course. The earliest metastases occur in the obturator lymph nodes, and then to iliac and periaortic lymph nodes. Metastases to the lung reflect further lymphatic spread through the thoracic duct and dissemination from the prostatic venous plexus to the inferior vena cava. Bony metastases, particularly to the vertebral column (Fig. 23-46), ribs and pelvic bones, are painful and difficult to manage.

 CLINICAL FEATURES: Current screening programs for prostate cancer use digital rectal examination in combination with serum PSA levels. PSA is a glycoprotein produced by the prostate. It is a serine protease involved in liquifying seminal ejaculate. It maintains a baseline serum level in men. Serum levels are increased by prostate inflammation, hypertrophy and neoplasia. Patients with elevated serum PSA levels are typically evaluated further by needle biopsies. *Preoperative PSA levels correlate with cancer volume.* Since most prostate cancers are asymptomatic, PSA screening is the most common detection method. Uncommonly, patients with prostate cancer present with

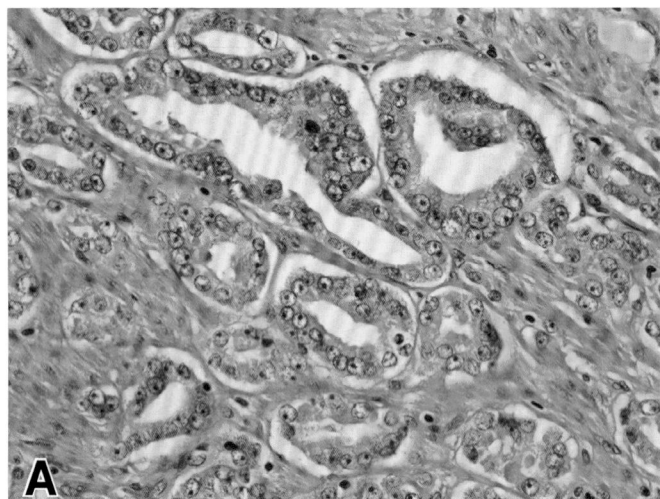

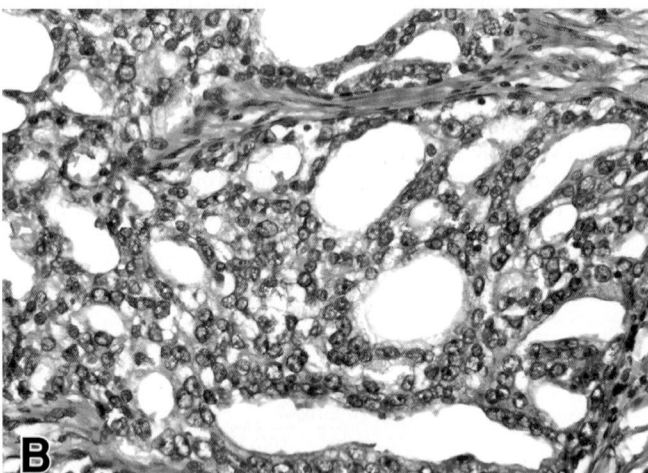

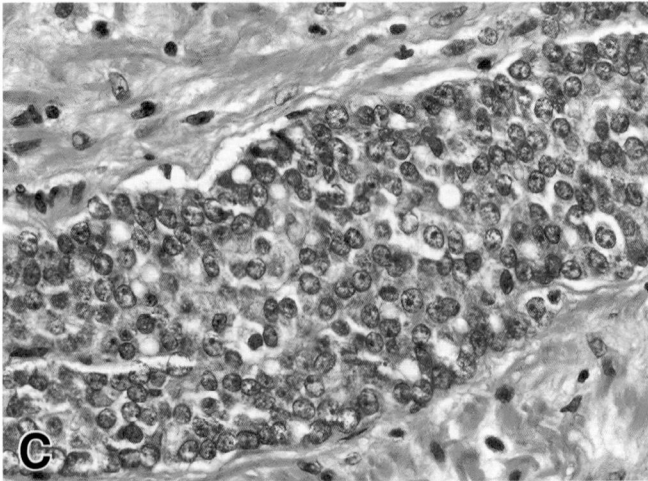

FIGURE 23-45. Gleason grading system. A. Gleason grade 1. **B.** Gleason grade 3. **C.** Gleason grade 5.

bladder outlet obstruction or symptoms referable to metastatic tumor.

At present, guidelines for prostate cancer screening are in flux. Widespread screening leads to more cancer diagnoses and treatment. With treatment come side effects and quality-of-life issues. Given that several large epidemiologic

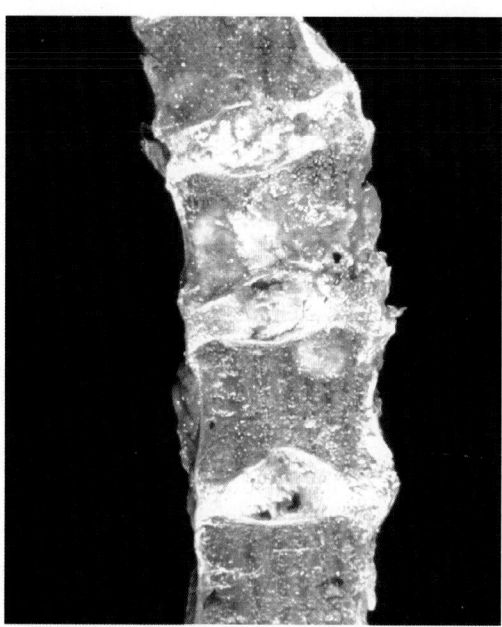

FIGURE 23-46. Prostatic carcinoma metastatic to the spine. The vertebral bodies contain several osteoblastic metastases.

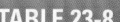

TABLE 23-8
TNM STAGING OF PROSTATIC CARCINOMA
T—Primary Tumor
T1 No clinically detectable tumor
T1a Histologic tumor found in 5% or less of tissue examined
T1b Histologic tumor found in more than 5% of tissue examined
T2 Tumor confined to the prostate
T2a Tumor in one lobe only
T2b Tumor in both lobes
T3 Tumor extends through the capsule
T3a Extracapsular extension only
T3b Tumor extends into seminal vesicles
T4 Tumor invades adjacent structures other than seminal vesicles
N—Regional Lymph Nodes
N0 No regional lymph node involvement
N1 Regional lymph node metastases present
M—Distant Metastases
M0 No distant metastases
M1 Distant metastases present

studies report conflicting results with regard to the benefit of active prostate cancer therapy, the high frequency of side effects that occur with aggressive screening and treatment (e.g., incontinence, impotence) cannot be ignored. To this end, the U.S. Preventive Service Task Force (USPSTF) was convened to examine the relevant published literature. It concluded that there was insufficient evidence to recommend routine prostate cancer screening (and, by default, therapy). This position remains controversial. Other national organizations such as the American College of Physicians and the American Urological Association have adopted less extreme guidelines, recommending individualized patient evaluation and selective screening.

The principles of clinical staging (TNM) of prostate cancer are shown in Fig. 23-47 and Table 23-8. At initial presentation, 10% of prostate cancers are stage T1. In patients with

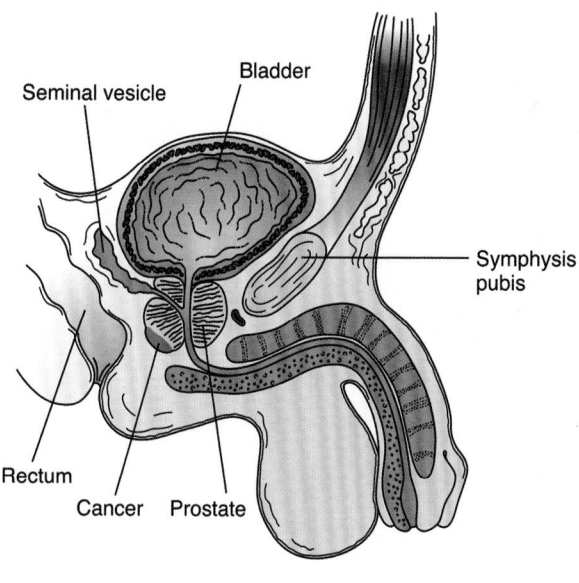

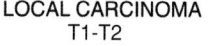

LOCAL CARCINOMA
T1-T2

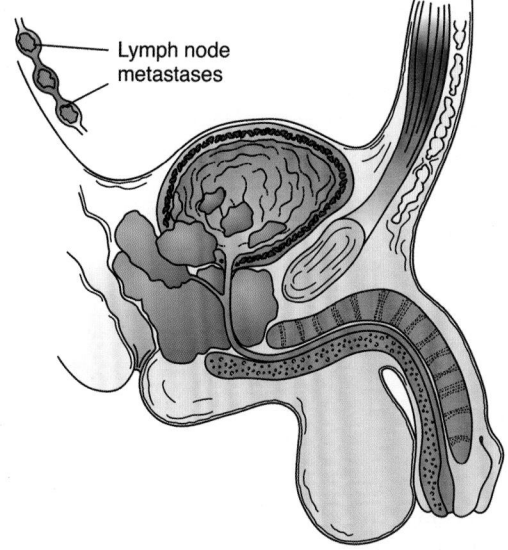

EXTENSIVE CARCINOMA
T3-T4

FIGURE 23-47. Staging of prostatic carcinoma. Tumor–node–metastasis (TNM) system is most widely used for staging of prostate carcinoma. Stage T1 and T2 tumors are localized to the prostate, whereas stage T3 and T4 tumors have spread outside the prostate.

tumors clinically judged to be localized to the prostate (stage T2), 60% show microscopic evidence of capsular penetration or seminal vesicle invasion (stage T3). Metastases are found in lymph nodes, bones, lung and liver, in order of decreasing frequency. Widespread tumor dissemination (carcinomatosis), with pneumonia or sepsis, is the most common cause of death.

The immunohistochemical demonstration of **PSA** in metastatic tumors is useful in identifying the prostate as the primary site of a tumor. PSA is also detectable in the serum of patients with prostate cancer. A rising serum PSA level is an indicator of recurrent disease after therapy. A new marker for prostate carcinoma, **α-methylacyl-CoA racemase** (AMCAR), is also useful for identifying prostatic adenocarcinoma inside the gland as well as in metastatic sites. **Serum alkaline phosphatase** levels are elevated in patients with osteoblastic bony metastases, because this enzyme is released from osteoblasts that are forming new bone at a site of metastasis.

Therapy for prostate cancer is highly controversial, owing to recent studies that suggest that many tumors may best be left alone and considerable difficulty in distinguishing between the tumors that are likely to benefit from treatment and those that are not. However, treatment generally depends on tumor stage. Patients with stage T1 and T2 cancers are treated by radical prostatectomy, radiofrequency ablation, cryogenic procedures or radiation therapy. Radiation therapy may be either external beam or implanted radioactive seeds (brachytherapy). In stage T3 tumors, radiation therapy, combined with androgen deprivation therapy, is the treatment of choice, acknowledging that half of these patients have occult pelvic lymph node metastases (and possibly further systemic dissemination), which cannot be cured by surgical means. Patients with low-grade, low-volume tumors may opt to be managed by active surveillance only.

For patients with metastatic disease or whose tumors progress clinically, traditional chemotherapy combined with androgen deprivation is the main strategy. Bone metastases can be treated using local radiation, bisphosphonates and supplements of calcium and vitamin D.

The 5-year survival rates depend on stage and Gleason grade (Fig. 23-44). Using staging data, survival is as follows: stages T1 and T2, 90%; stage T3, 40%; and stage T4, 10%.

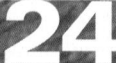
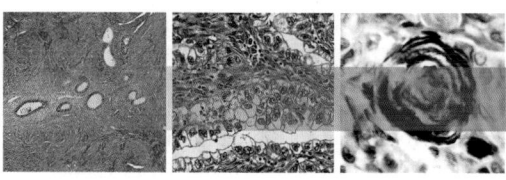

The Female Reproductive System and Peritoneum

George L. Mutter ▪ Jaime Prat

EMBRYOLOGY

The gonadal anlage forms as a swelling of the embryonic urogenital ridge, initially in an indifferent state. The gonad is derived from mesoderm except for the germ cells, which are of extraembryonic (yolk sac) origin. Both sex chromosomes and autosomal chromosomes determine whether gonadal stromal cells will differentiate into testis or ovary. If the gonadal stroma is male, a gene on the Y chromosome (sex-determining region Y [SRY]) interacts with the primitive gonad to initiate development of a testis. An ovary develops if gonadal stroma is female and there is no stimulus to form a testis. Ovaries and testes become histologically distinct by about day 40.

Wolffian (mesonephric) ducts begin to develop at about day 25, regardless of the embryo's sex. If stimulated by testosterone (secreted by Leydig cells starting about day 70), the ducts differentiate into vas deferens, epididymis and seminal vesicle. If not stimulated by day 84, the ducts regress and remain as vestigial rests in the female. They may form cysts in the cervix or vagina **(mesonephric cyst)**.

Müllerian (paramesonephric) ducts, the anlage of the fallopian tubes, uterus and vaginal wall, appear at about day 37 as funnel-shaped openings of celomic epithelium. They develop into paired, undifferentiated tubes, using the wolffian ducts as "guide wires" to reach the area of the future hymen. If a wolffian duct is absent, as in renal agenesis, the vagina and cervix are almost always abnormal or absent. At day 54, müllerian ducts fuse into a straight uterovaginal canal.

A central tenet of genital tract development in both sexes is that müllerian tubes develop along female lines unless specifically impeded by embryonic testicular factors. In males, Sertoli cells in developing testes produce **antimüllerian hormone,** also called **müllerian-inhibiting substance,** which causes müllerian ducts to regress.

External genitalia assume masculine form if testosterone is converted locally to dihydrotestosterone. Otherwise (i.e., relative estrogen excess), female external genitalia persist. The genital tubercle develops into the clitoris, genital folds into the labia minora and genital swellings into the labia majora. The basic layout of the female genital tract is established by day 120.

GENITAL INFECTIONS

Genital Infections Are Commonly Sexually Transmitted

Infectious diseases of the female genital tract are common and are caused by many organisms (Table 24-1; also see Chapter 9). Most of the important infectious diseases of the female genital tract are sexually transmitted.

Bacterial Infections

Gonorrhea

Gonorrhea is caused by *Neisseria gonorrhoeae,* a fastidious, gram-negative diplococcus. A million cases of gonorrhea occur yearly in the United States. The infection is a frequent cause of acute salpingitis and pelvic inflammatory disease (PID) (Fig. 24-1).

 **ETIOLOGIC FACTORS AND PATHOLOGY:** The organisms ascend through the cervix and endometrial cavity, where they cause **acute endometritis.** They then attach to mucosal cells in the fallopian tube and elicit acute inflammation, which is confined to the mucosal surface **(acute salpingitis).** Infection may then spread to the ovary, sometimes causing a **tubo-ovarian abscess.** Pelvic and abdominal cavities may be affected, leading to subdiaphragmatic and pelvic abscesses.

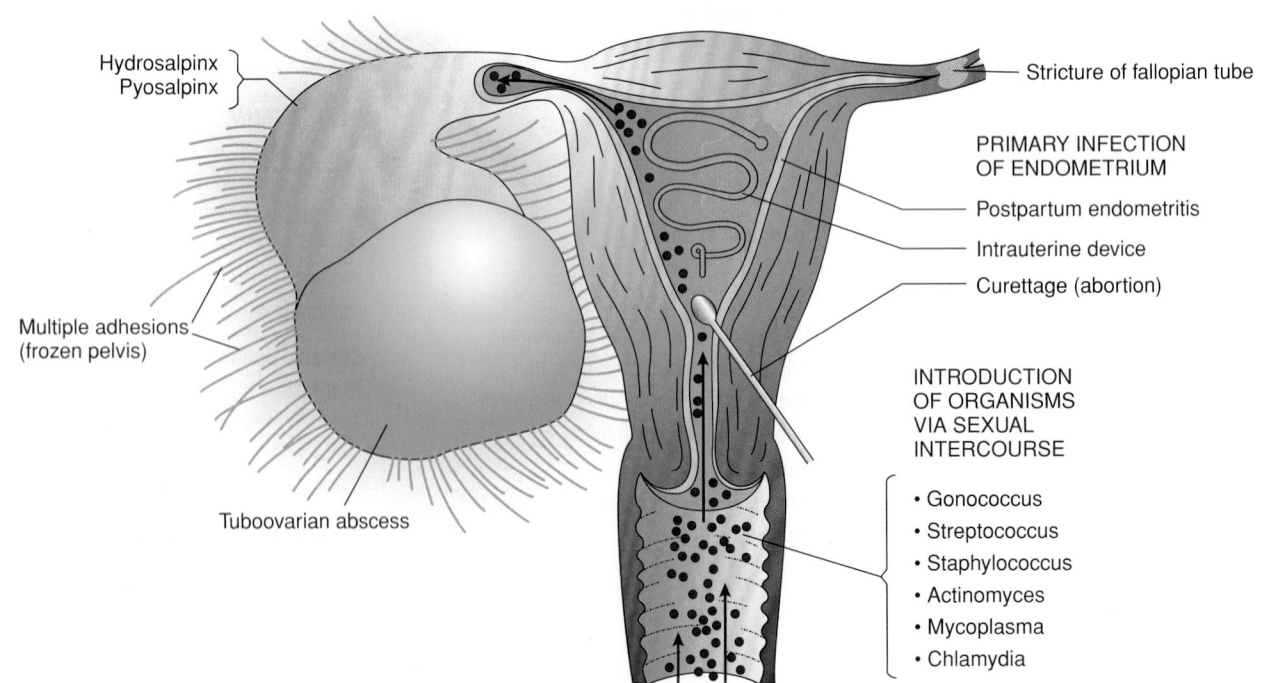

FIGURE 24-1. Pelvic inflammatory disease.

TABLE 24-1

INFECTIOUS DISEASES OF THE FEMALE GENITAL TRACT

Organism	Disease	Diagnostic Feature
Sexually Transmitted Diseases		
Gram-negative rods and cocci		
Calymmatobacterium granulomatis	*Granuloma inguinale*	Donovan body
Gardnerella vaginalis	*Gardnerella infection*	Clue cell
Haemophilus ducreyi	Chancroid (soft chancre)	
Neisseria gonorrhoeae	Gonorrhea	Gram-negative diplococcus
Spirochetes		
Treponema pallidum	Syphilis	Spirochete
Mycoplasmas		
Mycoplasma hominis	Nonspecific vaginitis	
Ureaplasma urealyticum	Nonspecific vaginitis	
Rickettsiae		
Chlamydia trachomatis types D–K	Various forms of pelvic inflammatory disease (PID)	
Chlamydia trachomatis type L_{1-3}	Lymphogranuloma venereum	
Viruses		
Human papillomavirus (HPV)	Condyloma acuminatum/planum Neoplastic potential	Koilocyte
Types 6, 11, 40, 42, 43, 44, 57	Low risk	Low-grade squamous intraepithelial lesion (LSIL)
Types 16, 18, 31, 33, 35, 39, 45, 51, 52, 56, 58, 66	High risk	High-grade squamous intraepithelial lesion (HSIL)
Herpes simplex type 2	Herpes genitalis	Multinucleated giant cell with intranuclear homogenization and inclusion bodies
Cytomegalovirus (CMV)	Cytomegalic inclusion disease	Bulbous intranuclear inclusion body
Molluscum contagiosum	Molluscum infection	Molluscum body
Protozoa		
Trichomonas vaginalis	Trichomoniasis	Trichomonad
Selected Nonsexually Transmitted Diseases		
Actinomyces and related organisms		
Actinomyces israelii	PID (one of many organisms)	Sulphur granules
Mycobacterium tuberculosis	Tuberculosis	Necrotizing granulomas
Fungi		
Candida albicans	Candidiasis	*Candida* sp.

Systemic complications of gonorrhea include septicemia and septic arthritis. At all sites of infection, the organisms induce purulent inflammatory reactions that rarely resolve completely. Dense fibrous adhesions often remain, distorting and destroying the plicae of the fallopian tube and frequently leading to sterility.

Syphilis

Syphilis (see Chapter 9) is caused by *Treponema pallidum,* a thin, motile spirochete. Spread is via sexual contact with an infected person or transplacental spread (congenital syphilis). *T. pallidum* penetrates small cuts in the skin or normal mucosal surfaces. Untreated, syphilis persists, often waxing and waning, through three stages.

- In the **primary stage,** a **chancre** usually appears after about 3 weeks at the portal of bacterial entry. It is a painless, indurated papule, 1 cm to several centimeters in diameter, surrounded by an inflammatory cuff that breaks down to form an ulcer. The lesion may persist for 2–6 weeks. It then heals spontaneously.
- **Secondary syphilis** appears after a latent period of several weeks to months and features low-grade fever, headache, malaise, lymphadenopathy and highly infectious lesions called **condylomata lata** (syphilitic warts). These secondary lesions heal after 2–6 weeks and symptoms disappear spontaneously.
- The **tertiary stage** develops any time thereafter and may entail severe damage to the cardiovascular and nervous systems.

 PATHOLOGY: The hallmark of syphilis in biopsy specimens is a dense inflammatory infiltrate with lymphocytes and plasma cells, particularly adjacent to blood vessels. Silver impregnation techniques (Warthin-Starry stain or its modifications) help demonstrate the spirochetes. The more advanced stages of disease show greater obliterative endarteritis and subsequent tissue destruction.

Granuloma Inguinale

Granuloma inguinale is caused by *Calymmatobacterium granulomatis,* a sexually transmitted, gram-negative, encapsulated rod. The disease occurs with equal frequency in women and men.

 PATHOLOGY: The primary lesion begins as a painless, ulcerated nodule involving genital, inguinal or perianal skin. The organisms invade through skin abrasions and spread initially by direct extension, destroying skin and underlying tissues. Extensive local spread and lymphatic permeation occur later. Vacuolated macrophages teem with characteristic intracellular bacteria **(Donovan bodies).** The organism, best seen with the Wright stain, resembles a closed safety pin. Hyperplasia of overlying squamous epithelium may be exuberant enough to be misinterpreted as a squamous cell carcinoma. Relapses after antibiotic therapy are common.

Chancroid

Chancroid, also called **soft chancre,** is caused by *Haemophilus ducreyi,* a gram-negative bacillus. It is rare in the United States but is common in underdeveloped countries.

 PATHOLOGY: Single or sometimes multiple small, vesiculopustular lesions appear on the cervix, vagina, vulva or perianal region 3–5 days after sexual contact with an infected partner. At this stage examination shows granulomatous inflammation. The lesion may rupture to form a painful, purulent ulcer that bleeds easily. Inguinal lymphadenopathy, fever, chills and malaise may occur. A major complication is scarring during the healing phase, which may cause urethral stenosis.

Gardnerella

Sexual transmission of *Gardnerella vaginalis,* a gram-negative coccobacillus, causes many cases of "nonspecific vaginitis." Since the organism does not penetrate the mucosa, it causes no inflammation and biopsies appear normal. A wet mount specimen of a vaginal discharge or a Papanicolaou-stained smear (Pap smear) can identify the bacteria. **Clue cells,** squamous cells covered by coccobacilli, are pathognomonic.

Mycoplasma

Mycoplasmas (see Chapter 9) are minute pleomorphic organisms that resemble the so-called L bacterial forms but differ by having no cell wall. They are common oropharyngeal and urogenital tract commensals and colonize the lower genital tract through sexual contact. *Ureaplasma urealyticum* can be isolated from the lower genital tract in 40% of healthy women. It may cause infertility and lead to adverse effects on pregnancy and perinatal infections. *Mycoplasma hominis* is found in the lower genital tract of 5% of healthy women and causes a small proportion of cases of symptomatic cervicitis and vaginitis. *M. hominis* is often isolated in association with *G. vaginalis* or *Trichomonas vaginalis* infection. Although the role of mycoplasma in genital tract infections is not completely understood, the organisms are encountered in PID, acute salpingitis, spontaneous abortion and puerperal fever. Affected tissue is usually unremarkable histologically.

Chlamydia Infections

Chlamydia trachomatis is a common, venereally transmitted gram-negative obligate intracellular rickettsia. Fifteen serotypes are known. *C. trachomatis* causes several disorders in women, men and infants. It has been found in the genital tracts of about 8% of asymptomatic women and 20% of women with symptoms of lower genital tract infection. Chlamydial disease is easily confused with gonorrhea, as the symptoms of both diseases are similar.

 PATHOLOGY: Serotypes D through K cause the more common genital infections. Cervical mucosa is severely inflamed, and endocervical and metaplastic squamous cells contain small inclusion bodies. Cytologically, perinuclear intracytoplasmic inclusions with distinct borders and intracytoplasmic **coccoid bodies** are seen. Complications include ascending infection of the endometrium, fallopian tube and ovary, which may result in tubal occlusion and infertility. Chlamydia may also infect Bartholin glands and cause acute urethritis. Infants delivered vaginally to infected mothers may develop conjunctivitis, otitis media and pneumonia.

Lymphogranuloma Venereum

Lymphogranuloma venereum is a venereal infection of men and women, endemic in tropical countries. It is caused by the L form of *C. trachomatis,* serotypes L1 through L3.

PATHOLOGY: After a few days to a month, a small painless vesicle forms at the site of inoculation. It heals rapidly and often is not even noticed. In the second stage, inguinal lymph nodes become enlarged and may rupture to form suppurative fistulas. Perirectal lymph nodes in women become matted and painful. In untreated patients, a third stage may appear after latency lasting several years. In this phase, scarring causes lymphatic obstruction, resulting in genital elephantiasis and rectal strictures. Infected tissues in the second and third stages show necrotizing granulomas and neutrophil infiltrates. Inclusion bodies within macrophages may also be seen.

Viral Infections

Human Papillomavirus

Human papillomavirus (HPV) is a DNA virus that infects genital skin and mucosal surfaces to produce wart-like lesions referred to as **condylomata acuminatum** or flat lesions known as **squamous intraepithelial lesions (SILs)**. Over 100 HPV serotypes are known, one third of which cause genital tract lesions. The median time from infection to first detection of HPV is 3 months. In the United States, as many as 2/3 of women graduating college have genital HPV infections, which result from sexual contact with an infected person. Even in women who have had only one sexual partner, the risk of cervical HPV by 3 years after first intercourse is 50%. HPV prevalence among women 14–59 years old exceeds 25%. About 20 million people are currently infected with HPV in this country; serotypes 6 and 11 account for over 80% of visible condylomata.

Several strains of HPV are the major etiologic factors for squamous cell cancer in the female lower genital tract, as well as anal and oropharyngeal cancers in both sexes. Types 16, 18, 31 and 45 are most often linked to squamous intraepithelial neoplasia and invasive cancer (see below). Vaccines to prevent infection with high-risk HPV serotypes 6, 11, 16 and 18 have been available since 2006 and are the reason for the lower infection rates in teenage girls.

Most cases of HPV are diagnosed by cervical Pap smear. Recent tests directly detect HPV DNA. Treatment is based on the histology of lesions (low vs. high grade), which predicts those at greatest risk for progression to carcinoma.

 PATHOLOGY: Lesions in the vulva, perianal region, perineum, vagina and cervix caused by HPV infection are separated into low and high grades based on the appearance of the affected epithelium, which may be flat or exophytic. The warty form of low-grade squamous intraepithelial lesion (LSIL) is known as condylomata acuminatum. Acuminate warts are generally caused by low-cancer-risk viral subtypes and may present as papules, plaques or nodules, which eventually become spiked or cauliflower-like excrescences (Fig. 24-2A). LSIL is characterized by koilocytes (from the Greek *koilos*, "hollow"), epithelial cells with a perinuclear halo and a wrinkled nucleus bearing HPV particles (Fig. 24-2B). Viral DNA typically remains episomal. Extensive virus replication causes cytoplasmic injury, creating koilocytes (Fig. 24-2C). High-grade squamous intraepithelial lesions (HSILs) are discussed below.

Herpesvirus

Herpes simplex type 2 is a very large double-stranded DNA virus that commonly causes sexually transmitted genital infections. After an incubation period of 1–3 weeks, small vesicles develop on the vulva and erode into painful ulcers. Similar lesions occur in the vagina and cervix. Epithelial cells adjacent to intraepithelial vesicles show ballooning degeneration and many contain large nuclei with eosinophilic viral inclusions.

Herpesvirus infections follow relapsing, remitting courses. While latent, the virus resides in spinal (sacral) ganglia. If it reactivates during pregnancy, passage through the birth canal may transmit the virus to the newborn infant, often with fatal consequences. Active vaginal herpetic lesions at the time of delivery are therefore an indication for Cesarean section.

Cytomegalovirus

Cytomegalovirus (CMV) is a ubiquitous double-stranded DNA virus of the *Herpesvirus* family. More than 80% of people over the age of 35 have antibodies to CMV. Several lines of evidence suggest that many cases are sexually transmitted: (1) seroprevalence of CMV has risen in young adults, (2) the virus is recovered more often from cervical secretions and semen than from any other body sites and (3) viral titers in semen are 100,000 times higher than in urine. Still, CMV only rarely causes genital infections in women. Infection in the endometrium may result in spontaneous abortion or infection of the newborn. Infected cells exhibit characteristic large, eosinophilic, intranuclear inclusions and, occasionally, cytoplasmic inclusions.

Molluscum Contagiosum

Molluscum contagiosum (see Chapter 28) is a highly contagious double-stranded DNA poxvirus. Infection leads to multiple smooth, gray-white nodules that are centrally umbilicated and exude a cheesy material. Lesions occur predominantly in the genital region but may be found elsewhere as well. Large, cytoplasmic viral inclusions **(molluscum bodies)** are seen in infected epithelial cells. Most lesions regress spontaneously, but untreated ones may persist for years.

Trichomoniasis

T. vaginalis is a large, pear-shaped, flagellated protozoan that often causes vaginitis. It is transmitted sexually, and 25% of infected women are asymptomatic carriers. Infection causes a heavy, yellow-gray, thick, foamy discharge with severe itching, dyspareunia (painful intercourse) and dysuria (painful urination). The motile trichomonads are identified on wet mount preparations and may also be demonstrated in Pap smears.

Pelvic Inflammatory Disease

PID is infection of pelvic organs due to extension of one of several microorganisms above the uterine corpus (Fig. 24-1). Ascending infection results in bilateral acute salpingitis, pyosalpinx and tuboovarian abscesses. **N. gonorrhoeae *and* Chlamydia *are the main organisms responsible for PID, but most infections are polymicrobial.* PID is less common in monogamous women than in others. Occasionally, it occurs after postpartum endometritis or as a complication of endometrial curettage.

 CLINICAL FEATURES: Patients with PID typically present with lower abdominal pain. Physical examination reveals bilateral adnexal tenderness

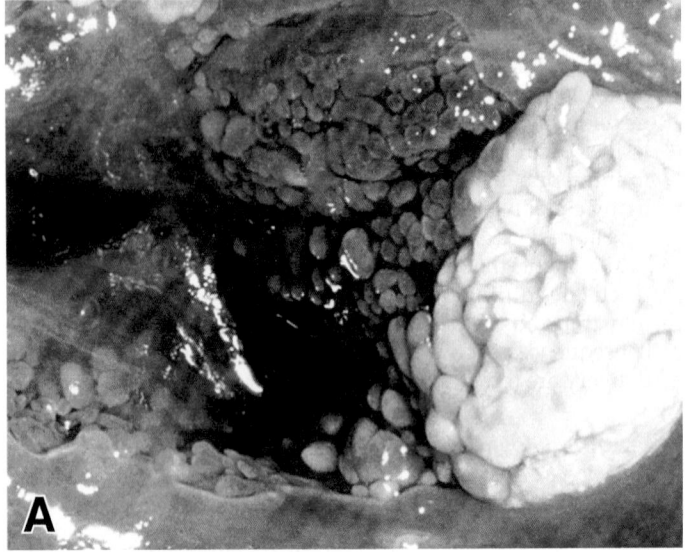

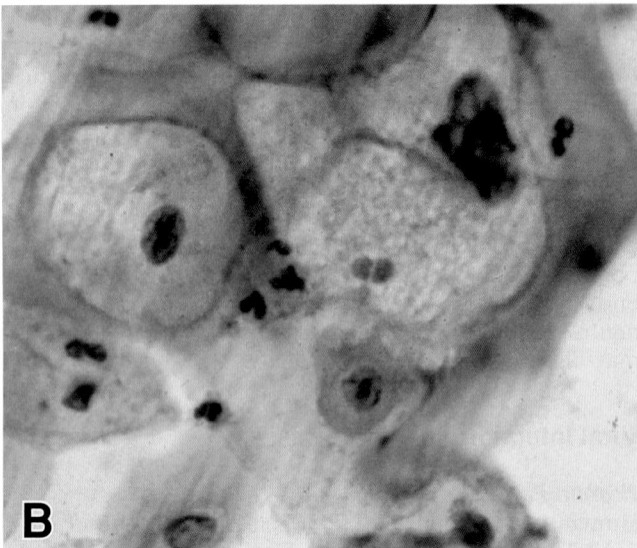

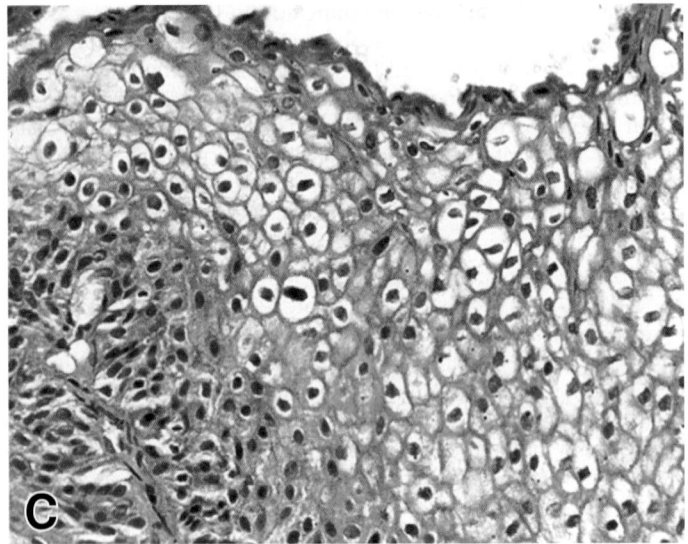

FIGURE 24-2. Human papillomavirus-induced condylomatous infections. A. Condyloma acuminatum on the cervix, visible with the naked eye as cauliflower-like excrescences. **B.** A cervical smear contains characteristic koilocytes, with a perinuclear halo and a wrinkled nucleus that contains viral particles. **C.** Biopsy of the condyloma shows koilocytes with perinuclear halos and significant nuclear pleomorphism and altered chromatin density.

and marked discomfort when the cervix is manipulated (chandelier sign). Complications of PID include (1) rupture of a tuboovarian abscess, which may result in life-threatening peritonitis; (2) infertility from scarring of the healed tubal plicae; (3) increased rates of ectopic pregnancy; and (4) intestinal obstruction from fibrous bands and adhesions.

Some Genital Infections Are Not Transmitted Sexually

Tuberculosis

Mycobacterium tuberculosis may infect any part of the female genital tract. Genital tuberculosis occurs in 1% of infertile women in the United States and in over 10% of such women in less developed countries. Detecting acid-fast bacilli (AFB) confirms the diagnosis.

PATHOLOGY:
TUBERCULOUS SALPINGITIS: Salpingitis is usually the initial lesion of tuberculous genital infection,

due to hematogenous dissemination from the respiratory tract. Tuberculous salpingitis results in fibrinous adhesions and scarring of the fallopian tube. These complications lead to multiple functional abnormalities (e.g., infertility, ectopic gestation, pelvic pain). The tubes may become nodular. **Pyosalpinx** (fallopian tube distended with pus) and **hydrosalpinx** (fluid-filled tube) are late sequelae, and the adjacent ovary may become infected.

TUBERCULOUS ENDOMETRITIS: Endometritis complicates half the cases of tuberculous salpingitis. Noncaseating, poorly formed granulomas with rare giant cells are typical. Although the endometrium may show well-formed granulomas with caseous necrosis and characteristic Langhans giant cells, menstrual shedding limits the time during which such mature granulomas may develop.

Candidiasis

Ten percent of women are asymptomatic carriers of fungi in the vulva and vagina, *Candida albicans* being the most common offender. Only 2% present with clinically apparent candidal vulvovaginitis, although the risk is greatly increased by diabetes mellitus, oral contraceptive use and pregnancy. Infection causes vulvar itching and a white discharge. Clinical examination reveals firmly adherent, small white plaques on mucous membranes ("thrush"). Biopsy shows submucosal edema and chronic inflammation. The fungi do not penetrate epithelium; the white patches are foci of desquamated, necrotic epithelial cells containing cellular debris; bacterial flora; candidal spores; and pseudohyphae. Characteristic spores and pseudohyphae in a wet mount preparation or with a Pap stain are diagnostic. Untreated infections wax and wane and often disappear after delivery.

Actinomycosis

Genital tract actinomycosis is uncommon but is increasingly reported in association with use of intrauterine devices (IUDs). *Actinomyces israelii,* the causative organism, is a gram-positive rod found in 4% of normal genital tracts. It enters the uterine cavity via the tail of the IUD; ascends to the fallopian tube, ovary and broad ligaments; and forms a tuboovarian abscess. Suppurating lesions display drainage tracts that contain dense microcolonies of organisms ("sulfur granules"). Actinomycosis results in extensive fibrosis and scarring of the female genital tract.

Toxic Shock Syndrome Is Due to Vaginal Staphylococcal Infection

Toxic shock syndrome is an acute, sometimes fatal disorder characterized by fever, shock and a desquamative erythematous rash. In addition, vomiting, diarrhea, myalgias, neurologic signs and thrombocytopenia are common. Certain strains of *Staphylococcus aureus* release an exotoxin called **toxic shock syndrome toxin-1,** which impairs the ability of mononuclear phagocytes to clear other potentially toxic substances, such as endotoxin. Pathologic alterations are characteristic of shock, and lesions of disseminated intravascular coagulation are usually prominent. Toxic shock syndrome was first recognized when long-acting tampons were introduced, allowing sufficient time for the staphylococci to proliferate. Contraceptive "sponges" were also associated. The incidence of toxic shock syndrome has decreased markedly since recognition of the role of tampons in promoting colonization of the vagina by *S. aureus.*

Vulva

ANATOMY

The vulva is composed of the mons pubis, labia majora and minora, clitoris and vestibule. At puberty, the mons pubis and lateral borders of the labia majora acquire increased subcutaneous fat and grow coarse hair. Sebaceous and apocrine glands in these regions develop concomitantly. The paired external openings of the paraurethral glands **(Skene glands)** flank the urethral meatus. **Bartholin glands,** just posterolateral to the introitus, are branching, mucus-secreting, tubuloalveolar glands drained by a short duct

lined by transitional epithelium. In addition, microscopic mucous glands are scattered throughout the area bounded by the labia minora. Inguinal and femoral lymph nodes provide primary lymph drainage routes, except for the clitoris (the homolog of the penis), which shares the lymphatic drainage of the urethra.

DEVELOPMENTAL ANOMALIES AND CYSTS

ECTOPIC BREAST TISSUE: Small, isolated nodules of ectopic breast tissue may extend in the "milk line" to the vulva and enlarge during pregnancy.

BARTHOLIN DUCT CYST: The paired Bartholin glands produce a clear mucoid secretion that continuously lubricates the vestibular surface. The ducts are prone to obstruction and consequent cyst formation (Fig. 24-3). Cyst infection may lead to **abscess formation**. Bartholin gland abscess was formerly associated with gonorrhea, but staphylococci, chlamydia and anaerobes are now more frequently the cause. Treatment consists of incision, drainage, marsupialization and appropriate antibiotics.

FOLLICULAR CYSTS: Follicular cysts recapitulate the most distal portion of the hair follicle. Also called **epithelial inclusion cysts** or **keratinous cysts,** follicular cysts frequently appear on the vulva, especially the labia majora. They contain a white cheesy material and typically are lined by stratified squamous epithelium.

MUCINOUS CYSTS: Vulvar mucinous glands occasionally become obstructed and develop cysts. Mucinous columnar cells line the cyst and may become infected.

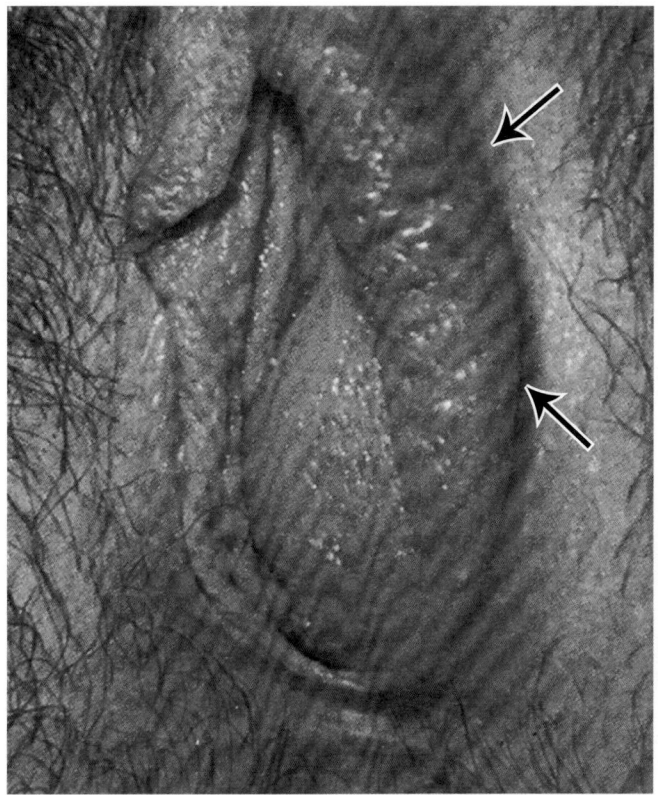

FIGURE 24-3. Bartholin gland cyst. The 4-cm lesion (*arrows*) is posterior to the vaginal introitus.

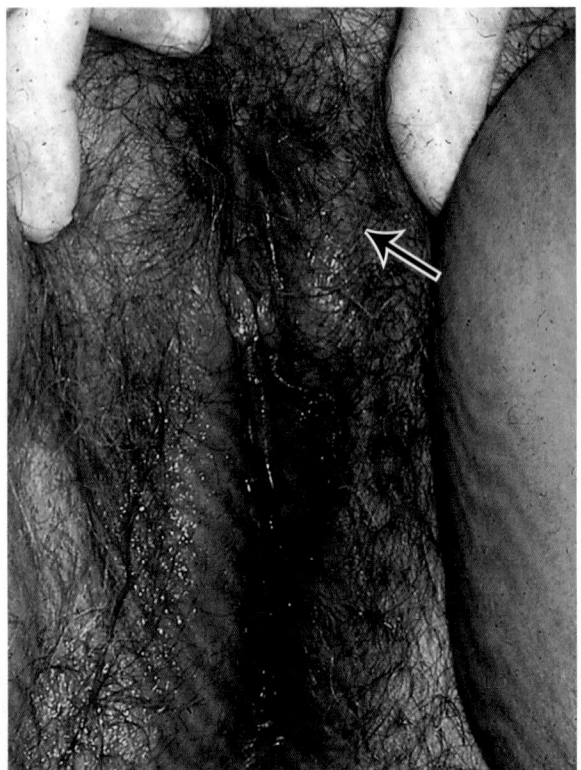

FIGURE 24-4. Vulvar acute dermatitis (eczema). Erythema, edema and weeping vesicles (*arrow*) are present.

DERMATOSES

Vulvar Acute Dermatitis Appears as Reddened Vesiculated Skin

 PATHOLOGY: As vesicles rupture (Fig. 24-4), the fluid forms a crust on the skin surface. The epidermis contains various inflammatory cells, and spongiotic areas form vesicles that rupture to produce the exudative lesions. The dermis shows a perivascular lymphocytic infiltrate and edema, with separation of collagen fibers. Dilated lymphatics and capillaries are typical.

The most common endogenous types of acute dermatitis are **atopic (hypersensitivity) dermatitis** and **seborrheic dermatitis,** seen as a scaly macular eruption. Dermatitides with exogenous causes include irritant dermatitis (e.g., urine on the vulvar skin) and contact allergic dermatitis (type 4 delayed hypersensitivity reaction) and are manifest as either acute or chronic dermatitis.

Chronic Dermatitis, or Lichen Simplex Chronicus, Is the End Stage of Many Vulvar Inflammatory Diseases

Vulvar chronic dermatitis (Fig. 24-5) follows many diseases that are clinically pruritic and thus subject to repeated scratching in their active phase. These include lichen planus, psoriasis and lichen sclerosus (see Chapter 28). The skin is thickened and white with exaggerated markings ("lichenification") as a result of marked hyperkeratosis. Scaling is generally present, and excoriations due to recent scratching are often seen.

LICHEN SCLEROSUS: Lichen sclerosus is an inflammatory disease associated with autoimmune disorders such as vitiligo, pernicious anemia and thyroiditis. Autoimmune etiology of lichen sclerosus is further suggested by the presence of activated T cells in the dermis.

  PATHOLOGY AND CLINICAL FEATURES: The condition is characterized by white plaques and atrophic skin with a parchment-like or crinkled appearance and, occasionally, marked contracture of vulvar tissues (Fig. 24-6A). Hyperkeratosis, loss of rete ridges, epithelial thinning with flattening of rete pegs, cytoplasmic vacuolation of the basal layer and a homogeneous, acellular zone in the upper dermis are seen (Fig. 24-6B). A band of lymphocytes with few plasma cells typically underlies this layer. The disease develops insidiously and is progressive, often causing itching and dyspareunia. Women with symptomatic lichen sclerosus have a 15% chance of developing squamous cell carcinoma.

BENIGN TUMORS

HIDRADENOMA: This benign apocrine sweat gland tumor appears chiefly in the labia majora as a well-circumscribed nodule, rarely larger than 1 cm. Microscopically, it is composed of papillary tubules and acini lined by two layers of cells: an inner layer of apocrine columnar cells and an outer one of myoepithelial cells.

SYRINGOMA: An adenoma of eccrine glands, syringoma manifests as a flesh-colored papule within the dermis of labia majora. This asymptomatic tumor is composed of a proliferation of small ducts embedded in a dense

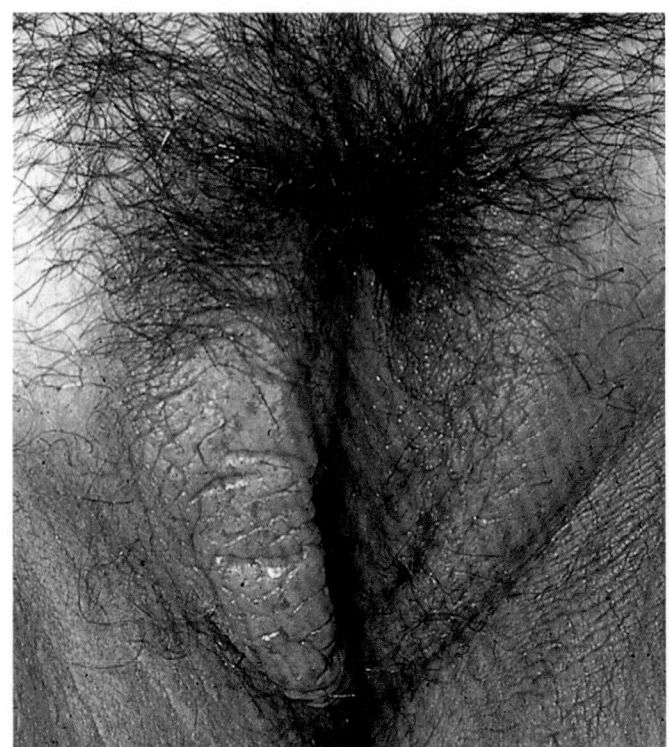

FIGURE 24-5. Lichen simplex chronicus of the right labium majus. There is thickening and accentuation of skin markings, with surface excoriation due to recent scratching.

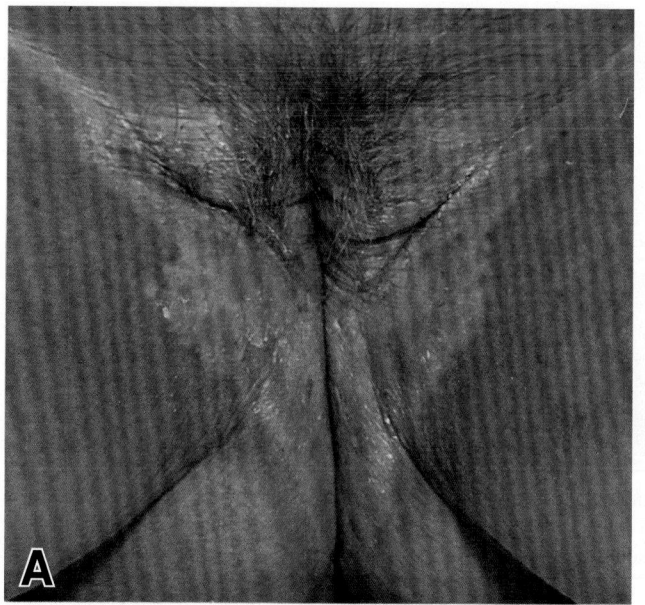
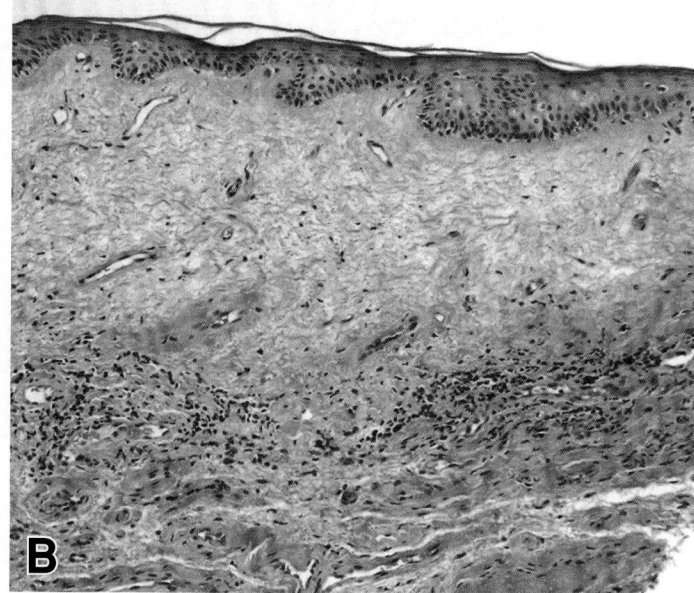

FIGURE 24-6. Lichen sclerosus of vulva. A. The sharply demarcated white lesion affects the vulva and perineum. **B.** The epidermis is thin and exhibits hyperkeratosis and a lack of the normal rete pattern. The dermis displays an acellular, homogeneous zone overlying a mild chronic inflammatory infiltrate.

fibrous stroma (see Chapter 28). Duct walls have two layers of cells: an inner layer of serous cells and an outer one of myoepithelial cells. The lumen contains amorphous eosinophilic material.

CONNECTIVE TISSUE TUMORS: **Senile hemangiomas** (cherry hemangiomas) are small, purple skin papules, which may bleed following surface trauma. **Lobular capillary hemangioma** (formerly called pyogenic granuloma), previously thought to be a reaction to superficial wound infection, is a variant of hemangioma. Secondary infection occurs, as the surface of the lesion is fragile and easily disrupted. Soft tissue tumors found elsewhere in the body also occur in the vulva, including granular cell tumor, leiomyoma, fibroma, lipoma and histiocytoma.

PIGMENTED VULVAR LESIONS: **Lentigo** occurs in about 10% of women and presents as small macules. **Nevi** and **seborrheic keratosis** also occur in this area (Chapter 28).

MALIGNANT TUMORS AND PREMALIGNANT CONDITIONS

Vulvar Intraepithelial Neoplasia Is a Precursor of Invasive Squamous Cell Carcinoma

Vulvar carcinoma, mostly squamous cell carcinoma, accounts for 3% of all female genital cancers and occurs mainly in women over age 60. These tumors are divided into keratinizing squamous cell carcinomas unrelated to HPV (>70% of cases) and warty basaloid carcinomas associated with high-risk HPV (<25% of cases). Classic vulvar intraepithelial neoplasia (VIN) lesions are also known as high-grade vulvar squamous intraepithelial lesions (vulvar HSILs).

 **ETIOLOGIC FACTORS AND CLINICAL FEATURES:** Keratinizing squamous carcinomas frequently develop in older women (mean age, 76 years), sometimes in the

context of long-standing lichen sclerosus. The precursor lesion is called **differentiated vulvar intraepithelial neoplasia (dVIN)** (Fig. 24-7A), which carries a high risk of cancer development. Carcinomas develop as nodules or masses in a background of "leukoplakia" (*white plaques,* a nonspecific, descriptive term). Cases of lichen sclerosus, differentiated VIN and invasive squamous cell carcinoma with identical p53 gene mutations have been reported. p53 gene mutation, however, is an uncommon late event in vulvar carcinogenesis.

By contrast, the less common HPV-associated warty and basaloid carcinomas develop from a precursor lesion called **classic VIN** (Fig. 24-7B). Since 1980, there has been a 5–10-fold increase in classic VIN in women under age 40, typically related to **HPV 16**. HPV-associated VIN lesions have a low risk of progression to invasive carcinomas (6%), except in older or immunosuppressed women. Lesions associated with oncogenic HPV types generally demonstrate activated p16. Women with VIN may have squamous neoplasms similar to VIN elsewhere in the lower genital tract.

 PATHOLOGY: VIN reflects a spectrum of neoplastic changes from minimal to severe cellular atypia with differing pathogenesis as described above. These lesions may be single or multiple, and macular, papular or plaque-like. Histologic grades of VIN I, II and III correspond to mild, moderate and severe dysplasia, respectively. However, grade III (which includes squamous cell carcinoma in situ [CIS]) is by far the most common. Differentiated VIN shows severe nuclear atypia of the basal layer with striking epithelial maturation in the superficial layers (Fig. 24-7A). Keratinocytes of the latter contain rounded nuclei with enlarged nucleoli and ample eosinophilic cytoplasm with prominent intercellular bridges. Rete pegs often contain keratin pearls.

Terminology for HPV-related lesions has recently been standardized throughout the anogenital tract along the lines

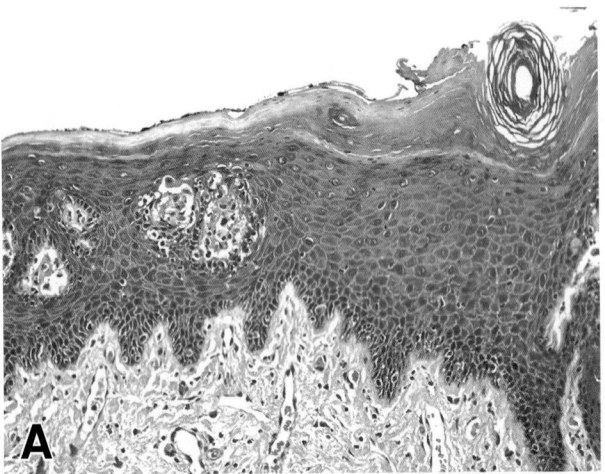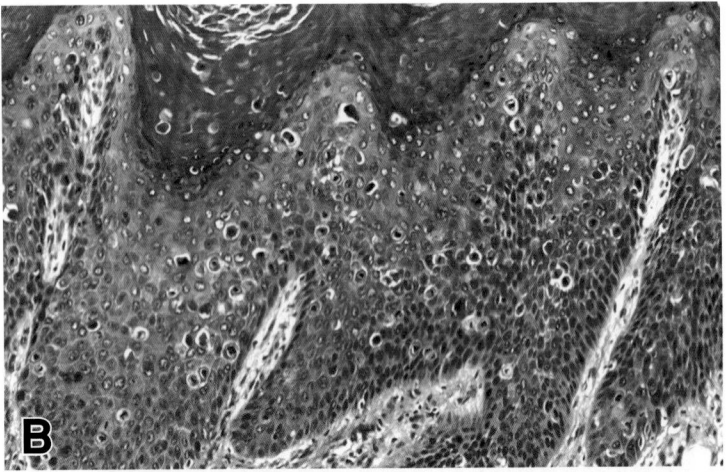

FIGURE 24-7. Vulvar intraepithelial neoplasia (VIN). A. Differentiated VIN is not associated with human papillomavirus (HPV) and demonstrates atypia accentuated in the basal and parabasal layers. There is striking epithelial maturation in the superficial layers. **B.** Classic VIN is caused by HPV and includes features of full-thickness atypia, numerous mitoses and often, as in this example, hyperkeratosis.

of what has been applied to the cervix: LSIL and HSIL. This has not been adopted universally, and there is the additional complication that most vulvar squamous precancerous lesions are not HPV related (differentiated VIN). In the vulva, LSILs include acuminate warts and bland flat lesions that may only have rare diagnostic koilocytes. As in comparable lesions in the cervix (see below), criteria used in establishing the grade of classic VIN include (1) nuclear size and atypia, (2) number and severity of atypical mitoses and (3) loss of cytoplasmic differentiation toward the epithelial surface. In the undifferentiated form seen in younger women, the entire epithelium consists of cells with highly atypical nuclei and negligible cytoplasm. Mitoses, often atypical, are common (Fig. 24-7B). **Bowen disease,** a term still used in the dermatologic literature, is a synonym for VIN III.

Keratinizing squamous cell carcinomas usually follow differentiated VIN. Two thirds of larger tumors are exophytic (Fig. 24-8A); the remainder are ulcerative and endophytic. The tumor is composed of invasive nests of malignant squamous epithelium with central keratin pearls (Fig. 24-8B). The

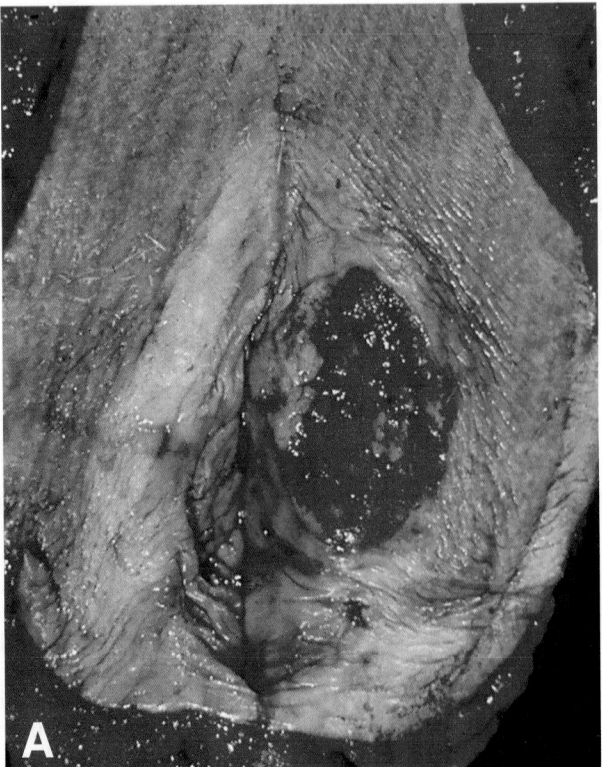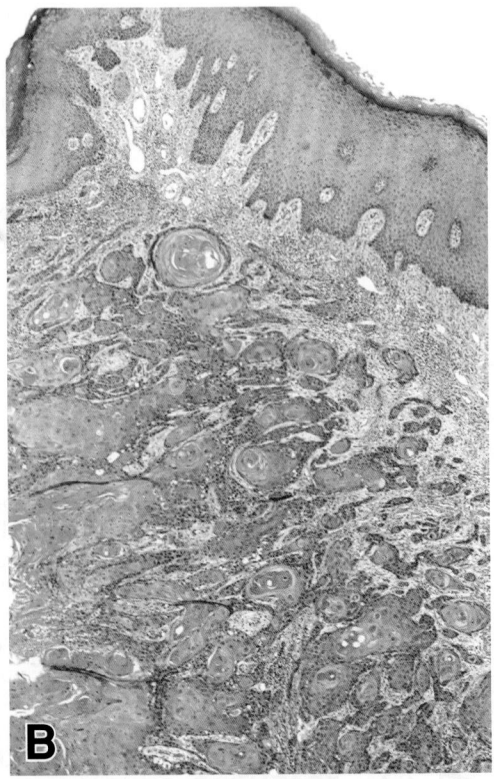

FIGURE 24-8. Squamous cell carcinoma of vulva. A. The tumor is situated in an extensive area of lichen sclerosus (*white*). **B.** Nests of neoplastic squamous cells, some with keratin pearls, are evident in this well-differentiated tumor.

tumors grow slowly, extending to contiguous skin, vagina and rectum. They metastasize initially to superficial inguinal lymph nodes and then to deep inguinal, femoral and pelvic lymph nodes.

 CLINICAL FEATURES: Most patients with VIN present with vulvar itching and burning with raised, well-defined skin lesions of variable sizes, which may be pink, red, brown or white. Carcinomas, but not VIN, may develop ulceration, bleeding and secondary infection. Spontaneous regression of VIN has been reported, most often in younger women.

Prognosis for patients with vulvar cancer is generally good, with 70% overall 5-year survival. Tumor grade, size, location and, most importantly, the number of lymph node metastases predict survival. Two thirds of women with inguinal node metastases survive 5 years, but only 1/4 of those with pelvic node metastases live that long. Better-differentiated tumors have a better mean survival, approaching 90% if nodes are negative.

Verrucous Carcinoma Is a Well-Differentiated Squamous Cancer

Vulvar verrucous carcinoma is a distinct variety of squamous cell carcinoma that grows as a large fungating mass resembling a giant condyloma acuminatum. HPV, usually type 6 or 11, is commonly involved. The tumor is very well differentiated, with large nests of squamous cells with abundant cytoplasm and small, bland nuclei. Squamous pearls are common and mitoses are rare. The tumor invades along broad fronts, and lymphocytes and plasma cells often heavily infiltrate the stromal interface. Verrucous carcinomas rarely metastasize. Wide local surgical excision is the treatment of choice, but other forms of therapy (cryosurgery and retinoids) have been used successfully.

Basal Cell Carcinoma

Basal cell carcinomas of the vulva are identical to those in the skin. They are not associated with HPV, rarely metastasize and are usually cured by surgical excision.

Malignant Melanoma

Although uncommon, malignant melanoma is the second most frequent cancer of the vulva (5%). It occurs in the sixth and seventh decades but is occasionally found in younger women. It has biological and microscopic characteristics of melanoma occurring elsewhere in the body. It is highly aggressive, and the prognosis is poor.

Extramammary Paget Disease Resembles Similar Tumors of the Breast and Elsewhere

The disorder usually occurs on the labia majora in older women. Women with Paget disease of the vulva complain of pruritus or a burning sensation for many years.

 PATHOLOGY: The lesion is large, red, moist and sharply demarcated. Diagnostic cells (Paget cells) may arise in the epidermis or epidermally derived adnexa. They have pale, vacuolated cytoplasm (Fig. 24-9) with abundant glycosaminoglycans; they stain with periodic acid–Schiff (PAS) and mucicarmine and expresses carcinoembryonic antigen (CEA). They appear as large single cells or, less often, as clusters of cells that lack intercellular bridges and are usually confined to the epidermis.

Intraepidermal Paget disease may be present for many years and is often far more extensive throughout the epidermis than preoperative biopsies indicate. Unlike Paget disease of the breast, which is almost always associated

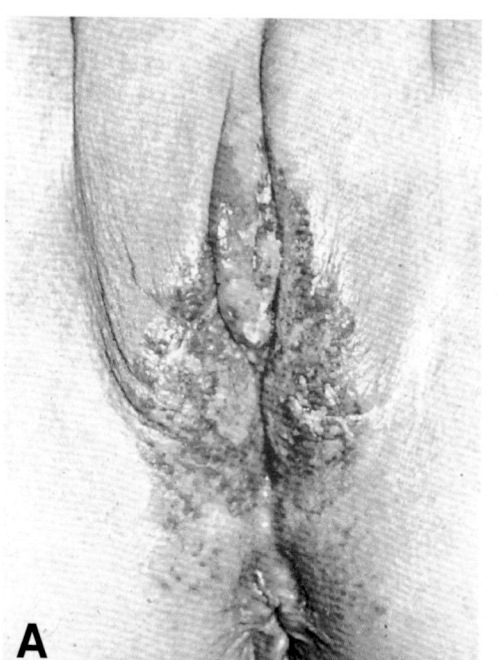
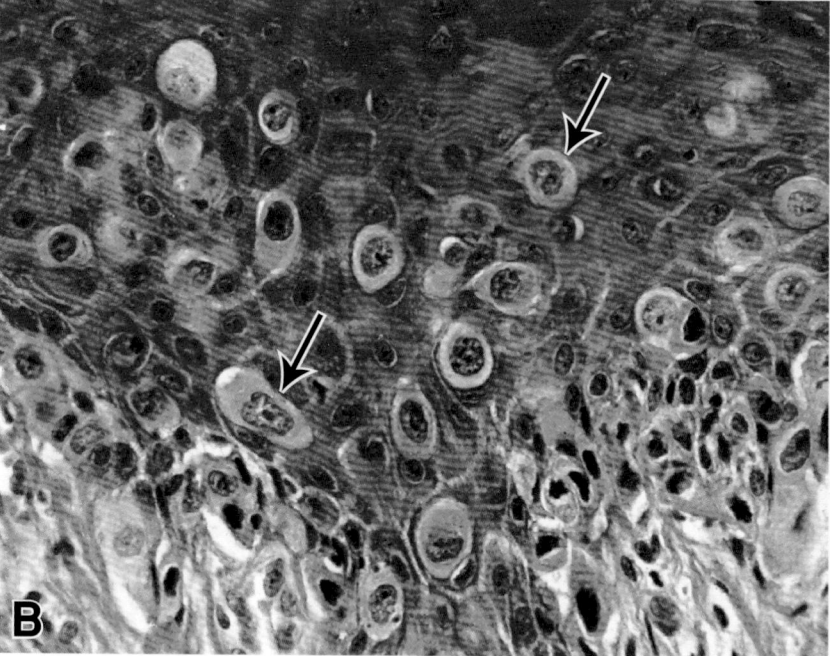

FIGURE 24-9. Paget disease of the vulva. A. The lesion is red, moist and sharply demarcated. **B.** Individual Paget cells (*arrows*), characterized by an abundant pale cytoplasm, infiltrate the epithelium and are interspersed among normal keratinocytes.

with underlying duct carcinoma, extramammary Paget disease is only rarely associated with carcinoma of the skin adnexa. Metastases occur rarely, so treatment requires only wide local excision or simple vulvectomy.

Vagina

ANATOMY

The vagina extends from the uterus to the vestibule of the vulva and is lined by hormone-responsive squamous epithelium. Estrogens stimulate, and progestogens inhibit, vaginal epithelial proliferation and maturation. Thus, in the secretory phase of the menstrual cycle or during pregnancy, when progesterone levels are high, intermediate cells, rather than superficial ones, predominate in vaginal smears. Maturing epithelial cells accumulate glycogen, giving their cytoplasm a clear appearance.

Lymph drains through the lateral perivaginal plexus. Lymphatics from the vaginal vault and upper vagina join branches from the cervix, to drain into pelvic and then paraaortic nodes. The lower vagina also drains to inguinal and femoral nodes.

NONNEOPLASTIC CONDITIONS AND BENIGN TUMORS

Congenital Anomalies of the Vagina Are Rare

Congenital absence of the vagina is generally associated with anomalies of the uterus and urinary tract. If there is a functional uterus, absence of a vagina may lead to accumulation of menstrual blood in the uterus.

Septate vagina results from failure of embryonic müllerian ducts to fuse properly, and the resulting median wall does not resorb.

Vaginal atresia and imperforate hymen prevent the vaginal embryonic lining from maturing from müllerian to squamous epithelium, which can cause vaginal adenosis.

Diminished Estrogen Stimulation Causes Atrophic Vaginitis

Atrophic vaginitis is thinning and atrophy of the vaginal epithelium. The thinned epithelium is a poor barrier to infections or abrasions. This occurs most commonly in postmenopausal women with low estrogen levels. Dyspareunia and vaginal spotting are common symptoms.

Vaginal Adenosis Occurred in Females Exposed to Diethylstilbestrol in Utero

In vaginal adenosis, the glandular epithelium that normally lines the embryonic vagina fails to be replaced during fetal life by squamous epithelium. Use of diethylstilbestrol (DES) to prevent miscarriages in women who were prone to repetitive abortions led, in the 1970s, to a substantial increase in this disorder in daughters of those women. Between the 10th and 18th weeks of gestation, upgrowth of squamous epithelium from the urogenital sinus replaces the glandular (müllerian) linings of the vagina and exocervix. DES exposure during this critical time arrests this process and some glandular tissue (i.e., adenosis) remains.

Adenosis manifests as red, granular patches on the vaginal mucosa, which microscopically are composed of mucinous columnar cells (resembling those lining the endocervix) and ciliated cells (like those lining the endometrium and fallopian tubes). Many of these lesions disappear as young women grow older. Rare cases of **clear cell adenocarcinoma** of the vagina (Fig. 24-10) have also occurred in the daughters of women treated with DES, typically in the upper third of the vagina. Clear cell adenocarcinomas are almost invariably curable when small and asymptomatic, but in more advanced stages, may spread by hematogenous or lymphatic routes.

Fibroepithelial Polyp

Vaginal polyps are uncommon benign growths with a connective tissue core and an outer lining of vaginal squamous epithelium. They are usually single, gray-white and smaller than 1 cm in diameter. Simple excision is usually curative.

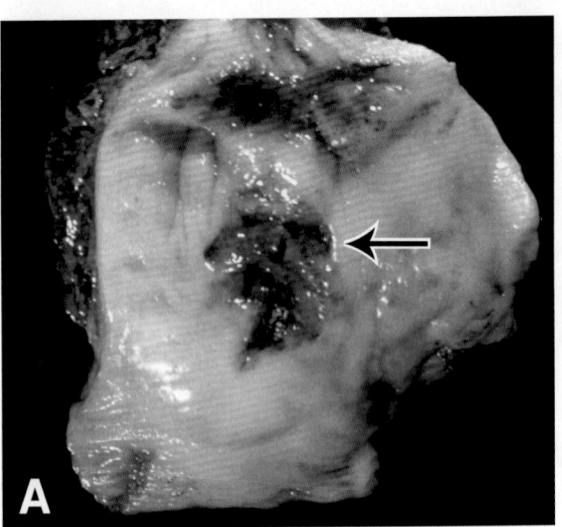

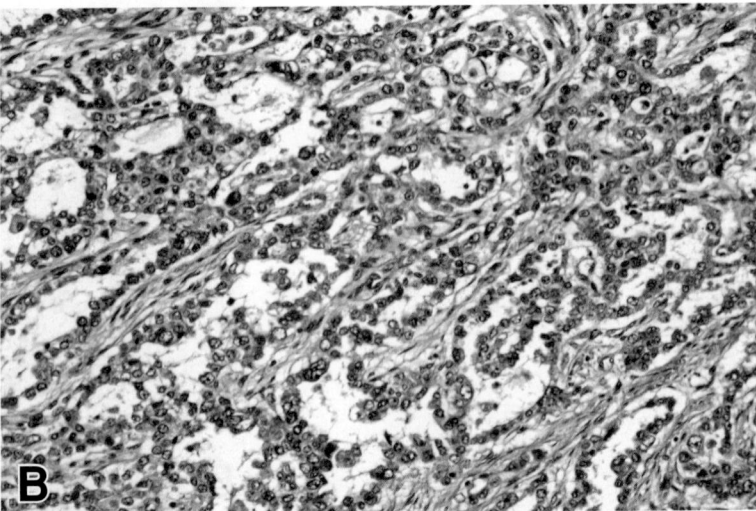

FIGURE 24-10. Clear cell adenocarcinoma of the vagina (in utero exposure to diethylstilbestrol [DES]). A. The tumor has arisen on the upper third of the anterior wall (*arrow*), corresponding to the most frequent site of adenosis. **B.** Microscopically, tubular glands are lined by hobnail cells.

Benign Mesenchymal Tumors

Most benign vaginal tumors resemble those elsewhere in the female genital tract (e.g., leiomyomas, rhabdomyomas and neurofibromas). These are solid submucosal tumors usually less than 2 cm in diameter.

MALIGNANT TUMORS OF THE VAGINA

Primary malignant tumors of the vagina are uncommon, constituting about 2% of all genital tract tumors. **Most (80%) vaginal malignancies represent metastatic spread.** The most common symptoms are vaginal discharge and bleeding during coitus, but advanced tumors may cause pelvic or abdominal pain and edema of the legs. Tumors confined to the vagina are usually treated by radical hysterectomy and vaginectomy.

Over 90% of Primary Vaginal Cancers Are Squamous Carcinomas

It is generally a disease of older women, with peak incidence between the ages of 60 and 70. It is most common in the anterior wall of the upper third of the vagina, where it usually grows as an exophytic mass. High-grade **vaginal intraepithelial lesion** (vaginal HSIL), a term replacing both "vaginal dysplasia" and "carcinoma in situ," frequently precedes invasive carcinoma. Vaginal squamous cell carcinoma may develop some years after cervical or vulvar carcinoma, suggesting a carcinogenic field effect in the lower genital tract, related to HPV infection.

Since most preinvasive and early invasive cancers are clinically silent, routine use of vaginal cytology is the most effective method to detect squamous carcinoma of the vagina. Prognosis is related to the extent of tumor spread at the time of discovery. Five-year survival in patients with tumors confined to the vagina (stage I) is 80%, whereas it is only 20% for those with extensive spread (stages III/IV).

Rhabdomyosarcoma Is a Rare Vaginal Tumor in Children

This tumor typically consists of confluent polypoid masses resembling a bunch of grapes, and hence may be called sarcoma botryoides (from the Greek *botrys*, "grapes") (Fig. 24-11). It occurs almost exclusively in girls under 4 years old. It arises in the lamina propria of the vagina and

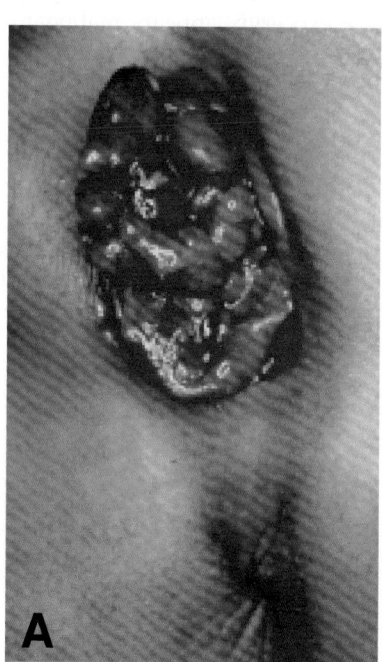
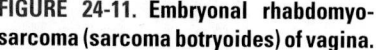
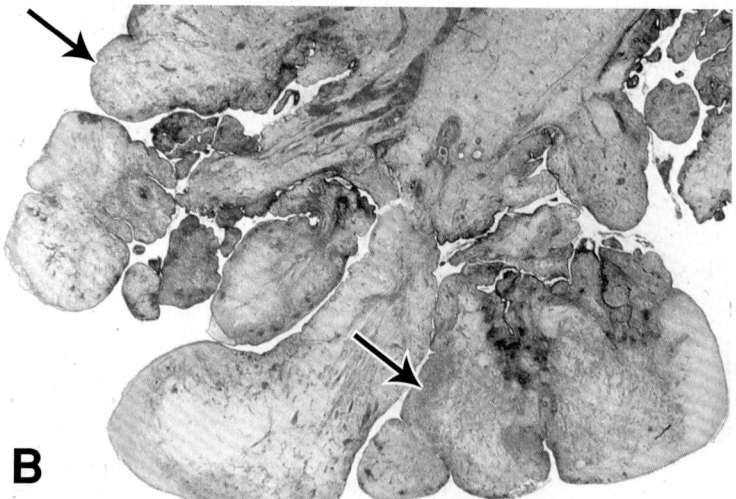
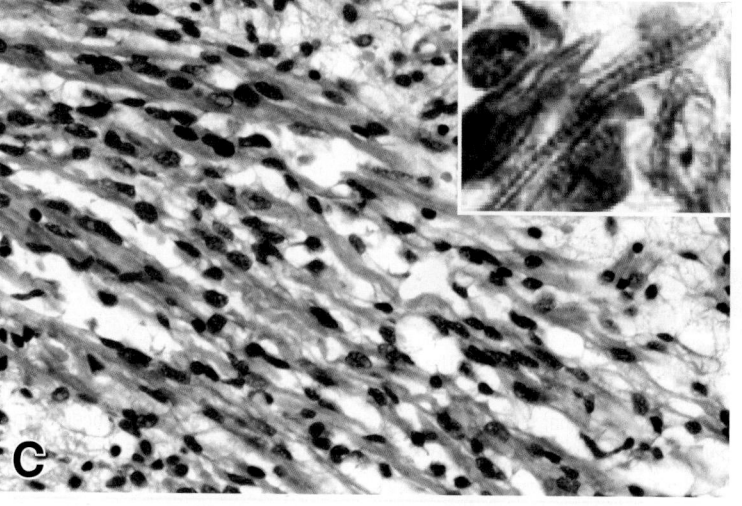

FIGURE 24-11. Embryonal rhabdomyosarcoma (sarcoma botryoides) of vagina. A. The grape-like tumor protrudes through the introitus. **B.** A section of the tumor shows a dense layer of neoplastic stroma termed the cambium layer (*arrows*) beneath the surface epithelium of the vagina. A loose neoplastic stroma is present beneath the cambium layer. **C.** The tumor cells are composed of elongated, primitive rhabdomyoblasts, with cross-striations seen at high magnification in the inset.

consists of primitive spindle rhabdomyoblasts (Fig. 24-11C), some of which show cross-striations. Myosin and actin myofibrils are often demonstrable. A dense zone of round rhabdomyoblasts (the cambium layer) is present beneath the vaginal epithelium (Fig. 24-11B). Deep to this layer, the stroma is myxomatous and shows fewer neoplastic rhabdomyoblasts. The tumor is usually detected because of spotting on the child's diaper. Tumors under 3 cm in greatest dimension tend to be localized and may be cured by wide excision and chemotherapy. Larger tumors often spread to adjacent structures, regional lymph nodes or distant sites. Even in advanced cases, half of patients survive with radical surgery and chemotherapy.

Cervix

ANATOMY

The cervix (from the Latin *collare*, "neck") is the inferior part of the uterus that connects the corpus to the vagina (Fig. 24-12). Its exposed portion (the **exocervix, ectocervix** or **portio vaginalis**) protrudes into the upper vagina and is covered by glycogen-rich squamous epithelium. The **endocervix** is the canal that leads to the endometrial cavity. It is lined by longitudinal mucosal ridges made of fibrovascular cores lined by a single layer of mucinous columnar cells. Occasionally, the outlet of an endocervical gland becomes blocked and mucin is retained, which produces cystic dilations of these glands, termed **nabothian cysts**. The **external os** is the *macroscopic* junction between the exocervix and endocervix. The **squamocolumnar junction** is the *microscopic* junction of the squamous and mucinous columnar epithelia. The area between the endocervix and endometrial cavity is called the **isthmus** or **lower uterine segment**.

The exocervix remodels continuously throughout life. During embryonic development, upward migration of squamous cells meets columnar epithelium of the endocervix to form the initial squamocolumnar junction (Fig. 24-13). In some young women, this "original" squamocolumnar junction is located at the internal os. In most, however, the columnar epithelium extends onto the exocervix, in which case, the areas of the exocervix lined by columnar epithelium are termed **endocervical ectropion** and appear by colposcopic examination as reddish discolorations. With age, the columnar epithelium of the ectropion undergoes squamous metaplasia and a new squamocolumnar junction is formed at the internal os.

The area between the distalmost squamocolumnar junction and the external os is called the **transformation zone**. Immature squamous epithelium of this zone displays progressive nuclear maturation and increasing amounts of glycogen-free cytoplasm toward the surface. Colposcopy shows a thin white membrane, which eventually becomes thicker and whiter as the squamous epithelium matures (Figs. 24-13 and 24-14). As cells accumulate glycogen, they become indistinguishable from normal squamous epithelium lining the exocervix. The transformation zone is the site of cervical squamous carcinoma (see below).

Examination of the transformation zone by iodine staining is the basis of the **Schiller iodine test**. Normal mature (glycogen-rich) squamous cells lining the exocervix stain with iodine and the exocervix appears mahogany brown. If they are immature (glycogen poor), no iodine staining occurs and the exocervix is pale.

CERVICITIS

Inflammation of the cervix is common and is related to constant exposure to bacterial flora in the vagina. Acute and chronic cervicitis are caused by many organisms, particularly

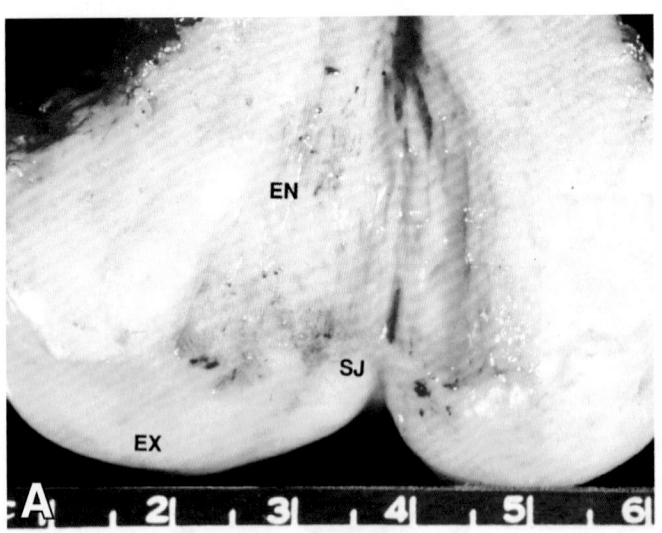
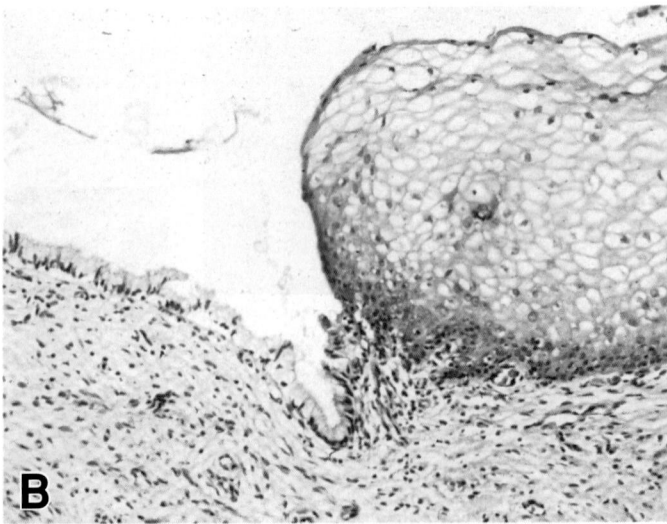

FIGURE 24-12. Anatomy of the cervix. A. The cervix has been opened to show the endocervix (EN), squamocolumnar junction (SJ) and exocervix (EX). The thick layer of squamous cells covering the exocervix accounts for its white color. **B.** A microscopic view of the squamocolumnar junction. The endocervix is lined by a single layer of columnar mucus-producing cells that abruptly meets the exocervix lined by mature squamous cells. *Note:* In specimens in which the squamocolumnar junction is on the ectocervix or in the endocervical canal, the region between it and the external os is called the *transformation zone* (Fig. 24-13).

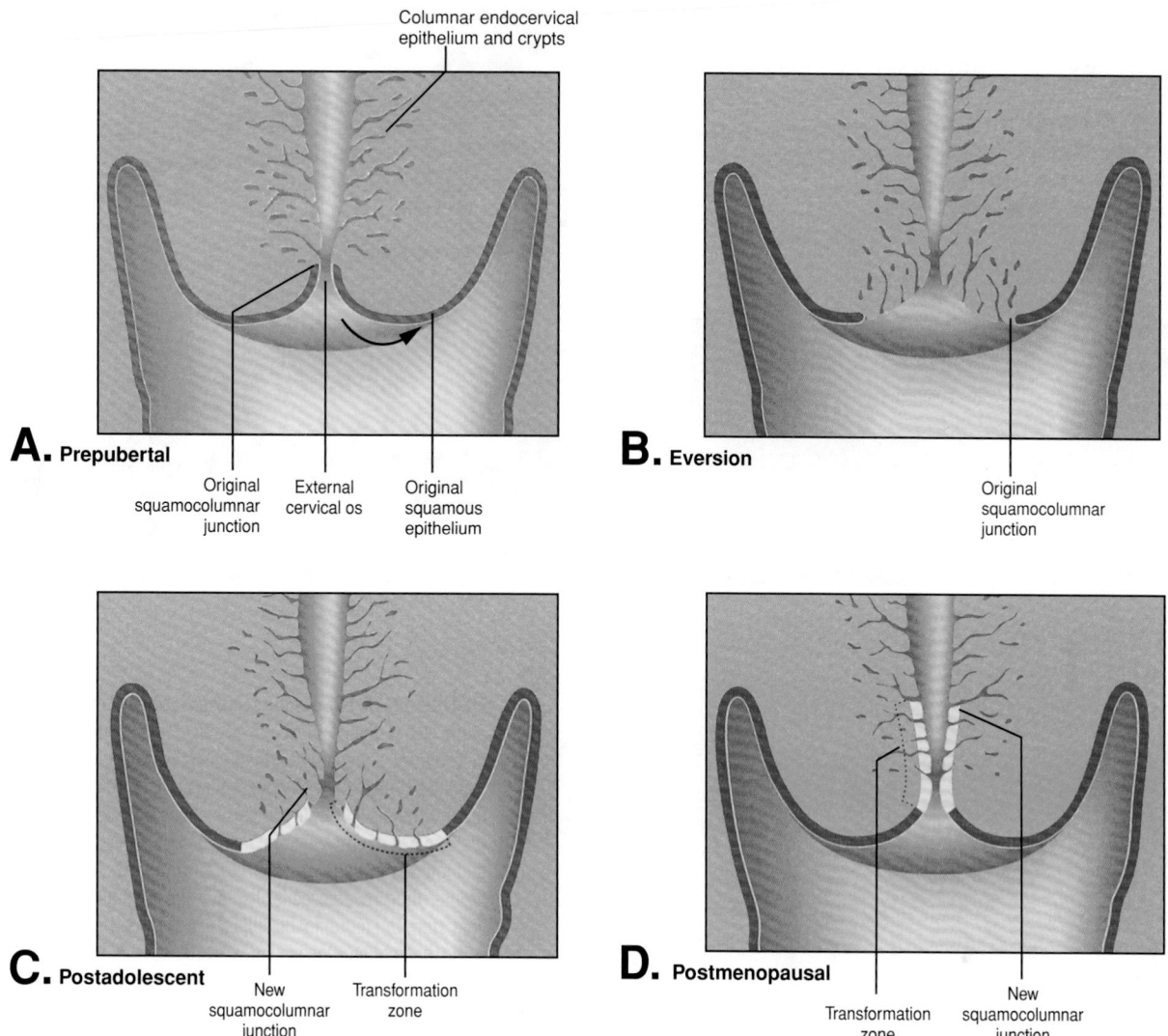

FIGURE 24-13. The transformation zone of the cervix. A. Prepubertal cervix. The squamocolumnar junction is situated at the external cervical os. The arrow shows the direction of the movement that takes place as a result of the increase in bulk of the cervix during adolescence. **B. The process of eversion.** On completion, endocervical columnar tissue lies on the vaginal surface of the cervix and is exposed to the vaginal environment. **C. Postadolescent cervix.** The acidity of the vaginal environment is one of the factors that encourages squamous metaplastic change, replacing the exposed columnar epithelium with squamous epithelium. **D. Postmenopausal cervix.** At this time, cervical inversion occurs. This phenomenon is the reverse of eversion, which was so important in adolescence. The transformation zone is now drawn into the cervical canal, often making it inaccessible to colposcopic examination.

endogenous vaginal aerobes and anaerobes, *Streptococcus*, *Staphylococcus* and *Enterococcus*. Other specific organisms include *C. trachomatis*, *N. gonorrhoeae* and occasionally herpes simplex type 2. Some agents are sexually transmitted; others may be introduced by foreign bodies, such as residual fragments of tampons and pessaries.

PATHOLOGY: In **acute cervicitis,** the cervix is grossly red, swollen and edematous, with copious pus "dripping" from the external os. Microscopically, the tissues exhibit extensive polymorphonuclear leukocyte infiltration and stromal edema.

Chronic cervicitis is more common. The cervical mucosa is hyperemic (Fig. 24-15) and may show true epithelial erosions. The stroma is infiltrated, principally by lymphocytes and plasma cells. Metaplastic squamous epithelium of the transformation zone may extend into endocervical glands,

forming clusters of squamous epithelium, which must be differentiated from carcinoma.

BENIGN TUMORS AND TUMOR-LIKE CONDITIONS OF THE CERVIX

Endocervical Polyps Are Usually Benign

Endocervical polyps are the most common cervical growths (Fig. 24-16). They appear as single smooth or lobulated masses, usually under 3 cm in greatest dimension. They typically manifest as vaginal bleeding or discharge. The lining epithelium is mucinous, with variable squamous metaplasia, but may feature erosions and granulation tissue if women are symptomatic. Simple excision or curettage is curative. Cancer rarely arises in an endocervical polyp (0.2% of cases).

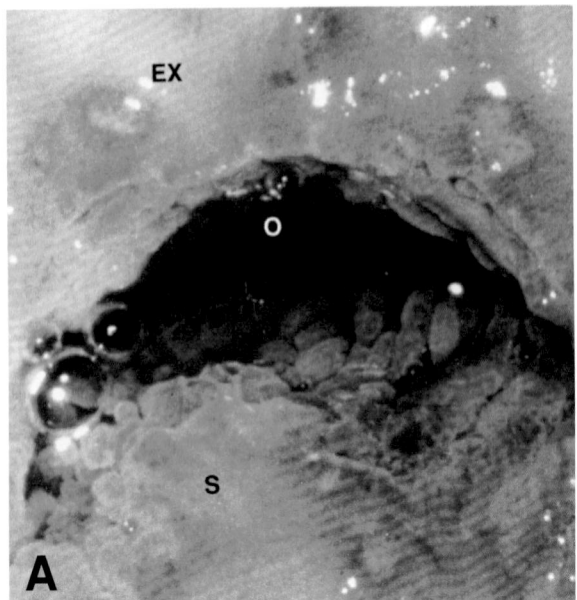
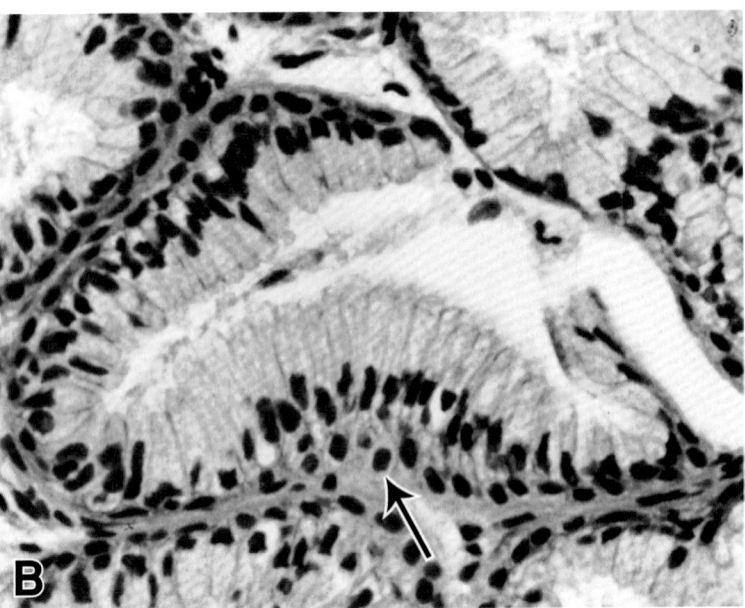
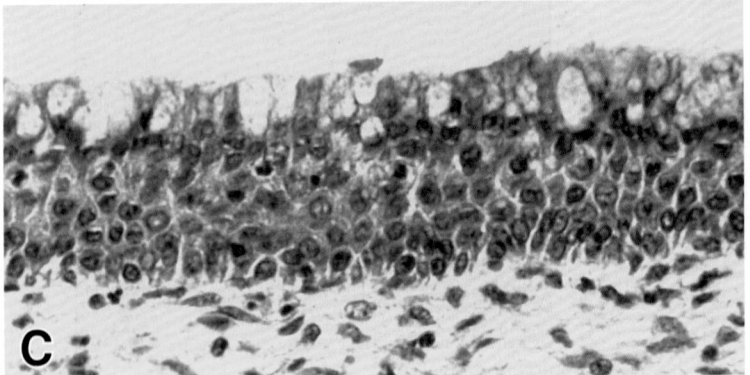

FIGURE 24-14. Squamous metaplasia in the transformation zone. A. In this colposcopic view of the cervix, a white area of metaplastic squamous epithelium (S) is situated between the exocervix (EX) and the mucinous endocervix (EN), which terminates at the internal os (O). **B.** In the early stages of squamous metaplasia of the transformation zone, the reserve cells, which normally constitute a single layer, begin to proliferate (*arrow*). **C.** At a later stage, the proliferating reserve cells displace the glandular epithelium. As a final step, the metaplastic cells mature into glycogen-rich squamous cells, resembling those in Fig. 24-12B.

Microglandular Hyperplasia Reflects Progestational Stimulation

Cervical microglandular hyperplasia is a benign condition showing closely packed vacuolated glands lacking intervening stroma and mixed with a neutrophilic infiltrate. The glands vary in size and are lined by a flattened-to-cuboidal epithelium (Fig. 24-17). Nuclei are uniform, and mitoses are rare. Squamous metaplasia and reserve cell hyperplasia are common. It should not be confused with well-differentiated adenocarcinoma. Microglandular hyperplasia is usually asymptomatic and, because it is typically associated with progestin stimulation, it usually occurs during pregnancy, in the postpartum period and in women taking oral contraceptives.

Leiomyomas Can Cause Cervical Bleeding

Cervical leiomyomas can prolapse into the endocervical canal and cause uterine contractions and pain resembling the early phases of labor. The appearance is similar to that of uterine leiomyomas (see below).

SQUAMOUS CELL NEOPLASIA

Fifty years ago, cervical cancer was the leading cause of cancer death in American women. The introduction and widespread use of cytologic screening decreased cervical carcinoma by 50%–85% in Western countries. It is now the sixth most common female cancer in the United States, and mortality has fallen by 70%. Worldwide, however, cervical cancer remains the second most common cancer in women.

Squamous Intraepithelial Lesions Are Precursors of Invasive Cancer

SILs of the cervix are the effects of human papilloma virus and are designated as low grade (LSILs) or high grade (HSILs) based on the corresponding infecting viral subtype and risk of progression to invasive squamous cell carcinoma (Fig. 24-18). Squamous precancer terminology was standardized across all anogenital sites in 2012 by the Lower Anogenital Squamous Terminology (LAST) group under the sponsorship of the College of American Pathologists, although legacy terms of cervical intraepithelial neoplasia (CIN), dysplasia and CIS are commonly used interchangeably.

Cervical SIL carries a risk for **malignant transformation** that varies between low- and high-grade subtypes (Figs. 24-18 and 24-19). The disease spectrum is primarily driven by the nature of the infecting virus, with each class demonstrating its own disease spectrum. The grades of SIL are:

- LSIL: CIN-1: mild dysplasia
- HSIL: CIN-2, moderate dysplasia; CIN-3, severe dysplasia, carcinoma in situ

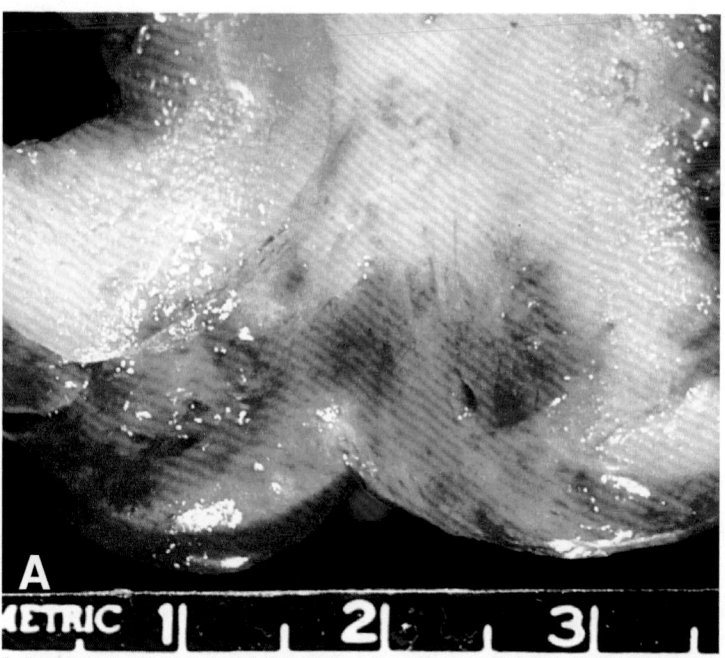
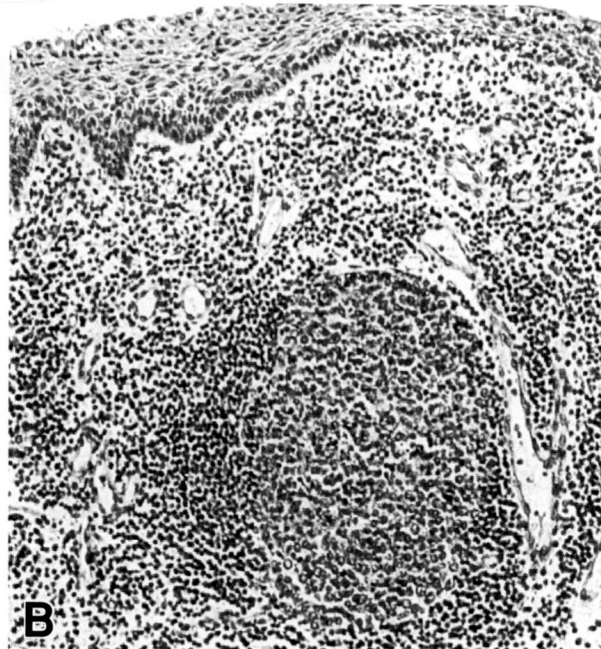

FIGURE 24-15. Chronic cervicitis. A. The cervix has been opened to reveal the reddened exocervix. **B.** Microscopic examination discloses chronic inflammation and the formation of a lymphoid follicle.

LSIL rarely progresses in severity and commonly disappears (CIN-1, mild dysplasia). HSIL describes more severe histologic lesions (CIN-2 and CIN-3), which tend to progress and require treatment. Early phases of infection with all HPV types likely involve episomal viral propagation throughout a polyclonal epithelial field, with an LSIL cytology. Oncogenic types of HPV are prone to subsequent genomic integration of virus and promote monoclonal outgrowth of cells driven by transforming viral proteins (E6/E7) with progression to HSIL.

EPIDEMIOLOGY AND MOLECULAR PATHOGENESIS: Epidemiologic features of SIL and invasive cancer are similar. Cervical cancer usually manifests in women 40–60 years old (mean 54), but SIL generally occurs before age 40. *The critical factor is HPV infection, which correlates with multiple sexual partners and early age at first coitus.* Thus, SIL is essentially a **sexually transmitted disease**. Smoking increases the incidence of cancer of the cervix, but the mechanism is obscure.

HPV infection leads to SIL and cervical cancer (Fig. 24-19). In LSIL, HPV is episomal and replicates freely to cause cell death. Huge numbers of virus must accumulate in the cytoplasm before being visible as a koilocyte. In most cases of HSIL, viral DNA integrates into the cell genome. Proteins encoded by HPV-16 E6 and E7 genes bind and inactivate p53 and Rb proteins, respectively, and mitigate their tumor suppressor functions (see Chapter 5). Once HPV integrates into host DNA, copies of intact virus do not accumulate and koilocytes are absent in many cases of high-grade dysplasia and all invasive cancers.

Roughly 85% of LSIL lesions have low-risk HPV. Genital warts (condylomata acuminata) of the cervix often contain

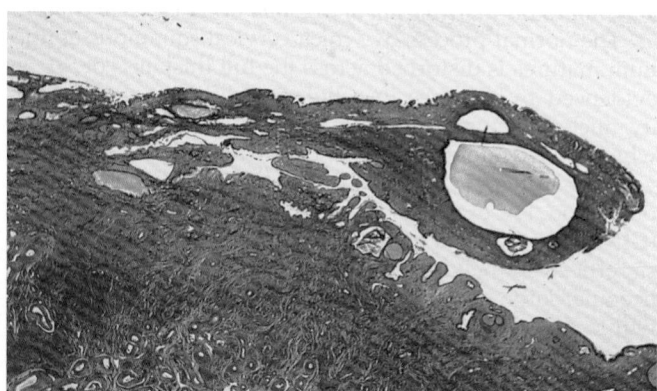

FIGURE 24-16. Endocervical polyp. An epithelial lining covers a fibrovascular core.

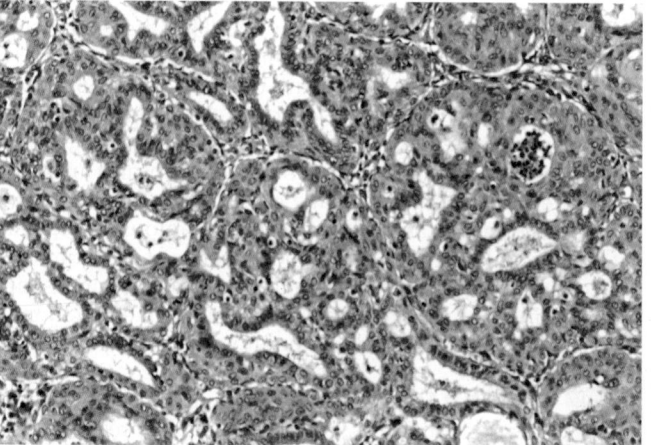

FIGURE 24-17. Microglandular hyperplasia. Small proliferated glands are admixed with a neutrophilic infiltrate.

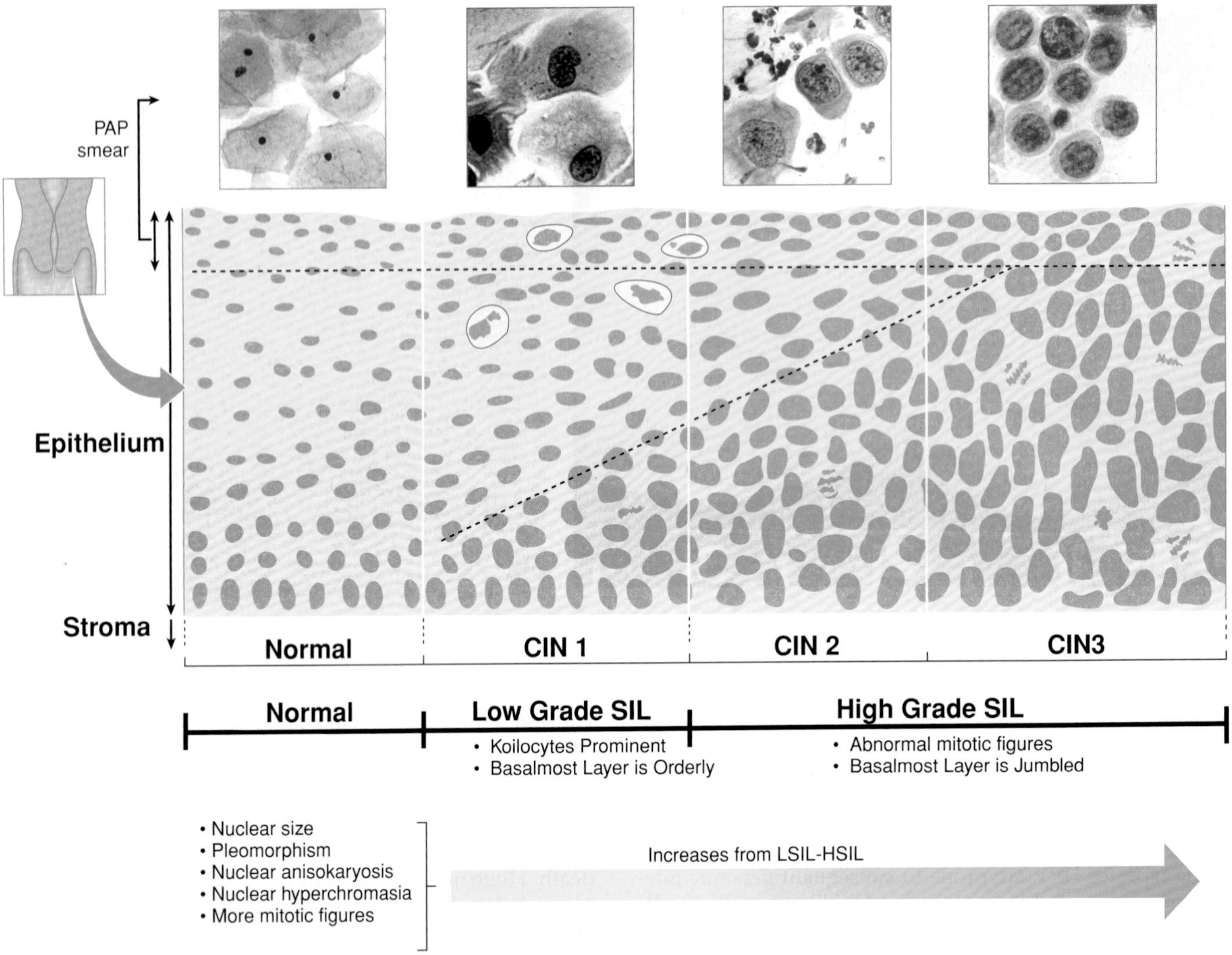

PAP
smear

Epithelium

Stroma

| Normal | CIN 1 | CIN 2 | CIN3 |

| Normal | Low Grade SIL | High Grade SIL |

Low Grade SIL
- Koilocytes Prominent
- Basalmost Layer is Orderly

High Grade SIL
- Abnormal mitotic figures
- Basalmost Layer is Jumbled

- Nuclear size
- Pleomorphism
- Nuclear anisokaryosis
- Nuclear hyperchromasia
- More mitotic figures

Increases from LSIL-HSIL

FIGURE 24-18. The Bethesda system for designation of premalignant cervical disease as squamous intraepithelial lesions (SILs). This chart integrates multiple aspects across the normal–LSIL (low-grade squamous intraepithelial lesion), and LSIL–HSIL (high-grade squamous intraepithelial lesion) interfaces, which correspond to therapeutic thresholds. It lists the qualitative and quantitative features that distinguish low-cancer-risk (LSIL) from high-cancer-risk (HSIL) lesions, which are generally caused by different subtypes of human papillomavirus. It also illustrates approximate counterparts for the legacy cervical intraepithelial neoplasia (CIN) system, which was based on a model of continuous progression rather than dichotomous viral subtypes. Finally, the scheme illustrates the corresponding cytologic smear resulting from exfoliation of the most superficial cells, indicating that even in the mildest disease state, abnormal cells reach the surface and are shed.

HPV-6 or -11, both considered low-risk HPV types. By contrast, cells in HSIL usually contain HPV types 16, 18, 31, 33, 35, 39, 45, 51, 52, 56, 58, 59 and 68. **HPV types 16 and 18** are found in 70% of invasive cancers; other high-risk types account for another 25%.

Hormonally induced eversion of the cervix and an acidic vaginal environment encourage development of the transformation zone. Without HPV, benign squamous metaplasia is the eventual outcome. But in the presence of HPV or other carcinogenic agents, transformation zone stem cells are diverted into SIL and may progress to invasive carcinoma, depending on the subtype and unknown host factors.

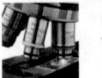 **PATHOLOGY:** The HPV-susceptible cell type has been identified as a cytokeratin 7–expressing stem cell located in the region of the cervical transformation zone between the columnar endocervix and squamous exocervix. *It is the location of the transformation zone and its*

component cell types on the exposed portion of the cervix that determines the distribution of SIL, and hence cervical cancer.

The normal process by which cervical squamous epithelium matures is disturbed across the full thickness of SIL, as evidenced by changes in cellularity, differentiation, polarity, nuclear features and mitotic activity. While the height to which the basaloid cells extend upward in the epithelium generally differs between LSIL and HSIL, this is an oversimplification. For example, the most dramatic changes in **LSIL (CIN-1)** occur not in the base, but rather in koilocytes of the superficial epithelium, which show ballooned cytoplasm and irregular large nuclei caused by episomal virus propagation within differentiated squamous cells that are absent in the base. Features in the basal region related to genomic integration of virus in propagating basal cells are prominent in **HSIL (CIN-2/-3)**. These include disorganization of basal cell alignment along the basement membrane and nuclear changes that persist as cells are pushed upward in the epithelium.

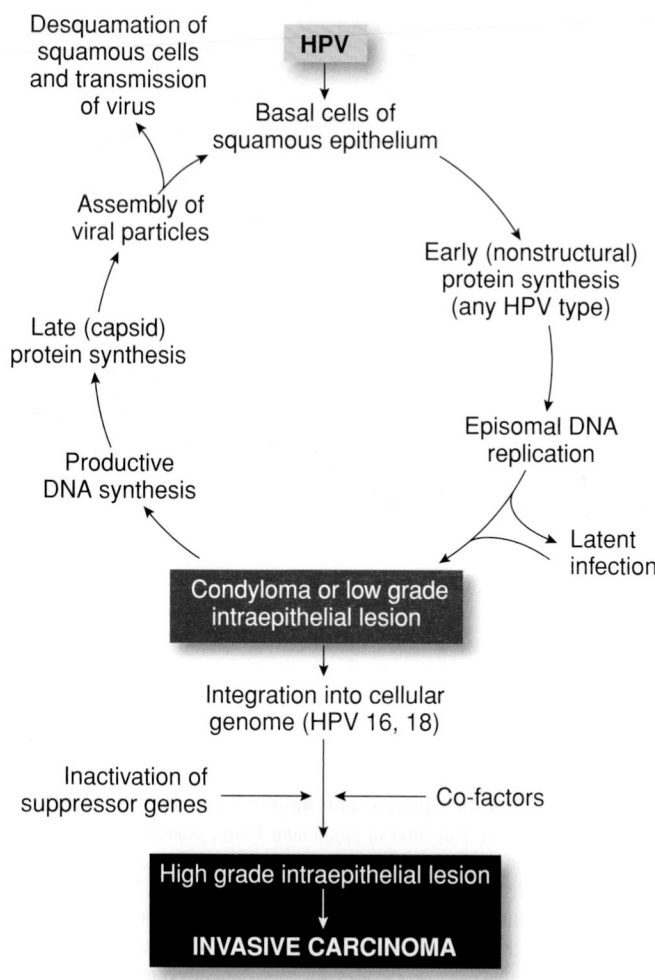

FIGURE 24-19. Role of human papillomavirus (HPV) in the pathogenesis of cervical neoplasia.

Abnormal mitotic figures, pathognomonic of chromosomal aneuploidy, may also be present in HSILs. Thus, grading of individual lesions as HSIL and LSIL requires consideration of all features described in Fig. 24-18. The differing histologic changes of LSIL and HSIL are shown in Fig. 24-20.

Since abnormal cells are present throughout the epithelium in women with SIL, they are shed into the Pap smear. Nuclear abnormalities and the degree of cytoplasmic differentiation in exfoliated abnormal cells are used to identify SIL and subclassify it as LSIL or HSIL. That this distinction can usually be made in shed cells indicates that morphologic differences between HSIL and LSIL are reflected in superficial as well as deep aspects of the epithelium. But while the Pap smear is an exquisitely sensitive screen for SIL lesions, it is only a screen. Definitive classification is best made in a histologic specimen where the full epithelium can be assessed.

Altered vasculature and epithelial changes in cervical SIL can be seen on colposcopic examination. Mosaicism (irregular surface resembling inlaid woodwork) (Fig. 24-21) and vascular punctation are two patterns most often seen in HSIL. The oncogenic process occurs more often on the anterior than the posterior cervical lip and often involves the endocervical glands.

 CLINICAL FEATURES: The mean age at which women develop SIL has declined over the past few decades and is now 25–30 years. Seventy percent of cases of LSIL regress, 6% progress to HSIL and less than 1% become invasive cancer. Progression of HSIL to invasive squamous carcinoma occurs with greater frequency and over a shorter interval, but the exact figures vary with intervening management. ***Ten to 20% of cases of HSIL progress to invasive carcinoma if untreated.***

Biopsy is indicated when SIL is discovered on Pap smear. Targeted biopsies may be visually directed by colposcopy, or the entire transformation zone can be removed by a wire "loop" electrosurgical excision procedure (LEEP). LEEP may fulfill both diagnostic and therapeutic functions. Diagnostic endocervical curettage also helps determine the extent of endocervical involvement. Women with LSIL are often followed conservatively (i.e., repeated Pap smears plus close follow-up), although some gynecologists advocate local ablative treatment. High-grade lesions are treated by ablation methods determined by their anatomic distribution. LEEP may be sufficient, if margins are negative. Cervical conization (removal of a cone of tissue around the external os), cryosurgery and (rarely) hysterectomy may also be done. Follow-up smears and clinical examinations should continue for life, as vaginal or vulvar squamous cancer may develop later.

Superficially Invasive Squamous Cell Carcinoma Is the Earliest Stage of Invasive Cervical Cancer

In this setting, stromal invasion usually arises from overlying HSIL. About 7% of specimens removed for CIS show focal superficially invasive cancer. Superficially invasive disease is based on width and depth of invasion, defined by the International Federation of Gynecology and Obstetrics (FIGO) as follows (Table 24-2):

- Invasion less than 3 mm from the basement membrane point of origin
- Less than or equal to 7-mm maximum lateral extension

The earliest recognizable invasive changes are tiny irregular epithelial buds emanating from the base of HSILs (Fig. 24-22), previously called "microinvasive" (Fig. 24-23). These small (<1 mm) tongues of neoplastic epithelial cells do not affect the prognosis of HSILs; hence, both can be treated similarly with conservative surgery. The LAST consensus group further limits use of the term "superficially invasive squamous cell carcinoma" to tumors that are not grossly visible. Conization or simple hysterectomy generally cures superficially invasive squamous cell carcinomas.

If the maximum dimensions described above are exceeded, the lesion is no longer considered "superficially invasive," but rather "invasive" squamous cell carcinoma of the cervix (Fig. 24-22; see below). The FIGO clinical staging criteria (Table 24-2) are widely used to guide management of gynecologic malignancies.

Invasive Squamous Cell Carcinoma Remains Common Worldwide

 **EPIDEMIOLOGY:** Squamous cell carcinoma is by far the most common type of cervical cancer. In the United States (Table 24-3), roughly 12,000 new

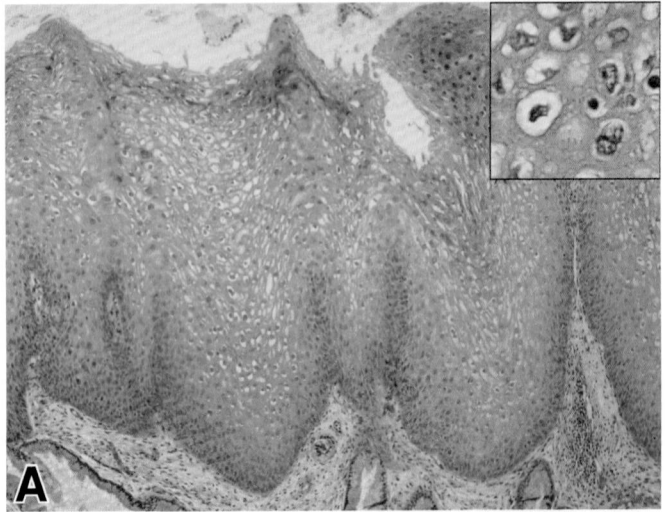

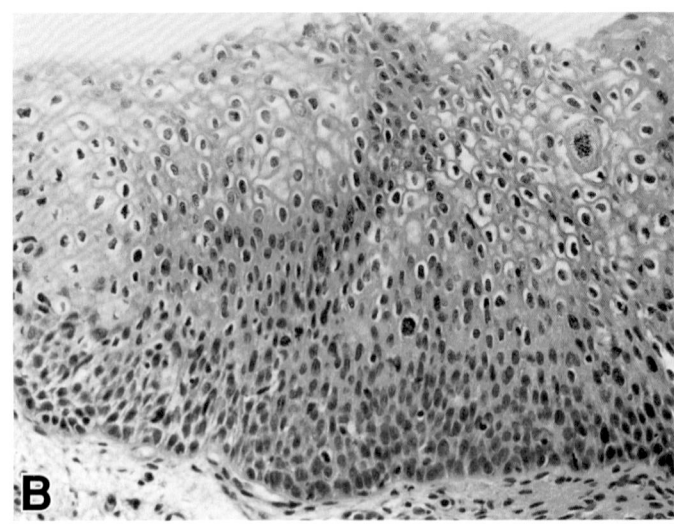

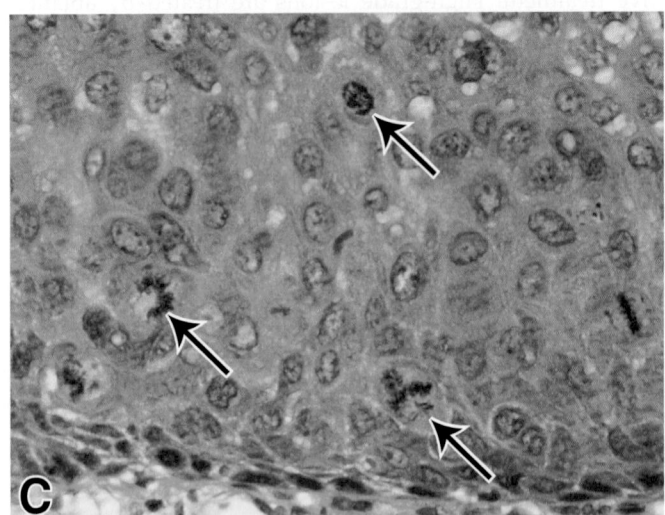

FIGURE 24-20. Cervical squamous intraepithelial lesions (SILs). A. Low-grade SIL (LSIL/CIN-1): The cervical epithelium shows pronounced vacuolated koilocytes (*inset*) in the upper epithelium and a thin basal zone that maintains polarity against the basement membrane. **B.** High-grade SIL (HSIL/CIN-2/-3): Basal cells with integrated HPV proliferate as neoplastic clones through the entire epithelium. Basal cells are disorganized and extend upward to a higher level without differentiation. Koilocytes may occur but are infrequent. **C.** Atypical mitoses (*arrows*) in this HSIL indicate an aneuploid genotype, seen with high-risk viruses. Horseshoe, multipolar and unequal metaphases are seen.

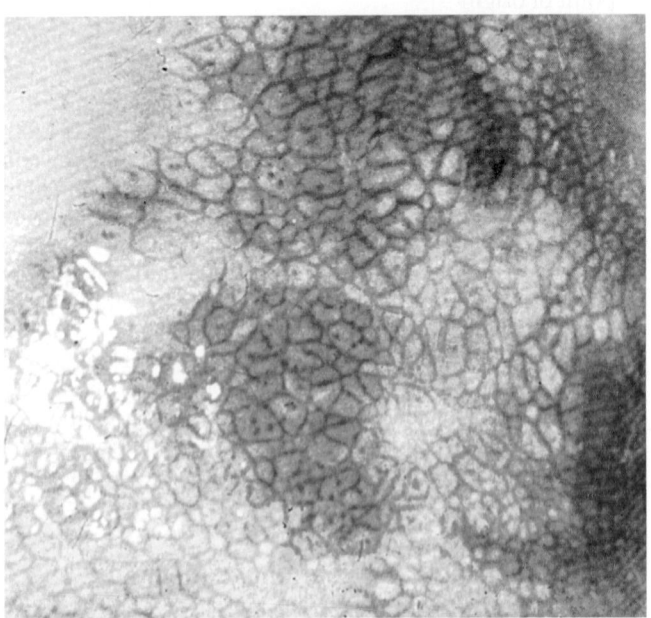

FIGURE 24-21. High-grade squamous intraepithelial lesion (HSIL) of the cervix. Examination with the colposcope discloses a mosaic pattern resembling inlaid woodwork.

cases occur annually, which is less than either endometrial or ovarian cancer. However, in underdeveloped areas, where cytologic screening is less available, cervical squamous cancer is still a major cause of cancer death. The HPV vaccine (often termed the **cervical cancer vaccine**) decreases individual risk of cervical cancer by 97%. Vaccinated women have reduced rates of both HPV-associated precancers and invasive cervical cancer.

 PATHOLOGY: Early stages of cervical cancer are often poorly defined, granular, eroded lesions or nodular and exophytic masses (Fig. 24-24A). If the tumor resides mainly within the endocervical canal, it can be an endophytic mass that infiltrates stroma and causes diffuse enlargement and hardening of the cervix. Most tumors are nonkeratinizing, with solid nests of large malignant squamous cells and no more than individual cell keratinization. Most remaining cancers show nests of keratinized cells in concentric whorls, so-called keratin pearls (Fig. 24-24B). The least common, and most aggressive, tumor is small cell carcinoma. It consists of infiltrating masses of small, cohesive, nonkeratinized, malignant cells, and has the worst prognosis.

Cervical cancer spreads by direct extension or through lymphatic vessels (Fig. 24-25) and only rarely by the hematogenous route. Local extension into surrounding tissues

TABLE 24-2

FIGO (2009) STAGING OF TUMORS OF THE UTERINE CERVIX

Stage	Anatomic Distribution
Stage I	Carcinoma confined to the uterus
IA	Invasive carcinoma that can be diagnosed only by microscopy, with deepest invasion ≤5 mm and largest extension ≤7 mm
IA1	Measured stromal invasion of ≤3.0 mm in depth and extension of ≤7.0 mm
IA2	Measured stromal invasion of >3.0 mm and <5.0 mm with an extension of not more than 7.0 mm
IB	Clinically visible lesions limited to the cervix uteri or preclinical cancers greater than stage IA
Stage II	Tumor invades beyond the uterus, but not to the pelvic wall or to the lower third of the vagina
IIA	Without parametrial invasion
IIB	With obvious parametrial invasion
Stage III	Tumor extends to the pelvic wall and/or involves lower third of the vagina and/or causes hydronephrosis or nonfunctioning kidney
IIIA	Tumor involves lower third of the vagina, with no extension to the pelvic wall
IIIB	Tumor extension to the pelvic wall and/or hydronephrosis or nonfunctioning kidney
Stage IV	Tumor has extended beyond the true pelvis or has involved (biopsy proven) the mucosa of the bladder or rectum
IVA	Spread to adjacent organs
IVB	Spread to distant organs

FIGO = International Federation of Gynecology and Obstetrics.

TABLE 24-3

INCIDENCE OF GYNECOLOGIC CANCER IN THE UNITED STATES (2013, ESTIMATED)

	New Cases		Death	
	Cases	%[a]	Cases	%[a]
Endometrium	49,560	6	8190	3
Ovary	22,240	3	14,030	5
Cervix, invasive	12,340	2	4030	2
Vulva, invasive	4700	<1	990	<1
Vagina and other, invasive	2890	<1	840	<1

[a]% = percentage of all cases of cancer in females.
American Cancer Society Statistics.

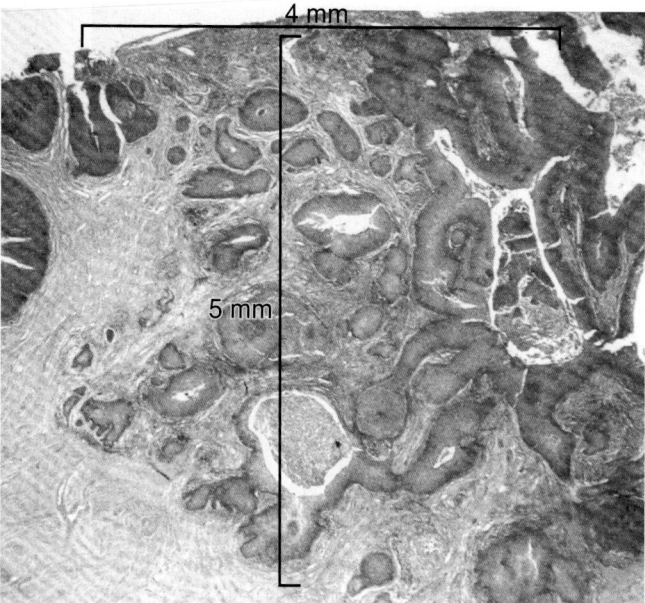

FIGURE 24-22. Invasive squamous cell carcinoma. The tumor invades 5 mm deep and 4 mm wide, exceeding the 3-mm depth limit placed on superficially invasive tumors.

(parametrium) (stage IIIB) may result in **ureteral compression** and cause clinical complications of hydroureter, hydronephrosis and renal failure, the most common cause of death (50% of patients). Bladder and rectal involvement (stage IVA) may lead to fistula formation. Lymphatic spread leads to metastases in paracervical, hypogastric and external iliac nodes. Overall, tumor growth and spread are relatively slow; the average age for patients with stage 0 tumor (HSIL) is 35–40 years; for stage IA, 43 years; and for stage IV, 57 years.

CLINICAL FEATURES: In early stages of cervical cancer, patients complain most often of vaginal bleeding after intercourse or douching. With more

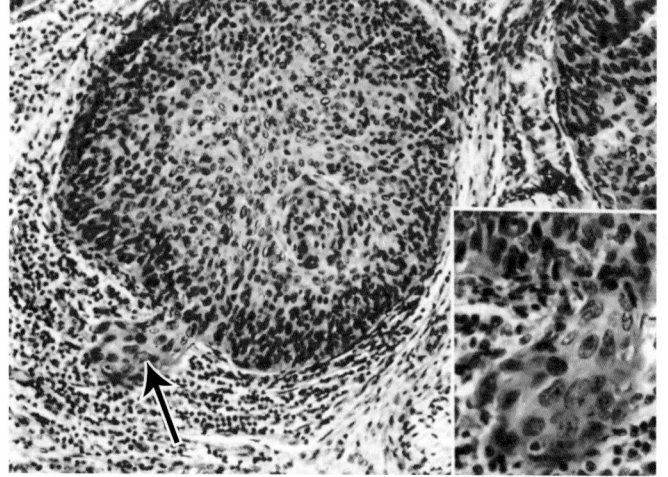

FIGURE 24-23. Early ("microinvasive") stromal invasion in a superficially invasive squamous cell carcinoma. Section of the cervix shows that high-grade squamous intraepithelial lesion (HSIL) in an endocervical gland has broken through the basement membrane (*arrow*) to invade the stroma. **Inset.** A higher-power view of the early invasive focus.

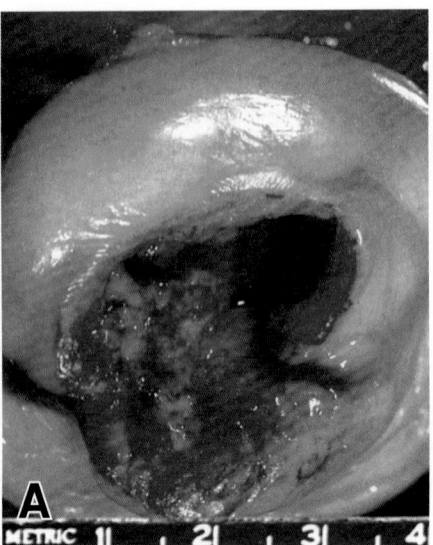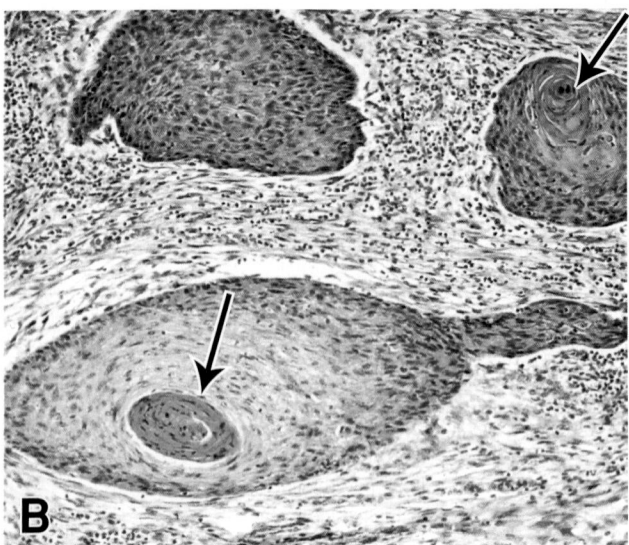

FIGURE 24-24. Squamous cell cancer. A. The cervix is distorted by the presence of an exophytic, ulcerated squamous cell carcinoma. **B.** The keratinizing pattern of the tumor is manifested as whorls of keratinized cells ("keratin pearls") (*arrows*).

advanced tumors, symptoms are referable to the route and degree of spread. The Pap smear remains the most reliable screening test for detecting cervical cancer.

The anatomic stage of cervical cancer is the best predictor of survival (Tables 24-2 and 24-3): 5-year survival is 90% in stage I; 75% in II; 35% in III; and 10% in VI, for an overall 5-year survival rate of 60%. About 15% of patients develop recurrences on the vaginal wall, bladder, pelvis or rectum within 2 years of therapy. Radical hysterectomy is favored for localized tumor, especially in younger women; radiation therapy or combinations of the two are used for more advanced tumors.

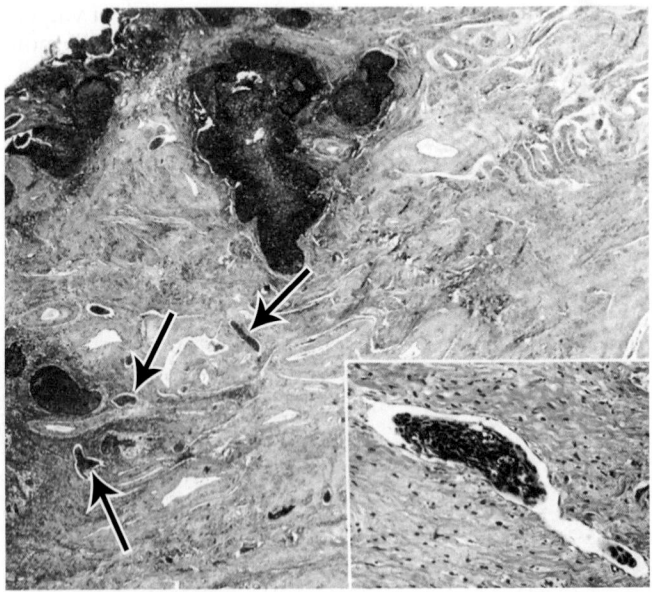

FIGURE 24-25. Squamous cell cancer of the cervix with lymphatic invasion. Low magnification shows a squamous cell carcinoma that has invaded the stroma and permeated the lymphatics (*arrows*). **Inset.** A high-power view of lymphatic invasion.

Endocervical Adenocarcinoma Accounts for 20% of Malignant Cervical Tumors

The incidence of cervical adenocarcinoma has increased recently, with a mean age of 56 years at presentation. Most tumors are of endocervical cell (mucinous) type, but the various subtypes have little bearing on overall survival. Adenocarcinoma shares epidemiologic factors with squamous carcinoma of the cervix and spreads similarly. They are often associated with adenocarcinoma in situ and contain HPV types 16 or 18.

PATHOLOGY:

ADENOCARCINOMA IN SITU: Also called **cervical glandular intraepithelial neoplasia,** this lesion generally arises at the squamocolumnar junction and extends into the endocervical canal. It displays tall columnar cells with eosinophilic or mucinous cytoplasm, sometimes resembling goblet cells. The pattern of spread and involvement of endocervical glands resemble those of cervical SIL. Adenocarcinoma in situ typically is intraepithelial, maintaining normal endocervical gland architecture. The cells show slight enlargement, atypical hyperchromatic nuclei, increased nuclear-to-cytoplasmic ratio and variable mitoses. Abrupt transitions help distinguish neoplastic from neighboring normal endocervical cells. Squamous HSIL occurs in 40% of cases of adenocarcinoma in situ.

INVASIVE ADENOCARCINOMA: This tumor typically presents as a fungating polypoid (Fig. 24-26A) or papillary mass. Exophytic tumors often have a papillary pattern (Fig. 24-26B), whereas endophytic ones display tubular or glandular patterns. Poorly differentiated tumors are predominantly composed of solid sheets of cells.

Adenocarcinoma of the endocervix spreads by local invasion and lymphatic metastases, but overall survival is somewhat worse than for squamous carcinoma. Treatment is similar to that for squamous carcinoma.

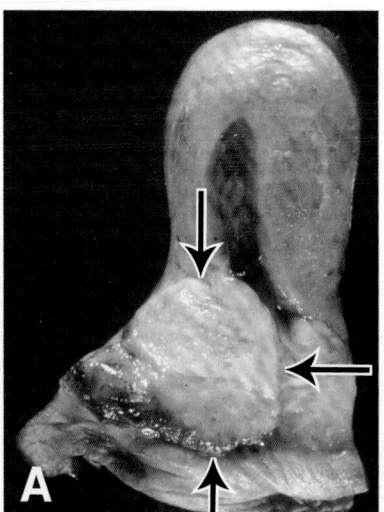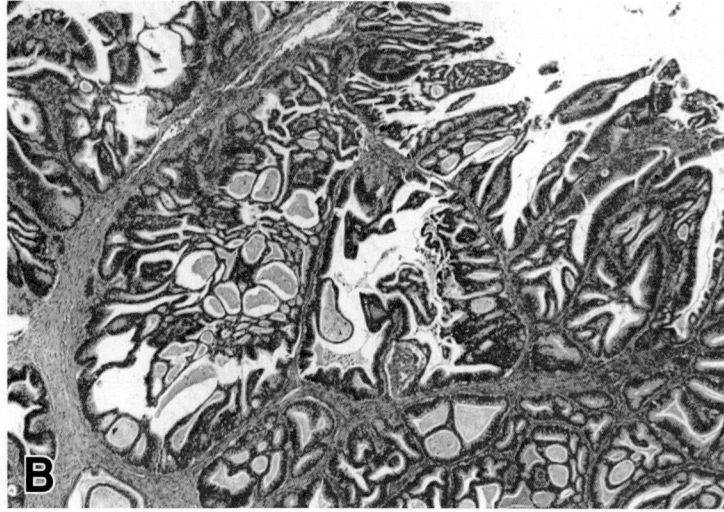

FIGURE 24-26. Endocervical adenocarcinoma. A. The endocervical tumor appears as a polypoid mass (*arrows*). **B.** Microscopic view of endocervical adenocarcinoma showing a papillary pattern of growth.

Uterus

ANATOMY

The uterine corpus (body) is smaller than the cervix at birth and during childhood but increases rapidly in size after puberty. The endometrium is composed of glands and stroma. It is thin at birth, when it consists of a continuous surface of cuboidal epithelium that dips to line a few sparse tubular glands. After puberty, it thickens. The superficial two thirds, the "zona functionalis," responds to hormones and is shed with each menstrual phase. The deepest third, the basal layer, is the germinative portion that regenerates a new functional zone with each cycle.

The endometrium is supplied by arcuate arteries that traverse the outer myometrium and give off two sets of vessels, one to the myometrium and the other, the radial arteries, to the endometrium. In turn, the radial arteries branch into two types of vessels. The basal arteries supply the basal endometrium and the spiral arteries nourish the superficial two thirds.

THE MENSTRUAL CYCLE

Normal endometrium undergoes sequential changes that support growth of implanted fertilized ova (zygotes) (Fig. 24-27). If conception does not occur, the endometrium is shed, and then regenerated to support a fertilized ovum in the next cycle.

MENSTRUAL PHASE: Without a blastocyst to secrete human chorionic gonadotropin (hCG), ovarian granulosa and thecal cells degenerate. Progesterone levels fall. The endometrium becomes desiccated, spiral arteries collapse and stroma disintegrates. Menses start at day 28, last 3–7 days and is composed of about 35 mL of blood. The denuded surface is regenerated by extension of the residual glandular epithelium.

PROLIFERATIVE PHASE: The endometrium is under estrogenic stimulation during days 3–15 of the menstrual cycle. Tubular to coiled glands in the functional zone are evenly distributed and supported by a cellular, monomorphic stroma (Fig. 24-27A). Glands are narrow early in the proliferative phase but coil and increase slightly in caliber over time. Columnar cells lining tubules increase from one layer in thickness to a mitotically active pseudostratified epithelium. The glands secrete a watery alkaline fluid that facilitates passage of sperm through the endometrium into the fallopian tubes. The stroma is also mitotically active. Spiral arteries are narrow and inconspicuous.

SECRETORY PHASE: Ovulation occurs about 14 days after the last menstrual period. The graafian follicle that discharged its ovum becomes a corpus luteum. Granulosa cells of the corpus luteum secrete progesterone, which transforms the endometrium from a proliferative to a secretory state.

- **Days 17–19 (postovulatory days 3–5):** Endometrial glands enlarge, dilate and become more coiled. The lining cells develop abundant and prominent, glycogen-rich, subnuclear vacuoles (day 17). Over the next several days, these cells produce copious secretions that support the zygote as it develops early chorionic villi capable of invading the endometrium.
- **Days 20–22 (postovulatory days 6–8):** The endometrium displays prominent stromal edema. Glands have homogenous cytoplasm with a few discrete vacuoles and are dilated and more tortuous.
- **Day 23 (postovulatory day 9):** Stromal cells surrounding spiral arterioles enlarge and exhibit large, round, vesicular nuclei and abundant eosinophilic cytoplasm ("vascular cuffing"). With time, these cells become more extensively distributed until they fill the functionalis. They are precursors of the decidual cells of pregnancy and are referred to as "predecidua."
- **Day 27 (postovulatory day 13):** The entire stroma is now predecidualized and ready for menstruation. Tubular glands continue to dilate and develop serrated (sawtoothed) borders.

ATROPHIC ENDOMETRIUM: After menopause, the number of glands and quantity of stroma diminish.

Day of Cycle		3—15	15–16	17	18	19–22	23	24–25	26–27	1—2
Post-ovulatory day			1–2	3	4	5–8	9	10–11	12–13	14+
Cycle phases		Proliferative	Interval	Early secretory		Mid-secretory			Late secretory	Menstrual
Key feature		Mitoses	Mitoses and subnuclear vacuoles	Maximum subnuclear vacuoles	Subnuclear vacuoles present	Stromal edema	Focal predecidua around spiral arteries	Patchy predecidua	Extensive predecidua	Stromal crumbling
Microscopic features of functional zone	Stroma	Loose stroma. Mitoses	Same as proliferative	Loose stroma. Scanty mitoses	Loose stroma	Stromal edema	Focal predecidua around spiral arteries. Edema prominent	Predecidua throughout stroma. Some edema	Extensive predecidua. Prominent granulated lymphocytes	Stromal crumbling. Hemorrhage
	Glands	Straight to tightly coiled tubules. Mitoses	Some subnuclear vacuoles, otherwise as proliferative	Extensive subnuclear vacuoles	Dilated glands. Some subnuclear vacuoles	Dilated glands with irregular outline. Luminal secretion		`Saw tooth' glands	Prominent 'saw tooth' glands	Disrupted glands. Secretory exhaustion. Regenerating epithelium
Appearances		A				B			C	

FIGURE 24-27. Main histologic features of the endometrial phases of the normal menstrual cycle. A. Proliferative phase. Straight tubular glands are embedded in a cellular monomorphic stroma. **B.** Secretory phase, day 24. Dilated tortuous glands with serrated borders are situated in a predecidual stroma. **C.** Menstrual endometrium. Fragmented glands, dissolution of the stroma and numerous neutrophils are evident.

Remaining glands have a thin epithelium and the stroma contains abundant collagen. Glands of the atrophic endometrium are often quite dilated, and this condition is called **senile cystic atrophy of the endometrium**.

ENDOMETRIUM OF PREGNANCY

The corpus luteum of pregnancy requires continuous stimulation by hCG secreted by placental trophoblast of the developing embryo. Trophoblast begins to develop at about day 23. Under hCG stimulation, the corpus luteum increases its progesterone output, stimulating secretion of fluid by endometrial glands. In the hypersecretory endometrium of pregnancy, highly dilated glands are lined by cells with abundant glycogen. These features can persist for up to 8 weeks after delivery.

The hypersecretory response may be exaggerated with intrauterine pregnancy, ectopic pregnancy or trophoblastic disease. Glandular cell nuclei may enlarge and appear bulbous and polyploid, owing to DNA replication without cell division. These nuclei protrude beyond the apparent cellular cytoplasmic limits into the gland lumen, an appearance referred to as the **Arias-Stella phenomenon** (Fig. 24-28). Enlarged nuclei are polyploid rather than aneuploid, a condition sometimes seen in adenocarcinoma.

CONGENITAL ANOMALIES OF THE UTERUS

Congenital anomalies of the uterus are rare.

- **Congenital absence of the uterus (agenesis)** reflects failure of müllerian ducts to develop. Since elongation of these ducts during embryonic life requires the wolffian

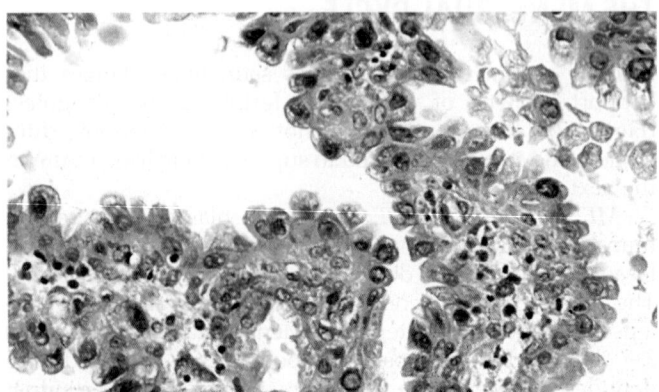

FIGURE 24-28. Arias-Stella reaction of pregnancy associated with human chorionic gonadotropin (hCG) stimulation. A section of endometrium shows enlarged, bulbous nuclei that protrude into the gland lumen.

ducts as guides, uterine agenesis is almost always accompanied by other urogenital tract anomalies and agenesis of the vagina and fallopian tubes.

- **Uterus didelphys** is a double uterus, due to failure of the two müllerian ducts to fuse in early embryonic life. A double vagina commonly accompanies this anomaly.
- **Uterus duplex bicornis** is a uterus with a common fused wall between two distinct endometrial cavities. The common wall between the apposed müllerian ducts fails to degenerate to form a single uterine cavity.
- **Uterus septus** is a single uterus with a partial septum, due to incomplete resorption of the wall of the fused müllerian ducts. These patients have increased risk for habitual abortion.
- **Bicornuate uterus** refers to a uterus with two cornua (horns) and a common cervix. Didelphic and bicornuate uterine fusion defects increase the risk of premature birth only slightly.

ENDOMETRITIS

In endometritis, or an inflamed endometrium, there is an abnormal inflammatory infiltrate in the endometrium. It must be distinguished from the normal presence of neutrophils during menstruation and mild lymphocytic infiltrates at other times. In most cases of endometritis, findings are nonspecific and rarely point to a specific cause.

ACUTE ENDOMETRITIS: This condition is defined as the abnormal presence of polymorphonuclear leukocytes in the endometrium. Most cases result from an ascending infection from the cervix (e.g., after the usually impervious cervical barrier is compromised by abortion, delivery or medical instrumentation). Curettage is diagnostic and often curative, because it removes necrotic tissue that has served as the nidus of the ongoing infection. Nowadays, the condition is of little significance, although it was quite dangerous before antibiotics.

CHRONIC ENDOMETRITIS: Although lymphocytes and lymphoid follicles occur occasionally in normal endometrium, plasma cells in the endometrium are diagnostic of chronic endometritis (Fig. 24-29). The disorder is associated with IUDs, PID and retained products of conception after an abortion or delivery. Without a culture, the pathologic findings alone do not distinguish between infective and noninfective causes. Patients usually complain of bleeding and/or pelvic pain. The condition is generally self-limited.

PYOMETRA: Defined as pus in the endometrial cavity, pyometra is associated with gross anatomic defects such as fistulous tracts between bowel and uterine cavity, bulky or perforating malignancies or cervical stenosis. Long-standing pyometra may rarely be associated with development of endometrial squamous cell cancer.

TRAUMATIC LESIONS

INTRAUTERINE DEVICE: IUDs predispose to (1) increased menstrual flow, (2) uterine perforation and (3) spontaneous abortion if conception occurs with the IUD in place. However, IUD use reduces endometrial cancer risk by half. Much of the adverse publicity about IUDs relates to early devices. Only 1% of women who desire contraception now use an IUD.

INTRAUTERINE ADHESIONS (ASHERMAN SYNDROME): Intrauterine fibrous adhesions sometimes develop after curettage, particularly for postpartum complications or therapeutic abortion. These bands traverse, but do not necessarily obliterate, the endometrial cavity. Additional complications include amenorrhea or, in the event of a subsequent pregnancy, increased abortion rates, preterm labor and placenta accreta.

ADENOMYOSIS

Adenomyosis is the presence of endometrial glands and stroma within the myometrium. Pain, dysmenorrhea or menorrhagia correlate with adenomyosis if the glands are 1 mm or more beneath the endometrial myometrial junction, with more severe symptoms as glands penetrate more deeply into the myometrium. Pain occurs as foci of adenomyosis enlarge when blood is entrapped during menses. One fifth of all uteri surgically removed show some adenomyosis.

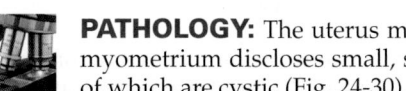 **PATHOLOGY:** The uterus may be enlarged. The myometrium discloses small, soft, tan areas, some of which are cystic (Fig. 24-30). Microscopic examination shows glands lined by proliferative to inactive endometrium and surrounded by endometrial stroma with varying degrees of fibrosis. Secretory changes are rare, except during pregnancy or in patients treated with progestins. The adjacent myometrium is often hypertrophic and nodular. The uterus may also become enlarged from cyclic bleeding into these foci. Extension of hyperplastic or neoplastic endometrium from the endometrial functionalis into adenomyotic foci may occur.

 CLINICAL FEATURES: Many patients with adenomyosis are asymptomatic, although pelvic pain, dysfunctional uterine bleeding, dysmenorrhea and dyspareunia are common. These symptoms appear in parous women of reproductive age and regress after menopause. The cause of adenomyosis remains unknown.

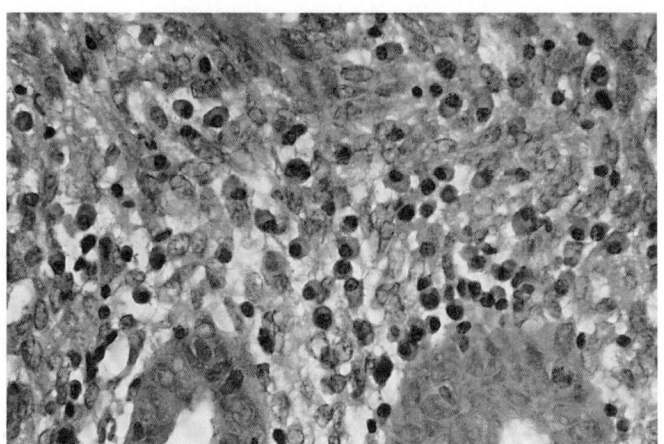

FIGURE 24-29. Chronic endometritis. The inflammatory infiltrate is composed largely of lymphocytes and plasma cells.

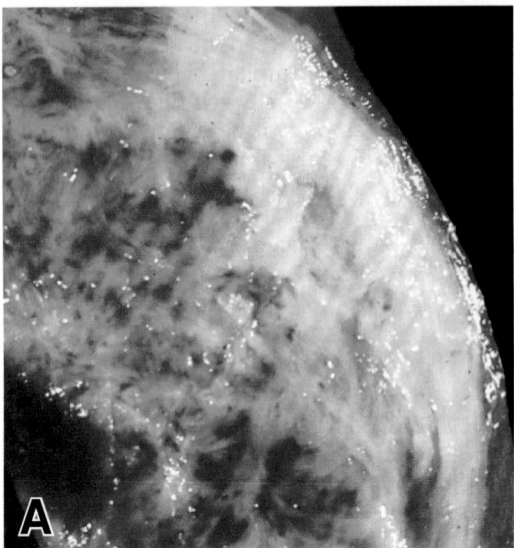
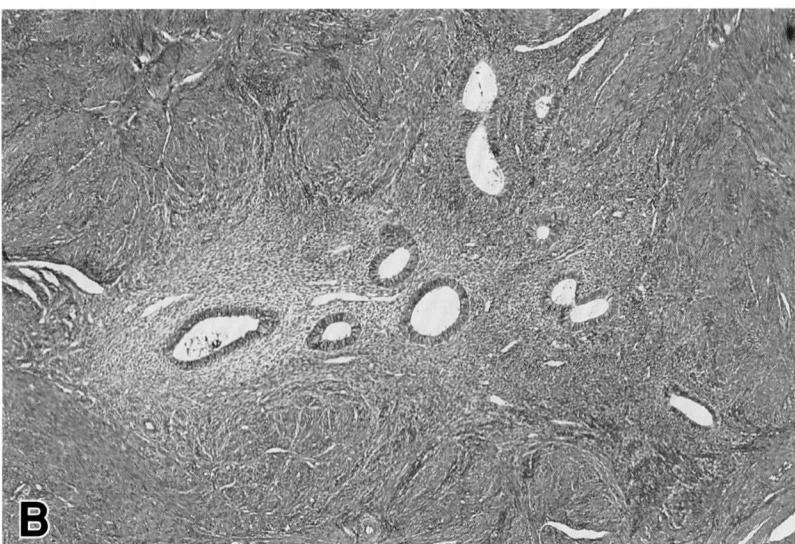

FIGURE 24-30. Adenomyosis. A. The cut surface of the uterus reveals small, red areas corresponding to endometrial glands in the myometrium. **B.** A microscopic view shows an endometrial gland and stroma in the myometrium.

HORMONAL EFFECTS

Contraceptive Steroids Prevent Pregnancy and Many Gynecologic Cancers

Oral contraceptive agents induce endometrial changes depending on the types, potencies and dosages of estrogens and progestins in individual formulations. Combined preparations generally contain potent progestins and weak estrogens. Pseudodecidual change thus appears early and overshadows the weak glandular growth. After several cycles, endometrial glands atrophy. Newer contraceptive combinations contain lower doses of hormones and elicit less change. Women who use contraceptives containing progestational agents have significantly lower rates of endometrial and ovarian cancer, reflecting the growth-inhibiting properties of progesterone and fewer ovulations (see below).

Dysfunctional Uterine Bleeding Occurs during or between Menstrual Periods

Dysfunctional bleeding is one of the most common gynecologic disorders of women of reproductive age but is still poorly understood. Its causes lie outside the uterus. Most cases are related to a disturbance of the hypothalamic–pituitary–ovarian axis (Table 24-4). Ovarian dysfunction also occurs, especially in the presence of anovulation.

Some causes of menstrual irregularity are intrinsic to the uterus and are not considered dysfunctional. These include (1) growths (e.g., carcinoma, endometrial intraepithelial neoplasia [EIN], submucosal leiomyomata and polyps), (2) inflammation (e.g., endometritis), (3) pregnancy (e.g., complications of intrauterine or ectopic pregnancy) and (4) the effects of IUDs (Table 24-4).

Anovulatory Bleeding Is the Most Common Form of Dysfunctional Bleeding

Anovulatory bleeding is a complex syndrome of many causes that manifests as the absence of ovulation during

TABLE 24-4	
CAUSES OF ABNORMAL UTERINE BLEEDING (INCLUDING UTERINE AND EXTRAUTERINE CAUSES)	
Newborn	**Maternal Estrogen**
Childhood	Iatrogenic (trauma, foreign body, infection of vagina)
	Vaginal neoplasms (sarcoma botryoides)
	Ovarian tumors (functional)
Adolescence	Hypothalamic immaturity
	Psychogenic and nutritional problems
	Inadequate luteal function
Reproductive age	Anovulatory
	Central: psychogenic, stress
	Systemic: nutritional and endocrine disease
	Gonadal: functional tumors
	End-organ: benign endometrial hyperplasia
	Pregnancy: ectopic, retained placenta, abortion, mole
	Ovulatory
	Organic: neoplasia, infections (PID), leiomyomas
	Polymenorrhea: short follicular or luteal phases
	Iatrogenic: anticoagulants, IUD
Menopause	Irregular shedding
Postmenopause	Carcinoma, EIN, benign hyperplasias, polyps, leiomyomata

EIN = endometrial intraepithelial neoplasia; IUD = intrauterine device; PID = pelvic inflammatory disease.

the reproductive years. It occurs most often at either end of reproductive life (i.e., menarche and menopause).

 **ETIOLOGIC FACTORS AND PATHO-LOGY:** In an anovulatory cycle, failure of ovulation leads to excessive and prolonged estrogen stimulation, without a postovulatory rise in progesterone. As a result, the endometrium remains in a proliferative state dominated by a disordered, cystic glandular appearance and excessive bulk. Lacking progesterone, the spiral arteries of the endometrium do not develop normally. "Breakthrough bleeding" can occur from damage to these fragile spiral arterioles. Thrombosis causes local tissue breakdown resembling that of menstrual endometrium, which the patient experiences as symptomatic bleeding out of synchrony with other areas of the endometrium. Elevated estrogen levels usually decline, either through delayed ovulation or involution of the stimulatory follicle. If the decline is rapid, the endometrium undergoes a heavy synchronized menstrual flow.

Luteal Phase Defect Is Caused by Inadequate Progesterone

Luteal phase defect results in an abnormally short cycle in which menses occur 6–9 days after the surge of luteinizing hormone (LH) associated with ovulation. It occurs when a corpus luteum develops improperly or regresses prematurely. Luteal phase defects are responsible for 3% of cases of infertility and must be considered in assessing infertility or in analysis of abnormal uterine bleeding. A biopsy showing an endometrium over 2 days out of synchrony with the chronologic day of the menstrual cycle confirms the diagnosis.

ENDOMETRIAL TUMORS

Endometrial Polyps Are Benign Stromal Neoplasms

Polyps occur mostly in the perimenopausal period and not before menarche. They are monoclonal outgrowths of endometrial stromal cells altered by chromosomal translocation, with secondary induction of polyclonal glandular elements. Stroma and glands of endometrial polyps respond poorly to hormonal stimulation and do not slough upon menstruation.

 PATHOLOGY: Most endometrial polyps arise in the fundus (Fig. 24-31) but can be found anywhere within the endometrium. They vary from several millimeters to growths filling the entire endometrial cavity. Most are solitary, but 20% are multiple. Polyp cores are composed of (1) endometrial glands, often cystically dilated and hyperplastic; (2) fibrous endometrial stroma; and (3) thick-walled, coiled, dilated blood vessels, derived from a straight artery that normally would have supplied the basal zone of the endometrium. Cores are covered by endometrial epithelium, usually out of cycle from adjacent normal endometrium.

 CLINICAL FEATURES: Endometrial polyps typically present with intermenstrual bleeding, owing to surface ulceration or hemorrhagic infarction. Since bleeding in an older woman may indicate endometrial cancer, this sign must be thoroughly evaluated. Endometrial polyps are not ordinarily precancerous, but up to 0.5% harbor adenocarcinoma.

Endometrial Hyperplasia Is Two Diseases, One of Which Is Neoplastic

The 2014 WHO classification of endometrial hyperplasias divides lesions into etiologic subgroups based on cancer risk and treatment options. **Nonatypical endometrial hyperplasia** is a functionally normal endometrium that responds to an abnormal hormonal state of excess estrogen; **endometrial intraepithelial neoplasia** (also called **atypical endometrial hyperplasia**) is composed of mutated precancerous cells that grow as a neoplastic clone.

- **Nonatypical hyperplasia:** Nonatypical endometrial hyperplasia is a spectrum of changes, dependant upon the duration and dose of estrogen exposure. Glands are irregularly distributed and punctuated by cysts, creating

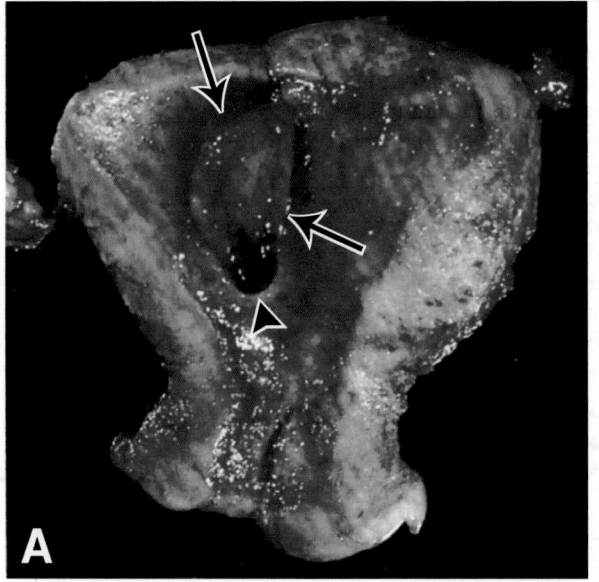 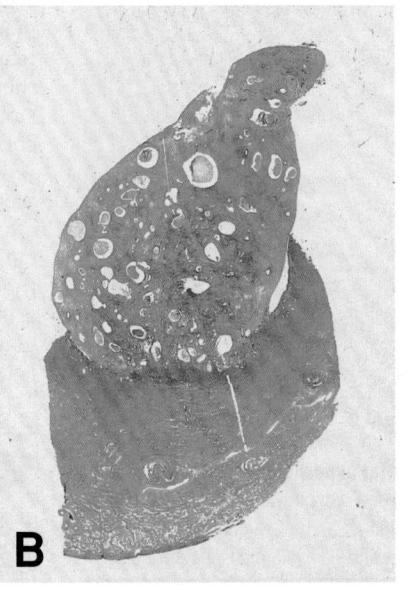

FIGURE 24-31. Endometrial polyp. A. A single polyp (*arrows*) extends into the endometrial cavity. The necrotic tip (*arrowhead*) is responsible for clinical bleeding. **B.** On microscopic section, a polyp exhibits slightly dilated endometrial glands embedded in a markedly fibrous stroma.

a variably increased ratio of glands to stroma. Cytologic change, when it occurs, is most often metaplastic and distributed in a scattered, nongeographic or random fashion. Adenocarcinoma develops in 1%–3%.

■ **EIN (atypical hyperplasia):** Endometrial intraepithelial neoplasia, or atypical endometrial hyperplasia, is a clonal outgrowth of genetically altered endometrial glands with an increased risk of future endometrioid endometrial carcinoma through malignant transformation. EIN is composed of crowded aggregates of cytologically altered tubular or slightly branching glands. Within the geographic confines of the lesion, the area of glands exceeds that of stroma, with altered cytology compared to residual background normal glands, which may be adjacent to and/or admixed with the lesion. Thirty-seven percent of patients with EIN will develop adenocarcinoma, almost always of the endometrioid type.

Nonatypical Endometrial Hyperplasia Is Caused by Abnormal Estrogenic Stimulation

It is characterized by diffuse architectural and randomly distributed cytologic changes (Fig. 24-32). Estrogenic stimulation of the endometrium beyond the normal 2-week proliferative phase causes progressive changes associated with a 2–10-fold increased risk of endometrial cancer. Aside from women with coexisting EIN (see below), it is not possible to estimate cancer risk in these patients by a single histologic examination. Endometrial histopathology varies greatly as a function of the sequence and tempo of hormonal stimulation.

 PATHOLOGY: Nonatypical endometrial hyperplasia affects the entire endometrium, in which remodeling of glands and stroma creates an irregular density of commingled cystic, slightly branching and tubular glands. The earliest changes are isolated cystic expansion of scattered proliferative glands without a substantial change in gland density, often designated **persistent**

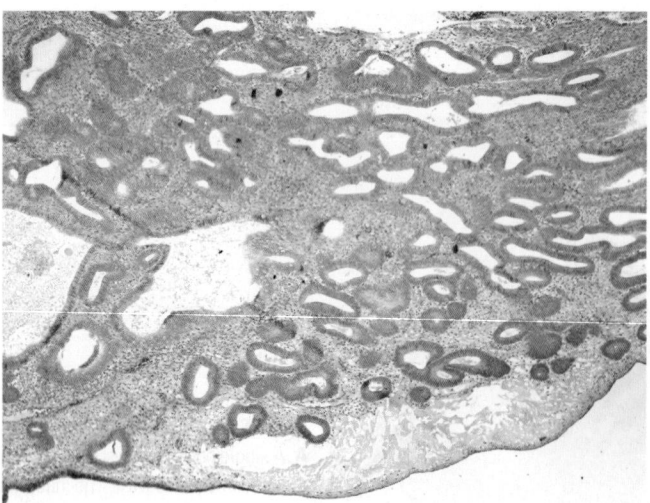

FIGURE 24-32. Nonatypical endometrial hyperplasia. Proliferative endometrial glands are irregularly distributed and randomly dilated. Gland density varies locally, but crowded and uncrowded areas have a consistent cytology throughout. This is a benign endometrium altered by unopposed estrogen.

proliferative or **disordered proliferative** endometrium. Morphologic transition to **nonatypical endometrial hyperplasia** is gradual and arbitrarily defined but can be said to occur when gland density becomes irregular throughout, with some regions having more glands than stroma.

As long as circulating estrogens persist, glands remain proliferative. Scattered glands may develop tubal differentiation with cilia formation. With increasing estrogen exposure, stromal breakdown and resultant gland collapse occur, often associated with fibrin vascular thrombi. Although prototypically an estrogenic lesion, architectural and metaplastic changes can persist after gradual weaning from a hyperestrogenic state. Sudden loss of estrogen leads to massive shedding with attendant heavy menses.

 **CLINICAL FEATURES:** Nonatypical endometrial hyperplasia may result from anovulatory cycles, polycystic ovary syndrome, an estrogen-producing tumor, estrogen administration or obesity. In such cases, therapy for the primary cause may alleviate estrogenic stimulation. Large doses of progestins can produce temporary symptomatic relief or objective remission, depending on persistence of the underlying hormonal condition. Short-term risk of endometrial cancer is low, if extensive sampling of the endometrium shows no EIN. Long-term risks of refractory nonatypical endometrial hyperplasia are best assessed by repeat biopsy.

Endometrial Intraepithelial Neoplasia Is a Clonal Precancer

EIN is a monoclonal neoplastic growth of genetically altered cells with greatly increased risk of becoming endometrioid type of endometrial adenocarcinoma (Fig. 24-33). It shows a continuity of acquired genetic markers upon transformation into a malignant phase. EIN and nonatypical endometrial hyperplasia coexist in many patients but have different histologies. Systemic hormonal factors are relevant to both, as they can be positive or negative selection factors for mutated cells in an EIN lesion.

 PATHOLOGY: EIN lesions begin at a single point and then expand centripetally as proliferating neoplastic glands that displace and separate normal glands. The densely crowded EIN glands differ cytologically from the background endometrium, have areas exceeding their stromal areas and measure more than 1 mm in dimension in a single fragment. A key diagnostic feature is the coordination of cytologic changes within the topographical region of crowded glands. Such changes are evident by comparison with flanking normal glands and usually include alterations in nuclear size, shape and texture and altered cytoplasmic differentiation. Eventually, EIN lesions overrun the entire endometrial compartment, but carcinoma can arise at any time. Malignant transformation is evident when glands develop solid, cribriform or maze-like patterns characteristic of adenocarcinoma.

 CLINICAL FEATURES: Women newly diagnosed with EIN have a 37% chance of having endometrial cancer diagnosed within 1 year. In most cases, cancer is probably present at the time of the initial biopsy, lending credence to the clinical adage "not cancer but better out." After excluding women with concurrent cancer

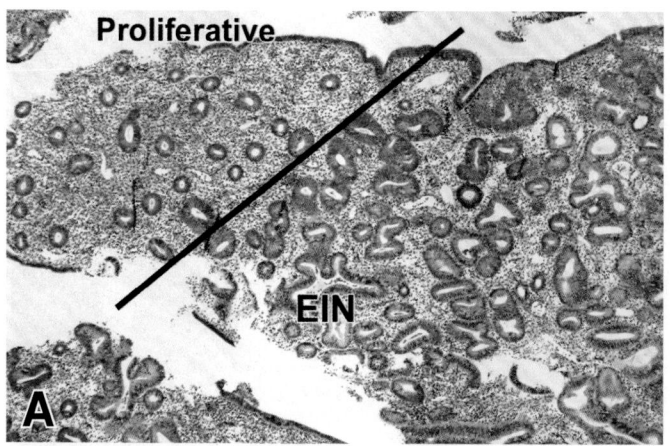
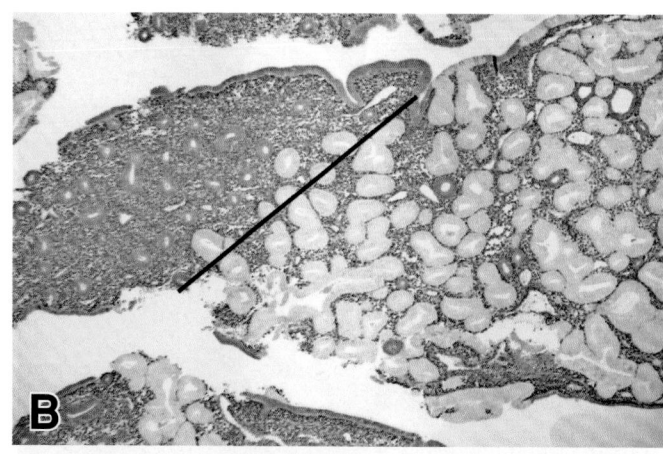

FIGURE 24-33. Endometrial intraepithelial neoplasia (EIN, atypical endometrial hyperplasia). A. Tight clusters of cytologically altered neoplastic endometrial glands with abundant cytoplasm and rounded nuclei (*right*) are offset from the background endometrium (*left*) in this geographic focus of EIN. Measurement across the perimeter of this aggregate of individual tubular glands exceeds 1 mm, and features of adenocarcinoma such as cribriform, maze-like, or solid architecture are lacking. **B.** Glands affected by EIN show loss of PTEN expression by immunohistochemistry (loss of brown staining).

and only looking at those with a cancer-free interval of 1 year, EIN-positive patients have a 45-fold increased risk of developing of endometrial cancer.

The goals of management are to rule out concurrent and prevent future cancer. Hysterectomy, usually the therapy of choice, meets both goals if a woman does not want more children. Those who want more children or are poor operative risks may be treated with progestins.

There Are two Main Types of Endometrial Adenocarcinoma

 **EPIDEMIOLOGY:** Endometrial carcinoma is the 4th most frequent cancer in American women and the most common gynecologic cancer (Table 24-5). It caused 8200 deaths in the United States in 2013 (3% of all cancers in women). Incidence of this cancer was stable from 1950 to 1970, but by 1975 it had increased by 40%, possibly related to use of estrogens for easing symptoms of menopause. By

1985, rates had returned nearly to 1950 levels, a trend that correlated with use of lower doses of estrogen, incorporation of progestins (estrogen antagonists) into estrogen replacement regimens and increased surveillance of women treated with estrogens.

The incidence of endometrial cancer varies with age, from 12 cases per 100,000 women at age 40 to 7-fold higher in 60-year-olds. Three quarters of women with endometrial cancer are postmenopausal. The median age at diagnosis is 63.

Endometrial carcinoma is broadly grouped into two histologic types (Fig. 24-34 and Table 24-5). Type I tumors (about 80%), endometrioid carcinomas, often arise from EIN precursors and are associated with estrogenic stimulation. They occur mainly in pre- or perimenopausal women and are associated with obesity, hyperlipidemia, anovulation, infertility and late menopause. Most endometrioid carcinomas are confined to the uterus and follow a favorable course. In contrast, type II tumors (about 10%) are nonendometrioid, largely papillary serous carcinomas, arising occasionally in endometrial polyps. A preinvasive form of disease, serous endometrial intraepithelial carcinoma (serous EIC, not to be confused with EIN) can metastasize to the peritoneum by exfoliation and surface spread. Although serous EIC can exhibit malignant behavior, it is not generally considered a precancerous lesion. Type II tumors are not associated with estrogen stimulation or hyperplasia, readily invade myometrium and vascular spaces and are highly lethal. The molecular alterations of endometrioid (type I) carcinomas are different from those of the nonendometrioid (type II) carcinomas.

These tumors overlap in clinical, pathologic, immunohistochemical and molecular characteristics. Some nonendometrioid (type II) carcinomas may arise from preexisting endometrioid carcinomas and share pathologic and molecular features of both types I and II endometrial carcinomas. The type II tumor category consists primarily of serous carcinomas but also includes rarer clear cell carcinoma and carcinosarcoma histotypes that have distinct molecular and clinical features.

Endometrial cancer occurs in association with a higher incidence of both breast and ovarian cancer in closely related women, suggesting a genetic predisposition. It is also the

TABLE 24-5

CLINICOPATHOLOGIC FEATURES OF ENDOMETRIAL CARCINOMA

	Type I: Endometrioid Carcinoma	Type II: Serous Carcinoma
Age	Pre- and perimenopausal	Postmenopausal
Unopposed estrogen	Present	Absent
Hyperplasia precursor	Present	Absent
Grade	Low	High
Myometrial invasion	Superficial	Deep
Growth behavior	Stable	Progressive
Genetic alterations	Microsatellite instability, PTEN, PIK3CA, β-catenin	p53 mutations, loss of heterozygosity (LOH)

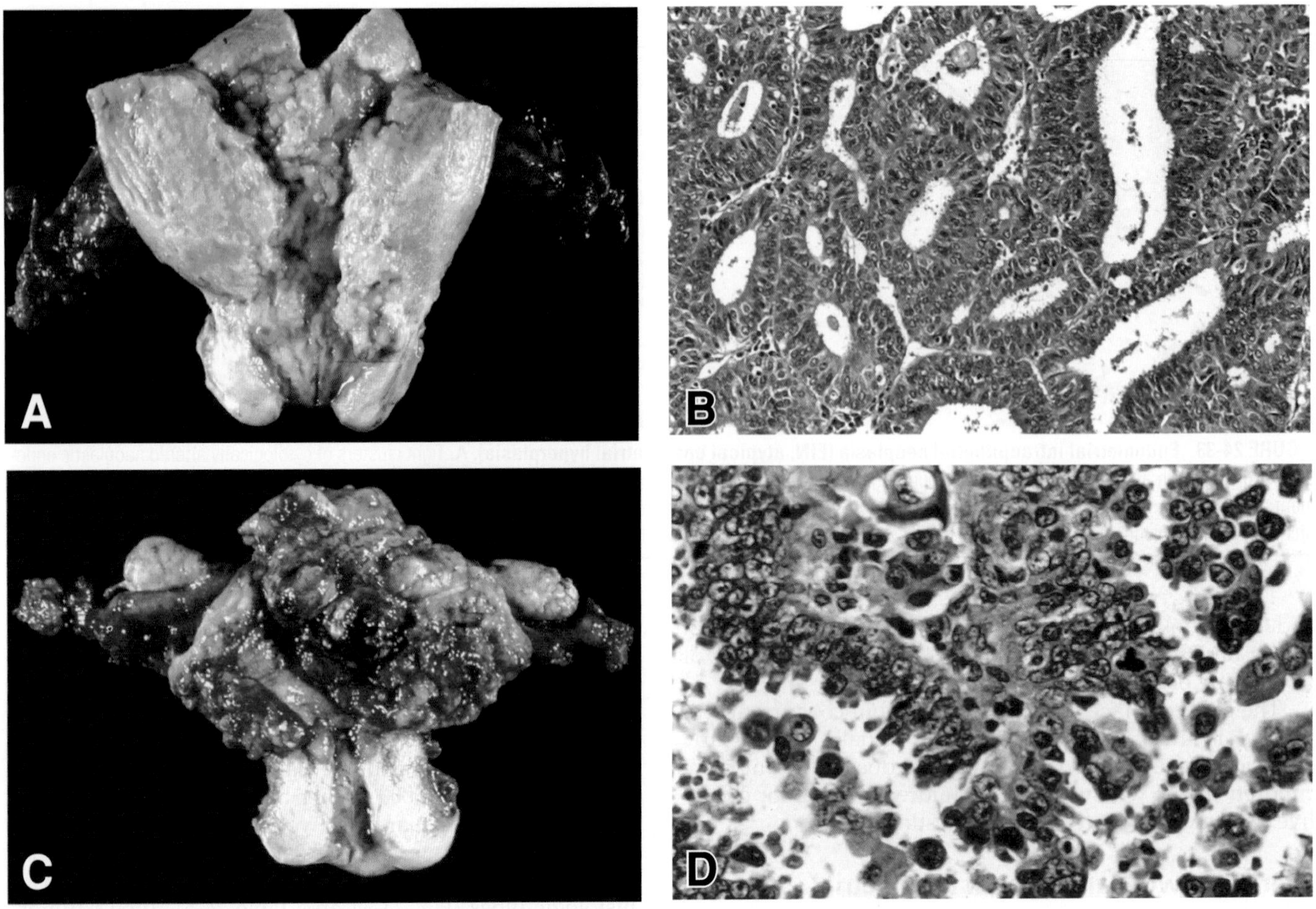

FIGURE 24-34. Adenocarcinoma of the endometrium. A, B. Endometrioid carcinoma. Polypoid tumor with only superficial myometrial invasion. Well-differentiated (grade 1) adenocarcinoma. The neoplastic glands resemble normal endometrial glands. **C, D. Nonendometrioid carcinoma.** Large hemorrhagic and necrotic tumor with deep myometrial invasion. Serous carcinoma (severe cytologic atypia) exhibiting stratification of anaplastic tumor cells and abnormal mitoses.

most common extracolonic cancer in women with hereditary nonpolyposis colon cancer syndrome, a defect in DNA mismatch repair (see Chapter 19) that is also associated with breast and ovarian cancers.

MOLECULAR PATHOGENESIS: A dualistic model of endometrial carcinogenesis has been proposed in which normal endometrial cells transform into endometrioid carcinoma by accumulating mutations in oncogenes and tumor suppressor genes. The most commonly affected genes and mechanisms of genetic damage differ between endometrioid (type I) and nonendometrioid (type II) cancers.

Genetic alterations accumulate in the type I carcinoma pathway, during the transition from normal to EIN to endometrioid carcinoma (Fig. 24-35). These may occur over a period of years and involve a combination of small-scale deletions, point mutations and epigenetic modifications of cells that maintain normal or near-normal karyotypes. *PTEN* is the most often inactivated tumor suppressor gene in endometrial tumorigenesis (2/3 of cases), resulting from deletion, mutation and/or promoter hypermethylation (Figs. 24-33 and 24-35). *PIK3CA* is the most commonly activated oncogene (by mutation, in up to 39% of cases) in endometrial carcinoma. *PTEN* inactivation frees the PI3K-Akt pathway, evading apoptosis and resulting in tumor growth

advantage; *PIK3CA* mutations are rarely seen in such cases. Other frequently mutated genes include *KRAS* (10%–30%) and β-catenin (*CTNNB1*) with nuclear protein accumulation (25%–38%). *TP53* mutations are rare (5%–10%). In a quarter of sporadic tumors, a specific type of genetic damage,

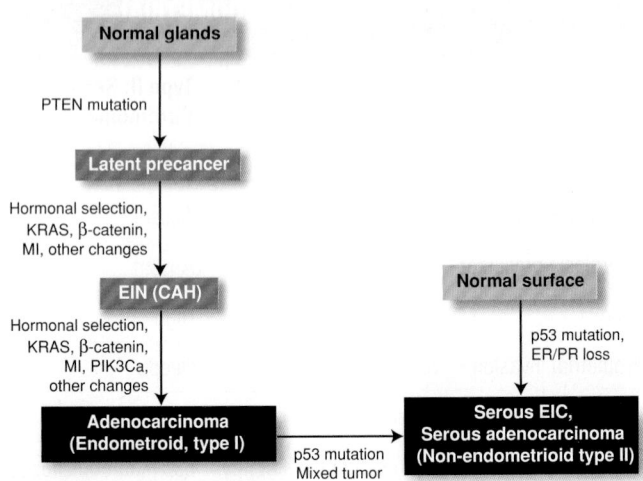

FIGURE 24-35. From endometrial hyperplasia to endometrioid carcinoma: molecular and genetic events. MI, microsatellite instability.

microsatellite instability (MSI), results from promoter hypermethylation of *MLH1* and leads to microsatellite instability and accelerated mutation in several critical target genes involved in apoptosis, cell proliferation and differentiation. The wide range of resultant mutations, in both microsatellite-stable and -unstable endometrioid tumors, creates genetically heterogeneous tumors.

Over 90% of type II nonendometrioid carcinomas have p53 mutations, and 80% lose estrogen and progesterone receptors. Mechanisms of DNA damage are different from endometrioid tumors. MSI is rare (<5%), and gross structural and numerical chromosomes abnormalities are more common. Nonendometrioid carcinomas may also develop from endometrioid tumors via p53 mutations and other means.

 PATHOLOGY: Endometrial cancer grows in diffuse or exophytic patterns (Fig. 24-34). Regardless of its site of origin, the tumor often tends to involve multiple areas. Large tumors are usually hemorrhagic and necrotic.

ENDOMETRIOID ADENOCARCINOMA OF THE ENDOMETRIUM: This type of endometrial cancer, composed entirely of glandular cells, is the most common histologic variant (80%–85%). The FIGO system divides this tumor into three grades depending on the ratio of glandular to solid elements, the latter signifying poorer differentiation (Fig. 24-36).

■ **Grade 1:** Well differentiated; almost only neoplastic glands, with minimal (<5%) solid areas

■ **Grade 2:** Moderately differentiated; 5%–50% of malignant epithelium forms glands
■ **Grade 3:** Poorly differentiated; large (>50%) areas of solid tumor

Nuclei of endometrial adenocarcinoma range from bland to markedly pleomorphic, usually with prominent nucleoli. Mitoses are abundant and may be abnormal in less differentiated tumors. Tumor cells that grow in solid sheets are generally poorly differentiated. The FIGO system also defines stages of endometrial cancer (Table 24-6).

ENDOMETRIOID ADENOCARCINOMA, WITH SQUAMOUS DIFFERENTIATION: One third of endometrial carcinomas contain squamous cells as well as glands. If the squamous element shows only minimal atypia, the tumor is a **well-differentiated adenocarcinoma with squamous differentiation** (previously, **adenoacanthoma**) (Fig. 24-37). If the squamous element appears malignant, the tumor is **poorly differentiated adenocarcinoma with squamous differentiation** (also known as **adenosquamous carcinoma**). These variants represent 22% and 7% of all endometrial cancers, respectively.

ENDOMETRIOID ADENOCARCINOMA, SECRETORY TYPE: This variant usually occurs in premenopausal women. It is an extremely well-differentiated but otherwise typical endometrial adenocarcinoma. Large subnuclear vacuoles of glycogen occur in some cases owing to progesterone stimulation. Secretory carcinoma, perhaps because it is very well differentiated, has the most favorable prognosis.

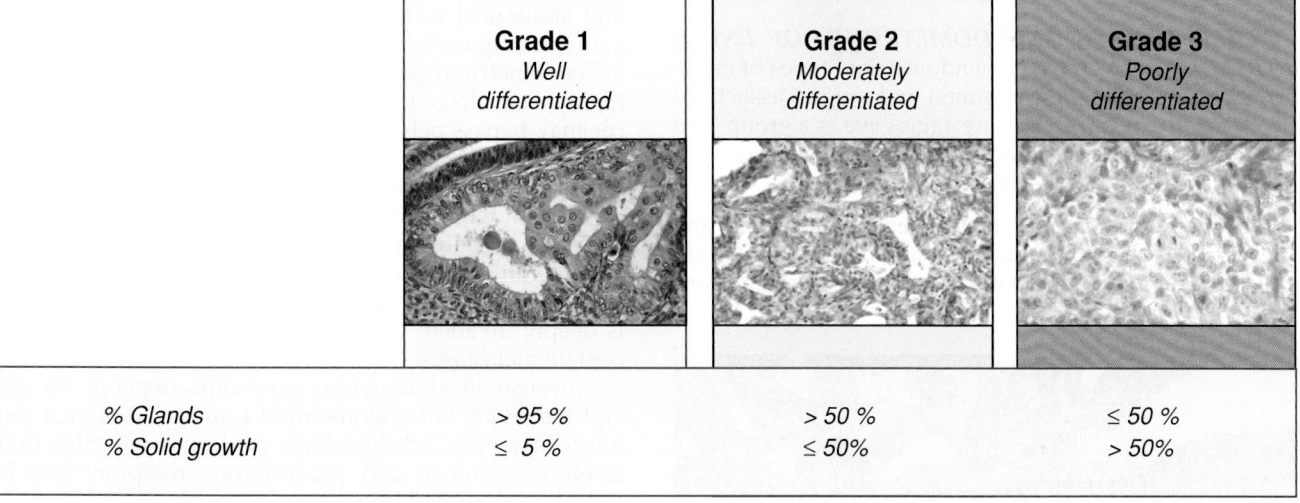

	Grade 1	Grade 2	Grade 3
% Glands	> 95 %	> 50 %	≤ 50 %
% Solid growth	≤ 5 %	≤ 50%	> 50%

Significant
NUCLEAR ATYPIA
if present
increases the grade

Nuclear atypia
Round nuclei
Variation in shape and size
Variation in staining
Hyperchromasia
Coarsely clumped chromatin
Prominent nucleoli
Frequent mitoses
Abnormal mitoses

FIGURE 24-36. Grading of endometrial adenocarcinoma. The grade depends primarily on the architectural pattern, but significant nuclear atypia changes a grade 1 tumor to grade 2, and a grade 2 tumor to grade 3. Nuclear atypia is characterized by round nuclei; variation in shape, size and staining; hyperchromasia; coarsely clumped chromating; prominent nucleoli; and frequent and abnormal mitoses. Significant nuclear atypia if present increases the tumor grade.

TABLE 24-6

FIGO (2009) STAGING OF CANCER OF THE ENDOMETRIUM

Stage	Anatomic Distribution
Stage I	Tumor confined to the corpus uteri
IA	No myometrial invasion or invasion <50% of myometrium thickness
IB	Tumor invades ≥50% of myometrium thickness
Stage II	Tumor invades cervical stroma but does not extend beyond the uterus
Stage III	Local and/or regional spread of the tumor
IIIA	Tumor invades the serosa of the corpus uteri and/or adnexa
IIIB	Vaginal and/or parametrial involvement
IIIC	Metastases to pelvic and/or para-aortic lymph nodes
Stage IV	Tumor invades bladder and/or bowel mucosa, and/or distant metastases
IVA	Tumor invasion of bladder and/or bowel mucosa
IVB	Distant metastases, including intra-abdominal metastases and/or inguinal lymph nodes

FIGO = International Federation of Gynecology and Obstetrics.

OTHER TYPES (NONENDOMETRIOID) OF ENDO-METRIAL CARCINOMA: Nonendometrioid types of endometrial carcinoma are less common and are not associated with estrogen exposure. They are aggressive as a group, and histologic grading is not clinically useful or separately diagnosed, as all cases are considered high grade.

- **Serous adenocarcinoma** histologically resembles, and behaves like, serous adenocarcinoma of the ovary (Fig. 24-34D). It often shows transtubal spread to peri-

toneal surfaces. An in situ form is termed "serous endometrial intraepithelial carcinoma" (serous EIC), not to be confused with EIN, described earlier.

- **Clear cell adenocarcinoma** is a tumor of older women. It contains large cells with abundant cytoplasmic glycogen ("clear cells") or cells with bulbous nuclei that line glandular lumens ("hobnail cells") (Fig. 24-38A). Serous and clear cell carcinomas have poor prognoses.

- **Carcinosarcoma (malignant mixed mesodermal tumor):** In this highly malignant tumor (Fig. 24-38B), pleomorphic **epithelial** cells comingle with areas showing **mesenchymal** differentiation (Fig. 24-38C). These mixed neoplasms are derived from a common clone believed to be of epithelial origin. Prognosis is determined by the presence of a mesenchymal component admixed with the malignant epithelial component, rather than the specific type of mesenchymal histology displayed. Overall 5-year survival is 25%.

Most endometrial carcinomas arise in the uterine corpus, but a small proportion originate in the lower uterine segment (isthmus). These tumors often occur in women under the age of 50 and are often high grade and deeply invasive.

 CLINICAL FEATURES: Endometrial cancers usually occur in peri- or postmenopausal women. The chief complaint is commonly abnormal uterine bleeding, especially in the early stages of tumor growth confined to the endometrium. Unfortunately, cervicovaginal cytologic screening does not efficiently detect early endometrial cancer. Fractional curettage is needed to assess spread to the cervix, whereas peritoneal washing detects tubal reflux and abdominal contamination. Transvaginal ultrasound is valuable diagnostically in postmenopausal patients in whom an endometrium greater than 5 mm thick is considered highly suspicious. Unlike cervical cancer, endometrial cancer may bypass pelvic lymph nodes and spread directly to para-aortic nodes. Patients with advanced cancers may also have pulmonary metastases (40% of cases with metastases).

Women with well-differentiated cancers confined to the endometrium are usually treated by simple hysterectomy. Postoperative radiation is considered if the tumor is poorly differentiated or nonendometrioid in type, the myometrium is deeply invaded, the cervix is involved or lymph nodes contain metastases.

Survival in endometrial carcinoma depends on stage and histotype. For endometrioid tumors, additional prognostic factors include histologic grade and age. High tumor levels of estrogen and progesterone receptors and low mitotic rates correlate with a better prognosis. Actuarial survival for all patients with endometrial cancer following treatment is 80% after 2 years, decreasing to 65% after 10 years. Tumors that have penetrated the myometrium or invaded lymphatics are more likely to have spread beyond the uterus. Endometrial cancers involving the cervix have a poorer prognosis. Spread outside the uterus carries the worst outlook (Table 24-7).

Fewer than 2% of Uterine Cancers Are Endometrial Stromal Tumors

Some endometrial stromal tumors are pure sarcomas; in others, sarcomatous (stromal) and epithelial elements are intermingled. The nomenclature of these tumor types, the

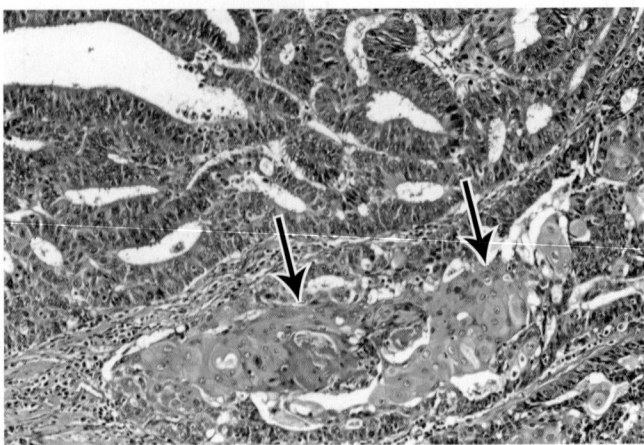

FIGURE 24-37. Squamous differentiation in endometrioid adenocarcinoma of the endometrium. The well-differentiated squamous cells (*arrows*) show minimal atypia. The pattern has been called adenoacanthoma when the squamous cells form squamous morules and nest among glands.

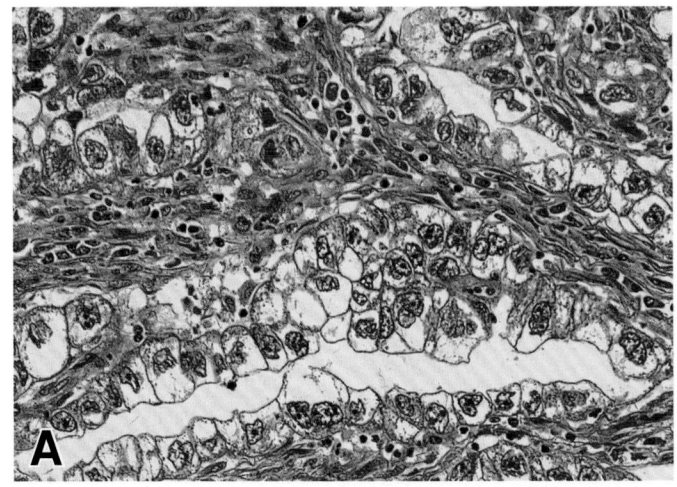

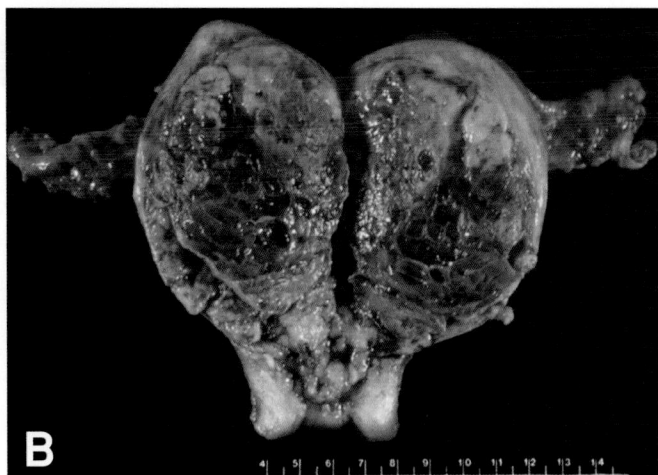

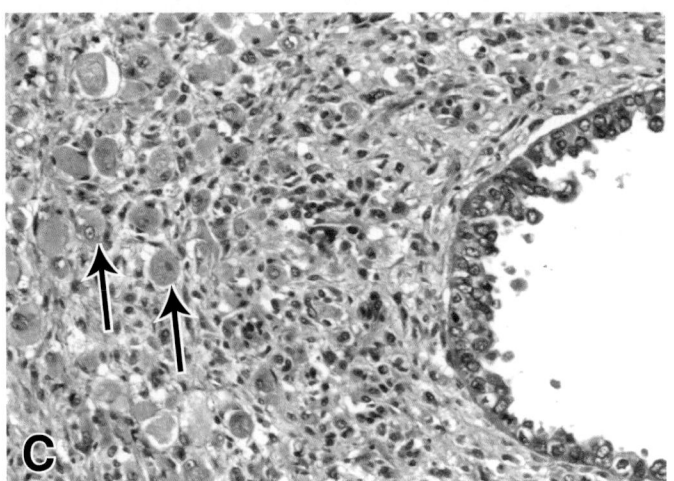

FIGURE 24-38. Nonendometrioid types of endometrial adenocarcinoma. A. Clear cell endometrial adenocarcinoma. The clear appearance of the cytoplasm is due to the dissolution of glycogen when the specimen was processed for microscopic examination. Hobnail cells with bulbous nuclei line glandular lumina. **B.** Carcinosarcoma (malignant mixed müllerian tumor). Solid, partially cystic and necrotic mass that expands the uterine cavity. **C.** Rhabdomyoblasts (heterologous elements, *arrows*) appear as pleomorphic, rounded cells with ample eosinophilic cytoplasm adjacent to malignant epithelium.

spectrum of their histologic components and the correlation of each tumor type with its potential for malignant behavior are presented in Table 24-8.

Endometrial Stromal Sarcoma

Pure stromal tumors are divided into two major categories, based on whether the tumor margin is expansile or infiltrating. Expansile lesions that do not invade are **benign stromal nodules,** which have little clinical significance. Tumors with infiltrating margins are termed **stromal sarcomas** and are classified into low-grade (most common) and high-grade categories.

PATHOLOGY: Low-grade endometrial stromal sarcomas may be polypoid and fill the endometrial cavity, or they may diffusely invade the myometrium. Large masses of spindle cells with scant cytoplasm dissect the myometrium and invade vascular channels (Fig. 24-39). Tumor cells resemble endometrial stromal cells in the proliferative phase and show little or no cytologic atypia and low mitotic activity. Expression of CD-10 and estrogen

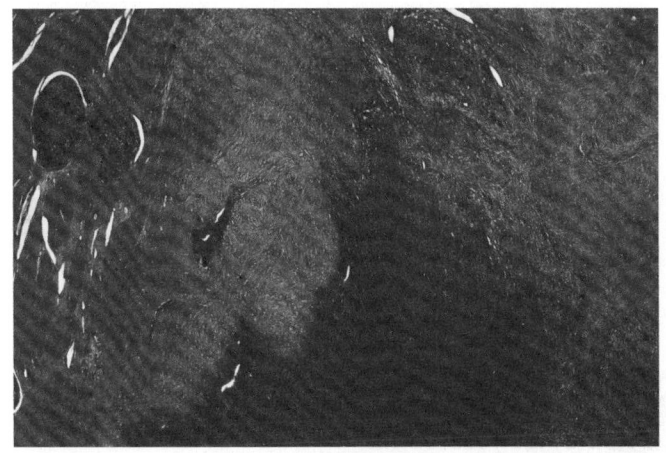

FIGURE 24-39. Endometrial stromal sarcoma, low grade. The myometrium is irregularly invaded by the tumor, which invades vascular spaces.

TABLE 24-7

STAGE, GRADE AND SURVIVAL FOR ENDOMETRIAL CANCER

Stage	5-Year Survival (%)		
	G-1[a]	G-2	G-3
I	90	69	52
II	80	42	12
III, IV	25	33	17

[a]G = FIGO (International Federation of Gynecology and Obstetrics) grade.

TABLE 24-8

NOMENCLATURE OF UTERINE TUMORS

Tumor	Epithelium	Stroma	Clinical Behavior
Epithelium and Stroma			
Endometrial polyp	Polyclonal benign	Neoplastic	Benign
Nonatypical endometrial hyperplasia	Polyclonal benign	Polyclonal benign	Benign
Endometrial intraepithelial neoplasia	Neoplastic	—	Premalignant
Endometrial adenocarcinoma	Neoplastic	—	Malignant
Endometrial stromal nodule	—	Neoplastic	Benign
Endometrial stromal sarcoma	—	Neoplastic	Low-grade malignant
Undifferentiated sarcoma	—	Neoplastic	Malignant
Adenosarcoma	Unknown	Neoplastic	Low-grade malignant
Carcinosarcoma	Neoplastic	Neoplastic, transformed epithelial cells	Malignant
Smooth Muscle			
Leiomyoma	—	Neoplastic	Benign
Cellular leiomyoma	—	Neoplastic	Benign
Intravenous leiomyomatosis	—	Neoplastic	Locally aggressive
Leiomyosarcoma	—	Neoplastic	Malignant

and progesterone receptors (ER and PR) helps confirm the diagnosis. Most low-grade endometrial stromal sarcomas harbor t(7;17)(p21;q15), which results in a fusion between JAZF1 and SUZ12. By contrast, the high-grade endometrial stromal sarcomas, characterized by the recurrent aberration t(10;17)(q22;p13), exhibit an atypical round cell (predominant) and a low-grade spindle cell component. CD10, ER and PR are negative, but cyclin D1 is strongly positive. Higher-grade sarcomas originating in the endometrium lose all antigenic and morphologic resemblance to endometrial stroma and are thus designated as **undifferentiated uterine sarcoma**.

CLINICAL FEATURES: Many years may elapse before low-grade endometrial stromal sarcomas recur clinically, and metastases may occur even if the original tumor was confined to the uterus at initial surgery. Recurrences usually involve the pelvis first, followed by lung metastases. Prolonged survival and even cure are feasible, despite metastases. By contrast, high-grade endometrial stromal and undifferentiated uterine sarcomas recur early, generally with widespread metastases, even if there had been little myometrial invasion. Low-grade endometrial stromal sarcomas can be successfully treated with surgery and progestin therapy, with an expectation of 90% survival 10 years after diagnosis.

Uterine Adenosarcoma

Uterine (müllerian) adenosarcoma is a distinctive low-grade tumor with benign glandular epithelium and malignant

stroma (Fig. 24-40). It differs from carcinosarcoma, in which both epithelial and stromal elements are malignant (see above).

Adenosarcoma typically presents as a polypoid mass within the endometrial cavity. The glandular epithelium resembles proliferative phase endometrial glands, but occasionally squamous epithelium and mucinous-type epithelium are seen. The stroma is cellular, may exhibit mitotic activity, is often densest about the glandular epithelium (periglandular cuffing) and resembles endometrial stromal

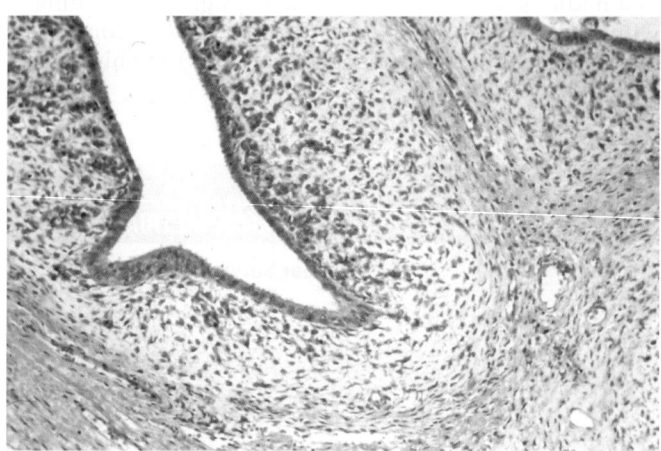

FIGURE 24-40. Adenosarcoma. There is periglandular cuffing by atypical stromal cells with mitotic activity.

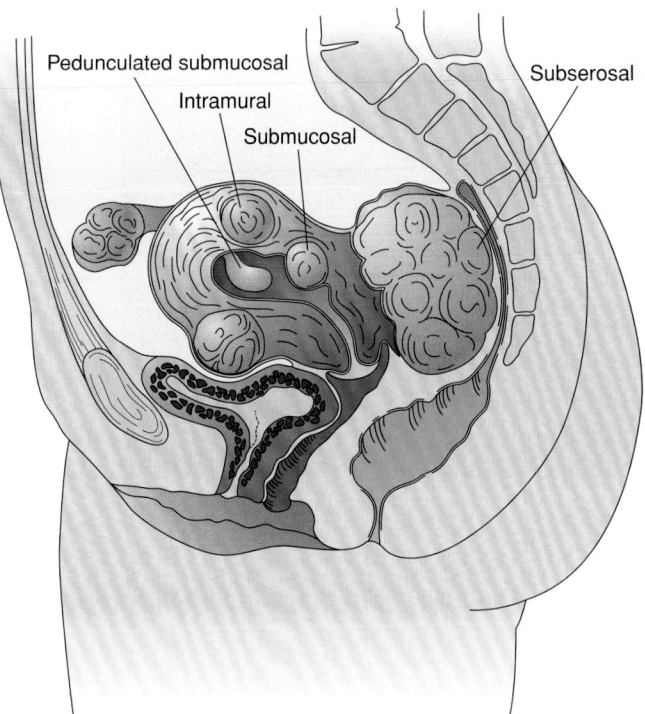

FIGURE 24-41. Leiomyomas of the uterus. The leiomyomas are intramural, submucosal (a pedunculated one appearing in the form of an endometrial polyp) and subserosal (one compressing the bladder and the other the rectum).

cells in the proliferative phase of the cycle. One fourth of patients with adenosarcoma eventually succumb to local recurrence or metastatic spread. In these patients, myometrial invasion and/or high-grade sarcomatous overgrowth usually occur.

Leiomyomas Are the Most Common Female Genital Tract Tumors

Leiomyomas, benign tumors of smooth muscle origin, are colloquially known as "myomas" or "fibroids." Including minute tumors, leiomyomas occur in 75% of women over age 30. They are rare before age 20, and most regress after

menopause. Although often multiple, each tumor is monoclonal (see Chapter 5). Estrogen promotes their growth but does not initiate them.

 PATHOLOGY: Grossly, leiomyomas are firm, pale gray, whorled and without encapsulation (Figs. 24-41 and 24-42). They vary from 1 mm to over 30 cm in diameter. Their cut surface bulges, and borders are smooth and distinct from neighboring myometrium. Most leiomyomas are intramural, but some are submucosal, subserosal or pedunculated. Many, especially larger ones, show areas of degenerative hyalinization that are sharply demarcated from adjacent normal myometrium. Leiomyomas show little mitotic activity (<4 mitoses per 10 high-power fields [HPFs]), lack nuclear atypia and geographical necrosis and have little or no malignant potential. A **"mitotically active leiomyoma"** is one that shows brisk mitotic activity but is relatively small, is sharply demarcated from adjacent normal myometrium and lacks both geographical necrosis and significant cellular atypia. It is usually benign.

Microscopically, leiomyomas exhibit interlacing fascicles of uniform spindle cells containing elongated nuclei with blunt ends (Fig. 24-42B). Cytoplasm is abundant, eosinophilic and fibrillar. The cells of leiomyomas and adjacent normal myometrium are cytologically identical, but leiomyomas are easily distinguished by their circumscription, nodularity and denser cellularity.

 CLINICAL FEATURES: Submucosal leiomyomas may cause bleeding owing to ulceration of thinned, overlying endometrium, or become pedunculated and protrude through the cervical os, eliciting cramping pains. Many intramural leiomyomas are symptomatic because of their sheer bulk, and large ones may interfere with bowel or bladder function or cause dystocia in labor. Pedunculated leiomyomas on the uterine serosa may interfere with the function of neighboring viscera. Leiomyomas may also infarct and become painful if they undergo torsion.

Leiomyomas usually grow slowly but occasionally enlarge rapidly during pregnancy. Large symptomatic leiomyomas are removed by myomectomy or hysterectomy. Ablation by arterial thrombosis has also been used recently.

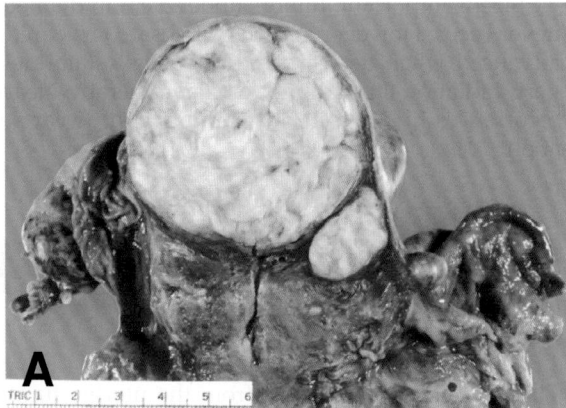
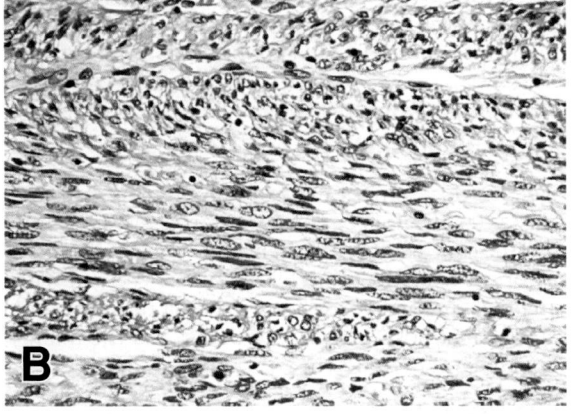

FIGURE 24-42. Leiomyoma of the uterus. A. A bisected uterus displays a prominent, sharply circumscribed, fleshy tumor. **B.** Microscopically, smooth muscle cells intertwine in bundles, some of which are cut longitudinally (elongated nuclei) and others transversely.

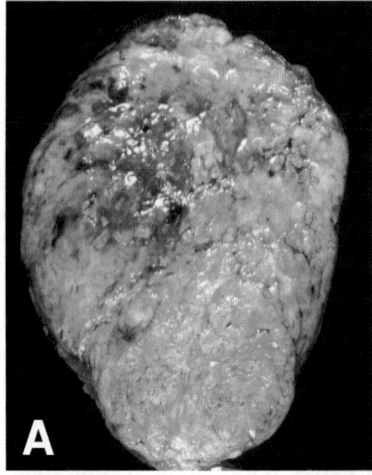

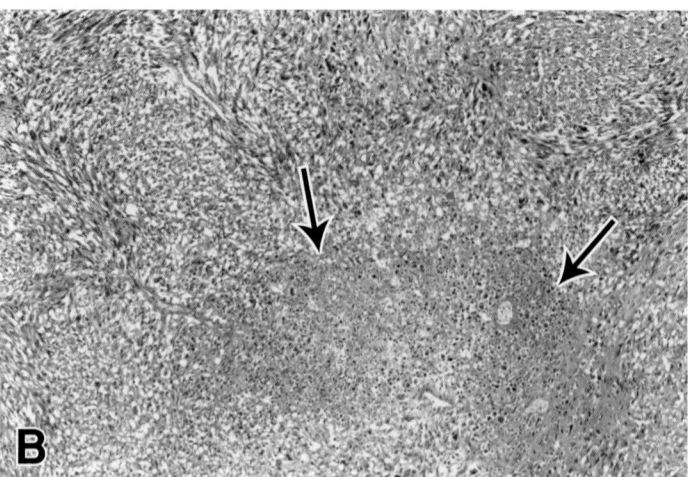

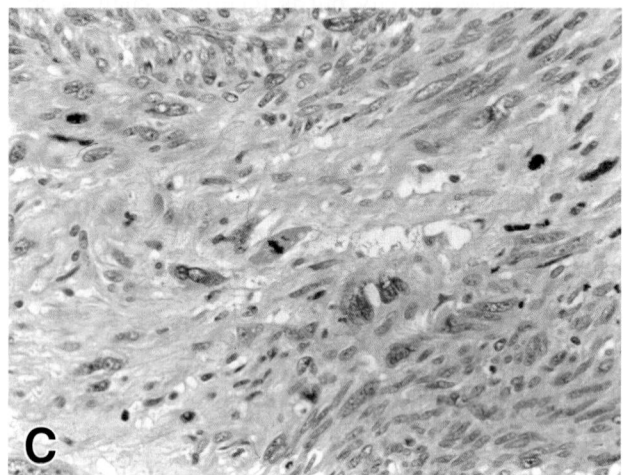

FIGURE 24-43. Leiomyosarcoma of the uterus. **A.** The uterus has been opened to reveal a large, soft leiomyosarcoma with extensive necrosis that replaces the entire myometrium. **B.** A zone of coagulative tumor necrosis (*arrows*) appears demarcated from the viable tumor. **C.** The tumor shows considerable nuclear atypia and abundant mitotic activity.

Intravenous Leiomyomatosis Does Not Metastasize

Intravenous leiomyomatosis is a rare condition in which benign smooth muscle grows within uterine and pelvic veins. It may develop after vascular invasion by a uterine leiomyoma or from growth of venous smooth muscle. At surgery, it appears as worm-like extensions near the external uterine surface or as projections into uterine veins in the broad ligament. Although they may grow extensively inside blood vessels, these neoplasms do not metastasize. Rare fatalities have resulted from direct extension of leiomyomas from pelvic veins into the inferior vena cava and right atrium. Treatment consists of total abdominal hysterectomy.

Leiomyosarcomas Are Very Rare Compared to Leiomyomas

Leiomyosarcoma is a smooth muscle malignancy whose incidence is 1/1000th of its benign counterpart. It accounts for 2% of uterine cancers. Its pathogenesis is uncertain, but at least some appear to arise within leiomyomas. Women with leiomyosarcomas are on average more than a decade older (age above 50) than those with leiomyomas, and the malignant tumors are larger (10–15 cm vs. 3–5 cm) (Fig. 24-43A).

 PATHOLOGY: Leiomyosarcoma should be suspected when an apparent leiomyoma is soft, shows areas of necrosis on gross examination, has irregular borders (invasion of adjacent myometrium) or fails to protrude above the surface when cut. Evidence that a uterine smooth muscle tumor is a leiomyosarcoma includes (1) presence of geographical necrosis with a sharp transition from viable tumor (Fig. 24-43B); (2) 10 or more mitoses per 10 HPFs (Fig. 24-43C), if the tumor is more than 5 cm in diameter; (3) 5 or more mitoses per 10 HPFs, with geographical necrosis and diffuse cytoplasmic/nuclear atypia; and (4) myxoid and epithelioid smooth muscle tumors with 5 or more mitoses per 10 HPFs.

Size is important: tumors under 5 cm in diameter almost never recur. However, most leiomyosarcomas are large and advanced when detected and are usually fatal despite surgery, radiation therapy and/or chemotherapy. Nearly half of recurrences first present in the lung, and 5-year survival is about 20%.

Fallopian Tube

ANATOMY

The fallopian tubes extend from the uterine fundus to the ovaries. An interstitial portion, the **isthmus,** lies within the cornua of the uterus and connects the uterine cavity with the straight portion of the tube. As the tube extends to the ovary, it increases in diameter to form the **ampulla,** which merges with the **infundibulum**. The fimbriated end opens like the bell of a trumpet and has finger-like extensions that envelop the ovary. The lining cells are ciliated and are important in transport of ova.

SALPINGITIS

Salpingitis is inflammation of the fallopian tubes, typically due to infections ascending from the lower genital tract. The most common causative organisms are *N. gonorrhoeae, Escherichia coli, Chlamydia* and *Mycoplasma,* and most infections are polymicrobial. Acute episodes of salpingitis (particularly if due to chlamydia) may be asymptomatic. A fallopian tube damaged by prior infection is very susceptible to reinfection. In most cases, chronic salpingitis develops only after repeated episodes of acute salpingitis.

 PATHOLOGY AND CLINICAL FEATURES: In acute salpingitis, there is marked neutrophil infiltration, edema and congestion of mucosal folds (plicae). In chronic salpingitis, the inflammatory infiltrate is mainly lymphocytes and plasma cells; edema and congestion are usually minimal. In late stages, the fallopian tube may seal and become distended with pus **(pyosalpinx)** or a transudate **(hydrosalpinx)**.

The fallopian tube allows infections from the lower genital tract to ascend to the peritoneal cavity, leading to peritonitis and PID. Fibrinous adhesions between the fallopian tube serosa and surrounding peritoneal surfaces organize into thin fibrous bands ("violin string" adhesions). The adjacent ovary may also be involved, sometimes as a **tuboovarian abscess**. Destruction of the fallopian tube epithelium or deposition of fibrin on its surface leads to fibrin bridges connecting the plicae to one another. In severe chronic salpingitis, dense adhesions cause the end of the tube to become blunted and clubbed. A blocked lumen may lead to hydrosalpinx or pyosalpinx. The damage wrought by chronic salpingitis may also impair tubal motility and passage of sperm, resulting in **infertility**. Chronic salpingitis is a common cause of **ectopic pregnancy,** since adherent mucosal plicae create pockets in which ova are entrapped.

ECTOPIC PREGNANCY

Ectopic pregnancy is implantation of a fertilized ovum outside the endometrium. The frequency of ectopic pregnancy in the United States has increased 3-fold, to 1.5% of live births, during the past two decades, although mortality has sharply declined. **Over 95% of such pregnancies are in the fallopian tube, mostly in the distal and middle thirds.**

 PATHOLOGY: Ectopic pregnancy results when passage of a conceptus along a fallopian tube is impeded, for example, by mucosal adhesions or abnormal tubal motility due to inflammatory disease or endometriosis. The trophoblast readily penetrates the tubal mucosa and musculature. Blood from the tubal implantation site enters the peritoneum, causing abdominal pain. Ectopic pregnancy is also associated with anomalous uterine bleeding

after a period of amenorrhea and Arias-Stella cells in the endometrium. The thin tubal wall usually ruptures by the 12th week of gestation. *Tubal rupture is life-threatening as it can lead to rapid exsanguination.*

Rupture of the tube's interstitial portion produces greater intra-abdominal hemorrhage than rupture in other locations because vasculature there is richer and rupture occurs later in gestation. In the isthmus, the tube ruptures early (within the first 6 weeks), because its thick muscular wall does not allow much distention. Tubal pregnancies in the ampulla tend to be of longer duration, since the distensible tubal wall can accommodate a growing pregnancy for a longer time.

Ectopic pregnancy must be treated promptly with surgery or chemotherapy. Administration of methotrexate terminates ectopic pregnancy and is used when the conceptus is smaller than 4 cm.

FALLOPIAN TUBE TUMORS

Benign tumors arising within the fallopian tube are rare. The most common is the small, circumscribed **adenomatoid tumor,** which is of mesothelial origin. It arises in the mesosalpinx and shows benign mesothelial cells that line slit-like spaces.

Thorough evaluation of the fallopian tube in women at heightened hereditary risk for "ovarian" cancer (*BRCA* mutation) has shown that many resultant cancers arise in the tubal fimbria as **serous tubal intraepithelial carcinoma** (STIC). The tubal fimbria have also been shown to be an early site of involvement of some sporadic (nonhereditary) serous adenocarcinomas. STIC lesions are physically small, often grossly inapparent and composed of mitotically active regions of atypical epithelium expressing mutant *TP53*. An unknown proportion of **high-grade pelvic serous adenocarcinomas** previously classified as ovarian or peritoneal primary tumors may in fact be tubal carcinomas metastatic to those sites. This revised biological model of pelvic serous carcinogenesis has identified new targets for prevention (the fallopian tube). Clinical tumor staging at these sites has been revised to consider ovarian and tubal carcinomas in an integrated fashion (Table 24-9).

Fallopian tube involvement by metastases or implants from adjacent ovarian and uterine neoplasms also occurs. Most primary malignancies are adenocarcinomas, with peak incidence among 50- to 60-year-olds.

Ovary

ANATOMY AND EMBRYOLOGY

The ovaries are paired organs that flank the uterus. They are attached to the posterior surface of the broad ligament in a shallow peritoneal fossa between the external iliac vessels and the ureter. Each ovary has an epithelial surface, a mesenchymal stroma containing steroid-producing cells and germ cells, an outer cortex and an inner medulla.

Ovaries appear early in fetal life as swellings of the genital ridges. At the 19th gestational day, germ cells migrate from the primitive yolk sac to the gonads and multiply by mitotic division. By the 40th day, ovaries and testes are

TABLE 24-9

FIGO (2012) STAGING OF CANCER OF THE OVARY, FALLOPIAN TUBE AND PERITONEUM

Stage	Anatomic Distribution
Stage I	Tumor confined to ovaries or fallopian tube(s)
IA	Tumor limited to one ovary (capsule intact) or fallopian tube Surface free of tumor and washings negative
IB	Tumor limited to both ovaries (capsules intact) or fallopian tubes Surface free of tumor and washings negative
IC	Tumor limited to one or both ovaries or fallopian tubes, with any of the following:
IC1	Surgical spill intraoperatively
IC2	Capsule ruptured before surgery or tumor on ovarian or fallopian tube surface
IC3	Malignant cells in the ascites or peritoneal washings
Stage II	Tumor involves one or both ovaries or fallopian tubes with pelvic extension (below pelvic brim) or primary peritoneal cancer
IIA	Extension and/or implants on the uterus and/or fallopian tubes and/or ovaries
IIB	Extension to other pelvic intraperitoneal tissues
Stage III	Cytologically or histologically confirmed spread to the peritoneum outside the pelvis and/or metastasis to the retroperitoneal lymph nodes
IIIA	Metastasis to the retroperitoneal lymph nodes with or without microscopic peritoneal involvement beyond the pelvis
IIIA1	Positive retroperitoneal lymph nodes only (cytologically or histologically proven)
IIIA1 (i)	Nodal metastasis ≤10 mm in greatest dimension
IIIA1 (ii)	Nodal metastasis >10 mm in greatest dimension
IIIA2	Microscopic extrapelvic (above the pelvic brim) peritoneal involvement with or without positive retroperitoneal lymph nodes
IIIB	Macroscopic peritoneal metastases beyond the pelvic brim ≤2 cm in greatest dimension with or without positive retroperitoneal nodes
IIIC	Macroscopic peritoneal metastases beyond the pelvic brim >2 cm in greatest dimension with or without positive retroperitoneal nodes
Stage IV	Distant metastasis excluding peritoneal metastases
IVA	Pleural effusion with positive cytology
IVB	Metastases to extra-abdominal organs (including inguinal lymph nodes and lymph nodes outside of abdominal cavity)

FIGO = International Federation of Gynecology and Obstetrics.

histologically distinct. Toward the third trimester of fetal life, germ cells stop multiplying and instead continue to develop by meiosis. Of 1 million primordial follicles present at birth, only 70% remain by puberty and fewer than 15% persist to age 25 years. Only some 450 ova are actually shed during a woman's average 35-year reproductive lifetime.

The ovarian cortex mesenchyme consists of spindle-shaped, fibroblast-like cells. These give rise to granulosa and theca cells, which form a functional unit about each ovum (theca interna and theca externa). The complex of a germ cell and supporting granulosa cells is known first as a **primordial follicle**. During the reproductive period, a dominant follicle develops every month into a **graafian follicle,** which then ruptures during ovulation. Ovulation itself is often associated with mild cramping pain, which, if severe, is called **mittelschmerz** (i.e., midcycle pain). It is frequently confused with appendicitis. After ovulation, the follicle granulosa cells luteinize, with hypertrophy and lipid accumulation. They then secrete progesterone in addition to estrogens. The collapsed follicle turns bright yellow and becomes the **corpus luteum** (yellow body).

Cells of ovarian stromal origin include hilus cells and those resembling luteinized cells of the theca interna, both of which respond to pituitary hormones. These specialized cells make and secrete both androgens and estrogens, which stimulate proliferation in end-organs (e.g., uterus). They inhibit hypothalamic function by negative feedback loops.

CYSTIC LESIONS OF THE OVARIES

Cysts usually arise from invaginated surface epithelium (serous cysts) and are the most common cause of enlarged ovaries. Almost all of the rest derive from ovarian follicles.

Follicle Cysts Tend to Be Asymptomatic

Follicle cysts are thin-walled, fluid-filled structures lined internally by granulosa cells and externally by theca interna cells. They occur at any age up to menopause, are unilocular and may be single or multiple, unilateral or bilateral. They arise from ovarian follicles and are probably related to abnormalities in pituitary gonadotropin release.

 PATHOLOGY: Follicle cysts rarely exceed 5 cm. In an unstimulated state, the granulosa cells of the cyst have uniform, round nuclei and little cytoplasm. Thecal cells are small and spindle shaped. Occasionally, the layers may be luteinized, and the lumen wall contains fluid high in estrogen or progesterone. If the cyst persists, hormonal output can cause precocious puberty in a child and menstrual irregularities in an adult. The only significant complication is mild intraperitoneal bleeding (Fig. 24-44).

Corpus Luteum Cysts Can Bleed

A corpus luteum cyst results from delayed resolution of a corpus luteum's central cavity. Continued progesterone synthesis by the luteal cyst leads to menstrual irregularities. Rupture of a cyst can cause mild hemorrhage into the abdominal cavity. A corpus luteum cyst is typically unilocular, 3–5 cm in size with a yellow wall. Cyst contents vary

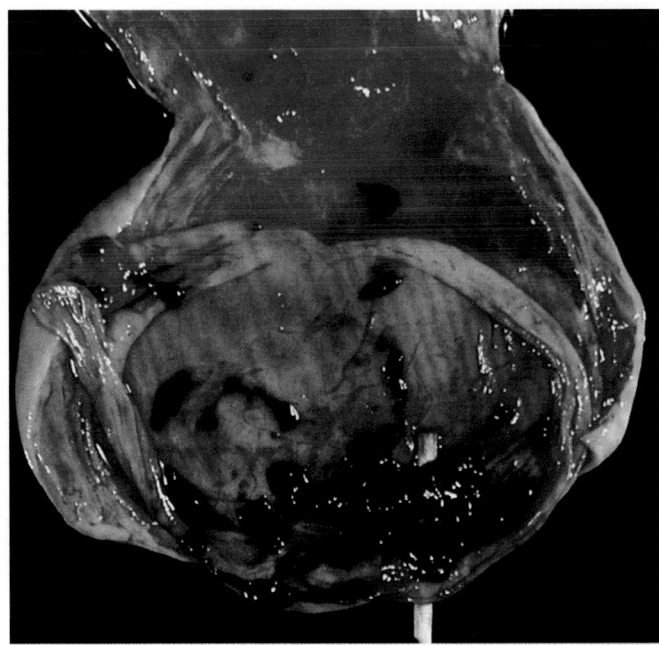

FIGURE 24-44. Follicle cyst of the ovary. The rupture of this thin-walled follicular cyst (dowel stick) led to intra-abdominal hemorrhage.

from serosanguineous fluid to clotted blood. Microscopic examination shows numerous large, luteinized granulosa cells. The condition is self-limited.

Theca Lutein Cysts Relate to High Gonadotropin Levels

Theca lutein cysts, also called *hyperreactio luteinalis,* are often multiple and bilateral. They are associated with high levels of circulating gonadotropin (as in pregnancy, hydatidiform mole, choriocarcinoma or exogenous gonadotropin therapy) or physical impediments (dense adhesions, cortical fibrosis) to ovulation. Excessive gonadotropin levels lead to exaggerated stimulation of the theca interna and extensive cyst formation.

 PATHOLOGY: Multiple thin-walled cysts filled with clear fluid and a markedly luteinized layer of theca interna replace both ovaries. Ovarian parenchyma shows edema and foci of luteinized stromal cells. Intra-abdominal hemorrhage due to torsion or rupture of the cyst may require surgical intervention.

POLYCYSTIC OVARY SYNDROME

Polycystic ovary syndrome, or **Stein-Leventhal syndrome,** reflects (1) excess secretion of androgenic hormones, (2) persistent anovulation and (3) many small subcapsular ovarian cysts. It was first described as a syndrome of **secondary amenorrhea, hirsutism and obesity,** but clinical presentations are now known to be far more variable and include amenorrheic women who appear otherwise normal and, even rarely, have ovaries lacking polycystic features. *This condition is a common cause of infertility: up to 7% of women experience polycystic ovary syndrome.*

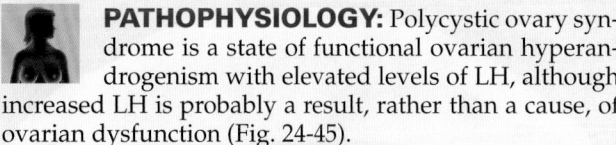 **PATHOPHYSIOLOGY:** Polycystic ovary syndrome is a state of functional ovarian hyperandrogenism with elevated levels of LH, although increased LH is probably a result, rather than a cause, of ovarian dysfunction (Fig. 24-45).

1. The central abnormality is thought to be increased ovarian production of androgens, although adrenal hypersecretion of androgens may also occur. The rate-limiting enzyme in androgen biosynthesis, cytochrome $P450_{c17\alpha}$ (17α-hydroxylase), expressed in both the ovary and the adrenal gland, is abnormally regulated.

2. Excess ovarian androgens act locally to cause (1) premature follicular atresia, (2) multiple follicular cysts and (3) a persistent anovulatory state. Impaired follicular maturation results in decreased secretion of progesterone. Peripherally, hyperandrogenism leads to hirsutism, acne and male-pattern (androgen-dependent) alopecia. Affected patients may have high serum levels of androgens, such as testosterone, androstenedione and dehydroepiandrosterone sulfate. But there are individual variations and some patients have normal androgen levels.

3. Excess androgens are converted to estrogens in peripheral adipose tissue, an effect that is exaggerated by obesity. Acyclic estrogen production and progesterone deficiency increase pituitary secretion of LH.

4. Women with polycystic ovary syndrome exhibit marked peripheral insulin resistance, out of proportion to the degree of obesity. The mechanism appears to involve a post–insulin-receptor defect, possibly related to decreased expression of a glucose transporter. In any event, the resulting hyperinsulinemia seems to contribute to increased ovarian hypersecretion of androgens and direct stimulation of pituitary LH production.

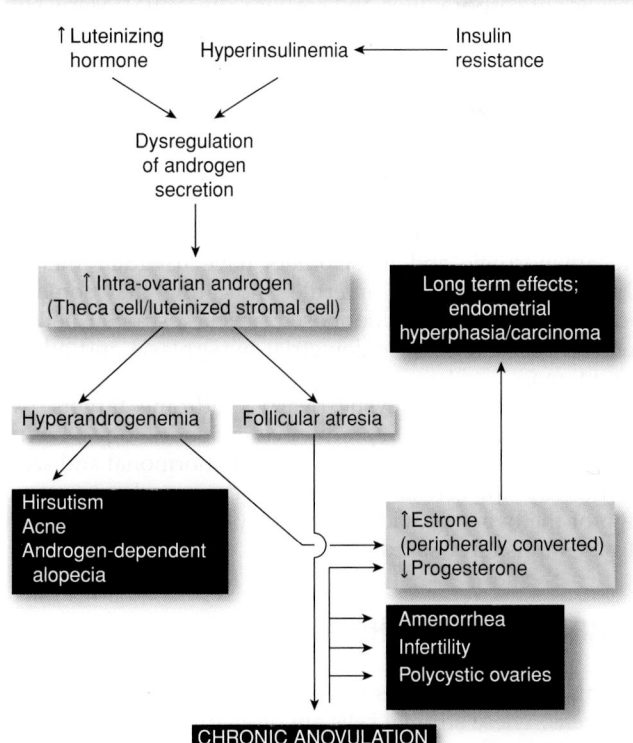

FIGURE 24-45. Pathogenesis of polycystic ovary syndrome.

THE FEMALE REPRODUCTIVE SYSTEM

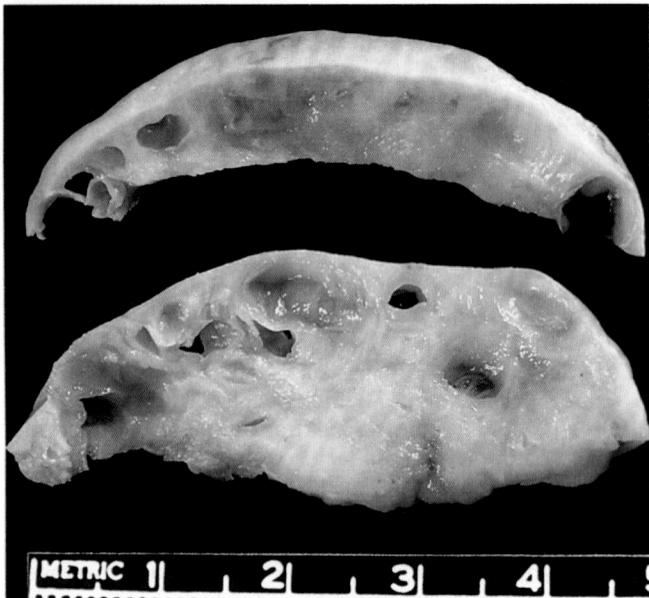

FIGURE 24-46. Polycystic disease of the ovary. Cut sections of an ovary show numerous cysts embedded in a sclerotic stroma.

 PATHOLOGY: Both ovaries are enlarged. The surface is smooth, owing to lack of ovulation. On cut section, the cortex is thickened and contains numerous theca lutein–type cysts, typically 2–8 mm in diameter, arranged peripherally around a dense core of stroma or scattered throughout an expanded stroma (Fig. 24-46). Microscopic features include (1) numerous follicles in early developmental stages; (2) follicular atresia; (3) increased stroma, occasionally with luteinized cells (hyperthecosis); and (4) features of anovulation (thick, smooth capsule and absence of corpora lutea and corpora albicantia). Many subcapsular cysts show thick zones of theca interna, in which some cells may be luteinized.

 CLINICAL FEATURES: *Nearly three quarters of women with anovulatory infertility have polycystic ovary syndrome.* Patients are typically in their 20s and tell of early obesity, menstrual problems and hirsutism. Half of women with polycystic ovary syndrome are amenorrheic and most others have irregular menses. Only 75% are actually infertile, indicating that some do occasionally ovulate. Unopposed acyclic estrogen activity increases incidence of endometrial hyperplasia and adenocarcinoma.

Treatment of polycystic ovary syndrome targets two common problems in reproductive endocrinology—hirsutism and anovulation. Therapy is mostly hormonal and seeks to interrupt the constant excess of androgens. Wedge resection of the ovary provides temporary remission of the syndrome but is rarely used today.

STROMAL HYPERTHECOSIS

Stromal hyperthecosis is focal luteinization of ovarian stromal cells. These stromal cells are often functional and cause **virilization**. The condition is most common in postmenopausal women and, in a microscopic form, is found in one third of postmenopausal ovaries.

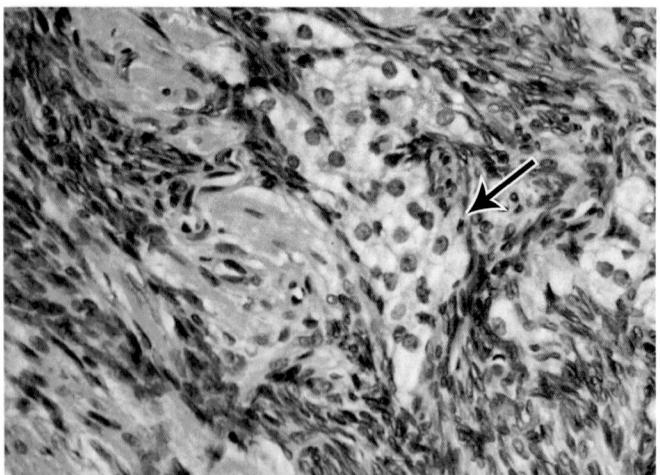

FIGURE 24-47. Hyperthecosis of the ovary. Nests of luteinized (lipid-rich) stromal cells are present (*arrow*).

 PATHOLOGY: If stromal hyperthecosis is detected clinically, usually owing to masculinizing signs, both ovaries may be enlarged, sometimes up to 8 cm in greatest dimension. The serosa is smooth, and the cut surface is homogeneous, firm and brown to yellow. Single nests or nodules of luteinized stromal cells with deeply eosinophilic, often vacuolated cytoplasm are seen in the cortex or medulla (Fig. 24-47). Luteinized cells have a large central nucleus and a prominent nucleolus, features shared with all hormonally active stromal cells in the ovary.

OVARIAN TUMORS

There are many types of ovarian tumors including benign, borderline and malignant ones. About two thirds occur in women of reproductive age; less than 5% develop in children. Approximately 80% are benign. Almost 90% of malignant and borderline tumors are diagnosed after the age of 40 years.

Ovarian tumors are classified by the ovarian cell type of origin (Fig. 24-48). Most are **common epithelial tumors** (approximately 60%) that arise directly or indirectly from müllerian epithelium. Other important groups are germ cell tumors (30%), sex cord/stromal tumors (8%) and tumors metastatic to the ovary. In the Western world, common epithelial tumors account for about 90% of ovarian malignancies, serous adenocarcinoma being the most common among these.

Ovarian cancer is the second most frequent gynecologic malignancy after endometrial cancer and carries a higher mortality rate than all other female genital cancers combined (Table 24-3). As it is difficult to detect at a curable stage, over three fourths of patients have tumor spread to the pelvis or abdomen at the time of diagnosis. Approximately 22,000 new cases of ovarian cancer are diagnosed each year in the United States, and more than 14,000 women die from the disease (Table 24-3). Lifetime risk of developing ovarian cancer is 2%. These tumors predominate in women older than 60 years but may occur in younger women with a family history of the disease.

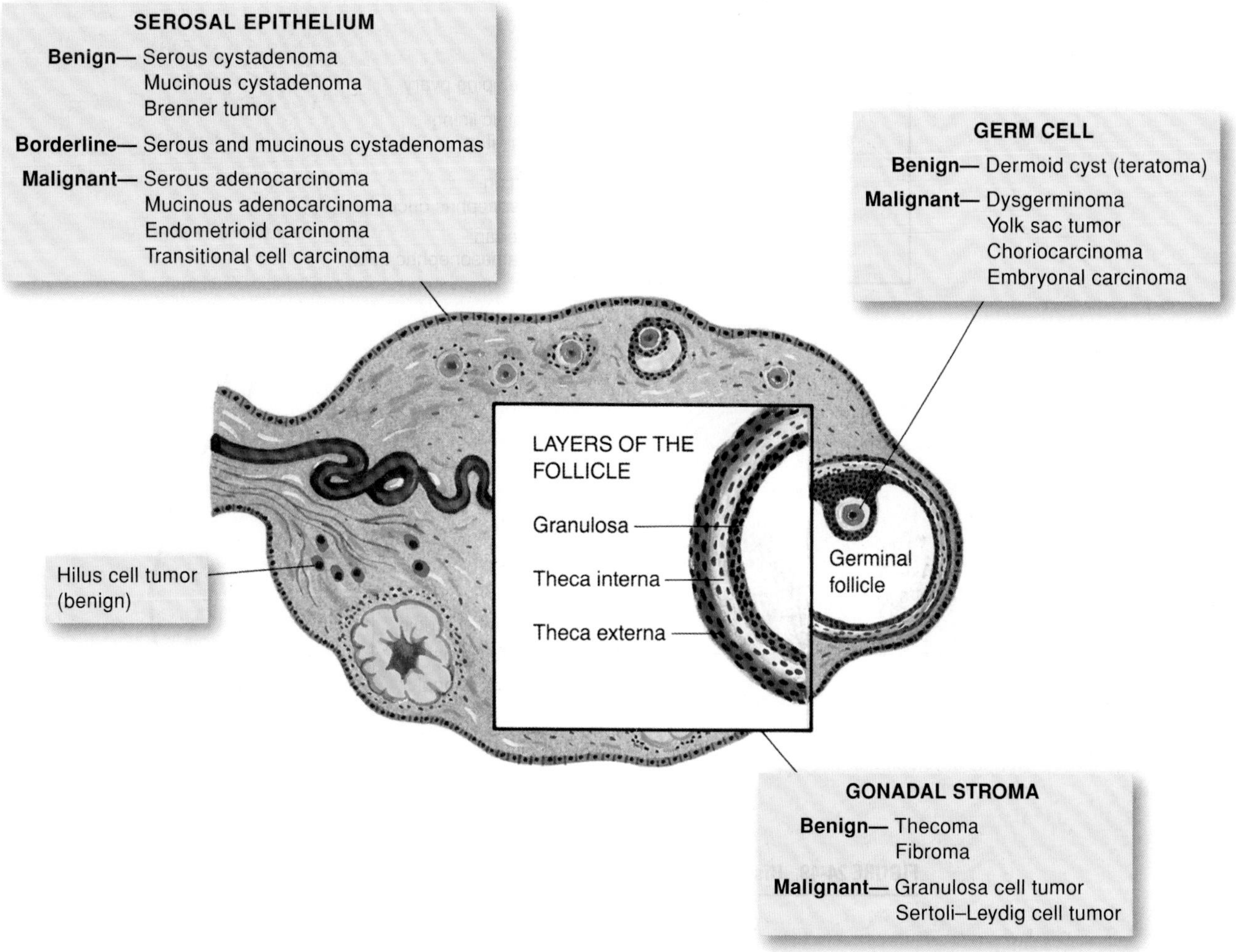

SEROSAL EPITHELIUM

Benign— Serous cystadenoma
Mucinous cystadenoma
Brenner tumor

Borderline— Serous and mucinous cystadenomas

Malignant— Serous adenocarcinoma
Mucinous adenocarcinoma
Endometrioid carcinoma
Transitional cell carcinoma

GERM CELL

Benign— Dermoid cyst (teratoma)

Malignant— Dysgerminoma
Yolk sac tumor
Choriocarcinoma
Embryonal carcinoma

LAYERS OF THE FOLLICLE

Granulosa

Theca interna

Theca externa

Germinal follicle

Hilus cell tumor (benign)

GONADAL STROMA

Benign— Thecoma
Fibroma

Malignant— Granulosa cell tumor
Sertoli–Leydig cell tumor

FIGURE 24-48. Classification of ovarian neoplasms based on cell of origin.

Epithelial Tumors Account for Over 90% of Ovarian Cancers

Tumors of common epithelial origin are broadly classified, according to cell proliferation, degree of nuclear atypia and presence or absence of stromal invasion: (1) **benign,** (2) of **borderline malignancy** (also called **low malignant potential**) and (3) **malignant** (Fig. 24-49).

  **MOLECULAR PATHOGENESIS AND ETIOLOGIC FACTORS:** Common epithelial neoplasms are apparently related to repeated disruption and repair of the epithelial surface resulting from cyclic or "incessant" ovulation. Thus, tumors occur most commonly in nulliparous women and least often in women in whom ovulation has been suppressed (e.g., by pregnancy or oral contraceptives). Persistent, high concentrations of pituitary gonadotropins after menopause may stimulate surface epithelial cells, promoting accumulation of genetic changes and carcinogenesis. Irritants, such as talc or asbestos, transported up the reproductive tract to the ovaries have also been implicated.

Common epithelial tumors, particularly serous carcinomas, are thought to arise from ovarian surface epithelium (mesothelium) or serosa. During embryonic life, the celomic cavity is lined by mesothelium, parts of which specialize to form the serosal epithelium covering the gonadal ridge. The same mesothelial lining gives rise to müllerian ducts, from which the fallopian tubes, uterus and vagina arise (Fig. 24-50). Thus, as the ovary develops, the surface epithelium may extend into the ovarian stroma to form glands and cysts, and in some cases, these inclusion cysts become neoplastic and show a variety of müllerian-type differentiations (Fig. 24-49).

Approximately 10% of patients with high-grade serous carcinoma (HGSC) have a family history of ovarian cancer. If a first-degree relative had ovarian cancer, a woman's risk of developing ovarian cancer is increased 3.5-fold. Women with a history of ovarian carcinoma are also at greater risk for breast cancer and vice versa. Defects in repair genes implicated in hereditary breast cancers, *BRCA1* and *BRCA2*, are incriminated in familial ovarian cancers as well. Ovarian carcinomas arising in patients with germline *BRCA1* or *BRCA2* mutations are almost invariably high-grade serous type. Women with *BRCA1* mutations tend to develop ovarian cancers at younger ages than those who develop sporadic ovarian tumors, but *BRCA1*–related tumors have better prognoses. The traditional view that HGSCs arise exclusively from ovarian surface epithelium or epithelial inclusion cysts has been challenged recently by the identification,

THE FEMALE REPRODUCTIVE SYSTEM

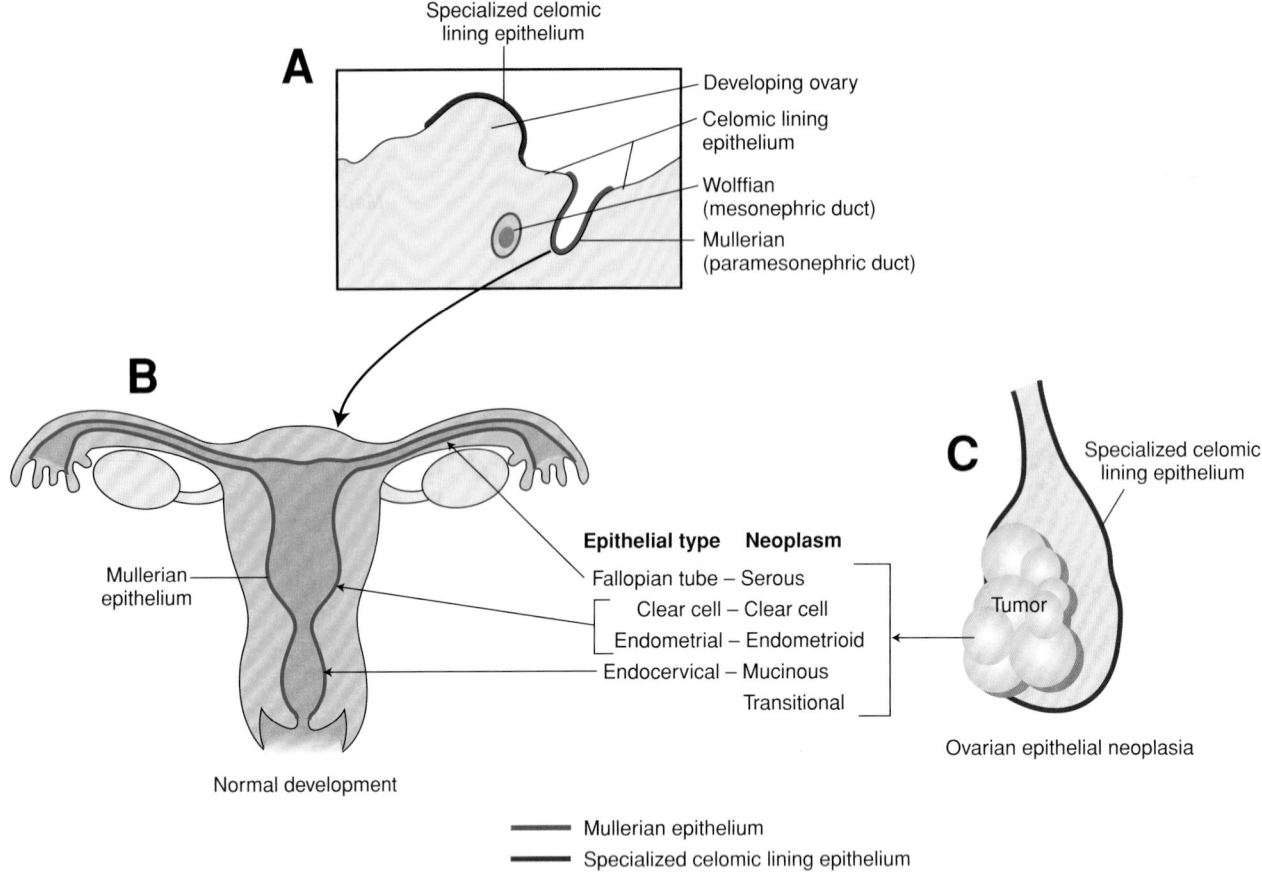

FIGURE 24-49. Histogenesis of ovarian epithelial/stromal tumors.

FIGURE 24-50. The müllerian relations of epithelial/stromal tumors of the ovaries.

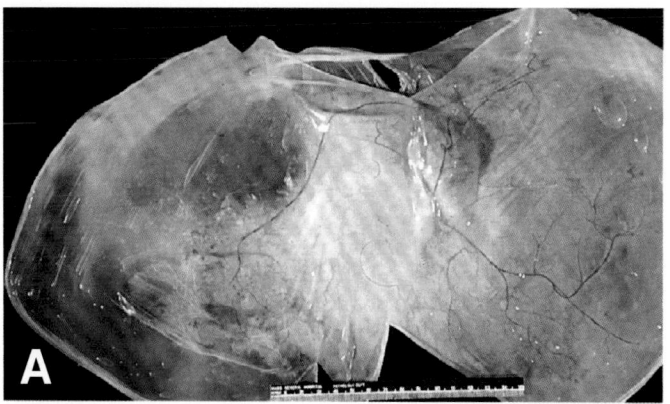
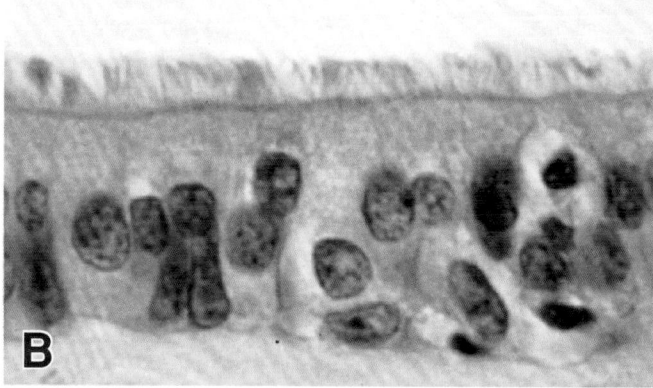

FIGURE 24-51. Serous cystadenoma of the ovary. A. Gross appearance of serous cystadenoma of the ovary. The fluid has been removed from this huge unilocular serous cystadenoma. The wall is thin and translucent. **B.** On microscopic examination, the cyst is lined by a single layer of ciliated tubal-type epithelium.

in women with *BRCA1* or *BRCA2* germline mutations, of serous tubal intraepithelial carcinoma (STIC) in the distal fimbriated end of the fallopian tube as a malignant lesion related to advanced HGSC. Currently, the relative proportion of HGSC of ovarian and tubal derivation is unknown mainly because the primary site is obscured in advanced stage cancers. As for endometrial carcinoma, women with hereditary nonpolyposis colon cancer (HNPCC) are also at greater risk for ovarian cancer. Most endometrioid and clear cell carcinomas of the ovary are thought to originate from ovarian endometriosis.

 PATHOLOGY: In order of decreasing frequency, the **common epithelial tumors** are:

- **Serous tumors** that resemble fallopian tube epithelium
- **Mucinous tumors** that mimic the mucosa of the endocervix
- **Endometrioid tumors** that are similar to the glands of the endometrium
- **Clear cell tumors** with glycogen-rich cells like endometrial glands in pregnancy
- **Transitional cell tumors** that resemble the mucosa of the bladder
- **Mixed tumors**

Cystadenomas

Common benign epithelial tumors are almost always serous or mucinous adenomas and generally arise in women 20–60 years old. These tumors are frequently large, often 15–30 cm in diameter. Some, particularly mucinous ones, reach massive proportions, exceeding 50 cm in diameter, and may mimic the appearance of a term pregnancy. Benign epithelial tumors are typically cystic, hence the term **cystadenoma**. Serous cystadenomas are more often bilateral (15%) than mucinous cystadenomas and tend to be unilocular (Fig. 24-51). By contrast, **mucinous tumors** usually show hundreds of small cysts (locules) (Fig. 24-52). Unlike their malignant counterparts, benign ovarian epithelial tumors tend to have thin walls and lack solid areas. A single layer of tall columnar epithelium lines the cysts. Papillae, if present, have a fibrovascular core covered by a layer of tall columnar epithelium identical to the cyst lining.

Transitional Cell Tumor (Brenner Tumor)

The typical Brenner tumor is benign and occurs at all ages. Half of cases present in women over the age of 50. Size varies from microscopic foci to masses 8 cm or more in diameter.

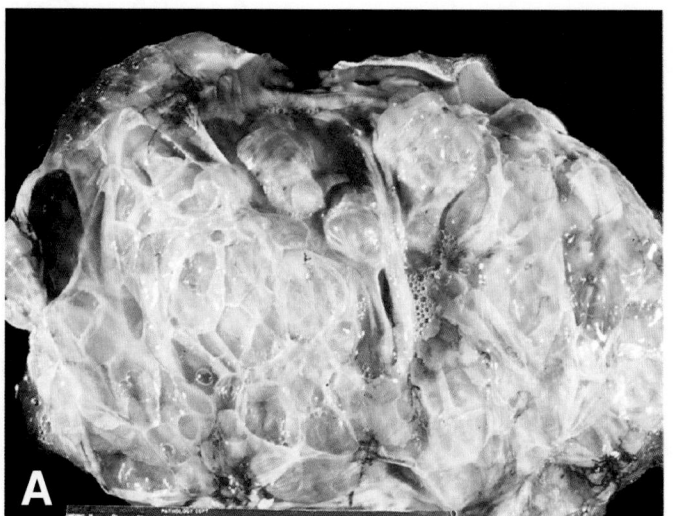
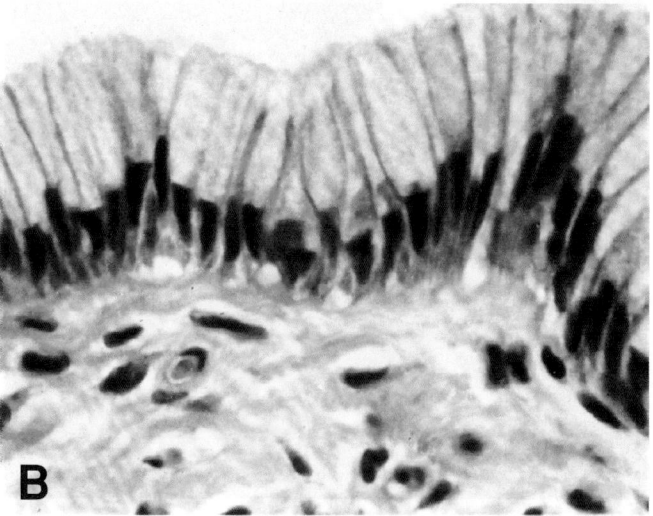

FIGURE 24-52. Mucinous cystadenoma of the ovary. A. The tumor is characterized by numerous cysts filled with thick, viscous fluid. **B.** A single layer of mucinous epithelial cells lines the cyst.

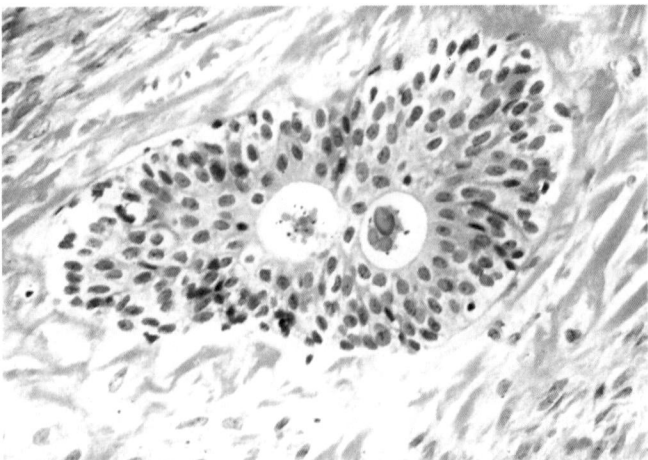

FIGURE 24-53. Brenner tumor. A nest of transitional-like cells is embedded in a dense, fibrous stroma.

Brenner tumors are adenofibromas, typically showing solid nests of transitional-like (urothelium-like) cells encased in a dense, fibrous stroma (Fig. 24-53). Epithelial nests are often cavitated and the most superficial epithelial cells may exhibit mucinous differentiation.

Borderline Tumors (Tumors of Low Malignant Potential)

"Borderline tumors" are a well-defined group of ovarian tumors characterized by epithelial cell proliferation and nuclear atypia but not destructive stromal invasion. Despite histologic features suggesting aggressiveness, they share an excellent prognosis. Serous borderline tumors generally occur in women 20–50 years old (average, 46 years) but are also seen in older women. Surgical cure is almost always possible if the tumor is confined to the ovaries. Even if it has spread to the pelvis or abdomen, 80% of patients are alive after 5 years. Although there is a significant rate of late recurrence, tumors rarely recur beyond 10 years. Late progression

to low-grade serous carcinoma occurs in approximately 7% of cases.

Serous tumors of borderline malignancy are more commonly bilateral (34%) than mucinous ones (6%) or other types. The tumors vary in size, although mucinous ones may be gigantic. In serous tumors of borderline malignancy, papillary projections, ranging from fine and exuberant to grape-like clusters arising from the cyst wall, are common (Fig. 24-54). These structures resemble papillary fronds in benign cystadenomas, but they show (1) epithelial stratification, (2) moderate nuclear atypia and (3) mitotic activity. The same criteria apply to borderline mucinous tumors, although papillary projections are less conspicuous. *By definition, the presence of more than focal microinvasion (i.e., discrete nests of epithelial cells <3 mm into the ovarian stroma) identifies a tumor as low-grade invasive serous carcinoma, rather than a borderline tumor.* However, borderline tumors with lymph node metastases or peritoneal implants (Fig. 24-55), whether noninvasive or invasive, are still "borderline," reflecting the fact that this well-defined category carries a far better prognosis than usual adenocarcinomas. The presence of ovarian surface excrescences does not seem to predict progression of disease.

Malignant Epithelial Tumors

Carcinomas of the ovary are most common in women 40–60 years old and are rare under the age of 35. Based on light microscopy and molecular genetics, ovarian carcinomas are classified into five main subtypes (Table 24-10), which, in descending order of frequency, are high-grade serous carcinomas (>70%), endometrioid carcinomas (10%), clear cell carcinomas (10%), mucinous carcinomas (3%–4%) and low-grade serous carcinomas (<5%). These subtypes, which account for 98% of ovarian carcinomas, can be reproducibly diagnosed and identified as diseases based on differences in epidemiologic and genetic risk factors, precursor lesions, patterns of spread, molecular events during oncogenesis, responses to chemotherapy and outcomes. Advances in subtype-specific management of ovarian cancer make accurate subtype assignment increasingly important.

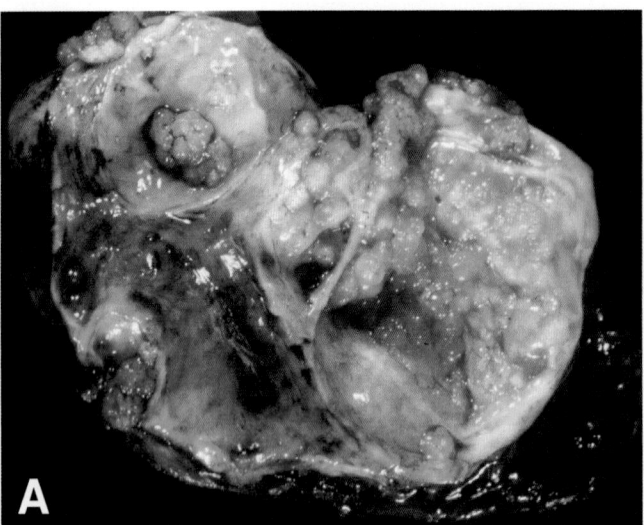

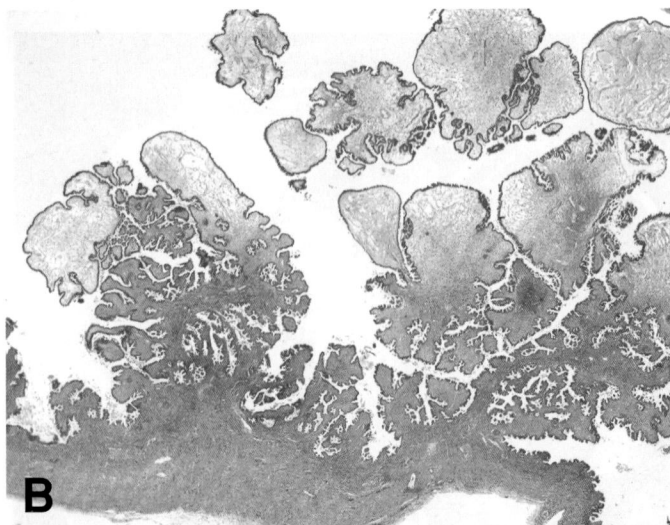

FIGURE 24-54. Serous cystic borderline tumor. A. The inner surface of the cysts is partly covered by closely packed papillae (endophytic growth). **B.** Microscopic view of the papillary tumor. The papillae show hierarchical and complex branching without stromal invasion. Some papillae have fibroedematous stalks.

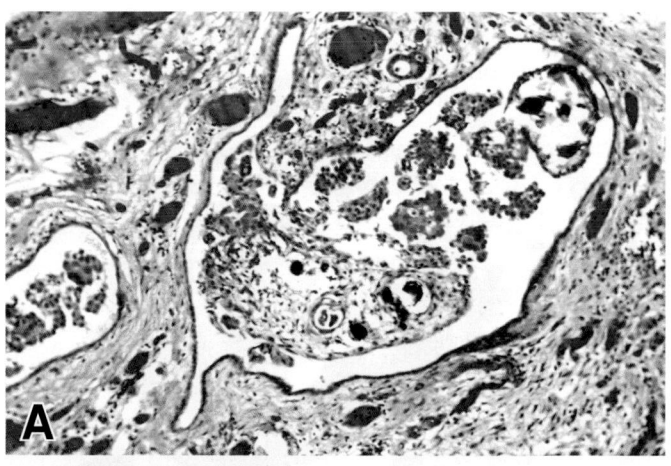

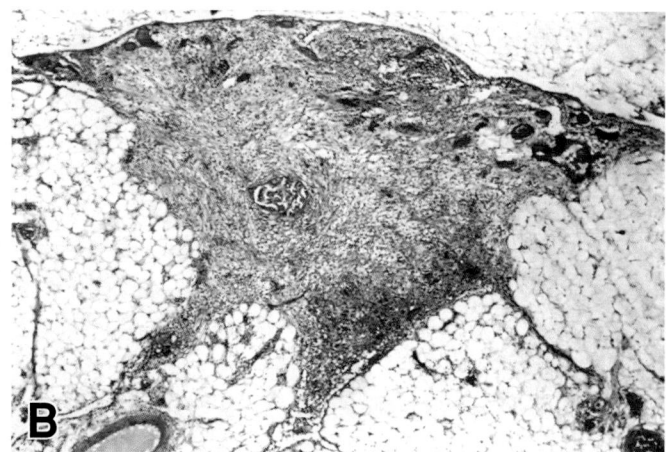

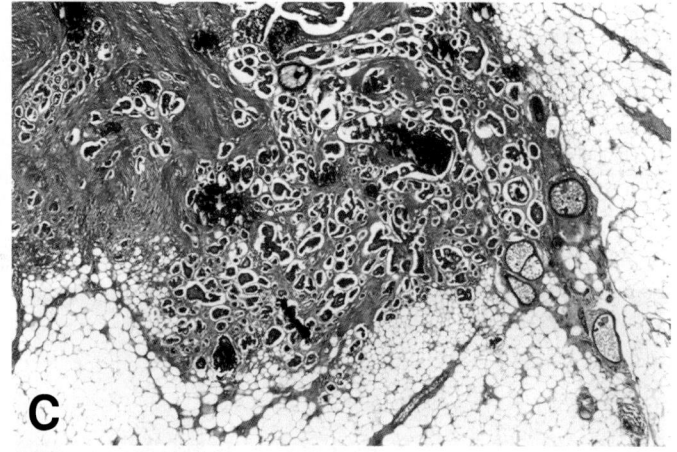

FIGURE 24-55. Peritoneal implants of serous borderline tumor. A. Noninvasive epithelial implant within a smoothly contoured invagination of the peritoneum. The epithelial proliferation contains psammoma bodies and resembles the primary ovarian tumor. **B.** Noninvasive desmoplastic implant. The implant invaginates between adjacent lobules of omental fat. A few nests of tumor cells are present within a loose fibroblastic stroma. **C.** Invasive omental implant. The tumor glands and papillae appear disorderly distributed within a dense fibrous stroma and resemble a low-grade serous carcinoma.

SEROUS ADENOCARCINOMAS:

MOLECULAR PATHOGENESIS: Low-grade and high-grade serous carcinomas are fundamentally different tumors. Whereas low-grade tumors are frequently associated with serous borderline tumors and have mutations of *KRAS* or *BRAF* oncogenes, high-grade serous carcinomas appear to arise de novo without identifiable precursor lesions and have a high frequency of mutations in *p53*, but not in *KRAS* or *BRAF*. Interestingly,

TABLE 24-10

MAIN SUBTYPES OF OVARIAN CARCINOMA

	Low-Grade Serous	High-Grade Serous	Clear Cell	Endometrioid	Mucinous
Usual stage at diagnosis	Early or advanced	Advanced	Early	Early	Early
Presumed tissue of origin/precursor lesion	Serous borderline tumor	Fallopian tube or tubal metaplasia in inclusions of ovarian surface epithelium	Endometriosis, adenofibroma	Endometriosis, adenofibroma	Adenoma–borderline–carcinoma sequence; teratoma
Genetic risk	?	BRCA1/2	?	HNPCC	?
Significant molecular abnormalities	BRAF or K-ras	p53 and pRb pathways	HNF-1β	PTEN, β-catenin, K-ras MI	K-ras
Proliferation	Low	High	Low	Low	Intermediate
Response to primary chemotherapy	26%–28%	80%	15%	?	15%
Prognosis	Favorable	Poor	Intermediate	Favorable	Favorable

HNF-1β = hepatocyte nuclear factor-1β; HNPCC = hereditary nonpolyposis colon cancer.

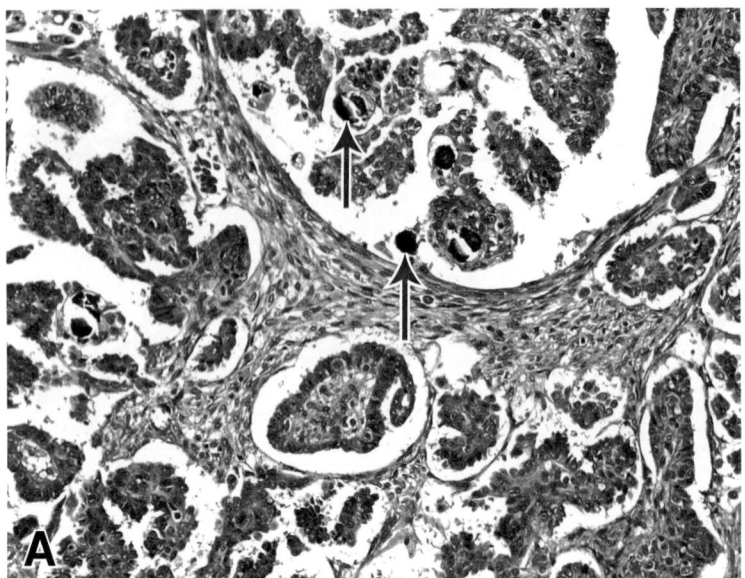
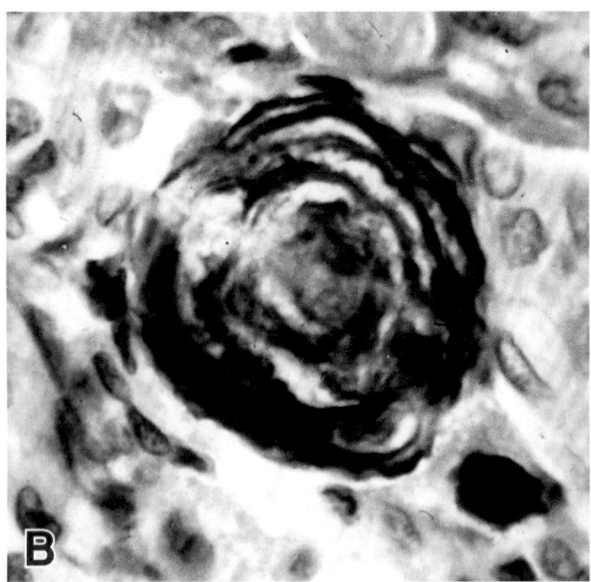

FIGURE 24-56. Low-grade serous carcinoma. A. The nests of tumor cells are disorderly distributed and appear surrounded by clefts. In contrast to high-grade serous carcinoma, the nuclei are low grade. Psammoma bodies (*arrows*) are seen. **B.** A higher-power view shows the laminated structure of a psammoma body.

carcinomas arising in patients with germline *BRCA1* or *BRCA2* mutations (hereditary ovarian cancers) are almost invariably the high-grade serous type and commonly have *p53* mutations. A significant number of *BRCA1*- or *BRCA2*-related tumors arise from epithelium of the fimbriated end of the fallopian tube, suggesting that at least some sporadic high-grade ovarian and "primary" peritoneal serous carcinomas may actually develop from the distal fallopian tube and "spill over" onto adjacent tissues.

PATHOLOGY: Low-grade serous carcinomas are characterized by irregular invasion of the ovary by small, tight nests of tumor cells with variable desmoplasia (Fig. 24-56). Nuclear uniformity is the principal criterion for distinguishing low- and high-grade serous carcinomas. Low-grade serous carcinomas rarely progress to high-grade tumors.

High-grade serous carcinomas (often called "cystadenocarcinoma") are mainly solid, multinodular masses, usually with necrosis and hemorrhage (Fig. 24-57A). Once a tumor has reached 10–15 cm, it has often spread beyond the ovary and seeded the peritoneum. Two thirds of serous cancers with extraovarian spread are bilateral. High-grade serous cancers typically show obvious stromal invasion. Most tumors have a high nuclear grade with irregularly branching, highly cellular papillae with little or no stromal support and slit-like glandular lumens within more solid areas (Fig. 24-57B). The mitotic rate is very high. Psammoma bodies are often present.

MUCINOUS ADENOCARCINOMA:

MOLECULAR PATHOGENESIS: Mucinous ovarian tumors are often heterogeneous. Benign, borderline, noninvasive and invasive carcinoma components may coexist within the same tumor. Such a morphologic continuum suggests progression from cystadenoma

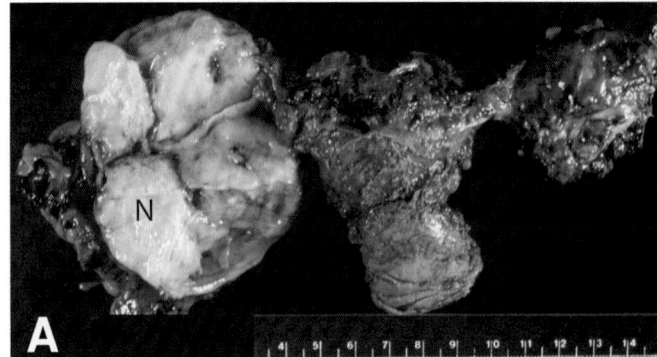
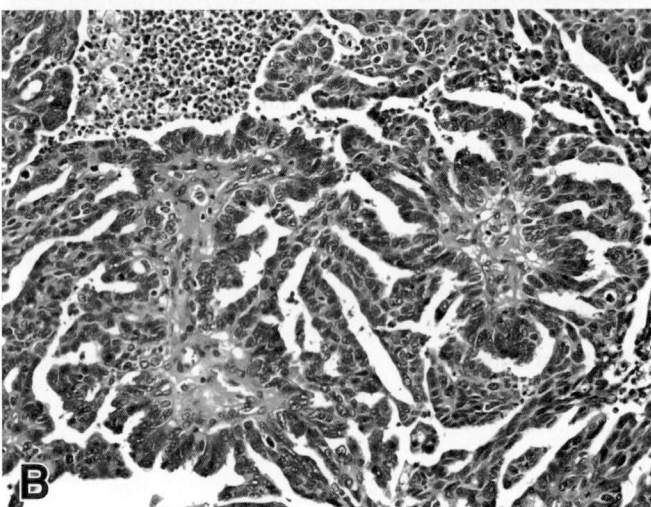

FIGURE 24-57. High-grade serous cystadenocarcinoma. A. In addition to cysts (*left*), the ovary is enlarged by a solid tumor that exhibits extensive necrosis (N). **B.** Microscopic examination shows complex papillae, lined by atypical nuclei, forming glomeruloid structures.

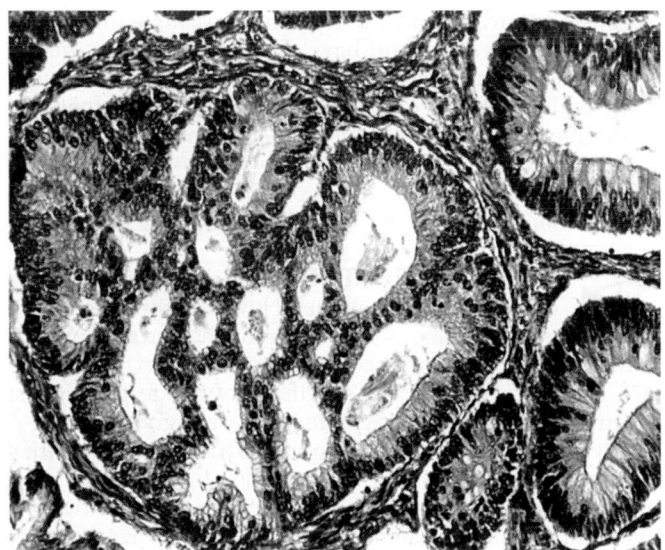

FIGURE 24-58. Mucinous cystadenocarcinoma. The malignant glands are arranged in a cribriform pattern and are composed of mucin-producing columnar cells.

and borderline tumor to noninvasive, microinvasive and invasive carcinomas. This hypothesis is supported by a similar progression in the incidence of *KRAS* mutations in mucinous tumors: 56% of cystadenomas and 85% of carcinomas express mutated *KRAS*, with borderline tumors being intermediate.

 PATHOLOGY: Mucinous carcinomas are usually large, unilateral, multilocular or unilocular cystic masses containing mucinous fluid. They often include papillary and solid areas that may be soft and mucoid or firm, hemorrhagic and necrotic. Since these tumors are bilateral in only 5% of cases, finding bilateral or unilateral mucinous tumors smaller than 10 cm raises suspicion of metastatic mucinous carcinoma from the gastrointestinal tract or elsewhere.

The category of mucinous borderline tumor with intraepithelial carcinoma is reserved for tumors that lack architectural features of invasive carcinoma but focally show unequivocal malignant cells lining glandular spaces. Mucinous borderline tumors with intraepithelial carcinoma have a very low likelihood of recurrence.

Mucinous adenocarcinomas may be further subdivided into (1) **expansile** or **confluent glandular pattern,** lacking destructive stromal invasion (Fig. 24-58) but there are back-to-back or complex malignant glands have minimal or no intervening stroma, and (2) **infiltrative,** with obvious glandular stromal invasion. The expansile pattern appears to have a more favorable prognosis than the infiltrative type. The combination of extensive, infiltrative stromal invasion; high nuclear grade; and tumor rupture should be considered a strong predictor of recurrence for stage I mucinous adenocarcinomas.

Pseudomyxoma peritonei is a clinical condition of abundant gelatinous or mucinous ascites in the peritoneum, fibrous adhesions and frequently mucinous tumors involving the ovaries. The appendix is involved by a similar mucinous tumor in 60% of the cases and appears normal in the remaining 40%. In most cases, the ovarian tumors are metastases from the appendiceal lesions. Concordant *KRAS* mutations have been found in both the appendiceal and ovarian tumors of individual patients.

ENDOMETRIOID ADENOCARCINOMA: Endometrioid adenocarcinoma histologically resembles its endometrial counterpart (Fig. 24-59A), may have areas of squamous differentiation and is second only to serous adenocarcinoma in frequency. It accounts for 10% of all ovarian cancers. These tumors occur most commonly after menopause. Unlike serous and mucinous neoplasms, most endometrioid tumors are malignant. Up to one half of these cancers are bilateral and, at diagnosis, most tumors are confined either to the ovary or within the pelvis.

MOLECULAR PATHOGENESIS: Endometrioid carcinomas are thought to arise by malignant transformation of endometriosis, and not ovarian surface epithelium (Fig. 24-59B). AT-rich interactive domain 1A gene (*ARID1A*) mutations have been implicated not only in endometrioid and clear cell carcinomas but also in adjacent endometriosis. *ARID1A* behaves as a tumor suppressor. Lack

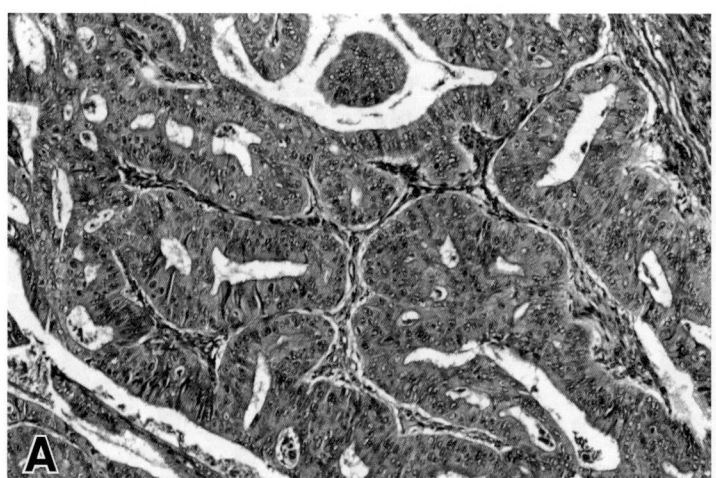
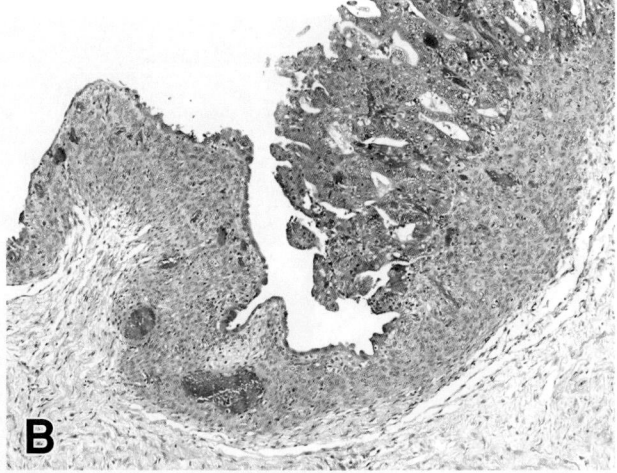

FIGURE 24-59. Endometrioid adenocarcinoma. A. The crowded neoplastic glands are lined by stratified non–mucin-containing epithelium. Nuclear atypia is moderate to severe. **B.** Endometrioid adenocarcinoma (*right*) arising in endometriosis. Note the stromal cells of endometriosis.

of expression of the BAF250 protein, encoded by *ARID1A,* may increase risk of developing clear cell or endometrioid ovarian cancer. Other common genetic abnormalities in sporadic endometrioid carcinoma of the ovary are somatic mutations of β-catenin (*CTNNB1*) and *PTEN* genes and microsatellite instability. Endometrioid borderline tumors also have β-catenin mutations.

 PATHOLOGY: Endometrioid carcinomas vary from 2 cm to more than 30 cm. Most are largely solid with areas of necrosis, although they may be cystic. Endometrioid tumors are graded like their endometrial counterparts. Between 15% and 20% of patients with endometrioid carcinoma of the ovary also harbor an endometrial cancer. If ovarian and endometrial cancers coexist, they generally arise independently, although one may be metastatic from the other. This distinction has important prognostic implications. Various molecular methods including loss of heterozygosity (LOH), gene mutation and clonal X-inactivation analysis can be helpful. The 5-year survival exceeds 85% in synchronous tumors. As with all malignant epithelial tumors of the ovary, prognosis depends on the stage at which it presents.

CLEAR CELL ADENOCARCINOMA: This enigmatic ovarian cancer is closely related to endometrioid adenocarcinoma and often occurs in association with endometriosis (Fig. 24-60A). It constitutes 5%–10% of all ovarian cancers usually occurring after menopause.

Roughly half of clear cell carcinomas (46%–57%) carry *ARID1A* mutations and lack BAF250 protein. Other common genetic abnormalities are inactivating *PTEN* mutations and activating *PIK3CA* mutations. Hepatocyte nuclear factor-1β (HNF-1β) regulates several specific genes in clear cell carcinoma, including dipeptidyl peptidase IV (glycogen synthesis), osteopontin (progesterone-regulated endometrial secretory protein), angiotensin-converting enzyme 2 (ferritin induction, iron deposition, antiapoptosis), annexin 4 (paclitaxel resistance) and UGT1A1 (detoxification).

Although patients typically present with stage I or II disease, clear cell carcinomas have a poor prognosis compared with other low-stage ovarian carcinomas. Tumors range in size from 2 to 30 cm, and 40% are bilateral. Most are partially cystic and show necrosis and hemorrhage in the solid areas.

Clear cell ovarian adenocarcinomas resemble their counterparts in the vagina and have sheets or tubules of malignant cells with clear cytoplasm (Fig. 24-60B). In the tubular form, malignant cells often display bulbous nuclei that protrude into the lumen of the tubule ("hobnail cell"), resembling an Arias-Stella reaction in gestational endometrium (Fig. 24-28). The clinical course parallels that of endometrioid carcinoma.

 CLINICAL FEATURES: Most ovarian tumors do not secrete hormones. However, the cancer antigen, CA-125, is detectable in the serum in about half of epithelial tumors confined to the ovary and about 90% that have spread. The specificity of this test is highest when combined with transvaginal ultrasonography.

Ovarian masses rarely produce symptoms until they become large and distend the abdomen to cause pain, pelvic pressure or compression of regional organs. By the time ovarian cancers are diagnosed, many have metastasized to (i.e., implanted on) the surfaces of the pelvis, abdominal organs or bladder. Evaluation of a patient with an epithelial ovarian cancer requires knowledge of staging, grading and routes of tumor spread. For example, ovarian tumors have a tendency to implant in the peritoneal cavity on the diaphragm, paracolic gutters and omentum. Lymphatic spread preferentially involves para-aortic lymph nodes near the origin of the renal arteries and to a lesser extent to external iliac (pelvic) or inguinal lymph nodes. In addition to local symptoms, metastatic cancers may cause ascites, weakness, weight loss and cachexia.

Survival in patients with malignant ovarian tumors is generally poor. The most important prognostic index is the surgical stage of the tumor at the time of detection (Table 24-9). Overall, 5-year survival is only 35%, because more than half of tumors have spread to the abdominal cavity (stage III) or elsewhere by the time they are discovered. Prognostic indices for epithelial tumors also include grade, histologic type and the size of the residual neoplasm.

Surgery, which removes the primary tumor, establishes the diagnosis and determines the extent of spread, is the mainstay of therapy. The peritoneal surfaces, omentum, liver, subdiaphragmatic recesses and all abdominal regions

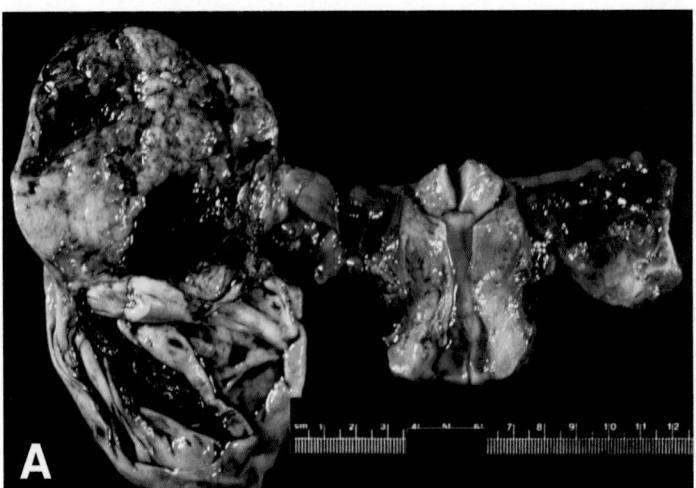

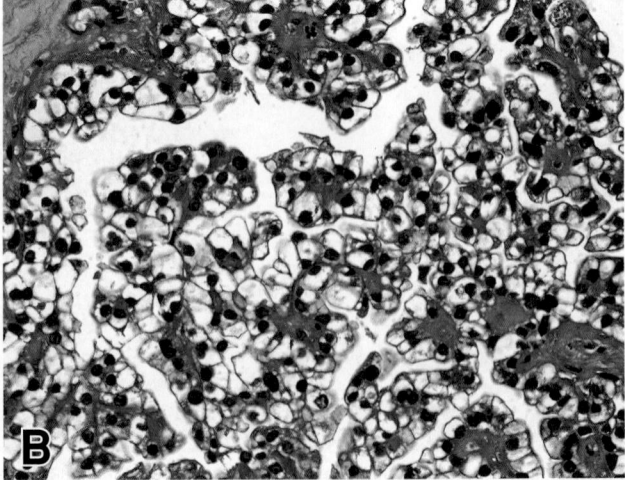

FIGURE 24-60. Clear cell adenocarcinoma. A. Clear cell adenocarcinoma arising as an ovarian mass in a large, hemorrhagic endometriotic cyst. **B.** The clear cells are polyhedral and have eccentric, hyperchromatic nuclei without prominent nucleoli.

must be visualized, and as much metastatic tumor removed as possible. Adjuvant chemotherapy is used to treat distant occult sites of tumor spread.

At some time after the initial operation, another exploratory (second-look) laparotomy may be used to assess effectiveness of therapy. Even if no residual disease is apparent, one third of older patients still develop recurrences. Risk factors for recurrence are (1) high stage, (2) high grade and (3) more than 2 cm of residual disease remaining after the primary operation.

Germ Cell Tumors Tend to Be Benign in Adults and Malignant in Children

Tumors derived from germ cells make up 1/4 of ovarian tumors. In adult women, ovarian germ cell tumors are virtually all benign (mature cystic teratoma, dermoid cyst), but in children and young adults, they are largely cancerous. *In children, germ cell tumors are the most common ovarian cancer (60%); they are rare after menopause.*

Neoplastic germ cells may differentiate along several lines (Fig. 24-61):

- **Dysgerminomas** are composed of neoplastic germ cells, similar to oogonia of fetal ovaries.
- **Teratomas** differentiate toward somatic (embryonic or adult) tissues.
- **Yolk sac tumors** form extraembryonic endodermal and mesenchymal tissue.
- **Choriocarcinomas** feature cells similar to those covering the placental villi.

Germ cell tumors in infants tend to be solid and immature (e.g., yolk sac tumor and immature teratoma). Tumors in young adults show greater differentiation, as in mature cystic teratoma. Malignant germ cell tumors in women older than 40 years usually result from transformation of a component of a benign cystic teratoma.

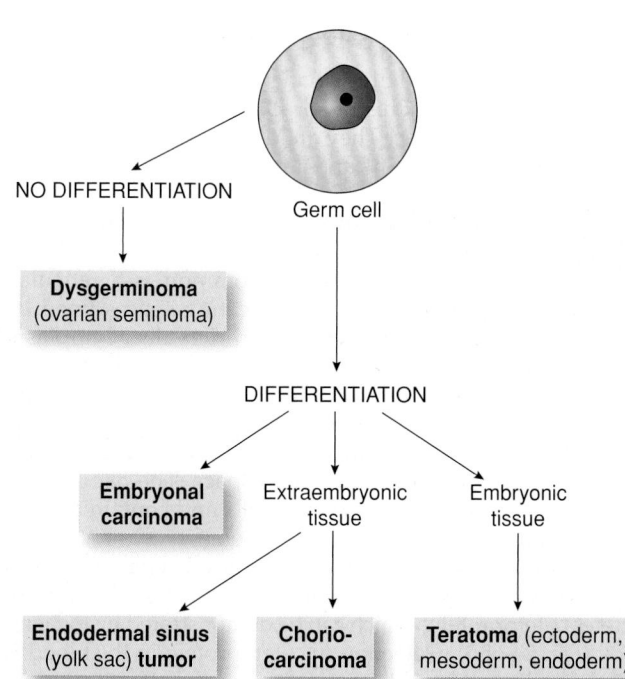

FIGURE 24-61. Classification of germ cell tumors of the ovary.

(Diagram labels:)
Germ cell
NO DIFFERENTIATION
Dysgerminoma (ovarian seminoma)
DIFFERENTIATION
Embryonal carcinoma
Extraembryonic tissue
Embryonic tissue
Endodermal sinus (yolk sac) **tumor**
Chorio-carcinoma
Teratoma (ectoderm, mesoderm, endoderm)

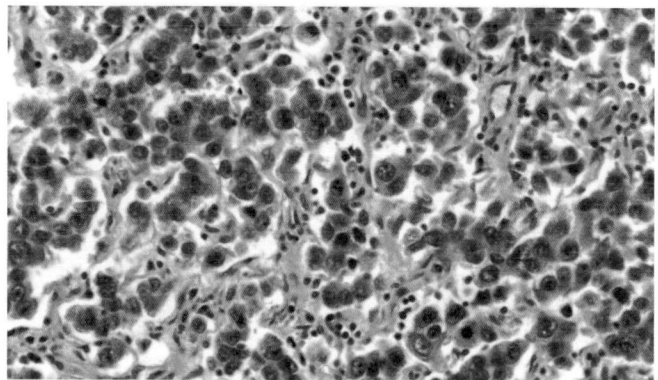

FIGURE 24-62. Dysgerminoma. The neoplastic germ cells are distributed in nests separated by delicate fibrous septa. The stroma contains lymphocytes.

Malignant germ cell tumors are very aggressive. Solid ovarian germ cell tumors were once always fatal, but now over 80% of patients survive with chemotherapy.

Dysgerminoma

Dysgerminoma, the ovarian counterpart of testicular seminoma, is composed of primordial germ cells. It accounts for less than 2% of ovarian cancers in all women, but constitutes 10% in women younger than 20 years. Most patients are between 10 and 30. The tumors are bilateral in about 15% of cases.

PATHOLOGY: Dysgerminomas are often large and firm and have a bosselated external surface. The cut surface is soft and fleshy. They contain large nests of monotonously uniform tumor cells that have clear glycogen-filled cytoplasm and irregularly flattened central nuclei (Fig. 24-62). Fibrous septa containing lymphocytes traverse the tumor.

Dysgerminomas are treated surgically; 5-year survival for patients with stage I tumor approaches 100%. Because the tumor is highly radiosensitive and also responsive to chemotherapy, even higher-stage tumors have 5-year survival rates exceeding 80%.

Teratoma

Teratoma is a tumor of germ cell origin that differentiates toward somatic structures. Most contain tissues from at least two, and usually all three, embryonic layers.

MATURE TERATOMA (MATURE CYSTIC TERATOMA, DERMOID CYST): This benign neoplasm accounts for 1/4 of all ovarian tumors, with peak incidence in the third decade. Mature teratomas develop by **parthenogenesis**. Haploid (postmeiotic) germ cells endoreduplicate to give rise to diploid genetically female tumor cells (46,XX).

PATHOLOGY: Mature teratomas are cystic and almost all contain skin, sebaceous glands and hair follicles (Fig. 24-63). Half have smooth muscle, sweat glands, cartilage, bone, teeth and respiratory epithelium. Other tissues, like gut, thyroid and brain, are seen less often. If present, nodular foci in the cyst wall ("mammary tubercles" or "Rokitansky nodules") contain tissue elements of all three germ cell layers: (1) ectoderm (e.g., skin, glia), (2) mesoderm (e.g., smooth muscle, cartilage) and (3) endoderm (e.g., respiratory epithelium).

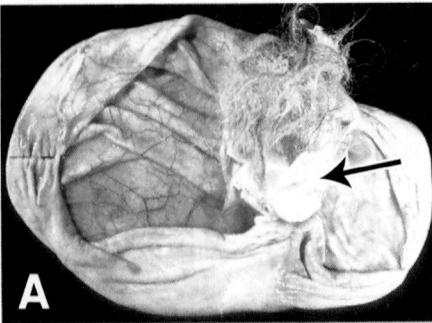

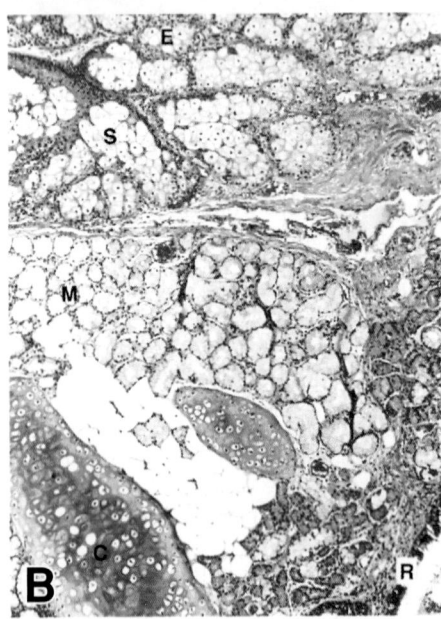

FIGURE 24-63. Mature cystic teratoma of the ovary. A. A mature cystic teratoma has been opened to reveal a solid knob (*arrow*) from which hair projects. **B.** A photomicrograph of the solid knob shows epidermal and respiratory components. Tissue resembling the skin exhibits an epidermis (E) with underlying sebaceous glands (S). The respiratory tissue consists of mucous glands (M), cartilage (C) and respiratory epithelium (R).

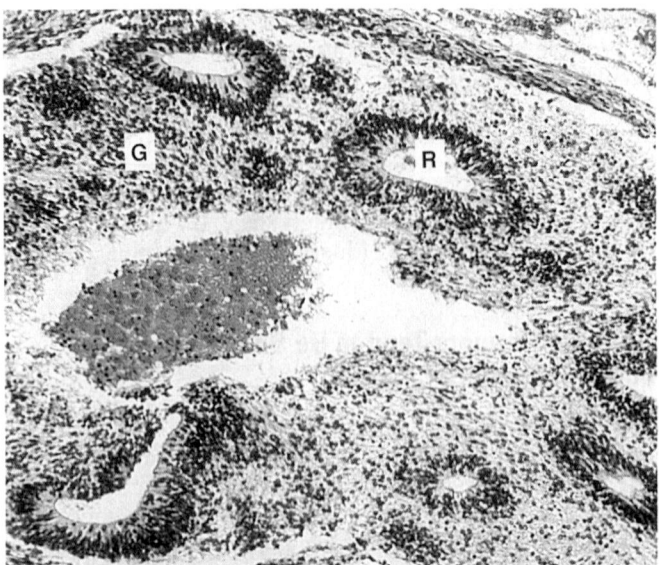

FIGURE 24-64. Immature teratoma of the ovary. Immature neural tissue exhibits rosettes (R) with multilayered nuclei. Embryonal glia (G) display densely packed, atypical nuclei.

Struma ovarii is a cystic lesion with mainly thyroid tissue (5%–20% of mature cystic teratomas). Rarely hyperthyroidism has occurred with struma ovarii.

Very few (1%) dermoid cysts become malignant. These cancers usually occur in older women and correspond to the tumors that arise in other differentiated tissues of the body. Three fourths of cancers that arise in dermoid cysts are squamous cell carcinomas. The remainder are carcinoid tumors, basal cell carcinomas, thyroid cancers and others. Rarely, functional gut derivatives may cause carcinoid syndrome. The prognosis of patients with malignancies in mature cystic teratoma is related largely to the stage of the cancer.

IMMATURE TERATOMA: Immature teratomas of the ovary contain elements derived from the three germ layers. However, unlike mature cystic teratomas, immature teratomas contain embryonal tissues. These tumors account for 20% of malignant tumors at all sites in women under the age of 20 but become progressively less common in older women.

 PATHOLOGY: Immature teratomas are predominantly solid and lobulated, with numerous small cysts. Solid areas may contain grossly recognizable

immature bone and cartilage. Multiple tumor components are usually seen, including those differentiating toward nerve (neuroepithelial rosettes and immature glia) (Fig. 24-64), glands and other structures found in mature cystic teratomas. Grading is based on the amount of immature tissue present. Metastases of immature teratomas are composed of embryonal, usually stromal, tissues. By contrast, rare metastases of mature cystic teratomas resemble epithelial adult-type malignancies.

Survival reflects tumor grade. Well-differentiated immature teratomas have a good prognosis, but high-grade tumors (mainly embryonal tissue) are often lethal.

Yolk Sac Tumor (Primitive Endodermal Tumor)

Yolk sac tumors are highly malignant tumors of women under the age of 30 that histologically resemble mesenchyme of the primitive yolk sac. They are the second most common malignant germ cell tumors and are almost always unilateral.

 PATHOLOGY: Yolk sac tumors are large, with extensive necrosis and hemorrhage. Several patterns are seen. The most common is a reticular, honeycombed structure of communicating spaces lined by primitive epithelial cells with glycogen-rich, clear cytoplasm and large hyperchromatic nuclei (primitive endoderm). Glomerular or **Schiller-Duval bodies** (Fig. 24-65A) are found sparingly in a few tumors but are characteristic. They consist of papillae that protrude into a space lined by tumor cells, resembling the glomerular Bowman space. The papillae are covered by a mantle of embryonal cells and contain a fibrovascular core and a central blood vessel.

Yolk sac tumor should not be confused with embryonal cell carcinoma, which is common in the testis. The former secretes α-fetoprotein, which can be demonstrated histochemically (Fig. 24-65B). Detection of α-fetoprotein in the blood is useful for diagnosis and for monitoring the effectiveness of therapy. Although once uniformly fatal, 5-year survival with chemotherapy for stage I yolk sac tumors now exceeds 80%.

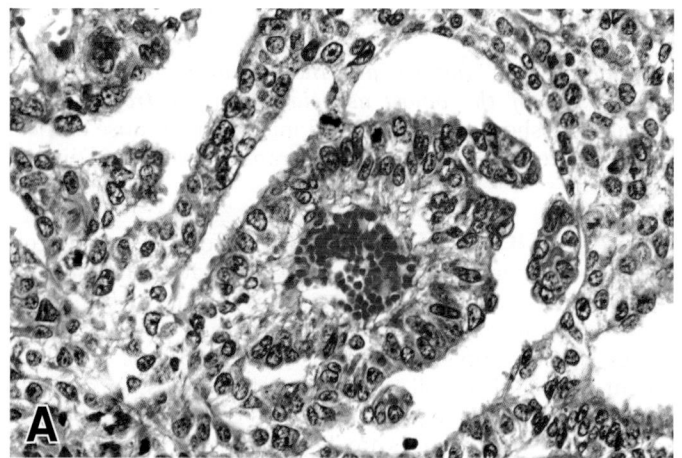
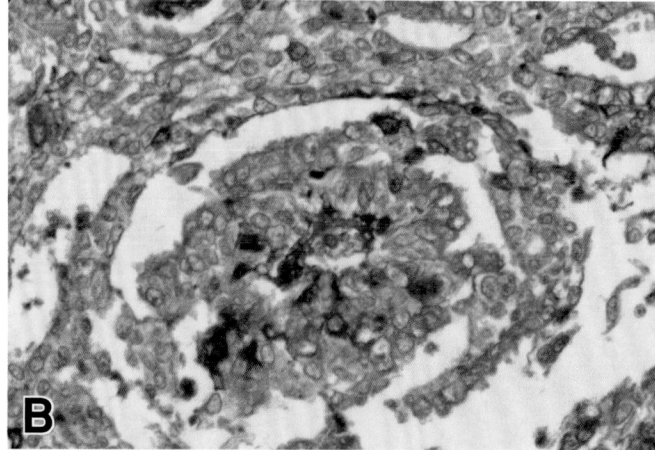

FIGURE 24-65. Yolk sac tumor of the ovary. A. Glomeruloid Schiller-Duval body that resembles the endodermal sinuses of the rodent placenta and consists of a papilla protruding into a space lined by tumor cells. **B.** Strong immunoreaction for α-fetoprotein.

Choriocarcinoma

Choriocarcinoma of the ovary is a rare tumor that mimics the epithelial covering of placental villi, namely, cytotrophoblast and syncytiotrophoblast. If it arises before puberty or together with another germ cell tumor, it most likely is of germ cell origin. Young girls may show precocious sexual development, menstrual irregularities or rapid breast enlargement. In women of reproductive age, however, it may also be a metastasis from an intrauterine gestational tumor.

 PATHOLOGY: Choriocarcinoma is unilateral, solid and widely hemorrhagic. Microscopically, it shows a mixture of malignant cytotrophoblast and syncytiotrophoblast (see placenta, choriocarcinoma, below). The syncytial cells secrete hCG, which accounts for the frequent finding of a positive pregnancy test result. Bilateral theca lutein cysts, a result of hCG stimulation, may also be found. Serial serum hCG determinations are useful both for diagnosis and follow-up. The tumor is highly aggressive but responds to chemotherapy.

Gonadoblastoma

Gonadoblastoma is a rare ovarian tumor that is distinctively associated with gonadal dysgenesis, especially in women who bear a Y chromosome. It occurs in phenotypic women under 30 years of age, although 20% are found in phenotypic men with cryptorchidism, hypospadias and female internal sex organs. Most affected women are virilized and suffer from primary amenorrhea and developmental abnormalities of the genitalia. Cellular nests show a mixture of germ cells and sex cord derivatives that resemble immature Sertoli and granulosa cells, suggesting that the tumor is an in situ form of germinoma. In half of cases, it is overgrown by dysgerminoma. Gonadoblastomas do not metastasize, but their overgrowths do.

Sex Cord/Stromal Tumors Are Clinically Functional

Tumors of sex cord and stroma originate from either primitive sex cords or from mesenchymal stroma of developing gonads. They represent 10% of ovarian tumors, vary from benign to low-grade malignant and may differentiate toward female (granulosa and theca cells) or male (Sertoli and Leydig cells) structures.

Fibroma

Fibromas account for 75% of all stromal tumors and 7% of all ovarian tumors. They occur at all ages, peaking in the perimenopausal period, and are almost always benign.

 PATHOLOGY: Tumors are solid, firm and white (Fig. 24-66). The cells resemble the stroma of the normal ovarian cortex, being well-differentiated spindle cells, with variable amounts of collagen. Half of the larger tumors are associated with ascites and, rarely, with ascites and pleural effusions **(Meigs syndrome)**.

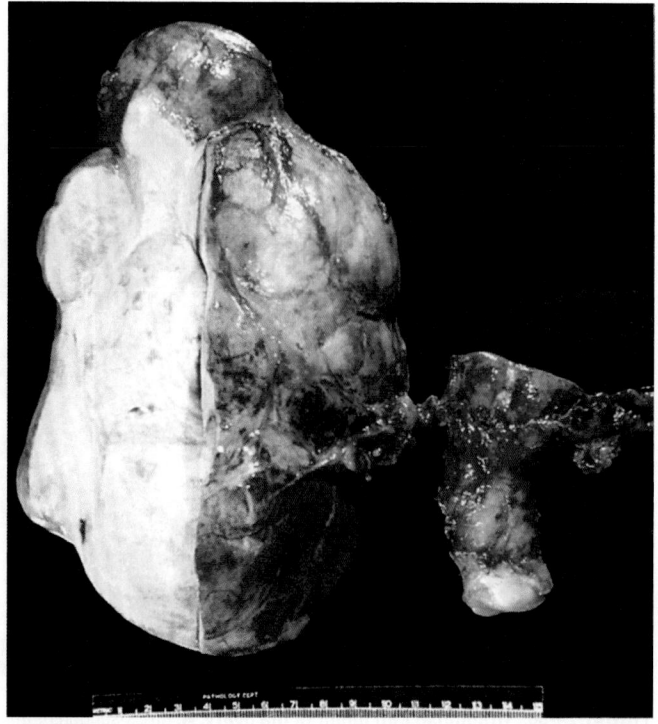

FIGURE 24-66. Fibroma of the ovary. The ovary is conspicuously enlarged by a firm, white, bosselated tumor.

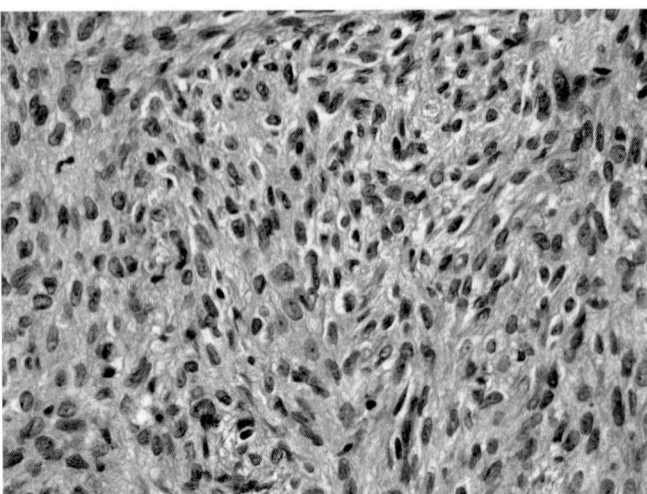

FIGURE 24-67. Thecoma of the ovary. Oblong cells are invested by collagen. The cytoplasm contains lipid.

Thecoma

Thecomas are functional ovarian tumors of postmenopausal women and are almost always benign. They are closely related to fibromas, but additionally contain varying amounts of steroidogenic cells that in many cases produce estrogens or androgen.

 PATHOLOGY: Thecomas are solid, mostly 5–10 cm in diameter. Cut section is yellow, owing to the many lipid-laden theca cells, which are large and oblong to round, with lipid-rich vacuolated cytoplasm (Fig. 24-67). Bands of hyalinized collagen separate nests of theca cells.

Because they produce estrogen, thecomas in premenopausal women may cause irregular menstrual cycles and breast enlargement. Endometrial hyperplasia and cancer are well-recognized complications.

Granulosa Cell Tumor

Granulosa cell tumors are the prototypical functional neoplasms of the ovary associated with estrogen secretion. They should be considered malignant because of their potential for local spread and the rare occurrence of distant metastases.

 **ETIOLOGIC FACTORS:** Most granulosa cell tumors occur after menopause (adult form) and are unusual before puberty. A juvenile form in children and young women has distinct clinical and pathologic features (hyperestrinism and precocious puberty). Development of granulosa cell tumors is linked to loss of oocytes. Oocytes appear to regulate granulosa cells, and tumorigenesis occurs when follicles are disorganized or atretic.

 PATHOLOGY: Adult-type granulosa cell tumors, like most ovarian tumors, are large and focally cystic to solid. The cut surface shows yellow areas, owing to lipid-rich luteinized granulosa cells, white zones of stroma and focal hemorrhages (Fig. 24-68). Granulosa cell tumors show diverse growth patterns: (1) diffuse (sarcomatoid), (2) insular (islands of cells) or (3) trabecular (anastomotic bands of granulosa cells). Random nuclear arrangement about a central degenerative space **(Call-Exner bodies)** gives a characteristic follicular pattern (Fig. 24-68B). Tumor cells are typically spindle shaped and have a cleaved, elongated nucleus (coffee bean appearance). They secrete **inhibin**, a protein that suppresses pituitary release of follicle-stimulating hormone (FSH). These tumors can also express **calretinin**, a primarily neuronal protein, which suggests possible neural differentiation or derivation for these neoplasms.

 CLINICAL FEATURES: *Three fourths of granulosa cell tumors secrete estrogens.* Thus, endometrial hyperplasia is a common presenting sign. EIN or endometrial adenocarcinoma may develop if a functioning granulosa cell tumor remains undetected. At diagnosis,

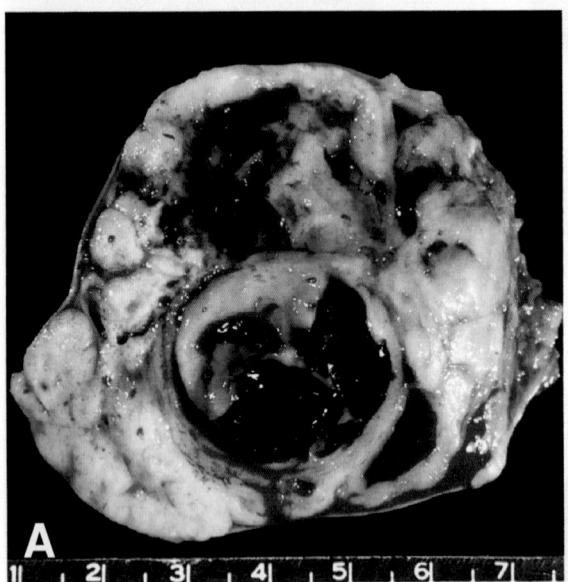

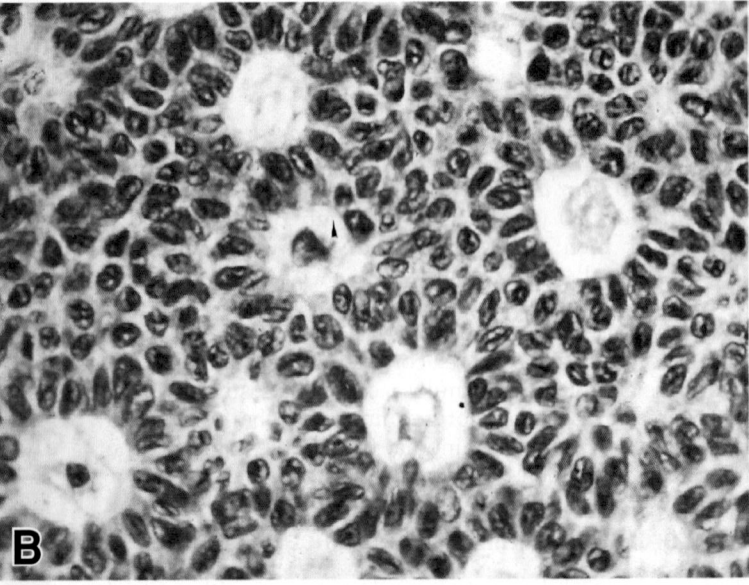

FIGURE 24-68. Granulosa cell tumor of the ovary. A. Cross-section of the enlarged ovary shows a variegated solid tumor with focal hemorrhages. The yellow areas represent collections of lipid-laden luteinized granulosa cells. **B.** The orientation of tumor cells about central spaces results in the characteristic follicular pattern (Call-Exner bodies).

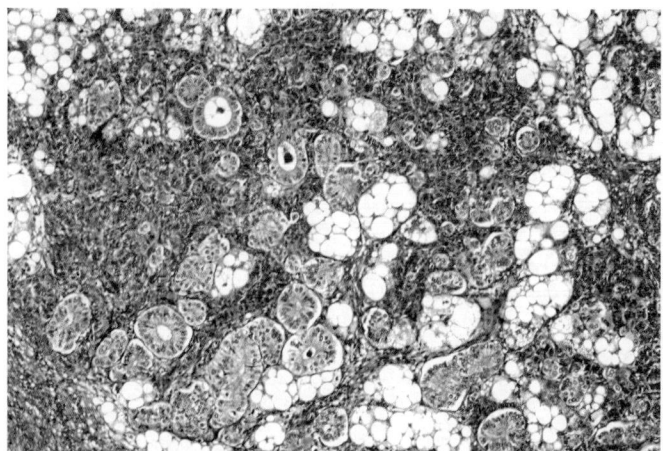

FIGURE 24-69. Sertoli-Leydig cell tumor, well differentiated. The hollow tubules are lined by mature Sertoli cells. The intervening stroma contains numerous Leydig cells with vacuolated cytoplasm.

90% of granulosa cell tumors are within the ovary (stage I). Over 90% of these patients survive 10 years. Tumors that have extended into the pelvis and lower abdomen have a poorer prognosis. Late recurrence 5–10 years after surgical removal is not uncommon and is usually fatal.

Sertoli-Leydig Cell Tumors

Ovarian Sertoli-Leydig cell tumors (**arrhenoblastoma** or **androblastoma**) are rare androgen-secreting mesenchymal neoplasms of low malignant potential that resemble embryonic testis. Tumor cells typically secrete weak androgens (dehydroepiandrosterone), so tumors are usually quite large before patients complain of masculinization. Sertoli-Leydig cell tumors occur at all ages but are most common in young women of childbearing age.

 PATHOLOGY: Sertoli-Leydig cell tumors are unilateral, usually 5–15 cm, and tend to be lobulated, solid and brown to yellow. They vary from well to poorly differentiated and some contain heterologous elements

(e.g., mucinous glands and, rarely, even cartilage). Large Leydig cells have abundant eosinophilic cytoplasm and a central round to oval nucleus with a prominent nucleolus. Tumor cells are embedded in a sarcomatoid stroma (Fig. 24-69). The stroma in some areas often differentiates into immature solid tubules of embryonic Sertoli cells.

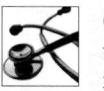 **CLINICAL FEATURES:** Nearly half of all patients with Sertoli-Leydig cell tumors exhibit signs of virilization: hirsutism, male escutcheon, enlarged clitoris and deepened voice. Initial signs are often defeminization, manifested as breast atrophy, amenorrhea and loss of hip fat. Once the tumor is removed, these signs disappear or lessen. Well-differentiated tumors are virtually always cured by surgical resection, but poorly differentiated ones may metastasize.

Steroid Cell Tumor

Steroid cell tumors of the ovary, also called **lipid cell** or **lipoid cell tumors,** are composed of cells that resemble lutein cells, Leydig cells and adrenal cortical cells. Most steroid cell tumors are hormonally active, usually with androgenic manifestations. Some secrete testosterone; others synthesize weaker androgens. **Hilus cell tumor** is a specialized form of steroid cell tumor that is typically a benign neoplasm of Leydig cells. It arises in the hilus of the ovary, usually after menopause. Because it secretes testosterone, the most potent of the common androgens, masculinizing signs are frequent (75%), even with small tumors. Most hilus cell tumors contain "crystalloids of Reinke" (rod-like cytoplasmic structures).

Tumors Metastatic to the Ovary May Mimic a Primary Tumor

About 3% of cancers found in the ovaries arise elsewhere, mostly in the breast, large intestine, endometrium and stomach, in descending order. These tumors vary from microscopic lesions to large masses. Those from the breast are usually tiny and are seen in 10% of ovaries removed prophylactically in cases of advanced breast cancer. Metastatic tumors large enough to cause symptoms originate most often in the colon (Fig. 24-70). Commonly, the tumor cells

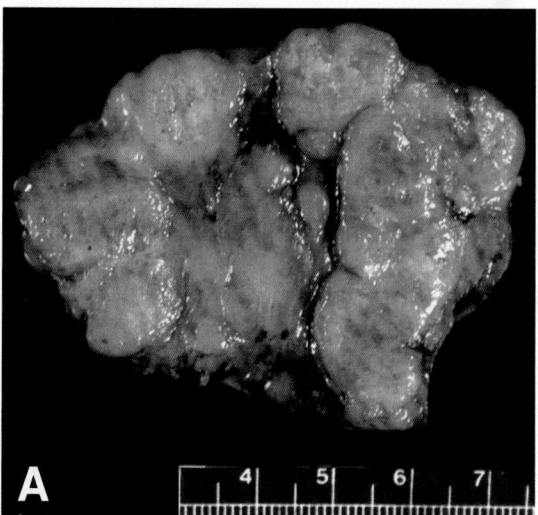
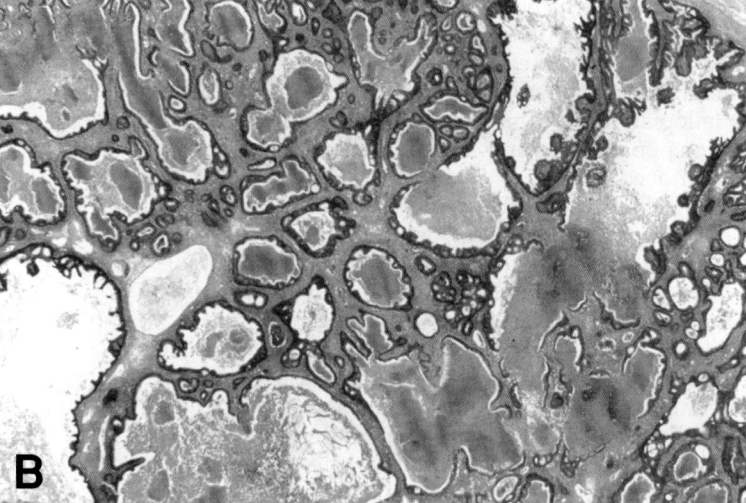

FIGURE 24-70. Metastatic adenocarcinoma from colon. A. The ovary is replaced by multinodular tumor. The sectioned surface appears solid. **B.** Microscopically, the tumor shows a garland-like glandular pattern with focal segmental necrosis and abundant necrotic debris.

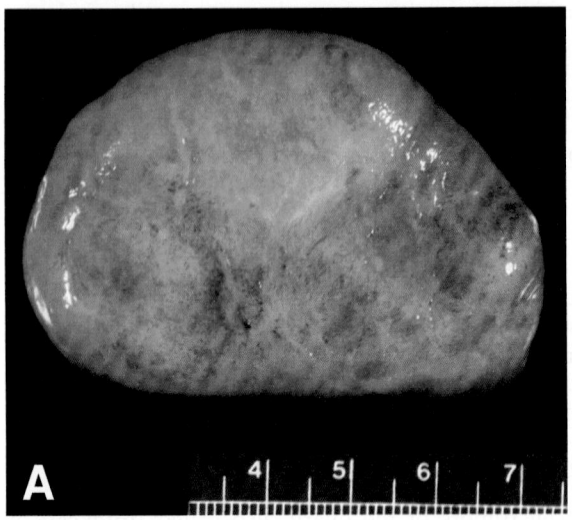
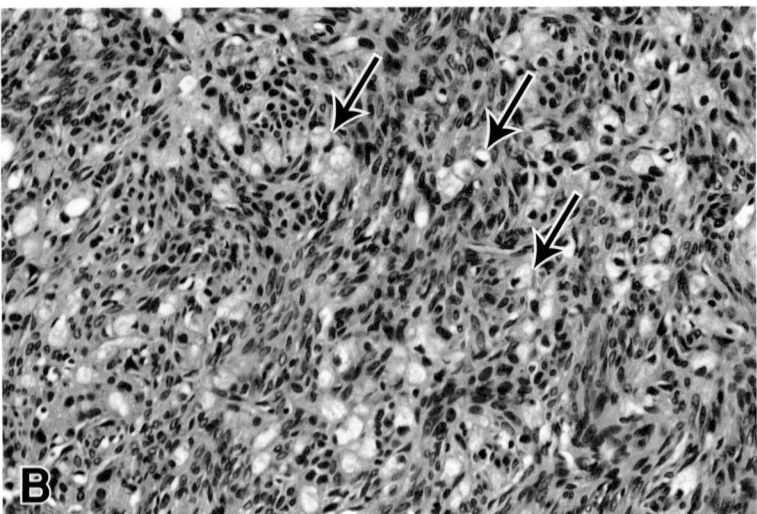

FIGURE 24-71. Krukenberg tumor. A. The ovary is enlarged and the cut surface appears solid, pale yellow and partially hemorrhagic. **B.** A microscopic section of **A** reveals mucinous (signet-ring) cells (clear cells, *arrows*) infiltrating the ovarian stroma.

stimulate ovarian stroma to differentiate into hormonally active cells (luteinized stromal cells), leading to androgenic and sometimes estrogenic symptoms.

Krukenberg tumors are metastases to the ovary, composed of nests of mucin-filled "signet-ring" cells in a cellular stroma derived from the ovary (Fig. 24-71). The stomach is the primary site in 75% of cases and most of the rest are from the colon.

Bilateral ovarian involvement and multinodularity suggest a metastatic carcinoma, and both ovaries are grossly involved in 75% of cases. Even an ovary that appears uninvolved grossly may contain surface implants or minute foci of tumor within the parenchyma. Thus, when metastasis to one ovary is documented, the other should also be removed.

Peritoneum

The peritoneum is a nearly continuous membrane that lines the peritoneal cavity and separates viscera from the abdominal wall. In men, the peritoneum is a closed system. In women, it is an "open system" interrupted in the pelvis by the fallopian tubes, which provide a final conduit for transmission of pathogens and chemicals from the genital tract to the peritoneal cavity.

The cells that line the peritoneal cavity and those that form the serosa of the ovary are both of celomic epithelial origin. *Thus, it is not clear whether tumors and tumor-like lesions of peritoneum and ovary (i.e., müllerian epithelial lesions) are the same entity in both locations.*

Many inflammatory lesions involve the peritoneum. Granulomatous peritonitis develops as a response to foreign materials such as sutures, surgical glove powder or contrast media. Exposure to intestinal contents after perforation (e.g., in Crohn disease or diverticulitis); rupture of a mature cystic teratoma (dermoid cyst) of the ovary; and, of course, tuberculosis can also cause peritoneal inflammation. Reactive mesothelial proliferation occurs with the slightest irritation. Peritonitis is discussed in Chapter 19.

ENDOMETRIOSIS

Endometriosis is the presence of benign endometrial glands and stroma outside the uterus. It afflicts 5%–10% of women of reproductive age and regresses after natural or artificial menopause. The mean age at diagnosis is the late 20s to early 30s, although it may appear any time after menarche. Sites most frequently involved are the ovaries (>60%), other uterine adnexa (uterine ligaments, rectovaginal septum, pouch of Douglas) and the pelvic peritoneum covering the uterus, fallopian tubes, rectosigmoid colon and bladder (Fig. 24-72). Endometriosis can be even more widespread and occasionally affects the cervix, vagina, perineum, bladder and umbilicus. Even pelvic lymph nodes may contain foci of endometriosis. Rarely, distant areas such as lungs, pleura, small bowel, kidneys and bones contain lesions.

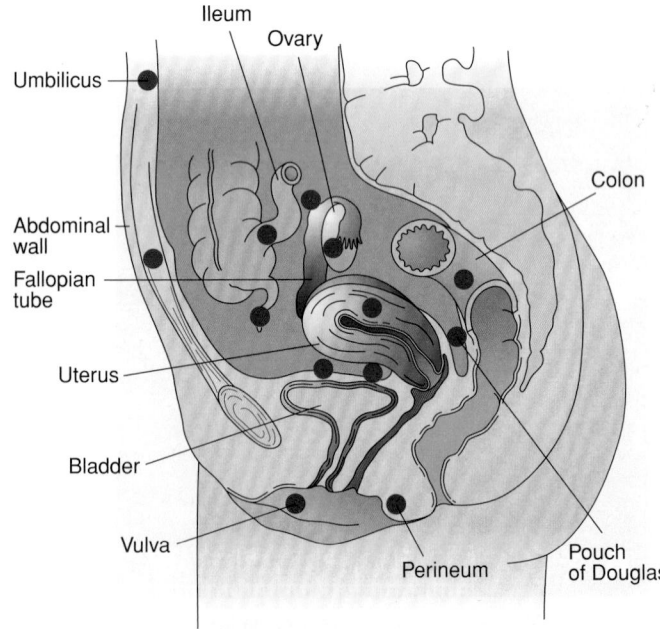

FIGURE 24-72. Sites of endometriosis.

 **PATHOPHYSIOLOGY:** The pathogenesis of endometriosis is uncertain. Several theories, not necessarily mutually exclusive, are proposed:

1. **Transplantation** of endometrial fragments to ectopic sites
2. **Metaplasia** of the multipotential celomic peritoneum
3. **Induction** of undifferentiated mesenchyme in ectopic sites to form lesions after exposure to substances released from shed endometrium

TRANSPLANTATION: The most widely accepted theory holds that menstrual endometrium refluxes through the fallopian tubes and implants at ectopic sites. It is known that retrograde menstruation through the fallopian tubes occurs in 90% of women. A mechanism involving lymphatic and hematogenous dissemination would explain endometriosis in lymph nodes and at distant organ sites like the lungs and kidneys. The observation that pulmonary endometriosis occurs almost exclusively in women who have had uterine surgery supports this contention.

CELOMIC METAPLASIA: This theory proposes that endometriosis arises by endometrial metaplasia of peritoneal serosa or serosa-like structures. Thus, if appropriately stimulated, the pelvic peritoneum may differentiate into any type of müllerian epithelium.

INDUCTION THEORY: This concept suggests that something secreted by the endometrium makes endometrial epithelium and stroma develop in ectopic sites.

 PATHOLOGY: The earliest lesions of endometriosis may be yellow-red stains, reflecting breakdown of blood products. Red lesions, which also occur early in the disease, are actively growing foci of endometriosis (Fig. 24-73). Operative specimens usually contain black lesions showing some degree of resolution. These 1–5-mm foci on the ovary and peritoneal surfaces are called "mulberry" nodules. With repeated cycles of hemorrhage and subsequent fibrosis, affected surfaces may scar and become grossly brown ("powder burns"). Over time, fibrous adhesions may become more pronounced and lead to complications, such as intestinal obstruction. Repeated hemorrhage in the ovaries may turn endometriotic foci into cysts up to 15 cm in diameter containing inspissated, chocolate-colored material ("chocolate cysts").

Endometriosis is characterized by ectopic normal endometrial glands and stroma (Fig. 24-73). Occasionally, healed foci may contain only fibrous tissue and hemosiderin-laden macrophages, which by themselves are not diagnostic. Immunohistochemical demonstration of CD-10 can be diagnostic.

 CLINICAL FEATURES: Symptoms of endometriosis depend on where implants are located. Dysmenorrhea, caused by implants on uterosacral ligaments, is common. Lesions swell just before or during menstruation, producing pelvic pain. Half of women with dysmenorrhea have endometriosis. Other symptoms include dyspareunia and cyclical abdominal pain.

Infertility is the primary complaint in a third of women with endometriosis (Fig. 24-74). The hormonal milieu in a woman who does not achieve pregnancy encourages development of endometriosis. In turn, once endometriosis develops, it contributes to the infertile state and a vicious circle is established. Conversely, pregnancy may alleviate the disease. Conservative surgery to restore pelvic anatomy helps many women with endometriosis to become pregnant.

Malignancy occurs in about 1%–2% of cases of endometriosis (Fig. 24-60). Clear cell and endometrioid tumors are the most frequent forms. Adenosarcoma, although rare, is the most common sarcoma.

MESOTHELIAL TUMORS

Mesothelial tumors range from benign to multicentric aggressive malignancies.

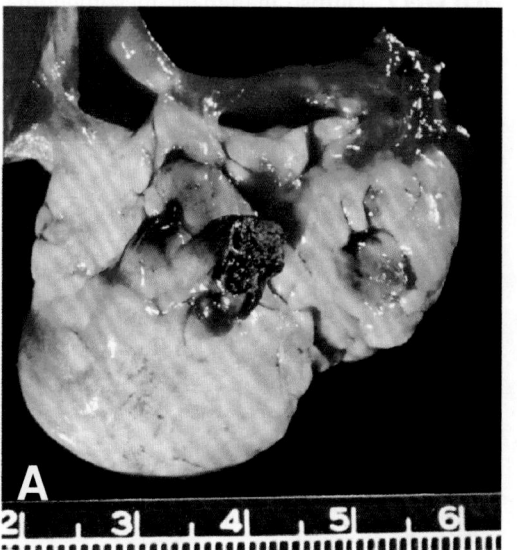
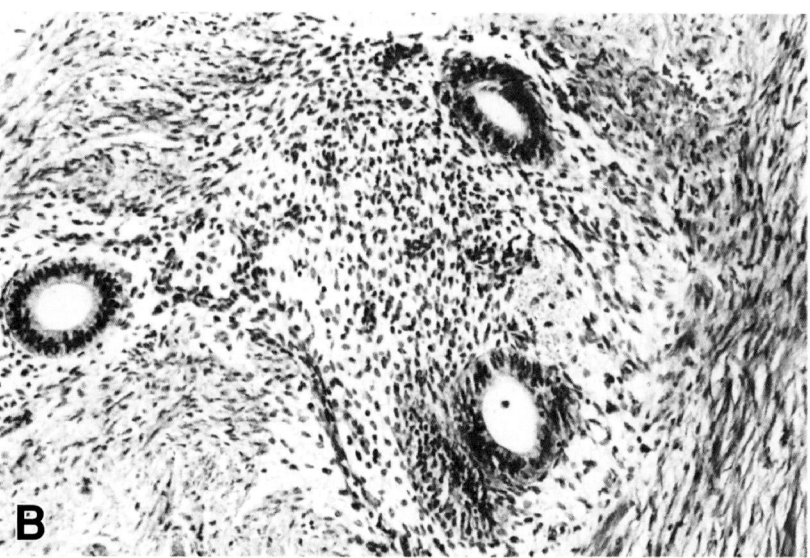

FIGURE 24-73. Endometriosis. A. Implants of endometriosis on the ovary appear as red-blue nodules. **B.** A microscopic section shows endometrial glands and stroma in the ovary.

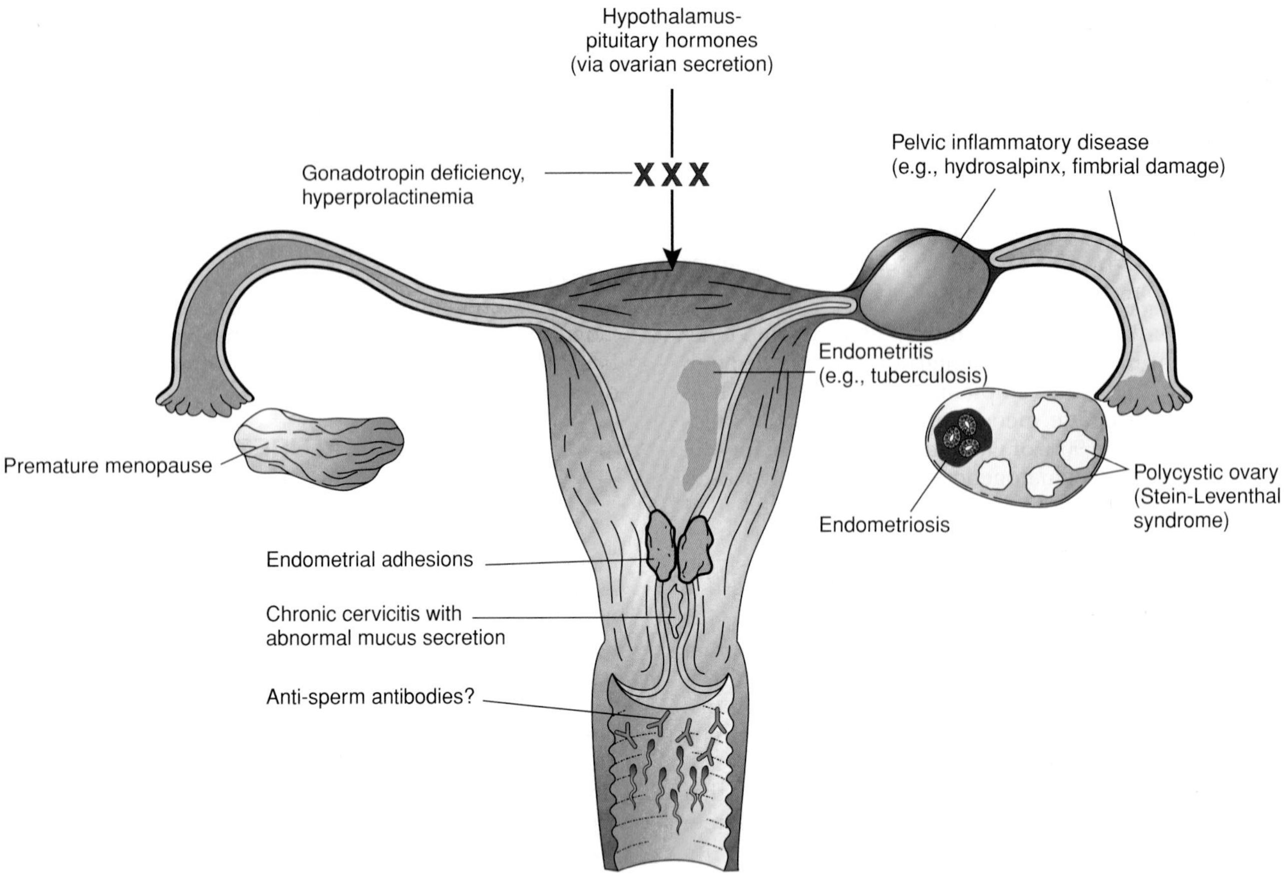

Hypothalamus-
pituitary hormones
(via ovarian secretion)

Gonadotropin deficiency,
hyperprolactinemia

X X X

Pelvic inflammatory disease
(e.g., hydrosalpinx, fimbrial damage)

Endometritis
(e.g., tuberculosis)

Premature menopause

Polycystic ovary
(Stein-Leventhal
syndrome)

Endometriosis

Endometrial adhesions

Chronic cervicitis with
abnormal mucus secretion

Anti-sperm antibodies?

FIGURE 24-74. Causes of acquired infertility.

Adenomatoid Tumors Are Benign Mesothelial Neoplasms, Mainly of Fallopian Tubes

It is encountered in the fallopian tubes and in subserosal tissue of the uterine corpus near the fallopian tubes. It is rare elsewhere in the peritoneum.

Well-Differentiated Papillary Mesotheliomas Are Benign

Well-differentiated papillary mesotheliomas are rare in women of reproductive age. They are typically asymptomatic and usually found incidentally at operation. These tumors are solitary, small, broad-based, wart-like polypoid or nodular excrescences with a single layer of small bland cuboidal cells covering thick papillae (Fig. 24-75). They often resemble serous epithelial tumors of the ovary, but the two are treated differently.

Diffuse Peritoneal Malignant Mesotheliomas Are Invariably Fatal

These tumors arise from peritoneal mesothelium. They are rare in women and constitute only a small proportion of all malignant mesotheliomas, most of which are pleural. They must be distinguished from serous adenocarcinomas, including those arising from the peritoneal surface itself and those metastatic from the ovary, because they are treated differently and have much different survival rates. Most patients

are middle-aged or postmenopausal with nonspecific symptoms such as ascites, abdominal discomfort, digestive disturbances and weight loss. Unlike pleural tumors, asbestos exposure is uncommon in women with peritoneal mesothelioma, but up to 2 million fibers per gram wet weight have been reported in some tumors.

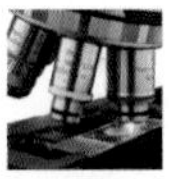

 PATHOLOGY: Diffuse malignant mesothelioma extensively involves and thickens the peritoneum and serosa of the various abdominal and pelvic

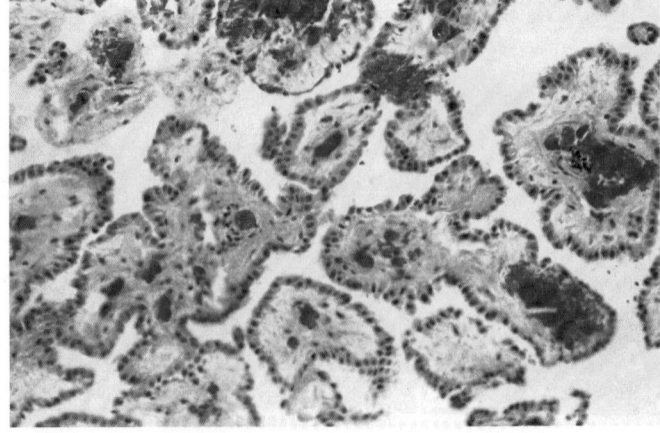

FIGURE 24-75. Well-differentiated peritoneal mesothelioma. Cuboidal epithelium lines papillae.

organs. It has a tubulopapillary to solid pattern. Unlike pleural mesothelioma, the sarcomatoid type is rare. The epithelial variant displays polygonal or cuboidal neoplastic cells with abundant cytoplasm. Thrombomodulin, calretinin, cytokeratin 5/6 and HBME-1 are markers of malignant mesothelioma, whereas CA-125, CEA and estrogen and progesterone receptors (ER and PR) are markers of ovarian epithelial tumors. No effective treatment is available.

SEROUS TUMORS (PRIMARY AND METASTATIC)

Unlike the ovary, which features a wide range of tumors, serous tumors are virtually the only type found in the peritoneum. Mucinous tumors in the peritoneum are metastases from a primary cancer of the appendix or ovary.

Serous Tumors of Borderline Malignancy Resemble the Corresponding Ovarian Neoplasms

Most serous borderline tumors in the peritoneum are metastases from the ovary, but some may be primary in the peritoneum. In the latter case, serous peritoneal tumors without invasion are usually benign; those that are invasive carry a worse prognosis.

 PATHOLOGY: Whether in the ovary or the peritoneum, borderline serous tumors are characterized by papillary processes, small clusters of cells, cell stratification, detached cellular clusters, nuclear atypia and mitotic activity in the absence of invasion. Implants appear as fine granularities or small nodules with clusters of blunt papillae or glandular structures, often having complex cellular tufts (Fig. 24-76). Psammoma bodies are common and may fill the core of the papillae. Mild to severe cytologic atypia with some stratification is common but is substantially less than that seen in adenocarcinoma.

Serous Adenocarcinoma Occurs in Women with Normal Ovaries

The frequency of serous adenocarcinoma arising de novo in the peritoneum is estimated as 10% of its counterpart in the ovary. The mean age of women with this tumor is 50–65 years. The diagnosis of a primary peritoneal tumor requires demonstration of normal ovaries. Abdominal pain and ascites are frequent presentations. Like ovarian cancer, serous adenocarcinoma primarily in the peritoneum may have a familial basis and can metastasize to distant locations.

PSEUDOMYXOMA PERITONEI

Pseudomyxoma peritonei is the accumulation of jelly-like mucus in the pelvis or peritoneum. Previously interpreted as spread from mucinous ovarian tumors, pseudomyxoma peritonei is now understood to derive largely from mucus-producing adenocarcinomas of the appendix.

 PATHOLOGY: The condition may be extensive and appear as semisolid gelatin covering all abdominal structures, or there may be little more than a slightly thickened gelatinous coat over a focal area of bowel or omentum. The appendix is commonly enlarged or adherent to an omentum covered with the gelatinous material. Within the gelatin are strips of very well-differentiated, intestinal-type, mucinous epithelium (Fig. 24-77). If only isolated foci are present, the epithelium may be so well differentiated that it resembles a simple mucinous adenoma. Cribriform patterns or other histologic features of malignancy, such as signet-ring cells or glands, are seen on occasion and warrant a diagnosis of adenocarcinoma.

Low-grade tumors are usually treated for cure, which entails aggressive surgical debulking and intraperitoneal chemotherapy. The 5-year survival is under 50%.

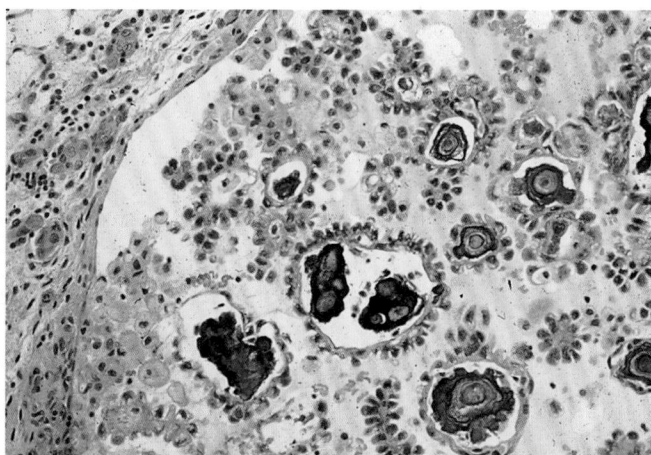

FIGURE 24-76. Noninvasive implants of borderline serous tumor on the peritoneum. The tumor exhibits epithelial tufts and psammoma bodies (compare to Fig. 24-56B).

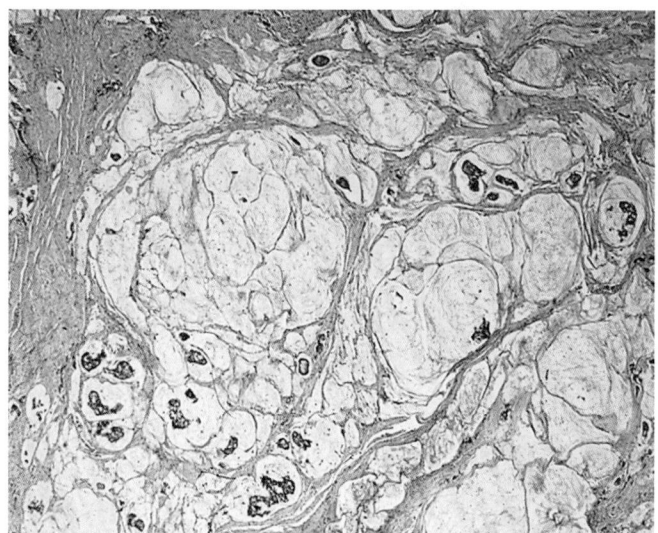

FIGURE 24-77. Pseudomyxoma peritonei. Multiple clusters of tumor cells are present in the mucinous material.

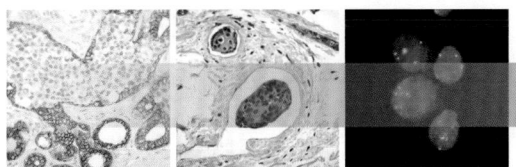

25

The Breast

Anna Marie Mulligan ■ Frances P. O'Malley

DEVELOPMENT, ANATOMY AND PHYSIOLOGIC CHANGE

During embryologic development, the human breast first appears at about the 5th week, when ectodermal thickenings—the mammary ridges, or "milk lines"—extend from the axilla to the medial part of the thigh. Regression occurs except in the 4th intercostal space, where the breast will later develop. By the 9th week of gestation, solid epithelial cords grow from the epidermal layer into the underlying mesenchyme. From about the 20th to 32nd weeks of gestation, these solid cellular invaginations canalize and form a network of about 15–25 branching, primary, mammary ducts under the influence of maternal hormones. Near the end of gestation, the breast responds to maternal and placental steroid hormones and to prolactin. These produce secretory activity, and breast development may be transiently prominent in male and female newborns before returning to the inactive state. Further breast development accelerates at puberty, when ducts begin to elongate and branch (Fig. 25-1A). Estrogen and progesterone cause the terminal end buds and connective tissue stroma to proliferate, differentiate and remodel to form the terminal duct lobular unit (TDLU) of the adult breast (Fig. 25-1B).

The breasts are on the upper chest wall between the 2nd and the 6th ribs. They extend medially to the sternum and laterally to the anterior axillary line, although the tail may extend farther into the axilla. Each breast is composed of skin, subcutaneous adipose tissue and the functional component composed of ducts, lobules and stroma. Collecting ducts, through which milk is secreted, open at the nipple. The nipple–areolar complex is centrally placed and contains abundant sensory nerves and sebaceous and apocrine glands. The nipple consists mainly of dense fibrous tissue mixed with smooth muscle. The latter gives the nipple its erectile capability and contributes to expression of milk. Pigmentation increases in the nipple and areola at puberty and increases further during pregnancy. Stratified squamous epithelium that lines the nipple skin extends superficially into the collecting duct before it transitions abruptly to glandular epithelium. The latter contains an inner luminal secretory epithelial cell layer and an outer myoepithelial cell layer.

Just beneath the nipple, collecting ducts dilate to form lactiferous sinuses, which subdivide into 15–25 lobes with segmental and subsegmental ducts. These terminate in the TDLU, where milk is made. The TDLU consists of (1) terminal ductules or acini, whose epithelium differentiates into secretory acini in pregnant or lactating glands; (2) the intralobular collecting duct; and (3) specialized intralobular stroma (Fig. 25-1B).

The TDLU is a dynamic structure that changes cyclically during the menstrual cycle. These periodic alterations include epithelial proliferation and apoptosis, as well as changes in intralobular stroma. In the follicular phase of the menstrual cycle, terminal ducts are few and are lined by a simple, two-cell layer of epithelium with surrounding myoepithelium. After ovulation, mitoses increase in the luminal epithelium, as do acini and edema of the intralobular stroma. Myoepithelial cells become more prominent, owing to cytoplasmic accumulation of glycogen. These changes

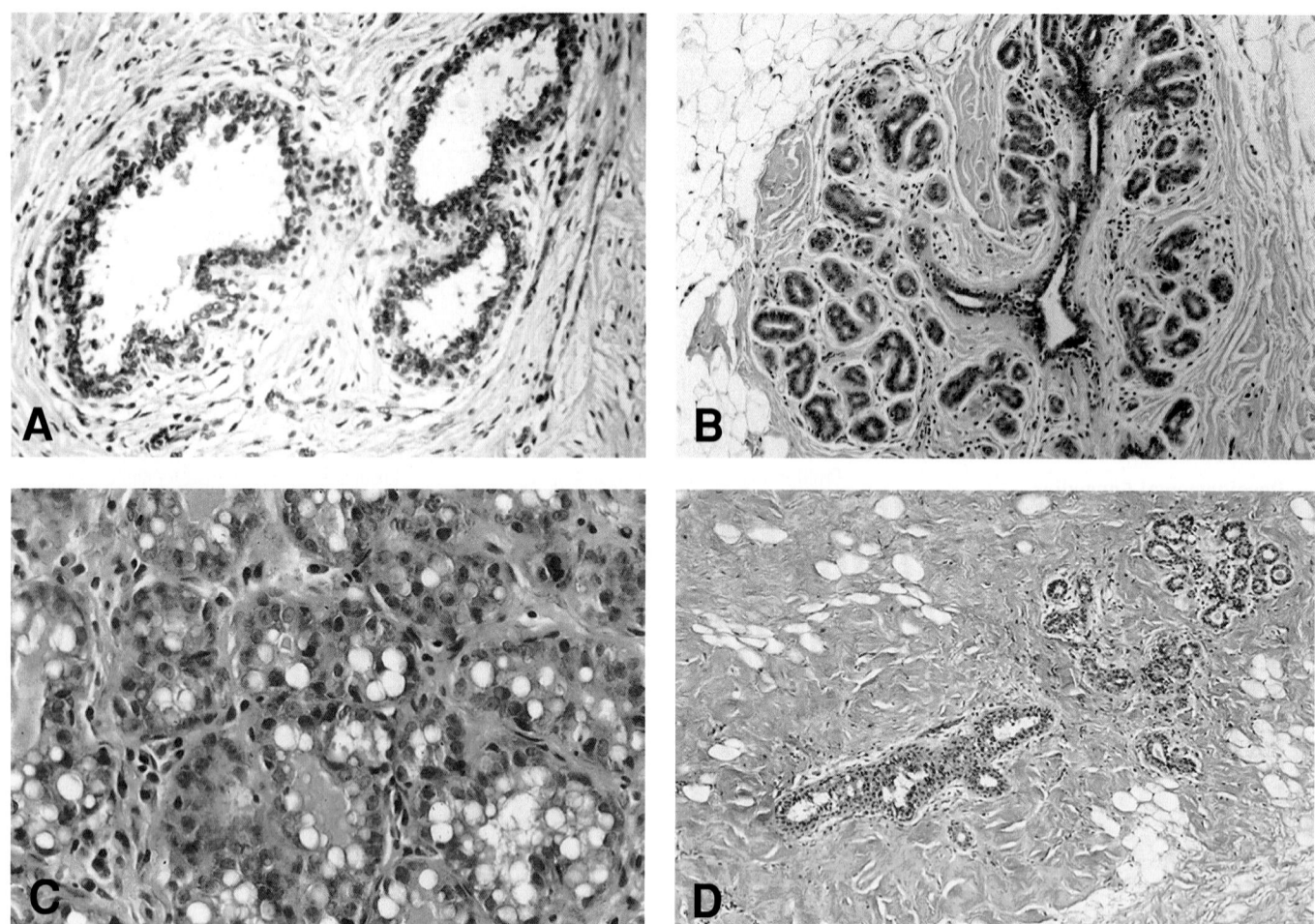

FIGURE 25-1. Normal breast architecture at various ages. A. Adolescent breast. Large and intermediate-size ducts are seen within a dense fibrous stroma. No lobular units are present. **B. Postpubertal breast.** The terminal duct lobular unit consists of small ductules arrayed around an intralobular duct. The two-cell-layered epithelium shows no secretory or mitotic activity. The intralobular stroma is dense and confluent with the interlobular stroma. **C. Lactating breast.** The terminal duct lobular units are conspicuously enlarged, with inapparent interlobular and intralobular stroma. The individual terminal ducts, now termed acini, show prominent epithelial secretory activity (cytoplasmic vacuolization). The acinar lumina contain secretory material. **D. Postmenopausal breast.** The terminal duct lobular units are absent. The remaining intermediate ducts and larger ducts are commonly dilated.

may cause progressive fullness of the breast and tenderness. The TDLUs return to their follicular phase state during menses, when declining estrogen and progesterone levels cause apoptosis. At this time, lymphocytes infiltrate the intralobular stroma.

Full functional breast development only occurs with the hormonal changes of pregnancy and lactation. In pregnancy, glandular tissue increases markedly, compared to fibrous and fatty connective tissue. Early in pregnancy the TDLU grows rapidly. Stromal vascularity and chronic inflammatory cells increase. In later pregnancy, lobular epithelial cells start to become vacuolated owing to increased secretion into distended lobular units. This effect becomes more pronounced with lactation (Fig. 25-1C). At the end of lactation, the gland involutes dramatically, as pronounced cell death and tissue remodeling eventually the breast returns to its prepregnancy state.

In menopause, TDLUs atrophy, but large and intermediate-sized ducts persist (Fig. 25-1D). Fat predominates over fibrous tissue, but the latter typically cuffs the remaining ducts. Fat increases as a percentage of total breast mass as the woman ages.

Outside of the TDLU, nonspecialized collagenous connective tissue and fat make up the bulk of the breast tissue. Intralobular stroma is more cellular than is interlobular stroma. Mucopolysaccharides in extracellular matrix are also more abundant, and a few lymphocytes, plasma cells, mast cells and macrophages are present.

The breast is very vascular and contains a complex lymphatic network, draining mainly into axillary lymph nodes, with a minority communicating with internal mammary nodes.

DEVELOPMENTAL ABNORMALITIES

Complete bilateral or unilateral absence of breast development occurs rarely, but hypoplasia is more common. Minor asymmetry between breasts occurs frequently. Less often, breasts may be markedly different in size owing to hypoplasia of one breast or unusual enlargement of the other **(juvenile hypertrophy)**. However, the latter is usually bilateral. Unless there is an underlying hormonal abnormality, juvenile breast hypertrophy regresses spontaneously.

The most common anomaly of breast development is **supernumerary nipples,** or **polythelia,** with or without associated breast tissue **(polymastia),** which results from persistent epidermal thickenings. These mostly occur along the milk line, which extends from the axilla to the groin, but other sites may rarely be involved. Congenitally **inverted nipple** is due to failure of nipple eversion in development, usually unilaterally.

INFLAMMATORY DISEASES OF THE BREAST

Acute Mastitis Is a Common Complication of Breast Feeding

Acute mastitis occurs mostly early in the postpartum period and reflects bacterial infection, usually with *Staphylococcus* or *Streptococcus.* Patients have pain, swelling or redness, often with fever and malaise. Cracks in the skin or lactational stasis predispose to infection. If minor, mastitis usually resolves with antibiotics and continued lactation. If it is severe or untreated, abscesses or systemic infection may occur.

Periductal Mastitis of Lactiferous Ducts Is Painful

The disease is unrelated to lactation, age or history of pregnancy. It presents with a painful subareolar mass and overlying erythema. The large majority of patients are cigarette smokers. Nipple ducts show keratinizing squamous metaplasia. A keratin plug can become trapped and lead to duct rupture. Keratin debris spilling into the stroma then elicits a foreign body, chronic, inflammatory response, which may become secondarily infected. Recurrences are common and can lead to fistulas. Surgical excision is curative.

Granulomatous Mastitis Has Diverse Etiologies

Granulomatous inflammation (Fig. 25-2) of the breast can be caused by mycobacteria, parasites, fungi or foreign material. **Tuberculosis** of the breast is rare in Western countries but

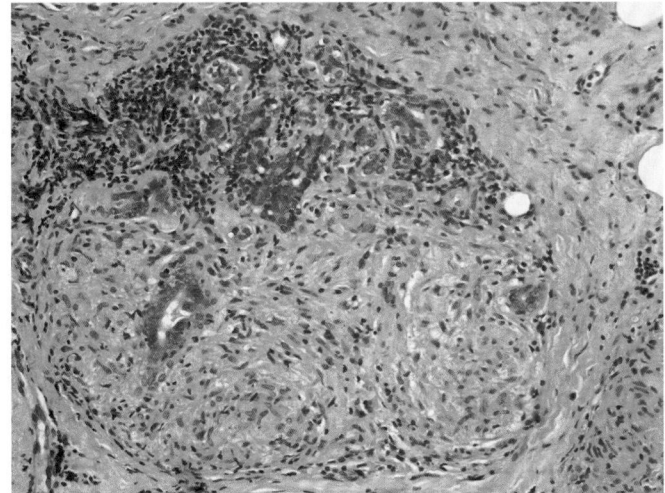

FIGURE 25-2. Breast lobule showing florid granulomatous inflammation characterized by collections of epithelioid histiocytes.

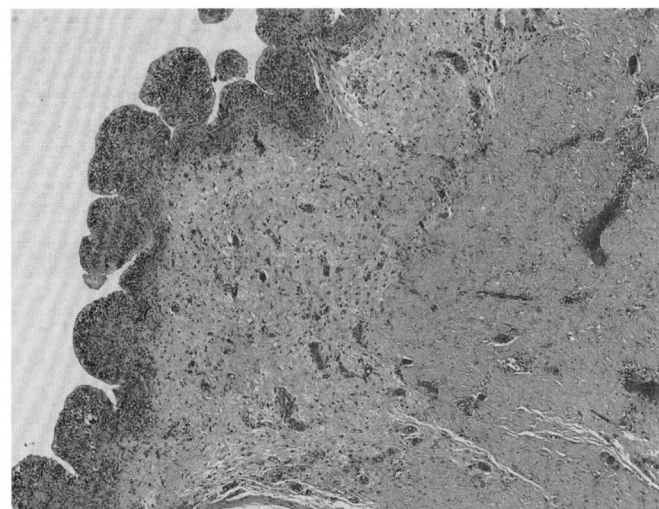

FIGURE 25-3. Capsule around breast implant showing synovial metaplasia with papillary hyperplasia and chronic inflammation.

more common in developing countries, where the infection is endemic. Patients typically present with a mass or sinus that may be mistaken clinically for invasive carcinoma. Other organisms that cause granulomas are discussed in Chapter 9. **Sarcoidosis** rarely involves the breast, but when it does, it presents as single or multiple breast masses.

Silicone gel can leak from breast implants and cause foreign body granulomatous inflammation, with a fibrous capsule. In severe cases, this may cause skin retraction, nipple inversion and formation of hard masses, which may simulate or obscure a malignancy. Draining lymph nodes may enlarge, owing to spread of vacuolated histiocytes containing refractile particles. The use of saline, rather than silicone, in implants has greatly reduced implant-associated granulomatous mastitis.

 PATHOLOGY: On gross sectioning, the breast tissue after rupture of an implant is firm and may be gritty if calcification is present. Fat necrosis and foreign body giant cell reaction, with varying degrees of inflammation and fibrosis, are characteristic. During tissue processing, the silicone is largely lost from the tissue, leaving behind clear spaces. These spaces, and the macrophages, may contain birefringent particles. The capsule is formed by a band of frequently calcified, collagenized fibrous tissue. Some capsules around implants develop synovial metaplasia: a lining that resembles synovium, with or without papillary hyperplasia (Fig. 25-3).

Idiopathic granulomatous mastitis is rare. It typically occurs in women 20–40 years old who have recently been pregnant. It may be bilateral in up to 25% of patients. The granulomas in this setting are centered within lobules, with frequent superimposed acute inflammation and microabscesses (Fig. 25-4).

Sclerosing Lymphocytic Lobulitis Is an Autoimmune Reaction

Sclerosing lymphocytic lobulitis, also called **lymphocytic** or **fibrous mastopathy,** is uncommon. It is often associated with other autoimmune diseases, in particular type 1 diabetes mellitus and Hashimoto thyroiditis. Clinically, most

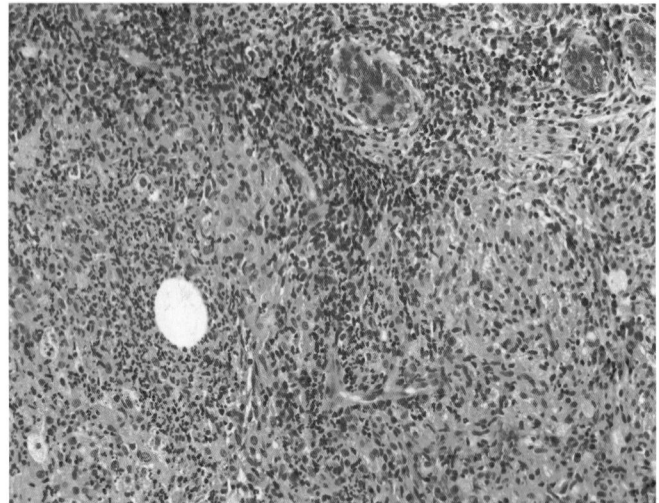

FIGURE 25-4. Granulomatous inflammation centered on a breast lobule with a prominent acute inflammatory cell infiltrate. The histologic appearances are in keeping with a diagnosis of idiopathic granulomatous mastitis.

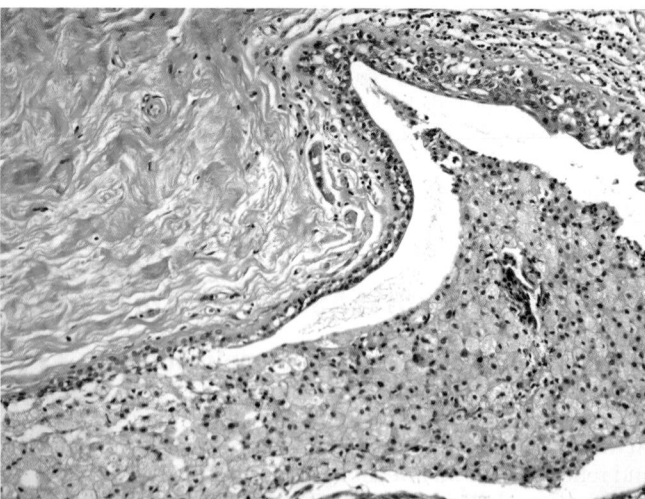

FIGURE 25-6. Duct ectasia. Dilated duct filled with foamy histiocytes. The duct epithelium is focally infiltrated by histiocytes and chronic inflammation of the periductal stroma is present.

patients exhibit a hard mass, which may be tender and sometimes bilateral. Circumscribed aggregates of small lymphocytes surround lobules, ducts and vessels, and lobular atrophy, basement membrane thickening and fibrosis are evident (Fig. 25-5). Interlobular stroma shows dense fibrosis and epithelioid myofibroblasts.

Duct Ectasia May Lead to Duct Rupture

Duct ectasia is common and is characterized by dilation and periductal inflammation, with fibrosis of large and intermediate breast ducts, which contain inspissated material. Peri- or postmenopausal women are more likely to be symptomatic, complaining of a serous or bloody discharge, mass or pain. As disease progresses, duct wall fibrosis may cause the nipple to retract. Episodes of acute inflammation are occasionally complicated by abscess or sinus formation.

Dilated ducts contain amorphous debris and foamy macrophages (Fig. 25-6). The lining epithelium and periductal stroma have inflammatory cells and foamy macrophages. Duct rupture incites a chronic inflammatory response, often with foreign body granulomas. Over time, fibrosis increases, with or without obliteration of ducts.

Fat Necrosis Often Mimics Cancer

Like carcinoma of the breast, fat necrosis often presents as a hard mass, frequently with associated skin tethering. Some patients may give a history of trauma. Necrotic fat cells, acute inflammation, cholesterol clefts and hemorrhage are evident early in the course of fat necrosis. Foamy macrophages and multinucleated giant cells that engulf lipid droplets then gradually accumulate (Fig. 25-7). With time, fibrosis and dystrophic calcification develop.

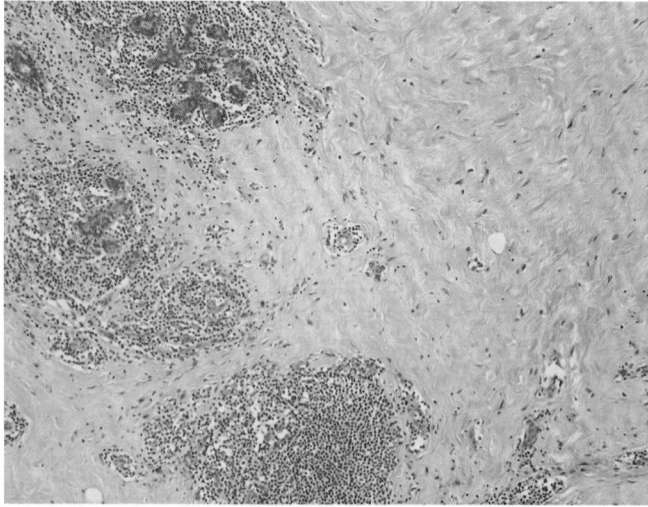

FIGURE 25-5. Prominent periductal and perivascular lymphocytic infiltration in a dense fibrous stroma, characteristic of sclerosing lymphocytic lobulitis.

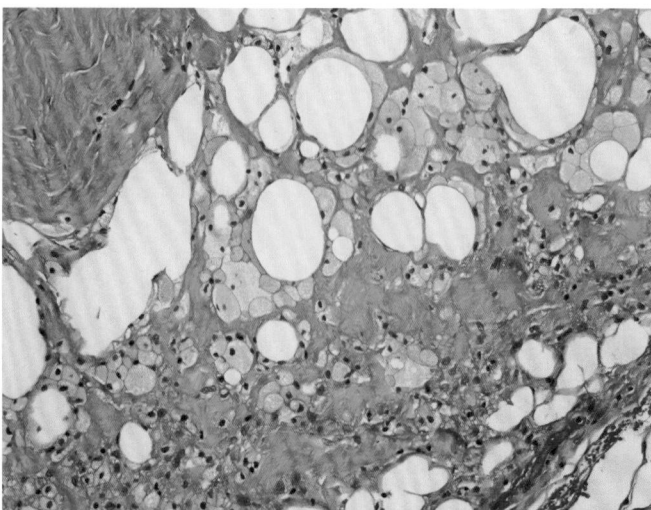

FIGURE 25-7. Fat necrosis. Necrotic fat cells with abundant foamy histiocytes.

BENIGN EPITHELIAL LESIONS

Benign epithelial lesions can be classified based on their risk of subsequent cancer development. Lesions not associated with increased risk are **nonproliferative breast changes** (e.g., fibrocystic change). **Proliferative disease without atypia** entails 1.5–2-fold increased risk of developing carcinoma over 5–15 years and is classified simply as **proliferative breast disease**. **Proliferative lesions with atypia** involve even greater relative risk (4–5-fold). Such patients require close clinical monitoring. Patients at high risk may consider medical treatment options (e.g., estrogen antagonists).

Fibrocystic Change Is an Exaggerated Physiologic Response

Fibrocystic change (FCC) is a nonproliferative change that includes gross and microscopic cysts, apocrine metaplasia, mild epithelial hyperplasia and an increase in fibrous stroma. FCC affects over one third of women 20–50 years old, then declines after menopause. Most women with FCC are asymptomatic, but some present with nodularity and, occasionally, pain. FCC is typically multifocal and bilateral.

 PATHOLOGY: The breast tissue in FCC consists grossly of firm fibrofatty tissue within which are multiple clear cysts or "blue dome" cysts (Fig. 25-8A). The latter contain a dark, thin fluid that imparts a blue color to unopened cysts. Cysts vary from 1 mm to several centimeters and may lack epithelial lining or be lined by attenuated epithelium and myoepithelium (Fig. 25-8C). Their lining may include apocrine-type cells, which are large and have abundant, granular, eosinophilic cytoplasm and a basally located nucleus (Fig. 25-8D). Surrounding stroma is often sclerotic. Inflammation may be due to cyst rupture. Mild "usual" ductal hyperplasia (see below) is frequent, with no

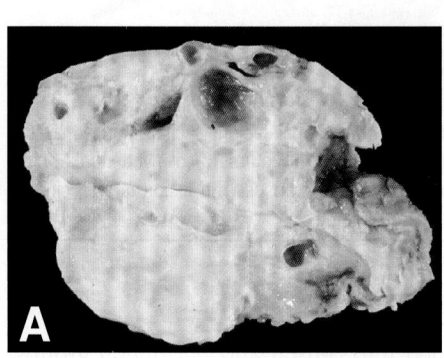

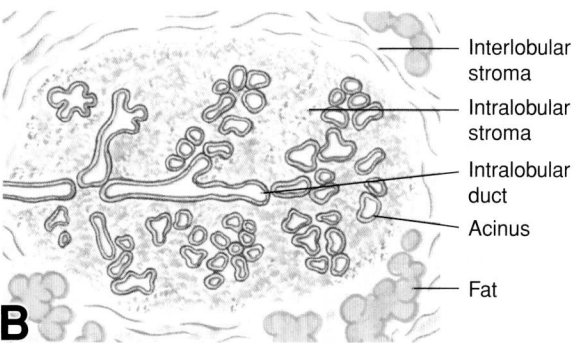

Interlobular stroma

Intralobular stroma

Intralobular duct

Acinus

Fat

Terminal duct lobular unit

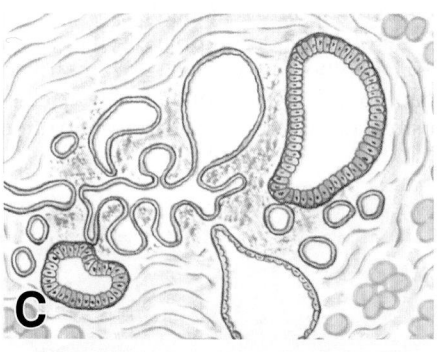

Nonproliferative fibrocystic change

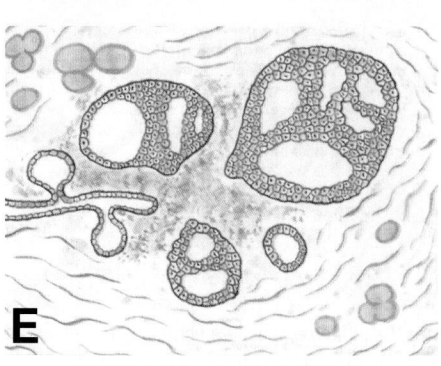

Proliferative breast disease

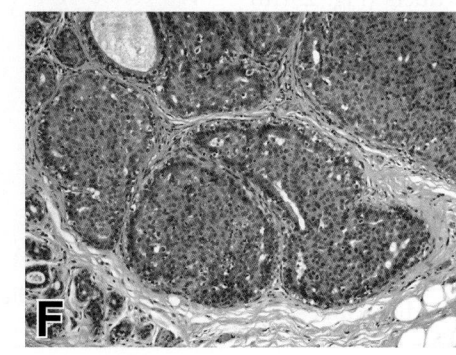

FIGURE 25-8. Fibrocystic change. A. Cysts of various sizes are dispersed in dense, fibrous connective tissue. Some of the cysts are large and contain old blood-tinged proteinaceous debris. **B. Normal terminal duct lobular unit. C. Nonproliferative fibrocystic change** combines cystic dilation of the terminal ducts with varying degrees of apocrine metaplasia of the epithelium and increased fibrous stroma. **D. Apocrine metaplasia.** Epithelial cells have apocrine features with eosinophilic cytoplasm. **E. Proliferative breast disease.** Terminal duct dilation and intraductal epithelial hyperplasia are present. **F. Florid epithelial hyperplasia of usual type.** The epithelium within the ducts proliferates and almost fills the duct lumen, with residual "secondary" spaces remaining as peripheral slit-like spaces. Cytoplasmic borders are indistinct and the nuclei appear round to oval and frequently overlap, resulting in a streaming pattern.

more than 3–4 cell layers above the basement membrane (Fig. 25-8C). Acini are increased in number and size, lined by columnar cells and frequently contain calcifications.

Proliferative Breast Disease Variably Increases Risk of Cancer

Usual Epithelial Hyperplasia

Usual epithelial hyperplasia within ducts or lobules is typified by increased cellularity, relative to the basement membrane (Fig. 25-8E, F). There may be more than 4 cell layers, often bridging across duct lumens. Nuclei may be so oriented as to present a streaming pattern. Secondary spaces are slit-like, irregular and typically peripheral in location. Both luminal and basal epithelial cells proliferate, the latter expressing high–molecular-weight ("basal") cytokeratins. Usual epithelial hyperplasia does not show consistent genetic alterations, and the characteristic alterations seen in atypical duct hyperplasia and low-grade ductal carcinoma in situ are absent (see below).

Sclerosing Adenosis

In sclerosing adenosis (SA), the TDLU shows disordered epithelial, myoepithelial and stromal components. Lesions vary from microscopic foci to masses that may be palpable and that may be mistaken clinically and radiologically for carcinoma. SA often calcifies and may be targeted for core biopsies. It is not a precursor of invasive cancer but is grouped with proliferative lesions without atypia for risk assessment purposes.

 PATHOLOGY: SA lesions show disorderly proliferation of ducts, tubules and intralobular stromal cells, resulting in distortion and expansion of lobules and obliterating duct spaces (Fig. 25-9). A lobulocentric architecture is maintained. In cases that are difficult to distinguish from invasive carcinoma, immunohistochemistry can highlight the preservation of myoepithelial cells around distorted ducts.

Radial Scar/Complex Sclerosing Lesion

Radial scar is a benign sclerosing lesion with a central fibroelastotic scar and peripheral radiating ducts and lobules. If over 1 cm, they are called complex sclerosing lesions. Larger lesions may be seen mammographically as stellate or spiculated structures with radiolucent central areas that may be difficult to distinguish from cancer.

 PATHOLOGY: Radial scars are characterized by central fibroelastotic cores, within which are found entrapped and distorted small ducts (Fig. 25-10). At the edges, radiating ducts and lobules show diverse benign alterations. Occasionally, atypical hyperplasia or carcinoma may be present.

 CLINICAL FEATURES: Radial scars carry a twofold increase in breast cancer risk, which is even greater in women with coexisting proliferative disease, with and without atypia. This increased risk pertains to both ipsilateral and contralateral breasts, indicating that radial scars are markers of generally increased susceptibility to breast cancer. Since cancer can occur in radial scars, surgical excision is recommended.

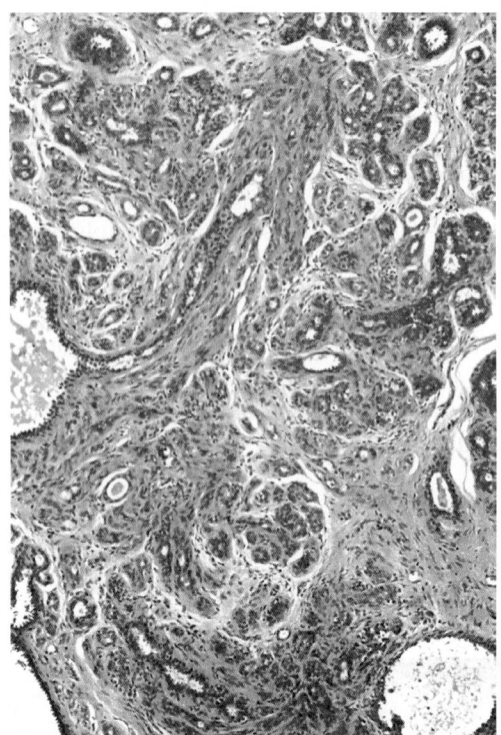

FIGURE 25-9. Sclerosing adenosis. This lesion is characterized by the proliferation of small, abortive, duct-like structures, and myoepithelial cells expand and distort the lobule in which it arises. The lesion is well circumscribed, in contrast to a cancerous lesion.

Intraductal Papilloma

Papillomas are divided into central and peripheral groups. Central papillomas arise in large lactiferous ducts and tend to be solitary. Peripheral papillomas originate in terminal duct lobular units and are usually multiple. Patients may present with a mass lesion or an often bloody nipple discharge. On mammography, central papillomas are well-circumscribed masses; peripheral papillomas are identified often as clustered calcifications or small nodular masses. Ultrasound often

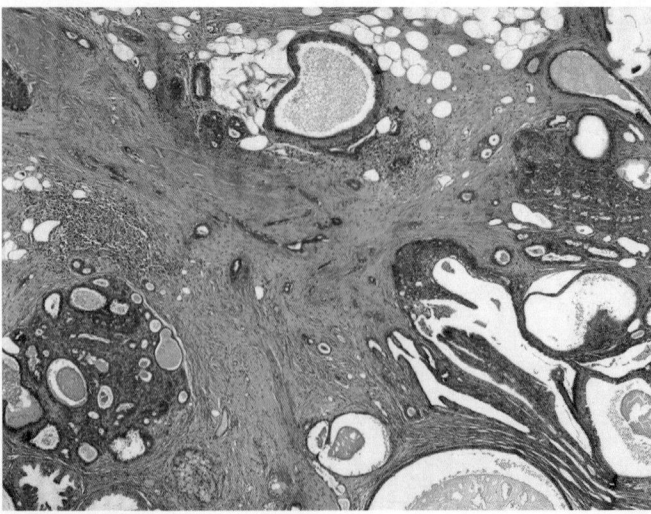

FIGURE 25-10. Radial scar. Angulated glands in a fibroelastotic center are surrounded by a radial distribution of benign ducts and apocrine cysts.

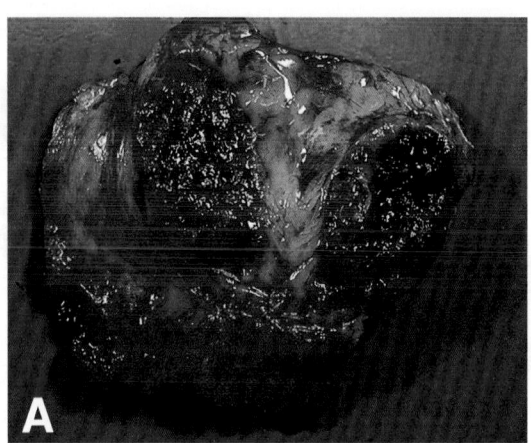
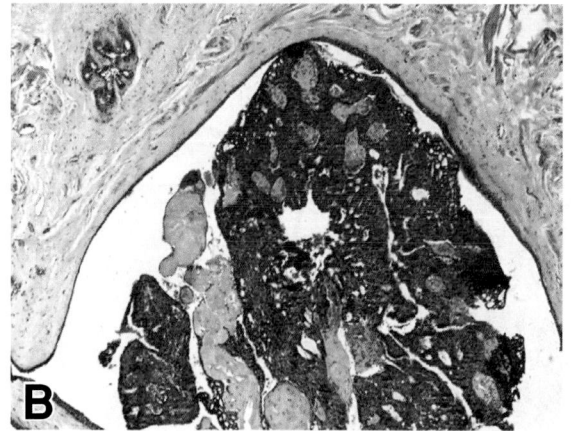

FIGURE 25-11. Intraductal papilloma. A. A large papillary mass is seen within dilated ducts. **B.** A photomicrograph shows a benign papillary growth in a subareolar duct.

shows larger lesions as well-defined hypoechoic masses, with solid and cystic components, near dilated ducts.

 PATHOLOGY: Papillomas vary from microscopic foci to masses several centimeters across (Fig. 25-11A). Larger lesions frequently show foci of hemorrhage or necrosis. Dilated duct spaces contain multiple branching papillae with fibrovascular cores. These are lined by a layer of myoepithelium, on which one or more layers of epithelium lie (Fig. 25-11B). Florid epithelial hyperplasia of usual type or atypical ductal hyperplasia may be present (Fig. 25-12). Papillomas often contain areas of apocrine change and, less often, squamous metaplasia. Sclerosis of papillae or duct walls is variable, but it may be marked and can entrap and distort benign epithelium at the periphery, mimicking an invasive process.

CLINICAL FEATURES: Peripheral papillomas are more often associated with concurrent or subsequent breast cancer. The relative risk of a malignancy

is 2-fold in patients with central papillomas and 3-fold if papillomas are peripheral. If there is atypia within these lesions, relative risks are 5- and 7-fold, respectively. If a papilloma is found on core biopsy, excision is generally recommended because atypia or carcinoma may coexist in areas not sampled in the biopsy.

Proliferative Disease with Atypia Is Composed of a Heterogeneous Group of Breast Lesions

Atypical Ductal Hyperplasia

PATHOLOGY: Atypical ductal hyperplasia (ADH) is an intraductal epithelial proliferation with a dual population of low-grade neoplastic epithelial cells and benign cells. The benign population may comprise normal lining cells or proliferating cells showing epithelial hyperplasia of usual type. The neoplastic population consists of monomorphic small cells that are evenly spaced, with well-defined cytoplasmic borders and round, hyperchromatic, uniform nuclei. These form architecturally complex structures, such as micropapillae, rigid bridges, bars, solid sheets or cribriform arrays (Fig. 25-13). If the duct is completely filled by neoplastic cells, and if two duct spaces extending at least 2 mm are involved, the lesion is considered low-grade ductal carcinoma in situ (DCIS). If these criteria are not met, most pathologists would designate the lesion ADH.

MOLECULAR PATHOGENESIS: One third to 1/2 of ADH lesions show no genetic changes. The others, however, show alterations that overlap with low-grade DCIS. Common patterns of genetic alterations in proliferative breast lesions are summarized in Table 25-1.

In patients with ADH, the relative risk of subsequent breast cancer is increased 4–5-fold compared to age-matched controls. Cancers occur in ipsilateral and contralateral breasts equally frequently. This raises the important question as to the extent to which these lesions are precursors of invasive malignancies, or whether they may on occasion represent nonprogressing lesions that are products of similar processes that also produce invasive cancers. Hormonal therapy may be used to reduce the risk of developing breast cancer.

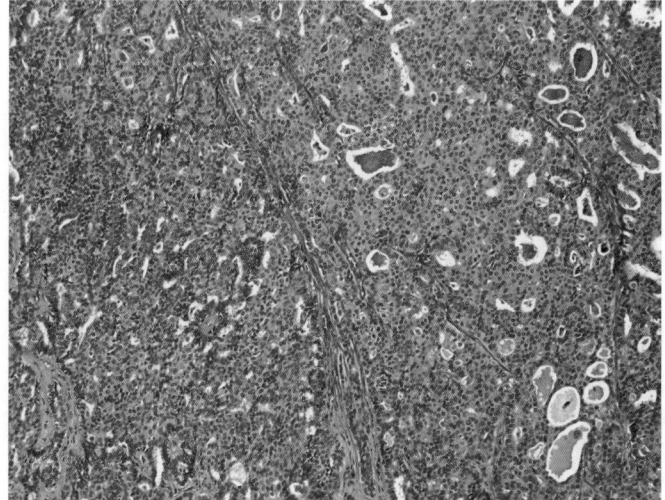

FIGURE 25-12. Intraductal papilloma with focus (on right of image) showing low-grade cytologic atypia and architectural atypia in keeping with atypical ductal hyperplasia occurring within a papilloma (atypical papilloma).

THE BREAST

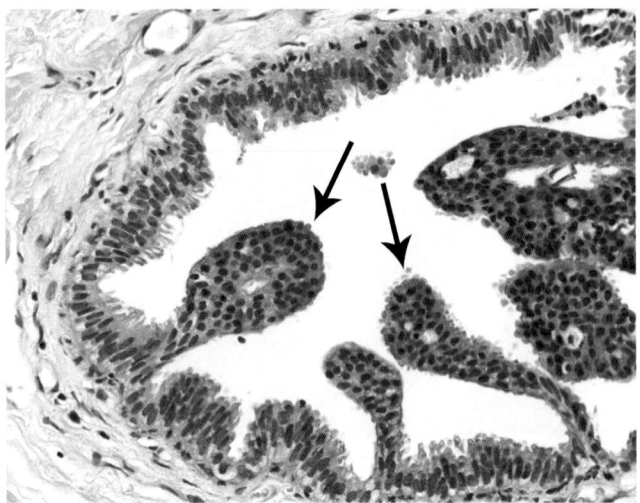

FIGURE 25-13. Atypical ductal hyperplasia (ADH). Micropapillae (*arrows*) project into the duct lumen and consist of cells with an increased nuclear-to-cytoplasmic ratio and nuclear hyperchromasia. Residual benign columnar cells are seen lining the duct.

Atypical Lobular Hyperplasia

Atypical lobular hyperplasia (ALH) is usually an incidental finding in a biopsy or excision performed for something else. In ALH, cells are indistinguishable from those seen in lobular carcinoma in situ (LCIS; see below), but the degree of involvement of the TDLU is less in ALH than in LCIS; fewer acini are involved and less than 50% within the lobule are distended (Fig. 25-14A). As in LCIS, cells of ALH can spread in a pagetoid fashion to involve ducts (Fig. 25-14B). ALH morphology and associated risk of subsequent breast cancer are discussed below.

Flat Epithelial Atypia

Flat epithelial atypia (FEA) describes a lesion of TDLUs in which acini are variably dilated, lined by one or several layers

FIGURE 25-15. Flat epithelial atypia. The terminal duct lobular unit (TDLU) is enlarged as a result of dilatation of the lobular acini. These are lined by one to two layers of epithelial cells showing low-grade cytologic atypia. Nuclei appear round with variably conspicuous nucleoli, and loss of their basal location (loss of polarity) is seen. Architectural complexity is not a feature.

of epithelial cells, with low-grade cytologic atypia. It presents as round, nonbranching mammographic microcalcifications.

PATHOLOGY: Variably distended acini lined by cuboidal to columnar epithelial cells distend the TDLU (Fig. 25-15). Cells show uniform round nuclei and a slight increase in the nuclear-to-cytoplasmic ratio. Cell polarity is lost, and nucleoli are variably prominent. Architectural complexity, such as micropapillae, bridges, bars or cribriform structures, is absent.

FEA may coexist with ADH, DCIS, ALH/LCIS and invasive carcinoma, particularly tubular carcinoma. The cells of FEA are similar in morphology to coexisting in situ and invasive carcinoma. Furthermore, loss of heterozygosity (LOH) is present in most cases, in patterns that are shared with

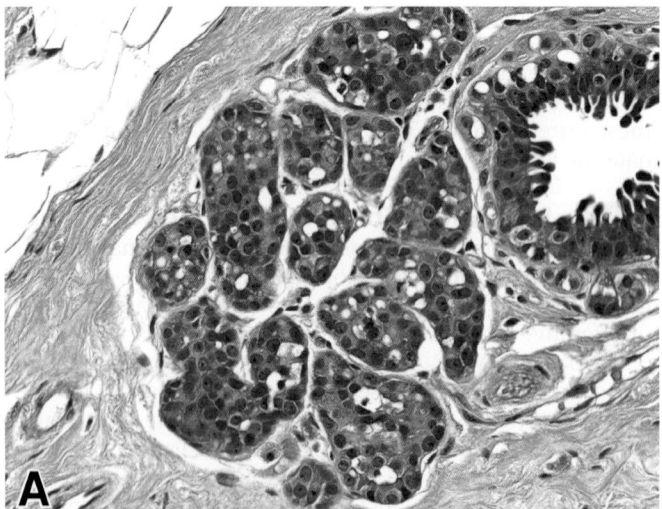

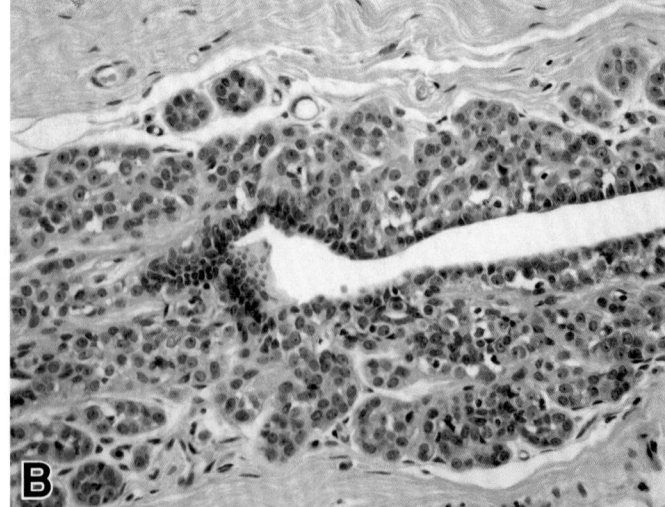

FIGURE 25-14. A. Atypical lobular hyperplasia (ALH). There is minimal distension of the lobular acini by a uniform population of cells with intracytoplasmic lumina and round nuclei containing small nucleoli. **B. Pagetoid spread** of lobular neoplastic cells into the terminal duct. Here the atypical cells lie beneath an attenuated surface layer of luminal epithelial cells.

TABLE 25-1

COMMON GENETIC ALTERATIONS ASSOCIATED WITH BREAST LESIONS

Lesion Type	Other	Alteration
ADH	Loss	16q
	Gain	17p
Phyllodes tumors	Gain	1q
	Loss	13
Familial adenomatous polyposis	Mutation	*APC*, β-catenin
	Loss	5q
Familial breast cancer, high penetrance		*BRCA1, BRCA2*
	Li-Fraumeni	*TP53*
	Cowden	*PTEN*
	Hereditary diffuse gastric cancer	*CDH1*
	Peutz-Jeghers	*STK11*
Familial breast cancer, low penetrance	Ataxia telangiectasia	*ATM*
	Li-Fraumeni variant	*CHEK2*
Low-grade DCIS	Gain	1q
	Loss	16q
High-grade DCIS	Gain	17q, 8q, 5p
	Loss	11q, 14q, 8p, 13q
	Amplifications	17, 6, 8, 11
Encapsulated papillary carcinoma		LOH, 16q, 1q
Lobular neoplasia	Gain	1q, 6q
	Loss	16p, 16q (especially 16q22.1), 17p, 22q
Pleomorphic LCIS	Gains and losses	Same as lobular neoplasia
	Amplification	8q24, 17q12
	LOH	16q22.1, p53, *HER2, BRCA1*
Invasive ductal NST, low grade	Loss	16q
	Gain	1q, 16p
Invasive ductal NST, high grade		Heterogeneous and aneuploid
Invasive lobular carcinoma	Loss	16q
	Gain	1q, 16p
Invasive lobular carcinoma, high grade		Same as invasive lobular carcinoma
	Amplification	8q24, 17q12, 20q13
Tubular carcinoma	Loss	16q (8p, 3p, 11q)
	Gain	1q, 16p
Medullary carcinoma	Mutations (acquired)	*TP53, BRCA1*
	Epigenetic inactivation	*BRCA1*
Micropapillary	Gain	8q, 17q, 20q
	Loss	6q, 13q
Metaplastic carcinoma	Mutations	*TP53*
Male breast cancer	Inherited mutations	*BRCA2*
	Acquired mutations	*TP53, PTEN, CHEK2*

ADH = atypical ductal hyperplasia; DCIS = ductal carcinoma in situ; LCIS = lobular carcinoma in situ; LOH = loss of heterozygosity; NST = no specific type.

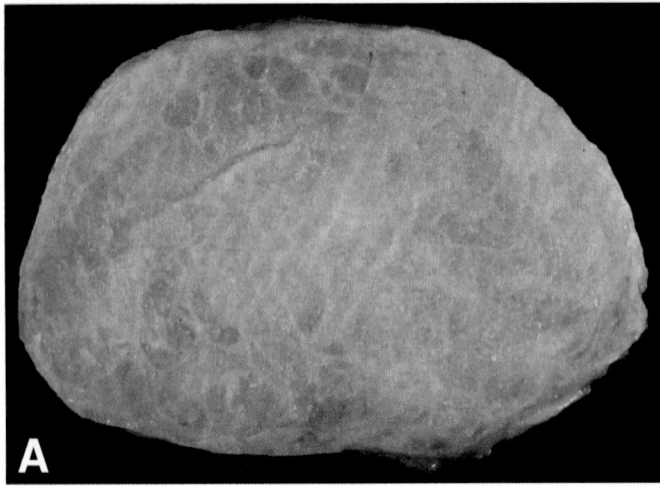
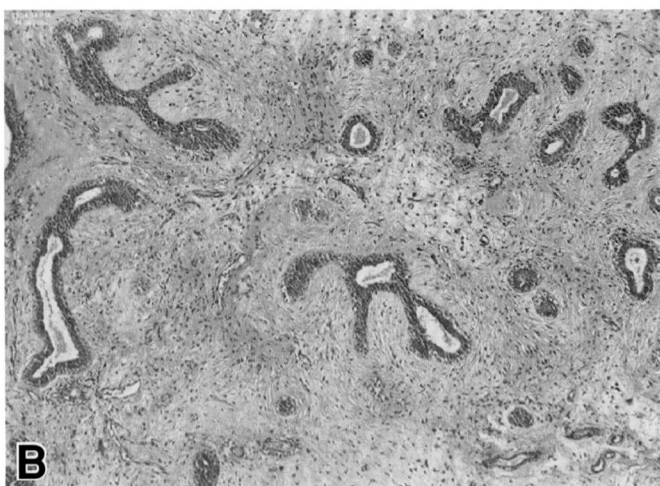

FIGURE 25-16. Fibroadenoma. A. Surgical specimen. This well-circumscribed tumor was easily enucleated from the surrounding tissue. The cut surface is characteristically glistening tannish-white and has a septate appearance. **B.** Microscopic section. Elongated epithelial duct structures are situated within a loose, myxoid stroma.

coexistent DCIS or invasive carcinoma. The characteristic 16q loss seen in low-grade DCIS and invasive carcinoma is the most frequently detected recurrent change in FEA.

Limited clinical outcome data in patients with FEA suggest that local recurrence and progression to invasive carcinoma are uncommon.

FIBROEPITHELIAL LESIONS

These arise from intralobular stroma and contain both stromal and epithelial elements.

Fibroadenomas Have Benign Epithelium and Stroma

Fibroadenomas are common, mobile, painless, breast lumps that most often affect 20- to 35-year-old women. Clinically silent lesions are particularly common and are usually identified by mammography. These are typically well-defined solitary masses, which may be calcified. However, they can be multiple and bilateral, most often in Afro-Caribbean women.

 PATHOLOGY: Fibroadenomas are round or ovoid and rubbery (Fig. 25-16A) and are sharply demarcated from surrounding breast tissue. Most are less than 3 cm, but they can rarely be much larger (up to 20 cm) in young women or adolescents. Fibroadenomas have two components: stroma and epithelium (Fig. 25-16B). The stroma typically contains spindle cells and shows variable, but usually low, cellularity. In younger women, the stroma is often myxoid. With age, stroma may be denser and can calcify. The epithelial component is formed from normal TDLU constituents; epithelial and myoepithelial layers are preserved. The relationship of the stroma to the epithelium is typically uniform throughout. Two patterns are known. In the **intracanalicular** pattern, stromal growth compresses ducts into curvilinear slits. The **pericanalicular** pattern is characterized by ducts that maintain a tubular configuration, surrounded by stromal proliferation. These growth patterns have no prognostic import.

The epithelial component of a fibroadenoma often shows hyperplasia, especially in young women. Rarely, atypical ductal hyperplasia, lobular neoplasia or DCIS can occur within fibroadenomas. Complex fibroadenomas show benign changes, including epithelial calcifications, sclerosing adenosis (Fig. 25-17), papillary apocrine change or cysts greater than 3 mm.

Variants of fibroadenoma include **tubular adenoma,** in which small tubular structures are surrounded by a loosely cellular vascularized stroma (Fig. 25-18), and **juvenile fibroadenoma,** which are most common in adolescents (Fig. 25-19). These grow rapidly and may reach 20 cm, causing clinical concern. Juvenile fibroadenomas resemble fibroadenomas histologically, but with more cellular stroma.

Fibroadenomas are surgically excised if they are of clinical or radiologic concern. They can recur, but not often. There is no risk of subsequent breast cancer in the vast majority of cases.

Phyllodes Tumor

These tumors make up less than 1% of breast tumors. They have epithelial and stromal components, the latter being neoplastic. The name is derived from the Greek word *phyllos,* meaning "leaf," because they show a leaf-like growth

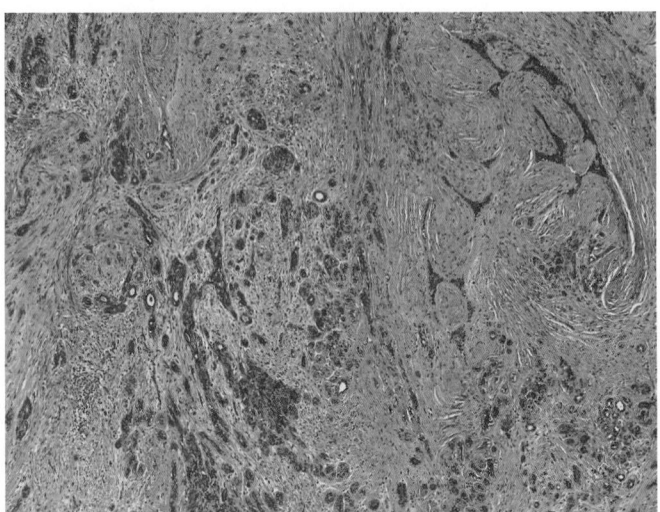

FIGURE 25-17. Fibroadenoma involved by sclerosing adenosis.

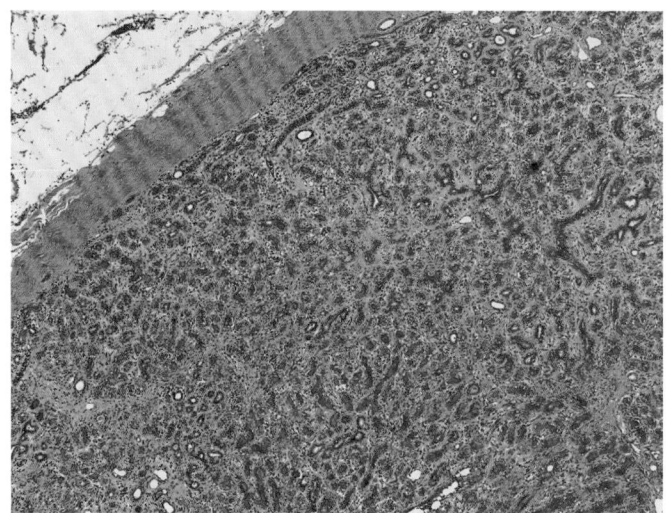

FIGURE 25-18. Tubular adenoma. Well-circumscribed fibroepithelial lesion with closely packed round tubules showing little intervening stroma.

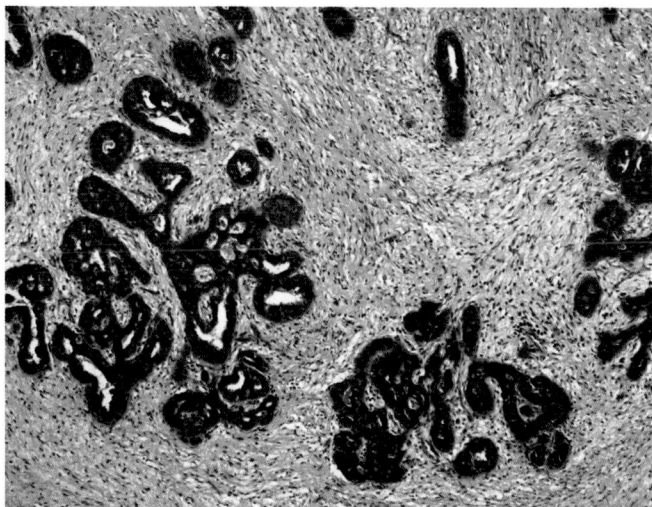

FIGURE 25-19. Juvenile fibroadenoma. The stroma shows hypercellularity, although mitoses and cellular atypia are not features. Epithelial hyperplasia of usual type is present in the glands.

pattern. They can occur at any age but are most common in the 6th decade. Phyllodes tumors present as rapidly growing breast masses and on mammography are well circumscribed or lobulated. Ultrasound may show internal hyperechoic areas in a hypoechoic mass.

PATHOLOGY: Phyllodes tumors vary in size from a few centimeters across to 20 cm. **Benign** phyllodes tumors are sharply circumscribed. Their cut surfaces are firm, glistening and grayish white. Clefts may be prominent. Malignant lesions often show infiltrative margins. On microscopy, fronds of hypercellular stroma lead to formation of leaf-like structures, which project into cystic spaces (Fig. 25-20). These spaces are lined by a dual layer of benign epithelium and myoepithelium. The stroma ranges from benign and hypercellular to frankly sarcomatous. Most phyllodes tumors are benign and have mild or moderately hypercellular stroma with mild cytologic atypia and few mitoses. In **malignant** phyllodes tumors, stroma is very hypercellular, with considerable pleomorphism, abundant

mitoses (>10 per 10 HPFs) and stromal overgrowth. Malignant heterologous elements, such as bone, cartilage or fat, may be present. Those tumors that are not clearly benign or malignant are called **borderline**.

MOLECULAR PATHOGENESIS: The epithelium in phyllodes tumors appears to influence stromal growth. The tumors upregulate transcriptionally active β-catenin and downstream effectors such as cyclin D1 via the Wnt pathway. Altered karyotypes may occur with malignant progression (Table 25-1).

The main risk of benign phyllodes tumors is local recurrence, which happens 20% of the time, rather than metastasis. The best predictor of recurrence is completeness of excision; thus, a rim of normal tissue should be excised with these tumors. Recurrence is more common with malignant lesions. Metastases are rare overall, but up to 25% of high-grade malignant phyllodes tumors may disseminate. *Only stromal components are seen in metastases.* Axillary lymph node metastases are very rare.

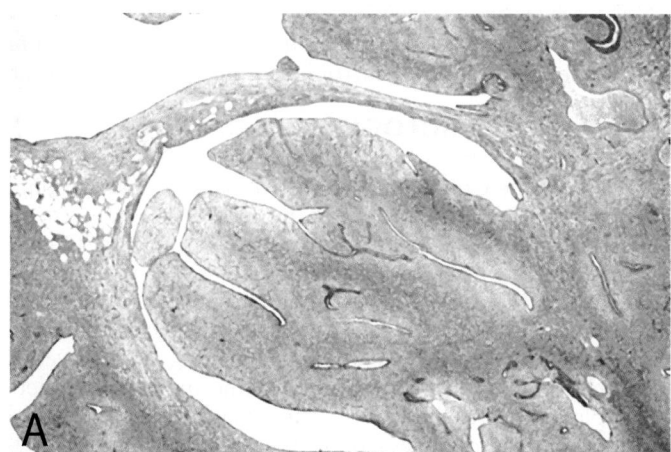

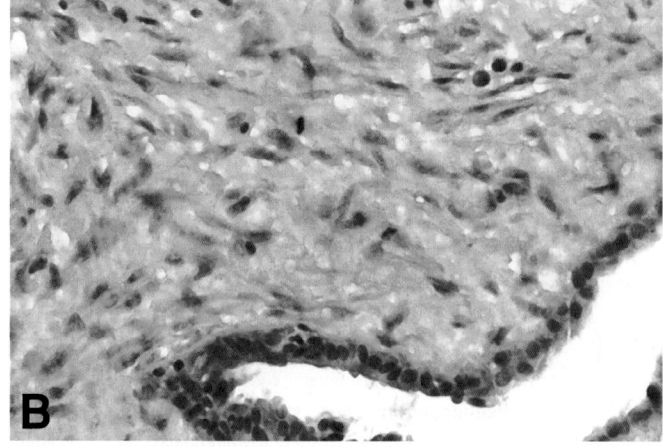

FIGURE 25-20. Phyllodes tumor. A. A polypoid tumor with a leaf-like pattern expands a duct. **B.** The stromal component adjacent to ductal epithelium is similar to a fibroadenoma, but is more cellular. The residual ductal structure is benign.

STROMAL LESIONS

Stromal lesions arise from nonspecialized interlobular stroma. Mesenchymal lesions that occur outside the breast, such as lipomas or vascular tumors, can occur here. Stromal lesions specific to the breast, such as pseudoangiomatous stromal hyperplasia and myofibroblastoma, are also found.

Pseudoangiomatous Stromal Hyperplasia Mimics a Vascular Lesion

Pseudoangiomatous stromal hyperplasia (PASH) is a benign process that is usually found incidentally in biopsies done for other reasons. It occasionally presents as a painless, circumscribed mass with a homogeneous cut surface. It commonly occurs in gynecomastia. Most female patients are premenopausal, suggesting that hormonal factors may play a role in PASH development and growth.

 PATHOLOGY: PASH lesions are circumscribed, with homogeneous tan cut surfaces. They vary from 1 to 7 cm. Interanastomosing spaces, which rarely contain red blood cells, are seen in dense collagenous stroma (Fig. 25-21). Myofibroblasts close to these spaces mimic endothelial cells. True vascular channels may occur in the stroma.

Fibromatosis Consists of Fibroblasts and Myofibroblasts

Fibromatosis can be locally aggressive but does not metastasize. The lesions present predominantly as unilateral, painless, firm to hard masses. Most patients are in their 40s, but any age group may be affected. Mammography shows a stellate mass, mimicking carcinoma.

 **MOLECULAR PATHOGENESIS:** Fibromatosis is usually sporadic but is rarely seen in association with familial adenomatous polyposis (FAP)

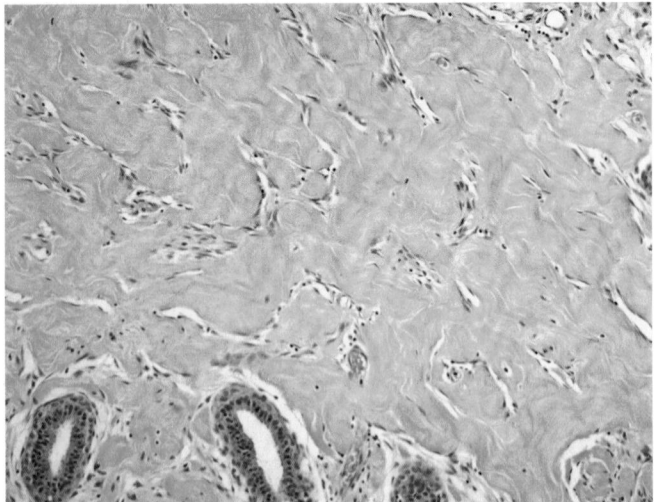

FIGURE 25-21. Pseudoangiomatous stromal hyperplasia. Slit-like spaces within a collagenized stroma are seen. Myofibroblasts are distributed singly at the margins of the spaces, resembling endothelial cells. True capillaries are also evident.

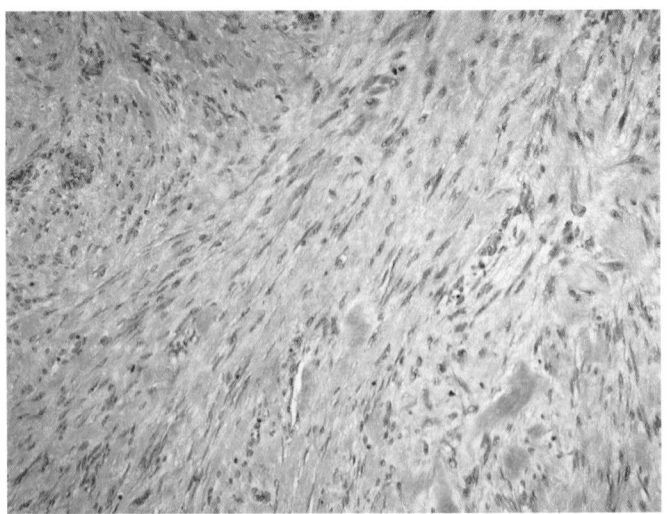

FIGURE 25-22. Fibromatosis. Interlacing bundles of spindle cells, without nuclear atypia, are present with focal bands of collagen.

and Gardner syndrome. FAP is caused by mutations in the adenomatous polyposis coli (*APC*) gene, which negatively regulates nuclear translocation of β-catenin. Sporadic and FAP-associated lesions show genetic alterations in APC or β-catenin, affecting the APC/β-catenin pathway (Table 25-1). Breast fibromatosis may also occur during pregnancy, but hormonal factors are not thought to contribute to the pathogenesis.

 PATHOLOGY: Grossly, fibromatosis is poorly defined and firm, with infiltrative margins. Sizes vary from less than 1 cm to greater than 10 cm. Broad sweeping fascicles and interlacing bundles of bland-appearing spindle or oval cells characterize fibromatosis (Fig. 25-22). Collagen may be prominent. Adjacent normal breast tissue is infiltrated by proliferating spindle cells, and collections of lymphocytes are common at the periphery. There is no cellular atypia, and mitotic figures are rare (<3 per 10 HPFs).

CARCINOMA OF THE BREAST

Breast cancer is the most common malignancy of women in the United States; its mortality is second only to lung cancer.

 **EPIDEMIOLOGY:** The incidence of breast cancer has slowly increased over the past 50 years. Women in the United States have a 1 in 9 risk of developing breast cancer; however, as this represents lifetime risk, it overestimates actual risk for an individual woman. One in 5 women with breast cancer will die from it. Age-specific incidence rates increase dramatically after age 40. In industrialized countries with high rates of breast cancer, incidence continues to increase with age, finally plateauing at 75–80 years. In some populations, including Hispanic and black women, that plateau is reached at a younger age. Breast cancer is uncommon before the age of 35 in all populations. The incidence of estrogen receptor (ER)–negative cancers increases rapidly until age 50, after which it flattens or decreases. By contrast, ER-positive breast cancer continues to rise after that

age. Thus, peak ages of onset for ER-negative and ER-positive breast cancers are 50 and 70, respectively.

Breast cancer occurs 4–5 times more commonly in Western industrialized countries than in the developing world. Risks in daughters and granddaughters of women who migrated from countries of low incidence to Western countries increase with successive generations.

Widespread use of screening mammography in the 1980s led to a sharp increase in the proportion of diagnoses of noninvasive breast lesions (i.e., DCIS). The frequency of small invasive cancers has also increased. However, although widespread screening mammography greatly increased detection of early breast cancers, it has not appreciably decreased the incidence of late-stage breast cancers. Overall mortality has declined from 30% to 20%, and stage-specific mortality has also improved. Improved therapies have contributed greatly to the decline in breast cancer mortality.

 **ETIOLOGIC FACTORS:** Multiple risk factors for breast cancer have been identified, some of which cannot be modified and some of which are amenable to change (Table 25-2). Women can be stratified by level of breast cancer risk. Those who carry a germline *BRCA* mutation (see below) or who have a history of chest radiation are considered high risk; women who have had multiple family members with breast cancer or who have multiple risk factors are at moderate risk.

Nonmodifiable risk factors include age, race (greatest in non-Hispanic white population), family history, genetic factors (germline mutations in *BRCA1* or *BRCA2*), breast density and early age at menarche. Modifiable risk factors are late age at first live birth, diet, high body mass index, alcohol consumption and use of exogenous hormones.

SPORADIC BREAST CANCER: Only about 25% of sporadic breast cancers have identifiable risk factors. Factors affecting the hormonal milieu modify breast cancer risk.

■ *The majority of breast cancers are stimulated by estrogen.* Cumulative lifetime exposure to estrogen determines the level of this risk. As such, early menarche (younger than 11 years), late menopause and older age at first term pregnancy increase risk. Pregnancy before age 20 is protective; nulliparity and deferring childbearing until after 35 years of age are associated with a two- to threefold increased relative risk. Longer lactation reduces risk of breast cancer. Oophorectomy before age of 35, but not afterward, dramatically lowers risk of breast cancer. Antiestrogens, including tamoxifen and aromatase inhibitors, decrease the development of ER-positive breast cancer. Oral contraceptives do not increase breast cancer risk, although hormone replacement therapy (HRT) increases risk slightly, 1.2–1.7 times.

■ **Radiation** increases risk of breast cancer, as documented in survivors of the atomic bomb and in women who received irradiation for Hodgkin lymphoma. Irradiation earlier in life (i.e., in childhood or adolescence) poses the greatest risk; exposure after the age of 40 years has not been shown to increase incidence.

■ The influence of **dietary fat** on breast cancer risk has been extensively studied, and there are limited data to suggest that total fat may increase risk of breast cancer after menopause. However, the risk, if existent, is likely to be small. The effect is postulated to occur through modifying levels of circulating estrogens. Prospective studies of the effects of carbohydrates have not shown consistent associations with breast cancer risk.

■ **Alcohol consumption** consistently predicts higher breast cancer rates. Results from the Nurses' Health Study showed that even low levels of alcohol consumption (3–6 drinks per week) were associated with a minute increase in breast cancer risk (relative risk 1.15). The most relevant measure was cumulative average alcohol consumption over long periods of time, and both drinking earlier and later in adult life were independently associated with breast cancer risk. An association with binge drinking was also found.

■ Postmenopausal women who are **overweight** or **obese** are at greater risk for breast cancer. Central adiposity has been positively associated with risk. Interestingly, obesity appears to have an opposite effect on breast cancer risk among premenopausal women.

■ **Smoking.** Active smoking, particularly if begun at an early age and continuing for a long time, confers increased risk for development of breast cancer. The magnitude of that increased risk is approximately 20%. This risk is strongly associated with a polymorphism at the *NAT2* gene site (N-acetyltransferase 2). One phenotype determined by this locus (slow acetylator) is associated with greater risk of smoking-related breast cancer. Risk of breast cancer associated with environmental smoking is less well established, but some agencies have concluded that younger, mainly premenopausal, nonsmoking women with significant exposure for extended times may have increased risk of breast cancer.

■ Mammographic breast density reflects the proportions of stroma and epithelium rather than fat in breasts. Patients with **denser breasts** (i.e., ≥75% density) have a four- to fivefold greater risk of breast cancer. Density is influenced by age, parity, body mass index and menopausal status, although genetic factors may also play a role.

■ Higher levels of **physical activity** are associated with a reduction in breast cancer risk, with most studies showing evidence of a dose-response relationship. The benefit of activity is independent of race or ethnicity.

TABLE 25-2	
RISK FACTORS FOR BREAST CANCER DEVELOPMENT	
Not Modifiable	**Modifiable**
Age	Body mass index
BRCA germline mutations	Diet
Family history	Alcohol
Chest radiation	Exogenous estrogen
Race/ethnicity	Exercise
Height	Smoking
Age at menarche	Reproductive history
Age at menopause	Age at first full-term delivery
Breast density	Lactation
Atypia on prior breast biopsy	

- Prior breast biopsies showing **atypical hyperplasia** or **nonatypical proliferative breast disease** increase relative risk of 4 to 5 times and 1.5 to 2 times, respectively (see above). Women with a previous breast cancer have a 10-fold increased risk of developing a second primary tumor in the ipsilateral or contralateral breast. Hormonal treatment with antiestrogens decreases this risk.

MOLECULAR PATHOGENESIS:

FAMILIAL BREAST CANCER: The strongest association with increased risk for breast cancer is a family history of breast cancer at a young age in first-degree relatives. The risk is greater if the relative was affected at a young age or had bilateral breast cancer. Familial disease accounts for 10% of breast cancers. Two high-risk breast cancer susceptibility genes, *BRCA1* and *BRCA2*, account for 20%–50% of familial tumors. Some inherited breast cancer susceptibility is part of more generalized familial cancer susceptibility syndromes (Table 25-1). Common inherited polymorphisms have been identified through genome-wide association studies, but the 20 common low-risk alleles identified thus far account for less than 5% of familial risk.

BRCA1 and *BRCA2* are tumor suppressor genes that display an autosomal dominant pattern of inheritance with variable penetrance. *BRCA1*, on chromosome 17q21, is involved in DNA repair, transcriptional regulation, chromatin remodeling and protein ubiquitination. Germline mutations in *BRCA1* confer a lifetime breast cancer risk of between 37% and 85% by age 70 years, with over half of the cancers occurring before age 50. In women older than 70 years, *BRCA1* germline mutations account for less than 2% of cancers; however, 30% of cancers in women under 45 years of age occur in mutation carriers. Carriers are also at significantly increased risk of other cancers, most notably ovarian cancer, with a lifetime risk of 15%–40%. Incidence of cancers of the cervix, endometrium, fallopian tube and stomach is elevated, and prostate cancer is more common in male carriers. About 0.1% of the population has *BRCA1* germline mutations, but rates are higher in Ashkenazi Jews and French Canadians. Breast cancers that develop in patients with germline mutations are typically high-grade, ductal carcinomas, of no special type; however, they show many of the features present in medullary-like cancers, with pushing margins, prominent inflammatory responses, absent tubule formation, high mitotic counts and significant nuclear pleomorphism (Fig. 25-23). In *BRCA1* carriers, the majority of cancers are negative for ER, progesterone receptor (PR) and human epidermal growth factor receptor 2 (HER2), and p53 mutations are more common. Young age at onset is typical.

Germline mutations in *BRCA2*, located on chromosome 13q12, are associated with a 30%–40% lifetime risk of developing breast cancer and an increased risk of ovarian cancer. Moreover, there is an increased incidence of uveal tract and skin melanomas and cancers of the pancreas and biliary tract. Male carriers of *BRCA2* mutations are also at risk for breast and prostatic cancers. Women mostly develop high-grade invasive ductal tumors of no special type. Unlike *BRCA1*-associated cancers, *BRCA2*-related cancers are more commonly ER and PR than are BRCA1 cancers. HER2 gene amplification is rare.

MAMMARY STEM CELLS: Self-renewal of mammary stem cells involves a diverse network of regulatory pathways including Notch, Hedgehog, Wnt/β-catenin, epidermal

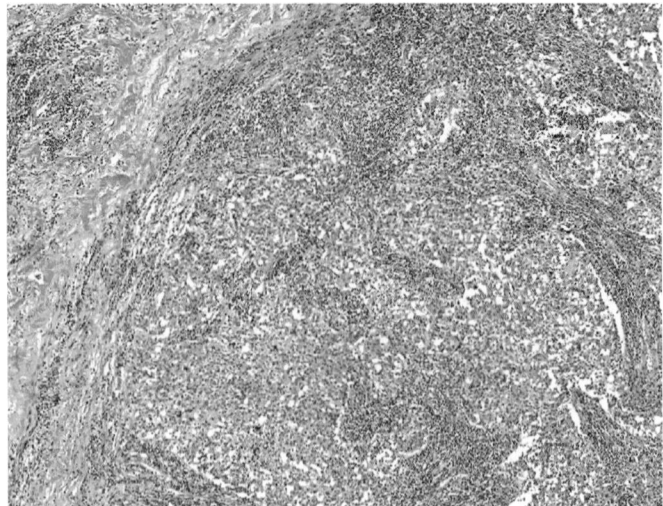

FIGURE 25-23. *BRCA1*-associated breast cancer. High-grade invasive ductal carcinoma, no special type, characterized by pushing margins and a prominent lymphocytic infiltrate.

growth factor receptor (EGFR), transforming growth factor-β (TGF-β), integrins and ER/PR, among others. Current anticancer therapies mostly fail to eradicate stem cell clones and instead favor expansion of the stem cell pool or select for resistant clones. Eradicating these cells may greatly influence breast cancer survival.

Carcinoma In Situ May Be a Non-obligate Precursor of Invasive Cancer

Carcinoma of the breast may be **in situ** (confined by the gland's basement membrane) or **invasive,** in which the malignant cells have infiltrated through the basement membrane into adjacent breast stroma. Further subclassification is based on morphology, immunohistochemistry and molecular profiling. Of women with biopsy-proven DCIS who received no further therapy, 20%–30% subsequently developed invasive cancer.

Ductal Carcinoma In Situ

DCIS identifies a heterogeneous group of lesions that vary in their architectural and cytologic features, as well as in their natural history. These abnormalities are considered nonobligate precursors of invasive carcinoma, the chance of progressing to invasion varying with the histologic subtype, grade and extent. The incidence of DCIS has soared with the advent of widespread screening mammography in the mid-1980s. It once represented about 5% of breast cancers beforehand, and now accounts for 25% of breast cancers in screened populations. Because this increased detection of DCIS has not been associated with decreased incidence of advanced breast cancers, the link between the lesions categorized as DCIS and invasive breast cancer is unclear.

MOLECULAR PATHOGENESIS: In some cases, DCIS may be a precursor of invasive breast carcinoma. Thus, DCIS is often seen together with invasive carcinomas. In those cases, noninvasive tumors and

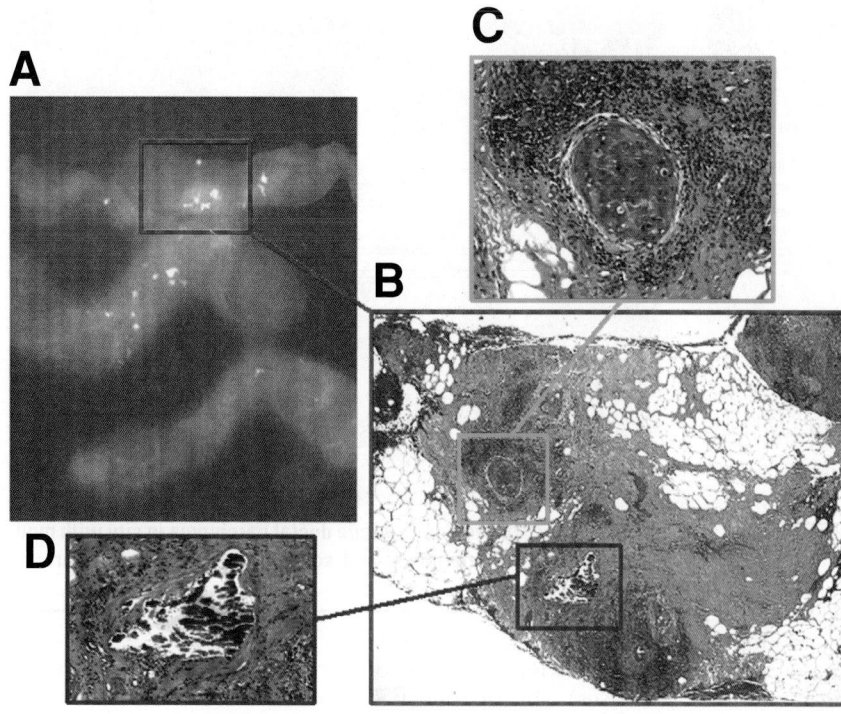

FIGURE 25-24. Ductal carcinoma in situ. A. Specimen radiograph of core biopsy shows linear and punctate atypical calcifications that are highly suspicious for cancer. **B.** Low-power photomicrograph showing high-grade in situ ductal carcinoma. **C.** High-power image of a duct expanded by in situ ductal carcinoma. **D.** High-power photomicrograph of tissue calcification.

their invasive counterparts may show similar cytologic appearance and nuclear grade. Also, DCIS and invasive carcinoma share distinct molecular and cytogenetic alterations. The mechanisms governing any such suggested progression of DCIS to invasive carcinoma, however, are poorly understood.

Further, molecular analyses have shown differences in the numbers and types of chromosomal changes in low- and high-grade DCIS (Table 25-1). Intermediate-grade DCIS shares alterations of both groups. Invasive carcinomas occurring in association with DCIS share grade and molecular alterations. Low-grade and high-grade DCIS are therefore fundamentally distinct entities, and one does not appear to evolve into the other. The same appears to be true for low- and high-grade invasive cancer. *Multiple pathways of carcinogenesis and progression are likely.*

PATHOLOGY: DCIS predominantly involves ducts but can extend into lobules and is characterized by a proliferation of malignant epithelial cells showing a range of histologic features (Fig. 25-24). Growth patterns may be cribriform, micropapillary, papillary, solid and comedo types, and multiple architectural patterns can coexist in one lesion. More important prognostically is the nuclear grade: low, intermediate and high, although heterogeneity in grade is not uncommon.

- **High-grade DCIS** is composed of large, pleomorphic cells with marked variation in size and shape. The cells have abundant cytoplasm, irregular nuclei with prominent nucleoli and coarse chromatin. They proliferate rapidly. Intraductal necrosis is common (Fig. 25-25) and appears grossly as distended ducts with white necrotic material resembling comedos, hence the term **comedo necrosis**. The cellular necrotic debris often undergoes dystrophic calcification, which may be seen on mammography as linear, branching calcifications. The cells remain in duct spaces, but periductal chronic inflammation and formation of new vessels may be present. DCIS spreads through the duct system and often extends beyond clinically detected borders, making clear margins difficult to obtain. Cells with high nuclear grade can be seen with any of the above growth patterns.

- **Low-grade DCIS:** At the other end of the histologic spectrum, in low-grade DCIS cells are uniform, small and evenly spaced, with round, regular hyperchromatic nuclei (Fig. 25-26). Mitoses are infrequent. Micropapillary or cribriform growth predominates, and solid growth patterns are less common. Although necrosis is uncommon, foci of either punctate or comedo necrosis can be seen.

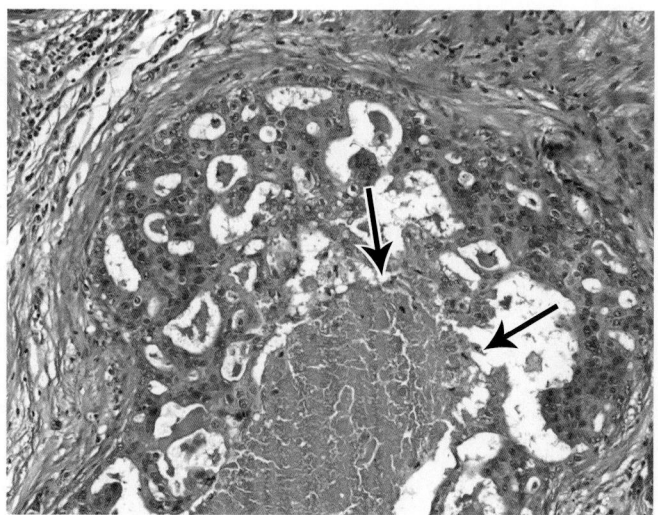

FIGURE 25-25. Ductal carcinoma in situ (DCIS) with comedo necrosis. Intraductal carcinoma with a cribriform architecture and central comedo necrosis (*arrows*).

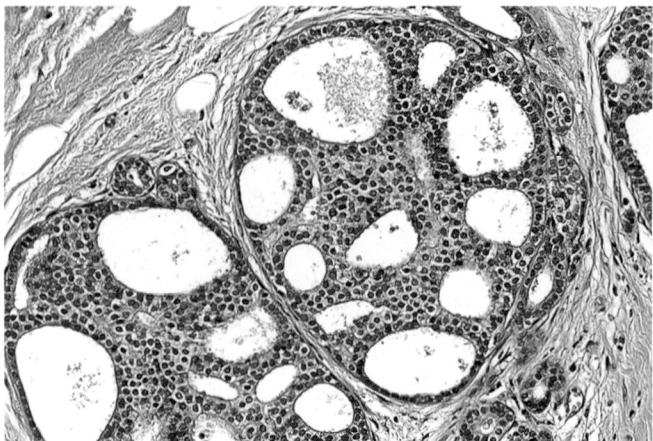

FIGURE 25-26. Ductal carcinoma in situ noncomedo type. A cribriform arrangement of tumor cells is evident.

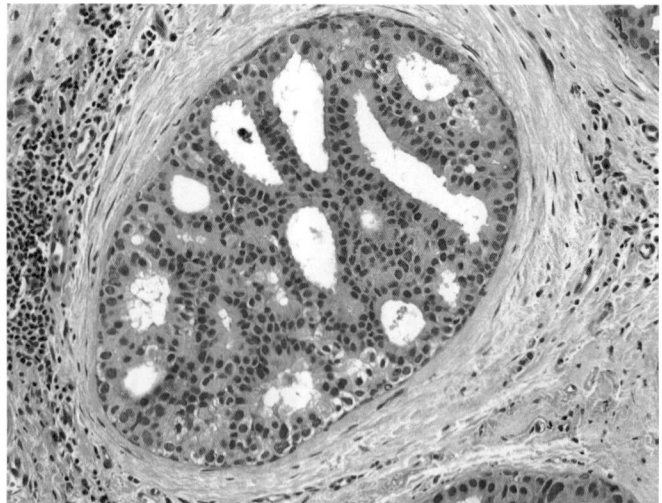

FIGURE 25-27. Intermediate-grade ductal carcinoma in situ with moderate nuclear pleomorphism and some polarization of cells around secondary spaces.

- **Intermediate-grade DCIS:** Intermediate-grade DCIS falls between high- and low-grade DCIS. Cells show moderate pleomorphism but maintain some degree of polarization (Fig. 25-27). Solid or cribriform growth is typical.
- **Microinvasive carcinoma:** This pattern is defined as one or more foci of invasive carcinoma, none of which exceed 1 mm in diameter (Fig. 25-28). *This lesion typically occurs in the setting of high-grade DCIS.*

Immunohistochemistry may occasionally be required to aid in the diagnosis of DCIS. DCIS is distinguished from epithelial hyperplasia of usual type because, in contrast to the latter, DCIS lacks high–molecular-weight cytokeratin staining. Still, some high-grade DCIS may express "basal," high–molecular-weight cytokeratins. Stains for myoepithelial cell markers (smooth muscle myosin heavy chain, calponin, p63, etc.) will confirm that the lesion is in situ and help in cases with foci suspicious for microinvasion.

Low- and intermediate-grade DCIS typically show strong diffuse staining for ER. High-grade lesions show less frequent ER staining but often overexpress HER2 (up to 60% of cases). This frequency is greater than what is seen in invasive carcinoma. Currently, ER is the only biomarker assessed in routine clinical practice.

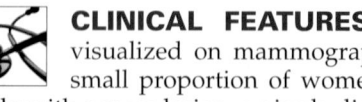 **CLINICAL FEATURES:** DCIS is most often visualized on mammography as calcifications. A small proportion of women present symptomatically with a mass lesion, a nipple discharge or Paget disease of the nipple (see below).

DCIS is treated by surgical excision. Breast-conserving surgery is possible in many cases, and adjuvant radiation reduces the risk of recurrence. When tumors recur, they do so at the site of the previous surgery and are invasive carcinomas 50% of the time. Lymph node metastases occur in less than 1% of patients with DCIS. In such cases, foci of invasion may have been missed when examining the

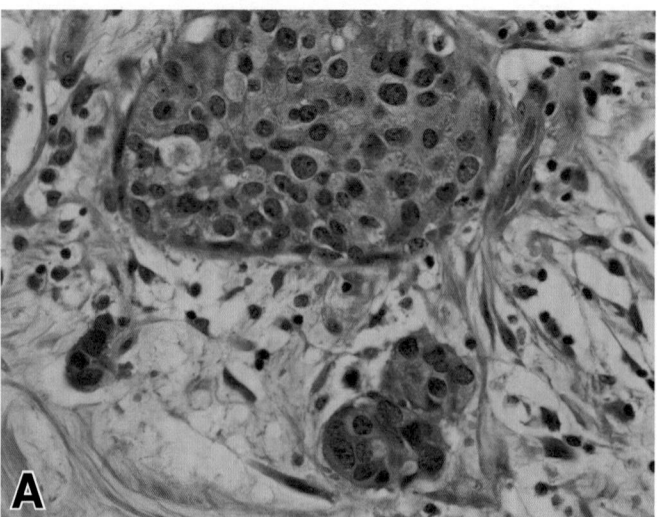

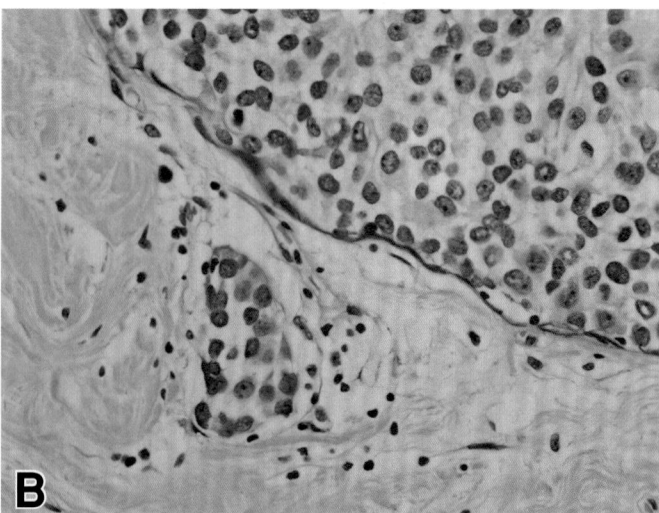

FIGURE 25-28. Ductal carcinoma in situ (DCIS) **(A)** with focus of microinvasive carcinoma. **(B)** Immunohistochemical staining with smooth muscle myosin heavy chain confirms the absence of a myoepithelial cell layer around the small stromal cluster.

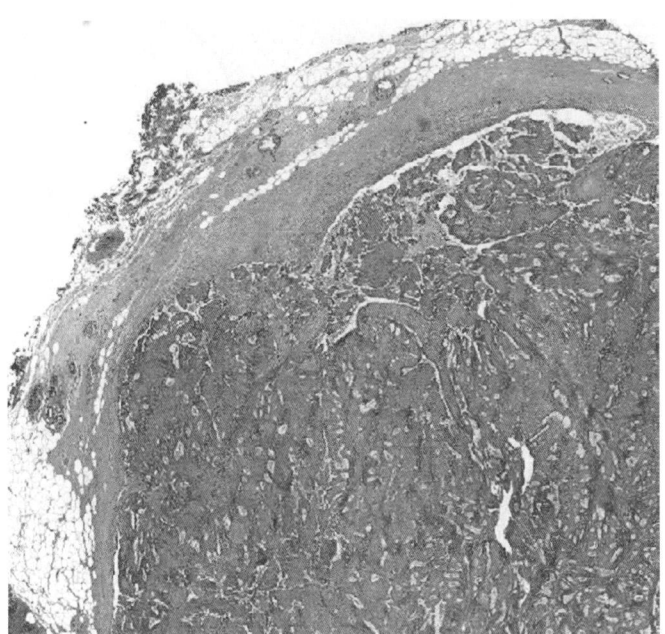

FIGURE 25-29. Encapsulated papillary carcinoma. Fibrovascular cores lined by malignant epithelial cells, without an intervening myoepithelial cell layer. The edge of the tumor has a pushing front, without evidence of stromal invasion.

primary lesions. Antihormone therapy reduces the risk of recurrence or progression for DCIS, which may be the case for hormone receptor–positive cases only. In all, the critical prognostic factors for patients with DCIS include lesion size, nuclear grade, the presence of comedo necrosis and margin status. Cancer-specific mortality is extremely low, with 1.0%–2.6% dying from invasive cancer 8–10 years after diagnosis of DCIS.

Encapsulated Papillary Carcinoma Is an Indolent Tumor

Encapsulated papillary carcinoma covers lesions previously called intracystic or encysted papillary carcinoma. These lesions have no myoepithelial cells at their periphery, and their true nature (i.e., whether they are truly in situ or, perhaps, invasive) is unclear. They are well-circumscribed, partially cystic, frequently hemorrhagic, solid masses. A capsule surrounds fibrovascular cores that are lined by one or more layers of malignant epithelial cells, with no intervening myoepithelial cell layer (Fig. 25-29). The cells are usually low to intermediate grade. At its edge, the tumor has a smooth pushing border, although frank stromal invasion can be present; this is typically invasive carcinoma of no special type.

Limited data show that these tumors have genetic alterations involving LOH at 16q and 1q. These tumors are not aggressive and metastases are rare. While controversial, the current approach is to stage them as Tis disease. If there is a component of conventional invasive carcinoma, the tumor stage should be based on the extent of the invasive component.

Paget Disease of the Nipple Reflects Extension of DCIS or Invasive Cancer

In Paget disease of the nipple, malignant glandular cells penetrate the epidermis of the nipple and areola. It is invariably associated with underlying DCIS, with or without invasive ductal carcinoma. This disease is rare, occurring in 1%–4% of breast cancers.

Paget disease presents as erythema or an eczematous change to the nipple and areola (Fig. 25-30A), sometimes with nipple retraction. Half of patients have palpable masses.

Malignant glandular epithelial cells are present in the epidermis, singly or in small groups (Fig. 25-30B). They

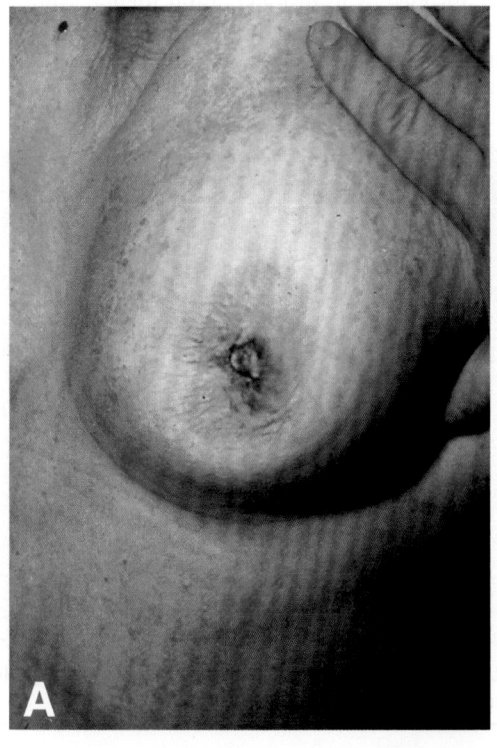

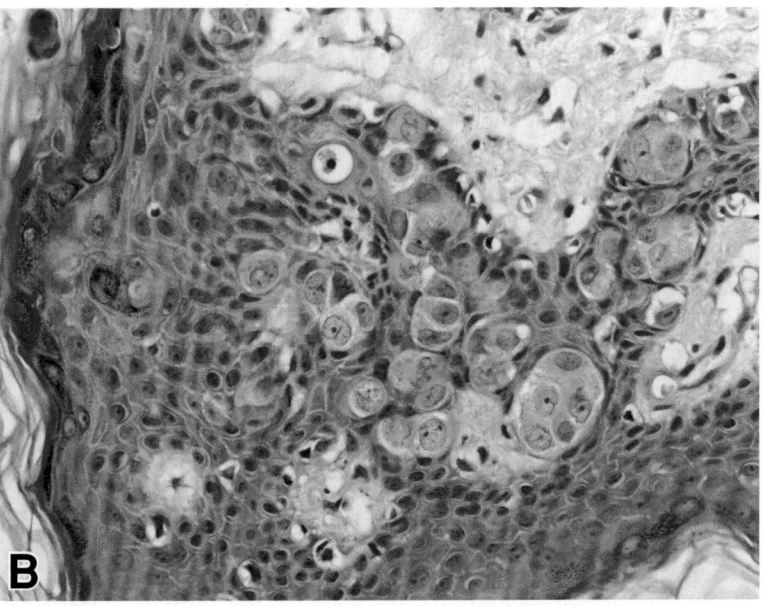

FIGURE 25-30. Paget disease of the nipple. A. An erythematous, scaly, and weeping "eczema" involves the nipple. **B.** The epidermis contains clusters of ductal-type carcinoma cells that are larger and have more abundant pale cytoplasm (*arrows*) than surrounding keratinocytes.

are large, with abundant cytoplasm that contains mucin globules, and pleomorphic nuclei with prominent nucleoli. These cells express epithelial membrane antigen (EMA) and low–molecular-weight cytokeratins. They almost always overexpress HER2. ER and PR are also positive in 40% and 30% of cases, respectively. Paget cells genetically resemble underlying tumor cells in the vast majority of cases. Prognosis is a function of the stage of the underlying breast cancer and not the presence of Paget cells.

Lobular Neoplasia Encompasses LCIS and ALH

Both ALH and LCIS (see above) reflect the same atypical proliferations of loosely cohesive epithelial cells, but they differ in the relative risk of developing breast cancer.

 **EPIDEMIOLOGY:** Since LCIS is generally asymptomatic, its true incidence is unknown. Estimated incidence is 1%–4%. It is bilateral in up to 30% of patients and multicentric in 85%. ALH and LCIS are best considered to be risk factors: the cancers that develop are typically not at the same site as these lesions and may be in the contralateral breast. Relative risk of subsequent cancer is 3–5.5-fold for ALH and 7–10-fold for LCIS. For LCIS, this means an absolute risk of 1%–2% per year and a lifetime risk of 30%–40%. Some evidence supports a precursor role for these lesions, albeit not an obligate one: a disproportionately high number of tumors that develop are invasive lobular carcinoma, and 2/3 occur in the ipsilateral breast. Furthermore, coexistent LCIS and invasive lobular carcinomas often show the same genetic changes, suggesting that at least some LCISs are precursors to invasive carcinoma.

 MOLECULAR PATHOGENESIS: Studies have identified genetic and karyotypic abnormalities in LCIS and ALH (Table 25-1). These studies have identified recurrent 16q22.1 loss in LCIS, ALH and invasive lobular carcinoma, for which the target gene encodes E-cadherin. This protein plays an essential role in cell adhesion and in cell cycle regulation through the β-catenin/Wnt pathway. Patients with germline mutations in this gene are at a high risk of developing lobular breast carcinoma and gastric signet ring cell carcinoma. Pleomorphic LCIS shares recurrent genomic alterations with classic LCIS (Table 25-1) but also harbors greater genomic instability.

PATHOLOGY: LCIS rarely appears grossly or with mammography: associated calcifications may present in nonneoplastic luminal epithelial cells. Also, rare variants, such as pleomorphic LCIS and classic LCIS with comedo necrosis, and dystrophic calcification with central necrosis, are detectable on mammography.

The cells of LCIS are monotonous and small, with round regular nuclei and minute nucleoli, although larger cells with conspicuous nucleoli occasionally dominate (Fig. 25-31). Cytoplasmic mucin vacuoles may be surrounded by a distinct halo. Unlike DCIS, the cells of LCIS do not form complex patterns but rather make solid clusters that pack and distend lobular acini. The growth pattern is loosely cohesive or dishesive. Gaps between individual cells reflect loss of cell–cell adhesion (see above). Pagetoid spread of lobular neoplastic cells is common in LCIS, where the cells track along beneath ductal luminal epithelial cells.

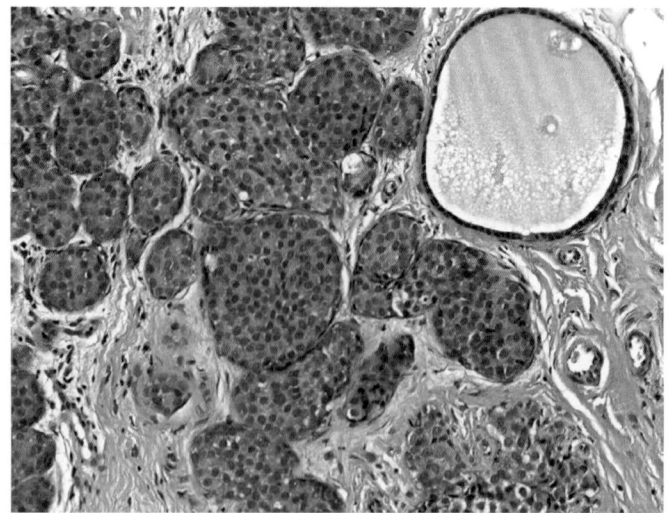

FIGURE 25-31. Lobular carcinoma in situ. The lumina of the terminal duct lobular units are distended by tumor cells, which exhibit round nuclei and small nucleoli. Cytoplasmic mucin vacuoles are present.

ALH and LCIS are diagnosed by the degree of filling and distention of acini. In LCIS, at least 50% of acini in a lobular unit are completely involved and distended by the atypical cell population, in contrast to less than 50% in ALH. LCIS rarely shows comedo necrosis, but when it does, the comedo necrosis greatly distends the involved spaces. Constituent cells retain the cytologic features of classic LCIS (Fig. 25-32).

Pleomorphic LCIS shows moderate to marked variation in nuclear size and shape and nuclear hyperchromasia. Nucleoli and mitotic figures are variably prominent (Fig. 25-33). Central comedo necrosis, often with microcalcifications, is typical. These are rare in classic LCIS.

Distinguishing LCIS from low-grade solid DCIS may be difficult. The absence of immunostaining for E-cadherin in LCIS and ALH may help make that distinction (Fig. 25-34), as DCIS cells retain cell membrane staining for E-cadherin.

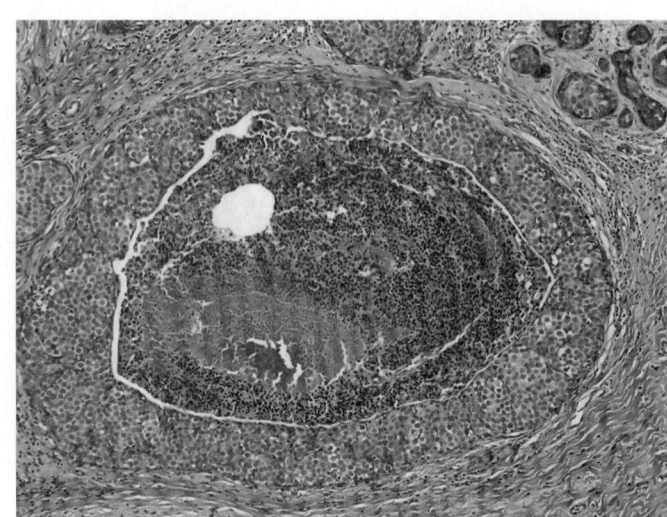

FIGURE 25-32. Lobular carcinoma in situ showing classic nuclear features but central expansile comedo necrosis.

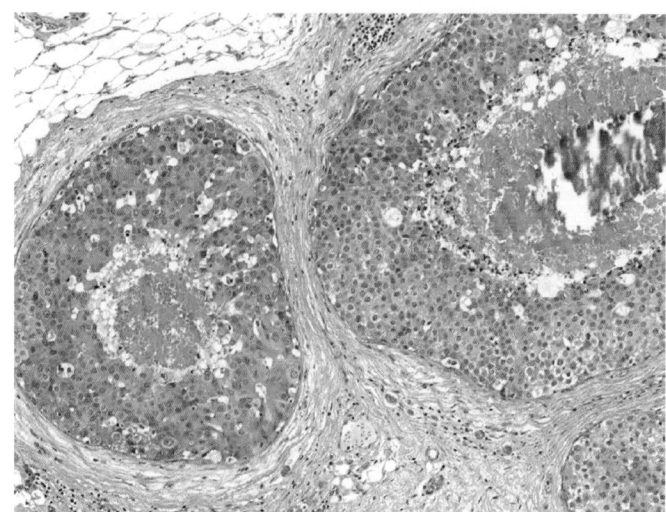

FIGURE 25-33. Pleomorphic lobular carcinoma in situ (PLCIS). A dyshesive population of markedly atypical epithelial cells with central comedo necrosis fill and distend the ducts. Dissociation of the neoplastic cells gives rise to spaces that may be misinterpreted as secondary spaces. E-cadherin expression was absent.

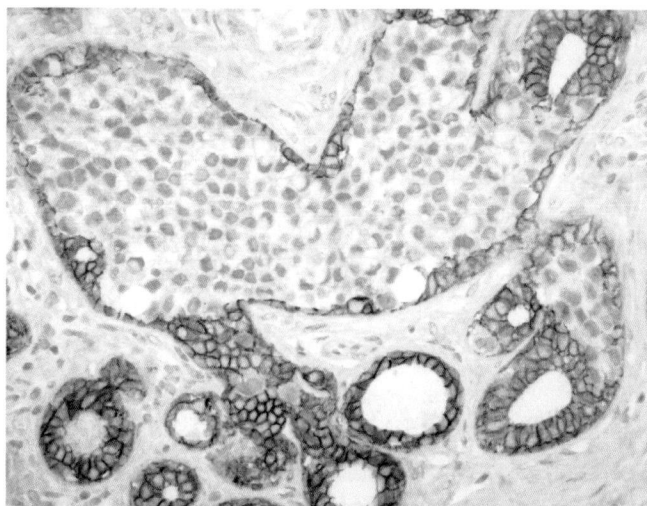

FIGURE 25-34. E-cadherin in lobular carcinoma in situ (LCIS). Membranous E-cadherin expression is seen in residual luminal epithelial cells, but the lobular neoplastic cells should show loss of staining.

CLINICAL FEATURES: The management of a patient with LCIS is controversial. For classic LCIS, many authorities would opt for no further surgical management. However, adjuvant hormonal therapy may be considered, and lifelong follow-up is required. Variant LCIS (pleomorphic, or classic LCIS with comedo necrosis), may require surgical excision with clear margins, plus, possibly, adjuvant radiation therapy.

Invasive Breast Carcinoma Is Derived from the TDLU

Breast cancer can occur anywhere in the breast but is most common in the upper outer quadrant. Patients most often have an ill-defined breast mass, which may be adherent to the skin or underlying muscle. Nonpalpable asymptomatic tumors are usually detected by mammography. These mostly appear radiologically as a spiculated mass or architectural distortion, with or without associated microcalcifications.

Most breast cancers are classified as carcinomas of no special type (NST). The remainder are special types of carcinomas or have mixed morphologic features.

Invasive Ductal Carcinoma, No Special Type

Of invasive breast cancers, 50%–70% fall in this category. These tumors are a heterogeneous group that do not show characteristics of a specific or "special" histologic type. The term "invasive carcinoma of no special type (ductal NST)" is preferred by the World Health Organization (WHO) Working Group.

Ductal NSTs present as irregular, dense masses on mammography or ultrasound (Fig. 25-35A). They are usually moderately or poorly defined, are nodular or stellate, and have firm to hard cut surfaces (Fig. 25-35B). Tumor cells form trabeculae, sheets, nests and glands (Fig. 25-35C). Nuclear pleomorphism and mitotic counts vary. Surrounding stroma varies from desmoplastic to collagenous. Higher-grade lesions may show

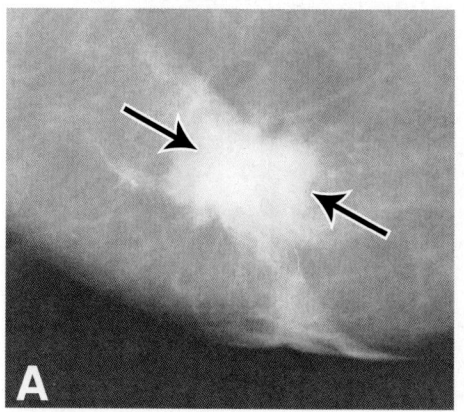
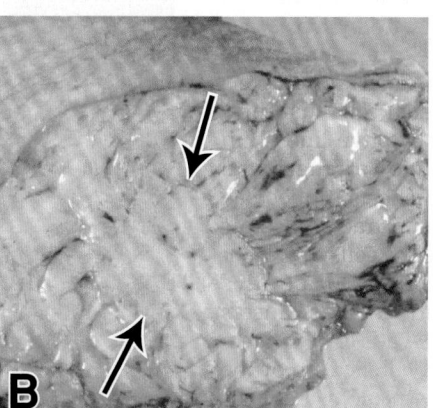
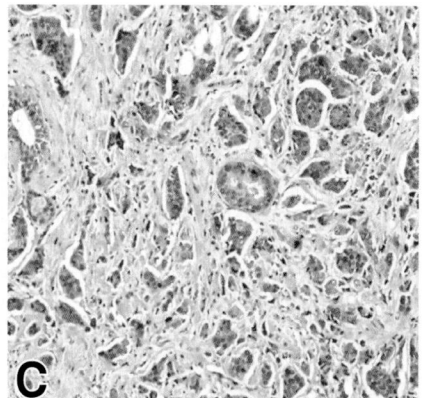

FIGURE 25-35. Carcinoma of the breast. A. Mammogram. An irregularly shaped, dense mass (*arrows*) is seen in this otherwise fatty breast. **B.** Mastectomy specimen. The irregular white, firm mass in the center is surrounded by fatty tissue. **C.** Photomicrograph showing irregular cords and nests of invasive ductal carcinoma cells invading stroma.

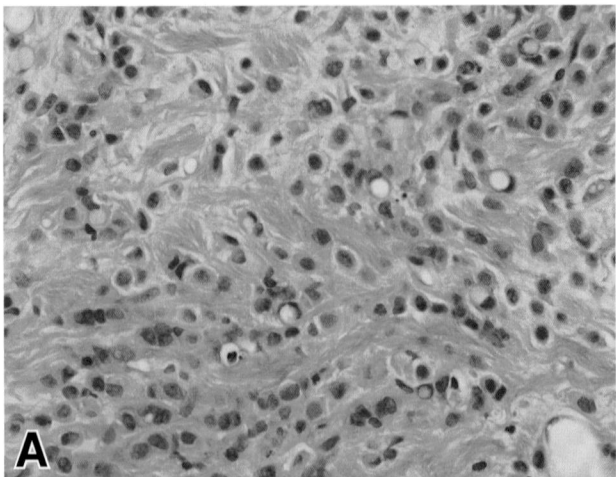
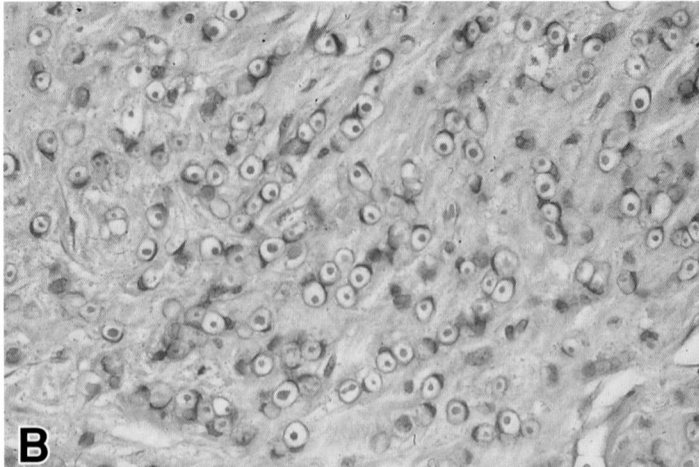

FIGURE 25-36. Lobular carcinoma. A. Invasive lobular carcinoma. In contrast to invasive ductal carcinoma, the cells of lobular carcinoma tend to form single strands that invade between collagen fibers in a diffuse pattern. The tumor cells are similar to those seen in lobular carcinoma in situ. **B. Signet ring carcinoma.** The tumor cells contain large amounts of clear mucin.

tumor necrosis. If a special-type component makes up over 50% of the tumor, the tumor is considered mixed (i.e., ductal with special-type features). DCIS is present in up to 80% of cases and is typically of the same nuclear grade as the invasive component.

Most ductal NSTs (75%) are ER positive, and 15% are HER2 positive. Specific genetic lesions or alterations are associated with a particular histologic type or grade in some cases. Low-grade invasive NSTs are usually diploid or near diploid, with trends in chromosomal variations (Table 25-1), while high-grade tumors tend to be less easily categorized. Since deletions of 16q are found in only about 1/3 of low-grade NSTs, progression from low- to high-grade cancer is probably relatively uncommon.

Overall, 35%–50% of patients with ductal NSTs survive 10 years, varying according to grade, tumor and lymph node stage and the presence of lymphovascular invasion.

Invasive Lobular Carcinoma

Invasive lobular carcinoma is the second most common form of invasive breast cancer, accounting for 5%–15% of all invasive carcinomas. Because stromal desmoplasia and fibrosis may be minimal, patients often have clinically silent disease grossly and by mammography, or may present with a poorly defined thickening of the breast. Lobular cancers characteristically show dishesive malignant epithelial cells that infiltrate the stroma diffusely (Fig. 25-36). They often line up in a row and may show a periductal "targetoid" arrangement. They do not form ducts, but rather solid sheets, trabeculae or nests. Neoplastic cells typically contain intracytoplasmic lumina and eccentric nuclei and resemble the cells of LCIS.

Invasive lobular carcinomas are more often ER positive than are ductal NSTs, although high-grade lobular cancers may lack ER and overexpress HER2. E-cadherin expression is usually low or absent, reflecting biallelic loss of the tumor suppressor gene that encodes this protein. Patterns of genetic changes in invasive lobular carcinoma differ from those in ductal carcinomas (Table 25-1).

These carcinomas tend to spread to the peritoneum, retroperitoneum, ovary and uterus, leptomeninges and gastrointestinal tract (Fig. 25-37). Matched for grade and stage, their prognosis is similar to that of ductal NST cancers.

Tubular Carcinoma

Tubular carcinomas represent 1%–2% of invasive breast cancers. Mammography detects this tumor disproportionately frequently. Tubular carcinomas are well-defined stellate masses whose cellular composition is almost entirely open and angulated tubules, lined by a single layer of mildly atypical epithelial cells (Fig. 25-38A). Over 95% of tubular carcinomas are ER positive and HER2 negative. Tubular carcinomas share some patterns of karyotypic changes with other tumor types (Table 25-1). Lymph node metastases are rare, and patients with tubular carcinomas have an excellent prognosis.

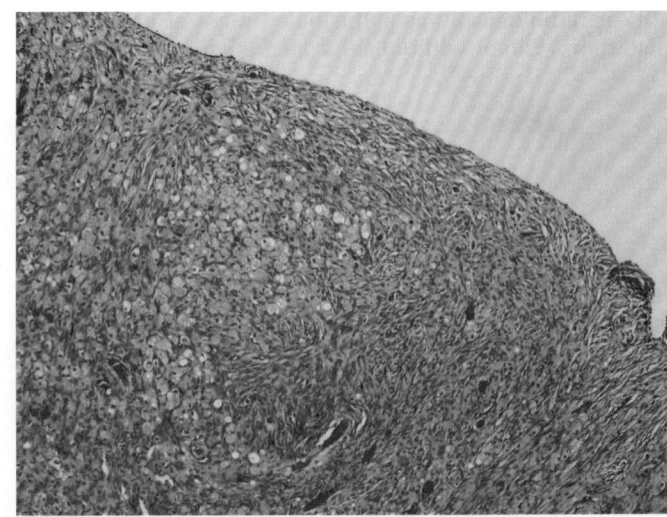

FIGURE 25-37. Ovary showing metastatic lobular carcinoma characterized by dyshesive cells with eccentric nuclei and intracytoplasmic lumens.

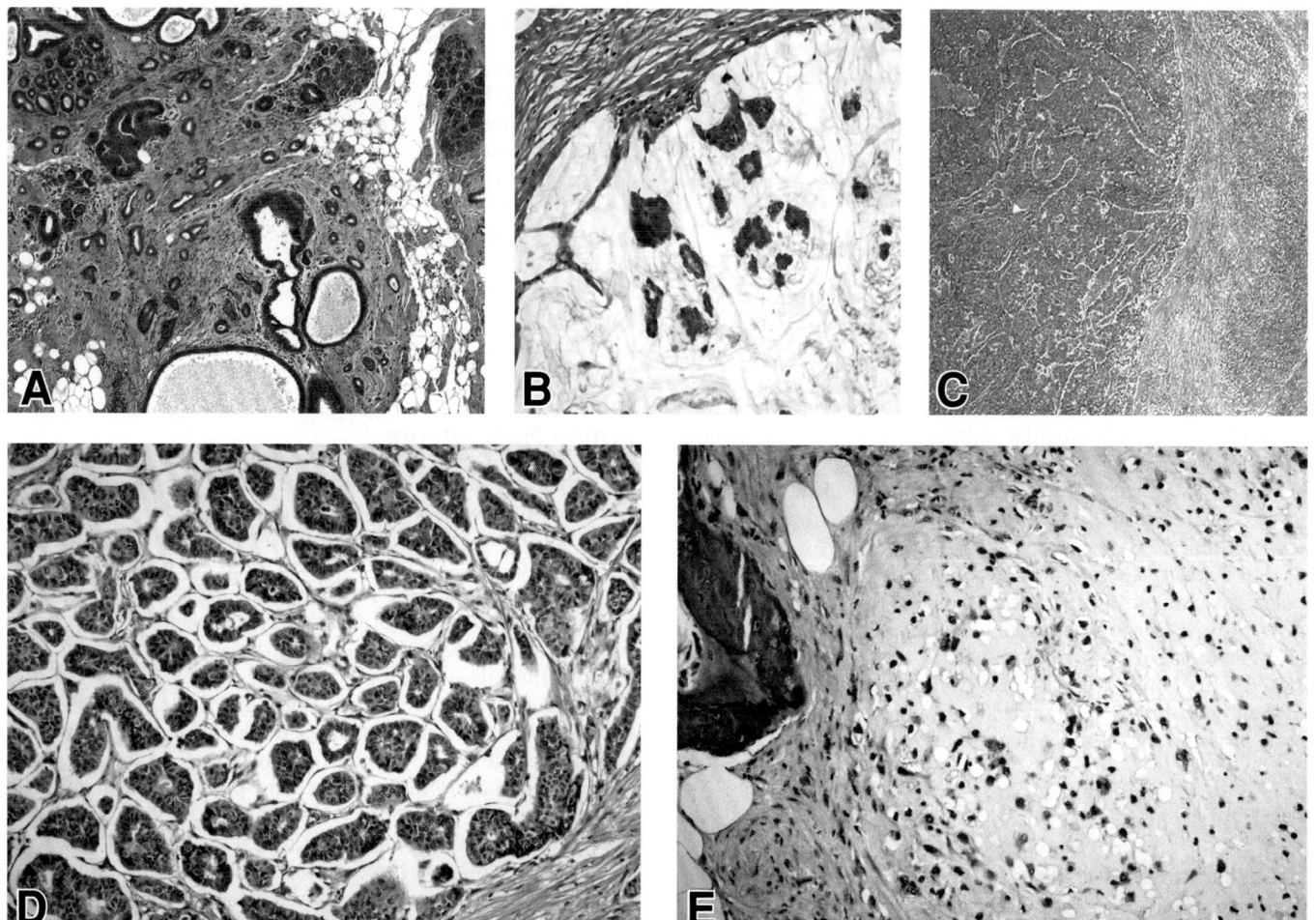

FIGURE 25-38. Patterns of breast carcinoma. A. Tubular carcinoma. Open and angulated malignant glands are dispersed between normal lobules and show extension into fat. A single layer of epithelium lines the tubules, and myoepithelial cells are absent. **B. Mucinous carcinoma.** Clusters of malignant cells float in large pools of extracellular mucin. **C. Medullary carcinoma.** The malignant cells are pleomorphic and grow in solid sheets, forming a blunt margin. There is no gland formation. Numerous mitoses are present. The tumor is surrounded by a dense lymphocytic infiltrate. **D. Micropapillary carcinoma.** Sponge-like pattern of empty spaces containing glands and small clusters of malignant epithelium. Focal serration of the outer borders of the glands is seen. **E. Metaplastic carcinoma.** Cartilaginous and osseus matrix in a metaplastic carcinoma with heterologous elements. Elsewhere, foci of poorly differentiated adenocarcinoma were seen.

Mucinous Carcinoma

Patients with mucinous carcinoma are typically older than those with other tumor types. These tumors, which make up 1%–6% of breast cancers, are well circumscribed, with a gelatinous texture. Low-grade malignant epithelial cells form acini, nests or trabeculae, which appear to float in pools of extracellular mucin (Fig. 25-38B). The malignant epithelial cells do not invade stroma directly. Pure mucinous carcinomas show little genomic instability or recurrent amplifications. They are uniformly of low histologic grade. Most are ER positive and HER2 negative. Patients with pure mucinous carcinoma have an excellent prognosis.

Carcinomas with Medullary Features

Classic medullary carcinomas are exceptionally rare, although other types of carcinoma may show medullary features. Almost 1/2 of patients are younger than 50. Medullary tumors are well circumscribed and soft, and include all of the following: (1) grade 2–3 nuclei; (2) circumscribed, pushing margins;

(3) syncytial growth pattern in greater than 75% of the tumor; (4) a moderate or marked lymphoplasmacytic infiltrate; and (5) no tubule formation (Fig. 25-38C). DCIS is an uncommon concomitant. Medullary cancers are typically ER, PR and HER2 negative ("triple negative") and have characteristic patterns of genetic changes (Table 25-1). While tumors arising in patients with *BRCA1* germline mutations often show medullary features, only 13% of tumors with medullary features are associated with this mutation.

The prognosis for pure medullary carcinoma is better than for high-grade ductal NST tumors, and lymph node metastases occur less frequently. Most women who die from their disease do so within 5 years of diagnosis.

Micropapillary Carcinoma

Pure micropapillary carcinoma occurs rarely, but micropapillary areas are more often admixed with ductal NST carcinoma. In these tumors, malignant epithelial nests or acini are surrounded by a clear space (Fig. 25-38D). As micropapillary tumors invade lymphatic vessels and metastasize to lymph nodes readily, recognizing even a minor component of micropapillary carcinoma is important. The high frequency of lymph node metastases notwithstanding, it is unknown if micropapillary tumors have an inherently poorer prognosis.

The vast majority of micropapillary carcinomas are ER and PR positive. Up to 1/3 show HER2 positivity. Common genetic changes seen in these tumors are shown in Table 25-1.

Metaplastic Carcinoma

Metaplastic carcinomas are heterogeneous tumors with malignant spindle cells, squamous cell carcinoma or heterologous elements, such as bone or cartilage (Fig. 25-38E). Adenocarcinoma may be absent, but cytokeratin immunostains are at least focally present. These tumors typically cluster with the basal molecular subgroup on gene expression profiling (see below).

Metaplastic tumors are usually ER and HER2 negative and show complex patterns of chromosomal gains and losses (Table 25-1).

Subtypes of metaplastic carcinomas are associated with better or worse prognosis when compared with ductal NSTs. Low-grade, fibromatosis-like, metaplastic carcinoma and low-grade adenosquamous metaplastic carcinoma are associated with a favorable outcome. Other metaplastic subtypes respond poorly to adjuvant chemotherapy and fare worse than other forms of triple-negative breast cancer.

PROGNOSTIC FACTORS

Breast Cancer Staging

Breast cancer survival is strongly influenced by tumor stage, expressed as the TNM classification (tumor [T], regional lymph nodes [N] and distant metastasis [M]) (Table 25-3). Breast cancer spreads by direct extension (e.g., to chest wall); via lymphatics to axillary, internal mammary and infra- and supraclavicular lymph nodes; and hematogenously to distant sites.

TABLE 25-3
PATHOLOGIC TUMOR STAGING

pTis	Carcinoma in situ (ductal or lobar) or Paget disease without invasive carcinoma
pT1mic	Microinvasion (≤1 mm)
pT1a	Invasive tumor >1 mm but ≤5 mm
pT1b	Invasive tumor >5 mm but ≤1 cm
pT1c	Invasive tumor >1 cm but ≤2 cm
pT2	Invasive tumor >2 cm but ≤5 cm
pT3	Invasive tumor >5 cm
pT4	Edema or tumor ulcerating through skin or satellite skin nodules and/or chest wall invasion[a] or inflammatory breast carcinoma

[a]Does not include invasion of the pectoralis muscle.
Data from Edge SB, Byrd DR, Compton CC, et al., eds. AJCC Cancer Staging Manual, 7th ed. New York: Springer, 2009.

Tumor Size

Prognosis varies with tumor size (T in the TNM protocol): patients with larger tumors show poorer survival. In assessing tumor size, only the invasive part is considered. Some locally advanced tumors are staged T4, based on skin or chest wall invasion, regardless of tumor size.

"Inflammatory breast cancer" has a particularly poor prognosis. This tumor features edema, erythema, induration, warmth and tenderness of overlying skin, resulting in an orange peel–like ("peau d'orange") appearance. Arm edema and pain may also occur, probably because of lymphatic obstruction by tumor. These findings correspond to tumor invasion of dermal lymphatic vessels.

Lymph Node Status

The presence or absence of axillary lymph node metastases is a key prognostic indicator for patients with breast cancer and requires pathologic evaluation of surgically resected lymph nodes. Axillary dissection risks significant postoperative morbidity (i.e., lymphedema and nerve damage). Sentinel lymph node (SLN) biopsy reduces this risk. This procedure requires injection of a dye and radioactive isotope and involves intraoperative lymphatic mapping of the draining or "sentinel" lymph node, the node most likely to contain breast cancer metastases. If it is negative, axillary dissection can safely be avoided. Immunohistochemical staining may help to identify cytokeratin-positive epithelial cells that may not be seen otherwise. Such detailed SLN evaluation has improved detection of micrometastases (>0.02 cm, <0.2 cm or >200 cells) and isolated tumor cells. The actual impact on prognosis of small metastases is small compared with node-negative women. Thus, there is a general consensus that there is little value in performing additional levels or immunohistochemical studies on SLNs.

Distant Metastases

Distant metastases portend a poor prognosis. Breast cancers metastasize to bone, which is where metastatic disease presents in 25% of cases. Of women who die from their disease, 70% eventually develop bone involvement. Smaller percentages of patients have other metastases, usually to lung, liver, central nervous system (CNS), skin and adrenal glands.

Tumor Grade

Histopathologic grading of breast tumors is one of the critical components of decision making. The Nottingham grading system, also called the modified Bloom and Richardson method, is most widely used. It combines scores for tubule formation, nuclear pleomorphism and mitotic count into a final grade of 1, 2 or 3 for low-, intermediate- and high-grade carcinomas, respectively (Fig. 25-39). Patients with grade 1 tumors have significantly better survival than those with grade 2 or grade 3 tumors.

Other Prognostic Features

- **Lymphovascular invasion (LVI):** Finding tumor cells within lymphovascular spaces correlates well with lymph node metastases (Fig. 25-40) and is a poor prognostic sign. If both LVI and nodal metastases are present, prognosis is worse than either alone. Furthermore, LVI is present in

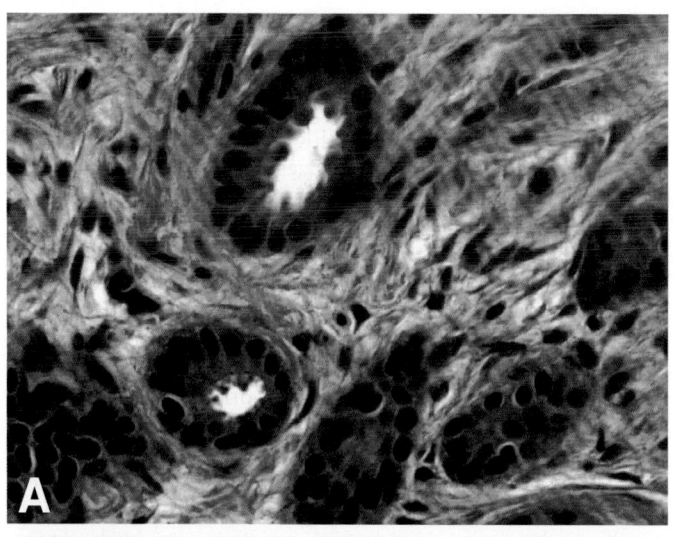

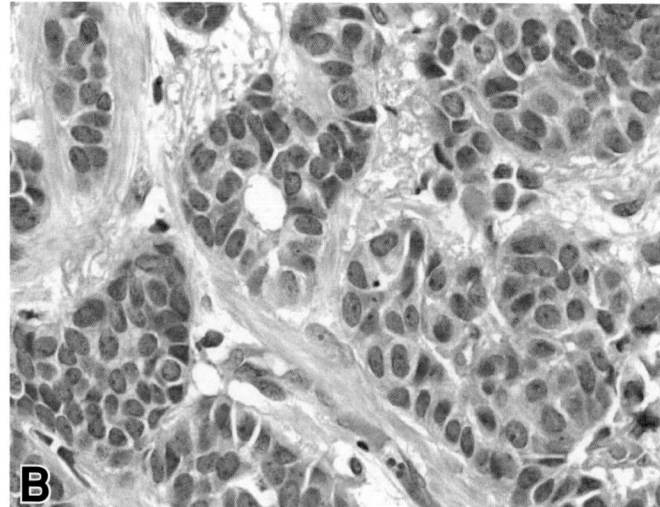

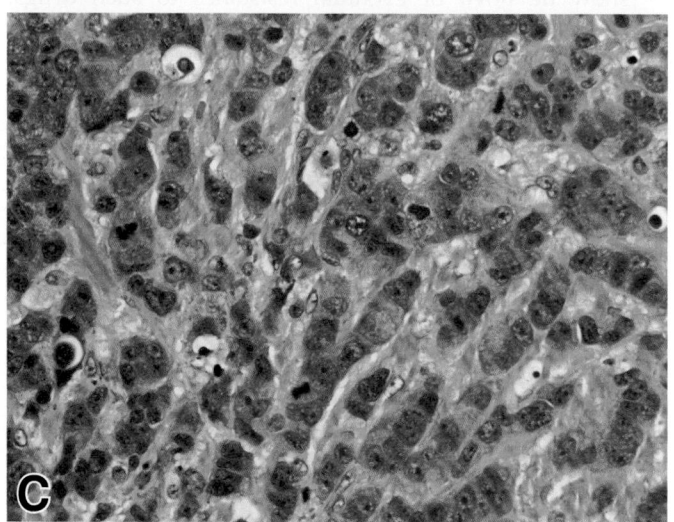

FIGURE 25-39. Tumor histologic grade. A. Low-grade invasive carcinoma showing good tubule formation, mild nuclear pleomorphism and inconspicuous mitoses. **B. Moderately differentiated** carcinoma with less tubule formation, moderate nuclear pleomorphism and variably prominent mitoses. **C. Poorly differentiated** carcinoma showing absent tubule formation, marked nuclear pleomorphism and frequent mitotic figures.

15% of patients without axillary nodal metastases and is a more important prognostic factor in this group.

- **Proliferative index and ploidy:** Tumors with high prolif-erative indices have worse prognoses. Several parameters are used to assess proliferation in breast cancers, including

(1) mitotic index, assessed histologically; (2) the propor-tion of cells in S phase of the cell cycle by flow cytometry; (3) immunohistochemical staining for proteins (Ki67) expressed by actively proliferating cells (Fig. 25-41); and (4) thymidine labeling index. Cell cycle analysis can also

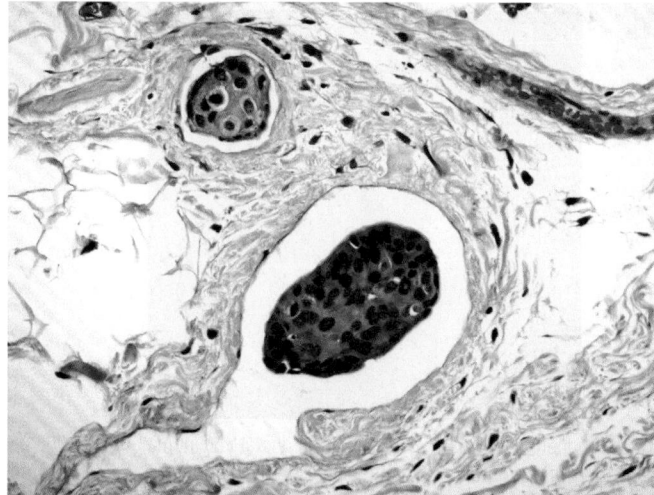

FIGURE 25-40. Lymphovascular invasion. Endothelial cell–lined lym-phatic channels containing tumor emboli.

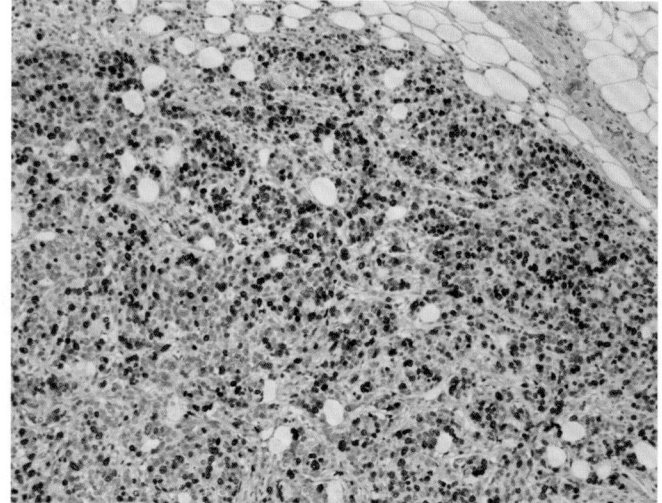

FIGURE 25-41. Ki67 staining (using MIB1 clone) in invasive carci-noma. This example shows a high percentage of cell nuclei staining.

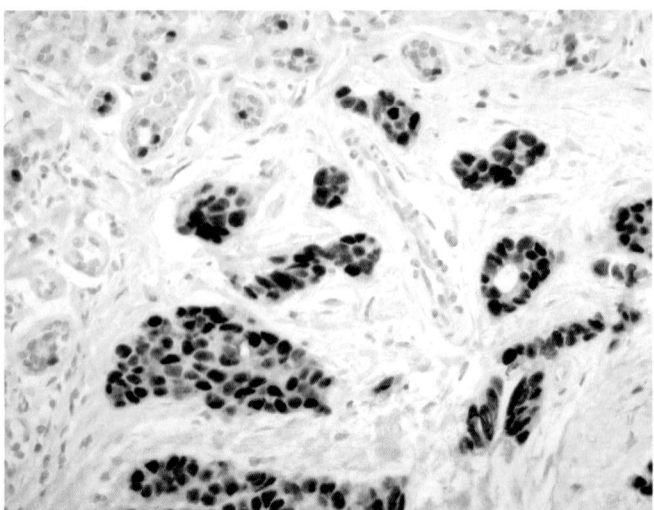

FIGURE 25-42. Estrogen receptor (ER). Strong nuclear positivity for estrogen receptor in this moderately differentiated invasive ductal carcinoma (immunohistochemical stain). Staining in normal breast lobules is seen in the upper left-hand corner.

detect aneuploidy, which occurs in 2/3 of breast cancers and confers a poorer prognosis. Notably, much of the prognostic impact of multigene predictor signatures (discussed below) comes from proliferation genes.

■ **Response to neoadjuvant therapy:** In patients who receive systemic treatment before surgery (neoadjuvant therapy), the response to the therapy is a strong prognostic factor. Patients who show complete pathologic responses (i.e., who lack pathologic evidence of residual breast or nodal disease) have an excellent long-term survival. Poorly differentiated tumors with high proliferation indices are more likely to respond to neoadjuvant treatment than low-grade cancers. A pathologically complete response occurs in 10%–30% of patients, little or no response in 10%–15% of patients and partial response in the remainder.

■ **Estrogen and progesterone receptors:** Steroid receptor proteins are expressed by benign breast epithelium and 70%–80% of breast cancers (ER > PR). ER and PR status is determined by immunohistochemistry, which uses antibodies to detect these nuclear receptors (Fig. 25-42). Hormone receptor positivity is defined as greater than or equal to 1% staining tumor cells. ER and PR bind their respective ligands (estrogen and progesterone) and stimulate cell growth. The greatest value of assessing hormone receptor status in breast cancer is its predictive ability. Patients with ER/PR-negative tumors are unlikely to respond to hormonal therapies with antiestrogens. On the other hand, ER/PR-positive tumors show a greater probability of response.

■ **HER2:** Overexpression or gene amplification (see Chapter 5) of HER2 occurs in 15%–20% of newly diagnosed breast cancers. HER2 positivity is an adverse prognostic factor irrespective of lymph node status. However, these patients may be treated with monoclonal antibodies or tyrosine kinase inhibitors that target HER2. As with hormone receptor status, many patients who express HER2 show de novo or eventual resistance to such drugs. Immunohistochemistry detects cell membrane expression of the protein, and in situ hybridization identifies gene amplification (Fig. 25-43).

Molecular Subtypes

Microarray gene expression profiling and other techniques have identified a set of genes, an "intrinsic gene list," of which several molecular subgroups (Table 25-4) appear to predict clinical outcome and response to therapy.

■ **Luminal A:** The luminal groups (A and B) are characterized by gene expression patterns similar to normal breast luminal epithelial cells, including low–molecular-weight cytokeratins 8/18, ER and ER-associated genes. Luminal A tumors are typically low grade and have an excellent prognosis.

■ **Luminal B** tumors also express ER and ER-associated genes but are usually higher grade than are luminal A tumors. They exhibit higher proliferative indices and have a poorer prognosis. Although they respond better to chemotherapy than do luminal A tumors, both luminal subtypes generally give poor responses.

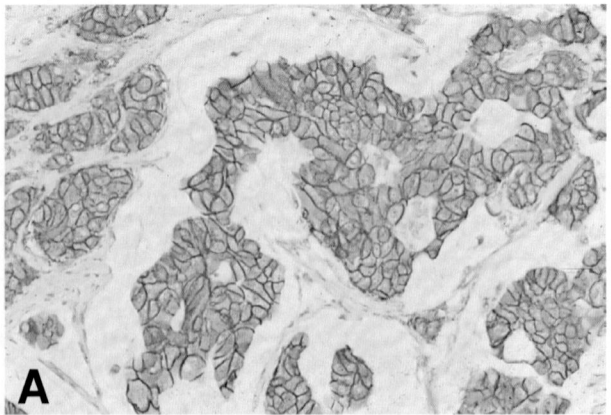
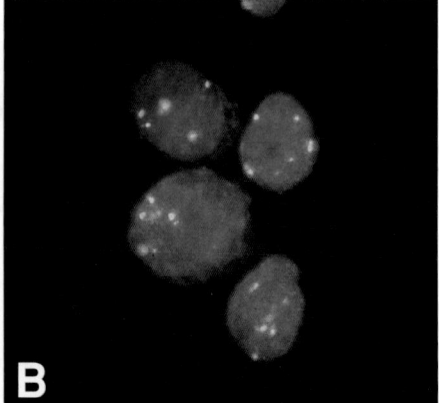

FIGURE 25-43. HER2/neu abnormalities in a breast cancer. A. Immunoperoxide staining of an invasive ductal carcinoma shows overexpression of the *HER2* (erbB-2) protein. **B.** Fluorescence in situ hybridization (FISH) methodology identifies the gene copies of *HER2* (erbB-2) in cancer cells. The *HER2* probe is red, and a normal cell should have two copies. More than two copies indicates *HER2* gene amplification. The green probe identifies the centromeric region of chromosome 17.

TABLE 25-4

MOLECULAR SUBTYPES OF BREAST CANCER

Molecular Subgroup	ER	PR	HER2	Proliferation Index	Other	Prognosis	Treatment
Luminal A	+	+	−	Low	CK8/18	Excellent	Hormonal
Luminal B	+	+	−/+	Moderate	CK8/18	Intermediate	Hormonal and chemotherapy
HER2+	−	−	+	High	AR	Poor	Trastuzumab Anthracyclines
Basal	−	−	−	Very high	CK5/6, CK14, vimentin, EGFR, c-kit	Poor	Platinum- and anthracycline-based chemo-therapy ?PARP inhibitors

+ positive; − negative; −/+ sometimes positive; AR = androgen receptor; ER = estrogen receptor; PARP = poly(adenosine diphosphate-ribose) polymerase; PR = progesterone receptor.

■ **HER2:** Tumors that overexpress HER2 express genes in the HER2 pathway and with ER negativity. These tumors behave aggressively, but targeting HER2 with an antibody, trastuzumab, has significantly increased patient longevity.

■ **Basal-like cancers:** These highly aggressive tumors constitute 10%–20% of invasive breast carcinomas. They are mainly ER and HER2 negative. Their name derives from their consistent expression of genes in the basal or myoepithelial cells of the breast, including high–molecular-weight cytokeratins 5/6, 14 and 17; caveolins 1 and 2; nestin; p63; and EGFR. These tumors are distinctive, with high nuclear grade, many mitoses, pushing margins, central areas of necrosis or fibrosis and a lymphocytic infiltrate. Cancers with medullary features and metaplastic carcinomas are typically basal-like. Most cancers arising in patients with germline *BRCA1* mutations are basal-like.

Additional subtypes of ER-negative breast cancers have also emerged: **molecular apocrine, claudin low** and **interferon rich. Molecular apocrine** tumors are androgen receptor positive and frequently HER2 positive. They demonstrate prominent apocrine features, with abundant eosinophilic cytoplasm and prominent nucleoli. **Claudin-low** tumors show high levels of expression of genes involved in epithelial-to-mesenchymal transition, including vimentin, Snail and TWIST, and down-regulation of genes involved in cell adhesion (E-cadherin, claudins 3, 4 and 7). These tumors also display stem cell–like features. Tumors of the **interferon-rich** subtype express high levels of interferon-regulated genes, including *STAT1*. The clinical importance of these additional subgroups has yet to be elucidated.

Gene Expression Profiling Prognostic Assays

A large proportion of patients with breast cancer are treated with adjuvant chemotherapy; yet not all will benefit from this therapy. In recent years, gene expression profiling prognostic assays have been developed. Commercially available approaches quantify messenger RNA (mRNA) levels for a panel of genes. One example is the **21-gene recurrence score,** which is based on the mRNA levels of 21 genes and performed using formalin-fixed, paraffin-embedded tumor tissue. The genes evaluated include 16 cancer-related genes and 5 reference genes. Analysis of respective gene expression levels leads to a "recurrence score," which is reported as reflecting low, high or intermediate risk of developing distant recurrence at 10 years after 5 years of tamoxifen (antiestrogen) therapy. The test has been shown to predict benefit from tamoxifen for patients with cancers with low- or intermediate-risk recurrence scores and benefit from chemotherapy for patients with high-risk recurrence scores.

The **70-gene prognostic signature** is a microarray-based multigene assay requiring fresh or frozen tumor samples. It is used to assess prognosis in invasive breast cancer based on expression levels of 70 cancer-related genes and 1800 reference genes. Results are reported as low or high risk for distant metastases at 10 years without adjuvant treatment and, thus, identify patients in whom withholding chemotherapy may be warranted. Importantly, *in guiding treatment decisions and evaluating prognosis, these tools complement, but do not replace, histopathology and clinical analyses.*

Genetic analysis has demonstrated that breast cancers are markedly heterogeneous, and only a few gene mutations are actually present in a high percentage of tumors (see Chapter 5). These include *PTEN, PIK3CA* and *TP53.* Analysis of matched primary and metastatic tumors shows that tumors are largely mosaics of subclones of cancer cells, and metastases may derive from genetically distinct subpopulations in the primary tumor (see Chapter 5).

Primary Therapy of Breast Cancer Almost Always Involves Surgery

Breast-conserving surgery (i.e., lumpectomy or quadrantectomy) is often used. Wider excision may be needed in patients with bulky disease. As indicated above, sentinel lymph node sampling often replaces more extensive axillary lymph node chain removal, and axillary lymph node dissection is reserved for patients in whom the SLN is positive for tumor. Postoperative radiation therapy is commonly used as well.

Systemic therapies (i.e., hormonal, chemotherapy and targeted molecular modalities) are often considered essential in managing patients with breast cancer. Patients with the worst prognoses usually gain most from such systemic therapies. Targeted therapies rely on the presence of particular targets in the tumor (e.g., ER, PR and HER2).

THE MALE BREAST

Gynecomastia Is Enlargement of the Male Breast

Male breast tissue has receptors for androgens, estrogens and progesterone. Estrogen stimulates duct development and

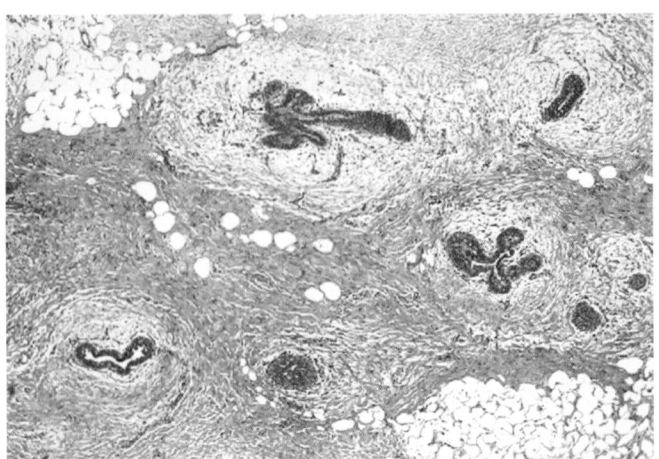

FIGURE 25-44. Gynecomastia. There is proliferation of branching, intermediate-sized ducts. The ductal epithelium is hyperplastic, and mitoses are present. A concomitant increase in the surrounding fibrous tissue causes a palpable mass.

progesterone stimulates lobular development in the presence of luteinizing hormone, follicle-stimulating hormone and growth hormone. Androgens antagonize the effects of estrogen. Testosterone can be converted to estradiol by the enzyme aromatase, which is especially present in adipose tissue.

Physiologic gynecomastia occurs in most neonates, owing to circulating maternal and placental estrogen and progesterone. Transient gynecomastia also affects over half of boys during puberty, because estrogen production peaks earlier than that of testosterone. With increasing age, free testosterone decreases and adipose tissue expands, increasing the prevalence of breast enlargement.

Gynecomastia is benign enlargement of the male breast, with proliferation of ductal and stromal elements. It is due to relatively decreased androgens or increased estrogen effect. Breast enlargement due to adipose tissue is called **pseudogynecomastia**. Nonphysiologic gynecomastia results from drugs or disorders associated with low testosterone levels, high conversion of testosterone to estrogens, elevated estrogen levels and increased sex hormone–binding globulin levels that lower free testosterone. It may occur in patients with hyperthyroidism, cirrhosis, renal failure, chronic lung disease and certain hormone-producing tumors, including Leydig and Sertoli cell tumors, testicular germ cell tumors and cancers of the liver and lung. Drugs implicated in gynecomastia include digitalis, cimetidine, spironolactone, marijuana and tricyclic antidepressants. Klinefelter syndrome is the most common chromosomal disorder associated with gynecomastia.

Gynecomastia presents as a rubbery discrete mass or ill-defined area of induration that may display either a florid or fibrous phase (Fig. 25-44). The florid phase typically occurs

early, within 6 months of onset. It is characterized by epithelial hyperplasia with flat or micropapillary architecture. Periductal stroma is hypercellular and edematous, with increased vascularity and chronic inflammation.

The fibrous phase is seen after 1 year or more. It lacks epithelial proliferation, and the stroma is more collagenous. Mixtures of both phases may be seen. Pseudoangiomatous stromal hyperplasia may be seen in either phase.

Male Breast Cancers Often Reflect Hyperestrogen States

 **EPIDEMIOLOGY:** These tumors make up 1% of breast cancers in the United States. In sub-Saharan Africa, they make up 7%–14% of breast cancers, the difference possibly reflecting endemic diseases causing liver damage and hence hyperestrogenism. In the United States, rates are highest in black men, intermediate in non-Hispanic white men and Asian-Pacific Islanders and lowest in Hispanic men. The mean age at presentation is 65.

The risk of breast cancer is greater in high-estrogen states. Men with Klinefelter syndrome have a 58-fold higher risk than normal men and an absolute risk of up to 3%. Male–female transsexuals following castration and high-dose estrogen and men treated with estrogen for prostate cancer also are at greater risk.

Men with breast cancer inherit germline mutations in *BRCA2* and show other gene mutation patterns that are similar to some observed in breast cancers in women (Table 25-1). Ionizing radiation has been implicated, being seen in Japanese men after nuclear fallout and in patients treated with therapeutic chest irradiation at a young age.

 PATHOLOGY: Most breast cancers in males are invasive carcinoma, NST; however, papillary carcinoma is disproportionately represented in men. Lobular carcinoma is rare. Ninety percent of cancers are ER and PR positive. Androgen receptor positivity is frequently seen.

 CLINICAL FEATURES: Most patients present with a painless lump. Nipple involvement, including retraction, discharge or ulceration, is an early event. Paget disease is a presenting feature in 1% of affected men.

Management of men with breast cancer largely reflects results of clinical studies done in women: simple mastectomy and sentinel lymph node biopsy or axillary dissection. Postoperative radiation may be given for large tumors or for close margins. Hormonal therapy with tamoxifen is frequently administered. There is limited experience in the treatment of male breast cancer with aromatase inhibitors. Adjuvant chemotherapy with or without trastuzumab may be indicated, depending on the aggressiveness of the disease and HER2 status, respectively.

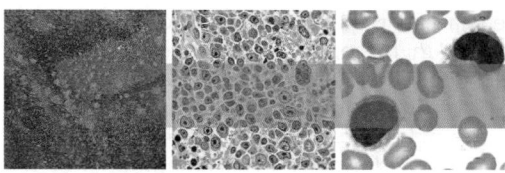

26

Hematopathology

Riccardo Valdez ▪ Mary Zutter ▪ Shauying Li ▪ Alina Dulau Florea

Bone and Normal Myelopoietic Cells

EMBRYOLOGY

The origin of hematopoietic stem cells (HSCs) is controversial, but they likely arise in the mesoderm of the intraembryonic aorta/gonad mesonephros region and/or the yolk. Blood cell formation shifts from the yolk sac to the fetal liver around the 3rd month of embryogenesis. HSCs and erythroid precursors make up most of the hematopoietic tissue during the early stages of blood cell formation in the fetal liver, but production of megakaryocytes and mature neutrophils soon follows. A switch from the production of red blood cell embryonic hemoglobins to fetal hemoglobins also occurs during the hepatic phase of erythropoiesis.

Hematopoietic stem cells migrate from the liver to the bone marrow around the 4th month of embryogenesis, and by the 26th week of intrauterine life, the bone marrow has become the main hematopoietic organ. At birth, hematopoiesis becomes fully established in the marrow and virtually ceases in the liver.

From birth to puberty, all skeletal bone marrow is densely packed with hematopoietic tissue (red marrow) that can produce all blood cell types. Red marrow is subsequently largely confined to the proximal epiphyseal regions of humeri and femurs and the flat bones (skull, scapula, clavicles, sternum, ribs, vertebrae, pelvis). In adults, adipose tissue (inactive "yellow marrow") occupies most available space in medullary cavities of the skeleton. The bone marrow in the axial skeleton continues to be active until old age, when resorption of cancellous bone enlarges marrow cavities and leads to further fatty replacement. Remarkably, in healthy individuals, peripheral blood counts are maintained normally even as amounts of red marrow decline.

Local expansion of hematopoietic progenitors in red (cellular) marrow and reactivation of peripheral yellow marrow allow the hematopoietic system to meet physiologic demands for increased blood cell formation. If the hematopoietic system cannot respond to stress/demand, there is probably an abnormality of one or more hematopoietic lineages. Reactivation of hepatic and splenic hematopoiesis rarely occurs in adult life. *Significant extramedullary hematopoiesis in adulthood usually suggests a clonal (malignant) disorder, rather than a reactive process.*

BONE MARROW

Hematopoietic Cells Derive from Multipotent Stem Cells

Bone marrow consists of a complex network of solid cords separated by sinusoids (Fig. 26-1). These cords contain stromal and hematopoietic cells, knitted together by extracellular matrix. A semipermeable barrier between sinusoids and cords consists of an endothelial cell layer, a thin basement membrane and an outer layer of interrupted reticular adventitial cells. The latter branch extensively throughout

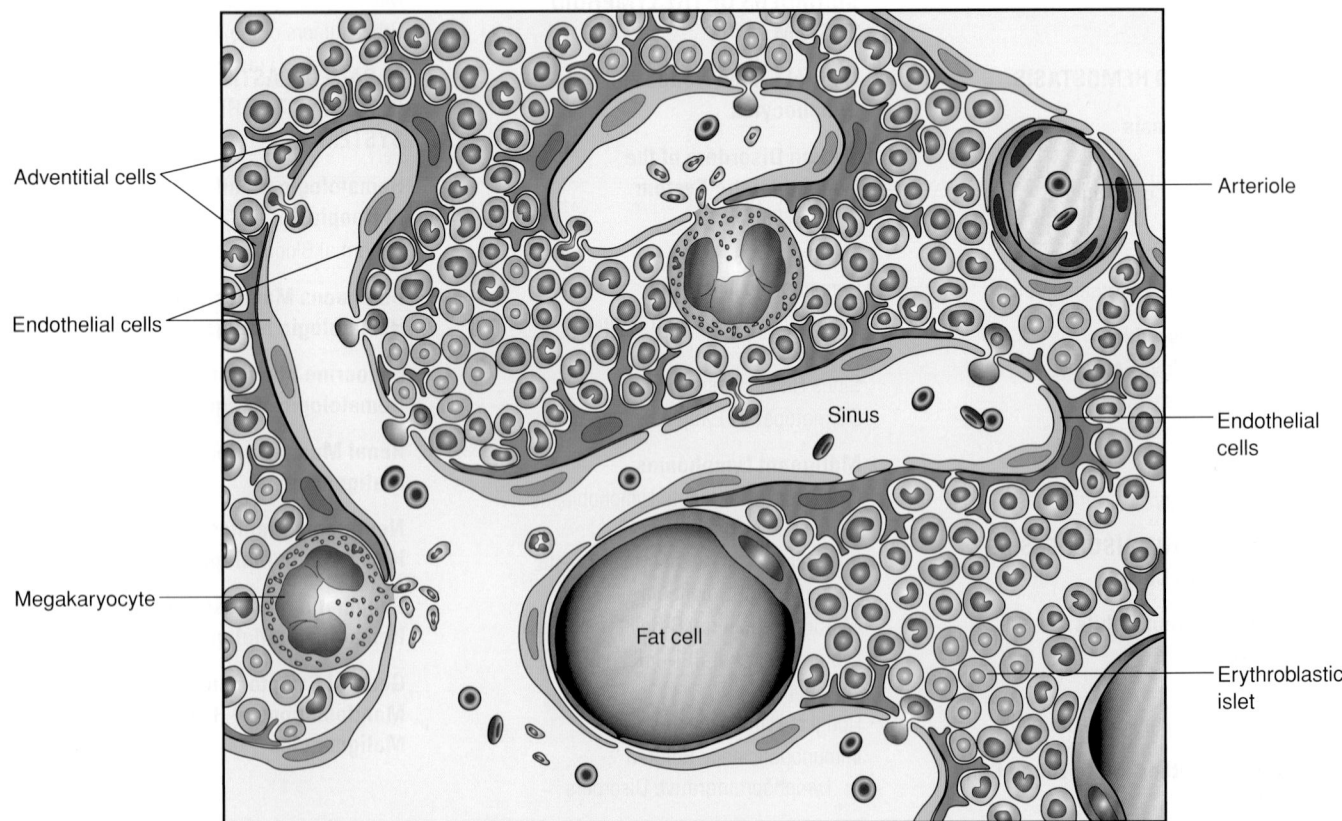

FIGURE 26-1. Structure of normal bone marrow. The sinusoids represent the major point of egress of hematopoietic cells from the bone marrow. Note that the bone marrow does not have lymphatic channels.

the cords and help anchor stromal and hematopoietic cells. Bone marrow stromal cells include macrophages, endothelial cells, lymphocytes and fibroblasts.

Islands of erythroblasts, usually in concentric rings around a macrophage that stores excess iron, are present within the cords. The erythroid islands lie close to sinusoid walls, as do megakaryocytes. Granulocyte precursors are deeper in the cords, adjacent to the bony trabeculae.

STEM CELLS: Pluripotent HSCs are a self-perpetuating pool, in which self-renewal balances differentiation and exit (Fig. 26-2). These stem cells are admixed with progenitor and more mature hematopoietic cells, with HSCs representing only a small proportion of total hematopoietic cell mass. They are small, mononuclear and difficult to identify by microscopy. HSCs are semidormant (noncycling) cells that differentiate to progenitor cells of specific lineages as needed. When marrow elements are injected into irradiated mice, stem cells form visible colonies in the spleen (**"colony-forming unit, spleen" [CFU-S]**). In bone marrow cultures, stem cells form colonies containing **multipotential cells** called granulocyte, erythroid, macrophage and megakaryocyte elements (**CFU-GEMM**) and lymphoid precursor cells (**CFU-L**).

PROGENITOR CELLS: Like stem cells, progenitor cells are small to medium-sized mononuclear cells that resemble mature lymphocytes. In culture, they give rise to colonies of differentiated progeny. Progenitor cells committed to red blood cell production forms luxuriant burst-shaped colonies (**"burst-forming unit, erythroid" [BFU-E]**). Each subsequent generation of BFU-E makes smaller colonies, until a final progenitor cell, the "colony-forming unit, erythroid" (**CFU-E**), produces only a small clone of mature erythroblasts.

Granulocytic and **monocytic** cell lines derive from a single progenitor cell. This cell, named "colony-forming unit, granulocyte-monocyte" (**CFU-GM**), makes a colony with both granulocytic and monocytic cells. As the cell matures, its progeny are increasingly committed to polymorphonuclear leukocytes (**CFU-G**) or monocyte/macrophages (**CFU-M**). **Eosinophils** and **basophils** also have specific progenitor cells (**CFU-Eo** and **CFU-Ba,** respectively). "Megakaryocytic progenitor cells" (**CFU-Meg**) produce colonies in vitro consisting of four to eight megakaryocytes.

GROWTH FACTORS: Bone marrow hematopoiesis responds to fluctuating needs for blood cells and maintains the size of the circulating blood cell mass. Growth factors mediate this responsiveness by regulating the rate of cellular proliferation, primarily in the progenitor cell compartment (Fig. 26-2).

- **Stem cell factor** (SCF, or c-KIT ligand) and **Flt3 ligand** (Flt3L) support survival and proliferation of pluripotent stem cells, CFU-GEMM and various progenitor cells.
- **Interleukin (IL)-3** and **granulocyte-macrophage colony-stimulating factor (GM-CSF)** are important for proliferation of CFU-GEMM and multiple CFUs.
- **Granulocyte colony-stimulating factor (G-CSF)** and **macrophage colony-stimulating factor (M-CSF)** promote granulocyte and monocyte maturation from CFU-G and CFU-M, respectively.
- **Erythropoietin (EPO),** released by renal interstitial peritubular cells in response to hypoxia, activates erythroid progenitor cells.
- **Thrombopoietin (TPO)** facilitates production and maturation of megakaryocytes.

- *Deficiencies in one or more blood cell populations (e.g., postchemotherapy pancytopenia, especially neutropenia, stem cell mobilization prior to bone marrow transplantation, renal failure; see below) respond to treatment with several growth factors, mainly GM-CSF, G-CSF and EPO. EPO and other factors stimulate the EPO receptor and are used illicitly to enhance performance for endurance sports.*

PRECURSOR CELLS: Progenitor cells mature into precursor cells, or **blasts**. *Starting at the precursor stage, and continuing beyond, cells are morphologically recognizable in terms of their lineage.* Maturation of precursor cells to mature cells entails progressive nuclear changes and cytoplasmic maturation to reflect cellular functions (e.g., oxygen carriage in red blood cells, cytotoxic enzymes in neutrophils). In parallel, lineage-related cell surface proteins/antigens appear. The latter help to identify both cell types and stages of maturation.

- **Erythroid precursor cells:** The **proerythroblast** is the first stage in red blood cell maturation. Like other committed blast cells, proerythroblasts are relatively few in number, compared to the more mature red cell forms. Proerythroblasts have intensely basophilic (blue) cytoplasm with a large round nucleus, fine open chromatin and visible nucleoli. Maturation in the erythroid series is marked by a progressive decrease in nuclear size, increased nuclear chromatin density and progressive hemoglobinization of the cytoplasm. In the process, the cytosol gradually changes from blue to pink. All erythrocytes express glycophorin, which helps to define erythroid lineage. **Orthochromatic erythroblasts** then banish their nuclei to create **reticulocytes,** whose cytosol has mitochondria and hemoglobin-producing polyribosomes. These reticulocytes represent the final stage of erythroid cell maturation in the bone marrow. After they leave the bone marrow, reticulocytes lose the capacity for aerobic metabolism and hemoglobin synthesis, and become mature erythrocytes within 1–2 days.
- **Granulocytic precursors: Myeloblasts** have round to oval nuclei with delicate chromatin, multiple visible nucleoli and a blue-gray cytoplasm. **Promyelocytes,** the next stage, have similar nuclei, but their cytoplasm contains primary (azurophilic) granules. Maturation from **promyelocytes** to mature **neutrophils** involves (1) progressive nuclear chromatin condensation, (2) increasing nuclear lobulation and (3) the appearance of secondary (specific) granules. **Basophils** and **eosinophils** derive from specific progenitor and precursor cells and are distinguished by their secondary granules. Granulocyte precursors express CD13 and CD33 and progressively lose CD34 as they mature.
- **Monocytic precursor cells:** Parallel formation of monocytes from monoblasts also involves a nuclear condensation process, but with less nuclear lobation. Cytoplasm becomes gray, with only a few pink or purple granules. *After monocytes leave the blood, they join the mononuclear phagocyte system.* They may evolve further, depending on tissue location, function as a **phagocyte** (fixed or wandering) or immunoregulatory activity (dendritic reticulum cells, Langerhans cells).
- **Megakaryocytic precursors:** Marrow megakaryocytes mature into big multilobed cells by endomitotic division. After reaching a certain ploidy, the cytosol becomes

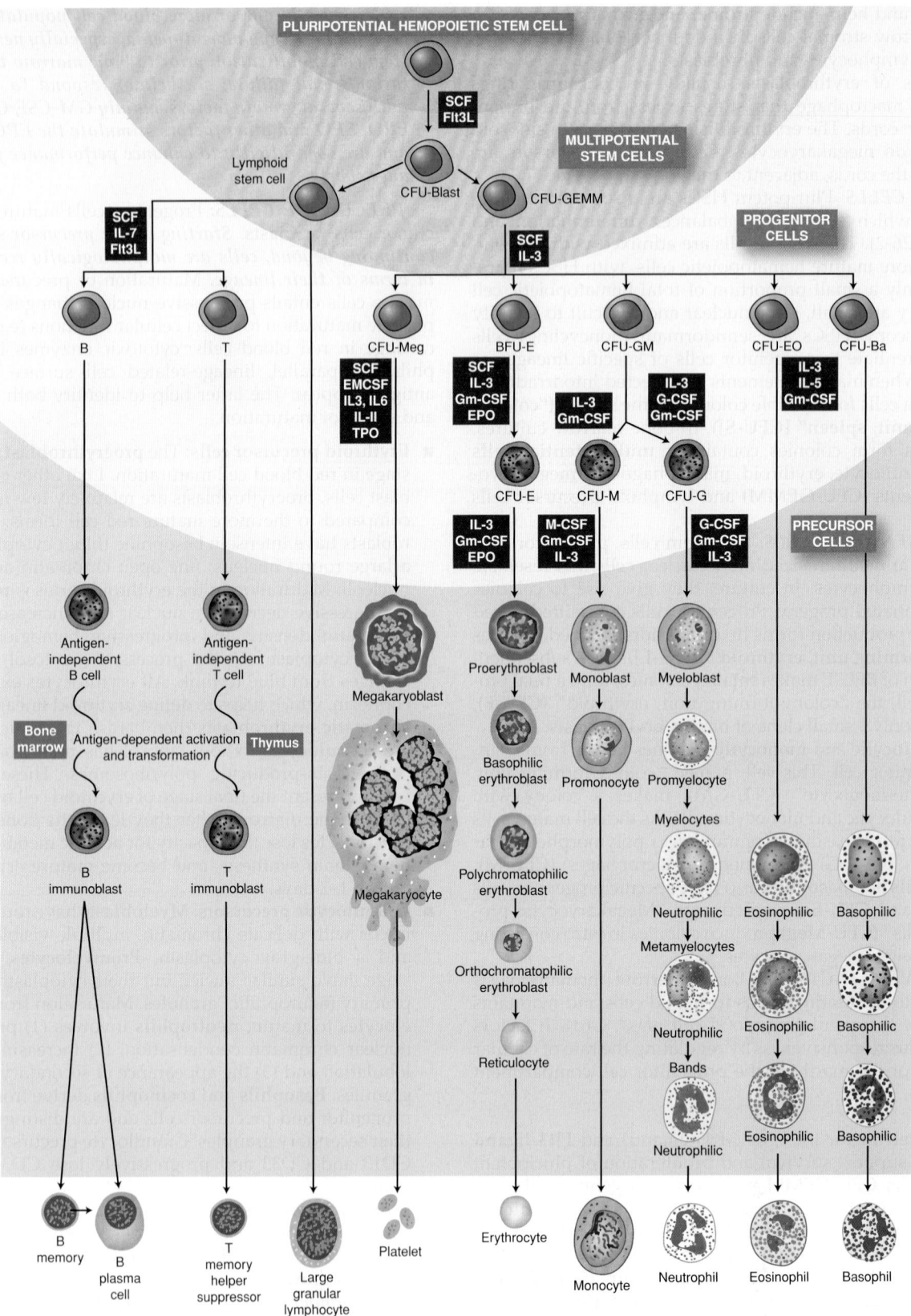

FIGURE 26-2. Cellular differentiation and maturation of the lymphoid and myeloid components of the hematopoietic system. Only the precursor cells (blasts and maturing cells) are identifiable by light microscopic evaluation of the bone marrow. *BFU* = burst-forming unit; *CFU* = colony-forming unit (*Ba* = basophils; *E* = erythroid; *Eo* = eosinophils; *G* = polymorphonuclear leukocytes; *GM* = granulocyte-monocyte; *M* = monocyte/macrophages; *Meg* = megakaryocytic); *EPO* = erythropoietin; *GM-CSF* = granulocyte-macrophage colony-stimulating factor; *IL* = interleukin; *NK* = natural killer; *SCF* = stem cell factor; *TPO* = thrombopoietin.

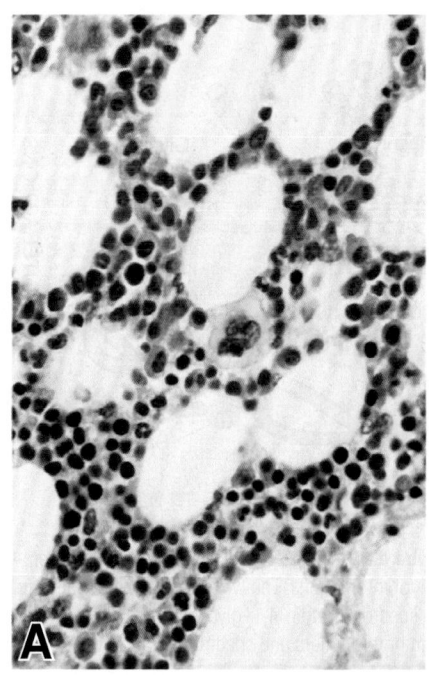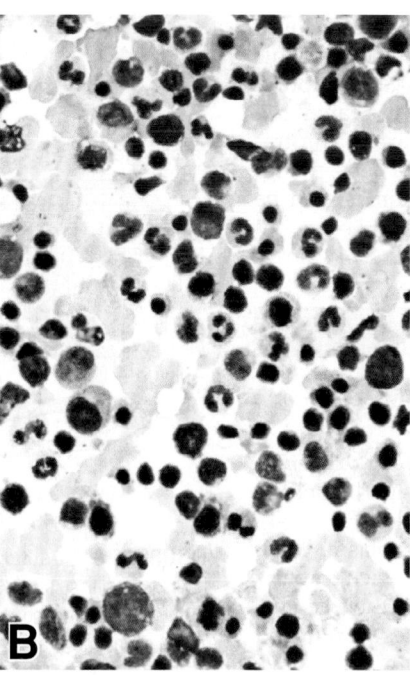

FIGURE 26-3. Normal bone marrow. A. Tissue section showing the normal relationship of cellular hematopoietic elements to fat cells, a normal myeloid-to-erythroid ratio (2:1) and a megakaryocyte in the center of the field (hematoxylin and eosin stain). **B.** Bone marrow aspirate smear from the same patient demonstrating normal hematopoietic elements in varying stages of differentiation (Wright-Giemsa stain).

stippled and azurophilic, eventually to be released into the sinusoids as long, platelet-containing ribbons. Some intact megakaryocytes are also released, and platelet production occurs after they localize in the pulmonary microcirculation.

RELEASE FROM THE MARROW: After they mature, hematopoietic cells leave the bone marrow through the sinusoids and enter the blood (Figs. 26-1 and 26-2). *Hematopoietic homeostasis is highly regulated by cell-cell interactions in the bone marrow and/or by both stimulatory and inhibitory cytokines.* The cellular release mechanism in the bone marrow responds to the needs of the peripheral circulation and can quickly provide a boost of mature cells in an emergency (e.g., red blood cells and/or reticulocytes during acute hemorrhage or neutrophils in acute infection).

Biopsy and Aspirate Smear Allow Complementary Analyses of Bone Marrow

The posterior iliac crest (or, rarely, the sternum) is the most common source of bone marrow for analysis in adults. In infants, the anterior tibia may also be used. Bone marrow core biopsy sections allow evaluation of the amount of hematopoietic elements and marrow architecture (Fig. 26-3A), while the several bone marrow cell lineages are identified and evaluated in stained smears made from aspirated liquid bone marrow (Fig. 26-3B). The ratio of hematopoietic cells to fat is the **cellularity,** which varies with age. In a normal middle-aged adult, about half of bone marrow core biopsy volume is adipocytes; the other half is actively dividing and differentiating hematopoietic cells. Marrow cellularity is higher in children and lower in the elderly.

Bone marrow cellularity mostly consists of maturing granulocyte precursors, erythroid precursors and megakaryocytes, called **trilineage hematopoiesis.** The ratio of myeloid to erythroid cells (i.e., the **M:E ratio**) is normally 2:1 to 5:1 (Table 26-1). There are usually 2–5 megakaryocytes per high-power field. Monocytic cells, lymphocytes and plasma cells are normally present in low numbers. Normal bone marrow has less than 3% plasma cells, up to 20% lymphocytes and only rare mast cells and macrophages. Blasts are usually less than 3% of marrow cells in normal adults.

Changes in the normal number and distribution of mature cells compared to immature cells are **left shifts**. These can occur in reactive and neoplastic processes. *The number of blasts in the bone marrow helps to distinguish these two broad categories, as reactive states do not significantly increase the numbers of blasts in the marrow.* In addition to evaluating cellularity and the proportions of the various cell types, bone marrow examination also enables assessment for evidence of normal maturation of hematopoietic precursors. *Dyssynchronization or aberration in the highly regulated process of nuclear and cytoplasmic maturation is evidence of bone marrow disease.*

TABLE 26-1
NORMAL ADULT BONE MARROW (AGE 18–70 YEARS)
Fat-to-cell ratio: 50:50 ± 15%
Myeloid-to-erythroid ratio: 2:1 to 5:1
Cell distribution (% surface area) 　Fat cells: 35%–65% 　Erythroid series: 10%–20% 　Granulocytic (myeloid) series: 40%–65%
Megakaryocytes: 2–5/high-power field
Plasma cells: <3% of nucleated cells
Lymphocytes: <20% of nucleated cells
No fibrosis

Iron metabolism and storage also can be tested by staining the bone marrow aspirate with Prussian blue. Using this stain, storage and sideroblastic iron granules can be found within the cytoplasm of macrophages and nucleated red blood cell precursors, respectively. Finally, marrow infiltration by abnormal cells, such as metastatic tumor cells, malignant hematopoietic cells or infectious granulomas, can be identified.

Red Blood Cells

NORMAL STRUCTURE AND FUNCTION

Red blood cells (RBCs), or erythrocytes, transport oxygen to tissues. Mature RBCs are nonnucleated 7- to 8-μm biconcave disks, similar in size to small lymphocyte nuclei (Fig. 26-4). They are round with reddish, eosinophilic cytoplasm. Their main cytoplasmic component is hemoglobin, which imparts the red color. Because they are biconcave disks, their centers tend to be paler than their outer rims. Erythrocytes are released from the marrow as reticulocytes, which are larger and have more diffusely basophilic gray cytoplasm than mature RBCs. These cells still synthesize hemoglobin, and the ribosomes needed for this process impart the **polychromatophilia**.

RBC membranes are attached to an underlying cytoskeletal network (Fig. 26-5). Transmembrane receptors, channels and anchors for other membrane components insert into the lipid bilayer, as does the underlying cytoskeleton. *Carbohydrate groups added to some membrane proteins lead to formation of different red cell antigen groups.* The erythrocyte cytoskeleton contains interconnected spectrin dimers and other stabilizing proteins (ankyrin, actin, band 4.1), which allow the cells to deform their shape, which may be necessary from time to time. *Changes in this membrane–cytoskeletal unit that lead to increased cell rigidity cause premature destruction of circulating RBCs.*

Hemoglobin accounts for the oxygen-carrying capacity of RBCs. Each hemoglobin molecule has 4 heme groups and 4 globin chains and, when fully saturated, transports 4 molecules of oxygen. The heme part of the molecule consists of a porphyrin ring (protoporphyrin IX), with one ferrous ion (Fe^{2+}). The globin portion of the molecule has pairs of two

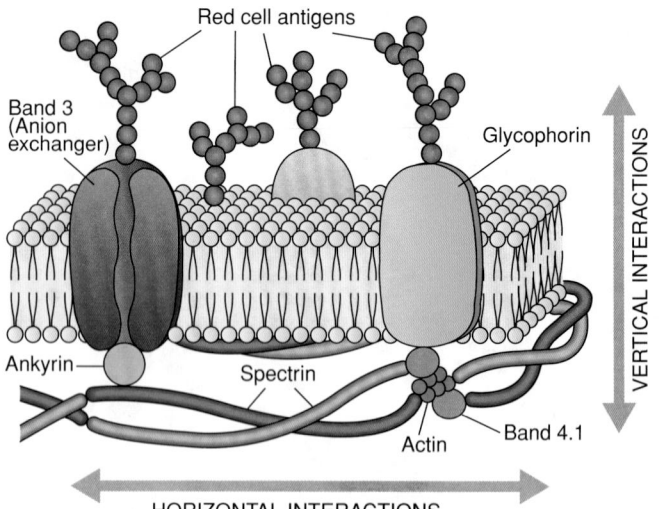

FIGURE 26-5. Structure of the erythrocyte plasma membrane. The membrane is stabilized by a number of interactions. The two vertical interactions are spectrin-ankyrin–band 3 and spectrin-protein 4.1–glycophorin. The two horizontal connections are spectrin heterodimers and spectrin-actin–protein 4.1.

different protein chains. The most abundant normal form, hemoglobin A, has two alpha (α)- and two beta (β)-globin chains. Hemoglobins F and A_2 are normally present in minor amounts in healthy adults. Both have two α-chains each. In addition, hemoglobin F has two gamma (γ)- and hemoglobin A_2 has two delta (δ)-globin chains, instead of β-globin chains. Synthesis and assembly of each hemoglobin molecule requires multiple biochemical steps that require distinct enzymes.

Each heme group interacts with a hydrophobic pocket of one globin chain, and the entire molecule has a globular tertiary structure. Deoxygenated hemoglobin has low oxygen affinity and requires increased oxygen tension for heme–oxygen binding to occur. After this initial interaction, hemoglobin molecules undergo conformational change, which facilitates subsequent oxygen binding to the remaining heme groups. Progressive increase in oxygen affinity is reflected in the sigmoid shape of the oxygen dissociation curve (Fig. 26-6).

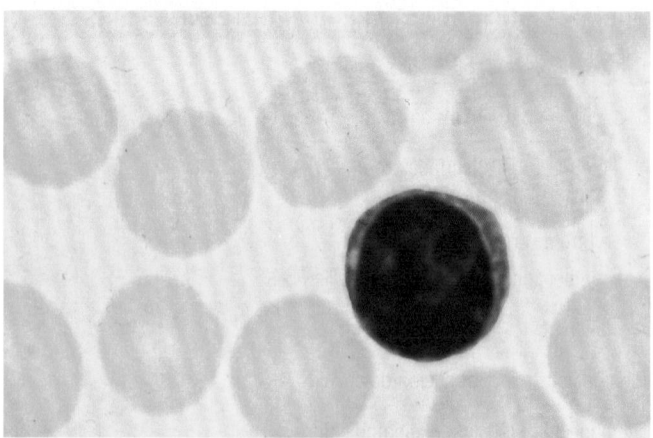

FIGURE 26-4. Normal red blood cells are approximately the same size as the nucleus of a small lymphocyte (approximately 7 μm).

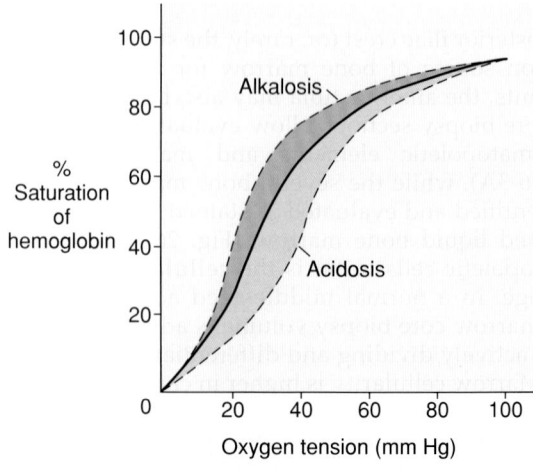

FIGURE 26-6. Oxygen dissociation curve of hemoglobin. With decreasing pH (acidosis), the oxygen affinity declines (shifts right); with increasing pH (alkalosis), the affinity increases (shifts left).

TABLE 26-2
COMPLETE BLOOD COUNT (CBC): NORMAL ADULT VALUES

Erythrocytes

Hemoglobin	Male, 14–18 g/dL
	Female, 12–16 g/dL
Hematocrit	Male, 40%–54%
	Female, 35%–47%
Red blood cell (RBC) count	Male, $4.5–6 \times 10^6/\mu L$
	Female, $4–5.5 \times 10^6/\mu L$
Reticulocytes	0.5%–2.5%
Indices	
Mean corpuscular volume	82–100 μm^3
Mean corpuscular hemoglobin	27–34 pg
Mean corpuscular hemoglobin concentration	32%–36%

	Absolute Count/µL	Differential Count (%)
Leukocytes		
White blood cells (WBCs)	4000–11,000	
Neutrophil granulocytes	1800–7000	50–60
Neutrophil bands	0–700	2–4
Lymphocytes	1500–4000	30–40
Monocytes	0–800	1–9
Basophils	0–200	0–1
Eosinophils	0–450	0–3

Platelets

Quantitative normal value: 150,000–400,000/µL

Qualitative estimation on smear: Number of platelets/oil immersion field × 10,000 = estimated platelet count

Normal ratio of RBC to platelets = 15:1 to 20:1

Acidosis shifts the slope of the oxygen dissociation curve to the right, which increases tissue oxygen delivery. Increased 2,3-diphosphoglycerate (2,3-DPG) (a product of an alternate pathway of glycolysis) has the same effect. Alkalosis shifts the curve to the left, increasing oxygen binding.

The average life span of blood erythrocytes is 120 days. Changes in membrane proteins and phospholipids appear in aged red cells and are likely signals for erythrocyte removal by mononuclear phagocytes.

The erythroid component of the blood is best analyzed by a complete blood count (CBC) plus microscopic examination of a blood smear (Table 26-2). The CBC measures hemoglobin (Hgb), RBC count and mean corpuscular volume (MCV). Additional calculated parameters include **hematocrit** (Hct = MCV × RBC), **mean corpuscular hemoglobin** (MCH = Hgb/RBC) and **mean corpuscular hemoglobin concentration** (MCHC = Hgb/Hct). Variability in RBC size, or red cell distribution width (RDW), is also derived. Reticulocytes can be accurately quantitated using supravital dyes that stain their cytoplasmic ribosome aggregates.

ANEMIA

Anemia is reduced circulating erythrocyte mass and is diagnosed as low hemoglobin, hematocrit (Hct) or RBC count. Anemia leads to decreased oxygen transport by the blood and ultimately tissue hypoxia.

Anemias Are Classified by Morphology or Pathophysiology

Morphologic classification of anemia is based on RBC appearance, as defined by automated blood counters and microscopy. RBC size (generally measured by analyzers) is reflected in the MCV, which divides anemias into three groups: (1) **microcytic** (decreased MCV), (2) **normocytic** and (3) **macrocytic** (increased MCV) (Table 26-3). Abnormally shaped RBCs **(poikilocytes)** are seen on blood smears in many anemias, and poikilocyte characteristics can aid in diagnosis (Fig. 26-7).

Pathophysiologic classification of anemia includes 4 groups (Table 26-4):

1. **Acute blood loss**
2. **Decreased production** of red cells by the bone marrow, either by **stem cell or progenitor cell defects**
3. **Ineffective hematopoiesis** with reduced release of erythrocytes from marrow
4. **Increased RBC destruction** outside the marrow, either **intracorpuscular** or **extracorpuscular**

In anemias with increased RBC destruction, circulating reticulocytes are elevated **(reticulocytosis)** as a response to hypoxia. This is different from the other groups.

TABLE 26-3
MORPHOLOGIC CLASSIFICATION OF ANEMIA

Macrocytic

Nutritional deficiency	Hypothyroidism
Alcohol use	Reticulocytosis
Liver disease	Primary bone marrow disease

Microcytic

Iron deficiency
Thalassemias
Sideroblastic

Normocytic

Anemia of chronic disease/inflammation
Anemia of renal disease
Acute blood loss

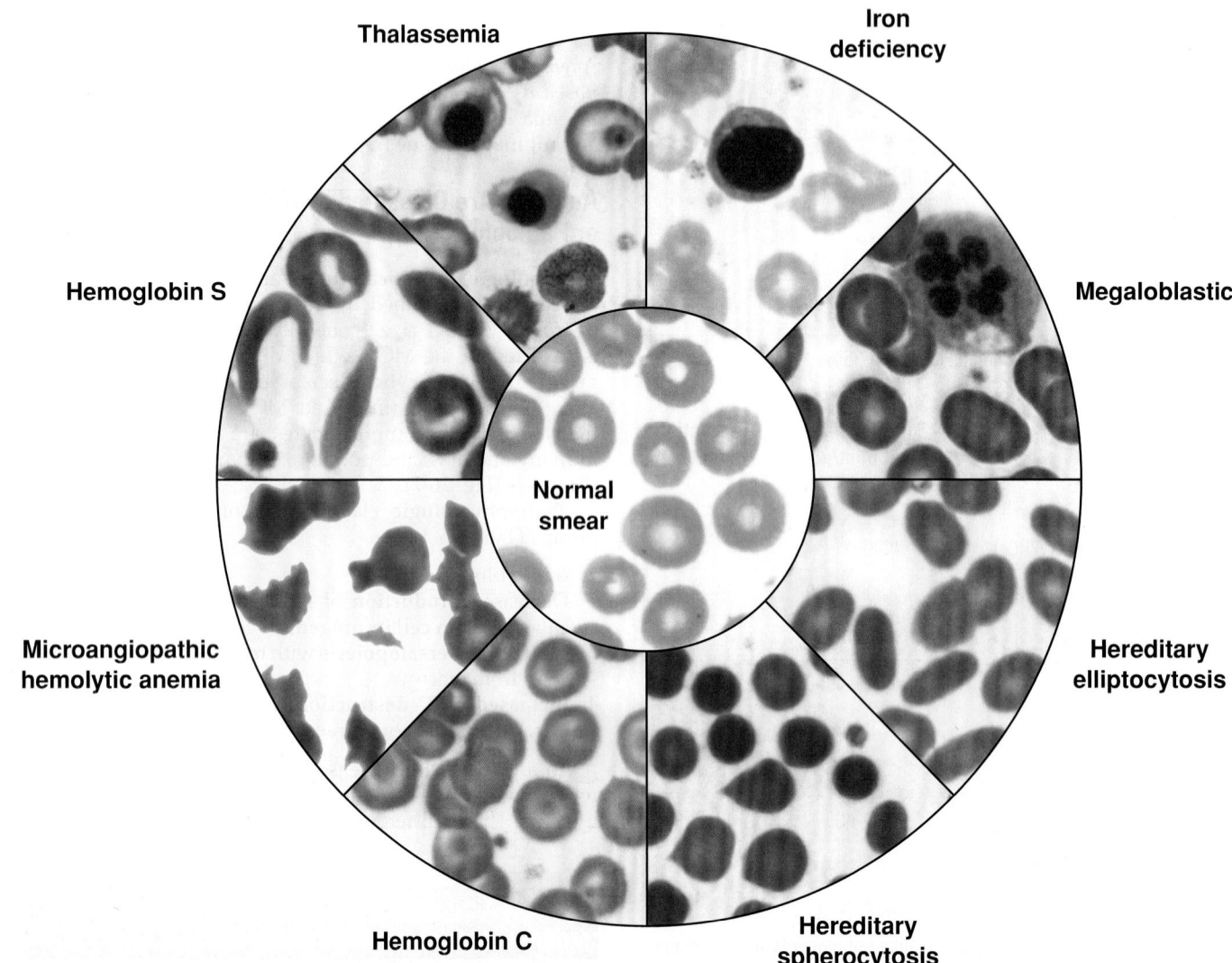

FIGURE 26-7. Abnormal red blood cell morphologies associated with various types of anemia. The morphology of normal erythrocytes is shown in the center. **Clockwise from 12:00:A. Iron deficiency (disturbance in hemoglobin synthesis; lack of iron):** Hypochromic, microcytic erythrocytes. A small lymphocyte is present for comparison. **B. Megaloblastic anemia (disturbance in DNA synthesis, most often caused by deficiency of vitamin B$_{12}$ or folic acid):** Oval macrocytes, some irregularly shaped cells and hypersegmented neutrophils. **C. Hereditary elliptocytosis (membrane defect):** Elliptocytes. **D. Hereditary spherocytosis (membrane defect):** Spherocytes lacking central pallor. **E. Hemoglobin C disease (abnormal globin chain):** Target cells. **F. Microangiopathic hemolysis (mechanical damage to erythrocytes;** disseminated intravascular coagulation [DIC], thrombocytic thrombocytopenic purpura [TTP], heart valve prosthesis sequela): Schistocytes/fragments. **G. Sickle cell (hemoglobin S) disease (abnormal globin chain):** Sickle cells. **H. Thalassemia (disturbance in hemoglobin synthesis):** Hypochromic, microcytic erythrocytes; poikilocytosis; basophilic stippling; target cells, nucleated red blood cells (RBCs).

TABLE 26-4	
PATHOPHYSIOLOGIC CLASSIFICATION OF ANEMIA	
Acute Blood Loss	
Decreased Production	
Stem Cell and Progenitor Cell Defects	
Iron deficiency	Leukemia
Anemia of chronic disease	Myelodysplastic syndromes
Aplastic anemia	Marrow infiltration
Pure red cell aplasia	Lead poisoning
Paroxysmal nocturnal hemoglobinuria	Anemia of renal disease
Ineffective Hematopoiesis	
Megaloblastic anemia	Thalassemia
Myelodysplastic syndromes	
Increased Destruction	
Intracorpuscular	
Membrane defect	Hemoglobinopathies
Enzyme defect	
Extracorpuscular	
Immunologic	
Autoimmune	Alloimmune
Nonimmunologic	
Mechanical	Infectious
Hypersplenism	Chemical

 CLINICAL FEATURES: In the face of anemia, there are several compensatory mechanisms to enhance oxygen delivery to tissues:

- Increased cardiac output
- Increased respiratory rate
- Shunting of blood flow to provide increased tissue perfusion of vital organs
- Decreased hemoglobin–oxygen affinity
- Increased marrow erythrocyte production due to EPO stimulation

Clinical signs and symptoms (tachycardia, shortness of breath, systolic murmurs) may reflect these compensatory processes. If anemia is severe (i.e., hemoglobin <7 g/dL), tissue hypoxia is uncompensated and additional clinical findings may include easy fatigability, faintness, angina and dyspnea on exertion.

Acute Blood Loss Leads to Normocytic Normochromic Anemia

Acute anemia reflects blood loss from the intravascular compartment.

 PATHOLOGY AND CLINICAL FEATURES: Initial signs of acute blood loss reflect volume depletion and decreased tissue perfusion. Since whole blood is lost, the severity of the anemia may not be appreciated at first. Within 24–48 hours after significant hemorrhage, however, fluid is mobilized from extravascular locations into the intravascular space to restore overall blood volume. This is when the extent of the anemia becomes apparent, since red cell replacement is not as rapid. If the underlying bleeding is stopped, EPO-driven bone marrow erythroid hyperplasia will gradually correct the anemia. The blood smear shows no specific abnormalities, but polychromasia occurs during the recovery phase.

Decreased Red Blood Cell Production Often Reflects Impaired Erythrocyte Precursor Development

Some disorders in which RBC production is decreased are inherited or acquired diseases of hematopoietic stem cells or of their committed derivatives. These are discussed below under HSC diseases.

Iron-Deficiency Anemia

Iron deficiency interferes with normal heme (hemoglobin) synthesis and leads to impaired erythropoiesis and anemia. Iron deficiency is the most common cause of anemia worldwide.

 **ETIOLOGIC FACTORS:** The normal Western adult diet contains about 20 mg of iron, 1–2 mg of which is absorbed by the duodenum and proximal jejunum (see Chapter 20). The rate of iron absorption is regulated by normal losses, but anemia (especially with ineffective erythropoiesis) triggers increased intestinal absorption and may ultimately lead to iron overload. About 85% of absorbed iron is transported by a carrier protein, transferrin, to be incorporated into developing red cells via transferrin receptors on their surface. As senescent red cells are removed from circulation, hemoglobin is broken down into its components, and iron is recycled. Excess iron is stored as **hemosiderin** and **ferritin**. Hemosiderin is large aggregates of iron with a disorganized structure; ferritin is complexed with protein (apoferritin) and appears highly organized.

Many underlying conditions cause iron deficiency. In infants and children, dietary iron may be insufficient for growth and development. Iron need also increases during **pregnancy** and **lactation**. In adults, iron deficiency typically results from **chronic blood loss** or, less often, **intravascular hemolysis.** Two milliliters of whole blood contains 1 mg of iron, which is lost with bleeding. In women of reproductive age, **gynecologic blood loss** (menstruation, parturition, vaginal bleeding) is most common. In postmenopausal women and men, unexplained iron deficiency should prompt a search for gastrointestinal **tumors** or **vascular lesions,** as this is the most common site of chronic blood loss.

 PATHOLOGY: Iron deficiency causes a microcytic, hypochromic anemia (Fig. 26-8). Variation in RBC size (**anisocytosis**) and shape (**poikilocytosis**) is reflected in increased RDW. **Ovalocytes** may be found; some of these are very thin and are called **pencil cells.** Iron

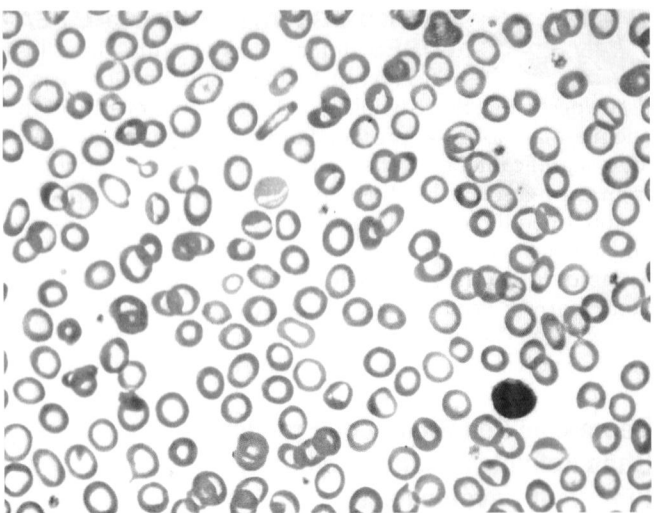

FIGURE 26-8. Microcytic hypochromic anemia caused by iron deficiency. Red blood cells (RBCs) are significantly smaller than the nucleus of a small lymphocyte, and they have increased central pallor (normal central pallor is about one third of the RBC diameter).

deficiency causes an RBC production defect, so marrow erythroid hyperplasia occurs but blood reticulocytosis does not. Prussian blue staining shows that iron storage and erythroid iron are absent.

Serum iron and ferritin levels are low in iron deficiency, while total iron-binding capacity (TIBC) is increased (because of increased serum transferrin levels). As a result, transferrin saturation is conspicuously lowered (often <5%).

 CLINICAL FEATURES: The symptoms of iron deficiency are those of anemia in general. With advanced disease, a smooth and glistening tongue **(atrophic glossitis)** and inflammation at the corners of the mouth **(angular stomatitis)** may occur, as may a spoon-shaped deformity of the fingernails **(koilonychia)**. Treatment requires correcting the source of chronic blood loss and oral or parenteral iron supplementation.

Anemia of Chronic Disease

Anemia of chronic disease occurs in chronic inflammatory and malignant conditions.

PATHOPHYSIOLOGY: Chronic disease causes ineffective use of iron from macrophage stores in bone marrow. This results in a functional iron deficiency, even though iron stores may be normal or even increased. Other factors that may contribute to anemia are shorter RBC life span, blunted renal EPO response to tissue hypoxia and poor bone marrow response to erythropoietin. Inflammatory cytokines (lactoferrin, IL-1, tumor necrosis factor-α [TNF-α] and interferon) may inhibit iron mobilization.

 **PATHOLOGY:** Anemia of chronic disease is mild to moderate; red cells are often normocytic and normochromic, but can be microcytic. In marrow

aspirates, Prussian blue shows normal or increased iron in macrophages, but reduced erythroid iron. Serum iron levels tend to be low. However, unlike iron-deficiency anemia, TIBC also tends to be decreased (as is serum albumin). Reticulocyte counts are not appropriately increased for the degree of anemia. Successful treatment of the underlying disease restores normal hemoglobin levels.

Anemia of Renal Disease

 PATHOPHYSIOLOGY: In some patients with chronic renal diseases, **decreased renal production of EPO** leads to anemia. The severity of anemia is proportional to the extent of renal insufficiency. Administration of recombinant EPO is the treatment of choice. A "uremic toxin," which suppresses erythroid precursors, and a minor hemolytic component may contribute to the anemia of chronic renal disease.

 **PATHOLOGY:** Anemia of chronic renal disease is normocytic and normochromic. Erythrocytes with scalloped cell membranes may sometimes be seen **(Burr cells)**. If the renal insufficiency is due to malignant hypertension, red cells may be fragmented and form schistocytes.

Anemia Associated with Marrow Infiltration (Myelophthisic Anemia)

Myelophthisic anemia is a hypoproliferative anemia associated with marrow infiltration.

 ETIOLOGIC FACTORS: Any infiltrative process (e.g., myelofibrosis, hematologic malignancies, metastatic carcinoma or granulomatous disease) may replace normal hematopoietic elements and cause anemia (and often leukopenia and thrombocytopenia). In an attempt to maintain blood cell production, extramedullary hematopoiesis may develop, mostly in the spleen and liver.

PATHOLOGY: Bone marrow infiltration causes moderate to severe normocytic anemia, with aniso-poikilocytosis and teardrop cells. Circulating immature granulocytes and nucleated erythrocytes **(leukoerythroblastosis)** are common.

Anemia of Lead Poisoning

Lead poisoning results in anemia by interfering with several enzymes involved in heme synthesis (see Chapter 8).

In Ineffective Red Cell Production, There Are Fewer Circulating Erythrocytes

Various anemias reflect abnormal erythrocyte production caused by ineffective hematopoiesis. In these cases, the bone marrow erythrocyte precursor pool is expanded. Thus, sufficient erythroid precursors are formed in the bone marrow, but erythrocytes do not enter the circulation.

Megaloblastic Anemias

Megaloblastic anemias are caused by impaired DNA synthesis, usually because of vitamin B$_{12}$ or folic acid deficiency.

  **PATHOPHYSIOLOGY AND ETIOLOGIC FACTORS:** Megaloblastic anemia defines a group of diseases characterized by hallmark megaloblasts. Impaired DNA synthesis leads to abnormal nuclear maturation. This in turn leads to ineffective erythrocyte maturation and anemia. All proliferating cell types, including myeloid precursors, and cervical and gastrointestinal mucosal cells are affected.

Megaloblastic anemia is most commonly due to B$_{12}$ or folate deficiency. Some chemotherapeutic agents (methotrexate, hydroxyurea) or antiretroviral drugs (5-azacytidine) may also be responsible. Inherited defects in purine or pyrimidine metabolism may rarely be involved.

Folate and B$_{12}$ are critical for normal DNA synthesis. Tetrahydrofolate is converted from methyl tetrahydrofolate by methyltransferase, with vitamin B$_{12}$ as a cofactor. Vitamin B$_{12}$ is also required for converting homocysteine to methionine. Using tetrahydrofolate as a cofactor, thymidylate synthetase converts uridylate to thymidylate (Fig. 26-9). Dihydrofolate reductase restores tetrahydrofolate.

With impaired DNA synthesis, nuclear development is delayed, but the cytoplasm matures normally. This leads to **nuclear-to-cytoplasmic asynchrony** and results in formation of large nucleated erythrocyte precursors **(megaloblasts)**. Since these megaloblasts do not mature enough to be released into the blood, they undergo intramedullary destruction. Released erythrocytes are macrocytic.

Vitamin B$_{12}$ (cyanocobalamin) cannot be synthesized by humans and must come from diet. It occurs in a variety of animal food sources and is produced by intestinal microorganisms. Proper vitamin B$_{12}$ absorption requires intrinsic factor, which is in the stomach (see Chapter 19) and protects vitamin B$_{12}$ from degradation by intestinal enzymes (Fig. 26-10). The intrinsic factor–vitamin B$_{12}$ complex is absorbed in the distal ileum via specific receptors. In the blood, the vitamin is transported by a group of proteins called **transcobalamins,** of which transcobalamin II is the most important. The daily usage of vitamin B$_{12}$ is 1 μg. Therefore, normal body stores of 1000–5000 μg provide several years of reserve.

Inadequate dietary intake of vitamin B$_{12}$ is rare and usually occurs only in strict vegetarians (vegans). *Most often, lack of intrinsic factor impairs its absorption.* Surgery that resects the gastric fundus removes the source of intrinsic factor.

Pernicious anemia, an autoimmune disorder in which patients develop antibodies against parietal cells and intrinsic factor (see Chapter 19), leads to intrinsic factor deficiency. Antiparietal cell antibodies also cause atrophic gastritis with achlorhydria. Primary intestinal disorders (inflammatory bowel disease) or previous intestinal surgery (ileal bypass) can impair vitamin B$_{12}$ absorption. Microbiologic competition (e.g., from bacterial overgrowth of a blind loop or infestation by a fish tapeworm, *Diphyllobothrium latum*) may lead to vitamin B$_{12}$ deficiency.

Folic acid is present in leafy vegetables, meat and eggs. Dietary folic acid exists in a polyglutamate form but

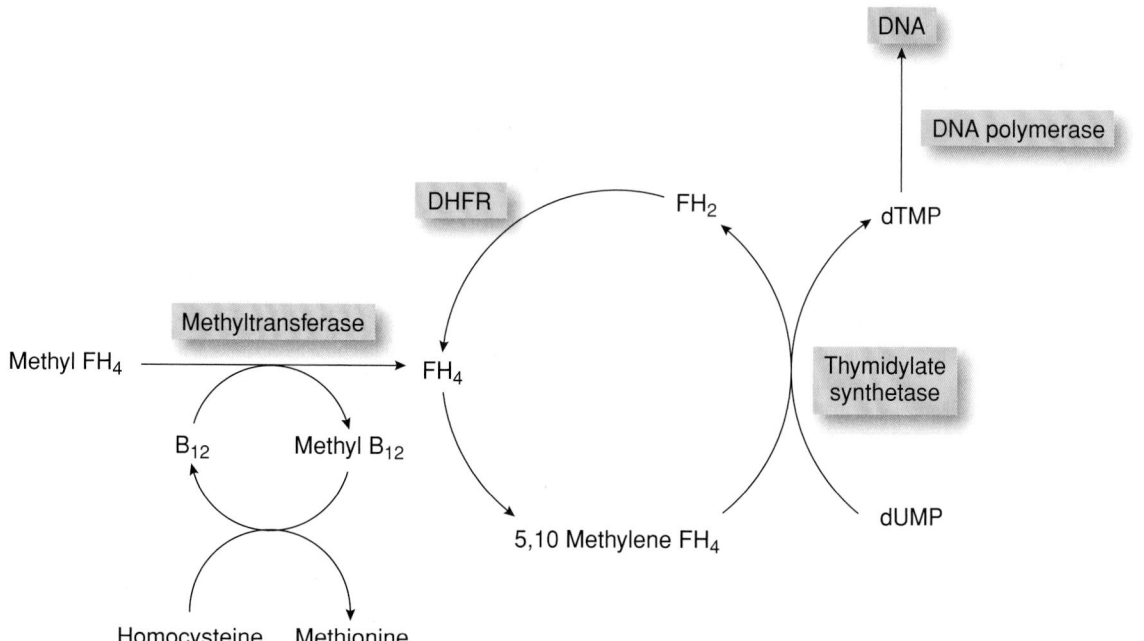

FIGURE 26-9. Relationship of folic acid to vitamin B$_{12}$. A 1-carbon transfer mediated by folic acid methylates dUMP to dTMP, which is then used for the synthesis of DNA. To enter this cycle, folate (methyl FH$_4$) is demethylated to FH$_4$, vitamin B$_{12}$ acting as the cofactor. Thus, both vitamin B$_{12}$ and folic acid deficiencies lead to impaired DNA synthesis and megaloblastic anemia. *DHFR* = dihydrofolate reductase; *dTMP* = deoxythymidine monophosphate; *dUMP* = deoxyuridine monophosphate; *FH$_2$* = dihydrofolate; *FH$_4$* = tetrahydrofolate.

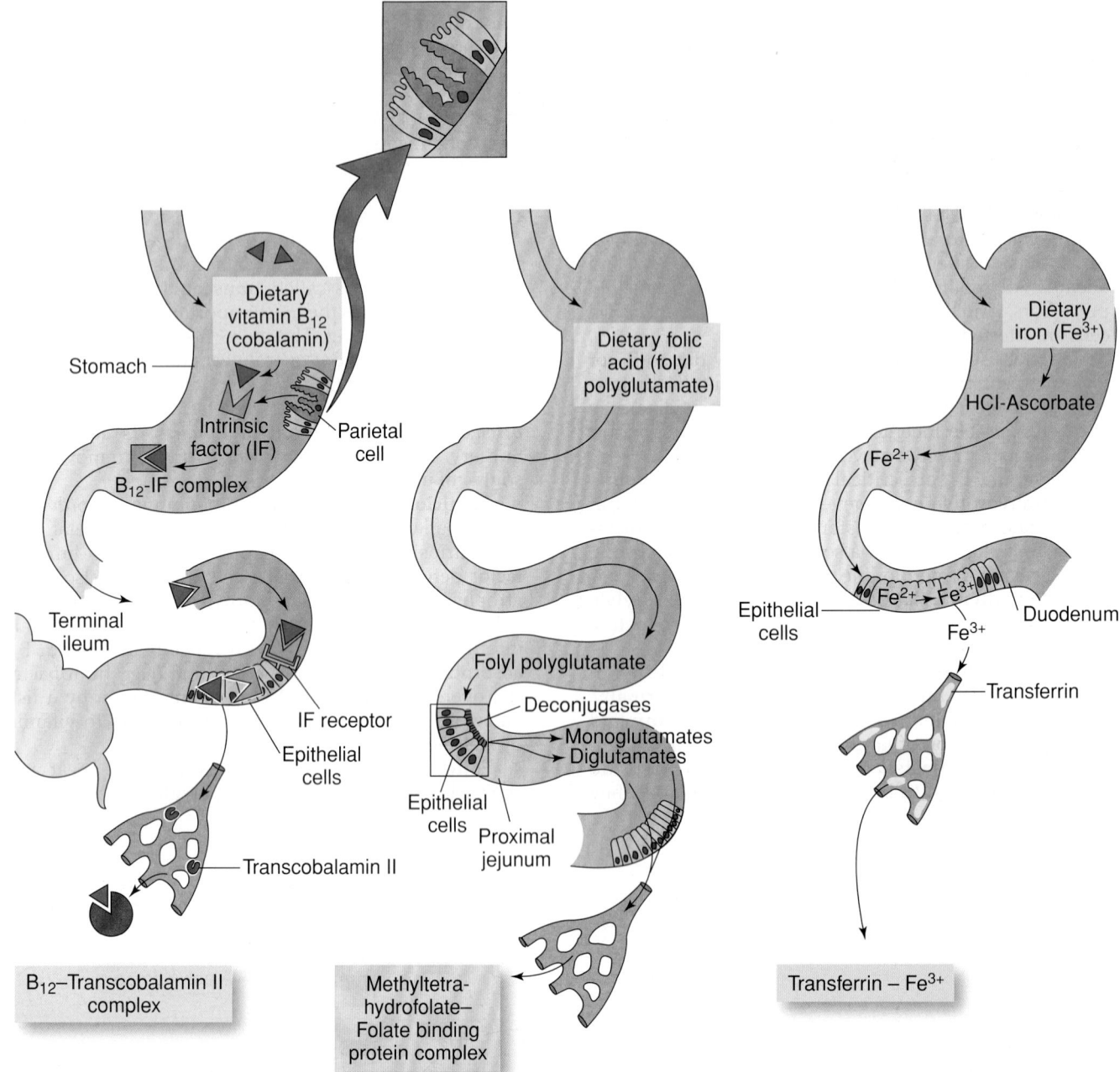

FIGURE 26-10. **Absorption of vitamin B$_{12}$,** folic acid and iron. Absorption of vitamin B$_{12}$ requires initial complexing with intrinsic factor (IF), which is produced by the parietal cells of the gastric mucosa. Absorption then occurs in the terminal ileum, where there are receptors for the IF–B$_{12}$ complex. Dietary folic acid is conjugated by conjugase enzymes to polyglutamate. Absorption occurs in the jejunum following deconjugation in the intestinal lumen. Reduction and methylation result in the generation of methyl tetrahydrofolate, which is then transported by folate-binding protein. Dietary ferric iron (Fe^{3+}) is reduced to ferrous iron (Fe^{2+}) in the stomach and absorbed principally in the duodenum. Iron is transported by transferrin in the circulation.

is deconjugated to monoglutamates in the intestines and absorbed primarily in the jejunum. Folate is then reduced and methylated to 5-methyl tetrahydrofolate, which is transported in the blood by folate-binding protein. The daily requirement for folate is about 50 µg. Body stores of folate average 2000–5000 µg, providing a few months' reserve before signs of deficiency develop.

The most common cause of folic acid deficiency is inadequate dietary intake. This occurs mostly in patients with poorly balanced diets (alcoholics, recluses). Demand for folic acid is increased in pregnancy, lactation, periods of rapid growth and chronic hemolytic disease. During these times, folate deficiency may occur unless folate supplementation is provided. Primary intestinal diseases (inflammatory bowel disease, sprue) may interfere with folic acid absorption. Various medications can also impair folic acid absorption (phenytoin) or metabolism (methotrexate).

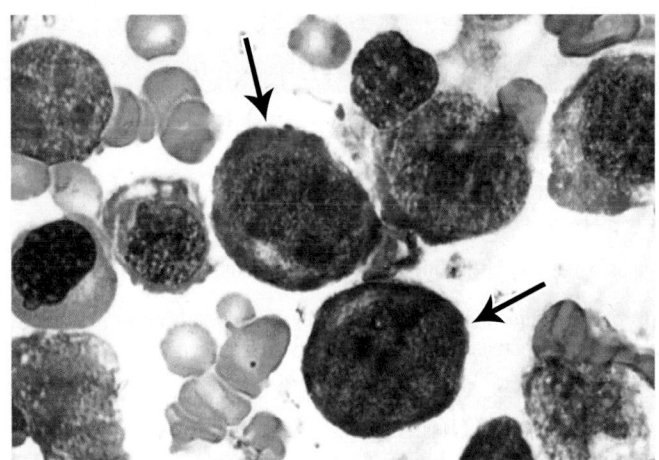

FIGURE 26-11. Megaloblastic anemia. A bone marrow aspirate from a patient with vitamin B_{12} deficiency (pernicious anemia) shows prominent megaloblastic erythroid precursors (*arrows*).

 PATHOLOGY: The hematologic manifestations of both folic acid and vitamin B_{12} deficiency are identical. Hematopoiesis in the bone marrow tends to be increased, but the marrow releases insufficient mature, functional cells because of increased intramedullary cell death. This is called **ineffective hematopoiesis**. RBC precursors show megaloblastic maturation, in which cells enlarge but the cytoplasm matures while the nucleus lags (Fig. 26-11). The myeloid series shows similar dyssynchrony, with giant bands and metamyelocytes, and hypersegmented nuclei in mature granulocytes. The megakaryocytes may also be large.

The magnitude of the anemia varies but may be severe. Erythrocytes are macrocytic and may be oval (oval macrocytes). Anisopoikilocytosis is usually prominent, sometimes with teardrop cells. Circulating neutrophils often show nuclear hypersegmentation (>5 lobes) (Fig. 26-12). Reticulocytes are not increased.

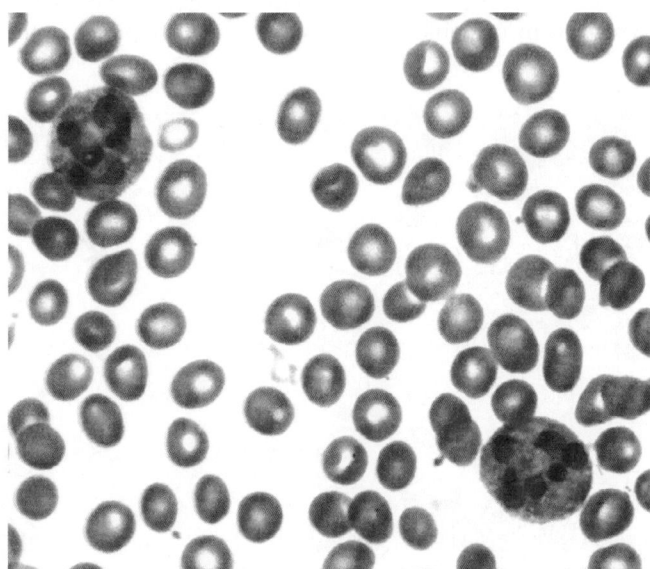

FIGURE 26-12. Hypersegmented granulocytes in a patient with vitamin B_{12} deficiency.

Folate and vitamin B_{12} deficiencies are usually distinguished by measuring serum levels of these vitamins. Occasionally, specific measurement of red cell folate provides more useful information than serum analyses. Because of massive intramedullary destruction of red cell precursors, serum levels of lactate dehydrogenase (LDH), especially isoenzyme 1, are conspicuously elevated.

The **Schilling test** can suggest the cause of B_{12} deficiency. It measures radiolabeled vitamin B_{12} absorption, with or without intrinsic factor. Urinary B_{12} is measured. However, this test is not commonly used. Elevated levels of homocysteine and methyl malonic acid may help diagnose vitamin B_{12} deficiency. Circulating antibodies against gastric parietal cells or intrinsic factor are present in cases of pernicious anemia. The former antibody is more often detected; the latter is more specific for pernicious anemia.

 **CLINICAL FEATURES:** The clinical presentation of megaloblastic anemia is similar, whether due to B_{12} or folate deficiency. In general, the latter develops more rapidly (months) than the former (years). The most important difference clinically is that B_{12} deficiency is complicated by neurologic symptoms, owing to posterior and lateral column demyelination in the spinal cord. This may cause sensory and motor deficiencies (see Chapters 8 and 32). Unless treated quickly, those neurologic symptoms may be irreversible. Folate deficiency involves no such complications.

Thalassemia

Thalassemias are congenital anemias caused by deficient globin chain synthesis. Depending on the affected globin chain, β-thalassemia (defective β-chain production), α-thalassemia (defective α-chain production) and δ/β-thalassemia result.

The basic defect is reduced or absent production of β-globin (in β-thalassemia) or α-globin (in α-thalassemia) chains. A minority of thalassemia cases have structural hemoglobin variants yielding unstable globins. Since α- and β-chains normally pair to form hemoglobin tetramers, the lack of one type of chain leads to unpaired normal globin chains in thalassemic erythrocytes. In β-thalassemia, the excess normal α-chains form an unstable structure that precipitates at the cell membrane. This makes the RBCs very fragile, so they are destroyed within the bone marrow. In α-thalassemia, β-chains are in excess (in extrauterine life). Resulting hemoglobin contains only β-chains. In intrauterine life, the excess of γ-chains yields a hemoglobin with only γ-chains. In both cases, there is excessive red blood cell destruction.

EPIDEMIOLOGY: Thalassemia is most common in the Mediterranean area, especially Italy and Greece. However, it has a wide distribution, particularly in areas where malaria has been endemic (Middle East, India, Southeast Asia, China). Heterozygosity for thalassemia may help protect against malaria and increase the reproductive potential of heterozygotes, which may explain how these diseases persist. In many geographic areas where thalassemia is common, other structural hemoglobin defects (e.g., hemoglobin S [HgbS]) are also frequent. This can lead to double heterozygosity (e.g., sickle thalassemia), which demonstrates features of both disorders.

TABLE 26-5

MAJOR FORMS OF HEMOGLOBIN AND THEIR CHAIN COMPOSITION

Type of Hemoglobin	Contribution of Globin Chains					Explanation
	α	β	γ	δ	ζ	
A	2	2				Principal normal hemoglobin (>95% of total) in postnatal life.
A₂	2			2		Usually <3% of total hemoglobin, but may be slightly increased in β-thalassemia.
F	2		2			Normal hemoglobin for most of intrauterine life. Production usually ends by early infancy; hemoglobin F is largely undetectable after 6 months of age. Persists in β-thalassemia.
H		4				Mainly seen in α-thalassemia, where deficiency of α-chains leads to hemoglobins composed of β-chain tetramers. Responsible for formation of Heinz bodies.
Bart's			4			Seen in babies with α-thalassemia. Heinz bodies seen.
Portland			2		2	Hemoglobin present very early in fetal life. May persist in very severe α-thalassemia.

There are 4 α genes, paired on each chromosome 16. Non-α genes are on chromosome 11, two γ, one δ and one β gene per chromosome. Embryonic globin genes zeta (ζ) (α equivalent) and epsilon (ε) (non-α equivalent) are on chromosomes 16 and 11. The most important different types of hemoglobin and the globin chains that contribute to each are presented in Table 26-5.

MOLECULAR PATHOGENESIS: Normal hemoglobin contains four globin chains: 2 α- and 2 non-α-chains. There are 3 normal hemoglobin variants, based on the nature of the non-α-chains (Fig. 26-13). *Adult hemoglobin is 95%–98% HgbA ($\alpha_2\beta_2$), plus small amounts of HgbF ($\alpha_2\gamma_2$) and A₂ ($\alpha_2\delta_2$).*

Thalassemias are generally classified by the affected globin chain. The two most clinically significant forms involve deficits of α- and β-chains. Thalassemias involving γ- and δ-globin chain synthesis occur but are not common.

β-Thalassemia

MOLECULAR PATHOGENESIS: β-Thalassemias are a heterogeneous group of disorders that are mostly caused by point mutations in the β-globin gene. Mutations may be in the gene's promoter region, a splice site or other coding regions, or may lead to creation of an inappropriate stop codon. The result is that transcription of the gene is entirely (β°) or partly (β⁺) suppressed. Occasionally, a mutation may also affect the adjacent δ-globin gene, leading to a β–δ-thalassemia.

PATHOLOGY AND CLINICAL FEATURES: Homozygous β-thalassemia (Cooley anemia) is characterized by moderate to severe, microcytic and hypochromic anemia (Figs. 26-14 and 26-15). There is a marked excess of α-chains, which form unstable tetramers (α_4) that precipitate in the

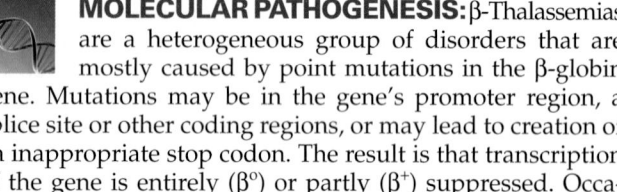
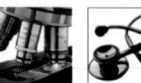
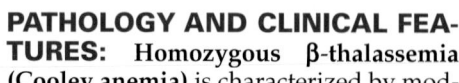

FIGURE 26-13. Hemoglobin assembly scheme using globin chains coded on chromosomes 11 and 16.

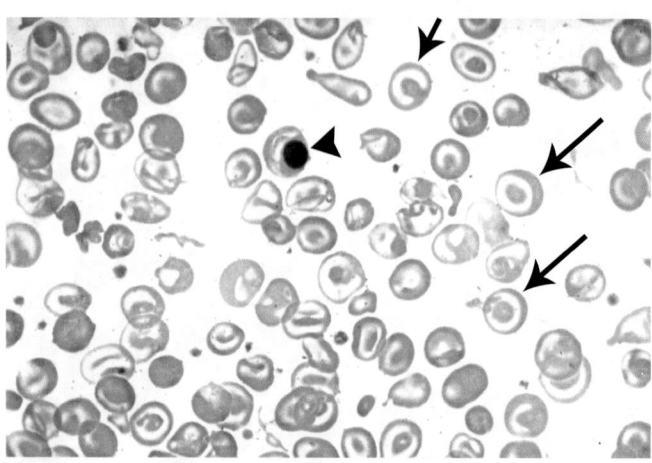

FIGURE 26-14. Thalassemia. The peripheral blood erythrocytes are hypochromic and microcytic and show anisopoikilocytosis with frequent target cells (*arrows*) and circulating nucleated red blood cells (*arrowhead*).

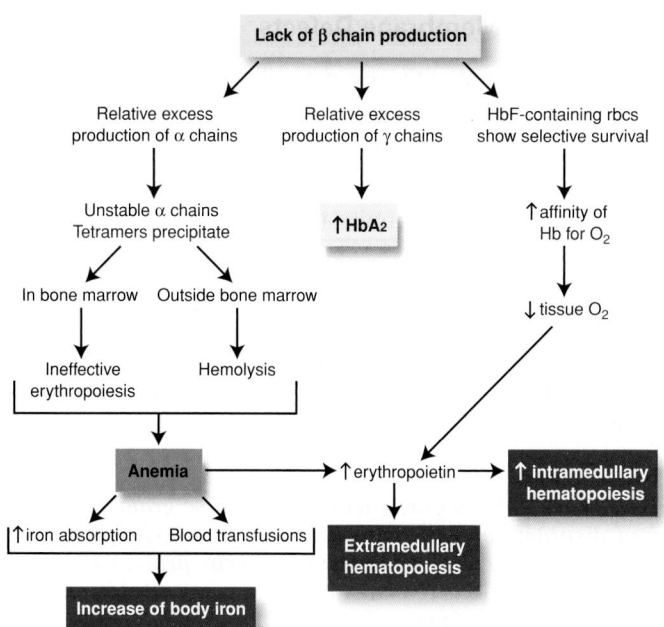

FIGURE 26-15. Pathogenesis of disease manifestations in β-thalassemia.

(especially after splenectomy). The increased oxygen affinity of HgbF, plus the underlying anemia, impairs oxygen delivery and elicits increased EPO. The latter causes marked bone marrow erythroid hyperplasia. The marrow space is expanded, causing facial and cranial bone deformities. Extramedullary hematopoiesis contributes to hepatosplenomegaly and may cause soft tissue masses.

Excess erythropoiesis stimulates iron absorption. This, together with repeated transfusions, causes iron overload. Excess iron deposition in tissues leads to morbidity and mortality in thalassemic patients and often requires aggressive chelation therapy.

Heterozygous β-thalassemia (heterozygous carrier of β-thalassemia) is associated with microcytosis and hypochromia. The degree of microcytosis is disproportionate to the severity of the anemia, which is generally mild or absent. Erythrocytosis (increased RBC count) with minimal anisocytosis (normal RDW) is common. Target cells, basophilic stippling, increased reticulocytes and a mild increase in HgbA₂ are present. Most patients are asymptomatic. Iron absorption is increased.

α-Thalassemia

MOLECULAR PATHOGENESIS: α-Thalassemias are most often due to gene deletions. More syndromes are clinically observed because of the potential number (up to four) of α-globin genes that may be affected. The genetics of the several α-thalassemias are illustrated in Fig. 26-16. α-Thalassemia is associated with excess β- or γ-chains, which can form the tetrameric HgbH (β_4) and Hgb Bart (γ_4). Hemoglobins H and Bart are both unstable and precipitate in the cytoplasm, forming Heinz bodies, but to a lesser degree than α_4 tetramers. Further, they have high oxygen affinities and cause decreased tissue oxygen delivery. The relative amount of these tetrameric hemoglobins depends on the number of α-genes involved and the patient's

cytoplasm of developing erythroid precursors. In the β⁰ type, most hemoglobin is fetal hemoglobin, although increased (5%–8%) HgbA₂ is also present. In the β₁ type, some HgbA may be present (depending on the nature of the underlying defect) and HgbA₂ is mildly increased. A modest increase in HgbA₂ is characteristic of all forms of β-thalassemia, as δ-globin genes are upregulated.

Blood smears show microcytosis, hypochromia and striking anisopoikilocytosis (uneven size and shape) with target cells, basophilic stippling and circulating normoblasts

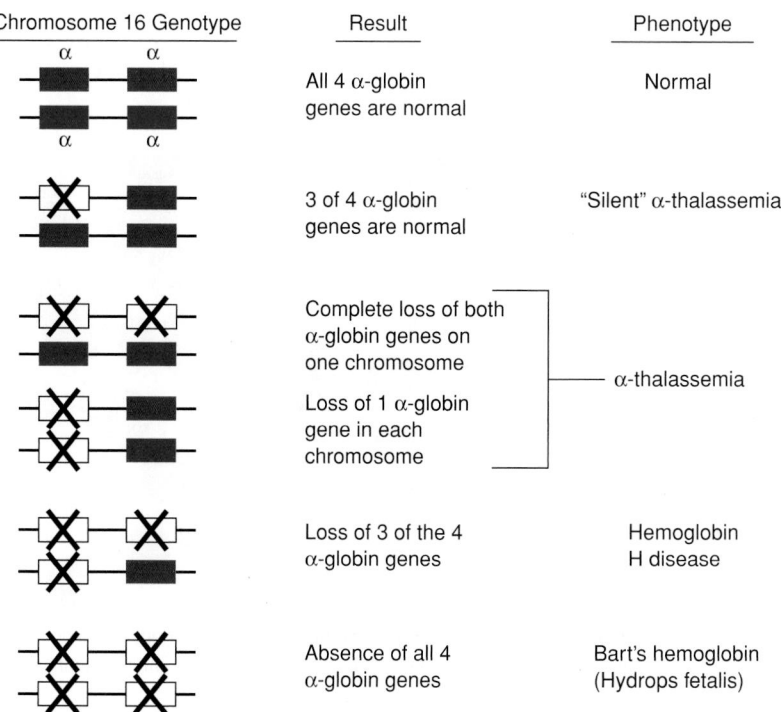

FIGURE 26-16. Genetics of α-globin deficiencies and their manifestations.

age. Because of the underlying impairment in hemoglobin synthesis, circulating red cells usually are microcytic and hypochromic.

PATHOLOGY AND CLINICAL FEATURES:

- **Silent carrier α-thalassemia** (one gene affected) is difficult to diagnose, because patients' only hematologic abnormality is small amounts of Hgb Bart, detectable only in infancy. There is no anemia; patients are asymptomatic.
- **α-Thalassemia trait** (two genes affected) is associated with a mild microcytic anemia. Like heterozygous β-thalassemia, the degree of microcytosis is disproportionately low compared to the degree of anemia. $HgbA_2$ is not increased, allowing distinction between α- and β-thalassemia traits. Up to 5% Hgb Bart can be seen during infancy.

 Two different genotypes are possible in heterozygous α-thalassemia. There may be a single gene deleted from each chromosome 16 or, alternatively, both genes may be deleted from the same chromosome 16. The former is more common in people of Mediterranean and African descent, while the latter occurs more often in Southeast Asia. Clinically, both genotypes present similarly, but homozygous α-thalassemia (see below) can only develop if both genes are deleted from the same chromosome.
- **Hemoglobin H disease** (3 genes affected) is associated with moderate microcytic anemia. Increased Hgb Bart (up to 25% in infancy) and variable levels of HgbH are seen. Both HgbH and Hgb Bart give characteristic patterns on hemoglobin electrophoresis, since they migrate faster than HgbA. Precipitated HgbH (Heinz bodies) also appears on supravital staining of blood smears.
- **Homozygous** (all 4 genes affected) **α-thalassemia,** also called α hydrops fetalis, is incompatible with life. Affected infants die in utero or shortly after birth with severe anemia, marked anisopoikilocytosis and large amounts of Hgb Bart. Severe impairment in tissue oxygen delivery is associated with heart failure and generalized edema. Massive hepatosplenomegaly is due to extramedullary hematopoiesis. A woman carrying a fetus with Hgb Bart has increased risk for obstetric complications, including eclampsia and postpartum bleeding.

Hemolytic Anemias Result from Increased Red Cell Destruction

Hemolysis (i.e., premature elimination of circulating RBCs) causes **hemolytic anemia**. These anemias are classified by the site of red cell destruction. In **extravascular hemolysis,** the monocyte/macrophage system in the spleen and, to a lesser extent, the liver is involved. In **intravascular hemolysis,** RBCs are destroyed while circulating.

 Hemolytic anemias are characterized by a compensatory increase in red cell production and release. In the blood, this manifests as red cell polychromasia because of increased reticulocytes. Other laboratory findings commonly associated with hemolysis include increased LDH (particularly isoenzyme 1) and unconjugated (indirect) bilirubin, decreased haptoglobin, free (extracellular) hemoglobin in the blood and urine, increased urobilinogen and urine hemosiderin.

Erythrocyte Membrane Defects

Erythrocyte membranes are normally remarkably deformable, which allows red cells to pass unimpaired through the microcirculation and splenic vasculature. The red cell membrane consists of a phospholipid bilayer linked to an underlying cytoskeleton, composed primarily of spectrin, a dimer of α- and β-subunits and other erythrocyte specific cytoskeletal components (Fig. 26-5). Ankyrin (band 2.1) anchors spectrin to transmembrane proteins (band 3, anion exchanger proteins), while spectrin is bound to actin and glycophorin by protein 4.1. *Alterations in any part of the red cell membrane can impair RBC plasticity, impacting the "vertical linkages" and rendering erythrocytes susceptible to hemolysis.*

Hereditary Spherocytosis

Hereditary spherocytosis (HS) is a diverse group of inherited disorders of RBC cytoskeletons, in which spectrin or another cytoskeletal component (ankyrin, protein 4.2, band 3) is deficient. HS is the most common congenital hemolytic anemia in Caucasians.

MOLECULAR PATHOGENESIS: Deficiency of any cytoskeletal protein leads to a **"vertical"** defect in red cell membranes, with the lipid bilayer uncoupled from the underlying cytoskeleton. The result is progressive loss of membrane surface area and **spherocyte** formation. These abnormal red cells are more rigid and fragile, and so cannot easily traverse splenic sinusoids. While circulating through the spleen, spherocytes lose additional surface membrane, are trapped and ultimately succumb to extravascular hemolysis. About 75% of HS cases are inherited as autosomal dominant traits. The rare recessive cases all involve a spectrin α-subunit.

PATHOLOGY: Most patients with HS have a moderate normocytic anemia. Conspicuous spherocytes that appear hyperchromic (no central pallor) are typical, along with polychromasia and reticulocytosis (Fig. 26-17). The bone marrow shows erythroid hyperplasia. Although typical spherocytes have

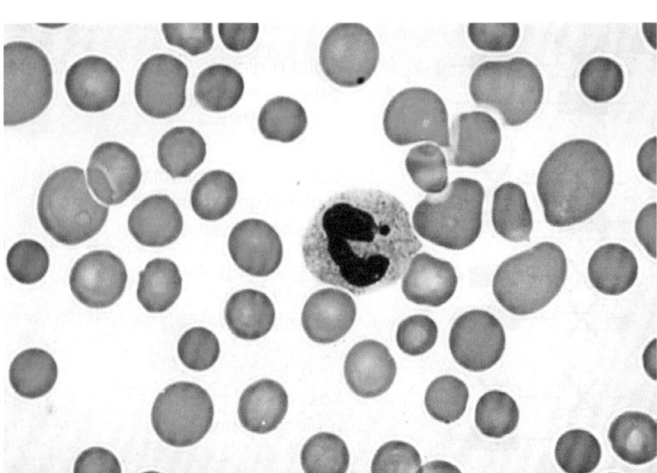

FIGURE 26-17. Hereditary spherocytosis. The peripheral blood smear shows frequent spherocytes with decreased diameter, intense staining and lack of central pallor (*arrows*).

low MCV because of membrane loss and cell dehydration, these patients may have normal mean MCV because of increased reticulocytes (which are larger than average red blood cells).

Spherocytes show greater **osmotic fragility** than normal erythrocytes. Laboratory findings are typical of hemolysis: decreased haptoglobin, increased indirect bilirubin, increased LDH.

 CLINICAL FEATURES: Most patients have splenomegaly caused by chronic extravascular hemolysis. They may appear jaundiced, and up to 50% develop cholelithiasis, with pigmented (bilirubin) gallstones. Despite chronic hemolysis, transfusion is not usually needed. An exception is a sudden decline in hemoglobin and reticulocytes, which heralds **aplastic crisis** (usually caused by infection by parvovirus B19). Anemia may also become more severe in so-called **hemolytic crisis,** when hemolysis accelerates transiently. Patients with HS can be managed effectively by splenectomy, although spherocytes still persist in the circulation. Splenectomy, however, renders patients more susceptible to certain infections, particularly with *Streptococcus* spp.

Hereditary Elliptocytosis
Hereditary elliptocytosis (HE) is a diverse group of inherited disorders affecting the erythrocyte cytoskeleton.

 **MOLECULAR PATHOGENESIS:** HE is characterized by elliptical or oval red blood cells. The most commonly described HE variants include defects in self-assembly of spectrin, spectrin–ankyrin binding, protein 4.1 and glycophorin C. RBCs have an area of central pallor, since there is no loss of the lipid bilayer (as seen in HS). Most forms of HE are autosomal dominant.

  PATHOLOGY AND CLINICAL FEATURES: HE is more common in malaria endemic regions of West Africa. Patients with HE usually have only mild normocytic anemia. Many are asymptomatic. Blood smears show many elliptocytes with only minimal reticulocytosis (Fig. 26-18). Generally, less hemolysis and subsequent anemia are seen than are seen

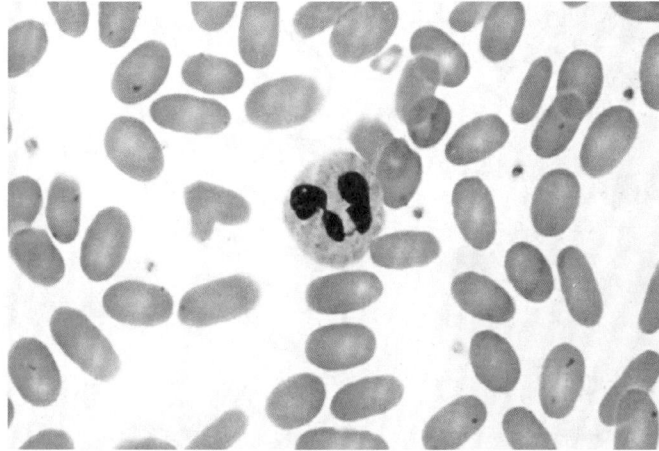

FIGURE 26-18. Hereditary elliptocytosis. A peripheral blood smear reveals that virtually all of the erythrocytes are elliptical with parallel sides.

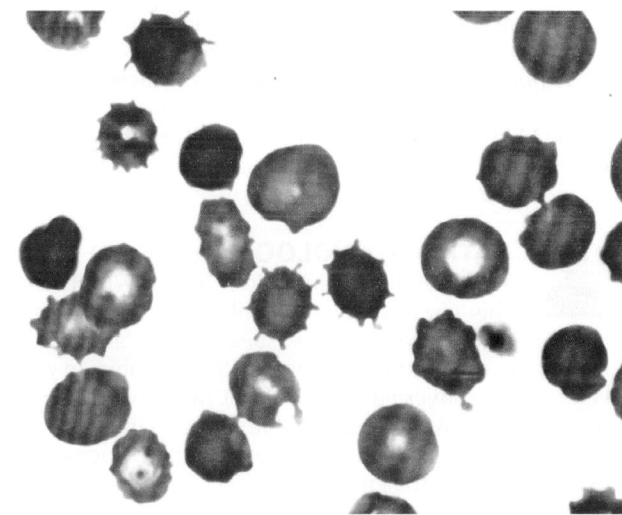

FIGURE 26-19. Acanthocytes. The red cells lack central pallor and display irregular spikes on the surface.

with HS. Occasional patients with more severe hemolysis may require splenectomy.

Acanthocytosis
Acanthocytosis results from a defect within the red cell membrane lipid bilayer and features irregularly spaced spiny projections of the surface, which may be associated with hemolysis.

 PATHOPHYSIOLOGY: The most common cause is chronic liver disease, in which increased free cholesterol deposits in cell membranes. Acanthocytes also occur in abetalipoproteinemia, an autosomal recessive disorder with lipid membrane abnormalities (see Chapter 19).

  PATHOLOGY AND CLINICAL FEATURES: Abnormalities in their lipid membranes cause erythrocytes to deform and develop irregular spiny surface projections and centrally dense cytoplasm (no central pallor) (Fig. 26-19). These **acanthocytes** (spur cells) should be distinguished from burr cells (crenated cells, **echinocytes**), which show more uniform membrane scalloping and keep their central pallor. Hemolysis and anemia in acanthocytosis are mild.

Enzyme Defects

Erythrocytes generate energy mainly by glycolysis. Inherited defects of enzymes in the glycolytic pathway can predispose circulating red cells to hemolysis. The most common enzyme defect involves glucose-6-phosphate dehydrogenase (G6PD), which catalyzes conversion of glucose-6-phosphate to 6-phosphogluconate. Deficiencies of other glycolytic enzymes are rare and autosomal recessive. Among these, pyruvate kinase deficiency is the most common. Clinically, these defects cause variable degrees of anemia and are classified as **hereditary nonspherocytic anemias**.

G6PD deficiency is an X-linked disease in which RBCs are abnormally sensitive to oxidative stress, which triggers hemolytic anemia. G6PD deficiency is most common in areas where malaria is historically endemic, notably Africa and the Mediterranean. The various G6PD mutations appear to protect somewhat against malaria.

PATHOPHYSIOLOGY: Since G6PD helps to recycle reduced glutathione, red cells deficient in this enzyme are susceptible to oxidative stress (e.g., infections, drugs or fava bean ingestion [favism]). Hemoglobin oxidation generates methemoglobin, in which Fe^{2+} ions are converted to ferric (Fe^{3+}). Methemoglobin cannot transport oxygen, is unstable and precipitates in the cytoplasm as Heinz bodies. These precipitates increase cell rigidity and lead to hemolysis.

PATHOLOGY: In quiescent periods, erythrocytes in G6PD deficiency appear normal. But, in a hemolytic episode precipitated by oxidative stress, Heinz bodies appear with supravital staining. Passage through the spleen may remove part of red blood cell membranes, to form so-called **bite cells**.

CLINICAL FEATURES: Full expression of G6PD deficiency is seen only in males; females are asymptomatic carriers. The A variant of G6PD is seen in 10%–15% of American blacks. It is associated with 10% of normal enzyme activity because of instability of the molecule. In affected patients, exposure to oxidant drugs, such as the antimalarial primaquine, may trigger hemolysis. In the Mediterranean type of G6PD mutation, enzyme activity is absent. Thus, exposure to oxidant stress sets off more sustained and severe hemolysis. Potentially lethal hemolysis may follow ingestion of fava beans **(favism)** in susceptible patients.

Hemoglobinopathies

Most clinically relevant hemoglobinopathies are caused by point mutations in the β-globin chain gene.

Sickle Cell Disease
In sickle cell disease, an abnormal hemoglobin, HgbS, causes RBCs to sickle upon deoxygenation.

EPIDEMIOLOGY: HgbS is most common in people of African ancestry, although the gene is also present in Mediterranean, Middle Eastern and Indian people. In some regions of Africa, up to 40% of the population is heterozygous for HgbS. Ten percent of American blacks are heterozygous and 1 in 650 is homozygous. Heterozygosity for HgbS may partially protect against falciparum malaria. Infected erythrocytes selectively sickle and are removed from the circulation by splenic and hepatic macrophages, effectively destroying the parasite.

MOLECULAR PATHOGENESIS: A point mutation in the gene for the β-globin chain gene substitutes valine for glutamic acid at the 6th amino acid. This single change makes an unstable molecule that polym-

erizes upon deoxygenation. Polymerization of HgbS transforms the cytoplasm into a rigid filamentous gel and produces less deformable sickled erythrocytes.

The rigidity of sickled erythrocytes obstructs the microcirculation, leading to tissue hypoxia and ischemic injury in many organs. The inflexibility of sickle cells also renders them susceptible to destruction (hemolysis) during passage through the spleen. Thus, the two primary manifestations of sickle cell disease are recurrent ischemic events and chronic extravascular hemolytic anemia.

At first, reoxygenation can reverse the sickling, but after several cycles of sickling and unsickling, the process becomes irreversible. Sickled erythrocytes also have changes in their membrane phospholipids, and so adhere more strongly to endothelial cells. This further impairs capillary blood flow.

People homozygous for HgbS show the full clinical picture of sickle cell disease. A sickling disorder also occurs in patients who are doubly heterozygous for two β-chain mutations (e.g., HgbSC disease, sickle/β-thalassemia). Heterozygotes for HgbS (sickle trait), however, do not develop red cell sickling, because their HgbA prevents HgbS polymerization. HgbF also interferes with HgbS polymerization, and patients who are homozygous for HgbS and have increased HgbF have a milder form of disease.

PATHOLOGY: Homozygous patients (HgbSS) have severe normocytic or macrocytic anemia. The macrocytosis reflects increased numbers of reticulocytes, owing to chronic hemolysis. Blood smears show marked anisopoikilocytosis and polychromasia. There are classic sickle cells and target cells, as well as other abnormally shaped erythrocytes (Fig. 26-20). Howell-Jolly bodies, which represent nuclear remnants, are evident in most patients beyond childhood and reflect hyposplenism because of ischemic loss of splenic tissue.

Electrophoretic analysis shows that HgbS accounts for 80%–95% of the total hemoglobin and HgbA is absent. HgbF and HgbA$_2$ make up the remaining hemoglobin.

CLINICAL FEATURES: Infants with SS hemoglobin are asymptomatic for their first 8–10 weeks of life, because they have high levels of HgbF.

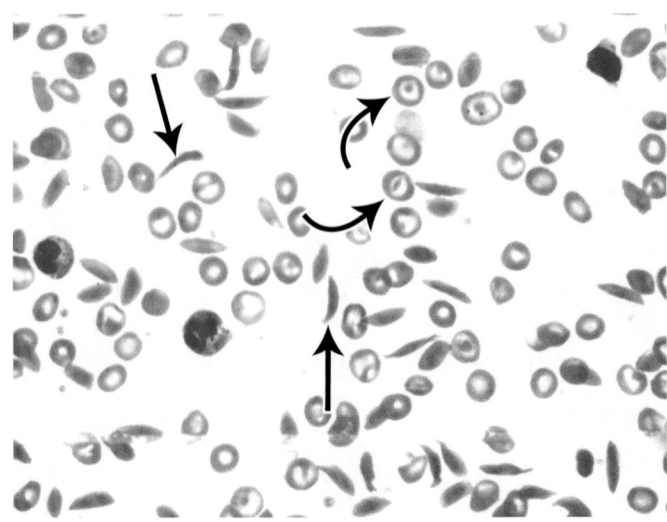

FIGURE 26-20. Sickle cell anemia. Sickled cells (*straight arrows*) and target cells (*curved arrows*) are evident in the blood smear.

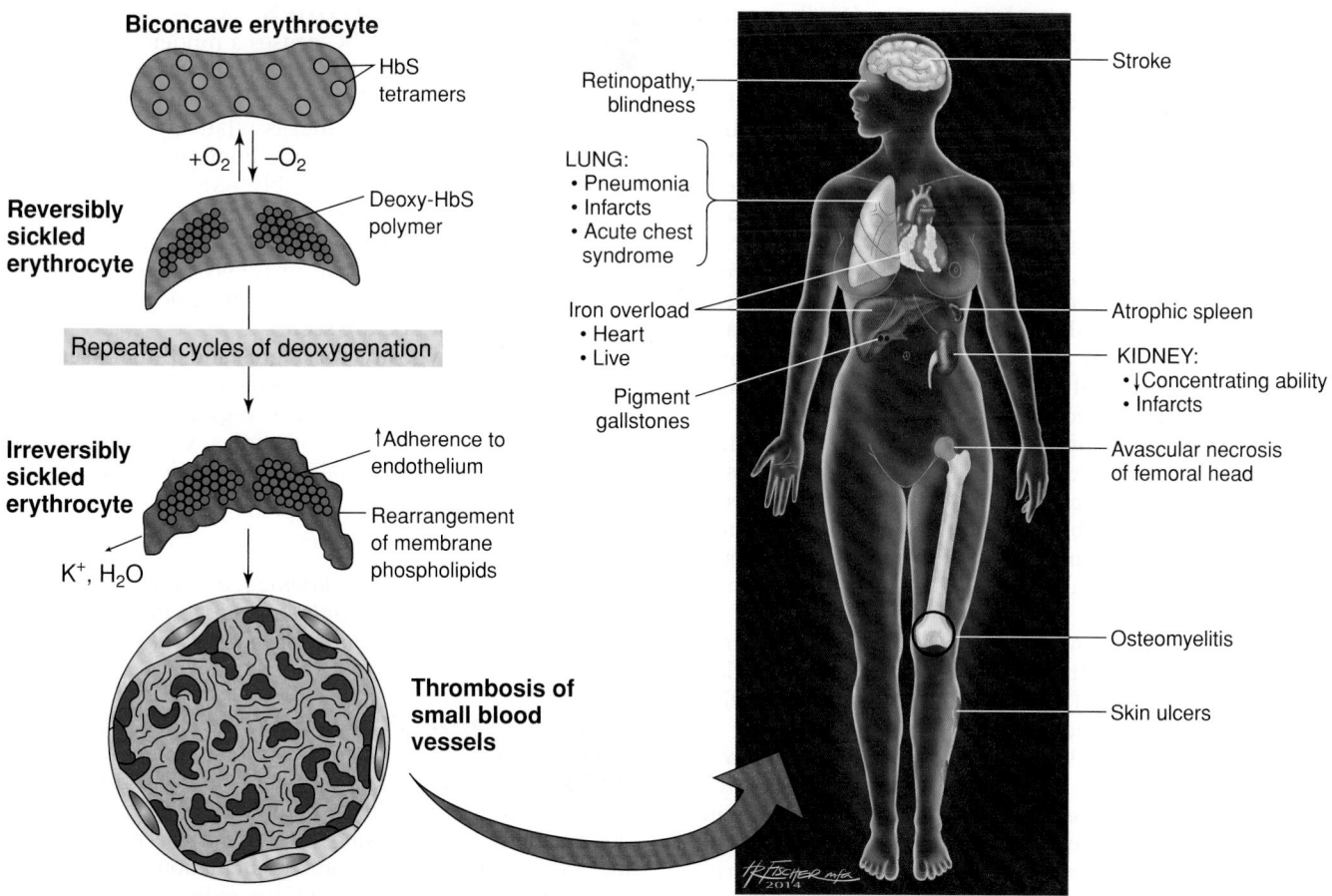

FIGURE 26-21. Pathogenesis of the vascular complications of sickle cell anemia. Substitution of valine for glutamic acid leads to an alteration in the surface charge of the hemoglobin molecule. Upon deoxygenation ($-O_2$), sickle hemoglobin (HbS) tetramers aggregate to form poorly soluble polymers. The erythrocytes change shape from a biconcave disk to a sickle form with the polymerization of HbS. This process is initially reversible upon reoxygenation ($+O_2$), but with repeated cycles of deoxygenation and reoxygenation, the erythrocytes become irreversibly sickled. Irreversibly sickled cells display a rearrangement of phospholipids between the outer and inner monolayers of the cell membrane, in particular an increase in aminophospholipids in the outer leaflet. Potassium (K^+) and water (H_2O) are lost from the cells. The erythrocytes are no longer deformable and are more adherent to endothelial cells, properties that predispose to thrombosis in small blood vessels. The resulting vascular occlusions lead to widespread ischemic complications.

Clinical symptoms first appear in children when synthesis of γ-globin chains declines. This decline is somewhat delayed in homozygous S patients. Although patients suffer from lifelong hemolysis, adaptation occurs over time and most may not require regular transfusions. Instead, the clinical picture is dominated by sequelae of repeated **vaso-occlusive disease**. In an attempt to minimize these complications by decreasing the amount of HgbS in circulation, a chronic exchange transfusion may be necessary. Sickle cell anemia is a systemic disorder and eventually impairs the functions of most organ systems and tissues (Fig. 26-21).

Patients with sickle cell disease develop episodic painful crises, which vary in number. Capillary occlusion leads to ischemia and hypoxic cell injury, which cause severe pain, especially in the chest, abdomen and bones. Painful crises can be triggered by various stimuli (e.g., underlying infection, acidosis or dehydration).

APLASTIC CRISIS: In aplastic crisis, the bone marrow fails to compensate for the high level of red cell loss. Hemoglobin levels drop rapidly, with no reticulocyte response. Parvovirus B19 is the most frequent cause of an aplastic crisis, although other viral and bacterial infections may also cause transient bone marrow suppression.

SEQUESTRATION CRISIS: In this case, sudden pooling of erythrocytes, especially in the spleen, decreases circulating blood volume and lowers hemoglobin levels. The etiology is unclear, but it occurs most often in young children who still have functioning spleens. This complication is followed by hypovolemic shock and is the most common cause of death early in life.

- **Heart:** Chronic demand for increased cardiac output may lead to cardiomegaly and congestive heart failure. In addition, obstruction of coronary microcirculation may cause myocardial ischemia. Myocyte function may also be impaired by excess iron deposition, owing to chronic hemolysis and repeated transfusions.

- **Lungs:** Up to 1/3 of patients with sickle cell anemia may rapidly lose respiratory function, with pulmonary infiltrates on chest radiography. This **acute chest syndrome** may be fatal. Pulmonary infarction may occur, and sickle cell patients are more susceptible to a variety of pulmonary infections.

- **Spleen:** Splenomegaly often occurs in childhood, but repeated splenic infarction leads to functional autosplenectomy. In most adults, only a small fibrous remnant of the spleen remains. The asplenic state renders the patient susceptible to infections with encapsulated bacteria, especially pneumococcus.

- **Brain:** Patients with sickle cell anemia develop neurologic complications related to vascular obstruction, including transient ischemic attacks, strokes and cerebral hemorrhages. Occlusion of retinal microvasculature may lead to retinal hemorrhage and detachment, proliferative retinopathy and blindness.
- **Kidney:** The hypoxic, acidotic and hypertonic environment in the renal medulla often leads to sickling there. This impairs the inability to form concentrated urine and causes renal infarcts and papillary necrosis. Men may develop priapism, which, if not treated promptly, may lead to permanent erectile dysfunction.
- **Liver:** As in any form of chronic hemolytic anemia, patients with sickle cell anemia have increased levels of unconjugated (indirect) bilirubin, which can predispose to pigmented bilirubin gallstones. Cholelithiasis may lead to cholecystitis and require cholecystectomy. Hepatomegaly and increased hepatic iron deposition are also seen.
- **Extremities:** Cutaneous ulcers over the lower extremities, especially near the ankles, are common and reflect obstruction of dermal capillaries. Children may develop "hand–foot syndrome," with self-limited swelling of the hands and feet because of underlying bone infarcts. Avascular necrosis of the femoral head requires corrective hip surgery. Sickle cell disease is also associated with increased incidence of osteomyelitis, particularly with *Salmonella typhimurium,* possibly because of the underlying impairment in splenic function.

Sickle Cell Trait
Heterozygosity for the HgbS mutation is called sickle cell trait.

 **PATHOPHYSIOLOGY:** In patients with sickle cell trait, the HgbA in their red cells prevents HgbS polymerization, so their erythrocytes do not normally sickle. However, under extreme conditions (e.g., high altitudes, deep-sea diving), their RBCs may sickle. Heterozygotes are clinically asymptomatic, do not develop hemolytic anemia and live normal life spans.

Double Heterozygosity for HgbS and Other Hemoglobinopathies
Some patients with a sickling disorder are actually heterozygous for both HgbS and other abnormal hemoglobins (e.g., HgbC or HgbD), or for thalassemia.

 PATHOPHYSIOLOGY: The presence of an additional abnormal hemoglobin or thalassemic gene does not prevent HgbS polymerization, and the clinical expression and severity of disease may be affected. People who are doubly heterozygous may have less frequent crises, higher baseline hemoglobin values, microcytic red cell indices or persistent splenomegaly into adult life.

 CLINICAL FEATURES: Double heterozygosity for HgbS and HgbC causes a milder sickle phenotype than does homozygosity for HgbS. These patients have episodic skeletal or abdominal pain. However, they develop a retinopathy that is relatively common and severe. They are also prone to undergo necrosis of their femoral heads. These features probably reflect the high blood viscosity conferred by HgbSC.

Blood smears from hemoglobin SC patients reveal mild reticulocytosis, target cells and relatively few sickled erythrocytes. However, red blood cells with hemoglobin crystals caused by hemoglobin C are seen.

Double heterozygosity for HgbS and β-thalassemia is either Hgb Sβ⁰ thalassemia, in which β-globin is absent, or Hgb Sβ⁺ thalassemia, in which β-globin is present but reduced. Hgb Sβ⁰ thalassemia is clinically similar to sickle cell disease in severity. Sβ⁺ thalassemia is milder than HgbSC disease.

Hemoglobin C Disease
HgbC disease results from homozygous inheritance of a structurally abnormal hemoglobin, which increases erythrocyte rigidity and causes mild chronic hemolysis.

 **PATHOPHYSIOLOGY:** In HgbC, lysine replaces glutamic acid at the sixth amino acid of β-globin. HgbC precipitates in erythrocyte cytoplasm, leading to cellular dehydration and decreased deformability. When passing through the spleen, the abnormal red cells are removed from the circulation, causing mild anemia and splenomegaly. HgbC has reduced oxygen affinity, so tissue oxygen delivery is increased. This mitigates the severity of disease. HgbC is mostly found in the same populations as HgbS, although it occurs less commonly.

PATHOLOGY: Homozygosity for HgbC disease (CC) causes a mild normocytic anemia. Hemoglobin may be unevenly distributed within red cells, and dense, rhomboidal crystals (precipitated HgbC) occur in some erythrocytes. Hemoglobin electrophoresis reveals no HgbA and greater than 90% HgbC.

Two to 3% of American blacks are heterozygous for HgbC and are asymptomatic (HgbC trait). In such people, about 40% of hemoglobin is HgbC. Red cell morphology is normal, except for some target cells.

Hemoglobin E Disease
HgbE disease is a result of homozygosity for a structurally abnormal hemoglobin, leading to a thalassemia-like defect that is associated with mild chronic hemolysis.

MOLECULAR PATHOGENESIS: In hemoglobin E, lysine substitutes for glutamic acid at position 26 of the β-globin chain. This is at a splice site in the gene, so the mutation results in a structurally abnormal molecule, decreased gene transcription and unstable β-globin messenger RNA (mRNA). The latter defects diminish synthesis of HgbE, creating a situation like that seen in thalassemia. HgbE is relatively unstable and may precipitate in the cell, leading to hemolysis. HgbE is most prevalent in Southeast Asia and globally is second in incidence only to HgbS. HgbE may help protect against malaria.

PATHOLOGY: Patients homozygous for HgbE (EE) have a mild microcytic anemia. MCV is decreased, and there is often erythrocytosis because of the thalassemia-like component. Their RBCs are microcytic and hypochromic and include target cells. More than 90% of hemoglobin is HgbE.

Other Hemoglobinopathies

Several hundred additional known hemoglobin variants result from mutations in α- or β-globin genes. These mutations may lead to structural abnormalities or to a functional derangement of the hemoglobin molecule.

 **PATHOPHYSIOLOGY:** Some mutations alter hemoglobin tertiary structure, destabilizing it and causing it to precipitate in the cytoplasm. As a group, these are **unstable hemoglobins** and are often named after the place where they were first discovered (e.g., hemoglobin Köln). Unstable hemoglobins precipitate and form Heinz bodies within erythrocytes that can be visualized with supravital staining. Heinz bodies bind to cell membranes, increasing their rigidity and leading to mild chronic hemolysis. Patients may suffer jaundice and splenomegaly.

Other hemoglobin mutations cause **abnormal oxygen affinity**. **Increased oxygen affinity** decreases tissue oxygen delivery. Resulting hypoxia elicits increased EPO production and bone marrow erythroid hyperplasia. This, in turn, causes erythrocytosis. Patients are mostly asymptomatic, but some may have symptoms related to hyperviscosity. Abnormal hemoglobins with **decreased oxygen affinity** readily release oxygen in tissues. EPO levels are low, and most patients have mild anemia. Because of increased deoxyhemoglobin, patients may appear cyanotic.

Immune and Autoimmune Hemolytic Anemias

In immune hemolytic anemias, red cell destruction (hemolysis) is caused by antibodies against erythrocyte surface antigens. The red cells themselves are intrinsically normal but are targets for immune-mediated attack. Immune hemolytic anemia can reflect auto- or alloantibodies, and the site of hemolysis may be **extravascular** or **intravascular.** The most common cause of anemia in the elderly is autoimmune hemolytic anemia associated with chronic lymphocytic leukemia and small lymphocytic lymphoma.

In autoimmune hemolytic anemia (AIHA), there are autoantibodies against red cells. Autoantibodies can be classified as either **warm** or **cold antibodies**.

Warm Antibody Autoimmune Hemolytic Anemia

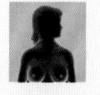 **PATHOPHYSIOLOGY:** Warm autoantibodies optimally bind their antigens at 37°C and account for 80% of cases of AIHA. They are usually immunoglobulin G (IgG) directed against erythrocyte membrane antigens, such as **Rh group proteins**. They do not bind complement, but "coat" red blood cells, and cause these RBCs to be removed by macrophages of the reticuloendothelial system (extravascular hemolysis), mainly in the spleen. Splenic macrophages have Fc receptors that recognize erythrocyte-bound warm antibodies and remove pieces of the membrane with attached antibody. Progressive membrane loss leads to formation of spherocytes, which ultimately undergo hemolysis.

Warm antibody AIHA affects women more than men. Half of cases are idiopathic. In the remaining cases, the antibody reflects an underlying condition (e.g., infection, collagen vascular disease, lymphoproliferative disorders and drug reactions).

Drug-induced warm antibodies arise by several different mechanisms (see Chapter 4). In the **hapten** mechanism, a drug such as penicillin attaches to RBC surfaces. With this modification, the red cell–drug complex elicits antibodies, some of which react with the erythrocyte itself. In the **immune complex** mechanism, a drug (like quinidine) reacts with specific circulating antibody to form immune complexes, which then bind to red cell membranes. In the **autoantibody** mechanism, a drug (e.g., α-methyldopa) elicits antibodies that cross-react with red cell membrane components. In hapten and immune-complex models, the drug is required for hemolysis, while in the autoantibody model, hemolysis occurs in the absence of the initiating drug.

  PATHOLOGY AND CLINICAL FEATURES: Warm antibody AIHA is associated with normocytic or occasionally macrocytic anemia, with spherocytes and polychromasia. Extravascular hemolysis leads to increased serum bilirubin, mostly unconjugated bilirubin; hemoglobinemia (free hemoglobin in the blood) and hemoglobinuria (hemoglobin in the urine) are uncommon. The direct antiglobulin (Coombs) test is usually positive and helps to distinguish immune from nonimmune spherocytosis. In the direct Coombs test, a patient's red cells are incubated with antihuman Ig. Agglutination indicates antibody is present on the cell surface. Warm antibody AIHA is treated with immunosuppression. Refractory cases may require splenectomy or transfusions.

Cold Antibody Autoimmune Hemolytic Anemia

Cold antibodies have maximal reactivity at 4°C. Some 20% of cases of AIHA are caused by cold IgM or IgG antibodies, which occur as cold agglutinins or hemolysins.

 PATHOPHYSIOLOGY: Cold agglutinins may be idiopathic or may be due to an underlying condition, mostly infections (Epstein-Barr virus [EBV], *Mycoplasma*) or lymphoproliferative disorders. Cold agglutinins are mostly IgMs directed against I/i antigens on red cells. At cooler temperatures in the peripheral circulation, these antibodies may bind and agglutinate red cells (Fig. 26-22). They may fix, then activate, complement to a variable extent.

The entire complement cascade may be activated (through the membrane attack complex). This process leads to intravascular hemolysis, resulting in hemoglobinemia, hemoglobinuria and decreased haptoglobin levels (free hemoglobin released into the circulation binds haptoglobin, which causes a decline in haptoglobin).

Alternatively, complement may only be activated through C3. In that case, complement-coated red cells are removed in the liver, because Kupffer cells have more complement receptors than do splenic macrophages.

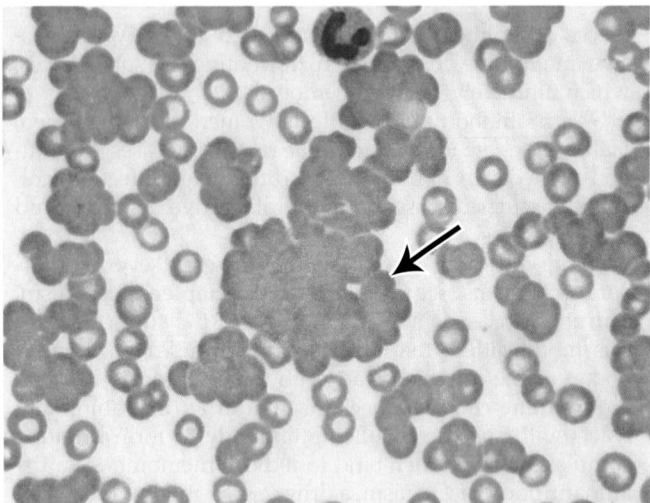

FIGURE 26-22. Red blood cell clumping (agglutination) caused by cold agglutinins (*arrow*). Note that this is not the same phenomenon as rouleaux formation.

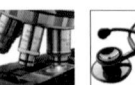 **PATHOLOGY AND CLINICAL FEATURES:** Cold agglutinins often are activated when blood cools to room temperature, and erythrocytes agglutinate in blood smears (Fig. 26-22). Agglutination leads to falsely low RBC counts and hematocrit (Hct), and falsely elevated MCV and MCHC. Warming a blood sample to 37°C before analysis corrects the spurious results. The direct Coombs test is positive but usually only for the presence of complement on red cells. Significant hemolysis is uncommon with cold agglutinins and patients are more likely to develop peripheral vascular symptoms (Raynaud phenomenon; see Chapter 11), owing to red cell agglutination with cold exposure.

Cold Hemolysin Disease (Paroxysmal Cold Hemoglobinuria)

PATHOPHYSIOLOGY: Cold hemolysins (Donath-Landsteiner antibodies) are usually biphasic IgGs directed against P antigens on red cells. Cold hemolysins have biphasic activity and rarely cause AIHA. The antibody binds to erythrocytes at low temperatures and fixes complement, but intravascular hemolysis does not occur at these temperatures. Because the antibody is IgG, red cells do not agglutinate. Upon warming to 37°C, the cold hemolysin remains attached, complement is activated and intravascular hemolysis occurs.

The clinical syndrome caused by cold hemolysins is **paroxysmal cold hemoglobinuria (PCH).** PCH most often follows viral illness. Immunosuppressive therapy and splenectomy are usually ineffective. Cold avoidance and supportive therapy such as RBC transfusions are required.

 PATHOLOGY: Patients with PCH may develop severe anemia, decreased haptoglobin levels and hemoglobinuria due to intravascular hemolysis. The direct Coombs test is positive for complement but may

be negative for IgG, since cold hemolysins may readily dissociate from red cells in vitro.

Hemolytic Transfusion Reactions

An **immediate hemolytic transfusion** reaction occurs when a patient with preformed alloantibodies receives grossly incompatible blood, usually because of a clerical error. Massive hemolysis of the transfused blood may cause severe complications, including hypotension, renal failure and death. Hemolytic transfusion reaction and hemolytic disease in the newborn (see below, Chapter 6) are examples of **alloimmune hemolytic anemia,** in which alloantibodies cause destruction of red cells.

Delayed hemolytic transfusion reactions usually involve antibodies to minor red cell antigens. After a first exposure to such antigens, antibody levels rise, but then may fall to become undetectable by routine pretransfusion screening. Subsequent reexposure to the offending antigen elicits an anamnestic antibody response; hemolysis occurs several days later. Delayed hemolytic transfusion reactions are usually less severe than immediate reactions and may be clinically undetectable. In both types of hemolytic transfusion reactions, the direct antiglobulin test is positive.

Hemolytic Disease of the Newborn

Hemolytic disease of the newborn (HDN) reflects incompatibility of blood types between a mother and her developing fetus; the mother lacks an antigen present on fetal RBCs. Maternal IgG alloantibodies can cross the placenta and cause hemolysis of fetal erythrocytes. Erythroblastosis is visible in peripheral blood smears (Fig. 26-23). Erythroblasts (immature red blood cells) are released from the fetal bone marrow in an effort to compensate for the RBC loss. HDN antibodies are mostly directed against ABO or Rh antigens.

With ABO-type HDN, the mother is type O and the fetus is usually type A. Naturally occurring maternal anti-A antibodies cause hemolysis in the fetus. No prior exposure through pregnancy or transfusion is required for hemolysis to develop. The anemia associated with ABO incompatibility is usually mild. Affected babies develop hyperbilirubinemia, spherocytosis and a positive direct antiglobulin test.

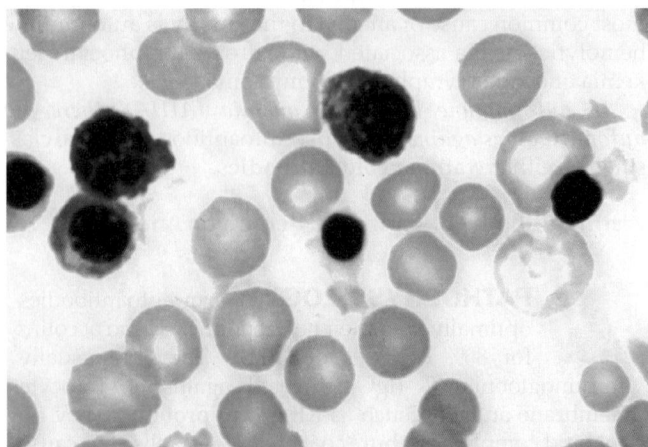

FIGURE 26-23. Hemolytic disease of the newborn (HDN). The presence of nucleated red blood cells in the peripheral blood is abnormal. They are often present in various types of hemolytic disorders, but are particularly numerous in HDN.

With Rh-type HDN, the mother is Rh negative and the fetus is Rh positive. The D antigen is most frequently involved, although minor Rh antigens can also cause disease. Prior maternal exposure occurs via previous pregnancy or transfusion. Disease severity varies, but hemolysis in Rh incompatibility is generally more significant than in ABO-type HDN. Severely affected fetuses may develop **hydrops fetalis,** with heart failure, generalized edema, ascites and intrauterine death (see Chapter 6). Fortunately, today most cases of D-related HDN are prevented by passive immunization of Rh-negative mothers during pregnancy with injections of Rh immune globulin. Laboratory findings are similar to those described above for ABO HDN.

Nonimmune Hemolytic Anemias

In nonimmune hemolytic anemias, factors other than antibodies to red cell antigens destroy RBCs (e.g., red cell fragmentation syndromes and "march" hemoglobinuria).

Mechanical Red Cell Fragmentation Syndromes (Microangiopathic Hemolytic Anemias)
In red cell fragmentation syndromes, intrinsically normal erythrocytes are damaged mechanically as they circulate in the blood (intravascular hemolysis).

 ETIOLOGIC FACTORS: In **thrombotic micro-angiopathic** hemolytic anemia, red cells are fragmented mechanically either by contact with an abnormal surface (e.g., prosthetic heart valve, synthetic vascular graft) or by altered small blood vessel endothelial surfaces associated with microthrombosis, fibrin deposition and platelet aggregation. As RBCs travel through such damaged vessels, these fibrin meshworks cause them to fragment (Fig. 26-7). Classic examples of microangiopathic hemolysis include **disseminated intravascular coagulation** (DIC), **thrombotic thrombocytopenic purpura** (TTP) and hemolytic–uremic syndrome (HUS). Altered blood flow, as occurs in malignant hypertension or vasculitis, may also lead to mechanical fragmentation of erythrocytes.

Long-distance running or walking ("march hemoglobinuria") or prolonged vigorous exercise can cause repetitive trauma to red cells and lead to hemolysis.

 PATHOLOGY: Laboratory findings in microangiopathic hemolytic anemia include a mild to moderate microcytic or normochromic anemia with appropriate reticulocyte response. Blood smears show fragmented erythrocytes (schistocytes) and polychromasia (Fig. 26-24). Abnormalities in coagulation and thrombocytopenia characterize DIC, while thrombocytopenia alone is seen in cases of TTP (see below).

Hypersplenism
A mild hemolytic anemia may develop in patients with hypersplenism and congestive splenomegaly. Splenomegaly causes pooling of blood and delayed transit of blood cells through the splenic circulation. Prolonged exposure of red cells to splenic macrophages may lead to their premature destruction.

  PATHOLOGY AND CLINICAL FEATURES: The anemia of hypersplenism shows no specific morphologic features. Leukopenia and thrombocytopenia are common and are

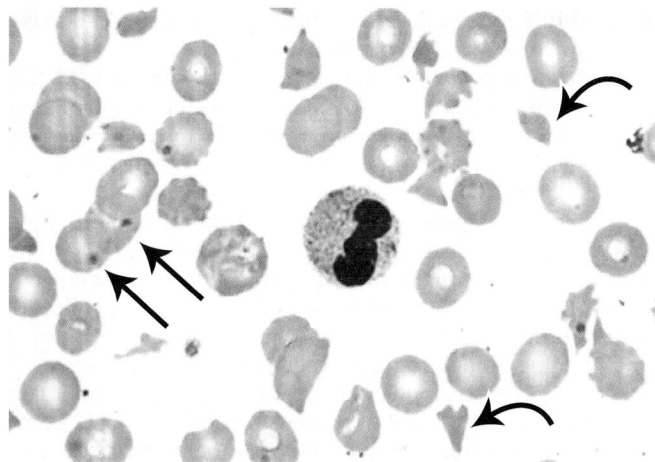

FIGURE 26-24. Microangiopathic hemolytic anemia (MAHA). Irregular, fragmented erythrocytes (schistocytes, *curved arrows*) are seen in the blood smear of a patient with disseminated intravascular coagulation. Howell-Jolly bodies are also present (*straight arrows*).

caused by sequestration of these elements in the enlarged spleen, not destruction. Bone marrow shows compensatory hyperplasia of all cell lines.

Other Hemolytic Anemias
Thermal burns lead to intravascular RBC hemolysis. Normal red cell membranes are disrupted and fragmented at temperatures over 49°C. Blood smears show schistocytes, microspherocytes and polychromasia. Direct Coombs tests are negative.

Infection can cause both pancytopenia and isolated anemia. Several **infectious microorganisms** specifically parasitize erythrocytes and can cause hemolysis. All species of *Plasmodium* have an intraerythrocytic life cycle, which causes RBC lysis when it is done (see Chapter 9). Infected red cells are also removed from circulation by splenic macrophages. *Babesiosis*, found in more temperate climates (northeastern United States), is also associated with hemolysis after the intraerythrocytic life cycle is over. In both cases, blood smears reveal the parasites within red cells.

POLYCYTHEMIA

Polycythemia (erythrocytosis) is an increase in RBC mass.

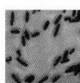 **ETIOLOGIC FACTORS:** Polycythemia is defined arbitrarily as an Hct greater than 54% in men and greater than 47% in women. Blood viscosity increases exponentially at Hcts over 50%, and cardiac function and peripheral blood flow may be impaired. If the Hct exceeds 60%, blood flow may be so compromised as to cause tissue hypoxia.

Polycythemia can be further divided on the basis of overall red cell mass into relative and absolute categories.

■ **Relative polycythemia** occurs in dehydration. Plasma volume is decreased, but red cell mass is normal. This is sometimes called Gaisböck syndrome, or spurious polycythemia: it is not a true increase in red cell mass, but rather a reflection of altered total blood volume.

- **Absolute polycythemia** is a true increase in red cell mass. It can be primary or secondary.
  - **Primary polycythemia,** or **polycythemia vera (PV),** is autonomous, EPO-independent proliferation of erythroid cells caused by an acquired, clonal, HSC disorder. PV is a chronic myeloproliferative disorder (see below).
  - **Secondary polycythemia** arises from EPO stimulation of erythropoiesis, usually to compensate for general tissue hypoxia. Tissue hypoxia may arise from chronic lung disease, cigarette smoking, residence at high altitudes, a right-to-left cardiac shunt or an abnormal hemoglobin with high oxygen affinity.

    Secondary polycythemia can also occur under certain circumstances unrelated to tissue hypoxia. Some tumors secrete ectopic EPO as a paraneoplastic syndrome (see below), particularly renal cell carcinoma, hepatocellular carcinoma, cerebellar hemangioblastoma and uterine leiomyoma. Some nonneoplastic conditions of the kidney may cause secondary polycythemia. Renal cysts or hydronephrosis may exert direct pressure on the kidney, leading to localized hypoxia and increasing EPO production. Some athletes use EPO to enhance their maximal exercise capacity.

Platelets and Hemostasis

NORMAL HEMOSTASIS

Normal hemostasis requires that platelets, endothelial cells, coagulation factors and endogenous anticoagulants and thrombolytics maintain a resting nonthrombotic state but that they can respond instantly to vascular damage and form a clot. After blood vessel injury, platelets adhere to the vascular endothelium to form a hemostatic plug. Activated platelets recruit and activate additional platelets to form a **platelet aggregate** and a **fibrin clot.** Fibrin stabilizes platelet aggregates after coagulation is activated.

Platelets Develop from Hematopoietic Stem Cells by Thrombopoiesis

A platelet count is $150–350 \times 10^3/\mu L$. To maintain this level requires continued proliferation, differentiation and release into the blood. Platelets are derived from megakaryocytes via the process of proplatelet formation and fragmentation. Thrombopoiesis requires the marrow microenvironment, plus stimulation by TPO. TPO is produced by the liver and binds the TPO receptor, c-Mpl, to stimulate megakaryocyte proliferation and differentiation. Mature megakaryocytes undergo proplatelet formation and fragmentation to release 1000–4000 anucleate platelets.

Morphology and Function

Platelets are small discoid cells, 2–3 μm in diameter (Fig. 26-25), with a life span of about 10 days. On Wright-stained smears they are pale blue with faint pink granules. They contain mitochondria, glycogen particles, dense granules and α granules. Dense granules contain adenosine

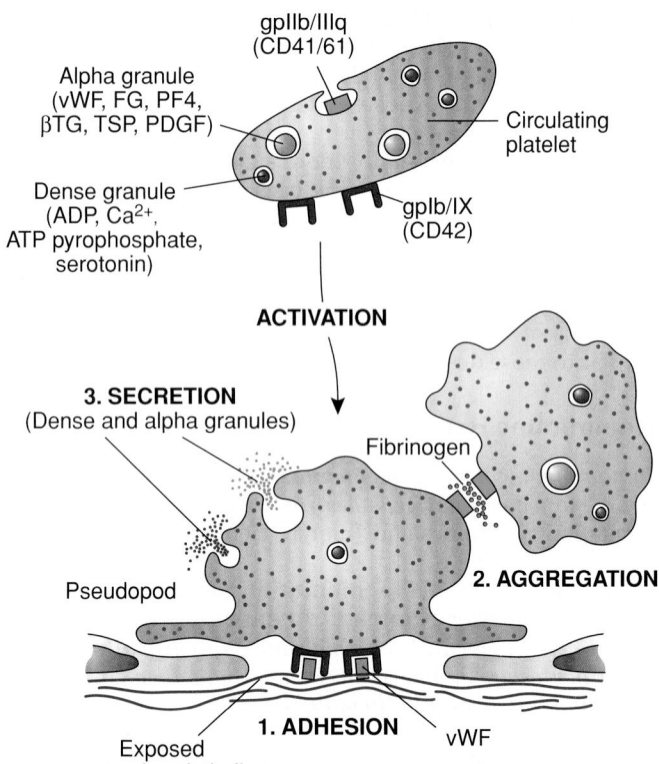

FIGURE 26-25. Platelet activation involves three overlapping mechanisms. 1. Adhesion to the exposed subendothelium is mediated by the binding of von Willebrand factor (vWF) to glycoprotein (Gp) Ib/IX (CD42) and is the initiation signal for activation. **2.** Exposure of Gp IIb/IIIa (CD41/61) to the fibrinogen (FG) receptor on the platelet surface allows for platelet aggregation. **3.** At the same time, platelets secrete their granule contents, which facilitates further activation. α-Granules contain vWF, fibrinogen, platelet factor 4 (PF4), thromboglobulin (TG), thrombospondin (TSP) and platelet-derived growth factor (PDGF).

diphosphate (ADP), a potent aggregating molecule; adenosine triphosphate (ATP); calcium; histamine; serotonin; and epinephrine. α Granules express the adhesive proteins P-selectin on their membranes and contain fibrinogen, von Willebrand factor (vWF), fibronectin and thrombospondin, as well as the chemokines platelet factor 4, neutrophil-activating peptide 2, platelet-derived growth factor (PDGF) and transforming growth factor-α (TGF-α).

Platelet Activation

When vascular endothelium is disrupted, platelets respond by creating a platelet plug to minimize bleeding. After contact with the extracellular matrix, particularly type I collagen, platelets undergo a sequence of steps of platelet activation (Fig. 26-25):

1. **Platelets adhere** to subendothelial matrix proteins with specific platelet surface glycoproteins (Gps). Major adhesive ligands include collagen (via the Gp Ia/IIa [$\alpha_2\beta_1$ integrin] and Gp VI receptors) and vWF (via Gp Ib/IX).
2. **Shape change,** from discoid to spherical to stellate, follows initial adhesion.
3. **Secretion of platelet granule contents from both the dense granules and α granules** results in the release of ADP, epinephrine, calcium, vWF and PDGF.

4. **Thromboxane A$_2$** is generated by cyclooxygenase 1.
5. **Membrane changes** expose P-selectin and procoagulant anionic phospholipids such as phosphatidylserine.
6. **Aggregation of platelets** occurs by fibrinogen receptor Gp IIb/IIIa cross-linking.

Each of these functional steps has specific consequences. Initial adhesion signals platelet activation. Secreted granule contents and thromboxane A$_2$ provide positive feedback to activate additional platelets via their surface receptors. The stellate shape projects the procoagulant membrane surface and activated Gp IIb/IIIa/fibrinogen to the site of interaction with coagulation factors and other platelets, respectively. *Thus, the surface of activated platelets is an optimal environment for propagating assembly of the coagulation–factor complex, including the prothrombinase complex. The resulting thrombin has many consequences, particularly further platelet activation.* Finally, P-selectin participates in binding leukocytes and localizing them to participate in healing, together with substances secreted by platelets such as PDGF. *As a result of these concerted steps, activated platelets form a strong primary plug and then an aggregate within a platelet–fibrin meshwork, which stops bleeding and begins healing.*

Activation of the Coagulation Cascade Completes Blood Clot Formation

Platelets and leukocytes circulate in an inactive state. Similarly, coagulation factors are present as inactive zymogen forms. Activation of platelets and coagulation factors is concerted and highly constrained in space and time, to prevent clots from spreading through the circulation. The localization of coagulation–factor complexes to activated surfaces of blood cells, especially platelets, accelerates activation of coagulation factors and avoids the many anticoagulant factors in plasma.

Activation of the coagulation cascade by damaged tissue exposes tissue factor and culminates in conversion of prothrombin (factor II) to thrombin (factor IIa), and generation of fibrin from fibrinogen (Fig. 26-26). Thrombin has additional roles. It activates both platelets and factors that sustain coagulation (see Chapter 16).

There are three essential procoagulant complexes and one anticoagulant complex (Figs. 26-26 and 26-27). *Generally, each active enzyme in the cascade is assisted by a cofactor and localized to a phospholipid surface (PL).*

PROCOAGULANT PATHWAYS: Factor Xa, together with its cofactor Va (Xa/Va complex), cleaves factor II (prothrombin) to IIa (thrombin). There are two complexes that activate factor X, the so-called Xase complexes.

1. The complex of **tissue factor (TF) and factor VIIa** initiates coagulation. Its activation is controlled by exposure to subendothelial cells or activated monocytes and endothelial cells. Microparticles derived from activated leukocytes and endothelial cells contribute to a pool of circulating TFs that participates in hemostasis and thrombosis. TF/VIIa/PL initiates factor X activation but is then rapidly shut off by **TF pathway inhibitor (TFPI)** (Fig. 26-27). The

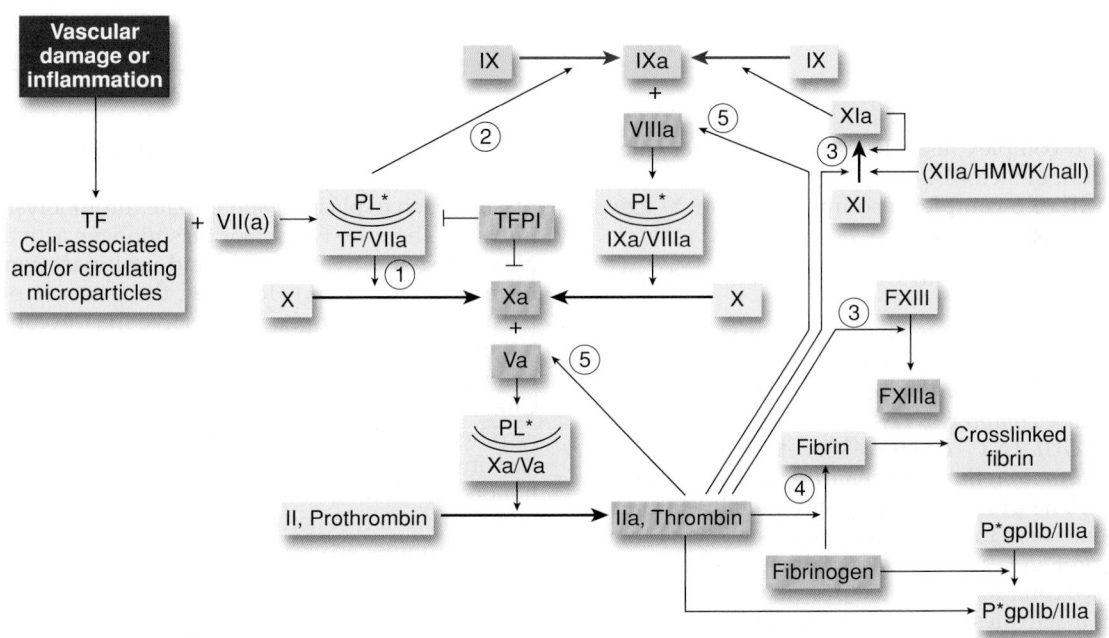

FIGURE 26-26. Hemostasis and thrombosis. Following injury to a vessel, rupture of an atherosclerotic plaque or the presence of major inflammation, coagulation is initiated when tissue factor (TF) binds to circulating factor VII, a small proportion of which is activated (VIIa). TF is located on cells (subendothelial or activated endothelial cells or leukocytes) or circulating microparticles. The TF/VIIa complex is activated by localizing to an activated phospholipid surface (PL*) such as that provided by activated platelets. TF/VIIa activates factor X to form Xa (*1*) and IX to form IXa (*2*). However, TF pathway inhibitor (TFPI) inhibits both (*1*) and (*2*). Sustained amplification is achieved through the actions of factors XI, IX and VIII. Factor XI is activated through the small amount of initial thrombin formed and, to a limited extent, by auto-activation or factor XIIa. Cofactors V and VIII, when activated by thrombin, form complexes with X (Xa/Va) and IX (IXa/VIIIa), respectively, on activated PL surfaces. Note the central and multiple roles for thrombin (*4*), which converts fibrinogen to fibrin, activates cofactors V and VIII (*5*), activates factors XI and XIII (*3*) and activates platelets. Fibrinogen binds to the Gp IIb/IIIa integrin receptor on activated platelets (P*). Note the extensive control in time and space of these concerted surface reactions. The combined result is the platelet–fibrin thrombus.

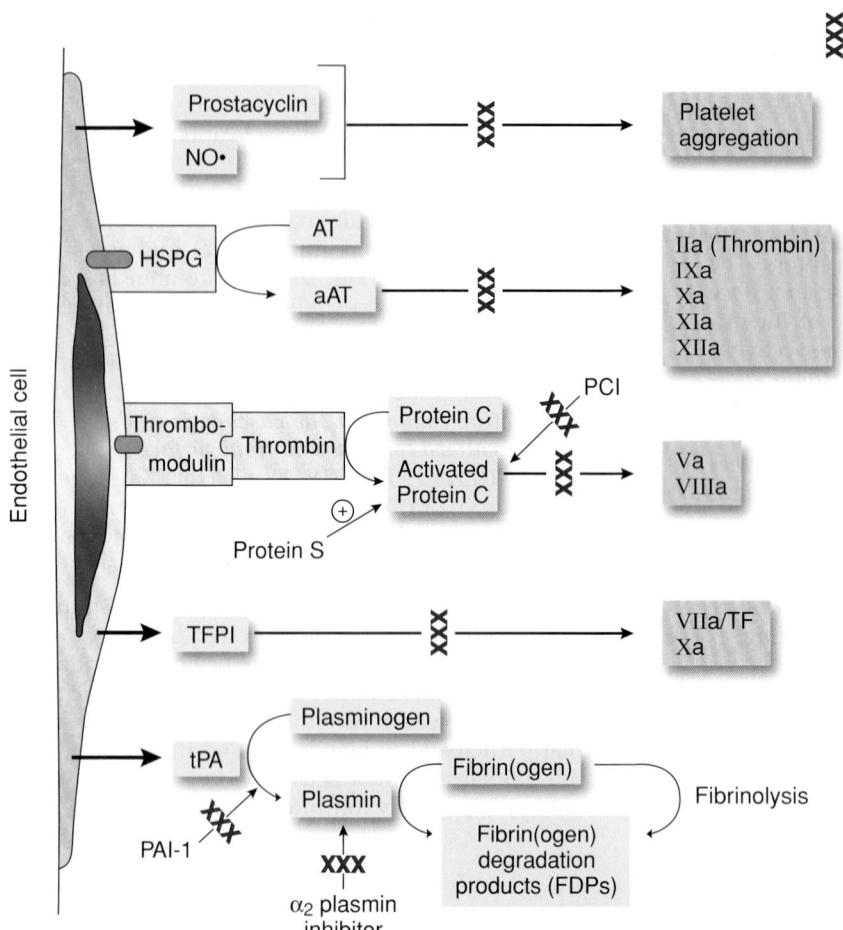

FIGURE 26-27. The role of endothelium in anticoagulation, platelet inhibition and thrombolysis. The endothelial cell plays a central role in the inhibition of various components of the clotting mechanism. Heparan sulfate proteoglycan potentiates the activation of antithrombin (AT) 15-fold. Thrombomodulin stimulates the activation of protein C by thrombin 30-fold. *HSPG* = heparan sulfate proteoglycan; *NO•* = nitric oxide; *PAI-I* = plasminogen activator inhibitor-I; *PCI* = protein C inhibitor; *tPA* = tissue plasminogen activator.

TF/VIIa/PL complex also cleaves and thus activates a small amount of factor IX.

2. The **IXa/VIIIa/PL complex** also initiates factor X activation, with ongoing activation of factor IX by XIa.

The coagulation pathways are presented in detail in Chapter 16.

Note that thrombin activates the Xase complexes by activating factors XI, VIII and V. *In summary, the three procoagulant complexes are the prothrombinase complex, Xa/Va/PL, and the two Xase complexes, TF/VIIa/PL and IXa/VIIIa/PL.*

ANTICOAGULANT PATHWAYS: An anticoagulant complex (α-thrombin–thrombomodulin) activates protein C (Fig. 26-27). The **protein C$_{ase}$ complex** contains thrombin and thrombomodulin in endothelial cell plasma membranes. Endothelial protein C receptor also participates in forming this cell surface complex. Activated protein C, with its cofactor protein S, inactivates the key cofactors VIIIa and Va, thus limiting further generation of Xa and IIa (see Chapter 16).

Antithrombin III inhibits thrombin activity. Antithrombin III also cleaves activated factors IXa, Xa, XIa and XIIa. In vivo this effect is accentuated by heparan sulfate proteoglycans and, most dramatically, by therapeutic administration of heparin.

Thrombolysis Is Mediated by Plasminogen Activation

After a thrombus is firmly established, its growth is curtailed further by removal of platelet-activating factors and

coagulation proteins. Endothelial cells near the thrombus produce plasminogen activators, which activate circulating plasminogen to plasmin and initiate thrombolysis (i.e., **fibrinolysis**). There are two major plasminogen activators, **tissue plasminogen activator** (t-PA) and **urokinase-type plasminogen activator** (u-PA). Together, the protease plasmin and the activity of macrophages dissolve the thrombus. Plasmin targets specific sites in the fibrin meshwork for degradation, helping to localize its activity to sites where it is needed (see Chapter 16).

The factors that limit clot formation are themselves limited in turn. Several naturally occurring inhibitors do the honors. Plasminogen activator inhibitor-I (PAI-I), antiplasmin and thrombin-activatable fibrinolysis inhibitor (TAFI) block plasminogen cleavage to plasmin and plasmin action.

Thrombolysis coincides with the start of wound repair (see Chapter 7). The latter involves fibroblasts and endothelial cells migrating and proliferating, secretion of new extracellular matrix and restoration of blood vessel patency. Angiogenesis (i.e., new blood vessels budding from existing ones) occurs in the setting of tissue ischemia or damage. Many products of coagulation and fibrinolysis are potent angiogenic agents.

Blood Vessels and Endothelial Cells Interact with Platelets

The above discussion highlights the many roles of endothelial cells in regulating platelets and coagulation (Fig. 26-27).

Endothelial cells rest on a basement membrane containing collagens, elastin, laminin, fibronectin, vWF and other structural and adhesive proteins. Subendothelial cells are a potent source of TF. When exposed, the intimal matrix is intensely thrombogenic. Its adhesive proteins bind corresponding platelet membrane glycoprotein receptors, which then adhere to the exposed matrix. TF binds circulating activated factor VIIa to activate factors X and IX (Fig. 26-26).

The endothelium provides a smooth, nonthrombogenic surface. It synthesizes anticoagulant molecules and prevents unstimulated platelets from adhering to, or penetrating, the endothelial barrier. Endothelial cells also synthesize prostacyclin, a potent vasodilator that also inhibits platelet activation. Nitric oxide (NO) exerts similar effects. These actions prevent clots from forming until injury to the endothelium exposes subendothelial tissue (see Chapters 2 and 16).

HEMOSTATIC DISORDERS

Defects in hemostasis occur when the balance of procoagulant and anticoagulant activities tilts toward one or the other. Such defects are either **hemostatic** disorders or **thrombotic** disorders. If hemostasis fails to restore an injured vessel's integrity, the result is **bleeding**. Inability to maintain the fluidity of blood causes **thrombosis**.

Clinical manifestations of hemorrhage associated with disorders of each component of the hemostatic system tend to be distinctive (Table 26-6). Platelet abnormalities result in both **petechiae** and purpuric hemorrhages in the skin and mucous membranes. Deficiencies of coagulation factors lead to hemorrhage into muscles, viscera and joint spaces. Disorders of the blood vessels usually cause **purpura**.

Hemostatic Disorders of Blood Vessels Reflect Dysfunction of Vascular or Extravascular Tissues

Dysfunction of the extravascular or vascular tissues may cause hemorrhages ranging from cosmetic blemishes to life-threatening blood loss.

Extravascular Dysfunction

SENILE PURPURA: The most common disorder in extravascular dysfunction, senile purpura, is age-related atrophy of supporting connective tissues. Senile purpura is associated with superficial, sharply demarcated, persistent purpuric spots on the forearms and other sun-exposed areas.

PURPURA SIMPLEX: A similar type of purpura occurs principally in women during menses. Purpura simplex occurs in the deep dermis and resolves quickly.

SCURVY: Vitamin C deficiency (scurvy) impairs collagen synthesis and leads to purpura (see Chapter 8). Perifollicular hemorrhages are characteristic.

Vascular Dysfunction

Deposition of immunoglobulin fragments in vessel walls occurs in **amyloidosis** (see Chapter 15), **cryoglobulinemia** and **other paraproteinemias** and can weaken vessel walls

TABLE 26-6
PRINCIPAL CAUSES OF BLEEDING

Vascular Disorders
- Senile purpura
- Purpura simplex
- Glucocorticoid excess
- Dysproteinemias
- Allergic (Henoch-Schönlein) purpura
- Hereditary hemorrhagic telangiectasia

Platelet Abnormalities
- Thrombocytopenia (see Table 26-7)
- Qualitative disorders
  - Inherited
    - Glycoprotein IIb/IIIa deficiency (Glanzmann thrombasthenia)
    - Glycoprotein Ib/IX/V deficiency (Bernard-Soulier syndrome)
    - Storage pool diseases (α and δ)
    - Abnormal arachidonic acid metabolism
  - Acquired
    - Uremia
    - Drugs
    - Cardiopulmonary bypass
    - Myeloproliferative disorders
    - Liver disease

Coagulation Factor Deficiencies
- Inherited
- von Willebrand disease
- Hemophilia A
- Hemophilia B
- Acquired
- Vitamin K deficiency/antagonism
- Liver disease
  - Disseminated intravascular coagulation

and cause purpura. Certain **arteritides** also injure vessel walls and may lead to hemorrhage (see Chapter 16).

Hereditary Hemorrhagic Telangiectasia (Rendu-Osler-Weber Syndrome)

Hereditary hemorrhagic telangiectasia (HHT) is an autosomal dominant disorder of blood vessel walls (venules and capillaries) in which arteriovenous malformations (AVMs) and telangiectases (dilated, tortuous small blood vessels) form in solid organs, mucous membranes and dermis. The incidence is 1–2 individuals per 10,000.

 **MOLECULAR PATHOGENESIS:** The underlying defect is dilation and thinning of vessel walls due to inadequate elastic tissue and smooth muscle. The disorder is caused by mutations in TGF-β family members, endoglin (*ENG*) or an activin receptor–like kinase 1 (*ALK1*).

CLINICAL FEATURES: At first, telangiectasias are punctate reddish spots on the lips and nose, up to 0.5 cm in diameter. They can remain as such or progress to arteriovenous malformations or aneurysmal dilations throughout the body. Patients with HHT have recurrent hemorrhages. These may occur spontaneously or after trivial trauma. As a consequence, patients also often are anemic. Bleeding may occur at the site of any lesion, but over 80% of patients have recurrent epistaxis, beginning at an early age. Later in life, gastrointestinal hemorrhage may be the dominant symptom. Arteriovenous fistulas in the lungs, brain and retina may lead to hemorrhage or clinically significant shunting of blood. Recurrent bleeding may limit patients' activities, but death from exsanguination is rare.

Allergic Purpura (Henoch-Schönlein Purpura)

Allergic purpura is a vascular disease that results from immunologic damage to blood vessel walls (see Chapter 22). In children, it often follows viral infections and is self-limited. In adults, it often reflects exposure to a variety of drugs and may be chronic.

PATHOLOGY: Henoch-Schönlein purpura is characterized by **leukocytoclastic vasculitis,** with perivascular infiltration of neutrophils and eosinophils, fibrinoid necrosis of vessel walls and platelet plugs in vascular lumens. IgA and complement complexes circulate in the blood and often deposit in vessel walls. Purpuric spots often accompany raised urticarial lesions. Cramps and bleeding indicate gastrointestinal involvement. If kidneys are affected, renal failure may ensue.

Platelet Disorders May Result from Insufficient Production, Excessive Destruction or Impaired Platelet Function

Patients may have histories of easy bruising; mucocutaneous bleeding, including gingival bleeding, epistaxis and menorrhagia; or life-threatening bleeds into the gastrointestinal (GI) tract, genitourinary tract and brain. Petechiae are characteristic of platelet disorders but may also accompany vascular diseases. They are nonblanching, red lesions less than 2 mm in diameter. They usually occur in the legs and dependent parts of the body, on the buccal mucosal and soft palate and at pressure points (waistband, wristwatch band). Platelet disorders reflect:

1. Decreased production
2. Increased destruction
3. Impaired function

Thrombocytopenia

Thrombocytopenia, defined as platelet counts under 150,000/μL, results from either decreased production or increased destruction. Manifestations of thrombocytopenia include spontaneous bleeding, prolonged bleeding time and normal prothrombin time (PT) and partial thromboplastin time (PTT). The lower the platelet count, the greater the risk of bleeding. Patients with less than 10,000 platelets/μL are at greatest risk of spontaneous hemorrhage (Table 26-7).

TABLE 26-7
PRINCIPAL CAUSES OF THROMBOCYTOPENIA

Decreased Production

Aplastic anemia

Bone marrow infiltration (neoplastic, fibrosis)

Bone marrow suppression by drugs or radiation

Ineffective Production

Megaloblastic anemia

Myelodysplasias

Increased Destruction

Immunologic (idiopathic, HIV, drugs, alloimmune, posttransfusion purpura, neonatal)

Nonimmunologic (DIC, TTP, HUS, vascular malformations, drugs)

Increased Sequestration

Splenomegaly

Dilutional

Blood and plasma transfusions

DIC = disseminated intravascular coagulation; HUS = hemolytic–uremic syndrome; TTP = thrombocytic thrombocytopenic purpura.

ETIOLOGIC FACTORS AND MOLECULAR PATHOGENESIS: Decreased **platelet production** can result from multiple congenital or acquired defects in megakaryocytopoiesis, including diseases that affect the marrow generally, abnormalities that selectively impair platelet production and defects that lead to ineffective megakaryocytopoiesis. Marrow infiltration with malignant cells or bone marrow failure (e.g., in patients with aplastic anemia or who received radiotherapy or chemotherapy) may cause pancytopenia, including thrombocytopenia. Certain viral infections, such as cytomegalovirus (CMV) and HIV, and certain drugs impair platelet production. (HIV may also increase platelet destruction; see below.) Megaloblastic anemia and myelodysplasia may cause thrombocytopenia due to ineffective megakaryopoiesis.

May-Hegglin anomaly is a congenital form of thrombocytopenia that entails decreased platelet production. It is the most common of a family of inherited thrombocytopenias called myosin heavy chain 9 (MYH9)-related platelet disorders. These disorders all result from mutations in the *MYH9* gene, which encodes a cytoskeletal contractile protein, nonmuscle myosin heavy chain IIA (NMMHC-IIA). There are 3 other overlapping disorders: Epstein syndrome, Fechtner syndrome and Sebastian platelet syndrome. These all lead to abnormal megakaryocyte maturation and abnormally large platelets (macrothrombocytopenia). Neutrophils are also slightly abnormal morphologically, with blue cytoplasmic inclusions (**Döhle-like bodies;** true Döhle bodies occur in acute infections).

Increased platelet destruction can result from immune-mediated damage with consequent removal of circulating platelets, as in idiopathic thrombocytopenic purpura and drug-induced thrombocytopenia. Or, excessive platelet destruction occurs by nonimmunologic conditions such as intravascular platelet aggregation (e.g., in TTP).

Abnormal platelet distribution, or pooling, is seen in disorders of the spleen and hypothermia.

Idiopathic (Autoimmune) Thrombocytopenic Purpura

Idiopathic thrombocytopenic purpura (ITP) is a syndrome in which antibodies against platelet or megakaryocytic antigens cause thrombocytopenia. It is, thus, more fittingly called **immune thrombocytopenic purpura**. ITP occurs in two forms: an acute, self-limited, hemorrhagic syndrome in children and a chronic bleeding disorder in adolescents and adults. The autoantibodies often recognize the platelet membrane glycoproteins, Gp IIb/IIIa or Ib/IX, which are involved in platelet adhesion and clot formation.

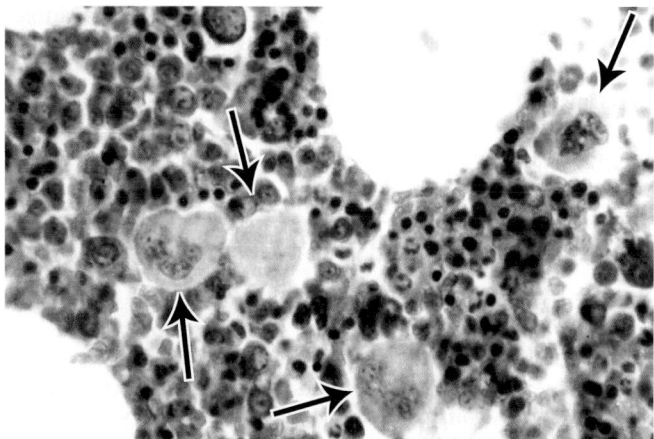

FIGURE 26-28. Idiopathic thrombocytopenic purpura. A section of the bone marrow reveals increased megakaryocytes (*arrows*).

 PATHOPHYSIOLOGY: Like autoimmune hemolytic anemia, ITP reflects antibody-mediated destruction of platelets or their precursors. In most cases, these are IgGs, but IgM antiplatelet antibodies also occur.

Acute ITP typically appears in children of either sex after a viral illness and is likely caused by virus-induced changes in platelet antigens that elicit autoantibodies. Complement bound at the surface lyses platelets in the blood or mediates their phagocytosis and destruction by splenic and hepatic macrophages.

Chronic ITP occurs mainly in adults (male-to-female ratio = 1:2.6) and may be associated with autoimmune (e.g., systemic lupus erythematosus) or malignant lymphoproliferative (e.g., chronic lymphocytic leukemia; see below) diseases. It is also common in people infected with HIV. The magnitude of thrombocytopenia in ITP reflects the balance between (1) levels of antiplatelet antibodies; (2) the extent to which platelet production in the marrow is impaired, as some antibodies may bind to megakaryocytes; and (3) expression of Fc and complement receptors at macrophage cell surfaces. This expression is upregulated in infection and pregnancy but is restored by certain drugs, for example, corticosteroids, danazol and intravenous γ-globulin, all of which are used to treat ITP.

 PATHOLOGY: In acute ITP, the platelet count is typically less than 20,000/μL. In chronic adult ITP, platelet counts vary from a few thousand to 100,000/μL. Peripheral blood smears show many large platelets, owing to accelerated release of young platelets by bone marrow actively engaged in platelet production. Bone marrow thus shows compensatory increases in megakaryocytes (Fig. 26-28). Platelets carry detectable IgG in more than 80% of patients with chronic ITP; in half of these, platelet-associated C3 is also detectable.

CLINICAL FEATURES: Children with **acute ITP** experience sudden onset of petechiae and purpura but are otherwise asymptomatic. Spontaneous recovery occurs within 6 months in over 80% of cases. The major threat (<1% of cases) is intracranial hemorrhage. Treatment is rarely necessary, but with serious disease,

corticosteroids and intravenous immunoglobulin may be needed. Glucocorticoids decrease antiplatelet antibody production and downregulate macrophage Fc receptors. γ-Globulin inhibits clearance of IgG-coated platelets from the circulation via multiple mechanisms.

Chronic ITP in adults manifests as bleeding episodes, such as epistaxis, menorrhagia or ecchymoses, and excessive bleeding after trauma and minor procedures (e.g., tooth extraction). Life-threatening hemorrhages are uncommon. Occasionally, asymptomatic people are discovered to have thrombocytopenia on a routine blood cell count. Most adults with chronic ITP improve with corticosteroids and intravenous γ-globulin. Danazol (a synthetic anabolic steroid) acts like glucocorticoids. In 70% of patients who do not respond adequately to drug therapy within 2–3 months, splenectomy produces complete or partial remission. For patients with severe ITP, ongoing studies are testing the efficacy of thrombopoietic agents that activate the TPO receptor.

Drug-Induced Autoimmune Thrombocytopenia

Many drugs cause immune-mediated platelet destruction: quinine, quinidine, heparin, sulfonamides, gold salts, antibiotics, sedatives, tranquilizers and anticonvulsants. The drugs often complex with a platelet-related protein to make a neoepitope that elicits antibody production. Chemotherapeutic agents, ethanol and thiazides cause thrombocytopenia by directly suppressing platelet production.

Heparin-induced thrombocytopenia (HIT) is a distinct type of drug-induced thrombocytopenia. There are two types of HIT. About 25% of patients experience mild, transient thrombocytopenia 2–5 days after heparin treatment starts. This mild form of HIT is self-limited, entails aggregation of platelets by nonimmune mechanisms and follows a relatively benign course.

Type II HIT is immunologically mediated, caused by acquired IgG antibodies against platelet factor 4–heparin complexes. It occurs in 1%–3% of patients treated with unfractionated heparin. After 4–10 days of therapy, these patients develop severe consumptive thrombocytopenia, platelet activation and thus a hypercoagulable state. Because this form of HIT entails hypercoagulability, platelet aggregation predisposes patients to arterial and venous thromboembolic events that may be lethal.

In both cases, the heparin functions seemingly paradoxically activate platelet aggregation. In type I HIT, it is the heparin itself that induces platelets to aggregate. In type II HIT, heparin acts as a hapten, binding platelet membranes and eliciting antibodies. These antibodies, in turn, trigger platelet aggregation. Thus, the principal complication of HIT is thrombosis.

Pregnancy-Associated Thrombocytopenia

Minimal thrombocytopenia occurs often during the third trimester of pregnancy, owing to dilution of platelets. Since platelet counts are usually above 100,000/μL, no special management is needed. Conversely, preeclampsia/eclampsia syndromes can result in maternal thrombocytopenia. A condition related to preeclampsia is called **HELLP** (hemolysis, elevated liver enzyme tests and low platelets; see Chapter 14). The latter two syndromes can be life-threatening.

Neonatal Thrombocytopenia

Neonatal thrombocytopenias are either **inherited** or **acquired**.

Inherited causes associated with increased platelet destruction include **Wiskott-Aldrich syndrome** (WAS), an X-linked recessive disorder caused by a defect in the Wiskott-Aldrich syndrome protein (*WASP*) gene. Affected boys have small platelets, eczema and immunodeficiency. A variant of WAS is **X-linked thrombocytopenia,** with mutations in the same gene, but which only involves thrombocytopenia. Other inherited defects associated with poor platelet production include amegakaryocytic thrombocytopenia, thrombocytopenia-absent radius syndrome and Fanconi anemia. Thrombocytopenia can also be seen in infants with trisomy 13, 18 or 21.

Fanconi anemia is an inherited, autosomal recessive, bone marrow failure disorder that often includes thrombocytopenia and RBC macrocytosis. The family of Fanconi genes mediate DNA double-strand break repair and genetic stability. There is a high incidence of malignancies as well as congenital anomalies, such as skin hypopigmentation and hyperpigmentation, short stature, microcephaly, microphthalmia and radial/thumb abnormalities (see Chapters 5 and 6).

Neonatal alloimmune thrombocytopenia (NAIT) is caused by increased destruction of platelets, because of alloimmunization to HPA-1a and other platelet-specific antigens that occurs during pregnancy. In NAIT, antibodies made by an HPA-1a–negative mother recognize a paternal HPA-1a–positive antigen on the fetus's platelets. The fetus or neonate, but not the mother, develops thrombocytopenia. NAIT predisposes to fetal and neonatal intracranial hemorrhage.

Nonimmune causes of thrombocytopenia in the neonate are like those in adults, with additional considerations such as birth asphyxia, hypoxic injury, sepsis and DIC, necrotizing enterocolitis, hemangiomas and thrombosis.

Posttransfusion Purpura

This complication of blood transfusion typically develops in women who are HPA-1 negative, and who were sensitized to HPA-1 as a result of previous pregnancies. It may also occur in men who have had previous blood transfusions. Thus, HPA-1–negative people may develop antibodies to HPA-1–positive platelets, after either pregnancy or transfusion with HPA-1–positive platelets. Any HPA-1–positive platelets infused thereafter are then destroyed by those antibodies. Curiously, the patient's own HPA-1–negative platelets are also destroyed. They may acquire the antigen passively or immune complexes may localize to the host platelet membranes. In any event, a self-limited thrombocytopenia occurs about a week after the transfusion.

Thrombotic Thrombocytopenic Purpura

Thrombotic microangiopathies (TMAs) are a heterogeneous group of syndromes that all cause thrombocytopenia, microangiopathic hemolytic anemia, neurologic symptoms, fever and renal impairment. TMAs include TTP and hemolytic–uremic syndrome. Their pathology reflects widespread platelet aggregation and deposition of hyaline thrombi in the microcirculation.

 **MOLECULAR PATHOGENESIS:** In TTP, platelet cross-linking by inappropriate vWF multimers from injured endothelial cells reflects altered cleavage of multimeric vWF multimers. vWF monomers are normally assembled into multimeric molecules of varying size (up to millions of daltons) within endothelial cells and released locally in response to endothelial stimulation. ADAMTS13 is a metalloprotease that normally cleaves large vWF multimers. *In TTP, ADAMTS13 is deficient, causing ultra-large vWF multimers to accumulate. These multimers bind platelets, which form thrombi in the microvasculature, depleting platelets and causing thrombocytopenia.* ADAMTS13 is genetically absent or defective in familial TTP because of mutations of the *ADAMTS13* gene. The protein is inactivated by autoantibodies in idiopathic TTP. Prophylactic plasma infusion, which replaces the missing *ADAMTS13,* is most effective in familial forms of TTP, and plasma exchange is preferred in acquired types.

Although most cases arise in otherwise normal people, TTP may also complicate systemic diseases such as autoimmune collagen vascular disorders (systemic lupus erythematosus, rheumatoid arthritis, Sjögren syndrome), drug-induced hypersensitivity reactions and malignant hypertension. It has also been triggered by infections, cancer chemotherapy, bone marrow transplantation and pregnancy in HELLP syndrome (see Chapter 12).

Other TMA disorders are much less well understood.

 PATHOLOGY: In TTP, periodic acid–Schiff (PAS)-positive hyaline microthrombi deposit in arterioles and capillaries throughout the body, mainly in the heart, brain and kidneys (Fig. 26-29). These microthrombi contain platelet aggregates, fibrin and a few erythrocytes and leukocytes. Unlike immune-mediated vasculitis, there is no inflammation in TTP. Fragmented erythrocytes (schistocytes) always appear in peripheral blood smears (Fig. 26-30) and are caused by RBC shearing in vessels narrowed by thrombi. RBC polychromasia is also a feature and reflects an increase in reticulocytes in response to anemia. Hemolysis increases serum LDH and unconjugated bilirubin levels.

 CLINICAL FEATURES: TTP may occur at any age but is most common in women in the 4th and 5th decades. It may be chronic and recurrent for years or, more frequently, occur as an acute, fulminant disease that is often fatal. Most patients present with neurologic

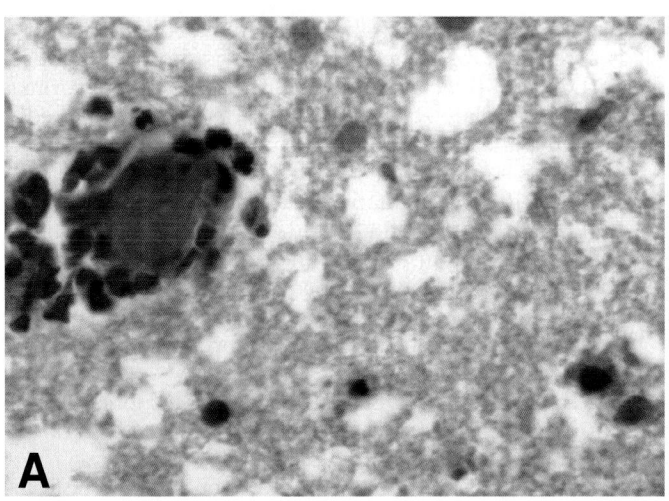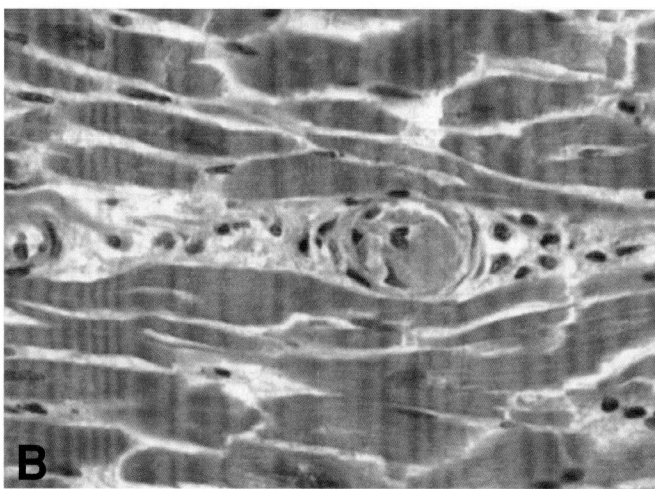

FIGURE 26-29. Thrombotic thrombocytopenic purpura. Microthrombi are present in the brain **(A)** and heart **(B)** of a patient who died of thrombotic thrombocytopenic purpura.

symptoms, including seizures, focal weakness, aphasia and alterations in consciousness. Widespread purpura is often present and vaginal bleeding may occur in women. Hemolytic anemia is a constant feature; hemoglobin levels are often below 6 g/dL. Jaundice caused by hemolysis may be severe. Renal dysfunction includes proteinuria, hematuria and mild renal insufficiency.

More than half of patients with TTP have platelet counts below 20,000/μL. Despite the presence of aggregated platelets, the coagulation cascade is not activated. Thus, PT, PTT and fibrinogen all remain normal. These parameters distinguish this syndrome from DIC (see below). With plasma infusion and plasmapheresis, about 89% of patients survive this once almost uniformly fatal disease.

Hemolytic–Uremic Syndrome

HUS is a thrombotic microangiopathy that resembles TTP, but its pathogenesis is entirely different. HUS is characterized

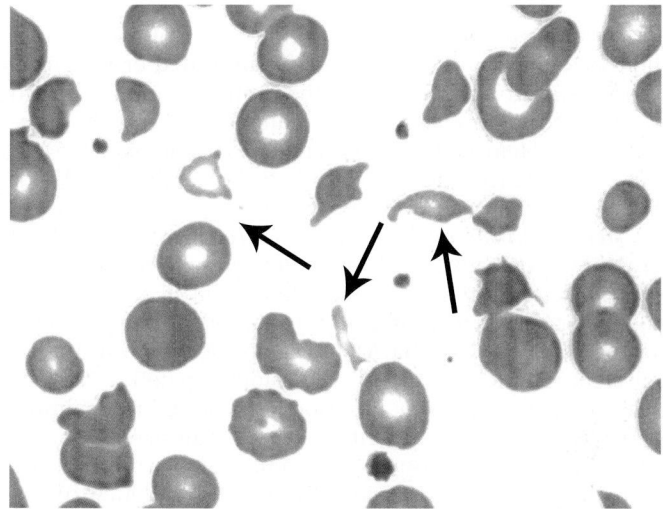

FIGURE 26-30. Microangiopathic hemolytic anemia. Numerous schistocytes (*arrows*) are present in a patient with thrombotic thrombocytopenic purpura.

by thrombocytopenia, microangiopathic hemolysis and acute renal failure.

Classic HUS occurs in children, usually after an acute infectious hemorrhagic gastroenteritis caused by *E. coli* strain O157:H7 or *Shigella dysenteriae* (see Chapter 22). Production of a Shiga-like toxin damages vascular endothelium and activates platelets. Fibrinogen then binds activated platelet Gp IIb/IIIa complex and platelets aggregate. In HUS, aggregated platelet thrombi are primarily in the renal microvasculature. Kidney failure, rather than neurologic abnormalities, is the main clinical feature.

Splenic Sequestration of Platelets

Many patients with splenomegaly, irrespective of the cause, show **hypersplenism**. This syndrome includes sequestration of platelets in the spleen. One third of platelets are normally stored temporarily in the spleen, but in massive splenomegaly, up to 90% of the total platelet pool may be sequestered in that organ. Interestingly, platelet life span is normal, or only slightly reduced. Thrombocytopenia associated with hypersplenism is rarely severe and by itself does not produce a hemorrhagic diathesis.

Other Causes of Thrombocytopenia

Vascular malformations, including hemangiomas and arteriovenous malformations, can cause thrombocytopenia. Platelet consumption due to hemangiomas has been called the **Kasabach-Merritt syndrome**. Platelet loss occurs in patients who have massive hemorrhage, such as in bleeding from a peptic ulcer or during surgery with heavy blood loss. Transfused blood does not contain viable platelets because it is stored at 4°C before administration. Thus, thrombocytopenia occurs in transfused patients because of platelet loss and dilution. Platelet transfusion may prevent this development.

Hereditary Disorders of Platelets

Bernard-Soulier Syndrome (Giant Platelet Syndrome)
Bernard-Soulier syndrome is an autosomal recessive disorder in which platelets have a quantitative or qualitative

defect in the membrane glycoprotein complex (Gp Ib/ IX [CD42] and sometimes Gp V) that serves as a receptor for vWF. The complex helps mediate platelet adhesion to vWF in injured subendothelial tissues. In Bernard-Soulier syndrome, platelets vary widely in size and shape, and the diagnosis is suggested by the combination of *thrombocytopenia and giant platelets* on a blood smear.

The syndrome manifests in infancy or childhood with a bleeding pattern characteristic of *abnormal platelet function*: ecchymoses, epistaxis and gingival bleeding. At a later age, traumatic hemorrhage, gastrointestinal bleeding and menorrhagia occur. Many patients have only a mild bleeding disorder, but others suffer more severe hemorrhage that requires frequent platelet transfusions and that may even be fatal.

Glanzmann Thrombasthenia

Glanzmann thrombasthenia is an autosomal recessive defect in platelet aggregation caused by a quantitative or qualitative abnormality in the glycoprotein complex IIb/ IIIa (CD41/61). In normal platelets, this complex is activated during platelet adhesion. It acts as a receptor for fibrinogen and vWF, to mediate platelet aggregation and generate a solid plug. The IIb/IIIa complex is also linked to platelet cytoskeleton and transmits the force of contraction to adherent fibrin, which promotes clot retraction. In Glanzmann thrombasthenia, the impaired aggregation and clot retraction hampers hemostasis and causes bleeding, despite a normal platelet count.

The disease becomes clinically apparent shortly after birth when an infant has mucocutaneous or gingival hemorrhage, epistaxis or bleeding after circumcision. Later, patients may suffer unexpected hemorrhage after trauma or surgery. Disease severity varies, and only a few patients experience life-threatening hemorrhage. Platelet transfusions correct the condition temporarily.

α Storage Pool Disease (Gray Platelet Syndrome)

α Storage pool disease is a rare inherited disease in which platelets lack morphologically recognizable α granules. The defect is in granule membranes, which are abnormal. Thrombocytopenia is common; platelets are large and pale. The bleeding diathesis tends to be mild.

δ Storage Pool Disease

This heterogeneous illness affects platelet-dense granules. It is sometimes associated with other multisystem hereditary disorders, including Chédiak-Higashi syndrome or Hermansky-Pudlak syndrome (both of which include oculocutaneous albinism). Bleeding manifestations are mild to moderate.

Acquired Qualitative Platelet Disorders

Several acquired disorders may impair platelet function (Table 26-7).

- **Drugs:** Various drugs can limit platelet activity. Aspirin irreversibly acetylates cyclooxygenase (COX), primarily COX-1. It thus blocks production of platelet thromboxane A_2, which is important for platelet aggregation. Platelets cannot synthesize cyclooxygenase, so the aspirin effect lasts for the life span of platelets (7–10 days). Nonsteroidal analgesics, such as indomethacin or ibuprofen, impair platelet function, but as their inhibition of cyclooxygenase is reversible, their effect on platelets is short. Antibiotics, particularly β-lactams (penicillin and cephalosporins), can cause platelet dysfunction. Ticlopidine markedly impairs platelet function and is used to treat thromboembolic disease. However, it may cause TTP.
- **Renal failure:** Qualitative platelet defects leading to prolonged bleeding times and a tendency toward hemorrhage may complicate kidney disease. These platelet abnormalities are heterogeneous and are aggravated by uremic anemia. Reestablishing a normal hematocrit using EPO may return bleeding time to normal without affecting the azotemia.
- **Cardiopulmonary bypass:** Use of extracorporeal circuit during bypass surgery may impair platelet function by activating and fragmenting platelets.
- **Hematologic malignancies:** Platelet dysfunction in chronic myeloproliferative neoplasms and myelodysplastic syndromes reflects intrinsic platelet defects. In dysproteinemias, platelets are coated with plasma paraprotein, impairing function.

Thrombocytosis

Reactive Thrombocytosis

Increases in platelet counts occur in association with (1) iron-deficiency anemia, especially in children; (2) splenectomy; (3) cancer; and (4) chronic inflammatory disorders. Reactive thrombocytosis is rarely symptomatic, but it may trigger thrombotic episodes, especially in patients bedridden after splenectomy.

Clonal Thrombocytosis

Myeloproliferative neoplasms (see below) such as polycythemia vera and essential thrombocythemia entail malignant proliferations of megakaryocytes. Resulting increases in circulating platelets may lead to episodic thrombosis or bleeding.

Coagulopathies Are Caused by Deficient or Abnormal Coagulation Factors

Quantitative and qualitative disorders of all of the coagulation factors are known, and may be **inherited** or **acquired**. Most result from deficiency of the protein factor, leading to inadequate hemostasis and concomitant bleeding. Occasionally the protein factor is present but dysfunctional. Only hereditary deficiencies of factor VIII (hemophilia A), factor IX (hemophilia B) and vWF are common.

Hemophilia is an X-linked recessive disorder of blood clotting that results in delayed bleeding along with joint and muscle bleeding. Classic hemophilia is actually two distinct diseases resulting from mutations in the genes for **factor VIII (hemophilia A)** and **factor IX (hemophilia B)**.

Hemophilia is one of the oldest genetic diseases recorded, having been described in the Talmud almost 2000 years ago: male infants of Jewish families that had a history of fatal bleeding after circumcision were excused from this ritual. Transmission of a bleeding tendency to boys from unaffected mothers has been known for 200 years. Dissemination of hemophilia throughout Europe's royal families by Queen Victoria's daughters highlighted this disease.

Hemophilia A (Factor VIII Deficiency)

MOLECULAR PATHOGENESIS: *Hemophilia A is the most common X-linked inherited bleeding disorder (1 per 5000–10,000 males).* The gene for factor VIII was cloned in 1984. Causative mutations in the very large factor VIII gene at the tip of the long arm of the X chromosome (Xq28) include deletions, inversions, point mutations and insertions. Each family with a history of hemophilia actually harbors a different mutation (private mutant allele). In half of cases, hemophilia A can be traced through many generations, but the other half represent de novo mutations arising within two generations of the index case. In most cases of de novo mutations, an origin in the mother, maternal grandfather or maternal grandmother has been identified.

CLINICAL FEATURES: Patients with hemophilia A have mild, moderate or severe bleeding tendencies. In most, the severity of the illness parallels factor VIII activity in the blood. Half of patients have virtually no factor VIII activity and often suffer spontaneous bleeding. A third of patients, with 1%–5% of normal factor VIII activity, will only occasionally bleed spontaneously, but often do so after minor trauma. One fifth have factor VIII activity levels from 5% to 40% of normal and bleed only after significant trauma or surgery.

The most frequent complication of hemophilia A is a degenerative joint disease caused by repeated bleeding into many joints. Although uncommon, bleeding into the brain was formerly the most common cause of death. Hematuria, intestinal obstruction and respiratory obstruction may all occur with bleeding into the respective organs.

Management consists of factor VIII replacement, either prophylactically to prevent bleeding or therapeutically in response to bleeding episodes. The aim is to correct factor VIII levels to control bleeding and prevent long-term sequelae. Unfortunately, in the 1980s, many of these patients developed AIDS and viral hepatitis from contamination of pooled factor VIII preparations (from plasma-derived concentrates). Screening blood donors for HIV, heat treating purified factor VIII to inactivate HIV and, now, the use of human recombinant factor VIII have eliminated these complications. Screening to detect female carriers and prenatal diagnosis using DNA markers are highly accurate.

Hemophilia B

MOLECULAR PATHOGENESIS: *Hemophilia B is an X-linked inherited disorder of factor IX deficiency.* It is 1/4 as common as hemophilia A, at 1 in 20,000 male births, and accounts for 15% of cases of hemophilia. Factor IX is a vitamin K–dependent protein made in the liver. Many different mutations, from single base substitutions to gross deletions, may cause hemophilia B.

CLINICAL FEATURES: Bleeding manifestations in hemophilia B are like those of hemophilia A. Treatment relies on infusion of purified or recombinant factor IX concentrates.

von Willebrand Disease

von Willebrand disease (vWD) is a heterogeneous complex of hereditary bleeding disorders related to deficiency or abnormality of vWF. Over 20 distinct subtypes are known. A simplified classification (see below) recognizes 3 major categories. Variable expression of vWF (especially type I) confounds estimates of prevalence, although some hold that vWD is the most common inherited coagulopathy (1%–2% of the population).

PATHOPHYSIOLOGY AND MOLECULAR PATHOGENESIS: vWF is an adhesive molecule made by endothelial cells and megakaryocytes as a 250-kd monomer. It polymerizes to form multimers with molecular weights in the millions. vWF is stored in cytoplasmic Weibel-Palade bodies of endothelial cells, from which it is released into subendothelial tissues and plasma. After endothelial insult, subendothelial vWF binds platelet glycoprotein receptors (Gp Ib/IX or CD42), triggering platelet adherence and sealing the injury (Fig. 26-31). vWF also binds Gp IIb/IIIa (CD41/61) to promote platelet aggregation. In plasma, it binds and protects factor VIII. In its absence, factor VIII activity is always impaired.

vWD is an autosomal disease, affecting men and women. The *vWF* gene on chromosome 12 is large and complex (180 kb with 52 exons). Three types of the disease are recognized, each of which is heterogeneous:

- **Type I vWD:** These variants constitute 75% of cases of vWD and are inherited as autosomal dominant traits with variable penetrance. Type I vWD is a **quantitative deficiency in vWF,** in which levels of **all** multimers are reduced, though their relative concentrations remain unchanged.
- **Type II vWD:** Qualitative defects in vWF characterize type II variants, which account for 20% of vWD. In type II disease, interactions of vWF and the blood vessel wall are defective. The plasma activities of both vWF and factor VIII are low. In type IIa, higher–molecular-weight multimers are **absent** from platelets and plasma. Type IIb, an **abnormal** vWF, has increased affinity for platelets and may cause thrombocytopenia.
- **Type III vWD:** This severe form of vWD is least common. It is inherited as an autosomal recessive trait, but some patients are compound heterozygotes with different mutations in the two vWF alleles. vWF activity is absent and plasma factor VIII levels are less than 10% of normal.

CLINICAL FEATURES: Except for type III, most cases of vWD entail only a mild bleeding diathesis. In contrast to hemophilia-related bleeding, patients with vWD show immediate, mucocutaneous bleeding such as easy bruising, epistaxis, GI bleeding and (in women) menorrhagia. The presenting symptom is often excessive hemorrhage after trauma or surgery. Patients with type III vWD may have life-threatening hemorrhage from the gut; hemarthroses like those in hemophilia are not unusual.

All forms of vWD respond well to vWF concentrates or cryoprecipitate. The vasopressin analog desmopressin (DDAVP) is the treatment of choice in types I and IIa, because it increases release of preformed vWF from endothelial storage pools. DDAVP intranasal sprays are now available.

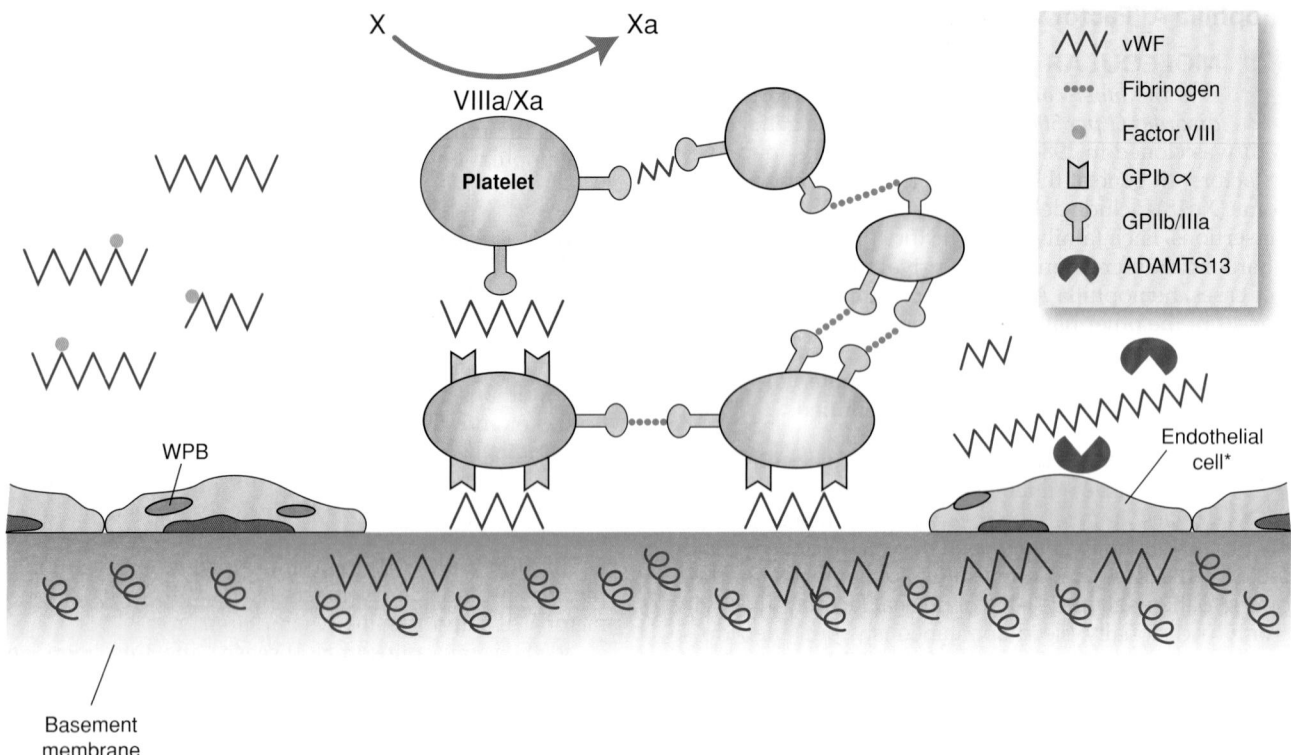

FIGURE 26-31. von Willebrand factor (vWF). vWF is stored in Weibel-Palade bodies (WPBs) of endothelial cells and is secreted from activated endothelial cells (*) into the subendothelial space. vWF is also secreted from platelet α granules. After endothelial injury, vWF binds to platelet glycoprotein (Gp) receptors Gp Ibα and promotes platelet adherence and protects factor VIII. Released vWF stabilizes platelet adhesion to the damaged vessel wall and promotes platelet–fibrin interactions. vWF also binds Gp IIB/IIA on the activated platelet surface to promote platelet aggregation. ADAMTS13 is the protease that cleaves ultralarge multimers of vWF.

Other Coagulation Factor Deficiencies

Deficiencies of all coagulation factor proteins, including factors VII, X, V, XI and II (prothrombin) and fibrinogen, have been reported in humans. As expected, the severity of bleeding usually correlates with the level of functional protein activity. Prolonged PT or PTT in patients who bleed excessively helps to identify a problem with coagulation factors. Factor-specific assays confirm the diagnosis. The thrombin time helps to screen for deficiency or dysfunction of fibrinogen. Deficiency of fibrinogen causes bleeding. By contrast, dysfibrinogenemia may cause bleeding but more often leads to thrombosis.

Liver Disease

Many coagulation factors are produced by the liver (e.g., II, V, VII, IX, X). In addition, the liver plays a key role in vitamin K absorption. Severe liver disease may impair secretion of coagulation factors, as a manifestation of the general protein synthetic defect. In this case, levels of all liver-synthesized coagulation factors are low, affecting the intrinsic and extrinsic pathways. PT and PTT are both prolonged.

Because vitamin K–dependent factors are disproportionately affected, in liver disease the PT is far more affected than the PTT. This is unlike DIC (see below).

Vitamin K Deficiency

Liver-derived coagulation factors depend on vitamin K as an essential cofactor in γ-carboxylation of glutamic acid residues to Gla residues. The secreted proteins are only functional if Gla residues are present. By contrast, factor V is made in the liver but does not require vitamin K. Thus, in vitamin K deficiency (see Chapter 8), activities of factors II, VII, IX and X are low but factor V activity is normal. Severe liver disease will, however, cause decreased activities of all of these factors.

 CLINICAL FEATURES: Levels of vitamin K are physiologically low in neonates, and it is standard practice to administer vitamin K to newborns to prevent hemorrhagic disease. In adults, vitamin K deficiency may reflect poor dietary intake. Since colonic bacteria produce the form of vitamin K that is best absorbed, prolonged antibiotic intake or large colonic resections may lead to vitamin K deficiency.

Inhibitors of Coagulation Factors

Acquired inhibitors of coagulation factors, **circulating anticoagulants,** are usually IgG autoantibodies. Most are directed against factor VIII and vWF, but rarely antibodies to any of the other coagulation factors can be present. In hereditary coagulation disorders, especially hemophilia, circulating anticoagulants arise because of administration of plasma concentrates containing the deficient factor. Anticoagulants also develop in some patients with autoimmune disorders (e.g., systemic lupus erythematosus, rheumatoid arthritis; see Chapter 11), presumably owing to abnormal immune regulation. Finally, acquired anticoagulants often appear in apparently normal people.

 CLINICAL FEATURES: Acquired anticoagulants may be asymptomatic laboratory findings, or they may cause life-threatening hemorrhage. These autoantibodies are difficult to eliminate, but 1/3 of patients remit spontaneously. Treatment includes plasma concentrates, corticosteroids and immunosuppression.

Disseminated Intravascular Coagulation

DIC is widespread intravascular activation of coagulation, generating thrombin and microvascular fibrin thrombi and triggering fibrinolysis. Platelets and clotting factors are consumed, so patients also tend to hemorrhage. DIC is serious and often fatal. It may complicate massive trauma, burns, sepsis (see Chapter 12) from diverse organisms and obstetric emergencies. It is also associated with metastatic cancer, hematopoietic malignancies, cardiovascular and liver disease and many other conditions.

 PATHOPHYSIOLOGY: DIC begins with activation of clotting cascades within the vascular compartment by tissue injury, endothelial damage or both. **Subsequent generation of substantial**

amounts of thrombin *(Fig. 26-32), combined with the failure of natural inhibitory mechanisms to neutralize thrombin, triggers DIC.* With consequent uncontrolled intravascular coagulation, the delicate balance between coagulation and fibrinolysis goes awry. This leads to consumption of clotting factors, platelets and fibrinogen and a consequent hemorrhagic diathesis.

Procoagulant TF is released into the circulation after many kinds of injury, including direct trauma, brain injury and obstetric accidents (e.g., premature separation of the placenta) (see Chapter 14). **Bacterial endotoxin** also stimulates macrophages to release TF (see Chapter 12). **Certain tumor cells** cause DIC by releasing TF. With activation of the clotting cascade, intravascular fibrin microthrombi deposit in the smallest blood vessels. Stimulation of the fibrinolytic system by fibrin generates fibrin split products, which possess anticoagulant properties and contribute to the bleeding diathesis.

Endothelial injury often plays an important role in the development of DIC. The anticoagulant properties of

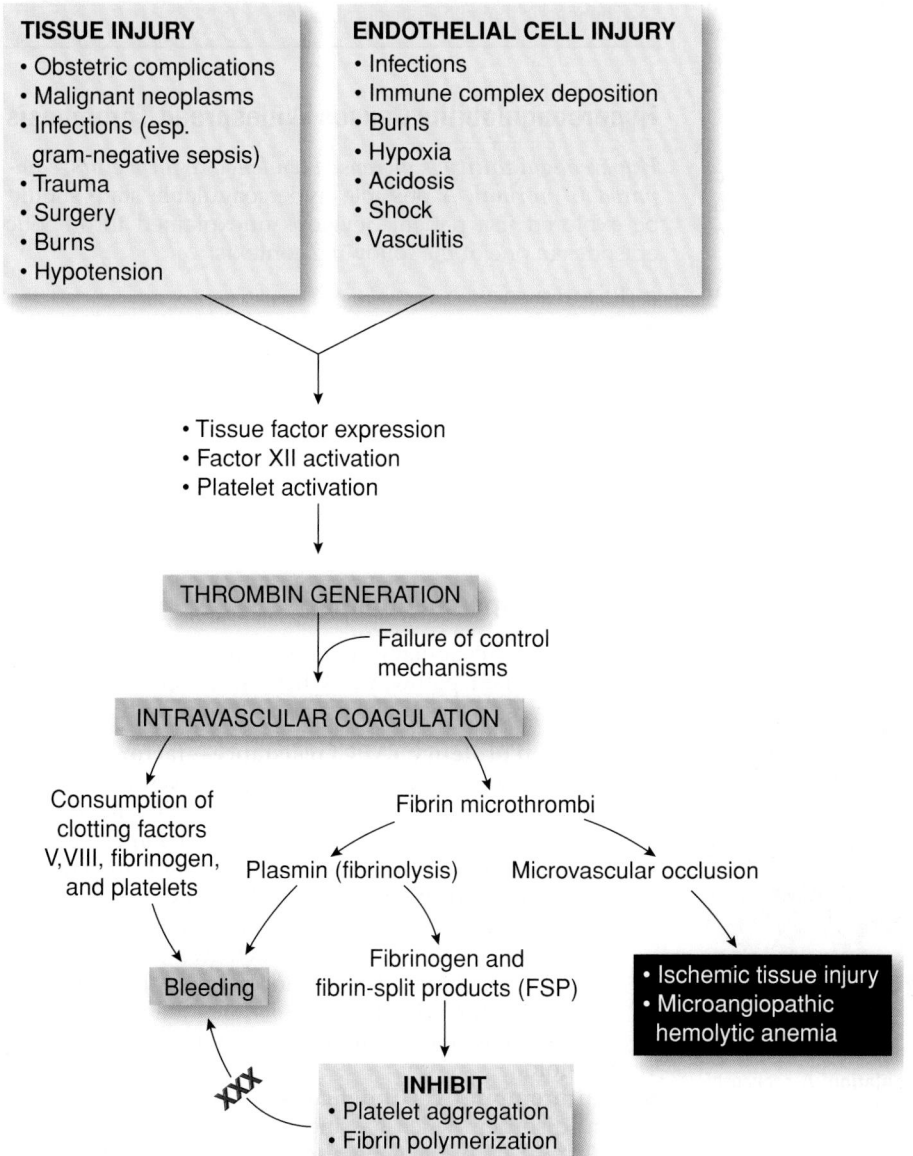

FIGURE 26-32. The pathophysiology of disseminated intravascular coagulation (DIC). The DIC syndrome is precipitated by tissue injury, endothelial cell injury or a combination of the two. These injuries trigger increased expression of tissue factor on cell surfaces and activation of clotting factors (including XII and V) and platelets. With the failure of normal control mechanisms, generation of thrombin leads to intravascular coagulation.

the endothelium (Fig. 26-27) are impaired by diverse injuries, including (1) TNF in Gram-negative sepsis; (2) other inflammatory mediators, such as activated complement, IL-1 or neutrophil proteases; (3) viral or rickettsial infections; and (4) trauma (e.g., burns). Thus, platelet aggregates form in the microvasculature.

 PATHOLOGY: Arterioles, capillaries and venules throughout the body are occluded by **microthrombi** made of fibrin and platelets (Fig. 26-33). However, because fibrinolysis is activated, these thrombi may no longer be visible at the time of autopsy. Microvascular obstruction is associated with widespread **ischemic changes,** particularly in the brain, kidneys, skin, lungs and GI tract. These organs are also sites of bleeding, which, in the case of the brain and gut, may be fatal.

Erythrocytes fragment **(schistocytes)** in passing through webs of intravascular fibrin, resulting in **microangiopathic hemolytic anemia**. Consumption of activated platelets leads to **thrombocytopenia,** while **depletion of clotting factors** causes prolonged PT and PTT and decreased plasma fibrinogen. Plasma fibrin split products prolong the thrombin time. Fibrinopeptide A and D-dimers are elevated (as markers of coagulation and fibrinolytic activation, respectively).

 CLINICAL FEATURES: DIC symptoms reflect both microvascular thrombosis and a bleeding tendency. Ischemic changes in the brain lead to seizures and coma. Depending on the severity of DIC, renal symptoms range from mild azotemia to fulminant acute renal failure. Acute respiratory distress syndrome (see Chapter 18) may supervene, and acute ulcers in the gut may bleed. The bleeding diathesis is evidenced by cerebral hemorrhage, ecchymoses and hematuria. Patients with DIC are treated with heparin anticoagulation to interrupt the cycle of intravascular coagulation, and replenishment of platelets and clotting factors to control the bleeding.

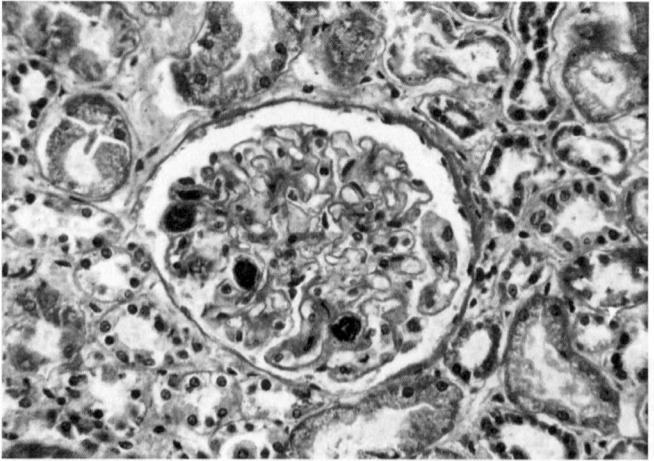

FIGURE 26-33. Disseminated intravascular coagulation. A section of a glomerulus stained with phosphotungstic acid hematoxylin (PTAH), which colors fibrin deep purple, demonstrates several microthrombi.

TABLE 26-8
PRINCIPAL CAUSES OF HYPERCOAGULABILITY

Inherited
Activated protein C resistance (factor V Leiden)
Antithrombin deficiency
Protein C deficiency
Protein S deficiency
Dysfibrinogenemias

Acquired
Lupus inhibitor
Malignancy
Nephrotic syndrome
Therapy
    Factor concentrates
    Heparin
    Oral contraceptives
Hyperlipidemia
Thrombotic thrombocytopenic purpura

Hypercoagulability Causes Widespread Thrombosis

Hypercoagulability is increased tendency to form clots, compared to normal. A possible hypercoagulable state should be explored if a patient develops unexplained thrombotic episodes in one of the following contexts:

- Recurrence
- Development at a young age
- Family history of thrombotic episodes
- Thrombosis in unusual anatomic locations
- Difficulty in controlling with anticoagulants

Disorders that enhance thrombosis are covered in Chapters 7, 16 and 17.

Hypercoagulable states are either inherited and acquired (Table 26-8).

Inherited Hypercoagulability

Inherited hypercoagulability reflects alterations in the natural anticoagulant pathways. A hereditary tendency to clot excessively, regardless of its origin, is **thrombophilia**.

- **Activated protein C (APC) resistance—factor V Leiden:** A point mutation in the *factor V* gene (factor V Leiden) renders it resistant to inhibition by APC. *Resistance APC action is the most common genetic hypercoagulability disorder. It accounts for up to 65% of patients with venous thrombosis.* The factor V Leiden mutation occurs worldwide, but more so in whites (up to 5% of the general population) and much less so in Africans (near 0%). Compared with normal people, heterozygotes for factor V Leiden have 7 times the risk for deep venous thrombosis. In homozygotes, the increased risk is 80-fold.

- **Antithrombin (ATIII) deficiency:** This autosomal dominant disorder, which has incomplete penetrance, occurs in 0.2%–0.4% of the general population and can result in either a quantitative or a qualitative effect on ATIII. The risk of a thrombotic event (usually venous) is 20%–80% in different families.

- **Protein C and protein S deficiencies:** Homozygous protein C deficiency causes life-threatening neonatal thrombosis with **purpura fulminans**. Up to 0.5% of the general population has heterozygous protein C deficiency, but many of them are symptom free. Clinically, deficiencies of proteins C and S resemble ATIII deficiency.
- **Other causes of hypercoagulability:** A genetic variant (G20210A) in the 3′-untranslated region of prothrombin mRNA is associated with thrombosis. The mechanism is unclear, but may involve excessively high prothrombin levels in people with this variant. Unusually high levels of fibrinogen and factors VII and VIII are associated with thrombosis. Again, how the elevated levels occur remains to be elucidated. Some dysfibrinogenemias are also associated with thrombosis.

Acquired Hypercoagulability

Venous stasis contributes to hypercoagulability associated with prolonged immobilization and congestive cardiac failure. Increased platelet activation probably accounts for excessive clotting in patients with myeloproliferative disorders, heparin-associated thrombocytopenia and TTP.

Antiphospholipid Antibody Syndrome

Antibodies against several negatively charged protein/phospholipid complexes are associated with antiphospholipid antibody syndrome. This is an autoimmune disorder that entails arterial and venous thrombosis, spontaneous abortions and immune-mediated thrombocytopenia or anemia.

In this syndrome, antibodies (mainly, but not exclusively, IgG) react with proteins that bind anionic phospholipids, such as phosphatidylserine (PS) or cardiolipin. These membrane lipids are only exposed when cells such as platelets are activated. Many plasma proteins and Gla domain–containing procoagulant proteins (e.g., prothrombin) bind to PS and related anionic phospholipids. Diagnosis entails detecting (1) lupus-type anticoagulant activity, (2) anticardiolipin antibodies and (3) antibodies to plasma protein β_2-glycosyl phosphatidylinositol (GPI). Anticardiolipin antibodies bind β_2-GPI in the presence of cardiolipin.

Lupus anticoagulants (a misnomer: these antibodies are not restricted to patients with systemic lupus erythematosus [see Chapter 11] and in fact cause increased coagulability) are antiphospholipid antibodies that occur in patients with systemic lupus erythematosus and other autoimmune conditions, or in otherwise asymptomatic people. Because they inhibit phospholipids, lupus anticoagulants prolong PTT in vitro, but these patients actually tend to be prone to hypercoagulability.

Antiphospholipid antibody syndrome is the leading acquired hematologic cause of thrombosis. Resulting thromboses may occur via several possible mechanisms, including platelet activation, endothelial cell activation and altered coagulation factor assembly on membranes. Thrombosis in the uteroplacental vasculature is the likely mechanism in recurrent fetal loss.

Nonmalignant Disorders of White Blood Cells

Chapters 2 through 4 discuss white blood cell structure and function.

DISORDERS OF NEUTROPHILS

Neutropenia Is an Absolute Neutrophil Count below 1500/µL

The clinical consequences of neutropenia depend entirely on the extent of neutropenia. In mild cases, absolute neutrophil counts (ANCs) are 1000–1500/µL; in moderate neutropenia, ANCs are 500–1000/µL. In severe cases, ANCs are less than 500/µL. In patients with mild neutropenia **(granulocytopenia)**, the number of neutrophils is adequate to defend against microorganisms. With moderate neutropenia, patients become vulnerable to microbial infections. In severe neutropenia, the risk of serious infection is high. **Agranulocytosis** is the virtual absence of neutrophils, caused by depletion of both the marginated pool and the bone marrow reserve.

Neutropenia reflects either decreased production or increased destruction of neutrophils (Table 26-9). Most cases are asymptomatic and unexplained, to which the term **chronic benign neutropenia** is applied. Sometimes, total granulocyte numbers are normal, but excessive neutrophils are stored in the marrow or marginated in blood vessels.

DECREASED NEUTROPHIL PRODUCTION: Radiation or chemotherapeutic drugs suppress normal hematopoiesis

TABLE 26-9

PRINCIPAL CAUSES OF NEUTROPENIA

Decreased Production
Irradiation
Drug induced (long and short term)
Viral infections
Congenital
Cyclic

Ineffective Production
Megaloblastic anemia
Myelodysplastic syndromes

Increased Destruction
Isoimmune neonatal
Autoimmune
　Idiopathic
　Drug induced
　Felty syndrome
　Systemic lupus erythematosus
　Dialysis (induced by complement activation)
　Splenic sequestration
　Increased margination

and so interfere with generation of neutrophils. Certain drugs, such as phenothiazines, phenylbutazone, antithyroid drugs and indomethacin, can cause **idiosyncratic** marrow suppression. Viral infection and alcohol intake may also suppress myelopoiesis.

 **MOLECULAR PATHOGENESIS:** Decreased granulocyte production can also result from constitutional genetic alterations in several rare hereditary disorders, including **Kostmann syndrome** and **infantile genetic agranulocytosis**. The genetic bases of several of these diseases are known. Mutations in the neutrophil elastase gene cause the most common form of congenital agranulocytosis. Mutations in *HAX*, a gene regulating apoptosis, are responsible for Kostmann syndrome. Ineffective myelopoiesis is involved in the neutropenia of megaloblastic anemias and myelodysplastic syndromes. In **cyclic neutropenia,** episodes recur regularly about every 21 days.

INCREASED PERIPHERAL DESTRUCTION OF GRANULOCYTES: Accelerated elimination of granulocytes is caused by:

- Increased consumption of neutrophils in overwhelming infections
- Increased sequestration in hypersplenism
- Increased destruction by antibodies

Many **drugs** can lead to immune-mediated neutrophil destruction, especially sulfonamides, phenylbutazone and indomethacin. The toxic effect results from attachment of circulating antigen–antibody complexes to granulocyte surfaces, with subsequent complement-mediated injury.

Neutropenia is common in AIDS patients and is multifactorial. Virus-induced depression of neutrophil production is aggravated by infectious consumption of neutrophils and often by antiretroviral drugs (e.g., zidovudine).

Neutrophilia Is an Absolute Neutrophil Count above 7000/μL

Neutrophilia has many causes (Table 26-10) and reflects (1) **increased mobilization** of neutrophils from bone marrow storage, (2) **enhanced release** from the peripheral blood marginal pool or (3) **stimulation of marrow granulopoiesis**. Increased mobilization of neutrophils from the marrow pool or from peripheral marginal pools occurs in settings of acute trauma or infections. Mild neutrophilia is seen in 20% of women in the third trimester of pregnancy, but the mechanism is poorly defined.

LEUKEMOID REACTION: In acute infections and occasionally in times of severe hemorrhage or acute hemolysis, white blood counts (and, implicitly, neutrophils) may be so high as to be mistaken for leukemia, especially chronic myeloid leukemia (CML). Such nonneoplastic increases in leukocyte counts are **leukemoid reactions**. Clues to the benign (or reactive) nature of a leukemoid reaction include the following: (1) the cells in the peripheral blood are usually segmented neutrophils and fewer neutrophilic myeloid precursors, (2) leukocyte alkaline phosphatase activity is high in a leukemoid reaction but low in CML, (3) white blood cell (WBC) counts are usually under 50,000/μL in reactive conditions and (4) reactive neutrophils often contain large blue cytoplasmic inclusions **(Döhle bodies)** or prominent blue-black granulation of the cytoplasm **(toxic granulation)**. If

TABLE 26-10
PRINCIPAL CAUSES OF NEUTROPHILIA
Infections
Primarily bacterial
Immunologic/Inflammatory
Rheumatoid arthritis
Rheumatic fever
Vasculitis
Neoplasia
Hemorrhage
Drugs
Glucocorticoids
Colony-stimulating factors (CSFs)
Lithium
Hereditary
CD18 deficiency
Metabolic
Acidosis
Uremia
Gout
Thyroid storm
Tissue Necrosis
Infarction
Trauma
Burns

uncertain, the absence of the Philadelphia chromosome (see below) or other cytogenetic abnormality supports a reactive, nonneoplastic diagnosis.

Qualitative Disorders of Neutrophils Are Associated with Impaired Function

If granulocyte functionality is impaired, resistance to infection may decrease despite a normal granulocyte count. Such rare hereditary disorders of granulocyte activity include chronic granulomatous disease, myeloperoxidase deficiency and Chédiak-Higashi syndrome (see Chapter 2).

DISORDERS OF OTHER WHITE BLOOD CELL SERIES

Eosinophilia Occurs with Allergic Reactions and Malignancies

Eosinophils differentiate in the bone marrow under the influence of eosinophil growth factors (e.g., IL-5). They circulate briefly in the blood, then migrate preferentially to the gut, respiratory tract and skin. Eosinophils respond to

TABLE 26-11

PRINCIPAL CAUSES OF EOSINOPHILIA

Allergic Disorders

Skin Diseases

Parasitic (Helminth) Infestations

Malignant Neoplasms

Hematopoietic

Solid tumors

Collagen Vascular Disorders

Miscellaneous

Hypereosinophilic syndromes

Eosinophilia–myalgia syndrome

Interleukin-2 therapy

chemotactic substances made by mast cells or are induced by persistent antigen–antibody complexes, such as occur in chronic parasitic, dermatologic and allergic conditions. The main causes of eosinophilia are listed in Table 26-11.

In **idiopathic hypereosinophilic syndrome,** circulating eosinophils exceed 1500/μL for more than 6 months without evident underlying disease. Eosinophil counts in this condition may reach 50,000–100,000/μL.

Hypereosinophilia may accompany mast cell disease (see below), tumors like Hodgkin or non-Hodgkin lymphoma or myeloproliferative disorders (see below). Some of these neoplasms are associated with platelet-derived growth factor receptor (PDGFR) or fibroblast growth factor receptor-1 (FGFR-1) gene rearrangements.

Regardless of the cause, accumulation of eosinophils in tissues often leads to necrosis, particularly in the myocardium, where it produces endomyocardial disease (see Chapter 17). Neurologic dysfunction may also develop. Eosinophil-mediated tissue injury is related to constituents of the eosinophil granules, particularly major basic protein and cationic protein (see Chapter 2).

The prognosis of untreated idiopathic hypereosinophilic syndrome is grave: only 10% of untreated patients survive 3 years. With aggressive corticosteroid therapy, 70% live over 5 years, even with cardiac involvement. If hypereosinophilia is associated with malignancy, prognosis depends on the course of tumor therapy (see below).

Basophilia Occurs in Allergic Reactions and Myeloproliferative Diseases

The basophil is the least abundant of all leukocytes. It differentiates in the bone marrow, circulates briefly in the blood and then passes into tissues. Its relationship to mast cells is controversial. Basophil granules contain several preformed inflammatory mediators, including histamine and chondroitin sulfate. When stimulated, these cells also synthesize leukotrienes and other mediators. Basophilia occurs most often in immediate-type hypersensitivity reactions and together with chronic myeloproliferative neoplasms. The major causes of basophilia are listed in Table 26-12.

Monocytosis Characterizes Both Malignant and Inflammatory Conditions

Monocytosis is defined as a peripheral blood monocyte count above 800/μL. The main causes include hematologic malignancies, immunologic and inflammatory conditions, infectious diseases and solid cancers. The former account for at least half of peripheral blood monocytoses. For example, monocytes may constitute a component of myeloproliferative neoplasms, or myelodysplastic/myeloproliferative neoplasms such as chronic myelomonocytic leukemia. In such cases, they may be either morphologically normal or immature and dysplastic cytologically. Peripheral blood monocytosis often occurs in neutropenic states, possibly as a compensatory mechanism. It may also accompany Hodgkin or non-Hodgkin lymphomas.

Proliferative Disorders of Mast Cells Release Inflammatory Mediators

Mast cell disorders are diverse and include many benign and malignant diseases. The benign, nonneoplastic, reactive conditions of mast cells are important to recognize and differentiate from the malignant syndromes. Mast cells derive from precursor cells in the bone marrow and are found in the connective tissues, usually in close proximity to blood vessels (see Chapter 2). Mast cell granules contain inflammatory mediators, such as histamine, heparin, eosinophil and neutrophil chemotactic factors and certain proteases. The symptoms of mast cell proliferative diseases are caused by release of these substances and include flushing, pruritus and hives. Secretion of heparin also causes bleeding from the nasopharynx or GI tract.

Reactive mast cell hyperplasia is a nonmalignant process that occurs in immediate- and delayed-type hypersensitivity reactions and in lymph nodes that drain the sites of

TABLE 26-12

PRINCIPAL CAUSES OF BASOPHILIA

Allergic (Drug, Food)

Inflammation

Juvenile rheumatoid arthritis

Ulcerative colitis

Infection

Viral (chickenpox, influenza)

Tuberculosis

Neoplasia

Myeloproliferative syndromes

Basophilic leukemia

Carcinoma

Endocrine

Diabetes mellitus

Myxedema

Estrogen administration

malignant tumors. It is also observed in Waldenström macroglobulinemia, in the bone marrow of women with postmenopausal osteoporosis, in myelodysplastic syndromes and after chemotherapy for leukemia.

Disorders of Hematopoietic Stem Cells

NONMALIGNANT STEM CELL DISORDERS

Disorders of HSC Failure May Manifest in Multiple Hematopoietic Series

Aplastic Anemia

Aplastic anemia is a disorder of pluripotential hematopoietic stem cells that leads to bone marrow failure. The marrow is hypocellular and all blood cell lineages are decreased **(pancytopenia)**.

  **PATHOPHYSIOLOGY AND ETIOLOGIC FACTORS:** Aplastic anemia is a rare heterogeneous disease that results from injury to hematopoietic stem cells. In 50%–70% of cases, there is no identifiable etiology (Table 26-13). In 10%–20% of cases, it is due to a marrow insult. In the rest of the cases, aplastic anemia is inherited. The inciting insult can be a predictable, dose-dependent, toxic injury (e.g., certain chemotherapeutic drugs, chemicals and ionizing radiation). Marrow damage can result from an idiosyncratic, dose-independent, immunologic injury, as occurs with idiopathic cases or after certain drug or viral exposures. The most common inherited cause of aplastic anemia is Fanconi anemia, as discussed below. Depending on its cause, stem cell injury may or may not be reversible.

In some patients, stem cell injury is an immune phenomenon: it responds clinically to antithymocyte globulin or other immunosuppressive agents. Other cases probably reflect an intrinsic abnormality of stem cells, as suggested by subsequent evolution of clonal stem cell disorders (paroxysmal nocturnal hemoglobinuria, myelodysplasia, acute leukemia).

 PATHOLOGY: The bone marrow in aplastic anemia shows variably reduced cellularity, depending on the clinical stage of the disease. Myeloid, erythroid and megakaryocytic lineages are decreased, with a relative increase in marrow lymphocytes and plasma cells. As marrow cellularity declines, there is a corresponding increase in fat (Fig. 26-34). Anemia, leukopenia (mainly granulocytopenia) and thrombocytopenia characterize aplastic anemia. Despite elevated EPO levels, reticulocytosis is absent, which underscores the underlying stem cell defect.

 CLINICAL FEATURES: Patients with aplastic anemia show signs and symptoms due to pancytopenia (i.e., weakness, fatigue, infection and bleeding).

TABLE 26-13
ETIOLOGY OF APLASTIC ANEMIA
Idiopathic (two thirds of cases)
Ionizing radiation
Drugs
Chemotherapeutic agents
Chloramphenicol
Anticonvulsants
Nonsteroidal anti-inflammatory agents
Gold
Chemicals
Benzene
Viruses
Hepatitis C virus (HCV)
Epstein-Barr virus (EBV)
HIV
Parvovirus B19
Hereditary
Fanconi anemia

For untreated aplastic anemia, the prognosis is grim, with a 3–6-month median survival. Only 20% live over 1 year. Immunosuppressive therapy often leads to transient remissions. Bone marrow or stem cell transplantation may be curative.

Fanconi Anemia

Fanconi anemia (FA) is the most common hereditary bone marrow failure syndrome. There are 15 associated genes known, labeled *FANC* (for Fanconi complementation group), followed by A, B, and so forth. The most commonly occurring mutants affect FANC genes A, C, G and D2. (FANCD1 is also BRCA2; see Chapters 5 and 25.) Affected patients may

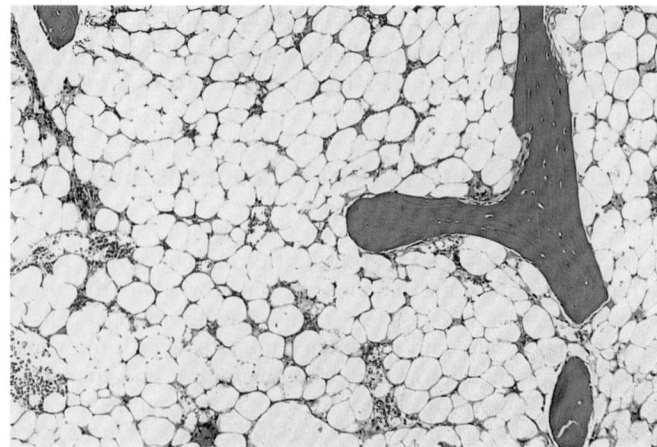

FIGURE 26-34. Aplastic anemia. The bone marrow consists largely of fat cells and lacks normal hematopoietic activity.

be obvious at birth or shortly afterward, as they often have abnormalities of their thumbs and radii, as well as cutaneous, renal and other malformations. Aggregate incidence of Fanconi anemia is less than 1 per 100,000 live births.

The underlying defect is in DNA repair, and in particular repair of cross-links between DNA strands, such as may occur during DNA duplication. Different members of the Fanconi gene family mediate key functions in this pathway and interact with other DNA damage/repair genes such as ATM, ATR and BRCA1 (see Chapter 5).

Aplastic anemia associated with Fanconi anemia usually occurs in the first decade and may be the sentinel event. All hematopoietic series are affected. It is important to distinguish FA patients from others with aplastic anemia, as Fanconi patients will not respond to immunosuppressive treatments used for people with idiopathic aplastic anemia. Androgens may be useful in treating bone marrow failure due to FA, but HSC transplantation is the treatment of choice. Unfortunately, the sensitivity of these patients to DNA damaging agents complicates pretransplant conditioning.

Long-term complications of Fanconi anemia, should patients survive hematopoietic failure events, include development of myelodysplastic syndromes and acute myelogenous leukemia (see below) during their teenage years or as young adults. As well, since the DNA repair defect affects all cells, FA patients are highly susceptible to developing epithelial tumors later in life.

Some HSC Disorders Affect One Series Preferentially

Pure Red Cell Aplasia

Pure red cell aplasia (PRCA) is selective marrow suppression of committed erythroid precursors. White blood cells and platelets are unaffected.

PATHOPHYSIOLOGY: PRCA most often results from immune suppression of red cell production, the etiology of which is unknown. On occasion, it is due to viral infection (parvovirus B19) or thymic lesions (e.g., thymoma, thymic hyperplasia). The P antigens on red cell membranes are receptors for parvovirus, which explains the restricted infection of erythroid precursors.

Diamond-Blackfan syndrome is a PRCA caused by de novo or inherited mutations in one of many ribosomal proteins. It manifests within the first 2 years of life with anemia, with or without physical abnormalities including cleft lip or palate, micrognathia, limb abnormalities and short stature. Anemia is caused by defective erythroid precursors that show a diminished response to erythropoietin and decreased erythroid burst- and colony-forming capacities.

PATHOLOGY: In PRCA, overall marrow cellularity is normal, but erythroid precursors are absent or are arrested at the erythroblast (pronormoblast) stage. In cases caused by parvovirus B19, proerythroblasts have intranuclear viral inclusions. Myeloid and megakaryocytic precursors are adequate in number and show normal maturation.

Patients with PRCA develop moderate to severe anemia, often with macrocytic indices. Despite increased EPO, there is no accompanying reticulocytosis.

CLINICAL FEATURES: Acquired PRCA manifests as an acute self-limited illness or a chronic relapsing process. **Acute self-limited PRCA** is often due to parvovirus B19. This condition may not be clinically apparent unless the patient suffers from an underlying chronic hemolytic anemia (e.g., hereditary spherocytosis, sickle cell anemia). Such cases may be complicated by an aplastic "crisis" (i.e., sudden worsening of anemia). Immunocompromised patients cannot clear parvovirus infection and anemia may be prolonged. **Chronic relapsing PRCA** may be idiopathic or associated with an underlying thymic lesion. In such cases, thymectomy may correct the anemia.

Diamond Blackfan syndrome is usually life-threatening owing to severe anemia and the gradual impact of iron overload. Some patients respond to glucocorticoids.

Paroxysmal Nocturnal Hemoglobinuria

Paroxysmal nocturnal hemoglobinuria (PNH) is an acquired clonal stem cell disorder characterized by episodic intravascular hemolytic anemia due to increased RBC sensitivity to complement-mediated lysis.

MOLECULAR PATHOGENESIS: The underlying defect in PNH involves somatic mutation of the *phosphatidylinositol glycan-class A (PIG-A)* gene, on the short arm of the X chromosome (Xp22.1) in HSCs (Table 26-14). This mutation disrupts synthesis of GPI, which normally anchors many proteins (e.g., CD14, CD16, CD55, CD59) to RBC membranes. Consequent loss of **decay acceleration factor** (CD55) and, more importantly, **membrane inhibitor of reactive lysis** (CD59) from their surfaces makes red blood cells more susceptible to lysis by complement. Leukocytes and platelets derived from the abnormal stem cells also lose GPI-linked membrane proteins.

PNH may develop as a primary disorder or evolve from preexisting aplastic anemia. Because the defect is clonal, it may progress to **myelodysplasia** or overt **acute leukemia** (see below). Some patients have several abnormal clonal erythrocyte populations, with varying susceptibility to complement.

PATHOLOGY: During hemolytic episodes, patients develop varyingly severe normocytic or macrocytic anemia, with an appropriate reticulocyte response. Because the hemolysis is intravascular, hemoglobinuria is present, and iron deficiency may develop over time from recurrent iron loss in the urine. *PNH is diagnosed by flow cytometric demonstration that blood cells lack GPI-anchored proteins.* Leukopenia and thrombocytopenia are frequent, and sensitivity to complement may lead to inappropriate platelet activation.

CLINICAL FEATURES: Patients may have intermittent intravascular hemolysis, although only a minority have it at night. Venous and arterial thrombosis, notably Budd-Chiari syndrome (hepatic vein thrombosis; see Chapter 20), are increased in PNH because of complement-mediated platelet activation. Thrombocytopenia may lead to bleeding. Treatment is supportive; bone marrow transplantation is curative.

TABLE 26-14

COMMON GENETIC ABNORMALITIES ASSOCIATED WITH MYELOID PROLIFERATIONS

Disease	Associated Genetic/Chromosomal Abnormality	Importance
Paroxysmal nocturnal hemoglobinuria (PNH)	PIG-A mutations	Characteristic of PNH
Chronic myeloid leukemia (CML)	t(9;22)(q34;q11) (Philadelphia chromosome)	Largely defines CML
	Trisomy 8; trisomy 19; isochromosome 17q; second Philadelphia chromosome	Occur in some cases in blast phase of CML
Polycythemia vera	Trisomy 8 or 9; del 20q; del 13q; del 9p	Associated in some cases
	JAK2 V617F	Seen in 95% of polycythemia vera cases
Primary myelofibrosis (PMF)	del(13)(q12–22)	Associated in some cases
	der(6)t(1;6)(q21–23;p21.3)	Strongly associated in some cases
	JAK2 V617F	Seen in 50% of PMF
Essential thrombocythemia (ET)	del 20q; trisomy 8	Diagnostically helpful if present
	JAK2 V617F	Seen in 40% of ET cases
	MPL mutations	Seen in rare cases of ET
Myelodysplastic syndromes	5q–	Suggests favorable prognosis
	7q–	Suggests unfavorable prognosis
Acute myelogenous leukemia (AML)	t(8;21)(q22;q22); inv(16)(p13;q22); t(16;16)(p13.1;q22); t(9;11)(p22;q23); t(6;9)(p3;q34); inv(3)(q21;q26.2)	Seen in some cases of AML with recurring chromosomal abnormalities
Acute promyelocytic leukemia (APL)	t(15;17)(q22;q12)	Defines APL
Acute monocytic leukemia (AMoL)	del(11q); t(9;11); t(11;19)	Seen in some cases of AMoL
Acute myelomonocytic leukemia (AMML)	inv(16)(p13;q22); del(16q)	Seen in some cases of AMML
Acute megakaryoblastic leukemia	t(1;22)(p13;q13)	Seen in some cases, particularly in children
Myeloid sarcoma	Translocations involving (11q23), NPM mutations	Seen in some cases, not unique to myeloid sarcomas

LEUKEMIAS AND MYELODYSPLASTIC SYNDROMES

Malignant leukocytes originate from either myeloid or lymphoid cells. Malignant proliferations of myeloid cells are derived from bone marrow cells and manifest as **acute myeloid leukemias, myelodysplastic syndromes** or **myeloproliferative neoplasms**. **Malignant lymphocytes** may arise anywhere there are lymphoid cells. World Health Organization (WHO) classifications are based on morphology, immunophenotype, cytogenetics and molecular abnormalities. In 2008, the WHO made significant changes to the classification of hematopoietic malignancies.

Myeloproliferative Neoplasms Are Clonal Stem Cell Disorders

Myeloproliferative neoplasms (MPNs) are clonal hematopoietic, stem cell disorders with unregulated, increased *proliferation of one or more myeloid lineages (granulocytes, erythrocytes, megakaryocytes or mast cells).* The WHO recognizes four well-established, and four additional, entities: **chronic myelogenous leukemia, BCR-ABL1 positive; polycythemia vera; primary myelofibrosis; essential thrombocythemia; chronic neutrophilic leukemia; chronic eosinophilic leukemia; mastocytosis; and unclassifiable myeloproliferative neoplasm** (Table 26-15).

Myeloproliferative neoplasms typically affect adults 40–80 years old. They are relatively uncommon, with a yearly incidence of 6–10 cases per 100,000. Radiation and benzene exposure are implicated in a few cases, but the etiology is largely unknown. There is also evidence of inherited predisposition to develop MPNs. Characteristic features of all subtypes include bone marrow hypercellularity with effective hematopoietic maturation and increased numbers of red cells, granulocytes and/or platelets. Bone marrow fibrosis of different degrees and splenomegaly often accompany MPNs. Specific oncogene mutations and/or translocations are diagnostic of certain myeloproliferative neoplasms (see below).

TABLE 26-15

MYELOPROLIFERATIVE NEOPLASMS[a]

	Chronic Myelogenous Leukemia, BCR-ABL1 Positive	Polycythemia Vera	Primary Myelofibrosis	Essential Thrombocythemia
Clinical Features				
Peak age range (years)	25–60	40–60	50–70	50–70
Splenomegaly	90%	75%	100%	30% (slight)
Hepatomegaly	50%	40%	80%	40% (slight)
Acute leukemic conversion	80%	5%–10%	5%–10%	2%–5%
Median survival (years)	3–4	13	5	>10
Bone Marrow				
Histopathology	Panhyperplasia (predominantly granulocytic)	Panhyperplasia (predominantly erythroid)	Panhyperplasia with fibrosis	Large megakaryocytes in clusters
M:E ratio	10:1 to 50:1	≤2:1	2:1 to 5:1	2:1 to 5:1
Fibrosis	<10%	15%–20%	90%–100%	<5%
Laboratory Findings				
Hemoglobin	Mild anemia	>20 g/dL	Mild anemia	Mild anemia
RBC morphology	Slight aniso- and poikilocytosis	Slight aniso- and poikilocytosis	Immature erythrocytes and marked aniso- and poikilocytosis	Hypochromic microcytes
Granulocytes	Moderate to markedly increased with spectrum of maturation	Normal to mildly increased; may show a few immature forms	Normal to moderately increased; some immature WBCs	Normal to slightly increased
Platelets	Normal to moderately increased	Normal to moderately increased	Increased to decreased	Markedly increased with abnormal forms
Genetics	Philadelphia chromosome: BCR/ABL gene rearrangement	JAK2 activating mutation	JAK2 activating mutation	JAK2 activating mutation

M:E ratio = ratio of myeloid to erythroid; RBC = red blood cell; WBC = white blood cell.
[a]Other myeloproliferative neoplasms include chronic neutrophilic leukemia, chronic eosinophilic leukemia, mastocytosis and myeloproliferative neoplasm, unclassifiable.

Chronic Myelogenous Leukemia

CML is derived from an abnormal pluripotent bone marrow stem cell and results in prominent neutrophilic leukocytosis over the full range of myeloid maturation. A **Philadelphia chromosome,** or molecular or cytogenetic demonstration of the *BCR/ABL* **fusion gene,** is required to establish the diagnosis. CML is the most common myeloproliferative neoplasm and accounts for 15%–20% of all cases of leukemia.

MOLECULAR PATHOGENESIS: The cause of CML is usually unknown. Radiation exposure and myelotoxic agents, such as benzene, have been implicated in a small number of cases. The leukemic cells represent clonal pluripotent stem cells that can differentiate along myeloid or lymphoid pathways; however, most cases show mainly granulocytic differentiation. Conventional cytogenetic and/or fluorescence in situ hybridization (FISH) techniques identify a reciprocal balanced translocation in 95% of cases. This translocation involves exchange of genetic material between chromosomes 9 and 22, resulting in a Philadelphia chromosome [t(9;22)(q34;q11)] (Table 26-14 and Fig. 26-35A). This chromosome itself is a derivative (shortened) chromosome 22 [der(22q)]. The *BCR* (breakpoint cluster region) gene on chromosome 22 is fused to the *ABL* gene on chromosome 9 to form a *BCR/ABL* fusion gene. A small number of cases have cryptic translocations involving 9q34 and 22q11 that cannot be identified by conventional cytogenetics. In these cases, *BCR/ABL* fusion is detected by FISH (Fig. 26-35B) or using molecular techniques, such as reverse transcriptase polymerase chain reaction (RT-PCR).

In the vast majority of cases, the abnormal BCR/ABL fusion gene encodes a 210-kd fusion protein (p210), which is

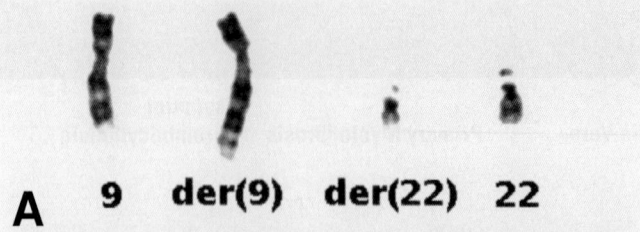

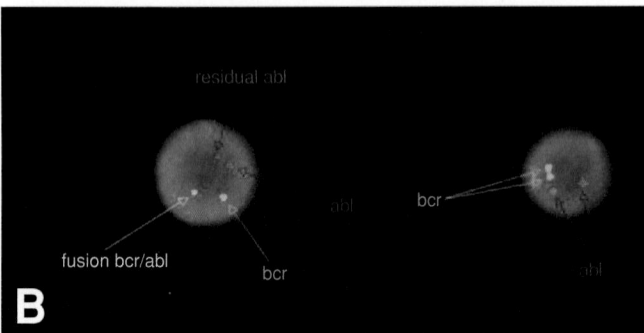

FIGURE 26-35. Chronic myelogenous leukemia. A. The Philadelphia chromosome der(22) is shown. **B.** Fluorescence in situ hybridization (FISH) in a patient with t(9;22) (Philadelphia chromosome)-positive chronic myeloid leukemia. *Right image.* A normal cell contains two separate bcr (chromosome 22) and abl (chromosome 9) genes. *Left image.* A leukemic cell with a fusion bcr/abl signal; residual abl signal; and two normal abl and bcr signals derived from normal chromosomes 9 and 22, respectively.

a constitutively active tyrosine kinase and is central to the pathogenesis of the neoplasm. This activated tyrosine kinase autophosphorylates and then activates downstream signaling pathways that trigger cell proliferation, differentiation, survival and adhesion. Much less commonly, the *BCR/ABL* fusion gene results from a breakage in the minor breakpoint cluster regions yielding alternative fusion proteins such as p190 and p230 (often associated with prominent neutrophilic maturation and/or thrombocytosis). While small amounts of p190 (often associated with monocytosis) fusion product occur in CML, this form of BCR/ABL is more often seen in **Philadelphia chromosome-positive acute lymphoblastic**

leukemia occurring outside the setting of CML. RT-PCR can determine the specific BCR/ABL product fusion present in the leukemic cells and can quantitate the fusion product. The latter is useful for monitoring patient responses to therapy. If there are additional chromosomal abnormalities (e.g., second Philadelphia chromosome, trisomy 8, etc.), they usually herald disease progression to clinically more aggressive phases.

PATHOLOGY: CML may present in **chronic, accelerated** or **blast phase**.

- **CML, chronic phase (CP):** patients have leukocytosis, consisting of neutrophils in all stages of maturation with a peak of myelocytes and mature neutrophils. By definition, blasts make up less than 10% of circulating or bone marrow leukocytes. Basophilia and eosinophilia are common. Platelets are normal or increased and may exceed $10^6/\mu L$. Bone marrow biopsies show hypercellularity, usually with total effacement of the marrow space by mostly myeloid cells and their precursors (Fig. 26-36). Megakaryocytes often form clusters and show abnormal morphologic features, including micromegakaryocytes and nuclear hypolobation. Reticulin fibers are normal or moderately increased.

- **CML, accelerated phase (AP):** AP represents disease progression from CML-CP. CML-AP is defined by one of the following criteria: (1) persistent or increasing WBC count unresponsive to therapy, (2) persistent or increasing splenomegaly unresponsive to therapy, (3) persistent thrombocytopenia or thrombocytosis unresponsive to therapy, (4) additional chromosomal abnormalities, (5) 20% or more blood basophils and (6) 10%–19% blasts in the blood or bone marrow.

- **CML, blast phase (BP):** Blast phase represents the evolution to acute leukemia and features (1) 20% or more blasts in the blood or bone marrow, (2) extramedullary proliferation of blasts (skin, lymph nodes, spleen, bone, brain) and (3) clusters of blasts in the bone marrow. Blast phase heralds a poor prognosis. In 70% of blast crises, the leukemic blasts show myeloid morphology and immunophenotype; in 30%, they are lymphoblasts, usually of B-cell precursor lymphoblast immunophenotype (expressing

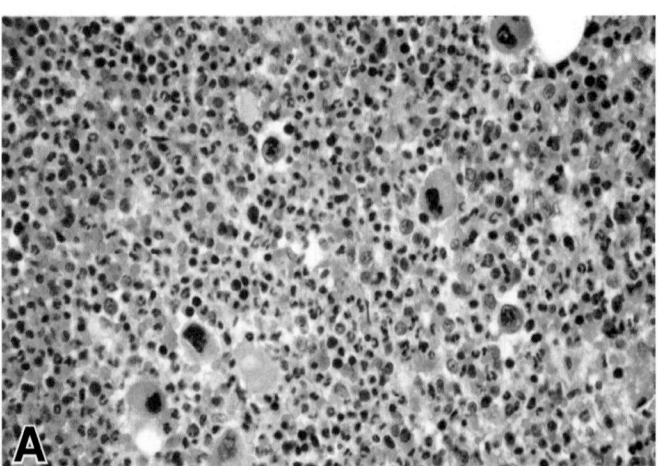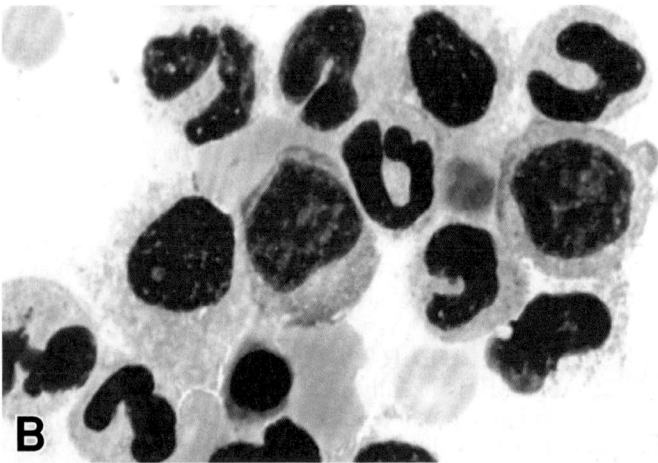

FIGURE 26-36. Chronic myelogenous leukemia. A. The bone marrow is conspicuously hypercellular because of an increase in granulocyte precursors, mature granulocytes and megakaryocytes. **B.** A smear of the bone marrow aspirate from the same patient reveals numerous granulocytes at various stages of development.

CD10, CD19, CD34 and terminal deoxynucleotidyl transferase [TdT]). In 80% of cases, transformation to accelerated phase or blast crisis entails additional cytogenetic alterations (Table 26-14).

CLINICAL FEATURES: Peak incidence is in the fifth and sixth decades, with a slight male predominance. Patients with CML report fatigue, anorexia, weight loss and vague abdominal discomfort caused by hepatosplenomegaly. Acute left upper quadrant pain is often a symptom of splenic infarction. Blood findings include mild to moderate anemia, leukocytosis and absolute basophilia. Peripheral granulocytes are markedly increased with a full maturation range with peaks in myelocytes and segmented neutrophils. Clinical deterioration often heralds blast phase.

CML is a model of targeted drug therapy in human malignancies. The drug imatinib, a tyrosine kinase inhibitor (TKI), blocks the ATP-binding site on *BCR/ABL* tyrosine kinase, and so inactivates it. Survival of 70%–90% is typical with imatinib. However, increasingly, subclones with point mutations within the ATP-binding pocket emerge and demonstrate resistance to imatinib. Second-generation TKIs and allogeneic bone marrow transplantation have greatly improved the outcome in CML patients.

Polycythemia Vera

PV is a myeloproliferative neoplasm arising from a clonal HSC and characterized by autonomous production of RBCs, not responsive to EPO. It is a clonal proliferation not only of erythroid elements but also of megakaryocytes and granulocytes in the bone marrow. As secondary polycythemia and other myeloproliferative neoplasms resemble PV both clinically and pathologically, the WHO established diagnostic criteria for polycythemia. A diagnosis of PV requires that both major criteria and one minor criterion, or the first major criterion and two minor criteria, be present. Major criteria include (1) increased RBC mass or Hgb greater than 18.5 g/dL in men or greater than 16.5 g/dL in women; and (2) V617F Janus kinase 2 (JAK2) mutation or a similar mutation of JAK2. Minor criteria include (1) no elevation of EPO; (2) hypercellular marrow with panmyelosis that includes erythroid, granulocytic and megakaryocytic hyperplasia; and (3) erythroid colony formation in vitro without growth factor stimulation (endogenous production).

 **PATHOPHYSIOLOGY AND MOLECULAR PATHOGENESIS:** PV derives from malignant transformation of a single stem cell with primary commitment to the erythroid lineage. Proliferation of the neoplastic clone occurs mainly in the bone marrow but may involve such extramedullary sites as the spleen, lymph nodes and liver **(myeloid metaplasia)**.

EPO is the primary regulator of erythropoiesis (see above), and its synthesis by the kidney is triggered by tissue hypoxia. The neoplastic erythroid progenitor cells of PV are sensitive to EPO, like their normal counterparts. In culture, they form luxuriant clusters of erythroid cells (BFU-E) when exposed to EPO. However, at the more mature colony-forming stage (CFU-E), cultured

PV neoplastic cells form erythroid colonies even without EPO stimulation. These autonomous erythroid colonies, "endogenous CFU-E," characterize PV throughout the disease and stand in contrast to normal erythroid progenitors, whose CFU-Es require added EPO ("exogenous CFU-E").

Autonomous (EPO-independent) proliferation of these PV cells gives them a proliferative advantage: the increased RBC mass suppresses EPO secretion and thus the proliferation of normal RBC progenitors. Serum EPO levels in PV are normal or low, while in secondary (functional) erythrocytosis EPO is increased.

Over 95% of patients with PV had a somatic mutation in JAK2 (V617F). This gain-of-function mutation occurs in the HSC and is found in all myeloid lineages. It makes daughter hematopoietic cells hypersensitive to growth factors and cytokines, including EPO. The JAK2 family of transcription factors plays a critical role in cytokine signaling in normal hematopoietic cells mainly by triggering signal transducers and activators of transcription (STAT) proteins. In vitro studies indicate that the activating JAK2 mutation confers proliferative and survival advantages to hematopoietic precursors. The JAK2 V617F mutation is not specific for PV: it occurs in other myeloproliferative neoplasms. Patients with the JAK2 mutation have a longer duration of disease and higher risk for bleeding complications and fibrosis.

Abnormal cytogenetic karyotypes occur in 20% of patients with PV, the most common of which are presented in Table 26-14. *The Philadelphia chromosome and BCR/ABL fusion protein do not occur in PV.*

PATHOLOGY: *Bone marrow in PV is hypercellular, and all elements—erythroid, granulocytic, megakaryocytic—are hyperplastic* (Table 26-15). Panmyelosis is characteristic but morphologic findings and clinical course vary, depending on the stage of disease. The three stages include prepolycythemic, overt polycythemic and postpolycythemic myelofibrosis phases. In pre- and polycythemic stages, erythroid precursors predominate, and the myeloid-to-erythroid ratio (M:E) is less than 2:1. Erythroid maturation is normal. The granulocyte series also shows normal maturation. Megakaryocytes are typically increased in number, are of variable size and tend to cluster. In over 95% of cases, marrow-stainable iron is decreased or absent. A mild to moderate increase in reticulin is common in the early stages. In the later stage of postpolycythemic myelofibrosis, or the "spent phase," erythropoiesis decreases and the marrow becomes replaced by reticulin and collagen fibrosis.

The spleen is typically enlarged, with prominent accumulation of erythrocytes in the red pulp cords and sinuses. In the polycythemic phase, there is minimal if any evidence of extramedullary hematopoiesis (EMH). However, EMH, with blood cell precursors outside the marrow, increases in the postpolycythemic myelofibrotic phase. Although the main site of extramedullary hematopoiesis is the spleen, liver and lymph nodes may also contain foci of erythroid precursors, immature granulocytes and megakaryocytes.

Blood hemoglobin concentrations may exceed 20 g/dL, and the Hct surpasses 60% (Table 26-14). Initially, there is mild to moderate leukocytosis (10,000–25,000/μL) in 2/3 of cases, and mild to moderate thrombocytosis (400,000–800,000/μL) in 1/2 of cases, often with abnormal platelet morphology. Anemia characterizes the later, spent phase of PV. Hyperuricemia and secondary gout may occur and are due to rapid cell turnover.

Peripheral blood smears in the polycythemic phase show crowding of usual normochromic, normocytic RBCs. Hypochromia and microcytosis occur if there is iron deficiency. Iron-deficiency anemia is common in PV, since stored iron is diverted to the erythropoiesis or is lost to phlebotomy or bleeding from the GI tract. In the later stages of PV, anemia develops and the peripheral blood shows a leukoerythroblastic picture, poikilocytosis with teardrop-shaped RBCs.

 CLINICAL FEATURES: In North America, 8–10 cases of PV per million present annually. The mean age at diagnosis is 60 years. Onset tends to be insidious, and symptoms are generally nonspecific, typically relating to the increased erythrocyte mass. Plethora and splenomegaly are early findings. Headache, dizziness and visual problems reflect hypertension and/or vascular disturbances in the brain and retina. Angina pectoris, from slowing of coronary blood flow, and intermittent claudication caused by sluggish peripheral blood flow in the lower extremities may be complaints. Gastric or duodenal ulcers may follow GI tract circulatory problems or, in part, histamine release by basophils. Major thrombotic complications, including stroke, myocardial infarction and deep vein thrombosis, occur in 20% of cases.

The clinical course of PV tends to proceed in the three phases described above. The **prepolycythemic phase** is the prodromal phase. It features borderline or mild erythrocytosis with mild erythroid hyperplasia, but not to the degree diagnostic of PV. The diagnosis can be rendered based on a low EPO level, JAK2 or similar mutation or endogenous erythroid colony formation. Later, when red cell mass is definitively increased, the polycythemic stage has been reached. In 10% of cases, the disease evolves to the postpolycythemic (spent) phase when excessive erythroid proliferation ceases, resulting in decreased erythrocyte mass and anemia. Another 10% of cases progress to myelofibrosis with extramedullary hematopoiesis, as in other MPNs **(postpolycythemic myelofibrosis)**. **Acute myelogenous leukemia (AML) or myelodysplasia** occurs in up to 15% of cases of PV and may in part be caused by treatment with ³²P or alkylating agents. Disease progression is often the result of karyotypic evolution and acquisition of complex chromosomal abnormalities.

Median survival with PV is 13 years. Specific causes of death related to the disease itself include thrombosis, hemorrhage, AML and the spent phase. Repeated phlebotomy or chemotherapy to reduce erythrocyte mass is effective management in most cases. JAK2 inhibitors have shown encouraging results.

Primary Myelofibrosis

Primary myelofibrosis (PMF) is a clonal myeloproliferative neoplasm in which prominent megakaryopoiesis and granulopoiesis accompany marrow fibrosis. Extramedullary hematopoiesis is present in fully developed disease.

 MOLECULAR PATHOGENESIS: As in other MPNs, exposures to benzene or radiation have occasionally been implicated in primary myelofibrosis (chronic idiopathic myelofibrosis). The neoplastic megakaryocytes in PMF produce PDGF and TGF-β, both of which are powerful fibroblast mitogens. Ultimately, although fibroblasts are not part of the clonal stem cell disorder, their stimulation by those cytokines causes the entire marrow space to be replaced by connective tissue. In the fibrotic phase, clonal stem cells enter the circulation to cause EMH at multiple sites, especially the spleen. Half of patients with PMF have the JAK2 V617F mutation, which is important in the pathogenesis of the disease. A minority of cases have mutations of *MPL*, which encodes the TPO receptor. Some chromosomal abnormalities suggest, but do not prove, PMF (Table 26-14).

 PATHOLOGY: PMF evolves through two stages, a prefibrotic and early stage, and a fibrotic stage. Most patients are diagnosed at the latter stage, but 30%–40% are first detected in a prefibrotic stage. The **prefibrotic stage** usually presents with unexplained thrombocytosis. The hypercellular bone marrow has minimal fibrosis and prominent neutrophilic and megakaryocytic proliferation. The megakaryocytes are densely clustered and atypically lobated with high a nuclear-to-cytoplasmic ratio. Some show "cloud-like" nuclei. In the **fibrotic stage,** the blood shows leukopenia or marked leukocytosis, with myeloid precursors and nucleated RBCs (leukoerythroblastosis) usually evident. The red cells exhibit poikilocytosis and teardrop forms (Fig. 26-37A). Bone marrow cellularity gradually decreases, and foci of hematopoiesis containing mostly atypical megakaryocytes alternate with hypo- or acellular regions. Conspicuous reticulin or collagen fibrosis in the marrow defines this stage (Fig. 26-37B). Extramedullary hematopoiesis leads to splenomegaly, hepatomegaly and lymphadenopathy, and may be seen in other organs.

The WHO requires 3 major criteria and 2 minor criteria for a diagnosis of PMF. Major criteria include megakaryocyte proliferation with or without fibrosis; absence of features of other well-defined MPNs; and a clonal genetic marker, such as *JAK2* mutation. Minor criteria include leukoerythroblastosis, elevated serum lactate dehydrogenase, anemia and splenomegaly.

 CLINICAL FEATURES: The annual incidence of idiopathic myelofibrosis is 0.5–1.5 per 100,000. Its peak incidence is in the seventh decade. A quarter of patients with idiopathic myelofibrosis are asymptomatic at diagnosis, the disease being detected by splenomegaly on physical examination or by identifying teardrop red cells or thrombocytosis. Early clinical symptoms are nonspecific and include fatigue, low-grade fever, night sweats and weight loss. Platelet function may be impaired and associated with either increased platelet aggregation and thrombosis or decreased platelet aggregation with a bleeding diathesis. Transformation to AML occurs in 5%–30% of cases (Table 26-14).

Essential Thrombocythemia

Essential thrombocythemia (ET) is an uncommon myeloproliferative neoplasm in which megakaryocytes proliferate without restraint. Blood platelet counts remain increased

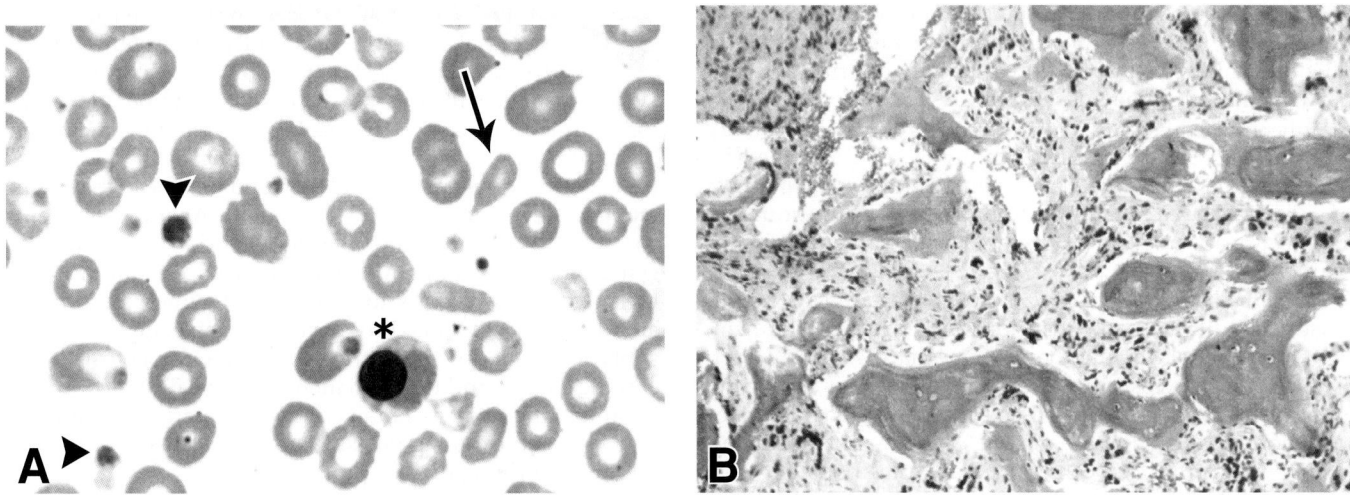

FIGURE 26-37. Chronic idiopathic myelofibrosis. A. Peripheral smear shows anisocytosis (red blood cells of different size), poikilocytosis with teardrop forms (*arrow*) and nucleated erythrocytes. Large to giant platelets are also present. **B.** A section of bone marrow shows collagenous fibrosis, osteosclerosis and numerous abnormal megakaryocytes.

(>450,000/μL), and recurrent episodes of thrombosis and hemorrhage are common. The disease affects middle-aged people, both genders equally (Table 26-14).

 MOLECULAR PATHOGENESIS: ET is a clonal disorder believed to derive from neoplastic transformation of a single HSC with principal, but not exclusive, commitment to megakaryocytic lineage. The disease features a marked proliferation of megakaryocytes, with up to a 15-fold or greater increase in platelet production and consequent marked thrombocytosis (sometimes >10^6/μL). About 40%–50% have a *JAK2* V617F mutation or other functionally similar abnormality. One to 2% of cases have an *MPL* gene mutation. Chromosomal abnormalities include deletion 20q and trisomy 8 and are identified in approximately 5%–10% of cases.

 PATHOLOGY: To diagnose ET, other chronic MPNs and reactive thrombocytosis must be excluded. Abnormalities of platelet function are common in primary thrombocythemia. Recurrent episodes of thrombosis in arteries or veins are attributed to severe thrombocytosis, and hemorrhage reflects defective platelet function. Thromboses in the spleen, with subsequent infarction, may cause splenic atrophy. Iron-deficiency anemia follows hemorrhage from GI or urogenital tracts. The bone marrow is normocellular or moderately hypercellular, with fewer fat cells (Fig. 26-38). Increased numbers of large, hyperlobulated, "stag-horn–shaped" megakaryocytes with abundant mature cytoplasm form cohesive clusters or sheets in the marrow. Marrow reticulin is normal or slightly increased. Post-ET myelofibrosis is rare. Iron stores are normal or low.

The spleen is mildly enlarged in 1/2 of cases of ET. Extramedullary hematopoiesis is common, but extensive myeloid metaplasia only occurs when myelofibrosis develops. The peripheral blood shows thrombocytosis.

 CLINICAL FEATURES: The clinical course of ET is indolent, with median survival exceeding 10–15 years. In untreated cases, thrombosis of large

arteries and veins is common, especially in the legs, heart, intestine and kidneys. Hemorrhage is less common, usually from mucosal surfaces, and is mild, not life-threatening. AML supervenes in up to 5% of cases. The disease is treated with platelet pheresis and myelosuppressive chemotherapy.

Mastocytosis

Mastocytosis is a clonal hematopoietic disorder in which neoplastic mast cells accumulate in certain tissues, mainly skin and bone marrow. Systemic neoplastic mast cell disorders are considered to be in the category of MPN. The distinct subtypes are characterized by tissue involvement and clinical manifestations.

CUTANEOUS MASTOCYTOSIS: This can present either as single or multiple lesions. In the former case, there is a tan-brown, cutaneous nodule in newborns; in the latter, there are several groups of skin nodules in young

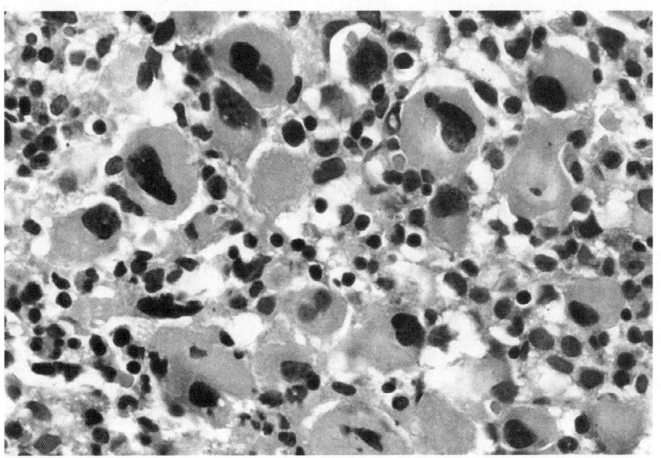

FIGURE 26-38. Essential thrombocythemia. A section of bone marrow exhibits a conspicuous increase in the number of megakaryocytes, which display atypical features and hypolobated forms.

children or disseminated brown-red macular or papular lesions. The most common type is **urticaria pigmentosa**. This presents as multiple, symmetrically distributed, tan-brown, cutaneous macules or papules, most commonly in infants and young children. The skin of the trunk is mostly affected, but any skin site may be involved. *There is a disseminated perivascular and periadnexal dermal infiltrate of spindle-shaped mast cells.* Spontaneous resolution usually occurs at puberty and systemic involvement does not happen.

SYSTEMIC MASTOCYTOSIS: This is a rare MPN, with mast cell infiltration of many organs, including the skin, lymph nodes, spleen, liver, bones, bone marrow and GI tract. Systemic mastocytosis has diverse manifestations, including an indolent form, a subtype associated with clonal hematologic non–mast cell lineage disease, an aggressive form and a leukemic form (mast cell leukemia). Transitions between these subtypes may occur. In most cases there is an activating mutation in the tyrosine kinase domain (D816V) of *c-kit* proto-oncogene. This underscores the neoplastic nature of this disorder. Skin lesions in the indolent form of systemic mastocytosis are clinically indistinguishable from those in cutaneous mastocytosis.

In mast cell leukemia, the bone marrow and peripheral blood show a significant increase in atypical mast cells (≥20% in the marrow) and depletion of fat and normal hematopoietic elements in the marrow. The circulating cells often exhibit cytologic atypia, including hypogranulation and/or nuclear irregularity, or less differentiated forms with blast-like morphology.

 PATHOLOGY: In systemic mastocytosis, lymph nodes are rarely involved and initially show perifollicular and perivascular infiltration by mast cells (Fig. 26-39). Compact aggregates of mast cells within the paracortical areas can also be seen. The spleen shows nodular aggregates of mast cells with accompanying dense fibrosis in both red and white pulp. In the liver, portal triads are involved first. Involvement of the bone marrow may be peritrabecular, perivascular or diffuse, and there is often accompanying fibrosis and eosinophilia.

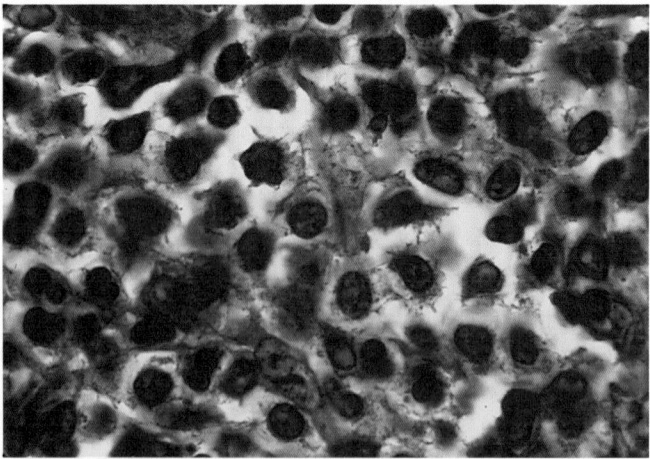

FIGURE 26-39. Mastocytosis. A section of lymph node shows effacement of the normal architecture by sheets of mast cells. The centrally situated nuclei are round to elongated, and occasionally indented. The cytoplasm is pale pink and finely granular.

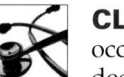 **CLINICAL FEATURES:** Systemic mastocytosis occurs at any age, but adults in the 6th and 7th decades are most commonly affected. Patients' symptoms reflect the overproduction of a number of mediators normally made by mast cells and basophils, including histamine, prostaglandin D_2 and thromboxane B_2. Most people experience gastrointestinal pain and diarrhea. The serum **tryptase** levels are usually elevated. Anaphylactic episodes—with pruritus, flushing, hypotension and asthmatic symptoms—are common. Extensive mast cell infiltration of the bone marrow leads to secondary anemia, neutropenia and thrombocytopenia. Prognosis is variable, depending on subtype. The indolent form of systemic mastocytosis has a chronic course, and half of patients survive 5 years or more. Symptomatic relief is obtained, at least partially, with H_1- and H_2-receptor antagonists. There is no effective therapy for the underlying disease process.

Myelodysplastic Syndromes Are Clonal Disorders of Ineffective Hematopoiesis

In myelodysplastic syndromes (MDSs), peripheral blood cytopenias accompany a hypercellular marrow with ineffective hematopoiesis. The latter entails dysplastic morphologies in one or more hematopoietic lineages and carries increased risk of transformation to AML. There is an apparent discrepancy between the paucity of peripheral blood elements and the hypercellularity in the bone marrow, which occurs because ineffective hematopoiesis leads to increased apoptosis in the marrow.

There are several subtypes of MDS, depending on whether dysplasia involves one or more cell lineages and the percentage of blasts in the blood or bone marrow. *All subtypes show refractory anemia and/or other cytopenia. Erythrocytosis, leukocytosis and thrombocytosis do not occur in MDS, unlike the MPNs (see above).* In MDS, there are less than 20% blasts in the blood or bone marrow, which is different from acute leukemias, in which blood or bone marrow have 20% blasts or greater. Progression of MDS to AML (i.e., progression from ineffective hematopoiesis to a proliferative state) occurs in 30%–40% of cases that usually have genetic instability. This progression coincides with more genetic abnormalities. Some low-grade MDS subsets have more stable clinical courses and do not progress, or progress rarely, to AML.

 **ETIOLOGIC FACTORS:** MDSs may be either primary (de novo) or secondary (therapy related). Patients with secondary MDSs usually have received radiation or chemotherapy (particularly alkylating agents or topoisomerase II inhibitors). Other risk factors include benzene exposure, cigarette smoking and congenital disorders such as Fanconi anemia or Kostmann syndrome.

 PATHOLOGY: Subclassification of MDS is based on whether one or more of the hematopoietic lineages show **dysplasia,** and on the percentage of myeloblasts. Dysplasia is most often seen in erythroid precursors, which show megaloblastoid changes, multinucleation, nuclear budding, bridging between nuclei and karyorrhexis (Fig. 26-40). Erythroid precursors with iron-laden mitochondria around the nuclei **(ringed sideroblasts)** occur in several subtypes of MDS (Fig. 26-41A). Dysgranulopoietic features include nuclear hyposegmentation (pseudo-Pelger-Huët cells)

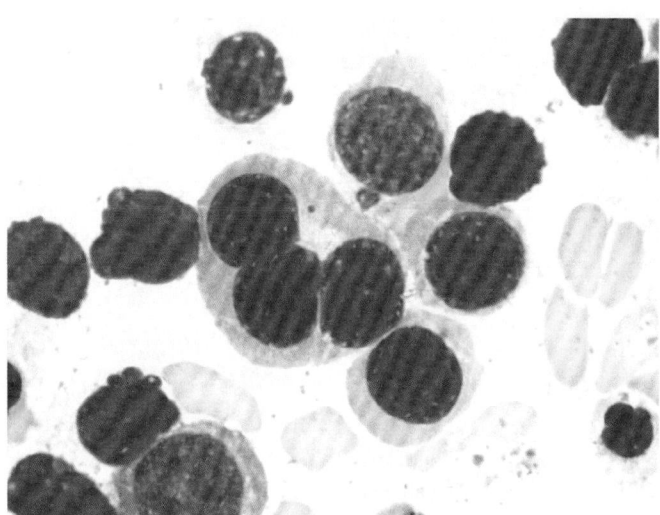

FIGURE 26-40. Myelodysplastic syndrome. Dysplastic, multinucleated, megaloblastoid erythroid precursors are shown.

and cytoplasmic hypogranulation. Dysplastic megakaryocytes may be mononuclear or hypolobated or show nuclear separation (Fig. 26-41B). Careful elucidation of the blast percentage is important in assigning an MDS subcategory and predicting the likely clinical course of the disease.

Cytogenetic and molecular studies are essential to diagnosing, treating and assessing prognosis of MDSs. Conventional cytogenetic tests identify clonal abnormalities in half of cases. If a patient has isolated deletion of the long arm of chromosome 5 (5q–), macrocytic anemia, megaloblastoid erythropoiesis with or without ringed sideroblasts and normal or increased platelets with monolobated megakaryocytes, that patient is likely to be an elderly woman and to have a more favorable prognosis. By contrast, deletion of chromosome 7 (7q–) has an unfavorable prognosis (Table 26-14). *More chromosomal abnormalities augur less favorable outcomes.*

Other techniques have identified additional recurrent mutations. Most of these involve genes encoding components of the epigenetic regulation or RNA spliceosome machinery (see Chapter 5). These findings suggest that epigenetic factors play a large role in the pathogenesis of MDS.

CLINICAL FEATURES: MDS usually occurs in older patients, with a median age of 70. The WHO classification of MDS subtypes is beyond the scope of this discussion. *However, in general, MDSs present with*

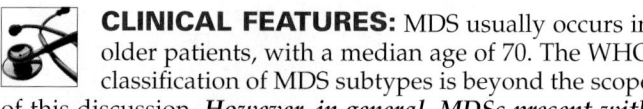
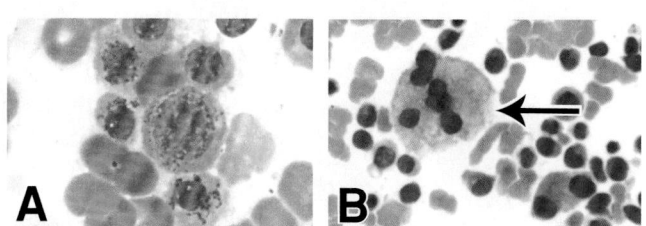

FIGURE 26-41. Myelodysplastic syndrome. A. Smear of a bone marrow aspirate stained with Prussian blue shows an erythroid precursor cell containing iron-laden mitochondria that encircle the nuclei (ringed sideroblast). **B.** Dysplastic megakaryocyte with nuclear separation (*arrow*).

symptoms related to peripheral blood cytopenias: weakness in anemia, recurrent infections in neutropenia and bleeding in thrombocytopenia. Up to 40% of patients with MDS progress to AML. Progression to AML and overall prognosis depend on the morphologic subtype of MDS. Increased numbers of blasts, complex cytogenetic abnormalities, certain specific mutations and increased cytopenia confer a worse prognosis.

Acute Myeloid Leukemia Is a Clonal Proliferation of Myeloblasts in the Marrow, with Their Subsequent Appearance in Blood and Possibly in Extramedullary Tissues

A diagnosis of AML requires greater than or equal to 20% myeloblasts in the blood or bone marrow. These criteria are relaxed in cases of several AML types with specific cytogenetic abnormalities (Table 26-14). AML with t(15;17) (q22;q12) is acute promyelocytic leukemia (APL). Such types are defined as AML regardless of blast cell count. If less than 20% blasts are present in AMLs without recurrent cytogenetic abnormalities, the disease should be classified in the MDS or MPN categories. There are 6 distinct types of AML (Table 26-16):

1. **AML with recurrent genetic abnormalities**
2. **AML with myelodysplasia-related changes**
3. **Therapy-related myeloid neoplasms**
4. **AML, not otherwise specified**
5. **Myeloid sarcoma**
6. **Myeloid proliferations related to Down syndrome**

Acute leukemias can derive from either myeloid (70%) or lymphoid (30%) lineages. The latter are discussed below under lymphoid malignancies.

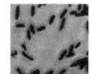 **ETIOLOGIC FACTORS:** Most cases of AML are of unknown etiology. Some cases are attributed to prior radiation, cytotoxic chemotherapy or benzene exposure. AML increased after the detonation of atomic bombs in Hiroshima and Nagasaki. Cigarette smoking doubles the risk for AML (see Chapter 8).

 PATHOLOGY: Malignant myeloblasts of AML are present in the bone marrow and, usually, in the blood. Typically, the malignant cells pack the bone marrow and displace normal hematopoietic cells (Fig. 26-42). Myeloblasts are medium-sized to large cells with round or slightly irregular nuclei and immature nuclear chromatin. Some cases show eosinophilic, slender cytoplasmic inclusions, *Auer rods*, which are coalesced primary granules (Fig. 26-43). Auer rods are specific for the myeloid lineage and preclude a diagnosis of lymphoblastic leukemia.

Immunophenotyping by flow cytometry, chromosomal analysis (cytogenetic studies) and molecular studies are essential for correct classification of AML. Myeloid antigens frequently expressed include CD13, CD15, CD33 and CD117 (*c-kit*), in addition to the progenitor cell marker CD34. AML with megakaryoblastic differentiation may show the platelet/megakaryocyte markers CD41 and CD61 (platelet Gp IIb/IIIa complex).

In addition, cytochemical staining, including myeloperoxidase, Sudan black and nonspecific esterase (NSE), remain helpful in classifying AML cases.

TABLE 26-16

WHO CLASSIFICATION OF ACUTE MYELOID LEUKEMIA (AML)

Acute Myeloid Leukemia with Recurrent Genetic Abnormalities

AML with t(8;21)(q22;q22); RUNX1-RUNX1T1

AML with abnormal bone marrow eosinophils inv(16)(p13q22) or t(16;16)(p13;q22); CBFβ/MYH11

Acute promyelocytic leukemia [AML with t(15;17)(q22;q12)(PML/RARα] and variants **(M3)**

AML with (9;11)(p22;q23); MLLT3-MLL

AML with t(6;9)(p23;q34); DEK-NUP214

AML with inv(3)(q21q24.2) or t(3;3)(q21;126.2); RPN1-EVI1

AML (megakaryoblastic) with t(1;22)(p13;q13); RBM15-MKL1

AML with gene mutations (NPM1, CEBPA, FLT3, etc.)

Acute Myeloid Leukemia with Myelodysplasia-Related Changes

Following a myelodysplastic syndrome or myelodysplastic syndrome/myeloproliferative disorder

Without antecedent myelodysplastic syndrome

Therapy-Related Myeloid Neoplasms

Alkylating agent related

Topoisomerase type II inhibitor related (some may be lymphoid)

Other types

Acute Myeloid Leukemia Not Otherwise Categorized

AML minimally differentiated **(M0)**

AML without maturation **(M1)**

AML with maturation **(M2)**

Acute myelomonocytic leukemia **(M4)**

Acute monoblastic and monocytic leukemia **(M5)**

Acute erythroid leukemia **(M6)**

Acute megakaryoblastic leukemia **(M7)**
Acute basophilic leukemia
Acute panmyelosis with myelofibrosis

Myeloid Sarcoma

Myeloid Proliferations Related to Down Syndrome

PML = promyelocytic leukemia; RAR = retinoic acid receptor; WHO = World Health Organization.

 CLINICAL FEATURES: *Most cases of AML occur in adults, with a median age of 67 at onset. The major problems associated with AML reflect progressive accumulation in the marrow of immature myeloid cells that cannot differentiate and mature further.* Although leukemic myeloblasts divide more slowly than do normal hematopoietic precursor cells, they also undergo spontaneous cell death less often than normal cells. The expanded pool of abnormal leukemic blasts overwhelms the marrow and suppresses normal hematopoiesis. *As a result, the major clinical problems in AML are leukopenia, thrombocytopenia and anemia.* Infections, especially with opportunistic organisms (e.g., fungi), are common, as are cutaneous bleeding (petechiae and ecchymoses) and serosal hemorrhages over viscera. Untreated AML has a dismal prognosis. Chemotherapy leads to remission

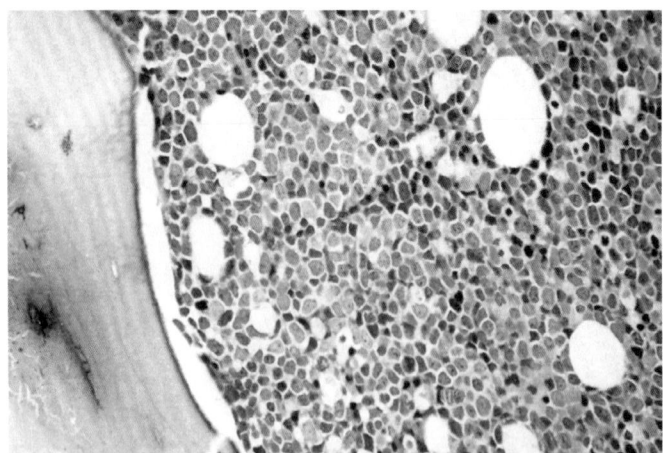

FIGURE 26-42. Acute myelogenous leukemia. A bone marrow section is hypercellular, resulting from effacement of the normal architecture by myeloblasts.

in over half of patients, but relapses are common and overall 5-year survival is under 30%. Bone marrow transplantation is a common mode of treatment for high-risk forms of AML and for AML in relapse.

Selected Acute Myeloid Leukemia Subtypes

AML WITH RECURRENT GENETIC ABNORMALITIES: There are multiple cytogenetic abnormalities associated with this category of AML (Table 26-14). These include AML with mutated *NPM1* or *CEBPA*.

AML with t(15;17)(q22;q12), which is **APL,** *is defined by a translocation involving the* promyelocytic leukemia 1 *(PML1) gene at 15q22 and the retinoic acid receptor-α (RARA) gene at 17q12.* APL mainly affects middle-aged patients and accounts for 5%–10% of AMLs.

APL is a paradigm for a molecularly defined disease in which the underlying genetic defect determines the type of treatment. The translocation results in the *PML/RARA* fusion gene that encodes a functional retinoic acid receptor. The

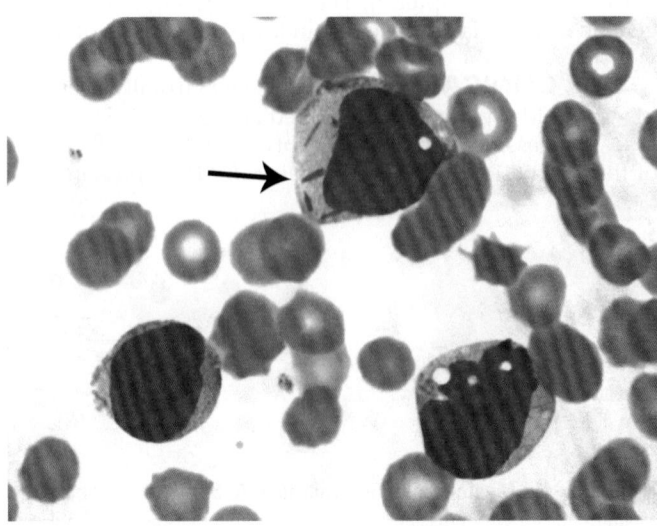

FIGURE 26-43. Acute promyelocytic leukemia. Auer rods are prominent (*arrow*).

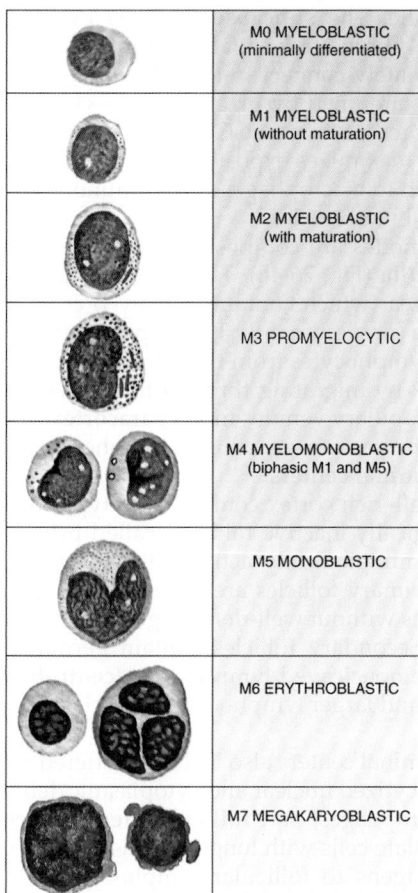

FIGURE 26-44. Morphology of acute myeloid leukemia (AML) in the traditional French-American-British (FAB) classification, now within the framework of the World Health Organization (WHO) classification "AML-not otherwise specified."

receptor can be targeted by all-*trans*-retinoic acid (ATRA), which causes tumor cells to mature. The bone marrow is packed with tumor cells with promyelocytic morphologic features. Auer rods may be abundant. Leukemic cells react strongly for myeloperoxidase or Sudan black. *Patients with APL frequently present with DIC.* Senescent leukemic cells degranulate and activate the coagulation cascade. Treatment with ATRA induces maturation of the tumor cells and prevents both degranulation and DIC. The prognosis for APL is more favorable than for all other AMLs.

THERAPY-RELATED MYELOID NEOPLASMS: Cytotoxic radiation or chemotherapy for a prior malignancy can induce mutational changes that lead to secondary hematopoietic neoplasms one to several years after treatment. This category includes AMLs, MDSs and MPNs related to prior mutagenic therapies. Alkylating agents and radiation most often give rise to myelodysplasia and subsequent AML after 5–10 years. In contrast, topoisomerase II inhibitors (epipodophyllotoxins) lead to overt AML with latencies of 1–5 years. Nearly all therapy-related MPNs have cytogenetic abnormalities and poor prognoses.

ACUTE MYELOID LEUKEMIA, NOT OTHERWISE SPECIFIED: This set of leukemias does not meet the characteristics of any of the other subtypes of AML. They are thus grouped based on the older French-American-British (FAB) classification. The WHO classification incorporates the FAB scheme (Fig. 26-44):

- **AML with minimally differentiation:** The leukemic cells are immature myeloblasts with no defining morphologic or cytochemical criteria of the myeloid lineage. Immunophenotyping by flow cytometry establishes the myeloid nature of the tumor cells. The prognosis is unfavorable.
- **AML without maturation:** Less than 10% of the myeloid cells are promyelocytes or more mature myeloid cells. This disease occurs most often in middle-aged people.
- **AML with maturation:** More than 10% maturing myeloid cells (promyelocytes and later) are present.
- **Acute myelomonocytic leukemia (AMML):** This tumor is composed of a mixture of neutrophils and their precursors, plus monocytes and their precursors. The latter make up 26%–80% of tumor cells. AMML accounts for 5%–10% of AMLs.
- **Acute monoblastic/monocytic leukemia (AMoL):** At least 80% of myeloid leukemic cells have monocytic differentiation, including monoblasts, abnormal promonocytes and monocytes. AMoL constitutes 5%–8% of AMLs and is seen in younger patients.
- **Acute erythroid leukemia:** Acute erythroid leukemias feature prominent erythroid proliferation. There are 2 subtypes. Erythroleukemia is defined by erythroid precursors making up greater than 50% of all nucleated cells in the bone marrow, and at least 20% of the remaining nonerythroid population are myeloblasts. The second type, pure erythroid leukemia, is characterized by neoplastic immature cells committed to erythroid lineage making up greater than 80% of the bone marrow nucleated cells. A rare, more chronic form of this disease (**erythremic myelosis** or **di Guglielmo syndrome**) has pure erythroblasts.
- **Acute megakaryoblastic leukemia (AMegL):** At least 50% of the blasts show a megakaryocytic immunophenotype.

MYELOID SARCOMA: **Myeloid sarcoma is an extramedullary solid tumor of myeloblasts or monoblasts** (Fig. 26-45).

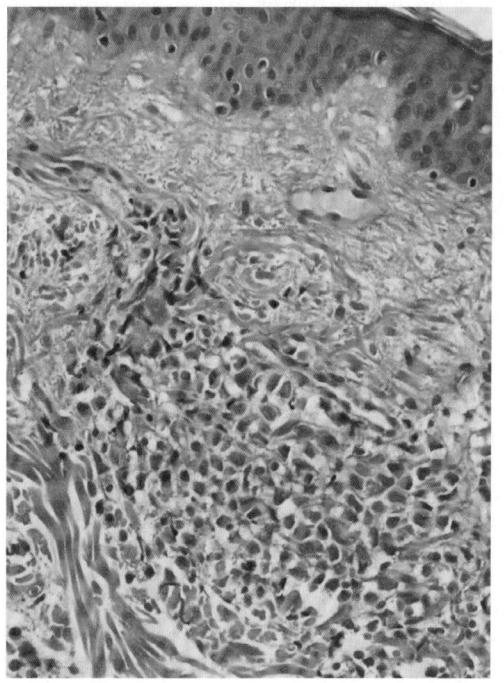

FIGURE 26-45. Myeloid sarcoma. The skin from a patient with acute monoblastic leukemia (leukemia cutis) shows neoplastic myeloid cells.

This entity is sometimes called a **chloroma** because of its greenish color, **granulocytic sarcoma** or **monoblastic sarcoma. Monoblastic differentiation** is uncommon and is most commonly associated with translocations involving the myelomonocytic leukemia (*MML*) gene (11q23). Myeloid sarcoma may evolve de novo or in association with AML, or it may represent the blast phase in myeloproliferative neoplasms. Prognosis is determined by the underlying leukemic process.

Disorders of the Lymphoid System

NORMAL LYMPH NODES AND LYMPHOCYTES

The lymphoid system consists of circulating T and B lymphocytes, natural killer cells (NK cells) and the secondary lymphoid organs, which mainly include the lymph nodes, spleen and thymus. In addition to the tonsils in the oro- and nasopharynx (Waldeyer ring), aggregates of organized lymphoid tissue known as mucosa-associated lymphoid tissue (MALT) are also present in extranodal sites, such as the gut, lungs and skin. Peyer patches in the terminal ileum are a prototypic example of MALT.

Lymphocytes in tonsils and Peyer patches arrive in those sites by migration through the tall endothelial cells of vessels, which are comparable to the postcapillary venules in lymph nodes. *MALT plays an important role in immunologic protection of the host in areas vulnerable to potential invaders.* IgA secretion is a key facet of this protection.

All three major types of lymphocytes (T cells, B cells and NK cells) develop from lymphoid stem cells in the bone marrow (Fig. 26-2). T cells mature and differentiate in the thymus. B cells undergo activation, transformation and selection in the lymph nodes and spleen. NK cells do not go through a thymic or lymph node education phase, but rather are released into the peripheral circulation, where they appear as large granular lymphocytes. All lymphocyte development entails a tightly controlled sequence of gene expression and silencing that leads to sequential gain and loss of nuclear material and changes cytoplasmic and/or surface antigen expression. *Patterns of antigenic expression identify the lineage and maturation stage of normal and neoplastic lymphoid cells* (see below and Chapter 4).

LYMPH NODES: Lymph nodes are located along lymphatic vessels throughout the body. Normal lymph nodes are typically round to bean shaped, and less than 1 cm. Larger nodes are considered clinically enlarged and may be abnormal microscopically. Lymph nodes are organized in regional collections, called chains or groups (e.g., cervical lymph node chain). Sometimes many nodes within a chain or group may be enlarged and/or matted together, often a feature of malignancy. Staging malignancies depends on identifying lymph node chains involved by tumor.

Individual lymph nodes are surrounded by a thin fibrous capsule with internally radiating trabeculae, which provides structural support (Fig. 26-46). Subjacent to the fibrous capsule sits the subcapsular sinus, which receives lymph fluid (potentially containing antigens) from **afferent lymphatic vessels** that penetrate the node at several points along the

outer capsule. The **subcapsular sinus** extends along the penetrating fibrous trabeculae, forming trabecular sinuses, which ultimately connect to the efferent lymphatic vessels. The sinuses are lined by macrophages, which are involved in antigen presentation (see Chapter 4). The arrangement of the sinuses maximizes exposure to foreign antigens present in the lymph to macrophages and immunoreactive lymphocytes in the lymph nodes.

Lymph nodes are composed of an **outer cortex** and an **inner medulla** (Fig. 26-46). The cortex is subdivided into a follicular area (which contains mostly B cells) and a paracortical area (predominantly T cells, plus many postcapillary venules). Lymphocytes from the circulation enter the lymph node cortex by migrating through the tall endothelial cells of the postcapillary venules in the **paracortex**. T cells tend to remain in the paracortex, while B lymphocytes home to the **follicle germinal centers**.

The B-cell–rich cortex contains two types of follicles: (1) immunologically inactive follicles, called **primary follicles**; and (2) immunologically active follicles, called **secondary follicles**. Primary follicles are cohesive aggregates of small lymphocytes without well-defined germinal centers or mantle zones. Secondary follicles contain germinal centers in which large noncleaved lymphocytes **(centroblasts)** mingle with small and larger lymphocytes with cleaved nuclei **(centrocytes)**.

The germinal centers also include scattered macrophages with phagocytized nuclear and cytoplasmic debris ("tingible body" macrophages) and **follicular dendritic cells (FDCs)** that are stellate cells with long cytoplasmic processes. FDCs present antigens to follicular lymphocytes. Macrophages, and to a lesser extent dendritic cells, provide growth factors for activated B cells.

The T-cell–rich paracortex, also known as the deep cortex or parafollicular area, is both between the B-cell follicles and deep to them. In addition to T cells, scattered macrophages and **interdigitating dendritic cells (IDCs)** are present in the paracortex. IDCs process and present antigens to T lymphocytes.

B-LYMPHOCYTE DEVELOPMENT: Normal **B-cell progenitor cells** arise in the bone marrow (Fig. 26-47) (called hematogones), where they are present in relatively low numbers. They have a similar phenotype to the cells of **precursor B-cell acute lymphoblastic leukemia (B-ALL):** both hematogones and B-ALL cells express the early B-cell surface antigens **CD10** (called common acute leukemia/lymphoma antigen [CALLA]) and **CD19,** and the nuclear enzyme **terminal deoxynucleotidyl transferase**. These cells largely lack CD20, a marker present at high levels on the more mature B-cell populations, and they also lack cell membrane Ig light (L) chains. Hematogones increase in number during viral infections and in bone marrow recovery after chemotherapy or stem cell transplantation.

A fraction of the bone marrow-derived progenitor B cells leave the marrow and home to lymph node germinal centers, where further development and selection occurs. Specifically, B cells with sufficient affinity for antigen survive the germinal center reaction and eventually leave the follicle compartment. As B lymphocytes mature, the genes for Ig heavy (H) chains are rearranged, leading to the synthesis of IgM antibodies. In precursor (progenitor) B cells, IgM is expressed in the cytoplasm. Mature B cells express the pan B-cell antigens CD19, CD20 and CD22, and surface Ig light and heavy chains. After activation and clonal expansion in

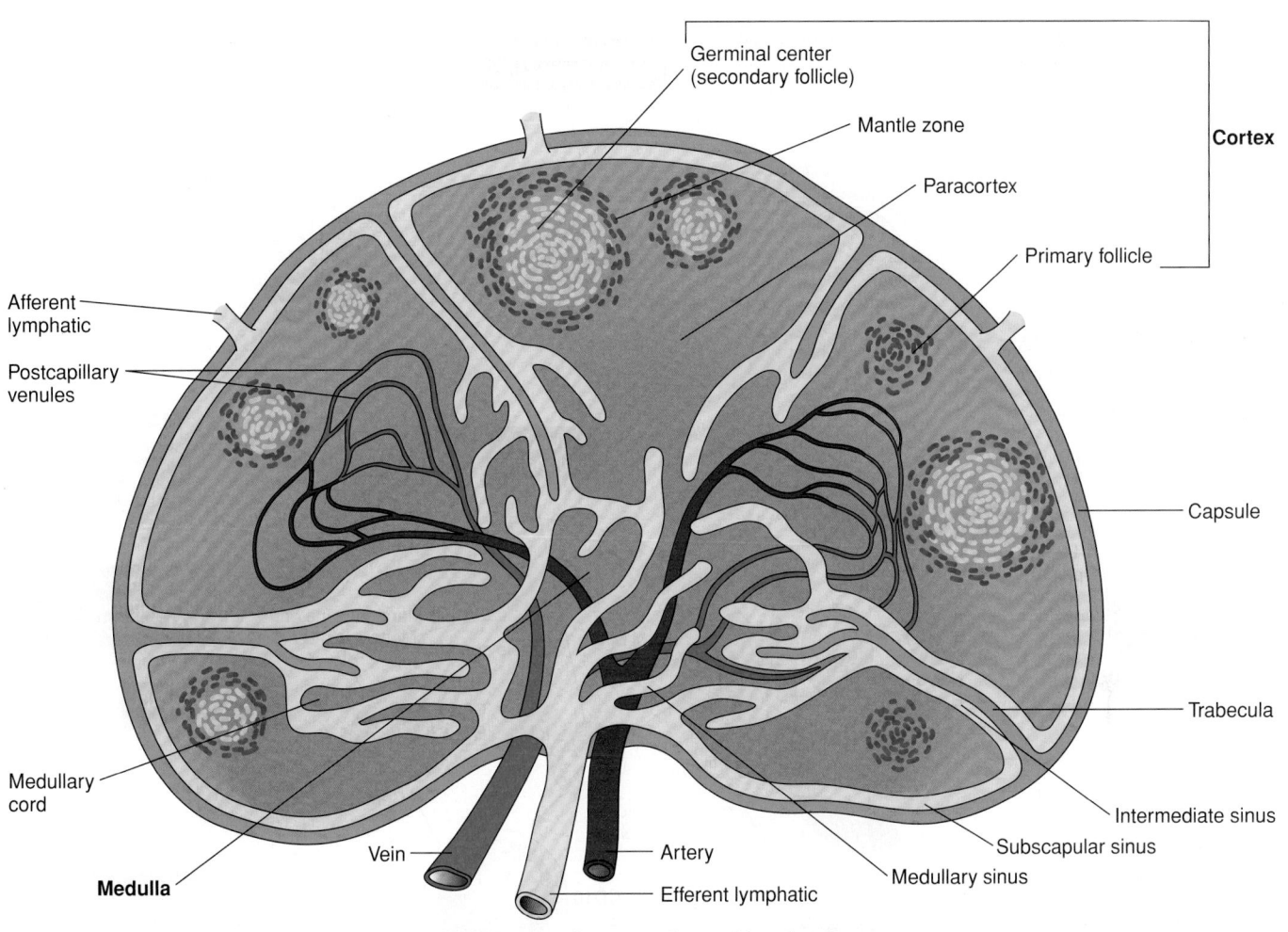

FIGURE 26-46. Structure of normal lymph node.

germinal centers, B cells migrate to the B-cell–dependent medullary cords of the lymph nodes. There, they become Ig-secreting **plasma cells,** or they exit the lymph nodes as **memory B cells**.

Plasma cells have eccentric nuclei with clumped chromatin marginated at the nuclear membrane, traditionally described as "clock-face chromatin." In their abundant blue-purple cytoplasm, plasma cells often have a clear paranuclear clear zone representing the Golgi complex. Plasma cells no longer normally express CD20 or surface Ig.

T LYMPHOCYTES: The lymphoid stem cells that migrate from the bone marrow to the thymus are exposed to a number of thymic hormones that induce sequential expression of pan T-cell surface antigens such as CD2, CD3, CD5 and CD7, and CD4 or CD8 (Fig. 26-48). *Recombination of T-cell receptor genes generates a diverse population of T cells, each of which can recognize a single antigen.* T cells that cannot bind a foreign antigen with high affinity and T cells that recognize self-antigens are eliminated via apoptosis. Once mature and educated, T cells leave the thymus to lymph nodes, spleen and peripheral blood to become **postthymic T cells**.

When exposed to foreign (nonself) receptor-specific antigen in the context of major histocompatibility complex (MHC) class II molecules, the CD4+ T cells become activated via release of mitogenic growth factors, such as IL-1 and IL-2. The antigens presented to T-helper cells are peptide fragments derived from partial digestion of foreign proteins by macrophages and/or other antigen-presenting cells. The T-helper cells in turn interact with B lymphocytes that express the same antigenic specificity and induce the latter to proliferate and differentiate into plasma cells. The latter produce antigen-specific antibody.

CD8+ cells are activated when their receptors recognize peptide antigens presented in association with MHC class I human leukocyte antigen (HLA) molecules. They then become suppressor/cytotoxic cells. CD8+ cells limit expansion of activated B cells and stop their immune response in a negative feedback response loop.

NATURAL KILLER AND CYTOTOXIC LYMPHOCYTES: A small subset of lymphocytes lack the usual T- or B-cell antigens. These are **natural killer cells**. NK cells are cytotoxic effectors that do not require antigen recognition to initiate their killing function. They are large lymphocytes with granular cytoplasm (i.e., **large granular lymphocytes**) (Fig. 26-49). They differ from mature T cells in that they lack surface CD3 and possess other surface antigens, such as CD16 and CD56.

Lymphocytes have diverse morphologies in stained peripheral blood and bone marrow smears, as well as in tissue sections. Like other blast cells, immature lymphoid cells have high nuclear-to-cytoplasmic ratios, fine chromatin and visible nucleoli. During maturation and differentiation,

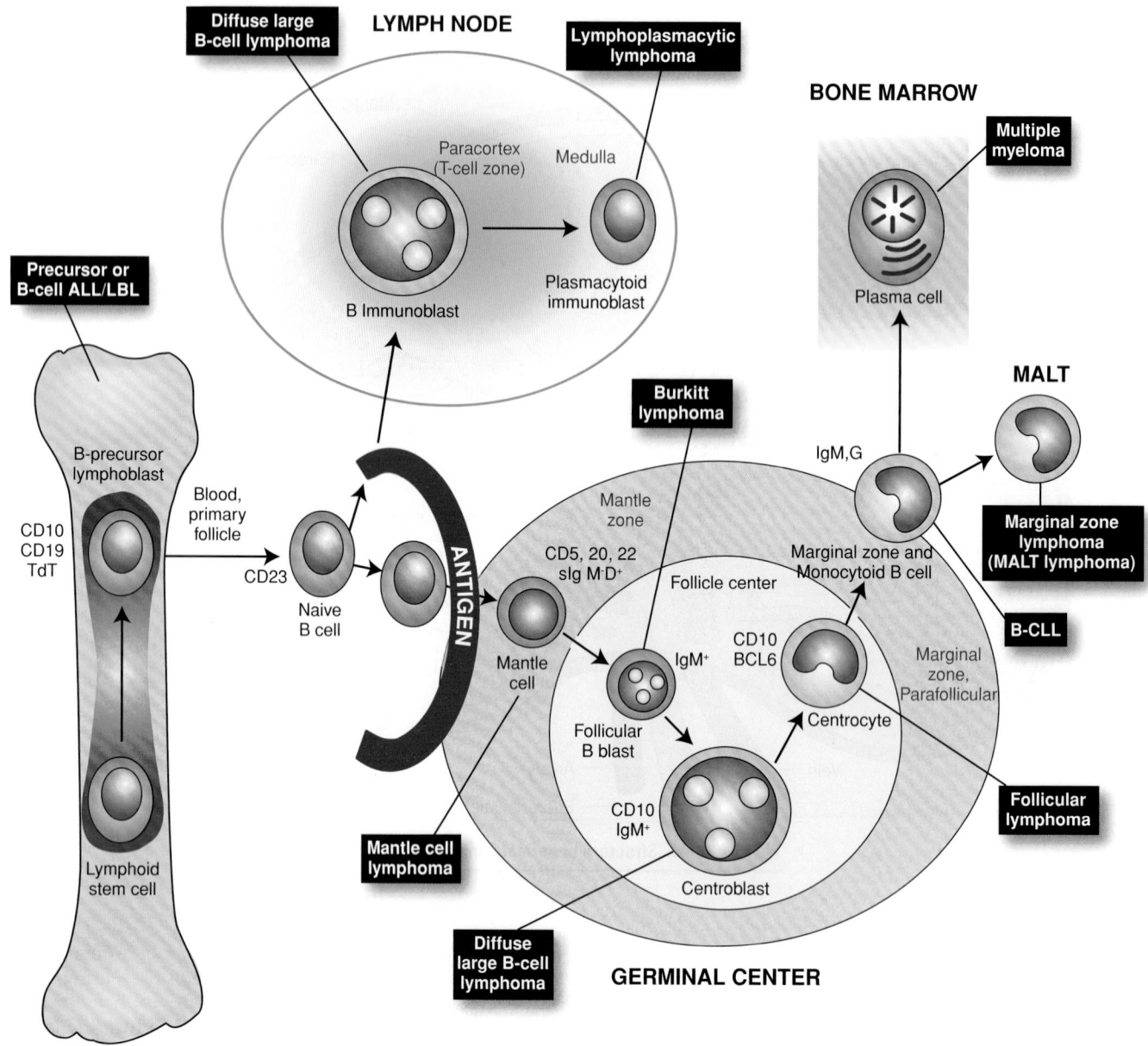

FIGURE 26-47. Pathway of normal B-cell differentiation and corresponding B-cell neoplasms. Following the lymphoid stem cell and precursor stage in the bone marrow, B cells mature into naive B lymphocytes and home to the secondary lymphoid organs (primarily lymph nodes). The germinal-center reaction represents an important turntable for immunoglobulin variable-region gene mutations, Ig heavy-chain switch and differentiation into plasma cells and memory B cells. Cluster designation (CD) markers are shown. B-cell immunoblasts and plasmacytoid immunoblasts reside in the T-cell–rich paracortex and medulla, respectively. Marginal zone B cells home to mucosa-associated lymphoid tissue (MALT) sites and bone marrow. Neoplastic transformation occurs at all phases of B-cell differentiation. *ALL/LBL* = acute lymphoblastic leukemia/lymphoma; *B-CLL* = B-cell chronic lymphocytic leukemia; *Ig* = immunoglobulin.

lymphoid cells can range from large to small, but they generally show more clumped nuclear chromatin and variable amounts of cytoplasm (with or without granules) compared to the immature (blast-like) cells. While a variety of cell sizes (including many large transformed or activated cells) are normally present in the secondary lymphoid organs, the lymphocytes that circulate in the blood and those in the bone marrow are mainly small and heterogeneous (Fig. 26-49).

In peripheral blood smears, transformed cytotoxic T cells are **variant lymphocytes** (sometimes called "atypical lymphocytes"). Variant lymphocytes tend to have abundant blue-gray cytoplasm and multiple nucleoli in Wright-Giemsa–stained smears. The same cells in tissue sections stained with hematoxylin and eosin have round to oval nuclei, one to several eosinophilic nucleoli apposed to their nuclear membranes and abundant clear to purple cytoplasm. *T and B cells appear identical in routinely stained smears or tissue sections. Precise identification and characterization of lymphoid cells requires flow cytometric or immunohistochemical analysis.* In the blood, 60%–80% of circulating lymphocytes are T cells, 10%–15% are B cells and the rest are NK cells.

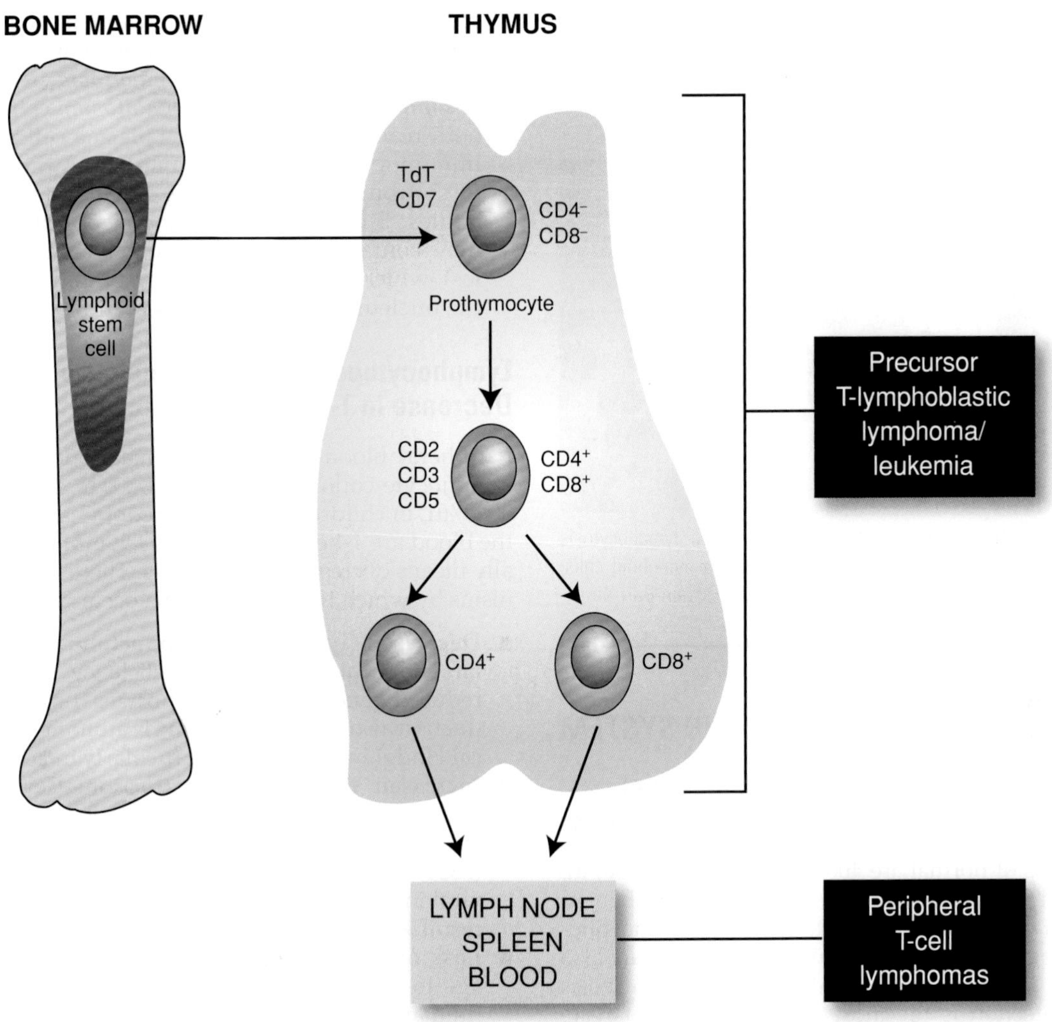

BONE MARROW   **THYMUS**

TdT
CD7

CD4⁻
CD8⁻

Lymphoid
stem
cell

Prothymocyte

CD2
CD3
CD5

CD4⁺
CD8⁺

CD4⁺

CD8⁺

**Precursor
T-lymphoblastic
lymphoma/
leukemia**

**LYMPH NODE
SPLEEN
BLOOD**

**Peripheral
T-cell
lymphomas**

FIGURE 26-48. Pathways of normal T-cell development and corresponding T-cell neoplasms. *CD* = cluster designation; *TdT* = terminal deoxynucleotidyl transferase.

Variant lymphocytes

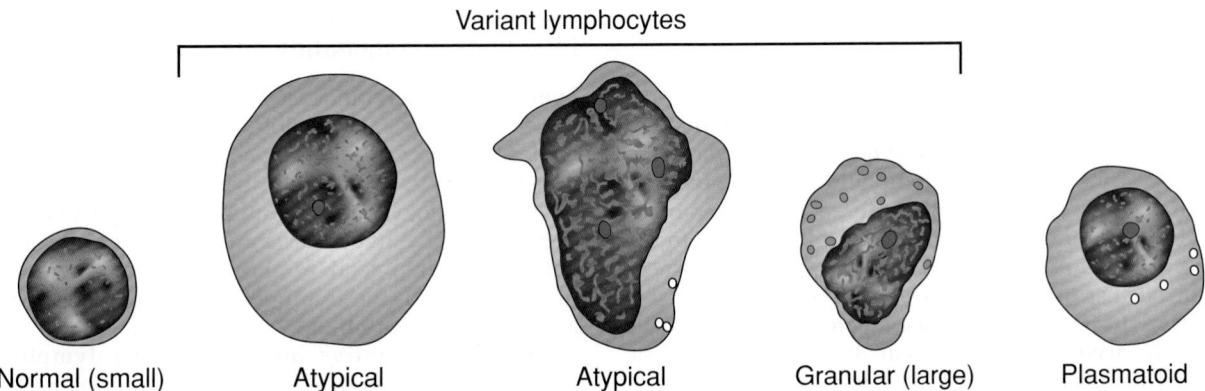

Normal (small)   Atypical   Atypical   Granular (large)   Plasmatoid

FIGURE 26-49. Lymphocyte morphology. The term "variant lymphocytes" covers atypical lymphocytes and large granular lymphocytes. **Atypical lymphocytes** are large and exhibit deep blue to pale gray cytoplasm; they are seen in benign reactive processes. **Large granular lymphocytes** are medium to large lymphoid cells with some pink cytoplasmic granules. They are suppressor T lymphocytes, some with natural killer (NK) function, and may be increased in benign or malignant disorders. **Plasmacytoid lymphocytes** have abundant blue cytoplasm and are seen in some reactive disorders.

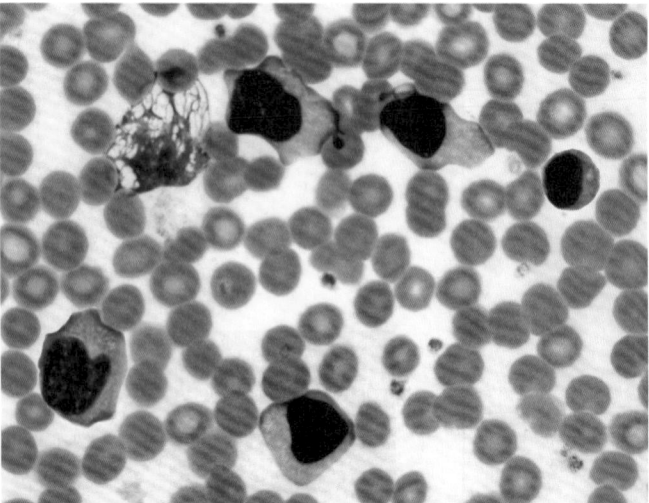

FIGURE 26-50. Infectious mononucleosis. An absolute lymphocytosis caused by a heterogeneous population of small and larger lymphoid cells, including atypical lymphocytes, is characteristic of this Ebstein-Barr virus–driven disorder.

BENIGN DISORDERS OF THE LYMPHOID SYSTEM

In Benign Lymphocytosis, Absolute Numbers of Circulating Lymphocytes Are Transiently Increased

The upper limits of normal are 4000/μL in adults, 7000/μL in children and 9000/μL in infants. Lymphocytes in benign lymphocytoses are usually reactive appearing and morphologically heterogeneous, but atypical lymphocytes may also be seen (Figs. 26-49 and 26-50). Infectious mononucleosis due to EBV infection is the most common cause of reactive lymphocytosis, but other viral infections can produce similar syndromes (e.g., CMV). Other less common causes of reactive lymphocytosis include pertussis, chronic bacterial infections such as tuberculosis and brucellosis, stress and cigarette smoking. Persistent absolute lymphocytosis, greater than 4000/μL, particularly in adults, raises suspicion for a lymphoproliferative disorder and deserves further evaluation.

Bone Marrow Plasmacytosis May Signify a Plasma Cell Disorder

- **Plasma cells in peripheral blood:** It is uncommon to find plasma cells in the blood. When seen, they are usually part of the spectrum of lymphoid cells in infectious mononucleosis–like syndromes caused by viruses other than EBV. The presence of circulating plasma cells in the blood of an adult raises suspicion for a plasma cell neoplasm, such as plasma cell myeloma (see below).
- **Reactive bone marrow plasmacytosis:** Plasma cells normally account for less than 3% of hematopoietic cells in the bone marrow. If they make up greater than 3% of bone marrow cells, plasmacytosis is diagnosed, and it may be polyclonal or monoclonal. In children and young adults, most plasmacytoses are caused by reactive conditions such as chronic infections or systemic inflammatory disorders. Autoimmune diseases are a particularly common cause of bone marrow

plasmacytosis, especially in women. A plasmacytosis can also accompany a metastatic neoplasm in the bone marrow. *Bone marrow plasmacytosis greater than 10% is typically associated with a plasma cell neoplasm.* In both reactive and neoplastic plasma cell proliferations, immunoglobulin may accumulate in the cytoplasm to form prominent eosinophilic globules, known as Russell bodies. Similarly, benign and neoplastic plasma cells may contain nuclear pseudoinclusions (Dutcher bodies), which represent immunoglobulin invaginated into the nucleus and seen in cross-section.

Lymphocytopenia Usually Reflects a Decrease in T-Helper Lymphocytes

Peripheral blood lymphocytopenia is defined as a blood lymphocyte count less than 1500/μL in adults or less than 3000/μL in children. Since the predominant lymphocytes in the blood are T-helper (CD4+) cells, lymphocytopenia generally means decreased CD4+ T cells. There are several mechanisms by which lymphocytopenia occurs:

- **Decreased lymphocyte production:** Several congenital and acquired immunodeficiency syndromes entail reduced generation of lymphocytes. Impaired T-cell production also occurs with some lymphomas, such as classical Hodgkin lymphoma, particularly in advanced stages.
- **Increased lymphocyte destruction:** Certain therapies, such as irradiation, chemotherapy, administration of antilymphocyte globulin, adrenocorticotropic hormone (ACTH) and corticosteroids, destroy lymphocytes. Some viral infections, particularly HIV, cause T-cell death, with resultant lymphopenia.
- **Loss of lymphocytes:** Disorders associated with damage to intestinal lymphatics can lead to loss of lymph fluid and lymphocytes into the gut lumen. Such diseases include protein-losing enteropathies, Whipple disease and conditions of increased central venous pressure (e.g., right-sided heart failure, chronic constrictive pericarditis). Immunologic damage to lymphocytes may occur in collagen vascular diseases, such as systemic lupus erythematosus.

Reactive Lymphoid Hyperplasia Is a Response to Diverse Stimuli, Including Infections, Inflammation and Tumors

Lymph nodes may undergo hyperplasia of all cellular components, or any combination of B cells, T cells and mononuclear phagocytes, in response to a variety of infectious, inflammatory and neoplastic disorders (Fig. 26-51).

The histology and magnitude of lymph node enlargement in reactive hyperplasia are functions of the age of the patient (children tend to show greater immunoreactivity than do adults), the immunologic competence of the host and the inciting stimulus.

Acute suppurative and necrotizing lymphadenitis occurs in lymph nodes that drain sites of acute bacterial or fungal infections. Such nodes enlarge rapidly because of edema and hyperemia, and are usually tender because the capsule becomes distended. Lymph node sinuses and stroma are infiltrated by neutrophils and variable numbers of bland macrophages. Well- or poorly defined granulomas are common, and necrosis can be focal and

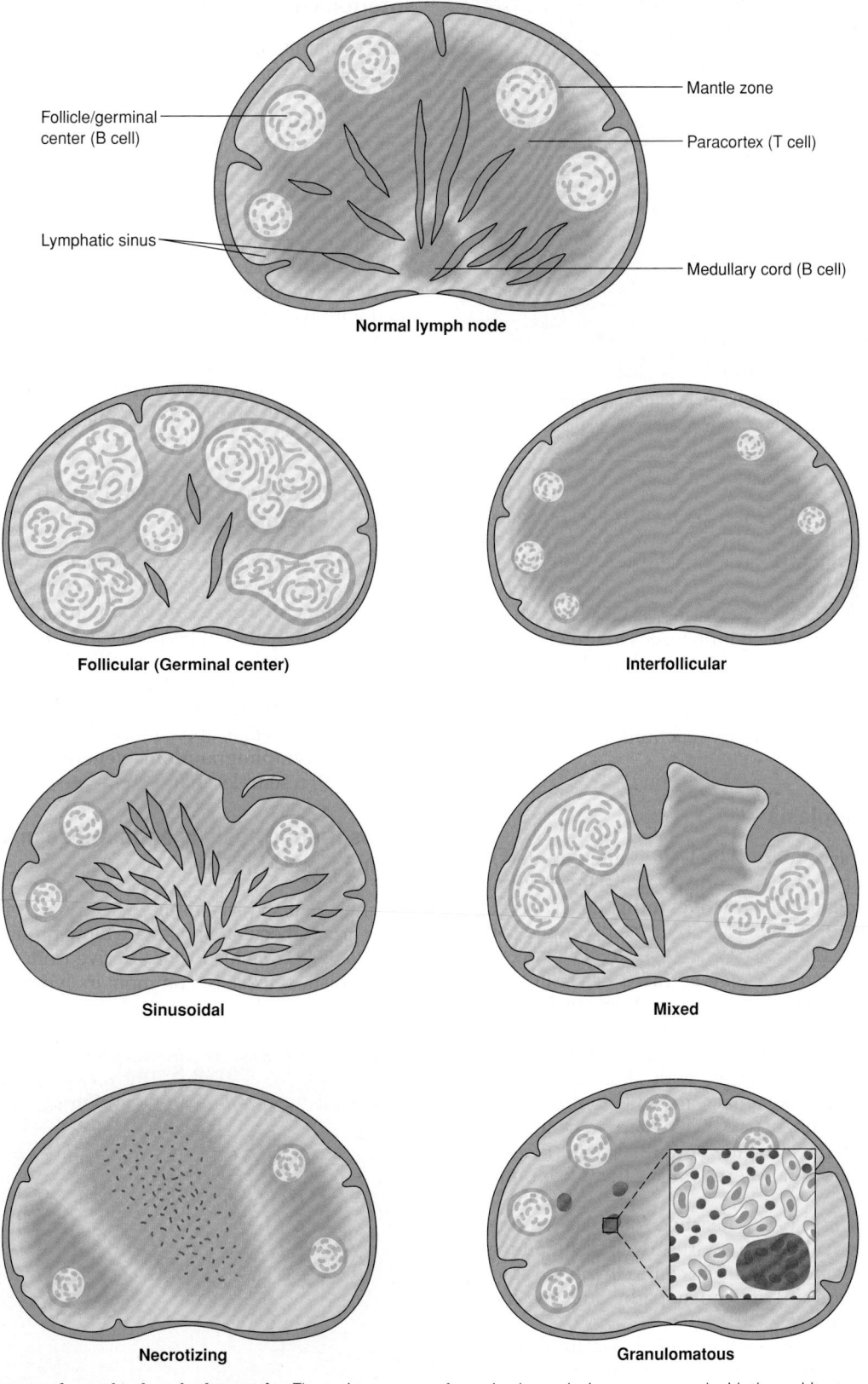

FIGURE 26-51. Patterns of reactive lymphadenopathy. The major patterns of reactive hyperplasia are contrasted with the architecture of a normal lymph node. **Follicular hyperplasia,** with an increased number of enlarged and irregularly shaped follicles, is characteristic of B-cell immunoreactivity. **Interfollicular hyperplasia** with expansion of the paracortex is typical of T-cell immunoreactivity. The **sinusoidal pattern** is typified by expansion of sinuses by bland macrophages. This patten is seen in reactive proliferations of the mononuclear–phagocyte system. A **mixed pattern** of follicular, interfollicular and sinusoidal hyperplasia is common in a variety of complex immune reactions. In **necrotizing lymphadenitis,** variable zones of necrosis are found within the lymph nodes, with or without the presence of neutrophils. Cohesive clusters of macrophages and occasional multinucleated giant cells are characteristic of the **granulomatous inflammation pattern**.

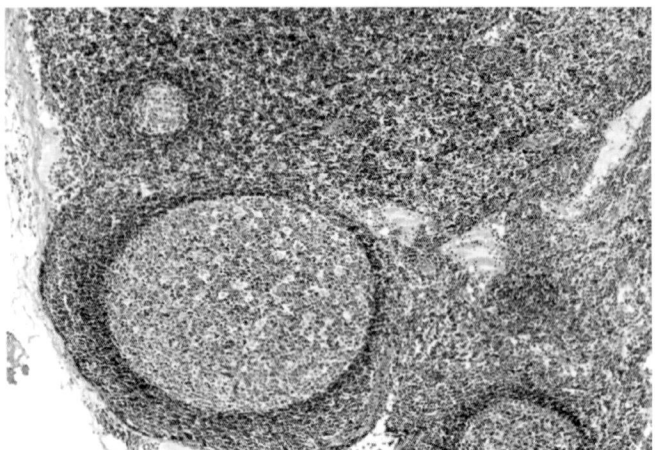

FIGURE 26-52. Lymph node with reactive follicular hyperplasia. A section of a hyperplastic lymph node shows prominent follicles (germinal centers) containing numerous macrophages with pale cytoplasm.

geographic or extensive. The location of the nodes involved in reactive lymphadenopathy often provides a clue to its cause. For example, posterior auricular lymph nodes are commonly enlarged in rubella infection; occipital lymph nodes in scalp infections; posterior cervical lymph nodes in toxoplasmosis; axillary lymph nodes in infections of the arms or chest wall; and inguinal lymph nodes in venereal infections and infections of the legs. Generalized lymphadenopathy may occur in systemic infections, hyperthyroidism, drug hypersensitivity reactions and autoimmune diseases.

Follicular Hyperplasia

Hyperplasia of secondary follicles (germinal centers) and plasmacytosis of medullary cords indicate B-cell immunoreactivity. In **nonspecific reactive follicular hyperplasia,** prominent hyperplastic follicles occur mainly in the cortices of the lymph node (Figs. 26-51 and 26-52). Follicles are round or irregularly shaped and may be fused or confluent. The activated B cells in these follicles range from small cells with irregular, cleaved nuclei to large immunoblasts. Many mitoses reflect rapid proliferation of activated B lymphocytes. Scattered benign macrophages, with abundant pale cytoplasm containing pyknotic nuclear and cytoplasmic debris, impart a characteristic "starry sky" pattern to benign follicle centers. A well-defined mantle of normal small B cells surrounds the follicles, sharply separating them from interfollicular regions.

The cause of nonspecific reactive follicular hyperplasia is often unknown, although a virus, drug or inflammatory process is often likely. The clinical course involves rapid and complete resolution of lymphadenopathy after the inciting stimulus disappears.

Reactive lymphadenopathy (either localized or generalized) due to follicular hyperplasia and interfollicular plasmacytosis is common in rheumatoid arthritis. It also occurs early in HIV infection. It is worth noting here that the lymph nodes in patients with HIV/AIDS show a high incidence of superimposed lymphomas (such as diffuse B-cell lymphoma, Burkitt lymphoma and classical Hodgkin lymphoma), Kaposi sarcoma or opportunistic infection (e.g., with atypical mycobacteria or CMV).

Interfollicular Hyperplasia

Interfollicular or diffuse hyperplasia of the deep cortex or paracortex is characteristic of T-lymphocyte immunoreactivity.

Nonspecific reactive interfollicular hyperplasia (Fig. 26-51) is most commonly caused by viral infections or immunologic reactions. Although the precise cause is often unknown, the condition usually resolves promptly. Interfollicular lymph node hyperplasia is common in viral diseases, including infectious mononucleosis, varicella-herpes zoster infection, measles and CMV lymphadenitis.

Systemic lupus erythematosus (SLE) is often associated with lymphadenopathy characterized by interfollicular hyperplasia with prominent immunoblasts and plasma cells, and variably pronounced necrosis. Arteriolitis with fibrinoid necrosis of vessel walls is common. Unlike acute suppurative and necrotizing lymphadenitis, neutrophils are absent in SLE-related lymphadenitis.

Mixed Patterns of Reactive Lymph Node Hyperplasia

Some infectious diseases are associated with mixed patterns of lymphoid hyperplasia, in which several different features are prominent. For example, in **toxoplasmosis,** one sees prominent follicular hyperplasia and small collections of epithelioid macrophages in interfollicular regions and around the hyperplastic follicles (Figs. 26-51 and 26-53). **Cat-scratch disease** elicits follicular hyperplasia and suppurative granulomas with a stellate appearance (Fig. 26-54). Lymphadenitis caused by **lymphogranuloma venereum** and **tularemia** (see Chapter 9) resembles that seen in cat-scratch disease.

Sinus Histiocytosis Is an Increase in Macrophages Lining Nodal Sinuses

In sinus histiocytosis, tissue macrophages in nodal subcapsular and trabecular sinuses are more prominent (Figs. 26-51 and 26-55). Sinus histiocytes derive from blood monocytes. Sinus histiocytosis is common in lymph nodes draining

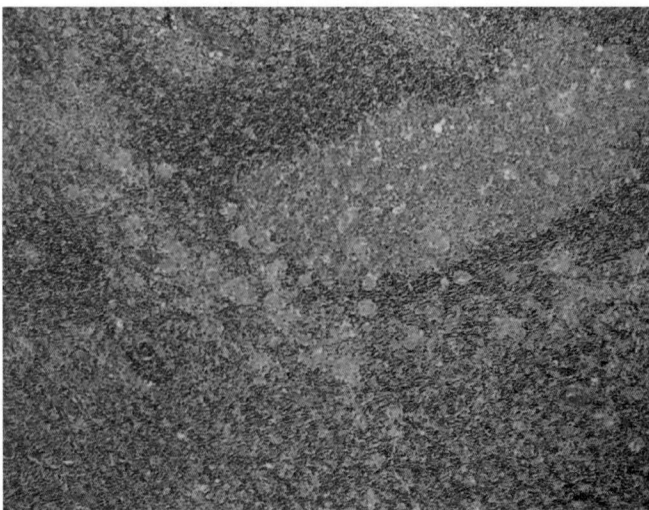

FIGURE 26-53. Toxoplasmosis. A section of a lymph node displays clusters of pink epithelioid macrophages and follicular hyperplasia.

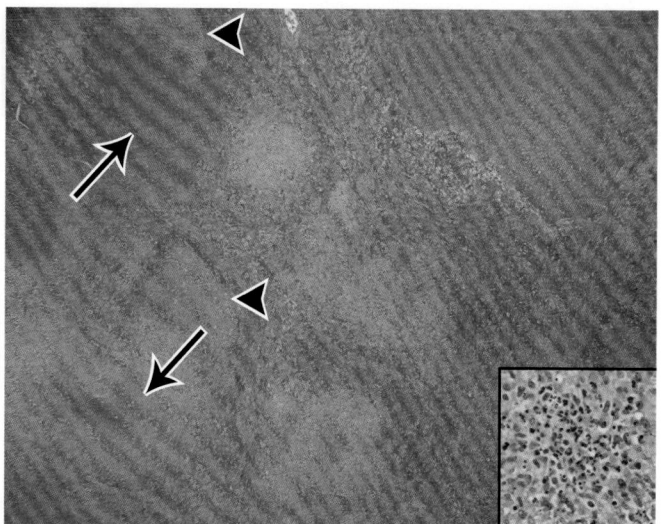

FIGURE 26-54. Cat-scratch disease. Follicular hyperplasia (*arrowheads*) is punctuated by irregularly shaped granulomas (*arrows*), which occasionally impinge on the germinal centers. **Inset.** The granulomas are composed of central cores of neutrophils with surrounding macrophages.

carcinomas and, less often, inflammatory and infectious foci. The nature of the phagocytic debris in the cytoplasm of such macrophages helps identify the origin of the process. For example, anthracotic pigment accumulates in macrophages in mediastinal lymph nodes showing sinus histiocytosis. Macrophages containing erythrocytes and hemosiderin pigment characterize autoimmune hemolytic anemias and sites draining hemorrhages.

Sinus histiocytosis may or may not cause lymph node enlargement. Common sinus histiocytosis should not be confused with **sinus histiocytosis with massive lymphadenopathy (Rosai-Dorfman disease),** in which prominent bilateral (usually cervical) lymphadenopathy reflects a marked expansion of lymph node sinuses by histocytes that have ingested intact lymphocytes (emperipolesis). Most

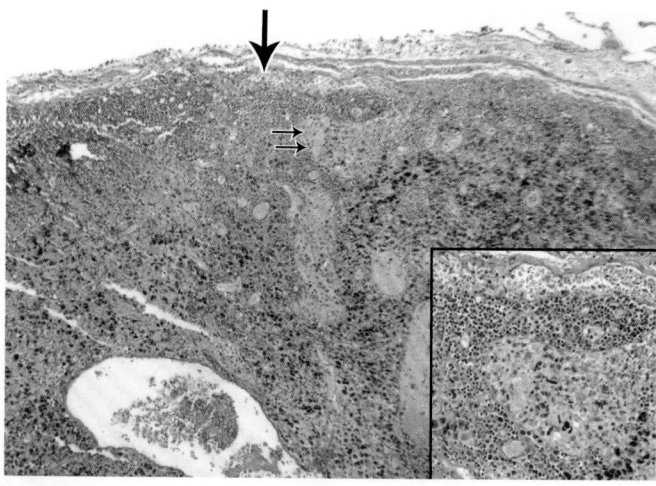

FIGURE 26-55. Sinus histiocytosis. In this hilar lymph node, macrophages are prominent in the subcapsular sinus (*single arrow*) and also in draining sinuses (*double arrows*). **Inset.** A higher-power view demonstrates the large, pink macrophages both at the bottom of the subcapsular sinus and in the draining sinus.

cases of Rosai-Dorfman disease occur in the second decade of life, and the disease is often associated with systemic findings including fever, leukocytosis and hypergammaglobulinemia.

Dermatopathic Lymphadenopathy Occurs in Chronic Dermatoses

Dermatopathic lymphadenopathy refers to paracortical T-cell proliferation caused by certain chronic skin diseases. Lipid, melanin and hemosiderin drain from the affected skin to the regional lymph nodes. The draining lymph nodes show an immune reaction to antigenic material arriving there from the skin, and mainly accumulating in paracortical macrophages. A heterogeneous cell population expands the paracortex. It consists of Langerhans cells, interdigitating reticulum cells and macrophages whose cytoplasm contains lipid or granular, brown, melanin pigment.

MALIGNANT LYMPHOMAS

Lymphomas are malignant proliferations of lymphocytes. B-cell, T-cell and NK-cell lymphomas may be **immature** (derived from precursor cells; lymphoblasts) or **mature** (derived from mature effector cells). The latter are more common. While all lymphomas are malignant, they show a wide spectrum of clinical behavior: some follow an indolent clinical course (and may not even require treatment), while others are very aggressive (and can cause death in a short time, if untreated).

Lymphomas mostly affect lymph nodes, but any tissue or organ may be involved (e.g., GI tract, thyroid, liver, skin, lungs, brain). If lymphoma cells are present in the peripheral blood and/or bone marrow, the tumor is "leukemic" or "peripheralized."

Beyond the broad categories of B-cell, T-cell and NK-cell types, lymphomas are further classified by their postulated cells of origin, normal cellular counterparts, immunophenotypes, molecular/genetic alterations, clinical features and morphology. Further, Hodgkin lymphomas (HLs) are classified separately from non-Hodgkin lymphomas (NHLs). The WHO classification of lymphoid tumors takes all of these parameters into account and is currently used by pathologists and clinicians alike. The major recognized types of B-, T-, and NK-cell lymphomas are shown in Tables 26-17 and 26-18. Selected examples are discussed in the following sections.

Precursor B-Cell Acute Lymphoblastic Leukemia/ Lymphoma Is a Malignancy of B Lymphoblasts

The malignant cells in precursor B-ALL and B-cell lymphoblastic lymphoma (B-LBL) are immature (precursor) cells, or **lymphoblasts**. If the B-lymphoblast proliferation involves the bone marrow and/or peripheral blood, it is **acute lymphoblastic leukemia**. But if it mainly involves extramedullary tissues (e.g., lymph nodes), it is called a **lymphoblastic lymphoma**.

EPIDEMIOLOGY: *Precursor B-cell ALL is the most common childhood leukemia.* Although the disease can present at any age, 75% of cases occur in children younger than age 6. The incidence of B-cell ALL

TABLE 26-17
WHO HISTOLOGIC CLASSIFICATION OF B-CELL NEOPLASMS

Precursor B-Cell Neoplasm

Precursor B-cell lymphoblastic leukemia/lymphoma

Mature B-Cell Neoplasms

Chronic lymphocytic leukemia/small lymphocytic lymphoma

B-cell prolymphocytic leukemia

Lymphoplasmacytic lymphoma

Splenic marginal zone lymphoma

Hairy cell leukemia

Plasma cell myeloma

Monoclonal gammopathy of undetermined significance (MGUS)

Solitary plasmacytoma of bone

Extraosseous plasmacytoma

Primary amyloidosis

Heavy-chain diseases

Extranodal marginal zone B-cell lymphoma of mucosa-associated lymphoid tissue (MALT lymphoma)

Nodal marginal zone B-cell lymphoma

Follicular lymphoma

Mantle cell lymphoma

Mediastinal (thymic) large B-cell lymphoma

Intravascular large B-cell lymphoma

Primary effusion lymphoma

Burkitt lymphoma/leukemia

WHO = World Health Organization.

TABLE 26-18
WHO HISTOLOGIC CLASSIFICATION OF T-CELL AND NK-CELL NEOPLASMS

Precursor T-Cell Neoplasm

Precursor T-cell lymphoblastic leukemia/lymphoma

Mature T-Cell Neoplasms

Leukemic/Disseminated

T-cell prolymphocytic leukemia

T-cell large granular lymphocytic leukemia

Aggressive NK-cell leukemia

Adult T-cell leukemia/lymphoma

Cutaneous

Mycosis fungoides

Sézary syndrome

Primary cutaneous anaplastic lymphoma

Large cell lymphoma

Lymphomatoid papulosis

Other Extranodal

Extranodal NK-/T-cell lymphoma, nasal type

Enteropathy-type T-cell lymphoma

Hepatosplenic T-cell lymphoma

Subcutaneous panniculitis-like T-cell lymphoma

Nodal

Angioimmunoblastic T-cell lymphoma

Peripheral T-cell lymphoma, unspecified

Anaplastic large cell lymphoma

Neoplasm of Uncertain Lineage and Stage of Differentiation

Blastic NK-cell lymphoma

NK = natural killer; WHO = World Health Organization.

is 1–4.75 per 100,000 people per year worldwide, and 1.65 per 100,000 people per year in the United States. Several environmental and genetic factors have been inculpated in the genesis of ALL, including Down syndrome, Bloom syndrome, ataxia-telangiectasia, neurofibromatosis type I, in utero exposure to ionizing radiation and solvents such as benzene. Most cases of precursor B-cell ALL are leukemic rather than lymphomatous at presentation, in contrast to its T-cell counterpart.

 **MOLECULAR PATHOGENESIS:** Chromosomal abnormalities are present in most cases of precursor B-cell ALL, including both numerical and structural abnormalities (Table 26-19). Translocations are common, including those involving chromosomes 9 and 22 (*BCR/ABL* fusion; Philadelphia chromosome), which tends to generate a smaller protein (p190) in childhood B-ALLs than in adult B-ALLs and CML (p210). Other chromosomal changes may impact prognosis (Table 26-19).

 PATHOLOGY: Lymphoblasts are small to medium-sized cells with high nucleus-to-cytoplasm ratios, fine chromatin, inconspicuous nucleoli and agranular cytoplasm (Fig. 26-56). The lymphoblasts typically make up greater than or equal to 20% of bone marrow cellularity, and variable numbers of blast cells circulate in the blood. Flow cytometry immunophenotyping is

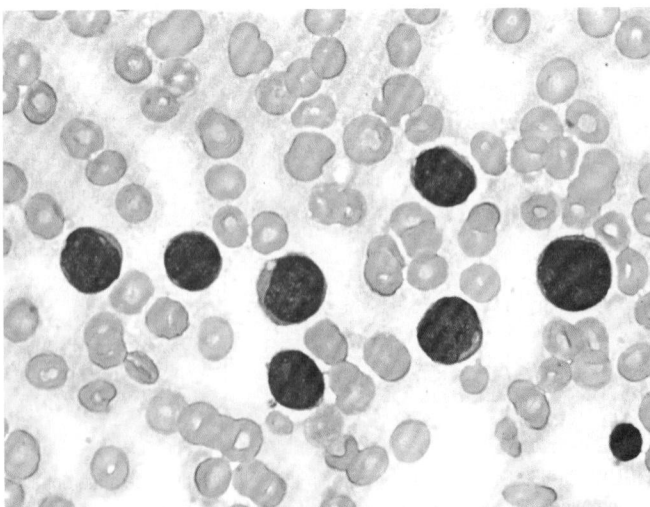

FIGURE 26-56. Acute lymphoblastic leukemia. The lymphoblasts in peripheral blood have irregular and indented nuclei with fine nuclear chromatin, visible nucleoli and variable amounts of agranular cytoplasm.

TABLE 26-19

COMMON GENETIC ABNORMALITIES ASSOCIATED WITH PROLIFERATIONS OF LYMPHOID CELLS

Disease	Associated Genetic/Chromosomal Abnormality	Importance
B-lymphoblastic leukemia/lymphoma	t(9;22) translocations involving *MLL* at 11q23	Children often make p190 bcr/abl, while adults make p210 bcr/abl from t(9;22)
	Hyperdiploidy	Better prognosis
	Hypodiploidy	Worse prognosis
T-lymphoblastic leukemia/lymphoma	TCR genes translocate to sites involving *MYC, TAL1, RBTN1, RBTN2, HOX11*	Disturbed transcriptional regulation results
B-cell chronic lymphocytic leukemia/ small lymphocytic lymphomas	del 13q12-14; frequent IgVH gene rearrangements	
	del 11q; trisomy 12; del 17p	17p locus encodes p53; these changes imply worse prognosis
Follicular lymphoma	t(14;18)(q32;q21)	Characteristic, leads to overexpression of Bcl-2
	Inactivation of p53; activation of *MYC*	Transformation to more aggressive phenotype
Mantle cell lymphoma	t(11;14)(q13;q32)	Primary genetic event, upregulates cyclin D1
	Mutation at 11q22-23	Inactivates *ATM*
Marginal zone lymphoma	t(11;18); t(1;14)	No longer responds to antibiotic treatment alone
	Mutations of IgV region genes; trisomy 3	
Diffuse large B-cell lymphoma	Rearrangements involving 3q27	3q27 carries *BCL6* locus
	t(14;18) rearrangements involving *MYC*	Tend to portend worse prognosis
Burkitt lymphoma	Rearrangements involving *MYC*: t(8;14) or t(2;8) or t(8;22)	Characteristic rearrangement
Plasma cell myeloma	Clonal rearrangements involving Ig H and L genes	
	Abnormalities of chromosome number	Poor prognosis
	IgH translocations with *cyclin D1, C-MAF, FGFR3, cyclin D3, MAFB*; monosomy or partial deletion of chromosome 13	
	t(4;14); t(14;16); t(14;20); del 17p	Poorer prognosis
Anaplastic large cell lymphoma	t(2;5) (involving anaplastic lymphoma kinase and *NPM* genes)	Tends to occur in younger patients, upregulates *ALK*, better prognosis

H = heavy; Ig = immunoglobulin; L = light; TCR = T-cell receptor.

needed to confirm the diagnosis. All cases show evidence of B-lymphoblast differentiation, but immunophenotypic patterns in precursor B-cell ALLs are variable and reflect the different stages of early B-cell maturation (Fig. 26-47). The earliest antigens that indicate B-cell differentiation are CD10, CD19 and TdT. B-cell neoplasms that express surface Ig are not considered precursor neoplasms since surface Ig expression is a feature of mature B cells.

 CLINICAL FEATURES: The leukemic cells of precursor B-cell ALL proliferate in the bone marrow and displace the normal marrow elements, resulting in anemia, thrombocytopenia and neutropenia. Organomegaly and central nervous system (CNS) involvement are common as the disease disseminates from the bone marrow. The rapidly growing tumor cells in the bone marrow cause bone pain and arthralgias, which may be the earliest presenting symptoms in children.

The prognosis for childhood precursor B-cell ALL is generally excellent with complete remission rates of greater than 90%. Among other variables, age younger than 1 year or older than 12 years, older adult onset and/or the presence of certain cytogenetic abnormalities [e.g., t(9;22), t(1;19), t(4;11), hypodiploidy] are poor prognostic indicators. All translocations involving the *MLL* gene at 11q23 are associated with a poor prognosis regardless of age.

The treatment includes chemotherapy or stem cell transplantation for patients with high-risk features or who are unresponsive to chemotherapy.

Precursor T-Cell Acute Lymphoblastic Leukemia/ Lymphoma Is a Neoplasm of T Lymphoblasts

Precursor T-cell acute lymphoblastic leukemia (T-ALL) and T-cell lymphoblastic lymphoma (T-LBL) are immature T-cell neoplasms. As with precursor B-ALL, the decision whether to call the tumor **leukemia** or **lymphoma** is often arbitrary.

 EPIDEMIOLOGY: Precursor T-cell ALL occurs at any age. It accounts for 15% of childhood ALL and affects adolescents more commonly than younger children. T-ALL is more common in males than females. In adults, 25% of acute lymphoblastic leukemias are precursor T-cell ALLs. Compared to its B-cell counterpart, precursor T-cell ALL is more likely to have a lymphomatous presentation.

 **MOLECULAR PATHOGENESIS:** The genes encoding the four T-cell receptor chains (α-, β-, γ-, δ-chains) often participate in chromosomal translocations with genes encoding transcription factors (Table 26-19). Juxtaposition of T-cell receptor loci to transcription factor genes often leads to disturbed transcriptional regulation.

 PATHOLOGY: The morphology of T lymphoblasts is like that of B lymphoblasts (Fig. 26-56). Immunophenotype in T-ALL reflects normal T-cell differentiation and maturation in the bone marrow and thymus (Fig. 26-48). The earliest T-cell antigen is CD7, followed by CD2 and CD5. During thymic differentiation, T cells become positive for CD1a and cytoplasmic CD3 (cCD3; CD3ε), CD4 and CD8. Like precursor B-cell ALL, lymphoblasts in most cases of T-cell ALL express TdT.

 CLINICAL FEATURES: The blood and bone marrow are almost always involved in precursor T-cell ALL. Presenting white blood cell counts are usually high, and a mediastinal mass or other tissue mass (lymphoma) is often present. Lymphadenopathy and organomegaly are common, as are pleural effusions. **Mediastinal adenopathy** occurs particularly often in adolescent males. The tumor usually grows rapidly, and patients with mediastinal involvement may present with respiratory distress because of compression of the central airways or superior vena cava syndrome. In general, precursor T-cell ALL has a worse prognosis than precursor B-cell ALL in children, but it has a slightly better outcome than B-ALL in adults.

Mature B-Cell Lymphomas Are the Most Common Type of Lymphoma in the Western World

Mature B-cell malignancies are clonal proliferations of differentiated B cells. As B cells progress through the steps of differentiation and maturation from naive B lymphocytes to plasma cells, lymphomas may arise at any point along the way (Fig. 26-47).

 EPIDEMIOLOGY: Mature B-cell lymphomas make up greater than 90% of lymphoid neoplasms worldwide. They are more common in developed countries, particularly the United States, Australia, New Zealand and western Europe, and their incidence is increasing. In the United States, the incidence of all lymphoid neoplasms is 34 cases per year per 100,000 people, of which B-cell lymphomas alone account for 26 per year per 100,000 people. The frequency of the specific types of B-cell lymphoma varies in different parts of the world. For example, Burkitt lymphoma is endemic in equatorial Africa (where it is the most common childhood malignancy), but it accounts for only 1%–2% of lymphomas in industrialized nations. Similarly, follicular lymphoma occurs more frequently in the United States and western Europe, compared to South America, eastern Europe and Asia. *Worldwide, the most common lymphomas are follicular lymphoma (29%) and diffuse large cell lymphoma (37%), exclusive of Hodgkin lymphoma and plasma cell myeloma (Table 26-20).*

Most mature B-cell lymphomas occur in the sixth and seventh decades of life. A variant of diffuse large B-cell lymphoma, mediastinal large B-cell lymphoma, is an exception, with a median age of 35. Mature B-cell lymphomas, other than Burkitt and diffuse large B-cell lymphomas, are distinctly uncommon in children.

Risk factors for development of B-cell lymphoma include abnormalities of the immune system (e.g., immunodeficiencies like AIDS or iatrogenic immunosuppression, and autoimmune diseases), certain infectious agents (e.g., EBV, hepatitis C, *Helicobacter pylori* and *Chlamydia*), environmental exposures (e.g., herbicides and pesticides) and even genetic polymorphisms in a number of immunoregulatory genes.

TABLE 26-20

FREQUENCY OF B- AND T-/NK-CELL LYMPHOMAS

Diagnosis	% of Total Cases
Diffuse large B-cell lymphoma	30.6
Follicular lymphoma	22.1
MALT lymphoma	7.6
Mature T-cell lymphomas (except ALCL)	7.6
Chronic lymphocytic leukemia/small lymphocytic lymphoma	6.7
Mantle cell lymphoma	6.0
Mediastinal large B-cell lymphoma	2.4
Anaplastic large cell lymphoma	2.4
Burkitt lymphoma	2.5
Nodal marginal zone lymphoma	1.8
Precursor T-cell lymphoblastic lymphoma	1.7
Lymphoplasmacytic lymphoma	1.2
Other types	7.4

ALCL = anaplastic large cell lymphoma; MALT = mucosa-associated lymphoid tissue; NK = natural killer.

PATHOPHYSIOLOGY: Most peripheral B-cell lymphomas occur without apparent cause; however, impairment of the immune system and certain infectious agents may give rise to certain types of lymphoma (Table 26-21). Immunodeficiency caused by HIV infection and therapeutic **immunosuppression in allograft recipients** favors development of large B-cell lymphoma or Burkitt lymphoma. Low-grade B-cell lymphomas tend to develop in patients with certain **autoimmune diseases**. For example, patients with Sjögren disease or Hashimoto thyroiditis (see Chapters 11, 27 and 29) may develop extranodal marginal zone B-cell lymphoma (MALT lymphoma). **Epstein-Barr virus** is linked to endemic Burkitt lymphoma, HIV-associated lymphomas and immunosuppression-related lymphomas. Human herpesvirus 8 (HHV-8) and hepatitis C virus also predispose to B lymphomas—primary effusion lymphoma and lymphoplasmacytic lymphoma associated with type 2 cryoglobulinemia, respectively. MALT lymphomas are often associated with gastric *H. pylori* infections (see Chapter 19) and often regress after antibiotic treatment.

As discussed earlier, lymphomas are classified according to their respective normal lymphocyte counterparts (Fig. 26-47). After the precursor stage, B cells undergo immunoglobulin *VDJ* gene rearrangements and mature to surface IgM- and IgD-positive naive B cells that often express CD5. These cells give rise to **mantle cell lymphoma**. Large activated B cells **(centroblasts)** home to germinal centers where they mature into smaller cells with cleaved nuclei **(centrocytes)**. Centroblasts and centrocytes express germinal center cell markers BCL-6 and CD10 and lack expression of Bcl-2 antiapoptotic protein. **Follicular lymphomas** derive from germinal center B cells and contain a mixture of centroblasts and centrocytes that overexpress Bcl-2, which gives them a survival advantage. **Burkitt lymphoma** and some diffuse large **B-cell lymphomas** also come from germinal center lymphocytes, with the latter known as germinal center–type B-cell lymphomas.

Late-stage memory B cells reside in marginal zones, the outermost compartment of lymphoid follicles. **Marginal zone lymphomas** include **splenic marginal zone lymphoma, nodal marginal zone lymphoma** and **MALT lymphomas**. The latter, particularly, involve extranodal sites such as the stomach and other mucosal tissues. Late-stage memory B cells can also give rise to a subset of chronic lymphocytic leukemia/small lymphocytic lymphomas **(CLL/SLL)**. Ultimately, some B cells differentiate into plasma cells. These are the only B cells to secrete antibodies, although they lack detectable cell surface immunoglobulins. Plasma cells home to the bone marrow, where they may give rise to **multiple myeloma**.

CLINICAL FEATURES: The various types of mature B-cell lymphoma may evolve aggressively, slowly or in between. Their behavior generally reflects their morphology, immunophenotype, genetic lesions and clinical presentation (including stage). *Usually, and with a few exceptions, mature B-cell lymphomas contain small lymphocytes and follow an indolent clinical*

TABLE 26-21
DISORDERS WITH INCREASED RISK OF SECONDARY MALIGNANT LYMPHOMA
Sjögren syndrome
Hashimoto thyroiditis
Renal and cardiac transplant recipients
AIDS
EBV infection
HHV-8 infection
Helicobacter pylori–positive gastritis
Hepatitis C
Congenital immune deficiency syndromes
Chediak-Higashi
Wiskott-Aldrich
Ataxia-telangiectasia
IgA deficiency
Severe combined immune deficiency
α Heavy-chain disease
Celiac disease
Hodgkin lymphoma (posttreatment)

EBV = Epstein-Barr virus; HHV = human herpesvirus; Ig = immunoglobulin.

course, while other B lymphomas, composed of mostly large cells, follow an aggressive course that would be rapidly fatal if untreated. Examples of indolent mature B-cell lymphomas include (but are not limited to) B-cell CLL/SLL, follicular lymphoma, extranodal marginal zone B-cell lymphoma (MALT lymphoma) and lymphoplasmacytic lymphoma; aggressive mature B-cell lymphomas include diffuse large B-cell lymphoma, Burkitt lymphoma and mantle cell lymphoma (MCL). The latter represents an important exception to the general rule of small cell morphology predicting indolent behavior (see below).

Ironically, although indolent lymphomas follow a prolonged clinical course, they are usually incurable using standard therapy. In contrast, aggressive lymphomas progress rapidly, but many are curable with conventional therapies. Unfortunately, not all lymphomas fall unequivocally into either category.

Our subsequent discussion of B-cell lymphomas follows the B-cell development paradigms outlined in Fig. 26-47.

B-Cell Chronic Lymphocytic Leukemia/Small Lymphocytic Lymphoma

B-cell CLL/SLL is a common, mature CD5⁺ B-cell tumor with a monomorphic population of mostly small lymphocytes with round to slightly irregular nuclear contours mixed with less abundant larger cells that have round nuclei and single basophilic nucleoli. These latter are called prolymphoycytes (in the blood) or paraimmunoblasts (in tissue). B-cell CLL/SLL may involve the blood, bone marrow, lymph nodes and/or extranodal sites. When the disease only affects the blood and bone marrow (leukemia), the term **CLL** is preferred. If, instead, lymphadenopathy or solid tumor masses predominate, **SLL** is the more fitting name. Since these two presentations are morphologically, phenotypically and genetically indistinguishable, they are often considered one entity, B-cell CLL/SLL. This tumor generally follows an indolent clinical course. MCL, another mature B-cell tumor that also expresses CD5, is more aggressive.

 **EPIDEMIOLOGY:** B-cell CLL is the most common form of leukemia in adults in the Western world. Its overall annual incidence is 2–6 cases per 100,000 people, but the incidence increases with age to 12.8 per 100,000 at age 65, which is the average age at diagnosis. Men develop CLL/SLL more frequently than women. SLL accounts for 7% of all non-Hodgkin lymphomas in tissue biopsies.

 **MOLECULAR PATHOGENESIS:** The vast majority of B-cell CLL/SLL tumors have cytogenetic abnormalities. The most common are shown in Table 26-19. Half of B-CLL cases do not show somatic mutations in Ig variable-region genes (i.e., unmutated *IgVH*), and so have the genotype of naive B cells. The other half have undergone *IgVH* gene rearrangement (i.e., mutated) and resemble postgerminal center B cells. Cases with unmutated immunoglobulin segments tend to behave more aggressively, for unknown reasons.

 PATHOLOGY: Lymph nodes involved by B-cell CLL/SLL are effaced by a proliferation of mostly small lymphocytes in a vaguely nodular or pseudofollicular to diffuse pattern (Fig. 26-57A). The blood shows absolute lymphocytosis composed mostly of small monotonous lymphocytes with round to slightly irregular nuclear contours and scant blue-gray cytoplasm (Fig. 26-57B). Peripheral smears also contain a large number of disrupted cells (smudge cells; Fig. 26-57B). The nuclear chromatin is clumped and often has a blotchy appearance resembling cracked mud; nucleoli are absent in the small cells.

In addition to the small cells, all cases also have some larger cells with round nuclear contours, less condensed chromatin, and a single prominent central nucleolus; these cells are known as prolymphocytes in the blood, and they usually account for less than 10% of total lymphocytes. In order to establish a diagnosis of B-CLL in the absence of tissue-based disease, the total number of circulating monoclonal B cells must exceed 5000/μL.

The vaguely nodular pattern of B-cell CLL/SLL (with noticeably light and darker staining areas) is most apparent at low magnification. Further examination of lighter-staining zones reveals so-called proliferation centers, which contain a small number of large cells called paraimmunoblasts (Fig. 26-57C). Large confluent sheets of paraimmunoblasts or other large lymphoid cells may represent transformation to diffuse large B-cell lymphoma (see below). B-cell CLL/SLL infiltrates the splenic white and red pulp and portal areas of the liver. Bone marrow involvement ranges from complete effacement of the marrow space to patchy interstitial or nonparatrabecular infiltrate of varying degree.

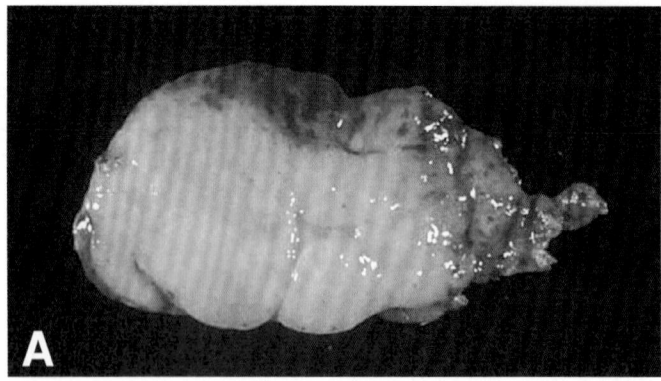

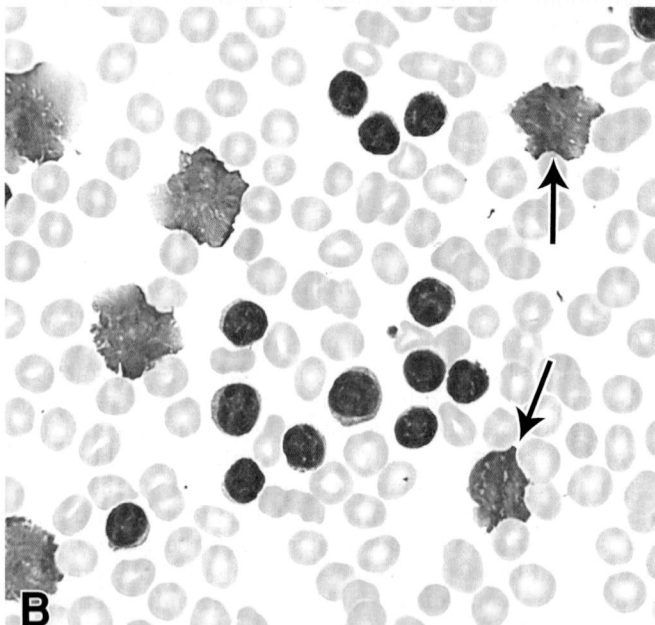

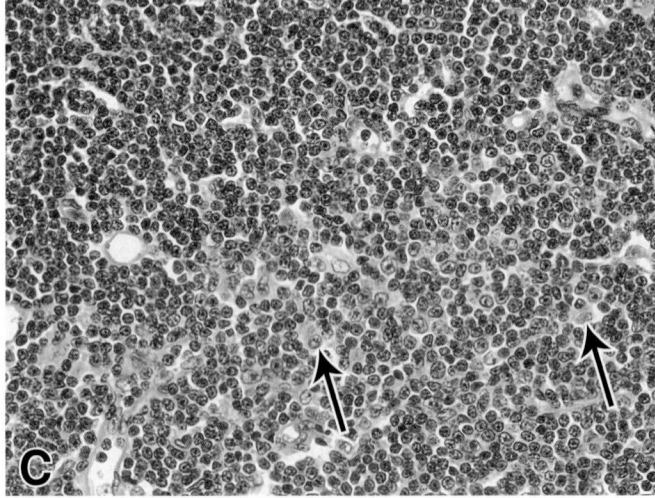

FIGURE 26-57. B-cell small lymphocytic lymphoma/chronic lymphocytic leukemia. A. Gross image of a bisected, enlarged lymph node shows the characteristic uniform, glistening, fish-flesh appearance seen in tissues involved by lymphoma. **B.** A smear of peripheral blood exhibits numerous small to medium-sized lymphocytes with clumped nuclear chromatin. Scattered smudge cells (osmotically fragile cells) are present (*arrows*). **C.** On microscopic examination, the nodal architecture is replaced by a diffuse proliferation of small lymphocytes admixed with a low number of larger cells known as paraimmunoblasts (*arrows*) found in scattered proliferation centers.

The immunophenotype of B-cell CLL/SLL is distinct. The neoplastic cells express pan B-cell antigens, including CD19, CD20, CD22 and CD79, as well as CD5, CD23 and surface immunoglobulin light chain. It is important to note that B-cell CLL/SLL cells show weaker CD20 and immunoglobulin light-chain expression compared to other mature B-cell neoplasms including mantle cell lymphoma, and these findings are diagnostically useful. B-cell CLL/SLL is negative for cyclin D1 and CD10. Some cases of B-cell CLL/SLL express CD38 and/or ZAP-70, and these markers serve as prognostic indicators often used in conjunction with other molecular and FISH tests to help predict individual patient outcome.

 CLINICAL FEATURES: Most patients with B-cell CLL/SLL are asymptomatic, and many cases are diagnosed incidentally. Often the first hint of the disease is an abnormal complete blood count showing absolute lymphocytosis. The total lymphocyte count is variable, but an absolute monoclonal B-cell count of at least 5000 cells/µL is needed to establish a diagnosis of CLL in the blood. Flow cytometry of the peripheral blood is sufficient to establish the diagnosis in most cases. The other peripheral counts may be normal or abnormal, and findings such as platelet count and hemoglobin level are used to stage the disease. Erythrocyte and platelet counts are initially normal, but as the disease advances, severe anemia, thrombocytopenia and even neutropenia can develop. A positive Coombs test occurs during the course of disease in up to 20% of patients and may be associated with immune-mediated hemolytic anemia. A small monoclonal paraprotein may be present in some patients, most of which are of the IgM heavy-chain type (in contrast to patients with multiple myeloma, who most often have IgG paraproteinemias).

Immune deficiencies, mainly of B cells but also of T cells, are common. The cause of B-cell dysfunction is unknown. Hypogammaglobulinemia occurs in 50%–75% of cases at some point during the disease; the degree of hypogammaglobulinemia generally correlates with disease stage and is responsible for infectious complications. Patients with B-CLL also have increased peripheral blood T cells (>3000/µL). $CD8^+$ T cells are increased, and $CD4^+$ cells correspondingly decreased, so that the $CD4^+/CD8^+$ ratio is low. The T cells, though increased in number, often show impaired delayed-type hypersensitivity reactivity, which may contribute to the increased risk of infection. The most common complicating infections are bacterial, then viral and fungal.

Median survival of patients with B-CLL/SLL is 4–6 years (untreated), but the disease course and prognosis are highly variable. For instance, patients with low disease burden can survive over 10 years, while others with extensive disease or poor prognostic features show rapid progression and may not survive more than 2 or 3 years. Certain molecular lesions suggest a worse prognosis (Table 26-19).

The survival of patients with B-CLL/SLL also reflects the risk of transformation or progression to a more aggressive B-cell tumor. *Transformation to prolymphocytic leukemia occurs in 15%–30% of cases and is the most common form of progression.* This type of transformation is heralded by worsening cytopenias, increasing splenomegaly and progressive increases in prolymphocytes in the blood or para-immunoblasts in lymph nodes or other tissues.

Transformation to diffuse large B-cell lymphoma, **Richter syndrome,** occurs in 10% of cases. This form of progression is marked by the appearance of a rapidly enlarging mass,

worsening of systemic symptoms and a high lactate dehydrogenase level in the serum. Other rare forms of transformation also occur, including a Hodgkin lymphoma or Hodgkin-like transformation, the latter occurring more frequently in patients treated with certain chemotherapeutic drugs. Most patients who undergo prolymphocytic or Richter transformation survive less than 1 year.

Asymptomatic patients with B-CLL/SLL who have stable lymphocyte counts may not need treatment. Multiagent chemotherapy and/or treatment with humanized monoclonal antibodies (e.g., Rituxan) is used in patients with high-stage or aggressive disease, but the disease generally remains incurable.

Follicular Lymphoma

Follicular lymphoma (FL) is a mature B-cell lymphoma of follicle center B cells (germinal center cells). FLs must have at least a partially follicular architecture to meet diagnostic criteria. The neoplastic cells are heterogeneous, with a mixture of small and large cleaved cells and centroblasts. This tumor's behavior may vary from indolent to aggressive. This largely reflects the histologic grade, which depends on the number of centroblasts in the neoplastic follicles.

 **EPIDEMIOLOGY:** FL is the second most common lymphoma worldwide, but it is the most common non-Hodgkin lymphoma in the United States, where it constitutes 20% of all adult lymphomas. It is mainly a disease of adults with a peak incidence in the sixth decade. It only rarely occurs in people under age 20, and is more common in women than men.

 MOLECULAR PATHOGENESIS: The t(14:18) is the characteristic genomic abnormality in FL. It occurs in up to 90% of grades 1 and 2 FLs (so-called low-grade follicular lymphomas; Table 26-19). It puts expression of the antiapoptotic protein, Bcl-2, under control of the IgH promoter, and results in Bcl-2 overexpression. *Bcl-2 protein is an inhibitor of apoptosis and provides a survival advantage to the lymphoma cells.* In addition to the *Bcl-2/IgH* rearrangement, several other genetic alterations have been found in FL, and some of them are associated with progression/transformation from the low-grade indolent forms to the more aggressive higher-grade form or diffuse large B-cell lymphoma (DLBCL) (Table 26-19).

PATHOLOGY: Lymph nodes (or other tissues) involved by follicular lymphoma have a distinctly nodular (follicular) pattern or a combination of nodular and diffuse architectural patterns (Fig. 26-58). The neoplastic follicles are present in high density, and are often in a back-to-back arrangement with little intervening paracortex. The neoplastic follicle centers (germinal centers) contain a mixture of small and large cells with irregular nuclear contours (centrocytes/cleaved cells) and scattered centroblasts, which have round nuclear contours and multiple nucleoli attached to the nuclear membrane.

Histologic grade helps to predict prognosis in FL. There are 3 such grades of FL, distinguished by the number of centroblasts per high-power field (Fig. 26-59). Diffuse areas occur in FL but generally do not affect prognosis unless they are composed of large B cells, in which case a diagnosis of concurrent DLBCL is made. The bone marrow is involved

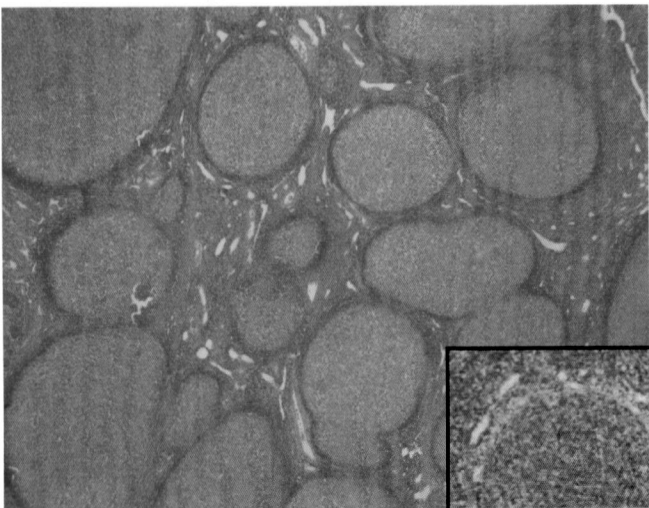

FIGURE 26-58. Follicular lymphoma. The normal lymph node architecture is replaced by malignant lymphoid follicles in a back-to-back pattern. **Inset.** Malignant lymphoid follicle germinal centers can be distinguished from normal/reactive germinal centers using immunohistochemistry for Bcl-2.

in 40%–60% of cases, in a characteristic paratrabecular pattern in most positive bone marrow core biopsies. Circulating follicular lymphoma cells are present in the blood in 10% of cases; they show prominent nuclear irregularity and deep nuclear clefts.

Follicular lymphomas express pan B-cell antigens including CD19, CD20, CD22, CD79a, PAX-5 and cell surface Ig, which in most cases contains only one type of light chain (κ or λ). In addition, FLs also express the germinal center cell markers CD10 and Bcl-6, as would be expected given that they originate from follicle centers. Unlike mantle cell lymphoma and B-cell CLL/SLL, FLs do not express CD5. Follicular lymphoma cells express Bcl-2 protein in over 90% of cases (Fig. 26-58, **inset**). The latter finding may help to distinguish FL from follicular hyperplasia, since the latter is negative for Bcl-2.

CLINICAL FEATURES: Most patients with follicular lymphomas present with generalized adenopathy. Over 80% have stage III or IV disease at the time of initial diagnosis. Extranodal presentations are relatively uncommon, compared to other B-cell lymphomas. The lymphadenopathy is painless and may have followed a waxing and waning course before the patient seeks medical attention. Some patients will report having fevers, fatigue and night sweats (B symptoms).

Most cases of FL follow an indolent clinical course. Therefore, and because the disease is usually incurable, treatment is not always needed at diagnosis. Overall median survival is 7–9 years, which does not improve dramatically with high-dose chemotherapy. As discussed above, the clinical course is linked to histologic grade, and progression/transformation to more aggressive disease may occur in 50% of cases.

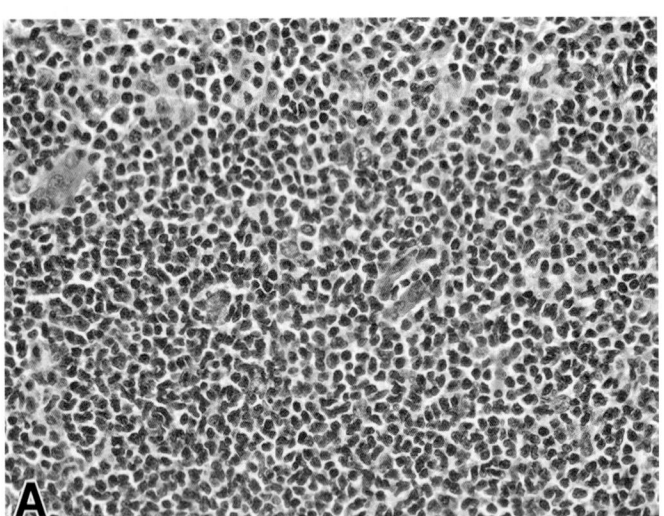

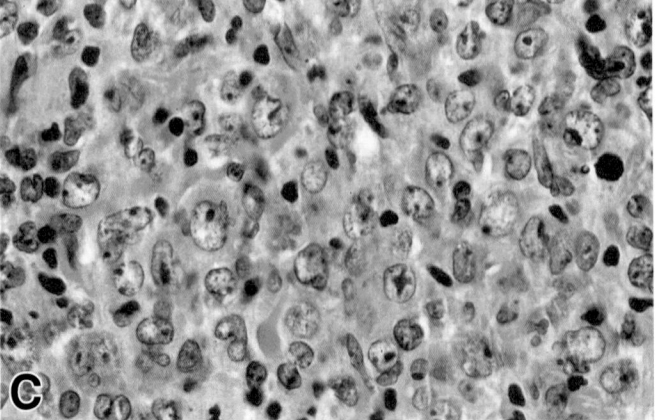

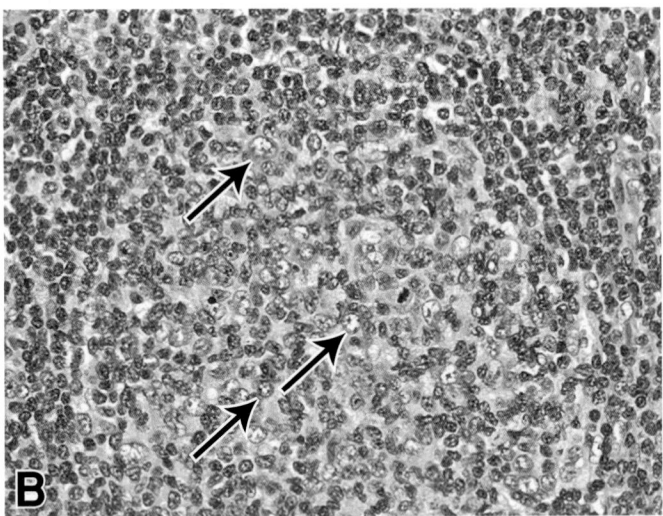

FIGURE 26-59. Follicular lymphoma grading. A. Follicular lymphoma, grade 1. The neoplastic follicles are composed of predominantly small cleaved cells (centrocytes) and only a few scattered centroblasts are present. **B. Follicular lymphoma, grade 2.** The neoplastic follicle shows a mixture of small and large cleaved cells and centroblasts characterized by multiple nucleoli (*arrows*). **C. Follicular lymphoma, grade 3.** The neoplastic follicle shows a predominance of centroblasts with only rare admixed centrocytes. The persistence of a follicular pattern helps distinguish this entity from diffuse large B-cell lymphoma.

Mantle Cell Lymphoma

Lymphomas of mantle cells (MCL) are CD5+ mature B-cell tumors presenting a picture of monotonous small- to medium-sized lymphocytes with irregular nuclear contours, like the normal lymphocytes of the mantle zone around germinal centers.

 **EPIDEMIOLOGY:** MCLs account for less than 10% of B-cell lymphomas. This is a disease of adults, with a median age of 60. MCL affects men twice as often as women; it does not occur in children.

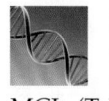 **MOLECULAR PATHOGENESIS:** The reciprocal chromosomal translocation t(11;14) is considered the primary genetic event in nearly all cases of MCL (Table 26-19). It causes overexpression of cyclin D1. Cyclin D1 drives cell cycle progression at the G_1-to-S-phase transition, by binding to Cdk4/6. This event leads to phosphorylation of retinoblastoma (Rb) and subsequent activation of transcription factors promoting cell cycle progression from the G_1 to S phase (see Chapter 5). Several other oncogenic changes may occur in MCL and are listed in Table 26-19.

 PATHOLOGY: Lymph nodes involved by MCL show a diffuse to vaguely nodular lymphoid infiltrate composed of small to medium-sized B cells with irregular nuclear contours. In some cases, MCL lymphocytes are round and resemble the cells of B-cell CLL/SLL, which is often in the differential diagnosis, especially since they also both aberrantly coexpress CD5. One of the characteristic features in typical cases of MCL is the striking monotony of the lymphoma cells with respect to size and shape (Fig. 26-60A). Unlike many other small B-cell lymphomas, large transformed cells and/or centroblasts are absent or rare. The presence of scattered epithelioid histiocytes and hyalinized small blood vessels completes the picture of typical cases.

There are 2 major variants: one with a more nodular-appearing pattern where the lymphoma cells surround the germinal centers (**mantle zone pattern**) and another where the cells are larger and resemble lymphoblasts (**blastic/blastoid variant**). The mantle zone pattern is thought to behave less aggressively than the typical type, while the blastic/blastoid variant is more aggressive. MCL is mainly a nodal-based disease, but it involves many different tissues and organs, particularly the spleen, bone marrow and GI tract. Multifocal mucosal involvement of the gut (mostly small intestine and colon) may produce a pattern known as **lymphomatous polyposis**.

Mantle cell lymphomas express the B-cell markers CD19 and CD20 and show surface light-chain restriction. The lymphoma cells are also positive for CD5, but they are negative for CD10 and CD23. *Importantly, MCL cells are positive for cyclin D1* (Fig. 26-60B). This immunophenotype, combined with the morphologic features, helps distinguish MCL from other small B-cell lymphomas with a more indolent course.

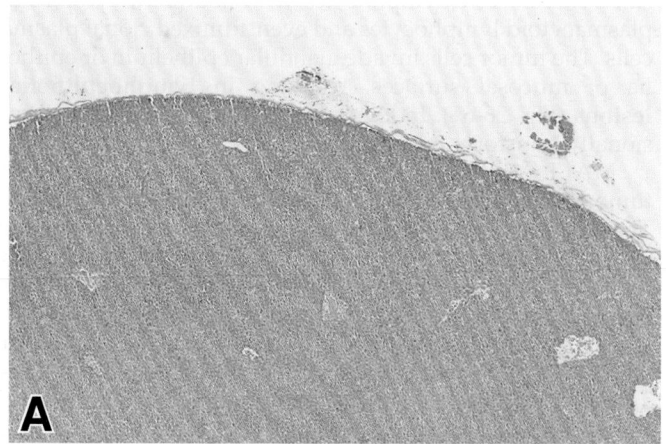

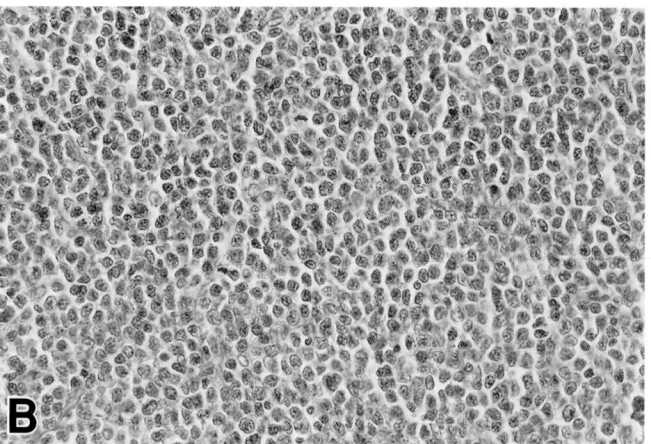

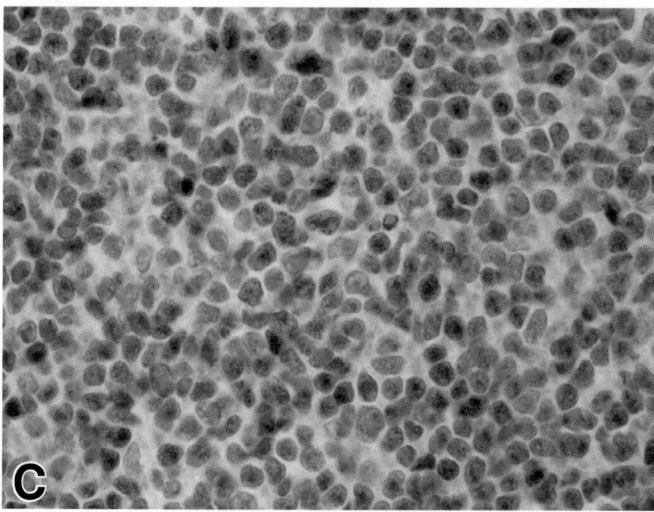

FIGURE 26-60. Mantle cell lymphoma (MCL). A. Lymph node architecture is completely effaced by a small lymphocytic infiltrate. **B.** At closer examination, the population of lymphocytes consists of monotonous, small cells with irregular nuclei. Unlike small lymphocytic lymphomas, MCL has very few admixed larger cells. **C.** A nuclear stain for Bcl-1 (cyclin D1) is positive. This finding correlates with the presence of t(11;14), the typical translocation in MCL.

 **CLINICAL FEATURES:** Most patients with MCL present with high-stage disease (III or IV). About 1/3 have peripheral blood involvement at diagnosis. Despite its small cell morphology, MCL is clinically aggressive and is considered incurable by standard chemotherapy. The median survival is 5 years for the typical type of MCL, and 3 years for the blastic/blastoid variant.

Marginal Zone Lymphomas

The marginal zone lymphomas are a heterogeneous group of mature B-cell tumors that arise in lymph nodes, spleen and extranodal tissues. The lymphoma cells are thought to arise from the marginal zone of the lymphoid follicle, which contains memory B cells that have gone through the germinal center reaction (postgerminal center). Regardless of the primary site of involvement, all marginal zone lymphomas share similar morphologic and immunophenotypic features. The prototypical marginal zone lymphomas are the extranodal marginal zone B-cell lymphomas arising in the mucosa-associated lymphoid tissues and called **MALT lymphomas** or **MALTomas**.

MALTomas are indolent B-cell lymphomas composed of a heterogeneous population of small B cells including centrocyte-like cells (marginal zone cells), monocytoid lymphocytes, small lymphocytes and scattered larger lymphoid cells resembling centroblasts and immunoblasts. These tumors often occur at extranodal sites, such as the GI tract, salivary glands, ocular adnexa, lungs and skin. Plasma cell differentiation is present in a variable proportion of cases.

 **EPIDEMIOLOGY:** MALT lymphomas account for 5%–10% of B-cell lymphomas and are the most common type of gastric lymphoma. Most cases occur in adults with a median age of 60; they are rare in children and young adults. There is a slight female predominance in part because they may occur at sites of autoimmune diseases (e.g., Sjögren syndrome, Hashimoto thyroiditis). Immunoproliferative small intestinal disease (IPSID), also called α-chain disease or **Mediterranean lymphoma,** is a subtype of MALT lymphoma that produces α heavy chains.

 **PATHOPHYSIOLOGY AND MOLECULAR PATHOGENESIS:** MALT lymphomas are monoclonal B-cell tumors that arise in the setting of chronic inflammation, most often due to autoimmunity or infection. What begins as a benign polyclonal reaction acquires mutations and/ or chromosomal lesions in B cells. T lymphocytes are necessary to maintain growth and survival of the neoplastic B cells. *The prototypical infection-driven MALToma is gastric lymphoma associated with* H. pylori *gastritis* (see Chapter 19). Gastric MALT lymphomas at their earliest phases of development may regress with antibiotic therapy to eradicate *H. pylori*. MALTomas that have progressed to acquire other chromosomal translocations (Table 26-19) no longer respond to antibiotic therapy alone. Dissemination to distant sites and/or transformation to diffuse large B-cell lymphoma occur as additional genetic lesions accrue. Similar progression, from polyclonal to monoclonal lymphoid infiltrates, occurs in EBV-related lymphomas.

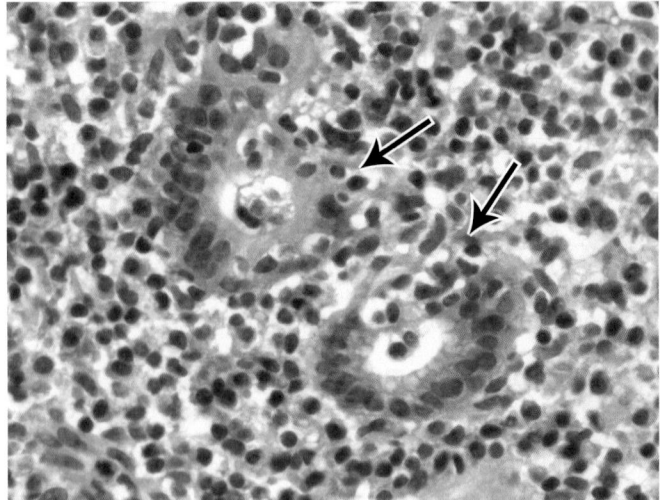

FIGURE 26-61. Mucosa-associated lymphoid tissue (MALT) lymphoma. A stomach biopsy showing the characteristic lymphoepithelial lesions seen in MALT lymphomas (*arrows*). The infiltrating lymphocytes are B cells.

 PATHOLOGY: Early-stage MALT lymphomas show increased marginal zone lymphocytes surrounding and infiltrating reactive B-cell follicles. The malignant B cells are heterogeneous and include varying proportions of small angulated lymphocytes, medium-sized monocytoid lymphocytes with abundant cytoplasm, plasmacytoid lymphocytes and even admixed clonal plasma cells. The tumor cells invade glandular epithelium or epithelia of mucosal surfaces, resulting in **lymphoepithelial lesions** (Fig. 26-61). Indolent MALT lymphomas may occasionally transform into large cell B-cell lymphomas.

MALTomas have no specific immunophenotype. Most tumor cells express IgM and show light-chain restriction. They express B-cell–associated antigens and are negative for CD5, CD23 and cyclin D1, which distinguishes them from B-CLL/SLLs and mantle cell lymphomas. Unlike follicular lymphomas, MALTomas do not express CD10.

MALT lymphomas typically show somatic mutation of variable-region genes. Common cytogenetic abnormalities are listed in Table 26-19 and, along with clonal *IgH* gene rearrangements, may help to establish the diagnosis if gastric infiltrates are subtle.

 **CLINICAL FEATURES:** Most MALT lymphomas involve the stomach or other mucosal sites, including the respiratory tract. They may also occur in the salivary glands, ocular adnexa, skin, thyroid and breast. These tumors may remain localized for prolonged periods and tend to follow an indolent clinical course. MALT lymphomas of the skin are sensitive to radiation therapy, and gastric MALTomas related to *H. pylori* infection often respond to antibiotic therapy alone. Transformation to diffuse large B-cell lymphoma may occur and is associated with more aggressive disease often requiring chemotherapy.

Lymphoplasmacytic Lymphoma

Lymphoplasmacytic lymphomas (LPLs) are relatively rare mature B-cell neoplasms containing small lymphocytes, plasmacytoid lymphocytes and plasma cells. They mainly involve the bone marrow, and occasionally spleen and lymph nodes. LPLs overlap considerably morphologically and immunophenotypically with MALT lymphomas, and distinction often depends in part on the site of involvement. Most LPLs produce a sizeable monoclonal serum paraprotein (usually of the IgM type), but such a finding is not required for diagnosis. A subset of patients with LPLs (and sometimes MALT lymphomas) develop the clinical syndrome of **Waldenström macroglobulinemia,** which can be associated with a **hyperviscosity syndrome**. The disease usually occurs in adults in their fifth to sixth decades, and there is a slight male predominance.

 PATHOLOGY: Bone marrows involved by LPL show a variably dense heterogeneous lymphoid infiltrate of small lymphocytes, plasmacytoid lymphocyte and mature plasma cells, in a diffuse and nonparatrabecular pattern. A few large transformed lymphoid cells are present in some cases. Lymphoplasmacytic cells with nuclear immunoglobulin pseudoinclusions (Dutcher bodies; see above) are common in tissue sections. Stained bone marrow aspirate smears show the cytologic features to advantage and also usually contain increased numbers of normal mast cells. Lymphoplasmacytic lymphoma cells may be present in the blood, but absolute lymphocytosis like CLL/SLL is rare. Affected lymph nodes show an interfollicular pattern of involvement, and nodal architecture is generally preserved.

Lymphoplasmacytic lymphomas express pan B-cell antigens and are negative for CD5, CD10, CD23 and cyclin D1. The plasma cell component expresses the plasma cell marker CD138. Plasma cell clonality is demonstrable in tissue sections using immunostains for κ and λ light chains. No specific chromosomal or oncogenic abnormalities are associated with LPL.

 CLINICAL FEATURES: Fatigue, weakness and weight loss are the most common presenting complaints of people with LPL. These nonspecific findings are usually related to anemia caused by marrow infiltration or immune-mediated hemolysis. About half of patients have lymphadenopathy and/or organomegaly at diagnosis. Most have a serum IgM paraprotein, although some may have a different isotype paraprotein (IgG, IgA) or none at all. Increased blood viscosity due to macroglobulinemia occurs in 30% of patients, and serum hyperviscosity may cause visual impairment, neurologic problems, bleeding and cryoglobulinemia. Therapeutic plasma exchange (plasmapheresis) is often necessary to control the complications of hyperviscosity syndrome until the patient receives more definitive therapy.

Lymphoplasmacytic lymphoma is an indolent disease that follows a progressive course. Median survival is 5–10 years. Like other small B-cell lymphomas, LPL is currently incurable. Transformation to diffuse large B-cell lymphoma may occur in a small proportion of patients and shortens survival considerably.

Hairy Cell Leukemia

Hairy cell leukemia (HCL) is a clonal B-cell neoplasm of small to medium-sized lymphocytes (with abundant pale cytoplasm and hair-like cell cytoplasmic protrusions) involving bone marrow and peripheral blood (Fig. 26-62A). The neoplastic cell is thought to arise from a postgerminal center–stage peripheral B cell (late activated memory B cell).

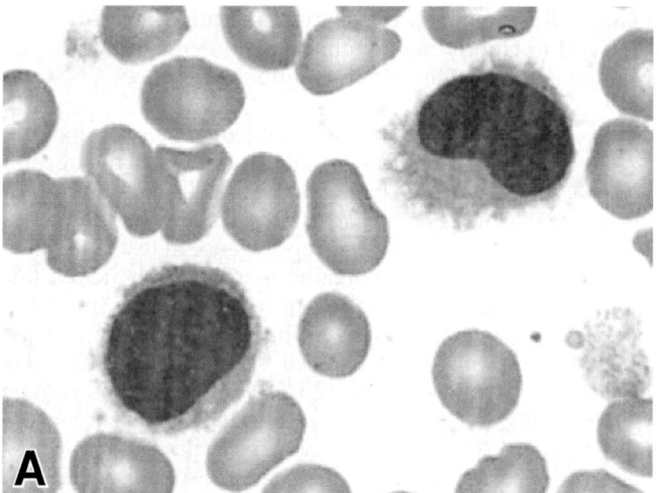
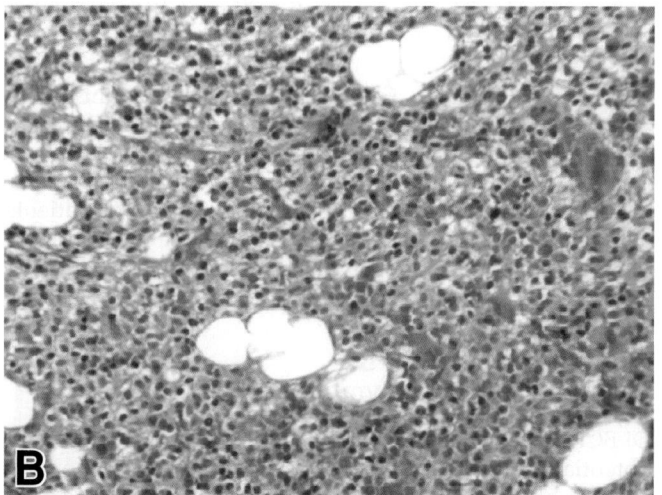
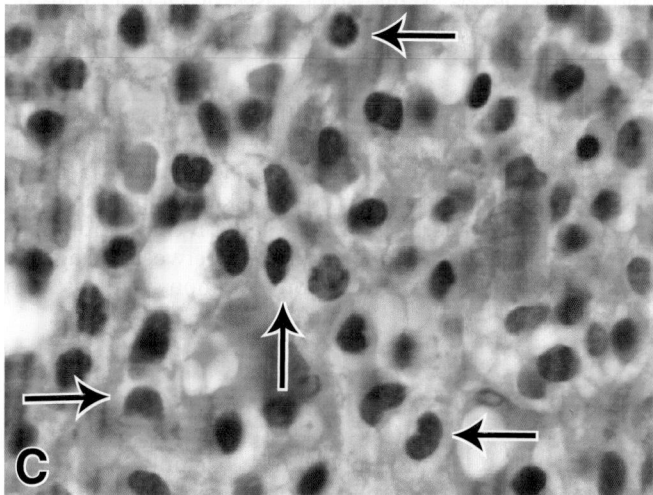

FIGURE 26-62. Hairy cell leukemia. A. Peripheral smear demonstrating "hairy" appearance of the leukemic cells in hairy cell leukemia. B. Bone marrow biopsy, showing infiltration of bone marrow by small to medium-sized lymphocytes with oval to reniform nuclei and pale cytoplasm with circumferential hair projections seen in peripheral blood and bone marrow aspirate smears. **C. Higher-power photomicrograph of the lymphocytes infiltrating the bone marrow in hairy cell leukemia.** Typical "fried egg" cells, with round-oval to kidney-shaped nuclei, are shown (*arrows*).

Hairy cell leukemia is uncommon and affects mainly middle-aged to elderly men, with a male-to-female ratio of 5:1. Marked splenomegaly at presentation is common.

 PATHOLOGY: Hairy cell leukemia shows subtle interstitial infiltrates that do not disturb the normal bone marrow architecture. The cells have abundant clear cytoplasm, compared to normal small lymphocytes, which gives them a "fried egg" appearance in tissue sections (Fig. 26-62B, C). HCL generally spares lymph nodes but involves both liver and spleen prominently. The immunophenotypic features of HCL are characteristic, allowing distinction from other small B-cell neoplasms. Hairy cells express the pan B-cell antigens CD19 and CD20, as well as CD11c, CD22, CD25 and CD103. Some cases may show variable expression of CD5, CD10 and even cyclin D1. The tumor cells produce tartrate-resistant acid phosphatase (TRAP), but immunophenotyping has largely replaced such cytochemical analysis in clinical practice. No specific cytogenetic abnormalities have been found in HCL.

 CLINICAL FEATURES: Most patients with HCL present with splenomegaly, leukopenia and monocytopenia or sometimes pancytopenia. Hepatomegaly is less common, and peripheral lymphadenopathy is rare. Infections are frequent, occurring in 1/3 of patients during their clinical course. HCL is otherwise indolent, and purine analogs such as deoxycoformycin or 2-chlorodeoxyadenosine (2-CDA) may provide complete and durable remissions.

Diffuse Large B-Cell Lymphoma

DLBCLs are a heterogeneous group of aggressive—but potentially curable—B-cell tumors. Their heterogeneity is evident at the morphologic, immunophenotypic, genetic and clinical levels. While some cases of DLBCL arise de novo, others represent transformation or progression from a more indolent type of lymphoma.

 **EPIDEMIOLOGY:** Diffuse large B-cell lymphomas are the most common B-cell lymphoma worldwide. They have been the single largest factor in the increasing incidence of non-Hodgkin lymphomas during the past few decades. Diffuse large B-cell lymphomas occur at all ages, but are most prevalent between the ages of 60 and 70. They are slightly more common in males than females.

  **PATHOPHYSIOLOGY AND MOLECULAR PATHOGENESIS:** The cause of DLBCL is unknown, but altered immune function is important, since a number of cases are associated with viral infections, such as EBV, HIV and rarely HHV-8. The frequency of EBV-positive cases is highest in immunosuppressed patients and in those older than age 50. Diverse pathogenetic mechanisms contribute to the development of DLBCL. A number of chromosomal rearrangements are seen in DLBCLs (Table 26-19). Some of these involve genes that directly or indirectly impair apoptosis and have substantial influence in prognosis. Some translocations overlap with characteristic FL rearrangements (Table 26-19).

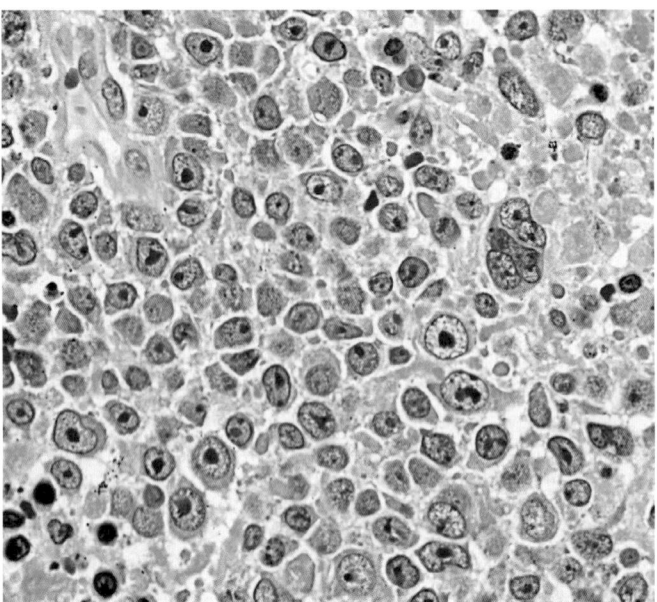

FIGURE 26-63. Diffuse large B-cell lymphoma. Sheets of large lymphoma cells with prominent nucleoli are present.

 PATHOLOGY: DLBCLs show diffuse proliferation of large neoplastic B cells (Fig. 26-63). The large lymphoma cells are comparable in size to the nucleus of a histiocyte (macrophage) or roughly twice the size of a normal lymphocyte. Morphologic variants include centroblastic, immunoblastic, T-cell/histiocyte rich and others. The malignant cells of DLBCL are sometimes pleomorphic and/or anaplastic appearing, or they may resemble cells seen in other malignant tumors, such as carcinoma, melanoma or seminoma. Immunohistochemical stains are therefore often necessary to establish the nature of the tumor. *While DLBCL most often involves lymph nodes, it commonly presents at extranodal sites, especially the GI tract.*

The immunophenotype of the malignant cells of DLBCL varies. Often, the cells express pan B-cell antigens, such as CD19 and CD20. However, owing to complete aberrant loss, downregulation or treatment effect, the lymphoma cells may not necessarily express these common markers. In that event, additional markers of B-cell differentiation such as CD22, CD79a and PAX-5 may be useful to distinguish DLBCL from other morphologically similar neoplasms. DLBCL cells may or may not express CD10 and BCL-6, markers of germinal center cell differentiation. They sometimes express CD5. Surface Ig light-chain restriction occurs most of the time. All cases are negative for TdT and cyclin D1, which distinguishes DLBCLs from B-cell lymphoblastic lymphoma (TdT positive) and MCL (cyclin D1), respectively.

 CLINICAL FEATURES: Patients with DLBCL most often present with a rapidly growing tumor in nodal and/or extranodal sites. One or more sites may be involved, but half of patients have limited disease (stage I or II) at presentation. Bone marrow involvement may occur but is usually a late event in this disease. Tumor cells rarely appear in the peripheral blood. Symptoms reflect the site(s) of involvement. For example, a large mass in the colon can cause obstruction or bowel perforation, while a rapidly growing mediastinal mass can impinge on the superior vena cava (SVC) to cause SVC syndrome. Systemic manifestations such as fever, fatigue and night sweats ("B symptoms") are not uncommon in patients with DLBCL.

These are aggressive neoplasms and are rapidly fatal if left untreated. Because these tumors generally proliferate quickly, however, they are sensitive to chemotherapeutic agents that target rapidly dividing cells. Complete remissions are achieved in 60%–80% of patients. The ultimate outcome depends on tumor stage: patients with limited disease at diagnosis do better compared to those with widespread (high-stage) disease.

Burkitt Lymphoma

Burkitt lymphoma (BL) is one of the most rapidly growing malignancies known. It is defined by a chromosomal translocation that activates the *MYC* oncogene (see Chapter 5). BLs often present at extranodal sites, contain a monomorphic population of medium-sized cells and tend to show involvement of the blood and/or bone marrow. The MYC translocation is highly characteristic, but is not specific to BL, and a combination of other diagnostic features is required to confirm the diagnosis.

 EPIDEMIOLOGY: BL occurs in three distinct variants, each with different clinical presentations, morphology and pathogenesis. In equatorial Africa and Papua, New Guinea, **endemic Burkitt lymphoma** is the most common childhood malignancy. Its peak incidence is in 4- to 7-year-olds, and it commonly involves the jaw, other facial bones and the abdominal viscera. **Sporadic BL** occurs worldwide and mainly affects children and young adults. In the Western world, BL is uncommon (1%–2% of lymphomas overall), but it accounts for 30%–50% of childhood lymphomas. The median age for adult patients is 30. Like most other B-cell lymphomas, BL afflicts males more than females. Unlike endemic BL, sporadic BL often presents as an abdominal mass involving the ileocecum. **Immunodeficiency-associated BL** mainly occurs in HIV-infected people and may be the initial manifestation of AIDS.

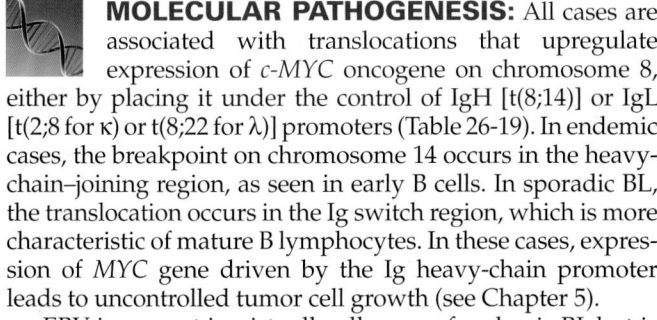 **MOLECULAR PATHOGENESIS:** All cases are associated with translocations that upregulate expression of *c-MYC* oncogene on chromosome 8, either by placing it under the control of IgH [t(8;14)] or IgL [t(2;8 for κ) or t(8;22 for λ)] promoters (Table 26-19). In endemic cases, the breakpoint on chromosome 14 occurs in the heavy-chain–joining region, as seen in early B cells. In sporadic BL, the translocation occurs in the Ig switch region, which is more characteristic of mature B lymphocytes. In these cases, expression of *MYC* gene driven by the Ig heavy-chain promoter leads to uncontrolled tumor cell growth (see Chapter 5).

EBV is present in virtually all cases of endemic BL but is responsible for less than 30% of sporadic and immunodeficiency-related cases. EBV-positive sporadic BL is associated with lower socioeconomic status. Many patients experience prodromal polyclonal B-cell activation caused by bacterial, viral or parasitic infections (e.g., malaria).

  CLINICAL FEATURES AND PATHOLOGY: BL typically produces extranodal tumors rather than lymphadenopathy. All variants of this lymphoma have a high risk for CNS involvement. The classic presentation for endemic BL is a destructive tumor in the jaws or other facial bones (Fig. 26-64A). Patients with sporadic BL typically present with abdominal

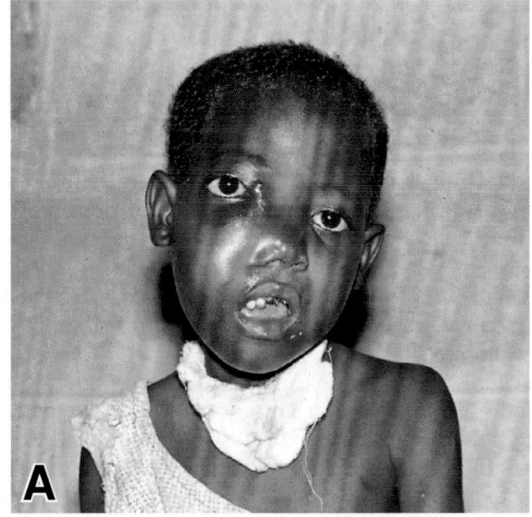

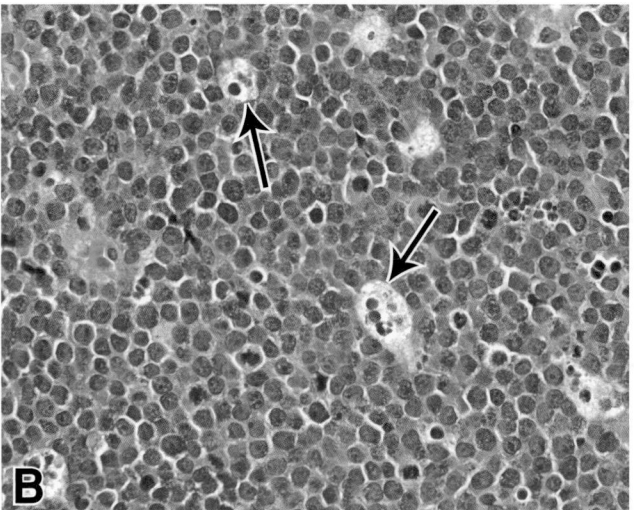

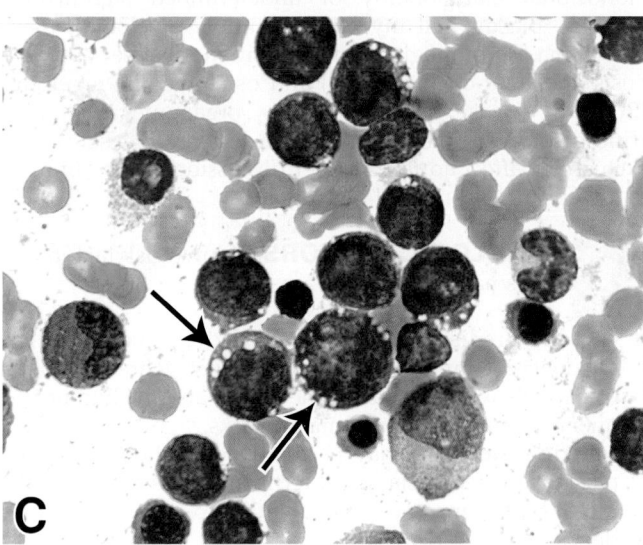

FIGURE 26-64. Burkitt lymphoma. A. A tumor of the jaw distorts the child's face. **B.** Lymph node is effaced by neoplastic lymphocytes with several starry-sky macrophages (*arrows*). **C.** Bone marrow aspirate smear showing typical cytologic features of Burkitt lymphoma. Note the deeply basophilic cytoplasm and lipid vacuoles (*arrows*).

masses. All types may involve ovaries, kidneys and breast. Patients with sizable bulky tumors sometimes present with Burkitt leukemia and extensive bone marrow involvement.

BL cells are medium sized and lack significant cytologic atypia. Tissue sections reveal abundant mitotic figures, reflecting the extremely high proliferative rate in this tumor. Macrophages ingesting the cellular debris of apoptotic tumor cells are scattered throughout the tumor, imparting a "starry sky" microscopic appearance to the tumor (Fig. 26-64B). Aspirate smears stained with Wright-Giemsa show lipid vacuoles in the deeply basophilic tumor cell cytoplasm (Fig. 26-64C).

BL cells express surface IgM and immunoglobulin light chain and are positive for common B-cell antigens (CD19, CD20, CD22). They also express CD10 and BCL-6, which suggests that they originate from germinal centers. BL cells do not express TdT, helping to distinguish these tumors from precursor B-cell acute lymphoblastic leukemia/ lymphoma (see above).

All variants of BL are highly aggressive, and most patients have bulky extranodal tumors, high tumor burdens and disseminated disease (stage III or IV) at presentation. Because of its high proliferative rate, BL responds to intensive chemotherapy. Thus, up to 90% of people with early stage disease and 60%–80% of those with high-stage disease may be cured. Children and young adults with BL tend to fare better than adults. Tumor lysis syndrome can occur when therapy begins, as a result of rapid tumor cell death. This is a potentially lethal complication of treatment.

Plasma Cell Neoplasia

Plasma cell neoplasms result from clonal expansion of plasma cells, that is, terminally differentiated B lymphocytes that can produce a monoclonal paraprotein (**monoclonal gammopathy**). The major plasma cell neoplasms include monoclonal gammopathy of undetermined significance (MGUS), plasma cell myeloma (multiple myeloma), plasmacytoma, immunoglobulin deposition disease (amyloidosis and light-chain disease) and osteosclerotic myeloma (**POEMS disease:** polyneuropathy, organomegaly, endocrine disorders, myeloma and skin lesions). These almost exclusively affect adults. Further discussion will be limited to MGUS and plasma cell myeloma.

 **ETIOLOGIC FACTORS:** Known risk factors for plasma cell neoplasia are:

- **Genetic predisposition** is suggested by the increased incidence of multiple myeloma in first-degree relatives of patients with plasma cell neoplasia and the higher frequency of multiple myeloma in blacks.
- **Ionizing radiation** may be involved in the etiology of plasma cell neoplasia. Long-term survivors of the bombing of Hiroshima and Nagasaki had a 5-fold greater incidence of multiple myeloma.
- **Chronic antigenic stimulation** may be a risk factor. Some cases of multiple myeloma follow chronic infections, such as HIV and chronic osteomyelitis, and with chronic inflammatory disorders (e.g., rheumatoid arthritis). Antigenic stimulation leads to reactive, polyclonal proliferation of B cells, which may render them susceptible to a later mutagenic event, establishing a single malignant clone.

Monoclonal Gammopathy of Undetermined Significance

MGUS occurs in about 3% of people older than age 50 and in greater than 5% who are older than 70. Criteria for diagnosing MGUS include (1) monoclonal paraproteinemia of less than 3.0 g/dL; (2) less than 10% plasma cells in the bone marrow; (3) lack of end-organ damage (CRAB: hypercalcemia, renal insufficiency, anemia, bone lesions); and (4) exclusion of other B-cell neoplasms or diseases known to produce a monoclonal paraprotein (M-protein).

IgM MGUS is most often associated with a clone of immunoglobulin-secreting B cells and can progress to a small B-cell lymphoma with plasma cell differentiation such as lymphoplasmacytic lymphoma. Non-IgM MGUS is most often associated with clonal plasma cells and may progress to a bona fide malignant plasma cell neoplasm. Although non-IgM MGUS entails an expanded clone of antibody-secreting plasma cells with genetic lesions similar to those in multiple myeloma, it is a preneoplastic condition that becomes overt plasma cell neoplasia (e.g., multiple myeloma) in about 1% of affected patients per year.

Plasma Cell Myeloma

Plasma cell myeloma (PCM) is a malignancy of plasma cells, in which the serum and/or urine contain an M-protein. The disease is primarily bone marrow based and tends to be multifocal. PCM varies from asymptomatic and indolent to highly aggressive with leukemic involvement. Diagnosis requires a combination of clinical and laboratory findings, including radiographic studies.

 EPIDEMIOLOGY: PCM accounts for 10% of hematologic malignancies, with 22,000 cases reported annually in the United States. Its overall incidence is about 6 cases per 100,000 people. Men are more affected than women, and the disease is proportionately twice as common in blacks as in whites. Incidence of PCM increases with age, with the median age at diagnosis being 69 years. Over 90% of cases occur in people older than age 50. PCM does not affect children and is extremely rare in adults under age 30. There is a familial predisposition: people who have a first-degree relative with PCM have a 4-fold greater risk of developing the disease.

 PATHOLOGY: Plasma cell myeloma produces multifocal destructive bone lesions with a lytic or "punched out" radiographic appearance throughout the skeleton. The vertebral column, ribs, skull, pelvis, femurs, clavicles and scapulae are most commonly affected. Plasma cells focally fill the medullary cavity, erode cancellous bone and eventually destroy the bony cortex, causing pathologic fractures. The affected bone contains gelatinous red-brown soft tissue masses that are sharply demarcated from the surrounding normal tissue (Fig. 26-65). If the tumors breach the bony cortex, they may spread beyond the medullary cavity into surrounding soft tissues.

Pathologic examination of the bone marrow is essential in diagnosing PCM and shows interstitial clusters, distinct nodules and/or confluent sheets of plasma cells in bone marrow core biopsies. Because malignant plasma infiltrates in PCM affect the bone patchily, variable amounts of normal bone marrow are often present. Such marrow reserves are not, however, seen in all cases, and are less likely in advanced disease. PCM is likely if plasma cell infiltrates involve over 30% of the marrow volume and/or there are large confluent

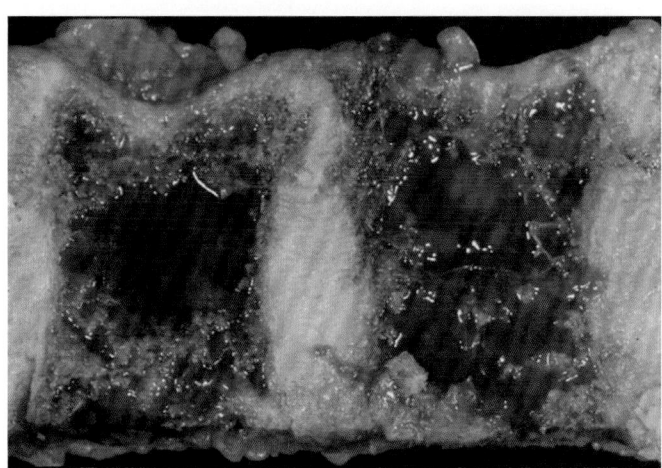

FIGURE 26-65. Plasma cell myeloma. Multiple lytic bone lesions are present in the vertebra. Bones such as this are prone to pathologic fracture.

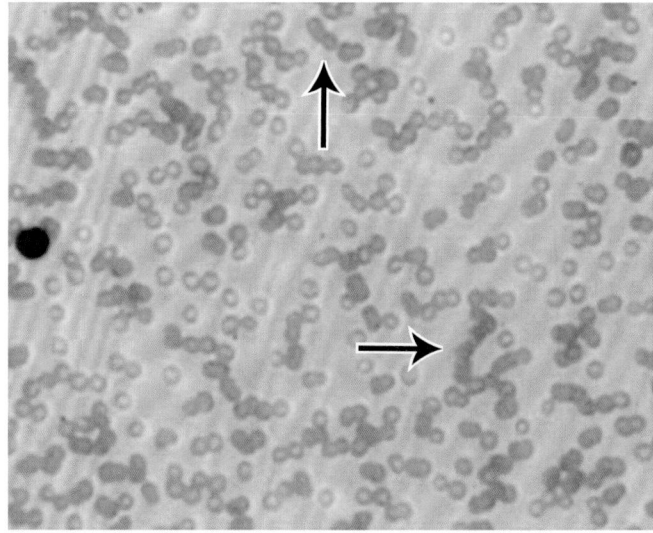

FIGURE 26-67. Plasma cell myeloma, rouleaux in peripheral blood. In plasma cell myeloma, the peripheral blood commonly shows red blood cells seemingly stacked on each other, like coins in a roll. These are rouleaux (*arrows*).

masses of plasma cells without admixed normal hematopoietic cells, even if other typical clinical and pathologic findings are absent.

Immunohistochemical stains for plasma cells (e.g., CD138) are very useful in assessing the degree and pattern of marrow infiltration. Bone marrow aspirate smears stained with Wright-Giemsa show variable plasmacytosis in PCM, again in part because the disease involves the marrow spottily. Myeloma plasma cells may resemble normal plasma cells (Fig. 26-66A), or they may show immature, plasmablastic or pleomorphic features (Fig. 26-66B). Cytoplasmic and nuclear inclusions, representing accumulated or partially degraded immunoglobulin, are occasionally present.

Erythrocyte rouleaux (Fig. 26-67) in peripheral blood smears reflect the type and quantity of circulating paraprotein. High levels of M-protein cause red blood cells to stick together end on end, like a stack of coins. Plasma cells may circulate in the blood in a minority of cases. Marked

peripheral blood plasmacytosis establishes a diagnosis of plasma cell leukemia. Renal disease occurs in more than 50% of cases (see Chapter 22).

Plasma cells in PCM usually express the B-cell marker CD79a, plasma cell markers CD38 and CD138 and monotypic *cytoplasmic* immunoglobulin. Unlike normal plasma cells, myeloma cells usually lack CD19, and unlike mature B cells, they do not express CD20. Aberrant expression of various markers such as CD56, CD117, CD52, CD10 and CD20 can occur in some cases. Occasional PCMs express cyclin D1 and have t(11;14) translocations; such cases must be distinguished from MCL. In most cases, the heavy chain in the monoclonal paraprotein is IgG or IgA. Rarely, it is IgD or IgE.

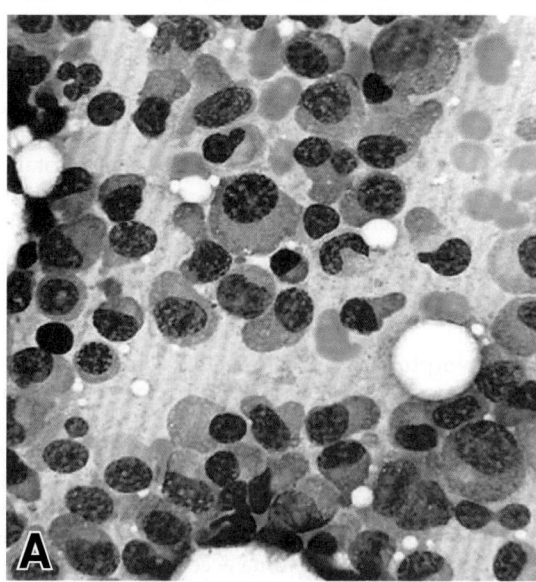 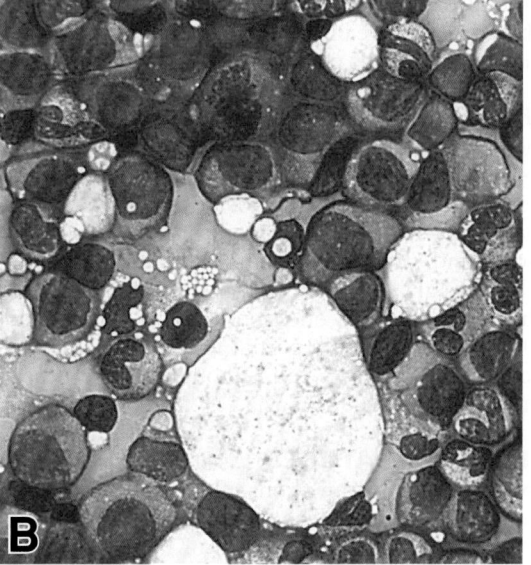

FIGURE 26-66. Plasma cell myeloma (PCM). Neoplastic plasma cells can show variable cytologic features ranging from normal-appearing cells (**A**) to cells resembling blasts (**B**). Total number, clonality and clinicopathologic findings help distinguish PCM from other plasma cell proliferations.

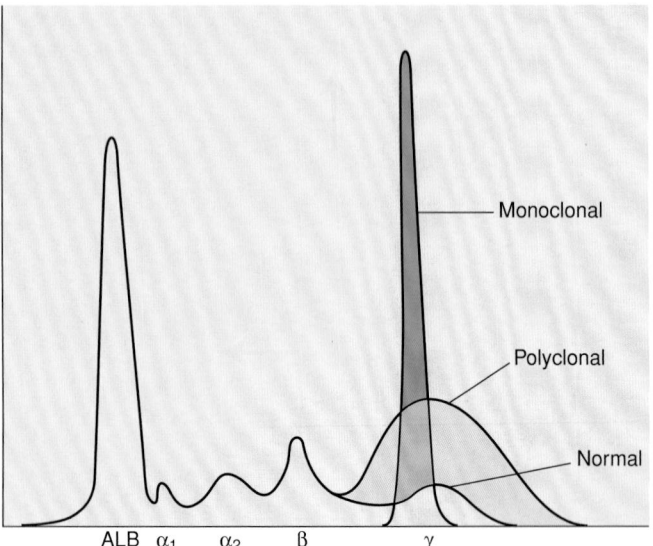

FIGURE 26-68. Abnormal serum protein electrophoretic patterns contrasted with a normal pattern. Polyclonal hypergammaglobulinemia, characteristic of benign reactive processes, shows a broad-based increase in immunoglobulins as a result of immunoglobulin secretion by myriad reactive plasma cells. Monoclonal gammopathy of unknown significance (MGUS) or plasma cell neoplasia shows a narrow peak, or spike, as a result of the homogeneity of the immunoglobulin molecules secreted by a single clone of aberrant plasma cells. *ALB* = albumin.

Immunoglobulins produced in 85% of cases are whole antibody molecules. However, the remaining 15% of myelomas only secrete light chains (**light-chain disease**). In some cases there is no detectable serum or urine paraprotein (nonsecreting myelomas). Laboratory assessment for monoclonal gammopathy entails serum (or urine) protein electrophoresis followed by immunofixation if a restricted protein (spike) is found (Fig. 26-68). The immunofixation test confirms the spike to be monoclonal κ or λ, and also identifies the heavy-chain type. IgGs account for 50% of cases, followed by IgA (20%), light chains only (20%) and IgD, IgE and biclonal (<10% combined). The type of M-component determines the course of the disease and its prognosis.

MOLECULAR PATHOGENESIS: All cases show clonal rearrangement of the Ig L- and H-chain genes. The pattern of somatic hypermutation in the variable regions of Ig heavy chains is consistent with the postgerminal center origin of the neoplastic cells in PCM. Both numerical and structural chromosomal abnormalities occur in PCM. The IgH gene frequently participates in translocations, involving diverse oncogenes (Table 26-19) and affecting 40% of cases. Loss or partial loss of one chromosome 13 occurs in 50% of cases and is thought to be an early genetic event in plasma cell neoplasia.

CLINICAL FEATURES: As stated above, diagnosis of PCM rests on a constellation of clinical and pathologic findings. The most important disorder to consider in the differential diagnosis of PCM is MGUS, which is a more common entity.

Symptomatic myeloma is characterized by end-organ damage (CRAB) in patients with serum or urine M-proteins plus clonal populations of plasma cells in the marrow.

Radiography reveals lytic bone lesions in 70% of cases; these lesions are often associated with bone pain and hypercalcemia. Pathologic bone fractures are common presenting manifestations of PCM. Bone destruction in multiple myeloma results from both progressive tumor growth and secretion of osteoclast-activating factor by malignant plasma cells. Osteoclasts may also be activated by IL-6, which is also increased in patients with PCM. Calcium released from injured or resorbed bone may precipitate in the kidneys (nephrocalcinosis) and impair renal function.

Monoclonal light-chain proteinuria can damage renal tubular epithelium and lead to kidney failure. M-proteins can suppress normal antibody responses, and so predispose to infectious complications. Anemia develops in 70% of patients, both because the neoplastic plasma cells displace normal bone marrow and because renal injury limits erythropoietin production. The serum and/or urine have detectable M-proteins in 97% of patients (see above), the isotype of which predicts disease progression:

- **IgG myelomas** are "typical" PCMs. Mean survivals are 3–4 years. Infectious complications are common.
- **IgA myelomas** cause serum hyperviscosity because IgA tends to form dimers.
- **IgD myelomas** are aggressive and tend to occur in middle-aged men. Mean survival is 1 year.
- **IgE myelomas** are uncommon and aggressive, and tend to occur in young adult men.
- **Light-chain disease** is an aggressive variant in which only κ or λ light chains are made. κ-Chain disease is twice as common as λ-chain disease, reflecting the normal ratio of κ and λ light chains in plasma cells. The serum protein pattern is normal until secondary renal disease prevents glomerular filtration of light chains.

While nonspecific, the finding of rouleaux in peripheral blood smears sometimes leads to initial serum protein analysis and subsequent diagnosis of a plasma cell disorder. *Additional findings and complications associated with PCM include amyloidosis, hyperviscosity syndrome, coagulation abnormalities, humoral immune deficiency and treatment-related myeloid malignancies (e.g., myelodysplasia and AML).*

Plasma cell myeloma remains an incurable disease; however, targeted therapies such as bortezomib, a proteasome inhibitor, portend increasingly better prognoses. Median survival is 3.75 years but is highly variable, ranging from less than 6 months to more than 10 years. Total disease burden (as reflected in serum β_2-microglobulin and albumin levels) and genetic abnormalities (Table 26-19) are the most accurate predictors of outcome.

Clinical Variants of Plasma Cell Myeloma

- **Asymptomatic myeloma** is a condition in which the diagnostic criteria for PCM are met, but the patient lacks detectable end-organ damage. This condition is like MGUS, which also shows a lack of clinical manifestations (i.e., CRAB), but it is more likely to progress to symptomatic PCM. Of patients who develop PCM, 8% were asymptomatic at first and so fall into this disease category.
- **Nonsecretory myeloma** accounts for 3% of cases of PCM. These patients lack detectable serum or urine M-protein. This occurs because the malignant plasma cells produce but cannot secrete immunoglobulin (85% of cases) or they simply do not synthesize any immunoglobulin at all (15%

of cases). Free Ig L chains are made in most of these cases, indicating that they are minimally secretory. The clinical features of nonsecretory PCM are otherwise similar to secretory PCM.

- **Plasma cell leukemia (PCL)** is an aggressive variant of PCM plasma cells and is represented by greater than 20% of circulating WBCs. At presentation, these patients often have widespread extramedullary involvement, especially of lymph nodes, spleen, liver, body cavities and cerebrospinal fluid. PCL may be the first presentation of a plasma cell tumor (primary), or it may evolve as a late complication of PCM (secondary). Many cases of PCL are IgD, IgE or light chain only. Abnormal cytogenetic karyotypes are common in PCL, as is the incidence of unfavorable genetic lesions. Plasma cell leukemia is therefore usually an aggressive disease with a short survival.

- **Solitary plasmacytoma of bone (osseous plasmacytoma)** presents as a single lytic skeletal lesion (most commonly in the ribs, vertebrae or pelvic bones) and accounts for 3%–5% of all plasma cell neoplasms. These patients most frequently present with pain at the tumor site or with a pathologic fracture. Between 1/4 and 3/4 have an M-protein, but these patients do not have clinical features of PCM and their bone marrow does not show plasmacytosis. *Plasmacytomas contain diffuse sheets of plasma cells with no normal hematopoietic elements.* Solitary osseous myelomas progress to multiple myeloma in 70% of cases. They may also undergo local extension or recurrence (15%), or extension to a distant skeletal site (15%). Local control with radiation therapy is often the first line of treatment. The median survival is 10 years.

- **Extramedullary (extraosseous) plasmacytomas** are localized plasma cell tumors that occur in tissues other than bone. Most (80%) arise in the upper respiratory tract, including nasal sinuses, nasopharynx and tonsils. The rest affect other soft tissue sites, such as lungs, breast and lymph nodes. Given their anatomic distribution, they must be distinguished from B-cell lymphoma with plasma cell differentiation such as MALT lymphomas. Extramedullary plasmacytoma can be definitively treated by surgery or local irradiation in most cases. Local recurrences occur in 1/4 of cases, and 15% progress to PCM.

- **Primary amyloidosis** is a complication of plasma cell tumors (or B-cell lymphomas with plasma cell differentiation) that secrete light-chain–type amyloid protein (AL amyloid; see Chapter 15). It is a disease of older adults with a median age of 65. Of patients with amyloidosis, 20% have PCM, but most only meet criteria for MGUS. Clinical presentations reflect organ sites where amyloid deposits are, resulting in organomegaly or organ dysfunction (e.g., congestive heart failure, nephrotic syndrome, malabsorption). Purpura, bone pain, peripheral neuropathy and carpal tunnel syndrome may be early signs of disease. An M-protein is seen in greater than 90% of cases, and most have λ light chains. Tissues infiltrated by amyloid have a dense lardaceous appearance. Median survival of patients with primary amyloidosis is 2 years from the time of diagnosis. Patients with PCM and amyloidosis fare worse than those with either alone. Amyloid-related cardiac disease is the most common cause of death.

Peripheral T-Cell and NK-Cell Lymphomas Originate in Postthymic T Cells

These are a heterogeneous group of mature lymphoid tumors that arise in lymphoid tissues outside of the thymus, such as lymph nodes, spleen, gut and skin (Fig. 26-48). They are relatively rare compared to B-cell lymphomas and generally have a poorer prognosis.

 EPIDEMIOLOGY: Mature T-cell neoplasms account for 12% of non-Hodgkin lymphomas worldwide. They are more common in Asia than in the Western world. Major risk factors for T-cell neoplasia include the prevalence of human T-cell leukemia virus type 1 (HTLV-1) and EBV, plus genetic predispositions to those viruses (see Chapter 5). HTLV-1 is endemic in southwestern Japan: 8%–10% of the population is seropositive, and lifetime risk for adult T-cell leukemia/lymphoma (ATLL) is 5%. EBV-associated T-cell lymphomas are more common in Asians than in other racial groups.

 PATHOLOGY: Peripheral T-cell and NK-cell neoplasms show variable morphologic features. Involved lymph nodes and other tissues are usually diffusely effaced by a heterogeneous population of malignant lymphoid cells. These vary from small to large, and from relatively bland or overtly anaplastic in appearance. Eosinophils and benign macrophages often comingle with the neoplastic T cells, probably recruited to the site of involvement by cytokines the lymphoma cells secrete. Some of these tumors show prominent vascularity.

Immunophenotypically, mature T-cell lymphomas express surface CD3, as well as a variable number of other pan T-cell antigens such as CD2, CD5 and CD7; CD4 or CD8; and either α–β or γ–δ T-cell receptor subunits. *Because α–β T cells are more common, most peripheral T-cell lymphomas are of the α–β type.* γ–δ T cells make up less than 5% of the T-cell repertoire and congregate at epithelial surfaces and in the splenic red pulp. γ–δ T cells do not express CD4, CD5 or CD8.

Some mature T-cell lymphomas have a **cytotoxic** phenotype and are positive for the granule-associated proteins perforin, granzyme B and T-cell intracellular antigen (TIA-1). Unlike immature T-cell neoplasms (such as T-cell lymphoblastic lymphoma), mature T-cell neoplasms lack TdT.

Natural killer cells lack surface CD3, but they do express the CD3 ε-subunit, which is intracellular. They also express other T-cell–associated markers including CD2, CD7, CD8, CD16 and CD56.

 **CLINICAL FEATURES:** Peripheral T-cell and NK-cell tumors are grouped clinically into **leukemic, nodal, extranodal** and **cutaneous** forms. *They are usually widely disseminated at presentation (high stage) and hence are generally more aggressive than are B-cell neoplasms.* Systemic manifestations such as fever, pruritus, eosinophilia, fever and weight loss are common. T- and NK-cell lymphomas are treated similarly to other aggressive lymphomas, with multiagent chemotherapy; however, most T-cell neoplasms respond poorly. Overall 5-year survival is 20%–30%.

Adult T-Cell Leukemia/Lymphoma

ATLL is caused by the human retrovirus **HTLV-1**. The normal counterparts of ATLL cells are mature, activated, CD4+ T cells.

 **EPIDEMIOLOGY:** In addition to southwestern Japan, ATLL is endemic in the Caribbean basin and parts of Central Africa. Worldwide, it accounts for 10% of mature T-cell neoplasms. Most cases are in people from endemic areas, but sporadic cases also occur elsewhere. The disease has a long latency period. Exposure to HTLV-1 occurs early in life in people who live in endemic regions. Still, ATLL only occurs in adults, with a mean age of 58. The virus may be transmitted in breast milk and via blood and blood products.

 PATHOLOGY: ATLL is usually widespread at presentation, often involving lymph nodes, spleen, bone marrow, peripheral blood and skin. The latter is the most common extralymphatic site of disease, and is affected in over 50% of cases. The neoplastic lymphoid cells vary widely in appearance (Fig. 26-69). They commonly have prominent nuclear convolutions and lobations, sometimes likened to flowers (flower cells). They express T-cell–associated antigens including CD2, CD3 and CD5, but usually lack CD7. Nearly all cases strongly express CD25, and most express CD4. *The tumor cells show clonal T-cell receptor gene rearrangements and have clonally integrated HTLV-1.* A viral protein, p40 (Tax), directs transcriptional activation of several genes in infected lymphocytes. While ATLL reflects infection with HTLV-1, infection alone is not sufficient for neoplastic transformation. Other genetic lesions are required to progress from lymphocyte infection to malignancy.

 CLINICAL FEATURES: ATLL is a systemic disease with multiorgan manifestations and peripheral leukocytosis. Acute, smoldering and chronic variants occur. Hypercalcemia, with or without lytic bone lesions, is typical. The skin is the most important extranodal site of involvement. Acute ATLL has a poor prognosis: most patients survive less than 1 year, despite aggressive systemic chemotherapy. Death frequently occurs from infectious complications, like those seen in HIV-infected patients. Chronic and smoldering forms have a somewhat better prognosis.

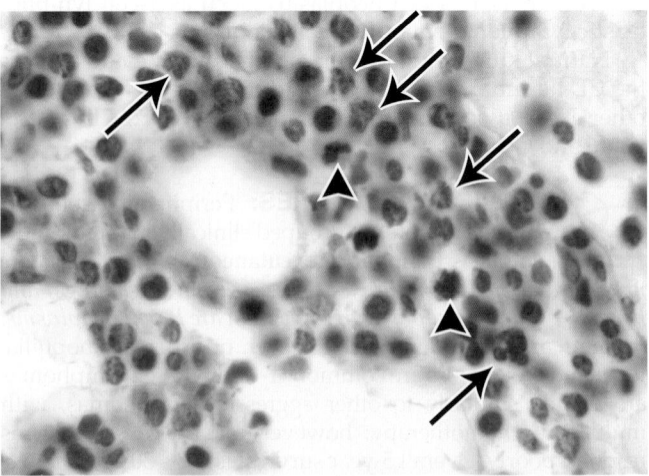

FIGURE 26-69. Adult T-cell leukemia/lymphoma (ATLL). This disease is characterized by proliferation of malignant T lymphocytes (here, in the bone marrow) with extremely irregular, knobby nuclei (*arrows*). The mitotic rate among the malignant cells is characteristically high (*arrowheads*).

Mycosis Fungoides and Sézary Syndrome

Mycosis fungoides (MF) is the most common form of primary cutaneous T-cell lymphoma (CTCL). It is characterized by infiltration of the epidermis by malignant CD4$^+$ (helper-type) T cells with marked nuclear folding. Sézary syndrome is a variant of MF, defined by a triad of erythroderma, generalized lymphadenopathy and circulating lymphoma cells in the blood (Sézary cells).

 EPIDEMIOLOGY: Mycosis fungoides occurs mainly in adults and the elderly. It affects men twice as often as women.

 CLINICAL FEATURES: MF is an indolent lymphoma that progresses slowly over years (and sometimes decades) from patches to plaques to mass lesions.

- The **premycotic or eczematous stage** lasts years and is difficult to distinguish from many benign chronic dermatoses. Skin biopsies may not be diagnostic of lymphoma, showing instead nonspecific perivascular and periadnexal lymphocytic infiltration with accompanying eosinophils and plasma cells.
- The **plaque stage** follows, with well-demarcated, raised cutaneous plaques. It is usually possible to diagnose MF at this stage (see below).
- In the **tumor stage,** there are raised cutaneous tumors, mostly on the face and in body folds. These tumors frequently ulcerate and may become secondarily infected. The name, **mycosis fungoides,** derives from these tumors' raised, fungating, mushroom-like appearance. Extracutaneous involvement is common, particularly of lymph nodes, spleen, liver, bone marrow and lungs.

The clinical stage (i.e., extent of disease) is the most important determinant of prognosis. Patients with limited disease generally have an excellent prognosis: their life expectancies are like those of the general population. Extracutaneous involvement augurs a poor prognosis. The 5-year survival in Sézary syndrome is 10%–20%.

 PATHOLOGY: The histologic features of MF vary with the stage of the disease (see Chapter 28). A superficial band-like infiltrate or lichenoid lymphoid infiltrate with early epidermotropism characterizes the initial patch stage.

The diagnostic plaque stage is marked by pronounced infiltration of the epidermis (epidermotropism). A dense band-like infiltrate of variably sized lymphoid cells fills the subepidermal space (Fig. 26-70). These cells have very irregular nuclear contours, reminiscent of the surface of the cerebral cortex (cerebriform nuclei). Such distinctive medium to large lymphoid cells with hyperchromatic cerebriform nuclei are called **mycosis cells,** and are typical. **Pautrier microabscesses** in intraepidermal clear spaces are highly characteristic but are not common.

Diffuse dermal infiltrates composed of small, medium and/or large lymphoma cells and loss of epidermotropism characterize the tumor stage. Identification of MF cells in extracutaneous sites such as lymph nodes may be difficult, and T-cell receptor gene rearrangement studies are necessary as an adjunct to the histologic evaluation.

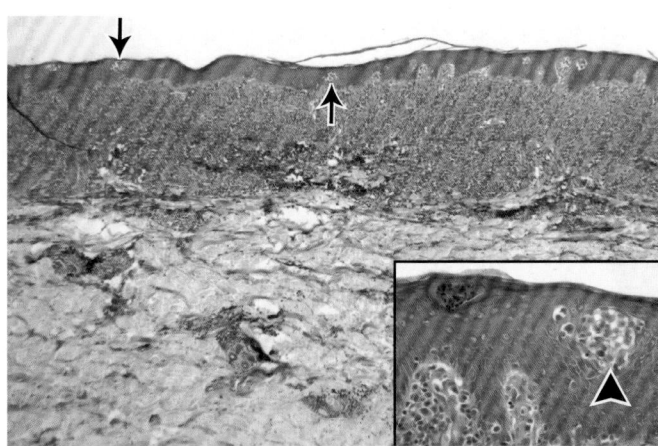

FIGURE 26-70. Mycosis fungoides, plaque phase. A diffuse infiltrate of neoplastic lymphocytes is present in the upper dermis and may occasionally invade the epidermis, as small Pautrier microabscesses (*arrows*). The lower dermis is often spared. A higher magnification of a Pautrier microabscess is shown in the inset (*arrowhead*).

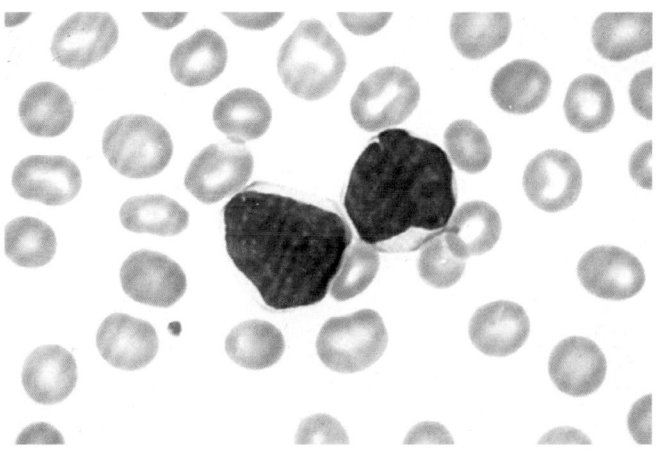

FIGURE 26-71. Sézary cells. Typical cells are medium to large with prominent nuclear convolutions resulting in a cerebriform appearance. This represents the leukemic phase of the cutaneous T-cell lymphoma, mycosis fungoides.

The characteristic cerebriform nuclei of Sézary cells aid in their identification in peripheral blood smears of patients with MF (Fig. 26-71).

The MF cells have a T-helper cell immunophenotype and generally express CD2, CD3, CD5, CD4 and T-cell receptor (TCR)-α,β. As in other mature T-cell lymphomas, CD7, the pan T-cell antigen, is absent. Clonal T-cell receptor gene rearrangements are common, which helps to distinguish subtle cases of MF from inflammatory dermatoses.

Anaplastic Large Cell Lymphoma

Anaplastic large cell lymphomas (ALCLs) are mature T-cell tumors that contain large pleomorphic cells that express the CD30 lymphoid activation marker. These lymphomas often involve both nodal and extranodal sites (frequently skin). This disease has a bimodal age distribution,

in which one peak occurs in young people and a second in older people.

MOLECULAR PATHOGENESIS: Some cases show translocations involving the *ALK* gene (Table 26-19) and have a relatively good prognosis. ALK-negative ALCLs tend to be more aggressive. Their prognosis is like that of unspecified types of peripheral T-cell lymphoma.

PATHOLOGY: The histology of ALCL is variable, but all cases have a population of cells with irregularly shaped nuclei (often horseshoe or kidney shaped) and abundant cytoplasm that often has a distinct eosinophilic area near the nucleus (Fig. 26-72). These cells, which are usually large, are diagnostic **hallmark cells** and express CD30. ALCL cells express several pan T-cell antigens

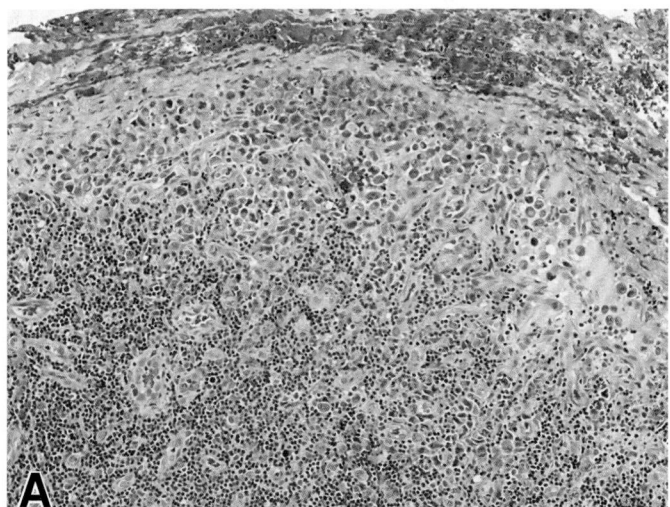

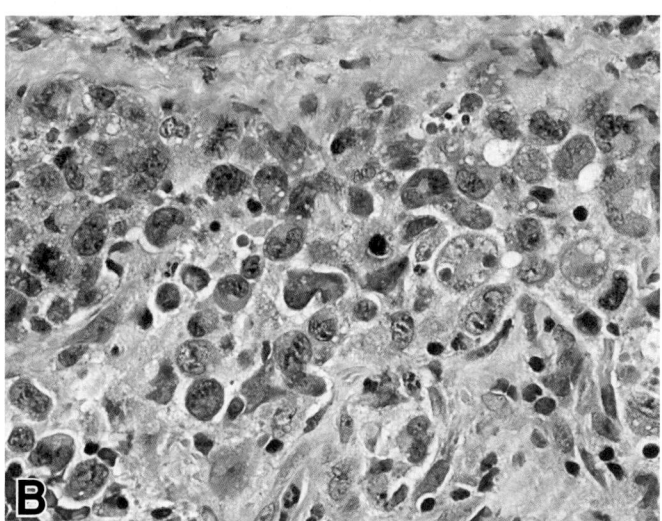

FIGURE 26-72. Anaplastic large cell lymphoma (ALCL). Partially effaced lymph node with accumulation of malignant cells in the subcapsular sinus. This common ALCL pattern may be confused with metastatic carcinoma. **Inset.** The intrasinusoidal lymphoma cells are large and pleomorphic. Cells with kidney-shaped nuclei and an eosinophilic zone near the nucleus are known as hallmark cells and are seen in all variants of ALCL.

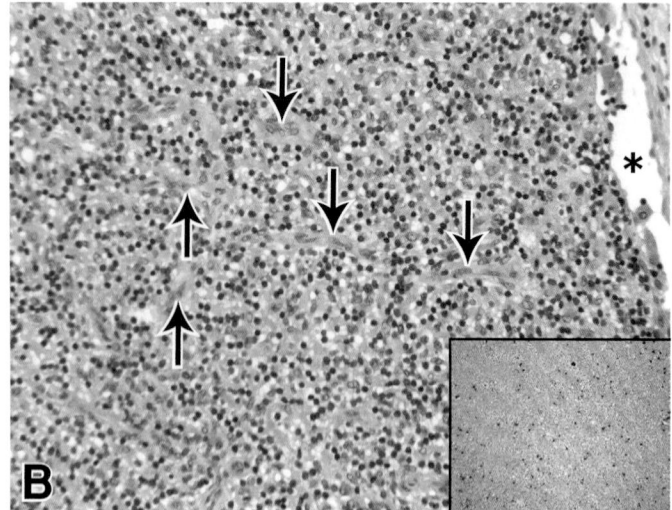

FIGURE 26-73. Angioimmunoblastic T-cell lymphoma. A. Complete effacement of lymph node architecture by an infiltrate that includes a mixture of neoplastic T cells, prominent blood vessels and Ebstein-Barr virus (EBV)-positive B lymphocytes. The lymph node capsule is at the top. **B.** Higher magnification showing the blood vessels (representative vessels are highlighted by *arrows*) and their prominent endothelial cells. The subcapsular sinus is identified (*). **Inset.** In situ hybridization for EBV transcript, demonstrating the scattered EBV-positive B lymphocytes scattered throughout the neoplastic T-cell proliferation.

and cytotoxic T-cell antigens (TIA-1, granzyme B), but most cases are negative for CD3. Over 90% of cases have T-cell receptor rearrangements, even if the tumor cells do not express T-cell antigens. ALK expression (see above) may also be useful in diagnosis.

CLINICAL FEATURES: Most patients have advanced disease (stage III or IV) at presentation. Peripheral and central lymphadenopathy are common, as are extranodal and bone marrow involvement. Patients often have B symptoms, especially fever. Overall 5-year survival with ALK-positive ALCL is 80%. This drops to 48% for patients with ALK-negative tumors.

Angioimmunoblastic T-Cell Lymphoma

Angioimmunoblastic T-cell lymphoma (AILT) is an aggressive peripheral (mature) T-cell lymphoma. Patients present with generalized adenopathy and symptoms consistent with a systemic disease process. Neoplastic T-cell infiltrates expand the paracortical regions of lymph nodes and are associated with a striking proliferation of high endothelial venules. EBV is present in nearly all cases, but the EBV infects only B cells, not the neoplastic T cells.

CLINICAL FEATURES: AILT occurs in adults and the elderly. At the outset, most patients have high-stage disease, generalized lymphadenopathy, hepatosplenomegaly, bone marrow involvement, hypergammaglobulinemia and body cavity effusions. A pruritic skin rash is also common. Other laboratory findings include cold agglutinins, hemolytic anemia, circulating immune complexes and rheumatoid factor. The tumor renders people with AILT immunodeficient, and the high incidence of EBV-positive B cells in these patients reflects their altered immune function. This is an aggressive lymphoma with a median survival of less than 3 years. Patients often die from infectious complications. Some patients develop a concomitant large B-cell lymphoma.

PATHOLOGY: Lymph nodes involved by AILT show partial or complete architectural effacement by a heterogeneous population of atypical small to medium-sized cells, in a setting of prominent, arborizing high endothelial venules. Some cases contain lymphoma cells with abundant clear cytoplasm and minimal atypia, and others show a population of atypical large lymphoid cells (Fig. 26-73). Tumor T cells express most pan T-cell antigens (CD2, CD3, CD5, CD7), plus CD4 in most cases. They also usually show a phenotype of follicular T-helper cells with expression of CD10, CXCL13 and PD-1. Clonal rearrangement of the T-cell receptor occurs in most AILTs, and a minority of cases also show clonal Ig gene rearrangement (reflecting a clonally expanded EBV-positive B-cell population, *not* T tumor cells).

In Classical Hodgkin Lymphomas an Inflammatory Background Accompanies Hodgkin and Reed-Sternberg Cells

Thomas Hodgkin of Guy's Hospital, London, first recognized and described these lymphomas in 1832, and the first descriptions of the distinctive malignant cell were by Sternberg in 1898 and Reed in 1902 (hence called Reed-Sternberg cells; Fig. 26-74). There are 2 types of HL: **classical Hodgkin lymphoma** and **nodular lymphocyte-predominant Hodgkin lymphoma**. Unlike the non-Hodgkin tumors discussed above, classical HLs usually arise in a single lymph node or lymph node chain and usually spread in a contiguous fashion, occur mostly in younger people and have relatively few neoplastic cells, amid a prominent mixed inflammatory cell background. *In the vast majority of cases, the neoplastic cells in HL are derivatives of germinal center B cells.*

EPIDEMIOLOGY AND ETIOLOGIC FACTORS: *HL is the most common malignancy of Americans between the ages of 10 and 30.* Some 8000 cases occur annually in the United States, an incidence of 3 per 100,000 people. It is

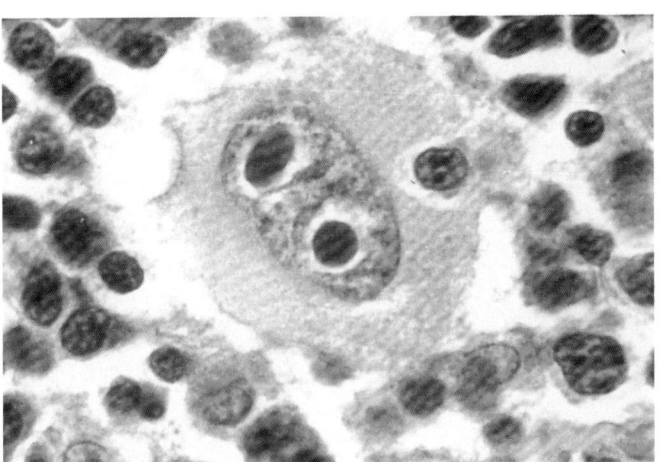

FIGURE 26-74. Classic Reed-Sternberg cell. Mirror-image nuclei contain large eosinophilic nucleoli.

slightly more common in men than in women (4:2.5) and in whites than in blacks (3.5:2).

The geographic variation in HL incidence and some clinicopathologic features that simulate an infectious process suggest a viral etiology. However, proof is lacking. Reports of several self-limited "mini-epidemics" of HL in children suggest possible horizontal transmission (i.e., by interpersonal contact) of an infectious agent. But these clusters are beguiling: such apparent case grouping is predictable on statistical grounds. Broader epidemiologic studies do not support a contagious etiology. A possible link between HL and EBV infection has been suggested. Young adults who have had EBV infectious mononucleosis have a 3-fold higher risk of developing HL, and the EBV genome is frequently identified in Reed-Sternberg cells.

Genetic factors may play a role in HL. Certain HLA subtypes, particularly HLA-B18, are more common in patients

with HL. Moreover, siblings of HL patients have a 7-fold increased risk of HL, which rises to 100-fold increased if they are monozygotic twins.

Immune status also seems to be a factor, at least in some cases. HL occurs more often in people with altered immunity or with autoimmune diseases, such as rheumatoid arthritis. Also, HL accounts for 7% of the malignancies seen in people with ataxia-telangiectasia, who develop cancer 100 times more often than the general population.

The fact that Hodgkin/Reed-Sternberg (HRS) cells are often less than 1% of the total cell content of affected tissues in HL has challenged investigators of HL pathogenesis. However, EBV is present in HRS cells in most patients with HL. EBV antigens may be present in HRS cells by immunohistochemistry or in situ hybridization (Fig. 26-75). However, this finding is variable: EBV occurs in 70%–80% of mixed-cellularity HL, but in less than 40% of nodular sclerosis HL.

Classical Hodgkin Lymphoma

This lymphoma, formerly called Hodgkin disease, is a B-cell neoplasm composed (in most cases) of mononuclear Hodgkin cells and multinucleate Reed-Sternberg (Fig. 26-74) cells in a reactive inflammatory cell milieu consisting of small lymphocytes (mostly T cells), plasma cells, bland histiocytes and eosinophils. Fibroblasts are variably prominent, with or without distinct bands of collagen fibrosis (Fig. 26-76). HRS cells are typically scattered and compose only a small fraction of the total cells in involved lymph nodes. Classical Hodgkin lymphomas are divided into 4 histologic subtypes, largely based on the nature of the associated inflammatory and fibroblastic background and the appearance of the HRS cells. These are (1) **nodular sclerosis,** (2) **mixed cellularity,** (3) **lymphocyte rich** and (4) **lymphocyte depleted.** HRS cells in all subtypes share similar immunophenotypes and genetic alterations. Treatment outcomes are about the same for all.

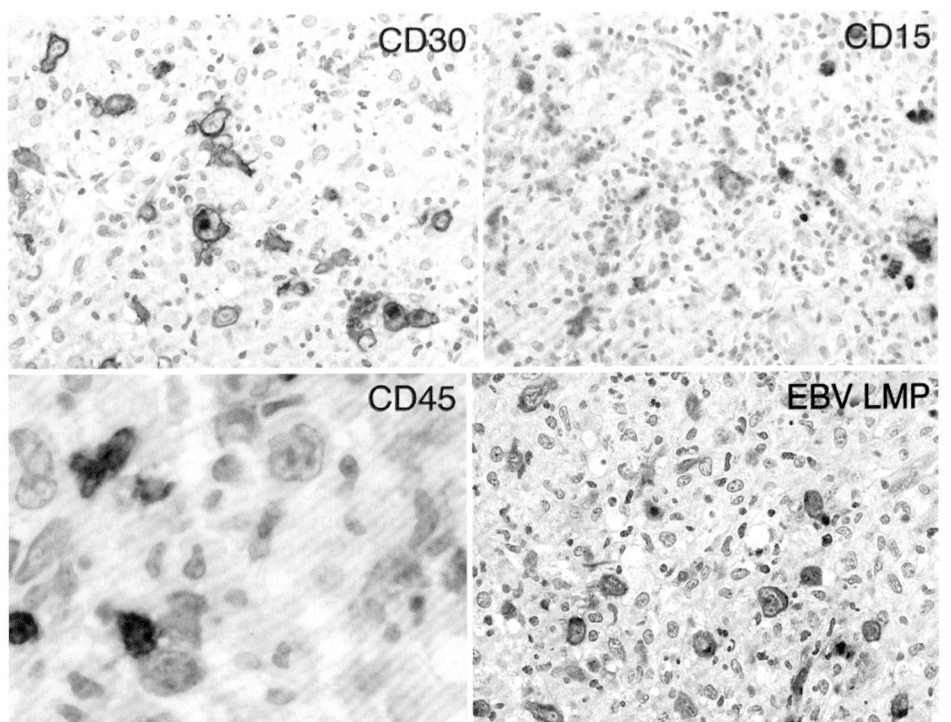

FIGURE 26-75. Reed-Sternberg and Hodgkin cells. The Hodgkin/Reed-Sternberg (HRS) cells are uniformly positive for CD30, CD15 and Epstein-Barr virus latent membrane protein antigen (EBV LMP) (immunohistochemistry; red chromogen). Common leukocyte antigen CD45 is not expressed on HRS cells.

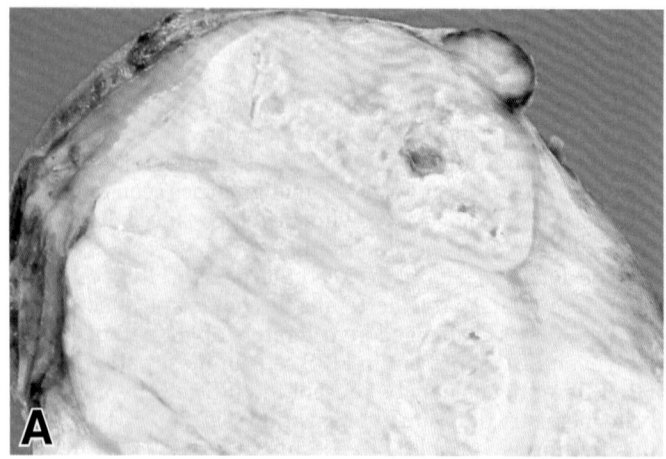

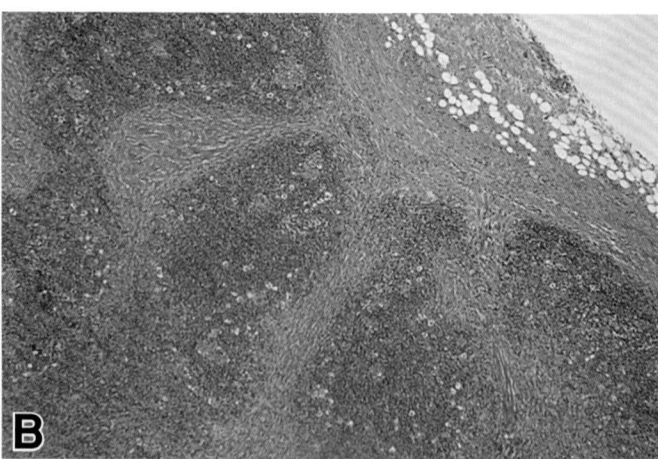

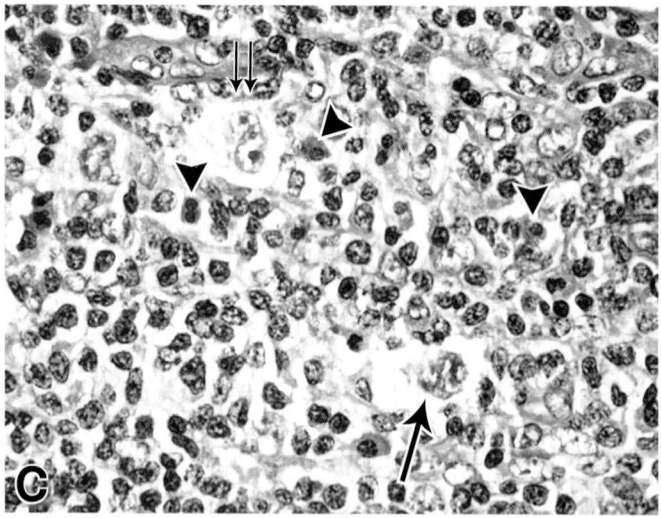

FIGURE 26-76. Nodular sclerosis Hodgkin lymphoma (NSHL). A. Gross photograph showing an enlarged lymph node with a thickened capsule and broad bands of fibrosis dividing the parenchyma into distinct nodules. Several foci of necrosis are evident (red-brown discolorations). **B.** A low-power photomicrograph demonstrates broad bands of fibrosis. There is a dense inflammatory background. Reed-Sternberg cells are rare. **C.** A photomicrograph of NSHL shows a mixed inflammatory background with eosinophils (*arrowheads*), Reed-Sternberg cells (*double arrow*) and lacunar cells (*arrow*).

 **EPIDEMIOLOGY:** Classical Hodgkin lymphomas represent 95% of HLs. The disease has a bimodal age distribution, with one peak at 15–35 years and another in older adults. People with a history of infectious mononucleosis caused by EBV have a higher incidence of classical HL.

 PATHOLOGY: Lymph nodes involved by classical HL show architectural effacement by a variable number of HRS cells in a mixed inflammatory cell background with variable amounts of fibrosis (sclerosis) (Fig. 26-76). Prototypical Reed-Sternberg cells are large with at least two nuclear lobes or nuclei and abundant light blue cytoplasm (Fig. 26-74). Their nuclei have irregular nuclear contours, prominent eosinophilic nucleoli and a perinuclear halo, giving the cells the appearance of "owl's eyes" or viral inclusions. HRS cells may undergo apoptosis, resulting in mummified-appearing cells with condensed cytoplasm and pyknotic nuclei. *Despite their unique appearance, the HRS cells may hide amid the dense reactive background, and typically account for 1%–3% of the cells in involved tissues.*

HRS cells express the lymphoid activation marker CD30 in nearly all cases (Fig. 26-75). They also express the macrophage/monocyte marker, CD15, in 85% of cases. Unlike B-cell non-Hodgkin lymphomas, HRS cells do not typically express such B-cell antigens as CD20 and CD79a, nor do they have CD45 (leukocyte common antigen).

The peculiar HRS immunophenotype, particularly the absence of definitive B-cell differentiation markers, caused decades of confusion about the origin of HRS cells. It was only with advanced molecular diagnostic techniques in the late 1990s that their relationship to clonal B cells of germinal center cell origin became clear. *A clonal Ig gene rearrangement occurs in greater than 98% of HRS cells.*

HRS cells produce cytokines that elicit characteristic tissue effects. The combined effects of IL-5 and eotaxin attract eosinophils, and IL-6 recruits plasma cells. TGF-β activates fibroblasts and may account for nodular fibrosis. Other growth factors and cytokines made by HRS cells include IL-2, -7, -9, -10 and -13.

Nodular Sclerosis Hodgkin Lymphoma

Nodular sclerosis Hodgkin lymphoma (NSHL) is characterized by a fibrous capsular thickening of involved lymph nodes, with bands of fibrosis extending from the capsule into the nodal cortex and forming nodules (Fig. 26-76A). **Lacunar cells** are helpful in diagnosis but result from a retraction artifact in formaldehyde-fixed tissue (Fig. 26-76C). The nodules contain the mixed inflammatory cell population described above and variable numbers of classical HRS and lacunar cells. NSHL subtype accounts for 70% of cases of classical HL and most often affects 15- to 30-year-olds. Over 80% of patients have mediastinal involvement, with bulky disease in over half of these. B symptoms (Table 26-22) occur in up to 40% of patients. Bone marrow involvement and association

TABLE 26-22
ANN ARBOR STAGING SYSTEM FOR HODGKIN DISEASE

Stage I A or B[a]	I	Involvement of a single lymph node region
		or
	I$_E$	A single extralymphatic organ or site
Stage II A or B	II	Involvement of two or more lymph node regions on the same side of the diaphragm
		or
	II$_E$	With localized contiguous involvement of an extralymphatic organ site
Stage III A or B	III	Involvement of lymph node regions on both sides of the diaphragm
		or
	III$_E$	With localized contiguous involvement of an extralymphatic organ or site
		or
	III$_S$	With involvement of spleen
		or
	III$_{ES}$	Both extralymphatic organ or site and spleen involvement
Stage IV A or B	IV	Diffuse or disseminated involvement of one or more extralymphatic organs with or without associated lymph node involvement

[a]A = asymptomatic; B = presence of constitutional symptoms (fever, night sweats and weight loss exceeding 10% of baseline body weight in preceding 6 months).

with EBV are low, relative to other types. NSHL has a better prognosis than the other subtypes.

Mixed Cellularity Hodgkin Lymphoma
In mixed cellularity Hodgkin lymphoma (MCHL), HRS cells are present amid a mixed inflammatory background of eosinophils, neutrophils, macrophages and plasma cells (Fig. 26-77),

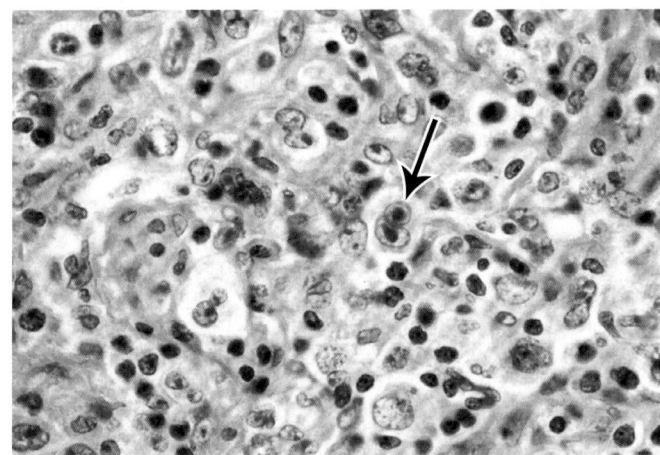

FIGURE 26-77. Mixed cellularity Hodgkin lymphoma. A photomicrograph of a lymph node shows classic, binucleated and mononuclear Reed-Sternberg cells (*arrow*) in a mixed inflammatory background that includes many small lymphocytes (T cells). Note the absence of fibrotic bands, which helps distinguish this subtype from nodular sclerosis Hodgkin lymphoma.

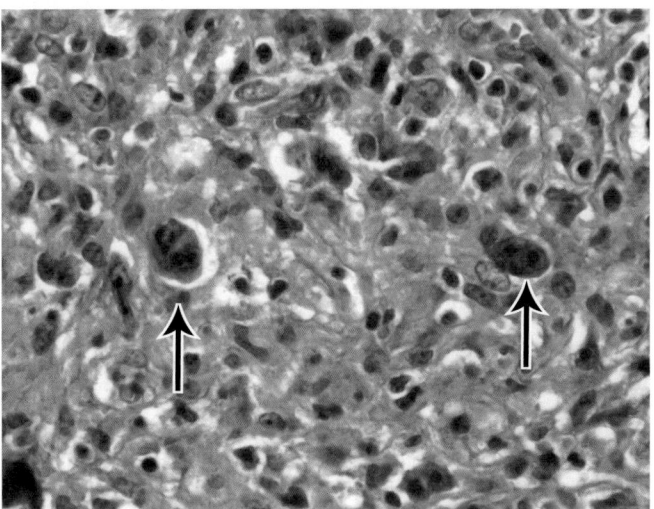

FIGURE 26-78. Lymphocyte-depleted Hodgkin lymphoma. Two Hodgkin/Reed-Sternberg cells are seen (*arrows*). The number of reactive lymphocytes in the fibrotic background is markedly reduced. The differential diagnosis in cases like this includes large cell lymphoma.

but there is a lack of the nodular fibrosis of NSHL. MCHL represents 1/4 of classical HLs. *It is the most frequent subtype in HIV-1–infected patients and shows the highest association with EBV.* MCHL is most common in the 4th and 5th decades. Cervical lymph nodes are the most common initial site of involvement; unlike NSHL, mediastinal involvement is uncommon in MCHL. The prognosis for patients with MCHL is similar to that for patients with NSHL.

Lymphocyte-Rich Hodgkin Lymphoma
In lymphocyte-rich Hodgkin lymphoma (LRHL), classical HRS cells are surrounded by a nodular (or rarely diffuse) lymphoid infiltrate of small B cells. Hallmarks of other forms—eosinophils, neutrophils and sclerosis—are absent. This subtype accounts for only 5% of classical HL and tends to occur in older people. Patients generally present with low-stage disease, without B symptoms. Overall survival for LRHL is better than for all other subtypes of classical HL, and similar to that seen in nodular lymphocyte-predominant HL (see below).

Lymphocyte-Depleted Hodgkin Lymphoma
Lymphocyte-depleted Hodgkin lymphoma (LDHL) is the least common subtype of classical HL, affecting less than 1% of HL patients. In LDHL, HRS cells predominate; background lymphocytes are largely absent (Fig. 26-78). Typical patients with LDHL are 30- to 40-year-old men. This subtype is also often associated with concomitant HIV infection. Involvement of retroperitoneal lymph nodes, which is rare in other subtypes, is not uncommon in LDHL, nor is infiltration of abdominal organs and bone marrow. Patients with associated HIV infection fare worse, but in others the disease course and outcome are like those in the other subtypes. Distinction from non-Hodgkin lymphoma may be more difficult with this subtype of classical HL.

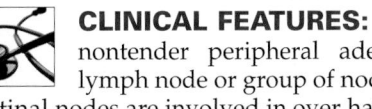 **CLINICAL FEATURES:** HL usually presents as nontender peripheral adenopathy in a single lymph node or group of nodes. Cervical and mediastinal nodes are involved in over half of cases. The anterior mediastinum is frequently involved, especially in the

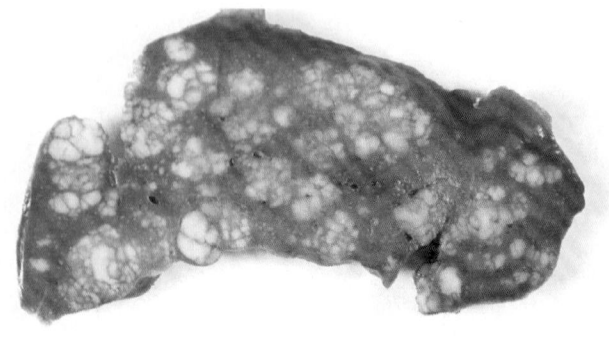

FIGURE 26-79. Hodgkin lymphoma involving the spleen. Multiple masses replace the normal splenic parenchyma. Laparotomy and splenectomy are no longer routinely performed for diagnostic and staging purposes.

nodular sclerosis type. Less commonly, axillary, inguinal and retroperitoneal lymph nodes are affected. Peripheral lymph node groups, such as antecubital, popliteal and mesenteric lymph nodes, are usually spared. Initially, HL spreads predictably between contiguous lymph node groups via efferent lymphatics. As it progresses, spread becomes less predictable because of vascular invasion and hematogenous dissemination (Fig. 26-79).

Constitutional ("B") symptoms are present in 40% of HL patients. These include low-grade fever, which may be cyclical (Pel-Ebstein fever); night sweats; and weight loss over 10% of body weight. Pruritus may occur as the disease progresses. For unknown reasons, drinking alcoholic beverages induces pain at involved sites in 10% of patients.

Patients with HL often have deficient T-lymphocyte function. Subtle defects of delayed-type hypersensitivity, which can be detected in most patients even at the time of initial diagnosis, often get worse as the disease progresses. Anergy to skin test antigens occurs early in HL. Such immune dysfunction is in addition to the immunosuppressive side effects of therapy. Absolute lymphocytopenia (<1500 cells/µL) is present in half of cases, most often those with advanced HL. Humoral immunity is usually intact until late in the course of the disease.

HL prognosis depends mainly on the patient's age and anatomic extent (stage) of the disease. Good prognostic factors include (1) younger age, (2) lower clinical stage (localized disease) and (3) absence of B signs and symptoms. The comprehensive Ann Arbor Staging System (Table 26-22) relies on clinical evaluation and radiographic and pathologic findings (including bone marrow biopsy) to assign stage.

Complications of HL include compromise of vital organs by enlarging tumor and secondary infections due to both primary defects in delayed-type hypersensitivity and immunosuppressive effects of therapy. Development of second malignancies after therapy is of special concern, and eventually affects over 15% of patients. AML develops in 5% of patients; aggressive large cell lymphomas occur somewhat less often.

Nodular Lymphocyte-Predominant Hodgkin Lymphoma

Nodular lymphocyte-predominant Hodgkin lymphoma (NLPHL) is different from classical HL discussed above.

While classified as an HL, its immunomorphologic, clinical and pathologic features more resemble indolent B-cell non-Hodgkin lymphomas than they do classical HL. In NLPHL, the characteristic cells are Hodgkin variants called **L&H cells** (for lymphocyte and histiocytic cells), or "popcorn" cells, because of their characteristic appearance. As in classical HL, these neoplastic cells are infrequent in tissues with NLPHL.

This is also a tumor of germinal center B-cell origin. Unlike classical HL, lymphoma cells in NLPHL express specific B-cell lineage antigens (CD20, CD79a, surface Ig) and are negative for CD15 and CD30. Clonal Ig gene rearrangement occurs in almost all cases. Rearranged immunoglobulin heavy-chain genes show a high degree of somatic hypermutation in the variable region, which indicates that they most likely derive from germinal center B cells.

NLPHL represents about 5% of HLs. It mainly affects men 30–50 years old. However, NLPHL also occurs in younger people, including children. It is typically localized at the time of diagnosis (i.e., stage I). Cervical, axillary or inguinal lymph nodes are common sites of disease. Unlike classical HL, mediastinal, splenic and bone marrow involvement is rare. Visceral involvement is also uncommon. This form of HL tends to skip anatomic lymph node regions (i.e., noncontiguous spread). Only 20% of cases present with B signs and symptoms. These tumors follow an indolent clinical course and are rarely fatal. The 10-year survival for patients with low-stage disease (stage I or II) is greater than 80%. However, outcomes are worse for patients with more advanced disease. Complications include recurrences, which are common, and progression to diffuse large B-cell lymphoma, which occurs in 3%–5% of cases.

Lymphoproliferative Disorders Are Associated with Immune Deficiencies

While several of the non-Hodgkin and Hodgkin lymphomas occur in patients with immune dysfunction, a specific group of lymphoproliferative diseases associated with immunodeficiency is also recognized. These develop against a background of primary immune defects (e.g., CD40 ligand and CD40 deficiencies, common variable immunodeficiency, Wiskott-Aldrich syndrome, ataxia-telangiectasia, Nijmegen breakage syndrome, X-linked lymphoproliferative disorder), lesions associated with HIV infection, posttransplant lymphoproliferative disorders and immune deficiency–associated lymphoproliferative disorders due to other iatrogenic immunosuppression.

Posttransplant Lymphoproliferative Disorders

Posttransplant lymphoproliferative disorders (PTLDs) occur in people who are treated with immunosuppressive regimens because they have received solid organ, bone marrow or stem cell allografts. PTLDs are either lymphoid or plasmacytic, and range from proliferations resembling infectious mononucleosis to overt large cell lymphomas, which are mostly B-cell type. Occasional PTLDs have T-cell phenotypes, and some resemble Hodgkin lymphomas or plasma cell neoplasms. *Most of these disorders reflect Epstein-Barr virus infection, and the key risk factor is seronegativity for EBV at the time of transplantation.*

EPIDEMIOLOGY: Several factors increase the risk of developing PTLD. These include patient characteristics, allograft types and immunosuppressive regimens, which may vary from institution to institution. The incidence of PTLD most closely parallels the extent of immunosuppression. Patients with renal allografts have the lowest frequency of PTLD (<1%), while those who receive heart/lung or intestinal allografts have the highest (>5%). Patients with stem cell or bone marrow allografts have a low risk of PTLD (1%). The risk in these individuals reflects the degree of HLA matching: unrelated or HLA-mismatched transplants are linked to higher rates of PTLD. PTLD is more common in children, probably because they are more often EBV naive than are adults.

 **MOLECULAR PATHOGENESIS:** Most cases are caused by EBV, with an average latency period of less than 1 year. However, EBV-negative cases may evolve 5 years or more after transplantation. In solid organ recipients, host lymphocytes become infected with EBV, but in bone marrow or stem cell allograft recipients, PTLD is often caused by infected *donor* lymphocytes.

 PATHOLOGY: The histology of PTLD is diverse and includes:

- **Early lesions:** These are characterized by plasmacytic hyperplasia or infectious mononucleosis–like changes. They tend to occur in younger patients, particularly those without prior EBV infection. Early lesions involve lymph nodes or tonsils and adenoids more often than true extranodal sites. These lesions usually regress spontaneously, or with a reduction in immunosuppression; however, some infectious mononucleosis–like lesions may occasionally be fatal. Early lesions can evolve into other PTLDs over time.
- **Polymorphic PTLD:** These lesions contain heterogeneous cellular populations, including immunoblasts, plasma cells and small to medium-sized lymphocytes (Fig. 26-80).

The atypical lymphoplasmacytic and immunoblastic proliferation tends to efface lymph node architecture and/or form destructive extranodal masses. This type of PTLD is most common in children and frequently follows primary EBV infection. Its clinical presentation is indistinguishable from other types of PTLD. Variable numbers of cases regress with reduction in immunosuppression, but others progress and require cytotoxic chemotherapy for lymphoma. The atypical cells in polymorphic PTLD show clonally rearranged immunoglobulin genes, although detectable clones are less prominent compared to the level seen in monomorphic PTLD (see below).

- **Monomorphic PTLD:** These are proliferations of transformed monoclonal B lymphocytes or plasma cells that qualify as diffuse large B-cell lymphomas, or less commonly Burkitt lymphomas or plasma cell myelomas/plasmacytomas. This type of PTLD presents similarly to other lymphomas or plasma cell neoplasms. Virtually all cases show clonal Ig gene rearrangements; most have clonal EBV genomes. Cytogenetic abnormalities are common. The majority require treatment for lymphoma; this type of PTLD does not typically respond to reduction in immunosuppression like other PTLD types discussed above.
- **Classical Hodgkin lymphoma–type PTLD:** This rare type of PTLD occurs more often in renal transplant patients, is almost always EBV positive and resembles classical HL (see above).

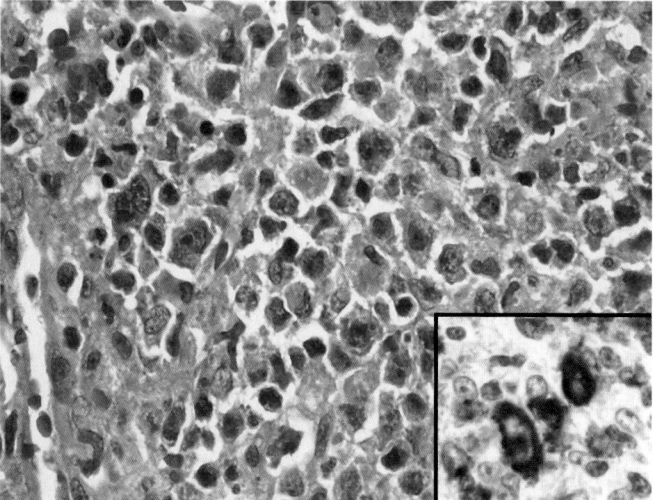 **CLINICAL FEATURES:** Patients with PTLD present with nonspecific symptoms, such as lethargy, malaise, weight loss and fever. Lymphadenopathy and allograft dysfunction are also common. Some patients, mostly children, may have symptoms of airway obstruction because of enlarged tonsils. In addition to lymph nodes and tonsils, PTLDs commonly involve extranodal sites, particularly the gut, lungs and liver. Moreover, PTLDs frequently involve the allograft itself, which may cause diagnostic confusion since allograft rejection can present similarly, both clinically and histologically. The prognosis of PTLD varies and depends largely on the type of lesion. Early lesions (see above) tend to regress with reduction in immunosuppression, without graft loss. Other forms that more closely resemble lymphomas may also regress when immunosuppression is reduced, but many of these require additional cytotoxic therapy, such as anti-CD20 (rituximab), chemotherapy or both. Bone marrow/stem cell allograft recipients tend to show a higher mortality from PTLD than do solid organ allograft recipients. Mortality may be lower in children than in adults. EBV viral load monitoring of seronegative patients is common practice in many transplant centers and has decreased the incidence of disseminated PTLD.

Iatrogenic Immunodeficiency-Associated Lymphoproliferative Disorders

These disorders mostly occur in patients receiving immunosuppressive drugs for autoimmune diseases or other conditions (excluding transplantation). Lymphoid proliferations in this group of patients resemble those in patients with PTLD, and vary from polymorphic disorders to outright diffuse large B-cell lymphoma, peripheral T-cell lymphoma

FIGURE 26-80. Posttransplant lymphoproliferative disorder (PTLD). Polymorphic-type PTLD is characterized by a heterogenous population of atypical lymphocytes with clonal immunoglobulin gene rearrangements. **Inset.** Atypical lymphocytes are positive for Ebstein-Barr virus latent membrane protein (EBV LMP) by immunohistochemistry.

or classical HLs. Methotrexate, which has long been used to treat rheumatoid arthritis (RA), was the first immunosuppressive agent reported to be associated with lymphoproliferative disorders. Newer agents used to treat RA, such as the TNF-α antagonists, also increase the risk of lymphoma, compared to healthy age-matched people. Like most PTLDs, the iatrogenic lymphoproliferative disorders are often associated with EBV, but EBV is not the only important risk factor. Chronic antigenic stimulation, with consequent lymphocytic proliferation, caused by the underlying inflammatory disease, plus the patient's genetic background, also affects lymphoma development. Close to 50% of cases have an extranodal presentation, with the GI tract, skin, liver, spleen, lung, kidney, thyroid gland, bone marrow and soft tissue commonly involved. The remaining clinical features are like those in lymphomas that occur in immunocompetent patients.

Many of these tumors resemble diffuse large B-cell lymphomas or classical HLs. Like PTLDs, iatrogenic lymphoproliferative disorders often respond, at least partially, to withdrawal of immunosuppressive medication. Most such responses occur in cases with EBV-positive cells. Overall survival of patients with DLBCL in this setting is 50%.

HISTIOCYTIC DISORDERS

Histiocytic Proliferations May Be Neoplastic or Nonneoplastic

Among the nonneoplastic disorders are Rosai-Dorfman disease (sinus histiocytosis with massive lymphadenopathy; see above), storage disorders such as Niemann-Pick disease, Gaucher disease and Tangier disease (see Chapter 6) and hemophagocytic syndromes.

Hemophagocytic Disorders

All hematophagocytic disorders have in common an immunologic defect that results in immune dysregulation, with consequent increases in certain cytokines. The result is inadequately regulated T-cell and macrophage activation. NK cells are normal in number but do not regulate antigen-presenting cells effectively. This leads to uncontrolled activation of CD8+ T cells. Proinflammatory cytokines (see Chapter 4), such as TNF-α, IL-6 and interferon-γ (IFN-γ), are increased.

Hemophagocytic syndromes may be genetic or acquired. Diagnosis requires a combination of clinical and pathologic criteria: (1) fever over 38.5°C, (2) splenomegaly, (3) anemia, (4) thrombocytopenia, (5) hypertriglyceridemia and (6) hypofibrinogenemia, accompanied by hemophagocytosis in bone marrow, spleen or lymph nodes. In these organs, one may find macrophages engulfing normal hematopoietic cells (Fig. 26-81).

Inherited hemophagocytic syndromes commonly involve mutations of the *PFR1* gene and typically present in children. They are associated with activation and proliferation of benign macrophages, hemophagocytosis, systemic symptoms (fever, etc.) and circulating cytopenias affecting one or more hematopoietic series. Cellular immune defects may also accompany these clinical manifestations.

Acquired hemophagocytic syndromes occur in several settings. These include viral infections (primary infections with EBV, CMV, HIV, parvovirus), malaria, *E. coli*

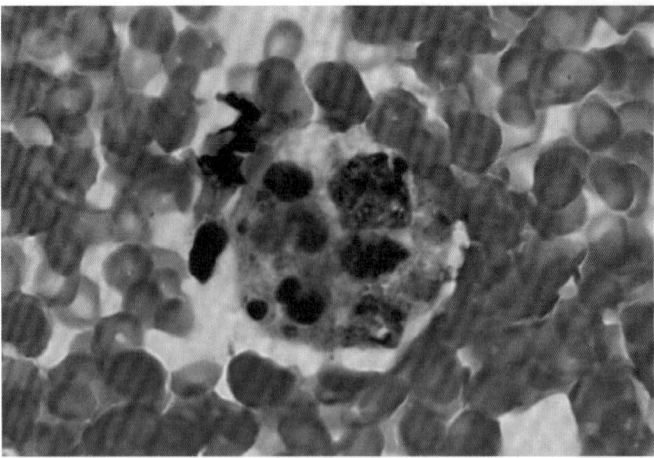

FIGURE 26-81. Hemophagocytic syndrome. This disorder is characterized morphologically by phagocytosis of hematopoietic cells by tissue macrophages. Shown here is a macrophage engulfing bone marrow cells.

and histoplasmosis. Hematologic malignancies such as T-cell and NK-cell lymphomas may underlie hemophagocytic diseases. Autoimmune diseases (juvenile rheumatoid arthritis, systemic lupus erythematosus) are also occasionally implicated.

Histiocytic Neoplasms Are Rare Tumors Derived from Macrophages, Dendritic Cells or Histiocytes

The true incidence of these tumors is unknown as many were poorly recognized and characterized until recently. Their clinical and pathologic features are broad and vary from indolent to aggressive. This group of neoplasms includes **Langerhans cell histiocytosis (LCH), histiocytic sarcoma** and **follicular and interdigitating dendritic cell sarcomas.** Only the former will be discussed.

Langerhans Cell Histiocytosis Is a Neoplastic Proliferation of Langerhans Cells That Occurs Mainly in Children

LCH represents a spectrum of uncommon Langerhans cell proliferations. Disorders arising from these cells span the gamut from asymptomatic involvement at a single site, such as bone or lymph nodes, to aggressive systemic multiorgan disease. Langerhans cells are mononuclear phagocytes derived from precursor cells in the bone marrow. They are present in the epidermis, lymph nodes, spleen, thymus and mucosal tissues, and their role is to ingest, process and present antigens to T cells. In lymph nodes, Langerhans cells are called interdigitating reticulum cells (IDCs).

The etiology and pathogenesis of LCHs are unknown. Langerhans cells in all forms of LCH are clonal, which strongly suggests that these are neoplastic diseases. LCHs mostly affect infants, children and young adults. The extent of disease and rate of progression correlate inversely with age at presentation. There were once eponyms attached to various presentations of LCH, but these terms are now used infrequently.

The least aggressive form is called **eosinophilic granuloma**. It is a localized, usually self-limited, disorder, usually involving one bone or, less often, lymph nodes, skin and

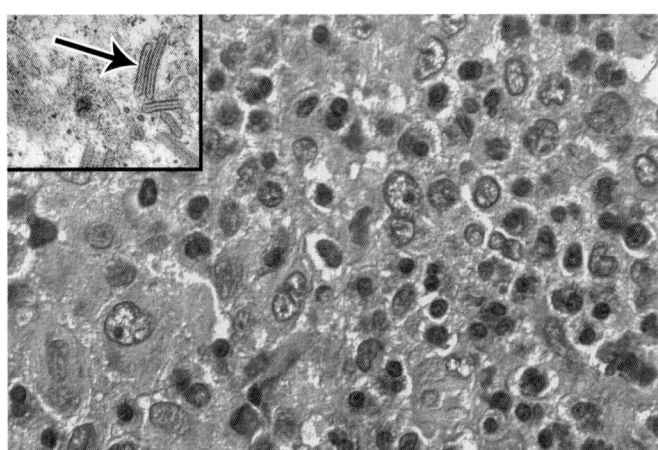

FIGURE 26-82. Eosinophilic granuloma. A section of an affected rib shows proliferated Langerhans cells and numerous eosinophils. **Inset.** Electron micrograph showing a Birbeck granule (*arrow*) in Langerhans histiocytosis.

lungs. This form of LCH affects older children (5–10 years old) and young adults (under 30), mostly males. Eosinophilic granuloma represents 75% of LCH.

In some cases, these lesions present as a multifocal, typically indolent disorder, localized to one organ system, largely bone. Children ages 2–5 generally present with multiple bony lesions that may be associated with soft tissue masses. This was once called **Hand-Schüller-Christian disease**.

The rarest of all forms of these diseases (<10% of cases) is an acute, disseminated variant that usually occurs in infants and children under age 2. There is no sex predominance. Skin lesions, hepatosplenomegaly, lymphadenopathy and bone lesions, along with pancytopenia, are typical. In older literature, this was **Letterer-Siwe** disease.

 PATHOLOGY: Despite their clinical heterogeneity, LCHs share common histopathologies (Fig. 26-82). The cells accumulate in an environment with eosinophils, histiocytes and small lymphocytes. Langerhans cells are large (15–25 μm), with grooved nuclei, delicate vesicular chromatin and small nucleoli. These cells contain distinctive rod-shaped or tubular cytoplasmic inclusions with dense cores and a double outer sheath, called Birbeck granules. One end of these granules is bulbous, in which case they resemble tennis rackets. Cell markers are identical to those of epidermal Langerhans cells, and include S-100 protein and CD1a.

 CLINICAL FEATURES: Clinical manifestations of LCH reflect the sites involved. Skin involvement, mainly in the Letterer-Siwe variant, resembles seborrheic or eczematoid dermatitis, and is most prominent on the scalp, face and trunk. Otitis media is common. Patients show painless localized or generalized lymphadenopathy and hepatosplenomegaly. Lytic lesions of bone cause pain or tenderness to palpation (see Chapter 30). Proptosis (protrusion of the eyeball) may reflect infiltration of the orbit. Diabetes insipidus occurs if the hypothalamic–pituitary axis is affected. *The classic triad of diabetes insipidus, proptosis and defects in membranous bones occurs in only 15% of cases of Hand-Schüller-Christian disease.*

Prognosis in LCH depends mainly on age at presentation, extent of disease and rate of progression. The disorder is usually self-limited and benign in older people (eosinophilic granuloma), while children under 2 years (Letterer-Siwe disease) tend to do poorly. Rarely, LCH follows an aggressive clinical course like a malignant tumor.

Spleen

ANATOMY AND FUNCTION

The spleen is a lymphoid organ that plays a major role in blood filtration, removing abnormal or senescent cells, immune complexes and opsonized bacteria. A normal spleen weighs 100–170 g and is not palpable on physical examination. The spleen's supporting structure includes a fibrous capsule, radiating fibrous trabeculae and a delicate stromal framework of reticulum fibers (Fig. 26-83). The splenic artery enters at the hilum and branches into trabecular arteries, following the course of the fibrous trabeculae. The organ is subdivided into areas of red and white pulp. This division is useful, since most diseases affect either one or the other.

THE WHITE PULP: The lymphoid tissue of the spleen, the white pulp, contains masses of T and B lymphocytes, ensheathing a central artery. The T-cell domain is in the periarteriolar lymphoid sheath; the B-cell domain has follicles and a perifollicular marginal zone. Arising from the central artery, follicular arteries enter B-cell follicles and end in marginal sinuses at the junction between the white and red pulp. Circulating lymphocytes exit the vascular system from the marginal sinus and travel to their respective B-cell and T-cell domains. Lymphocytes leave the white pulp and enter the red pulp by way of the same marginal sinuses.

As part of the peripheral lymphoid system, effector B and T cells of the white pulp carry out immunologic functions for the circulatory system like the immunologic functions of lymph nodes. The white pulp is (1) the source of protection from blood-borne infection, (2) a major site for synthesis of opsonizing IgM antibody and (3) a source of lymphocyte and plasma cell production.

THE RED PULP: The red pulp contains a network of stromal cords and vascular sinuses. Blood from the penicilliary arteries empties directly into the sinuses (closed circulation), then drains into trabecular veins, and ultimately into the splenic vein. A small fraction (5%–10%) is diverted into splenic cords (open circulation) and slowly percolates through a meshwork studded with phagocytic macrophages. Blood then reenters the sinusoids through narrow slits made of longitudinally oriented, slender endothelial cells and radially oriented ring fibers.

The red pulp is mainly a filter that screens and eliminates defective or foreign cells. In the splenic cords, mononuclear phagocytes scrutinize erythrocytes, which must be deformable enough to traverse the narrow interstices between the lining endothelial cells. The red blood cells must also be able to withstand hypoxia, hypoglycemia and acidosis that characterize the stromal cord microenvironment. Splenic macrophages identify and eliminate senescent and damaged erythrocytes. The spleen normally removes half of aged erythrocytes; the liver, bone marrow and other organs deal with the rest. After phagocytosing and breaking down erythrocytes, macrophages first store the resulting iron as hemosiderin. This pigment then binds to transferrin, leaves the macrophages and travels to the bone marrow to be reused in erythropoiesis.

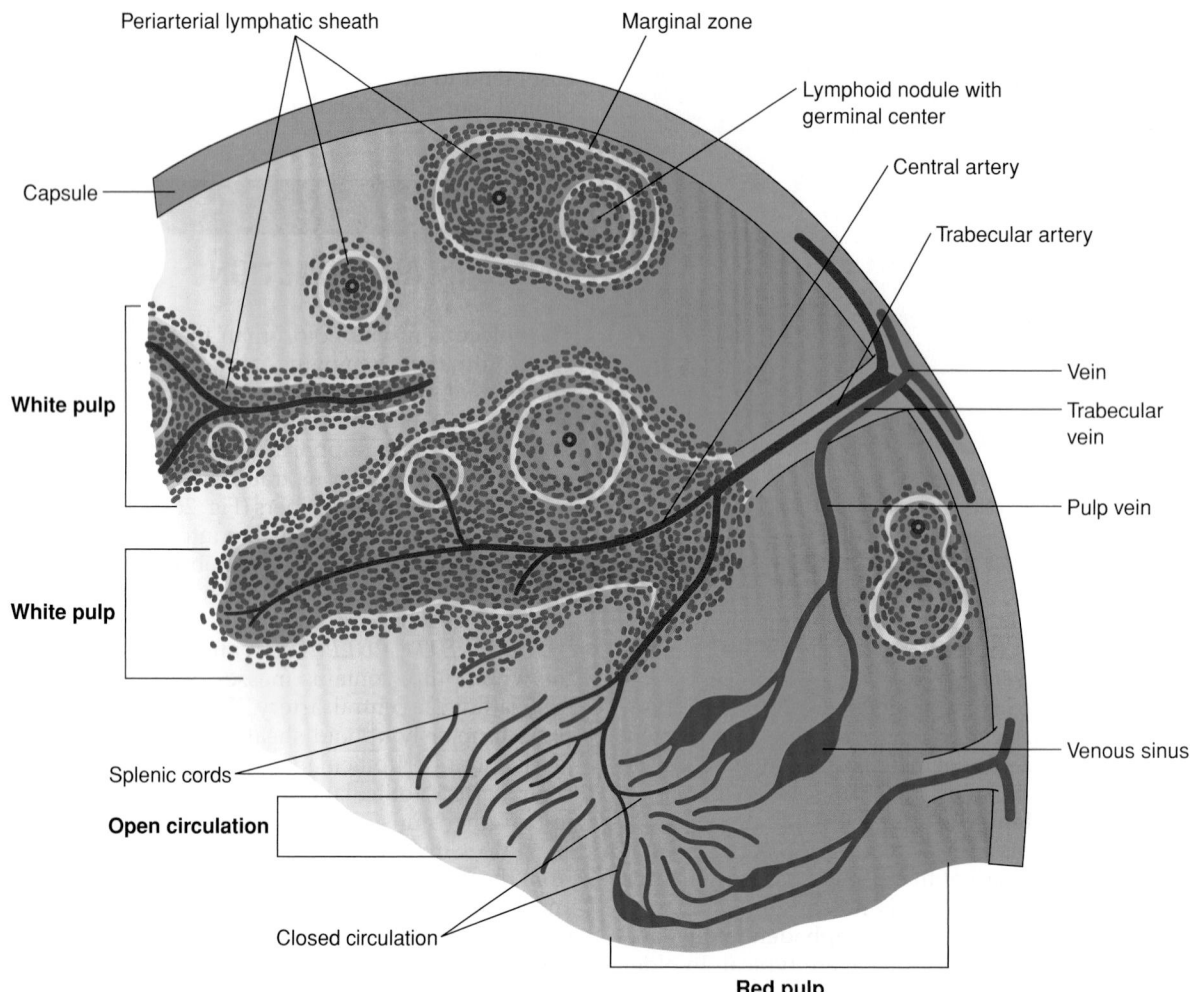

FIGURE 26-83. Structure of the normal spleen.

Splenic macrophages can also identify abnormal erythrocyte inclusions, such as Howell-Jolly bodies (remnants of nuclear DNA), Heinz bodies (denatured hemoglobin) and siderotic granules (iron), and remove them without destroying the erythrocytes.

Some membrane lipids of maturing erythrocytes are removed in the red pulp. Without this function, such as after splenectomy, red blood cell membrane may accumulate, relative to the amount of hemoglobin. This leads to central pooling of hemoglobin and a "target cell" appearance.

Most normal erythrocytes survive, as do granulocytes and platelets. They ultimately enter trabecular veins and leave the hilum via the splenic vein. One third of the blood platelet pool and a small fraction of granulocytes normally reside, undamaged, in the spleen. The spleen does not significantly sequester erythrocytes, however. Splenectomy, then, is followed only by increases in platelet and granulocyte counts.

DISORDERS OF THE SPLEEN

Hypersplenism is a functional disorder, which (see hemolytic anemia, above) features anemia, leukopenia, thrombocytopenia and compensatory bone marrow hyperplasia. In **hyposplenism,** normal splenic functions are impaired by disease or are absent after splenectomy. The spleen's normal filtering function is gone, which increases risk of severe bacteremia and causes mild leukocytosis and thrombocytosis. Nuclear remnants and Howell-Jolly bodies are present in many of circulating erythrocytes.

Asplenia, congenital absence of the spleen, occurs once in 40,000 births, and often accompanies other congenital anomalies. Acquired asplenia occurs in young adults with sickle cell anemia, after a period of hypersplenism. In these patients, multiple infarctions eventually lead to splenic atrophy and hyposplenism. Episodic infarction is often painful because of secondary fibrinous perisplenitis. Without the spleen to sequester erythrocytes and remove redundant materials from them, excess membrane and intracellular debris persist, and many red cells assume target shapes and carry nuclear remnants, Howell-Jolly bodies or even intact nuclei.

Accessory spleens are common congenital anomalies and occur in 1/6 of pediatric splenectomies. They are usually solitary and involve the splenic hilum, the tail of the pancreas or the gastrosplenic ligament. After splenectomy, accessory spleens may enlarge, but they rarely become large enough to replace the functions of a lost spleen. Other congenital anomalies of the spleen include polysplenia with multiple small splenic masses, fusion, hamartomas and cysts.

Reactive Splenomegaly

The spleen is a key member of both lymphopoietic and mononuclear phagocyte systems. Thus, splenomegaly is common in many unrelated benign and malignant diseases (Table 26-23). Acute splenitis occurs in many blood-borne infections: the spleen becomes congested, with red and white pulp infiltrated by neutrophils and plasma cells. In most cases the spleen is moderately enlarged (400 g).

In acute and chronic parasitemias, the red pulp may be engorged with parasites and their breakdown products. The spleen is often massively enlarged in chronic malaria (up to 10 kg). It shows fibrous thickening of the capsule and trabeculae, with slate gray to black coloration of the pulp because of phagocytosed malarial pigment (hematin).

In infectious mononucleosis, half of patients have splenomegaly, which may rarely lead to potentially fatal splenic rupture. Reactive lymphocytes infiltrate the capsular and trabecular systems and blood vessels, weaken the spleen's supporting structure and predispose the spleen to traumatic rupture in infectious mononucleosis. A polymorphic population of T and B immunoblasts, which may include large multinucleated forms, permeates the red pulp cords and sinuses.

In chronic inflammatory disorders, splenomegaly reflects white pulp hyperplasia. Germinal centers are prominent, as in rheumatoid arthritis, and the red pulp has a parallel increase in mononuclear phagocytes, immunoblasts, plasma cells and eosinophils. In systemic lupus erythematosus, fibrinoid necrosis of the capsule and concentric, or "onion skin," thickening of penicilliary arteries and central arterioles of the white pulp occur.

Congestive Splenomegaly

Chronic passive congestion of the spleen causes splenomegaly and hypersplenism. This occurs most often in patients with portal hypertension due to cirrhosis, thrombosis of the portal or splenic veins or right-sided heart failure. Splenic congestion also complicates hereditary hemolytic anemias and hemoglobinopathies. Common inherited causes of hemolytic anemia include hereditary spherocytosis and elliptocytosis, thalassemia and sickle cells anemia. Erythrocytes in these conditions are inflexible, so they become trapped as they attempt to pass through splenic cords.

The Spleen in Sickle Cell Anemia

The spleen is modestly enlarged (300–700 g), with a thickened, fibrotic capsule. Focal accentuation of the capsular fibrosis leads to a "sugar-coated" appearance. The cut surface is firm, and the color varies from pink to deep red, depending on the extent of fibrosis. Venous sinuses are distended with red cells and surrounded by hemosiderin-laden macrophages. Later, because of hypoxia and infarcts, splenic parenchyma becomes fibrotic, and the red pulp is hypocellular. Foci of old hemorrhage persist as Gamna-Gandy bodies, fibrotic nodules containing iron and calcium salts encrusted on collagenous and elastic fibers. The white pulp tends to be atrophic.

Infiltrative Splenomegaly

The spleen may be enlarged owing to increased cellularity or deposition of extracellular material, as in amyloidosis. Splenic macrophages accumulate in chronic infections, hemolytic anemias and a variety of storage diseases (see Chapter 6). Diverse neoplastic and reactive bone marrow diseases lead to extramedullary hematopoiesis and corresponding increases in spleen size. Malignant cells may infiltrate the spleen in hematologic proliferative disorders, such as leukemias and lymphomas, and in virus-associated hemophagocytic syndrome.

Splenomegaly Caused by Cysts and Tumors

Splenic cysts are rare. Most are actually pseudocysts, lined by fibrous walls. These represent the residues of old hemorrhage or infarction. Hydatid, or echinococcal, cysts are the most common cysts worldwide, in areas endemic for *Echinococcus granulosus* (see Chapter 9). They are quite rare in the United States.

Primary splenic neoplasms are also rare. Vascular tumors are the most common nonhematopoietic neoplasms that involve the spleen. They include benign tumors such as hemangiomas and lymphangiomas. The former are usually of the

TABLE 26-23
PRINCIPAL CAUSES OF SPLENOMEGALY

Infections
  Acute
  Subacute
  Chronic

Immunologic Inflammatory Disorders
  Felty syndrome
  Lupus erythematosus
  Sarcoidosis
  Amyloidosis
  Thyroiditis

Hemolytic Anemias

Immune Thrombocytopenia

Splenic Vein Hypertension
  Cirrhosis
  Splenic or portal vein thrombosis or stenosis
  Right-sided cardiac failure

Primary or Metastatic Neoplasm
  Leukemia
  Lymphoma
  Hodgkin disease
  Myeloproliferative syndromes
  Sarcoma
  Carcinoma

Storage Diseases
  Gaucher
  Niemann-Pick
  Mucopolysaccharidoses

cavernous variety, with large endothelial-lined spaces. They may vary from minute foci to lesions that occupy most of the spleen. The vascular spaces in hemangiomas contain erythrocytes; in lymphangiomas they have lymph. Other benign tumors include littoral cell angiomas and hemangioendotheliomas.

The most common primary malignant tumor of the spleen is the hemangiosarcoma. Splenic hemangiosarcomas are rare, highly malignant neoplasms of vascular endothelial cells that tend to metastasize to the liver via the portal drainage. Other malignancies, such as malignant lymphomas or HL, usually affect the spleen as part of generalized disease. Despite its large blood supply and filtering function, the spleen is only rarely involved by metastatic solid tumors, and then only in the setting of wildly metastatic cancers.

Thymus

The thymus elaborates many factors (thymic hormones) that play key roles in maturation of the immune system and development of immune tolerance. On this basis, we discuss certain entities associated with thymus abnormalities in this chapter.

ANATOMY AND FUNCTION

The thymus derives embryologically from the 3rd pair of pharyngeal pouches, with an inconstant contribution from the 4th pair. The organ is irregularly pyramidal. Its base is located inferiorly and its two lobes fuse in the midline. Its fibrous capsule extends into the parenchyma, forming septa that delimit lobules. The thymus is largest, relative to total body size and weight at birth, when it averages about 15 g. It continues to grow until puberty, and may then weigh 30–40 g.

Thymic lobules have outer cortices and inner medullas. The former consist of densely packed lymphocytes, which in this location are called thymocytes. Thymocytes mingle with a few epithelial and mesenchymal cells. The medulla has many more epithelial cells and fewer thymocytes. Hassall corpuscles are medullary structures that are focally keratinized, concentric aggregates of epithelial cells characteristic of the thymus.

The thymus is the key site for T-lymphocyte differentiation (see Chapter 4). It also has a small population of neuroendocrine cells, which may explain how neuroendocrine tumors arise in this organ. There is also a complement of myoid cells, which resemble striated muscle cells but are nevertheless regarded as epithelial cells. Their function is uncertain.

Beginning at puberty, the thymus starts to involute and continues to diminish in size into adulthood. Initially, cortical thymocytes are decreased relative to epithelial cells. Eventually, the thymus is little more than islands of epithelial cells depleted of lymphocytes and aggregates of Hassall corpuscles separated by adipose tissue.

AGENESIS AND DYSPLASIA

Alterations in the thymus vary from complete absence (agenesis) or severe hypoplasia to a situation in which the thymus is small but has normal architecture. Some small glands may show thymic dysplasia, in which there are no thymocytes, few if any Hassall corpuscles and only epithelial components. Various developmental anomalies are associated with immune deficiencies (see Chapter 4) and hematologic disorders.

- **Severe combined immunodeficiency (SCID)** represents a group of genetically distinct syndromes all characterized by defects of both T- and B-cell functions and associated with severe thymic dysplasia. Both X-linked and autosomal recessive inheritance may be involved. SCID can be caused by mutations in at least 10 different genes. The most common form is the X-linked type, caused by mutations in *IL-2RG,* a cytokine receptor gene. Common autosomal recessive inherited forms include adenosine deaminase deficiency and IL-7Ra.

- **Chromosome 22q11.2 deletion syndrome** (DiGeorge, velocardiofacial, Shprintzen, conotruncal anomaly face and Cayler syndromes) is a spectrum of overlapping conditions caused by 22q11.2 deletions. It is one of the most common (of 180 at least) genetic syndromes associated with variable clinical manifestations. Patients with DiGeorge syndrome fail to develop their 3rd and 4th branchial pouches, resulting in thymic and parathyroid agenesis or hypoplasia, congenital heart defects, dysmorphic facies and other congenital anomalies. As a result, patients have hypocalcemia and deficient cellular immunity, with a particular susceptibility to *Candida* infections. These patients are also at increased risk for psychotic illnesses. Endocrine abnormalities include hypocalcemia, thyroid dysfunction and short stature. The diagnosis, suspected on clinical grounds, can be readily established by FISH analysis.

- In **Nezelof syndrome,** lymphopenia, hypoplastic lymphoid tissue, abnormal thymus architecture and abnormal T-cell function are the rule. It resembles DiGeorge syndrome, save for the lack of parathyroid and cardiac manifestations.

- **Wiskott-Aldrich syndrome** is an X-linked, recessive immunodeficiency caused by mutations in the *WAS* gene. This syndrome entails a hypoplastic thymus, recurrent infections, eczema and thrombocytopenia (see Chapter 4). Patients are highly susceptible to lymphoid malignancies and autoimmune disorders.

- **Reticular dysgenesis (RD)** is a very rare, severe immune deficiency characterized by a vestigial thymus and developmental failure of bone marrow stem cells. It results in lymphopenia, granulocytopenia and death, either in utero or in the neonatal period. The defect in RD is not known.

- **Swiss-type hypogammaglobulinemia** is an autosomal recessive disorder with severe thymic hypoplasia or dysplasia. Infants with this condition have no lymphocytes or Hassall corpuscles in the thymus and die within a few years from infection. In this disease, thymic anlage in the neck fail to descend into the mediastinum.

- **Ataxia-telangiectasia (A-T)** is an autosomal recessive cerebellar ataxia associated with immunodeficiency, telangiectasia, increased sensitivity to ionizing radiation and frequent occurrence of lymphoma. The involuted thymus lacks epithelial differentiation and Hassall corpuscles. Classic A-T results from two truncating *ATM* gene mutations that cause complete loss of ATM protein kinase (see Chapter 5).

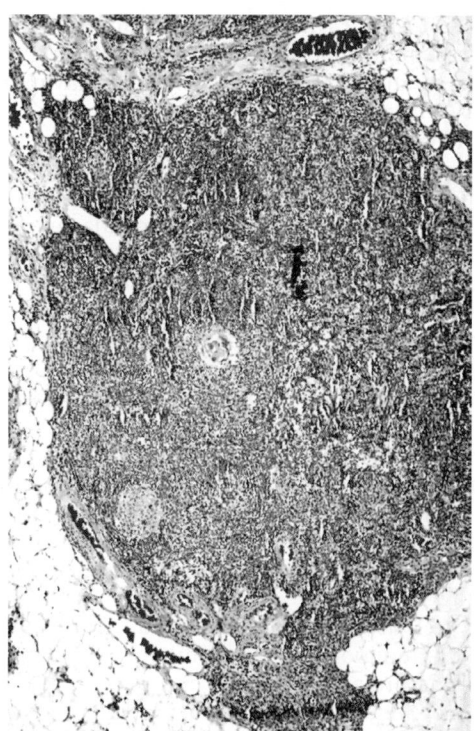

FIGURE 26-84. Thymic hyperplasia. This thymus removed from a patient with myasthenia gravis shows lymphoid follicles with germinal centers.

THYMIC HYPERPLASIA

Thymic hyperplasia is the presence of lymphoid follicles in the thymus, regardless of the size of the gland (Fig. 26-84). The total weight of the thymus is usually in the normal range, but may be slightly increased. The follicles contain germinal centers, composed largely of B lymphocytes that produce IgM and IgD. These follicles tend to occupy and distort the medullary zones.

Thymic hyperplasia occurs in 2/3 of patients with myasthenia gravis (see Chapter 31). Interestingly, thymic epithelial and myoid cells contain nicotinic acetylcholine receptor protein, which may stimulate the development of antibodies against that receptor. Thymic follicular hyperplasia also occurs in other autoimmune diseases, such as Graves disease, Addison disease, systemic lupus erythematosus, scleroderma and rheumatoid arthritis.

THYMOMA

Thymomas are neoplasms of thymic epithelial cells. They almost always occur in adult life and most (80%) are benign.

PATHOLOGY: Most thymomas are in the antero-superior mediastinum, although a few may occur elsewhere where thymic tissue is present, such as the neck, middle and posterior mediastinum and pulmonary hilus. Benign thymomas are irregularly shaped masses that vary from a few centimeters to 15 cm or more. They are encapsulated, firm and gray to yellow tumors that are divided into lobules by fibrous septa (Fig. 26-85). Large thymomas may have foci of hemorrhage, necrosis and cystic degeneration. Sometimes, the entire thymoma is cystic and

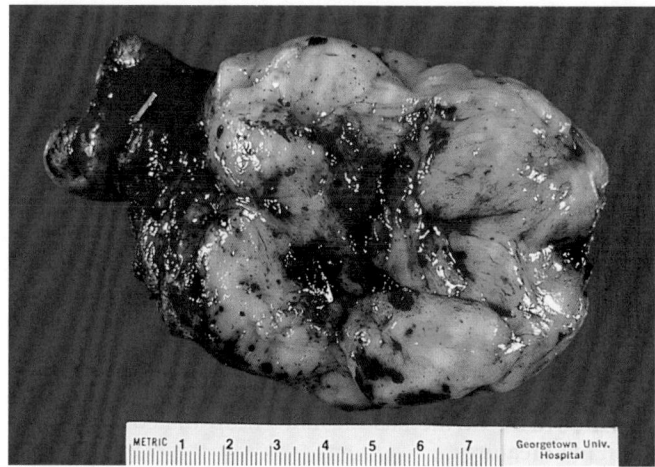

FIGURE 26-85. Thymoma. The tumor in cross-section is whitish and has a bulging surface with areas of hemorrhage. Note the attached portion of normal thymus.

multiple sections are required to identify the true nature of the lesion.

Thymomas contain a mixture of neoplastic epithelial cells and nontumorous lymphocytes (Fig. 26-86). The proportions of these elements vary from case to case, and even among different lobules. The epithelial cells are plump or spindle shaped, with vesicular nuclei. In cases in which epithelial cells predominate, they may show organoid differentiation, including perivascular spaces with lymphocytes and macrophages, tumor cell rosettes and whorls suggesting abortive Hassall corpuscles.

MYASTHENIA GRAVIS: Fifteen percent of patients with myasthenia gravis have thymomas. Conversely, 1/3 to 1/2 of patients with thymomas develop myasthenia gravis. This coincident occurrence of thymomas and myasthenia gravis is more common in men older than age 50.

When thymoma is associated with myasthenic symptoms, the epithelial cells are plump, rather than spindly. Antigens related to the nicotinic acetylcholine receptor also occur in thymomas. Thymic hyperplasia is almost always present in the nontumorous thymic tissue, and lymphoid follicles may even be present in the thymoma itself.

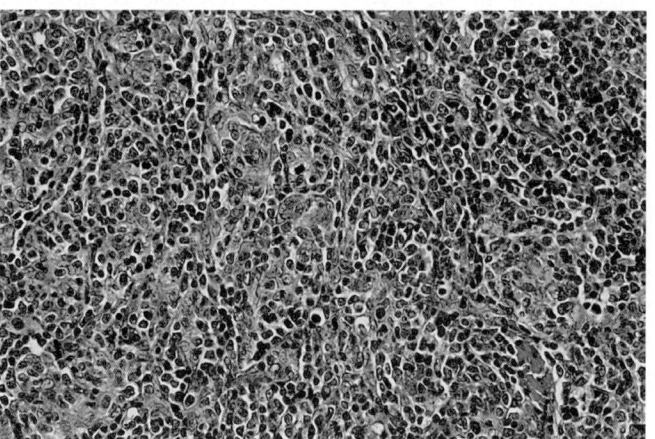

FIGURE 26-86. Microscopic features of thymomas. The tumor consists of a mixture of neoplastic epithelial cells and nontumorous lymphocytes.

OTHER ASSOCIATED DISEASES: Thymomas are associated with many other immune disorders. Over 10% of patients have hypogammaglobulinemia and 5% have erythroid hypoplasia. In these patients, unlike those with myasthenia gravis, the epithelial component of the thymoma is spindle shaped. Other associated diseases include myocarditis, dermatomyositis, rheumatoid arthritis, lupus erythematosus, scleroderma and Sjögren syndrome. Certain malignant tumors may also occur with thymoma, including T-cell leukemia/lymphoma and multiple myeloma.

Malignant Thymomas Invade Locally and May Metastasize

One fourth of thymomas are not encapsulated and show malignant features.

 PATHOLOGY: Type I malignant thymoma is the most common cancer of the thymus, and is virtually indistinguishable histologically from encapsulated, benign thymomas. However, it penetrates the capsule, implants on pleural or pericardial surfaces and metastasizes to lymph nodes, lung, liver and bone.

Type II malignant thymoma is a very uncommon invasive tumor, also called thymic carcinoma. Its morphology is highly variable and it resembles squamous carcinomas, lymphoepithelioma-like carcinomas (identical to those in the oropharynx; see Chapter 29), sarcomatoid variants (carcinosarcoma) and other rare patterns. These variants share a distinct epithelial appearance and a mediastinal tumor that lacks this feature is probably not thymic carcinoma.

 CLINICAL FEATURES: Malignant thymomas are treated by surgical excision and radiation. Chemotherapy is added in cases with distant metastases. The prognosis for benign thymoma is excellent. The presence or absence of myasthenic symptoms has little prognostic value. For type I malignant thymomas, the prognosis correlates with the extent of disease. Most patients with type II thymomas die within 5 years of diagnosis.

Other Tumors of the Thymus Are Uncommon

NEUROENDOCRINE TUMORS: Several neuroendocrine tumors arise in the thymus. These resemble comparable tumors elsewhere, clinically and pathologically, and include carcinoids (typical and atypical) and carcinomas (small and large cell). Neuroendocrine tumors express cytokeratins (AE1/AE3, CAM5.2) and endocrine markers (synaptophysin, chromogranin, NSE). They may produce ACTH and cause Cushing syndrome. Interestingly, many thymic neuroendocrine tumors lack expression of thyroid transcription factor 1 (TTF-1).

CARCINOID: Thymic carcinoid tumors are malignant. They tend to invade locally and metastasize widely, although they may be cured by local excision if they are well circumscribed. While 1/3 of these patients show Cushing syndrome, carcinoid syndrome is exceedingly rare. Thymic carcinoid tumors occur sporadically, in familial forms, and in the syndromes of multiple endocrine neoplasia (MEN)-1 and -2A. They may also accompany neurofibromatosis type I. Most thymic carcinoids are atypical (intermediate category) with frequent mitoses and/or necrosis.

SMALL CELL CARCINOMA: Small cell carcinomas (SCCs), indistinguishable from those in the lung, may also arise in the thymus. In them, SCC elements may mingle with squamous cell carcinomas.

GERM CELL TUMORS: Thymic germ cell tumors account for 20% of mediastinal tumors. It is felt that they arise from cells left behind when germ cells migrate during embryogenesis. The histologies of mediastinal germ cell tumors are like those in the gonads (see Chapters 23 and 24). Mature cystic teratomas are most common. Seminomas, embryonal carcinomas, endodermal sinus tumors, teratocarcinomas, immature teratomas and choriocarcinomas all occur. Mixed germ cell histologies are common.

Mediastinal germ cell tumors may on occasion show somatic-type malignant components of sarcoma, carcinoma or hematologic malignancies. Save for mature cystic teratoma, which affects both sexes equally, the other tumors occur mostly in males. Thymic seminomas arise only in men. Prognosis is like that for comparable gonadal tumors, although mediastinal nonseminomatous germ cell tumors are more aggressive.

Other lesions include benign and malignant stromal tumors. Thymolipomas are benign, well-circumscribed masses of mature adipose tissue and unremarkable thymic parenchyma. Thymic stromal sarcomas are low-grade malignant mesenchymal tumors with variable morphology, but frequently of a liposarcomatous nature.

Nonneoplastic masses include thymic, mesothelial and enteric-type cysts.

Paraneoplastic Syndromes Involving the Hematopoietic System

Paraneoplastic syndromes are tumor-associated clinical manifestations that occur distant to the tumor and are caused by the secretion of tumor cell products such as hormones, cytokines, growth factors and tumor antigens. They may precede, coexist or follow the diagnosis of underlying malignancy. Occasionally, they may be the first signs of tumor relapse. Rarely, they can even present when patients are in remission. Their clinical manifestations are diverse, depending on the organ/system involved, and early recognition of these syndromes may facilitate a timely diagnosis of malignancy. The most effective management of paraneoplastic syndromes in the setting of hematologic malignancies remains the treatment of the underlying malignancy.

The following are paraneoplastic syndromes commonly associated with hematologic disorders, grouped by organ system in which the manifestations occur.

HEMATOLOGIC MANIFESTATIONS OF NEOPLASIA

Abnormalities in Peripheral Blood Cell Counts Occur in Several Hematologic Malignancies

These may be identified before the diagnosis of malignancy is made, or they may be apparent at the time of diagnosis.

Autoimmune hemolytic anemia presents similar to idiopathic hemolytic anemia, with elevated LDH, unconjugated bilirubin and reticulocyte count and low serum haptoglobin. Direct antiglobulin test (DAT) is positive (IgG). The antibody specificity is against red blood cell antigens, owing to immune dysregulation resulting in the loss of tolerance to self-antigens (in this case, red cell antigens) in the setting of malignancy. CLL is a frequent hematologic malignancy associated with AIHA, but NHLs and HLs can also be the cause.

Immune thrombocytopenia presents with petechiae, bleeding and bruising. The antibody specificity is unknown. Among the most frequent hematologic malignancies, CLL and B-cell lymphomas are on top of the list.

AIHA occurring in combination with ITP is called **Evans syndrome**. If drugs, infections or connective tissue diseases are ruled out, evaluation for a lymphoproliferative disorder needs to be done.

Cancer-related **microangiopathic hemolytic anemia** (CRMAHA) is a Coombs-negative hemolytic anemia with schistocytes and thrombocytopenia. Among lymphomas, CRMAHA was described in Hodgkin lymphoma, diffuse large B-cell lymphoma, intravascular lymphoma, myeloma and rare cases of hairy cell leukemia. Treatment with fresh frozen plasma or plasmapheresis, which is usually effective in TTP and HUS, is rarely effective, but early chemotherapy may be efficacious and prolong survival.

Paraneoplastic leukocytosis with predominant neutrophilia and increased serum levels of G-CSF is attributed to release of cytokines (G-CSF and TNF-α) by tumor cells. Paraneoplastic leukocytosis has been reported in different malignancies of lung, gastrointestinal and genitourinary tract, multiple myeloma, Hodgkin lymphoma and anaplastic large cell lymphoma. Although some studies claimed that the presence of paraneoplastic leukocytosis with malignancies portends a poor prognosis, it is not clear if the association of paraneoplastic leukocytosis and lymphomas has the same impact on prognosis.

Eosinophilia without leukocytosis has been described in Hodgkin lymphoma and T-cell lymphoma.

Paraneoplastic leukocytosis has been described in multiple myeloma, Hodgkin lymphoma and anaplastic large cell lymphoma, and is characterized by neutrophilia in the absence of infection and elevated serum G-CSF levels. It is considered to be the consequence of intratumor G-CSF production.

Deep vein thrombosis can be a paraneoplastic manifestation of lymphomas.

CUTANEOUS MANIFESTATIONS OF HEMATOLOGIC MALIGNANCIES

Paraneoplastic pemphigus (PNP) is a mucocutaneous disease presenting with painful oral and mucosal ulcerations, with concomitant blistering skin lesions. In addition, ocular (conjunctivitis), lung (in the form of bronchiolitis obliterans) and nervous system involvement can occur. Therefore, PNP is considered a severe form of autoimmune multiorgan syndrome. The disease, immunologic in nature, is initiated by an occult or overt neoplasm, which elicits an immune response in the form of autoantibody production. The autoantibodies are directed against cell surface adhesion molecules (mainly plakin family proteins and desmogleins). Hematologic neoplasms or disorders are associated with 84% of the cases:

non-Hodgkin lymphomas, chronic lymphocytic leukemia, Castleman disease, dendritic cell tumors (sarcomas) and thymomas. Histopathologic evaluation reveals intraepidermal acantholysis, necrotic keratinocytes and vacuolar interface changes. In PNP, patients' serum contains autoantibodies that recognize proteins in the epithelium. Direct immunofluorescence shows intercellular and basement membrane staining for IgG and complement. Indirect immunofluorescence detects serum antibodies that bind to cell surfaces of stratified squamous epithelia. Response to treatment is generally poor, with high mortality rates.

Sweet syndrome is an acute febrile neutrophilic dermatosis characterized by abrupt onset of papular skin lesions, accompanied by systemic symptoms: fever, arthralgia, malaise, headache and myalgia. Laboratory abnormalities, if present, consist of elevated erythrocyte sedimentation rate and peripheral leukocytosis with neutrophilia. The lesions show dermal edema and dense superficial dermal infiltrate of mature neutrophils, with or without lymphocytes and histiocytes (Fig. 26-87). As a paraneoplastic syndrome preceding or accompanying hematologic malignancies, Sweet syndrome is seen mostly in acute myeloid leukemia and myelodysplastic syndromes. It occurs as well, albeit less commonly, in patients with lymphoid malignancies (hairy cell leukemia, Hodgkin and non-Hodgkin lymphomas).

Pyoderma gangrenosum is an ulcerative skin disease, most frequently associated with inflammatory bowel disease and rheumatoid arthritis. When associated with myelodysplastic syndrome, myeloma or leukemia, the presentation can be atypical, with vesiculobullous lesions and atypical distribution. The mechanism is not known, but numerous cytokines (TNF-α, IFN-γ, G-CSF, IL-6, IL-1β) are elevated.

Vasculitides, which manifest as acute-onset rashes, can be paraneoplastic manifestations of malignancies including myeloid leukemias, lymphomas and hairy cell leukemia. Several pathogenic mechanisms have been proposed: tumor-associated antigens mediate vascular damage, either directly or indirectly through formation of immune

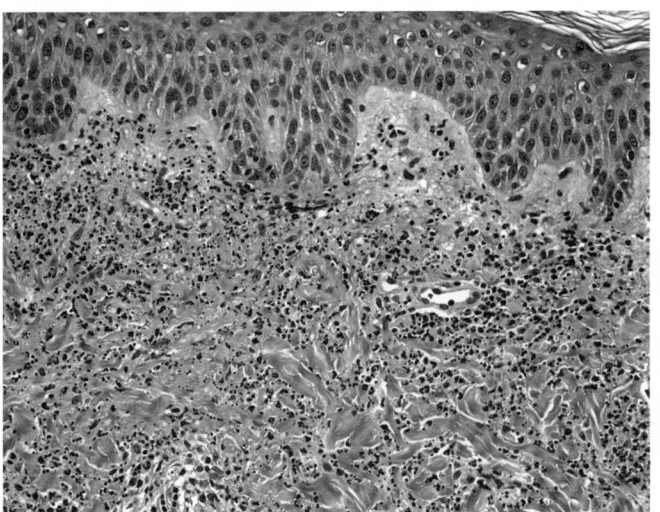

FIGURE 26-87. Sweet syndrome. Skin biopsy in a patient with Sweet syndrome, which developed clinically 4 months before myelodysplastic syndrome became evident. There is a dense neutrophilic infiltrate in the upper and mid-dermis, sparing the epidermis and without evidence of vasculitis.

HEMATOPATHOLOGY

complexes; direct vascular damage occurs by antibodies formed against leukemic cells. Examples of these include cutaneous leukocytoclastic vasculitis, which is the most common vasculitis associated with hematologic malignancies. Others (polyarteritis nodosa, Churg-Strauss syndrome, microscopic polyangiitis, granulomatous polyangiitis and Henoch-Schönlein purpura) are described in detail in Chapter 17.

Eczema and **erythema nodosum** have also been described in lymphomas.

ENDOCRINE MANIFESTATIONS OF HEMATOLOGIC MALIGNANCIES

Hypercalcemia has been described in patients with Hodgkin lymphoma. The mechanisms are either secretion of parathormone-related peptide by tumor cells or excess calcitriol produced by reactive macrophages infiltrating neoplastic lymph nodes.

Hypoglycemia of nonpancreatic causes including lymphomas (non–insulin-secreting tumors) is the result of hypersecretion of insulin-like growth factors (IGF-I and IGF-II) by tumor cells. Endocrinologic causes for hypoglycemia need to be excluded. Laboratory tests detect low levels of blood glucose and C peptide.

RENAL MANIFESTATIONS OF HEMATOLOGIC MALIGNANCIES

Paraneoplastic glomerular diseases often occur in lymphomas.

Minimal change disease (MCD) presents with heavy proteinuria at the level of nephrotic syndrome, in the absence of glomerular lesions on light microscopy. At the ultrastructural level (electron microscopy), glomerular epithelial cells show alterations of their foot processes, which normally regulate protein permeability. MCD can have multiple etiologies. Among malignancies, Hodgkin lymphoma is the most common. The pathophysiology is incompletely understood but involves dysfunctional podocytes due to cytokine production by infiltrated lymphocytes and macrophages.

Membranoproliferative glomerulonephritis (MPGN) and **membranous glomerulonephritis (MGN)** can be paraneoplastic manifestations of CLL and Hodgkin and non-Hodgkin lymphoma.

Focal segmental glomerulosclerosis (FSGS) presents with proteinuria, nephrotic syndrome, arterial hypertension and progressive renal insufficiency. Glomerular lesions are focal (only some glomeruli are affected) and segmental (portions of the glomeruli are affected), and commonly, tubular atrophy and interstitial fibrosis also occur.

NEUROLOGIC MANIFESTATIONS OF HEMATOLOGIC MALIGNANCIES

Paraneoplastic neurologic syndromes (PNSs) are caused by specific autoimmune responses to antigens produced by tumor cells, which mimic or are identical to antigens normally restricted to neurons. Specific antibodies are present in approximately 60% of patients with paraneoplastic syndromes of the CNS, in both serum and cerebrospinal fluid. If antibodies are not found, the differential diagnosis is extensive, since each of the following disorders can be caused by nonneoplastic conditions such as toxins, infections, vitamin deficiencies and metabolic or autoimmune disorders. Management includes treatment of the tumor and immunosuppression.

Paraneoplastic cerebellar degeneration starts with dizziness, vertigo, ataxia and dysarthria. It is mediated by specific antibodies (anti-Tr, anti-GAD, anti-mGLuR1). Among hematologic malignancies, Hodgkin lymphomas have a higher prevalence.

Limbic encephalitis presents with short-term memory loss, seizures, confusion, sleeping problems, psychiatric symptoms, irritability or depression. Although this condition is more common in nonhematopoietic tumors (non–small cell lung cancer), it may also be seen in lymphomas, both Hodgkin (associated with anti-Tr antibodies) and non-Hodgkin (serum anti-Ma2 antibodies).

Paraneoplastic encephalomyelitis is an immune-mediated inflammatory disorder that presents as a subacute sensory neuronopathy. Specific antibodies described are anti-Hu.

Paraneoplastic involvement of the peripheral nervous system, although rare, can occur in lymphomas. Careful differential diagnosis is important since neuropathies due to direct root infiltration by tumor, amyloid deposition or chemotherapy-induced neuropathy are not infrequent. Clinical manifestations include **chronic inflammatory demyelinating polyradiculopathy (CIDP), sensory-motor neuropathy, Guillain-Barré syndrome, myotonia and inclusion body myositis.**

RHEUMATIC MANIFESTATIONS OF HEMATOLOGIC MALIGNANCIES

Malignant neoplasms are associated with a large variety of paraneoplastic rheumatologic syndromes, and the most common malignancies are carcinomas of the lung, GI tract and prostate. Lymphomas and leukemias are rare players. As with other paraneoplastic disorders, a direct anatomic relationship between the malignant tumor and the sites of manifestation needs to be excluded.

Paraneoplastic polyarthritis, presenting as acute or chronic forms affecting both large and small joints, was described in several cases of B-cell lymphoma and acute leukemias of both lymphoid and myeloid lineage. In most cases, treatment of the underlying malignancy is followed by remission of the rheumatologic disorder.

Dermatomyositis (DM) and **polymyositis (PM)** may constitute paraneoplastic myopathies. They manifest with severe muscle weakness, skin manifestation, respiratory muscle weakness and dysphagia, and their clinical course parallels the course of malignancy. The risk of malignancy associated with DM is very high, while the risk of cancer associated with PM is smaller. DM is more commonly associated with solid tumors (adenocarcinomas of the lung, ovary, uterine cervix, stomach, colon, pancreas) and rarely with lymphoma. Paraneoplastic PM is associated with lymphoma.

Systemic lupus erythematosus is often idiopathic, but can be associated with malignancies. Patients present with fatigue, myalgia, rash and arthritis. Laboratory tests show antibodies including antinuclear antibody (ANA), Sm and double-stranded DNA (dsDNA).

Sjögren syndrome, which clinically presents with keratoconjunctivitis sicca and xerostomia (dryness of eyes and mouth), can be a paraneoplastic manifestation of non-Hodgkin lymphoma or chronic lymphocytic leukemia. In these cases, in addition to serum autoantibodies such as ANA, Ro/SSA and La/SSB, flow cytometry or molecular studies will detect abnormal, clonal B-cell populations.

GENERAL SYMPTOMATOLOGIC MANIFESTATIONS OF HEMATOLOGIC MALIGNANCIES

Paraneoplastic pruritus, defined as itch lasting more than 6 weeks, occurs early during the clinical evidence of malignancy or precedes clinical signs of malignancy by weeks or months. According to some studies, generalized pruritus is caused by malignancy in less than 10% of cases. Lymphoma and leukemia are the most common malignancies. The pathophysiologic mechanisms remain poorly understood.

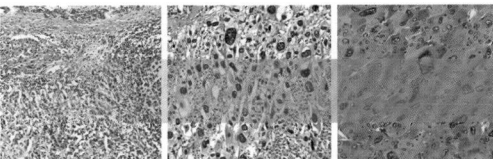

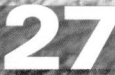

The Endocrine System

Maria J. Merino

The main function of the endocrine system is communication. Although the nervous and endocrine systems use some of the same soluble mediators and sometimes overlap functionally, the endocrine system is unique in its ability to communicate at a distance using soluble mediators, hormones.

The term **hormone** (from the Greek, *horman*, "set in motion") applies to chemicals secreted by "ductless" (i.e., endocrine) glands into the circulation, which carries it to the target organ. Many hormones, such as thyroid hormone, corticosteroids and pituitary hormones, fit this definition. However, some traditionally recognized hormones, such as

Endocrine (e.g., insulin, ACTH, parathyroid hormone)

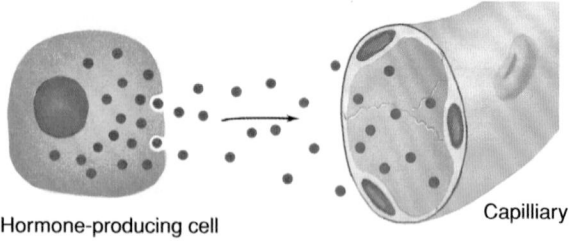

Hormone-producing cell   Capilliary

Paracrine (e.g., somatostatin, bombesin)

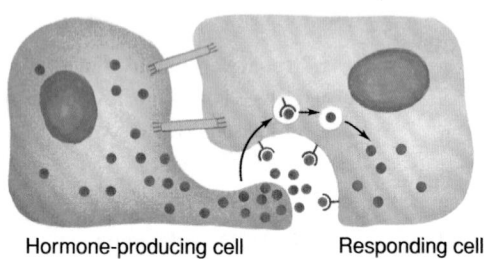

Hormone-producing cell   Responding cell

Synaptic (e.g., acetylcholine, dopamine)

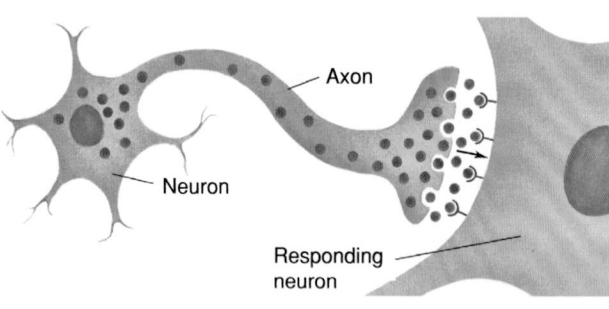

Axon

Neuron

Responding neuron

Neuroendocrine (e.g., vasopressin, epinephrine)

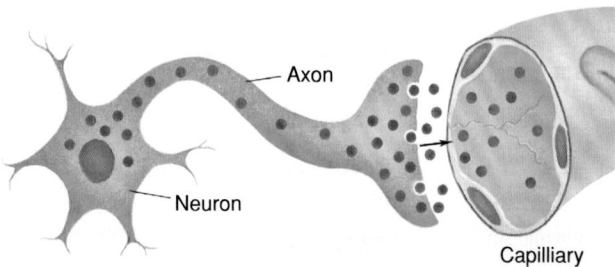

Axon

Neuron

Capilliary

FIGURE 27-1. Mechanisms of chemically mediated cell-to-cell communication. Biological messages may be transmitted by mechanisms other than the classic endocrine pathway via the circulation. These include paracrine, synaptic and neuroendocrine modes of communication.

catecholamines, are produced in multiple sites and may act either locally or through the circulation. Other mediators function only in restricted circulation compartments: hypothalamic hormones only act on the pituitary and reach it via portal tributaries without entering the systemic circulation. Finally, many hormones exert their effects in the very tissues that make them, such as müllerian-inhibiting substance. These diverse chemically mediated cell-to-cell communications are summarized in Fig. 27-1.

To qualify as a hormone, a chemical messenger must bind a receptor, whether on a cell's surface or inside it. Hormones act either on the final effector target or on other glands that in turn produce other hormones. For instance, thyroid-stimulating hormone (TSH) is released by the pituitary and promotes thyroid hormone secretion by the thyroid gland. Thyroid hormone, then, directly affects many types of peripheral cells. Diseases of the endocrine system may entail too little or too much hormone secretion. Target tissue insensitivity may simulate the clinical picture of hormone underproduction.

Pituitary Gland

ANATOMY

The pituitary gland, or the hypophysis, is a small gland that weighs 0.5 g and measures $1.3 \times 0.9 \times 0.5$ cm. It sits at the base of the brain in a bony cavity called the sella turcica, within the sphenoid bone.

Anatomically, it is composed of two lobes. The anterior lobe, or **adenohypophysis,** arises from the ectoderm, makes up 80% of the gland and is populated by epithelial cells. The posterior lobe, or **neurohypophysis,** originates from neuroectoderm as a prolongation of the hypothalamus (Fig. 27-2). The gland is near the optic chiasm and cranial nerves III, IV, V and VI; thus, pituitary enlargement may alter vision or cause palsies by impinging on various cranial nerves.

The anterior lobe develops from **Rathke's pouch,** an endodermal evagination from the developing oral cavity. Along its migration tract, this craniopharyngeal duct may leave intrasphenoidal squamous epithelial rests that may later give rise to tumors known as **craniopharyngiomas.** The neurohypophysis (posterior lobe) begins as a downward projection of the brain and remains connected to the

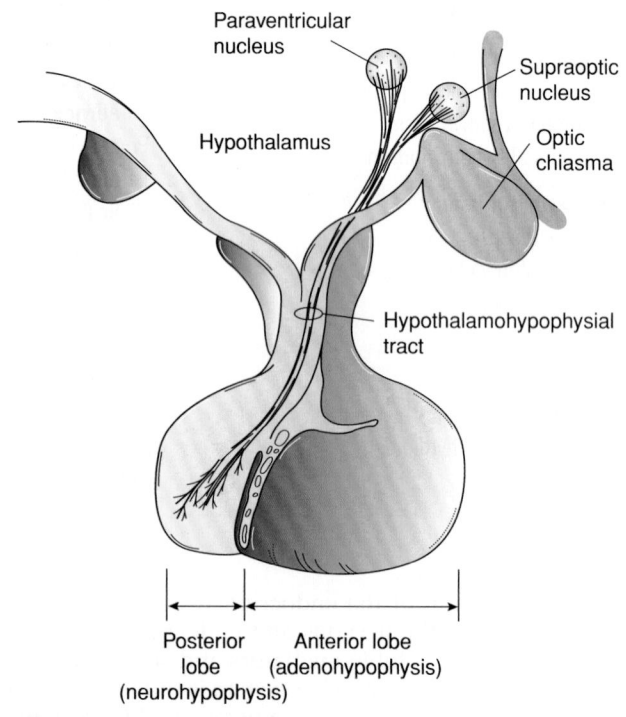

Paraventricular nucleus

Supraoptic nucleus

Hypothalamus

Optic chiasma

Hypothalamohypophysial tract

Posterior lobe (neurohypophysis)   Anterior lobe (adenohypophysis)

FIGURE 27-2. The pituitary gland.

hypothalamus by the hypophyseal stalk. Flanked on either side by the anterior and posterior lobes is a vestigial intermediate lobe, containing a few cystic cavities lined by cuboidal or columnar epithelium and considered as part of the anterior pituitary in humans.

The pituitary has a dual circulation. It has a complex portal system that originates in the hypothalamus, and a separate arterial and venous blood supply. The hypophysial portal system transports stimulatory and inhibitory hypothalamic-releasing hormones to the anterior pituitary. Venous drainage from the pituitary follows the cavernous sinus to both inferior petrosal sinuses.

Axons and unmyelinated nerve fibers from the hypothalamus proceed along the pituitary stalk to the neurohypophysis and are the nerve supply of the posterior lobe. These nerves regulate secretion of **arginine vasopressin (antidiuretic hormone [ADH])** and **oxytocin,** which are made in the hypothalamus, stored in the posterior lobe and later released into the systemic circulation.

The cells of the anterior pituitary are arranged in cords or nests in a highly vascular stroma. These cells were classically divided into two groups of equal number: stainable and unstainable cells, based on their hematoxylin and eosin (H&E) staining properties. The latter cells are **chromophobes** and have minimal to no hormone content. The cytoplasmic granules of stainable cells appeared acidophilic (eosinophilic) (40%), which contain polypeptide hormones, and basophilic (10%), which contain glycoprotein hormones. However, granules' tinctorial properties do not reflect their functions, so this histologic classification has been superseded by a system that identifies cells by the hormones they secrete, as identified by immunochemical staining (Fig. 27-3). The hormone-producing cells in the anterior pituitary are:

- **Corticotrophs:** These basophilic cells secrete **proopiomelanocortin (POMC)** and its derivatives including **adrenocorticotropic hormone (ACTH, corticotropin),** which controls adrenal secretion of **corticosteroids, melanocyte-stimulating hormone (MSH), lipotropic hormone (LPH)** and **endorphins.** In cases of glucocorticoid excess,

corticotrophs may undergo an alteration called Crooke's hyaline change. Basophilic corticotrophs of the **pars intermedia** may cluster and spread deep into the posterior lobe, a phenomenon called "basophil invasion."

- **Lactotrophs:** These acidophilic cells secrete **prolactin,** which is essential for lactation and other metabolic activities.
- **Somatotrophs:** These acidophilic cells produce and secrete growth hormone and constitute half of the hormone-producing cells of the adenohypophysis.
- **Thyrotrophs:** TSH is produced by pale basophilic or amphophilic cells, which make up only 5% of the cells of the anterior lobe.
- **Gonadotrophs: Follicle-stimulating hormone (FSH)** and **luteinizing hormone (LH)** are secreted by the same basophilic cell. FSH stimulates Graafian follicle formation in the ovary. LH induces ovulation and formation of corpora lutea.

The posterior lobe of the pituitary contains **pituicytes,** modified glial cells with no secretory function, axon terminals and unmyelinated nerve fibers containing ADH and oxytocin. Both of these hormones are formed in neurons in the hypothalamus and transported along axons to the neurohypophysis. A rich network of capillaries surrounds the axon terminals and facilitates hormone release into the vasculature. ADH promotes water resorption from distal renal tubules; oxytocin stimulates contraction of the pregnant uterus at term and also of cells around lactiferous ducts in the breasts.

HYPOPITUITARISM

Hypopituitarism is a rare disorder in which the pituitary secretes insufficient amounts of one or more hormones. It has many causes and various clinical presentations. Most often, only one or a few pituitary hormones are deficient. Occasionally **panhypopituitarism** occurs, in which the gland fails totally. The effects of hypopituitarism vary with the extent of the loss, specific hormones involved and age of the patient. In general, symptoms relate to deficient function of the thyroid and adrenal glands and the reproductive system. In children, growth retardation and delayed puberty are additional problems.

PITUITARY TUMORS: Over half of hypopituitarism in adults is caused by pituitary tumors, usually adenomas. The tumor itself may be functional, but symptoms of hypopituitarism often result because the tumor compresses adjacent tissue.

SHEEHAN SYNDROME: In this condition, ischemic necrosis of the pituitary causes panhypopituitarism. It is often caused by severe hypotension from postpartum hemorrhage or, rarely, without massive bleeding or after normal delivery. The pituitary is particularly vulnerable during pregnancy, because of reduced blood flow associated with its enlargement at this time. The result of the damage to the gland is permanent underproduction of essential pituitary hormones (hypopituitarism). Agalactia, amenorrhea, hypothyroidism and adrenocortical insufficiency are important consequences (Fig. 27-4). Treatment of Sheehan syndrome is hormone replacement therapy. This syndrome has become rare in developed countries.

PITUITARY APOPLEXY: Hemorrhage and/or infarction can occur in a normal pituitary, but at least half of cases occur

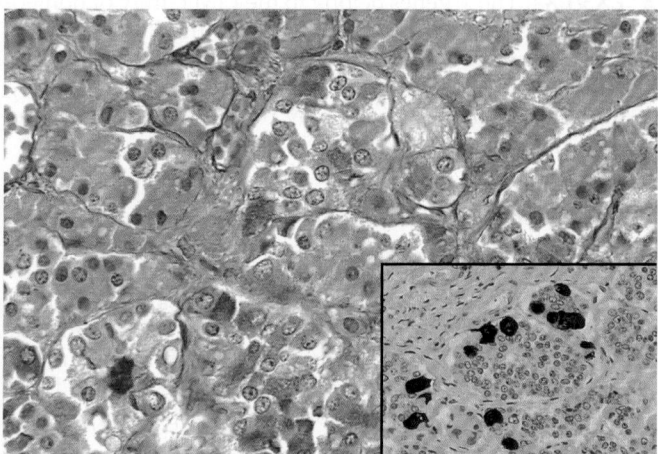

FIGURE 27-3. Normal anterior lobe of pituitary. In a periodic acid–Schiff (PAS)–orange G stain, the cytoplasm of somatotropic and prolactin-secreting cells takes up the orange G stain. Most of the cells with a lavender cytoplasm produce adrenocorticotropic hormone (ACTH) (corticotropes). An immunohistochemical stain (*inset*) demonstrates cells that synthesize growth hormone (somatotropes).

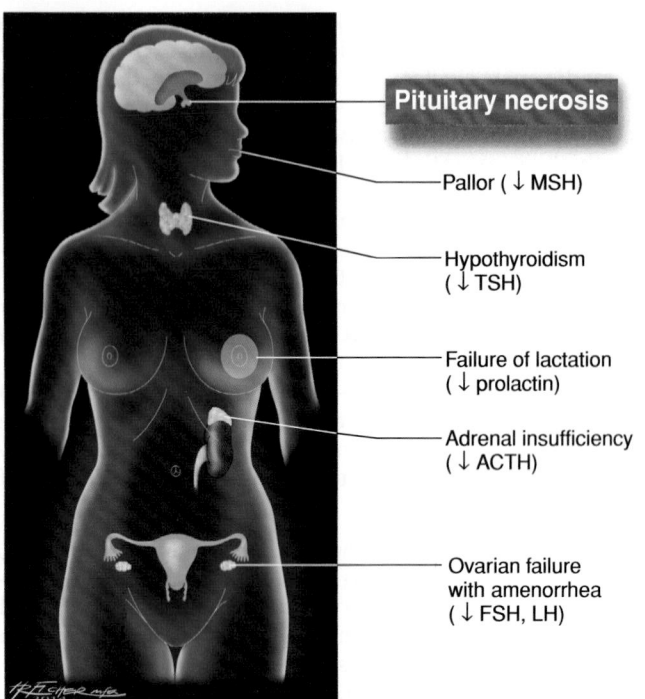

FIGURE 27-4. Major clinical manifestations of panhypopituitarism.
ACTH = adrenocorticotropic hormone; *FSH* = follicle-stimulating hormone;
LH = luteinizing hormone; *MSH* = melanocyte-stimulating hormone; *TSH* =
thyroid-stimulating hormone.

in association with endocrinologically inactive adenomas.
On occasion, pituitary apoplexy leads to hypopituitarism.
The initial symptoms include headaches and associated
visual problems.

IATROGENIC HYPOPITUITARISM: Radiation damage
to the hypothalamic–pituitary axis or neurosurgical procedures may cause neuroendocrine abnormalities, including
hypopituitarism.

TRAUMA: Traumatic brain injury entails significant risk
to the pituitary gland, with potential development of diabetes, hypopituitarism and other endocrinopathies.

INFILTRATIVE DISEASES: Bacterial and viral infections
may lead to inflammation, which can damage the gland.
The process can be primary if only the gland is involved or
secondary if it is associated with an underlying systemic
condition such as fungal or tuberculous infection. Involvement of the hypothalamic–pituitary axis in Langerhans cell
histiocytosis (see Chapter 26) causes endocrine abnormalities including diabetes insipidus in 5%–50% of patients and
panhypopituitarism in 5%–20%. Panhypopituitarism may
occur in hemochromatosis (see Chapter 20), owing to iron
deposition in the pituitary.

**GENETIC ABNORMALITIES OF PITUITARY DEVEL-
OPMENT:** Congenital growth hormone deficiency constitutes a unique group of disorders. It may occur in isolation,
in **isolated growth hormone deficiency** (IGHD), or together
with other pituitary hormone deficiencies. There are 4 types
of familial and sporadic IGHD, differentiated by the severity of the condition, inheritance pattern and causative gene.
Inheritance can be autosomal recessive (AR), autosomal
dominant (AD) or X-linked recessive. Inherited IGHD is
linked to mutations, including deletions, amino acid substitutions and splice site mutations, in the genes for **human
growth hormone** (GH) or growth hormone–releasing hormone (GHRH) receptor. This syndrome is caused by mutations in one of at least three genes. Isolated growth hormone
deficiency types IA and II are caused by mutations in the
GH1 gene. Type IB is caused by mutations in either the *GH1*
or *GHRHR* gene. Type III is caused by mutations in the *BTK*
gene. When no gene is identified as a cause of the disease,
it is called idiopathic. Recombinant GH is the treatment of
choice for children with this disorder.

There are several mutations targeting transcription factors during embryogenesis:

- **Pit-1:** Pit-1 is a POU homeodomain transcription factor
  important for **pituitary** development and expression of
  somatotrophs, lactotrophs and thyrotrophs. It is encoded
  by the *POU1F1* gene on human chromosome 3p11. Mutations in this gene appear to cause combined pituitary hormone deficiency (CPHD) with low levels or absence of
  GH, prolactin (PRL) and TSH.
- **PROP1 (5q):** Prop 1 is a pituitary specific paired-like
  homeo-domain transcription factor. Mutations of *PROP1*
  inactivate LH, FSH, GH, PRL and TSH. This trait is inherited as an autosomal recessive condition.
- **HESX1 (3p21):** This gene is a member of the paired-like
  class of homeobox genes important for optic nerve and
  pituitary development. Its expression begins before that
  of other developmental genes. Mutations of the *HESX1*
  gene occur in patients with septo-optic dysplasia, a
  rare congenital anomaly with midline forebrain abnormalities, optic nerve hypoplasia and hypopituitarism.
  Endocrinopathies are characterized by growth hormone
  deficiency followed by TSH and ACTH deficiency. This
  mutation is also associated with **Pickardt syndrome,** an
  uncommon form of tertiary hypothyroidism caused by
  abnormalities in the portal veins connecting the pituitary
  with the hypothalamus.
- **PITX2:** This gene is expressed in the fetal pituitary and
  in most cells of the adult gland. Mutations are associated
  with **Rieger syndrome,** an autosomal dominant condition with variable phenotypic expression including pituitary abnormalities.
- **LX3/LX4:** These genes belong to the LIM family of homeobox genes that are expressed early in the Rathke pouch.
  LHX3 is on chromosome 9q. Its mutations are associated
  with GH, TSH, LH, FSH and PRL deficiencies. Rarely,
  mutation of the *LX4* gene may present as GH, TSH and
  ACTH deficiency.

**GROWTH HORMONE INSENSITIVITY (LARON
SYNDROME):** *Laron dwarfism is a rare,* autosomal recessive
disorder characterized *by short stature due to extreme resistance to GH because of abnormalities in growth hormone receptor* (GHR). These dwarfs tend to be obese and have high
serum GH levels, but low concentrations of insulin-like
growth factor-I (IGF-I). Laron syndrome occurs mainly in
people of Mediterranean origin, such as Sephardic Jews.
The same lesion is responsible for dwarfism in African
pygmies.

Laron syndrome is caused by more than 30 *GHR* mutations, all of which involve the receptor's extracellular
domain. Clinical presentations are heterogeneous, and most
cases are unique to particular families or geographic areas.
Since GH exerts its effects by promoting IGF-I secretion,
IGF-I is effective replacement therapy for Laron syndrome,
mimicking most effects ascribed to GH itself. It is believed

that patients with this syndrome may have lower incidences of cancer and diabetes (see Chapters 5 and 13).

ISOLATED GONADOTROPIN DEFICIENCY (KALL-MANN SYNDROME): Kallmann syndrome is characterized by hypogonadotropic hypogonadism (due to gonadotropin-releasing hormone [GnRH] deficiency) and anosmia (absent sense of smell). Cleft lip/palate and other anomalies may also be present. Kallmann syndrome is usually diagnosed at puberty because of a delay in the appearance of secondary sex characteristics. It is likely to occur 3–5 times more often in males than females (1:8000). Most cases are sporadic, but there are familial forms, some of which are X-linked, while others are autosomal dominant or recessive. X-linked Kallmann syndrome (KAL1) involves mutations of the *KAL1* gene (Xp23.3), which encodes an extracellular matrix component with putative antiprotease activity and cell adhesion function. As a result, neurons destined to secrete GnRH fail to migrate from their origin in the olfactory anlage to their normal hypothalamic location. The autosomal dominant form of the disease (KAL2) is associated with mutations of the gene encoding fibroblast growth factor receptor 1 (FGFR1, at 8p11). A third form of Kallmann syndrome (KAL3) appears to be autosomal recessive, but the affected gene is unknown.

EMPTY SELLA SYNDROME: This is primarily a radiologic term for an enlarged sella containing a thin, flattened pituitary at the base (Fig. 27-5). It is due to a congenitally defective or absent diaphragma sella, which permits transmission of cerebrospinal fluid pressure into the sella. Empty sella syndrome can cause various degrees of pituitary dysfunction and endocrine abnormalities. It has been linked to both pituitary and nonpituitary causes and can result from pituitary gland regression after an injury, surgery or radiation therapy. Endocrine disturbances include hyperprolactinemia, oligomenorrhea or amenorrhea, frank hypopituitarism, acromegaly, diabetes insipidus and Cushing syndrome.

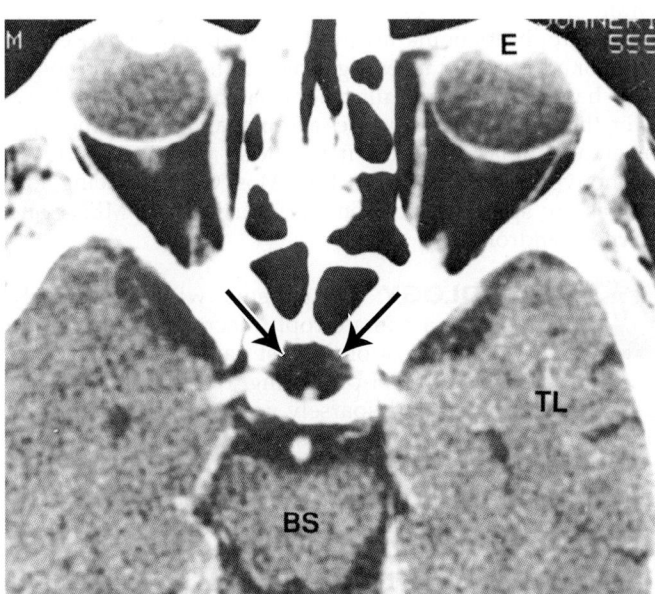

FIGURE 27-5. Empty sella syndrome. A computed tomography (CT) scan of the cranium in an axial section demonstrates an empty sella turcica (*arrows*). *BS* = brainstem; *E* = eye; *TL* = temporal lobe.

Cell Type	Hormone	Frequency (%)
Lactotrope	Prolactin	26
Null cell	None	17
Corticotrope	ACTH (corticotropin)	15
Somatotrope	Growth hormone	14
Plurihormonal	Multiple	13
Gonadotrope	FSH, LH	8
Oncocytoma	None	6
Thyrotrope	TSH	1

TABLE 27-1
FREQUENCY OF ADENOMAS OF THE ANTERIOR PITUITARY

ACTH = adrenocorticotropic hormone; FSH = follicle-stimulating hormone; LH = luteinizing hormone; TSH = thyroid-stimulating hormone.

PITUITARY ADENOMAS

Pituitary adenomas are benign tumors of the anterior lobe of the pituitary. They often cause excess secretion of one or more pituitary hormones and corresponding endocrine hyperfunction (Table 27-1). Pituitary adenomas occur in both sexes. They are more common in adults and rare in children. **PRL-producing adenomas** are the most common hormone-secreting tumors of adults and children. **Gonadotroph adenomas** are more frequent in the elderly. Small, apparently **nonfunctioning pituitary adenomas** are found incidentally in as many as 27% of adult autopsies.

 **ETIOLOGY AND MOLECULAR PATHOGENESIS:** The etiology of pituitary adenomas is obscure, but it is clear that hormonal, environmental and genetic factors are involved. Rarely, they occur in the context of multiple endocrine neoplasia (MEN) type 1, a hereditary syndrome in which patients develop pituitary adenomas, parathyroid hyperplasia or adenoma and islet cell adenomas of the pancreas (see Chapter 21). There is no evidence that *MEN1* mutations are involved in sporadic pituitary tumorigenesis.

Acquired activating mutations in the stimulatory subunit of the G_s protein that activates adenylyl cyclase have been reported in 40% of growth hormone–secreting pituitary adenomas. More specifically, elevation of intracellular cyclic adenosine 3′,5′-monophosphate (cAMP) levels is thought to stimulate hypersecretion of GH and cell proliferation. Some human pituitary tumors express a kinase-containing variant of fibroblast growth factor/receptor (FGFR4), which causes pituitary tumor formation in transgenic mice. Mutations or overexpression of a number of regulatory genes have been described in a number of pituitary adenomas, including *cyclin D₁, CREB, ras* and *pituitary tumor transforming* gene.

Patients with **Carney syndrome** can develop GH- and prolactin-producing pituitary tumors. Other syndromes associated with pituitary tumors include **McCune-Albright** and **familial acromegaly.**

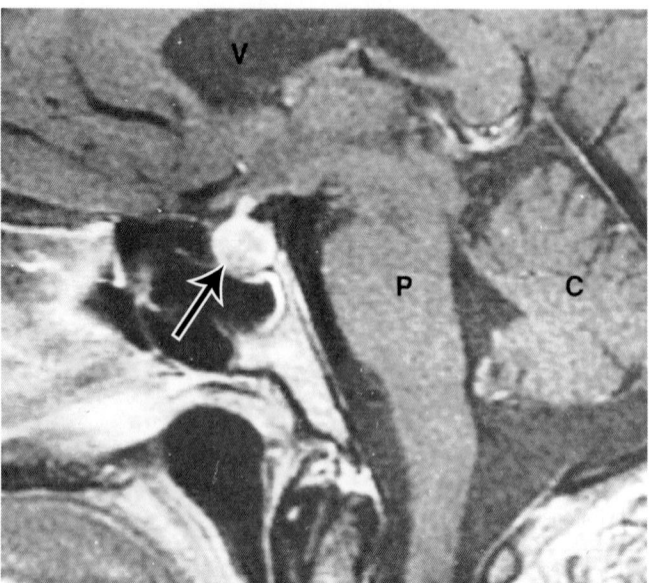

FIGURE 27-6. Pituitary adenoma. A magnetic resonance sagittal view of the brain shows a distinct pituitary tumor (*arrow*). C = cerebellum; P = pons; V = lateral ventricle.

 PATHOLOGY: Pituitary adenomas were traditionally classified as either acidophil, basophil or chromophobe adenomas depending on how constituent cells stained. Acidophil adenomas were associated with overproduction of GH, basophil adenomas with ACTH and chromophobe adenomas with no endocrine hyperfunction. Since H&E staining properties of the tumor cells do not correlate with the type of hormone secreted, pituitary adenomas are now classified by the hormone(s) they produce. The 2004 World Health Organization (WHO) classification of pituitary lesions accounts for histologic, histochemical, immunohistochemical and electron microscopic features.

Pituitary adenomas range from small lesions that do not enlarge the gland to expansive tumors that erode the sella turcica and impinge on adjacent cranial structures (Fig. 27-6). In general, adenomas less than 10 mm are called microadenomas; larger tumors are macroadenomas. Microadenomas are not symptomatic until they secrete hormones. Macroadenomas tend to cause local compression, by virtue of their size, and systemic manifestations, owing to overproduction of hormones.

 CLINICAL FEATURES: In general, symptoms reflect the hormone produced. Pituitary macroadenomas may compress the optic chiasm, causing severe headaches, bitemporal hemianopsia and loss of central vision. Oculomotor palsies occur when a tumor invades the cavernous sinuses. Large adenomas may invade the hypothalamus, interfere with normal hypothalamic input to the pituitary and lead to loss of temperature regulation, hyperphagia and hormonal syndromes. Symptoms of hypopituitarism may be present but difficult to recognize.

Hyperprolactinemia Is the Most Common Endocrinopathy Caused by Pituitary Adenomas

Almost half of pituitary microadenomas contain PRL, but many fewer actually secrete this hormone. PRL-producing tumors are most often symptomatic in young women, but more than half of macroadenomas that secrete PRL are in men. This difference in sex distribution is related to the more frequent occurrence of endocrine symptoms in women. The true incidence in unselected autopsies is similar in both sexes. In general, larger adenomas secrete more PRL. These are the most common pituitary adenomas, comprising 1/4 of the gland's benign tumors. They are mostly in the lateral or posterior parts of the pituitary gland.

 PATHOLOGY: Lactotroph adenomas tend to be chromophobic and contain spheroid nuclei with prominent nucleoli. They are sparsely granulated and may show diffuse or papillary growth patterns. Endocrine amyloid (see Chapter 15) and psammoma bodies (calcospherites) occur but are not pathognomonic. Lactotroph adenomas stain for PRL in a dot-like "Golgi pattern" by immunohistochemistry.

 CLINICAL FEATURES: In women, functional lactotroph adenomas lead to amenorrhea, galactorrhea and infertility. The consistently elevated blood PRL levels inhibit the surge of pituitary LH necessary for ovulation. Men tend to suffer from decreased libido and impotence. Functional lactotroph microadenomas are successfully treated with dopamine agonists (bromocriptine) to inhibit PRL secretion, but macroadenomas may require surgery or radiation therapy. Excess PRL secretion may be caused by factors other than pituitary adenomas, including pregnancy, lactation, administration of certain drugs or pressure on the hypothalamus by other tumors. They can occur in children and adolescents, in whom symptoms depend on the patient's age. Radiologically, they are mostly microadenomas and are frequently part of MEN1. The prognosis of these patients is good.

Somatotrope Adenomas Secrete Growth Hormone

Dramatic changes result from excess GH secretion. A somatotroph adenoma arising before epiphyses close in a child or adolescent causes **gigantism**. After long bone epiphyses have fused and adult height has been attained, however, the same tumor produces **acromegaly**. Most tumors are macroadenomas and cause mass effects and tumor-induced adenohypophyseal hypofunction. Most GH-producing adenomas are sporadic, but some arise as part of MEN1 and Carney syndrome.

PATHOLOGY: Of patients with acromegaly, 75% have a somatotroph macroadenoma within the gland. Most of the rest have microadenomas. Variants of isolated GH-producing tumors include the densely granulated and sparsely granulated somatotroph adenomas. Densely granulated somatotroph adenomas are composed of acidophilic cells with granular cytoplasm and a diffuse growth pattern (Fig. 27-7). They show strong, diffuse immunohistochemical reactivity for GH and low proliferative indices. Acidophilic somatotroph adenomas usually grow slowly and remain within the sella. Sparsely granulated adenomas have small chromophobe cells with characteristic spheroid cytoplasmic inclusions, called "fibrous bodies," that contain keratin intermediate filaments, especially keratin 8. The chromophobic variant tends

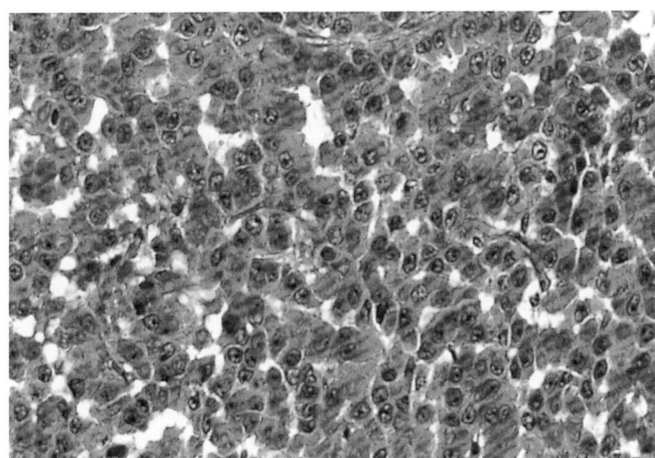

FIGURE 27-7. Pituitary somatotrope adenoma from a man with acromegaly. The tumor cells are arranged in thin cords and ribbons.

to grow faster and to invade. It also shows cellular and nuclear pleomorphism.

In mixed somatotroph–lactotroph adenomas (rare), the two cell types elaborate GH and PRL, respectively. Mammosomatotroph adenomas are monomorphous with a single cell type expressing both GH and PRL. **Acidophil stem cell adenomas** are monomorphous, slightly acidophilic tumors with nuclear pleomorphism and large cytoplasmic vacuoles. Key features include giant mitochondria, keratin 8–positive fibrous bodies and misplaced exocytosis. This subtype is clinically more aggressive.

 CLINICAL FEATURES: Acromegaly is uncommon, with an annual incidence of 3 cases per million. Over many years, patients with acromegaly gradually develop coarse facial features (Fig. 27-8), with overgrowth of the mandible (prognathism) and maxilla, increased space between upper incisor teeth and a thickened nose. Their hands, feet and heads often become enlarged.

Acromegaly has serious complications. Cardiovascular, cerebrovascular and respiratory deaths are increased. Most acromegalics have neurologic and musculoskeletal symptoms, including headaches, paresthesias, arthralgias and muscle weakness. One third have hypertension, and even half of normotensive acromegalics have increased left ventricular mass and are at risk for congestive heart failure. Visceral hypertrophy is common. Diabetes occurs in up to 20%, and hypercalciuria and renal stones develop in another 20%. Half of acromegalics have hyperprolactinemia severe enough to be symptomatic (see above).

Treatment for somatotroph adenomas is usually transsphenoidal hypophysectomy, after which circulating GH levels may decline to normal levels within hours. Radiation therapy is an alternative if surgery is contraindicated. A long-acting analog of somatostatin, an antagonist of GH, is a useful therapeutic adjunct. Most of these tumors are associated with good prognosis.

Corticotrope Adenomas Produce ACTH

ACTH excess induces adrenal cortical hypersecretion, causing **Cushing disease** (see below). In most cases, these

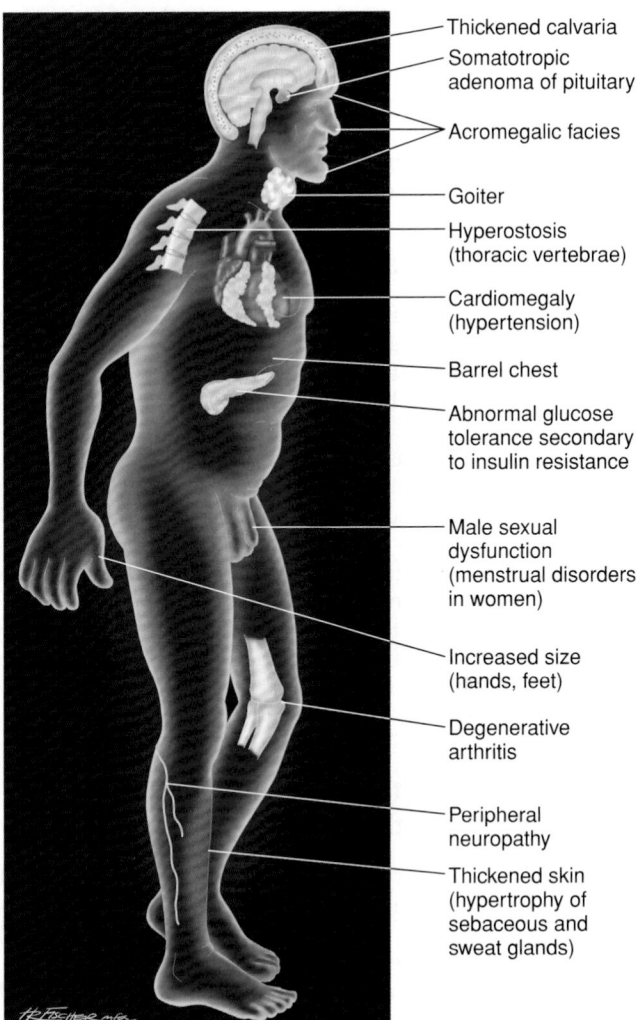

FIGURE 27-8. Clinical manifestations of acromegaly.

tumors are intrasellar microadenomas that are intensely basophilic and periodic acid–Schiff (PAS) positive. Immunohistochemistry shows ACTH and related peptides, such as endorphins and lipotropin. A few functional corticotroph adenomas are chromophobic and more aggressive than their basophilic counterparts and may show pleomorphic features and apoptosis. The proliferative index can be variable.

By electron microscopy, basophilic adenomas contain many secretory granules and perinuclear bundles of fine, keratin-positive, intermediate filaments (type I filaments). These filaments may be abundant enough to be visible by light microscopy as **Crooke hyalinization,** which reflects suppression of ACTH secretion by high levels of circulating cortisol. **Crooke adenomas** represent ACTH-producing tumors with massive cell hyaline deposition.

The prognosis of these patients depends on the severity of the symptoms.

Gonadotrope Adenomas Secrete LH and FSH

Most of these tumors are hormonally inactive macroadenomas and are detected either incidentally or because of local compressive effects due to suprasellar extension. Clinical presentations include headache, visual disturbance and hypopituitarism.

In general, gonadotrope adenomas are chromophobic and PAS negative and grow in a diffuse pattern. They proliferate slowly. Tumor cells are strongly immunopositive for FSH, LH or both. Treatment is surgical resection. Prognosis depends on the results of the surgery.

Thyrotrope Adenomas Produce TSH

These are the rarest of pituitary adenomas. They come to medical attention when there are symptoms of hyperthyroidism, goiter or a pituitary mass lesion. Circulating TSH and thyroid hormone levels are usually elevated, which is unique to this tumor. Thyrotroph adenomas are predominantly macroadenomas and can be invasive and fibrotic. They are chromophobic, with polyhedral or columnar cells that form collars around blood vessels. They stain for α- and β-TSH and tend to have high proliferative indices. By electron microscopy, secretory granules are often arranged in a single row just subjacent to the plasma membrane.

Patients with long-standing hypothyroidism may develop hyperplasia of pituitary thyrotrophs (thyroid deficiency cells), presumably due to inadequate feedback inhibition by thyroid hormones.

Nonfunctional Pituitary Adenomas Do Not Cause Endocrinopathies

One quarter of pituitary tumors removed surgically do not secrete excess hormones. They are slowly growing macroadenomas that occur in older people and come to medical attention because of their mass effect.

Null cell adenomas are usually chromophobic and arise in the adenohypophysis, are PAS negative and grow in a pseudopapillary pattern. Tumor cells are negative or sparsely positive for all anterior pituitary hormones. They are typically immunopositive for chromogranin A and synaptophysin.

Oncocytomas are variants of nonfunctional null cell adenoma, containing enlarged, eosinophilic and often granular cells. They are typically large at presentation and may extend outside the sella. Visual impairment and symptoms of hypopituitarism are common. The neoplastic cells of oncocytomas are packed with mitochondria but are otherwise similar to other null cell adenomas.

Silent adenomas differ from other nonfunctional pituitary adenomas in appearing well differentiated ultrastructurally. They are often immunoreactive for ACTH and other hormones.

PLURIHORMONAL ADENOMAS: These unusual adenomas produce a variety of pituitary hormones. The most frequent combinations include GH, PRL and one or more glycoprotein hormone subunits. The aggressive subtype 3 has a unique ultrastructural profile and expresses PRL and TSH staining.

PITUITARY CARCINOMAS: It is not possible to distinguish between pituitary adenomas and carcinomas on morphologic grounds. Pituitary carcinomas spread to cerebrospinal and/or extracranial sites. When functional, they primarily secrete PRL or ACTH.

Imaging reveals a tumor extending beyond the sella turcica. The tumors are very rare and their prognosis is poor.

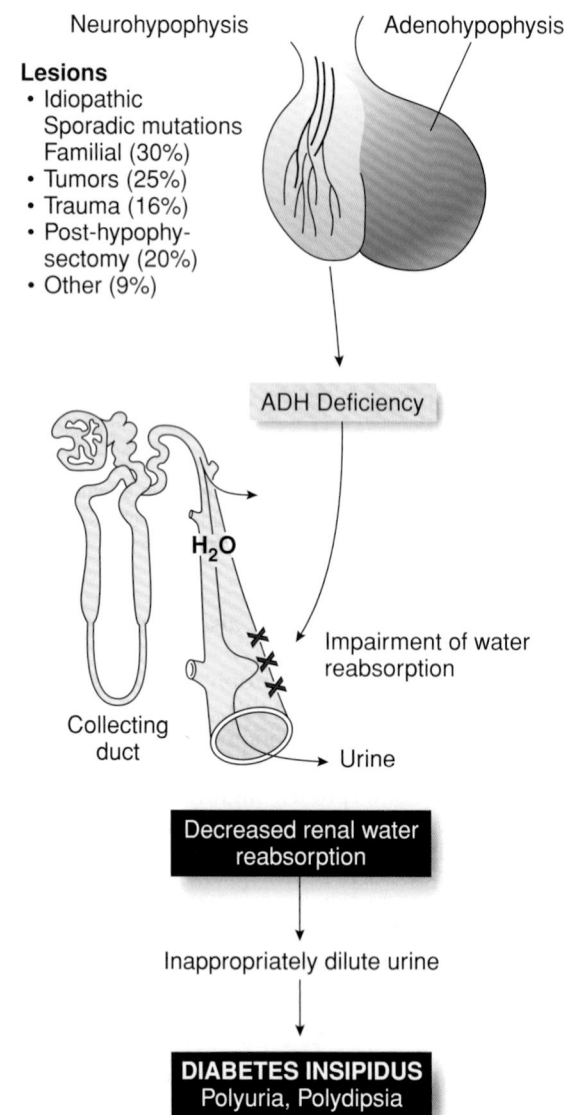

FIGURE 27-9. Mechanism of diabetes insipidus.

POSTERIOR PITUITARY

Central diabetes insipidus (Fig. 27-9) is the only significant disease associated with the posterior pituitary. Affected patients cannot concentrate their urine and so have chronic water diuresis (polyuria), thirst and polydipsia because they lack sufficient ADH (vasopressin). ADH is secreted by the posterior pituitary under the influence of the hypothalamus. One third of cases of central diabetes insipidus are of unknown etiology or can be attributed to sporadic or familial mutations in the vasopressin–neurophysin II gene. Currently, there are over 35 mutations known in familial neurohypophysial diabetes insipidus. Mutations or deletions in the vasopressin V2 receptor (Xq28) and the vasopressin-sensitive aquaporin-2 water channel genes may cause **nephrogenic diabetes insipidus**.

One fourth of cases of central diabetes insipidus are associated with brain tumors, particularly **craniopharyngiomas** (Fig. 27-10; see Chapter 32). These tumors arise above the sella turcica from remnants of the Rathke pouch and invade

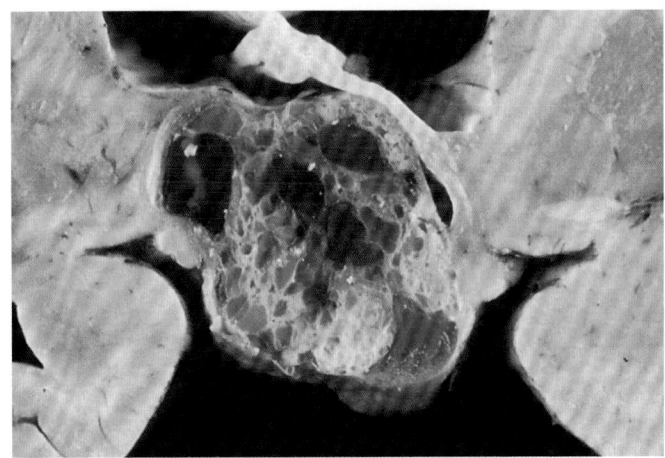

FIGURE 27-10. Craniopharyngioma. Coronal section of the brain shows a large, cystic tumor mass replacing the midline structures in the region of the hypothalamus.

and compress adjacent tissues. Trauma and hypophysectomy for anterior pituitary tumors account for most remaining cases of diabetes insipidus. Less often, localized hemorrhage or infarction, Langerhans cell histiocytosis (see Chapter 26) or granulomatous infiltrates involve the posterior pituitary stalk or body. Polyuria may be controlled by powdered posterior pituitary or vasopressin given as snuff. A syndrome of inappropriate ADH secretion (SIADH) may be caused by paraneoplastic secretion of ADH by tumors (see below).

HYPOTHALAMIC–PITUITARY AXIS

The hypothalamus, pituitary stalk and pituitary gland constitute an anatomically and functionally integrated "neuroendocrine system." Hypothalamic neurons secrete factors that stimulate the anterior pituitary (Table 27-2). Secretion of

TABLE 27-2

HORMONES OF THE HYPOTHALAMIC–PITUITARY–TARGET GLAND AXIS

Hypothalamus	Pituitary	Target Gland	Peripheral Inhibitory Hormone
CRH	ACTH	Adrenal	Corticosteroids
TRH	TSH	Thyroid	T_3, T_4
GHRH	Growth hormone	Varied	IGF-I
Somatostatin	Growth hormone	Varied	IGF-I
LHRH	LH	Gonads	Estradiol, testosterone
	FSH	Gonads	Inhibin, estradiol, testosterone
Dopamine	Prolactin	Breast	Unknown

ACTH = adrenocorticotropic hormone; CRH = corticotropin (ACTH)-releasing hormone; GHRH = growth hormone–releasing hormone; IGF-I = insulin-like growth factor-I; LHRH = luteinizing hormone–releasing hormone; T_3 = triiodothyronine; T_4 = tetraiodothyronine (thyroxine); TRH = thyrotropin-releasing hormone.

these hypothalamic factors is, in turn, antagonized by hormones made in peripheral target organs, thus completing a feedback loop. There are also specific hypothalamic inhibitory hormones. For example, dopamine inhibits pituitary PRL secretion.

The hypothalamus may be damaged by primary and metastatic tumors, viral infections and granulomatous inflammations, as well as degenerative and hereditary disorders. Hypothalamic dysfunction may also occur without an identifiable anatomic abnormality. Diverse conditions result from disturbances of hypothalamic function and include, among others, hypogonadism, precocious puberty, amenorrhea and eating disorders (obesity or anorexia). Some pituitary disorders characterized by increased or decreased hormone secretion have their origin in hypothalamic dysfunction.

Thyroid Gland

ANATOMY

The thyroid is one of the largest endocrine organs. It appears as early as 24 days of fetal development. The primitive thyroid descends to its eventual location in the lower anterior neck by elongation of its tubular attachment to the tongue, the thyroglossal duct, which then atrophies around the 7th week of life. The adult thyroid has two lobes connected by an isthmus and is below the thyroid cartilage anterior to the trachea. Each lobe is about 4 cm in greatest dimension. The gland weighs 25–35 g. Its cut surface has a glistening, light brown, lobulated appearance. In its early development, the gland contains cords of cells that will become the follicles or acini that make up the functional units of the thyroid gland. Follicles average 200 µm and are formed by a single row of cuboidal cells surrounded by a delicate basement membrane. A thyroid lobule contains 20–40 follicles. These are supplied by a lobular artery and sustained by a diffuse mesh of fibrous stroma, lymphatics and connective tissue. Follicles eventually become filled by an eosinophilic, proteinaceous **colloid**. This substance represents secreted thyroglobulin, from which active thyroid hormones are released.

Immunohistochemical staining for thyroglobulin has become a powerful marker to identify follicular cells. Thyroid transcription factor-1 (TTF1) is another marker utilized to identify follicular epithelium.

In addition to follicular epithelial cells, the thyroid also contains **parafollicular** or **C cells** in the lateral aspects of the upper portion of both thyroid lobes, close to the follicles. These cells probably derive from neural crest and are more prominent in children. They produce **calcitonin,** a calcium-lowering hormone, and can also secrete smaller amounts of other peptides such as serotonin and somatostatin. C cells are difficult to identify using routine stains but are readily seen by immunostaining for calcitonin or neuroendocrine markers such as chromogranin and synaptophysin.

THYROID FUNCTION

The main function of the **follicular cells** in the thyroid gland is to make the thyroid hormones **triiodothyronine** (T_3) and tetraiodothyronine (**thyroxine,** T_4). T_4 is principally a prohormone; the major effector of thyroid function is T_3. These molecules are formed by iodination of tyrosines in thyroglobulin by follicular cells. Iodinated thyroglobulin is then secreted into the follicle lumen. Alone among endocrine glands, the thyroid can store a large amount of preformed hormone.

On demand, follicular cells reabsorb thyroglobulin, liberate T_4 and T_3 by proteolytic cleavage and release them into the blood. Most secreted hormone is T_4, which is deiodinated in peripheral tissues to its more active form, T_3. Thyroid hormones in the blood are both free and bound to thyronine-binding globulin (TBG). Peripheral cells take up only free hormone, which binds to nuclear receptors and initiates specific protein synthesis.

Thyroid hormone affects almost all organs. It stimulates basal metabolic rate and metabolism of carbohydrates, lipids and proteins. It increases body heat and hepatic glucose production by increasing gluconeogenesis and glycogenolysis. It promotes synthesis of many structural proteins, enzymes and other hormones. Glucose use, fatty acid synthesis in the liver and adipose tissue lipolysis all increase. In general, thyroid hormone upregulates overall metabolic activities, both anabolic and catabolic.

Thyroid structure and function are mainly governed by pituitary TSH. In turn, thyroid hormone suppresses TSH secretion, to complete a feedback loop. Normal thyroid hormone production requires an adequate dietary supply of iodine.

CONGENITAL ANOMALIES

THYROID AGENESIS: Complete absence of thyroid tissue (athyrosis) is a rare congenital abnormality, usually not discovered until several weeks after birth because maternal thyroid hormone supplies the fetus through the placenta.

ECTOPIC THYROID: Thyroid tissue may occur outside the thyroid gland in several locations, as a result of abnormal migration during development. Such ectopic thyroid tissues are functionally normal and can produce thyroid hormone. Malignant tumors may develop in them.

LATERAL ABERRANT THYROID: This term describes the presence of thyroid tissue located lateral to the jugular veins, but not in lymph nodes. Ectopic thyroid tissue may occur in lymph nodes and soft tissue adjacent to the normal gland. The origin of lateral aberrant thyroid is controversial. Some hold that all of these cases actually represent well-differentiated metastases from occult thyroid cancers; others see them as embryonal rests lateral to the thyroid. If the aberrant thyroid tissue is histologically malignant (see below), then the lesion should be considered a metastasis.

LINGUAL THYROID: If the thyroid fails to descend during embryogenesis, it stays at its origin, as a nodule at the base of the tongue. This happens more in females and usually is found because of difficulty in swallowing, speaking or breathing. Removal may lead to total hypothyroidism. These tissues resemble normal thyroid histologically.

HETEROTOPIC THYROID TISSUE: Nests of thyroid tissue may be found anywhere along the gland's pathway of descent into the lower neck. Thyroid tissue may also occur in the pericardium or mediastinum.

THYROGLOSSAL DUCT CYST: Failure of a thyroglossal duct to involute completely can result in a cystic, fluid-filled remnant anywhere along the duct's route. This condition affects patients in all age groups. It presents as cystic masses of variable size (1–4 cm) often in the middle of the neck and attached to the hyoid bone or soft tissues. The cysts can be lined by squamous or respiratory-type epithelium and contain variable amounts of thyroid tissue. Malignancies can develop in these cysts, usually papillary carcinomas. Surgical excision is curative, and portions of the hyoid bone should be removed to avoid recurrences.

NONTOXIC GOITER

Goiter is thyroid gland enlargement, either nodular or diffuse. It is classified according to its function.

Nontoxic goiter (from the Latin, guttur, *"throat"), also called simple, colloid or multinodular goiter or nodular hyperplasia, is thyroid enlargement without functional, inflammatory or neoplastic changes.* Thus, patients with nontoxic goiter are euthyroid and do not have thyroiditis (see below). The disease is far more common in women than in men (8:1). Diffuse goiter is frequent in adolescence and during pregnancy, while the multinodular type usually occurs in people older than 50 years.

In nontoxic goiter, the capacity of the thyroid to produce thyroid leads to enlargement of the gland, which maintains the euthyroid state.

PATHOPHYSIOLOGY: The cause of the decrease in thyroid hormone production is unknown. However, in some endemic cases decreased hormone production is caused by low iodine content in drinking water. The thyroid gland can enlarge during pregnancy and during the course of inflammatory conditions. Goiters can develop in patients receiving a variety of medications such as sulfonamides or having an excess of iodine intake.

MOLECULAR PATHOGENESIS: Simple nodular thyroid enlargement tends to be familial, suggesting a genetic factor in the disorder. Indeed, mutations in the thyroglobulin gene occur in a number of families who have simple goiter. Linkage analysis studies identified two chromosomal regions (MNG-1 in chromosome 14q, and Xp22) as possible loci for multinodular goiter. These nodules may be either monoclonal or polyclonal. Recently, thyroid-stimulating hormone receptor (*TSHR*) gene D727E has been related to the development of nodular goiter.

PATHOLOGY: Nontoxic goiters range from double the size of a normal gland (40 g) to massive thyroid weighing hundreds of grams (Fig. 27-11).

Diffuse nontoxic goiter characterizes the early stages of the disease. The gland is diffusely enlarged, with hypertrophy and hyperplasia of follicular epithelial cells. On occasion, the epithelium is papillary. At this stage, follicles contain decreased colloid.

Multinodular nontoxic goiter reflects more chronic disease. The enlarged gland becomes increasingly nodular, and the cut surface typically shows many irregular nodules. When these nodules contain large amounts of colloid, the thyroid tends to be soft, glistening and reddish. These

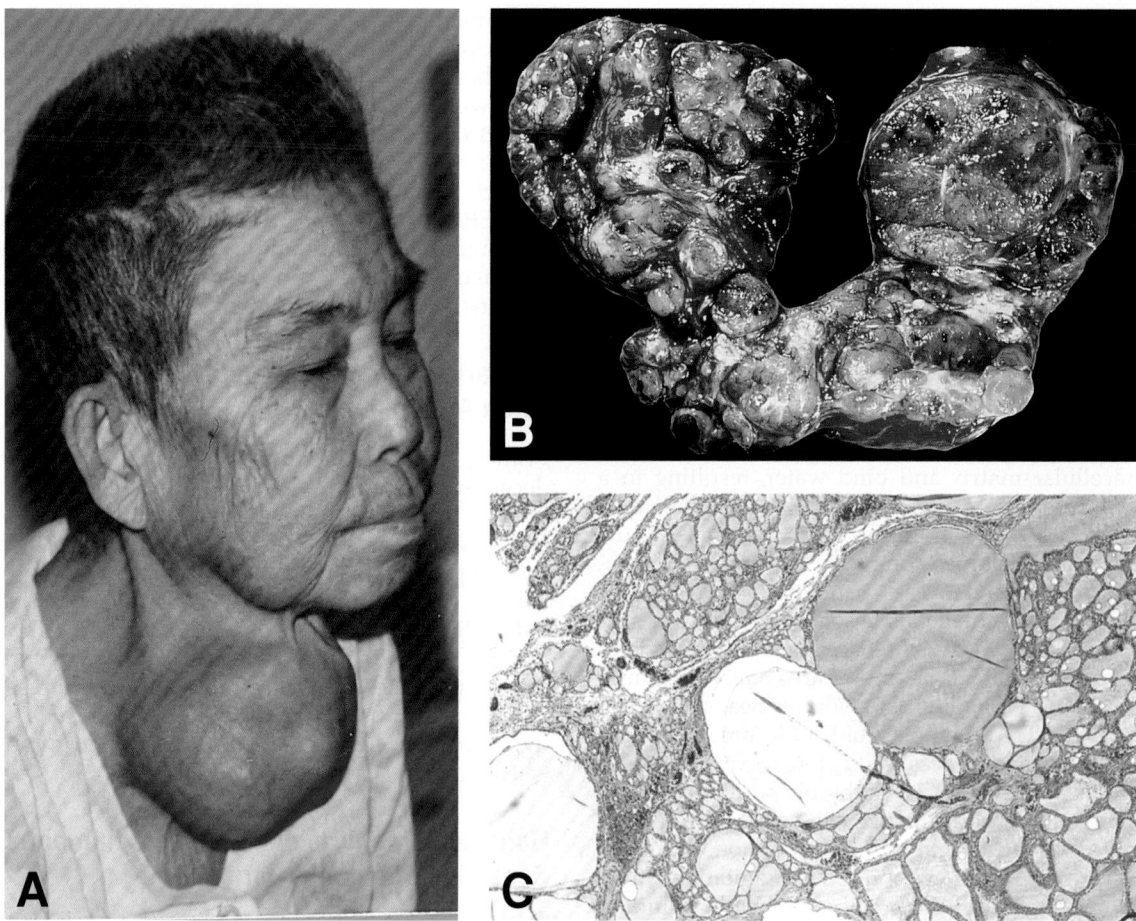

FIGURE 27-11. Nontoxic goiter. A. In a middle-aged woman with nontoxic goiter, the thyroid has enlarged to produce a conspicuous neck mass. **B.** Coronal section of the enlarged thyroid gland shows numerous irregular nodules, some with cystic and old hemorrhage. **C.** Microscopic view of one of the macroscopic nodules shows marked variation in the size of the follicles.

nodules vary considerably in size and shape. Some are distended with colloid; others are collapsed. Large colloid-containing follicles may fuse to form even larger "colloid cysts." Lining epithelial cells are flat to cuboidal and are occasionally arrayed as papillae that project into the follicular lumen. Hemosiderin deposition and cholesterol granulomas are evidence of old hemorrhage. Individual follicles or groups of follicles are separated by dense fibrosis and dystrophic calcifications. Hemorrhage and chronic inflammation are common.

 CLINICAL FEATURES: Patients with nontoxic goiter are typically asymptomatic and come to medical attention because of a mass in the neck. Large goiters may compress structures in the neck. Thus, they may cause dysphagia (esophagus), inspiratory stridor (trachea), venous congestion of the head and face (neck veins) or hoarseness (recurrent laryngeal nerve). Hemorrhage into a nodule or cyst leads to local pain. Patients are euthyroid: blood T_4, T_3 and (usually) TSH are normal.

Nontoxic goiters are most commonly treated with thyroid hormone to reduce TSH levels and, thus, the stimulus to thyroid growth. Older patients often have low TSH levels, so further suppression by exogenous thyroid hormone may be ineffective. In them, radioactive iodine therapy is indicated. Surgery is ordinarily contraindicated but may be necessary

if local obstructive symptoms become troublesome. Many patients with nontoxic goiter eventually develop hyperthyroidism, in which case the term **toxic multinodular goiter** is applied (see below).

HYPOTHYROIDISM

Hypothyroidism is the clinical manifestations of thyroid hormone deficiency. It can be the consequence of three general processes:

- **Defective thyroid hormone synthesis,** with compensatory goitrogenesis (goitrous hypothyroidism)
- **Inadequate thyroid parenchyma function,** usually due to thyroiditis, surgical resection of the gland or therapeutic radioiodine administration
- **Inadequate secretion of TSH** by the pituitary or of thyroid-releasing hormone (TRH) by the hypothalamus

Other causes include pregnancy (postpartum thyroiditis), congenital conditions and certain medications such as lithium.

 **MOLECULAR PATHOGENESIS:** Defects in thyroidal H_2O_2 generation have been identified in some patients with congenital hypothyroidism.

These include loss-of-function mutations in *DUOX2* and *DUOXA2* genes. Also, cloning of the *NIS* gene has allowed examination of the molecular basis of congenital hypothyroidism due to iodide transport defect (ITD). Inactivation of Kif3a leads to altered G-protein–coupled receptor expression, which may also cause hypothyroidism.

 CLINICAL FEATURES: Symptoms of hypothyroidism reflect decreased circulating thyroid hormone (Fig. 27-12). They develop insidiously. Often the first manifestations are tiredness, lethargy, sensitivity to cold and inability to concentrate. Many organ systems are affected, but all are hypofunctional. Hypothyroidism is treated effectively with thyroid hormone.

SKIN: Cutaneous signs are almost universal in patients with clinical hypothyroidism. Proteoglycans accumulate in the extracellular matrix and bind water, resulting in a peculiar form of edema called **myxedema**. Myxedematous patients have boggy facies, puffy eyelids, edema of the hands and feet and enlarged tongues. Thickening of laryngeal mucous membranes causes patients to be hoarse. A pale, cool skin reflects cutaneous vasoconstriction. The skin is also dry and coarse, because sebaceous and sweat gland secretions are inadequate. Ecchymoses are common because of increased capillary fragility. Skin wounds heal slowly.

NERVOUS SYSTEM: Hypothyroidism in pregnancy has grave neurologic consequences for the fetus, expressed after birth as cretinism (see below). Hypothyroid adults are lethargic and somnolent and show memory loss and slowed mental processes. Psychiatric symptoms are common, including paranoid ideation and depression. Severe agitation, **myxedema madness,** may develop. Sensory defects, including deafness and night blindness, occur. Cerebellar ataxia may appear and tendon reflexes are slow. The brain shows mucinous accumulations in nerve fibers and in the cerebellum.

HEART: In early hypothyroidism, heart rate and stroke volume are reduced, resulting in decreased cardiac output.

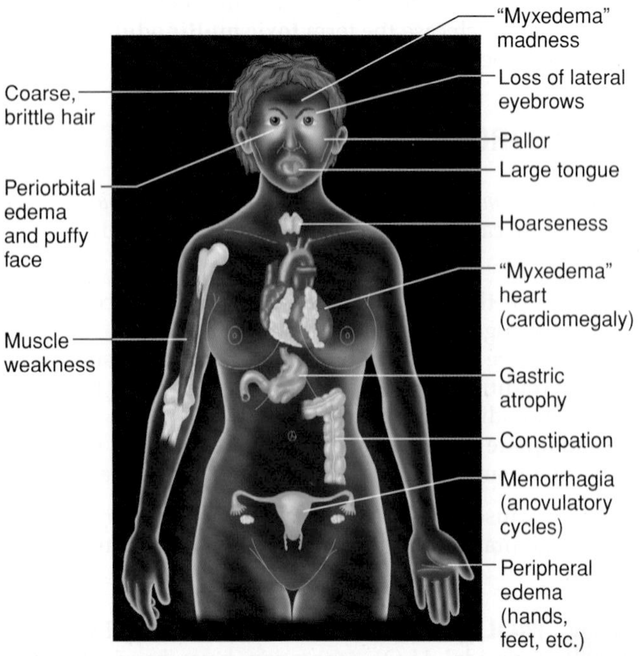

In untreated hypothyroidism, so-called **myxedema heart** develops, with cardiac dilatation and pericardial effusion. Such hearts are flabby and show interstitial edema and myocyte swelling. Coronary atherosclerosis is common.

GASTROINTESTINAL (GI) TRACT: Constipation, due to decreased peristalsis, is common and may be severe enough to lead to fecal impaction (**myxedema megacolon**).

REPRODUCTIVE SYSTEM: Women with hypothyroidism suffer ovulatory failure, progesterone deficiency and irregular and excessive menstrual bleeding. In men, erectile dysfunction and oligospermia are common.

Primary (Idiopathic) Hypothyroidism Is Often Autoimmune

Primary hypothyroidism is most common in the 5th and 6th decades. Like most thyroid disorders, it is more common in women than in men. Circulating antibodies to thyroid antigens are present in 75% of patients, suggesting that these cases represent an end stage of autoimmune thyroiditis (see below). Nongoitrous hypothyroidism may also result from antibodies that block TSH or TSH receptor without activating the thyroid. Some cases of primary hypothyroidism are part of the **multiglandular autoimmune syndrome,** including insulin-dependent diabetes, pernicious anemia, hypoparathyroidism, adrenal atrophy and hypogonadism (see below).

Goitrous Hypothyroidism Reflects Inadequate Secretion of Thyroid Hormone

There are a number of conditions in which thyroid enlargement (goiter) accompanies hypothyroidism. The etiology of goitrous hypothyroidism includes iodine deficiency, antithyroid agents (drugs or dietary goitrogens), long-term iodide intake and various hereditary defects in thyroid hormone synthesis. *The evolution of the pathology of goitrous hypothyroidism is like that described above for nontoxic goiter.*

Endemic Goiter

Endemic goiter is goitrous hypothyroidism due to dietary iodine deficiency in areas with a high prevalence of the disease. Salt water and seafood are rich sources of iodides. Thus, goiters are (or were) common far inland—for example, the Great Lakes area of the United States, alpine Europe, central Africa, parts of China and the Himalayas. The availability of iodized salt has eliminated endemic goiter in many areas. Still, over 200 million people worldwide have endemic goiters.

Pathologic evolution of endemic goiter is like that of nontoxic goiter (see above). However, unlike the latter, endemic goiter rarely causes hyperthyroidism. Iodine treatment may reverse the early, diffuse stage of endemic goiter but has little effect on a fully developed multinodular goiter. Replacement therapy with thyroid hormone is indicated. Local symptoms may necessitate surgical resection.

Goiter Induced by Antithyroid Agents

A number of drugs and naturally occurring chemicals in foods suppress thyroid hormone synthesis and so are goitrogenic. Such goiters may or may not be associated with hypothyroidism. Common goitrogenic drugs include **lithium,**

Coarse, brittle hair

Periorbital edema and puffy face

Muscle weakness

"Myxedema" madness

Loss of lateral eyebrows

Pallor

Large tongue

Hoarseness

"Myxedema" heart (cardiomegaly)

Gastric atrophy

Constipation

Menorrhagia (anovulatory cycles)

Peripheral edema (hands, feet, etc.)

FIGURE 27-12. Dominant clinical manifestations of hypothyroidism.

which is used to manage manic depressive states; phenylbutazone; and *p*-aminosalicylic acid. Certain cruciferous vegetables (turnips, rutabaga, cassava) contain goitrogens and can potentiate an iodine-deficient diet to produce goitrous hypothyroidism.

Iodide-Induced Goiter

Goiter and/or hypothyroidism may occur in people who consume large amounts of iodide, either as a medicinal component (potassium iodide–containing expectorants) or in foods rich in it (e.g., seaweed in Japan). In most cases, iodide-induced goiter develops in the context of preexisting thyroid disease, such as thyroiditis. Women given large doses of iodine during pregnancy may deliver goitrous infants.

Congenital Hypothyroidism Is Also Called Cretinism

Cretinism may be endemic, sporadic or familial and occurs twice as often in girls as boys. In nonendemic regions, 90% of cases result from developmental defects of the thyroid (**thyroid dysgenesis**). The remainder mainly reflect inherited metabolic defects, including mutations in genes for TRH and its receptor, TSH and its receptor, sodium–iodide symporter, thyroglobulin and thyroid oxidase.

 CLINICAL FEATURES: Symptoms of congenital hypothyroidism start in the early weeks of life. Infants are apathetic and sluggish. Their abdomens are large and often show umbilical hernias. Body temperatures are often below 35°C (95°F), and the skin is pale and cold. Refractory anemia and dilated hearts are common. By 6 months, the clinical syndrome of congenital hypothyroidism is well developed. Mental retardation, stunted growth (due to defective osseous maturation) and characteristic facies are evident. Serum T_4 and T_3 are low and TSH levels are high (unless the problem involves defective TSH secretion).

Prompt thyroid hormone replacement therapy is needed to prevent mental retardation and stunted growth. Although treatment may prevent dwarfism, its effects on mental development are more variable. Children in whom hypothyroidism is detected early with neonatal screening respond well to thyroid hormone treatment and are apparently normal mentally. Delayed treatment leads to irreversible brain damage.

Endemic cretinism is congenital hypothyroidism in areas of endemic goiter. Both parents are usually goitrous. The disease encompasses two overlapping clinical presentations, a neurologic syndrome and a predominantly hypothyroid one.

- **Neurologic cretinism** features mental retardation, ataxia, spasticity and deaf-mutism. In the pure form of neurologic cretinism, children may be of normal stature and virtually euthyroid. Iodine deficiency in the first trimester of pregnancy may damage a developing nervous system (see Chapter 12) independently of its effect on thyroid hormone production.
- **Hypothyroid cretinism** is thought to arise from iodine deficiency in late fetal life and in the neonatal period. The clinical course in these children is similar to that of other forms of congenital hypothyroidism.

Treatment is aimed at replacing the lacking thyroid hormone. Levothyroxine is the most common medication used.

HYPERTHYROIDISM

Hyperthyroidism is the clinical syndrome of excessive circulating thyroid hormone. In general, signs and symptoms of hyperthyroidism reflect a hypermetabolic state of target tissues. Prolonged hypersecretion of thyroid hormone can result from abnormal thyroid stimulator (Graves disease), intrinsic thyroid disease (toxic multinodular goiter or functional adenoma) and excess TSH production by a pituitary adenoma (rare).

Graves Disease Is the Most Common Cause of Hyperthyroidism in Young Adults

Also known as diffuse toxic goiter and **Basedow disease** in continental Europe, Graves disease is an autoimmune disease characterized by diffuse goiter, hyperthyroidism, exophthalmos (Fig. 27-13), tachycardia, weight loss and dermopathy. It is the most prevalent autoimmune disease in the United States, affecting 0.5%–1% of the population under age 40. Graves disease can also affect children.

 PATHOPHYSIOLOGY: The cause of Graves disease is not fully understood and seems to involve an interplay between immune mechanisms, heredity, sex and possibly emotional factors.

IMMUNE MECHANISMS: Patients have immunoglobulin G (IgG) antibodies that bind to specific domains of the plasma membrane TSH receptor (Fig. 27-14). These antibodies act as agonists; that is, they stimulate the TSH receptor and activate adenylyl cyclase, increasing thyroid hormone secretion. Under such continued stimulation, the thyroid becomes diffusely hyperplastic and highly vascular.

Elaboration of thyroid-stimulating antibodies requires thyroid-specific helper (CD4$^+$) T cells that recognize multiple

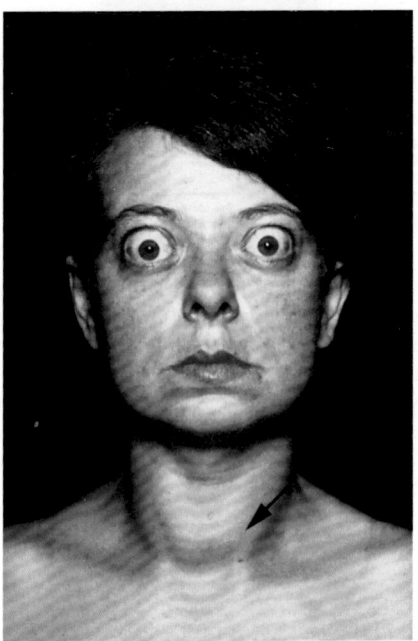

FIGURE 27-13. **Graves disease.** A young woman with hyperthyroidism displays a mass in the neck and exophthalmos.

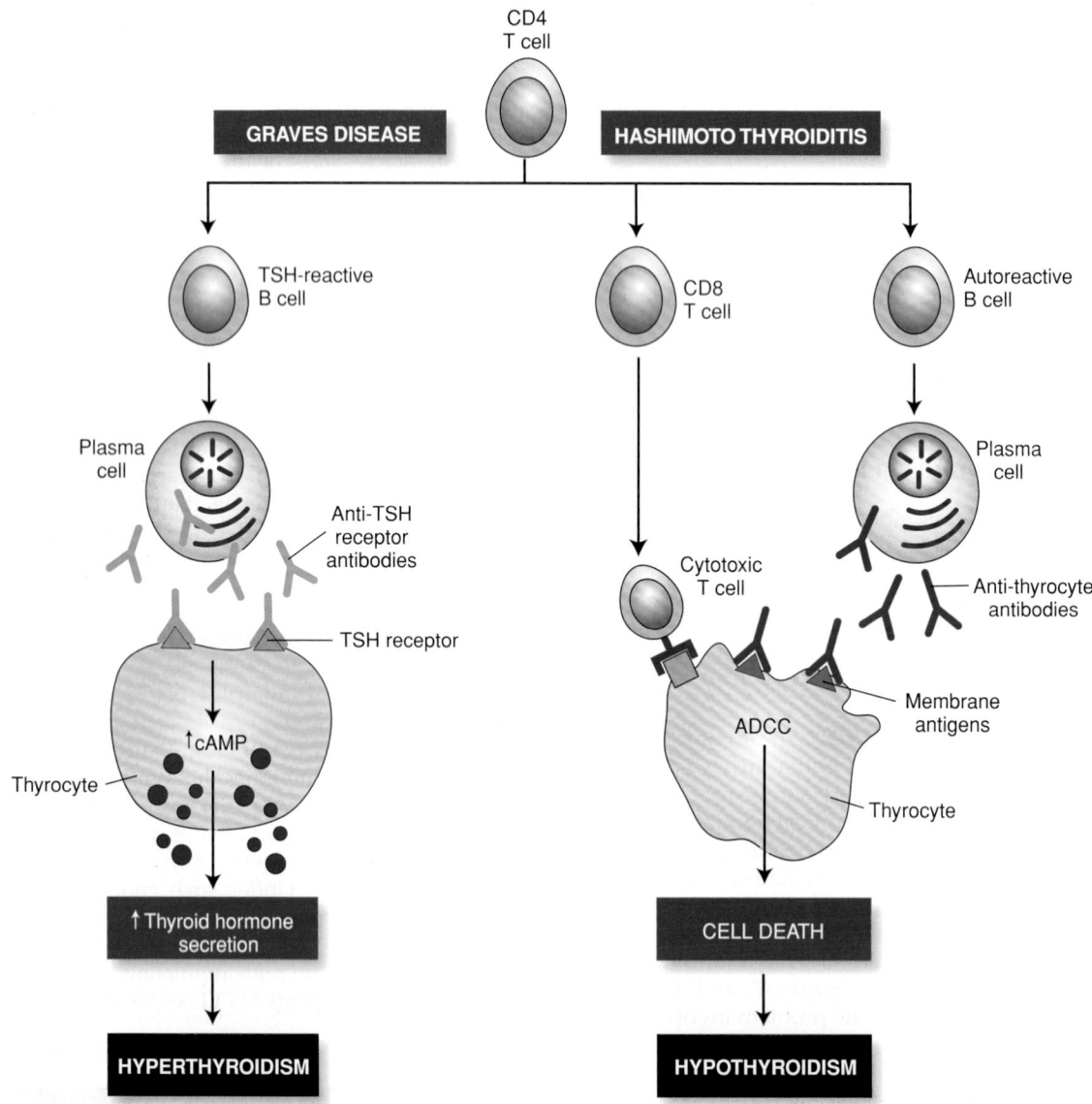

FIGURE 27-14. Immune mechanisms of Graves disease and Hashimoto thyroiditis. CD4$^+$ T cells stimulate antibody production by autoreactive B cells. Anti–thyroid-stimulating hormone (TSH) receptor antibodies stimulate thyroid hormone synthesis in Graves disease. Antibodies induce thyrocyte cell death in Hashimoto thyroiditis by complement-dependent cytotoxicity and antibody-dependent cell-mediated cytotoxicity (ADCC). Thyrocyte death also results from attack by CD8$^+$ (cytotoxic) T cells. *cAMP* = cyclic adenosine 3′,5′-monophosphate.

TSH receptor epitopes and stimulate autoreactive B cells. These then produce thyroid-stimulating immunoglobulins.

Graves autoantibodies are heterogeneous, and those that stimulate thyroid hormone secretion are only one component. Other antibodies seem to be cytotoxic and may cause the thyroid failure that often follows long-standing Graves disease. These include antibodies against thyroglobulin, thyroid peroxidase and the sodium–iodide symporter, all of which may also play roles in the pathogenesis of chronic lymphocytic thyroiditis (Hashimoto disease; see below). Patients with Graves disease have decreased levels of suppressor CD8$^+$ cells, which may play a role in the lack of immune tolerance.

SEX: Like other autoimmune diseases, Graves disease is far more common (7–10-fold) in women than in men.

It tends to arise during periods of hormonal imbalance, including puberty, pregnancy and menopause. Men with Graves disease are usually older, and although the degree of thyroid hyperfunction is often greater in men than in women, symptoms tend to be less severe in men.

EMOTIONAL INFLUENCES: Endocrinologists have long observed that onset of Graves disease often follows a period of emotional stress, such as separation anxiety, death of a loved one or injury in an accident. Quantitative data are lacking.

SMOKING: Smoking increases risk of Graves disease, and particularly the severity of the eye disease in patients who develop ophthalmopathy.

OPHTHALMOPATHY: Exophthalmos (protrusion of eyeballs) is a common feature of Graves disease (Fig. 27-13), but its occurrence and severity correlate poorly with levels of thyroid hormone. A combination of humoral and cell-mediated immune mechanisms is probably involved. T lymphocytes sensitized to antigens shared by thyroid follicular cells and orbital fibroblasts (possibly TSH receptor) accumulate around the eye, where they secrete cytokines that activate fibroblasts. There is also evidence for systemic or local production of antibodies that stimulate orbital fibroblasts to proliferate and produce collagen and glycosaminoglycans.

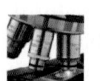 **MOLECULAR PATHOGENESIS:** The strongest risk factor for Graves disease is a positive family history. No single gene is responsible or is necessary for Graves disease: the concordance rate in monozygotic twins is only 30%–50%, while in dizygotic twins it is merely 5%. Thus, both genetic and environmental factors are probably involved. With respect to the genetic contribution, human leukocyte antigen (HLA) class II molecules exposed on thyrocytes (e.g., HLA-DR3, HLA-DQA1) have been established as susceptibility loci, with a number of loci carrying a relative risk of Graves disease of up to 4. Graves disease is also associated with polymorphism of cytotoxic T-lymphocyte antigen-4 (CTLA-4) on chromosome 2q33, which indicates the importance of autoreactive T cells. Patients with Graves disease and their relatives have a much higher incidence of other autoimmune diseases (e.g., pernicious anemia and Hashimoto thyroiditis). Asymptomatic, first-degree relatives of these patients may also show increased ^{131}I uptake. White patients with Graves disease more often express HLA-B8 and HLA-DR3, while Chinese patients are more likely to be positive for HLA-Bw46, and Japanese ones for HLA-Bw35.

A new polymorphic gene family is called the major histocompatibility complex class I chain-related gene A (MICA). The genotype MICA A5 may be regarded as a risk factor for Graves disease. The genotype MICA A6/A9 may prevent the disease.

A cluster of single nucleotide polymorphism (SNPs) occurring at Xq21.1 suggest the possibility of an X-linked risk locus for Graves disease.

 PATHOLOGY: The thyroid is symmetrically enlarged, usually 35–100 g. Cut surfaces are firm and dark red. The tan translucence of normal thyroid, which is due to stored colloid, is notably absent. There are diffuse follicular hyperplasia and increased vascularity. Thyroid epithelial cells are tall and columnar and array themselves on papillae that project into the lumens of the follicles but lack fibrovascular cores. This papillary proliferation may be misdiagnosed as papillary carcinoma. However, the nucleus is hyperchromatic—and not clear as it is in cancer (see below). Thyroid colloid tends to be depleted and appears pale, scalloped or "moth-eaten" where it abuts the epithelial cells (Fig. 27-15). Scattered B and T lymphocytes and plasma cells infiltrate the interstitial tissue, and B cells may even form germinal follicles. T cells predominate, however. Hyperplastic follicles may occur outside the gland's capsule and in adjacent muscle.

Therapy with antithyroid medication (e.g., methimazole or propylthiouracil) commonly results in increased thyroid hyperplasia and complete lack of colloid.

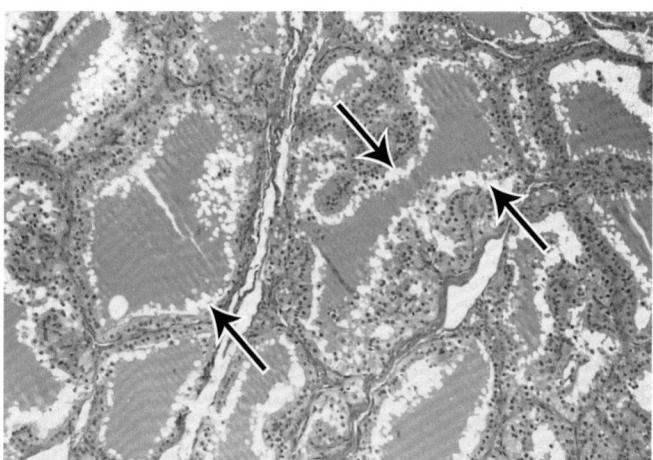

FIGURE 27-15. Graves disease. The follicles are lined by hyperplastic, tall columnar cells. Colloid is pink and scalloped at the periphery adjacent to the follicular cells.

Exophthalmos is caused by enlargement of orbital extraocular muscles. These muscles themselves are normal but are swollen by mucinous edema, accumulation of fibroblasts and lymphocyte infiltration. The increased orbital contents displace the eye forward **(proptosis)**.

The skin shows deposition of acid mucopolysaccharides in the dermis.

CLINICAL FEATURES: Patients with Graves disease note gradual onset of nonspecific symptoms, such as nervousness, emotional lability, tremor, weakness and weight loss (Fig. 27-16). They tolerate heat poorly, seek cooler environments, tend to sweat profusely and may report palpitations. Excess thyroid hormone reduces systemic vascular resistance, enhances cardiac contractility and increases heart rate. In patients with preexisting heart disease, congestive heart failure may ensue.

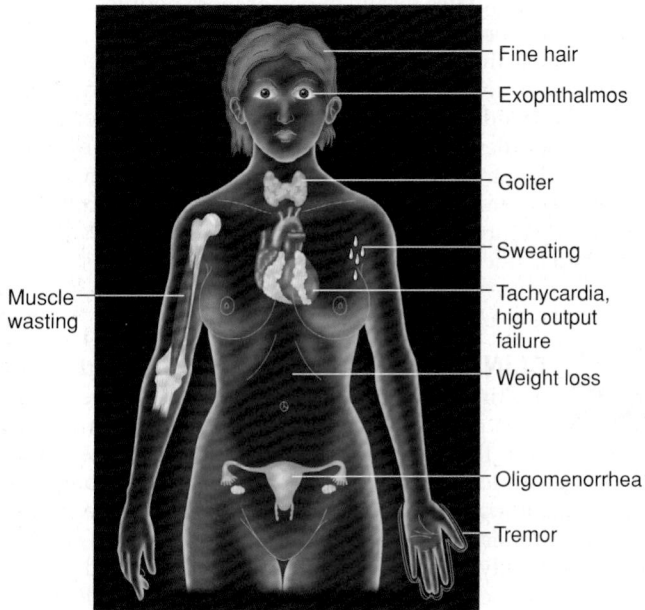

FIGURE 27-16. Major clinical manifestations of Graves disease.

Women develop oligomenorrhea, which may progress to amenorrhea.

They have symmetrically enlarged thyroids, often with an audible bruit and a palpable thrill. Proptosis and retraction of the eyelids expose the sclera above the superior margin of the limbus. The skin is warm and moist. Some patients show **Graves dermopathy,** a peculiar pretibial edema caused by accumulation of fluid and glycosaminoglycans. The diagnosis is confirmed by increased thyroid radioactive iodine uptake and elevated serum of T_4 and T_3. Serum TSH is very low.

The clinical course is characterized by exacerbations and remissions. Untreated, hyperthyroidism may eventually lead to progressive thyroid failure and hypothyroidism. Treatment depends on many individual factors and includes antithyroid medication such as thioisocyanate, destruction of thyroid tissue with radioactive iodine and adjunctive therapy with corticosteroids and adrenergic antagonists. Surgical ablation is uncommon. Unfortunately, even if hyperthyroidism is relieved, exophthalmos often persists and may even worsen.

Toxic Multinodular Goiter Results from Functionally Autonomous Thyroid Nodules

Many patients with nontoxic multinodular goiter, usually over the age of 50, eventually develop a toxic form of the disease. Toxic goiter is more common in women (10:1).

  PATHOPHYSIOLOGY AND PATHOLOGY: The mechanisms by which nontoxic multinodular goiter assumes functional autonomy are not clear, but there are two patterns. In some patients, iodine uptake is diffuse and not affected by administration of thyroid hormone. In them, the thyroid shows groups of small hyperplastic follicles mixed with other nodules of varying size that appear to be inactive. In the second pattern, radiolabeled iodine accumulates focally in one or more nodules. These hyperfunctional nodules suppress the rest of the gland. Exogenous thyroid hormone produces no further suppression of iodine uptake, although previously inactive areas respond to TSH by sequestering iodine. The functional nodules show large hyperplastic follicles resembling adenomas and clearly distinct from the inactive areas. The functional nodules are not neoplastic, but the clinical picture is like that of a normal thyroid with a single hyperfunctioning adenoma.

 CLINICAL FEATURES: Patients with toxic multinodular goiter often have less severe symptoms of hyperthyroidism than those with Graves disease, and they do not develop exophthalmos. Since patients with toxic goiter tend to be older, cardiac complications, including atrial fibrillation and congestive heart failure, may dominate the clinical presentation. Serum T_4 and T_3 levels are only minimally high, and radiolabeled iodine uptake may be normal or only slightly elevated. Radiolabeled iodine after a course of antithyroid therapy is the most common therapy.

Toxic Adenoma Is a Functional Neoplasm

Toxic adenoma is a solitary, hyperfunctioning, benign follicular tumor in an otherwise normal thyroid. It is an uncommon cause of hyperthyroidism. Such tumors display autonomous function independent of TSH and are not suppressed by exogenous thyroid hormone. A toxic adenoma eventually suppresses the rest of the thyroid, which then atrophies. ^{131}I scintiscans show a solitary focus of iodine uptake ("hot nodule") in a background of minimal uptake. Many, but not all, toxic adenomas have a variety of somatic activating mutations of the TSH receptor gene, leading to constitutive upregulation of the cAMP cascade and less commonly the inositol phosphate–diacylglycerol system.

 CLINICAL FEATURES: Toxic thyroid adenoma is most common in the 4th and 5th decades. Symptoms of hyperthyroidism usually begin when the adenoma is about 3 cm. Spontaneous necrosis and hemorrhage within an adenoma may relieve the hyperthyroidism. In that event, the rest of the gland resumes its normal function and the adenoma becomes a "cold" nodule simulating thyroid cancer in a scintigram.

Since the normal thyroid tissue is suppressed, toxic adenomas are treated effectively with radiolabeled iodine. Large nodules may be excised surgically, especially in young patients to minimize risk of thyroid cancer that may occur many years after radiolabeled iodine administration.

THYROIDITIS

Thyroiditis is a heterogeneous group of inflammatory disorders of the thyroid gland, including those caused by autoimmune mechanisms and infectious agents.

Acute Thyroiditis Is Caused by Bacterial or Fungal Infections

The disease usually develops during a systemic infection that reaches the thyroid by hematogenous spread. It occurs in patients of all ages, but children, the elderly or immunocompromised patients are most commonly affected.

Patients present with fever, chills, malaise and a painful, swollen neck. Infection may involve one lobe or the entire gland. There is diffuse acute and chronic inflammation with focal microabscess formation. Rarely, the infection may spread into the trachea, mediastinum and esophagus. The prognosis is excellent when the infection is promptly treated with antibiotics.

 **ETIOLOGIC FACTORS:** The most common causative organisms are streptococcus, staphylococcus and pneumococcus. Other causes include fungi and cytomegalovirus (CMV). Tuberculous thyroiditis is rare but can occur in immunosuppressed patients.

Chronic Autoimmune Thyroiditis (Hashimoto Thyroiditis) Is the Most Common Cause of Goitrous Hypothyroidism in the United States

Hashimoto thyroiditis (HT) is usually part of the spectrum of autoimmune diseases. It can affect several family members who often also suffer other autoimmune conditions such as lupus, Graves disease, arteritis and scleroderma (see Chapter 11).

 MOLECULAR PATHOGENESIS: The pathogenesis of HT involves cellular and humoral immunity. The autoimmune process in HT arises from activation of CD4 (helper) T lymphocytes sensitized to thyroid antigens (Fig. 27-14). Helper T-cell activation may be initiated by viral or bacterial infection.

In turn, these CD4$^+$ cells stimulate proliferation of autoreactive cytotoxic (CD8$^+$) T cells, which attack thyrocytes. The activated lymphocytes secrete interferon-γ, causing thyrocytes to express MHC class II molecules (HLA-DR, -DP, -DQ), thus expanding the autoreactive T-cell population. These effects account for the striking accumulation of lymphocytes in the glands of patients with autoimmune thyroiditis.

Activated CD4 cells also recruit autoreactive B cells to produce antibodies against thyroid antigens. These include antibodies against thyroid microsomal peroxidase (95%), thyroglobulin (60%) and TSH receptor. Cytotoxic antibodies that fix complement have been described in some patients, and antibody-dependent cell-mediated cytotoxicity (ADCC) may contribute to thyroid injury. Unlike the anti-TSH receptor antibodies in Graves disease, which stimulate thyroid function, antibodies in HT block TSH action. Such blocking antibodies have been described in 10% of patients with goitrous autoimmune thyroiditis and in 20% of those with end-stage atrophy of the gland. Half of all first-degree relatives of patients with this condition have antithyroid antibodies, which are apparently transmitted as a dominant trait. Moreover, both Graves disease and chronic autoimmune thyroiditis are described in these family members. A familial tendency for HT is further suggested by the higher prevalence of other autoimmune diseases in patients and their relatives, including MEN syndrome type 2, insulin-dependent diabetes, pernicious anemia, Addison disease and myasthenia gravis. The high incidence of autoimmunity and thyroiditis in people with Down syndrome and familial Alzheimer disease has attracted attention to genes on chromosome 21,

but none have yet been identified as causes of these disorders. Interestingly, half of adult patients with Turner syndrome, especially those with an X isochromosome, exhibit antithyroid antibodies, and a third develop hypothyroidism. Only association with HLA and CTLA-4 genes has been seen consistently, but how these contribute to autoimmune thyroiditis remains obscure. The *HLA-DR5* gene has been implicated in families with thyroid disorders.

HT is most common where **iodine intake** is greatest, for example, Japan and the United States. In iodine-deficient areas, iodine supplementation significantly increases the prevalence of chronic inflammation of the thyroid and the presence of thyroid autoantibodies.

 PATHOLOGY: The gland in patients with HT is diffusely enlarged and firm, weighing 60–200 g. The cut surface is pale tan and fleshy with a vaguely nodular pattern (Fig. 27-17). The capsule is intact; perithyroid tissues are not involved. The thyroid shows a conspicuous infiltrate of lymphocytes and plasma cells, with destruction and atrophy of follicles and oxyphilic metaplasia of follicular epithelial cells **(Hürthle** or **Askanazy cells)**. Lymphoid follicles, often with germinal centers, are present. The Askanazy cells are filled with mitochondria and often show nuclear atypia, which may be mistaken for cancer. Interstitial fibrosis is variable and is conspicuous in 10% of cases (fibrous variant). The thyroid eventually undergoes atrophy in some patients, who are left with a small, fibrotic gland infiltrated by lymphocytes. Thyroid lymphoma is a rare complication of HT.

CLINICAL FEATURES: HT mainly affects women between 30 and 50 years old, but no age group is spared. Patients may present with nonspecific symptoms such as fatigue, depression and fibromyalgia. Clinically they may have diffuse thyroid enlargement and either mild hyperthyroidism or hypothyroidism. Most patients note gradual onset of a goiter, although sometimes the gland enlarges rapidly. Eventually, 1/3 to 1/2 of patients progress to an overt hypothyroid state, the risk of which is much greater among men than women. Rarely, hyperthyroidism may occur

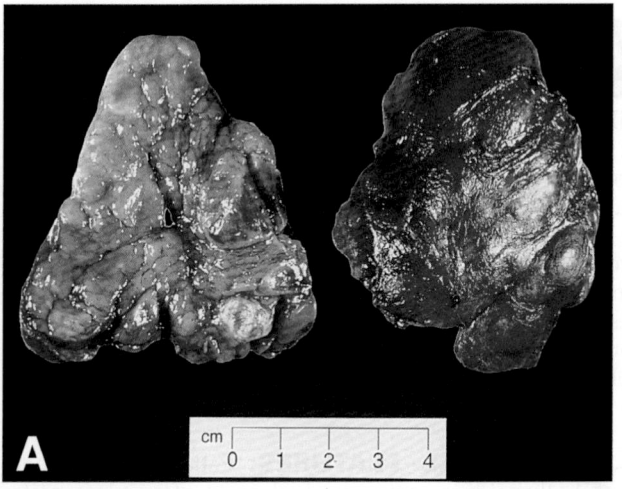 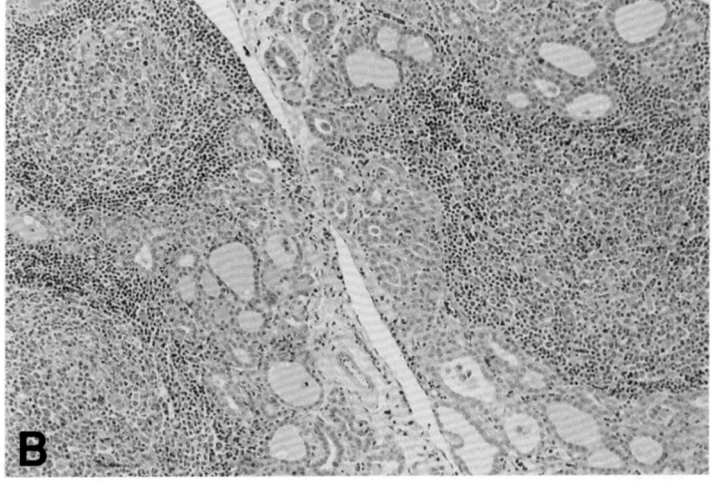

FIGURE 27-17. Chronic autoimmune (Hashimoto) thyroiditis. The thyroid gland is symmetrically enlarged and coarsely nodular. **A.** A coronal section of the right lobe shows irregular nodules and an intact capsule. **B.** A microscopic section of the thyroid reveals a conspicuous chronic inflammatory infiltrate and many atrophic thyroid follicles. The inflammatory cells form prominent lymphoid follicles with germinal centers.

(hashitoxicosis). The diagnosis of HT is now made by identifying circulating antithyroid antibodies (which occur in 95% of patients), **antithyroid peroxidase antibodies (anti-TPO)** and **antimicrosomal, antithyroglobulin** and cell membrane antibodies. Such patients show low levels of T_4, elevated serum thyrotropin and thyroxine index and elevated TSH. HT may frequently coexist with papillary cancer

Many patients need no therapy. Thyroid hormone is given to treat hypothyroidism and decrease the size of the gland. Surgery is reserved for patients who do not respond to suppressive hormone therapy or with troublesome pressure symptoms.

Subacute Thyroiditis (de Quervain, Granulomatous or Giant Cell Thyroiditis) Is Caused by a Viral Infection

Subacute thyroiditis, also known as granulomatous, de Quervain or nonsuppurative thyroiditis, is an uncommon, self-limited disorder characterized by granulomatous inflammation. It typically occurs after upper respiratory viral infections, such as with influenza virus, adenovirus, echovirus or coxsackievirus. Mumps virus has also been incriminated in some cases. de Quervain thyroiditis principally affects women 30–50 years old. The true incidence of subacute thyroiditis is unknown since many infectious thyroiditides have been reported under this name.

 **PATHOLOGY:** The thyroid is enlarged to 40–60 g. Its cut surface is firm and pale. Acute inflammation, often with microabscesses, is followed by a patchy infiltrate of lymphocytes, plasma cells and macrophages throughout the thyroid. Destruction of follicles releases colloid, which elicits a conspicuous granulomatous reaction (Fig. 27-18). Abundant foreign body–type multinucleated giant cells, often containing colloid, are present. Fibrosis may follow resolution of the inflammatory reaction, but normal thyroid architecture is usually restored.

 CLINICAL FEATURES: Patients with subacute thyroiditis typically notice pain in the anterior neck, sometimes with fever, malaise, fatigue and pain in the neck or radiating to the jaw. Other patients

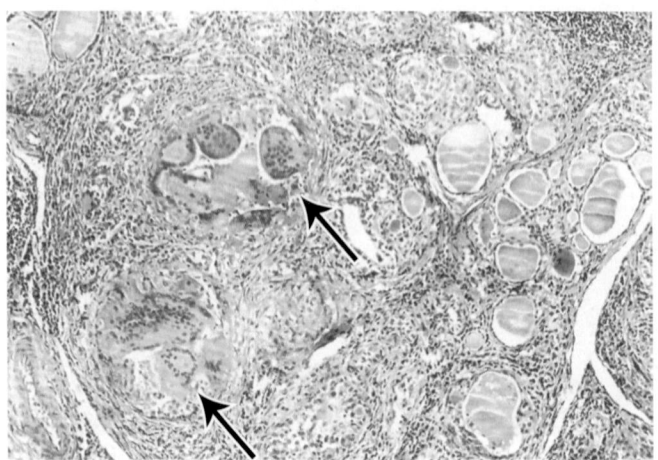

FIGURE 27-18. Subacute thyroiditis. The release of colloid into the interstitial tissue has elicited a prominent granulomatous reaction, with numerous foreign body giant cells (*arrows*).

follow a mild course with only minimal symptoms. The disorder is often mistaken for pharyngitis, as it follows respiratory infections and patients complain of hoarseness and dysphagia. On examination, the thyroid is moderately enlarged and exquisitely tender. Subacute thyroiditis generally resolves within a few months without any clinical sequelae. Iodine uptake is usually suppressed in the early stages of the disease.

Release of preformed thyroid hormone by destruction of the follicles often raises serum T_4 and T_3, which may be high enough to cause transient clinical hyperthyroidism. The consequent suppression of TSH leads to decreased radiolabeled iodine uptake. This phase is followed by decreased serum T_4 and T_3 levels, but as inflammation resolves, a euthyroid state returns. There may be low levels of antithyroid antibodies.

Silent Thyroiditis Causes Transient Hyperthyroidism

In silent thyroiditis, also called **painless subacute thyroiditis** or **lymphocytic thyroiditis,** patients experience painless thyroid enlargement, self-limited hyperthyroidism and destruction of gland parenchyma with lymphocytic infiltration. Thus, it resembles subacute thyroiditis clinically but is closer to HT pathologically. *Silent thyroiditis differs from the latter by the lack of antithyroid antibodies or other evidence of autoimmune thyroiditis.* However, association with HLA-DR3 has been reported. As in subacute thyroiditis, the hyperthyroid state reflects release of preformed thyroid hormone from the injured gland.

Silent thyroiditis mainly affects women, often in the postpartum period, causing hyperthyroidism that usually persists for 2–4 months. Treatment is symptomatic, and most patients become euthyroid.

Riedel Thyroiditis Causes Fibrosis of the Thyroid

The "thyroiditis" in Riedel thyroiditis is something of a misnomer, as this rare disease also involves extrathyroidal soft tissues of the neck and often progressive fibrosis in other locations, including the retroperitoneum, mediastinum and orbit. Riedel thyroiditis is mainly a disease of middle age. The female-to-male ratio is 3:1. Riedel thyroiditis is considered to be a manifestation of IgG4-related systemic disease.

 PATHOLOGY: Part or all of the thyroid is stony hard and "woody." The process is usually asymmetric and often affects only one lobe. The fibrous infiltrate extends into the thyroid gland and other tissues of the neck, including skeletal muscle and nerves. It may also surround and infiltrate lymph nodes and parathyroid glands. The surgeon may have extreme difficulty identifying a tissue plane. Dense, hyalinized fibrous tissue and chronic inflammation are present throughout involved portions of the thyroid (Fig. 27-19). Eosinophils may be also present. Follicles are normal in unaffected parts of the gland. Fibrosis surrounds and infiltrates other tissues, including skeletal muscle, nerves, fat, blood vessels and, sometimes, the parathyroids.

 CLINICAL FEATURES: Patients with Riedel thyroiditis notice gradual onset of painless goiter and present with a hard thyroid mass. They may also have fibrosing lesions at other sites, such as the retroperitoneum, mediastinum and retro-orbital tissues. Immunophenotyping shows mostly T cells with few B cells. Symptoms

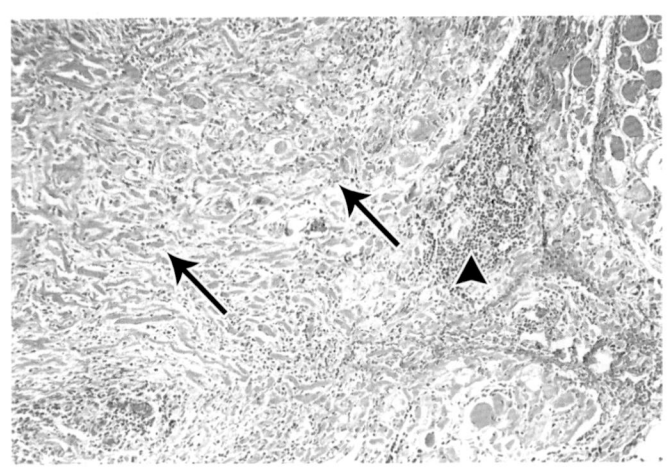

FIGURE 27-19. Riedel thyroiditis. The thyroid parenchyma is largely replaced by dense, hyalinized fibrous tissue (*arrows*) and a chronic inflammatory infiltrate (*arrowhead*).

may be due to compression of neck organs: the trachea (stridor), esophagus (dysphagia) and recurrent laryngeal nerve (hoarseness). Unusual cases may involve the entire thyroid and cause hypothyroidism. Treatment is primarily surgical to relieve symptomatic compression of local structures.

FOLLICULAR ADENOMA OF THE THYROID

Follicular adenomas are benign neoplasms with follicular differentiation. They are the most common thyroid tumors and typically present in euthyroid people as solitary "cold" nodules (i.e., that do not take up radioiodine). Follicular adenomas occur frequently in iodine-deficient areas. They can also occur in irradiated glands and as part of Cowden syndrome (see Chapter 5). Adenomas are solitary encapsulated neoplasms in which cells are arranged in follicles that resemble normal adult thyroid tissue or mimic stages in the gland's embryonic development. Multiple adenomas may occur. Up to 90% of palpable, solitary follicular lesions are actually the dominant nodule in a multinodular goiter. Thus, follicular adenomas are correspondingly uncommon. These are most common in the 4th and 5th decades, with a female-to-male ratio of 7:1. The clonal origin of follicular adenomas has been established.

 PATHOLOGY: Follicular adenomas are solitary, circumscribed, 1–3-cm nodules that protrude from the surface of the thyroid. They are completely enclosed by a thin fibrous capsule. The tumor cut surface is soft and paler than the surrounding gland. Hemorrhage, fibrosis and cystic change are common. There are several distinctive histologic patterns (Fig. 27-20). These variants are of no particular clinical or prognostic significance, but it is

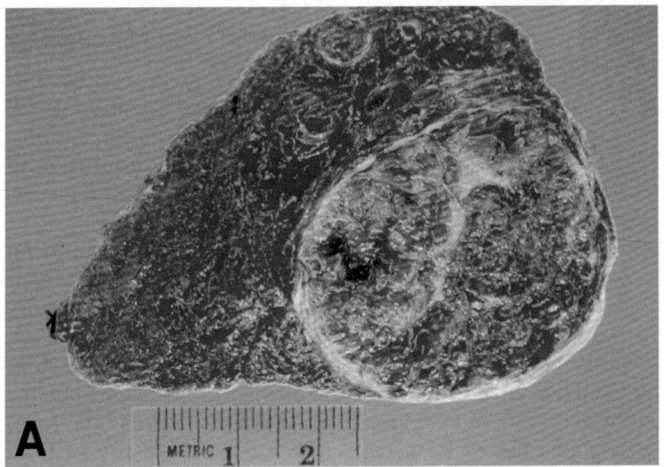

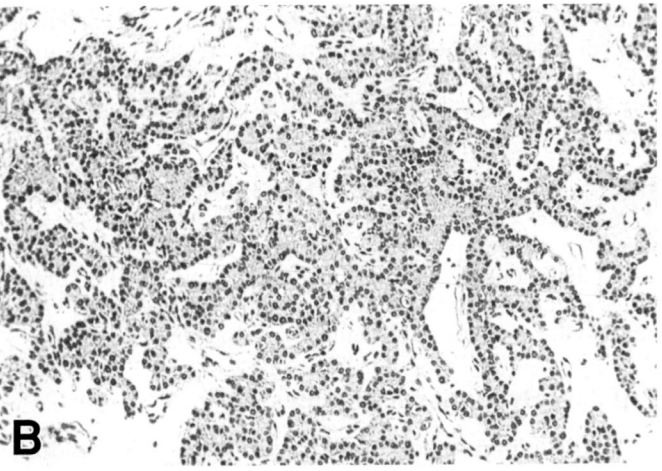

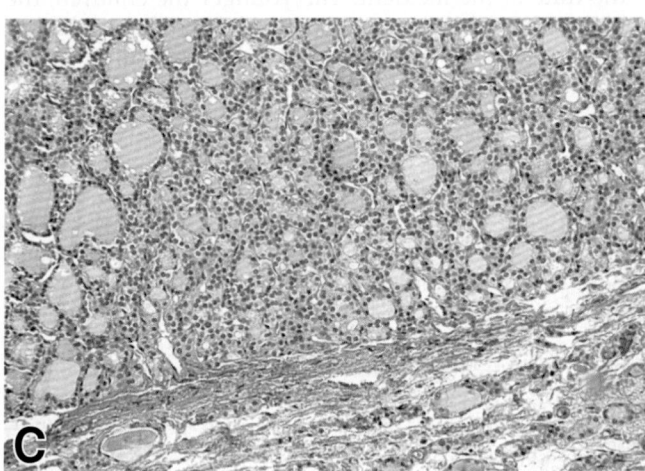

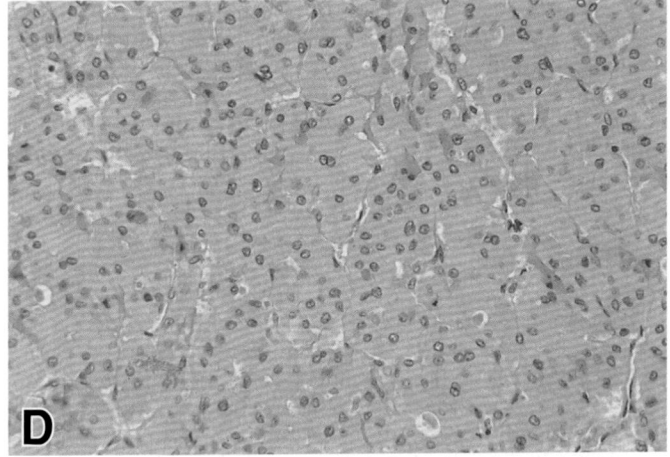

FIGURE 27-20. Follicular adenoma. A. Colloid adenoma. The cut surface of an encapsulated mass reveals hemorrhage, fibrosis and cystic change. **B.** Embryonal adenoma. The tumor features a trabecular pattern with poorly formed follicles that contain little if any colloid. **C.** Fetal adenoma. A regular pattern of small follicles is noted. **D.** Hürthle cell adenoma. The tumor is composed of cells with small, regular nuclei and abundant eosinophilic cytoplasm.

helpful to recognize them so as not to confuse them with thyroid malignancies.

- **Embryonal adenomas** have trabecular patterns, in which poorly formed follicles contain little or no colloid (Fig. 27-20B).
- **Fetal adenomas** contain cells like those of embryonal adenomas, but arranged in microfollicles with little colloid (Fig. 27-20C).
- **Simple adenomas** contain mature follicles with a normal amount of colloid.
- **Colloid adenomas** resemble simple adenomas except with larger follicles that contain more abundant colloid (Fig. 27-20A).
- **Hürthle (oncocytic) cell adenomas** are solid tumors characterized by oxyphil cells, small follicles and scanty colloid (Fig. 27-20D). These lesions frequently undergo infarction after fine-needle aspiration procedures.
- **Atypical adenomas** are follicular tumors with mitoses, excessive cellularity, nuclear atypism or equivocal capsular invasion, but for which a diagnosis of carcinoma cannot be established with certainty.

Differentiation between follicular adenoma and adenomatoid nodules may be difficult. However, adenomatoid nodules lack the fibrous delicate capsule seen in adenomas. Follicular adenomas stain negative for CK19, which can be useful to distinguish them from other papillary tumors.

These benign lesions should be differentiated from follicular carcinomas, which usually have thicker capsules. Careful evaluation of the capsule for capsular or vascular invasion is mandatory to make this distinction. *Malignancies can develop in association with or within benign nodules.* Surgical lobectomy to remove the lesion is curative.

 **MOLECULAR PATHOGENESIS:** Adenomas are clonal in over 60% of cases. Other molecular alterations include trisomy 7; translocations in 19q13; deletions in chromosomes 3p, 10 and 13; and sometimes **mutations in the RAS oncogene**. The oncocytic variant may have alterations in mitochondrial DNA.

Papillary Hyperplastic Nodules

Papillary hyperplastic nodules occur mainly in children and young women. They are solitary, well circumscribed and well encapsulated, and contain papillae of different sizes. Stalks of papillae may contain small follicles. The papillae themselves are lined by cuboidal cells with characteristic follicular nuclei (i.e., dense with dispersed chromatin). The center of nodules is often cystic and can contain colloid-like material. These lesions are often misdiagnosed as papillary cancer.

THYROID CANCER

Thyroid malignancies account for 0.4% of cancer deaths in the United States, with 10,000 new cases diagnosed each year. Mortality from thyroid cancer exceeds that from malignant tumors of all other endocrine organs.

The difficulty of distinguishing clinically between nonneoplastic lesions, benign tumors and thyroid cancer is a major clinical and pathologic concern. Thyroid nodules occur in 1%–10% of the population, but thyroid cancers represent only 1% of all cancers. A single nodule has up to a 12% probability of being malignant, and those odds decrease significantly (3%) if a nodule is palpable.

Most cases of thyroid carcinoma occur between the 3rd and 7th decades, but they do not spare children. These tumors occur in women 2.5-fold more often than in men. However, thyroid cancer is more aggressive in older males.

Fine-needle aspiration biopsy of thyroid nodules makes a diagnosis in most cases. Prognosis is a function of the tumor morphology, and clinical courses may range from virtually benign to rapidly fatal. Fortunately, the latter is uncommon.

Thyroid radioscintigraphy is helpful, since hyperfunctioning nodules are usually benign. "Cold" or nonfunctioning nodules, although more often malignant, may also be benign.

Papillary Thyroid Carcinoma Is the Most Common Thyroid Cancer

Papillary thyroid carcinoma (PTC) accounts for up to 90% of sporadic thyroid cancers in the United States. It occurs most often between the ages of 20 and 50, with a female-to-male ratio of 3:1. However, it may arise at any age, even in children: it is the most common thyroid tumor type in children and young adolescents. Elderly men have a worse prognosis with PTC.

  **ETIOLOGIC FACTORS AND MOLECULAR PATHOGENESIS:** The etiology of PTC is uncertain, but there are several potentially important connections.

- **Iodine excess:** PTC has been produced in animals by administering excess iodine. In endemic goiter regions, addition of iodine to the diet increased the proportion of thyroid cancers showing papillary, as compared with follicular, morphology.
- **Radiation:** External radiation to the neck of children and adults increases the incidence of later PTC. Survivors of atomic bomb explosions in Japan suffered more papillary cancers than would otherwise be expected. Children living in contaminated areas surrounding Chernobyl, the site in Ukraine of a nuclear reactor catastrophe in 1986, had substantially (almost 100-fold) higher rates of PTC, especially if they were under 15 at the time of the incident. The younger the children, the higher the risk, because younger children have a higher uptake of radioactive iodine. It is known that radiation produces DNA double-strand breaks (see Chapters 5 and 8), leading to mutations and translocations including RET rearrangements. On the other hand, treatment with radiolabeled iodine does not increase the risk of this tumor.
- **Genetic factors:** First-degree relatives of PTC patients have a 4–10-fold greater risk for PTC than the general population. Concordance for PTC has been described in monozygotic twins. A familial form of PTC accounts for some 5% of all cases, but the genes responsible have not been identified. Familial thyroid cancers may be more aggressive tumors, with increased frequency of lymph node metastases. PTC also occurs in association with familial polyposis syndrome (*APC* gene; see Chapter 5).
- **Somatic mutations:** Somatic rearrangements of *RET* proto-oncogene on chromosome 10 (10q11.2) are common in PTC, and 60% of such tumors in children exposed to

radiation from the Chernobyl accident showed this mutation. The same mutation occurs after external radiation to the thyroid. These rearrangements cause the tyrosine kinase domain of *RET* to fuse to various other genes, creating *RET/PTC* fusion oncogenes. The frequency of *RET/PTC* rearrangements in PTC varies geographically, from none in Korea to 2% in Saudi Arabia and 60% in the United States and Great Britain. The incidence of *RET/PTC* rearrangements also varies with age, being higher in children and young adults. Many types of RET/PTC are known, the most common of which is RET/PTC3. RET/PTC2 occurs less often and accounts for less than 5% of such rearrangements. RET/PTC3 is common in the tall cell variant of PTC, which is considered an aggressive PTC subtype.

- **Illegitimate recombination** involving the *NTRK1* gene on chromosome 1 with another gene (*TPM3*) on the same chromosome also occurs in some PTCs. *NTRK1* encodes a tyrosine kinase that is a high-affinity nerve growth factor receptor (*NGFR*). TRK rearrangements occur in 10% of PTCs.

- **BRAF mutations:** Point mutations of the *BRAF* gene are present in up to 70% of papillary thyroid cancers. This mutation is linked to specific characteristics of PTC that predict tumor behavior and progression. This *BRAF* mutation occurs particularly in PTC and PTC-derived anaplastic thyroid cancer. Differences between *BRAF*-positive and *BRAF*-negative PTC are distinct, suggesting that *BRAF* mutations can be used as a molecular prognostic factor. The BRAFV600E mutation occurs in some types of microcarcinomas.

- **RAS mutations:** *RAS* proto-oncogene mutations are present in 10% of PTCs. However, the number of PTCs with *RAS* mutations may be increasing, and approaching 25%.

 PATHOLOGY: PTCs vary from microscopic lesions to tumors larger than a normal gland. Serial sections of ostensibly normal thyroids obtained at autopsy have revealed a high proportion of papillary cancers that measure less than 1 mm across, but lymph node metastases in such cases are distinctly uncommon. Papillary cancers may occur in either lobe or the isthmus. They are firm, solid and white-yellowish, with irregular and infiltrative borders. Lesions may be multiple and are occasionally encapsulated (Fig. 27-21A).

Branching papillae contain a central fibrovascular core and a single or stratified lining of cuboidal to columnar cells (Fig. 27-21B). There are usually irregularly shaped or tubular neoplastic follicles, but relative proportions of papillary and follicular elements vary greatly. Nuclear atypia is an important diagnostic feature and includes clear **(ground-glass** or **Orphan Annie)** nuclei, eosinophilic pseudoinclusions (which are invaginations of cytoplasm into the nucleus) and nuclear grooves. Many papillary cancers show dense fibrosis. Calcospherites *(psammoma bodies)* are virtually diagnostic of papillary carcinoma: they are rare in other conditions and are present in half of PTCs. The stroma may be infiltrated by lymphocytes and Langerhans cells. In over 3/4 of cases of PTC, careful sectioning of a resected thyroid reveals multiple microscopic foci of tumor. It is not clear, though, whether these reflect multifocal origin of the tumor or lymphatic spread from a solitary primary. Vascular invasion is uncommon.

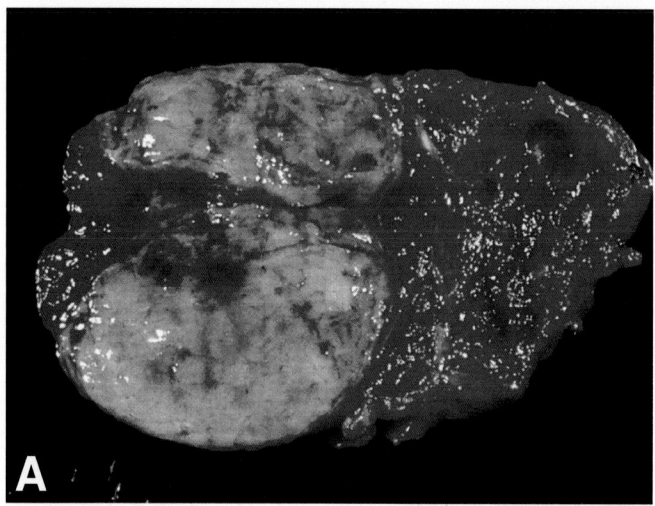

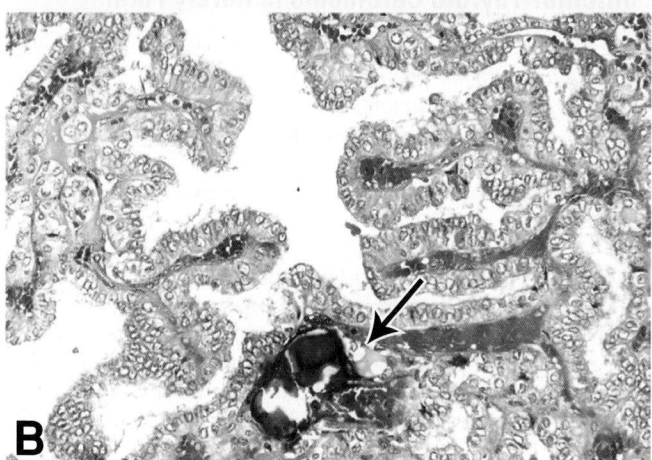

FIGURE 27-21. Papillary carcinoma of the thyroid. A. The cut surface of a surgically resected thyroid displays a circumscribed pale tan mass with foci of cystic change. **B.** Branching papillae are lined by neoplastic columnar epithelium with clear nuclei. A calcospherite, or psammoma body, is evident.

Several morphologic types of papillary carcinoma are known, some associated with good prognosis such as **microcarcinoma** (≤1 cm, not requiring further treatment), **follicular variant** of papillary cancer, **encapsulated** and the **papillary** or most common type. The **diffuse sclerosis, tall cell** and **columnar** variants have worse prognoses.

PTC typically invades lymphatics and spreads to regional cervical lymph nodes. Lymph node metastases vary from tiny foci in otherwise normal lymph nodes to large masses that dwarf the primary lesion. Direct extension of PTC into soft tissues of the neck occurs in 1/4 of cases. Hematogenous metastases are less common than in other types of thyroid cancer, but they do happen occasionally, mostly to the lungs.

 CLINICAL FEATURES: PTC generally presents as (1) a painless, palpable nodule in an otherwise normal gland; (2) a nodule with enlarged cervical lymph nodes; or (3) cervical lymphadenopathy without a palpable thyroid nodule. Tumors over 0.5 cm are usually cold areas in thyroid scintiscans.

In general, the prognosis of PTC is excellent, and life expectancy for these patients differs little from that of the general population. The prognosis is more serious in men over 50 years, but in children, the outlook is good even if there are lung metastases. PTC tends to be more aggressive in men than in women.

As a rule, larger primary tumors are more aggressive, and direct extension into adjacent soft tissues portends a poorer prognosis. The relative proportions of papillary and follicular elements do not affect prognosis, but less differentiated tumors behave worse. The presence of metastases to cervical nodes at the time of surgery does not change the prognosis, as less than 10% of such patients die of the tumor. In fatal cases of PTC, death is caused principally by metastases to the lungs or brain or by obstruction of the trachea or esophagus.

Therapies include surgery (lobectomy or total thyroidectomy) with or without neck dissection, followed by administration of radioiodine.

Follicular Thyroid Carcinoma Is Rarely Fatal

Follicular thyroid carcinoma (FTC) is a purely follicular malignant tumor with no papillary or other elements. It makes up 15%–20% of thyroid tumors. Most patients are older than 40 and female (3:1). FTC is extremely rare in children. However, in areas where iodine is added to salt, as in the United States, FTC is uncommon, representing as few as 5% of thyroid cancers.

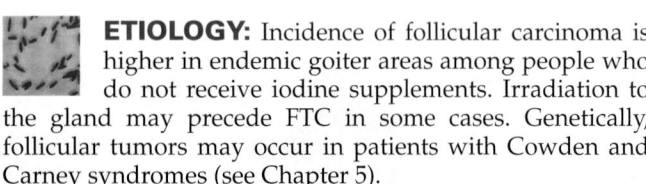

ETIOLOGY: Incidence of follicular carcinoma is higher in endemic goiter areas among people who do not receive iodine supplements. Irradiation to the gland may precede FTC in some cases. Genetically, follicular tumors may occur in patients with Cowden and Carney syndromes (see Chapter 5).

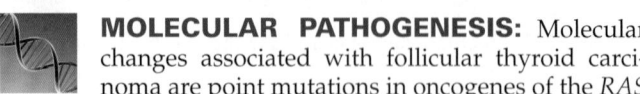

MOLECULAR PATHOGENESIS: Molecular changes associated with follicular thyroid carcinoma are point mutations in oncogenes of the *RAS* family (*NRAS, KRAS, HRAS*), which occur in 20%–45% of the tumors, and *PAX8/PPARγ* (paired box 8/peroxisome proliferator-activated receptor γ) rearrangement with a t(2;3)(q13;p25) translocation, affecting 20%–40% of patients. The latter seems to be more common in low-grade FTC with vascular invasion. However, the prevalence of PAX8-PPARγ may be lower than previously noted, and correlation with invasiveness and influence on prognosis are unclear. Mutations of *TP53* tumor suppressor and *PTEN* do occur and may play a role in tumor progression. Cytogenetic studies have shown imbalances in several chromosomes including 3p, 7q, 11, 10q and others.

Follicular tumors with oncocytic morphology have chromosomal changes and abnormalities in mitochondrial DNA like other thyroid tumors with oncocytic features.

PATHOLOGY: Follicular cancers vary in size, are yellow-tan and have thick white fibrous capsules. Areas of hemorrhage and necrosis and foci of cystic degeneration are not uncommon. FTCs are subdivided into minimally invasive and widely invasive variants.

Minimally invasive FTCs are well-defined, encapsulated tumors. They are soft and pale tan to pink, and bulge from within their capsules. Most resemble follicular adenomas, although they tend more to microfollicular or trabecular patterns. Hemorrhagic necrosis may occur in their centers. Mitoses are common, which distinguishes follicular cancers

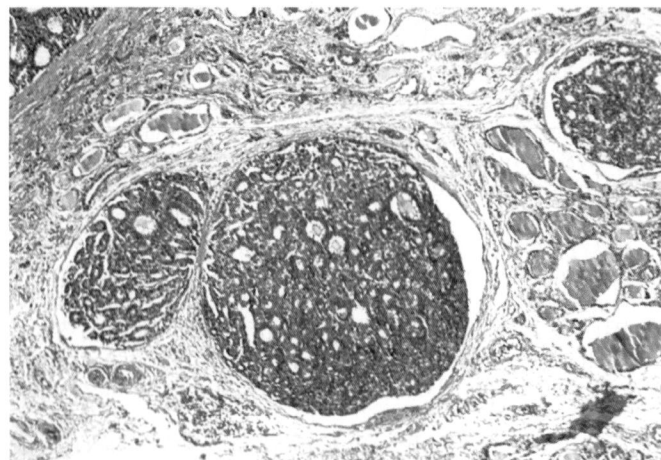

FIGURE 27-22. Follicular carcinoma of the thyroid. A microfollicular tumor has invaded veins in the thyroid parenchyma.

from benign adenomas. The main difference from adenomas is at the border between the tumor capsule and normal parenchyma. In minimally invasive cancers, tumor extends into, but not entirely through, the capsule or shows areas of vascular invasion.

Invasive FTC usually presents few diagnostic problems, since it extends through its capsule or shows vascular invasion (Fig. 27-22), often within or adjacent to the capsule. The tumor may also extend into surrounding soft tissues. Proliferative markers such as Ki67 may in some instances assist in the diagnosis. These tumors stain positively for thyroglobulin and TTF1.

Oncocytic (Hürthle cell) carcinomas are tumors of follicular derivation composed mainly (>75%) of oncocytes. The criteria for malignancy are the same as for follicular cancer: capsular and vascular invasion. These tumors account for 4%–5% of thyroid malignancies and tend to behave more aggressively than regular follicular cancer.

FTC differs from PTC in that its metastases are bloodborne, not lymphatic, and go mainly to the lung and bones of the shoulder, pelvic girdle, sternum and skull.

CLINICAL FEATURES: Most follicular cancers present as solitary palpable nodules or enlarged thyroids. However, in some cases, the presenting sign is a pathologic fracture through a bony metastasis or a pulmonary lesion. Both primary tumors and metastases take up radiolabeled iodine, but thyroid scintiscans may show a cold nodule, as the normal thyroid accumulates iodine more efficiently. Nonetheless, the tumors' affinity for ^{131}I may be used therapeutically. Minimally invasive follicular tumors have a cure rate of at least 95%, compared with a survival of about 50% for the widely invasive form. FTC is treated with unilateral lobectomy. Metastases can be treated with radioiodine.

Medullary Thyroid Carcinoma Is Derived from C Cells of the Thyroid

Medullary thyroid carcinomas (MTC) make up not more than 5% of thyroid cancers. Their cells originate from the branchial pouches. They secrete multiple hormones, including calcitonin, serotonin, ACTH and somatostatin.

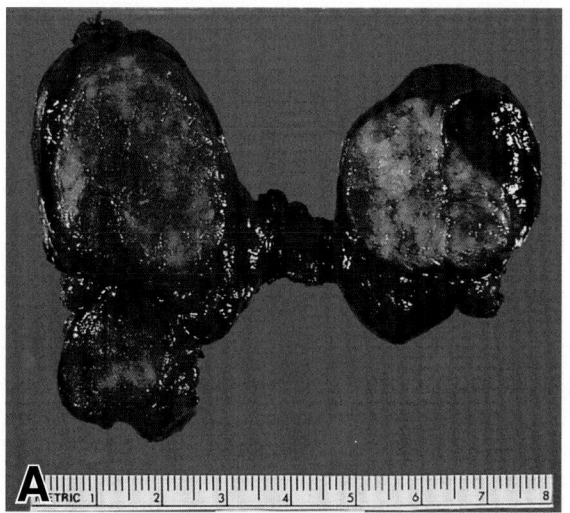

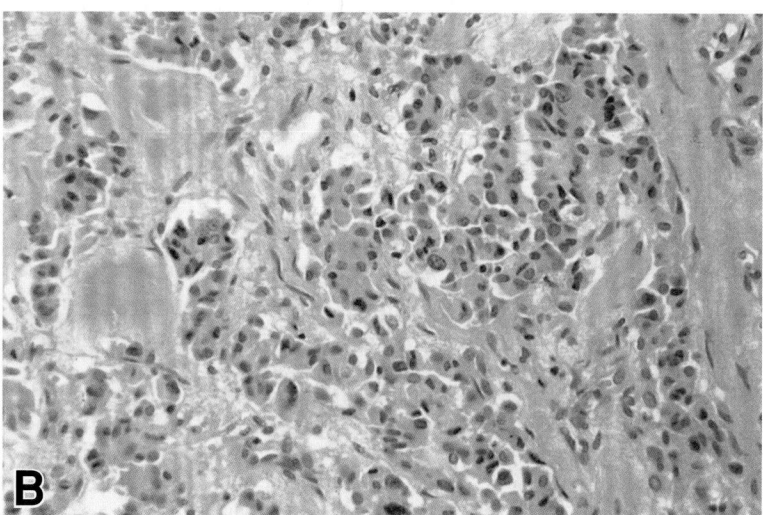

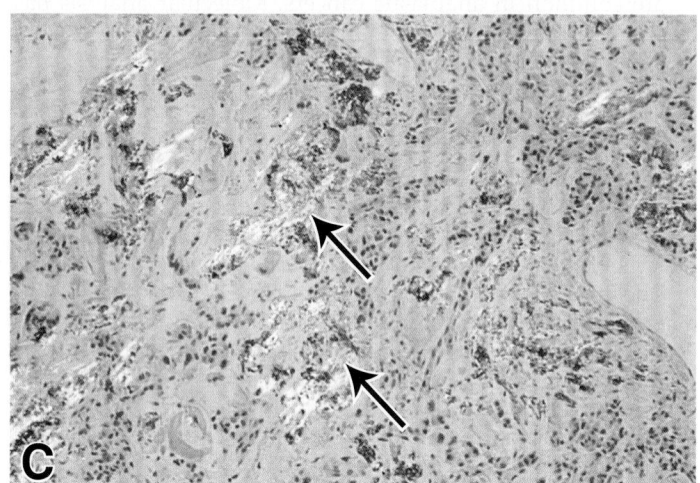

FIGURE 27-23. Medullary thyroid carcinoma. A. Coronal section of a total thyroid resection shows bilateral involvement by a firm, pale tumor. **B.** The tumor features nests of polygonal cells embedded in a collagenous framework. The connective tissue septa contain eosinophilic amyloid. **C.** A section stained with Congo red and viewed under polarized light demonstrates the pale green birefringence (*arrows*) of amyloid.

ETIOLOGY: The disease occurs in sporadic and familial forms, the latter accounting for **25%** of cases. Patients with familial forms of medullary carcinoma often have MEN type 2B or 2A. Tumors in patients with MEN type 2B occur in infancy; those in type 2A develop in adolescents. In familial cases, inheritance is autosomal dominant, and the sex distribution is equal. Sporadic cases present later in life and show slight female predominance (3:2). There are no known etiologic factors.

MOLECULAR PATHOGENESIS: Somatic mutations in *RET* proto-oncogene on chromosome 10 are present in 25%–70% of sporadic MTCs. Most of these are at codon 918 (ATG to ACG) in the tyrosine kinase domain of Ret protein and portend a poorer prognosis than in tumors without *RET* mutations. Other *RET* mutations at codons 768, 790, 791 and 804 may also occur. *RET* is discussed more fully in the section on MEN syndromes (below).

MTCs may show loss of heterozygosity involving several chromosomes such as 1p, 3p, 3q, 11p, 13q, 22q and others.

PATHOLOGY: These tumors tend to arise in the superior portion of the thyroid, which is the region richest in C cells. In the setting of MEN type 2, tumors are often multicentric and bilateral. MTCs are not encapsulated but are usually circumscribed. Cut surfaces are firm and grayish white. MTC histologies are highly variable. Characteristically, these tumors are solid with polygonal, granular cells separated by a highly vascular stroma (Fig. 27-23). However, architectural patterns and appearances of the cells are highly variable. *A conspicuous feature is stromal amyloid, representing deposition of procalcitonin.* Nests of tumor cells are embedded in a hyalinized collagenous framework. Focal calcification is often present and may be extensive enough to be detected radiologically. Besides amyloid, medullary carcinoma may contain mucin, melanin and many polypeptide hormones. Invasion into adjacent tissues is common.

By electron microscopy, the neoplastic C cells have dense-core secretory granules that are positive for several endocrine markers, including calcitonin, synaptophysin, chromogranin and neuron-specific enolase. Almost all of these tumors express carcinoembryonic antigen (CEA). Many are also positive for ACTH, serotonin, substance P, glucagon, insulin and human chorionic gonadotropin (hCG).

MTCs extend by direct invasion into soft tissues. They metastasize to regional lymph nodes and to lung, liver and bone. Sometimes, the initial presentation may be as metastatic disease. Metastases resemble primary tumors and also contain amyloid.

The precursor lesion of familial MTCs is C-cell hyperplasia. C-cell hyperplasia is composed of clusters of C cells with clear cytoplasm located near follicular cells. These nests of cells express calcitonin. *RET* mutations may occur in these early lesions. Thus, patients with MEN types 2A and 2B (see section on adrenal medulla) who are at risk for MTC are monitored by periodic measurements of serum calcitonin, CEA and sometimes chromogranin. If these are elevated, the patient receives a total thyroidectomy.

 CLINICAL FEATURES: Patients with MTC often suffer symptoms related to endocrine secretion, including carcinoid syndrome (serotonin) and Cushing syndrome (ACTH). Watery diarrhea in 1/3 of patients is caused by secretion of vasoactive intestinal peptide, prostaglandins and several kinins. In cases of familial MTC, patients may have hyperparathyroidism, episodic hypertension and other symptoms reflecting secretion of catecholamines by pheochromocytoma.

MTCs usually present as firm thyroid masses or cervical lymphadenopathy. By scintiscan, they are cold nodules. Treatment is total thyroidectomy, but tumors often recur locally. Thyroidectomies are also often performed in children belonging to families with known *RET* mutations and familial syndromes. Overall survival of patients with MTC is 86% at 5 years and 65% at 10 years. Prognosis depends on age (women do better), tumor size and stage. Other prognostic parameters include histologic type, mitotic count, necrosis and amount of calcitonin present. Other factors suggesting an ominous course include advanced age, advanced stage, prior neck surgery and associated MEN2B. Patients under 5 years old with MEN2A often undergo surgery to improve survival. All patients with MTC (whether familial or sporadic) should be tested for *RET* mutations; if they are positive, family members should also be tested.

Treatment is total thyroidectomy, but tumors recur locally in 1/3 of patients. Several new molecular targeted therapies with a tyrosine kinase inhibitor (vandetanib) have shown promising results in clinical trials for medullary thyroid cancer, with increased median progression-free survival.

Anaplastic (Undifferentiated) Thyroid Carcinoma Is Usually Fatal

Anaplastic thyroid cancer is a highly malignant tumor that mostly afflicts women (female-to-male ratio, 4:1) over age 60. This tumor constitutes 10% of thyroid cancers and is more common in areas endemic for goiter. In fact, overall, at least half of patients suffer from long-standing goiter. Many patients with anaplastic carcinoma also have histories of lower-grade thyroid cancers. Thus, the anaplastic variant probably often represents transformation of a benign or low-grade thyroid neoplasm into a more poorly differentiated, more aggressive cancer. External radiation appears to increase the risk of such an event.

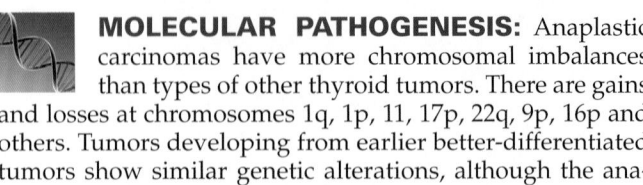 **MOLECULAR PATHOGENESIS:** Anaplastic carcinomas have more chromosomal imbalances than types of other thyroid tumors. There are gains and losses at chromosomes 1q, 1p, 11, 17p, 22q, 9p, 16p and others. Tumors developing from earlier better-differentiated tumors show similar genetic alterations, although the anaplastic component may have higher mutation rates.

Mutations in *TP53*, which encodes *p53* tumor suppressor, are common in anaplastic cancers. Molecular analysis has shown the following mutations in anaplastic tumors: *RAS*, 60%; *TP53*, 48%; *RET/PTC*, 4%; *BRAF*, 23%; *PTEN*, 16%; and *PI3KCA*, 24%. Genetic alterations may sometimes overlap. Mutations in *PAX8* also occur.

 PATHOLOGY: Anaplastic carcinoma of the thyroid presents as large poorly circumscribed masses in the gland, frequently extending into the soft tissues of the neck. The cut surface is hard and grayish white. The most common histologic pattern is a sarcoma-like proliferation of bizarre spindle and giant cells, with polyploid nuclei, many mitoses, necrosis and stromal fibrosis (Fig. 27-24). Other patterns include epithelial and giant cell differentiation. The tumor tends to invade veins and arteries, often occluding them and producing foci of infarction and necrosis within the tumor.

Immunohistochemistry in many cases is positive for cytokeratins and epithelial membrane antigen (EMA). However, TTF1 is negative.

 CLINICAL FEATURES: Anaplastic carcinomas compress and destroy local structures. Accordingly, the tumor presents as a rapidly enlarging neck mass, with symptoms such as dysphagia, hoarseness,

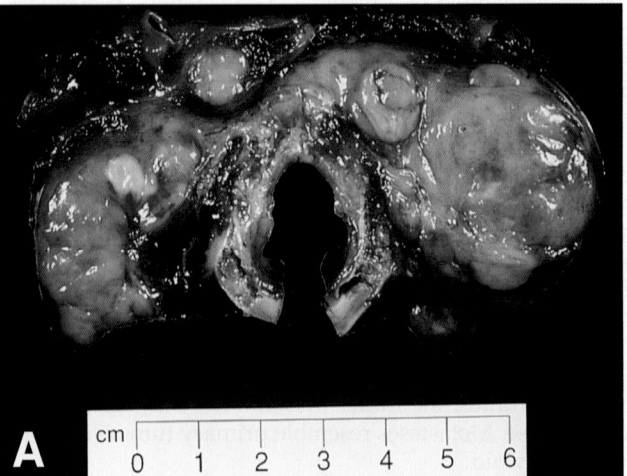
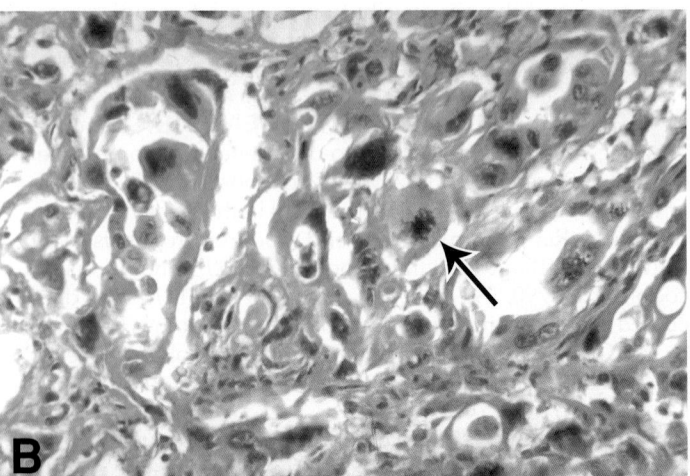

FIGURE 27-24. Anaplastic carcinoma of the thyroid. A. The tumor in transverse section partially surrounds the trachea and extends into the adjacent soft tissue. **B.** The tumor is composed of bizarre spindle and giant cells with polyploid nuclei and prominent mitotic activity (*arrow*).

dyspnea and enlargement of cervical nodes. Dysphagia and dyspnea are caused by tracheal compression or invasion. The prognosis is dismal, and widespread metastases are common. Under 10% of patients survive 5 years. Treatment with radiation and chemotherapy has had little success.

Lymphomas of the Thyroid Are Largely B-Cell Tumors

Lymphomas originating in the thyroid account for 2% of thyroid malignancies. Most, if not all, B lymphomas arise in glands with chronic thyroiditis. In fact, in regions where thyroiditis is frequent, up to 10% of thyroid malignancies are lymphomas.

Patients present with dyspnea, hoarseness and a mass in the neck. Like chronic thyroiditis, thyroid lymphoma occurs more commonly in women than in men (4:1), but the mean age at presentation (7th decade) is older. Their histology is similar to that of lymphomas at other sites; the most common subtype is the diffuse B large cell type.

Patients with thyroid lymphoma should be staged and treated as primary nodal lymphomas. Treatment with chemotherapy is similar to that for comparable nodal lymphomas. The prognosis of thyroid lymphomas of the MALT type (mantle zone lymphomas) is more favorable than those of some other B-cell types (see Chapter 26).

Parathyroid Glands

ANATOMY AND PHYSIOLOGY

The parathyroid glands are derivatives of branchial clefts III and IV. Most people have 4 glands, but numbers vary from 1 to 12. Normally, they are on the posterior thyroid surface, but they occasionally occur intrathyroidally or in ectopic locations such as mediastinum, pericardium or near the recurrent laryngeal nerve.

They are the size and color of a grain of saffron-cooked rice. All glands combined weigh about 130 mg. Individual gland weights vary considerably, but anything over 50 mg probably represents enlargement. They measure 4–6 mm in length. About 3/4 of the cells are chief and oxyphil cells, the remainder being fat cells scattered throughout the parenchyma. The amount of fat varies throughout life and it appears after puberty.

Chief cells secrete parathyroid hormone (PTH) and PTH-related protein. They are polyhedral cells with pale, eosinophilic-to-amphophilic cytoplasm that contains glycogen and fat droplets. Electron microscopy reveals cytoplasmic membrane-bound secretory granules. These cells stain positively for cytokeratins, chromogranin A and synaptophysin. Chief cells are the most sensitive to calcium concentrations. **Clear cells** are chief cells whose cytoplasm is packed with glycogen. **Oxyphil cells** appear after puberty, are larger than chief cells and have deeply eosinophilic cytoplasm, owing to many mitochondria. They have no secretory granules and do not secrete PTH.

The parathyroids respond to blood levels of ionized calcium and magnesium. In turn, PTH controls plasma calcium. Magnesium, a cation closely related to calcium, acts as a brake on PTH secretion. PTH is degraded in the liver and kidney. Other PTH functions also include regulation of renal phosphate excretion, increased tubular and intestinal reabsorption of calcium and bone resorption.

HYPOPARATHYROIDISM

Hypoparathyroidism results from decreased secretion of PTH or end-organ insensitivity to it (pseudohypoparathyroidism), whether congenital or acquired. It is clinically characterized by hypocalcemia and hyperphosphatemia.

Hypoparathyroidism Is Most Often Due to Surgical Removal of the Parathyroids at the Time of Thyroidectomy

The symptoms of hypoparathyroidism relate to hypocalcemia. Increased neuromuscular excitability may cause mild tingling in the hands and feet, severe muscle cramps, tetany, laryngeal stridor and convulsions. Neuropsychiatric manifestations include depression, paranoia and psychoses. High cerebrospinal fluid pressure and papilledema may mimic a brain tumor. Patients with all forms of hypoparathyroidism are successfully treated with vitamin D and calcium supplementation. Of patients undergoing surgery for primary hyperparathyroidism, 1% develop irreversible hypoparathyroidism. Radioactive iodine therapy can also cause hypoparathyroidism.

Familial hypoparathyroidism is a rare disease that can be inherited as autosomal dominant, X-linked recessive or autosomal recessive. It may also be part of a polyglandular syndrome that includes adrenal insufficiency and mucocutaneous candidiasis (see below). Hypoparathyroidism can occur with other congenital abnormalities as in DiGeorge syndrome (see Chapter 4), in which there is agenesis of the parathyroid glands. **Familial isolated hypoparathyroidism** has variable inheritance patterns, is rare and reflects deficient PTH secretion. Mutations in *GCM2* exon 3 may be responsible for some cases of congenital hypoparathyroidism. **Idiopathic hypoparathyroidism** is a heterogeneous group of rare disorders, sporadic and familial, that share deficient secretion of PTH.

Pseudohypoparathyroidism Reflects Target Organ Insensitivity to PTH

This group of hereditary conditions is characterized by hypocalcemia, hyperphosphatemia, increased serum concentration of parathyroid hormone and lack of response to PTH. It reflects mutation of the *GNAS1* gene on chromosome 20q, resulting in low activity of G_s, the G protein that couples hormone receptors to adenyl cyclase. Consequently, in renal tubular epithelium, cAMP production in response to PTH is impaired, causing inadequate calcium resorption from glomerular filtrate. Patients with pseudohypoparathyroidism (PHP) are also often resistant to other cAMP-coupled hormones, including TSH, glucagon, FSH and LH. These patients have a characteristic phenotype **(Albright hereditary osteodystrophy),** including short stature, obesity, mental retardation, subcutaneous calcification and a number of congenital anomalies of bone, particularly abnormally short metacarpals and metatarsals (Fig. 27-25). There are 3 forms of the disease: PHP type 1a, PHP type 1b and pseudopseudohypoparathyroidism (pseudo-PHP).

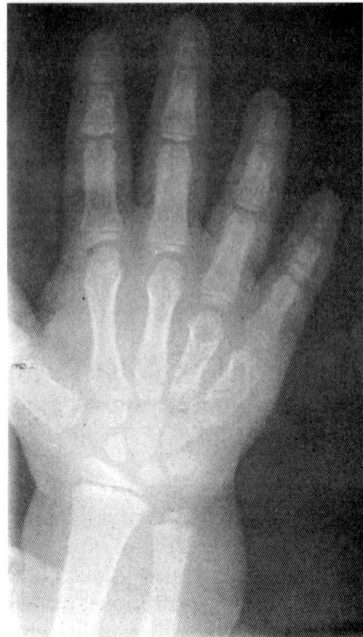

FIGURE 27-25. Pseudohypoparathyroidism. A radiograph of the hand reveals the characteristic shortness of the fourth and fifth metacarpal bones.

Some of those with pseudohypoparathyroidism have normal G$_S$ activity and a normal phenotype. The basis for their resistance to PTH is unclear.

Pseudopseudohypoparathyroidism reads like a typographical error, but it refers to rare cases in which the phenotype of Albright hereditary osteodystrophy is associated with normal cAMP response to PTH. These patients also have reduced G$_S$ activity like that reported in cases of pseudohypoparathyroidism. This condition is not caused by *GNAS1* mutations, but a candidate gene maps to a nearby part of chromosome 20.

PRIMARY HYPERPARATHYROIDISM

Primary Hyperparathyroidism Is Caused by Excessive PTH Secretion

In primary hyperparathyroidism, PTH production persists without intestinal or renal parathyroid gland stimulation. This condition is rare, with a probable incidence of 1 in 1000, and is most common in women in the 5th decade.

Patients present with hypercalcemia, hypophosphatemia, nephrolithiasis and bone disease. Some are asymptomatic and the only clinical finding is elevated serum calcium.

 **ETIOLOGY:** Hyperparathyroidism may be due to a parathyroid adenoma (80%–90%), hyperplasia involving all parathyroids (10%–15%) or (rarely) parathyroid carcinoma (1%–5%). PTH can be sporadic or part of familial syndromes such as MEN1 or MEN2A. Other associations include mutations in *HRPT2* and *CASR*.

Parathyroid Adenomas Account for Most Cases of Hyperparathyroidism

Solitary parathyroid adenomas cause 85% of primary hyperparathyroidism.

 **MOLECULAR PATHOGENESIS:** Parathyroid adenomas are monoclonal proliferations that arise sporadically or (20%) in the context of MEN1 (see below). In a small minority of cases of sporadic adenomas, the gene for cyclin D1 (*PRAD1*) has undergone rearrangement and the protein is overexpressed. This proto-oncogene is on chromosome 11 and shows breakpoints at 11q13 and 11p15. Comparative genomic hybridization studies of parathyroid adenomas have shown gains or losses in chromosomes 11q13, 11q23, 13q and 15q. Loss of heterozygosity at the MEN1 locus of 11q13 occurs in 20%–40% of adenomas with somatic mutations. *HRPT2* on chromosome 1q is the cause of the familial hyperparathyroidism–jaw tumor syndrome.

 PATHOLOGY: Parathyroid adenomas are circumscribed, red-brown, 1–3-cm solitary masses, weighing 0.05–200 g. Hemorrhagic areas are common, and cystic changes are occasionally noted. Adenomas show sheets of neoplastic chief cells in a rich capillary network. A rim of normal parathyroid tissue is usually evident outside the capsule and distinguishes adenomas from parathyroid hyperplasias (Fig. 27-26). Adenoma cells mostly resemble normal chief cells. Immunostaining for PTH documents the tumor's activity. The other parathyroid glands tend to be atrophic. Surgical removal of the tumor relieves the symptoms of hyperparathyroidism. Most parathyroid adenomas only involve one gland, but one patient may rarely harbor two. Adenomas can also occur within the thyroid gland or in ectopic parathyroid tissue. Proliferative markers such as MiB1 show scant proliferation. A proliferative index over 5% should raise the possibility of an atypical gland or cancer.

Primary Parathyroid Hyperplasia Causes 15% of Hyperparathyroidism

About 75% of parathyroid hyperplasias occur in women. Of these, 20% involve familial hyperparathyroidism or MEN syndromes (MEN types 1, 2A). A third of sporadic primary parathyroid hyperplasias are monoclonal, suggesting neoplastic proliferation. In such instances, both chief cell hyperplasia and multiple small adenomas occur in the same gland. Factors associated with sporadic primary hyperparathyroidism include external radiation and lithium ingestion.

 PATHOLOGY: All 4 parathyroid glands are enlarged, with combined weights from less than 1 g to 10 g. In half of patients, one gland may be noticeably larger than the others, which may complicate the distinction from adenoma. In hyperplastic glands, the normal glandular adipose tissue is replaced by hyperplastic chief cells arranged in sheets or trabecular or follicular patterns (Fig. 27-27). Scattered oxyphil cells are common, and small foci of adipose tissue may remain. An important feature that distinguishes hyperplasia from adenoma is that hyperplasias lack cellular pleomorphism.

Parathyroid Carcinomas Account for 1% of Hyperparathyroidism

Parathyroid carcinomas are rare. They affect both sexes, mainly between the ages of 30 and 60. They are usually functioning tumors, and most patients present with symptoms of hyperparathyroidism. Hypercalcemia in these patients is often severe, with serum calciums in excess of 14 mg/dL.

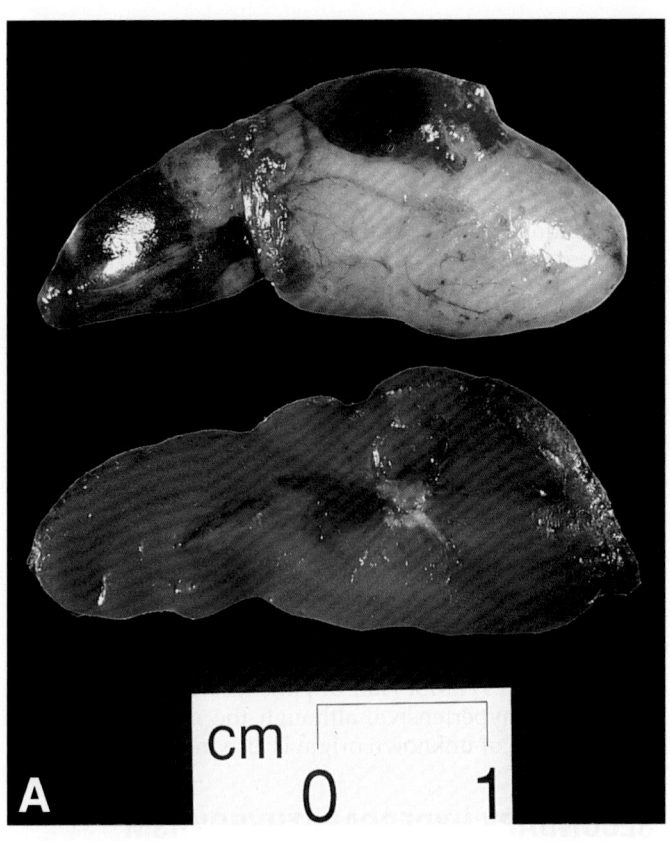

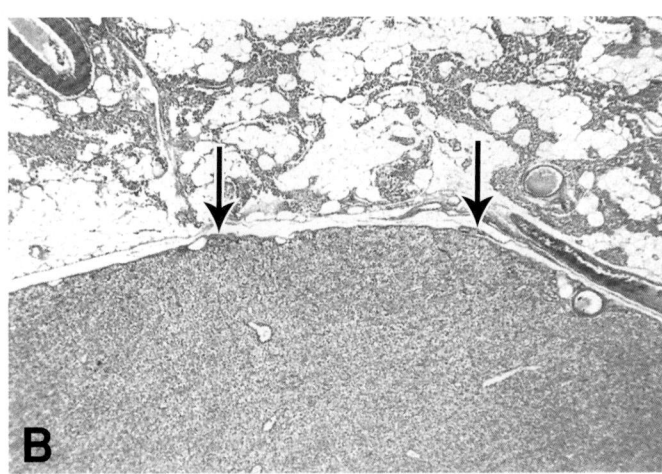

FIGURE 27-26. Parathyroid adenoma. A. External (*top*) and cross-section views (*bottom*) show a tan fleshy tumor. **B.** The tumor consists of sheets of neoplastic chief cells and is separated from normal parenchyma by a thin capsule (*arrows*).

ETIOLOGY: The etiology of these tumors is not known. Neck radiation and hereditary syndromes with histories of parathyroid adenomas are risk factors. Other syndromes of increased risk include hyperparathyroidism–jaw tumor syndrome and familial isolated hyperparathyroidism.

MOLECULAR PATHOGENESIS: Like functioning parathyroid adenomas, some parathyroid carcinomas overexpress cyclin D_1, suggesting that deregulation of this proto-oncogene may be important in parathyroid neoplasia in general. Most parathyroid carcinomas lack retinoblastoma protein (pRb; see Chapter 5), which

is present in most adenomas. Losses in chromosome 13q and mutations of *HRPT2* occur. This tumor suppressor gene, at chromosome 1q25-31, is responsible for the hyperparathyroidism–jaw tumor syndrome. It encodes parafibromin, expression of which is low or absent in hyperparathyroid–jaw tumor syndrome and in carcinomas.

PATHOLOGY: Parathyroid carcinomas tend to be larger than adenomas and appear as lobulated, firm, tannish, unencapsulated masses. They often adhere to surrounding soft tissues. Most carcinomas show trabecular cell arrangements, with significant mitotic activity and thick fibrous bands. Tumors occasionally invade capsules or blood vessels. The cellular atypia that occurs often in parathyroid adenomas is rare in carcinomas. Proliferative markers such as MiB1 show a high proliferative index. Other markers suggestive of parathyroid malignancy include increased expression of galectin 3, loss of *APC* and negative staining for parafibromin.

Treatment of PTH carcinoma includes surgery and, when invasive disease or metastases are present, chemotherapy and radiation therapy. After surgical removal, local recurrence is common: about 1/3 of patients develop metastases to regional lymph nodes, lungs, liver and bone. If fatal, death is most often due to hyperparathyroidism rather than carcinomatosis. Ten-year survival is 50%.

Clinical Features of Hyperparathyroidism are Highly Variable

CLINICAL FEATURES: Some patients with hyperparathyroidism have asymptomatic hypercalcemia, detected on routine blood analysis. Others show florid systemic, renal and skeletal disease (Fig. 27-28).

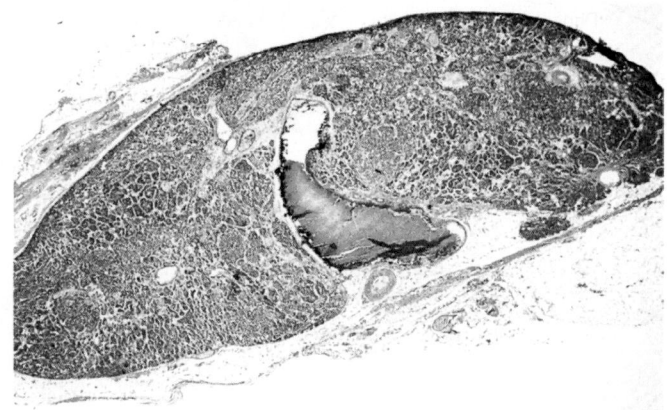

FIGURE 27-27. Primary parathyroid hyperplasia. The normal adipose tissue of the gland has been replaced by sheets and trabeculae of hyperplastic chief cells.

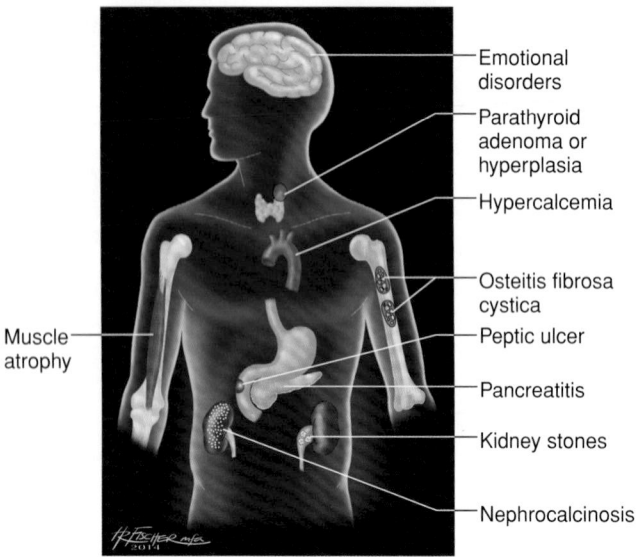

FIGURE 27-28. Major clinical features of hyperparathyroidism.

Hypercalcemia and hypophosphatemia are typical. High PTH levels cause excessive calcium loss from bones and enhanced calcium resorption by renal tubules. PTH also stimulates production of the activated form of vitamin D (1,25[OH]$_2$D) by renal tubules, thus increasing intestinal calcium absorption. The actions of PTH on the kidney, together with hypercalcemia, lead to hypophosphatemia. Common symptoms include nausea, vomiting, fatigue, weight loss, anorexia, polyuria and polydipsia. A neck mass is palpable in many patients. Other systems affected are:

SKELETAL SYSTEM: The classic bone lesions of hyperparathyroidism, **osteitis fibrosa cystica** (see Chapter 30),

occur in a minority of patients who have an accelerated and serious form of the disease. These patients present with bone pain, bone cysts, pathologic fractures and localized bone swellings (brown tumors, epulis of the jaw). Chondrocalcinosis may be a complication of hyperparathyroidism.

KIDNEY: Renal colic due to kidney stones brings 10% of patients with primary hyperparathyroidism to medical attention. Nephrocalcinosis, observed radiologically as diffuse renal calcification, may also occur (see Chapter 22). Polyuria is caused by hypercalciuria and leads to polydipsia.

NERVOUS SYSTEM: Psychiatric changes are common. They include depression, emotional lability, poor mentation and memory defects. Reflexes are hyperactive. Peripheral neuropathy with skeletal muscle type 2 fiber atrophy leads to weakness.

GI TRACT: Peptic ulcer disease is increased in patients with hyperparathyroidism, possibly because hypercalcemia increases serum gastrin, thus stimulating gastric acid secretion. Peptic ulcers in MEN1, which includes parathyroid hyperplasia or adenoma, may be secondary to Zollinger-Ellison syndrome (see Chapter 21). Hypercalcemia may also cause constipation and chronic pancreatitis by means not well understood.

OTHER SYSTEMS: Half of patients with hyperparathyroidism are hypertensive, although the mechanism is not clear. Anemia of unknown origin is also frequent.

SECONDARY HYPERPARATHYROIDISM

Secondary parathyroid hyperplasia occurs mainly in patients with chronic renal failure, but also in association with vitamin D deficiency, intestinal malabsorption, Fanconi syndrome and renal tubular acidosis (Fig. 27-29). Chronic hypocalcemia due to renal retention of phosphate,

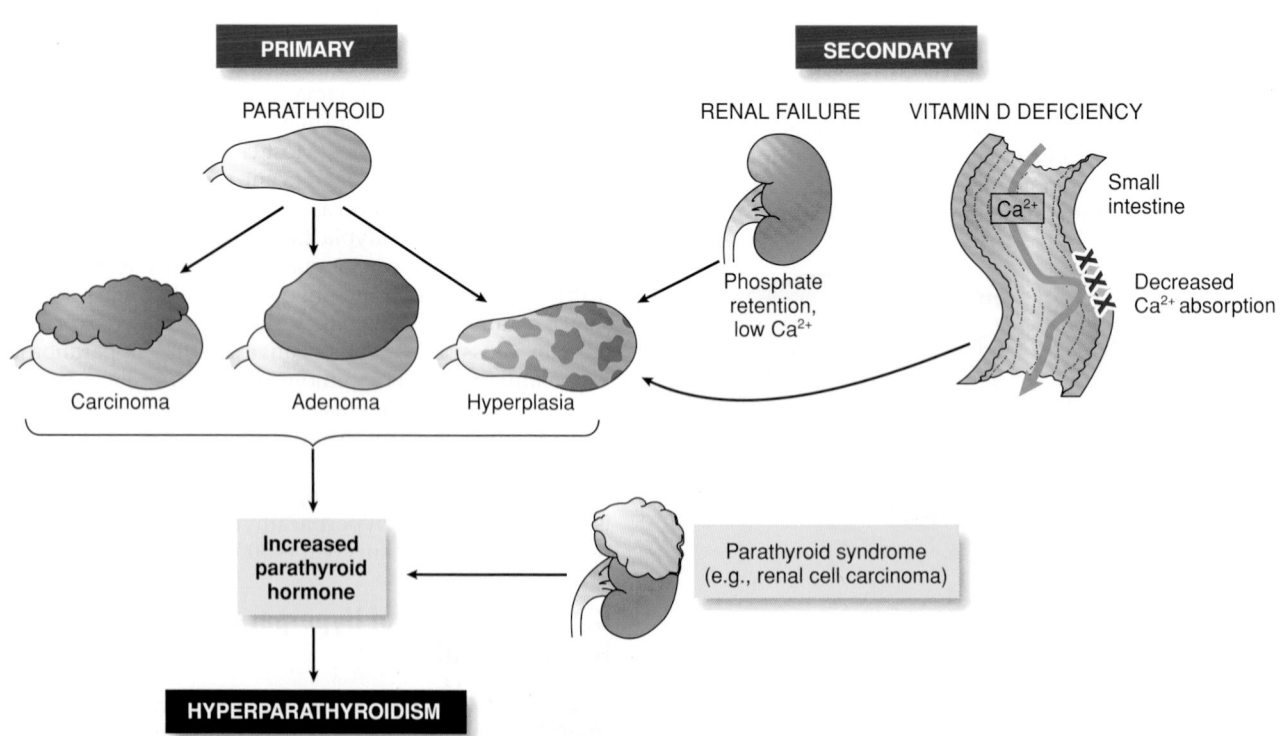

FIGURE 27-29. Major pathogenetic pathways leading to clinical primary and secondary hyperparathyroidism.

inadequate 1,25(OH)$_2$D production by diseased kidneys and some skeletal resistance to PTH all cause compensatory PTH hypersecretion.

Secondary hyperplasia of all parathyroids leads to excess levels of PTH, which produces the main clinical manifestations of skeletal pain and deformities, osteomalacia and osteitis fibrosis cystica and osseous manifestations of hyperparathyroidism, called **renal osteodystrophy** (see Chapter 30).

Pain, swelling and joint stiffness may be due to calcium deposits around joints. The parathyroids in secondary hyperplasia resemble those in primary chief cell hyperplasia. Treatment is surgical removal of the enlarged glands, with or without reimplantation.

Tertiary hyperparathyroidism is autonomous parathyroid hyperplasia following long-standing secondary hyperplasia because of renal failure. In such cases, parathyroid hyperplasia may not regress after renal transplantation, and parathyroidectomy is required. Two thirds of patients with long-standing uremia have monoclonal hyperplastic parathyroid proliferations.

Adrenal Cortex

ANATOMY

Each adrenal (or suprarenal) gland contains two independent endocrine organs: the cortex and the medulla. They are distinct anatomically, functionally and embryologically. The cortex arises from celomic mesenchymal cells near the urogenital ridge and secretes steroid hormones such as aldosterone, cortisol and testosterone. The medulla arises from neuroectoderm invading fetal adrenal glands. It produces catecholamines.

Adult adrenal glands are pyramidal organs above each kidney, found anteriorly in the retroperitoneum. Each gland is 4–6 cm in greatest dimension and weighs **4–6 g**. The adrenal glands secrete steroid hormones or corticosteroids, regulate metabolism and immune system function and aid in responses to stress. Grossly, and on cut section, the cortex has a characteristic yellow color because of lipid deposits. The medulla is paler gray-tan. The cortex contains 3 layers or zones:

- The **zona glomerulosa** is the outermost layer. There, aldosterone production is stimulated by angiotensin and potassium and inhibited by atrial natriuretic peptide and somatostatin. The zona glomerulosa makes up 15% of the cortex, with indistinct spherical nests of cells with dark-staining nuclei and moderate numbers of cytoplasmic fat droplets.
- The **zona fasciculata** makes up 75% of the cortex and produces glucocorticoids, such as cortisol. It is not distinctly separated from the zona glomerulosa. This zone contains radial cords of larger cells, each with a small nucleus and a large, foamy, clear cytoplasm, representing stored lipid.
- The **zona reticularis** secretes androgens and is the innermost layer, adjacent to the medulla. Irregular anastomosing cords are composed of compact smaller cells with a lipid-poor, slightly granular eosinophilic cytoplasm and bland nuclei.

Electron microscopy shows that adrenal cortical cells have abundant smooth endoplasmic reticulum and many mitochondria with lamellar cristae, which is common for steroid-producing cells.

The medulla is in the center of the gland, surrounded by cortex. It secretes norepinephrine and adrenaline.

Ectopic adrenal tissue can occur in many places outside the gland, since the cells migrate alongside the gonads. Common locations include the retroperitoneum, the broad ligament near the ovary, near the epididymis, the kidney and the liver. Ectopic adrenal tissue contains only cortex, not medulla. Small nodules of adrenocortical cells often occur in the fibroadipose tissue that surrounds the adrenal gland.

Congenital Adrenal Hypoplasia

This condition is quite rare and may accompany renal agenesis. It has been reported in association with infant death syndrome and with hypogonadotrophic hypogonadism in adolescents. It is X linked, caused by mutations in the *DAX-1* gene at Xp21.

CONGENITAL ADRENAL HYPERPLASIA

 **ETIOLOGY AND PATHOPHYSIOLOGY:** *Congenital adrenal hyperplasia (CAH) results from several autosomal recessive enzyme defects in the biosynthesis of cortisol from cholesterol* (Fig. 27-30). Deficiencies vary from mild to complete lack of cortisol. In general, impaired corticosteroid synthesis leads to unopposed action of ACTH and therefore adrenal hyperplasia. CAH occurs equally in males and females and is the most common cause of ambiguous genitalia in newborn girls (Fig. 27-31A).

 PATHOLOGY: Adrenal glands are enlarged, weighing as much as 30 g (Fig. 27-31B). Their cut surfaces are soft, tan to brown and either diffusely enlarged or nodular. The cortex is widened between the medulla and zona glomerulosa (Fig. 27-31C). The hyperplastic zone is filled by compact, granular, eosinophilic cells. In most cases, the zona glomerulosa is also hyperplastic, but not to the extent of the other zones, especially the zona fasciculata. Ectopic adrenal tissues or nodules may be also hyperplastic, and if stimulation persists, adenomas can develop.

21-Hydroxylase, or P450$_{C21}$, Deficiency Is the Major Cause of CAH

It is responsible for up to 90% of cases. The gene for P450$_{C21}$ (CYP21) is linked to the *MHC* locus on the short arm of chromosome 6 (6p21.3) and is closely associated with *HLA-B* and *C4A* and *C4B* complement genes. The incidence of CAH varies from 1 in 10,000 among whites to 1 in 500 in Alaskan Eskimos.

P450$_{C21}$ is a microsomal enzyme that converts 17-hydroxyprogesterone to 11-deoxycortisol. A deficiency in this enzymatic activity limits cortisol biosynthesis. Accumulated precursors are instead converted to androgens.

 CLINICAL FEATURES: Clinical manifestations are the result of cortisol or accumulation of steroids that may need to be synthesized in different pathways. There are different forms of CAH: 1, "classic"; 2, "nonclassic," a milder form that usually develops in late childhood or early adulthood; and 3, "cryptic," in which the

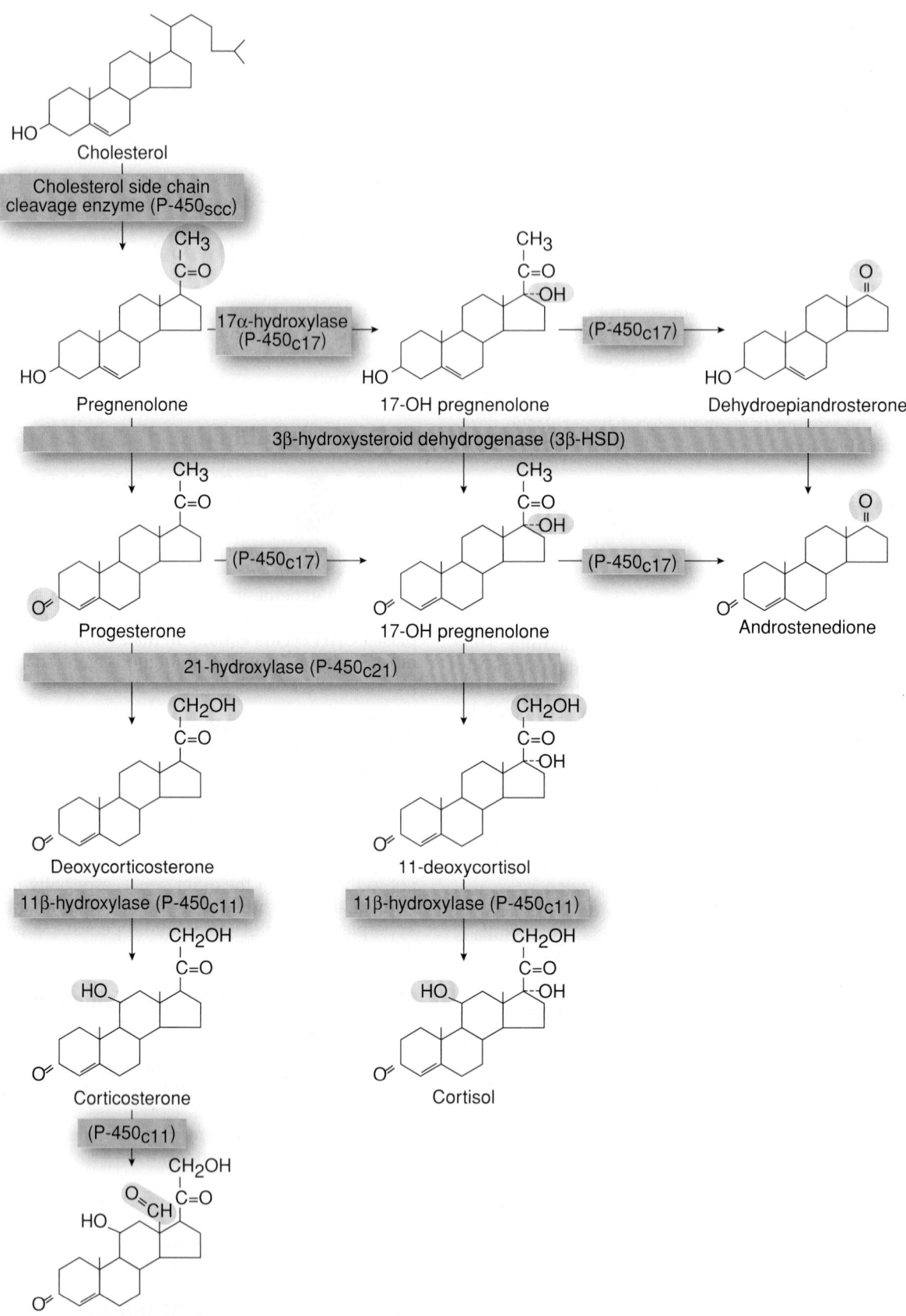

FIGURE 27-30. Biosynthetic pathways in the synthesis of adrenal corticosteroids.

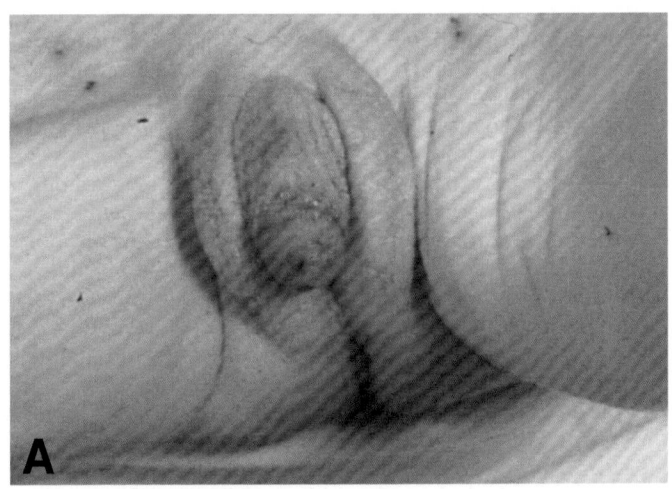

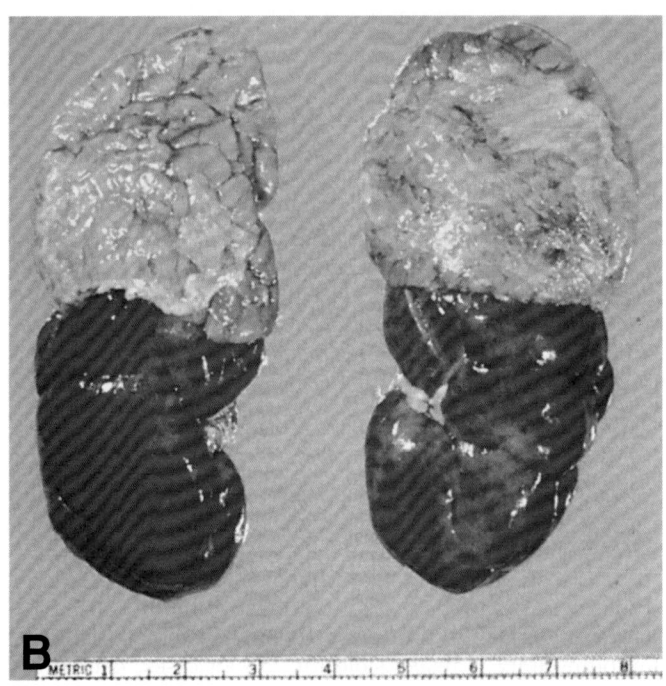

FIGURE 27-31. Congenital adrenal hyperplasia. A. A female infant is markedly virilized with hypertrophy of the clitoris and partial fusion of labioscrotal folds. **B.** A 7-week-old male died of severe salt-wasting congenital adrenal hyperplasia. At autopsy, both adrenal glands were markedly enlarged. **C.** A microscopic view shows a widened cortex containing compact eosinophilic cells.

biochemical abnormalities occur but patients do not have symptoms.

Classic CAH, the more severe form of the disease, is usually detected in infancy and is caused by $P450_{C21}$ deficiency. Two variants affect newborns. One is simple virilizing CAH; the other is a salt-wasting form that is linked to HLA-Bw47. There is also a less severe late-onset (nonclassic) variant. Mutations that result in complete inactivation of 21-hydroxylase lead to salt-wasting CAH, while those that reduce activity to 2% cause simple virilizing CAH. Late-onset CAH is intermediate.

SIMPLE VIRILIZING CAH: Female infants show pseudohermaphroditism; males have no abnormalities of the sexual organs. Conversion of cortisol precursors into adrenal androgens is amplified by the ACTH-dependent increase in the size of the gland. Female newborns exposed to a large excess of adrenal androgens in utero are born with fused labia, an enlarged clitoris and a urogenital sinus that may be mistaken for a penile urethra (Fig. 27-31A). As a result, the infant may be mislabeled as male.

Female external genitalia are not necessarily abnormal at birth, but infant girls may develop a syndrome of androgen excess, with clitoral enlargement and pubic hair. Infant boys exhibit sexual precocity. Eventually, the high levels of adrenal androgens lead to premature closure of epiphyses and short stature. Adult women with CAH tend to be infertile because elevated levels of androgens and progestogens interfere with the hypothalamic–pituitary–gonadal axis, disturb the menstrual cycle and inhibit ovulation. Men with CAH may be fertile, but some have azoospermia.

SALT-WASTING CAH: Owing to 21-hydroxylase deficiency, aldosterone synthesis may be impaired. Hypoaldosteronism then develops in the first few weeks of life in 2/3 of cases of CAH. Hyponatremia, hyperkalemia, dehydration, hypotension and increased renin secretion are typical. These may be rapidly fatal if not treated (Fig. 21-31B).

Therapy for both infantile variants of CAH caused by $P450_{C21}$ deficiency includes glucocorticoids and mineralocorticoids to suppress ACTH and replace steroids.

Reconstructive surgery may be necessary for virilized girls with ambiguous genitalia.

LATE-ONSET CAH: Patients with nonclassic variants of 21-hydroxylase deficiency show no abnormalities at birth but develop virilizing symptoms at puberty. In young women, late-onset CAH may closely resemble polycystic ovary syndrome (see Chapter 24). Most young men with the disorder are asymptomatic. This form of CAH is probably more common than is classic CAH, particularly among Ashkenazi Jews, Italians and people from the former Yugoslavia. Treatment is directed toward providing glucocorticoids to reduce hyperplasia and overproduction of androgens or mineralocorticoids.

11β-Hydroxylase Deficiency Causes 5% of CAH

This disorder is uncommon in the general population, but among Jews of Iranian or Moroccan ancestry in Israel, it is the most common cause of CAH. It is inherited as an autosomal recessive trait. The gene for 11β-hydroxylase is on chromosome 8q21-22 and so is unrelated to the *HLA* locus. 11β-Hydroxylase catalyzes terminal hydroxylation in cortisol biosynthesis. In addition to the androgenic complications of CAH, high levels of 11-deoxycortisol, which is a weak mineralocorticoid, often cause sodium retention and accompanying hypertension.

Rare forms of CAH include deficiencies of several enzymes of adrenocorticosteroid biosynthesis pathways. These lead to diverse combinations of electrolyte abnormalities and anomalies of the sex organs. Treatment of such conditions is lifelong glucocorticoid replacement sufficient to prevent adrenal insufficiency.

ADRENAL CORTICAL INSUFFICIENCY

Deficient production of adrenal cortical hormones can result from (1) adrenal gland destruction, (2) pituitary or hypothalamic dysfunction with decreased ACTH production or (3) chronic corticosteroid therapy.

Primary Chronic Adrenal Insufficiency (Addison Disease) Often Reflects Autoimmune Destruction of the Adrenal

Addison disease is a fatal wasting disorder caused by failure of the adrenal glands to produce glucocorticoids, mineralocorticoids and androgens. It causes weakness, weight loss, muscle pain, gastrointestinal symptoms, hypotension, electrolyte imbalance and hyperpigmentation. Some patients may have cravings for salt or salty foods.

PATHOPHYSIOLOGY: When Addison described primary adrenal insufficiency in 1855, the most common cause of the syndrome was tuberculosis involving the adrenal glands. Worldwide, tuberculosis is probably still the most common cause of chronic adrenal insufficiency, but in Western societies, autoimmunity is responsible for 75% of cases. Autoimmune adrenalitis may be an isolated disorder or a part of two different polyglandular autoimmune syndromes. Sporadic cases may in fact be variants of type II polyglandular autoimmune syndrome (see below). Other causes of adrenal destruction include metastatic carcinoma, amyloidosis, hemorrhage, sarcoidosis and fungal infections. In idiopathic Addison disease, the biochemical defect of adrenoleukodystrophy (see Chapter 32) is common. Rarely, adrenal insufficiency is due to congenital adrenal hypoplasia or familial glucocorticoid deficiency (defective ACTH receptor).

The autoimmune pathogenesis of most cases of Addison disease is supported by:

- Lymphoid infiltrates in the adrenal gland
- Circulating antibodies to adrenal antigens
- Abnormal cell-mediated immunity
- Associations with other autoimmune endocrinopathies
- Genetic linkage with *HLA* loci

IMMUNE MECHANISMS: Antiadrenal antibodies that react with tissue from all three zones of the adrenal cortex are present in 2/3 of patients with chronic adrenal insufficiency that could not be attributed to a specific cause. The major autoantigens are adrenal steroidogenic enzymes, particularly P450$_{C21}$. In Addison disease, autoantibodies do occur, but cell-mediated immunity is probably predominantly to blame. Increased numbers of Ia+ T lymphocytes and decreased suppressor T-cell function are reported in blood from patients with the disorder.

POLYENDOCRINE SYNDROMES: Half of patients with autoimmune adrenal insufficiency suffer from other autoimmune endocrine diseases. These are grouped into two polyendocrine syndromes.

Type I polyendocrine autoimmune syndrome or **candidiasis–hypoparathyroidism–Addison disease syndrome** is a rare autosomal recessive condition with a slight female predominance. It is seen in older children and adolescents. In addition to adrenal insufficiency, most (60%) patients also have hypoparathyroidism and chronic mucocutaneous candidiasis. Insulin-dependent diabetes (type 1) is common. Premature ovarian failure, hypothyroidism, infertility, malabsorption syndromes, pernicious anemia, chronic hepatitis, alopecia totalis and vitiligo are also frequent.

Type I polyendocrine disease is prevalent among Finns and Iranian Jews. The gene associated with it is *AIRE* (autoimmune regulator; see Chapter 11) on chromosome 21q22. *AIRE* is expressed in thymus, lymph nodes and fetal liver, all of which are involved in immune system maturation and immune tolerance. Like the common form of autoimmune Addison disease, sera from patients with type I polyendocrine disease recognize steroidogenic autoantigens and other targets.

Type II polyendocrine autoimmune syndrome (Schmidt syndrome) is more common than type I and always includes adrenal insufficiency. Women are affected twice as often as men. The disorder usually presents in young adults, ages 20–40. Half of cases are familial, but several modes of inheritance are known. HT and occasionally Graves disease occur in over 2/3 of cases. Insulin-dependent diabetes mellitus and premature ovarian failure are common. Rarely, other autoimmune diseases are present. This condition is considered as a polygenic disorder linked to HLA-DR3. Patients have a specific human leukocyte antigen genotype (*DQ2, DQ8* and *DRB1*0404*).

GENETIC FACTORS: Half of patients with autoimmune adrenal insufficiency as part of a polyendocrine syndrome have family histories of autoimmune endocrinopathy. If Addison disease occurs alone, 1/3 have an affected relative. Cases that are part of polyglandular syndrome type I are not linked to any *HLA* alleles. Otherwise, there is strong linkage between autoimmune adrenalitis and HLA-B8, HLA-DR3 and HLA-DR4.

PATHOLOGY: Over 90% of the adrenal gland must be destroyed in order for chronic adrenal insufficiency to be symptomatic. If specific infectious, neoplastic or metabolic disorders are involved, there is corresponding evidence of the underlying disorder in the adrenals. Autoimmune adrenalitis leads to pale, irregular, shrunken glands, weighing 2–3 g or less. The medulla is intact but surrounded by fibrous tissue with small islands of atrophic cortical cells (Fig. 27-32). Depending on the stage of the disease, variably intense lymphoid infiltrates, mainly T cells, may occur.

CLINICAL FEATURES: Addison's original description of the clinical features of chronic adrenal insufficiency still applies to untreated cases. Patients had "general languor and debility, remarkable feebleness of the heart's action, irritability of the stomach and a peculiar change of the colour of the skin." Typically, the first symptom is insidious onset of weakness, which may become so profound that a patient is bedridden. Anorexia and weight loss are always present. A diffuse, tan pigmentation usually develops on the skin, and dark patches may appear on the mucous membranes. This hyperpigmentation is related to pituitary POMC stimulation of skin melanocytes. Hypotension, with blood pressures around 80/50 mm Hg, is the rule. A variety of

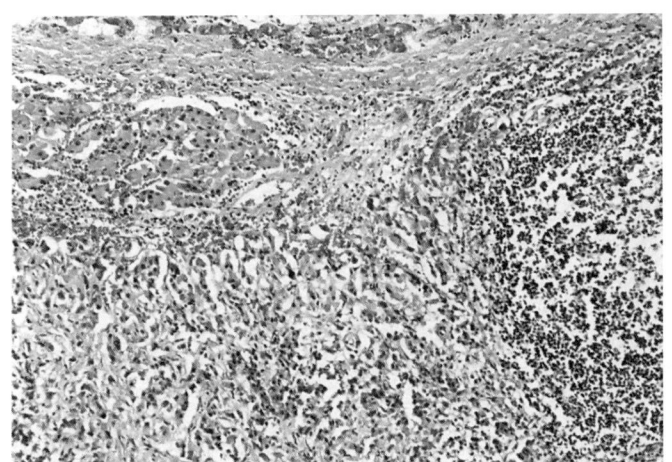

FIGURE 27-32. Autoimmune adrenalitis. A section of the adrenal gland from a patient with Addison disease shows chronic inflammation and fibrosis in the cortex, an island of residual atrophic cortical cells and an intact medulla.

GI symptoms, including vomiting, diarrhea and abdominal pain, affect most patients and may be the presenting complaint. Patients with Addison disease often show marked personality changes and even organic brain syndromes.

Deficient mineralocorticoid secretion, together with other metabolic derangements, leads to low serum sodium and high potassium levels. The absence of glucocorticoids leads to lymphocytosis and mild eosinophilia. The diagnosis is made by measuring corticosteroid blood levels after ACTH stimulation. With glucocorticoid and mineralocorticoid replacement, patients live normal lives.

Acute Adrenal Insufficiency Is a Life-Threatening Emergency

In acute adrenal insufficiency, or adrenal crisis, there is sudden loss of adrenal cortical function. Symptoms relate more to mineralocorticoid deficiency than to inadequate glucocorticoids. Adrenal crisis occurs in three settings:

- Abrupt withdrawal of corticosteroid therapy in patients with adrenal atrophy due to long-term steroid administration. This is the most common cause of acute adrenal insufficiency.
- Stress of infection or surgery may precipitate sudden, devastating worsening of chronic adrenal insufficiency.
- *Waterhouse-Friderichsen syndrome is acute, bilateral, hemorrhagic infarction of the adrenal cortex, most often secondary to meningococcus or* Pseudomonas *septicemia* (see Chapter 7). Adrenal hemorrhage in these circumstances is thought to be a local manifestation of a generalized Shwartzman reaction with disseminated intravascular coagulation. Acute adrenal insufficiency due to adrenal hemorrhage is also seen in newborns subjected to birth trauma.

CLINICAL FEATURES: The initial manifestations of adrenal crisis are usually hypotension and shock. Nonspecific symptoms commonly include weakness, vomiting, abdominal pain and lethargy, which may progress to coma. Typically in Waterhouse-Friderichsen syndrome, a young person suddenly develops hypotension and shock, abdominal or back pain, fever and purpura.

Adrenal crisis is almost always fatal unless diagnosed quickly and prompt and aggressive therapy is instituted with corticosteroids and supportive measures.

Secondary Adrenal Insufficiency Reflects Lack of ACTH

Destruction of the pituitary and consequent panhypopituitarism (see above) result in secondary adrenal insufficiency. Causes include pituitary tumors, craniopharyngioma, empty sella syndrome and pituitary infarction. Trauma, surgery and radiation therapy may also cause loss of pituitary function. Isolated ACTH deficiency is often associated with autoimmune endocrinopathies.

Any disorder that interferes with secretion of corticotropin (ACTH)-releasing hormone (CRH) by the hypothalamus (e.g., tumors, sarcoidosis) can lead to inadequate ACTH secretion. The fact that patients can secrete glucocorticoids in response to ACTH distinguishes this from primary adrenal insufficiency. Pigment and electrolyte abnormalities are typically absent in secondary adrenal insufficiency because these processes are not regulated by ACTH.

ADRENAL HYPERFUNCTION

Excess corticosteroid secretion occurs in adrenal hyperplasia or neoplasia (Fig. 27-33). Such hyperfunction may take one of two forms: **hypercortisolism** (Cushing syndrome) or **hyperaldosteronism** (Conn syndrome), for the two major classes of adrenal steroids.

Early in the 20th century, the neurosurgeon Harvey Cushing associated "painful obesity, hypertrichosis and amenorrhea" with the presence of a pituitary tumor. The combination of pituitary hyperfunction plus the signs and symptoms of chronic glucocorticoid excess was called Cushing disease. This constellation of clinical features due to high glucocorticoid levels can also result from adrenal tumors, ectopic ACTH or CRH secretion by tumors or exogenous corticosteroid administration. *Hypercortisolism from any cause is now called* **Cushing syndrome***; the term* **Cushing disease** *is reserved for excessive ACTH secretion by pituitary corticotrope tumors.*

The most common cause of Cushing syndrome in the United States is chronic corticosteroid administration to treat immune and inflammatory disorders. The second most common cause is paraneoplastic syndromes associated with nonpituitary cancers that inappropriately produce ACTH (see below). Cushing disease is 5-fold more common than the type of Cushing syndrome associated with adrenal tumors.

ACTH-Dependent Adrenal Hyperfunction Is of Pituitary Origin, or Ectopic

PATHOPHYSIOLOGY: Women, usually ages 25–45, are 5 times more likely than men to develop Cushing disease. Excessive ACTH secretion leads to adrenal cortical hyperplasia. ACTH-dependent adrenal hyperfunction results from:

- Ectopic ACTH production by a nonpituitary tumor
- Primary hypersecretion of ACTH by the pituitary (Cushing disease)

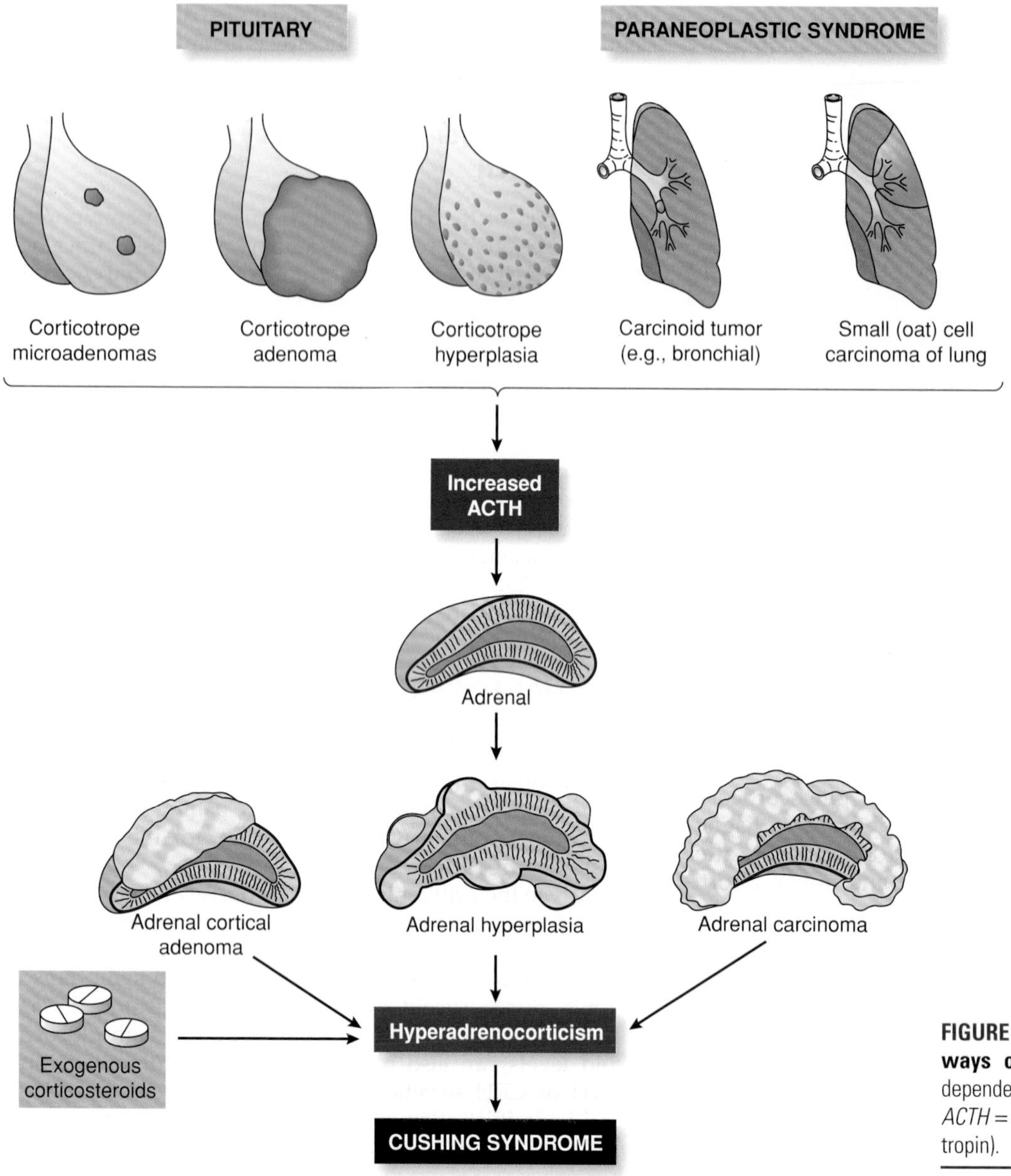

PITUITARY

PARANEOPLASTIC SYNDROME

Corticotrope
microadenomas

Corticotrope
adenoma

Corticotrope
hyperplasia

Carcinoid tumor
(e.g., bronchial)

Small (oat) cell
carcinoma of lung

**Increased
ACTH**

Adrenal

Adrenal cortical
adenoma

Adrenal hyperplasia

Adrenal carcinoma

Exogenous
corticosteroids

Hyperadrenocorticism

CUSHING SYNDROME

FIGURE 27-33. The pathogenetic pathways of Cushing syndrome. The ACTH-dependent pathway is called Cushing disease. *ACTH* = adrenocorticotropic hormone (corticotropin).

- Inappropriate secretion of CRH by tumors arising outside the hypothalamus, with secondary pituitary hypersecretion of ACTH

ECTOPIC PRODUCTION OF ACTH: Inappropriate ACTH secretion by a malignant tumor accounts for most cases of ACTH-dependent hyperadrenalism. Cancers of the lung, particularly small cell carcinoma, are responsible for over half of the cases of ectopic ACTH syndrome. The remainder are mainly due to carcinoids and neural crest tumors (pheochromocytomas, neuroblastomas, medullary thyroid carcinomas), thymomas and islet cell tumors of the pancreas.

PRIMARY HYPERSECRETION OF ACTH: Cushing disease usually results from pituitary corticotrope microadenomas, although it may be due to a macroadenoma or, rarely, diffuse corticotrope hyperplasia. Adenomas are clearly monoclonal, arising from one progenitor cell, but corticotrope hyperplasia reflects chronic CRH hypersecretion.

ECTOPIC CRH PRODUCTION: Ectopic CRH syndrome is like ectopic ACTH syndrome, except that the tumor secretes CRH. In turn, CRH stimulates pituitary ACTH secretion, leading to adrenal hyperplasia.

 PATHOLOGY: Cushing disease is characterized by bilateral, diffuse (75%) or nodular (25%) adrenal hyperplasia. Each gland usually weighs 8–10 g but may weigh as much as 20 g.

In **diffuse adrenal hyperplasia,** the cortex is grossly visible and broadened, with an inner brown layer and a yellow, lipid-rich cap. The inner third of the cortex is composed of a compact cell layer. The outer zone, corresponding to the zona fasciculata, has large clear cells packed with lipid. The zona glomerulosa varies: it may sometimes be prominent and at other times difficult to identify.

Nodular adrenal hyperplasia is limited to grossly visible nodules up to 2.5 cm (microscopic nodules are common in diffuse hyperplasia). Bilateral, multiple nodules compress the overlying cortex, and intervening parenchyma shows diffuse hyperplasia. However, nodular hyperplasia may be asymmetric and the two glands may differ significantly in weight. Hyperplastic nodules contain large, lipid-laden, clear cells.

ACTH-Independent Adrenal Hyperfunction Is Caused by Adrenal Tumors

In adults, the incidence of adrenal carcinoma peaks at age 40, and that of adenoma a decade later. In children, adrenal carcinomas account for half of cases of Cushing syndrome; 15% are caused by adenoma. At all ages, the female-to-male ratio is 4:1.

Adrenal Adenomas

Adrenal adenomas derive from the cortex. They produce SF-1Ad4BP, a binding protein secreted by adrenocortical cells. The incidence of these lesions is unknown because they are so often asymptomatic. Adenomas are frequently identified as part of syndromes such as MEN1, Carney complex and McCune Albright syndrome. Adenomas can produce hormones, the most common being cortisol and aldosterone.

 **PATHOLOGY:** A typical adenoma is 1–4 cm, encapsulated, firm, yellow and slightly lobulated (Fig. 27-34). These tumors usually weigh 10–50 g, although they may reach 100 g. Cut surfaces are mottled yellow and brown, and occasionally black, owing to lipofuscin pigment deposition. A thin rim of compressed normal adrenal cortex surrounds the tumor. Necrosis and calcifications are rare. Adenomas show clear, lipid-laden (fasciculata type) cells arranged in sheets or nests. They are often interspersed with clusters of compact, lipid-depleted, eosinophilic (reticularis type) cells. Large tumors may have myelolipomatous foci or calcification. The cortex of the involved, contralateral gland is generally atrophic or may show small micronodules.

Nonfunctional adrenal cortical adenomas occur in as many as 5% of adult autopsies, but less than 10% of surgically removed benign adrenal tumors are hormonally silent.

Nonfunctional adenomas are pathologically identical to their functional counterparts.

Adrenal Cortical Carcinomas

Adrenal cortical carcinomas (ACCs) are rare and aggressive tumors that have an incidence of 1 case per million per year. Sixty percent of adrenal cortical carcinomas are functional and secrete glucocorticoids and androgens. They occur more in women and have a poor prognosis. Computed tomography scans show a mass, usually larger than 5 cm. Positron emission tomography scanning with 18-fluorodeoxyglucose is useful to identify the primary tumor and its metastasis. Median survival is 30 months. The tumor metastasizes to lung, liver and lymph nodes. Local recurrences are common.

 ETIOLOGIC FACTORS: The etiology of these cancers is not known. Most cases are sporadic, but ACCs occur in association with Li-Fraumeni and Beckwith-Wiedemann syndromes and congenital adrenal hyperplasia.

 MOLECULAR PATHOGENESIS: No specific genetic alterations are characteristic for ACCs. However, overexpression of IGF-II in sporadic tumors; duplication of the paternal allele; and loss of heterozygosity at 11p15, 17p13 (p53 locus), 1p, 3p and 9p all occur in these tumors. Some tumors overexpress epidermal growth factor receptor and p21 and p16 genes (see Chapter 5). Diverse chromosomal gains and losses can occur, and rarely there can be alterations in other genes such as *RAS*, *RET* and *ATR1*. CXCL10 and CDH2 are downregulated. ACCs have shown MiR483-3p overexpression (68%) in comparison with adenomas (12%).

PATHOLOGY: The tumors vary in weight and may reach up to 5 kg. Improvements in diagnostic imaging have helped to identify smaller tumors at earlier stages. ACCs are soft, circumscribed, lobulated and bulky (Fig. 27-35). Cut surfaces are variegated pink, brown or yellow, often with necrosis, hemorrhage and cystic change. Local invasion is common, and remnants of normal adrenal are difficult to identify. The diagnosis of ACC is based on the

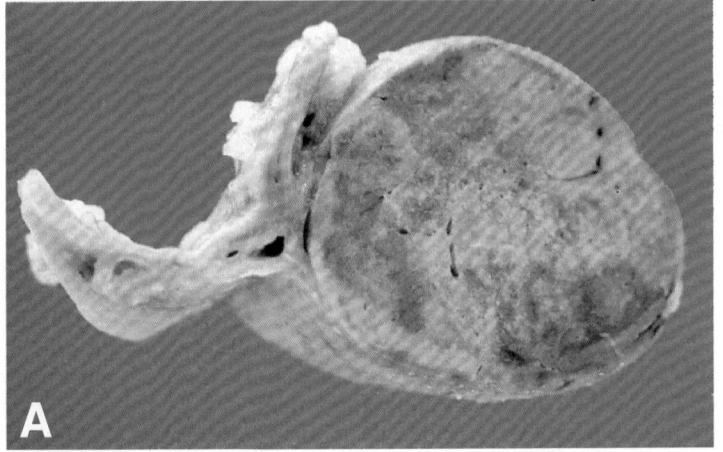

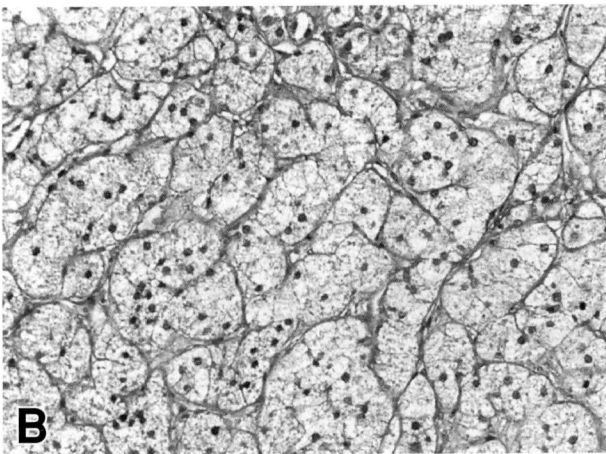

FIGURE 27-34. Adrenal adenoma. A. The cut surface of an adrenal tumor removed from a patient with Cushing syndrome is a mottled yellow with a rim of compressed normal adrenal tissue. **B.** A microscopic view reveals nests of clear, lipid-laden cells.

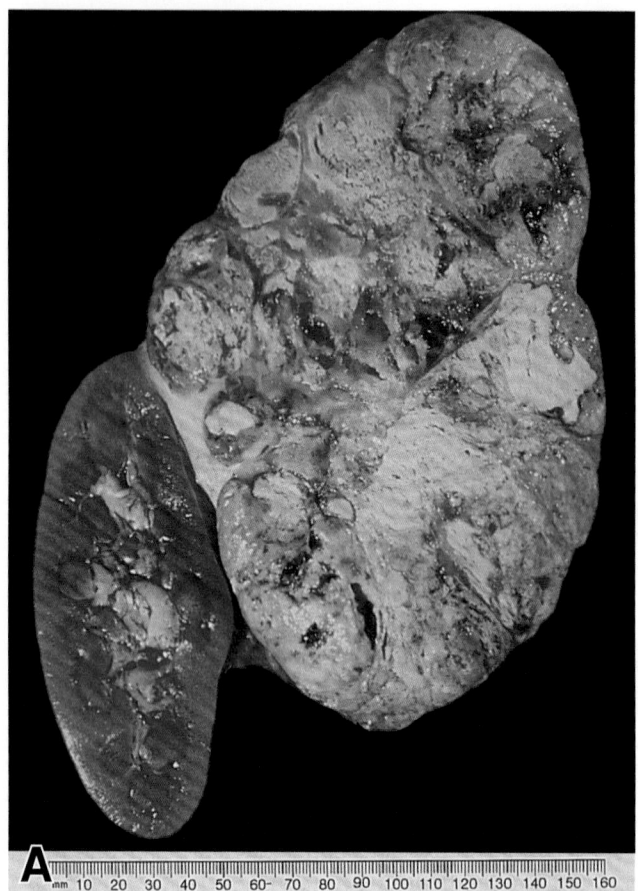

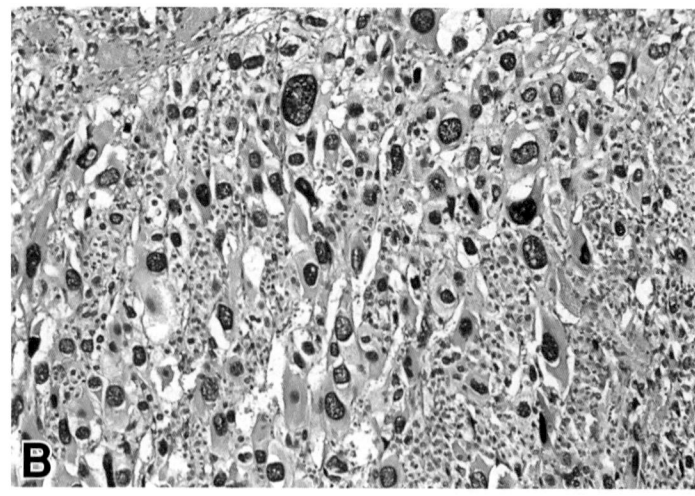

FIGURE 27-35. Adrenal cortical carcinoma. A. The bulky tumor on section is yellow to tan with areas of necrosis and cystic degeneration. **B.** A microscopic section demonstrates marked anisocytosis and nuclear pleomorphism.

modified criteria described by Weiss, which include mitotic figures (>5 per 50 high-power fields), clear cell cytoplasm, necrosis, nuclear pleomorphism, atypical mitosis, capsular or vascular invasion and diffuse architecture. In functional carcinomas, the contralateral adrenal cortex is atrophic. ACCs stain positively for synaptophysin, inhibin, MelanA/MART1, calretinin and CAM 5.2.

Most adrenal cortical carcinomas cannot be resected completely, and micrometastases in other organs are almost always already present. Surgery and adrenalectomy, followed by adjuvant therapy with mitotane plus radiation, offer the best hope of delaying tumor recurrence. Metastases to lung, liver and bone are common. The 5-year survival for patients with ACC limited to the adrenal gland is better (65%) than for patients with distant metastases (18%).

Nonfunctional adrenal cortical carcinomas tend to be highly malignant and often weigh more than 1 kg. They are morphologically identical to functional cancers.

Other Causes of ACTH-Independent Cushing Syndrome Include Chronic Corticosteroid Administration and Bilateral Micronodular Hyperplasia

Many immunologic and inflammatory diseases are treated with glucocorticoids, thus constituting by far the most common cause of Cushing syndrome. The synthetic hormones ordinarily used (e.g., dexamethasone, prednisone) have only glucocorticoid activity and little or no mineralocorticoid or androgen effect. Thus, hypertension and hirsutism, features common in Cushing syndrome due to adrenal hyperplasia or neoplasia, are usually absent in this iatrogenic disorder.

Bilateral adrenal cortical micronodular hyperplasia (Carney complex or **primary pigmented nodular adrenocortical disease)** is a rare cause of ACTH-independent Cushing syndrome, usually in children or young adults. Half have an autosomal dominant disease with pigmented skin lesions over much of their bodies, a variety of myxomas, testicular (Leydig cell) tumors and pituitary somatotrope adenomas. The adrenals contain small, brown or black nodules, up to 0.5 cm, with large eosinophilic cells laden with lipofuscin granules. The lesions appear as primary pigmented nodular adrenocortical disease (PPNAD). Half of patients with Carney complex carry mutations in a tumor suppressor gene (17q22-24), *PRKAR1A*, that encodes a regulatory subunit of protein kinase A. Another gene at 2p16 also is linked to the disease.

Clinical Features of Cushing Syndrome Are Seen in Many Organs

CLINICAL FEATURES: The manifestations of Cushing syndrome (Fig. 27-36) depend on the degree and duration of excessive corticosteroid levels, as well as on levels of adrenal androgens and mineralocorticoids. Most (70%) patients are females, and fewer than 20% of cases occur before puberty.

OBESITY: Typically, the patient notes gradual onset of obesity of the face (moon face), neck (buffalo hump), trunk and abdomen (Fig. 27-37). The extremities are characteristically unaffected or even wasted.

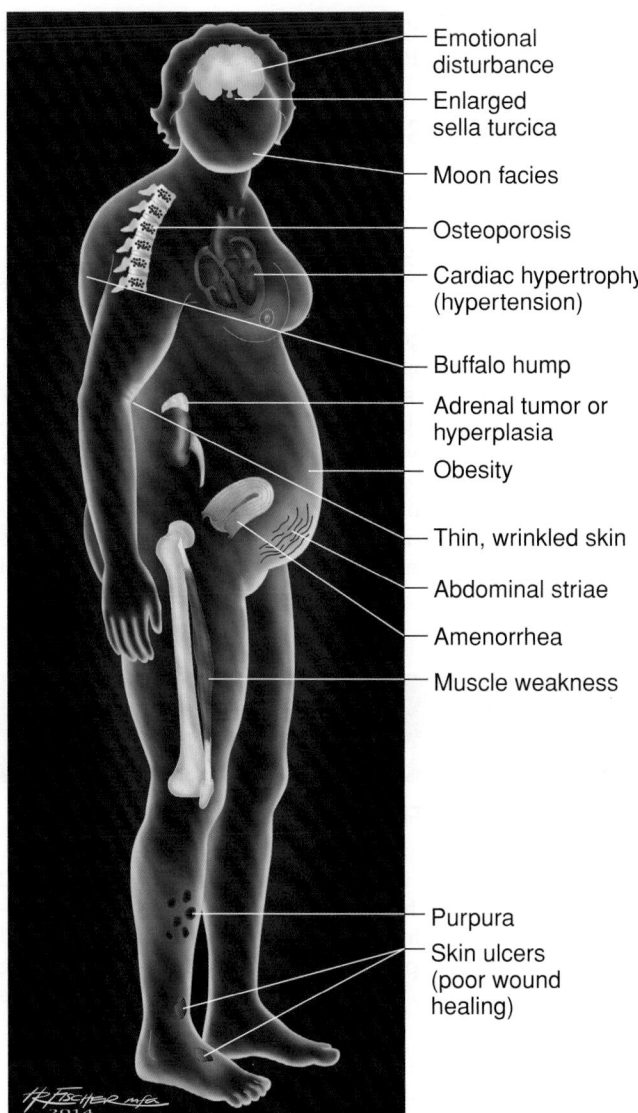

FIGURE 27-36. **Major clinical manifestations of Cushing syndrome.**

Emotional disturbance
Enlarged sella turcica
Moon facies
Osteoporosis
Cardiac hypertrophy (hypertension)
Buffalo hump
Adrenal tumor or hyperplasia
Obesity
Thin, wrinkled skin
Abdominal striae
Amenorrhea
Muscle weakness
Purpura
Skin ulcers (poor wound healing)

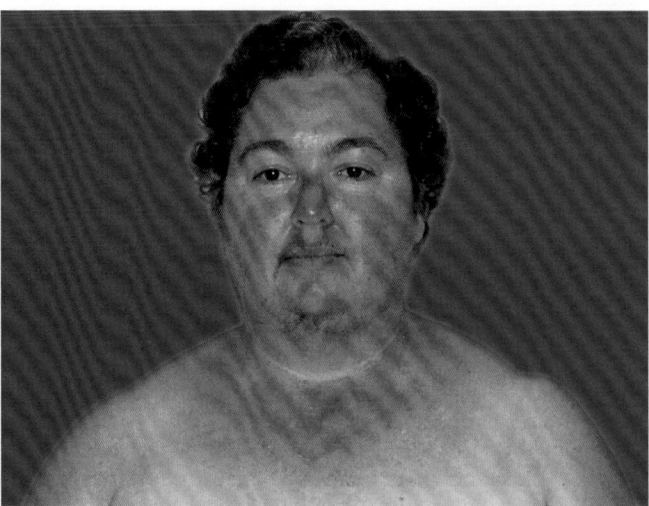

FIGURE 27-37. **Cushing syndrome.** A woman who had a pituitary adenoma that produced adrenocorticotropic hormone (ACTH) exhibits a moon face, buffalo hump, increased facial hair and thinning of the scalp hair.

SKIN: The skin is atrophic. Subcutaneous fat is decreased. The abdomen and other areas of fat deposition are prominent, stretching the skin thin and producing purplish striae. These represent venous channels that are visible through the attenuated dermis. Hyperpigmentation, similar to, but less severe than, that in Addison disease, may occur because of pituitary POMC hypersecretion. Acanthosis nigricans is increased in Cushing syndrome.

MUSCULOSKELETAL SYSTEM: Increased bone resorption causes osteoporosis. Back pain is common, and up to 1/5 of patients have radiologic evidence of vertebral compression fractures. Fractures of ribs and occasionally long bones may occur. Proximal muscle wasting **(steroid myopathy)** causes weakness, which may be so severe that the patient cannot rise from sitting or climb a flight of stairs.

CARDIOVASCULAR SYSTEM: Hypertension is common in Cushing syndrome, often reflecting excessive mineralocorticoid activity. In older patients, congestive heart failure may also result.

SECONDARY SEX CHARACTERISTICS: Women with Cushing syndrome tend to be virilized, with increased facial hair, thinning of scalp hair, acne and oligomenorrhea. Excess glucocorticoids in men cause erectile dysfunction, and both sexes experience decreased libido.

EYES: One fourth of patients have increased intraocular pressure, which may be a problem if there had been preexisting glaucoma.

GLUCOSE INTOLERANCE: Stimulation of gluconeogenesis by glucocorticoids leads to glucose intolerance and hyperinsulinemia. Diabetes mellitus develops in 15% of patients, usually in those with a family history of diabetes.

PSYCHOLOGICAL CHANGES: Most patients with Cushing syndrome, both endogenous and iatrogenic, undergo distinct personality changes. These include irritability, emotional lability, depression and paranoia. Disturbed mentation may be so severe that patients may become suicidal.

LABORATORY FINDINGS: Half of patients exhibit an absolute lymphopenia, and 1/3 have abnormally low eosinophil counts. Hypercalciuria is common, but serum calcium levels remain unchanged. Serum cholesterol and triglyceride levels are frequently elevated.

In all forms of Cushing syndrome, glucocorticoid levels are increased. The dexamethasone suppression test distinguishes ACTH-dependent and ACTH-independent forms of Cushing syndrome. Dexamethasone suppresses pituitary ACTH secretion, and hence hypercortisolism, but it is without effect on adrenal tumors.

Cushing syndrome is treated by (1) removal (surgery or irradiation) of pituitary, adrenal or ectopic ACTH-producing tumors; (2) stopping corticosteroid therapy; or (3) giving adrenal enzyme inhibitors (e.g., aminoglutethimide, ketoconazole, metapyrone). Except for ectopic ACTH syndrome and adrenal carcinoma, in which patients die of cancer rather than of hypercortisolism, Cushing syndrome is highly curable.

Primary Aldosteronism (Conn Syndrome) Leads to Hypertension and Hypokalemia

Excess secretion of aldosterone occurs with adrenal adenomas or hyperplasia. Such overproduction causes potassium to be lost in the urine and sodium retained.

Aldosterone-secreting adenomas are more common in women than in men (3:1) and usually occur between the ages of 30 and 50 years.

 MOLECULAR PATHOGENESIS: Most (75%) primary aldosteronism is due to solitary adrenal adenomas (aldosteronoma). In 1/4 of cases, adrenal hyperplasia is responsible. The rest reflect bilateral adrenal zona glomerulosa hyperplasia. Only a few cases of primary aldosteronism are caused by adrenal carcinomas.

There are 3 types of familial hyperaldosteronism. **Type I (glucocorticoid suppressible)** is an autosomal dominant disease caused by abnormal fusion of two genes, *CYP11B1* and *CYP11B2*, on chromosome 8. In these cases, hypertension generally appears in childhood. ACTH-responsive regulators of the 11β-hydroxylase gene fuse to the aldosterone synthase gene and create a hybrid constitutively active gene in the zona fasciculata. Bilateral hyperplasia of this zone results. By suppressing ACTH release, glucocorticoids prevent type I disease, which also responds to glucocorticoids.

In contrast, adrenal cortical adenomas are usually responsible for **type II familial hyperaldosteronism,** which therefore does not turn off with glucocorticoid administration. In type II, hypertension usually appears in early adulthood. **Type III hyperaldosteronism** is characterized by marked adrenal enlargement. Patients suffer childhood onset of severe hypertension that eventually may damage the heart and kidneys.

The underlying genetic defect(s) in familial hyperaldosteronism type II and type III are unknown. Early-onset hypertension and severe target organ damage are hallmarks of the heritable forms.

Aldosterone hypersecretion enhances renal tubular sodium reabsorption, thus increasing body sodium. Hypertension results not only from retention of sodium and consequent volume expansion but also from increased peripheral vascular resistance. Hypokalemia reflects aldosterone-induced loss of potassium in the distal renal tubule.

 PATHOLOGY: Most aldosterone-secreting adenomas measure less than 3 cm, weigh less than 6 g and are yellow. However, their sizes vary, and tumors up to 50 g may occur. The dominant cells are clear, lipid rich like the zona fasciculata and arranged in cords or alveoli. There is little nuclear pleomorphism. In contrast to cortisol-producing adenomas, the nontumorous cortex in cases of hyperaldosteronism is not atrophic, because aldosterone does not inhibit ACTH secretion by the pituitary.

If bilateral nodular adrenal hyperplasia causes Conn syndrome, adrenals contain yellow cortical nodules, usually less than 2 cm. These are formed by clear cells that show no nuclear pleomorphism.

CLINICAL FEATURES: Most patients with primary aldosteronism present with asymptomatic diastolic hypertension. Skeletal muscle weakness and fatigue are caused by potassium depletion. Polyuria and polydipsia result from impaired renal concentrating capacity, probably due to hypokalemia. Metabolic alkalosis and an alkaline urine are common.

Primary aldosteronism caused by an adenoma is curable by surgical removal of the tumor. Dietary sodium restriction and treatment with the aldosterone antagonist spironolactone are also frequently effective. Bilateral adrenal hyperplasia in Conn syndrome is treated medically with aldosterone antagonists, and sometimes with dexamethasone in the case of glucocorticoid-suppressible hyperaldosteronism.

MISCELLANEOUS ADRENAL TUMORS

Adrenal myelolipomas are mixtures of mature adipose tissue and hematopoietic marrow, notable because they may be very large. They rarely cause hypertension.

Adrenal cysts are rare. Most are actually pseudocysts derived from degeneration in benign adrenal tumors or resolution of hemorrhage. In some cases, they represent remnants of an underlying vascular lesion.

Metastatic cancers to the adrenal glands usually originate in the lungs or breast, or may be malignant melanomas. The glands may be unilaterally or bilaterally hugely enlarged, up to 20–45 g. They are largely replaced by cancer, often with necrosis and hemorrhage. Usually, enough functional adrenal cortex remains so that Addison disease does not develop, particularly in view of the limited survival of these patients.

Adrenal Medulla and Paraganglia

ANATOMY AND FUNCTION

The adrenal medulla is entirely surrounded by the adrenal cortex and accounts for 10% of the gland's weight. It consists of neuroendocrine cells, or **chromaffin cells,** derived from the primitive pheochromoblasts of the developing sympathetic nervous system (Fig. 27-38). Chromaffin cells

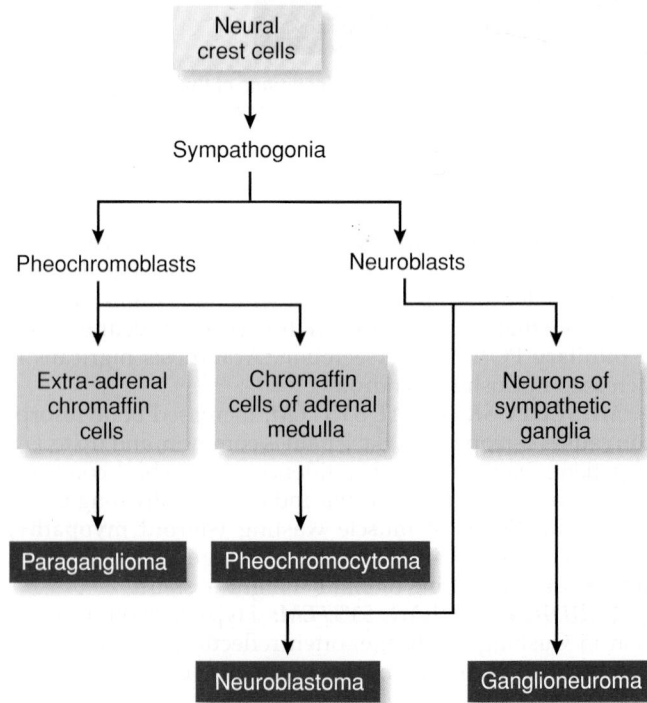

FIGURE 27-38. Histogenesis of tumors of the adrenal medulla and extra-adrenal sympathetic nervous system.

are so named because catecholamines in their cytoplasmic granules bind chromium salts and darken on oxidation by potassium dichromate. These cells are also present at extra-adrenal sympathetic nervous system sites, such as the preaortic sympathetic plexuses and paravertebral sympathetic chain.

Chromaffin cells appear as nests of small polyhedral cells with pale amphophilic cytoplasm and vesicular nuclei. The cells of the adrenal medulla have many electron-dense, 100–300-nm chromaffin (catecholamine-containing) granules, resembling those of sympathetic nerve endings. Epinephrine accounts for 85% of the content of these granules, with the remainder being norepinephrine and other noncatecholamine hormones. Interspersed among the chromaffin cells are postganglionic neurons and small autonomic nerve fibers. Stored catecholamines are secreted on sympathetic stimulation as a response to stress (exercise, cold, fasting, trauma) or emotional excitation accompanying fear and anger.

The adrenal medulla is supplied by arterial and portal venous circulations that originate in the zona reticularis of the cortex. Most of the blood to the hormonally active cells of the medulla is from the portal system. The medulla is innervated from the splanchnic nerves by cholinergic preganglionic sympathetic neurons.

PHEOCHROMOCYTOMA

Pheochromocytomas Are Rare Catecholamine-Secreting Tumors of Chromaffin Cells of the Adrenal Medulla and Elsewhere

Pheochromocytoma may arise in extra-adrenal sites, in which case they are called **paragangliomas**. Other catecholamine-producing tumors (e.g., chemodectoma and ganglioneuroma) may also cause a syndrome like that caused by pheochromocytomas.

Pheochromocytomas are rare tumors, somewhat more common in women than in men. They may occur at any age, including infancy, but are uncommon after age 60. *The presenting symptoms reflect sustained or episodic hypertension.* Other symptoms include headaches, pallor, anxiety and cardiac arrhythmias. Although they account for less than 0.1% of cases of hypertension, pheochromocytomas should be considered in evaluating any hypertensive patient. If detected early, they are amenable to surgical resection, but if left untreated, patients can die of complications of prolonged hypertension. Most pheochromocytomas are unexpected findings at autopsy, indicating that some curable cases of hypertension escaped clinical detection. Imaging using iodine-metaiodobenzylguanidine (I-MIBG), an analog of guanethidine that identifies several neuroendocrine tumors, may be useful in locating these tumors. Bilateral tumors strongly suggest familial disease.

PATHOPHYSIOLOGY: Pheochromocytomas are mostly sporadic. A minority are inherited, either alone or as part of hereditary syndromes, such as MEN types 2A or 2B, **paraganglioma-pheochromocytoma syndrome,** von Hippel-Lindau disease, neurofibromatosis type 1 or McCune-Albright syndrome.

The features of autosomal dominant MEN syndromes are (Fig. 27-39):

- **MEN type 1 (Wermer syndrome)** includes (1) pituitary adenoma, (2) parathyroid hyperplasia or adenoma and (3) islet cell tumors of the pancreas (e.g., insulinomas, gastrinomas). The pancreatic tumors tend to be multicentric and more malignant than in sporadic cases. Most (2/3) patients have adenomas of two or more endocrine organs, and 20% develop tumors of three or more. Carcinoid, adrenocortical and lipoid tumors may also occur in MEN1. Almost all people with MEN type 1 (>95%) have primary hyperparathyroidism. Mutation of the *MEN1* tumor suppressor gene (chromosome 11q13) is responsible. This gene encodes a nuclear protein, **menin,** which is thought to interact with the transcription factor junD.

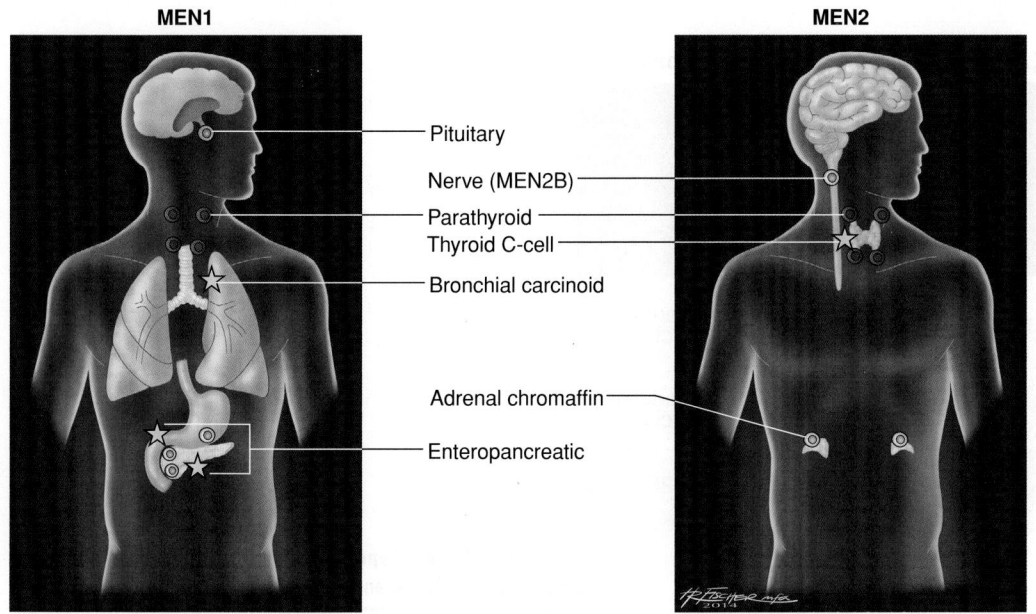

MEN1

- Pituitary
- Nerve (MEN2B)
- Parathyroid
- Thyroid C-cell
- Bronchial carcinoid
- Adrenal chromaffin
- Enteropancreatic

MEN2

FIGURE 27-39. Multiple endocrine neoplasia (MEN) syndromes. The locations of the most common endocrine tumors in hereditary MEN syndromes types 1 and 2 are shown.

- **MEN type 2 syndromes** almost always include MTCs, and pheochromocytoma is included in half.

MEN2A (SIPPLE SYNDROME): Most (95%) MEN2 patients are classified as type 2A. In addition to MTC and pheochromocytoma, 1/3 of patients show hyperparathyroidism due to parathyroid hyperplasia or adenomas. Several neural crest tumors may occur in MEN type 2A, including gliomas, glioblastomas and meningiomas. Hirschsprung disease is also associated with MEN type 2A.

MEN2B: This disorder resembles MEN2A, but it develops about 10 years earlier and rarely includes parathyroid disease. The **mucosal neuroma syndrome** (ganglioneuromas of the conjunctiva, oral cavity, larynx and gut) is a feature of MEN2B. Mucosal neuromas are always present, but only half of patients express the full phenotype. Many patients have a habitus resembling that of Marfan syndrome.

FAMILIAL MEDULLARY THYROID CARCINOMA: There are families who have at least 4 members with this tumor but no evidence of other features of MEN2.

Adrenal medullary hyperplasia occurs in some patients with MEN2A or -2B. Just as C-cell hyperplasia precedes medullary thyroid carcinomas, adrenal medullary hyperplasia may precede pheochromocytomas in these cases. Lesions are usually less than 1 cm. In these cases, an enlarged adrenal shows an expanded medulla. Chromaffin cells are larger than normal and are arranged in distinct nests or cords.

The *RET* proto-oncogene on chromosome 10q11.2 is responsible for MEN2 syndromes. *RET* encodes a transmembrane tyrosine kinase receptor whose ligands are glia-derived growth factor and neurturin. Several germline, missense and activating mutations in the cysteine-rich extracellular domain of RET occur in 95% of families with MEN2A, and in 85% of those with familial thyroid carcinomas (Fig. 27-40). The most common mutation (codon 634) constitu-

tively activates the receptor by promoting its dimerization, which recapitulates the result of ligand binding.

A point mutation at codon 918 of the tyrosine kinase domain of *RET* is present in 95% of patients with MEN2B. This mutation constitutively activates the receptor's tyrosine kinase function and also causes it to phosphorylate substrates ordinarily preferred by other kinases (e.g., c-*src* and c-*abl*).

Identification of RET *mutations confirms the diagnosis of MEN2 and identifies family members who are asymptomatic.* People with *RET* mutations are screened for thyroid cancer, pheochromocytoma and hyperparathyroidism between ages 6 and 35 and are offered prophylactic thyroidectomy.

Somatic mutations in *RET* occur in 10%–20% of cases of sporadic pheochromocytomas. In addition, some sporadic pheochromocytomas have mutations in the von Hippel-Lindau (*VHL*) and neurofibromatosis type 1 (*NF1*) genes.

 PATHOLOGY: In sporadic pheochromocytomas, 80% of tumors are unilateral, 10% are bilateral and 10% are in extraadrenal locations; 10% are malignant and 10% occur in children. Tumors occurring in the context of MEN are usually bilateral. Tumors vary from 1 cm to large masses of more than 2 kg. Most are 5–6 cm and weigh 80–100 g.

Pheochromocytomas tend to be encapsulated, spongy and reddish, with prominent central scars, hemorrhage and foci of cystic degeneration (Fig. 27-41A). Their histology is highly variable. Typically, circumscribed nests **(zellballen)** of polyhedral to fusiform neoplastic cells contain granular, amphophilic or basophilic cytoplasm and vesicular nuclei. Eosinophilic cytoplasmic globules are common. Cellular pleomorphism may be prominent, including multinucleated

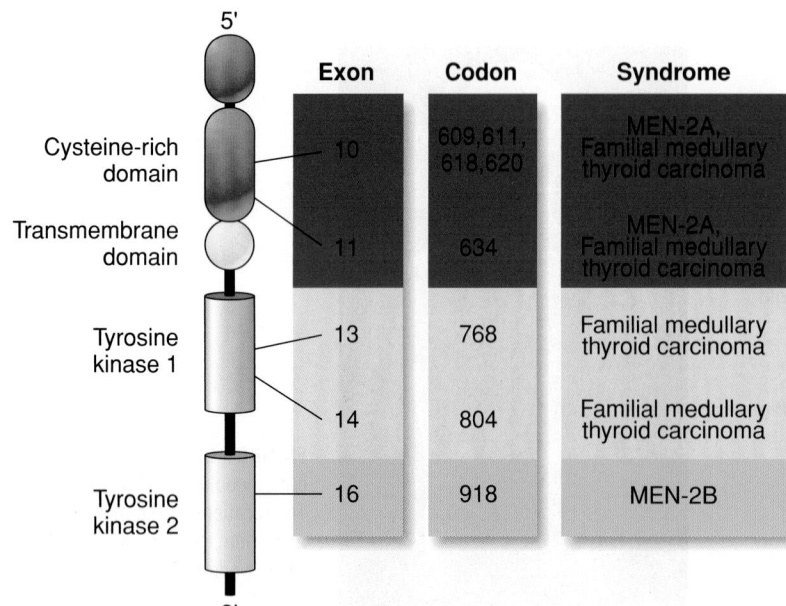

FIGURE 27-40. Representative RET proto-oncogene mutations in multiple endocrine neoplasia type 2 (MEN2).

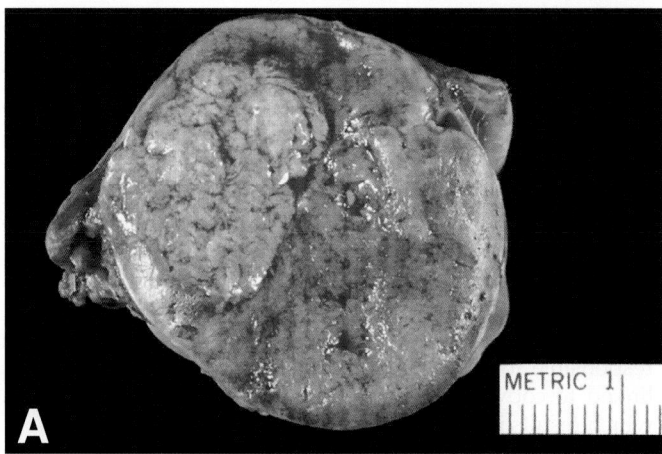

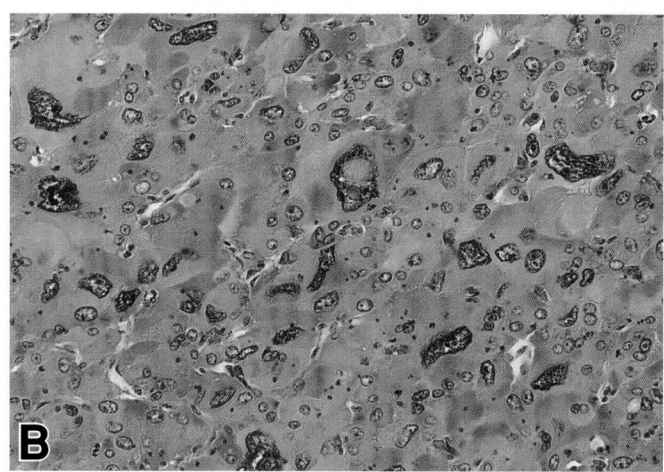

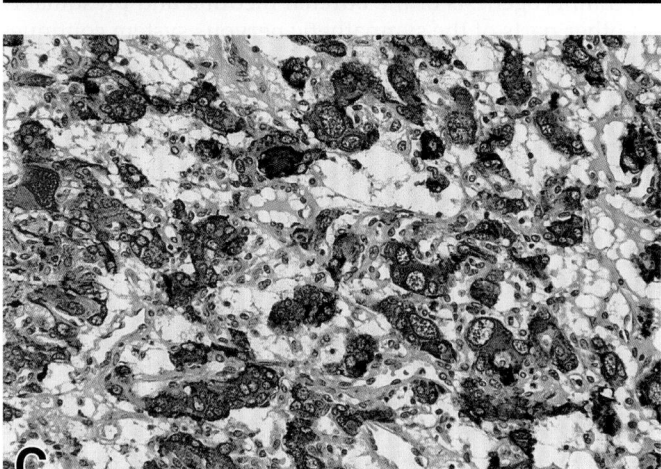

FIGURE 27-41. Pheochromocytoma. A. The cut surface of an adrenal tumor from a patient with episodic hypertension is reddish brown with a prominent area of fibrosis. Foci of hemorrhage and cystic degeneration are evident. **B.** A photomicrograph of the tumor shows polyhedral tumor cells with ample finely granular cytoplasm. Note the enlarged hyperchromatic nuclei. **C.** Many of the tumor cells show positive immunohistochemical staining for chromogranin A, a marker of neuroendocrine differentiation.

tumor giant cells (Fig. 27-41B). Tumors are highly vascular, with many capillaries. Trabecular or solid patterns, with only indistinct **zellballen,** are uncommon.

Electron microscopy shows membrane-bound, dense core granules, corresponding to stored catecholamines. Immunostains attest to the neuroendocrine nature of the tumor and show neuron-specific enolase, chromogranin (Fig. 27-41C) and synaptophysin.

Of adrenal pheochromocytomas, 5%–10% are malignant. Malignancy is more common among extra-adrenal tumors. *Only a tumor's behavior (i.e., metastases), and not its histology, defines malignancy: both benign and malignant pheochromocytomas show mitoses, cellular pleomorphism, capsular or vascular invasion and necrosis.* The tumors spread most often to regional lymph nodes, bone, lung and liver.

 CLINICAL FEATURES: With few exceptions, the clinical features of pheochromocytomas are caused by catecholamine release by the tumor. Patients may come to medical attention because of (1) asymptomatic hypertension discovered on routine physical examination; (2) symptomatic hypertension resistant to antihypertensive therapy; (3) malignant hypertension (e.g., encephalopathy, papilledema, proteinuria); (4) myocardial infarction or aortic dissection; or (5) paroxysms of convulsions, anxiety or hyperventilation.

Typically, episodic catecholamine release leads to paroxysms or crises, of up to several hours, with severe throbbing headache, sweating, palpitations, tachycardia, abdominal

pain and vomiting. Blood pressure may be elevated, often to an extreme degree. Paroxysms can be triggered by activities that place pressure on the abdominal contents (including the tumor), such as exercise, lifting, bending or vigorous abdominal palpation. Anxiety may occur during a paroxysm but is not an initiating factor.

Over 90% of patients with pheochromocytoma show hypertension. It is sustained in 2/3 of them and so resembles essential hypertension. In these patients, blood pressure rises to even higher levels during paroxysms. In the others, hypertension is episodic. Episodic hypertension may become sustained and evolves into malignant hypertension in many untreated patients.

There are other consequences of high catecholamine levels. Orthostatic hypotension results from decreased plasma volume and poor postural tone. Increased basal metabolism, sweating, heat intolerance and weight loss may mimic hyperthyroidism. Angina and myocardial infarction occur in the absence of coronary artery disease. The cardiac complications reflect myocardial necrosis caused by elevated catecholamine levels *(catecholamine cardiomyopathy)*.

Increased urinary levels of catecholamine metabolites, particularly vanillylmandelic acid (VMA), metanephrine and unconjugated catecholamines, help to confirm that a patient has a pheochromocytoma. Treatment for pheochromocytoma is surgical removal. β-Adrenergic blocking agents may help control hypertensive crises, and β-adrenergic receptor antagonists are helpful adjuncts.

Paragangliomas Are Pheochromocytomas Arising at Extra-Adrenal Sites

Paragangliomas may arise in paraganglia in any location, including the retroperitoneum, neck and bladder. They are frequently familial and inherited as autosomal dominant traits, with germline mutations in *SDHB, SDHC,* **SDHA** or *SDHD* genes.

Carotid body tumors are prototypical paragangliomas. They arise at the carotid bifurcation and form palpable masses in the neck. Interestingly, carotid body tumors are 10-fold more common in people living at high altitude than in those at sea level, suggesting that these tumors reflect hyperplastic responses to prolonged carotid body sensing of hypoxia.

Autosomal dominant transmission of paragangliomas occurs in some families, and **hereditary paraganglioma** was the first hereditary tumor syndrome reported to be caused by a germline mutation in a gene encoding a mitochondrial protein. It is linked to the *SDHD* gene (11q23), which encodes a subunit of cytochrome B that may participate in oxygen sensing. All affected patients, whether male or female, inherit the disease from their fathers. *SDHB*-related syndromes are associated with malignant pheochromocytomas that metastasize to distant organs such as lung and bone.

NEUROBLASTOMA

Neuroblastomas are embryonal malignant tumors of neural crest origin. They originate in the adrenal medulla, paravertebral sympathetic ganglia and sympathetic paraganglia and are composed of neoplastic neuroblasts. Neuroblasts derive from primitive sympathogonia and are an intermediate stage in the development of sympathetic ganglion neurons (Fig. 27-38). *These are the most common solid extracranial neoplasms of childhood, accounting for up to 10% of childhood cancers and 15% of cancer deaths in children.* Overall incidence peaks in the first 3 years and is 1 in 7000.

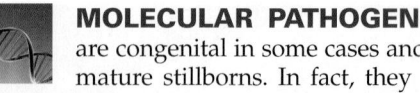 **MOLECULAR PATHOGENESIS:** The tumors are congenital in some cases and even occur in premature stillborns. In fact, they account for half of cancers diagnosed in the first month of life. Adolescents or adults may rarely develop them. Although neuroblastomas are sporadic, a few instances are familial. Those genetically predisposed to this disease usually have multifocal tumors at an early age and follow autosomal dominant inheritance. The short arm of chromosome 16 appears to be the affected locus. These tumors may occur with neurofibromatosis type 1, Beckwith-Wiedemann syndrome and Hirschsprung disease. Germline mutations in *PHOX2A* or *KIF1B* genes may be responsible for familial cases. These tumors have also been linked to copy number variations within the *NBPF10* gene, which results in the 1q21.1 deletion syndrome.

Embryogenesis of the adrenal medulla and presumably of other parts of the sympathetic nervous system continues during the first year of life. Persistence and transformation of these embryonal structures may be related to the pathogenesis of these tumors. Neuroblastomas carry frequent deletions on chromosome 1 (1p35-36), with unbalanced translocation with 17q. Extrachromosomal double minutes and homogeneously staining regions (HSRs) occur on chromosome 2. The HSRs represent amplification of N-*myc* (*MYCN*), which is a key determinant of tumor aggressiveness. The locus on chromosome 1 may suppress N-*myc* amplification.

 PATHOLOGY: Neuroblastomas can arise at any site with neural crest–derived cells (i.e., from the posterior cranial fossa to the coccyx). One third are in the adrenal, another 1/3 elsewhere in the abdomen and 20% in the posterior mediastinum.

The tumors vary from minute, barely discernible nodules to tumors readily palpable through the abdominal wall. They are round, irregularly lobulated masses that may weigh 50–150 g or more (Fig. 27-42A). Their cut surfaces are soft, friable and variegated maroon in color. Necrosis, hemorrhage, calcification and cystic change are common.

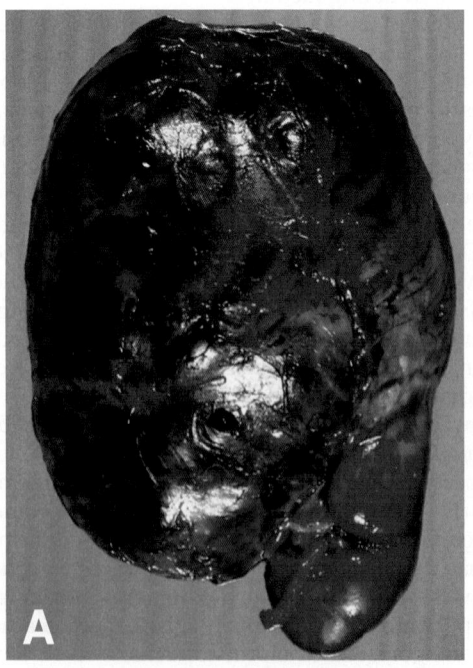

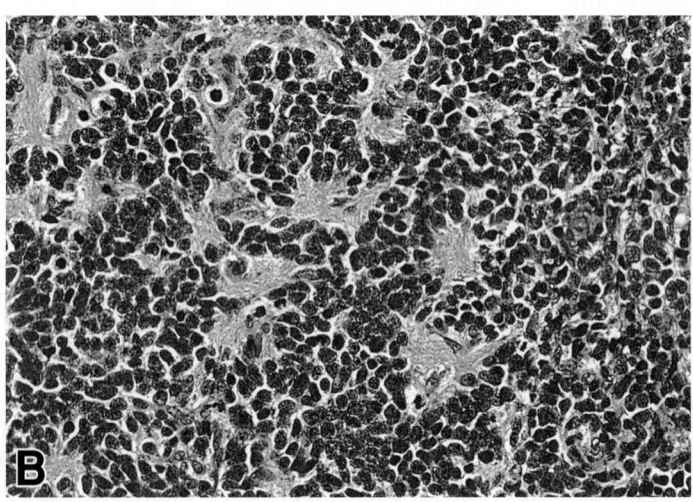

FIGURE 27-42. Neuroblastoma. A. A large, lobulated, hemorrhagic and cystic tumor, adherent to the upper pole of the kidney, was removed from a child who presented with an abdominal mass. **B.** A photomicrograph illustrates the characteristic rosettes, formed by small, regular, dark tumor cells arranged around a central, pale fibrillar core.

Neuroblastic tumors are classified as belonging to 1 of 4 categories:

- **Neuroblastoma** (Schwannian stroma poor)
- **Ganglioneuroblastoma, intermixed** (Schwannian stroma rich)
- **Ganglioneuroma** (Schwannian stroma dominant)
- **Ganglioneuroblastoma, nodular** (composite Schwannian stroma rich/stroma dominant and stroma poor).

Each category may have one or more subtypes.

Neuroblastomas contain dense sheets of small, round to fusiform cells with scant cytoplasm and hyperchromatic nuclei, resembling lymphocytes. There is limited or no Schwannian proliferation, and mitoses are frequent. Characteristic Homer Wright rosettes are defined by a rim of dark tumor cells in a circumferential arrangement around a central pale fibrillar core (Fig. 27-42B). By electron microscopy, malignant neuroblasts show peripheral dendritic processes with longitudinally oriented microtubules and neurosecretory granules and filaments.

Neuroblastomas readily infiltrate surrounding structures and metastasize to regional lymph nodes, liver, lungs, bones and other sites. The tumors may differentiate into ganglioneuromas (see below).

CLINICAL FEATURES: Clinical presentations are highly variable, reflecting the many sites where the primary tumors may develop and metastasize. The first sign is often an enlarging abdomen in a young child. Examination discloses a firm, irregular, nontender mass. Metastases may enlarge the liver and cause ascites. Marked irritability may reflect pain from bony metastases. Respiratory distress accompanies large masses in the thorax, and tumors in the pelvis may obstruct the bowel or ureters. Spinal cord compression may lead to gait disturbance and sphincter dysfunction. Tumor secretion of vasoactive intestinal peptide may cause diarrhea. Some patients show paraneoplastic opsoclonus-myoclonus syndrome, which usually indicates an excellent prognosis, although some may develop permanent neurologic deficits.

Urinary catecholamines and their metabolites are almost invariably elevated, particularly **norepinephrine, VMA, homovanillic acid** (HVA) and **dopamine**.

Several factors are useful in predicting the outcome of neuroblastomas:

- **Age:** Age at diagnosis is one of the most important predictors of survival. Children under 1 year old have better prognoses than do older patients with the same stage of disease. Spontaneous tumor regression occurs commonly at this age.
- **Site:** Extra-adrenal tumors tend to be better differentiated and so less aggressive.
- **Stage:** Survival is 90% in stage I (tumor confined to the organ of origin) and decreases to less than 3% in stage IV (widespread metastases). An exception is stage IVS (special), in which tumors lack the characteristic chromosomal abnormalities. Even with liver and bone marrow metastases, patients with stage IVS may undergo spontaneous remissions and have 60%–90% survival.
- **Tumor histology:** Low-grade (better-differentiated) tumors do better than high-grade (undifferentiated) tumors. If the **VMA/HVA ratio** is less than 1, the tumor is deficient in dopamine β-hydroxylase and likely to be more aggressive.

- **DNA ploidy:** A DNA index near the diploid/tetraploid range is unfavorable, but hyperdiploid or near-triploid neuroblastomas have a good prognosis. DNA ploidy has less prognostic value in patients older than 2 years.
- **Genomic alterations:** *MYCN* amplification occurs in 20%–25% of cases and suggests poor outcome. Tumors with *MYCN* amplification often have chromosome 1p deletions (especially del 1p36.3). Allelic gain of 17q implies more aggressiveness.

Neuroblastomas can express several tyrosine kinase neurotropin receptors: TrkA, TrkB and TrkC. High levels of TrkA correlate with younger age, lower stage, absence of *MYCN* amplification and favorable prognosis. Conversely, TrkB expression correlates with an invasive phenotype, high-risk disease and chemoresistance. TrkC occurs in lower-stage tumors. High-level expression of *EPHB6, CD44, EFNB2* and *EFNB3* correlates with good clinical outcome.

Prognosis also correlates with cytogenetic findings:

- Lack of significant chromosome changes portends excellent survival.
- Tumors with any chromosome copy number changes tend to relapse.
- Tumors with segmental alterations, *MYCN* amplification, 1p and 11q deletions and 1q gain imply overall poor survival.

Localized neuroblastomas are treated by surgical resection alone. Patients with disseminated tumors receive chemotherapy and sometimes irradiation.

Ganglioneuromas Are Mature Variants of Neuroblastic Tumors

Ganglioneuromas, like neuroblastomas, are tumors of neural crest origin. They occur in older children and young adults. *Ganglioneuromas are benign and arise in sympathetic ganglia, typically in the posterior mediastinum.* Up to 30% of these tumors develop in the adrenal medulla. In keeping with their degree of differentiation, ganglioneuromas do not manifest chromosomal abnormalities characteristic of neuroblastomas (see above).

PATHOLOGY: Ganglioneuromas are well encapsulated, with myxoid, glistening cut surfaces. They show well-differentiated, mature ganglion cells associated with spindle cells in a loose, abundant fibrillar stroma (Fig. 27-43). The fibrils represent neurites extending from tumor cell bodies. Cytoplasmic processes of ganglion cells contain neurosecretory granules and may form synaptic junctions. Typical neuroendocrine substances, such as neuron-specific enolase and certain peptide hormones, are abundant. Neuroblastomas may differentiate into a ganglioneuromas.

Pineal Gland

ANATOMY AND FUNCTION

The pineal gland resembles a 5–7-mm minute pine cone. It is below the posterior edge of the corpus callosum, suspended from the roof of the third ventricle over the superior colliculi. The pineal has a lobulated architecture, compartmentalized

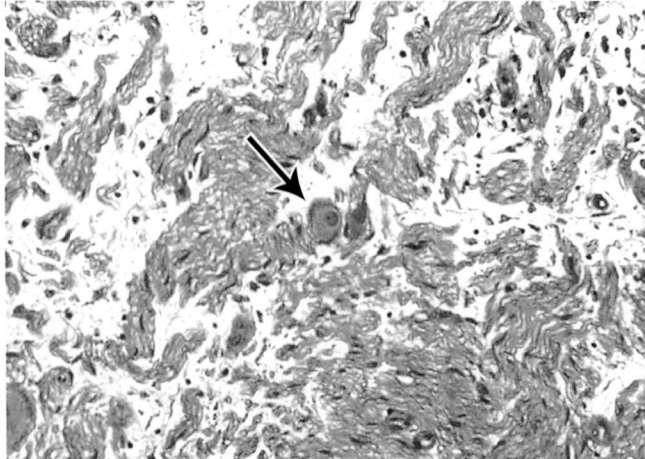

FIGURE 27-43. Ganglioneuroma. A photomicrograph shows mature ganglion cells (*arrow*) interspersed among wavy spindle cells embedded in a myxoid matrix.

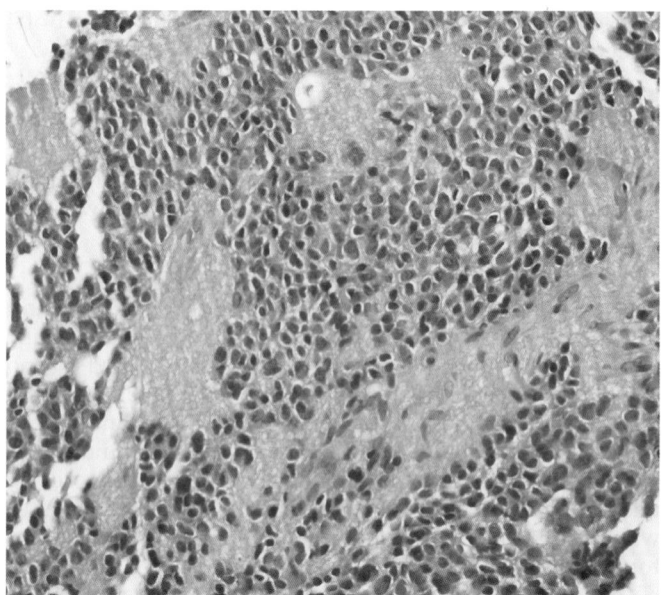

FIGURE 27-44. Pineocytoma. A photomicrograph shows nests of tumor cells with round nuclei and eosinophilic cytoplasm separated by connective tissue.

by fibrovascular septa, with cords and clusters of large epithelial-like cells, **pinealocytes**. These have modified photosensory and neuroendocrine functions. Astrocytes make up 10% of pineal gland cellularity.

The pineal gland produces several neurotransmitters, of which **melatonin** is among the most abundant. Since melatonin levels are distinctly higher at night than during waking hours, it may act as a sleep inducer.

Serotonin and several other substances are also produced by the pineal. The most significant of these is arginine vasotocin, a hormone that has important antigonadotropic activity. Melatonin may be a releasing factor for arginine vasotocin.

Beginning at about the time of puberty, calcifications (corpora arenacea or "brain sand") develop in the pineal gland, as visualized in autopsy specimens or by various radiographic techniques. These mineralized concretions accumulate increasingly with age and are accompanied by cystic degeneration and gliosis.

NEOPLASMS

Tumors of the pineal gland are rare. They represent less than 1% of brain tumors. Pineal tumors include neoplasms (1) originating from the pineal parenchyma, presumably from pinealocytes; (2) in the pineal gland region **(astrocytomas)** but derived from cells other than pinealocytes; and, rarely, (3) metastasis from other sites.

 PATHOLOGY:

■ **Germ cell tumors:** These are the most common pineal neoplasms. They apparently derive from misplaced germ cells. Of these, 60% are germinomas, or dysgerminomas, indistinguishable from their gonadal counterparts. Germ cell tumors are often immunopositive for placental alkaline phosphatase, CD117/c-kit and OCT4.

■ **Pineocytomas:** These benign tumors are solid, well-circumscribed masses that replace the pineal body. Small tumor cells with round nuclei and eosinophilic

cytoplasm grow in nests and rosettes separated by thin strands of connective tissue (Fig. 27-44). They resemble paragangliomas, but pineocytomas lack neurosecretory granules.

■ **Pineoblastomas:** These highly malignant tumors are extremely rare and occur in young adults. Soft masses, often with hemorrhagic and necrotic areas, invade and infiltrate surrounding structures. Pineoblastomas consist of clusters of densely packed small oval cells, with dark nuclei and scanty cytoplasm, resembling medulloblastomas or neuroblastomas and with rosette formation. Mitoses are abundant. These tumors are immunopositive for synaptophysin and negative for glial fibrillary acidic protein. Metastasis to the central nervous system and spine are common.

 CLINICAL FEATURES: Regardless of histologic type, pineal gland tumors present with signs and symptoms owing to their impact on surrounding structures, including headaches and visual and behavioral disturbances. In children, these tumors may precipitate precocious puberty, especially in boys. The prognosis of pineoblastoma is poor. However, even benign pineal tumors and nonneoplastic pineal cysts carry guarded prognoses and pose a great threat to life, because they are difficult to excise surgically.

PARANEOPLASTIC SYNDROMES WITH ENDOCRINE FUNCTION

Tumors May Produce Ectopic Peptide Hormones with Systemic Effects

Malignant tumors may produce diverse peptide hormones whose secretion is not under normal regulatory control. Most of these hormones are normally present in the brain, gastrointestinal tract or endocrine organs. Their inappropriate secretion can cause a variety of effects.

CUSHING SYNDROME: Ectopic secretion of ACTH by a tumor leads to features of Cushing syndrome, including hypokalemia, hyperglycemia, hypertension and muscle weakness. ACTH production is most commonly seen with cancers of the lung, particularly small cell carcinoma. It also complicates carcinoid tumors and other neuroendocrine tumors, such as pheochromocytoma, neuroblastoma and medullary thyroid carcinoma.

INAPPROPRIATE ANTIDIURESIS: Production of arginine vasopressin (ADH) by a tumor may cause sodium and water retention to such an extent that it is manifested as water intoxication, resulting in altered mental status, seizures, coma and sometimes death. The tumor that most often produces this syndrome is small cell lung carcinoma. It is also reported with carcinomas of the prostate, gastrointestinal tract and pancreas and with thymomas, lymphomas and Hodgkin disease.

HYPERCALCEMIA: A paraneoplastic complication that afflicts 10% of cancer patients, hypercalcemia is usually caused by metastatic disease of bone. However, in about one tenth of cases, it occurs in the absence of bony metastases. The most common cause of paraneoplastic hypercalcemia is the secretion of a parathormone-like peptide by an epithelial tumor, usually squamous cell lung carcinoma or breast adenocarcinoma. In multiple myeloma and lymphomas, hypercalcemia is attributed to the secretion of osteoclast-activating factor. Other mechanisms of hypercalcemia involve the production of prostaglandins, active metabolites of vitamin D, transforming growth factor-α (TGF-α) and TGF-β.

HYPOCALCEMIA: Cancer-induced hypocalcemia is actually more common than hypercalcemia and complicates osteoblastic metastases from cancers of the lung, breast and prostate. The cause of hypocalcemia is not known. Low calcium levels have been reported in association with calcitonin-secreting medullary carcinoma of the thyroid.

GONADOTROPIC SYNDROMES: Gonadotropins may be secreted by germ cell tumors, gestational trophoblastic tumors (choriocarcinoma, hydatidiform mole) and pituitary tumors. Less commonly, gonadotropin secretion is observed with hepatoblastomas in children and cancers of the lung, colon, breast and pancreas in adults. High gonadotropin levels lead to precocious puberty in children, gynecomastia in men and oligomenorrhea in premenopausal women.

HYPOGLYCEMIA: The best-understood cause of hypoglycemia associated with tumors is excessive insulin production by pancreatic islet cell tumors (see Chapter 21). Other tumors, especially large mesotheliomas, fibrosarcomas and primary hepatocellular carcinoma, are associated with hypoglycemia. The cause of hypoglycemia in nonendocrine tumors is not established, but the most likely candidate is production of somatomedins (IGFs), a family of peptides normally made by the liver, under regulation by growth hormone.

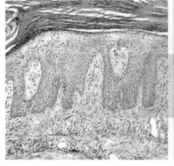
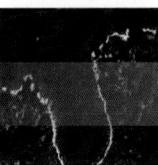
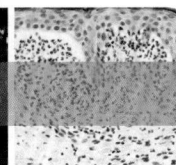

28

The Skin

Ronnie M. Abraham ■ Emily Y. Chu ■ David E. Elder

The skin is an optimal organ for studying fundamental principles of pathology because lesions on its surface are readily apparent and easily biopsied. Most classes of disease manifest in the skin. Some diseases, such as the blistering diseases, are mainly present in the skin.

Considering the imperatives of appearance in human interactions, a changed appearance of the skin may at times be the most important feature of cutaneous disease. Many cutaneous diseases have only minor symptoms, and some have no symptoms at all. Few are life-threatening, and many are self-limited. However, even self-limited, asymptomatic cutaneous diseases are often of great concern to the patient. For example, the symptoms of acne are systemically minor, but the disease can change a life. Although scalp hair is unneeded, baldness may cause considerable distress. Vitiligo, a completely asymptomatic, progressive, depigmentation disorder, often creates emotional havoc for an otherwise normal person of color.

ANATOMY AND PHYSIOLOGY OF THE SKIN

The skin is a protective barrier; microorganisms find it almost impossible to penetrate intact epidermis from the outside, and water loss is limited from the inside. The organ is vital in regulating temperature and protecting against ultraviolet (UV) light. Diverse sensory receptors communicate details of the immediate environment. The skin plays a prominent role in immune regulation through its associated lymphoid tissues, which include lymphocytes and antigen-presenting cells that travel between the skin and regional lymph nodes via the lymphatics and bloodstream. Keratinocytes, Langerhans cells, mast cells, lymphocytes and macrophages all participate in immune responses. Epidermal keratinocytes produce many cytokines, notably interleukin-1α (IL-1α) and IL-1β eicosanoids and melanocortin. The ability of keratinocytes to participate in immunity, inflammation and pigment production by melanocytes is necessary in an organ relentlessly exposed to the external environment. Langerhans cells, the dendritic antigen-presenting cells of the skin, are bone marrow–derived, epidermal immigrant cells. They are central to development and regulation of contact hypersensitivity, allograft rejection and graft-versus-host disease.

KERATINOCYTES: The epidermis is a multilayered sheet of keratin-producing cells. It forms undulating folds at the interface with the dermis, called dermal papillae. A progressive change in morphology occurs from the replicating

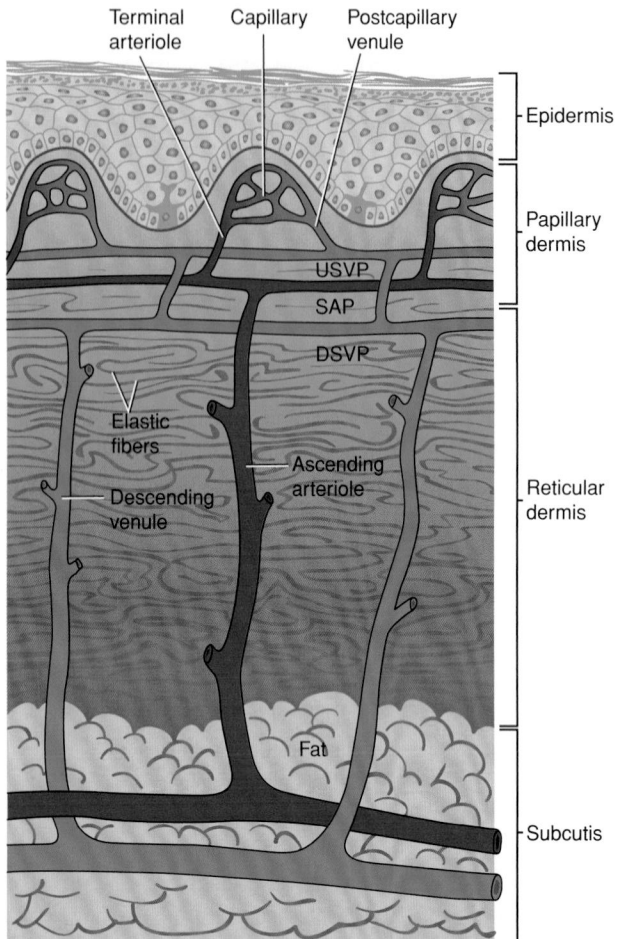

FIGURE 28-1. The dermis and its vasculature. The dermis is divided into two distinct anatomic regions. The papillary dermis with its vascular plexus and the epidermis usually react together in diseases that are primarily limited to the skin. The reticular dermis and the subcutis are altered in association with systemic diseases that manifest in the skin. *DSVP* = deep superficial venular plexus; *SAP* = superficial arterial plexus; *USVP* = upper superficial venular plexus.

columnar cells of the basal layer **(stratum basalis)** through the spinous layer **(stratum spinosum)** and the granular layer **(stratum granulosum)** to the nonviable flattened cells of the cornified layer **(stratum corneum)** (Figs. 28-1 and 28-2). The basal cells harbor most of the mitotic activity of the epidermis. As keratinocytes approach the surface, they lose their nuclei and form flattened plates of dead cells on the outer boundary of the skin (the cornified or keratin layer). Keratinocytes synthesize a sulfur-poor, filamentous **tonofibril,** which is related to the keratin molecules of the stratum corneum. Tonofibrils are composed of varying blends of acidic and basic intermediate keratin filaments; they result in over 30 different keratins that are responsible for structures such as the stratum corneum, hair and nails. Bundles of tonofibrils converge on, and terminate at, the plasma membrane in attachment plates called **desmosomes** (Fig. 28-3).

Keratinocytes are also distinguished by two other structural products: "keratohyaline granules" and **"Odland bodies."** Keratohyaline granules are the defining feature of the granular layer and are composed of a histidine-rich, electron-dense, basophilic protein—profilaggrin—which is associated with intermediate filaments. Odland bodies, also known as keratinosomes or membrane-coating granules, are the only structurally distinctive, epidermal secretory product (Fig. 28-3). They form in the outer spinous and granular layers and discharge their contents into intercellular spaces, appearing there as lamellar masses parallel to the surface of the skin. Odland bodies and the discharged lamellated products are most obvious in the outer granular layer and are related to epidermal barrier function.

The epidermis harbors immigrant cells of neuroectodermal and mesenchymal origin that do not synthesize keratin but which have their own highly distinctive organelles. Their numbers vary among the several different levels of the epidermis. Two of these cells, **melanocytes** and **Langerhans cells,** are dendritic. The third, the **Merkel cell,** is associated with a terminal neuronal axon (Fig. 28-2).

MELANOCYTES: Melanocytes are dendritic cells of neural crest origin that largely determine skin color. They lie in the basal layer of the epidermis, separated from the dermis by the epidermal basement membrane zone. A single melanocyte may supply dendrites to over 30 keratinocytes (Fig. 28-4).

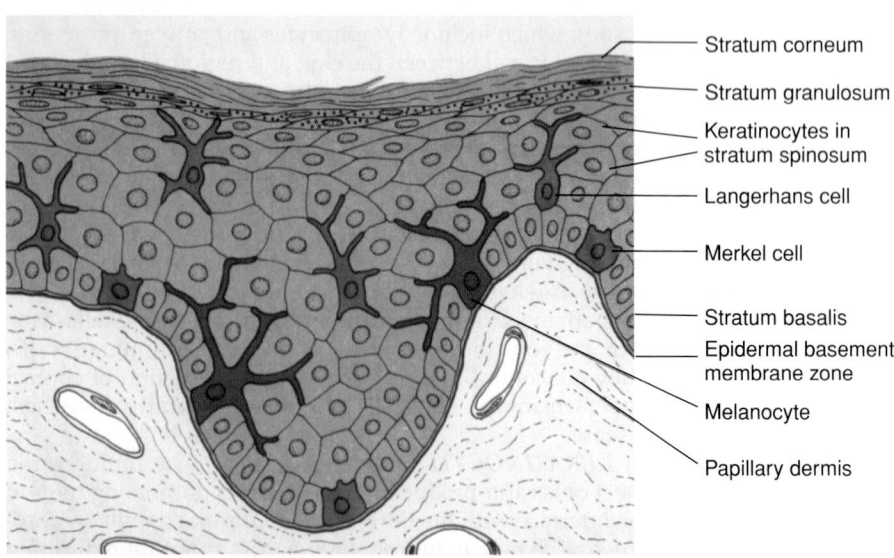

FIGURE 28-2. Normal epidermis and the epidermal immigrant cells. Keratinocytes form the multilayered epidermis, protecting against water loss and bacterial invasion. Melanocytes provide color as well as protection against ultraviolet radiation. Langerhans cells are among the cells responsible for the skin's function as an immunologic organ. Merkel cells may represent one of the enablers of tactile function of the skin.

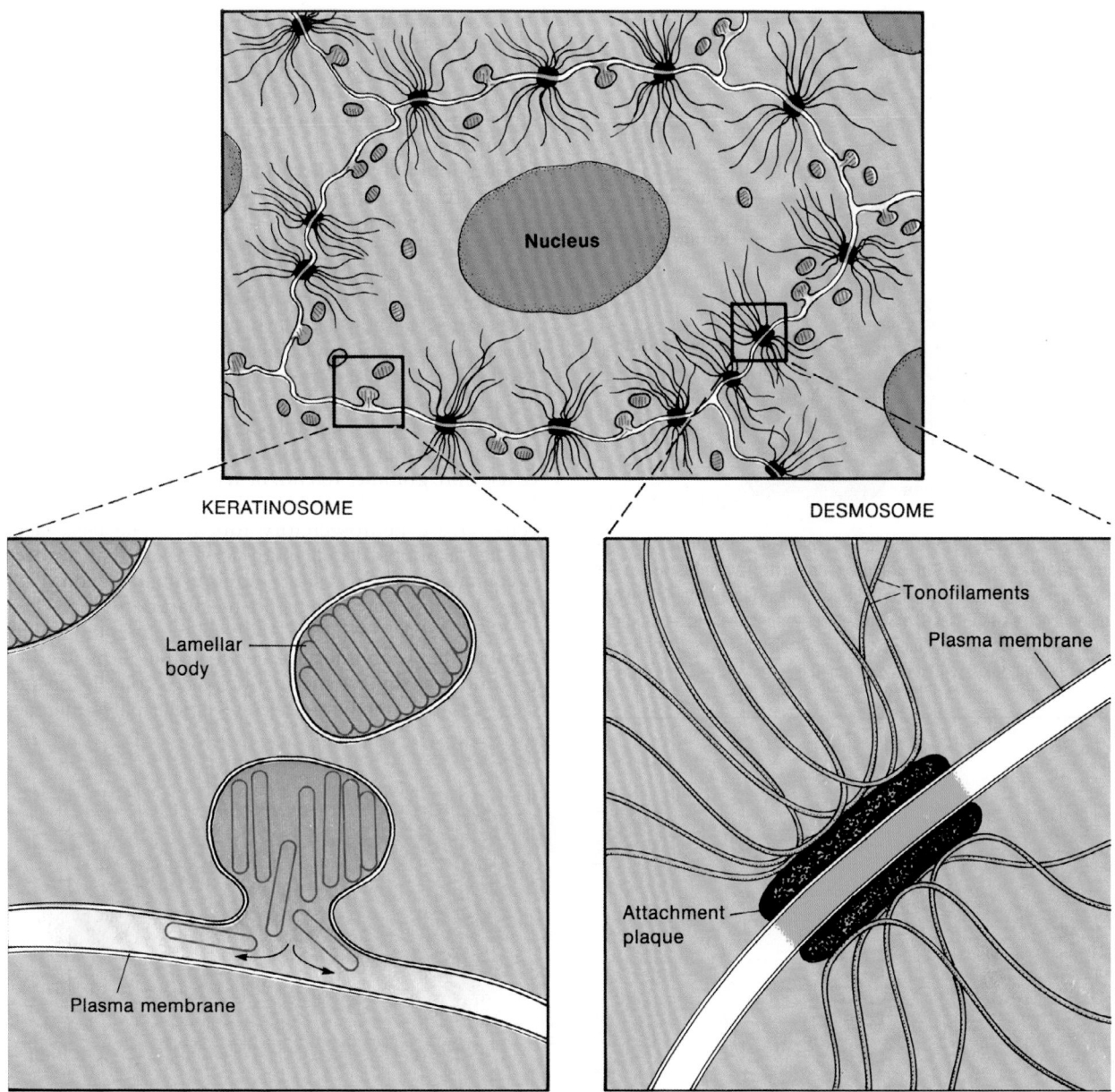

FIGURE 28-3. The keratinocyte, keratinosome and desmosome. The keratinocyte cytoplasm is dominated by delicate keratin fibrils, the tonofilaments. These are part of the cytoskeleton of the cell and loop within the attachment plaque of the desmosome. The lamellar body of the keratinocyte extrudes its contents into the intercellular space. This material probably has a role in cellular cohesion.

The **melanosome** is a cytoplasmic membrane–bound complex in which melanin is synthesized. When melanin synthesis is active, melanosomes contain filaments in parallel arrays along the long axis of the organelle (Fig. 28-4). As they mature, melanosomes' orderly internal structure is progressively obliterated, and they become electron-opaque granules. These are transferred to keratinocytes, where they form a supranuclear cap, protecting the nuclear material from ultraviolet light.

Skin color is largely based on the number, size and packaging of melanosomes in keratinocytes. In hair and epidermal keratinocytes, melanins are packaged and absorb and reflect visible light, thus forming the integumentary colors.

LANGERHANS CELLS: These cells arrive in embryonic skin in the last month of the first trimester, following the melanocytes by a month. These human leukocyte antigen (HLA)-DR–positive cells allow skin to recognize and process antigens, and so become a part of the immune system. These cells are uncommon in the dermis but are distributed throughout the nucleated layers of the epidermis, where they constitute about 4% of the cells. They are difficult to see by routine light microscopy because their cytoplasm is translucent and is formed of a perikaryon and dendrites. Langerhans cells do not have specialized attachments to the apposed keratinocytes. In electron micrographs, their cytoplasm contains a moderate number of specialized organelles, **Birbeck granules**. In two dimensions, these structures appear to be racquet shaped, but three-dimensional reconstruction shows them to be cup shaped (Fig. 28-5). These unique organelles are derived from the plasma membrane and probably participate in antigen presentation by Langerhans cells (antigenic material being internalized into Birbeck granules).

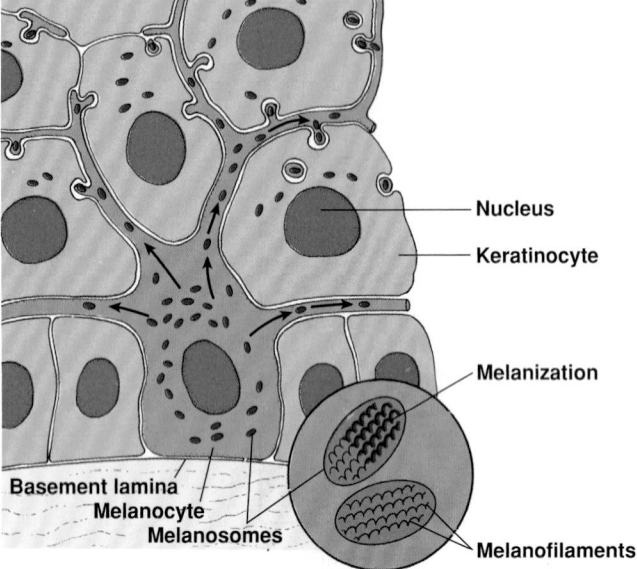

FIGURE 28-4. A melanocyte supplies over 30 keratinocytes with melanin granules by way of complex dendritic cytoplasmic extensions. Melanin granules are transferred to keratinocytes and come to lie in a supranuclear cap, a site indicating their protective function. Pigment granules are actually formed in the melanocytes within distinctive organelles—the melanosomes. Pigment is synthesized on small filaments within this organelle (*inset*).

In Langerhans cell histiocytoses, Birbeck granules attach to the plasma membrane of proliferating cells and communicate directly with the extracellular space. Furthermore, they have a fuzzy coat of clathrin, a feature of "coated pits," suggesting a relationship to receptor-mediated antigen processing and recognition. Langerhans cells express major histocompatibility complex I (MHC-I), MHC-II and receptors for Fc IgG and Fc IgE. They express CD1a and, less specifically, S-100 protein.

MERKEL CELLS: Although sometimes classified as "immigrant" cells, Merkel cells may be specialized basal keratinocytes. They form desmosomes with keratinocytes and express keratins similarly to keratinocytes. They project short, blunt cytoplasmic fingers into adjacent keratinocytes. Merkel cells do not appear in all areas of the epidermis but are seen in special regions such as the lips, oral cavity, external root sheaths of hair follicles and palmar skin of the digits. They have a distinctive organelle, a membrane-bound, dense-core granule, 100 nm or wider (Fig. 28-6). Immunohistochemical and ultrastructural studies suggest that Merkel cells have a neurosecretory function. The basal aspect of the cell is apposed to a small nerve plate that connects to a myelinated axon by a short, nonmyelinated axon. This complex structure may be a tactile mechanoreceptor.

BASEMENT MEMBRANE: The basement membrane zone (BMZ) is an interface between the dermis and epidermis and is as diverse in function as it is complex in structure (Fig. 28-7). It mediates dermal–epidermal adherence and

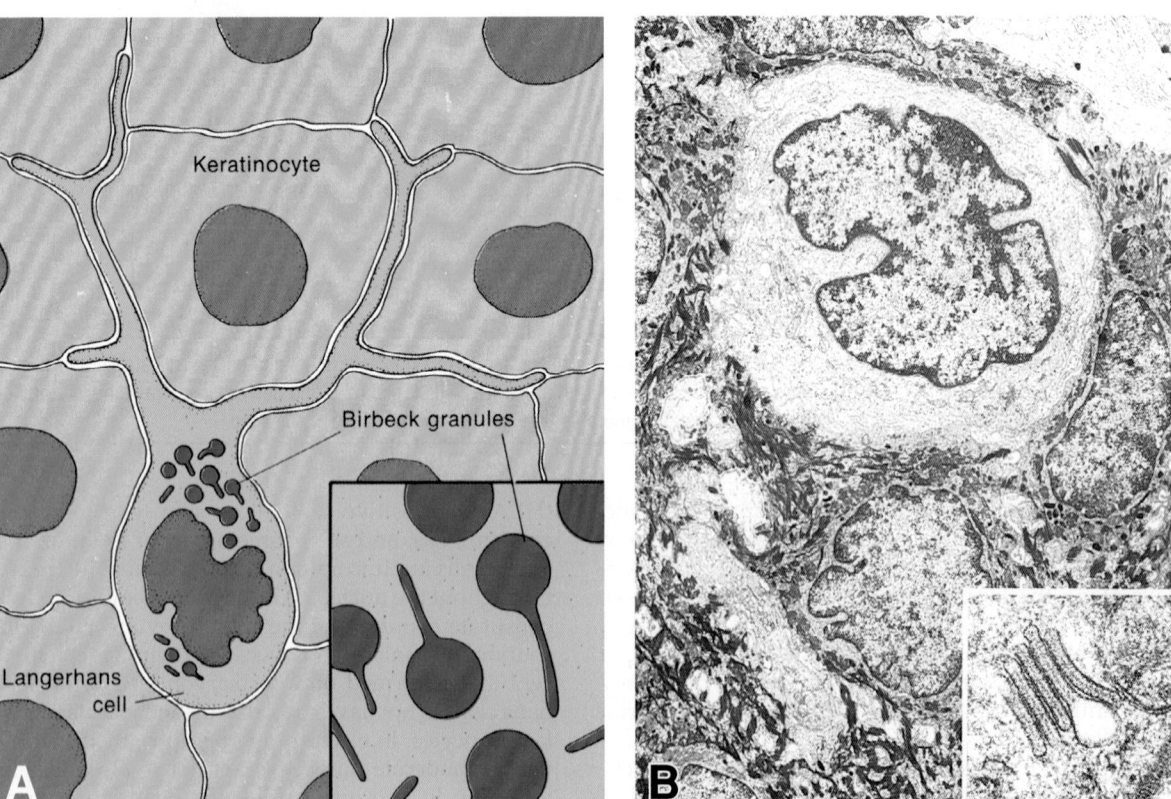

FIGURE 28-5. The dendritic Langerhans cell can recognize and process antigens. A. The unique racket-shaped organelles, called *Birbeck granules*, may be important in antigen presentation. **B.** An electron micrograph of a Langerhans cell shows a high-power view of the racket-shaped organelles (*inset*). The Langerhans cell body (*mid-upper portion*) is pale compared to the surrounding keratinocytes, whose cytoplasm contains electron-dense packets of tonofilaments. A dendrite is present (*arrow*).

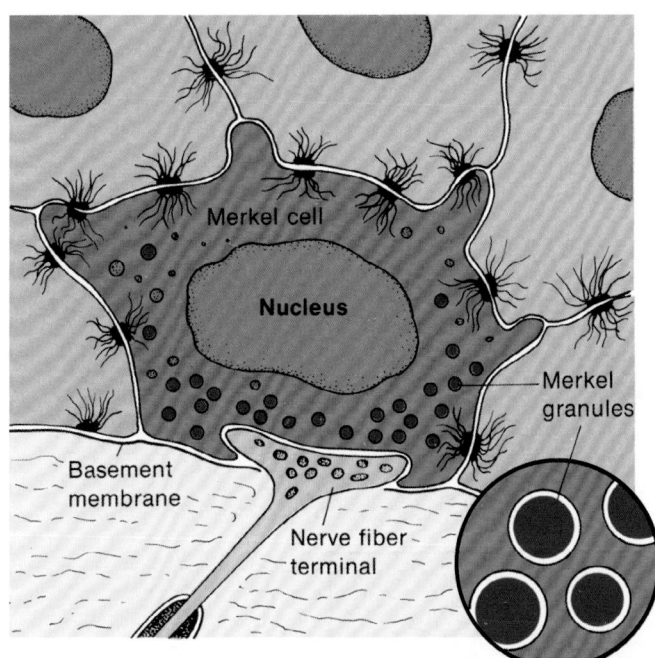

FIGURE 28-6. The Merkel cell, which differs from other immigrant cells, forms desmosomes with keratinocytes and is attached to a small nerve plate (nerve fiber terminal). The membrane-delimited, dense core granule is distinctive (*inset*).

probably acts as a selective macromolecular filter as well. It is also a site of immunoglobulin and complement deposition in certain cutaneous diseases. Most structures of the BMZ are elaborated by epidermal cells. The basal lamina is the primary organizational feature of the BMZ and is responsible for epithelial cell polarity as well as some keratin gene expression. Ultrastructurally, the basal lamina includes:

- **Deep aspects of basal keratinocytes** including plasma membrane and tonofilaments, which attach to the deep face of the hemidesmosome
- **Hemidesmosome,** with its subdesmosomal dense plate
- **Anchoring filaments,** which extend from subdesmosomal dense plates across the lamina lucida and insert into the lamina densa
- **Lamina lucida,** an electron-lucent layer containing adherence proteins
- **Lamina densa,** composed principally of type IV collagen
- **Anchoring fibrils,** which are arrays of type VII collagen extending from the inner face of the lamina densa for a short distance into the papillary dermis
- **Microfibrils,** which feature delicate, long, elastic fibrils that blend with the underlying elastic fibrillary system of the skin

Certain antigenic components have been identified in the BMZ, some of which play identified roles in cutaneous disease, particularly blistering disorders. **Laminin** is a glycoprotein in the lamina lucida and lamina densa of all BMZs. It helps to organize BMZ macromolecules and promotes cell attachment to extracellular matrix. Laminin binds **type IV collagen**.

Bullous pemphigoid (BP) antigens were identified with antibodies from patients with the blistering disorder BP (see below). The antigens BPAG1 and BPAG2 **(type XVII collagen)** are normal constituents of the dermal–epidermal junction but are absent in BMZs around adnexal structures and blood vessels. These BP antigens localize in hemidesmosomes and cytoplasm of basal keratinocytes. Type IV collagen, in the lamina densa of all BMZs, is the most superficial component of the complex collagen fiber network of the dermis. It is important in dermal–epidermal attachment. **Type VII collagen** is present on the deep aspect of the basal lamina in anchoring fibrils. Anchoring fibril antigens (AF-1 and AF-2) reside within anchoring fibrils and possibly within the lower lamina densa.

The **dermis** is a complex organization of connective tissue deep to the BMZ, containing mostly collagen, which is embedded in a ground substance rich in hyaluronic acid. The dermis has two zones:

PAPILLARY DERMIS: The papillary dermis is a narrow zone just below the BMZ of the epidermis. It has a pale pink eosinophilic appearance and has little organization when viewed with the light microscope (Figs. 28-1 and 28-2). Delicate collagen fibrils are the most apparent structures. This delicate connective tissue extends into the dermal papillae, and also as a sheath about blood vessels, nerves and adnexal structures. This entire network of collagen is known as the **adventitial dermis**.

The papillary dermis is generally altered in epidermal diseases and disorders affecting the superficial vascular bed. The epidermis, papillary dermis and superficial vascular bed react jointly and influence each other in complex ways. Some primary skin diseases with few, if any, systemic manifestations, such as psoriasis and lichen planus, involve these superficial structures.

RETICULAR DERMIS: The reticular dermis is deep to the papillary dermis and contains most of the dermal collagen, which is organized into coarse bundles and associated with elastic fibers (Fig. 28-1). The reticular dermis and subcutis (also recognized as a cutaneous structure) are less common sites of pathologic change. If they are diseased, it is often as a manifestation of systemic disease (e.g., scleroderma [progressive systemic sclerosis] and erythema nodosum).

CUTANEOUS VASCULATURE: Circulating blood in the skin has a number of functions. The skin, via its vascular network, is important in temperature regulation. Many aspects of cutaneous inflammation involve the superficial cutaneous vasculature.

An ascending arteriole arises from arteries in the subcutis and directly crosses much of the reticular dermis (Fig. 28-1). In the outer part of the reticular dermis, in conjunction with other similar ascending arterioles, a superficial arteriolar plexus is formed. A terminal arteriole extends from this plexus into each dermal papilla, where an arterial capillary is formed. The arterial capillary makes a U-turn and on its descent becomes a venous capillary and then a postcapillary venule. These venules join to form a complex venular plexus in the reticular dermis, just under the papillary dermis. The venular end of this vascular structure is important in cutaneous inflammatory responses.

Cutaneous lymphatic vessels form a random network, starting as lymphatic capillaries near the epidermis. A superficial lymphatic plexus then sends forth lymphatic channels to drain to regional lymph nodes. Lymphatic channels are involved in drainage of tissue fluids and metastasis of cutaneous cancers, especially malignant melanoma. Cutaneous lymphatics have, at best, an incomplete basal lamina.

Mast cells are derived from bone marrow and are normally present around dermal venules. They release vasoactive

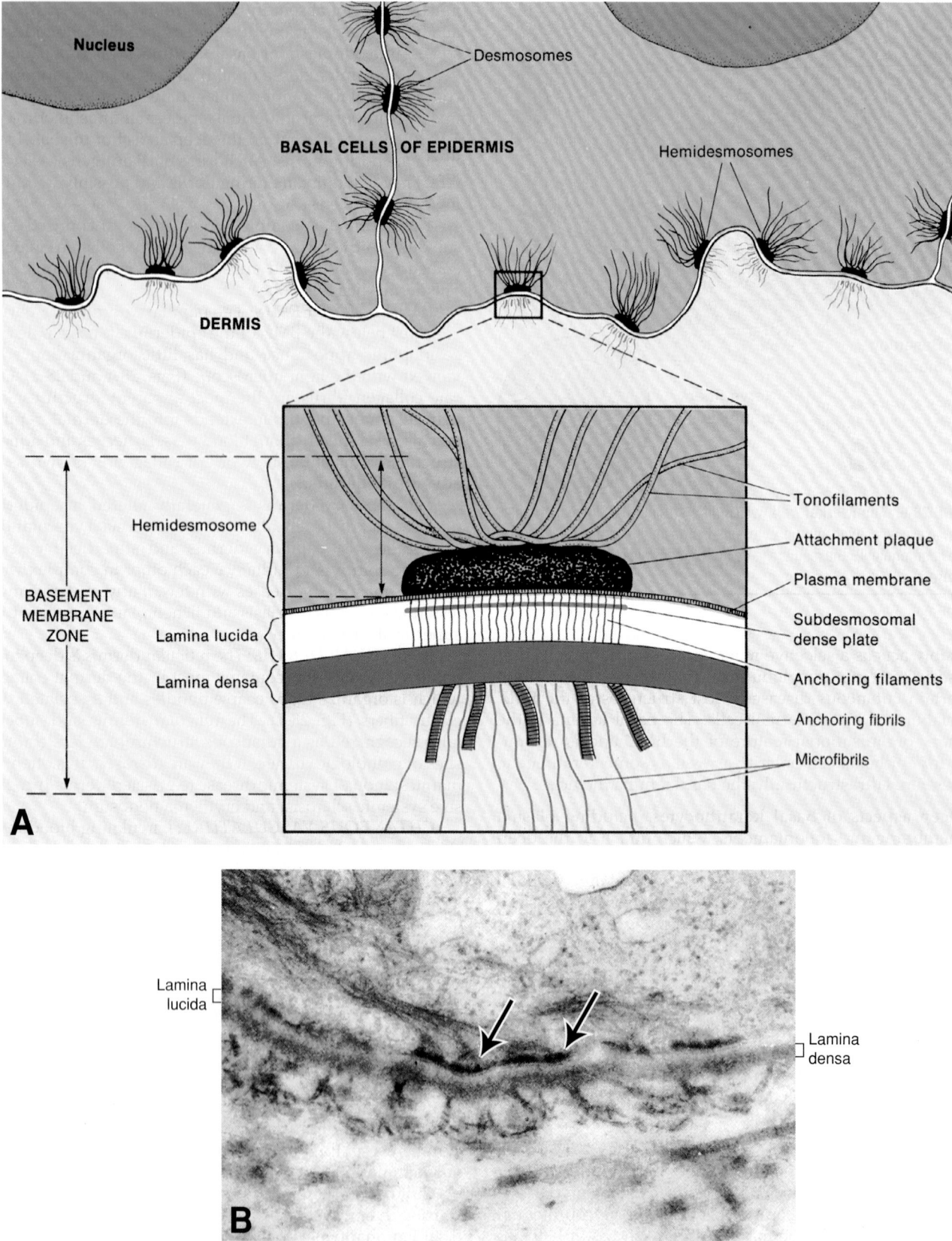

FIGURE 28-7. The dermal–epidermal interface and the basement membrane zone. A. This epithelial–mesenchymal interface is the site of the basement membrane zone, a complex structure that is mostly synthesized by the basal cells of the epidermis. Each of its complex structures is a site of change in specific disease, from tonofilaments and attachment plaques of basal cells to anchoring fibrils and microfibrils. **B.** An electron micrograph shows the hemidesmosomal attachment plaques with their inserting tonofilaments (*arrow*). The subdesmosomal dense plates, the lamina lucida, the lamina densa and the subjacent anchoring fibrils are well demonstrated.

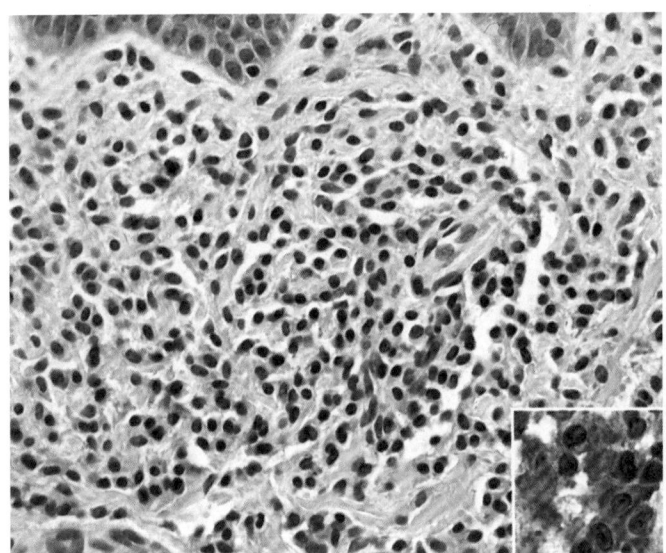

FIGURE 28-8. Urticaria pigmentosa. Mast cells fill and expand the papillary dermis. The cytoplasm of mast cells contains chloracetate esterase–rich granules, giving them a red hue in this Leder stain (*inset*), a useful distinguishing feature.

and chemotactic substances, mediate all types of inflammation and proliferate in a spectrum of diseases, called **urticaria pigmentosa** (Fig. 28-8).

HAIR FOLLICLES: Hair follicles originate in the primitive epidermis. They grow downward through the dermis and upward through the epidermis. Growing hairs of the scalp and beard have bulbs of epithelial and mesenchymal tissue firmly embedded in the subcutis. A vertical cross-section of a bulb reveals a cap of actively dividing, keratin-synthesizing cells that become arrayed in layers that join at the top of the bulb to form the cylindrical hair shaft. The differentiating hairs form the roof of the epithelial bulb and interact with an island of melanocytes that contribute melanin to the passing keratinocytes. This process results in hair color. The colored keratinocytes lose their nuclei as they form the final product, the cylindrical hair shaft. Curly hair is formed from angulated bulbs; straight hair develops from round bulbs.

THE HAIR CYCLE: Hair grows in a cyclical fashion. At any given time, 90% of hairs are normally in the actively growing, or **anagen,** phase. These are interspersed with hairs that show no evidence of active growth, **telogen** hairs. Hairs in the process of ceasing growth, **catagen** hairs, still have hair shafts. Catagen hairs end in the lower reticular dermis as slightly widened club-like structures, each surrounded by a rim of nucleated keratinocytes. Hair bulbs are no longer evident, and the lamina densa around the catagen hair is strikingly thickened.

As the **telogen** phase (resting follicle) is reached, the end of the hair retreats to the level of the arrector pili muscle. The hair shaft may be missing: it is no longer tethered at the base and leaves only a remnant of the original follicle. However, a delicate vascularized mesenchymal tract, the telogen tract, extends from the attenuated tip. At the top of this tract, an early anagen hair forms again from follicular stem cells. With growth, it follows the delicate pathway through the reticular dermis into the panniculus, there forming a mature anagen follicle and a new hair.

ALOPECIA: Alopecia, commonly known as baldness, is loss of hair. **Androgenetic alopecia,** or **common alopecia,** affects both men and women and results from a complex and poorly understood interaction of heritable and hormonal factors. Men castrated before puberty retain scalp hair and fail to grow a beard. On the other hand, administering testosterone to such castrated men results in growth of a beard and may lead to male-pattern baldness. Loss of scalp hair leads to replacement of large terminal hair follicles by tiny "vellus" hair follicles, the source of the delicate "fuzz" on the cheeks of women and the upper cheeks of men.

Growing hair is a site of active mitosis. Many systemic diseases inhibit hair mitosis and give rise to alopecia. If the condition passes, mitotic activity is renewed and hair regrows. If a patient is treated with potent antimitotic drugs (e.g., chemotherapy), hair follicles stop growth, hair is lost and a telogen follicle follows. When therapy stops, hair cycling resumes. Almost any kind of follicular inflammation can trigger the telogen phase. The synchronous onset of telogen in multiple follicles may result in rapid hair loss, called "telogen effluvium." If fibrosis distorts the telogen tract (the regrowth pathway), scarring alopecia with permanent loss of that follicle is the result.

Alopecia areata is a circumscribed area of hair loss, usually on the scalp, although other body areas may be involved. Brisk lymphocytic infiltrates around the hair bulb result in formation of telogen hairs and hair loss. Alopecia areata may actually result from several diseases. This histologic pattern and the association of this phenomenon with the inheritance of HLA class II alleles (especially HLA-DQ3) have been interpreted as evidence for an autoimmune etiology. Generally, scarring does not occur and hair may regrow normally after varying time periods. **Alopecia totalis** is an autoimmune disease that causes loss of all body hair. Aside from cosmetic problems, it is harmless.

VELLUS HAIRS: These fine hairs may play a role in touch perception in many mammals, but in humans they have no function. Vellus hairs are diminutive anagen hairs, with a small active bulb high in the reticular dermis, together with small sebaceous glands.

SEBACEOUS FOLLICLES: These structures develop with puberty and are the sites of **acne.** Sebaceous follicles have a minute vellus hair at the base. The central face has large sebaceous glands that dwarf the vellus hairs and fill the follicular canal with sebum.

DISEASES OF THE EPIDERMIS

Ichthyoses Feature Epidermal Thickening and Scales

Ichthyosiform dermatoses, many of which are heritable, are diverse diseases showing striking thickening of the stratum corneum. The term **ichthyosis** reflects the similarity of the diseased skin to coarse, fish-like scales (Fig. 28-9). Several rare ichthyoses are associated with other abnormalities, such as abnormal lipid metabolism, neurologic or bone diseases and cancer.

 **MOLECULAR PATHOGENESIS:** Three general defects are involved in the excessive epidermal cornification of ichthyoses:

- **Increased cohesiveness** of the cells of the stratum corneum, possibly reflecting altered lipid metabolism

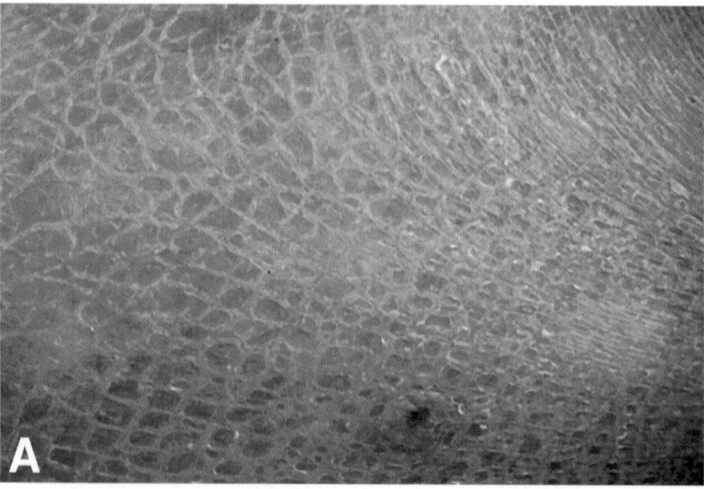
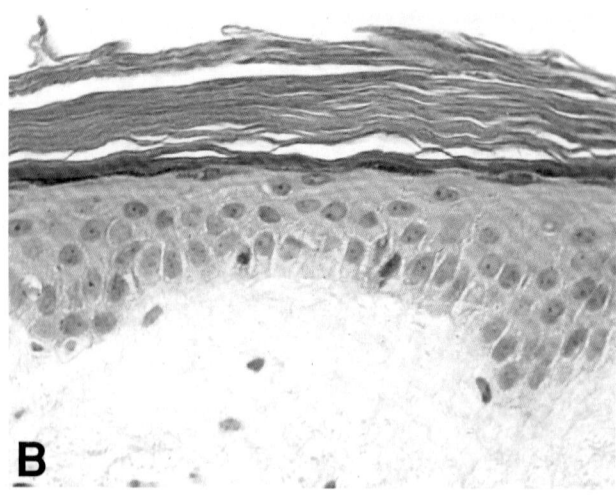

FIGURE 28-9. Ichthyosis vulgaris. A. Noninflammatory fish-like scales are evident on the thigh of a patient with a strong family history of ichthyosis vulgaris. **B.** There is disproportionate thickening of the stratum corneum relative to the normal thickness of the nucleated epidermal layer. The stratum granulosum is thin and focally absent.

- **Abnormal keratinization,** manifested as impaired tonofilament formation and keratohyaline synthesis and as excessive cornification
- **Increased basal cell proliferation,** associated with a decrease in transit time of keratinocytes across the epidermis

 PATHOLOGY: In all ichthyoses (with the possible exception of lamellar ichthyosis), the stratum corneum is disproportionately thick compared to the nucleated epidermal layers. Virtually all diseases characterized by thickening of the nucleated epidermal layers also exhibit hyperkeratosis. For example, chronic scratching or rubbing of normal skin causes a thickened epidermis, hyperkeratosis and dermal fibrosis, a condition known as **lichen simplex chronicus.** In this entity, the nucleated epidermis and stratum corneum may each be 3-fold thicker than normal. By contrast, in ichthyosis, the stratum corneum may be five times thicker than normal, but it overlies a disproportionately thin nucleated epidermis.

Ichthyosis Vulgaris

Ichthyosis vulgaris is an autosomal dominant disorder of keratinization characterized by hyperkeratosis and reduced or absent epidermal keratohyaline granules (Fig. 28-10). Scaly skin results from increased cohesiveness of the stratum corneum. The attenuated stratum granulosum is a single layer with small, defective keratohyaline granules. *Decreased or absent synthesis of* profilaggrin, *a keratin filament "glue," is responsible for these defects.*

Ichthyosis vulgaris is the prototype of disproportionate corneal thickening. The stratum corneum is loose and has a basket-weave appearance, which differs from normal only in amount. The granular layer is greatly diminished and often appears absent (Fig. 28-9B). Ultrastructurally, keratohyaline granules are small and sponge-like, which indicates defective synthesis. Basal and spinous layers appear normal. Thus, the primary defect in ichthyosis vulgaris is in the granular and cornified layers, the epidermal zones responsible for the final stage of keratinization and cornification.

 CLINICAL FEATURES: Ichthyosis vulgaris is the most common of the ichthyoses. It begins in early childhood, often in people with family histories of this condition. Small white scales occur on the extensor surfaces of extremities and on the trunk and face. The disease is lifelong, but most patients can be maintained free of scales with topical treatment.

States similar to ichthyosis vulgaris may accompany other diseases or may follow certain drugs. Ichthyosis may occur with lymphomas, especially Hodgkin disease, other cancers, systemic granulomatous disorders and connective tissue disease. Drugs may produce ichthyosis by interfering with similar pathways of lipid metabolism.

X-Linked Ichthyosis

This is a heritable epidermal disorder that, in recessive form, is characterized by delayed dissolution of desmosomal disks in the stratum corneum, owing to deficiency of steroid sulfatase. Steroid sulfatase normally degrades the Odland body product, cholesterol sulfate, which provides cellular adhesion in the lower stratum corneum. Failure of steroid sulfatase action on cholesterol sulfate leads to persistent cohesion of the stratum corneum, but in this disease the granular layer is preserved.

Epidermolytic Hyperkeratosis

This congenital, autosomal dominant ichthyosis features generalized erythroderma, ichthyosiform skin and blistering and is thus also known as "bullous congenital ichthyosiform erythroderma."

 **MOLECULAR PATHOGENESIS:** This *disease results from mutations in the K1 or K10 keratin genes (chromosomes 12 and 17, respectively), which encode the keratins in the suprabasal epidermis.* These mutations cause faulty assembly of keratin tonofilaments and impair their insertion into desmosomes. Cytoskeleton development is impaired, resulting in epidermal "lysis" and a tendency to form vesicles.

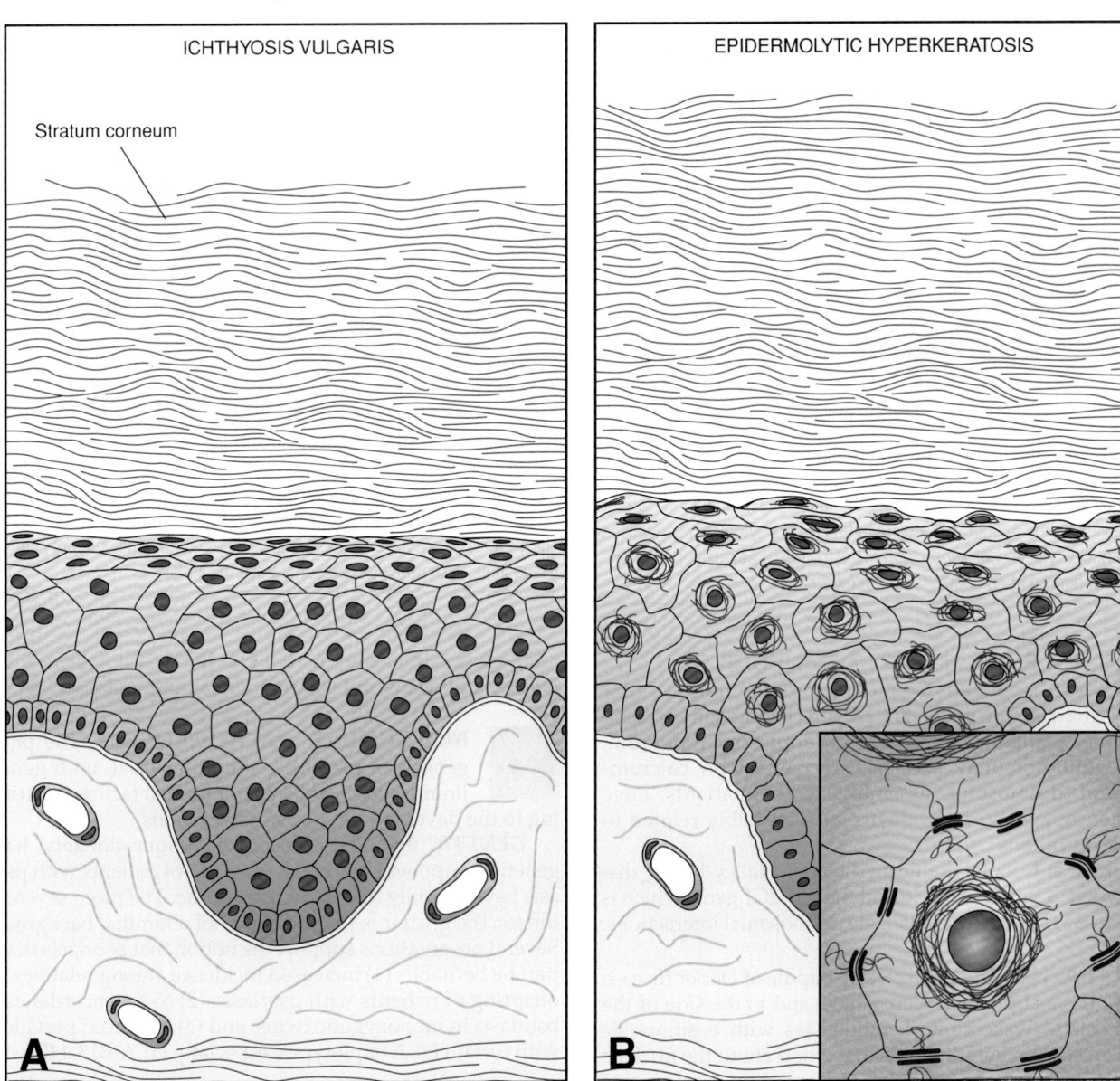

FIGURE 28-10. A. Ichthyosis vulgaris. B. Epidermolytic hyperkeratosis. Both diseases are characterized by thickening of the stratum corneum relative to the nucleated layers. Epidermolytic hyperkeratosis is characterized by abnormal keratin synthesis, manifested by whorled keratin filaments about the nucleus (*inset*).

In epidermolytic hyperkeratosis, suprabasal keratinocytes contain thick, eosinophilic tonofilaments that whorl around the nucleus in a concentric fashion (Fig. 28-11). The cytoplasm has a clear zone (vacuolization) around the perinuclear tonofilaments, but these filaments again condense at the outer margins of the cell. Enlarged keratohyaline granules are present. The stratum corneum is disproportionately thickened (Fig. 28-10).

CLINICAL FEATURES: Epidermolytic hyperkeratosis manifests with blistering at or shortly after birth. It may be generalized or localized to only several areas of the body. Lesions tend to appear dark and even verrucous. Other than cosmetic disfigurement, the major problem is secondary bacterial infection.

Lamellar Ichthyosis

This autosomal recessive congenital disorder of cornification is characterized by severe and generalized ichthyosis. Typically, increased cohesiveness of the stratum corneum is accompanied by numerous keratinosomes and an abnormally large amount of intercellular substance. *The disease is genetically heterogeneous but is often caused by mutations in the gene encoding transglutaminase 1 (TGM1; chromosome 14q11), resulting in defective lamellar body secretion.*

Darier Disease Is an Autosomal Dominant Disorder of Keratinization

Also called **keratosis follicularis,** this disease is characterized by multifocal keratoses.

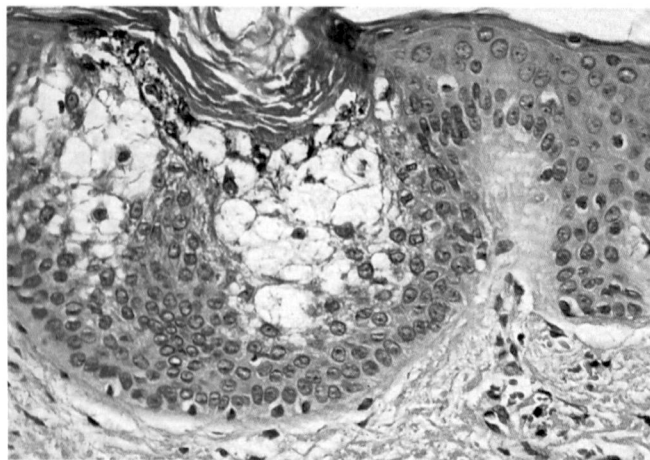

FIGURE 28-11. Epidermolytic hyperkeratosis. The keratinocytes of the stratum spinosum have clumped tonofilaments. As a result, their cytoplasm is relatively clear. In the outer stratum spinosum, the clumped fibrils are further compacted and whorl about the nuclei, resulting in dark cytoplasm condensed about the nuclei. These cells separate from each other to produce epidermolysis. A normal portion of epidermis is seen on the *right*.

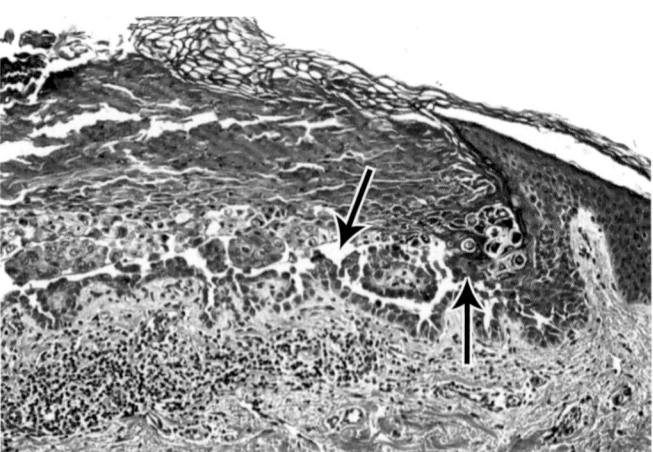

FIGURE 28-12. Darier disease. Virtually the entire epidermis exhibits focal acantholytic dyskeratosis. A small portion of normal epidermis is present (*right*). In the lesion, there is a suprabasal cleft (*arrows*) with a few dyshesive (acantholytic) keratinocytes surmounted by hyperkeratosis and parakeratosis. The cleft is not a vesicle because true vesicles contain inflammatory cells and tissue fluid. Dyskeratosis is present above the cleft.

MOLECULAR PATHOGENESIS: Darier disease is linked to a defect in the intercellular matrix. The gene, *ATP2A2* on chromosome 12q23-24, encodes a calcium pump of the endoplasmic reticulum, and its mutation may exert a direct effect on calcium-dependent desmosome assembly. These patients have many neuropsychiatric problems, also probably related to *ATP2A2* mutations.

A similar autosomal dominant disorder, Hailey-Hailey disease, involves chromosome 3q and the ATP2C1 gene, which is also believed to govern keratinocyte desmosomal interactions.

PATHOLOGY: The warty papule of Darier disease has a suprabasal cleft. Above and to the side of the cleft, dyskeratotic keratinocytes with eosinophilic cytoplasm contain keratin fibrils that whorl about the nucleus (Fig. 28-12). The roof of the cleft is formed by a column of compact keratotic material. Similar lesions may occur as an isolated scaly nodule called a "warty dyskeratoma." In the previously mentioned Hailey-Hailey disease, lesions resemble those of Darier disease, albeit with more acantholysis, or keratinocyte dyshesion. This condition is presumably caused by this altered desmosome function, which results in a characteristic "dilapidated brick wall" appearance (Fig. 28-13).

CLINICAL FEATURES: Darier disease first appears late in childhood or in adolescence as skin-colored papules that later become crusted. Affected areas have many warty elevations, 2–4 mm in diameter, largely on the chest, nasolabial folds, back, scalp, forehead, ears and groin.

Psoriasis Is a Proliferative Skin Disease with Persistent Epidermal Hyperplasia

Psoriasis is a chronic, frequently familial disorder that features large, erythematous, scaly plaques, commonly on extensor cutaneous surfaces. It affects 1%–2% of the population worldwide. Psoriasis may arise at any age but shows a peak in late

adolescence. Interestingly, the condition is not seen among Native Americans and is infrequent among Asians.

MOLECULAR PATHOGENESIS: The pathogenesis of psoriasis is multifactorial, with genetic, immunologic and environmental factors contributing to the development of psoriatic lesions.

GENETIC FACTORS: Psoriasis unquestionably has a genetic component, although only 1/3 of patients with psoriasis have a family history of the disease. The more severe the illness, the greater is the likelihood of a familial background. Several observations support the notion that psoriasis may in part be heritable: (1) increased incidence among relatives and offspring of patients with psoriasis; (2) 65% concordance for psoriasis in monozygotic twins; and (3) increased prevalence with certain HLA haplotypes, especially HLA-B13, HLA-B17,

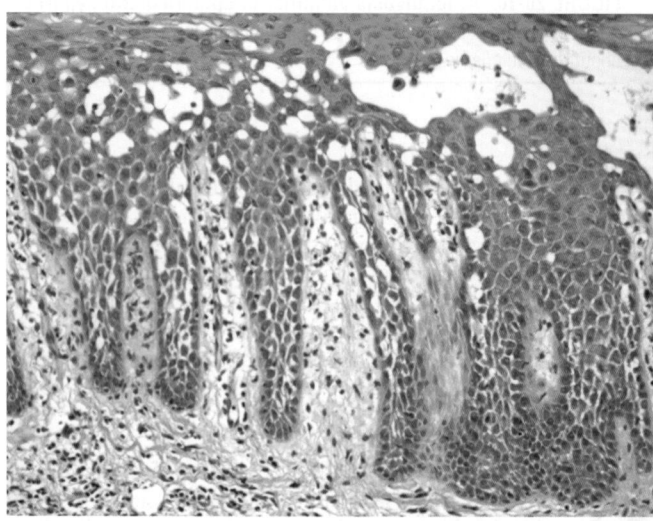

FIGURE 28-13. Hailey-Hailey disease. Hailey-Hailey disease shows acantholysis of the epidermis with dyskeratosis of keratinocytes, yielding a characteristic "dilapidated brick wall" appearance on histology.

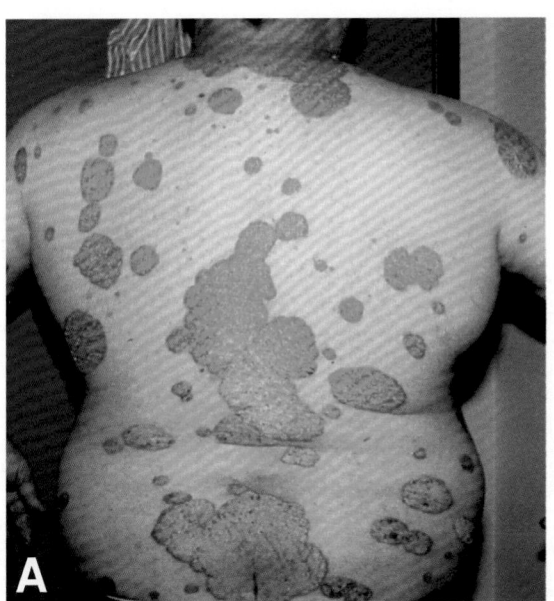
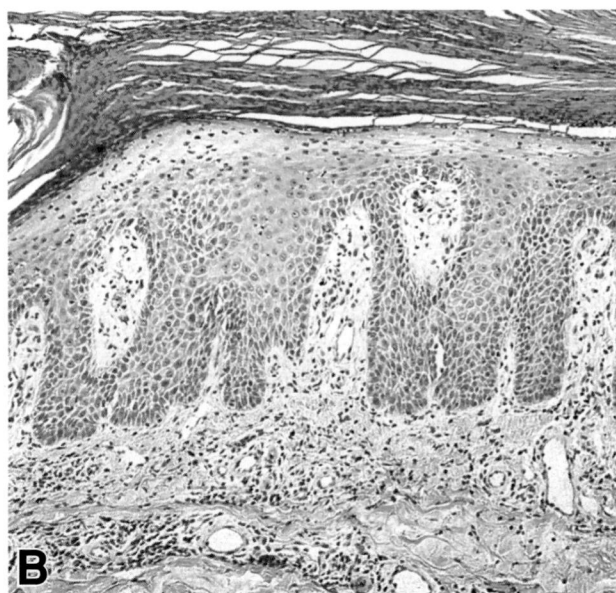

FIGURE 28-14. Psoriasis. This disorder is the prototype of psoriasiform epidermal hyperplasia. **A.** A patient with psoriasis shows large, confluent, sharply demarcated, erythematous plaques on the trunk. **B.** Microscopic examination of a lesion demonstrates that the rete ridges are uniformly elongated, as are the dermal papillae, giving an interlocking pattern of alternately reversed "clubs." The dermal papillae are edematous and reside beneath a thinned epidermis (suprapapillary thinning). There is striking parakeratosis, which is the scale observed clinically.

HLA-Bw57 and particularly HLA-Cw6. In fact, people with HLA-Cw6 are 10–15 times more likely to develop psoriasis than the general population. A 300-kb segment in the MHC-I region of chromosome 6p21, PSORS1, is felt to be a major genetic determinant of susceptibility.

IMMUNOLOGIC FACTORS: T lymphocytes are crucial to the pathogenesis of psoriatic lesions. T_H1 and T_H17 cells, subtypes of CD4$^+$ T cells, appear to drive the inflammatory response and subsequent dermatosis. These subsets of T cells, in addition to effector CD8$^+$ T cells and antigen-presenting dendritic cells, secrete proinflammatory cytokines, such as IL-12, IL-17, IL-22, IL-23, interferon-γ (IFN-γ) and tumor necrosis factor-α (TNF-α), as well as keratinocyte growth factors. The combination of these proinflammatory cytokines and epidermal growth factors likely causes the constellation of changes seen in psoriasis. For these reasons, therapeutics targeting cytokines, such as TNF-α inhibitors, or those targeting IL-12, IL-17 and IL-23 are currently being used.

ENVIRONMENTAL FACTORS: Clinical lesions may occur anywhere on the skin. Stimuli such as physical injury ("Köbner phenomenon"), infection, certain drugs and photosensitivity may produce psoriatic lesions in apparently normal skin. The pathogenesis of psoriatic plaques may be appreciated by contrasting the effect of chronic cutaneous trauma in people with and without psoriasis. Chronic irritation of normal skin, as in repeated rubbing, produces a tough, scaly, cutaneous plaque that is clinically and histologically psoriasiform. However, the lesion disappears when the trauma ceases. In psoriatic patients, even less trauma generates psoriatic plaques that may persist for years after an initial injury.

 PATHOLOGY: The most distinctive pathology is at the edges of chronic psoriatic plaques. The epidermis is thickened, with **hyperkeratosis** and

parakeratosis (persistence of nuclei in cells of the stratum corneum, which occurs with increased epidermal turnover). Parakeratosis may be circumscribed and focal, or it may be diffuse, in which case the granular layer is diminished or absent. The nucleated layers of the epidermis are thickened severalfold in the rete pegs and are frequently thinner over dermal papillae (Fig. 28-14). In turn, the papillae are elongated and appear as sections of cones, with their apices toward the dermis. In chronic lesions, dermal papillae may appear as bulbous "clubs" with short handles (Figs. 28-14 and 28-15). The rete ridges of the epidermis have a profile reciprocal to that of the dermal papillae, resulting in interlocked dermal and epidermal "clubs," with alternately reversed polarity. Capillaries of dermal papillae are dilated and tortuous (Fig. 28-15). In very early lesions, changes may be limited to capillary dilation, with a few neutrophils "squirting" into the epidermis. Epidermal hyperplasia and hyperkeratosis occur mainly in chronic lesions.

Ultrastructurally, the capillaries are venule-like; neutrophils may emerge at their tips and migrate into the epidermis above the apices of the papillae. Neutrophils may become localized in the epidermal spinous layer or in small microabscesses (of Munro) in the stratum corneum and may be associated with limited areas of parakeratosis (Fig. 28-16). The dermis below the papillae contains variable mononuclear inflammation, mostly lymphocytes, around the superficial vascular plexus. The inflammatory process does not extend into the subjacent reticular dermis.

The psoriasiform histology is common in cutaneous pathology. Seborrheic dermatitis, reaction to chronic trauma (lichen simplex chronicus), subacute and chronic spongiotic dermatitis (eczema) and cutaneous T-cell lymphoma (mycosis fungoides) all may exhibit such change. However, these usually do not mimic psoriasis precisely.

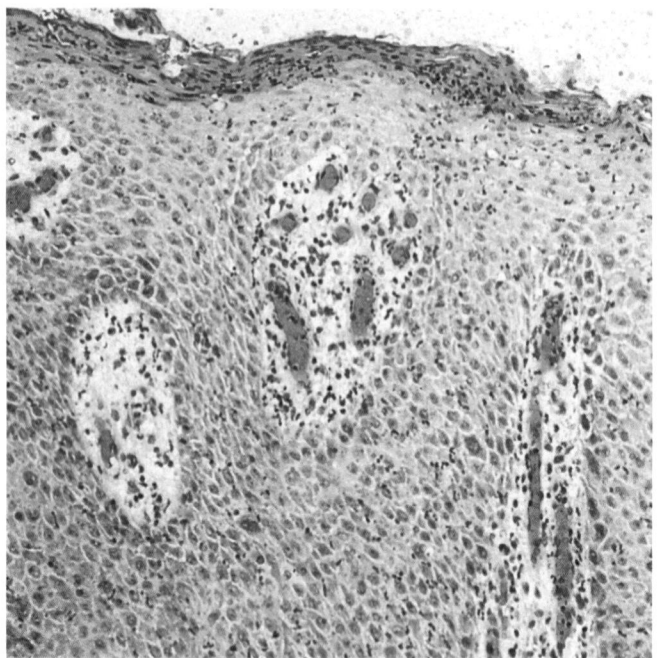

FIGURE 28-15. Psoriasis. The clubbed papillae contain tortuous dilated venules. The prominent venules are part of the venulization of capillaries, which may be of histogenetic importance in psoriasis. The papilla to the *right* has one cross-section of its superficial capillary venule loop, which is normal. The papilla in the *center* shows numerous cross-sections of its venule, indicating striking tortuosity.

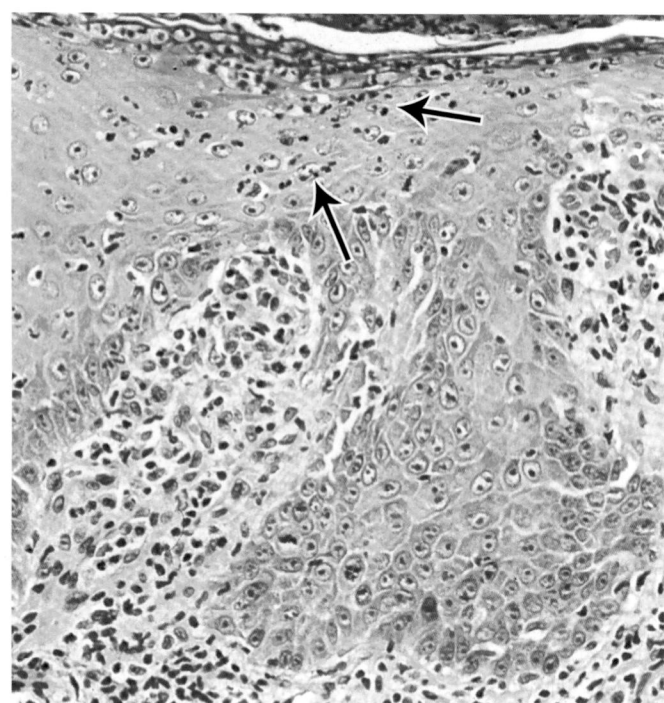

FIGURE 28-16. Psoriasis. Neutrophils migrate into the epidermis, emerging from the venulized capillaries at the tips of the dermal papillae. They migrate to the upper stratum spinosum and stratum corneum (*arrows*). In some forms of psoriasis, pustules are common clinical lesions.

CLINICAL FEATURES: The initial presentation of psoriasis is variable and disease activity is intermittent. Familial psoriasis tends to be more severe than sporadic types, but disease severity varies from annoying scaly lesions over the elbows to a serious debilitating disorder involving most of the skin and often associated with arthritis. A single lesion of psoriasis may be a small focus of scaly erythema or an enormous confluent plaque covering much of the trunk (Fig. 28-14A). A typical plaque is 4–5 cm, sharply demarcated at its margin and covered by a surface of silvery scales. If the scales are detached, pinpoint foci of bleeding from the dilated capillaries in the dermal papillae dot the underlying glossy erythematous surface ("Auspitz sign").

Seronegative arthritis develops in 7% of patients with psoriasis. The tendency to arthropathy is linked to several HLA haplotypes, particularly HLA-B27. Psoriatic arthritis closely resembles its rheumatoid counterpart, but it is usually milder and causes little disability.

In some variations of the disease, neutrophilic pustules (of Kogoj) dominate **(pustular psoriasis).** Severe intractable psoriasis has been observed in some patients with AIDS.

Psoriasis has long been treated with coal tar or wood tar derivatives and anthralin, a strong reducing agent. Topical and systemic corticosteroids have also been used. Severe, generalized psoriasis justifies systemic treatment with methotrexate. Phototherapy ("PUVA") after administration of psoralens, a UV-absorbing compound that binds to DNA, is often effective. Synthetic vitamin A and vitamin D derivatives have also been used. More recently, treatments that target immunologic and inflammatory mediators have been used, such as anticytokine therapeutics (see above), with promising results.

Pemphigus Vulgaris Is a Blistering Disease Due to Antibodies to Keratinocytes

Dyshesive disorders are cutaneous diseases in which blisters form because of diminished cohesiveness between epidermal keratinocytes. Pemphigus vulgaris (PV) (Greek, *pemphix,* "bubble"), the prototype of dyshesive diseases, is a chronic, blistering skin disorder that is most common in people 40–60 years old but is seen at all ages, including children. All races are susceptible, but people of Jewish or Mediterranean heritage are at greatest risk.

MOLECULAR PATHOGENESIS: PV is an autoimmune disease: patients have circulating IgG against an epidermal surface antigen, **desmoglein 3,** a desmosomal protein. Antigen–antibody union results in dyshesion, which is augmented by release of plasminogen activator and, hence, activation of plasmin. This proteolytic enzyme acts on the intercellular substance and may be the dominant factor in dyshesion. Internalization of pemphigus antigen–antibody complexes, disappearance of attachment plaques and retraction of perinuclear tonofilaments may all act in concert with proteinases to cause dyshesion and vesiculation (Fig. 28-17). Blisters in PV are intraepidermal. In other blistering disorders that affect the basement membrane zone, discussed below, subepidermal blisters are formed.

PATHOLOGY: The outer epidermal layers separate from the basal layer. This suprabasal dyshesion results in a blister with an intact basal layer as

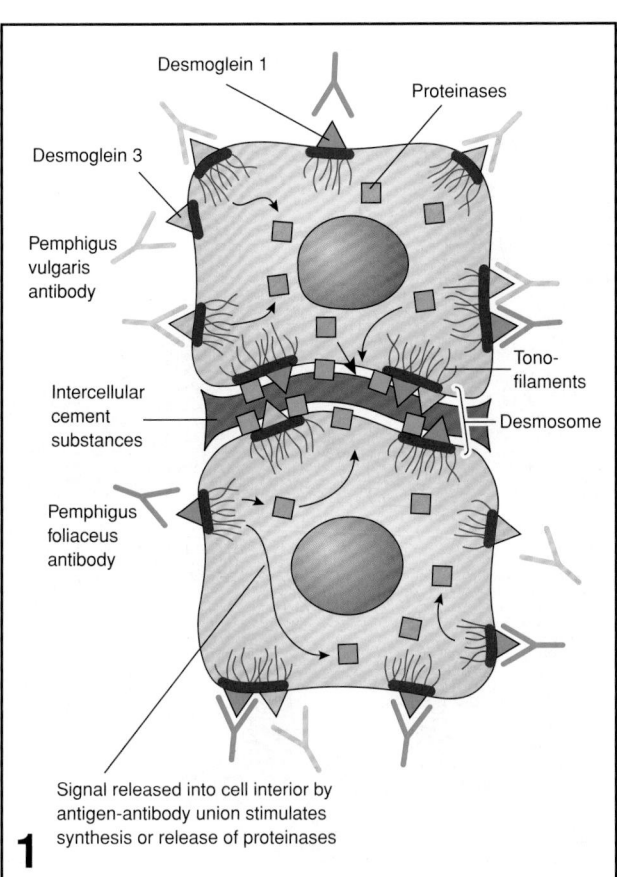

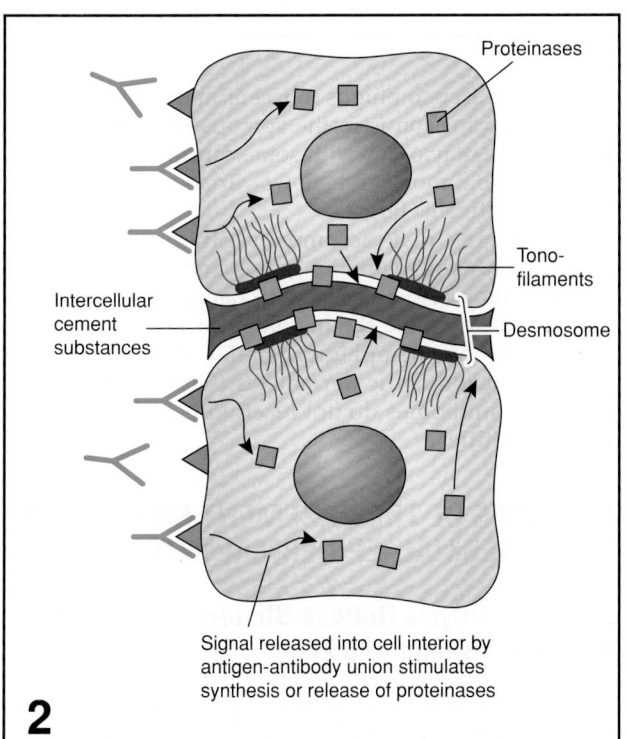

FIGURE 28-17. Pemphigus vulgaris. A pathogenetic mechanism of suprabasal dyshesion is shown. **1.** A circulating autoantibody binds to an antigen on the outer leaflet of the plasma membrane (desmosome) of the keratinocyte, especially in the basal regions. **2.** Antigen–antibody union results in release of a proteinase (plasmin). **3.** The proteinase interacts with intercellular cement, initiating dyshesion. (*continued*)

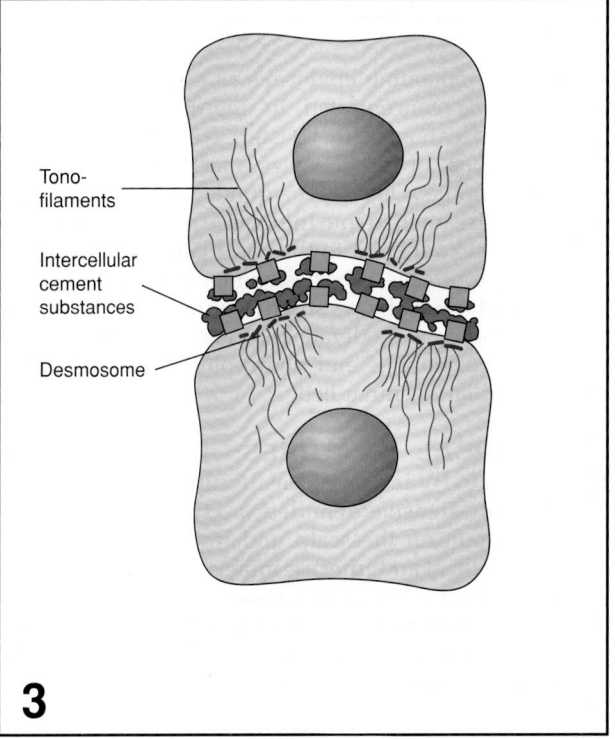

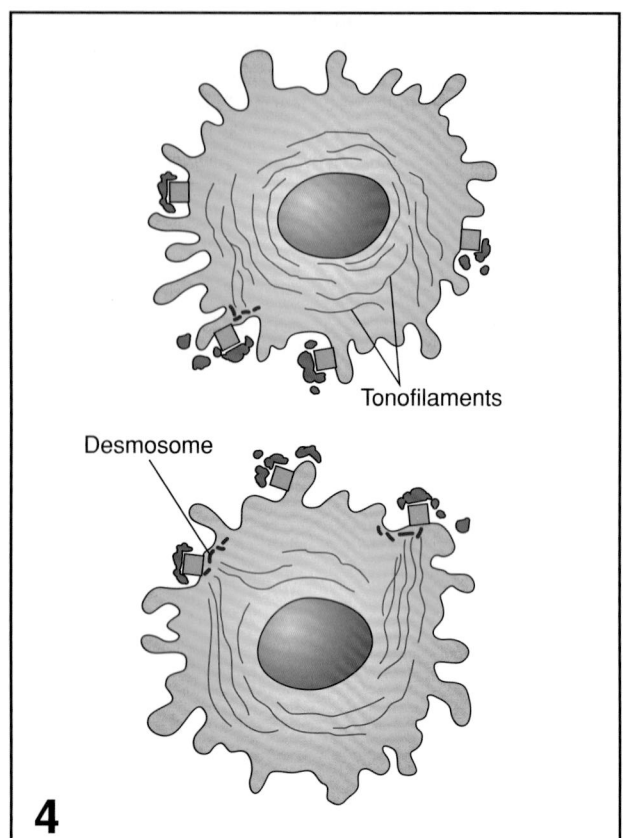

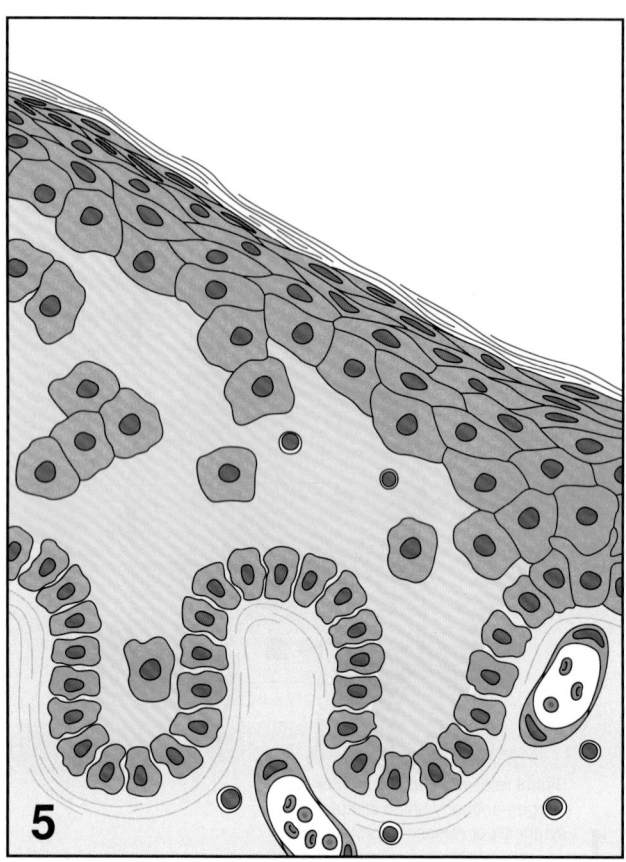

FIGURE 28-17. (*Continued*) **4.** Desmosomes deteriorate, tonofilaments clump about the nucleus, the cells round up and separation is complete. **5.** A vesicle, which is usually suprabasal, forms. Alternatively, acantholysis may occur by direct interference with desmosomal and adherence junction attachments.

a floor and the remaining epidermis as a roof (Fig. 28-18). Desmoglein 3 is concentrated in the lower epidermis, explaining the location of the blister. The blister contains moderate numbers of lymphocytes, macrophages, eosinophils and neutrophils. Distinctive, rounded keratinocytes, or acantholytic cells, are shed into the vesicle during dyshesion. Basal cells remain adherent to the basal lamina and form a layer of "tombstone cells." Dyshesion may extend along dermal adnexa and is not always strictly suprabasal. The subjacent dermis shows a moderate infiltrate of lymphocytes, macrophages, eosinophils and neutrophils, predominantly around the capillary venular bed.

 CLINICAL FEATURES: The characteristic lesion of PV is a large, easily ruptured blister that leaves extensive denuded or crusted areas. They are most common on the scalp and mucous membranes and in periumbilical and intertriginous areas. Without corticosteroid treatment, PV is progressive and usually fatal. Much of the skin surface may become denuded. Immunosuppression is also useful for maintenance therapy. With appropriate treatment, the 10-year mortality rate for PV is less than 10%.

Other diseases caused by dyshesion that have pathogenetic mechanisms like PV include **pemphigus foliaceus, pemphigus erythematosus** and **drug-induced pemphigus** (mostly associated with penicillamine or captopril). In pemphigus foliaceus, antibodies against **desmoglein 1,** a desmosomal protein, cause dyshesion in the outer spinous and granular epidermal layers (vs. suprabasal dyshesion in PV)

(Fig. 28-19). In pemphigus foliaceus and pemphigus erythematosus, dyshesion is in the spinous layer. **Paraneoplastic pemphigus** may occur with some cancers, usually lymphoproliferative tumors, and shows variable patterns of dyshesion and antigenic targets.

Pemphigus may accompany other autoimmune diseases, such as myasthenia gravis and lupus erythematosus, and may also be seen with benign thymomas. Other diseases may mimic the histology of PV, namely, familial benign chronic pemphigus (Hailey-Hailey disease) and transient acantholytic dermatosis (Grover disease). However, IgG antibodies do not react with epidermal antigens in these entities.

DISEASES OF THE BASEMENT MEMBRANE ZONE (DERMAL–EPIDERMAL INTERFACE)

In Epidermolysis Bullosa Blisters Form in the Basement Membrane Zone

Epidermolysis bullosa (EB) is a heterogeneous group of disorders loosely bound by their hereditary nature and by a tendency to form blisters at the sites of minor trauma. The clinical spectrum ranges from a minor annoyance to a widespread, life-threatening blistering disease. *These blisters are almost always present at birth or shortly thereafter.* The classification of these disorders is based on a combination of clinical features and site of blister formation in the BMZ. The different mechanisms of blister

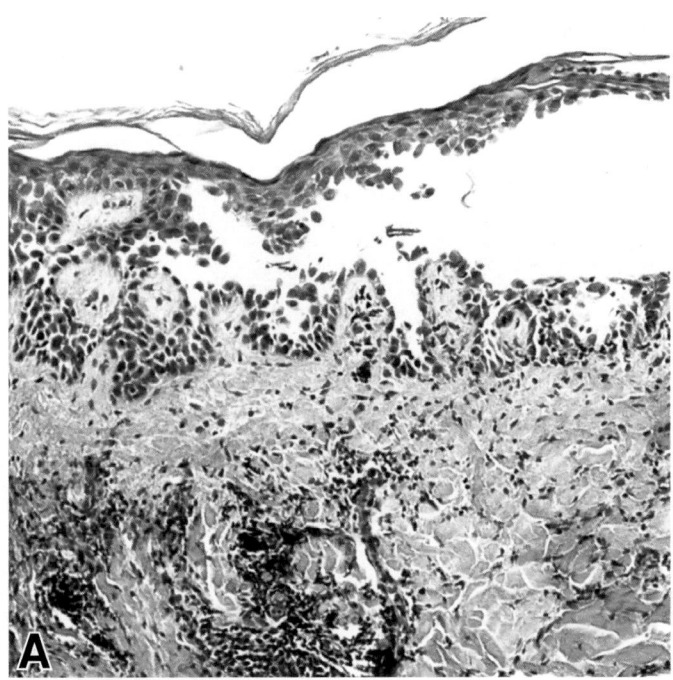
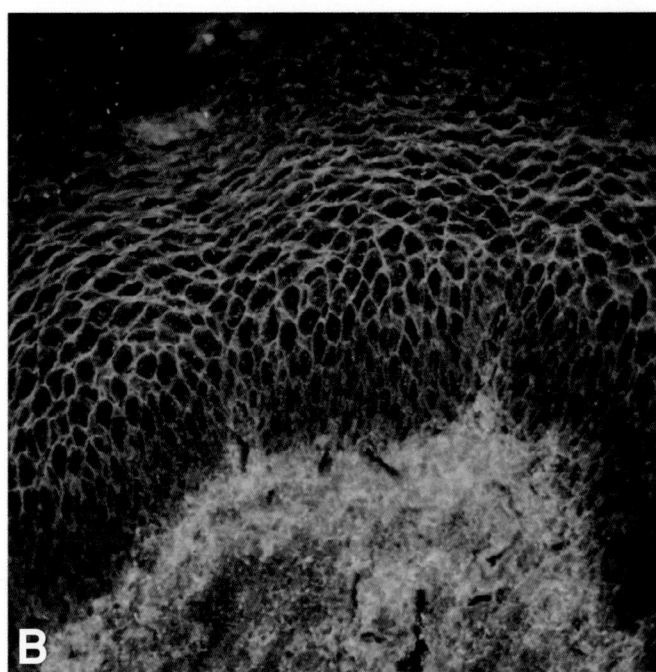

FIGURE 28-18. Pemphigus vulgaris. A. Suprabasal dyshesion leads to an intraepidermal blister containing acantholytic keratinocytes. The basal keratinocytes are slightly separated from each other and totally separated from the stratum spinosum. The basal keratinocytes are firmly attached to the epidermal basement membrane zone. **B.** Direct immunofluorescence examination of perilesional skin reveals antibodies, usually of the immunoglobulin G (IgG) type, deposited in the intercellular substance of the epidermis, yielding a lace-like pattern outlining the keratinocytes.

formation underlie each of the four major categories of EB (Fig. 28-20).

Epidermolytic Epidermolysis Bullosa

This disorder, also known as **EB simplex,** is a group of autosomal dominant and autosomal recessive skin diseases in which blisters form owing to disruption of basal keratinocytes. Blisters develop after minor trauma, such as merely rubbing the skin, but heal without scarring (thus the term

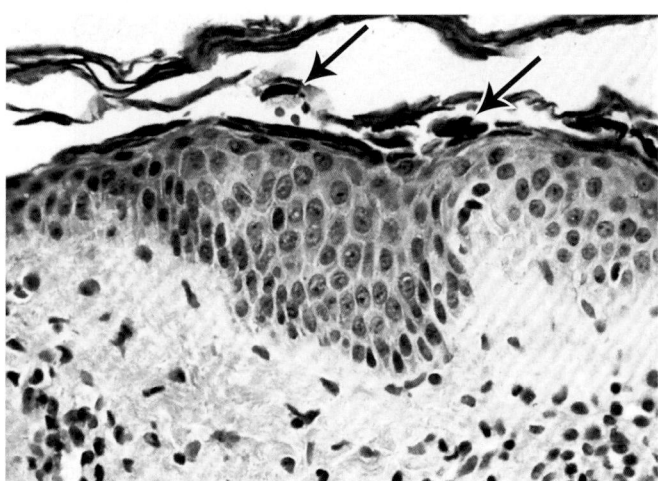

FIGURE 28-19. Pemphigus foliaceus. The dyshesion develops in the outer stratum spinosum and stratum granulosum. (Compare with that of pemphigus vulgaris, Fig. 24-18.) Dyshesive and dyskeratotic keratinocytes of the stratum granulosum (*arrows*) are important hallmarks.

"simplex"). Epidermolytic EB is cosmetically disturbing and sometimes debilitating but is not life-threatening.

 **MOLECULAR PATHOGENESIS:** Epidermolytic EB has been attributed to mutations of genes encoding cytokeratin intermediate filaments (12q11-13, 17q21), which provide mechanical stability to the epidermis. Cytolysis of basal keratinocytes causes the blisters in the epidermolytic variety of EB. Initially, small, subnuclear, cytoplasmic vacuoles develop, enlarge and coalesce. They reflect abnormalities in keratins 5 and 14, which aggregate about the keratinocyte nuclei. The plasma membrane ruptures when the large vacuole reaches it, after which the cell is lysed.

PATHOLOGY: An intraepidermal vesicle results from lysis of several basal keratinocytes. The roof of the vesicle is an almost intact epidermis with a fragmented basal layer. The vesicle floor shows bits of basal cell cytoplasm attached to the lamina densa, which appears as a well-preserved pink line at the base of the vesicle. Inflammatory cells are sparse.

Junctional Epidermolysis Bullosa

This type of EB is a group of autosomal recessive skin diseases in which blisters form within the lamina lucida. Clinical expression ranges from a benign disease with no effect on life span to a severe condition that may be fatal within the first 2 years of life. There may be associated abnormalities of the nails and teeth.

MOLECULAR PATHOGENESIS: In the severe form, mutations in the genes for certain isoforms of laminin and the integrins are reported (1q25-31,

EPIDERMOLYTIC EB

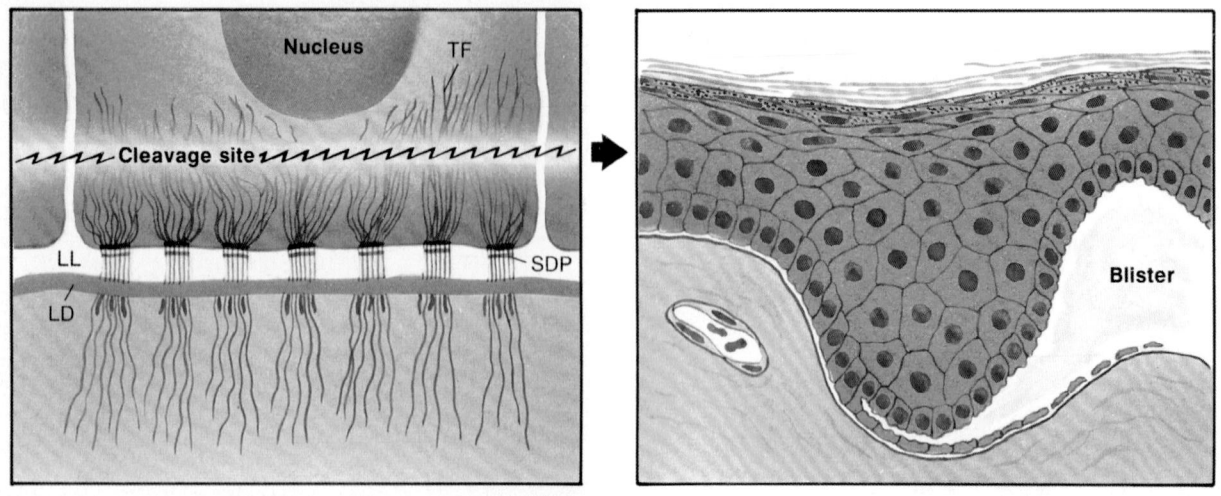

JUNCTIONAL EB

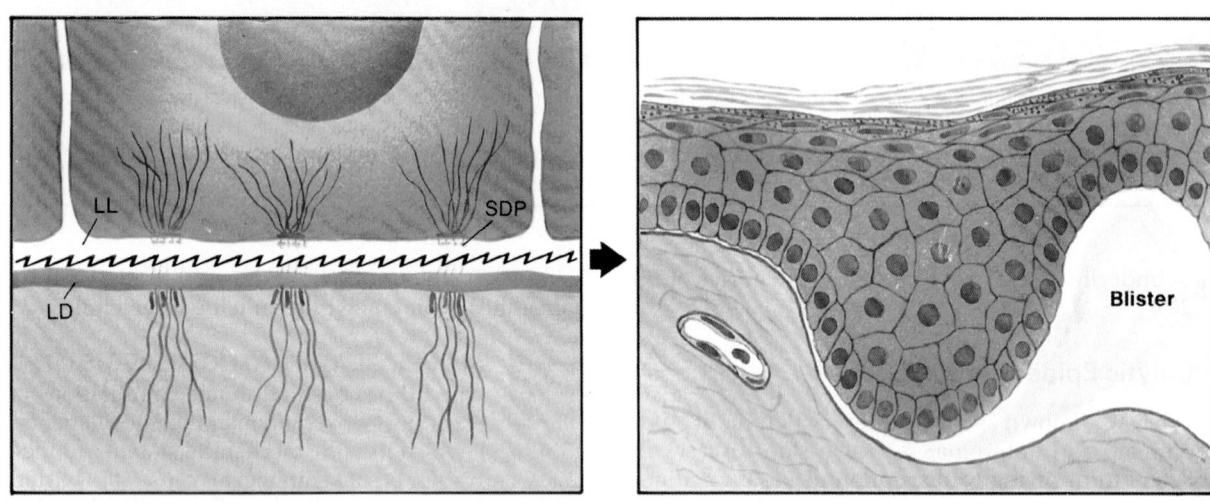

DERMOLYTIC EB

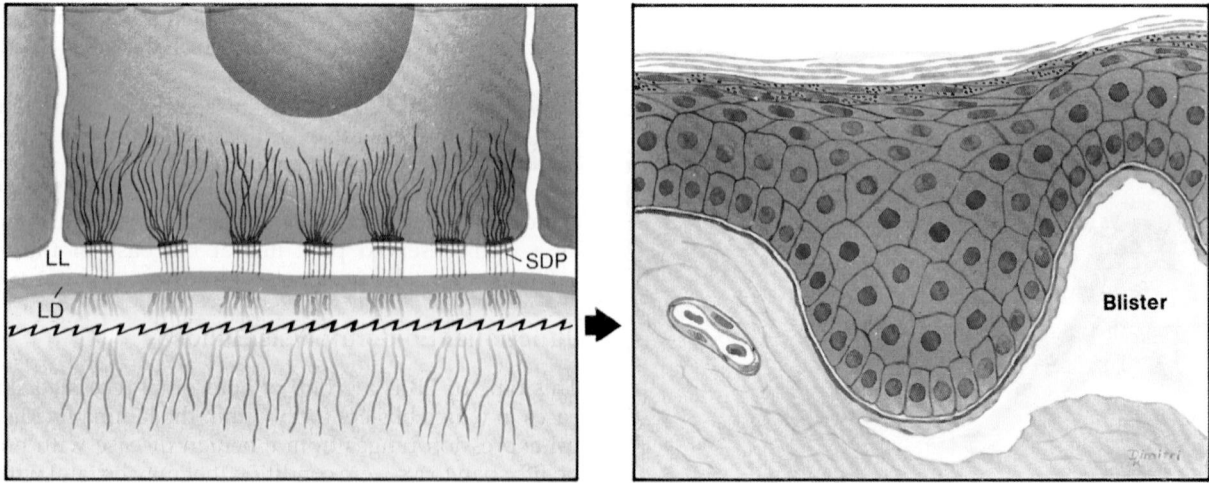

FIGURE 28-20. Epidermolysis bullosa (EB). Three distinct mechanisms of blister formation are shown. Electron microscopic images are diagrammed on the *left;* light microscopic images are on the *right.* **Epidermolytic EB** is caused by disintegration of the lowermost regions of the epidermal basal cells. The bottom portions of the basal cells cleave, and the remainder of the epidermis lifts away. Small fragments of basal cells remain attached to the basement membrane zone. **Junctional EB** is characterized by cleavage in the lamina lucida. **Dermolytic EB** is associated with rudimentary and fragmented anchoring fibrils. The entire basement membrane zone and epidermis split away from the dermis in relationship to these flawed anchoring fibrils. *LL* = lamina lucida; *LD* = lamina densa; *SDP* = subdesmosomal dense plate.

1q3, 18q11). The benign form reflects mutations in the gene for type XVII collagen (1q32, 10q23). Both types heal without scarring but may cause residual atrophy of the skin.

 PATHOLOGY: An intact epidermis forms the roof of the vesicle in junctional EB. Plasma membranes of basal keratinocytes are unchanged. The vesicle floor is an intact lamina densa, as in epidermolytic EB, but there are no attached fragments of basal cell cytoplasm. The blister is thus within the lamina lucida. Both lesional and uninvolved skin shows fewer basal hemidesmosomes, which have poorly developed attachment plaques and subbasal dense plates.

Dermolytic Epidermolysis Bullosa

Also known as **dystrophic EB,** dermolytic EB is a group of autosomal dominant and autosomal recessive diseases in which blisters are immediately deep to the lamina densa. The recessive variant is more severe. In both types, healed blisters show atrophic ("dystrophic") scarring. Nails and teeth may be involved.

 **MOLECULAR PATHOGENESIS:** Dermolytic EB is attributed to a defect in anchoring fibrils. These fibrils are abnormally arranged and reduced in number in apparently normal skin of affected newborns. The basic defect is a mutation in the gene for collagen type VII (3p21). Anchoring fibrils make up a net in the upper dermis, through which collagen types I and III fibers course. This structure anchors the epidermis to the underlying dermis. Its disruption results in subepidermal bullae arising in the sublamina densa zone.

 PATHOLOGY: The vesicle roof is normal epidermis with an attached, intact lamina lucida and lamina densa. The base of the vesicle is the outer part of the papillary dermis. Ultrastructurally, there are fewer anchoring fibrils in the dominant type and virtually none in the recessive form. A corresponding decrease in anchoring fibril proteins AF-1 and AF-2 occurs in the two variants.

Kindler Syndrome

This type of EB shows autosomal recessive transmission and blisters with mixed cleavage planes. Distinctive clinical findings that differentiate it from other inherited EB types include poikiloderma (mottled pigmentation of the skin) and photosensitivity.

 **MOLECULAR PATHOGENESIS:** This entity results from a mutation in FERMT1 (20p12), which encodes kindlin-1, a protein involved in adhesion between basal keratinocytes.

Bullous Pemphigoid Is a Subepidermal Blistering Disease Caused by Autoantibodies against Basement Membrane Proteins

BP is a common, autoimmune, blistering disease, which has clinical similarities to PV (hence the term "pemphigoid"), but which lacks acantholysis. The disease is most common in the later decades of life and affects all races and both genders.

 **MOLECULAR PATHOGENESIS:** Like PV, BP is an autoimmune disease, but here complement-fixing IgG antibodies are against BPAG1 and BPAG2 basement membrane proteins. BPAG1 is a 230-kd protein in the intracellular portion of the basal cell hemidesmosome. BPAG2 is a 180-kd protein that traverses the plasma membrane and extends into the upper lamina lucida. The antigen–antibody complex may injure the basal cell plasma membrane via the C5b–C9 membrane attack complex (see Chapter 4). This damage may in turn interfere with elaboration of adherence factors by basal keratinocytes. More importantly, anaphylatoxins C3a and C5a are released in complement activation. They trigger mast cell degranulation and release of factors chemotactic for eosinophils, neutrophils and lymphocytes. Levels of IL-5 and eotaxin, which play significant roles in recruitment and function of eosinophils, are elevated in the blister fluid of patients with BP. Eosinophil granules contain tissue-damaging substances, including eosinophil peroxidase and major basic protein. These molecules, together with neutrophil and mast cell proteases, cause dermal–epidermal separation within the lamina lucida (Fig. 28-21).

 PATHOLOGY: The blisters of BP are subepidermal; the roof is intact epidermis and the base is the lamina densa of the BMZ (Fig. 28-22). The blisters contain many eosinophils, plus fibrin, lymphocytes and neutrophils. In BP, apparently normal skin shows migration of mast cells from the venule toward the epidermis. With the onset of erythema, eosinophils appear in the upper dermis and may be arrayed along the epidermal BMZ. Ultrastructurally, dermal–epidermal separation begins with disruption of anchoring filaments of the lamina lucida. Immunofluorescence shows linear deposition of C3 and IgG at the epidermal BMZ and serum antibodies against BPAG1 and BPAG2 (Fig. 28-23).

 CLINICAL FEATURES: The blisters of BP are large and tense and may appear on normal-appearing skin or on an erythematous base (Fig. 28-22). The medial thighs and flexor aspects of the forearms are commonly affected, but the groin, axillae and other cutaneous sites may also develop blisters. The disease is self-limited but chronic, and the patient's general health is usually unaffected. Systemic glucocorticoid treatment greatly shortens the course of the disease.

Table 28-1 summarizes the molecular pathogenesis of the discussed immunobullous disorders as well acantholytic disorders.

Dermatitis Herpetiformis Reflects Gluten Sensitivity and Immune Complex Deposition

Dermatitis herpetiformis (DH) is an intensely pruritic eruption with urticaria-like plaques and small subepidermal vesicles over the extensor surfaces of the body.

 **MOLECULAR PATHOGENESIS:** It accompanies gluten sensitivity in patients with HLA-B8, HLA-DR3 and HLA-DQw2 haplotypes. Although gluten-sensitive enteropathy may be subclinical, most patients will show features of celiac disease on small intestinal biopsy. Gluten is a protein in wheat, barley, rye and oats. DH cutaneous lesions reflect granular deposits of IgA, mainly

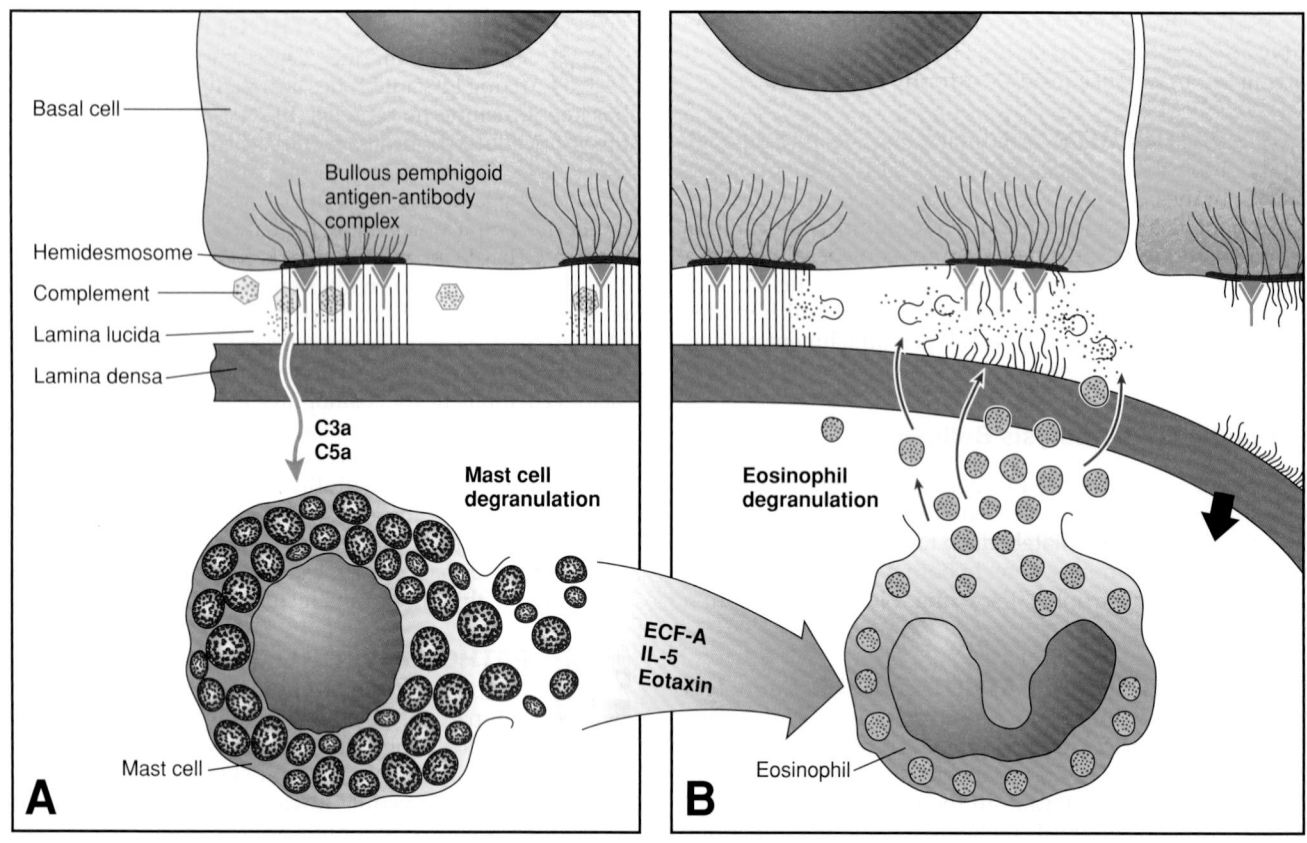

FIGURE 28-21. Bullous pemphigoid (BP). Pathogenetic mechanisms of blister formation are outlined. A circulating antibody to an apparently normal glycoprotein—BP antigen—in the lamina lucida precipitates the pathogenetic events in bullous pemphigoid. **A.** Antigen–antibody union activates complement, and the anaphylatoxins C3a and C5a are produced. These degranulate mast cells, resulting in the release of eosinophilic chemotactic factors. **B, C.** The tissue-damaging substances of eosinophilic granules cause vesicle formation at the lamina lucida, with some breakdown of the lamina densa. *ECF-A* = eosinophil chemotactic factor-A.

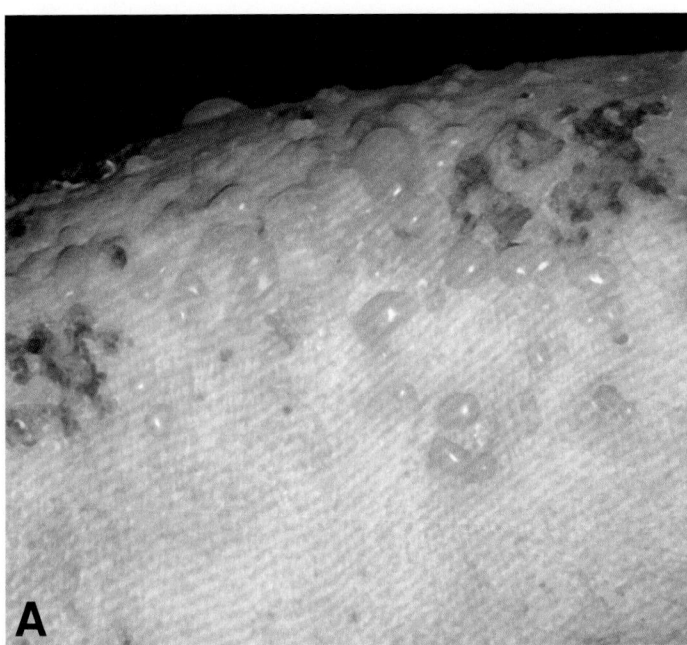
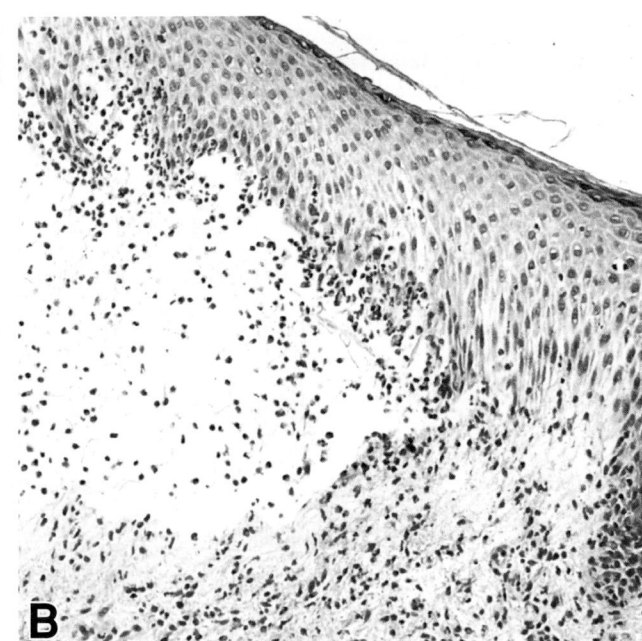

FIGURE 28-22. Bullous pemphigoid. A. The skin shows multiple tense bullae on an erythematous base and erosions, distributed primarily on the medial thighs and trunk. **B.** A subepidermal blister has an edematous papillary dermis as its base. The roof of the blister consists of the intact, entire epidermis, including the stratum basalis. Inflammatory cells, fibrin and fluid fill the blister.

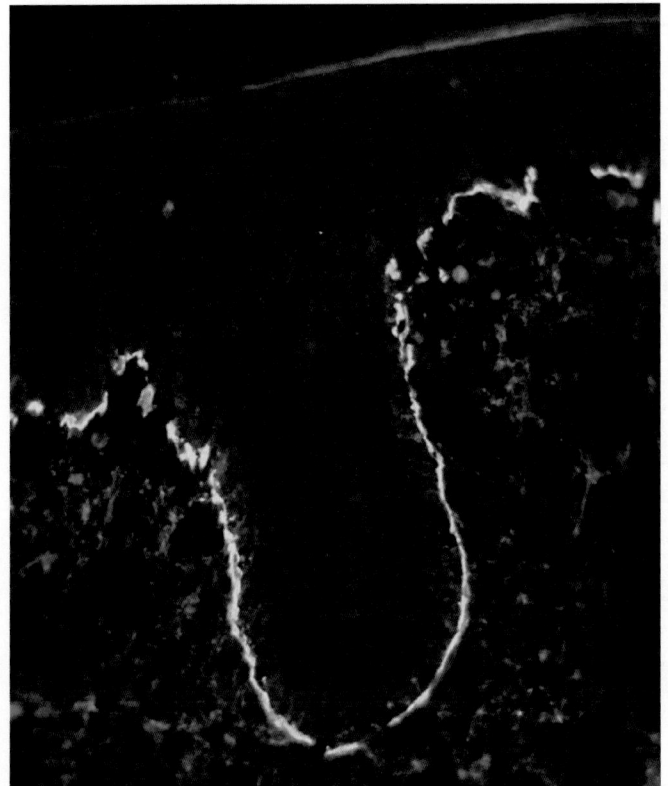

FIGURE 28-23. Bullous pemphigoid. Direct immunofluorescence study discloses linear deposition of immunoglobulin G (IgG) (and C3) along the dermal–epidermal junction. Ultrastructurally, these antibodies and complement are present in the lamina lucida.

at the tips of dermal papillae (Fig. 28-24). Such IgA immune complexes are more prominent in perilesional skin than in normal-appearing skin. Gluten-free diets control the disease; reintroduction of gluten provokes new lesions.

Genetically predisposed patients may develop IgA antibodies to components of gluten in the intestines. Resulting IgA complexes then gain access to the circulation and deposit in the dermal papillae (Fig. 28-24). Patients with DH have increased levels of IgA autoantibodies to tissue transglutaminase, suggesting that there is a dermal autoantigen related to tissue transglutaminase. Antibodies to smooth muscle endomysium are also increased in many patients with DH.

IgA immune complexes do not activate complement efficiently (alternate pathway), and few neutrophils are attracted to the site. However, those neutrophils that do accumulate elaborate leukotrienes, which attract more neutrophils. The neutrophils release lysosomal enzymes that degrade laminin and type IV collagen, cleaving the epidermis from the dermis and eventually causing blisters (Fig. 28-24).

CLINICAL FEATURES: The lesions of DH are especially prominent over the elbows, knees and buttocks (Fig. 28-25A). These intensely pruritic vesicles may become grouped similarly to those of herpes simplex infections (hence, "herpetiformis") and are almost invariably rubbed until broken. Thus, patients may present with only crusted lesions and no intact vesicles. DH is of varying severity and characterized by remissions, but it is disturbingly chronic. Healing lesions often leave scars. Besides a gluten-free diet, dapsone or sulfapyridine may control the signs and symptoms of DH by an unknown mechanism. An increased risk of lymphoproliferative disorders and systemic lupus erythematosus has been reported.

TABLE 28-1

PATHOGENESIS OF IMMUNOBULLOUS AND ACANTHOLYTIC DISORDERS

Condition	Pathogenetic Mechanism	Gene Target	Result
Bullous pemphigoid	Autoantibody against basal cell hemidesmosome	BPAG1, BPAG2	Subepidermal blister
Pemphigus vulgaris	Autoantibody against desmosomal proteins	Desmoglein 1, 3	Intraepidermal blister
Pemphigus foliaceous	Autoantibody against desmosomal proteins	Desmoglein 1	Intraepidermal blister
Epidermolysis bullosa (EB) simplex	Molecular defect in cytokeratin intermediate filaments	KRT5 KRT14	Intraepidermal blister
Junctional EB	Molecular defect in laminin, integrins, collagen	LAMA3, LAMB3, LAMC2, ITGB4, COL17A1	Blister within lamina densa
Dermolytic EB	Molecular defect in anchoring fibrils	COL7A1	Blister below lamina densa
Kindler syndrome	Molecular defect in basal keratinocyte adhesion	KIND1	Blistering, photosensitivity
Darier disease	Molecular defect in keratinocyte adhesion	ATP2A2	Acantholysis, dyskeratosis
Hailey-Hailey disease	Molecular defect in keratinocyte adhesion	ATP2C1	Acantholysis, dyskeratosis

PATHOLOGY: A delicate perivenular lymphocytic infiltrate appears first, together with a row of neutrophils just deep to the lamina densa in the dermal papillae. During the next 12 hours, neutrophils aggregate in clusters of 10–25 at the tips of the dermal papillae to create a diagnostic histologic appearance.

There are two related mechanisms of dermal–epidermal separation. One is associated with the sheet-like spread of a layer or two of neutrophils at the dermal–epidermal interface. In this case, the whole epidermis detaches from the papillary dermis (Fig. 28-25B). The vesicle roof contains the epidermis; the floor is composed of the lamina densa and

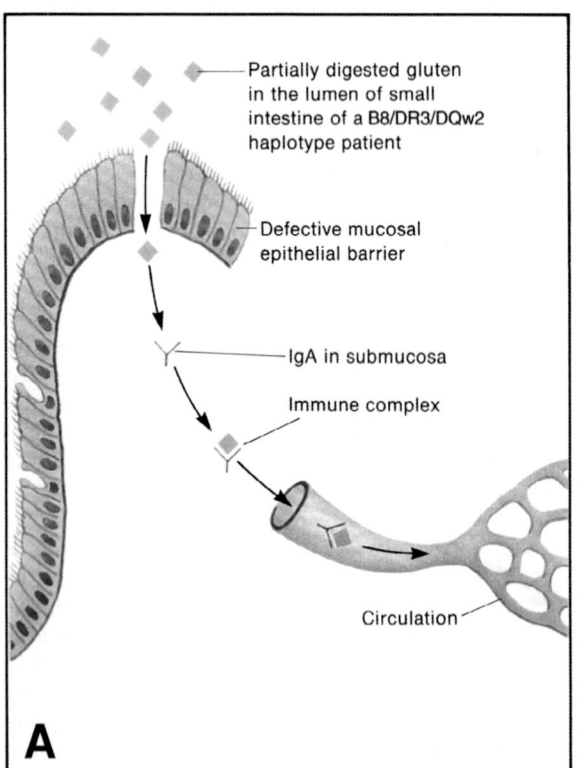

1. Formation of immune complexes in submucosa of small intestine. Passage of immune complexes into **the circulation.**

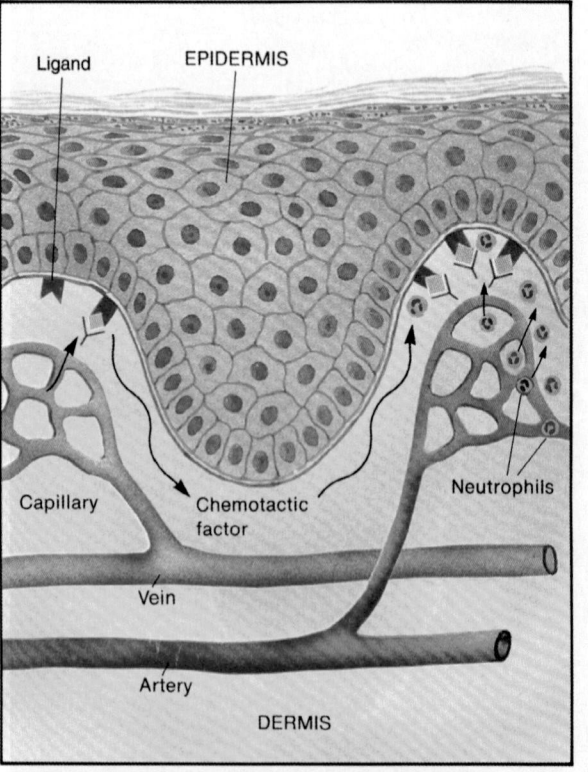

2. Ligand–immune complex union releases neutrophil chemotactic factor. Neutrophils migrate to the tips of the papillae.

FIGURE 28-24. Dermatitis herpetiformis. Proposed pathogenesis for cutaneous lesions. The disease is initiated in the small intestine and is likely expressed in the skin because of the presence of a ligand immediately deep to the lamina densa. *IgA* = immunoglobulin A.

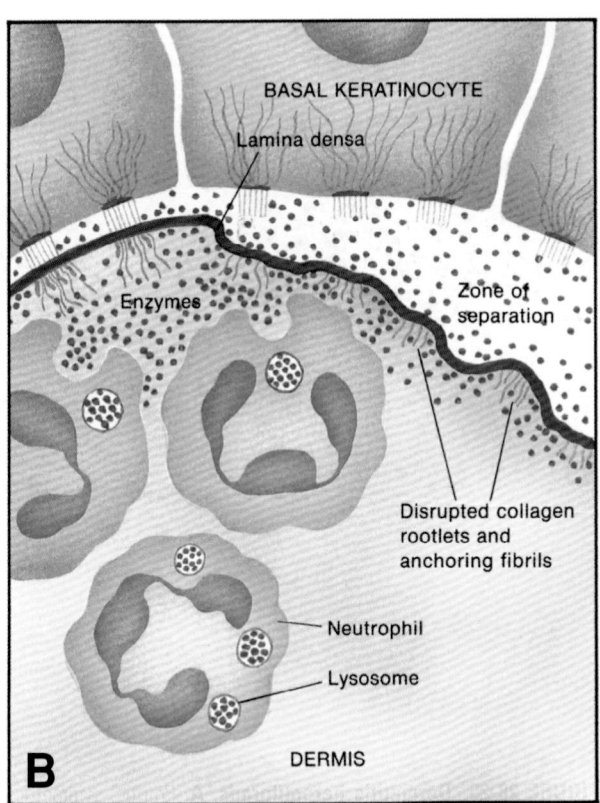

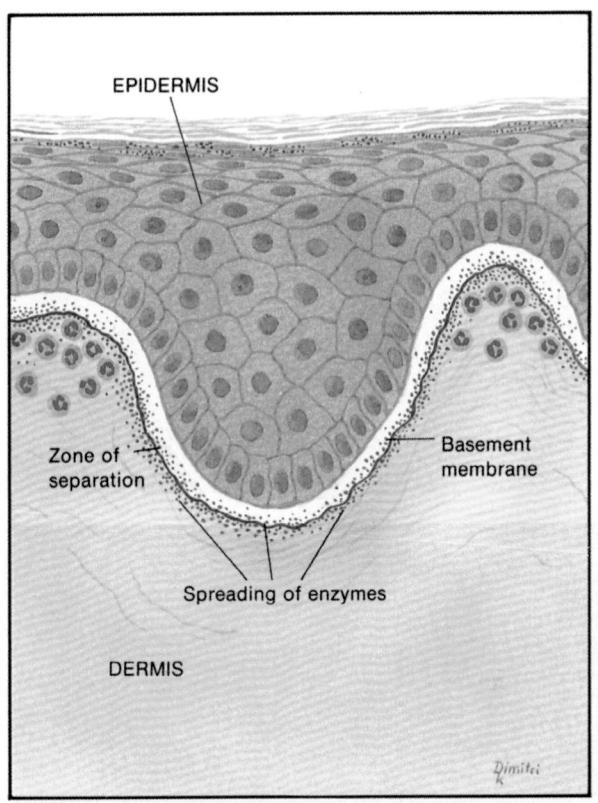

3. Dissolution of basal rootlets and anchoring fibrils by enzymes released by neutrophils. Early dermo-epidermal separation.

4. Concentration of neutrophils at the tips of the papillae. Spreading of enzymes along basement membrane. Lifting away of lamina densa.

FIGURE 28-24. (*Continued*)

the papillary dermis. Unlike BP, eosinophils are uncommon early in the course of DH. In the second route of vesicle formation, many neutrophils accumulate rapidly in the tips of the dermal papillae. Release of their lysosomal enzymes into the superficial portion of the dermal papillae uncouples the epidermis from the dermis at the tips of dermal papillae, disrupts the BMZ in the lamina lucida and superficial part of the papillae and tears the epidermis across the adjacent rete ridges. Roofs of resulting vesicles have alternating tears across their epidermal covering, and their floors show residual epidermal pegs alternating with the basal half of dermal papillae. In both cases, granular IgA is deposited at the dermoepidermal junction (Fig. 28-25C).

Erythema Multiforme Is Often a Reaction to a Drug or Infection

Erythema multiforme (EM) is an acute, self-limited disorder that varies from a few annular or ring-like and targetoid erythematous macules and blisters (EM minor) to a life-threatening, widespread ulceration of the skin and mucous membranes (EM major; Stevens-Johnson syndrome). *It is usually a reaction to a drug or an infectious agent, in particular, herpes simplex virus infection.*

ETIOLOGIC FACTORS: A long list of agents may provoke EM, including herpesvirus, *Mycoplasma* and sulfonamides, but precipitating factors are identified in only half of cases. In postherpetic EM, viral antigens, IgM and C3 deposit perivascularly, and at the

epidermal BMZ. The combination of infiltrating lymphocytes and antigen–antibody complexes within the lesions suggests that humoral and cellular hypersensitivity are both involved.

PATHOLOGY: The dermis in EM shows a sparse lymphocyte infiltrate about the superficial vascular bed and at the dermal–epidermal interface. The characteristic morphologic feature in the epidermis is apoptotic ("dyskeratotic") keratinocytes, with pyknotic nuclei and eosinophilic cytoplasm. Apoptosis may be extensive and associated with a subepidermal vesicle, whose roof is an almost completely necrotic epidermis. Because of the acute onset of the disease, in most cases there is little or no change in the stratum corneum. The dermis shows perivascular lymphocytic infiltrate, without eosinophils.

CLINICAL FEATURES: The characteristic "target" or "iris" lesions of EM have a central, dark red zone, occasionally with a blister, surrounded by a paler area (Fig. 28-26). In turn, the latter is encompassed by a peripheral red rim. Urticarial plaques are common. The presence of vesicles and bullae usually predicts a more severe course. EM is a common condition, with a peak incidence in the second and third decades of life. It is occasionally encountered in association with other presumably immunologic cutaneous disorders, including erythema nodosum, toxic epidermal necrolysis and necrotizing vasculitis. **Stevens-Johnson syndrome** and **toxic epidermal necrolysis** (TEN) refer to unusually severe forms of EM that involve mucosal surfaces and internal organs and are frequently fatal.

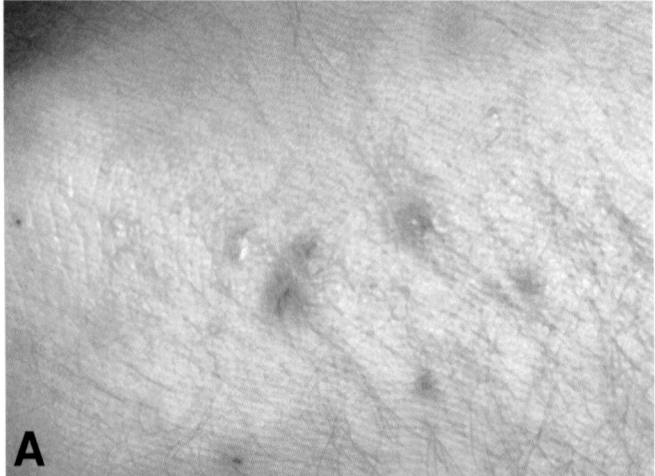

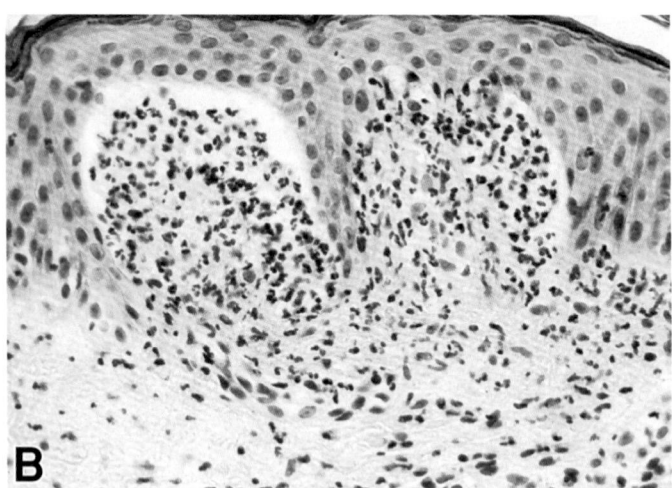

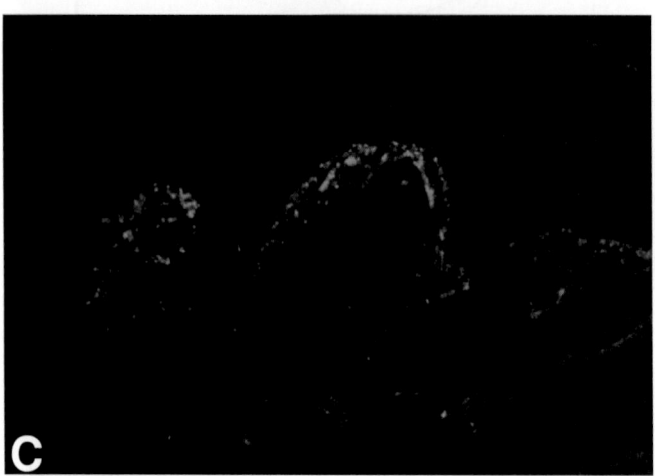

FIGURE 28-25. Dermatitis herpetiformis. A. Pruritic, symmetric, grouped vesicles on an erythematous base are seen on the elbows and knees. **B.** Dermal papillary abscesses of neutrophils with vesicle formation at the dermal–epidermal junction are characteristic. **C.** Direct immunofluorescence reveals immunoglobulin A (IgA) deposited in dermal papillae in association with (but not necessarily directly upon) anchoring fibrils and elastic tissue fibers. This is the site of neutrophil infiltration and subepidermal vesicle formation.

Systemic Lupus Erythematosus Is Characterized by Autoantibodies and Immune Complexes That Deposit in the Skin

Cutaneous involvement in systemic lupus erythematosus (SLE; see Chapter 11) may be severe and cosmetically devastating but is not life-threatening. However, the nature and pattern of immune reactants in the skin are an excellent guide to the likelihood of systemic disease.

PATHOPHYSIOLOGY: Immune complexes are present in both lesional and normal-appearing skin in SLE. Deposition of immune reactants along the epidermal BMZ of normal-appearing skin is important in making the diagnosis. Epidermal injury seems to be initiated by exogenous agents such as UV light and perpetuated by cell-mediated immune reactions, similar to those in graft-versus-host disease. The manifestations of epidermal injury include vacuolization of basal keratinocytes, hyperkeratosis and diminished epidermal thickness, release of DNA and other nuclear and cytoplasmic antigens to the circulation and deposition of DNA and other antigens in the epidermal BMZ (lamina densa and immediately subjacent dermis) (Fig. 28-27). Thus, epidermal injury, local immune complex formation, deposition of circulating immune complexes and lymphocyte-induced cellular injury all seem to act in concert.

The various forms of cutaneous lupus are classified according to their chronicity, but considerable overlap in features is possible. There is an inverse relationship between the prominence of skin lesions and the extent of systemic disease.

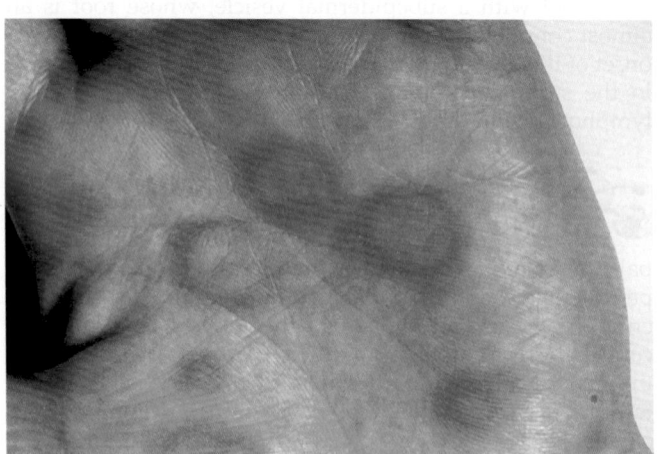

FIGURE 28-26. Erythema multiforme. Steroid-responsive "target" papules, characterized by central bullae with surrounding erythema, appeared after antibiotic therapy.

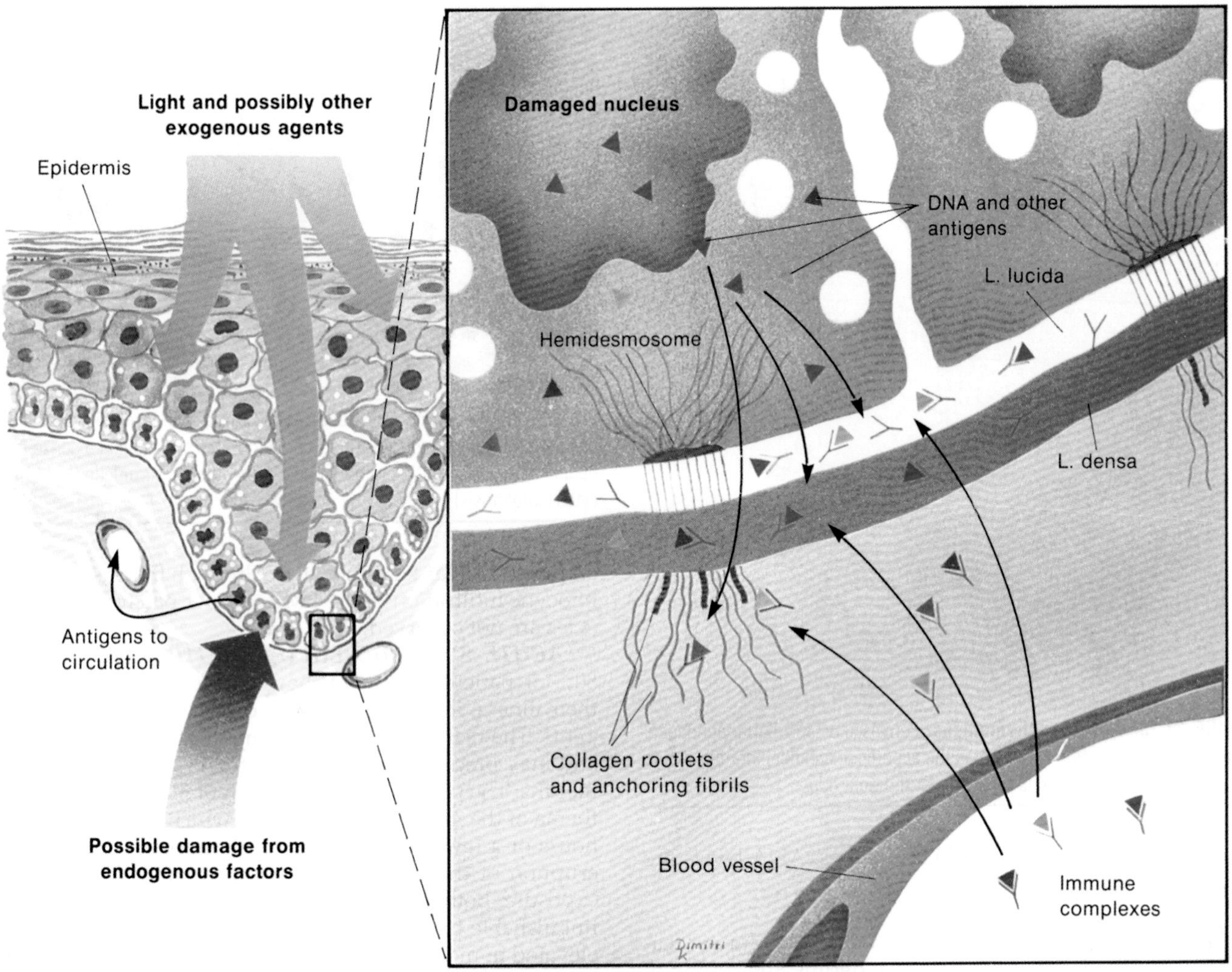

FIGURE 28-27. Lupus erythematosus. A cell-mediated immune reaction leads to epidermal cellular damage when initiated by light or other exogenous agents as well as endogenous ones. Such injury releases a large number of antigens, some of which may return to the skin in the form of immune complexes. Immune complexes are also formed in the skin by a reaction of local DNA with antibody that may also be deposited beneath the epidermal basement membrane zone. *L* = lamina.

CHRONIC CUTANEOUS (DISCOID) LUPUS ERYTHE-MATOSUS: This form of lupus is usually limited to the skin. It generally affects skin above the neck, on the face (especially the malar area), scalp and ears. Lesions begin as slightly elevated violaceous papules with a rough scale of keratin. They enlarge to assume a disc shape, with a hyperkeratotic margin and a depigmented center. The cutaneous lesions may culminate in disfiguring scars. Elevated circulating antinuclear antibody (ANA) levels are seen in under 10% of patients.

PATHOLOGY: In discoid lupus, nucleated epidermal layers are modestly thickened or somewhat thin. Hyperkeratosis, without prominent parakeratosis, and plugging of hair follicles are prominent. The rete–papillae pattern of the dermal–epidermal interface is partially effaced. Basal keratinocytes are vacuolated, and eosinophilic apoptotic bodies are noted. The lamina densa is greatly thickened and reduplicated. On periodic acid–Schiff (PAS) staining, multiple layers of lamina densa extend into the subjacent dermis. The excessive quantity of lamina densa, a product of the basal keratinocytes, reflects a response of basal cells to damage. These changes all suggest that injury to basal kerati-

nocytes is an essential pathogenetic characteristic of skin disease associated with lupus (Figs. 28-28, 28-29 and 28-30).

The basal keratinocytes and BMZ contain a diffuse lymphocytic infiltrate that penetrates the basal layer focally. Deeper in the dermis, dense patches of helper and cytotoxic/suppressor T lymphocytes, often with plasma cells, are commonly found around skin appendages. Immune complexes are mainly deep to the lamina densa but also occur as granular deposits on the lamina densa and within the lamina lucida. This pattern contrasts with that of BP in which there are only two antigens, both in the lamina lucida and characterized by a linear staining pattern.

SUBACUTE CUTANEOUS LUPUS ERYTHEMATOSUS: This disorder primarily afflicts young and middle-aged white women. Unlike discoid lupus, subacute cutaneous lupus may also involve the musculoskeletal system and kidneys. Initially, scaly erythematous papules develop and then enlarge into psoriasiform or annular lesions, which may fuse. Skin changes occur in the upper chest, upper back and extensor surfaces of the arms, suggesting that light exposure plays a role in the pathogenesis of the disorder. Significant scarring does not occur. About 70% of patients

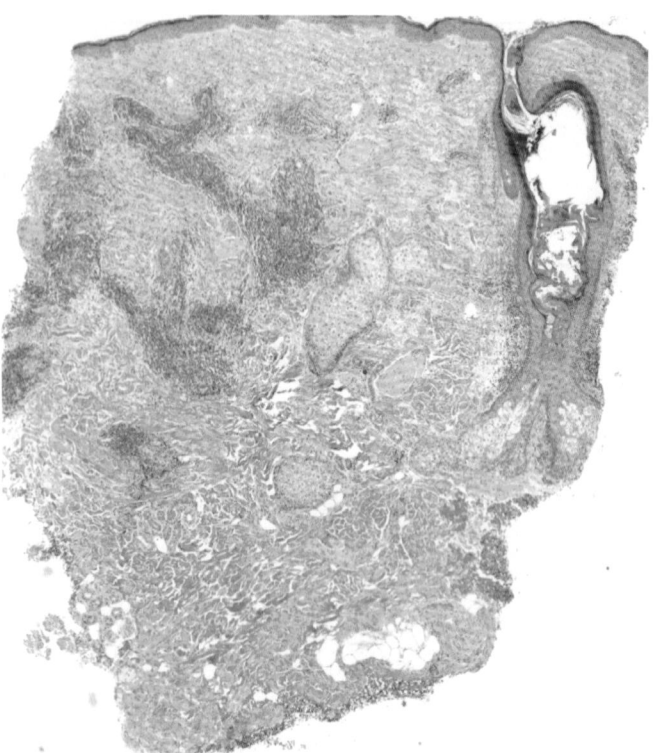

FIGURE 28-28. Lupus erythematosus. Perivascular and periappendageal lymphocytic inflammation is present in the superficial and deep dermis. A hair follicle plugged with keratin is present near the right edge.

have circulating anti-Ro (SS-A) antibodies. ANA levels are elevated in 70%.

PATHOLOGY: Subacute cutaneous lupus features edema of the papillary dermis, thickening of the lamina densa and prominent vacuolar degen-

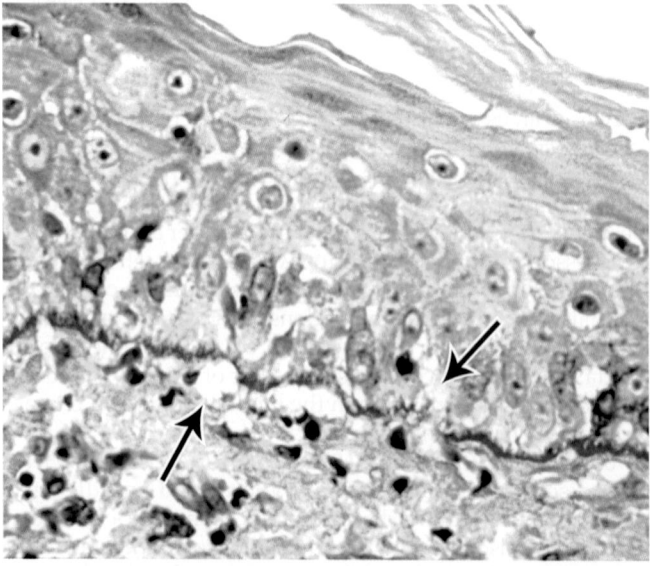

FIGURE 28-29. Lupus erythematosus. Basal cell necrosis with resultant basal keratinocytic migration and synthesis of new basement membrane zone leads to thickening of the epidermal basement membrane zone (BMZ), as evident in this periodic acid–Schiff (PAS) stain. Notice the vacuoles (*arrows*) on either side of the BMZ, an indicator of cellular injury.

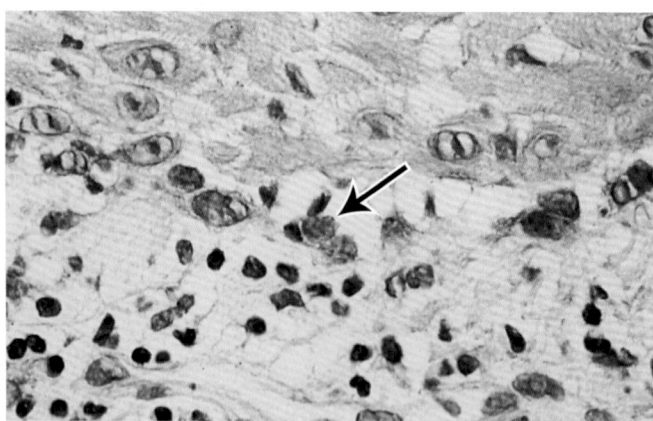

FIGURE 28-30. Lupus erythematosus. An active lesion shows striking basal vacuolization, with keratinocyte necrosis (*arrow*) forming a dense eosinophilic body (apoptotic/fibrillary/colloid body) that is surrounded by lymphocytes (satellitosis).

eration of basilar keratinocytes. Although there is some lymphocytic infiltration of the BMZ, deeper patches of lymphocytes are not observed.

ACUTE SYSTEMIC LUPUS ERYTHEMATOSUS: Over 80% of patients with SLE have acute skin disease during their illness, in association with disease of the kidneys and joints. The rash is often the first manifestation of the disease and may precede the onset of systemic symptoms by a few months. The typical "butterfly" rash of SLE is a delicate erythema of the malar area of the face, which may pass in a few hours or a few days. Many patients have a maculopapular eruption of the chest and extremities, often following sun exposure. Both rashes heal without scarring. Lesions indistinguishable from discoid lupus may occur. ANA levels are elevated in more than 90% of patients.

PATHOLOGY: The earliest malar blush of acute cutaneous lupus may show only edema of the papillary dermis. More often, changes are like those in the subacute form of lupus. The histopathologic picture of lupus can be indistinguishable from other connective tissue diseases such as dermatomyositis. In **bullous SLE,** blisters may occur subepidermally and beneath the lamina densa. An autoantibody against type VII collagen in this location, which is a component of anchoring fibrils, is deposited and is associated with an infiltrate of neutrophils at the junction.

Lichen Planus Is a Cell-Mediated Immune Reaction at the Dermal–Epidermal Junction

"Lichenoid" tissue reactions are so named because the clinical lesions resemble certain lichens that form scaly growths on rocks or tree trunks. Lichenoid infiltrates are characterized by a band-like congregation of lymphocytes that obscures the dermal–epidermal junction. Epidermal turnover is decreased, leading to hyperkeratosis without parakeratosis. Lichen planus (LP) is the prototypic disorder of this group, which includes entities such as lichen nitidus and lichenoid drug eruptions.

ETIOLOGIC FACTORS: The etiology of LP is unknown. It is occasionally familial and may also accompany autoimmune disorders, such as SLE

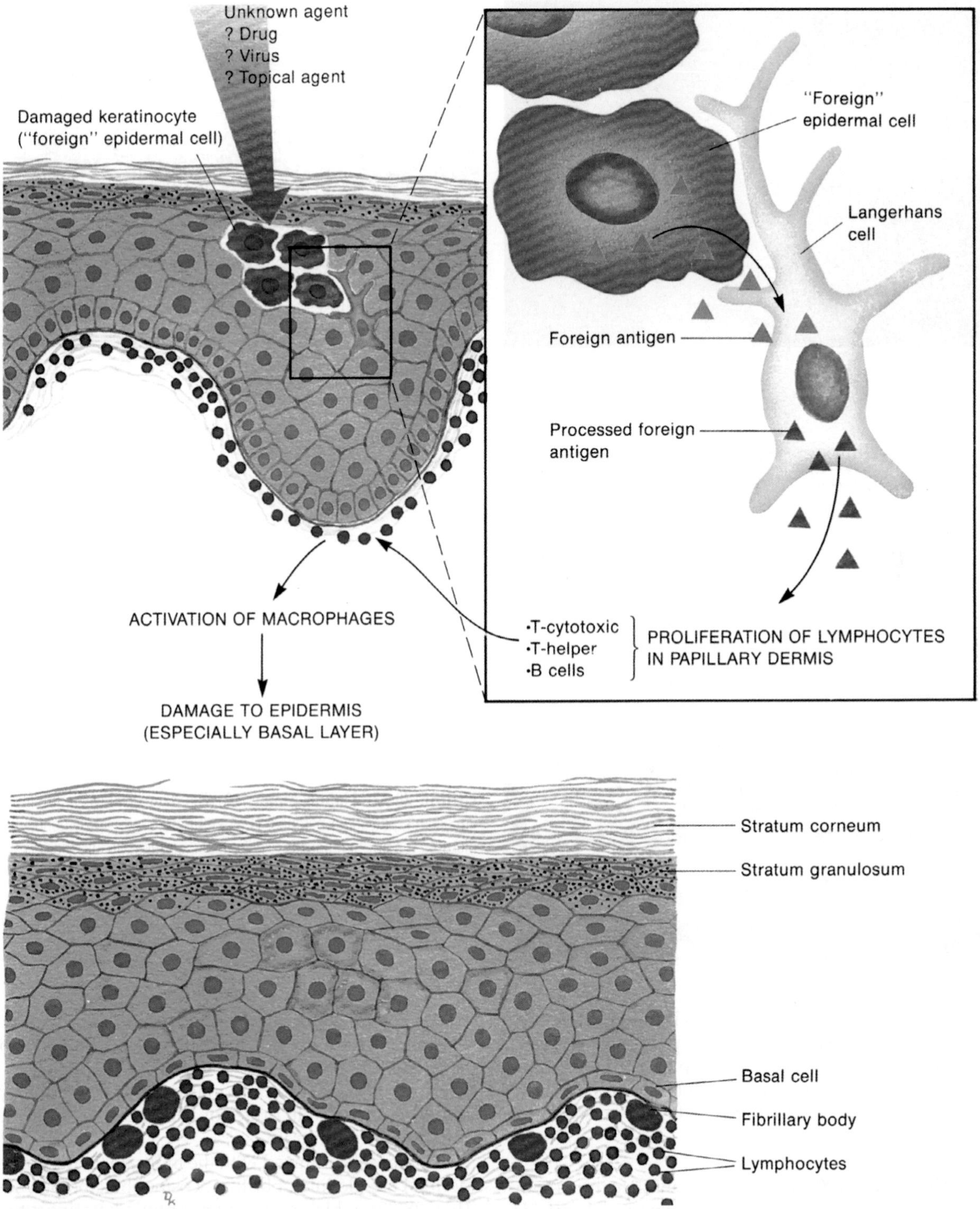

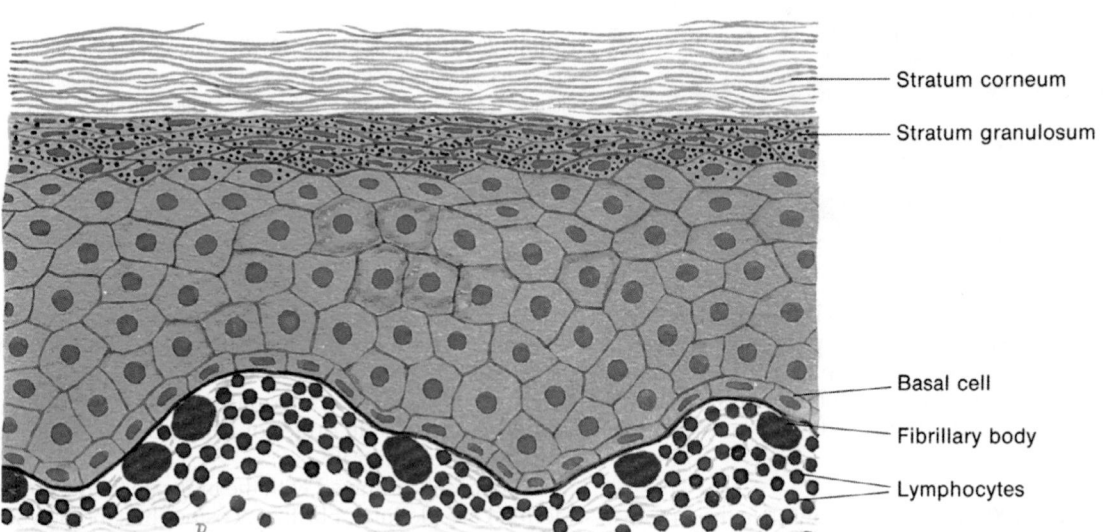

FIGURE 28-31. Lichen planus. Pathogenetic mechanisms are outlined. The disease is apparently initiated by epidermal injury. This injury causes some epidermal cells to be treated as "foreign." The antigens of such cells are processed by Langerhans cells. The processed antigen induces lymphocytic proliferation and macrophage activation. Macrophages, along with T lymphocytes, kill the epidermal basal cells, resulting in a reactive epidermal proliferation and the formation of fibrillary bodies.

and myasthenia gravis. LP is more common in patients with ulcerative colitis. Some drugs—gold, chlorothiazide and chloroquine—may induce lichenoid reactions. External agents such as photographic chemicals may evoke a lichenoid response. LP-like lesions often occur in later stages of chronic graft-versus-host disease. Thus, it seems that immunologic mechanisms play a role in the pathogenesis of LP (Fig. 28-31). The presence of apoptotic bodies and reduced epidermal cell turnover suggest that the lesions of LP result from basal layer cell destruction, creating reduced

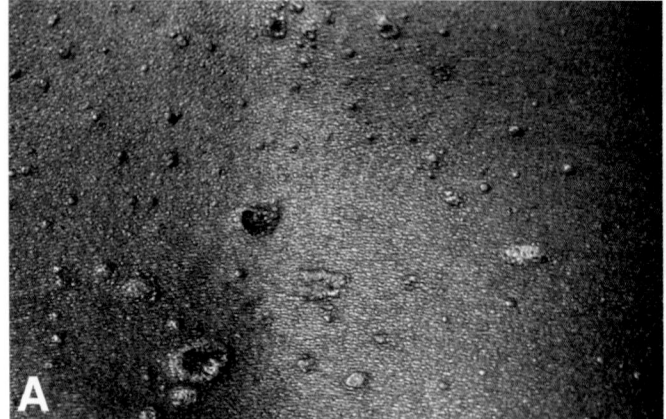

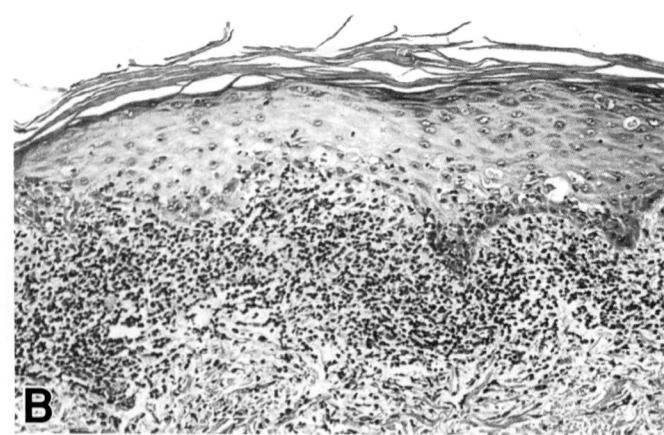

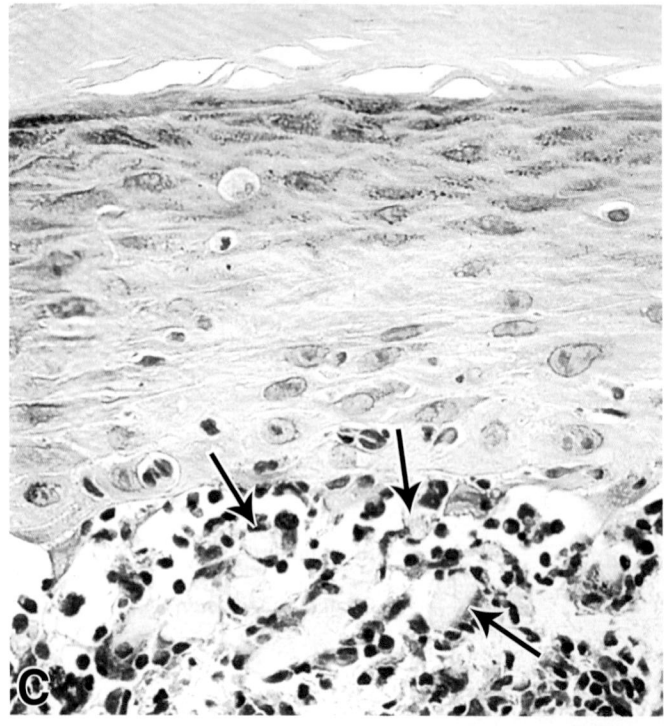

FIGURE 28-32. Lichen planus. A. The skin displays multiple flat-topped violaceous polygonal papules. **B.** A cell-rich, band-like, lymphocytic infiltrate disrupts the stratum basalis. Unlike lupus erythematosus, there is usually epidermal hyperplasia, hyperkeratosis and wedge-like hypergranulosis. **C.** Hypergranulosis and loss of rete ridges are noted. The site of pathologic injury is at the dermal–epidermal junction where there is a striking infiltrate of lymphocytes, many of which surround apoptotic keratinocytes (*arrows*).

and subsequent reactive epidermal proliferation. Evidence suggests that LP is a delayed type of hypersensitivity reaction (see Chapter 4), initiated and amplified by cytokines such as IFN-γ and IL-6, produced both by infiltrating lymphocytes and by stimulated keratinocytes. LP may coexist with hepatitis C infection.

PATHOLOGY: The epidermis in LP features compact hyperkeratosis with little or no parakeratosis, the lack of which correlates with reduced epidermal turnover associated with damage to basal keratinocytes. The stratum granulosum is thickened, frequently in a distinctive, focal, wedge-shaped pattern, with the base of the wedge abutting the stratum corneum. The stratum spinosum is variably thickened.

The distinctive pathology of LP is at the dermal–epidermal interface. The basal row of cuboidal cells is replaced by flattened or polygonal keratinocytes. The undulating interface between the dermal papillae and the rounded profiles of the rete ridges is obscured by a dense infiltrate of helper/inducer lymphocytes and macrophages, many of the latter

containing melanin pigment **(melanophages)** (Fig. 28-32). Plasma cells are absent; their presence in association with basal keratinocyte atypia would suggest a lichenoid actinic keratosis, a form of epidermal dysplasia. Sharply pointed ("saw-toothed") rete ridges of keratinocytes project into the inflammatory infiltrate.

Commonly admixed with the infiltrate (in the epidermis or dermis) are globular, fibrillary, eosinophilic bodies, 15–20 μm (Fig. 28-32), which represent apoptotic keratinocytes. These structures are variably called *apoptotic, colloid, Civatte* or *fibrillary bodies, or dyskeratotic cells*. The fibrils within the apoptotic bodies are keratin filaments. Epidermal Langerhans cells are increased early in LP.

CLINICAL FEATURES: LP is a chronic eruption with violaceous, flat-topped papules, usually on the flexor surfaces of the wrists (Fig. 28-32A). White patches or streaks may also be present on oral mucous membranes (Wickham striae). The pruritic lesions usually resolve in less than a year but may occasionally persist longer.

INFLAMMATORY DISEASES OF THE SUPERFICIAL AND DEEP VASCULAR BED

Urticaria and Angioedema Are IgE-Dependent Hypersensitivity Reactions

These reactions are initiated by degranulation of mast cells sensitized to a specific antigen. **Urticaria** ("hives") are raised, pale, well-demarcated pruritic papules and plaques that appear and disappear within a few hours. The lesions represent edema of the superficial dermis. **Angioedema** is a condition in which the edema involves the deeper dermis or subcutis, resulting in an egg-like swelling. Both entities have a rapid onset and range in severity from simply annoying lesions to life-threatening anaphylactic reactions. The mainstays of treatment are avoiding the offending agent and prompt administration of antihistamines.

Dermatographism is a linear hive with a rich pink flare produced by briskly stroking the skin. It occurs in 4% of the population. It represents an exaggerated IgE-dependent response. One may write on the skin of such individuals and create a hive in the form of a legible word.

 ETIOLOGIC FACTORS: Most cases of urticaria are IgE dependent and reflect exaggerated venule permeability due to mast cell degranulation. An almost endless list of materials may react with IgE antibodies on the surface of the mast cell. Urticaria may occur in both atopic and nonatopic people. Atopic patients have intensely pruritic skin eruptions, a family history of similar eruptions and a personal or family history of allergies. They commonly have elevated circulating IgE.

When mast cells degranulate and release their vasoactive mediators, cutaneous venules respond initially by becoming more permeable. This leads to rapidly forming edema. If the reaction persists, inflammatory cells are attracted to the area, causing an urticarial plaque (lasting more than a day).

Hereditary angioedema is a serious autosomal dominant disorder caused by mutation of the C1-esterase inhibitor.

 PATHOLOGY: In urticaria, collagen fibers and fibrils are splayed apart by excess fluid. Lymphatic vessels are dilated; venules show margination of neutrophils and eosinophils. Vessels are cuffed by a few lymphocytes. In persistent urticaria, lymphocytes and eosinophils are increased, but neutrophils are sparse.

Cutaneous Necrotizing Vasculitis Is an Immune Reaction with Neutrophil Inflammation of Vessel Walls

Cutaneous necrotizing vasculitis (CNV) presents as **"palpable purpura"** and has also been called **allergic cutaneous vasculitis, leukocytoclastic vasculitis** and **hypersensitivity angiitis.**

 ETIOLOGIC FACTORS: In CNV, circulating immune complexes deposit in vessel walls at sites of injuries, at branch points where turbulence is increased or where venous circulation is slowed, as in the lower extremities. Elaborated C5a complement component attracts neutrophils, which degranulate and release lysosomal

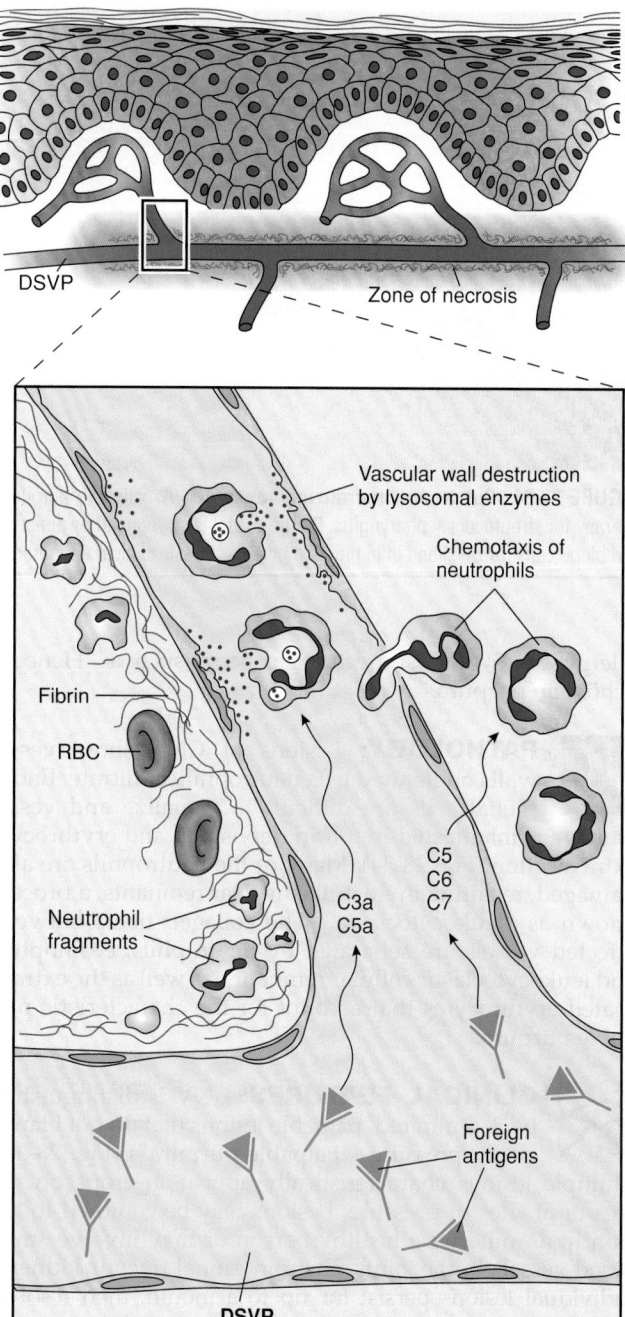

FIGURE 28-33. Cutaneous necrotizing vasculitis. The pathogenesis of vessel damage is depicted. The site of the vascular pathology is indicated in the *upper diagram*. Circulating immune complexes activate complement. There is neutrophilic chemotaxis (*C5a*) and neutrophilic destruction. Vascular damage occurs, with extravasation of erythrocytes, fibrin deposition and leukocytoclasia. *DSVP* = deep superficial venular plexus; *RBC* = red blood cell.

enzymes, causing endothelial damage and fibrin deposition (Fig. 28-33).

CNV may be primary, without a known precipitating event in about half of the cases, or associated with a specific infectious agent (e.g., hepatitis B or C viruses [HBV, HCV]). It may also be a secondary process in a variety of chronic diseases, such as rheumatoid arthritis, SLE and ulcerative colitis. CNV may also be associated with (1) underlying malignancies such as lymphoma, (2) a drug or some other

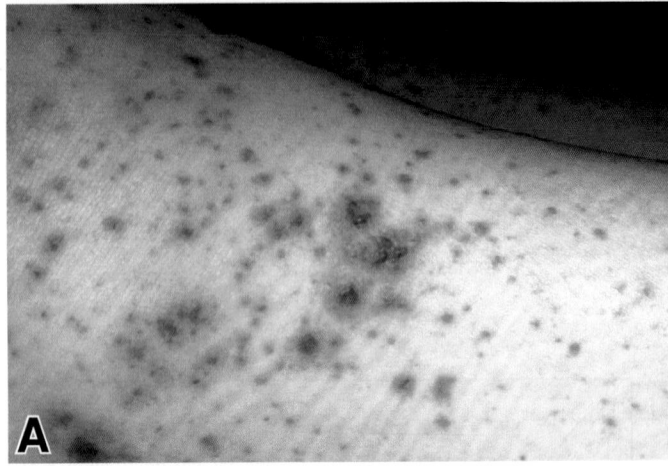
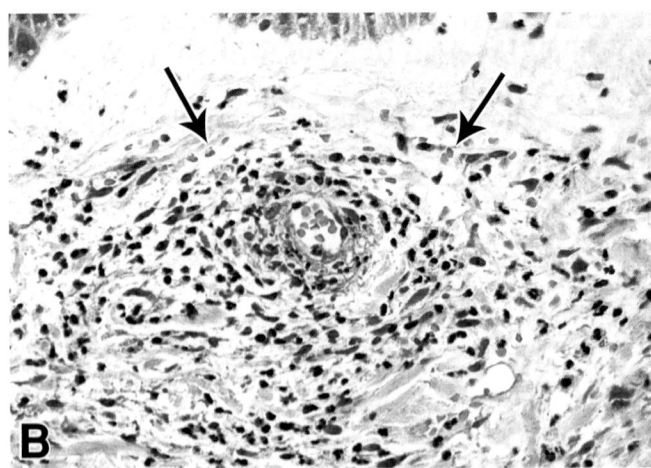

FIGURE 28-34. Cutaneous necrotizing vasculitis. A. Palpable purpuric tender papules on the legs of a 25-year-old woman. The condition resolved after therapy for streptococcal pharyngitis. **B.** The vessel is surrounded by pink fibrin and neutrophils, many of which have disintegrated (leukocytoclasis). Extravasated red blood cells (*arrows*) and inflammation give the classic clinical appearance of "palpable purpura."

allergy or (3) a postinfectious process such as Henoch-Schönlein purpura.

 PATHOLOGY: Lesions of CNV show vessel walls obliterated by a neutrophilic infiltrate. Endothelial cells are difficult to visualize and vessel damage is manifested by fibrin deposition and erythrocyte extravasation (Fig. 28-34). Many of the neutrophils are also damaged, resulting in dust-like nuclear remnants, a process known as "leukocytoclasia." The collagen fibers between affected vessels are separated by neutrophils, eosinophils and leukocytoclastic cellular remnants, as well as the extravasated erythrocytes that account for the characteristic palpable purpura.

 CLINICAL FEATURES: CNV is distinguished by 2–4-mm red, palpable lesions that do not blanch under pressure ("palpable purpura") (Fig. 28-34). Multiple lesions characteristically appear in crops on the legs or at sites of pressure. Lesions may be confined to the skin in an otherwise healthy person or may involve small blood vessels in the joints, gastrointestinal tract or kidneys. Individual lesions persist for up to a month, then resolve, leaving hyperpigmentation or atrophic scars. Despite removal of the offending agent, episodes of CNV may recur.

Allergic Contact Dermatitis Is Cell-Mediated Hypersensitivity to Exogenous Sensitizing Agents

Members of the *Rhus* genus of plants are common sensitizing agents, so that 90% of the population of the United States is sensitive to the common offenders: *Rhus radicans* (poison ivy), *Rhus diversiloba* (poison oak) and *Rhus vernix* (poison sumac). These plant dermatitides are so well known that the resultant disease is commonly labeled according to the offending plant. Patients state, "I have poison ivy" and go to physicians for relief rather than for diagnosis.

 **ETIOLOGIC FACTORS:** The offending plant contains low–molecular-weight **haptens** (see Chapter 4), in particular, oleoresins. They are active in

sensitization only when they combine with a carrier protein. This likely happens at the cell membrane of the Langerhans cell in the **sensitization phase,** a process that has been studied as a prototype of antigenic sensitization in delayed-type hypersensitivity (DTH). Formation of a **hapten–carrier complex** requires about 1 hour, after which it is processed as an antigen by Langerhans cells. These cells carry the antigen through the lymphatics to regional lymph nodes and present it to CD4$^+$ T cells (Fig. 28-35). After 5–7 days, some of these T lymphocytes recognize the antigen, become activated, multiply and circulate in the blood as memory cells. Some migrate to the skin, ready to react with the antigen if they encounter it. IL-1, made by Langerhans cells, supports proliferation of CD4$^+$ T$_H$1 cells, the effectors of DTH.

In the **elicitation phase,** specifically sensitized T lymphocytes in the circulation enter the skin. At the site of antigen challenge, Langerhans cells, endothelial cells, perivascular dendritic cells and monocytes process the antigen and present it to the specifically sensitized T cells, which then migrate into the epidermis. Cytokine production causes accumulation of more T cells and macrophages, which are responsible for epidermal cell injury.

 **PATHOLOGY:** Allergic contact dermatitis is a type of **spongiotic dermatitis**. In the 24 hours after reexposure to the offending plant (elicitation phase), lymphocytes and macrophages congregate about superficial venules and extend into the epidermis. Epidermal keratinocytes are partially separated by the edema fluid, creating a sponge-like appearance **(spongiosis)** (Fig. 28-36). The stratum corneum contains coagulated eosinophilic fluid and plasma proteins. Later, many mononuclear inflammatory cells and eosinophils accumulate. Vesicles containing lymphocytes and macrophages are present, and abundant eosinophilic coagulated fluid accrues in the stratum corneum.

 CLINICAL FEATURES: At first contact with poison ivy, for example, there is no immediate reaction. Five to 7 days after a reexposure, the site of contact becomes intensely pruritic. Then, erythema and small vesicles rapidly develop (Fig. 28-36). Over the next few

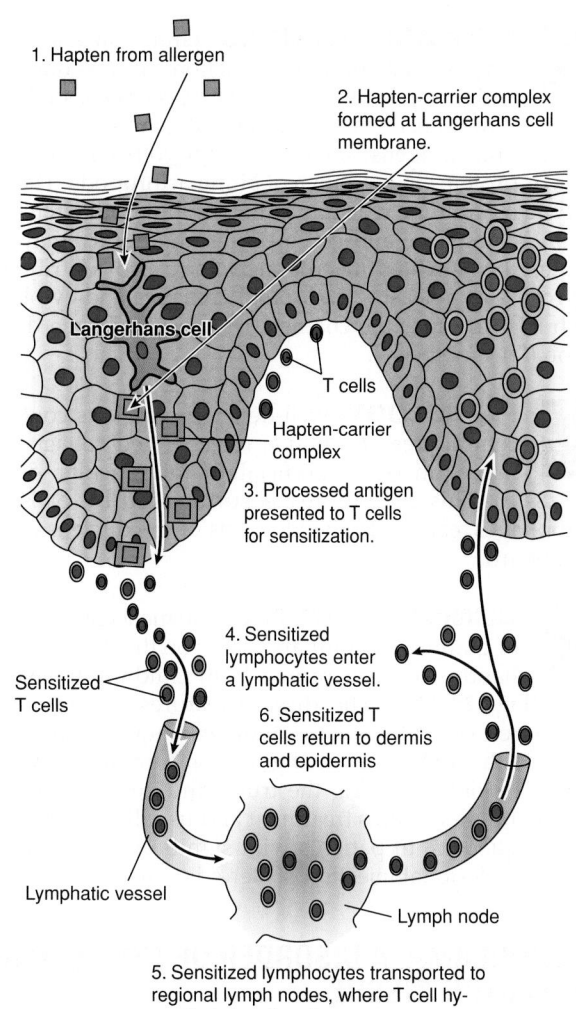

1. Hapten from allergen

2. Hapten-carrier complex formed at Langerhans cell membrane.

Langerhans cell

T cells

Hapten-carrier complex

3. Processed antigen presented to T cells for sensitization.

4. Sensitized lymphocytes enter a lymphatic vessel.

Sensitized T cells

6. Sensitized T cells return to dermis and epidermis

Lymphatic vessel

Lymph node

5. Sensitized lymphocytes transported to regional lymph nodes, where T cell hyperplasia is induced

FIGURE 28-35. Allergic contact dermatitis. Pathogenetic mechanisms are shown.

days, the area enlarges, becomes fiery red, develops vesicles and exudes a large amount of clear proteinaceous fluid. Pruritus is intense. The entire process lasts about 3 weeks. Exudation gradually subsides and the area is covered by an irregular crust that eventually falls off. Pruritus diminishes and healing occurs without scarring.

When a sensitized patient again comes into contact with poison ivy, the process is faster. Lesions appear within 1–2 days, spread rapidly and produce the same clinical appearance. However, the reaction is usually more intense. Lesions again clear in about 3 weeks. Allergic contact dermatitis responds to topical or systemic corticosteroids.

Granulomatous Dermatitis Is a Response to Indigestible Antigens

Granulomas, generally defined as localized collections of epithelioid macrophages (see Chapter 1), form in response to insoluble or slowly released antigens that produce either a focal nonallergic response or an allergic response in sensitized people. Implicated antigens include foreign substances implanted accidentally into the skin (e.g., silicone in breast implants) or endogenous antigens such as keratin. Other common causes include mycobacterial and other infections and granuloma annulare. Often, for example, in sarcoidosis and granuloma annulare, an inciting antigen may not be known. Phagocytosis of the foreign particulate matter, or processing of protein antigens, is central to activation of tissue macrophages, as they become the characteristic granulomatous epithelioid cells.

Sarcoidosis Is a Systemic Disease That May Lead to Skin Lesions

Sarcoidosis is a granulomatous disorder of unknown etiology that mainly affects the lungs but may also involve the skin, lymph nodes, spleen, eyes and other organs. Sarcoidal granulomas are the classic epithelioid cell type, without

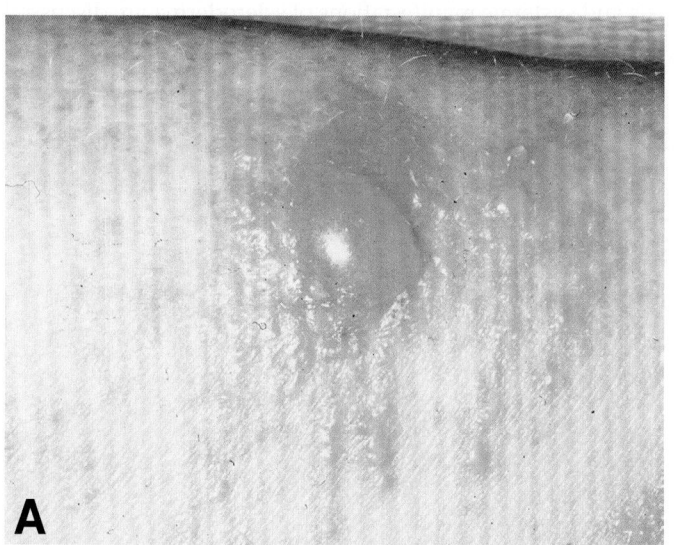

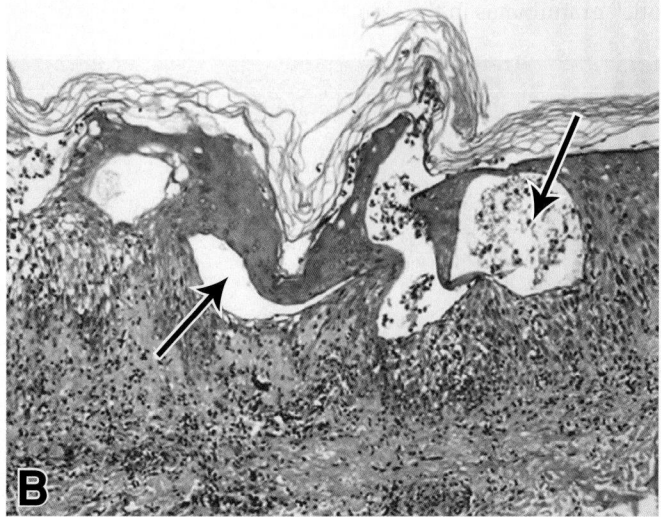

FIGURE 28-36. Allergic contact dermatitis. A. Vesicles and bullae developed on the volar forearm after application of perfume. **B.** Epidermal spongiosis and spongiotic vesicles (*arrows*) are present in this biopsy of "poison ivy." Infiltrating lymphocytes are apparent in the epidermis, where they effect the cell-mediated delayed hypersensitivity reaction.

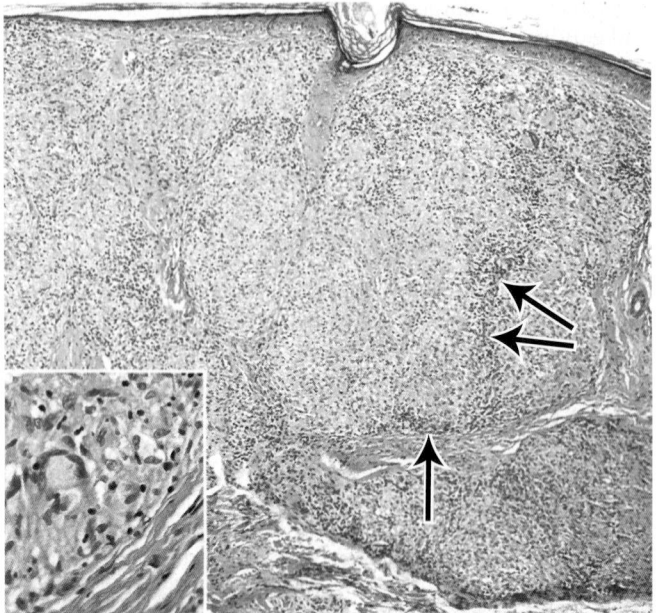

FIGURE 28-37. Sarcoidosis. Numerous large granulomas fill the reticular dermis. Around some of the granulomas are small cuffs of lymphocytes (*arrows*). The granulomas are composed of epithelioid macrophages, some of which are multinucleated (*inset*).

necrosis (Fig. 28-37). Cutaneous manifestations of sarcoidosis are asymptomatic papules, plaques and nodules in the dermis and subcutis. Some dermal plaques may be annular, and those that involve the subcutis appear as irregular nodules. In severe cases, cutaneous lesions may be so prominent that they simulate a diffusely infiltrative neoplasm.

Granuloma Annulare Is a Reaction to an Unknown Antigen

Granuloma annulare is a benign, self-limited disorder of unknown etiology, characterized by palisading "necrobiotic" granulomas in the skin.

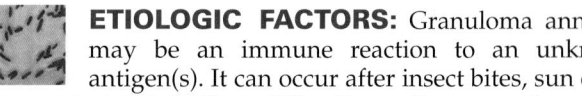 **ETIOLOGIC FACTORS:** Granuloma annulare may be an immune reaction to an unknown antigen(s). It can occur after insect bites, sun exposure and viral infections. Offending antigens are thought to include viral antigens, altered dermal collagen or elastic fibers, or proteins in the saliva of biting arthropods. The precise type of immune reaction is unclear, but both circulating immune complexes and cell-mediated immunity may participate. The activated macrophages may also contribute to the process by releasing lysosomal enzymes and cytokines, which in turn cause the characteristic focal collagen degeneration ("necrobiosis").

 PATHOLOGY: Well-developed lesions contain a central area of acellular degenerated collagen and mucin in the superficial to midreticular dermis (Fig. 28-38). This central area is surrounded by palisaded macrophages, each with the long axis of the nucleus radiating outward.

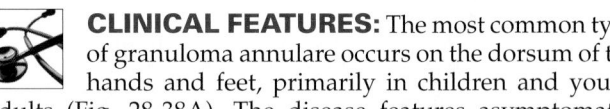 **CLINICAL FEATURES:** The most common type of granuloma annulare occurs on the dorsum of the hands and feet, primarily in children and young adults (Fig. 28-38A). The disease features asymptomatic, skin-colored or erythematous annular plaques. About 15% of patients have disseminated granuloma annulare, with 10 or more lesions involving the trunk and neck. Granuloma annulare rarely requires treatment and usually has no medical consequences. In patients with significant cosmetic disfigurement, lesional injection of steroids is usually effective.

SCLERODERMA: A DISORDER OF THE DERMAL CONNECTIVE TISSUE

Scleroderma (Greek, *skleros,* "hard") also displays variable structural and functional involvement of internal organs, including the kidneys, lungs, heart, esophagus and small intestine. **Morphea** is similar to scleroderma but involves only patchy, circumscribed areas of the skin. The pathogenesis and systemic manifestations of scleroderma are discussed elsewhere (see Chapters 4 and 12).

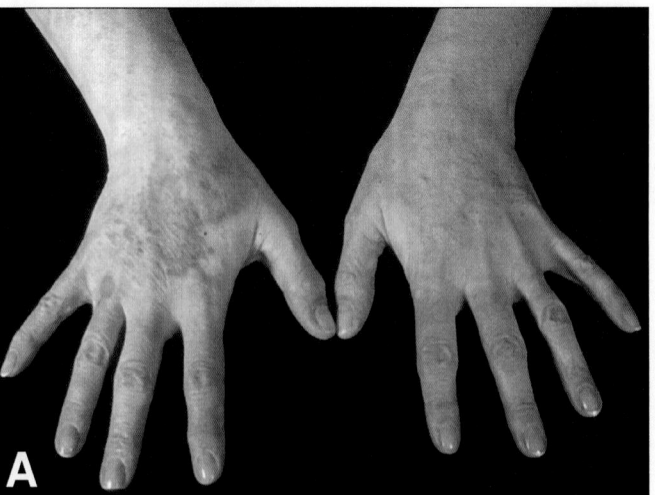

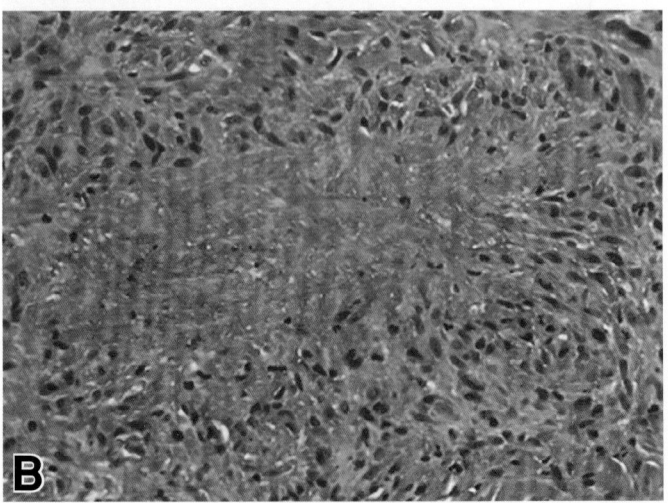

FIGURE 28-38. Granuloma annulare. A. The skin exhibits a typical annular plaque on the dorsal right hand. **B.** A central area of acellular degenerated collagen is surrounded by palisaded macrophages with the long axes of their nuclei radiating outward.

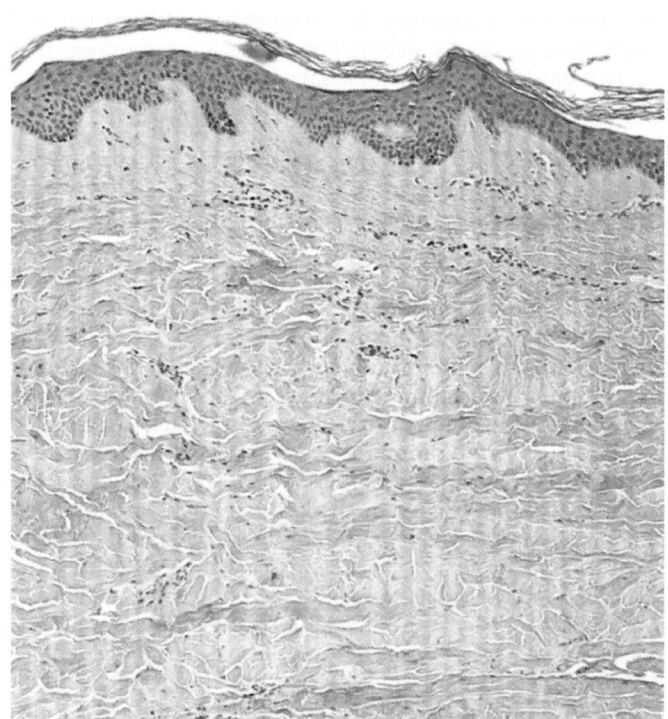

FIGURE 28-39. Scleroderma. The dermis is characterized by large, reticular collagen bundles that are oriented parallel to the epidermis. The large size and loss of basket-weave pattern of these collagen bundles are abnormal. No appendages are apparent because these structures have been destroyed.

 PATHOLOGY: The initial cutaneous lesions of scleroderma are in the lower reticular dermis, but eventually the entire reticular dermis and even the papillary dermis are involved. There is diminished space among collagen bundles in the reticular dermis and a tendency for the collagen bundles to be enlarged, hypocellular and parallel to each other. A patchy lymphocytic infiltrate containing a few plasma cells is common and may also be present in the underlying subcutaneous tissue. Sweat ducts are entrapped in the thickened fibrous tissue, and the fat that is usually around them is lost. Hair follicles are completely obliterated (Fig. 28-39). In late stages of the disease, large areas of subcutaneous fat are replaced by newly formed collagen.

CLINICAL FEATURES: Scleroderma shows a peak incidence in people 30–50 years old. Women are afflicted 4 times as often as men. Patients with early scleroderma usually present with Raynaud phenomenon or nonpitting edema of the hands or fingers. Affected areas become hard and tense. The skin of the face becomes mask-like and expressionless, and the skin around the mouth exhibits radial furrows. In late stages of the disease, the skin over large parts of the body is thickened, densely fibrotic and fixed to the underlying tissue. Prognosis is related to the extent of disease in visceral organs, particularly the lung and kidney.

INFLAMMATORY DISORDERS OF THE PANNICULUS

Panniculitis denotes a diverse group of diseases characterized by inflammation, mainly in the subcutis (panniculus).

The disorders gathered under the umbrella of panniculitis are classified according to the location of the inflammation. **Septal panniculitis** is inflammation in connective tissue septa, while **lobular panniculitis** entails involvement of fat lobules. These two entities may occur with or without accompanying vasculitis.

Erythema Nodosum Is Related to Toxic and Infectious Agents

Erythema nodosum (EN) is a cutaneous disorder that manifests as nonsuppurative, self-limited, tender nodules over extensor surfaces of the legs. It has a peak incidence in the third decade of life and is 3 times more common in women than in men.

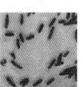 **ETIOLOGIC FACTORS:** EN is triggered by a variety of agents, such as drugs and microorganisms, and accompanies a number of benign and malignant systemic diseases. Common infections complicated by EN include streptococcal diseases (especially in children), tuberculosis and *Yersinia* infection. In endemic areas, deep fungal infections (blastomycosis, histoplasmosis, coccidioidomycosis) are common causes. EN also frequently occurs after acute respiratory tract infections of unknown etiology, but which are likely viral. The agents most commonly implicated in drug-induced EN are sulfonamides and oral contraceptives. Finally, people with Crohn disease and ulcerative colitis may develop EN.

It is thought that EN represents an immunologic response to foreign antigens, although the evidence is indirect. For example, patients with tuberculosis or coccidioidomycosis do not develop EN until skin tests for reactions to antigens of those infectious agents become positive, and testing with Frei antigen for lymphogranuloma venereum may itself induce EN. The early acute inflammation suggests that EN may be a response to complement activation, with resulting neutrophil chemotaxis. Subsequent chronic inflammation, foreign body giant cells and fibrosis are due to adipose tissue necrosis at the interface of septa and lobules.

 PATHOLOGY: Early EN lesions are in the fibrous septa of the subcutaneous tissue, where neutrophilic inflammation is associated with extravasation of erythrocytes. In chronic lesions, the septa are widened, with focal collections of giant cell macrophages around small areas of altered collagen and an ill-defined lymphocytic infiltrate (Fig. 28-40). Giant cells and inflammatory cells extend into the lobule from the interface between the septum and the fat lobule.

 CLINICAL FEATURES: EN typically manifests acutely on the anterior aspects of the legs as dome-shaped, exquisitely tender, erythematous nodules. These eventually become firm and less tender and disappear in 3–6 weeks. As some nodules heal, others may arise, but all lesions resolve without residual scarring within 6 weeks.

Erythema Induratum Is Often Associated with *Mycobacterium tuberculosis*

Erythema induratum (EI) refers to chronic, recurrent subcutaneous nodules or plaques on the legs, predominantly in

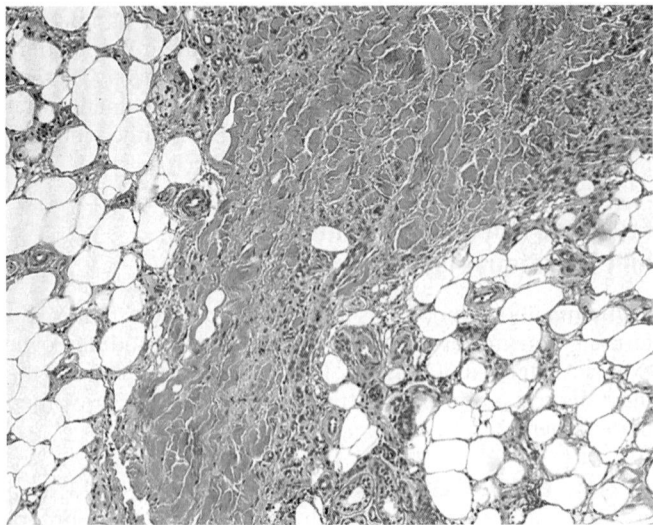

FIGURE 28-40. Erythema nodosum. The reticular dermis is present in the *upper right*. Within the panniculus is a widened septum (*extending through the middle of the field*). Lymphocytes and macrophages are present at its interface with the adipose tissue lobules. The vessels palisading along the interface of the septum are infiltrated by lymphocytes.

women. EI was traditionally considered a "tuberculid" (i.e., a hypersensitivity reaction to mycobacteria or associated antigens, but at a distant site). Although lesional tissue does not yield mycobacteria in culture or in laboratory animals, specific *Mycobacterium tuberculosis* DNA is present in greater than 75% of skin biopsies with EI.

 PATHOLOGY: In contrast to EN, which is a septal panniculitis, EI is a lobular panniculitis initially, secondary to a vasculitis that produces ischemic necrosis of the fat lobule. The panniculus exhibits a dense, chronic inflammation within lobules, which can form prominent tuberculoid granulomas or areas of coagulative necrosis. Septa around the lobules are relatively spared. Vascular changes are usually extensive and include (1) prominent infiltration of small and medium-sized arteries and veins by a dense lymphoid or granulomatous infiltrate; (2) endothelial swelling, which may progress to thrombosis; and (3) fibrous thickening of the intima. Thus, sometimes this condition is called "nodular vasculitis." Extensive ischemic necrosis provokes subsequent ulceration of the overlying epidermis. Eventually, lesions heal by fibrosis.

 CLINICAL FEATURES: Patients with EI present with recurrent, tender, erythematous, subcutaneous nodules on the legs, particularly the calves (as opposed to the shins, which are the usual location of EN). Lesions tend to ulcerate and heal with an atrophic scar. The course may last many years. Systemic steroids are usually necessary to control the disease.

Acne Vulgaris Is a Disorder of the Pilosebaceous Unit

Acne vulgaris is a self-limited, inflammatory disorder of sebaceous follicles that typically afflicts adolescents, results in intermittent formation of discrete papular or pustular lesions

and may lead to scarring. It is cosmetically disfiguring and often psychologically debilitating. Acne is so common that many regard it as a "rite of passage" through adolescence. In some cases, acne extends to the third decade.

 **ETIOLOGIC FACTORS AND PATHOLOGY:** The development of acne is related to (1) excessive hormonally induced production of sebum, (2) abnormal cornification of portions of the follicular epithelium, (3) a response to the anaerobic diphtheroid *Propionibacterium acnes* and (4) follicle rupture and subsequent inflammation. The sebaceous follicle contains a vellus hair and prominent sebaceous glands. Changes in hormonal status at puberty generate sebum production in the follicle and altered cornification in the neck of the sebaceous follicle (infundibulum). These effects lead to dilation of the follicular canal. Another round of excessive sebum production is associated with desquamation of squamous cells and accretion of keratinous debris, providing a rich environment for *P. acnes* proliferation. These combined changes produce a distended, plugged follicle: a **comedone**. Neutrophils attracted to the area by chemotactic factors released by *P. acnes* release hydrolytic enzymes to form a follicular abscess **(pustule)**. They also attack the follicle wall, thus permitting escape of sebum, keratin and bacteria into perifollicular tissue, where they stimulate further acute inflammation and a perifollicular abscess (Fig. 28-41). The development of allergy to *P. acnes* intensifies the inflammatory response. Fully evolved lesions show intense neutrophilic inflammation surrounding a ruptured sebaceous follicle. In addition, abundant macrophages, lymphocytes and foreign body giant cells accumulate in response to sebaceous follicle rupture.

 CLINICAL FEATURES: Acne vulgaris features a variety of skin lesions in different stages of development, including comedones, papules, pustules, nodules, cysts and pitted scars. Comedones, the primary noninflammatory lesions of acne, are either open **(blackheads)** or closed **(whiteheads)**. More advanced inflammatory lesions vary from small, erythematous papules to large, tender, purulent nodules and cysts.

Acne vulgaris is treated with topical cleansing and keratolytic and antibacterial agents. Severe cases are managed with topical vitamin A, systemic antibiotics or synthetic oral retinoids (isotretinoin).

INFECTIONS AND INFESTATIONS

The skin is under constant assault from countless marauders and is an effective but imperfect barrier against them; bacteria, fungi, viruses, parasites and insects sometimes penetrate this first line of defense.

Impetigo Is a Cutaneous Infection by Staphylococci or Streptococci

Superficial bacterial infections of the skin, known as **impetigo,** occur mostly in children, who are often infected through minor breaks in the skin. Adults tend to contract impetigo after an underlying disease process compromises the barrier function of the skin. Honey-colored crusted erosions or

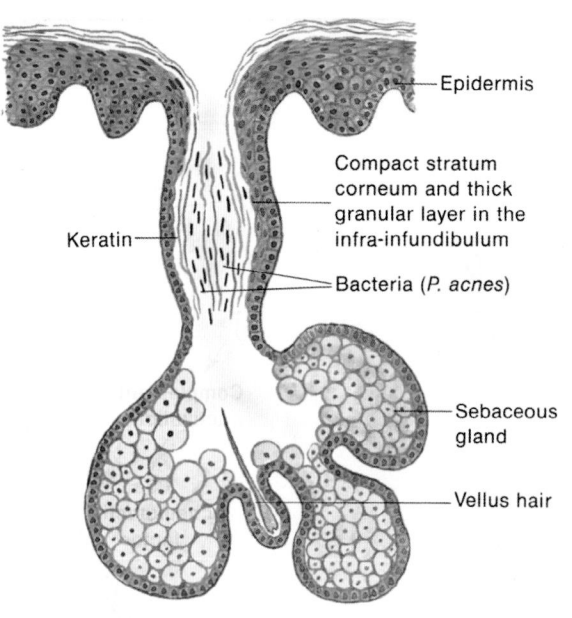

A. MICRODOMEDONE

Epidermis

Compact stratum corneum and thick granular layer in the infra-infundibulum

Keratin

Bacteria (*P. acnes*)

Sebaceous gland

Vellus hair

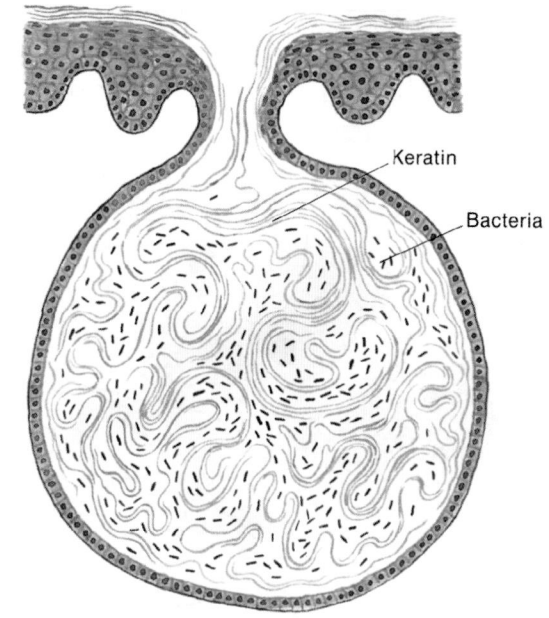

B. CLOSED COMEDONE

Keratin

Bacteria

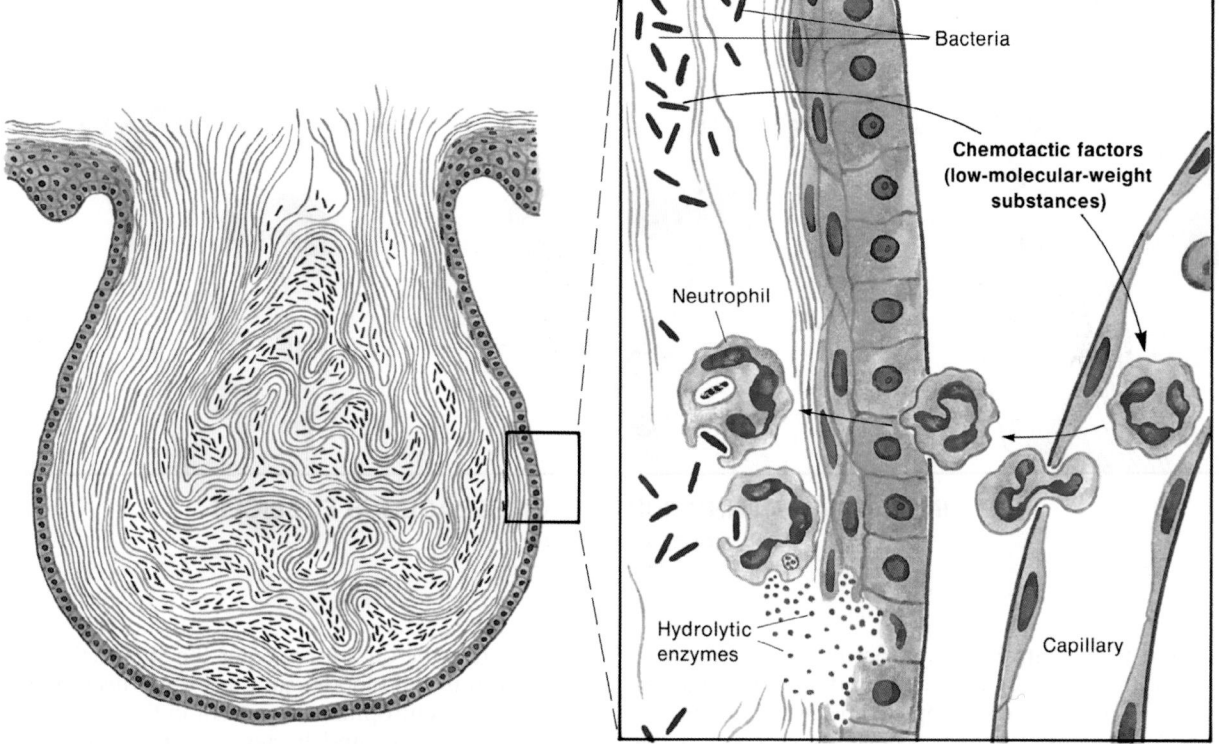

C. OPEN COMEDONE

D. INVASION OF FOLLICLE BY NEUTROPHILS

Bacteria

Chemotactic factors (low-molecular-weight substances)

Neutrophil

Hydrolytic enzymes

Capillary

FIGURE 28-41. Acne vulgaris. The pathogenesis of follicular distention, rupture and inflammation is depicted. Acne is a disease of the follicular canal of a sebaceous follicle. A compact stratum corneum and a thickened granular layer in the infrainfundibulum are the beginning of the formation of a comedone. Microcomedones **(A)** and closed **(B)** and open **(C)** comedones form. Excessive sebum secretion occurs, and the bacterium *Propionibacterium acnes* proliferates. The organism produces chemotactic factors, leading to neutrophil migration into the intact comedone. Neutrophilic enzymes are released, and the comedone ruptures, inducing a cycle of chemotaxis and intense neutrophilic inflammation **(D, E)**. (*continued*)

THE SKIN

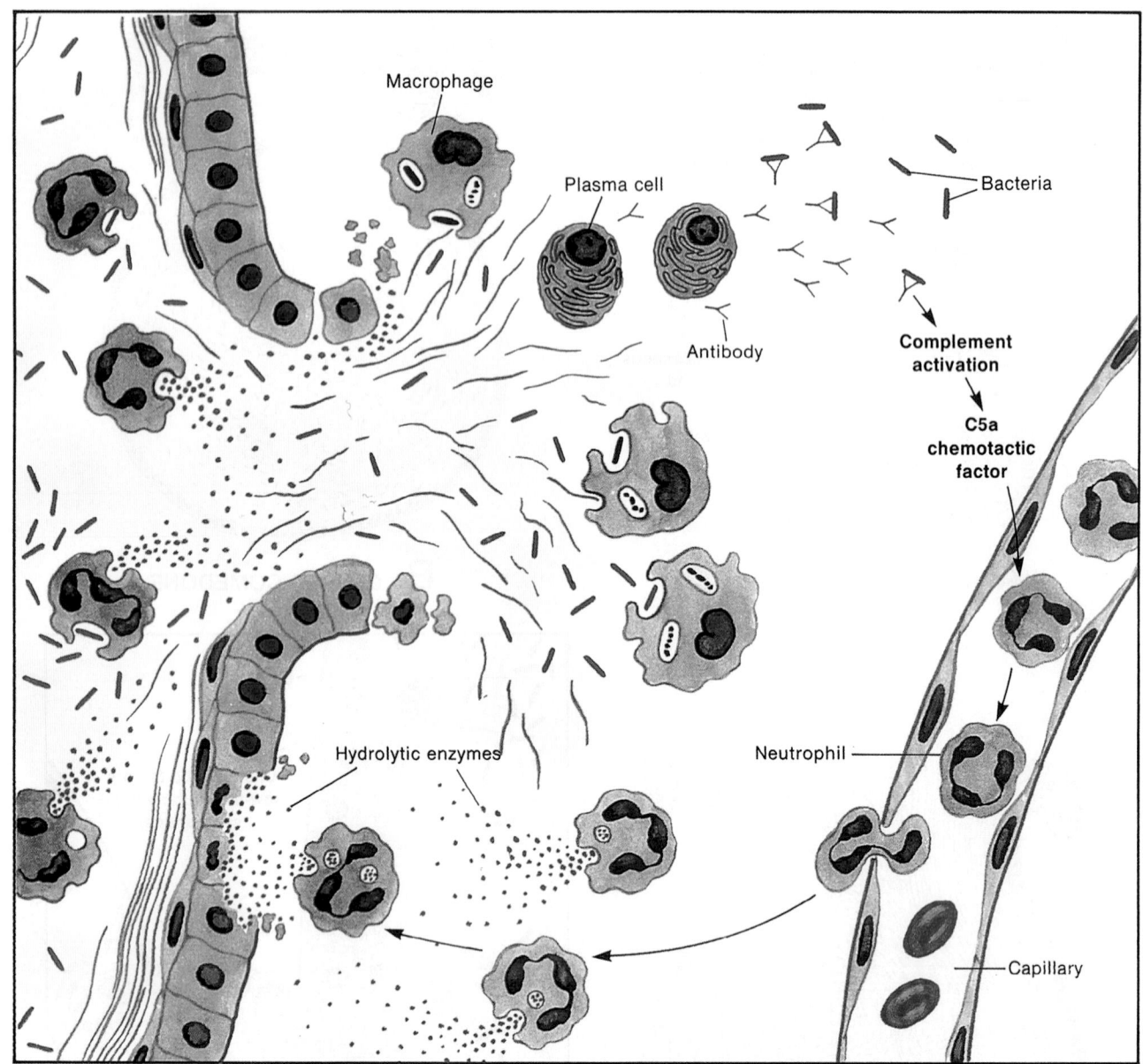

E. **INFLAMMATION AND RUPTURE OF SEBACEOUS FOLLICLE**

FIGURE 28-41. (*Continued*)

ulcers, often with central healing, occur most commonly on exposed areas such as the face, hands and extremities (Fig. 28-42). A combination of topical and systemic antimicrobial agents against staphylococci or streptococci is the mainstay of therapy.

PATHOLOGY: Neutrophils accumulate beneath the stratum corneum. Bacteria may be visualized with special stains. Vesicles or bullae form and eventually rupture, allowing a thin, seropurulent discharge to appear. This discharge dries and forms the characteristic layers of exudate containing neutrophils and cell debris. Reactive epidermal changes (spongiosis, elongation of rete ridges) and superficial dermal inflammation are usually present. **Ecthyma** is more typically caused by *Pseudomonas aeruginosa* (ecthyma gangrenosum) and several other organisms. It

occurs when the organisms enter the superficial aspects of the skin from the bloodstream to form a necrotizing ulcerated lesion. Neutrophils are present in the floor of the ulcer and in the dermis, and bacteria are often seen migrating through vessel walls.

Superficial Fungal Infections Are Caused by Dermatophytes

Dermatophytes are fungi that can infect nonviable keratinized epithelium, including stratum corneum, nails and hair. They synthesize keratinases that digest keratin and provide themselves with sustenance. Superficial fungal infections are often caused by a change in the skin microenvironment, which allows overgrowth of transient or resident flora. For example, use of immunosuppressive agents such as topical or

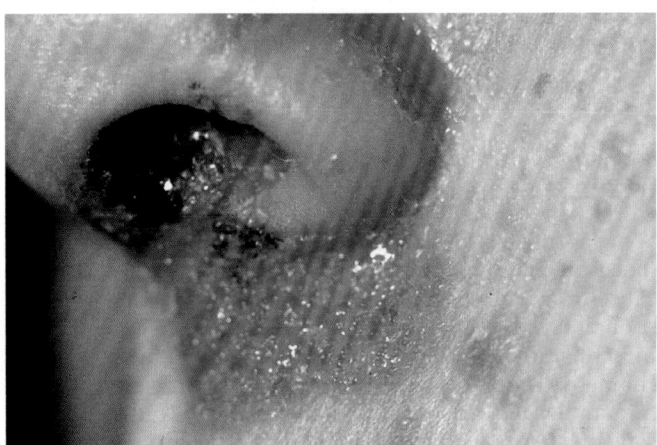

FIGURE 28-42. Impetigo contagiosa. Honey-colored crusts secondary to rupture of vesicopustules are seen in the nasal area of a child, an area commonly colonized by *Staphylococcus aureus.*

systemic glucocorticoids may impair cell-mediated immune responses that normally eliminate dermatophytes. Excessive sweating or occlusion of a body part may provide an environment that "tips the balance" between fungal proliferation and elimination in favor of proliferation.

Of the 10 or so dermatophyte species that often cause human cutaneous infection, *Trichophyton rubrum* is the most common. A superficial dermatophyte infection is called a dermatophytosis, tinea or ringworm. The tineas have distinctive clinical features depending on the site of infection. They are divided as follows: (1) **tinea capitis** (scalp; "ringworm"), (2) **tinea barbae** (beard), (3) **tinea faciei** (face), (4) **tinea corporis** (trunk, legs, arms or neck, excluding the feet, hands and groin), (5) **tinea manus** (hands), (6) **tinea pedis** (feet; "athlete's foot"; Fig. 28-43A), (7) **tinea cruris** (groin, pubic area and thigh; "jock itch") and (8) **tinea unguium** (nails; "onychomycosis").

Other causes of superficial fungal infections are *Candida* sp. and *Malassezia furfur. Candida* sp. require a warm, moist environment in which to flourish, such as that found when a baby's bottom is encased in a wet diaper. *M. furfur* needs a moist, lipid-rich environment. **Tinea versicolor,** caused by *M. furfur,* is more common in young adults when sebum production is greatest. Variably sized, pigmented, sharply demarcated, round or oval macules with fine scales are present, predominantly on the upper trunk.

Special stains such as PAS show budding yeast and hyphal forms in the most superficial layers of the stratum corneum. Hyperkeratosis, epidermal hyperplasia and chronic perivascular inflammation are noted in the dermis (Fig. 28-43B, C).

Deep Fungal Infections May Reflect Dissemination of Pulmonary Infections

Most invasive or systemic fungal infections arise from inhalation of aerosolized material contaminated with organisms such as *Histoplasma* or *Blastomyces.* A primary pulmonary

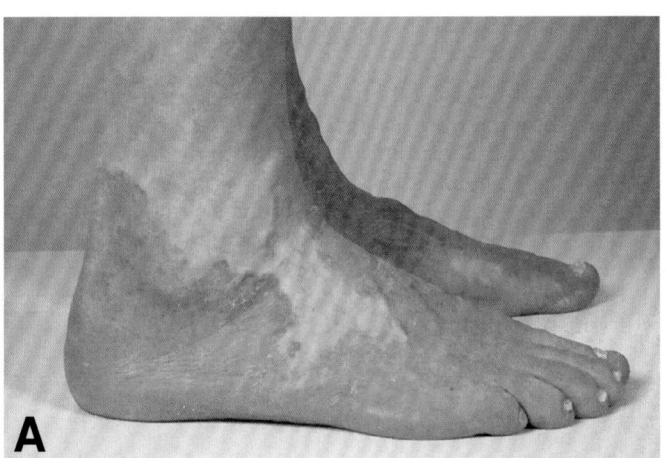

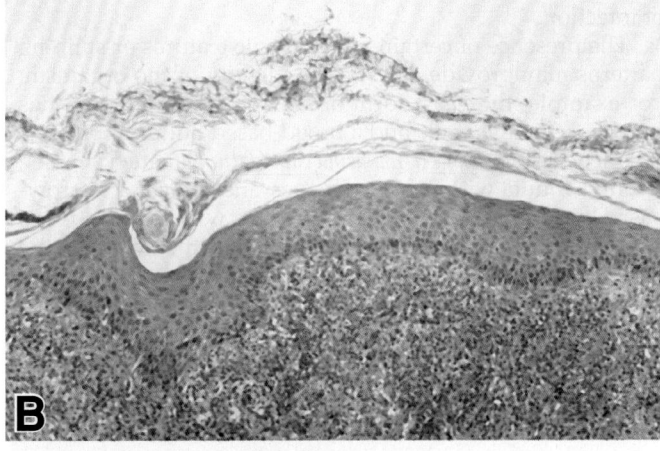

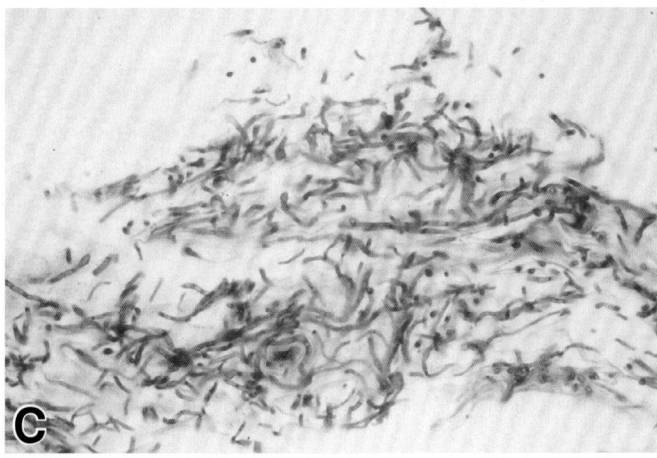

FIGURE 28-43. Dermatophytosis. A. Tinea pedis. A leading edge of scale and erythema in a moccasin distribution characterizes this infection, most commonly caused by *Trichophyton rubrum.* **B.** A dense inflammatory infiltrate is present in the epidermis and dermis and is associated with the presence of fungal hyphae in the stratum corneum. **C.** A higher-power view of the fungal hyphae in the stratum corneum.

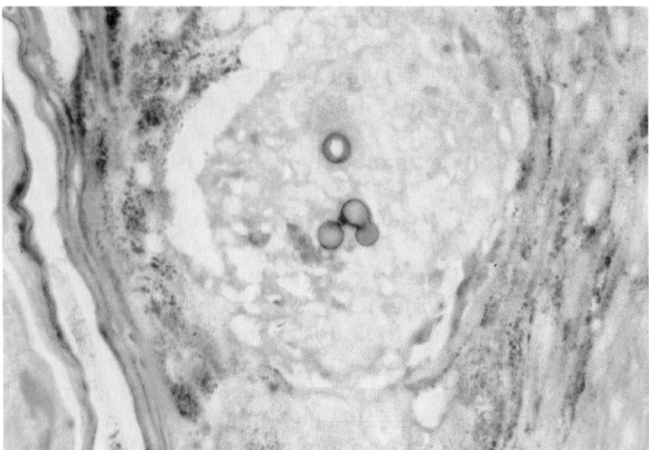

FIGURE 28-44. Blastomycosis. A Gomori methenamine silver stain highlights the organisms, which are thick-walled spores 8–15 microns in diameter. One of the organisms demonstrates broad-based budding.

infection may then spread to the skin or mucosa. Locally invasive fungal infections of the skin are rare and usually arise from traumatic implantation of organisms such as *Sporothrix* or *Fonsecaea*. An underlying immunocompromised state increases the likelihood of dissemination of fungal organisms.

Deep extension of a local cutaneous infection often causes a chancre-like lesion at the site of implantation. Intervening lymphatic vessels may be indurated and thickened. Nodules and ulcers, especially if bilateral, suggest an internal source of infection.

The presence of certain morphologic features or staining patterns may provide clues to the identity of the organism. For example, the yeast form of *Blastomyces dermatitidis* has notably refractile walls and a broad-based budding pattern, but the yeast form of *Histoplasma capsulatum* is much smaller, is often found within macrophages and shows a narrow-based budding pattern. Staining a smear with India ink, or a tissue biopsy with mucicarmine, may show the thick capsule characteristic of the yeast *Cryptococcus neoformans*. Marked epidermal hyperplasia, intraepidermal microabscesses and

suppurative granulomatous inflammation in the dermis is often associated with these deep-seated fungal infections (Fig. 28-44).

Viral Skin Infections Cause Diverse Clinical Manifestations

Some viruses (see Chapter 9), such as the poxvirus **molluscum contagiosum** or **human papillomaviruses** (HPVs), cause transient benign epithelial proliferations that resolve spontaneously. Others (e.g., measles or *parvovirus* [**erythema infectiosum**]) produce febrile illnesses with self-limited cutaneous eruptions **(exanthems)**. Primary infection by most **human herpesviruses** is often asymptomatic but results in a state of latent infection. Upon reactivation, the virus causes a painful, vesicular eruption.

Molluscum contagiosum is a common infection among children and sexually active adults. It is self-limited and is easily spread by direct contact. Firm, dome-shaped, smooth-surfaced papules with a characteristic central umbilication are usually found on the face, trunk and anogenital area. Epidermal cells contain large intracytoplasmic inclusion bodies ("molluscum bodies") within cup-shaped areas that also exhibit verrucous (papillomatous) epidermal hyperplasia. Numerous viral particles are present within these inclusion bodies (Fig. 28-45).

Arthropod Infestations Produce Pruritic Skin Lesions

Mites and lice, other insects and spiders cause local lesions that may be very pruritic.

- *Scabies* is a severely pruritic, eczematous dermatitis caused by the mite *Sarcoptes scabei*. The female mite burrows beneath the stratum corneum on the fingers, wrists, trunk and genital skin (Fig. 28-46). Intense lymphocytic and eosinophilic dermatitis is induced as a hypersensitivity reaction to the mite and its eggs and feces.
- *Pediculosis,* another pruritic dermatosis, may be caused by a variety of human lice. Eggs ("nits") of the lice may be found attached to hair shafts.

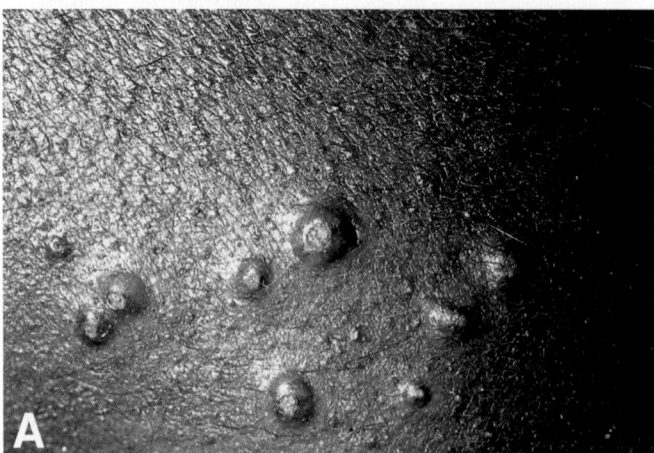
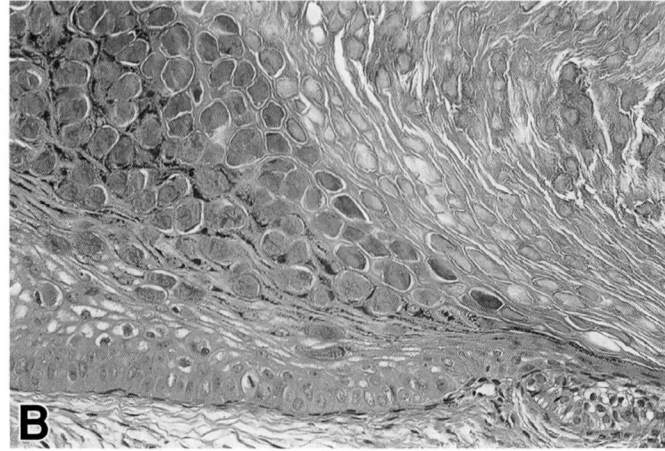

FIGURE 28-45. Molluscum contagiosum. A. Multiple umbilicated papules in an HIV-positive patient. **B.** The keratinocytes that are infected with this poxvirus show large eosinophilic cytoplasmic inclusions called "molluscum bodies."

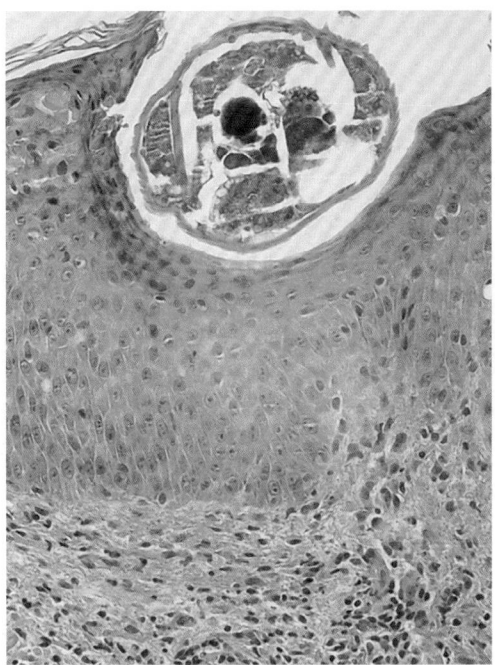

FIGURE 28-46. Scabetic nodule. A scabies mite is present in the stratum corneum.

■ **Biting insects** produce lesions that vary from small, pruritic papules to large, weeping nodules. The reaction varies with the arthropod species and host immune response. For example, tick bites tend to be large, with a striking lymphocytic and eosinophilic infiltrate. Lymphoid follicles may also form. Flea bites are usually urticarial, with a scant neutrophilic infiltrate. The venoms injected by arthropods such as the brown recluse spider may give rise to severe local tissue necrosis.

PRIMARY NEOPLASMS OF THE SKIN

Common Acquired Melanocytic Nevi (Moles) Are Localized Benign Neoplastic Proliferations of Melanocytes within the Epidermis or Dermis

 **ETIOLOGIC FACTORS:** Most people, regardless of skin color, develop 10–50 nevi on their skin. The total number depends on light exposure and innate susceptibility. Except for occasional cosmetic significance, nevi are important mainly in relation to melanoma, as markers of individuals at increased risk of developing melanoma, as potential precursors of melanoma and as stimulants of melanoma. Even though 30% of melanomas arise in relation to a nevus, nevi are much more common than melanomas, and most are stable or undergo senescence over time. Thus, wholesale excision of nevi is not effective as a means of preventing melanoma.

Black skin can develop nevi, but less commonly. Those nevi that develop in the skin of darkly pigmented people are usually not associated with an increased risk of melanoma or progression to melanoma. However, the risk of melanoma on the palms of the hands, the soles of the feet or the genital skin is the same in all races. Nevi, like melanomas, do not ordinarily develop in areas protected from light by

at least two layers of clothing, such as the buttocks. There is an unequivocal causal relationship between exposure to ultraviolet light and melanocytic nevi (and malignant melanoma), but the relationship is complex. Some people with fair skin form relatively few nevi, but those with dark skin occasionally develop numerous nevi. The ability to form nevi is partly under genetic control and has been correlated with polymorphic variants of the melanocortin receptor and with subsequent variation in the ratio of pheomelanin to eumelanin. These are the pigments associated with red and brown hair, respectively, and also with susceptibility to burning and tanning. There are at least two distinguishable profiles of individuals at risk for melanoma. One group prototypically has skin that may burn but can tan and has an increased number of nevi. The other group consists of red-haired, blue-eyed people with milk-white skin, who are exquisitely sensitive to light and do not tan well. However, they form freckles and do not develop a significant number of nevi. In addition, many patients with melanoma may have overlapping features.

 MOLECULAR PATHOGENESIS: A majority of nevi have recently been found to have an activating mutation of the oncogene *BRAF,* which can lead to growth stimulation through the mitogen-activated protein kinase (MAPK) pathway. However, after an initial period of growth, nevi are stable lesions that may regress or senesce. Such senescence is mediated by increased activity of p16, which is encoded by the gene *CDKN2A* on chromosome 9p21 and is an inhibitor of cyclin-dependent kinase 4 (CDK4). The p16 protein suppresses cell proliferation and promotes end-stage differentiation of the nevus cells (see Chapter 5).

Epidemiologic studies have shown melanocytic nevi to be strong risk markers for development of melanomas. Someone with 100 or more nevi that are 2–5 mm has a 3-fold greater risk of developing melanoma than a person with fewer than 25 similar nevi. Patients with clinically atypical-appearing nevi or histologically proven dysplastic nevi are at even greater risk for melanoma. Only 10 or more such clinically atypical or dysplastic nevi may be associated with a 12-fold increased risk for melanoma. As nevi are very common and melanomas are not, the risk of progression of any one nevus is small.

Melanocytic nevi begin to appear between the first and second years of life and continue to emerge for the first two decades of life. A nevus first appears as a small tan dot no bigger than 1–2 mm. During the next 3–4 years, the dot enlarges to become a uniform tan to brown circular or oval area. The peripheral outline usually remains regular. When it reaches 4–5 mm in diameter, it is flat or slightly elevated, stops enlarging peripherally and is sharply demarcated from surrounding normal skin. Over the next 10 years, the lesion elevates and its color pales to the point of becoming a tan tag-like protrusion. For the next decade or two, it gradually flattens and the skin may approximate a normal appearance. In most people, the number of nevi gradually decreases over time. Notably, many melanoma patients tend to retain increased numbers of nevi, including atypical ones, in the later decades of life.

PATHOLOGY: At the inception of a melanocytic nevus, melanocytes are increased in the basal epidermis, with subsequent hyperpigmentation. They

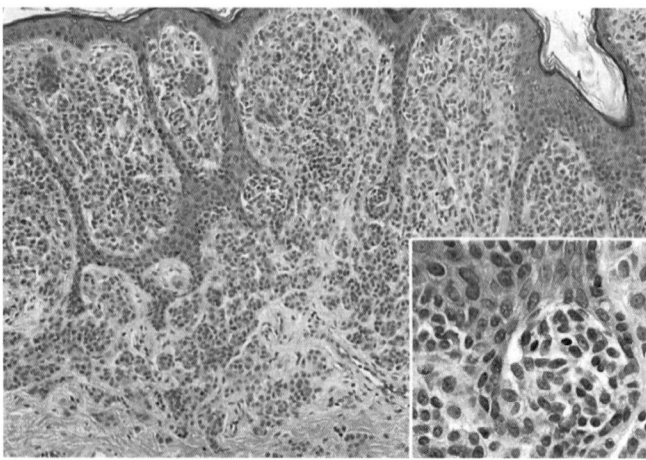

FIGURE 28-47. Compound melanocytic nevus. Melanocytes are present as nests within the epidermis and dermis. An intraepidermal nest of melanocytes is surrounded by keratinocytes (*inset*).

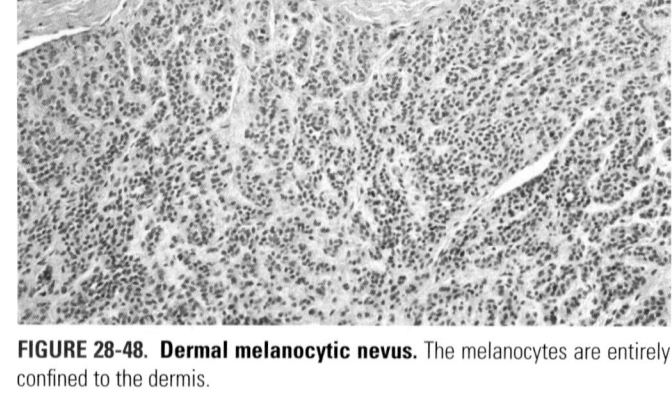

FIGURE 28-48. Dermal melanocytic nevus. The melanocytes are entirely confined to the dermis.

eventually form nests, frequently at tips of rete ridges, and then migrate into the dermis where they form small clusters. As the lesion becomes elevated, the dermal nevus cells begin to differentiate in a manner reminiscent of Schwann cells (melanocytes like Schwann cells are derived from embryonic neural crest), an evolution that gradually encompasses the entire dermal component, leaving a core of delicate neuromesenchyme. The nevus may eventually flatten and possibly even disappear. The histologic classification of melanocytic nevi reflects their evolution:

- **Junctional nevus:** Melanocytes form nests at the tips of epidermal rete ridges. They are then by definition known as "nevus cells," and they also tend to lose their dendritic morphology and retain pigment in their cytoplasm.
- **Compound nevus:** Nests of melanocytes are seen in the epidermis and some of the cells have migrated into the dermis (Fig. 28-47).
- **Dermal nevus:** Intraepidermal melanocytic growth has ceased and melanocytes are present only in the dermis (Fig. 28-48). Pigment tends to be lost at this stage, but the presence of a residual nested architecture is an important clue to the diagnosis of a nevus versus another tumor.

Dysplastic (Atypical) Nevi Are Risk Markers for Melanoma

An increased number of total nevi is a significant risk factor for melanoma, as is the presence of large nevi. Some common acquired nevi do not follow the pattern of growth, differentiation and disappearance described above and are called "dysplastic nevi." These are especially strong risk factors. Such lesions persist and are often larger than 5 mm. They may show foci of aberrant melanocytic growth and become larger and somewhat irregular peripherally (although less so than melanomas). The peripheral area is flat (macular) and extends symmetrically from the parent nevus. Some clinically dysplastic nevi are entirely macular.

Dysplastic nevi were first described in melanoma kindreds, families in which there is a greatly increased incidence of melanoma. In these families and in general population members, patients with dysplastic nevi are at increased risk of developing melanoma. Not all patients with dysplastic

nevi will develop melanomas, and not all melanomas occur in patients with dysplastic nevi. The magnitude of this risk varies with the number of nevi and is especially high in patients with a prior melanoma or family history of melanoma. The genetics of dysplastic nevi are not completely understood, and contributions from multiple genes are likely.

Melanocytic Dysplasia Features Architectural Disorder and Cytologic Atypia

Dysplastic nevi are characterized by junctional proliferation of nevoid to epithelioid melanocytes arranged singly and in nests, with nests predominating. These lesions occur mainly near the dermal–epidermal junction and at the tips and sides of elongated rete ridges. A band of eosinophilic connective tissue ("concentric eosinophilic fibroplasia") is seen around the rete ridges. Horizontal nests of lesional cells extend from some rete to adjacent rete ("bridging"). As these architectural features become more prominent, melanocytes with large atypical nuclei that are reminiscent of malignant cells may also appear in the areas of architectural disorder, remaining a minority population and constituting "random cytologic atypia." The combination of architectural disorder and cytologic atypia together defines a dysplastic nevus (Figs. 28-49 and 28-50). Areas of dysplasia may also be associated with a subjacent lymphocytic infiltrate. More than 1/3 of malignant melanomas have precursor nevi, most of which show melanocytic dysplasia. However, most dysplastic nevi are stable and never progress to melanoma. In other words, dysplastic nevi are much more common in the population than melanomas. Between 7% and 20% of the population has at least one dysplastic nevus, depending on the diagnostic criteria applied. In this regard, controversy about the significance of dysplastic nevi largely reflects diagnostic variation. Moderate and severe histologic dysplasia, but not mild dysplasia, is associated with increased risk of developing melanoma. Mild histologic dysplasia may thus be considered, like prostatic intraepithelial neoplasia type I (PIN I) in the prostate or mild dysplasia in the uterine cervix, to be a common lesion of little or no prognostic or diagnostic significance.

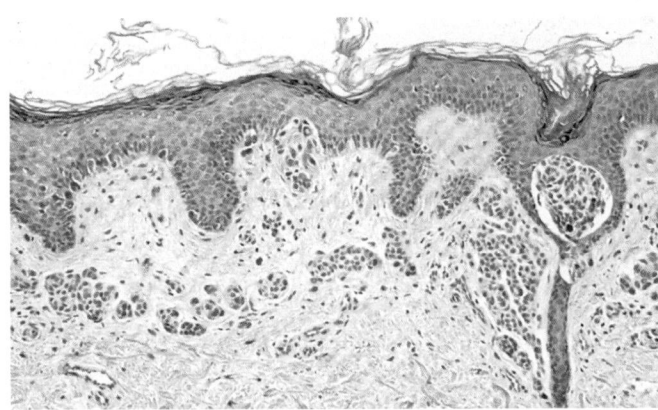

FIGURE 28-49. Compound nevus with melanocytic dysplasia. On the *right*, a compound nevus is apparent with both intraepidermal and dermal components. To the *left*, within the epidermis, are single, atypical melanocytes within the basal layer, as well as incipient lamellar fibroplasia. Dermal melanocytes are present *below*.

The Prognosis of Malignant Melanoma Reflects the Depth of Invasion

Malignant melanoma is a neoplasm of melanocytes. The term "melanoma" in current practice is synonymous with "malignant melanoma." Malignant melanoma, although not one of the most common cancers overall, is a leading cause of cancer mortality in young adults. It is rare in adolescence and exceedingly rare in childhood. Melanomas may progress through two major stages. In the "radial growth phase" (RGP), the lesion spreads (as viewed clinically) along the radii of an imperfect circle in the skin but remains superficial and thin (as measured by micrometer in the method originally described by Breslow). In the "vertical growth phase" (VGP), there is a focal area in which the lesion expands in a more or less spherical manner to form a tumor mass, with increasing Breslow thickness. Melanomas are dependent, to a greater or lesser extent, on an activated oncogene, *BRAF,* which is also mutated in benign nevi. The histopathologic subtypes of melanoma, discussed below, are related to the particular oncogenes involved in their pathogenesis. Loss of p16 (and in some cases other tumor suppressors) is common in melanomas and leads to unrestrained proliferation and the potential for future progression "from bad to worse."

The incidence of malignant melanoma is increasing rapidly. It is estimated that over 1% of children born today will develop malignant melanoma. The prognosis of most melanomas is excellent if lesions are recognized and excised before entering a vertical growth phase. However, a patient is at increased risk of dying from metastatic disease if the tumor exceeds a critical depth in the dermis.

Radial Growth Phase Melanoma

The most common type of melanoma is **superficial spreading melanoma,** which can present in the radial growth phase

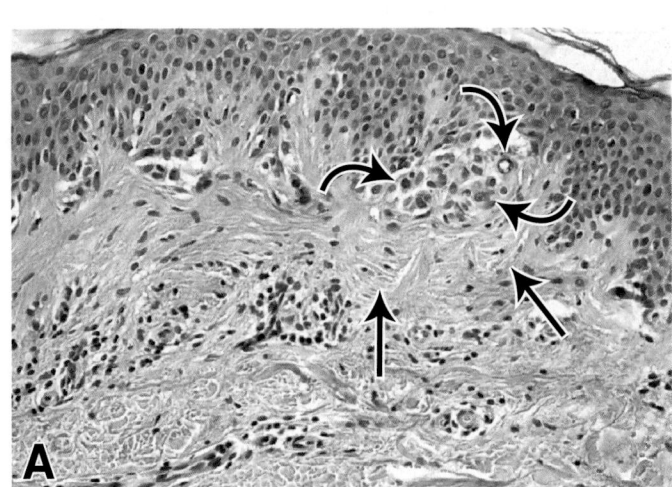

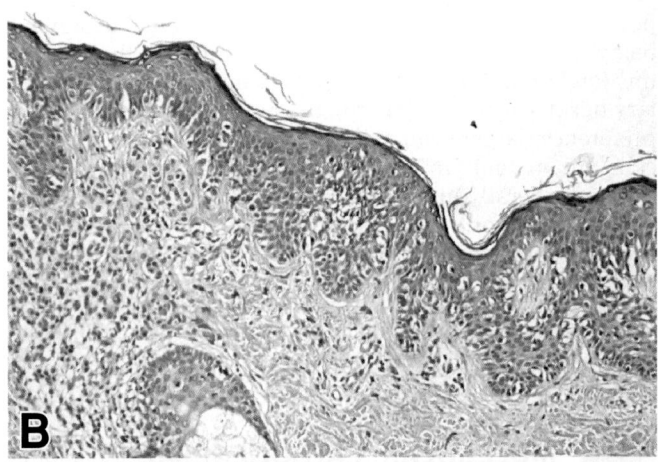

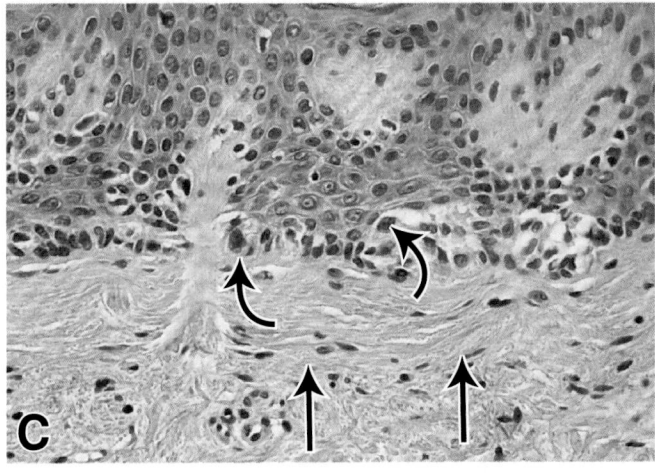

FIGURE 28-50. Dysplastic nevus. A. There is bridging of rete ridges by nests of melanocytes, melanocytes with cytologic atypia (*curved arrows*), lamellar fibroplasia (*straight arrows*) and a scant perivascular lymphocytic infiltrate. **B.** To the *left* is a zone containing typical dermal nevus cells of a compound melanocytic nevus. In the epidermis on the *right* is a proliferation of atypical melanocytes with lamellar fibroplasia. This photomicrograph is taken from the junction of the papular and macular components of this dysplastic nevus. Dysplasia usually develops in the macular portion, which takes up most of the field. **C.** Irregular melanocytic nests resting above lamellar fibroplasia (*straight arrows*) exhibit large epithelioid melanocytes with atypia (*curved arrows*).

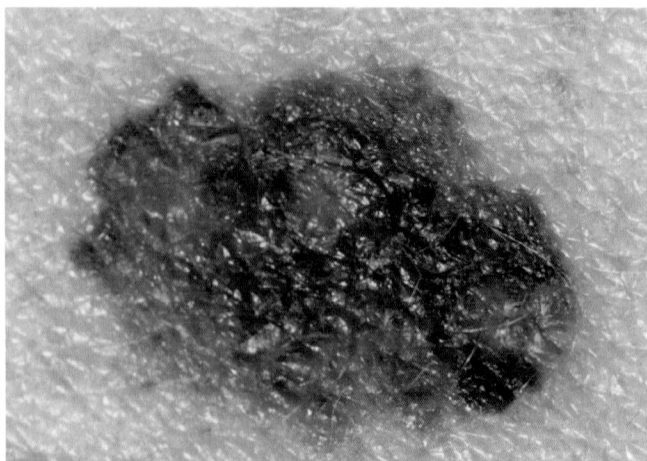

FIGURE 28-51. The clinical appearance of the radial growth phase in malignant melanoma of the superficial spreading type. The larger diameter is 1.8 cm.

or vertical growth phase (Fig. 28-51). Excision for histologic examination is the gold standard for diagnosis of melanoma of any sort.

PATHOLOGY: In a superficial spreading melanoma, large, often pigmented epithelioid melanocytes are dispersed in nests and as individual cells through the entire thickness of the epidermis ("pagetoid scatter") and not just along the basal layer (as occurs in nevi and in lentiginous forms of melanoma described below). These melanocytes may be limited to the epidermis **(melanoma in situ)** or they may invade into the papillary dermis. In the radial growth phase, no nest has growth preference (larger size) over the other nests (Fig. 28-52), so cells grow evenly in all directions: upward in the epidermis, peripherally in the epidermis and downward into the dermis **(invasion)**. Mitoses are not seen in dermal melanocytes (except when the vertical growth phase is present) but may be present in the epidermal component. These lesions enlarge at the periphery, hence the term **radial**. A brisk lymphocytic infiltrate typically accompanies melanocytes in the radial growth phase. Such lesions rarely metastasize.

MOLECULAR PATHOGENESIS: Melanoma has several different genetic mutations implicated in its pathogenesis, involving many different molecular pathways. As with nevi, activating *BRAF* mutations are seen in 40%–50% of melanomas, and *NRAS* mutations are seen in 10%–20%. These kinases both utilize the MAPK pathway, which regulates cell proliferation. Upstream from both NRAS and BRAF is the receptor tyrosine kinase c-Kit, for which mutations account for only 1% of melanomas overall. However, it is the most common mutation seen in acral and mucosal subtypes, and often in lentigo maligna melanoma. Downstream from NRAS is the phosphatidylinositol-3-kinase (PI3K)/AKT pathway, which regulates cell survival and is suppressed by PTEN (see Chapter 5). In this context, PTEN mutations occur in 60% of cases. Mutations in *CDKN2A* are common in sporadic and familial melanomas and account for 30% of cases overall. CDKN2A encodes two tumor suppressors, including $p16^{INK4A}$, which inhibits

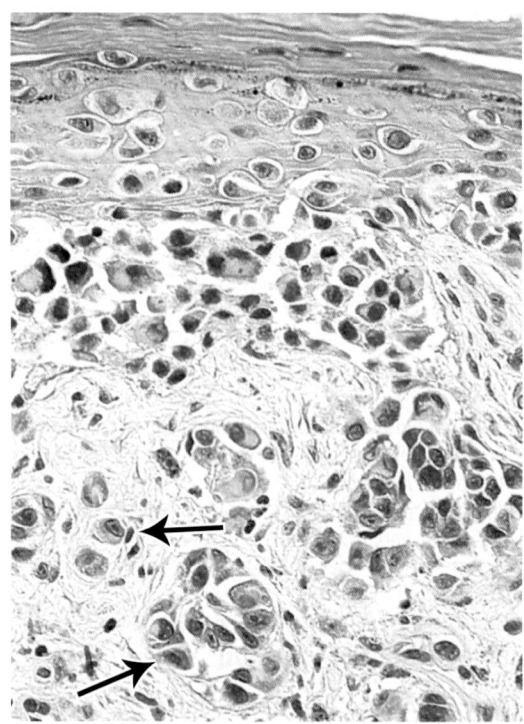

FIGURE 28-52. Malignant melanoma, superficial spreading type, radial growth phase. Melanocytes grow singly within the epidermis at all levels and as large, irregularly sized nests at the dermal–epidermal junction. Tumor cells are present in the papillary dermis (*arrows*), but no nest shows preferential growth over the others.

CDK4, and CDK6. p16 function may be impaired by other mechanisms, in addition to mutations of its gene. As many of the same activating mutations occur in both benign nevi and melanomas, malignancy most likely entails a combination of these mutations, inactivation of senescence genes (like p16) and other still unidentified alterations.

The increased understanding of melanoma molecular mechanisms has spurred the developments of targeted therapies aimed at inhibiting particular genetic pathways, including tyrosine kinase inhibitors of Kit and BRAF inhibitors, with many more in clinical development (Fig. 28-53).

CLINICAL FEATURES: Superficial spreading melanoma (SSM) usually follows a history of intermittent sun exposure and sunburn. Early melanomas in the radial growth phase have slightly elevated and palpable borders. The neoplasm is usually variably and haphazardly pigmented. Some parts are black or dark brown, while other areas may be lighter brown, possibly mixed with pink or light blue tints. The entire lesion is sometimes purely dark brown (Fig. 28-51). With regard to lesions that are eventually documented to be melanoma, patients often state that a change occurred in a nevus. Such alterations can include itching, increase in size, darkening or bleeding and oozing, though the latter signs tend to appear later. With or without such observations on the part of the patient, any lesion that prompts clinical suspicion of melanoma warrants an excisional biopsy. The "ABCDE rule" is a convenient mnemonic to help recognize changes in nevi that should prompt patients to seek medical attention: **a**symmetry of shape, **b**order irregularity, **c**olor variation and a **d**iameter more than

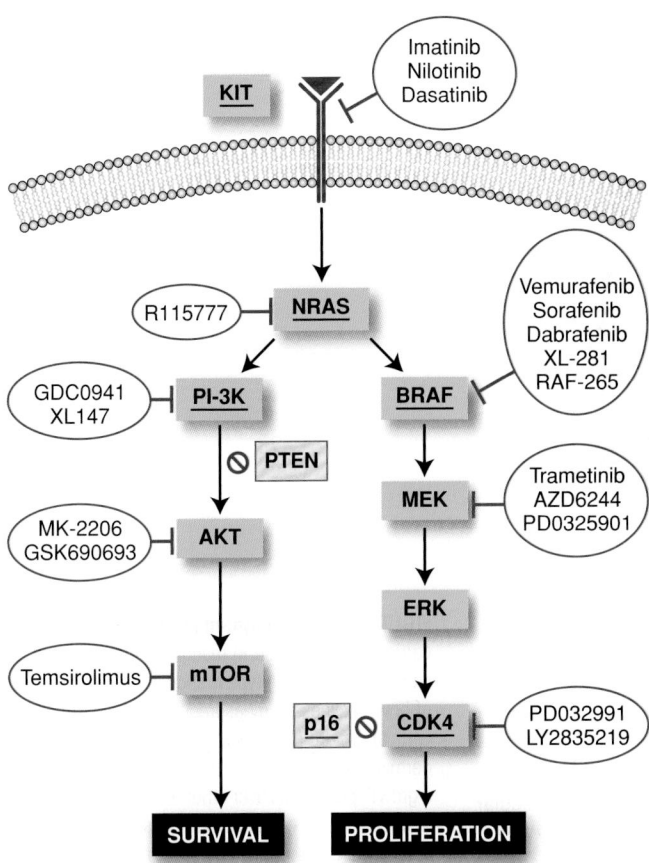

FIGURE 28-53. Simplified melanoma genetic pathway schema. Mitogen-activated protein kinase (MAPK) and phosphatidylinositol-3-kinase (PI3K)/AKT pathways are depicted, which regulate cell proliferation and cell survival, respectively. Red ovals contain examples of targeted therapeutic agents currently in use or in clinical trials. Underlined genes are ones with proven mutations in melanoma.

6 mm. The letter "E" can stand for "**e**levation" or more importantly "**e**volution." However, not all early melanomas exhibit these attributes, and any changing lesion should be evaluated for excisional biopsy.

Vertical Growth Phase Melanoma

After a variable time (usually 1–2 years), the character of growth begins to change. Melanocytes exhibit mitotic activity in both the epidermal and dermal components and grow as expanding spheroid nodules in the dermis (Fig. 28-54). The net direction of growth tends to be perpendicular to that of the radial growth phase, hence **vertical** (Figs. 28-54, 28-55 and 28-56).

 PATHOLOGY: The vertical growth phase is usually characterized by:

- The cellular aggregate that characterizes the vertical growth phase is larger than the clusters of melanocytes that form the epidermal and dermal (invasive) components of the radial growth phase. Invasion can occur in both the radial growth phase and vertical growth phase, but the dominant direction of tumor growth shifts from

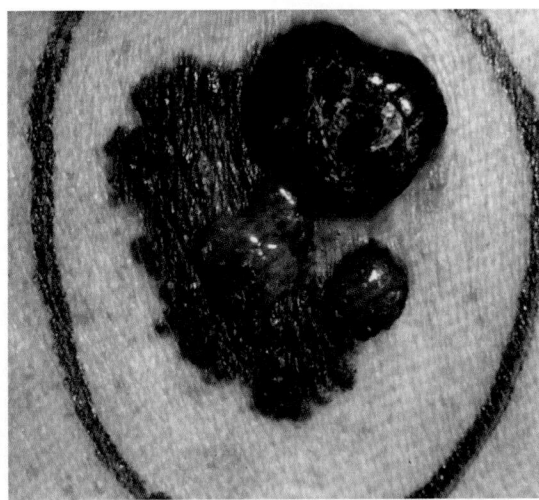

FIGURE 28-54. Malignant melanoma. The superficial spreading type is represented by the relatively flat, dark, brown–black portion of the tumor. Three areas in this lesion are characteristic of the vertical growth phase. All are nodular in configuration; two have a pink coloration, and the largest is a rich, ebony black.

the epidermis to the dermis in the vertical growth phase. This property of expansile growth in the dermis is called *tumorigenicity.*

- Mitotic figures are common in the vertical growth phase and, along with tumorigenicity, form one of its two defining attributes.
- Markers of cell cycle progression, such as Ki-67, and the phosphohistone mitosis markers increase in cells of the vertical growth phase.
- The melanocytes tend to look different from those of the radial growth phase. For example, they may contain little or no pigment, while the cells in the radial growth phase are melanotic.
- Tumors that involve the reticular dermis are usually considered to be in the vertical growth phase.

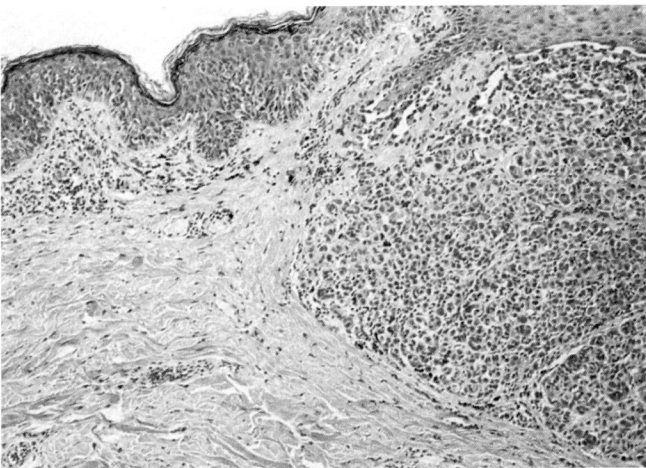

FIGURE 28-55. Malignant melanoma, superficial spreading type, vertical growth phase. Vertical growth is manifested by the distinct spheroid tumor nodule to the *right.* This focus of melanocytes clearly has a growth advantage (larger size of the aggregate) over nests in the adjacent radial growth phase (*left*).

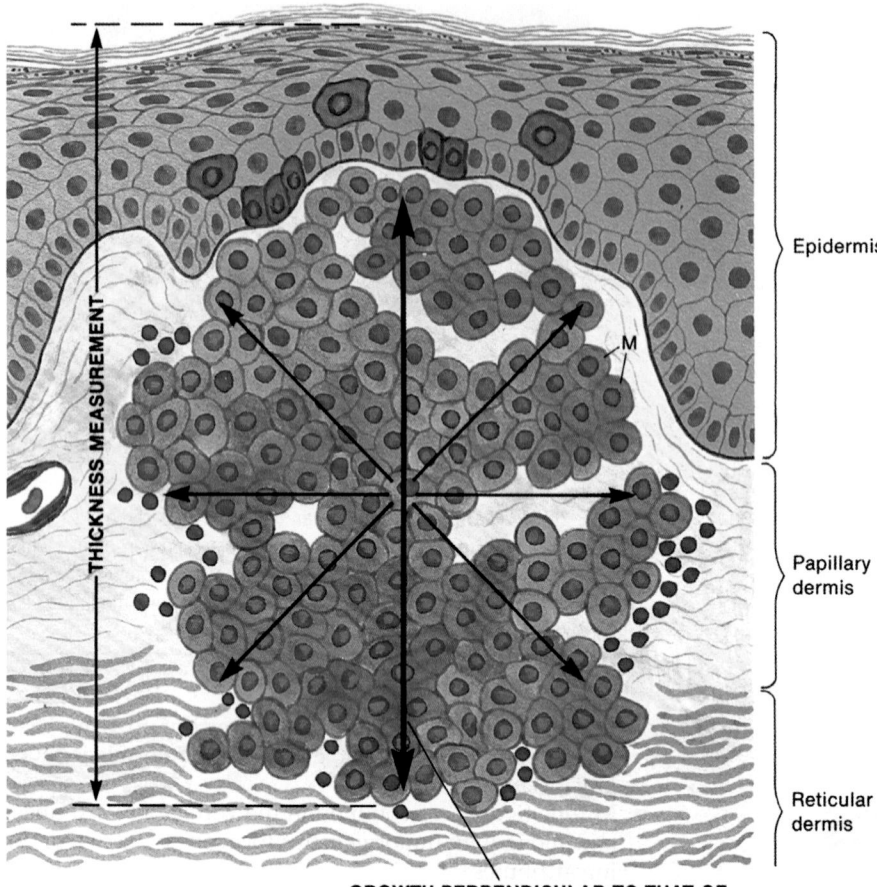

THICKNESS MEASUREMENT

Epidermis

Papillary dermis

Reticular dermis

M

GROWTH PERPENDICULAR TO THAT OF RADIAL GROWTH PHASE

FIGURE 28-56. Malignant melanoma. The evolved vertical growth phase in malignant melanoma of the superficial spreading type is shown, with an indication of how thickness is measured. In this illustration, the vertical growth phase has extended into the reticular dermis. Small nodules of tumor cells that clearly have a growth preference over other tumor cells are a manifestation of the vertical growth phase. Thickness measurements (*arrows*) are taken from the most superficial aspect of the granular layer across the tumor at its thickest point (to its deepest point of invasion).

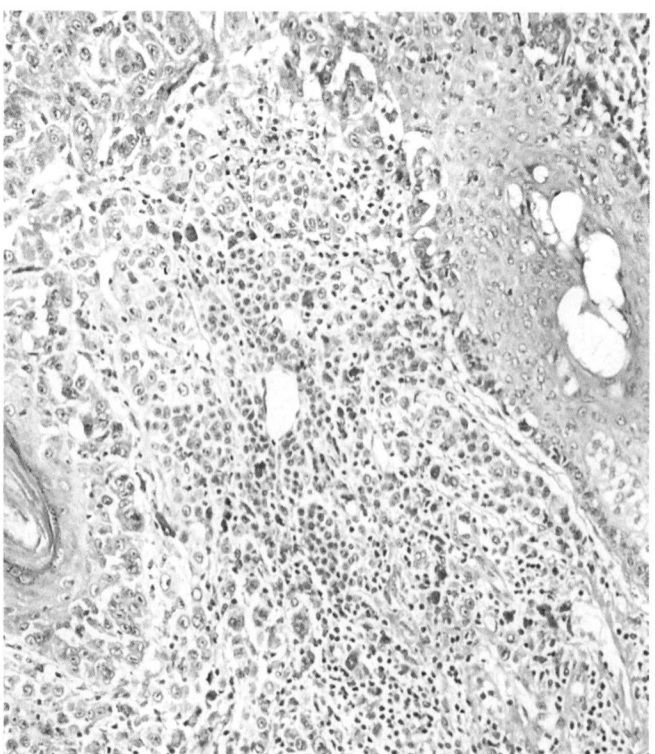

FIGURE 28-57. Malignant melanoma, vertical growth phase. The host response consists of lymphocytes infiltrating amid the melanocytes ("tumor-infiltrating lymphocytes").

- Host response (i.e., lymphocytic inflammation; Fig. 28-57) may be absent or reduced at the base of the vertical growth phase, compared to the radial growth phase.

   Not all tumors in the vertical growth phase possess the propensity to metastasize. Thus, vertical growth phase melanomas less than 1 mm thick that lack mitoses rarely metastasize. The risk of metastasis can be predicted, albeit imperfectly, through the use of prognostic models.

Nodular Melanoma

Occasionally, a melanoma "bypasses" the stepwise tumor progression described above and manifests all of its malignant characteristics in the initial lesion. Nodular melanoma is an uncommon form of the tumor (10%), which appears as a circumscribed, elevated, spheroidal nodule. It does not develop through a radial growth phase but is in the vertical growth phase when initially observed (Fig. 28-58). Nodular melanoma is composed of one or more nodules of cells that grow in an expansile fashion in the dermis (Fig. 28-59). These lesions lack most of the ABCD criteria. They may be advanced in thickness, and thus at high risk of metastasis at the time of diagnosis, despite being often small in diameter, symmetric and homogeneous in color.

Lentigo Maligna Melanoma

Lentigo maligna melanoma, also known as **Hutchinson melanotic freckle,** is a large, pigmented macule that occurs

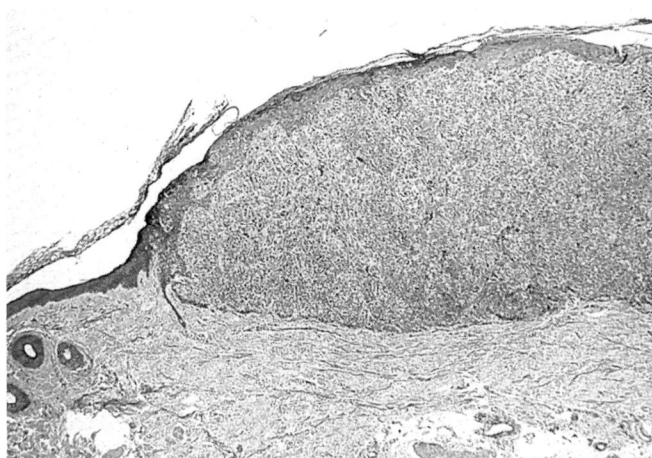

FIGURE 28-58. Malignant melanoma, nodular type. Intraepidermal growth is essentially absent. There is no radial growth lateral to the nodule. This tumor expands the papillary dermis and distorts the reticular dermal junction; it is therefore level III.

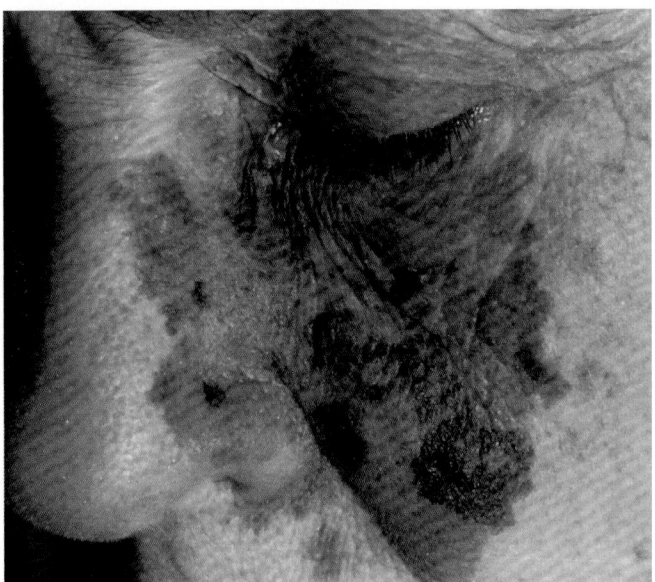

FIGURE 28-60. Malignant melanoma of the lentigo maligna type, radial growth phase.

on sun-damaged skin. It develops almost exclusively in fair-skinned, usually elderly whites, often with a history of being outdoor workers. Because it occurs on exposed body surfaces, often without history of acute sunburn injury, it is probably related to chronic ultraviolet light exposure. Lentigo maligna melanoma, like acral and mucosal melanomas (see below), is less likely than superficial spreading melanoma to be associated with mutations of *B-RAF*, while *NRAS* mutations are more common. Some of these melanomas have activating mutations of the receptor tyrosine kinase c-Kit and may be responsive, at least for a time, to c-Kit inhibitors.

PATHOLOGY: In the radial growth phase, lentigo maligna melanoma (LMM) is a flat, irregular, brown to black patch that may cover a large part of the face or dorsal hands (Fig. 28-60). The cells of the radial growth phase are predominantly in the basal layer, often forming contiguous rows of atypical single melanocytes, but occasionally forming small nests that hang down into the papillary dermis (Fig. 28-61). Although cells of the radial growth phase of LMM vary in size, they tend to be smaller and less pigmented than those of SSM and are usually associated with effacement of rete ridges and thinning of the epidermis. The subjacent dermis often shows a modest

lymphocytic infiltrate and, with only rare exceptions, solar degeneration of the connective tissue.

The clinical appearance of LMM in the vertical growth phase is shown in Fig. 28-62. Histologically, the cells in this phase tend to be spindle shaped. They occasionally provoke a connective tissue response to form a firm plaque **(desmoplastic melanoma),** which may mimic a scar or a neuroma and be difficult to diagnose histologically. Cells of the vertical growth phase, in any melanoma but especially in LMM and other lentiginous melanomas, may also grow along small nerves ("neurotropism").

Acral Lentiginous Melanoma

Acral lentiginous melanoma occurs with about equal frequency in all races. It is thus the most common form of

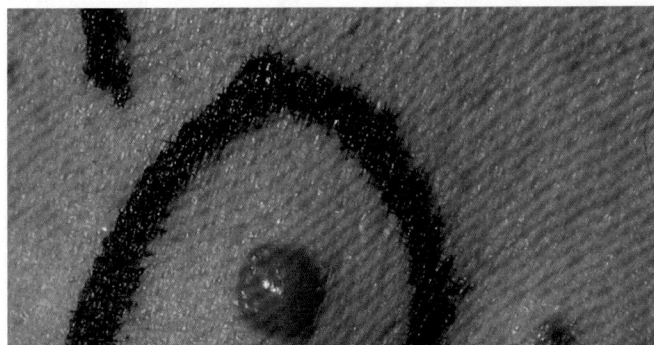

FIGURE 28-59. Malignant melanoma of the nodular type. The primary focus of growth of this 0.5-cm lesion is in the dermis.

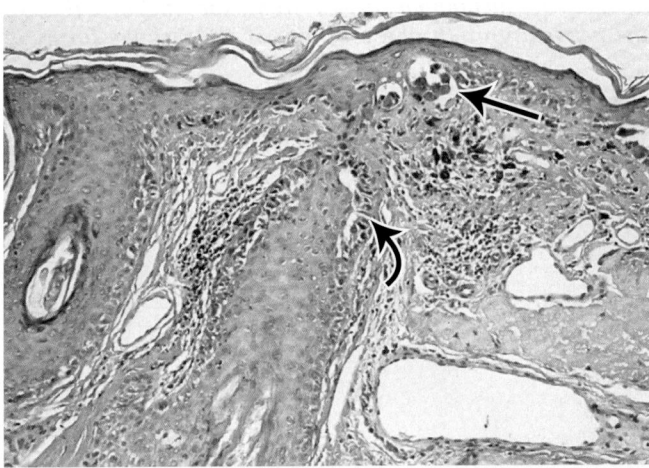

FIGURE 28-61. Lentigo maligna. Atypical melanocytes grow mostly at the dermal–epidermal interface (*straight arrow*), with extension down the external root sheath of follicles (*curved arrow*). Upward growth of melanocytes is much less prominent than in malignant melanoma of the superficial spreading type.

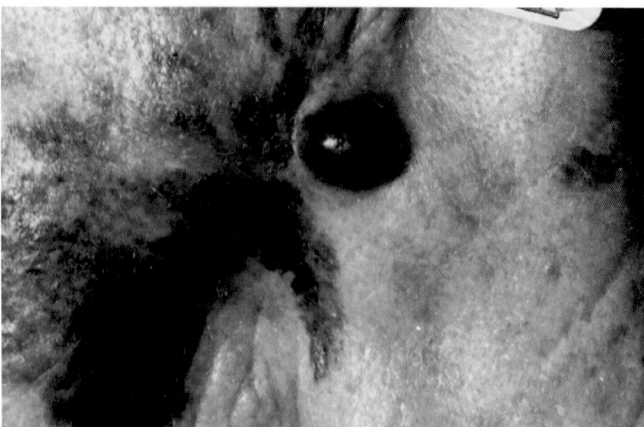

FIGURE 28-62. Lentigo maligna. The clinical appearance of the radial and vertical growth phase in malignant melanoma of the lentigo maligna type is shown. The lesion is 1 cm in diameter.

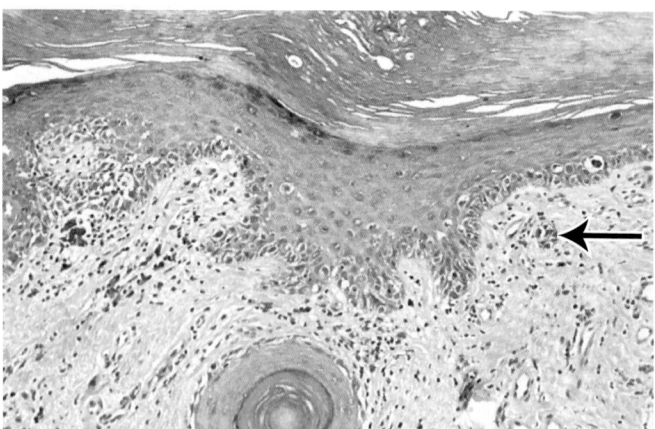

FIGURE 28-64. Malignant melanoma, acral lentiginous type, principally intraepidermal radial growth. Atypical melanocytes are present along the dermal–epidermal junction. A small dermal nest of atypical melanocytes is present (*arrow*).

melanoma in dark-skinned people. As the name implies, it is generally limited to palms, soles and subungual regions. The World Health Organization classifies "acral melanoma" to include not only lentiginous but all forms of melanoma in acral skin. Increased copy numbers and often mutations of the cell cycle marker cyclin D are common findings in these lesions.

 PATHOLOGY: In the radial growth phase, acral lentiginous melanoma forms an irregular, brown to black patch that covers a part of the palm or sole or arises under a nail, usually on a thumb or great toe (Fig. 28-63). Tumor cells are confined mostly to the basal layer of the epidermis and tend to maintain long dendrites (Figs. 28-64 and 28-65). A brisk lichenoid lymphocytic infiltrate is often seen.

The vertical growth phase (Figs. 28-66 and 28-67) is like that of lentigo maligna melanoma, in that it commonly consists of spindle cells and occasionally includes desmoplasia and neurotropism.

Metastatic Melanoma

Metastatic melanoma arises from the melanocytes of the vertical growth phase of any of the various forms of

melanoma. Initial metastases usually involve regional lymph nodes, although hematogenous spread to organs is also possible. When the latter occurs, metastases are unusually widespread in comparison with other neoplasms; virtually any organ may be involved. Metastatic melanomas may remain dormant and clinically undetectable for long periods after the apparently successful excision of a primary melanoma, only to reappear years later (see Chapter 5).

Staging and Prognosis of Melanoma

The prognosis of a patient with a melanoma is based on:

TUMOR THICKNESS: Tumor thickness, originally described by Breslow, is the strongest prognostic variable for melanomas that are apparently confined to their primary sites (stages 1 and 2 in the staging system of the American Joint Committee on Cancer [AJCC]). The "Breslow thickness" of a melanoma is measured from the most superficial aspect of the stratum granulosum to the point of maximal thickness (Fig. 28-56). Outcome may be predicted with some

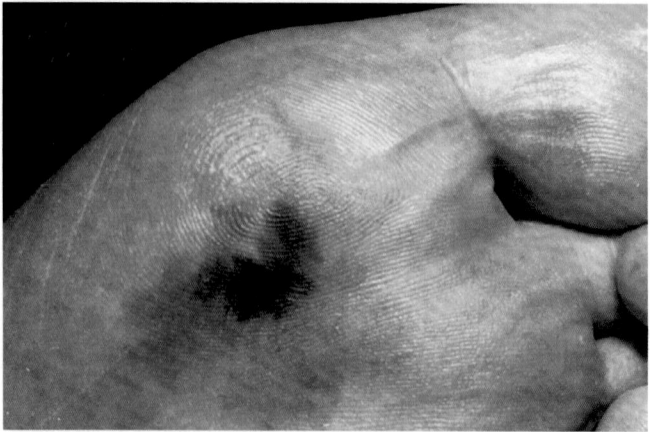

FIGURE 28-63. Malignant melanoma, acral lentiginous type (radial growth phase). The clinical appearance of the sole of the foot is depicted.

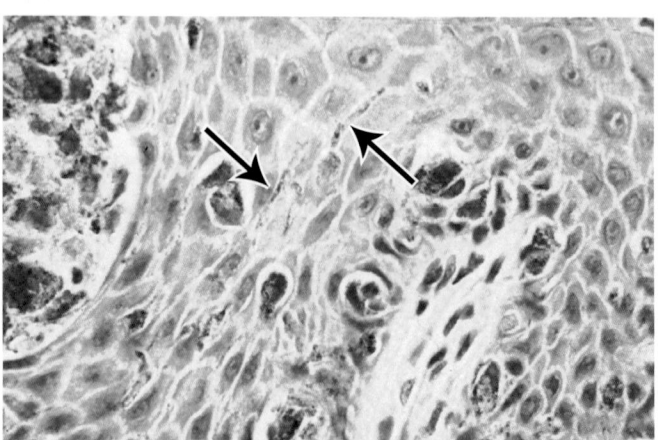

FIGURE 28-65. Malignant melanoma, acral lentiginous type. Large melanocytes with prominent dendrites (*arrows*) are present in the basilar region of the epidermis. The tumor cells contain numerous melanosomes, making the perinuclear and dendritic cytoplasms brown.

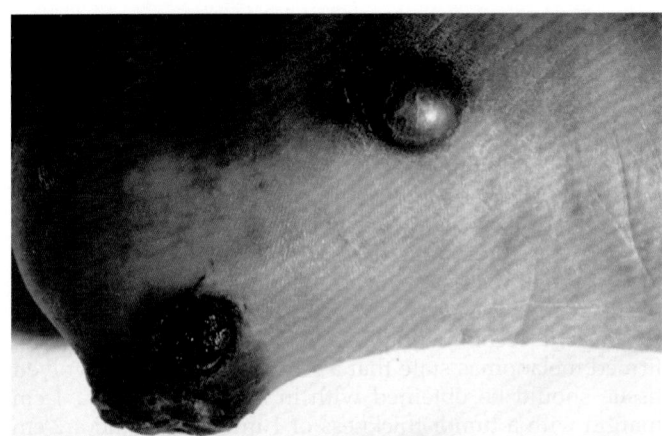

FIGURE 28-66. Malignant melanoma, acral lentiginous type. The lesion on the heel is the primary tumor. The flat portion represents the radial growth phase, while the elevated portion indicates the vertical growth phase. The dark nodule on the instep is a metastasis.

TABLE 28-2

TUMOR THICKNESS AS SOLE PREDICTOR OF OUTCOME 10 YEARS AFTER DEFINITIVE THERAPY OF PRIMARY MELANOMA

Thickness (mm)	Survival (%)
≤1	83–88
1.01–2	64–79
2.01–4	51–64
>4	32–54

accuracy by dividing tumors based on thickness. Cutoffs occur at 1-mm intervals, although the 0.76-mm cutoff originally proposed by Breslow still has merit for optimal separation of the lowest-risk melanomas. Prognosis up to 10 years after removal of the primary lesion may then be estimated from Table 28-2.

ULCERATION: Ulceration in a primary melanoma is associated with decreased survival. In one study, survival rates were 66% and 92% for patients with and without ulceration, respectively. Ulceration is a stage modifier in the AJCC system; its presence raises a lesion to the next stage in each thickness group.

DERMAL MITOTIC RATE: For tumor cells in the vertical growth phase, the mitotic rate correlates well with survival. Survival becomes progressively worse as the mitotic rate increases. The 5-year survival is 99% for patients whose tumors show no mitoses, 85% if the mitotic rate is 0.1–6.0/mm^2 and 68% with greater than 6 mitoses/mm^2. Mitogenicity, or the presence of any mitoses in the dermis, is a risk factor for recurrence in otherwise early-stage ("thin") melanomas and is a modifier of stage 1 (melanomas of thickness <1 mm).

LYMPHOCYTIC INFILTRATE: Interaction of lymphocytes with tumor cells in the vertical growth phase is an important prognostic indicator. Lymphocytes are said to be "infiltrative" when they actually penetrate and disrupt the tumor, frequently forming rosettes around tumor cells (Figs. 28-57 and 28-68). If tumor-infiltrating lymphocytes (TILs) are present throughout the vertical growth phase or are seen across the entire base of the vertical growth phase, the infiltrate is said to be "brisk." The more prevalent the TILs, the better is the prognosis. However, this and the other attributes listed below are not included in the AJCC staging system, which is the current standard of care.

LOCATION: Melanomas on the extremities have a better prognosis than those on the head, neck or trunk (axial).

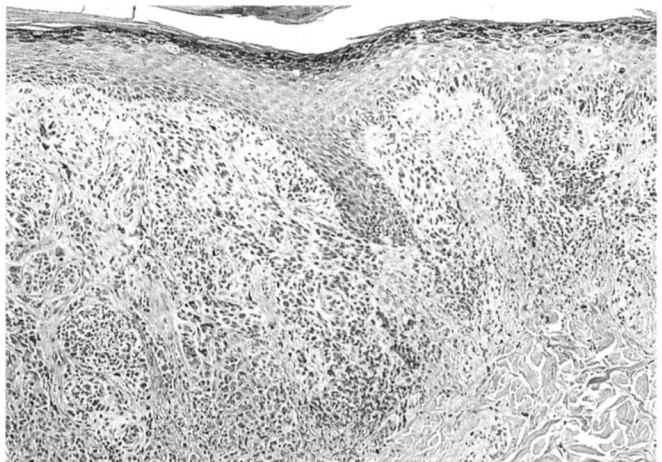

FIGURE 28-67. Malignant melanoma, acral lentiginous type, vertical growth phase. On the *left* is confluent growth of atypical dermal melanocytes filling and expanding the papillary dermis.

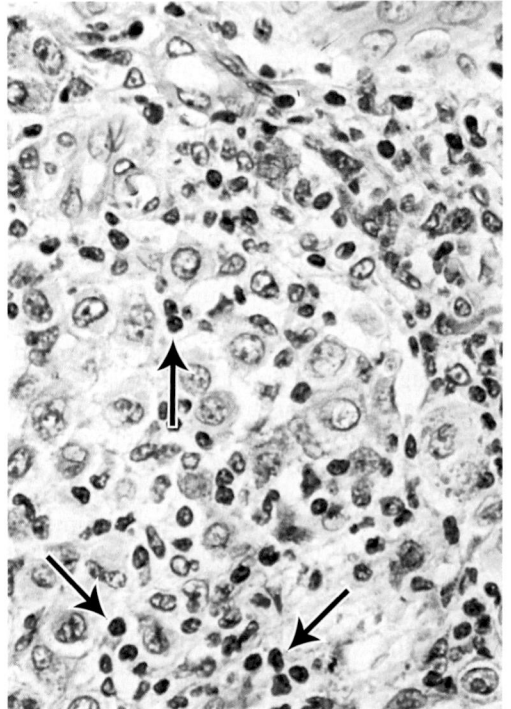

FIGURE 28-68. Malignant melanoma, vertical growth phase. Numerous tumor-infiltrating lymphocytes are arranged among individual tumor cells.

However, melanomas on the sole of the foot or the subungual region have a prognosis similar to, or worse than, axial lesions.

SEX: For every site and thickness, women have better prognoses than men. For example, women with axial melanomas 0.8–1.7 mm thick have almost 90% 10-year survival after excision of the lesion, while the comparable figure in men is 60%.

REGRESSION: Many primary melanomas show some spontaneous regression in the radial growth phase component, indicated clinically by a color change to blue-white or white. Such regression entails a widened papillary dermis, containing melanophages and a lymphocytic infiltrate, with no melanoma cells in the epidermis overlying these dermal changes. The prognostic significance of partial regression is unclear: many studies suggest that it reflects a worse prognosis, but the issue is not settled.

LEVELS OF INVASION: The Clark level system describes the degree of tumor penetration within the anatomic layers of the skin The Clark levels are not as accurate as tumor thickness in predicting risk of metastasis and are not included in the AJCC system. However, levels have prognostic significance in some subsets of cases.

- **Level I:** Tumor cells are entirely above the basement membrane (in situ).
- **Level II:** Invasive cells are present only in the papillary dermis without filling or expanding it (radial growth phase).
- **Level III:** The tumor has usually entered the vertical growth phase and impinges on the reticular dermis, forming small expansile nodules that expand and fill the papillary dermis.
- **Level IV:** Tumor cells invade between the collagen bundles of the reticular dermis.
- **Level V:** The tumor extends into the subcutaneous fat.

LYMPHATIC INVASION: Although intuitively important, this property has not been included in prognostic models because it is rarely seen in routine sections. There is recent evidence that lymphatic invasion may be more common than previously thought when enhanced detection techniques are used, and that it is prognostically significant.

STAGE: The stage of the disease is the most important single factor influencing a patient's survival. Metastasis to regional lymph nodes is now determined routinely by sentinel lymph node staging, which involves biopsy of a single node that lies first in the regional node drainage pattern. Lymph node involvement suggests an estimated 40% decrease in 5-year survival, compared with patients with clinically localized tumors. The number of involved lymph nodes is also highly predictive of prognosis. Patients with 1 positive node have a 10-year survival of 40%, compared with 25% with 2–4 positive nodes, and 15% with 5 or more nodes involved.

The tumor–node–metastasis (TNM) system of tumor staging incorporates features of the primary tumor, regional lymph nodes and soft tissues and distant metastases. The **T** (primary tumor) attributes of tumor thickness, presence or absence of ulceration and mitogenicity are classified histologically after excision of the melanoma. Numbers of lymph nodes with metastatic tumor and characterization of this tumor as micrometastasis or macrometastasis are a large part of the **N** (node) classification. **Micrometastases** are nodal metastases diagnosed after sentinel or elective lymphadenectomy; **macrometastasis** are clinically detectable nodal

metastases confirmed by therapeutic lymphadenectomy. The term "submicroscopic" metastasis has been proposed for sentinel node involvement below certain thresholds of size and penetration into the node. The **M (metastasis)** properties incorporate results of evaluation for distant metastases at various anatomic sites. TNM classification is based primarily on thickness and modified by ulceration and mitogenicity. For localized primary melanomas and for regional and systemic metastatic disease, it helps define the pathologic stage of disease, which in turn reflects the probability of survival.

Current recommendations regarding excision of confirmed melanomas state that a 5-mm margin of uninvolved tissue should be obtained with in situ melanoma, a 1-cm margin with a tumor thickness of 1 mm or less and a 2-cm margin with a tumor thickness greater than 1 mm or with Clark level IV or greater with any thickness. However, many clinicians would use a 1-cm margin, at least for tumors in the lower end of these ranges, and margins are typically adjusted so as to spare important structures, such as the eyes. Sentinel lymph node sampling is generally considered with tumor thickness greater than 1 mm or with other risk factors, including ulceration or mitogenicity (dermal mitotic activity), especially in tumors thicker than 0.75 mm. If metastatic disease ensues, targeted therapeutics, such as BRAF inhibitors, can be employed. Immunomodulatory drugs are also used, such as antibodies to CTLA-4 (cytotoxic T-lymphocyte antigen 4) and PD-1 (programmed cell death 1), to boost immune responses against malignancy.

Benign Tumors of Melanocytes May Mimic Melanoma

Congenital Melanocytic Nevus

About 1% of white children are born with some form of pigmented skin lesion, sometimes as inconspicuous as a small patch of pale tan hyperpigmentation. Much more rarely, the trunk or an extremity is covered by a large pigmented patch or plaque that is cosmetically deforming ("giant hairy" or "garment" nevus). Such areas display a striking increase in intraepidermal and dermal melanocytes, which may extend deep into the subcutaneous tissue. Malignant melanomas may develop in these large congenital melanocytic nevi, although not in the majority of cases. These melanomas may occur in childhood. Attempts are sometimes made to remove these large lesions, but their size may make surgical removal problematic.

Spitz Nevus/Tumor

Spitz tumors (also known as spindle and epithelioid cell nevi) occur in children or adolescents and, less often, in adults. They are elevated, spheroid, pink, smooth nodules, usually on the head or neck. Spitz tumors grow rapidly, reaching 3–5 mm in 6 months or less. Lesions are composed of large spindle or epithelioid melanocytes in the epidermis and dermis (Fig. 28-69). The cells, although to some extent stereotypic, are so atypical that an incorrect diagnosis of melanoma may be made, even though melanoma is rare in childhood. Most Spitz tumors are benign and are called Spitz nevi. A few have metastasized, although usually not beyond regional nodes. Therefore, the prognosis is to some extent uncertain,

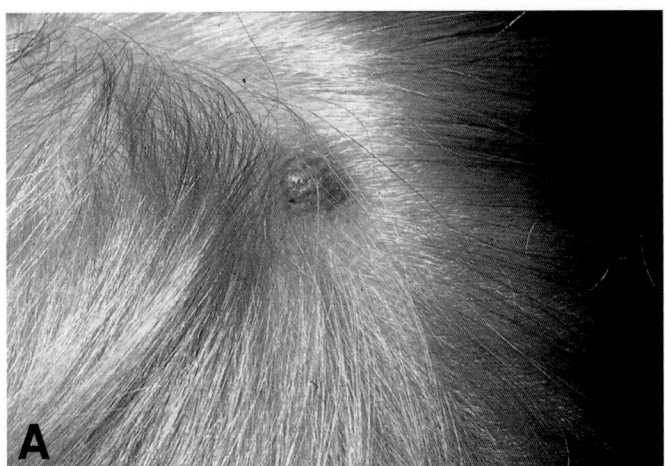
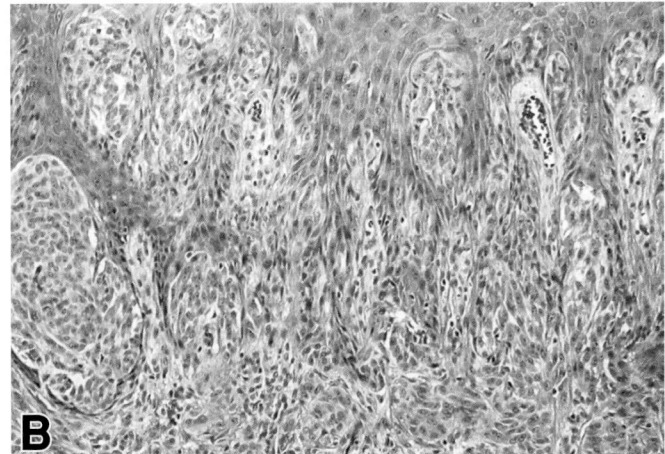

FIGURE 28-69. Spindle and epithelioid cell (Spitz) nevus. A. A symmetric pink nodule appeared suddenly in a child but then remained stable for several weeks until it was excised. **B.** Spitz tumors are composed of large melanocytes with prominent nuclei. Within a hyperplastic epidermis, the melanocytes are present in large nests. Even though the cells are large and, at first glance, suggest melanoma, they are much more uniform than the cells of most malignant melanomas.

especially in adults. Sometimes in these lesions, as in other rare categories of melanocytic tumors, a descriptive diagnosis, such as "melanocytic tumor of uncertain malignant potential" (MELTUMP), is all that can be rendered. Genomic studies that look for copy number variation in the tumor cell nuclei can provide additional information that may be of assistance in decision making regarding therapy. Most Spitz tumors have fusion gene rearrangements forming constitutively activated chimeric oncogenes, rather than the point mutations of oncogenes that are the rule in melanomas.

Blue Nevus

Blue nevi appear in childhood or late adolescence as dark blue, gray or black, firm, well-demarcated papules or nodules on the dorsal hands or feet or on the buttocks, scalp or face. Their clinical appearance may prompt an excisional biopsy to rule out nodular melanoma. Melanin-containing melanocytes with long, thin dendrites are present in the superficial to middermis, where they are often admixed with numerous melanin-containing macrophages (Fig. 28-70).

There are also rare examples of "cellular blue nevi" and "malignant blue nevi."

Freckle and Lentigo

Freckles, or **ephelides,** are small, brown macules that occur on sun-exposed skin, especially in people with fair skin (Fig. 28-71). They usually appear at about age 5. The pigmentation of a freckle deepens with exposure to sunlight and fades when light exposure ceases. A **lentigo** is a discrete, brown macule that appears at any age and on any part of the body (though a **solar lentigo,** or "liver spot," appears at an older age after long-term sun exposure) (Fig. 28-72). Unlike ephelides, the pigmentation of a lentigo does not depend on sun exposure. Ephelides show hyperpigmentation of basal keratinocytes without concomitant increases in the number of melanocytes. Lentigines, on the other hand, display elongated rete ridges, increased melanin pigment in both basal keratinocytes and melanocytes and increased melanocytes. Larger lesions may need to be biopsied to rule out lentigo maligna melanoma.

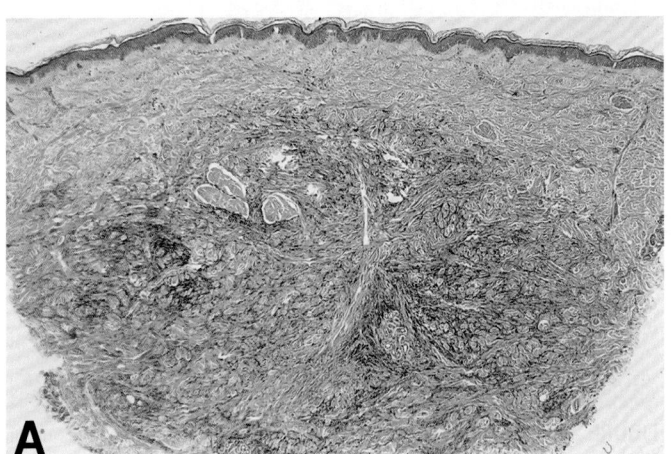
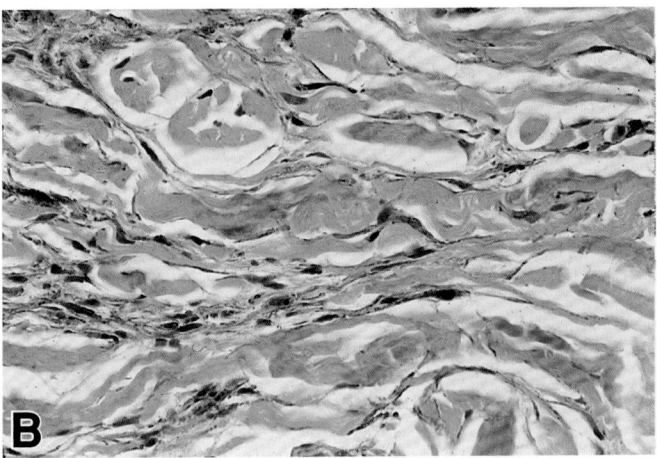

FIGURE 28-70. Blue nevus. A. Within the dermis there is a poorly defined but symmetric spindle cell proliferation that is dark brown. **B.** The lesion is composed of elongated cells with heavily pigmented dendrites and small bland nuclei.

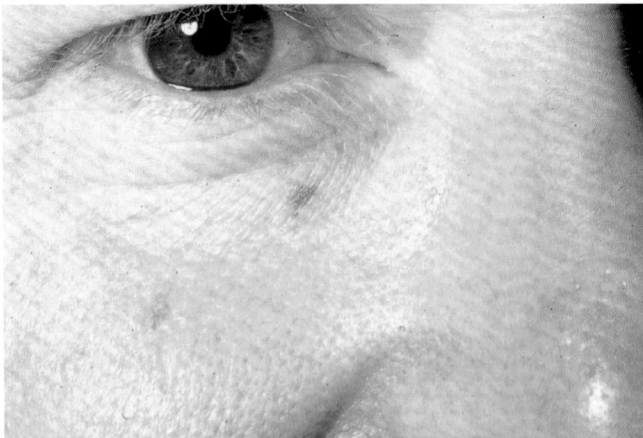

FIGURE 28-71. Freckle. A fair-complexioned man has a prominent brown macule that darkens in sunlight.

Lentigines, often called freckles by the public and by clinicians, are strong risk factors for melanoma, acting synergistically with nevi, dysplastic nevi and other risk factors. Their prevalence is strongly related to polymorphisms of the melanocortin receptor gene (*MC1R*, which has been named the "freckle gene").

Verrucae Are Warts Caused by Human Papillomavirus

Verrucae are cutaneous tumors. They are elevated, circumscribed, symmetric, epidermal proliferations that often appear papillary. *HPV is the cause of verrucae.*

 PATHOLOGY:

- **Verruca vulgaris,** or the **common wart,** is an elevated papule with a verrucous (papillomatous) surface. A papilla, the defining feature of a papilloma, is a finger of connective tissue usually containing a vessel, covered by a glove of epithelium. Such lesions may be single or multiple and occur most on the dorsal surfaces of the hands or on the face.

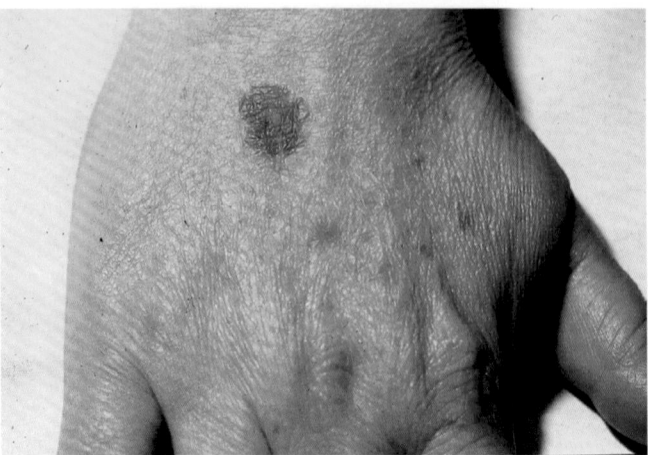

FIGURE 28-72. Lentigo. A 1-cm irregular patch of slightly variegated hyperpigmentation is present with a background of chronic solar damage.

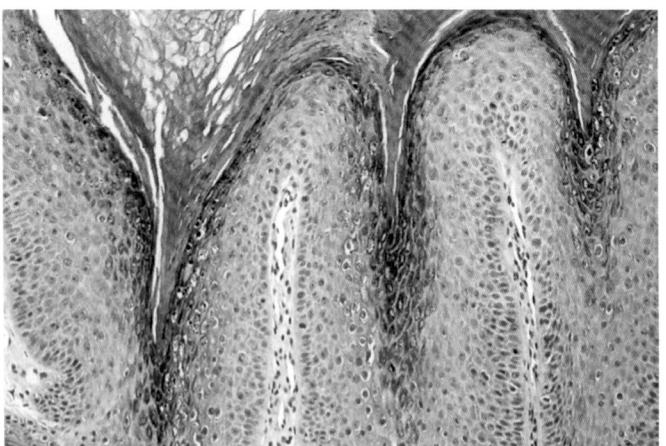

FIGURE 28-73. Verruca vulgaris. Verruca vulgaris is the prototype of papillary epidermal hyperplasia. Squamous epithelial-lined fronds have fibrovascular cores. The blood vessels within the cores extend close to the surface of verrucae, which makes them susceptible to traumatic hemorrhage and the resultant black "seeds" that patients observe.

Verruca vulgaris displays hyperkeratosis and papillary epidermal hyperplasia (Fig. 28-73). **Koilocytes** (i.e., enlarged keratinocytes with a pyknotic nucleus surrounded by a halo-like cleared area) are seen within the upper epidermis. Viral inclusions are difficult to identify (Fig. 28-74). HPV, especially serotypes 2 and 4, are commonly found in verruca vulgaris. There is no malignant potential.

- **Plantar warts** are benign, frequently painful, hyperkeratotic nodules on the soles of the feet. Occasionally, similar lesions appear on the palms of the hands **(palmar warts).** Plantar warts are endophytic or exophytic, papillary, squamous epithelial proliferations. The cells contain abundant cytoplasmic inclusions that resemble the darker-staining keratohyaline granules. The nuclei of keratinocytes near the base of these warts also contain pink nuclear inclusions. HPV type 1 is the etiologic agent.
- **Verruca plana,** or "flat warts," are small flat papules that typically appear on the face. They display slight elongation

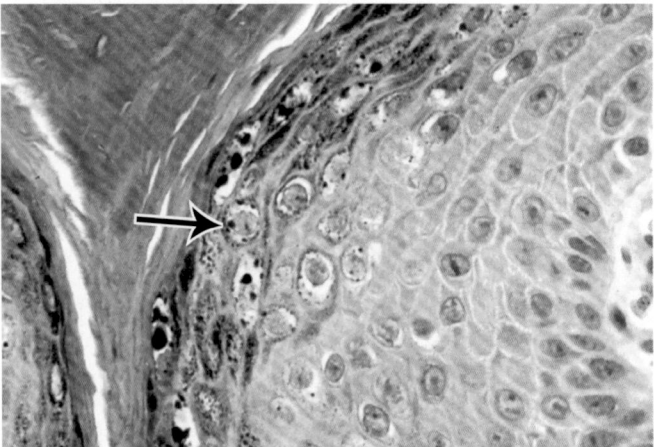

FIGURE 28-74. Verruca vulgaris. Characteristic cytopathic changes occur in the outer portion of the stratum spinosum and stratum granulosum, in which there is perinuclear vacuolization and prominent keratohyaline granules, with homogeneous blue inclusions (*arrow*).

of rete ridges (acanthosis), striking hypergranulosis and superficial koilocyte formation. HPV types 3 and 10 often elicit these lesions. The lesions do not progress to cancer.

- **Condyloma acuminatum** is a venereally transmitted wart usually caused by HPV serotypes 6 and 11 and occurring primarily around the genitalia. These are papillary squamous proliferations. Koilocytosis and an almost continuous cap of parakeratosis are usually present. Squamous carcinomas may develop, especially when HPV types 16 and 18 are involved.
- **Bowenoid papulosis,** also caused by HPV types 16 and 18, is characterized by multiple hyperpigmented papules on the genitalia. Lesions may be histologically identical to squamous cell carcinoma (SCC) in situ in that they display disordered epithelial maturation and scattered keratinocyte atypia. The lesions also exhibit parakeratosis and irregular acanthosis. Although Bowenoid papulosis often regresses, it may progress to dysplasia or malignancy.
- **Epidermodysplasia verruciformis** is a rare autosomal recessive disease characterized by impaired cell-mediated immunity and subsequent enhanced susceptibility to HPV infection. Warts similar to those of verruca plana, with confluence into patches, are widespread. It first appears in childhood, and squamous cell carcinoma develops in 30%–60% of patients. HPV types 5, 8, 9 and 47 are most common.

Keratosis Is a Benign Horny Growth Composed of Keratinocytes

Seborrheic Keratosis

Seborrheic keratoses are scaly, frequently pigmented, elevated papules or plaques with scales that are easily rubbed off. They are common later in life but their etiology is unknown. Seborrheic keratoses tend to be familial. Clinically and microscopically, they appear "pasted on" and contain broad anastomosing cords of mature stratified squamous epithelium, forming papillae and associated with small cysts of keratin (horn cysts) (Fig. 28-75). Seborrheic keratoses are innocuous but are a cosmetic nuisance. The sudden appearance of many seborrheic keratoses may be associated with internal malignancies ("sign of Leser-Trélat"), especially gastric adenocarcinoma.

Actinic Keratosis

Actinic keratoses ("from the sun's rays") are keratinocytic neoplasms that develop in sun-damaged skin as circumscribed keratotic patches or plaques, commonly on the backs of the hands or the face. The stratum corneum is no longer loose and basket-weaved but is replaced by a dense parakeratotic scale. The basal keratinocytes show significant atypia (Fig. 28-76). Actinic keratoses may evolve into squamous carcinomas in situ and finally into invasive cancers, but most are stable and many regress.

Keratoacanthoma

Keratoacanthomas are rapidly growing keratotic papules on sun-exposed skin that develop over 3–6 weeks into crater-like nodules. They reach a maximum size of 2–3 cm. Spontaneous regression usually follows within 6–12 months, leaving an atrophic scar. Some lesions may cause considerable damage before they regress, and some fail to regress. Keratoacanthomas are considered by some to be self-resolving variants of squamous cell carcinoma.

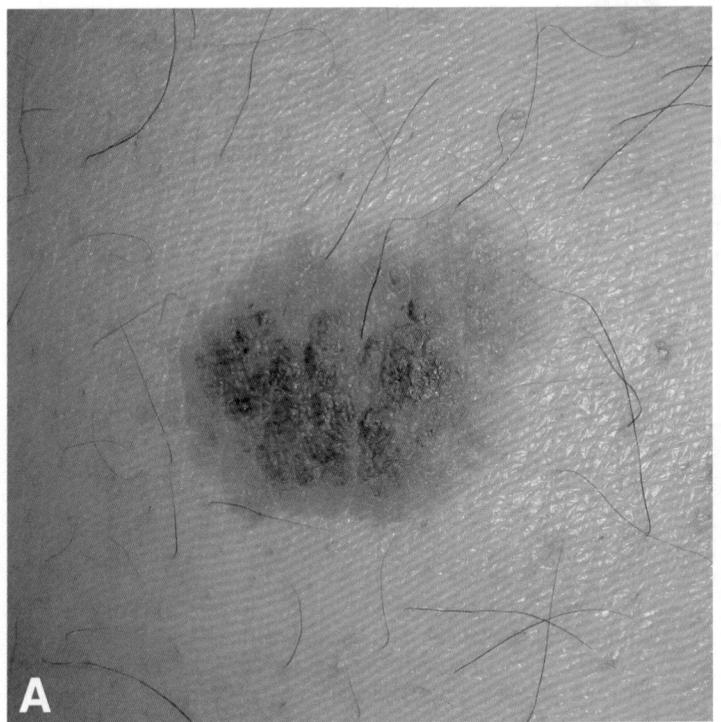
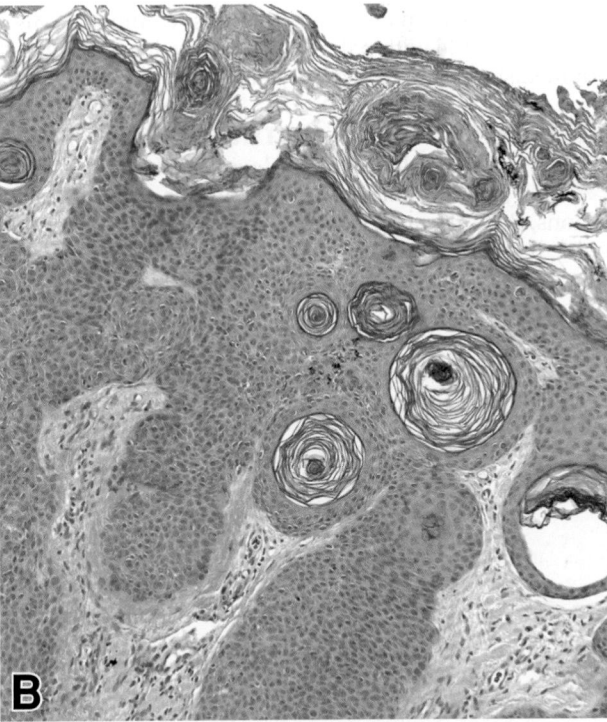

FIGURE 28-75. Seborrheic keratosis. A. Sharply defined, "stuck-on" brown lesions are a common presentation. **B.** Broad anastomosing cords of mature stratified squamous epithelium are associated with small keratin cysts.

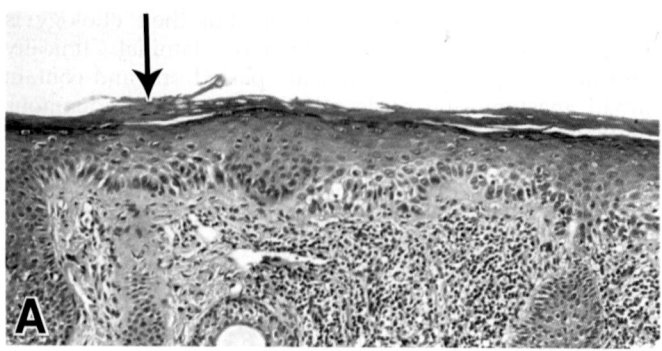
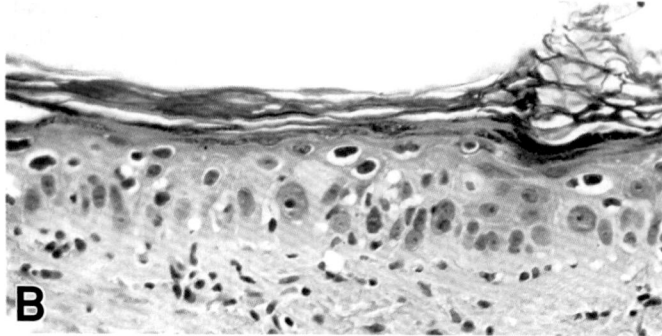

FIGURE 28-76. Actinic keratosis. A. A low-power view reveals cytologic atypia within the stratum basalis and lower stratum spinosum with loss of polarity. A lichenoid, band-like, lymphocytic infiltrate is frequently present. Parakeratosis is present here only in a small focus (*arrow*). **B.** High-power examination of an actinic keratosis reveals striking cytologic atypia of the basal keratinocytes, the hallmark of actinic keratoses.

PATHOLOGY: Histologically, keratoacanthomas are endophytic proliferations of keratinocytes. The lesion is cup shaped, with a central, keratin-filled umbilication and overhanging ("buttressing") epidermal edges (Fig. 28-77). At the base of the keratin, keratinocytes are large and have abundant homogeneous, eosinophilic ("glassy") cytoplasm. At the lower aspect of the lesion, irregular tongues of squamous epithelium infiltrate the collagen of the reticular dermis. Older lesions show active fibroplasia in the dermis around these tongues. There may be focal lichenoid inflammation, and the dermis may be markedly infiltrated with neutrophils, lymphocytes and eosinophils. Microabscesses of neutrophils and entrapped dermal elastic fibers are often present within the lesion.

Basal Cell Carcinoma Is a Locally Invasive Epidermal Neoplasm

Basal cell carcinoma (BCC) is the most common malignant tumor in people with pale skin. It may be locally aggressive, but metastases are exceedingly rare.

MOLECULAR PATHOGENESIS: *BCC usually develops on sun-damaged skin of people with fair skin and freckles.* However, unlike squamous lesions, BCC also arises on areas not exposed to intense sunlight. It is unusual to find BCC on the fingers and dorsal surfaces of the hands. The tumor is thought to derive from pluripotential cells in the basal layer of the epidermis, more specifically, in the bulge region of the hair follicle.

In several heritable syndromes, BCC originates on skin that has had little light exposure. In **nevoid BCC syndrome,** multiple tumors occur in the context of a complex multisystem disease. The syndrome also includes pits (dyskeratoses) on the palms and soles, mandibular cysts, hypertelorism and a predisposition to other neoplasms, including medulloblastoma. The BCCs of this syndrome appear at a young age and may number in the hundreds.

Germline mutations in the *PTCH* tumor suppressor gene on chromosome 9q22 cause nevoid BCC syndrome. Somatic mutations in *PTCH* have been implicated in up to 90% of sporadic BCCs and may be targeted in therapy of advanced lesions.

PATHOLOGY: BCCs contain nests of deeply basophilic epithelial cells with narrow rims of cytoplasm that are attached to the epidermis and protrude into the subjacent papillary dermis (Fig. 28-78). At least in early lesions, there is typically a specialized loose mucinous stroma containing fibroblasts and lymphocytes. Clefting artifact between the epithelial cells of the tumor and the stroma may sometimes help to distinguish BCC from

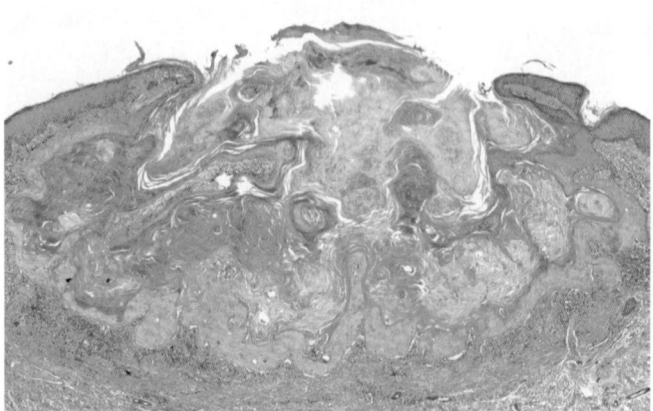

FIGURE 28-77. Keratoacanthoma. A keratin-filled crater (*center*) is lined by glassy proliferating keratinocytes.

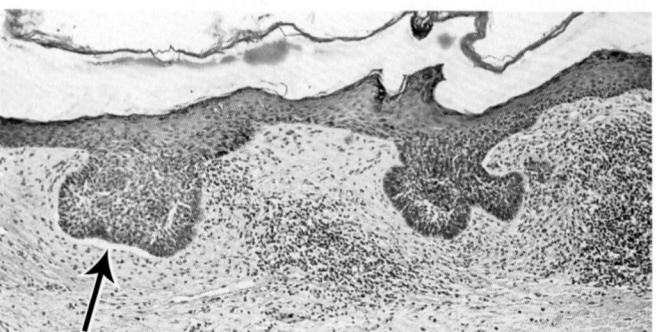

FIGURE 28-78. Basal cell carcinoma, superficial type. Buds of atypical basaloid keratinocytes extend from the overlying epidermis into the papillary dermis. The peripheral keratinocytes mimic the stratum basalis by palisading. The separation artifact (*arrow*) is present because of poorly formed basement membrane components and the hyaluronic acid-rich stroma that contains collagenase.

other adnexal neoplasms with basaloid cell proliferation. The central part of each nest contains closely packed keratinocytes that are slightly smaller than normal epidermal basal keratinocytes and show occasional apoptosis and mitoses. The periphery of each nest shows an organized layer of polarized, columnar keratinocytes, with the long axis of each cell perpendicular to the surrounding stroma ("peripheral palisading"). **Superficial, multicentric BCC** is composed of apparently isolated, but actually interconnected, nests that usually remain confined to the papillary dermis and manifest clinically as a spreading plaque. **Nodulocystic BCC** is also attached to the epidermis and exhibits the same cytologic and architectural features as the superficial type of BCC but grows more deeply into the dermis. Usually, tumor cells of the dermal islands are associated with a mucinous ground substance and are surrounded by an array of fibroblasts and lymphocytes. An important distinction is between BCCs with pushing borders and those with an infiltrative pattern, because the latter may be more likely to recur locally and to progress. Infiltrating BCCs with particularly dense sclerotic stroma are called **morpheaform BCCs** because of a clinical resemblance to lesions of localized scleroderma (also known as "morphea").

 CLINICAL FEATURES: Common forms of BCC include:

- **Pearly papule** is the prototypic nodulocystic type of lesion, so named because it resembles a 2–3-mm pearl (Fig. 28-79). It is covered by tightly stretched epidermis and is laced with small, delicate, branching vessels (telangiectasia).
- **Rodent ulcer** is a small crater in the center of the pearl.
- **Superficial BCC** appears as a scaly, red, sharply demarcated plaque.
- **Morpheaform BCC** is a pale, firm, scar-like tumor that is ill-defined on and especially beneath the skin surface, making it particularly difficult to eradicate.
- **Pigmented BCC** may grossly resemble malignant melanoma. The pigment comes from reactive melanocytes that populate the tumor.

Treatment of BCC usually involves various excision or eradication procedures.

Cells of Squamous Cell Carcinomas May Resemble Differentiated Keratinocytes

SCCs are second only to BCCs in skin cancer incidence. SCCs are most common on sun-damaged skin of fair individuals with light hair and freckles, and often originate in actinic keratoses. They are exceedingly rare on normal black skin.

 ETIOLOGIC FACTORS: SCCs have multiple causes, UV light being the most common, but also including ionizing radiation, chemical carcinogens and HPV. SCCs arising in sun-damaged skin metastasize rarely (<2%). They may also arise in chronic scarring processes, such as osteomyelitis sinus tracts, burn scars ("Marjolin ulcers") and areas of radiation dermatitis. In these settings, they metastasize more often. Over 90% of SCCs, and many actinic keratoses, have mutated *TP53* genes.

 PATHOLOGY: SCC is composed of tumor cells that mimic epidermal stratum spinosum in varying degrees and extend into the subjacent dermis (Fig. 28-80). The edges of many tumors show changes typical of actinic keratosis, namely, a variably thickened epidermis with parakeratosis and significant atypia of basal keratinocytes.

 CLINICAL FEATURES: SCCs characteristically arise in chronically sun-exposed areas such as the backs of the hands, face, lips and ears (Fig. 28-80A). Early lesions are small, scaly or ulcerated, erythematous papules, which may be pruritic. They are usually treated by excision, or sometimes by electrosurgery, topical chemotherapy or radiation therapy.

Merkel Cell Carcinomas Are Aggressive Tumors of Neurosecretory Cells That Show Epithelial Differentiation

These are typically solitary, dome-shaped, red to violaceous nodules or indurated plaques on the skin of the head and neck in elderly white patients. Merkel cell carcinomas

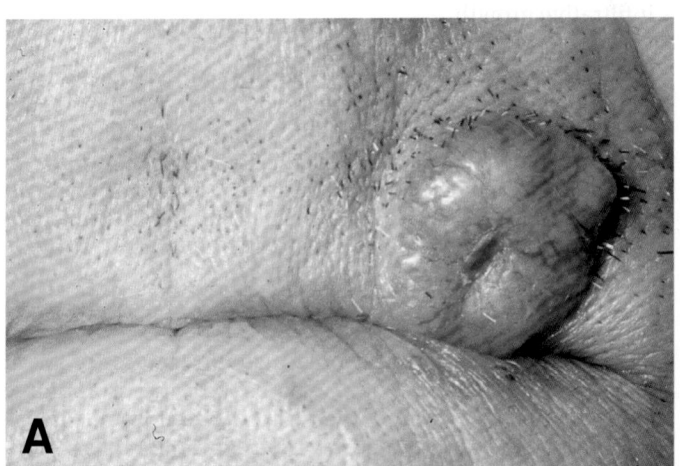
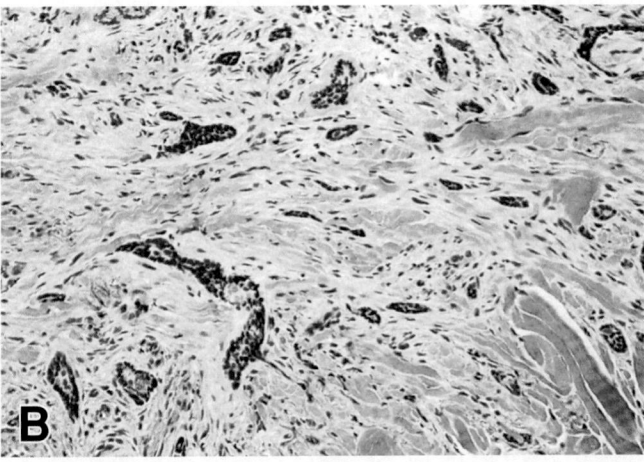

FIGURE 28-79. Basal cell carcinoma (BCC). A. Pearly papule: the tumor exhibits typical rolled pearly borders with telangiectases and central ulceration. **B.** Microscopic examination of morpheaform BCC shows a sclerosing and infiltrative lesion. Irregularly branching strands of tumor cells permeate the dermis, with induction of a cellular, fibroblastic, hyaluronic acid–rich stroma.

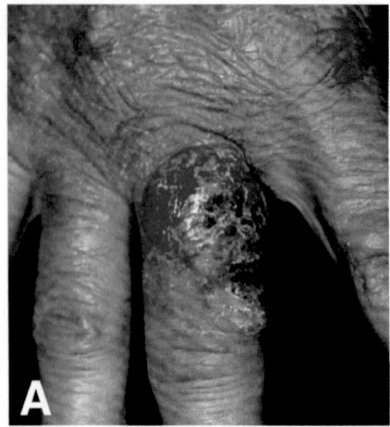
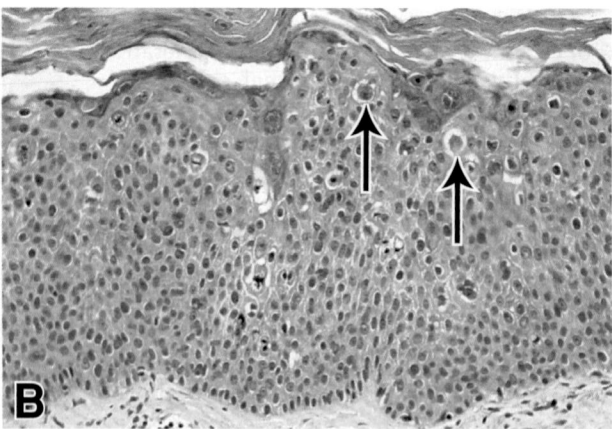

FIGURE 28-80. Squamous cell carcinoma. A. An ulcerated, encrusted and infiltrating lesion is seen on the sun-exposed dorsal aspect of a finger. **B.** A microscopic view of the periphery of the lesion shows squamous cell carcinoma in situ. The entire epidermis is replaced by atypical keratinocytes. Mitoses are apparent, as is apoptosis (*arrows*).

(MCCs) are aggressive tumors that are lethal in 25%–70% of patients within 5 years.

 PATHOLOGY: Most MCCs have large nests of undifferentiated cells that resemble small cell carcinoma of the lung (Fig. 28-81). Peripherally, the tumors may show a trabecular pattern. Nuclear chromatin is dense and evenly distributed, cytoplasm is scant and mitotic figures and nuclear fragments are common. Cytokeratin 20 is distributed in a "perinuclear dot" cytoplasmic pattern. Tumor cells also express neuroendocrine markers such as chromogranin and synaptophysin.

MOLECULAR PATHOGENESIS: The genome of Merkel cell polyoma virus (MCV) is present in 75% of MCCs and may play a role in tumorigenesis. However, MCV is a common virus and association with MCCs is still speculative (see Chapter 5). Tumorigenicity is associated with a truncating mutation of the MCV *Tag* gene.

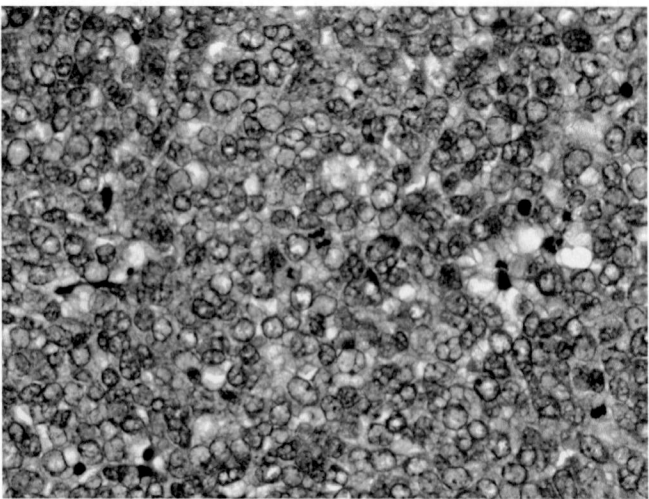

FIGURE 28-81. Merkel cell carcinoma. The tumor is composed of solid nests of undifferentiated cells that resemble small cell carcinoma of the lung.

Adnexal Tumors Differentiate toward Skin Appendages

Adnexal tumors appear as elevated small skin nodules that often occur in people with family histories of similar tumors. The lesions often appear at puberty. Although most are benign, malignant behavior is sometimes observed.

Sebaceous Neoplasms

Sebaceous neoplasms, including sebaceous adenomas, sebaceous epitheliomas (sebaceomas) and sebaceous carcinomas, are all tumors of sebaceous gland derivation. Clinically, sebaceous adenomas and epitheliomas are small, slow-growing papules or nodules commonly on the head and neck. Sebaceous carcinomas, however, often present larger than 1 cm and have a predilection for periocular sites. Histopathologically, sebaceous adenomas show a well-circumscribed proliferation of sebaceous lobules, primarily composed of mature sebocytes with some germinative basaloid cells. Sebaceous epitheliomas have a preponderance of germinative cells. Sebaceous carcinomas show histologic signs of malignancy, such as severe cytologic atypia, high mitotic activity and infiltrative growth.

MOLECULAR PATHOGENESIS: Patients with Muir-Torre syndrome, a variant of hereditary non-polyposis colorectal carcinoma (HNPCC), present with sebaceous neoplasms. HNPCC (or Lynch syndrome) is associated with inherited germline defects in mismatch repair genes such MLH1, MSH2 and MSH6 (Fig. 28-82). See Chapters 5 and 19 for more about HNPCC.

Cylindroma

Cylindromas are adnexal neoplasms with features of sweat gland differentiation. They may be solitary or multiple elevated nodules around the scalp. An autosomal dominant, heritable variant features multiple tumors. Occasionally, they become large and cluster about the head ("turban tumors"). Cylindromas show sharply circumscribed nests of deeply basophilic cells surrounded by a hyalinized, thickened BMZ (Fig. 28-83).

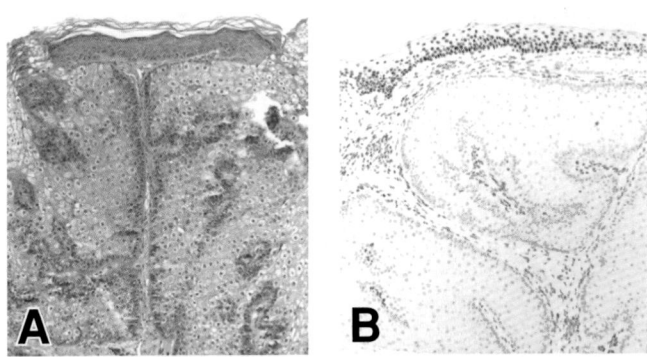

FIGURE 28-82. Sebaceous Adenoma. A. Microscopic view of sebaceous adenoma showing large sebaceous lobules composed primarily of clear sebocytes lined by basaloid germinative cells. **B.** Immunohistochemical staining for mismatch repair protein MSH6 shows loss of nuclear staining in the neoplastic sebaceous cells with intact staining in the benign surface epithelium and in intermixed dermal fibroblasts, indicating this patient may have Muir-Torre syndrome.

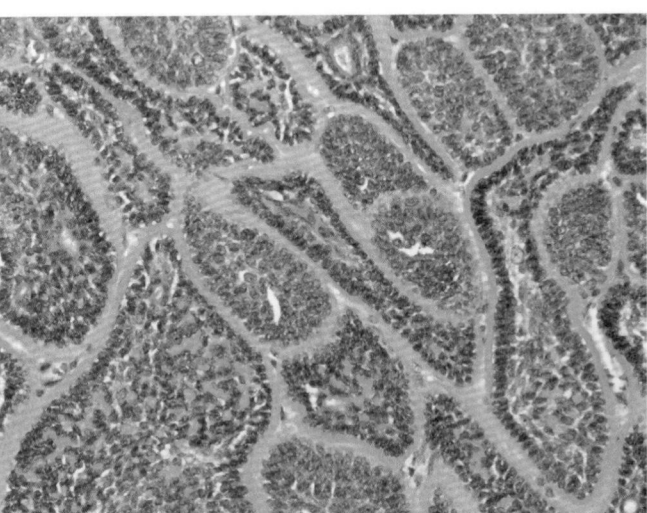

FIGURE 28-83. Cylindroma. Sharply circumscribed islands of basophilic epithelial cells reside in a jigsaw puzzle–like array. Dense eosinophilic hyaline sheaths surround each island.

Syringoma

Syringomas typically occur about the eyelid and upper cheek as small, elevated, flesh-colored papules. Small ducts resembling intraepidermal portions of eccrine sweat ducts are seen (Fig. 28-84).

Poroma

Poroma is a common, solitary neoplasm histologically similar to seborrheic keratosis but with narrow ductal lumina and occasional cystic spaces. The pattern has been interpreted as eccrine sweat gland differentiation. These tumors are firm, raised lesions, usually less than 2 cm in diameter, that develop on the sole or sides of the foot or on the hands or fingers. Poromas extend from the lower portion of the epidermis into the dermis as broad, anastomosing bands of uniform, cuboidal cells. Occasional malignant lesions with similar differentiation are called **porocarcinomas**.

Trichoepithelioma

Trichoepithelioma is a neoplasm that differentiates toward hair structures. It is usually a solitary lesion, but in "multiple

trichoepithelioma syndrome," it occurs as an autosomal dominant trait. Lesions begin to appear at puberty, on the face, scalp, neck and upper trunk. Trichoepitheliomas resemble basal cell carcinomas but contain many "horn cysts" (keratinized centers surrounded by basophilic epithelial cells).

Fibrohistiocytic Tumors of the Skin Show a Varied Spectrum of Differentiation

Dermatofibroma

Dermatofibroma is a common, benign tumor of fibroblast-like cells and macrophages. The former are the neoplastic cells. These tumors occur on the extremities as dome-shaped, firm nodules with ill-defined borders and pink to dark brown pigmentation. They rarely exceed 5 mm. The papillary and reticular dermis are replaced by fibrous tissue that forms ill-defined small cartwheels, with small central vascular spaces (Fig. 28-85). The tumors are not well demarcated and blend

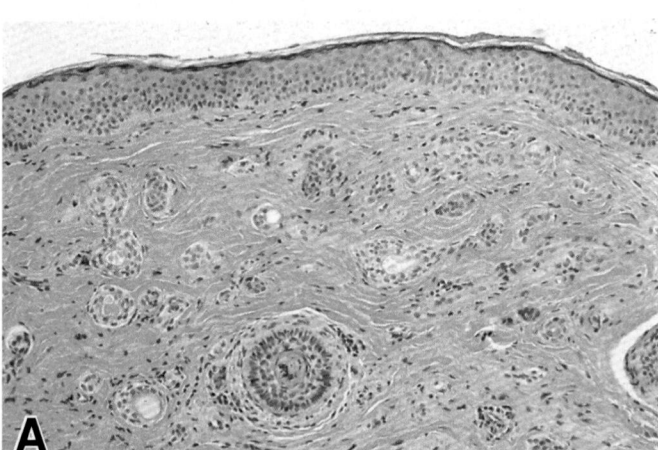

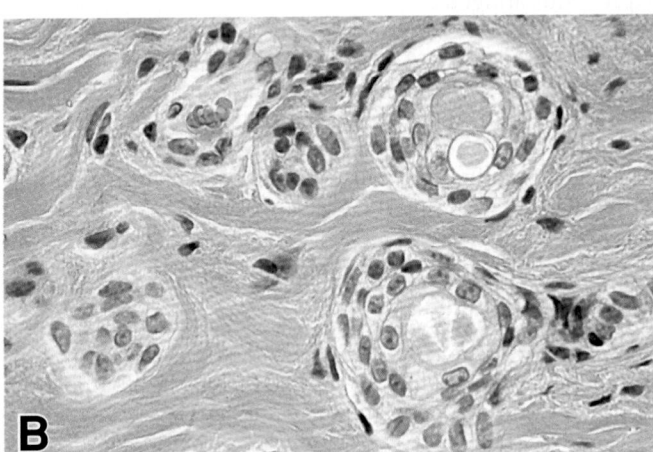

FIGURE 28-84. Syringoma. A. Within the upper dermis is an epithelial proliferation forming ducts, tubules and solid islands amid a dense fibrous stroma. **B.** The ductal differentiation closely mimics that of the straight dermal eccrine duct, with a central lumen and cuticle formation.

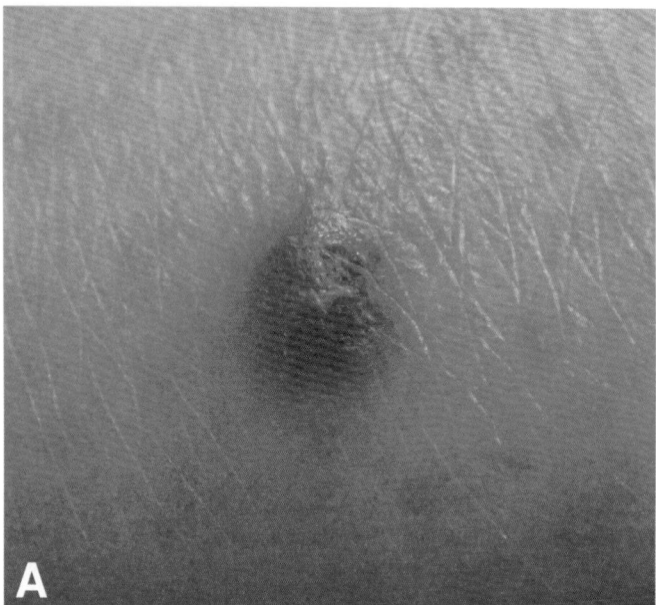
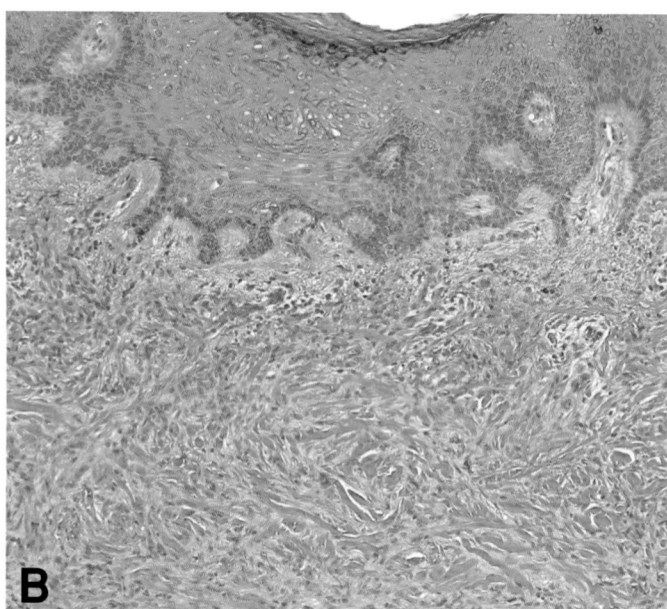

FIGURE 28-85. Dermatofibroma. A. A brown dome-shaped nodule occurring on the lower leg is a common clinical presentation. **B.** Fibrous tissue replaces the dermis and forms poorly defined cartwheels, with overlying epidermal hyperplasia and basaloid proliferation, resembling basal cell carcinoma.

into the surrounding dermis. The overlying epidermis is hyperplastic and often hyperpigmented.

Dermatofibrosarcoma Protuberans

Dermatofibrosarcoma protuberans (DFSP), a tumor with intermediate malignant potential, is a slowly growing nodule or indurated plaque that appears mostly on the trunk of young adults. Local recurrence after attempted complete excision is common, but metastases are rare. The most common histologic pattern is a poorly circumscribed, monotonous population of spindle cells arranged in a dense "storiform" (pinwheel-like) array (Fig. 28-86). The tumor extends into the subcutis along fat septa and interstices, creating an infiltrative, honeycomb-like pattern. Tumor cells display CD34, a marker of endothelial cells, and some neural tumor cells, as well as dermal fibroblast-like dendritic cells, the probable cell of origin. Positivity for CD34 may help distinguish this tumor from a dermatofibroma, which does not express this antigen.

 MOLECULAR PATHOGENESIS: More than 90% of DFSPs have a chromosomal translocation t(17;22), which fuses the collagen gene (*COL1A1*) with the *PDGF-B* gene. This balanced translocation creates a fusion gene product that causes transcriptional upregulation of the *PDGF-B* gene and increased neoplastic growth.

Mycosis Fungoides Is a Variant of Cutaneous T-Cell Lymphoma

The etiology of mycosis fungoides (MF) is unknown, but this malignancy of helper T cells (CD4⁺) may be a pathologic response to chronic exposure to an antigen.

PATHOLOGY: In the early stages of the disease, delicate, erythematous plaques appear, often by the buttocks. These plaques show psoriasiform

changes in the epidermis. The early inflammatory cell infiltrates in the dermis are polymorphic and are often not diagnostic of MF.

Skin involvement becomes progressively more prominent and infiltrative (Fig. 28-87). The most important histologic feature of MF is the presence of lymphocytes in the epidermis ("epidermotropism"). In later stages, the dermal infiltrate becomes dense to the point of forming tumor nodules. Increasing numbers of atypical lymphocytes that display hyperchromatic, convoluted ("cerebriform") nuclei are seen in the papillary dermis and epidermis. Circumscribed nests of these atypical lymphocytes ("Pautrier microabscesses") eventually involve the epidermis. T-cell receptor gene rearrangement studies show a clonal cell population.

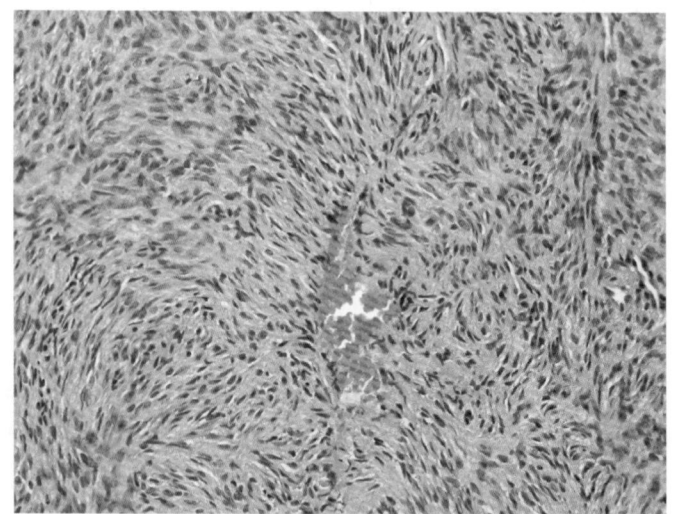

FIGURE 28-86. Dermatofibrosarcoma protuberans. Tumor cells form small cartwheels with central vascular spaces.

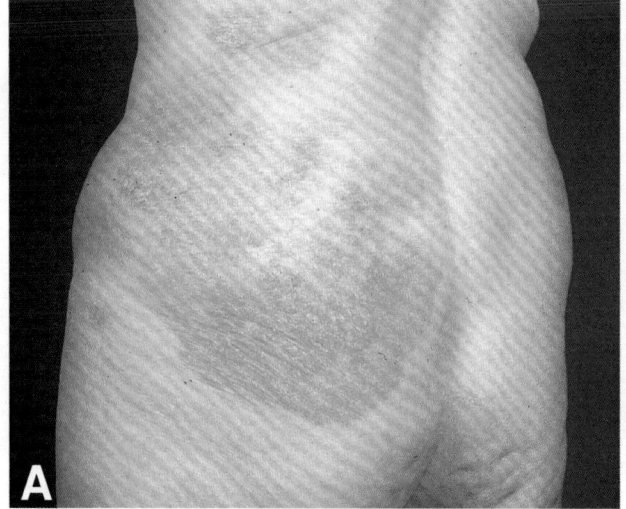

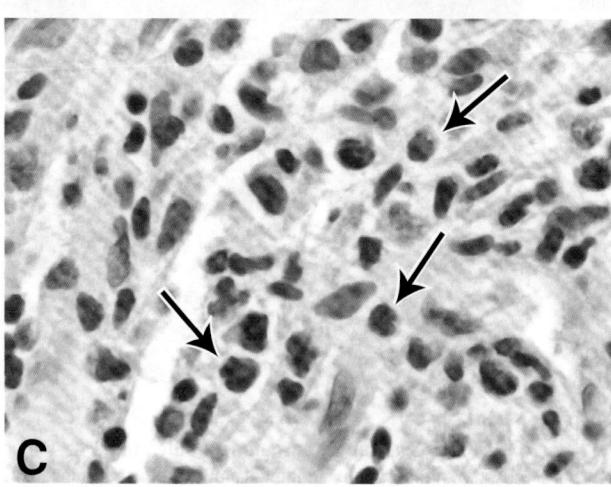

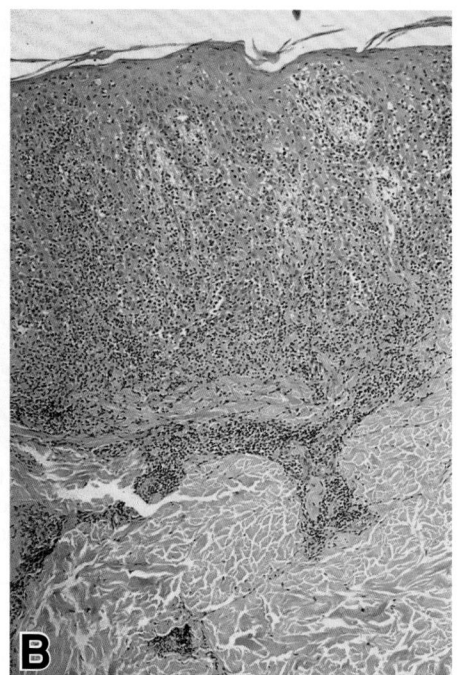

FIGURE 28-87. Mycosis fungoides. A. A 66-year-old woman presented with a 30-year history of erythematous scaly patches and plaques with telangiectases, atrophy and pigmentation. **B.** An atypical infiltrate of lymphocytes expands the papillary dermis and extends into the epidermis ("epidermotropism"). **C.** Some of the lymphocytes display hyperchromatic and convoluted ("cerebriform") nuclei (*arrows*).

Sézary syndrome is the systemic dissemination of MF. The characteristic feature is the presence of cerebriform lymphocytes in the peripheral blood.

 CLINICAL FEATURES: MF affects older people, has a slight male predominance and preferentially affects blacks over whites. It is classically divided into 3 stages: patch, plaque and tumor. In the patch stage, which may persist for months, eruptions consist of scaly, erythematous macules that may be slightly indurated. They usually involve the lower abdomen, buttocks and upper thighs as well as women's breasts, and can mimic other dermatitides such as psoriasis or eczema (Fig. 28-87A). Plaque-stage lesions are more infiltrated and circumscribed. As these coalesce, involvement becomes more widespread. Large, variably shaped tumor nodules can form on existing indurated plaques or on apparently normal skin. Spread to lymph nodes or visceral involvement portends reduced survival. Therapy includes UV light, topical nitrogen mustard and electron beam therapy.

HIV Infection Is Associated with Various Skin Diseases

Kaposi Sarcoma

This malignant tumor of endothelial cells of blood vessels was once seen only in older people of Mediterranean descent or in Africans. With the advent of HIV infection, Kaposi sarcoma (KS) is most often seen in patients with AIDS. *Human herpesvirus 8 (HHV8) is the etiologic agent of KS.*

 PATHOLOGY: All cases of Kaposi sarcoma, whether associated with HIV or not, evolve through three stages: patch, plaque and nodule. In the patch stage, a subtle proliferation of irregular vascular channels, lined by a single layer of mildly atypical endothelial cells, radiates from preexisting blood vessels and extends almost imperceptibly into the surrounding reticular dermis. Extravasated red blood cells, hemosiderin deposition and a sparse inflammatory infiltrate of lymphocytes and plasma cells are common.

In the plaque stage (Fig. 28-88), the entire reticular dermis is involved, with frequent extension into the subcutis and formation of bundles of spindle cells. In the nodule stage (Fig. 28-89), well-circumscribed dermal nodules are composed of anastomosing fascicles of spindle cells surrounding numerous slit-like spaces. HHV8 nuclear expression can be readily demonstrated with an immunohistochemical stain.

Bacillary Angiomatosis

Bacillary angiomatosis is a pseudoneoplastic proliferation of capillaries that arises in response to infection with *Bartonella* species. Patients with late-stage AIDS are at risk for

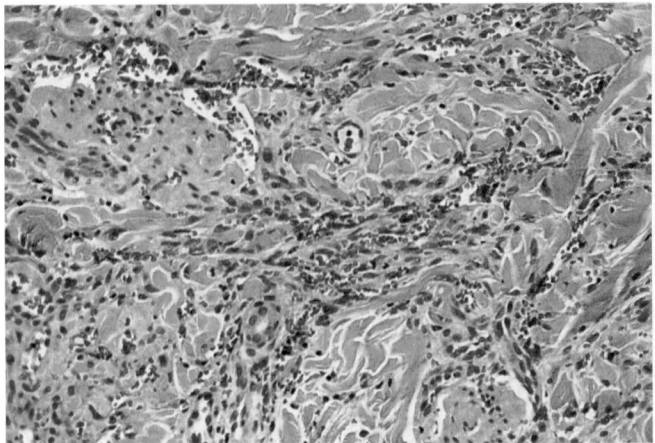

FIGURE 28-88. Kaposi sarcoma, plaque stage. Extending along the vascular arcades and amid reticular dermal collagen is a proliferation of endothelial cells. They form delicate vascular channels filled with red blood cells. Some endothelial cells are not canalized (have not formed lumina).

infection with these organisms. The proliferative lesions are red to brown papules, often in large numbers, and may be confused with Kaposi sarcoma. Silver impregnation stains show dense masses of bacilli within the basophilic deposits. Lesions clear with antibiotic treatment.

Eosinophilic Folliculitis

Eosinophilic folliculitis (EF) is a chronic pruritic eruption of papules, centered on hair follicles. Patients infected with HIV are a distinct population that displays EF, although variants that are not related to HIV infection occur in other populations. Lesions are most often on the trunk and proximal extremities. An infiltrate of lymphocytes, macrophages and many eosinophils is present in the intrafollicular and perifollicular areas and around dermal blood vessels.

PARANEOPLASTIC SYNDROMES INVOLVING THE SKIN

Diverse dermatologic manifestations may complicate internal malignancies, often preceding detection of the tumor itself. Pigmented lesions and keratoses are well-recognized paraneoplastic effects.

■ **Acanthosis nigricans** is marked by hyperkeratosis and pigmentation of the axilla, neck, flexures and anogenital region. *It is of particular interest because more than half of patients with acanthosis nigricans have cancer.* The development of the disease may precede, accompany or follow the detection of the cancer. Over 90% of cases occur in association with gastrointestinal carcinomas, and more than half accompany cancers of the stomach.

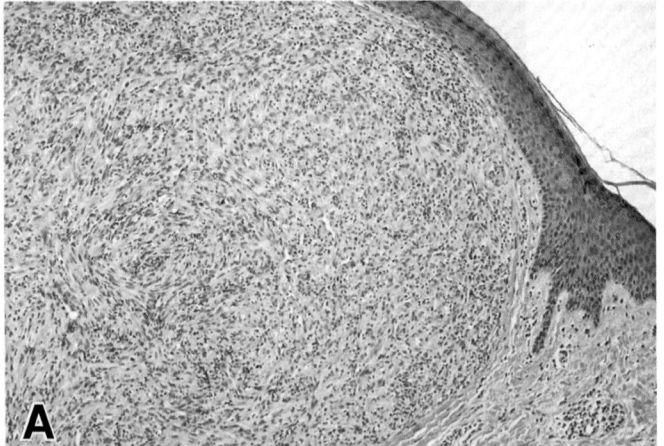

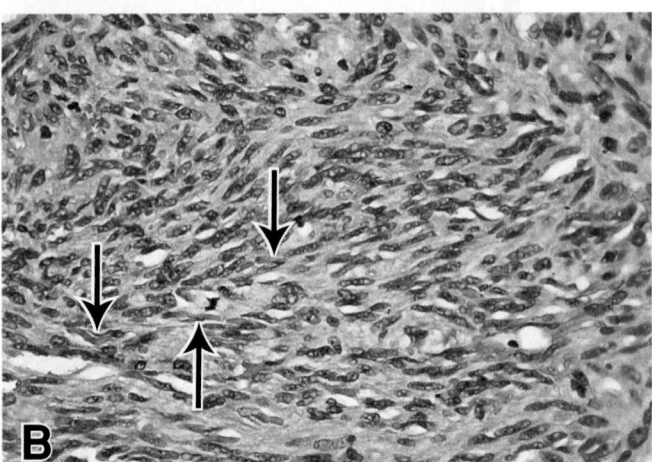

FIGURE 28-89. Kaposi sarcoma, nodule stage. A. A large nodule is composed of proliferating endothelial cells forming fascicles and vascular spaces. **B.** A higher-power view shows cytologic atypia of the spindle cells. Red blood cells appear agglutinated (*arrows*). The endothelial cells, in which the agglutinated red blood cells are present, form slit-like spaces.

■ **Dermatomyositis or polymyositis** has a five- to sevenfold greater incidence in cancer patients than in the general population. The association is most conspicuous in affected men older than 50 years, among whom more than 70% have cancer. In most cases, the muscle disorder and cancer present within a year of each other. In men, lung and gastrointestinal cancers are most often associated with dermatomyositis, whereas in women, the most common association is with breast cancer.
■ **Sweet syndrome** is a combination of elevated neutrophil count, acute fever and painful red plaques in the anus, neck and face. About 1/5 of cases occur with malignancies, particularly those of the hematopoietic system (see Chapter 26).

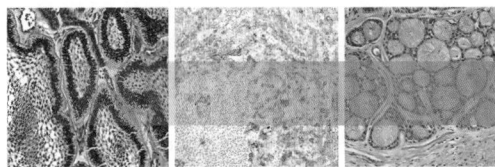

The Head and Neck

Diane L. Carlson

Oral Cavity

The oral cavity extends from the lips to the pharynx (Fig. 29-1). Its boundaries are:

- The vermilion border of the lips (anterior)
- A line from the junction of the hard and soft palate to the circumvallate papillae of the tongue (posterior)
- The hard palate until its junction with the soft palate (superior)
- The anterior two thirds of the tongue to the line of the circumvallate papillae (inferior)
- The buccal mucosa of the cheeks (lateral)

The oral mucosa consists of keratinized epithelia of the attached gingiva, hard palate mucosa and specialized keratinized gustatory mucosa of the dorsum of the tongue. It also includes nonkeratinized mucosal surfaces of the inner lip and inner cheek, the nonattached, movable gingiva that continues into the maxillary and mandibular sulci, ventral tongue, floor of the mouth, soft palate and tonsillar pillars.

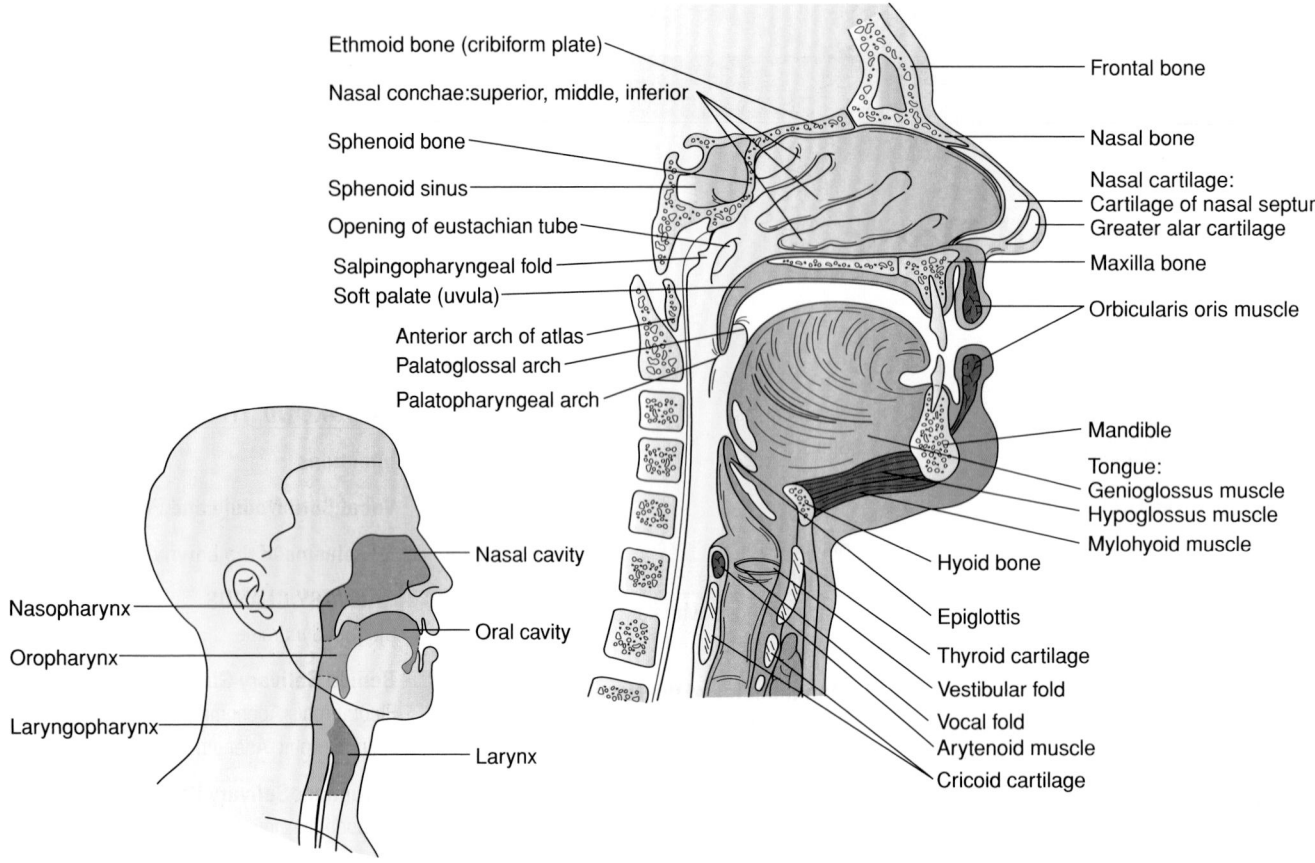

FIGURE 29-1. Structure of the oral cavity, oropharynx and larynx. Schematic diagram of the oral cavity, palate, oropharynx and larynx.

The epithelium is three to four times the thickness of epidermis. Under the epithelium is a lamina propria of fibrous tissue and blood vessels, beneath which is the densely fibrous periosteum of the hard palate or the alveolus of the maxilla and mandible. The term **submucosa** is sometimes loosely applied to the deep connective tissue just above the muscle layer, in which the minor salivary glands are often embedded.

Minor salivary glands are scattered throughout the oral cavity as unencapsulated small lobules within the mucosa and submucosa. There are mucous glands in the lamina propria, particularly in the posterior hard palatal mucosa. Minor salivary glands of pure mucous type exist in the anterior ventral portion of the tongue (called Blandin, or Nunn, glands). Serous salivary glands lie near circumvallate papillae on the posterior and lateral tongue (von Ebner glands). Mixed mucoserous and mainly mucous glands predominate in the rest of the oral cavity. There are minor salivary glands in the retromolar mandibular ridge, but not the anterior hard palate or gingiva.

The anterior two thirds of the dorsum of the tongue is covered by keratinized stratified squamous epithelium that is specialized to form **filiform papillae** (pointed projections of keratin). Between these are **fungiform papillae,** mushroom-shaped mucosal elevations containing taste buds. **Circumvallate papillae** separate the anterior 2/3 of the tongue from the posterior 1/3 and contain taste buds at their base. The final group is the **foliate papillae,** in the posterior lateral tongue in a series of ridges. Each taste bud is a barrel-shaped collection of modified epithelial cells that

extend vertically from the basal lamina to the epithelial surface, opening via a taste pore.

DEVELOPMENTAL ANOMALIES

FACIAL CLEFTS: If facial structures fail to fuse in the 7th week of embryonic life, facial clefts form. The most common of these is cleft upper lip **(harelip)**. It may be unilateral or bilateral and often occurs in association with cleft palate (see Chapter 6).

Crouzon syndrome (craniofacial dysostosis) and **Apert syndrome** (acrocephalosyndactyly) are autosomal dominant disorders associated with craniosynostosis (premature fusion of the cranial sutures). This can lead to **brachycephaly** (flat head), **scaphocephaly** or **dolichocephaly** (the head is disproportionately long and narrow or "boat" shaped) or **trigonocephaly** (triangular shaped). Severe craniosynostosis may result in **Kleeblattschädel deformity** ("cloverleaf" skull). *Both syndromes reflect mutations in fibroblast growth factor receptor 2 (FGFR2), on the long arm of chromosome 10.*

MOLECULAR PATHOGENESIS: The FGFR2 gene encodes a transmembrane protein that, upon binding its ligands, signals to induce bone maturation. In **Apert syndrome,** a mutant FGFR2 protein is produced, which promotes premature bone fusion in the calvarial (skull) bones.

HAMARTOMAS AND CHORISTOMAS: These lesions are common in the oral cavity. **Fordyce granules** are aggregates of

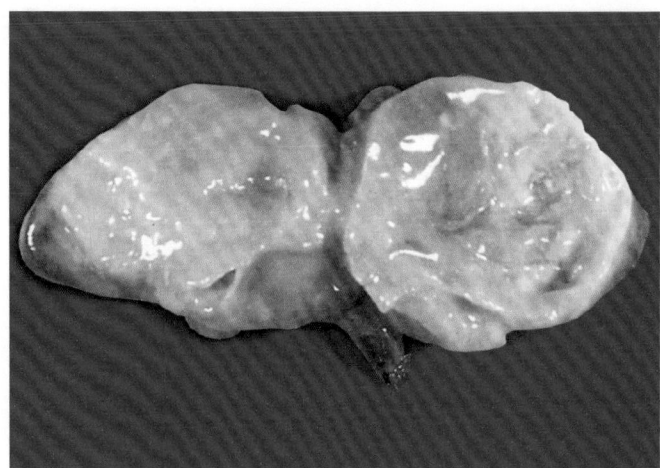

FIGURE 29-2. Branchial cleft cyst. Most of these cysts arise from the second branchial cleft and occur laterally in the neck. The cysts have a thin wall, contain turbid fluid and are lined by stratified squamous or respiratory-type epithelium.

sebaceous glands in the oral cavity **(choristoma)**. They occur on the buccal mucosa, lingual surface and lip in 70%–95% of adults; rarely, they coalesce to form mass lesions.

Abnormal descent of the thyroid during development may create submucosal foci of **ectopic thyroid** between the tongue and suprasternal notch. The base of the tongue between the foramen cecum and epiglottis is the most common site for ectopic thyroid **(lingual thyroid)**. Over 75% of patients with lingual thyroid lack a cervical thyroid ("total migration failure"). Thus, surgically removing a lingual thyroid may lead to hypothyroidism and stunted physical growth and mental development **(cretinism;** see Chapter 6). In fact, 70% of patients with symptomatic lingual thyroid are hypothyroid and 10% suffer from cretinism. Malignancies in ectopic thyroid glands are rare but are generally papillary thyroid carcinomas. The absence of a normally descended thyroid may also affect parathyroid gland development and localization.

Thyroglossal duct cysts result from persistence and cystic dilatation of the thyroglossal duct midline in the neck. The anomaly usually occurs above the thyroid isthmus but below the hyoid bone. Patients, usually under age 40, present clinically with a palpable 4–5-cm midline nodule, *which moves up and down upon swallowing.* Surgery is the treatment of choice. Malignancies, mostly papillary thyroid carcinomas, arise in up to 1% of thyroglossal duct cysts.

BRANCHIAL CLEFT CYST: Branchial cleft cysts originate from branchial arch remnants. They occur in the lateral anterior neck or parotid gland, mostly in young adults, and contain thin, watery fluid and mucoid or gelatinous material (Fig. 29-2). These cysts are usually lined by squamous epithelium, with occasional foci of ciliated respiratory or pseudostratified columnar epithelium.

INFECTIONS OF THE ORAL CAVITY

Bacteria and spirochetes, are present normally in the oral cavity and are generally harmless. If the mucosa is injured or immunity is impaired, otherwise normal oral flora may become pathogenic (see Chapter 9 for further discussion).

These terms are used to describe localized inflammation of the oral cavity:

- **Cheilitis** (lips)
- **Gingivitis** (gum)
- **Glossitis** (tongue)
- **Stomatitis** (oral mucosa)

Bacterial and Fungal Infections of the Oral Cavity May Involve Both Commensal and Invasive Species

SCARLET FEVER: Scarlet fever is mainly a disease of children, caused by several strains of β-hemolytic streptococci (*Streptococcus pyogenes*). Damage to vascular endothelium by the erythrogenic toxin results in a rash on the skin and oral mucosa. The tongue acquires a white coating, through which the hyperemic fungiform papillae project as small red knobs ("strawberry tongue"). Untreated scarlet fever can lead to glomerulonephritis and heart disease (**acute rheumatic fever;** see Chapters 11 and 16).

APHTHOUS STOMATITIS (CANKER SORES): Aphthous stomatitis is a common disease characterized by painful, recurrent, solitary or multiple, small ulcers of oral mucosa. Its cause is unknown, although various etiologies have been suggested. The lesion is a shallow ulcer covered by a fibrinopurulent exudate, with underlying mononuclear and polymorphonuclear inflammation. The lesions heal without scarring.

ACUTE NECROTIZING ULCERATIVE GINGIVITIS (VINCENT ANGINA): Vincent angina is an acute necrotizing ulcerative gingivitis caused by infection with two symbiotic organisms, a fusiform bacillus and a spirochete (*Borrelia vincentii*). The term **fusospirochetosis** is used for this infection. These organisms are found in the mouths of many healthy people, suggesting that other factors are involved, particularly decreased resistance to infection due to inadequate nutrition, immunodeficiency or poor oral hygiene. Vincent angina is characterized by punched-out erosions of the interdental papillae. The process tends to spread and eventually involves all gingival margins, which become covered by a necrotic pseudomembrane.

Noma (cancrum oris) is a severe fusospirochetal infection in people who are malnourished, debilitated from infections or weakened by blood dyscrasias. It features rapidly spreading gangrene of oral and facial tissues. Large masses of tissue slough and leave the bones exposed, especially in children (see Chapter 9).

LUDWIG ANGINA: Ludwig angina is a rapidly spreading cellulitis originating in the submaxillary or sublingual space but extending to involve both. Several aerobic and anaerobic oral bacteria have been implicated. Ludwig angina is a potentially life-threatening inflammatory process. It is uncommon in developed countries except in patients with chronic illnesses associated with immunosuppression.

Ludwig angina is most often related to dental extraction or trauma to the floor of the mouth. After extraction of a tooth, hairline fractures may occur in the lingual cortex of the mandible, providing microorganisms ready access to the submaxillary space. Infection may dissect into the parapharyngeal space along fascial planes and from there into the carotid sheath. A mycotic internal carotid artery aneurysm may result, erosion of which may cause massive hemorrhage. The inflammation may also dissect into the superior mediastinum to involve the pleural space and pericardium.

DIPHTHERIA: Infection with *Corynebacterium diphtheriae* is characterized by a patchy pseudomembrane, which often begins on the tonsils and pharynx but may also involve the soft palate, gingiva or buccal mucosa (see Chapter 9).

TUBERCULOSIS: Primary tuberculosis of the oral mucosa is rare. Most lesions spread from the lung, with bacilli carried in sputum and entering small breaks in the mucosa. There, they produce irregular, painful ulcers, mostly on the tongue. Caseating granulomatous inflammation is typical.

SYPHILIS: Primary syphilitic chancres may form on the lips, tongue or oropharyngeal mucosa after contact with an infectious lesion (see Chapter 9). Regional lymphadenitis follows and heals by itself in a few weeks. A diffuse mucocutaneous eruption of the secondary stage follows. Syphilitic lesions in the oral mucosa are multiple gray-white patches overlying ulcerated surfaces. They may remit and also recur spontaneously. **Gummas** on the palate and tongue may appear years after initial infection as firm nodular masses that ulcerate and may cause palatal perforation.

ACTINOMYCOSIS: Actinomycetes are common denizens of the oral cavity in healthy people. Invasive actinomycosis is most often caused by *Actinomyces bovis,* but *Actinomyces israelii* is sometimes seen. The organisms produce chronic granulomatous inflammation and abscesses that drain by fistula formation, with suppurative infection containing characteristic yellow "sulfur granules." In cervicofacial actinomycosis, soft tissue infection may extend to adjacent bones, most often to the mandible.

CANDIDIASIS: Also called **thrush** or **moniliasis,** oral candidiasis is caused by *Candida albicans* (see Chapter 9), which is common on the surfaces of the oral cavity, gastrointestinal tract and vagina. To cause disease, the fungus must penetrate tissues, albeit superficially. Oral candidiasis is mostly seen in diabetics and people with compromised immune systems. The incidence in patients with AIDS is 40%–90%. Lesions are white, slightly elevated, soft patches that consist mainly of fungal hyphae.

Oral Viral Diseases Are Mostly Recurrent Herpesvirus Infections

HERPES SIMPLEX VIRUS TYPE 1: Herpes labialis (cold sores, fever blisters) and herpetic stomatitis are caused by herpes simplex virus (HSV) type 1 and are among the most common viral infections of the lips and oral mucosa in children and young adults. Transmission is via aerosol, and the virus can be recovered from saliva of infected people. Disease starts with painful inflammation of affected mucosa, followed shortly by formation of vesicles. These result from "ballooning degeneration" of epithelial cells, some of which show intranuclear inclusions (Fig. 29-3). The vesicles rupture to form shallow, painful, 1–10-mm ulcers, which heal spontaneously without scarring.

Once HSV enters the body, it remains dormant in the trigeminal ganglion until stresses such as trauma, allergy, menstruation, pregnancy, exposure to ultraviolet light and other viral infections reactivate it. Recurrent oral cavity vesicles almost invariably develop on a mucosa that is tightly bound to periosteum, for example, the hard palate.

HUMAN PAPILLOMAVIRUS (HPV)–RELATED DISEASES: The HPV family of viruses (see Chapter 9) causes epithelial proliferations including papillomas (e.g., sinonasal, Schneiderian papillomas and other papillomas of upper

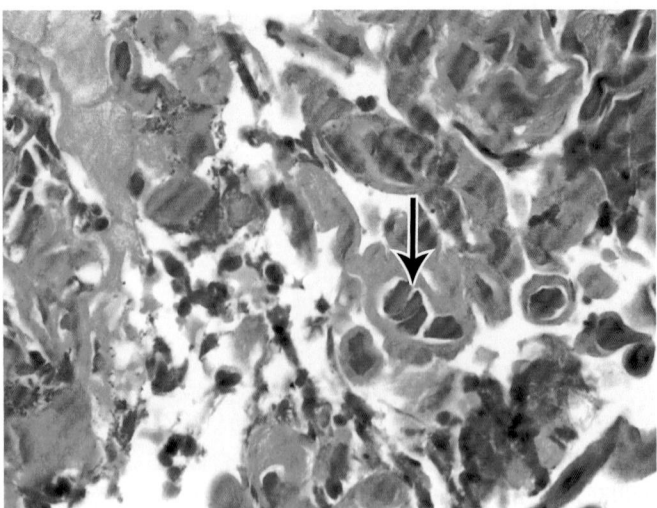

FIGURE 29-3. Herpes simplex virus type 1. A biopsy from a nonhealing ulcer on the tongue demonstrates intranuclear viral inclusions (*arrow*) within squamous cells infected by the virus.

aerodigestive tract sites). "High-risk" HPV, mainly types 16 and 18, as well as 31, 33 and 35, is strongly associated with oropharyngeal squamous cell carcinoma (see below).

EPSTEIN BARR VIRUS–RELATED DISEASES: Epstein-Barr virus (EBV) is a member of the *Herpesvirus* family that causes oral hairy leukoplakia, various lymphoid diseases (see Chapter 20) and epithelial cancers in the nose and pharynx (see below).

HUMAN HERPES VIRUS 8 (HHV8): HHV8 is associated with **Kaposi sarcoma** (KS). This tumor occurs most often in the skin (see Chapter 24) but can also involve, among other places, the tongue and oral cavity. These tumors resemble their cutaneous counterparts (Fig. 29-4). Immunosuppressed patients (e.g., transplant recipients or patients infected with HIV-1) are at very high risk for this disease. It is also seen in

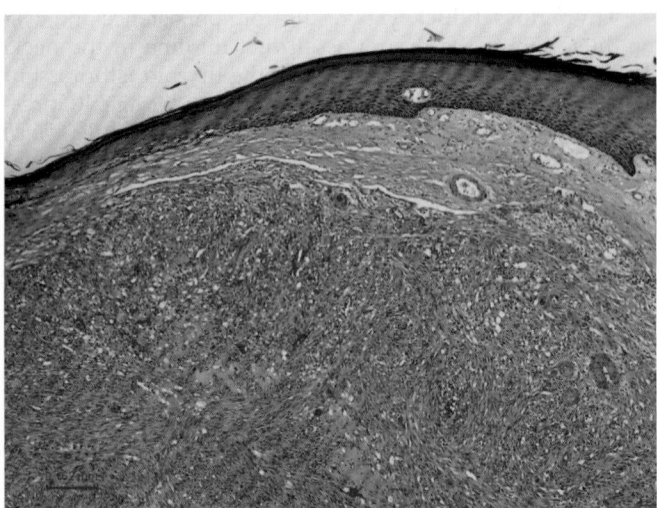

FIGURE 29-4. Kaposi sarcoma. This palate biopsy demonstrates an intact overlying squamous mucosa. Within the underlying lamina propria, there is a malignant spindle cell proliferation forming slit-like spaces filled with extravasated red blood cells.

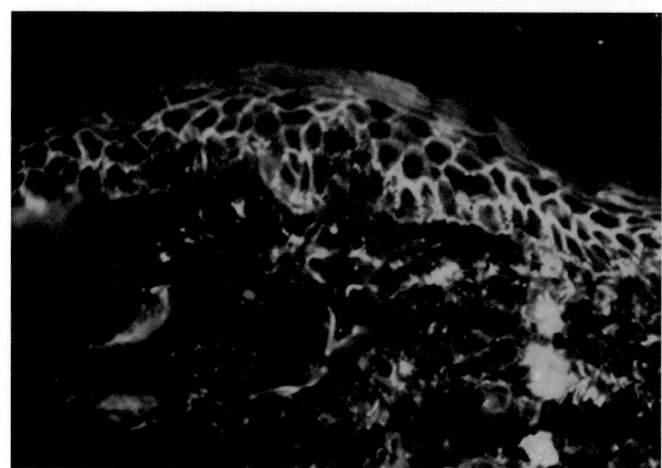

FIGURE 29-5. Pemphigus vulgaris. Direct immunofluorescence of auto-IgG antibodies demonstrates a lace-like pattern of reactivity. The antidesmoglein autoantibodies produced induce acantholysis, leading to vesicle formation in the oral cavity and the skin.

elderly men of Mediterranean/East European descent and in non–HIV-infected middle-aged adults and children in equatorial Africa.

 **MOLECULAR PATHOGENESIS:** Details of herpesvirus molecular pathogenesis are presented in Chapter 9.

OTHER VIRAL INFECTIONS: Coxsackievirus causes **herpangina,** an acute vesicular oropharyngitis. A brief infection confers lasting immunity. **Cytomegalovirus** (CMV) infection typically presents with surface ulceration. Other virus infections that involve the oral mucosa include measles, rubella, chickenpox and herpes zoster.

Bullous Lesions of the Oral Cavity Resemble Those in the Skin

PEMPHIGUS VULGARIS: Autoantibodies against desmogleins disrupt intercellular bridges between squamous cells

in the skin and oral mucosa, causing the blisters, or *bullae,* of **pemphigus vulgaris**. The oral cavity is often the site of initial presentation, with cutaneous bullae developing later. These blisters are very fragile and rupture so easily that one sees scabs more often than intact bullae. The disease occurs primarily in adults between 30 and 60 years old and is the most common type of pemphigus (*vulgaris* comes from the Latin meaning "common" or "derived from the common people"). This disease can be life-threatening. The diagnosis is made by observing an immunofluorescence pattern of a lace-like outline of the epidermal cells (Fig. 29-5). Treatment is with steroids or other immunosuppressive agents.

BULLOUS PEMPHIGOID: Clinically, this disease resembles pemphigus, but in bullous pemphigoid the autoantibodies are directed against the epidermal basement membrane. On immunofluorescence, one sees a line along the base of the epidermis. Resulting bullae are subepidermal, and thus less fragile than in pemphigus vulgaris. This is a disease of older patients and does not usually manifest in the mouth; the bullae are less delicate and less likely to get infected as they do not rupture as easily. Rarely, pemphigus may be caused by medications.

BENIGN TUMORS

Benign tumors found elsewhere in the body (e.g., nevi, fibromas, hemangiomas, lymphangiomas and squamous papillomas) are seen also in the oral cavity. Trauma may lead to ulceration of the lesions, causing bleeding or infection.

PAPILLOMA: Squamous papillomas are benign, exophytic epithelial tumors with branching fronds of squamous epithelium and fibrovascular cores (Fig. 29-6A). They are the most common benign oral cavity neoplasms and have been associated with HPV types 6 and 11, which are low-risk serotypes *not* associated with malignancy (Fig. 29-6B). They occur mainly in the third to fifth decades. The tongue, palate, buccal mucosa, tonsil and uvula are most often involved.

BENIGN MINOR SALIVARY GLAND TUMORS: **Pleomorphic adenoma** (benign mixed tumor) is the most common oral salivary gland tumor (see below). Monomorphic adenomas such as myoepithelioma or oncocytoma are less

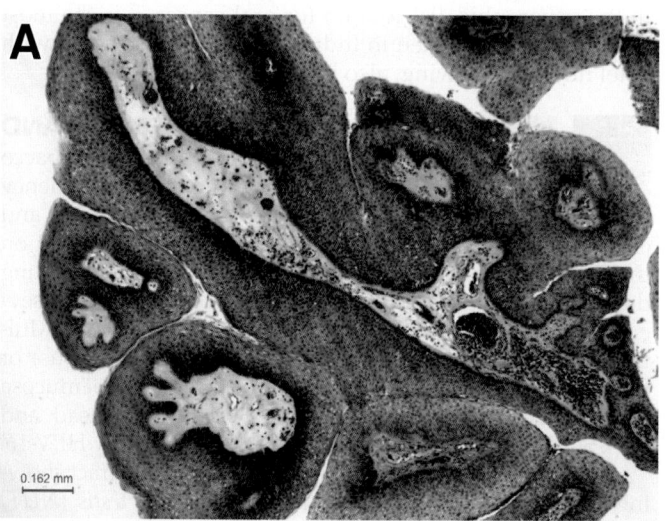
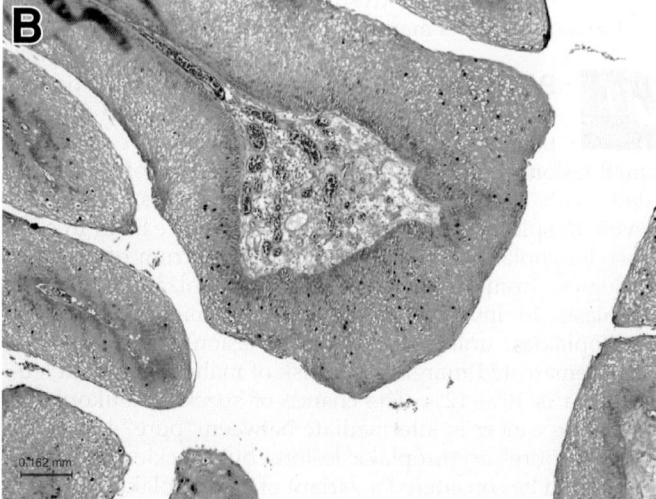

FIGURE 29-6. A. Squamous papilloma. This exophytic frond-like papillary tumor grew off of the patient's uvula. **B. In situ hybridization** for low-risk human papillomavirus (LR-HPV) demonstrates nuclear localization.

common. Benign mesenchymal tumors that may occur in the oral cavity include hemangiomas, leiomyomas and lipomas.

LOBULAR CAPILLARY HEMANGIOMA (PYOGENIC GRANULOMA; PREGNANCY TUMOR): Lobular capillary hemangiomas are benign polypoid capillary hemangiomas that occur mainly on the skin, mucous membranes and, most often, gingiva. The term "pyogenic granuloma" is a misnomer: it is neither infectious nor granulomatous. In the mouth, they are elevated, soft, red or purple lesions, from a few millimeters to a centimeter, with smooth, lobulated, ulcerated surfaces. They show lobules or clusters of submucosal vessels, with central capillaries and smaller ramifying tributaries. In time, the lesions may become less vascular and resemble fibromas.

An identical lesion in the gingiva **(pregnancy tumor)** may occur in pregnant women near the end of the third trimester. It may or may not regress after delivery.

PRENEOPLASTIC OR PRECURSOR EPITHELIAL LESIONS

Premalignant lesions of the upper aerodigestive tract include leukoplakia, erythroplakia or speckled leukoplakia, the terms describing a white, red or mixed white/red lesion, respectively. *Leukoplakia (from the Greek, leukos, "white," and plax, "plaque") is an asymptomatic white lesion on the surface of a mucous membrane*. It affects both sexes equally, mostly after the third decade. Some of these lesions may become squamous cell carcinomas (SCCs). Diverse diseases appear clinically as leukoplakia, including several keratoses and squamous carcinoma in situ. *Thus, leukoplakia is a descriptive clinical term, not a pathologic diagnosis.* Other diseases may also have white plaques on the oral mucosa (e.g., candidiasis, lichen planus, psoriasis, syphilis).

The causes of leukoplakia include tobacco use, alcoholism and local irritation. The same factors also appear to be important in the etiology of oral carcinoma.

Erythroplakia is the red equivalent of leukoplakia but occurs less often. Red areas associated with leukoplakic lesions are **speckled leukoplakia (speckled mucosa; erythroleukoplakia)**. Erythroplakia may represent moderate to severe dysplasia or carcinoma. However, not all red erythroplakic lesions indicate dysplasia/carcinoma, as many red oral mucosal lesions may be inflammatory.

 PATHOLOGY: Leukoplakia (Fig. 29-7) occurs mostly on the buccal mucosa, tongue and floor of the mouth. Plaques may be solitary or multiple, small lesions to large patches. Erythroplakia is often associated with ominous histopathologic features, including severe dysplasia, carcinoma in situ or invasive SCC. In contrast, leukoplakic lesions may show a spectrum of histopathologies, from increased surface keratinization without dysplasia to invasive keratinizing squamous carcinoma. Leukoplakias, unlike erythroplakic lesions, tend to show well-demarcated margins. The risk of malignancy with leukoplakia is 10%–12%. The chance of speckled leukoplakia becoming cancer is intermediate between "pure" leukoplakic and "pure" erythroplakic lesions, but speckled leukoplakia should be considered a variant of erythroplakia.

Oral hairy leukoplakia has shaggy parakeratosis and edema, with or without associated inflammation. It occurs mainly in people who are HIV-1 positive, usually with

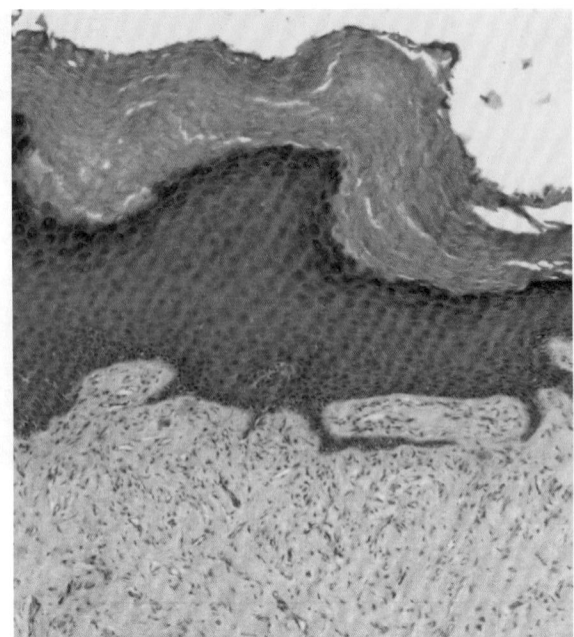

FIGURE 29-7. Leukoplakia. The lesion was seen as a white patch on the buccal mucosa of a heavy smoker. Histologically, epithelial hyperplasia and hyperkeratosis are evident.

associated candidiasis. The EBV-infected squamous cells are seen just beneath the keratin layer and have dense central eosinophilic inclusions and vacuolated cytoplasm. Oral hairy leukoplakia and candidiasis reflect immune status and together suggest low CD4$^+$ lymphocyte counts and high viral load.

SQUAMOUS CELL CARCINOMA

SCCs are the most common malignant tumors of the oral mucosa and may occur at any site. In the United States, there are over 40,000 cases yearly, most often involving the tongue, then, in descending order: the floor of the mouth, alveolar mucosa, palate and buccal mucosa. The male-to-female ratio is 2:1 for the gums but 10:1 for the lip. There is wide variation in the geographic distribution for oral cancer: it is the most common cancer of men in India, where it is associated with betel nut quid chewing, also known as *pan*.

 **MOLECULAR PATHOGENESIS AND ETIOLOGIC FACTORS:** Use of tobacco products, alcoholism, iron deficiency (Plummer-Vinson syndrome), Fanconi anemia, physical and chemical irritants, chewing of betel nuts, ultraviolet light on the lips and poor oral hygiene (craggy teeth and ill-fitting dentures), all predispose to oral SCC. Not surprisingly, several of these factors are also connected with leukoplakia. Multiple separate SCCs may be simultaneous (synchronous) or they may occur at intervals (metachronous) in the oral mucosa ("field cancerization"). Worldwide, 35%–50% of head and neck SCCs are associated with high-risk HPV, mostly HPV-16.

Midline carcinomas of the upper aerodigestive tract showing rearrangement of the *nuclear protein of the testis (NUT)* gene (NUT midline carcinoma) were first seen in children but have been identified increasingly in adults. These tumors have a balanced translocation (t15;19), creating a BRD4-NUT

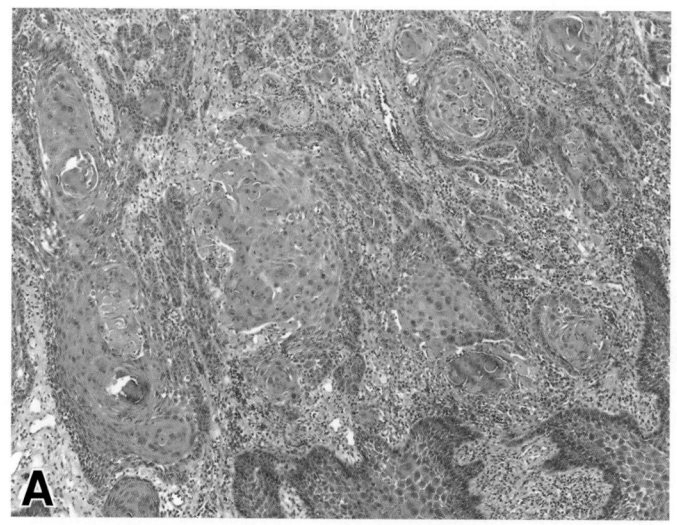

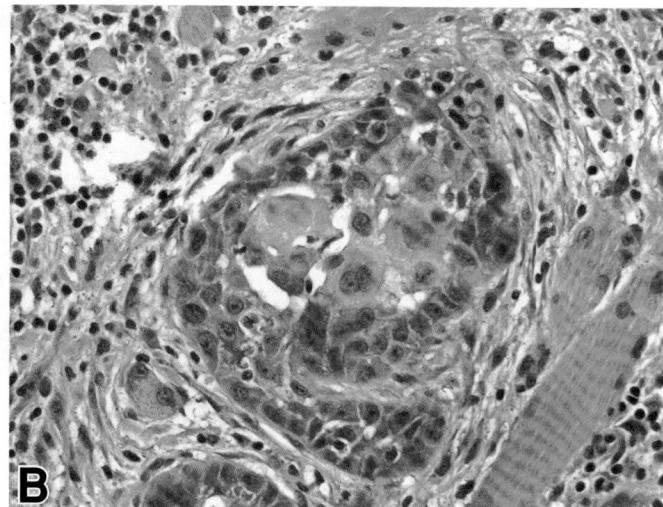

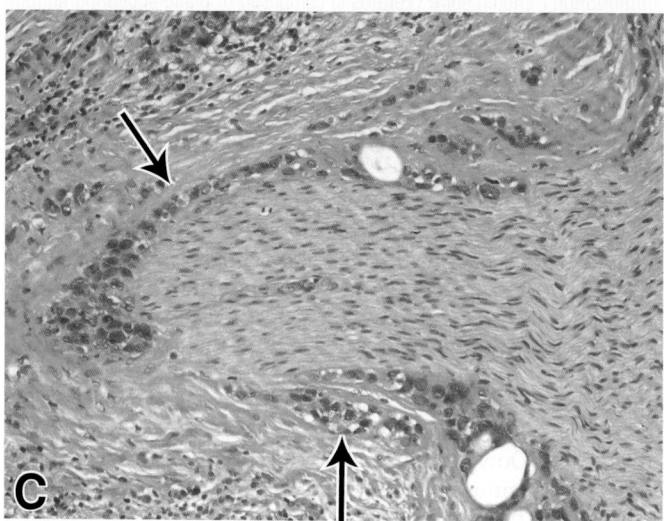

FIGURE 29-8. Squamous cell carcinoma. A. An infiltrative neoplasm is composed of cohesive nests of tumor. **B.** A less differentiated tumor displays cells with pleomorphic nuclei, prominent nucleoli, brightly eosinophilic cytoplasm indicating keratinization and intercellular bridges connecting adjacent cells. **C.** Perineural invasion by squamous cell carcinoma. Tumor surrounds a nerve (*arrows*).

oncogene. They tend to occur in midline structures of the upper aerodigestive tract (e.g., sinonasal tract) and non–head and neck sites (e.g., mediastinum) but may be away from the midline (e.g., parotid gland). NUT midline carcinomas are mainly undifferentiated or poorly differentiated SCCs.

 PATHOLOGY: *Invasive oral cavity SCC resembles the same tumor in other sites. It is generally preceded by carcinoma in situ.* It ranges from well to poorly differentiated, plus undifferentiated and sarcomatoid variants. Well-differentiated, or grade I, tumors are frequently keratinizing (Fig. 29-8). At the other end of the spectrum, tumors may be so poorly differentiated that their origin is difficult to determine.

Oral SCC mainly metastasizes to submandibular, superficial and deep cervical lymph nodes, and at autopsy 18% of these patients have axillary metastases. More than half of patients who die of head and neck SCC have distant, bloodborne metastases, most often in lungs, liver and bones.

Local recurrence is predicted by a tumor's pattern of infiltration: single-cell invasion is less favorable than a broad, "pushing" border. Other prognostic factors include depth of tumor invasion, perineural invasion and lymphovascular tumor emboli. Negative resection margins are important in local and regional control of the tumor.

Verrucous carcinomas (VCs) are highly differentiated variants of squamous cell carcinoma that generally occur in the sixth and seventh decades; they are locally destructive but do not usually metastasize. They may arise anywhere in this region but are most common on the buccal mucosa, gingiva and larynx. These tumors are usually white, warty to fungating, or exophytic and generally have broad bases (Fig. 29-9A). They are composed of benign-appearing squamous epithelium (without dysplasia or atypia), with marked surface keratinization and a pushing border of bulbous rete pegs (Fig. 29-9B). These tumors carry a good prognosis if completely removed.

MALIGNANT MINOR SALIVARY GLAND NEOPLASMS

About 50% of intraoral minor salivary gland tumors are malignant. These include mucoepidermoid carcinomas, adenoid cystic carcinomas and polymorphous low-grade adenocarcinomas (see below). Some tumors that are more common malignancies of major salivary glands occur uncommonly in minor salivary glands (e.g., acinic cell adenocarcinoma), while low-grade adenocarcinoma and clear cell carcinoma are more common in the palate than in major salivary glands.

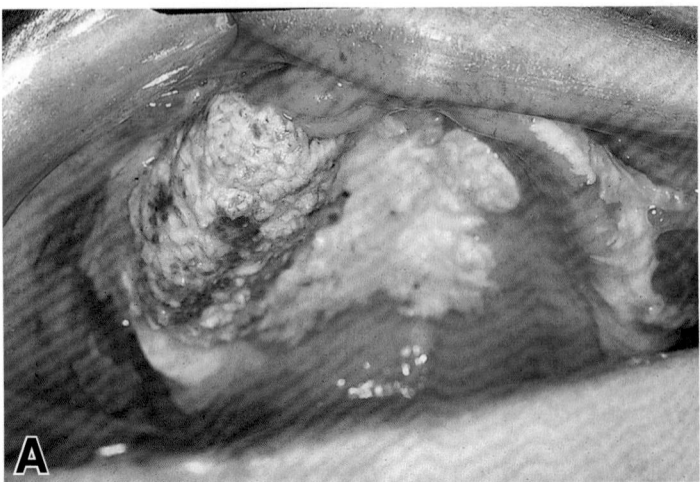
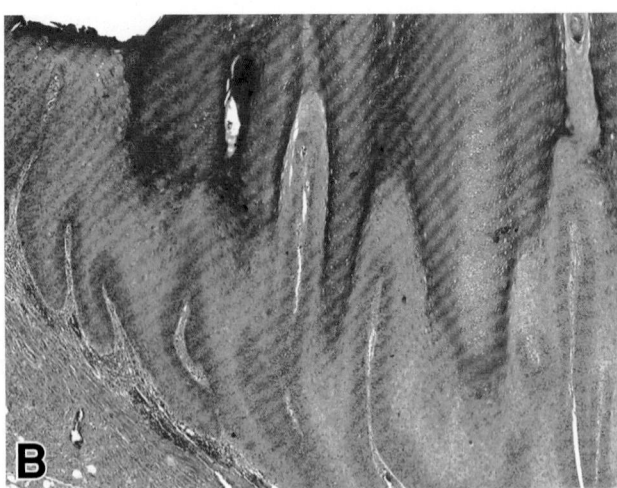

FIGURE 29-9. Verrucous carcinoma. A. The tumor is white with an exophytic appearance involving the alveolar ridge. Note the confluent flat white (leukoplakic) appearance of the palate. **B.** Microscopically, there is prominent surface keratinization ("church-spire" keratosis) composed of bland-appearing uniform squamous cells without dysplasia, and broad or bulbous rete pegs with a pushing margin into the submucosa.

BENIGN DISEASES OF THE LIPS

The lips are affected by many degenerative, inflammatory and proliferative processes. Some of these, particularly those expressed in the skin and mucous membranes, are systemic; others reflect localized disease. A **mucocele** is a mucus-filled cystic lesion associated with minor salivary glands that is probably caused by trauma (Fig. 29-10).

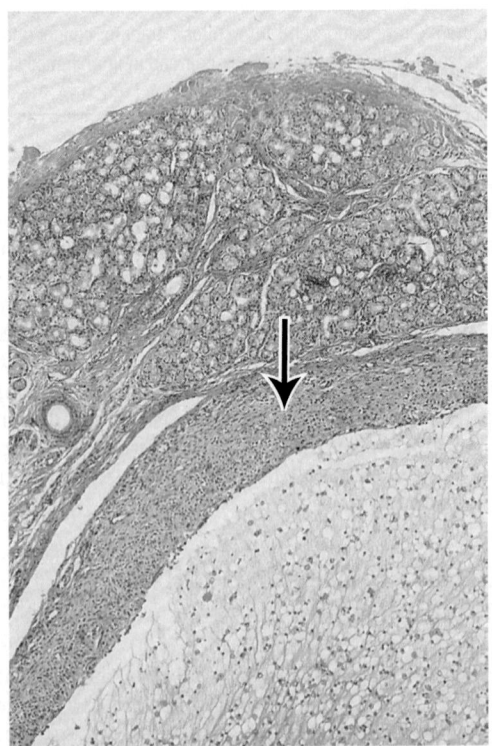

FIGURE 29-10. Mucocele of lower lip. This cystic lesion is associated with the minor salivary glands and is probably caused by trauma that permits escape of mucus. The cyst has a fibrous wall and is lined by granulation tissue (*arrow*). The lumen is filled with mucus that contains numerous macrophages.

BENIGN DISEASES OF THE TONGUE

MACROGLOSSIA: All parts of the tongue may be involved in localized or systemic diseases, some of which can cause tongue enlargement. If present at birth, macroglossia is usually due to diffuse lymphangioma (Fig. 29-11) or hemangioma, although it may rarely be caused by congenital neurofibromatosis or true muscle hypertrophy. An enlarged tongue that protrudes from the mouth occurs in congenital hypothyroidism, Hurler syndrome, glycogen storage disease type II (Pompe disease), Beckwith-Wiedemann syndrome and Down syndrome. Acquired macroglossia may be due to amyloidosis, acromegaly, or infiltration or lymphatic obstruction by tumors.

GLOSSITIS: Inflammation of the tongue can be caused by infectious or chemical agents, physical effects or systemic diseases. Some forms of glossitis reflect vitamin deficiencies of, for example, vitamin B_{12}, riboflavin, niacin (B_3) and pyridoxine (B_6).

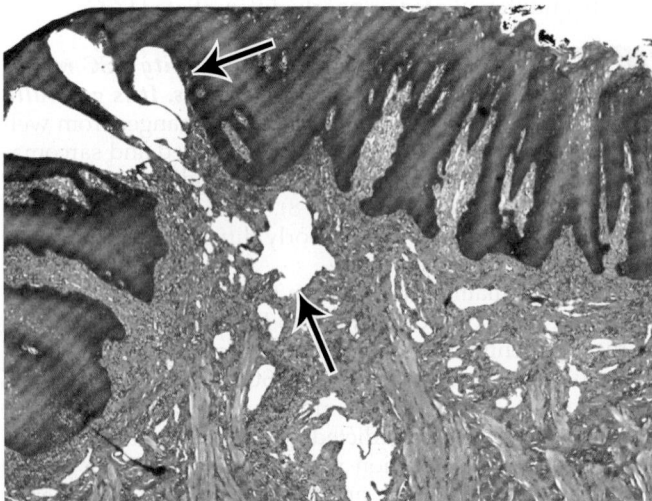

FIGURE 29-11. Lymphangioma of the tongue. Submucosal dilated lymphatics (*arrows*) splay skeletal muscle fibers.

DENTAL CARIES (TOOTH DECAY)

Caries is the most common chronic disease of the calcified tissues of teeth, affecting both sexes and every age group. Its incidence has plummeted with modern civilization.

 ETIOLOGIC FACTORS: The interactions of several factors cause caries:

BACTERIA: Dental caries is a chronic infectious disease of tooth enamel, dentin and cementum, the guilty organisms being part of the normal oral flora. Tooth surfaces are colonized by many microorganisms. Unless the surfaces are cleaned thoroughly and frequently, bacterial colonies coalesce into a soft mass known as **dental plaque**.

Carious lesions occur because acids produced from food residues by microorganisms on tooth surfaces leach the minerals in teeth. The culprits include streptococci, lactobacilli and actinomyces in the oral flora. Indirect evidence points strongly to *Streptococcus mutans* as the primary etiologic agent that initiates caries.

SALIVA: Saliva has a high buffering capacity that helps neutralize microbially produced acids in the mouth. It also contains bacteriostatic factors such as lysozyme, lactoferrin, lactoperoxidases and secretory immunoglobulins. **Xerostomia** (chronically dry mouth due to lack of saliva), which may be iatrogenic, for example, due to surgery or radiation therapy, results in rampant caries.

DIETARY FACTORS: One of the most important factors in the pathogenesis of caries is a high-carbohydrate diet. Roughage in raw and unrefined foods necessitates heavy mastication, which cleanses the teeth. By contrast, soft and refined foods tend to stick to the teeth and also require less chewing.

FLUORIDE: Fluoride protects from caries. It is incorporated into the crystal lattice structure of enamel, where it forms fluoroapatite, which is less acid soluble than is the apatite of enamel. Many communities fluoridated their drinking water, leading to huge reductions in dental caries in those children whose teeth were formed while they drank fluoride-containing water.

PATHOLOGY: Caries begins with disintegration of enamel prisms after decalcification of the interprismatic substance, events that lead to accumulation of debris and microorganisms (Fig. 29-12). These changes produce a small pit or fissure in the enamel. When the process reaches the dentinoenamel junction, it spreads laterally and also penetrates the dentin along the dentinal tubules. A substantial cavity then forms in the dentin, producing a flask-shaped lesion with a narrow orifice. Dentin decalcification causes the destroyed dentinal tubules to coalesce. Only when the vascular pulp of the tooth is invaded, does an inflammatory reaction **(pulpitis)** appear, accompanied for the first time by pain.

PERIODONTAL DISEASE

The gingiva (gum) is the part of the oral mucosa that surrounds the teeth. It ends in a thin edge (free gingiva) that adheres closely to teeth. A periodontal ligament of collagen fibers holds teeth in position in the socket (alveolus) of the jawbone. These structures form the periodontium.

Periodontal diseases are acute and chronic disorders of the soft tissues around the teeth, which eventually erode the supporting bone. Chronic periodontal disease typically occurs in adults with poor oral hygiene but may develop even in people with apparently impeccable habits who have strong family histories of periodontal disease. It causes more loss of teeth in adults than does any other disease, including caries.

Periodontal disease occurs when bacteria accumulate under the gingiva in the periodontal pocket. The mass of

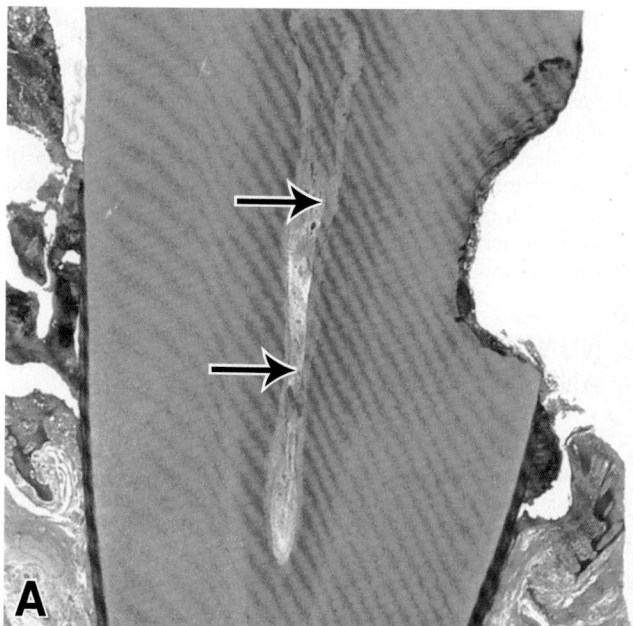

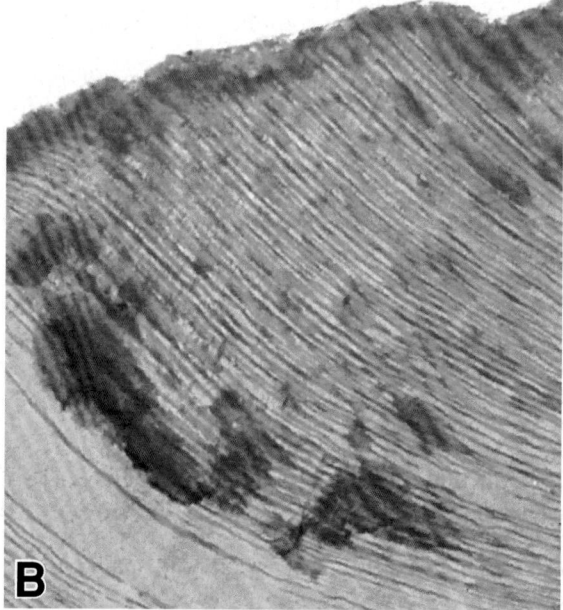

FIGURE 29-12. Dental caries. A. A large cavity close to the gingival margin is illustrated. *Arrows* indicate band of secondary dentin that lines the pulp chamber. This newly formed dentin is opposite the area of tooth destruction and was produced by the stimulated odontoblasts. **B.** Deposits of debris cover the surface. Bacterial colonies (*dark purple*) have extended into dentinal canals.

bacteria adhering to the tooth surface **(dental plaque)** ages, mineralizes and forms **calculus (tartar)**. Adult periodontitis is mostly associated with *Bacteroides gingivalis, Bacteroides intermedius, Actinomyces* sp. and *Haemophilus* sp., although other microorganisms may also participate.

Inflammation often starts as a marginal gingivitis. Untreated, it progresses to chronic periodontitis, in which the chronic inflammation weakens and destroys the periodontium, causing loosening and eventual loss of teeth.

Hematologic disorders may affect oral tissues. Agranulocytosis may lead to necrotizing ulcers anywhere in the oral and pharyngeal mucosa, but especially in the gingiva. Infectious mononucleosis often causes gingivitis and stomatitis, with exudation and ulceration. Acute and chronic leukemias of all types cause oral lesions. In **acute monocytic leukemia,** 80% of patients have gingivitis, gingival hyperplasia, petechiae and hemorrhage. Necrosis and ulceration of the gingiva lead to severe superimposed infection, which may cause loss of teeth and alveolar bone. A hemorrhagic diathesis may be reflected in gingival hemorrhage.

Mild scurvy (vitamin C deficiency; see Chapter 8) affects the marginal and interdental gingiva, which become swollen and bright red and bleed and ulcerate readily. Hemorrhage into the periodontal membrane causes loosening and loss of teeth.

ODONTOGENIC CYSTS AND TUMORS

Odontogenic cysts may be inflammatory or developmental. Most common are **radicular (apical, periodontal) cysts,** involving tooth apices, usually after infection of the dental pulp.

Dentigerous cysts are associated with the crowns of impacted, embedded or unerupted teeth, most often involving mandibular and maxillary third molars. They form after the crown has completely developed; fluid accumulates between the crown and overlying enamel epithelium. Dentigerous cysts may be complicated by ameloblastoma or SCC.

Ameloblastomas are tumors of odontogenic epithelia and are the most common clinically significant odontogenic tumors. They are slow growing and locally invasive, generally following a benign clinical course, even as they can be locally destructive. Most arise in the mandibular ramus or molar area, maxilla or floor of the nasal cavity. The tumors grow slowly as central lesions of bone, showing a characteristic "soap bubble" radiographic appearance. Ameloblastomas resemble the enamel organ in its various stages of differentiation, and a single tumor may show several histologic patterns. Thus, tumor cells resemble ameloblasts at the edges of epithelial nests or cords, where columnar cells are oriented perpendicularly to the basement membrane (Fig. 29-13). The prognosis is favorable, but incompletely excised tumors recur. Some may metastasize and yet remain histologically benign **(metastasizing ameloblastoma)**.

Ameloblastic carcinomas are frankly malignant, with atypia, necrosis, nuclear pleomorphism and abundant mitoses. Nuclei of ameloblastomas may show aberrant β-catenin expression. An APC gene missense mutation, which plays a role in colon cancer, may also participate in the pathogenesis of odontogenic tumors.

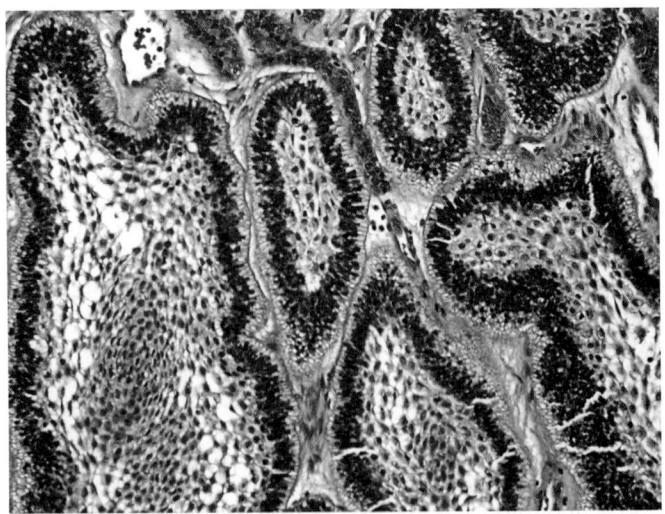

FIGURE 29-13. Ameloblastoma. A common histologic pattern is characterized by islands of odontogenic epithelium with a central stellate reticulum-like area, surrounded by basal cells with a "picket fence" appearance, due to subnuclear vacuoles.

Nasal Cavity and Paranasal Sinuses

ANATOMY: The **nostril apertures** (anterior nares) lead into the **nasal vestibule,** a space lined by skin that contains hairs and sebaceous glands. Beyond the nares, the median septum divides the nasal cavity into two symmetric chambers, the **nasal fossae.** Each nasal fossa has an **olfactory region,** consisting of the superior nasal concha and the opposed part of the septum, and a **respiratory region,** which is the rest of the cavity. Laterally, the inferior, middle and superior nasal conchae **(turbinates)** overhang the corresponding nasal passages or meatus.

The paranasal sinuses are paired air spaces that communicate with the nasal cavity. The respiratory portion of the nasal cavity is covered by ciliated, columnar epithelium with interspersed goblet cells.

These anatomic interrelations determine routes of disease spread (Fig. 29-14). Infections can spread to maxillary, ethmoid, frontal and sphenoid sinuses, causing intraorbital and intracranial disease. The vein of Vesalius, medial to the foramen ovale, puts the cavernous sinus at risk.

NONNEOPLASTIC DISEASES OF THE NOSE AND NASAL VESTIBULE

Virtually all diseases of the skin can occur on the external nose, including lesions due to solar damage (e.g., actinic keratosis, basal cell carcinoma, SCC and malignant melanoma). The many sebaceous glands of the nose are commonly affected in acne vulgaris.

Rosacea is a chronic skin disorder of the cheeks, nose, chin and central forehead, characterized by telangiectasias, flushing, erythema, papules, pustules, rhinophyma and ocular manifestations (Fig. 29-15). Bacteria (e.g., *Bacillus oleronius* and *Staphylococcus epidermidis*), as well as Demodex mites, have all been implicated. Inflammation is central to

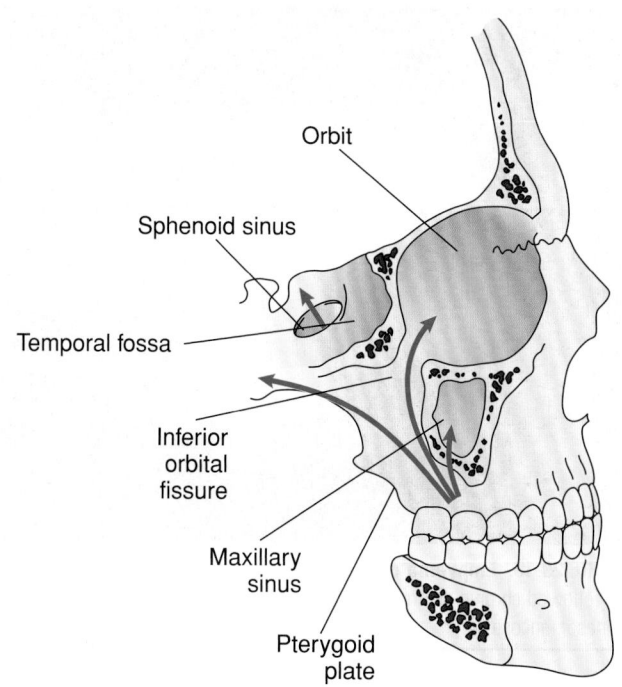

FIGURE 29-14. Pathways of infection to the intracranial cavity. Osseous pathways of infection from the jaws. *Arrows* indicate the direction of spread from the teeth to the maxillary sinus and through the inferior orbital fissure to the orbit. A deeper route is along the lateral pterygoid lamina up to the base of the skull, where, medial to the foramen ovale, a small aperture admits the vein of Vesalius. Through this small vein, the pterygoid plexus communicates with the cavernous sinus.

this disease, although the initiating factors and etiology of rosacea remain unknown. Antibiotics, such as tetracycline and metronidazole, are common therapies.

Rhinophyma is a protuberant bulbous mass on the nose caused by marked hyperplasia of sebaceous glands and chronic inflammation of the skin in acne rosacea.

Nosebleed (epistaxis) is most often due to trauma but has many causes, including hypertension, diverse hematologic abnormalities, inflammatory conditions and nasal mucosal tumors. Epistaxis often originates in a triangular area of the anterior nasal septum called "Little area," where the epidermis is thin and the anterior ethmoid, greater palatine, sphenopalatine and superior labial arteries anastomose to form the **Kiesselbach plexus.** Many dilated blood vessels, or telangiectasias, are often apparent. Ulcers and perforations, which may be caused by various diseases or by trauma to the septum, occur here (Table 29-1).

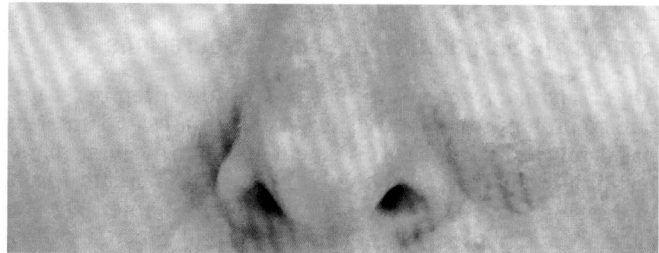

FIGURE 29-15. Rosacea. Typically characterized by erythema over the bridge of the nose and cheeks, as well as pustules and papules.

TABLE 29-1
CAUSES OF NASAL SEPTUM PERFORATION
Trauma
Specific infections (tuberculosis, syphilis, leprosy)
Wegener granulomatosis
Lupus erythematosus
Chronic exposure to dust (containing arsenic, chromium, copper, etc.)
Cocaine abuse
Malignant tumors

NONNEOPLASTIC DISEASES OF THE NASAL CAVITY AND SINUSES

Rhinitis Is Usually Viral or Allergic

Rhinitis is inflammation of the mucous membranes of the nasal cavity and sinuses. Its causes range from the common cold to unusual infections such as diphtheria, anthrax or glanders (see Chapter 9).

VIRAL RHINITIS: The most common cause of acute rhinitis is viral infection, especially the common cold **(acute coryza).** The virus replicates in epithelial cells, and degenerating epithelial cells are shed. The mucosa is edematous and engorged, infiltrated by neutrophils and mononuclear cells. Clinically, mucosal swelling is felt as nasal stuffiness. Abundant mucus secretion and increased vascular permeability lead to **rhinorrhea** (free discharge of a thin watery mucus).

Secondary infection caused by normal nasal and pharyngeal flora may follow viral rhinitis by a few days. The abundant serous discharge then becomes mucopurulent, after which the surface epithelium is shed. Once inflammation subsides, the epithelium regenerates rapidly.

ALLERGIC RHINITIS (HAY FEVER): Allergens are constantly present in our environment, and sensitivity to any one of them can cause allergic rhinitis. Allergic rhinitis may be acute and seasonal, or chronic and perennial.

 **MOLECULAR PATHOGENESIS:** Plasma cells of the nasal mucosa produce immunoglobulin E (IgE), which is bound by mast cells in the nasal mucosa. When air-borne allergens (e.g., pollens, molds, animal dander) deposit there, they activate IgE bound to mast cells or free in nasal secretions specifically directed against those allergens. Thus triggered, mast cells release cytoplasmic granules that contain diverse chemical mediators and enzymes. Some mediators are preformed and thus act rapidly (e.g., histamine); others (such as heparin or trypsin) elute slowly from the granule matrix; still others (e.g., leukotrienes) are newly synthesized. An immediate, rapid response ensues. It is followed by a prolonged inflammatory reaction as the various mediators exert their effects, causing the signs and symptoms of allergic rhinitis. Many of these responses are due to histamine, acting through its H_1 receptor.

PATHOLOGY: Vasodilators increase vascular permeability to cause edema of the nasal mucosa, especially of the inferior turbinates. Many eosinophils may be seen in the nasal mucosa or secretions. The late phase of mast cell–mediated reactions is associated with persistent mucosal edema and manifests clinically as nasal obstruction.

CHRONIC RHINITIS: Repeated bouts of acute rhinitis may lead to chronic rhinitis. In this condition, the nasal mucosa is thickened by persistent hyperemia, mucous gland hyperplasia and infiltration with lymphocytes and plasma cells.

Inflammatory Polyps Are Nonneoplastic Swellings

These polyps arise in the nose and sinuses, mostly from the lateral nasal wall or ethmoid recess. They may be unilateral or bilateral, single or multiple. Symptoms include nasal obstruction, rhinorrhea and headaches. Multiple etiologies are responsible, including allergy, cystic fibrosis, infections, diabetes mellitus and aspirin intolerance. These polyps are lined by respiratory epithelium and have mucous glands within a loose mucoid stroma, containing plasma cells, lymphocytes and eosinophils.

Sinusitis Is Inflammation of the Mucous Membranes

It usually reflects bacterial infections of the paranasal sinuses.

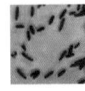 **ETIOLOGIC FACTORS:** Any condition (inflammation, neoplasm, foreign body) that interferes with sinus drainage or aeration renders it susceptible to infection. If a sinus ostium is blocked, secretions or exudate accumulate behind the obstruction.

Acute sinusitis is a disorder of less than 3 weeks' duration, largely caused by extension of infection from the nasal mucosa. *Haemophilus influenzae* and *Branhamella catarrhalis* are the most common organisms. Maxillary sinusitis may also be caused by odontogenic infections: bacteria from the roots of the first and second molars penetrate the thin bony plate that separates them from the floor of the maxillary sinus. Incomplete resolution of infection or recurrent acute sinusitis may lead to chronic sinusitis, in which the purulent exudate almost always includes anaerobic bacteria.

 PATHOLOGY: Complications of acute or chronic sinusitis may include:

- **Mucocele:** Mucocele is an accumulation of mucous secretions in a nasal sinus. If infected, a mucocele may cause a sinus to fill with mucopurulent exudate, called a **pyocele**. Purulent exudation in a sinus is **empyema** (Fig. 29-16). Mucoceles occur most often in the anterior compartments ("cells") of frontal and ethmoid sinuses. They develop slowly and the pressure of their expansion causes bone resorption. Mucoceles of anterior ethmoid or frontal sinuses may be large enough to displace the contents of the orbit and occasionally, erode into the central nervous system.
- **Osteomyelitis:** Suppurative infection of nasal sinus walls may spread through Volkmann canals to the periosteum, producing periostitis and subperiosteal abscess. If these

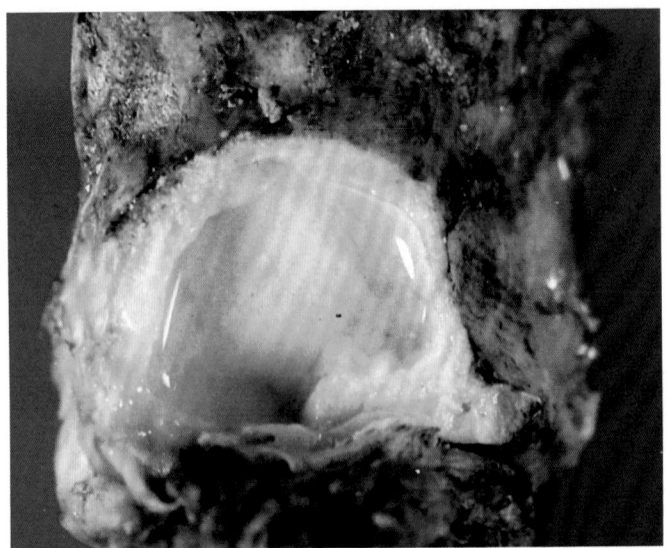

FIGURE 29-16. Empyema of the maxillary sinus (sagittal section). Infection followed chronic obstruction of the orifice caused by adenocarcinoma of the nasal mucosa.

occur on the orbital side of the bone, an orbital cellulitis or abscess forms. Overlying skin is often markedly edematous, and subcutaneous cellulitis or a subcutaneous abscess also may develop. Osteomyelitis also may spread rapidly between the outer and inner tables of the skull.
- **Septic thrombophlebitis:** Sinus infections that penetrate the bone may spread to frontal and diploe venous systems. Resulting septic thrombophlebitis may involve the cavernous venous sinus through the superior ophthalmic veins and is a potentially life-threatening condition.
- **Intracranial infections:** Sinusitis may also spread infection to the cranial cavity. Lesions include epidural, subdural and cerebral abscesses and purulent leptomeningitis. Spread may be via lymphatics and veins and need not involve extensive destruction of bone.

Syphilis May Destroy the Nasal Bridge

Primary chancres in the nose are rare, but mucosal lesions of secondary syphilis are common in the nose and nasopharynx. In tertiary syphilis, inflammation may involve large portions of the nasal mucosa, underlying cartilage and bone. Perichondrial or periosteal gummas may destroy nasal cartilage and bone, causing the nasal bridge to collapse and producing "saddle nose." Destruction of nasal bony walls may also lead to perforation of the nasal septum, hard palate, wall of the orbit or maxillary sinus.

Leprosy Is Spread through Nasal Secretions

Mycobacterium leprae multiplies best at lower temperatures and so prefers cooler body sites, like the nares and anterior nasal mucosa. Nasal involvement is often the first manifestation of leprosy. Tuberculoid and intermediate forms of leprosy account for most cases (see Chapter 9). The skin around the nares and anterior nasal mucosa shows nodules, ulceration or perforations. Nasal involvement is important as leprosy is spread via nasal secretions teeming with bacilli.

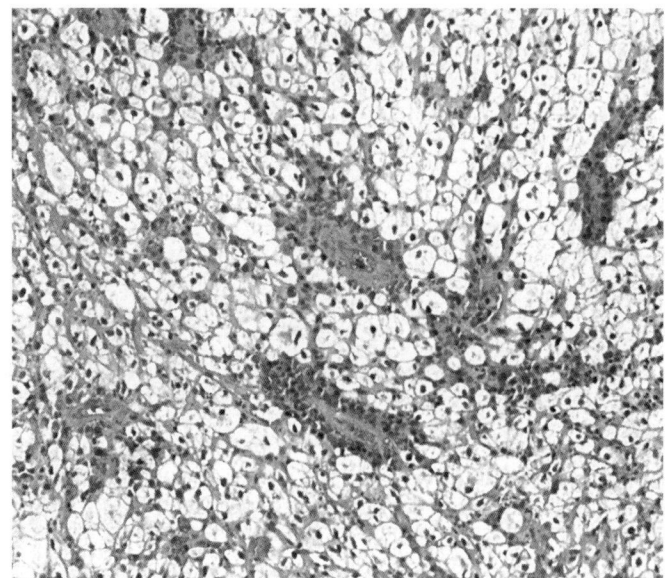

FIGURE 29-17. Rhinoscleroma. Granulation tissue contains numerous foamy macrophages (Mikulicz cells).

Rhinoscleroma (Scleroma) Is a Chronic Bacterial Infection

Rhinoscleroma is a chronic inflammatory process caused by a gram-negative diplobacillus, *Klebsiella rhinoscleromatis*. It begins in the nose and usually remains localized there but may extend slowly into the nasopharynx, larynx and trachea. It rarely involves other sites, such as the paranasal sinuses, orbital tissues, skin, lips, oral mucosa, cervical lymph nodes and gastrointestinal tract. Scleroma is endemic in parts of the Mediterranean basin, Asia, Africa and Latin America. Indigenous cases also occur in the United States. It affects both sexes and any age, and often reflects poor personal hygiene.

 PATHOLOGY: Infected tissues are firm, thickened, irregularly nodular and often ulcerated. The granulation tissue is very rich in plasma cells, lymphocytes and foamy macrophages (Fig. 29-17). Characteristic large macrophages or Mikulicz cells, contain masses of phagocytosed bacilli. The disease is treatable with antibiotics.

Most Fungal Infections of the Nose and Sinuses Are Opportunistic

Pathogenic fungi may involve the nose and paranasal sinuses as part of cutaneous or mucocutaneous infection, particularly in a setting of immunodeficiency (see Chapter 9).

Candidiasis is the most common fungus infection of the nasal mucosa. It usually accompanies oral and pharyngeal candidiasis **(thrush)**. **Aspergillosis** is uncommon, and when it occurs it generally involves a paranasal sinus. Fungi may disseminate to venous sinuses, meninges and the brain. Aspergillosis of the sinonasal tract may be noninvasive or invasive, including angioinvasive. Noninvasive aspergillus sinusitis includes **allergic fungal sinusitis** (AFS) and **sinus mycetoma** (so-called fungus ball).

Allergic Fungal Sinusitis

Allergic fungal sinusitis (AFS) reflects hypersensitivity to fungal antigens, such as allergic bronchopulmonary aspergillosis (see Chapter 12). AFS occurs at all ages but is most common in children or young adults, especially those who are atopic or immunologically "hypercompetent." Any sinus may be affected, but maxillary and ethmoid sinuses are most often involved.

Fungus balls, or **aspergillomas,** occur in immunologically normal patients, usually with chronic sinusitis and poor drainage. In this setting, fungi proliferate to form a dense mass of hyphae that causes nasal obstruction. Evidence of bone destruction and ocular symptoms may be present.

Invasive Fungal Sinusitis

Invasive fungal sinusitis usually affects immunocompromised patients (Fig. 29-18). In the rare **rhinocerebral aspergillosis,** the organisms penetrate venous sinuses and spread to the meninges and brain. Few patients survive.

Mucormycosis is a potentially life-threatening infection, particularly in diabetic and immunosuppressed patients. It typically involves the nasopharynx but can invade the skin, bone, orbit and brain.

Nasal **rhinosporidiosis** is caused by the fungus *Rhinosporidium seeberi*. The disease is endemic in Sri Lanka and parts of India, and Central and South America. Affected nasal mucosa contains vascular polyploid masses that show marked chronic inflammation and characteristic spherical 50–350-μm-diameter sporangia.

Leishmaniasis (Also Known as Kala-Azar)

Mucocutaneous leishmaniasis, due to *Leishmania braziliensis*, commonly affects the nose (see Chapter 9). The nasal disease, known as **espundia,** occurs in Central and South America. Initial skin sores heal within a few months, to be followed in some patients by mucocutaneous lesions of the nose or upper lip months or years later. Infection most likely spreads by nasal contact with contaminated fingers. Early

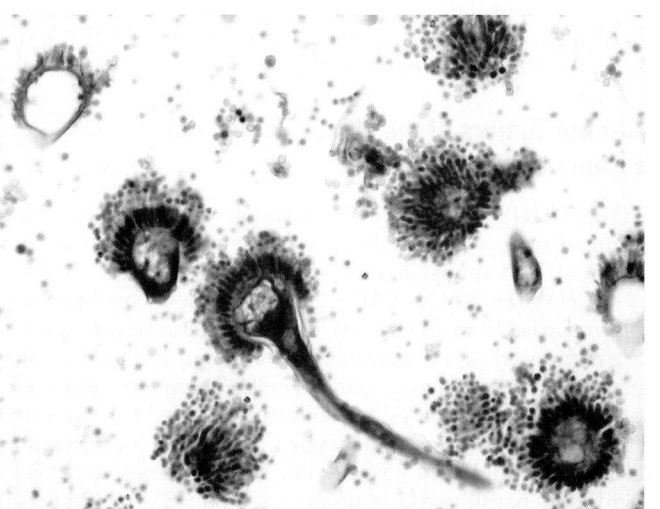

FIGURE 29-18. Aspergillus. A green, nasal mass in a patient with lymphoma demonstrated abundant fruiting bodies.

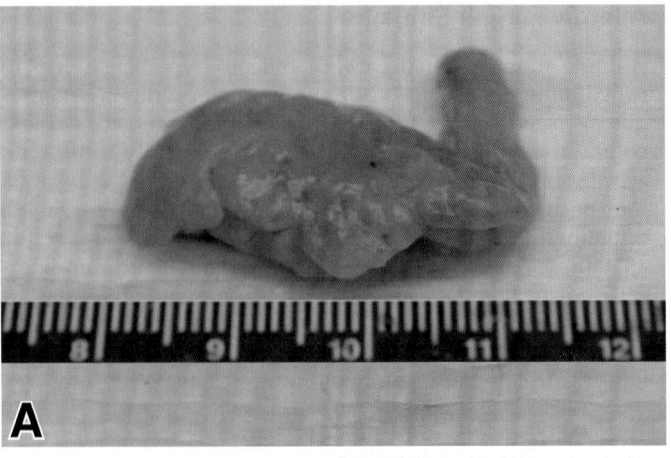

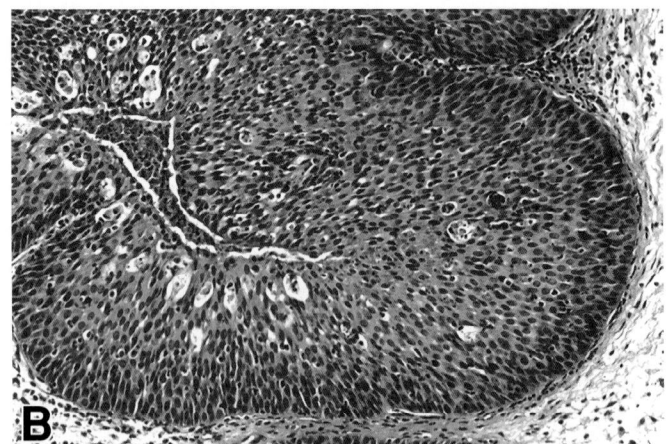

FIGURE 29-19. Sinonasal inverted papilloma. A. Gross photograph of sinonasal inverted papilloma. **B.** Epithelial nests are growing downward (inverted) into the submucosa. They are composed of a uniform cellular proliferation, which displays an inflammatory cell infiltrate and scattered microcysts.

in infection, the mucosa has polypoid inflammatory lesions, and superficial ulcers with macrophages contain parasites. Later, tuberculoid granulomatous responses develop, with few recognizable parasites. Bacterial infection may supervene and lead to soft tissue destruction and collapse of the anterior cartilaginous nasal septum.

Granulomatosis with Polyangiitis Is a Systemic Disease That Affects the Nose and Lower Airways

 PATHOLOGY: This condition, once called Wegener granulomatosis, may affect many organs (see Chapters 10, 12 and 16). The sinonasal tract may be the only involved site, or it may be part of systemic disease. Septal perforation and mucosal ulceration may be followed by slowly progressive destruction of the nose and paranasal sinuses, leading to a saddle nose deformity. Constitutional symptoms, such as fever, malaise and weight loss, may accompany resulting "runny nose," sinusitis and nosebleeds. Nasal lesions show ischemic-type necrosis, vasculitis, mixed chronic inflammation, scattered multinucleated giant cells and microabscesses. Well-formed granulomas are not seen. Elevated serum antineutrophil cytoplasmic antibodies (ANCAs; see Chapter 4) and proteinase 3 (PR3) are associated with active disease.

Benign Tumors of the Nasal Cavity and Paranasal Sinuses

SQUAMOUS PAPILLOMA: This is the most common benign tumor of the nasal cavity. It resembles a wart (verruca vulgaris) and almost always occurs in the nasal vestibule.

SCHNEIDERIAN PAPILLOMAS: These benign neoplasms arise from the sinonasal (Schneiderian) mucosa and are composed of a squamous or columnar epithelial proliferation with associated mucous cells. There are three morphologically distinct lesions collectively called Schneiderian papillomas: **inverted, oncocytic** (cylindrical or columnar cell) and **fungiform** (exophytic, septal) papillomas. Schneiderian papillomas represent less than 5% of sinonasal tract tumors (Fig. 29-19A).

INVERTED PAPILLOMA: This tumor involves the lateral nasal wall and may spread to the paranasal sinuses.

Inverted papillomas occur mainly in middle-aged people. As the name implies, they show inversion of surface epithelium into underlying stroma (Fig. 29-19B). HPV types 6 and 11 and, rarely, types 16, 18, 33, 40, or 57 are detected but are of uncertain significance. Although benign, these tumors may erode bone by pressure. Surgical resection must extend beyond the boundaries of grossly visible lesions, or they may recur. In 5% of cases, inverted papillomas give rise to SCC.

MALIGNANCIES OF THE NASAL CAVITY AND PARANASAL SINUSES

SCC Is Often Associated with Occupational Risk Factors

Over half of cancers of the nasal cavity and paranasal sinuses arise in the maxillary sinus antrum, one third in the nasal cavity, 10% in the ethmoid sinus and 1% in sphenoid and frontal sinuses (Fig. 29-20). Most are keratinizing or nonkeratinizing SCCs (Table 29-2). Some 15% are adenocarcinomas, or undifferentiated carcinomas.

TABLE 29-2
VARIANTS OF SQUAMOUS CELL CARCINOMA
Acantholytic squamous cell carcinoma
Adenosquamous carcinoma
Basaloid squamous cell carcinoma
Carcinoma cuniculatum
Papillary squamous cell carcinoma
Spindle cell squamous carcinoma
Verrucous carcinoma
Lymphoepithelial carcinoma (non-nasopharyngeal)

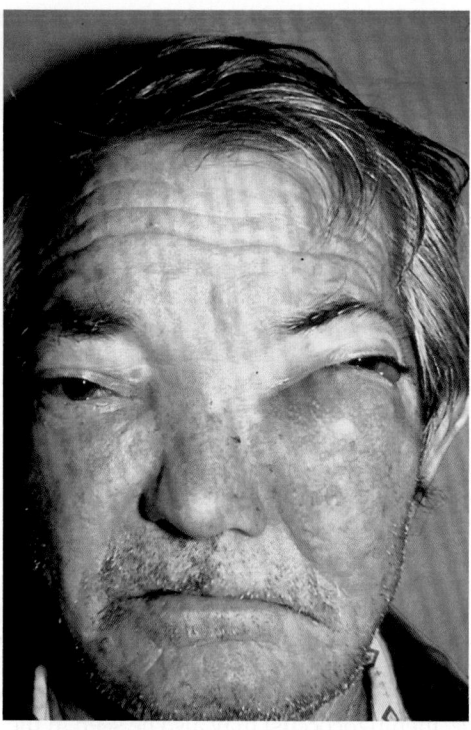

FIGURE 29-20. Squamous cell carcinoma of the maxillary sinus caused an obvious facial deformity, owing to invasion outside the confines of the sinus. Involvement of the orbit and facial nerve is evident. The latter is defined by drooping of the mouth to the side of the facial nerve paralysis.

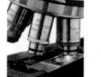 **ETIOLOGY:** Several industrial chemicals may cause cancer of the nose and sinuses, including nickel, chromium and aromatic hydrocarbons. Occupational settings reportedly with increased risk for cancer of the nose and sinuses (but for which a specific chemical agent is not identified) are woodworking in the furniture industry, use of cutting oils and leather textile industries.

Nickel workers are prone to SCCs, mostly from the middle turbinate, with latencies from 2 to over 30 years. Most other occupational exposures mainly lead to adenocarcinomas and occur mostly in the maxillary and ethmoid sinuses. Because of these occupational risk factors, cancers of the nose and sinuses occur far more often in men and after age 50. These tumors grow relentlessly and invade adjacent structures but typically do not metastasize. Survival is usually only a few years.

Olfactory Neuroblastoma Is of Neural Crest Origin

This tumor, also called esthesioneuroblastoma, is uncommon. It has a slight male predominance and occurs in people between 3 years of age and in the ninth decade but a bimodal distribution in the second and sixth decades are most common.

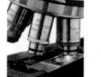 **PATHOLOGY:** This cancer arises from the olfactory mucosa covering the superior third of the nasal septum, cribriform plate (Fig. 29-21A) and superior turbinate. It is usually polypoid and highly vascular and shows diverse histologies, depending on the amount of intercellular neurofibrillary material. Tumor

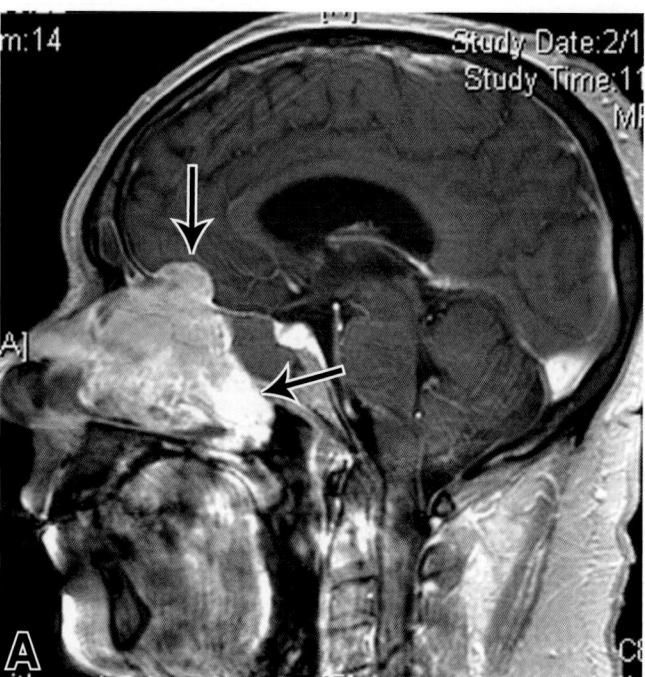

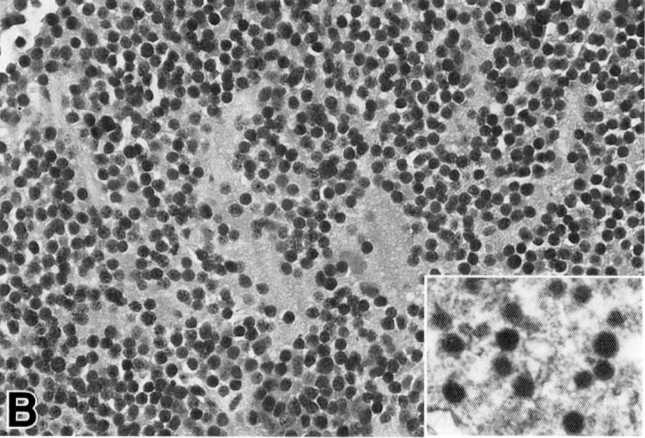

FIGURE 29-21. Olfactory neuroblastoma. A. Sagittal T1 postcontrast magnetic resonance image (MRI) demonstrates a hyperintense mass (*arrows*) arising from the cribriform plate and filling the nasal cavity. **B.** The tumor is composed of small round cells with hyperchromatic nuclei and a background eosinophilic stroma representing neurofibrillary matrix. *Inset.* An electron micrograph shows intracytoplasmic, secretory-type, membrane-bound granules with dense cores.

cells are slightly larger than lymphocytes, with round nuclei and inconspicuous cytoplasm (Fig. 29-21B). They may form pseudorosettes (Homer Wright rosettes) or true neural rosettes (Flexner-Wintersteiner rosettes). The World Health Organization (2005) adopted a four-tiered grading system, based on lobular architecture, mitosis, necrosis, nuclear pleomorphism, fibrillary matrix and rosettes. Olfactory neuroblastomas express synaptophysin and neuron-specific enolase (NSE) but not cytokeratin and epithelial membrane antigen (EMA). S-100 protein often surrounds nests or lobules **(sustentacular cells),** mostly in lower-grade tumors. The cells of olfactory neuroblastomas have intracytoplasmic neurosecretory granules like those of neuroblastomas at other sites.

THE HEAD AND NECK

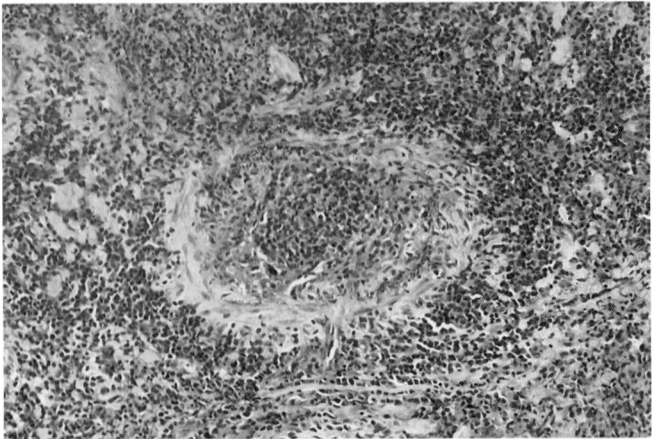

FIGURE 29-22. Angiocentric natural killer (NK)/T-cell lymphoma. A malignant cellular infiltrate growing around and into a medium-sized blood vessel with disruption of the external elastic membrane and occlusion of the vessel lumen.

 CLINICAL FEATURES: Olfactory neuroblastomas invade and destroy bony structures slowly. They spread readily via lymphatics to regional and distant lymph nodes. Hematogenous spread occurs less often. Prognosis usually corresponds to tumor grade. Complete removal is critical, and craniofacial resection with chemotherapy and/or radiation therapy provides 85% 5-year survival.

Nasal-Type Angiocentric Natural Killer/T-Cell Lymphoma Is Highly Lethal

These tumors, once called **lethal midline granulomas,** midline malignant reticulosis and polymorphic reticulosis, are now recognized as malignant lymphomas.

 PATHOLOGY: The characteristic lymphoid infiltrate is necrotizing and polymorphic. Similar infiltrates may occur in the upper airways, lungs and alimentary tract, but any organ can be involved. Tumor cells surround small to medium-sized blood vessels (angiocentric); infiltrate through their walls (angioinvasion), often occluding vessel lumens like a thrombus; and cause necrosis in adjacent tissues (ischemic type) (Fig. 29-22). *EBV infection is associated with this type of lymphoma.*

 CLINICAL FEATURES: Nasal-type natural killer (NK)/T-cell lymphoma usually begins insidiously as nonspecific rhinitis or sinusitis. Gradually, the nasal mucosa is focally swollen, indurated and eventually ulcerated. Ulcers are covered by a black crust, under which cartilage and bone are eroded, causing defects of the nasal septum, hard palate and nasopharynx, with serious functional consequences. The skin of the midface is often involved. Half of patients have localized disease, but wide dissemination is common. Death is due to secondary bacterial infection, aspiration pneumonia or hemorrhage from eroded large blood vessels. These lymphomas are, at least initially, radiosensitive, and remission with cytotoxic agents has also been reported.

Nasopharynx and Oropharynx

ANATOMY: The nasopharynx is continuous anteriorly with the nasal cavities; its roof is formed by the body of the sphenoid bone and its posterior wall by the cervical vertebrae. Eustachian tube openings are on the lateral walls of the nasopharynx. In newborns, it is covered by pseudostratified ciliated columnar epithelium. With advancing age, the nasopharynx is replaced by a stratified squamous epithelium over large areas (80%). The mucosa has many mucous glands and abundant lymphoid tissue.

Waldeyer ring *is a circular band of lymphoid tissue at the opening of the oropharynx into the respiratory and digestive tracts.* Lymphoid tissue on the superior posterior wall forms the nasopharyngeal tonsils, which, when hyperplastic, are called **adenoids.** The palatine tonsils are lateral, where the pharynx connects with the oral cavity. They are covered by stratified squamous epithelium, which lines infoldings **(tonsillar crypts)** into the lymphoid tissue. Crypts normally contain desquamated epithelium, lymphocytes, some neutrophils and saprophytic organisms, such as bacteria, *Candida* and actinomycetes. Pathogens (e.g., *Corynebacterium diphtheriae,* meningococcus) may also be seen in the pharynx of healthy people.

Waldeyer ring is well developed in children and its follicles have germinal centers. In fact, the tonsils represent the largest collections of B lymphocytes in a normal child. Pharyngeal lymphoid tissue diminishes considerably by adulthood. It gradually involutes with age but does not totally disappear.

PHARYNGEAL LYMPHOID HYPOPLASIA AND HYPERPLASIA

Bruton sex-linked agammaglobulinemia (see Chapter 4) affects only males, who have minimal or no lymphoid tissue in their tonsils, pharynx and intestines (Peyer patches and appendix). They have a normally developed thymus.

Atrophy of pharyngeal lymphoid tissue is common in chronically immunosuppressed patients. Local radiation therapy also causes marked loss of lymphoid tissue in the Waldeyer ring.

Hyperplasia of nasopharyngeal lymphoid tissue follows infections or chronic irritation due to dust, smoke and fumes. Tonsils may enlarge in some primary immunodeficiencies (dysgammaglobulinemia type I or nodular lymphoid hyperplasia), presumably reflecting an adaptive response by the immune system.

INFECTIONS

Pharyngitis and tonsillitis are among the most common diseases of the head and neck. Nasopharyngeal inflammation occurs mainly in children but is also common in adolescents and young adults. Viral or bacterial infections may be limited to the palatine tonsils but may also involve nasopharyngeal tonsils or adjacent pharyngeal mucosa, often as part of a general upper respiratory tract infection. Viruses are the usual culprits: influenza, parainfluenza, adenovirus, respiratory syncytial virus and rhinovirus, spread by droplet or by direct contact.

S. pyogenes is the most important cause of pharyngitis and tonsillitis, because it may cause serious suppurative and nonsuppurative sequelae. **Diphtheria** still produces pharyngitis in some countries. These infections are characterized by an exudate or, in the case of diphtheria, a pseudomembrane on the tonsils and pharynx.

Acute tonsillitis is usually due to *S. pyogenes* (group A β-hemolytic streptococci). In **follicular tonsillitis,** pinpoint exudates may be extruded from the crypts.

In **pseudomembranous tonsillitis,** a necrotic mucosa is covered by a coat of exudate, as in diphtheria or **Vincent angina**. The latter is caused by fusiform bacilli and spirochetes that are part of the normal oral flora. They become pathogenic when local or systemic resistance is low (e.g., after mucosal injury or in malnutrition).

Recurrent or chronic tonsillitis is not as common as once believed, and enlarged tonsils in children do not necessarily signify chronic tonsillitis. However, repeated infections can cause tonsils and adenoids to enlarge and obstruct air passages. Repeated streptococcal tonsillitis may lead to rheumatic fever or glomerulonephritis in children, who may benefit from tonsillectomy.

Peritonsillar abscesses (quinsy) are collections of pus behind the posterior capsule of the tonsil, usually due to α- and β-hemolytic streptococci. About one third of patients have histories of tonsillitis. Untreated, such abscesses may be life-threatening since (1) aided by gravity, they may dissect inferiorly to the pyriform sinus to obstruct, or rupture into, the airway; (2) they may extend laterally into the parapharyngeal space (parapharyngeal abscess) and weaken the carotid artery wall; or (3) they may penetrate along the carotid sheath inferiorly into the mediastinum or, superiorly, to the base of the skull or cranial cavity, with disastrous consequences.

Infectious mononucleosis (mostly due to EBV) often presents with exudative tonsillitis, pharyngitis and posterior cervical lymphadenopathy. **Adenoids** represent chronic inflammatory hyperplasia of pharyngeal lymphoid tissue. This condition is often accompanied by chronic tonsillitis or rhinitis, almost always in children. Enlarged adenoids may partly or completely obstruct the eustachian tube, leading to otitis media.

NEOPLASMS

Nasopharyngeal Angiofibroma Is a Tumor of Adolescent Boys

These tumors, once called "juvenile nasopharyngeal angiofibromas," are uncommon, highly vascular neoplasms of the nasopharynx. They are histologically benign but locally aggressive. These tumors most often arise in adolescent males but are not restricted to this age group.

 PATHOLOGY: Angiofibromas are multinodular, lobulated or smooth pink-white masses, which may show surface ulceration and obvious blood vessels (Fig. 29-23A). They typically arise in the submucosa of the **posterolateral nasal wall** and tend to expand into adjacent structures, causing local mass effects. These tumors may grow into fissures and foramina of the skull or destroy bone and spread into adjacent structures, such as the nasal

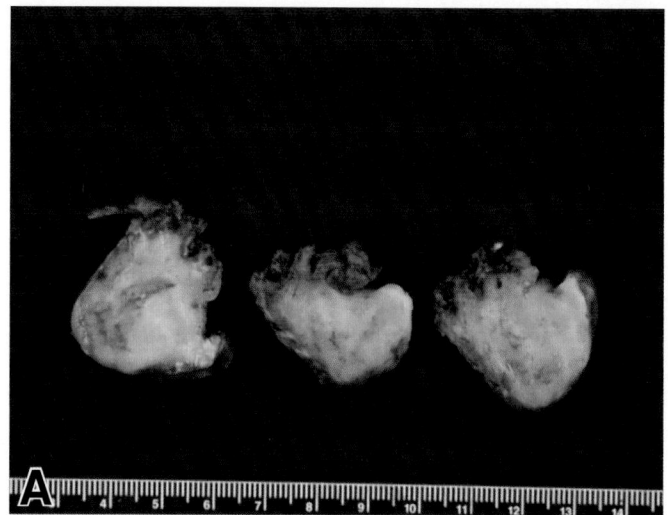
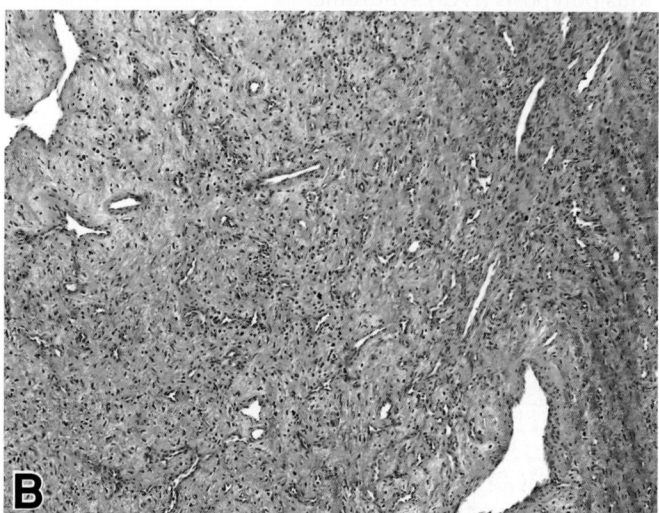
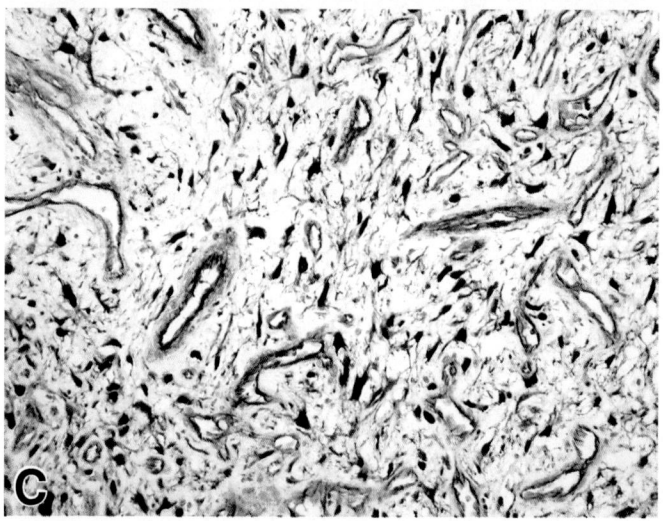

FIGURE 29-23. Nasopharyngeal angiofibroma. A. The cut surface of the tumor appears dense and spongy. **B.** Microscopically, it is composed of slit-like vascular structures in a collagenous stroma. **C.** Immunohistochemistry for β-catenin demonstrates aberrant nuclear labeling.

cavity, paranasal sinuses, orbit, middle cranial fossa or pterygomaxillary fossa.

Angiofibromas have vascular and stromal components (Fig. 29-23B). Blood vessels vary in size and shape; the smooth muscle in their walls is not layered, but rather arranged irregularly. Stromal fibroblasts express aberrant nuclear β-catenin (Fig. 29-23C).

 CLINICAL FEATURES: Many angiofibromas regress spontaneously after puberty. They respond to estrogen therapy, and so may be hormonally regulated and androgen dependent. Vessel wall defects preclude vasoconstriction, leading to brisk bleeding after trauma. Biopsies may thus be dangerous and are contraindicated. Radiation therapy is also effective. Preoperative embolization may be used to reduce vascularity prior to surgery. There is a familial tendency for these tumors; they occur 25 times more often in patients with familial adenomatous polyposis (FAP) syndrome.

Oropharyngeal SCCs Are Usually Associated with HPV

In the United States, 80% of oropharyngeal SCCs are associated with high-risk HPV serotypes. These cancers, called HPV-associated head and neck squamous cell carcinomas (HPV-HNSCCs), arise mainly from palatine and lingual tonsils and are nonkeratinizing tumors of the basaloid cell type (Fig. 29-24A). Such tumors may be small and difficult to detect and often present as metastatic cancer in a cervical lymph node.

Compared to non–HPV-HNSCCs, HPV-HNSCCs tend to occur in younger people without the risk factors for HNSCC as often seen in older patients (i.e., smoking, alcohol). HPV-HNSCCs also are radiosensitive and have better overall better prognosis than non–HPV-associated HNSCCs (Fig. 29-24B,C).

The pathogenetic roles played by cancer-associated HPV serotypes and their associated proteins are described elsewhere (see Chapters 5 and 18).

Nasopharyngeal Carcinoma Is Related to Epstein-Barr Virus

Nasopharyngeal carcinoma (NPC) is divided into keratinizing and nonkeratinizing types. The latter are associated with EBV infection and may be differentiated or undifferentiated.

 **EPIDEMIOLOGY:** *Undifferentiated nonkeratinizing carcinomas are particularly common in southeast Asia and parts of Africa.* By far the most

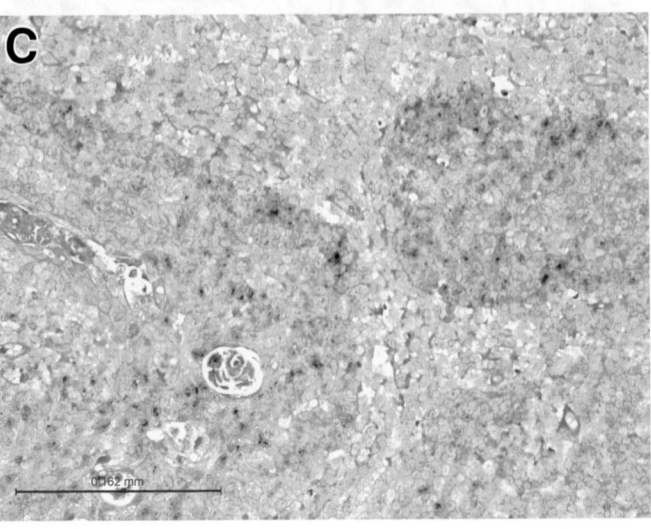

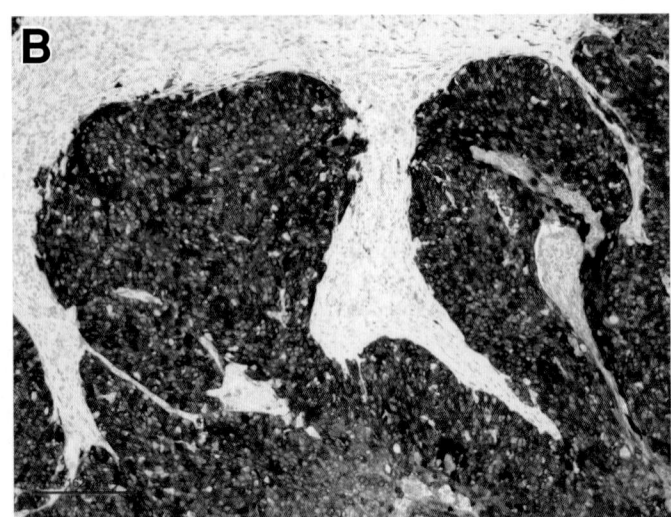

FIGURE 29-24. Human papillomavirus (HPV)-associated squamous cell carcinoma of the tonsil. A. Nests of invasive carcinoma are positive for p16 immunohistochemistry **(B)**. **C.** In situ hybridization for high-risk HPV (including types 16 and 18) demonstrates nuclear localization (blue dots).

common cancer of the nasopharynx, NPC is the most common of all cancers in China. In Hong Kong, it represents 18% of all malignancies, compared with 0.25% worldwide. Chinese born in the United States have a 20-fold greater mortality from this tumor than do other ethnicities.

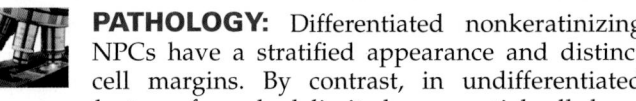 **MOLECULAR PATHOGENESIS:** Environmental risk factors for NPC have remained elusive. The A2/sin human leukocyte antigen (HLA) profile is more common in Chinese patients, suggesting a genetic susceptibility. Frequent deletions in several chromosomes, in particular 3p, 9p and 14q, occur in NPCs.

About 85% of patients with NPC have antibodies to EBV. The virus genomes are detected in 75%–100% of nonkeratinizing and undifferentiated types of NPC. EBV is more variable in keratinizing NPCs (see Chapters 5 and 9 for more detail).

PATHOLOGY: Differentiated nonkeratinizing NPCs have a stratified appearance and distinct cell margins. By contrast, in undifferentiated tumors, clusters of poorly delimited or syncytial cells have large oval nuclei and scant eosinophilic cytoplasm (Fig. 29-25A). Lymphoid infiltrates may be prominent in undifferentiated tumors, accounting for the obsolete (and misleading) term "lymphoepithelioma." Both subtypes express cytokeratin (Fig. 29-25B), but not hematologic or lymphoid markers. In situ hybridization studies usually identify EBV DNA (Fig. 29-25C).

CLINICAL FEATURES: Owing to their location, most NPCs are asymptomatic for a long time and in half of patients first present as palpable cervical lymph node metastases. Even then, many patients still have no complaints referable to the nasopharynx. Tumors invade nearby regions, such as the parapharyngeal space, orbit and cranial cavity, causing neurologic symptoms and hearing disturbances. Invasion of the base of the skull leads to cranial nerve involvement. Tumors in the fossa of Rosenmüller and the lateral wall of the nasopharynx cause symptoms referable to the middle ear. Eustachian tube obstruction is common. The abundant local lymphatic network gives rise to frequent and early metastases to cervical lymph nodes.

Nasopharyngeal undifferentiated carcinoma is radiosensitive, and most patients with tumors restricted to the nasopharynx survive 5 years or more. Cranial nerve involvement or metastases to cervical lymph nodes or beyond portend poor survival.

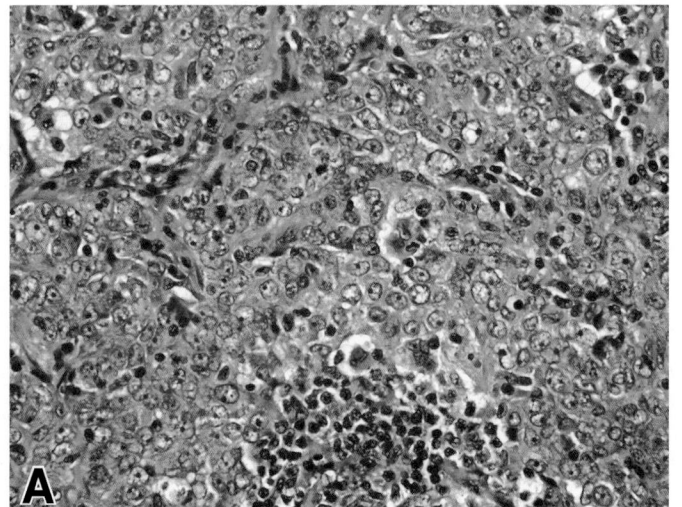

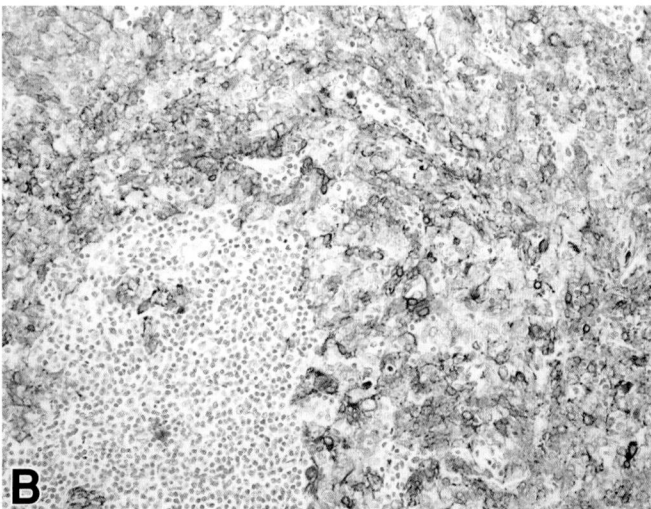

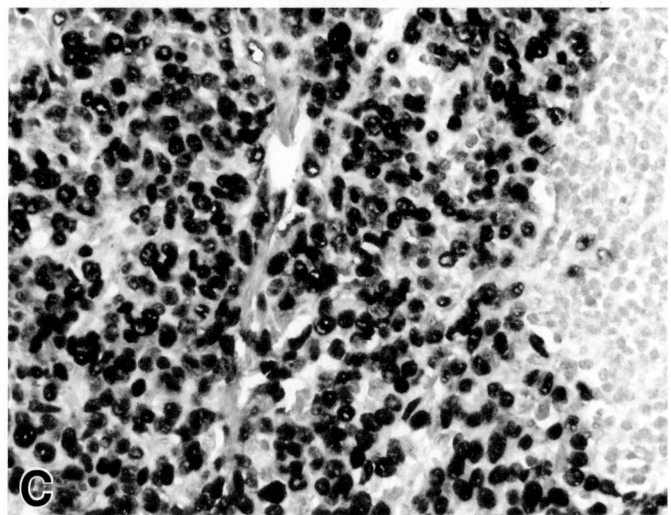

FIGURE 29-25. Nasopharyngeal nonkeratinizing carcinoma, undifferentiated type. **A.** The cells have large nuclei and prominent eosinophilic nucleoli. **B.** The cells are cytokeratin positive (by immunohistochemistry), indicating an epithelial cell proliferation. **C.** In situ hybridization for Epstein-Barr virus (EBER-ISH).

Lymphomas of the Waldeyer Ring Are Mostly Diffuse B-Cell Tumors

Lymphomas account for 5% of head and neck cancers. The Waldeyer ring is by far the most common site of origin of lymphoma in this region: the palatine tonsils first, then the nasopharynx and base of the tongue. These lymphomas are histologically diffuse (90%), and over half are large cell lymphomas. In the United States and Asia, the vast majority are of B-cell origin.

Most Extramedullary Plasmacytomas Occur in the Head and Neck

These tumors occur in the nasopharynx, nasal cavity and paranasal sinuses and behave like other extramedullary plasmacytomas. Head and neck plasmacytomas may remain localized or may evolve into systemic plasma cell myelomas (see Chapter 20).

Chordomas Are Derived from Remnants of Embryonic Notochord

Chordomas are uncommon cancers in people under age 40. In the cranial region, they originate from the area of the sphenooccipital synchondrosis or **clivus,** and in one third of cases, they extend into the nasopharynx. These tumors have large vacuolated **(physaliferous)** cells, surrounded by abundant intercellular matrix (Fig. 29-26). Chordomas grow slowly, but they infiltrate bone and are difficult to excise completely by surgery. Patients with cranial region chordomas rarely survive over 5 years.

Other Malignancies of the Nasopharynx Are Rare

They may derive from various components of mucosa or adjacent supportive soft tissues and skeleton. **Embryonal rhabdomyosarcomas** (Fig. 29-27) are highly malignant tumors of pharyngeal tissues of young children. They invade contiguous structures and metastasize via

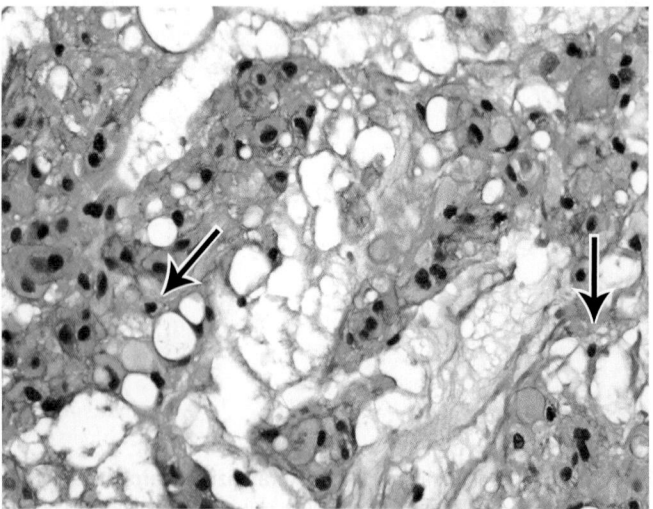

FIGURE 29-26. Chordoma. Large vacuolated (physaliferous) tumor cells (*arrows*) are evident.

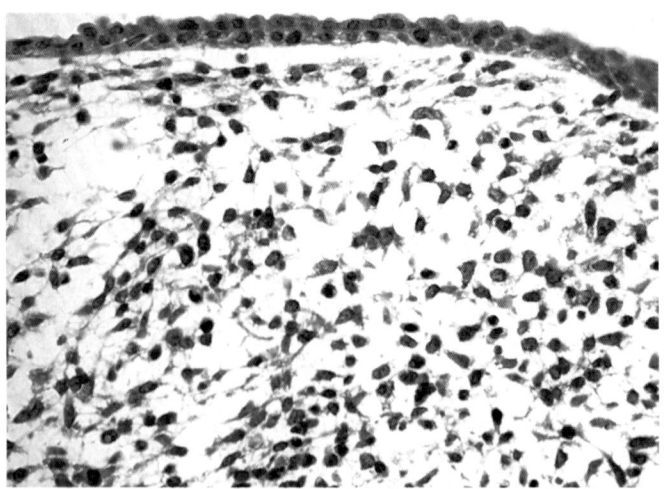

FIGURE 29-27. Embryonal rhabdomyosarcoma from a 3-year-old girl. This highly malignant tumor arose in the parapharyngeal space and invaded the adjacent structures. The oval or tadpole-shaped tumor cells under the epithelium have hyperchromatic, eccentric nuclei and immunohistochemical and ultrastructural features of rhabdomyoblasts.

the bloodstream and lymphatics. Nasopharyngeal **Kaposi sarcomas** may occur in patients with AIDS, in association with HHV8.

Larynx and Hypopharynx

INFECTIONS

EPIGLOTTITIS: Inflammation of the epiglottis is most commonly caused by *H. influenzae* type B. It occurs in infants and young children and may be a life-threatening emergency. Swelling of an acutely inflamed epiglottis may obstruct airflow. Inspiratory stridor (loud wheezing on inspiration) and the onset of cyanosis may indicate airway obstruction so severe as to require tracheostomy.

CROUP: Croup is a laryngotracheobronchitis of young children who have symptoms of inspiratory stridor, cough and hoarseness, due to varying degrees of laryngeal obstruction. It is a complication of an upper respiratory infection, with marked laryngeal edema and a "barking cough." This was once a deadly complication of diphtheria. However, antibiotics and immunizations have helped prevent or treat it, and today, it is most commonly caused by the parainfluenza viruses.

VOCAL CORD NODULE AND POLYP

Also called *singer's nodules,* these are stromal reactions related to inflammation and/or trauma. They may be seen in all age groups but are most common between the third and sixth decades (Fig. 29-28). Symptoms related to vocal cord polyps and nodules are similar: hoarseness or voice changes ("cracking" of the voice). Lesions occur after voice abuse, infection (laryngitis), excessive alcohol consumption,

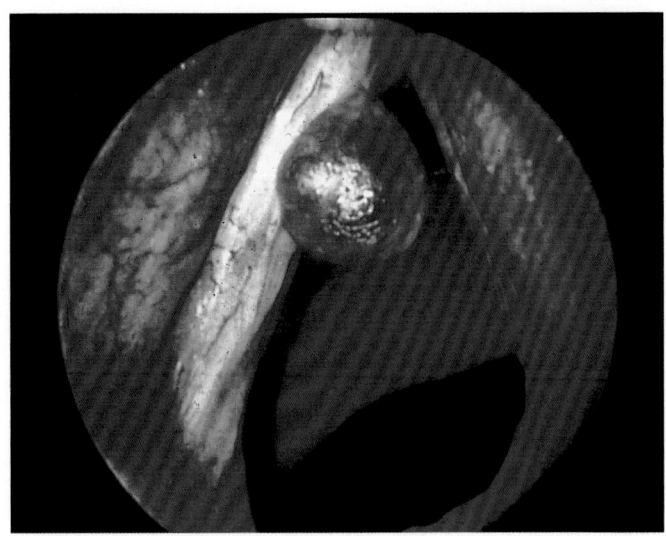

FIGURE 29-28. Vocal cord polyp. A solitary polypoid lesion with a glistening appearance is seen arising from the true vocal cord.

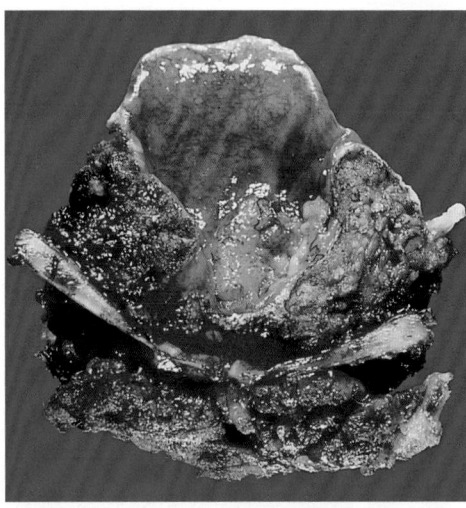

FIGURE 29-29. Supraglottic laryngectomy specimen for squamous cell carcinoma. The carcinoma appears as an irregular raised granular-appearing area in the right supraglottic larynx.

smoking or endocrine dysfunction (e.g., hypothyroidism). Histologies vary from a myxoid, edematous, fibroblastic stroma in early stages to a hyalinized, densely fibrotic stroma later.

NEOPLASMS OF THE LARYNX

SQUAMOUS PAPILLOMA AND PAPILLOMATOSIS: These papillomas are solitary or multiple papillary growths of the mature squamous cells that line the surface of fibrovascular cores. They may be multiple in children or adolescents **(juvenile laryngeal papillomatosis)** and may extend into the trachea and bronchi. HPV, especially serotypes 6 and 11, are the main causes. The condition may cause life-threatening respiratory obstruction and, rarely, evolve into overt SCC, particularly in smokers or after radiation therapy. Surgical excision may not be curative, as the viral infection is often widespread, and these tumors tend to recur over many years. Solitary laryngeal squamous papilloma occurs in adults, mostly men, and is usually cured surgically.

SQUAMOUS CELL CARCINOMA: Almost all laryngeal cancers are SCCs, predominantly in men, most of whom smoke cigarettes. HPV is found in a quarter of cases.

■ **Glottic carcinoma** is limited to one or both true vocal cords and accounts for 2/3 of laryngeal SCCs. It metastasizes late to lymph nodes and has a good prognosis.
■ **Supraglottic carcinomas** arise in the ventricle, false cords or epiglottis and, by definition, do not involve the true cords. Up to 1/3 of laryngeal cancers arise in this location. Nodal metastases are more common than in glottic tumors.
■ **Transglottic carcinoma** by definition involves true and false cords (Fig. 29-29). It spreads to lymph nodes and often requires total laryngectomy.
■ **Infraglottic carcinomas** are uncommon. Found below the true cords or involving the true cords with infraglottic extension and frequent extension into the trachea, they commonly spread to lymph nodes. Total laryngectomy is usually required.

CHONDROSARCOMA: Chondrosarcomas account for 75% of nonepithelial laryngeal malignancies. In the larynx, they grow as exophytic, polypoid masses and can cause airway obstruction. Most patients are men in their 70s. It also occurs in the nasopharynx, mandible, maxilla and nasal and paranasal sinuses. Patients present with hoarseness, airway obstruction and dyspnea.

Salivary Glands

The salivary glands develop as buds of oral ectoderm. They are tubuloalveolar structures that secrete saliva. Major salivary glands are paired organs. Parotid glands secrete serous saliva, and submandibular and sublingual glands make mixed serous and mucous saliva. Minor salivary glands are widespread under the mucosa of the lips, cheeks, palate and tongue. Lymph nodes are normally embedded in the parotid gland and may be involved in inflammatory, reactive, proliferative or malignant processes.

XEROSTOMIA: Xerostomia is chronic mouth dryness due to lack of saliva and has many causes. Diseases that involve major salivary glands and lead to xerostomia include mumps, Sjögren syndrome, sarcoidosis, radiation-induced atrophy (Fig. 29-30) and drug sensitivity (e.g., antihistamines, tricyclic antidepressants, phenothiazines).

SIALORRHEA: Increased salivary flow is associated with many conditions, including acute inflammation of the oral cavity (e.g., as in aphthous stomatitis), Parkinson disease, rabies, mental retardation, nausea and pregnancy.

ENLARGEMENT: Unilateral enlargement of major salivary glands is usually caused by cysts, inflammation or neoplasms. Bilateral enlargement is due to inflammation (mumps, Sjögren syndrome; see below), granulomatous disease (sarcoidosis) or diffuse neoplastic involvement (leukemia or lymphoma).

SIALOLITHIASIS: Calcific stones in salivary gland ducts mostly occur in the submandibular gland. They obstruct ducts, leading to inflammation distally.

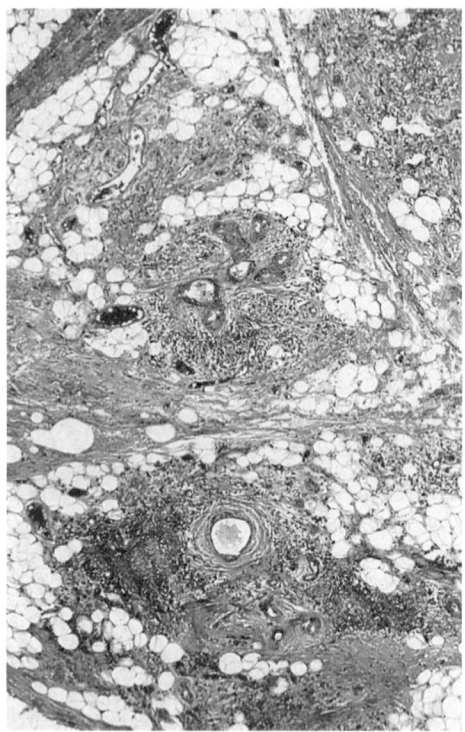

FIGURE 29-30. Chronic sialadenitis. Severe chronic inflammation and marked atrophy of the submandibular gland are present after irradiation of an adjacent oral cancer. The atrophic acini have been replaced by fat.

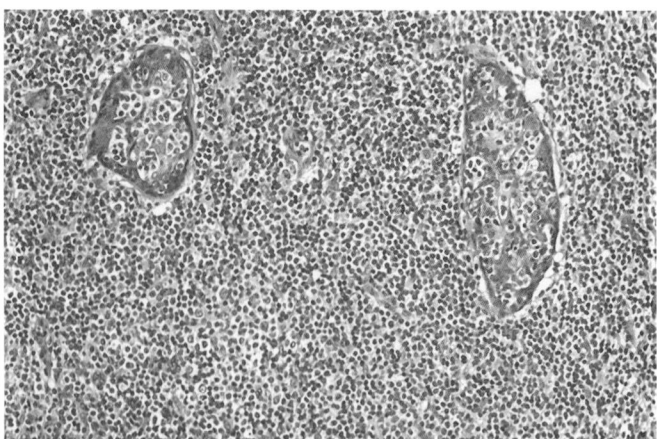

FIGURE 29-31. Sjögren syndrome. There is infiltration of the involved salivary gland by a mixed chronic inflammatory cell infiltrate. Extension of the infiltrate into epithelial (ductal) structures results in metaplasia and characteristic epimyoepithelial islands.

sialadenitis; Fig. 29-31). Similar changes occur in the lacrimal glands and minor salivary glands. Focal lymphocytic sialadenitis is also present in minor salivary glands. Late in the course of the disease, affected glands become atrophic, with fibrosis and fatty infiltration of the parenchyma. Lymphocytes in Sjögren syndrome may show restricted immunoglobulin types but may remain localized, without invasion.

PAROTITIS: Bacteria (usually *Staphylococcus aureus*) may ascend from the oral cavity when salivary flow is reduced and cause acute suppurative parotitis. It is most often seen in debilitated or postoperative patients. Salivary duct stricture or obstruction by stones may cause acute or chronic parotitis. Stagnant secretions serve as a medium for retrograde bacterial invasion.

Epidemic parotitis (mumps) is an acute viral disease of the parotid glands that spreads via infected saliva. Submandibular and sublingual glands also may be affected. Involved glands have dense lymphocytic and macrophage infiltrates, epithelial degeneration and necrosis.

Sjögren Syndrome Is a Systemic Autoimmune Disease Affecting the Salivary and Lacrimal Glands

The disease may be limited to these sites, or it may be associated with a systemic autoimmune disease (see Chapter 11). In the salivary glands, it leads to xerostomia. Involvement of the lacrimal glands results in dry eyes **(keratoconjunctivitis sicca)**. The pathogenesis and clinical features of Sjögren syndrome are discussed in Chapters 11 and 4.

 PATHOLOGY: In Sjögren syndrome, parotid glands, and sometimes submandibular glands, are enlarged unilaterally or bilaterally, but their lobulation is preserved. Initial periductal chronic inflammation gradually extends into the acini, until the glands are completely replaced by a sea of polyclonal lymphocytes, immunoblasts, germinal centers and plasma cells. Proliferating myoepithelial cells surround remnants of damaged ducts and form so-called epimyoepithelial islands **(lymphoepithelial**

BENIGN SALIVARY GLAND NEOPLASMS

Pleomorphic Adenoma Is the Most Common Salivary Gland Tumor

These neoplasms, also called **mixed tumors,** are benign proliferations with admixed epithelial and stromal elements. Two thirds of major salivary gland tumors, and about half of those in the minor glands, are pleomorphic adenomas. These tumors occur nine times more often in the parotid than in the submandibular gland and usually arise in the superficial lobe of the former. Middle-aged people and women are most affected.

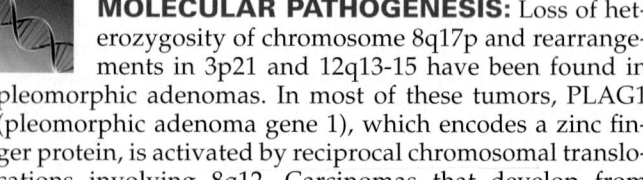 **MOLECULAR PATHOGENESIS:** Loss of heterozygosity of chromosome 8q17p and rearrangements in 3p21 and 12q13-15 have been found in pleomorphic adenomas. In most of these tumors, PLAG1 (pleomorphic adenoma gene 1), which encodes a zinc finger protein, is activated by reciprocal chromosomal translocations involving 8q12. Carcinomas that develop from pleomorphic adenomas may have 8q12 rearrangements, alterations in 12q13-15 and mutations in *HMGIC* and *MDM2* genes.

 PATHOLOGY: Pleomorphic adenomas are slowly growing, painless, movable, firm masses with smooth surfaces (Fig. 29-32). Those arising deep in the parotid may grow between the ramus of the mandible, the styloid process and the stylomandibular ligament into the parapharyngeal space and appear as swellings

ground substance that resembles cartilaginous, myxoid or mucoid material.

 CLINICAL FEATURES: Pleomorphic adenomas have fibrous capsules. As they grow, surrounding fibrous tissue condenses around them. The tumors expand and often protrude focally into adjacent tissues, becoming nodular and occasionally forming "podocytes" (Fig. 29-31B). These tumor projections can be missed if a tumor is not carefully excised with its capsule intact, plus an adequate margin of gland parenchyma. Tumor implanted during surgery or tumor nodules left behind continue to grow and recur in scars from previous operations. Recurrences usually represent local regrowth, not malignancy. Definitive surgery may necessitate sacrificing the facial nerve.

Carcinomas may rarely arise in pleomorphic adenomas (**carcinoma ex pleomorphic adenoma**). In this case, the tumor that was present for many years then begins to grow rapidly or becomes painful. Such carcinomas are most frequently high-grade malignancies set in otherwise benign pleomorphic adenomas. However, virtually any type of salivary gland malignancy may occur in this setting, including mucoepidermoid or adenoid cystic carcinomas. If the malignancy is confined to the tumor capsule and does not invade the adjacent salivary gland, it is considered **in situ** or **noninvasive carcinoma ex pleomorphic adenoma**. If the cancer invades beyond the tumor capsule but not more than 1.5 mm, it is called **minimally invasive carcinoma ex pleomorphic adenoma**. These entities have an excellent prognosis. However, tumors invading beyond 1.5 mm (i.e., *widely invasive tumor*) act aggressively, recur often, metastasize and have a poor prognosis.

Monomorphic Adenomas Represent 5%–10% of Benign Salivary Gland Tumors

In monomorphic adenomas, the epithelium is arranged in a regular, usually glandular, pattern with no mesenchymal component. Monomorphic adenomas include (1) Warthin tumors, (2) basal cell adenomas, (3) oxyphilic adenomas or

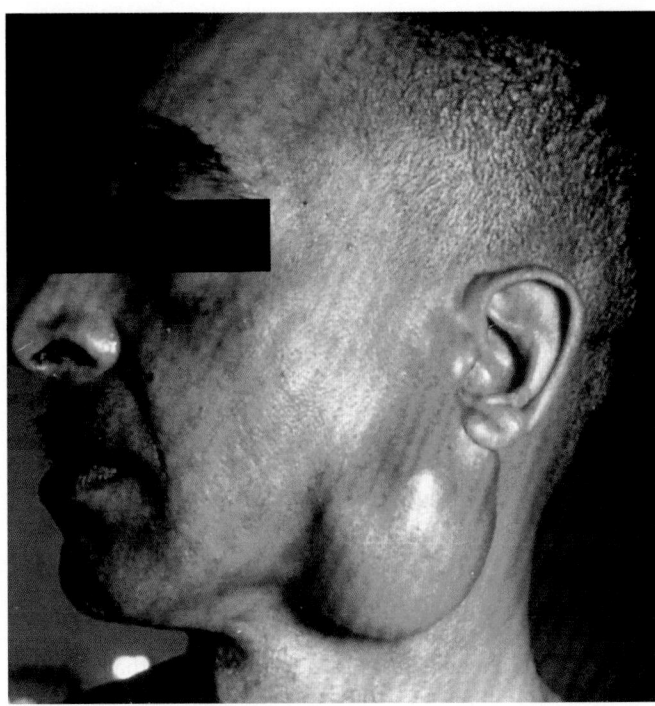

FIGURE 29-32. Pleomorphic adenoma of the parotid. A conspicuous tumor mass is seen at the angle of the jaw.

of the lateral pharyngeal or tonsillar regions. These tumors show epithelial tissue mingled with myxoid, mucoid or chondroid areas (Fig. 29-33A), hence the older term **benign mixed tumor**. However, the neoplasm is considered to be of epithelial origin.

The epithelial component consists of myoepithelial and ductal cells. The cells that line the ducts form tubules or small cystic structures and contain clear fluid or eosinophilic, periodic acid–Schiff (PAS)-positive material. Around ductal epithelial cells are smaller myoepithelial cells, which are the main cellular component. These cells form well-defined sheaths, cords or nests and are often separated by a cellular

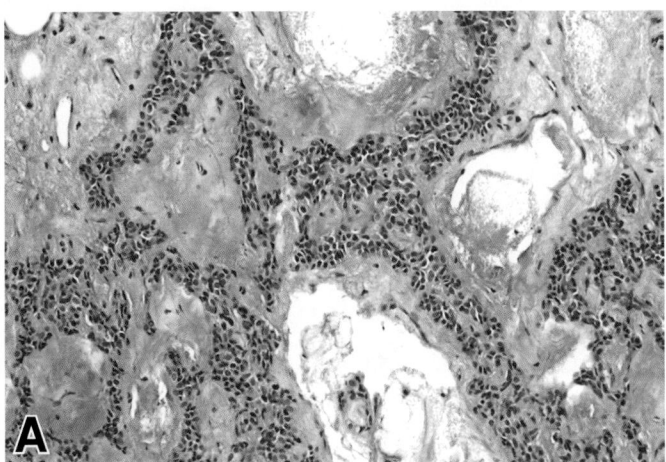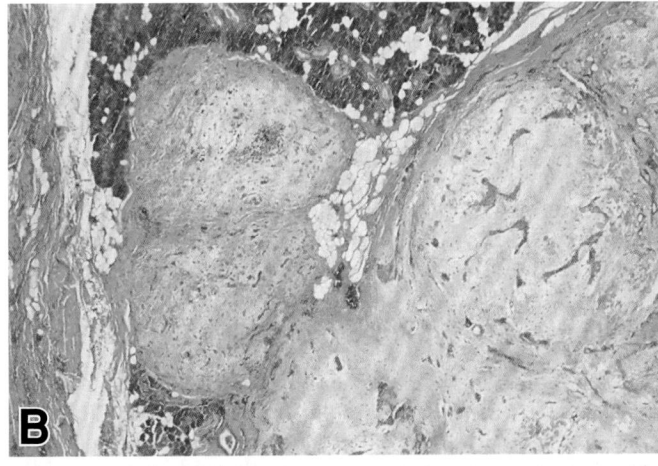

FIGURE 29-33. Pleomorphic adenoma of the parotid gland. A. Cellular components of pleomorphic adenomas include an admixture of glands and myoepithelial cells within a chondromyxoid stroma. **B.** The tumor contains characteristic myxoid and chondroid portions. The tumor is partly encapsulated, but a nodule protruding into the parotid gland lacks a capsule. If such nodules are not included in the resection, the tumor will recur.

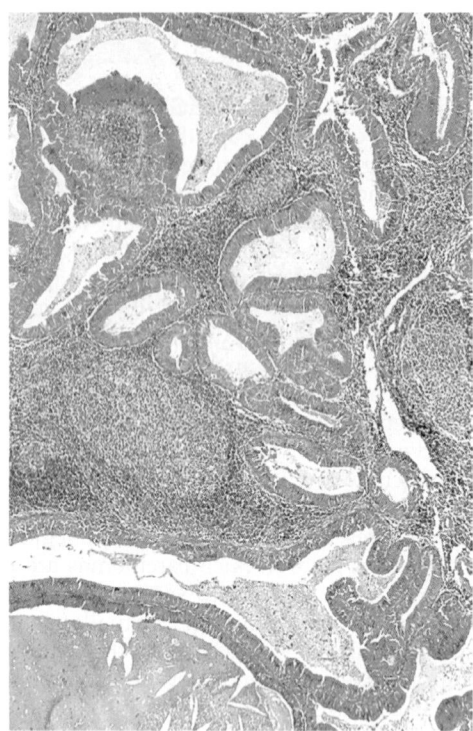

FIGURE 29-34. Warthin tumor. Cystic spaces and duct-like structures are lined by oncocytes. Follicular lymphoid tissue is present.

oncocytomas, (4) canalicular adenomas, (5) myoepitheliomas and (6) clear cell adenomas.

Warthin Tumor (Papillary Cystadenoma Lymphomatosum)

Warthin tumors are the most common monomorphic adenomas. They are benign parotid gland neoplasms composed of cystic glandular spaces within dense lymphoid tissue. Clearly benign, they may be bilateral (15% of cases) or multifocal within one gland. These are the only salivary gland tumors that are more common in men than in women. They generally occur after age 30, and most arise after age 50.

 PATHOLOGY: Warthin tumors have glandular spaces that tend to become cystic, with papillary projections. The cysts are lined by eosinophilic epithelial cells (oncocytes), surrounded by dense lymphoid tissue with germinal centers (Fig. 29-34).

The histogenesis of this tumor is uncertain. Lymph nodes are normally found in the parotid gland and its immediate vicinity and usually contain a few ducts or small islands of salivary gland tissue. Warthin tumors may arise from proliferation of these salivary gland inclusions.

Oncocytoma (Oxyphil Adenoma)

Oncocytes are benign epithelial cells swollen with mitochondria, which impart a granular appearance to the cytoplasm. They are normally scattered or in small clusters among epithelial cells of various organs (e.g., thyroid, parathyroid). Oncocytes first appear in early adulthood and increase in number with age. Rare adenomas of nests or cords of oncocytes occur in parotid glands of the elderly.

MALIGNANT SALIVARY GLAND TUMORS

Salivary gland tumors account for 5% of all head and neck cancers. Most (75%) arise in the parotid glands, 10% in the submandibular glands and 15% in the minor salivary glands of the upper aerodigestive tract. Malignancies of the sublingual glands are rare.

Mucoepidermoid Carcinomas Show Mixed Cell Populations

Mucoepidermoid carcinomas (MECs) derive from ductal epithelium, which has a great potential for metaplasia. They account for 5%–10% of major salivary gland tumors and 10% of tumors in minor salivary glands. Over half of MECs in the major glands arise in the parotid. Among minor salivary glands, they develop mostly in the palate. Most MECs arise in adult women but may occur in adolescents.

 **MOLECULAR PATHOGENESIS:** Over 60% of MECs are characterized by a t(11;19)(q21-22;p13) translocation (Fig. 29-35). This recombination generates a fusion gene (**MECT1–MAML2** fusion) that disrupts NOTCH signaling.

 PATHOLOGY: Mucoepidermoid carcinomas grow slowly and present as firm, painless masses. Low-grade tumors contain irregular solid, duct-like and cystic spaces that include squamous cells, mucus-secreting cells and intermediate cells (Fig. 29-36). Intermediate-grade tumors tend to grow in more solid patterns, with more epidermoid and intermediate cells and fewer mucus-secreting cells. High-grade MECs are very pleomorphic, with minimal differentiation, save for scattered glandular cells.

 CLINICAL FEATURES: Even low-grade mucoepidermoid carcinomas may metastasize, but over 90% of patients survive 5 years, regardless of the primary site. Survival with high-grade tumors is much

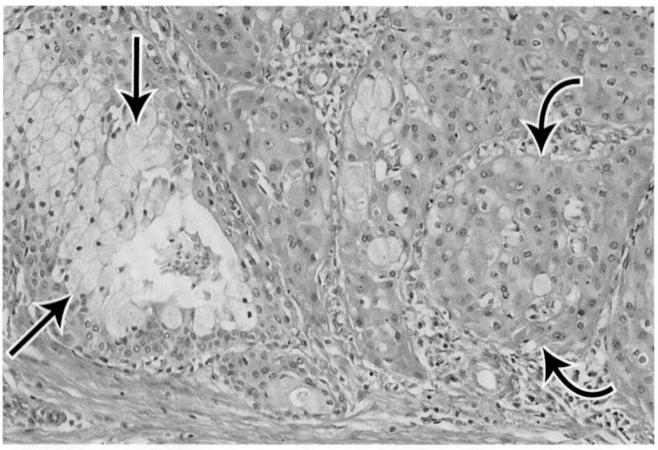

FIGURE 29-35. Mucoepidermoid carcinoma is characterized by an admixture of mucocytes (*straight arrows*), epidermoid cells (*curved arrows*) and intermediate cells. The mucocytes are clustered and have a clear cytoplasm with eccentrically situated nuclei. Epidermoid cells are squamous-like cells but lack keratinization and intercellular bridges. Intermediate cells (best seen at *lower left*) are smaller than epidermoid cells.

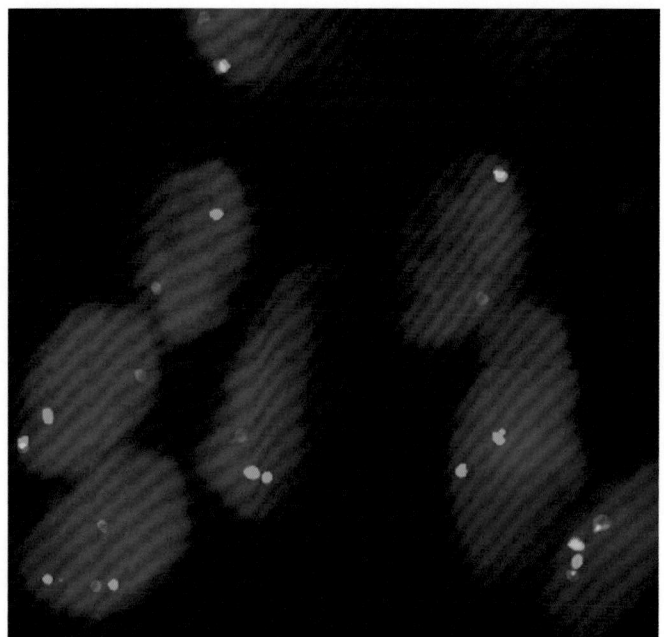

FIGURE 29-36. Mucoepidermoid carcinoma fluorescence in situ hybridization (FISH) MAML2-positive case. The green and red break-apart probes are both designed for the *MAML2* gene of chromosome 11. Yellow signals are essentially interpreted as an intact *MAML2* gene, whereas the solitary green and red probes are consistent with gene disruption or translocation. *Photograph courtesy of Dr. Joaquin Garcia, Mayo Clinic.*

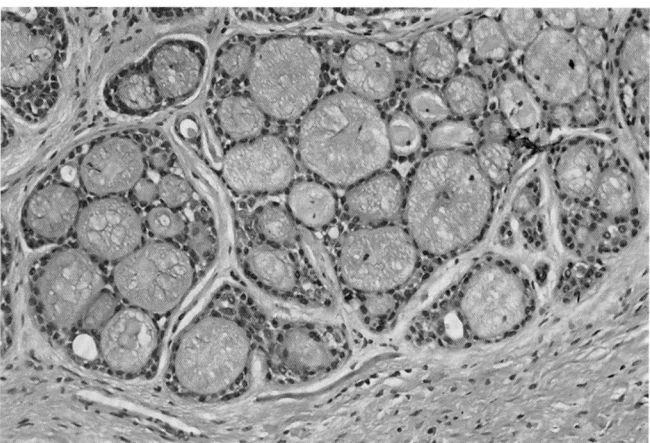

FIGURE 29-37. Adenoid cystic carcinoma showing cribriform growth in which cyst-like spaces are filled with basophilic material. The cyst spaces are really pseudocysts surrounded by myoepithelial cells.

worse (20%–40%). Treatment is dictated by grade; low-grade tumors are treated surgically, but high-grade tumors require both surgery and radiation therapy.

Adenoid Cystic Carcinomas Invade Locally and Often Recur After Resection

Adenoid cystic carcinomas (ACCs) tend to grow slowly. One third of ACCs arise in the major salivary glands and two thirds in the minor ones. They represent 5% of major salivary gland tumors and 20% of those of the minor salivary glands. ACCs may occur not only in the oral cavity but also in the lacrimal glands, nasopharynx, nasal cavity, paranasal sinuses and lower respiratory tract. They are most common in people 40–60 years old.

   MOLECULAR PATHOGENESIS: ACCs consistently demonstrate t(6;9) translocations and chromosome 6 deletions. The translocation t(6;9) (q22-23;p23-24) results in a novel fusion of the MYB proto-oncogene with NFIB, a transcription factor.

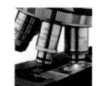   **PATHOLOGY:** ACCs show variable histology. The tumor cells are small, have scant cytoplasm and grow in solid sheets or as small groups, strands or columns. Within these structures, tumor cells interconnect to enclose cystic spaces, resulting in solid, tubular or cribriform (sieve-like) patterns (Fig. 29-37). Grading ACCs depends on the proportions of tubular and cribriform patterns, with over 30% solid growth defining "high grade." Such high-grade tumors have a 5-year survival rate of about 15%. Tumor cells produce a homogeneous basement membrane material that gives them the characteristic "cylindromatous" appearance.

ACCs probably arise from cells that differentiate toward intercalated ducts and myoepithelium. *They tend to infiltrate perineural spaces and thus are often painful.* Most do not metastasize for years, but they are often diagnosed late, are difficult to eradicate completely and have a poor long-term prognosis.

Acinic Cell Adenocarcinomas Arise from Secretory Cells

These uncommon parotid tumors (10% of salivary gland tumors) arise occasionally in other salivary glands. They occur mainly in young men ages 20–30 years. Acinic cell carcinomas are encapsulated, round masses, usually under 3 cm, and may be cystic. They are composed of uniform cells with a small central nucleus and abundant basophilic cytoplasm, similar to the secretory (acinic) cells of normal salivary glands (Fig. 29-38). They may spread to regional lymph nodes. Most

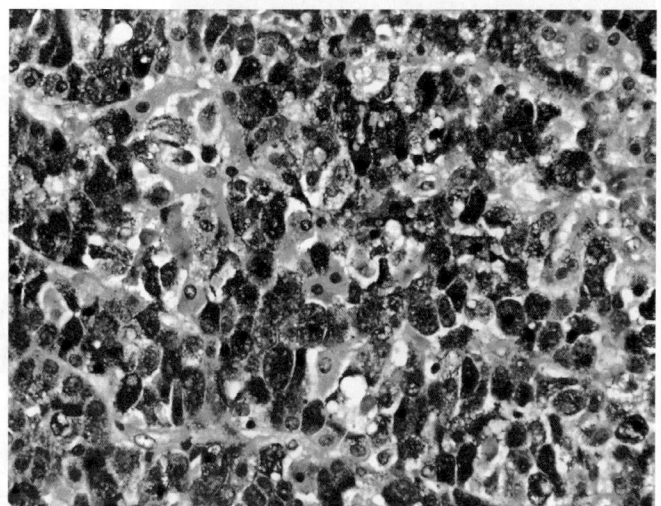

FIGURE 29-38. Acinic cell adenocarcinoma. This tumor demonstrates a solid growth pattern and is composed of basophilic cells with abundant cytoplasm filled with zymogen granules.

(90%) patients survive 5 years with surgery, but 1/3 experience local recurrences. Only half survive for 20 years.

Mammary Analog Secretory Carcinomas Resemble ACCs

These tumors compose a distinct histological entity. They have an associated unique translocation t(12;15)(p13;q25) that leads to the ETV6–NTRK3 fusion oncogene. Mammary analog secretory carcinomas mainly arise in the parotid gland.

The Ear

EXTERNAL EAR

ANATOMY: The outer portion of the external ear includes the auricle or pinna, leading into the external auditory canal. The external auditory canal or meatus extends from the concha medially to the tympanic membrane (eardrum). Its lateral wall is cartilage and connective tissue, and its medial wall is bone. The eardrum sits obliquely at the end of the external auditory canal, sloping medially from above downward and from behind forward, separating the external ear and the middle ear.

The auricle is composed of keratinizing, stratified squamous epithelium with associated adnexa (hair follicles, sebaceous glands, eccrine sweat glands). The outer third of the external auditory canal also has ceruminal glands, modified apocrine glands that replace the eccrine glands of the auricular dermis. They produce cerumen and contain clusters of cuboidal cells with eosinophilic cytoplasm, often with granular, golden yellow pigment and secretory droplets by their luminal border. Peripheral to the secretory cells are flattened myoepithelial cells. Ceruminal gland ducts end in

hair follicles or on the skin. The inner portion of the external auditory canal has no adnexa. The eardrum is airtight. Its outer surface is squamous epithelium, continuous with the skin of the external ear canal. Its inner surface is lined by cuboidal epithelium. Between these two is a middle layer of dense fibrous tissue.

KELOIDS: Keloids are very common on the ear lobes after piercing for earrings or other trauma (see Chapter 3). They are much more common in blacks and Asians than in whites. Keloids can attain considerable size and tend to recur. They are composed of thick, hyalinized bundles of collagen in the deep dermis (see Chapter 3).

CAULIFLOWER EARS: These deformities are particularly common in wrestlers and boxers and result from repeated mechanical trauma to the external ear. Blows to the ears cause subperichondrial hematomas, which organize and deform the ears.

RELAPSING POLYCHONDRITIS: This rare, chronic disorder of unknown origin is characterized by intermittent inflammation that destroys hyaline, elastic or fibrocartilage of the ears, nose, larynx, tracheobronchial tree, ribs and joints.

The etiology of relapsing polychondritis is obscure; immune mechanisms are suspected. During acute attacks, patients may have serum antibodies to cartilage, type II collagen and chondroitin sulfate. Immune complexes can be detected in involved cartilage. Relapsing polychondritis may occur alone or with other connective tissue diseases. Noncartilaginous tissues, such as the sclera and cardiac valves, also may be affected. Aortic involvement can lead to fatal rupture of the aorta.

 PATHOLOGY: The perichondrium is infiltrated by lymphocytes, plasma cells and neutrophils, which also extend into the adjacent cartilage (Fig. 29-39). Chondrocytes die. The cartilaginous matrix degenerates and fragments. Ultimately, the cartilage is destroyed and replaced by granulation tissue and fibrosis.

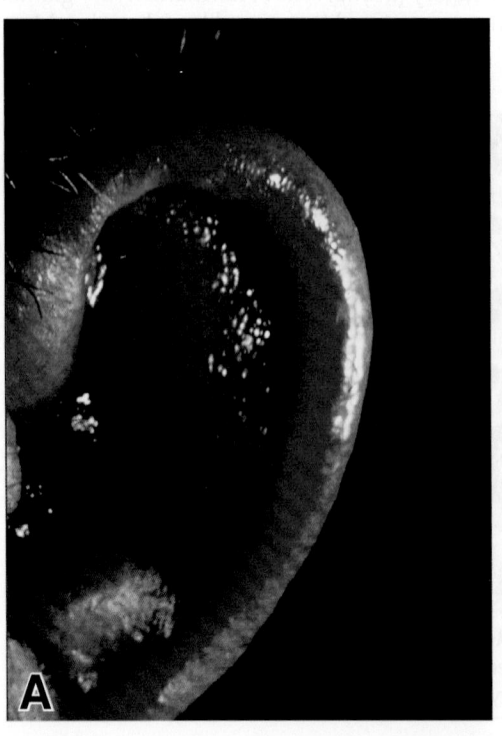
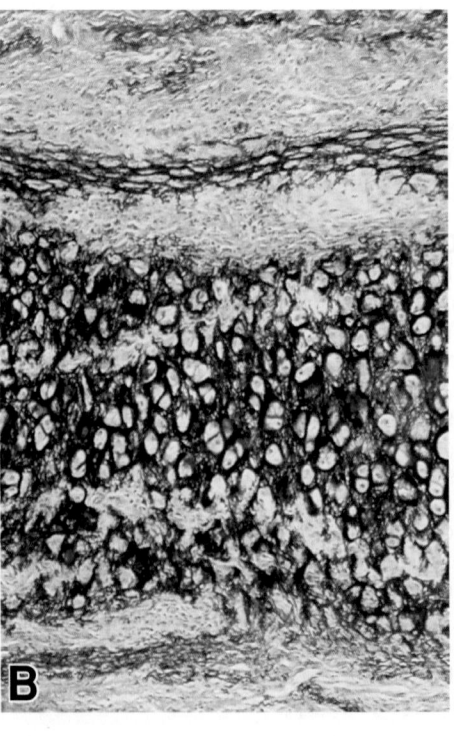

FIGURE 29-39. Relapsing polychondritis. A. The ear is beefy red. **B.** The perichondrium and elastic cartilage are infiltrated and partially destroyed by inflammatory cells and replaced by fibrosis.

"MALIGNANT" OTITIS EXTERNA: This infection of the external auditory canal is caused by *Pseudomonas aeruginosa.* Infection may spread through the skin and cartilage to cause mastoiditis or osteomyelitis of the skull, venous sinus thrombosis, meningitis and death. Malignant otitis externa occurs mainly in elderly diabetics but also in patients with blood dyscrasias (e.g., leukemia, granulocytopenia).

AURAL POLYPS: These benign inflammatory lesions arise in the external ear canal or extrude into the canal from the middle ear. Aural polyps are ulcerated, inflamed granulation tissue, which bleeds readily. Those arising in the middle ear result from chronic otitis media.

NEOPLASMS: Benign and malignant tumors of the external ear include the gamut of skin-related neoplasms: squamous papillomas, seborrheic keratosis, basal cell carcinoma, SCC and benign and malignant adnexal tumors.

Ceruminal gland tumors are unique to this area. Benign tumors include ceruminal gland adenomas and salivary gland–type tumors (e.g., pleomorphic and monomorphic adenomas). Malignant tumors include adenocarcinoma and malignant salivary gland–type tumors (e.g., adenoid cystic and mucoepidermoid carcinomas).

MIDDLE EAR

ANATOMY: The middle ear, or tympanic cavity, is an oblong space in the temporal bone lined by a mucous membrane. Together with the mastoid air sinuses, it forms a closed mucosal compartment, also called the **middle ear cleft.** Most of its lateral wall is the tympanic membrane. Anteriorly, the eustachian tube connects the middle ear to the nasopharynx. This air passage allows air pressure on both sides of the tympanic membrane to equalize. The three auditory ossicles—the malleus, incus and stapes—are a chain that connects the tympanic membrane with the oval window located at the medial wall of the tympanic cavity. They conduct sound across the middle ear. Free motion of the ossicles, mainly the stapes in the oval window, is more important for hearing than is an intact tympanic membrane. The middle ear opens posteriorly into the mastoid antrum, a honeycomb of small, aerated, bony compartments (air cells) lined by a thin mucous membrane continuous with that of the middle ear.

Otitis Media Often Follows Obstruction of the Eustachian Tube

Otitis media is inflammation of the middle ear. It usually results from upper respiratory tract infections that spread from the nasopharynx. Obstruction of the eustachian tube is important in production of middle ear effusions. When the pharyngeal end of the eustachian tube is swollen, air cannot enter the tube. Air in the middle ear is absorbed through the mucosa, and negative pressure causes transudation of plasma and occasional bleeding. Antibiotics usually cure or suppress the condition.

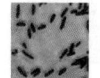 **ETIOLOGY:** Acute otitis media may be due to viral or bacterial infection or sterile obstruction of the eustachian tube. Viral otitis media may resolve without suppuration or lead to secondary invasion by pus-forming bacteria. Microorganisms ascend from the nasopharynx, through the eustachian tube, to the middle ear.

Otitis media almost invariably penetrates through the mastoid antrum into the mastoid cells.

ACUTE SEROUS OTITIS MEDIA: Obstruction of the eustachian tube may result from sudden changes in atmospheric pressure (e.g., during flying in an aircraft or deep-sea diving). This effect is particularly severe if there is an upper respiratory tract infection, acute allergic reaction or viral or bacterial infection at the eustachian tube orifice. Inflammation may also occur without bacterial invasion of the middle ear. Over half of children in the United States have at least one bout of serous otitis media before their third birthday. Repeated otitis media in early childhood often leads to residual (usually sterile) fluid in the middle ear, which contributes to unsuspected hearing loss.

CHRONIC SEROUS OTITIS MEDIA: The same conditions that cause acute obstruction of the eustachian tube also cause recurrent or chronic middle ear serous effusions. Carcinoma of the nasopharynx may cause chronic serous otitis media in adults and should be suspected if a unilateral middle ear effusion occurs in an adult.

 PATHOLOGY: In chronic serous otitis media, mucus-producing (goblet) cell metaplasia may be seen in the mucosal lining of the middle ear. Hemorrhage (e.g., in the mastoid cells) may accompany acute obstruction. Extravasation of blood and degradation of erythrocytes liberate cholesterol. Cholesterol crystals stimulate a foreign body response and granulation tissue, called a **cholesterol granuloma.** If large, these granulomas may destroy tissue in the mastoid or antrum. If they are allowed to persist for many months, the granulation tissue may become fibrotic, which may eventually lead to complete obliteration of the middle ear and mastoid by fibrous tissue.

ACUTE SUPPURATIVE OTITIS MEDIA: One of the most common infections of childhood, acute suppurative otitis media, is caused by pyogenic bacteria that invade the middle ear, usually via the eustachian tube. The most common culprit in all age groups (30%–40%) is *Streptococcus pneumoniae* (pneumococcus). *H. influenzae* causes about 20% of cases, but less often with increasing age. An accumulating purulent exudate in the middle ear may rupture the eardrum, causing a purulent discharge. In most cases, infection is self-limited and may heal even without therapy.

ACUTE MASTOIDITIS: Infection of the mastoid bone was once a common complication of acute otitis media, before the advent of antibiotics. It is still seen, rarely, if otitis media is not treated adequately. Mastoid air cells are filled with pus, and their thin osseous intercellular walls are destroyed. If the infection spreads to contiguous structures, serious complications may ensue (Fig. 29-40).

CHRONIC SUPPURATIVE OTITIS MEDIA AND MASTOIDITIS: Neglected or recurrent middle ear and mastoid infections may lead to chronic inflammation of the mucosa or destruction of the periosteum of the ossicles (Fig. 29-41). Chronic otitis media occurs much more commonly in people who have had ear disease in early childhood, which may have arrested normal development of the air cells in the mastoid.

 PATHOLOGY: Inflammation tends to be insidious, persistent and destructive. In chronic otitis media, by definition, the eardrum is always perforated. Painless discharge **(otorrhea)** and variable hearing

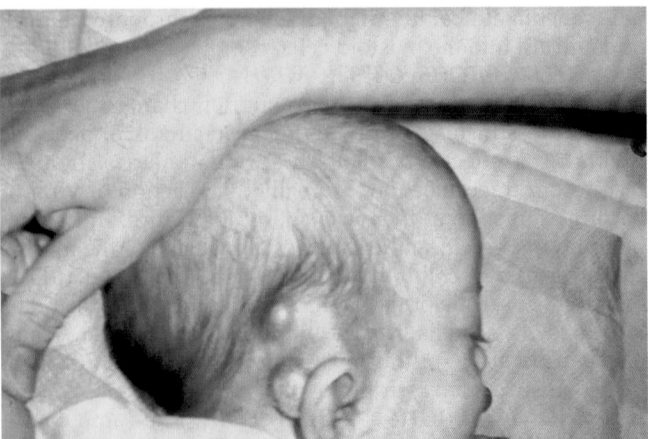

FIGURE 29-40. Acute mastoiditis. An unusual complication of otitis media, acute mastoiditis, appears as large bulging lesions above the child's ear.

loss are constant symptoms. Exuberant granulation tissue may form polyps, which can extend through the perforated eardrum into the external ear canal.

A **cholesteatoma** is a mass of accumulated keratin and squamous mucosa due to growth of squamous epithelium from the external ear canal through a perforated eardrum into the middle ear. There, it continues to produce keratin. Cholesteatomas are identical to epidermal inclusion cysts. They are surrounded by granulation tissue and fibrosis. The keratin mass often becomes infected and protects bacteria from antibiotics. The main dangers of cholesteatoma arise from bony erosion, which may destroy important contiguous structures (e.g., auditory ossicles, facial nerve, labyrinth).

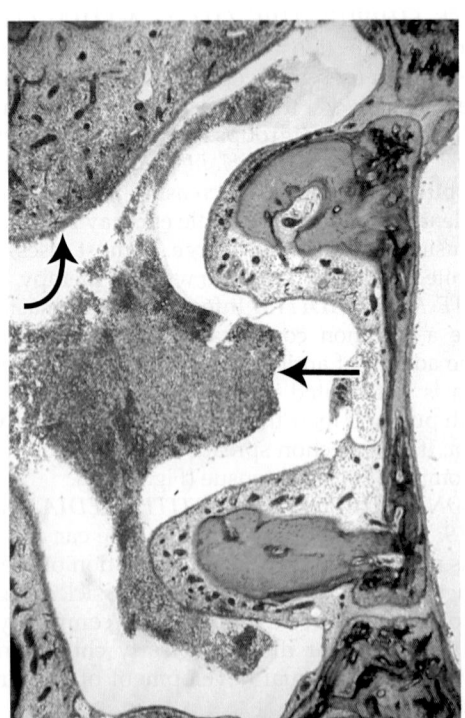

FIGURE 29-41. Chronic suppurative otitis media. A purulent exudate (*straight arrow*) is present in the middle ear cavity. The entire mucosa (*curved arrow*) is thickened by chronic inflammation and granulation tissue. The footplate and the crura of the stapes are at right.

COMPLICATIONS OF ACUTE AND CHRONIC OTITIS MEDIA: Antibiotic therapy has fortunately made complications of otitis media uncommon. However, suppurative middle ear infections may still cause these serious complications:

- Destruction of the facial nerve
- Deep cervical or subperiosteal abscess, if cortical bone of the mastoid process is eroded
- Petrositis, when infection spreads to the petrous temporal bone through the chain of air cells
- Suppurative labyrinthitis, due to infection of the internal ear
- Epidural, subdural or cerebral abscess, when infection extends through the inner table of the mastoid bone
- Meningitis, when infection reaches the meninges
- Sigmoid sinus thrombophlebitis, if infection traverses the dura to the posterior cranial fossa

Jugulotympanic Paragangliomas Arise from Middle Ear Paraganglia

Jugulotympanic paragangliomas are the most common benign tumors of the middle ear. They grow slowly but, over years, may destroy the middle ear and extend into the internal ear and cranial cavity. Metastases are rare.

Middle ear paragangliomas resemble those arising elsewhere, with characteristic lobules of cells in richly vascular connective tissue (Fig. 29-42). Paraganglial cells are of neural crest origin and contain varying amounts of catecholamines, mostly epinephrine and norepinephrine.

INTERNAL EAR

ANATOMY: The petrous portion of the temporal bone contains the labyrinth, which shelters the end organs for hearing **(cochlea)** and equilibrium **(vestibular labyrinth).** The complex cavities of the osseous labyrinth contain the **membranous labyrinth,** a series of communicating membranous sacs and ducts. The osseous labyrinth connects to the subarachnoid space via the cochlear aqueduct. It is filled with perilymph, a clear fluid that mingles with cerebrospinal

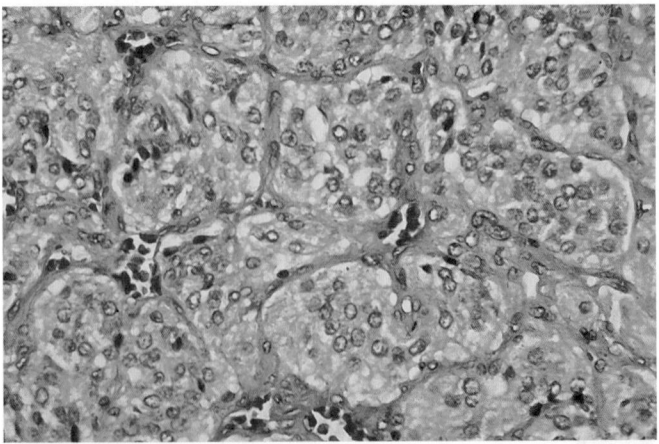

FIGURE 29-42. Jugulotympanic paraganglioma. Tumor cell nests are composed of cells with ill-defined cell borders and prominent eosinophilic cytoplasm (chief cells).

fluid. The membranous labyrinth contains a different fluid, the endolymph, which circulates in a closed system. Because there are no barriers between the cochlear and vestibular labyrinths, injury or disease of the inner ear frequently affects both hearing and equilibrium.

The **cochlea** is coiled upon itself like a snail shell and makes 2-1/2 turns. It has three compartments: two that contain perilymph and a third (the cochlear duct) with endolymph. The cochlear duct encompasses the end organ of hearing, **the organ of Corti,** which rests on the basement membrane and is arranged as a spiral, with three rows of outer hair cells and a row of inner hair cells. When hairs of these neuroepithelial cells are bent or distorted by vibration, the mechanical force is converted into electrochemical impulses and interpreted in the temporal cortex as sound. The vestibular part of the membranous labyrinth consists of the utricle, saccule and semicircular canals, each with specialized neuroepithelium that determines equilibrium.

Otosclerosis Is Formation of New Spongy Bone about the Stapes

Otosclerosis causes progressive deafness. *It is an autosomal dominant hereditary defect and is the most common cause of conductive hearing loss in young and middle-aged adults in the United States.* This disorder affects 10% of white and 1% of black adult Americans, although 90% of cases are asymptomatic. The female-to-male ratio is 2:1, and both ears are usually affected.

 PATHOLOGY: Although any part of the petrous bone may be affected, otosclerotic bone tends to form at particular points. The most frequent (85%) site is immediately anterior to the oval window. The focus of sclerotic bone extends posteriorly and may infiltrate and replace the stapes, progressively immobilizing the footplate of the stapes. The developing bony ankylosis is functionally manifested as a slowly progressive conductive hearing loss.

Otosclerosis begins with resorption of bone and formation of highly cellular fibrous tissue, with wide vascular spaces and osteoclasts. The resorbed bone is later replaced by immature bone, which, with repeated remodeling, becomes mature (Fig. 29-43). Otosclerosis is treated by surgical mobilization of the auditory ossicles.

Ménière Disease Is a Triad of Vertigo, Sensorineural Hearing Loss and Tinnitus

Several etiologies have been suggested, but the cause of **Ménière disease** is uncertain. About 45,500 new cases are diagnosed in the United States annually. Viral etiologies, vascular causes and, possibly, autoimmune mechanisms have all been suggested. Tinnitus is usually unilateral and is most frequent between 40 and 60 years of age. A familial association suggests an underlying genetic predisposition.

 PATHOLOGY: The earliest change is dilatation of the cochlear duct and saccule. As the disease **(hydrops)** progresses, the entire endolymphatic system dilates and the membranous wall may tear (Fig. 29-44). Ruptures can be followed by collapse of the membranous labyrinth, but atrophy of sensory and neural

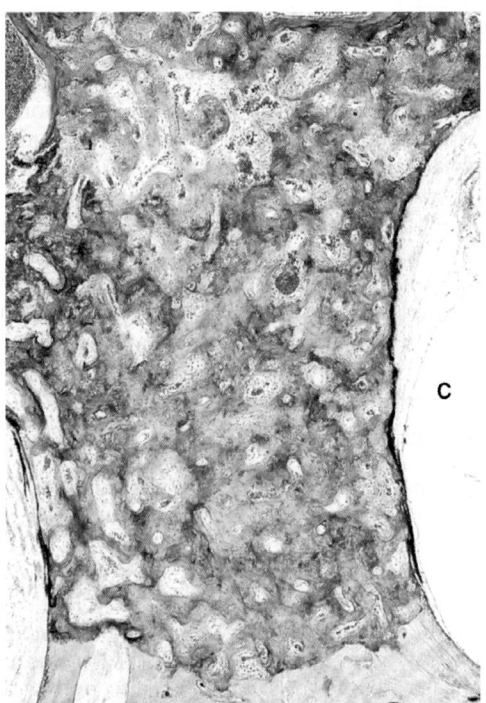

FIGURE 29-43. Otosclerosis. In the lateral wall of the cochlea, the basophilic and more vascular bone is well demarcated. *C* = organ of Corti.

structures is rare. Symptoms occur when endolymphatic hydrops causes rupture, and endolymph escapes into the perilymph.

 CLINICAL FEATURES: Attacks of vertigo, often with incapacitating nausea and vomiting, last less than 24 hours. Weeks or months go by before another episode. In time, remissions become longer. Hearing loss recovers between attacks but later may become permanent. Ménière disease may improve with a low-salt diet and diuretics.

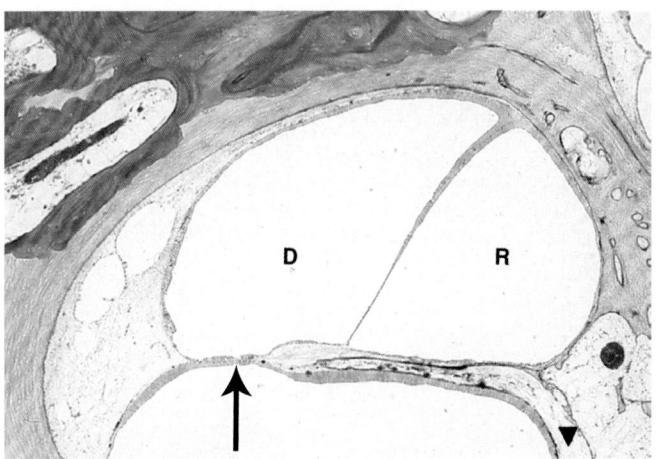

FIGURE 29-44. Ménière disease. The cochlear duct (D) is markedly distended, and the Reissner membrane (R) is pushed back by endolymphatic hydrops. Neither the organ of Corti (*arrow*) nor the spiral ganglion (*arrowhead*) is in its usual location.

Labyrinthine Toxicity Is a Cause of Drug-Induced Deafness

Aminoglycoside antibiotics are the most common ototoxic drugs, producing irreversible damage to vestibular or cochlear sensory cells. Other antibiotics, diuretics, antimalarials and salicylates may also lead to transient or permanent sensorineural hearing loss. Among antineoplastic drugs, cisplatin causes temporary or permanent hearing loss.

The labyrinth of the developing embryo is very sensitive to some drugs. Maternal use of antimalarials and other drugs may cause congenital deafness.

Viral Labyrinthitis Can Result in Congenital Deafness

Viral infections may cause inner ear disorders, particularly deafness. This is mostly due to viral invasion of the labyrinth. CMV and rubella are the best-known prenatal viral infections that cause congenital deafness via maternal-to-fetal transmission.

Mumps is the most common postnatal viral cause of deafness. It can cause rapid hearing loss, which is unilateral in 80% of cases. By contrast, prenatal infection of the labyrinth with rubella is usually bilateral, with permanent loss of cochlear and vestibular function. A number of other viruses are suspected to cause labyrinthitis, including influenza and parainfluenza viruses, EBV, herpesviruses and adenoviruses. Such cases show severe damage to the organ of Corti, with almost total loss of inner and outer hair cells.

Acoustic Trauma

Noise-induced hearing loss is a significant problem in industrialized countries. Occupational or recreational exposure to loud noises may impair hearing temporarily or permanently, as in people exposed to jet engines or loud music. The external hair cells of the organ of Corti are damaged earliest. Loss of sensory hairs is followed by deformation, swelling and disintegration of the hair cells.

Schwannoma Is the Most Common Tumor of the Inner Ear

SCHWANNOMA: Nearly all schwannomas in the internal auditory canal arise from the vestibular nerves. Vestibular schwannomas, which account for about 10% of all intracranial tumors, are slow growing and encapsulated. Larger tumors protrude from the internal auditory meatus into the cerebellopontine angle and may deform the brainstem and adjacent cerebellum. Schwannomas cause slowly progressive vestibular and auditory symptoms. In neurofibromatosis type 2 (NF-2; see Chapter 28), bilateral vestibular schwannomas identical to other vestibular schwannomas occur frequently.

MENINGIOMA: Meningiomas of the cerebellopontine angle originate from the meningothelial cells in the arachnoid villi. The favored sites for these tumors are the sphenoid ridge and petrous pyramid. Meningiomas may extend into the adjacent temporal bone or dural sinuses (see Chapter 28).

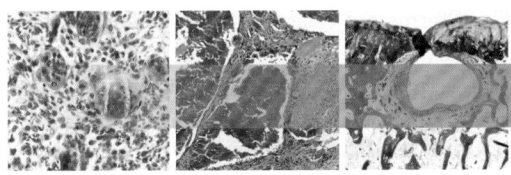

30

Bones, Joints and Soft Tissue

Roberto A. Garcia ▪ Elizabeth G. Demicco ▪ Michael J. Klein ▪ Alan L. Schiller

Bones

The functions of bone are mechanical, mineral storage and hematopoietic. Mechanical functions of bone include protection for the brain, spinal cord and chest organs; rigid internal support for limbs; and deployment as lever arms in the skeletal muscle. Bone is the principal reservoir for calcium and stores other ions such as phosphate, sodium and magnesium. The bones also serve as hosts for hematopoietic bone marrow.

The mechanical properties of bone are related to its construction and internal architecture. Although extremely light, it has high tensile strength. This combination of strength and light weight results from its hollow tubular shape, layering of bone tissue and internal buttressing of the matrix.

The term **bone** can refer to both an organ and a tissue. The "organ" is composed of bone tissue, cartilage, fat, marrow elements, vessels, nerves and fibrous tissue. Bone "tissue" is described in microscopic terms and is defined by the relation of its collagen and mineral structure to the bone cells.

ANATOMY

Macroscopically, two types of bone are recognized:

- **Cortical bone** is dense, compact bone, whose outer shell defines the shape of the bone. It composes 80% of the skeleton. Because of its density, its functions are mainly biomechanical.
- **Coarse cancellous bone** (also called **spongy, trabecular** or **medullary bone**) is found at the ends of long bones within the medullary canal. Cancellous bone has a high surface-to-volume ratio and contains many more bone cells per unit volume than cortical bone. **Changes in the rate of bone turnover are manifested principally in cancellous bone.**

All bones contain both cancellous and cortical elements (Fig. 30-1), but their proportions differ. The body or shaft of a long tubular bone, such as the femur, is composed of cortical bone and its marrow is mainly fat. Toward the ends of the femur, the cortex becomes thin and coarse cancellous bone becomes the predominant structure. By contrast, the skull is formed by outer and inner tables of compact bone, with only a small amount of cancellous bone within the marrow space, called the **diploë.**

The anatomy of bone is defined in relation to a transverse cartilage plate, which is present in the growing child. This structure is the **growth plate,** the **epiphyseal cartilage plate** or **the physis** (Fig. 30-2A–C). The terms **epiphysis, metaphysis** and **diaphysis** are defined in relation to the growth plate.

- **The epiphysis** is the area of the bone that extends from the subarticular bone plate to the base of the growth plate.
- **The metaphysis** contains coarse cancellous bone and is the region from the side of the growth plate facing away from the joint to the area where the bone develops its fluted or funnel shape.
- **The diaphysis** corresponds to the body or shaft of the bone and is the zone between the two metaphyses in a long tubular bone.

The metaphysis blends into the diaphysis and is the area where coarse cancellous bone dissipates. This area of bone is particularly important in hematogenous infections, tumors and skeletal malformations.

Two additional terms are essential to an understanding of bone organization:

- **Endochondral ossification** is the process by which bone tissue replaces cartilage.
- **Intramembranous ossification** refers to the mechanism by which bone tissue supplants membranous or fibrous tissue laid down by the periosteum.

All bones are formed by at least some intramembranous ossification. Some bones (e.g., the calvaria of the skull) are forged purely by intramembranous ossification. Because bone tumors tend to recapitulate their embryologic origins, it is not surprising that cartilaginous tumors of the frontal bone have not been seen, because the calvaria of the skull do not originate from cartilage.

The Bone Marrow Resides in the Marrow Space, or Medullary Canal

The marrow space is enclosed by cortical bone. It is supported by a delicate connective tissue framework that enmeshes marrow cells and blood vessels. Three types of marrow are evident to the naked eye:

- **Red marrow** corresponds to hematopoietic tissue and is found in virtually all bones at birth. At adolescence, it is confined to the axial skeleton, which includes the skull, vertebrae, sternum, ribs, scapulae, clavicles, pelvis and proximal humerus and femur. Its presence may also be pathologic, depending on the patient's age and the site of the marrow. For example, red marrow in the femoral diaphysis of a 55-year-old man is abnormal and may reflect underlying disease, such as leukemia.
- **Yellow marrow** is fat tissue and is found in the limb bones. In a normally hematopoietic area, such as a vertebral body, yellow marrow is abnormal at any age.
- **Gray or white marrow** is deficient in hematopoietic elements and is often fibrotic. *It is always a pathologic tissue in a nongrowing adult bone or in areas distant from the growth plate in a child.*

Blood Supply Enters Bone through Specialized Canals

The long tubular bones are provided with blood from two sources and contain canals to supply the tissues.

- **Nutrient arteries** enter bone through a nutrient foramen and supply the marrow space and the internal one third to one half of the cortex.
- **Perforating arteries** are small straight vessels that extend inward from periosteal arteries on the external surface of the periosteum (the fibrous capsule of the bone). Perforating arteries anastomose in the cortex with branches from nutrient arteries coming from the marrow space.
- **Haversian canals** are spaces in cortical bone that course parallel to the long axis of the bone for a short distance and then branch and communicate with other similar canals. Each canal contains one or two blood vessels, lymphatics and some nerve fibers (Fig. 30-2D).
- **Volkmann canals** (Fig. 30-2E) are spaces within the cortex that run perpendicular to the long axis of the cortex to connect adjacent Haversian canals. Volkmann canals also contain blood vessels.

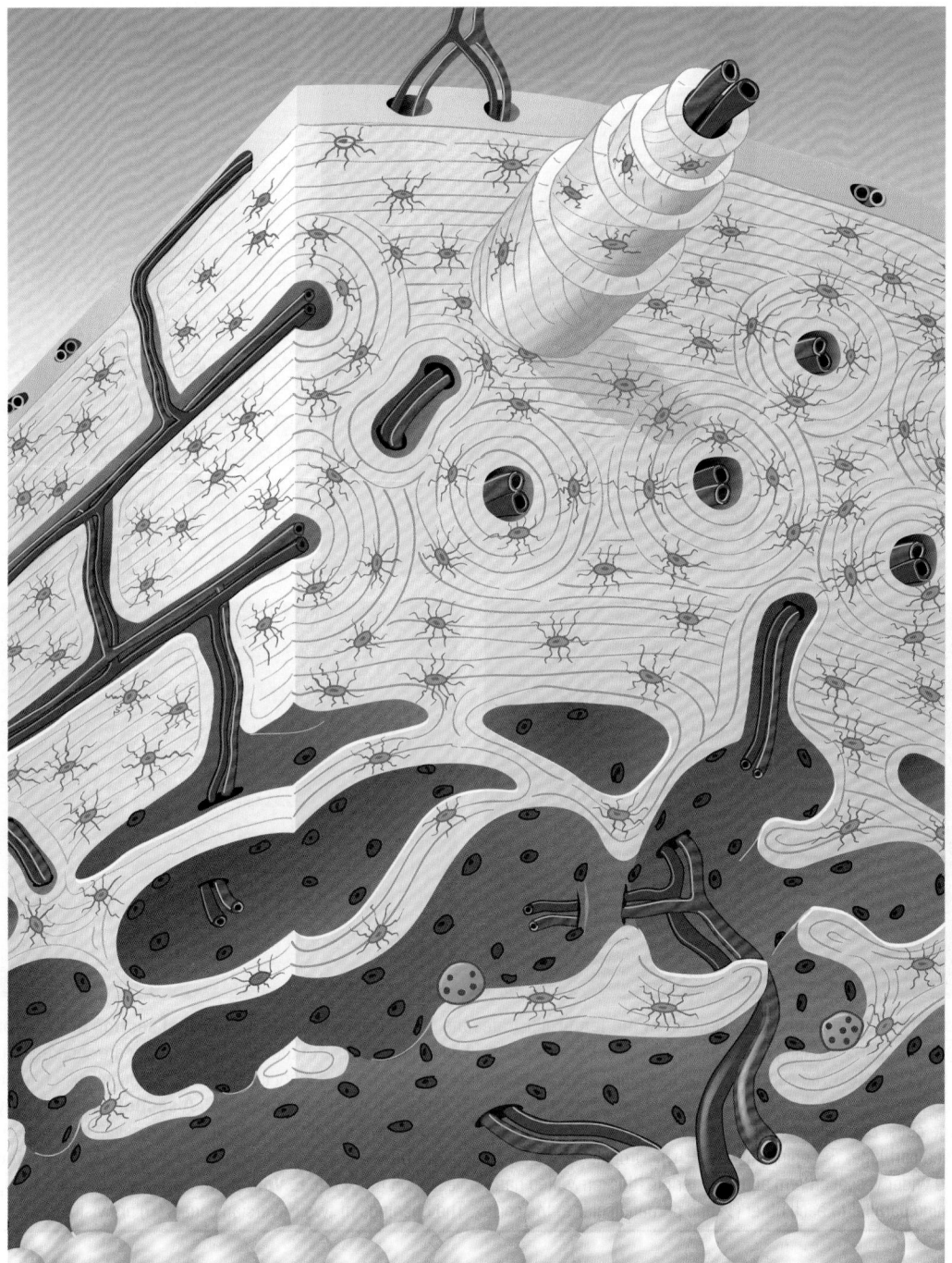

FIGURE 30-1. Anatomy of bone. A schematic representation of cortical and trabecular bone. The longitudinal section (*left*) shows the vasculature entering the periosteum via the periosteal perforating arteries and coursing through the bone perpendicular to the long axis in Volkmann canals. The vessels that proceed longitudinally, or parallel to the long axis, are located in Haversian canals. Each artery is accompanied by a vein. Within the cortex, osteocytes reside in lacunae, and their cell processes extend into the canaliculi. The cross-sectional view (*right*) illustrates the various types of lamellar bone in the cortex. Circumferential lamellar bone is located adjacent to the periosteum and borders the marrow space. Concentric lamellar bone surrounds the central Haversian canals to form an **osteon**. Each layer of the concentric lamellar bone displays a change in the pitch of the collagen fibers, such that each layer has a different arrangement of collagen. The interstitial lamellar bone occupies the space between osteons. The marrow space is filled with fat, and its trabecular bone is contiguous with the cortex. Multinucleated osteoclasts are present, and palisaded osteoblasts surround the bone surfaces. The perforating arteries from the periosteum and the nutrient artery from the marrow space communicate within the cortex via Haversian and Volkmann canals.

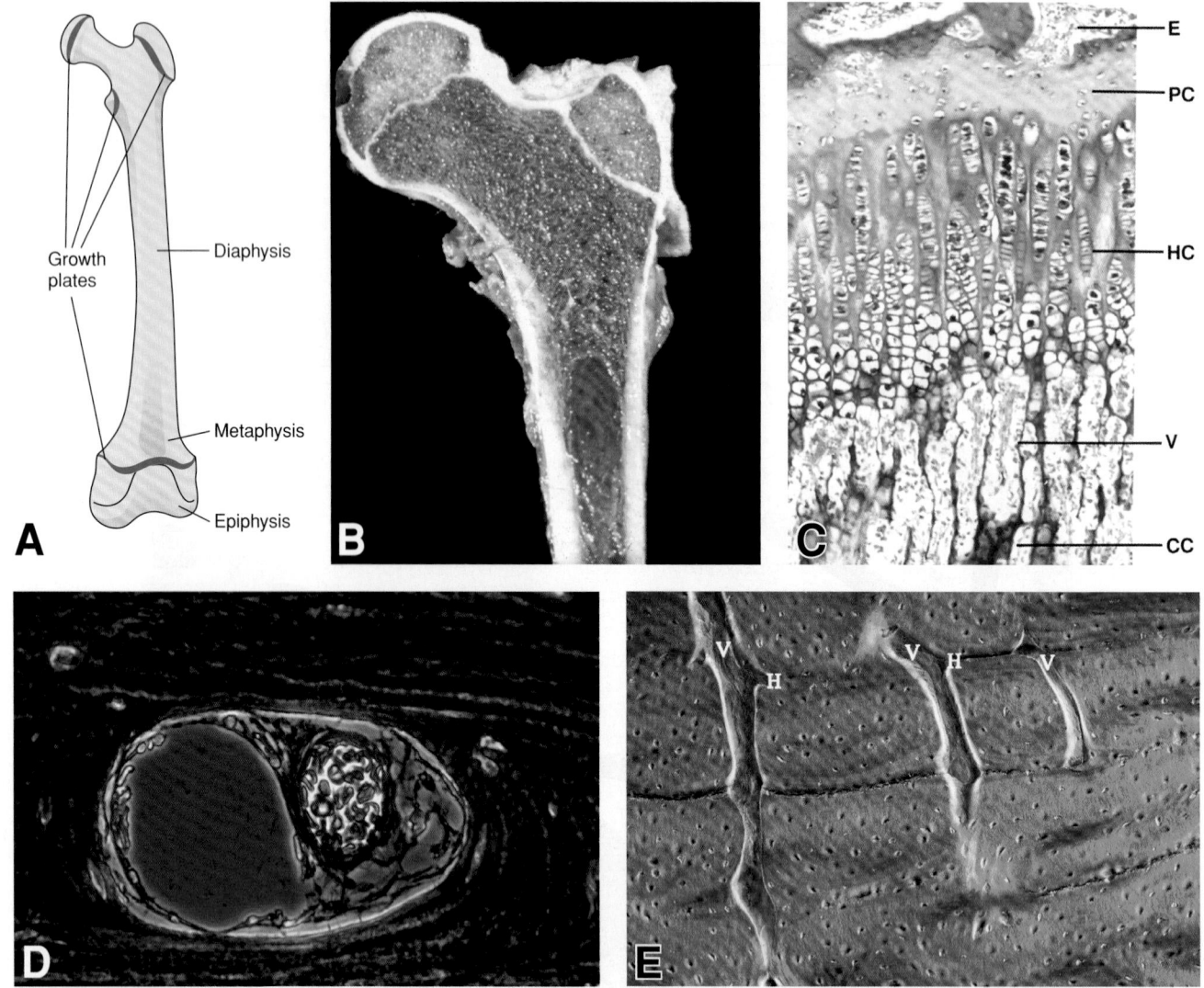

FIGURE 30-2. Anatomy of a long bone. A. Diagram of the femur illustrates the various compartments. **B. Coronal section of the proximal femur** illustrates the various anatomic parts of a long bone. The epiphysis of the femoral head and the apophysis of the greater trochanter are separated from the metaphysis by their respective growth plates. The cortex and the medullary cavity are well visualized. The medullary cavity contains cancellous bone until the metaphysis narrows into the diaphysis (shaft) of the bone, which is almost completely devoid of bone and filled with marrow. **C. A section of the epiphysis** with a zone of proliferating cartilage cells. Beneath this zone, the hypertrophic cartilage cells are arrayed in columns. At the *bottom*, the calcifying matrix is invaded by blood vessels. *CC* = calcified cartilage; *E* = epiphysis; *HC* = hypertrophic cartilage; *PC* = proliferative cartilage; *V* = vascular invasion. **D. Haversian canal** containing a venule (thin-walled wider vessel on *left*) and an arteriole (thicker-walled narrow vessel on the *right*). **E. Volkmann canals.** In this photograph, three Volkmann canals are seen running parallel to each other (*V*) and perpendicular to the cortex. The openings of two Haversian canals (*H*) are visible.

Each artery has its paired vein and, perhaps, free nerve endings. Venous drainage proceeds from the cortex outward to the periosteal veins, or inward into the marrow space and out the nutrient veins.

Periosteum Covers All Bones and Can Form Bone

The periosteum is the fibrous tissue that envelopes the outer surface of the bone and demarcates it from the surrounding soft tissue. It is connected to the bone by collagenous fibers called **Sharpey fibers**. The internal layer of the periosteum, the **cambium layer,** is applied to the surface of the bone and consists of loosely arranged collagenous bundles, with spindle-shaped connective tissue cells and a network of thin elastic fibers. The outer **fibrous layer** is contiguous with soft tissue planes and fascia. It is composed of dense connective tissue containing

blood vessels. The inner cambium layer is responsible for the process of intramembranous ossification and formation of the cortex. If the periosteum is irritated (e.g., infection, trauma or tumor), it can produce a significant amount of reactive bone that can be seen radiographically and in certain circumstances may reflect the biological potential of the underlying lesion.

Bone Matrix Is Organic and Heavily Mineralized

Bone tissue is composed of cells (10% by weight), a mineralized phase (hydroxyapatite crystals, representing 60% of the total tissue) and an organic matrix (30%). *Thus, except for its cells, bone is a biphasic structure composed of an organic and an inorganic matrix.*

The **mineralized matrix** consists of poorly crystalline hydroxyapatite, $Ca_{10}(PO_4)_6(OH)_2$. Because of its net negative charge, it can neutralize substantial amounts of acid. Other important ions in bone are carbonate, citrate, fluoride, chloride, sodium, magnesium, potassium and strontium.

The **organic matrix** consists of 88% type I collagen, 10% other proteins and 1%–2% lipids and glycosaminoglycans. *Thus, type I collagen basically defines the organic matrix.* Other proteins include:

- **Osteocalcin** is produced by osteoblasts. Blood levels of this protein are a useful marker of bone formation.
- **Osteopontin** and **sialoprotein** are bone matrix proteins containing the amino acid sequence *Arg-Gly-Asp*, which is recognized by **integrins**. Thus, osteopontin and bone sialoprotein probably help anchor cells to the bone matrix.

The Cells of the Bone Are Responsible for Maintaining Its Structure

There are four types of cells in bone tissue, each of which has specific functions related to the formation, resorption and remodeling of bone:

OSTEOPROGENITOR CELL: The osteoprogenitor cell, which differentiates ultimately into osteoblasts and osteocytes, is itself derived from a primitive stem cell. The stem cell can develop into adipocytes, myoblasts, fibroblasts or osteoblasts. Osteoprogenitor cells are found in marrow, periosteum and all supporting structures within the marrow cavity. They are not readily recognized by light microscopy as they are small, nonspecific, stellate or spindle-shaped cells. In response to an appropriate signal, the osteoprogenitor cell gives rise to an osteoblast. Osteoblast commitment and differentiation are controlled by complex activities involving signal transduction and transcriptional regulation of gene expression (e.g., Wnt signaling pathway, Runx2 and bone morphogenic proteins).

OSTEOBLAST: Osteoblasts are the protein-synthesizing cells that produce and mineralize bone tissue. They are derived from mesenchymal progenitors that also give rise to chondrocytes, myocytes, adipocytes and fibroblasts. These large mononuclear and polygonal cells are arrayed in a line along the bone surface (Fig. 30-3A). Underlying the layer of osteoblasts is a thin, eosinophilic zone of organic bone matrix that has not yet been mineralized, called **osteoid**. The time from the deposition of osteoid to its mineralization is known as the **mineralization lag time** (approximately 12 days). The protein synthetic capacity of osteoblasts is reflected in its abundant endoplasmic reticulum, prominent Golgi apparatus and mitochondria with calcium-containing granules.

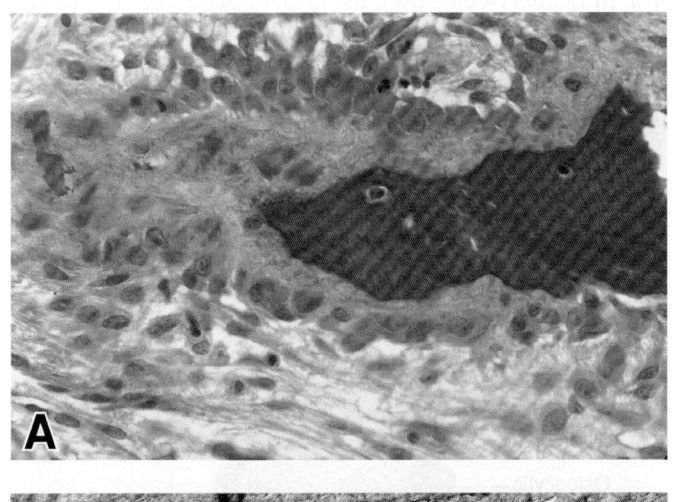

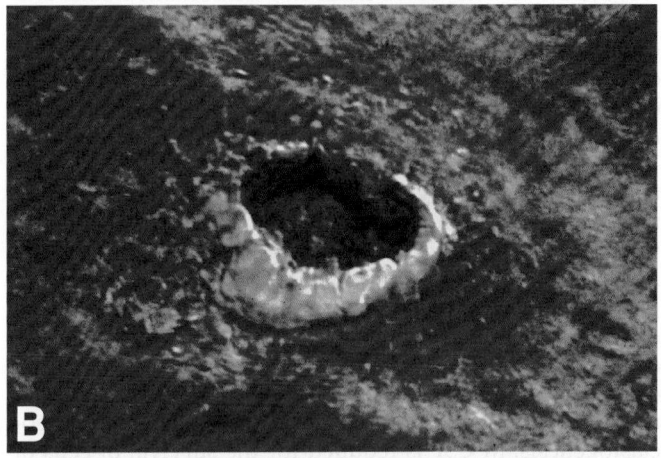

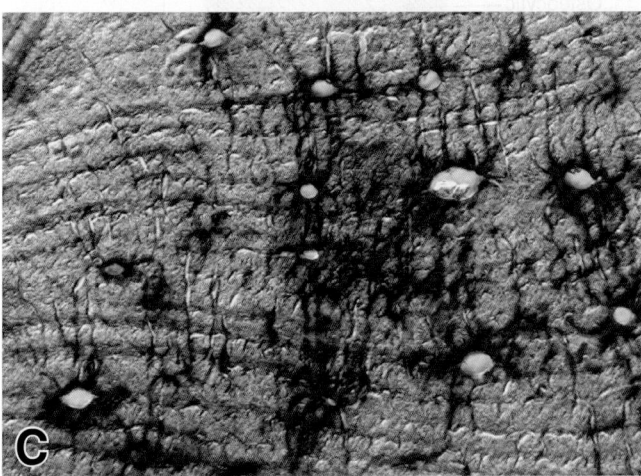

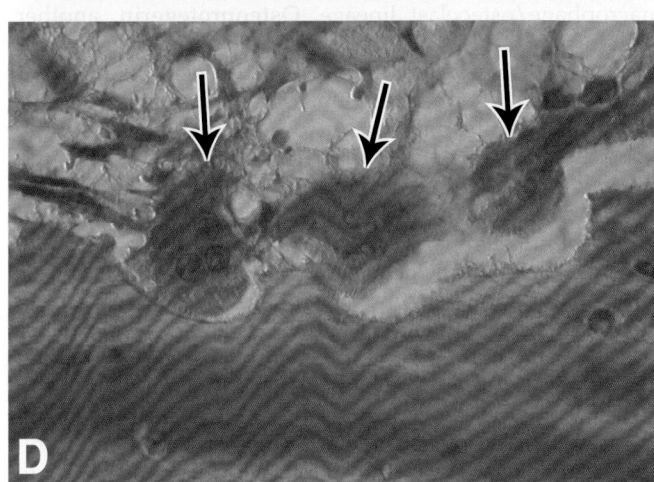

FIGURE 30-3. The cells of bones. A. A **developing bone spicule** demonstrates a prominent layer of plump osteoblasts lining the pink osteoid seam. The dark purple layer beneath the osteoid seam is mineralized bone. **B. Osteocytes.** Osteocytes represent trapped osteoblasts surrounded by bone matrix. The space surrounding the cell is called a **lacuna.** At this power, a few cytoplasmic extensions of the cell can be seen extending into narrow channels in the bone, called **canaliculi. C.** The extensive **intercommunication of osteocyte processes** via their canalicular network in cortical bone is visible in this section. **D. Osteoclasts.** These are multinucleated giant cells (*arrows*) found on bone surfaces within small scalloped reabsorption pits, called **Howship lacunae.**

Cytoplasmic processes that extend into the osteoid contact cells embedded in the matrix called **osteocytes**. The syncytium of osteocytes and osteoblasts probably prevents bone calcium (99% of the body's calcium) from equilibrating with the general extracellular space. When an osteoblast is inactive, it flattens on the surface of bone tissue. It contains alkaline phosphatase, manufactures osteocalcin and expresses parathyroid hormone (PTH) receptors. Collagenase secreted by osteoblasts may also facilitate osteoclastic activity. Finally, a number of growth factors, including transforming growth factor-β (TGF-β), insulin-like growth factor-I (IGF-I), IGF-2, platelet-derived growth factor (PDGF), interleukin-1 (IL-1), fibroblast growth factor (FGF) and tumor necrosis factor-α (TNF-α), are produced by osteoblasts and are important in regulating bone growth and differentiation. Furthermore, the osteoblast possesses surface receptors for various hormones (e.g., PTH, vitamin D, estrogen, glucocorticoids, etc.), as well as for cytokines and growth factors. *The osteoblast ultimately controls the activation, maturation and differentiation of the osteoclast through a paracrine cell signaling mechanism (see Osteoclast below).*

OSTEOCYTE: The osteocyte is an osteoblast that is completely embedded in bone matrix and is isolated in a lacuna (Fig. 30-3B). Osteocytes deposit small quantities of bone around lacunae, but with time, they lose the capacity for protein synthesis. They have small hyperchromatic nuclei and numerous processes that extend through bony canals called **canaliculi,** which communicate with those from other osteocytes and osteoblasts (Fig. 30-3C). *The osteocytes may be the bone cells that recognize and respond to mechanical forces and are important regulators of bone remodeling.*

OSTEOCLAST: Osteoclasts are the exclusive bone-resorptive cells. They are of hematopoietic origin, being members of the monocyte/macrophage family. Three major factors are required for osteoclastogenesis: (1) TNF-related receptor RANK (receptor activator for nuclear factor-κB [NFκB]), (2) RANK ligand (RANKL) and (3) macrophage colony-stimulating factor (M-CSF). RANK is expressed by osteoclast precursors. RANKL and M-CSF are produced by osteoblasts and stromal cells. Binding of RANKL to RANK activates NFκB signaling, which leads to increased osteoclastogenesis. M-CSF is required for the survival of cells of macrophage/osteoclast lineage. **Osteoprotegerin,** another protein produced by osteoblasts and also a member of the TNF family, blocks the interaction between RANK and RANKL and consequently inhibits osteoclastogenesis.

Osteoclasts are multinucleated cells that contain many lysosomes and are rich in hydrolytic enzymes. They are found in small depressions on bone surfaces called **Howship lacunae** (Fig. 30-3D). By electron microscopy, they form a polarized ruffled plasmalemmal membrane (Fig. 30-4) when the cell is in contact with and is actively degrading bone. Osteoclastic resorption is a multistep process that involves attachment of the cell to bone by integrins. A tight gasket-like seal isolates an extracellular compartment that forms between bone and the osteoclast ruffled membrane. A proton pump then acidifies this compartment to a pH of 4.5, in effect creating a giant extracellular lysosome. This proton-rich environment mobilizes bone mineral, thus exposing the organic bone matrix to degradation by lysosomal enzymes. Degraded fragments of bone are transported to the opposite side of the osteoclasts and then released to the extracellular space.

Although the machinery of an osteoclast is superbly suited for bone resorption, it functions only if the matrix

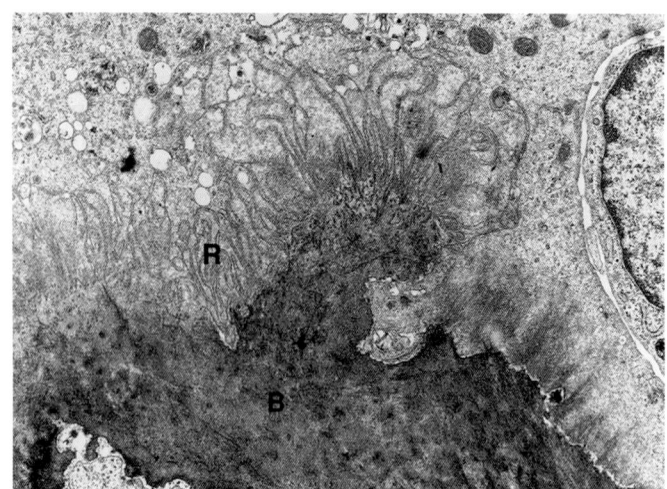

FIGURE 30-4. Osteoclast. An electron micrograph shows the ruffled membrane (*R*), which consists of a complex infolding of the plasma membrane juxtaposed to bone (*B*).

is mineralized. *In fact, any bone that is lined by osteoid or unmineralized cartilage is protected from osteoclastic activity.* In rickets (see below), the growth plate does not calcify normally; it thus grows without osteoclastic resorption and becomes very thick.

Constant bone remodeling is a normal part of skeletal maintenance (Fig. 30-5). It is initiated by activation of the cytokine receptor RANK on osteoclasts. Soluble factors released during bone resorption and PTH aid in recruitment of osteoblasts to the site and their activation to form new bone. Osteoclasts possess receptors for **calcitonin,** which inhibits osteoclast activity. *Thus, bone remodeling involves*

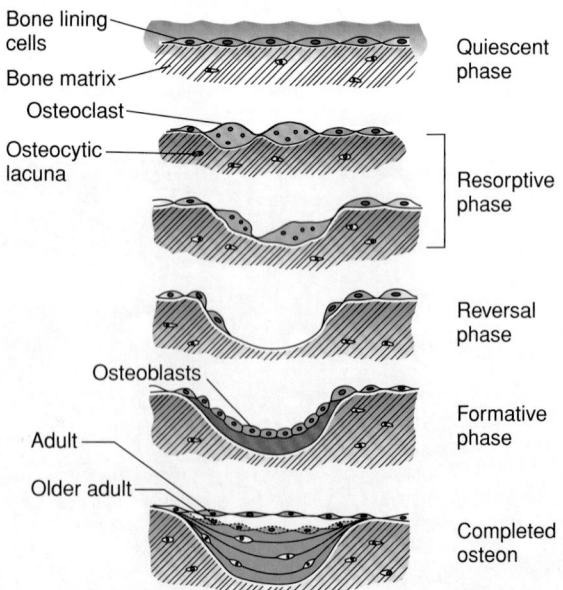

FIGURE 30-5. Bone-remodeling sequence. Bone remodeling is initiated by the appearance of osteoclasts on a bone surface previously lined by fusiform cells. After development of a resorption bay, osteoclasts are replaced by osteoblasts, which deposit new bone. The bone loss that attends aging (senile osteoporosis) is due to incomplete filling of resorption bays.

replacing old bone with newly formed bone via the functional coupling of osteoclasts and osteoblasts, called the bone-remodeling unit. Bone remodeling enables bone to adapt to mechanical stress, maintain its strength and regulate calcium homeostasis.

There Are Two Types of Bone Tissue: Lamellar Bone and Woven Bone

Both may be mineralized or unmineralized. Unmineralized bone is called **osteoid**.

Lamellar Bone

Lamellar bone is made slowly and is highly organized. As the stronger bone tissue, it forms the adult skeleton. *Anything other than lamellar bone in the adult skeleton is abnormal.* Lamellar bone is defined by (1) a parallel arrangement of type I collagen fibers, (2) few osteocytes in the matrix and (3) uniform osteocytes in lacunae parallel to the long axis

of the collagen fibers. There are four types of lamellar bone (Fig. 30-6):

- **Circumferential bone** forms the outer periosteal and inner endosteal lamellar envelopes of the cortex.
- **Concentric lamellar bone** is arranged around the Haversian canals. In two dimensions, concentric lamellar bone and its Haversian artery and vein constitute the **osteon** (Fig. 30-1). In three dimensions, osteons make up the **Haversian system**. These cylinders of bone around Haversian canals run parallel to the long axis of the cortex and are the strongest bone made. The osteons form only if there is appropriate stress. Thus, a paralyzed limb has a cortex composed exclusively of poorly formed Haversian systems and circumferential lamellar bone.
- **Interstitial lamellar bone** represents remnants of either circumferential or concentric lamellar bone that have been remodeled and are wedged between the osteons.
- **Trabecular lamellar bone** forms the coarse cancellous bone of the medullary cavity. It exhibits plates of lamellar bone perforated by marrow spaces.

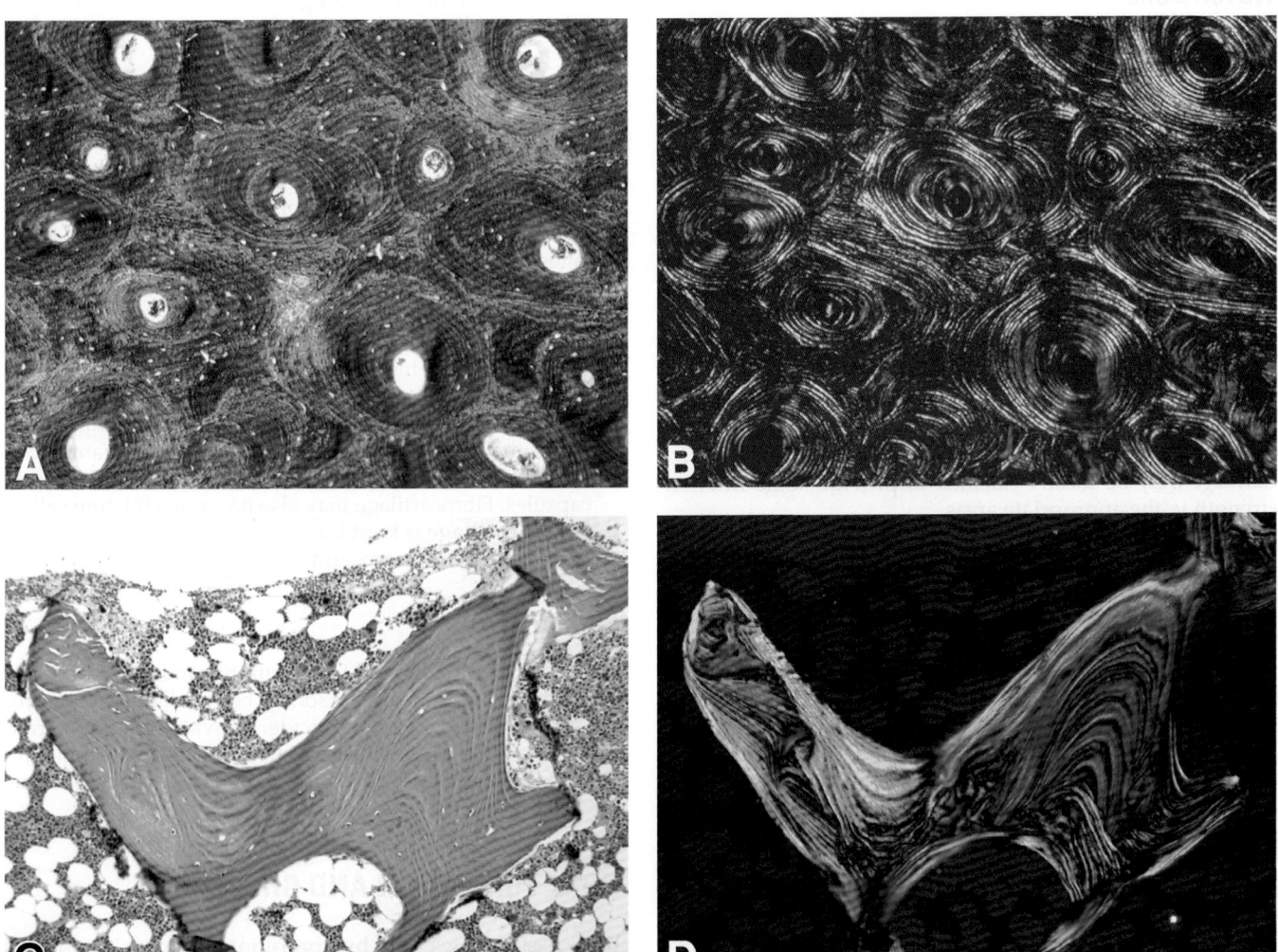

FIGURE 30-6. Cortical lamellar bone. A. Lamellae of the compacta (cortex) are arranged concentrically about Haversian canals. **B.** The same field in polarized light shows the alternating light and dark layered arrangement of the collagen fibers. **C. Lamellae of the spongiosa** in a single mature trabecula are shown in a bright field view. **D.** Polarized light demonstrates that the lamellae are arranged in light and dark layers, but these layers are in long plates rather than in a concentric arrangement.

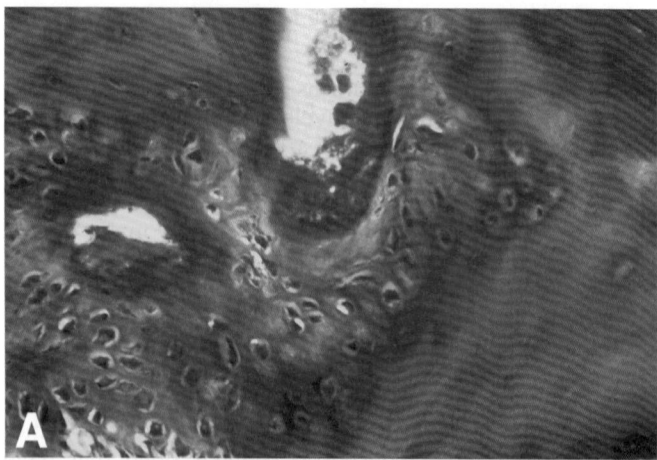
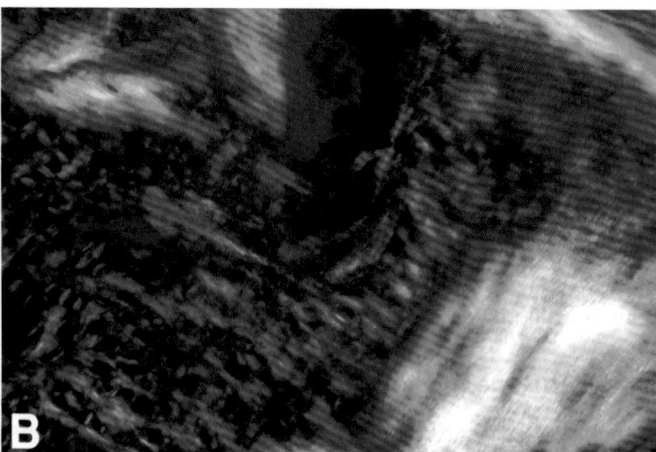

FIGURE 30-7. Woven bone. A. In this section, the woven bone constitutes early fracture repair. Note that in the area of new bone, there are many osteocytes that vary in size but are mainly large with prominent lacunae (compare with area of lamellar bone at *lower right*). **B.** This is the same section viewed in polarized light. Note that the collagen fibers are disposed in a pattern resembling the loose fiber pattern of coarsely woven burlap.

Woven Bone

Woven bone is identified by (1) an irregular arrangement of type I collagen fibers, hence the term *woven*; (2) numerous osteocytes in the matrix; and (3) variation in osteocyte size and shape (Fig. 30-7A,B).

Woven bone is deposited more rapidly than lamellar bone. It is haphazardly arranged and of low tensile strength, serving as a temporary scaffolding for support. It is not surprising that woven bone is found in the developing fetus, in areas surrounding tumors and infections and as part of a healing fracture. *Its presence in the adult skeleton is always abnormal and indicates that reactive tissue has been produced in response to some stress in the bone.*

Cartilage, Unlike Bone, Contains No Blood Vessels, Nerves or Lymphatics

Cartilage may be focally calcified to provide some internal strength in the appropriate areas.

Cartilage Matrix

Like bone, cartilage may be viewed as an organic and inorganic biphasic material. The inorganic phase is composed of calcium hydroxyapatite crystals, equivalent to those found in bone matrix. However, the organic matrix is quite different from that of bone. Essentially, cartilage is a hyperhydrated structure, with water forming some 80% of its weight. The remaining 20% is composed principally of two types of macromolecules, type II collagen and proteoglycans. The water content is extremely important in the function of articular cartilage as it enhances the resilience and lubrication of the joint. Proteoglycans are complex macromolecules composed of a central linear protein core, to which long side arms of polysaccharides, called **glycosaminoglycans,** are attached. These molecules are polyanionic because of the regular presence of carboxyl groups and sulfates along the molecules. Cartilage glycosaminoglycans comprise three long-chain, unbranched, repeating, polydimeric saccharides: chondroitin-4-sulfate, chondroitin-6-sulfate and keratan sulfate. The chondroitin sulfates are the most abundant, accounting for 55%–90% of the cartilage matrix, depending on the age of the tissue.

Types of Cartilage

There are three types of cartilage:

- **Hyaline cartilage:** This is the prototypic cartilage, constituting the articular cartilage of joints; cartilaginous anlage of developing bones; growth plates; costochondral cartilages; cartilages of the trachea, bronchi and larynx; and nasal cartilages. Hyaline cartilage is the most common cartilage in tumors, in fracture callus and in areas of relative avascularity.
- **Fibrocartilage:** This tissue is essentially hyaline cartilage that contains numerous type I collagen fibers for tensile and structural strength. It is found in the annulus fibrosus of the intervertebral disk, tendinous and ligamentous insertions, menisci, symphysis pubis and insertions of joint capsules. Fibrocartilage may also occur in a fracture callus.
- **Elastic cartilage** is found in the epiglottis, in the arytenoid cartilages of the larynx and in the external ear.

Chondrocytes

Chondrocytes are derived from primitive mesenchymal cells that are similar to the precursors of bone cells. The chondroblast gives rise to the chondrocyte. Activation of SOX9 transcription factor is essential for chondrocyte formation, and SOX9 is expressed in cartilaginous neoplasms. As in bone, the cell that resorbs calcified cartilage is the osteoclast.

BONE FORMATION AND GROWTH

Bone tissue grows only by appositional growth, defined as deposition of new matrix on a preexisting surface by adjacent surface osteoblasts. By contrast, virtually all other tissues, especially cartilage, increase by interstitial cell proliferation within the matrix as well as by appositional growth.

Bone development in the fetus follows a stereotyped sequence. Most of the skeleton (except the calvaria and clavicles) develops from cartilage anlagen present during fetal development. This cartilage is eventually resorbed and replaced by bone by **endochondral ossification**. Development of bone can be illustrated by using a limb as an example.

The Process of Primary Ossification Follows a Defined Temporal Sequence

1. **Cartilage anlage:** By 5 weeks of gestation, a thin layer of mesenchymal cells forms between the ectoderm and endoderm of the limb bud and condenses into a core of hyaline cartilage. This cartilaginous anlage is the precursor of the future long bone of that limb. The fibrous capsule of the cartilage anlage is called a **perichondrium**. The width of the cartilaginous anlage is increased by appositional growth of chondroblasts, which deposit cartilage matrix on the internal surface of the perichondrium. At the same time, the anlage increases in length by both appositional and interstitial growth of the chondrocytes. At this stage, the long "bone" is actually composed of cartilage.
2. **The primary center of ossification:** The vascular bed increases, and the perichondrium deposits woven bone on the surface of the cartilage core at the midportion of the future bone. This circumferential sleeve of woven bone is the primary center of ossification, because it is the first bone tissue to be formed. The perichondrium then becomes **periosteum** (Fig. 30-8A).
3. **Cylinderization:** Within the cartilaginous anlage, chondrocytes form proliferating columns, which eventually undergo focal calcification. Calcification is the signal for osteoclastic resorption and invasion of vessels into the cartilaginous mass. Thus, the earliest endochondral ossification occurs after the cartilage is hollowed out from the center of the anlage. This "cavitation" of the cartilaginous core forms the future marrow space. The progressive hollowing of the diaphysis is **cylinderization**.
4. **Primary spongiosum:** The swollen, hypertrophied chondrocytes within the central cartilage begin to die. Capillary invasion increases. The surfaces of the calcified cartilage cores become enveloped by woven bone

laid down by osteoblasts, which arrive through the pluripotential mesenchymal tissue that enters with the capillaries. This cartilaginous core, surrounded by woven bone, is called **primary spongiosum**, or **primary trabecula**. It is the first bone formed after the replacement of cartilage.

Cavitation continues along the future diaphysis toward each end of the bone. Meanwhile, the bone enlarges in width by appositional bone growth from the ever-increasing periosteal sleeve, which makes additional woven bone for the future cortex.

In Secondary Ossification, Cartilage Is Stimulated and Transformed into Bone

Programmed events similar to those in the primary spongiosum take place in the cartilaginous ends of the future bone. Resting (reserve) cartilage is stimulated to become columns of proliferating cartilage, which then progress to hypertrophied chondrocytes and, eventually, calcified cartilage.

1. **The secondary center of ossification** (Fig. 30-8B): Also called the **epiphyseal center of ossification,** this structure is formed at the ends of the bone when cartilage is resorbed. The centrifugal enlargement of the secondary ossification is called **hemispherization** and occurs simultaneously with the longitudinal development of the marrow cavity of the diaphysis.
2. **Formation of the growth plate:** As the bony ends expand during hemispherization and cylinderization occurs in the future diaphysis, a zone of cartilage is trapped between the end of the bone and the diaphysis. This cartilage is destined to be the **growth plate** (Fig. 30-9A), which is a layer of modified cartilage between the diaphysis and epiphysis. Its structure is essentially unchanged from early fetal life to skeletal maturity. *The growth plate controls the longitudinal growth of bones and ultimately determines adult height.*
3. **Structure of the growth plate:** The chondrocytes of the growth plate are arranged in vertical rows, which, in three

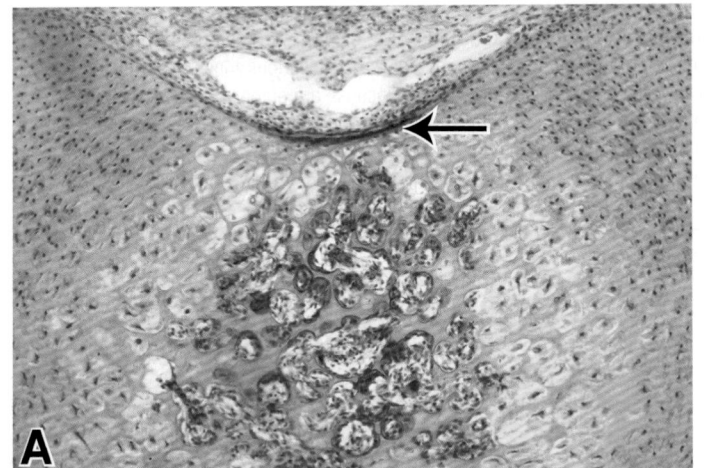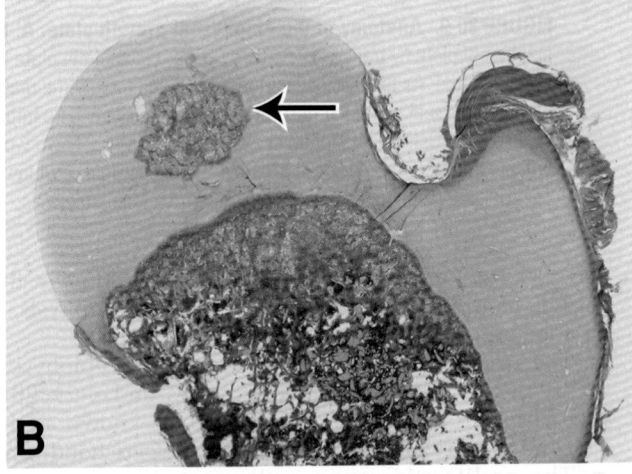

FIGURE 30-8. Primary ossification. A. This section of a short tubular bone demonstrates the first true bone tissue deposited on the outside of the midshaft of the cartilage model along with very early hollowing of the center of the cartilage model to form mixed spicules of cartilage and bone (primary spongiosa). **B.** The **secondary ossification center** is demonstrated in this femoral head.

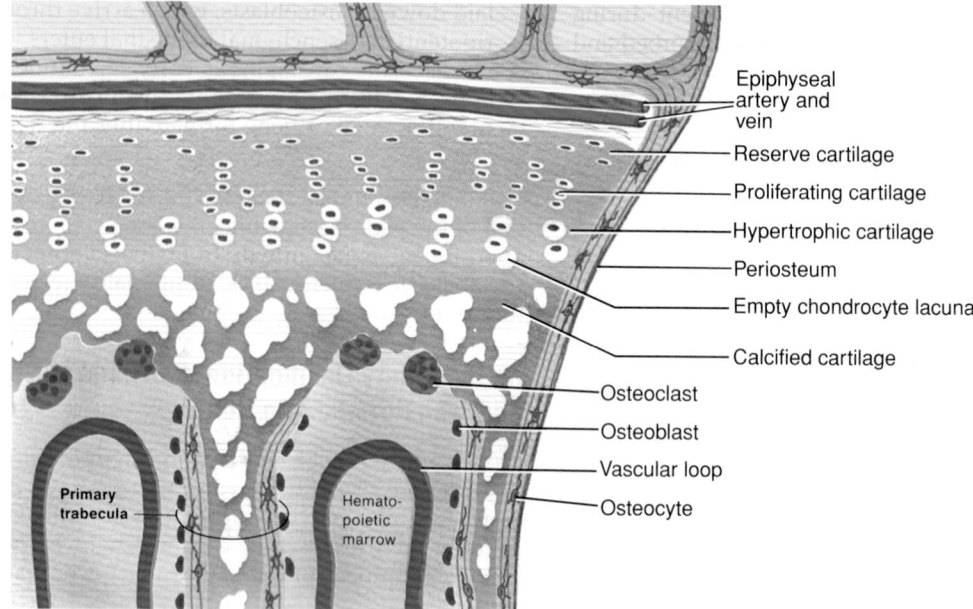

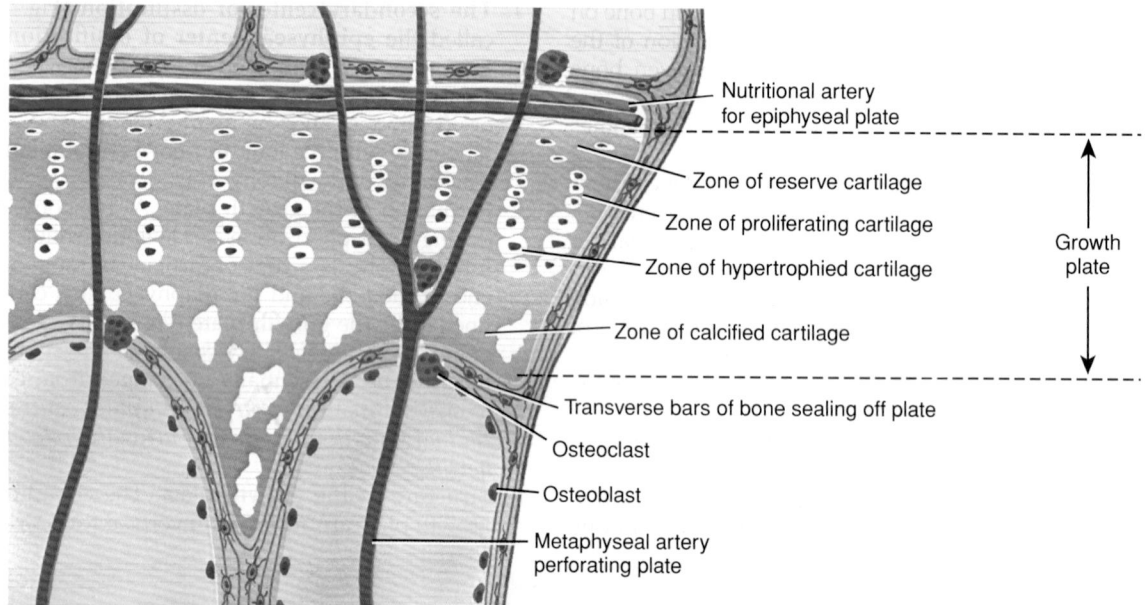

FIGURE 30-9. Anatomy of the epiphyseal growth plate. A. Normal growing epiphyseal plate. The epiphysis is separated from the epiphyseal plate by transverse plates of bone that seal the plate so that it grows only toward the metaphysis. The various zones of cartilage are illustrated. As the calcified cartilage migrates toward the metaphysis, the chondrocytes die, and the lacunae are empty. At the interface of the epiphyseal plate and the metaphysis, osteoclasts bore into the calcified cartilage, accompanied by a capillary loop from the metaphyseal vessels. Osteoblasts follow the osteoclasts and lay down woven bone on the cartilage core, thereby forming the primary spongiosum or primary trabeculae. **B. Normal closure.** The epiphyseal cartilage has ceased to grow, and metaphyseal vessels penetrate the cartilage plate. Transverse bars of bone separate the plate from the metaphysis.

dimensions, are really helices. Viewed longitudinally, the growth plate, proceeding from epiphysis to metaphysis, is divided into zones (Figs. 30-2B and 30-9).

- **The reserve (resting) zone** is supplied by epiphyseal arteries and has small chondrocytes and very little matrix. An additional peripheral zone, known as the **zone of Ranvier,** lies directly under the perichondrium.
- **The proliferative zone** is the next deeper zone, in which active proliferation of chondrocytes occurs both longitudinally and transversely, although the main growth thrust is longitudinal. In a very active growth

plate, proliferative zones account for over half the thickness of the growth plate.

- **The hypertrophic zone** is next and demonstrates a substantial increase in chondrocyte size. The intercellular matrix is prominent, and a dense zone, the **territorial matrix,** surrounds chondrocytes.
- **The zone of calcification** is the cartilaginous zone closest to the metaphysis, where the matrix becomes mineralized.
- **The zone of ossification** is the area where a coating of bone is laid down on the surface of the calcified

cartilage. Capillaries grow into the calcified cartilage and give access to osteoclasts, which resorb much of the calcified matrix. Residual vertical walls of calcified cartilage act as scaffolding for the deposition of bone.

The molecular mechanisms governing endochondral growth are beginning to be understood. Parathyroid hormone–related protein (PTHrP) is secreted from perichondrial cells and chondrocytes and maintains chondrocyte proliferation. PTHrP deficiency leads to severe growth retardation and distorted growth plates. The developmental regulator Indian hedgehog (Ihh) is also involved in growth plate maturation by acting in conjunction with PTHrP. A third major factor involved in growth plate regulation is FGF. FGF receptor-3 (FGFR3) is expressed on proliferating chondrocytes, and its activation leads to inhibition of growth plate proliferation. Mutations of FGFR3 are associated with growth arrest (e.g., achondroplasia or other forms of dwarfism) or growth acceleration.

Formation of the Metaphysis Is Called Funnelization

It occurs at the ring of Delacroix, a periosteal cuff of bone surrounding the epiphyseal cartilage. A wave of periosteal osteoclasts resorbs the cortex, so that a fluted or funnel shape begins to appear. At the same time, endosteal osteoblastic bone is deposited to keep pace with, and offset, some of the osteoclastic resorption. The net result is the funnel or fluted shape of the bone.

The Growth Plate Is Normally Obliterated at a Specific Age for Each Bone

Closure of the growth plate (Fig. 30-9B) is induced by sex hormones and occurs earlier in girls than in boys. Renewal of chondrocytes slows and ultimately ceases. The entire plate is eventually replaced by bone. In some people, a transverse bony plate representing the site of closure can be seen on radiography.

DISORDERS OF THE GROWTH PLATE

Cretinism Leads to Defective Cartilage Maturation

Cretinism results from **maternal iodine deficiency** (see Chapter 27) and has profound effects on the skeleton. Thyroid hormone plays a role in regulating chondrocytes, osteoblasts and osteoclasts through production of cytokines and other factors involved in bone development and growth. Linear growth is severely impaired, resulting in dwarfism, with limbs disproportionately short in relation to the trunk. Delayed closure of the fontanelles of the skull causes an unusually large head. There is a delay in closure of the epiphyses, as well as radiologic stippling of these zones. Shedding of deciduous teeth and eruption of permanent teeth are retarded.

 PATHOLOGY: In cretinism, chondrocytes do not follow the orderly endochondral sequence. Instead, maturation of the hypertrophied zone is retarded, and the zone of proliferative cartilage is narrow. Endochondral ossification, therefore, does not proceed appropriately, and transverse bars of bone in the metaphysis seal off the growth plate. Although growth plates may remain open, the failure of endochondral ossification produces severe dwarfism. The misshapen epiphyses seen on radiography reflect incomplete penetration of the secondary centers of ossification of the epiphysis.

Morquio Syndrome Features Mucopolysaccharide Deposition in Chondrocytes

Many of the mucopolysaccharidoses (see Chapter 6) involve skeletal deformities, attributable to deposition of mucopolysaccharides (glycosaminoglycans) in developing bones. An example is Morquio syndrome (mucopolysaccharidosis type IV), which leads to a particularly severe form of dwarfism, in addition to dental defects, mental retardation, corneal opacities and increased urinary excretion of keratan sulfate.

Achondroplasia Is an Inherited Dwarfism Caused by Arrest of the Growth Plate

Achondroplasia refers to a syndrome of short-limbed dwarfism and macrocephaly and represents a failure of normal epiphyseal cartilage formation. It is the most common genetic form of dwarfism (1 in 15,000 live births) and is inherited as an autosomal dominant trait. Most cases represent new mutations. The mean adult height in achondroplasia is 131 cm (51 inches) in men and 125 cm (49 inches) in women. Achondroplastic dwarfs have normal mentation and average life spans. However, some patients develop severe kyphoscoliosis and its complications.

 **MOLECULAR PATHOGENESIS:** Achondroplasia is caused by an **activating** mutation in FGFR3 encoded on chromosome 4(p16.3). The mutation constitutively inhibits chondrocyte differentiation and proliferation, which retards growth plate development.

 PATHOLOGY: The growth plate in achondroplasia is greatly thinned, and the zone of proliferative cartilage is either absent or extensively attenuated (Fig. 30-10). The zone of provisional calcification, if present, undergoes endochondral ossification, but at a greatly reduced rate. A transverse bar of bone often seals off the growth plate, thus preventing further bone formation and causing dwarfism. Interestingly, the secondary centers of ossification and the articular cartilage are normal. Because intramembranous ossification is undisturbed, the periosteum functions normally and the bones become very short and thick. For the same reasons, the head of the dwarf appears unusually large, compared with the bones formed from the cartilage of the face. The spine is of normal length, but limbs are abnormally short.

Scurvy Results from Dietary Deficiency of Vitamin C

 **MOLECULAR PATHOGENESIS AND PATHOLOGY:** Hydroxyproline and hydroxylysine are important in stabilizing the helical structure of collagen and in cross-linking the tropocollagen fibers into the proper molecular structure of collagen. Vitamin C is a cofactor in hydroxylation of proline and lysine. The skeletal changes of scurvy reflect the lack of osteoblastic function. Woven bone is not formed because osteoblasts cannot produce and normally cross-link

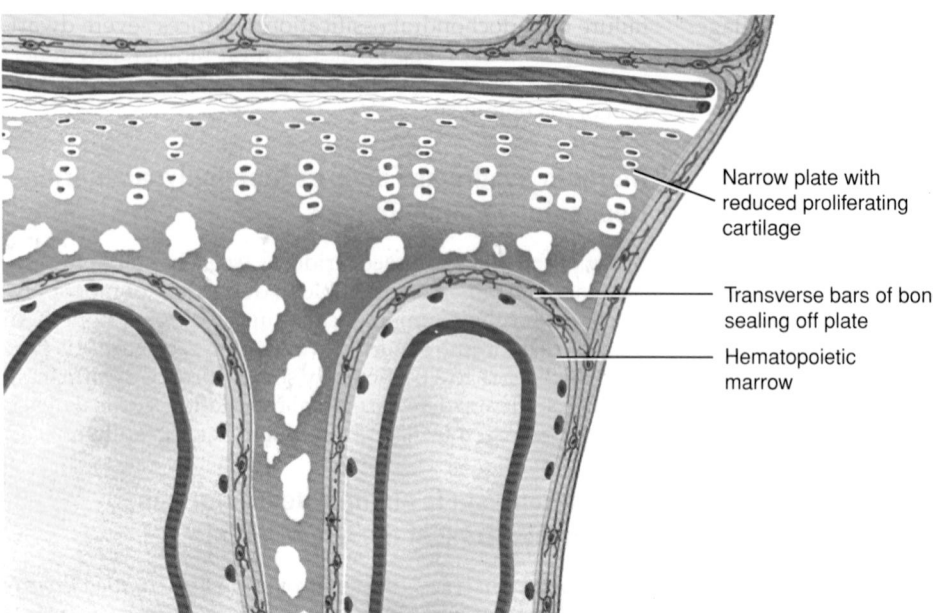

Narrow plate with reduced proliferating cartilage

Transverse bars of bone sealing off plate

Hematopoietic marrow

FIGURE 30-10. The epiphyseal growth plate of an achondroplastic dwarf. In achondroplasia, the epiphyseal plate is reduced in thickness, and the zones of proliferating cartilage are attenuated. Osteoclastic activity is inconspicuous, and the interface between the plate and the metaphysis is often sealed by transverse bars of bone that prevent further endochondral ossification. As a result, the bones are shortened.

collagen. Chondrocytes at the growth plate continue to grow. The zone of calcified cartilage may actually become more prominent, because it is more heavily calcified. Osteoclasts resorb this zone, but the primary spongiosum does not form properly, and there is irregular vascular perforation of the cartilage plate.

 CLINICAL FEATURES: Today, scurvy is a rare disease (see Chapter 8). Wound healing and bone growth are impaired in patients with scurvy. Furthermore, the basement membrane of capillaries is damaged by this condition and widespread capillary bleeding is common. Subperiosteal bleeding may occur, leading to joint and muscle pain.

Asymmetric Cartilage Growth Causes Spinal Disorders and Tumors

Asymmetric cartilage growth, such as occurs in patients with knock-knees and bowed legs, develops when one part of the growth plate, either medial or lateral, grows faster than the other. Most cases are hereditary, but mechanical forces such as trauma near the growth plate may stimulate one side to grow faster or in an asymmetric fashion. Aside from the cosmetic appearance, these conditions may require correction to prevent future incongruity, eventual loss of articular cartilage and joint destruction.

Scoliosis and Kyphosis

Scoliosis *is an abnormal lateral curvature of the spine, usually affecting adolescent girls.* **Kyphosis** *refers to an abnormal anteroposterior curvature.* When both conditions are present, the term **kyphoscoliosis** is used.

 **ETIOLOGIC FACTORS:** A vertebral body grows in length (height) from the endplates of the vertebrae, which correspond to the growth plates of long tubular bones. As in tubular bones, vertebral bodies

increase in width by appositional bone growth from the periosteum. In scoliosis, for unknown reasons, one portion of the endplate grows faster than the other, producing lateral curvature of the spine.

 CLINICAL FEATURES: The treatment is appropriate stress on the vertebral body through use of braces or internal fixation to straighten the spine. If kyphoscoliosis is severe, the patient may eventually develop chronic pulmonary disease, cor pulmonale and joint problems, particularly involving the hip.

Hemihypertrophy

Hemihypertrophy describes several conditions in which one limb's growth plate is stimulated to undergo rapid and prolonged endochondral ossification. That limb becomes much longer than the contralateral one. Infection in the metaphyseal area may stimulate the growth plate to grow rapidly. An arteriovenous malformation may also cause one growth plate to grow faster than its counterpart, as may fractures and tumors near the growth plate. In some cases, hemihypertrophy is part of an inherited syndrome. Children with isolated hemihypertrophy are at increased risk for neoplasms.

MODELING ABNORMALITIES

Osteopetrosis Is Characterized by Abnormally Dense Bone

Osteopetrosis, *also known as* **marble bone disease** *or* **Albers-Schönberg disease,** *is a heterogeneous group of rare inherited disorders in which skeletal mass is increased as a result of abnormally dense bone.* The most common autosomal recessive form is a severe, sometimes fatal disease affecting infants and children. Death of infants with this severe variant is attributable to marked anemia, cranial nerve entrapment, hydrocephalus and infection. A more benign form, transmitted as an autosomal dominant trait and seen in adulthood or adolescence, is associated with mild anemia or no symptoms at all.

 MOLECULAR PATHOGENESIS: *The sclerotic skeleton of osteopetrosis is the result of failed osteoclastic bone resorption.* The disease is caused by mutations in genes that govern osteoclast formation or function. The most common mutations cause defects in bone acidification, which is necessary for osteoclastic bone resorption. These include mutations in the *TCIRG1* gene (osteoclast proton pump; autosomal dominant); the *CLCN7* gene (osteoclast chloride channel; autosomal recessive); and the **carbonic anhydrase II** gene, autosomal recessive. Other mutations that cause osteopetrosis involve transcription factors or cytokines necessary for the osteoclast differentiation.

 PATHOLOGY: Because osteoclast function is arrested, osteopetrosis is characterized by (1) retention of the primary spongiosum with its cartilage cores, (2) lack of funnelization of the metaphysis and (3) a thickened cortex. The result is short, block-like, radiodense bones, hence the term **marble bone disease** (Fig. 30-11A). These bones are extremely radiopaque and weigh two to three times more than normal bone. However, they are basically weak because their structure is intrinsically disorganized and cannot remodel along lines of stress. The mineralized cartilage is also weak and friable, so that the bones in osteopetrosis fracture easily. Grossly, bones in osteopetrosis are widened in the metaphysis and diaphysis, causing the characteristic "Erlenmeyer flask" deformity (Fig. 30-11A,B). Histologically, the bone tissue is extremely irregular, and almost all areas contain a cartilage core (Fig. 30-11C). The marrow spaces become obliterated. Depending on the mutation, osteoclasts may be absent, present in normal numbers or even abundant. In the case of osteopetrosis characterized by normal or increased numbers of osteoclasts, the molecular defect lies in a gene involved in the function of osteoclasts, rather than in their formation.

 CLINICAL FEATURES: Suppression of hematopoiesis in osteopetrosis is due to replacement of the marrow by sheets of abnormal osteoclasts or extensive fibrosis. Marrow suppression in patients with the malignant form of osteopetrosis may be sufficiently severe to lead to severe anemia or pancytopenia. To compensate for loss of marrow hematopoiesis, extramedullary hematopoiesis occurs in the liver, spleen and lymph nodes, and these structures are enlarged. Narrowing of neural foramina causes cranial nerve involvement, and subsequent strangulation of nerves leads to blindness and deafness. Osteopetrosis can be treated by bone marrow transplantation, which gives rise to a new clone of functional osteoclasts.

Progressive Diaphyseal Dysplasia Features Thickened Long Bones

Progressive diaphyseal dysplasia (Camurati-Engelmann disease) is an autosomal dominant disorder of children in which cylinderization does not proceed appropriately, resulting in symmetric thickening and increased diameter of the diaphyses of long bones. It is due to increased bone formation linked to a mutation in the propeptide of TGF-β. The

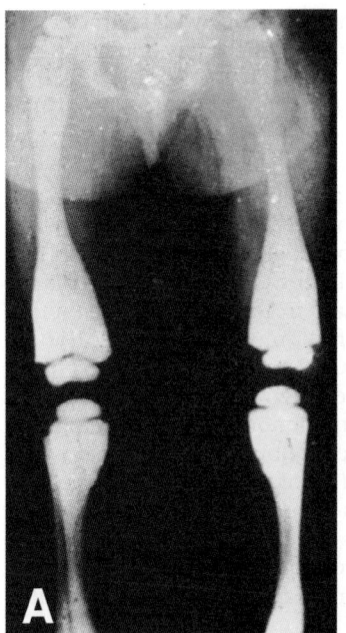
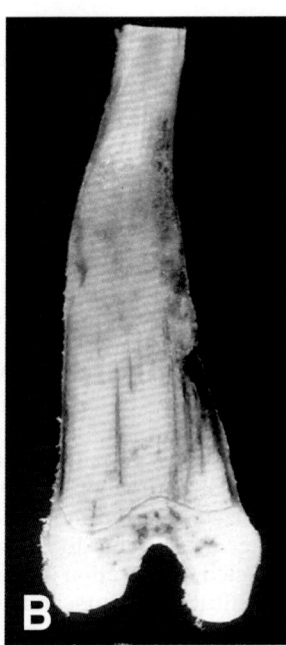
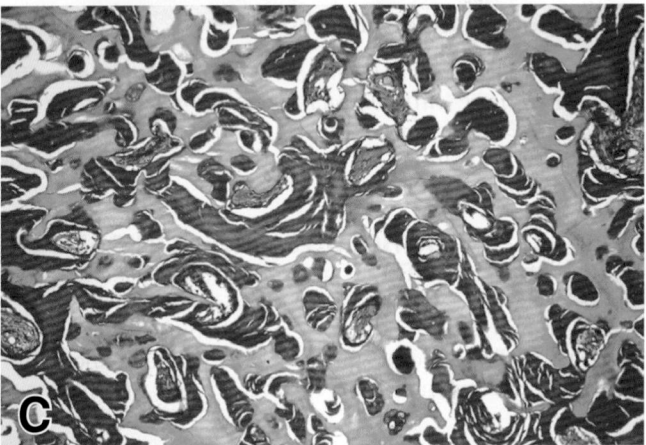

FIGURE 30-11. Osteopetrosis. A. A radiograph of a child shows markedly misshapen and dense bones of the lower extremities, characteristic of "marble bone disease." **B.** A gross specimen of the femur shows obliteration of the marrow space by dense bone. **C.** A photomicrograph of the bone of a child with autosomal recessive osteopetrosis demonstrates disorganization of bony trabeculae by retention of primary spongiosa (mixed spicules) and further obliteration of the marrow space by secondary spongiosa. The result is complete disorganization of the trabeculae and absence of marrow.

disease particularly affects the femur, tibia, fibula, radius and ulna. Patients have pain over the affected areas, fatigue, muscle wasting, atrophy and gait abnormalities.

DELAYED MATURATION OF BONE

Osteogenesis Imperfecta Is Characterized by Abnormal Type I Collagen

Osteogenesis imperfecta (OI) refers to a group of mainly autosomal dominant, heritable disorders of connective tissue, caused by mutations in the gene for type I collagen, affecting the skeleton, joints, ears, ligaments, teeth, sclerae and skin (see Chapter 6). There are four well-characterized types of OI, each different genetic structurally and clinically.

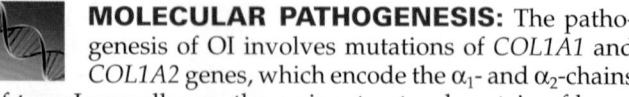 **MOLECULAR PATHOGENESIS:** The pathogenesis of OI involves mutations of *COL1A1* and *COL1A2* genes, which encode the α_1- and α_2-chains of type I procollagen, the major structural protein of bone. These genes are in chromosome 17 (17q21.3–q22) and chromosome 7 (7q21.3–q22), respectively. A point mutation that affects a glycine residue in either *COL1A1* or *COL1A2* is the most typical abnormality found in OI. While *COL1A1* mutations are seen in all types of OI, mutations of *COL1A2* are found in types II, III and IV OI. Mutations of *COL1A1* affect three fourths of the type I collagen molecules, with half of the molecules containing one abnormal pro–α_1-chain and one quarter containing two abnormal pro–α_1-chains. By contrast, mutations in *COL1A2* affect only half of the synthesized collagen molecules. The resulting phenotype will range from mild to lethal depending on which gene is affected, the location in the collagen triple helix at which the substitution occurs and which amino acid is substituted for glycine.

Osteogenesis Imperfecta Type I

OI type I is the mildest phenotype. It is inherited as an autosomal dominant trait, characterized by multiple fractures after birth, blue sclera and hearing abnormalities. In some patients, abnormalities of the teeth are also conspicuous (dentinogenesis imperfecta).

  PATHOLOGY AND CLINICAL FEATURES: Initial fractures usually occur after the infant begins to sit and walk. There may be hundreds of fractures a year with minor movement or trauma. On radiologic examination, bones are extremely thin, delicate and abnormally curved (Fig. 30-12A). The collagen

has reduced tensile strength and bone mineralization is abnormal. The combination of these abnormalities accounts for the brittleness of OI bone. In OI, insufficient bone is formed, leading to decreased cortical thickness and reduced trabecular bone. When a fracture occurs, the fracture callus may be extensive enough to resemble a tumor (Fig. 30-12B). As the child grows, fractures tend to decrease in severity and frequency, and stature is generally unaffected.

The sclerae are very thin, with a blue color attributable to the underlying choroid. Progressive hearing loss, which develops to total deafness in adulthood, results from fusion of the auditory ossicles. The joint laxity associated with the condition eventually leads to kyphoscoliosis and flat feet. Because of hypoplasia of the dentine and pulp, the teeth are misshapen and bluish yellow.

Osteogenesis Imperfecta Type II

OI type II is a lethal, autosomal dominant, perinatal disease. Affected infants are stillborn or die within a few days after birth, in a sense being crushed to death. They are markedly short in stature, with severe limb deformities. Almost all bones sustain fractures during delivery or during uterine contractions in labor. As in OI type I, sclerae are blue.

Osteogenesis Imperfecta Type III

OI type III is the progressive, most severely deforming type of disease and is characterized by many bone fractures, growth retardation and severe skeletal deformities. Inheritance is usually autosomal dominant, although (rarely) autosomal recessive forms are reported. Fractures are present at birth, but bones are less fragile than in the type II form. These patients eventually develop severe shortening of their stature because of progressive bone fractures and severe kyphoscoliosis. Although sclerae may be blue at birth, they become white shortly thereafter. Dental abnormalities are common.

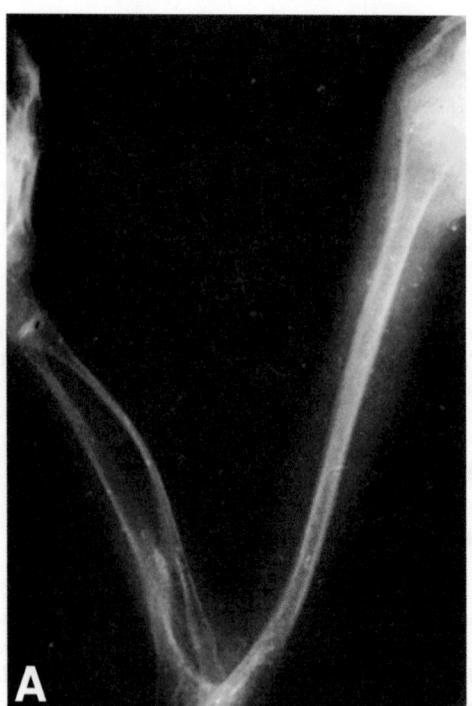

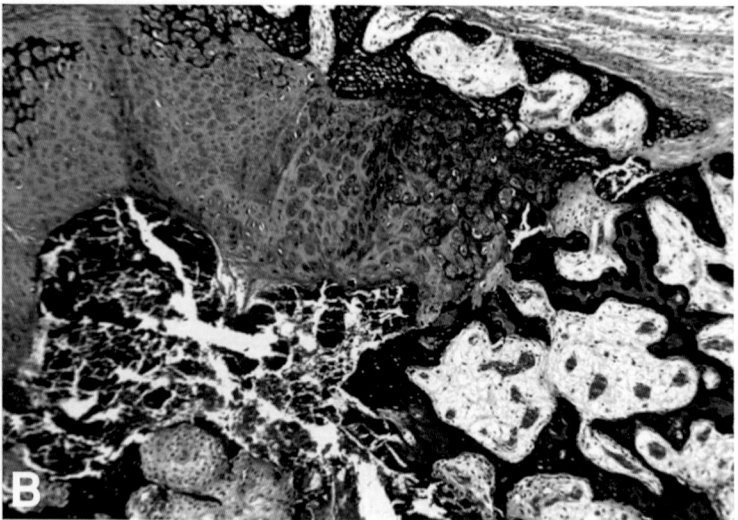

FIGURE 30-12. Osteogenesis imperfecta. A. A radiograph illustrates the markedly thin and attenuated humerus and bones of the forearm. There is a fracture callus in the proximal ulna. **B.** A photomicrograph of the fracture callus with prominent cartilage (*upper left*). The cortex is thin and composed of hypercellular woven bone.

Osteogenesis Imperfecta Type IV

OI type IV is similar to type I except that sclerae are normal. The condition is heterogeneous in presentation, and there may or may not be dental disease. In this disorder, abnormal cross-linkages of collagen result in thin, delicate and weak collagen fibrils. This inappropriate collagen does not allow the bone cortex to mature, so that at birth the cortex of the bone resembles that of a fetus. The cortex is composed of woven bone and small areas of lamellar bone. Over a period of years, the cortex matures, but this may not occur until adolescence or even later. In any event, the frequency of fractures tends to decrease over a long period. These patients are vigorously treated with orthopedic devices, including rods inserted into the medullary cavities to prevent the dwarfing effect of multiple fractures.

Additional types of OI (types V, VI, VII and VIII) have recently been identified from within the heterogeneous type IV group, based on distinct clinical, genetic and bone histologic features.

There is no single treatment for OI. Osteoprogenitor cells for bone marrow transplantation, growth factors, bisphosphonates and gene therapy to improve collagen synthesis have been undergoing clinical trials in an attempt to modify the course and severity of the disease. Because exuberant fracture callus occurs, it is not surprising that rare cases of OI have been interpreted as osteosarcoma.

FRACTURE

The most common bone lesion is a fracture, which is defined as a discontinuity of the bone. A force perpendicular to the long axis of the bone results in a **transverse fracture.** A force along the long axis of the bone yields a **compression fracture**. Torsional force results in **spiral fractures,** and combined tension and compression shear forces cause angulation and displacement of the fractured ends.

A force powerful enough to fracture a bone also injures adjacent soft tissues. In this situation, there is often (1) extensive muscle necrosis; (2) hemorrhage because of shearing of capillary beds and larger vessels of soft tissues; (3) tearing of tendinous insertions and ligamentous attachments; and (4) even nerve damage, caused by stretching or direct tearing of the nerve.

Fracture Healing Is Divided into Inflammatory, Reparative and Remodeling Phases

The duration of each phase (Fig. 30-13) depends on the patient's age, the site of fracture, the patient's overall health and nutritional status and the extent of soft tissue injury. Local factors, such as vascular supply and mechanical forces at the site, also play a role in healing. *In repairing a bone fracture, anything other than formation of bone tissue at the fracture site represents incomplete healing.*

 PATHOLOGY:

The Inflammatory Phase

In the first 1–2 days after a fracture, rupture of blood vessels in the periosteum and adjacent muscle and soft tissue leads to extensive hemorrhage. Extensive bone necrosis at the fracture site also occurs because of disruption of large vessels in the bone and interruption of cortical vessels (i.e., Volkmann and Haversian canals). *Dead bone is characterized by the absence of osteocytes and empty osteocyte lacunae.*

In 2–5 days, the hemorrhage forms a large clot, which must be resorbed so that the fracture can heal. Neovascularization begins to occur peripherally to this blood clot. By the end of the first week, most of the clot is organized by invasion of blood vessels and early fibrosis.

The earliest bone, which is invariably woven bone, is formed after 7 days. *This corresponds to the "scar" of bone.* Since bone formation requires a good blood supply, woven bone spicules begin to appear at the periphery of the clot. Pluripotential mesenchymal cells from the soft tissue and within the bone marrow give rise to the osteoblasts that synthesize woven bone. In most fractures, cartilage also is formed and is eventually resorbed by endochondral ossification. Granulation tissue containing bone or cartilage is called a **callus**. Woven bone also forms inside the marrow cavity at the edge of the blood clot because vascular tissue is also present in that location.

The Reparative Phase

The reparative phase follows the first week after a fracture and may last for months, depending on the degree of movement and the fixation of the fracture. By this time, acute inflammation has dissipated. Pluripotential cells differentiate into fibroblasts and osteoblasts. Repair proceeds from the periphery toward the center of the fracture site and accomplishes two objectives: (1) to organize and resorb the blood clot and, more importantly, (2) to neovascularize construction of the callus, which will eventually bridge the fracture site. Events leading to repair are as follows:

1. Armies of osteoclasts within the Haversian canals form **cutting cones** that bore into the cortex toward the fracture site. A new vessel accompanies the cutting cone, supplying nutrients to these cells and providing more pluripotential cells for cell renewal.
2. At the same time, the external callus, which is found on the surface of the bone and is formed from the periosteum and the soft tissue mesenchymal cells, continues to grow toward the fracture site.
3. Simultaneously, an endosteal or internal callus forms within the medullary cavity and grows outward toward the fracture site.
4. The cortical cutting cones reach the fracture site and the ends of the fractured bone begin to appear beveled and smooth, as the site is remodeled by osteoclasts.
5. The same is true of the endosteal surface of the cortex, as the internal callus works its way to the fracture site.
6. Where there are large areas of cartilage, new blood vessels invade the calcified cartilage, after which the endochondral sequence duplicates the normal formation of bone at the growth plate.

The Remodeling Phase

Several weeks after a fracture, the ingrowth of callus has sealed the bone ends and remodeling begins. In this phase, the bone is reorganized so that the original cortex is restored. Occasionally, the bone is strong enough to qualify as a clinically healed fracture, but biologically, the fracture may not

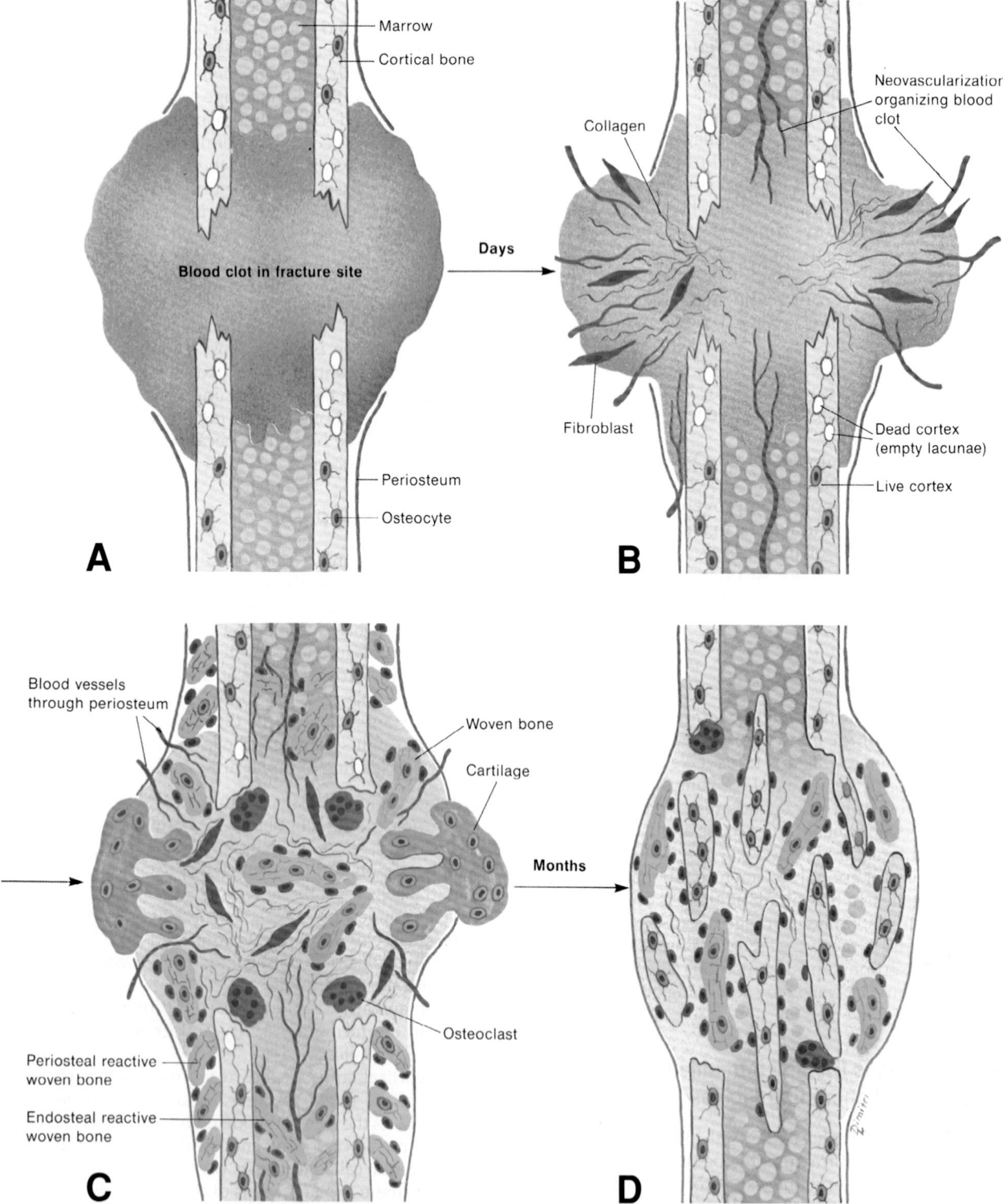

FIGURE 30-13. Healing of a fracture. A. Soon after a fracture is sustained, an extensive blood clot forms in the subperiosteum and soft tissue, as well as in the marrow cavity. The bone at the fracture site is jagged. **B.** The **inflammatory phase** of fracture healing is characterized by neovascularization and beginning organization of the blood clot. Because the osteocytes in the fracture site are dead, the lacunae are empty. The osteocytes of the cortex are necrotic well beyond the fracture site, owing to the traumatic interruption of the perforating arteries from the periosteum. **C.** The **reparative phase** of fracture healing is characterized by the formation of a callus of cartilage and woven bone near the fracture site. The jagged edges of the original cortex have been remodeled and eroded by osteoclasts. The marrow space has been revascularized and contains reactive woven bone, as does the periosteal area. **D.** In the **remodeling phase,** during which the cortex is revitalized, the reactive bone may be lamellar or woven. The new bone is organized along stress lines and mechanical forces. Extensive osteoclastic and osteoblastic cellular activity is maintained.

be truly healed and may continue to undergo remodeling for years. For instance, the callus of rib fractures may remain throughout life because the continual respiratory movement of the ribs shears blood vessels and preserves extensive cartilage callus. In a child, in whom the growth plates are still open, normal modeling of growing bone overtakes the callus, so that a fracture may not be recognizable in later life. Similarly, normal modeling in a child may correct the angulation of a bone at a fracture site. If a fracture is near the growth plate, differential growth rates of the growth plate also correct the angulation. In an adult, however, because the plates are closed, angulation often requires correction with external or internal devices.

Special Considerations

There are unusual nuances to fracture healing that deserve mention.

PRIMARY HEALING: A fracture does not necessarily result in bone displacement and soft tissue injury. For example, a drill hole in the bone cortex or a controlled fracture, such as an osteotomy created with a fine saw during orthopedic surgery, does not displace bone. In this situation, there is almost no soft tissue reaction and callus formation because the bone is rigidly fixed. The fracture callus grows directly into the fracture site by a process called **primary healing**. This results in rapid reconstitution of the cortex, including restoration of the Haversian systems. Similarly, if a fracture site is held in rigid alignment by metal screws and plates, there is also little external callus. The cortical cutting cones will then be prominent and will heal the fracture site quickly.

NONUNION: Failure of a fracture to heal is called **nonunion**. Causes of nonunion include interposition of soft tissues at the fracture site, excessive motion, infection, poor blood supply and other factors mentioned above. Continued movement at the unhealed fracture site may also lead to **pseudoarthrosis,** a condition in which tissue similar to that in the joint is formed. Pluripotential cells become histologically indistinguishable from synovial cells, secrete synovial fluid and form a joint-like structure. In such cases, the fracture never heals and the abnormal tissue must be removed surgically for the fracture to heal properly.

Stress Fractures Result from Microfractures

In these fractures, also known as **fatigue** *or* **march fractures**, *repeated microfractures eventually result in a true fracture through the bone cortex.*

 **ETIOLOGIC FACTORS:** A stress fracture occurs in bones in which the cortex has few osteons and forms only when stress is applied to the cortex. If the ill-prepared cortex (e.g., in the fifth metatarsal) undergoes repeated mechanical stress (e.g., from jogging, skiing or ballet dancing), the bone produces cutting cones in an attempt to implant osteons. If the stress continues and microfractures accumulate, periosteal and endosteal calluses develop to strengthen the bone while active remodeling takes place. An actual fracture occurs as the last event if the stresses are continually applied during remodeling.

 CLINICAL FEATURES: Stress fractures produce pain and swelling over the affected bone. *At the site of a future stress fracture, a callus forms before a fracture occurs.* When the actual fracture takes place, the pain becomes more severe. In the early stages of this condition, before the actual fracture, the radiologic appearance may resemble that of a tumor. A biopsy will show that the cortex is riddled with cutting cones for remodeling, which is also seen in the reactive bone at the edge of an invasive tumor.

OSTEONECROSIS (AVASCULAR NECROSIS, ASEPTIC NECROSIS)

Osteonecrosis refers to the death of bone and marrow in the absence of infection (Fig. 30-14). Causes of

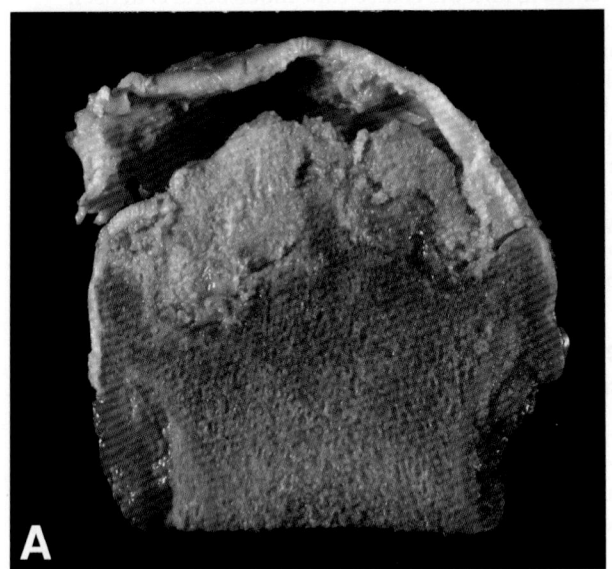 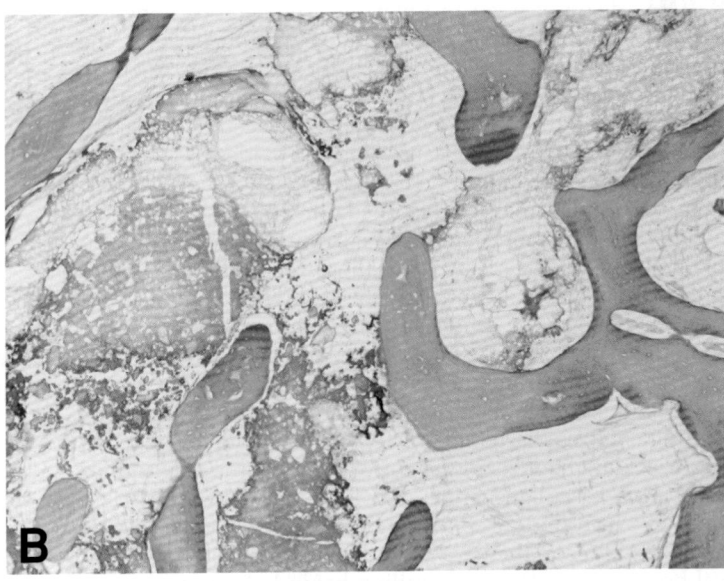

FIGURE 30-14. Osteonecrosis of the head of the femur. A coronal section shows a circumscribed area of subchondral infarction with partial detachment of the overlying articular cartilage and subarticular bone. **B.** Microscopically, the necrotic bone is characterized by empty lacunae and the necrotic marrow shows dystrophic calcification.

TABLE 30-1

CAUSES OF OSTEONECROSIS

Trauma, including fracture and surgery

Emboli, producing focal bone infarction

Systemic diseases, such as polycythemia, lupus erythematosus, Gaucher disease, sickle cell disease and gout

Radiation, either internal or external

Corticosteroid administration

Specific focal bone necrosis at various sites—for instance, in the head of the femur (Legg-Calvé-Perthes disease) or in the navicular bone (Köhler disease)

Organ transplantation, particularly renal, in patients with persistent hyperparathyroidism

Osteochondritis dissecans, a condition of unknown etiology in which a piece of articular cartilage and subchondral bone breaks off into a joint. It is thought that a focal area of bone necrosis occurs and eventually detaches.

Autografts and allografts

Thrombosis of local vessels secondary to the pressure of adjacent tumors or other space-occupying lesions

Idiopathic factors, as in the high incidence of osteonecrosis of the head and the femur in alcoholics. Necrotic bone heals differently in the cortex and in the underlying coarse cancellous bone.

osteonecrosis are listed in Table 30-1. Necrotic bone heals differently in the cortex than in the underlying coarse cancellous bone.

 PATHOLOGY: Osteonecrosis is characterized by death of bone and marrow. The necrotic bone has empty lacunae lacking osteocyte nuclei, and the marrow displays dystrophic calcification (Fig. 30-14B). Necrotic coarse cancellous bone heals by **creeping substitution,** in which the necrotic marrow is replaced by invading or creeping neovascular tissue, which provides the pluripotential cells needed for bone remodeling. Although necrotic bony trabeculae may be resorbed directly by osteoclastic activity, they are more commonly surrounded by new woven or lamellar bone generated by the osteoblastic activity of granulation tissue. Eventually, the sandwich composed of necrotic bone in the center and surrounding viable bone is remodeled by osteoclastic activity, and new bone is laid down through intramembranous bone formation.

Necrotic cortical bone is healed by a cutting cone. The cutting cone, as discussed above, forms by way of preexisting vascular channels in the cortex. The appropriate signals reach this vascular channel and stimulate neovascularization by surrounding pluripotential mesenchymal tissue. Osteoclasts make their way into the necrotic compact cortical bone, with osteoblasts trailing behind. As a result, tunnels bore their way into the necrotic cortex, leading to new bone formation. This is a slow process, and the bone is often laid down de novo as lamellar bone.

Legg-Calvé-Perthes disease is osteonecrosis in the femoral head in children; **idiopathic osteonecrosis** occurs in a similar location in adults. In both conditions, collapse of the femoral head may create joint incongruity and eventual severe osteoarthritis. Collapse of the subchondral bone results from several mechanisms:

- Necrotic bone may sustain stress fractures and compaction over a long period.
- The portion peripheral to the necrotic bone may undergo neovascularization. On radiologic examination, there is a lucent area surrounding the necrotic zone.
- The rigid articular cartilage and subchondral bone may actually crack as the subchondral necrotic zone collapses, producing a fracture.

A radiograph in avascular necrosis often shows the necrotic zone to be radiodense because of (1) relative osteoporosis in the surrounding viable bone compared with the unchanged necrotic bone; (2) addition of new bone through creeping substitution; (3) formation of calcium soaps, which arise as a result of the necrosis of marrow fat; and (4) actual compaction of the preexisting dead bone. Focal end-arterial vascular insufficiency may precede these events, as the necrotic zone tends to be wedge shaped.

REACTIVE BONE FORMATION

Reactive bone is intramembranous bone formed in response to stress on bone or soft tissue. Conditions such as tumors, infections, trauma or generalized or focal disease can stimulate bone formation.

 PATHOLOGY: The periosteum may respond with a so-called **sunburst** pattern (Fig. 30-15), as seen with certain tumors, or progressive layering of the periosteum, which yields an **onionskin pattern** of the cortex. The endosteal or the marrow surface may produce new bone, so that on radiologic studies, the cortex appears to be thickened, and the coarse cancellous bone is denser.

Reactive bone may be either woven or lamellar, depending on the rates of deposition of the reactive bone. Around an indolent infection, as in chronic osteomyelitis, reactive bone may be laid down de novo as lamellar bone from the periosteum. In this case, the bone has time to respond to the persistent stress. Similarly, a benign tumor may cause a lamellar bone reaction. By contrast, a rapidly enlarging tumor is more likely to promote woven bone. Invariably, reactive bone is of the intramembranous type, because it is derived from the periosteum or the endosteal tissue of the marrow.

Heterotopic Ossification Is Bone Formation outside the Skeletal System

Heterotopic ossification (HO) is formation of reactive bone (woven or lamellar) in extraskeletal sites such as the skin, subcutaneous tissue, skeletal muscle and fibroconnective tissue around joints. HO is not associated with any metabolic disease, reflected in the fact that patients have normal serum calcium and phosphorous levels. HO occurs in five major clinical settings: genetic, posttraumatic, neurogenic, postsurgical and as distinctive reactive lesions such as **myositis ossificans.** A genetic disorder known as **fibrodysplasia**

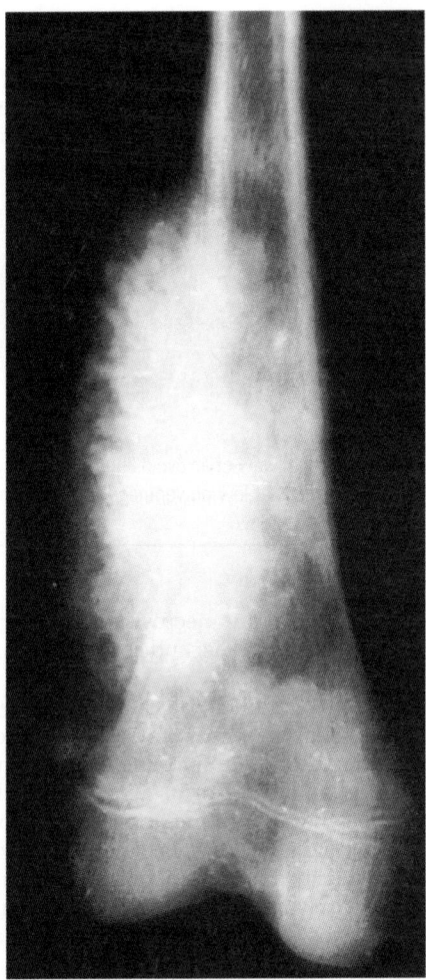

FIGURE 30-15. Reactive bone formation. A radiograph of a resected femur bearing an osteosarcoma shows a sunburst pattern of hyperdense new bone in the distal diaphysis and metaphysis. This radiodensity is due to woven bone produced by the sarcoma and the periosteal reaction of the host bone. The epiphyseal plate is represented as a transverse lucent line that separates the metaphysis from the epiphysis. The radiating radiodense bone extends beyond the periosteum into the soft tissues, obscuring the underlying bone architecture.

ossificans progressiva is characterized by massive deposits of bone around multiple joints. HO may form in hematomas or skeletal muscle after trauma. Neurogenic HO occurs in muscle and periarticular fibrous tissue at multiple sites in patients with head trauma, spinal cord injury or prolonged coma. HO can also form in periarticular soft tissue following joint surgery.

Heterotopic Calcification Is Deposition of Calcium Salts in Soft Tissues

Radiologically, heterotopic ossification and heterotopic calcification are usually distinctive. Bone formation is characterized by a spicular or trabeculated pattern, but heterotopic calcification has an irregular, splotchy, amorphous appearance. Heterotopic calcification tends to occur in necrotic soft tissue or in cartilage and on radiography is usually denser than bone. Heterotopic calcification appears in two forms:

- **Metastatic calcification** occurs when there is an increase in the calcium–phosphorus product. Thus, hypercalcemic

states or hyperphosphatemic conditions predispose normal soft tissues to calcification.
- **Dystrophic calcification** is seen in abnormal or damaged soft tissues (e.g., tumors), degenerative diseases such as arteriosclerosis and areas subjected to trauma. In addition, loss of neurologic function, as seen in quadriplegia and hemiplegia, predisposes the affected parts to soft tissue calcification.

Myositis Ossificans Is Formation of Reactive Bone in Muscle after Injury

Myositis ossificans is a distinctive form of heterotopic ossification that affects young people and, although it is entirely benign, often mimics a malignant neoplasm. It is a self-limited process and carries an excellent prognosis. Spontaneous regression has been observed. No treatment is required once the diagnosis is established.

 **ETIOLOGIC FACTORS:** The lesion typically results from blunt trauma to the muscle and soft tissues, usually of the lower limb. However, some cases occur spontaneously. Peripheral neovascularization and fibrosis at the site of damaged tissue, together with associated hemorrhage, leads in a short time to bone spicule formation. These changes are similar to those that occur at the initial hematoma in a healing fracture. Because myositis ossificans often occurs near a bone such as the femur or tibia, it may be misdiagnosed on radiography as a malignant bone-forming tumor.

 PATHOLOGY: Histologically, woven bone is formed within granulation tissue and reactive fibrous tissue (Fig. 30-16B). The center of an early lesion of myositis ossificans is characterized by proliferating fibroblasts and more peripheral osteoblastic cells that begin to form woven bone. The fibroblasts are often cytologically atypical and show abundant mitoses, a histologic appearance that also resembles a malignant tumor. *The key feature that distinguishes myositis ossificans from a neoplasm is that the bone matures peripherally, but in the center of the lesion it is immature or not formed at all.* The phenomenon of peripheral maturity with central immaturity, the **zonation effect**, clearly indicates a reactive process. In a well-developed lesion, this phenomenon may be seen radiographically (Fig. 30-16A). A neoplasm has an opposite zonation effect; the most mature tissue of the tumor is located centrally.

The growth pattern of myositis ossificans reflects the ingrowth of neovascular tissue from the periphery into the center of the damaged area. In the late stages, the lesion may contain cartilage and even lamellar bone. Thus, in a well-developed lesion, it may mimic a sesamoid bone in the soft tissue.

INFECTIONS

Osteomyelitis is Inflammation of Bone Secondary to Bacterial Infection

Any infectious agent may be responsible, but the most common pathogens are *Staphylococcus* sp. (60%–80%). Other organisms, such as *Escherichia coli*, *Neisseria gonorrhoeae*,

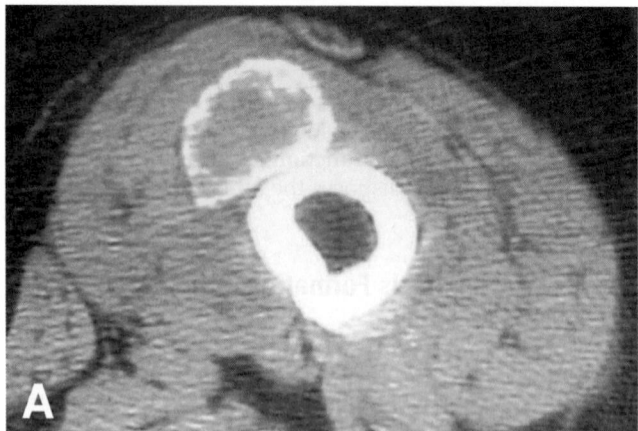
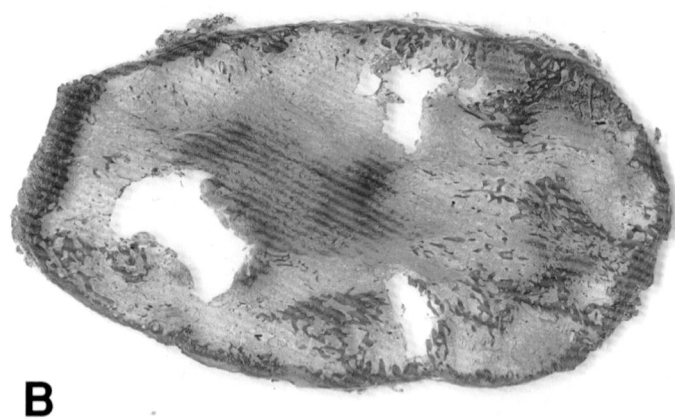

FIGURE 30-16. Myositis ossificans circumscripta. A. Computed tomography scan of the thigh shows an axial view of an ovoid, intramuscular mass adjacent to the femoral cortex with a radiolucent center and ossification that becomes denser at the periphery. **B.** The mass at low-power magnification with woven bone at the periphery and fibrous tissue in the center.

Haemophilus influenzae and *Salmonella* sp., are also seen. The organisms gain entry either via the bloodstream or by direct introduction into the bone.

Direct Penetration

Infection by direct penetration or extension of bacteria is now the most common cause of osteomyelitis in the United States. Bacterial organisms are introduced directly into bone by penetrating wounds, open fractures or surgery. Staphylococci and streptococci are still commonly incriminated, but in 25% of postoperative infections, anaerobic organisms are detected. Rarely, a gram-negative organism may seed a hip after a urologic or gastrointestinal surgical procedure or instrumentation.

Hematogenous Osteomyelitis

Infectious organisms may reach the bone from a focus elsewhere in the body through the bloodstream. Often the focus itself (e.g., a skin pustule or infected teeth and gums) poses little threat.

The most common sites affected by hematogenous osteomyelitis are the metaphyses of the long bones, such as in the knee, ankle and hip. The infection principally affects boys aged 5–15 years, but it is occasionally seen in older age groups as well. Drug addicts may develop hematogenous osteomyelitis from infected needles.

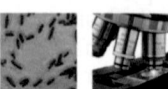 **ETIOLOGIC FACTORS AND PATHOLOGY:** Hematogenous osteomyelitis primarily affects the metaphyseal area because of the unique vascular supply in this region (Fig. 30-17). Normally, arterioles enter the calcified portion of the growth plate, form a loop, and then drain into the medullary cavity without establishing a capillary bed. This loop system permits slowing and sludging of blood flow, thus allowing bacteria enough time to penetrate blood vessel walls and establish infective foci within the marrow. If the organism is virulent and continues to proliferate, it creates increased pressure on the adjacent thin-walled vessels because they lie in a closed space, the marrow cavity. Such pressure further compromises the vascular supply in this

region and produces bone necrosis. The necrotic areas coalesce into an avascular zone, and so facilitate further bacterial proliferation.

If infection is not contained, pus and bacteria extend into the endosteal vascular channels that supply the cortex and spread throughout the Volkmann and Haversian canals of the cortex. Eventually, pus forms underneath the periosteum, shearing off the perforating arteries of the periosteum and further devitalizing the cortex. The pus flows between the periosteum and the cortex, isolating more bone from its blood supply, and may even invade the joint. Eventually, pus penetrates the periosteum and the skin to form a draining sinus (Fig. 30-17D and 30-18B). A sinus tract that extends from the cloaca (see below) to the skin may become epithelialized by epidermis that grows into the sinus tract. When this occurs, the sinus tract invariably remains open, continually draining pus, necrotic bone and bacteria.

Periosteal new bone formation and reactive bone formation in the marrow tend to wall off the infection. At the same time, osteoclastic activity resorbs bone. If the infection is virulent, this attempt to contain it is overwhelmed and it races through the bone, with virtually no bone formation but extensive bone necrosis. More commonly, pluripotential cells modulate into osteoblasts in an attempt to wall off the infection. Several lesions may develop:

- **Cloaca** is the hole formed in the bone during the formation of a draining sinus.
- **Sequestrum** is a fragment of necrotic bone that is embedded in the pus.
- **Brodie abscess** consists of reactive bone from the periosteum and the endosteum, which surrounds and contains the infection.
- **Involucrum** refers to a lesion in which periosteal new bone formation forms a sheath around the necrotic sequestrum. An involucrum that involves an entire bone may exist for several years before a patient seeks medical attention.

In very young children (1 year old or younger) afflicted with osteomyelitis, the adjacent joint is often involved (septic arthritis). This occurs because the periosteum is loosely attached to the cortex, and the metaphyseal vessels penetrate the open growth plate to join the epiphyseal vessels,

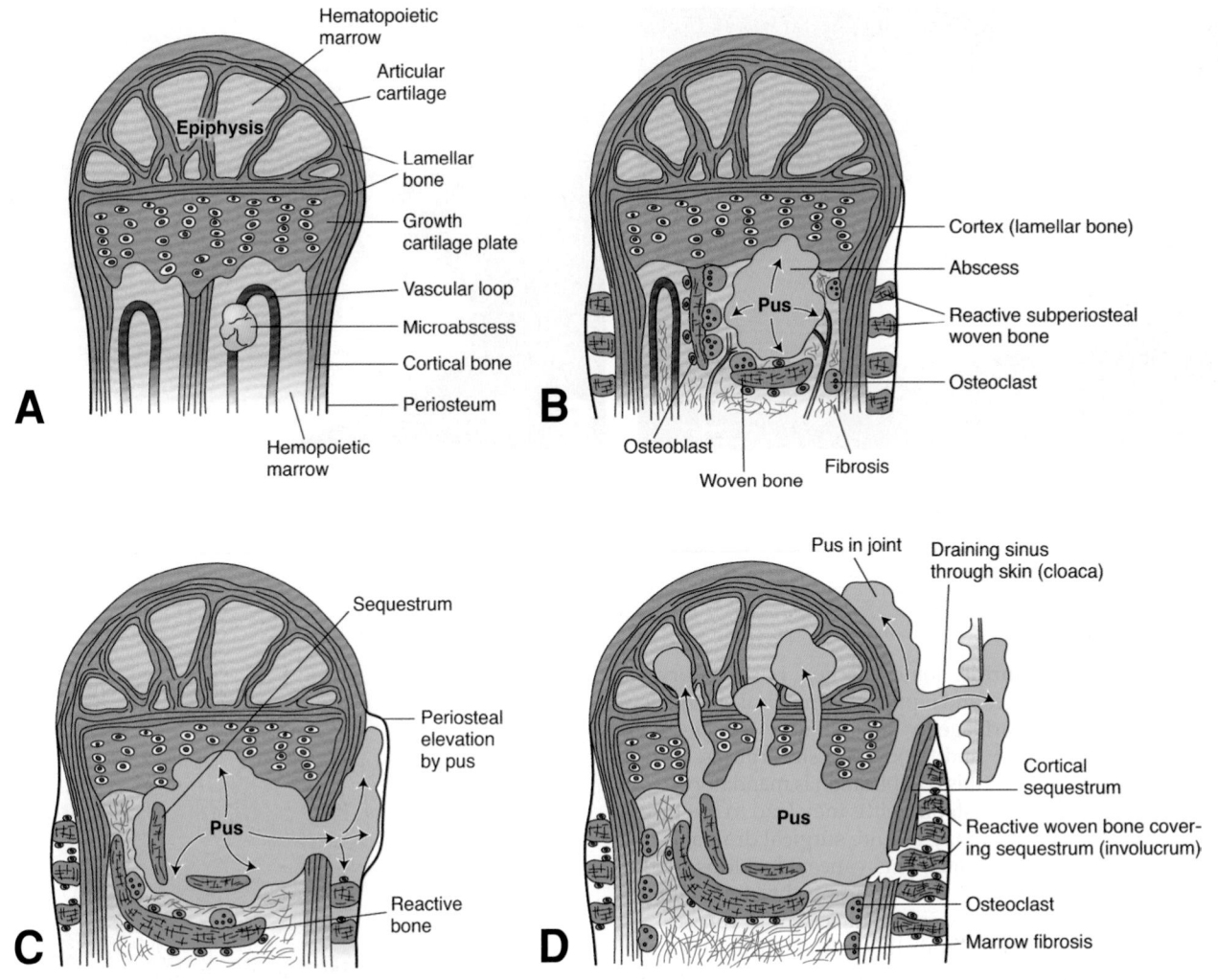

FIGURE 30-17. Pathogenesis of hematogenous osteomyelitis. A. The epiphysis, metaphysis and growth plate are normal. A small, septic microabscess is forming at the capillary loop. **B.** Expansion of the septic focus stimulates resorption of adjacent bony trabeculae. **Woven bone** begins to surround this focus. The abscess expands into the cartilage and stimulates reactive bone formation by the periosteum. **C.** The **abscess,** which continues to expand through the cortex into the subperiosteal tissue, shears off the perforating arteries that supply the cortex with blood, thereby leading to necrosis of the cortex. **D.** The extension of this process into the joint space, the epiphysis and the skin produces a **draining sinus.** The necrotic bone is called a **sequestrum.** The viable bone surrounding a sequestrum is termed the **involucrum.**

allowing the infectious organisms to reach the subchondral bone. From the age of 1 year to puberty, subperiosteal abscesses are common. Spread of infection to adjacent joints and subchondral bone regions also occur in adults.

Vertebral Osteomyelitis

In adults, osteomyelitis frequently involves vertebral bodies (Fig. 30-19). The intervertebral disk is not a barrier to bacterial osteomyelitis, particularly staphylococcal infection. Infections directly traverse the disk and travel from one vertebra to the next. Some investigators consider that the intervertebral disk is actually the primary source of infection, so-called diskitis. The disk expands with pus and is eventually destroyed as the pus bores into adjacent vertebral bodies.

Half or more of cases of vertebral osteomyelitis are caused by *Staphylococcus aureus.* Twenty percent involve *E. coli* and other enteric organisms, often originating from the urinary tract. *Salmonella* sp. are also seen in the vertebral bodies, as are *Brucella* sp. Predisposing factors are intravenous drug

abuse, upper urinary tract infections, urologic procedures and hematogenous spread of organisms from other sites. Back pain, with point tenderness over the area of infection, is associated with low-grade fever and an increased sedimentation rate.

Occasionally, a paravertebral abscess draining the bone may "point" and emerge in the groin or elsewhere. Vertebral osteomyelitis may lead to (1) vertebral collapse and paravertebral abscesses; (2) spinal epidural abscesses, with cord compression from the abscess or from displaced fragments of the infected bone; and (3) compression fractures of the vertebral body, leading to neurologic deficits.

Complications

The complications of osteomyelitis include:

■ **Septicemia:** Dissemination of organisms through the bloodstream may occur as a result of bone infection. It is unusual for osteomyelitis to result from septicemia.

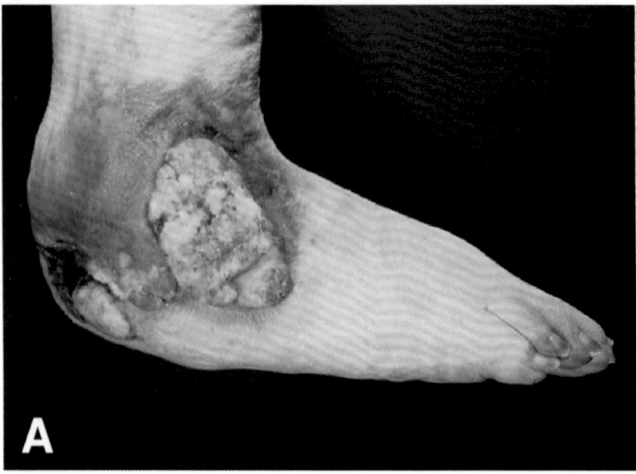
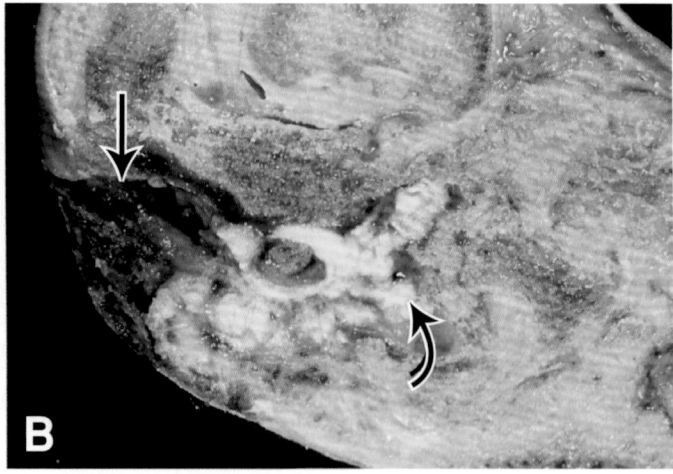

FIGURE 30-18. Chronic osteomyelitis. A. In this patient with chronic osteomyelitis, the skin overlying the infected bone is ulcerated and a draining sinus (*dark area*) is evident over the heel. **B.** After amputation of the foot, a sagittal section shows a draining sinus (*straight arrow*) that connects the infected bone with the surface of the ulcerated skin. The white tissue (*curved arrow*) is invasive squamous cell carcinoma, which arose in the skin.

- **Acute bacterial arthritis:** Joint infection is secondary to osteomyelitis at all ages and represents a medical emergency. Direct digestion of cartilage by inflammatory cells destroys the articular cartilage and produces osteoarthritis. Rapid intervention to prevent this complication is mandatory.
- **Pathologic fractures:** Osteomyelitis may lead to fractures, which heal poorly and may require surgical drainage.
- **Squamous cell carcinoma:** This cancer develops in the bone or the sinus tract of long-standing chronic osteomyelitis, often years after the initial infection. In such cases, squamous tissue arises from the epithelialization of the sinus tract and eventually undergoes malignant transformation (Fig. 30-18B).
- **Amyloidosis:** Amyloidosis used to be a common consequence of chronic osteomyelitis but is now rare in industrialized countries.
- **Chronic osteomyelitis:** Chronic osteomyelitis (Fig. 30-18) may follow acute osteomyelitis. It is difficult to treat, especially if it involves the entire bone, because necrotic bone or sequestra function as foreign bodies in avascular areas, and antibiotics do not reach the bacteria. Chronic osteomyelitis is, therefore, treated symptomatically with surgery or antibiotics for the duration of the patient's life.

CLINICAL FEATURES: Hematogenous osteomyelitis in children occurs as a sudden illness, with fever and systemic toxicity, or as a subacute illness in which local manifestations predominate. Swelling, erythema and tenderness over the involved bone are characteristic. The leukocyte count is often conspicuously increased, but it is normal in so many cases that absence of leukocytosis does not rule out the disease. Erythrocyte sedimentation rate and C-reactive protein are usually elevated but are not specific. Radiologic workup including radiography, computed tomography (CT), magnetic resonance imaging (MRI) and bone scan are very helpful. Bone biopsy is necessary for a definitive diagnosis, since it provides material for histologic examination, microbiological culture and antibiotic sensitivity.

The treatment depends on the stage of the infection. Early osteomyelitis is treated with intravenous antibiotics for 6 or more weeks. Surgery is used to drain and decompress

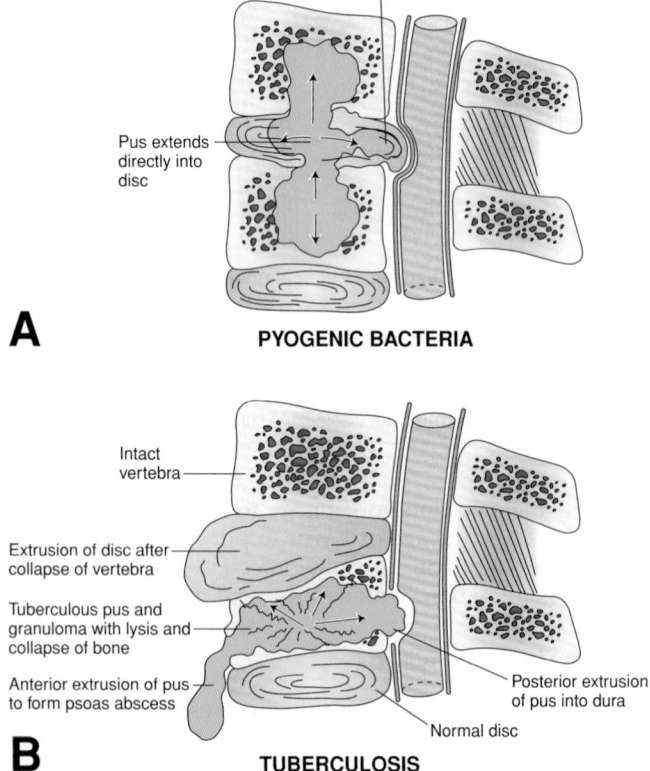

FIGURE 30-19. Osteomyelitis of the vertebral body. A. Bacterial osteomyelitis expands from one vertebral body to the next by direct invasion of the intervertebral disk and may actually push posteriorly into the spinal canal. The sequence of events in the marrow cavity is similar to that in a long bone. **B.** In **tuberculous osteomyelitis,** the bone is destroyed by resorption of bony trabeculae, which results in mechanical collapse of the vertebrae and extrusion of the intervertebral disk. Tuberculous organisms cannot penetrate the intervertebral disk directly; rather, they extend from one vertebra to the next after mechanical forces destroy and extrude the intervertebral disk.

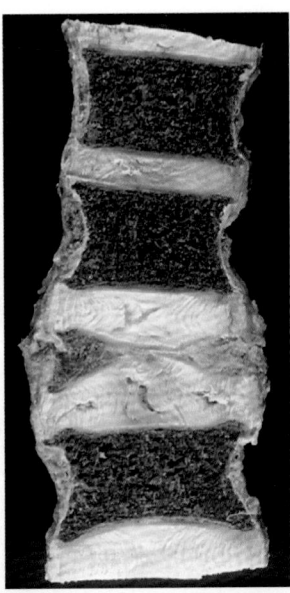

FIGURE 30-20. Tuberculous spondylitis (Pott disease). A vertebral body is almost completely replaced by tuberculous tissue. Note the preservation of the intervertebral disks.

the infection within the bone or to drain abscesses that do not respond to antibiotic therapy. In long-standing, chronic osteomyelitis, antibiotics alone are not curative and extensive surgical debridement of necrotic bone is often required.

Tuberculosis of Bone Represents Spread from a Primary Focus Elsewhere

Tuberculosis of bone usually originates in the lungs or lymph nodes (see Chapter 9). When the bone infection is caused by the rare bovine type of tubercle bacillus, the initial focus is often in the gut or tonsils. The mycobacteria spread to the bone hematogenously, and only rarely is there direct spread from the lungs or lymph nodes.

Tuberculous Spondylitis (Pott Disease)

Tuberculous spondylitis (i.e., infection of the spine) is a feared complication of childhood tuberculosis. The disease affects vertebral bodies, sparing the lamina, spines and adjacent vertebrae (Figs. 30-19B and 30-20). Thoracic vertebrae are usually affected, especially the 11th thoracic vertebra. The lumbar and cervical vertebrae are less often involved. As a result of currently available effective antibiotic treatment, Pott disease is now rare.

 PATHOLOGY: The pathology in tuberculous spondylitis is similar to tuberculosis at other sites. The granulomas first produce caseous necrosis of the bone marrow, which leads to slow resorption of bony trabeculae and, occasionally, to cystic spaces in the bone. Since there is little or no reactive bone formation, affected vertebrae tend to collapse, leading to kyphosis and scoliosis. The intervertebral disk is crushed and destroyed by the compression fracture, rather than by invasion of organisms. The typical "hunchback" of bygone days was often the victim of Pott disease.

If the infection ruptures into the soft tissue anteriorly, pus and necrotic debris drain along the spinal ligaments and form a **cold abscess** (i.e., an abscess lacking acute inflammation). A **psoas abscess** (Fig. 30-19B), which forms near

the lower lumbar vertebrae and dissects along the pelvis to emerge through the skin of the inguinal region as a draining sinus, may be the first manifestation of tuberculous spondylitis. Paraplegia results from vascular insufficiency of the spinal nerves, rather than from direct pressure.

Tuberculous Arthritis

Hematogenous spread of tuberculosis may bring organisms to the joint capsule, synovium or intracapsular portion of the bone. Tuberculosis induces granulomas in synovial tissue, which then becomes edematous and papillary and may fill the entire joint space. Massive destruction of the articular cartilage results from undermining granulation tissue in the bone. The destroyed joint is replaced by bone, an effect that produces an immovable joint **(bony ankylosis)**.

Tuberculous Osteomyelitis of the Long Bones

Infection of long bones is the least common bone manifestation of tuberculosis. This infection occurs near the joint, where it also produces arthritis. For unknown reasons, the greater trochanter of the femur is a common site for this disease.

Syphilis of Bone Is Today Rare

Syphilis causes a slowly progressive, chronic, inflammatory disease of bone, characterized by granulomas, necrosis and marked reactive bone formation. It may be acquired through sexual contact or transmitted transplacentally from mother to fetus (see Chapter 9). The bone changes in syphilis depend on the patient's age, endosteal and periosteal changes and the presence or absence of gummas.

Congenital Syphilis

 PATHOLOGY: Bone involvement in congenital syphilis may appear as early as the fifth month of gestation and is fully developed at birth. Spirochetes are ubiquitous in the epiphysis and periosteum, where they produce osteochondritis (epiphysitis) and periostitis, respectively (Fig. 30-21). In severe disease, an epiphysis may

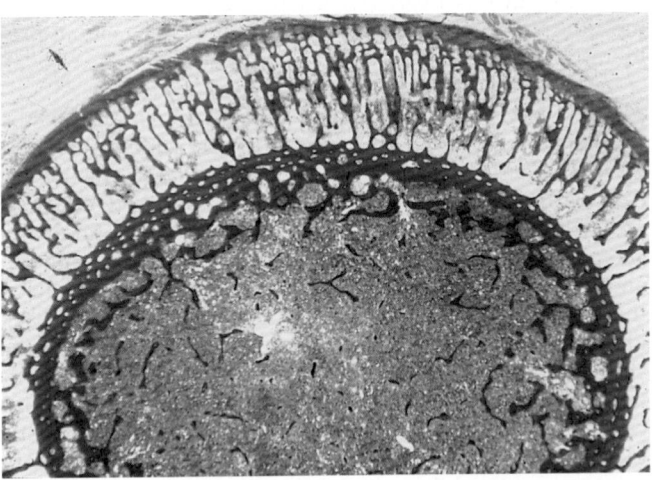

FIGURE 30-21. Congenital syphilis of bone. A cross-section of a tubular bone infected by syphilis shows marked periosteal new bone formation. The medullary cavity is filled with a lymphoplasmacytic infiltrate that replaces the normal marrow fat. The cortex is irregularly destroyed by osteoclastic resorption, a process that stimulates periosteal new bone formation.

become dislocated, leaving the child with a functionless limb (**pseudoparalysis of Parrot**).

The knee is most often affected by congenital syphilis. The growth plate is irregularly widened and displays a yellow discoloration. After the zone of calcified cartilage is destroyed, a sea of lymphocytes, plasma cells and spirochetes fills the marrow spaces. Because the periosteum is stimulated to produce reactive new bone, the thickness of the cortex may actually be doubled. The inflammatory infiltrate permeates the cortex through the Volkmann and Haversian canals and settles in the elevated periosteum. Ultimately, as the affected bones grow, they become short and deformed.

Acquired Syphilis

Acquired syphilis in adults produces lesions of the bone early in the tertiary stage, 2–5 years after inoculation of the organisms. Periostitis is predominant because the growth plates have already closed. The bones most commonly affected are the tibia, nose, palate and skull. Tibial lesions are marked by periostitis, with deposition of new bone on the medial and anterior aspects of the shaft, which leads to the **saber shin** deformity. The skull thickness also increases because of periosteal stimulation.

Gumma formation is seen most often in tertiary syphilis. Bone adjacent to gummas is slowly replaced by fibrous marrow. Ultimately, perforations occur through the cortex. The markedly irregular, thickened periosteal surfaces, which are perforated by pits and serpiginous ulcerations, are characteristic of syphilis. Lysis and collapse of nasal and palatal bones produce the classic **saddle nose**—perforation, destruction and collapse of the nasal septum (see Chapter 29).

LANGERHANS CELL HISTIOCYTOSIS

Langerhans cell histiocytosis (LCH) is a generic term (previously referred to as **histiocytosis X**) for three entities characterized by proliferation of Langerhans cells in various tissues: (1) **eosinophilic granuloma,** a localized form; (2) **Hand-Schüller-Christian disease,** a disseminated variant; and (3) **Letterer-Siwe disease,** a fulminant and often fatal generalized disease (see Chapter 26). Studies of X-chromosome inactivation have shown that LCH is a clonal proliferative disease.

 PATHOLOGY: The histologic appearance of the bones in all three variants of LCH is identical and is characterized by collections of large, histiocytic cells with pale, eosinophilic cytoplasm and convoluted or grooved nuclei (see Figs. 12-68 and 30-76). By immunohistochemistry, the histiocytic cells stain with CD1a, Langerin and S-100 protein. By electron microscopy these cells have the typical racquet-shaped, tubular structures, "Birbeck granules," which are seen in normal Langerhans cells of the skin (see Fig. 30-76, inset). There are many eosinophils throughout these lesions, occasionally forming collections called "eosinophilic abscesses." Multinucleated **osteoclastic** giant cells are often observed, as are chronic inflammatory cells and neutrophils.

The lesions of LCH may occur anywhere in the body, including bones, skin, brain, lungs, lymph nodes, liver and spleen. Radiologic findings in the bones in all three diseases are identical. The lesions may occur in the metaphysis or

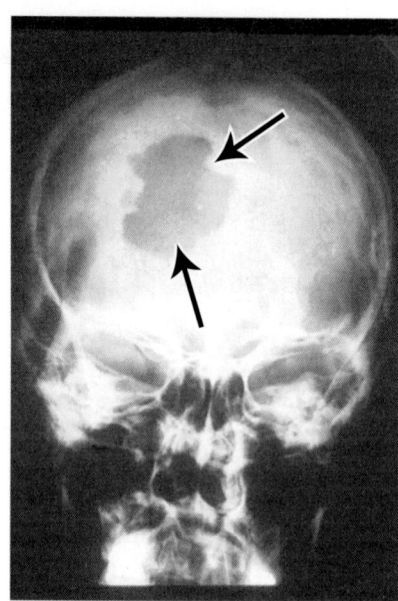

FIGURE 30-22. Eosinophilic granuloma. A radiograph of the skull shows a large, lytic lesion (*arrows*).

diaphysis of long bones, or in a flat bone, especially in the skull (Fig. 30-22). They are punched-out lytic defects, with virtually no reactive bone. Such lesions may precipitate fractures and periosteal callus formation.

Eosinophilic Granuloma Is a Self-Limited Disease

Eosinophilic granuloma, in either its solitary or multiple varieties, accounts for 70% of all cases of LCH. It is usually seen in the first two decades of life but occasionally occurs in older individuals. There are typically one or two lytic areas in bones of the axial or appendicular skeleton (Fig. 30-22) or the vertebrae. These lesions may cause mild pain or may be incidental findings on routine chest radiographs. Foci of disease in the lower thoracic or upper lumbar vertebrae may lead to collapse and pathologic fractures. Eventual recovery is the rule.

Hand-Schüller-Christian Disease Is a Multiorgan Disease of Childhood

Hand-Schüller-Christian disease occurs in children 2–5 years old and represents some 20% of all cases of LCH. The lesions are more widespread than in eosinophilic granuloma. Radiolucent bony lesions characterize the disorder, most frequently in the calvaria, ribs, pelvis and scapulae. Involvement of the jaw bone results in loss of teeth, evident radiologically as "floating teeth." Infiltration of the retroorbital space causes exophthalmos; infiltration of the hypothalamic stalk by Langerhans cells brings about diabetes insipidus. One fifth of patients have lymphadenopathy and lung infiltrates.

Crusty, red, weepy skin lesions occur at the hairline and on the extensor surfaces of the extremities, the abdomen and occasionally the soles of the feet. Deafness results from involvement of the external auditory canal and mastoid air cells. One third of affected patients have disease in the liver and spleen, and 40% have bone lesions, half of which involve the skull. Thus, the classic triad of Hand-Schüller-Christian disease, namely, **(1) radiolucent lesions of the skull, (2) diabetes insipidus and (3) exophthalmos,** occurs in only one third of patients.

Letterer-Siwe Disease Is an Aggressive, Potentially Fatal Disease of Infants

Letterer-Siwe disease accounts for 10% of cases of LCH. Affected children fail to thrive and become cachectic. Multiple organ involvement culminates in massive hepatosplenomegaly, lymphadenopathy, anemia, leukopenia and thrombocytopenia. Widely scattered, seborrheic skin lesions, which are often hemorrhagic, are usual. Bone lesions are not prominent initially, but progressive marrow replacement and pulmonary infiltration occasionally cause death.

 CLINICAL FEATURES: Eosinophilic granuloma is a self-limited disease, and most lesions disappear if left alone. A bone lesion may have to be curetted and packed with bone chips. Sometimes biopsy itself is enough to stimulate repair of the lytic lesion. A collapsed vertebra may actually reconstitute itself over time. Hand-Schüller-Christian disease may require radiation therapy for some bone and retro-orbital lesions. Diabetes insipidus seems to be irreversible, despite irradiation of the pituitary region. Drugs such as corticosteroids, cyclophosphamide and tumoricidal agents may also be used to treat Hand-Schüller-Christian disease. Aggressive chemotherapy for Letterer-Siwe disease seems to improve the prognosis.

Metabolic Bone Diseases

Metabolic bone diseases are defined as disorders of metabolism that result in secondary structural effects on the skeleton, including diminished bone mass due to decreased synthesis or increased destruction, reduced bone mineralization or both. Because metabolic bone diseases are systemic, a biopsy of any bone should reveal the abnormality, even though severity may differ in various parts of the skeleton (Fig. 30-23).

OSTEOPOROSIS

Osteoporosis is a metabolic bone disease in which normally mineralized bone is decreased in mass to the point that it no longer provides adequate mechanical support. Although osteoporosis reflects a number of causes, it is always characterized by loss of skeletal mass. Remaining bone has a normal ratio of mineralized to nonmineralized (i.e., osteoid) matrix. Bone loss and eventually fractures are the hallmarks of osteoporosis, regardless of the underlying causes (Fig. 30-24). The etiology for bone loss is diverse but includes menopause, smoking, vitamin D deficiency, low body mass index, hypogonadism, a sedentary lifestyle and glucocorticoid therapy.

 **EPIDEMIOLOGY:** Osteoporosis and its complications are huge public health problems that are expected to expand as life expectancy increases.

Bone mass normally peaks between the ages of 25 and 35 and begins to decline in the fifth or sixth decade. Bone loss with age occurs in all races, but because of higher peak bone mass, blacks are less prone to osteoporosis than are Asians and whites. Bone loss during normal aging in women has been divided into two phases: menopause and aging. The latter affects men as well as women. At a certain point, the loss of bone suffices to justify the label **osteoporosis** and renders weight-bearing bones susceptible to fractures. The most common fractures occur in the neck and intertrochanteric region of the femur (**hip fracture;** Fig. 30-24), vertebral bodies and distal radius (**Colles fracture**). In whites in the United States, 15% of people have had a hip fracture by the age of 80 years and 25% by age 90. Women have twice the risk of hip fracture as men, although among blacks and some Asian populations, the incidence is equal among the sexes. Compared with other osteoporotic fractures, hip fractures incur the greatest morbidity, mortality (up to 20% within a year) and direct medical costs. The female predominance of 8:1 is particularly striking for vertebral fractures. A subset of women in the early postmenopausal years is at particular risk of vertebral fractures, which are rare in middle-aged men. The propensity of men to sustain hip fractures as opposed to vertebral ones also reflects factors other than bone mass, such as loss of proprioception.

  **ETIOLOGIC FACTORS AND MOLECULAR PATHOGENESIS:** *Regardless of the cause of osteoporosis, it always reflects enhanced bone resorption relative to formation.* Thus, this family of diseases should be viewed in the context of the remodeling cycle. Bone resorption and bone formation exist simultaneously. All osteoblasts and osteoclasts belong to a unique temporary structure, known as the **basic multicellular unit** (BMU or **bone-remodeling unit**). The BMU is responsible for bone remodeling throughout life. Individuals younger than 35 or 40 years completely replace bone resorbed during the remodeling cycle. With age, less bone is replaced in resorption bays than is removed, leading to a small deficit at each remodeling site. Given the thousands of remodeling sites in the skeleton, net bone loss, even in a short time, can be substantial.

Osteoporosis is classified as either primary or secondary. **Primary osteoporosis,** by far the more common variety, is of uncertain origin and occurs principally in postmenopausal women (type 1) and elderly people of both sexes (type 2). **Secondary osteoporosis** is a disorder associated with a defined cause, including a variety of endocrine and genetic abnormalities.

Type 1 primary osteoporosis is due to an absolute increase in osteoclast activity. Since osteoclasts initiate bone remodeling, the number of remodeling sites increases in this state of enhanced osteoclast formation, a phenomenon known as **increased activation frequency.**

The increase in osteoclasts in the early postmenopausal skeleton is a direct result of estrogen withdrawal. The effects of lack of estrogen are not, however, targeted directly to the osteoclast, but rather to cells derived from marrow stroma, which secrete cytokines that recruit osteoclasts. These cytokines, which are believed to be estrogen sensitive, include IL-1 and IL-6, TNF and M-CSF.

Type 2 primary osteoporosis, also called **senile osteoporosis,** has a more complex pathogenesis than type 1. Type 2 osteoporosis generally appears after age 70 and reflects decreased

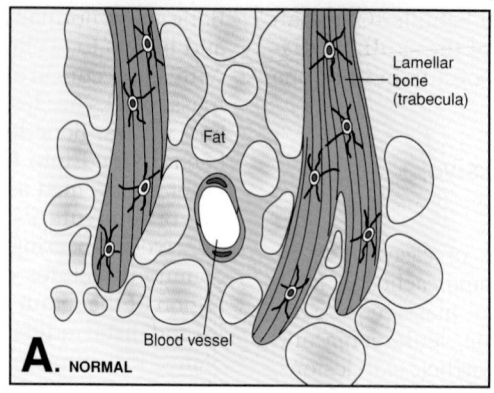

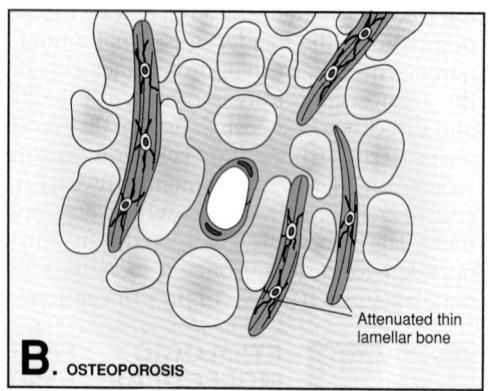

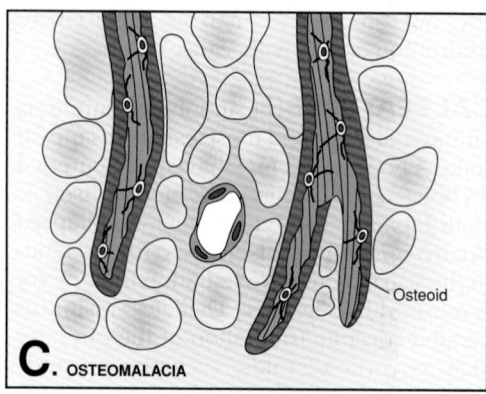

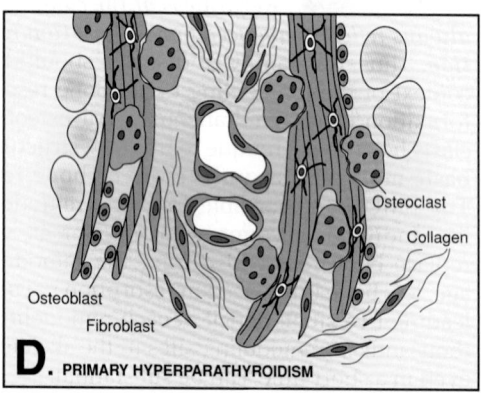

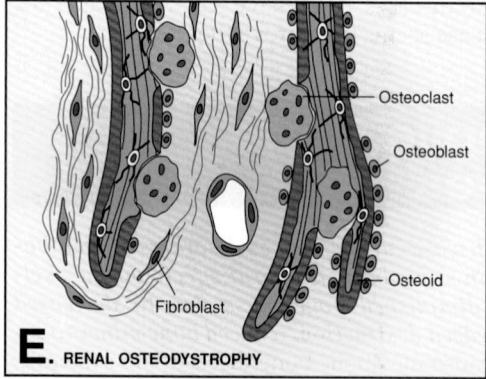

FIGURE 30-23. Metabolic bone diseases. A. Normal trabecular bone and fatty marrow. The trabecular bone is lamellar and contains evenly distributed osteocytes. **B. Osteoporosis.** The lamellar bone trabeculae are discontinuous and thin. **C. Osteomalacia.** The lamellar bone trabeculae have abnormal amounts of nonmineralized bone (osteoid). These osteoid seams are thickened and cover a larger than normal area of the trabecular bone surface. **D. Primary hyperparathyroidism.** The lamellar bone trabeculae are actively resorbed by numerous osteoclasts that bore into each trabecula. The appearance of osteoclasts dissecting into the trabeculae, a process termed **dissecting osteitis,** is diagnostic of hyperparathyroidism. Osteoblastic activity also is pronounced. The marrow is replaced by fibrous tissue adjacent to the trabeculae. **E. Renal osteodystrophy.** The morphologic appearance is similar to that of primary hyperparathyroidism, except that prominent osteoid covers the trabeculae. Osteoclasts do not resorb unmineralized bone, and wherever an osteoid seam is lacking, osteoclasts bore into the trabeculae. Osteoblastic activity is also prominent.

osteoblast function. Thus, although osteoclast activity is no longer increased, the number of osteoblasts and amount of bone produced per cell are insufficient to replace bone removed in the resorptive phase of the remodeling cycle.

Primary Osteoporosis Is Caused by a Number of Factors

Primary osteoporosis has been linked to a number of factors that influence peak bone mass and the rate of bone loss:

- **Genetic factors:** Environmental factors and an individual's genotype both play a role in determining peak bone mass and risk of osteoporosis. The development of clinically significant osteoporosis is related, in largest part, to the maximal amount of bone in a given person, referred to as the **peak bone mass.** In general, peak bone mass is greater in men than in women and in blacks than in whites or Asians. There is a higher concordance of peak bone mass in monozygotic than in dizygotic twins. Women of reproductive age whose mothers have postmenopausal

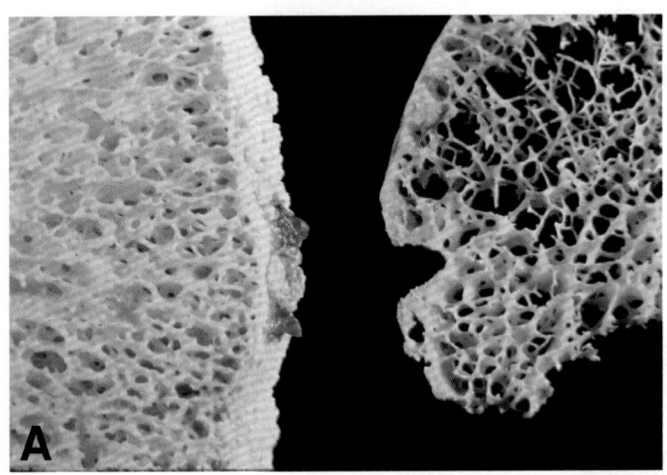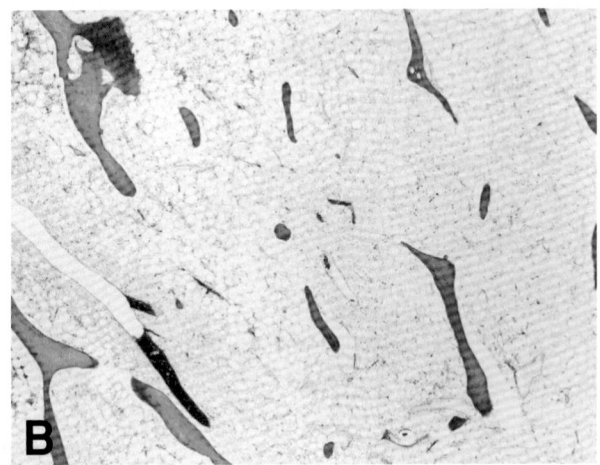

FIGURE 30-24. Osteoporosis. A. Femoral head of an 82-year-old female with osteoporosis and a femoral neck fracture (*right*) compared with a normal control cut to the same thickness (*left*). **B.** Microscopically, there is reduction in the size and thickness of bone trabeculae and loss of connectivity.

osteoporosis exhibit a lower bone mineral density (BMD) than do women in the general population. BMD is the most commonly used index for defining and studying osteoporosis. Genetic factors are thought to play an important role in regulating BMD. In fact, genetic variations explain as much as 70% of the variance in BMD. Sequence variance in the vitamin D receptor (VDR), *Col1A1* collagen gene, estrogen receptor-α (ESR1), IL-6 and low-density lipoprotein (LDL) receptor–related protein-5 (LRP5) are significantly associated with differences in BMD. Furthermore, VDR and IL-6 interact with environmental and hormonal factors (e.g., calcium intake, estrogen) to modulate BMD.

■ **Calcium intake:** The average calcium intake of postmenopausal women in the United States is below the recommended value of 800 mg/day. However, whether this apparent shortfall contributes to development of osteoporosis is controversial, in view of a number of studies to the contrary. Nevertheless, it has been recommended that both premenopausal and postmenopausal women increase the intake of calcium and vitamin D.

■ **Calcium absorption and vitamin D:** Calcium absorption by the intestine decreases with age. Because calcium absorption is largely under the control of vitamin D, attention has been directed to the role of this steroid hormone in osteoporosis. Compared with controls, people with osteoporosis have lower circulating levels of 1,25-dihydroxyvitamin D [1,25(OH)$_2$D], the active form of vitamin D that promotes calcium absorption in the intestine. This decrease has been attributed to age-related decreases in 1α-hydroxylase activity in the kidney, the enzyme that catalyzes formation of 1,25(OH)$_2$D. The lower 1α-hydroxylase activity has been attributed to diminished stimulation of the enzyme by PTH, as well as an age-related decrease in responses of renal tubules to PTH. Interestingly, giving estrogens to postmenopausal women with osteoporosis increases both circulating 1,25(OH)$_2$D and calcium absorption. It has been suggested that decreased 1α-hydroxylase activity in the kidney may stimulate PTH secretion, and so contribute to bone resorption.

■ **Exercise:** Physical activity is necessary to maintain bone mass, and athletes often have increased bone mass. By contrast, immobilization of a bone (e.g., prolonged bed rest, application of a cast) elicits accelerated bone loss.

The weightlessness of space flight results in severe bone loss (33% of trabecular bone mass in 25 weeks). Yet vigorous exercise in this setting does not seem to increase bone mass substantially or prevent osteoporosis.

■ **Environmental factors:** Cigarette smoking in women has been correlated with an increased incidence of osteoporosis. It is possible that the decreased level of active estrogens produced by smoking is responsible for this effect.

In summary, the two major determinants of primary osteoporosis are estrogen deficiency in postmenopausal women and the aging process in both sexes. The possible mechanisms for these effects are summarized in Fig. 30-25.

 PATHOLOGY: *The ratio of osteoid to mineralized bone is normal in individuals with osteoporosis.* Because of the abundance of cancellous bone in the spine, osteoporotic changes are generally most conspicuous there. In vertebral body fractures caused by osteoporosis, the vertebra is deformed, with anterior wedging and collapse. If the vertebral body is not fractured, there is a general outline of both endplates, with a virtual absence of cancellous bone.

Osteoporosis is characterized histologically by decreased thickness of the cortex and reduction in the number and size of trabeculae of the coarse cancellous bone (Fig. 30-24). Although senile osteoporosis tends to feature reduced trabecular thickness, postmenopausal osteoporosis exhibits disrupted connections between trabeculae. The loss of trabecular connectivity, which is attended by diminished biomechanical strength and ultimately provokes fracture, is due to perforation of trabeculae by resorbing osteoclasts in remodeling sites. In histologic sections, the loss of connectivity results in the appearance of "isolated" islands of bone (Figs. 30-23B and 30-24B).

 CLINICAL FEATURES: Postmenopausal osteoporosis is usually recognizable within 10 years after onset of the menopause; senile osteoporosis generally becomes symptomatic after age 70 years. Until recently, most patients were unaware of their disease until they had a fracture of a vertebra, hip or other bone. However, the use of sensitive screening techniques permits early

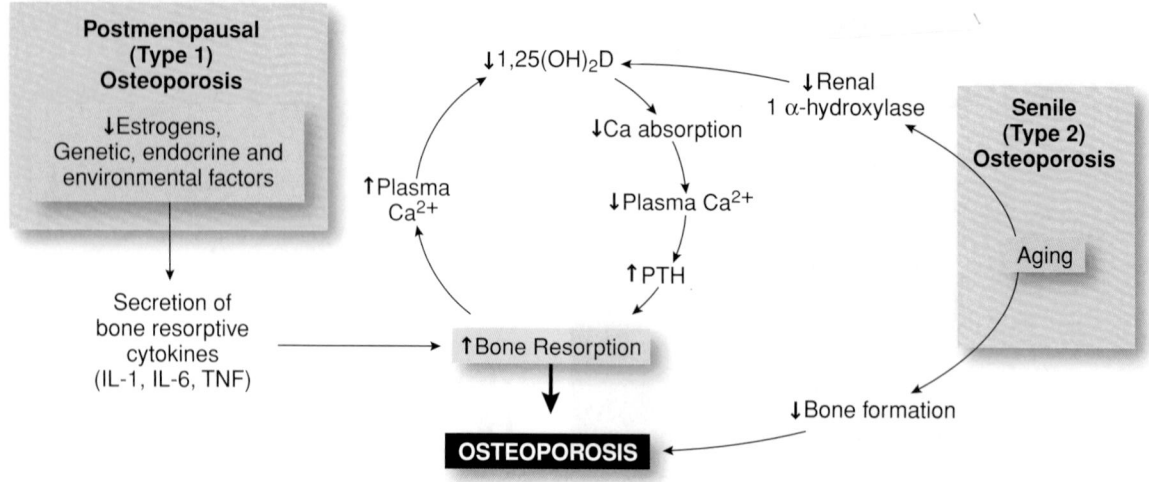

FIGURE 30-25. Pathogenesis of primary osteoporosis. Ca^{2+} = calcium; IL = interleukin; PTH = parathyroid hormone; TNF = tumor necrosis factor.

diagnosis. Vertebral body compression fractures often occur after trivial trauma or may even follow lifting a heavy object. With each compression fracture, the patient becomes shorter and develops kyphosis **(dowager's hump)**. Serum calcium and phosphorus levels remain normal.

Estrogen therapy is an effective yet controversial means of preventing postmenopausal osteoporosis. Because hormone treatment carries with it increased risks of breast and endometrial cancers, other bone-specific antiosteoporotic drugs have been developed. **Bisphosphonates** are currently the most popular therapeutic agents used. All successful antiosteoporotic agents thus far developed block or slow the rate of bone resorption but do not stimulate bone formation. Thus, the drugs may prevent disease progression but cannot cure a patient who already has osteoporosis. Dietary calcium supplementation in elderly patients reduces the risk of osteoporotic fractures by half.

Secondary Osteoporosis Reflects Extraosseous Metabolic Disorders

  **ETIOLOGIC FACTORS AND MOLE-CULAR PATHOGENESIS:** Causes of secondary osteoporosis include adverse effects of drug therapy, endocrine abnormalities, eating disorders, immobilization, marrow-related conditions, diseases of the gastrointestinal or biliary tracts, renal insufficiency and cancer.

- **Endocrine conditions:** The most common form of secondary osteoporosis is iatrogenic and results from corticosteroid administration. Bone loss may also result from an excess of endogenous glucocorticoids, as in Cushing disease (see Chapter 27). Corticosteroids inhibit osteoblastic activity, thus reducing bone formation. They also impair vitamin D–dependent intestinal calcium absorption, an effect that leads to increased secretion of PTH and enhanced bone resorption.

  Estrogen is a key hormone for maintaining bone mass, and its deficiency is the major cause of age-related bone loss in both sexes; estrogen deficiency or a low level of bioavailable estrogen decreases bone mass in elderly males. Its role in bone metabolism is focused on the role of proinflammatory cytokines: IL-1, IL-6, TNF-α, RANKL, granulocyte-macrophage colony-stimulating factor (GM-CSF), M-CSF and prostaglandin E_2 (PGE_2). It is thought that these cytokines act upon both osteoclasts and osteoblasts via mediation by estrogen receptors.

- **Hyperparathyroidism** induces osteoclast recruitment and increased osteoclastic activity, resulting in secondary osteoporosis (see below). In both sexes, hyperparathyroidism secondary to calcium malabsorption increases remodeling, worsening the cortical thinning and porosity and predisposing to hip fractures.

- **Hyperthyroidism** increases osteoclastic activity and causes accelerated turnover of bone. Although thyrotoxicosis is associated with some secondary osteoporosis, bone loss is limited.

- **Hypogonadism** in both men and women is accompanied by osteoporosis. In women with primary gonadal failure (Turner syndrome) or with secondary amenorrhea as a result of pituitary disease, estrogen deficiency is likely the cause. Hypogonadal men (e.g., Klinefelter syndrome, hemochromatosis) are at risk of osteoporosis because of a deficiency of anabolic androgens. Similarly, hypogonadism contributes to bone loss in 25% of elderly males. There is evidence of decreased bone density in androgen deprivation therapy for prostatic cancer.

- **Hematologic malignancies:** A variety of hematologic cancers, particularly multiple myeloma, are accompanied by significant bone loss. The malignant plasma cells of multiple myeloma secrete osteoclast-activating factor, which is presumably responsible for secondary osteoporosis. Some leukemias and lymphomas are also associated with osteoporosis. Even in the absence of skeletal metastases, some neoplasms (e.g., squamous cell carcinoma of lung) are associated with severe hypercalcemia due to bone resorption. Osteoclastic activity is enhanced in these patients, owing to secretion of PTH-related protein by the tumor (paraneoplastic syndrome).

- **Malabsorption:** Gastrointestinal and hepatic diseases that cause malabsorption often contribute to osteoporosis, probably because of impaired absorption of calcium, phosphate and vitamin D.

- **Alcoholism:** Chronic alcohol abuse also has been linked to development of osteoporosis. Alcohol is a direct inhibitor of osteoblasts and may also inhibit calcium absorption.

OSTEOMALACIA AND RICKETS

Osteomalacia (soft bones) *is a disorder of adults characterized by inadequate mineralization of newly formed bone matrix.* **Rickets** *refers to a similar disorder in children, in whom the growth plates (physes) are open.* Thus, children with rickets manifest defective mineralization not only of bone (osteomalacia) but also of the cartilaginous matrix of the growth plate. Diverse conditions associated with osteomalacia and rickets include abnormalities in vitamin D metabolism, phosphate deficiency states and defects in the mineralization process itself.

Vitamin D Metabolism Influences Bone Mineralization

MOLECULAR PATHOGENESIS: Vitamin D is ingested in food or synthesized in the skin from 7-dehydrocholesterol under the influence of ultraviolet light (Fig. 30-26). The vitamin is first hydroxylated in the liver to form its major circulating metabolite, 25-hydroxyvitamin D, then hydroxylated again in proximal renal tubules to produce the active hormone $1,25(OH)_2D$. Exposure to sunlight provides sufficient vitamin D for bone growth and mineralization, even if there is an inadequate dietary source.

Receptors for $1,25(OH)_2D$ are present not only in classic targets, such as intestine, bone and kidney, but also in many other cell types. This hormone is a general inducer of differentiation, for example, influencing maturation of hematopoietic and dermal cells, as well as many cancers. In the intestine, $1,25(OH)_2D$ stimulates calcium and phosphate absorption. It is also essential for osteoclast maturation. Regardless of mechanism, $1,25(OH)_2D$, in concert with PTH, maintains blood calcium and phosphate at levels that are required for proper mineralization of bone. *The key determinant of the formation of $1,25(OH)_2D$ is blood calcium concentration.* Decreases in blood calcium stimulate release of PTH, which augments renal synthesis of $1,25(OH)_2D$.

Hypovitaminosis D can result from (1) inadequate exposure to sunlight, (2) deficient dietary intake or (3) defective intestinal absorption. There are also hereditary and acquired disorders of vitamin D metabolism.

Dietary Deficiency of Vitamin D and Inadequate Exposure to Sunlight Cause Rickets

Rickets plagued some 85% of children in the industrial cities of the United States and Europe from the 17th century through the 19th century. These children had insufficient sun exposure, and their dietary intake of vitamin D was inadequate to avert hypovitaminosis D. Use of vitamin D–rich cod liver oil and later fortification of milk and other foods with vitamin D effectively ended widespread rickets in Western countries. However, nutritional vitamin D deficiency remains a problem elsewhere in the world, in the neglected elderly and in food faddists.

Intestinal Malabsorption Decreases the Availability of Vitamin D

In industrialized countries, diseases associated with intestinal malabsorption cause osteomalacia more often than does poor nutrition. *Intrinsic diseases of the small intestine, cholestatic disorders of the liver, biliary obstruction and chronic pancreatic insufficiency are the most frequent causes of osteomalacia in the United States.*

Malabsorption of vitamin D and calcium complicates a number of small-intestinal diseases, including celiac disease, Crohn disease, scleroderma and the postsurgical blind-loop syndrome. In obstructive jaundice, the lack of bile salts in the intestine impairs absorption of lipids and lipid-soluble substances, among which is fat-soluble vitamin D. Furthermore, hydroxylation of vitamin D is reduced in cases of severe liver damage. Oddly, biliary cirrhosis, a disease characterized by intestinal malabsorption and vitamin D deficiency, gives rise to osteoporosis rather than osteomalacia. Thus, vitamin D is essential not only for mineralization but also for the synthesis of bone collagen.

Disorders of Vitamin D Metabolism Are Inherited or Acquired

Vitamin D metabolism can be disturbed either by defective 1α-hydroxylation of vitamin D in the kidney or by

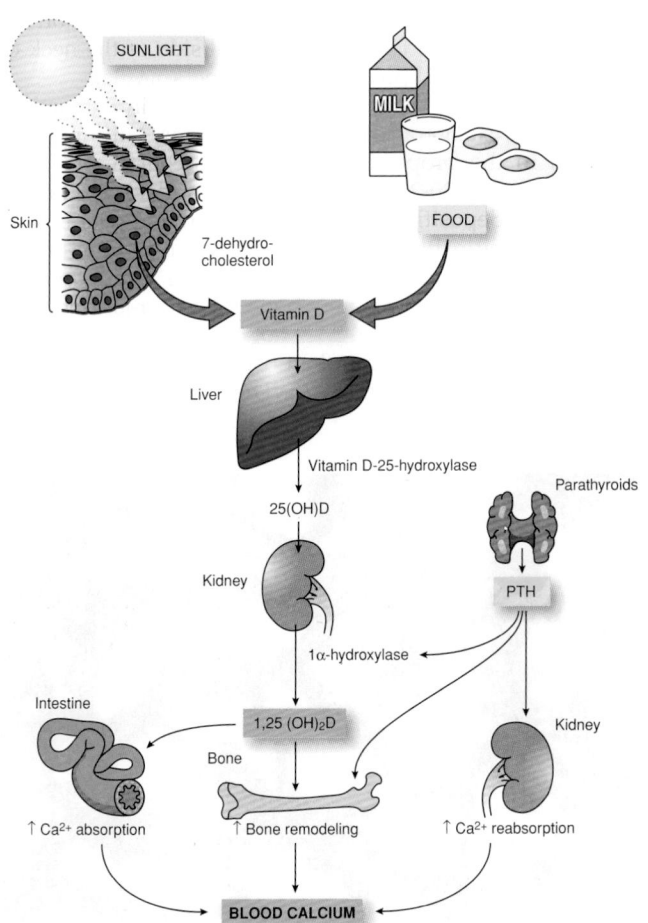

FIGURE 30-26. Metabolism of vitamin D and the regulation of blood calcium.

insensitivity of the target organ to 1,25(OH)$_2$D. Two autosomal recessive diseases associated with rickets are together known as **vitamin D–dependent rickets**.

- **Vitamin D–dependent rickets type I** results from an inherited deficiency of renal 1α-hydroxylase activity. The clinical and biochemical changes of rickets appear during the first year of life, and these children exhibit hypocalcemia, hypophosphatemia and high levels of serum PTH and alkaline phosphatase. The disease is controlled by the administration of 1,25(OH)$_2$D.
- **Vitamin D–dependent rickets type II** involves inherited mutations of the vitamin D receptor, so that end organs are insensitive to 1,25(OH)$_2$D. The disease usually manifests early in life but may appear at any time up to adolescence. Serum concentrations of 1,25(OH)$_2$D are very high. Patients do not respond to 1,25(OH)$_2$D but are helped by repeated intravenous administration of calcium.
- **Acquired alterations in vitamin D metabolism** include defective renal 1α-hydroxylation and end-organ insensitivity. Some of the causes of impaired α-hydroxylation are hypoparathyroidism, tumor-induced osteomalacia, chronic renal diseases and osteomalacia of old age. Osteomalacia occasionally complicates the treatment of epilepsy with anticonvulsant drugs, particularly phenobarbital and phenytoin. It is believed that these drugs block the action of 1,25(OH)$_2$D on target organs.

Renal Disorders of Phosphate Metabolism Interfere with Vitamin D Metabolism

Both rickets and osteomalacia may result from impaired reabsorption of phosphate by the proximal renal tubules, with resulting hypophosphatemia.

MOLECULAR PATHOGENESIS:

X-LINKED HYPOPHOSPHATEMIA: This condition, also known as **vitamin D–resistant rickets** or **phosphate diabetes,** is the most common type of hereditary rickets and is inherited as a dominant trait. Mutations in the *PHEX* (phosphate-regulating) gene on the X chromosome (Xp22) impair transport of phosphate across the luminal membrane of proximal renal tubular cells. The gene product of *PHEX* is a protease that inactivates fibroblast growth factor-23 (FGF23). Increased levels of FGF23 produced renal phosphate wasting. Although renal phosphate wasting is central to the disease, osteoblast function is also impaired. In boys, florid rickets appears during childhood, but girls often suffer only hypophosphatemia. Treatment consists of lifelong administration of phosphate and 1,25(OH)$_2$D. Microscopically, the bones of patients with X-linked hypophosphatemia show severe osteomalacia and wide osteoid seams. They also exhibit characteristic hypomineralized areas surrounding osteocytes, known as **halos**. The presence of these structures indicates that osteocytes are responsible for the terminal mineralization of bone.

FANCONI SYNDROMES: These inborn errors of metabolism are characterized by renal wastage of phosphate, glucose, bicarbonate and amino acids. They are all characterized by renal tubular acidosis and lead to rickets and osteomalacia. Fanconi syndromes include Wilson disease, tyrosinemia, galactosemia, glycogen storage disease and cystinosis. Renal tubular damage that leads to phosphate wastage may also

be acquired, as in lead or mercury intoxication, amyloidosis and Bence-Jones proteinuria.

TUMOR-ASSOCIATED OSTEOMALACIA: This disorder is a phosphate-wasting syndrome that is associated with predominantly benign and occasionally malignant tumors of soft tissue and bone. The typical laboratory features are hypophosphatemia, hyperphosphaturia, low serum concentrations of 1,25-(OH)$_2$D and elevated serum alkaline phosphatase. Oncogenic osteomalacia mimics the clinical phenotype of X-linked hypophosphatemia and autosomal dominant hypophosphatemia. The paraneoplastic phosphaturic factors secreted by the tumor, known as **phosphatonins,** cause renal tubular phosphate wasting and prevent tubular conversion of 25-hydroxyvitamin D into 1,25(OH)$_2$D. Phosphatonins thus appear to have the same effect as inherited mutations of the *PHEX* gene seen in X-linked hypophosphatemia. Removal of the primary tumor is often curative. FGF23 has been implicated as a phosphatonin. Overproduction of FGF23 by tumors results in renal phosphate wasting and tumor-associated osteomalacia.

PATHOLOGY:

OSTEOMALACIA: Osteomalacia, like osteoporosis, causes an osteopenic radiologic pattern. The only findings may be vertebral compression fractures and decreased bone thickness, as in osteoporosis. However, some specific findings may be seen in osteomalacia, including the pseudofractures of **Milkman-Looser syndrome.** These are radiolucent transverse defects that are most common on the concave side of a long bone, medial side of the neck of the femur, ischial and pubic rami, ribs and scapula.

Microscopically, defective mineralization in osteomalacia results in **exaggeration of osteoid seams,** both in thickness and in the proportion of trabecular surface covered (Figs. 30-23 and 30-27). Osteoid seams reflect a time lag between the deposition of collagen and the appearance of the calcium salt. Although adults add 1 μm of new matrix to the surfaces of bone every day, it requires approximately 10 days to mineralize this new bone. The normal thickness of osteoid seams, therefore, does not exceed 12 μm. Areas of pseudofracture display abundant osteoid and may function as stress points for true fractures. These areas do not evoke

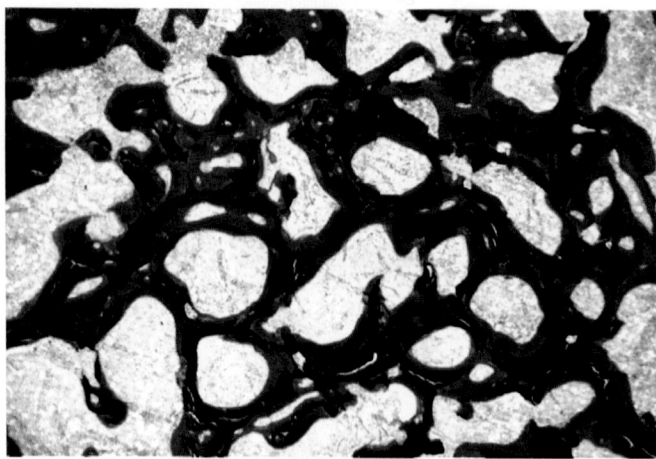

FIGURE 30-27. Osteomalacia. The surfaces of the bony trabeculae (*black*) are covered by a thicker than normal layer of osteoid (*red*) with the von Kossa stain, which colors calcified tissue black.

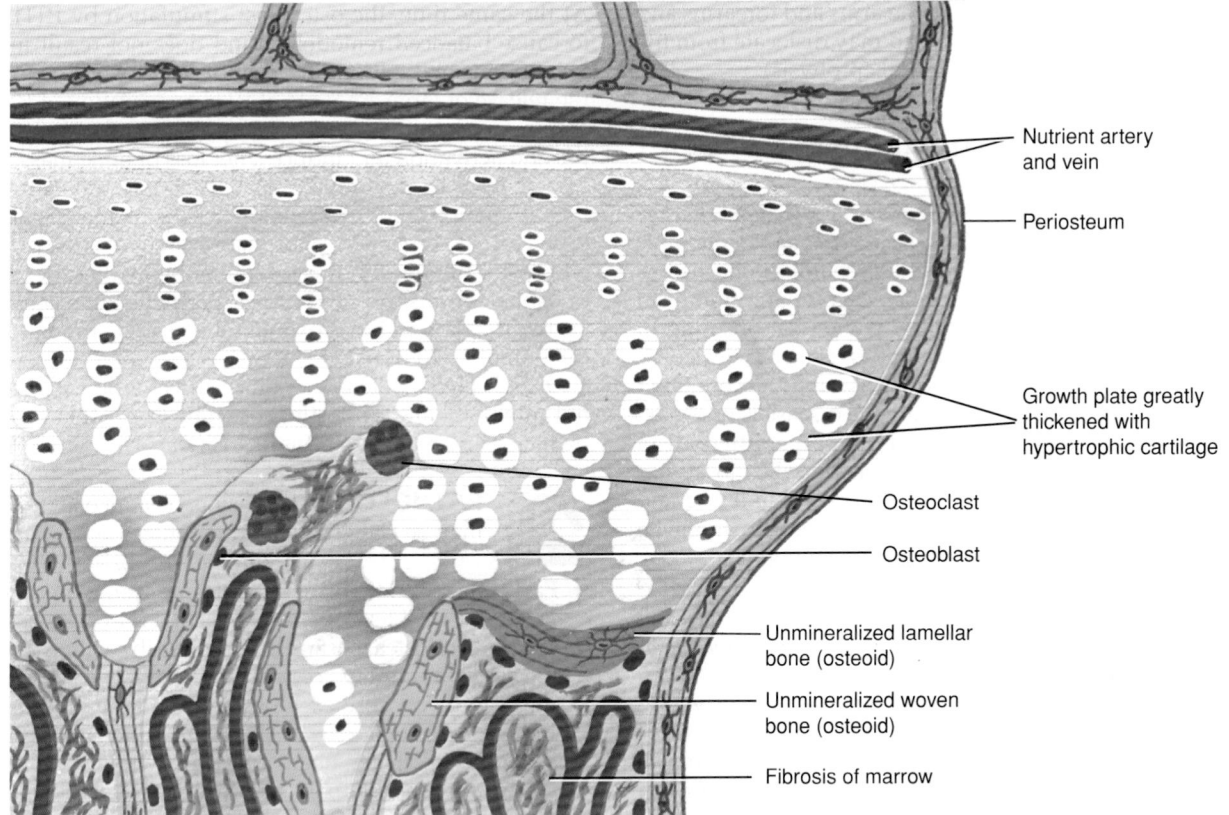

Nutrient artery and vein

Periosteum

Growth plate greatly thickened with hypertrophic cartilage

Osteoclast

Osteoblast

Unmineralized lamellar bone (osteoid)

Unmineralized woven bone (osteoid)

Fibrosis of marrow

FIGURE 30-28. The growth plate in rickets. The growth plate is thickened and disorganized, with a large zone of hypertrophic cartilage cells. Irregular perforation of the cartilage plate by osteoclasts occurs because there is little calcified cartilage. The woven bone on the surface of some of the primary trabeculae is unmineralized and therefore easily fractured. Such microfractures often lead to hemorrhage at the interface between the plate and the metaphysis.

formation of callus and do not extend through the entire diameter of the bone.

RICKETS: Rickets is a disease of children and thus causes extensive changes at the physeal plate (Fig. 30-28), which does not become adequately mineralized. The calcified cartilage and zones of hypertrophy and proliferative cartilage continue to grow because osteoclastic activity does not resorb the poorly mineralized growth plate cartilage. As a consequence, the growth plate is conspicuously thickened, irregular and lobulated. Endochondral ossification proceeds very slowly and preferentially at the peripheral portions of the metaphysis. The result is a flared, cup-shaped epiphysis. The largest part of the primary spongiosum is composed of lamellar or woven bone that, importantly, remains unmineralized.

Microscopically, the growth plate exhibits striking changes. The resting zone is normal, but the zones of proliferating cartilage are greatly distorted. The ordered progression of helix-forming chondrocytes is lost and is replaced by a disorderly profusion of cells separated by small amounts of matrix. Resulting lobulated masses of proliferating and hypertrophied cartilage are associated with increasing width of the growth plate, which may be 5–15 times the normal width. The zone of provisional calcification is poorly defined, and only a minimal amount of primary spongiosum is formed. Masses of proliferating cartilage extend into the metaphyseal region, without any apparent vascular invasion and with little osteoclastic activity.

CLINICAL FEATURES:
OSTEOMALACIA: Clinical diagnosis of osteomalacia is often difficult. Patients have nonspecific complaints, such as muscle weakness or diffuse aches and pains. In mild forms of the disease, only slowly progressive changes in bone are seen, and many patients are totally asymptomatic for years. In advanced cases, poorly localized bone pain and tenderness are common, especially in the spine, pelvis and proximal parts of the extremities. In such cases, the diagnosis may be made only after an acute fracture, the most common sites being the femoral neck, pubic ramus, spine or ribs. Muscular weakness and hypotonia lead to a waddling gait in severe cases, and some patients are unable to walk.

RICKETS: Children with rickets are apathetic and irritable and have short attention spans. They are content to be sedentary, assuming a "Buddha-like" posture. They are short, with characteristic changes of bones and teeth. Flattening of the skull, prominent frontal bones **(frontal bossing)** and conspicuous suture lines are typical. Delayed dentition is associated with severe dental caries and enamel defects. The chest has the classic **rachitic rosary** (a grossly beaded appearance of the costochondral junctions due to enlargement of the costal cartilages) and indentations of the lower ribs at the insertion of the diaphragm (Harrison groove). **Pectus carinatum** ("pigeon breast") reflects an outward curvature of the sternum.

The overall musculature is weak, and abdominal weakness generates a "potbelly." The limbs are shortened and deformed, with severe bowing of the arms and forearms and frequent fractures. The femoral head may dislocate from the growth plate (slipped capital femoral epiphysis).

PRIMARY HYPERPARATHYROIDISM

Primary hyperparathyroidism is a metabolic bone disease characterized by generalized bone resorption due to inappropriate secretion of PTH. Early in the 20th century, bone disease in patients diagnosed with primary hyperparathyroidism was often advanced and crippling. Owing to screening of hospitalized patients for abnormalities of serum calcium, severe primary hyperparathyroidism is rarely encountered nowadays and clinically significant bone disease is unusual.

The histologic changes of primary hyperparathyroidism are known as **osteitis fibrosa**. This term applies to all circumstances of markedly accelerated bone remodeling and may be seen in Paget disease, in hyperthyroidism and even in some patients with postmenopausal osteoporosis.

 **ETIOLOGIC FACTORS:** *Some 90% of cases of primary hyperparathyroidism are caused by one or more parathyroid adenomas. Hyperplasia of all four glands accounts for only 10%.* Because PTH promotes phosphate excretion in the urine and stimulates osteoclastic bone resorption, low serum phosphate and high serum calcium levels are characteristic. A familial type of primary hyperparathyroidism is associated with mutations in the calcium-sensing receptor (*CASR*) gene, located on chromosome 3 (3q13.3).

The effects of PTH are mediated by its effects on bone, kidney and (indirectly) intestine.

BONE: PTH mobilizes calcium from bone (the major reservoir of calcium in the body) by causing increased osteoclasis by extant osteoclasts and by recruitment of new osteoclasts from preosteoclastic mesenchymal cells. This action is indirect and is mediated by direct stimulation of osteoblasts by PTH. As a result, osteoblasts secrete RANKL, which then binds to RANK in osteoclasts and osteoclast precursors and results in bone resorption. Under physiologic circumstances, PTH secretion is shut down by increases in ionic calcium.

At the same time, the osteoblast stimulation by PTH tends to cause balanced remodeling and does not result in a net loss of bone mass. By contrast, under pathologic conditions, the release of large amounts of PTH and continued RANKL secretion prevent osteoclast apoptosis, prolong osteoclast life and activation and induce a net loss of bone mass.

KIDNEY: PTH stimulates reabsorption of calcium by the thick ascending and granular portions of the distal renal tubules. It also enhances phosphate excretion in the proximal and distal tubules by directly inhibiting sodium-dependent phosphate transport. PTH also augments the activity of 1α-hydroxylase in the proximal tubules and stimulates production of 1,25(OH)$_2$D.

INTESTINE: PTH does not act directly on the intestine, but rather enhances intestinal calcium absorption indirectly by increasing renal synthesis of 1,25(OH)$_2$D.

 PATHOLOGY: The histogenesis of osteitis fibrosa may be classified into three stages:

- **Early stage:** Initially osteoclasts are stimulated by the increased PTH levels to resorb bone. From the subperiosteal and endosteal surfaces, osteoclasts bore their way into the cortex as cutting cones. This process is called **dissecting osteitis** because each osteon is continually hollowed out by osteoclastic activity (Figs. 30-23 and 30-29A). At the same time, collagen fibers are laid down in the endosteal marrow and additional osteoclasts penetrate the bone. In contrast to myelofibrosis of hematologic origin, in which fibrous tissue is randomly distributed in the marrow space, the collagen of osteitis fibrosa is deposited adjacent to trabeculae. This observation suggests that the stromal cells depositing matrix material are osteoblast precursors.
- **Osteitis fibrosa:** In the second stage, the trabecular bone is resorbed and marrow is replaced by loose fibrosis, hemosiderin-laden macrophages, areas of hemorrhage from microfractures and reactive woven bone. These features constitute the "osteitis fibrosa" portion of the complex.
- **Osteitis fibrosa cystica:** As primary hyperparathyroidism progresses and hemorrhage continues, cystic degeneration ultimately occurs, evoking the final stage of the

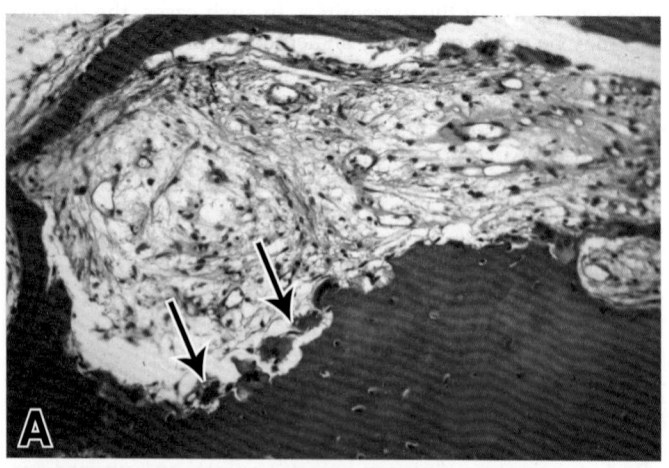

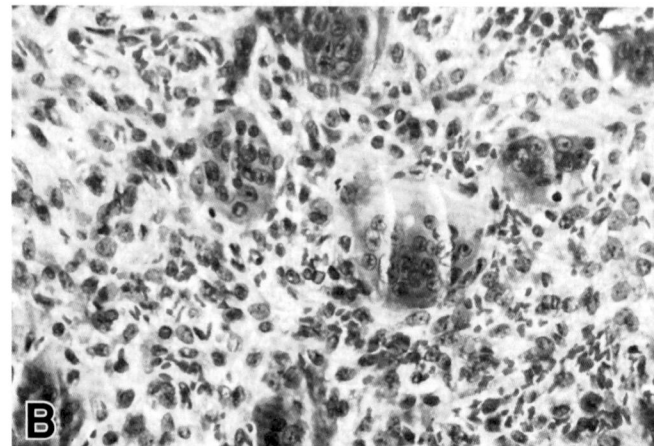

FIGURE 30-29. Primary hyperparathyroidism. A. Section through compact bone shows tunneling resorption of a Haversian canal. Numerous osteoclasts (*arrows*) and stromal fibrosis are evident. **B.** A section of tissue obtained from a "brown tumor" reveals numerous giant cells in a cellular fibrous stroma. Scattered erythrocytes are present throughout the tissue.

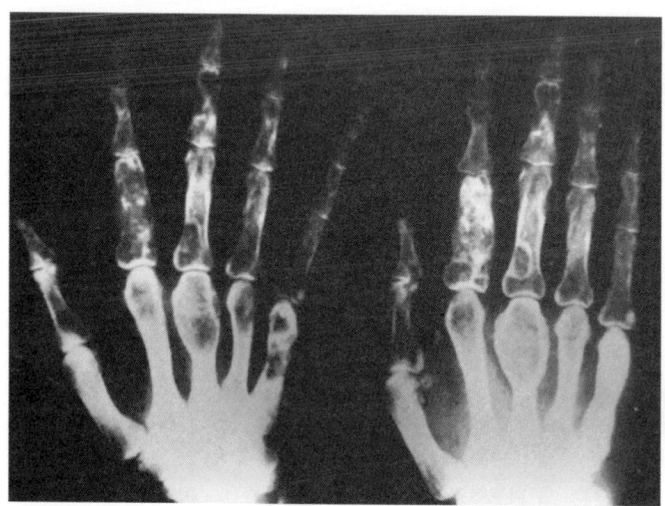

FIGURE 30-30. Primary hyperparathyroidism. A radiograph of the hands reveals bulbous swellings ("brown tumors") and numerous cavities, both representing bone resorption.

disease. The areas of fibrosis that contain reactive woven bone and hemosiderin-laden macrophages often display many osteoclastic giant cells. Because of its macroscopic appearance, this lesion has been dubbed **brown tumor** (Fig. 30-29B). This is not a neoplasm, but rather a repair reaction as an end stage of hyperparathyroidism.

The skeletal radiographs of most patients with primary hyperparathyroidism are normal. Some patients exhibit mottled bone cortices with an irregular frayed surface in the outer table of the skull, tufts of the terminal digits and shafts of the metacarpals (Fig. 30-30). A distinctive radiologic peculiarity, referred to as **subperiosteal bone resorption,** is evident in the subperiosteal outer surface of the cortex and reflects dissecting osteitis. Resorption around tooth sockets causes the lamina dura of the teeth to disappear, a well-known finding on radiography.

A classic feature of osteitis fibrosa cystica is the presence of multiple, localized, lytic lesions, which represent hemorrhagic cysts or masses of fibrous tissue. These eccentric and well-demarcated lesions are separated from the soft tissue by a periosteal shell of bone. The focal, tumor-like, lytic lesions always occur in the context of an abnormal skeleton produced by hyperparathyroidism. If a single lesion is examined in isolation, it may be mistaken for a primary giant cell neoplasm of bone.

 CLINICAL FEATURES: The symptoms of primary hyperparathyroidism are related to the abnormality of calcium homeostasis and have been summarized as "stones, bones, moans and groans." The "stones" refer to kidney stones and the "bones" to the skeletal changes. The "moans" describe psychiatric depression and other abnormalities associated with hypercalcemia. The "groans" characterize the gastrointestinal irregularities associated with a high serum calcium level.

Primary hyperparathyroidism is treated by surgical removal of the parathyroid adenomas. If parathyroid hyperplasia is the cause of the disease, three and a half glands are usually removed. The remaining fragment suffices to ensure that the patient does not develop hypocalcemia. After

surgery, the histologic appearance of the affected skeleton gradually normalizes.

RENAL OSTEODYSTROPHY

Renal osteodystrophy is a complex metabolic bone disease that occurs in the context of chronic renal failure. Severe renal osteodystrophy is most common in patients maintained on long-term dialysis, because they live long enough to develop conspicuous bone disease.

 **ETIOLOGIC FACTORS AND MOLECULAR PATHOGENESIS:** The pathogenesis of renal osteodystrophy is similar to that of osteomalacia, with secondary hyperparathyroidism exerting its influence by way of osteoclastic bone resorption (Fig. 30-23). The development of renal osteodystrophy is summarized as follows:

1. In chronic renal disease, a reduced glomerular filtration rate leads to retention of phosphate, leading to **hyperphosphatemia**. High serum phosphate levels drive down the serum calcium levels.
2. Tubular injury reduces 1α-hydroxylase activity, with a resulting deficiency of 1,25(OH)$_2$D.
3. Intestinal calcium absorption is, in turn, decreased, worsening the **hypocalcemia**.
4. Hypocalcemia stimulates **PTH production**. In fact, most patients with end-stage renal disease have substantial hyperparathyroidism. However, PTH does not effectively promote intestinal calcium absorption or renal tubular resorption of calcium because of failure to produce adequate 1,25(OH)$_2$D.
5. Perhaps because of hyperparathyroidism and hyperphosphatemia, a substantial proportion of patients with end-stage renal disease have increased bone mass. Renal osteosclerosis is particularly prominent in vertebrae where, owing to alternating bands of radiopaque and normally dense bone, the lesion is named "rugger jersey spine."
6. Osteomalacia may result from the disturbances of the vitamin D pathway.

The **adynamic variant of renal osteodystrophy (ARO)** is characterized by arrested bone remodeling. More than 40% of adults who are treated with hemodialysis and more than 50% of those who are treated with peritoneal dialysis have bone biopsy evidence of ARO. Adynamic bone is characterized microscopically by an overall reduction in cellular activity in bone, with fewer or absent osteoblasts and osteoclasts. These changes can be due either to direct inhibitory effects of systemic factors on osteoblast function or to indirect changes in osteoblast activity mediated through PTH-dependent mechanisms. Old bone accumulates because it is not remodeled, thus causing structural compromise of the skeleton and increased tendency to fractures.

 PATHOLOGY AND CLINICAL FEATURES: As a result of these effects of chronic renal failure, renal osteodystrophy is characterized by varying degrees of osteitis fibrosa, osteomalacia, osteosclerosis and adynamic bone disease (Fig. 30-31). Combinations of osteitis fibrosa and osteomalacia are particularly common. Hyperphosphatemic patients

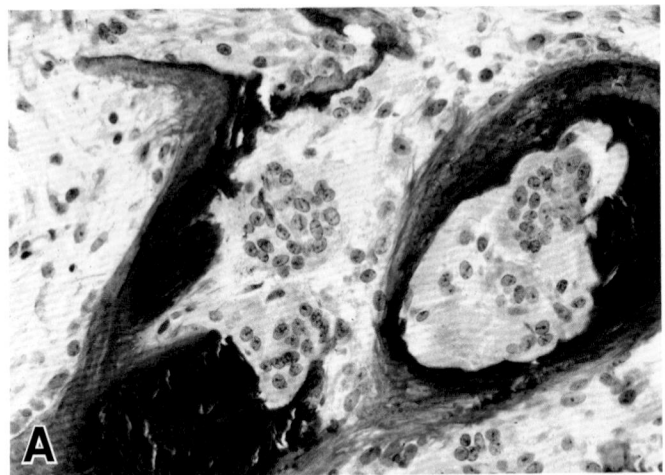

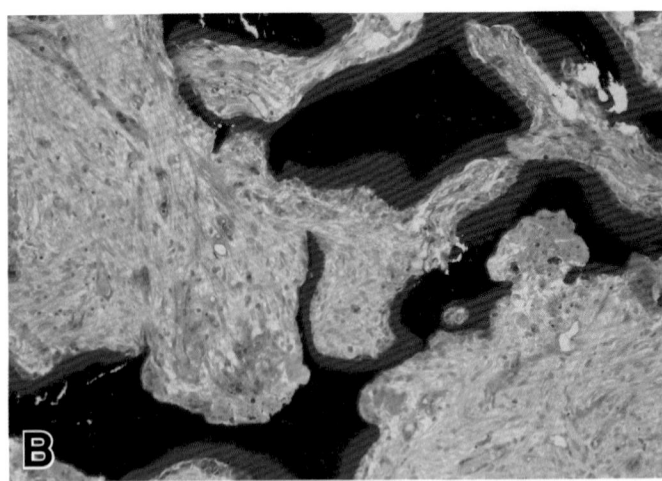

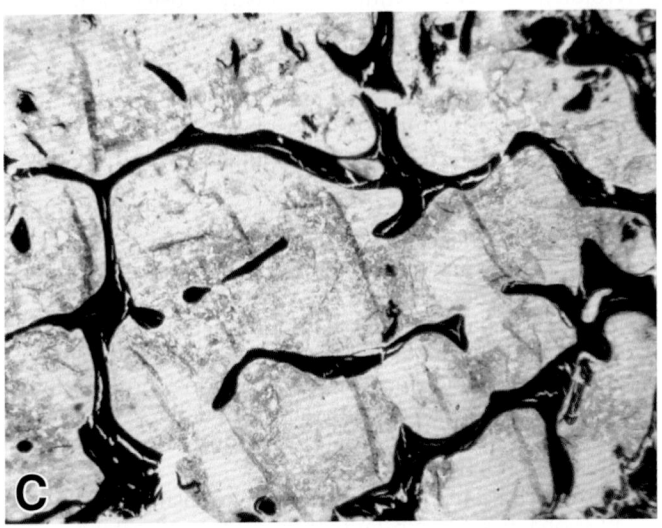

FIGURE 30-31. Renal osteodystrophy. A. Osteitis fibrosa. Several large multinucleated osteoclasts are resorbing these bone spicules, and the paraosseous tissue is fibrotic. Note that the osteoclastic resorption takes place only on the mineralized (*blue*) portions of the trabeculae. In this undecalcified section, the unmineralized bone (osteoid) appears *red*. **B. Osteomalacia.** This is a von Kossa stain prepared on an undecalcified section. The mineralized bone is *black* and the abundant osteoid appears *magenta*. Osteoid is thick and lines a large proportion of the bone surfaces. Surfaces not covered by the osteoid demonstrate scalloped Howship lacunae and contain abundant osteoclasts. **C. Adynamic bone disease** in which remodeling is attenuated, with a paucity of osteoblasts, osteoclasts and osteoid (von Kossa stain).

with terminal chronic renal disease may display metastatic calcification at various sites, including the eyes, skin, muscular coats of arteries and arterioles and periarticular soft tissues.

Management of renal osteodystrophy involves not only treatment of renal failure but also control of phosphate levels by appropriate drug therapy and infusions. Occasionally, parathyroidectomy is required to control hyperparathyroidism, and the administration of vitamin D may also be necessary.

PAGET DISEASE OF BONE

Paget disease is a chronic condition characterized by lesions of bone resulting from disordered remodeling, in which excessive bone resorption initially results in lytic lesions, to be followed by disorganized and excessive bone formation.

 **EPIDEMIOLOGY:** Paget disease generally affects men and women older than 50 years. In predisposed populations, 3% of the elderly manifest the disease. The disorder has an unusual worldwide distribution, afflicting populations of the British Isles and following their migrations throughout the world. People of English descent living in the United States, Australia, New Zealand and Canada have a high incidence of the disease. Northern Europeans have more Paget disease than southern Europeans.

The disorder is almost nonexistent in Asia and in the indigenous populations of Africa and South America. For unknown reasons, the incidence of Paget disease appears to have decreased worldwide over the last several decades.

MOLECULAR PATHOGENESIS: James Paget coined the term **osteitis deformans** for this disease over a century ago, but until recently its etiology has been obscure. Paget disease resembles a metabolic bone disease histologically and there is an increase in bone turnover in affected patients. However, its clinical tendency to involve one bone or only a few bones does not fulfill the definition of a metabolic disorder.

A hereditary predisposition has been suggested by reports of almost 100 families in whom Paget disease is transmitted as an autosomal dominant trait with incomplete penetrance that increases with age. There is evolving evidence that Paget disease and some related diseases are caused by mutations in genes encoding proteins in the RANK signaling pathway. Specifically, mutations in *Sequestosome 1 (SQSTM1)* have been found in familial and sporadic forms of Paget disease. The *SQSTM1* gene encodes a protein, also known as p62, which may act as a scaffold protein in the RANK signaling pathway. It is currently unknown how this mutated protein leads to accelerated osteoclast activity. Inactivation of *SQSTM1* causes defects in RANKL-induced osteoclastogenesis, suggesting a significant role of p62 in osteoclast function.

Some evidence indicates that Paget disease is of viral origin. Virtually all patients exhibit nuclear inclusions consistent with the structure of a virus in osteoclasts and osteoclast precursors. These inclusions are not found in any other skeletal disease other than giant cell tumors of bone. They consist of microfilaments in a paracrystalline array and have been compared with the inclusions in the brains of patients with subacute sclerosing encephalitis (see Chapter 32). This similarity has suggested that a slow virus may be involved (Fig. 30-32). Support for this hypothesis has come from the finding that the marrow of Paget disease patients contains paramyxovirus nucleocapsid transcripts. Infection of osteoclast precursor cells with paramyxovirus can increase expression of RANK and so increase osteoclastic activity. In addition, paramyxoviruses stimulate osteoblasts to produce IL-6, which contributes to osteoclastogenesis. Although a viral etiology seems plausible, actual live viruses have not been isolated from pagetic bone, and it is difficult to explain monostotic bone involvement by a systemic viral infection.

Overall, Paget disease is characterized by localized increases in osteoclast formation that lead to bone resorption and associated osteoblastic activity. The increased osteoclastogenic nature of the bone microenvironment is mediated by increases in IL-6 and the RANK signaling pathway. These are perturbed in Paget disease as a result of genetic factors such as *SQSTM1* mutations and possibly a slow virus infection that may serve as a catalyst for developing the pagetic phenotype in genetically predisposed individuals. The result is uncoupling of the normal osteoclast/osteoblast remodeling unit.

 PATHOLOGY: The lesions of Paget disease may be solitary (monostotic) or may involve multiple bones (polyostotic). They tend to localize to the bones of the axial skeleton, including the spine, skull and pelvis. The proximal femur and tibia may be involved in the polyostotic form of the disease. Solitary Paget disease rarely involves the humerus, but in polyostotic disease, lesions involving this bone are common.

Paget disease is an example of bone remodeling gone awry. The disease is triphasic:

1. **"Hot" or osteoclastic resorptive stage:** Radiologically, there is a characteristic, sharply defined, flame-shaped or wedge-shaped lysis of the cortex, which may mimic a tumor (Fig. 30-33A). Histologically, there is widespread **osteolysis** with marked osteoclastic resorption, marrow fibrosis and dilation of marrow sinusoids.
2. **Mixed stage of osteoblastic and osteoclastic activity:** By radiography, the bones are larger than normal. In fact, Paget disease is one of only two diseases that produce **larger than normal bones** (the other is fibrous dysplasia, discussed below). The cortex in the mixed phase is thickened, and the accentuation of the coarse cancellous bone makes the bone look heavy and enlarged (Fig. 30-33B,C). Involvement of vertebral bodies evokes a "picture frame" appearance (Fig. 30-33D), as cortices and endplates become greatly exaggerated compared to the coarse cancellous bone of the vertebral body. Although the bone is abnormal, the distorted, coarse cancellous bone and cortex still tend to align along stress lines. The pelvis is often thickened in the area of the acetabulum. Histologically, there is evidence of both increased osteoclastic and osteoblastic activity (Figs. 30-32 and 30-34B).

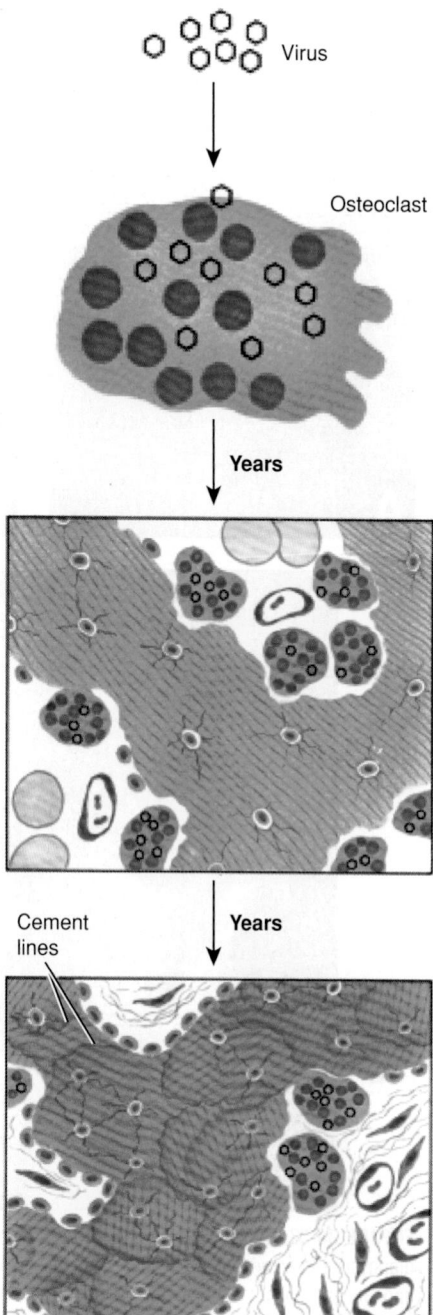

FIGURE 30-32. Hypothetical viral etiology of Paget disease of bone. A virus infects osteoclastic progenitors or osteoclasts in a genetically predisposed individual and stimulates osteoclastic activity, thereby leading to excessive resorption of bone. Over a period of years, the bone develops a characteristic mosaic pattern, produced by chaotically juxtaposed units of lamellar bone that form irregular cement lines. The adjacent marrow is often fibrotic, and there is a mixture of osteoclasts and osteoblasts on the surface of the bone.

3. **"Cold" or burnt-out stage:** This period is characterized histologically by little cellular activity and radiologically by thickened and disordered bones.

The disease need not progress through all three stages, and in polyostotic disease, various foci may appear in different stages.

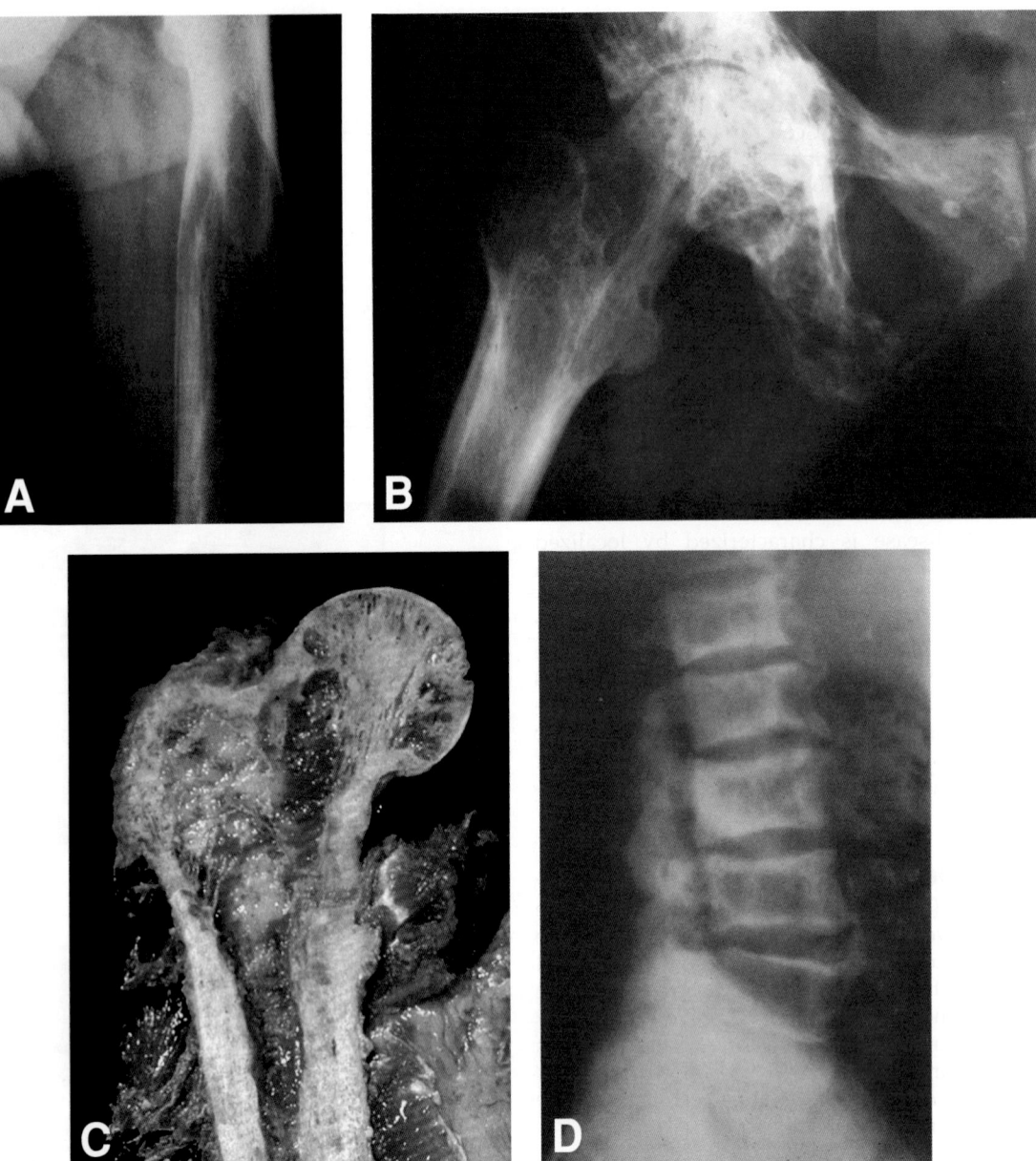

FIGURE 30-33. Paget disease. A. A radiograph of early Paget disease shows cortical dissolution, increased diameter of the diaphysis and an advancing, wedge-shaped area of cortical resorption ("flame sign"). Proximal to the edge of this wedge, the femur appears entirely normal. **B.** Later, Paget disease of the proximal femur and pelvis shows cortical disorganization and irregular coarse trabeculations. **C.** Gross specimen of proximal femur showing cortical thickening and coarse trabeculations of the femoral head and neck. **D.** Paget disease of the spine shows shortening and widening of the lumbar vertebral bodies. Their cortices and endplates are thickened and have a "picture frame" appearance.

The osteoclast is the pathologic cell of Paget disease, and its appearance is characteristic. While normal osteoclasts contain fewer than a dozen nuclei, those of Paget disease are huge and may have over 100 (Fig. 30-34B). Nuclei may contain intranuclear inclusions that contain virus-like particles (Fig. 30-34B,C).

Because active Paget disease is a disorder of accelerated remodeling, its histologic features are those of severe osteitis fibrosa. Numerous large osteoclasts, active osteoblasts and peritrabecular marrow fibrosis are encountered (Fig. 30-34B). The rapid remodeling occasions disruption of the trabecular architecture. Trabeculae are characteristically distorted and irregular, with a high surface-to-volume ratio. Bone collagen is often arranged in a woven rather than lamellar pattern.

With time, the lesions of Paget disease burn out and become inactive. The diagnostic hallmark of this stage is the abnormal arrangement of lamellar bone, in which islands of irregular bone formation resembling pieces of a jigsaw puzzle are separated by prominent irregular **cement lines** (Fig. 30-34A). The result is a **mosaic pattern** in the bone, which can be seen particularly well under polarized light. In the cortex of an affected bone, the osteons tend to be destroyed, and concentric lamellae are incomplete. Although the changes in lamellar bone are diagnostic, it is common to see woven bone as part of the pathologic process. In this

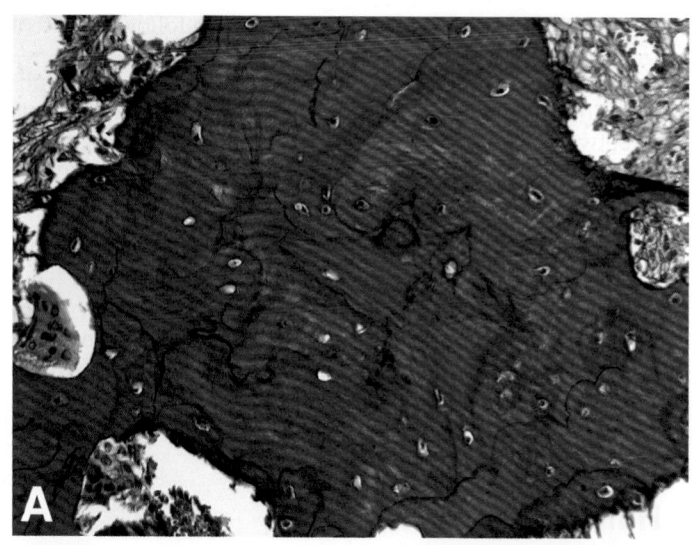

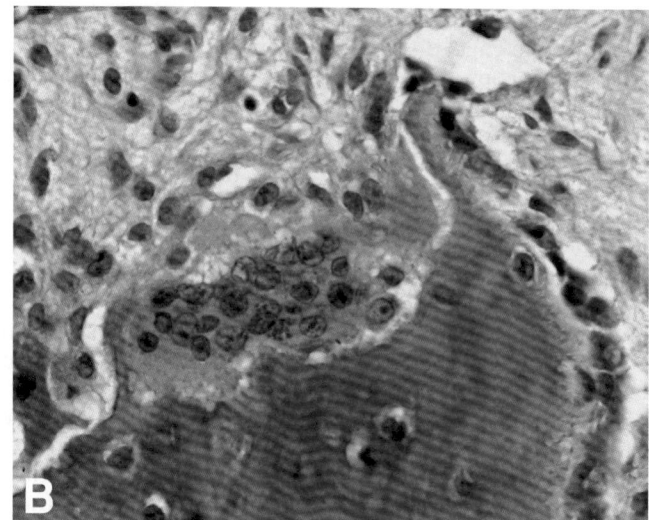

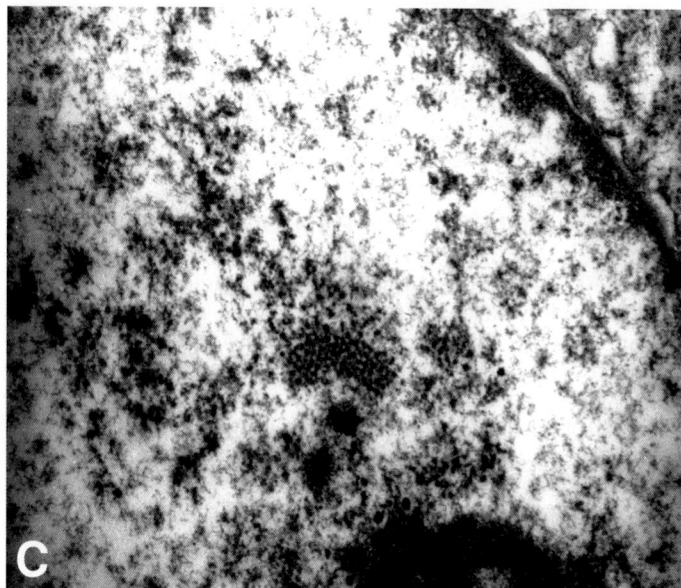

FIGURE 30-34. Paget disease. A. A section of bone shows prominent and irregular basophilic cement lines and numerous lining osteoclasts and osteoblasts. **B.** An osteoclast in pagetic bone contains many more nuclei than a usual osteoclast. A few of the nuclei contain eosinophilic intranuclear inclusion-like particles. **C.** On electron microscopy, the nuclei of the osteoclasts contain particles that resemble paramyxovirus in their shape and orientation.

situation, the woven bone is a reactive phenomenon, as in a microcallus, and represents a temporary bridge between islands of the mosaic bone of Paget disease.

 CLINICAL FEATURES: The most common focal symptom of Paget disease is pain in the affected bone, although its cause is not clear. The pain may be related to microfractures, stimulation of free nerve endings by dilated blood vessels adjacent to the bones or weight bearing in weaker bones. The diagnosis is primarily made by radiologic findings and bone biopsy is seldom necessary.

SKULL: Involvement of the skull is particularly common. The skull exhibits localized lysis, called **osteoporosis circumscripta,** generally in the frontal and parietal bones. Alternatively, there may be thickening of the outer and inner tables, which is most pronounced in the frontal and occipital bones. The skull becomes very heavy and may collapse over the C1 vertebra, compressing the brain and spinal cord. Hearing loss follows involvement of the middle ear ossicles and bony impingement on the eighth cranial nerve at the foramen. **Platybasia** (flattening of the base of the skull) impinges on the foramen magnum, compressing the medulla and upper spinal cord.

The jaws may be grossly misshapen and the teeth may fall out. Often, facial bones increase in size, especially the maxillary bones, producing the so-called **leontiasis ossea** (lion-like face).

PAGETIC STEAL: Occasionally, patients feel lightheaded, due to so-called pagetic steal. In this situation, blood is shunted from the internal carotid system to the bones rather than directed to the brain.

FRACTURES AND ARTHRITIS: Fractures are common in Paget disease, the bones snapping transversely like a piece of chalk. Incomplete fractures without displacement are called **infractions**. Involvement of the pelvis engenders hip problems. The loss of subchondral bone compliance causes secondary osteoarthritis and destruction of the articular cartilage.

HIGH-OUTPUT CARDIAC FAILURE: With extensive Paget disease, blood flow to the bones and subcutaneous tissue increases remarkably, requiring increased cardiac output. In the presence of underlying cardiac disease, it may be severe enough to result in cardiac failure.

SARCOMATOUS CHANGE: Neoplastic transformation may occur in Paget disease, usually in the femur, humerus or pelvis. This complication occurs in less than 1% of all cases and usually arises in patients with severe polyostotic disease. However, the incidence of bone sarcoma is 1000 times higher than that in the general population. Interestingly, the skull and vertebrae, the bones most commonly involved by Paget disease, rarely undergo sarcomatous change. Sarcomas are usually osteogenic but may be fibrosarcoma or chondrosarcoma. Their prognosis is very poor.

Serum calcium and phosphorus levels in Paget disease are normal, even though bone turnover increases more than 20-fold. Hypercalcemia is rare, but does occur if a patient is immobilized. The collagen structure of bone in Paget disease is entirely normal, but because of the accelerated bone turnover, levels of collagen breakdown products (hydroxyproline and hydroxylysine) increase in the serum and urine. Hydroxyproline excretion may reach 1000 mg/day (normal, <40 mg). The serum alkaline phosphatase level is the most useful laboratory test in diagnosing Paget disease. It increases enormously and correlates with osteoblastic activity. The alkaline phosphatase levels are disproportionately high with skull involvement but tend to be lower when only the pelvis is affected. A sudden increase in the activity of serum alkaline phosphatase may reflect sarcomatous change within a lesion.

Fortunately, most patients with Paget disease are asymptomatic and require no treatment. Fractures, osteoarthritis and other orthopedic complications are treated symptomatically. Drugs directed at hindering the abnormal osteoclast hyperfunction, including calcitonin and bisphosphonates, are useful.

GIANT CELL TUMOR: Giant cell tumor may arise in Paget disease. It is not a neoplasm but rather a reactive phenomenon similar to the "brown tumor" of hyperparathyroidism. Giant cell tumor is an overshoot of osteoclastic activity with an associated fibroblastic response. Radiation therapy has been used in the treatment of giant cell tumor but has been abandoned owing to a high incidence of malignant transformation.

GAUCHER DISEASE

This autosomal recessive hereditary storage disease is discussed in Chapter 6. We consider here only its skeletal manifestations. These include:

- **Failure of remodeling:** This is the most common, and least problematic, skeletal abnormality. Flaring is absent and funnelization and cylinderization are abnormal, giving rise to an Erlenmeyer flask shape of the distal femur and proximal tibia.
- **Bone crisis:** This rare but very painful event results from acute infarction of a large segment of one or more bones, often after an acute viral illness. There is insufficient bone blood flow owing to marrow infiltration by Gaucher cells. It lasts about 2 weeks and then gradually improves.
- **Localized and diffuse bone loss:** Radiolucent lesions with overlying cortical thinning are usually asymptomatic unless a fracture occurs at the site. These lesions are packed with Gaucher cells.
- **Osteosclerotic lesions:** These reflect increased bone formation, usually in the medullary cavity of the long bones

and pelvis. Reactive new bone formation following osteonecrosis may be involved.

- **Corticomedullary osteonecrosis:** This disabling complication of Gaucher disease is most common in patients between 8 and 35 years old. It mostly involves the femoral head or proximal humerus. Extensive marrow infiltration by Gaucher cells restricts adequate blood flow to the bone.
- **Pathologic fractures:** Vertebrae, long bones and even the pelvis may show spontaneous fractures, owing to bone necrosis or osteopenia.
- **Osteomyelitis and septic arthritis:** Commonly caused by coliform or anaerobic organisms, spread via bloodstream to the bones and joints of Gaucher patients is common, especially after surgery.

FIBROUS DYSPLASIA

Fibrous dysplasia is viewed as a developmental abnormality characterized by a disorganized mixture of fibrous and osseous elements in the medullary region of affected bones. It occurs in children and young adults and may affect one (monostotic) or multiple bones (polyostotic) or other systems (McCune-Albright syndrome).

 **MOLECULAR PATHOGENESIS:** Activating mutations in the *GNAS1* gene encoding the α subunit of the stimulatory $G_s\alpha$ protein, which is linked to adenyl cyclase, have been described in bone cells from patients with fibrous dysplasia and McCune-Albright syndrome. The result is constitutive activation of adenyl cyclase and increased levels of cyclic adenosine 3′,5′-monophosphate (cAMP), and so enhancing certain functions of the affected cells (e.g., c-*fos* and c-*jun* proto-oncogenes, IL-6 and IL-11).

 PATHOLOGY AND CLINICAL FEATURES:
MONOSTOTIC FIBROUS DYSPLASIA: Monostotic fibrous dysplasia is the most common form of the disease and is most often seen in the second and third decades, with no predilection for either sex. The bones commonly involved are the proximal femur, tibia, ribs and facial bones, although any bone may be affected. The disease may be asymptomatic or it may lead to a pathologic fracture.

POLYOSTOTIC FIBROUS DYSPLASIA: One fourth of patients with polyostotic fibrous dysplasia exhibit disease in more than half of the skeleton, including the facial bones. Symptoms usually are seen in childhood, and almost all patients have pathologic fractures, limb deformities or limblength discrepancies. Polyostotic fibrous dysplasia is more common in females. Sometimes the disease becomes quiescent at puberty, but pregnancy tends to stimulate the growth of lesions.

MCCUNE-ALBRIGHT SYNDROME: This condition is characterized by endocrine dysfunction, including acromegaly, Cushing syndrome, hyperthyroidism and vitamin D–resistant rickets. The most common endocrine abnormality is precocious puberty in girls (boys rarely have McCune-Albright syndrome). As a result, premature closure of the growth plates leads to abnormally short stature. The most common extraskeletal manifestations of McCune-Albright syndrome are characteristic skin lesions: pigmented macules

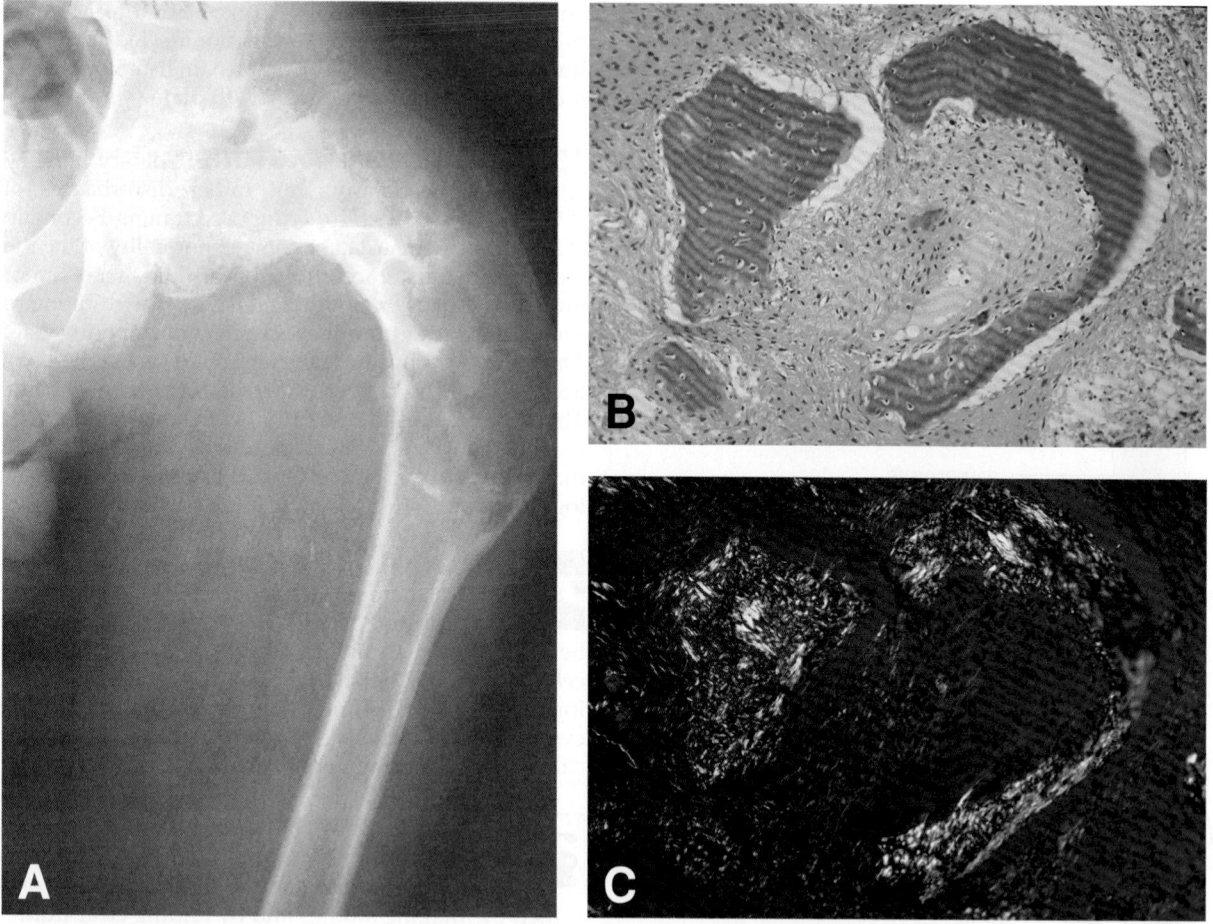

FIGURE 30-35. Fibrous dysplasia. A. A radiograph of the proximal femur shows the "shepherd's crook" deformity caused by fractures sustained over the years. Irregular, marginated, ground-glass lucencies are surrounded by reactive bone. The shaft has an appearance that has been likened to a soap bubble. **B.** Histologically, fibrous dysplasia consists of moderately cellular fibrous tissue in which irregular, curved spicules of woven bone develop without discernible appositional osteoblast activity. **C.** The same section in polarized light demonstrates not only that the spicules are woven but also that their fiber pattern extends imperceptibly into the fiber pattern of the surrounding stroma.

("café-au-lait" spots) with irregular ("coast of Maine") borders that do not cross the midline of the body and are usually located over the buttocks, back and sacrum. These often overlie the skeletal lesions.

Polyostotic fibrous dysplasia may also be associated with soft tissue myxomas **(Mazabraud syndrome)**. The radiographic features of fibrous dysplasia are distinctive. The bone lesion has a lucent ground-glass appearance with well-marginated borders and a thin cortex. The bone may be ballooned, deformed or enlarged, and involvement may be focal or may encompass the entire bone (Fig. 30-35A).

All forms of fibrous dysplasia have an identical histologic pattern (Fig. 30-35B,C). Benign fibroblastic tissue is arranged in a loose, whorled pattern. Irregularly arranged, purposeless spicules of woven bone that lack osteoblastic rimming are embedded in the fibrous tissue. In 10% of cases, irregular islands of hyaline cartilage are also present. Occasionally, cystic degeneration occurs, with hemosiderin-laden macrophages, hemorrhage and osteoclasts congregated about the cyst. Rarely (<1% of cases), malignant transformation (osteosarcoma, chondrosarcoma, fibrosarcoma) has been reported, but many of these cases involved prior radiation therapy. Treatment of fibrous dysplasia consists of curettage, repair of fractures and prevention of deformities.

BENIGN TUMORS OF BONE

Bone tumors of all kinds are uncommon but are nevertheless important neoplasms because many occur in children and young adults and are potentially lethal. A primary bone tumor may arise from any of the cellular elements of bone. Most neoplasms of bone occur near the metaphyseal area, and more than 80% of primary tumors are found in the distal femur or proximal tibia (Fig. 30-36). In a growing child, these areas show conspicuous growth activity.

Nonossifying Fibroma Is a Solitary Lesion of Childhood

Nonossifying fibroma, also called **fibrous cortical defect,** is a benign tumor that occurs in the metaphysis of a long bone, most commonly the tibia or femur. It is very common and may be present in as many as 25% of all children between the ages of 4 and 10 years, after which it characteristically regresses. Nonossifying fibroma is a developmental lesion and not a neoplasm. Most cases are asymptomatic, although pain or fracture through the thin cortex overlying the lesion occasionally calls attention to the condition. Multiple

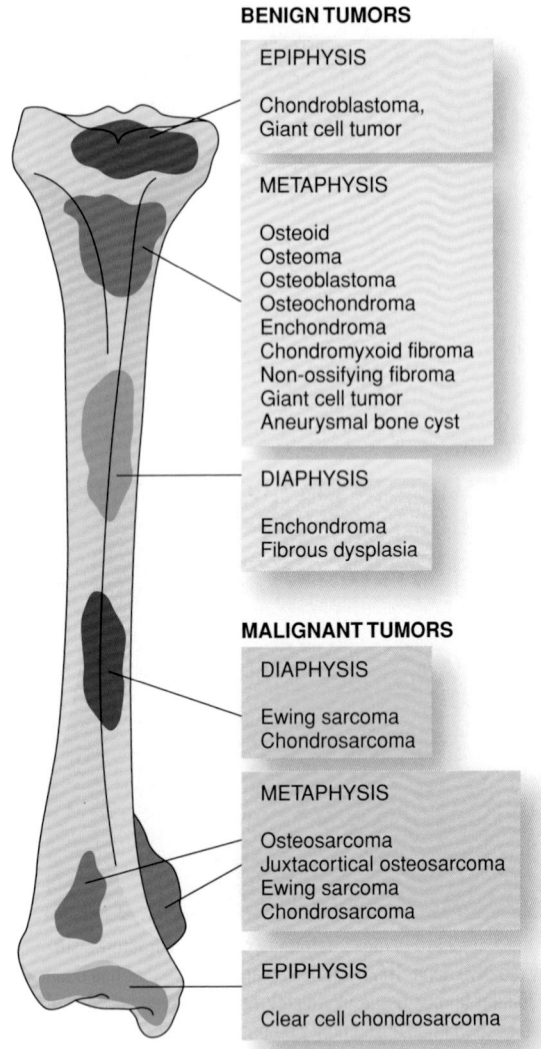

BENIGN TUMORS

EPIPHYSIS

Chondroblastoma,
Giant cell tumor

METAPHYSIS

Osteoid
Osteoma
Osteoblastoma
Osteochondroma
Enchondroma
Chondromyxoid fibroma
Non-ossifying fibroma
Giant cell tumor
Aneurysmal bone cyst

DIAPHYSIS

Enchondroma
Fibrous dysplasia

MALIGNANT TUMORS

DIAPHYSIS

Ewing sarcoma
Chondrosarcoma

METAPHYSIS

Osteosarcoma
Juxtacortical osteosarcoma
Ewing sarcoma
Chondrosarcoma

EPIPHYSIS

Clear cell chondrosarcoma

FIGURE 30-36. Location of primary bone tumors in long tubular bones.

ossifying fibromas may be seen with neurofibromatosis type 1 and in the **Jaffe-Campanacci syndrome (associated with café au lait spots)**.

 PATHOLOGY: Radiologically, nonossifying fibromas are characterized by a cortical, eccentric position and by well-demarcated, central lucent zones surrounded by scalloped, sclerotic margins (Fig. 30-37A). On gross examination, the lesion is granular and dark red to brown. Microscopically, bland spindle cells are arranged in an interlacing, whorled pattern, with scattered multinucleated giant cells and foamy macrophages (Fig. 30-37B). Spontaneous regression is common. Radiologic follow-up is sufficient management in most cases. The rare, symptomatic or expanded lesions that are prone to fracture are treated with curettage and bone grafting.

Solitary Bone Cyst Occurs in Children and Adolescents

Solitary, unicameral or simple bone cyst is a benign, fluid-filled, unilocular lesion. There is a male predilection (3:1),

and 80% occur in the first two decades of life. More than two thirds of all solitary bone cysts are located in the proximal humerus, proximal femur or proximal tibia, usually in the metaphysis adjacent to the growth plate.

 **ETIOLOGIC FACTORS:** Solitary bone cysts are not neoplasms but rather disturbances of bone growth with superimposed trauma. Secondary organization of a hematoma or some abnormality of the metaphyseal vessels causes accumulation of fluid. The "tumor" then grows by expansion of the fluid cavity. The resulting pressure causes bone resorption, mediated by neighboring osteoclasts. The process is slow, so that as the endosteal surface of the cortex is resorbed, a thin periosteal shell of new bone is laid down. This sequence results in a thin, well-marginated, radiolucent bone lesion (Fig. 30-38), which is never greater in diameter than the growth plate and is particularly susceptible to pathologic fracture.

 PATHOLOGY: Solitary bone cyst is not a true cyst since there is no distinct cell lining. It is rather lined by fibrous tissue, a few osteoclastic giant cells, hemosiderin-laden macrophages, chronic inflammatory cells and reactive bone. Osteoclasts are present in the advancing front of the cyst and allow expansion of the lesion. The cyst wall may contain characteristic masses of amorphous, calcified, fibrinous material resembling cementum.

 CLINICAL FEATURES: Most solitary bone cysts are entirely asymptomatic until a pathologic fracture calls attention to it. Once the diagnosis is confirmed by imaging studies and by finding clear fluid by needle aspiration, intralesional corticosteroids may be given. Currently, curettage and bone grafting are the preferred treatment of choice.

Aneurysmal Bone Cyst May Be Primary or Secondary

Aneurysmal bone cyst (ABC) is an uncommon, benign, expansive and often destructive lesion arising within a bone or on its surface. It occurs in children and young adults, with a peak incidence in the second decade. Although the lesion has been observed at every skeletal site, it is most frequent in the metaphysis of long bones and the vertebral column.

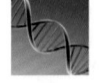 **MOLECULAR PATHOGENESIS:** The pathogenesis of ABC is controversial. Some cases represent cystic and hemorrhagic transformation of an underlying lesion, most commonly chondroblastoma, osteoblastoma, fibrous dysplasia, giant cell tumor and osteosarcoma ("secondary ABC"). Other cases of ABC have no detectable associated lesion ("primary ABC"). Primary ABC may be a true neoplasm, since it is associated with a recurring chromosomal translocation t(16;17)(q22;p13). This anomaly fuses the promoter region of the osteoblast cadherin 11 gene (*CDH11*) on chromosome 16q22 to the coding sequence of the ubiquitin protease (*USP6*) gene on chromosome 17p13. USP6 is thought to have a role in regulating actin remodeling. However, the possible mechanism of neoplastic transformation by upregulation of USP6 has not been elucidated.

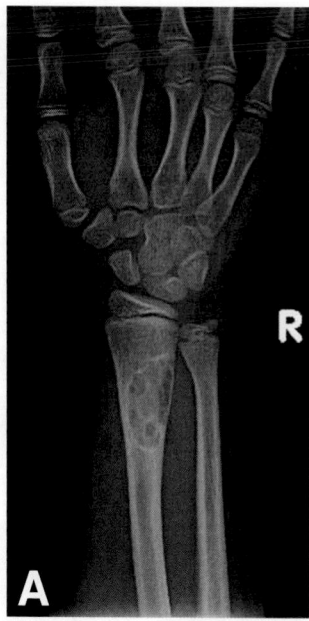
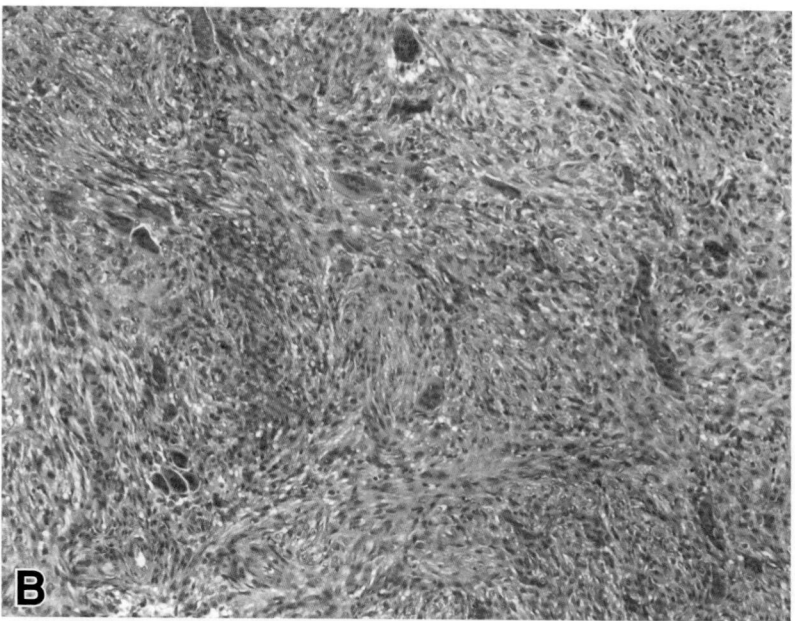

FIGURE 30-37. Nonossifying fibroma. A. A radiograph of the distal radius of a child with an eccentric, metaphyseal lytic lesion with scalloped and sclerotic margins. **B.** Microscopically, the lesion is composed of bland spindle cells arranged in interlacing fascicles, with scattered, multinucleated, osteoclast-type giant cells.

PATHOLOGY: The periosteum around an aneurysmal bone cyst is ballooned but intact. In the spine, the lesion may actually extend across more than one bone. By MRI, fluid-fluid levels may be seen as

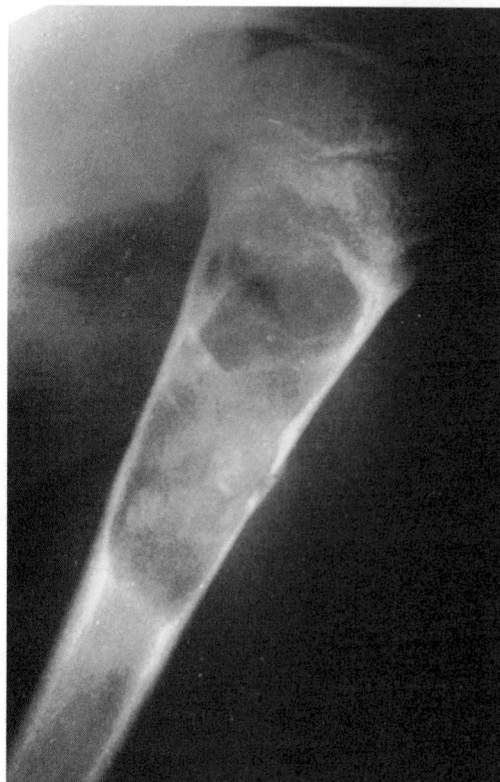

FIGURE 30-38. Solitary bone cyst. A radiograph of the proximal humerus of a child (note the epiphyseal plate) shows a large, well-demarcated, lytic epiphyseal and diaphyseal lesion. The cortex is thinned, but there is no cortical distortion or malformation of the shape of the bone.

blood cells separate from plasma (Fig. 30-39A). The cut surface of the cyst resembles a sponge permeated with blood and blood clots (Fig. 30-39B). The walls and septa are composed of moderately cellular fibrous tissue with multinucleated giant cells and reactive bone (Fig. 30-39C).

CLINICAL FEATURES: Although some aneurysmal bone cysts tend to grow slowly, most expand rapidly, and some are enormous. They usually manifest with pain and swelling, sometimes in relation to trauma, and often develop in a short period of time. A bone cyst may "blow out," that is, rupture and produce local hemorrhage. Treatment is usually excision and curettage with bone grafting. Recurrence rate is variable (20%–70%). At surgery, incising the cyst decreases its internal pressure, causing brisk bleeding that may be difficult to control. In sites such as the vertebral column or the pelvis, selective arterial embolization has been successful.

Osteoma Is a Benign Tumor Composed of Compact Cortical Bone

Osteoma is a benign, slow-growing tumor composed of cortical-type dense bone. These lesions can be divided into four major clinicopathologic subtypes: (1) calvarial and mandibular osteomas, (2) osteomas of the sinonasal and orbital bones, (3) bone islands occurring in medullary bone and (4) surface osteomas of long bones. Some osteomas are likely developmental or hamartomatous in nature. However, sinonasal osteomas may be benign osteoblastic neoplasms. Interestingly, multiple osteomas are associated with familial adenomatous polyposis in Gardner syndrome (see Chapter 19).

Osteoid Osteoma Is a Benign, Painful Lesion

Osteoid osteoma is composed of immature osseous tissue (the nidus) surrounded by a halo of dense reactive bone. The typical patient is between 5 and 25 years old. Boys are

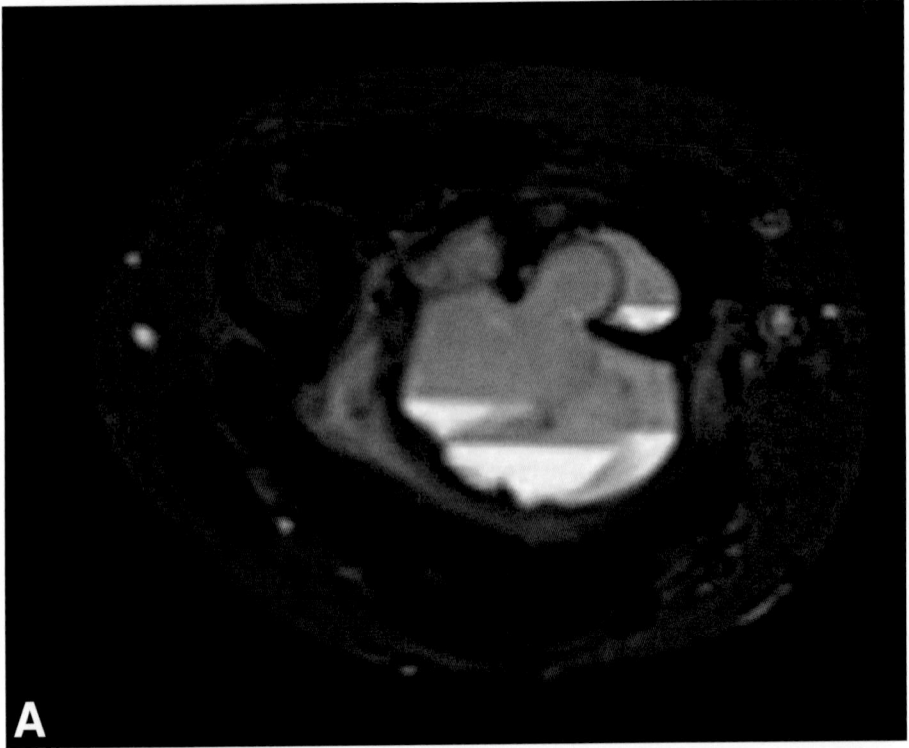

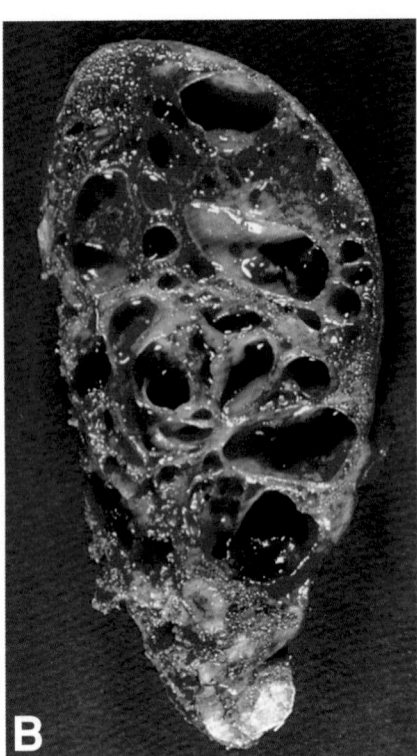

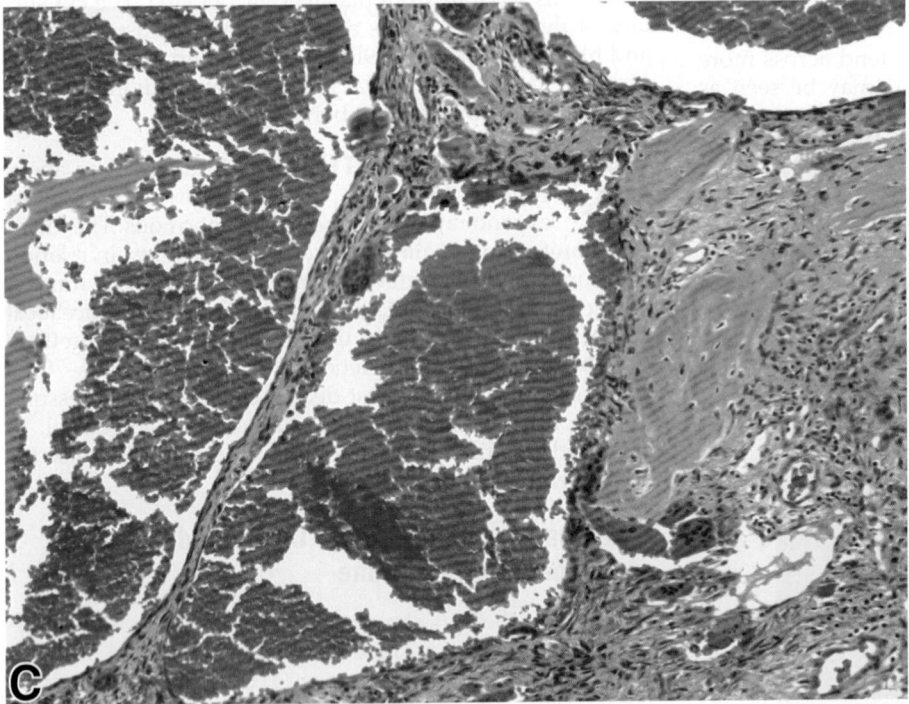

FIGURE 30-39. Aneurysmal bone cyst. A. A magnetic resonance image showing fluid-fluid levels. **B.** In cross-section, the lesion consists of a spongy mass containing multiple blood-filled cysts. Some of the septa between the cysts contain bony tissue. **C.** Microscopically, the blood-filled spaces are separated by cellular fibrous septa with scattered osteoclast-type giant cells and reactive bone.

affected more often than girls (3:1). The lesion frequently arises in the diaphyseal cortex of the tubular bones of the leg but may occur elsewhere. Osteoid osteomas have limited growth potential and do not metastasize.

 MOLECULAR PATHOGENESIS: Chromosomal analysis of a few osteoid osteomas has disclosed structural abnormalities of chromosome 22q13 and loss of part of 17q, which suggests that the lesions are neoplasms.

PATHOLOGY: Osteoid osteoma is a spherical, hyperemic tumor, about 1 cm in diameter, which is considerably softer than the surrounding bone (Fig. 30-40A) and easily enucleated at surgery. Microscopically, the center of the tumor (nidus) is composed of thin, irregular trabeculae of woven bone within a cellular and vascular fibrous stroma containing many osteoblasts and osteoclasts (Fig. 30-40B). The trabeculae are more mature in the center, which is often partially calcified. Reactive sclerotic bone surrounds the nidus.

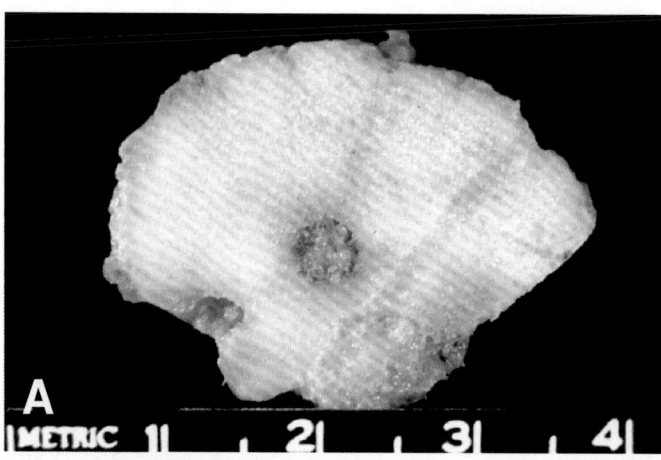
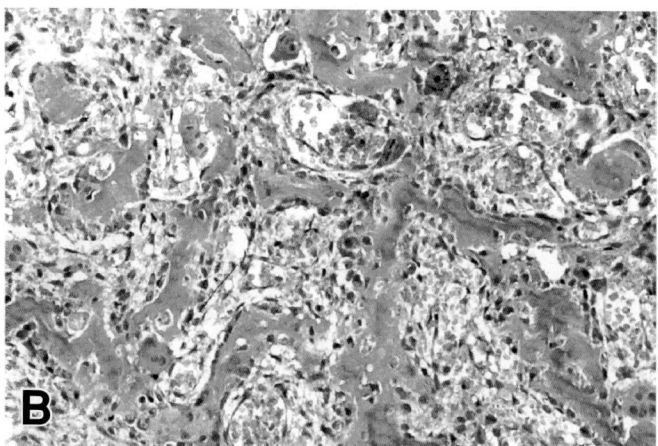

FIGURE 30-40. Osteoid osteoma. A. A gross specimen of an osteoid osteoma shows the central nidus, which is embedded in dense bone. **B.** A photomicrograph of the nidus reveals irregular trabeculae of woven bone surrounded by osteoblasts, osteoclasts and fibrovascular marrow.

 CLINICAL FEATURES: Pain is typically nocturnal and out of proportion to the size of the lesion. Interestingly, the pain is often exacerbated by drinking alcohol and promptly relieved by aspirin or other anti-inflammatory drugs, possibly because of the high prostaglandin content and abundant nerve fibers within the tumor. Surgical excision or radioablation (electric probe inserted into the tumor) is curative.

Osteoblastoma Is Usually Not Painful

Osteoblastoma is an uncommon, benign neoplasm that is histologically similar to osteoid osteoma but larger (usually >2 cm) and with a tendency to progressive growth. It is not accompanied by the characteristic nocturnal pain of osteoid osteoma, although dull pain sometimes occurs. It stimulates less bone reaction and appears mostly as a purely radiolucent lesion, with only a thin shell of surrounding bone. Osteoblastoma occurs in people between the ages of 10 and 35 years, is more common in males and mainly affects the spine and long bones. The histologic features of osteoblastoma are similar to those of osteoid osteoma. Secondary aneurysmal bone cysts may be seen. Curettage cures small osteoblastomas, but larger lesions require wide resection. Recurrences are uncommon and prognosis is excellent.

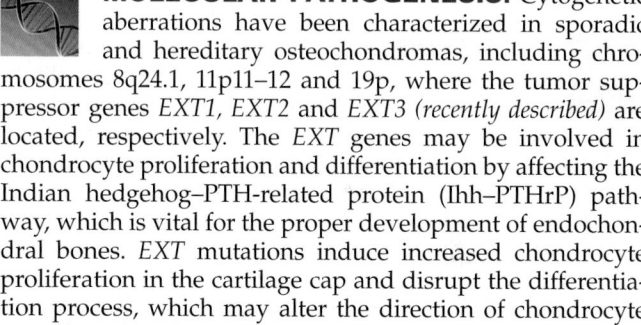 **MOLECULAR PATHOGENESIS:** Although several chromosomal and molecular abnormalities have been described in osteoblastoma, no consistent abnormality has emerged. Aneuploid to hyperdiploid karyotypes have been demonstrated. *MDM2* gene amplification and *TP53* gene deletion implicate cell cycle abnormalities in the pathogenesis of osteoblastoma.

Osteochondroma

Osteochondroma is a benign cartilaginous neoplasm consisting of a bony projection with a cartilaginous cap that arises on the surface of the bone. It occurs in bones formed by endochondral ossification and was viewed for many years as a developmental defect of the growth plate. Most are solitary but 15% are multiple and hereditary. Recently described gene mutations in solitary and multiple osteochondromas favor a neoplastic nature. Solitary osteochondroma is one of the most common benign bone tumors and is more frequent in young males. Most osteochondromas are asymptomatic, and some may need surgical excision if cosmetically displeasing or if they press upon an artery or nerve. Recurrence is very rare.

 MOLECULAR PATHOGENESIS: Cytogenetic aberrations have been characterized in sporadic and hereditary osteochondromas, including chromosomes 8q24.1, 11p11–12 and 19p, where the tumor suppressor genes *EXT1*, *EXT2* and *EXT3 (recently described)* are located, respectively. The *EXT* genes may be involved in chondrocyte proliferation and differentiation by affecting the Indian hedgehog–PTH-related protein (Ihh–PTHrP) pathway, which is vital for the proper development of endochondral bones. *EXT* mutations induce increased chondrocyte proliferation in the cartilage cap and disrupt the differentiation process, which may alter the direction of chondrocyte growth and lead to the development of osteochondromas.

PATHOLOGY: Osteochondromas tend to grow away from the nearest joint. In radiographs, the cartilaginous mass is in direct continuity with the parent bone and lacks an underlying cortex (Fig. 30-41A). The marrow cavity of the lesion is in continuity with that of the bone where it arose. The cartilage-capped, bony mass is surrounded by a surface fibrous membrane, which is the perichondrium. Histologically, the cap is composed of benign hyaline cartilage with active endochondral ossification, which is morphologically similar to that seen in the epiphyseal growth plate (Fig. 30-41B). The bony stalk is composed of cortical lamellar bone, and the medullary cavity contains lamellar bone trabeculae and fatty marrow.

HEREDITARY MULTIPLE OSTEOCHONDROMATOSIS: This inherited autosomal dominant disorder is characterized by multiple osteochondromas and associated skeletal deformities. Hereditary multiple osteochondromatosis (HMO) is one of the most common inherited musculoskeletal disorders and is caused by loss of *EXT1* or *EXT2* gene function (see Molecular Pathogenesis above). Although not as common as solitary osteochondroma, the heritable variety is not rare, with an incidence of about 1 in 50,000. It

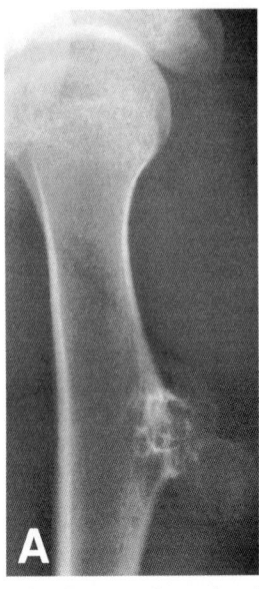
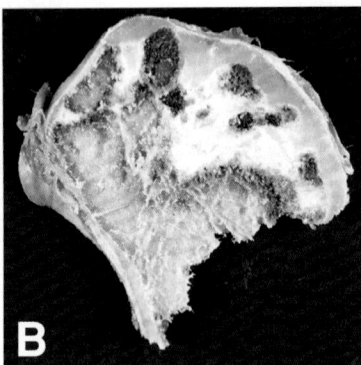
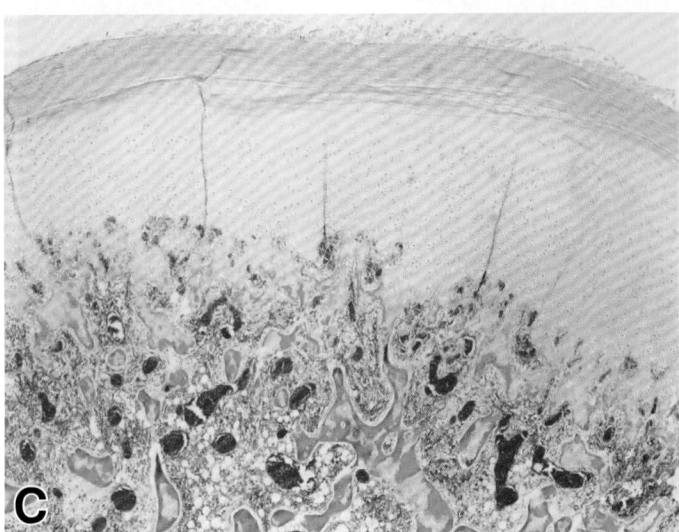

FIGURE 30-41. Osteochondroma. A. A radiograph of an osteochondroma of the humerus shows a lesion that is directly contiguous with the marrow space. **B.** The cross-section of an osteochondroma shows the cap of calcified cartilage overlying poorly organized cancellous bone. **C.** Microscopically, the cartilaginous cap is covered by a fibrous membrane (perichondrium) and undergoes endochondral ossification.

occurs predominantly in males, but because of its variable expression, a seemingly unaffected female from an afflicted family may transmit the disorder to her offspring.

 PATHOLOGY: Each individual lesion in multiple osteochondromatosis is identical to a solitary osteochondroma. In severe cases of hereditary osteochondromatosis, dwarfism may result because of lateral displacement of the longitudinal growth plate by the osteochondroma. Metacarpals may be shortened, and fixed pronation or supination may develop if the lesions occur in the forearm and interfere with wrist function. Further difficulties may be caused by unequal leg length and disturbed joint function because of encroaching osteochondromas. Chondrosarcoma is a rare complication.

Solitary Chondroma Is a Benign Intraosseus Tumor of Mature Hyaline Cartilage

Although their neoplastic nature has been questioned, these benign tumors, also called **enchondromas (because most are intramedullary),** may occasionally show chromosomal abnormalities suggesting that they are in fact neoplasms. They occur at any age, and many cases are entirely asymptomatic. Rarely, they arise on the bone surface under the periosteum, in which case they are regarded as periosteal or juxtacortical chondromas.

 PATHOLOGY: Most solitary enchondromas occur in the metacarpals and phalanges of the hands, the remainder being in almost any other tubular bone. The tumor is usually small and grows slowly. Radiologically, it appears as an intramedullary, well-delimited, radiolucent area, sometimes containing stippled calcifications (Fig. 30-42A). On gross examination, solitary enchondromas have the semitranslucent appearance of hyaline cartilage, often with a few calcified areas. Microscopically, the cartilaginous tissue is well differentiated with sparse

chondrocytes, extensive cartilaginous matrix and a lobular configuration (Fig. 30-42B). Asymptomatic enchondromas are best left untreated and followed radiographically. When pain or pathologic fracture occurs, curettage and bone grafting are the treatment of choice. Recurrences are uncommon.

Enchondromatosis Is Marked by Multiple Cartilaginous Tumors

Enchondromatosis, or Ollier disease, *is characterized by development of multiple cartilaginous masses that lead to bony deformities.* The condition is not strictly a disease of delayed maturation of bone; residual hyaline cartilage, anlage cartilage or cartilage from the growth plate does not undergo endochondral ossification and remains in the bones. As a consequence, bones show multiple, tumor-like masses of abnormally arranged hyaline cartilage (enchondromas), with zones of proliferative and hypertrophied cartilage (Fig. 30-43). These tumors tend to be located in the metaphyses. As growth continues, the enchondromas settle in the diaphysis of adolescents and adults.

Enchondromatosis is asymmetric and may cause bone deformities. There is a strong tendency for malignant transformation, mostly into chondrosarcoma. Therefore, a patient with enchondromatosis who has increasing pain or a lesion that is actively growing should be evaluated to rule out an underlying sarcoma.

Solitary enchondroma and enchondromas of Ollier disease are histologically similar, but the latter tend to be more cellular and atypical.

Maffucci syndrome is characterized by multiple enchondromas and cavernous or spindle cell hemangiomas of soft tissue. It usually manifests in early childhood and may lead to significant skeletal deformities. Chondrosarcoma develops in as many as half of all patients with Maffucci syndrome. The incidence of extraskeletal malignant tumors of different types (i.e., carcinomas, gliomas, etc.) is also greatly increased in patients with Maffucci syndrome.

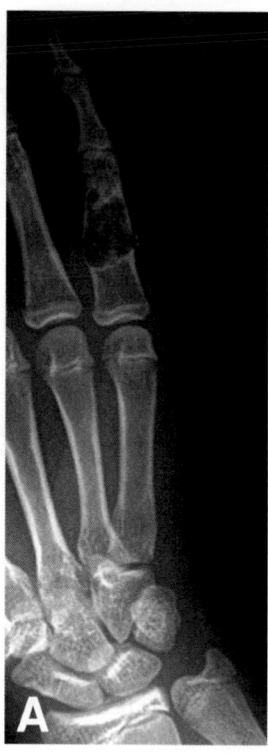

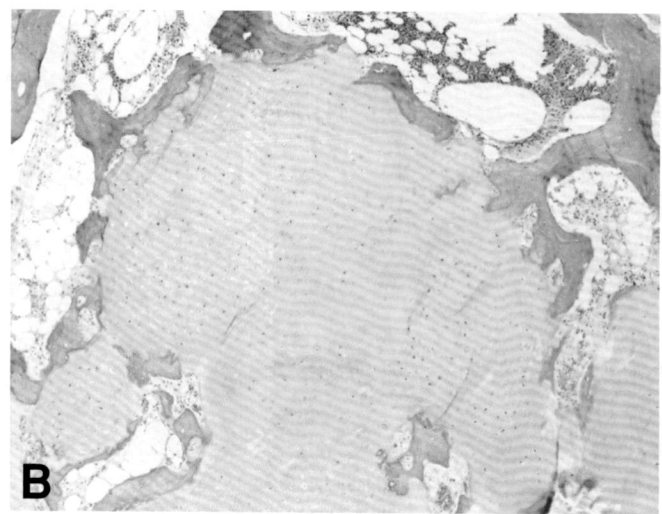

FIGURE 30-42. Enchondroma. A. An x-ray of an enchondroma demonstrates a well-demarcated, lytic lesion in the diaphysis of the proximal phalanx with internal calcification and associated pathologic fracture. **B.** Histologically, the tumor is composed of lobules of hypocellular hyaline cartilage without atypia.

MOLECULAR PATHOGENESIS: Most cases of enchondromatosis are sporadic, but a familial form, possibly with autosomal dominant inheritance, has been reported. Recent studies have disclosed mutations in the *PTHR1* gene, encoding a receptor for PTH and PTHrP, in some cases of enchondromatosis. The mutation results in a substitution in the receptor's extracellular domain, increasing cAMP signaling. The mutant receptor may delay chondrocyte differentiation by activating Hedgehog signaling, which results in the formation of the multiple cartilaginous masses characteristic of the disease.

Chondroblastoma Is a Benign Tumor of the Epiphyses of Long Bones

Chondroblastoma is an uncommon, chondrogenic tumor with predilection for epiphyses of the proximal femur, tibia and humerus. It is more common in males than in females (2:1), and 90% of cases occur in young people between the ages of 5 and 25.

MOLECULAR PATHOGENESIS: Genetic abnormalities suggest a neoplastic origin of chondroblastoma, including aneuploidy, abnormalities involving chromosomes 5 and 8 and mutations in the *p53* gene.

PATHOLOGY: Chondroblastoma grows slowly and on radiologic examination displays an eccentric, radiolucent appearance with sharply defined borders (Fig. 30-44A). On gross examination, the tumor is soft and compact with scattered gray or hemorrhagic areas. Microscopically, primitive chondroblasts are arranged as sheets of round to polyhedral cells that have well-defined cytoplasmic borders and large, ovoid nuclei, often with prominent nuclear grooves (Fig. 30-44B). Osteoclastic-type giant cells are frequently present. The usually scanty cartilage matrix is variably calcified and appears primitive. This accounts for the mottled pattern often seen in CT scans. Well-developed hyaline cartilage as seen in enchondroma is not found in chondroblastoma. The tumor causes bone

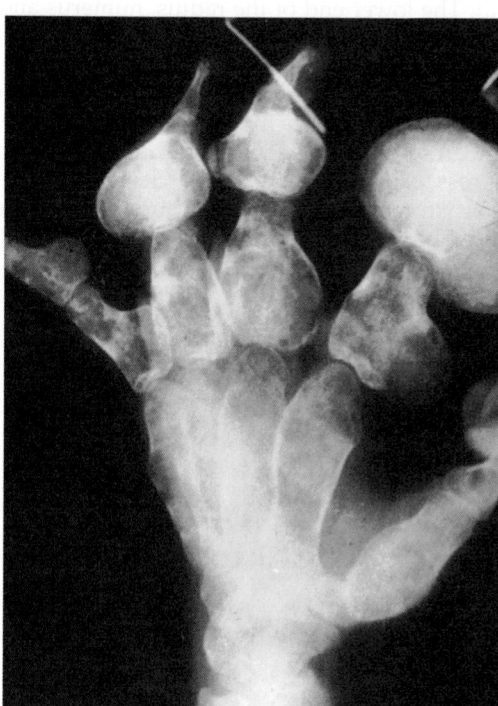

FIGURE 30-43. Multiple enchondromatosis (Ollier disease). A radiograph of the hand shows bulbous swellings that represent nodular masses composed of hyaline cartilage, which is sometimes admixed with more primitive myxoid cartilage.

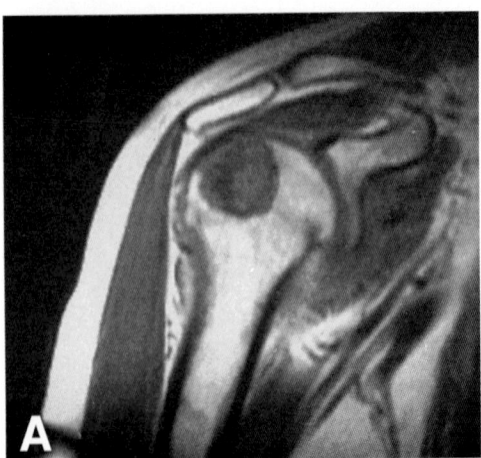
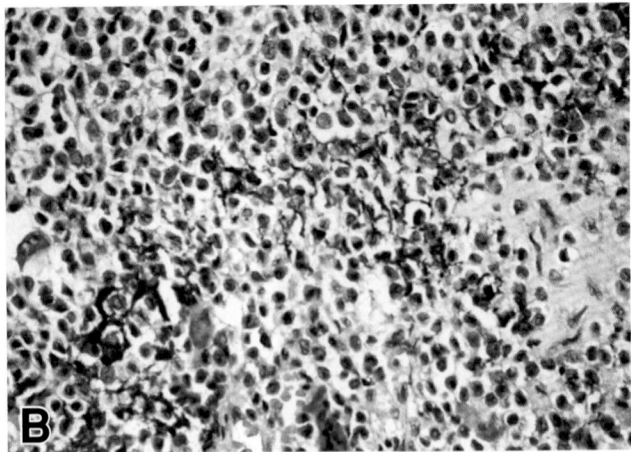

FIGURE 30-44. Chondroblastoma. A. A magnetic resonance image of the shoulder of a child shows a prominent lytic lesion of the head of the humerus that involves the epiphysis and extends across the epiphyseal plate. **B.** The histologic appearance of a chondroblastoma is defined by plump, round cells (chondroblasts) surrounded by a mineralized primitive chondroid matrix.

destruction by stimulating osteoclastic resorption. In fact, these neoplasms may perforate the cortex, although they remain confined by the periosteum.

 **CLINICAL FEATURES:** Because of its para-articular location, chondroblastoma tends to cause joint pain, with mild swelling and functional limitation of joint movement. If neglected, it may (rarely) attain a large size, destroy the epiphyseal area and invade the joint. Curettage is the treatment of choice, although in over 10% of cases, the tumor recurs.

Giant Cell Tumors of Bone Rarely Metastasize

Giant cell tumor (GCT) of bone is a benign, locally aggressive neoplasm characterized by the presence of osteoclastic, multinucleated giant cells, randomly and uniformly distributed in a background of proliferating mononuclear cells. It usually occurs in the third and fourth decades, has a slight predilection for women and seems to be more common in Asia than in Western countries. Paget disease may produce a giant cell reactive lesion that closely resembles a true GCT.

 MOLECULAR PATHOGENESIS: GCT is composed of numerous, large osteoclastic giant cells and two lineages of mononuclear cells. One population of mononuclear cells is believed to be of macrophage-monocyte origin and is likely nonneoplastic. The other has a preosteoblastic phenotype and is the neoplastic cell of GCT. These tumor cells produce RANKL and induce osteoclast formation (hence the large number of giant cells).

 PATHOLOGY: In most cases (90%), GCT of bone originates at the junction between the epiphysis and the metaphysis of a long bone, with more than half being situated in the knee area (distal femur and proximal tibia). The lower end of the radius, humerus and fibula are also occasionally involved. Radiologically, the tumor presents as an eccentric, expansile, lytic lesion with no matrix formation, which tends to be surrounded by a thin bony shell (Fig. 30-45A). Often, it has a multiloculated or "soap bubble" appearance, representing endosteal resorption of the bone.

On gross examination, GCT is clearly circumscribed and its cut surface is soft and light brown, without bone or calcification. Numerous hemorrhagic areas result in the

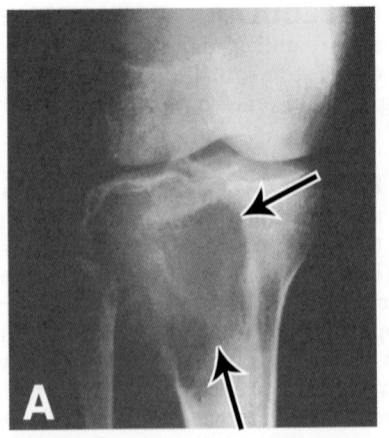
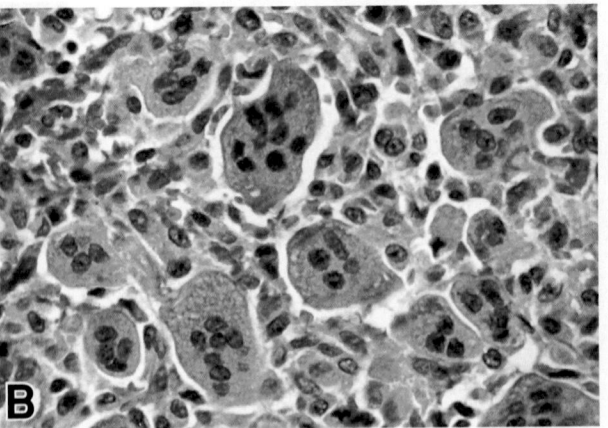

FIGURE 30-45. Giant cell tumor of bone. A. Radiograph of the proximal tibia shows an eccentric lytic lesion with virtually no new bone formation (*arrows*). The tumor extends to the subchondral bone plate and breaks through cortex into the soft tissue. **B.** Photomicrograph shows osteoclast-type giant cells and plump, oval, mononuclear cells. The nuclei of both types of cells are identical.

appearance of a sponge full of blood. In some cases, cystic cavities and necrotic areas are present. GCT is often limited by the periosteum, although aggressive forms penetrate the cortex and the periosteum, even reaching the joint capsule and the synovial membrane.

Microscopically, GCT exhibits two types of cells (Fig. 30-45B). The mononuclear ("stromal") cells are plump and oval, with large nuclei and scanty cytoplasm. Large osteoclastic giant cells, some with more than 100 nuclei, are scattered throughout the richly vascularized stroma. Diffuse interstitial hemorrhage is common. Secondary aneurysmal bone cyst may also be seen. On low-power examination, the tumor often appears as a syncytium of nuclei with poor demarcation of cytoplasmic borders and random distribution of the giant cells. It is evident that the mononuclear cells are the neoplastic and proliferative components of GCT (mitotic activity is common in the mononuclear cells but is not observed in the giant cells). Indeed, the diagnosis of malignancy in a GCT depends on the morphology of the mononuclear cells rather than that of the multinucleated cells.

 CLINICAL FEATURES: The vast majority of GCTs are considered benign, but locally aggressive tumors have the potential to recur locally after simple curettage and (rarely) metastasize to distant sites, particularly the lungs. Virtually all metastases have occurred after an initial surgical intervention and have the benign histology in appearance of the primary tumor. In contrast to patients with lung metastases from other malignant bone tumors, most of these patients enjoy an essentially normal life span, especially if the metastatic deposits are few and can be surgically removed. Thus, historical belief has been that local recurrence of the tumor reflects inadequate resection rather than biological aggressiveness and that distant metastases result from dislodgment of tumor fragments during surgery.

True malignancy in GCT is observed in 1% of cases as either a sarcomatous lesion arising in a typical GCT or as a pure sarcoma after a GCT has been curetted. Recurrence as pure sarcoma may occur spontaneously or after local radiation therapy.

GCTs manifest with pain, usually in the joint adjacent to the tumor. Microfractures and pathologic fractures are frequent, owing to thinning of the cortex. The tumor is treated with thorough curettage and bone grafting, although more aggressive management, including en bloc resection or even amputation, may be necessary. Local recurrence after simple curettage has been reported in one third to one half of cases, and 2%–5% metastasize to the lungs.

MALIGNANT TUMORS OF BONE

Osteosarcoma Is the Most Common Primary Malignant Bone Tumor

Osteosarcoma, or osteogenic sarcoma, is a highly malignant bone tumor characterized by formation of bone tissue by tumor cells. It represents one fifth of all bone cancers and is most frequent in adolescents between 10 and 20 years old, affecting boys more often than girls (2:1).

 **MOLECULAR PATHOGENESIS:** Conventional osteosarcoma has complex karyotypes, with multiple numerical and structural chromosomal aberrations. Osteosarcomas are associated with mutations in tumor suppressor genes; almost two thirds show mutations in the retinoblastoma (*Rb*) gene (see Chapter 5) and many have mutations in the *p53* gene. There are also many other chromosomal and molecular abnormalities pertaining to apoptosis, replicative potential, insensitivity to growth inhibitory signals and cell cycle regulation that contribute in some part to the development of the tumor. For example, amplification of *MDM2, CDK4* and *PRIM1,* as well as overexpression of *MET* and *FOS,* have been detected in a significant proportion of cases.

 **ETIOLOGIC FACTORS:** These tumors are more common in tall people. Interestingly, they occur more frequently in tall breeds of dogs. In older people, they usually occur in the context of Paget disease or radiation exposure. For example, radium watch dial painters, who wetted their brushes by licking them, developed osteosarcoma many years later, owing to radium depositing in their bones. Today, osteosarcoma can develop in adults and children previously subjected to external therapeutic radiation for some other tumor such as lymphoma. Several preexisting benign bone lesions are associated with an increased risk of developing osteosarcoma, including fibrous dysplasia, osteomyelitis and bone infarcts. Although trauma may call attention to an existing osteosarcoma, there is no evidence that it ever causes the tumor.

 PATHOLOGY: Osteosarcomas often arise near the knee, in the distal femur (Fig. 30-46A), proximal tibia or fibula, although any metaphyseal area of a long bone may be affected. The proximal humerus is the second most common site; 75% of tumors arise adjacent to the knee or shoulder.

Radiologic evidence of bone destruction and bone formation by osteosarcoma is characteristic, the latter representing neoplastic bone. Often, the periosteum produces an incomplete rim of reactive bone adjacent to the site where it is lifted from the cortical surface by the tumor. When this appears on a radiograph as a shell of bone intersecting the cortex at one end and open at the other end, it is referred to as **Codman triangle**. A "sunburst" periosteal reaction is also often superimposed (Fig. 30-15).

The gross appearance of osteosarcoma is highly variable, depending on the proportions of bone, cartilage, stroma and blood vessels. The cut surface may show any combination of hemorrhagic, cystic, soft and bony areas. The neoplastic tissue may invade and break through the cortex, spread into the marrow cavity, elevate or perforate the periosteum or grow into the epiphysis and even reach the joint space.

Histologic examination reveals malignant polygonal to spindled cells with osteoblastic differentiation, producing woven bone (Fig. 30-46B). The malignant cells have large hyperchromatic and pleomorphic nuclei, with a high nucleocytoplasmic ratio. Numerous mitoses, including atypical forms, are commonly seen. The tumor cells stain prominently for alkaline phosphatase, osteocalcin and osteonectin. The tumorous bone is laid down haphazardly and not aligned along stress lines. Often, foci of malignant cartilage or pleomorphic giant cells are intermixed. In areas of osteolysis, nonneoplastic osteoclasts are found at the advancing front of the tumor.

Osteosarcoma spreads through the bloodstream to the lungs. In fact, almost all patients (98%) who die of this

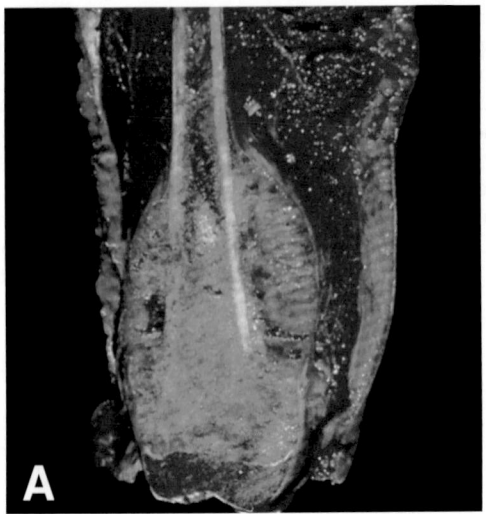
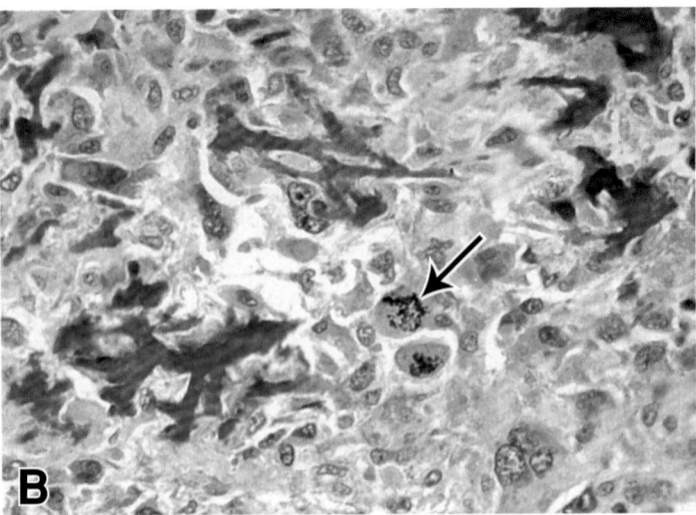

FIGURE 30-46. Osteosarcoma. A. The distal femur contains a dense osteoblastic malignant tumor that extends through the cortex into the soft tissue and the epiphysis. **B.** A photomicrograph reveals pleomorphic malignant cells, tumor giant cells and mitoses (*arrows*). The tumor cells produce woven bone that is focally calcified.

disease have lung metastases. Less commonly, the tumor metastasizes to other bones (35%), the pleura (33%) and the heart (20%).

CLINICAL FEATURES: Osteosarcoma presents with mild or intermittent pain around the involved area. As pain intensifies, the area becomes swollen and tender. The adjacent joint becomes functionally limited. Serum alkaline phosphatase is increased in half of patients and may decrease after amputation, only to increase again with recurrence or metastasis. Metastatic disease heralds rapid clinical deterioration and death.

Historically, osteosarcoma was treated exclusively by amputation or disarticulation of the involved limb, but the prognosis for 5-year survival did not exceed 20%. Today, standard therapy with preoperative chemotherapy and limb-sparing surgery gives 5-year disease-free rates from 60% to 80%. Resection of isolated pulmonary metastases may prolong survival.

Juxtacortical osteosarcoma is a rare variant of osteosarcoma that occurs on the surface of the bone, especially the lower posterior metaphysis of the femur (70% of cases). Unlike classic osteosarcoma, most patients are older than 25 years, and the tumor is more common in women. Juxtacortical osteosarcoma spares the deep cortex and medulla of the bone and grows external to the shaft. Usually, Codman triangle is not evident radiologically, because the periosteum is not elevated. Most juxtacortical osteosarcomas are low-grade lesions and do not require adjunctive chemotherapy. Surgical excision is the treatment of choice. The prognosis is good, with a 5-year survival of more than 80%.

Other rare variants of osteosarcoma include telangiectatic and small cell osteosarcoma, which are high-grade tumors, and low-grade intramedullary osteosarcoma.

Chondrosarcoma Is a Cartilaginous Malignancy Whose Grade Determines Prognosis

Chondrosarcoma is a malignant tumor of cartilage that arises from a preexisting cartilage rest or a preexisting lesion like an enchondroma. Some patients have a history of multiple enchondromas, solitary osteochondroma or hereditary multiple osteochondromas. Most have no known preexisting lesion. *Chondrosarcoma is the second most common primary malignant bone tumor and is more common in men than in women (2:1).* It is most frequently seen in the fourth to sixth decades (average age, 45 years).

MOLECULAR PATHOGENESIS: Numerous nonrandom chromosomal abnormalities have been discovered in chondrosarcoma. There probably is a different molecular mechanism resulting in tumor development between central chondrosarcoma and secondary peripheral chondrosarcoma (tumors arising in the cartilaginous cap of an osteochondroma; see below). The latter may develop by upregulation of PTHrP and Bcl-2 expression in an osteochondroma, along with mutations in other genes such as *p53* and nonspecific chromosomal abnormalities. Development of central chondrosarcoma is related, at least in part, to abnormalities of chromosome 9p12-22, which may involve the *CDKN2A* tumor suppressor gene. The transcription factor *SOX9*, which plays a critical role in normal chondrocyte development, is expressed in chondrosarcomas.

PATHOLOGY: Chondrosarcoma occurs in three anatomic variants:

CENTRAL CHONDROSARCOMA: This form arises in the medullary cavity of pelvic bones, ribs and long bones, although any site may be affected. Radiologically, poorly defined borders, a thickened shaft and perforation of the cortex characterize these tumors. There are usually stippled or ring-like radiopacities representing calcification or endochondral ossification in the tumor (Fig. 30-47A). Although central chondrosarcoma may penetrate the cortex, extension beyond the periosteum is uncommon. On gross examination, the neoplastic cartilaginous tissue is compressed inside the bone and exhibits areas of necrosis, cystic change and hemorrhage (Fig. 30-47B). The cortex of the bone and the intertrabecular spaces of the marrow are infiltrated by the tumor.

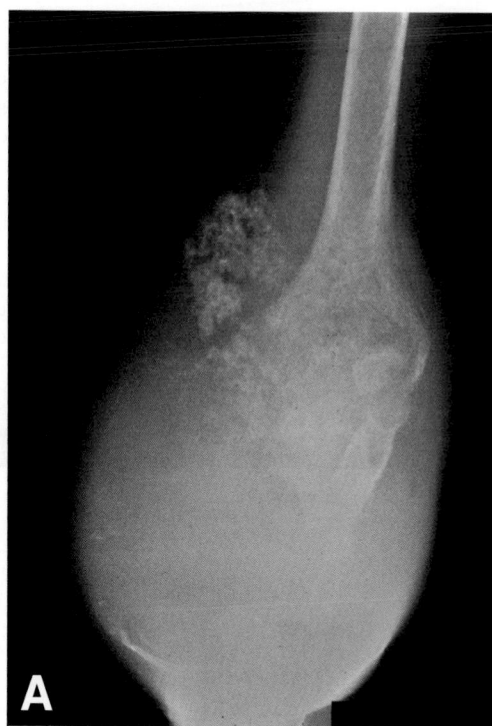

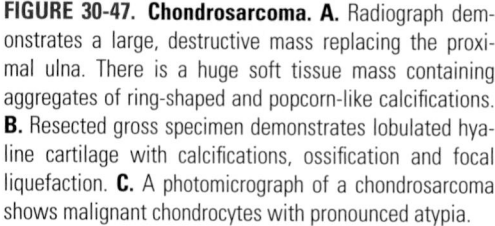

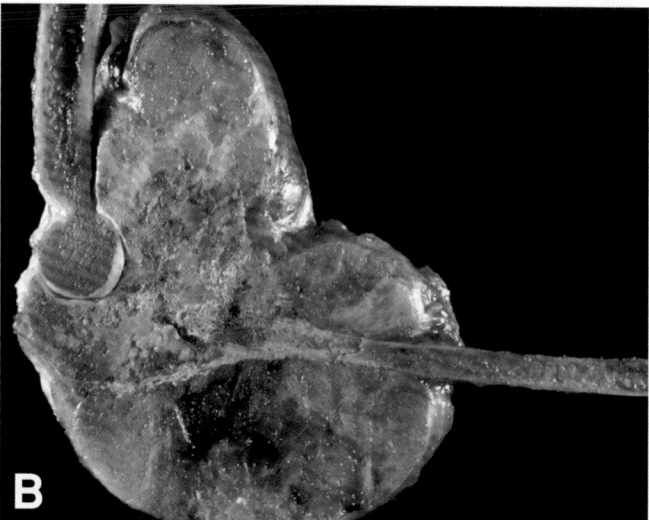

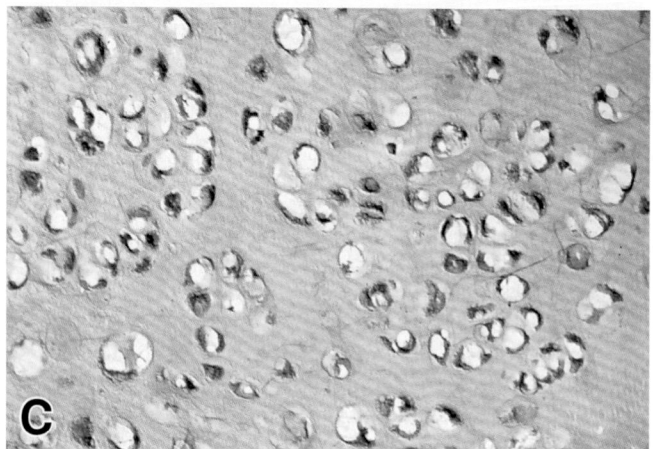

FIGURE 30-47. Chondrosarcoma. A. Radiograph demonstrates a large, destructive mass replacing the proximal ulna. There is a huge soft tissue mass containing aggregates of ring-shaped and popcorn-like calcifications. **B.** Resected gross specimen demonstrates lobulated hyaline cartilage with calcifications, ossification and focal liquefaction. **C.** A photomicrograph of a chondrosarcoma shows malignant chondrocytes with pronounced atypia.

Central chondrosarcoma begins with deep pain, which becomes more intense with time. The tumor is only rarely palpable, but in untreated cases, large masses may eventually form.

PERIPHERAL CHONDROSARCOMA: This variant is less common than the central variety of chondrosarcoma and arises outside the bone, almost always in the cartilaginous cap of an osteochondroma. It occurs after the age of 20 years and never before puberty. The most frequent location of peripheral chondrosarcoma is the pelvis, followed by the femur, vertebrae, sacrum, humerus and other long bones. It arises only rarely distal to the knee or elbow. Radiologically, characteristic radiopacities, representing calcification or ossification of the neoplastic cartilage, are virtually pathognomonic for the lesion. Macroscopically, peripheral chondrosarcoma tends to be a large bosselated mass that surrounds the base of an osteochondroma and invades and destroys the bone.

Peripheral chondrosarcoma is usually seen as a slowly growing mass. Expansion of the mass causes pain and local symptoms. In the pelvis, the lumbosacral plexus may be compressed, and tumors in the vertebrae may cause paraplegia.

JUXTACORTICAL CHONDROSARCOMA: This is the least common variety of chondrosarcoma and is similar to central chondrosarcoma in its predilection for middle-aged men. It tends to be situated in the metaphysis of long bones, lying on the outer surface of the cortex. Thus, it is probably periosteal or parosteal in origin. Radiologically, it may be entirely translucent or focally calcified. The symptoms of juxtacortical chondrosarcoma are dominated by swelling, with little accompanying pain.

Histologically, chondrosarcomas are composed of malignant cartilage cells in various stages of maturity (Fig. 30-47C). Occasionally, a well-differentiated chondrosarcoma is difficult to distinguish from a benign enchondroma on cytologic grounds alone. Zones of calcification are often conspicuous and are seen radiographically as splotches or bulky masses. Chondrosarcoma expands by stimulating osteoclastic resorption of bone and often breaks through the cortex. Most chondrosarcomas grow slowly, but hematogenous metastases to the lungs are common in poorly differentiated variants.

There is a positive correlation between histologic grade, morphologic features and the degree of karyotypic complexity. Trisomy 7 is associated with chondrosarcoma. Rearrangement of the short arm of chromosome 17 is associated with high-grade chondrosarcoma. Alterations of 12q13 are found in tumors that exhibit myxoid features.

OTHER VARIANTS OF CHONDROSARCOMA: The above forms of chondrosarcoma are all characterized by a hyaline cartilage matrix. Uncommon histopathologic variants of chondrosarcoma include **clear cell chondrosarcoma,** which occurs almost exclusively in the proximal epiphysis of the femur or humerus and is composed of chondrocytes with abundant clear cytoplasm, areas of woven trabecular bone and focal regions with a hyaline cartilage matrix. The prognosis for this tumor following complete excision is close to that of a conventional low-grade chondrosarcoma. **Dedifferentiated chondrosarcoma** is defined as a high-grade nonchondrogenic pleomorphic sarcoma (e.g., osteosarcoma or fibrosarcoma) arising in association with a low-grade conventional chondrosarcoma or enchondroma. This tumor usually arises in flat bones of the pelvis or long bones of the extremities and has a dismal prognosis, with less than 10% of patients surviving 5 years. Another variant is known as **mesenchymal chondrosarcoma** and is histologically characterized by two distinct components. The first is a high-grade

malignant, small, round, blue-cell tumor that resembles Ewing sarcoma. Sheets of these cells are interrupted by discrete islands of malignant hyaline cartilage histologically similar to conventional chondrosarcoma. The bones of the jaw and the chest wall are the most commonly affected sites. The prognosis for these tumors is poor.

CLINICAL FEATURES: Patients generally present with pain at the affected site. Chondrosarcoma is one of the few tumors in which microscopic grading has a significant prognostic value. The 5-year survival rate for low-grade conventional chondrosarcomas is

---

TABLE 30-2

SELECTED CHROMOSOMAL ABNORMALITIES IN SOFT TISSUE TUMORS

Tumor Type	Chromosomal Abnormality	Gene(s)
Fibroblastic Tumors		
Nodular fasciitis	t(17;22)(p13;q13)	*MYH9-USP6*
Congenital/infantile fibrosarcoma	t(12;15)(p13;q25)	*ETV6-NTRK3*
Dermatofibrosarcoma protuberans	t(17;22)(q21;q13)	*COLIA1-PDGFB*
Low-grade fibromyxoid sarcoma	t(7;16)(q33;p11)	*FUS-CREB3L2*
	t(11;16)(p11;p11)	*FUS-CREB3L1*
Sclerosing epithelioid fibrosarcoma	t(7;16)(p22;q24)	*FUS-CREB3L2*
Inflammatory myofibroblastic tumor	t(1;2)(q22;p23)	*TPM3-ALK*
	t(2;19)(p23;p13)	*TPM4-ALK*
	t(2;17)(p23;q23)	*CLTC-ALK*
	t(2;2)(p23;q13)	*RANBP2-ALK*
	t(2;11)(p23;p15)	*CARS-ALK*
	inv(2)(p23;q35)	*ATIC-ALK*
Lipogenic Tumors		
Well-differentiated liposarcoma/atypical lipomatous tumor/dedifferentiated liposarcoma	12q14-15 (ring chromosomes, giant marker chromosomes)	Amplification of *MDM2, CDK4, HMGA2, GLI, SAS*
Myxoid/round cell liposarcoma	t(12;16)(q13;p11)	*FUS-DD1T3*
	t(12;22)(q13;q12)	*EWSR1-DD1T3*
Myogenic Tumors		
Alveolar rhabdomyosarcoma	t(2;13)(q35;q14)	*PAX3-FKHR*
	t(1;13)(p36;q14)	*PAX7-FKHR*
	t(X;2)(q13;q35)	*PAX3-AFX*
Neuroectodermal Tumors		
Clear-cell sarcoma	t(12;22)(q13;q12)	*EWSR1-ATF1*
	t(2;22)(q33;q12)	*EWSR1-CREB1*
Ewing sarcoma; primitive neuroectodermal tumor (PNET)	t(11;12)(q24;q12)	*EWSR1-FLI1*
	t(21;22)(q22;q12)	*EWSR1-ERG*
	t(7;22)(p22;q12)	*EWSR1-ETV1*
	t(2;22)(q33;q12)	*EWSR1-FEV*
	t(16;21)(p11;q22)	*FUS-ERG*
	t(2;16)(q35;p11)	*FUS-FEV*
Synovial sarcoma	t(X;18)(p11;q11)	*SS18-SSX1, SSX2, SSX4*

80%, for moderate-grade tumors 50% and for high-grade tumors only 20%. Wide excision is the usual treatment, since response to radiation and chemotherapy is poor.

Ewing Sarcoma Is a Primitive Neuroectodermal Tumor of Childhood

Ewing sarcoma (EWS) is an uncommon malignant bone tumor composed of small, uniform, round cells (blue cells). It represents only 5% of all bone tumors and is found in children and adolescents, with two thirds of cases occurring in patients younger than 20 years. Boys are affected more often than girls (2:1). EWS is very rare in blacks. About 10%–20% of Ewing sarcomas are extraskeletal.

MOLECULAR PATHOGENESIS: EWS is thought to arise from primitive marrow elements or immature mesenchymal cells. Most (90%) of these tumors have a reciprocal translocation between chromosomes 11 and 22 [t(11;22)(q24;q12)], resulting in the fusion of the amino terminus of the *EWS1* gene to the carboxy terminus of the *FLI-1* gene, which encodes a transcription factor. The resulting fusion protein, EWS/FLI-1, is an aberrant transcription factor whose target genes are not yet fully identified. A less common translocation, t(21;22)(q22;q12), generates *EWS/ERG* gene fusion. Other alternate chromosomal rearrangements seen in EWS are listed in Table 30-2.

PATHOLOGY: EWS is primarily a tumor of the long bones in childhood, especially the humerus, tibia and femur, where it occurs as a midshaft or metaphyseal lesion. It tends to parallel the distribution of red marrow, so when it arises in the third decade or later, it affects the pelvis and spine. However, no bone is immune from involvement.

The radiographic findings are variable and depend on the interaction of the tumor with the host bone. There is often a destructive process in which the border between normal bone and the lesion is indistinct. Periosteal reaction and a soft tissue mass are also commonly seen (Fig. 30-48A). The onion-skin pattern of periosteal bone that is sometimes present on radiologic examination represents circumferential discontinuous layers of periosteal new bone associated with a lytic lesion in the medulla and endosteal surface of the cortex. Some patients present with fever and weakness as well as bone pain, so it is not surprising that their condition may be mistaken for osteomyelitis.

On gross examination, EWS is typically soft and grayish white, often studded by hemorrhagic foci and necrotic areas. The tumor may infiltrate the medullary spaces without destroying the bony trabeculae. It may also diffusely infiltrate the cortical bone or form nodules in which the bone is completely resorbed. In many cases, the tumor mass penetrates the periosteum and extends into the soft tissues.

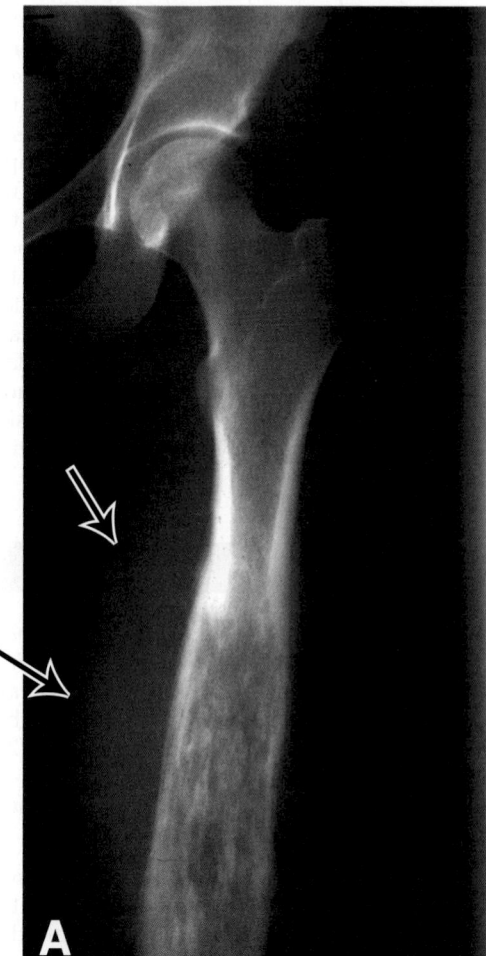

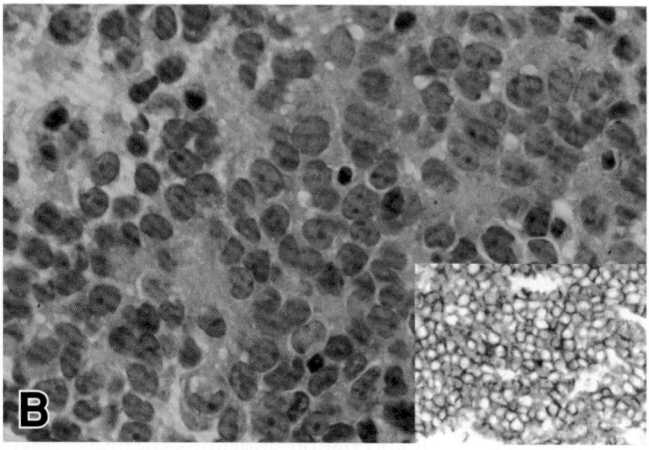

FIGURE 30-48. Ewing sarcoma. A. A clinical radiograph demonstrates expansile cortical destruction with poor circumscription and a delicate interrupted periosteal reaction (*arrows*). **B.** A biopsy specimen shows fairly uniform small cells with round, dark blue nuclei and poorly defined cytoplasm. Immunohistochemical stain for CD99 shows a membranous pattern (*inset*).

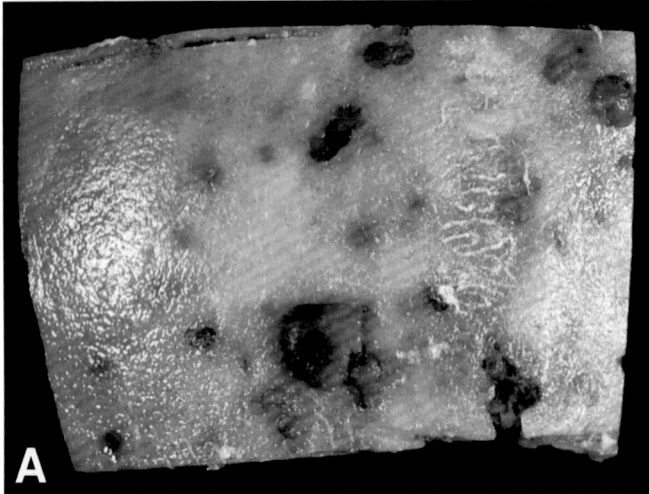
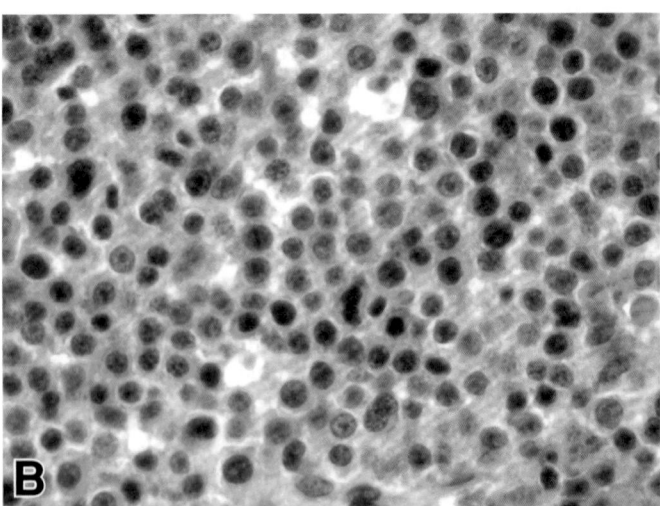

FIGURE 30-49. Multiple myeloma. A. A segment of the skull from a patient with multiple myeloma reveals numerous punched-out, lytic lesions. **B.** Microscopically, the lesions are composed of sheets of plasma cells with atypia, binucleation and discernible nucleoli.

Microscopically, EWS cells appear as sheets of closely packed, small, round cells with little cytoplasm, which are up to twice the size of a lymphocyte (Fig. 30-48B). Fibrous strands separate the sheets of cells into irregular nests. There is little or no interstitial stroma, and mitoses are frequent. In some areas, the neoplastic cells tend to form rosettes. An important diagnostic feature is the presence of substantial amounts of glycogen in the cytoplasm of the tumor cells, which is well visualized with the periodic acid–Schiff (PAS) stain. EWS cells also express characteristic antigens that can be detected by immunohistochemistry (Fig. 30-48B, *inset*), some of which are part of the translocation product (e.g., CD99 and FLI-1).

EWS metastasizes to many organs, including the lungs and brain. Other bones, especially the skull, are common sites for metastases (50%–75% of cases).

 CLINICAL FEATURES: EWS initially presents with mild pain, which becomes more intense and is followed by swelling of the affected area. Nonspecific symptoms, including fever and leukocytosis, commonly follow. In some cases, a soft tissue mass is encountered.

Although EWS prognosis used to be dismal, with current use of chemotherapy plus radiation and limb-sparing surgery, the 5-year disease-free survival is 60%–75% in the absence of metastases.

Multiple Myeloma Produces Lytic Lesions in Bone

Malignant plasma cell tumors may be either localized (plasmacytoma) or diffuse (see Chapter 26). Multiple myeloma occurs mostly in older people (average age, 65) and affects men twice as often as women. Because myeloma cells secrete cytokines that recruit osteoclasts, the lesions are unique in that they are almost exclusively lytic. The bones most frequently involved are the skull (Fig. 30-49A), spine, ribs, pelvis and femur. Pathologic fractures are common. On microscopic examination, sheets of plasma cells show varying degrees of maturity (Fig. 30-49B). Amyloid deposits, in both skeletal and extraskeletal sites, are seen in 10% of patients.

With newer therapeutic agents, the median survival of patients with multiple myeloma now is about 5 years. Death

is usually due to infection or renal failure. Solitary plasmacytoma has a better prognosis, with a 60% 5-year survival.

Metastatic Tumors Are the Most Common Malignant Tumors in Bone

In adults, most metastatic lesions to bone are carcinomas, particularly of the prostate, breast, lung, thyroid and kidney. In children, the most common bone metastases are from rhabdomyosarcoma, neuroblastoma, Wilms tumor and clear cell sarcoma of the kidney. It is estimated that skeletal metastases are found in at least 85% of cancer cases that have run their full clinical course. The vertebral column is the most common location in adults (Fig. 30-50A), and the appendicular skeleton is the most common site in children. Tumor cells usually arrive in the bone via the bloodstream; in the case of spinal metastases, the vertebral veins often transport them.

Some tumors (e.g., thyroid, gastrointestinal tract, kidney and neuroblastoma) produce mostly lytic lesions by stimulating osteoclasts (Fig. 30-50B). A few neoplasms (e.g., prostate, breast, lung, stomach) stimulate osteoblastic components to make bone, creating dense foci on radiographs (blastic or sclerotic lesions). However, most deposits of metastatic cancer in the bones have mixtures of both lytic and blastic elements.

Joints

A joint (or articulation) is a union between two or more bones, whose construction varies with the function of that joint. There are two types of joints: (1) a **synovial** or **diarthrodial joint,** which is a movable joint, such as the knee or elbow, that is lined by a synovial membrane; and (2) a **synarthrosis,** which is a joint that has little movement.

Synarthroses are further divided into four subclassifications:

- A **symphysis** is an articulation joined by fibrocartilaginous tissue and firm ligaments that allows little movement. Examples are the symphysis pubis and the ends of vertebral joints.

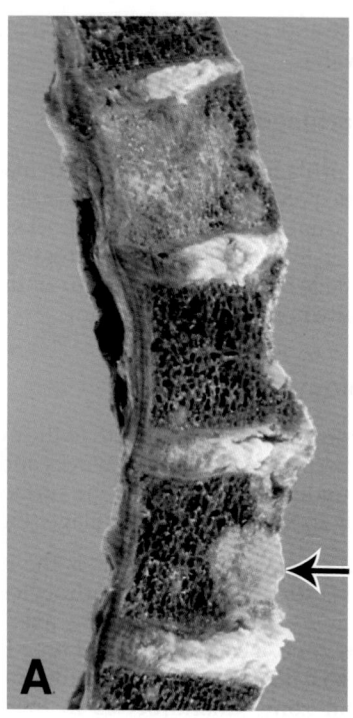

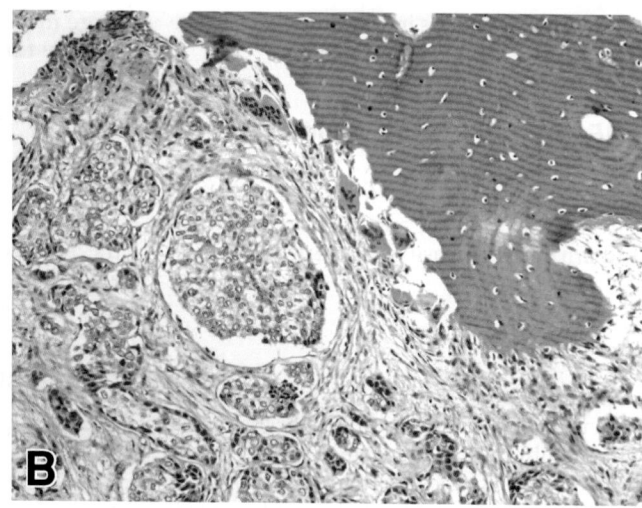

FIGURE 30-50. Metastatic carcinoma to bone. A. A section through the vertebral column reveals conspicuous tan nodules of metastatic tumor (*arrow*). **B.** Tumor-induced osteolysis. Breast cancer metastatic to bone recruits numerous osteoclasts, which resorb bone and lead to osteolytic lesions.

- A **synchondrosis** is found at the ends of bones and has articular cartilage but is not associated with synovium or a significant joint cavity (e.g., the sternal manubrial joint).
- A **syndesmosis** connects bones by fibrous tissue without any cartilaginous elements. The distal tibiofibular articulation and the cranial sutures are syndesmoses.
- A **synostosis** is a pathologic bony bridge between bones as, for example, in ankylosis of the spine.

Diseases of diarthrodial joints are among the oldest pathologic conditions known, having been found in the fossil bones of dinosaurs. One third of the population of the United States older than 50 years develop some form of clinically significant joint disease.

CLASSIFICATION OF SYNOVIAL JOINTS

The synovial, or diarthrodial, joints are classified according to the type of movement they permit.

- A **uniaxial joint** allows movement around only one axis. Examples include a hinge joint such as the elbow and a pivot (rotational) joint such as the radioulnar joint.
- A **biaxial joint** allows movement around two axes, as the condyloid joint of the wrist axis is oriented in the long diameter and the other along the short diameter of the articular surfaces. This allows four-way movement: flexion, extension, abduction and adduction. In a saddle joint, such as the carpometacarpal joint of the thumb, joint surfaces allow movement as in a condyloid joint.
- **Polyaxial joints** permit movement in virtually any axis. In a ball-and-socket joint, such as is found in the shoulder and hip, all movements, including rotation, are possible.
- A **plane joint**, represented by the patella, allows articular surfaces to glide over one another.

UNIT LOAD: **The concept of unit load is the most important principle in understanding joint function.** The unit load is the compressive force, expressed as kilograms per cubic centimeter of articular cartilage. It is fairly constant over the hip, knee and ankle (20–26 kg/cm^3 along the articular surfaces). Because the articular cartilage is injured if a load exceeds these values, several mechanisms protect a joint from exceeding the unit load.

Adjacent muscles are the major shock-absorbing structures that protect the joint. Deformation, even to the extent of microscopic fractures of the coarse cancellous bone, also helps protect the joint. Joint deformation allows the contact area to increase with increasing load. Diarthrodial joints may have intra-articular structures, such as ligaments and menisci. Menisci hold distributed force along the articular surface and allow two planes of motion, such as flexion and rotation. However, 90% or more of energy absorption across the knee joint is by active muscle contraction, and only 10% or less is by secondary mechanisms, such as by the coarse cancellous bone of the knee joint. A properly functioning joint also requires support from ligaments and tendons, periarticular connective tissues such as the joint capsule and nerves that provide proprioception. Thus, to protect the articular cartilage from forces that exceed the critical unit load, virtually any structure is sacrificed, even to the point of a bone fracture.

Once there is an insult to one component of the joint, the resulting dysfunction can lead to degeneration of other components of the joint. For example, knee ligament injuries sustained by athletes, such as a torn anterior cruciate ligament, can result in joint instability. Over time, this situation contributes to degeneration of articular cartilage, owing to changes in movement and load on the joint (secondary osteoarthritis).

ARTHRITIS: Arthritis refers to joint inflammation, usually accompanied by pain, swelling and sometimes change in structure. Arthritis is divided into two major forms: (1) **inflammatory arthritis** usually involves the synovium and is mediated by inflammatory cells (e.g., rheumatoid arthritis), and (2) **noninflammatory arthritis,** as featured in primary osteoarthritis, may involve cytokines in its pathogenesis (see below).

STRUCTURES OF THE SYNOVIAL JOINT

Movement plays a major role in joint formation. Lack of movement retards joint development and may cause **arthrogryposis,** a rare but crippling disease characterized by joint fusion.

Synovium

Synovial joints are partially lined on their internal aspects by the synovium. Synovial linings are not true membranes since they lack basement membranes to separate synovial lining cells from subsynovial tissue. The synovium is composed of one to three layers of lining cells and is made up of two cell types distinguishable only by electron microscopy. **Type A cells** are macrophages with lysosomal enzymes and dense bodies. **Type B cells** secrete hyaluronic acid. Synovial cell membranes are disposed in villi and microvilli, an arrangement that creates an enormous surface area. It is estimated that the knee alone has 100 m² of synovial lining.

The synovium controls (1) diffusion in and out of the joint; (2) ingestion of debris; (3) secretion of hyaluronate, immunoglobulins and lysosomal enzymes; and (4) lubrication of the joints by secreting glycoproteins. Synovial fluid is clear, sticky and viscous. It is present only in small amounts, not exceeding 1–4 mL, and is the main source of nourishment for chondrocytes of the articular cartilage, which lacks a blood supply. Synovial fluid is an ultrafiltrate that acts as a molecular sieve. It does not contain tissue thromboplastin and so cannot clot. Hyaluronate is a very large molecule and, because it is highly charged, has a high affinity for water.

Articular Cartilage

The hyaline cartilage that covers the articular ends of bones does not participate in endochondral ossification and is well suited for its dual role of absorbing shocks and lubricating the surfaces of movable joints. On gross examination, the articular cartilage is glistening, smooth, white and semirigid, and is generally not thicker than 6 mm.

Joint Histology

The articular surface appears smooth to the eye, but scanning electron microscopy reveals gentle waves and pits that correspond to the underlying lacunae of the surface chondrocytes. There are four zones in articular cartilage (Fig. 30-51).

- **Tangential** or **gliding zone:** This is the region closest to the articular surface, where chondrocytes are elongated, flattened and parallel to the long axis of the surface. Within this zone, a condensation of type II collagen fibers forms the so-called skin of the articular cartilage.
- **Transitional zone:** Chondrocytes in this slightly deeper zone are larger, ovoid and more randomly distributed than those in the tangential zone. The standard hyaline cartilage matrix is present, and by electron microscopy, the collagen fibers are arranged transverse to the articular surface.
- **Radial zone:** The next deeper zone is the radial zone, where chondrocytes are small and are arranged in short columns like those seen in the epiphyseal plate. In this area, collagen fibers are large and oriented perpendicular to the long axis of the articular surface.

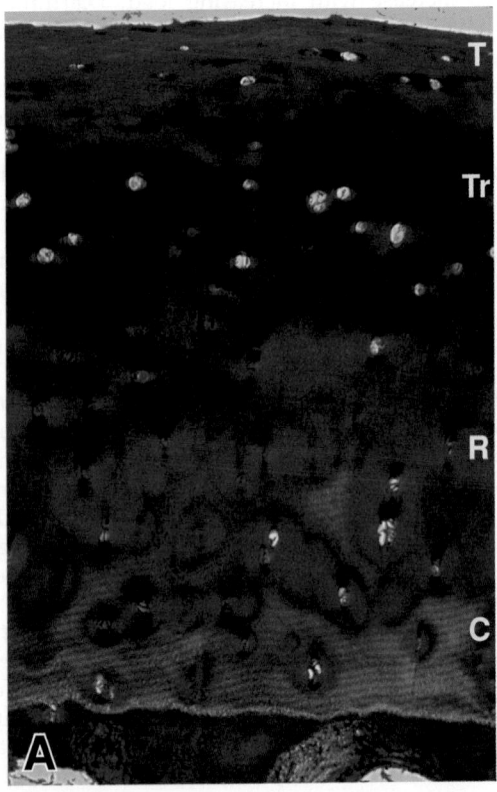

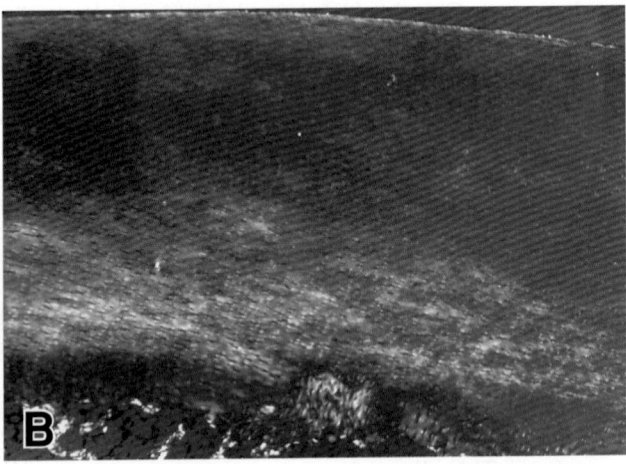

FIGURE 30-51. Articular hyaline cartilage. A. Demonstrating tangential zone (T), transitional zone (Tr), radial zone (R) and calcified zone (C). The chondrocyte lacunae change shape in conformation with the direction of the collagen arcades in the cartilage. **B.** Articular cartilage, polarized light. The tangential and radial zones have the highest concentration of collagen fibers and appear bright yellow.

- **Calcified zone:** Small chondrocytes and a heavily calcified matrix characterize the deepest region.

The calcified zone is separated from the radial zone by a transverse, undulating, heavily calcified "blue line" (evident on hematoxylin–eosin staining), called the **tidemark**. The tidemark is the interface between mineralized and unmineralized cartilage. Above the tidemark on the joint side, all of the cartilage is nourished by diffusion from the synovial fluid. Deep to the tidemark, the calcified cartilage is supplied by epiphyseal blood vessels.

The tidemark is the area where the cartilage cells are renewed. As a result of cell division, true articular chondrocytes migrate upward toward the joint surface. Cell division below the tidemark occurs in the calcified cartilage, if there is appropriate stimulation. For example, in acromegaly, when the epiphyseal plates have already closed, the bones may grow in minute increments, because growth hormone stimulates the calcified cartilage remnant of the epiphyseal cartilage anlage. Because the joints in acromegaly do not keep pace, joint incongruity leads to severe osteoarthritis. Deep to the calcified cartilage, the transverse bony plate, called the **subchondral bone plate,** supports the articular cartilage. It is directly contiguous with the coarse cancellous bone of the epiphysis.

OSTEOARTHRITIS

Osteoarthritis (OA), also known as degenerative joint disease (DJD), is a slowly progressive destruction of articular cartilage that affects weight-bearing joints and fingers of older individuals or the joints of younger people subjected to trauma. OA is the single most common form of joint disease and the major form of noninflammatory arthritis. It is a group of conditions that have in common the mechanical destruction of a joint.

In **primary OA,** destruction of joints results from intrinsic defects in the articular cartilage. The prevalence and severity of primary OA increase with age. About 4% of people aged 18–24 are affected, versus 85% of those 75–79 years. Before age 45, the disease mainly affects men. After age 55, OA is more common in women. Many cases of primary OA exhibit a familial clustering, suggesting a hereditary predisposition.

In primary OA, progressive degradation of articular cartilage leads to joint narrowing, subchondral bone thickening and eventually a nonfunctioning painful joint. Although OA is not primarily an inflammatory process, a mild inflammatory reaction may occur within the synovium.

Secondary OA has a known underlying cause, including congenital or acquired incongruity of joints, trauma, crystal deposits, infection, metabolic diseases, endocrinopathies, chronic inflammatory diseases, osteonecrosis and hemarthrosis.

Chondromalacia is a term applied to a subcategory of OA that affects the patellar surface of the femoral condyles of young people and produces pain and stiffness of the knee.

  ETIOLOGIC FACTORS:
INCREASED UNIT LOAD: Abnormal force on the cartilage may have many causes but is often attributable to incongruities of the joint. Thus, in congenital hip dysplasia, a fairly common abnormality, the socket of the

acetabulum is shallow, covering only 35% of the femoral head (normal, 50%). Less surface area is covered by articular cartilage, which thus bears an increased load. When the critical unit load is exceeded, chondrocyte death causes degradation of articular cartilage.

RESILIENCE OF THE ARTICULAR CARTILAGE: Because articular cartilage binds extensive amounts of water, it normally has a swelling pressure of at least 3 atmospheres. Disruption in water bonding leads to decreased resilience.

STIFFNESS OF SUBCHONDRAL COARSE CANCELLOUS BONE: The structure of bone adjacent to a joint is important in maintaining articular cartilage. Mechanical forces are not transferred to articular cartilage by normal stress, but rather are dissipated by microfractures of coarse cancellous bone. Damage to this structure results in an increased unit load on the cartilage because of an increase in the stiffness of subchondral bone (e.g., in Paget disease).

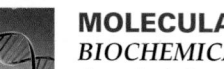 **MOLECULAR PATHOGENESIS:**
BIOCHEMICAL ABNORMALITIES: The biochemical changes of OA mainly involve proteoglycans. Proteoglycan content and aggregation decrease, and glycosaminoglycan chain length is reduced. Collagen fibers are thicker than normal and the water content of osteoarthritic cartilage increases. The reduction in proteoglycans allows more water to be bound to the collagen. Thus, osteoarthritic cartilage, or any cartilage that is fibrillated, swells more than normal cartilage.

Although matrix synthesis by chondrocytes is increased early in OA, protein synthesis eventually declines, suggesting that the cells reach a point at which they fail to respond to reparative stimuli. Similarly, chondrocytes in early osteoarthritic cartilage replicate, but cell replication diminishes with advanced disease. Acid cathepsin, which attacks the protein cores of the matrix macromolecules, increases in osteoarthritic cartilage. Collagenase is absent in normal cartilage but is found in osteoarthritic cartilage.

Chondrocyte apoptosis, decreased type II collagen synthesis and breakdown of extracellular matrix also occur and have been correlated with local increases in IL-1β and TNF-α. In turn, these cytokines induce increased production of matrix metalloproteinases (MMPs), nitric oxide and PGE$_2$. Mechanical stress appears to be the triggering factor for these signaling cascades.

Studies of identical twins have demonstrated genetic contributions to the prevalence of OA. Genetic analysis of patients with a type of familial, early-onset OA revealed a variety of mutations in the gene for type II collagen (*COL2A1*), the major collagen species of articular cartilage.

  PATHOLOGY: Joints commonly affected by OA are the proximal and distal interphalangeal joints, as well as the joints of the arms, knees, hips and cervical and lumbar spine. Radiologically, OA is characterized by (1) narrowing of the joint space, which represents the loss of articular cartilage; (2) increased thickness of the subchondral bone; (3) subchondral bone cysts; and (4) large peripheral growths of bone and cartilage, called **osteophytes** (Fig. 30-52). Histologic changes follow a well-described sequence.

1. First, loss of proteoglycans from the surface of the articular cartilage is seen histologically as decreased metachromatic staining. At the same time, empty lacunae in articular cartilage indicate that chondrocytes have died

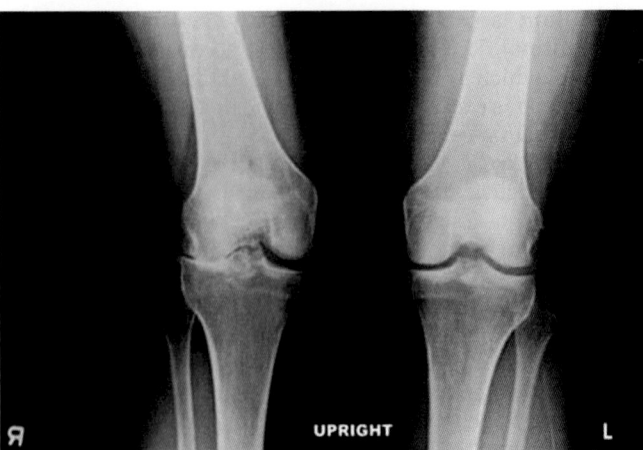

FIGURE 30-52. A radiograph of a patient with osteoarthritis of the right knee demonstrating marked narrowing of the joint space, increased density of subchondral bone and osteophyte formation laterally.

(Fig. 30-53A). Viable chondrocytes enlarge, aggregate into groups or clones (Fig. 30-53C) and become surrounded by basophilic staining matrix called the **territorial matrix**.

2. OA may arrest at this stage for many years before progressing to the next stage, which is characterized by fibrillation (i.e., development of surface cracks parallel to the long axis of the articular surface). These fibrillations may persist for many years before further progression occurs (Fig. 30-53B).

3. As fibrillations propagate, synovial fluid begins to flow into the defects. The cracks are progressively oriented more vertically, parallel to the long axis of the collagen fibrils. Synovial fluid penetrates deeper into the articular cartilage along these cracks. Eventually, pieces of articular cartilage break off and lodge in the synovium, inducing inflammation and a foreign body giant cell reaction. The result is a hyperemic and hypertrophied synovium.

4. As the crack extends down toward the tidemark and eventually crosses it, neovascularization from the epiphysis and subchondral bone extends into the area of the crack, inducing subchondral osteoclastic bone resorption (Fig. 30-53C). Adjacent osteoblastic activity also occurs and results in a thickening of the subchondral bone plate in the area of the crack. As neovascularization progressively extends into the area of the crack, mesenchymal cells invade and fibrocartilage forms as a poor substitute for the articular hyaline cartilage (Figs. 30-53D and 30-54A). These fibrocartilaginous plugs may persist, or they may be swept into the joint. The subchondral bone becomes exposed and burnished as it grinds against the opposite joint surface, which is undergoing the same process. These thick, shiny, smooth areas of subchondral bone are referred to as **eburnated** (ivory-like) bone.

5. In some areas, the eburnated bone cracks, allowing synovial fluid to extend from the joint surface into the subchondral bone marrow, where it eventually produces a **subchondral bone cyst** (Figs. 30-53E and 30-54B). These cysts increase in size as synovial fluid is forced into the space but cannot exit. Eventually, osteoclasts resorb bone and osteoblasts attempt to wall off the area. The result is a subchondral bone cyst filled with synovial fluid, with a well-marginated, reactive bone wall.

6. An osteophyte develops, usually in the lateral portions of the joint, when the mesenchymal tissue of the synovium differentiates into osteoblasts and chondroblasts to form a mass of cartilage and bone. Osteophytes are pearly grayish bone nodules on the periphery of the joint surface. These osteophytes, or bony spurs, also occur at lateral edges of intervertebral disks, extending from the adjacent vertebral bodies. They produce the "lipping" pattern seen on radiologic studies as OA of the spine. In the fingers, osteophytes at the distal interphalangeal joints are called **Heberden nodes**.

 CLINICAL FEATURES: The signs and symptoms of OA are functions of the location of the involved joints and the severity and duration of the joint deterioration. Physical findings vary. The involved joints may be enlarged, tender and boggy and may demonstrate crepitus. Deep, achy joint pain that follows activity and is relieved by rest is the clinical hallmark of OA. Pain is usually a sign of significant joint destruction and arises in the periarticular structures, since articular cartilage lacks a nerve supply. Discomfort also is caused by short periods of stiffness, which is frequently experienced in the morning or after periods of minimal activity. Restricted joint motion indicates severe disease and may result from joint or muscle contractures, intra-articular loose bodies, large osteophytes and loss of congruity of the joint surfaces.

At present, OA cannot be prevented or arrested. Therapy is directed at specific orthopedic conditions and includes exercise, weight loss and other supportive measures. In disabling osteoarthritis, joint replacement may be necessary.

NEUROPATHIC JOINT DISEASE (CHARCOT JOINT)

Neuropathic joint disease is a form of noninflammatory arthritis characterized by progressive joint destruction due to a primary neurologic disorder, such as peripheral neuropathy or central motor abnormality. In the mid-19th century, Jean-Martin Charcot described destruction of knee joints in patients with syphilitic tabes dorsalis (Charcot joint). *Today, the most common form of neuropathic joint disease is destruction of foot joints in people with diabetic peripheral neuropathy.* Destruction of shoulder or other upper extremity joints can occur in patients with syringomyelia, an abnormality affecting the cervical spinal cord.

Neuropathic joint disease can be viewed as a rapid and severe form of secondary OA in which a joint essentially fragments. Microscopically, there is marked destruction of articular cartilage and subchondral bone, inciting subchondral sclerosis, cyst formation and large amounts of cartilage and bone detritus within hyperplastic synovium. Although the pathogenesis remains uncertain, it is most likely that loss of innervation to the joint structures brings on a lack of proprioception and pain, abnormal joint mechanics and ultimately joint destruction.

RHEUMATOID ARTHRITIS

Rheumatoid arthritis (RA) is a systemic, chronic inflammatory disease in which chronic polyarthritis involves

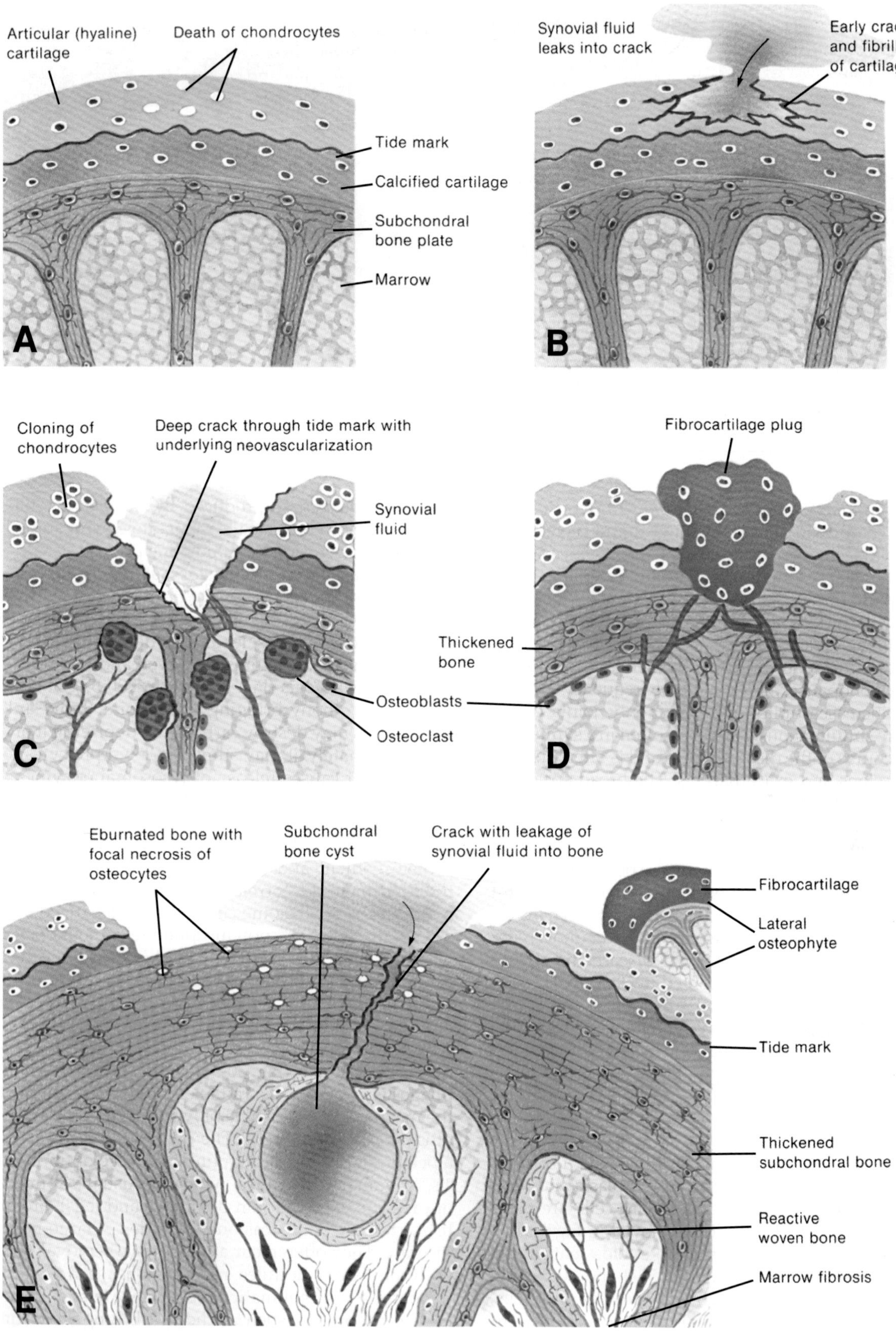

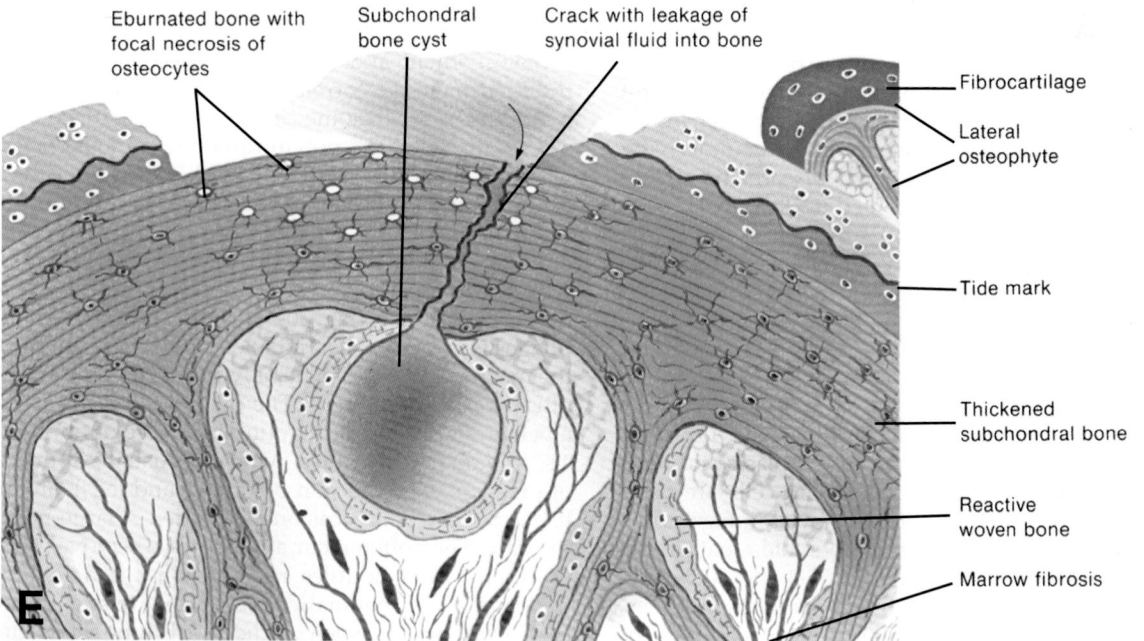

FIGURE 30-53. Histogenesis of osteoarthritis. A, B. The death of chondrocytes leads to a crack in the articular cartilage that is followed by an influx of synovial fluid and further loss and degeneration of cartilage. **C.** As a result of this process, cartilage is gradually worn away. Below the tidemark, new vessels grow in from the epiphysis, and fibrocartilage **(D)** is deposited. **E.** The fibrocartilage plug is not mechanically sufficient and may be worn away, thus exposing the subchondral bone plate, which becomes thickened and eburnated. If there is a crack in this region, synovial fluid leaks into the marrow space and produces a subchondral bone cyst. Focal regrowth of the articular surface leads to the formation of osteophytes.

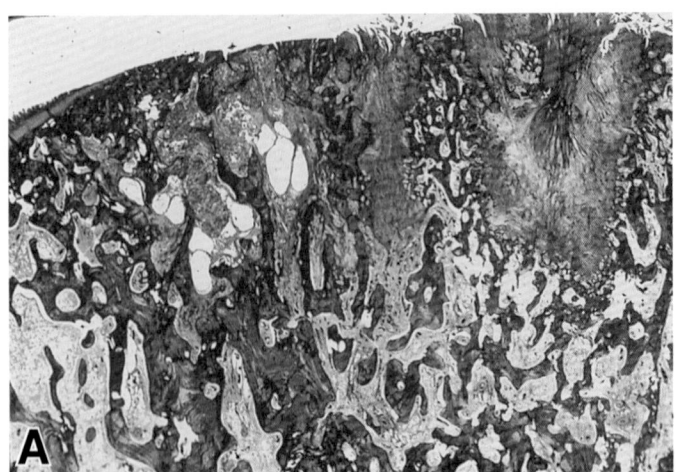
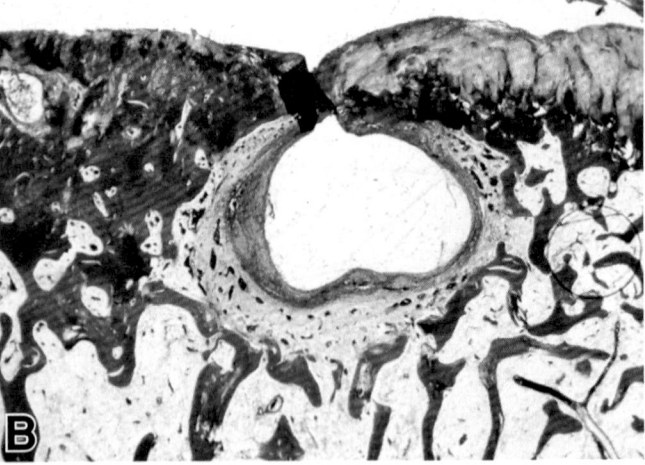

FIGURE 30-54. Osteoarthritis. A. A femoral head with osteoarthritis shows a fibrocartilaginous plug (*far right*) extending from the marrow onto the joint surface. Eburnated bone is present over the remaining surface. **B.** A section through the articular surface of an osteoarthritic joint demonstrates focal absence of the articular cartilage, thickening of subchondral bone (*left*) and a subchondral bone cyst.

diarthrodial joints, symmetrically and bilaterally (see Chapter 11). The proximal interphalangeal and metacarpophalangeal joints, elbows, knees, ankles and spine are most commonly affected. RA may occur at any age but usually begins in the third or fourth decade, and prevalence increases until age 70. The disease afflicts 1%–2% of the adult population, and its incidence is greater in women than in men (3:1). The excess incidence of RA in women is firmly established before menopause, after which the frequency for men and women increases uniformly. Commonly, joints of the extremities are simultaneously affected, often in a symmetric fashion. The course of the disease varies and is often punctuated by remissions and exacerbations. The broad spectrum of clinical manifestations ranges from barely discernible to severe, destructive, mutilating disease.

It is now thought that classic RA comprises a heterogeneous group of disorders. Patients who are persistently seronegative for rheumatoid factor probably have disease of a different etiology than those who are seropositive. There are also rheumatoid-like diseases associated with underlying conditions, such as inflammatory bowel disease and cirrhosis. The pathogenesis of RA is presented in Chapter 11.

PATHOLOGY: The early synovial changes of RA are edema and accumulation of plasma cells, lymphocytes and macrophages (Fig. 30-55-2). Vascularity increases, with exudation of fibrin into the joint space, which may result in small fibrin nodules that float in the joint **(rice bodies).**

PANNUS FORMATION: Synovial lining cells, normally only one to three layers thick, undergo hyperplasia and form layers 8–10 cells deep. Multinucleated giant cells are often found among the synovial cells. The synovial lining is thus thrown into numerous villi and frond-like folds that fill the peripheral recesses of the joint (Figs. 30-55-3 and 30-56A,B). This inflammatory synovium, which now contains mast cells, creeps over the surface of the articular cartilage and adjacent structures and is a **pannus** (cloak). Pannus covers the articular cartilage and isolates it from the synovial fluid (Fig. 30-55-4). Lymphocytes aggregate and eventually develop follicular centers (Figs. 30-55-3 and 30-56B). The pannus erodes the articular cartilage and adjacent bone, probably through the

action of collagenase produced by the pannus. Since PGE$_2$ and IL-1 are produced in the rheumatoid synovium, they may mediate bone erosion by stimulating osteoclasts.

The characteristic bone loss of RA is juxta-articular; that is, it is immediately adjacent to both sides of the joint. The pannus penetrates the subchondral bone; it may involve tendons and ligaments, leading to deformities and instabilities. Eventually, the joint is destroyed and undergoes fibrous fusion, or **ankylosis** (Fig. 30-55-5 and 30-57). Long-standing cases feature bony bridging of the joint **(bony ankylosis).** The pannus may destroy cartilage by depriving it of nourishment; alternately, it may stimulate T lymphocytes to secrete a factor that causes release of lysosomal enzymes. In turn, this process may lead to secondary OA.

Changes in synovial fluid include a massive increase in volume, increased turbidity and decreased viscosity. The protein content and the number of inflammatory cells in the fluid increase, correlating with the activity of the rheumatoid process. In some cases, the leukocyte count exceeds 50,000/μL, with 95% polymorphonuclear leukocytes.

RHEUMATOID NODULES: RA is a systemic disease that also involves tissues other than joints and tendons. A characteristic lesion, the "rheumatoid nodule," is found in extra-articular locations. It has a central core of fibrinoid necrosis, which is a mixture of fibrin and other proteins, such as degraded collagen (Fig. 30-58). A surrounding rim of macrophages is arranged in a radial or palisading fashion. Beyond the macrophages is a circle of lymphocytes, plasma cells and other mononuclear cells. The overall appearance resembles a peculiar granuloma surrounding a core of fibrinoid necrosis. Rheumatoid nodules, which are usually found in areas of pressure (e.g., the skin of elbows and legs), are movable, firm, rubbery and occasionally tender. A large nodule may ulcerate. They often recur after surgical removal.

Rheumatoid nodules may also be seen in lupus erythematous and rheumatic fever. They are sometimes found in visceral organs, such as the heart, lungs, intestinal tract and even the dura. Nodules in the bundle of His may cause cardiac arrhythmias; in the lungs, they produce fibrosis and even respiratory failure (see Chapter 18). RA also may be accompanied by **acute necrotizing vasculitis,** which can affect any organ.

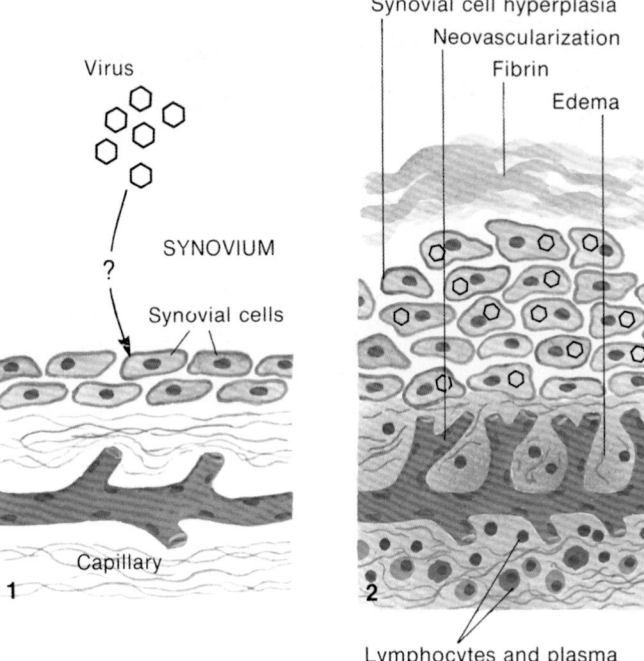

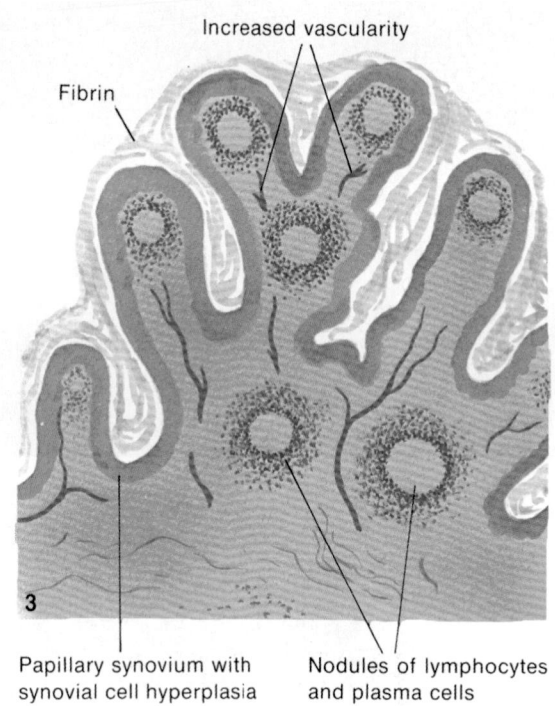

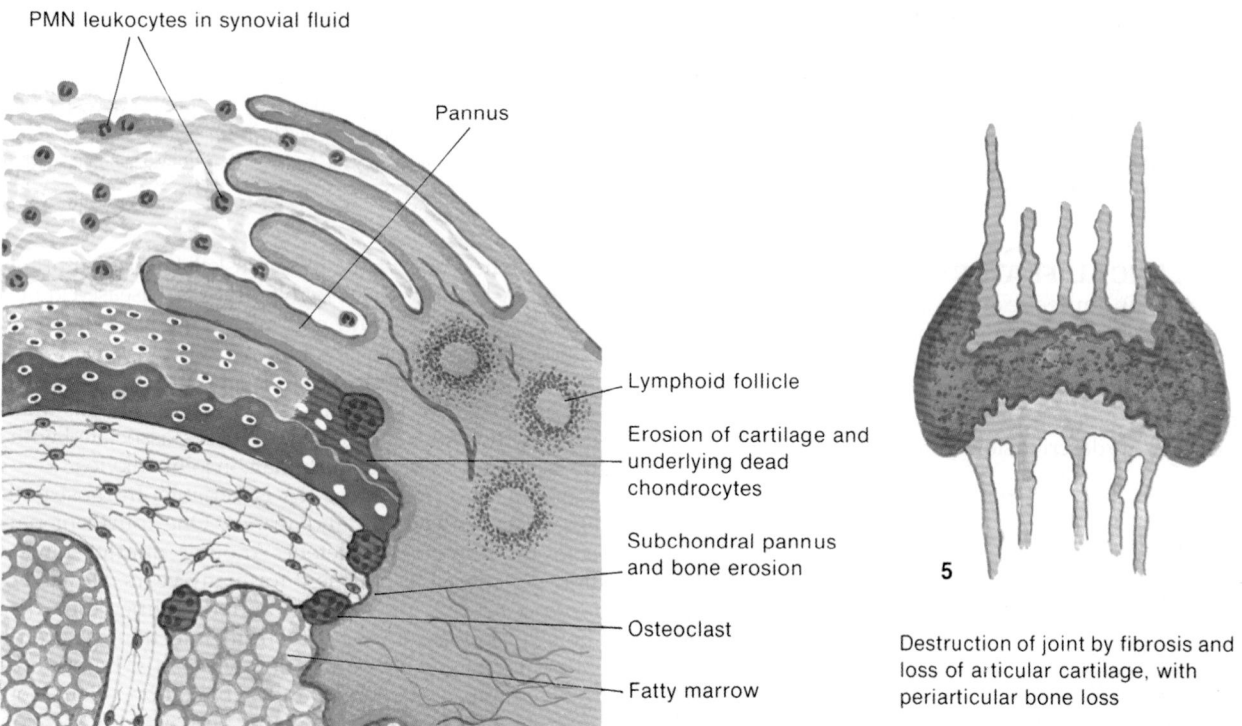

FIGURE 30-55. Histogenesis of rheumatoid arthritis. 1. A virus or an unknown stress may stimulate the synovial cells to proliferate. **2.** The influx of lymphocytes, plasma cells and mast cells, together with neovascularization and edema, leads to hypertrophy and hyperplasia of the synovium. **3.** Lymphoid nodules are prominent. **4.** Proliferating synovium extends into the joint space, burrows into the bone beneath the articular cartilage and covers the cartilage as a pannus. The articular cartilage is eventually destroyed by direct resorption or deprivation of its nutrient synovial fluid. The synovial tissue continues to proliferate in the subchondral region, as well as in the joint. **5.** Eventually, the joint is destroyed and becomes fused, a condition termed **ankylosis.**

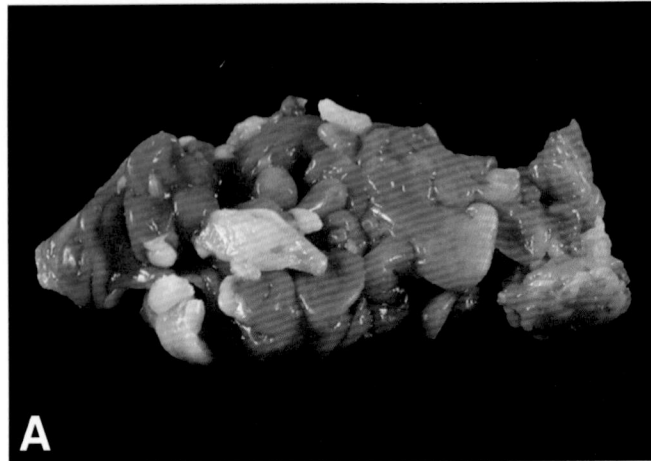

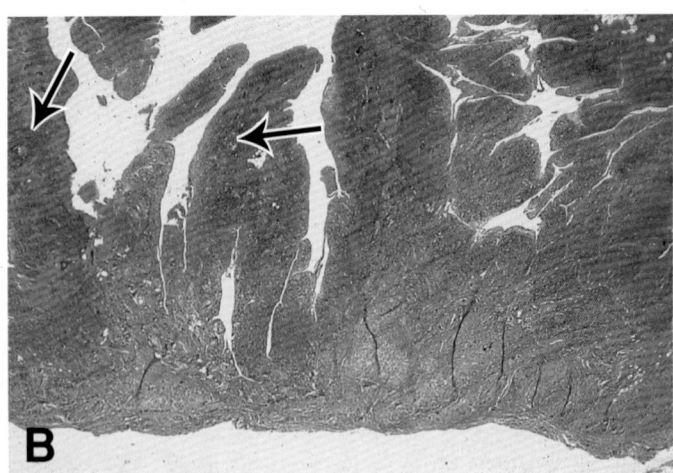

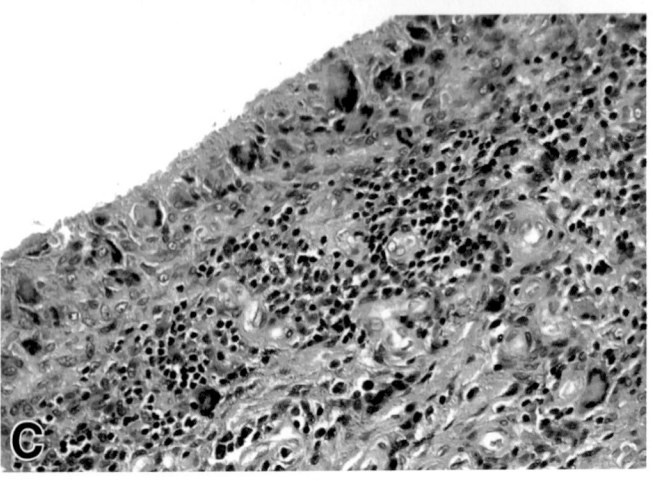

FIGURE 30-56. Rheumatoid arthritis. A. Hyperplastic synovium from a patient with rheumatoid arthritis shows numerous finger-like projections, with focal pale areas of fibrin deposition. The brownish color of the synovium reflects hemosiderin accumulation derived from old hemorrhage. **B.** A microscopic view reveals prominent lymphoid follicles (Allison-Ghormley bodies; *arrows*), synovial hyperplasia and hypertrophy, villous folds and thickening of the synovial membrane by fibrosis and inflammation. **C.** A higher-power view of the inflamed synovium demonstrates hyperplasia and hypertrophy of the lining cells. Numerous giant cells are on and below the surface. The stroma is chronically inflamed.

CLINICAL FEATURES: The clinical diagnosis of RA is imprecise and is based on a number of criteria, such as the number and types of joints involved, the presence of rheumatoid nodules and RF and radiographic features characteristic of the disease.

The onset of RA may be acute, slowly progressing or insidious. Most patients describe slowly developing fatigue, weight loss, weakness and vague musculoskeletal discomfort, which eventually localizes to the involved joints. Diseased joints tend to be warm, swollen and painful. The pain is heightened by motion and is most severe after periods of disuse. Unabated disease causes progressive destruction of the joint surfaces and periarticular structures. Eventually, patients manifest severe flexion and extension deformities, associated with joint subluxation, which may terminate in joint ankylosis.

The natural history of RA is variable. In most patients, disease activity waxes and wanes. One fourth of patients seem to recover completely. Another quarter have only slight functional impairment for many years. However, half develop serious progressive and disabling joint disease. There is increased mortality from infection, gastrointestinal hemorrhage and perforation, vasculitis, heart and lung involvement, amyloidosis and subluxation of the cervical spine. In fact, survival of patients with active RA is comparable to that in Hodgkin disease and diabetes.

Three types of drugs are used to suppress synovial inflammation and to induce a remission:

- **Nonsteroidal anti-inflammatory drugs (NSAIDs).**
- **Corticosteroids,** which have both anti-inflammatory and immunoregulatory activity.
- **Disease-modifying antirheumatic drugs (DMARDs),** which have been shown to alter the course of the disease and improve outcome. These include drugs such as methotrexate, leflunomide, cyclosporin, cyclophosphamide, azathioprine, sulfasalazine, gold salts, penicillamine,

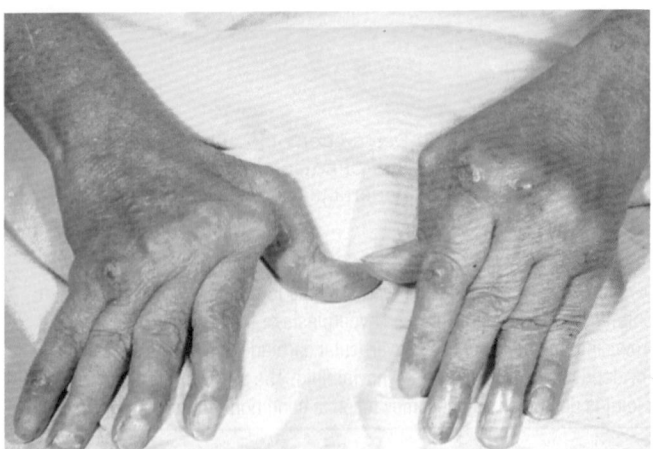

FIGURE 30-57. Rheumatoid arthritis. The hands of a patient with advanced arthritis show swelling of the metacarpophalangeal joints and the classic ulnar deviation of the fingers.

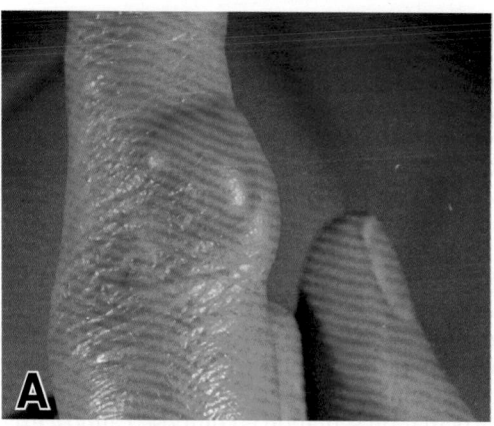
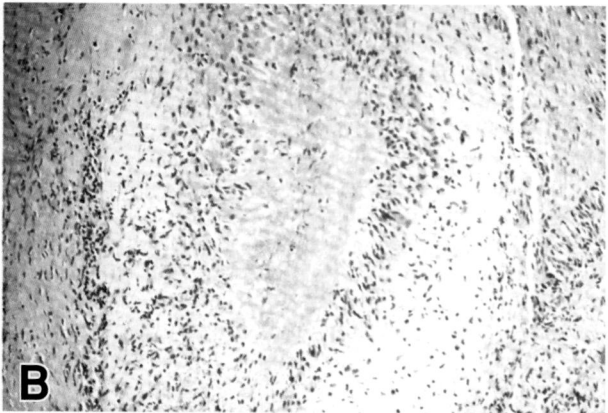

FIGURE 30-58. Rheumatoid nodule. A. A patient with rheumatoid arthritis has a subcutaneous mass on a digit. **B.** Microscopic view of a rheumatoid nodule shows a central area of necrosis surrounded by palisaded macrophages and a chronic inflammatory infiltrate.

antimalarial drugs (hydroxychloroquine), TNF inhibitors, T-cell costimulatory blockers, B-cell–depleting agents and IL-1 receptor antagonists. They are now recommended early in the course of the disease to prevent progression, induce remission and prevent joint deformities and functional disabilities.

Spondyloarthropathy Is a Seronegative Arthritis Mostly Linked to HLA-B27

A number of clinical entities were formerly classified as variants of RA but are now recognized to be distinct disorders. These forms of arthritis are now known as **spondyloarthropathies** and include ankylosing spondylitis, Reiter syndrome, psoriatic arthritis and arthritis associated with inflammatory bowel disease. They share several features:

- Seronegativity for RF and other serologic markers of RA
- Association with class I histocompatibility antigens, particularly human leukocyte antigen (HLA)-B27
- Sacroiliac and vertebral involvement
- Asymmetric involvement of only a few peripheral joints
- A tendency to inflammation of periarticular tendons and fascia
- Systemic involvement of other organs, especially uveitis, carditis and aortitis
- Preferential onset in young men

Ankylosing Spondylitis

Ankylosing spondylitis is an inflammatory arthropathy of the vertebral column and sacroiliac joints. It may be accompanied by asymmetric, peripheral arthritis (30% of patients) and systemic manifestations. It is most common in young men, with peak incidence at about age 20. Over 90% of patients have HLA-B27 (normal, 4%–8%), although the disorder affects only 1% of people with this haplotype.

 PATHOLOGY: Ankylosing spondylitis begins at the sacroiliac joints bilaterally, then ascends the spinal column by involving the small joints of the posterior elements of the spine. The result is destruction of these joints, after which the spine becomes fused posteriorly. The unburdened vertebral bodies become square and osteoporotic, because the main force of gravity is borne by the fused

posterior elements. In such cases, the intervertebral disk undergoes ossification and may disappear. Eventually, bony fusion of the vertebral bodies ensues (Fig. 30-59).

Although a few patients with ankylosing spondylitis rapidly develop crippling spinal disease, most are able to maintain their employment and live a normal life span. However, up to 5% of patients develop AA amyloidosis and uremia and a few manifest severe cardiac involvement.

Reactive Arthritis

Reactive arthritis (previously, Reiter syndrome) is a triad that includes (1) seronegative polyarthritis, (2) conjunctivitis/uveitis

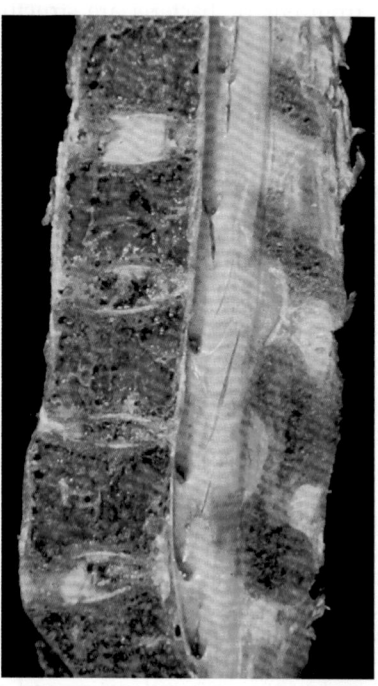

FIGURE 30-59. Ankylosing spondylitis. The vertebrae have been cut longitudinally. The vertebral bodies are square and have lost most of their trabecular bone, owing to osteoporosis from disuse. Bone bridges fuse one vertebral body to the next across the intervertebral disks. Portions of the intervertebral disk are replaced by bone marrow. Bony bridges also fuse the posterior elements **(ankylosis)**.

and (3) nonspecific urethritis. It occurs almost exclusively in men and usually follows venereal exposure or an episode of bacillary dysentery. As in ankylosing spondylitis, this syndrome is associated with HLA-B27 in 90% of patients. In fact, after an attack of dysentery, 20% of HLA-B27–positive men develop reactive arthritis.

The pathologic features of this syndrome are comparable to those of RA. More than half of patients develop mucocutaneous lesions similar to those of pustular psoriasis (**keratoderma blennorrhagica**) over the palms, soles and trunk. In most patients, the disease remits within a year, but in 20%, progressive arthritis develops, including ankylosing spondylitis.

Psoriatic Arthritis

Of all patients with psoriasis, particularly in those with severe disease, 7% develop an inflammatory seronegative arthritis. HLA-B27 has been linked to psoriatic spondylitis and inflammation of distal interphalangeal joints, and HLA-DR4 has been associated with a rheumatoid pattern of involvement. Joint disease is usually mild and slowly progressive, although a mutilating form is occasionally encountered.

Enteropathic Arthritis

Ulcerative colitis and Crohn disease are accompanied by seronegative peripheral arthritis in 20% of cases and spondylitis in 10%. This form of arthritis also is seen in patients with Whipple disease and after certain bacterial infections of the gut. No particular tissue type is associated with peripheral arthritis, but most patients with ankylosing spondylitis are HLA-B27 positive. It has been proposed that HLA-B27 and proteins from enteric bacteria are structurally related in a manner that affects antigen presentation to the T-cell receptor. Resection of the affected bowel in ulcerative colitis relieves the arthritis, but in Crohn disease, this complication often does not resolve.

Juvenile Arthritis Includes Any Inflammatory Arthritis in Children

Several different chronic arthritic conditions in children are included in this designation, also called **Still disease**. In addition to RA, many children with juvenile arthritis eventually develop ankylosing spondylitis, psoriatic arthritis and other connective tissue diseases.

- **Seropositive arthritis:** Fewer than 10% of children with arthritis are positive for RF and have a polyarticular presentation. Females predominate (80%) among children with seropositive Still disease, and in most cases (75%), antinuclear antibodies are present. HLA-D4 is often present, and more than half of the children eventually develop severe arthritis.
- **Polyarticular disease without systemic symptoms:** One fourth of juvenile arthritis patients (90% girls) have disease of several joints, are seronegative and do not manifest systemic symptoms. Fewer than 15% of these patients eventually develop severe arthritis.
- **Polyarticular disease with systemic symptoms:** Twenty percent of children with polyarticular arthritis have prominent systemic symptoms, which include high fever, rash, hepatosplenomegaly, lymphadenopathy, pleuritis,

pericarditis, anemia and leukocytosis. Most (60%) are boys who are negative for RF, and one fourth of all of these children are left with severe arthritis.
- **Pauciarticular arthritis:** Children with involvement of only a few large joints, such as the knee, ankle, elbow or hip girdle, account for half of all cases of juvenile arthritis and fall into two general groups. The larger group (80%) mainly comprises girls who are negative for RF but exhibit antinuclear antibodies and are positive for HLA-DR5, HLA-DRw6 or HLA-DRw8. Of these patients, one third have ocular disease, characterized by chronic iridocyclitis (inflammation of the iris and ciliary body). Only a small minority of these children have residual polyarthritis or ocular damage. The smaller group of children with a pauciarticular presentation is composed almost exclusively of boys, is negative for both RF and antinuclear bodies and is positive for HLA-B27 (75%). A few have acute iridocyclitis, which resolves spontaneously. Some of these boys subsequently develop ankylosing spondylitis.

LYME DISEASE

Lyme disease usually involves the knee or other large joints and is caused by the spirochete **Borrelia burgdorferi** *transmitted by the Ixodes tick* (see Chapter 9). Patients generally present with joint effusion and other manifestations of Lyme disease. Although there may be a transient arthritis with acute infection, some patients can develop chronic Lyme arthritis, which is microscopically identical to rheumatoid arthritis.

GOUT

Primary Gout Is a Disorder of Uric Acid Metabolism

Gout is a heterogeneous group of diseases collectively characterized by increased serum uric acid and urate crystal deposition in joints and kidneys. All such patients have hyperuricemia, but fewer than 15% of people with hyperuricemia have gout. It is characterized by acute and chronic arthritis. Gout is classified as primary or secondary, depending on the etiology of the hyperuricemia. In **primary gout**, hyperuricemia occurs without any other disease; **secondary gout** occurs in association with another illness that results in hyperuricemia. Of all cases of hyperuricemia, one third are primary and the remainder secondary.

 **MOLECULAR PATHOGENESIS:** Uric acid results from purine catabolism, due to either a high-purine diet or increased de novo synthesis. In humans, there is a tight balance between uric acid production and tissue deposition of urates. Uric acid is only eliminated in the urine. Thus, the blood uric acid level (normal, <7.0 mg/dL in men, <6.0 mg/dL in women) reflects the difference between the amount of purines ingested and synthesized and renal excretion. Gout can result from (1) overproduction of purines, (2) increased catabolism of nucleic acids due to greater cell turnover, (3) decreased salvage of free purine bases or (4) decreased urinary uric acid excretion (Fig. 30-60). A high dietary intake of purine-rich foods (e.g., meat) by an otherwise normal person does not lead to hyperuricemia and gout.

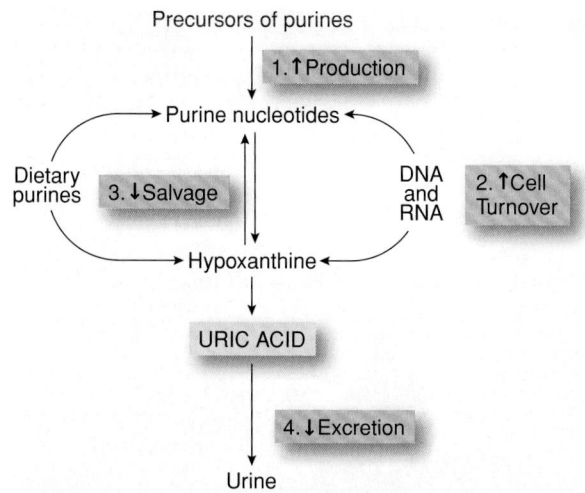

FIGURE 30-60. Pathogenesis of hyperuricemia and gout. Purine nucleotides are synthesized de novo from nonpurine precursors or derived from preformed purines in the diet. Purine nucleotides are catabolized to hypoxanthine or incorporated into nucleic acids. The degradation of nucleic acids and dietary purines also produces hypoxanthine. Hypoxanthine is converted to uric acid, which in turn is excreted into the urine. Hyperuricemia and gout result from (1) increased de novo purine synthesis, (2) increased cell turnover, (3) decreased salvage of dietary purines and hypoxanthine and (4) decreased uric acid excretion by the kidneys.

Most cases (85%) of idiopathic gout result from an as-yet-unexplained impairment of renal uric acid excretion. In the remainder, there is a primary overproduction of uric acid, but the underlying abnormality has been identified only in a minority of cases.

A *familial tendency* to gout has been recognized since the time of Galen. Hyperuricemia is common among relatives of patients with gout. It has been proposed that primary hyperuricemia in some people is inherited as an autosomal dominant trait with variable expression, in some as an X-linked abnormality and in others as instances of multifactorial inheritance. Precocious gout exhibits a strong familial tendency. The consensus today is that multiple genes control the level of serum uric acid.

Gout Can Be Due to Inborn Errors of Metabolism

The rate-limiting step in purine synthesis is condensation of glutamine with phosphoribosyl pyrophosphate (PP-ribose-P) to form phosphoribosylamine. Increased intracellular PP-ribose-P accelerates purine biosynthesis. PP-ribose-P, through the activity of hypoxanthine phosphoribosyl transferase (HPRT), also condenses with, and so salvages, purine bases (hypoxanthine and guanine) derived from the catabolism of nucleic acids. Although the specific cause of an abnormally high rate of urate production is not known, in most cases of primary gout, two inborn errors of metabolism are known to lead to elevated PP-ribose-P.

Lesch-Nyhan syndrome is an inherited, X-linked (Xq26-q27) deficiency of HPRT, a defect that leads to accumulation of PP-ribose-P, and in turn to enhanced purine synthesis. Children with this syndrome are clinically normal at birth but exhibit delays in development and neurologic dysfunction within the first year. Most are mentally retarded and exhibit self-mutilation. They are hyperuricemic and eventually develop gouty arthritis. In addition, obstructive nephropathy and hematologic abnormalities are often present.

Secondary Gout Often Results from DNA Turnover

A number of conditions result in hyperuricemia and secondary gout. As in primary gout, secondary hyperuricemia may reflect overproduction or decreased urinary excretion of uric acid. Increased production is most often associated with increased nucleic acid turnover, as seen in leukemias and lymphomas and after chemotherapy. Accelerated adenosine triphosphate (ATP) degradation may also lead to overproduction of uric acid and occurs in glycogen storage diseases and tissue hypoxia. Ethanol intake evokes secondary hyperuricemia, in part owing to accelerated ATP catabolism and (to a lesser degree) decreased renal excretion of uric acid. Reduced urate excretion may also result from primary renal disease. Dehydration and diuretics increase tubular reabsorption of uric acid and induce hyperuricemia. In fact, various drugs are implicated in 20% of patients with hyperuricemia.

Saturnine gout was described in 18th-century England, where this disease was prevalent among the upper classes with lead plumbing in their houses (Saturn is the symbol for lead). It is now recognized that these patients were afflicted with lead nephropathy. The Romans had a similar problem, because they drank from vessels containing lead.

 **EPIDEMIOLOGY:** Primary gout usually afflicts adult men; only 5% of cases occur in women. It is rare in children before puberty and in women during the reproductive years. Peak incidence is in the fifth decade. This sex distribution can be traced to the fact that at all ages, mean serum urate concentrations in women are lower than in men, although they increase after menopause. Many patients have a family history of gout, but environmental factors are also important. Positive correlations exist between the prevalence of hyperuricemia in a population and mean weight, protein intake, alcohol consumption, social class and intelligence. Thus, gout is a disease that exemplifies the interplay between genetic predisposition and environmental influences.

 PATHOLOGY: When sodium urate crystals precipitate from supersaturated body fluids, they absorb fibronectin, complement and a number of other proteins on their surfaces. Neutrophils that have ingested urate crystals release activated oxygen species and lysosomal enzymes, which mediate tissue injury and promote an inflammatory response.

The presence of long, needle-shaped crystals that are negatively birefringent under polarized light is diagnostic of gout (Fig. 30-61). Monosodium urate monohydrate crystals may be found intracellularly in leukocytes of the synovial fluid. A **tophus** is an extracellular soft tissue deposit of urate crystals surrounded by foreign body giant cells and an associated inflammatory response of mononuclear cells. These granuloma-like areas are found in cartilage, in any of the soft tissues around joints and even in the subchondral bone marrow adjacent to joints.

Macroscopically, any chalky white deposit on intraarticular surfaces, including articular cartilage, suggests gout. Radiologically, gouty arthritis exhibits characteristic, punched-out, juxta-articular, lytic ("rat bite") lesions that are

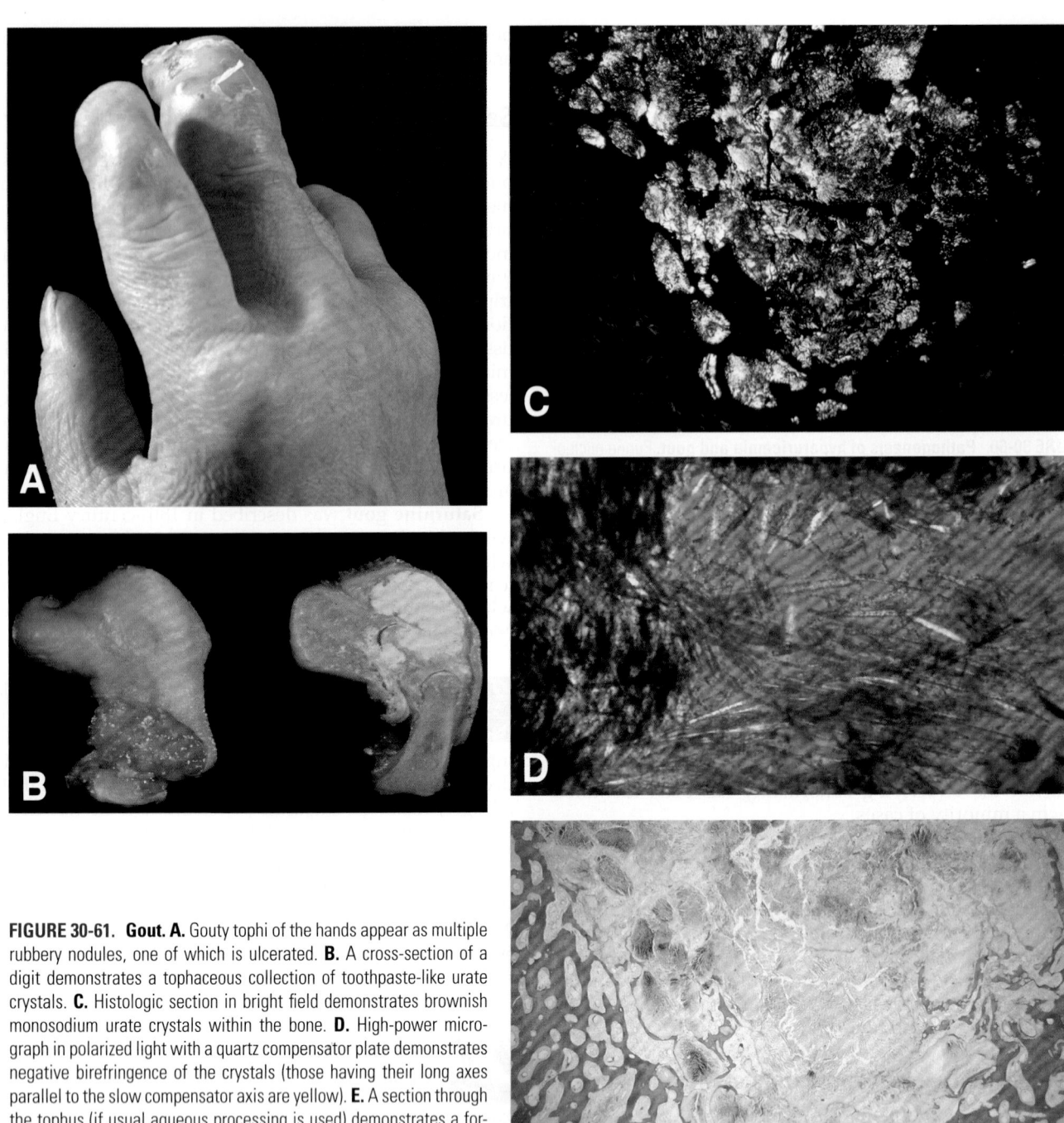

FIGURE 30-61. Gout. A. Gouty tophi of the hands appear as multiple rubbery nodules, one of which is ulcerated. **B.** A cross-section of a digit demonstrates a tophaceous collection of toothpaste-like urate crystals. **C.** Histologic section in bright field demonstrates brownish monosodium urate crystals within the bone. **D.** High-power micrograph in polarized light with a quartz compensator plate demonstrates negative birefringence of the crystals (those having their long axes parallel to the slow compensator axis are yellow). **E.** A section through the tophus (if usual aqueous processing is used) demonstrates a foreign body reaction around a pink, amorphous lesion from which the urate crystals have been dissolved during processing.

associated with only minimal reactive new bone (Fig. 30-62). In contrast to RA, there is no juxta-articular osteopenia in gout.

Renal urate deposits are between the tubules, especially at the apices of the medulla. These areas are grossly visible as small, shiny, golden-yellow, linear streaks in the medulla.

CLINICAL FEATURES: The clinical course of gout is divided into four stages: (1) asymptomatic hyperuricemia, (2) acute gouty arthritis, (3) intercritical gout and (4) chronic tophaceous gout. Renal stones may occur in any stage except the first. In most cases,

symptomatic gout appears before renal stones, which usually require 20–30 years of sustained hyperuricemia.

- **Asymptomatic hyperuricemia** often precedes clinically evident gout by many years.
- **Acute gouty arthritis** was well characterized by Thomas Sydenham, who described his own disease in the 1600s. It is a painful condition that usually involves one joint, without constitutional symptoms. Later in the course of the disease, polyarticular involvement with fever is common. At least half of patients are first seen with a painful and red first metatarsophalangeal joint (great toe), designated **"podagra."** Eventually, 90% of all patients have

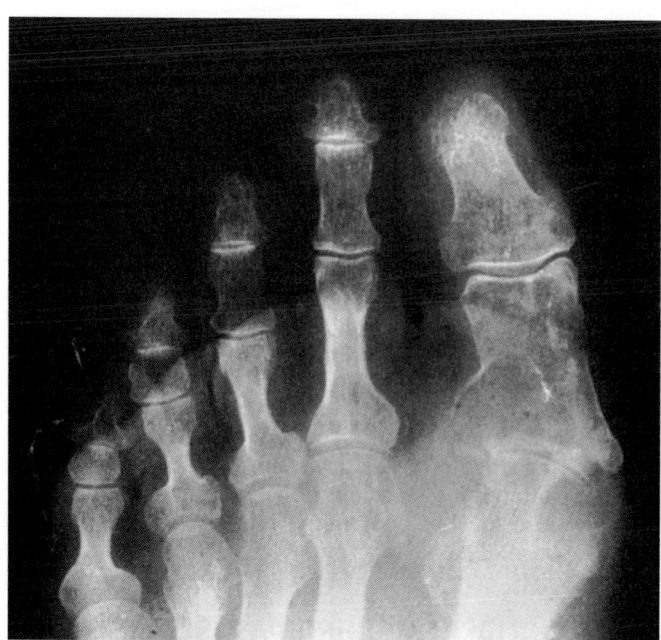

FIGURE 30-62. Gout. A radiograph of the first metatarsophalangeal joint shows a lytic lesion that destroys the joint space. There is an adjacent soft tissue tophus, as well as surrounding edema.

such an attack. Commonly, a gouty attack begins at night and is exquisitely painful, simulating an acute bacterial infection of the affected joint. A large meal or drinking alcoholic beverages may trigger an attack, but other specific events such as trauma, certain drugs and surgery may also be responsible. Even when untreated, acute attacks of gout are self-limited.

- The **intercritical period** is the asymptomatic interval between the initial acute attack and subsequent episodes. These periods may last up to 10 years, but later attacks tend to be increasingly severe, prolonged and polyarticular.
- **Tophaceous gout** eventually appears in the untreated patient in the form of tophi in the cartilage, synovial membranes, tendons and soft tissues.

Renal failure is responsible for 10% of deaths in patients with gout. One third of patients have mild albuminuria, reduced glomerular filtration and decreased renal concentrating ability. However, the contribution of urate nephropathy to chronic renal dysfunction is unclear, and hypertension, preexisting kidney disease and the intake of analgesic drugs may be more important. In patients with severe gout caused by inherited enzyme deficiencies and in those with a precocious presentation, urate nephropathy is a prominent feature of the clinical course. **Urate stones** are 10% of all renal calculi in the United States and up to 40% in Israel and Australia. The prevalence of urate stones correlates with the serum concentration of uric acid and affects 25% of gout patients. Patients also have an increased frequency of calcium-containing stones, in which case the uric acid may serve as a nidus for a calcium stone.

Treatment of gout is designed to (1) decrease the severity of acute attacks, (2) reduce serum urate, (3) prevent future attacks, (4) promote dissolution of urate deposits and (5) alkalinize the urine to prevent stone formation. The main drugs used to interrupt the inflammatory process, thus preventing or controlling the acute attack, are nonsteroidal anti-inflammatory agents. Colchicine has been used for hundreds of years and has been administered prophylactically during the intervals between gouty attacks to prevent recurrent episodes. Uricosuric drugs that interfere with urate reabsorption by the renal tubules are often useful.

Allopurinol is a competitive inhibitor of xanthine oxidase, the enzyme that converts xanthine and hypoxanthine to uric acid. This drug causes a prompt decrease in uricosemia and uricosuria and is used in people with renal insufficiency and those who are resistant to other uricosuric drugs. It also may be administered to patients undergoing chemotherapy for hematopoietic proliferative disorders, which increases the rate of urate production.

CALCIUM PYROPHOSPHATE DIHYDRATE DEPOSITION DISEASE (CHONDROCALCINOSIS AND PSEUDOGOUT)

Calcium pyrophosphate dihydrate (CPPD) deposition disease refers to the accumulation of this compound in synovial membranes (pseudogout), joint cartilage (chondrocalcinosis), ligaments and tendons. The disease can be idiopathic, associated with trauma, linked to a number of metabolic disorders or, in rare cases, hereditary.

CPPD deposition disease is principally a condition of old age; half of those over age 85 are afflicted. Most cases in the elderly are asymptomatic. Because fully two thirds of these patients manifest preexisting joint damage, it is believed that trauma and the aging process in cartilage promote nucleation of CPPD crystals. In asymptomatic cases, punctate or linear calcifications may be present in any fibrocartilage or hyaline cartilage surface. For example, radiography of the knee may disclose linear streaks that outline the menisci.

MOLECULAR PATHOGENESIS: The major predisposing abnormality in patients with CPPD deposition disease is an excessive level of inorganic pyrophosphate in the synovial fluid. This material derives from hydrolysis of nucleoside triphosphates in joint chondrocytes. Increased pyrophosphate levels in synovial fluid can result from either increased production or decreased catabolism.

CPPD deposition is commonly found in the knees after trauma and after surgical removal of the meniscus. Nucleotides released after injury to articular cartilage may act as substrates for nucleotide triphosphate pyrophosphohydrolase (NTP), thus increasing production of pyrophosphate. A number of other disorders are associated with deposition of CPPD crystals, including hyperparathyroidism, hypothyroidism, hemochromatosis, Wilson disease and ochronosis. Iron and copper are presumed to inhibit pyrophosphatase, accounting for decreased degradation of pyrophosphate.

Mutations in the *ANKH* gene cause familial autosomal dominant CPPD chondrocalcinosis. The *ANKH* gene is thought to encode a membrane pyrophosphate transporter that inhibits mineralization of several tissues including joints, articular cartilage and tendons. Mutated ANKH elevates intracellular pyrophosphate and reduces extracellular pyrophosphate.

Hypophosphatasia is a heritable condition in which activity of alkaline phosphatase (the enzyme that hydrolyzes pyrophosphate) in serum and tissue is deficient. As a result, pyrophosphate is not adequately metabolized and accumulates in synovial fluid.

  PATHOLOGY AND CLINICAL FEATURES: A minority of patients symptomatic with CPPD deposition disease are classified according to the nature of joint involvement.

■ **Pseudogout** refers to self-limited attacks of acute arthritis lasting from 1 day to 4 weeks and involving one or two joints. Some 25% of patients with CPPD deposition disease have an acute onset of gout-like symptoms manifesting as inflammation and swelling of the knees, ankles, wrists, elbows, hips or shoulders. Metatarsophalangeal joints, which are frequently affected in gout, are usually spared. The synovial fluid exhibits abundant leukocytes containing CPPD crystals.
■ **Pseudorheumatoid arthritis** is a variant of CPPD deposition disease in which multiple joints are chronically involved. The symptoms are mild and resemble those of RA.
■ **Pseudo-osteoarthritis** has symptoms similar to those of osteoarthritis.
■ **Pseudoneurotrophic disease** is characterized by joint destruction severe enough to resemble a neurotrophic joint.

On gross examination, CPPD deposits appear as chalky white areas on cartilaginous surfaces (Fig. 30-63A). Unlike needle-shaped urate crystals, they are stubby, short and rhomboid ("coffin shaped") and display weak birefringence under polarized light. In contrast to urate crystals, CPPD crystals do not dissolve in water and are easily found in tissue sections (Fig. 30-63B). Only a few mononuclear cells and macrophages surround foci of crystal deposition.

The treatment of CPPD is essentially symptomatic (pain control). Nonsteroidal anti-inflammatory drugs and steroids are commonly used.

CALCIUM HYDROXYAPATITE DEPOSITION DISEASE

Calcium hydroxyapatite deposition disease is an acute or chronic arthritis characterized by hydroxyapatite crystals within leukocytes and mononuclear cells in joint tissue and synovial fluid. Calcium hydroxyapatite (HA) is the major mineral of bone and teeth and is the compound deposited in dystrophic and metastatic calcification. HA crystals are frequently encountered in the synovial fluid of joints involved by osteoarthritis, but there is reason to believe that severe HA deposition is a distinct entity. The joints most frequently involved are the knee, shoulder, hip and fingers. Attacks may last several days.

HEMOPHILIA, HEMOCHROMATOSIS AND OCHRONOSIS

Hemophilia, hemochromatosis and ochronosis (see Chapter 6) all produce joint disease with degradation of the matrix and destruction of the articular cartilage.

■ **Hemophilia** gives rise to severe forms of arthritis because of extensive bleeding into joints (hemarthrosis), particularly the knees, elbows, ankles, shoulders and hips. In addition to the effects within the articular cartilage matrix, synovial proliferation also simulates RA.
■ **Hemochromatosis** is complicated by arthritis in half of affected patients. The hands, hips and knees may be involved in recurrent attacks.
■ **Ochronosis** is a rare, autosomal recessive disease caused by a defect in homogentisic acid oxidase. The deposition

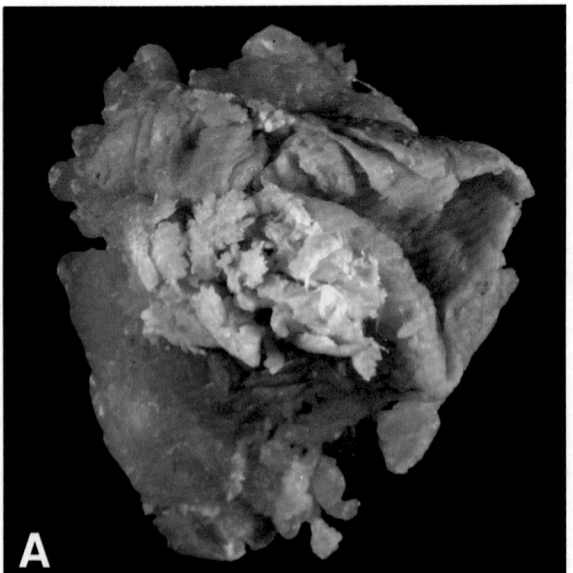

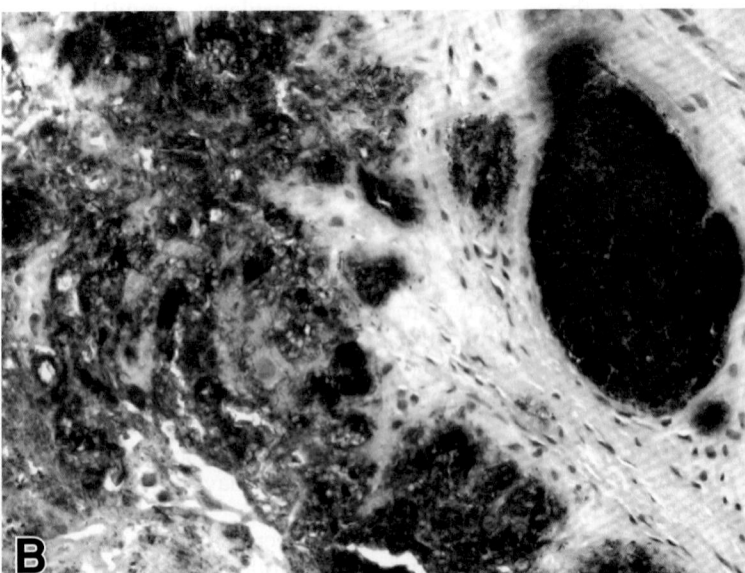

FIGURE 30-63. Calcium pyrophosphate dihydrate (CPPD) deposition disease. A. Gross specimen demonstrates chalky-white calcific material. **B.** Microscopically, the deposits are deep purple with discernible rhomboid-shaped crystals.

of ochronotic pigment in the cartilage of the joints, including the intervertebral disks, eventually causes them to become brittle and degenerate.

TUMORS AND TUMOR-LIKE LESIONS OF JOINTS

True neoplasms of the joints are rare. The most common malignant lesions of the synovium are metastatic carcinomas, particularly adenocarcinoma of the colon, breast and lung. Lymphoproliferative diseases (e.g., leukemia) may also involve the synovium, mimicking other conditions, such as RA. It is unusual for primary malignant bone tumors to extend into the joint, although they may invade the joint capsule from the soft tissues.

A Ganglion Is a Small Fluid-Filled Cyst

A ganglion is a thin-walled, simple cyst containing clear mucinous fluid, which occurs most commonly on the extensor surfaces of the hands and feet, especially the wrist. It is more common in women between the ages of 25 and 45 years. The cyst arises either from the synovium or from areas of myxoid change in the connective tissue, possibly after trauma. The wall is composed of fibrous tissue, and there is no cell lining. The lesion may be painful and can be readily removed surgically, although a blow with the family Bible was the traditional treatment for a ganglion on the dorsum of the wrist.

A **Baker cyst** is a herniation of the synovium of the knee joint into the popliteal space. It is most often seen in association with various forms of arthritis, in which the intra-articular pressure is increased. The cyst contains synovial fluid and microscopically demonstrates a synovial cell lining.

Synovial Chondromatosis Features Cartilage Nodules in a Joint

Synovial chondromatosis is a benign, self-limited disease in which hyaline cartilage nodules form in the synovium, detach from that structure and float in the synovial fluid, like grains of sand between gears. The chronic irritation produced by these "loose" bodies stimulates the synovium to secrete large amounts of synovial fluid and also causes bleeding in the synovial membrane. Synovial chondromatosis involves the large diarthrodial joints of young and middle-aged men, affecting the knee in most cases, but also the hip, elbow, shoulder, ankle and temporomandibular joints. Patients have pain, stiffness and locking of the joint, with associated bloody effusions.

Unlike cartilage that detaches from articular surfaces in osteoarthritis, in synovial chondromatosis the fragments of hyaline cartilage are formed de novo in the synovium (Fig. 30-64). They do not have a tidemark and thus differ morphologically from true articular cartilage. Occasionally, the cartilage nodules, while still in the synovium, undergo endochondral ossification, in which case the disease is called **synovial osteochondromatosis**. If these nodules detach, the bony portions undergo necrosis, but the cartilage fragments remain viable and enlarge because they are nourished by synovial fluid. The condition is treated by evacuating the joint and performing a synovectomy. Recurrence is seen in 15%–20% of the cases, but malignant transformation is rare.

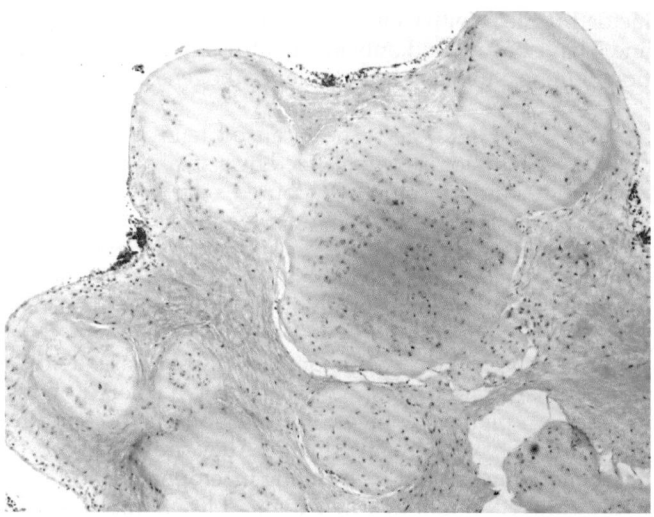

FIGURE 30-64. Synovial chondromatosis. Nodules of benign hyaline cartilage form in the synovium.

 **MOLECULAR PATHOGENESIS:** Dysregulation of Hedgehog signaling is a factor in the development of synovial chondromatosis in animal models and suggests that this disorder is a neoplasm. Clonal karyotypic abnormalities have been detected in a few cases of synovial chondromatosis, with diploid or near-diploid complements, chromosome 6 anomalies, rearrangements of 1p22 and 1p13 and extra copies of chromosome 5.

Tenosynovial Giant Cell Tumor Is a Benign Neoplasm of Synovial Lining

This is the most common neoplasm of the synovium and tendon sheath and occurs in a localized and a diffuse form. The lesions may be intra- or extra-articular.

- **Localized tenosynovial giant cell tumor or giant cell tumor of the tendon sheath** involves the hands and feet. In fact, it is the most common soft tissue tumor of the hand. It occurs mostly in young and middle-aged women (30–50 years) and involves flexor surfaces of the middle or index fingers. The tumor is usually well circumscribed and grows slowly.
- **Diffuse tenosynovial giant cell tumor or pigmented villonodular synovitis (PVNS)** is characterized by an ill-defined, exuberant proliferation of synovial lining cells arising from periarticular soft tissues, with extension into the subsynovial tissue. It involves a single joint, usually in young adults, and is seen equally in men and women. The most common site is the knee (80%), but it also occurs in the hip, ankle, calcaneocuboid joint, elbow and, less frequently, tendon sheaths of the fingers and toes.

MOLECULAR PATHOGENESIS: In the past, these lesions were regarded as reactive/inflammatory, but recurrent chromosomal aberrations have been described in both forms, supporting a neoplastic nature. Translocations involving the short arm of chromosome 1 have been detected, most commonly t(1;2)(p11;q35-36) or (p13;q37), with evidence of a fusion of colony-stimulating factor-1 (CSF-1) with COL6a3. Trisomies for chromosomes 5 and 7 have been found only in the diffuse form. The association of these anomalies with tumor pathogenesis is unclear.

 PATHOLOGY: The localized tenosynovial giant cell tumor is characterized by a small (<4 cm), multinodular, smooth-contoured, partially encapsulated, exophytic mass attached to a tendon sheath. The diffuse form is usually larger than 5 cm and poorly circumscribed. It invades the joint and erodes the bone (Fig. 30-65A). It may insinuate through joint capsules into soft tissue and encompass nerves and arteries, sometimes necessitating radical surgical excision. The synovium develops enlarged folds and nodular excrescences, which are brown colored owing to their iron pigment content (Fig. 30-65B). Microscopically, both tumors have similar histology. They are composed of bland mononuclear cells resembling macrophages, admixed with scattered multinucleated giant cells, fibroblasts and foam cells. Hemosiderin-laden macrophages reflect previous hemorrhage (Fig. 30-65C,D). The diffuse form exten-

sively infiltrates the surrounding tissue and frequently displays a villous configuration.

Treatment for these lesions is surgical excision. Radiation therapy has been used for unresectable cases. Amputation is occasionally necessary for local control. Tumors recur in 10%–20% of cases of localized tenosynovial giant cell tumor, in contrast to 40%–50% in the diffuse form. Metastases do not occur. A malignant counterpart has been described, but it is very rare.

Soft Tissue Tumors

Soft tissue tumors are mesenchymal neoplasms that may arise anywhere in the body but are most commonly found within skeletal muscle, fat, fibrous tissue or blood vessels. Tumors of peripheral nerves (see Chapter 32) and other tumors of neuroectodermal differentiation may be included in the category of soft tissue tumors. Malignant soft tissue tumors are rare, accounting for less than 1% of

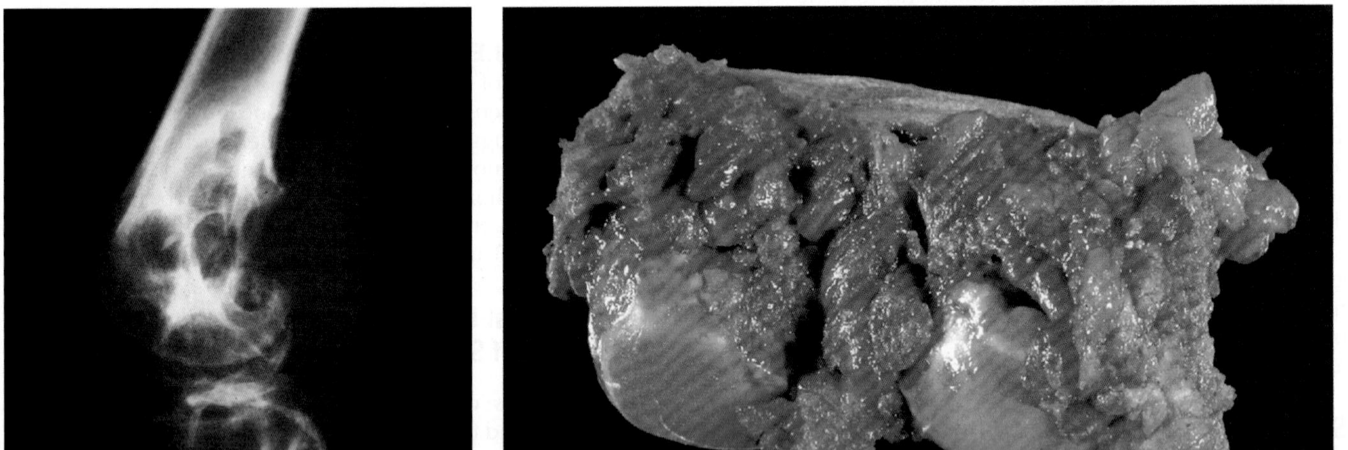

FIGURE 30-65. Pigmented villonodular synovitis. A. Radiograph of the knee demonstrates confluent erosions of the distal femur and proximal tibia and a soft tissue mass within the joint. **B.** Gross specimen shows massive destruction of the femoral condyles. Note brown color and nodular thickenings. **C.** Low-power microscopy demonstrates thickened villous synovium. **D.** At higher power, the cellular infiltrate mainly consists of mononuclear histiocytic synoviocytes, many of which contain brown hemosiderin pigment, and multinucleated giant cells.

all malignancies in the United States. Benign soft tissue neoplasms are 100 times more common than malignant ones.

Although soft tissue tumors may show evidence of differentiation toward a particular cell type (fibroblastic, adipocytic, vascular, myoid, etc.), they are thought to arise from pluripotent mesenchymal stem cells that reside in soft tissues and bone marrow. Not all soft tissue tumors can be readily classified by their line of differentiation. However, many do have characteristic and unique genomic abnormalities that are diagnostically useful (Table 30-2).

Soft tissue tumors may be benign, locally aggressive or malignant. Locally aggressive tumors invade and may recur locally (e.g., fibromatosis). Malignant soft tissue tumors (sarcomas) can metastasize via the bloodstream, usually to the lungs or bone. *Patients generally die of metastatic disease rather than local invasion at the primary tumor site.*

The ability to distinguish sarcoma from benign mimics is key to prognostication; outcome is predicated upon both tumor grade and stage. A number of published grading schemes exist, among which the Fédération National des Centres de Lutte Contre le Cancer (FNCLCC) system is one of the most widely accepted. In the FNCLCC system, grading is based on cellular phenotype (histologic tumor type and degree of differentiation), mitotic activity and presence of tumor necrosis as indicators of aggressive behavior. In addition, tumor size and depth (superficial vs. deep soft tissue) are regarded by some as the most important prognostic criteria in primary tumors. These criteria are combined with grade and metastatic status for overall staging and risk prediction.

A group of genetic disorders associated with soft tissue tumors includes neurofibromatosis type 1, tuberous sclerosis, Osler-Weber-Rendu disease, Li-Fraumeni syndrome and Gardner syndrome. Burns in childhood produce scars, which in rare instances lead to soft tissue fibroblastic tumors many years later. Radiation injury can also contribute to the development of sarcomas, in particular angiosarcoma, osteosarcoma or undifferentiated sarcoma, years after exposure. There is no evidence to support the association of trauma with the development of soft tissue tumors, and injury merely draws attention to a preexisting tumor.

A few important general principles relate to soft tissue tumors:

- Superficial tumors tend to be benign.
- Deep lesions are often malignant.
- Large tumors are more often malignant than small ones.
- Rapidly growing tumors are more likely to be malignant than tumors that develop slowly.
- Calcification may exist in both benign and malignant tumors.
- Benign tumors are relatively avascular, while most malignant ones are hypervascular.
- Some soft tissue tumors are classified on the basis of genetic or molecular findings.

TUMORS AND TUMOR-LIKE CONDITIONS OF FIBROUS ORIGIN

Nodular Fasciitis Is a Benign Lesion That May Mimic a Sarcoma

Nodular fasciitis is a rapidly growing but self-limited tumor that commonly affects superficial tissues of the forearm,

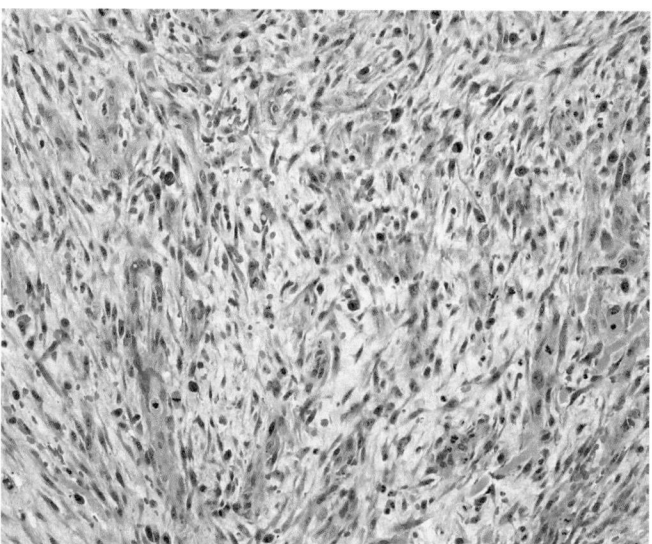

FIGURE 30-66. Nodular fasciitis. Elongated spindle and stellate cells are arranged haphazardly in a loose myxoid stroma, giving the lesion a "tissue culture–like" appearance. Extravasated erythrocytes and scattered lymphocytes are a common finding. Mitotic figures may be prominent.

trunk and back and is characterized by a t(17;22)(p13;q13) translocation. Most cases occur in young adults who present to medical attention following the rapid growth of the lesion. Histologically, nodular fasciitis may be mistaken for a sarcoma, because it is hypercellular and has abundant mitoses and numerous immature, spindle-shaped fibroblasts and myofibroblasts in a myxoid stroma (Fig. 30-66). While nodular fasciitis was long thought to be a posttraumatic reactive condition, the discovery of a recurrent translocation and associated chimeric fusion gene has resulted in a reclassification of this tumor as a form of neoplasia. *MYH-USP6* gene fusion results in overexpression of USP6, an oncogenic protein with possible roles in inflammation and proliferation. In addition, cytogenetic abnormalities involving chromosome 15 have been reported in some cases. The affected region on chromosome 15 codes for several proteins involved in tissue repair (e.g., FGF7) and oncogenesis. Despite these underlying genetic alterations, nodular fasciitis is self-limited and is cured by surgical excision.

Fibromatosis Is a Locally Aggressive Proliferation of Fibroblasts

Fibromatosis is a locally invasive, slowly growing mass that may occur virtually anywhere in the body. Although histologically similar, there are genetic distinctions between superficial and deep "aggressive" variants of fibromatosis. Fibromatosis does not metastasize, but surgical resection of deep tumors is often followed by local recurrence. Diabetics, alcoholics and epileptics have an increased incidence of fibromatosis, as do patients with familial adenomatous polyposis.

 **MOLECULAR PATHOGENESIS: Fibromatosis results from signaling alterations in the Wnt pathway.** Mutations involving *APC* or *CTNNB1* are present in deep aggressive fibromatosis (desmoid tumor) but have not been identified in superficial variants. Inactivating

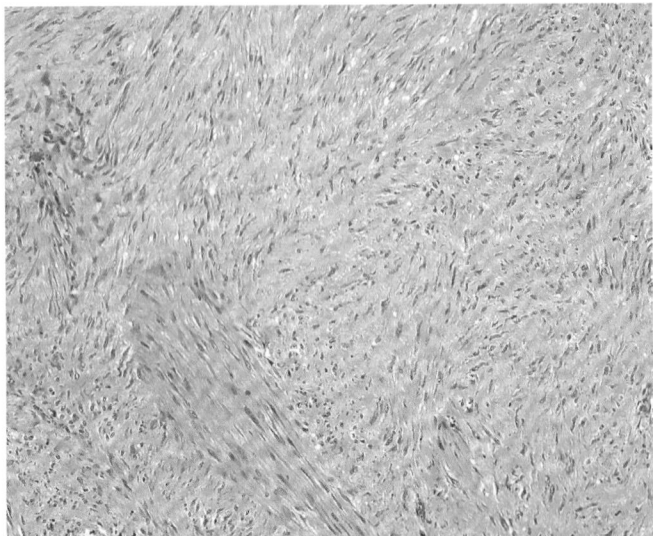

FIGURE 30-67. Fibromatosis. Microscopically, the lesion is composed of fascicles of bland spindle cells arrayed in long sweeping fascicles in a collagenous stroma.

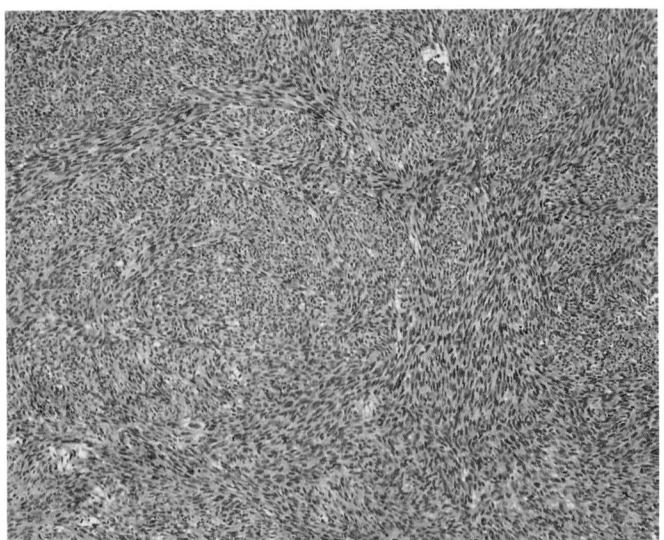

FIGURE 30-68. Fibrosarcoma. A photomicrograph demonstrates irregularly arranged malignant fibroblasts characterized by dark, irregular and elongated nuclei of varying sizes.

mutations in the *APC* gene are found mostly in cases of fibromatosis that are associated with familial adenomatous polyposis. The APC protein binds to β-catenin and enhances its degradation. Thus, loss of APC indirectly stabilizes β-catenin. β-Catenin in turn promotes Wnt pathway signaling, which modulates developmental genes and is thought to be important in the development of fibromatosis. Most sporadic cases of desmoid tumor have activating mutations in *CTNNB1*, the gene encoding β-catenin, which make it resistant to the inhibitory effect of APC. In short, mutations in both the *APC* and *CTNNB1* genes result in persistent stabilization of β-catenin.

 PATHOLOGY: On gross examination, the lesions of fibromatosis tend to be large, firm and whitish, with poorly demarcated borders and a whorled cut surface. Microscopic examination reveals sheets and interdigitating fascicles of benign-appearing spindle cells (fibroblasts) with little mitotic activity (Fig. 30-67). Because microscopic tongues of tumor extend between preexisting structures, surgical "shelling out" of the lesion is followed by recurrences in half of cases. Complete surgical excision is curative.

Specific forms of fibromatosis are identified by their characteristic locations:

- **Palmar fibromatosis** (Dupuytren contracture) is the most common form of fibromatosis. It affects 1%–2% of the general population but as many as 20% of people older than 65. In half of cases, the lesion is bilateral, and in 10% of cases, it is associated with fibromatosis in other locations. Fibrous nodules and cord-like bands in the palmar fascia eventually lead to flexion contractures of the fingers, particularly the fourth and fifth digits.
- **Plantar fibromatosis** is similar to palmar fibromatosis, except that it is less frequent and involves the plantar aponeurosis.
- **Penile fibromatosis** (Peyronie disease) is the least common of the localized fibromatoses. It is characterized by induration of, or a mass in, the penile shaft, causing it to

curve toward the affected side **(penile strabismus)**. The lesion leads to urethral obstruction and pain on erection.
- Deep aggressive fibromatosis (desmoid tumor) frequently involves fascia and muscular aponeuroses of the extremities or abdominal wall musculature. It may also arise in the mesentery. Lesions are highly infiltrative and difficult to resect completely, accounting for the high recurrence rates. Mesenteric fibromatosis is more commonly associated with APC mutations, whereas abdominal fibromatosis shows a predilection for women.

Fibrosarcoma Is a Malignant Tumor of Fibroblasts

Many subtypes of sarcoma show evidence of fibroblastic differentiation. Pure adult fibrosarcoma is a diagnosis of exclusion, which shows no characteristic cytogenetic abnormality and accounts for less than 3% of adult sarcomas. Congenital (infantile) fibrosarcoma is characterized by a chromosomal translocation, t(12;15)(p13;q26), that fuses the *ETV6* and *NTRK3* genes. Fibrosarcomas arise from deep connective tissue, such as fascia, scar tissue, periosteum and tendons. Macroscopically, the tumors are sharply demarcated and frequently exhibit necrosis and hemorrhage. They are characterized histologically by malignant-appearing fibroblasts (Fig. 30-68), which often form densely interlacing bundles and fascicles, producing a "herringbone" pattern. The prognosis for high-grade adult fibrosarcoma is guarded; the survival at 5 years is only 40% and at 10 years is 30%. Infantile fibrosarcoma rarely metastasizes, with a less than 5% mortality rate.

Other variants of fibroblastic sarcomas exist, including low-grade fibromyxoid sarcoma, myofibroblastic sarcoma and myxofibrosarcoma, among others, each with its own distinct pathologic features and clinical course.

Undifferentiated Pleomorphic Sarcoma (Malignant Fibrous Histiocytoma) Is a Diagnosis of Exclusion

Malignant fibrous histiocytoma (MFH) was historically considered to be a malignant soft tissue tumor with fibroblastic and histiocytic (macrophage) differentiation. More recently, it has been determined that the microscopic appearance of "MFH" may be seen in a phenotypically heterogeneous group of sarcomas generically called "undifferentiated pleomorphic sarcomas" (UPSs). Immunohistochemical, ultrastructural and, more recently, genomic studies have shown that the large majority of UPS represents the pleomorphic variants of liposarcoma, leiomyosarcoma or rhabdomyosarcoma. A small proportion of cases remain unclassifiable and may truly represent the most primitive undifferentiated form of sarcoma. Efforts to classify such tumors are important, as pleomorphic rhabdomyosarcoma or leiomyosarcoma may have a slightly worse prognosis. Collectively, UPS is the most common sarcoma in patients over the age of 40, but cases have been recorded at all ages. In half of the cases, tumors arise in the deep fascia or within skeletal muscle of the lower limbs. UPS has been reported in association with surgical scars and foreign bodies or after radiation treatment. At the molecular level, it shows highly complex chromosomal rearrangements, a phenotype associated with genomic instability. Several oncogenes may play a role in the pathogenesis of UPS, including *SAS, TP53, RB1* and *CDKN2A*, among others.

 PATHOLOGY: Adult UPSs are usually unencapsulated, gray-white or tan tumors that may have areas of hemorrhage and necrosis. Microscopically, the tumor displays a highly variable morphologic pattern, with areas of spindle-shaped cells arrayed in an irregularly whorled (storiform) pattern adjacent to fields with bizarre pleomorphic cells (Fig. 30-69). The spindle cells tend to be better differentiated and often show focal fibroblastic features. Mitoses are abundant. Often a nonneoplastic population of tumor-infiltrating inflammatory cells is seen, including xanthomatous cells, dendritic or histiocytic cells and a moderate chronic inflammatory reaction. Some tumors contain numerous tumor giant cells, which exhibit intense cytoplasmic eosinophilia. The extent of collagen deposition varies and sometimes dominates the microscopic pattern. Necrosis is often present and may be extensive. A few tumors reveal a conspicuous myxoid stroma. Immunohistochemical and ultrastructural studies are generally performed to establish a specific line of differentiation (smooth muscle, skeletal muscle, adipose tissue, etc.). If no such differentiation can be demonstrated, then the tumor can be considered to be an **undifferentiated pleomorphic sarcoma**.

The prognosis of adult undifferentiated pleomorphic sarcomas depends on the degree of cytologic atypia, the extent of mitotic activity and the degree of necrosis. Almost half of the patients develop a local recurrence after surgery, and a comparable proportion later manifest metastatic disease, particularly in the lungs. The overall 5-year survival range is about 50%.

Radiation-induced sarcomas are a form of adult undifferentiated pleomorphic sarcoma that arise in bone or soft tissue, usually 10–20 years after radiotherapy for a malignancy in that field. A typical story is development of UPS or osteosarcoma of a rib or vertebral body (uncommon sites for de novo osteosarcomas) after radiation to the thorax as treatment for mediastinal lymphoma or breast cancer. The incidence of postradiation sarcoma is low (<1% of irradiated patients).

TUMORS OF ADIPOSE TISSUE

Lipomas Are the Most Common Soft Tissue Mass and Closely Resemble Normal Fat

Composed of well-differentiated adipocytes, these benign, circumscribed tumors can originate at any site in the body that contains adipose tissue. Most occur in the subcutaneous tissues of the upper half of the body, especially the trunk and neck. Lipomas are seen mainly in adults, and patients with multiple tumors often have relatives with a similar history.

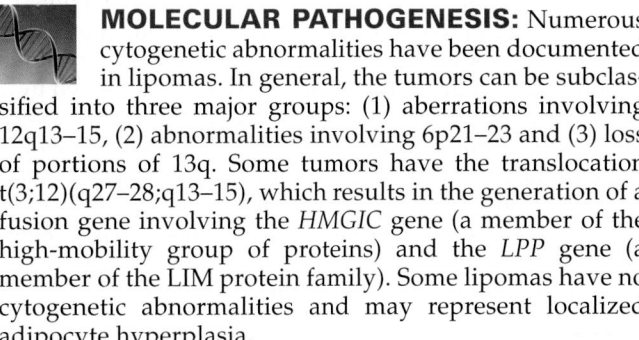 **MOLECULAR PATHOGENESIS:** Numerous cytogenetic abnormalities have been documented in lipomas. In general, the tumors can be subclassified into three major groups: (1) aberrations involving 12q13–15, (2) abnormalities involving 6p21–23 and (3) loss of portions of 13q. Some tumors have the translocation t(3;12)(q27–28;q13–15), which results in the generation of a fusion gene involving the *HMGIC* gene (a member of the high-mobility group of proteins) and the *LPP* gene (a member of the LIM protein family). Some lipomas have no cytogenetic abnormalities and may represent localized adipocyte hyperplasia.

 PATHOLOGY: On gross examination, lipomas are encapsulated, soft, yellow lesions that vary in size and may become very large. Deeper tumors are often poorly circumscribed. Histologically, a lipoma is often indistinguishable from normal adipose tissue (Fig. 30-70). Lipomas are adequately treated by simple local excision.

An **angiolipoma** is a small, well-circumscribed, subcutaneous lipoma with extensive vascular proliferation that usually occurs in the upper extremities and trunk of young adults. They are often multiple and painful.

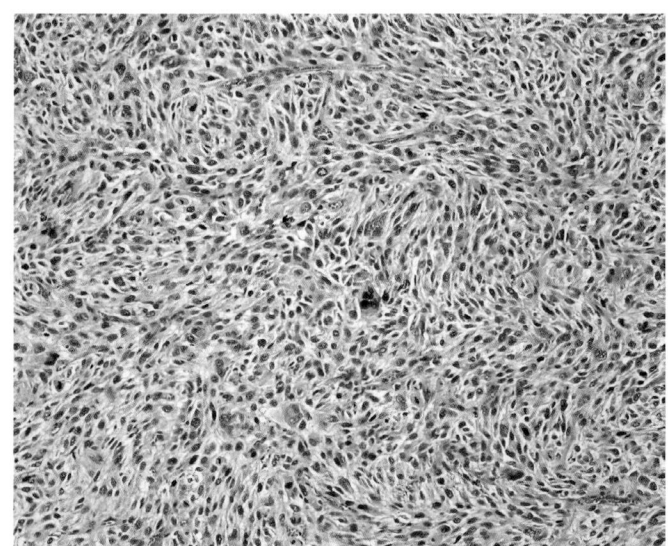

FIGURE 30-69. Undifferentiated pleomorphic sarcoma. An anaplastic tumor exhibits spindle cells, plump polygonal cells, bizarre tumor giant cells and scattered chronic inflammatory cells. This appearance can be seen in pleomorphic sarcomas with other lines of differentiation (e.g., pleomorphic liposarcoma).

FIGURE 30-70. Lipoma. The tumor is composed of mature adipocytes with small eccentric nuclei.

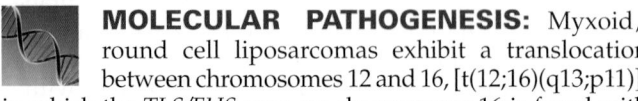

Liposarcomas Are the Second Most Common Sarcoma in Adults

Liposarcomas account for 25% of all malignant soft tissue tumors. The neoplasm arises after age 50 years and is most common in the deep thigh and retroperitoneum. They tend to grow slowly but may become extremely large. There are several subtypes of liposarcoma, including myxoid/round cell liposarcoma, well-differentiated liposarcoma and pleomorphic liposarcoma.

 MOLECULAR PATHOGENESIS: Myxoid/round cell liposarcomas exhibit a translocation between chromosomes 12 and 16, [t(12;16)(q13;p11)], in which the *TLS/FUS* gene on chromosome 16 is fused with the *DDIT3* gene on chromosome 12. The *TLS/FUS* gene product is a novel RNA-binding protein, with substantial homology to the EWS protein of Ewing sarcoma, while the DDIT3 protein is a transcriptional repressor. Atypical lipomatous tumors and well-differentiated liposarcomas are defined by a giant marker chromosome, or a supernumerary ring chromosome with amplification of the 12q14–15 region, which includes the *MDM2* and *CDK4* genes, among others. MDM2 is involved in regulating growth and signaling survival, in part by inhibition of p53 (see Chapter 5), while CDK4 is a regulatory factor promoting cell cycle progression. Pleomorphic liposarcomas have complex genomic rearrangements.

 PATHOLOGY: Gross appearances of liposarcoma subtypes vary depending on the proportions of adipose, mucinous and fibrous tissue. Well-differentiated tumors may resemble normal fat or may show fibrotic or gelatinous cut surfaces. Dedifferentiated or pleomorphic liposarcomas grossly can appear soft and gelatinous, with necrosis, hemorrhage and cysts. Lipoblasts may be seen microscopically in all types of liposarcoma *Lipoblasts are early adipocytes with univacuolated or multivacuolated cytoplasmic fat vesicles indenting the nucleus. While frequently seen in liposarcoma, lipoblasts may also be present in reactive or regenerative conditions*

and are neither necessary nor sufficient for the diagnosis of liposarcoma.

WELL-DIFFERENTIATED/DEDIFFERENTIATED LIPOSARCOMA: Well-differentiated liposarcomas typically measure 5–10 cm in diameter, although retroperitoneal tumors may reach gigantic proportions (i.e., 40 cm in diameter and weighing in excess of 20 kg). Well-differentiated liposarcomas are often composed of large amounts of mature fat, and therefore can be confused with lipomas if inadequately sampled. Sclerosis, prominent lymphoid aggregates or inflammatory infiltrates may also be seen. The defining feature of well-differentiated liposarcoma is the presence of atypical neoplastic stromal cells with large, irregular nuclei and hyperchromatic chromatin (Fig. 30-71). Dedifferentiated liposarcoma arises in preexisting well-differentiated tumors and is usually composed of a monotonous population of mitotically active spindle cells, although some tumors may be pleomorphic and resemble UPS.

MYXOID/ROUND CELL LIPOSARCOMA: These tumors most frequently arise in the proximal extremities but are exceedingly rare in the retroperitoneum. Microscopically, myxoid liposarcoma consists of univacuolated "signet ring" lipoblasts and variable amounts of primitive ovoid to round cells embedded in a vascularized myxoid stroma. Round cell liposarcoma represents a poorly differentiated form of myxoid liposarcoma and contains a high proportion of primitive round cells and a scant amount of myxoid stroma.

PLEOMORPHIC LIPOSARCOMA: Pleomorphic liposarcomas have a UPS-like histologic appearance with numerous large, bizarre tumor cells. However, they also contain lipoblasts.

Well-differentiated liposarcoma is known as atypical lipomatous tumor in the extremities, where complete resection results in low recurrence rates. Retroperitoneal tumors cannot be completely resected and frequently recur. Well-differentiated liposarcoma almost never metastasizes. Myxoid liposarcoma and differentiated liposarcoma have an intermediate risk of local recurrence and metastasis, whereas round cell and pleomorphic liposarcomas have a high frequency of local recurrence and metastasis. Pleomorphic liposarcoma has the worst outcome, with less than 20% 5-year survival rates, compared to greater than 70% for well-differentiated or pure myxoid variants.

RHABDOMYOSARCOMA

Rhabdomyosarcoma is a malignant tumor that displays features of striated muscle differentiation. It is uncommon in mature adults but is the most frequent soft tissue sarcoma of children and young adults.

 PATHOLOGY: Most cases of rhabdomyosarcoma can be classified in one of four subtypes. In addition to their light microscopic features, all subtypes of rhabdomyosarcoma show immunohistochemical evidence of skeletal muscle differentiation. Tumors may express nonspecific myoid markers, such as actin and desmin, but most demonstrate at least focal expression of skeletal muscle–specific markers, such as the transcription factors myogenin and MyoD1.

EMBRYONAL RHABDOMYOSARCOMA: This form is most common in children between 3 and 12 years old and frequently involves the head and neck, genitourinary tract and

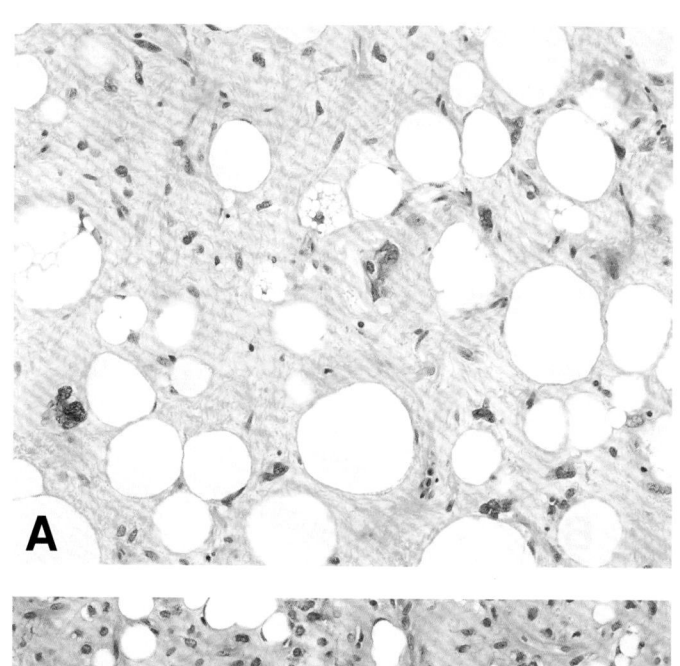

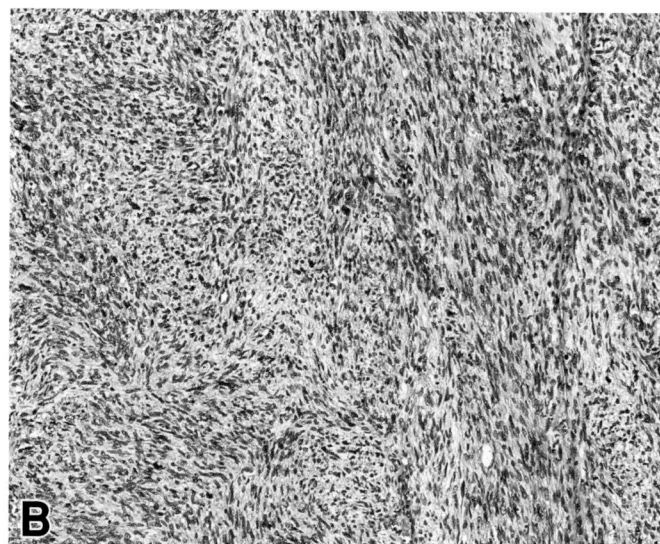

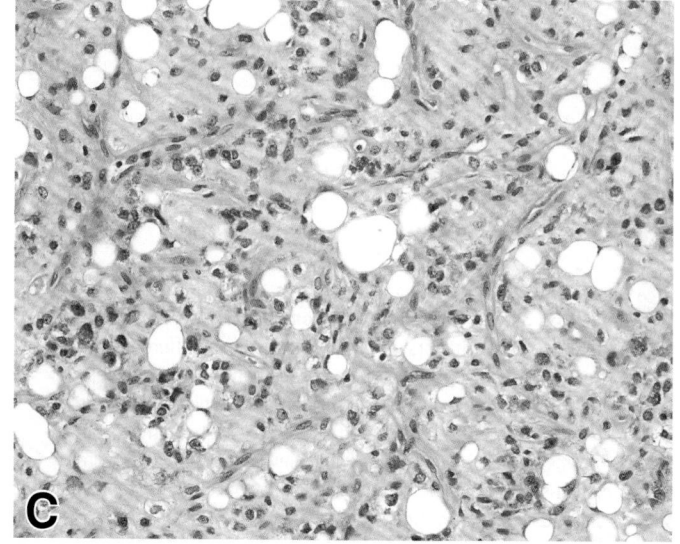

FIGURE 30-71. Liposarcoma. A. Well-differentiated liposarcoma. Atypical stromal cells with hyperchromatic enlarged nuclei are present within collagenous stroma surrounding mature adipocytes. Lipoblasts, with multiple cytoplasmic lipid vacuoles indenting the nucleus, are present but are not required for diagnosis. **B.** Dedifferentiated liposarcoma. The tumor is composed of a hypercellular proliferation of nondescript spindle cells, without evidence of lipogenic differentiation. **C.** Myxoid liposarcoma. The tumor is composed of a mixture of small round adipocyte precursors, univacuolated lipoblasts and mature adipocytes arrayed in a myxoid stroma with a prominent plexiform vascular network.

retroperitoneum. Its appearance varies from that of a highly differentiated tumor containing rhabdomyoblasts, with large eosinophilic cytoplasm and cross-striations (Fig. 30-72A), to that of a poorly differentiated small cell neoplasm.

BOTRYOID EMBRYONAL RHABDOMYOSARCOMA: This tumor, also known as **sarcoma botryoides,** is distinguished by the formation of polypoid, grape-like tumor masses. Microscopically, the malignant cells are scattered in an abundant myxoid stroma. Botryoid foci may occur in any type of embryonal rhabdomyosarcoma, but they are most common in tumors of hollow visceral organs, including the vagina (see Chapter 24) and urinary bladder.

ALVEOLAR RHABDOMYOSARCOMA: This neoplasm occurs less frequently than the embryonal type and principally affects young people between ages 10 and 25; rarely, it may be seen in elderly patients. It is most common in the upper and lower extremities, but it can also be distributed in the same sites as the embryonal type. Typically, club-shaped tumor cells are arranged in clumps that are outlined by fibrous septa. The loose arrangement of the cells in the center of the clusters generates an "alveolar" pattern (Fig. 30-72B). The tumor cells exhibit intense eosinophilia, and occasional multinucleated giant cells are identified. Malignant

rhabdomyoblasts, recognizable by their cross-striations, occur less commonly in the alveolar variant than in embryonal rhabdomyosarcoma, being present in only 25% of cases.

MOLECULAR PATHOGENESIS: Most alveolar rhabdomyosarcomas express *PAX3-FOXO1* or *PAX7-FOXO1* gene fusions, resulting from t(2;13)(q35;q14) or t(1;13)(p36;q14) translocations, respectively. In patients with localized tumors, the type of fusion does not correlate with the clinical outcome. However, in the presence of metastatic disease, *PAX3-FOXO1*–positive tumors have a worse prognosis than do *PAX7-FOXO1*–positive ones.

PLEOMORPHIC RHABDOMYOSARCOMA: The least common form of rhabdomyosarcoma is found in the skeletal muscles of older individuals, often in the thigh. This tumor differs from the other types of rhabdomyosarcoma in the pleomorphism of its irregularly arranged cells and can be categorized as a type of adult undifferentiated pleomorphic sarcoma. Large, granular, eosinophilic rhabdomyoblasts, together with multinucleated giant cells, are common. Cross-striations are virtually nonexistent.

The historically dismal prognosis associated with most rhabdomyosarcomas has improved in the past two decades

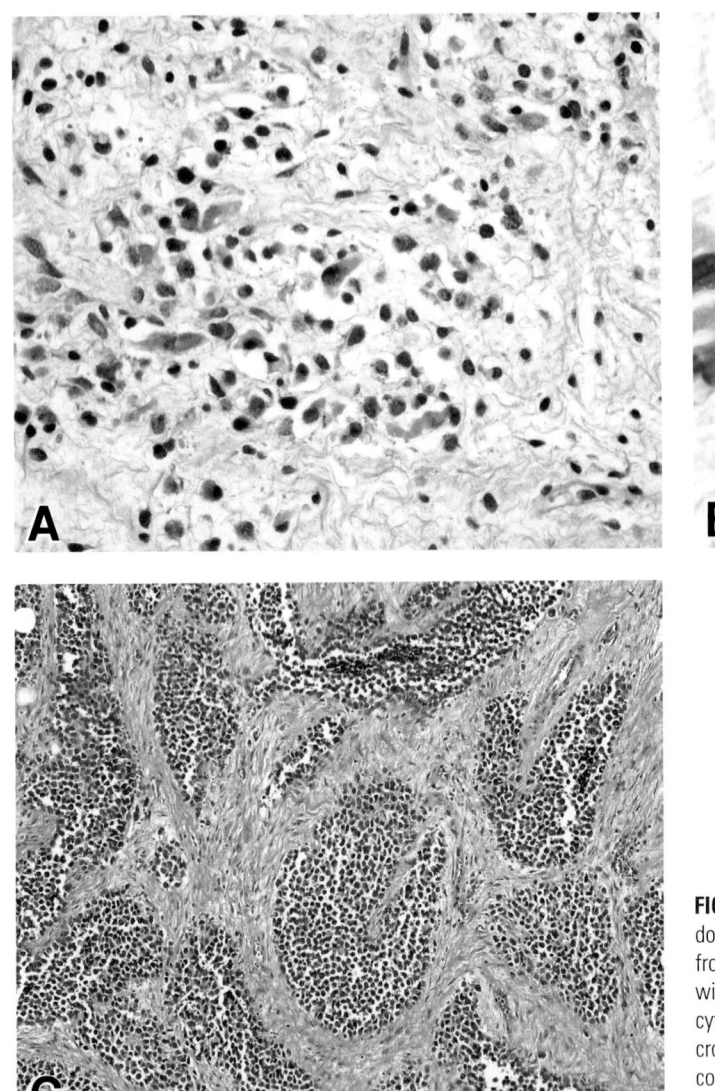

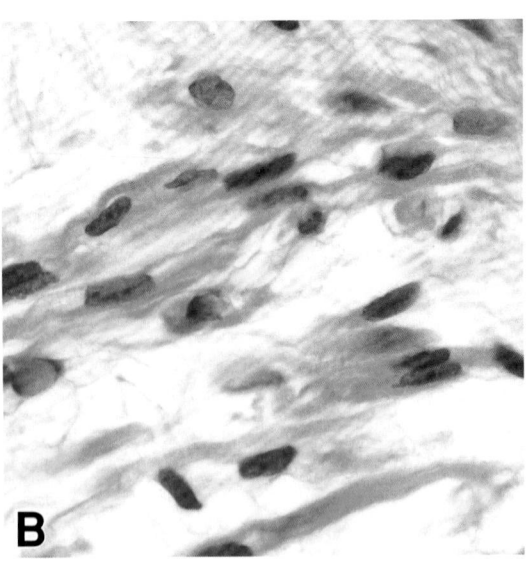

FIGURE 30-72. Rhabdomyosarcoma. A, B. Embryonal rhabdomyosarcoma. Tumors may show a spectrum of differentiation from **(A)** primitive small round cells and polyhedral tumor cells with enlarged, hyperchromatic nuclei and deeply eosinophilic cytoplasm to **(B)** differentiated strap cells with clearly visible cross-striations. **C.** Alveolar rhabdomyosarcoma. Tumors are composed of primitive small round cells, which are arranged in discohesive nests within a fibrous stroma.

as a result of the introduction of combined therapeutic modalities, including surgery, radiation therapy and chemotherapy. Today, more than 80% of patients with localized or regional disease are cured. Factors indicating a worse prognosis include age older than 10, tumor size greater than 5 cm, alveolar and pleomorphic histologic subtypes and advanced stage of disease.

SMOOTH MUSCLE TUMORS

These tumors are characterized histologically by fascicles of spindled cells with brightly eosinophilic cytoplasm, cylindrical nuclei and immunohistochemical expression of smooth muscle actin, muscle-specific actin and desmin.

LEIOMYOMA: This benign soft tissue tumor usually arises in sites associated with normal smooth muscle, including erector pili muscles in the dermis, blood vessel walls in subcutaneous or deep somatic tissues and the muscular wall of the esophagus or uterus. Leiomyomas appear as firm, gray-white, well-circumscribed nodules. Dermal or subcutaneous tumors may be painful. Microscopically, they are composed of intersecting fascicles of uniform spindled cells with cigar-shaped nuclei and very low mitotic activity. Some display prominent blood vessels (angiomyoma). Simple excision is curative.

LEIOMYOSARCOMA: This malignant soft tissue neoplasm is an uncommon tumor of adults that typically arises from the wall of blood vessels in the soft tissue of the extremities or in retroperitoneum. Macroscopically, leiomyosarcomas tend to be well circumscribed but are larger and softer than leiomyomas and often exhibit necrosis, hemorrhage and cystic degeneration. Histologically, the tumor cells are arranged in broad, intersecting fascicles. Well-differentiated tumor cells have elongated nuclei and eosinophilic cytoplasm; poorly differentiated ones show marked increased cellularity and severe cytologic atypia (Fig. 30-73). Leiomyosarcoma is differentiated from leiomyoma mainly by cellularity, atypia, mitotic activity and necrosis, which also indicates the prognosis. Most leiomyosarcomas eventually metastasize, although dissemination may occur as late as 15 or more years after resection of the primary tumor. Leiomyosarcomas have complex chromosomal rearrangements and numerous somatic mutations, but no characteristic alterations have been documented. Retroperitoneal tumors have a poor prognosis.

EBV-associated smooth muscle tumors are a distinctive subgroup of smooth muscle tumors that occur in

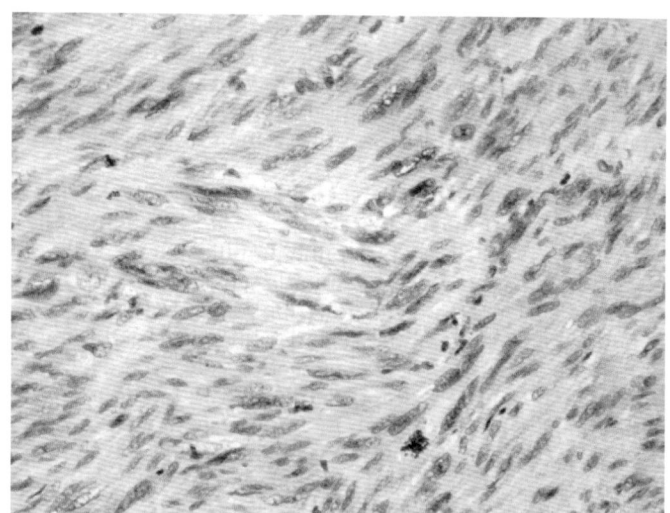

FIGURE 30-73. Leiomyosarcoma. The tumor is composed of spindle cells with elongated, hyperchromatic nuclei; a variable degree of pleomorphism; and frequent mitoses.

immunocompromised patients, mostly children and young adults who are infected with HIV or are status post–organ transplant. The tumors may be multifocal or multicentric. Their histologic appearance is variable and all display a degree of mitotic activity and numerous intralesional T lymphocytes. Death from these tumors is rare, but most patients have persistent disease.

VASCULAR TUMORS

Benign vascular tumors (hemangiomas) are among the most common soft tissue tumors and are the most frequent neoplasms of infancy and childhood. By contrast, angiosarcomas account for less than 1% of all sarcomas and are more common in older adults. Vascular tumors are discussed in detail in Chapter 16.

SYNOVIAL SARCOMA

Synovial sarcoma is a highly malignant soft tissue tumor characterized by translocations between chromosomes

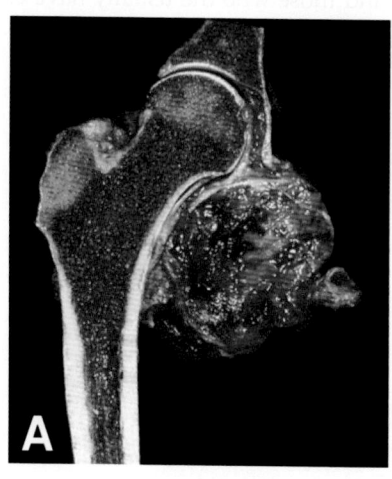

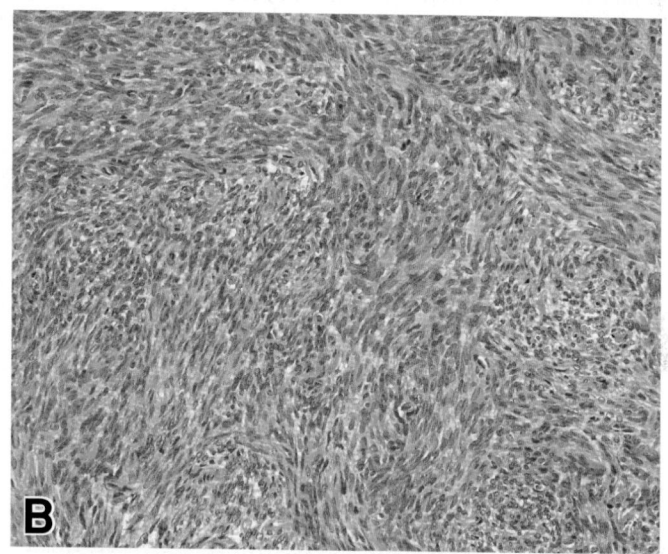

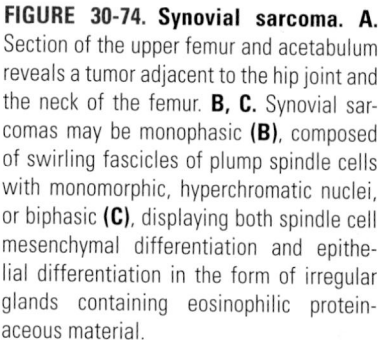

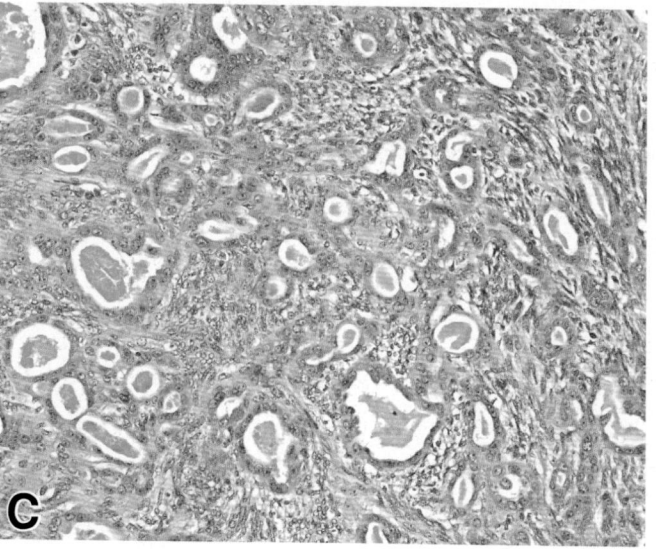

FIGURE 30-74. Synovial sarcoma. A. Section of the upper femur and acetabulum reveals a tumor adjacent to the hip joint and the neck of the femur. **B, C.** Synovial sarcomas may be monophasic **(B)**, composed of swirling fascicles of plump spindle cells with monomorphic, hyperchromatic nuclei, or biphasic **(C)**, displaying both spindle cell mesenchymal differentiation and epithelial differentiation in the form of irregular glands containing eosinophilic proteinaceous material.

X and 18. They may arise anywhere in the body but are commonly located in deep soft tissues near joints, tendon sheaths or joint capsules. Synovial sarcomas occur principally in young adults and usually present as a painful mass in the extremity.

Despite the name, synovial sarcomas neither arise from synovial tissues nor show synoviocyte differentiation. Expression of TLE1, a transcription factor associated with cell fate determination, is characteristic and may account for the dual epithelial and mesenchymal differentiation often seen in synovial sarcoma.

MOLECULAR PATHOGENESIS: Synovial sarcomas display a specific, balanced chromosomal translocation involving chromosomes X and 18 [t(x;18)(p11.2;q11.2)]. This translocation results in fusion of the *SS18/SYT* (synteny) gene on chromosome 18 to the *SSX* gene (a transcriptional repressor) on the X chromosome, leading to production of a hybrid protein, SS18-SSX1, SS18-SSX2 or, rarely, SS18-SSX4. The SS18-SSX2 protein is associated with a better prognosis if the disease is localized.

PATHOLOGY: On gross examination, synovial sarcomas are usually circumscribed, round or multilobular masses attached to tendons, tendon sheaths or the exterior wall of the joint capsule (Fig. 30-74A). The tumors tend to be surrounded by a glistening pseudocapsule and in many instances are cystic. Areas of hemorrhage, necrosis and calcification may be seen. They range from small nodules to masses of 15 cm or more in diameter, the average being 3–5 cm.

Microscopically, synovial sarcoma is classically described as having a **biphasic pattern** (Fig. 30-74B). Fluid-filled glandular spaces lined by epithelium-like tumor cells are embedded in a sarcomatous, spindle cell background. These elements vary in proportion, distribution and cellular differentiation, with the spindle cells usually considerably more numerous than the glandular elements. If the epithelial component is lacking, the tumor is referred to as **monophasic synovial sarcoma**. Although monophasic synovial sarcoma resembles fibrosarcoma, its atypical spindle cells are plumper and swirled with a "school of fish" appearance, rather than being arranged in a herringbone pattern. Calcifications may be conspicuous within the tumor. Poorly differentiated morphology imparts a poorer prognosis. Synovial sarcoma usually expresses cytokeratin or epithelial membrane antigen, further evidence of epithelial differentiation.

The recurrence rate of synovial sarcoma is high, and metastases occur in over 60% of cases. The 5-year survival rate is 50%, and those who die usually have extensive lung metastases.

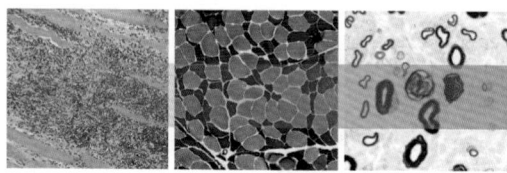

31

Skeletal Muscle and Peripheral Nervous System

Lawrence C. Kenyon ■ Thomas W. Bouldin

Skeletal Muscle

EMBRYOLOGY AND ANATOMY

The myoblast is a primitive cell that fuses with other myoblasts to form a cylindrical multinucleated myotube. The periphery of the myotube rapidly accumulates myofibrils, containing myosin and actin, which become arrayed in the cross-banded pattern characteristic of striated muscle (Fig. 31-1). The myofiber has a distinctive ultrastructural architecture (Fig. 31-2).

The myotube matures completely when it is innervated by the terminal axon of a lower motor neuron. Before innervation, the sarcolemma of the myotube contains diffusely distributed nicotinic receptors for acetylcholine on its surface membrane. Upon innervation, these receptors become highly concentrated at the motor endplate. An individual muscle fiber is innervated by only a single nerve ending, but each motor neuron innervates many muscle fibers. After innervation, the myofiber nuclei move from the center to arrange themselves in a regular pattern beneath the sarcolemma (Fig. 31-3A). Mature skeletal muscle cells are syncytia (multiple nuclei within a single cytoplasm) and can be several centimeters in length.

Muscle fibers responsible for movement are **extrafusal fibers,** while those in stretch receptors (muscle spindle organs, Fig. 31-3C) are **intrafusal fibers**. *In most primary myopathies, the damage affects extrafusal fibers but not intrafusal fibers.*

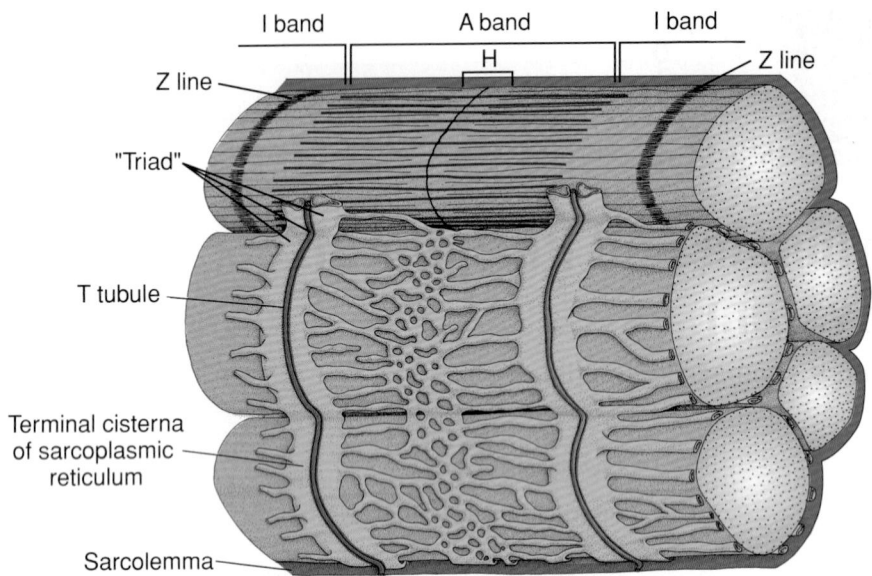

FIGURE 31-1. Normal striated muscle. Cross-striations of striated muscle are created by the arrangement of the myofilaments of the myofibril (compare to Fig. 31-2). The dark A band results from the thick myosin filaments and the thinner, partially overlapping actin filaments. In the middle portion of the myosin filaments where the actin does not overlap, there is a lighter band called the H zone or H band. In the middle of the H band, the center of each myosin filament thickens, forming intermolecular bridging with the adjacent myosin filament and giving rise to the M line (see Fig. 31-2). The finer actin filaments are anchored on the dark Z disk of the lighter I band. With contraction, the myosin filaments pull the actin filaments, causing the H zone to disappear, the I band to shrink and the A band to remain the same. The mitochondria are scattered throughout the sarcoplasm among the myofibrils. The endoplasmic reticulum (sarcoplasmic reticulum) forms an extensive, complex tubular network with periodic dilations (cisternae) around each myofibril. The cisternae are closely apposed to the transverse tubules, which are derived from the cell membrane (sarcolemma) and form a transverse network, which resembles chicken wire, around each myofibril, giving extensive communication between the internal and external environments. A triad consists of a T tubule and adjacent terminal cisternae of the sarcoplasmic reticulum.

Thus, muscle spindle organs, which are usually inconspicuous in routine histologic preparations, become relatively more prominent as extrafusal fibers disappear.

Myofiber Structure

The myofiber consists of distinct functional units (Figs. 31-1 and 31-2):

- **Sarcomere:** The functional myofibril unit, extending from one Z band to the next.
- **Z band:** A distinct electron-dense band that anchors the thin actin filaments.
- **I band:** Zone where actin filaments extend from the Z band into the A band.
- **A band:** Structure composed of the thick myosin filaments. Actin filaments overlap myosin filaments to a variable extent, depending on the degree of muscle contraction. The thin filaments form a hexagonal array around each thick filament (best seen in cross-section).
- **H zone:** Pale region in the midportion of the A band where actin filaments end.
- **M line:** Zone of intermolecular bridging and thickening of myosin filaments at the midline of the A band, which forms a thin, slightly darker electron-dense band.

During contraction, actin filaments slide past myosin filaments. The sliding actin filaments advance farther into the

A band, decreasing sarcomere length. As a result, the I band and H zone shorten, while the A band remains nearly constant. There are many filamentous proteins that make up the sarcomeres, and multiple proteins that anchor sarcomeres to the sarcolemma. These proteins may be mutated or abnormally regulated in muscular dystrophies (see below).

The **sarcoplasmic reticulum** surrounds each myofibril and forms an elaborate membranous network with irregular dilations (cisternae) juxtaposed to a transverse tubular network derived from the sarcolemma (Fig. 31-1). The **transverse tubular system** (T-tubule system) is arranged across the fiber like chicken wire, each ring wrapping around an individual myofibril. This arrangement allows an electrical stimulus to proceed along the muscle fiber surface and become diffusely and rapidly internalized via the transverse tubular system. The electrical signal is translated into a chemical signal between the transverse tubule and the cisternae of the sarcoplasmic reticulum. This process releases calcium from the sarcoplasmic reticulum into the vicinity of myofibrils, triggering muscle contraction.

The lower motor neurons and the fibers they innervate are the **motor units,** which vary in size. In limb muscles, one motor unit can include several hundred myofibers. By contrast, each motor unit of extraocular muscles may have only 20 myofibers. Eye muscles are also exceptional in that one fiber may have more than one motor endplate.

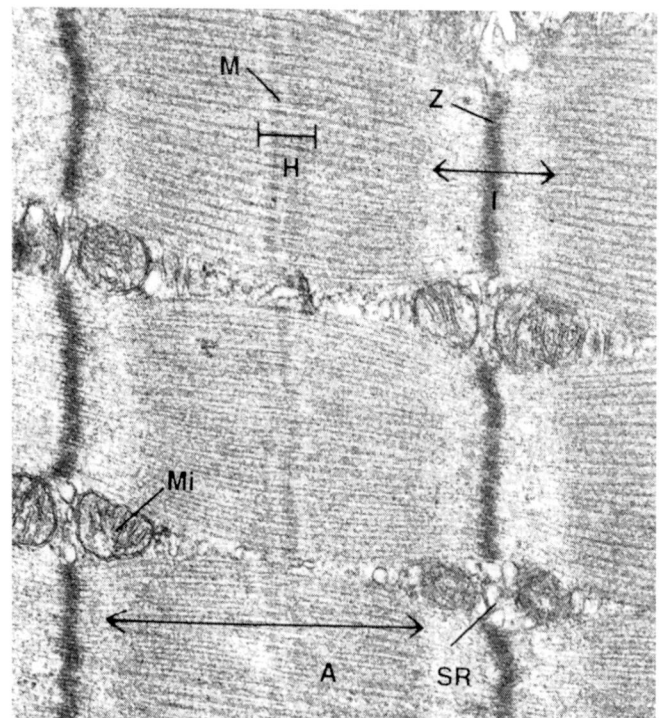

FIGURE 31-2. Normal muscle. This electron micrograph of the biceps muscle demonstrates the ultrastructure of the sarcomere. The thin dark band, the Z disk (*Z*), bisects the broad, pale I band (*I*), a zone composed of the thin actin filaments. The broad, dark band, made up of the thick myosin filaments and overlapping actin filaments, is the A band (*A*). The middle of the A band consists of the pale H zone (*H*), which in turn is bisected by a slightly darker M line (*M*), representing a zone of intermolecular bridging of myosin. Small membrane-bound vesicles compose the sarcoplasmic reticulum (*SR*) and the transverse tubules. Pairs of mitochondria (*Mi*) tend to be located between myofibrils at the level of the I bands.

Myofibers Are Classified as Slow Twitch or Fast Twitch

After innervation, a characteristic metabolic profile develops for different muscle fibers. Muscle fiber types are broadly classified by the rate of contraction and fatigueability, as type I or type II, or slow-twitch fibers and fast-twitch fibers, respectively. These can be further subdivided into slow twitch, fatigue resistant (type I); fast twitch, fatigue resistant (type IIA); and fast twitch, fatigue sensitive (type IIB). There are also type IIC fibers, which are an immature fiber type. In lower mammals, some muscles are deep red (type I), while others are pale (type II).

TYPE I FIBERS (RED, SLOW TWITCH): If a nerve stimulates a dark (red) muscle, the resulting contraction is slower and more prolonged than when a nerve excites a pale (white) muscle. For this reason, red muscles have been classified as "slow twitch." Type I fibers tend to have more mitochondria and more myoglobin, the red, oxygen-storing pigment. Krebs cycle enzymes and electron-transport-chain carrier proteins are all more abundant in slow-twitch muscle than in fast-twitch muscle. The alkaline histochemical reaction for myosin adenosine triphosphatase (ATPase) gives a crisp distinction between the two fiber types. Type I fibers stain poorly at high (alkaline) pH, but type II fibers stain darkly (Fig. 31-3B).

Functionally, type I muscles have a greater capacity for long, sustained contractions and resist fatigue. A training program that increases endurance produces little change in *size* of type I fibers, but conditioning of these fibers causes mitochondrial proliferation and increased capacity for generating energy.

TYPE II FIBERS (WHITE, FAST TWITCH): Stimulating type II fibers elicits faster, shorter and stronger contractions than with type I fibers. Glycogen, phosphorylase and other enzymes that produce energy by anaerobic glycolysis are present in higher concentrations in white muscle. Type II muscle fibers are used for rapid, brief contractions, and

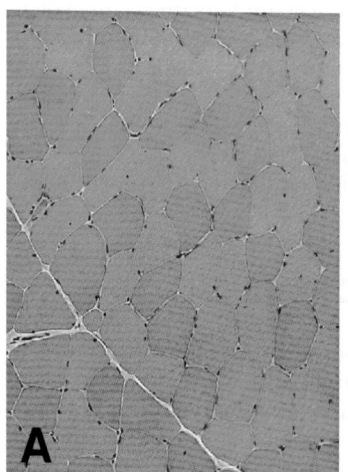
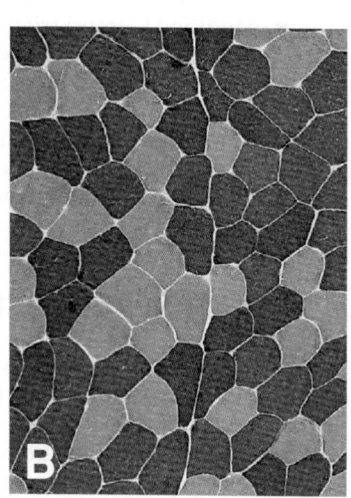
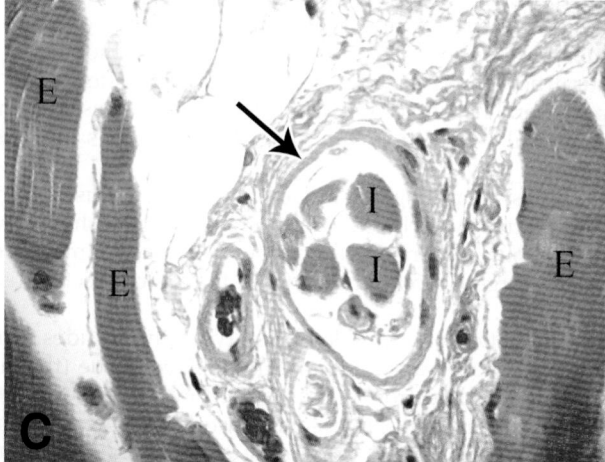

FIGURE 31-3. Normal muscle. A. Hematoxylin and eosin stain. In this transverse frozen section of the vastus lateralis, the polygonal myofibers are separated from each other by an indistinct, thin layer of connective tissue, the endomysium. The thicker band of connective tissue, the perimysium, demarcates a bundle or fascicle of fibers. All of the nuclei in this field are located at the periphery of the cells. Satellite cell nuclei are contained within the basement membrane of the muscle cell and cannot be distinguished from those of the myofibers by light microscopy. **B. Myofibrillar (myosin) ATPase.** Type I fibers are pale, at high (alkaline) pH; type II fibers are dark. Note the intermixture of fiber types. **C. Muscle spindle organ (stretch receptor).** The *arrow* marks the capsule of the muscle spindle organ. *I* = intrafusal fibers; *E* = extrafusal fibers.

hypertrophy during strength training. Type II fibers hypertrophy in response to androgenic steroids and undergo selective atrophy after disuse.

A good way to remember the distinction between fiber types is to consider a chicken. The breast muscles are pale (white) compared to those of the back or legs. The breast muscles are fast twitch since they pull down the wings during flight (granted, domesticated chickens have been bred to be too heavy to fly), while the darker muscles of the legs and back correspond to slow-twitch fibers since their function includes sustained contraction against gravity: standing and maintaining posture.

The lower motor neuron influences fiber type. During embryonic development, early muscle cells begin to express type-specific contractile proteins before muscle is innervated. Thus, the phenotype of a myofiber seems to be a programmed characteristic of the cell, rather than one induced by the nerve supply. However, the kind of innervation can alter the types of myofibers. For example, after denervation injury, reinnervation of a slow-twitch muscle (type I) by a nerve from a fast-twitch muscle (type II) causes the newly innervated type I fibers to resemble type II fibers. It is thought that the pattern or rate of discharge of lower motor neurons plays an important role in this process. Because lower motor neurons can determine fiber type, it follows that all muscle fibers in a given motor unit are of the same type. A cross-section of muscle stained with alkaline ATPase reaction (see above) shows a random mixture of fiber types (Fig. 31-3B), because motor units interdigitate extensively with each other.

In humans, no muscles are composed exclusively of one fiber type. However, proportions of fiber types vary from muscle to muscle. For example, the soleus muscle mainly contains (≥80%) type I fibers. The pattern of fiber types in a given muscle is apparently genetically determined and varies between people. Some evidence indicates that changing the use of a muscle through lengthy, intensive training may alter the pattern of muscle fiber types.

MUSCLE BIOPSY: Since normal muscle patterns are more constant within a specific muscle, the same muscles are biopsied from case to case. Samples from the quadriceps femoris or biceps brachii are suitable for biopsy diagnosis in most primary muscle diseases (myopathies). Biopsies of the sural nerve and gastrocnemius muscle are often done if a peripheral neuropathy is suspected. However, as some neuromuscular conditions are more focal, locations for muscle biopsies vary.

Biopsy sampling of a moderately affected muscle is most informative. Muscles that are uninvolved may show few or no pathologic changes, while very weak muscles may be end stage—largely replaced by fat and fibrous connective tissue (Fig. 31-4).

Evaluation of a muscle biopsy typically includes formalin-fixed, frozen and glutaraldehyde-fixed tissue (the latter for potential electron microscopy). Several frozen section histochemical stains are used, many of which measure enzymatic activity using colorimetric assays. Unlike immunohistochemical stains that tell whether a protein is present or not, histochemical stains allow visualization of an enzyme's function. Some of the usual histochemical reactions used to evaluate skeletal muscle are:

- **Nonspecific esterase:** Important for identifying denervation atrophy and the presence of neuromuscular junctions.

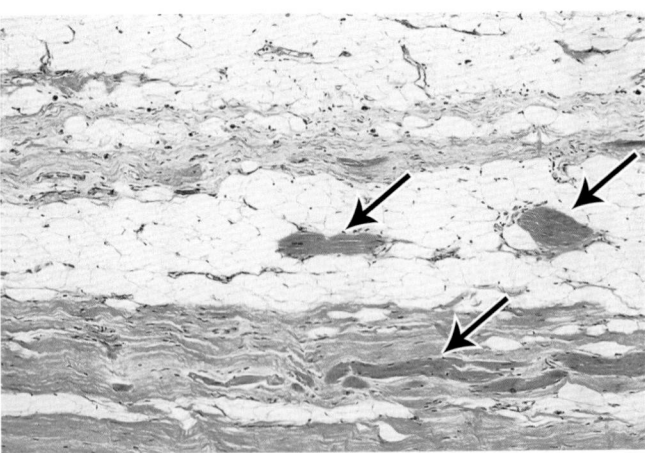

FIGURE 31-4. End-stage neuromuscular disease. In this section of the deltoid muscle stained by hematoxylin and eosin, skeletal muscle has been largely replaced by fibrofatty connective tissue. The few surviving muscle fibers have a deeper eosinophilia than does the abundant collagenous component (*arrows*).

- **NADH-tetrazolium reductase (NADH-TR):** Type I fibers appear dark owing to abundant mitochondria. This stain is useful in identifying central cores and signs of denervation.
- **Succinate dehydrogenase (SDH):** Sensitive histochemical index of mitochondrial proliferation due to mutations of mitochondrial DNA.
- **Cytochrome C oxidase:** Fibers containing abnormal mitochondria lacking the final enzyme of the electron transport chain will fail to stain.
- **Alkaline phosphatase:** Regenerating fibers are selectively stained.
- **Periodic acid–Schiff (PAS):** Helpful in identifying glycogen and diagnosing glycogen storage diseases (see below).
- **Oil red orcein (oil red O):** Marks neutral lipid and is particularly useful in assessing lipid storage myopathies such as carnitine deficiency (see below).
- **Modified Gomori trichrome stain:** Versatile stain in evaluating myopathies. It helps in assessing nemaline bodies, rimmed vacuoles of inclusion body myositis and "ragged red fibers" (see below).
- **Acid phosphatase stain:** Identifies lysosomal activity within muscle fibers and macrophages.
- **Myosin ATPase:** Depending on the pH, helps to differentiate fiber types.

GENERAL PATHOLOGIC REACTIONS

Necrosis is a common response of myofibers to injury in primary muscle diseases (**myopathies**). Widespread acute necrosis of skeletal muscle fibers (*rhabdomyolysis*) releases cytosolic proteins, including myoglobin, into the circulation, which may lead to myoglobinuria and cause acute renal failure. In many human myopathies, segmental necrosis occurs along the length of a fiber, with intact muscle flanking the site of damage (Fig. 31-5). The injury quickly elicits two responses: influx of blood-borne macrophages into the necrotic cytoplasm and activation of satellite cells, a population of dormant myoblasts nearby each fiber. As monocytes gradually phagocytose necrotic debris and remove it, satellite

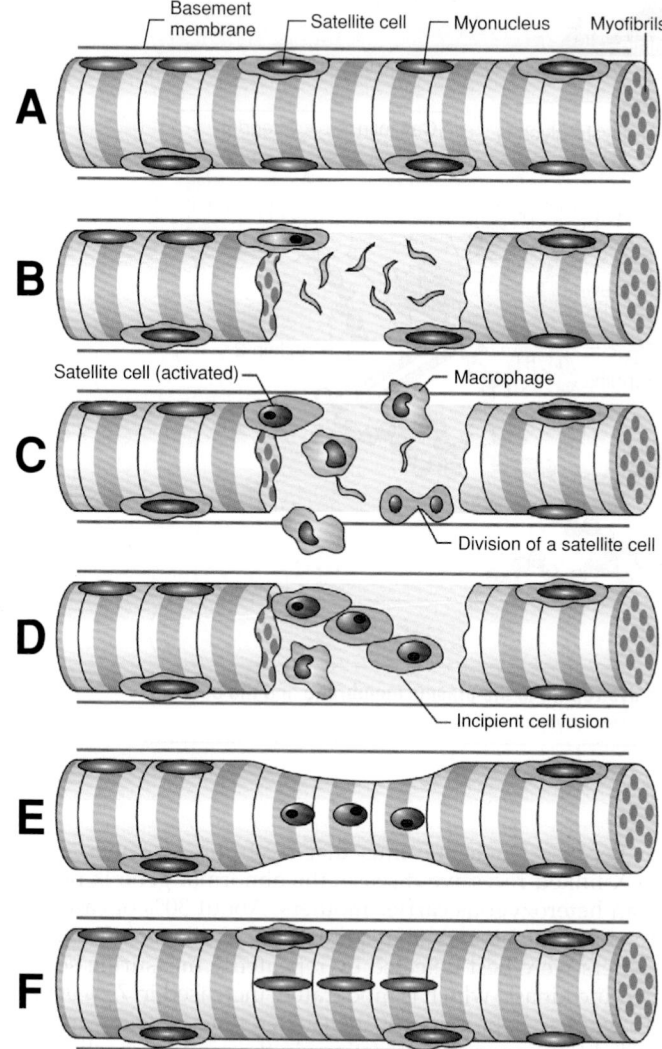

FIGURE 31-5. Segmental necrosis and regeneration of a muscle fiber. **A.** A normal muscle fiber contains myofibrils and subsarcolemmal nuclei and is covered by a basement membrane. Scattered satellite cells are situated on the surface of the sarcolemma, inside the basement membrane. These cells are dormant myoblasts, capable of proliferating and fusing to form differentiated fibers. They constitute 3%–5% of the nuclei, as observed in a cross-section of skeletal muscle. **B.** In many muscle diseases (e.g., Duchenne muscular dystrophy or polymyositis), injury to the muscle fiber causes segmental necrosis with disintegration of the sarcoplasm, leaving a preserved basement membrane and nerve supply (not shown). **C.** The damaged segment attracts circulating macrophages that penetrate the basement membrane and begin to digest and engulf the sarcoplasmic contents (myophagocytosis). Regenerative processes begin with the activation and proliferation of the satellite cells, forming myoblasts within the basement membrane. Macrophages gradually leave the site of injury with their load of debris. **D.** At a later stage, the myoblasts are aligned in close proximity to each other in the center of the fiber and begin to fuse. **E.** Regeneration of the fiber segment is prominent, as indicated by the large, pale, vesicular, centrally located nuclei. **F.** The fiber is nearly normal except for a few persistent central nuclei. Eventually, the normal state **(A)** is restored.

cells proliferate and become active myoblasts. Within 2 days, they begin to fuse to each other and to the ends of the intact fiber remnants, to form a joining multinucleated segment. This regenerating fiber is narrower than the parent fiber and has basophilic cytoplasm (owing to increased ribosomes)

and large, vesicular nuclei with prominent nucleoli arranged in long chains (see below).

Regeneration can restore normal structure and function of muscle fibers within a few weeks after a single episode of injury. With subacute or chronic disorders, fiber necrosis proceeds concurrently with fiber regeneration, gradually leading to atrophy of muscle fibers and fibrosis.

MUSCULAR DYSTROPHY

In the middle of the 19th century, physicians discovered that progressive weakness of voluntary muscles could be caused by either a disorder of the nervous system or primary muscle degeneration. The latter was called **muscular dystrophy**. It was found to be frequently hereditary (or at least familial) and relentlessly progressive. Muscles from these patients showed fiber necrosis, with regeneration, progressive fibrosis and infiltration by fatty tissue (Fig. 31-4). Little or no inflammation was seen. Subsequently, many variants of this type of muscle disease were found, and hereditary, progressive, noninflammatory degenerative conditions of muscle have been classified.

Duchenne and Becker Muscular Dystrophies Are Severe, Progressive, X-Linked Diseases

Duchenne muscular dystrophy is characterized by progressive degeneration of muscles, particularly in the pelvic and shoulder girdles. It is the most common noninflammatory myopathy in children. A milder form of the disease is known as **Becker muscular dystrophy** (see Chapter 6 for the genetics of both diseases). Serum creatine kinase is usually greatly increased in both conditions.

 **MOLECULAR PATHOGENESIS:** Duchenne and Becker muscular dystrophies are caused by several mutations in a large gene on the short arm of the X chromosome (Xp21). This gene encodes **dystrophin,** a 427-kd protein at the inner sarcolemma surface. Dystrophin links the subsarcolemmal cytoskeleton to the exterior of the cell via a transmembrane complex of proteins and glycoproteins that binds to laminin (Fig. 31-6). If it is absent or greatly decreased, often owing to deletions of the gene (Fig. 31-7), the normal interaction between the sarcolemma and extracellular matrix is absent. This may cause the observed increase in osmotic fragility of dystrophic muscle, excessive influx of calcium ions and release of soluble muscle enzymes such as creatine kinase into the serum. Breakdown of the sarcolemma precedes muscle cell necrosis, and the basal lamina seems to separate from the sarcolemma early in the course of Duchenne muscular dystrophy.

Dystrophin genes may show point mutations, deletions or duplications, leading to altered, usually truncated, proteins. Some mutated proteins may retain sufficient function to localize correctly to the muscle fiber surface but may distribute abnormally at the cell surface (Fig. 31-7). Such partly active proteins tend to produce less severe disease. Some patients have mutations affecting transmembrane proteins or glycoproteins that normally link the cytoskeleton and extracellular matrix (Table 31-1; Fig. 31-6). In them, dystrophin may be decreased or abnormally localized because its binding partners are abnormal, thus complicating diagnosis (see below).

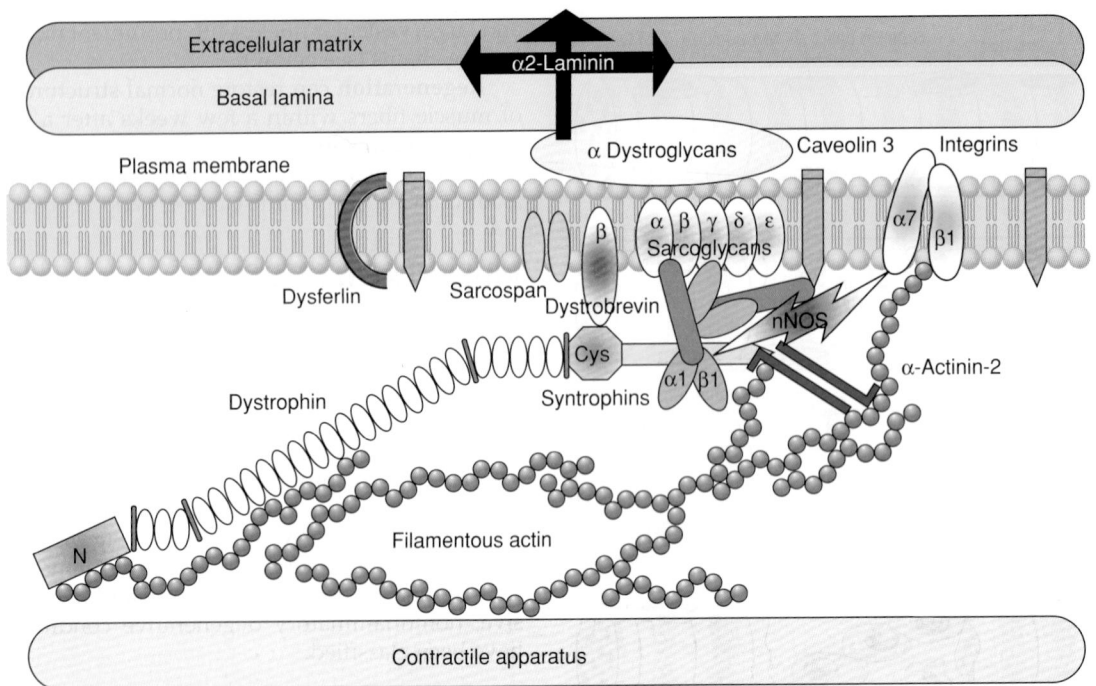

FIGURE 31-6. Diagrammatic representation of proteins linking dystrophin to the plasma membrane and the contractile apparatus. Several of these linking proteins are associated with known myopathies (Table 31-1).

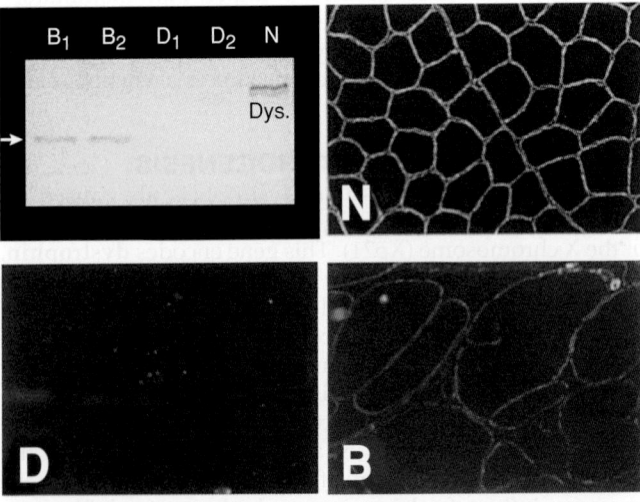

FIGURE 31-7. Dystrophin analysis in Duchenne and Becker muscular dystrophies. Immunofluorescence stain for dystrophin. The sections illustrate a normal subject (*N*), a patient with Duchenne muscular dystrophy (*D*) and one with Becker muscular dystrophy (*B*). Dystrophin is normally concentrated at the surface membrane of every muscle fiber, but in Duchenne muscular dystrophy, the protein is absent or is only barely detected in a small proportion of muscle fibers. Becker muscular dystrophy exhibits hypertrophic muscle fibers with reduced expression of dystrophin. The immunoblot (*upper left*) of normal muscle shows a band near the top of the gel corresponding to the 427-kd protein dystrophin. Dystrophin is undetectable in Duchenne muscular dystrophy (two patients, D_1, D_2). In Becker muscular dystrophy, a weaker band has migrated farther down the gel relative to the normal protein, and it corresponds to a smaller, truncated protein (two patients, B_1, B_2). The combined analysis (immunolocalization and immunoblot) of the dystrophin protein is diagnostic of this group of dystrophies (*dystrophinopathies*).

Because Duchenne muscular dystrophy is inherited as an X-linked recessive disease, the abnormal gene is passed from heterozygous carrier mothers. About 30% of cases are due to spontaneous somatic mutation. Until recently, female carriers were best detected by repeatedly measuring serum creatine kinase, which is moderately increased in 75% of heterozygotes. Expression of the carrier state is very variable, probably because of fluctuations in the random inactivation of the X chromosome. Dystrophin immunolocalization on muscle biopsy also identifies some carriers who show a characteristic mosaic pattern of deficient and normal myofibers. Molecular probes detect more than 2/3 of people who carry large deletions.

 PATHOLOGY: Duchenne muscular dystrophy causes relentless necrosis of muscle fibers, continuous effort at repair and regeneration and progressive fibrosis. Degeneration eventually outstrips the regenerative capacity of the muscle. The number of muscle fibers then progressively decreases, to be replaced by fibrofatty connective tissue. In the end stage, skeletal muscle fibers disappear almost completely (Fig. 31-4), but muscle spindle fibers (intrafusal fibers) are relatively spared.

Early in the disease, necrotic fibers and regenerating fibers tend to occur in small groups, together with scattered, large, hyalinized dark fibers. The latter are overly contracted and are thought to precede fiber necrosis (Figs. 31-8 and 31-9). Breakdown of the sarcolemma is one of the earliest ultrastructural changes. Macrophages invade necrotic fibers and reflect a scavenging function rather than an inflammatory process.

 CLINICAL FEATURES: Polymerase chain reaction (PCR) analysis of genomic DNA establishes the diagnosis of Duchenne dystrophy. In practice,

TABLE 31-1
LIMB-GIRDLE MUSCULAR DYSTROPHIES

Limb-Girdle Muscular Dystrophies[a]	Defective Protein	Subcellular Location
LGMD1A	Myotilin	Sarcomere
LGMDIB	Lamin	Nuclear envelope
LGMD1C	Caveolin 3	Sarcolemma
LGMD1D	?	
LGMD1E	?	
LGMD1F	?	
LGMD1G	?	
LGMD2A	Calpain 3	Sarcoplasm
LGMD2B/Miyoshi	Dysferlin	Sarcolemma
LGMD2C	γ-Sarcoglycan	Sarcolemma
LGMD2D	α-Sarcoglycan	Sarcolemma
LGMD2E	β-Sarcoglycan	Sarcolemma
LGMD2F	δ-Sarcoglycan	Sarcolemma
LGMD2G	Telethion	Sarcomere
LGMD2H	Trim32	Sarcoplasm
LGMD2I	Fukutin-related protein	Golgi
LGMD2J	Titin	Sarcomere
LGMD2K	POMT1	Endoplasmic reticulum
LGMD2L	Eukutin	Golgi
LGMD2M	DOMGnT1	Golgi

[a]LMGD1s show autosomal dominant inheritance, while LMGD2s show autosomal recessive inheritance.
Adapted from "Diseases of Muscle." In Love S, Louis DN, Ellison DW, eds. Greenfield's Neuropathology, 8th ed. New York: Oxford University Press, 2008.

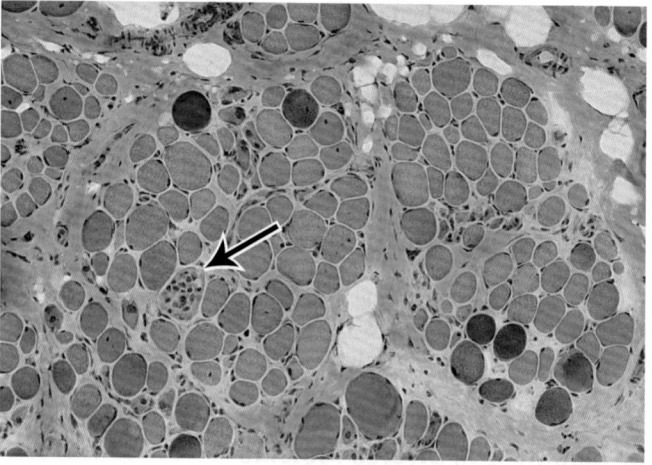

FIGURE 31-9. Duchenne muscular dystrophy. Modified Gomori trichrome stain. A section of vastus lateralis muscle shows necrotic muscle fibers, some of them invaded by macrophages (*arrow*). Dark-staining, enlarged fibers represent overly contracted fibers. Green amorphous material between the fascicles of muscle represents fibrosis. Calcium influx across the defective surface membrane overwhelms mechanisms that maintain a low resting Ca^{2+} concentration and triggers excessive contraction. There is conspicuous perimysial and endomysial fibrosis.

this method only detects large deletions of the gene. About 30% of patients have small rearrangements or point mutations and are evaluated by muscle biopsy, which shows little or no detectable dystrophin by immunoblot or immunohistochemistry. If there is an affected family member, prenatal diagnosis using chorionic villi may be useful.

Boys with Duchenne muscular dystrophy have markedly increased serum creatine kinase levels from birth and morphologically abnormal muscle, even in utero. Clinical weakness is not detectable during the first year but is usually evident by 3 or 4 years of age, mainly around pelvic and shoulder girdles (proximal muscle weakness). It progresses relentlessly. "Pseudohypertrophy" (enlargement of a muscle when muscle fibers are replaced by fibroadipose tissue) of calf muscles eventually develops. Patients are usually wheelchair bound by age 10 and bedridden by 15. Death is usually from complications of respiratory insufficiency caused by muscular weakness or cardiac arrhythmia due to

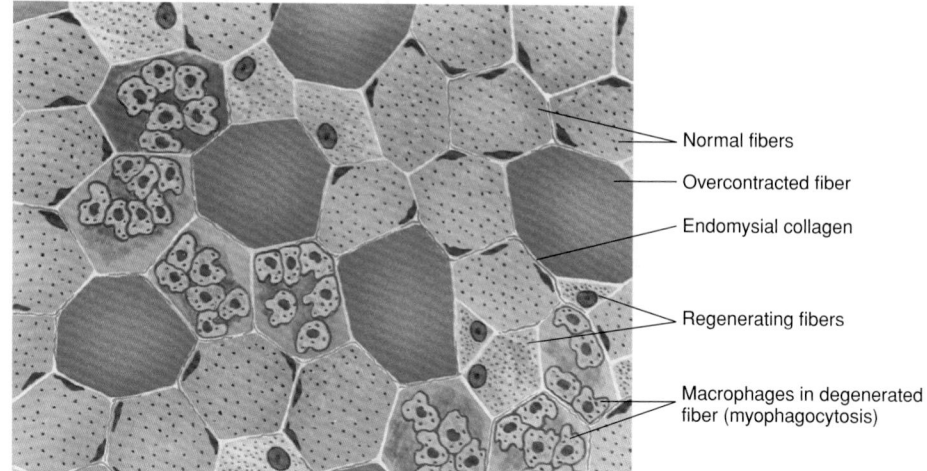

- Normal fibers
- Overcontracted fiber
- Endomysial collagen
- Regenerating fibers
- Macrophages in degenerated fiber (myophagocytosis)

FIGURE 31-8. Duchenne muscular dystrophy. The pathologic changes in skeletal muscle (illustration of modified Gomori trichrome stain). Some fibers are slightly larger and darker than normal. These represent overcontracted segments of sarcoplasm situated between degenerated segments. Other fibers are packed with macrophages (myophagocytosis), which remove degenerated sarcoplasm. Other fibers are smaller than normal and have granular sarcoplasm. These fibers have enlarged, vesicular nuclei with prominent nucleoli and represent regenerating fibers. Developing endomysial fibrosis is represented by the deposition of collagen around individual muscle fibers. The changes are those of a chronic, active noninflammatory myopathy.

myocardial involvement. Other extraskeletal manifestations include gastrointestinal dysfunction (from degeneration of smooth muscle) and intellectual impairment. Many boys with Duchenne dystrophy show variably severe mental retardation, apparently due to lack of dystrophin in the central nervous system (CNS).

While the clinical presentation of patients with Becker muscular dystrophy is typically milder and of later onset, affected individuals often have exercise intolerance with muscle cramping, occasional rhabdomyolysis and myoglobinuria. Unlike Duchenne muscular dystrophy, in which dystrophin is usually absent, in Becker dystrophy dystrophin is present as a truncated protein (Fig. 31-7).

Limb-Girdle Muscular Dystrophies Are Caused by Mutations in Diverse Proteins

Limb-girdle muscular dystrophies (LGMDs) are a group of disorders with several defective proteins and modes of inheritance (Table 31-1). Defects in many proteins have been implicated, but these patients show similar clinical features that include pelvic and shoulder girdle weakness. Onset may be in childhood or adulthood, with variable muscle weakness. Patients may have difficulty walking, running or rising from a sitting position. Cardiac involvement is common. The histology resembles all muscular dystrophies, but some variants show unusual features including inflammation (LGMD2B, Miyoshi myopathy) and rimmed vacuoles (LGMD1A) like those seen in inclusion body myositis (see below). As a result, proper diagnosis requires detailed clinical histories, plus immunohistochemical, immunoblotting and genetic tests. LGMD (2C through 2F) are also known as the sarcoglycanopathies (Fig. 31-6).

Congenital Muscular Dystrophies Present in the Perinatal Period

These diseases are characterized by hypotonia, weakness and contractures (Table 31-2). Depending on the variant, patients may also present with a leukoencephalopathy (white matter brain disease), brain malformations and eye involvement.

Pathologically, these diseases resemble other muscular dystrophies, with variable fibrosis and fatty infiltration of muscle. Many of these disorders reflect mutations in extracellular matrix proteins (e.g., collagens, laminin, integrins) or abnormal glycosylation of α-dystroglycan (α-dystroglycanopathies) and sarcoplasmic reticulum (rigid spine muscular dystrophy). Some affected proteins also cause certain limb-girdle muscular dystrophies, albeit with different mutations.

Nucleotide Repeat Syndromes May Cause Muscular Dystrophies

Several human genetic diseases are caused by abnormal numbers of intragenic oligonucleotide repeats. Myotonic dystrophy and oculopharyngeal muscular dystrophy are trinucleotide repeat syndromes with very different muscle pathologies. Both, however, exhibit "anticipation" (i.e., increasingly earlier ages at onset and more severe symptoms in successive generations, as numbers of repeats increase; see Chapter 6).

Myotonic Dystrophy Is the Most Common Adult Muscular Dystrophy

Myotonic dystrophy is an autosomal dominant disease characterized by slowed muscle relaxation (myotonia), progressive muscle weakness and wasting. Its prevalence is about 14 per 100,000, although minimally affected individuals are hard to diagnose, so this estimate may be low. Age at onset and severity of symptoms vary greatly. Myotonic dystrophy may be either adult onset or congenital.

 **MOLECULAR PATHOGENESIS:** The two forms of myotonic dystrophy (DM1, DM2) both follow autosomal dominant inheritance and reflect mutations in different genes. DM1 is due to expansion of a CTG repeat near the 3′ end of the DM protein

TABLE 31-2		
CONGENITAL MYOPATHIES CAUSED BY ABNORMALITIES IN THE SARCOLEMMA OR EXTRACELLULAR MATRIX		
Congenital Muscular Dystrophy (CMD)	**Protein**	**Location and/or Function of Protein**
Merosin-deficient CMD	Laminin α2	Extracellular matrix
Ullrich syndrome	Collagen VI	Extracellular matrix
Integrin α7 deficiency	Integrin α7	Plasma membrane
Fukuyama CMD	Fukutin	Possible substrate for glycosyltransferase
Muscle-eye-brain	POMGnT1 (*O*-mannose β-1,2-*N*-acetylglucosaminyl-tranferase	Glycosyltransferase
Walker-Warburg syndrome	POMT1 (protein-*O*-mannosyl-transferase) Fukutin-related protein	Glycosyltransferase Possible phosphor-sugar transferase
Rigid spine syndrome	Selenoprotein N1	Glycoprotein of the endoplasmic reticulum

Adapted from "Diseases of Muscle." In Love S, Louis DN, Ellison DW, eds. Greenfield's Neuropathology, 8th ed. New York: Oxford University Press, 2008.

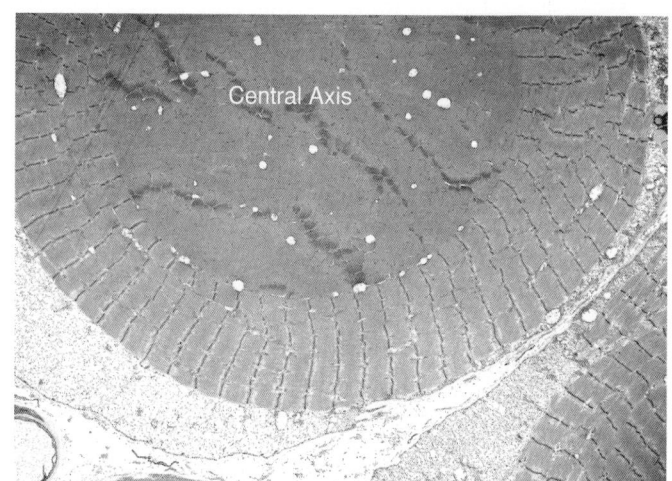

FIGURE 31-10. Ring fiber. Electron micrograph (magnification ×1900). The outer sarcomeres are oriented perpendicular to the axis of the myofiber.

kinase (DMPK) gene, which encodes a serine-threonine kinase. Normally, there are fewer than 30 copies of this repeat, but in minimally affected myotonic dystrophy patients, there may be 50 or more copies. The greater the number of repeats (sometimes as many as 4000), the more severe the disorder. The mechanism of injury brought about by expansion of CTG repeats in myotonic dystrophy, as in other trinucleotide repeat disorders, is not clearly understood at present (see Chapter 1). DM2 is caused by expansion of the tetranucleotide repeat CCTG in the first intron of the ZNF9 gene.

 PATHOLOGY: Pathology in adult myotonic dystrophy is highly variable, even in muscles from the same patient. Most patients show type I fiber atrophy and type II fiber hypertrophy. In contrast, most muscle disorders show relative type II fiber atrophy. Internally situated nuclei are a constant feature. The ATPase reaction shows many ring fibers, with circumferential concentration of heavily stained sarcoplasm. In these fibers, outer sarcomeres are circumferential, instead of their usual longitudinal arrangement along the fiber axis (Fig. 31-10). Necrosis and regeneration, although occasionally present, are not prominent (as they are in Duchenne muscular dystrophy).

Muscles in congenital myotonic dystrophy show myofiber atrophy, frequent central nuclei and failure of fiber differentiation. These features closely resemble those of the X-linked recessive type of myotubular myopathy (see below).

 CLINICAL FEATURES: People with DM1 experience slowly progressive muscle weakness and stiffness, principally in the distal limbs (proximal weakness is more common in DM2). Facial and neck weakness as well as ptosis are typical of DM1, but less common in DM2. Extraskeletal features sometimes present in myotonic dystrophy include frontal balding, gonadal atrophy, cataracts, personality degeneration and endocrine abnormalities. Cardiac arrhythmias and, less often, cardiomyopathy may occur. A few patients exhibit involvement of smooth muscle, with disorders of the gastrointestinal tract, gallbladder and uterus.

Diagnosis is based on clinical features, family history and characteristic electromyography, which exhibits myotonic

discharges. Identifying an expanded CTG repeat (DM1) or CCTG (DM2) is predictive in utero and can be diagnostic in patients.

Congenital myotonic dystrophy is seen only in children of women with DM1 who themselves show symptoms of myotonic dystrophy. Affected infants have severe muscle weakness at birth. Myotonia is inconspicuous or absent but appears in later childhood. Many of these patients suffer mental retardation. Congenital DM2 has not been identified.

Oculopharyngeal Muscular Dystrophy Usually Presents in Adults

Oculopharyngeal muscular dystrophy (OPMD) is typically diagnosed in middle age (over 45 years) and mostly shows autosomal dominant inheritance. However, an autosomal recessive form does exist. Patients develop slowly progressive eyelid ptosis and dysphagia and weakness of other muscle groups including the face and limbs. The autosomal dominant form is prevalent among French Canadians in Quebec and Bukhara Jews (formerly from central Asia), now living in Israel. Both autosomal dominant and recessive forms are due to abnormally increased numbers of GCG repeats in the poly(A) binding protein nuclear 1 gene (PABPN1), but differ in where these increased repeats are within the gene. Biopsies show intranuclear inclusions, rimmed vacuoles and filamentous inclusions similar to those in inclusion body myositis (see below). Unlike the latter, the intranuclear inclusions contain 8.5-nm filaments.

Facioscapulohumeral Muscular Dystrophy Usually Presents in Childhood

Facioscapulohumeral muscular dystrophy (FSHD) is a relatively common muscular dystrophy, inherited as an autosomal dominant disease that begins in childhood or young adulthood. Patients suffer from facial and shoulder girdle weakness. Scapular winging is prominent. Other muscles may also be affected. Life expectancy is usually normal, and extraskeletal involvement includes bundle branch block, hearing loss and retinal vasculopathy. FSHD is caused by deletion of part of a repetitive DNA fragment in the subtelomeric region of chromosome 4q: affected patients have fewer repeats than normal. Chronic inflammation is prominent, resembling an inflammatory myopathy such as polymyositis (see below), but does not correlate with the disease course. A detailed clinical history is essential to making the proper diagnosis; otherwise, a patient with muscle weakness and a lymphocytic inflammatory infiltrate could easily be misdiagnosed as suffering from polymyositis.

CONGENITAL MYOPATHIES

A newborn occasionally shows generalized hypotonia, with decreased deep tendon reflexes and muscle bulk. Many of these children have a difficult perinatal period because of pulmonary complications of weak respiration. Many of the muscle diseases already described are "congenital" in the sense that they are due to mutations present at birth. However, such disorders are not clinically evident until much later. In contrast, congenital myopathies, as described here, are evident at birth. Some have progressive "malignant"

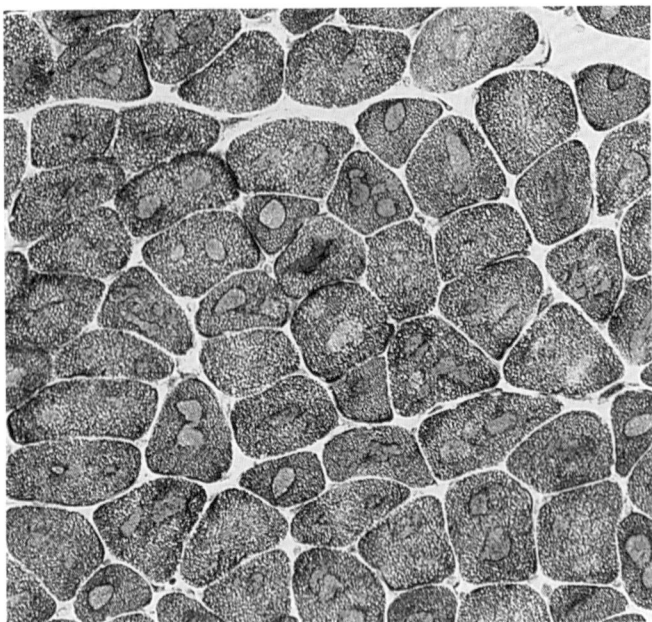

FIGURE 31-11. Central core disease. A section of vastus lateralis muscle stained for NADH-tetrazolium reductase shows a distinct circular zone of pallor in the center of most muscle fibers. A thin zone of excessive staining surrounds the core lesion. All of the myofibers in this case were type I, as demonstrated by the myofibrillar ATPase stain (not shown). Note the close resemblance of the core lesions to the target formations found in the muscle fibers of neurogenic disorders (Fig. 31-23).

hypotonia, which results in death within the first year of life, for example, **Werdnig-Hoffman disease** and **infantile acid maltase deficiency (Pompe disease)**.

In other hypotonic patients, hypotonia may persist with little or no progression. These people become ambulatory and live a normal life span, although sometimes with secondary skeletal complications of hypotonia such as severe scoliosis. Muscle from these patients rarely reveals distinctive structurally abnormal myofibers. Three of the most common forms of congenital myopathies are **central core disease** (Fig. 31-11), **nemaline (rod) myopathy** (Fig. 31-12)

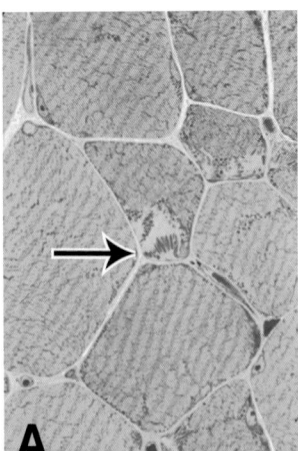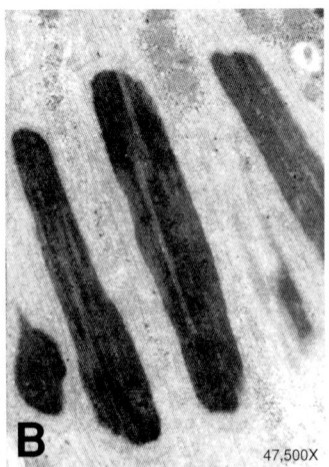

FIGURE 31-12. Rod (nemaline) myopathy. A. Muscle fibers contain dark aggregates of rods (toluidine blue, 1000×). **B.** An electron micrograph of the same biopsy shows that the structures are rod shaped organ are derived from the Z disk (47,500×).

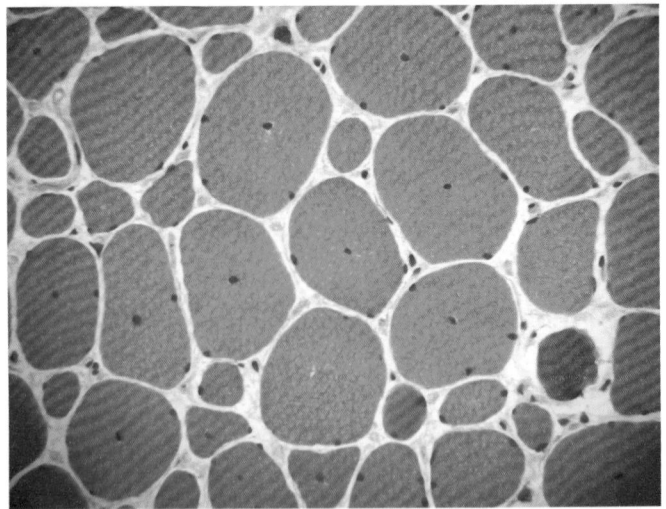

FIGURE 31-13. Central nuclear myopathy. Hematoxylin and eosin stain. Many muscle fibers contain a single central nucleus, and most of the affected muscle fibers are abnormally small. In addition, there are radiating spokes emanating from the central nuclei. These fibers resemble the late myotubular stage of fetal development of skeletal muscle.

and **central nuclear myopathy** (Fig. 31-13). All show congenital hypotonia, decreased deep tendon reflexes, decreased muscle bulk and delayed motor milestones. In all three conditions, abnormal muscle morphology is usually limited to type I fibers, with type I fiber predominance in some disorders and type I hypotrophy in others. Often, type I fibers are unusually predominant, or possibly, type II fibers fail to develop. There is no active myofiber necrosis or fibrosis, and patients have normal serum creatine kinase.

Central Core Disease Is an Autosomal Dominant Condition with Congenital Hypotonia and Proximal Muscle Weakness

 **MOLECULAR PATHOGENESIS:** Afflicted patients have decreased deep tendon reflexes and delayed motor development. The disease has been traced to a mutation on the long arm of chromosome 19 (19q13.1) that codes for the ryanodine receptor, the calcium release channel of the sarcoplasmic reticulum. Occasional cases are sporadic or show autosomal recessive inheritance. Typical patients become ambulatory, but muscle strength remains less than normal.

 PATHOLOGY: There is a striking predominance of type I fibers, often showing a central zone of degeneration with loss of NADH-TR reaction staining (Fig. 31-11) and extending the entire length of the fiber. By electron microscopy, mitochondria and other membranous organelles are lost in the central cores, with or without myofibril disorganization. Membranous organelles tend to condense around the margin of the central core. The periphery of the fiber is unremarkable.

Central core anomalies may resemble the target fibers seen in active denervating conditions (see below), although target fibers typically have dark rims around the areas of pallor and there is no evidence of denervation in central core disease.

Mutations of the ryanodine receptor 1 gene also cause **malignant hyperthermia,** a potentially fatal disorder that is triggered by succinylcholine and some anaesthetic agents, particularly halothane. It is characterized by hyperpyrexia and rhabdomyolysis (see Chapter 8). Central core disease and malignant hyperthermia may coexist in some patients, so patients with central core disease may be at risk for malignant hyperthermia. However, patients with malignant hyperthermia often have no abnormal histologic changes. Malignant hyperthermia is suspected by family history and confirmed by an in vitro caffeine-halothane contraction test.

Rod Myopathy Sarcoplasmic Inclusions Derive from Z Bands

Rod myopathy includes a group of diseases in which rod-like inclusions accumulate within skeletal muscle sarcoplasm. The tangled, thread-like appearance of the inclusions led to the original name, "nemaline" myopathy. In reality, they are clusters of rod-shaped structures.

 **MOLECULAR PATHOGENESIS:** Autosomal dominant and recessive inheritance is described. Genes responsible for rod myopathy include nebulin (most common), skeletal muscle α-actin, α- and β-tropomyosin and slow troponin T. Mutations in the ryanodine receptor gene may also lead to nemaline rod formation.

 PATHOLOGY: There is variable predominance of type I fibers containing rod-shaped structures in their sarcoplasm. Aggregates of these inclusions often occur in subsarcolemmal regions, near nuclei. They are brilliant, red to dark red, using modified Gomori trichrome stain, or blue on toluidine blue stain (Fig. 31-12A), but are often not visible with hematoxylin and eosin. The inclusions are rod shaped and arise from the Z band, which they resemble ultrastructurally (Fig. 31-12B).

Rods are described in several neuromuscular diseases, including denervation atrophy, muscular dystrophy and inflammatory myopathies. Experimental tenotomy (cutting a tendon) induces formation of rods in the muscle when the nerve supply remains intact. In rod myopathy, however, inclusions are the main pathologic feature. Other abnormalities (inflammation, denervation) are absent.

 CLINICAL FEATURES: In the classic congenital form of rod myopathy, patients show congenital hypotonia, delayed motor milestones of variable clinical severity and secondary skeletal changes such as kyphoscoliosis. Some exhibit severe involvement of muscles of the face, pharynx and neck. Later-onset (childhood and adult) forms tend to be associated with some muscle degeneration, increased serum creatine kinase levels and a slowly or nonprogressive course.

Central Nuclear Myopathy and Myotubular Myopathy Resemble the Myotubular Stage of Embryogenesis

 **MOLECULAR PATHOGENESIS AND CLINICAL FEATURES:** Central nuclear myopathy is a group of clinically and genetically heterogeneous inherited conditions in which skeletal muscle cells have centrally located nuclei. Autosomal recessive and autosomal dominant varieties are known. The latter tend to manifest in adolescence and show modestly increased serum creatine kinase. They progress slowly and, like rod myopathy, resemble the limb-girdle dystrophies (see above). Some patients exhibit a striking involvement of facial and extraocular musculature. Bilateral ptosis is almost always present. The gene responsible, dynamin 2, is involved in endocytosis, membrane trafficking and centrosome and actin assembly.

Myotubular myopathy is an X-linked disorder caused by myotubularin gene mutations. Myotubularin is a phosphatase expressed in most tissues and involved in phosphatidylinositol signaling. Clinically, myotubular myopathy is characterized by marked neonatal hypotonia and respiratory failure at birth. Pathologically, like central nuclear myopathy, there are centrally placed nuclei within both fiber types.

 PATHOLOGY: Biopsies show predominance of type I fibers (Fig. 31-13), many of which are small and round, with a single central nucleus (hence the name of the disease). They resemble the myotubular stage in skeletal muscle embryogenesis. This apparent immature state suggests a possible defect in the nerve supply to the muscle fiber because the lower motor neuron normally promotes subsequent maturation of the fiber. However, lower motor neurons in these patients, including motor endplates, are not demonstrably abnormal.

Later-onset forms of myotubular myopathy are characterized morphologically by more mature muscle fibers, in which fibers are larger, have more numerous myofibrils and display single central nuclei that appear more mature.

INFLAMMATORY MYOPATHIES

Inflammatory myopathies are a heterogeneous group of acquired disorders, all of which feature symmetric proximal muscle weakness, increased serum levels of muscle-derived enzymes and nonsuppurative inflammation of skeletal muscle.

These are uncommon diseases, the annual incidence being 1 in 100,000. *Dermatomyositis afflicts children and adults, but polymyositis almost always begins after 20 years of age.* Both disorders occur more often in females than males. In contrast, inclusion body myositis is usually a disease of men over age 50.

These myopathies are thought to have an autoimmune origin (see Chapter 11) because (1) they often occur in association with other autoimmune and connective tissues diseases, (2) the pathology suggests autoimmune cellular injury, (3) serum autoantibodies are detected and (4) polymyositis and dermatomyositis (but not inclusion body myositis) respond to immunosuppressive therapy. No specific target autoantigens in muscle or blood vessels have been identified, but antinuclear and anticytoplasmic antibodies against several different antigens exist in all.

The inflammatory myopathies are characterized by (1) the presence of inflammatory cells, (2) necrosis and phagocytosis of muscle fibers, (3) a mixture of regenerating and atrophic fibers and (4) fibrosis.

 CLINICAL FEATURES: All inflammatory myopathies manifest as insidious proximal and symmetric muscle weakness, gradually increasing over weeks to months. Patients have problems with simple activities that require use of proximal muscles, including lifting objects, climbing steps or combing hair. Dysphagia and difficulty in holding up the head reflect involvement of pharyngeal and neck-flexor muscles. Some patients with inclusion body myositis have distal muscle weakness of the limbs that equals or exceeds that of proximal muscles. In advanced cases, respiratory muscles may be affected. Interstitial lung disease may also compromise respiratory function in 10% of polymyositis and dermatomyositis patients. Myocardial involvement may also occur. Weakness progresses over weeks or months and leads to severe muscular wasting.

In Polymyositis Muscle Damage Is Mediated by Cytotoxic T Cells

 MOLECULAR PATHOGENESIS: In polymyositis, there is no detectable microangiopathy as is seen in dermatomyositis (see below). In these disorders, healthy muscle fibers are initially surrounded by CD8$^+$ T lymphocytes (Fig. 31-14) and macrophages, after which the fibers degenerate. Unlike normal muscle, muscle cells in inflammatory myopathies express major histocompatibility complex (MHC) I antigens. This aberrant expression promotes an autoimmune reaction.

The pathogenetic role of autoantibodies against nuclear antigens and cytoplasmic ribonucleoproteins in muscle injury is unknown. Polymyositis often has detectable anti-Jo-1, an antibody against histidyl-transfer RNA (tRNA) synthetase, with concomitant interstitial lung disease, Raynaud phenomenon and nonerosive arthritis.

Viral infections may precede polymyositis, but virus cultures of muscle are negative. An inflammatory myopathy may also occur in many cases of HIV-1 infection, but the role of the virus is unclear.

PATHOLOGY: Inflammatory cells infiltrate connective tissue mostly within fascicles (i.e., endomysial inflammation) and invade apparently

healthy muscle (Fig. 31-14). Angiopathy is absent. Isolated degenerating or regenerating fibers are scattered throughout fascicles. Perifascicular atrophy does not occur in polymyositis (see below).

Inclusion Body Myositis Is Characterized by β-Amyloid Deposits

Inclusion body myositis typically occurs in older patients (>50 years) and is the most common inflammatory myopathy of the elderly. It resembles polymyositis pathologically, showing single-fiber necrosis and regeneration, with predominantly endomysial cytotoxic T cells. Basophilic granular material is seen at the edge of vacuoles (rimmed vacuoles) within muscle fibers (Fig. 31-15A, B). These inclusions contain intracellular amyloid (Fig. 31-15C) that is immunoreactive for β-amyloid protein, the same type of amyloid as in senile plaques in Alzheimer disease. Other proteins associated with Alzheimer disease are also present including phosphorylated tau, α-synuclein, ubiquitin and presenilins (see Chapter 32). Parkin, which accumulates in hereditary Parkinson disease, and the prion precursor protein have also been localized to the inclusions.

The pathogenic role of these inclusions is unclear as similar neurodegenerative disease-associated protein accumulation has been observed in other rare myopathies (X-linked Emery-Dreifuss muscular dystrophy and myofibrillar myopathies) as well as in chronic denervation. By electron microscopy, the granules of rimmed vacuoles contain membranous whorls and adjacent distinctive filaments (Fig. 31-15D). Unique features of inclusion body myositis include Congo red–positive inclusions, the characteristic cytoplasmic (or rarely nuclear) filaments in muscle fibers and an inflammatory infiltrate, though the latter may be slight. An autosomal recessive hereditary form of the disease shows similar features but may present in late adolescence or adulthood. Despite the presence of inflammation, immunosuppressive therapy does not mitigate the disease, but intravenous immunoglobulin (IVIG) may be therapeutically useful.

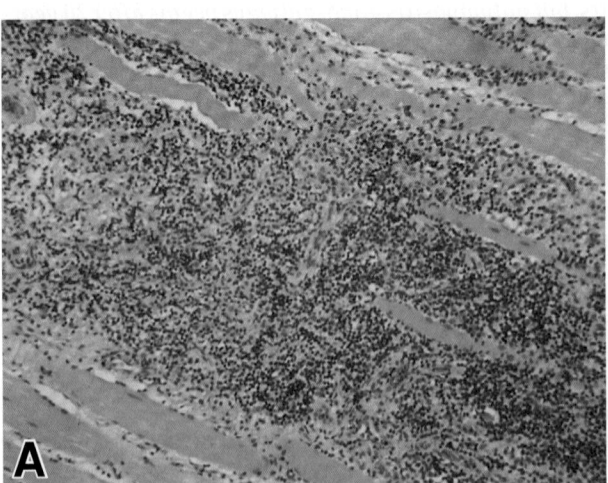
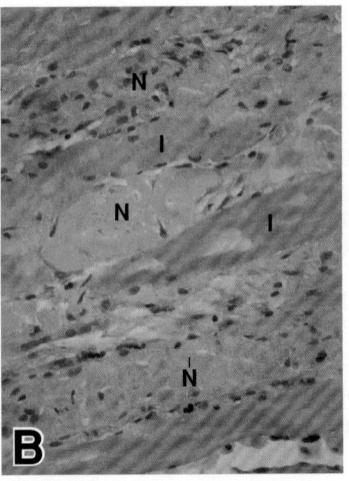
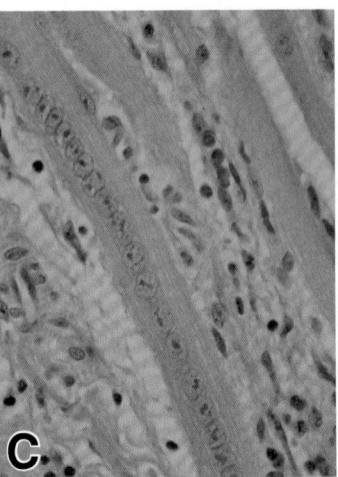

FIGURE 31-14. Polymyositis. A. Hematoxylin and eosin stain. A section of affected muscle shows an inflammatory myopathy. Mononuclear inflammatory cells infiltrate chiefly the endomysium. The field includes single-fiber necrosis. **B.** Region of healing inflammatory myopathy demonstrates intact fibers (*I*) and necrotic fibers (*N*). The uppermost necrotic fiber is heavily infiltrated with macrophages. **C.** Regenerating fiber displaying a linear array of enlarged centrally placed nuclei.

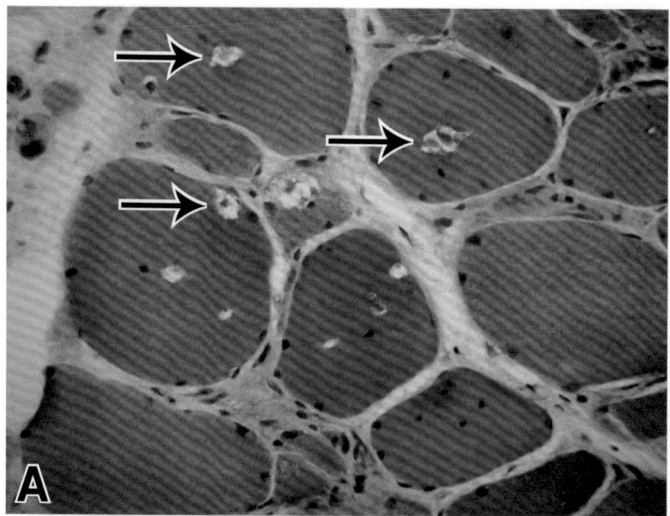
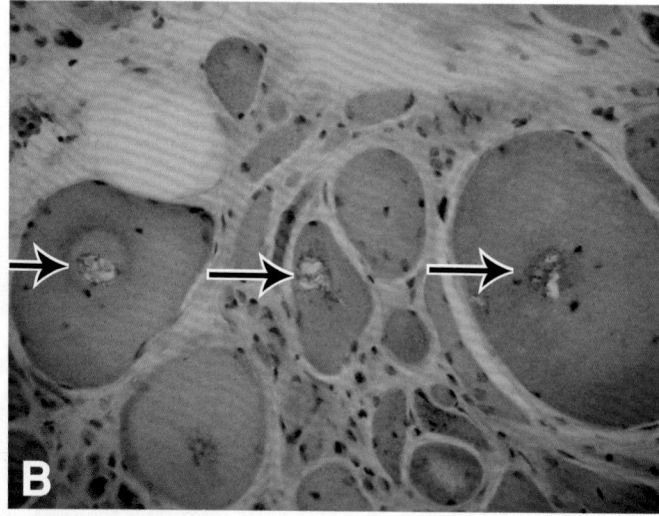
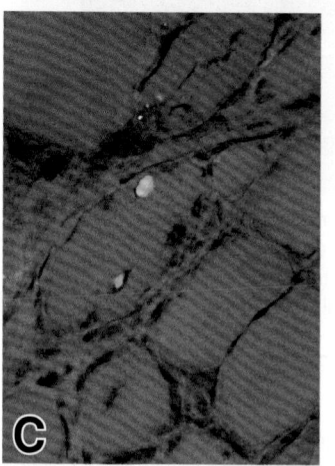
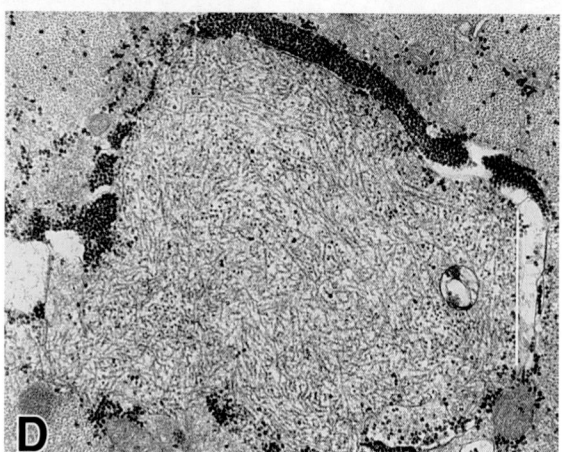

FIGURE 31-15. Inclusion body myositis (IBM). A. Hematoxylin and eosin stain (cryostat section). The features in IBM resemble those of polymyositis, but the muscle fibers also exhibit rimmed vacuoles (*arrows*) corresponding to enlarged lysosomes. **B.** Modified Gomori trichrome stain (cryostat section) shows granular basophilic rimming of vacuoles. **C.** Congo red stain. The inclusion has weak congophilia, but the color signal is strong because it has been enhanced by fluorescence excitation. **D.** An electron micrograph shows the characteristic filaments of the amyloid inclusions.

Dermatomyositis Is an Immune-Mediated Microangiopathy

Dermatomyositis differs from other myopathies in having a characteristic rash on the upper eyelids, face, trunk and sometimes elsewhere. It may occur alone or together with scleroderma, mixed connective tissue disease or other autoimmune conditions.

PATHOPHYSIOLOGY: This myopathy is characterized by (1) deposition of immune complexes of immunoglobulin G (IgG), IgM and complement components, including membrane attack complex C5b-9 in the walls of capillaries and other blood vessels; (2) microangiopathy with loss of capillaries; (3) signs of injury and atrophy of myofibers; and (4) perivascular infiltrates of B cells and CD4+ helper T cells (Fig. 31-16). These features suggest that muscle injury in dermatomyositis is mainly mediated by complement-fixing cytotoxic antibodies against skeletal muscle microvasculature. Complement deposition in capillary walls preceding inflammation or damage to muscle fibers is the most specific finding. This microangiopathy is thought to lead to ischemic injury of individual muscle fibers and eventually to fiber atrophy. True infarcts may result from involvement of larger intramuscular arteries. The rash clinically distinguishes dermatomyositis from the other inflammatory myopathies due to the same microangiopathy.

PATHOLOGY: B and T lymphocytes infiltrate around blood vessels and in perimysial connective tissue, with a high CD4+ (helper):CD8+ (cytotoxic/suppressor) T-cell ratio. Immune complexes, including IgG, IgM and complement C5-9 membrane attack complex, in the walls of blood vessels (Fig. 31-16, inset) are associated with the microangiopathy. Perifascicular atrophy (one or more layers of atrophic fibers at the periphery of fascicles) is pathognomonic (Fig. 31-16) even if inflammation is lacking. The perifascicular atrophy is due to relative hypoperfusion of perifascicular zones.

Vasculitis in Skeletal Muscle May be Part of Systemic Vasculitides

Vasculitis can be present in skeletal muscle in polyarteritis nodosa (PAN), granulomatosis with polyangiitis, collagen

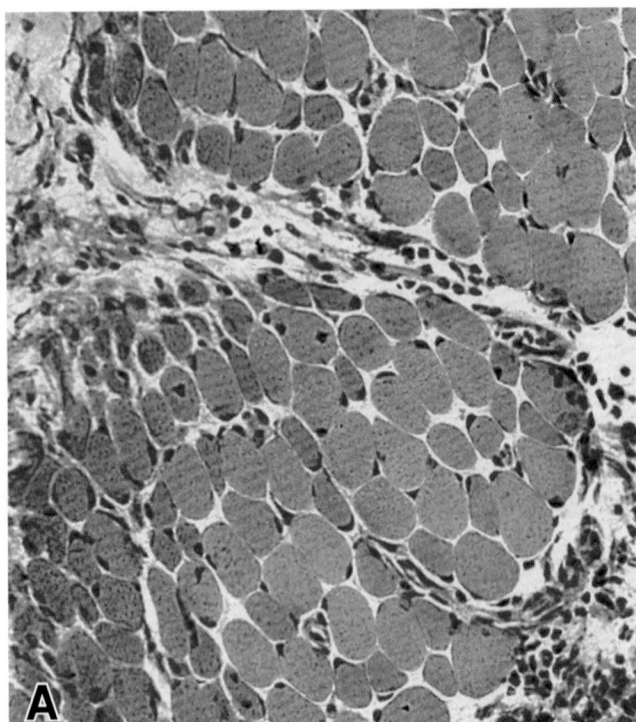
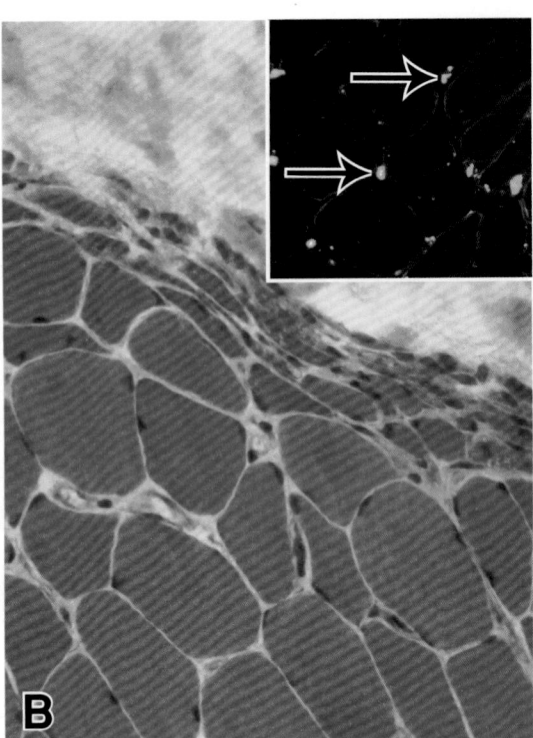

FIGURE 31-16. Dermatomyositis. A. Hematoxylin and eosin stain. The inflammatory cells infiltrate predominantly the perimysium rather than the endomysium. The periphery of muscle fascicles shows most of the muscle fiber atrophy and damage, resulting in a pattern of injury characteristic of dermatomyositis, termed *perifascicular atrophy*. **B.** High-magnification image of perifascicular atrophy demonstrating the flattening and shrinkage of fibers at the periphery of the fascicle. Immunofluorescence (*inset*) reveals that the walls of many capillaries display C5b-9 (membrane attack complex), reflecting the altered microvasculature typical of dermatomyositis.

vascular disease and immune-mediated hypersensitivity states. In such instances, skeletal muscle may show neurogenic changes (see below) secondary to nerve damage.

MYASTHENIA GRAVIS

Myasthenia gravis is an acquired autoimmune disease in which antibodies to the acetylcholine (Ach) receptor at the neuromuscular junction cause abnormal muscular fatigability. It occurs in all races and is twice as common in women as in men. The disease typically begins in young adults, but first presentations may vary from childhood to old age.

PATHOPHYSIOLOGY: In myasthenia gravis, antibodies bind the Ach receptor of the motor endplate. Complement activation leads to shedding of the Ach receptor–rich terminal portions of the folds of the neuromuscular junction. The bivalent IgG antibodies also cross-link receptor proteins that remain in the postsynaptic membrane. This accelerates Ach receptor endocytosis so much that the muscle cannot replace them. The combination of reduced postsynaptic membrane area, decreased numbers of Ach receptors per unit area and widened synaptic space impairs signal transmission and causes muscle weakness and abnormal fatigability. The antireceptor antibodies do not directly block Ach binding its receptor.

Most patients with myasthenia gravis have anti–Ach receptor antibodies and thymic hyperplasia. About 15% have an associated thymoma. Surgical removal of the hyperplastic thymic tissue or the thymoma often causes the myasthenia gravis to remit. Ach receptors are present on the surface of some thymic cells in thymoma and thymic hyperplasia. Thus, thymic T cells may trigger production of antireceptor antibodies.

PATHOLOGY: Light microscopy may reveal atrophy of type II muscle fibers and focal collections of lymphocytes within fascicles. However, electron microscopy shows that most muscle endplates are abnormal, even in muscles that are not weakened. Sarcolemmal secondary folds are simplified with breakdown, loss of the crests of the folds and widening of the clefts.

CLINICAL FEATURES: The clinical severity of the condition is quite variable, and symptoms tend to wax and wane as in other autoimmune diseases. Weakness of extraocular muscles is typically severe and causes ptosis and diplopia. Sometimes, myasthenia gravis may be limited to those muscles. More commonly, it progresses to other muscles (e.g., those associated with swallowing, the trunk and extremities). Patients with myasthenia gravis often have other autoimmune diseases.

The overall mortality from myasthenia gravis is about 10%, often because muscle weakness leads to respiratory insufficiency. In addition to thymectomy, corticosteroids, methotrexate and anticholinesterase drugs are used, alone or in combination. Plasmapheresis reduces anti–Ach receptor antibody titers, but any consequent clinical improvements are short-lived.

INHERITED METABOLIC DISEASES

Skeletal muscle is dramatically affected by many endocrine and metabolic diseases, such as Cushing syndrome, Addison disease, hypothyroidism, hyperthyroidism (see Chapter 27) and conditions associated with hepatic or renal failure. Only primary hereditary abnormalities in metabolism of skeletal muscle resulting in abnormal muscular function are discussed here.

Glycogen Storage Diseases Are Genetic Disorders with Variable Effects on Muscle

Glycogen storage diseases (glycogenoses) are autosomal recessive, inherited, metabolic disorders characterized by an inability to degrade glycogen (see Chapter 6). There are many glycogenoses, but only some of them affect skeletal muscle. Only the most important glycogenoses affecting skeletal muscle will be described.

Type II Glycogenosis (Acid Maltase [α-1,4-Glucosidase] Deficiency, Pompe Disease)

 MOLECULAR PATHOGENESIS: Various mutations affect muscle acid maltase activity and lead to distinctly different clinical syndromes. Acid maltase is a lysosomal enzyme that is expressed in all cells and participates in glycogen degradation. When the enzyme is deficient, glycogen is not broken down, accumulates within lysosomes and remains membrane bound (Fig. 31-17B).

PATHOLOGY: In all forms of glycogenosis due to acid maltase deficiency, the morphologic changes are distinctive and almost pathognomonic (Fig. 31-17A).

In the severe form, Pompe disease, muscle shows massive accumulation of membrane-bound glycogen. Myofilaments and other sarcoplasmic organelles disappear. There is very little regeneration, and apparently inactive satellite cells are present at the surfaces of muscle fibers that have been almost completely destroyed by the disease.

Late infantile, juvenile and adult-onset forms of type II glycogenosis are milder, with changes ranging from overt vacuolar myopathy to very subtle accumulation of membrane-bound glycogen particles only detectable by electron microscopy. Vacuoles seen by light microscopy are empty or contain glycogen.

 CLINICAL FEATURES: Pompe disease occurs in neonates or young infants and is the most extreme form of acid maltase deficiency. Patients have severe hypotonia and areflexia and clinically resemble patients with Werdnig-Hoffmann disease (see below). Some have enlarged tongues and cardiomegaly and die of cardiac failure, usually within their first 2 years. Many tissues are affected, but skeletal and cardiac muscle, the CNS and the liver are most involved. The serum creatine kinase level is slightly to moderately increased. Later-onset forms of the disease entail milder, but relentlessly progressive, myopathy. Glycogen accumulates in other organs, but clinical expression of the disorder is usually limited to muscle.

Type III Glycogenosis (Debranching Enzyme Deficiency, Cori Disease, Limit Dextrinosis, Amylo-1,6-Glucosidase Deficiency)

MOLECULAR PATHOGENESIS: Type III glycogenosis is a rare, autosomal recessive disease of children or adults. Because the debranching enzyme is absent, phosphorylase can hydrolyze 1,4-glycosidic linkages of the terminal glucose chains of glycogen, but not beyond branch points. Hepatomegaly and growth retardation are the rule. Muscle symptoms vary, and the most severe and consistent involvement is related to liver dysfunction in children.

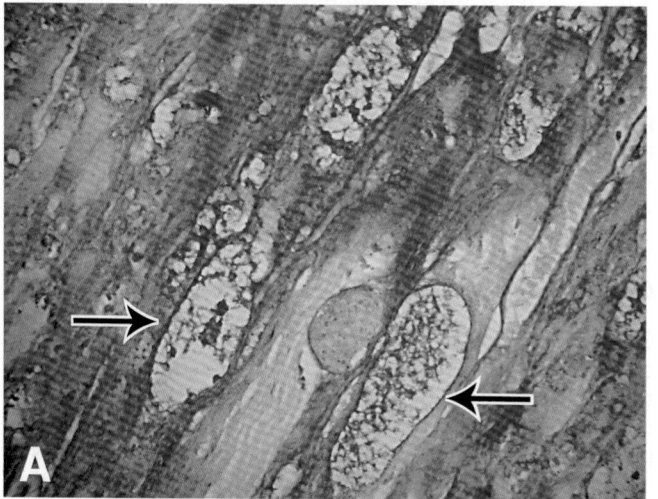
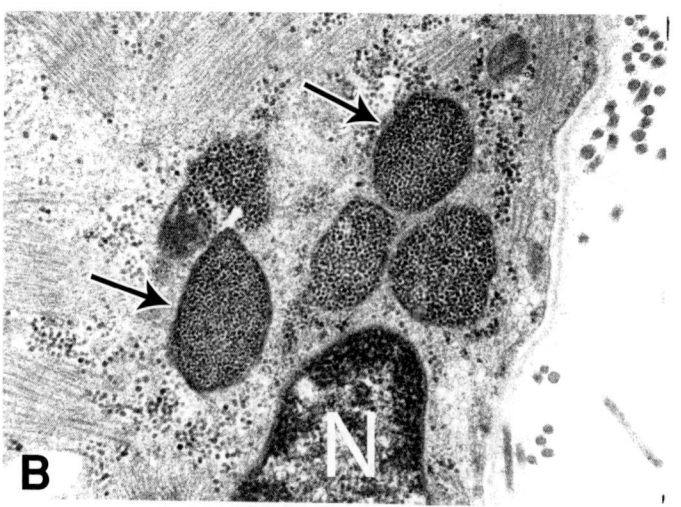

FIGURE 31-17. Acid maltase deficiency—adult onset. A. Periodic acid–Schiff (PAS) stain demonstrating large vacuoles filled with PAS-positive glycogen granules (*arrows*). **B.** Electron micrograph demonstrating membrane-bound glycogen granules (*arrows*). The structure marked *N* is a nucleus.

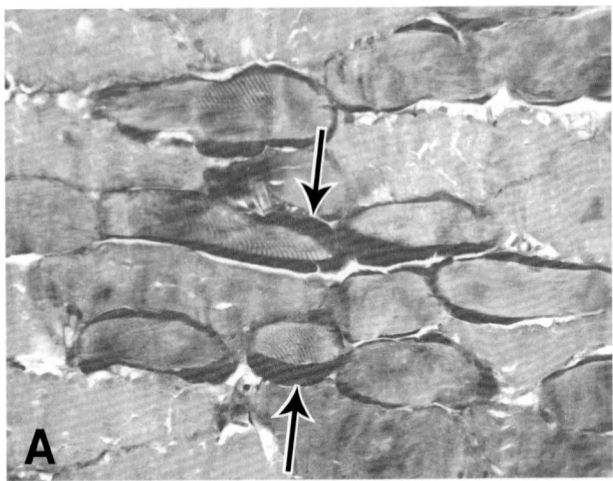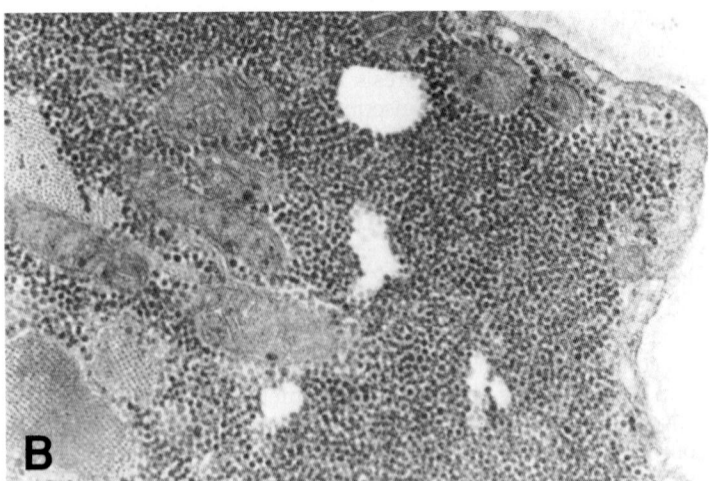

FIGURE 31-18. McArdle disease (myophosphorylase deficiency). A. Prominent periodic acid–Schiff (PAS)-positive glycogen accumulation in a subsarcolemmal distribution (*arrows*). **B.** An electron micrograph demonstrates an abnormal mass of glycogen particles just beneath the sarcolemma. The glycogen is not surrounded by a membrane, in contrast to the lysosomal glycogen storage of acid maltase deficiency.

Type V Glycogenosis (McArdle Disease, Myophosphorylase Deficiency)

 MOLECULAR PATHOGENESIS: Type V glycogenosis is a more common metabolic myopathy that is usually not progressive or severely debilitating. The deficient enzyme, myophosphorylase, is specific for skeletal muscle. Without this enzyme, skeletal muscle glycogen cannot be cleaved at 1,4-glycosidic chains to produce glucose for energy production during physical exertion. Thus, muscles cramp with exercise. Patients also cannot produce lactate during ischemic exercise, which is the basis for a metabolic test for the condition.

 PATHOLOGY: Tissue may appear completely normal, except for the absence of phosphorylase activity. However, there is usually subtle evidence of abnormal accumulation of glycogen granules within the sarcoplasm, mainly in the subsarcolemmal area (Fig. 31-18). The specific diagnosis can be made by a histochemical reaction for myophosphorylase but must be confirmed by biochemical assay of muscle enzyme activity or by DNA analysis. Electron microscopy will often demonstrate accumulation of non–membrane-bound glycogen.

 CLINICAL FEATURES: Myophosphorylase deficiency need not seriously interfere with patients' lives. However, prolonged, vigorous exercise can lead to widespread myofiber necrosis and release of soluble muscle proteins like creatine kinase and myoglobin into the blood. This can cause myoglobinuria and renal failure.

Muscle biopsy should be performed several weeks after an episode of symptoms to allow regeneration of the muscle.

Type VII Glycogenosis (Phosphofructokinase Deficiency, Tarui Disease)

 **MOLECULAR PATHOGENESIS:** Phosphofructokinase (PFK) deficiency is less common than McArdle disease but causes the same syndrome.

PFK converts fructose-6-phosphate to fructose-1,6-diphosphate and is a key enzyme in the Embden-Meyerhof pathway. In muscle, this enzyme has four identical subunits (M_4), while in erythrocytes, it has two different (M and L) subunits, each encoded separately. Genetic lack of the muscle subunit thus leads to complete absence of muscle PFK activity but reduces erythrocyte PFK by 50%. In red blood cells, the remaining active enzyme is composed of four normal L subunits.

Patients with type VII glycogenosis often have slight anemia or low-grade hemolysis, but muscle histology resembles that in McArdle disease, save that phosphorylase activity is present. By contrast, histochemistry shows little or no PFK. The diagnosis is substantiated by biochemical assay of enzyme activity in muscle.

Lipid Myopathies Are Caused by Defective Fat Metabolism

A muscle biopsy from a patient with exercise intolerance or muscle weakness may sometimes show excess neutral lipids. This occurs in several metabolic disorders of lipid metabolism, more than a dozen of which are known. In brief, lipid myopathies may involve deficiencies in (1) fatty acid transport into mitochondria (carnitine deficiency syndromes, carnitine palmityl transferase deficiency), (2) several enzymes that mediate β-oxidation of fatty acids, (3) respiratory chain enzymes and (4) triglyceride use. Only disorders involving carnitine metabolism are discussed here.

Carnitine Deficiency

Carnitine is synthesized in the liver and is present in large quantities in skeletal muscle. It is needed for long-chain fatty acid transport into mitochondria. Muscle carnitine deficiency is an autosomal recessive condition, with progressive proximal muscle weakness and atrophy, often with signs of denervation and peripheral neuropathy. Without carnitine, lipid droplets accumulate massively in the sarcoplasm outside mitochondria and are readily seen in muscle biopsies (Fig. 31-19). Sometimes oral carnitine therapy alleviates

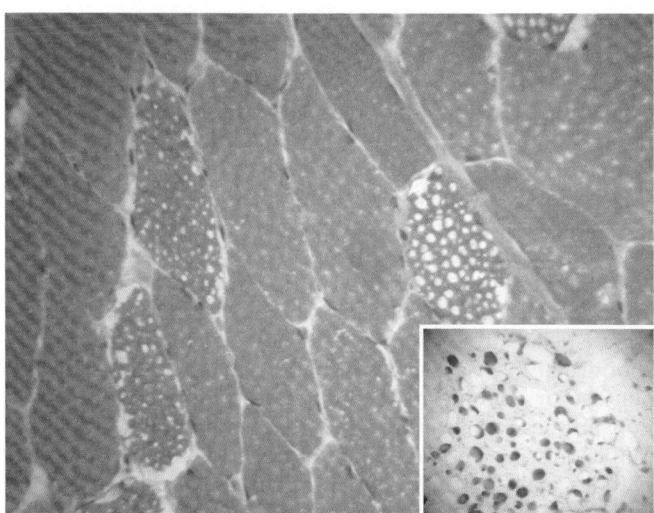

FIGURE 31-19. Lipid storage myopathy. Hematoxylin and eosin–stained frozen section. Numerous cytoplasmic vacuoles are present in the muscle fibers. Oil red-orcein stain (*inset*) demonstrates that the cytoplasmic vacuoles contain neutral lipid.

symptoms. Carnitine deficiency in skeletal muscle also occurs as part of a systemic disorder that can affect the CNS, heart and liver. Structural abnormalities of mitochondria may be present.

Carnitine Palmitoyltransferase Deficiency

Patients with carnitine palmitoyltransferase deficiency cannot metabolize long-chain fatty acids, owing to an inability to transport these lipids into mitochondria, where they undergo β-oxidation. After heavy exercise, these patients have muscular pain, which may progress to myoglobinuria. Prolonged fasting can produce the same symptoms. After such an episode, fibers regenerate and restore muscle structure. Biopsies are microscopically normal; the diagnosis requires biochemical assay for carnitine palmitoyltransferase activity.

In Mitochondrial Diseases Nuclear or Mitochondrial DNA May Be Mutated

Inherited defects of mitochondrial metabolism are uncommon but conceptually important disorders. Historically, diseases of muscle were recognized first and designated mitochondrial myopathies, but others affect both CNS and muscle and are known as **mitochondrial encephalomyopathies**. The nervous system, skeletal muscle, heart, kidney and other organs can be affected in different combinations as part of a multisystem disease.

Inherited diseases of mitochondria are divided into defects of **nuclear DNA** (nDNA) or **mitochondrial DNA** (mtDNA). Point mutations, deletions and duplications of mtDNA have been linked to several mitochondrial encephalomyopathies.

 MOLECULAR PATHOGENESIS: The genes for most mitochondrial proteins are in nDNA, but mtDNA encodes 13 of the 80 polypeptides in respiratory chain complexes. Defects in these proteins lead to mitochondrial encephalomyopathies.

Unlike Mendelian inheritance of nDNA genes, mtDNA diseases are transmitted in maternal mtDNA, since mtDNA derives only from the oocyte. The zygote and its daughter cells have many mitochondria, each of which contains maternally derived mtDNA. Mutations in this DNA are passed on randomly to later generations of cells. During fetal or later growth, some cells may thus contain only mutant genomes (mutant homoplasmy), others will have only normal genomes (wild-type homoplasmy) and still others receive mixed populations of mutant and normal mtDNA (heteroplasmy). Clinical expression of a disease due to a mutation in mtDNA depends on the proportion of the total content of mitochondrial genomes that is mutant. *The fraction of mutant mtDNA must exceed a critical value for a mitochondrial disease to be symptomatic.* This threshold varies in different organs and is related to cellular energy requirements.

 PATHOLOGY: In skeletal muscle, defects of mtDNA lead to accumulation of mitochondria, excessive numbers of which may appear as aggregates of reddish granular material in a subsarcolemmal location (underneath the myocyte plasma membrane) with modified Gomori trichrome stain (Fig. 31-20A). These are called **ragged red fibers** because these deposits have an irregular contour at the fiber periphery. Three subunits of complex IV (cytochrome oxidase) are encoded by mtDNA and are required for the assembled electron transport carrier to be functional. Pathogenic mutations of mtDNA may impair complex IV activity, so that ragged red fibers are often deficient in cytochrome oxidase activity (Fig. 31-20B). By contrast, they stain intensely for succinic dehydrogenase (SDH, complex II); this complex is exclusively encoded by nDNA (Fig. 31-20C). The increased SDH reflects mitochondrial proliferation. Such defects cause myofiber atrophy and accumulation of sarcoplasmic lipid and glycogen owing to impaired mitochondrial energy utilization. Ultrastructurally, mitochondria may display striking paracrystalline inclusions (Fig. 31-20D), ring-shaped mitochondria, spiral cristae and electron-dense deposits.

Increased ragged red fibers and cytochrome oxidase–negative fibers also occur in elderly patients with unexplained muscle weakness ("mitochondrial cytopathy of old age"), presumably because numbers of mutant mitochondria increase with age. Ragged red fibers, cytochrome oxidase–negative fibers and intramitochondrial paracrystalline inclusions may suggest a mitochondrial disorder but are not specific, as similar changes occur in some muscular dystrophies, in inclusion body myositis and after certain drugs. Conversely, the absence of such changes does not exclude a mitochondrial disorder.

CLINICAL FEATURES: Clinical presentations of encephalomyopathies vary, but diseases may begin in children or adults. Some patients start with muscle weakness and then develop brain disorders. Others present with CNS disease, with or without overt muscle weakness, even though muscle biopsy shows mitochondrial pathology. Other organs, such as the heart (arrhythmias), are often affected as part of a multisystem disorder. The number of known mitochondrial disorders is increasing rapidly. The discussion below of major mitochondrial myopathies is a small sample.

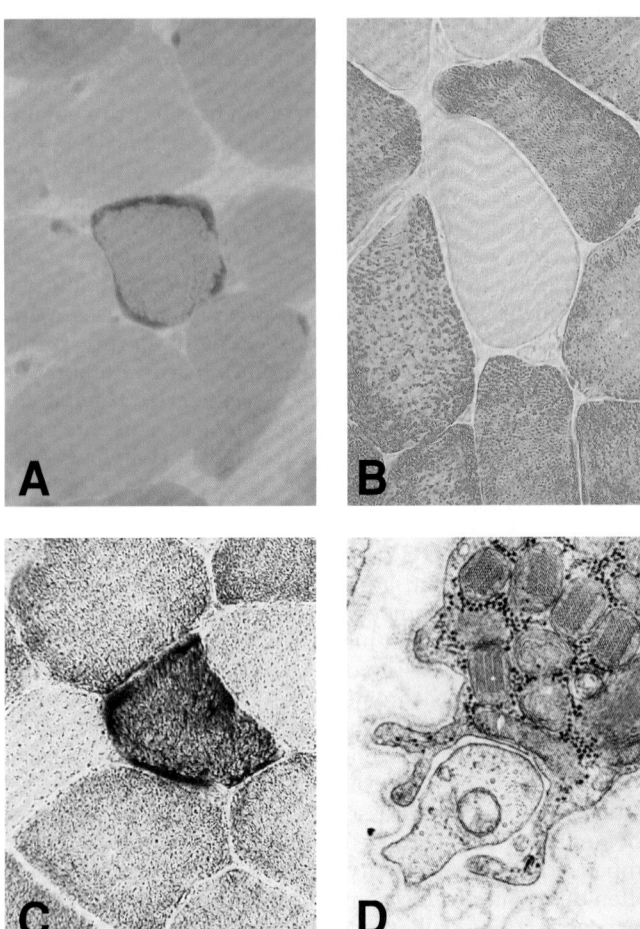

FIGURE 31-20. Mitochondrial myopathy caused by deletions of mitochondrial DNA (mtDNA). A. Modified Gomori trichrome. A ragged red fiber shows prominent proliferation of reddish, granular mitochondria, located chiefly in a subsarcolemmal region. **B.** A ragged red fiber displays lack of **histochemical staining for cytochrome oxidase** (central pale fiber). Three subunits of this electron-transport carrier are coded by mtDNA, and the mutations have interfered with function in this fiber. **C. Succinate dehydrogenase (SDH) stain.** A ragged red fiber shows overexpression of SDH, an enzyme that is entirely encoded by nuclear DNA (nDNA). **D.** An electron micrograph reveals mitochondria with ultrastructural abnormalities, including paracrystalline inclusions.

Three well-known neurologic syndromes include (1) **Kearns-Sayre syndrome** (progressive ophthalmoplegia, retinitis pigmentosum, cardiac arrhythmias, diabetes mellitus, cerebellar ataxia and multifocal neurodegeneration), (2) **MELAS** (mitochondrial myopathy, encephalopathy, lactic acidosis and stroke-like episodes) and (3) **MERRF** (myoclonic epilepsy and ragged red fibers). Most patients with Kearns-Sayre syndrome have large deletions of mtDNA that are usually nonfamilial. A related but clinically more benign condition, chronic progressive external ophthalmoplegia (CPEO), also has mitochondrial DNA deletions. Patients present with bilateral ptosis and weakness of eye muscles as in Kearns-Sayre syndrome. Such patients may progress to Kearns-Sayre syndrome. Clinically, the presence of cardiac arrhythmias in a CPEO patient predicts progression to Kearns-Sayre syndrome (KSS). The mitochondrial DNA deletions probably arise during oogenesis. All such affected

people are heteroplasmic (i.e., they have a mixture of mutant and normal mitochondria) and the phenotype depends on the distribution and relative numbers of mutant mitochondria at birth. Despite the presence of these congenital mutations, symptoms typically appear in adulthood. More severe forms (KSS) present in the second decade.

Progressive external ophthalmoplegia (PEO) is an autosomal dominant disorder characterized by ophthalmoparesis and exercise intolerance with onset typically between ages 20 and 40. These patients have multiple mtDNA deletions that are secondary to mutations in a number of nuclear-encoded genes such as in DNA polymerase-γ (which replicates mitochondrial DNA), as well as mutations in mitochondrial DNA helicase or adenine nucleotide translocator-1. Thus, mutations in these nuclear-encoded genes subsequently produce mitochondrial DNA deletions. PEO and CPEO are similar pathologically. MELAS and MERRF usually involve point mutations in mitochondrial genes for tRNAs, mostly—but not exclusively—leucine tRNA (MELAS) and lysine tRNA (MERRF). Mitochondrial genetic disorders like MELAS and MERRF are inherited from maternal mtDNA. Other syndromes affecting mitochondrial proteins encoded by nuclear genes show autosomal (such as PEO) or X-linked patterns of inheritance.

Myoadenylate Deaminase Deficiency Causes Mild Weakness

MOLECULAR PATHOGENESIS: There are large amounts of adenosine monophosphate deaminase (AMP-DA) in skeletal muscle, particularly in type II fibers. AMP-DA is important in regulating purine nucleotide cycles and maintaining the adenosine triphosphate–to–adenosine diphosphate (ATP:ADP) ratio during exercise. A group of patients with mild proximal muscle weakness and exercise intolerance completely lack AMP-DA activity. It is a common, autosomal recessive condition, seen in 1%–2% of all muscle biopsies. AMP-DA deficiency may thus not actually be a separate disease, but one that is unmasked by other neuromuscular diseases.

Familial Periodic Paralysis Reflects Impaired Electrolyte Flux

Familial periodic paralysis encompasses several autosomal dominant disorders in which episodic muscular weakness or even complete paralysis is followed by rapid recovery. These reflect abnormalities in sodium and potassium fluxes into and out of muscle cells. During an attack, muscle fiber surfaces do not propagate action potentials, although calcium entry into the muscle fiber causes contraction. Muscle biopsies during an attack show no detectable abnormalities of recent onset. Later, permanent mild myopathic changes and sarcoplasmic vacuoles appear. These vacuoles are dilated or remodeled sarcoplasmic reticulum and transverse tubules. In some cases, a distinct subpopulation of fibers (type IIB) contains numerous tubular aggregates derived from the tubular network of the sarcoplasmic reticulum.

MOLECULAR PATHOGENESIS: These dyskalemic episodic weakness syndromes include hypokalemic and hyperkalemic periodic paralysis. The former type is linked to mutations in several genes including a calcium channel (*CACNA1S*), a sodium channel (*SCN4A*) and a potassium channel (*KCNE3*). In the hyperkalemic form, the same sodium channel gene (*SCN4A*) is mutated, but the hyperkalemic form reflects a gain-of-function *SCN4A* mutation, while the hypokalemic form is due to a loss-of-function mutation in the same sodium channel gene. A previously described normokalemic periodic paralysis syndrome is now considered a variant of hyperkalemic periodic paralysis and demonstrates mutations in *SCN4A*.

RHABDOMYOLYSIS

Rhabdomyolysis is dissolution of skeletal muscle fibers and release of myoglobin into the blood. This may cause myoglobinuria and acute renal failure. The disorder may be acute, subacute or chronic. During acute rhabdomyolysis, muscles are swollen, tender and profoundly weak.

Episodes of rhabdomyolysis may be precipitated by diverse stimuli. They may complicate or follow bouts of influenza. Some patients develop rhabdomyolysis with apparently mild exercise and probably have some form of metabolic myopathy. A spectrum of muscle dysfunction, from pain (myalgia) to rhabdomyolysis, is also well known during treatment with statin cholesterol-lowering agents. Biopsies after recovery may show morphologically normal muscle. Rhabdomyolysis also may complicate heat stroke or malignant hyperthermia. Alcoholism is occasionally associated with either acute or chronic rhabdomyolysis.

Pathologically, rhabdomyolysis is an active, noninflammatory myopathy, with scattered muscle fiber necrosis and varying degrees of degeneration and regeneration. Macrophages, but no other inflammatory cells, are present in and around muscle fibers.

DENERVATION

The major differential diagnostic consideration in any patient with muscle weakness is whether the cause is myopathic or neurogenic. Myopathic conditions are those intrinsic to muscle and have been discussed above. Neurogenic causes of muscle weakness are due to denervation. The pathology of denervation reflects lesions of lower motor neurons and/or axons. Muscle biopsy detects lower motor neuron lesions, but patterns of denervation do not identify the cause of the lesion. The morphology may indicate whether denervation is recent or chronic but does not distinguish between, for example, amyotrophic lateral sclerosis, a disorder of motor neurons, and neuropathy due to diabetes mellitus. Lesions of upper motor neurons, as in multiple sclerosis or stroke, lead to paralysis and atrophy but leave lower motor neurons intact. Pathologic changes thus reflect nonspecific diffuse atrophy rather than denervation atrophy.

When a skeletal muscle fiber becomes separated from contact with its lower motor neuron, it invariably atrophies, owing to progressive loss of myofibrils. On cross-section, atrophic fibers are characteristically angular, as though compressed by surrounding normal muscle fibers (Fig. 31-21). If a fiber is not reinnervated, atrophy progresses to complete loss of myofibrils, with nuclei condensing into aggregates. In the end stage, muscle fibers disappear and are replaced chiefly by adipose tissue.

Early in denervation, fibers are irregularly scattered, angular and atrophic. As the disease progresses, these fibers are first seen in small clusters of several fibers, and then in progressively larger groups (Fig. 31-21B). They stain excessively darkly for nonspecific esterase (Fig. 31-22) and NADH-TR, in contrast to atrophy caused by disuse or wasting. Groups of denervated fibers include both type I and type II fibers: **denervating conditions are not selective for only one type of motor neuron**.

"Target fibers" (Fig. 31-23) are seen transiently in 20% of cases of denervation. This change occurs during or shortly after denervation or reinnervation and indicates that the process is active. The lesion consists of central pallor of the muscle fiber, which is surrounded by a condensed zone, in turn surrounded by a normal zone of sarcoplasm. Target fibers are difficult to see with hematoxylin and eosin stain, but the NADH-TR stain shows greatly reduced staining in the central zone, reflecting reduced or absent mitochondria.

Denervation is always followed by an effort at reinnervation. If denervation proceeds slowly, reinnervation may keep pace. New sprouting nerve endings make synaptic contact with the muscle fiber at the site of the previous motor end-plate. As in the myotubular phase of embryogenesis, nicotinic Ach receptors (extrajunctional receptors) cover muscle fibers soon after denervation. This denervated state induces sprouting of new nerve endings from adjacent surviving nerves. With reinnervation, extrajunctional receptors again disappear from the sarcolemma, except at the point of synaptic contact.

In a chronic denervating condition, reinnervation of each surviving motor unit gradually enlarges. As a specific type of lower motor neuron takes over innervation of a given field of fibers, fiber groups of one type are seen adjacent to groups of another type. This pattern, called **fiber-type grouping**, is pathognomonic of denervation followed by reinnervation (Fig. 31-21C).

Patients with striking fiber–type grouping often have symptoms of muscle cramping in addition to progressive muscular weakness. After a single episode of denervation, such as in poliomyelitis, reinnervation often leads to remarkable recovery of strength. Years later, one sees conspicuous-type grouping, with scattered pyknotic nuclear clumps. In such cases, there are neither angular atrophic fibers nor target fibers.

If denervation continues after development of fiber-type grouping, large motor units become atrophic. Such **grouped atrophy** (Fig. 31-21D) is characteristic of chronic denervating disorders such as amyotrophic lateral sclerosis (ALS).

Occasionally, one fiber type (either type I or type II) predominates over the other, in **type predominance**. There is frequently evidence of denervation. In such cases, reinnervation may favor one type of lower motor neuron over another.

Muscle fibers may uncommonly be lost or regenerate in neuropathic conditions. Then, muscle degeneration causes a modest increase in serum creatine kinase levels. This occurs in slowly progressive forms of spinal muscular atrophy (e.g., Kugelberg-Welander disease, Kennedy disease [X-linked spinobulbar muscular atrophy]).

Spinal Muscular Atrophy Reflects Progressive Degeneration of Anterior Horn Cells

This disease is, strictly speaking, not a primary muscle disorder but is usually included in discussions of skeletal muscle pathology since it represents a major consideration in the differential diagnosis of childhood or infantile weakness. *Spinal*

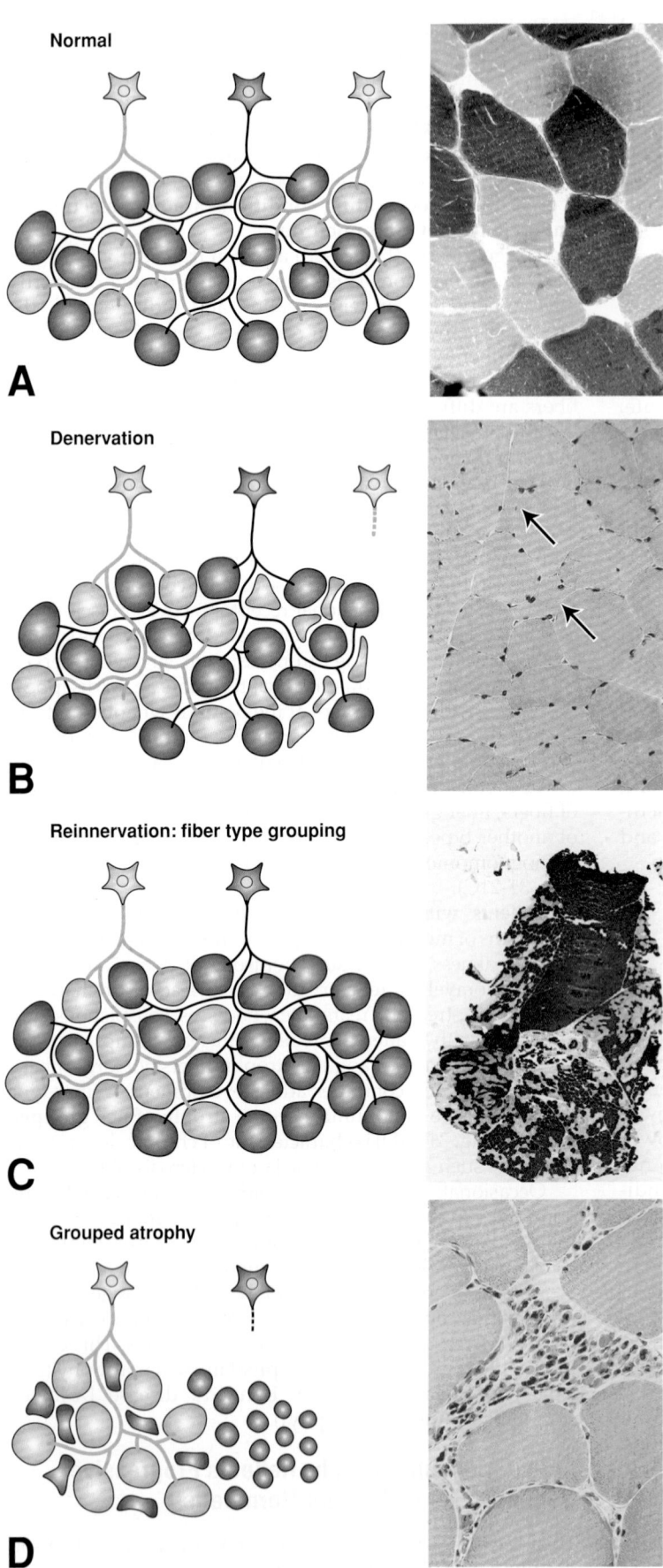

FIGURE 31-21. Denervation/reinnervation. A. As shown in the photomicrograph, the normal intermixed distribution of type I (*pale*) and type II (*dark*) muscle fibers is shown by staining for ATPase. In the drawing, two neurons (*pale*) innervate type I muscle fibers, and two neurons (*dark*) supply type II fibers. **B.** Denervation; hematoxylin and eosin stain. With early (mild) denervation, portions of the axonal tree degenerate, resulting in angular atrophy of scattered type I and II muscle fibers (*arrows*). **C.** Reinnervation; myofibrillar ATPase. As neurons degenerate, surviving neurons sprout more nerve endings and reinnervate some of the denervated fibers. These reinnervated fibers become either type I or type II, according to the type of neuron that reinnervates them. This process results in fewer, but larger, motor units and the appearance of clusters of fibers of one type adjacent to clusters of the other type, a pattern called "type grouping." The photomicrograph demonstrates type grouping. This field would appear normal except for a few atrophic fibers if it were stained with hematoxylin and eosin. **D.** With more advanced (severe, chronic) denervation, entire lower motor neurons or numerous axonal processes degenerate, causing small groups of angular atrophic fibers (grouped atrophy) to appear as illustrated in the photomicrograph.

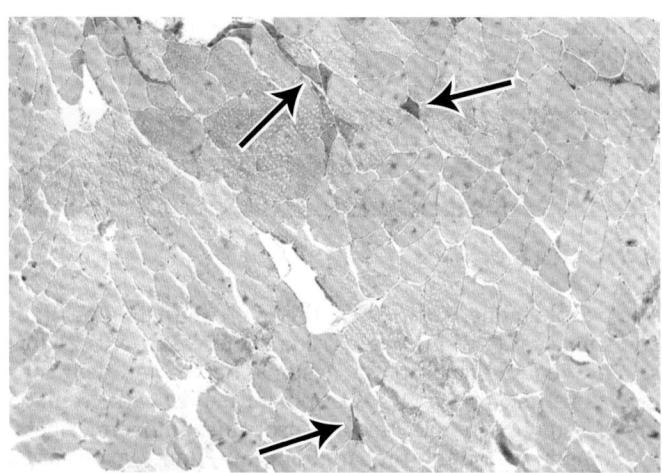

FIGURE 31-22. Denervation. In this frozen section of the biceps muscle subjected to the nonspecific esterase reaction, a few irregularly scattered, angular, atrophic fibers (*arrows*) are excessively dark stained. This pattern is highly characteristic of atrophy due to denervation.

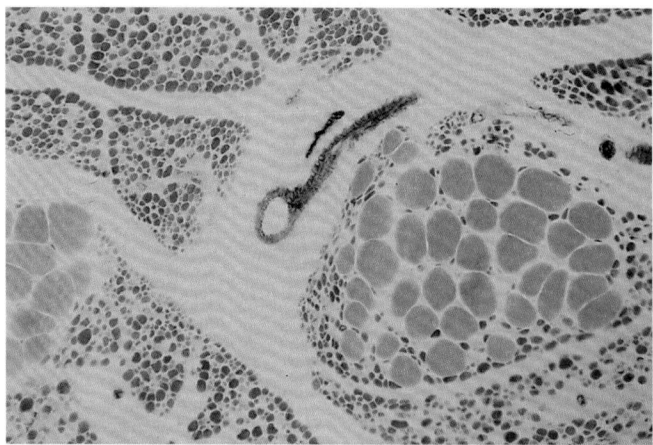

FIGURE 31-24. Werdnig-Hoffman disease (infantile spinal muscular atrophy). This cross-section of skeletal muscle stained for myofibrillar ATPase is derived from an infant with severe hypotonia. It shows groups of extremely atrophic, rounded type I and type II fibers and clusters of markedly hypertrophied pale type I fibers.

muscular atrophy (SMA) is the second most common lethal autosomal recessive disorder after cystic fibrosis. Childhood SMA is classified into type I **(Werdnig-Hoffmann disease)**, type II (intermediate) and type III **(Kugelberg-Welander disease)**. The survival motor neuron gene (5q11.2-13.3) is mutated in these related syndromes, mostly as a result of deletion.

WERDNIG-HOFFMANN DISEASE (INFANTILE SPINAL MUSCULAR ATROPHY): In *Werdnig-Hoffmann disease, infants show progressive and severe weakness* and seldom survive beyond 1 year of life. Denervation seems to begin in utero after motor units are established. The histology is virtually pathognomonic (Fig. 31-24). Groups of minute, rounded, atrophic fibers are still identifiable with the ATPase reaction as being either type I or type II. There are also fascicles of normal muscle fibers and almost invariably clusters

of hypertrophied type I fibers. In addition to the absent survival motor neuron gene, a second gene (neuronal apoptosis inhibitory protein gene) has also been implicated in the pathogenesis of Werdnig-Hoffmann disease.

KUGELBERG-WELANDER DISEASE (JUVENILE SPINAL MUSCULAR ATROPHY): **This variant is a later-onset form of SMA and is not necessarily progressive.** These patients had often been designated as having limb-girdle muscular dystrophy, but the electromyographic pattern of denervation helps to make the diagnosis. Muscle biopsies show type grouping and other evidence of a neurogenic disorder but can resemble a myopathy in a small sample because of coexisting necrotic fibers and regenerating fibers.

KENNEDY DISEASE (X-LINKED SPINOBULBAR MUSCULAR ATROPHY): An X-linked adult-onset form of spinobulbar muscular atrophy (Kennedy disease) is associated with trinucleotide repeat (CAG) expansion in the androgen receptor. As a result, anterior horn cells (motor neurons) degenerate, and the testes atrophy.

TYPE II FIBER ATROPHY

A commonly misinterpreted pathologic pattern in muscle biopsy specimens is atrophy from disuse, wasting, upper motor neuron disease and corticosteroid toxicity. This diffuse, nonspecific atrophy is a selective angular atrophy of type II fibers and may resemble denervation atrophy on hematoxylin and eosin stain. However, ATPase stains show that all angular atrophic fibers are type II (Fig. 31-25) and do not stain heavily by nonspecific esterase or NADH-TR reactions. Type II fiber atrophy is common and is often related to a more chronic problem.

STEROID MYOPATHY: Corticosteroid therapy can cause muscle weakness with type II atrophy. This may cause confusion clinically, as patients with polymyositis often receive large doses of corticosteroids. If such a patient's weakness worsens, the physician must decide if this development represents relapse of polymyositis, requiring more corticosteroids, or if it represents steroid myopathy, in which case steroid dosage should be reduced.

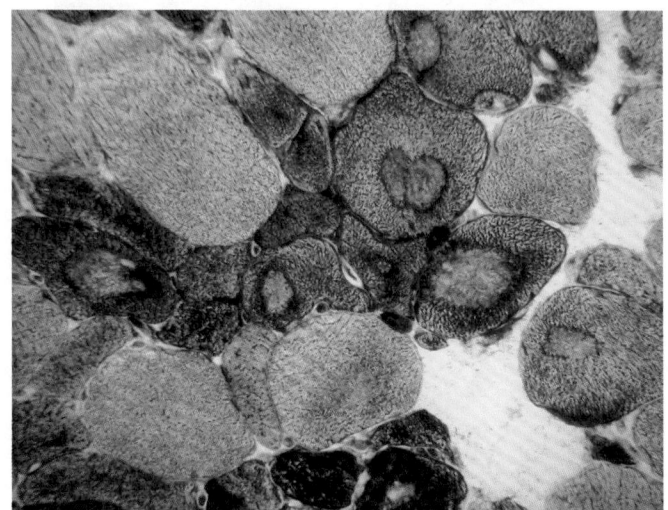

FIGURE 31-23. Target fiber. A cross-section of striated muscle treated with the NADH-tetrazolium reductase (NADH-TR) stain demonstrates several "target fibers," a characteristic feature of some cases of denervation. Because the enzyme reaction creates a product (formazan) that selectively fixes to membranous organelles, the centers of the target areas appear devoid of mitochondria and sarcoplasmic reticulum. The myofibrils may or may not be intact.

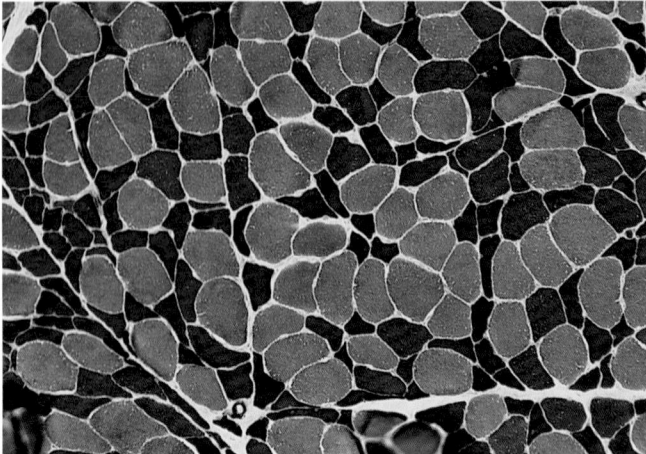

FIGURE 31-25. Type II fiber atrophy. This biopsy of the vastus lateralis muscle was taken from a 48-year-old man with proximal muscle weakness because of endogenous corticosteroid toxicity (Cushing syndrome). Virtually all of the angular atrophic fibers are type II. This form of atrophy closely mimics denervation atrophy when visualized with the hematoxylin and eosin stain.

Patients with corticosteroid toxicity do not have increased serum creatine kinase levels and biopsies show selective atrophy of type II fibers, without muscle fiber degeneration and inflammation. By contrast, in recurrent polymyositis, biopsy shows fiber degeneration and inflammation, with increased serum creatine kinase.

CRITICAL ILLNESS MYOPATHY

If patients on high-dose steroids and neuromuscular blocking agents experience severe weakness despite removal of paralyzing agents, they may have **critical illness myopathy**, also known as **myosin heavy-chain depletion syndrome**. These patients show loss of thick myosin filaments from muscle fibers (Fig. 31-26). The underlying mechanism of the myosin depletion is unclear, though myosin thick filaments

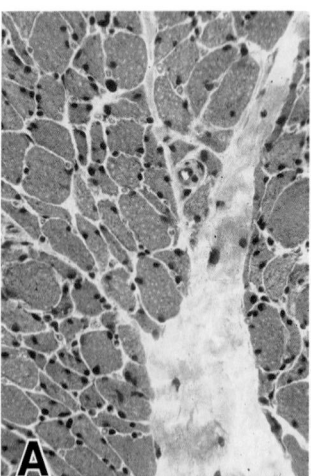
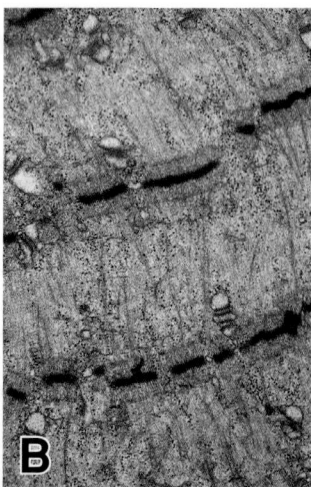

FIGURE 31-26. Critical illness myopathy. A. The condition frequently shows atrophic muscle with angular fibers (hematoxylin and eosin). **B.** By electron microscopy, there is marked loss of thick myosin filaments, while α-actin (thin) filaments are intact (compare to Fig. 31-2).

reappear with discontinuation of corticosteroids, and muscle strength returns.

The Peripheral Nervous System

ANATOMY

The peripheral nervous system (PNS) is external to the brain and spinal cord and includes (1) cranial nerves III–XII, (2) dorsal and ventral spinal roots, (3) spinal nerves and their continuations and (4) ganglia. Peripheral nerves carry somatic motor, somatic sensory, visceral sensory and autonomic fibers.

Somatic motor and preganglionic autonomic axons arise from neuronal cell bodies within the CNS. Sensory and postganglionic autonomic axons originate from neuronal cell bodies within ganglia located on cranial nerves, dorsal roots and autonomic nerves. Neurons, satellite cells of the ganglia and all Schwann cells are derived from neural crest.

Endoneurial connective tissue surrounds individual nerve fibers, which are bundled into fascicles by a **perineurial sheath**. Epineurial connective tissue binds the fascicles together and contains nutrient arteries. A blood-nerve barrier (BNB), located in endoneurial capillaries and the perineurial sheath, and analogous to the blood-brain barrier, protects peripheral nerves, but not ganglia. There are no lymphatic vessels in nerve fascicles.

Peripheral nerve axons may be myelinated or unmyelinated (Fig. 31-27). Myelinated axons are 1–20 μm in diameter.

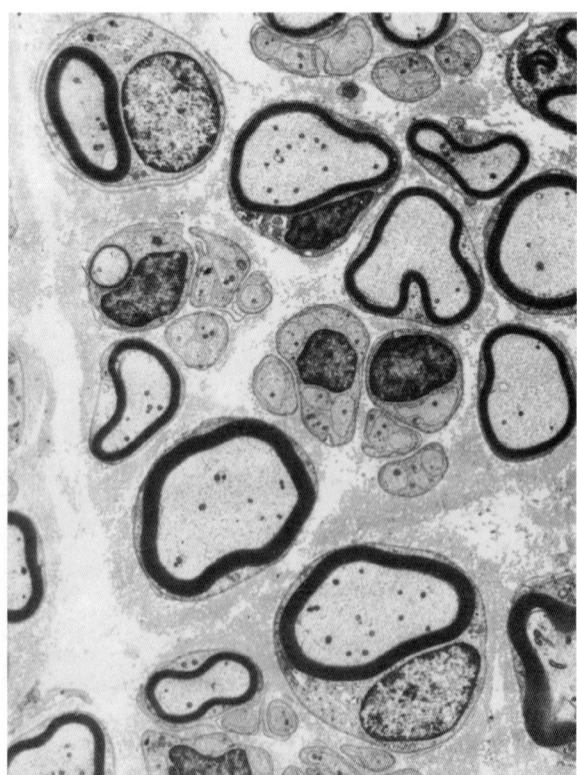

FIGURE 31-27. Structure of peripheral nerve. Electron micrograph of a peripheral nerve shows myelinated fibers interspersed with groups of unmyelinated fibers. Note that unlike myelinated axons, several unmyelinated axons may share a Schwann cell.

Unmyelinated ones, at 0.4–2.4 μm, are much smaller. Myelin is made from Schwann cell plasmalemma and is necessary for optimal nerve conduction. The lipids in Schwann cell–derived PNS myelin and oligodendrocyte-derived CNS myelin are similar, but their proteins differ substantially. Myelin protein zero (MPZ) and peripheral myelin protein 22 (PMP22) are only in the PNS. Schwann cells surround both myelinated and unmyelinated fibers. The axon determines whether the Schwann cell produces myelin. Myelin sheath thickness, internodal length (i.e., distance between two nodes of Ranvier) and conduction velocity are proportional to axonal diameter.

REACTIONS TO INJURY

Peripheral nerve fibers show only a limited number of reactions to injury (Fig. 31-28). The major types of nerve fiber damage are axonal degeneration and segmental demyelination. PNS fibers differ from those in the CNS by being able to regenerate and remyelinate to recover function.

Axonal Degeneration Reflects Injury to Axons or Neuronal Cell Bodies

Degeneration (necrosis) of the axon occurs in many neuropathies and may be limited to distal axons or involve both axons and neuronal cell bodies (Fig. 31-29A). Immediately after the axon degenerates, the myelin sheath breaks down and Schwann cells proliferate. The latter initiate myelin degradation, which is completed by macrophages that infiltrate the nerve within 3 days after axonal degeneration. If injury is restricted to the distal axon, regenerating axons may sprout within 1 week from the intact, proximal axonal stump. There are several types of axonal degeneration.

DISTAL AXONAL DEGENERATION: In many neuropathies, axon degeneration is initially limited to the distal ends of larger, longer fibers (**dying-back neuropathy** or **distal axonopathy**) (Fig. 31-28B). Peripheral neuropathies characterized by distal axonal degeneration typically present clinically as distal ("length-dependent" or "glove-and-stocking") neuropathies.

In this setting, neuron cell bodies and proximal axons stay intact. Axons may thus regenerate and nerve function

may return if the cause of the distal axonal degeneration is removed. This must occur before the dying-back degeneration reaches the proximal axon and causes the neuronal cell body to die. In some dying-back neuropathies, the axonal degeneration involves both the axon directed peripherally from the dorsal root ganglion neuron and the axon directed centrally to the spinal cord dorsal columns. These centrally

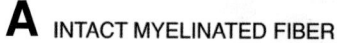
A INTACT MYELINATED FIBER

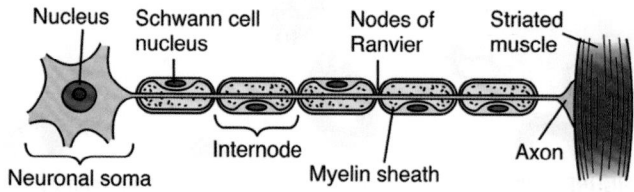

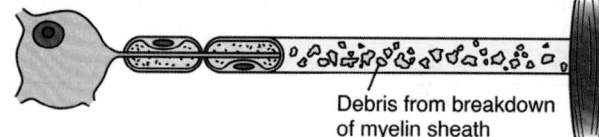
B DISTAL AXONAL DEGENERATION

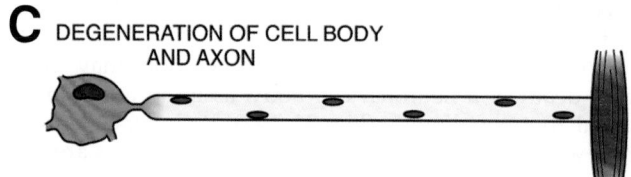
C DEGENERATION OF CELL BODY AND AXON

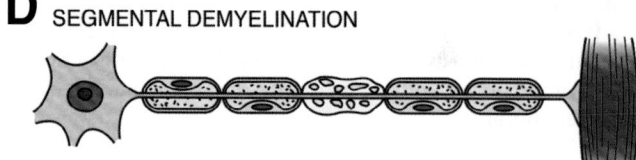
D SEGMENTAL DEMYELINATION

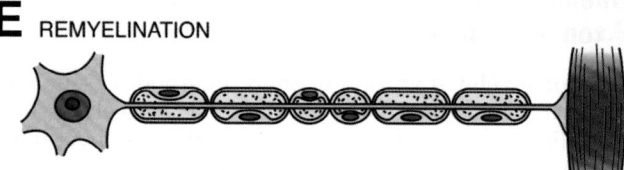
E REMYELINATION

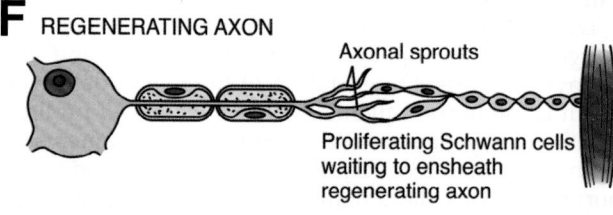
F REGENERATING AXON

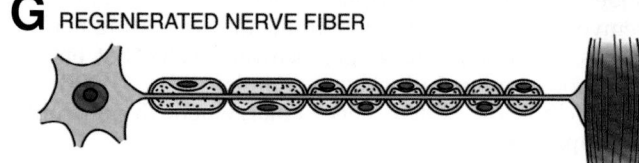
G REGENERATED NERVE FIBER

FIGURE 31-28. Basic responses of peripheral nerve fibers to injury. A. Intact myelinated fiber. The axon is insulated by the Schwann cell–derived myelin sheaths. **B. Distal axonal degeneration.** The distal axon has degenerated, and myelin sheaths associated with the distal axon have secondarily degenerated. The striated muscle shows denervation atrophy. **C. Degeneration of cell body and axon.** Degeneration involves the neuronal cell body and its entire axon. The myelin sheaths associated with the axon have also degenerated. **D. Segmental demyelination.** The myelin sheath associated with one Schwann cell has degenerated, leaving a segment of axon uncovered by myelin. The underlying axon remains intact. **E. Remyelination.** Proliferating Schwann cells cover the demyelinated segment of the axon and elaborate new myelin sheaths. The remyelinating Schwann cells have short internodal lengths. **F. Regenerating axon.** Regenerating axons sprout from the distal end of the disrupted axon. Ideally, the regenerating axons reinnervate the distal nerve stump, where they will be ensheathed and myelinated by Schwann cells of the distal stump. **G. Regenerated nerve fiber.** The regenerated portion of the axon is myelinated by Schwann cells with short internodal lengths. The striated muscle is reinnervated.

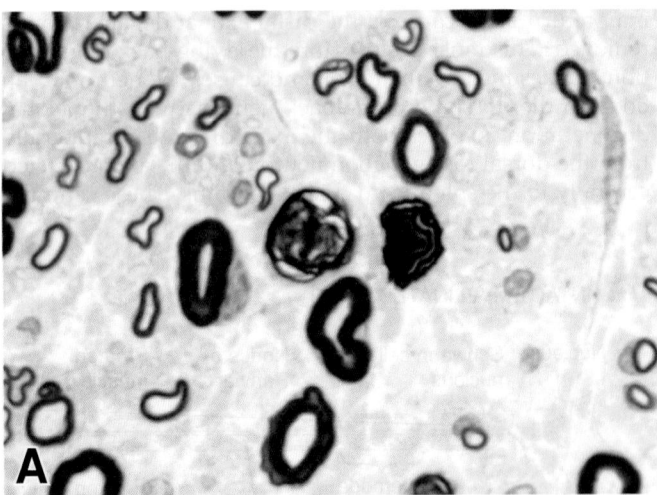
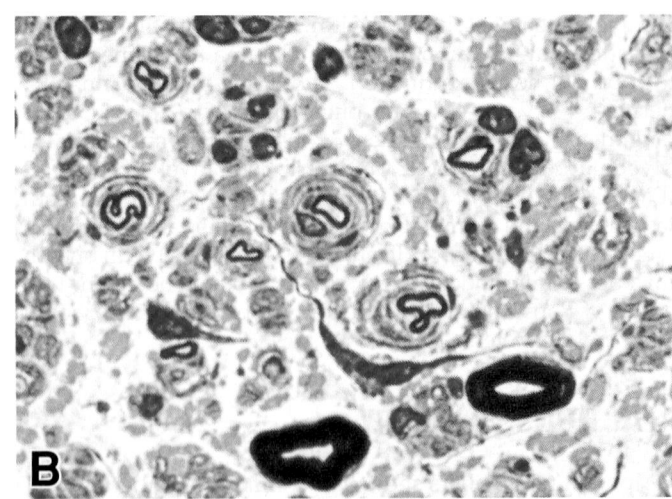

FIGURE 31-29. A. Axonal degeneration in an axonal neuropathy. Photomicrograph of a plastic-embedded cross-section of sural nerve shows two degenerating myelinated fibers in the center of the field. The degenerating fibers' axons are gone, and their myelin sheaths are reduced to rounded masses of myelin debris. In most axonal neuropathies, this axonal degeneration is limited to the distal axon. **B. Onion bulbs in chronic inflammatory demyelinating polyneuropathy.** Photomicrograph of a plastic-embedded cross-section of sural nerve shows several remyelinating axons with thin myelin sheaths in the center of the field. The remyelinating axons are surrounded by multiple concentric layers of Schwann cell cytoplasm, which resemble the concentric rings of a sectioned onion. Onion bulb formation is common in neuropathies with recurrent episodes of demyelination and remyelination.

directed axons, like other axons in the CNS, have little capacity for regeneration.

NEURONOPATHY: Axonal degeneration may result from death of a neuronal cell body, as in an autoimmune dorsal root ganglionitis (Fig. 31-28C). Peripheral neuropathies with selective damage to neuronal cell bodies are **neuronopathies** and are much rarer than distal axonopathies. Death of the neuronal cell body precludes axonal regeneration, making recovery impossible.

WALLERIAN DEGENERATION: This term describes axonal degeneration in a nerve distal to a transection or crush of the nerve. If the injury is not too proximal, the nerve may regenerate.

In Segmental Demyelination the Myelin Sheath Breaks Down but the Underlying Axon Remains Viable

Loss of myelin from one or more internodes (segments) along a myelinated fiber indicates Schwann cell dysfunction (Fig. 31-28D). This may be due either to direct injury to the Schwann cell or myelin sheath **(primary demyelination)** or to underlying axonal abnormalities **(secondary demyelination)**.

Loss of the myelin sheath does not cause the underlying axon to degenerate. Macrophages infiltrate the nerve and clear the myelin debris. Degeneration of the internodal myelin sheath is followed sequentially by Schwann cell proliferation, then remyelination of the demyelinated segments and finally functional recovery. Remyelinated internodes have shortened internodal lengths (Fig. 31-28E). Repeated episodes of segmental peripheral nerve demyelination and remyelination, as occurs in chronic demyelinating neuropathies, cause supernumerary Schwann cells that encircle the axons **(onion bulbs)** to accumulate (Fig. 31-29B) and cause clinically evident nerve enlargement **(hypertrophic neuropathy)**.

PERIPHERAL NEUROPATHIES

A peripheral neuropathy is a process that affects the function of one or more peripheral nerves. It may be restricted to the PNS, involve both the PNS and CNS or affect multiple organ systems. Peripheral neuropathies occur in all age groups and may be hereditary or acquired.

There are many causes of peripheral neuropathy (Table 31-3), but *diabetes mellitus is the most common cause of generalized peripheral neuropathy in the United States.* Other common causes include hereditary disorders, alcoholism, chronic renal failure, neurotoxic drugs, autoimmune diseases, paraproteinemia, nutritional deficiencies, infections, cancer and trauma.

 PATHOLOGY: Pathologic findings in most neuropathies are limited to axonal degeneration, segmental demyelination or both. If axonal degeneration predominates, the neuropathy is an **axonal neuropathy;** if segmental demyelination predominates, it is called a **demyelinating neuropathy.** *Most (80%–90%) neuropathies are axonal and of the dying-back type (distal axonal neuropathy).* Electrophysiologic studies often help to distinguish axonal and demyelinating neuropathies. Nerve conduction velocity is typically near normal in axonal neuropathies but is impaired in demyelinating neuropathies. The distinction between axonal and demyelinating neuropathies is useful clinically. Axonal neuropathies have many causes, but demyelinating neuropathies have a limited number of etiologies. The latter are most likely to be hereditary or immunologically mediated.

The histopathology of many neuropathies does not indicate the underlying cause, so that clinicopathologic correlation is usually needed to establish causation. Less often, a specific etiology may be seen, for example, necrotizing arteritis (vasculitic neuropathy), granulomatous inflammation (leprosy, sarcoid), amyloid deposits

TABLE 31-3

ETIOLOGIC CLASSIFICATION OF NEUROPATHIES

Immune-mediated neuropathies

Acute inflammatory demyelinating polyradiculoneuropathy (Guillain-Barré syndrome)

    Acute motor (and sensory) axonal neuropathy (axonal form of Guillain-Barré syndrome)

    Fisher syndrome

    Chronic inflammatory demyelinating polyradiculoneuropathy (CIDP)

    Multifocal motor neuropathy

    Dorsal root ganglionitis (sensory neuronopathy)

    Immunoglobulin M (IgM) paraproteinemia-associated demyelinating neuropathy

    Vasculitic neuropathy (systemic vasculitis, connective tissue disease, cryoglobulinemia)

Metabolic neuropathies

    Diabetic polyneuropathy and mononeuropathies

    Uremic neuropathy

    Critical illness polyneuropathy

    Hypothyroid neuropathy

    Acromegalic neuropathy

Nutritional neuropathies

    Neuropathy associated with deficiency of vitamin B_1, B_6, B_{12} or E

    Copper deficiency myeloneuropathy

Alcoholic neuropathy

Toxic and drug-induced neuropathies (see Table 31-4)

Amyloid neuropathy (AL amyloidosis and familial amyloid polyneuropathy)

Hereditary neuropathies (see Tables 31-5 and 31-6)

Neuropathies associated with infections

    Leprosy

    HIV

    Cytomegalovirus

    Hepatitis B and C (vasculitic neuropathy or CIDP)

    Herpes zoster

    Lyme disease

    Diphtheria (toxic neuropathy)

Paraneoplastic neuropathy

Sarcoid neuropathy

Radiation neuropathy

Traumatic neuropathy

Chronic idiopathic axonal polyneuropathy

(amyloid neuropathy), abnormalities of the myelin sheath (IgM paraproteinemic neuropathy, hereditary neuropathy with liability to pressure palsies) or abnormal accumulations within Schwann cells (leukodystrophy) or axons (giant axonal neuropathy).

 CLINICAL FEATURES: The major clinical manifestations of peripheral neuropathy are muscle weakness and atrophy, sensory loss, paresthesia, pain and autonomic dysfunction. Motor, sensory and autonomic functions may be equally or preferentially affected. Predominant involvement of large-diameter sensory fibers affects position and vibration sense, while injury to small-diameter fibers hinders pain and temperature sensation. A neuropathy may be acute (days to weeks), subacute (weeks to months) or chronic (months to years). It may affect one nerve (**mononeuropathy**) or several (**mononeuropathy multiplex**), dorsal root ganglia (**sensory neuronopathy**) or nerve roots (**radiculopathy**), and may involve multiple peripheral nerves (**polyneuropathy**), or nerve roots and peripheral nerves (**polyradiculoneuropathy**).

Peripheral Neuropathy Can Complicate Types 1 and 2 Diabetes Mellitus

Diabetic neuropathy may manifest as a distal sensorimotor polyneuropathy, autonomic neuropathy, mononeuropathy or mononeuropathy multiplex. The mononeuropathies may involve cranial nerves (cranial neuropathy), nerve roots or proximal peripheral nerves. *Distal, predominantly sensory, polyneuropathy is the most common form of diabetic neuropathy.*

 **ETIOLOGIC FACTORS:** How nerve fiber injury occurs in diabetes is unknown (see Chapter 13). It has long been held that the distal symmetric polyneuropathy is due to the metabolic abnormalities of diabetes, while the mononeuropathies are caused by nerve ischemia from small-vessel disease. However, local nerve ischemia also probably contributes to the symmetric polyneuropathy.

 PATHOLOGY: The distal symmetric polyneuropathy of diabetes is characterized by a mixture of axonal degeneration and segmental demyelination, with the former predominating. Axonal loss involves fibers of all sizes but may preferentially affect large myelinated fibers (**large-fiber neuropathy**) or small myelinated fibers and unmyelinated fibers (**small-fiber neuropathy**). Occasional neuronal loss in dorsal root ganglia and anterior horns most likely reflects centripetal progression of dying-back axonal degeneration, rather than a neuronopathy.

Uremic Neuropathy Often Complicates Chronic Renal Failure

Uremic neuropathy is a distal sensorimotor axonal polyneuropathy seen in half of patients with chronic renal failure, and causing both distal axonal degeneration and segmental demyelination. The former predominates and mainly affects large-diameter fibers. The mechanism is not known, but uremic neuropathy often stabilizes or improves with long-term dialysis and resolves after renal transplantation.

Critical Illness Polyneuropathy Develops in Many Severely Ill Patients

It is associated with sepsis and multiorgan failure. The acute, predominantly motor, neuropathy may first be apparent when a patient in the intensive care unit cannot be weaned from ventilatory support. A **critical illness myopathy** may also occur in these patients. The pathogenesis is obscure.

Neuropathy Is a Frequent Complication of Alcoholism

Alcoholic neuropathy is a distal sensorimotor axonal polyneuropathy, attributable to nutritional deficiencies and/or a direct toxic effect of ethanol on the PNS. Peripheral nerves show loss of nerve fibers from axonal degeneration of the dying-back type.

Nutritional Neuropathy Is an Axonal Polyneuropathy with Multiple Causes

Nutritional neuropathy is associated with deficiencies in vitamins (B_1, B_6, B_{12} or E) or copper. Copper deficiency may be a result of malnutrition, total parenteral nutrition, excessive ingestion of zinc or bariatric surgery. Isoniazid therapy for tuberculosis interferes with pyridoxine (vitamin B_6) metabolism and may cause vitamin B_6 deficiency neuropathy. It is unclear if the chronic axonal neuropathy sometimes seen in celiac disease is due to malnutrition or reflects the underlying autoimmune process.

Acute Inflammatory Demyelinating Polyradiculoneuropathy Is Immune Mediated

Acute inflammatory demyelinating polyradiculoneuropathy (AIDP) is an acquired, immune-mediated neuropathy that often follows bacterial, viral or mycoplasmal infections. It may also follow immunization or surgery. Usually, there is an antecedent upper respiratory or gastrointestinal infection. Commonly associated infectious agents include *Campylobacter jejuni*, cytomegalovirus, Epstein-Barr virus and *Mycoplasma pneumoniae*. AIDP is the most common cause in children and adults of the **Guillain-Barré syndrome,** which is an acute symmetric neuromuscular paralysis that often begins distally and ascends proximally. Sensory and autonomic disturbances may also occur, and 5% of cases present with ophthalmoplegia, ataxia and areflexia **(Fisher syndrome)**. Muscular paralysis may cause respiratory embarrassment, and autonomic involvement may lead to cardiac arrhythmias, hypotension or hypertension. The neuropathy begins to resolve 2–4 weeks after onset, and most patients recover. Characteristically, the cerebrospinal fluid (CSF) has increased protein but few white blood cells (albuminocytologic dissociation). The increased protein level is attributable to inflammation of spinal roots. The pathogenesis of the immunologically mediated demyelination is unknown.

AIDP may affect all levels of the PNS, including spinal roots (polyradiculoneuropathy), ganglia, craniospinal nerves and autonomic nerves. The distribution of lesions varies. Involved regions show endoneurial infiltrates of lymphocytes and macrophages, segmental demyelination and relative axonal sparing. Lymphoid infiltrates are often perivascular, but there is no true vasculitis. Macrophages are frequently adjacent to degenerating myelin sheaths and can strip off and phagocytose superficial myelin lamellae. Such macrophage-mediated demyelination is rare in other neuropathies.

Guillain-Barré syndrome may also be caused by an immune-mediated axonal neuropathy **(acute motor axonal neuropathy** or **acute motor and sensory axonal neuropathy)**. The axonal form of this disorder is much less common than the demyelinating type in North America and Europe but is more common in Asia. The axonal form often follows *C. jejuni* infection and shows serum antiganglioside antibodies (anti-GM_1 and others). Molecular mimicry between an antigenic component of the infectious agent and a component of the peripheral nerve may elicit a cross-reactive immune response that leads to axonal injury. Antiganglioside antibodies (anti-GQ1b and others) are also common in Fisher syndrome.

Chronic inflammatory demyelinating polyradiculoneuropathy (CIDP) is similar to AIDP but has a protracted course, with multiple relapses or slow continuous progression, and usually lacks evidence of antecedent infection. The neuropathy may occur sporadically (idiopathic CIDP) or be associated with paraproteinemia, HIV infection, chronic active hepatitis, connective tissue disease, inflammatory bowel disease or Hodgkin lymphoma. The demyelinating neuropathy is symmetric, sensorimotor and proximal and distal. Rarely, it may present as a multiple mononeuropathy **(multifocal acquired demyelinating sensory and motor neuropathy)**. Nerves and nerve roots in CIDP may show many onion bulbs owing to recurring episodes of demyelination, Schwann cell proliferation and remyelination (Fig. 31-29B). The pathogenesis of this immune-mediated neuropathy is obscure.

Multifocal motor neuropathy is a rare, slowly progressive, demyelinating mononeuropathy multiplex that may be mistaken clinically for motor neuron disease. There is often an associated increased titer of anti-GM_1 antibodies. This demyelinating neuropathy is immune mediated but is considered distinct from CIDP.

Dorsal Root Ganglionitis Is an Immune-Mediated Sensory Neuronopathy

This inflammatory ganglionopathy typically manifests as a subacute or chronic sensory polyneuropathy with sensory ataxia. The pathogenesis of this immune-mediated sensory neuronopathy is unknown. The disorder may occur sporadically **(idiopathic sensory neuronopathy),** in association with Sjögren syndrome or as a paraneoplastic sensory neuronopathy. The latter is often associated with anti-Hu antibodies (antineuronal autoantibodies) and may accompany a paraneoplastic encephalomyelitis. Dorsal root ganglia show infiltration by lymphocytes and loss of sensory neurons.

Vasculitis Causes Mononeuropathy Multiplex

Necrotizing arteritis may involve the epineurial arteries of nerves as a manifestation of systemic vasculitis (polyarteritis nodosa, Churg-Strauss syndrome, Wegener granulomatosis, microscopic polyangiitis), connective tissue disease (rheumatoid arthritis, systemic lupus erythematosus, Sjögren syndrome) or cryoglobulinemia, HIV infection or cancer. In

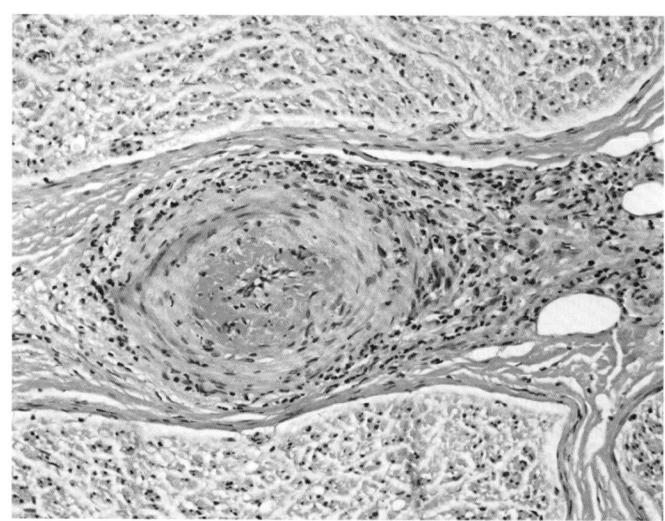

FIGURE 31-30. Vasculitic neuropathy in a patient with polyarteritis nodosa and mononeuropathy multiplex. Photomicrograph of a cross-section of a sural nerve reveals an inflamed epineurial artery with fibrinoid necrosis of its wall. The resultant nerve ischemia causes axonal degeneration.

one third of cases of vasculitic neuropathy, the necrotizing arteritis appears limited to the PNS **(nonsystemic vasculitic neuropathy)**. The ischemic neuropathy is characterized pathologically by axonal degeneration (Fig. 31-30).

Monoclonal Gammopathies May Cause Neuropathy

Monoclonal gammopathies, whether of undetermined significance (MGUS; see Chapter 26) or due to plasma cell myeloma, may cause amyloid neuropathy, cryoglobulinemia-associated vasculitic neuropathy or chronic demyelinating polyneuropathy. Chronic demyelinating polyneuropathy often occurs with an IgM MGUS or Waldenström macroglobulinemia, in which the IgM paraprotein binds myelin-associated glycoprotein (MAG). Anti-MAG antibodies may thus precipitate demyelination. Anti-MAG neuropathy is characterized by extensive segmental demyelination, a variable number of onion bulbs, axonal loss and a distinctive widening of myelin lamellae (Fig. 31-31).

Paraproteinemic neuropathy may rarely present as POEMS syndrome (polyneuropathy, organomegaly, endocrinopathy, monoclonal gammopathy and skin changes). Such patients show elevated serum levels of vascular endothelial growth factor (VEGF) and a plasma cell disorder.

Neuropathy Complicates Light-Chain and Familial Amyloidoses

In addition to its effects on sensory and motor nerves, amyloid infiltration of the PNS often leads to prominent autonomic dysfunction. The disorder may be hereditary but more often complicates light-chain amyloidosis (AL) in primary systemic amyloidosis or multiple myeloma. Familial amyloidosis is usually caused by a point mutation in the transthyretin gene (see Chapter 15), although mutations of the apolipoprotein A1 or gelsolin genes are inculpated in some cases.

Amyloid deposits in endoneurial and epineurial extracellular spaces and vascular walls in peripheral nerves, dorsal

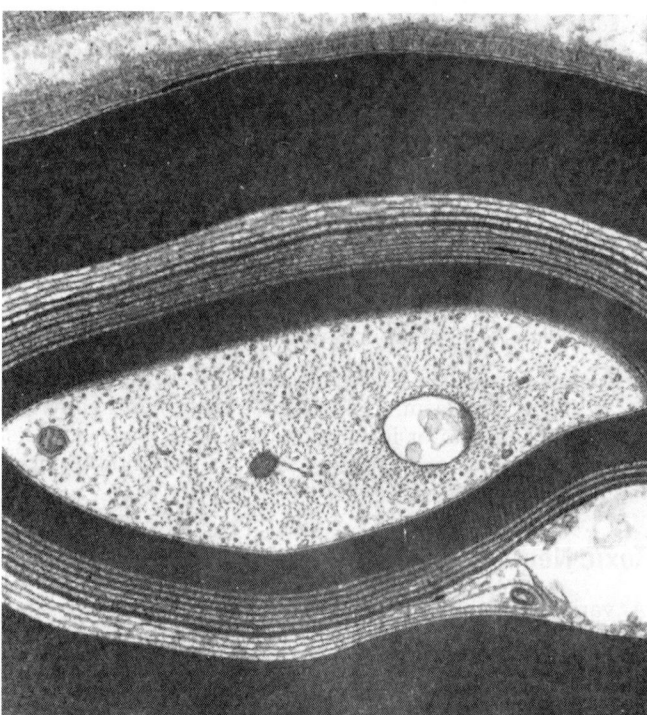

FIGURE 31-31. Anti–myelin-associated glycoprotein (MAG) IgM paraproteinemic demyelinating neuropathy. An electron micrograph shows a myelinated fiber with multiple, abnormally widely spaced, myelin lamellae from a patient with an IgM monoclonal gammopathy of unknown significance and a chronic demyelinating neuropathy. Widely spaced myelin is a characteristic ultrastructural feature of anti-MAG paraproteinemic neuropathy.

root ganglia and autonomic ganglia. Loss of myelinated and unmyelinated fibers ensues. Nerve-fiber damage may reflect direct mechanical injury of nerve fibers and ganglion cells by amyloid deposits, nerve ischemia caused by amyloid infiltration of vasa nervorum or both.

Systemic amyloidosis may also cause **carpal tunnel syndrome,** a chronic entrapment neuropathy of the median nerve at the wrist. Nerve entrapment results from amyloid infiltration of the flexor retinaculum. Carpal tunnel syndrome also occurs in many other settings, including occupational injuries, hypothyroidism, acromegaly, chronic renal failure (dialysis-related β_2-microglobulin amyloidosis), pregnancy and rheumatoid arthritis.

Paraneoplastic Neuropathies Often Precede Discovery of a Cancer

Paraneoplastic nervous system diseases include polyneuropathy, chronic encephalomyelitis, necrotizing myelopathy, cerebellar degeneration and the Eaton-Lambert syndrome. Several different clinicopathologic types of paraneoplastic neuropathy have been defined.

- **Paraneoplastic sensorimotor polyneuropathy:** This distal polyneuropathy is the most common paraneoplastic neuropathy. It is characterized by axonal degeneration and demyelination, mainly the former. The cause of the nerve-fiber degeneration is unknown.
- **Paraneoplastic sensory neuronopathy:** Less commonly, a paraneoplastic subacute sensory neuronopathy may be

caused by dorsal root ganglionitis. Similar chronic inflammatory changes may also occur in the CNS **(paraneoplastic encephalomyelitis)**. Small cell carcinoma of the lung is the usual culprit. The sensory neuronopathy and encephalitis are thought to be immune mediated, largely by anti-Hu antibodies.

- **Inflammatory demyelinating polyradiculoneuropathy:** Immune-mediated acute or chronic inflammatory demyelinating polyradiculoneuropathy may be associated with cancer.
- **Paraneoplastic vasculitic neuropathy:** Vasculitic neuropathy may rarely complicate cancer.

Not all paraneoplastic neuropathies reflect remote effects of a distant neoplasm. Tumors may cause neuropathy by direct compression or infiltration of nerves or nerve roots. Cancer therapies may induce toxic or radiation-induced neuropathies.

Toxic Neuropathy Is Often Iatrogenic

A variety of environmental agents and industrial compounds cause peripheral neuropathy (Table 31-4), but most

TABLE 31-4
AGENTS ASSOCIATED WITH TOXIC NEUROPATHY

Drugs	Environmental and Industrial Agents
Amiodarone	Acrylamide
Bortezomib	Allyl chloride
Colchicine	Arsenic
Dapsone	Buckthorn toxin
Disulfiram	Carbon disulfide
Gold salts	Chlordecone
Isoniazid	Dimethylaminopropionitrile
Metronidazole	Diphtheria toxin
Misonidazole	Ethylene oxide
Nitrofurantoin	n-Hexane (glue sniffing)
Nucleoside analogs (antiretrovirals)	Methyl n-butyl ketone
Paclitaxel (taxanes)	Lead
Phenytoin	Mercury
Platinum compounds	Methyl bromide
Podophyllin	Organophosphates
Pyridoxine (vitamin B_6)	Polychlorinated biphenyls
Suramin	Thallium
Thalidomide	Trichloroethylene
Vincristine	Vacor

TABLE 31-5
INHERITED DISEASES ASSOCIATED WITH NEUROPATHY

Ataxia-telangiectasia
Abetalipoproteinemia
Acute intermittent porphyria, hereditary coproporphyria, and variegate porphyria
Cerebrotendinous xanthomatosis
Fabry disease (α-galactosidase A deficiency)
Familial amyloid polyneuropathy (transthyretin, apolipoprotein A1, and gelsolin amyloidosis)
Friedreich ataxia
Giant axonal neuropathy
Hereditary motor and sensory neuropathies (Charcot-Marie-Tooth disease)
Hereditary motor neuropathies
Hereditary neuropathy with liability to pressure palsies
Hereditary sensory and autonomic neuropathies
Infantile neuroaxonal dystrophy
Leukodystrophies (metachromatic, globoid cell, and adrenoleukodystrophy)
Refsum disease (phytanic acid storage disease)
Tangier disease

cases of toxic neuropathy result from drugs. Almost all toxic neuropathies are characterized by axonal degeneration, usually of the dying-back type. Notable exceptions are platinum compounds and pyridoxine, which produce a sensory neuronopathy, and buckthorn toxin and diphtheria toxin, which produce a demyelinating neuropathy. People with hereditary neuropathy (see below) may be especially vulnerable to drug-induced peripheral neuropathy.

The Most Common Chronic Neuropathies in Children Are Hereditary

Many inherited diseases may manifest as peripheral neuropathies (Tables 31-5 and 31-6), with the neuropathy being the sole manifestation of a hereditary disease or a part of a multisystem disease.

Charcot-Marie-Tooth Disease

 MOLECULAR PATHOGENESIS: Charcot-Marie-Tooth disease (CMT) is a genetically and pathologically heterogeneous group of slowly progressive distal sensorimotor polyneuropathies that manifest in childhood or early adult life. It is the most common inherited neuropathy and among the most common inherited neurologic disorders, with a prevalence of 1 in 2500. CMT may be broadly divided into **demyelinating** and **axonal** types. **CMT1,** the most common form, is a chronic demyelinating

TABLE 31-6

CHARCOT-MARIE-TOOTH DISEASE (CMT) AND RELATED HEREDITARY MOTOR AND SENSORY NEUROPATHIES

Disease	Inheritance	Gene	Pathology
CMT1	Autosomal dominant	Peripheral myelin protein 22 (*PMP22*), myelin protein zero (*MPZ*) and others	Demyelinating neuropathy with onion bulbs; axonal loss also present
CMT2	Autosomal dominant	Mitofusin 2 and others	Axonal neuropathy
CMTX	X linked	Gap junction protein β1 (connexin 32)	Axonal loss, demyelination, and regenerating axons
Dejerine-Sottas syndrome (congenital hypomyelinating neuropathy)	Autosomal dominant or recessive	*PMP22, MPZ*, early growth response 2 (*EGR2*) and others	Demyelinating neuropathy with onion bulbs; axonal loss also present
Hereditary neuropathy with liability to pressure palsies (HNPP)	Autosomal dominant	*PMP22*	Demyelinating neuropathy with tomacula; axonal loss also present

polyneuropathy with onion bulbs and axonal loss. The less common **CMT2** variety shows distal axonal degeneration. CMT1 and CMT2 are autosomal dominant diseases. X-linked **(CMTX)** and autosomal recessive **(CMT4)** types are also described. Mutations in at least 30 different genes may cause a CMT phenotype. Classification is complex because mutations in diverse genes may produce the same phenotype, and different mutations in the same gene may lead to different phenotypes (Table 31-6). CMT1, the most common form, usually reflects heterozygous duplication of peripheral myelin protein 22 gene on chromosome 17. CMT2 is often caused by a mutation of the gene encoding a mitochondrial fusion protein, mitofusin 2. In CMTX, the gap junction protein β1 (connexin 32) gene on the X chromosome is altered.

Dejerine-Sottas syndrome (DSS, CMT3) resembles CMT1 but is much more severe, with onset in early infancy. Peripheral nerves show a severe demyelinating neuropathy with onion bulbs and axonal loss. Several genes are associated with this phenotype (Table 31-6).

Hereditary neuropathy with liability to pressure palsies (HNPP) typically manifests as recurrent mononeuropathies. Nerves show demyelination, distinctive sausage-shaped myelin sheath thickenings (tomacula) and axonal loss (tomaculous neuropathy). HNPP is associated with a heterozygous deletion of peripheral myelin protein 22 gene on chromosome 17.

Peripheral Neuropathies Commonly Complicate HIV-1 Infection

HIV-1 peripheral neuropathies may manifest clinically as a distal symmetric polyneuropathy, autonomic neuropathy, lumbosacral polyradiculopathy, mononeuropathy or mononeuropathy multiplex.

- **Distal symmetric polyneuropathy** is the most common type of neuropathy in HIV-positive patients. It usually occurs during the later stages of AIDS and is characterized by distal axonal degeneration. The pathogenesis of the axonal degeneration is obscure, and there is no effective therapy.
- **Inflammatory demyelinating polyradiculoneuropathy** in HIV-infected people may be acute (AIDP) or chronic (CIDP) and is immunologically mediated. It typically

occurs after HIV infection, before the onset of AIDS. The neuropathy often responds to plasmapheresis, intravenous γ-globulin or corticosteroids.

- **Cytomegalovirus infection** of the PNS is responsible for some of the mononeuropathies and lumbosacral polyradiculopathies associated with AIDS.
- **Vasculitic neuropathy** may be a mononeuropathy and mononeuropathy multiplex in some patients with AIDS.
- **Toxic neuropathies** occur with several drugs that are used to treat AIDS (Table 31-4). Such antiretroviral-induced axonal neuropathies resemble HIV-associated distal symmetric polyneuropathy clinically.
- **Diffuse infiltrative lymphocytosis syndrome** may be complicated by an acute or subacute axonal polyneuropathy. Peripheral nerve shows perivascular CD8+ lymphocytic infiltrates.

Chronic Idiopathic Axonal Polyneuropathy Occurs in Older Patients

No cause can be identified for peripheral neuropathy, even with careful investigation, in a quarter of patients, usually over age 50. Many of these patients have a slowly progressive, distal, sensory or sensorimotor, axonal polyneuropathy called chronic idiopathic axonal polyneuropathy (CIAP).

NERVE TRAUMA

Traumatic Neuromas Are Masses of Regenerating Axons and Scar Tissue

Traumatic neuromas form at the proximal stump of a nerve that has been disrupted physically. Within a week after transection of a peripheral nerve, regenerating axonal sprouts arise from the distal ends of the intact axons in the proximal nerve stump. If the severed ends of the proximal and distal nerve stumps are closely approximated, regenerating axonal sprouts may find and reinnervate the distal stump. Regenerating axons advance in the distal stump at a rate of about 1 mm/day. However, if the cut nerve ends are not closely apposed, or if there is an impediment (e.g., scar tissue) between the two stumps, regenerating sprouts may not reinnervate the distal stump. In that case, the regenerating axons grow haphazardly into the scar tissue at the end of the proximal stump to form a painful swelling: a **traumatic** or **amputation neuroma**.

Morton Neuroma Is a Painful Lesion in the Foot

Morton neuroma (plantar interdigital neuroma) is a sausage-shaped swelling of the plantar interdigital nerve between the second and third or third and fourth metatarsal bones. It is probably caused by repeated nerve compression, causing endoneurial, perineurial and epineurial fibrosis rather than a mass of regenerating axons. It thus is not a true neuroma. The fibrotic nerve also shows nerve fiber loss and areas of myxoid degeneration. Morton neuroma is particularly common in women who wear high heels.

TUMORS

Primary PNS tumors are of neuronal or nerve sheath origin. The former (e.g., neuroblastoma and ganglioneuroma) usually arise from the adrenal medulla or sympathetic ganglia. The common nerve sheath tumors are schwannoma and neurofibroma.

Schwannomas Are Benign Neoplasms of Schwann Cells

They are typically slowly growing, encapsulated tumors that originate in cranial nerves, spinal roots or peripheral nerves (Fig. 31-32A). Schwannomas usually occur in adults and rarely become malignant.

VESTIBULAR SCHWANNOMA (ACOUSTIC SCHWANNOMA): Intracranial schwannomas account for 8% of all primary intracranial tumors. Most arise from the vestibular branch of the eighth cranial nerve within the internal auditory canal or at the meatus. They cause unilateral, sensorineural hearing loss; tinnitus; and vestibular dysfunction. The slowly growing tumor enlarges the meatus, extends medially into the subarachnoid space of the cerebellopontine angle **(cerebellopontine angle tumor)** and compresses the fifth and seventh cranial nerves, brainstem and cerebellum. The posterior fossa mass may also lead to increased intracranial pressure, hydrocephalus and tonsillar herniation. Most vestibular schwannomas are unilateral and are not associated with neurofibromatosis (see Chapter 6). Bilateral vestibular schwannomas are a defining feature of NF2. Biallelic inactivation of the *NF2* gene, a tumor suppressor gene on chromosome 22, may also cause sporadic vestibular schwannomas.

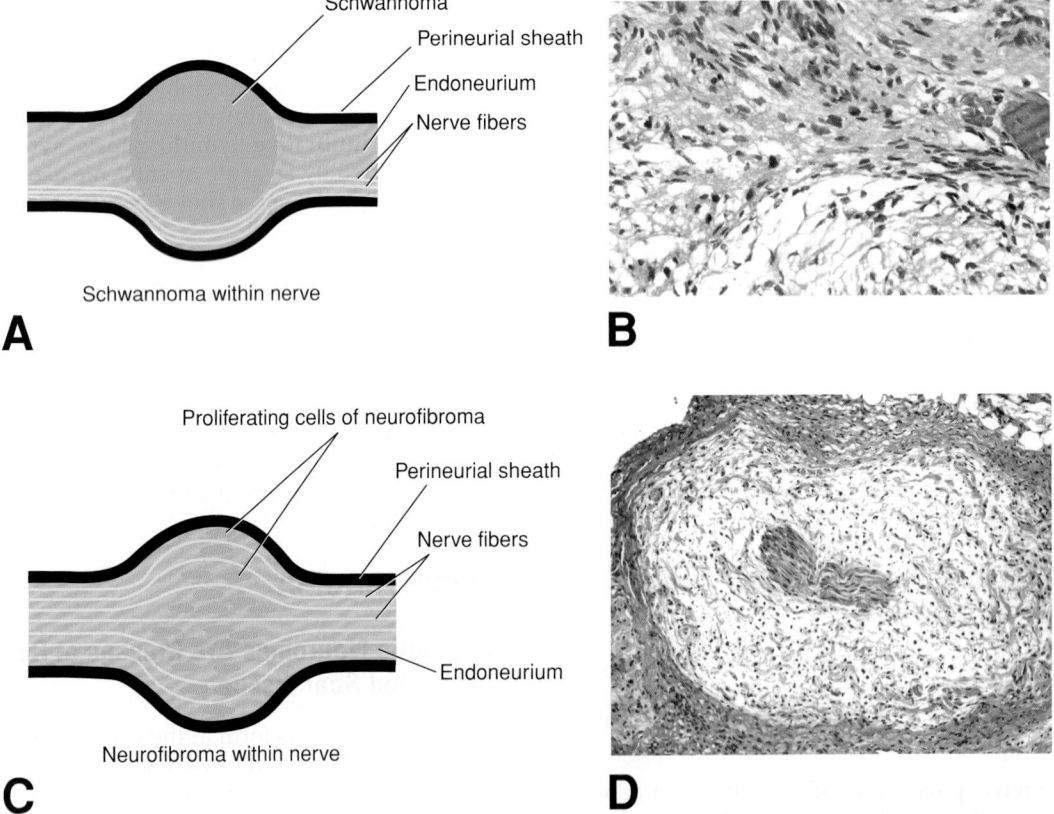

FIGURE 31-32. Growth patterns of schwannoma and neurofibroma within peripheral nerve. A. The cellular proliferation of the schwannoma is well circumscribed and pushes surviving nerve fibers to the periphery of the tumor. **B.** A photomicrograph of a schwannoma shows the characteristically abrupt transition between the compact Antoni type A histologic pattern (*top*) and the spongy Antoni type B histologic pattern (*bottom*). **C.** The cellular proliferation of the neurofibroma is interspersed among the surviving nerve fibers. **D.** Photomicrograph of neurofibroma shows that the proliferating spindle-shaped Schwann cells form small strands that course haphazardly through a myxoid matrix. A small cluster of surviving nerve fibers is in the center of the neurofibroma.

SPINAL AND PERIPHERAL SCHWANNOMAS: Spinal schwannomas are intradural, extramedullary tumors that arise most often from the dorsal (sensory) spinal roots. They produce radicular (root) pain and spinal cord compression. More peripherally located schwannomas usually arise on nerves of the head, neck and extremities.

 PATHOLOGY: Schwannomas tend to be oval and well demarcated and vary from a few millimeters to several centimeters. The nerve of origin, if large enough, may be identifiable. The cut surface is firm and tan to gray, often with focal hemorrhage, necrosis, xanthomatous change and cystic degeneration. The proliferating Schwann cells form two distinctive histologic patterns (Fig. 31-32B).

- **Antoni A pattern** is characterized by interwoven fascicles of spindle cells with elongated nuclei, eosinophilic cytoplasm and indistinct cytoplasmic borders. Nuclei may palisade (line up in a picket fence–like pattern) in areas to form structures known as **Verocay bodies**.
- **Antoni B pattern** has spindle or oval cells with indistinct cytoplasm in a loose, vacuolated matrix.

Degenerative changes in schwannomas are common and include collections of foam cells, recent or old hemorrhage, focal fibrosis and hyalinized blood vessels. Scattered atypical nuclei are frequently encountered in schwannomas, but mitotic figures are uncommon.

Neurofibromas May Be Sporadic or Part of Neurofibromatosis Type 1

Neurofibromas are benign, slowly growing tumors of peripheral nerve, composed of Schwann cells, perineurial-like cells and fibroblasts. *The Schwann cells are the neoplastic cells in these tumors.* Neurofibromas should be distinguished from schwannomas because the former are associated with NF1 and may become malignant peripheral nerve sheath tumors.

Neurofibromas may be solitary or multiple and may arise on any nerve. They occur in children and adults. They mostly involve skin, subcutis, major nerve plexuses, large deep nerve trunks, retroperitoneum and gastrointestinal tract. Most **solitary cutaneous neurofibromas** are not part of NF1 and do not degenerate into sarcomas. The presence of multiple neurofibromas or one large plexiform neurofibroma strongly suggests NF1 and should prompt a search for other stigmata of the disease.

 PATHOLOGY: Neurofibromas arising in large nerves are poorly circumscribed and fusiform (spindle shaped). A diffuse, intrafascicular growth of tumor within multiple nerve fascicles may so enlarge the fascicles that the nerve looks like a multistranded rope **(plexiform neurofibroma)**. Neurofibromas may involve long stretches of a nerve, making complete surgical excision impossible. When they arise from small nerves, the nerve of origin may not be apparent. Cutaneous neurofibromas originate from dermal nerves and are seen as soft nodular or pedunculated skin tumors.

These tumors are soft and light gray. Greatly enlarged, individual nerve fascicles of the plexiform neurofibroma may be prominent. Tumors arising in large nerves are characterized by endoneurial proliferation of spindle cells with

elongated nuclei, eosinophilic cytoplasm and indistinct cell borders (Fig. 31-32D). The proliferating spindle cells include Schwann cells, fibroblasts and perineurial-like cells. Mast cells are also increased. An extracellular myxoid matrix, wavy bands of collagen and residual nerve fibers are interspersed among the spindle cells. The nerve fibers coursing through a neurofibroma contrasts with the pattern in schwannomas, in which nerve fibers are pushed peripherally into the tumor capsule (compare Fig. 31-32A, C). The neurofibromatous proliferation often extends beyond the nerve fascicle into adjacent tissue.

Some 5% of NF1-associated plexiform neurofibromas become malignant peripheral nerve sheath tumors. Increased cellularity, nuclear atypia and mitotic figures herald malignant transformation.

Malignant Peripheral Nerve Sheath Tumor

Malignant peripheral nerve sheath tumor (MPNST) is a poorly differentiated, spindle cell sarcoma of peripheral nerve of uncertain histogenesis. It may arise de novo or from malignant transformation of a neurofibroma. MPNST is most common in adults and typically arises in larger nerves of the trunk or proximal limbs. About half occur in patients with neurofibromatosis. There is an increased incidence of MPNST at sites of previous irradiation.

MPNSTs are unencapsulated, fusiform enlargements of a nerve. The tumors resemble fibrosarcomas, with closely packed spindle cells, nuclear atypia, mitotic figures and, often, foci of necrosis. MPNSTs are prone to local recurrence and blood-borne metastasis.

PARANEOPLASTIC SYNDROMES INVOLVING MUSCLE AND PERIPHERAL NERVES

Neurologic disorders are common in cancer patients, usually resulting from metastases or from endocrine or electrolyte disturbances. Vascular, hemorrhagic and infectious conditions affecting the nervous system are also common. However, additional neurologic complications of malignancies are known and may appear before the underlying tumor is detected. Many of these are mediated by autoimmune mechanisms.

Sensory Neuropathy and Encephalomyeloneuritis

Patients afflicted with this paraneoplastic syndrome complain of numbness and paresthesias and, conversely, variably acute aching and pain. These may be focal, but often affect all extremities over time, and are often complicated by disorders of gait, confusion and weakness. This syndrome may occur in patients with small cell lung cancer (SCLC; see Chapter 12) and is caused by circulating antibodies against Hu, an RNA-binding protein. High titers of anti-Hu antibodies are almost exclusively detected in people with SCLC. Lymphocytic infiltration of dorsal root ganglia is seen. Symptoms tend to be treatable when the primary tumor is treated.

Paraneoplastic Autonomic Neuropathies

These are rare, but affect a quarter of patients with anti-Hu antibodies, and may be the initial presentation of the tumor. Systems affected, sometimes severely, include vascular tone, bowel and bladder. Antibodies against the nicotinic acetylcholine receptor are sometimes responsible.

Opsoclonus-Myoclonus

Nonvoluntary spasms of ocular and other muscles characterize this syndrome. Among children, about half of cases of this disorder are associated with neuroblastoma. About 10% of adults with opsoclonus-myoclonus will have a malignancy, most often Hodgkin lymphoma.

Diseases of Upper and Lower Motor Neurons

These syndromes may be paraneoplastic in origin. Diverse tumor associations have been reported, the most frequent being lymphoproliferative diseases and anti-Hu antibodies. Weakness is the most common presenting symptom. As many as 10% of patients presenting with amyotrophic lateral sclerosis have internal malignancies.

Subacute Motor Neuropathy

This is a disorder of the spinal cord, characterized by slowly developing lower motor neuron weakness without sensory changes. It is so strongly associated with cancer that an intensive search for an occult neoplasm, often a lymphoma, should be made in patients who present with these symptoms.

Peripheral Neuropathies

An array of peripheral neuropathies may be paraneoplastic in origin. Sensorimotor neuropathy, most likely attendant to lung cancer, is not associated with detectable antibodies. Some types of lymphoproliferative disorders associated with paraproteins, especially the sclerosing variant of plasma cell myeloma, may develop peripheral neuropathies.

Neuromuscular Junction Disorders

The most common association is with thymomas. About 15% of patients with myasthenia gravis have thymomas, and about half of patients with thymomas suffer from myasthenia gravis. Autoantibodies against the nicotinic acetylcholine receptor are the principal cause of this syndrome.

Eaton-Lambert Syndrome

This syndrome is a paraneoplastic disorder that manifests as muscle weakness, wasting and fatigability of proximal limbs and trunk. Also called **myasthenic–myopathic syndrome,** it is usually associated with small cell lung carcinoma, but may also occur with other malignancies, and rarely in the absence of underlying cancer. Neurophysiologic evidence suggests a defect in Ach release at nerve terminals. IgG from patients can transfer the disease to mice. The pathogenic IgG autoantibodies target voltage-sensitive calcium channels expressed in motor nerve terminals and in the cells of the lung cancer. These calcium channels are necessary for Ach release and are greatly reduced in presynaptic membranes in these patients, thus reducing neuromuscular transmission. Lambert-Eaton syndrome responds to corticosteroid treatment.

Dermatomyositis

Dermatomyositis (see above) in middle-aged men is associated with increased risk of epithelial cancer, mostly lung carcinoma. However, polymyositis and inclusion body myositis have a reduced risk of an associated malignancy.

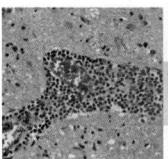
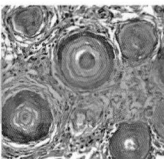
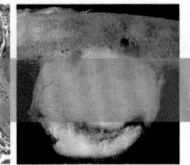
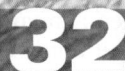

32

The Central Nervous System

Gregory N. Fuller ■ J. Clay Goodman

The Central Nervous System

The nervous system is the most complex organ system in the body. It is responsible for sensory processing and synthesis and motor control, and is the organ of thought, emotion and personality—in short, the basis of humanity itself. The vast majority of its operations occur without conscious supervision. Disorders of the central nervous system (CNS) strike at the core of our being as sentient organisms, and so inspire fear and dread. Diseases of the nervous system are common throughout the human life span and contribute substantially

to mortality and morbidity: stroke, Alzheimer disease, mental retardation, traumatic brain and spinal cord injury, meningitis and tumors.

TOPOGRAPHY: The functions of the nervous system have fine topographic localization, so that focal disease processes can produce myriad signs and symptoms that permit a skilled clinician to locate the affected site precisely. In addition, most neurons are organized in functional arrays, which, if damaged, cause some of the most vexing neurodegenerative and neuropsychiatric disorders. Selective vulnerability of different nervous system cells and CNS regions to specific disease processes is one of the most profound unresolved enigmas of neurologic illnesses. For example, Huntington disease primarily causes degeneration of neurons in the caudate nuclei; Parkinson disease targets the nigrostriatal system; amyotrophic lateral sclerosis (ALS) selectively singles out upper and lower motor neurons of the cerebrum, brainstem and spinal cord. Some infectious diseases prefer certain targets: poliomyelitis involves anterior horn cells of the spinal cord and motor nuclei of the brainstem, while herpes simplex virus preferentially affects the temporal lobes. Vascular and demyelinating diseases also have regional preferences within the CNS, as do some brain tumors. The basis of topographic vulnerability and protection for most such diseases is obscure.

AGE: The nervous system is affected by neurologic disorders throughout the life span, but individual diseases commonly affect selected age groups. Thus, inborn errors of metabolism such as Tay-Sachs disease, the leukodystrophies and several posterior fossa tumors mainly occur in childhood. Youthful reckless exuberance leads to a spike in traumatic brain and spinal cord injury in teens and young adults that subsides with maturity, only to return with the infirmities of age. Multiple sclerosis shows a strong preference for young adults, rarely beginning before puberty or after age 40. Neuropsychiatric disorders such as schizophrenia often appear in late adolescence and young adulthood when the brain undergoes striking neurodevelopmental changes. Huntington disease typically strikes youthful and middle-aged adults, while Parkinson disease and stroke occur late in life. Alzheimer disease tends to affect aged brains.

CELLS OF THE NERVOUS SYSTEM

The diversity and complexity of the CNS is reflected at all levels in its organization, from the morphologic and functional subspecialization of the many unique cellular constituents to the regional localization of sensory, motor and cognitive functions.

GRAY MATTER AND THE NEUROPIL: Gray matter includes all regions of the CNS rich in neurons: cerebral and cerebellar cortices, basal ganglia and central gray matter of the spinal cord. Gray matter consists of cell bodies (perikarya) of neurons and supporting glial cell nuclei, plus the intervening delicate interwoven meshwork of neuronal and glial cell processes, the **neuropil** (Fig. 32-1). Circumscribed collections of neuronal cell bodies that share a common functional task are referred to as "nuclei."

WHITE MATTER: White matter consists of compact bundles **(tracts, fascicles)** of myelinated axons with many oligodendrocytes and interspersed astrocytes (Fig. 32-2).

NEURONS: The morphology of neuronal subtypes in the gray matter varies due to functional subspecialization, ranging from large motor and primary sensory neurons to tiny "granular cell" neurons (Fig. 32-3A). For example, pigmented neurons, which occur only in specific brainstem nuclei, are distinguished by cytoplasmic brown neuromelanin pigment, a byproduct of catecholaminergic neurotransmitter synthesis (Fig. 32-3B). These clusters of pigmented catecholaminergic neurons are so dense as to be visible to the naked eye in the midbrain (substantia nigra) and pons (locus ceruleus).

ASTROCYTES: Astrocytes outnumber neurons at least 10:1 and play a critical supportive role in regulating the CNS microenvironment. They are also one of two primary CNS

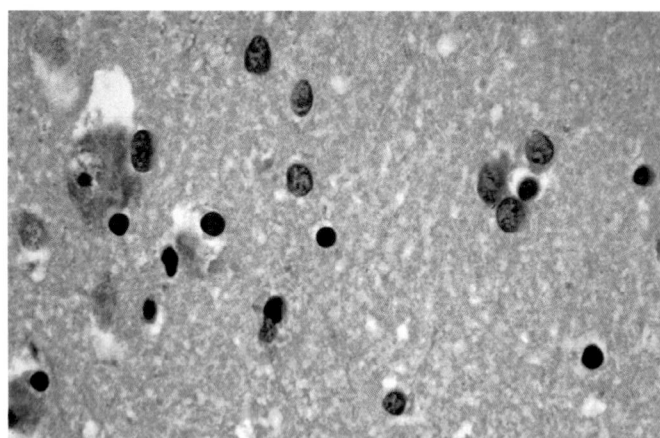

FIGURE 32-1. Gray matter and the neuropil. Gray matter by definition contains neuronal cell bodies. In addition, the nuclei of supporting glial cells, astrocytes and satellite oligodendroglia, are also present. The remaining finely fibrillar background meshwork is called the neuropil and consists of intimately intermingled axons, dendrites and astrocytic cytoplasmic processes.

cell types that respond to many CNS insults (the other being microglia). Astrocytes responding to acute injury upregulate synthesis of glial fibrillary acidic protein (GFAP) and assemble it into intracytoplasmic intermediate filaments, resulting in prominent cell bodies and cytoplasmic processes (Fig. 32-4A). With advancing age, astrocyte peripheral processes may accumulate spherical inclusion bodies, corpora amylacea. These are glucose polymers that are especially numerous in subpial, subependymal and perivascular sites and in olfactory tracts (Fig. 32-4B). Cytoplasmic strap-like densities, Rosenthal fibers (Fig. 32-4C), appear in longstanding astrogliosis as densely compacted glial intermediate filaments with entrapped cytosol proteins.

OLIGODENDROGLIA: Oligodendroglia produce and maintain CNS axon myelin sheaths, and so are CNS counterparts of Schwann cells in the peripheral nervous system.

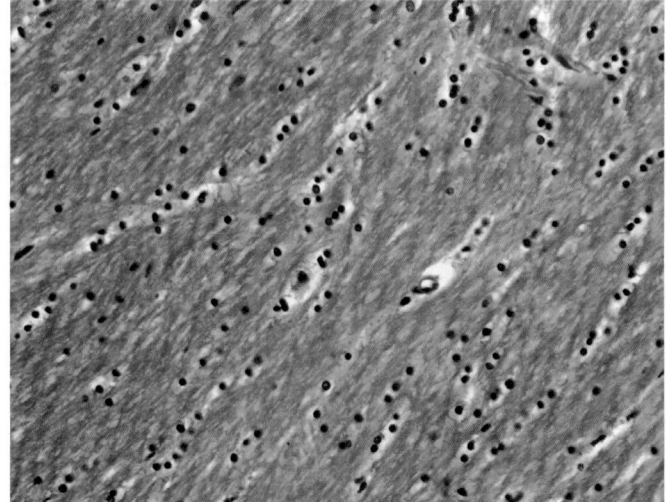

FIGURE 32-2. White matter. In contrast to gray matter, white matter is composed almost entirely of myelinated axons and the cells that produce and maintain their myelin sheaths, the oligodendroglia, whose small round nuclei are seen in between the fiber bundles.

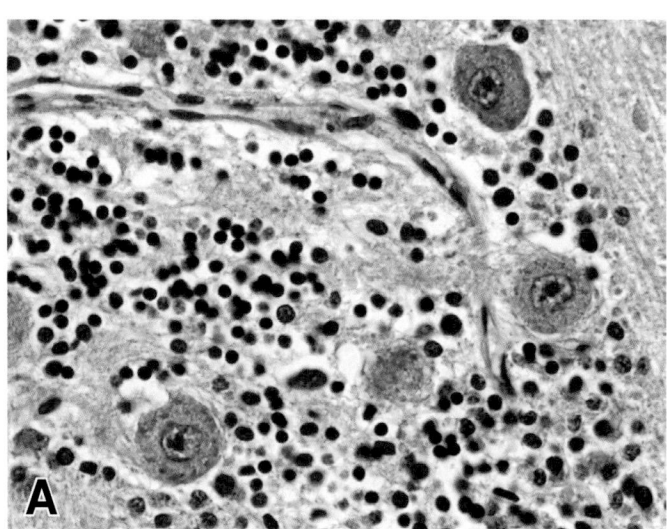 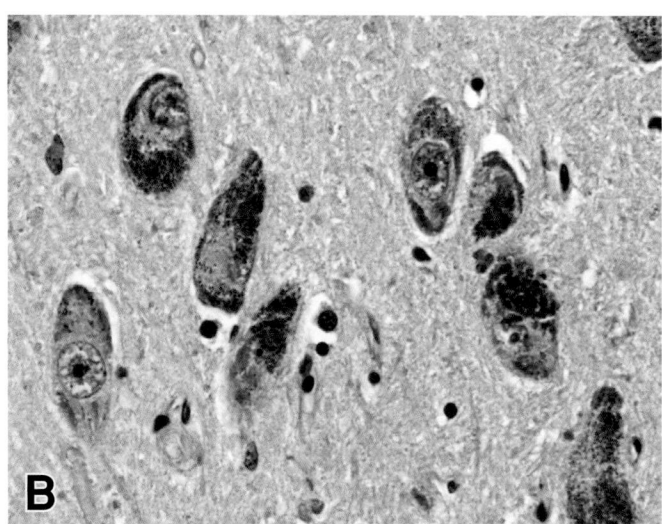

FIGURE 32-3. Neurons. A. The different neuronal populations of the central nervous system (CNS) subserve different functions, and this diversity is reflected in their morphology. Illustrative of the extremes are the large cell bodies of Purkinje cell neurons juxtaposed next to the diminutive granular cell neurons of the cerebellar cortex; the entire granular neuron cell body is not much bigger than the nucleolus of a Purkinje cell neuron! **B.** The pigmented catecholaminergic neurons with their prominent neuromelanin content serve as an additional, striking example of diversity in form and function among CNS neuronal populations.

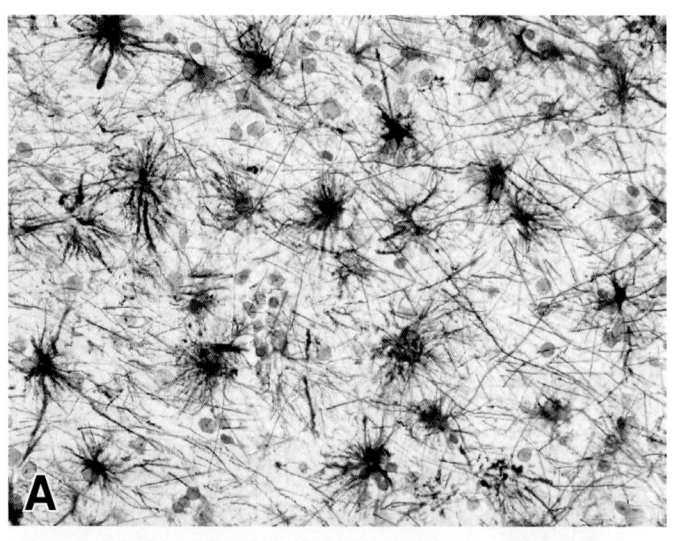 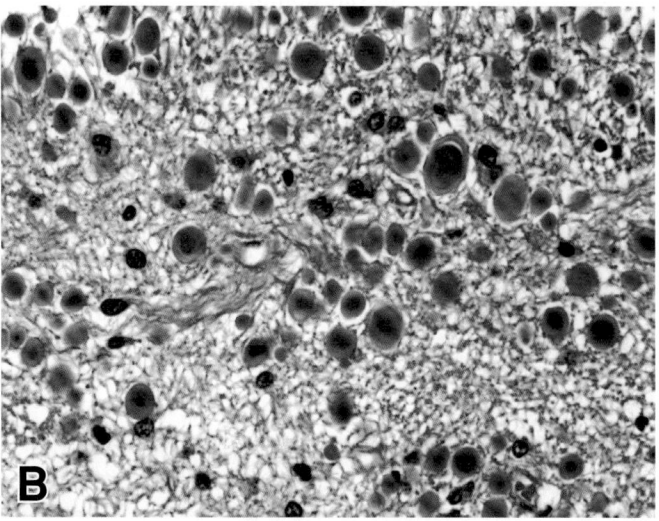

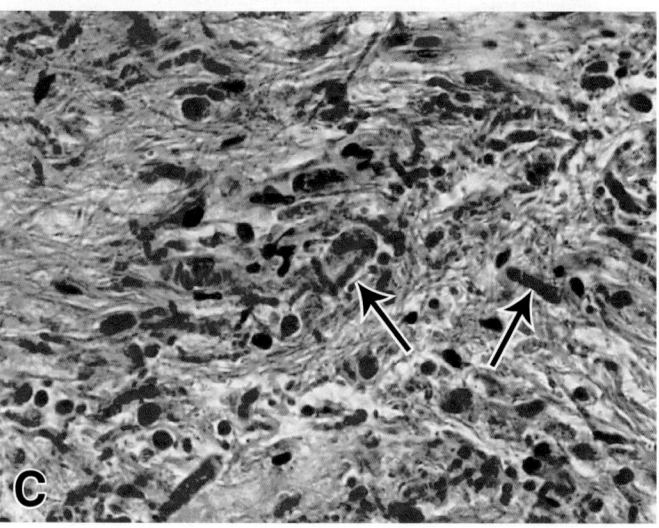

FIGURE 32-4. Astrocytes. A. Astrocytes have been called "the fibroblast of the central nervous system," referring to their role as the ubiquitous supporting cell of the brain and spinal cord that reacts to any pathologic insult. As seen in this immunostain directed against glial fibrillary acidic protein, astrocytes occupy adjacent domains and send cytoplasmic process radiating out in all directions to fill their individual fiefdoms. **B.** With advancing age, astrocytes are prone to develop glucose polymer inclusion bodies, called **corpora amylacea,** in the distal distribution of their cell processes, particularly around blood vessels and subjacent to the pia and ependyma. **C. Rosenthal fibers** are another astrocytic inclusion body formed as a response to long-standing astrogliosis; they are composed of densely compacted glial intermediate filaments together with entrapped cytosolic proteins (*arrows*).

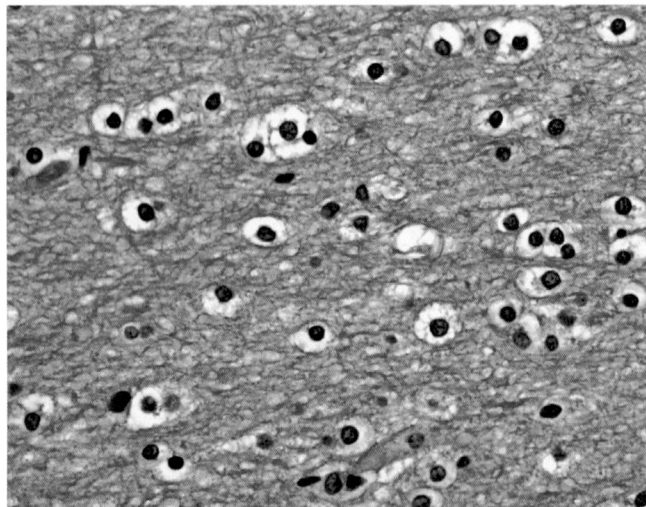

FIGURE 32-5. Oligodendroglia. Oligodendroglia are the myelin-forming glia of the central nervous system (CNS; including the optic "nerves," which are actually CNS tracts). On routine histologic imaging, oligodendroglia are easily recognized by their monotonous small dark round nuclei surrounded by a halo of vacuolated cytoplasm ("fried egg" appearance). This characteristic appearance is recapitulated in neoplastic oligodendrogliomas.

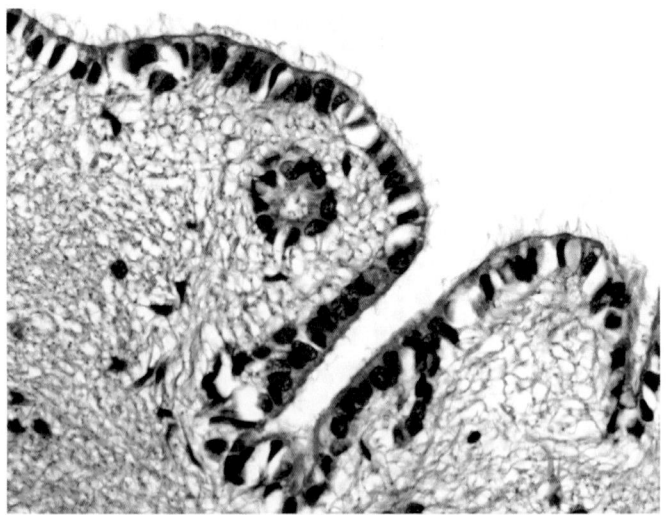

FIGURE 32-7. Ependyma. Ependymal cells form a ciliated cuboidal-to-columnar epithelium that lines the cerebral ventricles and spinal cord central canal. Ependymal cell clusters and true rosettes, as seen here, commonly are scattered beneath the ependymal lining.

Oligodendroglia cell bodies are dominated by uniform round nuclei that, in formalin-fixed paraffin-embedded tissue sections, are characteristically surrounded by only a small clear rim of vacuolated cytoplasm ("perinuclear halo") (Fig. 32-5).

MICROGLIA: Microglia are bone marrow–derived mononuclear phagocytes of the CNS. In health, they are inconspicuously distributed throughout the brain and spinal cord. But they respond quickly to CNS insults such as ischemia, trauma or viral infection by developing thin, elongated nuclei, migrating through the CNS and localizing to the site of injury (Fig. 32-6A,B).

EPENDYMA: The ependymal lining of the ventricular system forms a barrier between cerebrospinal fluid (CSF) and brain parenchyma and regulates fluid transfer between these two compartments. The normal ependyma is lined by ciliated cuboidal-to-columnar simple epithelium (Fig. 32-7).

SPECIALIZED REGIONS OF THE CENTRAL NERVOUS SYSTEM

CHOROID PLEXUS: The choroid plexus produces CSF. It is in the cerebral ventricles, including the temporal horns bilaterally, interventricular foramen of Monro, the roof of the third ventricle and the roof and lateral recesses of the fourth ventricle. The choroid plexus is composed of cuboidal epithelium (derived from embryologic ependyma) that covers a fibrovascular core (Fig. 32-8A). The highly vascular core

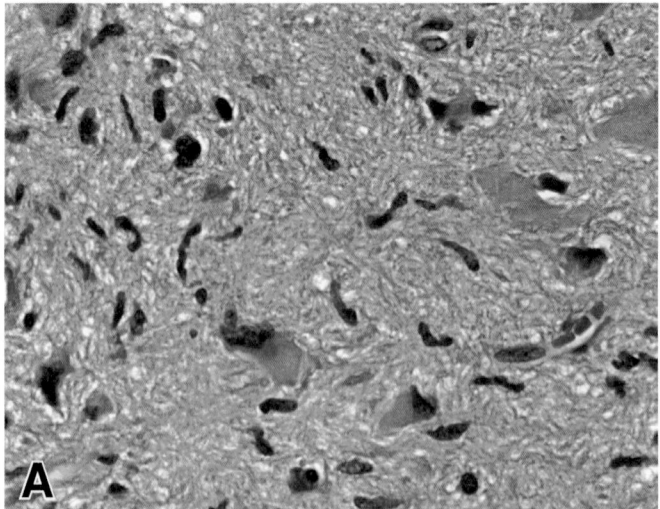

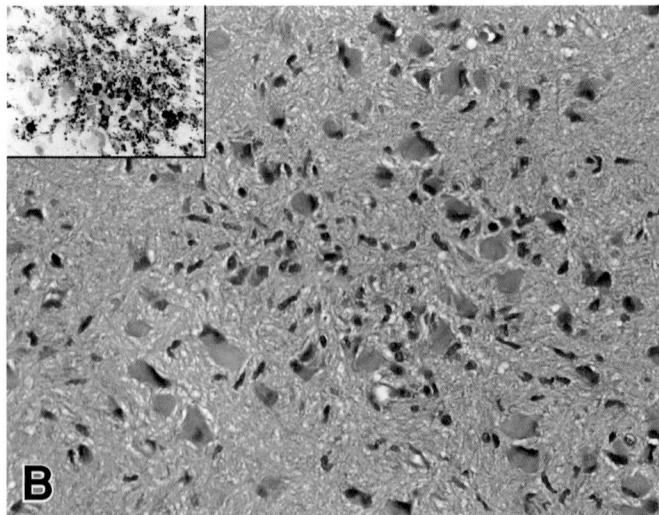

FIGURE 32-6. Microglia. A. Microglia are the resident representatives of the monocyte–macrophage system in the brain and spinal cord. While inconspicuous in normal healthy brain ("resting microglial"), they become very prominent when responding to central nervous system (CNS) injury and are easily recognized by their elongated nuclei ("rod cells"), which reflect their infiltrative phenotype. **B.** Actively migrating through CNS parenchyma, they commonly cluster around foci of disease; such collections are known as "microglial nodules." Microglia demonstrate strong immunohistochemical reactivity for the macrophage marker CD68 (*inset*).

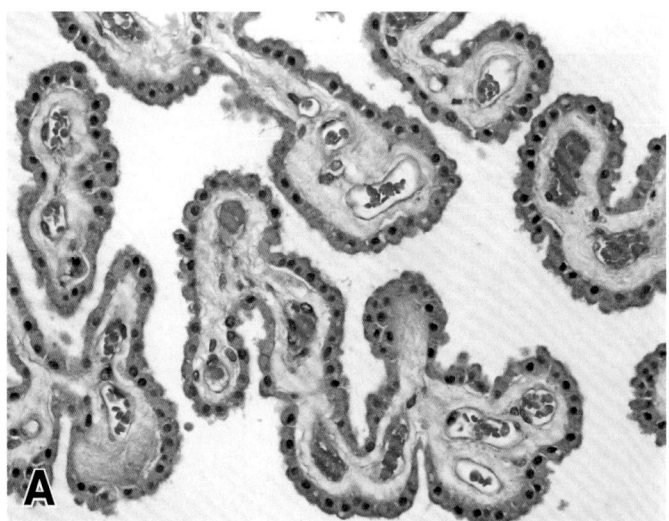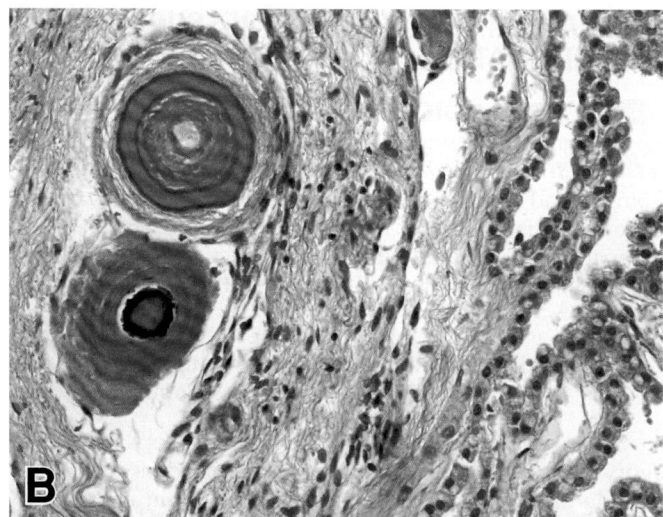

FIGURE 32-8. Choroid plexus. A. Choroid plexus is the central nervous system (CNS) organ responsible for producing cerebrospinal fluid and consists of innumerable papillae with a highly vascular core covered by cuboidal epithelium that is derived embryologically from the ependyma. **B.** The core also contains arachnoid (meningothelial) cell nests (by virtue of its embryologic derivation from the pia-arachnoid) that tend to mineralize with age, forming psammoma bodies (*B*).

is critical to CSF formation. It develops from leptomeninges (pia and arachnoid) and contains scattered nests of arachnoid (meningothelial) cells (Fig. 32-8B), hence the occasional "intraventricular" meningioma that is actually a choroid plexus meningioma.

MENINGES: Three layers of meninges cover and protect the CNS. The **dura** is the tough outer fibrous membrane. It is primarily collagen. Its outer surface is the inner periosteum of the cranial bones and its inner surface attaches weakly to the subjacent arachnoid via cell junctions. The two dural layers separate in several sites to form dural venous sinuses, the largest of which is the superior sagittal sinus. The underlying arachnoid is bound to the overlying dura by a loosely cohesive layer of cells, the **dural border cell (DBC) layer**.

This layer is the path of least resistance to pathogenic fluids, which easily dissect the weak intercellular junctions to form so-called subdural hematomas, hygromas and empyemas. The meningeal layer just beneath the DBC layer, the **arachnoid barrier cell (ABC) layer,** in contrast, forms a cohesive outer limiting membrane of the subarachnoid space via abundant intercellular junctions (desmosomes) that weld together elongated, interlacing arachnoid (meningothelial) cell processes. Whorls of arachnoid cells are common in thicker areas of the arachnoid (Fig. 32-9); this feature is often recapitulated in arachnoid tumors (meningiomas).

PINEAL GLAND: The pineal gland (see Chapter 27) contains pineal parenchymal cells (pineocytes), plus supporting glial cells (pineal astrocytes), arranged in cell clusters separated by collagenous septa (Fig. 32-10). Inconspicuous autonomic peripheral nerve fibers coming from cell bodies in the superior cervical ganglia provide sympathetic nervous system (noradrenergic) innervation.

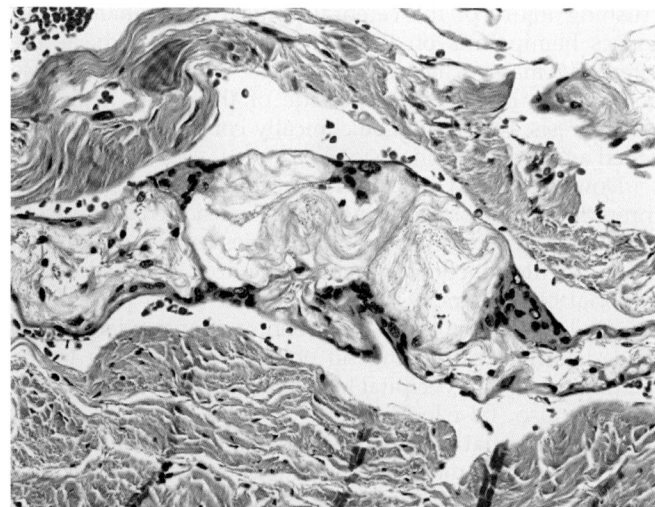

FIGURE 32-9. Arachnoid villi. The arachnoid membrane forms the outer boundary of the subarachnoid space and also protrudes into the dural venous sinuses, as seen here, to form arachnoid villi whose function is to return cerebrospinal fluid (CSF) into the venous circulatory system. The villi are covered by a layer of meningothelial cells, called arachnoid cap cells, that varies in thickness from a single cell to multilayered whorls.

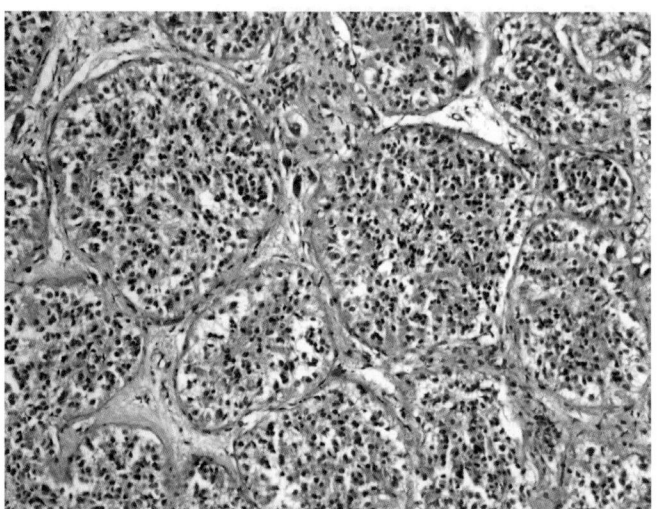

FIGURE 32-10. Pineal gland. The pineal is composed of pineal parenchymal cells (pineocytes) organized into lobules by fibrovascular septa.

INCREASED INTRACRANIAL PRESSURE AND HERNIATION

 **ETIOLOGIC FACTORS:** Pathophysiologically, the most important aspect of the brain is that it *lives in a closed box*! The brain, CSF and blood going to and from the brain occupy the intracranial space. In the adult, this is a rigidly fixed cavity. Any disease that takes up space does so at the expense of brain, CSF or blood. This is a verbal expression of the Monro-Kellie hypothesis that states:

$$\text{Intracranial volume} = \text{Volume}_{CNS} + \text{Volume}_{CSF} + \text{Volume}_{blood} + \text{Volume}_{lesion}$$

Space-occupying lesions may occur with every major category of disease except for degenerative disorders. Examples include brain tumors, abscesses, swollen brain contusions following trauma and stroke with brain swelling.

The immediate result of trying to fit more volume into the fixed space of the intracranial vault is increased intracranial pressure (ICP). The normal mean ICP is less than 200 mm H_2O or 15 mm Hg for a patient in the lateral decubitus position. The pressure can be measured by lumbar puncture or by an intracranial pressure transducer. As ICP increases, patients have headaches, confusion and drowsiness and may develop papilledema. To compensate, CSF volume is reduced; hence, the ventricles are compressed to small slits and sulci are effaced.

If a lesion takes up more space than a reduction in CSF volume can accommodate, blood flow then decreases. Such lower cerebral blood flow may have an immediate adverse impact as the brain is critically dependent upon uninterrupted supply of oxygen and nutrients. If the lesion expands further, the only structure remaining to "give" is the brain itself. The intracranial compartment is subdivided by the dura—the tentorium cerebelli divides the vault into supra- and infratentorial compartments; and the falx divides the supratentorial compartment into right and left compartments. Depending on where the space-occupying lesion is, the brain may be forced out of one compartment into another. Such shifts are called brain herniations.

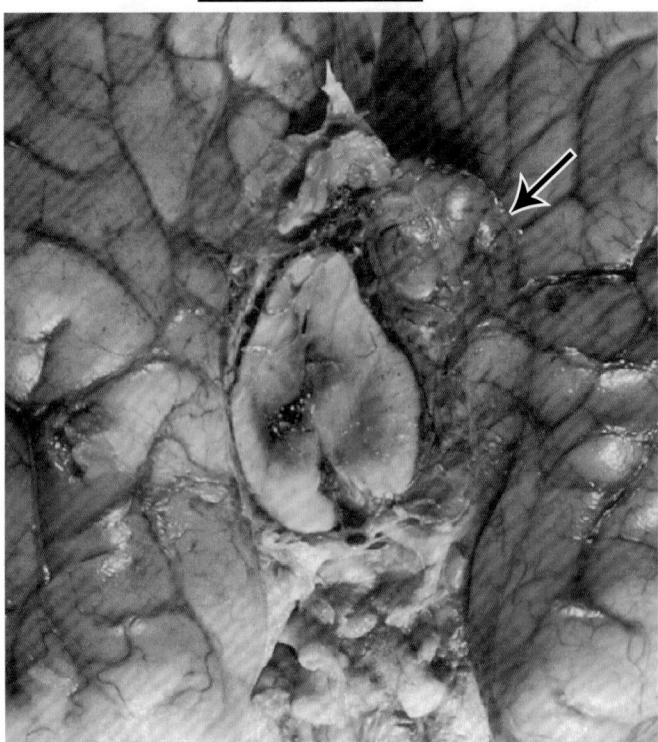

3.5 cm

FIGURE 32-11. Transtentorial herniation. The uncus (*arrow*) of the parahippocampal gyrus is herniated downward to displace the midbrain, resulting in distortion of the midbrain with increased anterior-to-posterior and diminished left-to-right dimensions. The oculomotor nerve may be compromised, leading to an ipsilateral third nerve palsy.

CLINICAL FEATURES:

CINGULATE HERNIATION: If a hemisphere is forced under the falx, the cingulate lobe is the first part of that hemisphere to be displaced. These situations are **subfalcine**, or **cingulate, herniations**. Someone experiencing such a herniation becomes confused and drowsy. The anterior cerebral artery is also displaced beneath the falx, so that infarction within this vessel's territory may occur, leading to contralateral lower extremity weakness and urinary incontinence.

UNCAL HERNIATION: If one hemisphere is forced from the supratentorial compartment toward the infratentorial compartment, the medial temporal lobe (the uncus) is the first portion of the hemisphere displaced; thus, this is an **uncal**, or **transtentorial, herniation** (Fig. 32-11). The ipsilateral oculomotor nerve (cranial nerve III) is crushed by the displaced temporal lobe, leading to ipsilateral pupillary dilatation and paresis of all extraocular muscles except the lateral rectus (cranial nerve VI) and superior oblique (cranial nerve IV). The unopposed action of the lateral rectus leads to the eye "looking" laterally. A dilated unresponsive or minimally responsive pupil indicates extreme danger and necessitates immediate measures to arrest the herniation.

As medial displacement continues, the midbrain shifts away from the displaced hemisphere, with the contralateral cerebral pedicle driven into the unyielding tentorium. This crushing injury of the cerebral pedicle **(Kernohan notch)** causes hemiparesis on the same side of the body as the offending mass. A hemispheric mass will normally cause hemiparesis on the opposite side of the body; ipsilateral hemiparesis, which may be clinically confusing, and this is called a "false localizing" sign.

Downward and medial displacement of a hemisphere through the tentorial opening may also lead to compression of one or both posterior cerebral arteries as they travel from the infratentorial compartment to the now crowded supratentorial compartment. This can impair blood flow to the occipital lobes, resulting in infarction with attendant visual field disturbances bearing no obvious relationship to the inciting mass. This occipital lobe infarction and its attendant signs are also "false localizing."

Uncal herniation syndrome is very ominous but is reversible with removal of the offending mass. Temporary measures to reduce intracranial pressure include intravenous mannitol to shrink the brain osmotically and hyperventilation to reduce PCO_2-inducing cerebral vasospasm and so decrease cerebral blood volume and thus pressure. These actions may gain enough time for definitive surgical treatment.

CENTRAL HERNIATION: If both hemispheres herniate transtentorially, **central herniation syndrome** results. Both

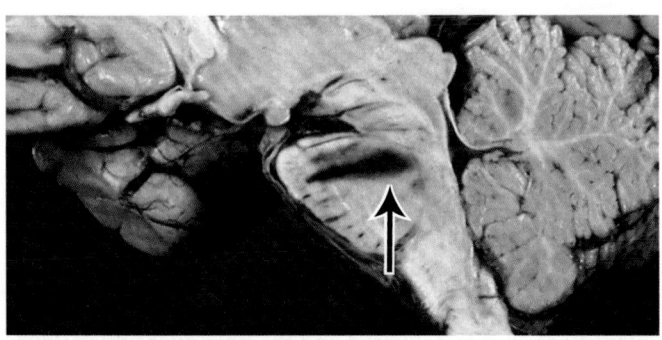

FIGURE 32-12. Duret hemorrhages (*arrow*) in a case of transtentorial herniation tend to be midline and to occupy the brainstem from the upper midbrain to midpons. (Courtesy of Dr. F. Stephen Vogel, Duke University.)

pupils dilate; flaccidity and coma ensue. The downward displacement of the brainstem may wrench vessels from their parenchymal beds within the midbrain and pons and cause multiple linear hemorrhages known as **Duret hemorrhages** or secondary hemorrhages of herniation (Fig. 32-12).

CEREBELLAR TONSILLAR HERNIATION: If the infratentorial compartment becomes crowded either from migrating supratentorial contents or from a mass arising in the infratentorial compartment, the brainstem and cerebellum may be forced through the foramen magnum. The compressed cerebellar tonsils and medulla may compress vital medullary centers and cause death. This bleak situation is **tonsillar herniation**.

FUNGUS CEREBRI: If there is a traumatic or surgical defect in the skull, the brain is under increased pressure and may ooze from the opening. This process is known as fungus cerebri.

Cerebral Edema May Occur Whenever Intracranial Pressure Increases

Cerebral edema can set up a self-perpetuating cycle in which increasing edema begets increasing pressure, which in turn begets more edema.

 **ETIOLOGIC FACTORS:** Cerebral edema is an absolute increase in brain water content. The amount of water in brain tissue is tightly controlled by the rates of CSF production, CSF outflow from the cranial vault and water flux across the blood-brain barrier. The blood-brain barrier (BBB) separates the brain from the blood so that only lipid-soluble molecules, or molecules that can access specialized transport systems, enter the brain. The structural basis of the BBB is endothelial cell tight junctions lining cerebral vessels. Water can enter the brain uncontrollably if the barrier is disrupted or if osmotic forces across it are sufficient to drive water into cerebral tissues. Three major forms of cerebral edema may occur:

- **Cytotoxic edema:** Water flows across an intact BBB by osmotic forces arising because cells within the brain fail to maintain osmotic homeostasis or because of systemic water overload. In either case, water is driven down its concentration gradient into cerebral tissues until osmotic equilibrium is reestablished.
- **Vasogenic edema:** The blood-brain barrier loosens, permitting uncontrolled entry of water into the tissues. *This*

is the most common cause of edema and occurs with neoplasms, abscesses, meningitis, hemorrhage, contusions and lead poisoning. A combination of cytotoxic and vasogenic edema is common in infarcts. The above processes may disrupt endothelial barrier activity, or the vessels formed in neoplasms may be defective from their inception. Vasogenic edema often responds dramatically to administration of corticosteroids, which restore barrier integrity even in tumors.

- **Interstitial edema:** While cytotoxic and vasogenic edema involve water fluxes across the endothelium, interstitial edema involves CSF overproduction or its failure to leave the cranial cavity, so that the fluid seeps across the ependymal lining of the ventricles and accumulates within the white matter.

Hydrocephalus Can Be Noncommunicating or Communicating

Hydrocephalus is accumulation of CSF within the ventricles, causing them to dilate (Fig. 32-13). When ventricular distension is sufficiently advanced, fluid will leak trans-ependymally into the white matter, causing interstitial edema. CSF accumulation can arise from (1) *overproduction of CSF, which is very rare,* occurring only in the context of tumors of the choroid plexus; and (2) *failure of CSF to leave the cranial vault, which is more common.* If the blockage occurs within the ventricular system itself, ventricles proximal to the block dilate, while those situated downstream from the block are spared. This is **obstructive, or noncommunicating, hydrocephalus.** The most frequent site of block is at the ventricular system's narrowest strait—the aqueduct of Sylvius connecting the third and fourth ventricles.

A block may occur after the CSF leaves the ventricular system and travels over the cerebral convexities to the arachnoid granulations that usher the fluid into the venous sinuses. Then, all the ventricles dilate. This is **communicating hydrocephalus,** meaning that ventricles are unobstructed in fluid flow. Communicating hydrocephalus may complicate subarachnoid hemorrhage or inflammation, resulting in arachnoid scarring, or may result from thrombosis of the dural venous sinuses themselves.

FIGURE 32-13. Hydrocephalus. Horizontal section of the brain from a patient who died of a brain tumor that obstructed the aqueduct of Sylvius shows marked dilation of the lateral ventricles.

CLINICAL FEATURES: The clinical features of hydrocephalus depend on the patient's age. In infants and children, before cranial sutures have fused, the head enlarges sometimes to grotesque proportions as the ventricles dilate. As hydrocephalus is common in infants and treatable by shunting, measurement of the head circumference is a fundamental part of the pediatric physical examination.

After sutures fuse, hydrocephalus cannot enlarge the head, but rather increases intracranial pressure. This causes headache, confusion, drowsiness, papilledema and vomiting. Ventricles enlarge at the expense of brain volume so that in advanced cases only a mantle of several millimeters' thickness remains. Remarkably, such individuals may retain substantial cognitive abilities, although spasticity may cloak the expression of this intelligence.

In older people, hydrocephalus may develop insidiously. Slow ventricular enlargement may appear clinically as progressive dementia, gait impairment and urinary incontinence as the long white matter fibers connecting portions of cortex to one another and lower motility centers are stretched apart by relentless expansion of the ventricles. This condition is usually accompanied by normal baseline intracranial pressure and so is called **normal-pressure hydrocephalus,** which may respond to shunting. If long-term CSF pressure is monitored, periodic waves of elevated intracranial pressure are seen.

All of the above forms of hydrocephalus result from disturbance of CSF dynamics and should be distinguished from **hydrocephalus ex vacuo,** which is compensatory ventricular enlargement due to loss of CNS tissue from other diseases. This occurs most often in diffuse cortical atrophy, but focal destruction such as occurs at the site of an old infarct may lead to focal compensatory ventricular enlargement.

TRAUMA

 **EPIDEMIOLOGY:** Physical injury to the brain, spinal cord and peripheral nervous system is a major cause of loss of life and productivity. Populations at highest risk for such injuries include children, men in late adolescence and early adulthood and the elderly. Such injuries are a signature of modern warfare, are the leading cause of death in childhood and young adulthood and are a major concern for participants in contact sports.

 **ETIOLOGIC FACTORS:** The brain and spinal cord are enclosed in protective bony cases that dissipate forces delivered to these delicate structures. However, evolutionary selection has not yet adequately responded to the need to survive motor vehicle crashes, personal assaults or dives into shallow pools. Injury to the nervous system results from the transfer of kinetic energy to the neural tissues—the degree of injury correlates with the quantity of energy delivered and the time over which it was delivered. This energy transfer may directly disrupt tissues in penetrating injuries, or the energy may be translated into movement and compression of neural structures within the skull or spinal canal in a closed injury. Extreme injury of the brain and cord is possible with minimal disruption of overlying tissues. Conversely, superficial tissues can sustain dramatic injury while the nervous system underneath remains unaltered.

Epidural Hematomas Are Often Fatal

Epidural hematomas usually result from blows to the head with skull fracture. Unless treated promptly, they can be fatal. The intracranial dura is securely bound to the inner aspect of the calvaria and so is analogous to the intracranial periosteum. The middle meningeal arteries reside in grooves in the inner table of the bone between the dura and the calvaria, and their branches splay across the temporal–parietal area. The temporal bone, being one of the thinnest bones of the skull, is particularly vulnerable to fracture. Seemingly minor trauma may fracture it, which may in turn lacerate branches of the middle meningeal artery, causing life-threatening epidural hemorrhage (Fig. 32-14).

 PATHOLOGY: Transection of the middle meningeal artery allows blood under arterial pressure to escape into the epidural space that separates the dura from the calvaria. The dura is tightly bound to the calvarium at the coronal sutures. Thus, epidural bleeding will not extend beyond the suture lines. This leads to a lens-shaped accumulation of fresh blood that stops at the coronal suture lines (Fig. 32-15).

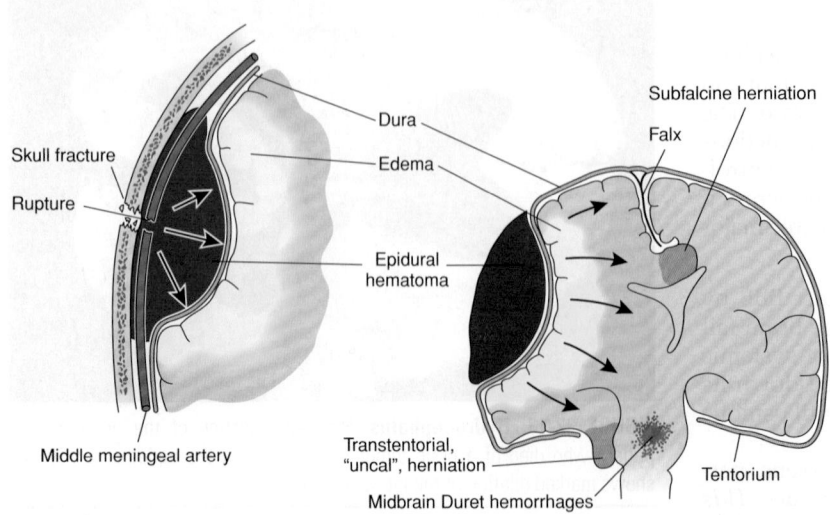

FIGURE 32-14. Development of an epidural hematoma. Laceration of a branch of the middle meningeal artery by the sharp bony edges of a skull fracture initiates bleeding under arterial pressure that dissects the dura from the calvaria and produces an expanding hematoma. After an asymptomatic interval of several hours, subfalcine and transtentorial herniation occur, and if the hematoma is not evacuated, lethal Duret hemorrhages will occur.

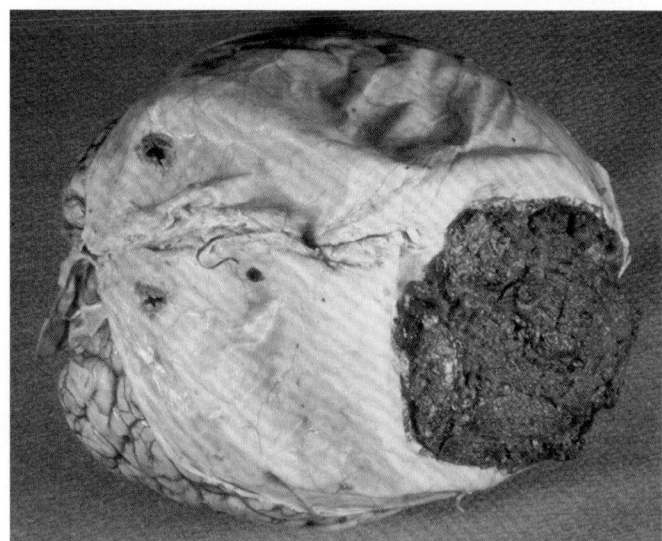

FIGURE 32-15. Epidural hematoma. A discoid mass of fresh hemorrhage overlies the dura covering frontal–parietal cortex but does not transgress the coronal sutures.

 CLINICAL FEATURES: Up to 1/3 of patients do not lose consciousness at the time of the precipitating injury and may have a "lucid interval" of unimpaired consciousness for several hours while epidural blood accumulates under arterial pressure. When the hematoma reaches 30–50 mL, symptoms of a space-occupying lesion appear. Epidural hematomas are invariably progressive and, when not recognized and evacuated, may be fatal in 24–48 hours.

Subdural Hematomas Develop More Slowly Than Epidural Hematomas

Subdural hematomas are a significant cause of death after head injuries from falls, assaults, vehicular accidents and sporting accidents. The hematomas expand more slowly than epidural hematomas, so their clinical tempo is slower, but once critical increased intracranial pressure is attained, clinical deterioration and death can occur with horrific rapidity.

PATHOLOGY: The cerebral hemispheres float in the CSF, tethered loosely by blood vessels and cranial nerves. Blood drains from cerebral hemispheres through veins that cross the subarachnoid space and arachnoid to breach the dura and enter the dural sinus. There is no true subdural space per se, but the inner layer of meningothelial cells of the dura has fewer tight junctions than those in the outer layers of the dura. Shearing forces will separate these cells, allowing blood to seep between them. Since bleeding in this situation is under low venous pressure, it is slow and may stop spontaneously from a local tamponade effect. The bleeding is within the dura itself and readily extends beyond the coronal sutures, causing a hematoma that can extend along the entire anterior to posterior dimensions of the calvarium (Fig. 32-16). Granulation tissue forms in reaction to the blood, and the delicate capillaries of this tissue may themselves leak. This leads to gradual accumulation of an ever enlarging subacute, and ultimately chronic, subdural hematoma.

The blood and granulation tissue are surrounded by a sheet of fibrous connective tissue—the "membranes" of a chronic subdural hematoma. Fibroblasts first create a membrane on the calvarial side of the hematoma, the **outer membrane**. Then they invade the subjacent hematoma to form a fibrous membrane subjacent to the blood clot. This **inner membrane** is visible in about 2 weeks (Fig. 32-17). A subdural hematoma may evolve in three ways. It may (1) be reabsorbed and leave only a small amount of telltale hemosiderin; (2) remain static, and perhaps calcify; or (3) enlarge as a result of recurrent microhemorrhages in the granulation tissue.

Expansion of the hematoma, and onset of symptoms, commonly results from rebleeding, usually within 6 months. Granulation tissue is fragile and so vulnerable to minor trauma, even that caused by shaking the head. Thus, subdural hematomas can rebleed and create a new hematoma subjacent to the outer membrane. Episodes of sporadic rebleeding expand these lesions periodically and at unpredictable intervals. Since the bleeding occurs in the inner dural border cell zone rather than an imaginary subdural space, no blood is seen in the CSF. In addition to granulation tissue and blood, other cellular constituents include plasma cells, lymphocytes and extramedullary hematopoiesis. These may contribute to the cellular dynamics of the subdural hematoma by releasing cytokines and causing cerebral edema in the underlying brain.

 CLINICAL FEATURES: Symptoms and signs of subdural hematomas are diverse. Stretching of meninges leads to headaches; pressure on the motor cortex produces contralateral weakness; and focal cortical irritation can initiate seizures. Subdural hematomas are bilateral in 15%–20% of cases, and these may impair cognitive function and lead to a mistaken diagnosis of dementia. Rebleeding with expansion may cause lethal transtentorial herniation (Fig. 32-16A).

Parenchymal Injuries Produce Variable Symptomatology

Traumatic brain and spinal cord injuries range in severity from temporary loss of function with little or no discernible structural damage in concussion, to intermediate damage with hemorrhage and necrosis of the tissue in contusions, to profound disruption of structure and function in lacerations.

Concussion

Concussion is transient loss of consciousness due to biomechanical forces acting on the CNS. A blow that causes an epidural hematoma does not necessarily produce a concussion. Consciousness depends on a functional brainstem reticular formation interacting with the cerebral hemispheres and is lost if either the reticular formation or both hemispheres are damaged. A classic example of concussion occurs in boxing, from a blow that deflects the head upward and posteriorly, often with a rotatory component. These motions impart quick rotational acceleration to the brainstem and cause dysfunction of reticular formation neurons. By contrast, a blow to the temporal–parietal area may cause a skull fracture and lethal epidural hematoma but may not cause loss of consciousness because lateral movement of the cerebral hemispheres does not occur.

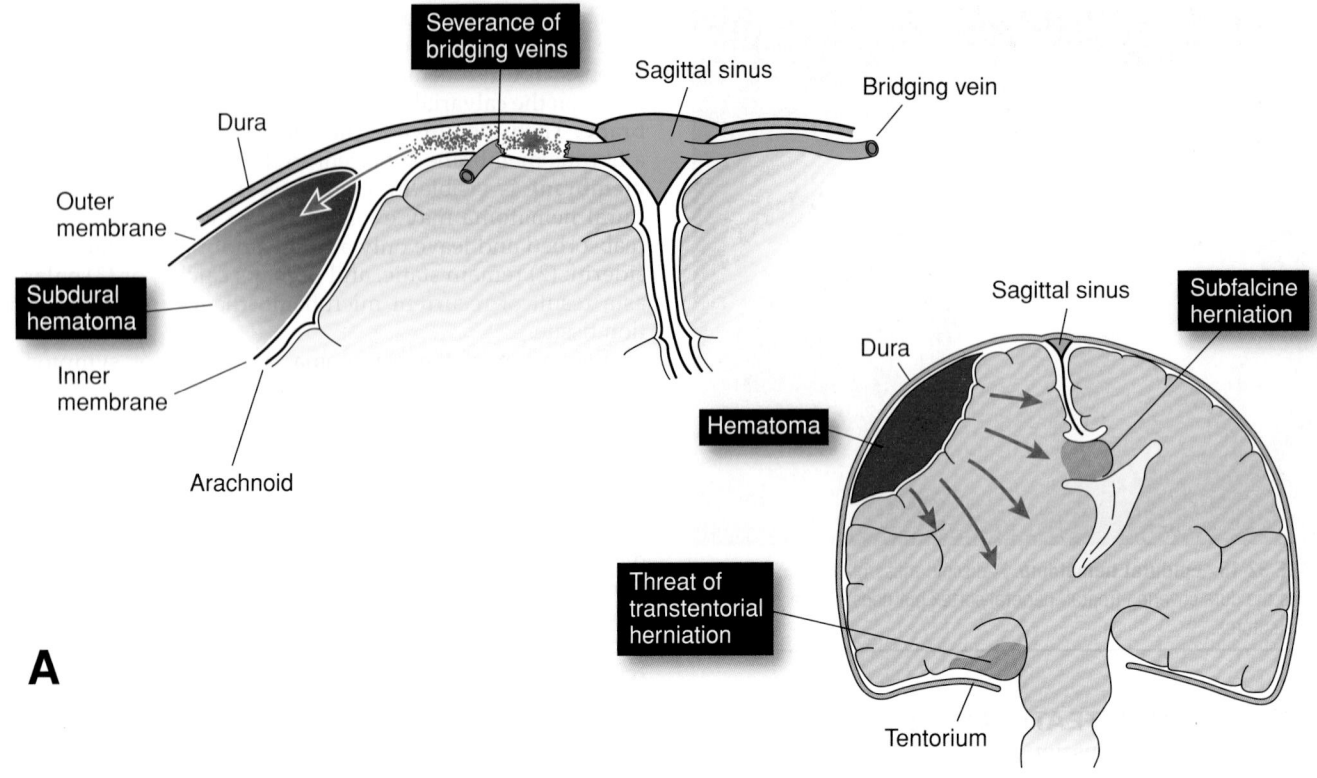

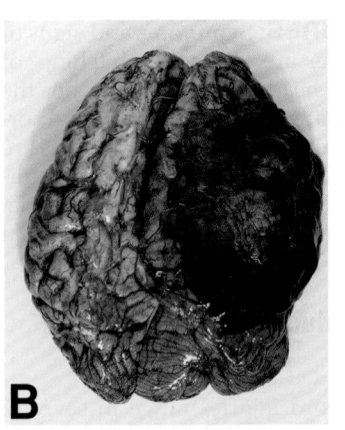

FIGURE 32-16. Development of a subdural hematoma. A. With head trauma, the dura moves with the skull, and the arachnoid moves with the cerebrum. As a result, the bridging veins are sheared as they cross between the dura and the arachnoid. Venous bleeding creates a hematoma in the expansile subdural space. Subsequent transtentorial herniation is life-threatening. **B.** The right hemisphere exhibits a large collection of blood in the "subdural space," owing to rupture of the bridging veins.

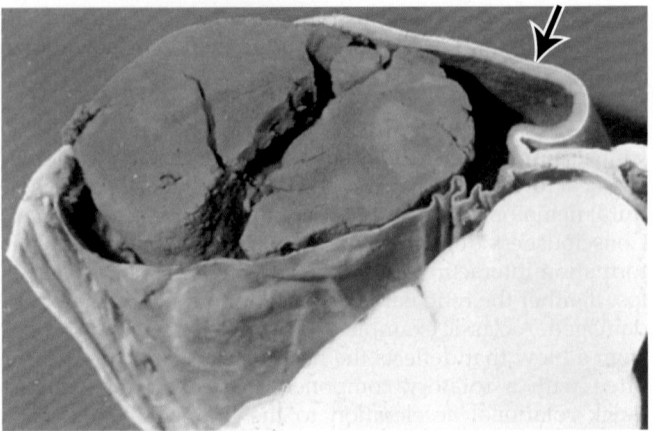

FIGURE 32-17. Chronic subdural hematoma with well-developed surrounding membranes. The thicker membrane (*arrow*) is the exterior membrane and the thinner membrane is adjacent to the brain. (Courtesy of Dr. F. Stephen Vogel, Duke University.)

Classically, concussion is not associated with gross neuropathology, and since the condition is not lethal, microscopic examination is not possible. Recent advances in diffusion tensor imaging suggest that axonal injury functionally disconnects the reticular activating system from the cerebral hemispheres. Axonal injury and disconnection may also account for cognitive and memory difficulties, vertigo and the feelings that "things are just not quite right" that bedevil people who have sustained "mild" traumatic brain injury.

Cerebral Contusion

 **ETIOLOGIC FACTORS:** A cerebral contusion is a brain bruise—an area of tissue disruption and blood seepage—usually when the brain strikes the irregular bony contours of the skull because of abrupt acceleration or deceleration. If a moving object strikes the head, acceleration will be imparted to the skull and its delicate cargo, the brain. In contrast, a fall results in an abrupt deceleration.

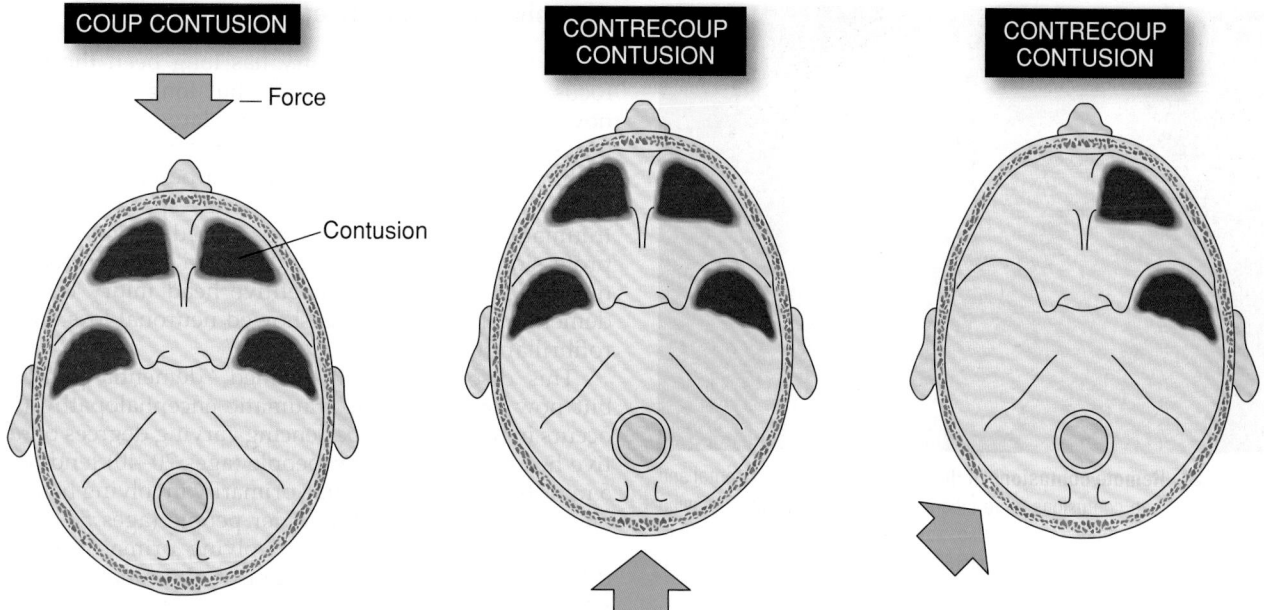

FIGURE 32-18. Biomechanics of cerebral contusion. The cerebral hemispheres float in the cerebrospinal fluid. Rapid deceleration or acceleration of the skull causes the cortex to impact forcefully into the anterior and middle fossae. The position of a contusion is determined by the direction of the force and the intracranial anatomy.

When a contusion occurs at a point of impact, the lesion is a **coup** injury (French, *coup* = "blow") (Fig. 32-18). If the side of the brain opposite the impact site strikes the skull, resulting contusions are contralateral to the point of initial contact (**contrecoup**). Coup injuries are maximal when the head is stationary and struck by an object, while contrecoup contusions are more severe when the head is in motion and abruptly stops. If an individual is struck by an assailant with a baseball bat, a large coup contusion will be present. In contrast, if a person falls off of a ladder, a large contrecoup contusion results.

PATHOLOGY: If the force of impact is mild, cerebral contusion is limited to the cortex and the crowns of gyri (Fig. 32-19A). Greater force destroys larger expanses of cortex, creating cavitary lesions that may extend into the white matter or lacerate the cortex, causing intraparenchymal hemorrhage (Fig. 32-19B). Together, edema and hemorrhage in a contusion may cause the contusion to expand over several days, which can become life-threatening as a result of increased intracranial pressure.

Contusions leave permanent marks on the brain. Bruised, necrotic tissue is phagocytosed by macrophages and eliminated in large part via the bloodstream. Astrocytosis then leads to local scar formation, which persists as telltale evidence of a prior contusion. Usually some residual hemosiderin imparts an orange brown hue to the old contusion (Fig. 32-20).

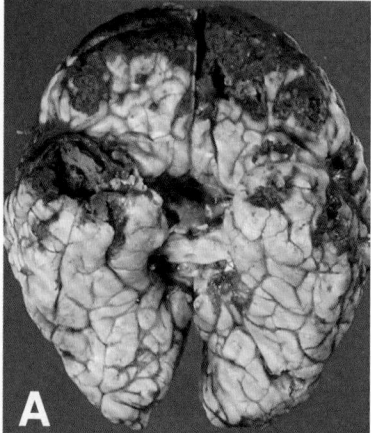
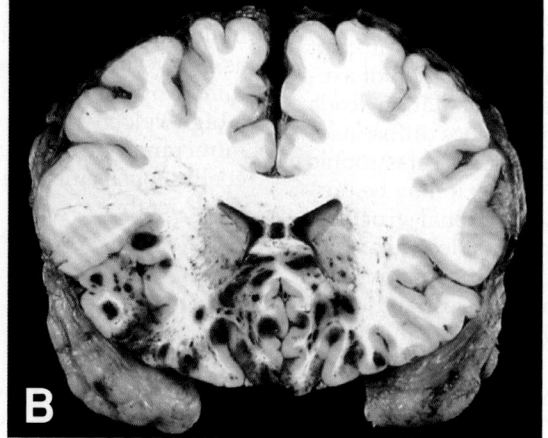
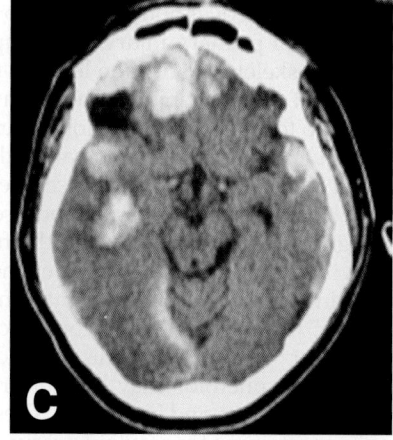

FIGURE 32-19. Acute contusions of the brain. A. After an automobile accident, the brain exhibits necrosis and hemorrhage involving the frontal and temporal lobes. **B.** In addition, there are some underlying white matter hemorrhages. **C.** Axial noncontrast computed tomography showing acute contusions in the basal frontal and temporal tips regions. The hemorrhage is the white signal in the frontal and temporal regions. (A and B Courtesy of Dr. F. Stephen Vogel, Duke University.)

THE CENTRAL NERVOUS SYSTEM

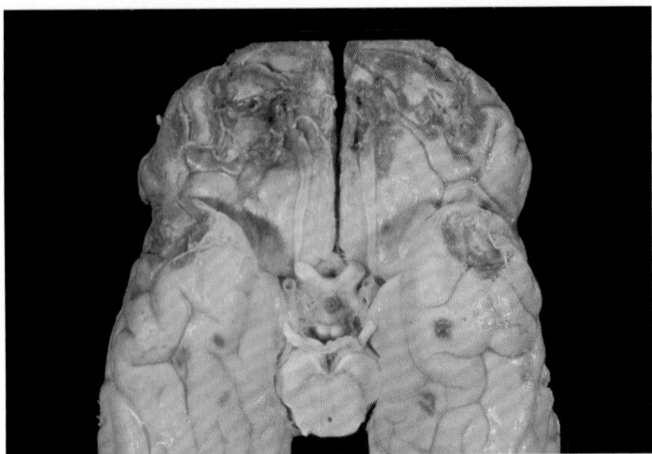

FIGURE 32-20. Remote contusions of the brain. Bilateral large frontal and smaller temporal tip contusions were cleared out by macrophages, leaving residual hemosiderin-stained divots. Also, note the involvement of the olfactory bulbs—anosmia (loss of sense of smell) is the most common cranial neuropathy following traumatic brain injury.

Diffuse Axonal Injury

Diffuse axonal injury (DAI) is a very common result of traumatic brain injury and may lead to severe neurologic deficits and coma in patients without gross hematomas, contusions or lacerations. Advances in imaging techniques allow better detection and quantification of these injuries, which are major contributors to morbidity and mortality. There is also increased interest in DAI as part of blast injuries.

 ETIOLOGIC FACTORS: The parasagittal cerebral hemispheres are anchored to arachnoid villi **(pacchionian granulations)**, while the lateral aspects of the cerebrum move more freely. This anatomic feature, together with the differential density of gray and white matter, allows for shearing forces between different brain regions, leading to axonal shearing injuries. Shearing injuries can distort or disrupt axons, causing immediate loss of function. Experimental studies indicate that diffuse axonal injury evolves over hours to days, so axons may be injured at the time of primary injury, with impaired axonal transport and cytoskeletal disruption leading to accumulation of axoplasm at sites of injury. Then, physical separation leads axons to form axonal retraction spheroids. Since diffuse axonal injury evolves over time, rather than being a catastrophic event leading to immediately severed axons, it may be possible to arrest its progression and preserve axonal structural integrity. If an injury is severe, the functional loss of axonal activity may immediately render the patient comatose, but imaging may show only small hemorrhages and focal edema, particularly in the corpus callosum and midbrain. However, more widely distributed axonal swelling and retraction spheroids may be seen in cerebral white matter, corpus callosum and brainstem. These can be highlighted by immunostaining for amyloid precursor protein (APP), which is normally transported along axons and accumulates at sites of injury where transport is impaired. Diffusion tensor imaging (DTI), a specialized magnetic resonance imaging (MRI) technique, detects and quantifies DAI.

Chronic Traumatic Encephalopathy

Acute traumatic brain injury has long been the primary focus of neurotrauma research, but long-term effects are now receiving overdue attention as large numbers of military service members return from Iraq and Afghanistan. In addition, the possible long-term neurodegenerative effects of repetitive head injury in sports—specifically chronic traumatic encephalopathy—has raised major concern in professional and amateur athletics. In 1928, it was recognized that boxers with repetitive head injury developed dementia and their brains showed neuronal loss and neurofibrillary tangles.

This disorder, initially named "dementia pugilistica" but now called chronic traumatic encephalopathy (CTE), occurs in nonboxers experiencing varying degrees of repetitive head injury. Younger people (ages 20–40) tend to have a rapidly progressive course primarily involving behavioral and mood changes, while older people (ages 50–70) have slower disease progression involving primarily cognitive difficulties. There is a spectrum of abnormalities in individuals with CTE.

 PATHOLOGY: The most distinctive finding is deposition of tau in neurons at the depths of sulci and around blood vessels. Abnormal tau accumulation occurs in many neurodegenerative diseases, including Alzheimer disease, frontotemporal lobar degeneration and progressive supranuclear palsy, among others, but it is the distribution of neurofibrillary tangles in CTE that is unique. CTE may represent a mechanistic bridge between acute injury and progressive neurodegenerative disease.

Penetrating Traumatic Brain Injury

 PATHOPHYSIOLOGY: Penetrating objects like bullets and knives enter the cranium and traverse the brain with variable velocities. If there is no direct damage to vital brain centers, hemorrhage is the immediate threat to life (Fig. 32-21).

The damage a projectile does depends on how much kinetic energy is involved ($E = mv^2$, where m = mass and v = velocity). Thus, projectile velocity is the key determinant of injury. The kinetic energy of a high-velocity bullet directly disrupts tissues by its own mass as well as by a centrifugal blast zone whose diameter is determined by the projectile's original kinetic energy. Thus, a high-velocity bullet can cause an explosive increase in intracranial pressure, which forcefully herniates the cerebellar tonsils into the foramen magnum, causing immediate death.

Spinal Cord Injury

 **ETIOLOGIC FACTORS:** Traumatic lesions of the spinal cord may result from direct injury by penetrating wounds (e.g., stab wounds, bullets) or indirect injury from vertebral fractures or displacement. The spinal cord may be contused not only at the site of injury but also above and below the point of trauma. Compromised arterial supply to the cord, with resulting infarction, may complicate traumatic injury.

A. HIGH-VELOCITY BULLET WOUND

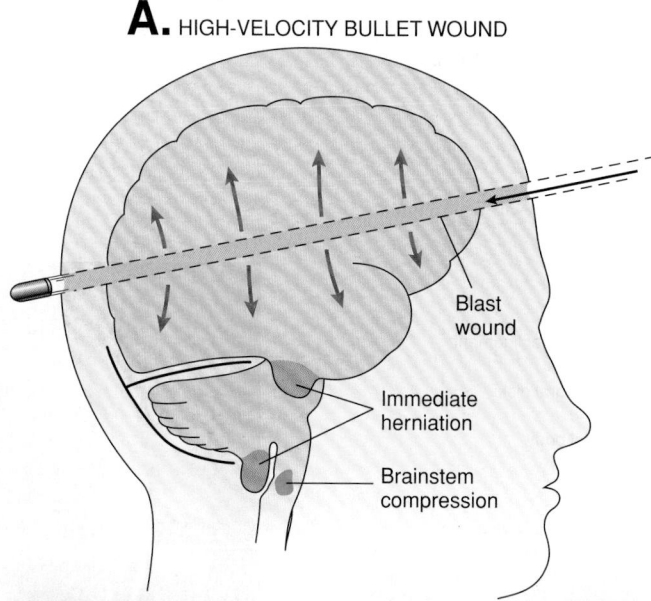

Blast wound

Immediate herniation

Brainstem compression

B. LOW-VELOCITY BULLET WOUND

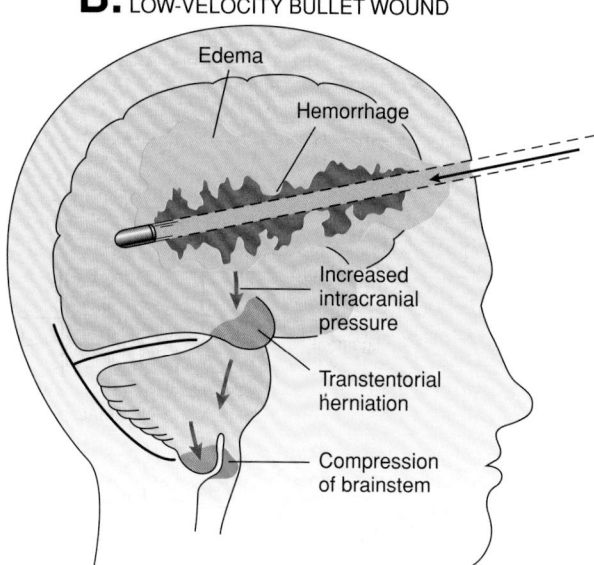

Edema

Hemorrhage

Increased intracranial pressure

Transtentorial herniation

Compression of brainstem

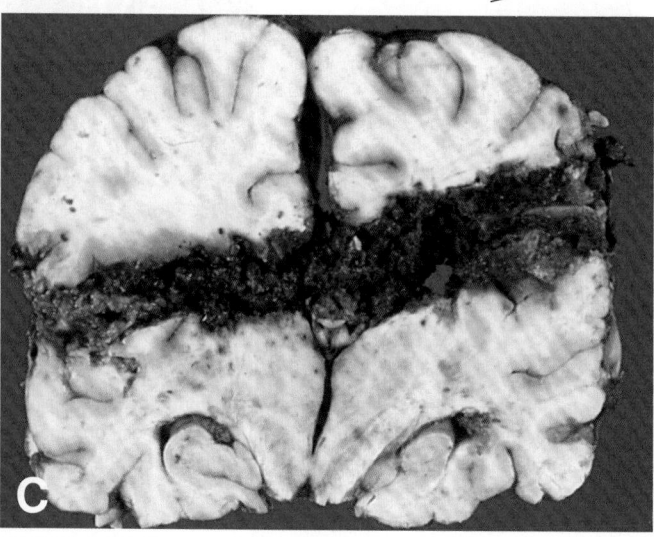

FIGURE 32-21. Consequences of high- and low-velocity bullet wounds. A. The "blast effect" of a high-velocity projectile causes an immediate increase in supratentorial pressure and results in death because of impaction of the cerebellum and medulla into the foramen magnum. **B.** A low-velocity projectile increases the pressure at a more gradual rate through hemorrhage and edema. **C. Bullet track in a through-and-through penetrating injury.** The "blast effect" of a high-velocity projectile causes an immediate increase in supratentorial pressure and may result in death because of impaction of the cerebellum and medulla into the foramen magnum. A lower-velocity projectile increases the pressure at a more gradual rate through hemorrhage and edema. (Courtesy of Dr. F. Stephen Vogel, Duke University.)

Vertebral bodies are separated by intravertebral disks and are stabilized in normal alignment by two longitudinal ligaments and the posterior bony processes. The anterior spinal ligament adheres to the ventral surface of the vertebral bodies, while the posterior spinal ligament is affixed to the dorsal vertebral column. After extreme flexion or extension, the angulation of the bony vertebral column brings the spinal cord forcefully into contact with bone or interferes with regional circulation.

The consequences of a spinal cord injury depend on the severity of the trauma. **Spinal cord concussion** is the mildest injury, with transient, reversible functional disturbance. **Contusion of the spinal cord** results from more severe trauma, varying from minor transient bruises to hemorrhagic spinal cord necrosis (Fig. 32-22). Spinal cord necrosis and edema due to severe contusion are **myelomalacia.** A hematoma within the cord is a **hematomyelia. Lacerations and transections of the spinal cord** are usually caused by penetrating wounds or severely displaced spinal fractures. They are irreversible and lead to complete loss of function below the spinal level of the injury. Whether paralysis affects only the legs **(paraplegia)** or all four extremities **(quadriplegia)** depends on the spinal level and extent of the injury. If even as little as 10%–15% of the cross-sectional diameter of the spinal cord is spared, functional recovery is much better than with complete transection.

Neurotrauma is a process, not an event. The initial transfer of kinetic injury sets into motion a cascade of secondary injury mechanisms. Mitigation of secondary injury and facilitation of recovery continue to be major thrusts in neurotrauma.

CEREBROVASCULAR DISORDERS

Stroke is the third leading cause of death in the United States, after myocardial infarction and cancer. As elsewhere, vascular disease can result from either vessel blockage, causing ischemia, or vascular leakage that results in hemorrhage. Vascular disorders of the nervous system lead to (1) globally or focally inadequate blood flow (ischemia), which, if sufficiently protracted, produces infarction; or (2) rupture of vascular structures that causes either intraparenchymal or subarachnoid hemorrhage.

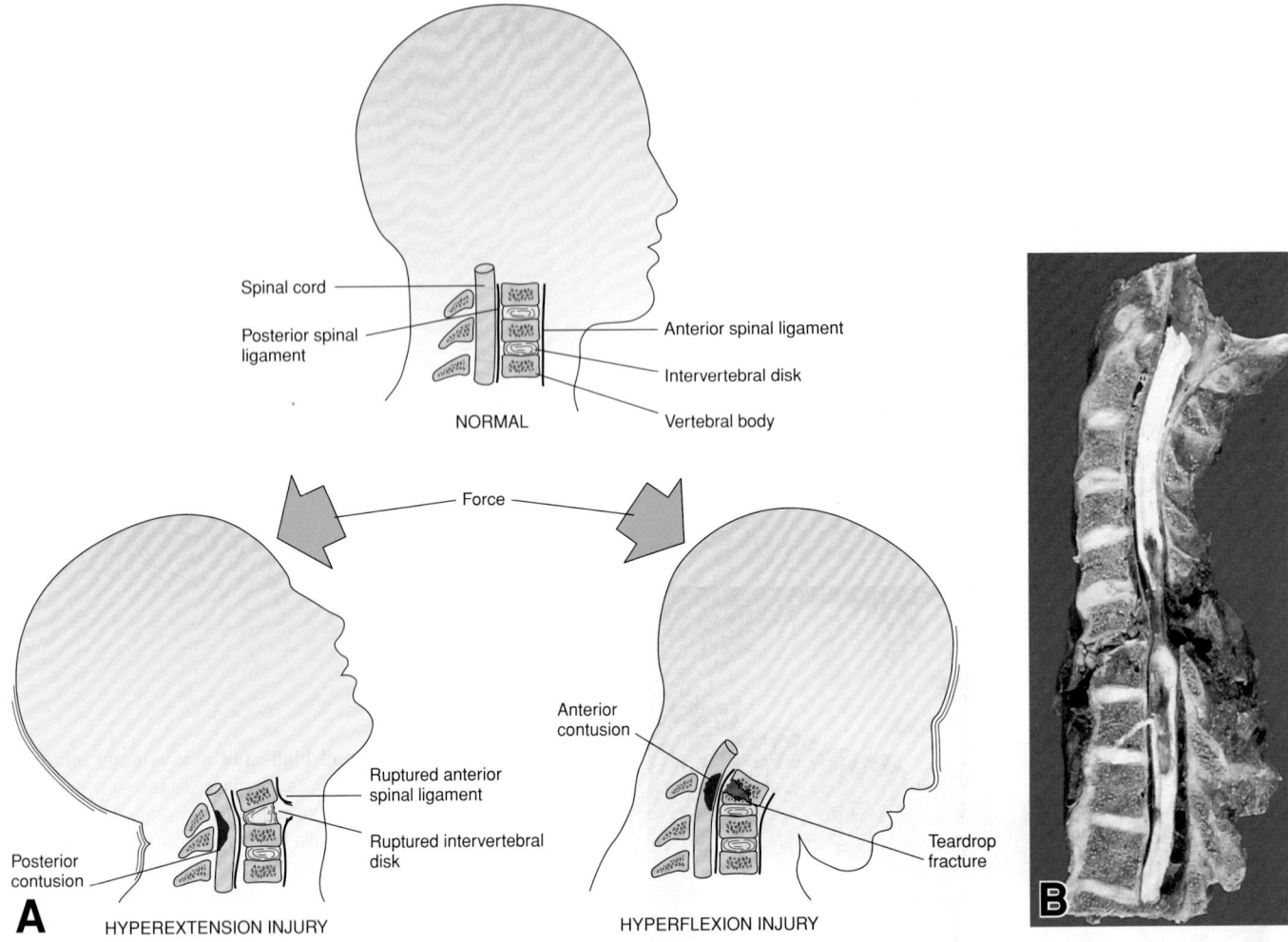

FIGURE 32-22. Spinal injury. A. Numerous different angles of force can be applied to the highly vulnerable cervical spine. Posterior (hyperextension) and anterior (hyperflexion) injuries are the most common. Hyperextension injury causes rupture of the anterior spinal ligament and excessive posterior angulation. Hyperflexion injury causes compression associated with a "teardrop" fracture of a vertebral body and produces excessive forward angulation of the cord. **B.** Fracture dislocation of the spinal column may result in spinal cord contusion, laceration, necrosis or frank transection. Preservation of a relatively small cross-sectional area of the spinal cord can have major beneficial effects on recovery. (Courtesy of Dr. F. Stephen Vogel, Duke University.)

Ischemic Stroke Often Follows Shock

ETIOLOGIC FACTORS: The brain receives about 20% of basal cardiac output. Aerobic glycolysis is virtually the sole source of energy of the mature brain. CNS glycogen reserves are meager and oxygen reserves are nil; hence, uninterrupted supply of oxygenated blood is essential for brain integrity. The brain's blood supply comes via paired internal carotid and vertebral arteries. The carotids, the "anterior circulation," supply most superficial and deep cerebral hemisphere structures; the vertebral arteries make up the "posterior circulation," feeding the brainstem, cerebellum and territory of the posterior cerebral arteries. The posterior and anterior circuits anastomose via the circle of Willis. This anastomotic network at the base of the brain is quite variable, but in some fortunate individuals, the blood supply of the brain is sufficiently redundant that complete blockage of two carotids and one vertebral can be asymptomatic. Despite these elaborate hemodynamic precautions, many people experience global or focal ischemia leading to cerebral infarction.

Global ischemia, which is usually due to cardiopulmonary arrest or extreme hypotension in severe shock, leads to widespread tissue injury, resulting in ischemic encephalopathy. If perfusion failure is brief (minutes), neurologic functions may quickly be restored with only transient postischemic confusion. Some patients may come back more slowly and suffer subtle higher intellectual function impairments, which may preclude complete resumption of societal activities. More severe injury may lead to dementia and spasticity. If the ischemic period is protracted, the patient may not regain consciousness and may show decorticate posturing and seizures and be in a coma indefinitely.

Although the entire brain is inadequately perfused, there is surprising focality to the pathologic alterations. Certain cell populations are most vulnerable to ischemic injury: the large neurons in the Sommer sector of the hippocampus, Purkinje cells of the cerebellum and neurons of layers 3 and 5 of the cerebral cortex (Fig. 32-23).

The basis of this selective vulnerability is not clear. It may be related to local metabolic requirements, hemodynamic factors and local neurotransmitters. When ischemia leads to brain energy failure, membranes depolarize, permitting uncontrolled release of the amino acid neurotransmitters glutamate and aspartate. These bind ligand-gated cation

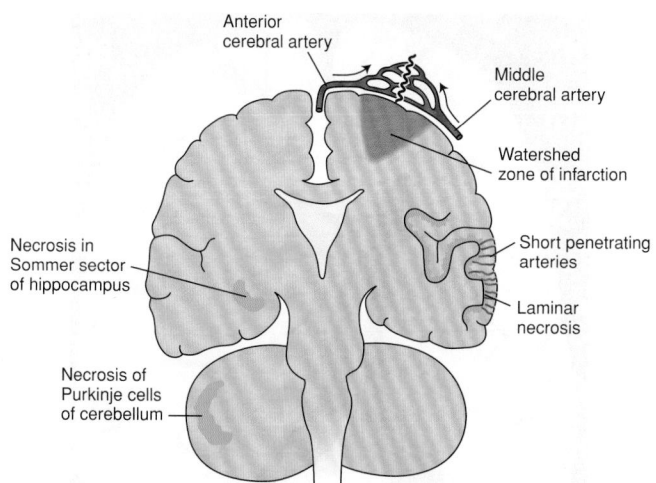

FIGURE 32-23. Mechanisms of injury in global ischemia. A global insult induces lesions that reflect the vascular architecture (watershed infarcts, laminar necrosis) and the selective vulnerability of individual neuronal systems (pyramidal cells of the Sommer sector, Purkinje cells, laminar necrosis). Both rheologic (blood flow) and neurochemical (excitotoxicity) factors may be operational in laminar necrosis.

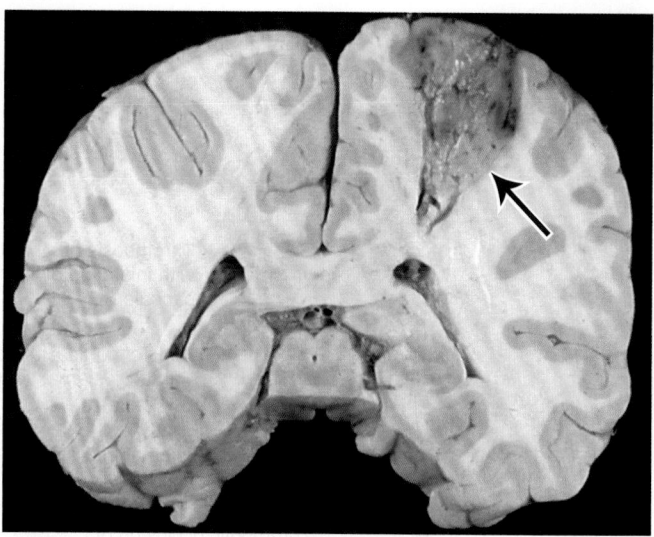

FIGURE 32-25. Watershed infarct. In global hypoperfusion, the most precarious perfusion zones are at the distal overlapping portions of the major cerebral vessels. Here an acute infarct is seen at the watershed of the anterior and middle cerebral arteries (*arrow*). (Courtesy of Dr. F. Stephen Vogel, Duke University.)

channels on postsynaptic cells, opening the floodgates for calcium and sodium entry. The latter depolarizes the cell membrane.

Calcium may activate intracellular proteases and quench mitochondrial energy production, propagating the energy failure and magnifying cellular injury. Injury done by abnormally released neurotransmitters is **excitotoxicity**, which may play a role in neurodegenerative disorders, epilepsy and stroke. In excitotoxicity, the areas of brain injury depend on the local use of toxic neurotransmitters. For example, high levels of amino acid neurotransmitters make the mid-cortex more vulnerable to ischemic injury, resulting in a mid-cortical band of necrosis with relatively preserved cortex in deep and superficial layers on either side of this band. As infarcted tissue is infiltrated by macrophages, it becomes grossly conspicuous as **laminar necrosis** (Fig. 32-24).

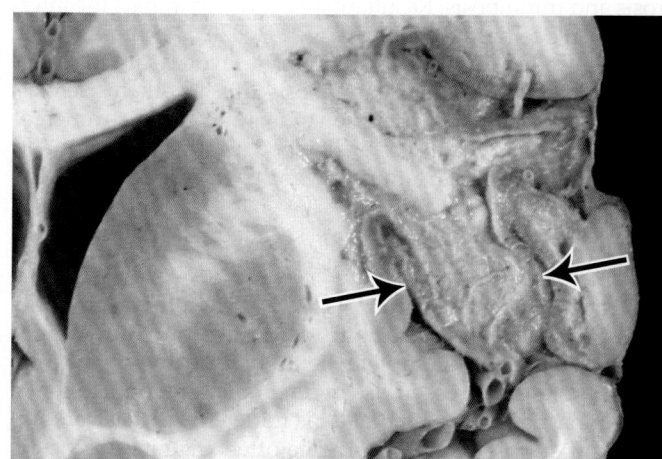

FIGURE 32-24. Laminar necrosis. A patient who suffered prolonged anoxia during a cardiac arrhythmia developed selective necrosis of layers in the cerebral cortex (*arrows*). (Courtesy of Dr. F. Stephen Vogel, Duke University.)

Hemodynamic factors cause **watershed** or **border-zone infarcts,** which occur at junctions of major arterial supply zones (Fig. 32-25). These zones are at the precarious distal regions of arterial supply. If perfusion pressure drops, these are the first areas affected. The classic border zone lies between the anterior and middle cerebral arteries' distal territories (Fig. 32-25). With global ischemia, this area in both hemispheres may be infarcted, leading to symmetric wedge-shaped parasagittal high-convexity infarcts.

Regional Ischemia Causes Localized Cerebral Infarction

Cerebrovascular occlusive disease remains a major cause of morbidity and death because atherosclerosis is ubiquitous and progressive. *Atherosclerosis predisposes to vascular thrombosis and embolism, both of which result in localized ischemia and subsequent cerebral infarction.*

 **ETIOLOGIC FACTORS:** Cerebral infarcts are usually designated **hemorrhagic** or **bland**. *In general, infarcts caused by emboli are hemorrhagic, while those due to local thrombosis are ischemic (i.e., bland).* Emboli occlude vascular flow abruptly, after which the distal segments of affected blood vessels lose integrity and leak blood into the region during reperfusion (Fig. 32-26A). Atherosclerotic plaques in the common and internal carotid arteries may lead to emboli. But the heart is also a rich source of emboli. These may derive from infected or defective valves, hypokinetic thrombogenic endocardial walls after myocardial infarction or atrial thrombi in atrial fibrillation, especially if there is associated mitral insufficiency. Fat emboli and deep vein thrombi from the systemic venous circulation may embolize paradoxically through a patent foramen ovale. Emboli of amniotic fluid or tumors (e.g., from atrial myxomas) occur but are rare.

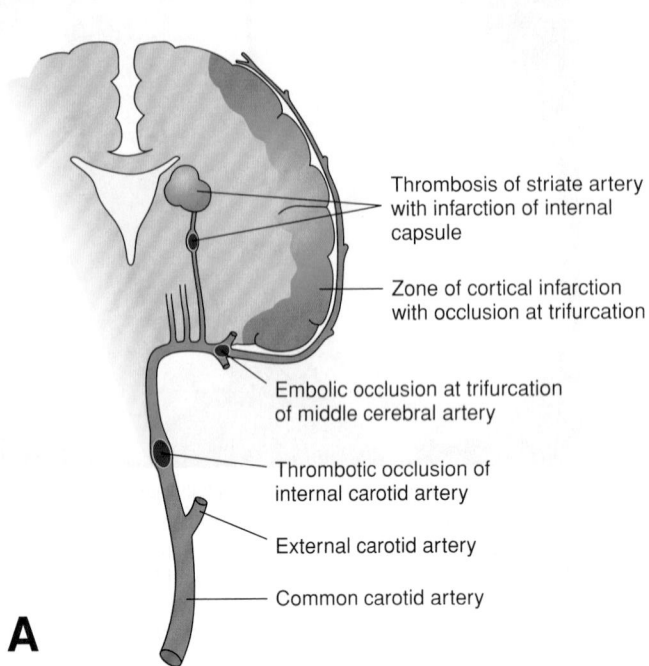

- Thrombosis of striate artery with infarction of internal capsule
- Zone of cortical infarction with occlusion at trifurcation
- Embolic occlusion at trifurcation of middle cerebral artery
- Thrombotic occlusion of internal carotid artery
- External carotid artery
- Common carotid artery

A

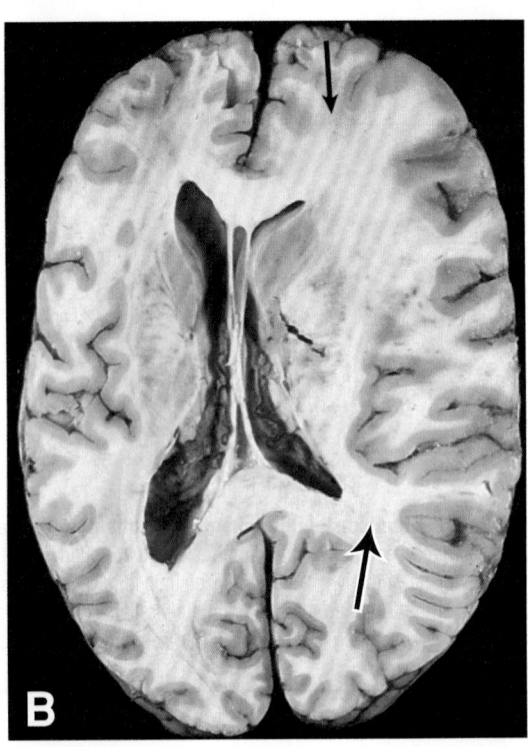

B

FIGURE 32-26. A. Distribution of cerebral infarcts. The normal distribution of the cerebral vasculature defines the pattern and size of infarcts and, consequently, their symptoms. Occlusion at the trifurcation causes cortical infarcts with motor and sensory loss and often aphasia. Occlusion of a striate branch transects the internal capsule and causes a motor deficit. **B. Acute middle cerebral artery distribution infarct.** An axial section of the brain of a patient who suffered thrombosis of the middle cerebral artery reveals a large infarct of the right hemisphere (*between arrows*) with swelling and focal dusky discoloration. (Courtesy of Dr. F. Stephen Vogel, Duke University.)

PATHOLOGY: Most infarcts caused by thrombosis are anemic or bland and are difficult to see grossly for several hours, after which softening and discoloration are increasingly prominent (Fig. 32-26B). Swelling and liquefaction follow within 3–5 days, when the patient is in danger from the mass effect of the infarct. The infarct then matures over weeks to months into a cystic space (Fig. 32-27), sometimes accompanied by compensatory ventricular enlargement. If blood flow is restored to a bland infarct, as may occur in embolic or compressive vascular disease, blood may seep into the softened tissues. This may cause a hemorrhagic infarct, which is readily discernible grossly and radiologically (Fig. 32-28).

As in other tissues, an orderly procession of pathologic changes allows estimation of an infarct's age. If a patient survives for minutes to several hours, no changes are seen. If the patient survives for 6–24 hours, the infarct is slightly discolored and softened with blurring of the border between gray and white matter. Shrunken eosinophilic neurons ("red neurons") with nuclear pyknosis are present in the infarct (Fig. 32-29). These changes become more pronounced as the infarct ages. By 24–72 hours, neutrophils infiltrate the tissue and blood vessels are prominent. The tissue is soft and edematous and may be sufficiently swollen to cause lethal mass effect.

By 3–4 days, macrophages replace neutrophils and clear debris in the infarct at a rate of about 1 mL per month. The infarct is now frankly mushy. In the second week, proliferating astrocytes join the macrophages. Over weeks to months, these astrocytes form a dense fibrillary glial meshwork around the dead tissue. The macrophages

dispose of debris in the infarct over weeks to months. Simultaneously, the infarct evolves into a glial lined cyst, crossed at points by delicate glial sheets and small vessels and invested with residual lipid and hemosiderin-laden macrophages.

CLINICAL FEATURES: The diversity of neurologic deficits caused by strokes reflects the functional eloquence of the brain. For example, the lengthy and slender striate arteries, which take origin from the proximal middle cerebral artery, are commonly occluded by atherosclerosis and thrombosis. Resultant infarcts often impact the internal capsule to produce hemiplegia (Fig. 32-26A). Similarly, the middle cerebral artery trifurcation is a favored site for lodgment of emboli and for thrombosis due to atherosclerosis. Middle cerebral artery occlusion at this site deprives much of the lateral hemispheric cortex of blood, producing motor and sensory deficits. If the dominant hemisphere is involved, aphasia may develop.

Localized ischemia may be associated with three distinct clinical syndromes:

■ **Transient ischemic attack (TIA)** is focal cerebral dysfunction, lasting under 24 hours, and often only a few minutes. Although complete neurologic recovery follows, TIA heralds increased risk of cerebral infarction. TIAs, like angina, are warnings that all is not well with the cerebral blood supply. Their occurrence often triggers diagnostic and therapeutic activity. A patient with TIAs is at risk for later cerebral infarction; about 1/3 of patients with TIAs will have a stroke within 5 years. The period of highest risk is the first 30 days after TIAs begin; in 1/3 of patients,

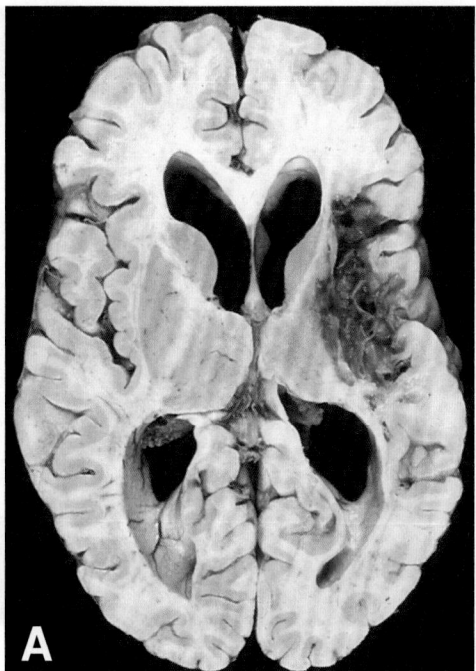
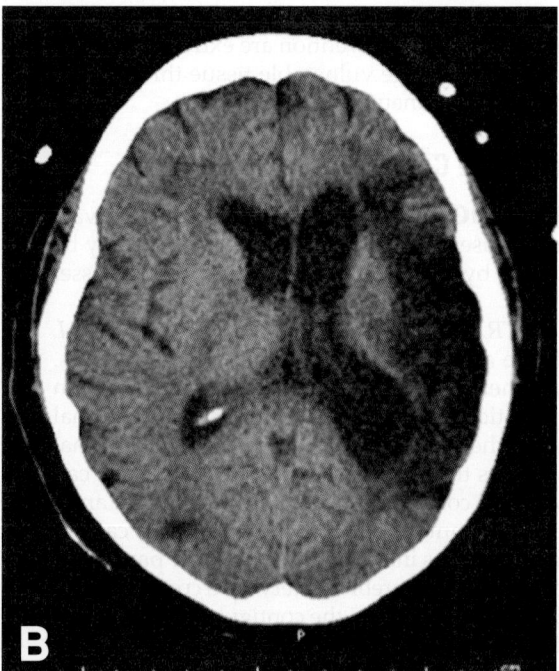

FIGURE 32-27. A. Remote middle cerebral artery distribution infarct. An axial section of the brain shows a remote middle cerebral artery distribution cystic infarct. The brain in Fig. 28-26B would transform to this state as a result of clearing out of the large infarct by macrophages. (Courtesy of Dr. F. Stephen Vogel, Duke University.) **B.** Axial noncontrast computed tomography showing a remote middle cerebral artery distribution infarct resulting from a cardiogenic embolus. Note the low signal in the middle cerebral artery territory and the compensatory enlargement of the ventricles.

the TIAs will simply continue; and about 1/3 of patients will have no more TIAs, nor will they suffer a stroke. *TIAs often are harbingers of a stroke, but many people (50%–85%) who develop cerebral infarcts never have a preceding TIA.* If a TIA lasts more than a few minutes, some tissue damage occurs as evidenced by MRI abnormalities on diffusion water inversion (DWI) sequences.

■ **Stroke in evolution** describes the often stuttering progression of neurologic symptoms as a patient is being observed. This clinically unstable situation reflects propagation of a thrombus in the carotid or basilar arteries and necessitates urgent treatment.

■ **Completed stroke** describes a stable or fixed neurologic deficit caused by a cerebral infarct. Two to three days after a completed stroke, there can be sufficient cerebral cytotoxic and vasogenic edema in the infarct that increased intracranial pressure and herniation become issues.

Our improved understanding of the basic pathophysiology of stroke has resulted in major advances in diagnosis and therapeutic intervention operating in a critical time window.

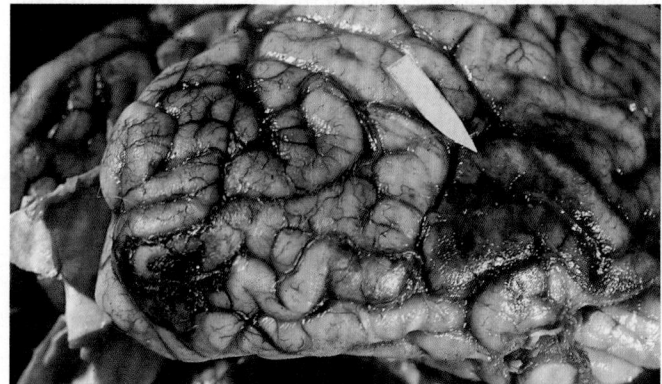

FIGURE 32-28. Hemorrhagic embolic infarct. Emboli from a carotid endarterectomy resulted in hemorrhagic infarcts in the territory of the middle cerebral artery (*arrow*). Such hemorrhagic infarcts may expand because of seepage of blood or frank hemorrhage and become life-threatening.

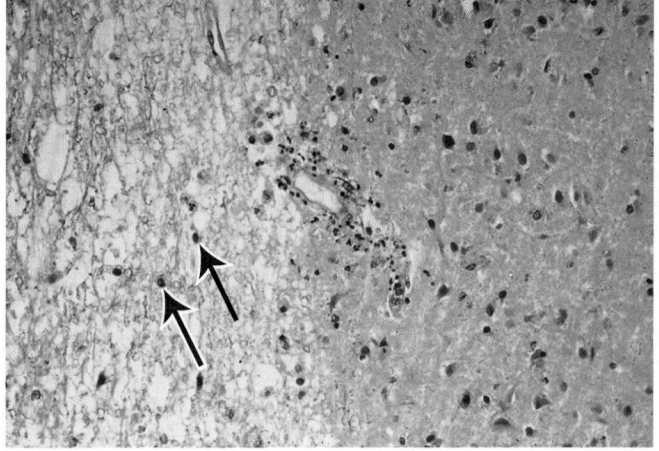

FIGURE 32-29. Acute cerebral infarct histopathology. An 18-hour-old cerebral infarct (*left*) shows edema, hypereosinophilic neurons and perivascular polymorphonuclear leukocytes. Pyknotic nuclei of dying neurons are shown (*arrows*).

Efforts directed at restoring circulation pharmacologically and through endovascular intervention are extremely promising, as are efforts to salvage vulnerable tissue through the use of neuroprotectant maneuvers.

Regional Occlusive Cerebrovascular Disease

 PATHOLOGY: The various occlusive cerebrovascular diseases that lead to cerebral infarcts may be classified by the caliber and nature of the vessel involved.

LARGE EXTRACRANIAL AND INTRACRANIAL ARTERIES: These arteries are often sites of atherosclerosis. Most notably, atherosclerotic plaques occur frequently in the common carotid artery at its bifurcation into external and internal branches. Occlusion or stenosis of an internal carotid artery affects the ipsilateral hemisphere, but this can be offset by variable collateral circulation through the anterior and posterior communicating arteries. Usually, carotid artery occlusion produces infarcts limited to all or part of the distribution of the middle cerebral artery. The consequences of large vessel disease depend on the configuration of the circle of Willis. Thus, a large anterior communicating artery can furnish collateral circulation to a frontal lobe whose blood supply is compromised by internal carotid artery occlusion. The middle cerebral artery is most often occluded by thrombosis complicating atherosclerosis in the circle of Willis. As a major stepdown in vascular caliber occurs at the trifurcation of the middle cerebral artery, this is the main site occluded by emboli.

While atherosclerosis is the primary substrate of ischemic stroke, both arterial dissection and vasculitis may also lead to stroke.

PARENCHYMAL ARTERIES AND ARTERIOLES: These vessels are less often severely atherosclerotic, but they are damaged by hypertension and can be narrowed by atherosclerosis. This causes small infarcts in the territories of the deep penetrating vessels. These **lacunar infarcts** are usually less than 15 mm. Depending on the functions of the small region supplied, symptoms can range from none to profound—contralateral hemiparesis from an infarct in the internal capsule or pure hemisensory loss caused by a thalamic lacunar infarct. When multiple, these minute infarcts can lead to impaired cognition, called **multiple infarct dementia**.

Hypertensive encephalopathy describes the acute neurologic complications of malignant hypertension. As in other affected organs, malignant hypertension can cause fibrinoid necrosis of small arteries and arterioles, as well as minute hemorrhages **(petechiae)**. Cerebral edema may complicate the vascular pathology. Hypertensive encephalopathy usually presents as headache and vomiting that progress to coma and death. With modern antihypertensive therapy, malignant hypertension is uncommon.

MICROCIRCULATION: Small emboli, composed, for example, of fat or air, may occlude capillaries. **Fat emboli,** usually from fractured bones, travel through cerebral vessels until the size of the emboli exceeds that of the blood vessel, at which point they lodge and block blood flow. The distal capillary endothelium becomes hypoxic and permeable, and petechiae develop, mostly in the white matter (Fig. 32-30). **Air emboli** liberate many bubbles that further fragment as they encounter vascular bifurcations, until they impede vascular flow in small blood vessels. In this

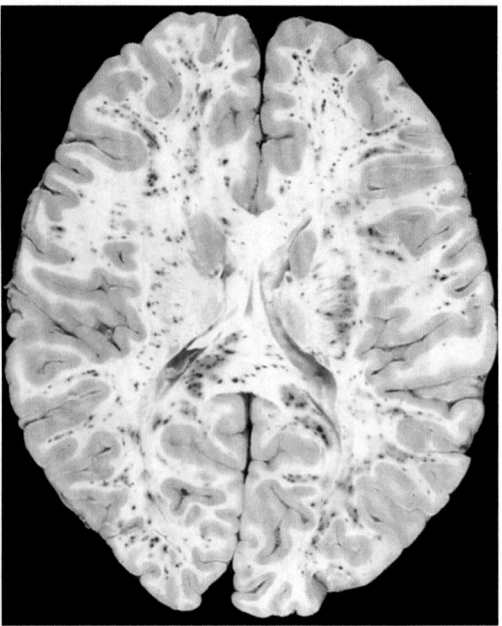

FIGURE 32-30. Fat emboli. An axial section of the brain in a patient with polytrauma with multiple bone fractures leading to cerebral fat emboli manifested by numerous small petechiae throughout the white matter where the small emboli lodge in the microcirculation. (Courtesy of Dr. F. Stephen Vogel, Duke University.)

situation, petechiae are less restricted to white matter than those caused by fat emboli.

VENOUS CIRCULATION: The cerebral veins empty into large venous sinuses, the largest of which is the sagittal sinus, which accommodates venous drainage from the superior aspects of the cerebral hemispheres. Venous sinus thrombosis in the brain is a potentially lethal complication of systemic dehydration, phlebitis caused by adjacent infections like mastoiditis, obstruction by a neoplasm such as a meningioma or sickle cell disease. Since venous obstruction causes stagnation upstream, abrupt sagittal sinus thrombosis leads to bilateral frontal lobe region hemorrhagic infarction (Fig. 32-31). More protracted occlusion of the sinus (e.g., due to invasion by a meningioma) allows recruitment of collateral circulation through the inferior sagittal sinus, which lies at the lower edge of the falx and empties into the straight sinus.

Intracranial Hemorrhage Can Be Intraparenchymal or in the Subarachnoid Space

 **ETIOLOGIC FACTORS:** Intraparenchymal hemorrhage is called intracerebral hemorrhage and usually results from rupture of small fragile vessels or vascular malformations. Subarachnoid hemorrhage is mostly caused by rupture of aneurysms or vascular malformations.

Intracerebral Hemorrhage

 PATHOLOGY: Cerebral hemorrhages that occur without trauma are usually caused by vascular malformations or are due to long-standing hypertension. **Hypertensive intracerebral hemorrhage (ICH)** occurs at preferential sites, which in order of frequency are

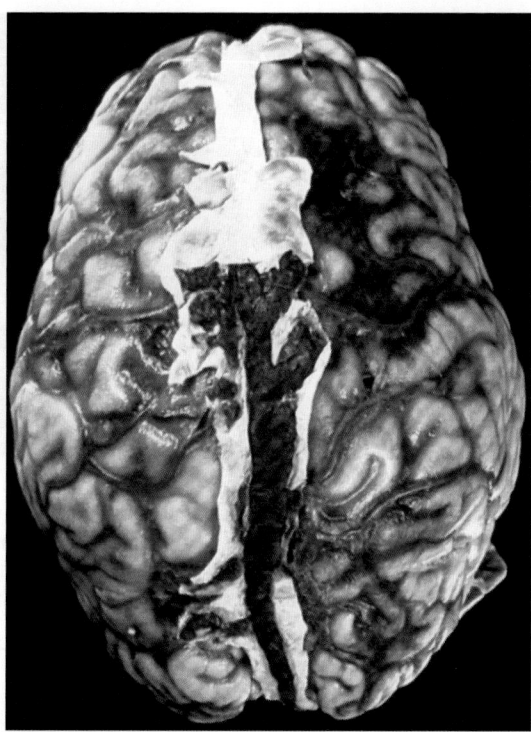

FIGURE 32-31. Superior sagittal sinus thrombosis. Upon opening of the superior sagittal sinus, a thrombus filling the sinus is seen. The thrombus impeded venous drainage of the cerebral hemisphere, leading to bilateral hemorrhagic infarcts of the cerebral hemispheres. Venous thrombosis is seen in hypercoagulable states such as dehydration, pregnancy, hereditary defects of thrombolysis, sickle cell disease or extension of an infection or neoplasm into the sinus. (Courtesy of Dr. F. Stephen Vogel, Duke University.)

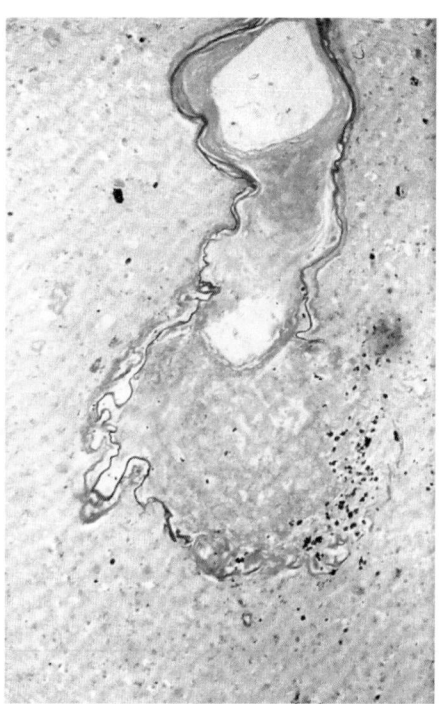

FIGURE 32-32. Charcot-Bouchard aneurysm. The combination of small penetrating cerebral vessels and high perfusion pressure leads to small microaneurysms that may rupture, leading to intracerebral hemorrhage. Effective treatment of hypertension reduces the formation of microaneurysms and the frequency of intracerebral hemorrhage. (Courtesy of Dr. F. Stephen Vogel, Duke University.)

(1) basal ganglia–thalamus (65%), (2) pons (15%) and (3) cerebellum (8%). Hypertensive ICH can also occur in the white matter of cerebral hemispheres, where it is called **lobar ICH**. Lobar ICH should suggest possible amyloid angiopathy, vascular malformation, coagulopathy or bleeding into a tumor, as well as simple hypertensive hemorrhage.

Hypertension compromises the integrity of cerebral arterioles by causing lipid and hyaline material to deposit in their walls: **lipohyalinosis**. Weakening of the wall leads to formation of **Charcot-Bouchard aneurysms,** which occur mainly along the trunk of an arteriole rather than sites where it bifurcates (Fig. 32-32).

 CLINICAL FEATURES: The onset of symptoms of a hypertensive cerebral hemorrhage is abrupt. A patient may clutch his head complaining of severe headache and lapse into coma. Basal ganglion hypertensive intracerebral hemorrhages may cause contralateral hemiparesis. If a hematoma progressively expands, as is common in the first day, death may occur when it reaches a critical volume of about 30 mL. An enlarging hematoma may cause death by transtentorial herniation. Rupture into a lateral ventricle may lead to massive intraventricular hemorrhage (Fig. 32-33).

INTRAVENTRICULAR HEMORRHAGE: Extension of the ICH into a ventricle rapidly distends the entire ventricular system with blood, including the fourth ventricle (Fig. 32-34). The blood may emerge from the foramina of Magendie and Luschka. Death may result from distention of the fourth ventricle and compression of vital centers in the

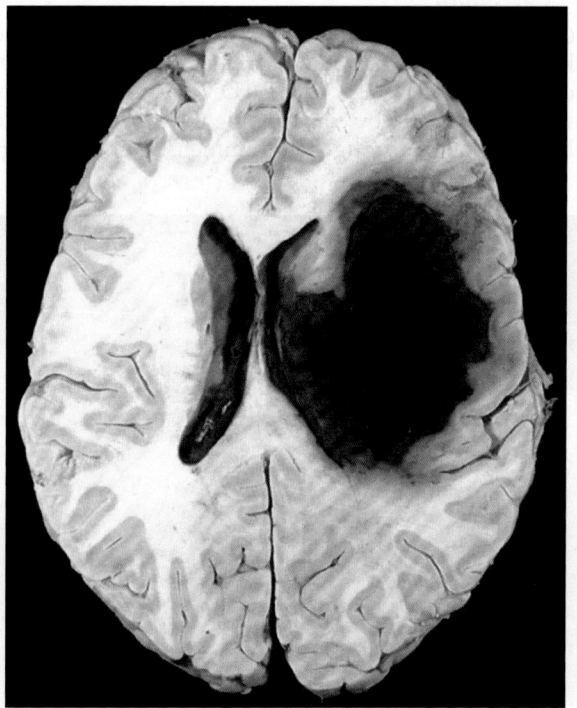

FIGURE 32-33. Intracerebral hemorrhage in the basal ganglia. A hypertensive patient bled into the basal ganglia, resulting in acute severe headache, contralateral hemiparesis and rapid decline in level of consciousness. The deep cerebral nuclei (basal ganglia) and thalamus are the most common locations of intracerebral hemorrhages. (Courtesy of Dr. F. Stephen Vogel, Duke University.)

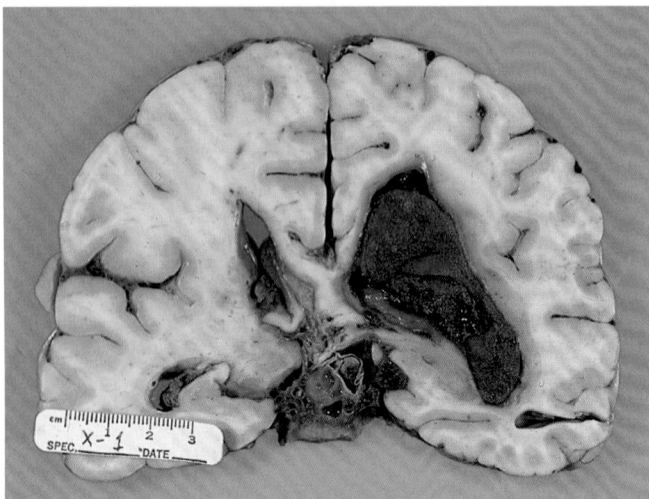

FIGURE 32-34. Intraventricular hemorrhage. A sagittal section of the brain shows ventricular chambers filled with blood that extended from a more anterior basal ganglionic intracerebral hemorrhage. The patient died rapidly from compression of the brainstem by blood in the fourth ventricle.

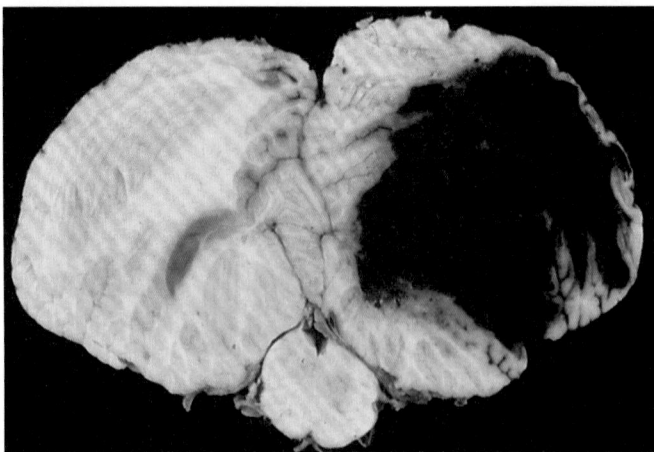

FIGURE 32-36. Cerebellar hemorrhage. Intracerebral hemorrhage in the cerebellum leads to acute-onset occipital headache, nausea, vomiting, vertigo and ataxia. If the hematoma expands rapidly, fatal compression of the medulla may ensue. Surgical evacuation of the cerebellar intracranial hemorrhage can be life saving and is a neurosurgical emergency. (Courtesy of Dr. F. Stephen Vogel, Duke University.)

medulla. Ventricular drainage allows reduction of intracranial pressure and removal of intraventricular blood.

PONTINE HEMORRHAGE: In this catastrophic event, loss of consciousness reflects damage to the reticular formation, an injury that overshadows all other specific cranial nerve deficits. The hemorrhage generally starts in the midpons (Fig. 32-35). It encroaches upon vital medullary centers with minimal enlargement, commonly causing death or severe disability.

CEREBELLAR HEMORRHAGE: Bleeding into the cerebellum leads to abrupt ataxia with a severe occipital headache and vomiting (Fig. 32-36). The expanding hematoma threatens life acutely by compressing the medulla or via cerebellar herniation through the foramen magnum. Surgical

evacuation of the hematoma is life saving and may leave few serious neurologic deficits, while surgical intervention for intracerebral hematomas in other locations has little or no demonstrated benefit.

Causes of spontaneous cerebral hemorrhages other than hypertension include leakage from an arteriovenous malformation, erosion of a blood vessel by a primary or secondary neoplasm, endothelial injury such as occurs in rickettsial infections, a bleeding diathesis or embolic infarction with consequent hemorrhage into the area of necrosis (hemorrhagic conversion).

AMYLOID ANGIOPATHY: This vascular change results from deposition of β-amyloid protein in vascular walls, rendering them weak and friable (Fig. 32-37). Small

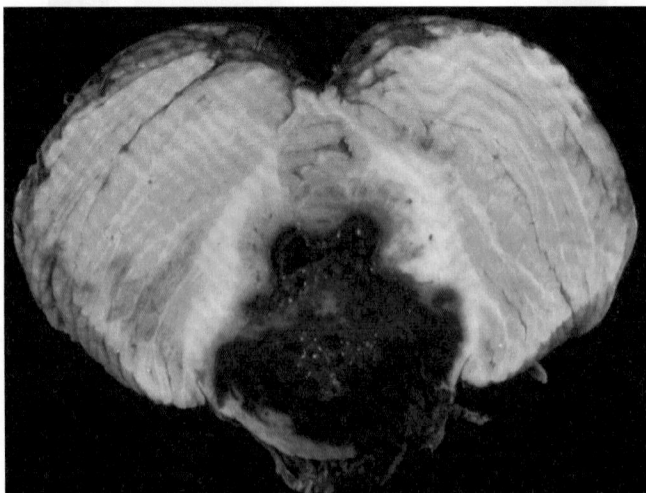

FIGURE 32-35. Pontine hemorrhage. Rupture of microaneurysms in the pons leads to rapid decline in level of consciousness as a result of disruption of the reticular activating system. Multiple cranial neuropathies, dysconjugate gaze, pupillary abnormalities, paralysis and dysregulation of respiration and cardiovascular systems are common. This is the second most common location of intracranial hemorrhage, and hemorrhage in the pons is often lethal. (Courtesy of Dr. F. Stephen Vogel, Duke University.)

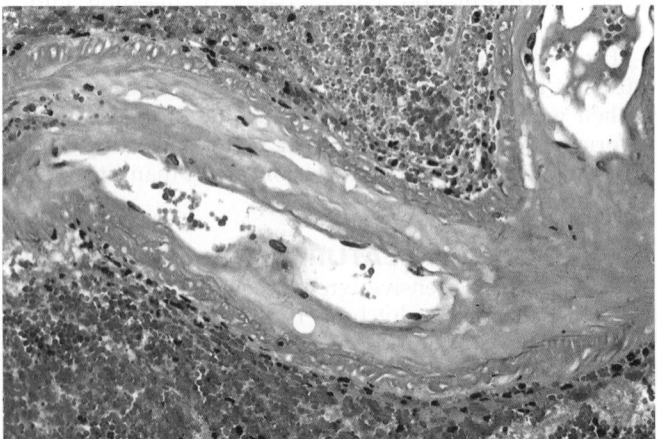

FIGURE 32-37. Amyloid angiopathy. While hypertension is the most common cause of intracerebral hemorrhage in the classic locations—basal ganglia and thalamus, pons and cerebellum—hemorrhage in the white matter of the cerebral hemispheres has a broader range of possible etiologies. These hemorrhages, called lobar hemorrhages, may be caused by amyloid angiopathy in which β-amyloid protein is deposited in the walls of vessels, rendering them weak and friable. This is the same protein as is involved in plaque formation in Alzheimer disease; amyloid angiopathy and Alzheimer disease frequently coexist.

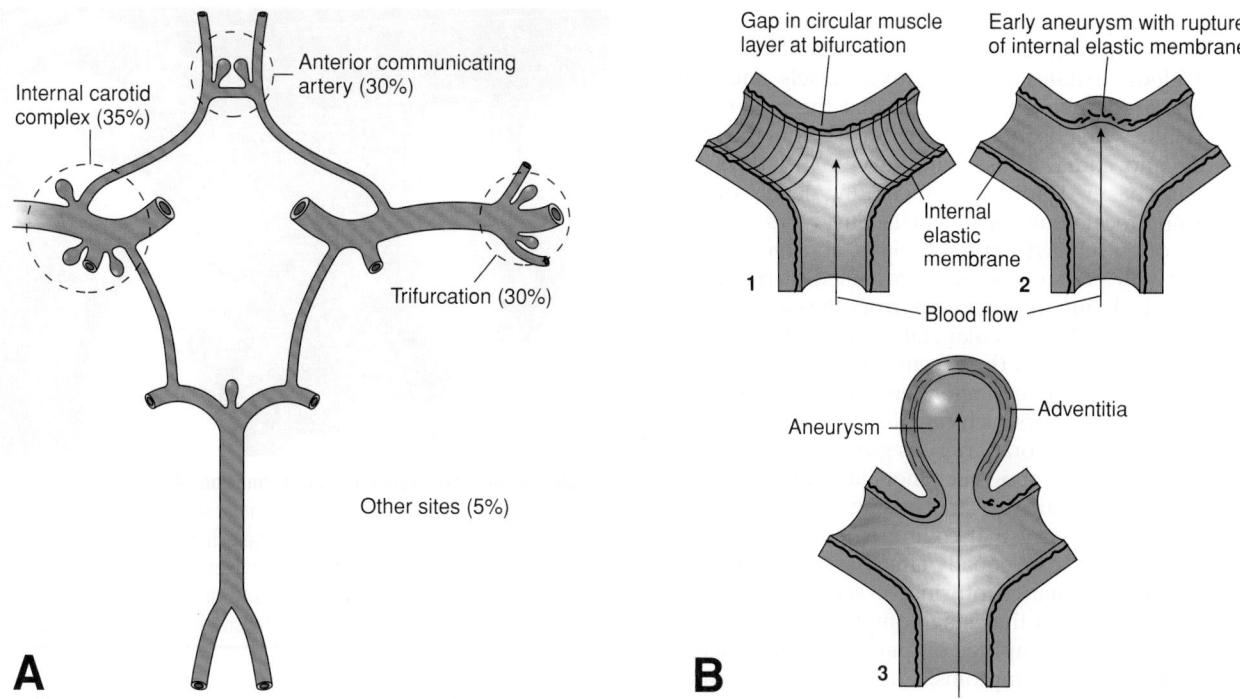

FIGURE 32-38. Pathophysiology of saccular aneurysm. A. The incidence of saccular aneurysms (berry aneurysms), which preferentially involve the proximal carotid tributaries, is shown. **B.** The lesion evolves as a result of blood under pressure acting on an early embryonic defect of the vascular wall at bifurcations.

intraparenchymal vessels in the lobar white matter are most affected, and their rupture may lead to lobar ICH. Amyloid angiopathy becomes more common with advancing age. It is an important cause of ICH in the elderly, in whom it may coexist with Alzheimer disease, in which β-amyloid protein processing is abnormal (see below).

Subarachnoid Hemorrhage

Intravascular pressure and weakness in arterial walls lead to formation of cerebral aneurysms that may rupture, leading to subarachnoid hemorrhage (SAH). Ruptured aneurysms cause about 85% of SAH, while vascular malformations account for 15%.

Saccular (Berry) Aneurysms

Saccular aneurysms are balloon-like outpouchings of cerebral arteries that may rupture to cause catastrophic subarachnoid hemorrhage. They tend to occur at branch points of the cerebral vasculature in or near the circle of Willis (Fig. 32-38).

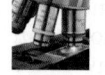 **PATHOLOGY:** When a developing blood vessel bifurcates into two branches, the muscularis layer may not adequately span the branch point. This leaves an area of congenital muscularis thinning, covered only by endothelium, the internal elastic membrane and a thin adventitia. Over time, pressure from the pulsatile blood flow from the parent vessel enlarges the defect. The internal elastic membrane may degenerate or fragment, after which a saccular aneurysm evolves that is precariously covered only by a layer of adventitia. Active vascular wall remodeling may contribute to the aneurysm's evolution.

More than 90% of saccular aneurysms occur at proximal branch points in the anterior circulation fed by the carotid system; however, some may arise on branches of the posterior circulation, particularly on the posterior communicating

and posterior cerebral arteries (Fig. 32-39). They are equally distributed at the junctions of the (1) anterior cerebral and anterior communicating arteries, (2) internal carotid–posterior communicating–anterior cerebral–anterior choroidal arteries and (3) trifurcation of the middle cerebral artery. In 15%–20% of cases, there are multiple aneurysms. The incidence of cerebral aneurysms is increased in polycystic kidney disease, coarctation of the aorta and Ehlers-Danlos syndrome.

 CLINICAL FEATURES: Rupture of a saccular aneurysm leads to life-threatening SAH, with 35% mortality due to the initial hemorrhage. Blood may

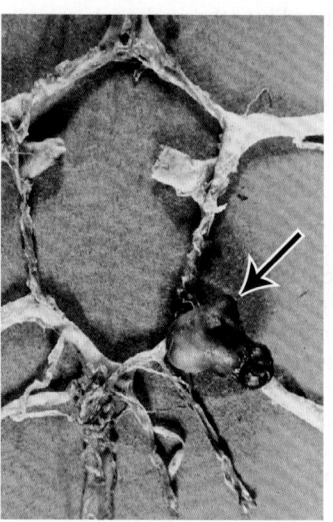

FIGURE 32-39. Berry aneurysm. A saccular aneurysm (*arrow*) arises from the posterior cerebral artery. The dark color is a result of subarachnoid blood from this aneurysm that ruptured.

jet under arterial pressure to produce intracerebral or intraventricular hemorrhage in up to 1/3 of patients. The subarachnoid blood irritates pain-sensitive vessels and dura, leading to a sudden severe headache that the patient may describe as "the worst headache in my life," before then lapsing rapidly into coma. Those who survive 3–4 days may develop vasospasm, leading to fluctuating levels of consciousness and focal neurologic deficits. Survivors of the initial episode often rebleed within 21 days, and half of those who rebleed will perish. Therapy is directed at preventing rebleeding by isolating the aneurysm from the circulation by surgical occlusion of the vascular stalk or neck that connects the sac of the aneurysm to the parent vessel. A metallic clip across the neck of the aneurysm renders the aneurysm bloodless. An endovascular approach can also be taken: a catheter inserted through the femoral artery is guided to the cerebral circulation. Thin thrombogenic metallic coils are then threaded into the aneurysm sac, causing the blood in the aneurysm to clot. Aneurysmal coiling is less invasive than clipping and appears to be equally effective and durable.

At times, rather than rupturing, a saccular aneurysm enlarges to form a mass that may compress cranial nerves and produce palsies or impinge on parenchymal structures and induce neurologic symptoms. Classically, for example, a posterior communicating artery aneurysm may compress the third cranial nerve, leading to an isolated oculomotor nerve palsy with dilated pupil.

Mycotic (Infectious) Aneurysms

Bacterial or fungal infections of an arterial wall may cause a focal dilatation called a mycotic aneurysm. These usually result from septic emboli originating in an infected cardiac valve. The embolus usually flows through the carotid circulation and lodges in the vasa vasorum of a distal branch of the middle cerebral artery, where microbes proliferate, induce inflammation and destroy the affected arterial wall. This forms an aneurysm. Mycotic aneurysms occur in the distal cerebral circulation, unlike saccular aneurysms, which occur proximally. Rupture of the aneurysm can cause intracerebral or subarachnoid hemorrhage. Alternatively, microorganisms may be released and produce a cerebral abscess or meningitis.

Atherosclerotic Aneurysms

Aneurysms caused by atherosclerosis occur mainly in major cerebral arteries (vertebral, basilar, internal carotid) that are favored sites of atherosclerosis. Fibrous replacement of the media and destruction of the internal elastic membrane weaken the arterial wall and cause aneurysmal dilation. As they enlarge, atherosclerotic aneurysms tend to be fusiform and elongate. An enlarging atherosclerotic aneurysm may compress cranial nerves or parenchyma, leading to focal neurologic deficits. Thus, atherosclerotic aneurysms of the basilar artery may encroach upon the cerebellopontine angle, compressing the eighth cranial nerve, and causing deafness and vertigo. Basilar aneurysms may compress cranial nerve V, leading to trigeminal neuralgia, or cranial nerve VII, leading to hemifacial spasm. Atherosclerotic aneurysms rarely rupture leading to subarachnoid hemorrhage, but intraplaque hemorrhage may lead to vascular occlusion or a complicated plaque may lead to arterial thrombosis and ischemic stroke.

Vascular Malformations

Vascular malformations arise during embryogenesis but evolve during angiogenesis, vascular remodeling and

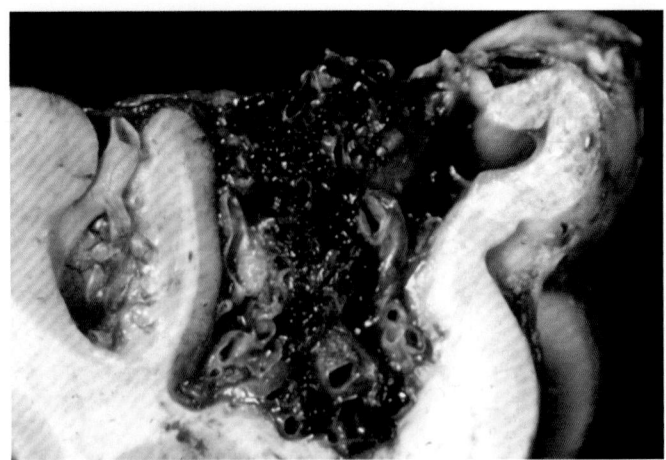

FIGURE 32-40. Arteriovenous malformation (AVM). A disorganized collection of arteries and veins is seen within the substance of the brain extending to the surface. AVMs may result in subarachnoid hemorrhage if they bleed on the surface or intraparenchymal hemorrhage if deeper vascular channels rupture. The hemorrhage is usually not as catastrophic as that seen in aneurysm subarachnoid hemorrhage or hypertensive intracerebral hemorrhage.

recruitment of vessels from normal parenchyma. They are named according to the nature of vascular channels in the malformation and the intervening neuroglial parenchyma that may be normal, gliotic or absent. Vascular malformations may bleed to cause subarachnoid or intraparenchymal hemorrhage or both. They may also irritate normal cerebral cortex, resulting in seizures, or they may divert blood flow from adjacent structures, leading to focal neurologic deficits.

ARTERIOVENOUS MALFORMATION: An arteriovenous malformation (AVM) is a tangle of arteries and veins of varying caliber and wall thickness separated by abnormal gliotic parenchyma (Fig. 32-40). The abnormal vessels form in embryogenesis from focal communications between cerebral arteries and veins without intervening capillaries. Resulting congeries of abnormal vessels are typically located in the cerebral cortex and the contiguous underlying white matter. AVMs enlarge with time and recruit vessels from adjacent tissue.

 CLINICAL FEATURES: Seizure disorders result from irritation of neural tissue; focal neurologic deficits caused by vascular steal; and intracranial hemorrhages, usually subarachnoid or intracerebral, which commonly arise in the second or third decades. The hemorrhage is not usually catastrophic but may be recurring.

CAVERNOUS ANGIOMA: Cavernous angiomas are wide, irregular, thin-walled vascular channels with no intervening neural parenchyma. They are less common than AVMs. Although most are asymptomatic, they may cause intracranial bleeding, seizures or focal neurologic disturbances. Cavernous angiomata may be multiple in 15%–20% of cases. Many patients have autosomal dominant cerebral cavernous malformations (CCMs), the most common form of which, CCM1, results from *krit* mutations.

TELANGIECTASIA: These are focal aggregates of uniformly dilated, thin-walled, small capillary-sized vessels with normal intervening neural parenchyma. They may very rarely initiate seizures but rupture only infrequently. Telangiectasias are usually discovered incidentally during imaging for other conditions or at autopsy.

VENOUS ANGIOMA: This malformation consists of a solitary or a few enlarged veins residing in normal parenchyma. They are distributed randomly in the spinal cord or brain and are generally asymptomatic.

There have been significant improvements in our understanding of molecular genetic mechanisms underlying vascular remodeling in aneurysm formation and growth, vascular malformations and small vessels exposed to chronic hypertension, so that major advances in the prevention and treatment of hemorrhagic stroke can be expected. Consequently, management of cerebrovascular disorders has moved from pessimistic nihilism toward a scientifically driven, clinically meaningful outlook.

CNS INFECTIONS

Many of the infections of the central nervous system are devastating or lethal if untreated. Their clinical course may be swift and ferocious or indolent and progressive, and can mimic many other disorders. Clinical vigilance, thorough diagnostic evaluation and emphatic therapeutic response, is essential for effective management. The clinical context of nervous system infections is crucial. Patients' age, socioeconomic situation, risky behaviors, immune status and travel history are critical in assessing infections of the CNS. AIDS, chemotherapy, economics, environmental change, bioterrorism, transglobal travel and immigration continue to change the face of infectious diseases.

Evaluation of CNS infections should include the location and extent of the infection, the nature of the host response and the inciting organism.

Empyema in the epidural or subdural space is usually related to trauma or spread from contiguous infection—usually bacterial—in the sinuses or ear.

In leptomeningitis **(meningitis),** the inflammatory response and most of the inciting organisms are in the subarachnoid space, floating in the CSF. The vigor of the inflammatory response may lead to parenchymal involvement including cerebral edema and vasculitis with thrombosis, hemorrhage or infarction. The war between host and organisms may involve the parenchyma, resulting in **cerebritis**. Long-term complications include effusions, obstruction of CSF flow with hydrocephalus and cranial neuropathies, particularly deafness from VIII nerve involvement.

Cerebritis is a purulent parenchymal infection that is usually bacterial or fungal. Brain tissue is soft and soupy and the borders of the infection cannot be easily discerned. If a host can contain the process, the cerebritis is walled off to form a brain abscess. Abscesses have many neutrophils within a necrotic core, surrounded by granulation tissue, a dense fibrovascular capsule and a gliotic rind.

Encephalitis, like cerebritis, is a parenchymal infection, but the term is usually reserved for viral infections with necrosis, perivascular lymphocytic cuffing and microglial nodules. Intranuclear or cytoplasmic viral inclusions may be seen, as may gliosis, demyelination and status spongiosus.

Different classes of infectious organisms produce distinctive host inflammatory responses. While not absolute, the inflammatory reaction provides clues about the inciting organism. Bacteria tend to induce vigorous polymorphonuclear (purulent) responses, while fungi and mycobacteria may elicit more indolent granulomatous reactions. In viral infections, lymphocytic responses predominate, while protozoa tend to incite lymphoplasmacytic infiltrates. Metazoan parasites generate eosinophilic and lymphocytic inflammation. Prions cause no inflammation but rather vigorous gliosis.

Bacterial Infections Produce Inflammation in the Subarachnoid Space

This response, called **leptomeningitis,** occurs between the pia and arachnoid layers of the meninges. The CSF filling this compartment is an excellent culture medium for most bacteria. The inflammatory response in the CSF to infections varies with the virulence of the organism and the tempo of the infection. Changes are detectable in CSF cellular constituents as well as glucose and protein concentrations. Organisms are sometimes visible microscopically in the CSF and can be definitively characterized by culture, antigenicity and in some cases polymerase chain reaction (PCR).

 CLINICAL FEATURES: The signs and symptoms of meningitis include headache, vomiting, fever, altered mental status and seizures. Classic signs of meningeal inflammation include neck rigidity, knee pain with hip flexion (Kernig sign) and knee/hip flexion when the neck is flexed (Brudzinski sign). At the extremes of age—newborn and senescence—clinical manifestations vary more widely. A newborn may have autonomic instability and fragmentary seizures, while the elderly may have altered mental status without fever or headache.

Bacterial Meningitis

 **ETIOLOGIC FACTORS:** Since most bacteria initiate purulent responses, the presence of neutrophils in the CSF is strong evidence of meningitis. CSF glucose will often be decreased and CSF protein elevated. The causes of bacterial meningitis depend on the age of the patient. Gram-negative *Escherichia coli* and β-hemolytic *Streptococcus* sp. predominate in neonates. In unvaccinated young children, *Haemophilus influenza* dominates, but vaccination programs against *H. influenzae* group B have changed the epidemiology, so that *Streptococcus pneumoniae* and *Neisseria meningitidis* are becoming more prevalent. *N. meningitidis* is most common in adolescence and early adult life. *S. pneumoniae* is most common thereafter. Routes of entry to the intracranial vault are shown in Fig. 32-41A.

ESCHERICHIA COLI: In newborns, whose resistance to gram-negative bacteria has not yet fully developed, *E. coli* is a major cause of meningitis. Transplacental transfer of maternal immunoglobulin (Ig) G protects newborns from many bacteria, but *E. coli* and similar gram-negative organisms require IgM for neutralization, and IgM does not cross the placenta. Thus, in infancy, gram-negative organisms quickly produce purulent meningitis with a high mortality.

HAEMOPHILUS INFLUENZAE: Environmental exposure to the gram-negative *H. influenzae* is somewhat delayed. Thus, the incidence of meningitis peaks from 3 months to 3 years. *H. influenza* meningitis has decreased in recent years (see above).

STREPTOCOCCUS PNEUMONIAE: Later in life, *Pneumococcus* is the main cause of meningitis. Patients with a history of basilar skull fracture with CSF leak have a high incidence of pneumococcal meningitis, which often recurs

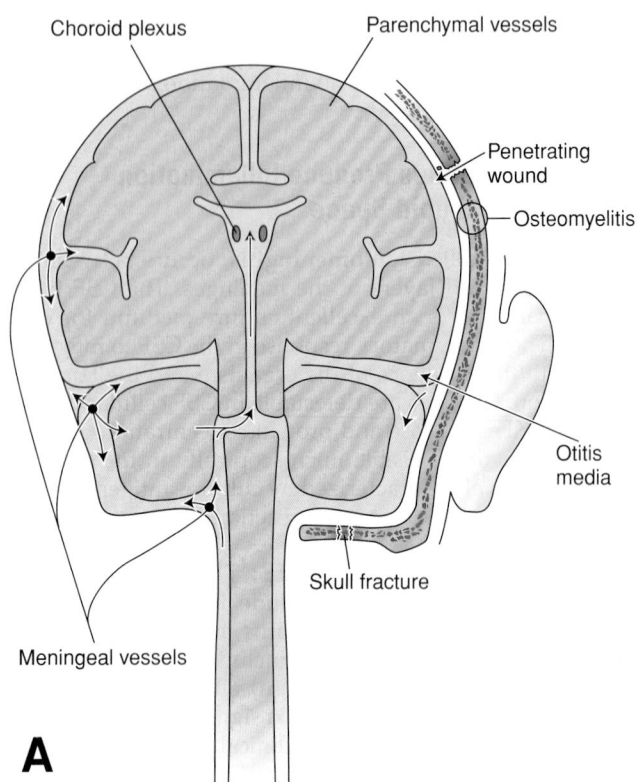

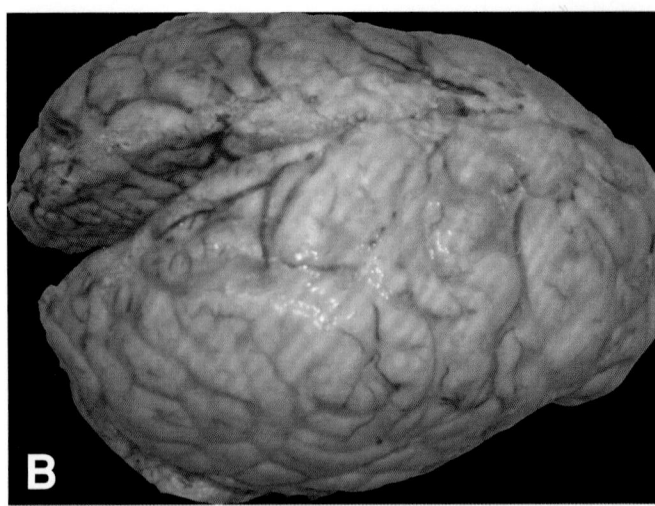

A

FIGURE 32-41. Purulent meningitis. A. Routes of entry of infectious organisms into the cranial cavity. B. A creamy exudate opacifies the leptomeninges in bacterial meningitis. The superficial veins are engorged and may develop thrombosis, and the arteries on the surface of the brain may also develop thrombosis, leading to infarcts.

after treatment. Alcoholics and patients who are asplenic are highly susceptible.

NEISSERIA MENINGITIDIS: The meningococcus resides in the nasopharynx, and airborne transmission in crowded places (e.g., schools or barracks) causes "epidemic meningitis." Initially, bacteremia causes fever, malaise and petechial rash, but intravascular coagulopathy may cause lethal adrenal hemorrhage **(Waterhouse-Friderichsen syndrome)**. Untreated meningococcal bacteremia can trigger acute fulminant meningitis. An available polyvalent vaccine is recommended for all young people and is extremely effective. There are, however, strains of *N. meningitidis* that are not covered by the vaccine. Unfortunately, vaccines are not widely available in many parts of the world. In 1996, sub-Saharan Africa experienced the largest epidemic of meningococcal meningitis in history, with over 250,000 cases and 25,000 deaths.

LISTERIA MONOCYTOGENES: Listerial meningitis is increasing in all ages and may account for up to 10% of bacterial meningitis. Its course is less fulminant than other bacterial meningitides and CSF cellular responses may be lymphocyte predominant.

BACILLUS ANTHRACIS: Anthrax produces a fulminant hemorrhagic meningitis in up to 50% of cases. During the bioterrorism attacks in 2001, the index case was diagnosed as a result of the presence of large gram-positive rods in the CSF. Anthrax is a readily weaponizable biological warfare agent.

 PATHOLOGY: In bacterial meningitis, an exudate of leukocytes and fibrin opacifies the arachnoid. This exudate varies from mild and equivocal to the naked eye to prominent enough to obscure blood vessels. Purulent exudates are most conspicuous over the cerebral hemispheres (Fig. 32-41B) but may extend to the base

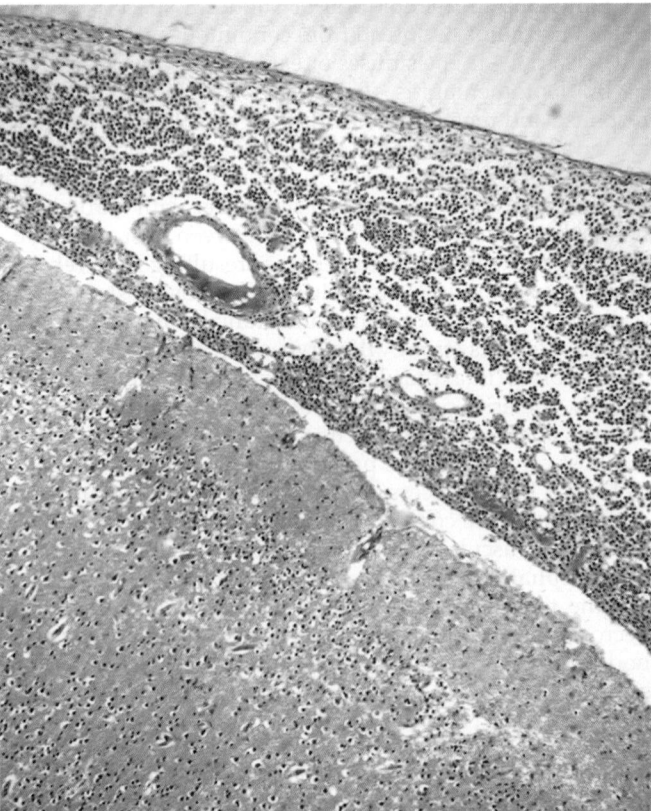

FIGURE 32-42. Bacterial meningitis. A microscopic section shows the accumulation of numerous neutrophils in the subarachnoid space.

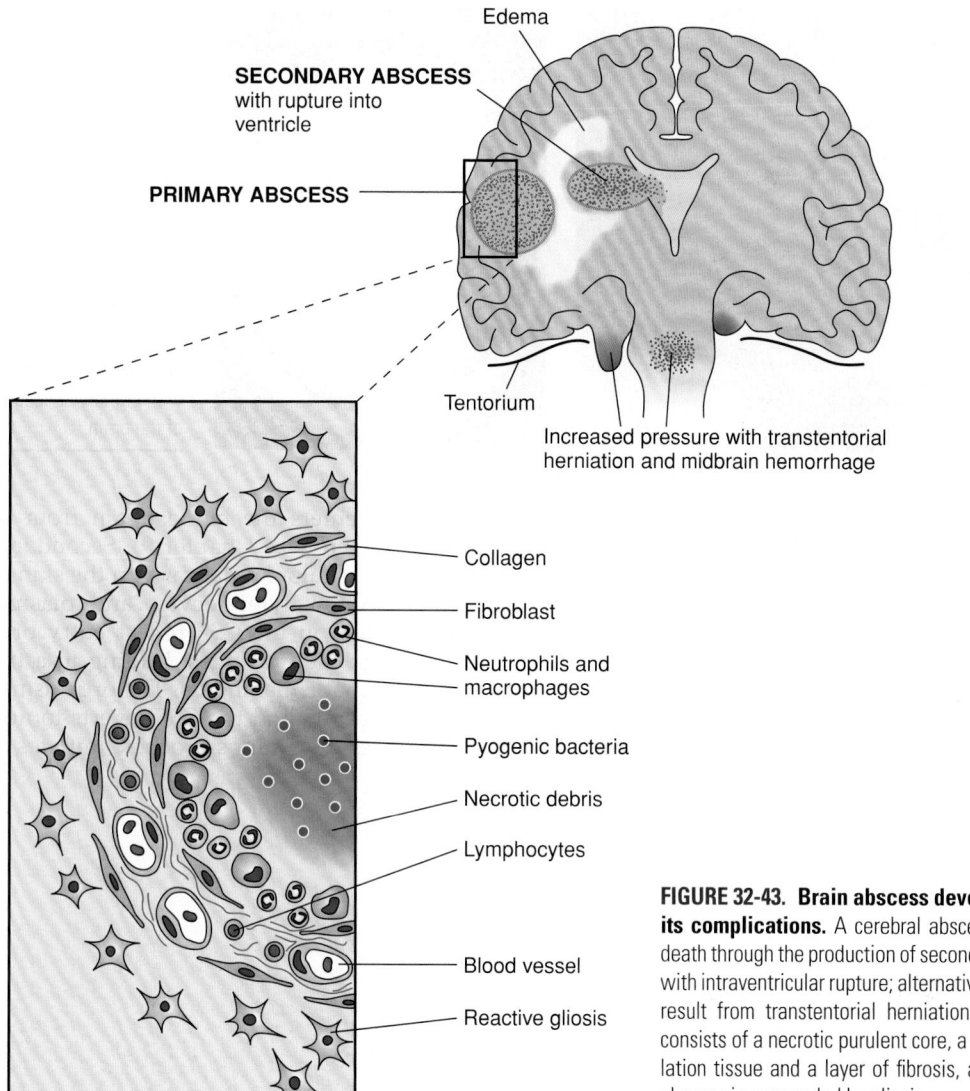

FIGURE 32-43. **Brain abscess development and its complications.** A cerebral abscess may cause death through the production of secondary abscesses with intraventricular rupture; alternatively, death may result from transtentorial herniation. The abscess consists of a necrotic purulent core, a layer of granulation tissue and a layer of fibrosis, and finally, the abscess is surrounded by gliosis.

of the brain and from intracranial to intraspinal and subarachnoid spaces. Cerebral abscesses rarely complicate meningitis. The pia forms sleeves around blood vessels that penetrate the brain **(Virchow-Robin spaces)** in continuity with the subarachnoid space. The subarachnoid space including the Virchow-Robin domain is usually packed with neutrophils and organisms (Fig. 32-42). A vigorous host response is essential to clear the infection, but significant vascular and neuropil damage results from cytotoxic substances such as free radicals and cytokines released by inflammatory cells. Those cells may compete with the brain for glucose; low CSF glucose in bacterial meningitis mostly reflects glucose consumption by inflammatory cells. Corticosteroids may be given with antibiotics to mitigate this host response–induced damage.

Cerebral Abscess

 PATHOLOGY: A localized intraparenchymal abscess begins when bacteria or fungi lodge in the neuropil and incite an acute inflammatory and edematous reaction called **cerebritis**. The tissue is soft and soupy, and within days, liquefactive necrosis causes an expanding mass that may threaten life by herniation or rupture into a ventricle (Fig. 32-43). Vigorous reactive astrogliosis is triggered, and fibroblasts make a rare appearance in the brain by invading from cerebral microvasculature to encapsulate the nascent abscess.

As the abscess matures over days to weeks, three layers surround a central core of purulent debris: (1) an inner layer of vigorous granulation tissue where host and microbes engage in open warfare; (2) a second layer of a dense meshwork of fibroblasts and collagen that forms a tough rind around the core and granulation tissue; and (3) finally a zone of intense astrogliosis, microglial activation and edema (Fig. 32-44). The granulation tissue layer lacks a blood-brain barrier and leaks contrast, to cause a smooth ring of enhancement.

If the abscess is not drained or treated with antibiotics, pressure builds within it that may extrude microbes into adjacent parenchyma to spawn "daughter" abscesses. Or, the abscess may rupture catastrophically into the ventricles. The bacteria that cause brain abscesses are often anaerobic or microaerophilic, and so may be difficult to culture. They often spread to the brain hematogenously from the heart or lungs; as showers of organisms repeatedly enter the circulation, abscesses are multiple in 15%–20% of cases.

THE CENTRAL NERVOUS SYSTEM

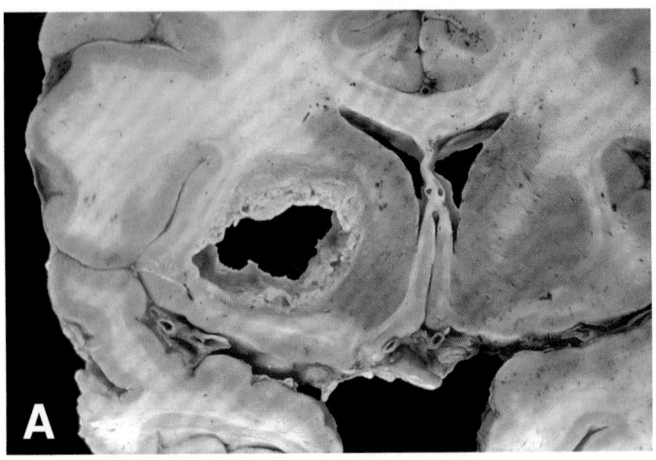

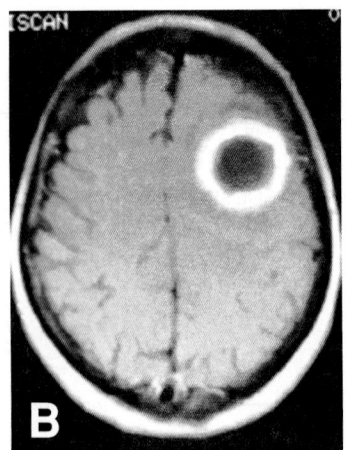

FIGURE 32-44. Cerebral abscess. A. A young man with bacterial endocarditis developed an abscess in the left basal ganglia. **B.** Axial contrast-enhanced computed tomography showing a smooth uniform ring of enhancement around a necrotic core of a brain abscess. A smooth ring-enhancing lesion is very suggestive of a brain abscess but may be seen with primary or secondary neoplasms of the brain.

Brain invasion may also be a result of contiguous spread from infected frontal or mastoid sinuses or neurosurgical wound infections.

Neurosyphilis

Syphilis is caused by a spirochete, *Treponema pallidum.* By aligning its transmission with host carnal impulses, *T. pallidum* has assured its status as a centuries-old scourge of mankind.

The organism enters the bloodstream from the primary lesion, the chancre (see Chapter 9). Secondary syphilis is heralded by a maculopapular rash on the skin and mucous membranes. A few lymphocytes and plasma cells and increased protein in the CSF reflect entry of bloodborne spirochetes into the meninges, leading to a transient and often asymptomatic meningitis. The organisms usually do not survive for long and the CSF reverts to normal. However, sometimes the errant spirochete initiates a meningeal

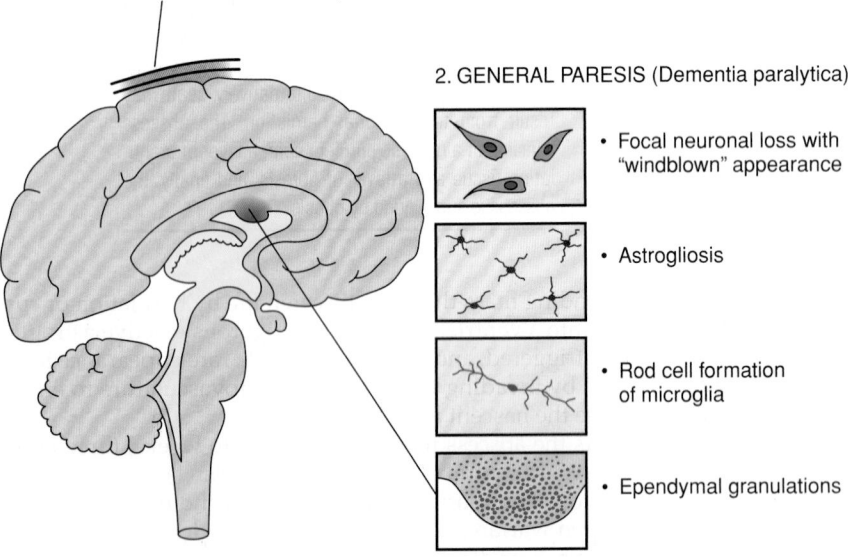

1. MENINGOVASCULAR SYPHILIS
- Thickened meninges
- Obliterative endarteritis with plasma cells

2. GENERAL PARESIS (Dementia paralytica)
- Focal neuronal loss with "windblown" appearance
- Astrogliosis
- Rod cell formation of microglia
- Ependymal granulations

3. TABES DORSALIS (Posterior column degeneration)

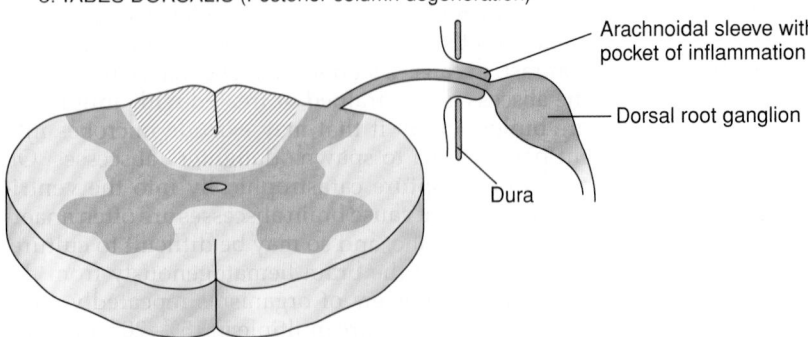

Arachnoidal sleeve with pocket of inflammation

Dorsal root ganglion

Dura

FIGURE 32-45. Involvement of the central nervous system in syphilis. Hallmarks of neurosyphilis are meningovascular inflammation leading to pachymeningitis and strokes caused by obliterative endarteritis, tabes dorsalis caused by inflammation of posterior roots and meninges, and intraparenchymal involvement leading to dementia.

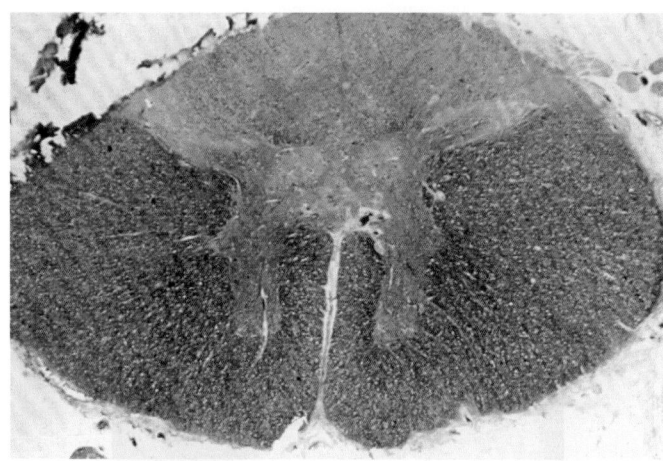

FIGURE 32-46. Tabes dorsalis. The spinal cord of a patient with tertiary syphilis displays posterior column degeneration (sliver impregnation stain). The patient would be unable to walk without visual cues because he has lost proprioception.

fibroblastic response, accompanied by obliterative endarteritis that induces multiple small cerebral cortex or brainstem infarcts. The classical eponymic brainstem strokes described in the 18th and 19th centuries were largely due to an obliterative syphilitic endarteritis. Plasma cells, the inflammatory hallmark of syphilis, surround arterioles of the cerebral cortex in meningovascular syphilis (Fig. 32-45).

Tabes Dorsalis

Tabes dorsalis is impairment of spinal dorsal column function, as manifested by loss of joint position sense and fine touch (Fig. 32-46). The dorsal nerve roots proximal to dorsal root ganglia are met by a conical sleeve of arachnoid filled with CSF, which can be the site of syphilitic inflammation. Fibrous tissue triggered by the inflammation constricts nerve roots, causing axonal (wallerian) degeneration. Since axons that course cephalad in the posterior columns do not synapse with intramedullary neurons, unlike spinothalamic afferents, wallerian degeneration initiated in the dorsal spinal nerves extends the length of the posterior

fasciculi. The patient loses position sense in the legs and comes to rely on visual cues for the position of his or her feet and legs in space. In darkness or with his or her eyes closed, the patient becomes unsteady and may even fall. This inability to remain standing with eyes closed is called a positive Romberg sign and reflects severe posterior column dysfunction.

Luetic Dementia

T. pallidum may remain latent in the brain for decades. The spirochetes replicate sluggishly and escape eradication, resulting in dementia and psychosis years after the initial infection. The morphologic features include focal loss of cortical neurons, disfigurement of residual nerve cells ("wind-blown appearance"), marked gliosis and conversion of microglia into elongated forms encrusted with iron ("rod cells") associated with nodular ependymitis.

Mycobacterial and Fungal Infections Elicit Granulomatous Responses

 PATHOLOGY: Mycobacterial and fungal infections progress more slowly than bacterial infections. Multinucleate giant cells are admixed with lymphocytes and plasma cells. Exudate tends to accumulate at the base of the brain, around the brainstem, rather than over the convexities as in bacterial meningitis.

 CLINICAL FEATURES: This chronic basilar meningitis may block CSF flow through the foramina of Magendie and Luschka, leading to hydrocephalus, headache, nausea and vomiting. Cranial nerve palsies can occur as these nerves traverse the exudate where they emerge from the brainstem.

Tuberculous Meningitis and Tuberculomas

 PATHOLOGY: Tuberculous meningitis is a chronic infection inciting a granulomatous host response with multinucleated giant cells and lymphocytes surrounding areas of caseous necrosis (Fig. 32-47).

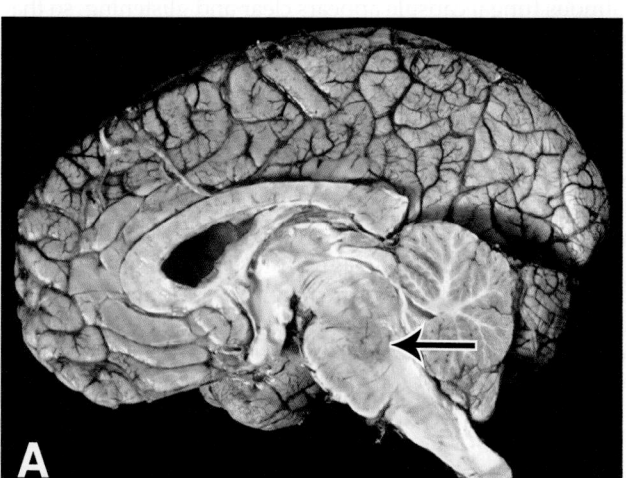

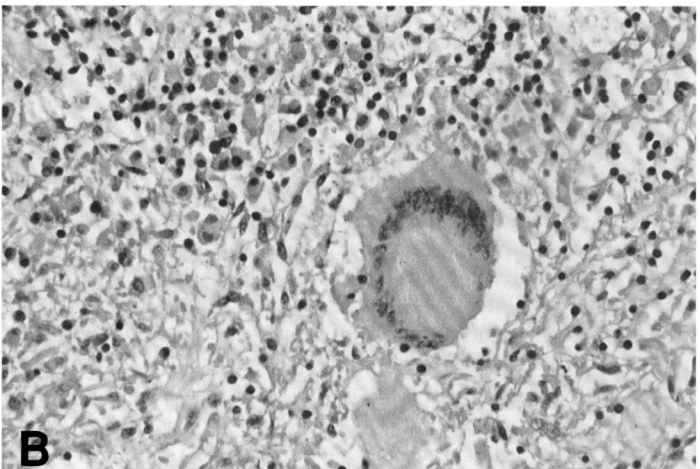

FIGURE 32-47. Tuberculoma. A. A focus of caseous necrosis is present in the pons and midbrain (*arrow*). **B.** A photomicrograph shows caseous necrosis, macrophages and Langhans giant cells in a tuberculoma. If the tuberculoma ruptures into the cerebrospinal fluid, tuberculous meningitis will ensue.

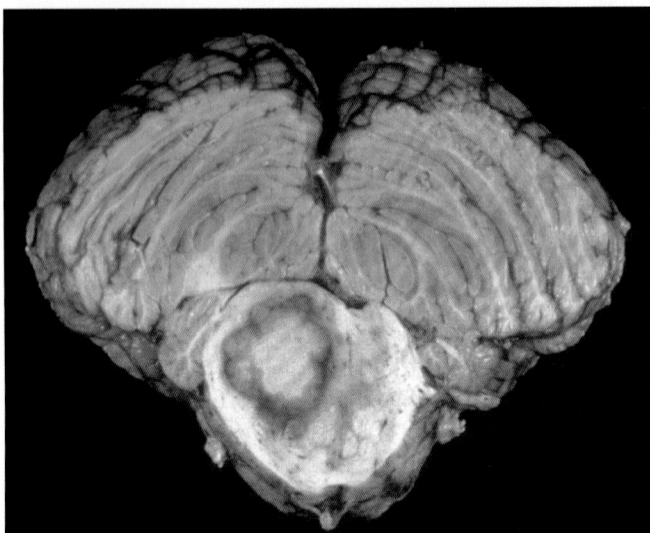

FIGURE 32-48. Tuberculoma. A focus of caseous necrosis is present in the pons and midbrain. In parts of the world where tuberculosis is endemic, tuberculomas are among the most common brain masses seen. (Courtesy of Dr. F. Stephen Vogel, Duke University.)

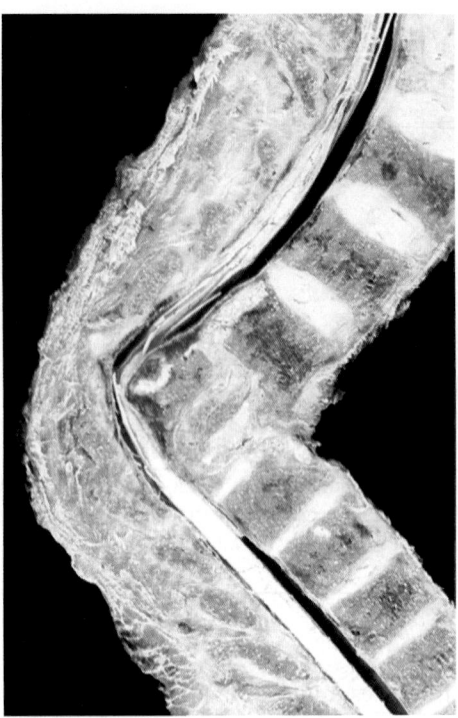

FIGURE 32-49. Pott disease. Tuberculosis involving the spinal column leads to slow vertebral collapse and acute angulation of the spine ("gibbus" deformity). Spinal cord compression may result, with myelopathic findings. (Courtesy of Dr. F. Stephen Vogel, Duke University.)

Like neurosyphilis, mycobacterial meningitis may lead to meningeal fibrosis, communicating hydrocephalus and arteritis that may cause infarcts. As tuberculous meningitis preferentially affects the base of the brain, these infarcts are usually in the distribution of the penetrating striate and brainstem arteries. Untreated tuberculous meningitis is usually fatal in 4–6 weeks but may progress faster in immunocompromised patients. Parenchymal tuberculosis produces **tuberculomas,** individual masses with central caseous necrosis surrounded by granulomatous inflammation (Fig. 32-48). In parts of the world where tuberculosis is endemic, mycobacterial granulomas are the most common brain masses. In childhood, these granulomas congregate in the posterior fossa, which is also the most common site of childhood brain tumors. Confluent tuberculomas occur in miliary tuberculosis. Tuberculous meningitis usually reflects hematogenous dissemination from an initial pulmonary focus, as intraparenchymal granulomas rupture into the CSF to produce meningitis. **Pott disease** is tuberculosis of the spine, in which epidural granulomatous inflammation destroys the bony spine, leading to spinal cord compression (Fig. 32-49).

Fungal Infections

Fungal infections of the CNS are often opportunistic, reflecting the indolent saprophytic lifestyle of these organisms, but a few fungi are sufficiently virulent to cause disease in immunocompetent people. Fungi invading tissue may be round to oval, often budding, yeast forms or branching hyphae. In some infections, yeast and hyphae both appear in infected tissues, facilitating tentative identification of fungi in tissue sections. However, ultimate speciation requires antigenic, PCR or culture confirmation.

Cryptococcus

EPIDEMIOLOGY: Cryptococci are the most common fungal causes of meningitis. *Cryptococcus* often acts opportunistically in immunocompromised

patients, but it can also establish meningitis in an immunologically competent host. *Cryptococcus neoformans* enters the host by inhalation. Birds are the major reservoir, and their inhaled fungus-laden excreta initiate a lung infection that may remain confined to the lungs or may disseminate to involve other organs including the brain.

PATHOLOGY: *C. neoformans* typically elicits granulomatous responses, with infectious foci appearing as discrete white meningeal nodules, about 1 mm. The organism may remain confined to the subarachnoid space, but infection sometimes spreads to the brain parenchyma. The gelatinous fungal capsule appears clear and glistening, so that microabscesses resemble soap bubbles (Fig. 32-50).

C. neoformans may be abundant, particularly in the Virchow-Robin spaces. An occasional multinucleated giant cell, sometimes with phagocytosed organisms, accompanies scant epithelioid cells and a few lymphocytes. The organisms are encapsulated, budding yeast forms that are large by fungal standards (5–15 μ) and have an external gelatinous capsule that looks like a clear halo. The organism can be highlighted by mixing contaminated CSF with India ink (Fig. 32-51). Its capsule shields the organism from host immune responses and accounts for the usually feeble inflammatory reaction. The capsule sheds specific antigens that can be detected in the CSF by the latex cryptococcal antigen test.

Coccidioidomycosis

Coccidioides immitis is endemic in arid regions of the Southwest and San Joaquin Valley in California. Initial pulmonary infection is usually asymptomatic and rarely spreads. It causes suppurative and granulomatous inflammation that

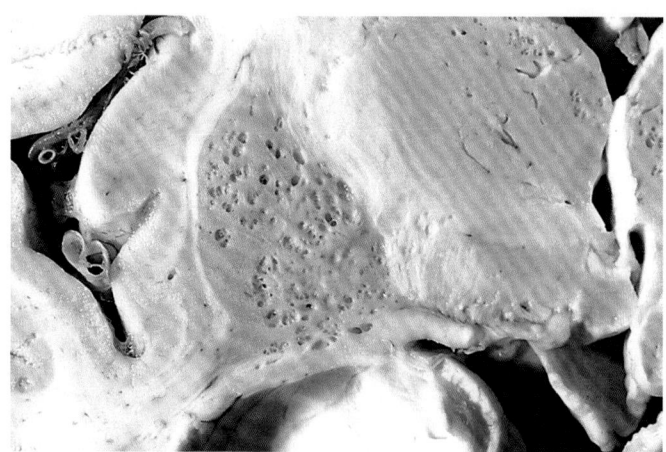

FIGURE 32-50. Cryptococcal "soap bubble" abscesses. The encapsulated organisms occur in great abundance in the Virchow-Robin space and in microabscesses within the parenchyma. The microbial capsule imparts a glistening clear appearance to these collections that has been likened to soap bubbles. (Courtesy of Dr. F. Stephen Vogel, Duke University.)

sometimes includes an arteritis that may be complicated by infarction. The organism appears in tissue as an eye-catching refractile endosporulating spherule.

Histoplasmosis

Histoplasma capsulatum is endemic in the Mississippi basin and usually causes asymptomatic pulmonary infections. Rare CNS dissemination of this tiny, intracytoplasmic yeast form residing in macrophages may occur. A chronic meningitis ensues in which the surface of the brain may be studded by small granulomata.

Blastomycosis

Blastomyces dermatitidis is an uncommon cause of mycotic meningitis. The organisms are broad-based budding yeasts.

Mucormycosis (Zygomycosis)

Fungi of the order *Mucorales* are angioinvasive, nonseptate, hyphal forms that mostly cause disease in

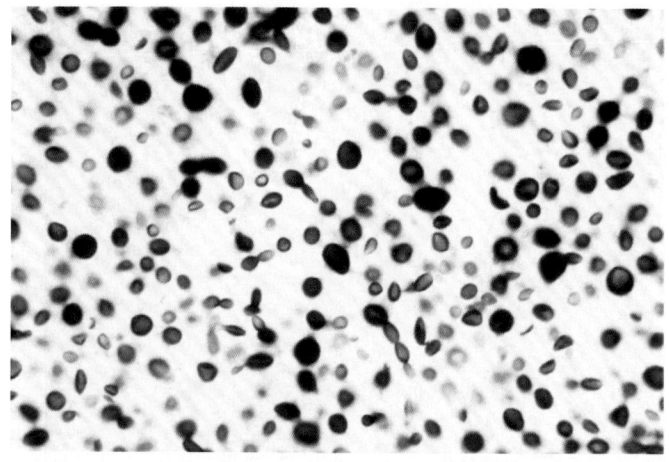

FIGURE 32-51. Cryptococcal meningitis. The cryptococcal organisms vary in size (5–15 microns in diameter), placing them among the largest of the yeast-form fungi (Gomori methenamine silver stain). They reproduce by budding. (Courtesy of Dr. F. Stephen Vogel, Duke University.)

immunocompromised people or those with poorly controlled diabetes. The large vessels at the skull base, orbit and neck are subject to invasion with occlusion and distal infarction. Black nasal mucosa indicating mucosal infarction is sometimes seen and can be used for diagnosis.

Aspergillosis

Aspergillus is an angiocentric septate hyphal fungus (usually, *Aspergillus fumigatus*) that mainly causes disease in immunocompromised hosts. Vascular involvement produces multiple gray necrotic abscesses within the parenchyma. The lung is the primary site of infection, but the brain is the second most commonly involved organ.

Candidiasis

Candida albicans is a ubiquitous opportunistic fungus that shows both yeast and pseudohyphae morphology in infected tissues. *Candida* produces many microabscesses, most often in immunocompromised patients. Systemic involvement is the rule, and in large hospital-based autopsy series, this is the most common systemic fungal infection.

Exserohilum rostratum: Infection from Contaminated Corticosteroid Injections

In 2012 and 2013, a serious epidemic of localized spinal and skull base fungal infections was traced to inadequate quality control in manufacturing of corticosteroids used for local articular, paraspinal and epidural spinal injections for pain. *Exserohilum rostratum,* a pigmented environmental fungus that rarely infects humans, was the culprit in most cases. It produced soft tissue and bone destruction with potential involvement of vertebral and basilar arteries. Approximately 700 patients were affected, with almost 60 deaths. This serious epidemic drew attention to inadequate quality control and nationwide dissemination of contaminated injectable compounds.

CNS Viral Infections Vary in Severity, Time Course and Resolution

The manifestations of viral infections of the CNS are remarkably diverse, ranging from non–life-threatening viral meningitis to more ominous viral encephalitis affecting the parenchyma. These diseases may unfold over a period of hours or span decades. In addition to producing infections, viruses have been implicated in some autoimmune and neurodegenerative diseases.

Viral Meningitis

Unlike bacterial meningitis, viral meningitis is usually benign and resolves without sequelae. The most common causative agents are enteroviruses (e.g., coxsackievirus B, echovirus), but mumps, lymphocytic choriomeningitis, Epstein-Barr and herpes simplex viruses cause many sporadic cases. Viral meningitis (mainly a disease of children and young adults) begins as a sudden febrile illness with a severe headache. The CSF contains excess lymphocytes and a slight increase in protein but, unlike bacterial meningitis, no decrease in CSF glucose.

Viral Encephalitis

The manifestations of viral infections of CNS parenchyma are clinically and pathologically heterogeneous (Fig. 32-52). For

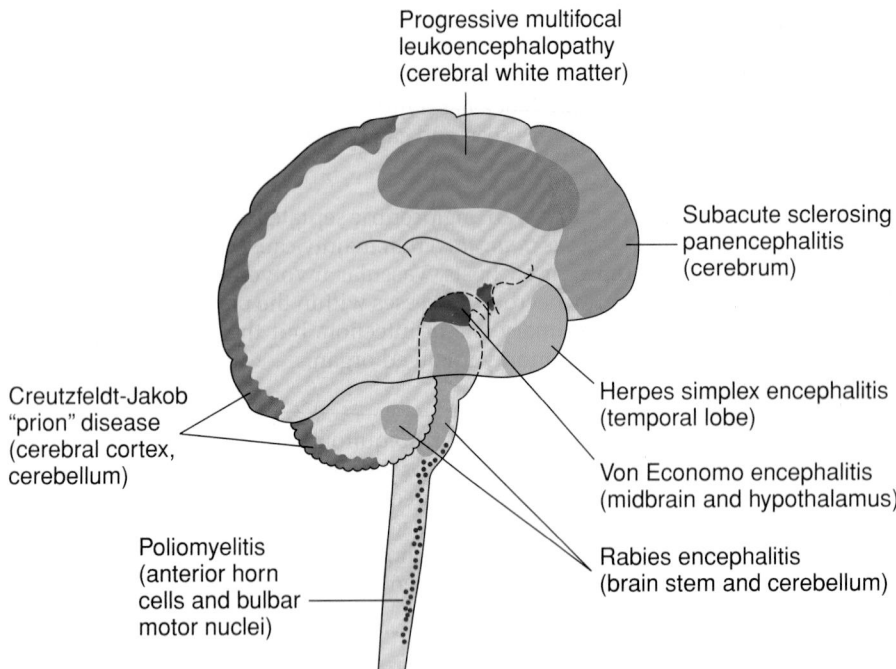

Progressive multifocal
leukoencephalopathy
(cerebral white matter)

Subacute sclerosing
panencephalitis
(cerebrum)

Creutzfeldt-Jakob
"prion" disease
(cerebral cortex,
cerebellum)

Herpes simplex encephalitis
(temporal lobe)

Von Economo encephalitis
(midbrain and hypothalamus)

Poliomyelitis
(anterior horn
cells and bulbar
motor nuclei)

Rabies encephalitis
(brain stem and cerebellum)

**FIGURE 32-52. Distribution of the lesions of
viral encephalitides.**

example, poliomyelitis affects spinal and brainstem motor neurons, while herpes simplex targets the temporal lobes. Subacute sclerosing panencephalitis involves the gray matter, while progressive multifocal leukoencephalopathy is a white matter disorder. The mechanisms of viral tropism may reflect binding of viruses to plasma membrane structure on specific CNS cells, the ability of viruses to remain latent or selective replication in specific intracellular microenvironments. Viruses may exploit axonal transport to travel to sites far distant from their point of entry, as exemplified by rabies and herpesviruses.

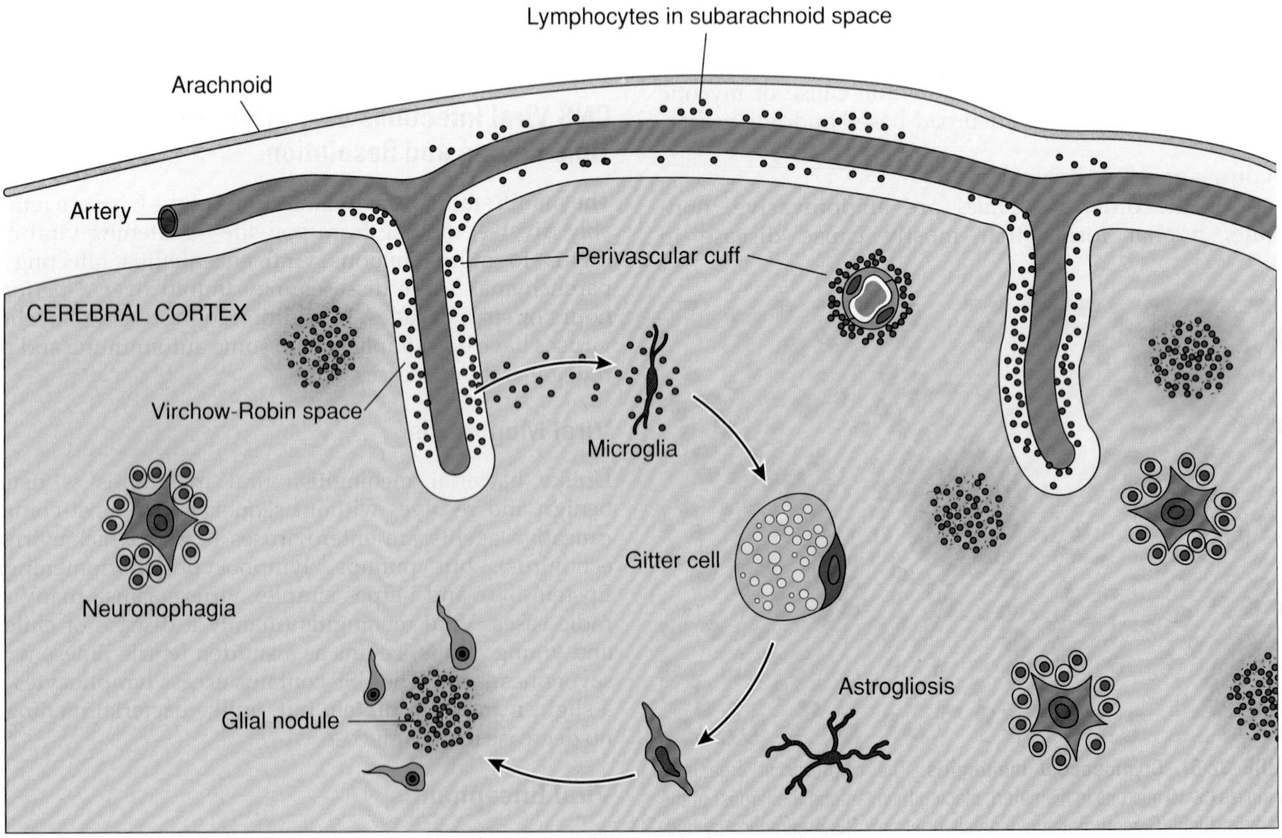

Lymphocytes in subarachnoid space

Arachnoid

Artery

Perivascular cuff

CEREBRAL CORTEX

Virchow-Robin space

Microglia

Gitter cell

Neuronophagia

Astrogliosis

Glial nodule

FIGURE 32-53. The lesions of viral encephalitis.

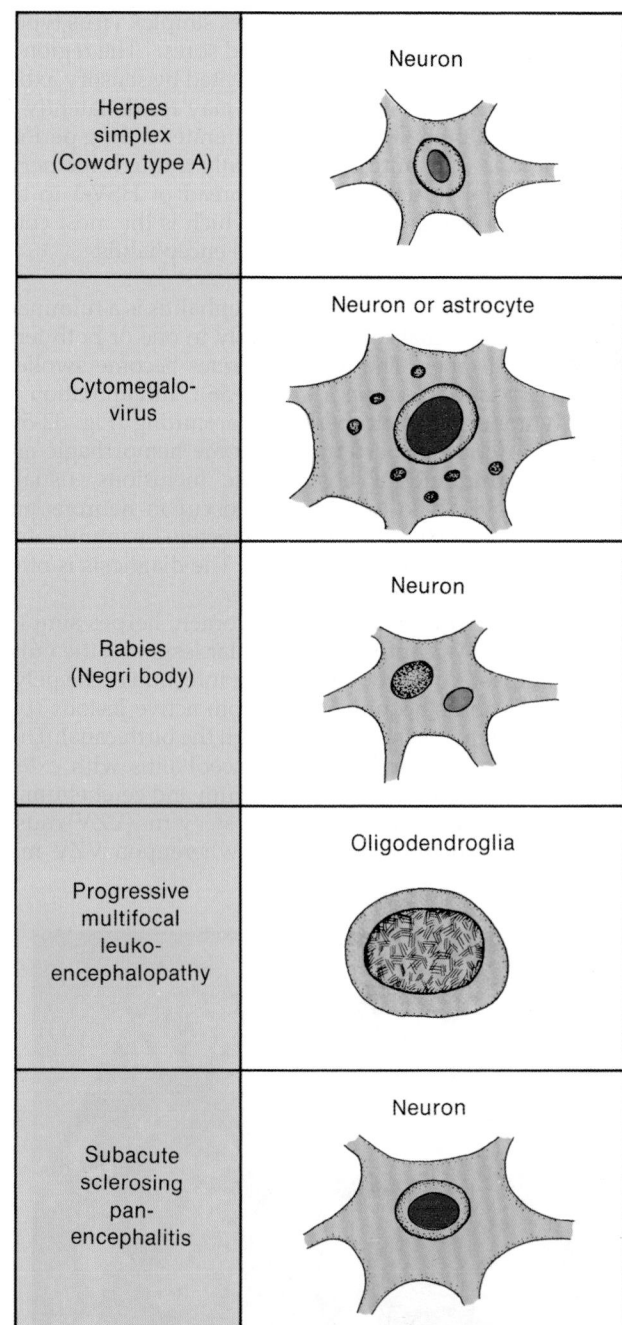

Herpes simplex (Cowdry type A)	Neuron
Cytomegalo-virus	Neuron or astrocyte
Rabies (Negri body)	Neuron
Progressive multifocal leuko-encephalopathy	Oligodendroglia
Subacute sclerosing pan-encephalitis	Neuron

FIGURE 32-54. Inclusion bodies in viral encephalitides.

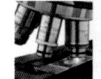 **PATHOLOGY:** Most CNS viral infections elicit perivascular lymphocytes, macrophage and microglial activation and gliosis (Fig. 32-53). These changes are not specific for viral infections, but the presence of viral inclusions strongly suggests a viral infection (Fig. 32-54). Such inclusion bodies do not occur with all viral infections. In situ hybridization, PCR and immunochemistry are most often used to establish a diagnosis.

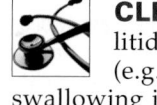 **CLINICAL FEATURES:** Most viral encephalitides begin abruptly. Specific neurologic deficits (e.g., paralysis of poliomyelitis, difficulty in swallowing in rabies) reflect the localization of the infection. Most encephalitides run a rapid course, but the tempo can vary. For example, the clinical course of subacute sclerosing panencephalitis may last years. Herpes simplex and varicella-zoster viruses may be latent in sensory ganglia for years, only to be reactivated decades after initial infection.

Poliomyelitis

The term **poliomyelitis** describes any inflammation of the gray matter of the spinal cord. In common usage it implies an infection by poliovirus, which is one of the enteroviruses. These are small, nonenveloped, single-stranded RNA viruses.

Historical evidence suggests that poliomyelitis has occurred in epidemics since antiquity. Affected people shed large amounts of virus in their stools, and spread is by the fecal–oral route.

 PATHOLOGY: Virus enters motor neurons via binding sites on their plasma membranes and replicates there. Infected cells may undergo chromatolysis, after which they are phagocytosed by macrophages (neuronophagia). Initial inflammatory responses briefly include neutrophils. Lymphocytes follow and surround blood vessels in the spinal cord and brainstem. The motor cortex usually shows no inflammation but may contain microglial nodules, which are focal collections of microglia and lymphocytes. Host immune responses to the virus, although limited, may halt progression of clinical disease. Sections of spinal cord in cases of healed poliomyelitis show loss of neurons, with secondary degeneration of corresponding ventral roots and peripheral nerves.

 CLINICAL FEATURES: Nonspecific symptoms such as fever, malaise and headache are followed in several days by signs of meningitis, and then by paralysis. In severe cases, the muscles of the neck, trunk and all four limbs may be rendered powerless. Paralysis of the respiratory muscles may be life-threatening. Patients with milder disease may show asymmetric and patchy paralysis, most often in the legs.

Improvement begins in about a week, and only some of the muscles affected at the outset may remain permanently paralyzed. Mortality is 5%–25%, with death usually due to respiratory failure. Development of effective vaccines in the 1950s has largely eliminated polio in most of the world. However, in parts of Asia and Africa, political instability have jeopardized vaccination programs. Recently, wild-type poliomyelitis has recurred in the Congo, where many people have not been vaccinated and are immunologically naïve, resulting in high case fatality rates.

Rabies

 **EPIDEMIOLOGY:** Rabies is an encephalitis caused by an enveloped, single-stranded RNA virus of the rhabdovirus group. Dogs, wolves, foxes and skunks are the main reservoirs, but bats and domestic animals, including cattle, goats and swine, also carry the disease. Rabies virus is transmitted to humans via contaminated saliva, introduced by a bite. In the United States, where dogs are routinely vaccinated against rabies, the few human rabies infections (1–5 per year) usually follow exposure to rabid bats. In areas of Asia, Africa and South America, however, rabies is endemic and most human

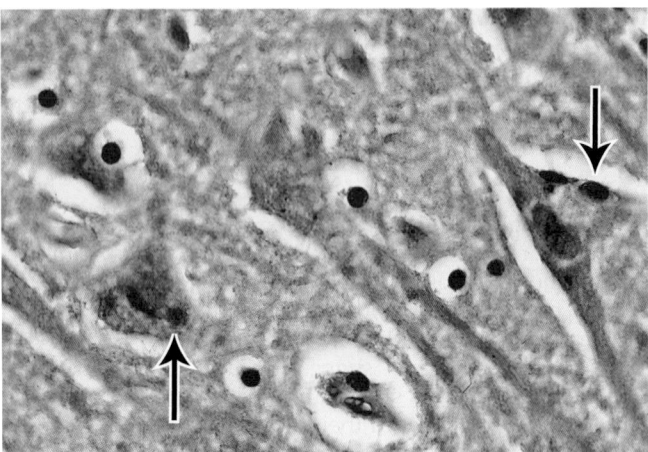

FIGURE 32-55. Negri body. Rabies encephalitis is characterized by round, eosinophilic cytoplasmic inclusions that resemble an erythrocyte (*arrows*).

infections come from dog bites. Rabies kills more than 50,000 people annually. Iatrogenic transmission has occurred, via corneal, solid organ and tendon transplants, and incubation periods may be extremely short or as mysteriously long as 18 months. Rabies is rare in industrialized countries, so the diagnosis may not be considered in potential organ donors. However, as the consequences of iatrogenic transmission of this uniformly fatal infection are so horrific, extreme caution is warranted in harvesting tissues from donors who die of strange or atypical neurologic disorders.

 PATHOLOGY: The virus enters a peripheral nerve and is transported by retrograde axoplasmic flow to the spinal cord and brain. Latent intervals vary in proportion to the distance of transport, from 10 days to as long as 3 months.

Perivascular lymphocytes, scattered neurons with chromatolysis and neuronophagia and microglial nodules are seen. Inflammation is mainly in the brainstem and affects the cerebellum and hypothalamus. Eosinophilic cytoplasmic viral inclusion bodies in the hippocampus, brainstem and cerebellar Purkinje cells **(Negri bodies)** confirm the diagnosis (Fig. 32-55).

CLINICAL FEATURES: Destruction of brainstem neurons by rabies virus initiates painful spasms of the throat, difficulty swallowing and a tendency to aspirate fluids that prompted the original name, "hydrophobia." Clinical symptoms also reflect a general encephalopathy, with irritability, agitation, seizures and delirium. In up to 15% of cases, rabies may present in the paralytic form resembling Guillain-Barré syndrome rather than the encephalopathic form. The CSF displays a typical viral response, including (1) a modest increase in lymphocytes, (2) a moderate increase in protein and (3) unaltered glucose and CSF pressure. Once symptoms develop, the illness relentlessly progresses to death within 1 to several weeks. Urgent rabies vaccination and hyperimmune globulin are administered for postexposure prophylaxis.

Herpes Viruses
Herpes viruses include herpes simplex (types 1 and 2), varicella-zoster virus, cytomegalovirus (CMV), Epstein-Barr virus (EBV) and simian B virus.

HERPES SIMPLEX TYPE 1: Herpes simplex virus type 1 (HSV-1) is largely responsible for "cold sores." The region of the vesicular lesion on the lip is innervated by sensory axons from the trigeminal ganglion. HSV-1 may reside latently in the trigeminal ganglion, where it proliferates during periods of stress and is transmitted centrifugally through the nerve trunk to the lip. Reactivation and spread of HSV-1 to the CNS results in herpes encephalitis, which is the most common sporadic (i.e., nonepidemic) viral encephalitis.

PATHOLOGY: Herpes encephalitis is a fulminant infection that localizes mainly in one or both temporal lobes. The temporal lobes become swollen, hemorrhagic and necrotic (Fig. 32-56). Inflammation is mainly lymphocytic, with perivascular cuffing (Fig. 32-57). The small arteries and arterioles become hemorrhagic and edematous. Intranuclear eosinophilic inclusions, usually surrounded by a halo (Cowdry A), occur in neurons and glial cells (Fig. 32-58). Viral protein detection by immunohistochemistry is diagnostically reliable. The diagnosis is often made by PCR of CSF and viral culture.

HERPES SIMPLEX TYPE 2: In women, herpes simplex virus type 2 (HSV-2) initiates a vesicular lesion on the vulva **(genital herpes),** coupled with a latent infection in the pelvic ganglia. Newborns acquire HSV-2 from active lesions (primary or recurrent) as they pass through the birth canal. They thereafter may develop fulminant encephalitis with extensive liquefactive necrosis in the cerebrum and cerebellum.

VARICELLA-ZOSTER: Varicella-zoster virus (VZV) causes childhood exanthem "chicken pox" whereupon VZV may

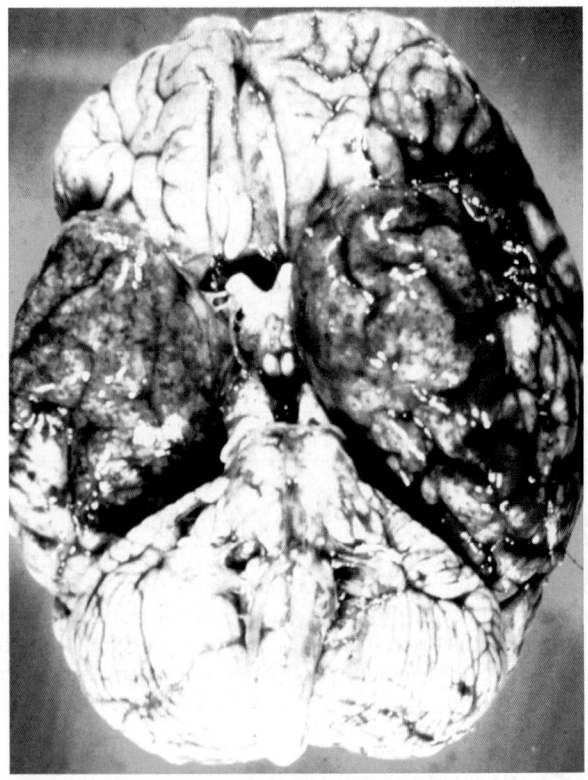

FIGURE 32-56. Herpes simplex encephalitis. Grossly, there are swollen hemorrhagic necrotic temporal lobes. The patient may experience memory disturbances and complex partial seizures as a result of this selective involvement of the temporal lobes. (Courtesy of Dr. F. Stephen Vogel, Duke University.)

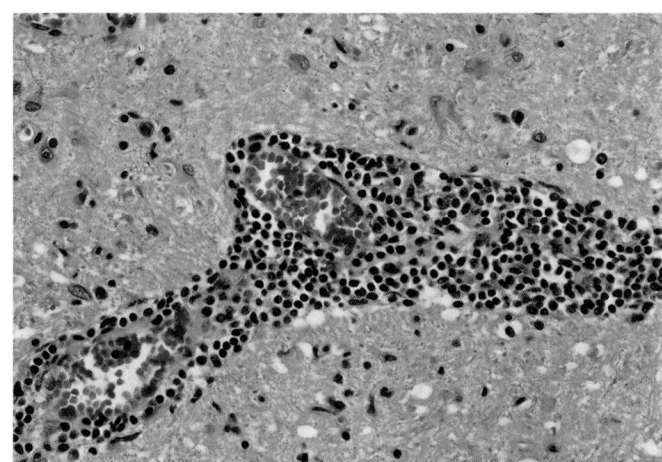

FIGURE 32-57. Herpes simplex encephalitis. Microscopically, the specimen exhibits pronounced perivascular lymphocytic inflammation. This finding indicates that active inflammation is present, but is not etiologically specific.

become latent in dorsal root ganglia. In later life, particularly after age 60, the virus may reactivate and be transported down the sensory axon to the skin, causing an exquisitely painful cutaneous vesicular eruption called "shingles" in the dermatome distribution of the dorsal root ganglion harboring the virus. The infection elicits only mild inflammation and rarely spreads to the CNS. Intranuclear Cowdry A inclusions like those of HSV are present.

Rarely, VZV may cause a fatal encephalitis, and the virus has been implicated in isolated giant cell arteritis of the CNS leading to stroke. "Shingles" reflects reemergence of latent infection by the VZV and may be the initial manifestation of immune dysfunction. The pain and vesicular eruption can be severe and disabling, but a VZV vaccine is now available and is recommended for individuals over 60 years of age.

CYTOMEGALOVIRUS: CMV crosses the placenta to induce encephalitis in utero. Lesions in the embryonic CNS are characterized by periventricular necrosis and calcification. Because of the proximity of these lesions to the

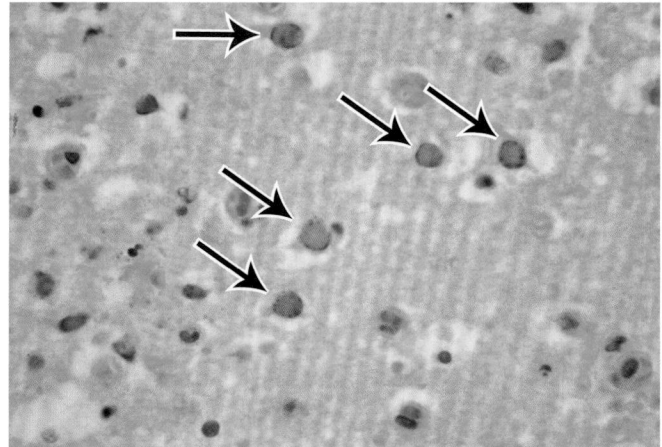

FIGURE 32-58. Herpes simplex encephalitis. The infected neurons display intranuclear, eosinophilic viral inclusions (Cowdry A inclusions) that fill the nuclei (*arrows*). The presence of these findings is extremely valuable in guiding diagnostic evaluation as a limited number of viruses produce Cowdry A inclusions.

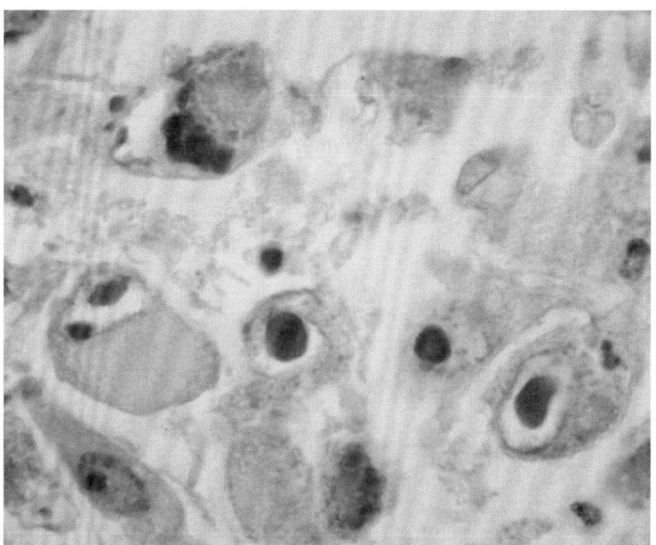

FIGURE 32-59. Cytomegalovirus ependymitis. Ependymal cells display large intranuclear inclusions in grotesquely enlarged infected cells.

third ventricle and the aqueduct, they may cause obstructive hydrocephalus. In adults, CMV encephalitis occurs in immunocompromised hosts. Eosinophilic nuclear and cytoplasmic viral inclusions are present in astrocytes and neurons, most conspicuously in enlarged nuclei, where they are sharply defined and surrounded by a halo (Fig. 32-59).

Arthropod-Borne Viral Encephalitis

 **EPIDEMIOLOGY:** Arthropod-borne viruses, or **arboviruses,** are transmitted between vertebrates by blood-sucking vectors (e.g., mosquitoes, ticks). The Togaviridae, Bunyaviridae and Flaviviridae include most of the arboviruses that cause human encephalitis. Arbovirus infections are zoonoses of animals; humans are infected when bitten by virus-harboring arthropods. Humans are not generally reservoirs, nor do they continue viral propagation. The various encephalitides caused by arboviruses are named principally for the location where they were first noted (Table 32-1), for example, Eastern, Western and Venezuelan equine encephalitis; St. Louis encephalitis; Japanese B encephalitis; California encephalitis; and West Nile encephalitis. The latter has numerically eclipsed all other arbovirus encephalitides in the United States since it first appeared in 1999. West Nile encephalitis epidemics continue to occur, underscoring the importance of mosquito control. Most cases of West Nile infection are asymptomatic, so most infections are unrecognized. As infection can be transmitted by blood transfusion, it is now necessary to screen blood for West Nile virus. Immunocompromised patients may have a fulminant course with the arboviral infections.

 PATHOLOGY: The lesions of the several arbovirus encephalitides resemble each other and vary from mild meningitis with scattered lymphocytes to severe inflammation of gray matter, thrombosis of small blood vessels and prominent necrosis. There are no inclusions in infected neurons. In necrotic foci, neuronophagia is evident, and if the patient survives, demyelination and

TABLE 32-1

INSECT-BORNE VIRAL ENCEPHALITIS

Virus	Insect Vector	Distribution
St. Louis encephalitis	Mosquito	North and South America
Western equine encephalitis	Mosquito	North and South America
Venezuelan equine encephalitis	Mosquito	North and South America
Eastern equine encephalitis	Mosquito	North America
California encephalitis	Mosquito	North America
Murray Valley encephalitis	Mosquito	Australia, New Papua
Japanese B encephalitis	Mosquito	Eastern and southeastern Asia
Tick-borne encephalitis	Tick	Eastern Europe, Scandinavia
West Nile encephalitis	Mosquito	Global

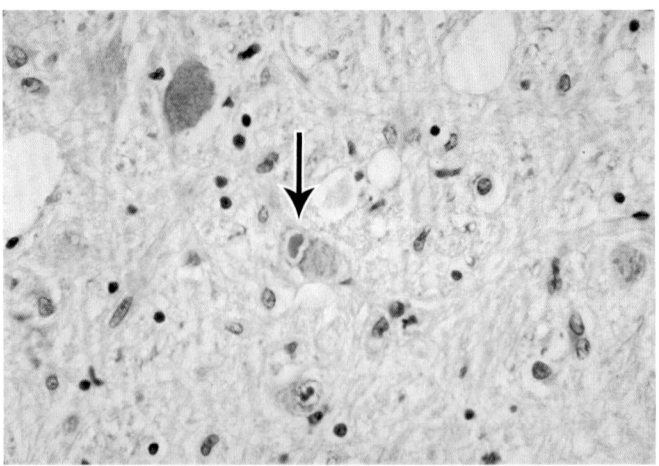

FIGURE 32-60. Subacute sclerosing panencephalitis. The brain shows loss of myelin and reactive gliosis. An intranuclear inclusion is present (*arrow*).

gliosis may develop. West Nile encephalitis has a tropism for the spinal cord and may produce a syndrome clinically indistinguishable from classical poliomyelitis.

 CLINICAL FEATURES: Arthropod-borne encephalitides share many features, but each has a different course. For example, Eastern equine encephalitis is commonly a more fulminant potentially lethal disease, but Venezuelan equine encephalitis tends to pursue a more benign course. Mild cases of arbovirus encephalitis may entail only a mild flu-like syndrome and may not be diagnosed as encephalitis. In more severe cases, onset is abrupt, often with high fever, headache, vomiting and meningeal signs, followed by lethargy and coma. Death is more likely at the extremes of age, and those who survive may be left with cognitive impairment and seizures.

Subacute Sclerosing Panencephalitis

 PATHOLOGY: Subacute sclerosing panencephalitis (SSPE) is a consequence of infection with the measles virus, and most patients have a history of measles. SSPE develops 6–8 years after the initial infection and is caused by a measles virus with defective expression of viral M (Matrix) protein. Nuclear inclusions occur in neurons and oligodendroglia, and marked gliosis affects gray and white matter, accompanied by patchy loss of myelin and ubiquitous perivascular lymphocytes and macrophages (Fig. 32-60). The intranuclear inclusions are basophilic, rimmed by a prominent halo. Affected neurons may have neurofibrillary tangles.

 CLINICAL FEATURES: SSPE is a chronic, lethal, viral infection of the brain caused by measles virus. First recognized in 1933 as "subacute inclusion-body encephalitis," SSPE has an insidious onset, mainly in childhood, with cognitive and behavioral decline

over months to years, ultimately leading to death. The CSF typically has increased antibody to measles virus. The course is protracted, and inflammation occurs mainly in cerebral gray matter. In adults, SSPE may follow a more rapid course.

Progressive Multifocal Leukoencephalopathy

Progressive multifocal leukoencephalopathy (PML) is an increasingly common infectious demyelinating disease caused by a ubiquitous polyoma virus that infects oligodendrocytes and leads to cytolysis and patchy multifocal demyelination. Astrocytes are also infected, but instead of dying, they show extreme pleomorphism.

 **ETIOLOGIC FACTORS:** JC virus is a polyoma virus, closely related to simian virus 40 (SV40). The "JC" derives from the initials of the first patient in whom the disease was described. Over 50% of people harbor JC virus, which resides in a latent state in the bone marrow after asymptomatic acquisition earlier in life. If the host becomes immunosuppressed, viremia ensues with specific neurovirulent viral strains.

 CLINICAL FEATURES: PML occurs mostly in immunocompromised patients and manifests as dementia, weakness, visual loss and ataxia, usually leading to death within 6 months. It is a terminal complication in immunosuppressed patients, such as those treated for cancer or lupus erythematosus, organ transplant recipients and especially people with AIDS. PML may complicate the use of drugs that inhibit T-cell adherence to endothelial cells as a treatment of immunologic disorders. Natalizumab is such a drug and was temporarily withdrawn from the market after the appearance of PML in patients treated for multiple sclerosis or Crohn disease. The drug has been reintroduced to clinical use with stringent guidelines.

 PATHOLOGY: Lesions typical of PML appear as widely scattered discrete foci of demyelination near the gray–white junction in the cerebral hemispheres and brainstem (Fig. 32-61). They are several millimeters and spherical, with a central area largely devoid of myelin. Axons are retained, a few oligodendrocytes are seen

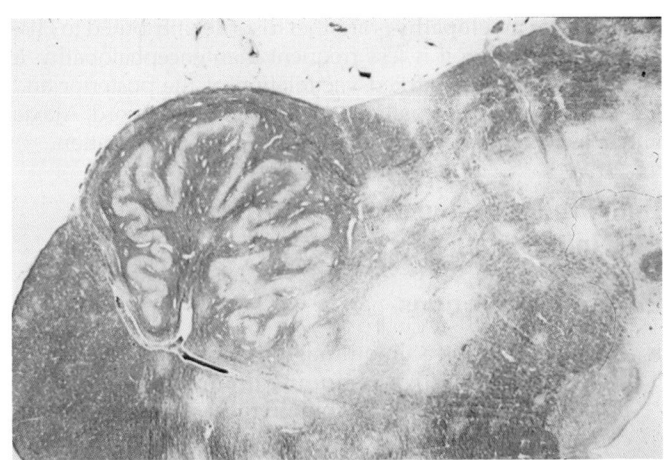

FIGURE 32-61. Progressive multifocal leukoencephalopathy. A Luxol fast blue stain of the medulla reveals severe patchy loss of myelin.

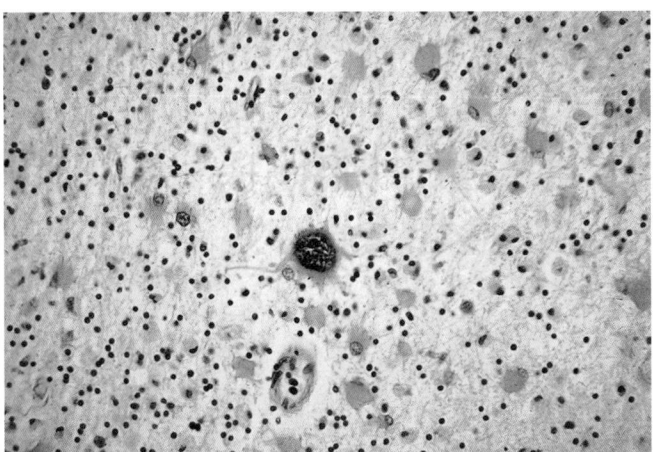

FIGURE 32-63. Progressive multifocal leukoencephalopathy (PML). A bizarre astrocyte is present (*center*) and may mimic neoplasia. The presence of macrophages and ground-glass inclusions should direct diagnostic consideration away from neoplasia and toward PML.

and the lesion is infiltrated by macrophages. At the edge of the demyelinated area, there are oligodendrocytes with enlarged nuclei occupied by homogeneously dense, hyperchromatic, "ground-glass" intranuclear inclusions lacking a halo. Electron microscopy discloses intranuclear, crystalline arrays of spherical 35–40-nm virions (Fig. 32-62). Infected astrocytes are highly pleomorphic, often with multiple irregular dark nuclei (Fig. 32-63). These astrocytes can be so pleomorphic as to suggest malignancy.

HIV

CNS disease is common in AIDS. Some patients have opportunistic CNS infections, such as toxoplasmosis, cytomegalovirus, herpes simplex or PML, or have EBV-driven primary CNS lymphoma (PCNSL). Cryptococcal meningitis is the most common fungal meningitis in AIDS patients, toxoplasmosis is the most common intracranial mass and PCNSL is the most common neoplasm. These are sentinels of AIDS; that is, any of these occurring in any patient should trigger diagnostic consideration of underlying AIDS. There are

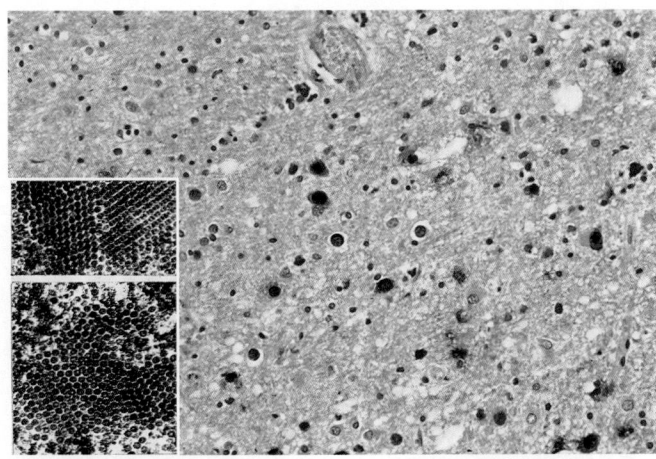

FIGURE 32-62. Progressive multifocal leukoencephalopathy. An immunohistochemical stain for JC virus demonstrates numerous infected oligodendroglia in the white matter. By electron microscopy, there are intranuclear paracrystalline arrays of viral particles (*insets*).

many other opportunistic nervous system infections that may complicate AIDS, and it is important to remember that the clinical presentation may be more fulminant or atypical than in immunocompetent individuals.

HIV Encephalopathy

Many AIDS patients have diffuse encephalopathy directly attributable to active CNS infection by HIV-1 retrovirus itself. This is variously called HIV encephalopathy (HIVE) or HIV-associated neurologic disease (HAND). Dementia was once the most common clinical manifestation of HIVE. It varies from mild to severe cognitive impairment with striking slowness of thought (bradyphrenia), often with marked bradykinesis mimicking Parkinson disease. CNS macrophages and microglial cells are productively infected by HIV-1. Infection of neurons and astrocytes is probably not clinically significant, but these cells are injured indirectly by neurotoxic viral proteins produced by infected cells or various cytokines, which cause oxidant-mediated cell injury.

The advent of highly active antiretroviral therapy (HAART) has dramatically extended the life span and quality of life of AIDS patients, including reducing opportunistic infections and primary CNS lymphoma. HAART drugs largely do not cross the blood-brain barrier, and since the virus enters the CNS via infected blood monocytes very soon after it enters the body, HAART has not altered the incidence of HAND. Rather, although frank dementia has become less common, a combination of sensory, motor and other defects causing minor cognitive motor disease (MCMD) affects as many as 30% of HIV-1–positive patients. As these people age, this prevalence increases by an additional approximately 5% of the HIV-1–positive population yearly. Initiation of HAART may also be complicated by immune reconstitution inflammatory syndrome (IRIS). In the brain, IRIS may lead to potentially lethal cerebral edema and exacerbation of focal symptoms and may contribute to fulminant HIVE.

 PATHOLOGY: HAND is characterized by mild cerebral atrophy, dilation of the lateral ventricles and slight prominence of gyri and sulci. Histologic

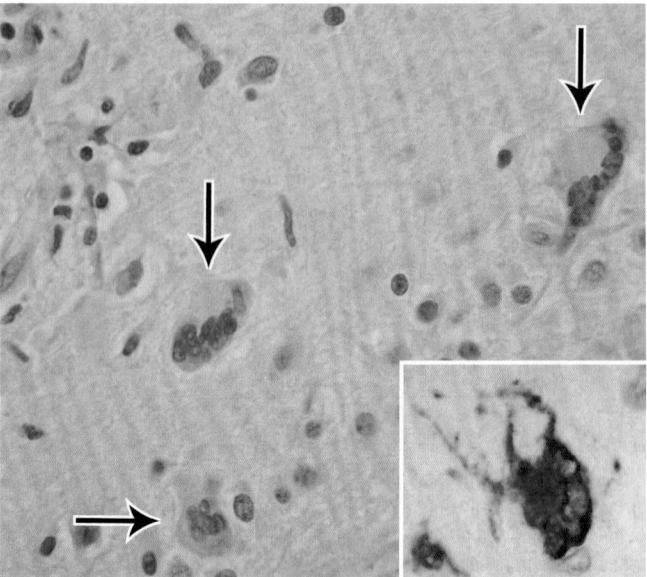

FIGURE 32-64. HIV encephalitis or encephalopathy (HIVE). Multinucleated giant cells (*arrows*) often in a perivascular location are characteristic of HIV encephalitis. *Inset.* Immunohistochemical stain for HIV anti-p24.

changes are usually in the subcortical gray and white matter. Multinucleated giant cells of monocyte/macrophage lineage are associated with microglial nodules (Fig. 32-64). In addition, myelin pallor, reflecting diffuse demyelination, intense astrogliosis and loss of neurons, is common (Fig. 32-65).

Vacuolar myelopathy is another disorder attributed to HIV infection, although it is less frequent than encephalopathy. It is characterized by marked vacuolation of the posterior and lateral columns, principally in the thoracic spinal cord. Ataxia and spastic paraparesis dominate the clinical presentation.

Both Protozoan and Metazoan Parasites May Infect the CNS

Protozoan Infections

- **Toxoplasmosis** is a ubiquitous protozoan to which most of us have protective immunity. Immunocompromised patients lose the ability to contain these organisms. Small comma-like tachyzoites and large polyorganismal cysts (bradyzoites) are seen in association with chronic inflammation, tissue necrosis and vasculitis. Toxoplasmosis is the most common cause of multiple intracranial masses in AIDS patients (Fig. 32-66).
- *Naegleria* **spp.,** especially *Naegleria fowleri,* cause primary amebic meningoencephalitis, a fulminant and rapidly fatal disease with diffuse brain swelling. The ameba infects the nasal cavities of people who swim in stagnant warm freshwater ponds or who irrigate their sinus passages with inadequately decontaminated water. They enter the brain by migrating up the olfactory bulb, through the cribriform plate. *Naegleria* trophozoites resemble macrophages (Fig. 32-67).
- *Acanthamoeba* produces granulomatous amoebic encephalitis, a subacute, usually fatal illness characterized by

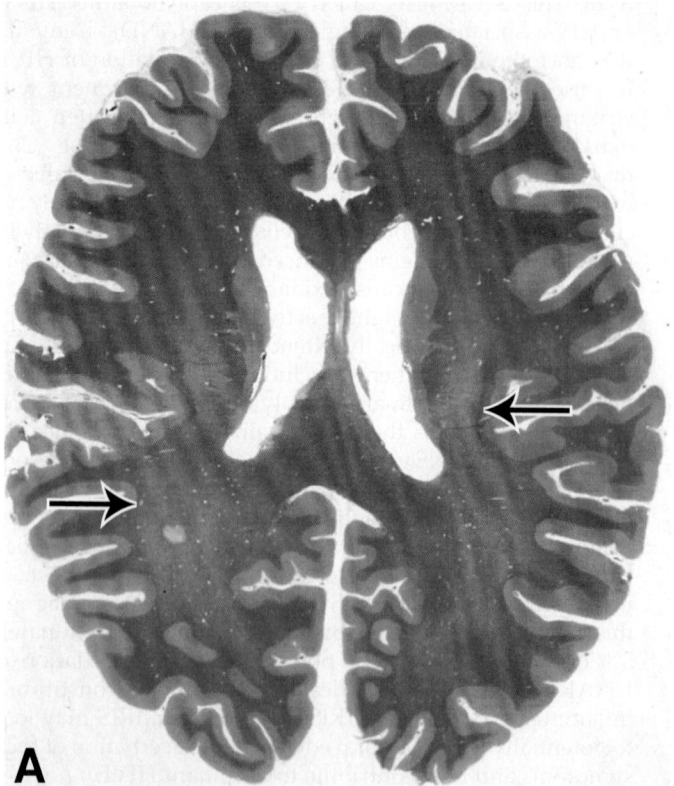

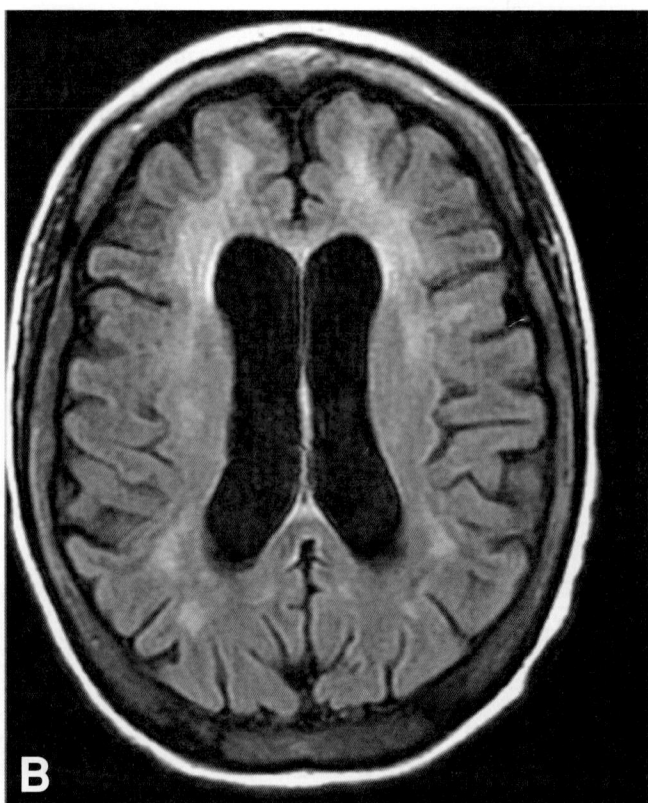

FIGURE 32-65. HIV encephalitis or encephalopathy (HIVE). A. An axial whole brain section in HIVE shows symmetric myelin pallor (*arrows*) caused by HIV-1. Demyelination caused by progressive multifocal leukoencephalopathy (PML) would be less symmetric and patchy. (Courtesy of Dr. F. Stephen Vogel, Duke University.) **B.** Axial magnetic resonance image showing bilateral white matter signal abnormalities in HIVE. The primary differential diagnosis is HIVE versus PML.

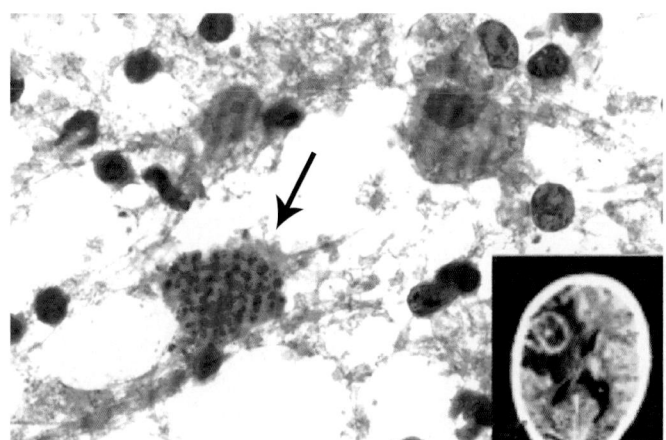

FIGURE 32-66. Toxoplasmosis in an HIV patient. This previously asymptomatic patient presented with an irregularly enhancing mass with surrounding edema that was initially thought to be a high-grade neoplasm. *Toxoplasma gondii* bradyzoites (*arrow*) are present in a necrotic inflammatory background. Toxoplasmosis is the most common mass lesion in patients with AIDS and is an indicator disease of HIV infection.

multiple granulomatous abscesses. This condition is usually seen in immunocompromised hosts.
- *Entamoeba histolytica* leads to amebic brain abscess by spread from a gastrointestinal or hepatic locus. Amebae in tissue sections can be difficult to distinguish from foamy macrophages.
- **CNS malaria** is most commonly caused by *Plasmodium falciparum.* During attacks of cerebral malaria, the CSF shows elevated protein and pressure but pleocytosis is uncommon. In fatal cases, the brain is diffusely swollen and may be otherwise unremarkable, but one may see microinfarcts with gliosis (Dürck granulomata) in white matter or many small hemorrhages. Infarcts and microhemorrhages may both arise from obstruction of blood flow in small vessels by parasitemia. Severity of cerebral malaria also reflects tumor necrosis factor-α release by host cells.

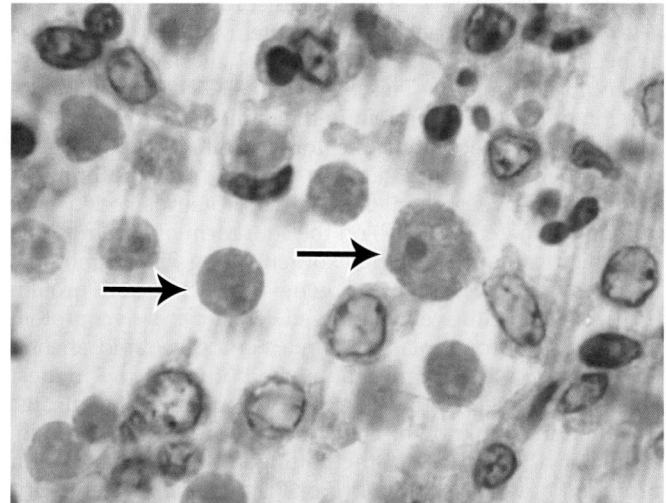

FIGURE 32-67. *Naegleria* **meningoencephalitis.** Amebic organisms (*arrows*) resemble macrophages but have much more prominent nucleoli.

- **Trypanosomal** infections include African sleeping sickness and American trypanosomiasis **(Chagas disease)**. Insect vectors transmit the disease. A meningoencephalitis may occur during the primary phase of infection. Reactivation of latent *Trypanosoma cruzi* produces multiple necrotic CNS lesions resembling toxoplasmosis and has been seen in people with AIDS and other forms of immunosuppression. Chagas disease is endemic in Central and South America, but 300,000–1,000,000 seropositive immigrants from those areas live in North America, and they are at risk for reactivation with immunosuppression.

Metazoan Infections of the Nervous System

- **Cysticercosis** caused by infection by *Taenia solium,* the pig tapeworm, may lead to multiple parasitic cysts up to 1 cm in the parenchyma, intraventricularly or in the basal cisterns. The intraparenchymal disease usually becomes symptomatic when the organism dies and is recognized immunologically by the host (Fig. 32-68). A peculiar form of this infection is racemose neurocysticercosis, in which grape-like clusters and sheets of worm tissues are made, without a fully formed worm. Racemose cysticercosis is essentially invertebrate tissue culture in the CSF and is resistant to therapy that is effective against intact parasites. Treatment of neurocysticercosis may lead to massive cerebral edema caused by massive host immune responses to the suddenly necrotic metazoan tissue. From a global health perspective, neurocysticercosis is one of the most common causes of epilepsy and intracranial mass lesions.
- **Echinococcosis** results from *Taenia echinococcus* or *Echinococcus granulosus,* the dog tapeworm, and produces cerebral cysts that are usually solitary and may be huge, in contrast to the smaller multiple cysts of cysticercosis. The brain lesion is frequently accompanied by hepatic cysts.
- **Trichinosis** is caused by *Trichinella spiralis* infection of skeletal and cardiac muscle, producing an acute eosinophilic myositis during the invasive phase. Larvae may then die and calcify, producing fibrosis and low-grade inflammation. The infection may rarely encroach on the CNS, producing lymphocytic-eosinophilic aseptic meningitis.

Prion Diseases (Spongiform Encephalopathies) Are Transmissible Neurodegenerative Diseases Caused by Modified Protein Particles

Prion diseases are characterized clinically by rapidly progressive ataxia and dementia and pathologically by accumulations of fibrillar or insoluble prion proteins, neuronal degeneration and vacuolization called **spongiform encephalopathy** (Fig. 32-69). The spongiform encephalopathies are biologically remarkable because the causative infectious agents, called **prions** (proteinaceous infectious particles), lack nucleic acids.

 **EPIDEMIOLOGY:** The classic spongiform encephalopathies in humans include kuru, Creutzfeldt-Jakob disease (CJD), Gerstmann-Sträussler-Scheinker syndrome (GSS) and fatal familial insomnia (Table 32-2). Similar diseases occur in animals, including scrapie in sheep and

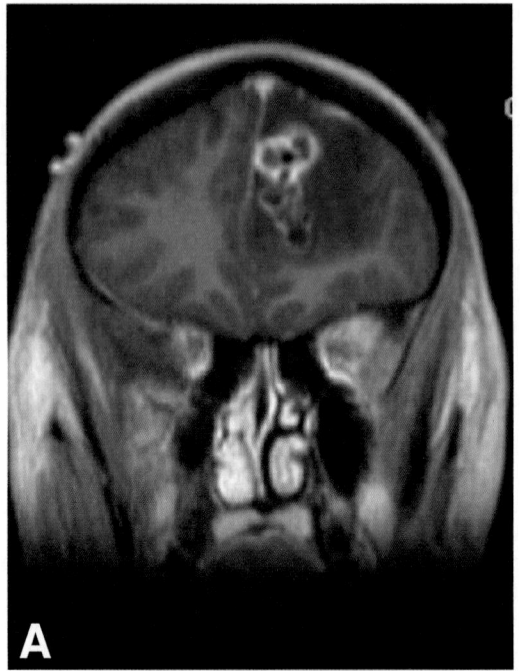

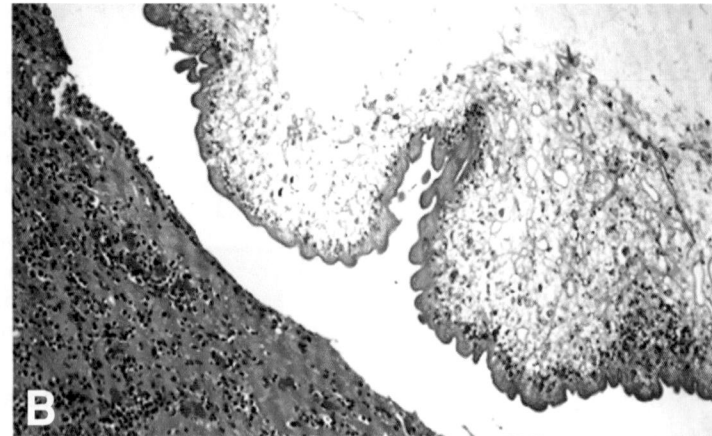

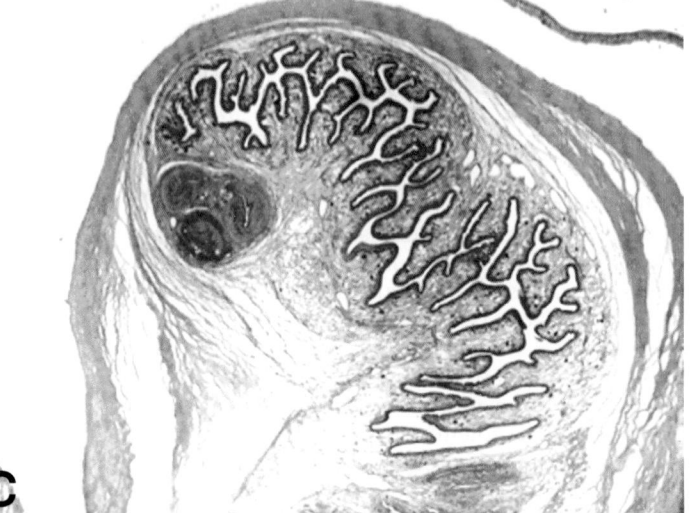

FIGURE 32-68. Neurocysticercosis. A. Radiographic appearance. Brain involvement by *Taenia solium* may result in solitary or multiple contrast-enhancing masses with surrounding edema. **B.** As the parasite begins to die and is detected by the host immune response, the lesions may become symptomatic. The corrugated cuticular surface forms an eosinophilic interface with inflamed adjacent brain. **C.** At low magnification, the worm scolex and gastrointestinal tract can sometimes be seen.

goats, bovine spongiform encephalopathy (BSE; mad cow disease), transmissible mink encephalopathy and chronic wasting disease in mule deer and elk. BSE is of particular interest because it resulted from inadvertent introduction of prion-contaminated feed to cattle, thus establishing that prions can be transmitted by the oral route. BSE is also

more easily transmitted and does not show the species selectivity of other prions. It decimated the cattle industry in the United Kingdom and spread to other regions of the world and to other species including zoo animals, pets and humans.

MOLECULAR PATHOGENESIS: The signal molecular event in prion disorders is conversion of a native α-helix–rich protein into a pathogenic β-sheet–rich isoform that tends to polymerize with subsequent fibril formation (Figs. 32-70 and 32-71). Uniquely, conversion of the native protein to the pathogenic form is autocatalyzed by the pathogenic form itself. The pathogenic protein begets more pathogenic protein from the limitless supply of native protein! The native protein is coded by a human prion gene (*PRNP*) on the short arm of chromosome 20, which contains a single exon encoding 254 amino acid residues. The normal prion gene product, prion protein (PrP), is a constitutively expressed cell surface glycoprotein that binds neuronal plasmalemma via a glycolipid anchor. PrP is made widely throughout the body, but the highest levels of PrP messenger RNA (mRNA) are in CNS neurons. Its function is unknown. The normal cellular prion protein, cellular PrP or PrP^C, and the pathogenic (infectious) prion protein, known as scrapie PrP or PrP^{SC}, have the same primary amino acid sequence but different tertiary structures and patterns of glycosylation. Specifically, PrP^C is rich in α-helix configuration, but the β-pleated sheet configuration

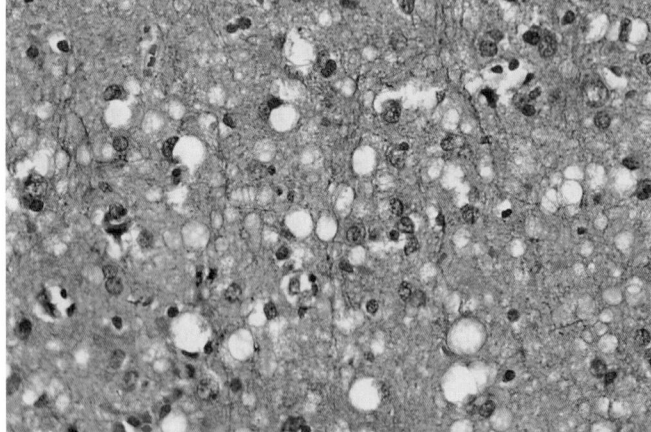

FIGURE 32-69. Creutzfeldt-Jakob disease. Spongiform degeneration of the gray matter is characterized by individual and clustered vacuoles, with no evidence of inflammation. (Courtesy of Dr. F. Stephen Vogel, Duke University.)

TABLE 32-2
PRION DISEASES

I. Human

A. Creutzfeldt-Jakob disease (CJD)

   1. Sporadic (85% of all CJD cases; incidence 1 per million worldwide)

   2. Inherited mutation of the prion gene, autosomal dominant transmission (15% of all CJD cases)

   3. Iatrogenic

      a. Hormone injection: human growth hormone, human pituitary gonadotropin

      b. Tissue grafts: dura mater, cornea, pericardium

      c. Medical devices: depth electrodes, surgical instruments (none definitely proven)

   4. New variant CJD (vCJD)

B. Gerstmann-Sträussler-Scheinker disease (GSS; inherited prion gene mutation, autosomal dominant transmission)

C. Fatal familial insomnia (FFI; inherited prion gene mutation, autosomal dominant transmission)

D. Kuru (confined to the Fore people of Papua New Guinea, formerly transmitted by cannibalistic funeral ritual)

II. Animal

A. Scrapie (sheep and goats)

B. Bovine spongiform encephalopathy (BSE; "mad cow disease")

C. Transmissible mink encephalopathy

D. Feline spongiform encephalopathy

E. Captive exotic ungulate spongiform encephalopathy (nyala, gemsbok, eland, Arabian oryx, greater kudu)

F. Chronic wasting disease of deer and elk

G. Experimental transmission to many species, including primates and transgenic mice

---

predominates in PrP^{SC}. The pathogenic conformation is extremely stable so that PrP^{SC} strongly resists conventional microbial decontamination methods. If PrP^{SC} enters the brain either through infectious transmission or by spontaneous misfolding of native protein, it will change other PrP^{C}

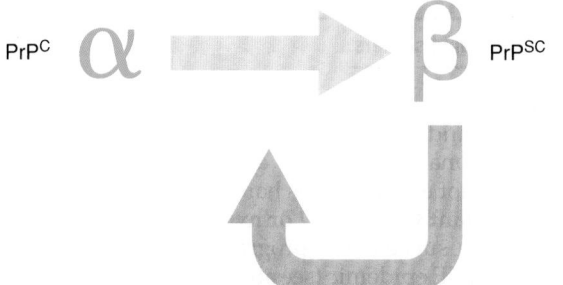

FIGURE 32-70. Creutzfeldt-Jakob disease. The unique mode of "reproduction" of the prion is the autocatalytic conversion of native α-helix–rich cellular prion protein into a β-sheet–rich pathogenic form that has a strong tendency toward aggregation.

proteins into pathogenic PrP^{SC}, leading to autocatalytic, exponentially expanding accretion of abnormal PrP^{SC}. The masses of PrP^{SC} compromise cell function and cause neurodegeneration by mechanisms that remain to be elucidated but may be similar to those of other neurodegenerative diseases characterized by fibrillogenesis.

All spongiform encephalopathies are transmissible, and inadvertent human transmission of CJD may follow administration of contaminated human pituitary growth hormone, corneal transplantation from a diseased donor, poorly sterilized neurosurgical instruments and surgical implantation of contaminated dura (Table 32-2).

 PATHOLOGY: Prion diseases entail neuron degeneration, gliosis, spongiform degeneration and accumulations of insoluble prions forming extracellular plaques. There are many small, clear, often confluent microcysts in the neuropil (Fig. 32-71). Lesions occur mostly in cortical gray matter but also involve deeper nuclei of the basal ganglia, thalamus, hypothalamus and cerebellum.

CLINICAL FEATURES: The several human prion diseases are distinct.

KURU: In 1956, a medical officer in New Guinea provided an account of kuru, a progressive, fatal neurologic disorder, in members of the isolated Fore tribe. The disease takes its name from the word "trembling" in their language. Transmission of kuru was linked to ritualistic funereal cannibalism in which women and children ate brains of deceased relatives.

Kuru was the first human prion disease shown to be transmissible. It attained epidemic proportions in the Fore people but was eliminated when cannibalism ceased. The initial and most prominent clinical feature of kuru is ataxia of the limbs and trunk, due to severe cerebellar involvement. In 70% of cases, insoluble, fibrillar prion proteins accumulate extracellularly in plaques. Spongiform change is present in both the cerebral hemispheres and cerebellum.

CREUTZFELDT-JAKOB DISEASE: CJD is the most common form of spongiform encephalopathy. Symptoms begin insidiously, but usually within 6 months to 3 years, patients exhibit severe dementia leading to death. Cerebellar involvement produces ataxia, which helps to distinguish CJD from Alzheimer disease. Myoclonus often occurs for some weeks to months during the afflicted person's decline. CJD is classified based on etiology: sporadic, familial, iatrogenic and new variant:

- **Sporadic CJD:** The sporadic form occurs worldwide, with an incidence of 1 per million, and accounts for 75% of CJD cases. The mode of acquisition is unknown; patients do not have the mutations associated with inherited forms of CJD or other prion diseases, and there is no history of iatrogenic exposure. A polymorphism in PRNP codon 129 confers differential susceptibility to CJD: homozygosity for either methionine (M) or valine (V) at this codon leads to disproportionate susceptibility to prion disorders, while heterozygotes (M/V) are resistant. Codon frequencies for the white population are 51% M/V, 37% M/M and 12% V/V.

- **Inherited CJD:** Familial CJD accounts for 15% of prion diseases, with an incidence of 1 in 10 million. Several different PRNP mutations are documented in various kindreds. In those cases, the PrP^{C} has a greater tendency to

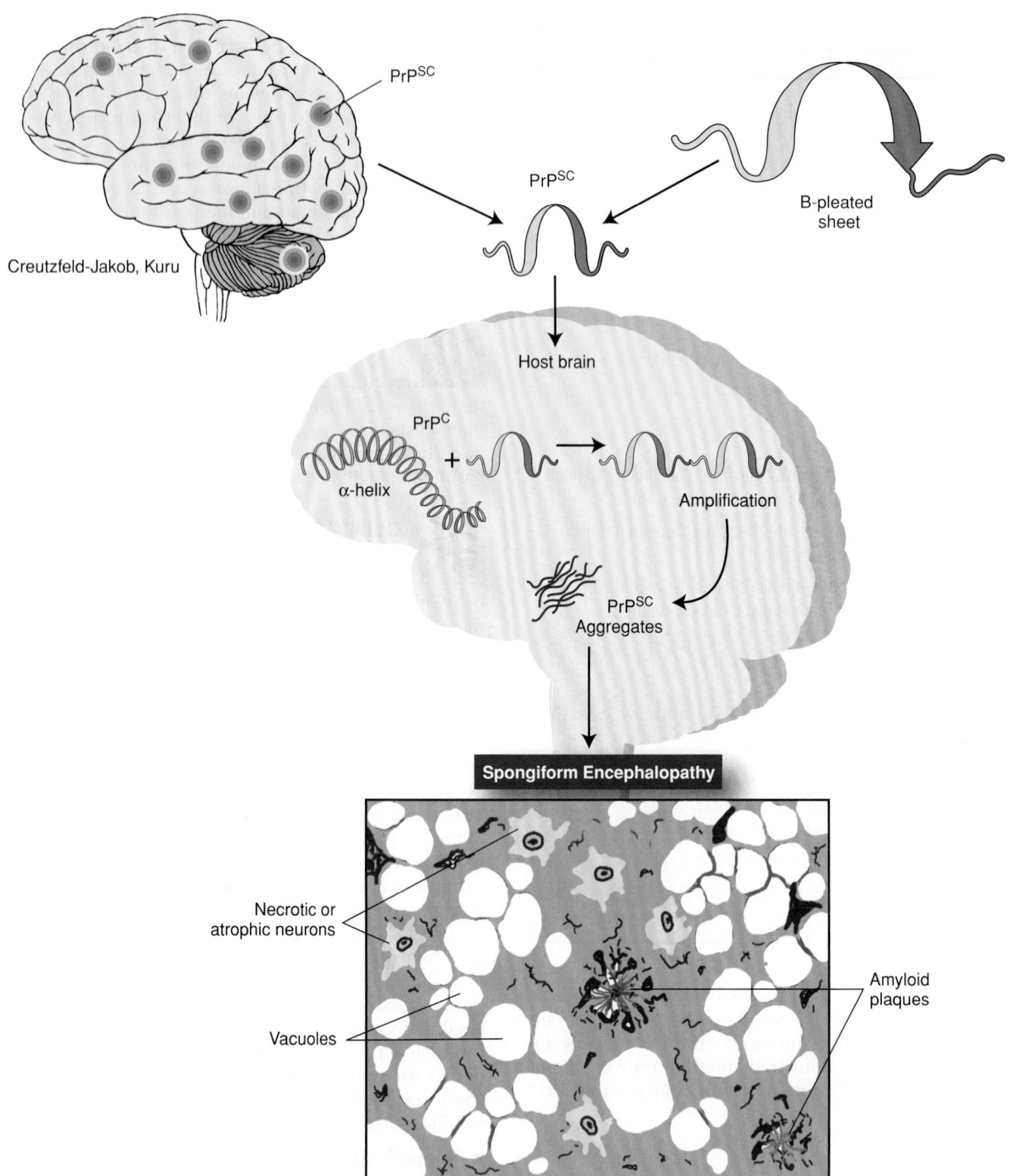

PrP^SC

PrP^SC

B-pleated
sheet

Creutzfeld-Jakob, Kuru

Host brain

PrP^C

α-helix

Amplification

PrP^SC
Aggregates

Spongiform Encephalopathy

Necrotic or
atrophic neurons

Amyloid
plaques

Vacuoles

FIGURE 32-71. Molecular pathogenesis of prion disorders.

misfold into the pathogenic isoform. The mutated PRNP causes familial CJD, fatal familial insomnia and Gerstmann-Sträussler-Scheinker disease.

■ **Iatrogenic CJD:** As listed in Table 32-2, several iatrogenic causes of CJD are known, but most causes for iatrogenic CJD now have been eliminated. Thus, recombinant human growth hormone has replaced human pituitary-derived preparations for therapy. When brain biopsies or autopsies are done in prion disease cases, special protocols are used to limit exposure of staff and patients to prions. Disposable instruments are used if possible, and

surfaces and instruments are treated with 2 N NaOH. Conventional autoclaving and most standard disinfectants do not eradicate this hardy infectious agent.

■ **New variant CJD (vCJD or nvCJD):** This form was identified by a surveillance program in the United Kingdom after the BSE epidemic (see above) between 1980 and 1996. A group of patients was identified that differed from other patients with sporadic CJD in several key characteristics, most importantly, age. The mean age at onset of symptoms for sporadic CJD is 65, but for vCJD it is 26. Also, vCJD patients had a longer duration of illness (median,

12 months vs. 4 months) and an atypical clinical presentation, including various behavioral changes or sensory disturbances (dysesthesias) and none of the usual electroencephalographic (EEG) findings of sporadic CJD. At autopsy, vCJD is characterized by prominent spongiform change in the basal ganglia and thalamus, and extensive PrP plaques in the cerebrum and cerebellum. The plaques are distinctive in that they resemble those of kuru. Finally, brains from vCJD patients contain much more PrP than brains of sporadic CJD patients. Physicochemical analysis showed different characteristics for vCJD PrP^{SC} from CJD PrP^{SC}, but similar to prions in BSE that were transmitted to mice and primates. Thus, BSE is considered to be the source of nvCJD. Current evidence suggests that vCJD cases have peaked and are declining. Essentially all vCJD cases were in codon 129 homozygotes (who are more susceptible), and a recent case in a heterozygote raises the unsettling specter of a longer incubation type of vCJD in this population. In addition, retrospective examination of surgical specimens of tonsils and appendices in the United Kingdom using PrP^{sc} has shown a significant number of asymptomatic individuals with pathogenic PrP that may become the nidus of a new epidemic of vCJD.

With globalization and diversification of economies, cultures and populations, a global perspective is essential in considering infectious diseases. New disorders can emerge and disseminate rapidly. Many of these infections have an impact on the nervous system, as we have seen with HIV and H1N1 influenza. Ease of movement leads to infections previously thought of as exotic or tropic occurring unexpectedly in industrialized countries. Larger populations rendered immunocompromised due to HIV, cancer or immunosuppressive therapies provide fertile grounds for clinically atypical neurologic infectious disease. Finally, there is the ever present danger of manmade biological agents being deployed.

DEMYELINATING DISEASES

Demyelinating diseases entail disruption of the myelin economy, including flawed manufacture (**dysmyelination**), destruction of myelin (**demyelination**) or disruption of myelin metabolism (**leukodystrophies**). Central myelin is made by oligodendrocytes, while peripheral myelin is made by Schwann cells (see Chapter 31). These two types of myelin differ biochemically. Operationally, the border between the CNS and the peripheral nervous system can be considered to be the point of transition between myelin made by oligodendrocytes and that made by Schwann cells. This transition usually occurs about 2–3 mm after a cranial nerve or spinal root exits the brainstem or spinal cord. Myelin disorders affect central or peripheral myelin, or both.

Multiple Sclerosis Is the Most Common Demyelinating Disease

 **EPIDEMIOLOGY:** Multiple sclerosis (MS) is a chronic demyelinating disease. With a prevalence of 1 per 1000, it is the most common chronic CNS disease of young adults in the United States. It is characterized by exacerbations and remissions over many years. It becomes symptomatic at a mean age of 30, and women are afflicted almost twice as often as men.

 **MOLECULAR PATHOGENESIS:** The etiology of MS is obscure, but genetic predisposition and immune dysfunction are probably involved. MS is mainly a disease of temperate climates. People who emigrate before age 15 from areas with a low prevalence to more temperate endemic areas assume the increased risk associated with their destinations, suggesting that environmental factors are important.

There are familial aggregates of the disease, with increased risk in second- and third-degree relatives of MS patients and 25% concordance for MS in monozygotic twins. Susceptibility is also linked to certain major histocompatibility complex (MHC) alleles (e.g., human leukocyte antigen [HLA]-DR2), implying that immune mechanisms are involved in the pathogenesis.

The lesions' microscopic appearance also suggests immune involvement. For example, chronic MS lesions show perivascular lymphocytes, macrophages and many CD4$^+$ as well as CD8$^+$ T cells (see Chapters 4 and 11). Moreover, CD4$^+$ T cells in the CSF of MS patients tend to be oligoclonal. Although no target antigen is established, data suggest an immune response to a specific CNS protein. Further support for immune mechanisms comes from an experimental antigen-specific, T-cell–mediated, autoimmune disease, **experimental allergic encephalitis (EAE)**. Injecting myelin basic protein into animals, including nonhuman primates, elicits a demyelinating disorder similar to MS. However, unlike MS, EAE is a monophasic illness.

Although an assortment of viruses have been implicated in the etiology of MS, to date there is no compelling evidence for the involvement of any infectious agent.

 PATHOLOGY: The demyelinated plaque is the hallmark of MS (Figs. 32-72 and 32-73). Plaques, rarely more than 2 cm, accumulate in great numbers in the brain and spinal cord (Fig. 32-74). They are discrete, with smoothly rounded contours, and are usually in white matter, although they may breach the gray matter. The lesions preferentially affect the optic nerves, chiasm, paraventricular white matter and spinal cord, but any part of the CNS may be involved.

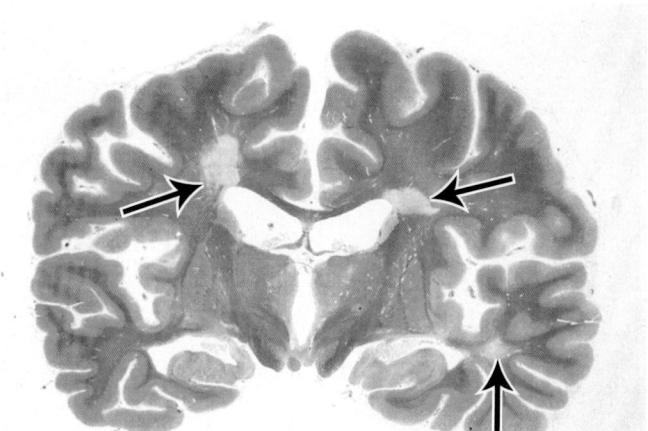

FIGURE 32-72. Multiple sclerosis. This myelin-stained coronal whole brain section of the brain of a patient with long-standing multiple sclerosis shows many areas of myelin loss—plaques (*arrows*)—with characteristic periventricular demyelination especially prominent at the superior angles of the lateral ventricles. (Courtesy of Dr. F. Stephen Vogel, Duke University.)

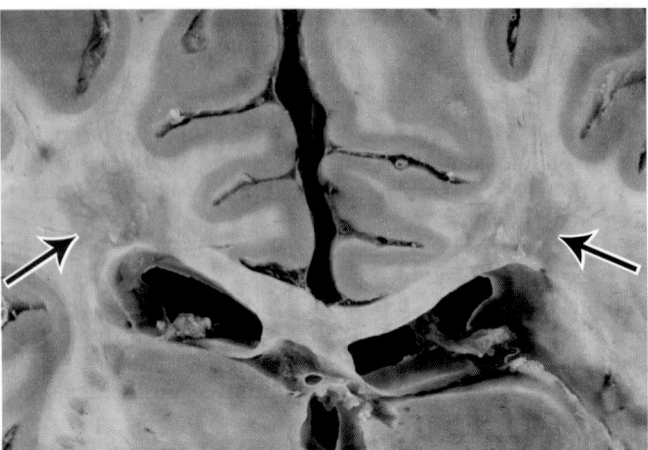

FIGURE 32-73. Multiple sclerosis. This fresh coronal section shows darker hues of the somewhat irregular periventricular plaques (*arrows*) reflecting the loss of myelin, which imparts the normal glistening white appearance of white matter.

Evolving plaques are marked by selective loss of myelin in regions of relative axonal preservation, lymphocytes clustering about small veins and arteries, influx of macrophages and considerable edema.

Neuronal bodies within plaques are remarkably spared, but axons may degenerate. Numbers of oligodendrocytes are moderately decreased. As plaques age, they become more discrete and less edematous. This sequence emphasizes the focal nature of the injury and its selectivity and severity, as demyelination is total within a plaque. Axons within plaques usually lose their myelin abruptly. Old MS plaques are dense and gliotic.

 CLINICAL FEATURES: MS usually begins in the third or fourth decades, after which patients experience abrupt episodes of clinical progression, separated by periods of relative stability. The essential clinical criterion for MS is dissemination of lesions in space and time; that is, multiple separate areas of the CNS must be affected at differing times. Our understanding of disease activity in MS has been revolutionized by use of serial MRI

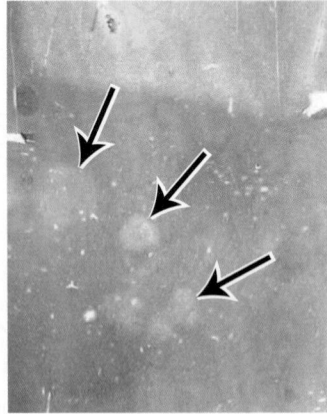

FIGURE 32-74. Multiple sclerosis. The subcortical white matter of a patient with multiple sclerosis showing multiple small irregular, partially confluent areas of demyelination (*arrows*). Normal intact myelin stains blue in this Luxol fast blue–stained section.

studies, which show ongoing disease activity despite apparent clinical quiescence. New plaques emerge and regress, only occasionally causing clinical manifestations. Contemporary diagnostic criteria for MS strongly incorporate periodic imaging to visualize plaques scattered in space and time. Thus, MS is an ongoing active process even between clinical exacerbations. The therapeutic focus is now suppression of ongoing disease activity using a variety of immune system modulators such as β-interferon, and MRI efficacy is an endpoint in drug trials and clinical management. Neuropathologic studies have confirmed increased inflammatory activity in brains of MS patients between exacerbations.

Many patients with MS pursue relapsing remitting clinical courses, but some suffer a relentless course without remissions. Each exacerbation reflects the formation of additional demyelinated MS plaques. MS typically begins with symptoms relating to lesions in the optic nerves, brainstem or spinal cord. Blurred vision or loss of vision in one eye as a result of optic neuritis is often the presenting complaint. When the initial lesion is in the brainstem, double vision and vertigo occur. In particular, internuclear ophthalmoplegia, caused by disruption of the medial longitudinal fasciculus, strongly suggests demyelinating disease when it occurs in a young person. Acute demyelination within the spinal cord is called **transverse myelitis** and produces weakness of one or both legs and sensory symptoms in the form of numbness in the lower extremities. Many of the initial symptoms are partially reversible within a few months.

Despite the fact that most patients have a chronic relapsing and remitting course, neurologic deficits accumulate gradually and relentlessly. Even in relatively quiescent plaques, there may be axonal attrition leading to irreversible lesions. In established cases, the degree of functional impairment is highly variable, ranging from minor disability to severe incapacity, with widespread paralysis, dysarthria, ataxia, severe visual defects, incontinence and dementia. Patients with severe disability usually die of respiratory paralysis or urinary tract infections. Most patients survive 20–30 years after the onset of symptoms.

Neuromyelitis Optica Is a Demyelinating Disease Common in Japan

Neuromyelitis optica (NMO) is a demyelinating disorder with a striking predilection for the optic nerves and spinal cord. Once regarded as a variant of MS, NMO is now recognized as resulting from autoantibodies against a water channel, aquaporin 4, and is thus pathophysiologically quite distinct from MS. It responds poorly to conventional MS therapy.

Postinfectious and Postvaccinal Encephalomyelitis Are Immune Responses to Viral Antigens

Some viral infections (e.g., measles, varicella, rubella) may rarely be followed in 3–21 days by an encephalomyelitis. The disease entails focal perivascular demyelination and conspicuous mononuclear cell infiltrates around small to medium-sized venules in brain and spinal cord white matter. It is suspected to be immune mediated, but its precise pathogenesis remains unclear. Onset of postinfectious encephalomyelitis is heralded by headache, vomiting, fever and meningismus that may be followed by paraplegia, incontinence and stupor. Up to 15%–20% of patients die.

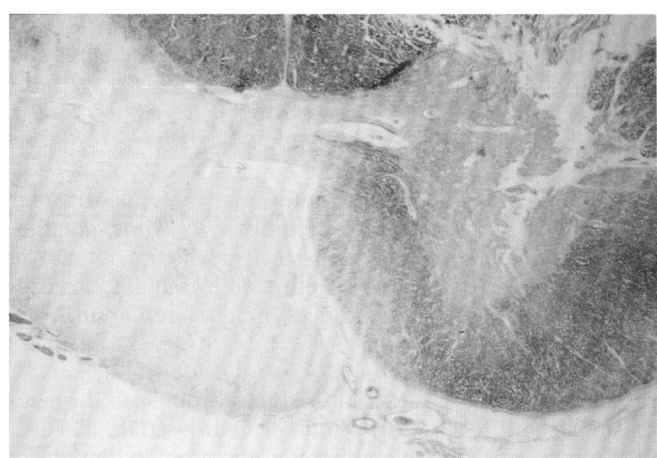

FIGURE 32-75. Postvaccinal encephalomyelitis involving the spinal cord with marked myelin loss in the lateral and anterior regions of the spinal cord on the left.

A similar syndrome, **postvaccinal encephalomyelitis,** may follow immunization against infectious agents (e.g., smallpox, rabies) (Fig. 32-75). Use of more-purified vaccines, free of cross-reacting antigenic contaminants, has dramatically reduced the frequency of this complication.

Chronic Lymphocytic Inflammation with Pontine Perivascular Enhancement Responsive to Steroids Affects the Brainstem

Chronic lymphocytic inflammation with pontine perivascular enhancement responsive to steroids (CLIPPERS) is a rare, newly described disorder with brainstem and cerebellar T-cell–predominant inflammation and demyelination. Patients have symmetric curvilinear gadolinium enhancement scattered throughout the pons and extending variably into the medulla, cerebellum, midbrain and occasionally spinal cord. Radiologic and clinical improvement occurs with high-dose glucocorticosteroid therapy, but patients routinely worsen after glucocorticosteroids are tapered and often require chronic glucocorticosteroid or other immunosuppressive therapy.

Leukodystrophies Are Inherited Defects of Myelin Biochemistry

These disorders often impact both central and peripheral myelin and usually manifest in infancy or childhood, although milder adult phenotypes may occur. Disruption of central myelin leads to blindness, spasticity and loss of developmental milestones, while loss of peripheral myelin leads to weakness and loss of reflexes.

Metachromatic Leukodystrophy

Metachromatic leukodystrophy (MLD), the most common leukodystrophy, is an autosomal recessive disorder characterized by accumulation of a cerebroside (galactosyl sulfatide) in the white matter of the brain and peripheral nerves. MLD predominates in infancy, but rare juvenile or adult cases are described. It is lethal within several years. A clinical trial using gene-corrected bone marrow transplantation has shown promise in preventing MLD progression.

 PATHOPHYSIOLOGY: MLD is caused by deficiency in arylsulfatase A activity. This lysosomal enzyme is involved in the degradation of myelin sulfatides. Accordingly, there is progressive accumulation of sulfatides within the lysosomes of myelin-forming Schwann cells and oligodendrocytes.

 PATHOLOGY: In MLD, the accumulated sulfatides form cytoplasmic spherical granules, 15–20 μ in diameter, which stain metachromatically with cresyl violet and toluidine blue. Normal staining is orthochromatic; that is, cresyl violet or toluidine blue stains tissue violet or blue. In metachromasia, the dye color shifts: tissue stained with cresyl violet or toluidine blue looks rusty brown to red. The brain shows diffuse myelin loss, accumulation of metachromatic material in white matter and astrogliosis. Demyelination of peripheral nerves is less severe.

Krabbe Disease

Krabbe disease is a rapidly progressive, fatal, autosomal recessive neurologic disorder caused by a deficiency of galactocerebroside β-galactosidase.

 PATHOLOGY: The brain is small, with widespread loss of myelin and preservation of the cerebral cortex. Astrogliosis is severe. Multinucleated "globoid cells" develop in the white matter and cluster around blood vessels, leading to the alternative name, **globoid cell leukodystrophy.** The globoid cells are multinucleated macrophages full of undigested galactocerebroside (galactosylceramide). These cells are up to 50 μ, with up to 20 peripheral nuclei. In end-stage disease, numbers of globoid cells decline, and in areas of severe myelin loss, only scattered globoid cells remain. Marbled areas of partial and total demyelination are present. By electron microscopy, the globoid cells contain crystalloid-like inclusions with straight or tubular profiles.

 CLINICAL FEATURES: Krabbe disease appears in infancy and progresses to death within 1–2 years. Severe motor, sensory and cognitive defects reflect diffuse involvement of the nervous system.

Adrenoleukodystrophy

 **MOLECULAR PATHOGENESIS:** Adrenoleukodystrophy (ALD) is an X-linked (Xq28) inherited disorder in which dysfunction of the adrenal cortex and nervous system demyelination are associated with high levels of saturated very-long-chain fatty acids (VLCFAs) in tissue and body fluids. The enzyme mutation in ALD impairs degradation of VLCFAs by preventing normal activation of free VLCFAs by the addition of coenzyme A (CoA). Disease reflects accumulation of abnormal cholesterol esters and VLCFA toxicity.

 PATHOLOGY: In the brain, there is confluent, bilaterally symmetric demyelination. The most severe lesions are in the subcortical white matter of the parieto-occipital region, which then extend rostrally (while sparing cortex) to result in severe loss of myelinated axons and oligodendrocytes. Gliosis and perivascular infiltrates of mononuclear cells (mostly lymphocytes) are prominent in affected areas. Scattered macrophages contain periodic acid–Schiff (PAS)-positive and sudanophilic material. Peripheral nerves are affected, but to a lesser degree than the brain. The adrenal glands are atrophic. Electron microscopy of cortical cells shows pathognomonic cytoplasmic, membrane-bound, curvilinear inclusions or clefts (lamellae) containing VLCFAs. Similar inclusions occur in Schwann cells and CNS macrophages.

 CLINICAL FEATURES: ALD occurs in children ages 3–10 years old, in whom neurologic symptoms precede signs of adrenal insufficiency. The disease progresses rapidly for 2–4 years, and the patient is quickly reduced to a vegetative state, which may persist for several years before death. Manipulation of dietary lipid composition and quantity using a 4:1 mixture of glycerol trioleate and glycerol trierucate ("Lorenzo's oil") reduces serum VLCFAs and slows progression of the disease in some cases. If the patient survives through childhood, the diet can be liberalized.

TOXIC AND METABOLIC DISORDERS

Given the enormous appetite of the brain for oxygen and amino acids and other metabolic morsels, it is not surprising that the brain is subject to malfunction as a result of lack or malutilization of essential substances, intoxication and hereditary metabolic diseases. These disorders are particularly important since correction of underlying metabolic derangements restores function. In most cases, these dysfunctions may be functionally profound but have no morphologic correlate; however, in some cases, pathologic changes occur.

Metabolic Storage Diseases Reflect Lack of Key Enzymes

Neuronal storage diseases are inherited enzyme defects in which normal metabolic products accumulate in lysosomes.

Unlike leukodystrophies, which produce blindness and spasticity, these diseases affect neurons to cause seizures and cognitive decline.

Tay-Sachs Disease

Tay-Sachs disease is a lethal, autosomal recessive disorder caused by deficiency of hexosaminidase A. Thus, ganglioside accumulates in CNS neurons. The disease is fatal in infancy and early childhood. Retinal involvement increases macular transparency and causes a **cherry-red spot** in the macula.

The brain is the major site of ganglioside storage, and it progressively enlarges in infancy. Lipid droplets in the cytoplasm distend CNS and peripheral neurons (Fig. 32-76A). Electron microscopy demonstrates the lipid within lysosomes as whorled "myelin figures" (Fig. 32-76B). The neural tissues develop diffuse astrogliosis. An affected infant appears normal at birth but by age 6 months shows delayed motor development. Thereafter, progressive deterioration leads to flaccid weakness, blindness and severe mental impairment. Death usually supervenes before the end of the second year.

Hurler Syndrome

Hurler syndrome is an autosomal recessive disturbance in glycosaminoglycan metabolism that results in intraneuronal accumulation of mucopolysaccharides. Clinical variants of this syndrome are distinguished by variable involvement of visceral organs and the nervous system. The disease is typically expressed in infancy or early childhood as reduced stature, corneal opacities, skeletal deformities and hepatosplenomegaly. The intraneuronal storage distends the cytoplasmic compartment and is accompanied by astrogliosis and progressive mental deterioration.

Gaucher Disease

Gaucher disease is an autosomal recessive genetic deficiency of glucocerebrosidase, leading to glucocerebroside accumulation, principally in macrophages. The CNS is most severely involved in infantile (type II) Gaucher disease.

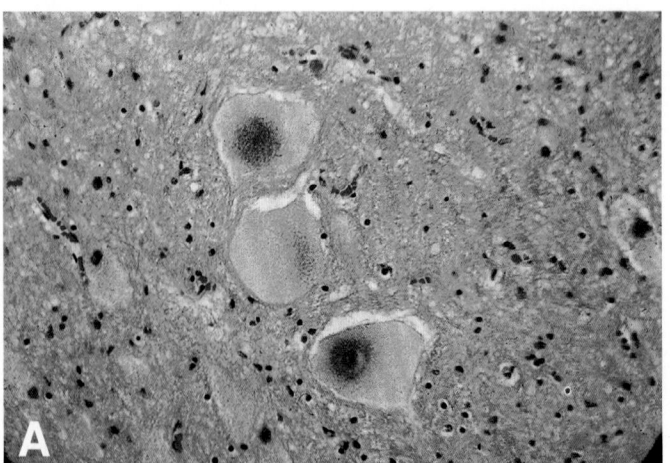
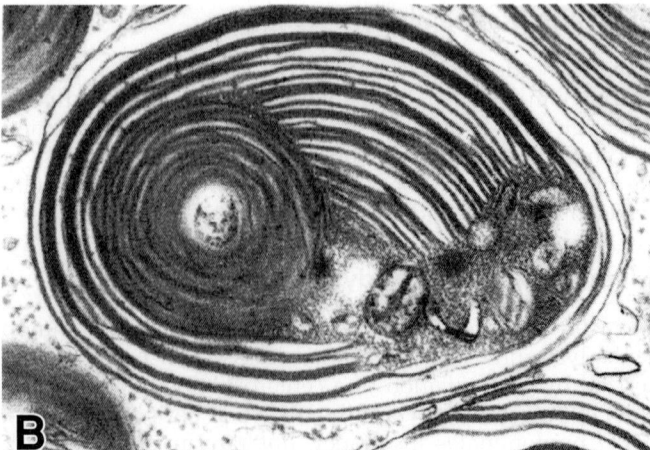

FIGURE 32-76. Tay-Sachs Disease A. The cytoplasm of the neurons is distended by the accumulation of eosinophilic storage material. **B.** Ultrastructurally, whorled "myelin bodies" composed of accumulated gangliosides are present within the cytoplasm.

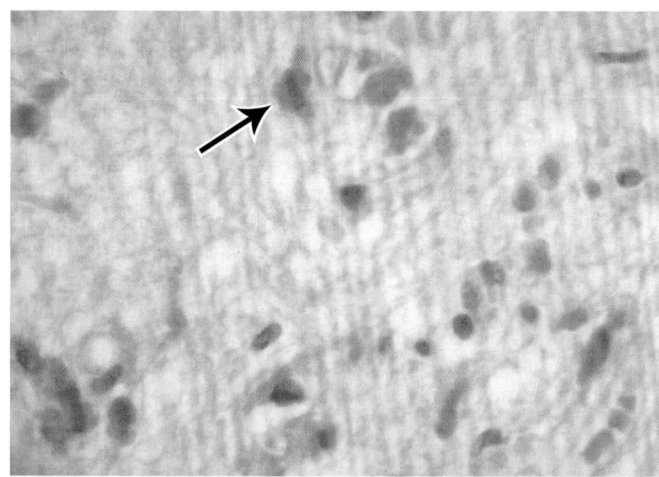

FIGURE 32-77. Alexander disease. This disease reflecting a mutation in the glial fibrillary acidic protein (GFAP) gene is characterized by accumulation of aggregated GFAP into eosinophilic bodies called Rosenthal fibers (*arrows*). Rosenthal fibers are seen in Alexander disease, in pilocytic astrocytoma and as a reaction adjacent to chronic compressive lesions.

Although intraneuronal accumulation of glucocerebroside is not conspicuous, neuronal loss is severe and is accompanied by diffuse astrogliosis. These infants fail to thrive and die at an early age.

Niemann-Pick Disease

Niemann-Pick disease is an autosomal recessive disorder in which a deficiency of sphingomyelinase leads to intraneuronal storage of sphingomyelin. Symptoms occur early, with failure of the infant to develop and thrive. The mononuclear phagocyte system is targeted for storage, but the nervous system may predominate symptomatically during infancy. The brain becomes atrophic, with marked astrogliosis. Retinal degeneration may produce a cherry-red spot, like that in Tay-Sachs disease.

Alexander Disease

Alexander disease is an astrocytic storage disease. It is an uncommon neurologic disorder of infants, children and rarely adults, and is characterized by a loss of myelin in the brain and striking eosinophilic collections of GFAP in astrocytic processes (Rosenthal fibers; Fig. 32-77). The Rosenthal fibers are abundant, particularly in a perivascular and subpial distribution. Clinically, children have psychomotor retardation, progressive dementia and paralysis and eventually die. The disease is caused by mutations in the gene encoding GFAP. It is not yet clear how this process impairs myelin formation and induces degeneration of oligodendrocytes and myelin.

Phenylketonuria Is a Deficiency in Phenylalanine Hydroxylase

Phenylketonuria (PKU) is an autosomal recessive disease (see Chapter 6) in which phenylalanine accumulates in blood and tissues because its conversion to tyrosine is blocked. Symptoms appear in the early months of life, with mental retardation, seizures and impaired physical development.

Treatment consists of restricting dietary phenylalanine. Untreated patients rarely obtain an IQ above 50, but those on the diet do well. Since the morbidity of PKU is preventable by a simple dietary restriction, all newborns are now screened for it. Although there are no consistent morphologic alterations, the brain may be underweight and deficient in myelination.

Wilson Disease Is an Autosomal Recessive Disorder of Copper Metabolism

Wilson disease, or **"hepatolenticular degeneration,"** affects the brain and the liver and is caused by mutations of the *WD* gene (see Chapter 20). Defective excretion of copper in the bile leads to copper deposition in the brain.

 CLINICAL FEATURES: Symptoms of cerebral involvement appear as a movement disorder with a tendency to choreoathetosis, usually in the second decade, but the disease may not become apparent until as late as the eighth decade. The movement disorder may be associated with psychosis. Before, during or after the appearance of neurologic symptoms, an insidiously developing cirrhosis may result in hepatic failure. Copper deposition in the limbus of the cornea produces a visible golden-brown band, the **Kayser-Fleischer ring,** seen on slit lamp examination.

The lenticular nuclei of the brain show a light golden discoloration, and 25% of cases have small cysts or clefts in the putamen or in deep layers of the neocortex. Mild neuron loss and gliosis are characteristic.

Some patients are "presymptomatic," never developing high enough levels of copper to accumulate in the brain or eyes or developing cirrhosis. Diagnosis is critical as Wilson disease is treatable, and failure to treat can lead to irreversible hepatic and CNS damage. Anyone presenting with a hyperkinetic movement disorder, particularly with onset in early adult life, in association with psychiatric or hepatic manifestations must be evaluated for Wilson disease.

Brain Dysfunction in Systemic Metabolic Disease Is Metabolic Encephalopathy

Such metabolic derangements may be caused by cardiopulmonary, renal, hepatic or endocrine diseases occurring singly or in combination. Clinically, patients show declining level of consciousness, starting with inattentiveness that may include rowdiness, progressing to lethargy and finally lack of arousal, regardless of level of stimulation. The change in consciousness may be accompanied by tremor, asterixis and changing multifocal neurologic signs. Computed tomography (CT) and MRI scans show no structural abnormality, and EEG shows progressive slowing of rhythmic cortical activity, sometimes accompanied by periodic high-amplitude discharges known as triphasic waves (which are seen most often in hepatic encephalopathy but are not specific for this condition). Biochemically, metabolic encephalopathy is characterized by lower cerebral glucose and oxygen utilization regardless of the underlying disorder. There are no specific morphologic features in metabolic encephalopathy, but presence of Alzheimer type II astrocytes suggests, but is not diagnostic of, hepatic encephalopathy.

Hepatic Encephalopathy

Hepatic encephalopathy is a common clinical expression of liver failure, with delirium, seizures and coma. Symptoms generally greatly exceed their morphologic correlates, which are restricted to the appearance of altered astroglia **(Alzheimer type II astrocytes)** with enlarged nuclei and marginated chromatin, especially in the thalamus.

Osmotic Demyelination Syndrome (Central Pontine Myelinolysis)

This is a rare demyelinating disorder of the pons, where discrete areas of selective demyelination occur (Fig. 32-78). Lesions often are too small to manifest clinically and are evident only at autopsy. In a few patients, quadriparesis, pseudobulbar palsy or locked-in syndrome may occur. Central pontine myelinolysis (CPM) arises from overly rapid correction of hyponatremia in alcoholics, malnourished people or patients with marked electrolyte instability, including those with renal failure and liver transplant recipients. Demyelination is not confined to the pons, and other extrapontine white matter areas may be involved; thus, CPM is now considered part of a broader disorder called osmotic demyelination syndrome. A classical corpus callosal demyelination process, called Marchiafava Bignami syndrome, is now considered to be part of osmotic demyelination, but internal capsule, corona radiata and cerebellar white matter tracts may be involved as well.

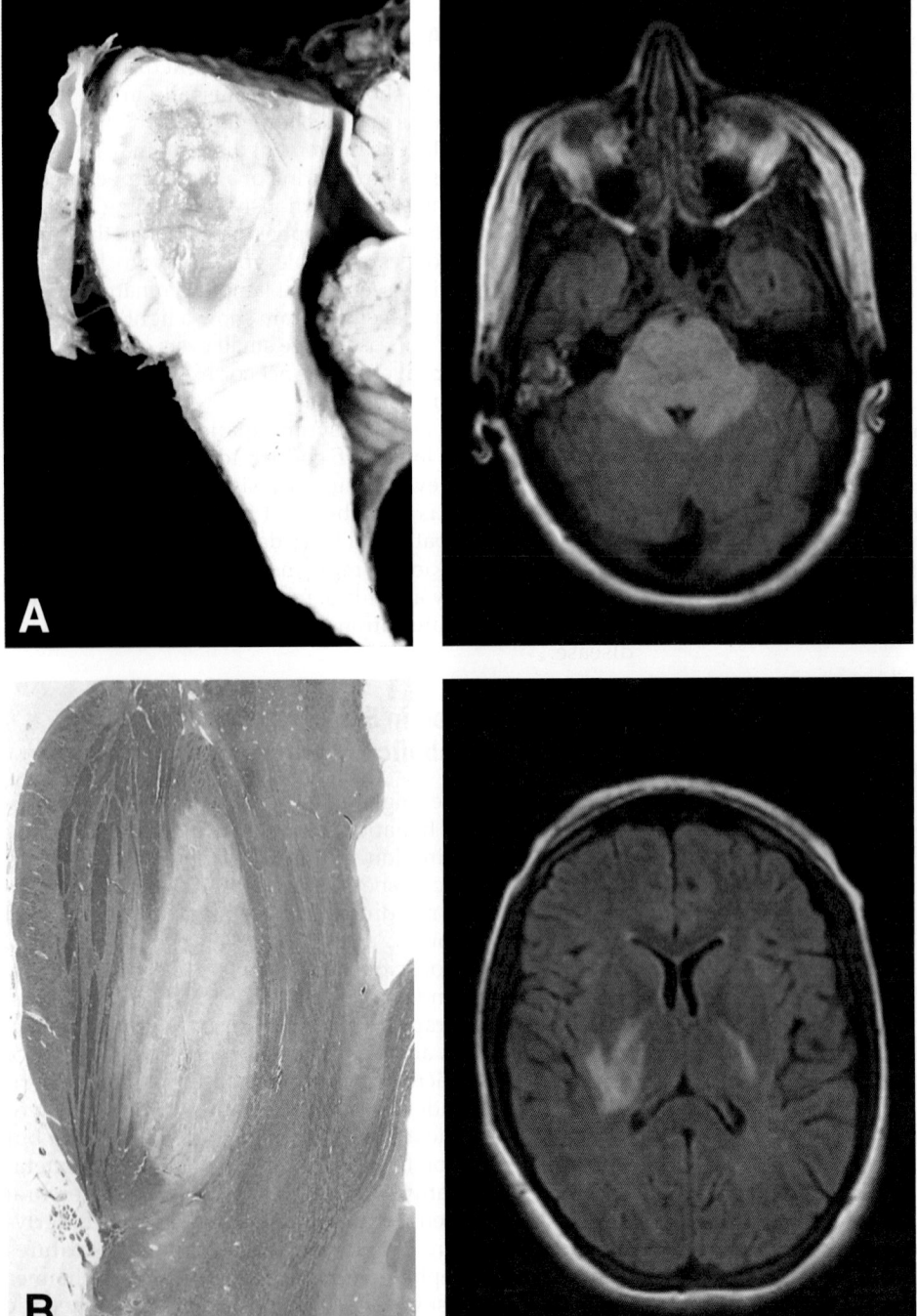

FIGURE 32-78. Osmotic demyelination syndrome with central pontine myelinolysis. A. This sagittal section of the brainstem shows a soft, discolored, midpontine lesion. **B.** A myelin-stained section reveals a sharply demarcated loss of myelin appearing as a pink ovoid zone. (A and B Courtesy of Dr. F. Stephen Vogel, Duke University.)

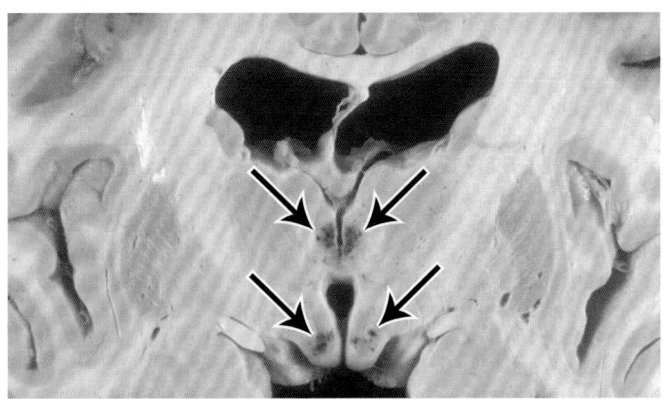

FIGURE 32-79. Wernicke encephalopathy. This coronal section shows hemorrhagic petechiae in the mamillary bodies and periventricular anterior thalamus (*arrows*). (Courtesy of Dr. F. Stephen Vogel, Duke University.)

Vitamin Deficiencies

Vitamin deficiencies and their systemic consequences are discussed in Chapter 8.

Wernicke Syndrome

Wernicke syndrome results from thiamine (vitamin B_1) deficiency and is characterized clinically by rapid onset of altered consciousness with dramatically impaired short-term memory, ophthalmoplegia and nystagmus. Lesions are seen in the hypothalamus and mamillary bodies, the periaqueductal regions of the midbrain and the pontine tegmentum (Fig. 32-79). The syndrome is most common in chronic alcoholics but may occur in others whose diets lack thiamine. It may progress rapidly to death, but it is reversed by administration of thiamine. In fatal cases, petechiae form around capillaries in the mamillary bodies, hypothalamus, periaqueductal region and floor of the fourth ventricle (Fig. 32-80). Over time, hemosiderin deposition identifies

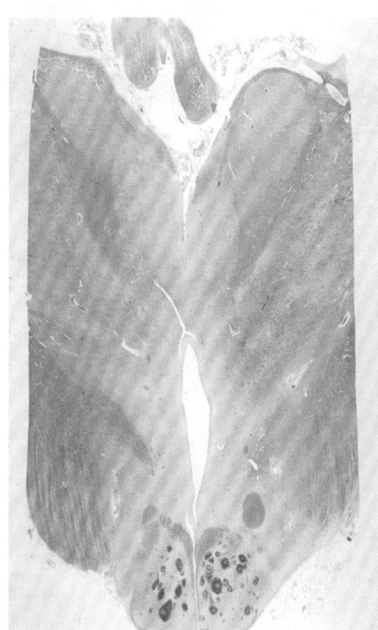

FIGURE 32-80. Wernicke encephalopathy with petechial hemorrhage in mammillary bodies. (Courtesy of Dr. F. Stephen Vogel, Duke University.)

regions where petechiae occurred. Neurons and myelin are generally spared, but mamillary body atrophy and capillary proliferation may be prominent.

Wernicke-Korsakoff syndrome is a state of disordered recent memory often compensated for by confabulation. It resembles Wernicke syndrome pathologically but may show degeneration of neurons in the medial–dorsal thalamic nucleus.

Many chronic alcoholics have cerebral atrophy of uncertain cause and for which the relative contributions of alcohol toxicity, malnutrition and other factors are not defined. Similar uncertainties prevail with regard to atrophy of the Purkinje and granular cells of the cerebellum. These changes are common in chronic alcoholism and are the cause of truncal ataxia, which persists during periods of sobriety.

Subacute Combined Degeneration

Subacute combined degeneration of the spinal cord results from vitamin B_{12} deficiency (pernicious anemia) and leads to lesions in the posterolateral portions of the spinal cord. Initially, there is symmetric myelin and axonal loss in the thoracic spinal cord. Astrogliosis is mild in the acute lesions, but with time, gliosis and atrophy develop, especially in the posterolateral areas of the cord.

A burning sensation in the soles of the feet and other paresthesias herald the onset of this rapidly progressive and poorly reversible neurologic disorder. Weakness emerges in all four limbs, then defective postural sensibility, incoordination and ataxia. Subacute combined degeneration may complicate a rare case of extensive gastric resection and other malabsorption syndromes. As vitamin B_{12} is not found in plants, some extreme vegetarians who eschew all animal products, even milk and eggs, develop subacute combined degeneration after many years on a restricted diet.

Iatrogenic, occupational or recreational exposure to the anesthetic gas nitrous oxide (N_2O) may lead to a clinically and morphologically indistinguishable condition. N_2O interferes with vitamin B_{12}–dependent enzymes. Hypocupric (low serum copper) myelopathy after bariatric surgery or zinc overdosage is also similar.

Intoxication

Neurotoxicology is a major aspect of contemporary neuropathology. The breadth of this area far exceeds the scope of this chapter, so we concentrate on the more common and better-understood toxic injuries to the brain.

ETHANOL: Acute and chronic alcohol intake has widespread harmful effects and more widespread societal repercussions owing to its behavioral consequences. Acute alcohol intoxication signs and symptoms correspond to dose-related blood level, such that 0.05–0.1 mg/dL is associated with disinhibition and motor impairment; 0.1–0.3 mg/dL with frank inebriation and ataxia; and 0.3–0.35 mg/dL with extreme intoxication and sleepiness, nausea and vomiting. Over 0.35 mg/dL is potentially lethal owing to respiratory depression and inability to protect the airway from aspiration. Lethal intoxication may tragically occur during competitive drinking among college students.

Chronic alcohol use is associated with neurologic complications caused by nutritional deficiencies, including Wernicke-Korsakoff syndrome and possibly peripheral neuropathy; liver failure with hepatic encephalopathy and non-Wilsonian hepatocerebral degeneration; and metabolic derangements including central pontine myelinolysis from rapid correction of hyponatremia (Fig. 32-81). Alcoholics may also develop

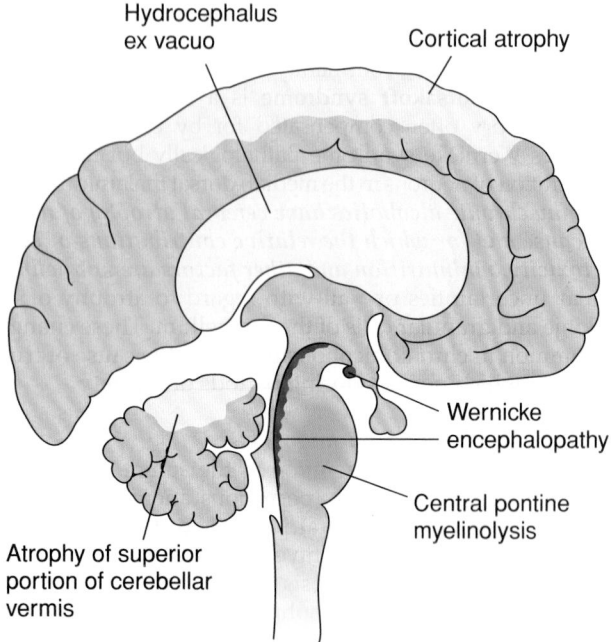

FIGURE 32-81. Regions of the brain with lesions associated with chronic ethanol abuse.

central necrosis of the corpus callosum or Marchiafava-Bignami disease (see above). This disease is part of the osmotic demyelination syndrome caused by overly rapid correction of hyponatremia. Less well understood is anterior superior vermal cerebellar degeneration, which occurs mainly in alcoholic men, presents with truncal ataxia and is grossly evident as atrophy of the vermis (Fig. 32-82).

METHANOL: In their quest for ethanol, alcoholics may from time to time drink methanol, which is oxidized to formaldehyde and formic acid. Patients dying of methanol intoxication have severe cerebral edema with hemorrhagic necrosis of the lateral putamen. Retinal edema and ganglion cell degeneration account for the blindness that afflicts these patients. Blindness may result from ingestion of as little as 4 mL, while a lethal dose is in the range of 8–10 mL of pure methanol, although usually 70–100 mL is consumed in fatal cases.

ETHYLENE GLYCOL: Similarly, ethylene glycol (automotive antifreeze) is sometimes consumed as an alternative to ethanol or by children or animals because of its sweet taste. Oxalate is its metabolic product. Severe organic acidosis may lead to coma and renal failure, and survivors may have residual neurologic deficits. Tissue oxalate crystal deposition may be seen.

CARBON MONOXIDE (CO): This colorless, odorless, tasteless gas is formed by incomplete combustion. CO binds hemoglobin far more avidly than oxygen. It thus displaces oxygen from hemoglobin, to form carboxyhemoglobin (COHb), which in turn reduces the oxygen-carrying capacity of blood. COHb is red and imparts a "cherry-red" hue to victims of CO poisoning. Severe intoxication causes almost pathognomonic bilateral liquefactive necrosis of the globus pallidus. Other areas of CNS ischemic injury may be seen. The mechanism of the selective globus pallidus injury is unclear, but the recent discovery that CO may act as a neurotransmitter suggests that areas rich in heme-iron (such as the basal ganglia) may use CO under physiologic conditions for cell-to-cell signaling. As in amino acid excitotoxicity (see above), an excess neurotransmitter such as CO might injure the areas where it normally plays a physiologic role.

METAL INTOXICATION OR DEFICIENCY: Many metals employed in industry and medicine can cause neurologic disease; additionally, the biocidal properties of some of these substances, such as arsenic and thallium, have made them favorite tools of murderers, suicidal individuals and pesticide users.

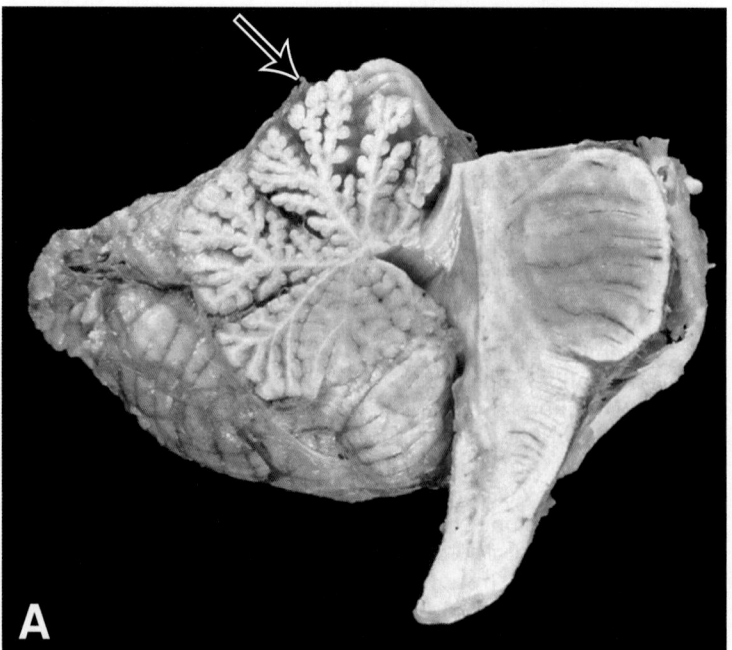
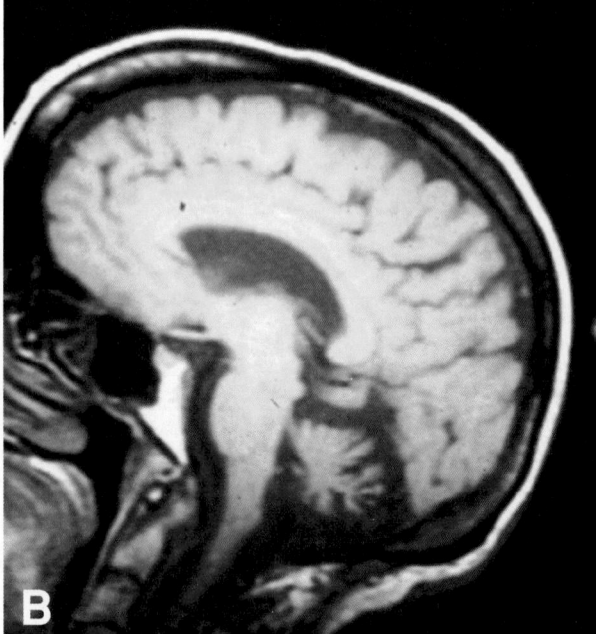

FIGURE 32-82. Chronic alcoholism. A. The superior and anterior portions of the cerebellar vermis are atrophic (*arrow*), leading to truncal ataxia. (Courtesy of Dr. F. Stephen Vogel, Duke University.) **B.** Coronal noncontrast computed tomography showing profound vermal atrophy in an alcoholic individual.

- **Lead:** Lead intoxication produces an edema-based encephalopathy in acute poisoning, especially in childhood. An amorphous exudate around microvessels may be seen, as may some vascular proliferation. Excess exposure in children may entail their ingesting lead-based paint, fishing sinkers and other lead weights. In adults, lead poisoning more commonly presents as a neuropathy rather than as an encephalopathy.
- **Mercury:** Chronic inorganic mercury intoxication may present with dementia, delirium, tremor, irritability and insomnia. Now rare, mercury poisoning in the 19th century decimated workers in cinnabar mines, hat manufacturing ("mad as a hatter"), mirror silvering plants and manufacturing of scientific instruments. Cerebellar atrophy with loss of Purkinje cells was seen.
- Organomercurial poisoning is now more prevalent. In Japan, in Minamata Bay, industrial mercuric chloride from the manufacture of vinyl chloride was dumped into the bay. The marine food chain concentrated the metal. Fishermen and local inhabitants then ate contaminated seafood. Many people were injured or died. These patients developed ataxia and blindness. Cerebellar and cerebrocortical atrophy occurred, with some cortical damage elsewhere. Congenital methylmercury neurotoxicity from in utero exposure results in severe mental retardation, athetosis, ataxia and spastic quadriparesis. Severe atrophy of the cerebrum with milder cerebellar atrophy is evident, with loss of the cortical lamellar organization perhaps indicating a defect in neuronal migration and organization in development.
- **Arsenic:** Arsenical intoxication manifests with gastrointestinal complaints including nausea, vomiting and diarrhea; cutaneous features including hyperkeratosis and increased pigmentation of the soles and palms and Mees lines on the nails; and a severe axonal neuropathy. In the brain, swelling and petechiae may be present. Long-term exposure has other risks (see Chapter 8).
- **Thallium:** Like arsenic, gastrointestinal disturbances are evident, with major cutaneous manifestations of late alopecia and Mees lines occasionally, and a severe axonal neuropathy.
- **Manganese:** Basal ganglionic damage producing parkinsonism is seen in manganese miners. This may be associated with a psychosis known as "manganese madness."

Metal deficiencies may also occur. For example, copper deficiency may follow bariatric surgery due to insufficient absorption or competitive malabsorption if the patient consumes excessive zinc or bismuth. Hypocupric myelopathy results with dorsal column and lateral column loss.

NEURODEGENERATIVE DISORDERS

Neurodegenerative disorders involve death of functionally related neurons; hence, these disorders can be classified by the primary functional system involved. **Cortical** degeneration leads to dementia, **basal ganglia** degeneration to movement disorders, **spinocerebellar** degeneration to ataxia and **motor neuron** degeneration to upper and lower motor neuron weakness. *Neuropathologically, there is loss of neurons in these systems. There are often characteristic cellular inclusions and extracellular protein accumulations in these disorders and variable glial and microglial activation.*

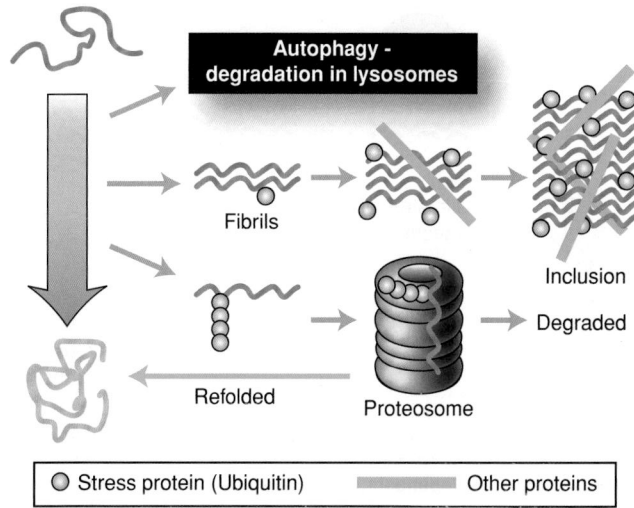

FIGURE 32-83. Possible fates of misfolded proteins. Many of the neurodegenerative diseases appear to be, at least in part, disorders of proteostasis, which consist of the cellular pathways that control protein synthesis, folding, trafficking, aggregation, disaggregation and degradation.

PATHOPHYSIOLOGY: Neurodegenerative disorders are classified according to which neuronal systems are most involved and the biochemistry of the proteins that accumulate in those cells.

Intracellular, and particularly intracytoplasmic, inclusions have a history that is inextricably bound to neurodegenerative disorders, as these engaging features of diseased cells were among the first histologic nervous system abnormalities recognized. We now understand them to be markers of cellular stress: cytoplasmic landfills made of abnormal cellular proteins and heat shock proteins. Abnormal protein homeostasis is probably central to the development of these disorders (Fig. 32-83; see Chapter 1).

When a cell is stressed, its intermediate filament network collapses into perinuclear bundles or clumps. This may reflect increased phosphorylation or proteolysis of these proteins due to calcium influx into the stressed cell. If the stress is not lethal, the cell deploys an adaptive **heat shock response**. The cell produces several proteins that may restore functional activity of partially denatured proteins or, if the insult is too severe to allow restoration, the proteins are polyubiquitinated for subsequent proteolysis. However, their highly stable β-pleated sheet structure leads to aggregation and prevents their effective removal by proteasomal or other means. Other stress proteins may include crystallin and a family of heat shock proteins. If the proteins conjugated to these stress proteins are not successfully degraded, the conjugated complexes aggregate as intracellular inclusions.

The inclusions in neurodegenerative disorders *reflect damaged native cellular proteins and their stress response conjugates.* Cells activate stress responses whenever they are damaged; thus, stress response inclusions do not identify the inciting insult, but rather indicate that cells are trying to protect themselves. Neuropathologic inclusions are made from relatively few permutations of cytoskeletal

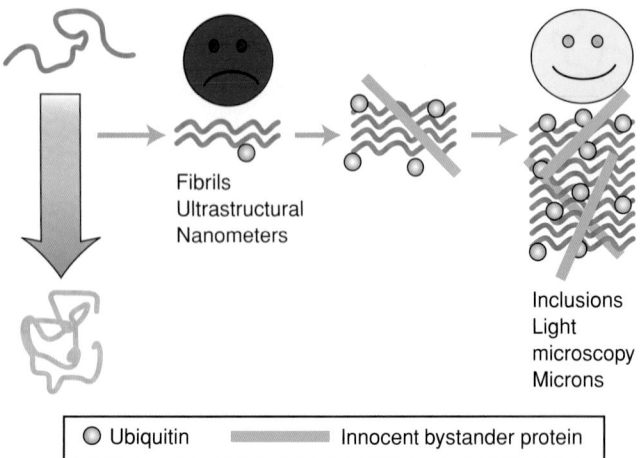

FIGURE 32-84. Fibrillogenesis and inclusions. Misfolded proteins with a tendency toward polymerization may form extremely cytotoxic fibrils that are only visible by electron microscopy. The cellular stress response may facilitate hyperaggregation to inclusions that are visible by light microscopy. Such inclusions may be considered "toxic landfills" and may be protective.

give limited data about the precise stress damaging the cell, their biochemical compositions often overlap and final diagnostic categorization depends on clinical data, immunohistochemical characterization of inclusions and analysis of the cell populations affected.

These protein aggregates may cause disease (Fig. 32-84; Table 32-3) by several routes. Sequestering protein or other macromolecules makes them unavailable for their normal functions. As aggregates enlarge, they may physically obstruct axons, dendrites or movement of material within the cytoplasm. They may also act as ubiquitin sinks, depleting cell ubiquitin that is needed to send misfolded proteins to be recycled. Thus, cellular protein recycling and homeostasis are impaired. As these proteins aggregate, they initially form ultrastructural fibrils that may be extremely cytotoxic. Thus, it appears that cellular stresses from a variety of causes may disrupt proteostasis and generate toxic fibrils that themselves can perpetuate and amplify the cellular stress.

Neurodegenerative disorders often begin focally and then spread in reasonably predictable ways throughout the CNS. This stereotypical dissemination likely involves abnormally folded pathogenic proteins recruiting and transforming native protein. This phenomenon is reminiscent of the molecular pathogenesis of prion diseases and is called "prion-like" protein misfolding or "templating."

At their core, the neurodegenerative diseases are largely disorders of proteostasis, involving impaired cellular pathways that control protein synthesis, folding, trafficking, aggregation, disaggregation and degradation. Because of this unifying theme, fundamental pathogenetic insights derived from one neurodegenerative disease may be generalizable to others.

and stress proteins—fewer, in fact, than the number of apparently discrete types of inclusions described. Ubiquitin is present in many intracellular inclusions. While itself not "diagnostic" of any particular disease, ubiquitin immunostaining is the most sensitive technique for detecting such aggregated proteins. Combined with the morphology, cellular distribution and clinical context, it may be helpful diagnostically. Available antibodies allow identification of ubiquitinated proteins: tau, neurofilament, α-synuclein and others. In summary, inclusions

TABLE 32-3			
REPRESENTATIVE NEURODEGENERATIVE DISEASES WITH FIBRILLOGENESIS			
Disease	**Lesion**	**Components**	**Location**
Alzheimer disease	Senile plaques	β-Amyloid	Extracellular
	Neurofibrillary tangles	Tau	Intracytoplasmic
Amyotrophic lateral sclerosis	Spheroids	Neurofilament	Intracytoplasmic
		Superoxide dismutase (SOD-1)	
		TDP43	
		FUS	
Dementia with Lewy bodies	Lewy bodies	α-Synuclein	Intracytoplasmic
Frontotemporal dementias	Neurofibrillary tangles	Tau	Intracytoplasmic
		TDP43, progranulin and other proteins	
Multiple system atrophy	Glial inclusions	α-Synuclein	Intracytoplasmic
Parkinson disease	Lewy bodies	α-Synuclein	Intracytoplasmic
Prion diseases	Prion deposits	Prions	Extracellular
Trinucleotide repeat diseases	Inclusions	Polyglutamine tracts	Intranuclear and cytoplasmic

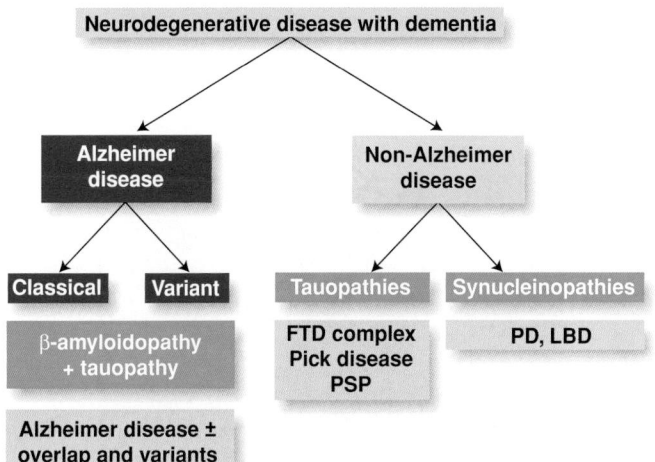

FIGURE 32-85. **Protein fibrillogenesis.** Molecular classification of the dementias and other neurodegenerative diseases now recognizes disorders based on the proteins that undergo fibrillogenesis. Alzheimer disease (AD) is a combination of a β-amyloidopathy and a tauopathy. Most of the frontotemporal lobar degenerations (FTDs) such as Pick disease and progressive supranuclear palsy (PSP) are pure tauopathies. Lewy body dementia (LBD) and Parkinson disease (PD) complex are α-synucleinopathies.

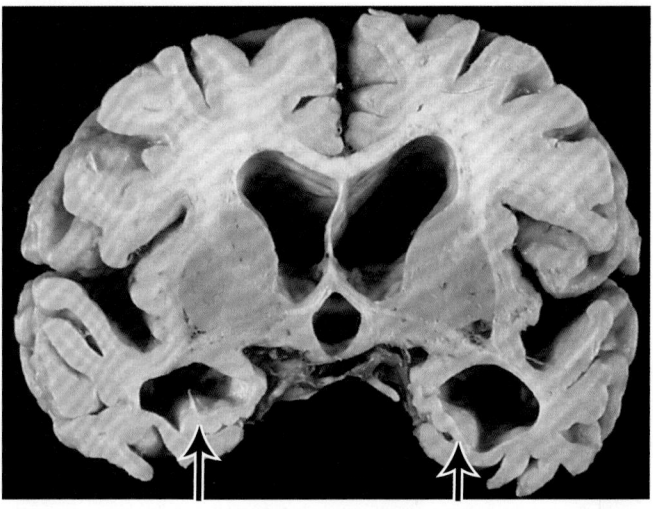

FIGURE 32-87. **Cerebral atrophy with hydrocephalus ex vacuo in Alzheimer disease.** Note also the severe atrophy of the hippocampus (*arrows*) leading to early memory disturbances in this disease. (Courtesy of Dr. F. Stephen Vogel, Duke University.)

There Are Three Major Cerebral Cortical Neurodegenerative Diseases

Their clinical and pathologic features are distinctive, as different polymerized proteins accumulate (Fig. 32-85). These cortical degenerations ultimately lead to dementia.

- **Alzheimer disease (AD)** accounts for the majority of neurodegenerative dementia. It is characterized by abnormal accumulation of two proteins: β-amyloid and tau.
- **Pick disease,** which is the prototypical frontotemporal lobar dementia, is characterized by accumulation of abnormal tau without β-amyloid.
- **Lewy body dementia** features accumulation of α-synuclein.

Alzheimer Disease

 **EPIDEMIOLOGY:** AD is an insidious progressive neurologic disorder characterized clinically by loss of memory, cognitive impairment and, eventually, dementia. Although Alzheimer's original patients were younger than 65 and suffered "presenile dementia," the term is now used for dementia at any age with characteristic pathologic changes. *It is the most common dementia in the elderly, accounting for over half of cases.* The prevalence of the condition is closely related to age. In patients younger than 65, Alzheimer disease affects at most 1%–2%, but it occurs in 40% or more of patients older than 85. Women are affected twice as often as men. Most cases are sporadic, but familial variants are reported.

 PATHOLOGY: AD brains show cortical atrophy with hydrocephalus ex vacuo (Figs. 32-86 and 32-87). Gyri narrow, sulci widen and cortical

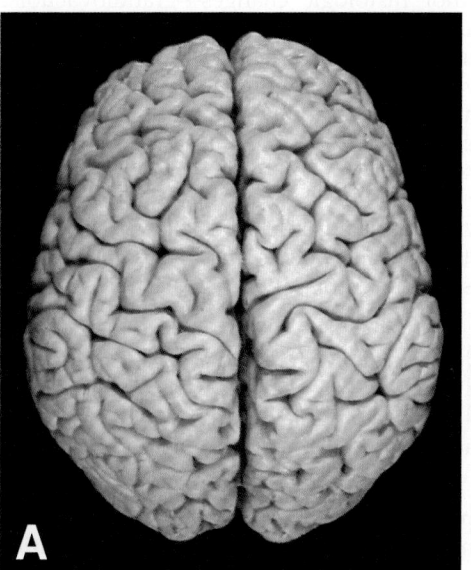

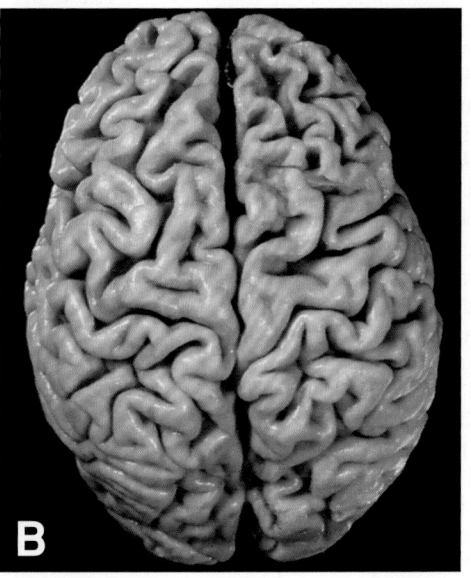

FIGURE 32-86. **Cortical atrophy.** A normal brain is shown on the left **(A)** and a brain with cortical atrophy caused by Alzheimer disease is shown on the right **(B)** with thinning of the gyri and prominent sulci. (Courtesy of Dr. F. Stephen Vogel, Duke University.)

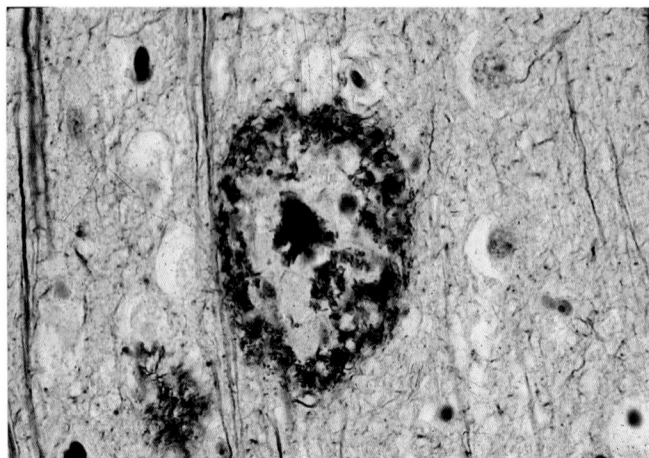

FIGURE 32-88. Neuritic plaques are extracellular accumulations of polymerized β-amyloid centrally with a rim of dystrophic neuritic processes. The number of plaques in the cerebral cortex does not correlate well with the severity of dementia in Alzheimer disease.

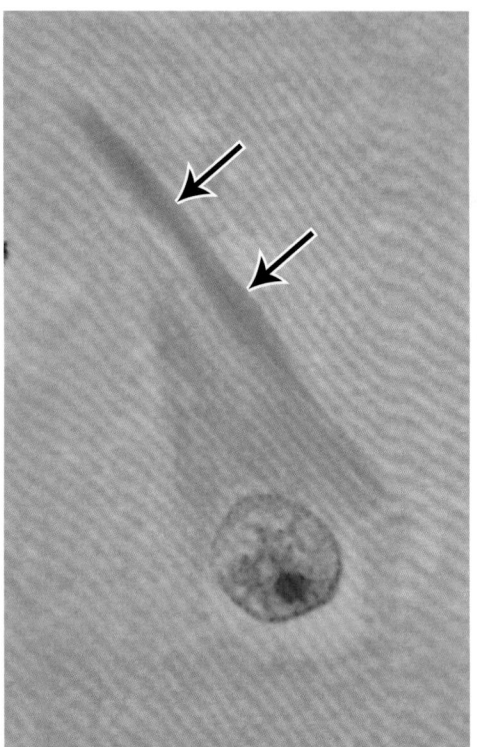

FIGURE 32-89. Neurofibrillary tangles are intracytoplasmic intraneuronal accumulations of polymerized hyperphosphorylated tau protein (*arrows*). The sites and degree of distribution of neurofibrillary tangles correlate with clinical symptoms.

atrophy is especially apparent in the parahippocampal regions. However, as the disease progresses, atrophy of temporal, frontal and parietal cortex becomes more severe.

Senile plaques and neurofibrillary tangles (NFTs) dominate the histology. Small numbers of plaques and tangles are common in elderly patients with mild forgetfulness and mild cognitive impairment, which in half of cases is a prodrome of AD.

NEURITIC PLAQUES: The most conspicuous histologic lesions, senile or neuritic plaques, are *extracellular* spherical deposits of β-amyloid several hundred microns in diameter. In end-stage disease, senile plaques occupy large volumes of affected cerebral gray matter (Fig. 32-88). They bind planar amyloid binding dyes such as Congo red and thioflavin S, and silver containing dyes (argentophilic), and are immunoreactive for β-amyloid protein (Aβ) at the core and periphery. They are surrounded by reactive astrocytes and microglia and display swollen distorted neuronal processes (dystrophic neurites). Detection of plaques is necessary to diagnose AD; their number and distribution do not correlate well with clinical disease severity.

NEUROFIBRILLARY TANGLES: NFTs are *intracytoplasmic* collections of polymerized tau filaments (Fig. 32-89). NFTs contain irregular bundles of fibrils that are positive by Congo red and thioflavin S and immunoreactive for tau. The tangles are paired, 10-nm-thick, helical filaments with abundant insoluble tau proteins. Their distribution correlates with the clinical severity of AD. Tangles in the entorhinal cortex and parahippocampal gyrus can be seen in asymptomatic people decades before the usual age of onset of AD and may represent the disease's earliest phases. As more temporal neocortex comes to possess tangles, mild cognitive impairment may develop. Finally, when large swaths of neocortex, deep nuclei and brainstem are involved, full-blown AD is present. As this concept of gradual accretion of neurofibrillary tangles is increasingly validated, efforts are increasingly directed at early diagnosis during the asymptomatic phase and development of drugs that will arrest progression.

NFTs are not unique to AD. They also occur in other neurodegenerative diseases including dementia pugilistica (punch drunk syndrome in boxers), postencephalitic

parkinsonism, Guam ALS/parkinsonism dementia complex, Pick disease, corticobasal degeneration, sporadic frontotemporal dementias and hereditary frontotemporal lobe dementia with parkinsonism associated with mutations on chromosome 17 (FTDP-17). Collectively, these hereditary and sporadic neurodegenerative diseases showing abnormal tau aggregation are called **tauopathies**. They may share common mechanisms of brain degeneration. *Alzheimer disease is both a tauopathy and a β-amyloidopathy, leading to intracellular and extracellular tangles and plaques, respectively, seen in this disorder.*

There are minor histologic changes—granulovacuolar degeneration and Hirano bodies—in AD and normal aging that can be visually arresting but lack diagnostic significance. **Granulovacuolar degeneration** is largely restricted to the cytoplasm of hippocampal pyramidal cells, where it is evident as circular clear zones containing basophilic and argentophilic granules (Fig. 32-90A). **Hirano bodies,** like granulovacuolar degeneration, occur almost exclusively in hippocampal pyramidal neurons, especially in their processes (Fig. 32-90B). Hirano bodies are 10–15-micron-thick eosinophilic rods composed of polymerized action.

  **PATHOPHYSIOLOGY AND MOLECULAR PATHOGENESIS:** The cause of AD is not known, but the origins of associated amyloid and NFTs are increasingly understood.

■ **β-Amyloid protein (Aβ):** Increasing evidence points to the importance of deposition of Aβ protein in **neuritic**

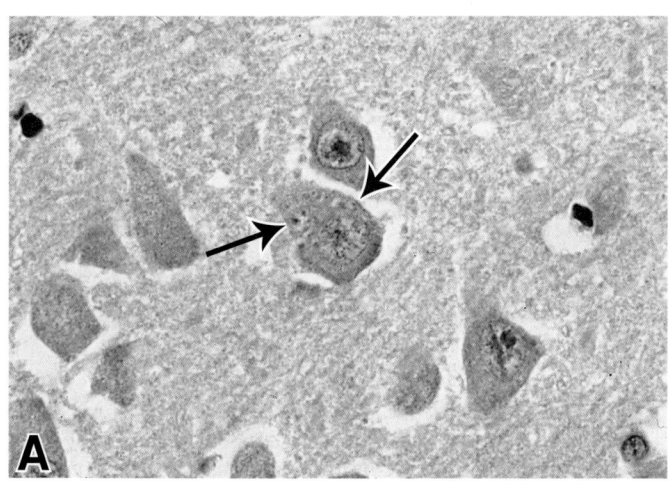
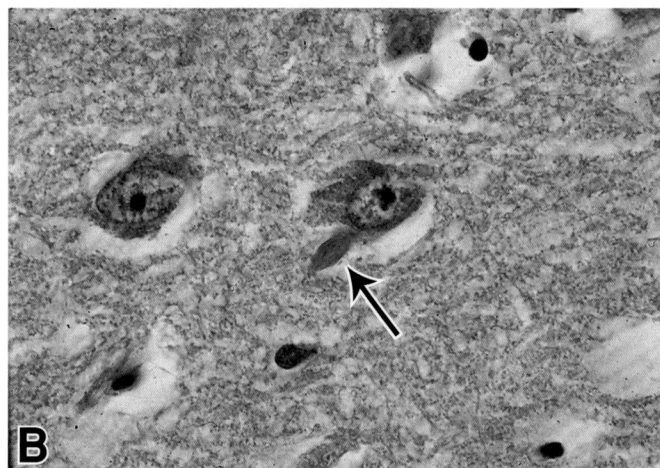

FIGURE 32-90. A. Granulovacuolar degeneration (*arrows*) is seen in hippocampal pyramidal neurons in both normal aging and Alzheimer disease. **B. Hirano bodies** are eosinophilic cytoplasmic accumulations of actin (*arrow*) seen in the cytoplasm of hippocampal pyramidal neurons in normal aging and Alzheimer disease.

plaques of Alzheimer disease. The core of these plaques contains a distinct form of Aβ peptide, which is mainly 42 amino acids long. Aβ is derived by proteolysis from a much larger (695 amino acids) membrane-spanning APP. Full-length APP has an extracellular region, a transmembrane sequence and a cytoplasmic domain. The region comprising Aβ anchors the amino-terminal portion of APP to the membrane. The physiologic functions of APP and Aβ remain obscure.

The normal degradation of APP involves proteolytic cleavage in the middle of the Aβ domain, to release a nonamyloidogenic fragment from the middle of the Aβ domain to the amino end of APP. Proteolysis at either end of the Aβ domain then releases intact and highly amyloidogenic Aβ that accumulates in senile plaques as amyloid fibrils.

Aβ deposition may be needed for Alzheimer disease to develop because:

1. Patients with **Down syndrome** (trisomy 21) develop clinical and pathologic features of Alzheimer disease, including deposition of Aβ in neuritic plaques, generally by age 40. The gene for APP is on chromosome 21, and the additional dose of the gene product in trisomy 21 may predispose to precocious accumulation of Aβ.
2. Some patients with familial Alzheimer disease carry mutant *APP* genes or mutant presenilin genes. These mutations lead to increased production of Aβ, the amyloidogenic part of APP.
3. Transgenic mice expressing mutant human *APP* genes develop senile plaques in the brain very similar to those of Alzheimer disease. However, these mice lack other critical features of Alzheimer disease, such as NFTs, and evidence of neurodegeneration, such as significant loss of neurons.

Neurons and glial cells are sites of APP synthesis in the brain, but Aβ also accumulates in cerebral blood vessel walls.

■ **Neurofibrillary tangles:** NFTs are paired helical filaments that contain tau abnormally phosphorylated at aberrant sites. The resultant protein does not associate with microtubules but instead aggregates to form paired helical filaments. Release of tau from microtubules may deprive cells of tau's microtubule-stabilizing effects, thus impairing axonal transport and compromising neuron function. Alternatively, fibril formation occurring as the hyperphosphorylated tau aggregates may itself be cytotoxic.

There are several genetic risk factors for AD. Mutations in the *APP* gene have been associated with early-onset familial variants of Alzheimer disease. Additional genetic associations (Table 32-4) involve apolipoprotein E (apoE) genotype and the genes for presenilin 1 (*PS1*) and 2 (*PS2*).

APOLIPOPROTEIN E: Apolipoprotein E (apoE) has long been known for its role in cholesterol metabolism. In 1993, it was reported that specific apoE isoforms confer differential susceptibility to sporadic and late-onset familial subtypes of AD. The human apoE gene is on chromosome 19 (19q13.2). The three common alleles—ε2, ε3 and ε4—all occur in North American apoE genotypes. Inheritance of the ε4 allele, particularly the homozygous ε4/ε4 genotype, confers increased risk of late-onset familial and sporadic AD. This genotype occurs in 2% of the population. Conversely, the ε2 allele may confer some protection. The age at which symptoms appear in late-onset AD also correlates with the ε4 allele, with ε4/ε4 homozygotes showing the earliest onset (younger than 70) and patients with the ε2 allele having the latest onset (older than 90). The ε4 allele also correlates with increased numbers of senile plaques in patients with Alzheimer disease, but the apoE genotype is not an absolute determinant of the disease and does not predict who will develop it. How these different apoE alleles influence the risk of Alzheimer disease remains poorly understood.

PRESENILIN: Two genes with significant homology are associated with different kindreds of familial AD. Mutations of the *PS1* gene, on chromosome 14, are linked to the most common form of autosomal dominant early-onset Alzheimer disease. The *PS2* gene on chromosome

TABLE 32-4

GENETIC FACTORS IN ALZHEIMER DISEASE

Gene	Chromosome	Disease Association
Amyloid precursor protein (*APP*)	21	Mutations of the *APP* gene are associated with early-onset familial Alzheimer disease
Presenilin 1 (*PS1*)	14	Mutations of the *PS1* gene are associated with early-onset familial Alzheimer disease
Presenilin 2 (*PS2*)	1	Mutations of the *PS2* gene are associated with Volga German familial Alzheimer disease
Apolipoprotein E (*apoE*)	19	Presence of the ε4 allele is associated with increased risk and younger age of onset of both inherited and sporadic forms of late-onset Alzheimer disease

1 is associated with Alzheimer disease in Volga German pedigrees (Table 32-4). Presenilin mutations occur in half of cases of inherited AD, compared with only a few percent for mutant *APP* genes. There is some evidence that mutant PS1 and PS2 proteins alter processing of β-APP to favor increased production and deposition of Aβ. Cell processing of APP releases Aβ fragments of varying lengths, but the Aβ42 variant seems to be especially amyloidogenic. It is the Aβ molecule whose production is enhanced by mutant *PS1*.

Proposed mechanisms leading to development of AD are shown in Fig. 32-91.

It is now recognized that AD evolves over a period of years, if not decades. In 2011, a National Institute on Aging/ Alzheimer Association (NIA/AA) consensus statement was released indicating at AD occurs in three stages:

1. **Presymptomatic:** The patient has no cognitive impairment. There is growing evidence, however, that extracellular β-amyloid is accumulating and tangles are beginning to form, especially in the hippocampus and adjacent temporal cortex.
2. **Mild cognitive impairment (MCI):** Patients experience mild deterioration of memory and cognitive function that worries the patient but does not interfere with daily living. A significant number of patients with MCI will go on to develop frank AD, but many do not. People with low levels of CSF β-amyloid 1-42 or high levels of amyloid load detected by positron emission tomography (PET) scanning appear more likely to progress to AD.
3. **Alzheimer disease:** These patients are frankly demented on clinical examination and neuropsychological evaluation. Activities of daily living are impaired.

In parallel with the development of these clinical consensus guidelines, new neuropathologic criteria for diagnosing AD were postulated. Neurofibrillary tangles, neuritic plaques and β-amyloid distribution are assessed in standardized sections. β-Amyloid distribution is assessed by immunohistochemistry and described as absent (A0), neocortical and allocortical only (A1), diencephalon and striatum (A2) and brainstem and cerebellum (A3). The distribution of neurofibrillary tangles is absent (B0), trans-entorhinal (B1), limbic system and hippocampus (B2) and neocortical and brainstem (B3). Numbers of neuritic plaques are absent (C0), sparse (C1), moderate (C2) or frequent (C3). These changes are then Ax, Bx and Cx, with higher values in each dimension corresponding to a higher probability of AD. Comorbidities such as vascular disease, hippocampal sclerosis and Lewy bodies are also described.

 CLINICAL FEATURES: Patients with AD come to medical attention because of gradual loss of memory and cognitive function, difficulty with language and changes in behavior. Those with mild cognitive impairment are increasingly being recognized, since they move on to full-blown dementia at a rate of about 15% per year. Alzheimer disease progresses inexorably, so that previously intelligent and productive people become demented, mute, incontinent and bedridden. Bronchopneumonia, urinary tract infections and pressure decubiti are common medical complications that lead to death.

Frontotemporal Lobar Degeneration: Pick Disease Complex

 CLINICAL FEATURES: The frontotemporal lobar degenerations (FTLDs) are mainly tauopathies in which the frontal and temporal lobes bear the early brunt of the disease. The prototype eponymic disorder of the FTLDs is **Pick disease,** which manifests clinically as loss of frontal executive function causing disinhibition, loss of judgment about social propriety and inability to plan or foresee the consequences of one's actions. Most cases are sporadic, although Pick disease kindreds have been described. Sporadic Pick disease becomes symptomatic in midadult life and progresses relentlessly to death in 3–10 years. A respected pillar of the community may be reduced to a vulgar, disheveled derelict as this tragedy unfolds. Unlike AD, which generally begins with memory difficulties, FTLD starts with disruptive, inappropriate behavior. These dementias converge clinically at the end.

 PATHOLOGY: Cortical atrophy is mostly in the frontotemporal regions in Pick disease (Fig. 32-92). The atrophy may attain extreme proportions, so that affected gyri are reduced to thin slivers **(knife-edge atrophy)**. The involved cortex is severely depleted of neurons and shows intense astrogliosis. Residual neurons have intensely argentophilic and tau-immunoreactive round cytoplasmic inclusions called **Pick bodies** (Fig. 32-93A,B). These are formed by densely aggregated straight tau filaments.

Pick disease is the prototypical FTLD, but there are others that only recently have begun to reveal their molecular secrets. In any cohort of patients with clinical FTLD, many have Pick disease, but a significant number do not. Often, their neurons are immunoreactive for ubiquitin, implying an as yet unidentified protein triggering an unfulfilled degradative response. These are classified at FTLD-U, the U for ubiquitin immunoreactivity. Several of these proteins have recently been identified.

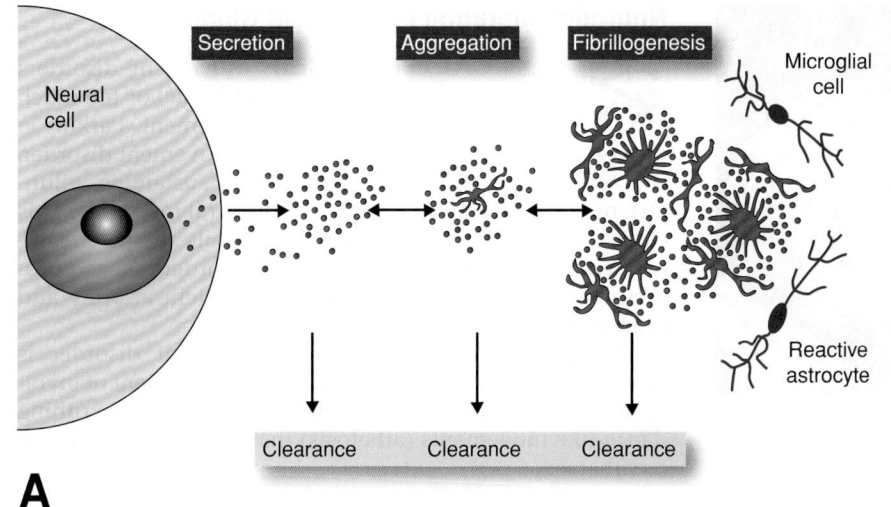

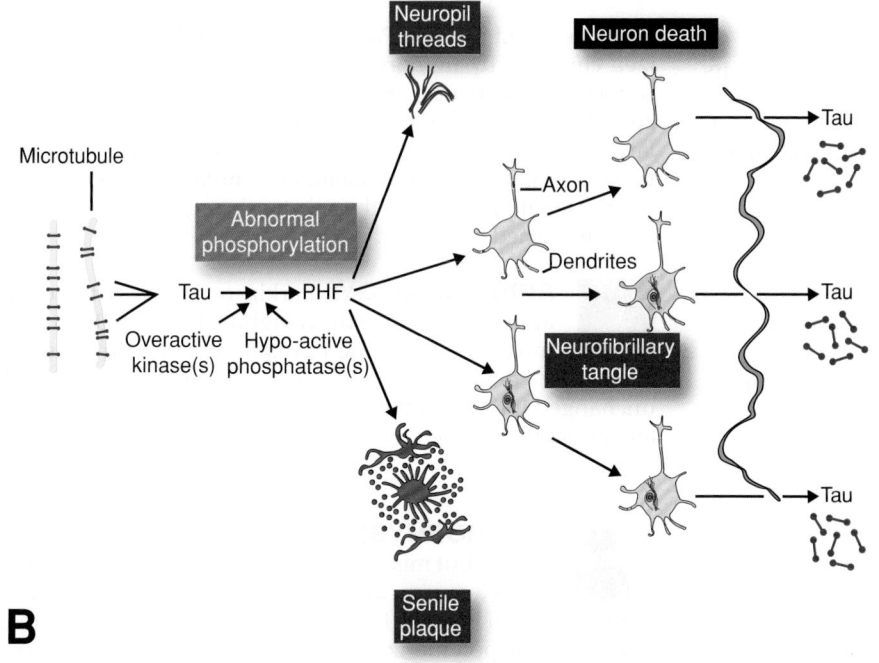

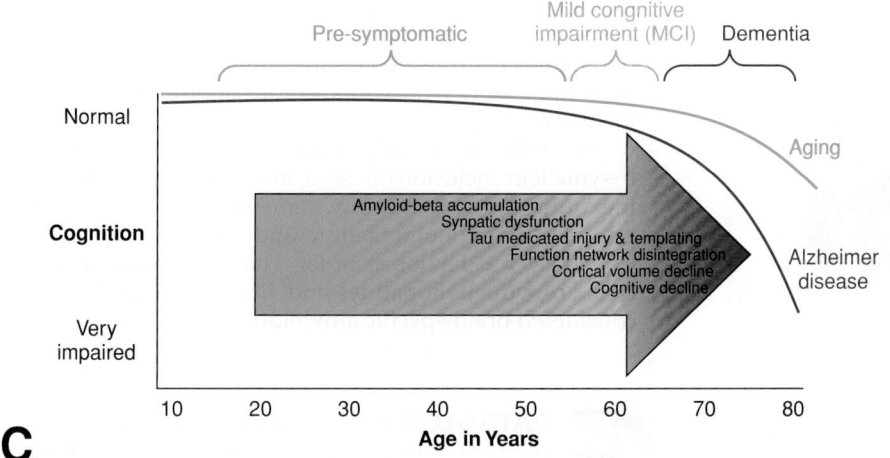

FIGURE 32-91. Mechanisms of amyloidosis and brain degeneration in Alzheimer disease. A. This schematic illustrates a hypothetical mechanism for the formation of senile plaques (SPs) from soluble Aβ peptides produced inside cells and secreted into the extracellular space. Amyloidogenic Aβ may encounter fibril-inducing cofactors and go on to form A fibrils to deposit in SPs (*far right*). SPs are surrounded by reactive astrocytes and microglial cells, which secrete cytokines that may contribute to the toxicity of the SPs. These steps may be reversible. Increasing Aβ clearance or reducing its production, as well as modulating the inflammatory response, may be effective therapeutic interventions for Alzheimer disease, in combination with therapies that target brain degeneration caused by neurofibrillary tangles (NFTs). **B.** This schematic illustrates a hypothetical mechanism leading to the conversion of normal human central nervous system (CNS) tau overlying two microtubules into paired helical filaments (PHFs). PHFs are generated in neuronal perikarya and their processes. Overactive kinase(s) or hypoactive phosphatase(s) may contribute to this effect. Abnormally phosphorylated tau forms PHFs in neuronal processes (neuropil threads) and neuronal perikarya (NFTs). Tau in PHFs loses the ability to bind microtubules, thus causing their depolymerization, disruption of axonal transport and degeneration of neurons. Accumulation of PHFs in neurons could exacerbate this process by physically blocking transport in neurons. The death of affected neurons would release tau and increase the levels of tau in the cerebrospinal fluid (CSF) of patients with Alzheimer disease. NFT formation may be reversible, and drugs that block NFT formation, reverse it or stabilize microtubules may be effective therapeutic interventions for Alzheimer disease. **C.** The National Institute on Aging/Alzheimer Association (NIA/AA) 2011 formulation on Alzheimer disease formally recognizes the temporal evolution of the disease from a long presymptomatic phase in which amyloid-β is accumulated and the pathophysiologic cascade is initiated. The pathogenic mechanisms interact to move the disease to mild cognitive impairment (MCI) and finally to frank dementia. Interventions during the symptomatic phase may be too late to fundamentally change the trajectory of the disease, and increased attention is being directed at the pr-symptomatic phase of the illness. This would be a primary prevention approach not unlike the highly successful presymptomatic intervention in myocardial infarction and stroke by exercise and control of hypertension and hyperlipidemia.

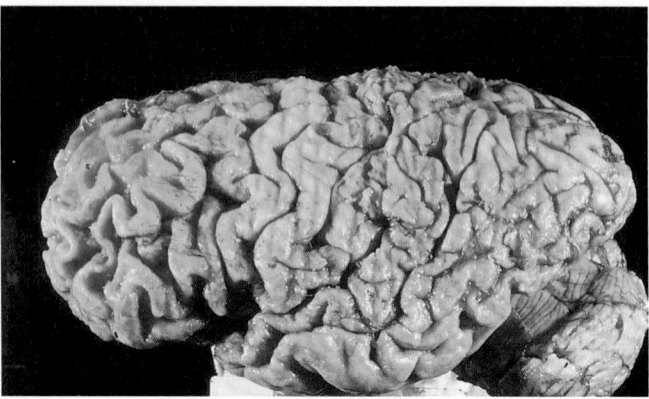

FIGURE 32-92. Severe cortical atrophy with marked frontotemporal atrophy is characteristic of the frontotemporal lobar degenerations, such as Pick disease, but may be seen in Alzheimer disease. Frontal atrophy correlates with loss of executive function, impaired judgment and disinhibition.

The protein TDP43 bears brief consideration, since its abnormal accumulation occurs in both FTLD and motor neuron disease. This molecular commonality coincides with the increasingly recognized coexistence of FTLD and motor neuron disease.

Lewy Body Dementia

Lewy body dementia (LBD), also known as Lewy body disease or diffuse Lewy body disease, is characterized by intracytoplasmic α-synuclein inclusions in a relatively small number of cortical neurons, mostly in the cingulate cortex. AD pathology may coexist with Lewy body inclusions at the end stage of the disease.

 **CLINICAL FEATURES:** LBD is distinctive in that cognitive function fluctuates greatly from day to day, subtle extrapyramidal manifestations may be present and the patient may experience fascinating well-formed visual hallucinations. LBD exists on a continuum with the other α-synucleinopathies that include Parkinson disease and multiple system atrophy.

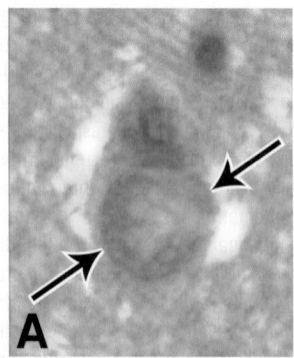 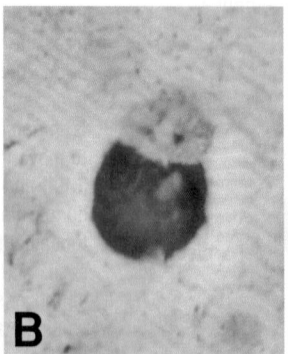

FIGURE 32-93. Pick bodies. A. In hematoxylin and eosin–stained sections, Pick bodies are basophilic, spherical, intracytoplasmic, intraneuronal aggregates of tau protein (*arrows*). They tend to be round rather than angular like the neurofibrillary tangles (NFTs) in Alzheimer disease, but like NFTs, they are argentophilic (silver impregnation) **(B)**.

Neurodegeneration of the Basal Ganglia

 CLINICAL FEATURES: Movement disorders may result in too little (**bradykinetic**) or too much involuntary (**hyperkinetic**) movement. Parkinson disease is the prototypical bradykinetic movement disorder, characterized by difficulty initiating and sustaining voluntary movement, resting tremor and postural instability. This clinical triad is **"parkinsonism,"** and while the most common cause is Parkinson disease, other disorders such as progressive supranuclear palsy, multiple system atrophy and even neuro-AIDS may result in parkinsonism.

The prototypical hyperkinetic movement disorder is Huntington disease, with progressive development of involuntary rapid twitching movements (chorea) and writhing dance-like movements (athetosis) that may conflate as choreoathetosis.

Parkinson Disease

First described in 1817, Parkinson disease (PD) is characterized clinically by tremors at rest, cogwheel rigidity, expressionless countenance, postural instability and, less often, cognitive impairment. Pathologically, neurons are lost, largely in the substantia nigra, and Lewy bodies, filamentous aggregates of α-synuclein, accumulate. Dopaminergic neurons that project from the substantia nigra to the striatum are diminished.

 EPIDEMIOLOGY: Parkinson disease typically appears in the sixth to eighth decades. It is common: 1%–2% of the population in North America eventually develops it. PD prevalence has remained unchanged for at least the past 40 years. No racial differences are apparent, but men are more affected than women.

PATHOPHYSIOLOGY: Most cases are sporadic, but missense mutations in the α-synuclein gene cause rare autosomal dominant, early-onset, familial PD. The finding that wild-type α-synuclein is the major polymerized protein in Lewy bodies led to consideration of fibrillogenesis as a major contributor to the pathogenesis of neurodegenerative diseases. Accumulating evidence suggests that oxidative stress due to auto-oxidation of catecholamines during melanin formation injures neurons in the substantia nigra by promoting misfolding of α-synuclein and formation of filamentous inclusions.

In addition to PD, accumulation of filamentous α-synuclein inclusions is seen in other diseases, including multiple system atrophy, dementia with Lewy bodies, progressive autonomic failure and rapid eye movement (REM) sleep behavior disorder. These disorders are now called **α-synucleinopathies** and, like the tauopathies, are considered brain-specific amyloidoses.

 PATHOLOGY: Brains of PD patients show loss of pigmentation in the substantia nigra and locus ceruleus (Fig. 32-94). Other brain regions are less affected. Pigmented neurons are scarce, and small extracellular deposits of melanin are derived from dying neurons.

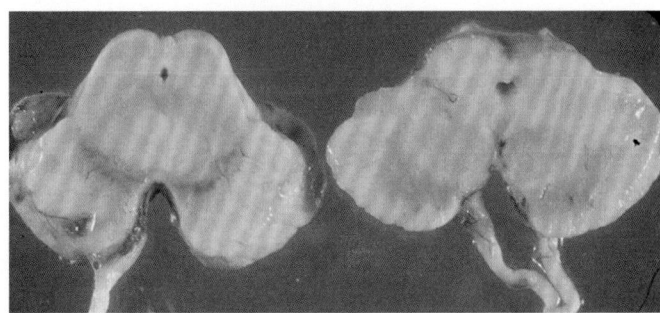

FIGURE 32-94. Parkinson disease. The normal substantia nigra on the left in an adult is heavily pigmented, while the substantia nigra in a patient with Parkinson disease has lost pigmented neurons and the nucleus now blends inconspicuously with the rest of the midbrain. The locus ceruleus in the pons is also depigmented (not shown). (Courtesy of Dr. F. Stephen Vogel, Duke University.)

Some residual neurons are atrophic, and a few contain Lewy bodies, which are spherical, eosinophilic cytoplasmic inclusions (Fig. 32-95). By electron microscopy, Lewy bodies show amyloid-like filaments of insoluble α-synuclein.

Other Disorders Causing Parkinsonism

PD is not the sole cause of parkinsonism. Other disorders share a common theme of loss of pigmented dopaminergic neurons in the substantia nigra. Normal aging is associated with some neuron loss in the substantia nigra and reduced dopamine levels, but these features are exaggerated in PD and these other causes of parkinsonism.

- **MPTP-induced parkinsonism** was discovered the late 1970s when there was an epidemic of parkinsonism among intravenous drug abusers that was ultimately

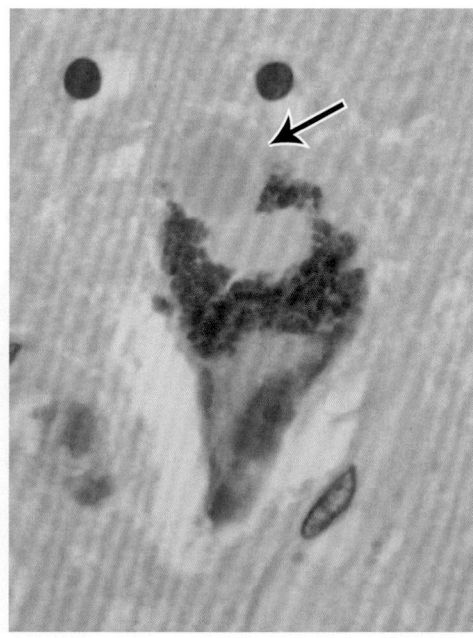

FIGURE 32-95. Lewy body in Parkinson disease. Examination of residual neurons in the substantia nigra show intracytoplasmic, intraneuronal, spherical eosinophilic inclusions composed of polymerized α-synuclein called Lewy bodies (*arrow*). These inclusions often have a thin clear halo.

linked to a toxic byproduct of the illicit synthesis of a meperidine (Demerol). That contaminant, 1-methyl-4-phenyl-1,2,3,6-tetrahydropyridine (MPTP), is turned by the brain's own monoamine oxidase into a highly reactive free radical.

- **Postinfectious parkinsonism** occurred after viral encephalitis (von Economo encephalitis) associated with the influenza pandemic after World War I and has not recurred to a major degree since. It was characterized by loss of substantia nigra neurons but no Lewy bodies being present. How this disorder develops is unknown, but there is concern that a similar combination of influenza antigens may lead to a recurrence of this epidemic. The 2009 H1N1 influenza virus, for example, was very similar antigenically to that seen in the earlier pandemic.

- **Striatonigral degeneration** is a rare disorder that closely mimics PD. At autopsy, the striatum (caudate and putamen) is visibly atrophied, with severe loss of neurons in this region. Changes in the substantia nigra and locus ceruleus are less severe. This condition may coexist with Shy-Drager disease (dysautonomia) and olivopontocerebellar atrophy (OPCA) as part of a unified disorder of **multiple system atrophy (MSA),** in which filamentous α-synuclein inclusions, known as **glial cytoplasmic inclusions,** accumulate primarily in oligodendroglia. They also occur to a lesser extent in neurons, where they resemble the Lewy bodies of Parkinson disease and Lewy body dementia.

- **Progressive supranuclear palsy (PSP)** is an uncommon disorder characterized by parkinsonism, severe postural instability with falls and progressive paralysis of vertical eye movements. Pathologic changes in the brain are more widespread than in PD, but the hallmark is atrophy of the midbrain tegmentum, leading to an exaggerated contribution of the cerebral peduncles to the profile of the midbrain in axial sections—a profile that is referred to by some as "Mickey Mouse" midbrain. Since the midbrain, as well as the substantia nigra, is the locus of integration of vertical eye movement, the combination of parkinsonism and vertical gaze dysfunction makes anatomic sense. PSP is a **tauopathy:** the sole inclusions are tau-rich NFTs. PSP spreads throughout the nervous system, and cognitive impairment complicates the disease course.

Huntington Disease

 **EPIDEMIOLOGY:** First described in 1872, Huntington disease (HD) is an autosomal dominant genetic disorder characterized by involuntary movements, deterioration of cognitive function and often severe emotional disturbances. It mainly affects whites of northwestern European ancestry, with an incidence of 1 in 20,000. Genealogic studies indicate that all cases derive from an original founder in northern Europe; the disease is very rare in Asia and Africa.

 CLINICAL FEATURES: Symptoms of HD usually begin by age 40, but 5% of patients with the disorder develop neurologic signs before age 20, and a similar proportion first present after age 60. Cognitive and emotional disturbances precede the onset of abnormal movements by several years in over half of patients. Once it develops, choreoathetosis may be incapacitating. Cortical involvement leads to a severe loss of cognitive function and intellectual deterioration, often accompanied by paranoia and delusions. The interval from the onset of symptoms to death averages 15 years.

 MOLECULAR PATHOGENESIS: The *HD* gene, on chromosome 4 (4p16.3), codes for the protein **huntingtin.** The aberration at this locus is expansion of a trinucleotide (CAG) repeat (see Chapter 6). The repeat is within a coding region of the gene and yields an altered protein, with a polyglutamine tract near the N-terminus. In agreement with the dominant mode of inheritance, the triplet expansion causes a toxic gain of function.

Huntingtin is widely expressed in tissues throughout the body and in all regions of the CNS by neurons and glia, but its function is unknown. As with other CAG repeat expansion diseases (see Chapter 6), the longer the CAG repeat, the more severe the disease phenotype and the earlier the age of clinical onset. In HD, CAG length is more unstable and tends to be longer when inherited from the father than in maternal transmission. As a result, transmission of the *HD* mutation from the father results in clinical disease some 3 years earlier than when it is passed on from the mother. Of children with juvenile-onset HD, the ratio of those who inherit the expanded CAG allele from their father to those who inherit it from their mother is 10:1.

PATHOLOGY: The frontal cortex is symmetrically and moderately atrophic, while the lateral ventricles are disproportionately large, owing to loss of the normal convex curvature of the caudate nuclei (Fig. 32-96). There is symmetric atrophy of the caudate nuclei, with lesser involvement of the putamen. Neuron populations of the caudate and putamen, especially the small neurons, are severely depleted, with accompanying astrogliosis. The cerebral cortical neurons are similarly, but less severely, lost. Huntingtin aggregates in neurons, mainly in nuclei, but also in neuronal processes, potentially impairing axodendritic transport. γ-Aminobutyric acid (GABA) and glutamic acid decarboxylase are markedly decreased.

Nucleotide Repeat Expansion Disorders

HD is one of an ever-increasing group of neurologic diseases that are nucleotide repeat expansion syndromes (see Chapter 6). These are not rare, but rather include the most

common cause of mental retardation in boys (fragile X syndrome), the most common adult-onset muscular dystrophy (myotonic dystrophy) and the most common hereditary spinocerebellar ataxia (Friedreich ataxia).

MOLECULAR PATHOGENESIS: Trinucleotide repeats are a normal feature of many genes, and expansion of the number of triplet repeats confers pathogenicity. Some triplet repeat diseases show only a small expansion compared with their normal counterparts (e.g., Huntington disease), but in others, the expansion is quite large (e.g., fragile X syndrome and Friedreich ataxia). This class of diseases includes examples of all forms of inheritance: X-linked, autosomal dominant and autosomal recessive. In most of the autosomal dominant CAG expansion disorders, the abnormal expansion is in the coding region of a gene and causes production of an abnormal protein. In other disorders, the expansion is in a noncoding part of the gene and may interfere with transcription or message processing. Resulting decreased protein levels constitute a loss-of-function mutation (as appears to be the case with GAA expansion in Friedreich ataxia). In myotonic dystrophy, a noncoding region expansion yields a transcript that interferes with correct mRNA splicing for multiple gene products, leading to the multiorgan multiprotein manifestations of this condition.

Spinocerebellar Neurodegeneration

The spinocerebellar ataxias are a heterogeneous group of genetic disorders that impact cerebellar inflow and outflow pathways, or the cerebellar parenchyma itself. The cerebellum plays a key role in helping the cerebral motor cortex and basal ganglia in motor functions, and in ensuring smooth performance of repetitive motor tasks such as playing the piano, riding a bicycle or speaking. Once the cerebellum is exposed to motor tasks, it acts as a repository of motor programs (i.e., a "motor memory").

Cerebellar dysfunction leads to ataxia—the inability to execute motor tasks smoothly, particularly those requiring rapid alternating movement or precise motor control. Ataxia may result from defects in the major cerebellar input pathways including the middle cerebellar peduncle, which conveys motor execution commands from the cerebral motor and premotor cortex, and the inferior cerebellar peduncle,

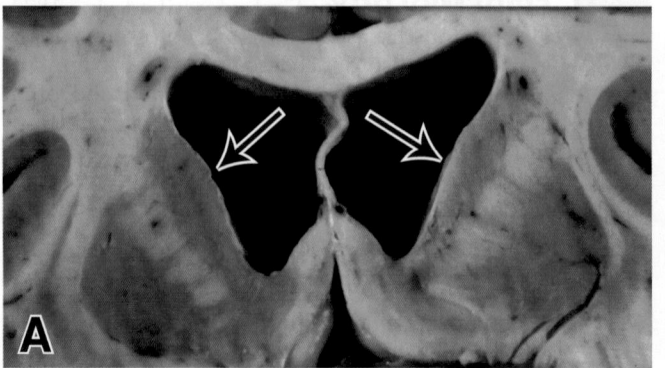
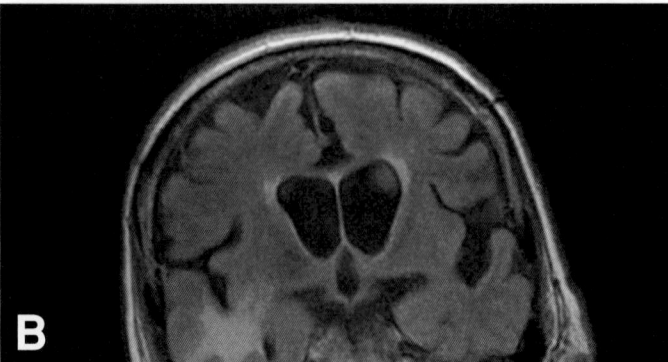

FIGURE 32-96. Huntington disease. A. The caudate nuclei (*arrows*) bilaterally are atrophic, leading to enlarged lateral ventricles. Some cortical atrophy is also seen, but it is usually not as severe as that seen in the primary cortical dementias such as Alzheimer and Pick disease. **B.** Axial magnetic resonance image showing the enlarged lateral ventricles accompanied by modest cortical atrophy. The square-shaped lateral ventricles of Huntington disease are sometimes called "box-car ventricles."

which receives proprioceptive data from the spinal cord via the spinocerebellar tracts. If the cerebellar parenchyma itself degenerates, ataxia will reflect a distribution congruent to the functional portion of the cerebellum involved—vermal degeneration leads to truncal ataxia, while cerebellar hemispheric degeneration leads to appendicular ataxia. Finally, the cerebral outflow—the dentatorubrothalamic pathway—may degenerate, leading to a peculiarly high-amplitude ataxia called "wing-beating ataxia."

Friedreich Ataxia

 EPIDEMIOLOGY: Friedreich ataxia is the most common inherited ataxia. Its prevalence in European populations is 1 in 50,000. Inheritance is autosomal recessive, but many cases arise sporadically without prior family history.

 CLINICAL FEATURES: Symptoms usually begin before age 25, followed by an unremittingly progressive course of about 30 years to death. Friedreich ataxia is a cerebellar inflow disorder with ataxia of both the upper and lower limbs, dysarthria, lower limb areflexia, extensor plantar reflexes and sensory loss reflecting concurrent degeneration of spinal long tracts. Common concomitants include deformities of the skeletal system (e.g., scoliosis, pes cavus), hypertrophic cardiomyopathy (which commonly causes death) and diabetes mellitus.

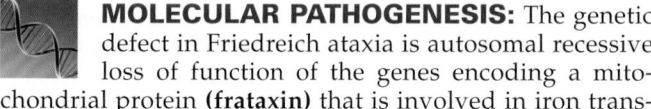 **MOLECULAR PATHOGENESIS:** The genetic defect in Friedreich ataxia is autosomal recessive loss of function of the genes encoding a mitochondrial protein **(frataxin)** that is involved in iron transport into mitochondria. In most cases the mutation is an unstable expansion of a trinucleotide (GAA) repeat in the first intron of this gene (9q13.3–21.1). The recessive pattern of inheritance means that both frataxin alleles must be lost—both may bear the trinucleotide repeat expansion. Or, one may have the repeat expansion while the other allele may be compromised by a different mutation. The expansion mutation may impede transcription or RNA processing. In unaffected people, levels of frataxin protein are highest in the heart and spinal cord. Lack of frataxin is thus probably responsible for neurologic and cardiac manifestations of Friedreich ataxia. The longer the repeat, the earlier the age of disease onset, the faster the rate of progression and the greater the frequency of hypertrophic cardiomyopathy.

 PATHOLOGY: The most prominent postmortem findings in Friedreich ataxia are in the spinal cord, which shows degeneration of the posterior columns, corticospinal pathways and spinocerebellar tracts (Fig. 32-97). Posterior column degeneration accounts for the sensory loss experienced by these patients and results from loss of the parent neuronal cell bodies in the dorsal root ganglia. In advanced cases, this degeneration appears grossly as shrinkage of dorsal spinal roots and posterior funiculi. Similarly, spinocerebellar tract atrophy, with attendant ataxia, follows neuronal degeneration in the dorsal nucleus of Clarke. The corticospinal tracts show the most pronounced degeneration more distally in the cord leading to weakness and release of the plantar extensor reflex.

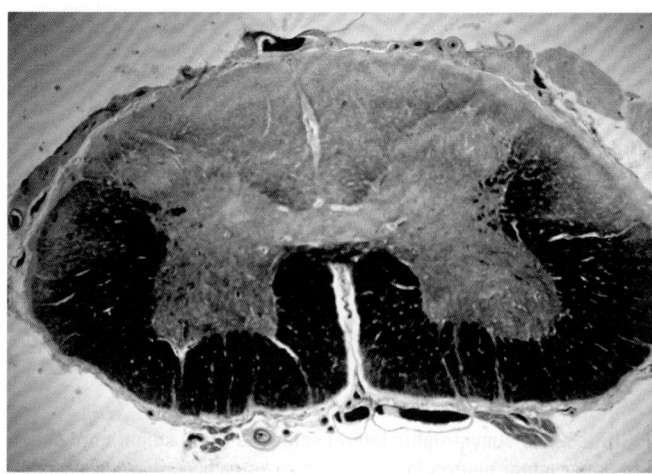

FIGURE 32-97. Friedreich ataxia. This is the most common hereditary ataxia. Myelin-stained sections show secondary degeneration of the dorsal columns, lateral corticospinal tracts and spinocerebellar tracts. This is predominantly an inflow ataxia and the cerebellum is usually not atrophic.

Amyotrophic Lateral Sclerosis Is the Most Common Motor Neuron Disease

Amyotrophic Lateral Sclerosis

ALS is a degenerative disease of upper and lower motor neurons of the brain and spinal cord, with progressive weakness and wasting of extremities and tongue, a sometimes confusing combination of hyperreflexia and hyporeflexia and eventual impairment of respiratory muscles.

 **EPIDEMIOLOGY:** It is a worldwide disease with an incidence of 1 in 100,000. It peaks in the fifth decade, and it is rare in people before age 35. There is a 1.5–2-fold excess of ALS in men. Restricted geographic areas with a particularly high incidence of ALS exist in Guam and parts of Japan and Papua New Guinea, but these cases differ from ALS in the rest of the world. Cases in the Chamorro people indigenous to Guam are characterized by abundant accumulations of tau-rich NFTs and are now classified as **tauopathies**. Moreover, ALS in Guam is part of a spectrum of disorders that includes dementia and parkinsonism.

 **MOLECULAR PATHOGENESIS:** Familial ALS cases, with an autosomal dominant pattern, account for 5% of ALS. The most common form has been associated with missense mutations in the gene that codes for the cytosolic form of the antioxidant enzyme superoxide dismutase (Cu/Zn SOD, or SOD1; see Chapter 1). Since SOD1 is a key free radical detoxifying enzyme, SOD1 mutations might lead to increased free radical damage. The extent to which enzyme activity is lost is unclear, but mutant SOD1 is more prone to aggregation than wild-type SOD1, so familial ALS may be a **protein conformational disorder**.

 PATHOLOGY: ALS affects lower motor neurons, including anterior horn cells of the spinal cord and the motor nuclei of the brainstem, especially the hypoglossal nuclei; and the upper motor neurons of the cerebral cortex. Loss of the upper motor neurons leads to

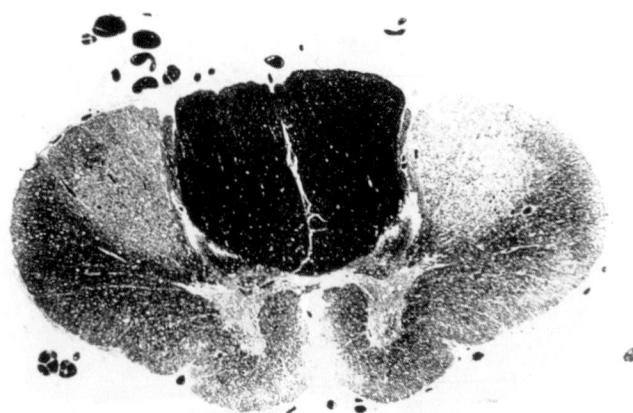

FIGURE 32-98. Amyotrophic lateral sclerosis (ALS) spinal cord showing upper motor neuron loss. Myelin-stained sections show degeneration of the lateral corticospinal tracts reflecting degeneration of the axons of the upper motor neurons originating in the motor strip of the cerebral cortex. Note the preservation of the dorsal columns, spinothalamic tracts and spinocerebellar pathways.

degeneration of their axons, with secondary demyelination visualized in myelin-stained axial sections of the spinal cord as loss of the lateral and anterior corticospinal pathways (Fig. 32-98).

The main histologic change in ALS is loss of large motor neurons, with mild gliosis (Fig. 32-99). This is most apparent in the anterior horns of the lumbar and cervical enlargements of the spinal cord, and the hypoglossal nuclei. There is also a loss of the giant pyramidal Betz cells in the cerebral motor cortex. The anterior nerve roots bearing the few remaining axons of the dying lower motor neurons become atrophic, and affected muscles are pale and shrunken, reflecting severe neurogenic atrophy.

CLINICAL FEATURES: ALS often begins asymmetrically as weakness and wasting of muscles of one hand. Irregular rapid involuntary contractions of small muscle groups (fasciculations) are characteristic and are felt to arise from hyperirritability of terminal

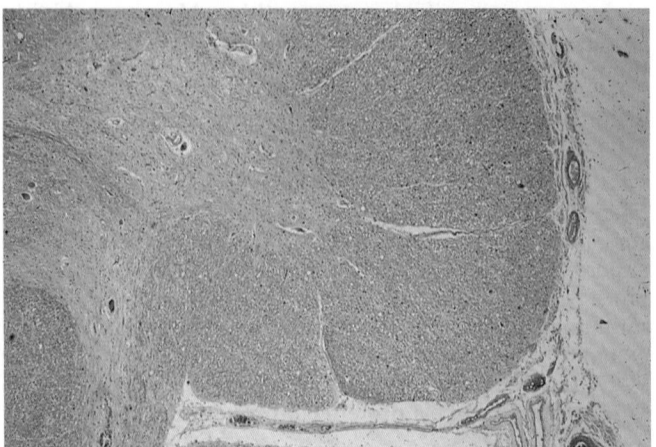

FIGURE 32-99. Amyotrophic lateral sclerosis (ALS) spinal cord showing lower motor neuron loss. The anterior horn of the spinal cord normally contains numerous very large lower motor neurons. In ALS, there is anterior horn cell loss and gliosis.

arborizations of dying lower motor neurons. The disease is inexorably progressive, with increasing weakness of the limbs leading to total disability. Speech may become unintelligible, and respiratory weakness supervenes. Despite the dramatic wasting of the body, intellectual capacity is preserved to the end, although some patients with ALS also suffer dementia of the frontotemporal lobar type. The clinical course does not usually exceed a decade.

Spinal muscular atrophy (Werdnig-Hoffman disease) is the second most common lethal autosomal recessive condition in white populations. It usually presents in infancy with extreme muscle weakness and atrophy due to severe loss of anterior horn cells. Death from respiratory failure or aspiration pneumonia usually occurs within a few months of diagnosis. Accurate diagnosis is critical for genetic risk management. This disorder results from a loss-of-function mutation of a neuronal apoptosis inhibitor protein resulting in neurons having an extremely low threshold for initiating programmed cell death.

Several neurodegenerative, infectious and vitamin deficiency disorders impact the spinal long tracts and are summarized in Fig. 32-100.

DEVELOPMENTAL MALFORMATIONS

CNS development unfolds according to a precise schedule, with each morphologic event being the foundation for those that follow. Thus, congenital anomalies reflect interruptions in the completion of developmental processes. *Congenital malformations are defined more by the timing than the specific nature of an insult.*

ETIOLOGIC FACTORS: There are 3 critical stages of CNS development: (1) neurulation, (2) segmentation and cleavage and (3) proliferation and migration. Neurulation consists of formation and closure of the neural tube and is complete by 4 weeks of gestation, often before a woman is aware that she is pregnant. This step establishes the cranial–caudal, dorsal–ventral and left–right axes of the embryo. From weeks 4 to 8, the neural tube segments into neighborhoods that will ultimately become the spinal cord, medulla, pons and cerebellum, midbrain, diencephalon and telencephalon. The diencephalon and telencephalon then split into the paired basal ganglia, thalami and cerebral hemispheres. By the end of 8 weeks of gestation, basic CNS architecture is established. For the rest of gestation and beyond into postnatal life, cell proliferation creates the *trillions* of neuroglia that ultimately populate the mature CNS. These cells are mostly born in the periventricular germinal matrix and must successfully migrate to their ultimate destinations. In humans, defects of proliferation and migration mainly impact the formation of cerebral cortex and cause mental retardation and seizures. Once neurons and glia reach their destinations, they must wire the brain correctly using axonal pathfinding and oligodendroglial myelination.

Defects of Neurulation Are the Neural Tube Defects

Anencephaly

Anencephaly is the congenital absence of all or part of the brain as a result of unsuccessful closure of the cephalad (anterior neuropore) portion of the neural tube.

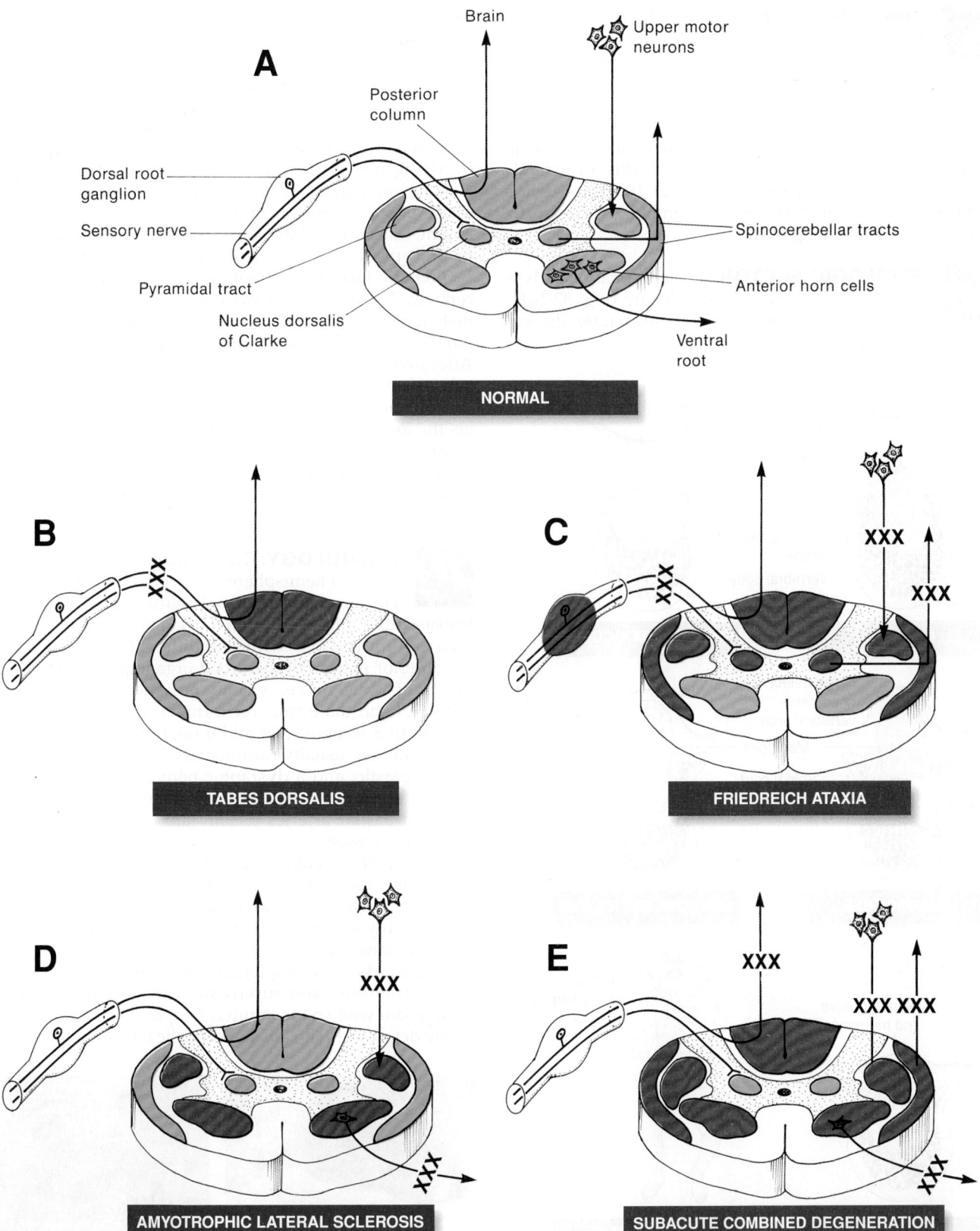

FIGURE 32-100. Tract degeneration in diseases of the spinal cord. Ascending (*blue*) sensory and descending (*green*) pathways travel through the spinal cord. These tracts may be differentially affected (*red*) depending on the nature of the underlying disease, as shown in this example of four diseases that we have considered.

 **EPIDEMIOLOGY:** Anencephaly is the second most common CNS malformation after spina bifida (0.5–2.0 per 1000 births, with females predominating) and is the most common lethal CNS malformation. Anencephalic fetuses are stillborn or die in the first few days of life.

Anencephaly is a multifactorial birth defect exhibiting geographic variation in incidence. In the United States, it occurs in 0.3 per 1000 live births and stillbirths. In Ireland, the frequency is 20-fold greater (5–6 per 1000). Incidence declines to 2–3 per 1000 among Irish immigrants to North America. It is rare among blacks.

 **ETIOLOGIC FACTORS:** Anencephaly is a dysraphic defect of neural tube closure (Fig. 32-101). Its concurrence with other neural tube defects (NTDs), such as spina bifida, suggests shared pathogenic mechanisms. During development, the neural plate invaginates and is transformed into the neural tube by fusion of the posterior surfaces. Mesenchymal tissue overlying the primitive neural tube then forms the skull and vertebral arches posterior to the spinal cord, while ectoderm forms the overlying skin. If the neural tube does not close, neither will the overlying bony structures of the cranium. The calvarium, skin and subcutaneous tissues will be absent in this region. The exposed brain is incompletely formed or even entirely absent. Most often, the base of the skull has only bits of neural and ependymal tissue and residues of meninges.

Genetic factors contribute to the pathogenesis of anencephaly. The anomaly is twice as common in female as in male fetuses, and it occurs with higher frequency in certain families. The risk of a second anencephalic fetus is 2%–5%. After two anencephalic fetuses, the risk reaches 25% for each subsequent pregnancy.

Folic acid supplied in the periconceptional period lowers the incidence of NTDs. In 1998, the U.S. Food and Drug Administration began requiring supplemental folate to be added to enriched flour, bread, cereals and some other products. This led to a significant decrease in the incidence of NTDs of all types (see Chapters 6 and 14).

 PATHOLOGY: The cranial vault is absent. The cerebral hemispheres are replaced by a highly vascularized, disorganized neuroglial tissue, the **cerebrovasculosa** (Fig. 32-102), on the flattened base of the skull. Two well-formed eyes with well-differentiated retinas mark the anterior margin of disturbed organogenesis. Short segments of optic nerves extend posteriorly. The posterior aspect of the malformation forms a variable transitional zone with a recognizable midbrain, but the brainstem and cerebellum are usually rudimentary. The upper spinal cord is hypoplastic, and a dysraphic bony posterior spinal column defect **(rachischisis)** may affect the cervical area. Vertebral and basilar arteries usually are identifiable amid the meningeal vessels.

The cerebrovasculosa typically contains islands of immature neural tissue. It also encloses cavities partly lined by ependyma, with or without choroid plexus. However, the mass mainly consists of abnormal vascular channels that vary considerably in size.

Two thirds of anencephalic fetuses die in utero; those that are alive at birth rarely survive more than a week. Screening of pregnant women for serum α-fetoprotein and ultrasonography detect virtually all anencephalic fetuses.

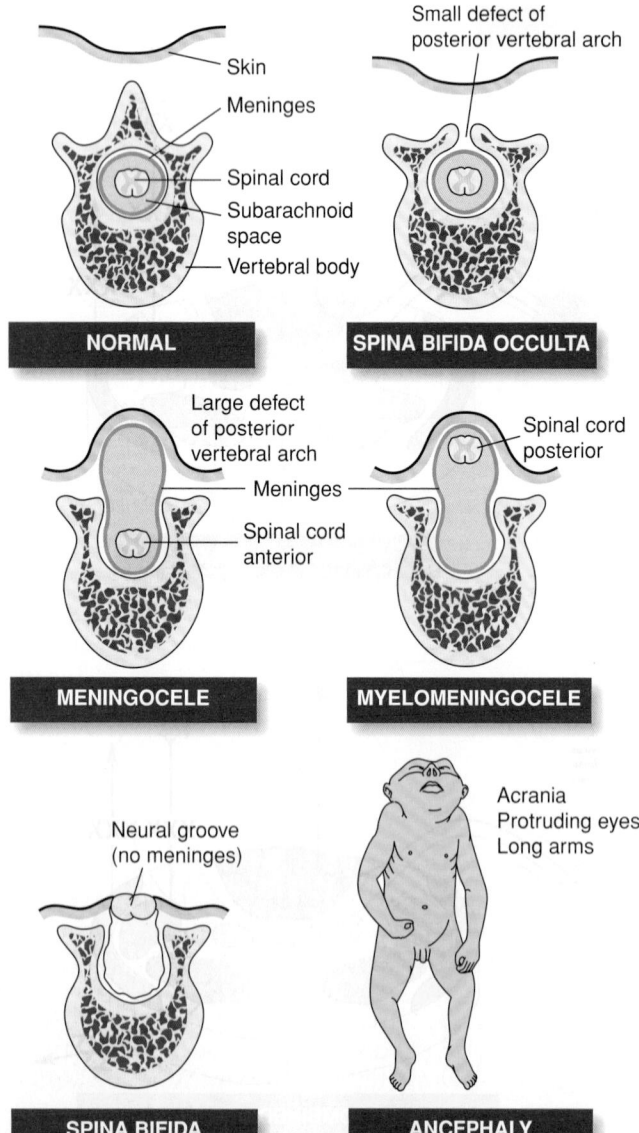

FIGURE 32-101. Defects of the neural tube. The first critical step in neural development is neurulation—formation and closure of the neural tube. Incomplete fusion of the neural tube and overlying bone, soft tissues or skin leads to several defects, varying from mild anomalies (e.g., spina bifida occulta) to severe anomalies (e.g., anencephaly).

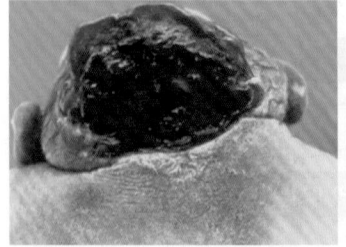 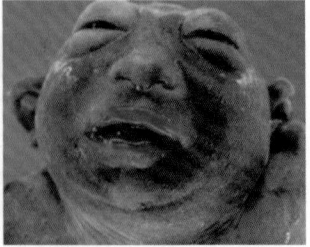

FIGURE 32-102. Anencephaly is the most severe defect of neurulation. The cerebral vault is absent (*right panel*), and the absence of a calvarium exposes a mass of vascularized tissue (cerebrovasculosa, *left panel*), in which there are rudimentary neuroectodermal structures. The lesion is bounded anteriorly by normally formed eyes and posteriorly by the brainstem.

Spina Bifida

Spina bifida is a group of NTDs that are due to failure of neural tube closure in the more caudal regions. These anomalies are usually in the lumbar region and vary in severity from asymptomatic to disabling. They are not usually lethal. Spina bifida results from an insult between the 25th and 30th days of gestation, reflecting the timing of neural tube closure. These anomalies are subclassified by the severity of the defect:

- **Spina bifida occulta:** This defect is restricted to the vertebral arches and is usually asymptomatic. It frequently manifests externally only by a dimple or small tuft of hair on the lower back.
- **Meningocele:** This condition features a greater bone and soft tissue defect that permits the meninges to protrude as a fluid-filled sac visible on the external surface of the back, in the midline. The sides of the sac are usually covered by a thin layer of skin. Its apex may be ulcerated, allowing microorganisms to enter the CSF.
- **Meningomyelocele:** This is an even more extensive defect that exposes the spinal canal and causes nerve roots (particularly those of the cauda equina) and spinal cord to be entrapped in an externally visible protruding CSF-filled sac (Fig. 32-103). Usually, the spinal cord is a flattened, ribbon-like structure. Severe neurologic consequences include lower extremity motor and sensory defects and compromise of bowel and bladder neurogenic control.
- **Rachischisis:** In this extreme defect, the spinal column is a gaping canal, often without a recognizable spinal cord (Fig. 32-104). Rachischisis is usually lethal and seen in abortuses.

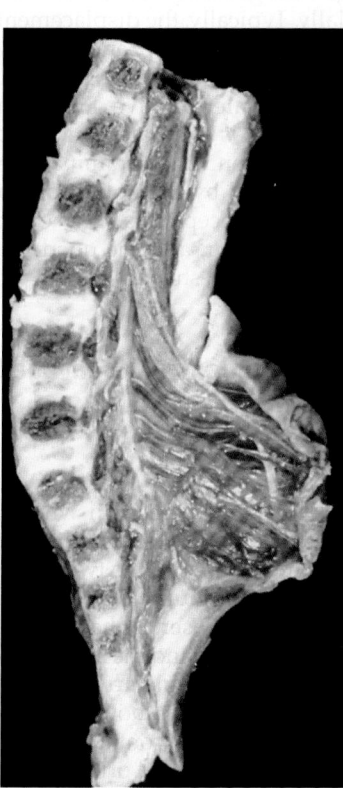

FIGURE 32-103. Meningomyelocele. This dysraphic defect, which is caused by lack of fusion of the spinal canal usually in the lumbar region, reveals disorganized spinal cord tissue with entrapment of nerve roots in a cerebrospinal fluid–filled sac. (Courtesy of Dr. F. Stephen Vogel, Duke University.)

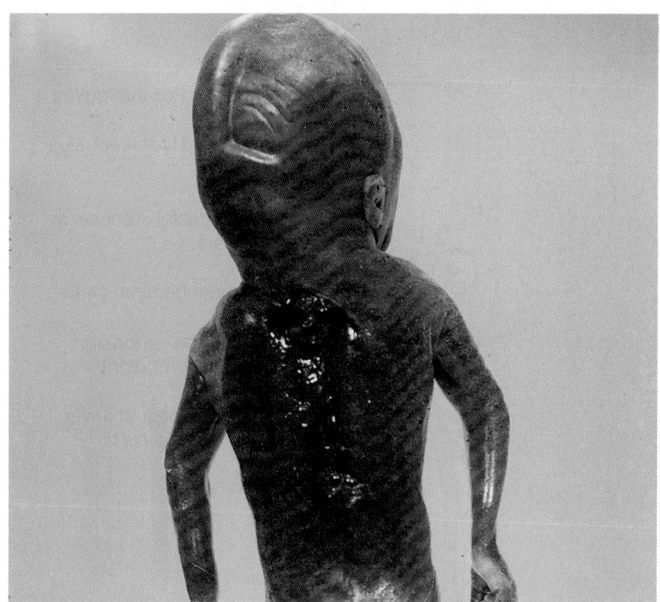

FIGURE 32-104. Rachischisis. A view of the vertebral column shows a bony, cutaneous defect with segmental thoracic absence of the spinal cord and overlying vertebral arches and soft tissues.

Spina bifida is induced readily in rats and chicks at the 8th to 9th gestational day by chemicals such as trypan blue or by hypervitaminosis A. It probably reflects failure of the neural tube to close, but this concept is not established. As mentioned above, maternal folate deficiency is implicated in NTDs. Some drugs, notably retinoids used for acne and valproic acid used to manage seizures, must be avoided by women of childbearing age because of their association with NTDs.

 CLINICAL FEATURES: Clinical neurologic deficits in NTDs range from no symptoms in spina bifida occulta to lower limb paralysis, sensory loss and incontinence in meningomyelocele. One must be aware of potential associated malformations such as Arnold-Chiari malformation, hydrocephalus, polymicrogyria and hydromyelia of the spinal central canal (see below).

Malformations of the Spinal Cord

Other spinal cord malformations that are less apparent at birth than NTDs include rare total **(dimyelia)** to partial duplication of spinal cord into two separate structures **(diastematomyelia)**. **Hydromyelia** is dilation of the central spinal cord canal.

Syringomyelia is a congenital malformation, a tubular cavitation (syrinx), which may or may not communicate with the central canal, that extends for variable distances within the spinal cord. Many cases represent congenital malformations, but the condition progresses slowly and usually first presents clinically in adults. Some cases of syringomyelia are not congenital but are caused by trauma, ischemia or tumors. The syrinx is filled with a clear fluid similar to CSF. **Syringobulbia** is a variant of syringomyelia in which the syrinx is located in the medulla.

 CLINICAL FEATURES: The symptoms of syringomyelia are present at the spinal level of the syrinx. At that point, the centrally located syrinx

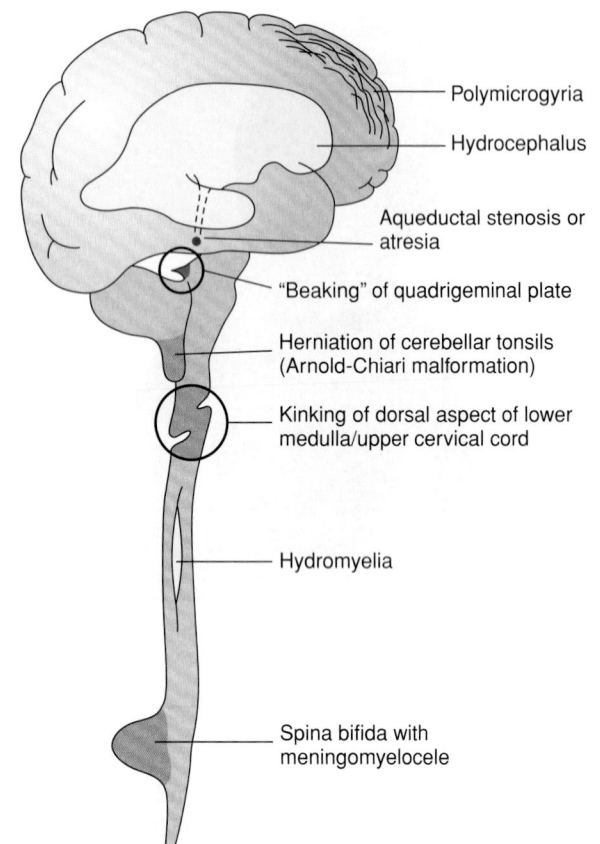

FIGURE 32-105. **Arnold-Chiari malformation and associated lesions.**

Labels in figure:
- Polymicrogyria
- Hydrocephalus
- Aqueductal stenosis or atresia
- "Beaking" of quadrigeminal plate
- Herniation of cerebellar tonsils (Arnold-Chiari malformation)
- Kinking of dorsal aspect of lower medulla/upper cervical cord
- Hydromyelia
- Spina bifida with meningomyelocele

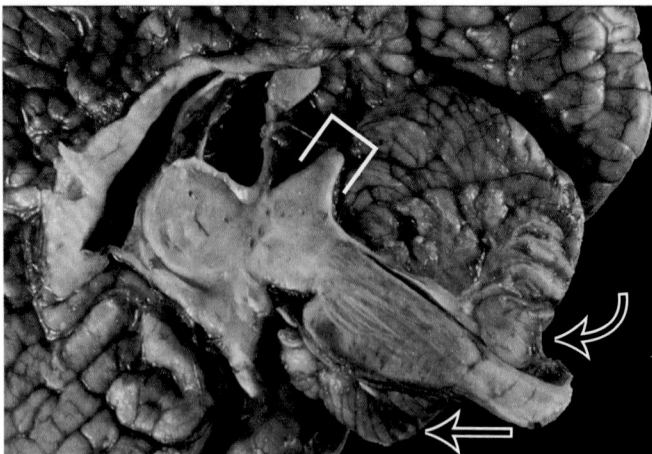

FIGURE 32-106. **Arnold-Chiari malformation.** The cerebellar vermis is herniated below the level of the foramen magnum (*arrow*). The downward displacement of the dorsal portion of the cord causes the obex of the fourth ventricle to occupy a position below the foramen magnum (*curved arrow*). The midbrain shows extreme "beaking" of the tectum with the four colliculi being replaced by a single pyramidal-shaped structure (*bracket*).

disrupts the segmentally crossing secondary axons of the spinothalamic pathway. This leads to loss of pain and thermal sensation bilaterally at the spinal level of the syrinx with relative sparing of fine touch and proprioception as well as motor pathways.

Arnold-Chiari Malformation

Arnold-Chiari malformation is a complex condition in which the brainstem and cerebellum are compacted into a shallow, bowl-shaped posterior fossa with a low-positioned tentorium. It is often associated with syringomyelia or a lumbosacral meningomyelocele. Symptoms depend on the severity of the defect (Fig. 32-105). *Since this malformation involves segmentation of the medulla and cerebellum as well as neural tube closure, it represents a defect of both neurulation and segmentation.*

 PATHOPHYSIOLOGY: The genesis of Arnold-Chiari malformation is obscure. It has spawned much speculation, but no one theory covers all features of the condition. One theory posits that a meningomyelocele anchors the lower end of the spinal cord, causing downward growth of the vertebral column, and creating traction on the medulla. This theory does not explain other facets of the malformation (curvature of the medulla, beaking of the quadrigeminal plate). Other proposals include increased intracranial pressure plus hydrocephalus or limited size of the posterior fossa.

PATHOLOGY: In Arnold-Chiari malformation, the caudal aspect of the cerebellar vermis is herniated through an enlarged foramen magnum and protrudes onto the dorsal cervical cord, often reaching C3–C5 (Fig. 32-106). The herniated tissue is held in position by thickened meninges and shows pressure atrophy (i.e., depletion of Purkinje and granular cells). The brainstem also is displaced caudally. Typically, the displacement is more exaggerated dorsally than ventrally, and landmarks (e.g., the obex of the fourth ventricle) are more caudal than ventral structures such as the inferior olive. From a lateral perspective, the lower medulla is angulated in its midsegment, creating a dorsal protrusion. The foramina of Magendie and Luschka are compressed by the bony ridge of the foramen magnum, causing hydrocephalus. The cerebellum is flattened to a discoid contour, and the quadrigeminal plate is often deformed by a "beak-shaped" dorsal protrusion of the inferior colliculi.

Defects of Segmentation and Cleavage Cause Loss of Key Structures

Holoprosencephaly

This represents a series of defects in which the interhemispheric fissure is absent or partly formed owing to a failure of the telencephalon to divide into the two hemispheres. Holoprosencephaly is a continuum: complete cleavage failure gives rise to **alobar holoprosencephaly,** partial failure leads to **lobar holoprosencephaly** and the subtlest form is failure of olfactory nerves to form, causing **arrhinencephaly**. In alobar holoprosencephaly, there is a bulbous horseshoe-shaped cortical dome consisting of fused frontal poles, across which the gyri show an irregular horizontal orientation (Fig. 32-107). A common ventricular chamber is created by lateral displacement of the posterior portions of the telencephalon. Bilobed caudate nuclei and thalami are prominent. In lobar holoprosencephaly, there is partial cleavage in the posterior portion of the telencephalon, but there remains a single gaping

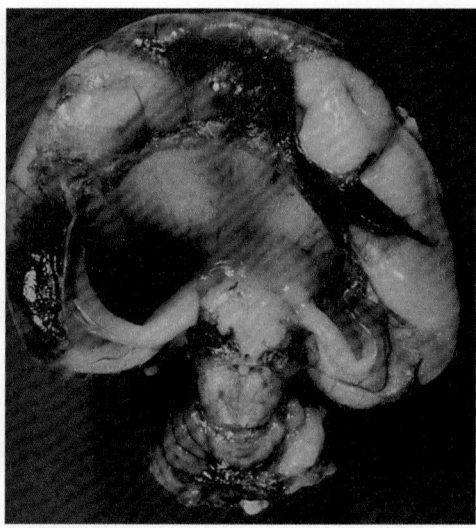

FIGURE 32-107. Holoprosencephaly. The brain exhibits a lack of separation of the hemispheres and a single large ventricle when viewed from an anterior perspective. No interhemispheric fissure is present; therefore, this is alobar holoprosencephaly.

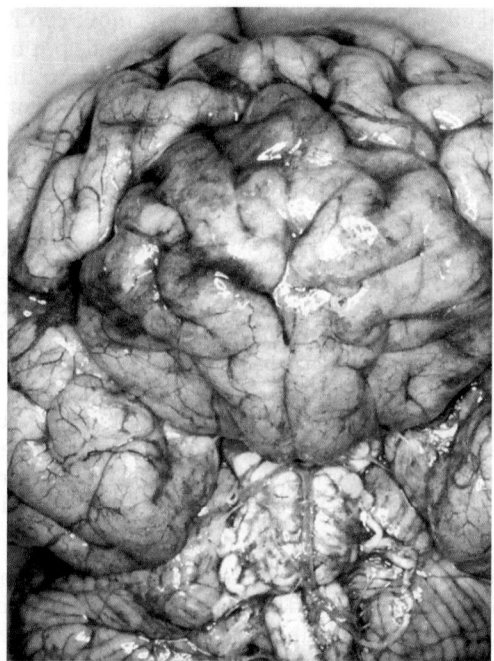

FIGURE 32-108. Arrhinencephaly is the least severe form of holoprosencephaly and consists grossly solely of absence of the olfactory bulbs and nerves, hence the name ("a," *without,* and "rhinencephaly," *nose brain*). There are usually more subtle microscopic abnormalities, and most of these individuals have some degree of mental retardation. (Courtesy of Dr. F. Stephen Vogel, Duke University.)

ventricular chamber. Holoprosencephaly is rarely compatible with life beyond a few weeks or months, and survival is associated with severe mental retardation and seizures.

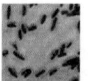 **MOLECULAR PATHOGENESIS:** About 25%–50% of patients with holoprosencephaly have numerical or structural chromosomal abnormalities. Monogenic holoprosencephaly is sometimes associated with mutations in *sonic hedgehog,* an important signaling molecule.

Arrhinencephaly

The absence of the olfactory tracts and bulbs (rhinencephalon) is the least severe of the holoprosencephaly defects (Fig. 32-108). It is clinically manifested by lack of a sense of smell **(anosmia)** and may be associated with mental retardation.

Agenesis of the Corpus Callosum

This anomaly is a regular feature of holoprosencephaly but can also be a solitary lesion. Lack of a corpus callosum does not entail significant loss of interhemispheric functional coordination, but it is associated with seizures. The corpus callosum physically tethers and functionally interconnects the hemispheres, so its absence permits the lateral ventricles to drift outward and upward, a radiographically diagnostic finding of "bat-wing" ventricles (Fig. 32-109).

Congenital Atresia of the Aqueduct of Sylvius

This is the most common cause of congenital obstructive hydrocephalus. It may result from deranged mesencephalic (midbrain) development and occurs in 1 in 1000 live births. The brain is enlarged owing to grotesque ventricular enlargement, with thinning of the cerebral cortex and stretching of white matter tracts. The midbrain may show multiple atretic channels or an aqueduct narrowed by gliosis, which may

result from developmental failure during segmentation or later in gestation as a result of transplacental transmission of infections that induce ependymitis.

Cortical Malformations Arise from Defects of Neuroglial Proliferation and Migration

ETIOLOGIC FACTORS: Neuroglial proliferation and migration begin in the first trimester of embryonic development and continue throughout

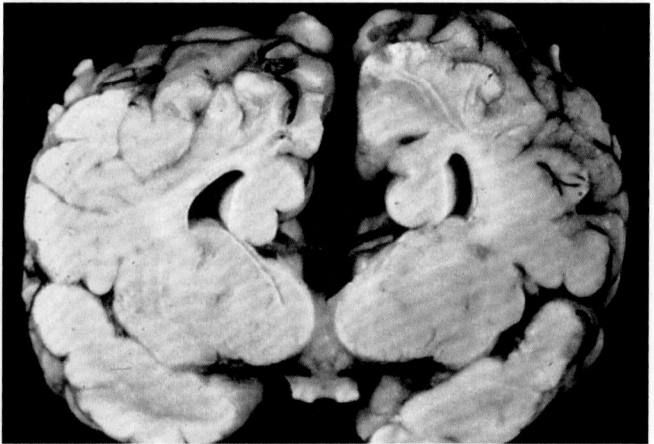

FIGURE 32-109. Congenital absence of the corpus callosum. A coronal section of the brain at the level of the thalamus reveals absence of the corpus callosum and "bat-wing" shape of the lateral ventricles. (Courtesy of Dr. F. Stephen Vogel, Duke University.)

prenatal life. Primitive neurons and glia move centrifugally from the periventricular germinal matrix to populate the cortex. The number and positions of neurons in the cortex determine the cortical infolding that creates sulci and gyri.

These disorders of cortical development thus reflect the nature and severity of disruption of gyral patterning. A cortical defect may be global or focal. Portions of the germinal matrix induce formation of specific overlying portions of the cerebral cortex; that is, there is a spatial destiny of neuroglial cells in a given region of germinal matrix. If a focal region of germinal matrix is destroyed or damaged, the cortical destination of the cells spawned in that region will reflect this damage. **Schizencephaly** is an example of such a failure of focal cortical development due to damage to the germinal matrix. Here, a patch of cortex is "missing." Cortex built from undamaged germinal matrix will be structurally normal. More global, often genetically determined defects of neuroglial proliferation and migration result in a more widespread and severe cortical defect, called lissencephaly, meaning "smooth brain."

- **Lissencephaly** is the most severe congenital disorder of cortical development. The cortical surface of the cerebral hemispheres is smooth or has imperfectly formed gyri. Some 60% of patients with lissencephaly show deletions in the region of the *LIS1* gene on chromosome 17p13.3, which encodes a protein involved in cytoskeletal dynamics that affects cell proliferation and motility. The white matter contains clusters of neurons that failed to reach the cortex.
- **Heterotopias** are focal disturbances in neuronal migration that lead to nodules of ectopic neurons and glia, usually in white matter. They are often associated with mental retardation and seizures and may be caused by maternal alcoholism.
- **Polymicrogyria** describes the presence of small and excessive gyri (Fig. 32-110). The brain surface appears to be textured with many small bumps.
- **Pachygyria** is a condition in which the gyri are reduced in number and unusually broad (Fig. 32-111).

Late-Term and Perinatal Insults May Lead to Severe Brain Damage

Sometimes the CNS develops successfully, only to suffer catastrophic damage late in pregnancy or in the perinatal

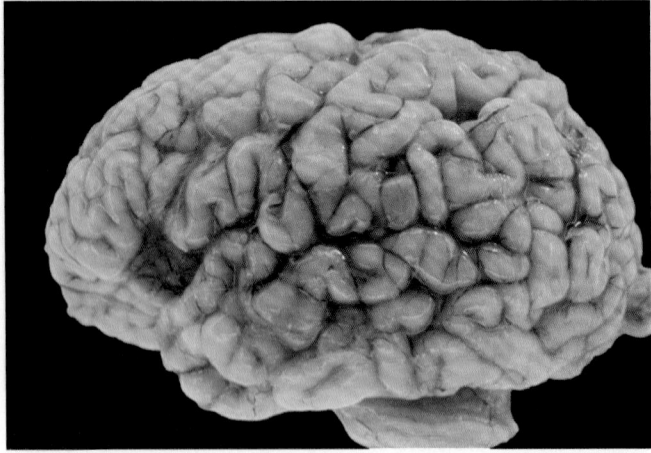

FIGURE 32-110. Polymicrogyria. The surface of the brain exhibits an excessive number of small, irregularly sized, randomly distributed gyral folds.

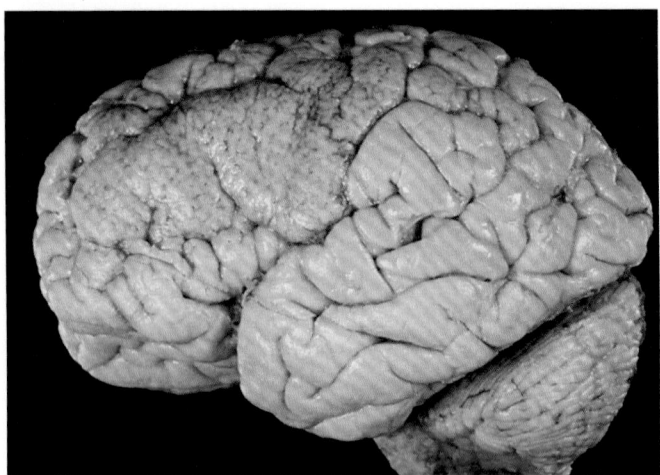

FIGURE 32-111. Pachygyria. Broad textured gyri are seen here in the superior frontal region, indicating a defect in cortical formation. (Courtesy of Dr. F. Stephen Vogel, Duke University.)

period. If the brain is deprived of blood or oxygen, the cerebral hemispheres may liquify, leaving a fluid-filled cranial cavity, a state called **hydranencephaly.** The head circumference reflects the largest size that the brain attained before the insult, and the head can be transilluminated as no tissue remains to block the passage of light through the cranial vault. The cranial sutures may override as the nascent brain degenerates.

Less severe, but still devastating, hypoxia/ischemia may lead to late-term and perinatal cerebral infarcts. Developing brains are unique bioenergetically. In adults, the gray matter receives 3 times the blood and consumes 3 times the oxygen as the white matter. In developing brains, the periventricular germinal matrix and streams of migrating neuroglia equalize bioenergetic demand, so that deep structures and cerebral cortex have similar huge energy and substrate requirements. The deep periventricular white matter is a watershed perfusion zone and is at highest risk for infarction. Thus, intrauterine or perinatal hypoxia ischemia may cause chalky white, sometimes calcific **periventricular leukomalacia.** Infarcted areas may undergo resorption, leading to **multicystic leukoencephalopathy,** with numerous interconnected cystic cavities deep in the white matter near the ventricles.

The germinal matrix is active during later phases of gestation but gradually involutes as term approaches. If a baby is born prematurely, its metabolically active germinal matrix is perfused by delicate capillaries floating in a frenzied sea of stem cells and newly spawned neuroglia. Such an infant is ill equipped for cerebrovascular regulation. These delicate vessels may be exposed to dramatic swings in perfusion pressure, leading to **germinal matrix hemorrhage.** Hemorrhage may remain confined to a small region of the germinal matrix or it may spread catastrophically as intraventricular hemorrhage. Germinal matrix hemorrhage is a major challenge in clinical management of premature newborns.

Congenital Defects May Be Associated with Chromosomal Abnormalities

Derangements of the larger autosomes, 1 through 12, are incompatible with sustained intrauterine life: affected fetuses are spontaneously aborted. Structural and functional abnormalities may be attributed to gross chromosomal derangements of the smaller autosomes (e.g., trisomies of chromosomes 13–15 and 21 [Down syndrome]). Trisomies 13 or 15 occur in 1 per 5000 births, with a modest female predominance. The congenital deformities involve the brain, facial features and extremities: holoprosencephaly, arrhinencephaly, microphthalmia, cyclopia, low-set ears, harelip and cleft palate. The extremities exhibit polydactyly and "rocker bottom" feet.

CENTRAL NERVOUS SYSTEM NEOPLASIA

Primary CNS cancers represent 1.5% of all primary malignant tumors. Metastatic tumors to the CNS are far more common than are primary tumors and are a major problem in clinical management. The broad spectrum of cellular constituents of the CNS—all of the diverse cell types that are represented in the CNS—is mirrored by the wide range of tumor types that arise within the brain and spinal cord and their overlying meninges. Over 130 different types of CNS neoplasms are recognized and formally codified by the World Health Organization (WHO), but most are very rare. By far the most common are meningiomas and gliomas, each of which accounts for 1/3 of CNS tumors (Table 32-5). While most brain tumors arise in adults, some are more common in childhood, the most prominent being medulloblastoma, pilocytic astrocytoma and diffuse pontine astrocytoma. Together, primary brain tumors are second only to leukemia as the most common childhood malignancy, and are the most common pediatric solid tumors.

Diagnosing a brain tumor entails generating a preoperative differential diagnosis of the most likely possibilities based on the patient's clinical information (Table 32-6), then obtaining a definitive tissue-based diagnosis by biopsy or resection. Further clinical management requires a definitive diagnosis. This approach integrates the key characteristics of different brain and spinal cord tumors and other kinds of diseases, plus the patient's age, the location of

TABLE 32-6
ESSENTIAL CLINICAL INFORMATION
Patient age and gender
Anatomic location and compartment of the lesion
Neuroimaging (computed tomography, magnetic resonance imaging) features
Nature and time course of presenting signs and symptoms
Relevant clinical history

the lesion, specific neuroimaging features, the nature and time course of preceding clinical signs and symptoms and major elements of the clinical history, such as the presence of a systemic primary tumor or of a tumor predisposition syndrome.

PATIENT AGE: Different types of brain tumors tend to arise at particular ages. The two most common brain tumors of childhood are medulloblastoma and pilocytic astrocytoma. Other, rarer tumors also tend to occur in children, such as diffuse pontine glioma, atypical teratoid/ rhabdoid tumor and choroid plexus carcinoma. Similarly, metastatic carcinomas from the lung, breast and colon mainly affect older adults. Still others have a peak incidence in young adulthood, such as ganglioglioma and central neurocytoma. Some tumors may be most common in adults but spare no age group: glioblastomas are the most common and most malignant gliomas and may occur at any time in life.

PATIENT GENDER: Most primary brain tumors are more common in males, with two notable exceptions being pituitary adenomas and meningiomas, which are more common in young adult and middle-aged to older adult women, respectively. Brain metastases of primary tumors elsewhere follow the gender patterns of incidence of those tumor types (e.g., breast, prostate).

ANATOMIC LOCATION AND COMPARTMENT OF THE LESION: Anatomic localization of brain lesions includes two components: the region of the CNS involved, such as the cerebrum, cerebellum or spinal cord, and the compartment(s). Examples of the latter include intraparenchymal (e.g., within the brain substance), intraventricular or intradural–extra-axial (within the spinal subarachnoid space). Such information greatly facilitates formulation of a differential diagnosis. Thus, intradural, extra-axial spinal cord masses would be meningioma and peripheral nerve sheath tumors; masses within a cerebral lateral ventricle are more likely to be choroid plexus papillomas, ependymomas or other tumors that frequent those haunts.

NEUROIMAGING FEATURES: Preoperative imaging of a CNS lesion provides critical data that bear directly on the differential diagnosis (Table 32-7; Fig. 32-112). The most obvious are the number and distribution of lesions, as noted above. The nature of the interface between the lesion and the surrounding brain is also important. For example, the borders of highly infiltrative tumors, such as fibrillary astrocytomas and lymphomas, are subtle and diffuse, but interfaces with the surrounding brain are much better circumscribed for metastases or minimally infiltrative primary tumors, such as pilocytic astrocytoma or ganglioglioma.

TABLE 32-5
MAJOR TYPES OF PRIMARY CENTRAL NERVOUS SYSTEM (CNS) TUMORS
Meningioma
Gliomas (including diffuse and circumscribed astrocytomas, oligodendroglioma, ependymoma, choroid plexus tumors, several rare glioma subtypes)
Medulloblastoma and other primitive neuroectodermal tumors
Craniopharyngioma
Germ cell tumors
Hemangioblastoma
Neuronal and mixed glioneuronal tumors
Pineal tumors
Primary CNS lymphoma

TABLE 32-7

MAJOR NEUROIMAGING (COMPUTED TOMOGRAPHY, MAGNETIC RESONANCE IMAGING) FEATURES

Anatomic location and compartment of the lesion(s)

Nature of the interface between the lesion and the surrounding parenchyma (e.g., sharply circumscribed vs. diffuse)

Presence or absence of enhancement following contrast agent administration

If contrast enhancing, the pattern of enhancement (e.g., solid uniform enhancement, ring enhancement around a central area of necrosis, C-shaped open ring enhancement, enhancing nodule within the wall of a cyst)

Vascularity, when contrast agents are given, is also helpful, since some tumor types, such as glioblastoma, meningioma, medulloblastoma and metastatic carcinomas, are more vascular, while others usually are not, such as low-grade diffuse fibrillary astrocytoma. Some tumor types tend to show relatively solid, even enhancement, such as meningiomas and primary CNS lymphoma, but for other types, ring enhancement around a central area of necrosis is typical, such as glioblastoma. Nontumor diseases, many of which mimic tumor radiologically, also often have characteristic enhancement patterns; for example, demyelinating pseudotumor frequently presents as a mass lesion with "open ring" or "C-shaped" enhancement, while cerebral abscesses typically show a very smooth-walled enhancing ring (Fig. 32-112).

NATURE AND TIME COURSE OF CLINICAL SIGNS AND SYMPTOMS: In general, a long history, such as several years of poorly controlled seizures, favors more indolent or

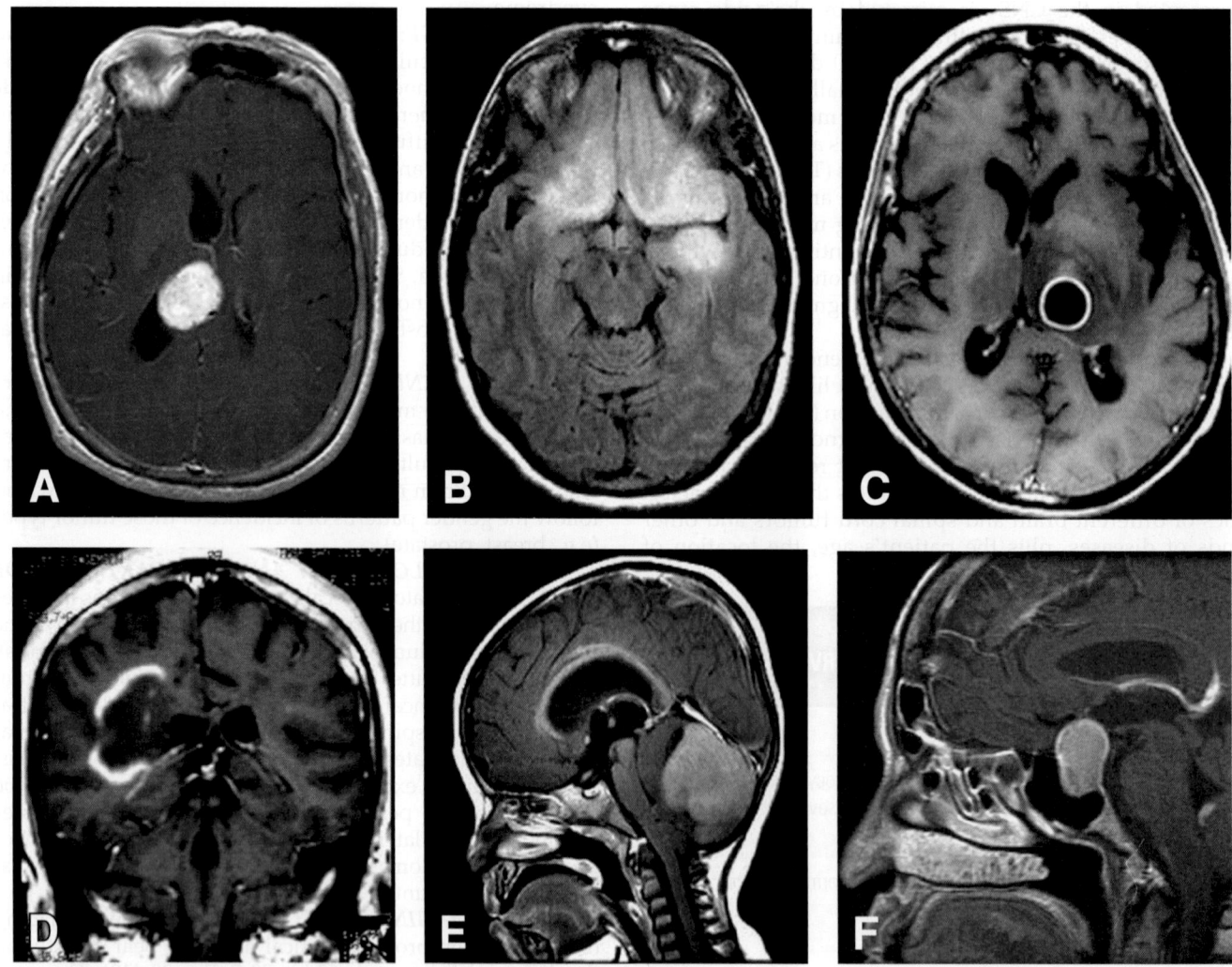

FIGURE 32-112. Neuroimaging—the modern pathologist's gross pathology. Contemporary neuroimaging techniques provide the first look at the "gross pathology" of a central nervous system lesion and constitute a rich source of information that can be utilized by the pathologist to formulate a refined differential diagnosis prior to surgical biopsy and tissue examination. Shown here are representative examples of magnetic resonance images that illustrate the highly informative features of six different brain lesions. **A.** A contrast-enhancing, circumscribed mass located within the lateral ventricle (choroid plexus meningioma). **B.** Diffuse hyperintensity involving both frontal lobes and the left temporal lobe (infiltrating glioma). **C.** Smooth-walled ring-enhancing mass in the left thalamus (pyogenic abscess). **D.** C-shaped open ring-enhancing lesion in the white matter of the right parietal lobe (demyelinating pseudotumor). **E.** Hyperintense midline mass of the cerebellar vermis and fourth ventricle (medulloblastoma). **F.** Contrast-enhancing midline mass of the sellar and suprasellar region (pituitary adenoma).

TABLE 32-8

MAJOR NERVOUS SYSTEM TUMOR PREDISPOSITION SYNDROMES

Syndrome	Chromosome Locus	Gene (protein)	Associated Nervous System Tumors
Neurofibromatosis type 1 (NF1)	17q11.2	*NF1* (neurofibromin)	Neurofibromas (dermal and plexiform) Malignant peripheral nerve sheath tumor (MPNST) Pilocytic astrocytoma ("optic glioma") Diffuse astrocytoma Glioblastoma
Neurofibromatosis type 2 (NF2)	22q12	*NF2* (merlin/schwanomin)	Vestibular schwannomas (bilateral) Other schwannomas Meningiomas (multiple) Meningioangiomatosis Ependymoma of spinal cord Diffuse astrocytoma
Schwannomatosis (sometimes referred to as "NF3")	Unknown	Unknown	Schwannomas (multiple, spinal roots, cranial nerves, skin, not vestibular)
von Hippel-Lindau (vHL)	3p25–26	*VHL* (pVHL)	Hemangioblastomas (multiple) of cerebellum, spinal cord, brainstem, retina, spinal peripheral nerve roots Endolymphatic sac tumor
Tuberous sclerosis complex	9q34 16p13.3	*TSC1* (hamartin) *TSC2* (tuberin)	Subependymal giant cell astrocytoma
Li-Fraumeni syndrome	17p13	*TP53* (TP53 protein)	Diffuse astrocytomas, including glioblastoma Medulloblastoma Choroid plexus papilloma Ependymoma Oligodendroglioma Meningioma
Cowden disease	10q23	*PTEN/MMAC1* (PTEN protein)	Dysplastic gangliocytoma of the cerebellum (Lhermitte-Duclos disease)
Turcot type 1 syndrome (mismatch repair [MMR]/hereditary nonpolyposis colon cancer [HNPCC]– associated Turcot)	3p21.3 2p16 5q11–q13 2q32 7p22	*MLH1* *MSH2* and *MSH6 MSH3* *PMS1* *PMS2* *APC* (APC protein)	Glioblastoma
Turcot type 2 syndrome (familial adenomatous polyposis [FAP]–associated Turcot)	5q21		Medulloblastoma
Nevoid basal cell carcinoma (Gorlin) syndrome	9q22.3	*PTCH* (Ptch protein)	Medulloblastoma
Rhabdoid tumor predisposition syndrome	22q11.2	*INI1* (INI1 protein)	Atypical teratoid/rhabdoid tumor

low-grade disease, while a relatively brief history, such as a 2-week history of headache, nausea and emesis and localizing signs, favors a higher grade and more aggressively expanding lesion.

RELEVANT CLINICAL HISTORY: Histories of, for example, previous non-CNS tumors, systemic diseases or tumor predisposition syndromes are also useful (Table 32-8).

GRADING OF CENTRAL NERVOUS SYSTEM TUMORS: Tumors in brain and spinal cord are commonly graded according to criteria established in the *WHO Classification of Tumours of the Central Nervous System.* Tumor grades according to WHO criteria range from I to IV, with I being the lowest grade and IV the most malignant. The subjective and ill-defined term "benign" should be used with extreme caution, if at all, with respect to CNS tumors, even WHO grade I tumors, because anatomic location, growth pattern and other factors can result in a clinical course for a grade I CNS tumor that entails considerable morbidity and even mortality. For example, most meningiomas are grade I. However, there are those that grow en plaque (flat and plaque-like) along the skull base and surround cranial nerves and blood vessels as they enter and exit the cranial cavity. These can be very difficult to treat surgically and often do not respond well to radiation or chemotherapy. As well, the vast majority of low-grade diffuse gliomas (WHO grade II) are ultimately fatal, even though they are the lowest grade for this subtype of glioma.

Meningiomas Are the Most Common Central Nervous System Tumors

Meningiomas are derived from the middle layer of arachnoid (meningothelial) cells that form the outer boundary of the subarachnoid space. Thus, the anatomic locations in which meningiomas arise parallel the distribution of the arachnoid membrane, and these tumors can arise at any CNS site where arachnoid cells are present—including at the dural venous sinuses (such as the superior sagittal sinus), at the cerebral convexity, at the skull base, around the optic nerve, around the spinal cord and even within the choroid plexus in the cerebral ventricles as mentioned earlier.

 **MOLECULAR PATHOGENESIS:** Meningiomas typically arise in one of three settings:

■ **Sporadic:** *The vast majority of meningiomas arise sporadically.* Many show loss, partial deletion or mutation of the *NF2* locus (22q12). Disturbances of this tumor suppressor gene may thus be involved not only in neurofibromatosis type 2 (NF2)-associated tumors but also in the origin of many sporadic meningiomas (and schwannomas).

■ **Iatrogenic:** Induction of meningiomas by radiation therapy generally involves a latent period of a decade or more and is directly related to radiation dosage. Low-dose scalp irradiation for tinea capitis was widely used until around 1960. The average interval between treatment and detection of a meningioma for such patients was 35 years. With higher radiation doses, such as are used for head and neck cancers, the interval may be as short as 5 years.

■ **Tumor predisposition syndromes:** Meningiomas also occur in conjunction with several genetic syndromes, most importantly NF2. Additional rare multiple meningioma syndromes have also been documented.

 PATHOLOGY: On MRI and gross examination, most meningiomas are well-circumscribed dura-based masses of variable size that compress, but do not invade, the underlying brain (Fig. 32-113A,B). The cut

TABLE 32-9

MENINGIOMA SUBTYPES

World Health Organization (WHO) Grade I: Benign Meningioma

Meningothelial

Fibrous

Transitional

Psammomatous

Angiomatous

Microcystic

Secretory

Lymphoplasmacyte rich

Metaplastic

WHO Grade II: Atypical Meningioma

Chordoid

Clear cell

WHO Grade III: Anaplastic (Malignant) Meningioma

Rhabdoid

Papillary

surface is fleshy and tan. The classic histologic hallmark of meningiomas is a whorled pattern, often in association with psammoma bodies (laminated, spherical calcospherites) (Fig. 32-113C,D). However, these tumors can show diverse morphologic patterns, and 13 subtypes are recognized by the WHO (Table 32-9). Most of these are WHO grade I, but two variants, clear cell and chordoid, behave more aggressively (WHO grade II), and two other variants, papillary and rhabdoid, are frankly anaplastic (WHO grade III). Meningiomas typically express epithelial membrane antigen (EMA) focally (Fig. 32-113C). They have many intercellular junctions, owing to their origin from the cohesive arachnoid barrier cell layer (Fig. 32-113E).

CLINICAL FEATURES: The indolent growth of most meningiomas enables them to enlarge slowly for years before becoming symptomatic. During that time, they displace the brain but do not infiltrate it (Fig. 32-114A,B). Patients often have seizures, particularly with tumors at parasagittal sites over the convexity of the hemispheres. In other locations, meningiomas compress a variety of functional structures. Thus, tumors of the olfactory groove produce anosmia; those in the suprasellar region cause visual deficits by compressing the optic chiasm; meningiomas in the cerebellopontine angle cause cranial nerve dysfunction; and those along the spinal cord compromise spinal nerve root and spinal cord function. Invasion of cranial bone, often accompanied by hyperostosis on CT scans, is relatively common, and growth through the calvarium may create a tumor mass beneath the scalp. In contrast, meningiomas rarely invade the underlying brain. Such aggressive behavior warrants upgrading to WHO grade II (atypical). Tumors that are not completely excised tend to recur, and some may undergo anaplastic progression over time. Anaplastic (malignant) meningiomas (WHO grade III) may also rarely arise de novo.

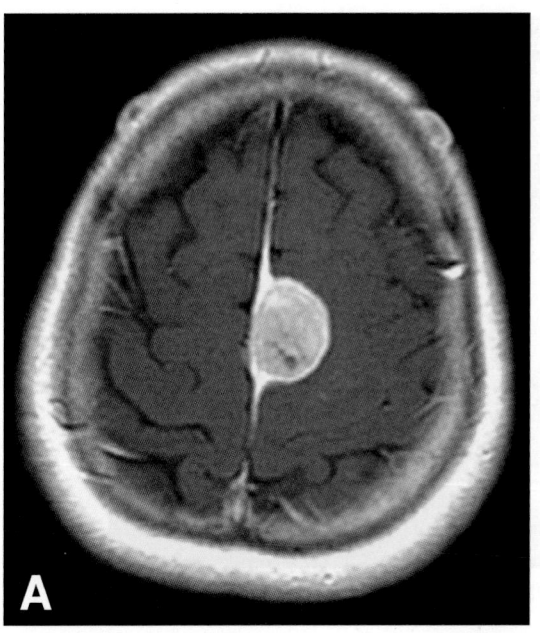

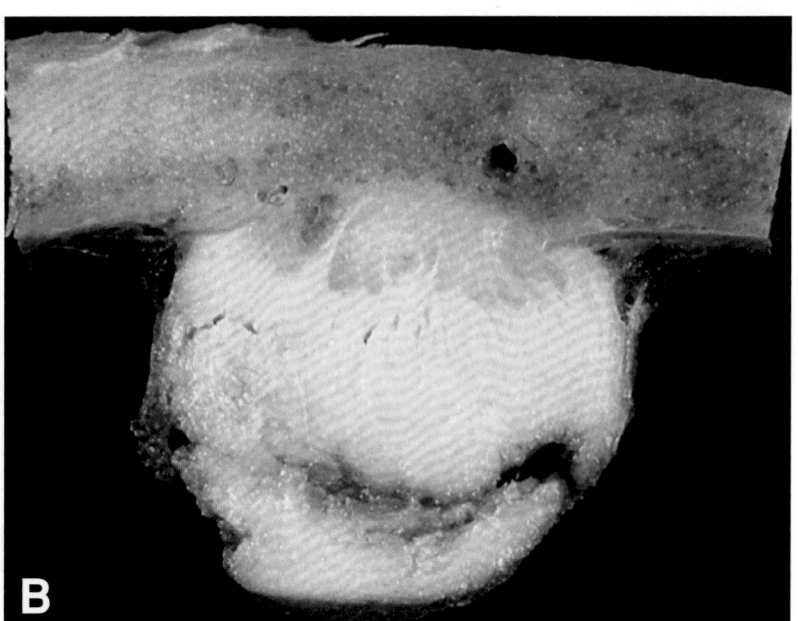

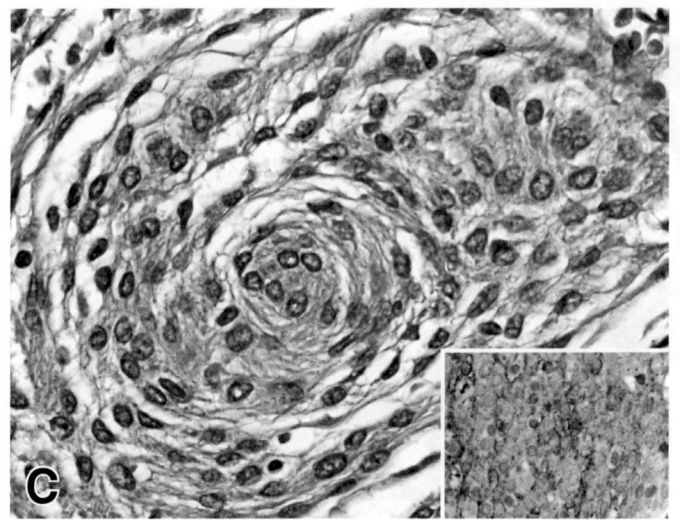

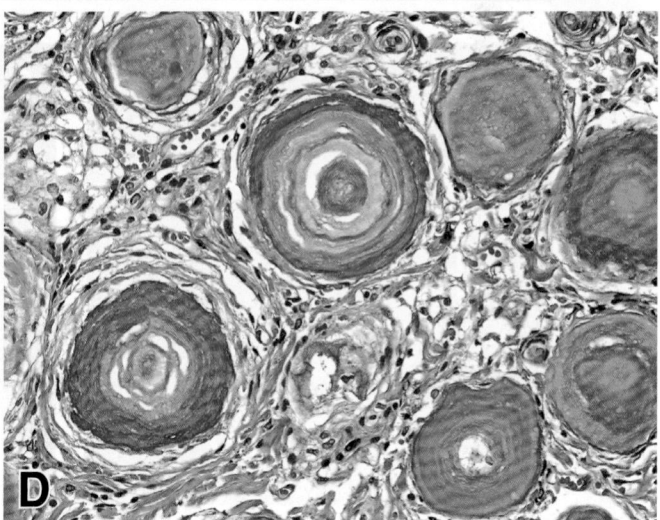

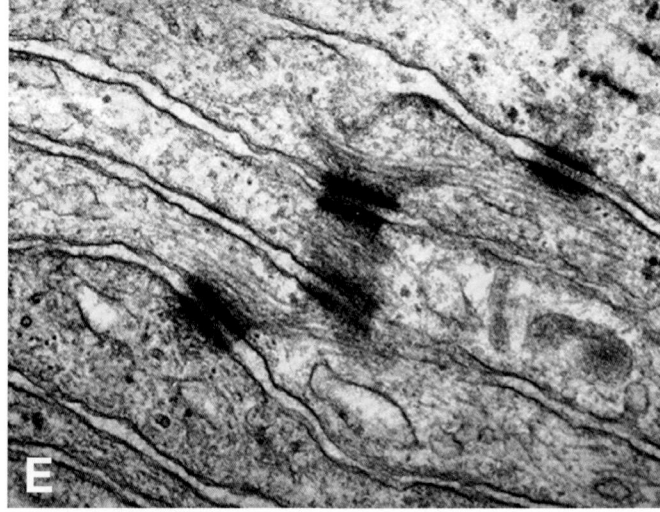

FIGURE 32-113. Meningioma. A. Magnetic resonance imaging showing a superficial dura-based circumscribed mass, with tapering enhancement of the dura adjacent to the site of tumor attachment ("dural tail"); the chief entity in the differential diagnosis for this magnetic resonance appearance is meningioma. **B.** Gross surgical specimen consisting of excised meningioma together with cranial bone and dura. (Courtesy of Dr. F. Stephen Vogel, Duke University.) **C. Histology of meningioma.** Note the whorled, bland, plump spindle cells. Meningiomas are immunopositive for epithelial membrane antigen, which is used as a diagnostic adjunct in difficult cases (*inset*). **D.** Prominent psammoma body formation, typical of the "psammomatous" subtype of meningioma. **E.** The ultrastructural hallmark of meningiomas is numerous intercellular junctions (desmosomes), which tightly bind adjacent meningioma cell processes together.

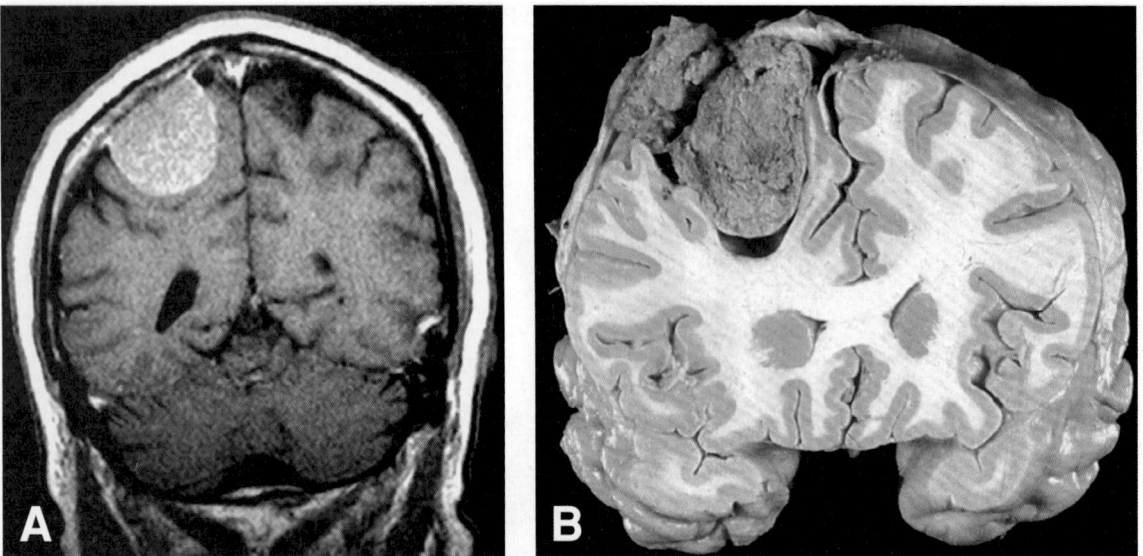

FIGURE 32-114. Meningioma. Meningiomas compress, but do not usually invade, the underlying brain. **A.** Magnetic resonance image. **B.** Gross specimen. (Courtesy of Dr. F. Stephen Vogel, Duke University.)

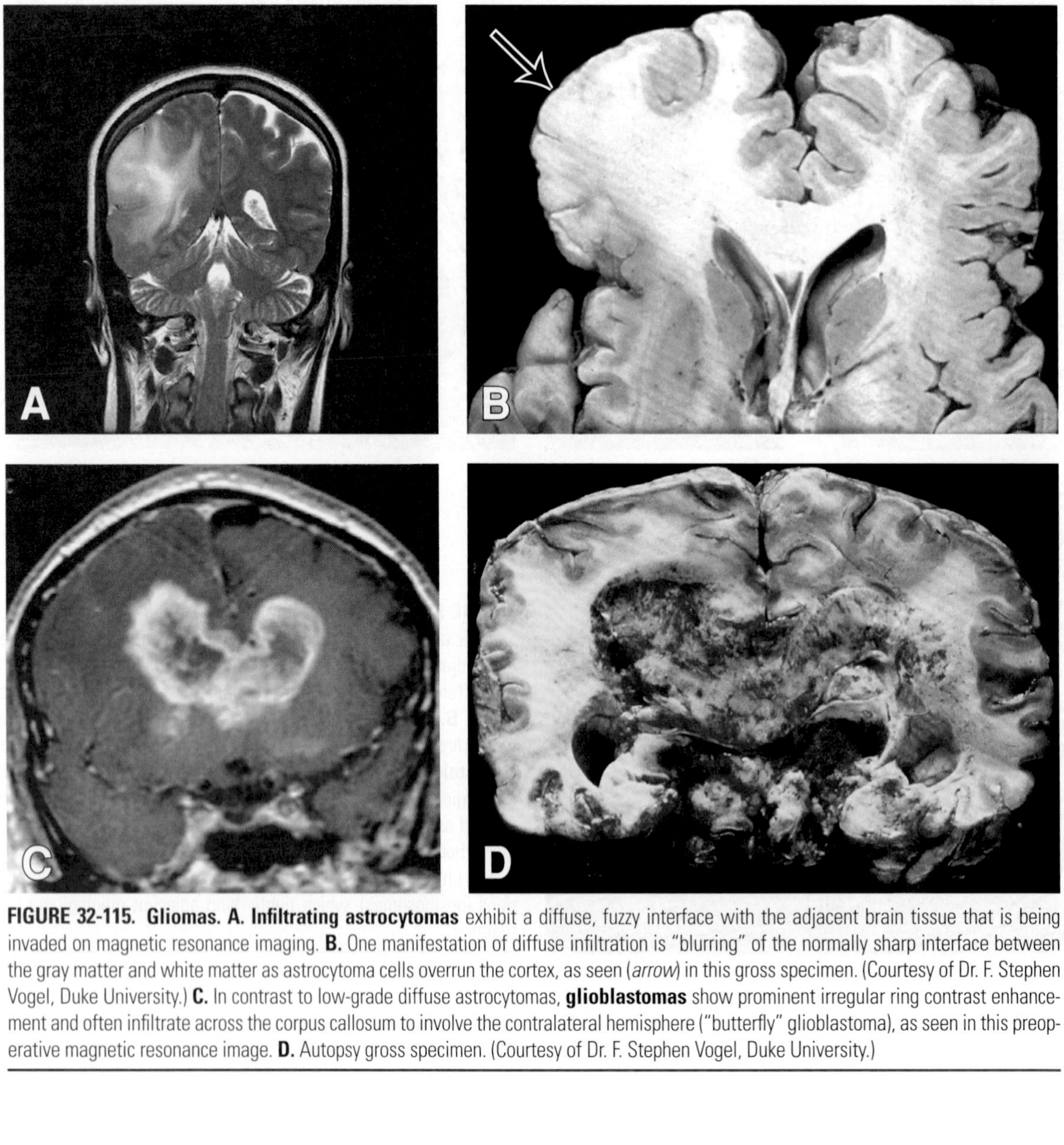

FIGURE 32-115. Gliomas. A. Infiltrating astrocytomas exhibit a diffuse, fuzzy interface with the adjacent brain tissue that is being invaded on magnetic resonance imaging. **B.** One manifestation of diffuse infiltration is "blurring" of the normally sharp interface between the gray matter and white matter as astrocytoma cells overrun the cortex, as seen (*arrow*) in this gross specimen. (Courtesy of Dr. F. Stephen Vogel, Duke University.) **C.** In contrast to low-grade diffuse astrocytomas, **glioblastomas** show prominent irregular ring contrast enhancement and often infiltrate across the corpus callosum to involve the contralateral hemisphere ("butterfly" glioblastoma), as seen in this preoperative magnetic resonance image. **D.** Autopsy gross specimen. (Courtesy of Dr. F. Stephen Vogel, Duke University.)

Astrocytomas Are the Most Common Primary Brain Tumors

They can be divided into two major categories based on how diffusely they infiltrate the brain parenchyma. *Diffuse astrocytomas* infiltrate the brain widely and include low-grade fibrillary astrocytoma, anaplastic astrocytoma and the most malignant astrocytic tumor, glioblastoma. Members of the other major category of astrocytomas typically do not infiltrate the CNS but rather are slowly enlarging, compact masses that cause symptoms by compressing adjacent structures. These include pilocytic astrocytoma, pleomorphic xanthoastrocytoma and subependymal giant cell astrocytomas.

Diffuse Astrocytoma

The most salient biological characteristic of diffuse astrocytomas, as the name implies, is the ability of individual tumor cells to infiltrate widely through brain and spinal cord parenchyma (Fig. 32-115). This property reaches its extreme in **gliomatosis cerebri (WHO grade III),** in which infiltrating glioma cells (usually astrocytes but occasionally oligodendroglia) involve at least three cerebral lobes, and often more, with infiltration into both hemispheres, the brainstem,

the cerebellum and even the spinal cord. Diffuse tumor infiltration of brain and spinal cord is a major reason there is little effective therapy for these tumors.

Glioblastoma typically presents as a large, ring-enhancing mass with an irregular central area of necrosis and prominent edema of surrounding white matter. The infiltrating component of glioblastomas often crosses to contralateral hemispheres via the corpus callosum; such cases are referred to as "butterfly" glioblastomas based on their appearance on coronal MRI (Fig. 32-115).

 PATHOLOGY: Low-grade fibrillary astrocytomas **(WHO grade II)** have well-differentiated astrocytic tumor cells with little nuclear atypia or cell proliferation. Gemistocytic astrocytoma is a distinctive subtype of low-grade astrocytoma in which the main population of cells has prominent globular cytoplasm filled with glial intermediate filaments (Fig. 32-116). Despite a deceptively bland appearance, diffuse astrocytomas often undergo anaplastic progression, usually over several years, into high-grade astrocytoma (anaplastic astrocytoma, WHO grade III) and, ultimately, into glioblastoma (WHO grade IV). This tendency for anaplastic progression is even more pronounced with the gemistocytic variant. **Anaplastic astrocytoma (WHO grade III)** is more cellular than low-grade fibrillary

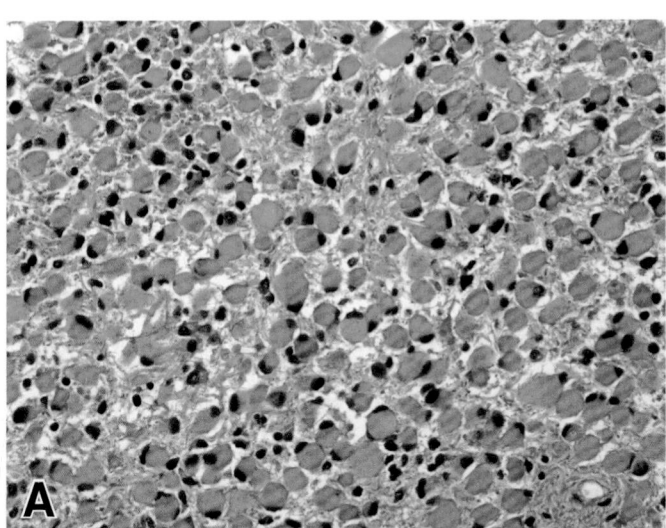

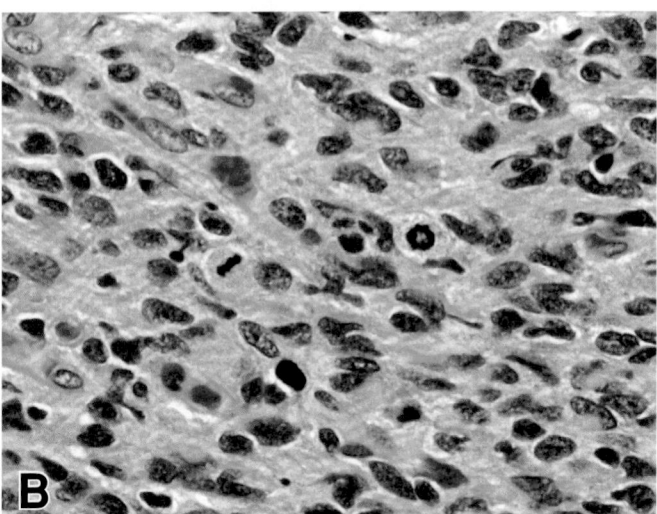

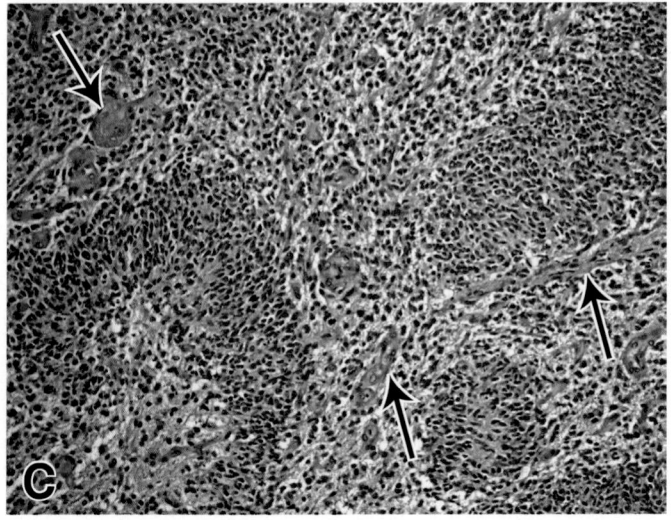

FIGURE 32-116. Diffuse astrocytoma histology. A. Gemistocytic astrocytomas are low-grade (World Health Organization [WHO] grade II) diffuse astrocytomas characterized by prominent globular cytoplasm. **B. Anaplastic astrocytoma (WHO grade III),** in contrast, is more cellular and more pleomorphic, in addition to having a higher proliferation rate. **C. Glioblastoma (WHO grade IV)** displays foci of tumor necrosis surrounded by hypercellular cuffs of tumor cells ("pseudopalisading necrosis") as well as vascular proliferation (*arrows*).

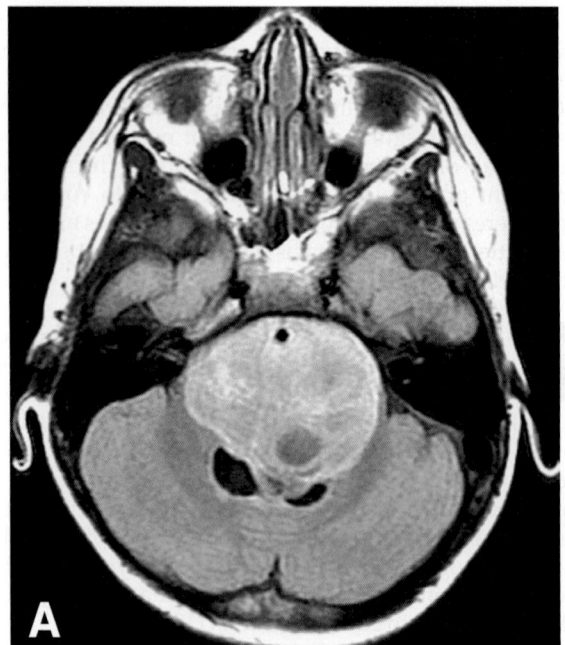 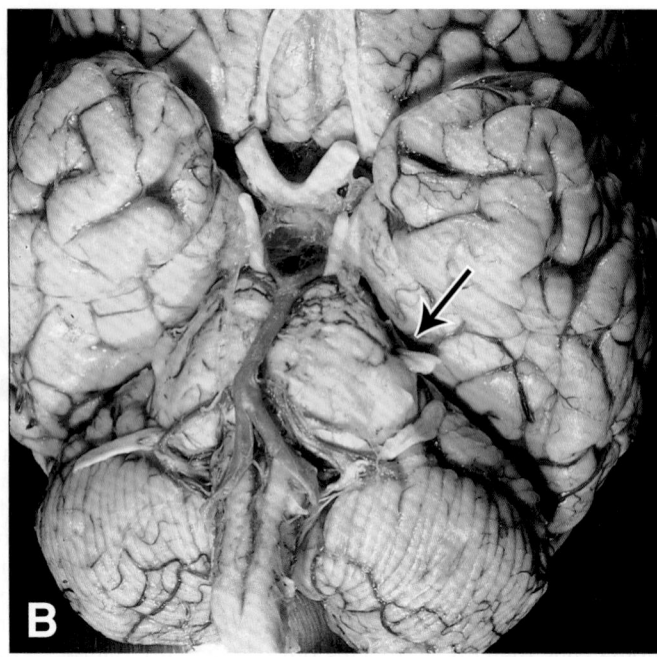

FIGURE 32-117. Diffuse pontine astrocytoma ("pontine glioma"). Diffuse astrocytomas of childhood, diffuse pontine astrocytomas infiltrate and expand the brainstem pons, often to the point of encircling the basilar artery. **A.** Magnetic resonance imaging. **B.** Autopsy gross specimen.

astrocytoma, and individual tumor cells are more pleomorphic (Fig. 32-116). Mitotic rates are elevated and mitoses are easily seen. Anaplastic astrocytomas typically progress to glioblastoma within a few years.

Glioblastoma multiforme (GBM; WHO grade IV) is the single most common primary malignant brain tumor. It accounts for about 20% of all CNS tumors. GBMs are cytologically highly pleomorphic, and constituent cells vary greatly in size and shape, with large bizarre nuclei and multinucleated cells. They may arise by anaplastic progression from lower-grade diffuse astrocytomas (secondary glioblastoma; 5% of GBMs) or, much more commonly, de novo (primary glioblastoma; 95% of GBMs). Although usually solitary, they may rarely present as two separate epicenters of enhancement within the brain. Such cases may closely mimic metastases radiologically, with biopsy providing a definitive diagnosis. Mitotic activity in GBMs is high; vascular proliferation and foci of tumor necrosis surrounded by a densely cellular cuff of tumor cells ("pseudopalisading necrosis") are characteristic (Fig. 32-116C).

Diffuse pontine astrocytoma (diffuse intrinsic pontine glioma; WHO grade II through IV) is a diffusely infiltrating astrocytoma that arises in, and expands, the pons of the brainstem of young children (Fig. 32-117). MRI plus clinical features are so distinctive that treatment is usually initiated without biopsy confirmation of the diagnosis. Their grade varies from II to IV, but despite aggressive treatment all cases are ultimately lethal, with infiltration and compromise of vital brainstem structures.

MOLECULAR PATHOGENESIS: *The vast majority of GBMs are sporadic,* but a minority arise in the setting of a genetic tumor predisposition syndrome (Table 32-8). Sporadic GBMs may arise de novo or via anaplastic progression from lower-grade astrocytoma (see above). Molecular characterization reveals differences

in the mutations seen in these two major classes. Primary GBMs show amplification of the epidermal growth factor receptor (*EGFR*) gene and mutation of the *PTEN* gene more often, but *TP53* is more often mutated in secondary GBMs. More recent molecular and genomic profiling studies have identified mutation of the isocitrate-dehydrogenase genes 1 or 2 (*IDH1, IDH2*), and especially *IDH1*, as a very common signature of low-grade (grade II) and anaplastic (grade III) diffuse gliomas and also of a majority of secondary GBMs that arise from these lower-grade tumors (see Chapter 5). Primary GBMs generally do not show *IDH* mutations. Other mutations in specific molecular subsets of GBM include deletion or mutation of the *NF1* gene and amplification of the *ERBB2* gene.

Similarly, molecular insight into the basis for resistance to treatment is also beginning to be understood. GBMs can be stratified into two groups based on whether the promotor for the DNA repair gene *MGMT* is methylated, and hence inactivated, or unmethylated, and so capable of repairing damage caused by alkylating agents used in chemotherapy. Patients with *MGMT* promotor methylation (inactivation) respond significantly better to treatment. Gliomas with both IDH mutation and 1p/19q whole arm codeletion have a more favorable prognosis and response to therapy; this molecular signature is considered a favorable predictive molecular marker.

Pilocytic Astrocytoma (WHO Grade I)

Pilocytic astrocytomas (PAs) are circumscribed gliomas that typically arise in children and young adults and expand very slowly. Unlike diffuse astrocytomas, PAs do not infiltrate brain or spinal cord parenchyma diffusely and rarely progress to higher-grade tumors. Common locations include the cerebellum, brainstem, optic nerves and third ventricular region. PAs are contrast enhancing, may be associated with

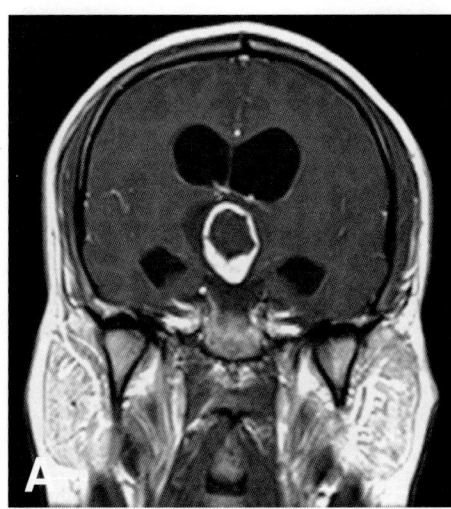
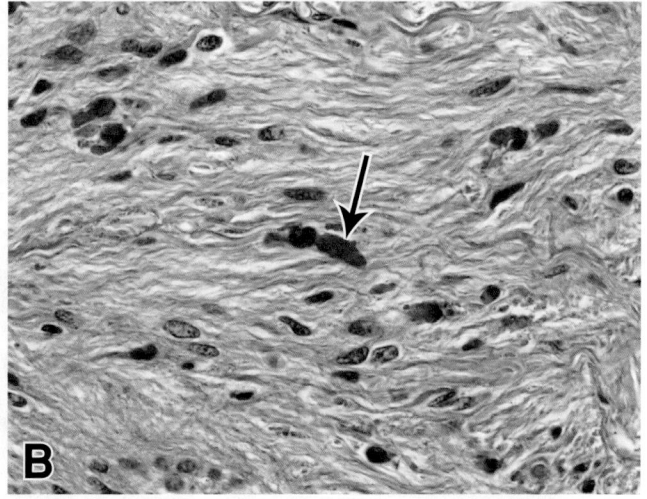

FIGURE 32-118. Pilocytic astrocytoma (World Health Organization grade I). A. Pilocytic astrocytomas are very low-grade circumscribed contrast-enhancing gliomas. **B.** Histologically, the neoplastic pilocytes ("hair cells") exhibit greatly elongated bipolar cytoplasmic processes that are prone to Rosenthal fiber formation (*arrow*).

a cystic component and are well circumscribed on preoperative imaging studies (Fig. 32-118).

PATHOLOGY: PAs consist of compact areas of tumor cells with elongated bipolar cytoplasmic processes (pilocytes) separated by prominent microcysts. The compact areas frequently have prominent **Rosenthal fibers,** a histologic hallmark of pilocytic astrocytoma. Vascular proliferation is typical and correlates with the contrast enhancement seen on preoperative MRI studies. Mitotic activity, vascular proliferation and foci of necrosis in pilocytic areas do not have the same kind of negative prognostic significance as in diffuse astrocytomas. In favorable anatomic locations, such as the cerebellum, surgical resection may be curative. **Pilomyxoid astrocytoma** (WHO grade II) is a recently recognized variant of PA, primarily arising in

the hypothalamic region, that exhibits a more aggressive clinical behavior.

Pleomorphic Xanthoastrocytoma (WHO Grade II)

Pleomorphic xanthoastrocytoma (PXA) is another circumscribed astrocytoma variant of children and young adults (Fig. 32-119A). There is usually a several-year history of poorly controlled seizure activity; the temporal lobe is the most common location. In favorable anatomic locations, PXAs, like PAs, are amenable to surgical resection, but incompletely resected tumors frequently recur. About 15% of these undergo anaplastic progression to high-grade diffuse astrocytoma. Up to 66% of PXAs harbor a *BRAF* V600E mutation, which may indicate a greater tendency for progression.

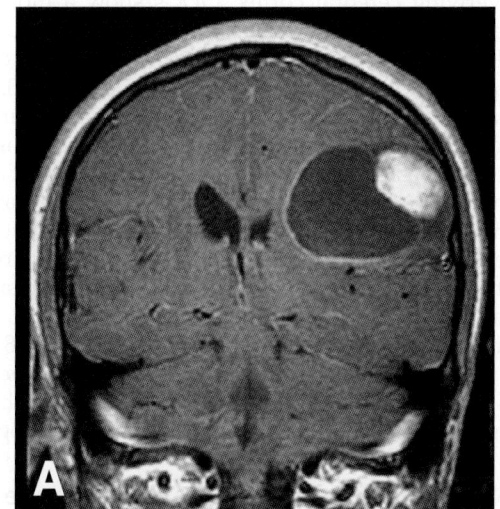
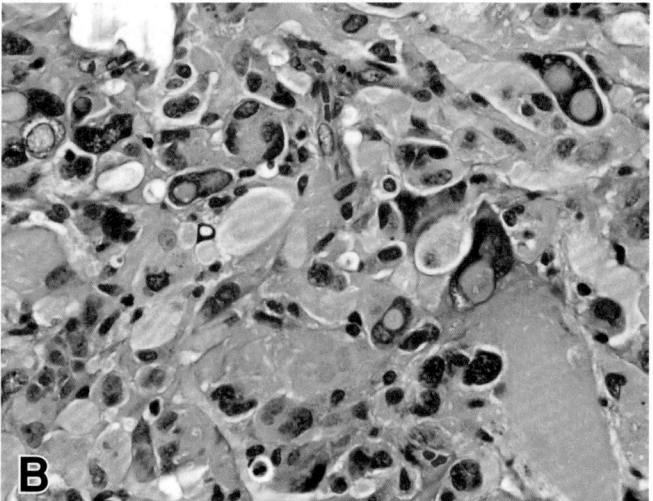

FIGURE 32-119. Pleomorphic xanthoastrocytoma (PXA). A. PXAs are low-grade (World Health Organization grade II) circumscribed astrocytomas that typically display a "cyst with enhancing mural nodule" pattern, similar to other low-grade tumors such as pilocytic astrocytoma and ganglioglioma, on imaging studies. **B.** Microscopically, PXAs superficially resemble giant cell glioblastoma, with strikingly bizarre giant cells (*B*), but pursue a much more indolent clinical course.

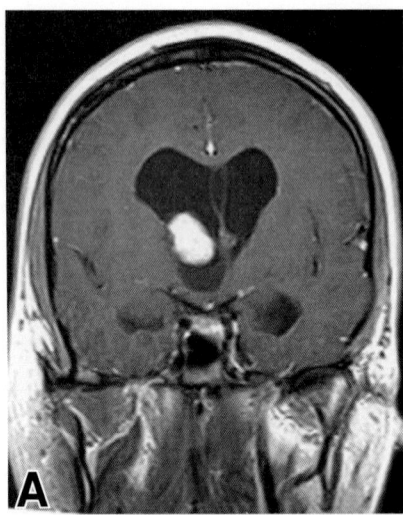
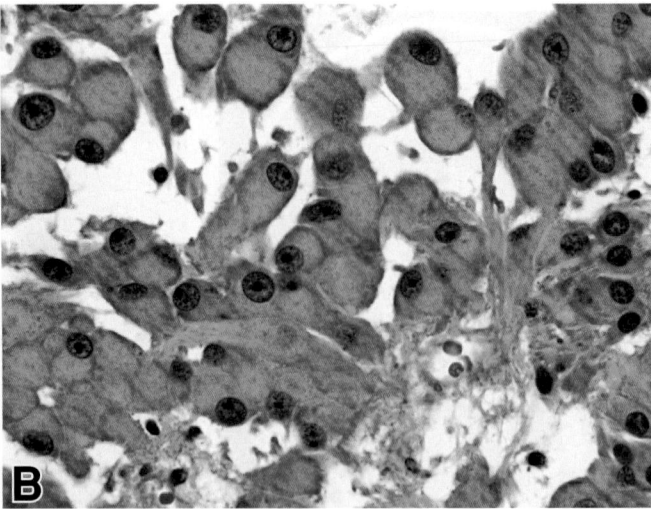

FIGURE 32-120. Subependymal giant cell astrocytoma (SEGA). A. This World Health Organization grade I astrocytoma arises within the lateral ventricle, often obstructing the interventricular foramen of Monro, resulting in obstructive hydrocephalus. **B.** Microscopically, SEGAs have globular eosinophilic cytoplasm and the nuclei often display single prominent nucleoli, thus mimicking gemistocytic astrocytoma or ganglion cell tumor. However, the anatomic location within the cerebral ventricle should preclude misdiagnosis.

 PATHOLOGY: PXA mimics giant cell glioblastoma in having strikingly pleomorphic tumor cells (Fig. 32-119B). Unlike GBM, however, mitotic activity is very low, and vascular proliferation and necrosis are usually absent. The characteristic eosinophilic granular bodies, which are also seen in other low-grade circumscribed tumors such as pilocytic astrocytoma and ganglioglioma, are a strong signature of PXA.

Subependymal Giant Cell Astrocytoma (WHO Grade I)

Subependymal giant cell astrocytoma (SEGA) is a very indolent low-grade glioma that arises from the wall of the lateral ventricle. It grows slowly within the ventricular cavity until it causes obstructive hydrocephalus with the attendant signs and symptoms of increased intracranial pressure by encroaching on the interventricular foramen of Monro (Fig. 32-120A). SEGAs are densely compact mixtures of very plump epithelioid cells, often with elongated spindle cells (Fig. 32-120B). Based only on histology, SEGAs could be misconstrued as gemistocytic astrocytomas or gangliogliomas, but their intraventricular location, as readily identified by preoperative imaging and the young patient age, helps to guide diagnosis. SEGAs are associated with **tuberous sclerosis** and may be the presenting feature in a child with otherwise inconspicuous stigmata of that disease. In keeping with its WHO grade I assignment and favorable location within the lateral ventricle, surgical resection of SEGA is curative. Tuberous sclerosis entails loss of TSC1 or TSC2 inhibition of the mammalian target of rapamycin (mTOR). Thus, pharmacologic inhibitors of the mTOR pathway can shrink SEGAs and provide a medical approach in the management of these patients.

Oligodendrogliomas (WHO Grade II) Are Often More Indolent Than Diffuse Astrocytomas

Like diffuse astrocytomas, oligodendrogliomas (ODGs) are highly infiltrative. However, their response to treatment and overall survival are much more favorable than for diffuse astrocytomas of similar grade, so ODGs must be distinguished from their diffuse astrocytic cousins.

MOLECULAR PATHOGENESIS: Translocation between chromosomes 1 and 19 is a characteristic ODG molecular signature. This translocation causes complete loss of the short arm of chromosome 1 (1p) and the long arm of chromosome 19 (19q). *Combined whole arm deletion of 1p and 19q is a favorable genetic signature in diffuse gliomas and correlates closely with classic ODG morphologic features.*

PATHOLOGY: Most ODGs arise in adults in the fourth and fifth decades, largely in the white matter of cerebral hemispheres. They commonly infiltrate into overlying cerebral cortex. ODGs show a monotonous population of cells with regular round nuclei surrounded by a small rim of clear cytoplasm ("perinuclear halo" or "fried egg" appearance) like normal oligodendroglia (Fig. 32-121A). This halo is a diagnostically useful artifact of specimen processing by formalin fixation and paraffin embedding. Other characteristic features of ODGs include a network of delicate, branching blood vessels ("chicken wire" pattern) and scattered microcalcifications. In areas of cortical infiltration, ODG cells tend to cluster around neuron cell bodies (perineuronal satellitosis) and blood vessels (perivascular satellitosis). They also form an infiltrating layer just beneath the pia (subpial growth). These features, described by Scherer in 1938, are still called "secondary structures of Scherer." Mitotic activity is inconspicuous in low-grade (WHO grade II) ODG, but these tumors recur and ultimately undergo anaplastic progression.

Anaplastic Oligodendroglioma (WHO Grade III)

Anaplastic oligodendroglioma differs from WHO grade II ODG by showing increased mitotic activity and microvascular proliferation. These may sometimes be accompanied by foci of tumor necrosis (Fig. 32-121B).

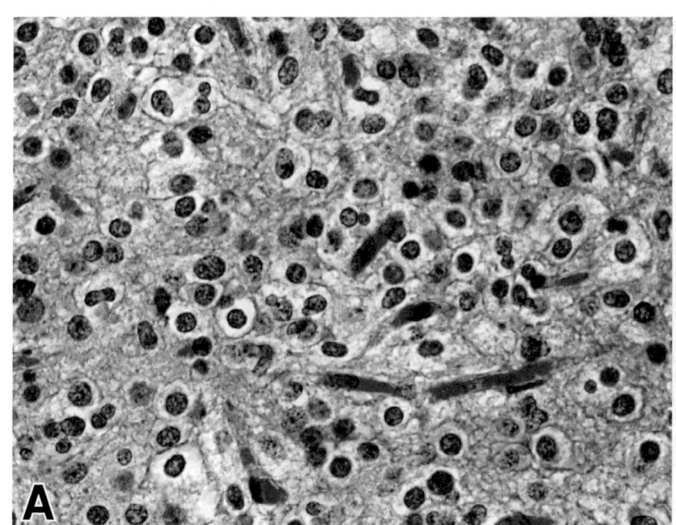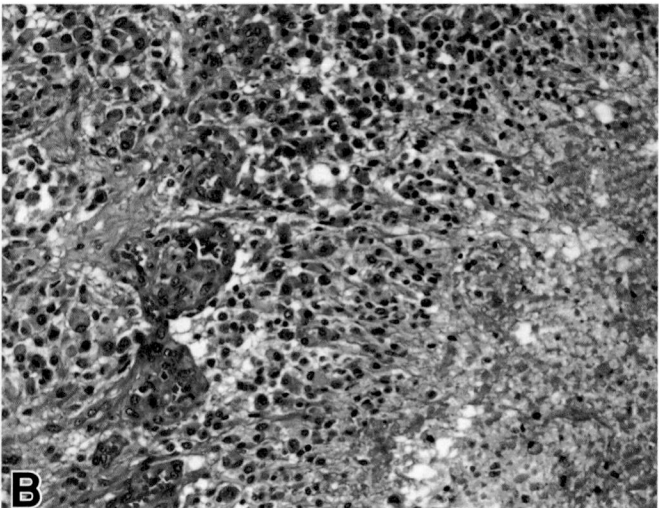

FIGURE 32-121. Oligodendroglioma. A. The cells of **low-grade oligodendroglioma** (World Health Organization grade II) closely resemble normal oligodendrocytes, with regular round nuclei surrounded by perinuclear halos. **B. Anaplastic oligodendroglioma** (AO) displays increased cellularity and brisk mitotic activity, with some tumors also developing foci of necrosis with tumor cell pseudopalisading.

Ependymomas (WHO Grade II) Derive from Ependymal Lining Cells

These are typically slow-growing tumors of children and young adults that originate in the cerebral ventricles or central canal of the spinal cord. In children, the posterior fossa fourth ventricle is the preferred location, while in adults most are in the supratentorial compartment and may arise in either the ventricle or in the cerebral hemisphere white matter. Ependymomas of the fourth ventricle tend to fill the ventricle and grow into the lateral recesses, occasionally even flowing through the lateral foramina of Luschka into the subarachnoid space (Fig. 32-122A,B). In the spinal cord, ependymomas are the most common intra-axial tumors, followed by diffuse astrocytoma.

 PATHOLOGY: Ependymomas grow as relatively circumscribed masses, and so are amenable to surgical resection. Their histologic hallmark is perivascular pseudorosettes, cuffs of radiating tumor cell cytoplasmic processes around vessels (Fig. 32-122C). True ependymal rosettes, in which tumor cells surround a central lumen, can also be seen but are rarer. Ependymomas express epithelial membrane antigen (EMA; Fig. 32-122C, *inset*) and GFAP (Fig. 32-122D, *inset*). GFAP reactivity is often strongest in perivascular pseudorosettes, and—unlike the membranous pattern of EMA expression in meningiomas—ependymoma EMA positivity is characteristically in a cytoplasmic dot-like and ring-like distribution. This pattern correlates with the presence of intercellular lumina filled with microvilli and cilia, sealed by intercellular junctional complexes at the ultrastructural level. **Anaplastic ependymoma (WHO grade III)** shows increased mitotic activity and microvascular proliferation.

Myxopapillary Ependymoma (WHO Grade I)

Myxopapillary ependymomas (MPEs) are unique low-grade variants of ependymoma that arise almost exclusively in the spinal cords of adults from ependymal remnants in the conus medullaris or filum terminale (Fig. 32-123A). These tumors slowly enlarge as discrete, well-circumscribed, elongated masses in the lumbar CSF cistern. They are covered by an outer layer of investing leptomeninges. Nests and ribbons of epithelioid and spindled ependymal tumor cells are interspersed between myxoid microcysts, and perivascular cuffs of myxoid material are also prominent (Fig. 32-123B). The immunophenotype is similar to other ependymomas: they express both glial (S-100, GFAP) and epithelial markers (EMA). Because of their circumscription and favorable anatomic location in the lumbar cistern, complete surgical resection is the treatment of choice. Microscopic breach of the pial "capsule" may occur in some tumors before surgery, so that locally disseminated tumor grows around nerve roots in the cauda equina. Such cases are difficult to treat with conventional irradiation or chemotherapy, as their slow rate of growth makes them relatively resistant to cell cycle inhibitors.

Subependymoma (WHO Grade I)

Subependymomas are indolent intraventricular gliomas of adults (rare cases may arise in the spinal cord). These tumors are often small and asymptomatic and are found incidentally on imaging studies or at autopsy. Occasionally, however, they enlarge to block the interventricular foramen of Monro or fourth ventricle outlet foramina, causing obstructive hydrocephalus (Fig. 32-124A). Subependymomas show scattered clusters of small uniform glial cell nuclei separated by large zones of fibrillary matrix formed by tumor cell cytoplasmic processes (Fig. 32-124B). Surgical resection is curative.

Choroid Plexus Tumors Originate from Choroid Plexus Epithelium

Unlike other common childhood brain tumors, which favor the posterior fossa (cerebellum, fourth ventricle and brainstem), **choroid plexus papillomas (CPPs; WHO grade I)** in children most commonly arise in the lateral ventricles (Fig. 32-125A). In adults, the fourth ventricle is preferred.

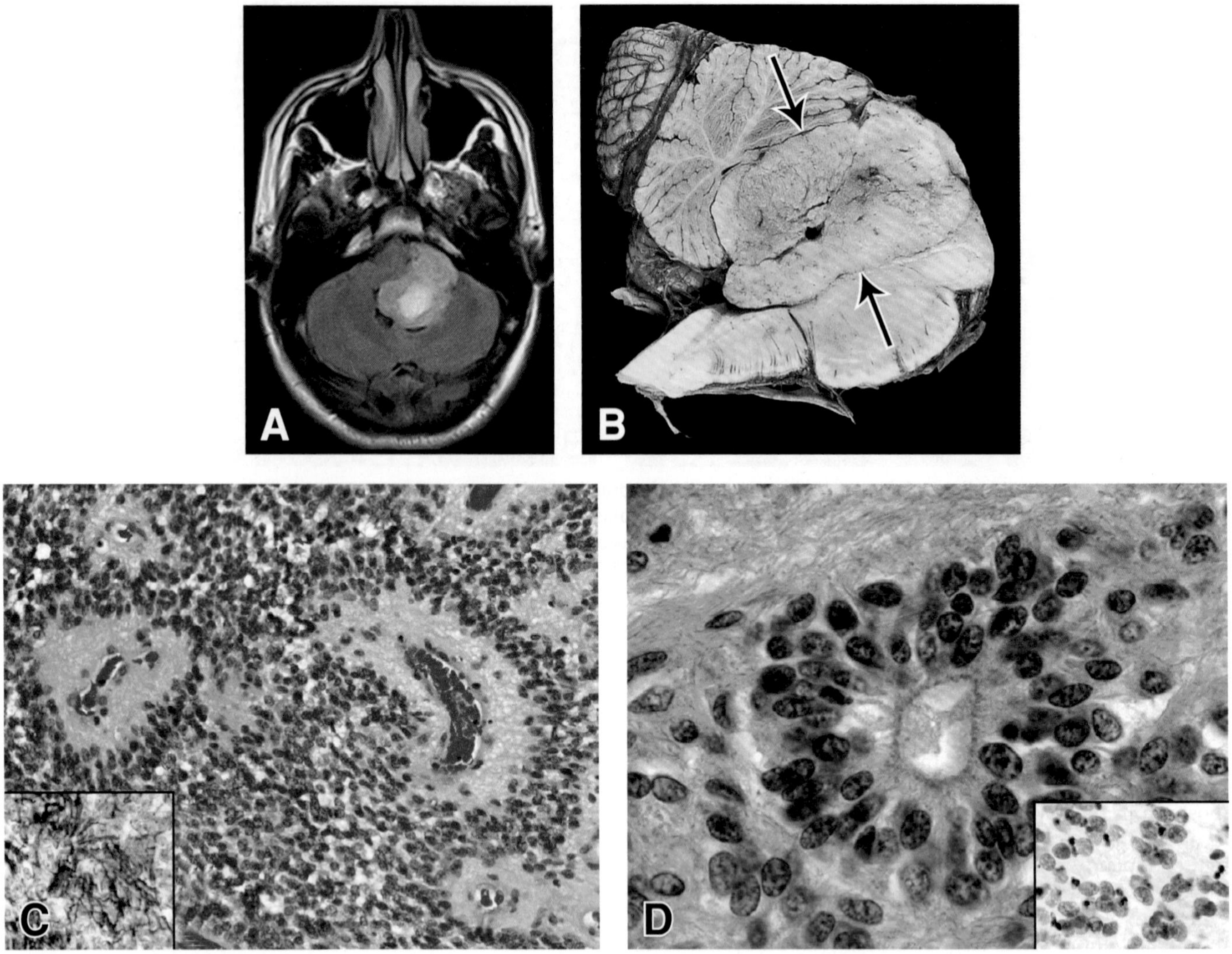

FIGURE 32-122. Ependymoma. A. Ependymomas can arise in the ventricles, the cerebral hemisphere or the spinal cord. Those located within the posterior fossa tend to grow through the ventricular outlet foramina (median foramen of Magendie and lateral foramina of Luschka) into the subarachnoid space, as seen in this magnetic resonance image. **B.** Autopsy gross specimen. Tumor is identified between the arrows. (Courtesy of Dr. F. Stephen Vogel, Duke University.) **C.** Microscopically, the hallmark of ependymomas is the perivascular pseudorosette. The immunophenotype of ependymoma includes dot-like and ring-like positivity for epithelial membrane antigen (*inset*). **D.** Well-formed true ependymal rosette with immunoreactivity of the glial marker glial fibrillary acidic protein (*inset*).

CPPs are benign and, given their location within ventricles, are potentially curable by surgery; however, CSF dissemination can occur, significantly worsening the prognosis in such cases.

 PATHOLOGY: CPP closely recapitulates the papillary architecture of normal choroid plexus, but the tumor cells tend to be more crowded together and commonly assume a columnar rather than cuboidal architecture (Fig. 32-125B). Their immunophenotype includes reactivity for glial markers (S-100, GFAP) and transthyretin (prealbumin). There are two higher-grade choroid plexus tumors: **atypical CPP (WHO grade II),** which has increased mitotic activity compared to grade I tumors, and **choroid plexus carcinoma (WHO grade III),** which show increased mitotic activity, loss of papillary architecture with a solid growth pattern and often marked nuclear atypia and cellular pleomorphism (Fig. 32-125C). The latter tumors can invade adjacent brain parenchyma and can also disseminate via the CSF.

The choroid plexus may also host several other types of neoplastic and nonneoplastic mass lesions, including "intraventricular" meningioma, metastatic carcinoma (especially renal cell carcinoma) and **xanthogranuloma** (a reactive mass lesion probably related to microhemorrhage, and showing prominent cholesterol clefts and multinucleated giant cell reaction).

Medulloblastoma and Other Primitive Neuroectodermal Tumors (WHO Grade IV) Are Largely Tumors of Children

Of the several different types of primitive neuroectodermal tumors (PNETs) recognized in the WHO classification, medulloblastoma (MB) is by far the most common. By definition, MBs arise in the cerebellum. Their peak incidence is at 7 years, but they also occur in 20–45-year-old adults. Childhood MBs commonly arise in the midline vermis, often expanding to fill the fourth ventricle (Fig. 32-126A).

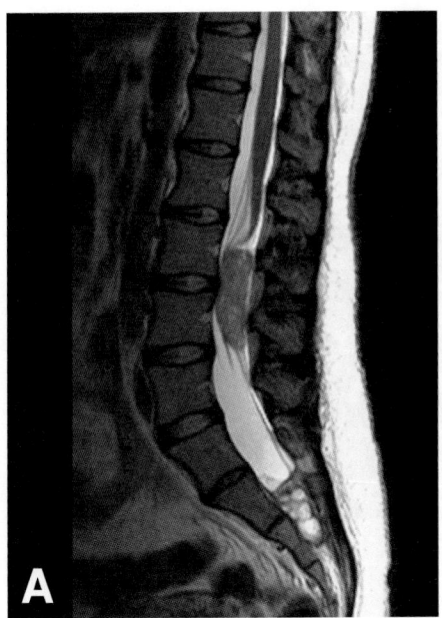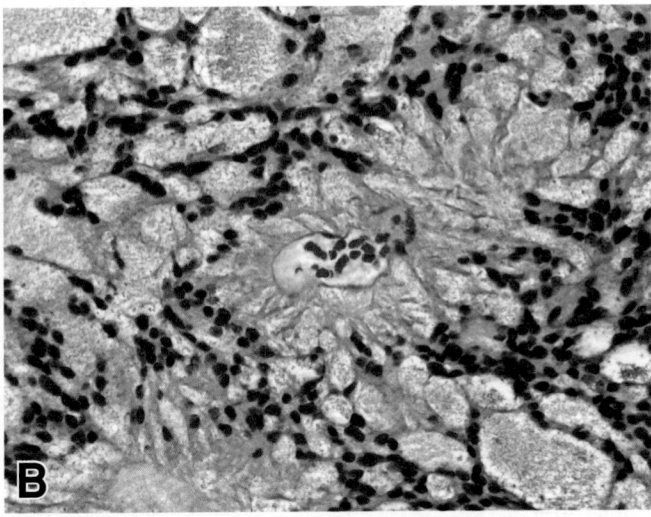

FIGURE 32-123. Myxopapillary ependymoma (MPE). A. MPEs are very low-grade (World Health Organization grade I) ependymal tumors that arise from remnants of the central canal in the spinal cord conus medullaris and filum terminale within the lumbar cistern. **B.** Histologically, prominent myxoid microcysts and perivascular myxoid cuffs separate nests and cords of ependymal cells.

The adult versions prefer the cerebellar hemispheres. There are, however, many exceptions in both children and adults. About 1/3 of patients have leptomeningeal spread, a negative prognostic factor, at the time of presentation. Only partial surgical resection, large cell or anaplastic morphology and amplification of the *MYCN* oncogene all portend poor prognosis.

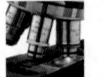 **CLINICAL FEATURES:** In addition to the common classic subtype, there are 4 recognized MB variants. Two of these, desmoplastic/nodular MB and MB with extensive nodularity, have better prognoses than does the classic subtype; the remaining two variants,

anaplastic and large cell, are the most aggressive varieties and have a worse prognosis. CSF dissemination is common and may be a presenting feature of the tumor. MBs sometimes metastasize to regional lymph nodes, lungs or bone and may disseminate, if provided the opportunity, via ventriculoperitoneal shunts.

PATHOLOGY: MBs are composed of sheets of densely packed malignant small cells with a high nucleus:cytoplasm ratio (Fig. 32-126B). Neuroblastic (Homer Wright–type) rosettes are present in 40% of cases. Mitotic activity is high. Desmoplastic/nodular MB superficially resembles lymph node tissue, with reticulin-free

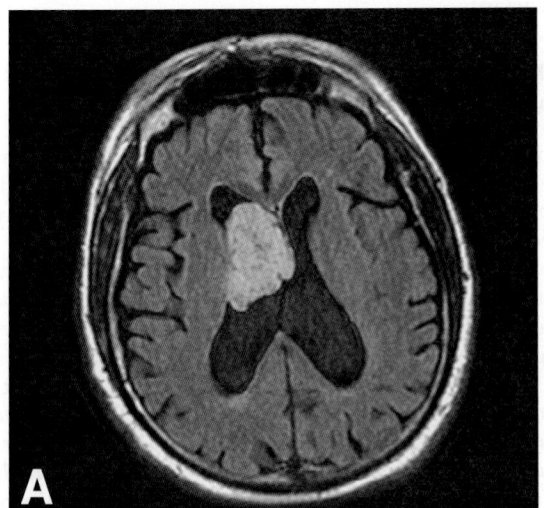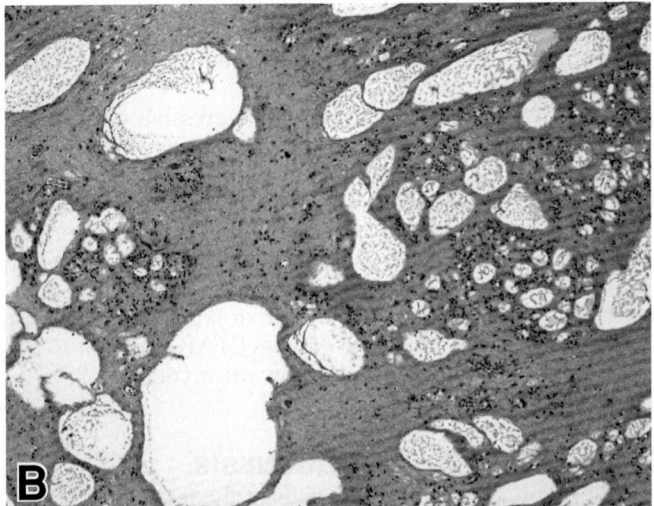

FIGURE 32-124. Subependymoma (SE). A. SE is another very low-grade (World Health Organization grade I) ependymal tumor that arises within the cerebral ventricle (shown in this magnetic resonance imaging scan) or very rarely within the spinal cord (not shown). **B.** Microscopically, SE consists of clusters of small, bland glial nuclei embedded within an abundant finely fibrillar matrix composed of tumor cell processes. Those examples located in the lateral ventricles tend to undergo microcystic degeneration as they enlarge.

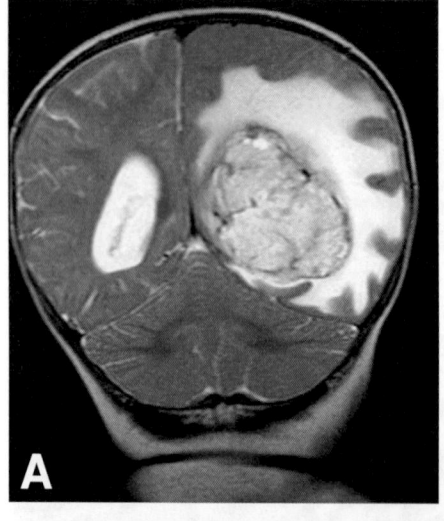

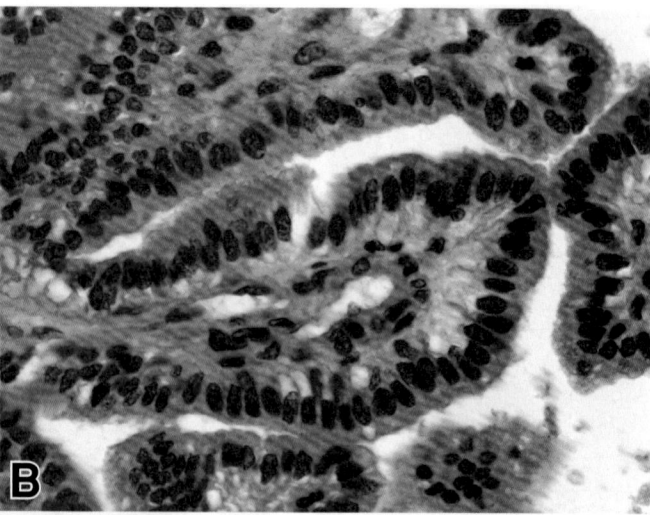

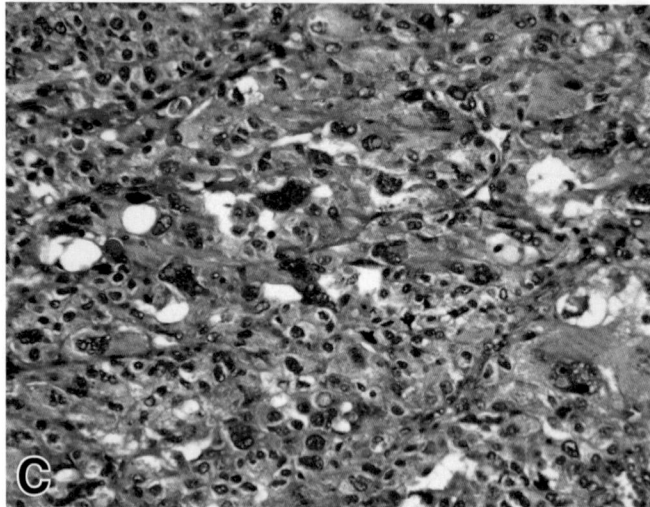

FIGURE 32-125. Choroid plexus papilloma (CPP) and carcinoma (CPC). A. CPP is a low-grade intraventricular tumor that arises from the fourth ventricular choroid plexus in adults and the lateral ventricular choroid plexus in children. **B.** Histologically, **CPP** retains the papillary architecture of choroid plexus, but the cells are more crowded and columnar rather than cuboidal. **C. CPC** is a high-grade tumor that differs from CPP in showing loss of papillary architecture, marked cellular pleomorphism, an increased proliferation rate and a more aggressive clinical course.

neurocytic islands ("pale islands") looking like germinal centers (Fig. 32-126C,D). This variant arises mainly in the cerebellar hemispheres of adults. The closely related MB with extensive nodularity is a tumor of infancy and has a distinctive multinodular appearance on imaging, as well as histologically.

Anaplastic MB and large cell MB are aggressive variants with overlapping morphologies (Fig. 32-126E). The former shows marked nuclear pleomorphism, nuclear molding and cell–cell wrapping. In contrast, the large cell variant has a monomorphous population of large cells whose nuclei have prominent nucleoli. Both variants have high proliferative rates and abundant apoptosis. Most MBs show neuronal differentiation, in the form of immunoreactivity for synaptophysin; some also express GFAP, like glial cells. Rare cases show differentiation toward myocytes or melanocytes.

MOLECULAR PATHOGENESIS: MB is thought to arise from stem cells of the fetal external granular layer and/or the periventricular germinal matrix. Molecular studies have implicated the *Wnt* and *sonic hedgehog (SHH)* signaling in tumor genesis. Differential activation of these pathways likely determines the MB subclass: the SHH pathway underlies desmoplastic/

nodular MB and MB with extensive nodularity variants. The Wnt pathway favors the classic and anaplastic/large cell variants.

Atypical Teratoid/Rhabdoid Tumor (WHO Grade IV) Shows Multilineage Differentiation

Atypical teratoid/rhabdoid tumor (ATRT) is a malignant tumor of early childhood with divergent differentiation along rhabdoid, epithelial, mesenchymal, neuronal and glial lines. The posterior fossa is most affected (75%), followed by the supratentorial compartment (25%). Rhabdoid cells, with eccentrically located nuclei and eosinophilic globular cytoplasm, rarely may compose the entire tumor (referred to as "CNS rhabdoid tumor") but most often are one component of a heterogeneous malignancy (Fig. 32-127). *Inactivation of the INI-1 (hSNF5/SMARCB1) tumor suppressor gene through mutation or deletion is the molecular hallmark of ATRT* and is detected as loss of immunostaining for INI1 protein (Fig. 32-127). Renal rhabdoid tumors (see Chapter 22) share the same genetic alteration as ATRT. Germline *INI1* mutations result in **rhabdoid tumor predisposition syndrome,** with CNS and systemic rhabdoid tumors in infancy.

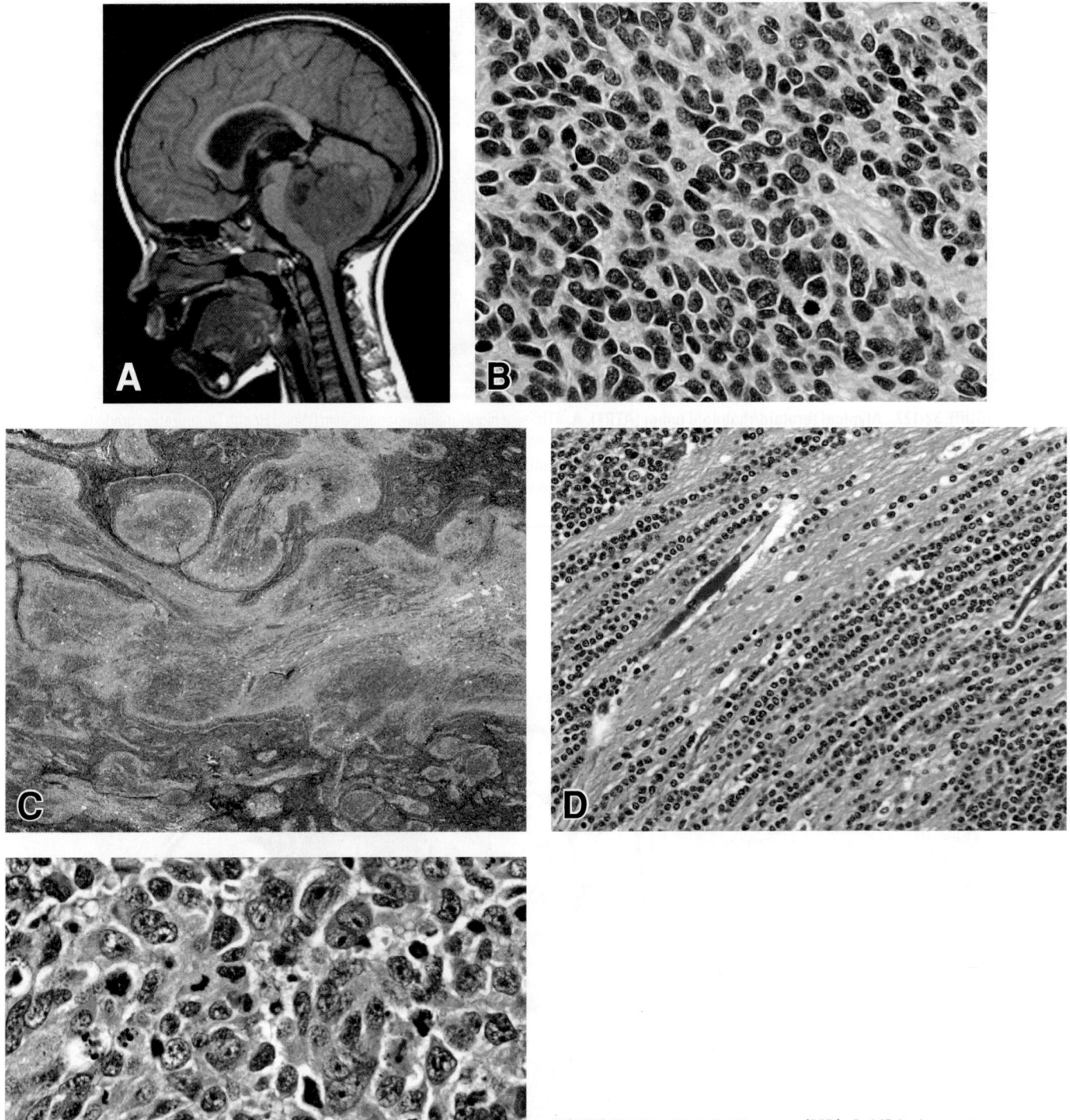

FIGURE 32-126. Medulloblastoma (MB). A. MB is the most common type of primitive neuroectodermal tumor and arises in the cerebellum. **B.** By light microscopy, MB is a "small blue cell" tumor. **C, D.** Two MB variants, desmoplastic/nodular MB and MB with extensive nodularity, have a better prognosis. **E.** Variants with large, anaplastic cells pursue a more aggressive clinical course.

Craniopharyngiomas (WHO Grade I) Arise in the Sella Turcica and Suprasellar Region

Craniopharyngioma (CP) is a circumscribed epithelial tumor, presumptively derived from Rathke cleft remnants. It arises mainly in children but also occurs in adults. These tumors typically show complex heterogeneous solid and cystic areas on imaging (Fig. 32-128A). Given the origin and expansile growth in the sellar/suprasellar region, CPs typically present with mixed endocrine and visual disturbances, due to compression of the pituitary below and optic chiasm above. Surgical resection is the preferred

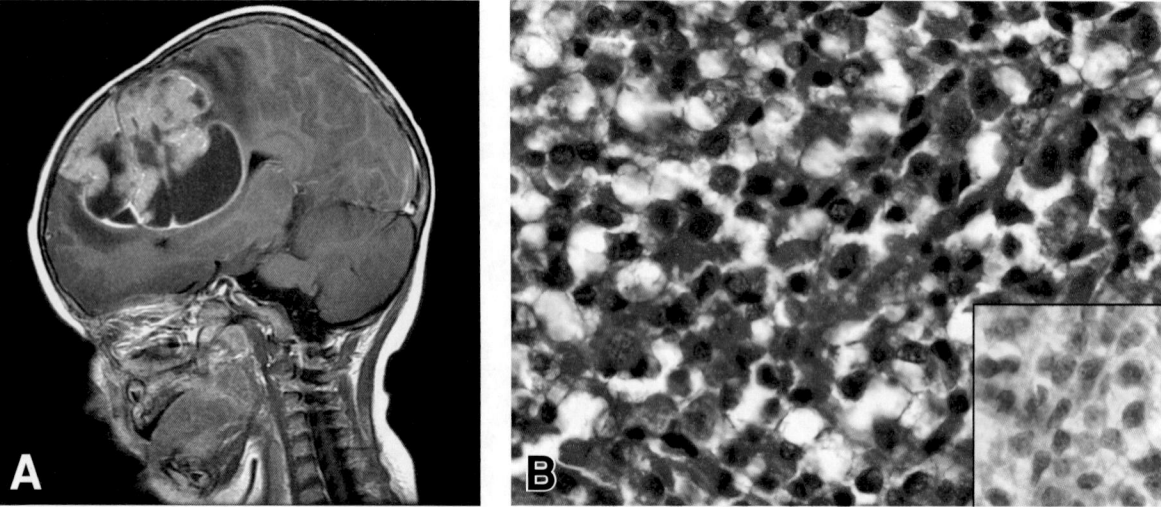

FIGURE 32-127. Atypical teratoid/rhabdoid tumor (ATRT). A. ATRT is a highly malignant neoplasm (World Health Organization grade IV) of early childhood that can arise in the cerebellum or, as illustrated here, in the cerebrum. **B.** The histologic features vary but usually include a rhabdoid cell component featuring plump hypereosinophilic cytoplasm. The molecular signature of ATRT is mutation or deletion of the *INI-1* gene, which can be detected as loss of immunostaining in tumor cell nuclei (*inset*); normal host cells, such as vascular endothelium, serve as positive internal control in this immunostain.

treatment; however, encroachment on the many vital structures in this area, including cranial nerves and blood vessels, often limits resectability, and residual tumor will recur inexorably.

 PATHOLOGY: There are two morphologic subtypes: **adamantinomatous** (by far the more common), which arises in children and adults, and the rarer **papillary**, which occurs almost exclusively

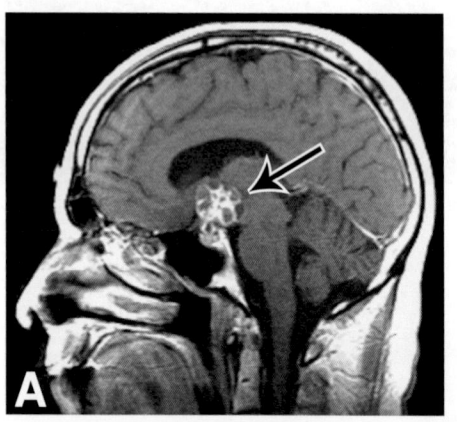

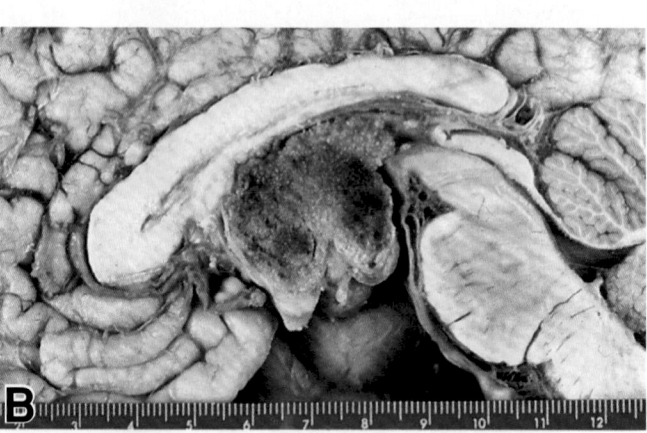

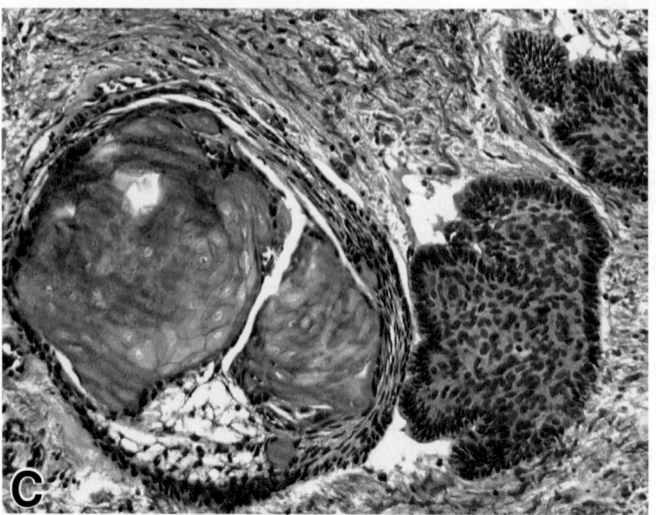

FIGURE 32-128. Craniopharyngioma. A. Craniopharyngiomas arise in the sellar/suprasellar region (*arrow*). **B.** Craniopharyngioma, gross photograph. (Courtesy of Dr. F. Stephen Vogel, Duke University.) **C.** Histologically, craniopharyngiomas are composed of squamous epithelium that displays a number of distinctive morphologic features, including peripheral palisaded nuclei and nodules of plump keratinocytes ("wet keratin") that are prone to calcify.

in adults. The former has distinctive morphology, including sheets of squamous epithelium with prominent peripheral palisading, hydropic degeneration of central areas of the epithelium ("stellate reticulum") and nodular aggregates of plump keratinocytes ("wet keratin") that tend to calcify (Fig. 32-128B). Long-standing compression of surrounding brain parenchyma may cause reactive piloid astrocytosis with prominent Rosenthal fibers. Papillary CP contains exclusively nonkeratinizing squamous epithelium. Its histologic appearance is very bland compared to the variegated morphology of the adamantinomatous subtype.

Germinoma (WHO Grade III) and Other CNS Germ Cell Tumors Often Involve the Pineal Gland

Germ cell tumors (GCTs) of the CNS most often arise in midline structures, especially the pineal gland and third ventricular region (Fig. 32-129A). **Germinomas** tend to have biphasic cell composition: large malignant cells are interspersed with swarms of small reactive lymphocytes (Fig. 32-129B). In some cases, a granulomatous response may predominate and obscure the neoplastic germ cell component. The tumors are characterized by strong immunoreactivity for OCT3/4 and c-kit, with focal positivity for placental alkaline phosphatase (PLAP) (Fig. 32-129C). In some cases, β-human chorionic gonadotropin (β-HCG) expression identifies isolated syncytiotrophoblastic cells. Pure germinomas are highly radiosensitive, and patients may receive radiation therapy, chemotherapy or a combination of both. Other germ cell tumors from the pineal region and at other CNS sites include **teratoma** (mature and immature), **yolk sac tumor, embryonal carcinoma** and **choriocarcinoma**.

After germinomas, teratomas are the most common of this group to occur as pure (nonmixed) tumors. The remaining GCTs are mostly **mixed germ cell tumors**. The prognosis for nongerminomatous GCTs is less favorable than for pure germinoma and largely depends on the extent of surgical resection.

Hemangioblastomas (WHO Grade I) Occur Most Often in the Cerebellum

Hemangioblastomas (HBs) are very vascular tumors that mainly arise in the cerebellum but may also occur in the spinal cord and brainstem, especially in von Hippel-Lindau disease. They are among a number of low-grade circumscribed CNS tumors that appear on preoperative imaging studies as cysts with enhancing mural nodules (Fig. 32-130A). They

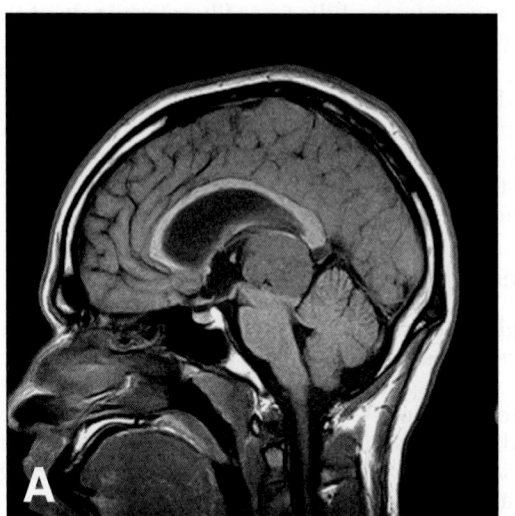

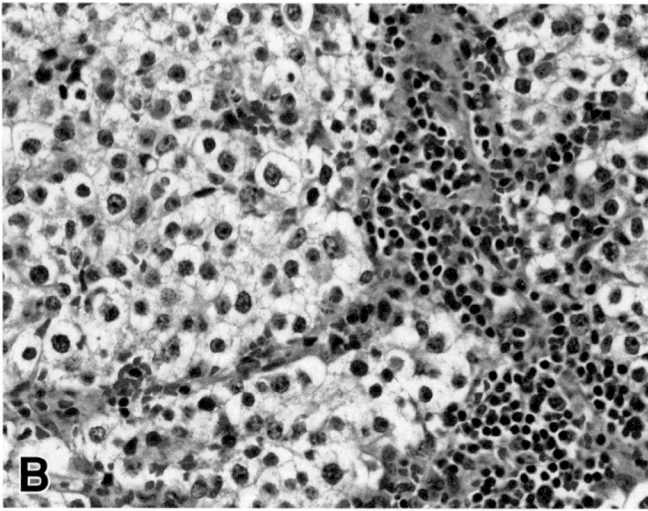

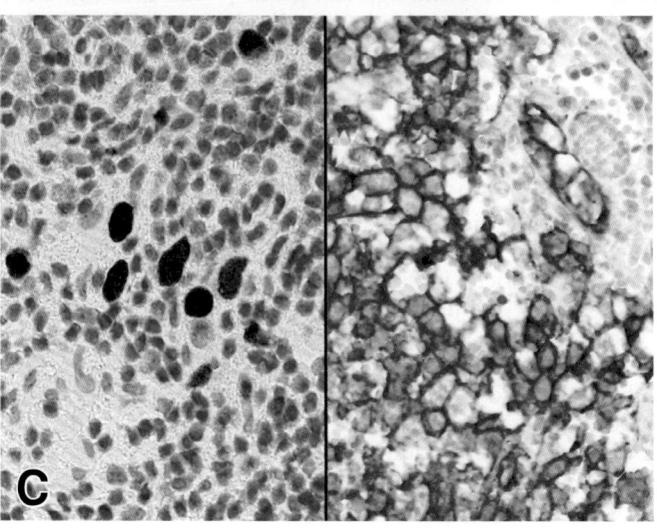

FIGURE 32-129. Germinoma. A. Germ cell tumors most commonly arise in the midline, such as in the pineal gland, as illustrated here. **B.** Microscopically, germinoma, the most common central nervous system germ cell tumor, exhibits a biphasic population of cells: very large germinoma tumor cells and small reactive lymphocytes. **C.** The germinoma immunophenotype includes diagnostically useful nuclear positivity for OCT3/4 (*left panel*) and cytoplasmic positivity for placental alkaline phosphatase (PLAP) (*right panel*).

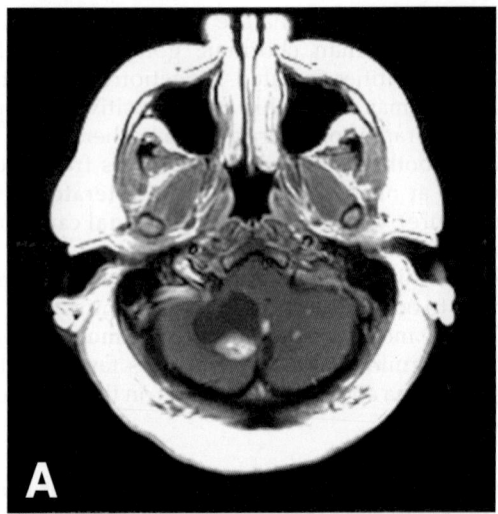
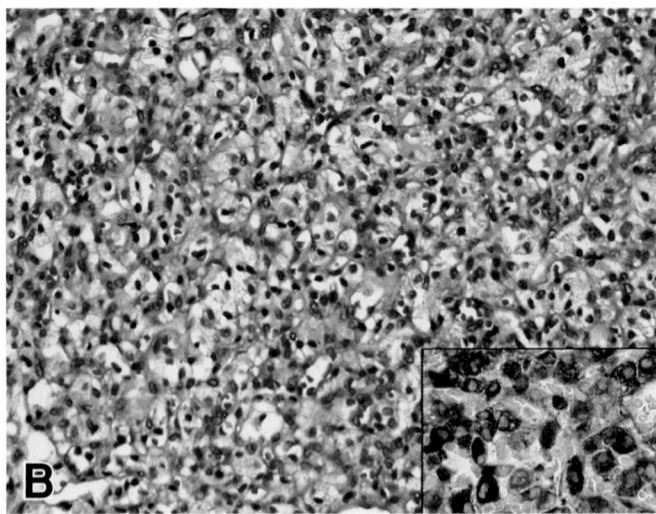

FIGURE 32-130. Hemangioblastoma (HB). A. HB most commonly arises in the cerebellum either sporadically or as part of von Hippel-Lindau disease. A common imaging presentation is as a cyst with a mural nodule. **B.** Microscopically, HB is a highly vascular neoplasm, with the neoplastic stromal cells enmeshed in a dense capillary network. The tumor cells of HB display strong cytoplasmic positivity for inhibin-α (*inset*).

usually present clinically as expanding masses in patients 20–40 years old. In 20% of cases, HBs secrete erythropoietin and induce secondary polycythemia. They can often be cured by surgical resection alone.

 PATHOLOGY: HBs have vacuolated stromal cells amid a dense capillary vasculature (Fig. 32-130B). The stromal cells are the neoplastic element and are immunoreactive for inhibin-α.

Tumors That Show Only Neuronal Differentiation Are Rare

All such tumors are low grade (WHO grade I or II). **Gangliocytoma (WHO grade I)** is a very well-differentiated, circumscribed tumor composed entirely of dysmorphic mature ganglion cells. The temporal lobe is a favored location. **Dysplastic gangliocytoma of the cerebellum (Lhermitte-Duclos disease; WHO grade I)** is a distinctive entity of the cerebellum, presenting with gross enlargement of the folia as easily seen on MRI and disorganized cerebellar cortical histology with large ganglion cells (derived from granular cell neurons). A layer of myelinated axons in the outermost molecular layer just beneath the pia is another distinctive feature. Half of patients have **Cowden syndrome** (see Chapter 5). Complete surgical resection is curative.

Central neurocytoma (CN; WHO grade II) and **extraventricular neurocytoma (WHO grade II)** are low-grade tumors of young adults that arise from the septum pellucidum, grow into the lateral ventricles and often extend into the third ventricle (Fig. 32-131A). CNs contain monomorphous round cells that look like oligodendrocytes (Fig. 32-131B) but, like neurons, strongly express synaptophysin. Extraventricular neurocytomas look and behave similarly but occur in the brain parenchyma rather than the ventricles. Surgery can be curative for small tumors, but partially resected tumors may recur, and central neurocytomas also have the potential for CSF dissemination.

Paraganglioma of the filum terminale (PFT; WHO grade I) is an uncommon neuroendocrine tumor that, like myxopapillary ependymoma, arises in the lumbar cistern from the conus medullaris or filum terminale of the spinal cord (Fig. 32-131C). Like paragangliomas elsewhere in the body, PFTs show compact acinar ("zellballen") architecture (Fig. 32-131D) and express such neuronal markers as synaptophysin and chromogranin. They often show ganglion cell differentiation. Most are "encapsulated" by an investing layer of leptomeninges and are cured by surgical excision.

Mixed Glioneuronal Tumors

Gangliogliomas (GGs; WHO grades I and III) are well-differentiated, circumscribed tumors of neoplastic ganglion cells, with a glioma component. The temporal lobe is its favored location. GGs are the most common tumors associated with chronic temporal lobe epilepsy (40% of tumor-associated temporal lobe epilepsy cases). Atypical ganglion cells are intermixed with the glioma element, usually astrocytoma. Although low grade (WHO grade I), GG can progress to **anaplastic ganglioglioma (WHO grade III)**. For either grade, prognosis depends on the extent of surgical resection.

Dysembryoplastic neuroepithelial tumors (DNETs; WHO grade I) are low-grade glioneuronal tumors arising superficially within the cerebral cortex of children (Fig. 32-132A). Their intracortical location correlates with the typical clinical history of long-standing seizures. They may also occur anteriorly in the frontal horn of the lateral ventricle, in association with the caudate nucleus and septum pellucidum. DNETs have multinodular architecture, with prominent nodular aggregates of small rounded oligodendroglial-like cells with interspersed neurons that appear to "float" within cystic spaces in the cortical parenchyma (Fig. 32-132B). These tumors resemble low-grade oligodendrogliomas but lack the latter's characteristic translocation. Foci of cortical dysplasia may occur in adjacent peritumoral cortex. Resection is curative.

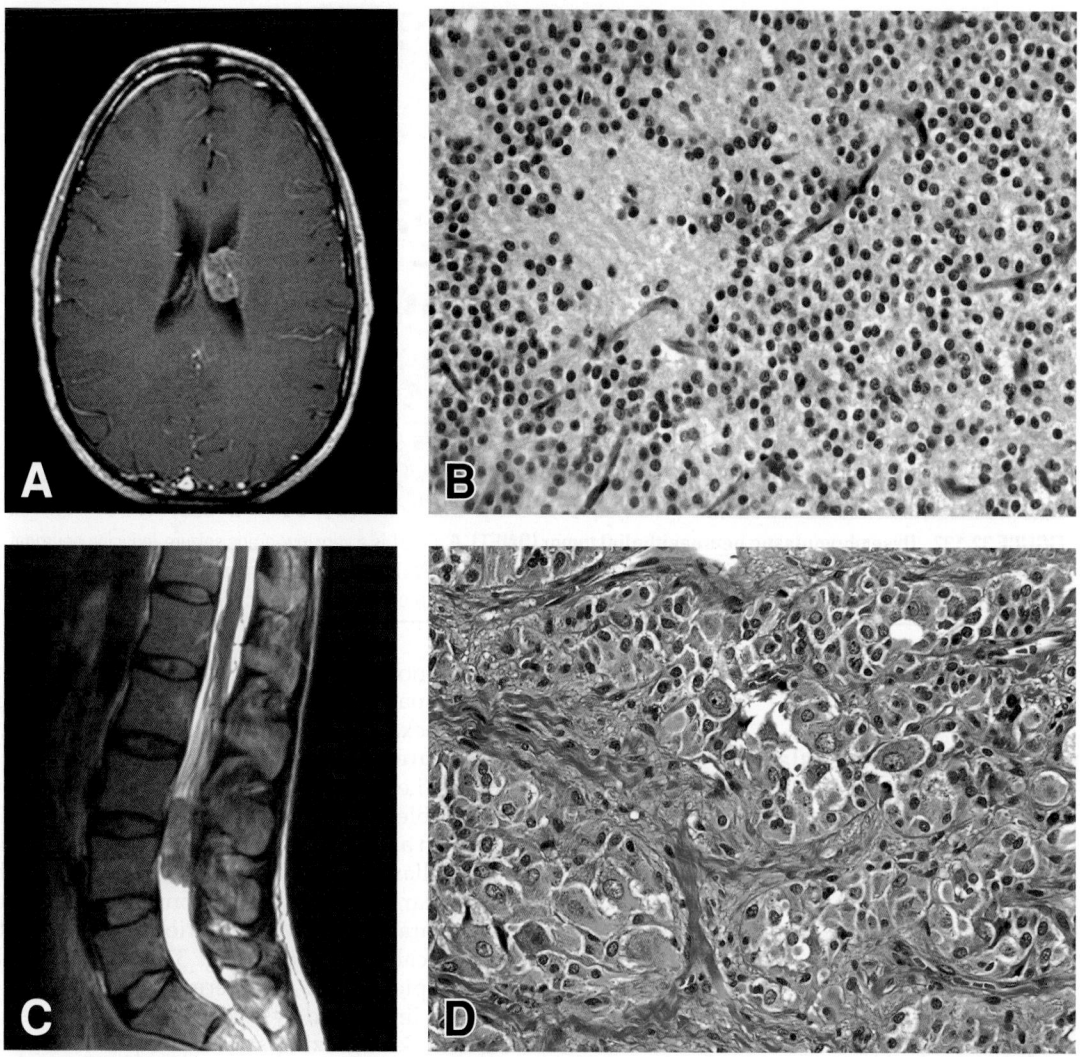

FIGURE 32-131. Neuronal and neuroendocrine tumors. A. Central nervous system neoplasms that exhibit purely neuronal/neuroendocrine differentiation are rare, and the vast majority are low grade. **Central neurocytoma** (CN) is a low-grade neuronal tumor of young adulthood that arises within the lateral ventricle. **B.** CN cells closely mimic oligodendroglioma (compare to Fig. 32-121A) but exhibit a neuronal immunophenotype, including immunoreactivity for synaptophysin. **C. Paraganglioma of the filum terminale** arises, as the name implies, from the distal spinal cord terminus within the lumbar cistern. **D.** Paraganglioma tumor cells exhibit a neuroendocrine phenotype, with strong reactivity for synaptophysin and chromogranin, and frank ganglion cell differentiation is seen in about 25% of cases.

Pineal Parenchymal Tumors Encompass a Spectrum of Clinical Behavior

Pineal parenchymal tumors (PPTs) range from the very low-grade **pineocytoma (WHO grade I)** to **pineoblastoma,** a highly malignant PNET **(WHO grade IV)**. Between these two extremes are **pineal parenchymal tumors of intermediate differentiation (PPTIDs; WHO grade II or III)**. These are discussed in Chapter 27.

Primary CNS Lymphomas Are Usually B-Cell Tumors

Systemic lymphomas often spread to the CNS, but lymphomas may also originate in the CNS. PCNSLs are tumors of adults and have increased in incidence in the last several decades in both immunocompromised and elderly immunocompetent patients. They may present with a wide variety of MRI patterns, including in superficial cortical, deep periventricular or cerebellar location, and may be solitary or multiple (Fig. 32-133A).

Definitive pathologic diagnosis is usually made by stereotactic biopsy; surgical resection does not aid survival or response to treatment. PCNSLs are composed of highly infiltrative neoplastic lymphocytes that show prominent invasion and expansion of blood vessel walls (Fig. 32-133B). The vast majority are large cell B-cell tumors and express CD20 and other B-cell markers (Fig. 32-133B). In immunocompromised individuals, PCNSL may be driven by Epstein-Barr virus, which can be detected by immunohistochemistry. They are highly sensitive to steroids, often shrinking dramatically after glucocorticoid treatment, but this response is temporary. In addition, steroid therapy can make histologic diagnosis of PCNSL extremely difficult because posttreatment biopsies may show only gliosis and reactive changes. Radiation and/or chemotherapy give a median survival of

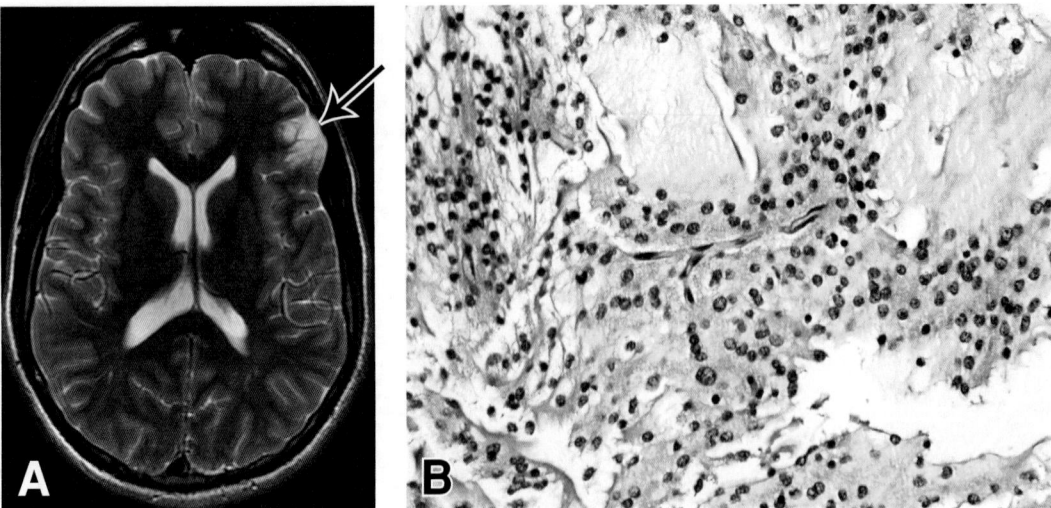

FIGURE 32-132.   Dysembryoplastic neuroepithelial tumor (DNET). A. DNET is a very low-grade seizure-inducing neuronal tumor of childhood that arises superficially within the cerebral cortex. **B.** DNET is composed of monotonous round cells that resemble oligodendroglia (*B*) but is not infiltrative and is potentially curable through surgical resection.

70% at 2 years and up to 45% at 5 years in immunocompetent patients.

Many Different Benign (Nonneoplastic) Cysts Occur in the CNS

These are listed in Table 32-10. Some are degenerative in nature and are usually incidental findings on neuroimaging studies done for other reasons, or at autopsy. Only very rarely do they cause clinical symptoms, such as **choroid plexus cysts** and **pineal gland cysts**. Others, such as **arachnoid cysts** and **ependymal cysts,** are largely asymptomatic but may occasionally require surgical fenestration of the cyst wall to release pressure and relieve mass effects on surrounding structures. The remaining group are primarily of developmental origin and relatively often may cause mass effects that require simple surgery as definitive treatment.

Diagnosis of specific cyst types depends on a combination of anatomic location and histology of the cyst wall lining. For example, three CNS cysts, **Rathke cyst, colloid cyst** and **neurenteric cyst,** share virtually identical epithelial linings (i.e., ciliated pseudostratified columnar epithelium with goblet cells) but are easily and confidently diagnosed based on anatomic location: Rathke cysts arise in the sellar/suprasellar region, colloid cysts in the roof of the third ventricle near the foramen of Monro and neurenteric cysts in the subarachnoid space anterior to the brainstem medulla or cervical spinal cord (Fig. 32-134). **Epithelial inclusion cysts** (epidermoid and dermoid cysts) are distinguished by their lining and cyst contents, with epidermoids showing only keratinizing stratified squamous epithelium and sheets of anucleate flattened squames for contents, and dermoids displaying a wall that includes dermal appendages, such as sebaceous glands and hair follicles, and contents that include not only anucleate squames but also matted hair (Fig. 32-134).

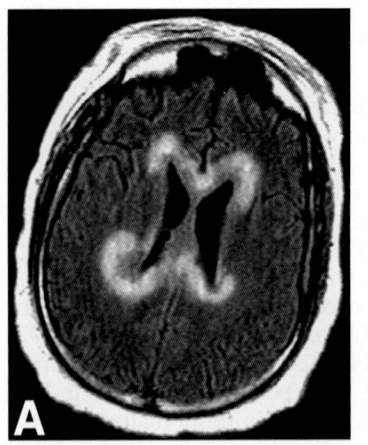
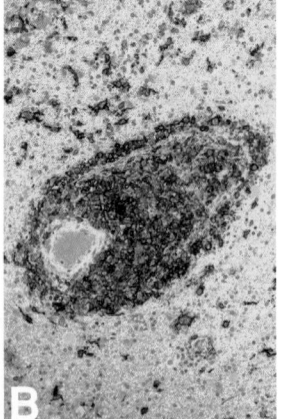

FIGURE 32-133.   Primary central nervous system lymphoma (PCNSL). A. One common clinical presentation of PCNSL is as a diffuse periventricular tumor lining the lateral ventricles. **B.** The vast majority of PCNSLs are of diffuse large B-cell phenotype and thus strongly express B-cell markers such as CD20. (Courtesy of Dr. F. Stephen Vogel, Duke University.)

TABLE 32-10
CENTRAL NERVOUS SYSTEM CYSTS
Choroid plexus cyst
Pineal cyst
Epidermoid cyst
Dermoid cyst
Arachnoid cyst
Ependymal cyst
Neurenteric (enterogenous) cyst
Rathke cyst
Colloid cyst

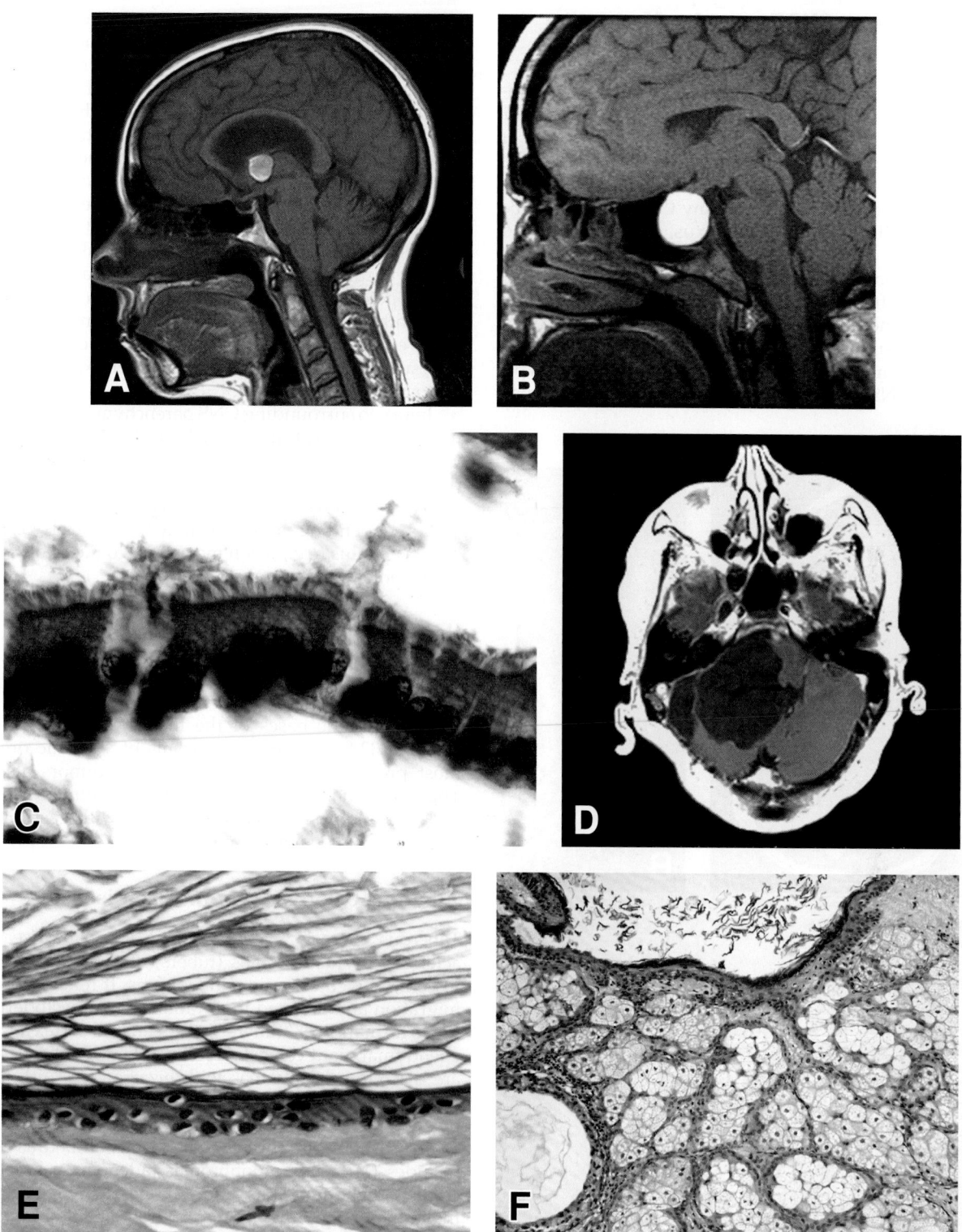

FIGURE 32-134. Cysts of the central nervous system. A. Colloid cysts arise in the rostral roof of the third ventricle. **B. Rathke cysts** are located in the sellar/suprasellar region. **C.** Both of these cysts exhibit a very similar epithelial lining, consisting of ciliated pseudostratified columnar epithelium with goblet cells. **D.** A favored anatomic site for **epidermoid cysts** is the cerebellopontine angle. **E.** Epidermoid cysts differ from dermoid cysts in that the lining of epidermoids is composed of only keratinizing squamous epithelium. **F.** Dermoids also include skin adnexal appendage structures, such as sebaceous glands and hair follicles.

The Most Common CNS Tumors Are Metastases from Elsewhere

Metastatic tumors far surpass primary CNS tumors in numbers, and malignancies metastatic to the CNS are major clinical problems. Autopsy series show that up to 25% of patients with systemic cancers have CNS metastases. The most common site for brain metastasis is at the gray–white junction of the cerebral cortex, but any CNS region may be affected, including the choroid plexus, pineal gland and pituitary gland.

The most common primary tumors to involve the CNS are lung (most frequent for both men and women), breast, melanoma, kidney and gastrointestinal tract. Over half of all metastatic disease cases involve multiple metastases (Fig. 32-135A), and metastatic patterns may reflect tumor type. For example, CNS metastases from cancers of gastrointestinal,

breast, prostate and uterine origin are frequently solitary, but those from lung carcinomas and melanomas are usually multiple. A rare extreme form of multiple metastasis, called military metastasis ("carcinomatous encephalitis"), in which innumerable minute metastases shower the brain, is most common with lung adenocarcinomas. Metastases to cranial bones and vertebrae usually originate in the prostate, breast, kidney, thyroid, lung or lymphoma/leukemia (acronym: "Pb KTL"—"lead kettle") (Fig. 32-135B). Isolated dural metastases most often represent spread from breast cancers, and single metastases to the leptomeninges and subarachnoid space usually occur with lung, breast and gastric adenocarcinomas; hematopoietic tumors; and melanomas. Prostate carcinomas frequently metastasize to the skull and spine but only rarely involve the brain parenchyma. For some very common cancers, such as carcinoma of the uterine cervix, CNS metastases are extremely rare.

Injury to surrounding CNS parenchyma due to metastatic tumors entails (1) tumor growth itself; (2) attendant elicited vasogenic edema in surrounding brain tissue; (3) hemorrhage in the tumor, which can be substantial (especially with melanomas, renal cell carcinomas and choriocarcinomas); and (4) depending on the location of metastasis, obstructive hydrocephalus (e.g., when metastases to the midbrain cause occlusion of the cerebral aqueduct).

Hereditary Intracranial Neoplasms Are Often Associated with Extracranial Tumors

Several hereditary disorders associated with CNS tumors and the genetic bases of the major syndromes are listed in Table 32-8. In some, neoplasms of systemic organs are most prominent, but nervous system tumors also occur. Thus, malignant gliomas occur in Li-Fraumeni syndrome, and medulloblastomas are associated with gastrointestinal tumors in Turcot syndrome.

Tuberous Sclerosis (Bourneville Disease)

Tuberous sclerosis is an autosomal dominant disease characterized by hamartomas (tubers) of the brain, retina and viscera, as well as various neoplasms. It reflects disordered migration and arrested maturation of neuroectoderm, leading to formation of "tubers" in the cerebral cortex and of subependymal giant cell astrocytomas (Fig. 32-120). The tubers are discrete cortical areas with bizarre cells with neuronal and glial features. The subependymal giant cell astrocytomas resemble "candle drippings."

In addition to intracranial lesions, tuberous sclerosis includes (1) facial angiofibromas (adenoma sebaceum), (2) cardiac rhabdomyomas and (3) mesenchymal tumors of the kidney (angiomyolipomas). Most patients have seizures and are mentally retarded. Mutations in *TSC1* and *TSC2* are responsible: *TSC1* (9q34) encodes a protein called hamartin, and *TSC2* (16p13) encodes tuberin, which is homologous to a GTPase-activating protein. Both are tumor suppressors (see Chapter 5).

Sturge-Weber Syndrome (Encephalofacial Angiomatosis)

Sturge-Weber syndrome is a rare, nonfamilial congenital disorder characterized by angiomas of the brain and face.

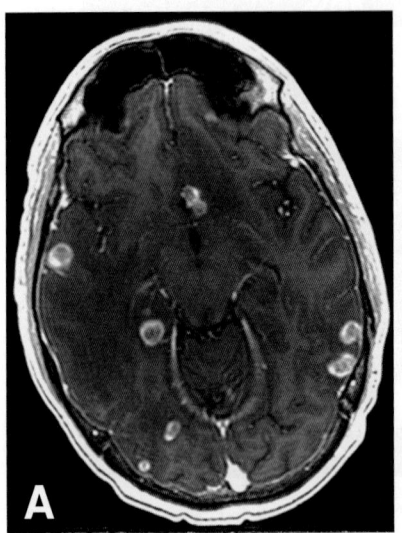
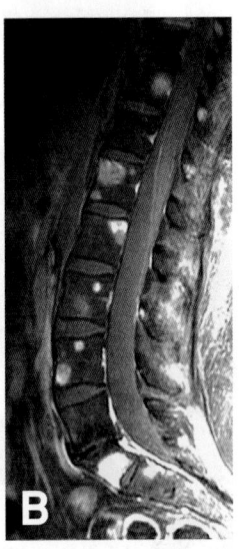
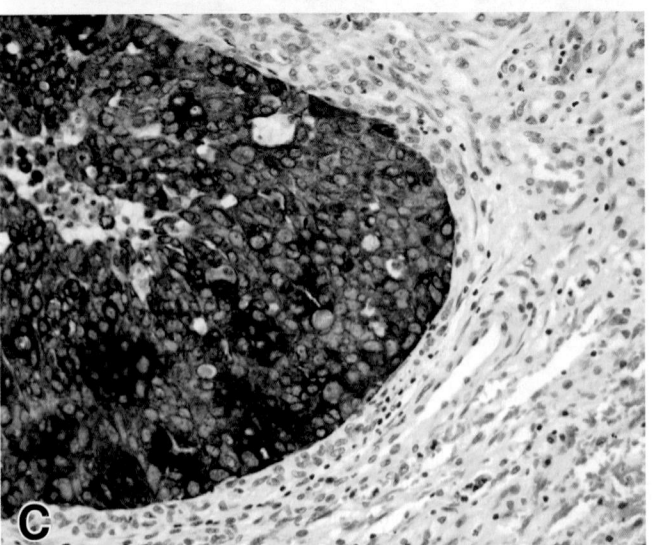

FIGURE 32-135. Metastatic disease. Metastases to the central nervous system commonly produce multiple lesions in both the brain **(A)** and spine **(B)**. **C.** Metastatic tumor masses typically show very sharp "pushing" borders with the adjacent brain tissue, as illustrated here with metastatic carcinoma immunostained for keratin.

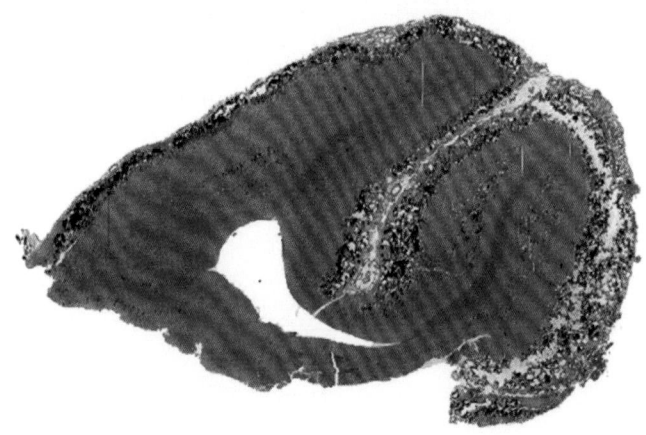

FIGURE 32-136. Sturge-Weber syndrome. Portion of cerebral cortex with overlying capillary angioma involving the leptomeninges and underlying cortical calcification (*purple*).

The facial lesion is usually unilateral and is called a **port wine stain (nevus flammeus)**. The leptomeninges contain large angiomas, which in severe cases may occupy an entire hemisphere. Cerebral calcification and atrophy often underlie the intracranial angiomas (Fig. 32-136). The link between angiomas of the face and brain may reflect the continuity of the embryologic vascular supply to the telencephalon, the eye and the overlying skin. In most instances, Sturge-Weber syndrome is associated with mental deficiency.

Paraneoplastic Syndromes Involving the Central Nervous System

AUTOIMMUNE TUMOR-ASSOCIATED SYNDROMES

Systemic benign or malignant tumors may occasionally elicit autoimmune attack on the nervous system. Paraneoplastic neurologic disorders occur when an immune response against a tumor antigen recognizes an antigen, usually a protein, on a nervous system cell **(onconeural antigens)**. Anti-onconeural antibodies can often be identified in a patient's serum or CSF. *Paraneoplastic manifestations may precede clinical signs of the primary tumor,* sometimes by years, and successful treatment of the cancer often results in resolution of the paraneoplastic syndrome associated with it.

The clinical signs and symptoms of a given syndrome depend on where the neurons that express the particular onconeural antigen are. In some cases, it is broadly expressed in neuron populations throughout the brain and spinal cord, and so results in a **diffuse encephalomyelitis**. A prominent example is the Hu antigen (see below), for which the most commonly associated cancer is small cell lung carcinoma (SCLC). In other cases, the antigen is more restricted, as in **cerebellar degeneration** resulting from immune attack against cerebellar Yo or Ri antigens, typically associated with breast or ovarian cancer, or **limbic encephalitis** targeting the Ma or Ma2 antigen, which is often associated with SCLC or testicular cancer.

Two major classes of neuron proteins are targets of paraneoplastic autoimmune attack: (1) **intracellular antigens,** such as Hu, Yo, Ri and Ma; and (2) **neuron cell surface antigens,** such as potassium channel proteins, and AMPA, GABA(B), glycine, glutamate and *N*-methyl-D-aspartic acid (NMDA) receptors. The latter exemplify the importance of clinical recognition and accurate diagnosis of paraneoplastic syndromes. Limbic encephalitis due to anti-NMDA receptor autoantibodies is potentially a lethal disease that can be completely cured by simple surgical resection of a triggering benign ovarian teratoma!

Manifestations of CNS-Directed Paraneoplastic Diseases

Limbic Encephalitis

This condition may mimic herpes encephalitis, with seizures, memory deficits and a predilection for temporal lobe involvement. Anti-Hu antibodies in SCLC are often the culprits, although other autoantibodies causing this syndrome may be associated with other tumors (e.g., testicular cancer). There are some forms involving antibodies to voltage-gated potassium channels, in which immune suppression, in addition to antineoplastic chemotherapy, may treat the CNS symptoms.

Progressive Cerebellar Degeneration

This paraneoplastic syndrome may be the presenting feature of an underlying malignancy and can be devastating. It occurs most often in association with breast cancer and, less often, Hodgkin lymphoma. Progressive cerebellar degeneration (PCD) often is caused by an antibody against a leucine zipper protein, Yo, although a number of other autoantibodies have been implicated. People afflicted with paraneoplastic PCD vary greatly in their responses to therapeutics, in part as a function of the particular autoantibody involved.

Vision Loss

Loss of sight may occur as an unusual paraneoplastic syndrome, most often caused by loss of retinal photoreceptors. SCLC is the tumor most often responsible, by virtue of eliciting an antibody against a photoreceptor antigen, recoverin.

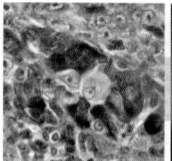
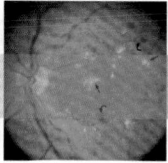
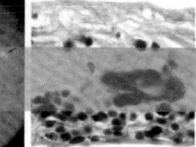

The Eye

Gordon K. Klintworth

PHYSICAL AND CHEMICAL INJURIES

Physical trauma to the eye commonly causes ecchymosis of the highly vascular eyelids (black eye); when this occurs, other parts of the eye also may be injured. Superficial disruptions of the corneal epithelium follow traumatic abrasions, prolonged wearing of a contact lens, foreign bodies on the eye and exposure to ultraviolet light. The eye is commonly injured by a variety of household and industrial caustic chemicals. The damage created depends on the nature of the chemical.

Blunt trauma increases intraorbital pressure momentarily and may cause the bones in the floor of the orbit to fracture into the maxillary sinus (**blowout fracture**). The inferior rectus muscle may become entrapped in such a fracture, thereby causing the eye to sink into the orbit (**enophthalmos**).

An array of foreign materials can injure the eye. Whereas small particles often lodge in superficial ocular tissues, some penetrate into or through the eye. A foreign particle may damage the eye during entry or because of secondary infection after the introduction of microorganisms. Some foreign bodies provoke a prominent acute inflammatory or granulomatous reaction. Others, such as those containing iron, cause retinal degeneration and even

discoloration of ocular tissues (**siderosis bulbi**), effects that may not be evident for several years. Other complications of ocular injuries include cataracts, retinal detachment and glaucoma.

THE EYELIDS

The important conditions affecting the eyelids include:

- **Blepharitis** is inflammation of the eyelids. It is common and sometimes produces an acute, red, tender, inflammatory mass.
- **Hordeolum (or sty)** refers to an acute, inflammatory, focal lesion of the eyelid. Acute inflammation involving the meibomian glands is termed an **internal hordeolum**, whereas acute folliculitis of the glands of Zeis is an **external hordeolum**.
- **Chalazion** is a granulomatous inflammation centered around the meibomian glands or the glands of Zeis. It is thought to represent a reaction to extruded lipid secretions and usually produces a painless swelling in the eyelid.
- **Xanthelasma** is a yellow plaque of lipid-containing macrophages, usually involving the nasal aspect of the

eyelids. It is often seen in older persons and patients with disorders of lipid metabolism (e.g., familial hypercholesterolemia, primary biliary cirrhosis).

THE ORBIT

Exophthalmos or Proptosis Is Abnormal Forward Protrusion of the Eyeball

The term **exophthalmos** is used mainly when the condition is bilateral; **proptosis** refers to a unilateral protrusion of the eye. Numerous conditions cause forward protrusion of the eye. The most common cause is thyroid disease, followed by orbital dermoid cysts and hemangiomas. Other orbital conditions can cause proptosis: various inflammatory lesions, lymphomas, developmental anomalies, vascular problems and neoplasms. Proptosis also results from lesions of the paranasal sinuses and intracranial cavity.

Exophthalmos of Hyperthyroidism Continues Despite Treatment

Exophthalmos caused by Graves disease may precede or follow other manifestations of thyroid dysfunction. Exophthalmos resulting from thyroid disease usually occurs in early adult life, especially in women (female-to-male ratio, 4:1). It may be severe and progressive, particularly in middle life, when exophthalmos no longer correlates well with the state of thyroid function. Dysthyroid exophthalmos may be associated with edema of the eyelids, chemosis (conjunctival edema) and limitation of ocular motion. Theories of the pathogenesis of hyperthyroidism-related exophthalmos are discussed in Chapter 27.

 CLINICAL FEATURES: Although exophthalmos of hyperthyroidism is usually bilateral, one eye may be involved earlier or more extensively than the other. Other ocular manifestations of hyperthyroidism include upper eyelid retraction (due to increased sympathetic tone) and a characteristic stare or apparent proptosis resulting from exposure of the conjunctiva above the corneoscleral limbus.

Complications of severe exophthalmos include several potentially blinding complications: corneal exposure with subsequent ulceration, and optic nerve compression. Paradoxically, thyroidectomy may increase the incidence and severity of exophthalmos associated with hyperthyroidism.

Inflammatory Pseudotumor Is a Chronic Idiopathic Inflammatory Condition

Inflammatory pseudotumor is associated with a variable degree of fibrosis. It is a common cause of proptosis and partial immobility of the eyeball.

THE CONJUNCTIVA

Conjunctival Hemorrhage May Follow Blunt Trauma, Anoxia or Severe Coughing

Conjunctival hemorrhages also occur spontaneously, often first noted on arising after sleep. They do not extend into the cornea because of the barrier imposed by the close apposition of corneal epithelium to the underlying substantia propria.

Conjunctivitis May Be Infectious or Allergic

Microorganisms lodging on the surface of the eye frequently cause conjunctivitis, keratitis (corneal inflammation) or a corneal ulcer. The conjunctiva, as well as other parts of the eye, may also become infected by hematogenous spread from a focus of infection elsewhere. Iatrogenic eye infections (e.g., with adenovirus) may follow ophthalmic manipulations, such as corneal grafts, intraocular implantation of lens prostheses or use of infected eyedrops or diagnostic instruments.

At some stage in life, virtually everyone has viral or bacterial conjunctivitis. This extremely common eye disease is characterized by hyperemic conjunctival blood vessels (pink eye). The inflammatory exudate that accumulates in the conjunctival sac commonly crusts, causing the eyelids to stick together in the morning. The conjunctival discharge may be purulent, fibrinous, serous or hemorrhagic. Participating inflammatory cells vary with the etiologic agent. As many allergens are seasonal, the allergic conjunctivitis they elicit tends to occur only at particular times of the year.

Trachoma

Trachoma is a chronic, contagious conjunctivitis caused by *Chlamydia trachomatis*. Various serotypes of *C. trachomatis* cause ocular, genital and systemic infections (trachoma, inclusion conjunctivitis and lymphogranuloma venereum; see Chapter 9).

 **EPIDEMIOLOGY:** About 500 million people are afflicted by trachoma, an acute, infectious, fibrosing keratoconjunctivitis caused by *C. trachomatis* (serotypes A, B and C). *This infection is the most common cause of blindness in the world and is especially prevalent in Asia, the Middle East and parts of Africa.* The disease has been eradicated in the United States and other developed countries. Trachoma is not very contagious, but overcrowding and poor hygienic conditions favor its transmission by fingers, fomites and flies. Spontaneous healing is common in children, but in adults, the disease progresses more rapidly and rarely heals without treatment.

 ETIOLOGIC FACTORS: An inflammatory reaction is generated by the immune system in response to *C. trachomatis*. Serial persistent or repetitive inflammatory reactions to different strains of the pathogen are believed to cause the serious cicatricial complications.

 PATHOLOGY: Trachoma is virtually always bilateral and involves the upper half of the conjunctiva more than the lower (Fig. 33-1). The cellular infiltrate is predominantly lymphocytic, and conjunctival lymph follicles with necrotic germinal centers are characteristic. Eventually lymphocytes and blood vessels invade the superior portion of the cornea between the epithelium and Bowman zone **(trachomatous pannus)**. Scarring of the conjunctiva and eyelids distorts the eyelids. On microscopic examination, the desquamated conjunctival epithelium

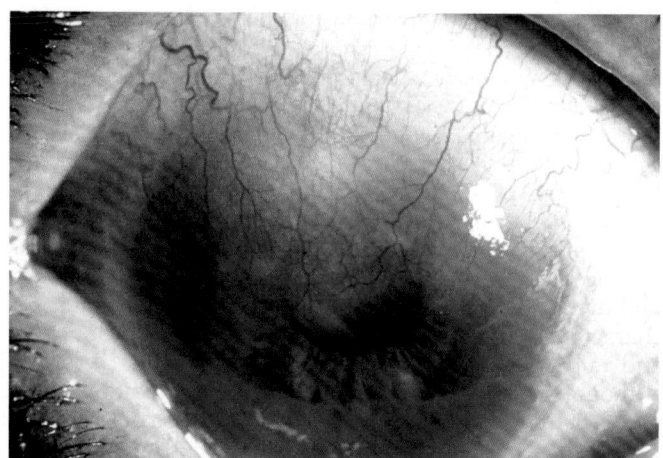

FIGURE 33-1. Trachoma. The cornea of a patient with severe trachoma shows extensive fibrovascular opacity **(pannus)** in the superior cornea.

exhibits glycogen-rich intracytoplasmic inclusion bodies and large macrophages containing nuclear fragments (Leber cells). Secondary bacterial infections occur commonly.

Other Chlamydial Infections

Chlamydia is responsible for a purulent conjunctivitis **(inclusion blennorrhea)** that develops in newborns, who become infected during passage through the birth canal. The infection is also acquired by swimming in nonchlorinated pools (swimming pool conjunctivitis) or from contact with discharges of infected urethra or cervix.

In adults and older children, *Chlamydia* causes a chronic follicular conjunctivitis with focal lymphoid hyperplasia **(inclusion conjunctivitis)**. In contrast to trachoma, the lower tarsal conjunctiva is involved. Scarring and necrosis do not develop, and keratitis is rare and mild.

Ophthalmia Neonatorum

Ophthalmia neonatorum is a severe, acute conjunctivitis with a copious purulent discharge, especially in the newborn, caused by **Neisseria gonorrhoeae.** The infection, which is a common cause of blindness in some parts of the world, is complicated by corneal ulceration, perforation, scarring and panophthalmitis. Infants usually become infected while passing through the birth canal of an infected mother. Other causative organisms for ophthalmia neonatorum include other pyogenic bacteria and *C. trachomatis.* Today, newborns are usually routinely treated with 5% Betadine eye drops.

Pinguecula and Pterygium

Pinguecula is a yellowish conjunctival lump usually located nasal to the corneoscleral limbus. It is the most common conjunctival lump. It consists of sun-damaged connective tissue identical to that in similarly injured skin (actinic elastosis; see Chapter 28).

Pterygium is a fold of vascularized conjunctiva that grows horizontally onto the cornea in the shape of an insect wing (hence the name). It is often associated with a pinguecula and frequently recurs after excision.

THE CORNEA

Herpes Simplex Virus Causes Corneal Ulcerations

Herpes simplex virus (HSV) has a predilection for corneal epithelium, where it causes keratitis, but it can invade corneal stroma and occasionally other ocular tissues.

PRIMARY INFECTION BY HERPES SIMPLEX VIRUS TYPE 1: Subclinical or undiagnosed localized ocular lesions are caused by HSV type 1 in childhood. These infections are accompanied by regional lymphadenopathy, systemic infection and fever. Except in newborns infected during passage through an infected mother's birth canal, HSV type 2 rarely causes ocular infection. When it does, it may produce widespread lesions of the cornea and retina. Most corneal lesions due to HSV are asymptomatic plaques of diseased epithelial cells that contain replicating virus. These usually heal without ulceration, but an acute unilateral follicular conjunctivitis may occur. Corneal ulcers appear after serum antibody levels increase.

REACTIVATION OF HERPES SIMPLEX VIRUS INFECTION: Latent in the trigeminal ganglion, HSV may pass down the nerves and reactivate the infection. Unlike primary HSV infection, reactivation disease is characterized by corneal ulceration and a more severe inflammatory reaction. Recurrence of corneal ulcers due to HSV may be precipitated by ultraviolet light, trauma, menstruation, emotional and physical stress, exposure to light or sunlight, vaccination and other factors.

 PATHOLOGY: HSV causes multiple, minute, discrete, intraepithelial corneal ulcers (superficial punctate keratopathy). Although some of these lesions heal, others enlarge and eventually coalesce to form linear or branching fissures (dendritic ulcers, from the Greek *dendron,* "tree"). The epithelium between the fissures desquamates, leading to sharply demarcated, irregular geographical ulcers. The corneal ulcers are readily visualized after the cornea is stained with fluorescein. Affected epithelial cells, which may become multinucleated, contain eosinophilic, intranuclear inclusion bodies (Lipschütz bodies).

The lesions of the corneal stroma vary in reactivated HSV infection. Typically, a central disc-shaped corneal opacity develops beneath the epithelium, owing to edema and minimal inflammation **(disciform keratitis).** The corneal stroma may become markedly thinned, and the Descemet membrane may bulge into it (descemetocele). Corneal perforation can also occur.

Onchocerciasis Leads to Blindness in Tropical Regions

The nematode *Onchocerca volvulus,* which is transmitted by bites of infected blackflies, is by far the most important helminthic infection of the eye (see Chapter 9). *This parasite accounts for blindness in at least half a million people in regions of Africa and Latin America in which it is endemic.* Microfilariae released from fertilized adult female worms migrate into the superficial cornea, bulbar conjunctiva, aqueous humor and other ocular tissues. The intracorneal microfilariae die and elicit an inflammatory response that leads to corneal opacification and visual impairment **(river blindness).** Less frequently, endophthalmitis, retinal lesions and optic atrophy occur. Treatment with ivermectin is highly effective.

Arcus Lipoides Is a White Arc Due to Lipid Deposition in the Peripheral Cornea

Formerly called **arcus senilis** because of its frequency in the elderly, arcus lipoides may also form an entire ring, in which case the term **annulus lipoides** is more appropriate. Although not necessarily associated with increased serum lipid levels, arcus lipoides accompanies certain disorders of lipid metabolism, and its presence alerts the perceptive clinician to the systemic disorder.

Band Keratopathy Is an Opaque Horizontal Band across the Cornea

The opacification in band keratopathy may contain calcium phosphate (**calcific band keratopathy**) or noncalcified protein (**chronic actinic keratopathy**).

In **calcific band keratopathy**, calcium phosphate deposits in a horizontal band across the superficial central cornea in conditions associated with hypercalcemia. However, the disorder most often occurs in the absence of hypercalcemia, as in chronic uveitis.

Chronic actinic keratopathy occurs worldwide but is most severe in regions in which people spend a considerable amount of time outdoors. Their unprotected eyes are exposed to excessive ultraviolet light, such as that reflected from desert, water or snow.

Noninflammatory Genetic Corneal Disorders Are Diverse

Most corneal dystrophies have an autosomal dominant or recessive mode of inheritance, but rare cases are X-linked recessive. Some of these diseases affect other parts of the body (e.g., Fabry disease, cystinosis, certain types of mucopolysaccharidosis and ichthyosis). Other conditions that primarily affect the cornea were traditionally called corneal dystrophies before the era of molecular genetics and were classified according to the primary corneal layer that is involved: (1) the outer layer composed of epithelium, basement membrane and Bowman layer; (2) the stroma; and (3) the endothelium and Descemet membrane, the basement membrane of the corneal endothelium. However, this classification is now considered somewhat artificial because many corneal dystrophies involve more than one layer.

EPITHELIAL DYSTROPHIES: The different epithelial dystrophies are characterized by a variety of distinct abnormalities, which include microcysts or accumulations of anomalous material within the cytoplasm of the corneal epithelium, defects in the epithelial basement membrane and deposition of a finely fibrillar substance in the Bowman layer. In some epithelial dystrophies, faulty desmosomes may permit adjacent epithelial cells to separate, leading to accumulation of fluid-filled microcysts. Loss of hemidesmosomes between the epithelium and Bowman layer leads to painful, recurrent erosions that begin in early childhood. Although there may be a slow decrease in visual acuity, epithelial dystrophies do not ordinarily cause blindness.

 **MOLECULAR PATHOGENESIS:** Patients with one disorder of the corneal epithelium (*Meesmann dystrophy*) have dominant mutations in the *KRT3* or *KRT12* genes, which encode keratin 3 and keratin 12, respectively. The

mutations result in aggregations of abnormal cytokeratin filaments and severely impair cytoskeletal function in the affected cells. In the rare bilateral, autosomal recessive corneal disorder *familial subepithelial corneal dystrophy,* wherein the *TACSTD2* gene is mutated, amyloid is found beneath the corneal epithelium in gelatinous drop-like deposits.

STROMAL DYSTROPHIES: The stromal corneal dystrophies are clear-cut entities in which different substances (amyloid, glycosaminoglycans, proteins or a variety of lipids) accumulate within corneal stroma because of inherited metabolic disorders. Each stromal dystrophy causes a characteristic form of corneal opacification. The age of onset and rate of progression vary with the particular disorder. Although clinical manifestations may be limited to the cornea, other tissues are involved in some of these disorders.

 **MOLECULAR PATHOGENESIS:** Several clinically and histopathologically different inherited corneal disorders, including the granular corneal dystrophies and most lattice corneal dystrophies, result from distinctly different mutations in the same gene, namely, the *TFGBI* gene. Another predominantly stromal corneal dystrophy (macular corneal dystrophy) results from a defect in the *CHST6* gene, which encodes a sulfotransferase that catalyzes sulfation of *N*-acetyl glucosamine and galactose in keratan sulfate. Other corneal stromal diseases are caused by mutations in the genes *PIP5K3* (fleck corneal dystrophy), *DCN* (congenital stromal corneal dystrophy) and *UBIAD1* (Schnyder corneal dystrophy).

 **MOLECULAR PATHOGENESIS:** *ENDOTHELIAL DYSTROPHIES:* Several different endothelial dystrophies are recognized, usually accompanied by abnormalities in the Descemet membrane. In *Fuchs endothelial corneal dystrophy,* wart-like excrescences form on the Descemet membrane (guttae), and progressive visual loss follows corneal edema and endothelial cell degeneration. Missense mutations in *COL8A2*, the gene encoding the α_2-chain of type VIII collagen, have been identified in some patients with early-onset Fuchs dystrophy and in ***posterior polymorphous corneal dystrophy***, both of which affect the corneal endothelium and Descemet membrane.

THE LENS

Cataracts Are Opacifications in the Crystalline Lens

Cataracts are a major cause of visual impairment and blindness throughout the world and are the outcome of numerous conditions.

ETIOLOGIC FACTORS: The most common cause of cataracts in the United States is advancing age (age-related cataract). Other cataracts are caused by diabetes, nutritional deficiencies (e.g., deficiencies in riboflavin or tryptophan), toxins (e.g., dinitrophenol, naphthalene, ergot), drugs (e.g., corticosteroids, topical phospholine iodide, phenothiazines) or physical agents (e.g., heat, ultraviolet light, trauma, intraocular surgery and ultrasound).

Cataracts may develop in ocular diseases such as uveitis, intraocular neoplasms, glaucoma, retinitis pigmentosa and retinal detachment. Cataracts also are associated with congenital rubella virus infection, some skin diseases (e.g., atopic dermatitis, scleroderma) and various systemic diseases.

 **MOLECULAR PATHOGENESIS:** A wide variety of cataracts result from genetic disorders, and some of them are associated with other ocular or systemic abnormalities. Cataracts can result from mutations in the heat shock transcription factor-4 (*HSF4*) gene and genes that encode specific lens proteins such as connexins (*GJA3, GJA8*), crystallins (a family of *CRY* genes), a beaded filament structural protein-2 (*BFSP2*), a putative cell-junction protein (*LIM2*) and aquaporin 0 (*MIP*). They also result from genetic mutations and chromosomal anomalies that cause numerous systemic diseases and syndromes.

 PATHOLOGY: In the development of cataracts, clefts appear between the lens fibers, and degenerated lens material accumulates in these spaces (morgagnian corpuscles, incipient cataract). Degenerated lens material exerts osmotic pressure, causing the damaged lens to imbibe water and swell. The swollen lens may obstruct the pupil and cause glaucoma (phacomorphic glaucoma).

In a *mature cataract* (Fig. 33-2), the entire lens degenerates, and the lenticular debris escapes into the aqueous humor through the lens capsule, diminishing the volume of the lens (hypermature cataract). After becoming engulfed by macrophages, the extruded lenticular material may obstruct aqueous outflow and produce glaucoma (phacolytic glaucoma). The compressed lens fibers in the center of the lens normally harden with aging (simple nuclear sclerotic cataract) and may become brown or black. If the peripheral part of the lens (lens cortex) becomes liquefied (morgagnian cataract), the sclerotic nucleus may sink within the lens by gravity.

Fortunately, cataractous lenses can be surgically removed, and optical devices can be provided to permit focusing of light on the retina (spectacles, contact lenses, implantation of prosthetic lenses).

Presbyopia Is a Failure of Accommodation as a Result of Aging

With this impairment of vision, the near point of distinct vision becomes located farther from the eye. At the equator

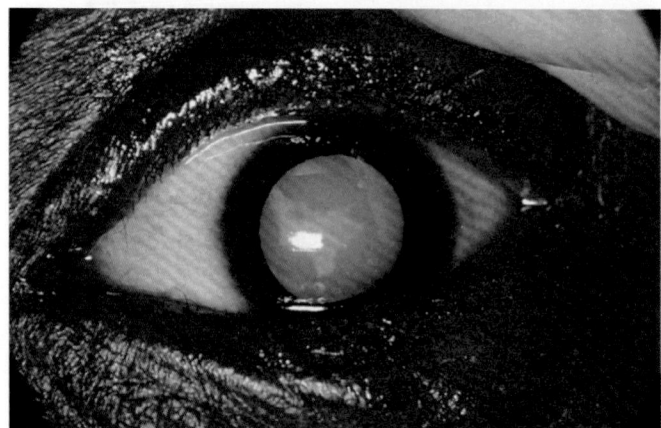

FIGURE 33-2. Cataract. The white appearance of the pupil in this eye is due to complete opacification of the lens ("mature cataract").

of the crystalline lens, the cuboidal subcapsular cells normally differentiate into elongated lens fibers throughout life. Once formed, these lens fibers persist indefinitely. Older fibers become displaced into the center of the lens, causing it to enlarge with age. After this process occurs over many years, the lens loses its elasticity. This effect interferes with the normal tendency of the lens to become spherical, and so diminishes the power of accommodation. As a result, most persons after age 40 years begin to have difficulty reading and require spectacles for near vision.

Phacoanaphylactic Endophthalmitis Is an Autoimmune Granulomatous Reaction to Lens Proteins

In this disorder, an inflammatory lesion occurs around or within the lens (or its remains) in an eye with a traumatized or cataractous lens and sometimes after surgical removal of a cataractous lens. A similar reaction may occur spontaneously in the contralateral eye months or years later. This autoimmune reaction to unique lens proteins, which are normally sequestered from the immune system, can be provoked experimentally by immunization with autologous lens material.

THE UVEA

A Variety of Inflammatory Conditions Affect the Uveal Tract

Inflammation of the uvea **(uveitis)** also encompasses inflammation of the iris **(iritis)**, the ciliary body **(cyclitis)** and the iris plus the ciliary body **(iridocyclitis)**. Inflammation of the iris and ciliary body typically causes a red eye, photophobia, moderate ocular pain, blurred vision, a pericorneal halo, ciliary flush and slight miosis. A flare is common in the anterior chamber on slit-lamp biomicroscopy, and keratic precipitates or a **hypopyon** (leukocytic exudate in the anterior chamber) also develops.

Peripheral anterior synechiae are adhesions between the peripheral iris and the anterior chamber angle. **Posterior synechiae** are adhesions that develop between the iris and the lens. Both types of synechiae are complications of iritis, and both can cause glaucoma.

Sympathetic Ophthalmitis Is an Autoimmune Uveitis

In sympathetic ophthalmitis, the entire uvea develops granulomatous inflammation after a latent period, in response to an injury in the other eye. Perforating ocular injury and prolapse of uveal tissue often lead to a progressive, bilateral, diffuse, granulomatous inflammation of the uvea. This uveitis develops in the originally injured eye (exciting eye) after a latent period of 4–8 weeks. The latent period may, however, be as short as 10 days or as long as many years. The uninjured eye (sympathizing eye) becomes affected at the same time as the injured eye, or shortly thereafter. Vitiligo and graying of the eyelashes sometimes accompanies the uveitis. Nodules containing reactive retinal pigment epithelium, macrophages and epithelioid cells commonly appear between the Bruch membrane **(lamina vitrea)** and retinal pigment epithelium **(Dalen-Fuchs nodules)**.

Experimental studies suggest that the antigen responsible for sympathetic ophthalmitis resides in the photoreceptors of the retina **(arrestin)**.

Sarcoidosis Commonly Affects the Eye

Ocular involvement occurs in one fourth to one third of patients with sarcoidosis and is often the initial clinical manifestation. Both eyes are usually affected, most often with a granulomatous uveitis. Although any ocular and orbital tissues may be involved, this granulomatous disease has a predilection for the anterior segment of the eye. Other ocular manifestations of sarcoidosis include calcific band

keratopathy, cataracts, retinal vascularization, vitreous hemorrhage and bilateral enlargement of the lacrimal and salivary glands **(Mikulicz syndrome)**.

THE RETINA

Retinal Hemorrhage May Occur in Both Local and Systemic Diseases

The important causes of retinal hemorrhages are hypertension, diabetes mellitus, central retinal vein occlusion, bleeding diatheses and trauma, including the "shaken baby

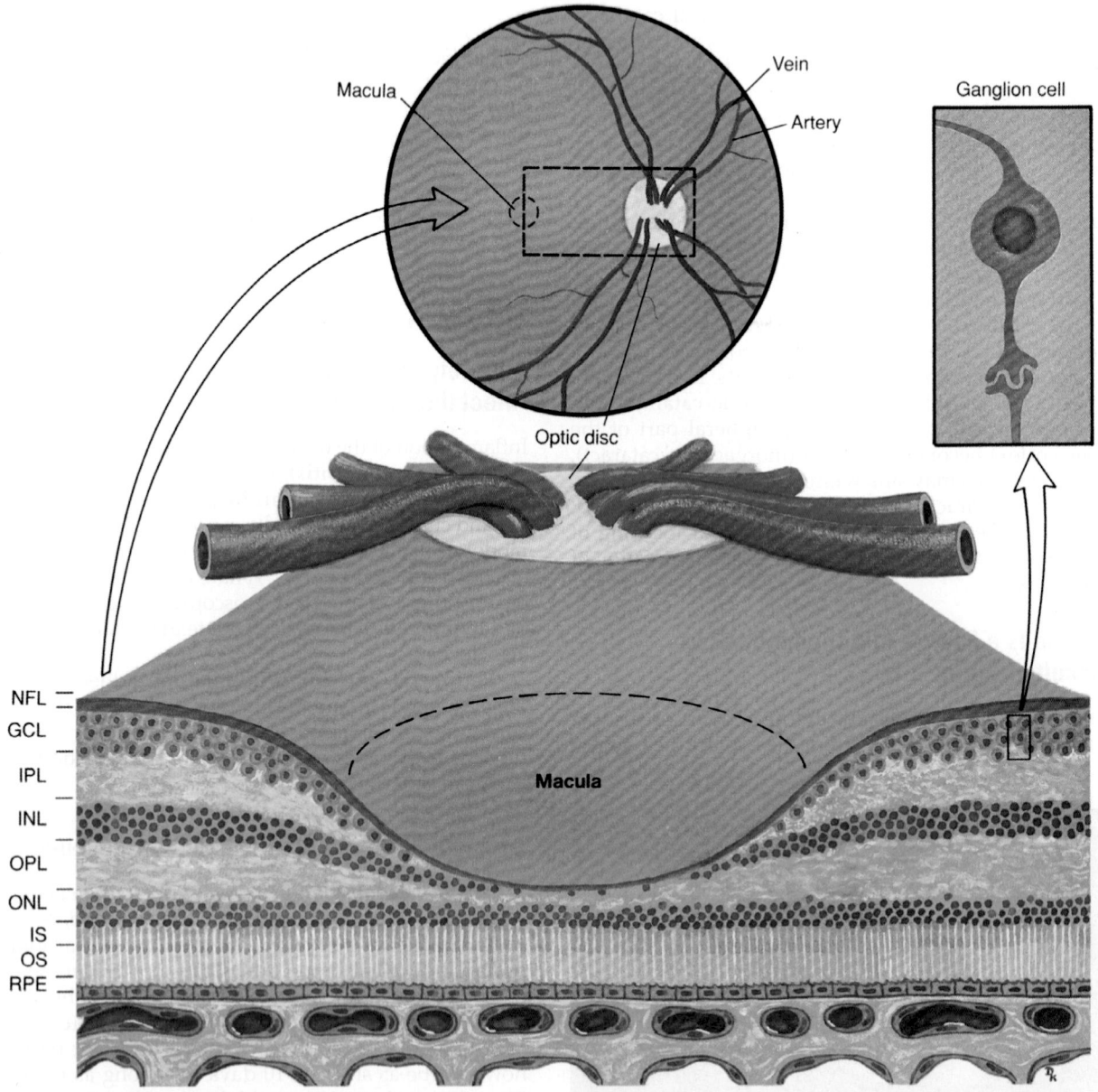

FIGURE 33-3. The normal retina. Constituents of the normal retina are arranged in distinct layers. These include the nerve fiber layer (*NFL*), ganglion cell layer (*GCL*), inner plexiform layer (*IPL*), inner nuclear layer (*INL*), outer plexiform layer (*OPL*), outer nuclear layer (*ONL*), inner segments (*IS*) and outer segments (*OS*) of the photoreceptors and the retinal pigment epithelium (*RPE*). The axons from the ganglion cells enter the nerve fiber layer and converge toward the optic nerve head. The inner retina contains arteries and veins. The retina is thinnest at the center of the macula, where bare photoreceptors rest on the retinal pigment epithelium. Only one cell thick in most of the retina, the ganglion cell layer is multilayered at the macula.

syndrome." Appearance varies with cause and location. Hemorrhages in the nerve fiber layer spread between axons and causes a flame-shaped appearance on funduscopy, whereas deep retinal hemorrhages tend to be round. When located between the retinal pigment epithelium and Bruch membrane, blood appears as a dark mass, which may resemble a melanoma.

After accidental or surgical perforation of the globe, choroidal hemorrhages may detach the choroid and displace the retina, vitreous body and lens through the wound.

Retinal Occlusive Vascular Disease Is an Important Cause of Blindness

Vascular occlusion results from thrombosis, embolism, stenosis (as in atherosclerosis), vascular compression, intravascular sludging or coagulation and vasoconstriction (e.g., in hypertensive retinopathy or migraine). Thrombosis of ocular vessels may accompany primary disease of these vessels, as in giant cell arteritis.

Certain disorders of the heart and major vessels, such as the carotid arteries, predispose to emboli that may lodge in the retina and are evident on funduscopic examination at points of vascular bifurcation. Within the optic nerve, emboli in the central retinal artery frequently lodge in the vessel where it passes though the scleral perforations **(lamina cribrosa)**.

 PATHOLOGY: The effect of vascular occlusion depends on the size of the vessel involved, the degree of resultant ischemia and the nature of the embolus. Small emboli often do not interfere with retinal function, whereas septic emboli may cause foci of ocular infection. Retinal ischemia due to any cause frequently leads to white fluffy patches that resemble cotton on ophthalmoscopic examination **(cotton-wool spots)**. These round spots, which are seldom wider than the optic nerve head, consist of aggregates of swollen axons in the nerve fiber layer of the retina. Affected axons contain numerous degenerated mitochondria and dense bodies related to the lysosomal system, which accumulate because of impaired axoplasmic flow. Histologically, in cross-section, individual swollen axons resemble cells (cytoid bodies). Cotton-wool spots are reversible if circulation is restored in time.

Central Retinal Artery Occlusion

Like neurons in the rest of the nervous system, those in the retina (Fig. 33-3) are extremely susceptible to hypoxia. Central retinal artery occlusion (Figs. 33-4 and 33-5) may follow thrombosis of the retinal artery, as in atherosclerosis or giant cell arteritis, or embolization to that blood vessel. Intracellular edema, manifested by retinal pallor, is prominent, especially in the macula, where ganglion cells are most numerous. The foveola, the center of the macula, stands out in sharp contrast as a prominent **cherry-red spot,** because of the underlying vascularized choroid. The lack of retinal circulation reduces retinal arterioles to delicate threads (Fig. 33-5).

Permanent blindness follows central retinal artery obstruction, unless the ischemia is of short duration. Unilateral blurred vision, lasting a few minutes **(amaurosis fugax),** occurs with small retinal emboli.

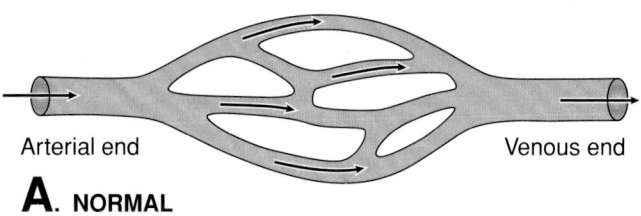

A. NORMAL

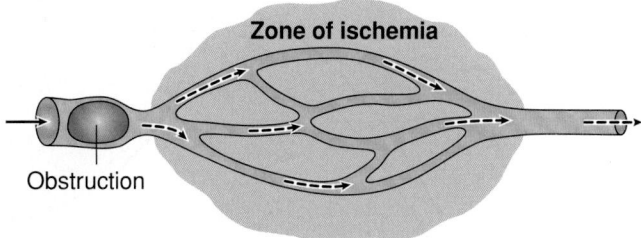

Neuronal functional impairment → Visual loss
Edema → Pallor

B. RETINAL ARTERIAL OCCLUSION

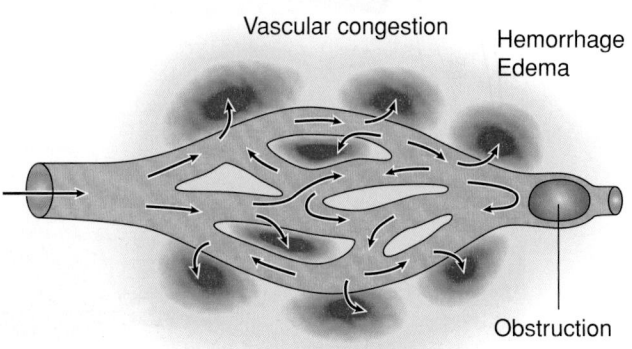

Mild ischemia: normal neuronal function

C. RETINAL VEIN OCCLUSION

FIGURE 33-4. Occlusion of the retinal artery and vein. A. In the retina, as in other parts of the body, blood normally flows through a capillary network. **B.** When the retinal arteries become occluded (e.g., with an embolus), a zone of retinal ischemia ensues. This is accompanied by impaired neuronal function and visual loss, and the ischemic retina becomes pale. Because the intravascular pressure within the ischemic tissue is low, hemorrhage is inconspicuous. **C.** With retinal vein occlusion, vascular congestion, hemorrhage and edema are prominent, whereas ischemia is mild and neuronal function remains intact.

Central Retinal Vein Occlusion

Central retinal vein occlusion results in flame-shaped hemorrhages in the nerve fiber layer of the retina, especially around the optic nerve head. The hemorrhages reflect the high intravascular pressure that dilates and ruptures the veins and collateral vessels (Fig. 33-6). Edema of the optic nerve head and retina occurs because absorption of interstitial fluid is impaired.

Vision is disturbed but may recover surprisingly well, considering the severity of the funduscopic changes. An intractable, closed-angle glaucoma, with severe pain and repeated hemorrhages, commonly ensues 2–3 months after central retinal vein occlusion (so-called 100-day glaucoma, thrombotic glaucoma or neovascular glaucoma). This distressing complication is caused by neovascularization of the

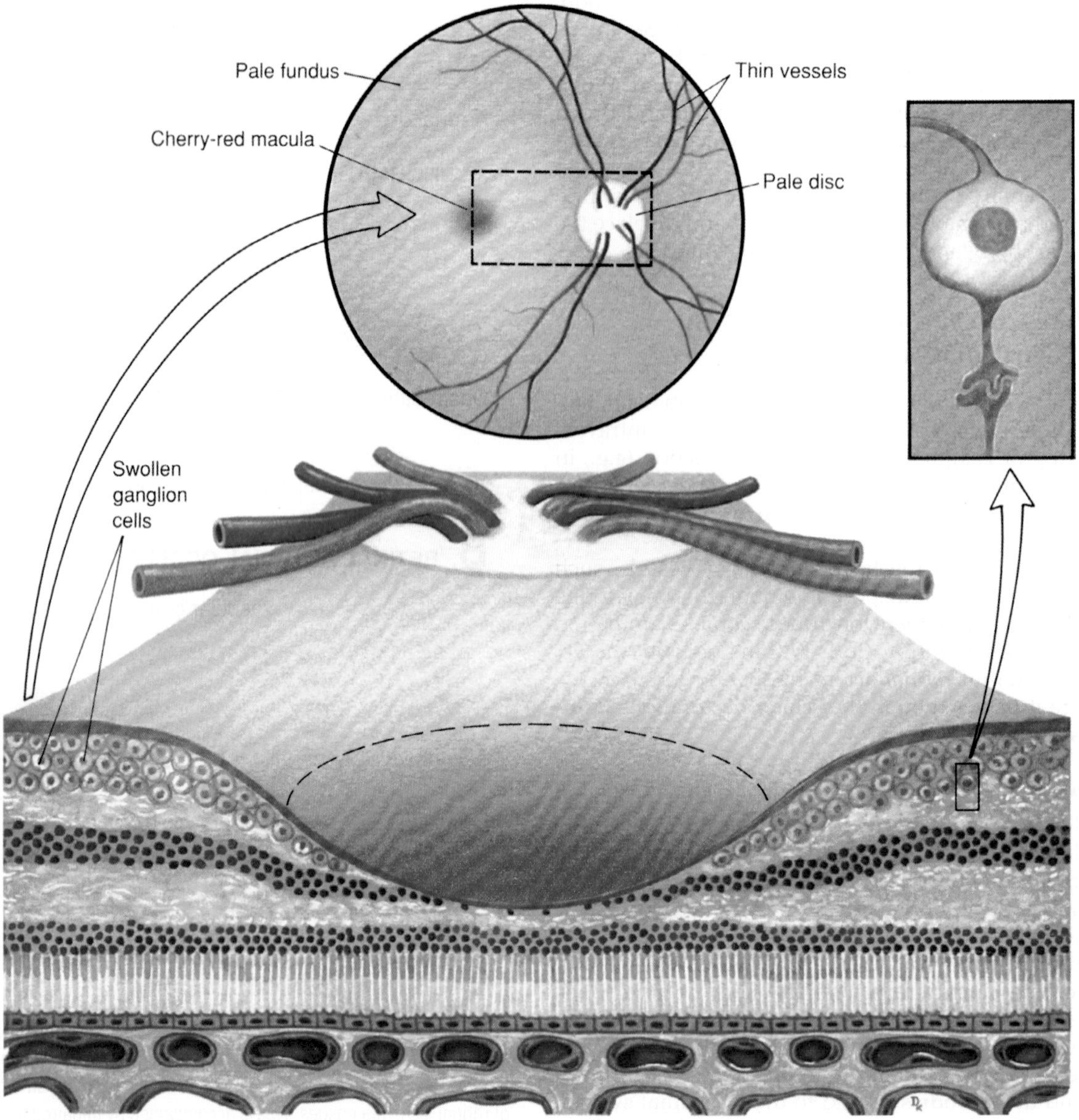

FIGURE 33-5. Central retinal artery occlusion. When the central retinal artery becomes occluded (e.g., with an embolus), the entire retina becomes edematous and pale. Decreased blood flow makes the retinal vessels less visible on funduscopic examination. The macula becomes cherry-red, owing to the prominent, but normal, underlying vasculature of the choroid.

iris and adhesions between the iris and the anterior chamber angle **(peripheral anterior synechiae)**.

Hypertensive Retinopathy Correlates with the Severity of Hypertension

Increased blood pressure commonly affects the retina, causing changes that can readily be seen with the ophthalmoscope (Figs. 33-7 and 33-8).

PATHOLOGY: Features of hypertensive retinopathy include:

- **Arteriolar narrowing**
- **Hemorrhages** in the retinal nerve fiber layer (flame-shaped hemorrhages)
- **Exudates,** including some that radiate from the center of the macula (macular star)

- Fluffy white bodies in the superficial retina **(cotton-wool spots)**
- **Microaneurysms**

In the eye, arteriolosclerosis accompanies long-standing hypertension and commonly affects the retinal and choroidal vessels. Lumina of the thickened retinal arterioles become narrowed, increasingly tortuous and of irregular caliber. At sites where arterioles cross veins, the latter appear kinked **(arteriovenous nicking)**. However, the venous diameter before the site of compression is not wider than that after it. The kinked appearance of the vein reflects sclerosis within the venous walls, because retinal arteries and veins share a common adventitia at sites of arteriovenous crossings, rather than compression by a taut sclerotic artery.

By funduscopy, abnormal retinal arterioles appear as parallel white lines at sites of vascular crossings **(arterial sheathing)**. Initially, the narrowed lumen of the retinal

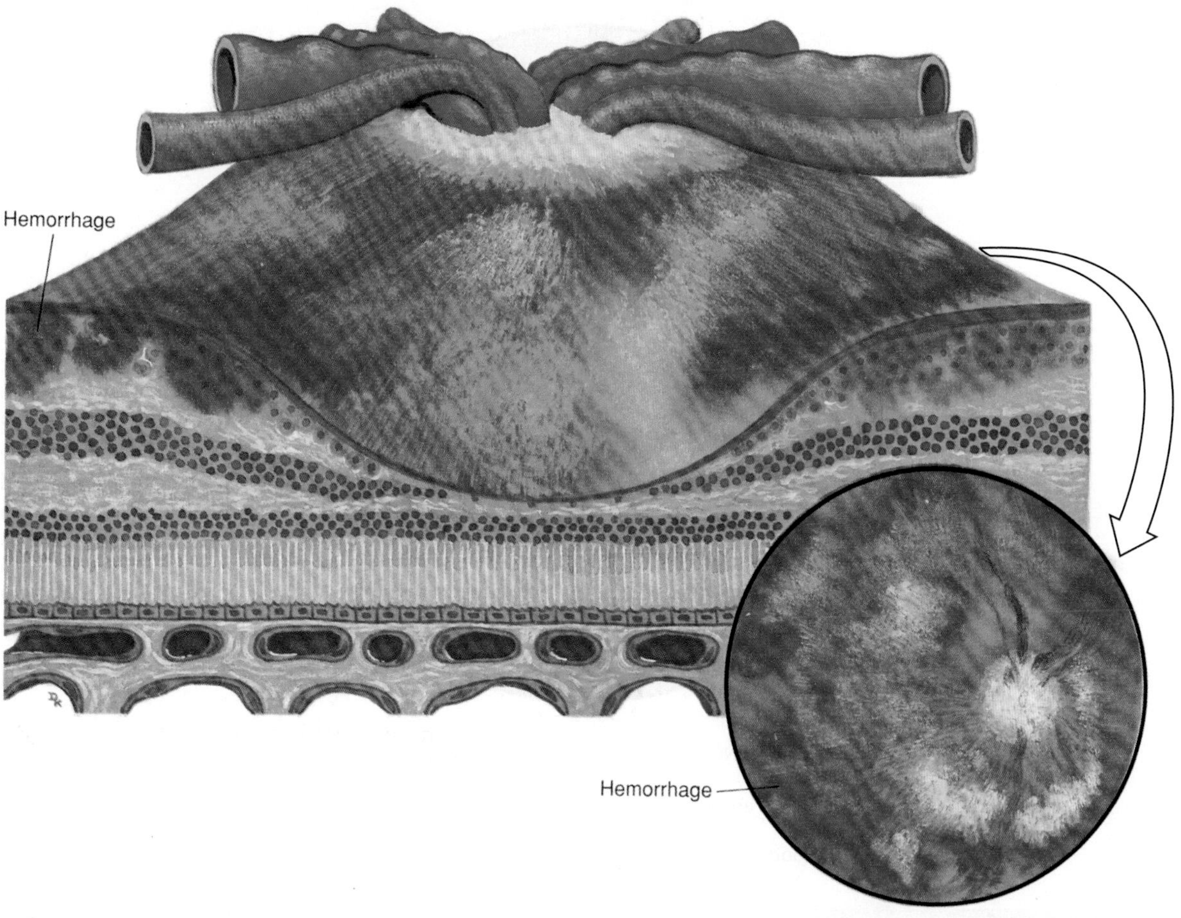

FIGURE 33-6. **Central retinal vein occlusion.** In contrast to central retinal artery occlusion, central retinal vein occlusion produces considerable vascular engorgement and retinal hemorrhage as a consequence of increased intravascular pressure.

vessels decreases the visibility of the blood column and makes it appear orange on ophthalmoscopic examination **(copper wiring)**. However, as the blood column eventually becomes completely obscured, light reflected from the sclerotic vessels appears as threads of silver wire **(silver wiring)**.

Small superficial or deep retinal hemorrhages often accompany retinal arteriolosclerosis. **Malignant hypertension** is characterized by necrotizing arteriolitis, with fibrinoid necrosis and thrombosis of precapillary retinal arterioles.

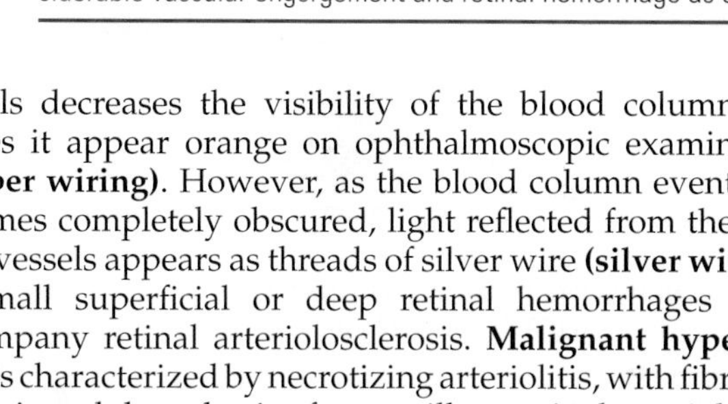

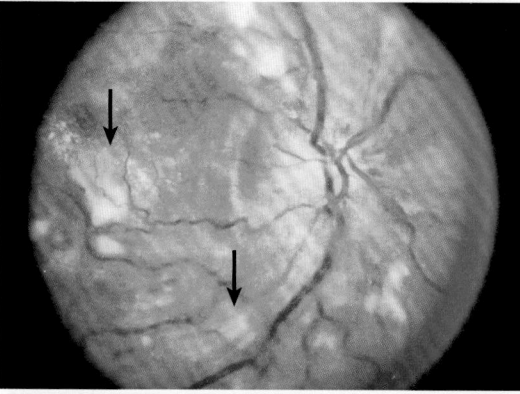

FIGURE 33-7. **Hypertensive retinopathy.** A photograph of the ocular fundus in a patient with extensive retinopathy. The optic nerve head is edematous; the retina contains numerous "cotton-wool spots" (*arrows*).

Diabetic Retinopathy Is Primarily a Vascular Disease

The eye is frequently involved in diabetes mellitus. Ocular symptoms occur in 20%–40% of diabetics and may even be evident at the time diabetes is diagnosed. Virtually all patients with type 1 (insulin-dependent) diabetes and many of those with type 2 (non–insulin-dependent) diabetes develop some background retinopathy (see below) within 5–15 years of the onset of diabetes (Figs. 33-9 to 33-11). The more dangerous **proliferative retinopathy** does not appear until at least 10 years of diabetes, after which its incidence increases rapidly and remains high for many years. *In type 1 diabetes, the frequency of proliferative retinopathy correlates with the degree of glycemic control; patients whose diabetes is better controlled develop retinopathy less frequently.* The relationship between retinal microvascular disease and blood glucose levels in type 2 diabetes is less clear, and other parameters (e.g., blood cholesterol levels, blood pressure) may play more of a role than blood glucose levels.

Retinal ischemia can account for most features of diabetic retinopathy, including the cotton-wool spots, capillary closure, microaneurysms and retinal neovascularization. Ischemia results from narrowing or occlusion of retinal arterioles (as from arteriolosclerosis or platelet and lipid thrombi) or from atherosclerosis of the central retinal or ophthalmic arteries.

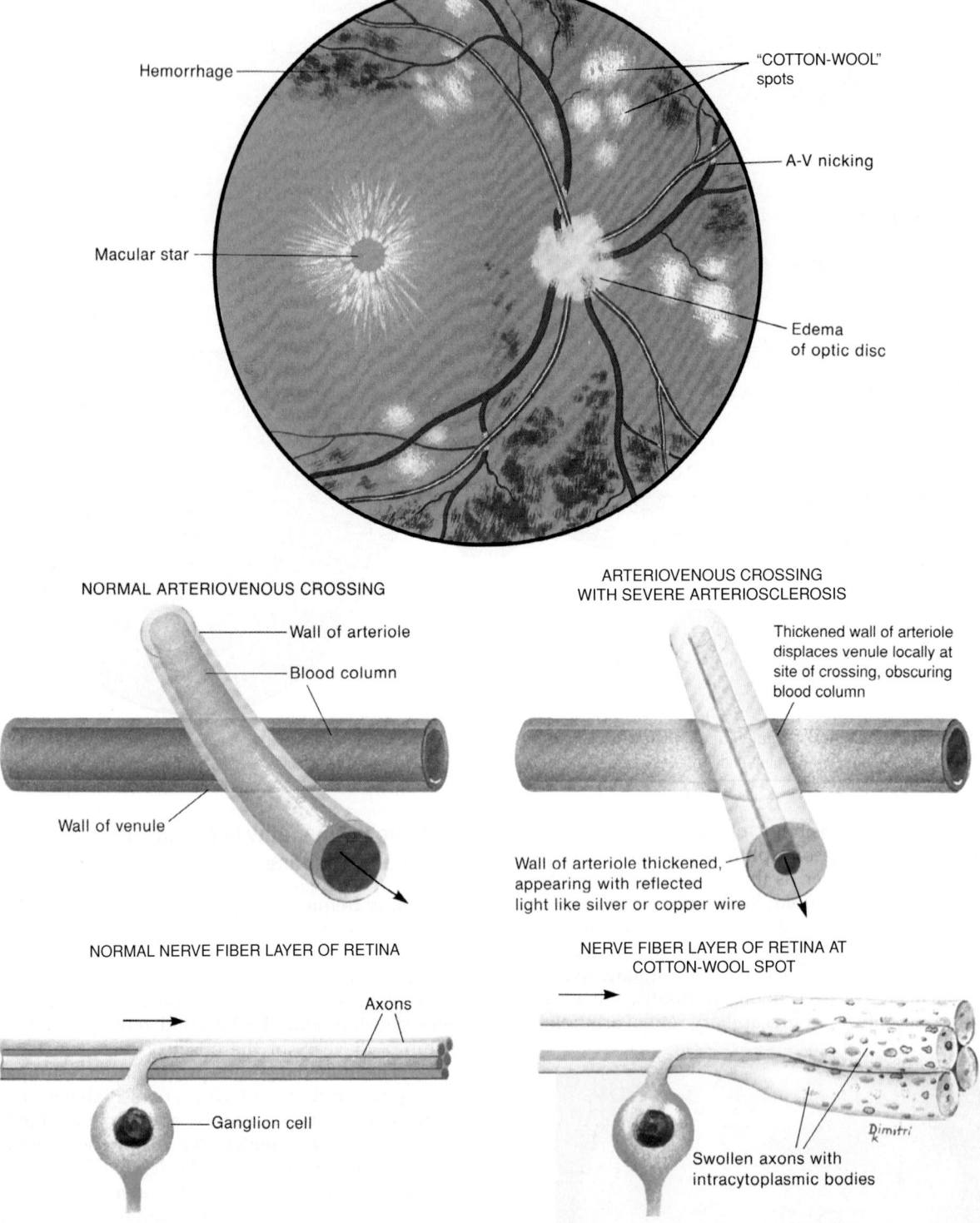

Hemorrhage

"COTTON-WOOL" spots

A-V nicking

Macular star

Edema of optic disc

NORMAL ARTERIOVENOUS CROSSING

Wall of arteriole

Blood column

Wall of venule

ARTERIOVENOUS CROSSING WITH SEVERE ARTERIOSCLEROSIS

Thickened wall of arteriole displaces venule locally at site of crossing, obscuring blood column

Wall of arteriole thickened, appearing with reflected light like silver or copper wire

NORMAL NERVE FIBER LAYER OF RETINA

Axons

Ganglion cell

NERVE FIBER LAYER OF RETINA AT COTTON-WOOL SPOT

Swollen axons with intracytoplasmic bodies

FIGURE 33-8. Hypertensive retinopathy. Various abnormalities develop within the retina in hypertension. The commonly associated arteriolosclerosis affects the appearance of the retinal microvasculature. Light reflected from the thickened arteriolar walls mimics silver or copper wire. Blood flow through the retinal venules is not well visualized at the sites of arteriolar–venular crossings. This effect is due to a thickening of the venular wall rather than to an impediment to blood flow caused by compression; the column of blood proximal to the compression is not wider than the part distal to the crossing. Impaired axoplasmic flow within the nerve fiber layer, caused by ischemia, results in swollen axons with cytoplasmic bodies. Such structures resemble cotton on funduscopy ("cotton-wool spots"). Hemorrhages are common in the retina, and exudates frequently form a star around the macula.

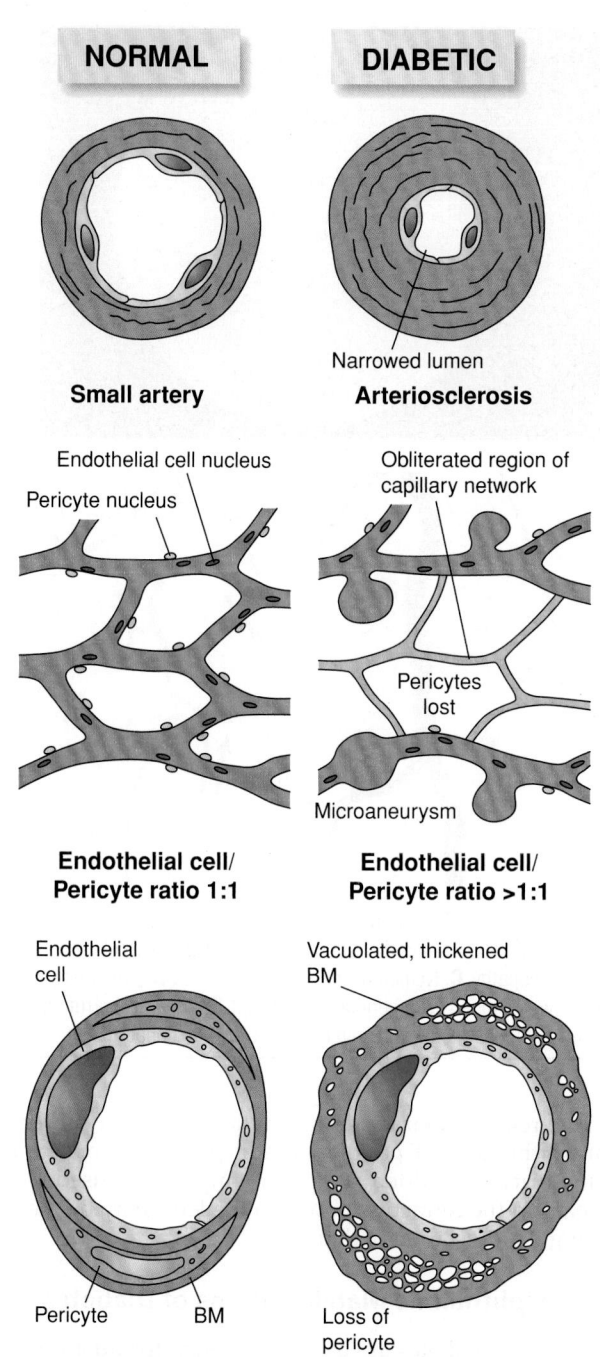

NORMAL

Small artery

DIABETIC

Narrowed lumen

Arteriosclerosis

Endothelial cell nucleus

Pericyte nucleus

Obliterated region of capillary network

Pericytes lost

Microaneurysm

Endothelial cell/ Pericyte ratio 1:1

Endothelial cell/ Pericyte ratio >1:1

Endothelial cell

Vacuolated, thickened BM

Pericyte   BM

Loss of pericyte

Retinal capillary

Retinal capillary

FIGURE 33-9. Diabetic retinopathy. In diabetic retinopathy, the microvasculature is abnormal. Arteriosclerosis narrows the lumen of the small arteries. Pericytes are lost, and the endothelial cell–to–pericyte ratio is greater than 1. Capillary microaneurysms are prominent, and portions of the capillary network become acellular and show no blood flow. The basement membrane (BM) of the retinal capillaries is thickened and vacuolated.

PATHOLOGY: The retinopathy of diabetes is characterized by background and proliferative stages.

BACKGROUND (NONPROLIFERATIVE) DIABETIC RETINOPATHY: This stage exhibits venous engorgement, small hemorrhages (dot and blot hemorrhages), capillary microaneurysms and exudates. These lesions usually do not impair vision unless associated with macular edema. The retinopathy begins at the posterior pole but eventually may involve the entire retina.

On funduscopy, the first discernible clinical abnormality in background diabetic retinopathy is engorged retinal veins, with localized sausage-shaped distentions, coils and loops. This is followed by small hemorrhages in the same areas, mostly in the inner nuclear and outer plexiform layers. With time, "waxy" exudates accumulate, chiefly in the vicinity of the microaneurysms. The retinopathy of elderly diabetic persons frequently displays numerous exudates **(exudative diabetic retinopathy),** which are not seen with type 1 diabetes. Because of the hyperlipoproteinemia of diabetics, the exudates are rich in lipid and thus appear yellowish **(waxy exudates).**

PROLIFERATIVE RETINOPATHY: After many years, diabetic retinopathy becomes proliferative. Delicate new blood vessels grow along with fibrous and glial tissue toward the vitreous body. Retinal neovascularization is a prominent feature of diabetic retinopathy and of other conditions caused by retinal ischemia. Tortuous new vessels first appear on the surface of the retina and optic nerve head and then grow into the vitreous cavity. The newly formed friable vessels bleed easily, and resultant vitreal hemorrhages obscure vision. Neovascularization is associated with proliferation and immigration of astrocytes, which grow around the new vessels to form delicate white veils (gliosis). The proliferating fibrovascular and glial tissue contracts, often causing retinal detachment and blindness. Frequently, features of hypertensive and arteriolosclerotic retinopathy are associated with diabetic retinopathy.

Diabetic retinopathy, glaucoma and age-related maculopathy are the leading causes of irreversible blindness in the United States. Blindness in diabetic retinopathy results when the macula is involved, but it also follows vitreous hemorrhage, retinal detachment and glaucoma. Once blindness ensues, it heralds an ominous future for the patient, because death from ischemic heart disease or renal failure often follows. In fact, the mean life expectancy in such cases is less than 6 years, and only one fifth of blind diabetics survive 10 years. Laser phototherapy and strict glycemic control early in the course of proliferative retinopathy have proved effective in controlling this complication.

Diabetic Iridopathy

In diabetics with severe retinopathy, a fibrovascular layer frequently grows along the anterior surface of the iris and in the anterior chamber angle. Because such iris neovascularization **(rubeosis iridis)** occurs in several conditions associated with retinal ischemia, it is believed to be due to an angiogenic factor produced by the ischemic retina.

PATHOLOGY: A fibrovascular membrane leads to adhesions between the iris and the cornea **(peripheral anterior synechiae)** and between the iris and lens **(posterior synechiae),** while traction by the fibrovascular membrane pulls the iris pigment epithelium around the pupillary margin **(ectropion uveae).** The friable new vessels on the iris bleed easily and cause **hyphema** (hemorrhage within the anterior chamber of the eye). Neovascularization of the iris is clinically important because it frequently culminates in a blind, painful eye, owing to secondary glaucoma **(neovascular glaucoma).**

THE EYE

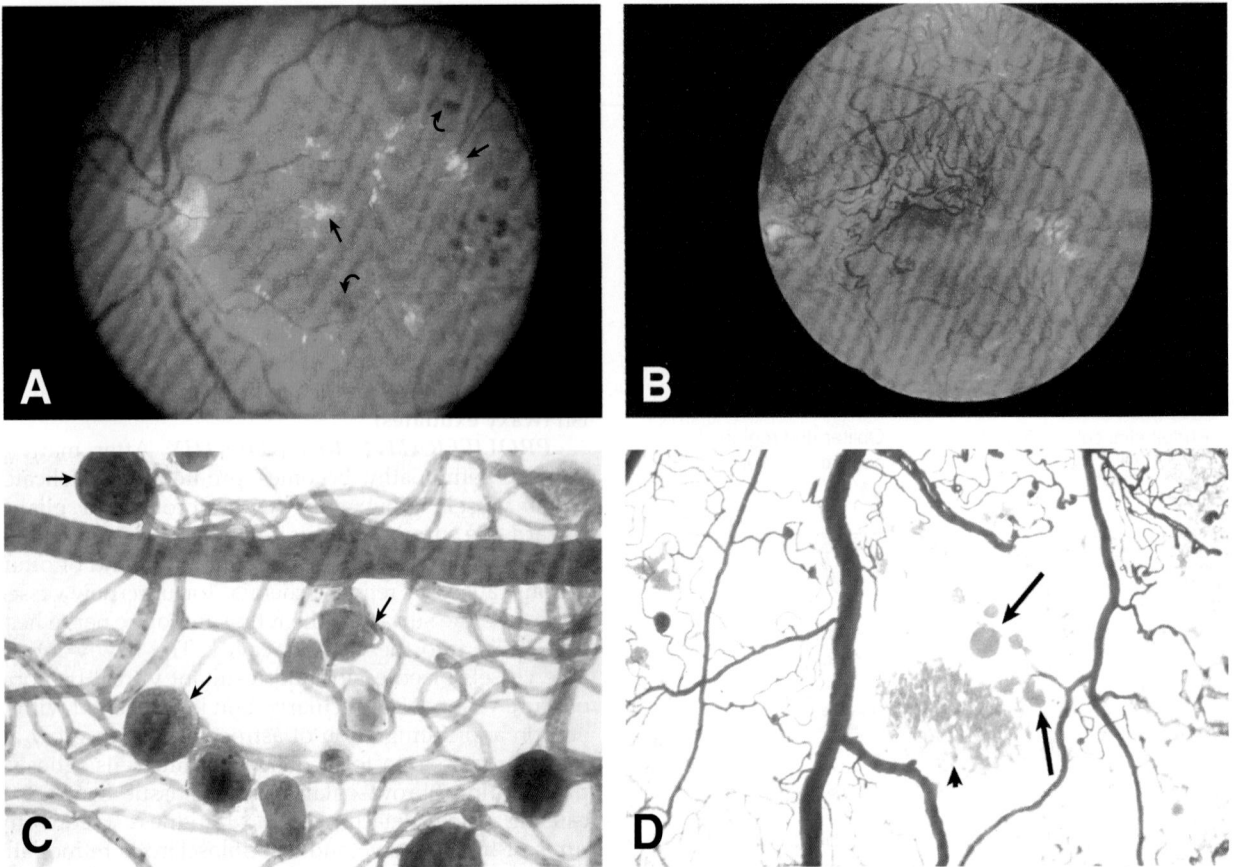

FIGURE 33-10.   Diabetic retinopathy. A. The ocular fundus in a patient with background diabetic retinopathy. Several yellowish "hard" exudates (*straight arrows*), which are rich in lipids, are evident, together with several relatively small retinal hemorrhages (*curved arrows*). **B.** A vascular frond (*top half*) has extended anteriorly to the retina in the eye with proliferative diabetic retinopathy. **C.** Numerous microaneurysms (*arrows*) are present in this flat preparation of a diabetic retina. **D.** This flat preparation from a diabetic was stained with periodic acid–Schiff (PAS) after the retinal vessels had been perfused with India ink. Microaneurysms (*arrows*) and an exudate (*arrowhead*) are evident in a region of retinal nonperfusion.

Hyperglycemia leads to glycogen storage in the pigmented epithelium of the iris, a phenomenon analogous to that produced in the renal tubules by glycosuria. When tissue sections of diabetic eyes are processed in the usual manner, the pigment epithelium of the iris sometimes contains numerous vacuoles, which imparts a lacy appearance. The vacuoles result from loss of glycogen during preparation of tissue sections. Glycogen storage within the iris pigment epithelium is thought to account for the scattering of iris pigment observed clinically in diabetic patients.

Diabetic Cataracts

Patients with type 1 diabetes often develop bilateral "snowflake" cataracts, a blanket of white needle-shaped opacities in the lens immediately beneath the anterior and posterior lens capsule. The opacities coalesce within a few weeks in adolescents, and within days in children, until the whole lens becomes opaque. Snowflake cataracts can be produced experimentally in young animals and result from an osmotic effect caused by an accumulation of sorbitol, the alcohol derived from glucose (see Chapter 13). The increased sorbitol content of the lens causes imbibition of water and enlargement of the lens.

Age-related cataracts occur in diabetics at an earlier age than in the general population and progress more rapidly to maturity. A sudden temporary myopia, caused by an increase in the refractive power in the lens, may be the presenting manifestation of diabetes.

Other Ophthalmic Manifestations of Diabetes

People with diabetes are at increased risk for inflammation of the anterior segment of the eye, phycomycosis (mucormycosis) of the orbit and primary open-angle glaucoma. They are also prone to the **Argyll Robertson pupil** (unequal and irregularly shaped pupils that react to accommodation but not to light). Cranial nerve palsies occur, especially of the oculomotor nerve. Some patients with long-standing diabetes develop recurrent corneal erosions, which are thought to be due to impaired innervation of the cornea.

The effects of diabetes mellitus on the eye are reviewed in Fig. 33-11.

Retinal Detachment Separates the Sensory Retina from the Pigment Epithelium

During fetal development, the space between the sensory retina and the retinal pigment epithelium is obliterated

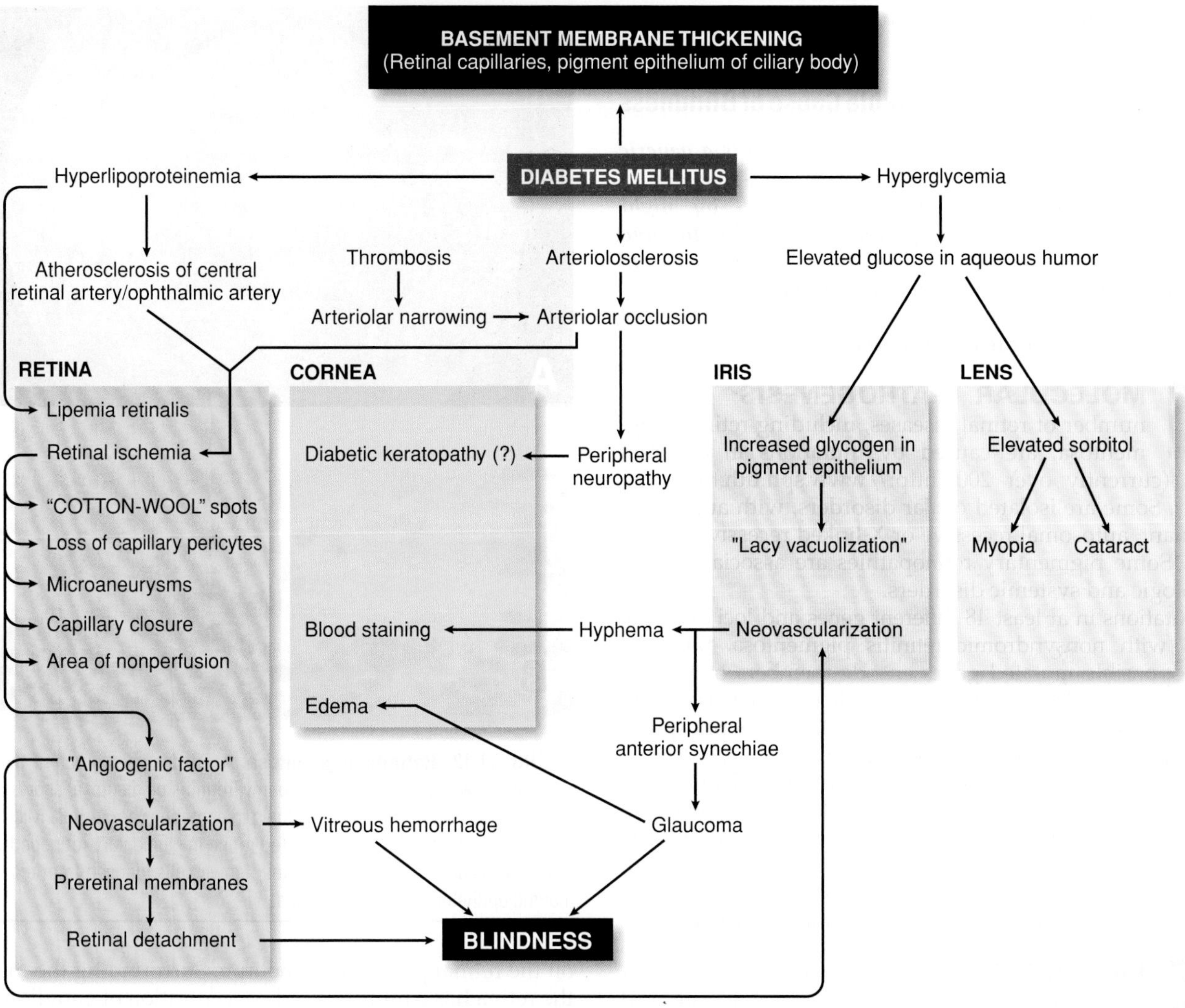

BASEMENT MEMBRANE THICKENING
(Retinal capillaries, pigment epithelium of ciliary body)

FIGURE 33-11. Effects of diabetes on the eye.

when these two layers become apposed. However, the sensory retina readily separates from the retinal pigment epithelium when fluid (liquid vitreous, hemorrhage or exudate) accumulates within the potential space between these structures. Such a separation is a common cause of visual impairment and blindness. Laser therapy and surgical approaches have greatly improved the prognosis for patients with detached retina.

ETIOLOGIC FACTORS: Retinal detachment follows intraocular hemorrhage (e.g., after trauma) and is a potential complication of cataract extractions and several other ocular operations. Factors predisposing to retinal detachment include retinal defects (due to trauma or certain retinal degenerations), vitreous traction, diminished pressure on the retina (e.g., after vitreous loss) and weakening of the fixation of the retina. Full-thickness holes in the retina are not complicated by retinal detachment unless liquid vitreous gains access to the potential space between the retina and the retinal pigment epithelium. Even then, some vitreoretinal traction seems to be necessary for retinal detachment to occur.

The photoreceptors and retinal pigment epithelium normally function as a unit. After they separate in a retinal detachment, oxygen and nutrients that normally reach the outer retina from the choroid must diffuse across a greater distance. This situation causes the photoreceptors to degenerate, after which cyst-like extracellular spaces appear within the retina.

 PATHOLOGY: Three varieties of retinal detachment are recognized: rhegmatogenous, tractional and exudative.

RHEGMATOGENOUS RETINAL DETACHMENT: This type of retinal detachment is associated with a retinal tear and also often with degenerative changes in the vitreous body or peripheral retina.

TRACTIONAL RETINAL DETACHMENT: In some cases of retinal detachment, the retina is pulled toward the center of the eye by adherent vitreoretinal adhesions, as occurs in proliferative diabetic retinopathy, in retinopathy of prematurity and after intraocular infection.

EXUDATIVE RETINAL DETACHMENT: Accumulation of fluid in the potential space between the sensory retina and the retinal pigment epithelium causes a detached retina in disorders such as choroiditis, choroidal hemangioma and choroidal melanoma.

Retinitis Pigmentosa Is a Heritable Cause of Blindness

Retinitis pigmentosa (pigmentary retinopathy) is a generic term that refers to a variety of bilateral, progressive, degenerative retinopathies characterized clinically by night blindness and constriction of peripheral visual fields and pathologically by loss of retinal photoreceptors (rods and cones) and pigment accumulation within the retina.

The term "retinitis" is a misnomer since inflammation of the retina is not a feature of this disease.

 **MOLECULAR PATHOGENESIS:** A large number of retinal diseases, including retinitis pigmentosa, are caused by mutations in different genes (currently over 200; http://www.sph.uth.tmc.edu/retnet). Some are isolated ocular disorders, with autosomal dominant, autosomal recessive or X-linked recessive inheritance. Some pigmentary retinopathies are associated with neurologic and systemic disorders.

Mutations in at least 48 different genes and loci are associated with nonsyndromic retinitis pigmentosa. Some of the responsible mutated genes encode members of the rod phototransduction cascade, such as rhodopsin (*RHO*) and rod photoreceptor cyclic guanosine 3′,5′-monophosphate (cGMP), phosphodiesterase α and β subunits (*PDE6A*, *PDE6B*) and photoreceptor structures such as peripherin. How defective proteins in the rod photoreceptors lead to retinitis pigmentosa and the eventual loss of cones remains incompletely understood, but presumably all responsible mutations ultimately cause the death of photoreceptors because of a convergence at a final common point in key metabolic pathways.

 PATHOLOGY: In retinitis pigmentosa, destruction of rods, and subsequently cones, is followed by migration of retinal pigment epithelial cells into the sensory retina (Fig. 33-12). Melanin appears within slender processes of spidery cells and accumulates mainly around small branching retinal blood vessels (especially in the equatorial portion of the retina), like spicules of bone. The retinal blood vessels then gradually attenuate, and the optic nerve head acquires a characteristic waxy pallor.

 CLINICAL FEATURES: The clinical manifestations of retinitis pigmentosa, including the appearance and distribution of the retinal pigmentation, vary with the causes of the retinopathy. Half of these patients have a family history of the disease. Those with autosomal recessive and X-linked disease are more severely affected and develop night blindness and peripheral field defects in childhood. Autosomal dominant forms of retinitis pigmentosa tend to be less severe, with symptoms beginning later in life. As the condition progresses, contraction of visual fields eventually leads to tunnel vision. Central vision is usually preserved until late in the course of the disease. In some cases, blindness follows macular involvement.

Macular Degeneration Is a Common Cause of Blindness in the Elderly

The center of the macula, the foveola, is the point of greatest visual acuity. In this area, a high concentration of cones rests

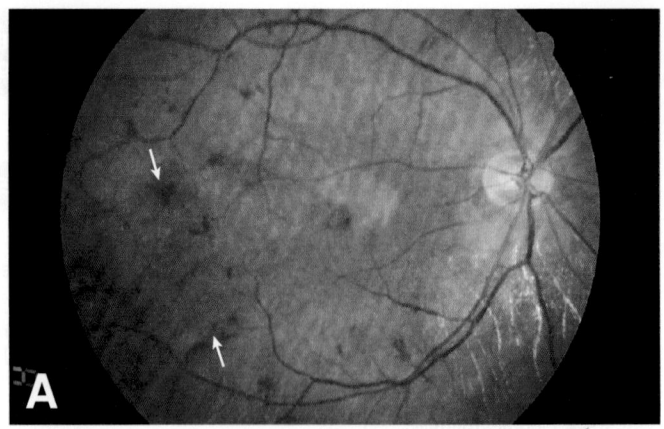

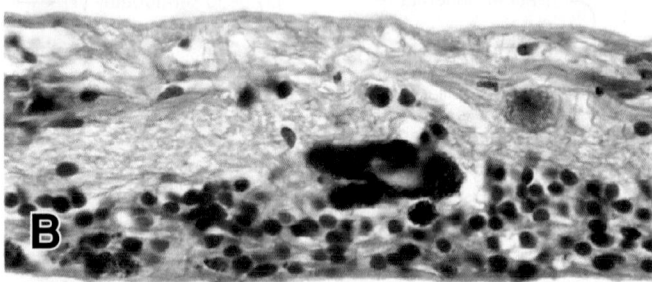

FIGURE 33-12. Retinitis pigmentosa. A. Fundus photograph of the retina of a patient with pigmentary retinopathy (retinitis pigmentosa) shows attenuated retinal vessels and foci of retinal pigmentation (*arrows*). **B.** Microscopic appearance of a severely degenerated retina in pigmentary retinopathy. Note the focal accumulations of pigmented, brown cells (derived from retinal pigmented epithelium) within the retina.

on the retinal pigment epithelium. Surrounding the macula, the retina has a multilayered concentration of ganglion cells. With aging, in certain drug toxicities (e.g., chloroquine) and in several inherited disorders, the macula degenerates, causing central vision to be impaired.

Age-related macular degeneration currently affects about 15 million people in the United States and is the most common cause of blindness among individuals of European descent older than age 65. Dry and wet forms of age-related macular degeneration are recognized. The wet variety of this disease accounts for 20% of cases and is associated with subretinal fibrovascular tissue and sometimes bleeding into the subretinal space. Laser photocoagulation and other intraocular antiangiogenic therapies are beneficial in this type of the disorder.

 ETIOLOGIC FACTORS: There is general agreement that age-related maculopathy is a multifactorial disease to which environmental and genetic factors contribute. Risk factors include advancing age, smoking, carotid/cardiovascular disease and elevated serum cholesterol levels.

 **MOLECULAR PATHOGENESIS:** A common missense variant of the *CFH* gene that encodes for complement factor H is a risk factor for about 50% of cases of age-related macular degeneration. A susceptibility to age-related macular degeneration has also been associated with mutations or single-nucleotide polymorphisms in *ABCA4* (formerly called *ABCR*), *FBLN5*,

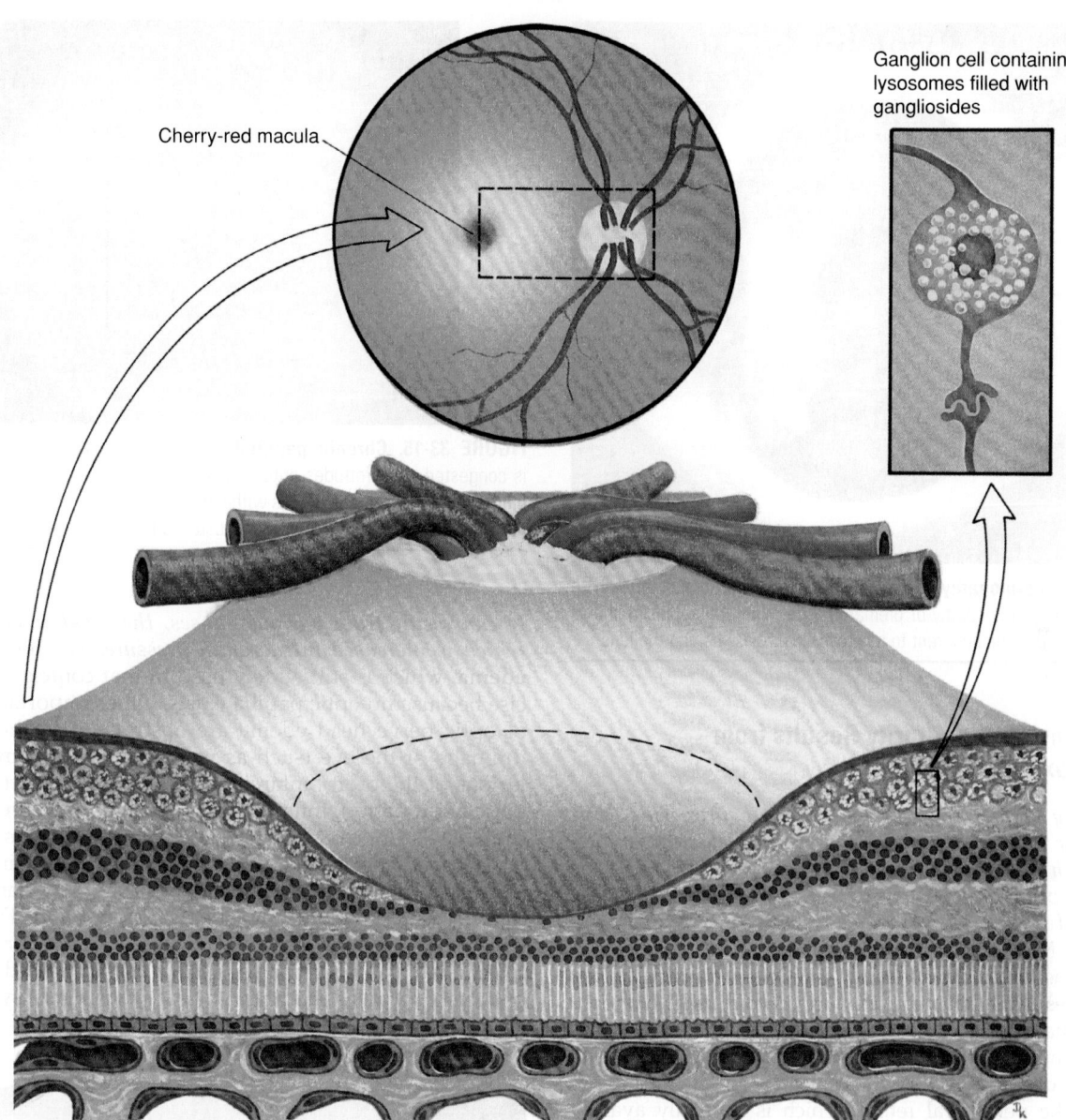

Ganglion cell containing
lysosomes filled with
gangliosides

Cherry-red macula

FIGURE 33-13. Cherry-red macula. A cherry-red spot appears at the macula in several lysosomal storage diseases that are characterized by intracytoplasmic accumulations within the retinal ganglion cells, such as Tay-Sachs disease, in which a particular ganglioside is stored (GM$_2$-ganglioside). The macula develops this appearance because the pallor created by the deposits within the multilayered ganglion cells enhances the visibility of the underlying normal choroidal vasculature.

FBLN6, C3, CST3, LOC387715, TLR4, ERCC6, RAXL1, HTRA1, CX3CR1 and *ESR1* genes and in a mitochondrial gene (*MTTL1*). *ABCA4* encodes a rod cell protein (rim protein) thought to be a transporter involved in molecular recycling. Mutations in this gene may allow degraded material **(drusen)** to accumulate and interfere with retinal function.

Lysosomal Storage Diseases Feature a Cherry-Red Spot at the Macula

In lysosomal storage diseases, including the gangliosidoses, myriad intracytoplasmic lysosomal inclusions within the multilayered ganglion cell layer of the macula impart a striking pallor to the affected retina. As a result, the central foveola appears bright red because of the underlying choroidal

vasculature (Fig. 33-13). As mentioned above, a cherry-red spot also occurs at the macula after central retinal artery occlusion because the pale, edematous retina highlights the subfoveolar vascular choroid.

Angioid Streaks Are Vessel-Like Fractures in the Bruch Membrane

Angioid streaks are seen when the posterior segment of the eye is examined clinically. This occurs when the Bruch membrane fractures, causing characteristic irregular lines that radiate beneath the retina from the optic nerve head **(angioid streaks)**. This happens spontaneously in a variety of systemic disorders, most commonly pseudoxanthoma elasticum, sickle cell disease and Paget disease of bone.

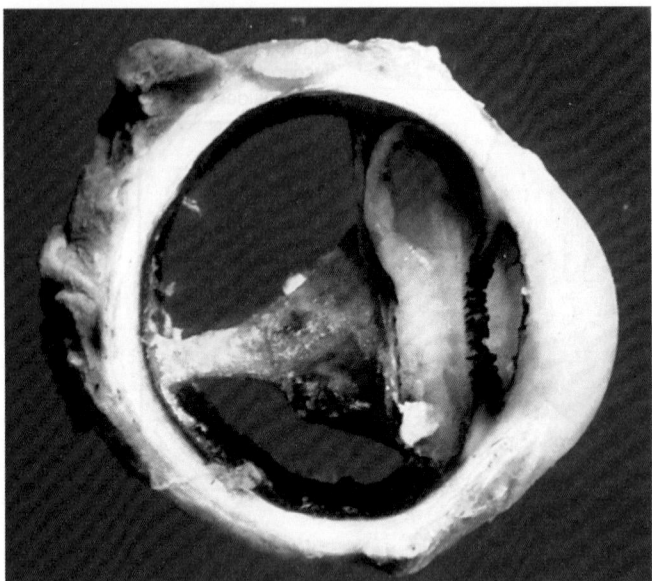

FIGURE 33-14. Retinopathy of prematurity. Horizontal section through an eye with advanced retinopathy of prematurity (retrolental fibroplasia) shows a totally detached retina adherent to a fibrovascular mass behind the lens.

Retinopathy of Prematurity Results from Oxygen Toxicity

Retinopathy of prematurity is a bilateral, iatrogenic, retinal disorder that occurs predominantly in premature infants treated with high levels of inspired oxygen after birth. The entity was originally called **retrolental fibroplasia** because of a mass of scarred tissue behind the lens in advanced cases (Fig. 33-14). More than a half century ago, retinopathy of prematurity was the leading cause of blindness in infants in the United States and many other developed countries. Retinopathy of prematurity is almost always restricted to premature infants administered high concentrations of oxygen. In such infants, the developing retinal blood vessels become obliterated, and the peripheral retina, which is normally avascular until the end of fetal life, does not vascularize. The more mature the retina, the less the vaso-obliterative effect of hyperoxia. When the infant eventually returns to ambient air, intense proliferation of vascular endothelium and glial cells begins at the junction of the avascular and vascularized portions of the retina. This becomes apparent 5–10 weeks after removal of the infant from the incubator and, as in diabetic retinopathy, is thought to result from the liberation of an angiogenic factor produced by the avascular and ischemic peripheral retina. This angiogenic factor is also believed to account for the neovascularization of the iris that sometimes accompanies retinopathy of prematurity. In 25% of cases, the retinopathy progresses to a scarring phase, characterized by retinal detachment, a fibrovascular mass behind the lens (retrolental) and blindness.

THE OPTIC NERVE

Optic Nerve Head Edema Often Reflects Increased Intracranial Pressure

Optic nerve head (optic disc) edema refers to swelling of the optic nerve head where the retinal axons leave the globe.

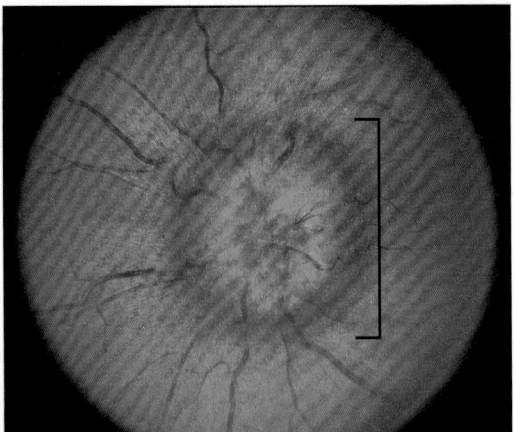

FIGURE 33-15. Chronic papilledema. The optic nerve head (*bracket*) is congested and protrudes anteriorly toward the interior of the eye. It has blurred margins, and the vessels within it are poorly seen. In contrast to acute papilledema, the veins are not so congested, and hemorrhage is not a feature.

It can result from various causes, the most important of which is increased intracranial pressure. The term **papilledema,** which is still widely used in that context, is imprecise because no optic papilla exists. Other important causes of optic nerve head edema are obstruction to the venous drainage of the eye (such as may occur with compressive lesions of the orbit), infarction of the optic nerve (ischemic optic neuropathy), inflammation of the optic nerve close to the eyeball (optic neuritis, papillitis) and multiple sclerosis.

Edema of the optic nerve head is characterized clinically by a swollen optic nerve head that displays blurred margins and dilated vessels (Fig. 33-15). Frequently, hemorrhages (Fig. 33-16), exudates and cotton-wool spots are seen, and concentric folds of the choroid and retina may surround the nerve head. Acutely, optic nerve head edema results in few, if any, visual symptoms. As the condition becomes established, swelling of the optic

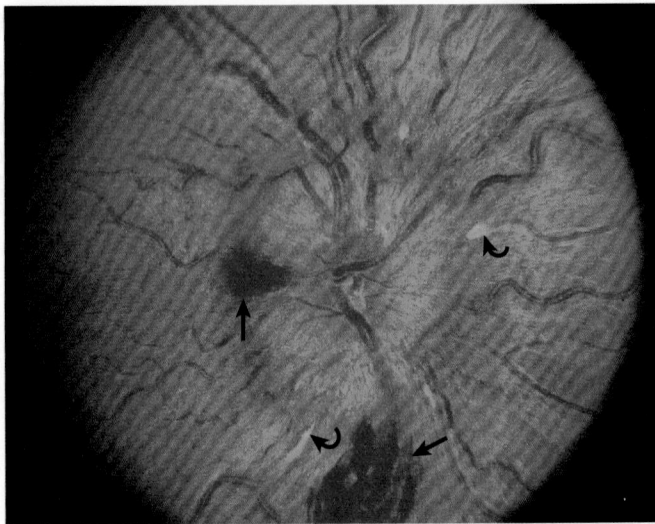

FIGURE 33-16. Hemorrhage in papilledema. The optic nerve head is markedly congested, with dilated veins and a blurred margin. A small hemorrhage is evident within the optic nerve head at its junction with the retina (*straight arrows*). Several small "cotton-wool spots" are present within the adjacent retina (*curved arrows*).

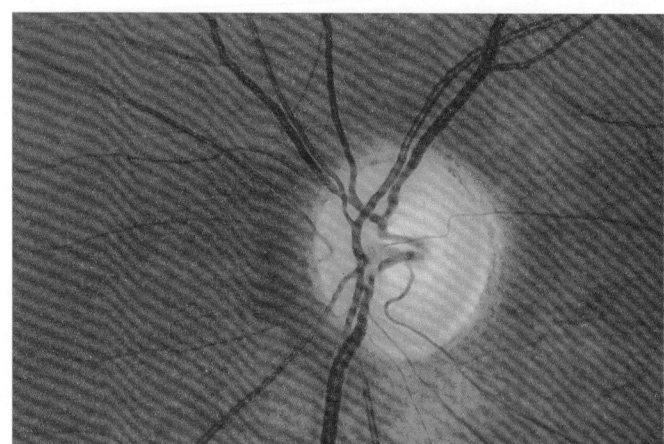

FIGURE 33-17. Optic atrophy. The margin of the optic nerve head is sharply demarcated from the adjacent retina. Because the myelinated axons in the optic nerve are markedly diminished, the optic nerve head appears much whiter than normal.

nerve head enlarges the normal blind spot. After many months, atrophic changes lead to loss of visual acuity.

Optic Atrophy Is a Thinning of the Optic Nerve Caused by Loss of Axons within Its Substance

The nerve axons within the optic nerve are lost in many conditions, including long-standing edema of the optic nerve head, optic neuritis, optic nerve compression, glaucoma and retinal degeneration.

 **ETIOLOGIC FACTORS:** Optic atrophy can also be caused by some drugs, such as ethambutol and isoniazid. The optic nerve head is usually flat and pale in optic atrophy (Fig. 33-17), but when this disorder follows glaucoma, the optic nerve head is excavated **(glaucomatous cupping)**.

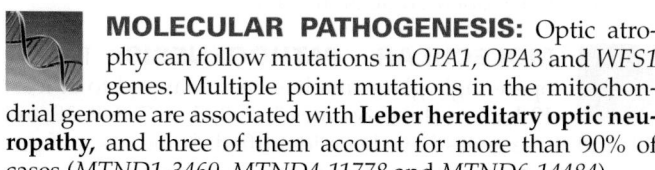 **MOLECULAR PATHOGENESIS:** Optic atrophy can follow mutations in *OPA1, OPA3* and *WFS1* genes. Multiple point mutations in the mitochondrial genome are associated with **Leber hereditary optic neuropathy,** and three of them account for more than 90% of cases (*MTND1-3460, MTND4-11778* and *MTND6-14484*).

GLAUCOMA

Glaucoma refers to a collection of disorders that feature an optic neuropathy accompanied by a characteristic progressive loss of visual field sensitivity and eventual excavation of the optic nerve head. In most cases, glaucoma is produced by increased intraocular pressure **(ocular hypertension)**; however, increased intraocular pressure does not necessarily cause glaucoma, and not all patients with glaucoma have elevated intraocular pressure.

After being produced by the ciliary body, the aqueous humor enters the posterior chamber (the space between the iris and the zonules) before passing through the pupil to the anterior chamber (between the iris and the cornea). From that site, it drains into veins by way of the trabecular meshwork and the canal of Schlemm (Fig. 33-18). A delicate balance

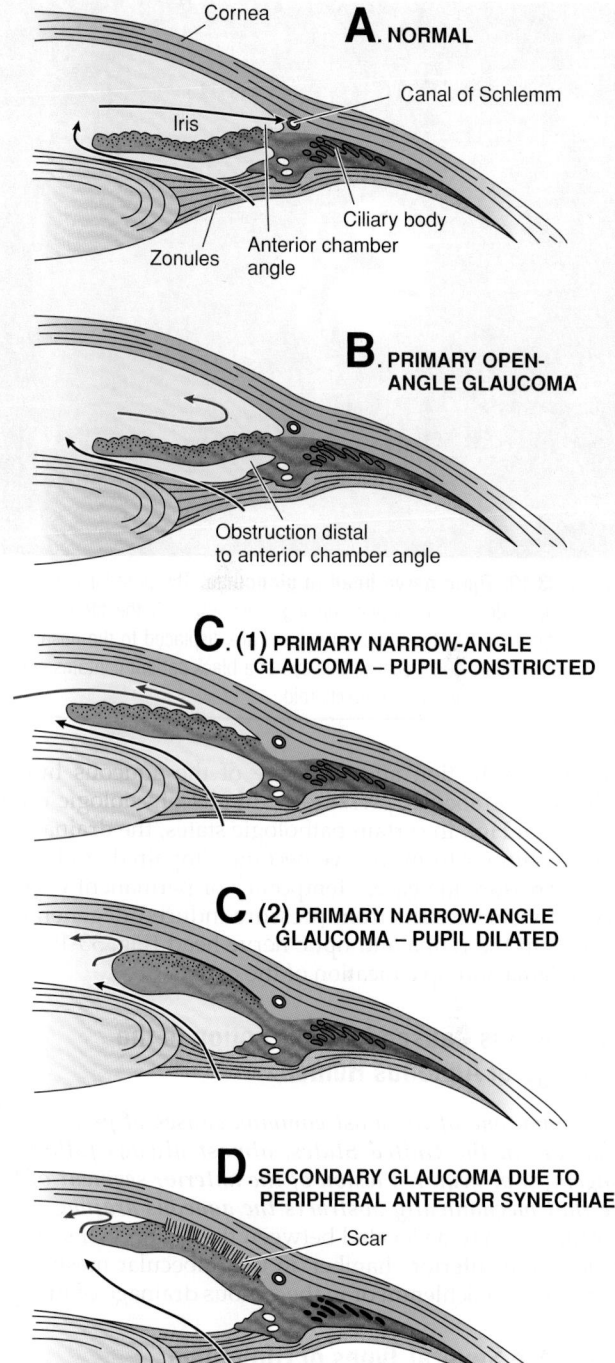

FIGURE 33-18. Pathogenesis of glaucoma. The anterior segment of the eye is affected differently in various forms of glaucoma. **A.** Structure of the normal eye. **B.** In primary open-angle glaucoma, the obstruction to the aqueous outflow is distal to the anterior chamber angle, and the anterior segment resembles that of the normal eye. **C.** In primary narrow-angle glaucoma, the anterior chamber angle is open, but narrower than normal when the pupil is constricted **(C1)**. When the pupil becomes dilated in such an eye, the thickened iris obstructs the anterior chamber angle **(C2)**, causing increased intraocular pressure. **D.** The anterior chamber angle can become obstructed by a variety of pathologic processes, including an adhesion between the iris and the posterior surface of the cornea **(peripheral anterior synechiae)**.

THE EYE

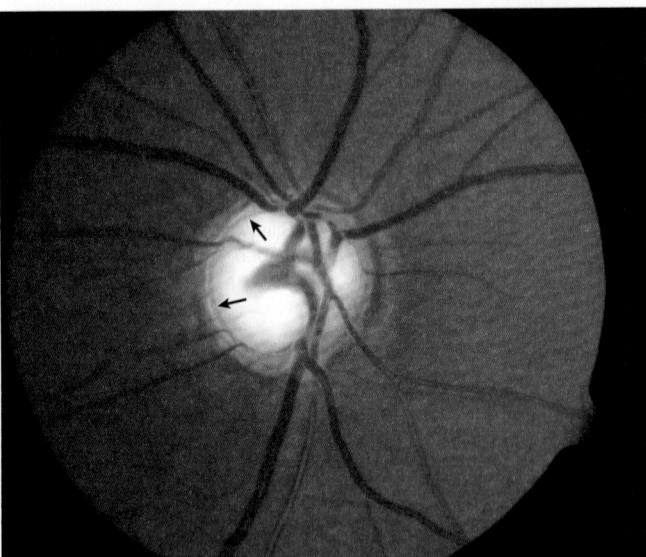

FIGURE 33-19. Optic nerve head in glaucoma. The anterior part of the optic nerve is depressed ("optic cupping"; *arrows*), and the blood vessels crossing the margin of the optic nerve head are displaced to the nasal side. The fundus appears dark because this eye of a black patient contains numerous pigmented melanocytes in the choroid.

between production and drainage of the aqueous humor maintains intraocular pressure within its physiologic range (10–20 mm Hg). In certain pathologic states, the drainage of aqueous humor from the eye becomes impaired, and intraocular pressure increases. Temporary or permanent impairment of vision results from pressure-induced degenerative changes in the retina and optic nerve head (Fig. 33-19) and from edema and opacification of the cornea.

Glaucoma Is Caused by Obstruction to the Drainage of Aqueous Humor

Glaucoma, one of the most common causes of preventable blindness in the United States, almost always follows a congenital or acquired lesion of the anterior segment of the eye that mechanically obstructs the aqueous drainage. The obstruction may be located between the iris and lens, in the angle of the anterior chamber, in the trabecular meshwork, in the canal of Schlemm or in the venous drainage of the eye.

There Are Several Types of Glaucoma

Congenital Glaucoma (Infantile Glaucoma, Buphthalmos)

Congenital glaucoma is caused by obstruction to aqueous drainage by developmental anomalies. This type of glaucoma develops even though intraocular pressure may not increase until early infancy or childhood. Most cases of congenital glaucoma occur in boys (65%), and an X-linked recessive mode of inheritance is common. The developmental anomaly usually involves both eyes and, although often limited to the angle of the anterior chamber, it may be accompanied by a variety of other ocular malformations. Congenital glaucoma is associated with a deep anterior chamber, corneal cloudiness, sensitivity to bright lights **(photophobia)**, excessive tearing and buphthalmos. The term **buphthalmos**

(from the Greek *bous*, "ox"; *ophthalmos*, "eye") describes the enlarged eyes of patients with congenital glaucoma that result from expansion caused by increased intraocular pressure beneath a pliable sclera.

 **MOLECULAR PATHOGENESIS:** Several genes for primary congenital glaucoma have been identified. Homozygous mutations in the cytochrome P4501B1 gene (*CYP1B1*) account for some cases of autosomal recessive primary infantile glaucoma. Congenital glaucoma associated with developmental anomalies of the eye (secondary congenital glaucoma) results from mutations in the fork-head transcription factor gene (*FOXC1*), pituitary homeobox 2 gene (*PITX2*) or paired box 6 gene (*PAX6*).

Adult-Onset Primary Glaucoma

Adult-onset primary glaucoma develops in a person with no apparent underlying eye disease. It is subdivided into **primary open-angle glaucoma** (in which the anterior chamber angle is open and appears normal) and **primary closed-angle glaucoma** (in which the anterior chamber is shallower than normal, and the angle is abnormally narrow) (Fig. 33-18).

Primary Open-Angle Glaucoma
Primary open-angle glaucoma is the most frequent type of glaucoma and a major cause of blindness in the United States. It affects 1%–3% of the population older than 40 years and occurs principally in the sixth decade. The angle of the anterior chamber is open and appears normal, but there is increased resistance to the outflow of the aqueous humor in the vicinity of the canal of Schlemm. The intraocular pressure increases insidiously and asymptomatically, and although almost always bilateral, one eye may be affected more severely than the other. With time, damage to the retina and optic nerve causes irreversible loss of vision.

 **ETIOLOGIC FACTORS:** Persons with diabetes mellitus and myopia have increased risk of primary open-angle glaucoma.

 **MOLECULAR PATHOGENESIS:** Primary open-angle glaucoma has been mapped to at least 13 loci on chromosomes 1, 2, 3, 5, 6, 7, 8, 9, 10 and 20, and three genes have been identified. Some cases of primary open-angle glaucoma are due to numerous different mutations in the *MYOC* (*TGRR*) gene on chromosome 1 (1q21-q31). Primary open-angle glaucoma can occur as a manifestation of the nail–patella syndrome, in association with mutations in the Lim homeobox transcription factor-1 (*LMX1B*) gene. Juvenile-onset primary open-angle glaucoma may result from mutations in the *CRYP1B1*, *FKHL7*, *MYOC* and *OPTN* genes.

Primary Closed-Angle Glaucoma
Primary closed-angle glaucoma, differentiated from open-angle glaucoma above, occurs after age 40 years. *It is the predominant form of primary glaucoma in adults living in Asia.*

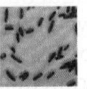 **ETIOLOGIC FACTORS:** The disorder afflicts persons whose peripheral iris is displaced anteriorly toward the trabecular meshwork, thereby creating an abnormally narrow anterior chamber angle. When the pupil is constricted (miotic), the iris remains stretched so

that the chamber angle is not occluded. However, when the pupil dilates (mydriasis), the iris obstructs the drainage of aqueous humor from the eye, resulting in sudden episodes of intraocular hypertension. This is accompanied by ocular pain, and halos or rings are seen around lights. In such persons, intraocular pressure may also increase if the pupil becomes blocked (e.g., by a swollen lens) and aqueous humor accumulates in the posterior chamber.

 MOLECULAR PATHOGENESIS: Primary closed-angle glaucoma has a familial predisposition, but in contrast to primary open-angle glaucoma, genetic loci have not yet been identified.

 CLINICAL FEATURES: *Acute closed-angle glaucoma is an ocular emergency, and it is essential to start ocular hypotensive treatment within the first 24–48 hours if vision is to be maintained.* Primary closed-angle glaucoma affects both eyes, but it may become apparent in one eye 2–5 years before it is noted in the other. The intraocular pressure is normal between attacks, but after many episodes, adhesions form between the iris and the trabecular meshwork and cornea **(peripheral anterior synechiae)** and accentuate the block to the outflow of aqueous humor.

Low-Tension Glaucoma

In low-tension glaucoma, the characteristic visual field defect and all of the ophthalmoscopic features of chronic open-angle glaucoma occur, but without increased intraocular pressure. The characteristic visual field defect and all of the ophthalmoscopic features of chronic simple (open-angle) glaucoma often occur in elderly people who do not show increased intraocular pressure.

 **ETIOLOGIC FACTORS:** Although some eyes may be hypersensitive to normal intraocular pressure, many cases of low-tension glaucoma probably represent an infarction of the optic nerve head. Susceptibility to normal tension glaucoma is associated with an intronic polymorphism of the *OPA1* gene, as well as with a mutation in the *OPTN* gene.

Secondary Glaucoma

In secondary glaucoma, anterior chamber angles may be open or closed. Because the underlying disorder is usually limited to one eye, secondary glaucoma tends to be unilateral. There are numerous causes of secondary glaucoma including inflammation, hemorrhage, neovascularization of the iris and adhesions.

Effects of Increased Intraocular Pressure

Prolonged ocular hypertension has several effects on the eye:

- In adults, increased intraocular pressure leads to a characteristic cupped excavation of the optic nerve head (glaucomatous cupping), accompanied by a nasal displacement of the retinal blood vessels. In infants, cupping of the optic nerve head tends to be less prominent (Fig. 33-19).
- The cornea or sclera bulges at weak points, such as sites of scars in the outer coat of the eye.

- Optic atrophy, with loss of axons, gliosis and thickening of the pial septa, follows the retinal degeneration and damage to the nerve fibers at the optic nerve head.
- The ganglion cell and nerve fiber layers of the retina degenerate, thereby impairing vision. The outer retina, which derives its nutrition from the underlying choroid, remains intact.
- When intraocular pressure is increased in a child younger than 3 years of age, the pliable eye sometimes enlarges extensively (buphthalmos). After the first few years of life, a rigid sclera prevents glaucomatous eyes from enlarging under the increased pressure.

MYOPIA

Myopia (also called "nearsightedness") is a refractive ocular abnormality in which light from the visualized object focuses at a point in front of the retina because of a longer than usual anteroposterior diameter of the eye. Myopia affects more than 70 million persons in the United States and is the most common clinically significant disorder of the eye. In Asia, it affects an even greater percentage of the population. Treatment requires refractive correction. In addition to glasses and contact lenses, refractive surgery using an excimer laser such as laser-assisted in situ keratomileusis (LASIK) and laser epithelial keratomileusis (LASEK) are popular. Myopia usually begins in young persons and varies in severity. A mild form (stationary or simple myopia) is generally nonprogressive after cessation of body growth, whereas a genetically determined "progressive myopia" is more severe.

 **ETIOLOGIC FACTORS AND MOLECULAR PATHOGENESIS:** There is strong evidence to implicate excessive accommodation from reading and other near work in childhood in the pathogenesis of myopia. In childhood, the vast majority of human eyes with myopia adjust their axial length to the refraction by the anterior segment of the eye **(emmetropization),** and studies in animal models indicate that emmetropization mechanisms elongate the eye. Some nonsyndromic inherited types have been mapped to 14 different loci on various chromosomes. Myopia is also a feature of several systemic diseases, including some disorders of fibrillin (Marfan syndrome), collagen (Stickler syndrome, Knobloch syndrome) and perlecan (Schwartz-Jampel syndrome type I).

PHTHISIS BULBI

Phthisis bulbi refers to a nonspecific, end-stage eye that is disorganized and atrophic. This condition (Fig. 33-20) is most common after trauma to, or inflammation of, the eye. Eyes afflicted with phthisis bulbi are often enucleated. The eye is small and often extremely hard owing to intraocular ossification. The choroid and ciliary body are separated from the sclera, which is thickened, wrinkled and indented owing to loss of intraocular pressure. The cornea is flattened, shrunken and opaque. Intraocular contents are disorganized by diffuse scarring and detachment of the sensory retina is invariably encountered. If present, the lens is displaced and

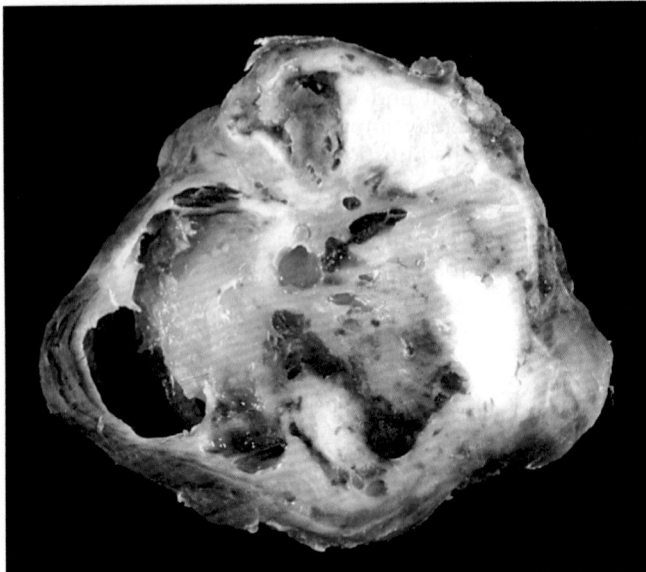

FIGURE 33-20. Phthisis bulbi. Section through an eye with phthisis bulbi, exemplifying the markedly disorganized nature of the intraocular contents of such atrophic disordered globes.

often calcified. A typical finding in phthisis bulbi is intraocular bone formation, which may be derived from the hyperplastic pigment epithelium.

OCULAR NEOPLASMS

The eye and adjacent structures contain a large number of cell types, and as one might expect, benign and malignant neoplasms arise from them. *Intraocular neoplasms arise mostly from immature retinal neurons (retinoblastoma) and uveal melanocytes (melanoma).* Although the retinal pigment epithelium often undergoes reactive proliferation, it seldom becomes neoplastic.

Malignant Melanoma Arises from Melanocytes in the Uvea

Malignant melanoma is the most common primary intraocular malignancy. It may arise from melanocytes in any part of the eye, the choroid being the most common site.

 PATHOLOGY: Choroidal melanomas are mostly circumscribed and commonly invade the Bruch membrane, causing a mushroom-shaped mass (Fig. 33-21). By contrast, some tumors are flat (diffuse melanoma) and cause a gradual deterioration of vision over many years. Some do not become apparent until extraocular dissemination has occurred. Orange lipofuscin pigment is sometimes evident over the surface of some choroidal melanomas.

Microscopically, uveal melanomas may be composed mainly of variable numbers of spindle-shaped cells without nucleoli (spindle A cells), spindle-shaped cells with prominent nucleoli (spindle B cells), polygonal cells with distinct cell borders and prominent nucleoli (epithelioid cells) or a fourth cell type that is similar to epithelioid cells but smaller with indistinct cell borders.

Melanomas of the ciliary body and iris may extend circumferentially around the globe (ring melanoma). Melanomas in the iris are usually diagnosed clinically one to two decades earlier than those in the choroid and ciliary body, perhaps because they are more easily seen and are often first observed by the patient.

Lymphatic spread does not occur because the eye has no lymphatic vessels. Aside from hematogenous spread, uveal melanomas disseminate by traversing the sclera to enter the orbital tissues, usually at sites where blood vessels and nerves pass through the sclera. The liver is a common site of metastases, and anecdotally, the diagnosis of metastatic ocular melanoma can be made intuitively by astute clinicians who discover an enlarged liver in a patient with a "glass eye."

 CLINICAL FEATURES: Intraocular melanomas may cause cataract, glaucoma, retinal detachment, inflammation and hemorrhage. The options for

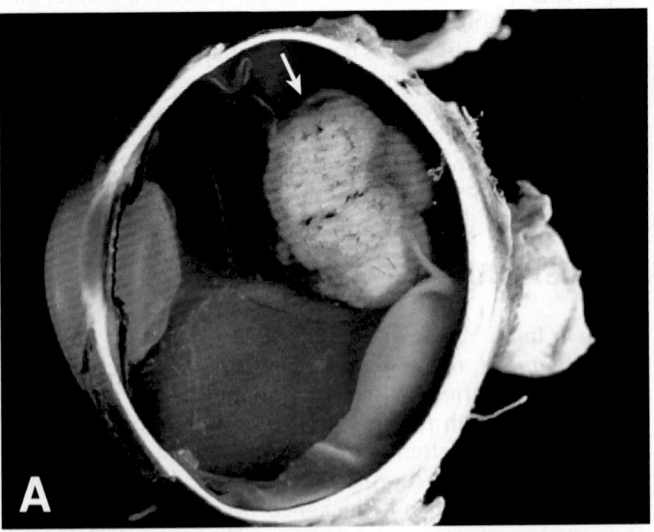

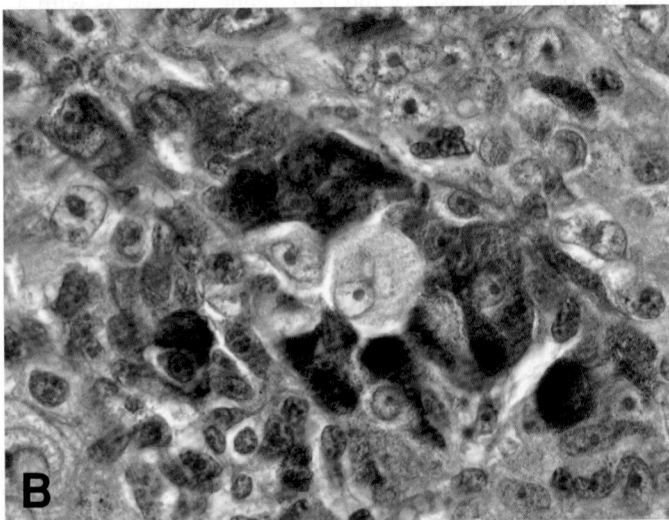

FIGURE 33-21. Malignant melanoma. A. A mushroom-shaped melanoma of the choroid is present in this eye (*arrow*). Choroidal melanomas commonly invade through the Bruch membrane and result in this appearance. **B.** Photomicrograph of a heavily pigmented melanoma of the choroid depicting epithelioid tumor cells with prominent nucleoli.

treating uveal melanomas include enucleation of the eye, radiotherapy and local excision. More than half of patients with uveal melanomas survive for 15 years after enucleation. Prognostic factors include tumor size, tumor location and cell type. Unfavorable indicators are tumor hyperploidy, high mitotic activity, high microvascular density, high tumor-infiltrating lymphocyte counts, chromosome 3 monosomy and high serum melanoma inhibitory activity protein. Deaths have been reported within 5 years from spindle A melanomas, but tumors composed purely of epithelioid cells have the worst prognosis.

Retinoblastomas Originate from Immature Neurons

Retinoblastoma is the most common intraocular malignant neoplasm of childhood, affecting 1 in 20,000 to 1 in 34,000 children. It occurs most frequently within the first 2 years of life and may even be found at birth. Most retinoblastomas occur sporadically and are unilateral. Some 6%–8% of retinoblastomas are inherited. Up to 25% of sporadic retinoblastomas and most inherited retinoblastomas are bilateral.

MOLECULAR PATHOGENESIS: Retinoblastomas are related to inherited or acquired deletions of, or mutations in, the retinoblastoma (*Rb*) tumor suppressor gene, located on the long arm of chromosome 13 (13q14) (see Chapter 5). Some patients with retinoblastoma have homologous genomic mutations in the *Rb* gene. Others have a single genomic mutation but the tumors possess an additional one.

PATHOLOGY: Some retinoblastomas grow toward the vitreous body and can be seen with an ophthalmoscope (**endophytic retinoblastoma**). Others extend between the sensory retina and the retinal pigment epithelium, thereby detaching the retina (**exophytic retinoblastoma**). A few retinoblastomas are both endophytic and exophytic. Rarely, a retinoblastoma spreads diffusely within the retina without forming an obvious mass (**diffuse retinoblastoma**). The retina often contains several distinct foci of tumor in the same eye, some of which represent a multifocal origin, whereas others are tumor implants from dissemination through the vitreous body.

Retinoblastoma is a cream-colored tumor that contains scattered, chalky white, calcified flecks within yellow necrotic zones (Fig. 33-22), which may be detected radiologically. The tumors are intensely cellular and display several morphologic patterns. In some instances, densely packed, round neoplastic cells with hyperchromatic nuclei, scant cytoplasm and abundant mitoses are randomly distributed. In other retinoblastomas, the cells are arranged radially around a central cavity (**Flexner-Wintersteiner rosettes**), as they differentiate toward photoreceptors. In some cases, the cellular arrangement resembles a fleur-de-lis (**fleurette**). Viable tumor cells align themselves around blood vessels, and necrotic areas with calcification are seen a short distance from the vascularized regions.

Retinoblastomas disseminate by several routes. They commonly extend into the optic nerve, from where they spread intracranially. They also invade blood vessels, especially in the highly vascular choroid, before metastasizing

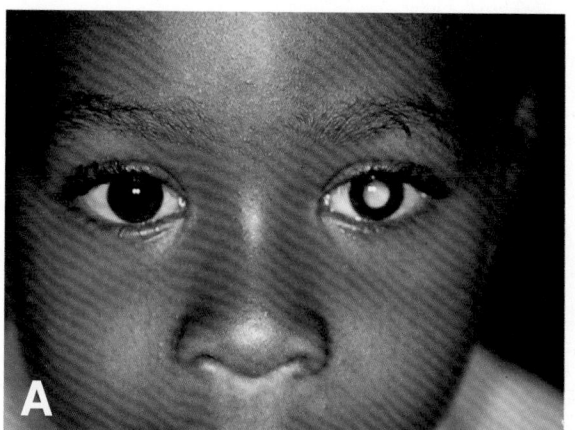

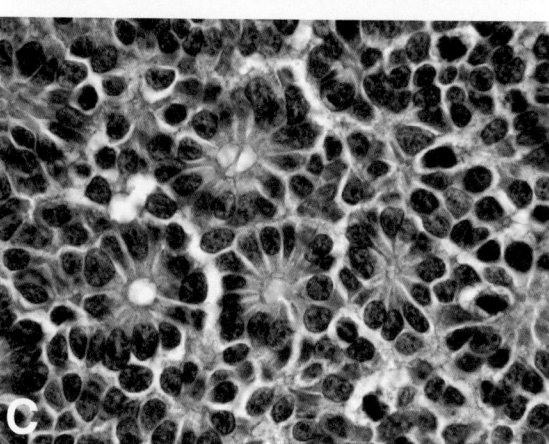

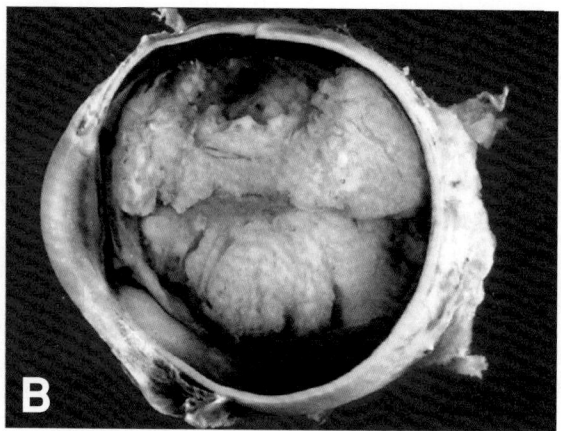

FIGURE 33-22. Retinoblastoma. A. The white pupil (leukocoria) in the left eye is the result of an intraocular retinoblastoma. **B.** This surgically excised eye is almost filled by a cream-colored intraocular retinoblastoma with calcified flecks. **C.** Light microscopic view of a retinoblastoma showing Flexner-Wintersteiner rosettes characterized by cells that are arranged around a central cavity.

hematogenously throughout the body. Bone marrow is a common site of blood-borne metastases, but surprisingly, the lung is rarely involved.

 CLINICAL FEATURES: Presenting signs include a white pupil (leukocoria), squint (strabismus), poor vision, spontaneous hyphema or a red, painful eye. Secondary glaucoma is a frequent complication. Light entering the eye commonly reflects a yellowish color similar to that from the tapetum of a cat (cat's eye reflex).

Retinoblastomas are almost always fatal if left untreated. However, with early diagnosis and modern therapy, survival is high (about 90%). Rarely, spontaneous regression occurs for reasons that remain unknown. Patients with inherited retinoblastomas, presumably as a consequence of the loss of *Rb* gene function, show increased susceptibility to other malignant tumors, including osteogenic sarcoma, Ewing sarcoma and pinealoblastoma.

Metastatic Tumors to the Eye Are More Common Than Primary Ocular Neoplasms

Sometimes an ocular metastasis may be the initial clinical manifestation of a cancer, but most cases are diagnosed only after death. Leukemias and cancers of the breast and lung usually metastasize to the posterior choroid and account for most cases of intraocular metastases. Neuroblastoma frequently metastasizes to the orbit in infancy and childhood. The orbit may be invaded by malignant neoplasms of the eyelid, conjunctiva, paranasal sinuses, nose, nasopharynx and intracranial cavity.

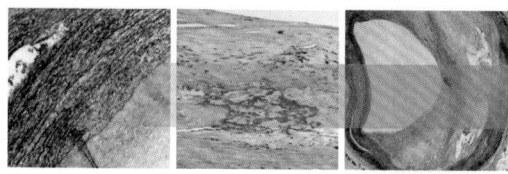

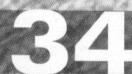

Forensic Pathology

Marc S. Micozzi

The Manner of Death
Cause of Death versus Mechanism of Death

Evidence Analyzed by the Forensic Pathologist
Traumatic Injuries
Sharp Force and Incised Wounds
Blunt Force Trauma
Death Occurring before a "Fatal" Accident

Determination of Timing and Order of Receiving Wounds
Asphyxiation

Accident versus Homicide versus Suicide
Cutting
Motor Vehicles
Gunshot Wounds
Drug Overdose

Hanging
Poisonings
Electrical Injury and Lightning Strikes

Timing of Death
Body Temperature
Lividity
Rigor
Decomposition
Disarticulation

Forensic pathology is the specialty in which pathological examinations and related investigations are conducted for the purposes of classifying the cause and manner of death. A related goal is the establishment of the time since death, which may range from minutes to days to years.

There are many observations of the deceased body that are made at the gross level and that cannot be documented by microscopic examination. Examples are the nature of traumatic injuries and the presence, location, size and extent of a pulmonary embolism. Whereas gross pathology is always part of the autopsy examination, the forensic pathologist may or may not pursue further microscopic examination, depending upon the nature of the case and the evidence. This chapter presents a summary of frequent problems in the practice of forensic pathology.

THE MANNER OF DEATH

The causes of death are multiple, but the manner is classified into only five categories: (1) accident, (2) homicide, (3) suicide, (4) natural and (5) undetermined/unclassified.

Most of the cases that fall under medical examiner jurisdiction actually support areas beyond or outside public safety. Only about 20% of cases are **homicides**. A rule of thumb is that the rate of **suicide** is double the rate of homicide (except in excessively violent, crime-ridden jurisdictions). In most locations, about 1/2 of **accidents** relate to motor vehicle accidents and traffic fatalities, whereas the other 1/2 are industrial accidents and those in the home or in recreational settings. In terms of **natural** causes of death occurring outside the presence of a treating physician, these investigations are often important in identifying acute or chronic threats to public health, such as infectious disease outbreaks, contaminated water supplies, accidental poisonings or other toxic exposures.

Cause of Death versus Mechanism of Death

Both resident and practicing physicians frequently complete a death certification incorrectly stating "cardiopulmonary" arrest as the cause of death. However, cardiopulmonary arrest is not a cause of death but a final common pathway whereby the underlying disease process finally leads to cessation of vital signs. The mechanism of cardiopulmonary arrest may be precipitated by (1) an event that causes respiratory arrest, evolving rapidly to cardiac arrest; (2) a fatal occurrence causing cardiac arrest, leading rapidly to respiratory arrest; or (3) a fatal central nervous system (CNS) injury that rapidly causes cessation of vital functions in both the heart and lungs. Through the intervention of respiratory ventilation therapy and cardiac electroversion, an otherwise fatal CNS event leading to "brain death" may not immediately cause physiologic death.

Causes of true sudden death, whereby an otherwise healthy ambulatory person suddenly "drops dead in his tracks," are relatively few. In the forensic context, a sudden gunshot wound (GSW) to the base of the brain will produce immediate cessation of vital functions; a similar wound to the heart can immobilize the organ. Medically, a pulmonary embolism may cause sudden death (see Chapter 7). A massive myocardial infarction brought about suddenly by coronary occlusion (see Chapter 7) may inactivate the conduction system and evoke an arrhythmia.

EVIDENCE ANALYZED BY THE FORENSIC PATHOLOGIST

Traumatic Injuries

Traumatic injuries result from incidents such as violent assaults upon one person by another, by encounters with

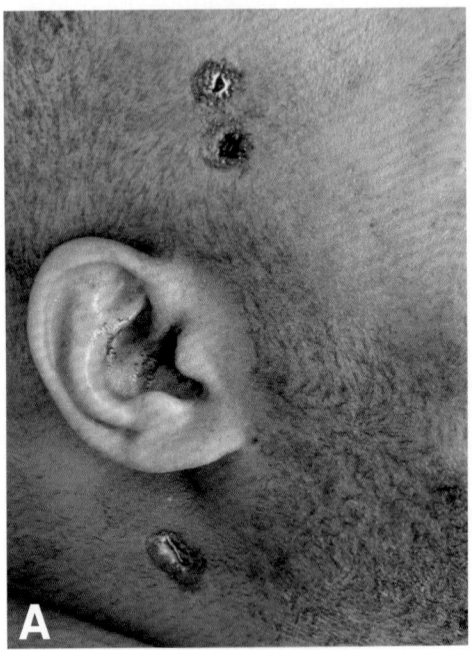
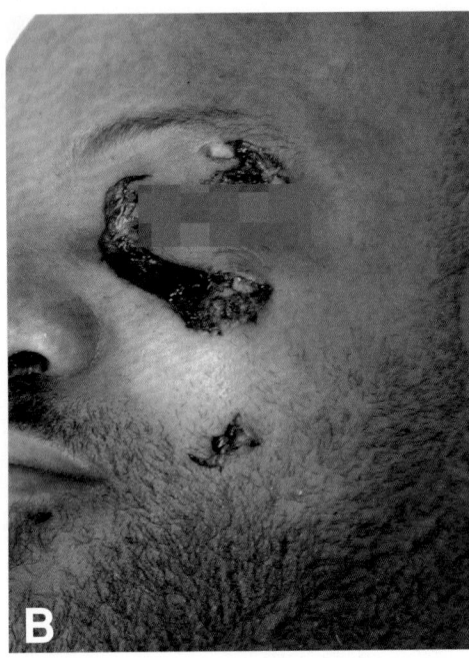

FIGURE 34-1. Entrance wounds **(A)** and exit wounds **(B)** on the right and left sides of the face, respectively, of this 39-year-old man with multiple gunshot wounds. The smaller entrances show a round to oval skin defect surrounded by abrasion rings. The exits are irregular lacerations, generally larger than the entrances, and lack a surrounding abrasion.

machinery at high velocity or by random physical forces and gravity. Fatal assaults are usually carried out with weapons such as (1) firearms, knives and other bladed weapons; (2) blunt objects of various kinds; and (3) occasionally only fists and other hard bodily surfaces such as feet, knees, elbows or even the forehead. Hard contact against a hard surface such as concrete is occasionally fatal.

Gunshot Wounds

GSWs actually represent only a small proportion of the work of a forensic pathologist. In densely populated areas, most fatal assaults with firearms involves handguns or small arms. Such weapons are really only useful at shorter ranges, and much of the forensic work involves identifying the distance between the muzzle of the firearm and the entrance wound.

There are basically two types of GSW, namely (1) penetrating wounds in which the projectile enters the body but does not exit and (2) perforating wounds in which the projectile passes through the body, creating both entrance and exit wounds (Fig. 34-1). Cases have been described in which a man supposedly died of natural causes and had been buried without an autopsy. An x-ray of the exhumed body later pointed out the presence of a projectile in the chest caviy.

Rifling

The barrels of modern firearms are rifled, and the markings or striations on the sides of the round projectile shaft can be compared to the weapon used in the assault. Test shots are fired into a tank of water and compared to the striations on a projectile recovered from the body. These markings can then be matched precisely.

Gunpowder residue may be recovered from the assailant if the hands are swabbed in a timely fashion. In the case of a suspected suicide by small firearm, one expects to find gunpowder remains on the dominant hand of the deceased.

Caliber

Small caliber wounds (e.g., a .22 caliber) can be fatal, especially in the case of head wounds. A small caliber projectile frequently penetrates the skull, but without the force to perforate the back of the skull, it may ricochet or "rattle around" within the skull, causing extensive brain damage. Likewise, the ability of a projectile to traverse and exit a body partially depends on whether or not it encounters bone, especially dense cortical bone, as in the mandible.

Notwithstanding the above considerations, the amount of damage caused by a projectile is directly related to its caliber (mass) and its velocity, thus momentum. The larger and heavier the projectile, the larger its momentum. Traveling at high velocity, a bullet transfers the force to the tissues of the body, causing tissue disruption. In the head, in addition to the focal injury in the path of the projectile, there is diffuse injury throughout the brain due to compression, stretching and tearing at the microscopic level, owing to the "shock wave" within an enclosed space. With penetrating wounds, exit wounds are larger and more irregular than the smaller and rounder entrance wounds.

Range

At extremely close range (contact wound), with the muzzle pressed against the skin, there may be stellate lesions, with star-shaped defects extending from the borders of the wound owing to expansion of hot gases from the barrel trapped in the enclosed space. There may also be a muzzle burn mark around the perimeter of the wound from heat of the metal (Fig. 34-2).

At close range, where the muzzle is separated from the surface of the skin, there tends to be stippling in a perimeter around the wound (Fig. 34-3). In this situation, the heated detritus that exits from the barrel along with the projectile reaches the surface of the skin. These particles expand out of the barrel of the firearm following the inverse square law for expanding particles from a point source; the perimeter of the stippling increases as the square of the distance from the

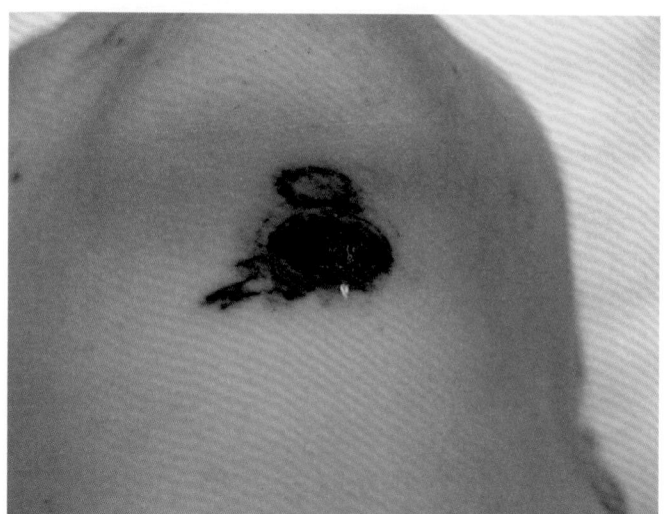

FIGURE 34-2. A muzzle imprint surrounds the entrance wound under the chin in a self-inflicted gunshot wound to the head.

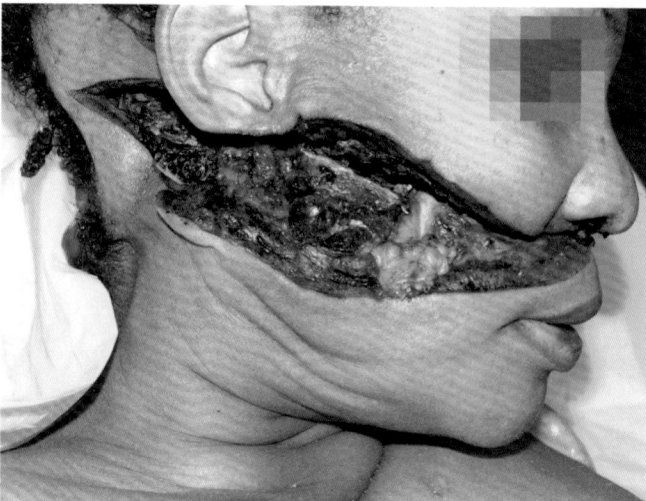

FIGURE 34-4. A single, deep-cutting wound using a samurai sword is on the right side of the face of this 34-year-old woman.

gun barrel increases. Ultimately, there comes a point where the particles do not reach the surface of the skin at all in a long- or mid-range wound.

The wounds caused by a shotgun (especially with a "sawed-off" or intentionally shortened barrel) also follow a pattern dictated by the inverse square law. The shotgun pellets describe a larger perimeter of entrance wounds as the distance from the barrel increases, owing to the dispersal of the pellets from the barrel of the shotgun.

Gunshot Wounds to the Head

GSWs to the head present a special case because projectiles enter a closed space. Energy, heat and gases expand rapidly within the skull, causing extensive damage beyond the actual pathway of the projectile. The expansion causes ejection of blood and tissue through both entrance and exit wounds. Another force that also occurs with blunt trauma to the skull, or when there is no exit wound, is the "contra-coup" injury on the contralateral side of the "coup" (strike or hit). This results in damage to the brain against the skull

opposite to the site of the blow or entry. Within the closed space of the skull, bleeding may be intracranial, epidural or subdural. The spinal cord is also within the enclosed space of the CNS and is enclosed by the bony vertebrae of the spine.

Sharp Force and Incised Wounds

Incised wounds are caused by bladed objects such as knives (Fig. 34-4). Features of entry wounds made by a knife are distinguished by whether there is a single- or double-edged blade. The former is distinguished by a sharp incision at one border of the wound and a blunt border at the opposite edge. If the knife enters the body up to the hilt, a mark may be left behind on the skin where the hilt impacted the skin. When a blade is inserted at an oblique angle, it causes a wound whose dimensions are wider than the maximum width of the blade.

A sharp force wound also includes incised wounds that result from sharp, round, pointed objects, such as an ice pick, knitting needle, sharp stick or bone, or even an icicle (which has the feature of making the evidence rapidly disappear). Although small in diameter, such wounds can be deadly.

Blunt Force Trauma

Blunt force trauma can be inflicted by any object with enough hardness, mass and momentum to damage tissues. Such assaults cause blunt force injuries, which may or may not break the surface of the skin, and which may cause external or internal bleeding. Because of the strength and resilience of the skin, sufficient force may be transmitted to the underlying tissues and organs to cause extensive injury, even when the skin remains unbroken.

When the skin surface is broken by blunt trauma, it may manifest as a puncture, abrasion, laceration, maceration or avulsion. If the surface of the skin is not broken, internal bleeding may still be extensive. Exsanguination can be caused either by bleeding out from the body or into internal body cavities.

Pattern Injury

Sometimes distinctive patterns on the skin can be matched to the surface of a blunt object ("pattern injuries"). Such

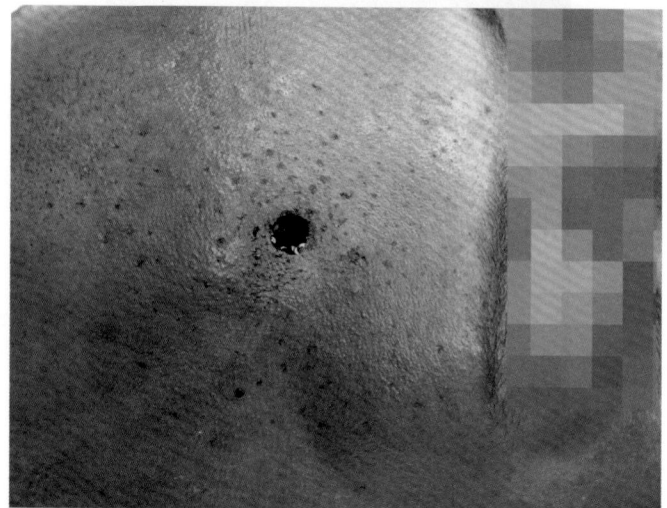

FIGURE 34-3. A close-range gunshot wound of entrance with surrounding stippling.

FORENSIC PATHOLOGY

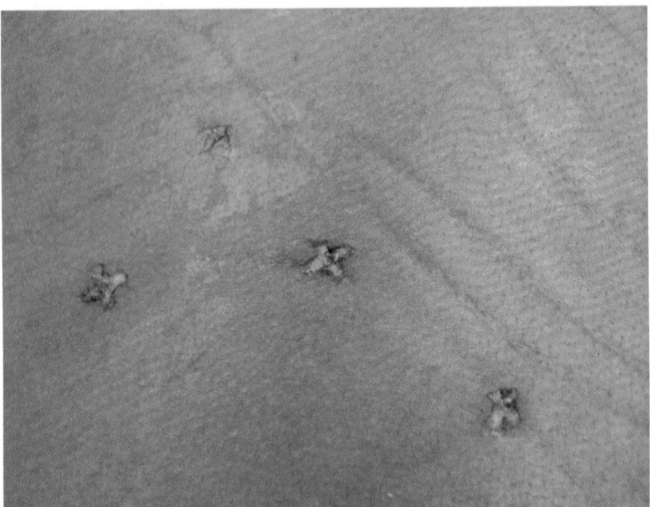

FIGURE 34-5. Four patterned punctures are present in this 35-year-old man stabbed with a Phillips-head screwdriver.

patterns include the shape of a waffle iron, the tread of a shoe and even uniquely distinguishing marks that match the weapon ("tool mark") to the type of hardware used (Fig. 34-5). Although the surface of a blunt object is firm and hard, the skin is elastic and may well be stretched out of shape owing to the application of force that leaves a "distorted" pattern, which may nonetheless still be matched properly. The scalp holds a pattern injury relatively well, as its skin covers a firm surface of bone.

Abrasions, Avulsions, Contusions, Incisions, Lacerations, Punctures

Other blunt force injuries may result from the encounter of the body with hard surfaces of machinery, with surfaces of a motor vehicle (Fig. 34-6) or with the ground.

When they break the surface of the skin, such wounds may include punctures, avulsions, abrasions and incisions.

Contusions

Whether or not the skin is broken from blunt force contact, a contusion (bruise) may develop in the underlying tissues. Contusions result from bleeding into the surrounding tissues by ruptured blood vessels. As the bleeding occurs into any enclosed space (e.g., a muscle or joint compartment, or connective tissues), swelling occurs, pressure increases and the back pressure helps to staunch further blood flow while clotting takes place. Since hemoglobin in red blood cells breaks down over time, contusions manifest various pigment colorations of black-blue, purple, green and yellow (Fig. 34-7). These variations assist in the timing of the bruise in a victim who survives injury.

Exsanguination

Where the surface of the skin and the underlying blood vessels are broken, the body may exsanguinate quickly because the heart continues to pump large quantities of blood through the wounds. Deeper injuries involving the arteries at high blood pressure are also capable of causing exsanguination. More superficial injuries involving only veins at lower blood

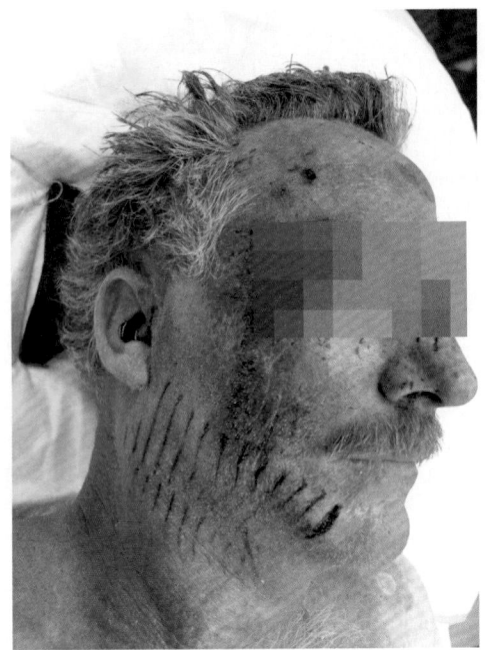

FIGURE 34-6. This individual was extricated from the truck that he was driving after hitting a tree. He was found lying on the floor of the truck with his feet facing the driver seat and his head against one of the pedals. The right side of the face is diffusely congested with a contusion over the cheek and a pattern abrasion (truck pedal imprint) on the lower side of the face.

pressure are not likely to cause exsanguination unless the injury covers extensive surfaces or blood loss is prolonged.

Internal Bleeding

If the skin surface is not broken, internal bleeding may still occur. Even at a relatively "bloodless" scene of the death,

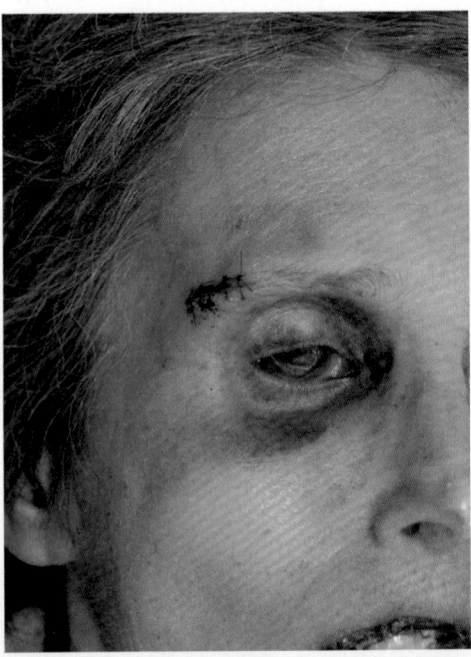

FIGURE 34-7. A sutured laceration present on the orbital ridge is surrounded by a healing contusion (with red, blue, yellow and green hues) in a patient with multiple sclerosis who suffered a fall 10 days before being pronounced dead.

body cavities may contain copious quantities of blood, resulting in exsanguination.

Death Occurring before a "Fatal" Accident

When a victim succumbs to sudden death prior to the time of blunt force injuries, bleeding will be minimal because the heart has stopped pumping prior to the occurrence of the wounds. For example, when a vehicle driver succumbs to sudden death from a heart attack or pulmonary embolism behind the wheel and then experiences a motor vehicle crash, multiple blunt injuries affect what is essentially a dead body. This may result in a bloodless scene despite extensive injuries.

Determination of Timing and Order of Receiving Wounds

A major issue is determining whether wounds contributed to death (homicide) or whether they were inflicted on the body after death (mayhem). Postmortem wounds are associated with minimal bleeding, as the heart has stopped pumping blood. In a deceased body, blood does not clot normally and the "dead" blood remains liquid. The appearance of postmortem injury itself is also relatively dry, tough and leathery compared to wounds inflicted on a still living body. Being able to determine the order and fatality of wounds is important when there are multiple assailants and when it can be determined that the first assailant committed homicide to a living victim whereas a subsequent one only committed mayhem on a deceased body.

Asphyxiation

Death by asphyxiation is a relatively slow process. During asphyxiation, the brain maintains consciousness for 2–3 minutes, at which point the victim may be expected to cease struggling. After an additional 2–3 minutes of asphyxiation, the brain dies from anoxia.

Strangulation: Ligature and Manual

The neck is a narrow structure that carries about 1/3 of the total blood volume at any given time to meet the high metabolic demands of the brain. Thus, it represents a convenient and efficient location for inducing asphyxiation by strangulation, either forcefully using the hands (manual) or by a ligature around the neck. In a homicidal assault by strangulation, there may be ligature marks around the neck; the hyoid bone, thyroid cartilage, cricoid cartilage and tracheal rings may (or may not) be broken. Petechial hemorrhages may occur in the eyes and elsewhere.

In addition to closing off the airway and causing asphyxiation, strangulation may compress the carotid arteries, directly cutting off blood flow to the brain. Extensive stress and stimulation to the carotid artery may also result in a reflex that induces cardiac arrhythmia.

To strangulate the neck structures, about 7 lb (3.2 kg) of pressure is required. Against a normal blood pressure of 120/80 mm Hg, the carotid artery is compressed by about 11–13 lb (5.0–5.9 kg) of pressure. The larynx is crushed by about 30 lb (13.6 kg) of pressure. These forces can be delivered by the hands (to a lean person) or by the elbow, knee or foot.

If a single blunt injury is applied by striking the neck with sufficient power to crush and collapse the larynx, suffocation and asphyxia will inexorably progress, whether or not any continued force is applied, because the airway has been cut off.

Asphyxiation by strangulation of the neck also occurs in judicial, suicidal and accidental hangings in autoerotic asphyxia. In a judicial hanging, the neck may be broken, causing instantaneous death due to injury to the cervical spine and CNS. If the hanging is not carried out "humanely," the neck may remain intact, and death eventually ensues from asphyxiation.

Petechial Hemorrhages

With asphyxiation (strangulation, drowning, fire/smoke inhalation), although the lungs continue to "breathe" or move, no oxygen enters the lungs. Thus, the heart continues to beat for several minutes and circulates unoxygenated blood. Sensitive cells in the peripheral blood vessels begin to die due to lack of oxygen, but the pumping heart pressures blood to rupture from the damaged capillaries for a short time, until the heart itself stops beating. The bleeding from the damaged blood vessels causes petechial hemorrhages. In the case of manual strangulation or suffocation, back pressure from cutting off circulation in the neck also contributes to petechiae. Such hemorrhages are typically observed in the conjunctivae of the eyes and in the pericardium.

Drownings: Asphyxiation and Hypothermia

Despite widespread aquatic safety measures in the United States, hundreds of drownings still occur each year in swimming pools and bathtubs. The fishing industry has the highest occupational death rates overall, often from drowning or hypothermia. In water, the body rapidly loses heat, causing death from hypothermia in minutes in freezing water and in up to a few hours in water at 40°–50°F (4°–10°C). Death may also result in water as warm as 70°–80°F (21°–27°C) when exposure is sufficiently prolonged.

A normal human body immersed in cold water will go through the following stages of reaction:

- **0–2 minutes:**
  Cold shock: Initial reaction, most likely to recover rapidly
- **5–15 minutes:**
  Motor incapacitation: Normal muscle movements maintained
- **Greater than 30 minutes:**
  Onset of hypothermia: Perceptions and sensations remain
- **Greater than 1 hour; up to 2 hours or more:** Loss of consciousness

Rates and Effects of Immersion Hypothermia

The ability to maintain consciousness, to survive and to maintain body functions in hypothermia is related to the time of immersion and the temperature of the water.

In cases of fatal drowning, water is usually present in the lungs. However, there are a minority of cases in which "dry drowning" occurs, owing to laryngeal spasm that closes off the lower respiratory system, causing asphyxiation with dry

TABLE 34-1

EFFECTS OF CARBON MONOXIDE POISONING

Carbon monoxide (CO) binds preferentially to hemoglobin, displacing oxygen and causing chemical asphyxia.

Blood Level of CO (hemoglobin concentrations)	Exposure	Effects
<10%	Tobacco smoking	None
10%–30%	Smoke/exhaust	Headache, dyspnea
30%–50%		Confusion, lethargy
50%–60%		Convulsions, coma
>60%		Death

lungs. Water enters the sinuses, and the presence of water in the sphenoid sinus is a typical sign of drowning.

Fires

Asphyxiation is a frequent cause of death in fire victims due to inhalation of carbon monoxide (Table 34-1) and other noxious combustion gases. Death from smoke inhalation usually occurs before thermal injuries occur or become fatal. The presence of soot in the airway of an outwardly burned body is a sign that the victim was alive and breathing at the time of the fire. The level of carbon monoxide in the blood is also a measure of smoke inhalation (Table 34-1).

When bodies are extensively damaged by fire, the tissues contract and the body assumes a "pugilistic" or defensive posture, drawing inward. This is not a conscious defensive pose but a postmortem artifact. Fire also sterilizes the body, resulting in reduced or absent postmortem decomposition and preservation of the remaining, albeit burned, tissues of the body.

ACCIDENT VERSUS HOMICIDE VERSUS SUICIDE

The rate of suicide is generally double the rate of homicides. Suicides occur by self-inflicted GSWs, asphyxiation by hanging (or rarely by drowning), intentional drug overdoses and a variety of other more rare means.

Cutting

Fatal exsanguination by cutting across the wrists is unusual despite many attempts, more commonly in females than in males. If cuts are made across the wrists, multiple strong tendons prevent the incision from reaching the larger blood vessels, and peripheral vasospasm and clotting minimize the blood loss. To be effective, as with the ancient Romans, consuming alcohol to dilate the peripheral blood vessels, cutting longitudinally and deeply between the tendons and being immersed in a warm bath to slow blood clotting are more successful in this regard. Incisions across the neck or throat are also effective for many of the same the reasons described in the earlier discussion of strangulation (Fig. 34-8). Fatal

neck incisions are often part of homicidal assaults; however, in a determined victim, they may also be suicidal.

Motor Vehicles

Vehicular suicide can occur when a driver intentionally precipitates a motor vehicle accident, such as by driving into a tree or telephone pole. Vehicular homicide can also occur when a victim is purposely assaulted, using a motor vehicle with intent to kill. Deaths in vehicles may also be natural deaths rather than accidents. As an example, a driver may suffer a fatal heart attack behind the wheel, which then precipitates a motor vehicle accident.

Gunshot Wounds

Among white males, a self-inflicted GSW to the head is the preferred method of suicide. Suicidal GSWs to other parts of the body are rare, although suicide by GSW in women is rare in general. Females generally prefer suicide by intentional drug overdose. Black and Hispanic males are less likely than white males to commit suicide.

Drug Overdose

With intentional overdose, the presence or absence of pill bottle(s) at the scene of death is not determinative. Victims often transfer the medication to another vessel before taking the fatal overdose. The presence or absence of pills in the stomach is also not necessarily determinative, depending upon the dosage, form and metabolism of the fatal drug(s).

Hanging

With respect to manual asphyxia, suicidal hanging can happen from rafters, fixtures, doorways or even the horizontal poles for hanging clothes in closets. It is not necessary for the feet to be unable to touch the ground for hangings to occur. A once-confusing circumstance of sexual asphyxia has now been understood. Males (and infrequently females) can

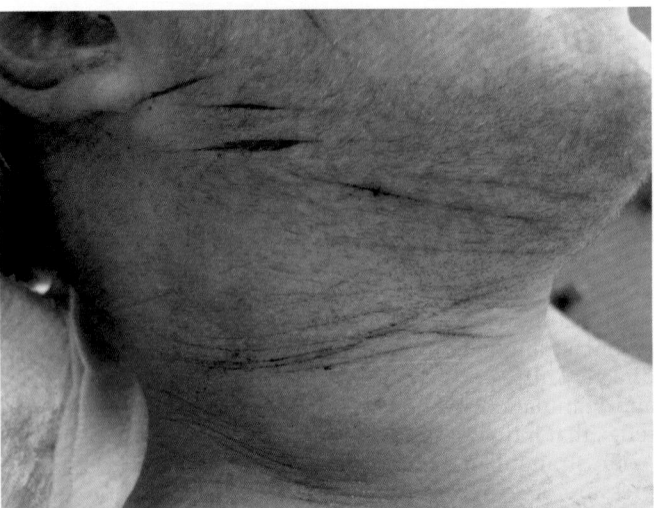

FIGURE 34-8. Multiple linear, parallel, superficial cutting wounds (hesitation wounds) in the right side of the face and neck of this 20-year-old man who died of self-inflicted sharp force injuries. Additional stab and cutting wounds were present in the chest, abdomen and wrists.

TABLE 34-2

ACUTE FATAL CHEMICAL POISONINGS

Chemical	Exposures	Toxicity
Benzene	Occupational-industrial, chemical manufacturing, solvent use, gasoline (3%)	Acute CNS and respiratory failure
Chloroform and carbon tetrachloride	Cleaning solvents	Depressant effects on CNS and heart Hepatic necrosis, fatty liver, liver failure
Cyanide/prussic acid (HCN)	Trace amounts in nuts and fruit seeds as natural pesticides (e.g., bitter almond [*Prunus amygdalus*])	Acute global anoxia; binds to mitochondrial cytochrome oxidase, arrests cellular respiration
Ethylene glycol	Antifreeze (ethanol substitute)	CNS depression and metabolic acidosis Oxalate urinary crystals and renal failure
Gasoline and kerosene	Accidental ingestion Inhalation of combustion products	Gastrointestinal Asphyxiation, carbon monoxide poisoning (see Table 34-1)
Methanol	Ethanol substitute	Metabolism to formaldehyde, then formic acid; blindness, seizures, coma
Trichlorethylene	Industrial solvent	CNS depression; minimal liver toxicity

devise various means for temporarily restricting blood supply to the brain to heighten autoerotic experience—the ensuing anoxia apparently leads to increased sexual sensation. On occasion, if the apparatus used involves being suspended in a kind of hanging, the victim may lose consciousness while masturbating and then imperceptibly proceed to suffer further strangulation and fatal asphyxia.

Poisonings

There are many natural and manufactured substances that may cause poisoning, fatal or nonfatal (Table 34-2). Poisonings can be caused by chemicals, drugs, plants or other biotoxins. In forensic medicine, it is important to determine whether fatal overdoses of drugs are accidental, homicidal or suicidal.

Both illicit and prescription drugs can be abused through intravenous injection. Heroin (synthetic acetyl morphine) is an opioid that does not occur in nature and is the prototype for intravenous drug abuse. Cocaine and amphetamines are also injected. These substances cause constriction of blood vessels, especially in the cerebral circulation, leading to anoxic brain injury. Fatal brain abscess may result from the introduction of infectious contaminants.

Talc is a noninfectious contaminant frequently introduced through illicit intravenous drugs. It is a nonactive filler used to "cut" (effectively diluting) the drug itself. Talc granulomas in the lungs present a characteristic appearance (see Chapter 8).

Plant poisonings are common as irritants to the skin or respiratory system. Rarely, ingestion of poisonous plants may be fatal in sufficient dose, especially with babies or children who may be unaware of the danger and for whom a smaller dose may be fatal. Biotoxins created by bacteria and fungi are responsible for gastrointestinal poisonings, causing fatal dehydration in circumstances where advanced medical care is not available (e.g., cholera). Other toxins cause

hepatocellular necrosis acutely, and liver cancer chronically, as with aflatoxins from Asia and Africa (see Chapter 14). So-called mycotoxins are in fashion as pseudoscience for causing any number of illnesses, from sick building syndrome to fatal fungal infections of the CNS. The science behind such claims is often not accepted by the courts as credible.

Chemical poisonings are the most common form of acute fatal poisonings and are summarized in Table 34-2.

Electrical Injury and Lightning Strikes

Exposure to household voltage, or high voltage, often in an occupational setting or during storms that cause downed electrical lines, may be fatal but leave barely perceptible evidence. Electrical currents can create cardiac arrhythmias and sudden death. Where the current exits the body, there may be a trace of thermal injury on the surface of the skin, which has a dry, leathery appearance (as observed in postmortem wounds, see below). Any overlying clothing may also show subtle tears and burns.

Usually, a fatal electrical shock is instantaneous, as the victim will let go or fall away from the source. When voltages are very high and contact is prolonged, there tends to be more extensive injury owing to the heat generated by resistance to the current in the body. Lightning strikes are a dramatic type of fatal electrical shock.

TIMING OF DEATH

Since the forensic pathologist invariably arrives after the time of death, he attempts to establish the interval between death and examination of the body. Over a period of hours, the medical examiner relies on *algor mortis* (body temperature), *livor mortis* (postmortem lividity) and *rigor mortis* (postmortem rigidity), all of which are influenced by environmental temperature and other factors.

Body Temperature

After death, normal body temperature falls at a predictable rate, if one takes into account the size of the body and the external temperature. The ability to retain heat by the body generally varies directly with increasing size, as the surface area of the body, through which heat is lost, is proportional to the square of the height. The mass or weight of the body, in which heat is retained, varies as the cube of the height. Factors that increase body temperature at the time of death require recalibration in estimating the time since death, for example, in people dying with a fever or from acute cocaine intoxication.

Lividity

Postmortem lividity results from passive pooling of blood into dependent areas owing to the effects of gravity. It presents as a distinctive red-purplish discoloration, unlike anything seen in life. The pattern of lividity indicates the position of the dead body and, depending on the presence of shifting patterns, whether a body was moved at certain intervals after death. Up to a period of 1–2 hours, lividity can be displaced with manual pressure (unfixed lividity), and the skin will blanche to a pale white color. After 3–4 hours, lividity becomes fixed and cannot be displaced by manual pressure.

Rigor

Postmortem rigidity (rigor mortis) is the result of a chemical reaction whereby muscle tissues irreversibly go through a process of contraction, causing the body and appendages to become stiff. Over the initial few hours, rigidity develops. Over several more hours, rigidity begins to pass away again and the body becomes lax. Once rigor passes, it does not return. Since it is a chemical process, it is accelerated by higher temperatures and retarded by lower ones. Rigor mortis starts from the top down—that is, it extends from the head and neck down to the arms and then the legs.

Decomposition

Postmortem decomposition is essentially a competition between decay from the outside-in and putrefaction from the inside-out. The process involves activity of aerobic decay organisms, such as bacteria and fungi, as well as insects. Putrefaction results from the activity of internal bacteria in the gastrointestinal tract that grow anaerobically after death. If the external environment is very hot, perceptible decay may ensue from the outside. But generally, in light of retained body temperature at the time of death, putrefaction predominates, causing decomposition from the inside to predominate.

Decomposition itself also presents a competition over time between desiccation and decay/putrefaction. In a very hot, arid environment, such as the sands of Egypt, a body may actually dry out before internal bacteria can bring about decomposition. Once a body is desiccated, it does not provide a fertile medium for bacterial growth, and the body becomes preserved, potentially for long periods of time. The ancient "secret" of Egyptian mummification lay in the removal of internal organs that harbored bacteria, together with exposing the body to desiccation.

As decomposition ensues, postmortem blood presents a fertile medium for bacterial growth. Wherever tissues are injured, bacterial decomposition is accelerated by the presence of blood in the wounds. Initially, below the skin, discoloration occurs along the distributions of blood vessels, as bacteria metabolize respiratory pigments to variously colored chemicals, appearing blue-green, yellow and purple-black. Another product of postmortem bacterial metabolism is the generation of decomposition gases, which accumulate under the skin. These expand areas of subdermal connective tissues, especially in the areolar looser tissues around the eyes, face and torso. These gases may also expel decomposition fluids (which may appear "bloody") from body orifices.

Disarticulation

As soft tissues decompose, after a period of weeks or months (depending upon seasonality, environmental temperatures and exposures) the skeleton becomes exposed to decay. Although the skeletal elements are usually preserved (and eventually over time the mineralized matrix becomes fossilized), there is a pattern by which skeletal elements become disarticulated from one another after soft tissues have disintegrated.

The first bone to disarticulate from the skeleton is the mandible. In addition to being highly recognizable as a human bone, it often carries specific information as to the identity of the deceased through dental work. Although the dense cortical bone and the teeth are very durable, they may not be found with the skeleton. The next articulation to be lost from the skeleton is the skull from the spinal column (which is otherwise held in place by the ribs). Separation of the skull from the skeleton can also prevent problems for the identification of the skeletal remains. Then, various bones of the arms and legs, hands and feet become disarticulated in a predictable sequence.

Specific acknowledgment is made for permission to use the following material:

Chapter 1, Figure 17. From Okazaki H, Scheithauer BW. Atlas of Neuropathology. New York: Gower Medical Publishing, 1988. By permission of the author.

Chapter 3, Figure 17. From Okazaki H, Scheithauer BW. Atlas of Neuropathology. New York: Gower Medical Publishing, 1988. By permission of the author.

Chapter 5, Figure 1C. From Bullough PG, Vigorita VJ. Atlas of Orthopaedic Pathology. New York: Gower Medical Publishing, 1984.

Chapter 5, Figure 10. From Bullough PG, Boachie-Adjei O. Atlas of Spinal Diseases. New York: Gower Medical Publishing, 1988. Copyright Lippincott Williams & Wilkins.

Chapter 5, Figure 63. From US Mortality Data, 1960 to 2005, US Mortality Volumes, 1930 to 1959. National Center for Health Statistics, Centers for Disease Control and Prevention, 2008.

Chapter 6, Figure 31. From Bullough PG, Vigorita VJ. Atlas of Orthopaedic Pathology. New York: Gower Medical Publishing, 1984.

Chapter 7, Figures 4 and 34. Courtesy of UBC Pulmonary Registry, St. Paul's Hospital.

Chapter 7, Figure 6. Courtesy of Dr. Charles Lee, University of British Columbia, Department of Pathology and Laboratory Medicine.

Chapter 7, Figures 7 and 16. Courtesy of Dr. Greg J. Davis, Department of Pathology, University of Kentucky College of Medicine.

Chapter 7, Figure 21. Courtesy of Dr. Sean Kelly, Office of Chief Medical Examiner of the City of New York.

Chapter 7, Figure 27. Courtesy of Dr. Ken Berry, Department of Pathology, St. Paul's Hospital.

Chapter 7, Figure 39. Courtesy of Dr. Alex Magil, Department of Pathology, St. Paul's Hospital.

Chapter 8, Figures 2 and 8. U.S. Department of Health and Human Services. The Health Consequences of Smoking: 50 Years of Progress. A Report of the Surgeon General. Atlanta, GA: U.S. Department of Health and Human Services, Centers for Disease Control and Prevention, National Center for Chronic Disease Prevention and Health Promotion, Office on Smoking and Health, 2014.

Chapter 8, Figure 13. From Okazaki H, Scheithauer BW. Atlas of Neuropathology. New York: Gower Medical Publishing, 1988. By permission of the author.

Chapter 8, Figure 15. From McKee PH. Pathology of the Skin. New York: Gower Medical Publishing, 1989. Copyright Lippincott Williams & Wilkins.

Chapter 8, Figure 29. From Shils ME, Shike M, Ross AC, et al., eds. Modern Nutrition in Health and Disease, 10th ed. Philadelphia: Lippincott Williams & Wilkins, 2006: Fig. 38.1C.

Chapter 8, Figure 33. From Shils ME, Shike M, Ross AC, et al., eds. Modern Nutrition in Health and Disease, 10th ed. Philadelphia: Lippincott Williams & Wilkins, 2006: Fig. 38.2C.

Chapter 9, Figures 21A, 21B, 28, 55A, 73, 87, 93, 94, 102A, and 102B. From Farrar WE, Wood MJ, Innes JA, Tubbs H. Infectious Diseases Text and Color Atlas, 2nd ed. New York: Gower Medical Publishing, 1992.

Chapter 10, Figure 5. Used with permission from Hisama FM, Bohr VA, Oshima J. WRN's Tenth Anniversary. Sci. Aging Knowl. Environ. 2006 (10), pe18 (2006).

Chapter 10, Figure 7. Courtesy of Dr. Richard Miller.

Chapter 13, Figure 3. Adapted with permission from Wu X, Williams KJ. NOX4 pathway as a source of selective insulin resistance and responsiveness. Arterioscler Thromb Vasc Biol. 2012;32:1236–1245.

Chapter 13, Figure 8. Adapted from Kendall DM, Bergenstal RM. © 2005 International Diabetes Center at Park Nicollet, Minneapolis, MN. All rights reserved. Used with permission.

Chapter 13, Figure 9. Redrawn from Pfeifer MA, Halter JB, Porte D. Insulin secretion in diabetes mellitus. Am. J. Med. 1981;70:579–588.

Chapter 13, Figure 16. Courtesy of the American Diabetes Association.

Chapter 14, Figure 37. Reprinted with permission from Stanley J. Robboy, MD, and Gynecologic Pathology Associates, Durham and Chapel Hill, North Carolina.

Chapter 18, Figure 40. From Travis WB, Colby TV, Koss MN, et al. Non-neoplastic Disorders of the Lower Respiratory Tract. Washington, DC: American Registry of Pathology, 2002.

Chapter 18, Figure 55. Courtesy of the Armed Forces Institute of Pathology.

Chapter 18, Figure 70. The authors would like to gratefully acknowledge Dr. Anthony Gal for the contribution of Figure 18-70.

Chapter 19, Figure 15. Courtesy of Dr. Cecilia M. Fenoglio-Preiser.

Chapter 19, Figures 61B and 66. From Mitros FA. Atlas of Gastrointestinal Pathology. New York: Gower Medical Publishing, 1988. Copyright Lippincott Williams & Wilkins.

Chapter 20, Figure 1. From Ross MH, Pawlina W. Histology: A Text and Atlas, 6th ed. Philadelphia: Lippincott Williams & Wilkins, 2011: 636.

Chapter 23, Figures 4 and 10. From Weiss MA, Mills SE. Atlas of Genitourinary Tract Diseases. New York: Gower Medical Publishers, 1988.

Chapter 23, Figure 17. From Bulock BA, Henze RL. Focus on Pathophysiology. Philadelphia: Lippincott Williams & Wilkins, 2000.

Chapter 24, Figures 4, 5, 16, 29, 31, 38A, 50, 76, and 77.   Reprinted with permission from Stanley J. Robboy, MD, and Gynecologic Pathology Associates, Durham and Chapel Hill, North Carolina.

Chapter 24, Figures 13, 18, 27, and 30A.   From Robboy SJ, Anderson MC, Russell P, eds. Pathology of the Female Reproductive Tract. London: Churchill-Livingstone, 2002: 111–112, 147, 167, 140, 203, 248, 322, 354.

Chapter 27, Figure 13.   Sandoz Pharmaceutical Corporation.

Chapter 28, Figures 9A, 22A, 25A (Courtesy W. Witmer), 26, 32A, 34A, 36A, 38A, 42, 43A, 44, 45, 46, 69A, 70, 71, 72, 79A, and 87A.   From Elder AD, Elenitsas R, Johnson BL, et al. Synopsis and Atlas of Lever's Histopathology of the Skin. Philadelphia: Lippincott Williams & Wilkins, 1999: p. 2, clin. fig. IA1; p. 163, clin. fig. IVE3; p. 167, clin. fig. IVE4.b; p. 124, clin. fig. IIIH1.a; p. 105, clin. fig. IIIF1.a; p. 115, clin. fig. IIIG1.a; p. 85, clin. fig. IIIB1a.a; p. 219, clin. fig. VE3.a; clin. fig. IVA2.b; p. 7, clin. fig. IC1; p. 212, fig. VD1.d; p. 51, clin. fig. IIE1.f and IIE1.1; p. 226, clin. fig. VE5.f; p. 283, clin. fig. VIB3.g; p. 280, clin. fig. VIB3.q and VIB3.s; p. 10, clin. fig. ID1.b; p. 31, clin. fig. IIC1.a; clin. fig. IIF2.a; p. 96, clin. fig. IIID1.d.

Chapter 30, Figures 18, 39B, 54B, 59, and 74A.   From Bullough PG. Atlas of Orthopaedic Pathology, 2nd ed. New York: Gower Medical Publishing, 1992. Copyright Lippincott Williams & Wilkins.

Chapter 31, Figure 1.   From Ross MH, Pawlina W. Histology: A Text and Atlas, 5th ed. Philadelphia: Lippincott Williams & Wilkins, 2006.

Chapter 31, Figure 6.   Redrawn from Karpati G. Structural and Molecular Basis of Skeletal Muscle Diseases. Basel: ISN Neuropath Press, 2002: 8, Fig. 2.

Chapter 32, Figures 12, 17, 19A, 19B, 21C, 22B, 24, 25, 26B, 27A, 30, 31, 32, 33, 35, 36, 48, 49, 50, 51, 56, 65A, 69, 72, 78A, 78B, 79, 80, 82A, 86A, 86B, 87, 94, 103, 108, 109, 111, 113B, 114B, 115B, 115D, 122B, 128B, and 133B.   Courtesy of Dr. F. Stephen Vogel, Duke University.

Chapter 34, Figures 1, 2, 3, 4, 5, 6, 7, and 8.   From Troncoso JC, Rubio A, Fowler DR. Essential Forensic Neuropathy. Baltimore: Lippincott Williams & Wilkins, 2010.

Note: Page numbers followed by f and t indicates figure and table respectively.

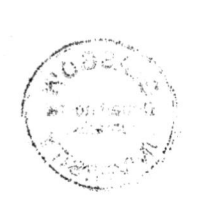